D0059812

Lists adverse reactions by body system

Details dosage adjustments needed for specific populations

Adjust-a-dose: Readjust dosage periodically for changes in child's weight.
➤ **Traumatic brain injury** ◆
Adults: 60 mg P.O. daily. Increase in 60-mg/day increments every third day until agitation ceases, adverse reactions occur, or the maxi-
___0 mg/day is reached.

propranolol hydrochloride   1227

ADVERSE REACTIONS
CNS: fatigue, lethargy, fever, vivid dreams, hallucinations, mental depression, light-headedness, dizziness, insomnia.
CV: hypotension, *bradycardia, heart fail-_____*, intermittent
_____ation, diar-

Lists potential interactions with other drugs, herbs, and lifestyle factors

INTERACTIONS
Drug-drug. *Aminophylline:* May antagonize beta-blocking effects of propranolol. Use together cautiously.
Amiodarone, diltiazem, verapamil: May cause hypotension, bradycardia, and increased depressant effect on myocardium. Use together cautiously.
Cardiac glycosides: May reduce the positive inotrope effect of the glycoside. Monitor patient for clinical effect.
Cimetidine, ciprofloxacin, fluconazole, fluoxetine, paroxetine: May inhibit metabolism of propranolol. Watch for increased beta-blocking effect.
Epinephrine: May cause severe vasoconstriction. Monitor BP and observe patient carefully.
Drug-herb. *Betel palm:* May decrease temperature-elevating effects and enhanced CNS effects.
Discourage use together.
Ma huang: May decrease antihypertensive effects. Discourage use together.
Drug-lifestyle. *Alcohol use:* May increase or decrease propranolol level. Discourage alcohol use.
Cocaine use: May increase angina-inducing
_____nt of this

Lists how results may be affected by taking drug

_____ol level.
_____st dosage
__ _____.

EFFECTS ON LAB TEST RESULTS
• May increase T_4, BUN, transaminase, alkaline phosphatase, potassium, and LDH levels. May decrease T_3 level.
• May decrease granulocyte count.

CONTRAINDICATIONS & CAUTIONS
Black Box Warning Abrupt withdrawal of drug may cause exacerbation of angina or MI. To discontinue drug, gradually reduce dosage over 1 to 2 weeks. If angina worsens or acute coronary insufficiency develops, resume therapy at least temporarily. Because CAD may be unrecognized, don't discontinue drug abruptly, even when taken for other indications. ■
• Contraindicated in patients with known hypersensitivity to drug, bronchial asthma, sinus bradycardia and heart block greater than first-degree, cardiogenic shock, and overt and decompensated heart failure (unless failure is secondary to a tachyarrhythmia that can be treated with propranolol).
Dialyzable drug: No.
⚠ **Overdose S&S:** Bradycardia, cardiac failure, hypotension, bronchospasm.

PREGNANCY-LACTATION-REPRODUCTION
• Drug is associated with fetal intrauterine growth retardation, and neonatal bradycardia, hypoglycemia and respiratory depression. If drug is used during pregnancy, ensure adequate monitoring of infants is available at birth.
• Use cautiously in breast-feeding women. Drug appears in breast milk with peak concentrations occurring 2 to 3 hours after oral doses. Monitor infants for signs and symptoms of beta blockade.

NURSING CONSIDERATIONS
• Drug masks common signs and symptoms of shock and hypoglycemia.
• Monitor black patients for expected therapeutic effects; dosage adjustments may be necessary.
🛈 **Alert:** Don't stop drug before surgery for pheochromocytoma. Before any surgical procedure, tell anesthesiologist that patient is receiving propranolol.
• **Look alike–sound alike:** Don't confuse propranolol with prasugrel or Pravachol. Don't confuse Inderal with Isordil, Adderall or Imuran.

PATIENT TEACHING
• Caution patient to continue taking this drug as prescribed, even when he's feeling well.

Easy-to-spot black box warnings

Indicates level of drug that can be reduced by dialysis

Identifies known signs and symptoms of overdose

Highlights pregnancy, lactation, and reproduction concerns

P

Points out critical information that can't be overlooked

Identifies drugs with similar appearance or name

Lists most important information patients should know

38th Edition

Nursing2018

DRUG

HANDBOOK®

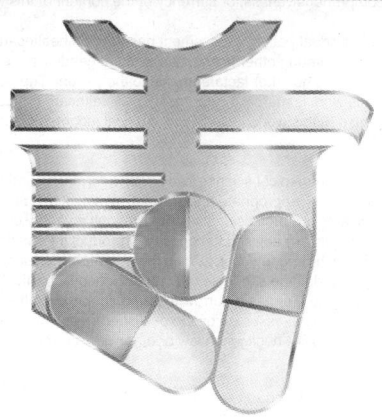

. Wolters Kluwer

Philadelphia · Baltimore · New York · London
Buenos Aires · Hong Kong · Sydney · Tokyo

Chief Nurse: Anne Dabrow Woods, DNP, RN, CRNP, ANP-BC, AGACNP-BC
Publisher: Jay Abramovitz
Clinical Director: Joan M. Robinson, RN, MSN
Clinical Project Manager: Lorraine Hallowell, RN, BSN, RVS
Clinical Editors: Janet Rader, RN, BSN; Dorothy Terry, RN; Leigh Ann Trujillo, RN, MSN
Product Director: David Moreau
Senior Product Manager: Diane Labus
Editor: Karen C. Comerford
Copy Editor: Mary T. Durkin
Editorial Assistants: Jeri O'Shea, Linda K. Ruhf
Art Director: Elaine Kasmer
Designer: Joseph John Clark
Senior Production Project Manager: Cynthia Rudy
Manufacturing Manager: Kathleen Brown
Production Services: Aptara, Inc.

9 8 7 6 5 4 3 2 1
Printed in China

NDH38-010517
ISSN: 0273-320X
ISBN-13: 978-1-4963-5359-7
ISBN-10: 1-4963-5359-5
ISBN-13: 978-1-4963-5360-3 (Canada)
ISBN-10: 1-4963-5360-9 (Canada)

LWW.com

Contents

Anatomy of a monograph ....inside front cover
Contributors and consultants... v
How to use *Nursing2018 Drug Handbook*® vi
Quick guide to special symbols, logos, and highlighted terms ix
Guide to abbreviations... x

General information

1. Drug actions, interactions, and reactions....................................... 1
2. Drug therapy across the lifespan.. 6
3. Safe drug administration.. 13
4. Selected therapeutic drug classifications 22

Alphabetical listing of drugs by generic name 60

New drugs 1575

Appendices 1621

1. Avoiding common drug errors: Best practices and prevention............ 1621
2. Pregnancy risk categories: The FDA's Final Rule............................. 1624
3. Controlled substance schedules... 1624
4. Abbreviations to avoid (The Joint Commission)............................... 1625
5. Pediatric drugs commonly involved in drug errors........................... 1626
6. Elder care medication tips 1628
7. Prescription drug abuse: Identifying and treating toxicity 1629
8. Understanding biosimilar drugs 1632
9. Nursing process: Patient safety during drug therapy....................... 1634
10. Serotonin syndrome: What you should know to protect
    your patient... 1635
11. Tumor lysis syndrome: A life-threatening emergency....................... 1636
12. Antidiarrheals: Indications and dosages....................................... 1637
13. Antidotes: Indications and dosages 1638
14. Selected biologicals and blood derivatives: Indications
    and dosages... 1644
15. Common combination drugs: Indications and dosages...................... 1651
16. Vaccines and toxoids: Indications and dosages 1666
17. Vitamins and minerals: Indications and dosages............................ 1673
18. Antacids: Indications and dosages.. 1680
19. Laxatives: Indications and dosages... 1682
20. Additional OTC drugs: Indications and dosages............................. 1686
21. Do not use: Dangerous abbreviations, symbols, and
    dose designations (ISMP Canada).. 1691
22. Decision tree: Deciding about medication administration 1692

23. Canadian National Drug Schedules..1693
24. Safe disposal of unused drugs: What patients need to know...............1694
25. Therapeutic drug monitoring guidelines 1696
26. Less commonly used drugs: Indications and dosages 1704
27. Additional new drugs: Indications and dosages 1752

Index **1753**

Contributors and consultants

Janine Barnaby, BS, RPh, BCOP
Manager, Hospital Outpatient Pharmacy
Lehigh Valley Hospital
Allentown, PA

David Bruch, BS, PharmD
Assistant Lecturer
University of Wyoming School of Pharmacy
Laramie

Lawrence Carey, PharmD
Associate Chair, Department of Pharmacy
    Practice
Temple University School of Pharmacy
Philadelphia, PA

Jason C. Cooper, PharmD
Clinical Pharmacist, MUSC Drug
    Information Center
Medical University of South Carolina
Charleston

Lana Gettman, PharmD
Assistant Professor
Harding University College of Pharmacy
Searcy, AR

Toshal Hallowell, PharmD
Pharmacist
Edward M. Kennedy Community Health
    Center
Worcester, MA

Lauren Hazelton, PharmD
Pharmacy Manager
Walgreens Pharmacy
Haddon Township, NJ

AnhThu Hoang, PharmD
Professor
Sheridan College
Brampton, Ontario

Rebecca Hoover, PharmD, MBA, BCPS
Assistant Professor, Director, Idaho Drug
    Information Center
Idaho State University
Pocatello

Olga Klibanov, PharmD, BCPS
Professor of Pharmacy
Wingate University
Wingate, NC

Jill Krabak, PharmD
Consultant Pharmacist
AlixaRx, Inc.
Plano, TX

Chung-Shien Lee, PharmD, BCPS, BCOP
Assistant Professor
St. John's University
Queens, NY

Hannah Livengood, PharmD
Staff/Clinical Pharmacist
Health Partners Plans
Philadelphia, PA

Kristy H. Lucas, PharmD, FCCP
Professor, Pharmacy Practice Department
University of Charleston School of Pharmacy
Charleston, WV

Michael A. Mancano, PharmD, RPh
Chairman, Department of Pharmacy Practice
Clinical Professor of Pharmacy Practice
Temple University School of Pharmacy
Philadelphia, PA

Melissa Max, PharmD, CDE, BC-ADM
Associate Professor of Pharmacy Practice
Harding University College of Pharmacy
Searcy, AR

Kimberly E. Ng, PharmD, BCPS
Assistant Professor
St. John's University
Queens, NY

Janet Rader, BSN, RN
Clinical Consultant
New Tripoli, PA

Melissa Rinaldi, PharmD
Clinical Pharmacist
Independence Blue Cross
Philadelphia, PA

Kerry Rinato, PharmD
Director of Pharmacy
Mountainview Hospital
Las Vegas, NV

Michele F. Shepherd, PharmD, MS, BCPS
Clinical Specialist
Abbott Northwestern General Medicine
    Associates
Edina, MN

Michelle Smith, PharmD, BCPS, CPE
Consultant
Havre, MT

James S. Wheeler, PharmD, BCPS
Assistant Professor of Clinical Pharmacy
University of Tennessee Health Science
    Center
College of Pharmacy
Nashville

How to use *Nursing2018 Drug Handbook*®

The best-selling nursing drug guide for more than 38 years, *Nursing Drug Handbook* is meticulously reviewed and updated annually by pharmacists and nurses to include the most current, relevant information that practicing nurses and students need to know to administer medications safely in any health care setting. As in previous editions, *Nursing2018 Drug Handbook* emphasizes nursing and safety aspects of drug administration without attempting to replace detailed pharmacology texts. Only the most essential information is included, and helpful graphic symbols, logos, and highlighting draw special attention to critical details that can't be overlooked. Recently redesigned, this new edition ensures easy readability and quick access to content that busy nurses need on the go.

New and outstanding features

The 38th edition provides a wealth of the latest drug information right at your fingertips:

- Tabbed "New Drugs" section—ensures quick access to all 29 complete drug monographs introduced in this edition, with helpful cross-references inserted alphabetically in the A-Z section, directing you to complete information on these recent FDA approvals
- Thoroughly updated text featuring generic, brand, and combination drugs; 745 comprehensive drug monographs; 31 generic drugs newly approved by the FDA—well over 4,000 clinical changes in all
- Pregnancy-Lactation-Reproduction header in each monograph—captures all relevant information in one convenient place
- Drug safety always at the forefront—includes a special chapter with newly added information about the Common Terminology Criteria for Adverse Events classification system used to describe the severity and toxicities related to cancer treatment, sections on preventing and treating I.V. vesicant extravasation injury and preventing hazardous drug exposure; in addition, you'll find numerous appendices covering drug safety guidelines, dosage alerts, best practices to avoid medication errors, pediatric drugs commonly involved in drug errors, and elder care medication tips
- New appendices on Prescription drug abuse: Identifying and treating toxicity, Understanding biosimilar drugs, and Safe disposal of unused drugs: What patients need to know
- Appendices covering Canadian drugs and safety concerns—Do Not Use list (ISMP Canada), decision tree, and the official Canadian National Drug Schedules
- Easy-to-spot icons and logos—Canadian drugs (maple leaf) and Do Not Crush logo—as well as Black Box Warnings and other special alerts
- Dialyzable drug logo under Contraindications & Cautions—indicates if drug levels can be reduced by hemodialysis and, if so, the percentage reduced
- Photoguide of more than 450 full-color, actual-sized tablets and capsules.

Introductory chapters

Chapter 1, "Drug actions, interactions, and reactions," explains how drugs work in the body. It provides a general overview of drug properties (absorption, distribution, metabolism, and excretion) and other significant factors affecting drug action (including protein binding, patient's age, underlying disease, dosage form, and route and timing of administration). Also discussed are drug interactions, adverse reactions, and toxic reactions. Chapter 2, "Drug therapy across the lifespan," discusses the danger associated with indiscriminate use of drugs during pregnancy and breast-feeding and the special precautions women should take when medications are necessary. This chapter also covers the unique challenges of giving drugs to children and elderly patients and offers practical suggestions on how to minimize problems with these special populations. Chapter 3, "Safe drug administration," explores the ongoing involvement of governmental and nongovernmental organizations weighing in on drug safety issues and the necessary measures nurses must take to prevent medication errors from occurring.

Chapter 4, "Selected drug classifications," summarizes the indications, actions, and contraindications and cautions of more than 60 drug classes represented in *Nursing2018 Drug Handbook*. Generic drugs within each class are also listed, allowing nurses to quickly identify and compare similar drugs when patients can't tolerate or don't respond to a particular drug.

Drug monographs

Each generic drug monograph in *Nursing2018 Drug Handbook* includes the most pertinent clinical information nurses must know to administer medications safely, monitor for potential interactions and adverse effects, implement necessary care measures, and provide appropriate patient teaching. Entries are arranged alphabetically, with the generic drug name prominently displayed—along with its "tall man" lettering (if applicable), pronunciation, corresponding brand (or trade) names, therapeutic class, and pharmacologic class—on a shaded background for quick and easy identification. Banners or symbols to identify drugs that warrant a special safety alert or drugs that appear in the color photoguide are also included in this highlighted area.

Specific information for each drug is then systematically organized under the headings below. Special icons and logos may be used throughout, as warranted, to point out the drug's safety concerns. For example, a clinical alert logo (🜚) provides important advice about life-threatening effects associated with the drug or its administration; a black box warning (**Black Box Warning**) represents a specific warning issued by the FDA. A special icon (🔵) indicates oral drug forms that shouldn't be crushed or chewed. (See *Anatomy of a monograph*, on the inside book cover, for a visual guide to the various symbols that may appear within a drug entry.)

Available forms

This section lists the preparations available for each drug (for example, tablets, capsules, solutions for injection) and specifies available dosage forms and strengths. Dosage strengths specifically available in Canada are designated with a maple leaf (🍁). Preparations that may be obtained over the counter, without a prescription, are marked with an open diamond (◇). Liquid formulations that contain alcohol are indicated with an asterisk (*).

Indications & dosages

General dosage information for adults and children is found in this section. Dosage instructions reflect current trends in therapeutics and can't be considered absolute or universal. For individual patients, dosage instructions must be considered in light of the patient's condition.

Indications and dosages that aren't approved by the FDA are followed by a closed diamond (◆). It should be noted that only highly evidence-based off-label uses are included in this edition. An ***Adjust-a-dose*** logo appearing within this section indicates the need for a special dosage adjustment for certain patients, such as elderly patients or those with renal or hepatic impairment. In some cases, a dosage adjustment may apply to all patient populations for all of the indications listed; this is marked accordingly.

Administration

Here, readers will find guidelines for safely administering drugs by all applicable routes, including P.O., I.V., I.M., subcutaneous, ophthalmic, inhalational, topical, rectal, vaginal, transdermal, and buccal. A special screened background highlights I.V. administration guidelines (including specific instructions on how to reconstitute, mix, and store I.V. medications) and potential I.V. incompatibilities.

Action

This section succinctly describes the mechanism of action—that is, how the drug provides its therapeutic effect. For example, although all antihypertensives lower blood pressure, they don't all do so by the same process. Also included, in table form, are the onset, peak (described in terms of effect or peak blood level), and duration of drug action for each route of administration, if data are available or applicable. Values listed are for patients with normal renal function unless otherwise specified. The drug's half-life is also provided when known.

Adverse reactions

In this section, adverse reactions to each drug are listed according to body system. Life-threatening reactions appear in ***bold italic*** type.

Interactions

Within this section, readers can find each drug's confirmed, clinically significant interactions (additive effects, potentiated effects, and antagonistic effects) with other drugs, herbs, foods, beverages, and lifestyle behaviors (such as alcohol use, sun exposure, or smoking). Interactions with a rapid onset are highlighted in color; interactions with a delayed onset are in **bold** type.

Drug interactions are listed under the drug that's adversely affected. For example, because magnesium trisilicate, an antacid ingredient, interacts with tetracycline to decrease tetracycline's absorption, this interaction is listed under tetracycline. To check on the possible effects of using two or more drugs simultaneously, refer to the interaction section for each drug.

Effects on lab test results
This section lists increased and decreased levels, counts, and other values in laboratory test results that may be caused by the drug's systemic effects. It also indicates false-positive, false-negative, and otherwise altered results of laboratory tests a drug may cause.

Contraindications & cautions
This section outlines any conditions or special circumstances, such as diseases or conditions, in which use of the drug is undesirable or for which the drug should be given with caution. When applicable, specific signs and symptoms of drug overdose are listed as the last bulleted item under this heading and highlighted by a special logo (⚠*Overdose S&S:*) for easy identification.

Pregnancy–lactation–reproduction
This section provides nurses with targeted, easy-to-understand safety information about each drug's use during pregnancy and breastfeeding. It also provides information about fertility effects, contraception recommendations, and enrollment information for registries that monitor drug safety during pregnancy.

Nursing considerations
Within this section, readers can find practical information on patient-monitoring techniques and suggestions for the prevention and treatment of adverse reactions as well as helpful tips on promoting patient comfort.

Patient teaching
Concise guidelines for explaining the drug's purpose, encouraging compliance, ensuring proper use and storage, and preventing or minimizing adverse reactions are included in this section.

Appendices and other helpful aids
Nursing2018 Drug Handbook includes 27 appendices that provide nurses and students with hands-on access to a wealth of supportive data and clinical information. You'll find three new

appendices in this edition: "Prescription drug abuse: Identifying and treating toxicity," "Understanding biosimilar drugs," and "Safe disposal of unused drugs: What patients need to know."

"Additional new drugs: Indications and dosages" introduces two brand-new FDA-approved drugs that couldn't be included as full monographs in time for publication of this edition.

A handy visual "Quick guide to special symbols, logos, and highlighted terms" and "Guide to abbreviations" immediately follow this "How to use" piece.

Photoguide to tablets and capsules
To enhance patient safety and help make drug identification easier, *Nursing2018 Drug Handbook* offers a 32-page full-color photoguide to the most commonly prescribed tablets and capsules. Shown in actual size, the drugs are arranged alphabetically by generic name for quick reference followed by the brand names and their most common dosage strengths. Below the name of each drug is a cross-reference to where information on the drug can be found in the book. Brand names of drugs that appear in the photoguide are shown in text with a special capsule symbol (✐). Page references to the drug photos appear in boldface type in the index (for example, **C12**).

Photos for certain brands were provided by the following companies for use in this book: Forest Pharmaceuticals, Inc. (Campral); Novartis Pharmaceuticals (Enablex); Sepracor, Inc. (Lunesta); Teva Pharmaceuticals (Azilect); and Pfizer (Sutent). Additional photos were provided by Jeff Sigler of SFI Medical Publishing.

Online Toolkit
A Toolkit containing a wide array of drug-related materials that practicing nurses and students can use on the job and for study—covering safety issues (such as an equianalgesic dosing chart), pharmacology, drug therapy guidelines, patient populations, and a host of other drug-specialty areas—can be found online at **NDHnow.com.** Included are a dosage calculator, drug safety and administration videos, pharmacology animations, English-Spanish translator, audio drug pronunciation guide, 325-question NCLEX®-style test, and access to free and discounted CE tests. Monthly FDA drug updates, drug warnings, and newsworthy drug information can also be accessed through this site.

Quick guide to special symbols, logos, and highlighted terms

The following symbols or highlighted features appear throughout drug monographs and select appendices in this edition.

Special symbols and logos	Usage or meaning
SAFETY ALERT!	Drug that presents a heightened avoidable danger
buPROPion	"Tall man" lettering for FDA-designated generic drug names prone to mix-ups
➤	Indication for drug
✳ *NEW INDICATION:*	New indication for drug
Adjust-a-dose:	Dosage adjustment needed for certain populations
Adjust-a-dose (for all indications):	Dosage adjustment needed for all indications
↻ *Alert:*	Clinical alert
♣	Available in Canada
◇	Over-the-counter (OTC)
◆	Off-label use
⌀	Appears in Photoguide
*	Liquid contains alcohol
⊘⃝	Drugs that shouldn't be crushed or chewed
Look alike–sound alike	Drugs with easily confused names
Black Box Warning	FDA black box warning
⚠ *Overdose S&S:*	Overdose signs & symptoms
Highlighted reactions and interactions	
life-threatening	Life-threatening reaction
rapid onset	Causes interaction with rapid onset
delayed onset	Causes interaction with delayed onset

Guide to abbreviations

ACE	angiotensin-converting enzyme	5-FU	fluorouracil	msec	millisecond
ADH	antidiuretic hormone	G	gauge	NNRTI	non-nucleoside reverse transcriptase inhibitor
ADHD	attention deficit hyperactivity disorder	g	gram		
		G6PD	glucose-6-phosphate dehydrogenase	NSAID	nonsteroidal anti-inflammatory drug
AEDs	antiepileptic drugs	GABA	gamma-aminobutyric acid	NSS	normal (0.9%) saline solution
AIDS	acquired immunodeficiency syndrome	GERD	gastroesophageal reflux disease		
				ODT	orally disintegrating tablet
ALT	alanine transaminase	GFR	glomerular filtration rate	OTC	over-the-counter
ANA	antinuclear antibody	GGT	gamma-glutamyltransferase	oz	ounce
ANC	absolute neutrophil count	GI	gastrointestinal	PABA	para-aminobenzoic acid
aPTT	activated partial thromboplastin time	gtt	drops	PCA	patient-controlled analgesia
		GU	genitourinary	PCI	percutaneous coronary intervention
ARB	angiotensin receptor blocker	GVHD	graft-versus-host disease		
ARDS	acute respiratory distress syndrome	H_1	histamine$_1$	PDE5	phosphodiesterase type 5
		H_2	histamine$_2$	PE	pulmonary embolus
AST	aspartate transaminase	Hb	hemoglobin	P.O.	by mouth
AV	atrioventricular	HBV	hepatitis B virus	PPI	proton pump inhibitor
b.i.d.	twice daily	HCV	hepatitis C virus	P.R.	by rectum
BMI	body mass index	HDL	high-density lipoprotein	p.r.n.	as needed
BP	blood pressure	HF	heart failure	PSA	prostate-specific antigen
BPH	benign prostatic hypertrophy	HIV	human immunodeficiency virus	PT	prothrombin time
				PTT	partial thromboplastin time
BSA	body surface area	HMG-CoA	3-hydroxy-3-methyl-glutaryl coenzyme A	PVC	premature ventricular contraction
BUN	blood urea nitrogen				
CABG	coronary artery bypass graft	HPA	hypothalamic-pituitary-adrenal	q.i.d.	four times daily
CAD	coronary artery disease			RA	rheumatoid arthritis
cAMP	cyclic 3′, 5′ adenosine monophosphate	HR	heart rate	RAAS	renin-angiotensin-aldosterone system
		ICP	intracranial pressure		
CBC	complete blood count	ICU	intensive care unit	RBC	red blood cell
CDAD	*Clostridium difficile*-associated diarrhea	I.D.	intradermal	RDA	recommended daily allowance
		I.M.	intramuscular		
CDC	Centers for Disease Control and Prevention	INR	International Normalized Ratio	REM	rapid eye movement
				RNA	ribonucleic acid
CK	creatine kinase	IOP	intraocular pressure	RSV	respiratory syncytial virus
CMV	cytomegalovirus	IPPB	intermittent positive-pressure breathing	SA	sinoatrial
CNS	central nervous system			sec	second
COPD	chronic obstructive pulmonary disease	ITP	idiopathic thrombocytopenic purpura	SIADH	syndrome of inappropriate antidiuretic hormone
CrCl	creatinine clearance	I.V.	intravenous	S.L.	sublingual
CSF	cerebrospinal fluid	kg	kilogram	SSNRI	selective serotonin and norepinephrine reuptake inhibitor
CT	computed tomography	L	liter		
CTCAE	Common Terminology Criteria for Adverse Events	lb	pound		
		LDH	lactate dehydrogenase	SSRI	selective serotonin reuptake inhibitor
CV	cardiovascular	LDL	low-density lipoprotein		
D_5W	dextrose 5% in water	LFTs	liver function tests	Subcut.	subcutaneous
DEHP	di(2-ethylhexyl) phthalate	LVEF	left ventricular ejection fraction	T_3	triiodothyronine
DIC	disseminated intravascular coagulation			T_4	thyroxine
		M	molar	TB	tuberculosis
dL	deciliter	m^2	square meter	TCA	tricyclic antidepressant
DMARD	disease-modifying antirheumatic drug	MAO	monoamine oxidase	TIA	transient ischemic attack
		mcg	microgram	t.i.d.	three times daily
DNA	deoxyribonucleic acid	mEq	milliequivalent	TNF	tumor necrosis factor
DPP-4	dipeptidyl peptidase-4	mg	milligram	TSH	thyroid-stimulating hormone
DVT	deep vein thrombosis	MI	myocardial infarction		
ECG	electrocardiogram	min	minute	tsp	teaspoon
EEG	electroencephalogram	mL	milliliter	ULN	upper limit of normal
EENT	eyes, ears, nose, throat	mm^3	cubic millimeter	URI	upper respiratory infection
ESRD	end-stage renal disease	mo	month	USP	United States Pharmacopeia
FDA	Food and Drug Administration	MRSA	methicillin-resistant *Staphylococcus aureus*	UTI	urinary tract infection
				VLDL	very low density lipoprotein
FSH	follicle-stimulating hormone	MS	multiple sclerosis	WBC	white blood cell
				wk	week

1

Drug actions, interactions, and reactions

Any drug a patient takes causes a series of physical and chemical events in his body. The first event, when a drug combines with cellular drug receptors, is the *drug action*. What happens next is the *drug effect*. Depending on the type of cellular drug receptors affected by a given drug, an effect can be local, systemic, or both. A systemic drug effect can follow a local effect. For example, when you apply a drug to the skin, it causes a local effect. But transdermal absorption of that drug can then produce a systemic effect. A local effect can also follow systemic absorption. For example, the peptic ulcer drug cimetidine produces a local effect after it's swallowed by blocking histamine receptors in the stomach's parietal cells. Diphenhydramine, on the other hand, causes a systemic effect by blocking histamine receptors throughout the body.

Drug properties

Drug absorption, distribution, metabolism, and excretion make up a drug's pharmacokinetics. These processes determine a drug's onset of action, peak concentration, duration of action, and bioavailability.

Absorption

Before a drug can act in the body, it must be absorbed into the bloodstream—usually after oral administration, the most common route. Before an oral drug can be absorbed, it must disintegrate into particles small enough to dissolve in GI secretions. Only after dissolving can the drug be absorbed. Most absorption of orally given drugs occurs in the small intestine because the mucosal villi provide extensive surface area. Once absorbed and circulated in the bloodstream, the drug is *bioavailable,* or ready to produce a drug effect. The speed of absorption and whether absorption is complete or partial depend on the drug's effects, dosage form, administration route, interactions with other substances in the GI tract, and various patient characteristics. Oral solutions and syrups bypass the need for disintegration and dissolution and are usually absorbed faster than solid dosage forms. Some tablets have enteric coatings to prevent disintegration in the acidic environment of the stomach; others have coatings of varying thickness that simply delay release of the drug.

Drugs given I.M. must first be absorbed through the muscle into the bloodstream. Rectal suppositories must dissolve to be absorbed through the rectal mucosa. Drugs given I.V. are injected directly into the bloodstream and are bioavailable completely and immediately.

Distribution

After absorption, a drug moves from the bloodstream into the fluids and tissues in the body, a movement known as *distribution.* The volume into which a drug is distributed is known as the *volume of distribution.* Individual patient variations can change the amount of drug distributed throughout the body. For example, in an edematous patient, a given dose is distributed into a larger volume than in a nonedematous patient. Occasionally, a dose is increased to account for this difference. In this case, the dose should be decreased after the edema is corrected. Conversely, a dose given to a dehydrated patient must be decreased to allow for its distribution into a much smaller volume. Patients who are very obese may present another problem when considering drug distribution. Some drugs—such as digoxin, gentamicin, and tobramycin—aren't well-distributed to fatty tissue. Sometimes, doses based on actual body weight may lead to overdose and serious toxicity. In these cases, doses must be based on lean body weight, or adjusted body weight, which may be estimated from mathematical formulas or actuarial tables that give average weight range for height.

Metabolism

Most drugs are metabolized in the liver. Hepatic diseases may affect the liver's metabolic functions and may increase or decrease a drug's usual metabolism. Closely monitor all patients with hepatic disease for drug effect and toxicity.

The rate at which a drug is metabolized varies from person to person. Some patients metabolize drugs so quickly that the drug levels in their blood and tissues prove therapeutically inadequate. In other patients, the rate of metabolism is so slow that ordinary doses can produce toxicity or prolonged duration of action.

Excretion

The body eliminates drugs by metabolism (usually hepatic) and excretion (usually renal). *Drug excretion* is the movement of a drug or its metabolites from the tissues back into circulation and from the circulation into the organs of excretion, where they're removed from the body. Most drugs are excreted by the kidneys, but some can be eliminated through the lungs, exocrine (sweat, salivary, or mammary) glands, liver, skin, or intestinal tract. Drugs also may be removed artificially by direct mechanical intervention, such as peritoneal dialysis or hemodialysis.

Other modifying factors

One important factor influencing a drug's action and effect is its tendency to bind to plasma proteins, especially albumin, and other tissue components. Because only a free, unbound drug molecule can act in the body, protein binding greatly influences the degree and duration of a drug's effect. Malnutrition, renal failure, and the presence of other protein-bound drugs can influence protein binding. When protein-binding behavior changes, the drug dosage may need to be adjusted accordingly.

The patient's age is another important factor. Elderly patients usually have decreased hepatic function, less muscle mass, diminished renal function, and lower albumin levels. These patients need lower doses and sometimes longer dosage intervals to avoid toxicity. Neonates have underdeveloped metabolic enzyme systems and inadequate renal function, so they need highly individualized dosages and careful monitoring.

Underlying disease also may affect drug action and effect. For example, acidosis may cause insulin resistance. Genetic diseases, such as G6PD deficiency and hepatic porphyria, may turn drugs into toxins, with serious consequences. Patients with G6PD deficiency may develop hemolytic anemia when given certain drugs, such as sulfonamides. A genetically susceptible patient can develop acute porphyria if given a barbiturate. A patient with a highly active hepatic enzyme system, such as a rapid acetylator, can develop hepatitis when treated with isoniazid because of the quick intrahepatic buildup of a toxic metabolite.

Drug administration issues

How a drug is given can also influence a drug's action in the body. The dosage form of a drug is important. Some tablets and capsules are too large to be easily swallowed by sick patients. An oral solution may be substituted, but it may produce higher drug levels than a tablet because the liquid is more easily and completely absorbed. When a potentially toxic drug (such as digoxin) is given in the liquid form, its increased absorption can cause toxicity. Sometimes a change in dosage form also requires a change in dosage.

Routes of administration aren't always interchangeable. For example, diazepam is readily absorbed P.O. but is slowly and erratically absorbed I.M. On the other hand, gentamicin must be given parenterally because oral administration results in drug levels too low to effectively treat systemic infections.

Improper storage can alter a drug's potency. Most drugs must be stored in tight containers protected from direct sunlight and extremes in temperature and humidity that can cause them to deteriorate. Some drugs require special storage conditions, such as refrigeration. Patients should be cautioned not to store drugs in a bathroom because of the constantly changing environment.

The timing of drug administration can be important. Sometimes, giving an oral drug during or shortly after a meal changes the amount of drug absorbed. This may not be significant and the presence of food in the GI tract may even be desirable with irritating drugs such as aspirin. But penicillins and tetracyclines shouldn't be taken at mealtimes because certain foods can inactivate them. If in doubt about the effect of food on a certain drug, the nurse should check with a pharmacist.

The nurse documents the patient's age, height, and weight. The prescriber will need this information when calculating the dosage for many drugs. This information should be recorded accurately on the patient's chart. The chart should also include all current laboratory data, especially results of renal and liver function studies, so the prescriber can adjust the dosage as needed.

The nurse also watches for metabolic changes and physiologic changes (such as depressed respiratory function, acidosis, or alkalosis) that might alter drug effect.

The nurse obtains a comprehensive family history from the patient or his family, asking about past reactions to drugs, possible genetic traits that might affect drug response, and the current use of other prescription and OTC drugs, illicit drugs, herbal supplements, and vitamin supplements. Multiple drug therapies can cause serious and fatal drug interactions and can dramatically change many drugs' effects.

Drug interactions

A *drug interaction* occurs when a drug given concomitantly with another drug alters the effect of either or both drugs. Usually the effect of one drug is increased or decreased. For instance, one drug may inhibit or stimulate the metabolism or excretion of the other or free it for further action by releasing the drug from protein-binding sites.

Combination therapy is based on drug interactions. One drug may be given to complement the effects of another. For example, imipenem and cilastatin are given together because cilastatin inhibits a renal enzyme that prevents inactivation of imipenem. In many cases, two drugs with similar actions are given together precisely because of the additive effect. For instance, acetaminophen and codeine are commonly given in combination because together they provide greater pain relief than if either is given alone.

Drug interactions are sometimes used to prevent or antagonize certain adverse reactions. The diuretics hydrochlorothiazide and spironolactone are often given together because the former is potassium-depleting and the latter potassium-sparing.

Not all drug interactions are beneficial. Many drugs interact to decrease efficacy or increase toxicity. An example of decreased efficacy occurs when a tetracycline is given with drugs or foods that contain calcium or magnesium (such as antacids or milk). These bind with tetracycline in the GI tract and cause inadequate drug absorption. An example of increased toxicity can be seen in a patient taking a diuretic and lithium. The diuretic may increase the lithium level, causing lithium toxicity. Avoid drug combinations that produce these effects, if possible.

Sometimes drug interactions occur after a drug that inhibits or increases the metabolism of another drug has been discontinued. After the drug is discontinued, the other drug's levels may increase or decrease, so the dosage may need adjustment.

Adverse reactions

Drugs cause adverse *effects;* patients have adverse *reactions.* An adverse reaction may be tolerated to obtain a therapeutic effect, or it may be hazardous and unacceptable. Some adverse reactions subside with continued use. For example, the drowsiness caused by paroxetine and the orthostatic hypotension caused by prazosin usually subside after several days, when the patient develops tolerance. But many adverse reactions are dose related and lessen or disappear only if the dosage is reduced. Most adverse reactions aren't therapeutically desirable, but a few can be put to clinical use. An example of this is the drowsiness caused by diphenhydramine, which makes it useful as a mild sedative.

Common Terminology Criteria for Adverse Events (CTCAE) are standardized definitions that describe adverse events that occur in the course of cancer therapy. An adverse event is considered any event that's unfavorable or has an unfavorable outcome to a patient due to a medication and not to the underlying condition of the patient. (See *Common Terminology Criteria for Adverse Events,* page 4.)

Drug hypersensitivity, or drug allergy, is the result of an antigen–antibody immune reaction that occurs in the body when a drug is given to a susceptible patient. Signs and symptoms of a drug allergy may include rash, itching, angioedema, or shortness of breath. One of the most dangerous of all drug hypersensitivities is penicillin allergy. In its most severe form, penicillin anaphylaxis can rapidly become fatal.

Rarely, idiosyncratic reactions occur. These reactions are highly unpredictable and unusual. One of the best known idiosyncratic adverse reactions is aspirin-induced asthma, which may be life-threatening. A more common idiosyncratic reaction is extreme sensitivity to very low doses of a drug or insensitivity to higher-than-normal doses.

To manage adverse reactions correctly, you need to be alert to even minor changes in the patient's clinical condition. Such changes may be an early warning of impending toxicity. Listen to the patient's complaints about his re-actions to a drug, and consider each objectively. You may be able to reduce adverse reactions in several ways. Dosage reduction can help. But, in many cases, so does a simple rescheduling of the dose. For example, the stimulation that pseudoephedrine may produce may be managed if it's given early in the day rather than at

The National Cancer Institute developed a classification system to grade and describe the severity of certain toxicities related to cancer treatment. This grading scale is used to manage the dosage and administration of the patient's chemotherapy and, in clinical trials, to provide standardized definitions of toxicities for scientific analysis. The Common Terminology Criteria for Adverse Events (CTCAE) classification is applied to blood, cardiac, fatigue, GI, hepatobiliary, infusion reaction and extravasation, kidney and urinary tract, lung, metabolic, neurologic, pain, psychiatric, and skin-related adverse events.

The CTCAE classification consists of five different grades that define the severity of the adverse events and describe them. Each grade has specific parameters related to the physiologic or anatomic system involved.

Grade 1: Mild; asymptomatic or mild symptoms with no intervention needed

Grade 2: Moderate; minimal local or noninvasive intervention indicated

Grade 3: Severe or medically significant but not immediately life-threatening; hospitalization or prolonged hospitalization stay indicated; disabling

Grade 4: Life-threatening; urgent intervention indicated

Grade 5: Death related to adverse event.

bedtime. Similarly, drowsiness from antihistamines or tranquilizers can be less important if these drugs are given at bedtime. Most importantly, your patient needs to be told which adverse reactions to expect so that he won't become worried or even stop taking the drug on his own. Always advise the patient to report adverse reactions to the prescriber immediately.

Your ability to recognize signs and symptoms of drug allergies or serious idiosyncratic reactions may save your patient's life. Ask each patient about the drugs he's taking currently or has taken in the past and whether he experienced any unusual reactions from taking them. If a patient claims to be allergic to a drug, ask him to tell you exactly what happens when he takes it. He may be calling a harmless adverse reaction such as upset stomach an allergic reaction, or he may have a true history of anaphylaxis. In either case, you and the prescriber need to be aware of the reaction. Record and report clinical changes throughout the patient's course of treatment. If you suspect a severe adverse reaction, withhold the drug until you can check with a pharmacist and the prescriber.

Toxic reactions

Chronic drug toxicities are usually caused by the cumulative effect and resulting buildup of the drug in the body. These effects may be extensions of the desired therapeutic effect. For example, standard doses of glyburide normalize the glucose level, but higher doses can produce hypoglycemia.

Drug toxicities may also occur when a drug level rises as a result of impaired metabolism or excretion. For example, hepatic dysfunction impairs the metabolism of amiodarone, raising its blood level. Similarly, renal dysfunction may cause digoxin toxicity because this drug is eliminated by the kidneys. Excessive dosage can also cause toxic levels. For instance, tinnitus is usually a sign that the safe dose of aspirin has been exceeded.

Many drug toxicities are predictable, dosage-related, and reversible upon dosage adjustment. So, monitor patients carefully for physiologic changes that might alter drug effect. Watch especially for hepatic and renal impairment. Warn the patient about signs of impending toxicity and tell him what to do if a toxic reaction occurs. Also, make sure to emphasize the importance of taking a drug exactly as prescribed. Warn the patient that serious problems could arise if he changes the dose or schedule or stops taking the drug without his prescriber's knowledge.

Pharmacogenetics

As a rule, prescribers typically follow a standardized approach to prescribing drugs. Although decisions are made with evidence-based approaches and the best of intentions, some result in the development of adverse drug reactions. It would be helpful to be able to accurately predict which patients will (and which will not) respond and to what degree when prescribed a certain drug. Pharmacogenetics—the study of how varied responses to a drug can be caused by genetic differences between individuals—attempts to do just this.

The first pharmacogenetic detection occurred when Pythagoras recognized the dangers of ingesting fava beans in 510 B.C., which eventually led to the discovery of G6PD in 1956. Shortly after, the term *pharmacogenetics* was coined and later defined as the study of variability in drug response due to heredity.

The goals of pharmacogenetics include identification of innovative drug targets, consideration of DNA sequence variation on drug effects, development of new agents, and optimization of drug efficacy while minimizing drug toxicity.

Pharmacogenetics considers the existence of polymorphisms, which are defined as genetic variations that occur in 1% or more of the population. If clinicians are able to predict which patients may express polymorphisms, they can provide targeted therapy. Researchers have learned that many polymorphisms involve cytochrome P450 (CYP450) isoenzymes.

Polymorphisms play a significant role in determining whether a drug will be predictably metabolized. Patients fall into one of four classes of metabolizers: extensive, ultrarapid, intermediate, and poor. Patients considered "extensive metabolizers" possess an overwhelming capacity to metabolize certain drugs and may exhibit therapeutic failure, whereas patients who are "poor metabolizers," such as those with G6PD deficiency, exhibit toxicities due to their inability to metabolize certain drugs. Ethnicity may also play a role in determining how patients are classified in regard to metabolism.

It's vital to recognize the importance of the CYP450 system. Approximately 60 CYP enzymes are found in humans, and many genes that encode for these enzymes are polymorphic. Polymorphism associated with CYP enzymes may be expressed via amino acid substitution (thereby reducing enzymatic activity) or by amplification or duplication of activity (thereby increasing enzymatic activity). It's thought that approximately one-third of all medications prescribed today are metabolized by CYP450, including tricyclic antidepressants, antiarrhythmics, beta-receptor antagonists, codeine, warfarin, phenytoin, and nicotine.

In addition, enzymes that metabolize cancer chemotherapy drugs, such as thiopurine S-methyltransferase, dihydropyrimidine dehydrogenase, and UDP-glucuronosyl transferase, can have therapeutic implications; for example, polymorphisms affecting these enzymes can result in serious adverse reactions, such as anemia and neurotoxicity. Finally, miscellaneous polymorphisms affecting drug transport proteins such as P-glycoprotein may affect drug response; this protein acts as a safety mechanism to remove toxins from cells and has a role in the distribution of cancer chemotherapy drugs, digoxin, cyclosporine, and protease inhibitors.

As a nurse, you need to be aware of the clinical ramifications of pharmacogenetics—having an effective knowledge of which drugs, diseases, or ethnic groups are affected by these variations can help you anticipate issues that may arise with patients under your care. For example, some Asian patients have a significant reduction in enzyme activity secondary to amino acid substitution and, therefore, exhibit slower metabolism of certain drugs compared to patients from other ethnic groups. The effect of this on clinical practice is seen in the dosing of rosuvastatin; patients of Asian descent are typically started at 5 mg/day P.O., whereas non-Asian patients are started at 10 mg/day. Giving a lower dose helps limit the development of serious adverse reactions in Asian patients.

Another example of how drug metabolism is affected by genetic polymorphism involves the drug warfarin. Studies have shown that CYP2C9, which is the primary enzyme responsible for warfarin metabolism, has two genetic variants. These variants are associated with up to an 80% decrease in enzymatic activity that can affect approximately 7% to 11% of patients. Patients with these variant genotypes have a 2.4 times increase in the risk of serious or life-threatening bleeding after normal doses of warfarin. Consequently, patients with these variants retain warfarin longer and need significantly lower maintenance dosages.

Fortunately, genetic testing for polymorphisms is available when issues such as these arise. Although testing isn't done for every patient, it can be helpful for those who seem to be refractory or overly sensitive to the effects of certain drugs (such as warfarin) or who meet other criteria (such as ethnicity).

2

Drug therapy across the lifespan

Drug therapy is a fact of life for millions of people of all ages, and certain aspects of a patient's life, such as age, growth, and development, can affect drug therapy.

Drugs and pregnancy

Drug administration during pregnancy has been a source of serious medical concern and controversy since the thalidomide tragedy of the late 1950s, when thousands of malformed infants were born after their mothers were given this mild sedative–hypnotic while pregnant. To identify drugs that may cause such teratogenic effects, preclinical drug studies include tests on pregnant laboratory animals. These studies may reveal gross teratogenicity but don't establish absolute safety. This is because different animal species react to drugs in different ways. Consequently, animal studies can't reveal all possible teratogenic effects in humans. For example, the preliminary studies on thalidomide gave no warning of teratogenic effects, and it was subsequently released for general use in Europe.

What about the placental barrier? Once thought to protect the fetus from drug effects, the placenta isn't much of a barrier at all. Almost every drug a pregnant woman takes crosses the placenta and enters the fetal circulation, except for drugs with exceptionally large molecular structures, such as heparin, the injectable anticoagulant. By this standard, heparin could be used in a pregnant woman without fear of harming the fetus, but even heparin carries a warning for cautious use during pregnancy. Conversely, just because a drug crosses the placenta doesn't necessarily mean it's harmful to the fetus.

One factor—stage of fetal development—seems clearly related to greater risk during pregnancy. During the first and third trimesters of pregnancy, the fetus is especially vulnerable to damage from maternal use of drugs. During these times, give *all* drugs with extreme caution.

Organogenesis—when fetal organs differentiate—occurs in the first trimester. This is the most sensitive period for drug-induced fetal malformation. Strongly advise your patient to avoid *all* self-prescribed drugs during early pregnancy.

Fetal sensitivity to drugs is also of special concern during the third trimester. At birth, after separation from his mother, the neonate must rely on his own metabolism to eliminate any remaining drug. Because his detoxifying systems aren't fully developed, any residual drug may take a long time to be metabolized and thus may induce prolonged toxic reactions. For this reason, discourage pregnant patients from taking drugs except when absolutely necessary and advised by their prescriber during the last 3 months of pregnancy.

In many circumstances, pregnant women must continue to take certain drugs. For example, a woman with a seizure disorder that is well-controlled with an anticonvulsant should keep taking the drug during pregnancy. Similarly, a pregnant woman with a bacterial infection must receive antibiotics. In such cases, the potential risk to the fetus is outweighed by the mother's medical needs, and drugs with lower teratogenic potential are used whenever possible.

Complying with the following general guidelines can prevent indiscriminate and harmful use of drugs in pregnancy:
• Before a drug is prescribed for a woman of childbearing potential, ask the date of her last menstrual period and whether she may be pregnant. If a drug is a known teratogen (for example, isotretinoin), some manufacturers may recommend special precautions to ensure that the drug isn't given to a woman of childbearing potential until pregnancy is ruled out and may require that contraceptives be used throughout the course of therapy.
• Caution a pregnant woman to avoid all drugs (including OTC drugs and herbs and supplements) except those essential to maintain her pregnancy and health—especially during the first and third trimesters.
• Topical drugs may be subject to the same warning against use during pregnancy. Many topically applied drugs can be absorbed in large enough amounts to be harmful to the fetus.
• When a pregnant woman needs a drug, use the safest drug in the lowest possible dose to minimize harm to the fetus.

• Instruct a pregnant woman to check with her prescriber before taking any drug.

• Encourage a pregnant woman to enroll in the pregnancy exposure registry for drugs that have one. Registries compile data on pregnancy outcomes to further define the risks of drug exposure in human pregnancies.

Drugs and breast-feeding

Many drugs a breast-feeding mother takes appear in breast milk. Drug levels in breast milk tend to be high when drug levels in maternal blood are high, especially after each dose. Advise the mother to breast-feed *before* taking each drug dose, not *after*. Also, in general, drugs with short half-lives are preferred because they peak quickly and are then eliminated and are less likely to be excreted in breast milk.

A mother who wants to breast-feed usually may continue to do so with her prescriber's advice. However, breast-feeding should be temporarily interrupted and replaced with bottle-feeding when the mother must take drugs such as a tetracycline, a sulfonamide (during the first 2 weeks postpartum), an oral anticoagulant, a drug that contains iodine, or an antineoplastic.

Caution the breast-feeding patient to protect her infant by not taking drugs indiscriminately. Instruct the mother to first check with her prescriber to be sure she's taking the safest drug at the lowest dose. Also instruct her to give her prescriber a list of all drugs and herbs she's currently taking.

Drug therapy in children

Providing drug therapy to infants, children, and adolescents is challenging. Physiologic differences between children and adults, including those involving vital organ maturity and body composition, significantly influence a drug's effectiveness.

Physiologic changes affecting drug action

As a child develops, the processes of absorption, distribution (including drug binding to plasma proteins), metabolism, and excretion undergo profound changes that affect drug dosage. To ensure optimal drug effect and minimal toxicity, consider these factors when giving drugs to a child.

Absorption

Drug absorption in children depends on the form of the drug, its physical properties, si-

multaneous ingestion of other drugs or food, physiologic changes, and concurrent disease.

The pH of neonatal gastric fluid is neutral or slightly acidic; it becomes more acidic as the infant matures, which affects drug absorption. For example, nafcillin and penicillin G are better absorbed in an infant than in an adult because of low gastric acidity.

Various infant formulas or milk products may increase gastric pH and impede absorption of acidic drugs. If possible and so advised, give a child oral drugs on an empty stomach.

Gastric emptying time and transit time through the small intestine—which takes longer in children than in adults—can affect absorption. Also, intestinal hypermotility (as occurs in patients with diarrhea) can diminish the drug's absorption.

A child's comparatively thin epidermis allows increased absorption of topical drugs.

Distribution

As with absorption, changes in body weight and physiology during childhood can significantly influence a drug's distribution and effects. In a premature infant, body fluid makes up about 85% of total body weight; in a full-term infant, it makes up 55% to 70%; in an adult, 50% to 55%. Extracellular fluid (mostly blood) constitutes 40% of a neonate's body weight, compared with 20% in an adult. Intracellular fluid remains fairly constant throughout life and has little effect on drug dosage.

Extracellular fluid volume influences a water-soluble drug's concentration and effect because most drugs travel through extracellular fluid to reach their receptors. Compared with adults, distribution volume in children is proportionately greater because their fluid-to-solid body weight proportion is larger.

Because the proportion of fat to lean body mass increases with age, the distribution of fat-soluble drugs is more limited in children than in adults. As a result, a drug's fat or water solubility affects the dosage for a child.

Plasma protein binding

A decrease in albumin level or intermolecular attraction between drug and plasma protein causes many drugs to be less bound to plasma proteins in infants than in adults.

Strongly protein-bound drugs may displace endogenous compounds, such as bilirubin or free fatty acids. Displacement of bound bilirubin can increase unbound bilirubin, which can lead to increased risk of kernicterus at normal bilirubin levels. Conversely, an endogenous compound may displace a weakly protein-bound drug.

Because only an unbound (free) drug molecule has a pharmacologic effect, a change in the ratio of a protein-bound to an unbound active drug can greatly influence the drug's effect.

Several diseases and disorders, such as nephrotic syndrome and malnutrition, can decrease plasma protein levels and increase the level of an unbound drug, which can either intensify the drug's effect or produce toxicity.

Metabolism

A neonate's ability to metabolize a drug depends on the integrity of the hepatic enzyme system, intrauterine exposure to the drug, and the nature of the drug itself.

Certain metabolic mechanisms are underdeveloped in neonates. Glucuronidation is a metabolic process that renders most drugs more water soluble, facilitating renal excretion. This process isn't developed enough to permit full pediatric doses of most drugs until the infant is 1 month of age. The use of chloramphenicol sodium succinate in a neonate may cause gray baby syndrome because the infant's immature liver can't metabolize the drug and toxic levels accumulate in the blood. Reduce the dosage in a neonate and periodically monitor drug levels. Conversely, intrauterine exposure to drugs may induce precocious development of hepatic enzyme mechanisms, increasing the infant's capacity to metabolize potentially harmful substances.

Older children can metabolize some drugs (theophylline, for example) more rapidly than adults. This ability may arise from their increased hepatic metabolic activity. Doses larger than those recommended for adults may be required.

Also, more than one drug given simultaneously to a child may change hepatic metabolism and initiate production of hepatic enzymes. Phenobarbital, for example, induces hepatic enzyme production and accelerates the metabolism of some drugs taken concomitantly.

Excretion

Renal excretion of a drug is the net result of glomerular filtration, active tubular secretion, and passive tubular reabsorption. Many drugs are excreted in the urine. The degree of renal development or presence of renal disease can greatly affect a child's dosage requirements because if a child can't excrete a drug renally, the drug may accumulate to toxic levels.

Physiologically, an infant's kidneys differ from an adult's because infants have a high resistance to blood flow and their kidneys receive a smaller proportion of cardiac output. Infants have incomplete glomerular and tubular development and short, incomplete loops of Henle. (A child's GFR reaches an adult value between ages 2½ and 5 months; his tubular secretion rate may reach an adult value between ages 7 and 12 months.) Infants also are less able to concentrate urine or reabsorb certain filtered compounds. The proximal tubules in infants also are less able to secrete organic acids.

Children and adults have diurnal variations in urine pH that correlate with sleep patterns. Changes in urine pH can affect the amount of drug excreted into the urine.

Special administration considerations

Biochemically, a drug displays the same mechanisms of action in all people. But the response to a drug can be affected by a child's age and size, as well as by the maturity of the target organ. To ensure optimal drug effect and minimal toxicity, consider the following factors when giving drugs to children.

Adjusting dosages for children

When calculating children's dosages, don't use formulas that modify adult dosages. A child isn't a scaled-down version of an adult. Base pediatric dosages on either body weight (mg/kg) or body surface area (mg/m^2).

Reevaluate dosages at regular intervals to ensure needed adjustments as the child develops. Although body surface area provides a useful standard for adults and older children, use the body weight method instead in premature or full-term infants. Don't exceed the maximum adult dosage when calculating amounts per kilogram of body weight (except with certain drugs, such as theophylline, if indicated).

Obtain an accurate maternal drug history, including prescription and nonprescription drugs, vitamins, herbs, or other health foods taken during pregnancy. Drugs passed into breast milk can have adverse effects on the breast-feeding infant. Before giving a drug to a breast-feeding mother, investigate its potential effects on the infant.

For example, a sulfonamide given to a breast-feeding mother for a UTI appears in breast milk and may cause kernicterus in an infant with low levels of unconjugated bilirubin. Also, high levels of isoniazid appear in the breast milk of a mother taking this drug. Because isoniazid is metabolized by the liver, the infant's immature hepatic enzyme mechanisms can't metabolize the drug, and he may develop CNS toxicity.

Giving oral drugs
Remember the following when giving oral drugs to a child:

If the patient is an infant, give drugs in liquid form, if possible. For accuracy, measure and give the preparation by oral syringe, never a parenteral syringe. It's very important to remove the syringe cap to keep the infant from aspirating it. Be sure to instruct parents to do the same. Never use a vial or cup. Lift the patient's head to prevent aspiration of the drug, and press down on his chin to prevent choking. You may also place the drug in a nipple and allow the infant to suck the contents.

If the patient is a toddler, explain how you're going to give him the drug. If possible, have the parents enlist the child's cooperation. Never call it "candy," even if it has a pleasant taste. Let the child drink a liquid drug from a calibrated medication cup rather than a spoon. It's easier and more accurate. If the preparation is available only in tablet form, crush and mix it with an appropriate vehicle, such as jelly or applesauce. (First, verify with a pharmacist that the tablet can be crushed and mixed without compromising its effectiveness.)

If the patient is an older child who can swallow a tablet or capsule by himself, have him place the drug on the back of his tongue and swallow it with water or nonacidic fruit juice, because milk and milk products may interfere with drug absorption.

Giving I.V. infusions
For I.V. infusions in infants, use a peripheral vein or a scalp vein in the temporal region. The scalp vein is safe because the needle isn't likely to dislodge. However, the hair must be clipped around the site, and the needle and infiltrated fluids may cause temporary disfigurement. For these reasons, scalp veins aren't used as commonly today as they were in the past.

The arms and legs are the most accessible insertion sites, but because children tend to move about, take these precautions:
• Protect the insertion site to keep the catheter or needle from being dislodged. Use a padded arm board to reduce the risk of dislodgment. Remove the arm board during range-of-motion exercises.
• Place the I.V. tubing clamp out of the child's reach. If extension tubing is used to allow the child greater mobility, securely tape the connection.
• Explain in simple terms to the child why he must be restrained while asleep, to alleviate anxiety and maintain trust.

During an infusion, monitor flow rates and check the child's condition and the insertion site at least every hour. Titrate the flow rate only while the patient is composed; crying and emotional upset can constrict blood vessels. Flow rate may vary if a pump isn't used. Flow should be adequate because some drugs (calcium, for example) can be irritating at low flow rates. Infants, small children, and children with compromised cardiopulmonary status are especially vulnerable to fluid overload with I.V. drug administration. To prevent this problem and help ensure that a limited amount of fluid is infused in a controlled manner, use a volume-control device in the I.V. tubing and an infusion pump or a syringe. Don't place more than 2 hours of I.V. fluid in the volume-control set at a time.

Giving I.M. injections
I.M. injections are preferred when a drug can't be given by other parenteral routes and rapid absorption is needed.

The vastus lateralis muscle is the preferred injection site in children age 2 and younger. For children ages 3 to 18, the deltoid muscle is the preferred site. Though rarely used in children, the ventrogluteal site can be used in certain circumstances, such as when the child's condition prevents administration in other sites. To select the correct needle size, consider the patient's age, muscle mass, nutritional status, and drug viscosity.

Record and rotate injection sites. Explain to the patient that the injection will hurt but that the drug will help him. Swaddle an infant or use an assistant during the injection, if needed, and comfort him afterward.

Giving topical drugs and inhalants
When you give a child a topical drug or inhalant, consider the following:

Use eardrops warmed to room temperature. Cold drops can cause pain and vertigo. To give drops, turn the patient on his side, with the affected ear up. If he's younger than age 3, pull the pinna down and back; if age 3 or older, pull the pinna up and back.

Avoid using inhalants in young children because it's difficult to get them to cooperate. Before you try to give a drug to an older child through a metered-dose inhaler, explain the inhaler to him. Then have him hold the inhaler upside down and close his lips around the mouthpiece. Have him exhale and pinch his nostrils shut. When he starts to inhale, release one dose of the drug into his mouth. Tell the patient to continue inhaling until his lungs feel full; then he can breathe normally and unpinch his nostrils. Most inhaled drugs aren't useful if the drug remains in the mouth or throat—if you doubt the patient's ability to use the inhaler correctly, don't use it. Devices, such as spacers or assist devices, may help. Check with a pharmacist, the prescriber, or a respiratory therapist.

Use topical corticosteroids cautiously because prolonged use in children may delay growth. When you apply topical corticosteroids to the diaper area of infants, don't cover the area with plastic or rubber pants, which act as an occlusive dressing and may enhance systemic absorption.

Giving parenteral nutrition
Give I.V. nutrition to patients who can't or won't take adequate food orally and to patients with hypermetabolic conditions who need supplementation. The latter group includes premature infants and children with burns or other major trauma, intractable diarrhea, malabsorption syndromes, GI abnormalities, emotional disorders (such as anorexia nervosa), and congenital abnormalities.

Before giving fat emulsions to infants and children, weigh the potential benefits against any possible risks. Fats—supplied as 10% or 20% lipid emulsions—are given both peripherally and centrally. Their use is limited by the child's ability to metabolize them. For example, an infant or child with a diseased liver can't efficiently metabolize fats.

Some fats, however, must be supplied both to prevent essential fatty acid deficiency and to permit normal growth and development.

A minimum of calories (2% to 4%) must be supplied as linoleic acid—an essential fatty acid found in lipids. Nevertheless, fat solutions may decrease oxygen perfusion and may adversely affect children with pulmonary disease. This risk can be minimized by supplying only the minimum fat needed for essential fatty acid requirements and not the usual intake of 40% to 50% of the child's total calories.

Fatty acids can also displace bilirubin bound to albumin, causing a rise in free, unconjugated bilirubin and an increased risk of kernicterus. Fat solutions may interfere with some bilirubin assays and cause falsely elevated bilirubin levels. To avoid this complication, draw a blood sample 4 hours after infusion of the lipid emulsion, or, if the emulsion is infused over 24 hours, be sure the laboratory is aware so that the blood samples can be centrifuged before the assay is performed.

Drug therapy in elderly patients

If you're giving drugs to elderly patients, you'll need to understand the physiologic and pharmacokinetic changes in this population that may affect drug dosage, cause common adverse reactions, or create compliance problems.

Physiologic changes affecting drug action

As a person ages, gradual physiologic changes occur. Some of these age-related changes may alter the therapeutic and toxic effects of drugs.

Body composition
Proportions of fat, lean tissue, and water in the body change with age. Total body mass and lean body mass tend to decrease, but the proportion of body fat tends to increase.

Body composition varies from person to person, and these changes in body composition affect the relationship between a drug's concentration and distribution in the body.

For example, a water-soluble drug such as gentamicin isn't distributed to fat. Because there's relatively more fat tissue and less lean tissue in an elderly person, more drug remains in the blood. Fat-soluble drugs tend to accumulate in older patients, resulting in prolonged half-lives and more pronounced effects.

Gastrointestinal function
In elderly patients, decreases in gastric acid secretion and GI motility slow the emptying of stomach contents and movement through the entire intestinal tract. Research suggests

that elderly patients may have more difficulty absorbing drugs than younger patients. This is an especially significant problem with drugs that have a narrow therapeutic range, such as digoxin, in which any change in absorption can be crucial.

Hepatic function

The liver's ability to metabolize certain drugs decreases with age. This decrease is caused by diminished blood flow to the liver, which results from an age-related decrease in cardiac output, and from the lessened activity of certain liver enzymes. When an elderly patient takes a sleep medication such as flurazepam, for example, the liver's reduced ability to metabolize the drug as well as the lipophilic property of the drug can produce residual effects the next morning.

Decreased hepatic function may result in more intense drug effects caused by higher levels, longer-lasting drug effects because of prolonged levels, and a greater risk of drug toxicity.

Renal function

An elderly person's renal function is usually sufficient to eliminate excess body fluid and waste, but the ability to eliminate some drugs may be reduced by 50% or more.

Many drugs commonly used by elderly patients, such as digoxin, are excreted primarily through the kidneys. If the kidneys' ability to excrete the drug is decreased, high blood levels may result. Digoxin toxicity can occur in elderly patients who don't receive a reduced digoxin dosage to accommodate decreased renal function.

Drug dosages can be modified to compensate for age-related decreases in renal function. Aided by results of laboratory tests, such as BUN and creatinine levels, adjust drug dosages so the patient receives therapeutic benefits without the risk of toxicity. It is important to remember that serum creatinine is a function of muscle mass and that most elderly people lose muscle mass as they age. An elderly patient can have significant renal impairment even with a serum creatinine level in the normal range. Also, observe the patient for signs and symptoms of toxicity. A patient taking digoxin, for example, may experience anorexia, nausea, vomiting, or confusion.

Special administration considerations

Aging is usually accompanied by a decline in organ function that can affect drug distribution and clearance. This physiologic decline is likely to be worsened by a disease or a chronic disorder. Together, these factors can significantly increase the risk of adverse reactions and drug toxicity, as well as noncompliance.

Adverse reactions

Compared with younger people, elderly patients experience twice as many adverse drug reactions, mostly from greater drug use, poor compliance, and physiologic changes.

Signs and symptoms of adverse drug reactions—including confusion, weakness, agitation, and lethargy—are often mistakenly attributed to senility or disease. If the adverse reaction isn't identified, the patient may continue to receive the drug. He may receive other, unnecessary drugs to treat complications caused by the original drug. This regimen can sometimes result in a pattern of inappropriate and excessive drug use.

Any drug can cause adverse reactions, but most of the serious reactions in the elderly are caused by relatively few drugs. Be particularly alert for toxicities resulting from diuretics, antihypertensives, digoxin, corticosteroids, anticoagulants, sleeping aids, and OTC drugs.

Diuretic toxicity

Because total body water content decreases with age, a normal dosage of a potassium-wasting diuretic, such as hydrochlorothiazide or furosemide, may result in fluid loss and even dehydration in an elderly patient.

These diuretics may deplete a patient's potassium level, making him feel weak, and they may raise blood uric acid and glucose levels, complicating gout and diabetes mellitus.

Antihypertensive toxicity

Many elderly patients experience light-headedness or fainting when taking antihypertensives, partly in response to atherosclerosis and decreased elasticity of the blood vessels. Antihypertensives can lower BP too rapidly, resulting in insufficient blood flow to the brain, which can cause dizziness, fainting, or even a stroke.

Consequently, dosages of antihypertensives must be carefully individualized. In elderly patients, aggressive treatment of high BP may be harmful. Treatment goals should be reasonable.

Elevated BP needs to be reduced more slowly in elderly patients.

Digoxin toxicity

As the body's renal function and rate of excretion decline, the digoxin level in the blood of an elderly patient may increase to the point of causing nausea, vomiting, diarrhea and, most seriously, cardiac arrhythmias. Monitor the patient's digoxin level and observe him for early signs and symptoms of toxicity, such as appetite loss, confusion, or depression.

Corticosteroid toxicity

Elderly patients taking a corticosteroid may experience short-term effects, including fluid retention and psychological effects ranging from mild euphoria to acute psychotic reactions. Long-term toxic effects, such as osteoporosis, can be especially severe in elderly patients who have been taking prednisone or related steroidal compounds for months or even years. To prevent serious toxicity, carefully monitor patients on long-term regimens. Observe them for subtle changes in appearance, mood, and mobility and for impaired healing and fluid and electrolyte disturbances.

Anticoagulant effects

Elderly patients taking an anticoagulant have an increased risk of bleeding, especially when they take NSAIDs at the same time. Be sure to evaluate all drugs the patient is taking for increased risk of bleeding. Because they are more likely to fall, they're also at increased risk. Monitor the patient's INR carefully, if applicable, and monitor for bruising and other signs of bleeding.

Sleeping aid toxicity

Sedatives and sleeping aids such as zolpidem may cause excessive sedation or drowsiness. Keep in mind that consumption of alcohol may increase CNS depressant effects, even if the sleeping aid was taken the previous evening. Use these drugs sparingly in elderly patients.

Over-the-counter drug toxicity

Prolonged ingestion of aspirin, aspirin-containing analgesics, and other OTC NSAIDs (such as ibuprofen, ketoprofen, and naproxen) may cause GI irritation—even ulcers—and gradual blood loss resulting in severe anemia. Prescription NSAIDs may cause similar problems. Both OTC and prescription NSAIDs can cause renal toxicity in older adults. Anemia from prolonged aspirin consumption can affect all age groups, but elderly patients may be less able to compensate because of their already reduced iron stores. These drugs should be used very carefully and at the lowest effective doses.

Acetaminophen is found in a variety of prescription and OTC products. Liver injury may occur from inadvertently taking excess acetaminophen from multiple sources.

Laxatives may cause diarrhea in elderly patients, who are extremely sensitive to drugs such as bisacodyl. Long-term oral use of mineral oil as a lubricating laxative may result in lipid pneumonia from aspiration of small residual oil droplets in the patient's mouth.

Antihistamines such as diphenhydramine have anticholinergic effects and can cause confusion and mental status changes; they are also more likely to cause dizziness, sedation, and hypotension in elderly patients. OTC decongestants can have systemic effects, such as hypertension, anxiety, insomnia, and agitation.

Noncompliance

Poor compliance can be a problem with patients of any age. Many hospitalizations result from noncompliance with a medical regimen. In elderly patients, factors linked to aging, such as diminished visual acuity, hearing loss, forgetfulness, the need for multiple drug therapy, and socioeconomic factors, can combine to make compliance a special problem. About one-third of elderly patients fail to comply with their prescribed drug therapy. They may fail to take prescribed doses or to follow the correct schedule. They may take drugs prescribed for previous disorders, stop drugs prematurely, or indiscriminately use drugs that are to be taken as needed. Elderly patients may also have multiple prescriptions for the same drug and inadvertently take an overdose.

Review the patient's drug regimen with him. Make sure he understands the dose amount, the time and frequency of doses, and why he's taking the drug. Also, explain in detail if a drug is to be taken with food, with water, or separate from other drugs. To verify the patient's understanding, ask him to repeat the instructions back to you.

Help the patient avoid drug therapy problems by suggesting that he use drug calendars, pill sorters, or other aids to help him comply. Refer him to the prescriber, a pharmacist, or social services if he needs further information or assistance with his drug therapy.

3

Safe drug administration

Medication therapy is a primary intervention for many illnesses. It greatly benefits many patients and yet is involved in many instances of unintended harm to patients and health care workers from either unintended consequences of therapy (adverse drug reactions or exposure to hazardous drugs) or medication-related errors (adverse drug events). (See *Preventing and treating I.V. vesicant extravasation injury,* page 14.) Medication errors are a significant cause of patient morbidity and mortality in the United States. In 1999, the Institute of Medicine (IOM) published its first Quality Chasm report, "To Err is Human: Building a Safer Health System," which reported that errors related to medications accounted for approximately 1 out of 131 outpatient deaths, 1 out of 854 inpatient deaths, and more than 7,000 deaths annually. Recent research indicates that the number of medication errors may actually be much higher. Of all sentinel events reviewed between 2004 and 2015 (9,581) by The Joint Commission (a nonprofit organization that seeks to improve public health care through the voluntary accreditation of health care institutions), approximately 475 events have been attributed to medication errors plus an additional 236 events were medication equipment–related.

Many governmental and nongovernmental organizations are dedicated to improving the safety of drug administration. One mission of the FDA, for example, is to protect the public health by assuring the safety, effectiveness, and security of human drugs, vaccines, and medical devices. In 2007, the Food and Drug Administration Amendments Act expanded the FDA's authority regarding assessing and communicating risks associated with drugs. One of the new provisions of the law granted the FDA authority to require drug manufacturers to submit Risk Evaluation and Mitigation Strategies (REMS). (See *Risk Evaluation and Mitigation Strategies,* page 15.) The U.S. Pharmacopeia (USP), a nonprofit, nongovernmental public health organization, sets official public standards for drugs and other health care products manufactured or sold in the United States. It also sets standards for the quality, purity, and strength of food ingredients and dietary supplements.

In 2005, The Patient Safety and Quality Improvement Act authorized the creation of patient safety organizations (PSOs) to improve the quality and safety of U.S. health care delivery. One of these PSOs, the Institute for Safe Medication Practices (ISMP), is a nonprofit organization entirely dedicated to preventing medication errors and using medications safely. In addition, The Joint Commission has established National Patient Safety Goals and standards to improve the safe use of medications in its accredited facilities.

The CDC has a number of campaigns and initiatives to promote medication safety by developing evidence-based policies and using collaborative interventions.

One important initiative of the CDC, FDA, and other organizations is to address the use and misuse of opioids in treating chronic pain (pain not related to cancer or palliative care that lasts longer than 3 months or past the time of normal tissue healing). Research from 2013 showed that approximately 1.9 million individuals in the United States misused or were dependent on prescription opioids, and from 1999 to 2014, 165,000 people died from opioid-related overdose. The death rate continues to increase.

The CDC has developed an evidence-based guideline, "CDC Guideline for Prescribing Opioids for Chronic Pain–United States, 2016" (www.cdc.gov/mmwr/volumes/65/rr/rr6501e1.htm?s_cid=rr6501e1_w), which addresses "1) when to initiate or continue opioids for chronic pain; 2) opioid selection, dosage, duration, follow-up, and discontinuation; and 3) assessing risk and addressing harms of opioid use." The CDC has also developed the "Checklist for Prescribing Opioids for Chronic Pain" (https://stacks.cdc.gov/view/cdc/38025), which provides guidance for primary care providers treating adults with chronic pain.

The FDA is developing a comprehensive action plan to reassess its approach to opioids and will focus on policies to reverse the opioid abuse epidemic while providing patients access to effective pain relief. The FDA opioid medication action plan includes reexamining the risks and benefits of opioids and their effects on public health, supporting alternative pain

Preventing and treating I.V. vesicant extravasation injury

Extravasation injuries occur when vesicant I.V. solutions or drugs—those with the potential to cause significant tissue injury (such as certain chemotherapy drugs, antibiotics, electrolyte solutions, vasopressors, and antiemetics)—accidentally escape from blood vessels into surrounding tissue (extravasate) during administration. Drugs or solutions that produce inflammation rather than serious or lasting tissue injury from extravasation are considered irritants. Extravasation injuries may occur when vesicants are given centrally or peripherally. Such injury can cause significant harm, including necrotic ulcers that may require surgical intervention, infection, loss of a limb or limb function, or complex regional pain syndrome.

Signs and symptoms of peripheral extravasation include:

- changes in I.V. site appearance (blanching, bruising) or temperature (coolness, erythema)
- pain, tightness, or itching at or surrounding the insertion site
- I.V. site fluid leakage
- numbness or tingling, diminished capillary refill, or decreased motor function in the extremity.

Signs and symptoms of central venous access device (CVAD) extravasation include:

- discomfort at the insertion site or along the CVAD path
- fluid leakage from the insertion site
- increased resistance to solution injection
- shoulder, neck, or chest edema.

Preventing extravasation

Use the following measures to prevent extravasation injuries:

- Know facility policy for administering vesicant drugs and solutions. Make sure you've been properly trained in prevention measures and extravasation recognition and management.
- When administering vesicants, know the specific antidote for the drug being given, and make sure that the antidote and equipment needed to manage extravasation are on hand. Some antidotes for vesicants and solutions include sodium thiosulfate for alkylating agents, hyaluronidase for electrolytes and antibiotics (nafcillin, vancomycin [Vancocin]), and phentolamine for vasopressors (dopamine, norepinephrine).

- Ensure that the I.V. access site or CVAD is patent before giving the drug. Make sure the insertion site is visible, and use an appropriate catheter stabilization device.
- Make sure the drug is given by the proper route according to facility policy. Most vesicants administered by continuous infusion should be given utilizing a CVAD. Know when an I.V. infusion pump device should and shouldn't be used.
- Frequently monitor the patient for extravasation signs and symptoms, and teach the patient to immediately report them.

Treating extravasation

- Follow facility policy for treatment of extravasation injury. Stop the drug, and aspirate any residual drug and blood from the I.V. catheter or CVAD.
- Estimate the amount of solution extravasated and notify the practitioner.
- If an antidote exists, prepare for administration through the existing I.V. catheter or CVAD. After administration, remove the peripheral I.V. catheter, but avoid pressure to the site.
- For extravasation from a CVAD, prepare the patient for a CT scan to assess catheter placement and fluid collection, if appropriate.
- For peripheral extravasation, prepare for subcutaneous injections of drug-specific antidote, if appropriate.
- Elevate the affected limb.
- Apply hot (for vasoconstrictors) or cold (for alkylating drugs) compresses, if ordered.
- Use a skin marker or photo for serial documentation of extravasation according to facility policy.
- Monitor the site for pain, erythema progression, induration, tissue necrosis, and possible compartment syndrome. Note that symptom development may be delayed for 48 hours.
- Document the date and time of the infusion, time when signs and symptoms were first noted, extravasation signs and symptoms, type and size of venous access device, estimated extravasation solution amount, treatment instituted, practitioner notification, and the patient's response to treatment. Patients with significant tissue damage may need surgery.

---

management options, consulting expert advisory committees for opioid new drug approvals and for appropriate opioid use in children, developing additional changes and warnings to opioid labeling information, updating REMS requirements, supporting the development of and expanding use of abuse-deterrent opioids, improving access to naloxone and other drug treatment options for opioid use disorders, and strengthening drug company requirements to provide postmarketing data on the long-term effects of opioid use.

Causes of medication errors

The National Coordinating Council for Medication Error Reporting and Prevention

Risk Evaluation and Mitigation Strategies

Risk Evaluation and Mitigation Strategies (REMS) is a risk management program that goes beyond the drug's package insert and is used when necessary to make certain that a drug's benefits outweigh its risks. The FDA can require a REMS at any stage of a drug's lifecycle (as part of a drug's New Drug Application or after approval as new safety information becomes available), and manufacturers who fail to comply with REMS requirements can face substantial monetary penalties.

When evaluating the necessity of REMS, the FDA takes into consideration such factors as:
- the number of patients most likely to use the drug
- the seriousness of the patient's disease
- the drug's benefit
- the projected duration of treatment
- the severity of known or potential adverse events
- whether the drug is a new molecular entity.

The FDA has issued an outline of specific components that manufacturers should use to develop a REMS proposal. These include the development of specific REMS goals and elements to ensure a drug's safe and appropriate use. The REMS must also describe how the manufacturer plans to evaluate whether the REMS goal is being met and the timetable for periodic assessments and reassessments. The results of the evaluations must be reported to the FDA, and the FDA may require that the REMS be modified and will determine if additional actions must be taken.

REMS may contain one or all of the following components:
- **Medication guide:** Written safety information for patients that must be distributed by the pharmacist to each patient receiving the drug
- **Communication plan:** Plan that includes the tools to teach health care professionals how to use the drug safely and appropriately
- **Elements to Assure Safe Use (EASU):** Specific requirements and elements to ensure safe use of the drug, including requirements that each patient be enrolled in a registry, that essential laboratory monitoring be performed, that the drug may only be prescribed by a prescriber with a specific certification, and that the drug may only be distributed by a specialty pharmacy
- **Implementation plan:** Plan that describes how the EASUs will be put into action.

(www.nccmerp.org/) defines a *medication error* as "any preventable event that may cause or lead to inappropriate medication use or patient harm while the medication is in the control of the health care professional, patient, or consumer. Such events may be related to professional practice, health care products, procedures, and systems, including prescribing; order communication; product labeling, packaging, and nomenclature; compounding; dispensing; distribution; administration; education; monitoring; and use."

Medication errors were once thought to be caused by lapses in an individual's practice. Traditionally, teaching nurses to administer drugs safely focused on the individual nurse's practice and the application of the "rights" of safe medication administration. (See *The eight "rights" of medication administration,* page 16.)

Although individual nursing practice is still an extremely important part of safe drug administration, the focus has widened. After medication errors had been systematically studied by numerous organizations who shared data, it became apparent that medication errors are complex events with multiple factors and are most often caused by failures within systems. As a result of these findings, research has shifted to preventing medication errors by identifying their root causes and then developing and validating evidence-based prevention strategies. Organizational processes, management decisions, inadequate medication administration protocols, staffing shortages, environmental conditions, poor communication, inadequate drug knowledge and resources, and individual mistakes or protocol violations may all contribute to drug errors.

The medication administration process

Medication errors can occur from medication administration process problems or within any one or more than one of the five stages of medication administration. Because up to 40% of a nurse's time may be spent in medication administration and nursing practice intersects multiple stages, nurses may often be involved in medication errors. Here are some of the types of errors that have been reported in each stage.

Stage 1: Ordering and prescribing
- Prescriber orders are incomplete or illegible.
- Contraindicated drugs (such as drugs to which the patient is allergic) are prescribed.
- The prescriber specifies the wrong drug, dose, route, frequency, or duration, or fails to specify the indication.

Traditionally, nurses have been taught the "five rights" of medication administration. These are broadly stated goals and practices to help individual nurses administer drugs safely.

1. The *right drug:* Check the drug label and verify that the drug and form to be given is the drug that was prescribed.
2. The *right patient:* Confirm the patient's identity by checking two patient identifiers.
3. The *right dose:* Verify that the dose and dosage form to be given are appropriate for the patient, and check the drug label with the prescriber's order.
4. The *right time:* Ensure that the drug is administered at the correct time and frequency.
5. The *right route:* Verify that the route by which the drug is to be given is specified by the prescriber and is appropriate for the patient.

In addition to the traditional "five rights" of individual practice, best-practice researchers have added three additional "rights":

6. The *right reason:* Verify that the drug prescribed is appropriate to treat the patient's condition.
7. The *right response:* Monitor the patient's response to the drug administered.
8. The *right documentation:* Completely and accurately document in the patient's medical record the drug administered; the monitoring of the patient, including his response; and other nursing interventions.

• Drugs are prescribed using inappropriate or inadequate verbal orders.

Stage 2: Transcribing and verifying
• An incorrect drug, dose, route, time, or frequency is transcribed into the medication administration record (MAR) by the pharmacist or nurse.
• Drug verification and documentation in the MAR by the pharmacist or nurse are inadequate.

Stage 3: Dispensing and delivery
• The prescribed drug is filled incorrectly.
• Failure to deliver the right drug to the right place for the right patient occurs.

Stage 4: Administering
• The wrong drug is given to the wrong patient by the nurse or other licensed professional.
• The wrong dose is calculated and given or infused by the nurse or other licensed professional.

• The right drug is incorrectly prepared (such as crushing a drug that shouldn't be crushed) and is given by the nurse or other licensed professional.
• The correct drug is administered by the wrong route (such as an oral drug that is injected I.V.) by the nurse or other licensed professional.
• The correct drug is given at the wrong time or frequency by the nurse or other licensed professional.

Stage 5: Monitoring and reporting
• Monitoring of the patient by the nurse before and after medication administration is inadequate.
• Documentation and reporting of the patient's condition by the nurse before and after medication administration are inadequate.
• Hand-off communication between licensed professionals is inadequate.
• Reporting of medication errors is inadequate.

Elements contributing to safer drug administration

Ensuring the safe delivery of medication involves a system-wide approach, and research has shown that improvements in communication, education, and prevention of hazardous drug exposure can facilitate the safe delivery of medication.

Communication improvements

Communication issues have been implicated in approximately 60% of reported medication errors. Communication can be improved in many ways throughout the medication administration process. The traditional nursing process "rights" of safe drug administration are still important components of safe drug administration, but even when protocols are followed exactly, some medication errors still occur. For example, a nurse who's exactly following the eight "rights" might administer a drug to which a patient is allergic if his allergy information is incomplete or undocumented or hasn't been communicated effectively. Appropriate communication among all members of the health care team, including nurses, is vitally important.

Many health care facilities have instituted measures to help standardize and organize appropriate communication. One tool commonly used is SBAR (Situation, Background, Assessment, and Recommendation); its purpose is to logically organize information to optimize proper communication among health care providers.

Each institution must have tools and policies in place for the documentation of medication administration. Each prescribed medication order must be clearly written or entered into an electronic medical chart system, and verbal orders must be used and documented according to facility policy. Each verbal order should be read back and verified with the prescriber before the drug is administered. The patient's condition must be monitored after each medication is given, and the patient's response and any nursing interventions must be documented appropriately. Clear communication through documentation is essential to safe practice.

The Joint Commission has developed goals and standards regarding medication reconciliation—the process of comparing a patient's medication regimen at every transition in his care (for example, on admission, upon discharge, and between care settings and levels). Medication reconciliation helps ensure that essential information about the patient's medication regimen is communicated to the health care team. Medication reconciliation helps prevent the inadvertent omission of needed medications, prevents medication duplication, and helps identify medications with potentially harmful interactions.

Education improvements

Lack of knowledge has been implicated in many medication errors; therefore, education about medications is essential to their safe administration. All health care team members involved in the process of medication administration, including the prescriber, pharmacist, and nurse, must have access to accurate information about each drug's indications, appropriate dosing regimen, appropriate route, appropriate frequency, possible drug interactions, appropriate monitoring, any cautions, and possible adverse effects. Each facility should have processes in place to educate staff and communicate important drug information.

Governmental and nongovernmental agencies are doing their part toward educating facilities, prescribers, and nurses. In 1995, the FDA established the black box warning system to alert prescribers to drugs with increased risks to patients. These boxed warnings are the strongest labeling requirements for drugs that can have serious reactions. The Joint Commission requires accredited health care facilities

to develop a list of abbreviations to avoid in all medication communications. The ISMP maintains a list of high-alert medications that may cause significant patient harm when given incorrectly. (Each facility should have protocols in place for administering high-alert medications with safeguards built into the process.) The FDA and ISMP have developed a list of drugs with similar names—sound-alike, look-alike (SALA) medications—that can be easily confused. Dissimilarities in each drug's name are highlighted with tall letters (so each name has mixed-case letters), making each drug less prone to mix-ups.

Patient education

Patients and their families should be active participants in the patient's care and should understand the patient's plan of care, including the purpose of newly prescribed medications. The patient and family need to be taught what to watch for, how the patient's condition will be monitored, and what signs and symptoms to report, and to report anything that doesn't seem right, including unfamiliar medications. Before administering a medication, the nurse needs to verify with the patient medication allergies or unusual past reactions to medications.

The following general teaching guidelines will help ensure that the patient receives the maximum therapeutic benefit from his medication regimen and will help him avoid adverse reactions, accidental overdose, and harmful changes in effectiveness.

• Instruct the patient to learn the brand names, generic name, and dosages of all drugs and supplements (such as herbs and vitamins) that he's taking.

• Tell the patient to notify the pharmacist and prescriber about everything he takes, including prescription drugs, OTC drugs, and herbal or other supplements, and about any drug allergies or reactions.

• Advise the patient to always read the label before taking a drug, to take it exactly as prescribed, and to never share prescription drugs.

• Warn the patient not to change brands of a drug without consulting the prescriber, to avoid harmful changes in effectiveness. For example, certain generic preparations aren't equivalent in effect to brand-name preparations of the same drug.

• Tell the patient to check the expiration date before taking a drug.

• Teach the patient how to safely discard drugs that are outdated or no longer needed.

• Caution the patient to keep all drugs safely out of the reach of children and pets.

• Advise the patient to store drugs in their original containers, at the proper temperature, and in areas where they won't be exposed to sunlight or excessive heat or humidity. Sunlight, heat, and humidity can cause drug deterioration and reduce a drug's effectiveness.

• Encourage the patient to report all suspected adverse or unusual reactions to the prescriber, and teach him proper techniques to monitor his condition (for example, how to obtain a resting HR before taking digoxin).

• Suggest that the patient have all prescriptions filled at the same pharmacy so that the pharmacist can warn against potentially harmful drug interactions.

• Tell the patient to report his complete medication history to all of his health care providers, including his dentist.

• Instruct the patient to call the prescriber, poison control center, or pharmacist immediately and to seek immediate medical attention if he or someone else has taken an overdose. The National Poison Control Center emergency phone number is 1-800-222-1222. Tell the patient to keep this and other emergency numbers handy at all times.

• Advise the patient to make sure he has a sufficient supply of drugs when traveling. He should carry them with him in their original containers and not pack them in luggage. Also, recommend that he carry a letter from his prescriber authorizing the use of a drug, especially if the drug is a controlled substance.

• Encourage the patient to keep a wallet card that lists all his medications, including the dose, route, frequency, and indication.

Improvements in preventing hazardous drug exposure

The CDC estimates that 8 million U.S. health care workers are potentially exposed to hazardous drugs in the workplace. Hazardous drugs, as defined by the American Society of Health-System Pharmacists and the National Institute for Occupational Safety and Health (NIOSH), have one or more of the following characteristics:

• carcinogenicity (cause cancer)

• teratogenicity (cause defects in the developing fetus) or cause other developmental toxicities

• reproductive toxicity

• organ toxicity at low doses

• genotoxicity (cause damage to DNA)

• a structure and toxicity profile that mimics that of existing hazardous drugs.

The NIOSH list of antineoplastics and other hazardous drugs can be found at www.cdc.gov/niosh/docs/2014-138/pdfs/2014-138_v3.pdf. Health care workers can be exposed to hazardous drugs through inhalation, ingestion, skin contact/absorption, or injection; exposure is most likely from skin contact/absorption or inhalation. Potential exposure can occur in many ways, such as:

• preparing drugs for administration (reconstituting powdered drugs, crushing tablets for oral liquids, compounding powders, or counting out oral doses from multidose bottles)

• administering hazardous drugs I.M., I.V., or subcutaneously

• directly contacting drugs on the contaminated exteriors of drug vials, on drug-contaminated work surfaces, and on I.V. tubing and syringes

• handling body fluids that contain drugs or drug-contaminated dressings, linens, or waste

• transporting hazardous drugs

• removing and disposing of personal protective equipment (PPE)

• cleaning contaminated work spaces and spills.

Protecting workers and minimizing exposure

Protecting health care workers and minimizing their exposure to hazardous drugs can be achieved through engineering and administrative controls and use of appropriate PPE.

Engineering controls include:

• class II or III biological safety cabinets (also known as *vertical flow hoods* or *ventilated cabinets*) for hazardous drug preparation

• closed-system drug transfer devices

• needleless systems.

Administrative controls include:

• implementing training, retraining, and testing programs to educate and monitor staff about best practices to prevent hazardous drug exposure

• developing and implementing management policies and protocols to reduce staff risk

• using monitoring programs to identify hazardous drugs and staff exposure or development of early disease.

Appropriate use of PPE includes:

• making sure PPE fits and is used and disposed of properly, following facility policies and protocols

• selecting PPE based on assessment of the potential for hazardous drug exposure:
– Gloves: Select gloves appropriate for the potential exposure. Double gloving may be necessary depending on the potential exposure. Polyvinyl chloride exam gloves offer little hazardous drug protection. Look for test information provided by the glove manufacturer showing resistance to specific hazardous drugs.
– Gowns: These should be long-sleeved, with tight-fitting cuffs. Disposable gowns coated with laminate materials provide better protection than noncoated gowns. Refer to the manufacturer for permeation information. Don't reuse gowns; change gowns immediately after a spill or splash.
– Respirators: A properly fit-tested certified N-95 respirator or surgical N-95 respirator provides protection from most airborne particles. Other types of respirators may be necessary to protect from airborne gases. Surgical masks don't provide adequate respiratory protection from drug exposure.
– Face shields: Using face shields with goggles protects against splashes to the face and eyes. Full-face respirators also provide protection. Face shields or eye glasses with side shields don't provide full eye and face protection.
– Sleeve, hair, and shoe covers: These covers help provide additional protection. They may be required in certain environments such as drug-compounding areas.

Strategies for reducing error rates
In addition to improvements in communication and education, other strategies that have helped reduce medication administration error rates include:
• providing adequate nurse-to-patient staffing ratios
• designing drug preparation areas as safety zones that promote making correct choices during the medication administration process according to drug importance, frequency of use, and sequence of use
• improving the medication administration environment (reduce noise to 50 dB, improve lighting to at least 100 foot-candles, obtain nonglare computer screens)
• developing and using protocols that reduce distractions for nursing staff directly involved in administering medications
• dispensing medications in unit-dose or unit-of-use packaging

• restricting high-alert drugs and administration routes (limiting their number, variety, and concentration in patient care areas). For example, remove all neuromuscular blockers from units where patients aren't normally intubated. Remove highly concentrated electrolytes from unit stock in patient care units. Remove concentrated oral opioids from unit stock and dispensing cabinets. Apply additional strong warnings to drug labels. Make sure emergency equipment is always available.
• switching from I.V. to oral or subcutaneous forms as soon as possible
• dispensing I.V. and epidural infusions only from the pharmacy
• labeling all medications both on and off the sterile field
• posting drug information in patient care units and having drug information available for all health care providers at the point of care; using infusion rate and dosing charts in patient care areas
• avoiding unapproved abbreviations
• using leading zeros; for example, use "0.5 mg" rather than ".5 mg"
• avoiding trailing zeros; for example, use "5 mg" rather than "5.0 mg"
• requiring that medication orders be prescribed by metric weight, not by volume (for example, in mg/kg not mL). Never rely on a patient's stated or historical weight. Weigh patients as soon as possible and measure and document actual weights only in metric units in all electronic and written formats.
• establishing protocols and checklists to double-check and document unusual drugs, dosages, or regimens
• always recalculating doses before giving drugs to children or neonates. Make sure that the dose formula is included for calculating the dose. Have a second clinician (preferably a pharmacist) double-check the calculations.
• making sure each patient is monitored appropriately before and after drug administration. Have appropriate monitoring equipment (cardiac monitors, capnography, pulse oximeters) available as needed.

Using technology to promote safety
Technology is becoming an increasingly important part of providing safer drug administration. The goal of medication administration technology is to enhance individual practice and

help build safeguards into the medication administration process. Information about ISMP and safe medication practices can be found at http://ismp.org/.

Computerized provider order entry

In computerized provider order entry (CPOE), the prescriber enters the medication orders into a computerized record, thus eliminating errors due to illegible handwriting. Such safeguards as immediate order checking for errors (such as incorrect dosing or routes of administration) and drug interactions, allergy checks, and administration protocols can be built into the system. Orders can be immediately transmitted to the appropriate department and can also be linked to drug information databases. CPOE can be used to monitor how drugs are utilized and can provide data for quality improvement.

Bar codes

Bar-code technology is widely used and was initially developed to help control and track inventory for industry. The use of this technology for safer drug administration, dispensing, inventory control, and drug storage and preparation has been endorsed by the IOM, The Joint Commission, Agency for Healthcare Research and Quality, and ISMP. With this technology, the patient wears a bar-code identifier on a wristband; the medication also has a bar code that uses the medication's own unique National Drug Code to identify the name, dose, manufacturer, and type of packaging. The nurse scans the bar code using an optical scanner, verifying the patient's identity and medication. The system supports but does not replace the traditional "rights" of safe medication.

Bar-code systems have been shown to reduce medication errors, but they aren't without disadvantages. For example, they don't save time in the medication administration process. Problems with the technology can cause delays in treatment. Wristbands can become unreadable due to wear, and scanners can malfunction. These problems may tempt nurses to develop dangerous shortcuts, such as attaching patients' wristbands to clipboards or giving the patient the medication first and then scanning his wristband.

Automated dispensing cabinets

Automated dispensing cabinets (ADCs) are computer-controlled medication distribution systems in the patient care unit or ancillary department that are used to store, track, and dispense medications. ADCs can provide nurses with near-total access to medications needed in their patient care area and promote the control and security of medications. They electronically track the use of drugs such as controlled substances. They may have bar-code capabilities for restocking and correct medication selection, and can be programmed to provide safeguards such as drug safety alerts. ADCs can be linked with external databases and billing systems to increase the efficiency of drug dispensing and billing.

"Smart" pumps

From 2005 through 2009, the FDA received 56,000 reports of adverse events and 500 deaths linked to infusion pumps. Currently, there are initiatives to improve infusion systems and technology. "Smart" I.V. pumps can have such features as programmable drug libraries and dosage limits, can perform automatic calculations, have dose-error reduction software, and can be programmed to signal dosage alerts. ISMP recommends administering high-alert I.V. medications using programmable infusion pumps with dose error-reduction software. They can be integrated with bar-code and CPOE technologies and can be wireless. Smart pumps can help alert nurses when incorrect dosages have been selected or to dosages that may exceed recommended levels.

Smart pumps can't detect all problems with I.V. drug infusions, however. For example, an incorrect drug can be selected from the library database and, with some pumps, it's possible to override safety alerts. Other infusion pump problems include software defects and failure of built-in safety alarms. Some pumps have ambiguous on-screen directions that can lead to dosing errors. The FDA recommends reporting all infusion-related adverse events, planning ahead in case a pump fails, labeling the channels and tubing to prevent errors, checking all settings, and monitoring patients for signs and symptoms of infusion problems. Nurses should perform independent calculation of all doses and infusion rates and not rely solely on the pump. It's essential to double-check each dose calculation. Nurses shouldn't bypass pump alarms, and must verify that the pump is functioning properly before beginning an infusion.

Other technologies

Using oral syringes that don't have luer-locks to administer oral or enteral medications helps prevent oral or enteral medications from being administered via the wrong route. (The ISMP has reported cases in which oral medications were drawn into parenteral syringes and inadvertently injected into I.V. lines, resulting in patient deaths.) Utilizing special tubing that doesn't have side ports for epidural medication administration prevents inadvertent injection of an incorrect drug into the epidural catheter. Certain drugs such as vincristine should always be dispensed in a minibag (25 to 50 mL) of solution and never in a syringe, to avoid accidental intrathecal instead of I.V. administration. Oral liquid dosing devices, such as syringes, cups, and droppers, should display the metric scale only.

Reporting medication errors

Clearly, medication errors are a major threat to patient safety. Only by sharing and analyzing data and performing more research can evidence-based quality improvements be developed and validated. Several agencies and organizations provide voluntary reporting systems to study the causes and prevalence of medication errors. The FDA has its Adverse Event Reporting System, which is part of the MedWatch program. The USP maintains MEDMARX (a national database utilized to lower the incidence of hospital medication errors) and the Medication Errors Reporting Program. In addition, the USP works with the ISMP to compile voluntary reports of medication errors. The reports are analyzed by these watchdog agencies, and information is published about their findings. Nurses should be encouraged to report medication errors and "near misses" and to help identify problems within systems.

Selected therapeutic drug classifications

Alkylating drugs
bendamustine hydrochloride
busulfan
carboplatin
carmustine
chlorambucil
cisplatin
cyclophosphamide
dacarbazine
ifosfamide
lomustine
melphalan
oxaliplatin
temozolomide
thiotepa

INDICATIONS
➤ **Various tumors, especially those with large volume and slow cell-turnover rate**

ACTION
Alkylating drugs appear to act independently of a specific cell-cycle phase. These polyfunctional compounds can be divided chemically into five groups: nitrogen mustards, ethylene amines, alkyl sulfonates, triazines, and nitrosoureas. Highly reactive, they primarily target nucleic acids and form links with the nuclei of different molecules. This allows the drugs to cross-link double-stranded DNA and to prevent strands from separating for replication, which may contribute to these drugs' ability to destroy cells.

ADVERSE REACTIONS
The most common adverse reactions are bone marrow depression, chills, diarrhea, fever, flank pain, hair loss, leukopenia, nausea, redness or pain at the injection site, sore throat, swelling of the feet or lower legs, thrombocytopenia, secondary leukemia, infertility, and vomiting.

CONTRAINDICATIONS & CAUTIONS
Black Box Warning Refer to individual drug monographs for black box warnings. ■
• Contraindicated in patients hypersensitive to these drugs.
• Use cautiously in patients receiving other cell-destroying drugs or radiation.

• In pregnant women, use only when potential benefits to the mother outweigh known risks to the fetus. Breast-feeding women should stop breast-feeding during therapy because drugs are found in breast milk. In children, safety and effectiveness of many alkylating drugs haven't been established. Elderly patients are at increased risk for adverse reactions; monitor closely.

Alpha blockers (peripherally acting)
alfuzosin hydrochloride
doxazosin mesylate
phentolamine mesylate
prazosin hydrochloride
silodosin
tamsulosin hydrochloride
terazosin hydrochloride

INDICATIONS
➤ **Hypertension, or mild to moderate urinary obstruction in men with BPH**

ACTION
Selective alpha blockers decrease vascular resistance and increase vein capacity, thereby lowering BP and causing nasal and scleroconjunctival congestion, ptosis, orthostatic and exercise hypotension, mild to moderate miosis, interference with ejaculation, and pink, warm skin. They also relax nonvascular smooth muscle, especially in the prostate capsule, which reduces urinary problems in men with BPH. Because alpha$_1$ blockers don't block alpha$_2$ receptors, they don't cause transmitter overflow.

Nonselective alpha blockers antagonize both alpha$_1$ and alpha$_2$ receptors. Generally, alpha blockade results in tachycardia, palpitations, and increased renin secretion because of abnormally large amounts of norepinephrine (from transmitter overflow) released from adrenergic nerve endings as a result of the blockade of alpha$_1$ and alpha$_2$ receptors. Norepinephrine's effects are counterproductive to the major uses of nonselective alpha blockers.

ADVERSE REACTIONS

Alpha blockers may cause severe orthostatic hypotension and syncope, especially with the first few doses, an effect commonly called the *first-dose effect*. The most common adverse effects of alpha$_1$ blockade are dizziness, headache, drowsiness, somnolence, and malaise. These drugs also may cause tachycardia, palpitations, fluid retention (from excess renin secretion), nasal and ocular congestion, and aggravation of respiratory tract infection.

CONTRAINDICATIONS & CAUTIONS

• Contraindicated in patients with hypersensitivity to these drugs or any of their components. Also contraindicated in combination therapy with PDE5 inhibitors (sildenafil, tadalafil, vardenafil) due to increased risk of priapism. Tadalafil may be taken with tamsulosin 0.4 mg daily. Discontinue if symptoms of angina or coronary insufficiency occur. May cause hypotension and increased risk of syncope. Use cautiously. Alfuzosin is contraindicated in patients with moderate or severe hepatic insufficiency and when administered with potent CYP3A4 inhibitors.

• In pregnant or breast-feeding women, use cautiously. In children, the safety and effectiveness of many alpha blockers haven't been established; use cautiously. In elderly patients, hypotensive effects may be more pronounced.

Alzheimer disease drugs

donepezil hydrochloride
galantamine hydrobromide
memantine hydrochloride
rivastigmine tartrate

INDICATIONS

➤ **Treatment of mild to moderate dementia of the Alzheimer type**

ACTION

Current theories attribute signs and symptoms of Alzheimer disease to a deficiency of cholinergic neurotransmission. It's suggested that these drugs improve cholinergic function by increasing acetylcholine levels through reversible inhibition of its hydrolysis by cholinesterase. Memantine is an N-methyl-D-aspartate (NMDA) receptor antagonist. Persistent activation of the NMDA receptors is thought to contribute to the symptoms of Alzheimer disease. No evidence indicates that these drugs alter the course of the underlying disease process.

ADVERSE REACTIONS

Weight loss, diarrhea, anorexia, nausea, vomiting, dizziness, headache, bradyarrhythmias; hypertension and constipation (memantine).

CONTRAINDICATIONS & CAUTIONS

• Contraindicated in patients hypersensitive to any of the drug components.

• May exaggerate neuromuscular blocking effects of succinylcholine-type and similar neuromuscular blocking agents used during anesthesia.

• Use cautiously with concomitant drugs that slow HR. There is an increased risk for heart block.

• Use cautiously with NSAIDs because the drugs increase gastric acid secretion. There is increased risk of developing ulcers and active or occult GI bleeding.

• Use cautiously in patients with moderate hepatic or renal impairment. Some drugs aren't recommended in severe hepatic impairment or severe renal impairment (CrCl less than 9 mL/minute). Refer to manufacturer's instructions for use and dosage adjustments for patients with renal impairment.

• Use cautiously in patients with a history of asthma or COPD.

Aminoglycosides

amikacin sulfate
gentamicin sulfate
neomycin sulfate
tobramycin sulfate

INDICATIONS

➤ **Septicemia; postoperative, pulmonary, intra-abdominal, and urinary tract infections; skin, soft-tissue, bone, and joint infections; aerobic gram-negative bacillary meningitis not susceptible to other antibiotics; serious staphylococcal, *Pseudomonas aeruginosa*, and *Klebsiella* infections; enterococcal infections; nosocomial pneumonia; TB; initial empirical therapy in febrile, leukopenic patients**

ACTION

Aminoglycosides are bactericidal. They bind directly and irreversibly to 30S ribosomal subunits, inhibiting bacterial protein synthesis.

DRUG CLASSES

They're active against many aerobic gram-negative and some aerobic gram-positive organisms and can be used in combination with other antibiotics for short courses of therapy.

ADVERSE REACTIONS
Ototoxicity and nephrotoxicity are the most serious complications. Neuromuscular blockade also may occur. Oral forms (neomycin) most commonly cause diarrhea, nausea, and vomiting. Parenteral drugs may cause vein irritation, phlebitis, and sterile abscess.

CONTRAINDICATIONS & CAUTIONS
Black Box Warning Refer to individual drug monographs for black box warnings. ■
• Contraindicated in patients hypersensitive to these drugs.
Black Box Warning Aminoglycosides are associated with significant nephrotoxicity and ototoxicity. Toxicity may develop even with conventional doses, particularly in patients with prerenal azotemia or impaired renal function. Evidence of renal function impairment or ototoxicity requires drug discontinuation or appropriate dosage adjustments. When possible, monitor serum drug concentrations. Avoid use with other ototoxic, neurotoxic, or nephrotoxic drugs. Aminoglycosides can cause fetal harm when administered to pregnant women. ■
• Use cautiously in patients with a neuromuscular disorder and in those taking neuromuscular blockers.
• Use at lower dosages in patients with renal impairment.
• In pregnant women, use cautiously. Safety hasn't been established in breast-feeding women. In neonates and premature infants, the half-life of aminoglycosides is prolonged because of immature renal systems. In infants and children, dosage adjustment may be needed. Elderly patients have an increased risk of nephrotoxicity and commonly need a lower dose and longer dosage intervals; they're also susceptible to ototoxicity and superinfection.

Angiotensin-converting enzyme inhibitors
benazepril hydrochloride
captopril
enalaprilat
enalapril maleate
fosinopril sodium
lisinopril
moexipril hydrochloride
perindopril erbumine
quinapril hydrochloride
ramipril
trandolapril

INDICATIONS
➤ **Hypertension, HF, left ventricular dysfunction (LVD), MI, and diabetic nephropathy**

ACTION
ACE inhibitors prevent conversion of angiotensin I to angiotensin II, a potent vasoconstrictor. Besides decreasing vasoconstriction and thus reducing peripheral arterial resistance, inhibiting angiotensin II decreases adrenocortical secretion of aldosterone. This reduces sodium and water retention and extracellular fluid volume. ACE inhibition also causes increased levels of bradykinin, which results in vasodilation. This decreases HR and systemic vascular resistance.

ADVERSE REACTIONS
The most common adverse effects of therapeutic doses are angioedema of the face and limbs, dry cough, dysgeusia, fatigue, headache, hyperkalemia, hypotension, proteinuria, rash, and tachycardia. Severe hypotension may occur at toxic drug levels.

CONTRAINDICATIONS & CAUTIONS
• Contraindicated in patients hypersensitive to these drugs.
Black Box Warning When pregnancy is detected, discontinue drug as soon as possible. Drugs that act directly on the renin-angiotensin system can cause fetal injury and death. ■
• Use cautiously in patients with impaired renal function or serious autoimmune disease and in those taking other drugs known to decrease WBC count or immune response.
• Women of childbearing potential taking ACE inhibitors should report suspected pregnancy immediately to the prescriber. High risks of fetal morbidity and mortality are linked to ACE inhibitors, especially in the second and third trimesters. Some ACE inhibitors appear in breast milk. To avoid adverse effects in infants, instruct patient to stop breast-feeding during therapy. Safe use in children hasn't been established for all products; for use in children, refer to manufacturer's instructions for individual products. Elderly patients may

need lower doses because of impaired drug clearance.

Antacids
aluminum hydroxide
calcium carbonate
magnesium hydroxide
magnesium oxide
sodium bicarbonate

INDICATIONS
➤ **Gastric hyperacidity; hyperphosphatemia (aluminum hydroxide); hypomagnesemia (magnesium oxide); postmenopausal hypocalcemia (calcium carbonate)**

ACTION
Antacids reduce the total acid load in the GI tract and elevate gastric pH to reduce pepsin activity. They also strengthen the gastric mucosal barrier and increase esophageal sphincter tone. Aluminum-containing antacids bind with phosphate ions in the intestine to form insoluble aluminum phosphate, which is excreted in feces. Calcium helps to prevent or treat negative calcium balance and bone loss in osteoporosis.

ADVERSE REACTIONS
Antacids containing aluminum may cause aluminum intoxication, constipation, hypophosphatemia, intestinal obstruction, and osteomalacia. Antacids containing magnesium may cause diarrhea or hypermagnesemia (in renal failure). Calcium carbonate, magnesium oxide, and sodium bicarbonate may cause constipation, milk-alkali syndrome, or rebound hyperacidity.

CONTRAINDICATIONS & CAUTIONS
• Calcium carbonate and magnesium oxide are contraindicated in patients with severe renal disease. Sodium bicarbonate is contraindicated in patients with hypertension, renal disease, or edema; in those who are vomiting; in those receiving diuretics or continuous GI suction; and in those on sodium-restricted diets.
• In patients with mild renal impairment, give magnesium oxide cautiously.
• Give aluminum preparations and calcium carbonate cautiously in elderly patients; in those receiving antidiarrheals, antispasmodics, or anticholinergics; and in those with dehydration, fluid restriction, chronic renal disease, or suspected intestinal absorption problems.

• Pregnant and breast-feeding women should consult their prescriber before using antacids. Serious adverse effects from changes in fluid and electrolyte balance are more likely in infants; monitor them closely. Elderly patients have an increased risk of adverse reactions; monitor them closely.

Antianginals
ranolazine

Beta blockers
atenolol
bisoprolol fumarate
metoprolol
nadolol
propranolol hydrochloride

Calcium channel blockers
amlodipine besylate
diltiazem hydrochloride
niCARdipine hydrochloride
NIFEdipine
verapamil hydrochloride

Nitrates
isosorbide dinitrate
isosorbide mononitrate
nitroglycerin

INDICATIONS
➤ **Moderate to severe angina (beta blockers); classic, effort-induced angina and Prinzmetal angina (calcium channel blockers); recurrent angina (long-acting nitrates and topical, transdermal, transmucosal, and oral extended-release nitroglycerin); acute angina (S.L. nitroglycerin and S.L. or chewable isosorbide dinitrate); unstable angina (I.V. nitroglycerin); chronic angina (ranolazine)**

ACTION
The mechanism of action of ranolazine's antianginal effects hasn't been determined. Beta blockers decrease catecholamine-induced increases in HR, BP, and myocardial contraction. Calcium channel blockers inhibit the flow of calcium through muscle cells, which dilates coronary arteries and decreases systemic vascular resistance, known as *afterload.* Nitrates decrease afterload and left ventricular end-diastolic pressure, or *preload,* and increase blood flow through collateral coronary vessels.

DRUG CLASSES

ADVERSE REACTIONS

Ranolazine may cause QT-interval prolongation, dizziness, constipation, and nausea. Beta blockers may cause bradycardia, cough, diarrhea, disturbing dreams, dizziness, dyspnea, fatigue, fever, HF, hypotension, lethargy, nausea, peripheral edema, and wheezing. Calcium channel blockers may cause bradycardia, confusion, constipation, depression, diarrhea, dizziness, dyspepsia, edema, elevated liver enzyme levels (transient), fatigue, flushing, headache, hypotension, insomnia, nervousness, and rash. Nitrates may cause flushing, headache, orthostatic hypotension, reflex tachycardia, rash, syncope, and vomiting.

CONTRAINDICATIONS & CAUTIONS

• Contraindicated in patients hypersensitive to these drugs.

Black Box Warning Abrupt discontinuation of beta blocker therapy has been associated with angina exacerbation and, in some cases, MI and ventricular arrhythmias. When discontinuation of beta blockers is planned, gradually reduce dosage over at least a few weeks. ∎

• Ranolazine is contraindicated in patients taking strong inhibitors of CYP3A or inducers of CYP3A and in those with clinically significant hepatic impairment. Beta blockers are contraindicated in patients with cardiogenic shock, sinus bradycardia, heart block greater than first degree, or bronchial asthma. Calcium channel blockers are contraindicated in patients with severe hypotension or heart block greater than first degree (except with functioning pacemaker). Nitrates are contraindicated in patients with severe anemia, cerebral hemorrhage, head trauma, or glaucoma, and in patients using PDE5 inhibitors (sildenafil, tadalafil, vardenafil).

• Use beta blockers cautiously in patients with nonallergic bronchospastic disorders, diabetes mellitus, or impaired hepatic or renal function. Use calcium channel blockers cautiously in those with hepatic or renal impairment, bradycardia, HF, or cardiogenic shock. Use nitrates cautiously in those with hypotension or recent MI.

• In pregnant women, use beta blockers cautiously. Recommendations for breast-feeding vary by drug; use beta blockers and calcium channel blockers cautiously. In children, safety and effectiveness haven't been established. Check with the prescriber before giving these drugs to children. Elderly patients have an increased risk of adverse reactions; use cautiously.

Antiarrhythmics

adenosine
dronedarone

Class IA
disopyramide
procainamide hydrochloride
quinidine gluconate
quinidine sulfate

Class IB
lidocaine hydrochloride
mexiletine hydrochloride

Class IC
flecainide acetate
propafenone hydrochloride

Class II (beta blockers)
esmolol hydrochloride
sotalol hydrochloride

Class III
amiodarone hydrochloride
dofetilide
ibutilide fumarate
sotalol hydrochloride

Class IV (calcium channel blockers)
diltiazem hydrochloride
verapamil hydrochloride

INDICATIONS

➤ Atrial and ventricular arrhythmias

ACTION

Class I drugs reduce the inward current carried by sodium ions, which stabilizes neuronal cardiac membranes. Class IA drugs depress phase 0, prolong the action potential, and stabilize cardiac membranes. Class IB drugs depress phase 0, shorten the action potential, and stabilize cardiac membranes. Class IC drugs block the transport of sodium ions, which decreases conduction velocity but not repolarization rate. Class II drugs decrease HR, myocardial contractility, BP, and AV node conduction. Class III drugs prolong the repolarization phase. Class IV drugs decrease myocardial contractility and oxygen demand by inhibiting calcium ion influx; they also dilate coronary arteries and arterioles.

ADVERSE REACTIONS

Most antiarrhythmics can aggravate existing arrhythmias or cause new ones. They also may produce CNS disturbances, such as dizziness or fatigue; GI problems, such as nausea, vomiting, or altered bowel elimination; hypersensitivity reactions; and hypotension. Some antiarrhythmics may worsen HF. Class II drugs may cause bronchoconstriction.

CONTRAINDICATIONS & CAUTIONS

Black Box Warning Refer to individual drug monographs for black box warnings. ■
• Contraindicated in patients hypersensitive to these drugs.
• Many antiarrhythmics are contraindicated or require cautious use in patients with cardiogenic shock, digitalis toxicity, and second- or third-degree heart block (unless patient has a pacemaker or implantable cardioverter-defibrillator).
• In pregnant women, use only if potential benefits to the mother outweigh risks to the fetus. In breast-feeding women, use cautiously; many antiarrhythmics appear in breast milk. Monitor closely in children because they have an increased risk of adverse reactions. Use cautiously in elderly patients, who may exhibit physiologic alterations in CV system.

Antibiotic antineoplastics

bleomycin sulfate
DAUNOrubicin hydrochloride
DOXOrubicin hydrochloride
epirubicin hydrochloride
idarubicin hydrochloride
mitomycin

INDICATIONS

➤ **Various tumors**

ACTION

Although classified as antibiotics, these drugs destroy cells, thus ruling out their use as antimicrobials alone. They interfere with proliferation of malignant cells in several ways. Their action may be specific to cell-cycle phase, not specific to cell-cycle phase, or both. Some of these drugs act like alkylating drugs or antimetabolites. By binding to or creating complexes with

DNA, antibiotic antineoplastics directly or indirectly inhibit DNA, RNA, and protein synthesis.

ADVERSE REACTIONS

The most common adverse reactions include anxiety, bone marrow depression, chills, confusion, diarrhea, fever, flank or joint pain, hair loss, nausea, redness or pain at the injection site, sore throat, swelling of the feet or lower legs, vomiting, and cardiomyopathy.

CONTRAINDICATIONS & CAUTIONS

Black Box Warning Refer to individual drug monographs for black box warnings. ■
• Contraindicated in patients hypersensitive to these drugs.
• In pregnant women, avoid antineoplastics. Breast-feeding during therapy isn't recommended. In children, safety and effectiveness of some drugs haven't been established; use cautiously. Use cautiously in elderly patients because of their increased risk of adverse reactions.

Anticholinergics

atropine sulfate
benztropine mesylate
dicyclomine hydrochloride
scopolamine

INDICATIONS

➤ **Prevention of motion sickness, preoperative reduction of secretions and blockage of cardiac reflexes, adjunctive treatment of peptic ulcers and other GI disorders, blockage of cholinomimetic effects of cholinesterase inhibitors or other drugs, and (for benztropine) various spastic conditions, including acute dystonic reactions, muscle rigidity, parkinsonism, and extrapyramidal disorders**

ACTION

Anticholinergics competitively antagonize the actions of acetylcholine and other cholinergic agonists at muscarinic receptors.

ADVERSE REACTIONS

Therapeutic doses commonly cause blurred vision, constipation, cycloplegia, decreased sweating or anhidrosis, dry mouth, headache, mydriasis, palpitations, tachycardia, urinary hesitancy, and urine retention. These reactions usually disappear when therapy stops.

DRUG CLASSES

Toxicity can cause signs and symptoms resembling psychosis (disorientation, confusion, hallucinations, delusions, anxiety, agitation, and restlessness); dilated, nonreactive pupils; blurred vision; hot, dry, flushed skin; dry mucous membranes; dysphagia; decreased or absent bowel sounds; urine retention; hyperthermia; tachycardia; hypertension; and increased respirations.

CONTRAINDICATIONS & CAUTIONS
• Contraindicated in patients hypersensitive to these drugs and in those with angle-closure glaucoma, renal or GI obstructive disease, reflux esophagitis, or myasthenia gravis.
• Use cautiously in patients with heart disease, GI infection, open-angle glaucoma, prostatic hypertrophy, hypertension, hyperthyroidism, ulcerative colitis, autonomic neuropathy, or hiatal hernia with reflux esophagitis.
• In pregnant women, safe use hasn't been established. In breast-feeding women, avoid anticholinergics because they may decrease milk production; some may appear in breast milk and cause infant toxicity. In children, safety and effectiveness haven't been established. Patients older than age 40 may be more sensitive to these drugs. In elderly patients, use cautiously and give a reduced dosage, as indicated.

Anticoagulants
Coumarin derivative
warfarin sodium

Heparin derivative
heparin sodium

Low-molecular-weight heparins
dalteparin sodium
enoxaparin sodium

Selective factor Xa inhibitors
apixaban
edoxaban
fondaparinux sodium
rivaroxaban

Thrombin inhibitors
argatroban
bivalirudin
dabigatran etexilate mesylate
desirudin

INDICATIONS
➤ PE, DVT, thrombus, DIC, unstable angina, MI, atrial fibrillation, heparin-induced thrombocytopenia, heparin-induced thrombosis–thrombocytopenia syndrome

ACTION
Heparin derivatives accelerate formation of an antithrombin–thrombin complex. They inactivate thrombin and prevent conversion of fibrinogen to fibrin. The coumarin derivative warfarin inhibits vitamin K–dependent activation of clotting factors II, VII, IX, and X, which are formed in the liver. Thrombin inhibitors directly bind to thrombin and inhibit its action. Selective factor Xa inhibitors directly bind to factor Xa.

ADVERSE REACTIONS
Anticoagulants commonly cause bleeding and may cause hypersensitivity reactions. Warfarin may cause agranulocytosis, alopecia (long-term use), anorexia, dermatitis, fever, nausea, tissue necrosis or gangrene, urticaria, and vomiting. Heparin derivatives may cause thrombocytopenia and may increase liver enzyme levels. Nonhemorrhagic adverse reactions associated with thrombin inhibitors may include back pain, bradycardia, and hypotension.

CONTRAINDICATIONS & CAUTIONS
Black Box Warning Refer to individual drug monographs for black box warnings. ■
• Contraindicated in patients hypersensitive to these drugs or any of their components; in patients with aneurysm, active bleeding, CV hemorrhage, hemorrhagic blood dyscrasias, hemophilia, severe hypertension, pericardial effusions, or pericarditis; and in patients undergoing major surgery, neurosurgery, neuraxial anesthesia, spinal puncture, or ophthalmic surgery.
• Heparin formulations are contraindicated in patients with history of heparin-induced thrombocytopenia and heparin-induced thrombosis–thrombocytopenia syndrome.
• Use cautiously in patients with severe diabetes, renal impairment, severe trauma, ulcerations, or vasculitis.
• Most anticoagulants (except warfarin) may be used in pregnancy only if the potential benefit to the mother outweighs the potential risk to the fetus. In pregnant women and those who have just had a threatened or complete spontaneous abortion, warfarin is contraindicated. Women

should avoid breast-feeding during therapy. Infants, especially neonates, may be more susceptible to anticoagulants because of vitamin K deficiency. Elderly patients are at greater risk for hemorrhage because of altered hemostatic mechanisms or age-related deterioration of hepatic and renal functions.

Anticonvulsants

carbamazepine
clobazam
clonazepam
diazepam
ezogabine
felbamate
fosphenytoin sodium
gabapentin
lacosamide
lamotrigine
levetiracetam
magnesium sulfate
oxcarbazepine
phenytoin sodium
phenytoin sodium (extended)
primidone
rufinamide
tiagabine hydrochloride
topiramate
valproate sodium
valproic acid
vigabatrin
zonisamide

INDICATIONS
➤ **Seizure disorders; acute, isolated seizures not caused by seizure disorders; status epilepticus; prevention of seizures after trauma or craniotomy; neuropathic pain**

ACTION
Anticonvulsants include six classes of drugs: selected hydantoin derivatives, barbiturates, benzodiazepines, succinimides, iminostilbene derivatives (carbamazepine), and carboxylic acid derivatives. Magnesium sulfate is a miscellaneous anticonvulsant. Some hydantoin derivatives and carbamazepine inhibit the spread of seizure activity in the motor cortex. Some barbiturates and succinimides limit seizure activity by increasing the threshold for motor cortex stimuli. Selected benzodiazepines and carboxylic acid derivatives may increase inhibition of GABA in brain neurons. Magnesium sulfate

interferes with the release of acetylcholine at the myoneural junction.

ADVERSE REACTIONS
Anticonvulsants can cause adverse CNS effects, such as ataxia, confusion, somnolence, and tremor. Many anticonvulsants also cause CV disorders, such as arrhythmias and hypotension; GI effects, such as vomiting; and hematologic disorders, such as agranulocytosis, bone marrow depression, leukopenia, and thrombocytopenia. Stevens-Johnson syndrome, other severe rashes, and abnormal LFT results may also occur.

CONTRAINDICATIONS & CAUTIONS
Black Box Warning Refer to individual drug monographs for black box warnings. ∎
• Contraindicated in patients hypersensitive to these drugs.
• Carbamazepine is contraindicated within 14 days of MAO inhibitor use.
• Use cautiously in patients with blood dyscrasias. Also, use barbiturates cautiously in patients with suicidal ideation.
• In pregnant women, therapy may continue despite the fetal risks caused by some anticonvulsants. Refer to manufacturer's instructions for each product for use during pregnancy and breast-feeding. Children, especially young ones, are sensitive to the CNS depression of some anticonvulsants; use cautiously. Elderly patients are sensitive to CNS effects and may require lower doses. Also, some anticonvulsants may take longer to be eliminated because of decreased renal function, and parenteral use is more likely to cause apnea, hypotension, bradycardia, and cardiac arrest.

Antidepressants, tricyclic

amitriptyline hydrochloride
clomiPRAMINE hydrochloride
desipramine hydrochloride
doxepin hydrochloride
imipramine hydrochloride
imipramine pamoate
nortriptyline hydrochloride
protriptyline hydrochloride

INDICATIONS
➤ **Depression, anxiety (doxepin), obsessive-compulsive disorder (clomipramine), enuresis in children older than age 6 (imipramine), neuropathic pain**

DRUG CLASSES

ACTION
TCAs may inhibit reuptake of norepinephrine and serotonin in CNS nerve terminals (presynaptic neurons), thus enhancing the concentration and activity of neurotransmitters in the synaptic cleft. TCAs also exert antihistaminic, sedative, anticholinergic, vasodilatory, and quinidine-like effects.

ADVERSE REACTIONS
Adverse reactions include anticholinergic effects, orthostatic hypotension, and sedation. The tertiary amines (amitriptyline, doxepin, and imipramine) exert the strongest sedative effects; tolerance usually develops in a few weeks. TCAs may cause CV effects such as T-wave abnormalities, conduction disturbances, and arrhythmias.

CONTRAINDICATIONS & CAUTIONS
Black Box Warning Antidepressants can increase the risk of suicidal thinking and behavior. Appropriately monitor patients of all ages who are started on antidepressant therapy, and observe closely for clinical worsening, suicidality, or unusual changes in behavior. Advise families and caregivers of the need for close observation and communication with the prescriber. ∎
• Contraindicated in patients hypersensitive to these drugs and in patients with urine retention or angle-closure glaucoma.
• TCAs are contraindicated within 2 weeks of MAO inhibitor therapy.
• Use cautiously in patients with suicidal tendencies, schizophrenia, paranoia, seizure disorders, CV disease, or impaired hepatic function.
• In pregnant and breast-feeding women, safety hasn't been established; use cautiously. In children younger than age 12, TCAs aren't recommended except for imipramine, which is used for enuresis in children age 6 and older. Elderly patients are more sensitive to therapeutic and adverse effects; they need lower dosages.

Antidiabetics
acarbose
albiglutide
alogliptin
canagliflozin
dapagliflozin propanediol
dulaglutide
empagliflozin
exenatide
glimepiride
glipiZIDE
glyBURIDE
linagliptin
liraglutide
metformin hydrochloride
miglitol
nateglinide
pioglitazone hydrochloride
pramlintide acetate
repaglinide
rosiglitazone maleate
saxagliptin
sitagliptin phosphate

INDICATIONS
➤ **Mild to moderately severe, stable, non-ketotic, type 2 diabetes mellitus that can't be controlled by diet alone**

ACTION
Oral antidiabetics come in several types. Sulfonylureas are sulfonamide derivatives that aren't antibacterial. They lower glucose levels by stimulating insulin release from the pancreas. These drugs work only in the presence of functioning beta cells in the islet tissue of the pancreas. After prolonged administration, they produce hypoglycemia by acting outside of the pancreas, resulting in effects that include reduced glucose production by the liver and enhanced peripheral sensitivity to insulin. The latter may result from an increased number of insulin receptors or from changes after insulin binding.

Meglitinides, such as nateglinide and repaglinide, are nonsulfonylurea antidiabetics that stimulate the release of insulin from the pancreas.

Metformin decreases hepatic glucose production, reduces intestinal glucose absorption, and improves insulin sensitivity by increasing peripheral glucose uptake and utilization. With metformin therapy, insulin secretion remains unchanged, and fasting insulin levels and all-day insulin response may decrease.

Alpha-glucosidase inhibitors, such as acarbose and miglitol, delay digestion of carbohydrates, resulting in a smaller rise in glucose levels. Pramlintide, a human amylin analogue, slows the rate at which food leaves the stomach, decreasing postprandial increase in glucose level, and reduces appetite.

Rosiglitazone and pioglitazone are thiazolidinediones, which lower glucose levels by improving insulin sensitivity. They are potent and highly selective agonists for receptors found in insulin-sensitive tissues, such as adipose tissue, skeletal muscle, and liver.

DPP-4 inhibitors (such as linagliptin, sitagliptin) increase insulin release by inhibiting the enzyme DPP-4. Sodium–glucose cotransporter 2 inhibitors (such as dapagliflozin, empagliflozin) reduce reabsorption of filtered glucose and lower plasma glucose concentration by increasing urinary excretion of glucose.

Glucagonlike peptide 1 receptor agonists (albiglutide, dulaglutide, and others) increase insulin secretion from pancreatic beta cells, suppress glucagon secretion, and slow gastric emptying.

ADVERSE REACTIONS

❸ *Alert:* All antidiabetics have the potential to cause severe hypoglycemia.

Sulfonylureas cause dose-related reactions that usually respond to decreased dosage: anorexia, headache, heartburn, nausea, paresthesia, vomiting, and weakness.

The most serious adverse reaction linked to metformin is lactic acidosis. It's a rare effect and is most likely to occur in patients with renal dysfunction. Other reactions to metformin include dermatitis, GI upset, megaloblastic anemia, rash, and unpleasant or metallic taste.

Thiazolidinediones may cause fluid retention leading to or exacerbating HF. Alpha-glucosidase inhibitors can cause abdominal pain, diarrhea, and flatulence.

Sodium–glucose cotransporter 2 inhibitors may cause hypotension and abnormal renal function and increase risk of UTIs.

DPP-4 inhibitors may cause GI reactions and antibody formation.

CONTRAINDICATIONS & CAUTIONS

Black Box Warning Refer to individual drug monographs for black box warnings. ∎
- Contraindicated in patients hypersensitive to these drugs, in patients with history of allergic reaction to sulfonamide derivatives (glimepiride), and in patients with diabetic ketoacidosis with or without coma. Metformin is also contraindicated in patients with renal disease or metabolic acidosis and generally should be avoided in patients with hepatic disease.
- Use sulfonylureas cautiously in patients with renal or hepatic disease or history of sulfonamide antibiotic hypersensitivity. Use metformin cautiously in patients with adrenal

or pituitary insufficiency and in debilitated and malnourished patients. Alpha-glucosidase inhibitors should be used cautiously in patients with mild to moderate renal insufficiency. Thiazolidinediones aren't recommended in patients with edema, HF, or liver disease.
- DPP-4 inhibitors may increase the risk of pancreatitis and are contraindicated in patients with a personal or family history of medullary thyroid cancer and in patients with multiple endocrine neoplasia syndrome type 2.
- In pregnant or breast-feeding women, use is contraindicated. Oral antidiabetics appear in small amounts in breast milk and may cause hypoglycemia in the infant. In children, oral antidiabetics aren't effective in type 1 diabetes mellitus. Elderly patients may be more sensitive to these drugs, usually need lower dosages, and are more likely to develop neurologic symptoms of hypoglycemia; monitor these patients closely.

Antidiarrheals

bismuth subsalicylate
diphenoxylate hydrochloride–atropine sulfate
loperamide
octreotide acetate

INDICATIONS

➤ **Mild, acute, or chronic diarrhea; certain cancers that cause diarrhea (octreotide acetate)**

ACTION

Bismuth preparations may have a mild water-binding capacity, may absorb toxins, and provide a protective coating for the intestinal mucosa.

ADVERSE REACTIONS

Bismuth preparations may cause salicylism (with high doses) or temporary darkening of tongue and stools.

CONTRAINDICATIONS & CAUTIONS

- Contraindicated in patients hypersensitive to these drugs.
- Some antidiarrheals may appear in breast milk; check individual drugs for specific recommendations. For children or teenagers recovering from flu or chickenpox, consult prescriber before giving bismuth subsalicylate. For elderly

DRUG CLASSES

patients, use caution when giving antidiarrheal drugs.

Antiemetics

aprepitant
dimenhyDRINATE
dolasetron mesylate
dronabinol
fosaprepitant dimeglumine
granisetron hydrochloride
meclizine hydrochloride
metoclopramide hydrochloride
ondansetron hydrochloride
palonosetron hydrochloride
prochlorperazine
promethazine hydrochloride
rolapitant hydrochloride
scopolamine
trimethobenzamide hydrochloride

INDICATIONS
➤ **Nausea, vomiting, motion sickness, and vertigo**

ACTION
For antihistamines (dimenhydrinate, meclizine hydrochloride, trimethobenzamide), the mechanism of action is unclear. Phenothiazines (prochlorperazine, promethazine hydrochloride) work by blocking the dopaminergic receptors in the chemoreceptor trigger zone of the brain. Serotonin-receptor antagonists (dolasetron, granisetron, ondansetron) block serotonin stimulation centrally in the chemoreceptor trigger zone and peripherally in vagal nerve terminals.

ADVERSE REACTIONS
Antiemetics may cause asthenia, fatigue, dizziness, headache, insomnia, abdominal pain, anorexia, constipation, diarrhea, epigastric discomfort, gastritis, heartburn, nausea, vomiting, neutropenia, hiccups, tinnitus, dehydration, and fever. Metoclopramide may cause tardive dyskinesia. Rolapitant may cause neutropenia and anemia.

CONTRAINDICATIONS & CAUTIONS
Black Box Warning Refer to individual drug monographs for black box warnings. ∎
• Contraindicated in patients hypersensitive to any of the drug components.
• Contraindicated in severe vomiting until etiology of vomiting is established.

• Rolapitant is contraindicated in patients receiving thioridazine because of risk of torsades de pointes.
• Use cautiously in patients with tartrazine and sulfite sensitivities. Antiemetics may cause allergic-type reactions, including hives, itching, wheezing, asthma, and anaphylaxis.

Antifungals

amphotericin B lipid complex
amphotericin B liposomal
anidulafungin
caspofungin acetate
clotrimazole
econazole nitrate
efinaconazole
fluconazole
isavuconazonium sulfate
itraconazole
ketoconazole
luliconazole
micafungin sodium
miconazole nitrate
nystatin
posaconazole
sertaconazole nitrate
tavaborole
terbinafine hydrochloride
voriconazole

INDICATIONS
➤ **Various fungal infections**

ACTION
The amphotericin products bind to sterols in the fungal cell membrane, altering permeability and allowing intracellular components to leak out. These drugs usually inhibit fungal growth and multiplication, but if the level is high enough, the drugs can destroy fungi. Fluconazole, itraconazole, efinaconazole, ketoconazole, luliconazole, isavuconazonium, itraconazole, posaconazole, voriconazole, nystatin, and terbinafine interfere with sterol synthesis in fungal cells, damaging cell membranes and increasing permeability. Caspofungin inhibits the synthesis of an integral component of fungal cell walls. Tavaborole inhibits fungal protein synthesis.

ADVERSE REACTIONS
Fluconazole may cause transient elevations of liver enzymes, alkaline phosphatase, and bilirubin levels, as well as dizziness, nausea,

vomiting, abdominal pain, diarrhea, rash, headache, and hypokalemia. Adverse reactions to itraconazole include headache and nausea. The most common adverse reactions to ketoconazole are nausea and vomiting. Adverse reactions to voriconazole are uncommon. However, the drug may alter renal function and cause vision changes. Common adverse reactions to caspofungin include paresthesia, tachycardia, anorexia, anemia, pain, myalgia, tachypnea, chills, and sweating. Reactions to nystatin seldom occur, but may include diarrhea, nausea, vomiting, and abdominal pain. Terbinafine may cause abdominal pain, jaundice, diarrhea, flatulence, nausea, anaphylaxis, headache, rash, and vision disturbances. Efinaconazole, luliconazole, and tavaborole can cause local skin irritation.

CONTRAINDICATIONS & CAUTIONS
Black Box Warning Refer to individual drug monographs for black box warnings. ■
• Contraindicated in patients hypersensitive to any of the drug components.
• Administer I.V. amphotericin under close clinical observation. Acute infusion reactions can occur, including fever, shaking chills, hypotension, anorexia, nausea, vomiting, and tachypnea.
• Caspofungin is contraindicated with concomitant use of cyclosporine because of the possibility of elevated liver enzymes.
• Amphotericin drugs aren't interchangeable and are each prescribed differently.

Antihistamines
cetirizine hydrochloride
chlorpheniramine maleate
desloratadine
diphenhydrAMINE hydrochloride
fexofenadine hydrochloride
levocetirizine
loratadine
promethazine hydrochloride

INDICATIONS
➤ **Allergic rhinitis, urticaria, pruritus, vertigo, motion sickness, nausea and vomiting, sedation, dyskinesia, parkinsonism**

ACTION
Antihistamines are structurally related chemicals that compete with histamine for H_1-receptor sites on smooth muscle of bronchi, GI tract, and large blood vessels, binding to cellular receptors and preventing access to and subsequent activity of histamine. They don't directly alter histamine or prevent its release.

ADVERSE REACTIONS
First-generation antihistamines cause drowsiness and impaired motor function early in therapy. They also can cause blurred vision, constipation, and dry mouth and throat. Some antihistamines, such as promethazine, may cause cholestatic jaundice, which may be a hypersensitivity reaction, and may predispose patients to photosensitivity. Promethazine may also cause extrapyramidal reactions with high doses.

CONTRAINDICATIONS & CAUTIONS
Black Box Warning Refer to individual drug monographs for black box warnings. ■
• Contraindicated in patients hypersensitive to these drugs and in those with angle-closure glaucoma, stenosing peptic ulcer, pyloroduodenal obstruction, or bladder neck obstruction. Promethazine is contraindicated in those taking MAO inhibitors.
• In pregnant women, safe use hasn't been established. During breast-feeding, antihistamines shouldn't be used because many of these drugs appear in breast milk and may cause unusual excitability in the infant. Neonates, especially premature infants, may experience seizures. Children, especially those younger than age 6, may experience paradoxical hyperexcitability with restlessness, insomnia, nervousness, euphoria, tremors, and seizures; give cautiously. Elderly patients usually are more sensitive to the adverse effects of antihistamines, especially dizziness, sedation, hypotension, and urine retention; use cautiously and monitor these patients closely.

Antihypertensives
ACE inhibitors
benazepril hydrochloride
captopril
enalaprilat
enalapril maleate
fosinopril sodium
lisinopril
moexipril hydrochloride
perindopril erbumine
quinapril hydrochloride
ramipril
trandolapril

DRUG CLASSES

Angiotensin II receptor blockers
candesartan cilexetil
eprosartan mesylate
irbesartan
losartan potassium
olmesartan medoxomil
telmisartan
valsartan

Beta blockers
atenolol
bisoprolol fumarate
carvedilol
labetalol hydrochloride
metoprolol succinate
metoprolol tartrate
nadolol
propranolol hydrochloride

Calcium channel blockers
amlodipine besylate
diltiazem hydrochloride
felodipine
niCARdipine hydrochloride
NIFEdipine
nisoldipine
verapamil hydrochloride

Centrally acting alpha blockers (sympatholytics)
clonidine hydrochloride
guanfacine hydrochloride
methyldopa

Direct renin inhibitor
aliskiren

Peripherally acting alpha blockers
doxazosin mesylate
prazosin hydrochloride
terazosin hydrochloride

Vasodilators
hydrALAZINE hydrochloride
nitroglycerin
nitroprusside sodium

INDICATIONS
➤ **Essential and secondary hypertension**

ACTION
For information on the action of ACE inhibitors, alpha blockers, ARBs, beta blockers, calcium channel blockers, and diuretics, see their individual drug class entries. Centrally acting sympatholytics stimulate central alpha-adrenergic receptors, reducing cerebral sympathetic outflow, thereby decreasing peripheral vascular resistance and BP. Vasodilators act directly on smooth muscle to reduce BP.

ADVERSE REACTIONS
Antihypertensives commonly cause orthostatic changes in HR, headache, hypotension, nausea, and vomiting. Other reactions vary greatly among different drug types. Centrally acting sympatholytics may cause constipation, depression, dizziness, drowsiness, dry mouth, headache, palpitations, severe rebound hypertension, and sexual dysfunction; methyldopa also may cause aplastic anemia and thrombocytopenia. Vasodilators may cause ECG changes, diarrhea, dizziness, HF, palpitations, pruritus, and rash.

CONTRAINDICATIONS & CAUTIONS
Black Box Warning When pregnancy is detected in patients receiving ACE inhibitors, ARBs, or direct renin inhibitors, discontinue therapy as soon as possible. Drugs that act directly on the renin-angiotensin system can cause fetal injury and death. ■
Black Box Warning Abrupt discontinuation of beta blocker therapy has been associated with angina exacerbation and, in some cases, MI and ventricular arrhythmias. When discontinuation of beta blockers is planned, gradually reduce dosage over at least a few weeks. ■
Black Box Warning Refer to individual drug monographs for additional black box warnings. ■
• Contraindicated in patients hypersensitive to these drugs and in those with hypotension.
• Use cautiously in patients with hepatic or renal dysfunction.
• ACE inhibitors should be avoided in women of childbearing potential. Refer to each manufacturer's instructions for use in pregnancy. In breast-feeding women, refer to manufacturer's instructions for use as some antihypertensives appear in breast milk. In children, safety and effectiveness of many antihypertensives haven't been established; refer to individual manufacturer's instructions. Elderly patients are more susceptible to adverse reactions and may need lower maintenance doses; monitor these patients closely.

Antilipemics

alirocumab
atorvastatin calcium
cholestyramine
colesevelam hydrochloride
evolocumab
ezetimibe
fenofibrate
fluvastatin sodium
gemfibrozil
lovastatin
mipomersen sodium
pitavastatin
pravastatin sodium
rosuvastatin calcium
simvastatin

INDICATIONS
➤ **Hyperlipidemia, hypercholesterolemia**

ACTION
Antilipemics lower elevated lipid levels. Bile-sequestering drugs (cholestyramine, colesevelam) lower LDL level by forming insoluble complexes with bile salts, triggering cholesterol to leave the bloodstream and other storage areas to make new bile acids. Fibric acid derivatives (gemfibrozil) reduce cholesterol formation, increase sterol excretion, and decrease lipoprotein and triglyceride synthesis. HMG-CoA reductase inhibitors (atorvastatin, fluvastatin, lovastatin, pitavastatin, pravastatin, rosuvastatin, simvastatin) interfere with the activity of enzymes that generate cholesterol in the liver. Selective cholesterol absorption inhibitors (ezetimibe, evolocumab) inhibit cholesterol absorption by the small intestine, reducing hepatic cholesterol stores and increasing cholesterol clearance from the blood.

ADVERSE REACTIONS
Antilipemics commonly cause GI upset. Bile-sequestering drugs may cause bloating, cholelithiasis, constipation, and steatorrhea. Fibric acid derivatives may cause cholelithiasis and have other GI or CNS effects. Use of gemfibrozil with HMG-CoA reductase inhibitors may affect liver function or cause rash, pruritus, increased CK levels, rhabdomyolysis, and myopathy.

CONTRAINDICATIONS & CAUTIONS
• Contraindicated in patients hypersensitive to these drugs. Also, bile-sequestering drugs are contraindicated in patients with complete biliary obstruction. Fibric acid derivatives are contraindicated in patients with primary biliary cirrhosis or significant hepatic or renal dysfunction. HMG-CoA reductase inhibitors and cholesterol absorption inhibitors are contraindicated in patients with active liver disease or persistently elevated transaminase levels.
• Use bile-sequestering drugs cautiously in constipated patients. Use fibric acid derivatives cautiously in patients with peptic ulcer. Use HMG-CoA inhibitors cautiously in patients who consume large amounts of alcohol or who have a history of liver or renal disease.
• In pregnant women, use bile-sequestering drugs and fibric acid derivatives cautiously and avoid using HMG-CoA inhibitors. In breast-feeding women, avoid using fibric acid derivatives and HMG-CoA inhibitors; give bile-sequestering drugs cautiously. In children ages 10 to 17, certain antilipemics have been approved to treat heterozygous familial hypercholesterolemia. Elderly patients have an increased risk of severe constipation; use bile-sequestering drugs cautiously and monitor patients closely.

Antimetabolite antineoplastics

capecitabine
cytarabine
fludarabine phosphate
fluorouracil
gemcitabine
hydroxyurea
mercaptopurine
methotrexate
pemetrexed
pralatrexate
trifluridine–tipiracil hydrochloride

INDICATIONS
➤ **Various tumors and hematologic conditions**

ACTION
Antimetabolites are structurally similar to naturally occurring metabolites and can be divided into three subcategories: purine, pyrimidine, and folinic acid analogues. Most of these drugs interrupt cell reproduction at a specific phase of the cell cycle. Purine analogues are incorporated into DNA and RNA, interfering with nucleic acid synthesis (by miscoding)

DRUG CLASSES

and replication. They also may inhibit synthesis of purine bases through pseudofeedback mechanisms. Pyrimidine analogues inhibit enzymes in metabolic pathways that interfere with biosynthesis of uridine and thymine. Folic acid antagonists prevent conversion of folic acid to tetrahydrofolate by inhibiting the enzyme dihydrofolic acid reductase.

ADVERSE REACTIONS

The most common adverse effects include anxiety, bone marrow depression (anemia, leukopenia, thrombocytopenia), chills, diarrhea, fever, flank or joint pain, hair loss, nausea, redness or pain at injection site, stomatitis, swelling of the feet or lower legs, and vomiting.

CONTRAINDICATIONS & CAUTIONS

Black Box Warning Refer to individual drug monographs for black box warnings. ■
• Contraindicated in patients hypersensitive to these drugs.
• Most drugs can cause fetal harm and women exposed to them during pregnancy should be informed of the risks to the fetus. Breast-feeding isn't recommended for women taking these drugs. In children, safety and effectiveness of some drugs haven't been established. Elderly patients have an increased risk of adverse reactions; monitor them closely.

Antimigraine drugs

almotriptan malate
eletriptan hydrobromide
frovatriptan succinate
naratriptan hydrochloride
rizatriptan benzoate
sumatriptan succinate
zolmitriptan

INDICATIONS
➤ Migraines with or without aura

ACTION
The antimigraine drugs are serotonin 5-HT$_1$ agonists. These drugs constrict cranial vessels, inhibit neuropeptide release, and reduce transmission in the trigeminal nerve pathway.

ADVERSE REACTIONS
These drugs have a wide range of adverse reactions. These include weakness, drowsiness, tingling, warmth or hot sensations, flushing, nasal discomfort, visual disturbances, paresthe-

sia, dizziness, fatigue, somnolence, chest pain, weakness, dry mouth, dyspepsia, nausea, sweating, injection-site reactions, and neck, throat, or jaw pain. Intranasal sumatriptan can cause nasal or throat discomfort and taste disturbances.

CONTRAINDICATIONS & CAUTIONS
• Contraindicated in patients hypersensitive to any of the drug components.
• Contraindicated in patients with ischemic heart disease, angina, previous MI, uncontrolled hypertension or other significant underlying CV conditions, cerebrovascular disease, peripheral vascular disease, and ischemic bowel disease.
• Serotonin syndrome can occur, especially when used with other serotonergic drugs.

Antiparkinsonian drugs

amantadine hydrochloride
apomorphine hydrochloride
benztropine mesylate
bromocriptine mesylate
diphenhydrAMINE hydrochloride
entacapone
levodopa–carbidopa
levodopa–carbidopa–entacapone
pramipexole dihydrochloride
rasagiline mesylate
rOPINIRole hydrochloride
selegiline hydrochloride
tolcapone

INDICATIONS
➤ **Signs and symptoms of Parkinson disease and drug-induced extrapyramidal reactions**

ACTION
Antiparkinsonian drugs include synthetic anticholinergics, dopaminergics, and the antiviral amantadine. Anticholinergics probably prolong the action of dopamine by blocking its reuptake into presynaptic neurons and by suppressing central cholinergic activity. Dopaminergics act in the brain by increasing dopamine availability, thus improving motor function. Entacapone is a reversible inhibitor of peripheral catechol-*O*-methyltransferase (commonly known as COMT), which is responsible for elimination of various catecholamines, including dopamine. Blocking this pathway when giving levodopa–carbidopa should result in higher levels of levodopa, thereby allowing greater dopaminergic stimulation in the CNS and leading to a greater effect in treating parkinsonian

symptoms. Amantadine is thought to increase dopamine release in the substantia nigra.

ADVERSE REACTIONS

Anticholinergics may cause blurred vision, cycloplegia, constipation, decreased sweating or anhidrosis, dry mouth, headache, mydriasis, palpitations, tachycardia, and urinary hesitancy and urine retention. Dopaminergics may cause arrhythmias, confusion, disturbing dreams, dystonias, hallucinations, headache, muscle cramps, nausea, orthostatic hypotension, and vomiting. Amantadine also causes irritability, insomnia, and livedo reticularis (with prolonged use).

CONTRAINDICATIONS & CAUTIONS

Black Box Warning Refer to individual drug monographs for black box warnings. ∎
• Contraindicated in patients hypersensitive to these drugs.
• Use cautiously in patients with prostatic hyperplasia or tardive dyskinesia and in debilitated patients.
• Neuroleptic malignant-like syndrome involving muscle rigidity, increased body temperature, and mental status changes may occur with abrupt withdrawal of antiparkinsonian agents.
• In pregnant women, safe use hasn't been established. Antiparkinsonian agents may appear in breast milk; a decision should be made to stop the drug or stop breast-feeding, taking into account the importance of the drug to the mother. In children, safety and effectiveness haven't been established. Elderly patients have an increased risk for adverse reactions; monitor them closely.

Antiplatelet drugs

abciximab
cangrelor tetrasodium
cilostazol
clopidogrel bisulfate
dipyridamole
eptifibatide
prasugrel
ticagrelor
ticlopidine hydrochloride
tirofiban hydrochloride
vorapaxar sulfate

INDICATIONS

➤ **Reduction of thrombotic events by reducing platelet aggregation; adjunct to**
PCI, prevention of cardiac ischemic complications, or treatment of unstable angina not responding to conventional therapy when PCI is planned within 24 hours (abciximab); acute coronary syndrome and PCI (eptifibatide); acute coronary syndrome (tirofiban); non-ST-segment elevation acute coronary syndrome and ST-segment elevation MI, recent MI, recent stroke or peripheral vascular disease (clopidogrel, ticlopidine, and vorapaxar)

ACTION

The I.V. drugs abciximab, eptifibatide, and tirofiban antagonize the glycoprotein (GP)IIb/IIIa receptors located on platelets, which are involved in platelet aggregation. Clopidogrel, cangrelor, prasugrel, and ticagrelor are inhibitors of platelet aggregation that inhibit the binding of adenosine diphosphate (ADP) to its platelet receptor and the subsequent ADP-mediated activation of the GPIIb/IIIa complex. Ticlopidine inhibits the binding of fibrinogen to platelets. Vorapaxar inhibits thrombin-induced and thrombin receptor agonist peptide-induced platelet aggregation.

ADVERSE REACTIONS

The I.V. drugs can cause serious bleeding, thrombocytopenia, and anaphylaxis. The most common adverse reactions to the oral agents include anaphylaxis, rash, stomach pain, nausea, and headache. Ticlopidine may cause neutropenia and elevated alkaline phosphatase and serum transaminase levels. Prasugrel and ticagrelor can cause atrial fibrillation, dyspnea, cough, and hypotension.

CONTRAINDICATIONS & CAUTIONS

Black Box Warning Refer to individual drug monographs for black box warnings. ∎
• Contraindicated in patients hypersensitive to any of the drug components.
• Contraindicated in active bleeding, bleeding disorders, intracranial neoplasm, AV malformation or aneurysm, cerebrovascular accident (within 2 years), recent major surgery or trauma, severe uncontrolled hypertension, or thrombocytopenia.
• Avoid use of ticagrelor in patients with severe hepatic impairment.
• Because of its very long half-life, vorapaxar is effectively irreversible.

DRUG CLASSES

Antipsychotics

First generation
chlorproMAZINE hydrochloride
fluphenazine decanoate
fluphenazine hydrochloride
haloperidol
haloperidol decanoate
haloperidol lactate
loxapine hydrochloride
loxapine succinate
molindone hydrochloride
perphenazine
pimozide
prochlorperazine edisylate
prochlorperazine maleate
thioridazine hydrochloride
thiothixene hydrochloride
trifluoperazine hydrochloride

Second generation
aripiprazole
asenapine maleate
brexpiprazole
cariprazine hydrochloride
clozapine
iloperidone
lurasidone hydrochloride
olanzapine
olanzapine pamoate
paliperidone
paliperidone palmitate
quetiapine fumarate
risperiDONE
ziprasidone hydrochloride
ziprasidone mesylate

INDICATIONS
➤ **Schizophrenia (all but pimozide); schizoaffective disorder (paliperidone); psychosis, acute agitation, depression, or mania in bipolar I disorder; depression, hiccups (chlorpromazine); autism irritability (aripiprazole, risperidone); child hyperactivity and severe behavioral problems (chlorpromazine, haloperidol); acute intermittent porphyria (chlorpromazine); nausea, vomiting, anxiety, tetanus (chlorpromazine); Tourette syndrome (haloperidol, pimozide)**

ACTION
Antipsychotics block several neurotransmitters, particularly dopamine. The exact mechanism of action and ideal combination of targeted neurotransmitters remain unknown.

ADVERSE REACTIONS
First-generation antipsychotics may cause cardiac arrhythmias, cardiac arrest, hypotension, tachycardia, agitation, akathisia, seizures, dizziness, sedation, dystonia, headache, insomnia, neuroleptic malignant syndrome (NMS), extrapyramidal symptoms, tardive dyskinesia, photosensitivity, pruritus, anorexia, constipation, dry mouth, nausea, weight gain, amenorrhea, galactorrhea, gynecomastia, impotence, urine retention, blurred vision, and hyperthermia/hyperpyrexia.

Second-generation antipsychotics may cause akathisia, dizziness, drowsiness, extrapyramidal symptoms, headache, constipation, nausea, QT-interval prolongation, weight gain, hyperprolactinemia, dyslipidemia, hyperglycemia, and hyperthermia/hyperpyrexia.

CONTRAINDICATIONS & CAUTIONS
Black Box Warning Elderly patients with dementia-related psychosis treated with antipsychotics are at increased risk for death. Antipsychotics aren't approved for treatment of patients with dementia-related psychosis. ∎
Black Box Warning Refer to individual drug monographs for additional black box warnings. ∎
• Contraindicated in patients hypersensitive to drug.
• Use cautiously and observe for tardive dyskinesia, which may be irreversible.
• Use cautiously and watch for signs and symptoms of NMS (muscle rigidity, fever, delirium), especially with first-generation injectable antipsychotics.
• Use cautiously in depressed or agitated patients.
• Use cautiously with lithium because of risk of encephalopathic syndrome (weakness, lethargy, fever, confusion).
• Use cautiously in patients with MI, ischemic heart disease, HF, conduction abnormalities, or cerebrovascular disease, and in those at risk for hypotension.
• Use cautiously in patients with dyslipidemia or diabetes mellitus, particularly with second-generation antipsychotics.
• Use cautiously in patients with respiratory infections or chronic disorders because of increased pneumonia risk.

• Use cautiously in patients with blood dyscrasias.

• Use cautiously in patients with history of seizures.

• Use cautiously in patients with Parkinson disease or dementia with Lewy bodies.

• Use cautiously in patients with renal impairment; lower the dosage or discontinue drug if BUN level is abnormal.

• Risk in pregnancy is unknown; refer to manufacturer's instructions for use in pregnancy and breast-feeding. When used during the third trimester, there is an increased risk of extrapyramidal symptoms or withdrawal symptoms in the newborn that can be severe and require hospitalization.

• Patients taking antipsychotics should use caution when driving or performing hazardous work due to drowsiness.

Antirheumatics

abatacept
adalimumab
auranofin
infliximab
leflunomide

INDICATIONS
➤ RA, ankylosing spondylitis, Crohn disease, psoriatic arthritis

ACTION
Activated T lymphocytes are found in the synovium of patients with RA. Some drugs bind to TNF so it can't bind to a receptor and exert an effect. TNF plays an important role in pathologic inflammation and joint destruction.

ADVERSE REACTIONS
The most serious adverse reactions include serious infections and malignancies in patients treated with abatacept, adalimumab, infliximab, and leflunomide. The most common adverse reactions include rash, pruritus, hair loss, urticaria, nausea, vomiting, anorexia, flatulence, dyspepsia, anemia, leukopenia, thrombocytopenia, elevated liver enzymes, stomatitis, hypertension, headache, and hematuria.

CONTRAINDICATIONS & CAUTIONS
Black Box Warning Refer to individual drug monographs for black box warnings. ■

• Contraindicated in patients hypersensitive to any of the drug components.

• Use cautiously in patients receiving two antirheumatics with similar mechanisms of action.

• Use with caution in patients with a history of recurrent infections, COPD, CNS disorders, demyelinating disorders, HF, and immunosuppression.

Antituberculotics

bedaquiline fumarate
cycloserine
ethambutol hydrochloride
isoniazid
pyrazinamide
rifabutin
rifampin
rifapentine

INDICATIONS
➤ Acute pulmonary and extrapulmonary TB, acute UTIs

ACTION
Cycloserine and isoniazid inhibit cell-wall synthesis in susceptible strains of gram-positive and gram-negative bacteria, including *Mycobacterium tuberculosis*. Rifampin, rifapentine, and rifabutin inhibit DNA-dependent RNA polymerase activity in susceptible *M. tuberculosis* organisms. Ethambutol causes impaired cell metabolism. Bedaquiline inhibits an enzyme essential to generate energy in *M. tuberculosis* organisms. The mechanism of action for pyrazinamide is unknown.

ADVERSE REACTIONS
Adverse reactions primarily affect the GI tract, peripheral nervous system, and hepatic system. Use cautiously in patients with hepatic impairment. Isoniazid may precipitate seizures in patients with a seizure disorder and may produce optic or peripheral neuritis. Optic neuritis, blood dyscrasias, anaphylaxis, and hepatotoxicity may occur with ethambutol. Rifampin may cause epigastric pain, nausea, vomiting, flatulence, abdominal cramps, anorexia, and diarrhea. Cycloserine can cause seizures, confusion, dizziness, headache, and somnolence.

CONTRAINDICATIONS & CAUTIONS
• Contraindicated in patients hypersensitive to any of the drug components.

• Multidrug regimens should be used.

DRUG CLASSES

• Drugs should be discontinued or dosage reduced if patients develop signs of CNS toxicity, including convulsions, psychosis, somnolence, depression, confusion, hyperreflexia, headache, tremor, vertigo, paresis, or dysarthria.

Benzodiazepines

alprazolam
chlordiazepoxide hydrochloride
clobazam
clonazepam
diazepam
lorazepam
midazolam hydrochloride
oxazepam
temazepam
triazolam

INDICATIONS
➤ **Seizure disorders (clobazam, clonazepam, diazepam, midazolam, parenteral lorazepam); anxiety, tension, and insomnia (chlordiazepoxide, clonazepam, diazepam, lorazepam, oxazepam, temazepam, triazolam); conscious sedation or amnesia in surgery (diazepam, lorazepam, midazolam); skeletal muscle spasm and tremor (oral forms of chlordiazepoxide and diazepam); delirium**

ACTION
Benzodiazepines act selectively on polysynaptic neuronal pathways throughout the CNS. Precise sites and mechanisms of action aren't fully known. However, benzodiazepines enhance or facilitate the action of GABA, an inhibitory neurotransmitter in the CNS. These drugs appear to act at the limbic, thalamic, and hypothalamic levels of the CNS to produce anxiolytic, sedative, hypnotic, skeletal muscle relaxant, and anticonvulsant effects.

ADVERSE REACTIONS
Therapeutic dose may cause drowsiness, impaired motor function, constipation, diarrhea, vomiting, altered appetite, urinary changes, visual disturbances, and CV irregularities. Toxic dose may cause continuing problems with short-term memory, confusion, severe depression, shakiness, vertigo, slurred speech, staggering, bradycardia, shortness of breath, difficulty breathing, or severe weakness. Prolonged or frequent use can cause physical dependency and withdrawal syndrome when drug is stopped.

CONTRAINDICATIONS & CAUTIONS
Black Box Warning Refer to individual drug monographs for black box warnings. ∎
• Contraindicated in patients hypersensitive to these drugs, in those with acute angle-closure glaucoma, and in those with depressive neuroses or psychotic reactions in which anxiety isn't prominent.
• Avoid use in patients with suicidal tendencies and in patients with a history of drug abuse. If drug is necessary, monitor patient carefully.
• Abrupt discontinuation can trigger withdrawal symptoms; withdraw drug gradually.
• Use cautiously in patients with chronic pulmonary insufficiency or sleep apnea and in those with hepatic or renal insufficiency.
• In pregnant patients, benzodiazepines increase the risk of congenital malformation if taken in the first trimester. Use during labor may cause neonatal flaccidity. A neonate whose mother took a benzodiazepine during pregnancy may have withdrawal symptoms. Benzodiazepines appear in breast milk; women shouldn't breast-feed during therapy. In elderly patients, benzodiazepine elimination may be prolonged; consider a lower dosage or use of a shorter-acting agent.

Beta blockers

Beta$_1$-selective blockers
atenolol
betaxolol
bisoprolol fumarate
esmolol hydrochloride
metoprolol succinate
metoprolol tartrate

Beta$_1$ and beta$_2$ (nonselective) blockers
carvedilol (nonselective beta blocker and alpha$_1$ blocker)
labetalol hydrochloride (nonselective beta blocker and alpha$_1$ blocker)
nadolol
propranolol hydrochloride
sotalol hydrochloride
timolol maleate

INDICATIONS
➤ **Hypertension (most drugs), angina pectoris (atenolol, metoprolol, nadolol, and propranolol), arrhythmias (esmolol,**

propranolol, and sotalol), glaucoma (betaxolol and timolol), prevention of MI
(atenolol, metoprolol, propranolol),
prevention of recurrent migraine and
other vascular headaches (propranolol),
pheochromocytomas or essential tremors
(selected drugs), HF (atenolol, carvedilol,
metoprolol)

ACTION
Beta blockers compete with beta agonists
for available beta receptors; individual drugs
differ in their ability to affect beta receptors.
Some drugs are nonselective: they block beta$_1$
receptors in cardiac muscle and beta$_2$ receptors
in bronchial and vascular smooth muscle.
Several drugs are cardioselective and, in lower
doses, inhibit mainly beta$_1$ receptors. Some
beta blockers have intrinsic sympathomimetic
activity and stimulate and block beta receptors,
and thereby have less effect on slowing HR.
Others stabilize cardiac membranes, which
affects cardiac action potential.

ADVERSE REACTIONS
Therapeutic dose may cause bradycardia, dizziness, fatigue, and erectile dysfunction; some
may cause other CNS disturbances, such as
depression, hallucinations, memory loss, and
nightmares. Toxic dose can produce severe hypotension, bradycardia, HF, or bronchospasm.

CONTRAINDICATIONS & CAUTIONS
Black Box Warning Abrupt discontinuation
of beta blocker therapy has been associated with
angina exacerbation and, in some cases, MI and
ventricular arrhythmias. When discontinuation
of beta blockers is planned, gradually reduce
dosage over at least a few weeks. ▪
Black Box Warning Refer to individual
drug monographs for additional black box
warnings. ▪
• Contraindicated in patients hypersensitive
to these drugs and in those with cardiogenic
shock, sinus bradycardia, heart block greater
than first degree, or bronchial asthma.
• Beta blockers may mask signs and symptoms
of hypoglycemia (palpitations, tachycardia,
tremor).
• Use cautiously in patients with nonallergic
bronchospastic disorders, diabetes mellitus,
impaired hepatic or renal function, and HF.
• In pregnant women, use cautiously. Drugs
appear in breast milk. In children, safety and
effectiveness haven't been established; use

only if the benefits outweigh the risks. In elderly patients, use cautiously; patients may
need reduced maintenance doses because of
increased bioavailability, delayed metabolism,
and increased adverse effects.

Calcium channel blockers
amlodipine besylate
clevidipine butyrate
diltiazem hydrochloride
felodipine
isradipine
niCARdipine hydrochloride
NIFEdipine
niMODipine
nisoldipine
verapamil hydrochloride

INDICATIONS
➤ **Prinzmetal variant angina; chronic
stable angina; unstable angina; mild-to-
moderate hypertension; arrhythmias;
subarachnoid hemorrhage (nimodipine)**

ACTION
The main physiologic action of calcium channel blockers is to inhibit calcium influx across
the slow channels of myocardial and vascular
smooth muscle cells. By inhibiting calcium
flow into these cells, calcium channel blockers
reduce intracellular calcium levels. This, in
turn, dilates coronary arteries, peripheral arteries, and arterioles and slows cardiac conduction.
    When used to treat Prinzmetal variant
angina, calcium channel blockers inhibit coronary spasm, which then increases oxygen
delivery to the heart. Peripheral artery dilation
reduces afterload, which decreases myocardial
oxygen use. Inhibiting calcium flow into specialized cardiac conduction cells in the SA and
AV nodes slows conduction through the heart.
Verapamil and diltiazem have the greatest effect
on the AV node, which slows the ventricular
rate in atrial fibrillation or flutter and converts
supraventricular tachycardia to a normal sinus
rhythm.

ADVERSE REACTIONS
Verapamil may cause bradycardia, hypotension,
various degrees of heart block, and worsening
of HF after rapid I.V. delivery. Prolonged oral
verapamil therapy may cause constipation.
Nifedipine may cause flushing, headache,
heartburn, hypotension, light-headedness, and

DRUG CLASSES

peripheral edema. The most common adverse reactions to diltiazem are anorexia and nausea; it also may induce bradycardia, HF, peripheral edema, and various degrees of heart block.

CONTRAINDICATIONS & CAUTIONS
Black Box Warning Refer to individual drug monographs for black box warnings. ■
• Contraindicated in patients hypersensitive to these drugs and in those with second- or third-degree heart block (except those with a pacemaker) and cardiogenic shock. Use diltiazem and verapamil cautiously in patients with HF.

• In pregnant women, use cautiously and refer to individual manufacturer's instructions for use. Calcium channel blockers may appear in breast milk; instruct patient to stop breastfeeding during therapy. In neonates and infants, adverse hemodynamic effects of parenteral verapamil are possible, but safety and effectiveness of other calcium channel blockers haven't been established; avoid use, if possible. In elderly patients, the half-life of calcium channel blockers may be increased as a result of decreased clearance.

Cephalosporins

First generation
cefadroxil
cefazolin sodium
cephalexin

Second generation
cefoxitin sodium
cefprozil
cefuroxime axetil
cefuroxime sodium

Third generation
cefdinir
cefotaxime sodium
cefpodoxime proxetil
ceftazidime
ceftriaxone sodium

Fourth generation
cefepime hydrochloride

Fifth generation
ceftaroline fosamil

INDICATIONS
➤ **Infections of the lungs, skin, soft tissue, bones, joints, urinary and respiratory tracts, blood, abdomen, and heart; CNS infections caused by susceptible strains of *Neisseria meningitidis, Haemophilus influenzae*, and *Streptococcus pneumoniae*; meningitis caused by *Escherichia coli* or *Klebsiella*; infections that develop after surgical procedures classified as contaminated or potentially contaminated; penicillinase-producing *Neisseria gonorrhoeae*; otitis media and ampicillin-resistant middle ear infection caused by *H. influenzae***

ACTION
Cephalosporins are chemically and pharmacologically similar to penicillin; they act by inhibiting bacterial cell-wall synthesis, causing rapid cell destruction. Their sites of action are enzymes known as penicillin-binding proteins. The affinity of certain cephalosporins for these proteins in various microorganisms helps explain the differing actions of these drugs. They are bactericidal: they act against many aerobic gram-positive and gram-negative bacteria and some anaerobic bacteria but don't kill fungi or viruses.

First-generation cephalosporins act against many gram-positive cocci, including penicillinase-producing *Staphylococcus aureus* and *S. epidermidis, S. pneumoniae,* group B streptococci, and group A beta-hemolytic streptococci. Susceptible gram-negative organisms include *Klebsiella pneumoniae, E. coli, Proteus mirabilis,* and *Shigella.*

Second-generation cephalosporins are effective against all organisms susceptible to first-generation drugs and have additional activity against *Moraxella catarrhalis, H. influenzae, Enterobacter, Citrobacter, Providencia, Acinetobacter, Serratia,* and *Neisseria. Bacteroides fragilis* are susceptible to cefoxitin.

Third-generation cephalosporins are less active than first- and second-generation drugs against gram-positive bacteria but are more active against gram-negative organisms, including those resistant to first- and second-generation drugs. They have the greatest stability against beta-lactamases produced by gram-negative bacteria. Susceptible gram-negative organisms include *E. coli, Klebsiella, Enterobacter, Providencia, Acinetobacter, Serratia, Proteus, Morganella,* and *Neisseria.* Some third-generation drugs are active against *B. fragilis* and *Pseudomonas.*

The fourth-generation cephalosporin (cefepime hydrochloride) shows activity against a wide range of gram-positive and gram-negative bacteria. Cefepime exhibits resistance to beta-lactamases. Susceptible gram-negative bacteria include *Enterobacter, E. coli, K. pneumoniae, P. mirabilis,* and *Pseudomonas aeruginosa.* Susceptible gram-positive bacteria include *S. aureus, S. pneumoniae,* and *Streptococcus pyogenes.*

The fifth-generation cephalosporin (ceftaroline fosamil) has antimicrobial activity against gram-negative bacteria similar to third-generation cephalosporins. It is also active against gram-positive bacteria such as MRSA and methicillin-resistant *S. pneumoniae.*

ADVERSE REACTIONS

Many cephalosporins have similar adverse effects. Hypersensitivity reactions range from mild rashes, fever, and eosinophilia to fatal anaphylaxis and are more common in patients with penicillin allergy. Adverse GI reactions include abdominal pain, diarrhea, dyspepsia, glossitis, nausea, tenesmus, and vomiting. CDAD ranging in severity from mild to fatal colitis can occur during or after treatment ends. Hematologic reactions include positive direct and indirect antiglobulin on Coombs test, thrombocytopenia or thrombocythemia, transient neutropenia, and reversible leukopenia. Minimal elevation of LFT results occurs occasionally. Adverse renal effects may occur with any cephalosporin; they are most common in older patients, those with decreased renal function, and those taking other nephrotoxic drugs. Some products increase risk of arrhythmia, chest pain, hypotension, and hypertension.

Local venous pain and irritation are common after I.M. injection; these reactions occur more often with higher doses and long-term therapy. Bacterial and fungal superinfections may result from suppression of normal flora.

CONTRAINDICATIONS & CAUTIONS

• Contraindicated in patients hypersensitive to cephalosporins and related antibiotics.
• Use cautiously in patients with renal or hepatic impairment, history of GI disease, or allergy to penicillins.
• In pregnant women, use only when potential benefits outweigh potential fetal hazards; safety hasn't been definitively established. In breast-feeding women, use cautiously because drugs appear in breast milk. In neonates and infants, half-life is prolonged; use cautiously. Elderly patients are susceptible to superinfection and coagulopathies, commonly have renal impairment, and may need a lower dosage; use cautiously.

CNS stimulants
armodafinil
dexmethylphenidate hydrochloride
dextroamphetamine sulfate
doxapram hydrochloride
lisdexamfetamine dimesylate
methylphenidate hydrochloride
modafinil
phentermine hydrochloride

INDICATIONS
➤ **Stimulation of respiration in patients with drug-induced postanesthesia respiratory depression or CNS depression caused by overdose and as temporary measure in acute respiratory insufficiency (doxapram); obstructive sleep apnea (armodafinil, modafinil); narcolepsy (armodafinil, dextroamphetamine, methylphenidate, modafinil); shift-work sleep disorder (armodafinil, modafinil); obesity (phentermine); binge eating disorder (lisdexamfetamine); ADHD (dextroamphetamine, lisdexamfetamine, dexmethylphenidate, methylphenidate)**

ACTION
Doxapram produces respiratory stimulation through the peripheral carotid chemoreceptors. The exact mechanism of action of armodafinil and modafinil isn't known. Phentermine is a sympathomimetic amine. The exact mechanism of action in treating obesity isn't established. Dextroamphetamine, dexmethylphenidate, lisdexamfetamine, and methylphenidate promote nerve impulse transmission.

ADVERSE REACTIONS
Phentermine's adverse reactions are related to its stimulatory effect and include hypertension, palpitations, tachyarrhythmias, urticaria, constipation, diarrhea, dizziness, excitement, insomnia, tremor, and restlessness. Armodafinil and modafinil may cause severe rash, including Stevens-Johnson syndrome.

CONTRAINDICATIONS & CAUTIONS

Black Box Warning   Refer to individual drug monographs for black box warnings. ■

• Contraindicated in patients hypersensitive to any of the drug components.

• Use drugs cautiously in patients with a psychiatric illness.

• Be aware that drugs have the potential for abuse and misuse.

• Doxapram is contraindicated in epilepsy, seizure disorders, mechanical disorders of ventilation such as muscle paresis, flail chest, pneumothorax, asthma, pulmonary fibrosis, head injury, stroke, cerebral edema, uncompensated HF, severe coronary disease, and severe hypertension.

• Delay administration of doxapram in patients who have received general anesthesia utilizing a volatile agent until the volatile agent has been excreted. This will lessen the chance for arrhythmias, including ventricular tachycardia or ventricular fibrillation.

• Administer doxapram cautiously in patients taking MAO inhibitors or sympathomimetics because an added pressor effect may occur.

• Phentermine is contraindicated in agitated states, CV disease, history of drug abuse, severe hypertension, hyperthyroidism, and glaucoma.

• Dextroamphetamine, phentermine, lisdexamfetamine, dexmethylphenidate, and methylphenidate are contraindicated during or within 14 days after use of MAO inhibitors.

• Drugs can cause arrhythmias, hypertension, nervousness, and insomnia.

• Use lisdexamfetamine, dextroamphetamine, methylphenidate, dexmethylphenidate, and modafinil cautiously in patients with seizure disorder.

Corticosteroids

beclomethasone dipropionate
betamethasone
budesonide
ciclesonide
dexamethasone
dexamethasone sodium phosphate
fludrocortisone acetate
flunisolide
fluticasone propionate
hydrocortisone
hydrocortisone acetate
hydrocortisone butyrate
hydrocortisone cypionate
hydrocortisone probutate

hydrocortisone sodium succinate
hydrocortisone valerate
methylPREDNISolone
methylPREDNISolone acetate
methylPREDNISolone sodium succinate
mometasone furoate
prednisoLONE
prednisoLONE acetate
prednisoLONE sodium phosphate
predniSONE
triamcinolone

INDICATIONS

➤ **Hypersensitivity; inflammation, particularly of eye, nose, and respiratory tract; to initiate immunosuppression; replacement therapy in adrenocortical insufficiency, dermatologic diseases, respiratory disorders, and rheumatic disorders**

ACTION

Corticosteroids suppress cell-mediated and humoral immunity by reducing levels of leukocytes, monocytes, and eosinophils; by decreasing immunoglobulin binding to cell-surface receptors; and by inhibiting interleukin synthesis. They reduce inflammation by preventing hydrolytic enzyme release into the cells, preventing plasma exudation, suppressing polymorphonuclear leukocyte migration, and disrupting other inflammatory processes.

ADVERSE REACTIONS

Systemic corticosteroid therapy may suppress the hypothalamic-pituitary-adrenal (HPA) axis. Excessive use may cause cushingoid symptoms and various systemic disorders, such as diabetes and osteoporosis. Other effects may include dermatologic disorders, edema, euphoria, fluid and electrolyte imbalances, gastritis or GI irritation, hypertension, immunosuppression, increased appetite, insomnia, psychosis, and weight gain.

CONTRAINDICATIONS & CAUTIONS

• Contraindicated in patients hypersensitive to these drugs or any of their components and in those with systemic fungal infection.

• Use cautiously in patients with GI ulceration, renal disease, hypertension, osteoporosis, varicella, vaccinia, exanthem, diabetes mellitus, hypothyroidism, thromboembolic disorder, seizures, myasthenia gravis, HF, TB, ocular herpes simplex, hypoalbuminemia, emotional instability, or psychosis.

• In pregnant women, avoid use, if possible, because of fetal risk. If use during pregnancy is necessary, use the lowest effective dose for the shortest duration. Inhaled drugs are preferred for treating asthma during pregnancy. Women should stop breast-feeding because these drugs appear in breast milk and could cause serious adverse effects in infants. In children, long-term use should be avoided whenever possible because stunted growth may result. Elderly patients may have an increased risk of adverse reactions; monitor them closely.

Diuretics, loop
bumetanide
ethacrynate sodium
ethacrynic acid
furosemide
torsemide

INDICATIONS
➤ Edema from HF, hepatic cirrhosis, or nephrotic syndrome; mild-to-moderate hypertension; adjunctive treatment in acute pulmonary edema or hypertensive crisis

ACTION
Loop diuretics inhibit sodium and chloride reabsorption in the ascending loop of Henle, thus increasing excretion of sodium, chloride, and water. Like thiazide diuretics, loop diuretics increase excretion of potassium. Loop diuretics produce more diuresis and electrolyte loss than thiazide diuretics.

ADVERSE REACTIONS
Therapeutic dose commonly causes metabolic and electrolyte disturbances, particularly potassium depletion. It also may cause hyperglycemia, hyperuricemia, hypochloremic alkalosis, and hypomagnesemia. Rapid parenteral administration may cause hearing loss (including deafness) and tinnitus. High doses can produce profound diuresis, leading to hypovolemia and CV collapse. Photosensitivity also may occur.

CONTRAINDICATIONS & CAUTIONS
Black Box Warning Refer to individual drug monographs for black box warnings. ■
• Contraindicated in patients hypersensitive to these drugs and in patients with anuria, hepatic coma, or severe electrolyte depletion.

• Use cautiously in patients with severe renal disease. Also use cautiously in patients with severe hypersensitivity to sulfonamides because allergic reaction may occur.
• Use cautiously in pregnant women. Don't use in breast-feeding women. In neonates, use cautiously; the usual pediatric dose can be used, but dosage intervals should be extended. If needed in elderly patients, use a lower dose and monitor patient closely; these patients are more susceptible to drug-induced diuresis.

Diuretics, potassium-sparing
amiloride hydrochloride
eplerenone
spironolactone
triamterene

INDICATIONS
➤ Edema from hepatic cirrhosis, nephrotic syndrome, and HF; mild or moderate hypertension; diagnosis of primary hyperaldosteronism; aid in treatment of hypokalemia; prophylaxis of hypokalemia in patients taking cardiac glycosides

ACTION
Spironolactone and eplerenone competitively inhibit aldosterone at the distal renal tubules, also promoting sodium excretion and potassium retention.

ADVERSE REACTIONS
Hyperkalemia is the most serious adverse reaction; it could lead to arrhythmias. Other adverse reactions include nausea, vomiting, headache, weakness, fatigue, bowel disturbances, cough, and dyspnea.

CONTRAINDICATIONS & CAUTIONS
Black Box Warning Refer to individual drug monographs for black box warnings. ■
• Contraindicated in patients hypersensitive to spironolactone, in those taking other potassium-sparing diuretics or potassium supplements, and in those with anuria, acute or chronic renal insufficiency, severe hyperkalemia, or diabetic nephropathy.
• Use cautiously in patients with severe hepatic insufficiency because electrolyte imbalance may lead to hepatic encephalopathy, and in patients with diabetes, who are at increased risk for hyperkalemia.

DRUG CLASSES

• No controlled studies of use in pregnant women exist. Women who wish to breast-feed should consult the prescriber because drug may appear in breast milk. In children, use cautiously; they're more susceptible to hyperkalemia. In elderly and debilitated patients, observe closely and reduce dosage, if needed; they're more susceptible to drug-induced diuresis and hyperkalemia.

Diuretics, thiazide and thiazide-like

Thiazide
hydrochlorothiazide

Thiazide-like
indapamide
metolazone

INDICATIONS
➤ **Edema from right-sided HF, mild-to-moderate left-sided HF, or nephrotic syndrome; edema and ascites caused by hepatic cirrhosis; hypertension; diabetes insipidus, particularly nephrogenic diabetes insipidus**

ACTION
Thiazide and thiazide-like diuretics interfere with sodium transport across the tubules of the cortical diluting segment in the nephron, thereby increasing renal excretion of sodium, chloride, water, and potassium and decreasing calcium excretion.

Thiazide diuretics also exert an antihypertensive effect. Although the exact mechanism is unknown, direct arteriolar dilation may be partially responsible. In diabetes insipidus, thiazides cause a paradoxical decrease in urine volume and an increase in renal concentration of urine, possibly because of sodium depletion and decreased plasma volume. This increases water and sodium reabsorption in the kidneys.

ADVERSE REACTIONS
Therapeutic doses cause electrolyte and metabolic disturbances, most commonly potassium depletion. Other abnormalities include elevated cholesterol levels, hypercalcemia, hyperglycemia, hyperuricemia, hypochloremic alkalosis, hypomagnesemia, hyponatremia, and photosensitivity.

CONTRAINDICATIONS & CAUTIONS
Black Box Warning Refer to individual drug monographs for black box warnings. ■
• Contraindicated in patients hypersensitive to these drugs and in those with anuria.
• Use cautiously in patients with severe renal disease, impaired hepatic function, or progressive liver disease.
• Use cautiously in pregnant women. Drugs appear in breast milk; patient should either discontinue breast-feeding or discontinue drug. Safety and effectiveness haven't been established in children. If needed in elderly patients, reduce dosage and monitor patient closely; these patients are more susceptible to drug-induced diuresis.

Estrogens
esterified estrogens
estradiol
estradiol cypionate
estradiol hemihydrate
estradiol valerate
estrogens (conjugated)
estropipate

INDICATIONS
➤ **Prevention of moderate to severe vasomotor symptoms linked to menopause, such as hot flushes and dizziness; stimulation of vaginal tissue development, cornification, and secretory activity; inhibition of hormone-sensitive cancer growth; female hypogonadism; female castration; primary ovulation failure; ovulation control; prevention of conception**

ACTION
Estrogens promote the development and maintenance of the female reproductive system and secondary sexual characteristics. They inhibit the release of pituitary gonadotropins and have various metabolic effects, including retention of fluid and electrolytes, retention and deposition in bone of calcium and phosphorus, and mild anabolic activity.

Estrogens and estrogenic substances given as drugs have effects related to endogenous estrogen's mechanism of action. They can mimic the action of endogenous estrogen when used as replacement therapy and can inhibit ovulation or the growth of certain hormone-sensitive cancers.

ADVERSE REACTIONS

Acute adverse reactions include abdominal cramps; bloating caused by fluid and electrolyte retention; breast swelling and tenderness; changes in menstrual bleeding patterns, such as spotting and prolongation or absence of bleeding; headache; loss of appetite; loss of libido; nausea; photosensitivity; swollen feet or ankles; and weight gain.

Long-term effects include benign hepatomas, cholestatic jaundice, elevated BP (sometimes into the hypertensive range), endometrial carcinoma (rare), and thromboembolic disease (risk increases greatly with cigarette smoking, especially in women older than age 35).

CONTRAINDICATIONS & CAUTIONS

Black Box Warning Refer to individual drug monographs for black box warnings. ∎
• Contraindicated in women with thrombophlebitis or thromboembolic disorders, unexplained abnormal genital bleeding, or estrogen-dependent neoplasia.
• Use cautiously in patients with hypertension; metabolic bone disease; migraines; seizures; asthma; cardiac, renal, or hepatic impairment; blood dyscrasia; diabetes; family history of breast cancer; or fibrocystic disease.
• Contraindicated in pregnant or breast-feeding women. In adolescents whose bone growth isn't complete, use cautiously because of effects on epiphyseal closure. Postmenopausal women with a history of long-term estrogen use are at increased risk for endometrial cancer and stroke. Postmenopausal women also have increased risk for breast cancer, MI, stroke, and blood clots with long-term use of estrogen plus progestin.

Fluoroquinolones

ciprofloxacin
gatifloxacin
gemifloxacin mesylate
levofloxacin
moxifloxacin hydrochloride
ofloxacin

INDICATIONS

➤ **Bone and joint infection, bacterial bronchitis, endocervical and urethral chlamydial infection, bacterial gastroenteritis, endocervical and urethral gonorrhea, intra-abdominal infection, empirical** therapy for febrile neutropenia, pelvic inflammatory disease, bacterial pneumonia, bacterial prostatitis, acute sinusitis, skin and soft-tissue infection, typhoid fever, bacterial UTI (prevention and treatment), chancroid, meningococcal carriers, and bacterial septicemia caused by susceptible organisms; bacterial conjunctivitis (gatifloxacin)

ACTION

Fluoroquinolones produce a bactericidal effect by inhibiting intracellular DNA gyrase and topoisomerase IV, which prevents DNA replication. These enzymes are essential catalysts in the duplication, transcription, and repair of bacterial DNA.

Fluoroquinolones are broad-spectrum, systemic antibacterial drugs active against a wide range of aerobic gram-positive and gram-negative organisms. Gram-positive aerobic bacteria include *Staphylococcus aureus, S. epidermidis, S. hemolyticus, S. saprophyticus;* penicillinase- and non–penicillinase-producing staphylococci and some methicillin-resistant strains; *Streptococcus pneumoniae;* group A (beta) hemolytic streptococci *(S. pyogenes);* group B streptococci *(S. agalactiae);* viridans streptococci; groups C, F, and G streptococci and nonenterococcal group D streptococci; and *Enterococcus faecalis.* Fluoroquinolones are also effective against gram-negative aerobic bacteria, including, but not limited to, *Escherichia coli, Neisseria meningitidis* and most strains of penicillinase- and non–penicillinase-producing *Haemophilus ducreyi, H. influenzae, H. parainfluenzae, Moraxella catarrhalis, N. gonorrhoeae,* most clinically important *Enterobacteriaceae,* and *Vibrio parahaemolyticus.* Certain fluoroquinolones are active against *Chlamydia trachomatis, Legionella pneumophila, Mycobacterium avium-intracellulare, Mycoplasma hominis, M. pneumoniae,* and *Pseudomonas aeruginosa.*

ADVERSE REACTIONS

Adverse reactions that are rare but need medical attention include CNS stimulation (acute psychosis, agitation, hallucinations, tremors), hepatotoxicity, hypersensitivity reactions, interstitial nephritis, phlebitis, pseudomembranous colitis, and tendinitis or tendon rupture. Adverse reactions that need no medical attention unless they persist or become intolerable include CNS effects (dizziness, headache, nervousness, drowsiness, insomnia), GI reactions, and photosensitivity.

CONTRAINDICATIONS & CAUTIONS

Black Box Warning Fluoroquinolones are associated with increased risk of tendinitis and tendon rupture in all age-groups. The risk further increases in older patients (usually older than age 60), in patients taking corticosteroids, and in patients who have received kidney, heart, or lung transplants. For patients with sinusitis, bronchitis, and uncomplicated UTIs, use only if there are no alternative treatment options. ■

Black Box Warning Fluoroquinolones may exacerbate muscle weakness in persons with myasthenia gravis. Avoid use in patients with known history of myasthenia gravis. ■

• Contraindicated in patients hypersensitive to fluoroquinolones because serious, possibly fatal, reactions can occur.

• Most systemic fluoroquinolones can cause QT-interval prolongations. Avoid in patients with a history of QTc-interval prolongation or uncorrected electrolyte disorders (hypokalemia, hypomagnesemia) and in patients taking Class IA or Class III antiarrhythmics and other drugs that prolong the QT interval.

• Hypoglycemia may occur in patients with or without diabetes.

• Use cautiously in patients with known or suspected CNS disorders that predispose them to seizures or lower the seizure threshold, cerebral ischemia, severe hepatic dysfunction, or renal insufficiency.

• CDAD ranging in severity from mild to fatal colitis can occur during treatment or even more than 2 months after therapy ends.

• If phototoxicity occurs, drug should be discontinued.

• Refer to manufacturer's instructions for use during pregnancy and breast-feeding. In children, fluoroquinolones aren't recommended because they can cause joint problems. If needed in elderly patients, reduce dosage, because these patients are more likely to have reduced renal function.

Hematopoietic agents

darbepoetin alfa
epoetin alfa

INDICATIONS

➤ **Anemia associated with chronic renal failure, zidovudine therapy in patients with HIV, and cancer patients on chemotherapy; to reduce the need for allogeneic blood transfusions in surgical patients (epoetin alfa)**

ACTION

Epoetin alfa and darbepoetin alfa stimulate RBC production in the bone marrow.

ADVERSE REACTIONS

Hematopoietics may cause fatigue, headache, chest pain, hypertension, nausea, vomiting, diarrhea, mucositis, stomatitis, myalgias, fever, dyspnea, cough, sore throat, alopecia, rash, urticaria, seizures, and stinging at injection site.

CONTRAINDICATIONS & CAUTIONS

Black Box Warning Refer to individual drug monographs for black box warnings. ■

• Contraindicated in patients hypersensitive to any of the drug components or human albumin.

• Contraindicated in uncontrolled hypertension.

• Darbepoetin alfa and epoetin alfa shouldn't be used in patients with breast, non–small-cell lung, head and neck, lymphoid, and cervical cancers, or for the treatment of cancers with curative potential.

• Use cautiously in patients with cardiac disease, seizures, and porphyria.

Histamine₂-receptor antagonists

cimetidine
famotidine
nizatidine
ranitidine hydrochloride

INDICATIONS

➤ **Acute duodenal or gastric ulcer, Zollinger-Ellison syndrome, gastroesophageal reflux**

ACTION

H_2-receptor antagonists inhibit the action of H_2 receptors in gastric parietal cells, reducing gastric acid output and concentration, regardless of stimulants, such as histamine, food, insulin, and caffeine, or basal conditions.

ADVERSE REACTIONS

H_2-receptor antagonists rarely cause adverse reactions. Cardiac arrhythmias, dizziness, fatigue, gynecomastia, headache, mild and transient diarrhea, and thrombocytopenia are possible.

CONTRAINDICATIONS & CAUTIONS
• Contraindicated in patients hypersensitive to these drugs.
• Use cautiously in patients with impaired renal or hepatic function.
• In pregnant women, use cautiously. Refer to each manufacturer's instructions for use during breast-feeding as some drugs should not be used. Elderly patients have increased risk of adverse reactions, particularly those affecting the CNS; use cautiously.

Immunosuppressants
alefacept
anakinra
azathioprine
basiliximab
belimumab
certolizumab pegol
cycloSPORINE
etanercept
fingolimod
glatiramer acetate
infliximab
lymphocyte immune globulin
muromonab-CD3
mycophenolate mofetil
sirolimus
tacrolimus

INDICATIONS
➤ **Prevention of rejection in organ transplants and in the management of severe RA, MS, psoriasis, systemic lupus erythematosus**

ACTION
The exact mechanism of action is not fully known. Immunosuppressants act by suppressing cell-mediated hypersensitivity reactions and produce various alterations in antibody production, blocking the activity of interleukin, inhibiting helper T cells and suppressor T cells, and antagonizing the metabolism of purine, therefore inhibiting RNA and DNA structure and synthesis.

ADVERSE REACTIONS
Immunosuppressants may cause albuminuria, hematuria, proteinuria, renal failure, hepatotoxicity, oral *Candida* infections, gingival

hyperplasia, tremors, and headache. The most serious reactions include leukopenia, thrombocytopenia, and risk of secondary infection.

CONTRAINDICATIONS & CAUTIONS
Black Box Warning Refer to individual drug monographs for black box warnings. ■
• Contraindicated in patients hypersensitive to any of the drug components.
• Use cautiously in patients with severe renal disease, or severe hepatic disease.
• Refer to manufacturer's instructions for use in pregnancy and breast-feeding.

Inotropics
digoxin
milrinone

INDICATIONS
➤ **HF and supraventricular arrhythmias, including supraventricular tachycardia, atrial fibrillation, and atrial flutter (digoxin); short-term HF and patients awaiting heart transplantation (milrinone)**

ACTION
Inotropics help move calcium into the cells, which increases cardiac output by strengthening contractility. Digoxin also acts on the central nervous system to slow HR. Milrinone relaxes vascular smooth muscle, decreasing peripheral vascular resistance (afterload) and the amount of blood returning to the heart (preload).

ADVERSE REACTIONS
Inotropics may cause arrhythmias, nausea, vomiting, diarrhea, headache, fever, mental disturbances, visual changes, and chest pain. Milrinone may cause thrombocytopenia, hypotension, hypokalemia, and elevated liver enzymes.

CONTRAINDICATIONS & CAUTIONS
• Contraindicated in patients hypersensitive to any of the drug components.
• Digoxin is contraindicated in ventricular fibrillation.
• Use cautiously in patients with renal insufficiency because of the potential for toxicity.
• Use digoxin cautiously in patients with sinus node disease or AV block because of the potential for advanced heart block.

DRUG CLASSES

Laxatives

Bulk-forming
calcium polycarbophil
psyllium

Emollient
mineral oil

Hyperosmolar
glycerin
lactulose
lubiprostone
polyethylene glycol

Saline
magnesium citrate
magnesium hydroxide
magnesium sulfate
sodium phosphates

Stimulant
bisacodyl

Stool softener, stool surfactant
docusate calcium
docusate sodium

INDICATIONS
➤ **Constipation, irritable bowel syndrome, diverticulosis**

ACTION
Laxatives promote movement of intestinal contents through the colon and rectum in several ways: bulk-forming, emollient, hyperosmolar, and stimulant.

ADVERSE REACTIONS
All laxatives may cause flatulence, diarrhea, and abdominal disturbances. Bulk-forming laxatives may cause intestinal obstruction, impaction, or (rarely) esophageal obstruction. Emollient laxatives may irritate the throat. Hyperosmolar and saline laxatives may cause fluid and electrolyte imbalances. Stimulant laxatives may cause urine discoloration, malabsorption, and weight loss.

CONTRAINDICATIONS & CAUTIONS
• Contraindicated in patients with GI obstruction or perforation, toxic colitis, megacolon, nausea and vomiting, or acute surgical abdomen.

• Use cautiously in patients with rectal or anal conditions such as rectal bleeding or large hemorrhoids.
• For pregnant women and breast-feeding women, recommendations vary for individual drugs. Infants and children have an increased risk of fluid and electrolyte disturbances; use cautiously. In elderly patients, dependence is more likely to develop because of age-related changes in GI function. Monitor these patients closely.

Macrolide anti-infectives
azithromycin
clarithromycin
erythromycin ethylsuccinate
erythromycin lactobionate
erythromycin stearate
fidaxomicin

INDICATIONS
➤ **Various common infections**

ACTION
Inhibit RNA-dependent protein synthesis by acting on a small portion of the 50S ribosomal unit. They're active against *Staphylococcus aureus, Streptococcus pneumoniae, Streptococcus pyogenes, Streptococcus agalactiae, Moraxella catarrhalis, Chlamydia trachomatis, Mycoplasma pneumoniae, Haemophilus influenzae,* and *Neisseria gonorrhoeae.*

ADVERSE REACTIONS
These drugs may cause cardiac effects (prolonged QT interval, arrhythmias, torsades de pointes), nausea, vomiting, diarrhea, abdominal pain, palpitations, chest pain, vaginal candidiasis, nephritis, dizziness, headache, vertigo, somnolence, rash, and photosensitivity.

CONTRAINDICATIONS & CAUTIONS
• Contraindicated in patients hypersensitive to drug's components.
• CDAD ranging in severity from mild to fatal colitis can occur during treatment or even more than 2 months after therapy ends.

Neuromuscular blockers

atracurium besylate
cisatracurium besylate
pancuronium bromide
succinylcholine chloride

INDICATIONS
➤ To relax skeletal muscle during surgery, reduce intensity of muscle spasms in drug-induced or electrically induced seizures, and manage patients who are fighting mechanical ventilation

ACTION
Nondepolarizing blockers (atracurium, cisatracurium, and pancuronium) compete with acetylcholine at cholinergic receptor sites on the skeletal muscle membrane. This action blocks acetylcholine's neurotransmitter actions, preventing muscle contraction. Succinylcholine is a depolarizing blocker. This drug isn't inactivated by cholinesterase, thereby preventing repolarization of the motor endplate and causing muscle paralysis.

ADVERSE REACTIONS
Neuromuscular blockers may cause apnea, hypotension, hypertension, arrhythmias, tachycardia, bronchospasm, excessive bronchial or salivary secretions, and skin reactions.

CONTRAINDICATIONS & CAUTIONS
Black Box Warning Refer to individual drug monographs for black box warnings. ■
• Contraindicated in patients hypersensitive to any of the drug components.
• The drugs should be used only by personnel skilled in airway management and respiratory support.

Nonsteroidal anti-inflammatory drugs

aspirin
celecoxib
diclofenac epolamine
diclofenac potassium
diclofenac sodium
diflunisal
etodolac
ibuprofen
indomethacin
indomethacin sodium
ketoprofen
ketorolac tromethamine
nabumetone
naproxen
naproxen sodium

INDICATIONS
➤ Mild-to-moderate pain, inflammation, stiffness, swelling, or tenderness caused by headache, arthralgia, myalgia, neuralgia, dysmenorrhea, RA, juvenile arthritis, osteoarthritis, dental or surgical procedures, or patent ductus arteriosus

ACTION
The analgesic effect of NSAIDs may result from interference with the prostaglandins involved in pain. Prostaglandins appear to sensitize pain receptors to mechanical stimulation or to other chemical mediators. NSAIDs inhibit synthesis of prostaglandins peripherally and possibly centrally.

NSAIDs exert an anti-inflammatory effect that may result in part from inhibition of prostaglandin synthesis and release during inflammation. The exact mechanism isn't clear.

ADVERSE REACTIONS
Adverse reactions chiefly involve the GI tract, particularly erosion of the gastric mucosa. The most common symptoms are abdominal pain, dyspepsia, epigastric distress, heartburn, and nausea. CNS and skin reactions also may occur. Flank pain with other evidence of nephrotoxicity occurs occasionally. Fluid retention may aggravate hypertension or HF.

CONTRAINDICATIONS & CAUTIONS
Black Box Warning Refer to individual drug monographs for additional black box warnings. ■
Black Box Warning NSAIDs may increase risk of serious CV thrombotic events, MI, and stroke, which can be fatal, and are contraindicated after CABG surgery. ■
Black Box Warning NSAIDs increase risk of serious GI reactions, including inflammation, ulceration, and perforation of the stomach or intestines, which can be fatal. Elderly patients are at increased risk. ■
• Contraindicated in patients hypersensitive to these drugs.
⊙ *Alert:* MI or stroke can occur as early as the first week of using an NSAID. The risk appears higher with higher doses. Use the

DRUG CLASSES

lowest effective dose for the shortest duration possible.

❶ *Alert:* NSAIDs increase the risk of HF.

• Use cautiously in patients with HF, hypertension, risk of MI (except low-dose aspirin), fluid retention, renal insufficiency, or coagulation defects.

• Safe use in pregnant women hasn't been established. Use during the third trimester increases risk of premature closure of the ductus arteriosus. Patients older than age 60 may be more susceptible to toxic effects of NSAIDs because of decreased renal function.

Nucleoside reverse transcriptase inhibitors
abacavir sulfate
didanosine
emtricitabine
lamivudine
stavudine
tenofovir disoproxil fumarate
zidovudine

INDICATIONS
➤ **HIV infection, AIDS, prevention of maternal-fetal HIV transmission, prevention of HIV infection after occupational exposure (such as needle stick or mucous membrane or nonintact skin contact) or nonoccupational exposure to blood, genital secretions, or other potentially infectious body fluids of an HIV-infected person when there's substantial risk of transmission**

ACTION
Nucleoside reverse transcriptase inhibitors (NRTIs) inhibits DNA viral replication by chain termination, competitive inhibition of reverse transcriptase, or both.

ADVERSE REACTIONS
Because of the complexity of HIV infection, it's often difficult to distinguish between disease-related symptoms and adverse drug reactions. The most frequently reported adverse effects of NRTIs are anemia, leukopenia, and neutropenia. Thrombocytopenia is less common. Rare adverse effects of NRTIs are hepatotoxicity, myopathy, and neurotoxicity. Any of these adverse effects requires prompt medical attention.

Adverse effects that don't need medical attention unless they persist or are bothersome

include headache, insomnia, myalgias, nausea, or hyperpigmentation of nails.

CONTRAINDICATIONS & CAUTIONS
Black Box Warning Refer to individual drug monographs for black box warnings. ■

• Contraindicated in patients hypersensitive to these drugs and patients with moderate to severe hepatic impairment (abacavir) or pancreatitis (didanosine).

• Use cautiously in patients with mild hepatic impairment or risk factors for liver impairment, risk for pancreatitis (didanosine), or compromised bone marrow function (zidovudine).

• In pregnant women, use drug only if benefits outweigh risks. To reduce the risk of transmitting the virus, HIV-infected mothers shouldn't breast-feed. The pharmacokinetic and safety profiles of NRTIs are similar in children and adults. NRTIs may be used in children age 3 months and older, but the half-life may be prolonged in neonates. In elderly patients, elimination half-life may be prolonged.

Opioids
codeine phosphate
codeine sulfate
fentanyl citrate
hydromorphone hydrochloride
meperidine hydrochloride
methadone hydrochloride
morphine sulfate
nalbuphine hydrochloride
oxycodone hydrochloride
oxymorphone hydrochloride
pentazocine lactate

INDICATIONS
➤ **Moderate-to-severe pain from acute and some chronic disorders; management of pain severe enough to require daily, around-the-clock, long-term opioid treatment; dry, nonproductive cough (codeine); management of opioid dependence (methadone); anesthesia support; sedation**

ACTION
Opioids act as agonists at specific opioid-receptor binding sites in the CNS and other tissues, altering perception of pain.

ADVERSE REACTIONS

Respiratory and circulatory depression (including orthostatic hypotension) are the major hazards of opioids. Other adverse CNS effects include agitation, coma, depression, dizziness, dysphoria, euphoria, faintness, mental clouding, nervousness, restlessness, sedation, seizures, visual disturbances, and weakness. Adverse GI effects include biliary colic, constipation, nausea, and vomiting. Urine retention or hypersensitivity also may occur. Drug tolerance and psychological or physical dependence may follow prolonged use.

CONTRAINDICATIONS & CAUTIONS

Black Box Warning Refer to individual drug monographs for black box warnings. ∎

• Contraindicated in patients hypersensitive to these drugs and in those who have recently taken an MAO inhibitor. Also contraindicated in those with acute or severe bronchial asthma or respiratory depression.

⊖ Alert: When used concomitantly with serotonergic drugs, risk of serotonin syndrome increases.

⊖ Alert: Use may lead to rare but serious decrease in adrenal gland cortisol production and, with long-term use, to decreased sex hormone levels.

• Use cautiously in patients with head injury, increased ICP or increased IOP, hepatic or renal dysfunction, mental illness, emotional disturbances, or drug-seeking behaviors.

• In pregnant or breast-feeding women, use cautiously. Prolonged maternal use of opioids during pregnancy can cause neonatal withdrawal syndrome in the newborn, which may be life-threatening if not recognized and treated according to protocols developed by neonatology experts. Breast-feeding infants of women taking opioids may develop physical dependence. In children, safety and effectiveness of some opioids haven't been established. Elderly patients may be more sensitive to opioids, and lower doses are usually given.

Penicillins

Natural penicillins
penicillin G benzathine
penicillin G potassium
penicillin G procaine
penicillin G sodium
penicillin V potassium

Aminopenicillins
amoxicillin
amoxicillin–clavulanate potassium
ampicillin
ampicillin sodium–sulbactam sodium
ampicillin trihydrate

Extended-spectrum penicillins
piperacillin sodium–tazobactam sodium
ticarcillin disodium–clavulanate
  potassium

Penicillinase-resistant penicillins
nafcillin sodium

INDICATIONS

➤ **Streptococcal pneumonia; enterococcal and nonenterococcal group D endocarditis; diphtheria; anthrax; meningitis; tetanus; botulism; actinomycosis; syphilis; relapsing fever; Lyme disease; pneumococcal infections; rheumatic fever; bacterial endocarditis; neonatal group B streptococcal disease; septicemia; gynecologic infections; infections of urinary, respiratory, and GI tracts; infections of skin, soft tissue, bones, and joints**

ACTION

Generally bactericidal, penicillins inhibit synthesis of the bacterial cell wall, causing rapid cell destruction. They're most effective against fast-growing susceptible bacteria. Their sites of action are enzymes known as *penicillin-binding proteins* (PBPs). The affinity of certain penicillins for PBPs in various microorganisms helps explain the different activities of these drugs.

Susceptible aerobic gram-positive cocci include *Staphylococcus aureus;* nonenterococcal group D streptococci; groups A, B, D, G, H, K, L, and M streptococci; *Streptococcus viridans;* and *Enterococcus* (usually with an aminoglycoside). Susceptible aerobic gram-negative cocci include *Neisseria meningitidis* and non–penicillinase-producing *N. gonorrhoeae.*

Susceptible aerobic gram-positive bacilli include *Corynebacterium, Listeria,* and *Bacillus anthracis.* Susceptible anaerobes include *Peptococcus, Peptostreptococcus, Actinomyces, Clostridium, Fusobacterium, Veillonella,* and non–beta-lactamase–producing strains of *Streptococcus pneumoniae.* Susceptible spirochetes include *Treponema pallidum, T. pertenue,*

DRUG CLASSES

Leptospira, Borrelia recurrentis and, possibly, *B. burgdorferi.*

Aminopenicillins have uses against more organisms, including many gram-negative organisms. Like natural penicillins, aminopenicillins are vulnerable to inactivation by penicillinase. Susceptible organisms include *Escherichia coli, Proteus mirabilis, Shigella, Salmonella, S. pneumoniae, N. gonorrhoeae, Haemophilus influenzae, S. aureus, S. epidermidis* (non–penicillinase-producing *Staphylococcus*), and *Listeria monocytogenes.*

Extended-spectrum penicillins offer a wider range of bactericidal action than the other three classes and usually are given in combination with aminoglycosides. Susceptible strains include *Enterobacter, Klebsiella, Citrobacter, Serratia, Bacteroides fragilis, Pseudomonas aeruginosa, Proteus vulgaris, Providencia rettgeri,* and *Morganella morganii.* These penicillins are also vulnerable to beta-lactamase and penicillinases.

Penicillinase-resistant penicillins are semisynthetic penicillins designed to remain stable against hydrolysis by most staphylococcal penicillinases and thus are the drugs of choice against susceptible penicillinase-producing staphylococci. They also act against most organisms susceptible to natural penicillins.

ADVERSE REACTIONS

With all penicillins, hypersensitivity reactions range from mild rash, fever, and eosinophilia to fatal anaphylaxis. Hematologic reactions include hemolytic anemia, leukopenia, thrombocytopenia, and transient neutropenia. Certain adverse reactions are more common with specific classes. For example, bleeding episodes are usually seen with high doses of extended-spectrum penicillins, whereas GI adverse effects are most common with ampicillin. In patients with renal disease, high doses (especially of penicillin G) irritate the CNS, causing confusion, twitching, lethargy, dysphagia, seizures, and coma. Hepatotoxicity may occur with penicillinase-resistant penicillins, and hypokalemia and hypernatremia have been reported with extended-spectrum penicillins. Local irritation from parenteral therapy may be severe enough to warrant administration by subclavian or centrally placed catheter or stopping therapy.

CONTRAINDICATIONS & CAUTIONS

Black Box Warning Refer to individual drug monographs for black box warnings. ■

• Contraindicated in patients hypersensitive to these drugs.

• Use cautiously in patients with history of asthma or drug allergy, mononucleosis, renal impairment, CV diseases, hemorrhagic condition, or electrolyte imbalance.

• In pregnant women, use cautiously. For breast-feeding patients, recommendations vary depending on the drug. For children, dosage recommendations have been established for most penicillins. Elderly patients are susceptible to superinfection and renal impairment, which decreases excretion of penicillins; use cautiously and at a lower dosage.

• May cause CDAD requiring discontinuation of drug and treatment with vancomycin.

Phenothiazines

chlorproMAZINE hydrochloride
fluphenazine decanoate
perphenazine
prochlorperazine maleate
promethazine hydrochloride
thioridazine hydrochloride
thiothixene
trifluoperazine hydrochloride

INDICATIONS

➤ **Agitated psychotic states, hallucinations, manic-depressive illness, excessive motor and autonomic activity, nausea and vomiting, moderate anxiety, behavioral problems caused by chronic organic mental syndrome, tetanus, acute intermittent porphyria, intractable hiccups, itching; allergies (promethazine)**

ACTION

Phenothiazines are believed to function as dopamine antagonists by blocking postsynaptic dopamine receptors in various parts of the CNS. Their antiemetic effects result from blockage of the chemoreceptor trigger zone. They also produce varying degrees of anticholinergic effects and alpha-adrenergic–receptor blocking.

ADVERSE REACTIONS

Phenothiazines may produce extrapyramidal symptoms, such as dystonic movements, torticollis, oculogyric crises, and parkinsonian symptoms ranging from akathisia during early treatment to tardive dyskinesia after long-term use. A neuroleptic malignant syndrome resembling severe parkinsonism may occur, most often in young men taking fluphenazine.

Other adverse reactions include abdominal pain, agitation, anorexia, arrhythmias, confusion, constipation, dizziness, dry mouth, endocrine effects, fainting, hallucinations, hematologic disorders, local gastric irritation, nausea, orthostatic hypotension with reflex tachycardia, photosensitivity, seizures, skin eruptions, urine retention, visual disturbances, and vomiting. Promethazine injection can cause severe chemical irritation and tissue damage with such reactions as burning, pain, thrombophlebitis, tissue necrosis, and gangrene.

CONTRAINDICATIONS & CAUTIONS
Black Box Warning Refer to individual drug monographs for black box warnings. ∎
• Contraindicated in patients with CNS depression, bone marrow suppression, HF, circulatory collapse, coronary artery or cerebrovascular disorders, subcortical damage, or coma. Also contraindicated in patients receiving spinal and epidural anesthetics and adrenergic blockers.
• Use cautiously in debilitated patients and in those with hepatic, renal, or CV disease; respiratory disorders; hypocalcemia; seizure disorders; suspected brain tumor or intestinal obstruction; glaucoma; and prostatic hyperplasia.
• In pregnant women, use only if clearly necessary; safety hasn't been established. Women shouldn't breast-feed during therapy because most phenothiazines appear in breast milk and directly affect prolactin levels. For children younger than age 12, phenothiazines aren't recommended unless otherwise specified; use cautiously for nausea and vomiting. Acutely ill children, such as those with chickenpox, measles, CNS infections, or dehydration, have a greatly increased risk of dystonic reactions. Elderly patients are more sensitive to therapeutic and adverse effects, especially cardiac toxicity, tardive dyskinesia, and other extrapyramidal effects; use cautiously and give reduced doses, adjusting dosage to patient response.

Progestins
medroxyPROGESTERone acetate
norethindrone
norethindrone acetate

INDICATIONS
➤ **Amenorrhea, endometrial hyperplasia, abnormal uterine bleeding, endometriosis, contraception**

ACTION
Progestins transform proliferative endometrium into secretory endometrium.

ADVERSE REACTIONS
Progestins may cause amenorrhea, breakthrough bleeding, spotting, changes in menstrual flow, breast enlargement and tenderness, alterations in weight, and mood changes.

CONTRAINDICATIONS & CAUTIONS
Black Box Warning Refer to individual drug monographs for black box warnings. ∎
• Contraindicated in patients with impaired liver function or liver disease; known or suspected breast cancer; active DVT, PE, or history of these conditions; active or recent arterial thromboembolic disease; and undiagnosed vaginal bleeding. Also contraindicated in patients hypersensitive to the drug components.
• Use cautiously in patients with depression, epilepsy, migraine headaches, asthma, cardiac dysfunction, or renal dysfunction.
• In pregnant women, use is contraindicated. Use cautiously in breast-feeding women because detectable amounts of progestins have been identified in breast milk. Progestins aren't indicated in children.

Protease inhibitors
atazanavir sulfate
darunavir
fosamprenavir calcium
indinavir sulfate
lopinavir–ritonavir
nelfinavir mesylate
ritonavir
saquinavir mesylate
tipranavir

INDICATIONS
➤ **HIV infection and AIDS, postexposure prophylaxis**

ACTION
Protease inhibitors bind to the protease active site and inhibit HIV protease activity. This enzyme is required for the proteolysis of viral polyprotein precursors into individual

DRUG CLASSES

functional proteins found in infectious HIV. The net effect is formation of noninfectious, immature viral particles.

ADVERSE REACTIONS
The most common adverse effects, which require immediate medical attention, include kidney stones, pancreatitis, diabetes or hyperglycemia, ketoacidosis, and paresthesia.

Common adverse effects that don't need medical attention unless they persist or are bothersome include generalized weakness, GI disturbances, headache, insomnia, and taste disturbance. Less common adverse effects include dizziness and somnolence.

CONTRAINDICATIONS & CAUTIONS
Black Box Warning Refer to individual drug monographs for black box warnings. ∎
• Contraindicated in patients hypersensitive to these drugs or their components and in patients taking a drug highly dependent on CYP3A4 for metabolism.
• Use cautiously in patients with impaired hepatic or renal function and those with diabetes mellitus or hemophilia.
• In pregnant women, use drug only if benefits outweigh risks. To reduce the risk of transmitting HIV to the infant, HIV-infected mothers shouldn't breast-feed.

Proton pump inhibitors
dexlansoprazole
esomeprazole
lansoprazole
omeprazole
pantoprazole
rabeprazole

INDICATIONS
➤ **Duodenal ulcers, gastric ulcers, erosive esophagitis, and GERD; hypersecretory conditions (Zollinger-Ellison syndrome)**

ACTION
The drugs reduce stomach acid production by combining with hydrogen, potassium, and adenosine triphosphate in parietal cells of the stomach to block the last step in gastric acid secretion.

ADVERSE REACTIONS
PPIs may cause abdominal pain, diarrhea, constipation, flatulence, nausea, dry mouth,

headache, asthenia, URI, abnormal LFT results, and hyperglycemia.

CONTRAINDICATIONS & CAUTIONS
• Contraindicated in patients hypersensitive to the drug components.
• May increase risk of osteoporosis-related bone fractures and CDAD. Use lowest effective dose for the shortest duration.
• May increase risk of GI infections, hypomagnesemia and, with prolonged use, vitamin B_{12} deficiency.

Selective serotonin reuptake inhibitors
citalopram hydrobromide
escitalopram oxalate
fluoxetine hydrochloride
fluvoxamine maleate
paroxetine hydrochloride
sertraline hydrochloride

INDICATIONS
➤ **Major depression, obsessive-compulsive disorder, bulimia nervosa, premenstrual dysphoric disorders, panic disorders, posttraumatic stress disorder (sertraline)**

ACTION
SSRIs selectively inhibit the reuptake of serotonin with little or no effects on other neurotransmitters in the CNS, such as norepinephrine or dopamine.

ADVERSE REACTIONS
Common adverse effects include headache, tremor, dizziness, sleep disturbances, GI disturbances, and sexual dysfunction. Less common adverse effects include bleeding (ecchymoses, epistaxis), akathisia, breast tenderness or enlargement, extrapyramidal effects, dystonia, fever, hyponatremia, mania or hypomania, palpitations, serotonin syndrome, weight gain or loss, rash, urticaria, or pruritus.

CONTRAINDICATIONS & CAUTIONS
Black Box Warning Antidepressants can increase risk of suicidal thinking and behavior. Appropriately monitor patients of all ages who are started on antidepressant therapy; observe closely for clinical worsening, suicidality, or unusual behavior changes. Advise families and caregivers of the need for close observation and communication with the prescriber. ∎

• Contraindicated in patients hypersensitive to these drugs or their components and within 14 days of MAO inhibitor therapy.

• Use cautiously in patients with hepatic, renal, or cardiac insufficiency.

• In pregnant women, use drug only if benefits outweigh risks; use of certain SSRIs in the first trimester may cause birth defects. Neonates born to women who took an SSRI during the third trimester may develop complications that warrant prolonged hospitalization, respiratory support, and tube feeding. In breast-feeding women, use isn't recommended. SSRIs appear in breast milk and may cause diarrhea and sleep disturbance in neonates. However, risks and benefits to both the woman and infant must be considered. Children and adolescents may be more susceptible to increased suicidal tendencies when taking SSRIs or other antidepressants. Elderly patients may be more sensitive to the insomniac effects of SSRIs.

Skeletal muscle relaxants

baclofen
carisoprodol
cyclobenzaprine hydrochloride
dantrolene sodium
methocarbamol
orphenadrine citrate
tizanidine hydrochloride

INDICATIONS
➤ **Painful musculoskeletal disorders, muscle spasticity**

ACTION
Baclofen may reduce impulse transmission from the spinal cord to skeletal muscle. Carisoprodol, cyclobenzaprine, methocarbamol, orphenadrine, and tizanidine's mechanism of action is unclear. Dantrolene acts directly on skeletal muscle to decrease excitation and reduce muscle strength by interfering with intracellular calcium movement.

ADVERSE REACTIONS
Skeletal muscle relaxants may cause ataxia, confusion, depressed mood, dizziness, drowsiness, dry mouth, hallucinations, headache, hypotension, nervousness, tachycardia, tremor, and vertigo. Baclofen also may cause seizures with abrupt withdrawal.

CONTRAINDICATIONS & CAUTIONS
Black Box Warning Refer to individual drug monographs for black box warnings. ■

• Contraindicated in patients hypersensitive to these drugs.

• Use cautiously in patients with impaired renal or hepatic function.

• Refer to manufacturer's instructions for use in pregnant and breast-feeding patients. In children, recommendations vary. Elderly patients have an increased risk of adverse reactions; monitor them carefully.

Sulfonamides
sulfADIAZINE
sulfamethoxazole–trimethoprim

INDICATIONS
➤ **Bacterial infections, nocardiosis, toxoplasmosis, chloroquine-resistant *Plasmodium falciparum* malaria**

ACTION
Sulfonamides are bacteriostatic. They inhibit biosynthesis of tetrahydrofolic acid, which is needed for bacterial cell growth. They're active against some strains of staphylococci, streptococci, *Nocardia asteroides* and *N. brasiliensis, Clostridium tetani* and *C. perfringens, Bacillus anthracis, Escherichia coli,* and *Neisseria gonorrhoeae* and *N. meningitidis.* Sulfonamides are also active against organisms that cause UTIs, such as *E. coli, Proteus mirabilis* and *P. vulgaris, Klebsiella, Enterobacter,* and *Staphylococcus aureus,* and genital lesions caused by *Haemophilus ducreyi* (chancroid).

ADVERSE REACTIONS
Many adverse reactions stem from hypersensitivity, including bronchospasm, conjunctivitis, erythema multiforme, erythema nodosum, exfoliative dermatitis, fever, joint pain, pruritus, leukopenia, Lyell syndrome, photosensitivity, rash, Stevens-Johnson syndrome, and toxic epidermal necrolysis. GI reactions include anorexia, diarrhea, folic acid malabsorption, nausea, pancreatitis, stomatitis, and vomiting. Hematologic reactions include agranulocytosis, granulocytopenia, hypoprothrombinemia, thrombocytopenia and, in G6PD deficiency, hemolytic anemia. Renal effects usually result from crystalluria caused by precipitation of sulfonamide in the renal system.

DRUG CLASSES

CONTRAINDICATIONS & CAUTIONS
• Contraindicated in patients hypersensitive to these drugs.
• Use cautiously in patients with renal or hepatic impairment, bronchial asthma, severe allergy, or G6PD deficiency.
• In pregnant women at term and in breast-feeding women, use is contraindicated; sulfonamides appear in breast milk. Elderly patients are susceptible to bacterial and fungal superinfection and have an increased risk of folate deficiency anemia and adverse renal and hematologic effects.

Tetracyclines
doxycycline
doxycycline hyclate
doxycycline monohydrate
minocycline hydrochloride
tetracycline hydrochloride

INDICATIONS
➤ **Bacterial, protozoal, and rickettsial infections**

ACTION
Tetracyclines are bacteriostatic but may be bactericidal against certain organisms. They bind reversibly to 30S and 50S ribosomal subunits, which inhibits bacterial protein synthesis.

Susceptible gram-positive organisms include *Bacillus anthracis, Actinomyces israelii, Clostridium perfringens* and *C. tetani, Listeria monocytogenes,* and *Nocardia.*

Susceptible gram-negative organisms include *Neisseria meningitidis, Pasteurella multocida, Legionella pneumophila, Brucella* species, *Vibrio cholerae, Yersinia enterocolitica, Yersinia pestis, Bordetella pertussis, Haemophilus influenzae, Haemophilus ducreyi, Campylobacter fetus, Shigella* species, and many other common pathogens.

Other susceptible organisms include *Rickettsia akari, Rickettsia typhi, Rickettsia prowazekii,* and *Rickettsia tsutsugamushi; Coxiella burnetii; Chlamydia trachomatis* and *Chlamydia psittaci; Mycoplasma pneumoniae* and *Mycoplasma hominis; Leptospira* species; *Treponema pallidum* and *Treponema pertenue;* and *Borrelia recurrentis.*

ADVERSE REACTIONS
The most common adverse effects involve the GI tract and are dose related; they include abdominal discomfort; anorexia; bulky, loose stools; colitis; epigastric burning; flatulence; nausea; and vomiting. Superinfections also are common.

Photosensitivity reactions may be severe. Permanent discoloration of teeth occurs if drug is given during tooth formation in children younger than age 8.

CONTRAINDICATIONS & CAUTIONS
• Contraindicated in patients hypersensitive to these drugs.
• Use cautiously in patients with renal or hepatic impairment.
• Tetracyclines can cause fetal harm and shouldn't be used in pregnant women. Tetracyclines appear in breast milk; the decision to continue or discontinue breast-feeding should take into account benefits to the mother and risks to the infant. Children younger than age 8 shouldn't take tetracyclines; these drugs can cause permanent tooth discoloration, enamel hypoplasia, and a reversible decrease in bone calcification. Elderly patients may have decreased esophageal motility; use these drugs cautiously, and monitor patients for local irritation from slow passage of oral forms. Elderly patients also are more susceptible to superinfection.

Thrombolytics
alteplase
defibrotide sodium
reteplase
tenecteplase

INDICATIONS
➤ **To dissolve a preexisting clot or thrombus, often in acute or emergency situations**
➤ **Acute MI, acute ischemic stroke, PE, peripheral vascular occlusion; to restore patency to clotted grafts and I.V. access devices (alteplase); hepatic sinusoidal obstruction syndrome after hematopoietic stem cell transplant (defibrotide)**

ACTION
Thrombolytics convert plasminogen to plasmin, which lyses thrombi, and degrade fibrin, fibrinogen, and other plasma proteins.

ADVERSE REACTIONS
The most common adverse reactions are bleeding and allergic responses. Other adverse

reactions common to all are nausea, vomiting, fever, and hypotension.

CONTRAINDICATIONS & CAUTIONS
• Contraindicated in patients hypersensitive to components of drug and in combination with other fibrinolytics.
• Contraindicated in active bleeding, history of stroke, recent intracranial or intraspinal surgery or trauma, intracranial neoplasm, arteriovenous malformation or aneurysm, bleeding diathesis, or severe uncontrolled hypertension.

Vasopressors
DOBUTamine hydrochloride
DOPamine hydrochloride
ephedrine sulfate
norepinephrine bitartrate

INDICATIONS
➤ **Correction of hemodynamic imbalances present in cardiogenic shock due to MI, trauma, septicemia, cardiac surgical procedures, spinal anesthesia, drug reactions, renal failure, and HF**
➤ **Stokes-Adams syndrome with complete heart block, narcolepsy, and myasthenia gravis (ephedrine sulfate)**

ACTION
Dobutamine is a direct-acting inotrope whose primary activity results from stimulation of the beta receptors of the heart while producing mild chronotropic, hypertensive, arrhythmogenic, and vasodilatory effects. Dobutamine increases cardiac output by decreasing peripheral vascular resistance, reducing ventricular filling pressure, and increasing AV node conduction. Dopamine is a natural catecholamine, a precursor to norepinephrine in noradrenergic nerves, and a neurotransmitter in certain areas of the CNS. It produces positive chronotropic and inotropic effects on the myocardium, resulting in increased HR and cardiac contractility. This is accomplished by directly exerting an agonist action on beta-adrenoreceptors.

ADVERSE REACTIONS
Adverse reactions to vasopressors may include ventricular arrhythmias, tachycardia, angina, palpitations, cardiac conduction abnormalities, widened QRS complex, bradycardia, hypotension, hypertension, vasoconstriction, headache, anxiety, azotemia, dyspnea, phlebitis, peripheral cyanosis, and gangrene of the extremities. Difficult or painful urination can be seen with ephedrine. Less common are hypotension, thrombocytopenia, hypokalemia, and nausea.

CONTRAINDICATIONS & CAUTIONS
Black Box Warning Refer to individual drug monographs for black box warnings. ■
• Contraindicated in patients hypersensitive to any of the drug components.
• Contraindicated in patients with pheochromocytoma, uncorrected tachyarrhythmias, or ventricular fibrillation.
• Dobutamine is contraindicated in patients with idiopathic hypertrophic subaortic stenosis.
• Before treatment, hypovolemia should be corrected.
• Some vasopressors must be used cautiously in patients with a sulfite allergy, particularly asthmatic patients. Allergic-type reactions, including anaphylactic symptoms and severe asthmatic episodes, can occur.
• Infusion should be given into a large vein to prevent extravasation into surrounding tissue because this can cause tissue necrosis.
• Use with extreme caution in patients taking MAO inhibitors or who have been treated with MAO inhibitors 2 to 3 weeks before infusion. Patients taking dopamine will require substantially reduced dosages.
• Dopamine, ephedrine, and norepinephrine bitartrate shouldn't be used during cyclopropane and halothane anesthesia because of the risk of ventricular tachycardia or fibrillation.
• Use cautiously in patients with hyperthyroidism, bradycardia, partial heart block, myocardial disease, or severe arteriosclerosis.
• Give these drugs to pregnant women only if clearly indicated. Use caution when giving these drugs to breast-feeding women. Safety and effectiveness in children haven't been established.

DRUG CLASSES

abacavir sulfate
ah-BAK-ah-veer

Ziagen

Therapeutic class: Antiretrovirals
Pharmacologic class: Nucleoside
and nucleotide reverse transcriptase
inhibitors

AVAILABLE FORMS
Oral solution: 20 mg/mL
Tablets: 300 mg

INDICATIONS & DOSAGES
➤ **HIV-1 infection**
Adults: 300 mg P.O. b.i.d. or 600 mg P.O.
daily with other antiretrovirals.
Children ages 3 months and older: 8 mg/kg
P.O. b.i.d. up to maximum of 600 mg P.O.
daily, with other antiretrovirals.
Adjust-a-dose: In patients with mild hepatic
impairment (Child-Pugh score 5 to 6), give
200 mg (oral solution) P.O. b.i.d. Don't use
in patients with moderate to severe hepatic
impairment.

ADMINISTRATION
P.O.
• Drug is considered hazardous; use safe
handling and disposal precautions according
to facility policy.
• Always give drug with other antiretrovirals, never alone.
• Patient may take drug with or without
food.

ACTION
Converted intracellularly to the active
metabolite carbovir triphosphate, which
inhibits activity of HIV-1 reverse transcriptase, terminating viral DNA growth.

Route	Onset	Peak	Duration
P.O.	Unknown	Unknown	Unknown

Half-life: 1 to 2 hours.

ADVERSE REACTIONS
CNS: fever or chills, headache, insomnia
and sleep disorders, anxiety, depressive
disorders, malaise, fatigue, dizziness.
EENT: ear, nose, and throat infections.

GI: anorexia, diarrhea, nausea, vomiting.
Hepatic: *lactic acidosis.*
Skin: rash.
Other: *hypersensitivity reaction,*
redistribution/accumulation of body fat.

INTERACTIONS
Drug-drug. *Methadone:* May slightly
increase methadone elimination. Monitor
effectiveness; increase methadone dosage if
needed.
Drug-lifestyle. *Alcohol use:* May decrease
elimination of drug, increasing overall
exposure. Monitor alcohol consumption.
Discourage use together.

EFFECTS ON LAB TEST RESULTS
• May increase ALT, AST, amylase, CK,
glucose, and triglyceride levels.

CONTRAINDICATIONS & CAUTIONS
Black Box Warning Patients who carry
the HLA-B*5701 allele are at high risk for
hypersensitivity reactions; screen patients
before start of therapy and before reinitiating therapy in those with unknown status
who previously tolerated drug. ■
• Contraindicated in patients hypersensitive
to drug or its components.
• Contraindicated in patients with moderate
to severe hepatic impairment.
Black Box Warning Due to increased risk
of hepatotoxicity, use cautiously when giving drug to patients at risk for liver disease.
Lactic acidosis and severe hepatomegaly
with steatosis, including fatal cases, have
been reported with the use of nucleoside
analogues alone or in combination, including abacavir and other antiretrovirals. Stop
treatment with drug if events occur. ■
Dialyzable drug: Unknown.

PREGNANCY-LACTATION-REPRODUCTION
• Use cautiously in pregnant women because the effects are unknown. Use during
pregnancy only if potential benefits outweigh risk. Register pregnant women with
the Antiretroviral Pregnancy Registry at
1-800-258-4263.
• To avoid risk of postnatal transmission of
HIV-1 infection, the CDC recommends that
infected mothers not breast-feed.

Reactions in bold italics are *life-threatening*. Interactions may have a *rapid onset* or a *delayed onset*.

NURSING CONSIDERATIONS

• Women are more likely than men to experience lactic acidosis and severe hepatomegaly with steatosis. Obesity and prolonged nucleoside exposure may be risk factors.

Black Box Warning Drug can cause fatal hypersensitivity reactions with multiple organ involvement; if patient develops signs or symptoms of hypersensitivity (such as fever, rash, fatigue, achiness, generalized malaise, nausea, vomiting, diarrhea, abdominal pain, cough, dyspnea, or pharyngitis), stop drug and notify prescriber immediately. ■

Black Box Warning Don't restart drug or any abacavir-containing product after a hypersensitivity reaction, regardless of HLA-B*5701 status, because severe signs and symptoms will recur within hours and may include life-threatening hypotension and death. ■

• Because of a high rate of early virologic resistance, triple antiretroviral therapy with abacavir, lamivudine, and tenofovir shouldn't be used as a new treatment regimen for treatment-naive or pretreated patients. Monitor patients currently controlled with this combination and those who use this combination in addition to other antiretrovirals, and consider modification of therapy.

• Monitor patient for immune reconstitution syndrome. Inflammatory response to indolent or residual opportunistic infection (*Mycobacterium avium* infection, CMV, *Pneumocystis jiroveci* pneumonia, or TB) may occur during initial treatment; autoimmune disorders (Graves disease, polymyositis, and Guillain-Barré syndrome) may occur at any time after start of therapy.

• Assess for fat redistribution, which may appear as central obesity, dorsocervical fat enlargement (buffalo hump), peripheral wasting, facial wasting, breast enlargement, and cushingoid appearance. These signs have occurred in patients receiving antiretroviral therapy.

• Assess for CAD risk factors with antiretroviral use, and address modifiable risk factors (such as hypertension, hyperlipidemia, diabetes mellitus, and smoking).

• Drug may mildly elevate glucose level.

PATIENT TEACHING

• Inform patient that drug can cause a life-threatening hypersensitivity reaction. Warn patient who develops signs or symptoms of hypersensitivity (such as fever, rash, severe tiredness, achiness, a generally ill feeling, nausea, vomiting, diarrhea, stomach pain, cough, shortness of breath, or sore throat) to stop taking drug and notify prescriber immediately.

• Encourage patient to review information leaflet about drug with each new prescription and refill and to carry a warning card summarizing the signs and symptoms of hypersensitivity.

• Inform patient that drug doesn't cure HIV infection. Tell patient that drug doesn't reduce the risk of transmission of HIV to others through sexual contact or blood contamination and that its long-term effects are unknown.

• Caution patient not to stop anti-HIV medicines, even for a short time, because the virus count may increase and the virus may become harder to treat.

• Warn patient not to restart abacavir or other abacavir-containing drugs without being under medical care because of the risk of serious hypersensitivity reaction.

• Tell patient to take drug exactly as prescribed with or without food.

---

abatacept
uh-BAY-tuh-sept

Orencia

Therapeutic class: Antirheumatics
Pharmacologic class: Selective costimulation modulators

AVAILABLE FORMS

Lyophilized powder for injection: 250 mg single-use vial (25 mg/mL when reconstituted)
Solution for subcutaneous administration: 125 mg/mL

INDICATIONS & DOSAGES

➤ **To reduce signs and symptoms, induce major clinical response, inhibit disease progression and structural damage, and** improve physical function in patients with moderate to severe RA whose response to one or more DMARDs has been inadequate. Used alone or with other DMARDs (except TNF antagonists and anakinra)

Adults weighing more than 100 kg: 1 g I.V. over 30 minutes. Repeat 2 and 4 weeks after initial infusion and then every 4 weeks thereafter.

Adults weighing 60 to 100 kg: 750 mg I.V. over 30 minutes. Repeat 2 and 4 weeks after initial infusion and then every 4 weeks thereafter.

Adults weighing less than 60 kg: 500 mg I.V. over 30 minutes. Repeat 2 and 4 weeks after initial infusion and then every 4 weeks thereafter.

Adults (subcutaneous): 125 mg subcutaneously once weekly with or without I.V. loading dose. For patients receiving loading dose, give single I.V. dose based on weight. Then give 125 mg subcutaneously within a day, followed by 125 mg subcutaneously once weekly. Patients transferring from I.V. to subcutaneous form should receive the first subcutaneous dose instead of the next scheduled I.V. dose.

➤ **As monotherapy or with methotrexate to reduce signs and symptoms of moderately to severely active juvenile idiopathic arthritis**

Children ages 6 to 17 weighing 75 kg or more: Use adult dosing.

Children ages 6 to 17 weighing less than 75 kg: 10 mg/kg I.V. over 30 minutes. Repeat 2 and 4 weeks after initial infusion and then every 4 weeks thereafter. Maximum dose is 1,000 mg. Calculate dosing based on body weight before each dose is administered.

ADMINISTRATION

I.V.

▼ Reconstitute vial with 10 mL of sterile water for injection, using only the silicone-free disposable syringe provided, to yield 25 mg/mL. Use an 18G to 21G needle for preparation.

▼ Gently swirl contents until completely dissolved. Avoid vigorous shaking.

▼ Vent the vial with a needle to clear away foam.

▼ Solution should be clear and colorless to pale yellow. Don't use if opaque particles, discoloration, or other foreign particles are present.

▼ Further dilute solution to 100 mL total volume with NSS. Infuse over 30 minutes using an infusion set and a sterile, nonpyrogenic, low–protein-binding filter (pore size 0.2 to 1.2 micron).

▼ Store diluted solution at room temperature or refrigerate at 36° to 46° F (2° to 8° C). Complete infusion within 24 hours of reconstituting.

▼ **Incompatibilities:** Don't infuse in the same line with other I.V. drugs.

Subcutaneous

● Abatacept 125-mg/mL syringe isn't intended for I.V. administration.

● Remove prefilled syringe from refrigerator 30 to 60 minutes before administration so that it reaches room temperature.

● Abatacept should be clear and colorless to pale yellow; don't use if you observe particulate matter or discoloration.

● Rotate injection sites.

● Never inject into tender, bruised, red, or hard areas.

ACTION

Inhibits T-cell activation, decreases T-cell proliferation, and inhibits production of TNF-alpha, interferon-gamma, and interleukin-2.

Route	Onset	Peak	Duration
I.V., subcut.	Unknown	Unknown	Unknown

Half-life: I.V., 13 days; subcutaneous, 14.3 days.

ADVERSE REACTIONS

CNS: headache, dizziness, pyrexia.
CV: hypertension.
EENT: nasopharyngitis, rhinitis, sinusitis.
GI: nausea, diverticulitis, dyspepsia, diarrhea, abdominal pain.
GU: acute pyelonephritis, UTI.
Musculoskeletal: back pain, limb pain.
Respiratory: URI, bronchitis, cough, pneumonia, rhonchi, dyspnea.
Skin: cellulitis, rash.
Other: infections, *malignancies,* herpes simplex, influenza, infusion reactions, injection-site reaction.

INTERACTIONS

Drug-drug. *Anakinra, TNF antagonists:*
May increase risk of infection. Don't use
together.
Live-virus vaccines: May decrease effectiveness of vaccine. Avoid giving vaccines
during or for 3 months after abatacept
therapy.

EFFECTS ON LAB TEST RESULTS

• GDH-PQQ (glucose dehydrogenase
pyrroloquinoline quinone)–based glucose
monitoring systems may react with maltose
present in abatacept, causing falsely elevated blood glucose readings on the day of
infusion (I.V. form only).

CONTRAINDICATIONS & CAUTIONS

• Contraindicated in patients hypersensitive
to drug or its components.
• Rare cases of severe hypersensitivity
reactions have been reported. Reactions
may occur with the first dose or within
24 hours of infusion. Discontinue drug and
treat emergently if hypersensitivity occurs.
• Don't use in patients taking a TNF antagonist or anakinra.
• Use cautiously in patients with active
infection, history of chronic infections, or
underlying conditions that may predispose
patient to infection; scheduled elective
surgery; or COPD.
• Patients should be screened for viral hepatitis before starting therapy. Antirheumatic
treatment may cause reactivation of HBV.
• Patients who test positive for TB should
be treated before receiving drug.
Dialyzable drug: Unknown.

PREGNANCY-LACTATION-REPRODUCTION

• Use cautiously in pregnant women and
only if benefit to the mother justifies potential risk to the fetus.
• Register pregnant women with the pregnancy registry by calling 1-877-311-8972.
• It isn't known if drug appears in breast
milk. Patient should discontinue breast-
feeding or discontinue drug, taking into account the importance of drug to the mother.

NURSING CONSIDERATIONS

• Make sure patient has been screened for
TB before giving.

• Monitor patient, especially an older adult,
carefully for infections and malignancies.
• If patient develops a severe infection,
notify prescriber; therapy may need to be
stopped.
⊙ *Alert:* If patient has COPD, watch for
worsening respiratory status.
• Ensure the availability of appropriate
supportive measures to treat possible hypersensitivity reactions.
• Ensure that patients with juvenile idiopathic arthritis are up to date with all
immunizations before start of therapy.
• *Look alike–sound alike:* Don't confuse
Orencia with Oracea.

PATIENT TEACHING

• Instruct patient to have TB screening
before therapy.
• Tell patient to continue taking prescribed
arthritis drugs. Caution against taking
anakinra or TNF antagonists, such as etanercept, infliximab, or adalimumab.
• Tell patient to avoid exposure to infections.
• Tell patient to immediately report signs
and symptoms of infection, swollen face or
tongue, and difficulty breathing.
• Tell patient with COPD to report worsening signs and symptoms.
• Advise patient to avoid live-virus vaccines
during and for 3 months after therapy.
• Advise woman to consult prescriber if she
becomes pregnant or plans to breast-feed.
• Encourage pregnant patients to enroll in
pregnancy registry at 1-877-311-8972.
• Advise patient to contact prescriber before
taking any other drugs or herbal supplements.
• Remind patient to contact prescriber
before scheduling surgery.

SAFETY ALERT!

abiraterone acetate
a-by-RAY-ter-own

Zytiga

Therapeutic class: Antineoplastics
Pharmacologic class: Androgen biosynthesis inhibitors

AVAILABLE FORMS
Tablets ⓞⓝⓒ: 250 mg

INDICATIONS & DOSAGES
➤ **Metastatic, castration-resistant prostate cancer in combination with prednisone**
Adult men: 1,000 mg P.O. once daily. Use in combination with 5 mg prednisone P.O. b.i.d.
Adjust-a-dose: For patients with baseline moderate hepatic impairment (Child-Pugh class B), reduce starting dosage to 250 mg P.O. once daily. If hepatotoxicity develops during treatment (ALT or AST level greater than 5 × ULN or total bilirubin level greater than 3 × ULN), stop drug. Restart at 750 mg once daily after LFTs have shown a return to patient's baseline or the AST or ALT level is 2.5 × ULN or lower and total bilirubin level is 1.5 × ULN or lower. If hepatotoxicity recurs at a dosage of 750 mg once daily, stop drug and restart at 500 mg once daily using liver function guidelines above. Discontinue drug if hepatotoxicity recurs at the 500-mg once-daily dosage. Monitor liver function at least every 2 weeks for 3 months and monthly thereafter. Safety of abiraterone retreatment in patients who develop an AST or ALT level 20 × ULN or more or bilirubin level 10 × ULN or more is unknown.

ADMINISTRATION
P.O.
● Drug is hazardous: use safe handling and disposal precautions according to facility policy. Women who are pregnant or may become pregnant should wear gloves when handling tablets.
● Give tablets on an empty stomach; patient shouldn't eat for 2 hours before or 1 hour after receiving drug.
● Patient should swallow tablets whole with water and not crush or chew them.
● Store tablets at room temperature.

ACTION
Inhibits biosynthesis of androgen production and increases mineralocorticoid production by the adrenal glands.

Route	Onset	Peak	Duration
P.O.	Rapid	2 hr	Unknown

Half-life: 14.4 to 16.5 hours.

ADVERSE REACTIONS
CNS: fatigue, pyrexia, insomnia.
CV: edema, hot flushes, hypertension, *arrhythmias,* chest pain, *cardiac failure.*
EENT: nasopharyngitis.
GI: diarrhea, dyspepsia, constipation, vomiting.
GU: UTI, hematuria, urinary frequency, nocturia.
Hematologic: anemia, bruising.
Hepatic: *hepatotoxicity.*
Metabolic: *hypokalemia, hypophosphatemia, hyperglycemia,* hyperlipidemia, hypernatremia.
Musculoskeletal: joint swelling, joint discomfort, muscle discomfort, fractures.
Respiratory: URI, cough, dyspnea.
Skin: rash.
Other: falls.

INTERACTIONS
Drug-drug. *Dextromethorphan, thioridazine, other CYP2D6 substrates:* May inhibit metabolism of these drugs, causing higher levels. Avoid using together. If drugs must be used together, consider reducing dosage of CYP2D6 substrate drug.
Strong CYP3A4 inducers (such as carbamazepine, phenobarbital, phenytoin, rifabutin, rifampin, rifapentine): May decrease abiraterone level. If drugs must be used together, increase abiraterone dosage to 1,000 mg b.i.d. during concomitant use; decrease to 1,000 mg once daily if CYP3A4 inducer is discontinued.
Drug-food. *Any food:* May significantly increase drug absorption. Patient must take drug on an empty stomach.

Reactions in bold italics are *life-threatening*. Interactions may have a *rapid onset* or a *delayed onset*.

EFFECTS ON LAB TEST RESULTS
• May increase ALT, AST, bilirubin, alkaline phosphatase, glucose, cholesterol, and triglyceride levels.
• May decrease potassium, phosphate, Hb, and serum testosterone and other androgen levels.
• May decrease lymphocyte count.

CONTRAINDICATIONS & CAUTIONS
• Contraindicated in patients hypersensitive to drug or its components and in those with baseline severe hepatic impairment (Child-Pugh class C).
• Use cautiously in patients with a history of CV disease (HF, recent MI, ventricular arrhythmias) or liver disease.
• Safety in patients with LVEF of less than 50% or New York Heart Association Class III or IV HF hasn't been established.
• Because drug may harm a developing fetus, women who are pregnant or may become pregnant shouldn't handle drug without protection (gloves). It isn't known if drug or its metabolites are present in semen.
Dialyzable drug: Unknown.

PREGNANCY-LACTATION-REPRODUCTION
• Drug isn't indicated for use in women and is contraindicated in women who are pregnant, may become pregnant, or are breast-feeding.

NURSING CONSIDERATIONS
• Monitor ALT, AST, and bilirubin levels in all patients at baseline, every 2 weeks for first 3 months, then monthly thereafter. For patients with moderate hepatic impairment, measure at baseline, every week during first month of treatment, every 2 weeks for next 2 months, and monthly thereafter.
• Monitor LFTs frequently for elevated results and signs and symptoms of hepatotoxicity (malaise, jaundice, abdominal pain, nausea, and vomiting).
• Monitor patient with a history of CV disease at least monthly for hypertension, hypokalemia, and fluid retention. Control hypertension and correct hypokalemia before and during treatment.
• Monitor patient for signs and symptoms of adrenocortical insufficiency (chronic fatigue, loss of appetite, muscle weakness, weight loss, nausea, and vomiting). Patient may need an increased corticosteroid dosage before, during, and after stressful situations.

PATIENT TEACHING
• Teach patient to take drug on an empty stomach and not to eat for at least 2 hours before or 1 hour after taking drug. Advise patient to swallow tablets whole with water.
• Instruct patient that abiraterone and prednisone must be used together.
• Warn patient not to stop abiraterone, prednisone, or other chemotherapy drugs without consulting prescriber.
• Advise patient that if he misses a single dose of abiraterone or prednisone, he should take the regular dose the next day. If he misses more than one dose, he should inform his prescriber.
• Teach patient that periodic blood tests will be needed to monitor tolerance to therapy.
• Warn patient, female caregivers, and female sexual partners about risk of fetal harm from abiraterone therapy. Teach women who are pregnant or may become pregnant to wear gloves while handling drug.
• Teach patient and female sexual partners the importance of using condoms. Patient should use a condom and another effective birth control method if his partner is pregnant or of childbearing potential. Inform patient that these protective measures are required during treatment and for 1 week after treatment has ended.

acamprosate calcium
a-kam-PRO-sate

Therapeutic class: Alcohol deterrents
Pharmacologic class: Synthetic amino acid neurotransmitter analogues

AVAILABLE FORMS
Tablets (enteric-coated) ⓄⓃⒼ: 333 mg

INDICATIONS & DOSAGES
➤ **Adjunct to management of alcohol abstinence**
Adults: 666 mg P.O. t.i.d.
Adjust-a-dose: In patients with CrCl of 30 to 50 mL/minute, give 333 mg t.i.d. Do not use in patients with severe renal impairment (CrCl 30 mL/minute or less).

ADMINISTRATION
P.O.
- Don't crush or break tablets.
- Give drug without regard for food.

ACTION
Restores the balance of neuronal excitation and inhibition, probably by interacting with glutamate and GABA neurotransmitter systems, thus reducing alcohol dependence.

Route	Onset	Peak	Duration
P.O.	Unknown	3–8 hr	Unknown

Half-life: 20 to 33 hours.

ADVERSE REACTIONS
CNS: abnormal thinking, amnesia, anxiety, asthenia, depression, dizziness, headache, insomnia, migraine, paresthesia, somnolence, *suicidal thoughts,* syncope, tremor, pain.
CV: chest pain, hypertension, palpitations, peripheral edema, vasodilation.
EENT: abnormal vision, pharyngitis, rhinitis.
GI: abdominal pain, anorexia, constipation, diarrhea, dry mouth, dyspepsia, flatulence, increased appetite, nausea, taste disturbance, vomiting.
GU: erectile dysfunction.
Metabolic: weight gain.
Musculoskeletal: arthralgia, back pain, myalgia.
Respiratory: bronchitis, dyspnea, increased cough.
Skin: increased sweating, pruritus, rash.
Other: accidental injury, chills, decreased libido, flulike symptoms, infection.

INTERACTIONS
None significant.

EFFECTS ON LAB TEST RESULTS
- May increase ALT, AST, bilirubin, blood glucose, and uric acid levels. May decrease Hb level and hematocrit.
- May decrease platelet count.

CONTRAINDICATIONS & CAUTIONS
- Contraindicated in patients hypersensitive to drug or its components and in those with CrCl of 30 mL/minute or less.
- Use cautiously in elderly patients, patients with moderate renal impairment, and patients with a history of depression and suicidal thoughts or attempts.
Dialyzable drug: Unknown.
⚠ *Overdose S&S:* Diarrhea, hypercalcemia in chronic overdose.

PREGNANCY-LACTATION-REPRODUCTION
- Use cautiously in pregnant women and only if potential benefit justifies potential risk to the fetus.
- It isn't known if drug appears in breast milk. Use cautiously in breast-feeding women.

NURSING CONSIDERATIONS
- Use only after the patient successfully becomes abstinent from drinking.
- Drug doesn't eliminate or reduce withdrawal symptoms.
- Monitor patient for development of depression or suicidal thoughts.
- Drug doesn't cause alcohol aversion or a disulfiram-like reaction if used with alcohol.

PATIENT TEACHING
- Tell patient to continue the alcohol abstinence program, including counseling and support.
- Advise patient to notify his prescriber if he develops depression, anxiety, thoughts of suicide, or severe diarrhea.
- Caution patient's family or caregiver to watch for signs of depression or suicidal ideation.
- Tell patient that drug may be taken without regard to meals, but that taking it with meals may help him remember it.
- Tell patient not to crush, break, or chew the tablets but to swallow them whole.
- Advise women to use effective contraception while taking this drug. Tell patient to contact her prescriber if she becomes pregnant or plans to become pregnant.
- Explain that this drug may impair judgment, thinking, or motor skills. Urge patient to use caution when driving or performing hazardous activities until drug's effects are known.
- Tell patient to continue taking acamprosate and to contact his prescriber if he resumes drinking alcohol.

Reactions in bold italics are *life-threatening*. Interactions may have a *rapid onset* or a *delayed onset*.

acetaminophen (APAP, paracetamol)
a-seet-a-MIN-a-fen

Abenol✦ ◊, Acephen ◊, ACET✦ ◊, Aminofen ◊, APAP ◊, APAP Extra Strength ◊, Aphen ◊, Arthritis Pain Relief ◊, Atasol Forte✦ ◊, Beta Temp Childrens ◊, Children's Mapap Rapid Tabs ◊, Children's Silapap ◊, Chloraseptic Sore Throat ◊, Ed-APAP ◊, Febrol ◊, FeverAll Children's ◊, FeverAll Infants' ◊, Fortolin✦, Infants' Silapap ◊, Junior Mapap ◊, Little Fevers Fever/Pain Reliever ◊, Mapap Arthitis Pain ◊, Nortemp Infants ◊, Novo-Gesic✦ ◊, Ofirmev, Pediaphen✦ ◊, Pediatrix✦ ◊, Q-Pap Infants ◊, Rapid Action✦ ◊, Relief✦ ◊, Stanback Aspirin Free ◊, Taminol✦, Tempra Children's Syrup✦ ◊, Triaminic Fever Reducer ◊, Tylenol ◊, Tylenol Arthritis Pain ◊, Tylenol Extra Strength ◊, Tylenol Go Tabs Extra Strength ◊, Tylenol Jr. Meltaways ◊, Tylenol Sore Throat Daytime ◊, Vicks Custom Care Body Aches✦ ◊

Therapeutic class: Analgesics
Pharmacologic class: Para-aminophenol derivatives

AVAILABLE FORMS
Caplets: 500 mg ◊
Caplets (extended-release) ⓐ: 650 mg✦ ◊
Capsules: 325 mg ◊, 500 mg ◊
Drops: 80 mg/mL✦ ◊
Elixir: 160 mg/5 mL✦ ◊*
Gelcaps: 500 mg ◊
Injection: 10 mg/mL
Oral liquid: 160 mg/5 mL✦ ◊, 500 mg/ 5 mL ◊, 500 mg/15 mL ◊, 1,000 mg/30 mL
Oral solution: 80 mg/mL✦ ◊, 100 mg/mL, 160 mg/5 mL✦ ◊
Oral suspension: 80 mg/0.8 mL ◊, 160 mg/5 mL✦ ◊
Oral syrup: 160 mg/5mL ◊
Packets: 950 mg/pk

Suppositories: 80 mg ◊, 120 mg✦ ◊, 325 mg✦ ◊, 650 mg✦ ◊
Tablets: 325 mg✦ ◊, 500 mg✦ ◊, 650 mg ◊
Tablets (chewable): 80 mg ◊, 160 mg✦ ◊, 500 mg ◊
Tablets (dispersible): 80 mg ◊, 160 mg ◊
Tablets (extended-release) ⓐ: 650 mg ◊

INDICATIONS & DOSAGES
➤ **Mild pain or fever**
P.O.
Adults: 325 to 650 mg P.O. every 4 to 6 hours. Or, two extended-release caplets P.O. every 8 hours. Maximum, 3,250 mg daily unless under health care provider supervision when 4 g daily (immediate-release), may be used. For long-term therapy, don't exceed 2.6 g daily unless prescribed and monitored closely by health care provider.
Children older than age 12: 325 to 650 mg P.O. every 4 to 6 hours or 1,300 mg P.O. every 8 hours (extended-release) p.r.n. Maximum dose for immediate-release is 3,250 mg/24 hours unless under health care provider supervision, when up to 4 g/ 24 hours may be used. Maximum dose for extended-release is 3,900 mg/24 hours.
Children ages 6 to 11 (immediate-release): 325 mg P.O. every 4 to 6 hours. Maximum daily dose is 1,625 mg/day P.O. Don't use for more than 5 days unless directed by health care provider.
Children age 11 weighing 32.7 to 43.2 kg: 480 mg P.O. (oral suspension or chewable tablets) every 4 hours p.r.n. Maximum, five doses/day.
Children ages 9 to 10 weighing 27.3 to 32.6 kg: 400 mg P.O. (oral suspension or chewable tablets) every 4 hours p.r.n. Maximum, five doses/day.
Children ages 6 to 8 weighing 21.8 to 27.2 kg: 320 mg P.O. (oral suspension or chewable tablets) every 4 hours p.r.n. Maximum, five doses/day.
Children ages 4 to 5 weighing 16.4 to 21.7 kg: 240 mg P.O. (oral suspension or chewable tablets) every 4 hours p.r.n. Maximum, five doses/day.
Children ages 2 to 3 weighing 10.9 to 16.3 kg: 160 mg P.O. (oral suspension or

chewable tablets) every 4 hours p.r.n. Maximum, five doses/day.

Adjust-a-dose: For adults with GFR of 10 to 50 mL/minute/1.73 m^2, give every 6 hours; if GFR is less than 10 mL/minute/1.73 m^2, give every 8 hours. For patients receiving continuous renal replacement therapy, give every 6 hours. For infants, children, and adolescents with GFR less than 10 mL/minute/1.73 m^2, give every 8 hours. For infants, children, and adolescents receiving hemodialysis or peritoneal dialysis, give every 8 hours.

Rectal
Adults and children age 12 and older:
650 mg P.R. every 4 to 6 hours p.r.n. Maximum, 3.9 g daily. For long-term therapy, don't exceed 2.6 g daily unless prescribed and monitored closely by health care provider.
Children ages 6 to 11: 325 mg P.R. every 4 to 6 hours p.r.n. Maximum, 1,625 mg in 24 hours.
Children ages 3 to 6: 120 mg P.R. every 4 to 6 hours p.r.n. Maximum, 600 mg in 24 hours.
Children ages 1 to 3: 80 mg P.R. every 4 to 6 hours p.r.n. Maximum, 400 mg in 24 hours.
Children ages 6 to 11 months: 80 mg P.R. every 6 hours p.r.n. Maximum, 320 mg in 24 hours.

➤ **Mild to moderate pain; mild to moderate pain with adjunctive opioid analgesics; fever**
Adults and children age 13 and older weighing 50 kg or more: 1,000 mg I.V. every 6 hours or 650 mg I.V. every 4 hours. Maximum dose is 1,000 mg as a single dose and 4,000 mg/day.
Adults and children age 13 and older weighing less than 50 kg: 15 mg/kg I.V. every 6 hours or 12.5 mg/kg I.V. every 4 hours. Maximum dose is 15 mg/kg (up to 750 mg) as a single dose and 75 mg/kg (up to 3,750 mg)/day.
Children ages 2 to 12: 15 mg/kg I.V. every 6 hours or 12.5 mg/kg I.V. every 4 hours. Maximum dose is 15 mg/kg as a single dose and 75 mg/kg/day.
Adjust-a-dose: Longer dosing intervals and a reduced total daily dose may be warranted in patients with CrCl of 30 mL/minute or less.

ADMINISTRATION
P.O.
● Use liquid form for children and patients who have difficulty swallowing.
● Give drug without regard for food.
● Dispersible tablet should be allowed to dissolve in the mouth.
● Shake liquid formulations well before using.
● Give extended-release forms whole; don't crush, dissolve, or allow patient to chew extended-release forms.
I.V.
▼ Examine vial; don't use if particulate matter or discoloration is observed.
▼ For 1,000-mg dose, give by inserting a vented I.V. set through the septum of 100-mL vial.
▼ For doses less than 1,000 mg, withdraw appropriate dose and place into separate container before administration.
▼ Place small-volume pediatric doses of up to 60 mL in a syringe and use a syringe-pump.
▼ May administer without further dilution.
▼ Give over 15 minutes.
▼ Entire 100-mL vial isn't for use in patients weighing less than 50 kg.
▼ Monitor end of infusion to prevent possibility of air embolism.
▼ Use within 6 hours of penetrating vial seal.
▼ Vial is for single use only. Discard unused portion.
▼ **Incompatibilities:** Diazepam, chlorpromazine hydrochloride.
Rectal
● If suppository is too soft, refrigerate for 15 minutes or run under cold water in wrapper.

ACTION
Thought to produce analgesia by inhibiting prostaglandin and other substances that sensitize pain receptors. Drug may relieve fever through central action in the hypothalamic heat-regulating center.

Route	Onset	Peak	Duration
P.O.	Unknown	½–1 hr	3–4 hr
I.V.	Unknown	15 min	Unknown
P.R.	Unknown	1½–5 hr	Unknown

Half-life: P.O., 2 to 3 hours; I.V., 2.4 to 7 hours; P.R., 2 to 3 hours.

ADVERSE REACTIONS
CNS: agitation (I.V.), anxiety, fatigue, headache, insomnia, pyrexia.
CV: hypertension, hypotension, peripheral edema, periorbital edema, tachycardia (I.V.).
GI: nausea, vomiting, abdominal pain, diarrhea, constipation (I.V.).
GU: oliguria (I.V.).
Hematologic: hemolytic anemia, *leukopenia, neutropenia, pancytopenia, anemia.*
Hepatic: jaundice.
Metabolic: hypoalbuminemia (I.V.), *hypoglycemia, hypokalemia,* hypervolemia, *hypomagnesemia,* hypophosphatemia (I.V.).
Musculoskeletal: muscle spasms, extremity pain (I.V.).
Respiratory: abnormal breath sounds, dyspnea, *hypoxia,* atelectasis, pleural effusion, *pulmonary edema, stridor,* wheezing (I.V.).
Skin: rash, urticaria; infusion-site pain (I.V.), pruritus.

INTERACTIONS
Drug-drug. *Barbiturates, carbamazepine, hydantoins, rifampin, sulfinpyrazone:* High doses or long-term use of these drugs may reduce therapeutic effects and enhance hepatotoxic effects of acetaminophen. Avoid using together.
Busulfan: May increase busulfan level. Monitor patient closely.
Cholestyramine resin: May decrease acetaminophen absorption. Give at least 1 hour after acetaminophen or consider therapy change.
Dasatinib: May enhance hepatotoxic effects of dasatinib and increase acetaminophen level. Avoid use together.
Dofetilide, pimozide: May increase levels of these drugs. Monitor patient closely.
Imatinib, mipomersen: May increase hepatotoxic effects of these drugs. Monitor patient closely.
Isoniazid: May increase risk of acetaminophen adverse effects. Monitor patient closely.
Lamotrigine: Prolonged acetaminophen use may decrease lamotrigine level. Monitor patient for therapeutic effects; adjust lamotrigine dosage as needed.
Lomitapide: May increase lomitapide level. Limit maximum adult dose of lomitapide to 30 mg daily or consider therapy change.

Methemoglobinemia-associated agents (nitric oxide, prilocaine): May increase risk of significant methemoglobinemia. Avoid use together. Monitor patient closely for hypoxia or cyanosis if used together.
Metyrapone, probenecid: May increase acetaminophen level and risk of hepatotoxicity. Avoid use together.
Sorafenib: May increase levels of both drugs. Avoid use together.
Warfarin: May increase hypoprothrombinemic effects with long-term use with high doses of acetaminophen. Monitor INR closely.
Drug-lifestyle. *Alcohol use:* May increase risk of hepatic damage. Discourage use together.

EFFECTS ON LAB TEST RESULTS
• May increase AST level. May decrease glucose, potassium, phosphorus, magnesium, albumin, and Hb level and hematocrit.
• May decrease neutrophil, WBC, RBC, and platelet counts.
• May cause false-positive test result for urinary 5-hydroxyindoleacetic acid. May falsely decrease glucose level in home monitoring systems.

CONTRAINDICATIONS & CAUTIONS
Black Box Warning Drug can cause acute liver failure, which may require a liver transplant or cause death. Most cases of liver injury are associated with drug doses exceeding 4,000 mg/day and often involve more than one acetaminophen-containing product. ■
⚠ *Alert:* May cause serious, potentially fatal skin reactions, including Stevens-Johnson syndrome, toxic epidermal necrolysis, and acute generalized exanthematous pustulosis. Reaction may occur with first or subsequent use when acetaminophen is used as monotherapy or when it is one component of combination drug therapy. Monitor for reddening of the skin, rash, blisters, and detachment of the upper surface of the skin. Stop drug immediately if skin reaction is suspected.
• Contraindicated in patients hypersensitive to drug. I.V. form is contraindicated in patients with severe hepatic impairment or severe active liver disease.

• Use cautiously in patients with any type of liver disease, G6PD deficiency, chronic malnutrition, severe hypovolemia (dehydration, blood loss), or severe renal impairment (CrCl of 30 mL/minute or less).

• Use cautiously in patients with long-term alcohol use because therapeutic doses cause hepatotoxicity in these patients. Chronic alcoholics shouldn't take more than 2 g of acetaminophen every 24 hours.

Dialyzable drug: Unknown.

⚠ *Overdose S&S:* Stage 1 (up to 24 hours)—abdominal pain, diaphoresis, nausea, vomiting, malaise, pallor; stage 2 (24 to 36 hours)—right upper quadrant pain, elevated LFT results, prolonged PT; stage 3 (72 to 96 hours)—hepatic failure, encephalopathy, coma.

PREGNANCY-LACTATION-REPRODUCTION

• Use cautiously in pregnant and breast-feeding women. Embryo-fetal risk is very low.

• There are no studies of I.V. acetaminophen use in pregnant women. Use during pregnancy only if clearly needed.

NURSING CONSIDERATIONS

Black Box Warning Many OTC and prescription products contain acetaminophen; be aware of this when calculating total daily dose. ∎

Black Box Warning Use caution when prescribing, preparing, and administering I.V. acetaminophen to avoid dosing errors leading to accidental overdose and death. Be careful not to confuse dose in milligrams and dose in milliliters. Be sure to base dose on weight for patients weighing less than 50 kg, to properly program infusion pump, and to ensure that total daily dose of acetaminophen from all sources doesn't exceed maximum daily limit. ∎

• Consider reducing total daily dose and increasing dosing intervals in patients with hepatic or renal impairment.

PATIENT TEACHING

• Tell parents to consult prescriber before giving drug to children younger than age 2.

• Advise parents that drug is only for short-term use; urge them to consult prescriber if

giving to children for longer than 5 days or adults for longer than 10 days.

Black Box Warning Advise patient or caregiver that many OTC products contain acetaminophen and should be counted when calculating total daily dose. ∎

• Tell patient not to use for marked fever (temperature higher than 103.1° F [39.5° C]), fever persisting longer than 3 days, or recurrent fever unless directed by prescriber.

☝ *Alert:* Warn patient that high doses or unsupervised long-term use can cause liver damage. Excessive alcohol use may increase the risk of liver damage. Caution long-term alcoholics to limit drug to 2 g/day or less.

• Caution patient to contact health care provider if signs and symptoms of liver damage (illogical thinking, severe dyspepsia, jaundice, inability to eat, weakness) occur.

• Tell breast-feeding women that drug appears in breast milk in low levels. Drug may be used safely if therapy is short-term and doesn't exceed recommended doses.

☝ *Alert:* Warn patient to stop drug and seek medical attention immediately if rash or other reactions occurs while using acetaminophen.

acetylcysteine
a-se-teel-SIS-tay-een

Acetadote ✤, Parvolex ✤

Therapeutic class: Mucolytics
Pharmacologic class: L-cysteine derivatives

AVAILABLE FORMS

Inhalation solution: 10%, 20%
I.V. injection: 200 mg/mL

INDICATIONS & DOSAGES

➤ **Adjunctive therapy for abnormal viscid or thickened mucous secretions in patients with pneumonia, bronchitis, bronchiectasis, primary amyloidosis of the lung, tuberculosis, cystic fibrosis, emphysema, atelectasis, pulmonary complications of thoracic surgery, or CV surgery**

Adults and children: 1 to 2 mL 10% or 20% solution by direct instillation into trachea as often as every hour. Or, 1 to 10 mL of 20% solution or 2 to 20 mL of 10% solution by nebulization every 2 to 6 hours, p.r.n.

➤ **Diagnostic bronchial studies**
Adults and children: Two or three administrations of 1 to 2 mL of 20% solution or 2 to 4 mL of 10% solution by nebulization or intratracheal instillation before procedure.

➤ **Routine tracheostomy care**
Adults and children: 1 to 2 mL of 10% or 20% solution by direct instillation into tracheostomy every 1 to 4 hours.

➤ **Acetaminophen toxicity**
P.O.
Adults and children: Initially, 140 mg/kg P.O.; then 70 mg/kg P.O. every 4 hours for 17 doses (total).

I.V.
Adults and children weighing 41 to 100 kg: 150 mg/kg in 200 mL of diluent I.V. over 1 hour. Then, 50 mg/kg in 500 mL of diluent I.V. over 4 hours. Then, 100 mg/kg in 1,000 mL of diluent I.V. over 16 hours.
Adults and children weighing 21 to 40 kg: 150 mg/kg in 100 mL of diluent I.V. over 1 hour. Then, 50 mg/kg in 250 mL of diluent I.V. over 4 hours. Then, 100 mg/kg in 500 mL diluent I.V. over 16 hours.
Adults and children weighing 5 to 20 kg: 150 mg/kg in 3 mL/kg diluent I.V. over 1 hour. Then, 50 mg/kg in 7 mL/kg diluent I.V. over 4 hours. Then, 100 mg/kg in 14 mL/kg diluent I.V. over 16 hours.
Adjust-a-dose: Refer to manufacturer's instruction for dosing in patients weighing less than 40 kg and requiring fluid restriction.

ADMINISTRATION
P.O.
● The inhalation formulation is administered via the oral route. Dilute oral dose (used for acetaminophen overdose) with diet cola or other diet soft drinks or water. Dilute 20% solution to 5% (add 3 mL of diluent to each milliliter of drug). If patient vomits within 1 hour of receiving loading or maintenance dose, repeat dose. Use diluted solution within 1 hour.

● Drug smells strongly of sulfur. Mixing oral form with juice or cola improves its taste.
● Drug delivered through NG tube may be diluted with water.
● Store opened, undiluted oral solution in the refrigerator for up to 96 hours.

I.V.
▼ Drug may turn from a colorless liquid to a slight pink or purple color once the stopper is punctured. This color change doesn't affect the drug.
▼ Drug is hyperosmolar and is compatible with D₅W, half-NSS, and sterile water for injection.
▼ Adjust total volume given for patients who weigh less than 40 kg or who are fluid restricted.
▼ For patients who weigh 40 kg or more, dilute loading dose in 200 mL of D₅W, second dose in 500 mL, and third dose in 1,000 mL.
▼ For patients who weigh 25 to less than 40 kg, dilute loading dose in 100 mL, second dose in 250 mL, and third dose in 500 mL.
▼ For patients who weigh between 20 and 25 kg, dilute loading dose in 60 mL, second dose in 140 mL, and third dose in 280 mL.
▼ For patients who weigh between 15 and 20 kg, dilute loading dose in 45 mL, second dose in 105 mL, and third dose in 210 mL.
▼ For patients who weigh 10 to 15 kg, dilute loading dose in 30 mL, second dose in 70 mL, and third dose in 140 mL.
▼ Reconstituted solution is stable for 24 hours at room temperature.
▼ Vials contain no preservatives; discard after opening.
▼ **Incompatibilities:** Incompatible with rubber and metals, especially iron, copper, and nickel.

Inhalational
● Use plastic, glass, stainless steel, or another nonreactive metal when giving by nebulization. Hand-bulb nebulizers aren't recommended because output is too small and particle size too large.
● **Incompatibilities:** Physically or chemically incompatible with inhaled tetracyclines, erythromycin lactobionate,

---

amphotericin B, and ampicillin sodium. If given by aerosol inhalation, nebulize these drugs separately. Iodized oil, trypsin, and hydrogen peroxide are physically incompatible with acetylcysteine; don't add to nebulizer.

ACTION
Reduces the viscosity of pulmonary secretions by splitting disulfide linkages between mucoprotein molecular complexes. Also, restores liver stores of glutathione to treat acetaminophen toxicity.

Route	Onset	Peak	Duration
P.O., inhalation	Unknown	Unknown	Unknown
I.V.	Unknown	½–1 hr	Unknown

Half-life: P.O., inhalation, unknown; I.V., 5.6 hours.

ADVERSE REACTIONS
CNS: fever, drowsiness.
CV: chest tightness, flushing, tachycardia, edema.
EENT: rhinorrhea, pharyngitis, throat tightness.
GI: nausea, stomatitis, vomiting.
Respiratory: *bronchospasm,* cough, dyspnea, rhonchi.
Skin: clamminess, diaphoresis, pruritus, rash, urticaria.
Other: *anaphylactoid reaction,* chills.

INTERACTIONS
Drug-drug. *Activated charcoal:* May limit acetylcysteine's effectiveness. Avoid using activated charcoal before or with oral acetylcysteine.

EFFECTS ON LAB TEST RESULTS
None reported.

CONTRAINDICATIONS & CAUTIONS
• Contraindicated in patients hypersensitive to drug.
❶ *Alert:* Serious anaphylactoid reactions, including rash, hypotension, dyspnea, and wheezing, have been reported. Reactions usually occur 30 to 60 minutes after start of infusion and may require treatment and drug discontinuation.
• Use cautiously in elderly or debilitated patients with severe respiratory insufficiency. Use I.V. form cautiously in patients

with asthma or a history of bronchospasm, in those weighing less than 40 kg, and in patients requiring fluid restriction.
Dialyzable drug: Unknown.

PREGNANCY-LACTATION-REPRODUCTION
• There are no adequate and well-controlled studies in pregnant women. Use cautiously in pregnant women and only if clearly indicated.
• It's unknown if drug appears in breast milk. Use cautiously in breast-feeding women.

NURSING CONSIDERATIONS
• Monitor cough type and frequency.
❶ *Alert:* Monitor patient for bronchospasm, especially if he has asthma.
• Ingestion of more than 150 mg/kg of acetaminophen may cause hepatotoxicity. Measure acetaminophen level 4 hours after ingestion to determine risk of hepatotoxicity.
❶ *Alert:* Drug is used for acetaminophen overdose within 24 hours of ingestion. Start drug immediately; don't wait for results of acetaminophen level. Give within 10 hours of acetaminophen ingestion to minimize hepatic injury.
• For suspected acetaminophen overdose, obtain baseline AST, ALT, bilirubin, PT, BUN, creatinine, glucose, and electrolyte levels.
• Half-life elimination increases by 80% in patients with severe liver damage.
❶ *Alert:* Monitor patient receiving I.V. form for anaphylactoid reactions. Reactions involving more than simple skin flushing or erythema should be treated as anaphylactoid reactions. If anaphylactoid reaction occurs, stop infusion and treat reaction with antihistaminics and epinephrine if needed. Once anaphylaxis treatment starts, carefully restart infusion. If anaphylactoid symptoms return, stop drug.
• Facial erythema may occur within 30 to 60 minutes of start of I.V. infusion and usually resolves without stopping infusion.
• When acetaminophen level is below toxic level according to nomogram, stop therapy.
• The vial stopper doesn't contain natural rubber latex, dry natural rubber, or blends of natural rubber.

Reactions in bold italics are *life-threatening*. Interactions may have a *rapid onset* or a *delayed onset*.

• **Look alike–sound alike:** Don't confuse acetylcysteine with acetylcholine.

PATIENT TEACHING
• Warn patient that drug may have a foul taste or smell that may be distressing.
• For maximum effect, instruct patient to cough to clear his airway before aerosol administration.

acyclovir
ay-SYE-kloe-ver

Sitavig, Zovirax

acyclovir sodium
Zovirax

Therapeutic class: Antivirals
Pharmacologic class: Nucleosides and nucleotides

AVAILABLE FORMS
Capsules: 200 mg
Cream: 5%
Injection: 500 mg/vial, 1 g/vial
Ointment: 5%
Solution (I.V.): 50 mg/mL
Suspension: 200 mg/5 mL
Tablets: 400 mg, 800 mg
Tablets (buccal) ⓄⓃⒸ: 50 mg

INDICATIONS & DOSAGES
Adjust-a-dose (for all indications): For patients receiving the I.V. form, if CrCl is 25 to 50 mL/minute, give 100% of dose every 12 hours; if CrCl is 10 to 24 mL/minute, give 100% of dose every 24 hours; if CrCl is less than 10 mL/minute, give 50% of dose every 24 hours.

For patients receiving the P.O. form, if normal dose is 200 mg every 4 hours five times daily and CrCl is less than 10 mL/minute, give 200 mg P.O. every 12 hours. If normal dose is 400 mg every 12 hours and CrCl is less than 10 mL/minute, give 200 mg every 12 hours. If normal dose is 800 mg every 4 hours five times daily and CrCl is 10 to 25 mL/minute, give 800 mg every 8 hours; if CrCl is less than 10 mL/minute, give 800 mg every 12 hours.

For patients who require hemodialysis, give additional dose after each dialysis.
➤ **First and recurrent episodes of muco-cutaneous HSV (HSV-1 and HSV-2) infections in immunocompromised patients; severe first episodes of genital herpes in patients who aren't immunocompromised**
Adults and children age 12 and older: 5 mg/kg given I.V. over 1 hour every 8 hours for 7 days. Give for 5 to 7 days for severe first episode of genital herpes.
Children younger than age 12: 10 mg/kg I.V. over 1 hour every 8 hours for 7 days.
➤ **First genital herpes episode**
Adults: 200 mg P.O. every 4 hours while awake, five times daily. Continue for 10 days.
➤ **Initial genital herpes; limited, non-life-threatening mucocutaneous HSV infections in immunocompromised patients**
Adults and children age 12 and older: Cover all lesions every 3 hours six times daily for 7 days. Although dosage varies depending on total lesion area, use about ½-inch (1.3-cm) ribbon of ointment on each 4-inch (10-cm) square of surface area.
➤ **Intermittent therapy for recurrent genital herpes**
Adults: 200 mg P.O. every 4 hours while awake, five times daily. Continue for 5 days. Begin therapy at first sign of recurrence.
➤ **Long-term suppressive therapy for recurrent genital herpes**
Adults: 400 mg P.O. b.i.d. for up to 12 months. Or, 200 mg P.O. three to five times daily for up to 12 months.
➤ **Varicella zoster infections in immuno-compromised patients**
Adults and children age 12 and older: 10 mg/kg I.V. over 1 hour every 8 hours for 7 days. Dosage for obese patients is 10 mg/kg based on ideal body weight every 8 hours for 7 days. Don't exceed maximum dosage equivalent of 20 mg/kg every 8 hours.
Children younger than age 12: 10 mg/kg I.V. over 1 hour every 8 hours for 7 to 10 days.
➤ **Varicella (chickenpox) infection in immunocompetent patients**
Adults and children weighing more than 40 kg: 800 mg P.O. q.i.d. for 5 days.

Children age 2 and older weighing less than 40 kg: 20 mg/kg (maximum, 80 mg/kg/day) P.O. q.i.d. for 5 days. Start therapy as soon as symptoms appear.

➤ **Acute herpes zoster infection in immunocompetent patients**
Adults and children age 12 and older:
800 mg P.O. every 4 hours five times daily for 7 to 10 days.

➤ **Herpes simplex encephalitis**
Adults and children age 12 and older:
10 mg/kg I.V. over 1 hour every 8 hours for 10 days.
Children ages 3 months to 12 years: 20 mg/kg I.V. over 1 hour every 8 hours for 10 days.

➤ **Recurrent herpes labialis**
Adults and children age 12 and older: Apply cream five times daily for 4 days. Start therapy as early as possible after signs and symptoms occur.

➤ **Recurrent herpes labialis in immunocompetent patients**
Adults: 50-mg buccal tablet as a single dose to upper gum region within 1 hour after onset of prodromal symptoms and before appearance of signs of cold sore.

ADMINISTRATION
P.O.
● Give drug without regard for meals, but give with food if stomach irritation occurs.
● Patient should take drug as prescribed, even after he feels better.
Buccal
● Patients shouldn't chew, suck, crush, or swallow tablets.
● Apply with dry finger immediately after taking tablet out of blister pack.
● Place tablet just above incisor tooth on upper gum on the same side of the mouth as prodromal symptoms appeared.
● Hold tablet in place with slight pressure over upper lip for 30 seconds to ensure adhesion. Place rounded side to gum for comfort, but either side can be applied.
● Tablet will stay in place and dissolve gradually.
● Food and drink can be taken normally with tablet in place.
● Patients should avoid chewing gum, touching or pressing tablet, wearing upper denture, brushing teeth, or other activity that may interfere with adhesion.

● Patients should drink plenty of liquids in case of dry mouth.
● If buccal tablet doesn't adhere or falls off within first 6 hours, reposition same tablet immediately. If tablet doesn't adhere, place a new tablet.
● If patient swallows buccal tablet within first 6 hours, have patient drink a glass of water; then apply a new tablet.
● If buccal tablet falls out or patient swallows it after first 6 hours, don't reapply.
I.V.
▼ Solutions concentrated at 7 mg/mL or more may cause a higher risk of phlebitis.
▼ Encourage fluid intake because patient must be adequately hydrated during infusion.
▼ Bolus injection, dehydration (decreased urine output), renal disease, and use with other nephrotoxic drugs increase the risk of renal toxicity. Don't give by bolus injection.
▼ Give I.V. infusion over at least 1 hour to prevent renal tubular damage.
▼ Monitor intake and output, especially during the first 2 hours after administration.
◑ *Alert:* Don't give I.M. or subcutaneously.
▼ **Incompatibilities:** Amifostine, aztreonam, biological or colloidal solutions, cefepime, cisatracurium besylate, diltiazem hydrochloride, dobutamine hydrochloride, dopamine hydrochloride, fludarabine phosphate, foscarnet sodium, gemcitabine hydrochloride, idarubicin hydrochloride, levofloxacin, meperidine hydrochloride, meropenem, morphine sulfate, ondansetron hydrochloride, parabens, piperacillin sodium–tazobactam sodium, sargramostim, tacrolimus, vinorelbine tartrate.
Topical
● Apply with finger cot or rubber glove to prevent autoinoculation of other body sites and transmission of infection to others.
● Thoroughly cover all lesions.
● Topical form is for cutaneous use only; don't apply to eyes.

ACTION
Interferes with DNA synthesis and inhibits viral multiplication.

Reactions in bold italics are *life-threatening*. Interactions may have a *rapid onset* or a *delayed onset*.

Route	Onset	Peak	Duration
P.O.	Unknown	2½ hr	Unknown
Buccal	Unknown	8 hr (in saliva)	Unknown
I.V.	Immediate	Immediate	Unknown
Topical	Unknown	Unknown	Unknown

Half-life: 2 to 3½ hours with normal renal function; up to 19 hours with renal impairment.

ADVERSE REACTIONS

CNS: headache, malaise, *encephalopathic changes (including lethargy, obtunda-tion, tremor, confusion, hallucinations, agitation, seizures, coma).*
EENT: gum pain, canker sores (buccal tablets).
GI: nausea, vomiting, diarrhea.
GU: *acute renal failure,* hematuria.
Hematologic: *leukopenia, thrombocytope-nia,* thrombocytosis.
Skin: inflammation or phlebitis at injection site, rash, urticaria, eczema, dryness, pru-ritus, contact dermatitis, application-site reaction; mild pain, burning, or stinging (topical or buccal form); *Stevens-Johnson syndrome,* toxic epidermal necrolysis.
Other: *angioedema, anaphylaxis.*

INTERACTIONS

Drug-drug. *Hydantoins, valproic acid:* May decrease levels of these drugs. Monitor patient closely.
Probenecid: May increase acyclovir level. Monitor patient for possible toxicity.
Theophylline: May increase theophylline level. Monitor patient for toxicity.
Zidovudine: May cause drowsiness or lethargy. Use together cautiously.

EFFECTS ON LAB TEST RESULTS

• May increase BUN and creatinine levels.
• May decrease WBC count. May increase or decrease platelet count.

CONTRAINDICATIONS & CAUTIONS

• Contraindicated in patients hypersensitive to drug.
• Use cautiously in patients with neurologic problems, renal disease, or dehydration, and in those receiving other nephrotoxic drugs.
• Drug increases risk of thrombotic throm-bocytopenic purpura and hemolytic-uremic syndrome in immunocompromised patients, which can be fatal.

Dialyzable drug: Yes.
⚠ Overdose S&S: Agitation, coma, seizures, lethargy, elevated BUN and creatinine levels, renal failure.

PREGNANCY-LACTATION-REPRODUCTION

• Use cautiously in pregnant women and only if potential benefit outweighs potential risk to the fetus.
• Drug appears in breast milk. Women with active herpetic lesions near or on the breasts should avoid breast-feeding.

NURSING CONSIDERATIONS

• Start therapy as early as possible after signs or symptoms occur.
• Drug isn't a cure for herpes, but it helps improve signs and symptoms.
⚠ Alert: Long-term acyclovir use may result in nephrotoxicity. In patients with renal disease or dehydration and in those taking other nephrotoxic drugs, monitor renal function.
⚠ Alert: If signs and symptoms of extrava-sation occur, stop I.V. infusion immediately and notify prescriber. Hyaluronidase may need to be injected subcutaneously at ex-travasation site as an antidote.
• Encephalopathic changes are more likely to occur in patients with neurologic disor-ders and in those who have had neurologic reactions to cytotoxic drugs.
• *Look alike–sound alike:* Don't confuse acy-clovir sodium (Zovirax) with acetazolamide sodium (Diamox) vials, which may look alike. Don't confuse Zovirax with Zyvox.

PATIENT TEACHING

• Tell patient to take drug as prescribed, even after he feels better.
• Tell patient drug is effective in managing herpes infection but doesn't eliminate or cure it. Warn patient that drug won't prevent spread of infection to others.
• Tell patient to avoid sexual contact while visible lesions are present. Virus transmis-sion can occur during treatment.
• Teach patient about early signs and symp-toms of herpes infection (such as tingling, itching, or pain). Tell him to notify pre-scriber and get a prescription for drug before the infection fully develops. Early treatment is most effective.

adalimumab
ay-da-LIM-yoo-mab

Humira

Therapeutic class: Antiarthritics
Pharmacologic class: TNF blockers

AVAILABLE FORMS
Injection: 10 mg/0.2 mL, 20 mg/0.4 mL,
40 mg/0.8 mL as prefilled syringes or pens;
40 mg/0.8 mL single-use vial

INDICATIONS & DOSAGES
➤ **RA; psoriatic arthritis; ankylosing spondylitis**
Adults: 40 mg subcutaneously every
other week. Patient may continue to take
methotrexate, steroids, NSAIDs, salicylates,
analgesics, or other DMARDs during therapy. Patients with RA who aren't also taking
methotrexate may have the dose increased to
40 mg weekly, if needed.
➤ **Moderate to severe Crohn disease
when response to conventional therapy
is inadequate or when response to infliximab is lost or patient can't tolerate the
drug; moderate to severe active ulcerative colitis when response to immunosuppressants (such as corticosteroids,
azathioprine, or 6-mercaptopurine) is
inadequate**
Adults: Initially, 160 mg subcutaneously
on day 1 given as four 40-mg injections in
1 day or as two 40-mg injections per day for
two consecutive days; then 80 mg 2 weeks
later (day 15), followed by a maintenance
dose of 40 mg every other week starting
at week 4 (day 29). For ulcerative colitis,
only continue in patients who have shown
evidence of clinical remission by 8 weeks
(day 57) of therapy.
➤ **To reduce the signs and symptoms of
moderately to severely active polyarticular juvenile idiopathic arthritis**
*Children ages 2 to 17 weighing from 10 to
less than 15 kg:* 10 mg subcutaneously every
other week.
*Children ages 2 to 17 weighing between
15 and 30 kg:* 20 mg subcutaneously every
other week.
*Children ages 4 to 17 weighing 30 kg
or more:* 40 mg subcutaneously every

other week. Patients may continue to take
methotrexate, steroids, NSAIDs, and analgesics during therapy.
➤ **Moderate to severe chronic plaque
psoriasis**
Adults: 80 mg subcutaneously, followed by
40 mg subcutaneously every other week
starting 1 week after the initial dose. Treatment beyond 1 year has not been studied.
➤ **Crohn disease**
*Children age 6 and older weighing 40 kg
or more:* Initially, 160 mg subcutaneously
on day 1 given as four 40-mg injections on
1 day or as two 40-mg injections per day
for 2 consecutive days; then 80 mg 2 weeks
later (day 15), followed by a maintenance
dose of 40 mg every other week starting at
week 4 (day 29).
*Children age 6 and older weighing from
17 to less than 40 kg:* 80 mg subcutaneously
on day 1 as two injections, followed by
40 mg 2 weeks later (day 15), followed by
a maintenance dose of 20 mg every other
week starting at week 4 (day 29).
✳ *NEW INDICATION:* **Moderate to severe
hidradenitis suppurativa**
Adults: Initially, 160 mg subcutaneously
given as four 40-mg injections on day 1 or
as two 40-mg injections per day for two
consecutive days; then 80 mg (two 40-mg
injections) subcutaneously on day 15 followed by one 40-mg subcutaneous injection
on day 29; then one 40-mg injection every
week thereafter.
✳ *NEW INDICATION:* **Noninfectious
intermediate, posterior, and panuveitis**
Adults: 80 mg subcut. followed by 40 mg
subcut. every other week starting 1 week
after the initial dose.

ADMINISTRATION
Subcutaneous
● Inject subcutaneously into abdomen or
thigh at separate sites.
● Rotate injection sites.
● Don't give in an area that is bruised,
tender, red, or hard.
● May store at room temperature (max-
imum, 77° F [25° C]) for up to 14 days.
Discard after 14 days. Protect from light.
🜂 *Alert:* Needle caps of the 17G pen and
prefilled syringe contain latex.

Reactions in bold italics are *life-threatening*. Interactions may have a *rapid onset* or a ***delayed onset***.

ACTION

A recombinant human immunoglobulin
G₁ monoclonal antibody that blocks
human TNF-alpha. TNF-alpha partici-
pates in normal inflammatory and immune
responses and in the inflammation and joint
destruction of RA.

Route	Onset	Peak	Duration
Subcut.	Variable	Variable	Unknown

Half-life: 10 to 20 days.

ADVERSE REACTIONS

CNS: headache, syncope, hypertensive
encephalopathy, confusion, paresthesia,
subdural hematoma, tremor, myasthenia,
fever.
CV: *hemorrhage,* hypertension, arrhythmia,
atrial fibrillation, chest pain, CAD, cardiac
arrest, cardiac failure, MI, palpitations, pericardial effusion, pericarditis, tachycardia,
edema, thrombosis.
EENT: sinusitis, cataract.
GI: abdominal pain, nausea, cholecystitis,
cholelithiasis, esophagitis, gastroenteritis,
GI hemorrhage, vomiting, diverticulitis.
GU: hematuria, UTI, cystitis, kidney stones,
menstrual disorder.
Hematologic: *leukopenia, pancytopenia,
thrombocytopenia,* polycythemia, *agranulocytosis.*
Hepatic: hepatic necrosis.
Metabolic: hypercholesterolemia, hyperlipidemia, dehydration, ketosis.
Musculoskeletal: back pain, bone disorder, bone necrosis, joint disorder, muscle
cramps, synovitis, tendon disorder, pyogenic
arthritis.
Respiratory: URI, bronchitis, dyspnea,
decreased lung function, pleural effusion,
asthma, *bronchospasm,* pneumonia.
Skin: rash, injection-site reactions (erythema, itching, pain, swelling), alopecia,
cellulitis, erysipelas.
Other: accidental injury, *anaphylaxis,
malignancy,* allergic reactions, flulike
syndrome, parathyroid disorder.

INTERACTIONS

Drug-drug. *Abatacept, anakinra,
tocilizumab:* May increase risk of serious
infections and neutropenia. Don't use
together.

*CYP450 substrates with narrow therapeutic
index (cyclosporine, theophylline, warfarin):* May affect CYP450 substrate level.
Monitor levels closely when initiating or
discontinuing adalimumab; adjust CYP450
substrate dosage as needed.
Live-virus vaccines: No data are available
on secondary transmission of infection from
live-virus vaccines. Avoid using together.

EFFECTS ON LAB TEST RESULTS

• May increase CK, alkaline phosphatase,
and cholesterol levels.
• May decrease platelet and WBC counts.
• May cause positive ANA titer and development of antibodies.

CONTRAINDICATIONS & CAUTIONS

• Contraindicated in immunosuppressed
patients and in those with an active chronic
or localized infection.
❂ **Alert:** Anaphylaxis and angioneurotic
edema have been reported. If serious reaction occurs, discontinue drug immediately
and treat appropriately.
Black Box Warning Patients taking TNF-
alpha blockers are at increased risk for developing serious infections that can lead to
hospitalization or death. Most patients were
taking concomitant immunosuppressants,
such as methotrexate or corticosteroids.
Reported infections include *Legionella* and
Listeria infections, active TB, and invasive
fungal infections. Consider empirical antifungal therapy for patients at risk for invasive fungal infections who develop systemic
illness. Carefully consider risk and benefits
of therapy before starting drug in patients
with chronic or recurrent infections. ■
Black Box Warning Lymphoma and
other malignancies, some fatal, have
been reported in children and adolescents
treated with TNF blockers, including
adalimumab. ■
Black Box Warning Hepatosplenic
T-cell lymphoma, a rare type of T-cell lymphoma, has occurred in adolescents and
young adults with inflammatory bowel disease treated with TNF blockers, including
adalimumab. ■
• Use cautiously in patients with demyelinating disorders, a history of recurrent
infection, those with underlying conditions

that predispose them to infections, those who have lived in areas where TB and histoplasmosis are endemic, patients with HF, and elderly patients.
Dialyzable drug: Unknown.

PREGNANCY-LACTATION-REPRODUCTION
• Use during pregnancy only if clearly needed.
• Drug appears in breast milk. Use cautiously in breast-feeding women.

NURSING CONSIDERATIONS
• Give first dose under supervision of prescriber.
Black Box Warning Patient should be evaluated, and treated if necessary, for latent TB before starting adalimumab therapy. Closely monitor patient for possible development of TB even if he has tested negative before initiating therapy. ■
Black Box Warning Serious infections and sepsis, including TB and invasive fungal infections, may occur. If patient develops new infection during treatment, monitor him closely; if infection becomes serious, stop drug. ■
❸ *Alert:* Drug may increase the risk of malignancy. Patients with highly active RA may be at an increased risk for lymphoma.
❸ *Alert:* If patient develops anaphylaxis, a severe infection, other serious allergic reaction, or evidence of a lupuslike syndrome, stop drug.
• Drug may cause reactivation of HBV in chronic carriers.
❸ *Alert:* The needle cover contains latex and shouldn't be handled by those with latex sensitivity.
• *Look alike–sound alike:* Don't confuse Humira with Humulin or Humalog.

PATIENT TEACHING
• Tell patient to report all adverse reactions and any evidence of TB or other infection.
• Teach patient or caregiver how to give drug.
❸ *Alert:* Warn patient to seek immediate medical attention for symptoms of blood dyscrasias or infection, including fever, bruising, bleeding, and pallor.
• Tell patient to rotate injection sites and to avoid tender, bruised, red, or hard skin.

• Teach patient to dispose of used needles and syringes properly and not in the household trash or recyclables.
• Tell patient to refrigerate drug in its original container before use.

adefovir dipivoxil
ah-DEF-oh-veer

Hepsera

Therapeutic class: Antivirals
Pharmacologic class: Nucleosides and nucleotides

AVAILABLE FORMS
Tablets: 10 mg

INDICATIONS & DOSAGES
➤ **Chronic HBV infection**
Adults and children age 12 and older: 10 mg P.O. once daily.
Adjust-a-dose: In adult patients with CrCl of 30 to 49 mL/minute, give 10 mg P.O. every 48 hours. In patients with CrCl of 10 to 29 mL/minute, give 10 mg P.O. every 72 hours. In patients receiving hemodialysis, give 10 mg P.O. every 7 days, after dialysis session. There are no dose recommendations for adolescents with renal impairment.

ADMINISTRATION
P.O.
• Give drug without regard for meals.

ACTION
An acyclic nucleotide analogue that inhibits HBV reverse transcription via viral DNA chain termination.

Route	Onset	Peak	Duration
P.O.	Unknown	1–4 hr	Unknown

Half-life: 7½ hours.

ADVERSE REACTIONS
CNS: asthenia, headache.
GI: abdominal pain, diarrhea, dyspepsia, flatulence, nausea, vomiting.
GU: *renal failure, renal insufficiency.*
Hepatic: *hepatic failure,* hepatomegaly with steatosis, *severe acute exacerbation of hepatitis.*

Metabolic: *lactic acidosis.*
Skin: pruritus, rash.

INTERACTIONS
Drug-drug. *Ibuprofen:* May increase adefovir bioavailability. Monitor patient for adverse effects.
Nephrotoxic drugs (aminoglycosides, cyclosporine, NSAIDs, tacrolimus, vancomycin): May increase risk of nephrotoxicity. Use together cautiously.
Tenofovir disoproxil fumarate–containing products (Atripla, Complera, Stribild, Truvada): Use together increases risk for lactic acidosis and hepatotoxicity. Contraindicated for use together.

EFFECTS ON LAB TEST RESULTS
• May increase ALT, amylase, AST, CK, creatinine, and lactate levels. May decrease phosphorus level.

CONTRAINDICATIONS & CAUTIONS
• Contraindicated in patients hypersensitive to components of drug.
• Use cautiously in patients with renal dysfunction, in those receiving nephrotoxic drugs, and in those with known risk factors for hepatic disease.
• Use cautiously in elderly patients because they're more likely to have decreased renal and cardiac function.
• Safety and effectiveness in children younger than age 12 haven't been established.
Dialyzable drug: 35%.
⚠ *Overdose S&S:* GI adverse reactions.

PREGNANCY-LACTATION-REPRODUCTION
• Use cautiously in pregnant women and only if potential benefit to the mother justifies potential risk to the fetus.
• To monitor fetal outcomes of pregnant women exposed to drug, health care providers should register patients in the antiretroviral pregnancy registry (1-800-258-4263).
• It isn't known if drug appears in breast milk. Patient should discontinue breast-feeding or discontinue drug.

NURSING CONSIDERATIONS
Black Box Warning Due to increased risk of nephrotoxicity, monitor renal function, and adjust dosage if needed, especially in patients with renal dysfunction or those taking nephrotoxic drugs. ■
Black Box Warning Patients may develop lactic acidosis and severe hepatomegaly with steatosis during treatment. Women, obese patients, and those taking antiretrovirals are at higher risk. Monitor hepatic function. Stop drug, if needed. ■
Black Box Warning Stopping adefovir may cause severe worsening of hepatitis. Monitor hepatic function closely for at least several months in patients who stop antihepatitis B therapy. ■
• The ideal length of treatment hasn't been established.
Black Box Warning Offer patients HIV antibody testing; drug may promote resistance to antiretrovirals in patients with chronic HBV infection who also have unrecognized or untreated HIV infection. ■

PATIENT TEACHING
• Inform the patient that drug may be taken without regard to meals.
• Tell patient to immediately report weakness, muscle pain, trouble breathing, stomach pain with nausea and vomiting, dizziness, light-headedness, fast or irregular heartbeat, and feeling cold, especially in arms and legs.
• Warn patient not to stop taking this drug unless directed because it could cause hepatitis to become worse.
• Instruct woman to tell her prescriber if she becomes pregnant or is breast-feeding. It's unknown if drug appears in breast milk.

SAFETY ALERT!

adenosine
a-DEN-oh-seen

Adenocard

Therapeutic class: Antiarrhythmics
Pharmacologic class: Nucleosides

AVAILABLE FORMS
Injection: 3 mg/mL

INDICATIONS & DOSAGES

➤ **To convert paroxysmal supraventricular tachycardia (PSVT) to sinus rhythm**
Adults and children weighing 50 kg or more:
6 mg I.V. by rapid bolus injection over 1 to
2 seconds. If PSVT isn't eliminated in 1 to
2 minutes, give 12 mg by rapid I.V. push and
repeat, if needed.
Children weighing less than 50 kg: Initially,
0.05 to 0.1 mg/kg I.V. by rapid bolus injection followed by a saline flush. If PSVT isn't
eliminated in 1 to 2 minutes, give additional
bolus injections, increasing the amount given
in 0.05- to 0.1-mg/kg increments, followed
by a saline flush. Continue, as needed, until
conversion of the PSVT or a maximum single
dose of 0.3 mg/kg (up to 12 mg) is given.
➤ **Stress-testing diagnostic aid**
Adults: 140 mcg/kg/minute infused for
6 minutes (total dose of 0.84 mg/kg).

ADMINISTRATION

I.V.

▼ Don't give single doses exceeding 12 mg.

▼ Crystals may form if solution is cold;
gently warm solution to room temperature.
Don't use solutions that aren't clear.

▼ In adults, avoid giving drug through
a central line because more prolonged
asystole may occur.

▼ Give by rapid I.V. injection to ensure
drug action.

▼ Give directly into a vein, if possible.
When giving through an I.V. line, use the
port closest to the patient.

▼ Flush immediately and rapidly with NSS
to ensure that drug quickly reaches the
systemic circulation.

▼ Drug lacks preservatives. Discard unused portion. Don't refrigerate.

▼ **Incompatibilities:** Other I.V. drugs.

ACTION

Naturally occurring nucleoside that acts
on the AV node to slow conduction and
inhibit reentry pathways. Drug is also useful
in treating PSVTs, including those with
accessory bypass tracts (Wolff-Parkinson-
White syndrome).

Route	Onset	Peak	Duration
I.V.	Immediate	Immediate	Unknown

Half-life: Less than 10 seconds.

ADVERSE REACTIONS

CNS: dizziness, light-headedness, numbness, tingling in arms, headache.
CV: chest pressure, facial flushing, hypotension, arrhythmias, first- or second-degree
AV block.
EENT: throat, neck, or jaw discomfort.
GI: nausea.
Respiratory: dyspnea.

INTERACTIONS

Drug-drug. *Carbamazepine:* May cause
high-level heart block. Use together cautiously.
Digoxin, verapamil: May cause ventricular
fibrillation. Monitor ECG closely.
Dipyridamole: May increase adenosine's
effects. Adenosine dose may need to be
reduced. Use together cautiously.
Methylxanthines (caffeine, theophylline):
May decrease adenosine's effects. Adenosine dose may need to be increased, or patients may not respond to adenosine therapy.

EFFECTS ON LAB TEST RESULTS

None reported.

CONTRAINDICATIONS & CAUTIONS

● Contraindicated in patients hypersensitive
to drug.

● Contraindicated in those with second-
or third-degree heart block or sinus node
disease (such as sick sinus syndrome and
symptomatic bradycardia), except those
with a pacemaker.

● Use cautiously in patients with obstructive
lung disease not associated with bronchoconstriction (emphysema or bronchitis);
avoid use in those with bronchoconstriction
or bronchospasm (asthma).

● Drug may increase risk of seizures.

● Avoid use in patients with signs and symptoms of acute MI (unstable angina, CV instability). Drug may increase risk of serious
CV reaction (fatal or nonfatal cardiac arrest,
supraventricular tachycardia, MI). Make
sure appropriate emergency equipment is
readily available.

● Use cautiously in patients with autonomic
dysfunction, stenotic valvular heart disease,
pericarditis or pericardial effusions, stenotic
carotid artery disease with cerebrovascular
insufficiency, or uncorrected hypovolemia.

Drug may increase risk of hypotensive complications.
Dialyzable drug: Unknown.

PREGNANCY-LACTATION-REPRODUCTION

● No studies have been performed in pregnant women. Use in pregnant women only if clearly indicated.
● There are no well-controlled studies in breast-feeding women. Patient should discontinue breast-feeding or discontinue drug, taking into account importance of drug to the mother.

NURSING CONSIDERATIONS

❸ Alert: By decreasing conduction through the AV node, drug may produce first-, second-, or third-degree heart block. Patients who develop high-level heart block after a single dose shouldn't receive additional doses.
❸ Alert: New arrhythmias, including heart block and transient asystole, may develop; monitor cardiac rhythm and treat as indicated.
● Monitor BP closely. Discontinue drug in patients who develop persistent or symptomatic hypotension.
● Monitor patient for seizures during therapy.
❸ Alert: Don't confuse adenosine with adenosine phosphate.

PATIENT TEACHING

● Instruct patient to report adverse reactions promptly.
● Tell patient to report discomfort at I.V. site.
● Inform patient that he may experience flushing or chest pain lasting 1 to 2 minutes.

SAFETY ALERT!

ado-trastuzumab emtansine
ADD-oh tras-TOOZ-oo-mab em-TAN-seen

Kadcyla

Therapeutic class: Antineoplastics
Pharmacologic class: Antibody drug conjugates

AVAILABLE FORMS
Injection (lyophilized powder for solution): 100 mg, 160 mg in single-use vials

INDICATIONS & DOSAGES

➤ **HER2-positive, metastatic breast cancer in patients who previously received trastuzumab and a taxane, separately or in combination. Patients should have either received previous treatment for metastatic disease or developed recurrence during or within 6 months of completing adjuvant treatment**
Adults: 3.6 mg/kg I.V. every 21 days until disease progression or unacceptable toxicity occurs. Maximum dose is 3.6 mg/kg.
Adjust-a-dose: If dosage reductions are necessary for adverse events, the first dosage reduction is to 3 mg/kg; the second is to 2.4 mg/kg. If further reduction is necessary, discontinue drug. Don't re-escalate after dosage reduction is made.

For increased serum transaminase levels (AST/ALT) of more than 5 and up to 20 × ULN (grade 3), withhold dose until levels return to 5 × ULN or less (grade 2); then reduce by one dosage level. For AST or ALT of more than 20 × ULN, permanently discontinue drug.

For increased total bilirubin level of more than 1.5 and up to 3 × ULN (grade 2), withhold dose until total bilirubin level returns to less than 1.5 × ULN (grade 1); then treat at same dosage level. For increased total bilirubin level of more than 3 and up to 10 × ULN, withhold dose until level returns to grade 1; then reduce by one dosage level. For total bilirubin level of more than 10 × ULN, permanently discontinue drug.

For serum transaminase levels greater than 3 × ULN concomitant with total bilirubin level greater than 2 × ULN, discontinue drug.

For left ventricular dysfunction with LVEF of less than 40%, withhold drug and repeat LVEF assessment within 3 weeks. If LVEF remains less than 40%, discontinue drug. For LVEF of 40% to 45% when LVEF decrease is 10% or more from baseline, withhold drug and repeat LVEF assessment within 3 weeks. If LVEF hasn't recovered to within 10% of baseline, discontinue drug. For LVEF of 40% to 45% when the decrease is less than 10% from baseline, continue treatment and repeat LVEF assessment within 3 weeks. For LVEF of more than 45%, continue treatment. Discontinue drug for symptomatic HF.

For platelet count of 25,000/mm³ to less than 50,000/mm³ (grade 3), withhold drug until platelet count recovers to 75,000/mm³ or more (grade 1); then continue at same dosage level. For platelet count of less than 25,000/mm³ (grade 4), withhold drug until platelet count returns to 75,000/mm³ or more (grade 1); then reduce by one dosage level.

For grade 3 or 4 peripheral neuropathy, temporarily withhold drug until recovery to grade 2 or less.

ADMINISTRATION

I.V.

Black Box Warning Don't confuse this drug with trastuzumab (Herceptin). These drugs aren't interchangeable. ■

☉ *Alert:* The manufacturer recommends that the trade name be used and clearly recorded in the patient record to avoid confusion.

▼ Drug is considered hazardous; use safe handling and disposal precautions according to facility policy.

▼ To reconstitute, slowly inject 5 mL sterile water for injection into 100-mg vial or 8 mL sterile water for injection into 160-mg vial to yield concentration of 20 mg/mL.

▼ Swirl gently until dissolved. Don't shake. Solution should be colorless to pale brown.

▼ Add reconstituted dose to 250 mL of NSS in infusion bag and administer immediately through I.V. line containing 0.22-micron in-line nonprotein adsorptive polyethersulfone filter.

▼ Administer initial infusion over 90 minutes. Don't administer as I.V. push or bolus. Monitor patient for infusion-related reactions during administration and for 90 minutes after completion. Slow or interrupt infusion for infusion-related events. Discontinue drug if life-threatening infusion-related reactions occur.

▼ May administer subsequent infusions over 30 minutes if initial infusion was uneventful. Monitor patient during infusion and for 30 minutes after completion.

▼ Observe for subcutaneous infiltration during infusion.

▼ Give at dosage and rate patient tolerated at most recent infusion.

▼ If dose is delayed or missed, give as soon as possible; don't wait for next planned cycle.

▼ Reconstituted vials can be stored in refrigerator for 24 hours at 36° to 46° F (2° to 8° C). Don't freeze.

▼ **Incompatibilities:** Dextrose solution, other drugs.

ACTION

Drug contains both trastuzumab and DM1 (a microtubule inhibitor), linked by a covalent bond, and targets the HER2 receptor by combined mechanisms of trastuzumab and DM1. The recombinant monoclonal antibody, trastuzumab, binds to the HER2 receptor and intracellular lysosomal degradation releases the cytotoxic component, DM1, resulting in microtubule disruption and cell death.

Route	Onset	Peak	Duration
I.V.	Unknown	End of infusion	Unknown

Half-life: 4 days.

ADVERSE REACTIONS

CNS: chills, fatigue, headache, fever, asthenia, dizziness, peripheral neuropathy, insomnia.

CV: left ventricular dysfunction, edema, hypertension.

EENT: dry eye syndrome, blurred vision, conjunctivitis, increased lacrimation, epistaxis.

GI: nausea, constipation, stomatitis, abdominal pain, vomiting, diarrhea, dyspepsia, dry mouth, taste perversion.
GU: UTI.
Hematologic: *thrombocytopenia, neutropenia,* anemia, hemorrhage.
Hepatic: elevated transaminase levels, increased alkaline phosphatase level, increased bilirubin level.
Metabolic: *hypokalemia.*
Musculoskeletal: musculoskeletal pain, arthralgia, myalgia, weakness.
Respiratory: pneumonitis, dyspnea, cough.
Skin: pruritus, rash.
Other: chills, hypersensitivity reactions, infusion reaction.

INTERACTIONS
Drug-drug. *Strong CYP3A4 inhibitors (atazanavir, clarithromycin, indinavir, itraconazole, ketoconazole, nefazodone, nelfinavir, ritonavir, saquinavir, telithromycin, voriconazole):* May increase ado-trastuzumab level and potential toxicity. Avoid use together. If use together is necessary, stop inhibitor and delay treatment until inhibitor clears from patient's circulation, or monitor patient carefully for adverse effects.

EFFECTS ON LAB TEST RESULTS
• May increase bilirubin, AST, and ALT levels. May decrease potassium level.
• May decrease Hb level and platelet and neutrophil counts.

CONTRAINDICATIONS & CAUTIONS
• Contraindicated in patients hypersensitive to drug or its components.
• Use cautiously in patients with liver failure, risk of hepatotoxicity, symptomatic HF, serious cardiac arrhythmia, history of MI, or unstable angina.
• Avoid use in patients with history of trastuzumab hypersensitivity or infusion-related events.
• Discontinue drug in patients diagnosed with interstitial lung disease or pneumonitis.
• Patients with shortness of breath at rest due to advanced malignancy and comorbidities may be at increased risk for pulmonary toxicity.
• Use cautiously in patients taking anticoagulants and in those with preexisting thrombocytopenia. Patients of Asian ancestry may be at higher risk for thrombocytopenia.
Dialyzable drug: Unknown.
⚠ *Overdose S&S:* Thrombocytopenia, death.

PREGNANCY-LACTATION-REPRODUCTION
Black Box Warning Exposure to drug can result in embryo-fetal death or birth defects. ■
• Verify pregnancy status before start of therapy.
• Women of childbearing potential should use effective contraception during treatment and for 7 months after last dose.
◑ *Alert:* Advise patient to immediately inform her physician if she suspects or confirms pregnancy during therapy or within 7 months after last dose. Encourage patient to participate in MotHER Pregnancy Registry (1-800-690-6720).
• It isn't known if drug appears in breast milk. Patient should discontinue breast-feeding or discontinue drug.

NURSING CONSIDERATIONS
• Confirm HER2 testing with FDA-approved test by established laboratory. Only patients with HER2 protein overexpression should receive drug because these are the only patients studied for whom benefit has been shown.
• Infusion-related reactions, including hypersensitivity reactions, may occur. Closely monitor patient during and for 90 minutes after infusion for fever, chills, flushing, dyspnea, hypotension, wheezing, bronchospasm, or tachycardia. Slow or interrupt infusion as necessary. In most patients, these reactions resolve over the course of several hours to a day after the infusion is terminated.
• Monitor patient for extravasation, which may cause redness, tenderness, skin irritation, pain, or swelling at infusion site.
Black Box Warning Severe liver injury (including fatal liver damage, liver failure, and death) has been reported. Monitor serum transaminase and bilirubin levels before starting drug and before each dose. Dosage modifications or discontinuation of therapy may be necessary. ■

Black Box Warning Drug may significantly reduce LVEF. Assess LVEF before starting drug and every 3 months during treatment. Withhold or discontinue drug as clinically indicated. ∎

🔾 *Alert:* Permanently discontinue drug in patients diagnosed with interstitial lung disease or pneumonitis.

• Monitor platelet count before treatment and before each dose.

• Discontinue drug in patients diagnosed with nodular regenerative hyperplasia of the liver.

🔾 *Alert:* Asian patients may have increased incidence and severity of thrombocytopenia.

PATIENT TEACHING

• Inform patient that drug may cause severe liver damage that may be life-threatening.

• Tell patient to report unexplained nausea, vomiting, abdominal pain, jaundice, dark urine, generalized itchiness, or anorexia.

• Caution patient that drug may cause heart problems, with or without symptoms. Instruct patient to report new-onset or worsening of shortness of breath, cough, swelling of the ankles or legs, palpitations, weight gain of more than 2.27 kg in 24 hours, fatigue, dizziness, or loss of consciousness.

• Advise patient that drug may cause lung problems. Tell patient to report trouble breathing, cough, or tiredness.

• Alert patient that drug may cause low platelet count. Instruct patient to contact prescriber if excessive bleeding occurs.

• Warn patient that drug may cause nerve damage. Instruct patient to report numbness or tingling, burning or sharp pain, sensitivity to touch, lack of coordination, or muscle weakness or loss of muscle function.

Black Box Warning Inform patient that drug may cause birth defects and fetal death. Advise woman of childbearing potential to use effective contraception during treatment and for 7 months after last dose. ∎

🔾 *Alert:* Advise patient to immediately inform her physician if she suspects or confirms pregnancy during therapy. Encourage patient participation in MotHER Pregnancy Registry by contacting 1-800-690-6720.

• Inform breast-feeding patient that it isn't known if drug appears in breast milk and that she must discontinue either breast-feeding or drug.

---

albuterol sulfate
al-BYOO-ter-ole

AccuNeb, Airomir🍁, PHL-Salbutamol🍁, ProAir HFA, ProAir RespiClick, Proventil-HFA, Ventolin HFA, VoSpire ER

Therapeutic class: Bronchodilators
Pharmacologic class: Adrenergics

AVAILABLE FORMS
Inhalation aerosol: 100 mcg/actuation🍁, 108 mcg/actuation
Inhalation powder: 108 mcg/actuation
Oral solution: 0.4 mg/mL🍁
Solution for inhalation: 0.021% (0.63 mg/3 mL), 0.042% (1.25 mg/3 mL), 0.083% (2.5 mg/3 mL), 0.5 mg/mL🍁, 1 mg/mL🍁, 2 mg/mL🍁, 0.5% (5 mg/mL)
Syrup: 2 mg/5 mL
Tablets: 2 mg, 4 mg
Tablets (extended-release) ⓞⓝⓒ: 4 mg, 8 mg

INDICATIONS & DOSAGES
➤ **To prevent or treat bronchospasm in patients with reversible obstructive airway disease**
Tablets (extended-release)
Adults and children age 13 and older: 4 to 8 mg P.O. every 12 hours. Maximum, 32 mg daily.
Children ages 6 to 13: 4 mg P.O. every 12 hours. Maximum, 24 mg daily.
Tablets
Adults and children age 13 and older: 2 to 4 mg P.O. t.i.d. or q.i.d. Maximum, 32 mg daily.
Children ages 6 to 12: 2 mg P.O. t.i.d. or q.i.d. Maximum, 24 mg daily.
Children ages 2 to 5: 0.1 mg/kg P.O. t.i.d. Maximum, 12 mg/day.
Solution for inhalation
Adults and children age 13 and older: 2.5 mg t.i.d. or q.i.d. by nebulizer, given over 5 to 15 minutes. To prepare solution, use 0.5 mL of 0.5% solution diluted with 2.5 mL of NSS. Or, use 3 mL of 0.083% solution.

Children ages 2 to 12 weighing more than 15 kg: 2.5 mg by nebulizer given over 5 to 15 minutes t.i.d. or q.i.d., with subsequent doses adjusted to response. Don't exceed 2.5 mg t.i.d. or q.i.d.
Children ages 2 to 12 weighing 15 kg or less: 0.63 mg or 1.25 mg by nebulizer given over 5 to 15 minutes t.i.d. or q.i.d. with subsequent doses adjusted to response. Don't exceed 2.5 mg t.i.d. or q.i.d.
Syrup
Adults and children age 15 and older: 2 to 4 mg P.O. t.i.d. or q.i.d. Maximum, 32 mg daily.
Children ages 6 to 14: 2 mg P.O. t.i.d. or q.i.d. Maximum, 24 mg daily.
Children ages 2 to 5: Initially, 0.1 mg/kg P.O. t.i.d. Starting dose shouldn't exceed 2 mg t.i.d. Maximum, 12 mg daily.
Inhalation aerosol
Adults and children age 4 and older: 1 to 2 inhalations every 4 to 6 hours as needed. Regular use for maintenance therapy to control asthma symptoms isn't recommended.
Adjust-a-dose: For elderly patients and those sensitive to sympathomimetic amines, 2 mg P.O. t.i.d. or q.i.d. as oral tablets or syrup. Maximum, 32 mg daily.
Inhalational powder
Adults and children age 12 and older: 2 inhalations every 4 to 6 hours. In some patients, 1 inhalation every 4 hours may be sufficient.
➤ **To prevent exercise-induced bronchospasm (except ProAir RespiClick)**
Adults and children age 4 and older: 2 inhalations using the inhalation aerosol 15 minutes before exercise; up to 12 inhalations may be taken in 24 hours.
➤ **To prevent exercise-induced bronchospasm (ProAir RespiClick)**
Adults and children age 12 and older: 2 inhalations 15 to 30 minutes before exercise.
➤ **Hyperkalemia ♦**
Adults: 10 to 20 mg by nebulizer over 15 minutes, given with other recommended therapy.

ADMINISTRATION
P.O.
● When switching patient from regular to extended-release tablets, remember that a regular 2-mg tablet every 6 hours is equivalent to an extended-release 4-mg tablet every 12 hours.
● Give extend-release tablets whole; don't break or crush tablets or mix them with food.
Inhalational
● If more than 1 inhalation is ordered, wait at least 2 minutes between inhalations.
● Inhalation powder inhaler device doesn't require priming. Use spacer device to improve drug delivery, if appropriate. Don't use ProAir RespiClick with a spacer or volume holding chamber.
● Discard ProAir RespiClick 13 months after opening foil pouch, when dose counter displays "0," or after expiration date on product, whichever comes first.
● Shake the aerosol inhaler well before use and prime inhaler according to manufacturer's instructions before first use, when it has been dropped, or when it hasn't been used for more than 2 weeks.
● Keep cap on inhaler closed during storage.

ACTION
Relaxes bronchial, uterine, and vascular smooth muscle by stimulating beta$_2$ receptors.

Route	Onset	Peak	Duration
P.O.	15–30 min	2–3 hr	4–8 hr
P.O. (extended)	Unknown	6 hr	12 hr
Inhalation (aerosol)	5–15 min	30–120 min	3–4 hr
Inhalation (powder)	Rapid	30 min	3–4 hr

Half-life: Oral, 5 to 6 hours; inhalation aerosol, 6 hours; inhalation powder, 5 hours.

ADVERSE REACTIONS
CNS: tremor, nervousness, headache, hyperactivity, insomnia, dizziness, weakness, CNS stimulation, malaise.
CV: tachycardia, palpitations, hypertension, chest pain, lymphadenopathy.
EENT: conjunctivitis, otitis media, dry and irritated nose and throat (with inhaled form), nasal congestion, epistaxis, hoarseness, pharyngitis, rhinitis.
GI: nausea, vomiting, heartburn, anorexia, altered taste, increased appetite.
GU: UTI.
Metabolic: hypokalemia.

Musculoskeletal: muscle cramps, back pain.
Respiratory: *bronchospasm,* cough, wheezing, dyspnea, bronchitis, increased sputum.
Other: hypersensitivity reactions, flulike syndrome, cold symptoms.

INTERACTIONS
Drug-drug. *Antiarrhythmics (amiodarone, bretylium, disopyramide, dofetilide, procainamide, quinidine, sotalol), arsenic trioxide, chlorpromazine, dolasetron, droperidol, mefloquine, mesoridazine, moxifloxacin, pentamidine, pimozide, tacrolimus, thioridazine, ziprasidone:* May prolong QT interval and increase risk of life-threatening arrhythmias, including torsades de pointes. Monitor QT interval and patient.
CNS stimulants: May increase CNS stimulation. Avoid using together.
Digoxin: May decrease digoxin level. Monitor digoxin level closely.
Diuretics (furosemide, thiazides): May cause ECG changes and hypokalemia. Monitor potassium level. Use caution when administered with non-potassium-sparing diuretics.
Linezolid, MAO inhibitors, TCAs: May increase adverse CV effects. Consider alternative therapy. Monitor patient closely if used together.
Propranolol and other beta blockers: May cause mutual antagonism. Monitor patient carefully.
Theophyllines: May decrease theophylline plasma concentration. Adjust dosage as needed and monitor patient.

EFFECTS ON LAB TEST RESULTS
● May decrease potassium level.

CONTRAINDICATIONS & CAUTIONS
● Contraindicated in patients hypersensitive to drug or its ingredients.
● Use cautiously in patients with CV disorders (including coronary insufficiency and hypertension), hyperthyroidism, or diabetes mellitus and in those who are unusually responsive to adrenergics.
● Use extended-release tablets cautiously in patients with GI narrowing.
Dialyzable drug: Unknown.

⚠ *Overdose S&S:* Exaggeration of adverse reactions, seizures, angina, hypotension, hypertension, tachycardia, arrhythmias, nervousness, headache, tremor, dry mouth, palpitations, nausea, dizziness, fatigue, malaise, sleeplessness, hypokalemia, cardiac arrest.

PREGNANCY-LACTATION-REPRODUCTION
● There are no adequate and well-controlled studies in pregnant women. Use during pregnancy only if potential benefit justifies potential risk to the fetus.
● It isn't known if drug appears in breast milk. Use cautiously in breast-feeding women.

NURSING CONSIDERATIONS
● Drug may decrease sensitivity of spirometry used for diagnosis of asthma.
● Syrup contains no alcohol or sugar and may be taken by children as young as age 2.
● In children, syrup may rarely cause erythema multiforme or Stevens-Johnson syndrome.
● Monitor patient for effectiveness. Using drug alone may not be adequate to control asthma in some patients. Long-term control medications may be needed.
⊙ *Alert:* Drug may cause paradoxical bronchospasm. Monitor patient closely; discontinue drug immediately and use alternative therapy if paradoxical bronchospasm occurs. Bronchospasm with inhaled formulations frequently occurs with first use of new canister or vial.
⊙ *Alert:* Patient may use tablets and aerosol together. Monitor these patients closely for signs and symptoms of toxicity.
● *Look alike–sound alike:* Don't confuse albuterol with atenolol or Albutein. Don't confuse Salbutamol with salmeterol.

PATIENT TEACHING
● Warn patient about risk of paradoxical bronchospasm and to stop drug immediately if it occurs.
● Teach patient to perform oral inhalation correctly. Give the following instructions for using the metered-dose inhaler (MDI):
– Prime before first use, if not used for 2 weeks, or if MDI has been dropped.
– Shake the inhaler.

Reactions in bold italics are *life-threatening*. Interactions may have a *rapid onset* or a *delayed onset.*

– Clear nasal passages and throat.

– Breathe out, expelling as much air from lungs as possible.

– Place mouthpiece well into mouth, seal lips around mouthpiece, and inhale deeply as you release a dose from inhaler. Or, hold inhaler about 1 inch from open mouth; inhale while dose is released.

– Hold breath for several seconds, remove mouthpiece, and exhale slowly.

• If prescriber orders more than 1 inhalation, tell patient to wait at least 2 minutes before repeating procedure.

• Tell patient that use of a spacer device with appropriate inhaler may improve drug delivery to lungs.

• If patient is also using a corticosteroid inhaler, instruct him to use the bronchodilator first and then to wait about 5 minutes before using the corticosteroid.

• Tell patient to remove canister and wash aerosol inhaler with warm, soapy water at least once a week.

• Warn patient not to wash or place any part of powder inhaler in water. If mouthpiece needs cleaning, advise patient to gently wipe it with dry cloth or tissue.

• Advise patient not to use more than prescribed and not to increase dose or frequency without consulting physician. Fatalities have been reported from excessive use.

• Instruct patient to report worsening symptoms.

• Advise patient not to chew or crush extended-release tablets or mix them with food.

alectinib hydrochloride
See NEW DRUGS for information.

alendronate sodium
ah-LEN-dro-nate

Binosto, Fosamax✐

Therapeutic class: Antiosteoporotics
Pharmacologic class: Bisphosphonates

AVAILABLE FORMS
Oral solution: 70 mg/75 mL
Tablets: 5 mg, 10 mg, 35 mg, 40 mg, 70 mg
Tablets (effervescent): 70 mg

INDICATIONS & DOSAGES
➤ **Osteoporosis in postmenopausal women; to increase bone mass in men with osteoporosis**
Adults: 10 mg P.O. daily or 70-mg tablet or solution P.O. once weekly.
➤ **Paget disease of bone (osteitis deformans) (excluding Binosto and oral solution)**
Adults: 40 mg P.O. daily for 6 months.
➤ **To prevent osteoporosis in postmenopausal women (excluding Binosto and oral solution)**
Adults: 5 mg P.O. daily or 35-mg tablet P.O. once weekly.
➤ **Glucocorticoid-induced osteoporosis in patients receiving glucocorticoids in a daily dose equivalent to 7.5 mg or more of prednisone and who have low bone mineral density (excluding Binosto and oral solution)**
Adults: 5 mg P.O. daily. For postmenopausal women not receiving estrogen, recommended dose is 10 mg P.O. daily.

ADMINISTRATION
P.O.
• Give drug with 180 to 240 mL of water at least 30 minutes before patient's first food or drink of the day to facilitate delivery to the stomach.
• Dissolve effervescent tablet in 120 mL of plain room-temperature water.
• Give at least 60 mL of water after oral solution.
• Don't allow patient to lie down for 30 minutes after taking drug and until after first food of the day.

ACTION
Suppresses osteoclast activity on newly formed resorption surfaces, which reduces bone turnover. Bone formation exceeds resorption at remodeling sites, leading to progressive gains in bone mass.

Route	Onset	Peak	Duration
P.O.	Unknown	Unknown	Unknown

Half-life: More than 10 years.

ADVERSE REACTIONS
CNS: headache.

GI: abdominal pain, nausea, dyspepsia, constipation, diarrhea, flatulence, acid regurgitation, esophageal ulcer, vomiting, dysphagia, abdominal distention, gastritis, taste perversion, melena.
Musculoskeletal: pain.

INTERACTIONS

Drug-drug. *Antacids, calcium supplements, many oral drugs:* May interfere with absorption of alendronate. Instruct patient to wait at least 30 minutes after taking alendronate before taking other drug orally.
Aspirin, NSAIDs: May increase risk of upper GI adverse reactions with drug doses greater than 10 mg daily. Monitor patient closely.
Ranitidine (I.V. form): May increase availability of alendronate. Reduce dosage as needed.
Drug-food. *Any food:* May decrease absorption of drug. Advise patient to take with full glass of water at least 30 minutes before food, beverages, or ingestion of other drugs.

EFFECTS ON LAB TEST RESULTS
● May decrease calcium and phosphate levels.

CONTRAINDICATIONS & CAUTIONS
● Contraindicated in patients hypersensitive to drug and in those with hypocalcemia or abnormalities of the esophagus that delay esophageal emptying.
● Drug isn't recommended for patients with CrCl of less than 35 mL/minute.
◆ **Alert:** There may be an increased risk of atypical fractures of the thigh in patients treated with bisphosphonates.
● Contraindicated in patients unable to stand or sit upright for at least 30 minutes.
● Use cautiously in patients with active upper GI problems (dysphagia, symptomatic esophageal diseases, gastritis, duodenitis, ulcers) or mild to moderate renal insufficiency.
● Use cautiously in patients with known risk factors for osteonecrosis of the jaw (diagnosis of cancer; concomitant treatment with chemotherapy, radiotherapy, corticosteroids), poor oral hygiene, and comorbid disorders, such as preexisting dental disease, anemia, coagulopathy, or infection.

Dialyzable drug: No.
⚠ **Overdose S&S:** Hypocalcemia, hypophosphatemia, upset stomach, heartburn, esophagitis, gastritis, ulcer.

PREGNANCY-LACTATION-REPRODUCTION
● No data exist on fetal risk in humans, but there is a theoretical risk of fetal harm. Use during pregnancy only if potential benefit justifies potential risk to the fetus.
● It isn't known if drug appears in breast milk. Use cautiously in breast-feeding women.

NURSING CONSIDERATIONS
● Correct hypocalcemia and other disturbances of mineral metabolism (such as vitamin D deficiency) before therapy begins.
● When used to treat osteoporosis, disease may be confirmed by findings of low bone mass on diagnostic studies or by history of osteoporotic fracture.
● The recommended daily intake of vitamin D is 400 to 800 international units. Patients at risk for vitamin D deficiency, such as those who are chronically ill, who are nursing home bound, who have a GI malabsorption syndrome, or who are older than age 70, may require additional supplementation.
● In Paget disease, drug is indicated for patients with alkaline phosphatase level at least 2 × ULN, for those who are symptomatic, and for those at risk for future complications from the disease.
● Monitor patient's calcium and phosphate levels throughout therapy.
● Severe musculoskeletal pain has been associated with bisphosphonate use and may occur within days, months, or years of start of therapy. When drug is stopped, symptoms may resolve partially or completely.
● Patients who develop osteonecrosis of the jaw should receive care by an oral surgeon.
● Optimal length of treatment hasn't been determined. Reevaluate need for continued therapy periodically. Patients at low risk for fracture should be considered for discontinuation after 3 to 5 years of treatment.
● *Look alike–sound alike:* Don't confuse Fosamax with Flomax.

PATIENT TEACHING

• Stress importance of taking tablet only with 180 to 240 mL of water at least 30 minutes before ingesting anything else, including food, beverages, and other drugs. Tell patient that waiting longer than 30 minutes improves absorption.

• Warn patient not to lie down for at least 30 minutes after taking drug to facilitate delivery to stomach and to reduce risk of esophageal irritation.

• Tell patient who misses a once-weekly dose to take one dose on the morning after she remembers and then return to weekly dosing on the chosen day as originally scheduled.

• Advise patient to report adverse effects immediately, especially chest pain or difficulty swallowing.

• Advise patient to take supplemental calcium and vitamin D if dietary intake is inadequate.

• Tell patient about benefits of weight-bearing exercises in increasing bone mass. If applicable, explain importance of reducing or eliminating cigarette smoking and alcohol use.

---

alfuzosin hydrochloride
al-foo-ZOE-sin

Uroxatral✐, Xatral✦

Therapeutic class: BPH drugs
Pharmacologic class: Alpha$_1$ blockers

AVAILABLE FORMS
Tablets (extended-release) 🔴: 10 mg

INDICATIONS & DOSAGES
➤ **BPH**
Men: 10 mg P.O. immediately after same meal each day.

ADMINISTRATION
P.O.
• Give drug after same meal each day.
• Don't crush tablets.

ACTION
Selectively blocks alpha$_1$ receptors in the prostate, which relaxes the smooth muscles in the bladder neck and prostate, improving urine flow and reducing symptoms of BPH.

Route	Onset	Peak	Duration
P.O.	Unknown	8 hr	Unknown

Half-life: 10 hours.

ADVERSE REACTIONS
CNS: dizziness, fatigue, headache, pain.
EENT: pharyngitis, sinusitis.
GI: abdominal pain, constipation, dyspepsia, nausea.
GU: erectile dysfunction.
Respiratory: bronchitis, URI.

INTERACTIONS
Drug-drug. *Alpha-adrenergic antagonists (doxazosin, prazosin, silodosin, terazosin):* May increase risk of adverse events. Use with drug of same class is contraindicated.
Amiodarone: May increase alfuzosin plasma level and pharmacologic effects. Use with caution and monitor patient.
Antihypertensives (diltiazem), nitrates: May cause hypotension. Monitor BP and use together cautiously.
Beta blockers (atenolol): May cause hypotension and reduce HR. Monitor BP and HR for these effects.
Cimetidine: May increase alfuzosin level. Use together cautiously.
Moderate CYP3A4 inhibitors (diltiazem, verapamil): May increase alfuzosin level. Use cautiously together and monitor patient for adverse reactions.
Potent CYP3A4 inhibitors (itraconazole, ketoconazole, ritonavir): May inhibit hepatic metabolism of alfuzosin. Use together is contraindicated.

EFFECTS ON LAB TEST RESULTS
None reported.

CONTRAINDICATIONS & CAUTIONS
• Contraindicated in patients with moderate to severe hepatic impairment (Child-Pugh class B or C) and those hypersensitive to alfuzosin or its ingredients.
• Use cautiously in patients with severe renal insufficiency, QT-interval prolongation, or symptomatic hypotension and hypotensive responses to other drugs.

• Drug is associated with rare cases of priapism, which can lead to permanent erectile dysfunction if not treated promptly.
Dialyzable drug: Unknown.
⚠ *Overdose S&S:* Hypotension.

PREGNANCY-LACTATION-REPRODUCTION
• Not indicated for use in women. There are no studies in pregnant or breast-feeding women.

NURSING CONSIDERATIONS
• Don't use drug to treat hypertension.
• Asymptomatic orthostatic hypotension may develop within a few hours.
• Symptoms of BPH and prostate cancer are similar; rule out prostate cancer first.
• If angina pectoris develops or worsens, stop drug.
• Current or previous use of an alpha blocker may predispose the patient to intraoperative floppy iris syndrome during cataract surgery.

PATIENT TEACHING
• Tell patient to take drug just after the same meal each day.
• At start of therapy, warn patient about possible hypotension and explain that the drug may cause dizziness. Caution patient against performing hazardous activities until he knows how the drug affects him.
• Tell patient to avoid situations in which he could be injured if he became light-headed or fainted.
• Warn patient not to crush or chew tablets.
• Advise patient planning cataract surgery to alert his ophthalmologist about this drug and current or previous alpha blocker therapy.
• Caution patient that priapism (persistent, painful penile erection unrelated to sexual activity) has occurred rarely with drug use. Warn patient of risk of permanent impotence if priapism isn't treated properly and to seek medical attention promptly.

alirocumab
AL-i-rok-ue-mab

Praluent

Therapeutic class: Antilipemics
Pharmacologic class: Proprotein convertase subtilisin/kexin type 9 (PCSK9) antibody inhibitors

AVAILABLE FORMS
Injection: 75 mg/mL, 150 mg/mL in single-dose prefilled pens or syringes

INDICATIONS & DOSAGES
➤ **Adjunct to diet and maximally tolerated statin therapy for the treatment of heterozygous familial hypercholesterolemia or clinical atherosclerotic CV disease in patients who require additional lowering of LDL cholesterol (LDL-C) levels**
Adults: 75 mg subcutaneously every 2 weeks. If LDL-C response is inadequate (within 4 to 8 weeks), may increase dosage to maximum of 150 mg every 2 weeks.

ADMINISTRATION
Subcutaneous
• Don't give orally, I.V., or I.M.
• Allow drug to warm to room temperature (30 to 40 minutes) before use. Use as soon as possible after it has warmed. Don't shake.
• Don't use solution if discolored, if particulate matter is present, or if drug has been at room temperature for 24 hours or longer.
• Give dose subcutaneously into thigh, abdomen, or upper arm. Rotate injection sites with each dose.
• Don't inject into areas of skin disease or injury, such as sunburn, rashes, inflammation, or skin infections. Don't give with other injectable drugs at the same injection site.
• If a dose is missed, administer injection within 7 days from missed dose; then resume original schedule. If missed dose is beyond 7 days, skip dose and give next dose on the original schedule.
• Store in refrigerator. Don't freeze or expose to extreme heat.

ACTION
A monoclonal antibody that binds to the protein PCSK9, leaving more receptors available to remove LDL-C from the blood, thus lowering LDL levels.

Route	Onset	Peak	Duration
Subcut.	4–8 hr	3–7 days	Unknown

Half-life: 17 to 20 days; 12 days when given with a statin.

ADVERSE REACTIONS
EENT: nasopharyngitis, sinusitis.
GI: diarrhea.
GU: UTI.
Hepatic: elevated LFT values.
Musculoskeletal: muscle spasms, musculoskeletal pain, myalgia.
Respiratory: bronchitis, cough.
Skin: injection-site reactions (erythema/redness, itching, swelling, pain/tenderness), contusion.
Other: antidrug antibodies, hypersensitivity reactions, flulike symptoms.

INTERACTIONS
Belimumab: May enhance adverse effects of belimumab. Avoid combination.

EFFECTS ON LAB TEST RESULTS
● May decrease apolipoprotein B, LDL and non-HDL cholesterol, and total cholesterol levels.
● May increase AST and ALT levels.

CONTRAINDICATIONS & CAUTIONS
● Contraindicated in patients with a history of serious hypersensitivity reactions to drug or its components.
● Hypersensitivity reactions, including pruritus, rash, urticaria, hypersensitivity vasculitis, and other serious events requiring hospitalization, have been reported. Discontinue drug if signs or symptoms occur, treat appropriately, and monitor patient until signs and symptoms resolve.
● Use in patients with severe renal or hepatic impairment hasn't been studied.
● Safety and effectiveness in children haven't been established.
Dialyzable drug: Unknown.

PREGNANCY-LACTATION-REPRODUCTION
● There are no adequate studies of use in pregnant women, and it isn't known if drug appears in breast milk. Alirocumab, like other IgG antibodies, may cross the placental barrier and pass into breast milk. Before using drug in women who are pregnant or breast-feeding, consider maternal and fetal risks and benefits.

NURSING CONSIDERATIONS
● Measure LDL-C levels within 4 to 8 weeks of initiating or titrating drug to assess response; adjust dosage if needed.
● LDL-C levels of less than 25 mg/dL have occurred during clinical trials. Adverse consequences of long-term very low LDL-C levels aren't known.
● Patients who develop antidrug antibodies tend to have high incidence of injection-site reaction.
● *Look alike–sound alike:* Don't confuse alirocumab with alemtuzumab or Praluent with pravastatin.

PATIENT TEACHING
● Advise patient to discontinue drug and seek prompt medical attention if signs or symptoms of serious allergic reactions occur.
● Instruct patient on proper administration of drug.
● Counsel patient to store drug in the refrigerator; not to freeze, shake, or expose drug to extreme heat; and to discard drug if it has been kept at room temperature for 24 hours or longer.
● Inform patient that syringes and pens are for one-time use and shouldn't be reused. Demonstrate proper disposal.
● Inform patient that laboratory tests will be needed to monitor drug's effectiveness. Encourage patient to keep all health care appointments.

aliskiren hemifumarate
a-LIS-ke-ren

Rasilez ✤, Tekturna

Therapeutic class: Antihypertensives
Pharmacologic class: Renin inhibitors

AVAILABLE FORMS
Tablets: 150 mg, 300 mg

INDICATIONS & DOSAGES
➤ **Hypertension, alone or with other antihypertensives**
Adults: 150 mg P.O. daily; may increase to 300 mg P.O. daily.

ADMINISTRATION
P.O.
- Don't give drug with high-fat meal; may decrease drug's effectiveness.
- Give consistently at same time each day with or without meals. However, consistent administration with regard to meals is recommended.

ACTION
Inhibits conversion of angiotensin to angiotensin I, decreasing vasoconstriction and lowering BP.

Route	Onset	Peak	Duration
P.O.	Unknown	1–3 hr	Unknown

Half-life: 24 hours.

ADVERSE REACTIONS
CNS: headache, dizziness, fatigue, *seizures.*
CV: hypotension.
GI: abdominal pain, diarrhea, dyspepsia, gastroesophageal reflux.
Metabolic: hyperuricemia, *hyperkalemia.*
Respiratory: cough, URI.
Skin: rash.
Other: *angioedema.*

INTERACTIONS
Drug-drug. ⟳ *Alert: ACE inhibitors (benazepril, captopril, lisinopril, moexipril, perindopril, quinapril, ramipril, trandolapril), ARBs (azilsartan, candesartan, eprosartan, irbesartan, losartan, olmesartan, telmisartan, valsartan), other drugs that antagonize RAAS:* May increase risk of renal impairment, hypotension, and hyperkalemia. Concomitant use is contraindicated in diabetic patients. Avoid concomitant use in patients with moderate to severe renal impairment (GFR < 60 mL/minute).
Atorvastatin: May increase aliskiren levels. Use cautiously together.
CYP3A4/P-glycoprotein inhibitors (cyclosporine, itraconazole, ketoconazole, verapamil): May increase aliskiren concentration and risk of adverse reactions. Use with caution. Avoid concurrent use with cyclosporine or itraconazole.
Furosemide: May reduce furosemide peak levels. Monitor patient for effectiveness.
NSAIDs, potassium-sparing diuretics, potassium supplements: May increase risk of hyperkalemia. Use cautiously together.
Rifampin: May decrease aliskiren plasma concentration. Larger aliskiren doses may be needed.
Drug-food. *Grapefruit:* May decrease aliskiren plasma level. Advise patient to avoid grapefruit products.
High-fat meals: May substantially decrease plasma levels of drug. Monitor patient for effectiveness.

EFFECTS ON LAB TEST RESULTS
- May increase potassium, CK, BUN, uric acid, and serum creatinine levels.

CONTRAINDICATIONS & CAUTIONS
- Contraindicated in patients hypersensitive to drug or its components and in those with diabetes who are receiving ARBs or ACE inhibitors.
- Contraindicated in patients taking cyclosporine.
- Use cautiously in patients with history of angioedema, severe renal dysfunction (creatinine level of 1.7 mg/dL in women and 2 mg/dL in men, or GFR of less than 30 mL/minute), history of dialysis, nephrotic syndrome, or renovascular hypertension.
Dialyzable drug: No.
⚠ *Overdose S&S:* Hypotension.

PREGNANCY-LACTATION-REPRODUCTION
Black Box Warning Drug can cause fetal harm. Drugs that act on the renin-angiotensin system can cause injury and

---

Reactions in bold italics are *life-threatening*. Interactions may have a *rapid onset* or a ***delayed onset***.

death to the developing fetus. Discontinue drug as soon as possible once pregnancy is detected. ▪
• Women of childbearing potential should avoid becoming pregnant while taking drug.
• It isn't known if drug appears in breast milk. Patient should discontinue breast-feeding or discontinue drug.

NURSING CONSIDERATIONS
• Monitor BP for hypotension, especially if used in combination with other antihypertensives.
• Monitor potassium levels, especially in patients also taking ACE inhibitors.
❸ Alert: Rarely, angioedema may occur at any time during treatment. Discontinue drug for angioedema or anaphylaxis and don't readminister. Early emergency treatment is critical and may include antihistamines, steroids, and epinephrine.
• Monitor renal function. It's unknown how patients with significant renal disorders will respond to the use of this drug.
• Correct volume or salt depletion before giving drug or start therapy under close monitoring.
• Effect of any dose is usually seen within 2 weeks.
• Monitor patient for serious skin reactions (Stevens-Johnson syndrome, toxic epidermal necrolysis).

PATIENT TEACHING
• Instruct patient not to take drug with a high-fat meal because this may decrease drug's effectiveness.
• Instruct patient to monitor BP daily, if possible, and to report low readings, dizziness, and headaches to prescriber.
• Tell patient to immediately report swelling of the face or neck or difficulty breathing.
• Advise patient of need for regular laboratory tests to monitor for adverse effects.

allopurinol
al-oh-PURE-i-nole

Lopurin, Zyloprim✤

allopurinol sodium
Aloprim

Therapeutic class: Antigout drugs
Pharmacologic class: Xanthine oxidase inhibitors

AVAILABLE FORMS
allopurinol
Tablets (scored): 100 mg✤, 200 mg✤, 300 mg✤
allopurinol sodium
Injection: 500 mg/30-mL vial

INDICATIONS & DOSAGES
Adjust-a-dose (for all indications): If CrCl is 10 to 20 mL/minute, give 200 mg P.O. or I.V. daily; if CrCl is less than 10 mL/minute, give 100 mg P.O. or I.V. daily; if CrCl is less than 3 mL/minute, give a maximum of 100 mg P.O. or I.V. at extended intervals. If patient is receiving hemodialysis, give a 50% supplemental dose after dialysis.
➤ **Gout or hyperuricemia**
Adults: Mild gout, 200 to 300 mg P.O. daily; severe gout with large tophi, 400 to 600 mg P.O. daily. Maximum 800 mg daily. Dosage varies with severity of disease; can be given as single dose or divided, but doses greater than 300 mg should be divided.
➤ **Hyperuricemia caused by malignancies**
Adults and children older than age 10: 200 to 400 mg/m^2 daily I.V. as a single infusion or in equally divided doses every 6, 8, or 12 hours beginning 24 to 48 hours before initiation of chemotherapy. Maximum 600 mg daily.
Children age 10 and younger: Initially, 200 mg/m^2 daily I.V. as single infusion or in equally divided doses every 6, 8, or 12 hours beginning 24 to 48 hours before initiation of chemotherapy. Then titrate according to uric acid levels. For children ages 6 to 10, give 300 mg P.O. daily or in three divided doses; for children younger than age 6, give 150 mg P.O. daily.

✤Canada   ◇OTC   ◆Off-label use   ✐Photoguide   ⓓDo not crush   *Liquid contains alcohol.

➤ **To prevent uric acid nephropathy during cancer chemotherapy**
Adults: 600 to 800 mg P.O. daily for 2 to 3 days, with high fluid intake.
➤ **Recurrent calcium oxalate calculi**
Adults: 200 to 300 mg P.O. daily in single or divided doses.

ADMINISTRATION
P.O.
• Give drug with or immediately after meals to minimize GI upset.
I.V.
▼ When possible, initiate therapy 24 to 48 hours before the start of chemotherapy known to cause tumor lysis.
▼ Dissolve contents of each 30-mL vial in 25 mL of sterile water for injection.
▼ Dilute solution to desired concentration (no greater than 6 mg/mL) with NSS for injection or D₅W. Can give as a single daily infusion or in equally divided infusions at 6-, 8-, or 12-hour intervals. Rate of infusion depends on volume of infusate.
▼ Store solution at 68° to 77° F (20° to 25° C) and use within 10 hours. Don't use solution if it contains particulates or is discolored.
▼ **Incompatibilities:** Amikacin, amphotericin B, carmustine, cefotaxime, chlorpromazine, cimetidine, clindamycin phosphate, cytarabine, dacarbazine, daunorubicin, diphenhydramine, doxorubicin, doxycycline hyclate, droperidol, floxuridine, gentamicin, haloperidol lactate, hydroxyzine, idarubicin, imipenem–cilastatin sodium, mechlorethamine, meperidine, methylprednisolone sodium succinate, metoclopramide, minocycline, nalbuphine, netilmicin, ondansetron, prochlorperazine edisylate, promethazine, sodium bicarbonate (or solutions containing sodium bicarbonate), streptozocin, tobramycin sulfate, vinorelbine.

ACTION
Reduces uric acid production by inhibiting xanthine oxidase.

Route	Onset	Peak	Duration
P.O.	Unknown	1½ hr (allopurinol); 5 hr (oxypurinol)	1–2 wk
I.V.	Unknown	30 min	Unknown

Half-life: Allopurinol, 1 to 2 hours; oxypurinol, about 15 hours.

ADVERSE REACTIONS
GI: nausea, vomiting, abdominal pain, diarrhea.
GU: *renal failure.*
Musculoskeletal: acute gout attack.
Skin: rash, maculopapular rash.

INTERACTIONS
Drug-drug. *Amoxicillin, ampicillin:* May increase possibility of rash. Avoid using together.
Anticoagulants: May increase anticoagulant effect. Dosage may need to be adjusted.
Antineoplastics: May increase potential for bone marrow suppression. Monitor patient carefully.
Azathioprine, mercaptopurine: May increase levels of these drugs. Concomitant administration of 300 to 600 mg of oral allopurinol per day requires dosage reduction to ⅓ to ¼ of usual dose of azathioprine or mercaptopurine. Make subsequent dosage adjustments based on therapeutic response and appearance of toxic effects.
Chlorpropamide: May increase hypoglycemic effect. Avoid using together.
Ethacrynic acid, thiazide diuretics: May increase risk of allopurinol toxicity. Reduce allopurinol dosage, and monitor renal function closely.
Theophylline: May increase theophylline level. Adjust theophylline dosage as needed.
Uricosurics: May have additive effect. May be used to therapeutic advantage.
Drug-lifestyle. *Alcohol use:* May increase uric acid level. Discourage use together.

EFFECTS ON LAB TEST RESULTS
• May increase alkaline phosphatase, ALT, and AST levels.
• May increase eosinophil count. May decrease Hb level, hematocrit, and granulocyte and platelet counts.
• May increase or decrease WBC count.

CONTRAINDICATIONS & CAUTIONS
• Contraindicated in patients hypersensitive to drug.
Dialyzable drug: Yes.

PREGNANCY-LACTATION-REPRODUCTION
• Use in pregnancy only if clearly needed.
• It isn't known if drug appears in breast milk. Use cautiously in breast-feeding women.

NURSING CONSIDERATIONS
❸ *Alert:* Rash can be followed by more severe hypersensitivity reactions (Stevens-Johnson syndrome, vasculitis, irreversible hepatotoxicity), which can be fatal. Discontinue drug at first sign of rash.
• Monitor uric acid level to evaluate drug's effectiveness.
• Monitor fluid intake and output; daily urine output of at least 2 L and maintenance of neutral or slightly alkaline urine are desirable.
• Periodically monitor CBC and hepatic and renal function, especially at start of therapy.
• Optimal benefits may need 2 to 6 weeks of therapy. Because acute gout attacks may occur during this time, concurrent use of colchicine may be prescribed prophylactically.
• Don't restart drug in patients who have a severe reaction.
• *Look alike–sound alike:* Don't confuse Zyloprim with ZORprin or zolpidem.

PATIENT TEACHING
• To minimize GI adverse reactions, tell patient to take drug with or immediately after meals.
• Encourage patient to drink plenty of fluids while taking drug unless otherwise contraindicated.
• Drug may cause drowsiness; tell patient not to drive or perform hazardous tasks requiring mental alertness until CNS effects of drug are known.
• If patient is taking drug for recurrent calcium oxalate stones, advise him or her also to reduce his dietary intake of animal protein, sodium, refined sugars, oxalate-rich foods, and calcium.
• Tell patient to stop drug at first sign of rash, which may precede severe hypersensitivity or other adverse reactions. Rash is more common in patients taking diuretics and in those with renal disorders. Tell patient to report all adverse reactions.
• Advise patient to avoid alcohol during therapy.
• Teach patient importance of continuing drug even if asymptomatic.

almotriptan malate
al-moh-TRIP-tan

Axert

Therapeutic class: Antimigraine drugs
Pharmacologic class: Serotonin 5-HT$_1$ receptor agonists

AVAILABLE FORMS
Tablets: 6.25 mg, 12.5 mg

INDICATIONS & DOSAGES
➤ **Acute migraine with or without aura**
Adults and adolescents ages 12 to 17: 6.25-mg or 12.5-mg tablet P.O., with one additional dose after 2 hours if headache is unresolved or recurs. Maximum, two doses (total of 25 mg) within 24 hours.
Adjust-a-dose: For patients with hepatic or renal impairment, initially 6.25 mg, with maximum daily dose of 12.5 mg.

ADMINISTRATION
P.O.
• Give drug without regard for food.
• Give only one repeat dose within 24 hours, no sooner than 2 hours after first dose.

ACTION
May act as an agonist at serotonin receptors on extracerebral intracranial blood vessels, which constricts the affected vessels, inhibits neuropeptide release, and reduces pain transmission in the trigeminal pathways.

Route	Onset	Peak	Duration
P.O.	1–3 hr	1–3 hr	Unknown

Half-life: 3 to 4 hours.

ADVERSE REACTIONS
CNS: paresthesia, headache, dizziness, somnolence.
GI: nausea, vomiting, dry mouth.

INTERACTIONS
Drug-drug. *Antiemetics (5-HT$_3$ antagonists), antipsychotics, metazolone, methylene blue, metoclopramide, opioid analgesics, tramadol:* May increase serotonergic effects and serotonin syndrome. Monitor therapy.
CYP3A4 inhibitors (such as ketoconazole): May increase almotriptan level. Monitor patient for potential adverse reaction. May need to reduce dosage. Avoid concomitant use in patients with renal or hepatic impairment.
Ergot-containing drugs, serotonin 5-HT$_{1B/1D}$ agonists: May cause additive effects. Avoid using within 24 hours of almotriptan.
MAO inhibitors, verapamil: May increase almotriptan level. No dose adjustment is necessary.
SSNRIs, SSRIs: May cause additive serotonin effects, resulting in weakness, hyperreflexia, or incoordination. Monitor patient closely if given together.

EFFECTS ON LAB TEST RESULTS
None reported.

CONTRAINDICATIONS & CAUTIONS
• Contraindicated in patients hypersensitive to drug.
• Contraindicated in patients with angina pectoris, history of MI, silent ischemia, coronary artery vasospasm, Prinzmetal variant angina, or other CV disease; uncontrolled hypertension; peripheral vascular disease, including ischemic bowel disease; cerebrovascular disease (history of stroke or TIA); and hemiplegic or basilar migraine.
• Don't give within 24 hours after treatment with other 5-HT$_{1B/1D}$ agonists or ergot derivatives.
• Use cautiously in patients with renal or hepatic impairment and in those with cataracts because of the potential for corneal opacities.
• Use cautiously in patients with risk factors for CAD, such as obesity, diabetes, and family history of CAD.

• Use cautiously in patients with known hypersensitivity to sulfonamides.
• Drug isn't intended for migraine prophylaxis or treatment of cluster headaches.
Dialyzable drug: Unknown.
⚠ *Overdose S&S:* Hypertension, more serious CV symptoms.

PREGNANCY-LACTATION-REPRODUCTION
• Use during pregnancy only if potential benefit justifies potential fetal risk.
• It isn't known if drug appears in breast milk. Use cautiously in breast-feeding women.

NURSING CONSIDERATIONS
• Patients with renal or hepatic impairment should receive a reduced dosage.
• Repeat dose after 2 hours, if needed, and don't give more than two doses (or 25 mg) in 24 hours.
• Consider obtaining ECG with first dose of drug in patients with positive CAD risk factors.
• Assess patients with signs and symptoms of angina after almotriptan dose for CAD and Prinzmetal or variant angina, including ECG monitoring.
❂ *Alert:* Combining triptans with SSRIs or SSNRIs may cause serotonin syndrome. Signs and symptoms include restlessness, hallucinations, loss of coordination, rapid heartbeat, rapid changes in BP, increased body temperature, overactive reflexes, nausea, vomiting, and diarrhea. Serotonin syndrome occurs more often when starting or increasing the dose of a triptan, SSRI, or SSNRI.
• *Look alike–sound alike:* Don't confuse Axert with Antivert.

PATIENT TEACHING
• Tell patient that drug can be taken with or without food.
• Advise patient to take drug only when he's having a migraine; explain that drug isn't taken on a regular schedule.
• Advise patient to use only one repeat dose within 24 hours, no sooner than 2 hours after first dose.
• Advise patient that other commonly prescribed migraine drugs can interact with almotriptan.

- Advise patient to report chest or throat tightness, pain, or heaviness.
- Teach patient to avoid possible migraine triggers, such as cheese, chocolate, citrus fruits, caffeine, and alcohol.

SAFETY ALERT!

alogliptin benzoate
AL-oh-GLIP-tin

Nesina

Therapeutic class: Antidiabetics
Pharmacologic class: DPP-4 inhibitors

AVAILABLE FORMS
Tablets: 6.25 mg, 12.5 mg, 25 mg

INDICATIONS & DOSAGES
➤ **Adjunct to diet and exercise to improve glycemic control in adults with type 2 diabetes**
Adults: 25 mg P.O. daily.
Adjust-a-dose: For patients with moderate renal impairment (CrCl of 30 to less than 60 mL/minute), give 12.5 mg P.O. daily. For patients with severe renal impairment (CrCl of 15 to less than 30 mL/minute) and for those with ESRD (CrCl of less than 15 mL/minute) or requiring hemodialysis, give 6.25 mg P.O. daily.

ADMINISTRATION
P.O.
- Give without regard for food.
- Store at room temperature.

ACTION
Slows inactivation of incretin, which increases blood concentrations of incretin and reduces fasting or postprandial glucose in patients with type 2 diabetes.

Route	Onset	Peak	Duration
P.O.	Unknown	1–2 hr	Unknown

Half-life: 21 hours.

ADVERSE REACTIONS
CNS: headache.
EENT: nasopharyngitis.
Metabolic: *hypoglycemia.*
Respiratory: URI.

INTERACTIONS
Drug-drug. *ACE inhibitors:* May enhance the adverse effects of ACE inhibitor, especially angioedema. Monitor therapy.
Androgens (except danazol), pegvisomant: May enhance hypoglycemic effect. Monitor therapy.
Danazol, fluoroquinolones, thiazide diuretics: May diminish hypoglycemic effect. Monitor therapy.
Insulin, sulfonylureas: May enhance hypoglycemic activity. Adjust dosage of insulin or sulfonylurea.
MAO inhibitors, salicylates, SSRIs: May cause hypoglycemia. Monitor therapy.

EFFECTS ON LAB TEST RESULTS
- May decrease glucose level.

CONTRAINDICATIONS & CAUTIONS
- Contraindicated in patients hypersensitive to drug or its components and in those with type 1 diabetes mellitus or ketoacidosis.
- Use cautiously in patients with liver disease or injury, history of pancreatitis, gallstones, history of alcoholism, renal disease, or history of angioedema with another dipeptidyl peptidase-4 inhibitor.
- ☻ *Alert:* Use cautiously in patients with a history of HF or renal disease. Drug may increase risk of HF in these patients.
Dialyzable drug: No.

PREGNANCY-LACTATION-REPRODUCTION
- Use cautiously in pregnant women and only if clearly needed.
- It isn't known if drug appears in breast milk. Use cautiously in breast-feeding women.

NURSING CONSIDERATIONS
- ☻ *Alert:* Monitor patient for signs and symptoms of HF (shortness of breath, orthopnea, tiredness, weakness, fatigue, weight gain, peripheral or abdominal edema). Drug may need to be discontinued and other antidiabetics may be needed.
- Assess renal function at baseline and periodically during treatment.
- Monitor patient for hypersensitivity reactions, including Stevens-Johnson syndrome (rare). Stop drug immediately if hypersensitivity is suspected.

• Monitor patient for signs and symptoms (rare) of acute pancreatitis (severe abdominal pain that may radiate to the back, with or without vomiting).
• Assess LFTs before treatment. If liver injury (rare) is suspected during treatment (fatigue, anorexia, abdominal discomfort, dark urine, jaundice), obtain LFTs. If elevated LFT values are present, persist, or worsen, withhold drug and determine probable cause. Restart drug only if cause isn't alogliptin-related.
• Monitor blood glucose level if patient is receiving concurrent antidiabetic medications; adjust dosages of these medications if needed.
☻ Alert: May cause joint pain that can be severe and disabling. Report severe and persistent joint pain to prescriber; drug may need to be discontinued.

PATIENT TEACHING
☻ Alert: Instruct patient to immediately report signs and symptoms of HF. Patient shouldn't stop drug without first discussing with prescriber.
• Instruct patient to monitor blood glucose level carefully.
• Advise patient to report respiratory symptoms to prescriber.
• Caution patient to seek medical attention for signs and symptoms of pancreatitis (severe abdominal pain that may radiate to the back, with or without vomiting) or liver injury (fatigue, anorexia, abdominal discomfort, dark urine, or jaundice).

SAFETY ALERT!

alprazolam
al-PRAH-zoe-lam

Apo-Alpraz✸, Apo-Alpraz TS✸, Xanax◆, Xanax XR

Therapeutic class: Anxiolytics
Pharmacologic class: Benzodiazepines
Controlled substance schedule: IV

AVAILABLE FORMS
ODTs: 0.25 mg, 0.5 mg, 1 mg, 2 mg
Oral solution: 1 mg/mL (concentrate)
Tablets: 0.25 mg, 0.5 mg, 1 mg, 2 mg

Tablets (extended-release) ⓞⓝⓒ: 0.5 mg, 1 mg, 2 mg, 3 mg

INDICATIONS & DOSAGES
Adjust-a-dose (for all indications): For debilitated patients or those with advanced hepatic disease, usual first dose is 0.25 mg P.O. b.i.d. or t.i.d. For extended-release tablets, 0.5 mg P.O. once daily.
➤ **Anxiety**
Adults: Usual first dose, 0.25 to 0.5 mg (immediate-release) P.O. t.i.d. Maximum, 4 mg daily in divided doses.
Elderly patients: Usual first dose, 0.25 mg P.O. b.i.d. or t.i.d. Maximum, 4 mg daily in divided doses. For extended-release tablets, 0.5 mg P.O. once daily. May increase gradually as needed and tolerated.
➤ **Panic disorders**
Adults: 0.5 mg P.O. t.i.d., increased at intervals of 3 to 4 days in increments of no more than 1 mg/day. Maximum, 10 mg daily in divided doses. For extended-release tablets, start with 0.5 to 1 mg P.O. once daily. Increase by no more than 1 mg/day every 3 to 4 days. Maximum daily dose, 10 mg.
Elderly patients: Usual first dose, 0.25 mg (immediate-release) P.O. b.i.d. or t.i.d. Maximum, 4 mg daily in divided doses.

ADMINISTRATION
P.O.
• Don't break or crush extended-release tablets.
• Mix oral solution with liquids or semisolid food, such as water, juices, carbonated beverages, applesauce, and puddings. Use only calibrated dropper provided with this product.
• Use dry hands to remove ODTs from bottle. Discard cotton from inside bottle.
• Discard unused portion if breaking scored ODT.
• Patients treated with divided doses of immediate-release tablets can be switched to extended-release tablets at same total daily dose. Patients should take extended-release tablets in the morning.

ACTION
Unknown. Probably potentiates the effects of GABA, depresses the CNS, and suppresses the spread of seizure activity.

Route	Onset	Peak	Duration
P.O.	Unknown	1–2 hr	Unknown
P.O. (extended-release)	Unknown	Unknown	Unknown

Half-life: Immediate-release, 12 to 15 hours; extended-release, 11 to 16 hours.

ADVERSE REACTIONS

CNS: insomnia, irritability, dizziness, headache, anxiety, confusion, drowsiness, light-headedness, sedation, somnolence, difficulty speaking, impaired coordination, memory impairment, fatigue, depression, *suicide,* mental impairment, ataxia, paresthesia, dyskinesia, hypoesthesia, lethargy, vertigo, malaise, tremor, nervousness, restlessness, agitation, nightmare, syncope, akathisia, mania.
CV: palpitations, chest pain, hypotension.
EENT: allergic rhinitis, blurred vision, nasal congestion.
GI: diarrhea, dry mouth, constipation, nausea, increased or decreased appetite, anorexia, vomiting, dyspepsia, abdominal pain.
GU: dysmenorrhea, sexual dysfunction, premenstrual syndrome, difficulty urinating.
Metabolic: increased or decreased weight.
Musculoskeletal: arthralgia, myalgia, arm or leg pain, back pain, muscle rigidity, muscle cramps, muscle twitch.
Respiratory: URI, dyspnea, hyperventilation.
Skin: pruritus, increased sweating, dermatitis.
Other: influenza, injury, emergence of anxiety between doses, dependence, feeling warm, increased or decreased libido.

INTERACTIONS

Drug-drug. *Anticonvulsants, antidepressants, antihistamines, barbiturates, benzodiazepines, general anesthetics, narcotics, phenothiazines, protease inhibitors:* May increase CNS depressant effects. Avoid using together.
Carbamazepine: May induce alprazolam metabolism and may reduce therapeutic effects. May need to increase dose.
Cimetidine, fluoxetine, fluvoxamine, hormonal contraceptives: May increase alprazolam level. Use cautiously together, and consider alprazolam dosage reduction.
CYP3A strong inhibitors (atazanavir, clarithromycin, fluconazole, indinavir, itraconazole, ketoconazole, miconazole, nelfinavir, ritonavir, saquinavir, telithromycin, voriconazole), delavirdine: May increase and prolong alprazolam level, CNS depression, and psychomotor impairment. Use together is contraindicated.
Hydantoins (phenytoin): May decrease effects of alprazolam and increase hydantoin levels. Monitor patient closely.
Methadone: May significantly increase risk of respiratory depression. Use together cautiously.
Black Box Warning *Opioids:* May cause slow or difficult breathing, sedation, and death. Avoid use together. If use together is necessary, limit dosage and duration of each drug to the minimum necessary for desired effect. ∎
Rifamycins (rifampin): May decrease effects of alprazolam. Alprazolam dosage increase may be needed.
TCAs (amitriptyline, doxepin, imipramine, nortriptyline): May increase levels of these drugs. Monitor patient closely.
Drug-herb. *Kava, valerian root:* May increase sedation. Discourage use together. *St. John's wort:* May decrease drug level. Discourage use together.
Drug-food. *Grapefruit juice:* May increase drug level. Discourage use together.
Drug-lifestyle. *Alcohol use:* May cause additive CNS effects. Discourage use together. *Smoking:* May decrease effectiveness of drug. Monitor patient closely.

EFFECTS ON LAB TEST RESULTS

● May increase ALT and AST levels.

CONTRAINDICATIONS & CAUTIONS

● Contraindicated in patients hypersensitive to drug or other benzodiazepines and in those with acute angle-closure glaucoma.
Black Box Warning Opioid drugs should only be prescribed with benzodiazepines or other CNS depressants to patients for whom alternative treatment options are inadequate. ∎
● Use cautiously in patients with hepatic, renal, or pulmonary disease or history of substance abuse.

• Use cautiously in elderly patients.
Dialyzable drug: No.
⚠ *Overdose S&S:* Somnolence, confusion, impaired coordination, diminished reflexes, coma.

PREGNANCY-LACTATION-REPRODUCTION
• Drug may cause fetal harm. Use isn't recommended during pregnancy.
• Drug appears in breast milk. Use isn't recommended in breast-feeding women.

NURSING CONSIDERATIONS
• The optimum duration of therapy is unknown.
• Give smallest effective dose to prevent ataxia or oversedation, especially in elderly or debilitated patients.
⟳ *Alert:* Don't withdraw drug abruptly; withdrawal symptoms, including seizures, may occur. Gradually reduce dosage. Abuse or addiction is possible.
• Monitor hepatic, renal, and hematopoietic function periodically in patients receiving repeated or prolonged therapy.
• Closely monitor addiction-prone patients.
⟳ *Alert:* Panic disorder is associated with major depressive disorders and increased reports of suicide among untreated patients. Monitor patients with depression for suicidal ideation or plans for suicide.
• Consider giving same total daily dose of immediate-release formulation in divided doses more frequently in patients being treated for panic disorder who experience early-morning anxiety or anxiety symptoms between doses.
• *Look alike–sound alike:* Don't confuse alprazolam with alprostadil or lorazepam. Don't confuse Xanax with Fanapt, Zantac, Xopenex, or Tenex.

PATIENT TEACHING
Black Box Warning Caution the patient or the caregiver of a patient taking an opioid drug with a benzodiazepine, CNS depressant, or alcohol to seek immediate medical attention if the patient has symptoms of dizziness, light-headedness, extreme sleepiness, slowed or difficult breathing, or unresponsiveness. ■

• Warn patient to avoid hazardous activities that require alertness and good coordination until effects of drug are known.
• Tell patient to avoid use of alcohol while taking drug.
• Advise patient that smoking may decrease drug's effectiveness.
• Warn patient not to stop drug abruptly because withdrawal symptoms or seizures may occur.
• Tell patient to swallow extended-release tablets whole.
• Tell patient using ODT to remove it from bottle using dry hands and to immediately place it on his tongue where it will dissolve and can be swallowed with saliva.
• Tell patient taking half a scored ODT to discard the unused half.
• Advise patient to discard the cotton from the bottle of ODTs and keep it tightly sealed to prevent moisture from dissolving the tablets.
• Warn women to avoid use during pregnancy and breast-feeding and to report pregnancy to prescriber.

SAFETY ALERT!

alprostadil (injection)
al-PROSS-ta-dil

Prostin VR Pediatric

Therapeutic class: Prostaglandins
Pharmacologic class: Prostaglandins

AVAILABLE FORMS
Injection: 500 mcg/mL

INDICATIONS & DOSAGES
➤ **Palliative therapy for temporary maintenance of patency of ductus arteriosus until surgery can be performed**
Neonates: 0.05 to 0.1 mcg/kg/minute by I.V. infusion. When therapeutic response is achieved, reduce infusion rate to lowest dose that will maintain response. Maximum dose is 0.4 mcg/kg/minute. Or, give drug through umbilical artery catheter placed at ductal opening.

ADMINISTRATION

I.V.

▼ Dilute drug before giving. Prepare fresh solution daily; discard solution after 24 hours.

▼ For infusion, dilute 1 mL of concentrate labeled as containing 500 mcg in 25 to 250 mL NSS or D_5W injection to yield a solution containing 2 to 20 mcg/mL.

▼ When using a device with a volumetric infusion chamber, add appropriate volume of diluent to the chamber; then add 1 mL of alprostadil concentrate.

▼ During dilution, avoid direct contact between concentrate and wall of plastic volumetric infusion chamber because solution may become hazy. If this occurs, discard solution.

▼ Don't use diluents that contain benzyl alcohol. Fatal toxic syndrome may occur.

▼ Drug isn't recommended for direct injection or intermittent infusion. Give by continuous infusion using an infusion pump. Infuse through a large peripheral or central vein or through an umbilical artery catheter placed at the level of the ductus arteriosus. If flushing from peripheral vasodilation occurs, reposition catheter.

▼ Reduce infusion rate if patient develops fever or significant hypotension.

▼ **Incompatibilities:** None reported.

ACTION

Relaxes smooth muscle of ductus arteriosus.

Route	Onset	Peak	Duration
I.V.	20 min	1–2 hr	Length of infusion

Half-life: About 5 to 10 minutes.

ADVERSE REACTIONS

CNS: fever, *seizures.*
CV: flushing, *bradycardia, cardiac arrest,* edema, hypotension, tachycardia.
GI: diarrhea.
Hematologic: *DIC.*
Metabolic: hypokalemia.
Respiratory: *apnea.*
Other: *sepsis.*

INTERACTIONS

Drug-drug. *PDE5 inhibitors:* May increase toxic effects of alprostadil. Don't use together.

EFFECTS ON LAB TEST RESULTS

● May decrease potassium level.

CONTRAINDICATIONS & CAUTIONS

● Contraindicated in patients hypersensitive to drug. Use cautiously in patients hypersensitive to other drugs in this class.

● Contraindicated in neonates before making differential diagnosis between respiratory distress syndrome and cyanotic heart disease; also contraindicated in those with respiratory distress syndrome.

● Use cautiously in neonates with bleeding tendencies because drug inhibits platelet aggregation.

Dialyzable drug: Unknown.

⚠ *Overdose S&S:* Apnea, bradycardia, pyrexia, hypotension, flushing.

PREGNANCY-LACTATION-REPRODUCTION

● Not indicated for use in women.

NURSING CONSIDERATIONS

Black Box Warning Apnea is most often seen in neonates weighing less than 2 kg at birth and usually appears during the first hour of drug infusion. Monitor respiratory status and keep emergency ventilatory support available. ■

● In infants with restricted pulmonary blood flow, measure drug's effectiveness by monitoring blood oxygenation. In infants with restricted systemic blood flow, measure drug's effectiveness by monitoring systemic BP and blood pH.

● Monitor arterial pressure by umbilical artery catheter, auscultation, or Doppler transducer. If arterial pressure falls significantly, slow infusion rate.

● Carefully monitor neonates receiving drug at recommended doses for longer than 120 hours for gastric outlet obstruction and antral hyperplasia.

● *Alert:* CV and CNS adverse reactions occur more often in infants weighing less than 2 kg and in those receiving infusions for longer than 48 hours.

● *Alert:* Stop infusion immediately if overdose is suspected.

● *Look alike–sound alike:* Don't confuse alprostadil with alprazolam.

PATIENT TEACHING
● Tell parents why this drug is needed, and explain its use.
● Encourage parents to ask questions and express concerns.

SAFETY ALERT!

alteplase
al-ti-PLAZE

Activase, Cathflo Activase

Therapeutic class: Thrombolytics
Pharmacologic class: Enzymes

AVAILABLE FORMS
Cathflo Activase injection: 2-mg single-patient vials
Injection: 50-mg (29 million international units) vials, 100-mg (58 million international units) vials

INDICATIONS & DOSAGES
➤ **Lysis of thrombi obstructing coronary arteries in acute MI (Activase)**
3-hour infusion
Adults weighing 65 kg or more: 100 mg by I.V. infusion over 3 hours, as follows: 60 mg in first hour, 6 to 10 mg of which is given as a bolus over first 1 to 2 minutes. Then 20 mg/hour infused for 2 hours.
Adults weighing less than 65 kg: 1.25 mg/kg in a similar fashion: 60% in first hour, 10% of which is given as a bolus; then 20% of total dose per hour for 2 hours. Don't exceed total dose of 100 mg.
Accelerated infusion
Adults weighing more than 67 kg: 100 mg maximum total dose. Give 15 mg I.V. bolus over 1 to 2 minutes, followed by 50 mg infused over the next 30 minutes; then 35 mg infused over the next hour. Don't exceed total dose of 100 mg.
Adults weighing 67 kg or less: 15 mg I.V. bolus over 1 to 2 minutes, followed by 0.75 mg/kg (not to exceed 50 mg) infused over the next 30 minutes; then 0.5 mg/kg (not to exceed 35 mg) infused over the next hour. Don't exceed total dose of 100 mg.
➤ **To manage acute massive PE (Activase)**
Adults: 100 mg by I.V. infusion over 2 hours. Begin heparin at end of infusion when PTT

or thrombin time returns to twice normal or less. Don't exceed 100-mg dose. Higher doses may increase risk of intracranial bleeding.
➤ **Acute ischemic stroke (Activase)**
Adults: 0.9 mg/kg by I.V. infusion over 1 hour with 10% of total dose given as an initial I.V. bolus over 1 minute. Maximum total dose is 90 mg.
➤ **To restore function to central venous access devices (Cathflo Activase)**
Adults and children older than age 2: For patients weighing more than 30 kg, instill 2 mg in 2 mL sterile water into catheter. For patients weighing between 10 and 30 kg, instill 110% of the internal lumen volume of the catheter, not to exceed 2 mg in 2 mL sterile water. After 30 minutes of dwell time, assess catheter function by aspirating blood. If function is restored, aspirate 4 to 5 mL of blood in patients weighing 10 kg or 3 mL in patients weighing less than 10 kg to remove drug and residual clot, and gently irrigate the catheter with NSS. If catheter function isn't restored after 120 minutes, instill a second dose.

ADMINISTRATION
I.V.
▼ Immediately before use, reconstitute solution with unpreserved sterile water for injection. Check manufacturer's labeling for specific information.
▼ Don't use 50-mg vial if vacuum isn't present; 100-mg vials don't have a vacuum.
▼ Using an 18G needle, direct stream of sterile water at lyophilized cake. Don't shake.
▼ Slight foaming is common. Let it settle before giving drug. Solution should be colorless or pale yellow.
▼ Drug may be given reconstituted (at 1 mg/mL) or diluted with an equal volume of NSS or D_5W to yield 0.5 mg/mL.
▼ Give drug using a controlled infusion device.
▼ Discard any unused drug after 8 hours.
Cathflo Activase
▼ Assess the cause of catheter dysfunction before using drug. Possible causes of occlusion include catheter malposition, mechanical failure, constriction by a suture, and lipid deposits or drug precipitates

---

Reactions in bold italics are *life-threatening*. Interactions may have a *rapid onset* or a ***delayed onset***.

in the catheter lumen. Don't try to suction the catheter because you risk damaging the vessel wall or collapsing a soft-walled catheter.

▼ Reconstitute Cathflo Activase with 2.2 mL sterile water to yield 1 mg/mL. Dissolve completely to produce a colorless to pale yellow solution. Don't shake.

▼ Don't use excessive pressure while instilling drug into catheter; doing so could rupture the catheter or expel a clot into circulation.

▼ Solution is stable for up to 8 hours at room temperature.

▼ **Incompatibilities:** Bivalirudin, dobutamine, dopamine, heparin, morphine, nitroglycerin. Consult detailed reference for other specific incompatibilities.

ACTION

Converts plasminogen to plasmin by directly cleaving peptide bonds at two sites, causing fibrinolysis.

Route	Onset	Peak	Duration
I.V.	Unknown	Unknown	Unknown

Half-life: Less than 10 minutes.

ADVERSE REACTIONS

CNS: *cerebral hemorrhage,* fever.
CV: *arrhythmias,* hypotension, edema, *cholesterol embolization, venous thrombosis.*
GI: *bleeding (Cathflo Activase),* nausea, vomiting.
GU: *bleeding.*
Hematologic: *spontaneous bleeding.*
Skin: ecchymosis.
Other: *anaphylaxis, sepsis (Cathflo Activase),* bleeding at puncture sites, hypersensitivity reactions.

INTERACTIONS

Drug-drug. *Aspirin, clopidogrel, dipyridamole, drugs affecting platelet activity (abciximab), heparin, warfarin, anticoagulants:* May increase risk of bleeding. Monitor patient carefully.
Nitroglycerin: May decrease alteplase antigen level. Avoid using together. If use together is unavoidable, use the lowest effective dose of nitroglycerin.

EFFECTS ON LAB TEST RESULTS

● May alter coagulation and fibrinolytic test results.

CONTRAINDICATIONS & CAUTIONS

● Contraindicated in patients hypersensitive to drug or its components.
● Activase therapy for acute MI or PE is contraindicated in patients with active internal bleeding; history of stroke; recent intracranial or intraspinal surgery or trauma; intracranial neoplasm, AV malformation, or aneurysm; known bleeding diathesis; or severe uncontrolled hypertension.
● Activase therapy for acute ischemic stroke is contraindicated in patients with evidence of intracranial hemorrhage; suspected subarachnoid hemorrhage; recent (within 3 months) intracranial or intraspinal surgery; serious head trauma or previous stroke; history of intracranial hemorrhage; uncontrolled hypertension (BP greater than 185 mm Hg systolic or 110 mm Hg diastolic) at time of treatment; seizure at onset of stroke; active internal bleeding; intracranial neoplasm, AV malformation, or aneurysm; bleeding diathesis (which may include current use of oral anticoagulants, INR greater than 1.7, PT longer than 15 seconds, platelet count less than 100,000/mm^3, current use of direct thrombin inhibitors or direct factor Xa inhibitors with elevated sensitive laboratory tests, or patients who have received heparin within the previous 48 hours and who at presentation have a prolonged aPTT).
● In patients with acute ischemic stroke, Activase may be initiated before available coagulation study results. The infusion should be discontinued if either a pretreatment INR is greater than 1.7 or a prolonged aPTT is identified.
● Patients with severe neurologic deficits (National Institutes of Health Stroke Scale greater than 22) or who have major early infarct signs on a CT scan may have increased risk of bleeding.
● Use cautiously in patients having major surgery within 10 days (when bleeding is difficult to control because of its location) and in those with previous puncture of a noncompressible vessel; concomitant oral anticoagulant therapy; organ biopsy; trauma

(including cardiopulmonary resuscitation); GI or GU bleeding; cerebrovascular disease; systolic pressure of 175 mm Hg or higher or diastolic pressure of 110 mm Hg or higher; mitral stenosis, atrial fibrillation, or other conditions that may lead to left heart thrombus; acute pericarditis or subacute bacterial endocarditis; hemostatic defects caused by hepatic or renal impairment; septic thrombophlebitis; or diabetic hemorrhagic retinopathy.

• Use cautiously in patients receiving anticoagulants and in patients age 75 and older.
Dialyzable drug: Unknown.

PREGNANCY-LACTATION-REPRODUCTION
• Information related to use in pregnant women is limited; most guidelines consider pregnancy to be a relative contraindication. Drug shouldn't be withheld from pregnant women in life-threatening situations but should be avoided if safer alternatives are available.
• It isn't known if drug appears in breast milk. Use cautiously in breast-feeding women.

NURSING CONSIDERATIONS
⚠ *Alert:* When used for acute ischemic stroke, give drug within 3 hours after symptoms occur and only when intracranial bleeding has been ruled out.
• Drug may be given to menstruating women.
• To recannulize occluded coronary arteries and improve heart function, begin treatment as soon as possible after symptoms start.
• Anticoagulant and antiplatelet therapy is commonly started during or after treatment, to decrease risk of another thrombosis.
• Monitor vital signs and neurologic status carefully. Keep patient on strict bed rest.
• Coronary thrombolysis is linked with arrhythmias caused by reperfusion of ischemic myocardium. Such arrhythmias don't differ from those commonly linked with MI. Have antiarrhythmics readily available, and carefully monitor ECG.
• Avoid invasive procedures, I.M. injections, and nonessential handling of the patient during thrombolytic therapy. Perform essential venipunctures carefully. Closely monitor patient for signs of internal bleed-

ing, and frequently check all puncture sites. Bleeding is the most common adverse effect and may occur internally and at external puncture sites.
• If an arterial puncture is necessary during Activase infusion, use an arm vessel that can be manually compressed. Apply pressure for at least 30 minutes followed by a pressure dressing. Check the site regularly for bleeding.
• If uncontrollable bleeding occurs, stop infusion (and heparin) and notify prescriber.
• *Look alike–sound alike:* Don't confuse alteplase with Altace or Activase with Cathflo Activase or TNKase.

PATIENT TEACHING
• Explain use and administration of drug to patient and family.
• Tell patient to report adverse reactions promptly and to immediately report signs and symptoms of bleeding, urinary problems, abdominal pain, nausea, vomiting, confusion, severe headache, one-sided weakness, trouble speaking or thinking, visual disturbances, dizziness, passing out, chest pain, or catheter-site pain.

alvimopan
al-VIM-oh-pan

Entereg

Therapeutic class: Bowel restorative drugs
Pharmacologic class: Peripherally acting mu-opioid receptor antagonists

AVAILABLE FORMS
Capsules: 12 mg

INDICATIONS & DOSAGES
➤ **Acceleration of recovery after partial large- or small-bowel resection surgery with primary anastomosis**
Adults: 12 mg P.O. 30 minutes to 5 hours before surgery, followed by 12 mg P.O. b.i.d. beginning day after surgery, for maximum of 15 in-hospital doses (180 mg).

ADMINISTRATION
P.O.
• May give with or without food.

ACTION

Competitively and selectively binds to mu-opioid receptors in GI tract, preventing peripheral effects of opioids on GI motility and secretion and thereby shortening recovery time after surgery.

Route	Onset	Peak	Duration
P.O.	Rapid	2 hr	Unknown

Half-life: 10 to 18 hours.

ADVERSE REACTIONS

GI: dyspepsia.
GU: urine retention.
Hematologic: anemia.
Metabolic: hypokalemia.
Musculoskeletal: back pain.

INTERACTIONS

None.

EFFECTS ON LAB TEST RESULTS

None.

CONTRAINDICATIONS & CAUTIONS

Black Box Warning Alvimopan is available only for short-term (15 doses) use in hospitalized patients. Only hospitals that have registered in and met all requirements for the Entereg Access Support and Education (E.A.S.E.) program may use alvimopan. ■
• Contraindicated in patients who have taken opioids for more than 7 days immediately before taking this drug.
• Not recommended in patients with severe renal or hepatic impairment, pancreatic or gastric anastomosis, or complete GI obstruction, or after surgery to correct complete bowel obstruction.
• Use cautiously in patients with history of recent opioid use.
Black Box Warning An increased incidence of MI was seen in a clinical trial of patients taking alvimopan and treated with opioids for chronic noncancer pain; however, a causal relationship hasn't been established. ■
Dialyzable drug: Unknown.

PREGNANCY-LACTATION-REPRODUCTION

• Use during pregnancy only if clearly needed.

• It isn't known if drug appears in breast milk. Use cautiously in breast-feeding women.

NURSING CONSIDERATIONS

• Drug is available only to hospitals that enroll in the E.A.S.E. program (1-866-423-6567). Hospitals that enroll must educate staff about limiting use to inpatients for maximum of 15 doses.
• Monitor GI status closely.
• Closely monitor patients with history of opioid use for chronic pain; drug is associated with increased incidence of MI in these patients.
• To avoid increasing sensitivity, take careful drug history to rule out recent opioid use. Signs and symptoms of increased sensitivity include abdominal pain, nausea, vomiting, and diarrhea.
• ***Look alike–sound alike:*** Don't confuse alvimopan with almotriptan.

PATIENT TEACHING

• Tell patient to report previous use of opioids, including in the week before surgery.
• Instruct patient to report all adverse effects, such as diarrhea, abdominal pain, nausea, vomiting, muscle pain, weakness, severe constipation, abnormal heartbeat, urine retention, and chest pain.
• Explain that drug is to be used only while in the hospital, for no more than 7 days after surgery.

---

amantadine hydrochloride
a-MAN-ta-deen

Therapeutic class: Antivirals
Pharmacologic class: Synthetic cyclic primary amines

AVAILABLE FORMS

Capsules: 100 mg
Syrup: 50 mg/5 mL
Tablets: 100 mg

INDICATIONS & DOSAGES

Adjust-a-dose (for all indications): For patients with CrCl of 30 to 50 mL/minute, 200 mg the first day and 100 mg thereafter;

if CrCl is 15 to 29 mL/minute, 200 mg the first day and then 100 mg on alternate days; if CrCl is less than 15 mL/minute or if patient is receiving hemodialysis, 200 mg every 7 days.

➤ **Parkinson disease**
Adults: Initially, if used as monotherapy, 100 mg P.O. b.i.d. In patients with serious illness or in those already receiving high doses of other antiparkinsonians, begin dose at 100 mg P.O. once daily. Increase to 100 mg b.i.d. if needed after at least 1 week. Some patients may benefit from 400 mg daily in divided doses.

➤ **To prevent or treat symptoms of influenza type A virus and respiratory tract illnesses**
Children age 13 and older and adults up to age 65: 200 mg P.O. daily as a single dose or 100 mg P.O. b.i.d.
Children ages 9 to 12: 100 mg P.O. b.i.d.
Children ages 1 to 8: 4.4 to 8.8 mg/kg P.O. as a total daily dose given once daily or in two equally divided doses. Maximum daily dose is 150 mg.
Elderly patients: 100 mg P.O. once daily in patients older than age 65 with normal renal function.

Begin treatment within 24 to 48 hours after symptoms appear and continue for 24 to 48 hours after symptoms disappear (usually 2 to 7 days). Start prophylaxis as soon as possible after exposure and continue for at least 10 days after exposure. May continue prophylactic treatment up to 90 days for repeated or suspected exposures if influenza vaccine is unavailable. If used with influenza vaccine, continue dose for 2 to 3 weeks until antibody response to vaccine has developed. Refer to Advisory Committee on Immunization Practices guidelines for use during current influenza season (www.cdc.gov/vaccines/acip).

➤ **Drug-induced extrapyramidal reactions**
Adults: 100 mg P.O. b.i.d. May increase to 300 mg daily in divided doses.

ADMINISTRATION
P.O.
● Give without regard for food.

ACTION
May exert its antiparkinsonian effect by causing the release of dopamine in the substantia nigra. As an antiviral, may prevent release of viral nucleic acid into the host cell, reducing duration of fever and other systemic symptoms.

Route	Onset	Peak	Duration
P.O.	Unknown	1½–8 hr	Unknown

Half-life: About 10 to 25 hours; with renal dysfunction, as long as 10 days.

ADVERSE REACTIONS
CNS: dizziness, insomnia, irritability, lightheadedness, depression, fatigue, confusion, hallucinations, anxiety, ataxia, headache, nervousness, dream abnormalities, agitation, somnolence.
CV: *HF,* peripheral edema, orthostatic hypotension.
EENT: blurred vision.
GI: nausea, anorexia, constipation, vomiting, dry mouth, diarrhea.
Skin: livedo reticularis.

INTERACTIONS
Drug-drug. *Anticholinergics:* May increase anticholinergic effects. Use together cautiously; reduce dosage of anticholinergic before starting amantadine.
CNS stimulants: May increase CNS stimulation. Use together cautiously.
Quinidine, sulfamethoxazole–trimethoprim, thiazide diuretics, triamterene: May increase amantadine level, increasing the risk of toxicity. Use together cautiously.
Thioridazine: May worsen Parkinson disease tremor. Monitor patient closely.
Drug-herb. *Jimsonweed:* May adversely affect CV function. Discourage use together.
Drug-lifestyle. *Alcohol use:* May increase CNS effects, including dizziness, confusion, and orthostatic hypotension. Discourage use together.

EFFECTS ON LAB TEST RESULTS
● May increase CK, BUN, creatinine, alkaline phosphatase, LDH, bilirubin, GGT, AST, and ALT levels.

CONTRAINDICATIONS & CAUTIONS
• Contraindicated in patients hypersensitive to drug.
• Use cautiously in elderly patients and in patients with seizure disorders, psychosis, impulse control disorders, HF, peripheral edema, hepatic disease, mental illness, eczematoid rash, renal impairment, orthostatic hypotension, and CV disease.
• Avoid use in patients with untreated angle-closure glaucoma.
Dialyzable drug: No.
⚠ *Overdose S&S:* Arrhythmia, hypertension, tachycardia, pulmonary edema, respiratory distress, increased BUN level, decreased CrCl, renal insufficiency, insomnia, anxiety, aggressive behavior, hypertonia, hyperkinesia, tremor, confusion, disorientation, depersonalization, fear, delirium, hallucinations, psychotic reactions, lethargy, somnolence, coma, seizures, hyperthermia.

PREGNANCY-LACTATION-REPRODUCTION
• Drug may cause fetal harm. Use during pregnancy only if potential benefit justifies potential risk to the fetus.
• Drug appears in breast milk. Use isn't recommended in breast-feeding women.

NURSING CONSIDERATIONS
• Patients with Parkinson disease who don't respond to anticholinergics may respond to this drug.
🌢 *Alert:* Elderly patients are more susceptible to adverse neurologic effects. Monitor patient for mental status changes.
🌢 *Alert:* Suicidal ideation and attempts may occur in any patient, regardless of psychiatric history.
🌢 *Alert:* Sporadic cases of neuroleptic malignant syndrome have been reported with dosage reduction or drug withdrawal. Observe patient carefully when dosage is abruptly reduced or drug is discontinued.
• Drug can worsen mental problems in patients with a history of psychiatric disorders or substance abuse.
• Monitor renal function tests and LFTs.
• *Look alike–sound alike:* Don't confuse amantadine with amiodarone, rimantadine, or ranitidine.

PATIENT TEACHING
🌢 *Alert:* Tell patient to take drug exactly as prescribed because not doing so may result in serious adverse reactions or death.
• If insomnia occurs, tell patient to take drug several hours before bedtime.
• If patient gets dizzy when he stands up, instruct him not to stand or change positions too quickly.
• Instruct patient to notify prescriber of adverse reactions, especially dizziness, depression, anxiety, nausea, and urine retention.
• Caution patient to avoid activities that require mental alertness until effects of drug are known.
• Encourage patient with Parkinson disease to gradually increase his physical activity as his symptoms improve.
• Advise patient to avoid alcohol while taking drug.

SAFETY ALERT!

ambrisentan
am-bree-SEN-tan

Letairis, Volibris ✦

Therapeutic class: Antihypertensives
Pharmacologic class: Endothelin-receptor antagonists

AVAILABLE FORMS
Tablets ⓓⓝⓒ: 5 mg, 10 mg

INDICATIONS & DOSAGES
➤ **Pulmonary arterial hypertension (World Health Organization group 1) in patients with functional class II (with significant exertion) or III (with mild exertion) symptoms to improve exercise tolerance and decrease rate of clinical worsening, in combination with tadalafil**
Adults: 5 mg P.O. once daily; may increase to 10 mg P.O. once daily if tolerated.

ADMINISTRATION
P.O.
• Drug is considered hazardous: use safe handling and disposal precautions according to facility policy.

- Give without regard for food.
- Give whole; don't crush or split tablets.

ACTION

Blocks endothelin-1 receptors on vascular endothelin and smooth muscle. Stimulation of these receptors in smooth muscle cells is associated with vasoconstriction and pulmonary artery hypertension.

Route	Onset	Peak	Duration
P.O.	Rapid	2 hr	Unknown

Half-life: 9 hours.

ADVERSE REACTIONS

CNS: asthenia, dizziness, fatigue.
CV: peripheral edema, flushing, *HF.*
EENT: nasal congestion, sinusitis.
GI: nausea, vomiting.
Hematologic: anemia.
Hepatic: hepatic impairment.
Respiratory: *pulmonary arterial hypertension.*
Other: hypersensitivity reaction (*angioedema*), rash).

INTERACTIONS

Drug-drug. *Cyclosporine:* May increase ambrisentan levels. Use together cautiously. Limit ambrisentan dosage to 5 mg daily.
Rifampin: May increase ambrisentan area under the curve. Use together cautiously.
Drug-herb. *St. John's wort:* May decrease ambrisentan level. Avoid use together.
Drug-food. *Grapefruit juice:* May increase levels and effects of ambrisentan. Advise patient to avoid grapefruit products.

EFFECTS ON LAB TEST RESULTS

- May increase AST, ALT, and bilirubin levels.
- May decrease Hb level and hematocrit.

CONTRAINDICATIONS & CAUTIONS

- Contraindicated in patients hypersensitive to drug or its components and in those with idiopathic pulmonary fibrosis, including patients with pulmonary hypertension.
- Use cautiously in patients with mild hepatic impairment. Not recommended in patients with moderate or severe hepatic impairment.

- Use cautiously in those with renal impairment; drug hasn't been studied in those with severe renal impairment.
- **Alert:** Patients who develop acute pulmonary edema during initial treatment may have pulmonary veno-occlusive disease. Discontinue drug if pulmonary veno-occlusive disease is confirmed.
Dialyzable drug: Unknown.
Overdose S&S: Headache, flushing, dizziness, nausea, nasal congestion, hypotension.

PREGNANCY-LACTATION-REPRODUCTION

Black Box Warning May cause birth defects. Contraindicated in pregnant women. ∎
Black Box Warning Pregnancy must be excluded before therapy is begun. Obtain monthly pregnancy tests during treatment and 1 month after discontinuation. ∎
Black Box Warning Women of childbearing potential must use two reliable methods of contraception during treatment and for 1 month after treatment ends. ∎
Black Box Warning Because of risk of birth defects, ambrisentan is available only through the Letairis Risk Evaluation and Mitigation Strategy (REMS). Only registered prescribers and pharmacies may prescribe and dispense ambrisentan and only to patients enrolled in and meeting all the conditions of REMS at www.letairisrems.com or 1-866-664-5327. ∎
- It isn't known if drug appears in breast milk. Patient should discontinue breastfeeding or discontinue drug.

NURSING CONSIDERATIONS

- Treat women of childbearing potential only after negative pregnancy tests.
- Assess Hb level at initiation, at 1 month, and periodically thereafter. Use isn't recommended in patients with significant anemia.

PATIENT TEACHING

Black Box Warning Inform female patient that she'll need to have a pregnancy test done monthly and to report suspected pregnancy to her prescriber immediately. ∎
Alert: Teach woman of childbearing potential to use two reliable birth control methods unless she has had tubal sterilization or has a Copper T 380A intrauterine device (IUD) or an LNg 20 IUD inserted.

Reactions in bold italics are *life-threatening.* Interactions may have a *rapid onset* or a *delayed onset.*

- Tell patient that monthly blood tests will be done to monitor for adverse effects.
- Advise patient to take the tablet whole and not to split, crush, or chew it.

❶ Alert: Teach patient to notify prescriber immediately of signs or symptoms of liver injury, including anorexia, nausea, vomiting, fever, malaise, fatigue, right upper quadrant abdominal discomfort, itching, and jaundice.

- Tell the patient to report edema and weight gain.
- Inform male patient of potential for decreased sperm count.

amikacin sulfate
am-i-KAY-sin

Therapeutic class: Antibiotics
Pharmacologic class: Aminoglycosides

AVAILABLE FORMS
Injection: 50-mg/mL (pediatric) vial, 250-mg/mL vial, 250-mg/mL disposable syringe

INDICATIONS & DOSAGES
Adjust-a-dose (for all indications): For adults with impaired renal function, initially, 7.5 mg/kg I.M. or I.V. Subsequent doses and frequency determined by amikacin levels and renal function studies. For adults receiving hemodialysis, give supplemental doses of 50% of initial loading dose at end of each dialysis session. Monitor drug levels and adjust dosage accordingly.

➤ **Serious infections caused by sensitive strains of *Pseudomonas aeruginosa, Escherichia coli, Proteus, Klebsiella*, or *Staphylococcus***
Adults and children: Maximum dosage is 15 mg/kg/day I.M. or I.V. infusion, in divided doses every 8 to 12 hours, for 7 to 10 days.
Neonates: Initially, loading dose of 10 mg/kg I.V.; then 7.5 mg/kg every 12 hours for 7 to 10 days.

➤ **Uncomplicated UTI caused by organisms not susceptible to less toxic drugs**
Adults: 250 mg I.M. or I.V. b.i.d.

ADMINISTRATION
I.V.
▼ Obtain specimen for culture and sensitivity tests before giving first dose. Begin therapy while awaiting results.
▼ For adults, dilute I.V. drug in 100 to 200 mL of D_5W or NSS. For children, the amount of fluid will depend on the ordered dose.
▼ In adults and children, infuse over 30 to 60 minutes. In infants, infuse over 1 to 2 hours.
▼ After infusion, flush line with NSS or D_5W.
▼ **Incompatibilities:** Allopurinol, aminophylline, amphotericin B, ampicillin, azithromycin, bacitracin, cefazolin, ceftazidime, chlorothiazide sodium, cisplatin, heparin sodium, hetastarch in 0.9% sodium chloride, oxacillin, phenytoin, propofol, thiopental, vancomycin, vitamin B complex with vitamin C. Don't administer with other drugs.

I.M.
- Obtain specimen for culture and sensitivity tests before giving first dose. Begin therapy while awaiting results.
- Obtain blood for peak level 1 hour after I.M. injection and 30 minutes to 1 hour after I.V. infusion ends; for trough levels, draw blood just before next dose. Don't collect blood in a heparinized tube; heparin is incompatible with aminoglycosides.

ACTION
Inhibits protein synthesis by binding directly to the 30S ribosomal subunit; bactericidal.

Route	Onset	Peak	Duration
I.V.	Immediate	30 min	8–12 hr
I.M.	Unknown	1 hr	8–12 hr

Half-life: Adults, 2 hours; patients with severe renal damage, 17 to 150 hours.

ADVERSE REACTIONS
CNS: *neuromuscular blockade.*
EENT: ototoxicity.
GU: azotemia, *nephrotoxicity,* increase in urinary excretion of casts.
Respiratory: *apnea.*

INTERACTIONS
Drug-drug. `Black Box Warning` *Acyclovir, amphotericin B, bacitracin, cephaloridine, cisplatin, colistin, paromomycin, polymixin B, vancomycin, viomycin, other aminoglycosides:* May increase nephrotoxicity. Avoid use together and monitor renal function test results. ∎

Dimenhydrinate: May mask ototoxicity symptoms. Monitor patient's hearing.
`Black Box Warning` *General anesthetics:* May increase neuromuscular blockade. Monitor patient for increased effects. ∎
Indomethacin: May increase trough and peak amikacin levels. Avoid administering together. Monitor amikacin level.
`Black Box Warning` *I.V. loop diuretics (ethacrynic acid, furosemide):* May increase ototoxicity. Avoid use together and monitor patient's hearing. ∎
`Black Box Warning` *Neuromuscular blockers:* May increase effects of nondepolarizing muscle relaxants, including prolonged respiratory depression. Use together only when necessary, and expect to reduce dosage of nondepolarizing muscle relaxant. ∎
NSAIDs: May increase amikacin level. Avoid administering together.
Parenteral penicillins: May inactivate amikacin in vitro. Don't mix.

EFFECTS ON LAB TEST RESULTS
● May increase BUN, creatinine, nonprotein nitrogen, and urine urea levels.

CONTRAINDICATIONS & CAUTIONS
● Contraindicated in patients hypersensitive to drug or other aminoglycosides.
● Use cautiously in patients with sulfite sensitivity.
● Use cautiously in patients with impaired renal function, hypocalcemia, neuromuscular disorders (myasthenia gravis, parkinsonism), or hearing impairment; neonates and infants; and elderly patients.
● Drug can cause superinfection such as CDAD, which can be severe and can occur more than 2 months after therapy ends.
Dialyzable drug: Yes.
⚠ **Overdose S&S:** Nephrotoxicity, ototoxicity, neurotoxicity.

PREGNANCY-LACTATION-REPRODUCTION
● There are no well-controlled studies in pregnant women. Other aminoglycosides can cause fetal harm. Not recommended in pregnant women. If drug is used during pregnancy, or if patient becomes pregnant while taking drug, patient should be apprised of potential hazard to the fetus.
● Drug appears in breast milk. Not recommended in breast-feeding women.

NURSING CONSIDERATIONS
`Black Box Warning` Due to increased risk of ototoxicity, evaluate patient's hearing before and during therapy if he'll be receiving the drug for longer than 2 weeks. Notify prescriber if patient has tinnitus, vertigo, or hearing loss. ∎
`Black Box Warning` Weigh patient and review renal function studies before and periodically during therapy. ∎
● Correct dehydration before therapy because of increased risk of toxicity.
`Black Box Warning` Monitor serum amikacin peak and trough concentrations periodically during therapy. Peak drug levels greater than 35 mcg/mL and trough levels greater than 10 mcg/mL may be linked to a higher risk of toxicity. ∎
`Black Box Warning` Due to increased risk of nephrotoxicity, monitor renal function: urine output, specific gravity, urinalysis, BUN and creatinine levels, and CrCl. Report evidence of declining renal function to prescriber. Safe use for longer than 14 days hasn't been established. ∎
● Watch for signs and symptoms of superinfection (especially of upper respiratory tract), such as continued fever, chills, and increased pulse rate.
`Black Box Warning` Neuromuscular blockade and respiratory paralysis have been reported after aminoglycoside administration, especially in patients receiving anesthetics, neuromuscular blockers, or massive transfusions of citrate-anticoagulated blood. If blockade occurs, calcium salts may reverse these phenomena, but mechanical ventilation may be necessary. Monitor patient closely. ∎
● Therapy usually continues for 7 to 10 days. If no response occurs after 3 to

5 days, stop therapy and obtain new specimens for culture and sensitivity testing.
- *Look alike–sound alike:* Don't confuse amikacin with anakinra.

PATIENT TEACHING
- Instruct patient to promptly report all adverse reactions, especially changes in urine, weight gain, edema, hearing impairment, fever, diarrhea, and abdominal pain.
- Warn patient about risks to fetus if drug is taken during pregnancy and to report possible pregnancy to prescriber immediately.
- Encourage patient to maintain adequate fluid intake.

amiloride hydrochloride
a-MILL-oh-ride

Midamor✲

Therapeutic class: Diuretics
Pharmacologic class: Potassium-sparing diuretics

AVAILABLE FORMS
Tablets: 5 mg

INDICATIONS & DOSAGES
➤ **Hypertension; hypokalemia; edema of HF, usually in patients also taking thiazide or other potassium-wasting diuretics**
Adults: 5 mg P.O. daily, increased to 10 mg daily if needed. If hypokalemia persists with 10 mg, dosage can be increased to 15 mg, then 20 mg with careful monitoring of electrolyte levels.

ADMINISTRATION
P.O.
- Give with food to minimize GI upset.

ACTION
Inhibits sodium reabsorption and potassium excretion in the distal tubules.

Route	Onset	Peak	Duration
P.O.	2 hr	6–10 hr	24 hr

Half-life: 6 to 9 hours.

ADVERSE REACTIONS
CNS: dizziness, fatigue, headache, weakness, *encephalopathy.*
GI: abdominal pain, anorexia, appetite changes, constipation, diarrhea, nausea, vomiting.
GU: erectile dysfunction.
Metabolic: hyperkalemia.
Musculoskeletal: muscle cramps.
Respiratory: cough, dyspnea.

INTERACTIONS
Drug-drug. *ACE inhibitors, indomethacin, other potassium-sparing diuretics, potassium supplements:* May cause severe hyperkalemia. Avoid use together if possible. Monitor potassium level closely if using together.
Digoxin: May decrease digoxin clearance and decrease inotropic effects. Monitor digoxin level.
Lithium: May decrease lithium clearance, increasing risk of lithium toxicity. Monitor lithium level.
NSAIDs: May decrease diuretic effectiveness. Avoid use together.
Drug-food. *Foods high in potassium (such as bananas, oranges), salt substitutes containing potassium:* May cause hyperkalemia. Advise patient to choose diet carefully and to use low-potassium salt substitutes.

EFFECTS ON LAB TEST RESULTS
- May increase BUN and potassium levels. May decrease pH, Hb, and liver enzyme and sodium levels.
- May decrease neutrophil count.

CONTRAINDICATIONS & CAUTIONS
- Contraindicated in patients hypersensitive to drug, in those with potassium level greater than 5.5 mEq/L, and in those with anuria, acute or chronic renal insufficiency, or diabetic nephropathy.
- Contraindicated in patients receiving potassium supplementation or other potassium-sparing diuretics, such as spironolactone and triamterene.
- Use cautiously in patients with diabetes mellitus, cardiopulmonary disease, or severe hepatic insufficiency.

● Use cautiously in elderly or debilitated patients.
● Safety and effectiveness in children haven't been established.
Dialyzable drug: Unknown.
⚠ *Overdose S&S:* Dehydration, electrolyte imbalance.

PREGNANCY-LACTATION-REPRODUCTION
● Use during pregnancy only if clearly needed.
● It isn't known if drug appears in breast milk. Patient should discontinue breast-feeding or discontinue drug.

NURSING CONSIDERATIONS
● To prevent nausea, give with meals.
`Black Box Warning` Carefully monitor potassium level because of the risk of hyperkalemia, especially in patients with renal impairment or diabetes and in elderly patients. Monitor potassium level when drug is initiated, when diuretic dosages are adjusted, and during an illness that could affect renal function. Alert prescriber immediately if potassium level exceeds 5.5 mEq/L; expect to stop drug. ∎
● Drug may cause severe hyperkalemia after glucose tolerance testing in patients with diabetes; stop drug at least 3 days before testing.
● *Look alike–sound alike:* Don't confuse amiloride with amiodarone or amlodipine.

PATIENT TEACHING
● Instruct patient to take drug with food to minimize GI upset.
● Advise patient to avoid sudden posture changes and to rise slowly to avoid dizziness.
● Caution patient not to perform hazardous activities if adverse CNS reactions occur.
● To prevent serious hyperkalemia, warn patient to avoid eating potassium-rich foods, potassium-containing salt substitutes, and potassium supplements.
● Advise patient to report signs of hyperkalemia, such as tingling, muscle weakness, muscle cramps, fatigue, and limb paralysis.
● Instruct patient to check with prescriber before taking new prescriptions or OTC drugs.

SAFETY ALERT!

amiodarone hydrochloride
am-ee-OH-dah-rohn

Cordarone, Nexterone, Pacerone

Therapeutic class: Antiarrhythmics
Pharmacologic class: Benzofuran derivatives

AVAILABLE FORMS
Injection: 50 mg/mL, 150 mg/100 mL, 360 mg/200 mL
Tablets: 100 mg, 200 mg, 300 mg, 400 mg

INDICATIONS & DOSAGES
`Black Box Warning` Amiodarone is intended for use only in patients with life-threatening recurrent ventricular fibrillation or recurrent hemodynamically unstable ventricular tachycardia unresponsive to adequate doses of other antiarrhythmics or when alternative drugs can't be tolerated. ∎
➤ **Prevention of recurrent life-threatening ventricular arrhythmias, such as ventricular fibrillation or hemodynamically unstable ventricular tachycardia**
Adults: Give loading dose of 800 to 1,600 mg P.O. daily or divided into two equal doses daily for 1 to 3 weeks until first therapeutic response occurs; then 600 to 800 mg P.O. daily for 1 month, followed by maintenance dose of 400 mg P.O. daily or, for patients with severe GI intolerance, 200 mg P.O. b.i.d. Determine long-term maintenance dose according to antiarrhythmic effect.
   Or, give loading dose of 150 mg I.V. over 10 minutes (15 mg/minute); then 360 mg I.V. over next 6 hours (1 mg/minute), followed by 540 mg I.V. over next 18 hours (0.5 mg/minute). After first 24 hours, continue with maintenance I.V. infusion of 720 mg/24 hours (0.5 mg/minute).
   Maintenance infusion can continue cautiously for 2 to 3 weeks. To convert to oral form from I.V.: If I.V. infusion has been for less than 1 week, initial dose is 800 to 1,600 mg P.O. daily; if I.V. infusion has been from 1 to 3 weeks, initial dose is 600 to 800 mg P.O. daily; if I.V. infusion has been

more than 3 weeks, initial dose is 400 mg P.O. daily.

If breakthrough episodes of ventricular fibrillation or hemodynamically unstable ventricular tachycardia occur, may give supplemental infusions of 150 mg I.V. over 10 minutes.

ADMINISTRATION
P.O.
• Divide oral loading dose into two or three equal doses and give with meals to decrease GI intolerance. Give maintenance dose once daily or divide into two doses with meals to decrease GI intolerance.

I.V.
▼ Give drug I.V. only if continuous ECG and electrophysiologic monitoring are available.
▼ Mix first dose of 150 mg in 100 mL of D₅W solution.
▼ If infusion will last 2 hours or longer, mix solution in glass or polyolefin bottles.
▼ If concentration is 2 mg/mL or more, give drug through a central line. If possible, use a dedicated line.
▼ Use an in-line filter.
▼ Continuously monitor patient's cardiac status. If hypotension occurs, reduce infusion rate.
▼ I.V. amiodarone leaches out plasticizers from I.V. tubing and adsorbs to polyvinyl chloride (PVC) tubing, which can adversely affect male reproductive tract development in fetuses, infants, and toddlers when used at concentrations or flow rates outside of recommendations.
▼ **Incompatibilities:** Aminophylline, ampicillin sodium–sulbactam sodium, bivalirudin, cefazolin sodium, ceftazidime, digoxin, furosemide, heparin sodium, imipenem–cilastatin sodium, magnesium sulfate, nitroprusside sodium, NSS, piperacillin sodium, piperacillin–tazobactam sodium, quinidine gluconate, sodium bicarbonate, sodium phosphates.

ACTION
Effects result from blockade of potassium chloride, leading to a prolongation of action potential duration.

Route	Onset	Peak	Duration
P.O.	Variable	3–7 hr	Variable
I.V.	Unknown	Unknown	Variable

Half-life: 15 to 142 days.

ADVERSE REACTIONS
CNS: fatigue, malaise, tremor, peripheral neuropathy, ataxia, paresthesia, insomnia, sleep disturbances, headache, dizziness.
CV: hypotension, *asystole,* atrial fibrillation, *bradycardia, arrhythmias, HF, heart block, sinus arrest,* edema, flushing.
EENT: asymptomatic corneal microdeposits, visual disturbances, optic neuropathy or neuritis resulting in visual impairment, abnormal smell.
GI: nausea, vomiting, abnormal taste, anorexia, constipation, abdominal pain, diarrhea.
Hematologic: *coagulation abnormalities.*
Hepatic: *hepatic failure,* hepatic dysfunction.
Metabolic: hypothyroidism, hyperthyroidism.
Respiratory: *ARDS, severe pulmonary toxicity, pulmonary edema, eosinophilic pneumonitis.*
Skin: photosensitivity, solar dermatitis, blue-gray skin.
Other: decreased libido.

INTERACTIONS
Drug-drug. *Antiarrhythmics:* May reduce hepatic or renal clearance of certain antiarrhythmics, especially flecainide, procainamide, and quinidine. Use of amiodarone with other antiarrhythmics, especially mexiletine, propafenone, disopyramide, and procainamide, may induce torsades de pointes. Avoid using together.
Azole antifungals, disopyramide, pimozide: May increase the risk of arrhythmias, including torsades de pointes. Avoid using together.
Beta blockers, calcium channel blockers: May potentiate bradycardia, sinus arrest, and AV block; may increase hypotensive effect. Use together cautiously.
Cimetidine: May increase amiodarone level. Use together cautiously.
Cyclosporine: May increase cyclosporine level, resulting in an increase in the serum

creatinine level and renal toxicity. Monitor cyclosporine levels and renal function tests.
Dabigatran: May increase bleeding risk. Monitor patient closely.
Digoxin: May increase digoxin level 70% to 100%. Monitor digoxin level closely, and reduce digoxin dosage by half or stop drug completely when starting amiodarone therapy.
Fentanyl: May cause hypotension, bradycardia, and decreased cardiac output. Monitor patient closely.
Fluoroquinolones: May increase risk of arrhythmias, including torsades de pointes. Avoid using together.
HMG-CoA reductase inhibitors (such as simvastatin): May cause myopathy or rhabdomyolysis. Monitor patient carefully.
Loratadine, trazodone: May cause prolonged QT interval and torsades de pointes. Monitor closely.
Macrolide antibiotics (azithromycin, clarithromycin, erythromycin, telithromycin): May cause additive prolongation of the QT interval. Use with caution. Avoid use with telithromycin.
Methotrexate: May impair methotrexate metabolism, causing toxicity. Use together cautiously.
Phenytoin: May decrease phenytoin metabolism and amiodarone level. Monitor phenytoin level and adjust dosages of drugs if needed.
Protease inhibitors (amprenavir, atazanavir, indinavir, lopinavir–ritonavir, nelfinavir, ritonavir, saquinavir): May increase the risk of amiodarone toxicity. Use of ritonavir or nelfinavir with amiodarone is contraindicated. Use other protease inhibitors cautiously.
Quinidine: May increase quinidine level, causing life-threatening cardiac arrhythmias. Avoid using together, or monitor quinidine level closely if use together can't be avoided. Adjust quinidine dosage as needed.
Rifamycins: May decrease amiodarone level. Monitor patient closely.
Simvastatin: May cause myopathy and rhabdomyolysis with concomitant use. Simvastatin dosage shouldn't exceed 20 mg daily.
Theophylline: May increase theophylline level and cause toxicity. Monitor theophylline level.

Warfarin: May increase anticoagulant response, with the potential for serious or fatal bleeding. Decrease warfarin dosage 33% to 50% when starting amiodarone. Monitor patient closely.
St. John's wort: May decrease amiodarone levels. Discourage use together.
Drug-food. *Grapefruit juice:* May inhibit CYP3A4 metabolism of drug in the intestinal mucosa, causing increased levels and risk of toxicity. Discourage use together.
Drug-lifestyle. *Sun exposure:* May cause photosensitivity reaction. Advise patient to avoid excessive sunlight exposure and to take precautions while in the sun.

EFFECTS ON LAB TEST RESULTS
● May increase alkaline phosphatase, ALT, AST, GGT, reverse T_3, and T_4 levels. May decrease T_3 level.
● May increase total cholesterol and serum lipid levels.
● May prolong PT and increase INR.

CONTRAINDICATIONS & CAUTIONS
● Contraindicated in patients hypersensitive to drug or to iodine.
● Contraindicated in those with cardiogenic shock, second- or third-degree AV block, severe SA node disease resulting in bradycardia unless an artificial pacemaker is present, and in those for whom bradycardia has caused syncope.
● Use cautiously in patients receiving other antiarrhythmics. Upon starting amiodarone, attempt to gradually discontinue prior antiarrhythmics.
● Use cautiously in patients with pulmonary, hepatic, or thyroid disease.
🔊 **Alert:** Avoid use in patients with Wolff-Parkinson-White syndrome and preexcited atrial fibrillation or flutter.
Dialyzable drug: Unknown.
⚠ **Overdose S&S:** AV block, bradycardia, hypotension, cardiogenic shock, hepatotoxicity.

PREGNANCY-LACTATION-REPRODUCTION
● Drug may cause fetal harm. Use during pregnancy only to treat life-threatening or refractory arrhythmias.
● Drug appears in breast milk. Contraindicated in breast-feeding women.

Reactions in bold italics are *life-threatening*. Interactions may have a *rapid onset* or a ***delayed onset***.

NURSING CONSIDERATIONS

• Be aware of the high risk of adverse reactions.

• Obtain baseline pulmonary, liver, and thyroid function test results and baseline chest X-ray.

🔾 *Alert:* Drug may cause hyperthyroidism or hypothyroidism. Hyperthyroidism can result in fatal thyrotoxicosis or arrhythmia. If hyperthyroidism or hypothyroidism occurs, reduce dosage or discontinue drug. Thyroid nodules and thyroid cancer have been reported. Use cautiously in patients with thyroid disease. Monitor thyroid function during treatment, particularly in elderly patients and those with underlying thyroid dysfunction.

Black Box Warning Give loading doses in a hospital setting and with continuous ECG monitoring because of the slow onset of antiarrhythmic effect and the risk of life-threatening arrhythmias. ■

Black Box Warning Drug may pose life-threatening management problems in patients at risk for sudden death. Use only in patients with life-threatening, recurrent ventricular arrhythmias unresponsive to or intolerant of other antiarrhythmics or alternative drugs. ■

Black Box Warning Drug is highly toxic. Watch carefully for pulmonary toxicity. Risk increases in patients receiving doses over 400 mg/day. Liver injury is also common and is usually mild but has been fatal in a few cases. ■

• Watch for evidence of pneumonitis, exertional dyspnea, nonproductive cough, and pleuritic chest pain. Monitor pulmonary function tests and chest X-ray.

• Correct electrolyte imbalances before start of therapy and throughout treatment.

• Monitor liver and thyroid function test results and electrolyte levels, particularly potassium and magnesium.

• Monitor PT and INR if patient takes warfarin and digoxin level if he takes digoxin.

• Instill methylcellulose ophthalmic solution during amiodarone therapy to minimize corneal microdeposits. About 1 to 4 months after starting amiodarone, most patients develop corneal microdeposits, although 10% or less have vision disturbances. Regular ophthalmic examinations are advised.

• Monitor BP and HR and rhythm frequently. Perform continuous ECG monitoring when starting or changing dosage. Notify prescriber of significant change in assessment results.

🔾 *Alert:* Patients may continue to be at risk for drug-related adverse reactions or drug interactions after discontinuation of amiodarone.

🔾 *Alert:* May cause life-threatening or fatal reactions, including Stevens-Johnson syndrome and toxic epidermal necrolysis. Discontinue drug immediately if such signs or symptoms as progressive rash with blisters or mucosal lesions occur.

• Safety and effectiveness in children haven't been established. Life-threatening gasping syndrome may occur in neonates given I.V. solutions containing benzyl alcohol.

• During or after treatment with I.V. form, patient may be transferred to oral therapy.

• *Look alike–sound alike:* Don't confuse amiodarone with amiloride. Don't confuse Cordarone with Cardura.

PATIENT TEACHING

• Advise patient to wear sunscreen or protective clothing to prevent sensitivity reaction to the sun. Monitor patient for skin burning or tingling, followed by redness and blistering. Exposed skin may turn blue-gray.

• Advise patient to keep follow-up appointments, including eye exams and blood tests.

• Tell patient to report vision changes, weakness, "pins and needles" or numbness, poor coordination, weight change, heat or cold intolerance, neck swelling, progressive rash, or mucosal lesions.

• Tell patient to take oral drug with food if GI reactions occur.

• Inform patient that adverse effects of drug are more common at high doses and become more frequent with treatment lasting longer than 6 months, but are generally reversible when drug is stopped. Resolution of adverse reactions may take up to 4 months.

• Tell patient not to stop taking this medication without consulting with prescriber.

amitriptyline hydrochloride
a-mee-TRIP-ti-leen

Elavil ✤, Levate ✤

Therapeutic class: Antidepressants
Pharmacologic class: TCAs

AVAILABLE FORMS
Tablets: 10 mg, 25 mg, 50 mg, 75 mg,
100 mg, 150 mg

INDICATIONS & DOSAGES
➤ **Depression (outpatients)**
Adults: 75 mg P.O. daily in divided doses.
Or, 25 to 50 mg P.O. daily as single dose at
bedtime or in divided doses. May increase
by 25 to 50 mg, as needed, to a total of
150 mg/day. Make increases preferably in
late afternoon or at bedtime. Continue for at
least 3 months. Maintenance, 40 to 100 mg
daily.
Elderly patients and adolescents: 10 mg
P.O. t.i.d. and 20 mg at bedtime daily.
➤ **Depression (hospitalized patients)**
Adults: Initially, 100 mg P.O. daily. If necessary, gradually increase to 200 to 300 mg
daily. Maintenance dose is 40 to 100 mg
daily. Continue for at least 3 months.
➤ **Postherpetic neuralgia ◆**
Adults: 65 to 100 mg P.O. daily for at least
3 weeks.

ADMINISTRATION
P.O.
● Give drug without regard for food.

ACTION
Unknown. A TCA that increases the amount
of norepinephrine, serotonin, or both in
the CNS by blocking their reuptake by the
presynaptic neurons.

Route	Onset	Peak	Duration
P.O.	Unknown	2–5 hr	Unknown

Half-life: 13 to 36 hours.

ADVERSE REACTIONS
CNS: *stroke, seizures, coma,* ataxia, tremor,
peripheral neuropathy, anxiety, insomnia,
restlessness, drowsiness, dizziness, weakness, fatigue, headache, extrapyramidal
reactions, hallucinations, delusions, disorientation.
CV: orthostatic hypotension, tachycardia, *heart block, arrhythmias, MI,* ECG
changes, hypertension, edema, palpitations,
syncope.
EENT: blurred vision, mydriasis, increased
IOP, tinnitus.
GI: dry mouth, nausea, vomiting, anorexia,
epigastric pain, diarrhea, constipation,
paralytic ileus.
GU: urine retention, altered libido, erectile
dysfunction.
Hematologic: *agranulocytosis, thrombocytopenia, leukopenia,* eosinophilia.
Metabolic: *hypoglycemia,* hyperglycemia.
Skin: rash, urticaria, photosensitivity reac-
tions, diaphoresis.
Other: hypersensitivity reactions.

INTERACTIONS
Drug-drug. *Barbiturates:* May increase
amitriptyline metabolism. Consider therapy
modification.
CNS depressants: May enhance CNS depression. Avoid using together.
Cimetidine: May decrease TCA
metabolism. Monitor therapy.
Disulfiram: May increase pharmacologic
effects of amitriptyline. May cause acute
organic brain syndrome. Monitor patient.
Stop amitriptyline or decrease amitriptyline
dosage if an interaction is suspected.
Epinephrine, norepinephrine: May increase
hypertensive effect. Use together cautiously.
**Fluoxetine, fluvoxamine, hormonal con-
traceptives, paroxetine, sertraline:** May
increase TCA level. Consider therapy modification.
Linezolid, methylene blue: May cause serotonin syndrome. Avoid combination.
MAO inhibitors: May cause severe excitation, hyperpyrexia, or seizures, usually with
high doses. Avoid using within 14 days of
MAO inhibitor therapy.
Quinolones: May increase the risk of life-
threatening arrhythmias. Monitor therapy.
Drug-herb. *SAM-e, St. John's wort,
yohimbe:* May cause serotonin syndrome
and decrease amitriptyline level. Discourage
use together.
Drug-lifestyle. *Alcohol use:* May enhance
CNS depression. Discourage use together.

Smoking: May lower drug level. Watch for lack of effect.

Sun exposure: May increase risk of photosensitivity reactions. Advise patient to avoid excessive sunlight exposure.

EFFECTS ON LAB TEST RESULTS
• May increase or decrease glucose level.
• May increase eosinophil count and LFT values.
• May decrease granulocyte, platelet, and WBC counts.

CONTRAINDICATIONS & CAUTIONS
• Contraindicated in patients hypersensitive to drug, in those who have received an MAO inhibitor within the past 14 days, and in the acute MI recovery phase.
🟢 *Alert:* Concomitant use with linezolid or methylene blue can cause serotonin syndrome (fever, mental status changes, muscle twitching, excessive sweating, shivering or shaking, diarrhea, loss of coordination). Use drug with linezolid or methylene blue only for life-threatening or urgent conditions when the potential benefits outweigh the risks of toxicity.
Black Box Warning Drug isn't approved for use in children younger than age 12. ∎
• Use cautiously in patients with history of seizures, urine retention, angle-closure glaucoma, or increased IOP; in those with hyperthyroidism, CV disease, diabetes, or impaired liver function; and in those receiving thyroid drugs.
• Use cautiously in elderly patients and in patients with suicidal ideation.
• Use cautiously in those receiving electroconvulsive therapy.
Dialyzable drug: No.
⚠ *Overdose S&S:* Cardiac arrhythmias, severe hypotension, seizures, CNS depression, impaired myocardial contractility, confusion, disturbed concentration, transient visual hallucinations, dilated pupils, disorders of ocular motility, agitation, hyperactive reflexes, polyradiculoneuropathy, stupor, drowsiness, muscle rigidity, vomiting, hypothermia.

PREGNANCY-LACTATION-REPRODUCTION
• There are no adequate and well-controlled studies in pregnant women. Use during pregnancy only if potential benefit outweighs potential risk to the fetus.
• Drug appears in breast milk. Patient should discontinue breast-feeding or discontinue drug.

NURSING CONSIDERATIONS
Black Box Warning Drug may increase the risk of suicidal thinking and behavior in children, adolescents, and young adults with major depressive disorder or other psychiatric disorder. Don't use in children younger than age 12. ∎
🟢 *Alert:* If linezolid or methylene blue must be given, amitriptyline must be stopped and the patient should be monitored for serotonin toxicity for 2 weeks, or until 24 hours after the last dose of methylene blue or linezolid, whichever comes first. Treatment with amitriptyline may be resumed 24 hours after last dose of methylene blue or linezolid.
• Amitriptyline has strong anticholinergic effects and is one of the most sedating TCAs. Anticholinergic effects have rapid onset even though therapeutic effect is delayed for weeks.
• Elderly patients may have an increased sensitivity to anticholinergic effects of drug; sedating effects of drug may increase the risk of falls in this population.
• If signs or symptoms of psychosis occur or increase, expect prescriber to reduce dosage. Record mood changes. Monitor patient for suicidal tendencies and allow only minimum supply of drug.
• Because patients using TCAs may suffer hypertensive episodes during surgery, stop drug gradually several days before surgery.
• Monitor glucose level.
• Watch for nausea, headache, and malaise after abrupt withdrawal of long-term therapy; these symptoms don't indicate addiction.
• Don't withdraw drug abruptly.
• *Look alike–sound alike:* Don't confuse amitriptyline with nortriptyline or aminophylline. Don't confuse Elavil with Eldepryl or enalapril.

PATIENT TEACHING
Black Box Warning Advise families and caregivers to closely observe patient for increased suicidal thinking and behavior. ∎

🌢 *Alert:* Teach patient to recognize and immediately report symptoms of serotonin toxicity (fever, mental status changes, muscle twitching, excessive sweating, shivering or shaking, diarrhea, loss of coordination).

• Whenever possible, advise patient to take full dose at bedtime, but warn him of possible morning orthostatic hypotension.

• Tell patient to avoid alcohol during drug therapy.

• Advise patient to consult prescriber before taking other drugs.

• Warn patient to avoid activities that require alertness and good psychomotor coordination until CNS effects of drug are known. Drowsiness and dizziness usually subside after a few weeks.

• Inform patient that dry mouth may be relieved with sugarless hard candy or gum. Saliva substitutes may be useful.

• To prevent photosensitivity reactions, advise patient to use a sunblock, wear protective clothing, and avoid prolonged exposure to strong sunlight.

• Warn patient not to stop drug abruptly.

• Advise patient that it may take as long as 30 days to achieve full therapeutic effect.

---

amlodipine besylate
am-LOE-di-peen

Norvasc◆

Therapeutic class: Antihypertensives
Pharmacologic class: Calcium channel blockers

AVAILABLE FORMS
Tablets: 2.5 mg, 5 mg, 10 mg

INDICATIONS & DOSAGES
➤ **Chronic stable angina, vasospastic angina (Prinzmetal or variant angina); to reduce risk of hospitalization because of angina; to reduce risk of coronary revascularization procedure in patients with recently documented CAD by angiography and without HF or with LVEF less than 40%**
Adults: Initially, 5 to 10 mg P.O. daily. Most patients need 10 mg daily.
Elderly patients: Initially, 5 mg P.O. daily.

Adjust-a-dose: For patients who are small or frail or have hepatic insufficiency, initially, 5 mg P.O. daily.
➤ **Hypertension**
Adults: Initially, 5 mg P.O. daily. Dosage adjusted according to patient response and tolerance. Titration should occur over 7 to 14 days. Maximum daily dose is 10 mg.
Children ages 6 to 17: 2.5 to 5 mg P.O. once daily. Maximum dosage is 5 mg daily.
Elderly patients: Initially, 2.5 mg P.O. daily.
Adjust-a-dose: For patients who are small or frail, are taking other antihypertensives, or have hepatic insufficiency, initially, 2.5 mg P.O. daily.

ADMINISTRATION
P.O.
• Give without regard for food.

ACTION
Inhibits calcium ion influx across cardiac and smooth-muscle cells, dilates coronary arteries and arterioles, and decreases BP and myocardial oxygen demand.

Route	Onset	Peak	Duration
P.O.	Unknown	6–12 hr	24 hr

Half-life: 30 to 50 hours.

ADVERSE REACTIONS
CNS: headache, somnolence, fatigue, dizziness.
CV: edema, flushing, palpitations.
GI: nausea, abdominal pain.
Respiratory: *pulmonary edema,* dyspnea.
Skin: pruritus, rash.

INTERACTIONS
Drug-drug. *Conivaptan, CYP3A4 strong inhibitors (itraconazole, ketoconazole, ritonavir):* May increase amlodipine plasma concentration. Monitor patient for hypotension and edema.
Cyclosporine: May increase cyclosporine level. Monitor level and patient.
Simvastatin: May increase risk of myopathy, including rhabdomyolysis. Simvastatin dosage shouldn't exceed 20 mg daily.

EFFECTS ON LAB TEST RESULTS
None reported.

Reactions in bold italics are *life-threatening*. Interactions may have a *rapid onset* or a ***delayed onset***.

CONTRAINDICATIONS & CAUTIONS
• Contraindicated in patients hypersensitive to drug.
• Use cautiously in patients receiving other peripheral vasodilators, especially those with severe aortic stenosis or hypertrophic cardiomyopathy with outflow tract obstruction, and in patients with HF with reduced LVEF. Because drug is metabolized by the liver, use cautiously and in reduced dosage in patients with severe hepatic disease.
Dialyzable drug: No.
⚠ *Overdose S&S:* Marked peripheral vasodilation with hypotension and possibly reflex tachycardia.

PREGNANCY-LACTATION-REPRODUCTION
• Use in pregnancy only if potential benefit justifies the risk to the fetus. Other antihypertensives are preferred during pregnancy.
• It isn't known if drug appears in breast milk. Patient should discontinue breastfeeding or discontinue drug.

NURSING CONSIDERATIONS
⚕ *Alert:* Monitor patient carefully. Some patients, especially those with severe obstructive CAD, have developed increased frequency, duration, or severity of angina or acute MI after initiation of calcium channel blocker therapy or at time of dosage increase.
• Monitor BP frequently during initiation of therapy. Because drug-induced vasodilation has a gradual onset, acute hypotension is rare.
• Notify prescriber if signs of HF occur, such as swelling of hands and feet or shortness of breath.
⚕ *Alert:* Abrupt withdrawal of drug may increase frequency and duration of chest pain. Taper dose gradually under medical supervision.
• *Look alike–sound alike:* Don't confuse amlodipine with amiloride.

PATIENT TEACHING
• Caution patient to continue taking drug, even when he feels better.
• Tell patient S.L. nitroglycerin may be taken as needed when angina symptoms are acute. If patient continues nitrate therapy

during adjustment of amlodipine dosage, urge continued compliance.

---

amoxicillin
a-moks-i-SIL-in

Amox ✤, Amoxil, Apo-Amoxi ✤, Larotid, Moxatag, Novamoxin ✤

Therapeutic class: Antibiotics
Pharmacologic class: Aminopenicillins

AVAILABLE FORMS
Capsules: 250 mg, 500 mg
Oral suspension: 50 mg/mL (pediatric drops), 125 mg/5 mL, 200 mg/5 mL, 250 mg/5 mL, 400 mg/5 mL (after reconstitution)
Tablets: 500 mg, 875 mg
Tablets (chewable): 125 mg, 200 mg, 250 mg, 400 mg
Tablets (extended-release) ⓄⓃⒸ: 775 mg

INDICATIONS & DOSAGES
Adjust-a-dose (for all indications): Adults with GFR of less than 30 mL/minute shouldn't receive the 875-mg tablet. Adults with GFR of 10 to 30 mL/minute should receive 250 or 500 mg every 12 hours depending on the infection. Adults with GFR of less than 10 mL/minute should receive 250 or 500 mg every 24 hours depending on the severity of infection. Adults on hemodialysis should receive 250 or 500 mg every 24 hours with an extra dose both during and at the end of dialysis.
➤ **Mild to moderate infections of the ear, nose, and throat; skin and skin structure; or GU tract**
Adults and children weighing 40 kg or more: 500 mg P.O. every 12 hours or 250 mg P.O. every 8 hours.
Children older than age 3 months weighing less than 40 kg: 25 mg/kg/day P.O. divided every 12 hours or 20 mg/kg/day P.O. divided every 8 hours.
Neonates and infants up to age 3 months: Up to 30 mg/kg/day P.O. divided every 12 hours.
➤ **Mild to severe infections of the lower respiratory tract and severe infections of**

---

the ear, nose, and throat; skin and skin structure; or GU tract
Adults and children weighing 40 kg or more: 875 mg P.O. every 12 hours or 500 mg P.O. every 8 hours.
Children older than age 3 months weighing less than 40 kg: 45 mg/kg/day P.O. divided every 12 hours or 40 mg/kg/day P.O. divided every 8 hours.
Neonates and infants up to age 3 months: Up to 30 mg/kg/day P.O. divided every 12 hours.
➤ **Pharyngitis, tonsillitis, or both secondary to *Streptococcus pyogenes* infection**
Adults and children age 12 and older: 775-mg extended-release tablet P.O. once daily with a meal for 10 days.
➤ **Uncomplicated gonorrhea**
Adults and children weighing more than 45 kg: 3 g P.O. given as a single dose.
Children age 2 and older weighing less than 45 kg: 50 mg/kg to a maximum of 3 g P.O. with 25 mg/kg of probenecid, to a maximum of 1 g, as a single dose. Don't give probenecid to children younger than age 2.
➤ *Helicobacter pylori* **eradication to reduce risk of duodenal ulcer recurrence**
Adults: Amoxicillin 1 g with lansoprazole 30 mg P.O. every 8 hours for 14 days (dual therapy). Or, amoxicillin 1 g, clarithromycin 500 mg, and lansoprazole 30 mg, all given P.O. every 12 hours for 14 days (triple therapy).
➤ **Acute otitis media ♦**
Children age 6 and older with mild to moderate infection: 80 to 90 mg/kg P.O. daily for 5 to 7 days.
Children younger than age 6 and those with severe infection: 80 to 90 mg/kg P.O. daily for 10 days.

ADMINISTRATION
P.O.
● Before giving, ask patient about allergic reactions to penicillin. A negative history of penicillin allergy is no guarantee against allergic reaction.
● Obtain specimen for culture and sensitivity tests before giving first dose. Begin therapy while awaiting results.

● Give drug with or without food, except for extended-release tablets, which are given within 1 hour of finishing a meal.
● Don't crush or split extended-release tablets.
● For a child, place drops directly on child's tongue for swallowing or add to formula, milk, fruit juice, water, ginger ale, or other cold drink for immediate and complete consumption.
● Store reconstituted oral suspension in refrigerator, if possible. Be sure to check individual product labels for storage information.

ACTION
Inhibits cell-wall synthesis during bacterial multiplication.

Route	Onset	Peak	Duration
P.O.	Unknown	1–2 hr	6–8 hr

Half-life: 1 to 1½ hours (7½ hours in severe renal impairment).

ADVERSE REACTIONS
CNS: *seizures,* anxiety, confusion, agitation, dizziness, reversible hyperactivity, anxiety, insomnia, behavioral changes.
GI: diarrhea, nausea, ***pseudomembranous colitis,*** vomiting.
GU: interstitial nephritis, nephropathy.
Hematologic: *agranulocytosis, leukopenia, thrombocytopenia, thrombocytopenic purpura,* anemia, eosinophilia, hemolytic anemia.
Other: *anaphylaxis,* hypersensitivity reactions, overgrowth of nonsusceptible organisms.

INTERACTIONS
Drug-drug. *Beta blockers:* May potentiate anaphylactic reactions. Monitor patient.
Hormonal contraceptives: May decrease contraceptive effectiveness. Advise use of additional form of contraception during penicillin therapy.
Live-virus vaccines: May decrease effectiveness of live-virus vaccines. Concurrent use isn't recommended.
Methotrexate: May increase methotrexate serum concentration. Monitor patient closely for toxicity.

Reactions in bold italics are *life-threatening*. Interactions may have a *rapid onset* or a *delayed onset*.

Probenecid: May increase levels of amoxicillin and other penicillins. Probenecid may be used for this purpose.

Drug-herb. *Khat:* May decrease antimicrobial effect of certain penicillins. Discourage khat chewing, or tell patient to take drug 2 hours after khat chewing.

EFFECTS ON LAB TEST RESULTS
● May increase AST and ALT levels.
● May decrease Hb level.
● May increase eosinophil count. May decrease granulocyte, platelet, and WBC counts.
● May falsely decrease aminoglycoside level. May alter results of urine glucose tests that use cupric sulfate, such as Benedict reagent and Clinitest.
● May cause transient decrease in total conjugated estriol, estriol glucuronide, conjugated estrone, and estradiol in pregnant women.

CONTRAINDICATIONS & CAUTIONS
● Contraindicated in patients hypersensitive to drug or other penicillins.
● Use cautiously in patients with other drug allergies (especially to cephalosporins) because of possible cross-sensitivity.
● Use cautiously in those with mononucleosis because of high risk of maculopapular rash.
Dialyzable drug: Yes.
⚠ *Overdose S&S:* Oliguric renal failure.

PREGNANCY-LACTATION-REPRODUCTION
● Use during pregnancy only if clearly needed.
● Drug appears in breast milk. Use cautiously in breast-feeding women.

NURSING CONSIDERATIONS
● If large doses are given or if therapy is prolonged, bacterial or fungal superinfection may occur, especially in elderly, debilitated, or immunosuppressed patients.
● CDAD, ranging from mild diarrhea to fatal colitis, has been reported with nearly all antibacterial agents, including amoxicillin. Evaluate patient if diarrhea occurs.
● Amoxicillin usually causes fewer cases of diarrhea than ampicillin.

● ***Look alike–sound alike:*** Don't confuse amoxicillin with amoxapine.

PATIENT TEACHING
● Tell patient to take entire quantity of drug exactly as prescribed, even after he feels better.
● Instruct patient to take drug with or without food, except extended-release tablets, which are taken with a meal.
● Tell patient to swallow extended-release tablets whole and not to chew, crush, or split them.
● Tell patient to notify prescriber if rash, fever, or chills develop. A rash is the most common allergic reaction, especially if allopurinol is also being taken.
● Tell parent to place drops directly on child's tongue for swallowing or add to formula, milk, fruit juice, water, ginger ale, or other cold drink for immediate and complete consumption.

amoxicillin–clavulanate potassium
a-mox-i-SILL-in/KLAV-yu-lah-nate

Augmentin, Augmentin ES 600, Augmentin XR, Clavulin ✣

Therapeutic class: Antibiotics
Pharmacologic class: Aminopenicillins–beta-lactamase inhibitors

AVAILABLE FORMS
Oral suspension: 125 mg amoxicillin trihydrate, 31.25 mg clavulanic acid/5 mL (after reconstitution); 200 mg amoxicillin trihydrate, 28.5 mg clavulanic acid/5 mL (after reconstitution); 250 mg amoxicillin trihydrate, 62.5 mg clavulanic acid/5 mL (after reconstitution); 400 mg amoxicillin trihydrate, 57 mg clavulanic acid/5 mL (after reconstitution); 600 mg amoxicillin trihydrate, 42.9 mg clavulanic acid/5 mL (after reconstitution)
Tablets (chewable): 125 mg amoxicillin trihydrate, 31.25 mg clavulanic acid; 200 mg amoxicillin trihydrate, 28.5 mg clavulanic acid; 250 mg amoxicillin trihydrate, 62.5 mg clavulanic acid; 400 mg amoxicillin trihydrate, 57 mg clavulanic acid

Tablets (extended-release) ⓄⓉⒸ: 1,000 mg amoxicillin trihydrate, 62.5 mg clavulanic acid

Tablets (film-coated): 250 mg amoxicillin trihydrate, 125 mg clavulanic acid; 500 mg amoxicillin trihydrate, 125 mg clavulanic acid; 875 mg amoxicillin trihydrate, 125 mg clavulanic acid

INDICATIONS & DOSAGES

➤ **Recurrent or persistent acute otitis media caused by** *Streptococcus pneumoniae, Haemophilus influenzae,* **or** *Moraxella catarrhalis* **in patients exposed to antibiotics within the previous 3 months, who are age 2 or younger or in day-care facilities**

Children age 3 months and older:
90 mg/kg/day (600 mg amoxicillin/ 42.9 mg clavulanic acid/5 mL) P.O., based on amoxicillin component, every 12 hours for 10 days.

➤ **Lower respiratory tract infections, otitis media, sinusitis, skin and skin-structure infections, and UTIs caused by susceptible strains of gram-positive and gram-negative organisms**

Adults and children weighing 40 kg or more: 250 mg P.O., based on amoxicillin component, every 8 hours; or 500 mg every 12 hours. For more severe infections, 500 mg every 8 hours or 875 mg every 12 hours.

Children age 3 months and older and weighing less than 40 kg: 20 to 45 mg/kg P.O., based on amoxicillin component and severity of infection, daily in divided doses every 8 to 12 hours.

Children younger than age 3 months: 30 mg/kg/day P.O., based on amoxicillin component of the 125-mg/5-mL oral suspension, in divided doses every 12 hours.

Adjust-a-dose: Don't give the 875-mg tablet to patients with CrCl of less than 30 mL/minute. If CrCl is 10 to 30 mL/minute, give 250 to 500 mg P.O. every 12 hours. If CrCl is less than 10 mL/minute, give 250 to 500 mg P.O. every 24 hours. Give hemodialysis patients 250 to 500 mg P.O. every 24 hours with an additional dose both during and after dialysis.

➤ **Community-acquired pneumonia or acute bacterial sinusitis caused by** *H. influenzae, M. catarrhalis, H. parainfluenzae, Klebsiella pneumoniae,* **methicillin-susceptible** *Staphylococcus aureus,* **or** *S. pneumoniae* **with reduced susceptibility to penicillin**

Adults and children age 16 and older: 2,000 mg/125 mg Augmentin XR tablets every 12 hours for 7 to 10 days for pneumonia; 10 days for sinusitis.

Adjust-a-dose: In patients with CrCl less than 30 mL/minute and patients receiving hemodialysis, don't use Augmentin XR.

ADMINISTRATION
P.O.
• Before giving drug, ask patient about allergic reactions to penicillin. A negative history of penicillin allergy is no guarantee against an allergic reaction.
• Obtain specimen for culture and sensitivity tests before giving first dose. Begin therapy while awaiting results.
• Give drug at the start of a meal to enhance absorption.
• Give drug at least 1 hour before a bacteriostatic antibiotic.
• Avoid use of 250-mg tablet in children weighing less than 40 kg . Use chewable form instead.
• After reconstitution, refrigerate the oral suspension; discard after 10 days.

ACTION
Prevents bacterial cell-wall synthesis during replication. Increases amoxicillin's effectiveness by inactivating beta-lactamases, which destroy amoxicillin.

Route	Onset	Peak	Duration
P.O.	Unknown	1–2½ hr	6–8 hr
P.O. (600 mg amoxicillin/ 42.9 mg clavulanic acid)	Unknown	1–4 hr	Unknown
P.O. (Augmentin XR)	Unknown	1–6 hr	Unknown

Half-life: 1 to 1½ hours. For patients with severe renal impairment, 7½ hours for amoxicillin and 4½ hours for clavulanate.

ADVERSE REACTIONS

CNS: agitation, anxiety, behavioral changes, confusion, dizziness, insomnia, headache.

GI: nausea, vomiting, diarrhea, indigestion, gastritis, stomatitis, glossitis, black hairy tongue, enterocolitis, *pseudomembranous colitis,* mucocutaneous candidiasis, abdominal pain.

GU: vaginal candidiasis, vaginitis.

Hematologic: anemia, *thrombocytopenia, thrombocytopenic purpura,* eosinophilia, *leukopenia, agranulocytosis.*

Other: hypersensitivity reactions, *anaphylaxis,* pruritus, rash, urticaria, *angioedema,* overgrowth of nonsusceptible organisms, serum sickness–like reaction.

INTERACTIONS

Drug-drug. *Allopurinol:* May increase risk of rash. Monitor patient for rash.

Hormonal contraceptives: May decrease hormonal contraceptive effectiveness. Advise use of additional form of contraception during penicillin therapy.

Methotrexate: May increase risk of methotrexate toxicity. Monitor methotrexate levels.

Oral anticoagulants (warfarin): May prolong PT. Monitor PT closely during coadministration.

Probenecid: May increase levels of amoxicillin and other penicillins. Use together isn't recommended.

Tetracyclines: May reduce therapeutic action of penicillins. Avoid administering together.

Drug-herb. *Khat:* May decrease antimicrobial effect of certain penicillins. Discourage khat chewing, or tell patient to take amoxicillin 2 hours after khat chewing.

EFFECTS ON LAB TEST RESULTS

● May decrease platelet, leukocyte, and granulocyte counts. May increase or decrease eosinophil count.

● May falsely decrease aminoglycoside level.

● May alter results of urine glucose tests that use cupric sulfate, such as Benedict reagent and Clinitest.

CONTRAINDICATIONS & CAUTIONS

● Contraindicated in patients hypersensitive to drug or other penicillins and in those with a history of amoxicillin-related cholestatic jaundice or hepatic dysfunction.

● Use cautiously in patients with other drug allergies (especially to cephalosporins) because of possible cross-sensitivity.

● Augmentin XR is contraindicated in patients receiving hemodialysis and those with CrCl of less than 30 mL/minute.

● Use cautiously in patients with hepatic dysfunction.

● Drug may increase risk of hepatic dysfunction (hepatitis, cholestatic jaundice), especially in elderly patients, males, and patients on prolonged treatment.

● Don't give ampicillin-class antibiotics to patients with mononucleosis due to high incidence of erythematous rash.

Dialyzable drug: Yes.

⚠ Overdose S&S: Crystalluria, oliguric renal failure, GI symptoms, rash, hyperactivity or drowsiness.

PREGNANCY-LACTATION-REPRODUCTION

● Use during pregnancy only if clearly needed.

● Drug appears in breast milk. Use cautiously in breast-feeding women.

NURSING CONSIDERATIONS

● Each Augmentin XR tablet contains 29.3 mg (1.27 mEq) of sodium.

● Augmentin XR isn't indicated for treating infections caused by *S. pneumoniae* with penicillin minimum inhibitory concentration, or MIC, of 4 mcg/mL or greater.

● If large doses are given or therapy is prolonged, bacterial or fungal superinfection may occur, especially in elderly, debilitated, or immunosuppressed patients.

● CDAD, ranging from mild diarrhea to fatal colitis, has been reported with nearly all antibacterial agents, including amoxicillin–clavulanate. Evaluate patient if diarrhea occurs.

● Chewable tablets and powder for oral solution contain phenylalanine.

● Monitor LFTs periodically in patients with hepatic impairment. Discontinue drug if signs of hepatitis occur.

◑ Alert: Don't interchange the oral suspensions because of varying clavulanic acid contents.

• 600 mg amoxicillin/42.9 mg clavulanic acid/5 mL is intended only for children ages 3 months to 12 years with persistent or recurrent acute otitis media.

◑ Alert: Both 250- and 500-mg film-coated tablets contain the same amount of clavulanic acid (125 mg). Therefore, two 250-mg tablets aren't equivalent to one 500-mg tablet. Regular tablets aren't equivalent to Augmentin XR.

• This drug combination is particularly useful in clinical settings with a high prevalence of amoxicillin-resistant organisms.

• **Look alike–sound alike:** Don't confuse amoxicillin with amoxapine or Azulfidine.

PATIENT TEACHING

• Tell patient to take entire quantity of drug exactly as prescribed, even after feeling better.

• Instruct patient to take drug with food to prevent GI upset. If he's taking the oral suspension, tell him to keep drug refrigerated, to shake it well before taking it, and to discard remaining drug after 10 days.

• Tell patient to call prescriber if a rash occurs because rash is a sign of an allergic reaction.

SAFETY ALERT!

amphotericin B lipid complex
am-foe-TER-i-sin

Abelcet

Therapeutic class: Antifungals
Pharmacologic class: Polyene antibiotics

AVAILABLE FORMS
Suspension for injection: 100 mg/20-mL vial

INDICATIONS & DOSAGES
➤ **Invasive fungal infections, including *Aspergillus* and *Candida* species, in patients refractory to or intolerant of conventional amphotericin B therapy**

Adults and children: 5 mg/kg daily I.V. as a single infusion given at rate of 2.5 mg/kg/hour.

Adjust-a-dose: For patients with CrCl of less than 10 mL/minute, give 5 mg/kg every 24 to 36 hours.

ADMINISTRATION
I.V.
▼ To prepare, shake vial gently until there's no yellow sediment. Using aseptic technique, withdraw calculated dose into one or more 20-mL syringes using an 18G needle. More than one vial will be needed.

▼ Attach a 5-micron filter needle to syringe and inject dose into I.V. bag of D_5W. Volume of D_5W should be sufficient to yield 1 mg/mL (2 mg/mL for pediatric and CV patients). One filter needle can be used for up to four vials of amphotericin B lipid complex.

▼ Don't use an in-line filter.

▼ If infusing through an existing I.V. line, flush first with D_5W.

▼ Use an infusion pump, and give by continuous infusion at 2.5 mg/kg/hour.

▼ If infusion time exceeds 2 hours, mix contents by shaking infusion bag every 2 hours.

▼ Monitor vital signs closely. Fever, shaking chills, and hypotension may appear within 2 hours of starting infusion. Slowing infusion rate may decrease risk of infusion-related reactions.

▼ If severe respiratory distress occurs, stop infusion, provide supportive therapy for anaphylaxis, and notify prescriber. Don't restart drug.

▼ Reconstituted drug is stable up to 48 hours if refrigerated (36° to 46° F [2° to 8° C]) and up to 6 hours at room temperature.

▼ Discard any unused drug because it contains no preservative.

▼ **Incompatibilities:** Electrolytes, other I.V. drugs, saline solutions.

ACTION
Binds to sterols of fungal cell membranes, altering cell permeability and causing cell death.

Reactions in bold italics are *life-threatening*. Interactions may have a *rapid onset* or a **delayed onset**.

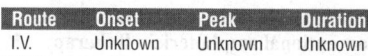
Route	Onset	Peak	Duration
I.V.	Unknown	Unknown	Unknown

Half-life: About 1 week.

ADVERSE REACTIONS
CNS: fever, headache, pain.
CV: *cardiac arrest,* chest pain, hypertension, hypotension.
GI: *GI hemorrhage,* abdominal pain, diarrhea, nausea, vomiting.
GU: *renal failure.*
Hematologic: *leukopenia, thrombocytopenia,* anemia.
Hepatic: hyperbilirubinemia.
Metabolic: hypokalemia.
Respiratory: *respiratory failure,* dyspnea, respiratory disorder.
Skin: rash.
Other: *multiple organ failure,* chills, *sepsis,* infection.

INTERACTIONS
Drug-drug. *Antineoplastics:* May increase risk of renal toxicity, bronchospasm, and hypotension. Use together cautiously.
Cardiac glycosides: May increase risk of digitalis toxicity from amphotericin B–induced hypokalemia. Monitor potassium level closely.
Clotrimazole, fluconazole, itraconazole, ketoconazole, miconazole: May counteract effects of amphotericin B by inducing fungal resistance. Monitor patient closely.
Corticosteroids, corticotropin: May enhance hypokalemia, which could lead to cardiac toxicity. Monitor electrolyte levels and cardiac function.
Cyclosporine: May increase renal toxicity. Monitor renal function test results closely.
Flucytosine: May increase risk of flucytosine toxicity from increased cellular uptake or impaired renal excretion. Use together cautiously.
Leukocyte transfusions: May increase risk of pulmonary reactions, such as acute dyspnea, tachypnea, hypoxemia, hemoptysis, and interstitial infiltrates. Don't coadminister.
Nephrotoxic drugs (such as aminoglycosides, pentamidine): May increase risk of renal toxicity. Use together cautiously and monitor renal function closely.

Skeletal muscle relaxants: May enhance skeletal muscle relaxant effects of amphotericin B–induced hypokalemia. Monitor potassium level closely.
Zidovudine: May increase myelotoxicity and nephrotoxicity. Monitor renal and hematologic function.

EFFECTS ON LAB TEST RESULTS
● May increase alkaline phosphatase, ALT, AST, bilirubin, BUN, creatinine, GGT, and LDH levels. May decrease Hb and magnesium and potassium levels.
● May decrease platelet and WBC counts.

CONTRAINDICATIONS & CAUTIONS
● Contraindicated in patients hypersensitive to amphotericin B or its components.
● Anaphylaxis can occur. If patient develops severe respiratory distress, discontinue infusion, treat appropriately, and don't restart drug.
● Use cautiously in patients with renal impairment. Adjust dosage based on patient's overall condition. Renal toxicity is more common at higher dosages.
Dialyzable drug: Unknown.
⚠ **Overdose S&S:** Cardiorespiratory arrest.

PREGNANCY-LACTATION-REPRODUCTION
● Use cautiously during pregnancy, taking into account importance of drug to the mother.
● It isn't known if drug appears in breast milk. Patient should discontinue breastfeeding or discontinue drug.

NURSING CONSIDERATIONS
❸ **Alert:** Different amphotericin B preparations aren't interchangeable, so dosages will vary. Confusing the preparations may cause permanent damage or death.
● Hydrate before infusion to reduce risk of nephrotoxicity.
● Monitor creatinine and electrolyte levels (especially magnesium and potassium), liver function, and CBC during therapy.
● Acute infusion reactions, including fever and chills, may occur 1 to 2 hours after start of infusion and are more common with first few doses. Infusion has rarely been associated with arrhythmias, hypotension, and shock.

● **Alert:** Immediately stop infusion if severe respiratory distress occurs. Patient shouldn't receive further infusions.

● **Look alike–sound alike:** Don't confuse amphotericin B with AmBisome.

PATIENT TEACHING

● Inform patient that he may develop fever, chills, nausea, and vomiting during infusion, but that these symptoms usually subside with subsequent doses.

● Instruct patient to report any redness or pain at infusion site.

● Teach patient to recognize and report to prescriber signs and symptoms of acute hypersensitivity, such as respiratory distress.

● Warn patient that therapy may take several months.

● Tell patient to expect frequent laboratory testing to monitor kidney and liver function.

SAFETY ALERT!

amphotericin B liposomal
am-foe-TER-i-sin

AmBisome

Therapeutic class: Antifungals
Pharmacologic class: Polyene antibiotics

AVAILABLE FORMS
Powder for injection: 50-mg vial

INDICATIONS & DOSAGES
Adjust-a-dose (for all indications): For patients with CrCl of less than 10 mL/minute, give 3 mg/kg I.V. every 24 hours. For adults receiving standard intermittent hemodialysis or continuous renal replacement therapy, give 3 to 5 mg/kg I.V. every 24 hours and after the dialysis session.

➤ **Empirical therapy for presumed fungal infection in febrile, neutropenic patients**
Adults and children: 3 mg/kg I.V. infusion over 2 hours daily.

➤ **Systemic fungal infections caused by *Aspergillus* species, *Candida* species, or *Cryptococcus* species refractory to conventional amphotericin B therapy; patients for whom renal impairment or**

unacceptable toxicity precludes use of conventional amphotericin B therapy
Adults and children: 3 to 5 mg/kg I.V. infusion over 2 hours daily.

➤ **Visceral leishmaniasis in immunocompetent patients**
Adults and children: 3 mg/kg I.V. infusion over 2 hours daily on days 1 to 5, day 14, and day 21. A repeat course of therapy may be beneficial if initial treatment fails to clear parasites.

➤ **Visceral leishmaniasis in immunocompromised patients**
Adults and children: 4 mg/kg I.V. infusion over 2 hours daily on days 1 to 5, day 10, day 17, day 24, day 31, and day 38.

➤ **Cryptococcal meningitis in patients with HIV infection**
Adults and children: 6 mg/kg/day I.V. infusion over 2 hours. Reduce infusion time to 1 hour if treatment is well tolerated, and increase infusion time if discomfort occurs.

➤ **Candidiasis (invasive) in HIV-exposed/ infected patients ◆**
Infants and children: 5 mg/kg/dose I.V. once daily.

➤ **Coccidioidomycosis in HIV-exposed/ infected patients with severe non-meningeal infection (diffuse pulmonary or extrathoracic, disseminated disease) ◆**
Adolescents: 4 to 6 mg/kg/day I.V. until clinical improvement.
Infants and children: 3 to 5 mg/kg/dose I.V. once daily.

ADMINISTRATION
I.V.

▼ Don't reconstitute with bacteriostatic water for injection, and don't allow bacteriostatic product in solution.

▼ Don't reconstitute with saline solutions, add saline solutions to reconstituted concentration, or mix with other drugs.

▼ Reconstitute each 50-mg vial with 12 mL of sterile water for injection to yield 4 mg/mL. A yellow, translucent suspension will form.

▼ After reconstitution, shake vial vigorously for 30 seconds or until particulate matter disperses.

▼ Dilute to 1 to 2 mg/mL by withdrawing calculated amount of reconstituted solution into a sterile syringe and injecting it through a 5-micron filter into an appropriate amount of D_5W. Use only one filter needle per vial. Concentrations of 0.2 to 0.5 mg/mL may provide sufficient volume of infusion for children.

▼ Flush existing I.V. line with D_5W before infusing drug. If this isn't possible, give drug through a separate line.

▼ Use a controlled infusion device and an in-line filter with a mean pore diameter of 1 micron or larger.

▼ Initially, infuse drug over at least 2 hours. If drug is tolerated well, reduce infusion time to 1 hour. If discomfort occurs, increase infusion time.

▼ Store unopened vial at 36° to 46° F (2° to 8° C). Store reconstituted drug for up to 24 hours at 36° to 46° F. Use within 6 hours of dilution with D_5W. Don't freeze.

▼ **Incompatibilities:** Other I.V. drugs, saline solutions.

ACTION
Binds to sterols of fungal cell membranes, altering cell permeability and causing cell death.

Route	Onset	Peak	Duration
I.V.	Unknown	Unknown	Unknown

Half-life: About 4 to 6 days.

ADVERSE REACTIONS
CNS: fever, anxiety, confusion, headache, insomnia, asthenia, pain.
CV: chest pain, hypotension, tachycardia, hypertension, edema, flushing.
EENT: epistaxis, rhinitis.
GI: anorexia, constipation, nausea, vomiting, abdominal pain, diarrhea, *GI hemorrhage.*
GU: hematuria, *renal failure.*
Hematologic: anemia, thrombocytopenia, leukopenia.
Hepatic: hyperbilirubinemia, *hepatotoxicity.*
Metabolic: hyperglycemia, hypernatremia, hyponatremia, hypocalcemia, hypokalemia, *hypomagnesemia.*
Musculoskeletal: back pain, weakness.
Respiratory: increased cough, dyspnea, hypoxia, pleural effusion, lung disorder, hyperventilation.
Skin: pruritus, rash, sweating.

Other: chills, infection, *anaphylaxis, sepsis,* blood product infusion reaction.

INTERACTIONS
Drug-drug. *Antineoplastics:* May enhance potential for renal toxicity, bronchospasm, and hypotension. Use together cautiously.
Cardiac glycosides: May increase risk of digitalis toxicity caused by amphotericin B–induced hypokalemia. Monitor potassium level closely.
Clotrimazole, fluconazole, ketoconazole, miconazole: May induce fungal resistance to amphotericin B. Use together cautiously.
Corticosteroids, corticotropin: May increase potassium depletion, which could cause cardiac dysfunction. Monitor electrolyte levels and cardiac function.
Flucytosine: May increase flucytosine toxicity by increasing cellular reuptake or impairing renal excretion of flucytosine. Use together cautiously.
Leukocyte transfusions: Increases risk of pulmonary toxicity. Don't use together.
Other nephrotoxic drugs, such as antibiotics and antineoplastics: May cause additive nephrotoxicity. Use together cautiously; monitor renal function closely.
Skeletal muscle relaxants (tubocurarine): May enhance effects of skeletal muscle relaxants resulting from amphotericin B–induced hypokalemia. Monitor potassium level.

EFFECTS ON LAB TEST RESULTS
● May increase alkaline phosphatase, ALT, AST, bilirubin, BUN, creatinine, GGT, glucose, LDH, and sodium levels. May decrease calcium, magnesium, and potassium levels.
● May decrease Hb and platelet count.

CONTRAINDICATIONS & CAUTIONS
● Contraindicated in patients hypersensitive to drug or its components.
● Use cautiously in patients with impaired renal function, in elderly patients, and in pregnant women.
Dialyzable drug: Unknown.
⚠ *Overdose S&S:* Cardiorespiratory arrest.

♣Canada   ◇OTC   ♦Off-label use   ✐Photoguide   ⬤Do not crush   *Liquid contains alcohol.

PREGNANCY-LACTATION-REPRODUCTION

● Use during pregnancy only if potential benefits outweigh potential risks to the fetus.
● It isn't known if drug appears in breast milk. Patient should discontinue breast-feeding or discontinue drug.

NURSING CONSIDERATIONS

● Patients also receiving chemotherapy or bone marrow transplantation are at greater risk for additional adverse reactions, including seizures, arrhythmias, and thrombocytopenia.
⊙ **Alert:** Different amphotericin B preparations aren't interchangeable, so dosages will vary. Confusing the preparations may cause permanent damage or death.
● Premedicate patient with antipyretics, antihistamines, antiemetics and corticosteroids.
● Hydrate before infusion to reduce the risk of nephrotoxicity.
● Monitor BUN, creatinine, and electrolyte levels (particularly magnesium and potassium), liver function, and CBC.
● Watch for signs and symptoms of hypokalemia (ECG changes, muscle weakness, cramping, drowsiness).
● Patients treated with this drug have a lower risk of chills, elevated BUN level, hypokalemia, hypertension, and vomiting than patients treated with conventional amphotericin B.
● Therapy may take several weeks or months.
● Observe patient closely for adverse reactions during infusion. If anaphylaxis occurs, stop infusion immediately, provide supportive therapy, and notify prescriber.
● **Look alike–sound alike:** Don't confuse amphotericin B liposomal with Abelcet.

PATIENT TEACHING

● Teach patient signs and symptoms of hypersensitivity, and stress importance of reporting them immediately.
● Warn patient that therapy may take several months; teach personal hygiene and other measures to prevent spread and recurrence of lesions.
● Instruct patient to report any adverse reactions that occur while receiving drug.

● Tell patient to watch for and report signs and symptoms of low blood potassium levels (muscle weakness, cramping, drowsiness).
● Advise patient that frequent laboratory testing will be needed.

ampicillin
am-pi-SIL-in

ampicillin sodium

Therapeutic class: Antibiotics
Pharmacologic class: Aminopenicillins

AVAILABLE FORMS
Capsules: 250 mg, 500 mg
Injection: 125 mg, 250 mg, 500 mg, 1 g, 2 g, 10 g
Oral suspension: 125 mg/5 mL, 250 mg/5 mL

INDICATIONS & DOSAGES
Adjust-a-dose (for all indications): When giving I.V. to patients with impaired renal function, use the following schedule: If CrCl is 10 to 50 mL/minute, give dose every 6 to 12 hours. If CrCl is less than 10 mL/minute, give dose every 12 to 24 hours. If patient is receiving intermittent hemodialysis three times a week, give 1 to 2 g every 12 to 24 hours. If the dose is given every 24 hours, administer after dialysis. If patient is receiving continuous ambulatory peritoneal dialysis, give 250 mg every 12 hours.
➤ **Respiratory tract infections**
Adults and children weighing more than 20 kg: 250 mg P.O. every 6 hours.
Children weighing 20 kg or less: 50 mg/kg/day P.O. in equally divided doses every 6 to 8 hours. Maximum dose is 250 mg q.i.d.
➤ **GI infections or GU infections (excluding gonorrhea)**
Adults and children weighing 20 kg or more: 500 mg P.O. every 6 hours. For severe infections, larger doses may be needed.
Children weighing less than 20 kg: 100 mg/kg/day P.O. in equally divided doses every 6 hours. Maximum dose is 500 mg q.i.d.

➤ **Uncomplicated gonorrhea**
Adults and children weighing more than 20 kg: 3.5 g P.O. with 1 g probenecid given as a single dose.

➤ **Bacterial meningitis or septicemia**
Adults: 150 to 200 mg/kg/day I.V. in divided doses every 3 to 4 hours. May be given I.M. after 3 days of I.V. therapy. Maximum recommended daily dose is 14 g.
Children: 150 to 200 mg/kg I.V. daily in divided doses every 3 to 4 hours. Give I.V. for 3 days; then give I.M.

➤ **GI infections and GU tract infections (including gonorrhea in females)**
Adults and children weighing 40 kg or more: 500 mg I.V. or I.M. every 6 hours.
Adults and children weighing less than 40 kg: 50 mg/kg/day I.V. or I.M. in equally divided doses every 6 to 8 hours.

➤ **Respiratory tract and soft-tissue infections**
Adults and children weighing 40 kg or more: 250 to 500 mg I.V. or I.M. every 6 hours.
Adults and children weighing less than 40 kg: 25 to 50 mg/kg/day I.V. or I.M. in equally divided doses every 6 to 8 hours.

➤ **Urethritis in males due to gonorrhea**
Adult men: Two doses of 500 mg each I.V. or I.M. at 8- to 12-hour intervals. May repeat or extend treatment if necessary.

ADMINISTRATION
P.O.
● Before giving drug, ask patient about allergic reactions to penicillin. A negative history of penicillin allergy is no guarantee against a future allergic reaction.
● Obtain specimen for culture and sensitivity tests before giving. Begin therapy while awaiting results.
● Give drug 1 to 2 hours before or 2 to 3 hours after meals. When given orally, drug may cause GI disturbances. Food may interfere with absorption.
● Give drug I.M. or I.V. if infection is severe or if patient can't take oral dose.

I.V.
▼ Before giving drug, ask patient about allergic reactions to penicillin. A negative history of penicillin allergy is no guarantee against a future allergic reaction.

▼ Obtain specimen for culture and sensitivity tests before giving. Begin therapy while awaiting results.
▼ Give drug I.M. or I.V. only if infection is severe or if patient can't take oral dose.
▼ Give drug intermittently to prevent vein irritation. Change site every 48 hours.
▼ For direct injection, reconstitute with bacteriostatic water for injection. Use 5 mL for 250-mg or 500-mg vials, 7.4 mL for 1-g vials, and 14.8 mL for 2-g vials. Give drug over 10 to 15 minutes to avoid seizures. Don't exceed 100 mg/minute.
▼ For intermittent infusion, dilute in 50 to 100 mL of NSS for injection. Give drug over 15 to 30 minutes.
▼ Use first dilution within 1 hour. Follow manufacturer's directions for stability data when drug is further diluted for I.V. infusion.
▼ **Incompatibilities:** Amphotericin B cholesteryl sulfate complex, caspofungin, ciprofloxacin, dextrose 5% in NSS, D_5W, $D_{10}W$, epinephrine, fat emulsion 10%, fenoldopam, fluconazole, hetastarch 6%, hydralazine, midazolam, nicardipine, ondansetron, lactated Ringer solution, sargramostim, verapamil, vinorelbine.

I.M.
● Before giving drug, ask patient about allergic reactions to penicillin. A negative history of penicillin allergy is no guarantee against a future allergic reaction.
● Obtain specimen for culture and sensitivity tests before giving. Begin therapy while awaiting results.
● Give drug I.M. or I.V. only if infection is severe or patient can't take oral dose.

ACTION
Inhibits cell-wall synthesis during bacterial multiplication.

Route	Onset	Peak	Duration
P.O.	Unknown	2 hr	6–8 hr
I.V.	Immediate	Immediate	Unknown
I.M.	Unknown	1 hr	Unknown

Half-life: 1 to 1.8 hours (10 to 24 hours in severe renal impairment).

ADVERSE REACTIONS
GI: diarrhea, nausea, *pseudomembranous colitis,* abdominal pain, black hairy tongue,

enterocolitis, gastritis, glossitis, stomatitis, vomiting.

Hematologic: *leukopenia, thrombocytopenia, thrombocytopenic purpura,* anemia, eosinophilia, hemolytic anemia, *agranulocytosis.*

Other: hypersensitivity reactions, overgrowth of nonsusceptible organisms.

INTERACTIONS

Drug-drug. *Allopurinol:* May increase risk of rash. Monitor patient for rash.

H_2 *antagonists, PPIs:* May decrease ampicillin absorption and level. Separate administration times. Monitor patient for continued antibiotic effectiveness.

Hormonal contraceptives: May decrease hormonal contraceptive effectiveness. Advise use of another form of contraception during therapy.

Live-virus vaccines: May decrease effectiveness of live-virus vaccines. Concurrent use isn't recommended.

Oral anticoagulants: May increase risk of bleeding. Monitor PT and INR.

Probenecid: May increase levels of ampicillin and other penicillins. Probenecid may be used for this purpose.

EFFECTS ON LAB TEST RESULTS

● May decrease Hb level.
● May increase eosinophil count. May decrease granulocyte, platelet, and WBC counts.
● May falsely decrease aminoglycoside level. May alter results of urine glucose tests that use cupric sulfate, such as Benedict reagent and Clinitest.

CONTRAINDICATIONS & CAUTIONS

● Contraindicated in patients hypersensitive to drug or other penicillins and in those with infections caused by penicillinase-producing organisms.
● Use cautiously in patients with other drug allergies (especially to cephalosporins) because of possible cross-sensitivity, and in those with mononucleosis because of high risk of maculopapular rash.
● Use cautiously in patients with renal impairment.

Dialyzable drug: Yes.

PREGNANCY-LACTATION-REPRODUCTION

● There are no adequate and well-controlled studies in pregnant women. Use during pregnancy only if clearly needed.
● Drug appears in breast milk. Use cautiously in breast-feeding women.

NURSING CONSIDERATIONS

● Monitor sodium level because each gram of ampicillin contains 2.9 mEq of sodium.
● If large doses are given or if therapy is prolonged, bacterial or fungal superinfection may occur, especially in elderly, debilitated, or immunosuppressed patients.
● Watch for signs and symptoms of hypersensitivity, such as erythematous maculopapular rash, urticaria, and anaphylaxis.
● In patients with impaired renal function, decrease dosage.
● Use lowest dosage compatible with effective treatment in neonates and infants because of incompletely developed renal function in these patients.
● Monitor patients for CDAD, which can be fatal and can occur even more than 2 months after therapy ends. Antibiotic may need to be stopped and other treatment begun.

PATIENT TEACHING

● Tell patient to take entire quantity of drug exactly as prescribed, even after he feels better.
● Instruct patient to take oral form on an empty stomach 1 hour before or 2 hours after meals.
● Inform patient to report all adverse reactions and to notify prescriber if rash, fever, or chills develop. A rash is the most common allergic reaction, especially if allopurinol is also being taken.
● Instruct patient to report diarrhea.

ampicillin sodium–sulbactam sodium

am-pi-SIL-in/sul-BAK-tam

Unasyn

Therapeutic class: Antibiotics
Pharmacologic class: Aminopenicillins–beta-lactamase inhibitors

AVAILABLE FORMS

Injection: Vials and piggyback vials containing 1.5 g (1 g ampicillin sodium and 0.5 g sulbactam sodium), 3 g (2 g ampicillin sodium and 1 g sulbactam sodium)

INDICATIONS & DOSAGES

Adjust-a-dose (for all indications): If CrCl in adults is 15 to 29 mL/minute, give 1.5 to 3 g every 12 hours; if CrCl is 5 to 14 mL/minute, give 1.5 to 3 g every 24 hours. Give dose after hemodialysis.

➤ **Intra-abdominal, gynecologic, and skin-structure infections caused by susceptible strains**

Adults: 1.5 to 3 g I.M. or I.V. every 6 hours. Don't exceed 4 g/day of sulbactam.

Children age 1 or older weighing 40 kg or more (skin and skin-structure infections only): 1.5 to 3 g I.V. or I.M. every 6 hours. Don't exceed 4 g/day sulbactam.

Children age 1 or older weighing less than 40 kg (skin and skin-structure infections only): 200 mg/kg/day I.V. in divided doses every 6 hours for no longer than 14 days.

ADMINISTRATION

I.V.
▼ Before giving drug, ask patient about allergic reactions to penicillin. A negative history of penicillin allergy is no guarantee against future allergic reaction.
▼ Obtain specimen for culture and sensitivity tests. Begin therapy while awaiting results.
▼ Reconstitute powder with one of these diluents: NSS, sterile water for injection, D$_5$W, lactated Ringer injection, M/6 sodium lactate, dextrose 5% in half-NSS for injection, or 10% invert sugar.

▼ After reconstitution, let vials stand for a few minutes so foam can dissipate. Inspect solution for particles.
▼ Give drug at least 1 hour before giving a bacteriostatic antibiotic.
▼ For infusion, dilute in 50 to 100 mL of compatible diluent and infuse over 15 to 30 minutes.
▼ Stability varies with diluent, temperature, and concentration of solution.
▼ **Incompatibilities:** Aminoglycosides.

I.M.
● Before giving drug, ask patient about allergic reactions to penicillin. A negative history of penicillin allergy is no guarantee against future allergic reaction.
● Obtain specimen for culture and sensitivity tests. Begin therapy while awaiting results.
● For I.M. injection, reconstitute with sterile water for injection or 0.5% or 2% lidocaine hydrochloride injection. Add 3.2 mL to a 1.5-g vial (or 6.4 mL to a 3-g vial) to yield 375 mg/mL. Give deep into muscle.
● I.M. injection may cause pain at injection site.
● In children, don't use I.M. route.

ACTION

Inhibits cell-wall synthesis during bacterial multiplication.

Route	Onset	Peak	Duration
I.V.	Immediate	15 min	Unknown
I.M.	Unknown	30–52 min	Unknown

Half-life: 1 to 1½ hours (10 to 24 hours in severe renal impairment).

ADVERSE REACTIONS

CV: thrombophlebitis.
GI: diarrhea.
Hematologic: *agranulocytosis, leukopenia, thrombocytopenia, thrombocytopenic purpura.*
Skin: pain at injection site, thrombophlebitis, rash, urticaria.
Other: hypersensitivity reactions.

INTERACTIONS

Drug-drug. *Allopurinol:* May increase risk of rash. Monitor patient for rash.
Hormonal contraceptives: May decrease hormonal contraceptive effectiveness.

Strongly advise use of another contraceptive during therapy.

Live-virus vaccines: May decrease effectiveness of live-virus vaccines. Use together isn't recommended.

Methotrexate: May increase methotrexate level, increasing risk of toxicity. Monitor methotrexate level.

Oral anticoagulants: May increase risk of bleeding. Monitor PT and INR.

Probenecid: May increase ampicillin level. Probenecid may be used for this purpose.

Tetracycline: May decrease effectiveness of ampicillin–sulbactam. Avoid coadministration if possible.

EFFECTS ON LAB TEST RESULTS

● May increase alkaline phosphatase, ALT, AST, bilirubin, BUN, CK, creatinine, GGT, and LDH levels. May decrease Hb level.

● May transiently decrease conjugated estriol, conjugated estrone, estradiol, and estriol glucuronide levels in pregnant women.

● May increase eosinophil count. May decrease granulocyte, platelet, and WBC counts.

● May alter results of urine glucose tests that use cupric sulfate, such as Benedict reagent and Clinitest.

CONTRAINDICATIONS & CAUTIONS

● Contraindicated in patients hypersensitive to drug or other penicillins, in those with sensitivity to multiple allergens, and in those with mononucleosis because of high risk of maculopapular rash.

● Contraindicated in patients with a history of cholestatic jaundice or hepatic dysfunction associated with ampicillin–sulbactam injection.

● Use cautiously in patients with other drug allergies (especially to cephalosporins) because of possible cross-sensitivity and in those with renal impairment.

Dialyzable drug: Yes.

⚠ *Overdose S&S:* Neuromuscular hyperexcitability, seizures.

PREGNANCY-LACTATION-REPRODUCTION

● There are no adequate and well-controlled studies in pregnant women. Use cautiously during pregnancy and only if clearly needed.

● Drug appears in breast milk. Use cautiously in breast-feeding women.

NURSING CONSIDERATIONS

● Dosage is expressed as total drug. Each 1.5-g vial contains 1 g ampicillin sodium and 0.5 g sulbactam sodium.

● In patients with impaired renal function, decrease dosage.

● Monitor LFT results during therapy, especially in patients with impaired liver function.

● If large doses are given or if therapy is prolonged, bacterial or fungal superinfection may occur, especially in elderly, debilitated, or immunosuppressed patients.

● Watch for signs and symptoms of hypersensitivity, such as erythematous maculopapular rash, urticaria, and anaphylaxis.

● Monitor for CDAD, which can be fatal. Antibiotic may need to be stopped and other treatment begun.

PATIENT TEACHING

● Tell patient to report rash, fever, or chills. A rash is the most common allergic reaction.

● Warn patient that I.M. injection may cause pain at injection site.

anakinra
ann-ACK-in-rah

Kineret

Therapeutic class: Immunomodulators
Pharmacologic class: Interleukin-1 receptor antagonists

AVAILABLE FORMS

Injection: 100 mg/0.67 mL in a prefilled glass syringe

INDICATIONS & DOSAGES

Adjust-a-dose (for all indications): In severe renal insufficiency or ESRD (CrCl less than 30 mL/minute), consider every-other-day dosing.

➤ **Neonatal-onset multisystem inflammatory disease (NOMID)**

Adults and children: Initially, 1 to 2 mg/kg subcutaneously once daily. May increase in 0.5- to 1-mg increments to maximum dosage of 8 mg/kg daily for adults or 7.6 mg/kg daily for children. Maintenance dosage is 3 to 4 mg/kg daily. May divide total daily dosage into two equal doses.

➤ To reduce signs and symptoms and slow progression of structural damage in moderately to severely active RA after one or more failures with DMARDs, alone or combined with DMARDs other than TNF blockers

Adults: 100 mg subcutaneously daily at the same time each day.

ADMINISTRATION

Subcutaneous

• Don't shake. Trace amounts of small, translucent to white amorphous particles may be visible.

🕙 *Alert:* Needle cover contains natural rubber and may cause allergic reactions in patients sensitive to latex.

• Inject entire contents of prefilled syringe.

• Give dose about the same time every day.

• When used for NOMID, once-daily administration is recommended, but the dose may be split into twice-daily administration.

• Store drug in the refrigerator at 35° to 46° F (2° to 8° C). Don't freeze or shake.

• Protect drug from light.

ACTION

A recombinant, nonglycosylated form of the human interleukin-1 receptor antagonist (IL-1Ra). The level of naturally occurring IL-1Ra in synovium and synovial fluid from patients with RA isn't enough to compete with the elevated level of locally produced IL-1. Anakinra blocks the biological activity of IL-1 by competitively inhibiting IL-1 from binding to the IL-1 receptor, which is expressed in various tissues and organs.

Route	Onset	Peak	Duration
Subcut.	Unknown	3–7 hr	Unknown

Half-life: 4 to 6 hours.

ADVERSE REACTIONS

CNS: headache, fever.
EENT: sinusitis, nasopharyngitis.
GI: abdominal pain, diarrhea, nausea, vomiting.
Hematologic: *neutropenia.*
Musculoskeletal: worsening of RA, arthralgia.
Respiratory: URI.
Skin: ecchymosis, injection-site reactions (erythema, inflammation, pain).

Other: infection (cellulitis, pneumonia, bone and joint), flulike symptoms.

INTERACTIONS

Drug-drug. *Etanercept, other TNF blockers:* May increase risk of severe infection. Use together isn't recommended.
Vaccines: May decrease effectiveness of vaccines or may increase risk of secondary transmission of infection with live-virus vaccines. Avoid using together.

EFFECTS ON LAB TEST RESULTS

• May increase eosinophil count. May decrease neutrophil, platelet, and WBC counts.

CONTRAINDICATIONS & CAUTIONS

• Contraindicated in patients hypersensitive to *Escherichia coli*–derived proteins or any components of the product, or in patients with active infections.

• Hypersensitivity and anaphylactic reactions can occur. Discontinue drug for severe reaction; begin appropriate therapy.

• Use drug cautiously in immunosuppressed patients, those with chronic infections, and in elderly patients.

• Safety and effectiveness in patients with juvenile RA haven't been established.
Dialyzable drug: No.

PREGNANCY-LACTATION-REPRODUCTION

• Use during pregnancy only if clearly needed.

• It isn't known if drug appears in breast milk. Use cautiously in breast-feeding women.

NURSING CONSIDERATIONS

• Don't start treatment if patient has active infection.

• Obtain neutrophil count before treatment, monthly for the first 3 months of treatment, and then quarterly for up to 1 year.

• Monitor patient for infections and injection-site reactions.

• Stop drug if a serious infection develops.

• Monitor patient for possible anaphylactic reaction.

• *Look alike–sound alike:* Don't confuse anakinra with amikacin or Kineret with Amikin.

PATIENT TEACHING
- Tell patient to store drug in refrigerator and not to freeze or expose to excessive heat. Advise letting drug come to room temperature before giving dose.
- Tell patient not to shake drug.
- Teach patient proper dosage, administration, and needle and syringe disposal.
- Urge patient to rotate injection sites.
- Review signs and symptoms of allergic and other adverse reactions, especially signs of serious infections. Urge patient to contact prescriber if they arise.
- Inform patient that injection-site reactions are common, usually mild, and typically last 14 to 28 days.
- Tell patient to avoid live-virus vaccines during therapy.

SAFETY ALERT!

anastrozole
an-AS-troh-zol

Arimidex⬦

Therapeutic class: Antineoplastics
Pharmacologic class: Aromatase inhibitors

AVAILABLE FORMS
Tablets: 1 mg

INDICATIONS & DOSAGES
➤ **First-line treatment of postmenopausal women with hormone receptor–positive or hormone receptor–unknown locally advanced or metastatic breast cancer; advanced breast cancer in postmenopausal women with disease progression after tamoxifen therapy; adjunctive treatment of postmenopausal women with hormone receptor–positive early breast cancer**
Adults: 1 mg P.O. daily.
➤ **Risk reduction for breast cancer in postmenopausal women ◆**
Adults: 1 mg P.O. daily for 5 years.

ADMINISTRATION
P.O.
- Drug is a potential teratogen. Follow safe handling procedures when preparing, administering, or dispensing.
- Give drug without regard for meals.

ACTION
A selective nonsteroidal aromatase inhibitor that significantly lowers estradiol levels, which inhibits breast cancer cell growth in postmenopausal women.

Route	Onset	Peak	Duration
P.O.	<24 hr	2 hr	<7 days

Half-life: 50 hours.

ADVERSE REACTIONS
CNS: headache, asthenia, pain, dizziness, depression, paresthesia, anxiety, insomnia, stroke.
CV: hot flashes, ***thromboembolic disease,*** chest pain, peripheral edema, hypertension, vasodilation, cardiac ischemia.
EENT: cataracts, pharyngitis, sinusitis.
GI: nausea, vomiting, diarrhea, constipation, abdominal pain, anorexia, dry mouth, dyspepsia.
GU: vaginal dryness, pelvic pain, UTI.
Metabolic: weight gain, increased appetite.
Musculoskeletal: bone pain, back pain, arthritis, arthralgia, osteoporosis, fractures.
Respiratory: dyspnea, bronchitis, cough.
Skin: rash, sweating.
Other: lymphedema, flulike symptoms.

INTERACTIONS
Drug-drug. *Estrogen:* May decrease pharmacologic action of anastrozole. Use together isn't recommended.
Tamoxifen: May reduce anastrozole plasma level. Don't use together.

EFFECTS ON LAB TEST RESULTS
- May increase liver enzyme and cholesterol levels.

CONTRAINDICATIONS & CAUTIONS
- Contraindicated in women who are or may be pregnant and in patients hypersensitive to drug or its components.
- Use cautiously in patients with preexisting ischemic heart disease.
Dialyzable drug: Unknown.

PREGNANCY-LACTATION-REPRODUCTION
- Drug can cause fetal harm. Contraindicated in women who are or may become pregnant.

• It isn't known if drug appears in breast milk. Patient should discontinue breast-feeding or discontinue drug.

NURSING CONSIDERATIONS
• Give drug under supervision of a pre-scriber experienced in use of antineoplastics.
• Patients with hormone receptor–negative disease and patients who didn't respond to previous tamoxifen therapy rarely respond to anastrozole.
• For patients with advanced breast cancer, continue anastrozole until tumor progresses.
• Monitor bone mineral density as indicated.
• Use drug only in postmenopausal women.
• Rule out pregnancy before starting drug.

PATIENT TEACHING
• Instruct patient to report adverse reactions, especially difficulty breathing, chest pain, or skin lesions or blisters.
• Tell patient to take medication at the same time each day.
• Stress need for follow-up care.
• Counsel women about risks of pregnancy during therapy.
• Tell patient that drug lowers estrogen level, which may lead to decreased bone strength and increased risk of fractures.

anidulafungin
ah-nid-doo-la-FUN-jin

Eraxis

Therapeutic class: Antifungals
Pharmacologic class: Echinocandins

AVAILABLE FORMS
Powder for injection: 50 mg/vial, 100 mg/vial with companion diluent

INDICATIONS & DOSAGES
➤ **Candidemia and other *Candida* infections (intra-abdominal abscess, peritonitis)**
Adults: A single 200-mg loading dose given by I.V. infusion at no more than 1.1 mg/minute on day 1; then 100 mg daily for at least 14 days after last positive culture result.
➤ **Esophageal candidiasis**
Adults: A single 100-mg loading dose given by I.V. infusion at no more than

1.1 mg/minute on day 1; then 50 mg daily for at least 14 days and for at least 7 days after symptoms resolve.

ADMINISTRATION
I.V.
▼ Obtain specimens for culture and sensitivity tests and baseline laboratory tests before starting therapy.
▼ Reconstitute each 50-mg vial with 15 mL of supplied diluent. Reconstitute each 100-mg vial with 30 mL of supplied diluent.
▼ Further dilute with D_5W or NSS.
▼ Add 50-mg dose (in 15 mL) to 50 mL of D_5W or NSS. Resulting volume is 65 mL. Add 100-mg dose (in 30 mL) to 100 mL of D_5W or NSS. Resulting volume is 130 mL. Add 200-mg dose (in 60 mL) to 200 mL of D_5W or NSS. Resulting volume is 260 mL.
▼ Don't infuse faster than 1.1 mg/minute. Minimum duration of infusion is 45 minutes for 50 mg, 90 minutes for 100 mg, and 180 minutes for 200 mg.
▼ Store at room temperature; don't freeze. Use reconstituted solution within 24 hours of preparation.
▼ **Incompatibilities:** Unknown. Only use supplied diluent to reconstitute and D_5W or NSS to further dilute.

ACTION
Inhibits glucan synthase, which in turn inhibits formation of 1,3-β-D-glucan, an essential component of fungal cell walls.

Route	Onset	Peak	Duration
I.V.	<24 hr	Unknown	Unknown

Half-life: 40 to 50 hours.

ADVERSE REACTIONS
CNS: headache, fever, confusion, depression, insomnia.
CV: *DVT,* hypotension, hypertension, edema, chest pain.
EENT: oral candidiasis.
GI: nausea, vomiting, diarrhea, constipation, abdominal pain, dyspepsia.
GU: UTI.
Hematologic: *leukocytosis, anemia.*
Metabolic: hypokalemia, *hyperkalemia,* hyperglycemia, *hypoglycemia,* hypomagnesemia, dehydration.

Musculoskeletal: back pain.
Respiratory: dyspnea, pleural effusion, cough, respiratory distress, pneumonia.
Skin: rash.
Other: histamine-mediated symptoms (bronchospasm, dyspnea, flushing, hypotension, pruritus, rash, urticaria), infection, sepsis.

INTERACTIONS
None reported.

EFFECTS ON LAB TEST RESULTS
• May increase AST, ALT, alkaline phosphatase, GGT, amylase, lipase, bilirubin, CK, creatinine, urea, calcium, glucose, and sodium levels.
• May decrease glucose and magnesium levels. May increase or decrease potassium level.
• May prolong PT and decrease platelet count or increase WBC count.

CONTRAINDICATIONS & CAUTIONS
• Contraindicated in patients hypersensitive to drug, other echinocandins, or any component of the drug.
• Anaphylaxis has been reported. If reaction occurs, discontinue drug and give appropriate treatment.
• Use cautiously in patients with hepatic impairment and in elderly patients.
• Safety and effectiveness in children haven't been established.
Dialyzable drug: No.

PREGNANCY-LACTATION-REPRODUCTION
• Use during pregnancy only if clearly needed.
• It isn't known if drug appears in breast milk. Use cautiously in breast-feeding women.

NURSING CONSIDERATIONS
• Use only the supplied diluent to reconstitute powder.
• To avoid histamine-mediated symptoms, such as rash, urticaria, flushing, itching, dyspnea, and hypotension, don't infuse faster than 1.1 mg/minute.
• Monitor patient closely for changes in liver function and blood cell counts during therapy.

• Notify prescriber about signs or symptoms of liver toxicity, such as dark urine, jaundice, abdominal pain, and fatigue.
• Patients with esophageal candidiasis who are HIV positive may need suppressive antifungal therapy after drug to prevent relapse.

PATIENT TEACHING
• Tell patient to immediately report rash, itching, trouble breathing, or other adverse effects during infusion.
• Explain that blood tests will be needed to monitor the drug's effects.

SAFETY ALERT!

apixaban
a-PIX-a-ban

Eliquis

Therapeutic class: Anticoagulants
Pharmacologic class: Factor Xa inhibitors

AVAILABLE FORMS
Tablets: 2.5 mg, 5 mg

INDICATIONS & DOSAGES
➤ **Reduction of risk of stroke and systemic embolism in patients with nonvalvular atrial fibrillation**
Adults: 5 mg P.O. b.i.d.
Adjust-a-dose: Reduce dosage to 2.5 mg b.i.d. in patients with any two of the following characteristics: age 80 or older, body weight 60 kg or less, or serum creatinine 1.5 mg/dL or greater.
➤ **DVT prophylaxis after hip or knee replacement surgery**
Adults: 2.5 mg P.O. b.i.d. beginning 12 to 24 hours after surgery. Continue for 35 days after hip replacement surgery or for 12 days after knee replacement surgery.
➤ **DVT and PE**
Adults: 10 mg P.O. daily for 7 days followed by 5 mg P.O. b.i.d.; then, to reduce risk of recurrence after 6 months of treatment, give 2.5 mg P.O. b.i.d.

ADMINISTRATION
P.O.
• May give without regard for food.

• If patient doesn't take dose at the scheduled time, he should take the dose as soon as possible on the same day, then resume twice-daily administration. Patient shouldn't double the dose to make up for a missed dose.

• May crush and suspend in 60 mL D_5W and give immediately through an NG tube if necessary.

• Store at room temperature.

ACTION

Selectively inhibits factor Xa, decreasing thrombin generation and thrombus development.

Route	Onset	Peak	Duration
P.O.	Unknown	3–4 hr	Unknown

Half-life: 12 hours.

ADVERSE REACTIONS

GI: nausea.
Hematologic: *major bleeding,* anemia, bruising.

INTERACTIONS

Drug-drug. *Aspirin and other antiplatelet agents/anticoagulants, heparin, NSAIDs, SNRIs, SSRIs, thrombolytics:* May increase bleeding risk. Avoid use together.
Enoxaparin, naproxen: May increase antifactor Xa activity. Avoid use together.
Strong dual inducers of CYP3A4 and P-glycoprotein (P-gp) (carbamazepine, phenytoin, rifampin): May decrease apixaban concentration. Avoid use together.
Strong dual inhibitors of CYP3A4 and P-gp (clarithromycin, itraconazole, ketoconazole, ritonavir): May increase apixaban concentration. Recommended dosage is 2.5 mg b.i.d.; avoid use together in patients already taking 2.5 mg b.i.d.
Voraxapar: May increase bleeding risk. Avoid use together.
Drug-herb. *Alfalfa, anise, bilberry:* May increase bleeding risk. Consider therapy modification.
St. John's wort: May decrease apixaban concentration. Discourage use together.
Drug-food. *Grapefruit juice:* May increase drug level and risk of bleeding. Use cautiously and monitor patient for bleeding.

EFFECTS ON LAB TEST RESULTS

• May increase LFT values.
• May prolong PT, INR, and aPTT.

CONTRAINDICATIONS & CAUTIONS

• Contraindicated in patients hypersensitive to drug or its components and in those with active pathological bleeding.
• Use cautiously in patients at risk for severe bleeding (especially those concomitantly taking drugs that affect hemostasis).
Black Box Warning Discontinuing drug increases risk of thrombotic events. If anticoagulation with apixaban must be discontinued for a reason other than pathological bleeding, strongly consider coverage with another anticoagulant. ∎
Black Box Warning Consider potential risk of epidural or spinal hematoma versus benefit in patients scheduled for spinal procedures, such as spinal or epidural anesthesia or spinal puncture. Hematomas may result in long-term or permanent paralysis. Risk may increase with use of indwelling epidural catheters, concomitant use of drugs that affect hemostasis (NSAIDs, platelet inhibitors, anticoagulants), history of traumatic or repeated epidural or spinal punctures, or history of spinal deformity or surgery. ∎
🔵 *Alert:* Discontinue apixaban at least 48 hours before elective surgery or invasive procedures with a moderate or high risk of unacceptable or clinically significant bleeding.
🔵 *Alert:* Discontinue apixaban at least 24 hours before elective surgery or invasive procedures with a low risk of bleeding or when the bleeding would be noncritical in location and easily controlled.
• Drug isn't recommended for patients with severe hepatic impairment or prosthetic heart valves.
• Bleeding risk is increased in patients with severe renal impairment.
Dialyzable drug: 14%.

PREGNANCY-LACTATION-REPRODUCTION

• Not recommended in pregnant women.
• It isn't known if drug appears in breast milk. Not recommended for breast-feeding women.

NURSING CONSIDERATIONS

● Monitor patient for bleeding. Discontinue drug if acute pathological bleeding occurs.

🔸 *Alert:* Promptly evaluate signs and symptom of blood loss. Drug can cause serious, potentially fatal bleeding.

Black Box Warning Monitor patients for neurologic impairment (midline back pain, sensory or motor deficits, such as numbness or weakness in lower limbs, bowel or bladder dysfunction). Treat impairment urgently. ■

🔸 *Alert:* Removal of indwelling epidural or intrathecal catheters should be delayed for at least 24 hours after last dose of apixaban. Next dose of apixaban should be given no earlier than 5 hours after catheter removal. Don't give drug for at least 48 hours after traumatic or repeated epidural or spinal punctures.

● Keep in mind that protamine sulfate and vitamin K have no effect on the activity of apixaban.

● When switching from warfarin to apixaban, discontinue warfarin and start apixaban when INR is below 2.0.

● If switching from apixaban to warfarin, discontinue apixaban and begin both a parenteral anticoagulant and warfarin at the time the next dose of apixaban would have been taken. Discontinue the parenteral anticoagulant when INR reaches an acceptable range.

● If switching between apixaban and anticoagulants other than warfarin, discontinue drug being taken and begin other drug at next scheduled dose.

PATIENT TEACHING

● Warn patient not to discontinue drug without first talking to prescriber, because of risk of clot formation and stroke.

● Tell patient to report all adverse reactions; caution patient that bruising or bleeding may occur more easily.

● Advise patient to report unusual bleeding.

● Instruct patient to inform all health care providers (including dentists) about taking this drug as well as other products known to affect bleeding (including nonprescription products, such as aspirin or NSAIDs) before scheduling surgery or medical or dental procedure and before taking any new drug.

● Tell female patient to inform practitioner if she is pregnant, plans to become pregnant, is breast-feeding, or intends to breast-feed during treatment.

---

apremilast
a-PRE-mi-last

Otezla

Therapeutic class: Antiarthritics
Pharmacologic class:
Phosphodiesterase-4 inhibitors

AVAILABLE FORMS

Tablets 🔵: 10 mg, 20 mg, 30 mg

INDICATIONS & DOSAGES

Adjust-a-dose (for all indications): In patients with severe renal impairment (CrCl less than 30 mL/minute), give doses according to a.m. schedule only (omit p.m. doses) from days 1 through 5. For day 6 and onward, give 30 mg once daily.

➤ **Active psoriatic arthritis; moderate to severe plaque psoriasis in patients who are candidates for phototherapy or systemic therapy**

Adults: Initially, 10 mg P.O. in a.m. on day 1; 10 mg P.O. b.i.d. (a.m. and p.m.) on day 2; 10 mg P.O. in a.m. and 20 mg P.O. in p.m. on day 3; 20 mg P.O. b.i.d. (a.m. and p.m.) on day 4; 20 mg P.O. in a.m. and 30 mg P.O. in p.m. on day 5; then 30 mg P.O. b.i.d. (a.m. and p.m.) on day 6 and thereafter.

ADMINISTRATION
P.O.

● Give without regard to meals.

● Don't crush, split, or allow patient to chew tablets.

● Store tablets at room temperature.

ACTION

Increases intracellular cAMP level. Its action in the treatment of psoriatic arthritis isn't well defined.

Route	Onset	Peak	Duration
P.O.	Unknown	2½ hr	Unknown

Half-life: 6 to 9 hours.

ADVERSE REACTIONS
CNS: headache, depression, fatigue, insomnia, migraine.
EENT: nasopharyngitis.
GI: anorexia, diarrhea, nausea, vomiting, upper abdominal pain, decreased appetite, dyspepsia.
Metabolic: weight loss.
Musculoskeletal: back pain.
Respiratory: URI, bronchitis.

INTERACTIONS
Drug-drug. *Strong CYP450 inducers (carbamazepine, phenobarbital, phenytoin, rifampin):* May decrease apremilast level, causing loss of effectiveness. Use together isn't recommended.
Drug-herb. *St. John's wort:* May decrease apremilast level. Consider therapy modification.

EFFECTS ON LAB TEST RESULTS
None reported.

CONTRAINDICATIONS & CAUTIONS
• Contraindicated in patients hypersensitive to drug or its components.
• Use cautiously in patients with history of depression or suicidal thoughts. Weigh risks and benefits of using drug in these patients.
• Use cautiously in patients with severe renal impairment.
• Safety and effectiveness in children haven't been established.
Dialyzable drug: Unknown.

PREGNANCY-LACTATION-REPRODUCTION
• Use cautiously in pregnant women and only if benefits outweigh risks to the fetus. Enroll pregnant patients in pregnancy exposure registry (1-877-311-8972) to monitor pregnancy outcomes.
• It isn't known if drug appears in breast milk. Use cautiously in breast-feeding women.

NURSING CONSIDERATIONS
• Titration to maintenance dose is intended to reduce GI symptoms with initial therapy.
• Monitor patient for depression or suicidal thoughts.
• Monitor patient regularly for unexplained or significant weight loss. Evaluate cause and consider discontinuing drug.

PATIENT TEACHING
• Explain to patient that drug may cause weight loss.
• Warn patient and caregivers to looks for signs and symptoms of depression or suicidal thoughts and to contact prescriber immediately if they occur.
• Instruct patient to titrate drug as directed to reduce GI symptoms.
• Advise patient that drug may be taken without regard to food and not to crush, chew, or split tablets.
• Educate patient on possible adverse effects of this drug, such as headache, diarrhea, nausea, vomiting, upper abdominal pain, weight loss, or infections in the nose, throat, or lungs.

aprepitant
ah-PRE-pit-ant

Emend

fosaprepitant dimeglumine
Emend

Therapeutic class: Antiemetics
Pharmacologic class: Substance P and neurokinin-1 receptor antagonists

AVAILABLE FORMS
Capsules: 40 mg, 80 mg, 125 mg
Injection: 150 mg
Powder for oral suspension (kit): 125 mg

INDICATIONS & DOSAGES
➤ **To prevent nausea and vomiting after highly emetogenic chemotherapy (including cisplatin) and moderately emetogenic chemotherapy, with a 5-HT$_3$ antagonist and a corticosteroid**
Adults and children age 12 and older (capsules): On day 1 of chemotherapy, 125 mg P.O. 1 hour before treatment; on days 2 and 3, give 80 mg P.O. 1 hour before chemotherapy and if no chemotherapy is scheduled, give in the morning. Or, a single dose of 150 mg I.V. over 20 to 30 minutes given 30 minutes before treatment.
Adults unable to swallow capsules and children age 6 months to younger than 12 years (oral suspension): On day 1 of chemotherapy, 3 mg/kg P.O. 1 hour before treatment; maximum dose, 125 mg. On days 2 and 3,

2 mg/kg P.O. 1 hour before chemotherapy and if no chemotherapy is scheduled, give in the morning; maximum dose, 80 mg.

➤ **To prevent postoperative nausea and vomiting**

Adults: 40 mg P.O. within 3 hours before induction of anesthesia.

ADMINISTRATION
P.O.
- Give drug without regard for food.
- Drug may be given with other antiemetics.
- Oral suspension should be prepared by a health care provider, but once prepared may be administered by a health care provider, patient, or caregiver.
- Refer to manufacturer's instructions for preparing oral suspension.
- Refrigerate prepared oral suspension until administered. May store at room temperature for up to 3 hours before use. Discard any dose remaining after 72 hours.

I.V.
▼ Reconstitute with 5 mL of NSS. Add the NSS along the vial wall to prevent foaming. Swirl gently and avoid shaking.
▼ Add entire volume to infusion bag containing 110 mL of NSS. Total volume will be 115 mL and final concentration is 1 mg/mL. If using the 150-mg vial, add the reconstituted volume to 145 mL. Total volume will be 150 mL and concentration will be 1 mg/mL.
▼ Gently invert the bag two to three times.
▼ Administer 150-mg dose over 20 to 30 minutes by I.V. infusion.
▼ Final solution is stable for 24 hours at ambient room temperature.
▼ **Incompatibilities:** Any solutions containing divalent cations (e.g., Ca^{2+}, Mg^{2+}), including lactated Ringer solution and Hartmann solution.

ACTION
Inhibits emesis by selectively antagonizing substance P and neurokinin-1 receptors in the brain; appears to be synergistic with 5-HT_3 antagonists and corticosteroids.

Route	Onset	Peak	Duration
P.O.	Unknown	4 hr	Unknown
I.V.	Unknown	Less than 30 min	Unknown

Half-life: 9 to 13 hours.

ADVERSE REACTIONS
CNS: asthenia, fatigue, dizziness, fever, headache, insomnia.
CV: *bradycardia,* hypertension, hypotension, dehydration.
EENT: mucous membrane disorder, tinnitus.
GI: anorexia, constipation, diarrhea, nausea, abdominal pain, epigastric pain, flatulence, gastritis, heartburn, vomiting.
GU: UTI.
Hematologic: *neutropenia,* anemia.
Respiratory: hiccups.
Skin: pruritus, infusion-site pain, infusion-site induration.
Other: dehydration, alopecia.

INTERACTIONS
Drug-drug. *Alprazolam, midazolam, triazolam:* May increase levels of these drugs. Watch for CNS effects, such as increased sedation. Decrease benzodiazepine dose by 50%.
Carbamazepine, phenytoin, rifampin, other CYP3A4 inducers: May decrease aprepitant level. Watch for decreased antiemetic effect.
Clarithromycin, diltiazem, erythromycin, itraconazole, ketoconazole, nefazodone, nelfinavir, ritonavir, troleandomycin, other CYP3A4 inhibitors: May increase aprepitant level and risk of toxicity. Use together cautiously.
Dexamethasone, methylprednisolone: May increase levels of these drugs and risk of toxicity. Decrease P.O. corticosteroid dose by 50%; decrease I.V. methylprednisolone dose by 25%.
Diltiazem: May increase diltiazem level. Monitor HR and BP. Avoid using together.
Docetaxel, etoposide, ifosfamide, imatinib, irinotecan, paclitaxel, vinorelbine, vinblastine, vincristine: May increase levels and risk of toxicity of these drugs. Use together cautiously.
Hormonal contraceptives: May decrease contraceptive effectiveness. Tell women to use additional birth control method during therapy.
Paroxetine: May decrease paroxetine and aprepitant effects. Monitor patient for effectiveness.
Phenytoin: May decrease phenytoin level. Monitor level carefully. Avoid using

---

Reactions in bold italics are ***life-threatening***. Interactions may have a *rapid onset* or a **delayed onset**.

together. Increase phenytoin dose as needed during therapy.

Pimozide: May increase pimozide level. Use together is contraindicated.

Tolbutamide: May decrease tolbutamide effects. Monitor glucose level.

Warfarin: May decrease warfarin effectiveness. Monitor INR carefully for 2 weeks after each aprepitant treatment.

Drug-herb. *St. John's wort:* May decrease antiemetic effects by inducing CYP3A4. Discourage use together.

Drug-food. *Grapefruit juice:* May increase drug level and risk of toxicity. Discourage use together.

EFFECTS ON LAB TEST RESULTS

• May increase alkaline phosphatase, AST, ALT, BUN, creatinine, glucose, and urine protein levels. May decrease sodium level.
• May increase RBC and WBC counts. May decrease neutrophil count.

CONTRAINDICATIONS & CAUTIONS

• Contraindicated in patients hypersensitive to fosaprepitant, aprepitant, or their components. Hypersensitivity reactions have been reported. Also contraindicated in patients taking pimozide.
• Use cautiously in patients receiving chemotherapy drugs metabolized mainly via CYP3A4 and in those with severe hepatic disease.
• Safety and effectiveness in children haven't been established.
Dialyzable drug: No.
⚠ *Overdose S&S:* Drowsiness, headache.

PREGNANCY-LACTATION-REPRODUCTION

• Use during pregnancy only if clearly needed.
• It isn't known if drug appears in breast milk. Patient should discontinue breast-feeding or discontinue drug.

NURSING CONSIDERATIONS

• Avoid giving drug for more than 3 days per chemotherapy cycle.
🔵 *Alert:* Fosaprepitant is given I.V. on day 1 only of a 3-day regimen.
🔵 *Alert:* Before giving drug, screen patient carefully for possible drug and herb interactions.

• Don't give drug for existing nausea or vomiting.
• Expect to give drug with other antiemetics to treat breakthrough emesis.
• Monitor CBC, LFT results, and creatinine level periodically during therapy.
• *Look alike–sound alike:* Don't confuse aprepitant (oral form) with fosaprepitant (I.V. form).

PATIENT TEACHING

• Advise patient to report all adverse reactions to prescriber.
• If nausea or vomiting occurs, instruct patient to take breakthrough antiemetics rather than more aprepitant.
• Urge patient to report use of any other drugs or herbs.
• Caution patient against taking drug with grapefruit juice.
• Advise woman who takes a hormonal contraceptive to use an additional form of birth control.
• Tell patient who takes warfarin that PT and INR will be monitored closely for 2 weeks after therapy starts.
• Teach patient to take drug 1 hour before chemotherapy, then daily in the morning or as directed.

arformoterol tartrate
arr-fohr-MOH-tur-ahl

Brovana

Therapeutic class: Bronchodilators
Pharmacologic class: Long-acting selective beta$_2$ agonists

AVAILABLE FORMS

Solution for inhalation: 15 mcg/2-mL vials

INDICATIONS & DOSAGES

➤ **Long-term maintenance treatment of bronchoconstriction in patients with COPD, including chronic bronchitis and emphysema**
Adults: 15 mcg inhaled b.i.d. (morning and evening) via nebulizer. Maximum dose is 30 mcg daily.

ADMINISTRATION
Inhalational
• Use only the recommended nebulizer and compressor for treatment.
• Don't mix with other drugs or solutions in the nebulizer.
• Store vials in the foil pouches in the refrigerator and use immediately after opening.

ACTION
Relaxes bronchial and cardiac smooth muscle by acting on beta$_2$-adrenergic receptors; stimulates the enzyme adenyl cyclase, which catalyzes the conversion from ATP to cAMP. This further relaxes bronchial smooth muscle and inhibits release of mediators (like histamine and leukotrienes) from mast cells.

Route	Onset	Peak	Duration
Inhalation	7–20 min	½–3 hr	Unknown

Half-life: 26 hours.

ADVERSE REACTIONS
CNS: pain, agitation, cerebral infarction, hypokinesia, paralysis, somnolence, tremor.
CV: chest pain, *AV block, atrial flutter, HF, MI, prolonged QT interval, supraventricular tachycardia,* inverted T wave, peripheral edema.
EENT: sinusitis.
GI: diarrhea, constipation, gastritis.
Metabolic: *hypoglycemia,* hypokalemia.
Musculoskeletal: back pain, leg cramps.
Respiratory: dyspnea, lung disorders, pulmonary or chest congestion, *bronchospasm.*
Skin: rash, dry skin, herpes simplex, skin discoloration, skin hypertrophy.
Other: hypersensitivity reaction, flulike syndrome.

INTERACTIONS
Drug-drug. *Aminophylline, corticosteroids (such as dexamethasone, prednisone), theophylline:* May increase risk of hypokalemia. Monitor patient's potassium level.
Beta blockers (such as metoprolol, atenolol): May decrease effectiveness of arformoterol and increase risk of bronchospasm. Avoid using together, if possible; otherwise, use with extreme caution.

Non–potassium-sparing diuretics (such as furosemide, hydrochlorothiazide): May increase risk of hypokalemia and ECG changes. Use cautiously together, and monitor patient's ECG and potassium level.
Other beta$_2$ agonists (such as albuterol, formoterol): May cause additive effects. Avoid using together.
QT interval-prolonging drugs (such as MAO inhibitors, TCAs): May increase risk of ventricular arrhythmias. Use cautiously together.

EFFECTS ON LAB TEST RESULTS
• May increase PSA levels. May decrease potassium levels. May increase or decrease glucose levels.

CONTRAINDICATIONS & CAUTIONS
• Contraindicated in patients hypersensitive to drug, formoterol, or any other components.
Black Box Warning Safe and effective use of arformoterol in patients with asthma hasn't been established. Arformoterol is contraindicated in patients with asthma who aren't using a long-term asthma control medication. ∎
• Don't use in patients with acutely deteriorating COPD.
• Use cautiously in patients with seizure disorder; diabetes; hypokalemia; thyrotoxicosis; hepatic insufficiency; or preexisting CV disease, including coronary insufficiency, arrhythmias, and hypertension; and in those unresponsive to sympathomimetic amines.
Dialyzable drug: Unknown.
⚠ *Overdose S&S:* Exaggeration of adverse reactions, hyperglycemia, hypertension, hypotension, metabolic acidosis, cardiac arrest.

PREGNANCY-LACTATION-REPRODUCTION
• There are no adequate and well-controlled studies in pregnant women. Use during pregnancy only if potential benefit justifies potential risk to the fetus.
• It isn't known if drug appears in breast milk. Use cautiously in breast-feeding women.

Reactions in bold italics are *life-threatening*. Interactions may have a *rapid onset* or a *delayed onset*.

A

NURSING CONSIDERATIONS

Black Box Warning Drug may increase risk of asthma-related death. ∎

☉ Alert: Make sure patient has a rescue inhaler, such as albuterol, to treat an acute asthma attack or bronchospasm.

☉ Alert: Notify prescriber if patient experiences decreasing control of symptoms or begins using his short-acting beta$_2$ agonist more often.

• If paradoxical bronchospasm occurs, stop drug immediately.

• Monitor BP, pulse, and ECG, as indicated.

• *Look alike–sound alike:* Don't confuse Brovana with Boniva.

PATIENT TEACHING

• Tell patient to store vials in foil pouches in refrigerator and use immediately after opening.

• Tell patient to use only recommended nebulizer and compressor for treatment and not to mix drug with other inhaled drugs or solutions.

☉ Alert: Warn patient that drug is for maintenance treatment only and shouldn't be used to stop an asthma attack or bronchospasm. For emergency treatment, use a short-acting rescue inhaler such as albuterol.

• Educate patient using a short-acting bronchodilator on a scheduled basis, to stop scheduled use and use only for rescue therapy.

☉ Alert: Warn patient that serious adverse effects, including death, can occur at higher than recommended doses. Warn patient not to take more inhalations than prescribed.

• Tell patient to stop drug immediately and obtain medical help if life-threatening bronchospasm, severe rash, or swelling in throat occurs.

• Inform patient that he may experience palpitations, chest pain, rapid heartbeat, tremors, or nervousness.

• Tell patient not to swallow the inhalation solution.

• Caution patient to notify prescriber if he notices a decrease in symptom control or more frequent use of his rescue inhaler.

SAFETY ALERT!

argatroban
ahr-GAH-troh-ban

Therapeutic class: Anticoagulants
Pharmacologic class: Direct thrombin inhibitors

AVAILABLE FORMS
Injection: 1 mg/mL, 100 mg/mL

INDICATIONS & DOSAGES

➤ **To prevent or treat thrombosis in patients with heparin-induced thrombocytopenia**
Adults without hepatic impairment:
2 mcg/kg/minute, given as a continuous I.V. infusion; adjust dose until the steady-state aPTT is 1½ to 3 times the initial baseline value, not to exceed 100 seconds; maximum dose 10 mcg/kg/minute. See current manufacturer's label for recommended doses and infusion rates.
Children: 0.75 mcg/kg/minute by I.V. infusion. Check aPTT after 2 hours and adjust dosage in 0.1- to 0.25-mcg/kg/minute increments to achieve target aPTT of 1½ to 3 times the baseline value, not to exceed 100 seconds.
Adjust-a-dose: For adults with moderate hepatic impairment, reduce first dose to 0.5 mcg/kg/minute, given as a continuous infusion. Monitor aPTT closely and adjust dosage as needed. For children with hepatic impairment, initial dose is 0.2 mcg/kg/minute. Adjust dosage in 0.05-mcg/kg/minute or lower increments. Monitor aPTT after 2 hours and adjust dosage as needed to achieve target aPTT.

➤ **Anticoagulation in patients with or at risk for heparin-induced thrombocytopenia during PCI**
Adults: 350 mcg/kg I.V. bolus over 3 to 5 minutes. Start a continuous I.V. infusion at 25 mcg/kg/minute. Check activated clotting time (ACT) 5 to 10 minutes after bolus dose is completed.

Adjust-a-dose: Use the following table to adjust dosage.

Activated clotting time	Additional I.V. bolus	Continuous I.V. infusion
<300 sec	150 mcg/kg	30 mcg/kg/min*
>450 sec	None needed	15 mcg/kg/min*

*Check ACT again after 5 to 10 minutes.

Once a therapeutic ACT (300 to 450 sec) has been achieved, continue this dose for the duration of the procedure. In case of dissection, impending abrupt closure, thrombus formation during the procedure, or inability to achieve or maintain an ACT exceeding 300 seconds, give an additional bolus of 150 mcg/kg and increase infusion rate to 40 mcg/kg/minute. Check ACT again after 5 to 10 minutes.

ADMINISTRATION

I.V.
▼ Before starting therapy, obtain a complete list of patient's prescription and OTC drugs and supplements, including herbs.
▼ Stop all parenteral anticoagulants before giving drug. Giving with antiplatelets, thrombolytics, and other anticoagulants may increase risk of bleeding.
▼ Before starting drug, get results of baseline coagulation tests, platelet count, Hb level, and hematocrit, and report any abnormalities to prescriber.
▼ Dilute in NSS, D$_5$W, or lactated Ringer injection to a final concentration of 1 mg/mL.
▼ Dilute each 2.5-mL vial 100-fold by mixing it with 250 mL of diluent.
▼ Mix the solution by repeated inversion of the diluent bag for 1 minute.
▼ Administer bolus over 3 to 5 minutes through large-bore I.V. line. Initiate infusion at 25 mcg/kg/minute.
▼ Don't expose solution to direct sunlight.
▼ Prepared solutions are stable for up to 24 hours at 77° F (25° C).
▼ **Incompatibilities:** Other I.V. drugs.

ACTION

Reversibly binds to the thrombin-active site and inhibits thrombin-catalyzed or -induced reactions: fibrin formation; coagulation factor V, VIII, and XIII activation; protein C activation; and platelet aggregation. May inhibit the action of free and clot-associated thrombin.

Route	Onset	Peak	Duration
I.V.	Rapid	1–3 hr	Duration of infusion

Half-life: 39 to 51 minutes.

ADVERSE REACTIONS

CNS: *cerebrovascular disorder, hemorrhage,* fever, pain, headache.
CV: *atrial fibrillation, cardiac arrest,* hypotension, *ventricular tachycardia,* chest pain, angina, *bradycardia, MI,* groin or brachial bleeding.
GI: abdominal pain, diarrhea, *GI bleeding,* nausea, vomiting.
GU: abnormal renal function, hematuria, UTI.
Hematologic: anemia, *bleeding.*
Respiratory: cough, dyspnea, pneumonia, hemoptysis.
Other: allergic reactions, brachial bleeding, infection, *sepsis.*

INTERACTIONS

Drug-drug. *Glycoprotein IIb and IIIa inhibitors (abciximab, eptifibatide, tirofiban), thrombolytics:* May increase risk of bleeding, including intracranial bleeding. Avoid using together. Safety and effectiveness of concurrent use hasn't been established.
Heparin: May increase risk of bleeding. Allow sufficient time for heparin's effect on aPTT to decrease before starting argatroban.
Warfarin: May prolong PT and INR and may increase risk of bleeding. Monitor patient closely.
Drug-herb. *Herbs with anticoagulant or antiplatelet properties (alfalfa, anise, bilberry, others):* May increase risk of bleeding. Discourage use together.

EFFECTS ON LAB TEST RESULTS

● May decrease Hb level and hematocrit.

CONTRAINDICATIONS & CAUTIONS

● Contraindicated in patients who have overt major bleeding or who are hypersensitive to drug or any of its components.
● Use cautiously in patients with hepatic disease or conditions that increase the risk of hemorrhage, such as severe hypertension.

Reactions in bold italics are *life-threatening*. Interactions may have a *rapid onset* or a *delayed onset*.

• Use cautiously in patients who have just had lumbar puncture, spinal anesthesia, or major surgery, especially of the brain, spinal cord, or eye; patients with hematologic conditions causing increased bleeding tendencies, such as congenital or acquired bleeding disorders; and patients with GI ulcers or other lesions.

• Use cautiously in critically ill patients; reduced dosages may be needed.

Dialyzable drug: No.

⚠ *Overdose S&S:* Excessive anticoagulation, with or without bleeding.

PREGNANCY-LACTATION-REPRODUCTION

• There are no adequate well-controlled studies in pregnant women. Use during pregnancy only if clearly needed.

• It isn't known if drug appears in breast milk. Patient should discontinue breast-feeding or discontinue drug.

NURSING CONSIDERATIONS

• Check aPTT 2 hours after giving drug; dose adjustments may be required to get a targeted aPTT of 1.5 to 3 times the baseline, no longer than 100 seconds. Steady state is achieved 1 to 3 hours after starting drug.

• Draw blood for additional ACT about every 20 to 30 minutes during prolonged PCI.

❸ *Alert:* Patients can hemorrhage from any site in body. Unexplained decreases in hematocrit or BP or other unexplained symptoms may signify a hemorrhagic event.

• To convert to oral anticoagulant therapy, give warfarin P.O. with argatroban at up to 2 mcg/kg/minute until INR exceeds 4 on combined therapy. After argatroban is stopped, repeat INR in 4 to 6 hours. If the repeat INR is less than desired therapeutic range, resume I.V. argatroban infusion. Repeat procedure daily until desired therapeutic range on warfarin alone is reached.

• *Look alike–sound alike:* Don't confuse argatroban with Aggrastat or Organan.

PATIENT TEACHING

• Tell patient that this drug can cause bleeding, and ask him to report any unusual bruising or bleeding (nosebleeds, bleeding gums) or tarry stools to the prescriber immediately.

• Advise patient to avoid activities that carry a risk of injury and to use a soft toothbrush and an electric razor during therapy.

• Advise patient to consult with prescriber before initiating any herbal therapy; many herbs have anticoagulant, antiplatelet, and fibrinolytic properties.

• Instruct patient to notify prescriber if he has wheezing, trouble breathing, or skin rash.

• Instruct woman who is pregnant, has recently delivered, or is breast-feeding to notify her prescriber.

• Tell patient to notify prescriber if he has GI ulcers or liver disease, or has had recent surgery, radiation treatment, falling episodes, or injury.

aripiprazole
air-eh-PIP-rah-zole

Abilify✒, Abilify Discmelt, Abilify Maintena

aripiprazole lauroxil
Aristada

Therapeutic class: Antipsychotics
Pharmacologic class: Quinolinone derivatives

AVAILABLE FORMS

Injection: 9.75 mg/1.3 mL (7.5 mg/mL) in a single-dose vial
ODTs: 10 mg, 15 mg
Oral solution: 1 mg/mL
Suspension for I.M. use (extended-release): 300 mg, 400 mg; 441 mg/1.6 mL, 662 mg/2.4 mL, 882 mg/3.2 mL in prefilled syringes
Tablets: 2 mg, 5 mg, 10 mg, 15 mg, 20 mg, 30 mg

INDICATIONS & DOSAGES

Adjust-a-dose (for all indications except adjunctive treatment of major depressive disorder): When using with CYP3A4 inhibitors, such as ketoconazole or clarithromycin, or CYP2D6 inhibitors, such as quinidine, fluoxetine, or paroxetine, give half the aripiprazole dose.

When using with drugs that are strong, moderate, or weak inhibitors of CYP3A4 and CYP2D6 or in patients who are poor

metabolizers of CYP2D6, give ¼ the aripiprazole dose. Return to original dosing
after the other drugs are stopped.

When using with CYP3A4 inducers such
as carbamazepine, double the aripiprazole
dose. When the CYP3A4 inducer is stopped,
reduce aripiprazole dose to 10 to 15 mg.

➤ **Schizophrenia (oral, Abilify Maintena)**
Adults: Initially, 10 to 15 mg P.O. daily; increase to maximum daily dose of 30 mg, if
needed, after at least 2 weeks. Responding
patients should be continued on the lowest dosage needed to maintain remission.
Patients should be periodically reassessed
to determine the need for maintenance
treatment.

Or, 400 mg (extended-release suspension) I.M. monthly. Maintenance dosage
is 400 mg I.M. monthly, no sooner than
26 days after previous injection. If adverse
reactions occur or for patients who are poor
metabolizers of CYP2D6, give 300 mg
I.M. monthly. If second or third doses
are missed and more than 4 but less than
5 weeks have elapsed since last injection,
give dose as soon as possible. If more than
5 weeks have elapsed, restart concomitant oral aripiprazole for 14 days with next
scheduled injection. If fourth or subsequent
doses are missed and more than 4 but less
than 6 weeks have elapsed since last injection, give dose as soon as possible. If
more than 6 weeks have elapsed, restart
concomitant oral aripiprazole for 14 days
with next scheduled injection.

*Adjust-a-dose (for extended-release sus-
pension):* For patients who are poor metabolizers of CYP2D6 and who are taking
concomitant CYP3A4 inhibitors, give
200 mg extended-release suspension. For
patients taking 400-mg I.M. dose who are
taking strong CYP2D6 or CYP3A4 inhibitors for more than 14 days, give 300 mg.
For patients taking 400-mg I.M. dose who
are taking CYP2D6 and CYP3A4 inhibitors
for more than 14 days, give 200 mg. For
patients taking 400-mg I.M. dose who are
taking CYP3A4 inducers for more than
14 days, avoid use. For patients taking
300-mg I.M. dose who are taking strong
CYP2D6 or CYP3A4 inhibitors for more
than 14 days, give 200 mg. For patients
taking 300-mg I.M. dose who are taking

CYP2D6 and CYP3A4 inhibitors for more
than 14 days, give 160 mg. Avoid use in
patients taking CYP3A4 inducers for more
than 14 days. If CYP2D6 or CYP3A4 inhibitor is withdrawn, dosage may need to be
increased.

Adolescents ages 13 to 17: Initially, 2 mg
P.O. daily; increase to 5 mg after 2 days,
then to recommended dose of 10 mg in
2 more days. May titrate to maximum daily
dose of 30 mg in 5-mg increments. Responding patients should be continued on
the lowest dosage needed to maintain remission. Patients should be periodically
reassessed to determine the need for maintenance treatment.

➤ **Schizophrenia (Aristada)**
Adults: Establish tolerability with oral
aripiprazole before initiating treatment
with aripiprazole lauroxil, which may take
up to 2 weeks. Base initial dose on current oral aripiprazole dose and administer
in conjunction with oral aripiprazole for
21 consecutive days. If current oral aripiprazole dose is 10 mg/day, give 441 mg I.M.
once per month. If current oral aripiprazole
dose is 15 mg/day, give 662 mg I.M. once
per month. If current oral aripiprazole dose
is 20 mg/day or more, give 882 mg I.M.
once every 4 to 6 weeks.

Adjust-a-dose: Adjust dosage as needed; if
a dose is required earlier than the recommended interval, don't administer earlier
than 14 days after the previous injection.
If a strong CYP3A4 inhibitor is initiated
for 2 weeks or more, reduce dose to the
next lower strength. If patient is receiving
882 mg every 6 weeks, give 441 mg every
4 weeks. If patient is a known poor metabolizer of CYP2D6, reduce dose to 441 mg
regardless of current dose. In patients receiving aripiprazole lauroxil 441 mg, no
dosage adjustment is necessary if tolerated.
If a strong CYP2D6 inhibitor is initiated
for 2 weeks or more, reduce dose to the
next lower strength. If patient is receiving
882 mg every 6 weeks, give 441 mg every
4 weeks. In patients receiving aripiprazole
lauroxil 441 mg, no dosage adjustment is
necessary if tolerated. In patients receiving aripiprazole lauroxil 662 or 882 mg,
avoid initiating both a strong CYP3A4 *plus*
a strong CYP2D6 inhibitor for 2 weeks or

---

more. If a CYP3A4 inducer is initiated for 2 weeks or more, increase the 441-mg dose to 662 mg.

➤ **Bipolar mania, including manic and mixed episodes, with or without psychotic features; adjunctive therapy with either lithium or valproate for treatment of manic and mixed episodes associated with bipolar I disorder with or without psychotic features**

Adults: Initially, 15 mg P.O. once daily as monotherapy or 10 to 15 mg P.O. once daily as adjunctive therapy with lithium or valproate. Target dose is 15 mg/day as monotherapy or adjunctive therapy. Dose can be increased to maximum of 30 mg/day based on clinical response. For maintenance, responding patients on monotherapy should be continued on the lowest dose needed to maintain remission. Patients should be periodically reassessed to determine the long-term usefulness of maintenance treatment.

Children ages 10 to 17: Initially, 2 mg P.O. daily; increase to 5 mg P.O. daily after 2 days, then to recommended dose of 10 mg in 2 more days. May titrate to maximum daily dose of 30 mg in 5-mg increments every 5 days. For maintenance, responding patients on monotherapy should be continued on the lowest dose needed to maintain remission. Patients should be periodically reassessed to determine the need for maintenance treatment.

➤ **Adjunctive treatment of major depressive disorder**

Adults: Initially, 2 to 5 mg P.O. daily. Dose range is 2 to 15 mg/day. Dosage adjustments of up to 5 mg/day should occur gradually, at intervals of no less than 1 week.

➤ **Agitation associated with schizophrenia or bipolar I disorder, mixed or manic**

Adults: 5.25 to 15 mg by deep I.M. injection. Recommended dose is 9.75 mg. May give a second dose after 2 hours, if needed. Safety of giving more frequently than every 2 hours or a total daily dose more than 30 mg isn't known. Switch to oral form as soon as possible.

➤ **Irritability associated with autistic disorder**

Children ages 6 to 17: Initially, 2 mg P.O. daily. Increase dosage to 5 mg/day, with

subsequent increases to 10 or 15 mg/day if needed. Dosage adjustments of up to 5 mg/day should occur gradually, at intervals of no less than 1 week.

➤ **Tourette disorder**

Children ages 6 to 18 weighing 50 kg or more: Initially, 2 mg/day P.O. for 2 days; then increase to 5 mg/day with a target dose of 10 mg/day on day 8. If optimal control of tics isn't achieved, increase by 5 mg/day at intervals of no less than 1 week to maximum of 20 mg/day.

Children ages 6 to 18 weighing less than 50 kg: Initially, 2 mg/day P.O. and increasing to target dose of 5 mg/day after 2 days. If optimal control of tics isn't achieved, increase to 10 mg/day. Adjust dosage at intervals of no less than 1 week.

ADMINISTRATION

P.O.
● Give drug without regard for food.
● Substitute the oral solution on a milligram-by-milligram basis for the 5-, 10-, 15-, or 20-mg tablets, up to 25 mg. Give patients taking 30-mg tablets 25 mg of solution.
● Keep ODTs in blister package until ready to use. Use dry hands to carefully peel open the foil backing and remove the tablet. Don't split tablet.
● Store oral solution in refrigerator; it can be used up to 6 months after opening.

I.M.
● Inject slowly and deep into the muscle mass. Use the deltoid muscle only for the 441-mg dose.
● Don't give I.V. or subcutaneously.
● Don't confuse I.M. formulations. They aren't interchangeable.

ACTION

Thought to exert partial agonist activity at dopamine 2 and 5-HT$_{1A}$ receptors and antagonist activity at 5-HT$_{2A}$ receptors.

Route	Onset	Peak	Duration
P.O.	Unknown	3–5 hr	Unknown
I.M.	Unknown	1–3 hr	Unknown

Half-life: About 75 hours in patients with normal metabolism; about 6 days in those who can't metabolize the drug through CYP2D6.

ADVERSE REACTIONS

CNS: headache, anxiety, insomnia, light-headedness, somnolence, akathisia, *increased suicide risk, neuroleptic malignant syndrome, seizures, suicidal thoughts,* extrapyramidal disorder (children), tremor, asthenia, depression, fatigue, dizziness, nervousness, hostility, manic behavior, confusion, abnormal gait, cogwheel rigidity, fever, tardive dyskinesia, restlessness, agitation.

CV: peripheral edema, chest pain, hypertension, tachycardia, orthostatic hypotension, *bradycardia.*

EENT: blurred vision, conjunctivitis, ear pain, rhinitis, increased salivation, nasopharyngitis.

GI: nausea, vomiting, constipation, anorexia, dry mouth, dyspepsia, diarrhea, abdominal pain, esophageal dysmotility, increased appetite.

GU: urinary incontinence.

Hematologic: ecchymosis, anemia.

Metabolic: weight gain, weight loss, hyperglycemia, hypercholesterolemia.

Musculoskeletal: neck pain, neck stiffness, muscle cramps, myalgia, extremity pain.

Respiratory: dyspnea, pneumonia, cough.

Skin: rash, dry skin, pruritus, sweating, ulcer.

Other: flulike syndrome.

INTERACTIONS

Drug-drug. *Antihypertensives:* May enhance antihypertensive effects. Monitor BP.

Benzodiazepines: May cause excessive sedation and orthostatic hypotension. Monitor patient closely (I.M. form).

Carbamazepine and other CYP3A4 inducers: May decrease levels and effectiveness of aripiprazole. Double the usual dose of aripiprazole, and monitor patient closely.

CNS depressants: May lead to enhanced CNS depression. Use together with caution.

Ketoconazole and other CYP3A4 inhibitors: May increase risk of serious toxic effects. Start treatment with half the usual dose of aripiprazole, and monitor patient closely.

Metoclopramide: May increase risk of extrapyramidal reactions. Use together is contraindicated.

Black Box Warning *Opioids:* May cause slow or difficult breathing, sedation, and death. Avoid use together. If use together is necessary, limit dosage and duration of each drug to the minimum necessary for desired effect. ∎

Potential CYP2D6 inhibitors (fluoxetine, paroxetine, quinidine): May increase levels and toxicity of aripiprazole. Give half the usual dose of aripiprazole (P.O.) or 25% the usual dose (I.M.).

Drug-food. *Grapefruit juice:* May increase drug level. Tell patient not to take drug with grapefruit juice.

Drug-lifestyle. *Alcohol use:* May increase CNS effects. Discourage use together.

EFFECTS ON LAB TEST RESULTS

● May increase CK and glucose levels.
● May decrease WBC count and ANC.

CONTRAINDICATIONS & CAUTIONS

● Contraindicated in patients hypersensitive to drug.

Black Box Warning Opioid drugs should only be prescribed with benzodiazepines or other CNS depressants to patients for whom alternative treatment options are inadequate. ∎

Black Box Warning Drug isn't approved for use in children with depression. ∎

Black Box Warning Elderly patients with dementia-related psychosis treated with atypical antipsychotics are at an increased risk for death. Abilify isn't approved for treatment of patients with dementia-related psychosis. ∎

● Use cautiously in patients with CV disease, cerebrovascular disease, or conditions that could predispose patient to hypotension, such as dehydration or hypovolemia.

● Life-threatening arrhythmias have occurred with therapeutic doses of antipsychotics.

● Use cautiously in patients with history of seizures or with conditions that lower the seizure threshold.

● Use cautiously in patients who engage in strenuous exercise, are exposed to extreme heat, take anticholinergics, or are susceptible to dehydration.

● Use cautiously in patients with Lewy body dementia or Parkinson disease; drug may aggravate motor disturbances.

Reactions in bold italics are *life-threatening*. Interactions may have a *rapid onset* or a *delayed onset.*

● Use cautiously in patients at risk for aspiration pneumonia, such as those with Alzheimer disease.

● Discontinue drug at first sign of blood dyscrasia or if ANC is less than $1,000/mm^3$.

Dialyzable drug: Unknown.

⚠ Overdose S&S: Somnolence, tremor, vomiting, acidosis, aggression, atrial fibrillation, bradycardia, coma, confusion, seizures, depressed level of consciousness, hypertension, hypokalemia, hypotension, increased AST and blood CK levels, lethargy, loss of consciousness, aspiration pneumonia, prolonged QRS complex, prolonged QT interval, respiratory arrest, status epilepticus, tachycardia.

PREGNANCY-LACTATION-REPRODUCTION

● Safety of atypical antipsychotic use in pregnant women hasn't been well studied; routine use isn't recommended. Use during pregnancy only if potential benefit justifies potential risk to the fetus.

● **Alert:** Neonates exposed to antipsychotics during the third trimester are at risk for developing extrapyramidal signs and symptoms (repetitive muscle movements of the face and body) and withdrawal signs and symptoms (agitation, abnormally increased or decreased muscle tone, tremors, sleepiness, severe difficulty breathing, difficulty feeding) after delivery.

● Enroll pregnant women exposed to aripiprazole in the National Pregnancy Registry for Atypical Antipsychotics (1-866-961-2388).

● Drug appears in breast milk. Use in breast-feeding women isn't recommended.

NURSING CONSIDERATIONS

● **Alert:** Neuroleptic malignant syndrome may occur. Monitor patient for hyperpyrexia, muscle rigidity, altered mental status, irregular pulse or BP, tachycardia, diaphoresis, and cardiac arrhythmias.

● If signs and symptoms of neuroleptic malignant syndrome occur, immediately stop drug and notify prescriber.

● Monitor patient for signs and symptoms of tardive dyskinesia. Elderly patients, especially women, are at highest risk for developing this adverse effect.

● **Alert:** Fatal cerebrovascular adverse events (stroke, TIA) may occur in elderly patients with dementia. Drug isn't safe or effective in these patients.

Black Box Warning Drug may increase the risk of suicidal thinking and behavior in children, adolescents, and young adults ages 18 to 24 during the first 2 months of treatment, especially in those with major depressive or other psychiatric disorder. ∎

● **Alert:** Hyperglycemia may occur. Monitor patient with diabetes regularly. Patient with risk factors for diabetes should undergo fasting blood glucose testing at baseline and periodically. Monitor all patients for symptoms of hyperglycemia, including increased hunger, thirst, frequent urination, and weakness. Hyperglycemia may resolve when patient stops taking drug.

● **Alert:** Monitor patient for symptoms of metabolic syndrome (significant weight gain and increased BMI, hypertension, hyperglycemia, hypercholesterolemia, and hypertriglyceridemia).

● **Alert:** Monitor patient for new or increasing compulsive or uncontrollable urges to gamble, binge eat, shop, and have sex. Dosage may need to be reduced or drug discontinued if urges occur.

● Monitor patients with clinically significant neutropenia for fever or other signs and symptoms of infection; treat promptly if they occur. Discontinue drug if ANC is less than $1,000/mm^3$.

● Treat patient with the smallest dose for the shortest time, and periodically reevaluate for need to continue.

● Give prescriptions only for small quantities of drug, to reduce risk of overdose.

● **Look alike–sound alike:** Don't confuse aripiprazole with rabeprazole, omeprazole, or pantoprazole.

PATIENT TEACHING

Black Box Warning Advise families and caregivers to closely observe patient for clinical worsening, suicidality, or unusual changes in behavior. ∎

Black Box Warning Caution the patient or the caregiver of a patient taking an opioid drug with a benzodiazepine, CNS depressants, or alcohol to seek immediate medical attention if the patient has symptoms of dizziness, light-headedness, extreme sleepiness, slowed or difficult breathing, or unresponsiveness. ■

ⓘ Alert: Advise patient and caregiver to notify prescriber if compulsive or uncontrollable urges occur.

ⓘ Alert: Caution patient not to stop drug without first discussing with prescriber.

• Tell patient to use caution while driving or operating hazardous machinery because psychoactive drugs may impair judgment, thinking, or motor skills.

• Tell patient that drug may be taken without regard to meals.

• Advise patients that grapefruit juice may interact with aripiprazole and to limit or avoid its use.

• Advise patient that gradual improvement in symptoms should occur over several weeks rather than immediately.

ⓘ Alert: Warn patient with phenylketonuria that ODTs contain phenylalanine.

• Tell patients to avoid alcohol use while taking drug.

• Advise patients to limit strenuous activity while taking drug to avoid dehydration.

• Tell patient to keep ODT in blister package until ready to use. Using dry hands, he should carefully peel open the foil backing and place tablet on tongue. Tell him not to split tablet.

• Tell patient to store oral solution in refrigerator, and that the solution can be used for up to 6 months after opening.

armodafinil
ar-moe-DAF-i-nil

Nuvigil

Therapeutic class: Stimulants
Pharmacologic class: CNS stimulants
Controlled substance schedule: IV

AVAILABLE FORMS
Tablets: 50 mg, 150 mg, 200 mg, 250 mg

INDICATIONS & DOSAGES
➤ **To improve wakefulness in patients with excessive sleepiness caused by narcolepsy, obstructive sleep apnea–hypoapnea syndrome (OSAHS), or shift-work sleep disorder**

Adults: 150 or 250 mg P.O. daily in morning. For OSAHS, doses exceeding 150 mg daily may not be more effective. For shift-work sleep disorder, 150 mg P.O. daily, 1 hour before start of shift.

Adjust-a-dose: Reduce dosage in patients with severe hepatic impairment, with or without cirrhosis. Consider lower doses in elderly patients.

ADMINISTRATION
P.O.
• Give drug consistently with or without food at same time each day. Food may delay effect of drug.

ACTION
Unknown. May be similar to sympathomimetics, such as amphetamine and methylphenidate. Also may inhibit dopamine reuptake.

Route	Onset	Peak	Duration
P.O.	Unknown	2 hr	Unknown

Half-life: 15 hours.

ADVERSE REACTIONS
CNS: agitation, anxiety, depression, dizziness, fatigue, headache, insomnia, migraine, nervousness, pain, paresthesia, pyrexia, tremor, disturbance in attention.
CV: increased BP, increased pulse rate, palpitations.
GI: abdominal pain, anorexia, constipation, diarrhea, dry mouth, dyspepsia, loose stools, nausea, vomiting, decreased appetite.
Respiratory: dyspnea, seasonal allergy.
Skin: contact dermatitis, hyperhidrosis, rash, *Stevens-Johnson syndrome.*
Other: allergic reactions, flulike illness, thirst.

INTERACTIONS
Drug-drug. *Drugs metabolized by CYP2C19 (diazepam, omeprazole, phenytoin, propranolol):* May increase levels of these drugs. Monitor patient and reduce doses as needed.
Drugs metabolized by CYP3A (cyclosporine, ethinyl estradiol, midazolam, triazolam): May decrease levels of these drugs. Adjust doses as needed.

Reactions in bold italics are *life-threatening*. Interactions may have a *rapid onset* or a *delayed onset*.

Drugs that induce CYP3A (carbamazepine, phenobarbital, rifampin): May decrease armodafinil level. Check drug level and adjust dose as needed.

Drugs that inhibit CYP3A (erythromycin, ketoconazole): May increase armodafinil level. Monitor patient carefully and decrease dose as needed.

Hormonal contraceptives: May decrease effectiveness of these drugs. Alternative or concomitant contraceptive methods are recommended during and for 1 month after armodafinil therapy.

Drug-food. *Any food:* May delay onset of action by several hours. Monitor effect and give drug consistently with or without food, at the same time daily.

Drug-lifestyle. *Alcohol use:* May counteract armodafinil's effect. Discourage use together.

EFFECTS ON LAB TEST RESULTS
• May increase GGT and alkaline phosphatase levels.

CONTRAINDICATIONS & CAUTIONS
• Contraindicated in patients hypersensitive to modafinil, armodafinil, or their inactive ingredients.
• Avoid use in patients with left ventricular hypertrophy and in those who have experienced mitral valve prolapse when drug is given with other CNS stimulants.
• Use cautiously in patients with a history of drug abuse or dependence.
🜂 *Alert:* Use cautiously in patients with psychosis, depression, or mania; drug may increase the risk of mania, delusion, hallucinations, and suicidal ideation.
• Use cautiously in patients with cardiac disease, Tourette syndrome, multiorgan hypersensitivity, severe hepatic impairment, or rash, including Stevens-Johnson syndrome.
• Use cautiously in elderly patients.
• Safety and effectiveness in patients younger than age 17 haven't been established.
Dialyzable drug: Unknown.
⚠ *Overdose S&S:* Excitation or agitation, insomnia, slight or moderate elevations in hemodynamic parameters, restlessness, disorientation, confusion, hallucinations, nausea, diarrhea, tachycardia, bradycardia, hypertension, chest pain.

PREGNANCY-LACTATION-REPRODUCTION
• Use in pregnancy only when benefit to mother outweighs risk to fetus.
• Register women exposed to drug in the Nuvigil Pregnancy Registry (1-866-404-4106).
• It isn't known if drug appears in breast milk. Use cautiously in breast-feeding women.

NURSING CONSIDERATIONS
• Obtain a thorough medication history to avoid potentially dangerous drug interactions.
• Obtain a complete cardiac history. Monitor patient for increased BP and pulse rate, ECG changes, chest pain, and arrhythmias.
• Monitor patient carefully for evidence of allergic reaction. If rash or other symptoms appear, stop drug immediately, notify prescriber, and monitor carefully.
• Monitor patients for signs and symptoms of misuse or abuse, especially those with a history of drug or stimulant abuse.
• Assess patient for abnormal level of sleepiness. Don't allow patient to engage in dangerous activities, such as driving, until effect of medication is known.
• Patients receiving continuous positive airway pressure therapy for OSAHS should continue its use regardless of armodafinil therapy.

PATIENT TEACHING
🜂 *Alert:* Instruct patient to stop taking drug and notify prescriber if rash, hives, mouth sores, blister, peeling skin, trouble swallowing or breathing, or other symptoms of allergic reaction occur.
• Tell patient not to perform hazardous tasks, such as driving, if he feels excessive sleepiness or until effects of drug are known.
• Tell patient to notify prescriber of all drugs he takes to avoid potentially dangerous drug interactions.
• Tell patient to take drug at the same time, with or without food, every day.
• Caution woman of childbearing potential taking hormonal contraceptives to use alternative or additional methods of contraception during and for 1 month after armodafinil therapy.

• Advise patient that taking drug with food may delay its effects.

• Urge patient to notify prescriber right away if she becomes pregnant or plans to breast-feed.

asenapine
a-SEN-uh-peen

Saphris

Therapeutic class: Antipsychotics
Pharmacologic class: Dopamine–serotonin antagonists

AVAILABLE FORMS
Tablets (sublingual) ⒪⒯⒞: 2.5 mg, 5 mg, 10 mg

INDICATIONS & DOSAGES
➤ **Acute schizophrenia**
Adults: 5 mg S.L. b.i.d. May increase up to 10 mg b.i.d. after 1 week based on tolerability.
➤ **Acute manic or mixed episodes associated with bipolar I disorder as monotherapy or as adjunctive therapy with either lithium or valproate**
Adults: For monotherapy, 10 mg S.L. b.i.d. For adjunctive therapy, 5 mg S.L. b.i.d. Dosage may be increased to a maximum of 10 mg S.L. b.i.d.
Adjust-a-dose: If adverse effects occur, reduce dosage to 5 mg b.i.d.
➤ **Acute manic or mixed episodes associated with bipolar I disorder as monotherapy**
Children ages 10 to 17: Initially, 2.5 mg S.L. b.i.d. May increase after 3 days to 5 mg b.i.d., then to 10 mg b.i.d. after 3 additional days based on tolerability.

ADMINISTRATION
P.O.
• Obtain BP before starting drug, and monitor pressure regularly. Watch for orthostatic hypotension.
• Make sure patient doesn't split, crush, chew, or swallow tablet.
• Peel back colored tab on tablet pack, gently remove tablet, place under patient's tongue, and allow to dissolve completely.
• Advise patient not to eat or drink for 10 minutes after taking drug.

ACTION
Unknown. May block dopamine and 5-HT$_2$ receptors.

Route	Onset	Peak	Duration
S.L.	Immediate	½–1 hr	Unknown

Half-life: 24 hours.

ADVERSE REACTIONS
CNS: akathisia, anxiety, depression, dizziness, extrapyramidal symptoms, fatigue, headache, insomnia, irritability, somnolence.
CV: hypertension, peripheral edema.
EENT: dry mouth, oral hypoesthesia, salivary hypersecretion, toothache.
GI: constipation, dyspepsia, increased appetite, stomach discomfort, taste perversion, vomiting.
Metabolic: weight gain.
Musculoskeletal: arthralgia, extremity pain.

INTERACTIONS
Drug-drug. *Alpha$_1$ blockers (such as doxazosin, terazosin):* May increase risk of hypotension. Use together cautiously.
Antiarrhythmics, class IA (procainamide, quinidine) and class III (amiodarone, sotalol); antibiotics (gatifloxacin, moxifloxacin); antipsychotics (chlorpromazine, thioridazine, ziprasidone); citalopram: May prolong QTc interval, leading to lethal arrhythmias such as torsades de pointes. Avoid use together.
Antidepressants (fluvoxamine, imipramine, paroxetine): May increase asenapine level. Use together cautiously. Reduce paroxetine dosage by half if using with asenapine.
CNS agents (opioids): May enhance CNS depression. Use with caution.
Dextromethorphan, paroxetine: May increase dextromethorphan and paroxetine levels. Use together cautiously.
Metoclopramide: May increase risk of extrapyramidal reactions. Avoid administering together.
Black Box Warning *Opioids:* May cause slow or difficult breathing, sedation, and death. Avoid use together. If use together is necessary, limit dosage and duration of each drug to the minimum necessary for desired effect. ∎
Drug-lifestyle. *Alcohol use:* May increase CNS effects. Discourage use together.

EFFECTS ON LAB TEST RESULTS
• May increase glucose, cholesterol, ALT, AST, and prolactin levels.
• May decrease WBC and neutrophil counts.

CONTRAINDICATIONS & CAUTIONS
Black Box Warning Elderly patients with dementia-related psychosis treated with atypical or conventional antipsychotics are at increased risk for death. Antipsychotics aren't approved for the treatment of dementia-related psychosis. ■
Black Box Warning Opioid drugs should only be prescribed with benzodiazepines or other CNS depressants to patients for whom alternative treatment options are inadequate. ■
☋ *Alert:* Don't administer drug to patients with a known hypersensitivity. Hypersensitivity reactions may occur as early as the first dose.
☋ *Alert:* Contraindicated in patients with severe hepatic failure (Child-Pugh class C).
☋ *Alert:* Avoid use in patients with conditions that may increase risk of torsades de pointes and in those taking other drugs that prolong QTc interval.
• Use cautiously in patients with or at risk for diabetes; in those with known CV or cerebrovascular disease, preexisting low WBC count, difficulty swallowing, history of leukopenia or neutropenia, Parkinson disease, or history of seizures or conditions that lower the seizure threshold; and in antipsychotic-naive patients.
• Don't use in patients at risk for aspiration pneumonia.
• Safety and effectiveness in children younger than age 10 haven't been established.
Dialyzable drug: Unknown.
⚠ *Overdose S&S:* Agitation, confusion, hypotension, circulatory collapse.

PREGNANCY-LACTATION-REPRODUCTION
• Drug may cause fetal harm. Safety of atypical antipsychotic use during pregnancy hasn't been well studied; routine use isn't recommended. Use during pregnancy only if potential benefit justifies potential risk to the fetus.
☋ *Alert:* Neonates exposed to antipsychotics during the third trimester are at risk for developing extrapyramidal signs and symptoms (repetitive muscle movements of the face and body) and withdrawal signs and symptoms (agitation, abnormally increased or decreased muscle tone, tremors, sleepiness, severe difficulty breathing, difficulty feeding) after delivery.
• Pregnant women exposed to asenapine should be enrolled in National Pregnancy Registry for Atypical Antipsychotics (1-866-961-2388).
• It isn't known if drug appears in breast milk. A decision should be made to discontinue breast-feeding or discontinue drug, taking into account risk to infant and importance of drug to mother.

NURSING CONSIDERATIONS
• Monitor ECG before and regularly during treatment for prolongation of QTc interval.
• Monitor patient for tardive dyskinesia, which may occur after prolonged use. It may disappear spontaneously or persist for life, despite stopping drug.
☋ *Alert:* Watch for signs and symptoms of neuroleptic malignant syndrome (extrapyramidal effects, hyperthermia, autonomic disturbance), which are rare but can be fatal. Discontinue drug immediately if they occur, and monitor patient closely.
• Monitor patient for serious allergic reactions (anaphylaxis, angioedema, hypotension, difficulty breathing, wheezing, swollen tongue, rash).
• Drug may alter glucose control in diabetics. Monitor glucose levels closely.
• Monitor CBC frequently during first few months of therapy in those with history of leukopenia or neutropenia. If WBC count decreases, monitor patient for signs and symptoms of infection; if infection occurs, discontinue drug in the absence of another cause.
• Obtain BP before starting drug, and monitor BP regularly. Watch for orthostatic hypotension.
• Monitor patient for dysphagia, which can lead to aspiration and aspiration pneumonia.
• Dispense lowest appropriate quantity of drug, to reduce risk of overdose.
• Monitor patient for abnormal body temperature regulation, especially if he exercises, is exposed to extreme heat, takes anticholinergics, or is dehydrated.

PATIENT TEACHING

Black Box Warning Caution the patient or the caregiver of a patient taking an opioid drug with a benzodiazepine, CNS depressant, or alcohol to seek immediate medical attention if the patient has symptoms of dizziness, light-headedness, extreme sleepiness, slowed or difficult breathing, or unresponsiveness. ■

• Instruct patient to peel back colored tab on tablet pack, gently remove tablet, place under the tongue, and allow to dissolve completely. Advise patient not to swallow tablet and not to eat or drink for 10 minutes after taking drug.

• Warn patient to avoid activities that require mental alertness, such as operating hazardous machinery or operating a motor vehicle, until drug's effects are known.

• Advise patient to contact prescriber if palpitations or rapid heartbeat occurs.

• Advise patient not to stand up quickly but to get up slowly from a sitting position to avoid dizziness.

• Inform patient that weight gain may occur.

• Warn patient against exposure to extreme heat because drug may impair body's ability to reduce temperature.

• Advise patient to avoid alcohol.

---

aspirin
(acetylsalicylic acid, ASA)
AS-pir-in

Asaphen✹ ◇, Asatab✹ ◇, Aspir-Low ◇, Aspir-81 ◇, Bayer Aspirin ◇, Durlaza, Ecotrin ◇, EcPirin ◇, Entrophen✹ ◇, Lowprin✹ ◇, Miniprin Low Dose ◇, Norwich ◇, Novasen✹ ◇, Rivasa✹ ◇, St. Joseph Aspirin ◇

Therapeutic class: NSAIDs
Pharmacologic class: Salicylates

AVAILABLE FORMS

Capsules: 325 mg ◇
Capsules (extended-release) **ONC**: 162.5 mg
Suppositories: 60 mg ◇, 120 mg ◇, 150 mg✹ ◇, 200 mg ◇, 300 mg ◇, 600 mg ◇, 650 mg✹ ◇
Tablets: 325 mg ◇, 500 mg ◇

Tablets (chewable): 80 mg✹ ◇, 81 mg ◇
Tablets (enteric-coated) **ONC**: 80 mg✹ ◇, 81 mg ◇, 162 mg✹ ◇, 325 mg ◇, 500 mg ◇, 975 mg✹ ◇

INDICATIONS & DOSAGES

➤ **RA, osteoarthritis, or other poly-arthritic or inflammatory conditions**
Adults: Initially, 3 g P.O. daily in divided doses. Increase as needed, with target plasma salicylate levels of 150 to 300 mcg/mL.

➤ **Juvenile RA**
Children: 90 to 130 mg/kg/day in divided doses. Increase as needed, with target plasma salicylate levels of 150 to 300 mcg/mL.

➤ **Mild pain or fever; spondylo-arthropathies**
Adults: and children older than age 12: 324 to 1,000 mg P.O. or P.R. every 4 hours p.r.n. Or, for delayed-release products, 1,300 mg P.O. followed by 650 to 1,300 mg P.O. every 8 hours. Maximum dose is 4,000 mg in 24 hours.
Children ages 2 to 11: 10 to 15 mg/kg/dose P.O. or P.R. every 4 hours up to 80 mg/kg daily.

➤ **Suspected acute MI**
Adults: Initial dose of 160 to 325 mg P.O. as soon as MI is suspected. Continue maintenance dose of 160 to 325 mg P.O. daily for 30 days after infarction. After 30 days, consider further therapy for prevention of MI.

➤ **To reduce risk of MI in patients with previous MI, unstable angina, and chronic stable angina pectoris**
Adults: 75 to 325 mg P.O. daily. Or, 162.5 mg extended-release capsule P.O. daily.

➤ **To reduce risk of recurrent TIAs and stroke or death in patients at risk**
Adults: 50 to 325 mg P.O. daily.

➤ **Acute ischemic stroke**
Adults: 50 to 325 mg P.O. daily, started within 48 hours of stroke onset; continue indefinitely.

➤ **CABG**
Adults: 325 mg P.O. daily starting 6 hours postprocedure.

➤ **Percutaneous transluminal coronary angioplasty**

Reactions in bold italics are *life-threatening*. Interactions may have a *rapid onset* or a *delayed onset*.

Adults: Initial dose of 325 mg P.O. 2 hours before surgery and then 160 to 325 mg P.O. daily.

➤ **Carotid endarterectomy**
Adults: 80 mg P.O. daily to 650 mg P.O. b.i.d. starting before surgery.

ADMINISTRATION
P.O.
• For patient with swallowing difficulties, crush non–enteric-coated aspirin and dissolve in soft food or liquid. Give liquid immediately after mixing because drug will break down rapidly.
• Give drug with food, milk, antacid, or large glass of water to reduce GI effects.
• Give enteric-coated or extended-release forms whole; don't crush or break these tablets.
• For acute MI, have patient chew tablet.
Rectal
• Refrigerate suppositories.

ACTION
Thought to produce analgesia and exert its anti-inflammatory effect by inhibiting prostaglandin and other substances that sensitize pain receptors. Drug may relieve fever through central action in the hypothalamic heat-regulating center. In low doses, drug also appears to interfere with clotting by keeping a platelet-aggregating substance from forming.

Route	Onset	Peak	Duration
P.O. (buffered)	5–30 min	1–2 hr	1–4 hr
P.O. (enteric-coated)	5–30 min	Variable	1–4 hr
P.O. (tablet)	5–30 min	25–40 min	1–4 hr
P.O. (extended-release)	Unknown	2 hr	4–8 hr
P.R.	Unknown	3–4 hr	Unknown

Half-life: 15 minutes to 6 hours (dose dependent).

ADVERSE REACTIONS
CNS: agitation, *cerebral edema, coma,* confusion, dizziness, headache, lethargy, *seizures, subdural or intracranial hemorrhage.*
CV: *arrhythmias,* hypotension, tachycardia.
EENT: tinnitus, hearing loss.
GI: nausea, *GI bleeding,* dyspepsia, GI distress, occult bleeding, *pancreatitis,* vomiting.

GU: *antepartum and postpartum bleeding,* interstitial nephritis, papillary necrosis, prolonged pregnancy and labor, proteinuria, renal insufficiency, renal failure.
Hematologic: prolonged bleeding time, *leukopenia, thrombocytopenia,* coagulopathy, *DIC.*
Hepatic: *hepatitis.*
Metabolic: dehydration, *hyperkalemia, metabolic acidosis,* respiratory alkalosis.
Skin: rash, bruising, urticaria, hives.
Other: *angioedema, Reye syndrome,* hypersensitivity reactions, low birth weight (infants), stillbirth.

INTERACTIONS
Drug-drug. *ACE inhibitors:* May decrease antihypertensive effects. Monitor BP closely.
Acetazolamide: May cause accumulation and toxicity of acetazolamide, resulting in CNS depression, metabolic acidosis, anorexia, and death. Administer together with caution and monitor patient for toxicity.
Ammonium chloride and other urine acidifiers: May increase levels of aspirin products. Watch for aspirin toxicity.
Antacids in high doses and other urine alkalinizers: May decrease levels of aspirin products. Watch for decreased aspirin effect.
Anticoagulants, antiplatelet agents: May increase risk of bleeding. Use with extreme caution if these drugs must be used together.
Beta blockers: May decrease antihypertensive effect. Avoid long-term aspirin use if patient is taking antihypertensives.
Corticosteroids: May enhance salicylate elimination and decrease drug level. Watch for decreased aspirin effect.
Diuretics: May decrease effectiveness of diuretics in patients with underlying renal or CV disease. Monitor patient for effectiveness.
Heparin: May increase risk of bleeding. Monitor coagulation studies and patient closely if used together.
Ibuprofen, other NSAIDs: May negate the antiplatelet effect of low-dose aspirin therapy. Patients using immediate-release aspirin (not enteric-coated) should take ibuprofen at least 30 minutes after or more than 8 hours before aspirin. Occasional use

of ibuprofen is unlikely to have a negative effect.

Influenza virus vaccine, live: Increased risk of Reye syndrome. Use together is contraindicated in children and adolescents.

Methotrexate: May increase risk of methotrexate toxicity. Avoid using together.

Oral antidiabetics: May increase hypoglycemic effect. Monitor patient closely.

Probenecid, sulfinpyrazone: May decrease uricosuric effect. Avoid using together.

Valproic acid: May increase valproic acid level. Avoid using together.

Drug-herb. *White willow:* Contains salicylates and may increase risk of adverse effects. Discourage use together.

Drug-food. *Caffeine:* May increase drug absorption. Watch for increased effects.

Drug-lifestyle. *Alcohol use:* May increase risk of GI bleeding. Discourage use together.

EFFECTS ON LAB TEST RESULTS
● May increase LFT values, BUN, creatinine, and potassium levels.
● May decrease platelet and WBC counts.
● May falsely increase protein-bound iodine level.
● May interfere with urine glucose analysis with Diastix, Chemstrip uG, Clinitest, and Benedict solution; with urinary 5-hydroxyindoleacetic acid and vanillylmandelic acid tests; and with Gerhardt test for urine acetoacetic acid.

CONTRAINDICATIONS & CAUTIONS
● Contraindicated in patients hypersensitive to drug and in those with NSAID-induced sensitivity reactions, G6PD deficiency, or bleeding disorders, such as hemophilia, von Willebrand disease, telangiectasia, bleeding ulcers, and hemorrhagic states.
● Use cautiously in patients with GI lesions, impaired renal function, hypoprothrombinemia, vitamin K deficiency, thrombocytopenia, or thrombotic thrombocytopenic purpura.
● Avoid use in patients with severe hepatic impairment or history of active peptic ulcer disease.
● **Alert:** Oral and rectal OTC products containing aspirin and nonaspirin salicylates shouldn't be given to children or teenagers who have or are recovering from chickenpox

or flulike symptoms with or without fever because of the risk of Reye syndrome.
● Safe use of extended-release capsules in children hasn't been established.
Dialyzable drug: Unknown.
⚠ **Overdose S&S:** Severe acid-base and electrolyte disturbance, hyperthermia, dehydration, tinnitus, vertigo, headache, confusion, drowsiness, diaphoresis, hyperventilation, vomiting, diarrhea.

PREGNANCY-LACTATION-REPRODUCTION
● Use in pregnancy only if clearly needed and specifically directed to do so by a physician. Avoid use during third trimester.
● Drug appears in breast milk. Breastfeeding women should avoid aspirin if possible.

NURSING CONSIDERATIONS
● For inflammatory conditions, rheumatic fever, and thrombosis, give aspirin on a schedule rather than as needed.
● Because enteric-coated tablets are slowly absorbed, they aren't suitable for rapid relief of acute pain, fever, or inflammation. They cause less GI bleeding and may be better suited for long-term therapy, such as for arthritis.
● For patients who can't tolerate oral drugs, ask prescriber about using aspirin rectal suppositories. Watch for rectal mucosal irritation or bleeding.
● Febrile, dehydrated children can develop toxicity rapidly.
● Monitor elderly patients closely because they may be more susceptible to aspirin's toxic effects.
● Monitor salicylate level. Therapeutic salicylate level for arthritis is 150 to 300 mcg/mL. Tinnitus may occur at levels above 200 mcg/mL, but this isn't a reliable indicator of toxicity, especially in very young patients and those older than age 60. With long-term therapy, severe toxic effects may occur with levels exceeding 400 mcg/mL.
● During prolonged therapy, assess hematocrit, Hb level, PT, INR, and renal function periodically.
● Drug irreversibly inhibits platelet aggregation. Stop drug 5 to 7 days before elective

surgery to allow time for production and
release of new platelets.
- Monitor patient for hypersensitivity reactions, such as anaphylaxis and asthma.
- *Look alike–sound alike:* Don't confuse aspirin with Asendin or Afrin.

PATIENT TEACHING
- Tell patient who's allergic to tartrazine to avoid aspirin.
- Advise patient on a low-salt diet that 1 tablet of buffered aspirin contains 553 mg of sodium.
- Advise patient to take drug with food, milk, antacid, or large glass of water to reduce GI reactions.
- Tell patient not to crush or chew enteric-coated or extended-release forms but to swallow them whole.
- Warn patient not to drink alcohol 2 hours before or 1 hour after taking extended-release capsule and not to take extra capsule to make up for a missed dose.
- Remind patient not to stop drug without first discussing with prescriber.
- Instruct patient to discard aspirin tablets that have a strong vinegar-like odor.
- Tell patient to consult prescriber if giving drug to children for longer than 5 days or adults for longer than 10 days.
- Advise patient receiving prolonged treatment with large doses of aspirin to watch for small, round, red pinprick spots; bleeding gums; and signs of GI bleeding; advise patient to drink plenty of fluids. Encourage use of a soft-bristled toothbrush.
- Because of the many drug interactions with aspirin, warn patient taking prescription drugs to check with prescriber or pharmacist before taking aspirin or OTC products containing aspirin.
- Ibuprofen can interfere with the antiplatelet effect of low-dose aspirin therapy, negating its effect. Teach patient how to safely use ibuprofen in relation to aspirin therapy.
- Urge pregnant women to avoid aspirin during last trimester of pregnancy unless specifically directed by prescriber.
- Drug is a leading cause of poisoning in children. Caution parents to keep drug out of reach of children. Encourage use of child-resistant containers.

atazanavir sulfate
ah-TAZ-ah-nah-veer

Reyataz

Therapeutic class: Antiretrovirals
Pharmacologic class: Protease inhibitors

AVAILABLE FORMS
Capsules: 150 mg, 200 mg, 300 mg
Oral powder: 50 mg

INDICATIONS & DOSAGES
Adjust-a-dose (for all indications): In patients with Child-Pugh class B hepatic insufficiency who haven't experienced prior virologic failure, reduce dosage to 300 mg P.O. once daily. Treatment-naive patients with ESRD who are on hemodialysis should receive atazanavir 300 mg with ritonavir 100 mg. Don't give to treatment-experienced patients on hemodialysis.
➤ **HIV-1 infection, with other antiretrovirals in treatment-experienced patients**
Adults: Give 300 mg (as one 300-mg capsule or two 150-mg capsules) once daily, plus 100 mg ritonavir once daily with food. Give patients also taking H_2-receptor antagonist (H2RA) and tenofovir 400 mg P.O. once daily, plus 100 mg ritonavir.
Children and adolescents ages 6 to younger than 18 who are treatment-experienced and receiving ritonavir: For patients weighing 40 kg or more, give 300 mg with ritonavir 100 mg P.O. once daily. For patients weighing 20 to 39 kg, give 200 mg with ritonavir 100 mg P.O. once daily. For patients weighing 15 to 19 kg, give 150 mg with ritonavir 100 mg P.O. once daily.
Children at least age 3 months and weighing at least 5 kg and less than 25 kg: For patients weighing 15 kg to less than 25 kg, give 250 mg P.O. immediately followed by 80 mg ritonavir daily. For patients weighing 5 kg to less than 15 kg, give 200 mg P.O. immediately followed by 80 mg ritonavir daily.
➤ **HIV-1 infection, with other antiretrovirals, in treatment-naive patients**
Adults: Recommended regimen is 300 mg P.O. once daily with ritonavir 100 mg. When drug is given with efavirenz, give atazanavir

400 mg and ritonavir 100 mg as a single daily dose with food and efavirenz on an empty stomach, preferably at bedtime. For adults unable to tolerate ritonavir, give 400 mg P.O. one daily.

Adolescents at least age 13 and weighing at least 40 kg who can't tolerate ritonavir: 400 mg P.O. once daily with food.

Children and adolescents ages 6 to younger than 18: For patients weighing 40 kg or more, give 300 mg with ritonavir 100 mg P.O. once daily. For patients weighing 20 kg to less than 40 kg, give 200 mg with ritonavir 100 mg P.O. once daily. For patients weighing 15 kg to less than 20 kg, give 150 mg with ritonavir 100 mg P.O. once daily.

Children at least age 3 months and weighing at least 5 kg and less than 25 kg: For patients weighing 15 kg to less than 25 kg, give 250 mg P.O. immediately followed by 80 mg ritonavir daily. For patients weighing 5 kg to less than 15 kg, give 200 mg P.O. immediately followed by 80 mg ritonavir daily.

Adjust-a-dose: In adults with mild hepatic impairment (Child-Pugh class A), give 400 mg P.O. daily; for moderate hepatic impairment (Child-Pugh class B), give 300 mg daily; for severe hepatic impairment (Child-Pugh class C), atazanavir with or without ritonavir isn't recommended.

➤ **HIV-1 infection, with other antiretrovirals, in pregnant patients**
Women: Give 300 mg P.O. daily with 100 mg ritonavir. For treatment-experienced patients during second or third trimester when given with either H2RA or tenofovir, give 400 mg P.O. daily with 100 mg ritonavir.

ADMINISTRATION
P.O.
- Give drug with food.
- Give to pregnant women only if potential benefit justifies risk to the fetus.
- Don't open capsules.
- Mix oral powder with food (such as applesauce or yogurt) or beverage (such as milk, infant formula, or water).
- When mixing with food, mix powder with a minimum of 1 tablespoon of food in small container and feed to child. Add additional

tablespoon of food to container, mix, and feed residual mixture to child.
- When mixing with beverage, mix powder with minimum of 30 mL of beverage and give to child to drink. Add additional 15 mL of beverage to the drinking cup, mix, and give to child to drink residual mixture. If water is used, also give food at same time.
- For young infants who can't eat solid food or drink from a cup, mix powder with 10 mL of infant formula in a medicine cup and draw up into oral syringe. Give to infant into either inner cheek. Pour additional 10 mL of formula into medicine cup and mix. Give residual mixture to infant in the same manner. Don't give in an infant bottle.
- Give entire dose of powder after mixing within 1 hour of preparation. Additional food may be given after dose is given.

ACTION
Inhibits viral maturation in HIV-1–infected cells, resulting in the formation of immature noninfectious viral particles.

Route	Onset	Peak	Duration
P.O.	Unknown	2–3 hr	Unknown

Half-life: About 8 to 9 hours.

ADVERSE REACTIONS
CNS: headache, depression, dizziness, fatigue, fever, insomnia, pain, peripheral neuropathy.
CV: prolonged PR interval, first- and second-degree heart block, peripheral edema.
EENT: nasal congestion, rhinorrhea, oropharyngeal pain.
GI: abdominal pain, diarrhea, nausea, vomiting.
Hematologic: *neutropenia.*
Hepatic: hyperbilirubinemia, jaundice.
Metabolic: lipodystrophy, hyperglycemia, *hypoglycemia.*
Musculoskeletal: arthralgia, back pain, myalgia.
Respiratory: increased cough, wheezing.
Skin: rash.

INTERACTIONS
Drug-drug. *Alfuzosin:* May increase alfuzosin plasma concentration, increasing risk of hypotension. Avoid use together.

Reactions in bold italics are *life-threatening*. Interactions may have a *rapid onset* or a *delayed onset*.

Antacids, buffered medications (didanosine buffered preparation): May reduce atazanavir plasma concentration. Administer atazanavir 2 hours before or 1 hour after these medications.

Antiarrhythmics (amiodarone, bepridil, systemic lidocaine, quinidine): May produce serious or life-threatening adverse reactions. Use cautiously. Monitor antiarrhythmic therapeutic concentration.

Anticoagulants (warfarin): May cause serious or life-threatening bleeding. Monitor INR.

Antifungals (itraconazole, ketoconazole, posaconazole, voriconazole): May increase risk of toxicity of both antifungal and atazanavir. Use cautiously when high doses of ketoconazole or itraconazole are administered with atazanavir and ritonavir. Administration of voriconazole with atazanavir and ritonavir isn't recommended.

Aripiprazole: May increase aripiprazole plasma concentration. Monitor patient and adjust aripiprazole dosage as needed when atazanavir is started or stopped.

Benzodiazepines (midazolam, triazolam): May increase plasma concentrations of these drugs. Oral midazolam and triazolam are contraindicated because of the potential for serious or life-threatening events, such as prolonged or increased sedation or respiratory depression. Use I.V. midazolam with caution and close monitoring.

Bosentan: May decrease atazanavir plasma concentration when administered without ritonavir; coadministration of atazanavir and bosentan without ritonavir isn't recommended. May increase bosentan plasma concentration. Adjust bosentan dose when used with atazanavir/ritonavir. Consider therapy modification.

Brentuximab: May increase brentuximab plasma concentration. Close monitoring is warranted. Adjust brentuximab dosage as needed.

Cabazitaxel: May increase cabazitaxel plasma concentration. Avoid administering together.

Calcium channel blockers (amlodipine, diltiazem, felodipine, nicardipine, nifedipine, verapamil): May prolong PR interval in some patients; use caution. Consider reducing diltiazem dosage by 50% and titrating dosages of other calcium channel blockers. Monitor ECG.

Carbamazepine: May increase carbamazepine level. May decrease atazanavir level, resulting in antiretroviral treatment failure. If coadministration can't be avoided, monitor patient closely. Consider alternative therapy for carbamazepine.

Cilostazol: May increase cilostazol plasma concentration. Consider reducing cilostazol dosage.

Clarithromycin: May prolong QTc interval; reduce clarithromycin dosage by 50%. Significantly reduces concentration of active metabolite (14-OH clarithromycin); consider alternative therapy for indications other than *Mycobacterium avium* complex.

Colchicine: May increase plasma concentrations of colchicine. Don't give colchicine and atazanavir together to patients with hepatic or renal impairment. In those with normal renal and hepatic function, reduce colchicine dose. Consider therapy modification.

Corticosteroids (fluticasone, prednisone): May increase corticosteroid plasma concentration. Monitor patient for signs and symptoms of adrenal insufficiency. Consider alternatives to fluticasone for long-term use.

Crizotinib, docetaxel, dronedarone, ixabepilone, ticagrelor, toremifene: May increase plasma concentration of these drugs. Avoid administering together.

Delavirdine: May increase atazanavir plasma concentration and decrease delavirdine plasma concentration. Atazanavir dosage reduction may be needed during coadministration of delavirdine. Delavirdine dosage increases may be required when administered with atazanavir. Closely monitor patient and adjust therapy as needed.

Didanosine (buffered): May decrease atazanavir concentration. Give atazanavir 2 hours before or 1 hour after buffered formulation of didanosine. Coadministration of enteric-coated didanosine capsules and atazanavir decreases didanosine exposure. Separate atazanavir and didanosine administration times.

Digoxin: May prolong PR interval. Use with caution.

Eletriptan: May increase eletriptan plasma concentration. Don't use eletriptan within 72 hours of atazanavir.

Eplerenone: May increase eplerenone plasma concentration. Avoid combination.

Ergot derivatives (dihydroergotamine, ergonovine, ergotamine, methylergonovine): May cause serious or life-threatening events such as acute ergot toxicity (peripheral vasospasm, ischemia of the extremities). Don't administer together.

Erlotinib: May increase erlotinib plasma concentration. Monitor clinical response and watch for adverse reactions. Adjust erlotinib dosage as needed.

Erythromycin: May increase erythromycin plasma concentration, increasing risk of sudden death from cardiac causes. Avoid concurrent use.

Eszopiclone: May increase eszopiclone plasma concentration. Monitor patient closely. Consider reducing eszopiclone dosage when administered with atazanavir.

Fluoxetine: May increase plasma concentrations of both drugs. Closely monitor patient for adverse reactions, including serotonin syndrome. Fluoxetine or atazanavir dosage reduction may be needed.

HMG-CoA reductase inhibitors (atorvastatin, lovastatin, rosuvastatin, simvastatin): May increase serum concentrations of these drugs, possibly increasing their toxicity, including rhabdomyolysis. Administration with simvastatin or lovastatin is contraindicated. If using atorvastatin or rosuvastatin, start with lowest possible dosage with careful monitoring. Consider pravastatin or fluvastatin in combination with atazanavir.

Hormonal contraceptives (ethinyl estradiol, norethindrone, norgestimate): Unboosted atazanavir may increase hormonal contraceptive plasma concentration. Ritonavir-boosted atazanavir may decrease hormonal contraceptive plasma concentration. Alternative methods of nonhormonal contraception are recommended.

H2RAs (famotidine): May decrease atazanavir plasma concentration, possibly causing development of resistance. Monitor patient.

Iloperidone: May increase iloperidone plasma concentration. Reduce iloperidone dosage by half when administering with

atazanavir. If atazanavir is discontinued, increase iloperidone dosage to original dosage.

Immunosuppressants (cyclosporine, sirolimus, tacrolimus): May increase levels of these drugs. Monitor immunosuppressant concentrations.

Irinotecan: May interfere with irinotecan metabolism, resulting in increased toxicity. Avoid use together.

Lurasidone: May increase lurasidone plasma concentration. Avoid use together.

Maraviroc: May increase maraviroc plasma concentration. Monitor patient response and adjust maraviroc dosage as needed.

mTOR inhibitors (everolimus, temsirolimus): May increase plasma concentrations of these drugs. If coadministration can't be avoided, monitor clinical response and adjust mTOR inhibitor dosage as needed.

Muscarinic receptor antagonists (darifenacin, fesoterodine, solifenacin, tolterodine): May increase plasma concentrations of these drugs. When atazanavir is coadministered, don't exceed the following dosages: darifenacin 7.5 mg daily, fesoterodine 4 mg daily, solifenacin 5 mg daily, and tolterodine 2 mg daily.

Nilotinib: May increase nilotinib plasma concentration. Avoid administering together. If atazanavir must be given with nilotinib, consider interrupting nilotinib therapy. Consult manufacturer's instructions for specific recommendations.

NNRTIs (efavirenz, nevirapine): May decrease atazanavir plasma level. In treatment-naive patients, administer atazanavir 400 mg and ritonavir 100 mg with efavirenz 600 mg. Don't administer atazanavir with efavirenz in treatment-experienced patients. Nevirapine may decrease atazanavir exposure; administering them together may increase nevirapine exposure. Use together is contraindicated.

Opioid analgesics (buprenorphine, fentanyl, oxycodone, sufentanil): May increase plasma concentration and half-life of opioid; reduced opioid dosage may be needed. Closely monitor respiratory function during opioid administration and for a longer period than usual after stopping opioid.

Reactions in bold italics are *life-threatening*. Interactions may have a *rapid onset* or a *delayed onset*.

Atazanavir without ritonavir shouldn't be administered with buprenorphine.

PDE5 inhibitors (sildenafil, tadalafil, vardenafil): Coadministration of atazanavir and sildenafil for pulmonary arterial hypertension is contraindicated. When sildenafil is used for erectile dysfunction, starting dose is 25 mg. Consider therapy modification.

Pimozide: May cause serious or life-threatening reactions (cardiac arrhythmias). Use is contraindicated.

Protease inhibitors (amprenavir, darunavir, fosamprenavir, indinavir, nelfinavir, ritonavir, saquinavir, tipranavir): Drug may increase concentration of other protease inhibitors. Atazanavir and indinavir are contraindicated together. Atazanavir/ritonavir isn't recommended with other protease inhibitors. Other combinations may require dosage changes. Consider therapy modification.

PPIs (omeprazole): Substantially decrease atazanavir plasma concentration, possibly causing development of resistance. In treatment-naive patients, administer PPI 12 hours before atazanavir dose. PPI shouldn't exceed dose equivalent to omeprazole 20 mg. Don't use PPIs in treatment-experienced patients receiving atazanavir.

Quetiapine: May increase quetiapine plasma concentration. Administer cautiously; closely monitor clinical response. Adjust quetiapine dosage as needed.

Raltegravir: May increase raltegravir plasma concentration. Closely monitor clinical response. Adjust raltegravir dosage as needed.

Ranolazine: Increases risk of dose-related QTc-interval prolongation, torsades de pointes–type arrhythmias, and sudden death. Avoid use together.

Rifabutin: May increase rifabutin blood level. Rifabutin dosage reduction of up to 75% (150 mg every other day or three times/week) is recommended.

Rifampin: May decrease atazanavir plasma concentration, possibly causing development of resistance. Use together is contraindicated.

Risperidone: May increase risperidone plasma concentration. Closely monitor clinical response. Adjust risperidone dosage as needed.

Romidepsin: May increase romidepsin plasma concentration, increasing risk of adverse reactions, including QT-interval prolongation. If use together can't be avoided, closely monitor clinical, laboratory, and ECG results. Adjust romidepsin dosage as needed.

Salmeterol: May increase salmeterol concentration, increasing risk of CV events, including QT-interval prolongation, palpitations, and sinus tachycardia. Use together isn't recommended.

Saxagliptin: May increase saxagliptin plasma concentration. Limit saxagliptin dosage to 2.5 mg daily.

TCAs (amitriptyline): May cause serious or life-threatening adverse reactions. Monitor TCA concentration.

Tenofovir: May decrease atazanavir area under the curve and minimum (trough) concentration. Don't administer atazanavir with tenofovir unless also administering ritonavir; administer as atazanavir 300 mg, ritonavir 100 mg, and tenofovir 300 mg. Atazanavir increases tenofovir concentration; watch for tenofovir-associated adverse reactions.

Tetracyclines (minocycline): May reduce atazanavir plasma concentration. Closely monitor atazanavir concentration and clinical response. Adjust atazanavir dosage as needed.

Trazodone: May increase trazodone plasma concentration. Use cautiously and reduce trazodone dosage.

Tyrosine kinase inhibitors (dasatinib, lapatinib, pazopanib, sorafenib, sunitinib): May increase protein-tyrosine kinase inhibitor plasma concentrations. If use together can't be avoided, closely monitor clinical response and adjust protein-tyrosine kinase inhibitor dosage as needed.

Vasopressin receptor antagonists (conivaptan, tolvaptan): May increase plasma concentration of these drugs. Coadministration is contraindicated.

Vemurafenib: May increase vemurafenib plasma concentration. Avoid combination.

Vilazodone: May increase vilazodone plasma concentration. Reduce vilazodone dosage to 20 mg in patients receiving atazanavir.

Vinca alkaloids (vinblastine, vincristine): May increase pharmacologic effects of these drugs and risk of toxicity (characterized by profound neutropenia or severe neuropathy). Consider temporarily suspending atazanavir in patients experiencing hematologic or GI toxicity during administration of atazanavir and vinca alkaloids. Or, reducing vinca alkaloid dosage may decrease toxicity.

Drug-herb. *St. John's wort:* May decrease drug level, reducing therapeutic effect and causing drug resistance. Avoid combination.

Drug-food. *Any food:* May increase bioavailability of drug. Tell patient to take drug with food.

EFFECTS ON LAB TEST RESULTS

• May increase ALT, AST, amylase, bilirubin, lipase, CK, glucose, triglyceride, and total cholesterol levels. May decrease glucose and Hb level.

• May decrease neutrophil and platelet counts.

CONTRAINDICATIONS & CAUTIONS

• Contraindicated in patients hypersensitive to drug or its ingredients.

• Contraindicated in patients taking drugs cleared mainly by CYP3A4 or drugs that can cause serious or life-threatening reactions at high levels (alfuzosin, dihydroergotamine, ergonovine, ergotamine, indinavir, irinotecan, lovastatin, methylergonovine, midazolam (P.O.), nevirapine, pimozide, rifampin, sildenafil (Revatio), St. John's wort, simvastatin, triazolam).

• Don't use in patients with Child-Pugh class C hepatic insufficiency.

• Use cautiously in patients with conduction system disease, hepatic impairment, diabetes, or hemophilia types A and B.

• Use cautiously in elderly patients because of the increased likelihood of other disease, additional drug therapy, and decreased hepatic, renal, or cardiac function.

Dialyzable drug: No.

⚠ **Overdose S&S:** Asymptomatic bifascicular block, PR-interval prolongation, jaundice.

PREGNANCY-LACTATION-REPRODUCTION

• Use during pregnancy only if potential benefit justifies potential risk to the fetus.

The U.S. Department of Health and Human Services Perinatal HIV Guidelines recommend atazanavir as a preferred protease inhibitor in antiretroviral-naive pregnant women when combined with low-dose ritonavir boosting. Enroll pregnant women in the Antiretroviral Pregnancy Registry at 1-800-258-4263.

• Drug appears in breast milk. Breast-feeding is contraindicated in HIV-infected mothers because of risk of postnatal transmission of HIV.

NURSING CONSIDERATIONS

🕄 **Alert:** Drug may prolong the PR interval. Monitor ECG, especially in patients with preexisting conduction system disease.

• Monitor patient for hyperglycemia and new-onset diabetes or worsened diabetes. Insulin and oral antidiabetic dosages may need adjustment.

• Monitor patient with HBV or HCV infection for elevated liver enzyme levels or hepatic decompensation.

• Monitor patient for immune reconstitution syndrome. Evaluate and treat indolent or residual opportunistic infections, such as CMV, *Pneumocystis jiroveci* pneumonia, or TB. Some autoimmune disorders, such as Graves disease, polymyositis, and Guillain-Barré syndrome, have also occurred, even after many months of treatment.

• Watch for life-threatening lactic acidosis syndrome and symptomatic hyperlactatemia, especially in women and obese patients.

• If the patient has hemophilia, watch for bleeding.

• Drug may cause nephrolithiasis or cholelithiasis. Evaluate patient for signs or symptoms of nephrolithiasis (flank pain) or cholelithiasis (abdominal pain, nausea, vomiting, jaundice); interrupt or discontinue drug as clinically indicated should signs or symptoms occur.

• Monitor patient for rash. Discontinue drug if rash occurs.

• Most patients have an asymptomatic increase in indirect bilirubin, possibly with yellowed skin or sclerae. This hyperbilirubinemia will resolve when therapy stops.

• Monitor liver enzyme levels before and periodically during treatment.

Reactions in bold italics are *life-threatening*. Interactions may have a *rapid onset* or a *delayed onset*.

• Although cross-resistance occurs among protease inhibitors, resistance to drug doesn't preclude use of other protease inhibitors.

۞ *Alert:* For patients with phenylketonuria, be aware that oral powder contains 35 mg of phenylalanine; capsules don't.

PATIENT TEACHING

• Urge patient to take drug with food every day and to take other antiretrovirals as prescribed.

• Explain that drug doesn't cure HIV infection and that the patient may develop opportunistic infections and other complications of HIV disease.

• Caution patient that drug doesn't reduce the risk of transmitting HIV to others.

• Tell patient that drug may cause altered or increased body fat, central obesity, buffalo hump, peripheral wasting, facial wasting, breast enlargement, and a cushingoid appearance.

• Tell patient to report yellowed skin or eyes, dizziness, or light-headedness.

• Caution patient not to take other prescriptions or OTC or herbal medicines without first consulting his prescriber.

SAFETY ALERT!

atenolol
a-TEN-o-loll

Tenormin ✔

Therapeutic class: Antihypertensives
Pharmacologic class: Beta blockers

AVAILABLE FORMS
Tablets: 25 mg, 50 mg, 100 mg

INDICATIONS & DOSAGES

Adjust-a-dose (for all indications): If CrCl is 15 to 35 mL/minute, maximum dose is 50 mg daily; if CrCl is below 15 mL/minute, maximum dose is 25 mg daily. Hemodialysis patients need 25 to 50 mg after each dialysis session. For elderly patients, initial dose is 25 mg P.O. daily.

➤ **Hypertension**
Adults: Initially, 25 to 50 mg P.O. daily alone or in combination with a diuretic as a single dose, increased to 100 mg once daily after 7 to 14 days. Dosages of more than 100 mg daily are unlikely to produce further benefit.

➤ **Angina pectoris**
Adults: 50 mg P.O. once daily, increased as needed to 100 mg daily after 7 days for optimal effect. Maximum, 200 mg daily.

➤ **Acute MI**
Adults: 100 mg P.O. daily or 50 mg b.i.d. for 6 to 9 days or until discharge from the hospital.

ADMINISTRATION
P.O.

• Check apical pulse before giving drug; if slower than 60 beats/minute, withhold drug and call prescriber.

• Give drug exactly as prescribed, at the same time each day.

ACTION

Selectively blocks beta$_1$-adrenergic receptors, decreases cardiac output and cardiac oxygen consumption, and depresses renin secretion.

Route	Onset	Peak	Duration
P.O.	1 hr	2–4 hr	24 hr

Half-life: 6 to 7 hours.

ADVERSE REACTIONS

CNS: depression, dizziness, fatigue, lethargy, vertigo, drowsiness, fever.
CV: hypotension, *bradycardia, HF, heart block,* intermittent claudication, atrial fibrillation, *supraventricular tachycardia, cardiac arrest, ventricular tachycardia.*
GI: nausea, diarrhea.
Musculoskeletal: leg pain.
Respiratory: *bronchospasm,* dyspnea, *PE,* wheezing.
Skin: rash.

INTERACTIONS

Drug-drug. *Aluminum salts:* May reduce bioavailability of atenolol. Separate doses by at least 2 hours.
Amiodarone: May increase risk of bradycardia, AV block, and myocardial depression. Monitor ECG and vital signs.
Antihypertensives: May increase hypotensive effect. Use together cautiously.

Anticholinergics (atropine, benztropine, oxybutynin), quinidine: May increase atenolol level. Monitor patient and adjust atenolol dosage as needed.

Calcium carbonate, calcium citrate: May decrease atenolol level. Monitor patient and adjust atenolol dosage as needed.

Calcium channel blockers, hydralazine, methyldopa: May cause additive hypotension and bradycardia. Adjust dosage as needed.

Cardiac glycosides, diltiazem, verapamil: May cause excessive bradycardia and increased depressant effect on myocardium. Use together cautiously.

Clonidine: May exacerbate rebound hypertension if clonidine is withdrawn. Atenolol should be withdrawn before clonidine by several days or added several days after clonidine is stopped.

Dolasetron: May decrease clearance of dolasetron and increase risk of toxicity. Monitor patient for toxicity.

Insulin, oral antidiabetics: May alter dosage requirements in previously stabilized diabetic patient. Observe patient carefully.

I.V. lidocaine: May reduce hepatic metabolism of lidocaine, increasing risk of toxicity. Give bolus doses of lidocaine at a slower rate and monitor lidocaine level.

NSAIDs: May decrease antihypertensive effects. Monitor BP.

Penicillins: May reduce bioavailability of atenolol. Monitor BP closely.

Prazosin: May increase the risk of orthostatic hypotension in the early phases of use together.

Reserpine: May cause hypotension or marked bradycardia. Use cautiously.

Rifamycins: May reduce effects of atenolol. Monitor BP.

Salicylates: May reduce effects of atenolol. Consider lowering salicylate dosage or changing to a nonsalicylate antiplatelet.

EFFECTS ON LAB TEST RESULTS

- May increase alkaline phosphatase, BUN, creatinine, glucose, LDH, potassium, AST, ALT, and uric acid levels. May decrease glucose level.
- May increase platelet count.

CONTRAINDICATIONS & CAUTIONS

- Contraindicated in patients hypersensitive to drug or its components.
- Contraindicated in patients with sinus bradycardia, heart block greater than first degree, overt cardiac failure, untreated pheochromocytoma, and cardiogenic shock.
- Contraindicated in patients with acute MI and HF who don't promptly respond to I.V. furosemide or equivalent therapy.
- Use cautiously in patients at risk for HF and in those with diabetes, hyperthyroidism, and impaired renal or hepatic function.
- Beta blockers shouldn't be routinely used in patients with bronchospastic disease. Atenolol may be used cautiously in patients who don't respond to or can't tolerate other antihypertensive treatment. Use lowest possible dosage and have bronchodilator available. Consider divided doses if atenolol dosage must be increased.
- Safe use in children hasn't been established.

Dialyzable drug: Yes.

⚠ *Overdose S&S:* Lethargy, decreased respiratory drive, wheezing, sinus pause, bradycardia.

PREGNANCY-LACTATION-REPRODUCTION

- Drug can cause fetal harm. Use cautiously in pregnant women.
- Drug appears in breast milk. Use cautiously in breast-feeding women.

NURSING CONSIDERATIONS

- Monitor BP, preferably just before next dose, to evaluate effectiveness.
- Monitor hemodialysis patients closely because of hypotension risk.
- Beta blockers may mask tachycardia caused by hyperthyroidism. In patients with suspected thyrotoxicosis, withdraw beta blocker gradually to avoid thyroid storm.
- Drug may mask signs and symptoms of hypoglycemia in diabetic patients.
- Drug may cause changes in exercise tolerance and ECG.
- Monitor patient for cardiac failure. Discontinue drug in patients who develop cardiac failure that doesn't respond to standard treatment.

Black Box Warning Avoid abrupt discontinuation of therapy. Withdraw drug gradually

to avoid serious adverse reactions, such as severe exacerbations of angina, MI, and ventricular arrhythmias even in patients treated only for hypertension. ■
● *Look alike–sound alike:* Don't confuse atenolol with timolol or albuterol.

PATIENT TEACHING
● Instruct patient to take drug exactly as prescribed, at the same time every day.
Black Box Warning Caution patient not to stop drug suddenly. ■
● Advise patient to report all adverse reactions to prescriber.
● Teach patient how to take his pulse. Tell him to withhold drug and call prescriber if pulse rate is below 60 beats/minute.
● Tell woman of childbearing potential to notify prescriber about planned, suspected, or known pregnancy.
● Advise breast-feeding mother to contact prescriber; drug isn't recommended for breast-feeding women.

atezolizumab
See NEW DRUGS for information.

atomoxetine hydrochloride
at-oh-MOKS-ah-teen

Strattera✐

Therapeutic class: ADHD drugs
Pharmacologic class: Selective norepinephrine reuptake inhibitors

AVAILABLE FORMS
Capsules ⓞⓣⓒ: 10 mg, 18 mg, 25 mg, 40 mg, 60 mg, 80 mg, 100 mg

INDICATIONS & DOSAGES
➤ **ADHD**
Adults, children older than age 6, and adolescents weighing more than 70 kg: Initially, 40 mg P.O. daily; increase after at least 3 days to a total of 80 mg/day P.O., as a single dose in the morning or two evenly divided doses in the morning and late afternoon or early evening. After 2 to 4 weeks, increase total dose to a maximum of 100 mg, if needed.

Children age 6 and older weighing 70 kg or less: Initially, 0.5 mg/kg P.O. daily; increase after a minimum of 3 days to a target total daily dose of 1.2 mg/kg P.O. as a single dose in the morning or two evenly divided doses in the morning and late afternoon or early evening. Don't exceed 1.4 mg/kg or 100 mg daily, whichever is less.
Adjust-a-dose: In patients with moderate hepatic impairment, reduce to 50% of the normal dose; in those with severe hepatic impairment, reduce to 25% of the normal dose. Poor metabolizers of CYP2D6 or those also receiving strong CYP2D6 inhibitors may require a reduced dose. In children weighing less than 70 kg, adjust dosage to 0.5 mg/kg daily and increase to 1.2 mg/kg daily if symptoms don't improve after 4 weeks and if first dose is tolerated. In children and adults weighing more than 70 kg, start at 40 mg daily and increase to 80 mg daily if symptoms don't improve after 4 weeks and if first dose is tolerated.

ADMINISTRATION
P.O.
● Give drug without regard for meals.
● Capsules should be swallowed whole and not opened.

ACTION
May be related to selective inhibition of the presynaptic norepinephrine transporter.

Route	Onset	Peak	Duration
P.O.	Rapid	1–2 hr	Unknown

Half-life: 5 hours; 24 hours in poor metabolizers.

ADVERSE REACTIONS
CNS: headache, insomnia, dizziness, somnolence, irritability, mood swings, fatigue, sedation, depression, tremor, early-morning awakening, paresthesia, abnormal dreams, sleep disorder, syncope, anxiety.
CV: orthostatic hypotension, tachycardia, hypertension, palpitations, hot flashes.
EENT: mydriasis, conjunctivitis, oropharyngeal pain, pharyngolaryngeal pain, sinus headache.
GI: abdominal pain, constipation, dyspepsia, nausea, vomiting, decreased appetite, dry mouth.

GU: urine retention, urinary hesitation, ejaculatory problems, difficulty in micturition, dysmenorrhea, erectile disturbance, erectile dysfunction, menstrual disorder, prostatitis.
Metabolic: weight loss.
Skin: pruritus, increased sweating, rash.
Other: decreased libido, chills.

INTERACTIONS
Drug-drug. *Albuterol:* May increase CV effects. Use together cautiously.
MAO inhibitors: May cause hyperthermia, rigidity, myoclonus, autonomic instability with possible rapid fluctuations of vital signs, and mental status changes. Avoid use within 2 weeks of MAO inhibitor.
Pressor agents: May increase BP. Use together cautiously.
Strong CYP2D6 inhibitors (paroxetine, fluoxetine, quinidine): May increase atomoxetine level. Reduce first dose. Increase to the usual target dose of 80 mg only if signs and symptoms fail to improve after 4 weeks and the initial dose is well tolerated.

EFFECTS ON LAB TEST RESULTS
None reported.

CONTRAINDICATIONS & CAUTIONS
● Contraindicated in patients hypersensitive to drug or its components; in those with serious heart problems, current or history of pheochromocytoma, or angle-closure glaucoma; in those who are intolerant of increased BP or HR; and in those who have taken an MAO inhibitor within the past 2 weeks.
● Use cautiously in patients with hypertension, tachycardia, hypotension, urine retention, or cerebrovascular disease.
● Safety and effectiveness in children younger than age 6 haven't been established.
Dialyzable drug: No.
⚠ *Overdose S&S:* Somnolence, agitation, hyperactivity, abnormal behavior, GI symptoms, mydriasis, tachycardia, dry mouth, prolonged QT interval, disorientation, hallucinations, seizures.

PREGNANCY-LACTATION-REPRODUCTION
● Don't use in pregnant women unless potential benefit justifies potential risk to the fetus. Women of childbearing potential should be advised to use effective contraception.
● It isn't known if drug appears in breast milk. Use cautiously in breast-feeding women.

NURSING CONSIDERATIONS
● Use drug as part of a total treatment program for ADHD, including psychological, educational, and social intervention. Drug may be discontinued without tapering.
● Monitor patients for the appearance or worsening of aggressive behavior or hostility, especially when treatment is initiated.
Black Box Warning Monitor children and adolescents closely for worsening of condition, agitation, irritability, suicidal thinking or behaviors, and unusual changes in behavior, especially the first few months of therapy or when dosage is increased or decreased. ∎
● Periodically monitor patients for changes in HR or BP.
● Assess patients carefully for cardiac disease, including family history of sudden death or ventricular arrhythmia. Evaluate patients with new cardiac symptoms promptly.
● Patients taking drug for extended periods must be reevaluated periodically to determine drug's usefulness.
● Monitor growth during treatment. If growth or weight gain is unsatisfactory, consider interrupting therapy.
🕒 *Alert:* Severe liver injury may occur and progress to liver failure. Notify prescriber of any sign of liver injury: yellowing of the skin or the sclera of the eyes, pruritus, dark urine, upper right-sided tenderness, or unexplained flulike syndrome.
● Monitor BP and pulse rate at baseline, after each dosage increase, and periodically during treatment.
● Monitor patient for urinary hesitancy, urine retention, or sexual dysfunction. Drug may increase risk of priapism.

PATIENT TEACHING
Black Box Warning Advise parents to call prescriber immediately about unusual behavior or suicidal thoughts. ∎

Reactions in bold italics are *life-threatening*. Interactions may have a *rapid onset* or a ***delayed onset***.

- Instruct patient to immediately report chest pain, shortness of breath, or fainting.
- Tell patient to use caution when operating a vehicle or machinery until the effects of drug are known.
- Warn male patient to seek prompt medical attention for an erection that lasts more than 4 hours.
- Inform patient that therapy may be interrupted periodically to check ADHD symptoms.
- Tell female patient who is pregnant, planning to become pregnant, or breast-feeding to consult prescriber before taking atomoxetine.

atorvastatin calcium
ah-TOR-va-stah-tin

Lipitor✒

Therapeutic class: Antilipemics
Pharmacologic class: HMG-CoA reductase inhibitors

AVAILABLE FORMS
Tablets ⊕: 10 mg, 20 mg, 40 mg, 80 mg

INDICATIONS & DOSAGES
➤ **In patients with clinically evident CAD, to reduce risk of nonfatal MI, fatal and nonfatal strokes, angina, HF, and revascularization procedures**
Adults: Initially, 10 to 20 mg P.O. daily. May increase based on patient response and tolerance; usual dosage, 10 to 80 mg P.O. daily.
➤ **To reduce risk of MI, stroke, angina, or revascularization procedures in patients with multiple risk factors for CAD but who don't yet have the disease**
Adults: 10 to 80 mg P.O. daily.
➤ **To reduce risk of MI or stroke in patients with type 2 diabetes and multiple risk factors for CAD but who don't yet have the disease**
Adults: 10 to 80 mg P.O. daily.
➤ **Adjunct to diet to reduce LDL, total cholesterol, apolipoprotein B, and triglyceride levels and to increase HDL levels in patients with primary hypercholesterolemia (heterozygous familial**

and nonfamilial) and mixed dyslipidemia (Fredrickson types IIa and IIb); adjunct to diet to reduce triglyceride level (Fredrickson type IV); primary dysbetalipoproteinemia (Fredrickson type III) in patients who don't respond adequately to diet**
Adults: Initially, 10 or 20 mg P.O. once daily. Patient who requires a reduction of more than 45% in LDL level may be started at 40 mg once daily. Increase dose, as needed, to maximum of 80 mg daily as single dose. Dosage based on lipid levels drawn within 2 to 4 weeks of starting therapy and after dosage adjustment.
➤ **Alone or as an adjunct to lipid-lowering treatments, such as LDL apheresis, to reduce total and LDL cholesterol in patients with homozygous familial hypercholesterolemia**
Adults: 10 to 80 mg P.O. once daily.
➤ **Heterozygous familial hypercholesterolemia in patients who don't respond adequately to dietary treatment**
Children ages 10 to 17 (girls should be 1 year postmenarche): Initially, 10 mg P.O. once daily. Adjustment intervals should be at least 4 weeks. Maximum daily dose is 20 mg.
➤ **Intensive lipid-lowering after an acute coronary syndrome event regardless of baseline LDL; noncardioembolic stroke/TIA (secondary prevention)** ◆
Adults: Initially, 80 mg P.O. once daily. Adjust dosage based on tolerability.

ADMINISTRATION
P.O.
- Give drug without regard for meals.

ACTION
Inhibits HMG-CoA reductase, an early (and rate-limiting) step in cholesterol biosynthesis.

Route	Onset	Peak	Duration
P.O.	Unknown	1–2 hr	Unknown

Half-life: 14 hours.

ADVERSE REACTIONS
CNS: insomnia.
EENT: nasopharyngitis, pharyngolaryngeal pain.

GI: abdominal pain, diarrhea, dyspepsia, flatulence, nausea.
GU: UTI.
Musculoskeletal: *rhabdomyolysis,* arthralgia, myalgia, extremity pain, muscle spasms, musculoskeletal pain.
Skin: rash.

INTERACTIONS
Drug-drug. *Amiodarone:* May increase risk of severe myopathy or rhabdomyolysis. Avoid use together or decrease atorvastatin dose.
Antacids, cholestyramine, colestipol: May decrease atorvastatin level. Separate administration times.
Colchicine, **diltiazem,** *fibric acid derivatives,* **nefazodone,** *niacin, protease inhibitors, tacrolimus,* **verapamil:** May decrease metabolism of HMG-CoA reductase inhibitors, increasing toxicity. Monitor patient for adverse effects and report unexplained muscle pain.
Cyclosporine, *telaprevir, tipranavir plus ritonavir:* May increase statin level and risk of myopathy and rhabdomyolysis. Avoid use together.
Darunavir and ritonavir, fosamprenavir, fosamprenavir and ritonavir, saquinavir and ritonavir: May increase atorvastatin level and risk of myopathy and rhabdomyolysis. Atorvastatin dosage shouldn't exceed 20 mg daily.
Digoxin: May increase digoxin level. Monitor digoxin level and patient for evidence of toxicity.
Fluconazole, itraconazole, ketoconazole, voriconazole: May increase atorvastatin level and adverse effects. Avoid using together or, if unavoidable, atorvastatin dosage shouldn't exceed 20 mg daily.
Gemfibrozil: May increase risk of myopathy/rhabdomyolysis. Avoid combination.
Hormonal contraceptives: May increase norethindrone and ethinyl estradiol levels. Consider increased drug levels when selecting an oral contraceptive.
Lopinavir and ritonavir: May increase statin level and risk of myopathy and rhabdomyolysis. Use together cautiously and at lowest atorvastatin dosage necessary.
Macrolides (azithromycin, clarithromycin, erythromycin, telithromycin): May increase atorvastatin level and risk of myopathy and rhabdomyolysis. Atorvastatin dosage shouldn't exceed 20 mg daily.
Nelfinavir: May increase statin level and risk of myopathy and rhabdomyolysis. Atorvastatin dosage shouldn't exceed 40 mg daily.
Drug-herb. *Jin bu huan, kava:* May increase risk of hepatotoxicity. Discourage use together.
Drug-food. *Grapefruit juice:* May increase drug levels when consumed in large quantities, increasing risk of adverse reactions. Discourage use together.

EFFECTS ON LAB TEST RESULTS
● May increase ALT, AST, and CK levels.

CONTRAINDICATIONS & CAUTIONS
● Contraindicated in patients hypersensitive to drug and in those with active liver disease or unexplained persistent elevations of transaminase levels.
● Some dosage forms contain polysorbate 80, which can cause delayed hypersensitivity reactions.
● Use cautiously in patients with hepatic impairment or heavy alcohol use, in patients with inadequately treated hypothyroidism, with other drugs associated with myopathy, and in elderly patients.
● Withhold or stop drug in patients at risk for renal failure caused by rhabdomyolysis resulting from trauma; in serious, acute conditions that suggest myopathy; and in major surgery, severe acute infection, hypotension, uncontrolled seizures, or severe metabolic, endocrine, or electrolyte disorders.
● Limit use in children to those older than age 9 with homozygous familial hypercholesterolemia.
Dialyzable drug: No.

PREGNANCY-LACTATION-REPRODUCTION
● Drug may cause fetal harm. Contraindicated in women who are pregnant or may become pregnant. Women of childbearing potential should be apprised of potential hazards to the fetus.
● It isn't known if drug appears in breast milk. Women taking atorvastatin shouldn't breast-feed.

NURSING CONSIDERATIONS

• Patient should follow a standard cholesterol-lowering diet before and during therapy.
• Before treatment, assess patient for underlying causes for hypercholesterolemia and obtain a baseline lipid profile. Obtain periodic LFT results and lipid levels before starting treatment and at 6 and 12 weeks after initiation, or after an increase in dosage and periodically thereafter.
• Watch for signs of myositis and myopathy (unexplained muscle pain, tenderness, weakness, malaise, dark urine, fever). Drug may need to be discontinued.
• *Look alike–sound alike:* Don't confuse atorvastatin with atomoxetine. Don't confuse Lipitor with Loniten, Levatol, or Zyrtec.

PATIENT TEACHING

• Teach patient about proper dietary management, weight control, and exercise. Explain their importance in controlling high fat levels.
• Warn patient to avoid alcohol.
• Tell patient to inform prescriber of all adverse reactions, such as muscle pain, malaise, and fever.
• Advise patient that drug can be taken at any time of day, without regard for meals.
 Alert: Tell female patient to stop drug and notify prescriber immediately if she is or may be pregnant or if she's breast-feeding.

---

atovaquone
a-TOE-va-kwon

Mepron

Therapeutic class: Antiprotozoals
Pharmacologic class: Ubiquinone analogues

AVAILABLE FORMS
Suspension: 750 mg/5 mL

INDICATIONS & DOSAGES
➤ **Acute, mild to moderate *Pneumocystis jiroveci* pneumonia in patients who can't tolerate sulfamethoxazole–trimethoprim**

Adults and adolescents ages 13 to 16: 750 mg (5 mL) P.O. b.i.d. with food for 21 days.
➤ **To prevent *P. jiroveci* pneumonia in patients who are unable to tolerate sulfamethoxazole–trimethoprim**
Adults and adolescents ages 13 to 16: 1,500 mg (10 mL) P.O. daily with food.

ADMINISTRATION
P.O.
• Taking with meals enhances absorption.
• Shake bottle gently before using.
• Give entire contents of foil pouch, which can be poured into a dosing spoon or cup or be taken directly into the mouth.

ACTION
May interfere with electron transport in protozoal mitochondria, inhibiting enzymes needed to synthesize nucleic acids and adenosine triphosphate.

Route	Onset	Peak	Duration
P.O.	Unknown	Unknown	Unknown

Half-life: 2 to 4 days.

ADVERSE REACTIONS
CNS: headache, insomnia, fever, pain, asthenia, anxiety, dizziness, depression.
CV: hypotension.
EENT: sinusitis, rhinitis.
GI: abdominal pain, nausea, diarrhea, oral candidiasis, vomiting, constipation, anorexia, dyspepsia, taste perversion.
Hematologic: *neutropenia,* anemia.
Metabolic: *hypoglycemia,* hyponatremia.
Musculoskeletal: myalgia.
Respiratory: cough, dyspnea.
Skin: rash, diaphoresis, pruritus.
Other: flulike syndrome.

INTERACTIONS
Drug-drug. *Metoclopramide:* May decrease atovaquone bioavailability. Use another antiemetic.
Rifabutin, rifampin: May decrease atovaquone's steady-state level. Avoid using together.
Tetracycline: May decrease atovaquone level. Monitor parasitemia.
Zidovudine: May elevate zidovudine level and lead to toxicity. Monitor closely.

EFFECTS ON LAB TEST RESULTS

• May increase glucose, amylase, alkaline phosphatase, ALT, and AST levels. May decrease Hb and sodium levels.
• May decrease neutrophil count.

CONTRAINDICATIONS & CAUTIONS

• Contraindicated in patients hypersensitive to drug.
• Serious hypersensitivity reactions have been reported.
• Use cautiously in patients with hepatic impairment.
• Use cautiously with other highly protein-bound drugs; if used together, assess patient for toxicity.
⚠ **Alert:** Patients with GI disorders may not absorb drug well and may not achieve adequate plasma levels. Consider parenteral therapy with alternative drugs.
Dialyzable drug: Unknown.
⚠ **Overdose S&S:** Methemoglobinemia, rash.

PREGNANCY-LACTATION-REPRODUCTION

• Use cautiously in pregnant women and only if potential benefit justifies potential risk to the fetus.
• It isn't known if drug appears in breast milk. Use cautiously in breast-feeding women.

NURSING CONSIDERATIONS

⚠ **Alert:** Monitor patient closely during therapy because of risk of pulmonary infection.
• Monitor patients with hepatic impairment closely.
• Monitor patient for GI disorders (nausea, vomiting, diarrhea) that might affect patient's ability to absorb drug.

PATIENT TEACHING

• Instruct patient to take drug with meals; food significantly enhances absorption.
• Stress importance of taking atovaquone as prescribed.
• Advise patient to report all adverse reactions and to immediately report nausea, vomiting, diarrhea, white mouth patches, flulike symptoms, dark urine, tiredness, lack of appetite, yellow skin, and light stools.

atovaquone–proguanil hydrochloride
a-TOE-va-kwon/pro-GWA-nil

Malarone, Malarone Pediatric

Therapeutic class: Antimalarials
Pharmacologic class: Hydroxynaphthoquinone and biguanide derivatives

AVAILABLE FORMS

Tablets (adult-strength): 250 mg atovaquone and 100 mg proguanil hydrochloride
Tablets (pediatric-strength): 62.5 mg atovaquone and 25 mg proguanil hydrochloride

INDICATIONS & DOSAGES

➤ **To prevent *Plasmodium falciparum* malaria, including in areas where chloroquine resistance has been reported**
Adults and children weighing more than 40 kg: 1 adult-strength tablet P.O. once daily with food or milk, beginning 1 or 2 days before entering a malaria-endemic area. Continue prophylactic treatment during stay and for 7 days after return.
Children weighing 31 to 40 kg: 3 pediatric-strength tablets P.O. once daily with food or milk, beginning 1 or 2 days before entering endemic area. Continue prophylactic treatment during stay and for 7 days after return.
Children weighing 21 to 30 kg: 2 pediatric-strength tablets P.O. once daily with food or milk, beginning 1 or 2 days before entering endemic area. Continue prophylactic treatment during stay and for 7 days after return.
Children weighing 11 to 20 kg: 1 pediatric-strength tablet P.O. daily with food or milk, beginning 1 or 2 days before entering endemic area. Continue prophylactic treatment during stay and for 7 days after return.
Adjust-a-dose: Don't use for malaria prophylaxis in patients with severe renal impairment (CrCl less than 30 mL/minute).
➤ **Acute, uncomplicated *P. falciparum* malaria**
Adults and children weighing more than 40 kg: 4 adult-strength tablets P.O. once daily, with food or milk, for 3 consecutive days.

Children weighing 31 to 40 kg: 3 adult-strength tablets P.O. once daily, with food or milk, for 3 consecutive days.
Children weighing 21 to 30 kg: 2 adult-strength tablets P.O. once daily, with food or milk, for 3 consecutive days.
Children weighing 11 to 20 kg: 1 adult-strength tablet P.O. once daily, with food or milk, for 3 consecutive days.
Children weighing 9 to 10 kg: 3 pediatric-strength tablets P.O. once daily, with food or milk, for 3 consecutive days.
Children weighing 5 to 8 kg: 2 pediatric-strength tablets P.O. once daily, with food or milk, for 3 consecutive days.

ADMINISTRATION
P.O.
● Give dose at same time each day, with food or milk.
● If child has difficulty swallowing tablets, parents may crush tablet and mix it in condensed milk.
● Store tablets at controlled room temperature of 59° to 86° F (15° to 30° C).

ACTION
Thought to interfere with nucleic acid replication in the malarial parasite. Atovaquone selectively inhibits mitochondrial electron transport in the parasite. Cycloguanil, an active metabolite of proguanil hydrochloride, inhibits dihydrofolate reductase. Atovaquone and cycloguanil are active against the erythrocytic and exoerythrocytic stages of *Plasmodium* species.

Route	Onset	Peak	Duration
P.O.	Unknown	Unknown	Unknown

Half-life: Atovaquone: 2 to 3 days in adults, 1 to 2 days in children; proguanil: 12 to 21 hours in adults and children.

ADVERSE REACTIONS
CNS: headache, asthenia, dizziness, dreams, insomnia.
GI: abdominal pain, nausea, vomiting, diarrhea, anorexia, dyspepsia, gastritis, oral ulcers.
Respiratory: cough.
Skin: pruritus.

INTERACTIONS
Drug-drug. *Metoclopramide:* May decrease atovaquone bioavailability. Use another antiemetic.
Rifabutin, rifampin: May decrease atovaquone level by about 50%. Avoid using together.
Tetracycline: May decrease atovaquone level by about 40%. Monitor patient with parasitemia closely.
Warfarin: May increase anticoagulation effect. Monitor INR.

EFFECTS ON LAB TEST RESULTS
● May increase alkaline phosphatase, ALT, and AST levels. May decrease Hb level and hematocrit.
● May decrease WBC count.

CONTRAINDICATIONS & CAUTIONS
● Contraindicated in patients hypersensitive to atovaquone, proguanil hydrochloride, or components of drug and in those with severe renal impairment or severe or complicated malaria.
● Use cautiously in patients who are vomiting.
● Use cautiously in elderly patients because they have a greater frequency of decreased renal, hepatic, and cardiac function.
● Safety and effectiveness haven't been established for prevention in children who weigh less than 11 kg or for treatment in children who weigh less than 5 kg.
Dialyzable drug: Unknown.
⚠ **Overdose S&S:** Rash, methemoglobinemia (atovaquone); epigastric discomfort, vomiting, reversible hair loss, scaling of the skin on the palms or soles, reversible aphthous ulceration, hematologic adverse effects (proguanil).

PREGNANCY-LACTATION-REPRODUCTION
● Use during pregnancy only if potential benefit justifies potential risk to the fetus.
● It isn't known if atovaquone appears in breast milk, but proguanil does appear in small amounts. Use cautiously in breast-feeding women.

NURSING CONSIDERATIONS

• Persistent diarrhea or vomiting may decrease drug absorption. Patients with these symptoms may need a different antimalarial.
• Monitor patients on prophylactic therapy for elevated liver enzyme levels, hepatitis, and hepatic failure.
• Treatment failure risk may increase in patients weighing more than 100 kg; monitor patients closely.

PATIENT TEACHING

• Tell patient to take dose at same time each day with food or milk.
• Tell parents that if child has difficulty swallowing tablets, to crush tablets and mix in condensed milk.
• Tell patient to repeat dose if he vomits within 1 hour.
• Advise patient to notify prescriber if he can't complete the course of therapy as prescribed.
• Instruct patient to supplement preventive antimalarial with use of protective clothing, bed nets, and insect repellents.

SAFETY ALERT!

atropine sulfate
AT-troe-peen

AtroPen

Therapeutic class: Antiarrhythmics
Pharmacologic class: Anticholinergics–belladonna alkaloids

AVAILABLE FORMS

Injection: 0.05 mg/mL, 0.1 mg/mL, 0.4 mg/mL, 0.8 mg/mL, 1 mg/mL
Prefilled auto-injectors: 0.25 mg, 0.5 mg, 1 mg, 2 mg

INDICATIONS & DOSAGES

➤ **Bradyarrhythmias**
Adults: Usually 0.4 to 1 mg I.V. push, repeated every 1 to 2 hours to maximum of 2 mg.
Children and adolescents: 0.01 to 0.03 mg/kg I.V.
➤ **Poisoning**
Adults and children weighing more than 41 kg: For anticholinesterase poisoning,

give at least 2 to 3 mg parenterally; repeat until signs of atropine intoxication appear. For muscarinic mushroom poisoning, give in doses sufficient to control parasympathetic signs before coma and CV collapse occur. When using the AtroPen, 2 mg I.M. is typically used for patients weighing more than 41 kg. More than one AtroPen may be needed until atropinization occurs. No more than three AtroPens should be used unless given under the supervision of a trained medical provider.
Children weighing 18 to 41 kg: AtroPen 1 mg I.M. per dose for one to three doses.
Children weighing 7 to 18 kg: AtroPen 0.5 mg I.M. per dose for one to three doses.
Infants weighing less than 7 kg: AtroPen 0.25 mg I.M. per dose for one to three doses.
➤ **Preoperatively to diminish secretions and block cardiac vagal reflexes**
Adults and children weighing 20 kg or more: 0.4 to 0.6 mg I.V., I.M., or subcutaneously 30 to 60 minutes before anesthesia.
Children weighing less than 20 kg: 0.01 mg/kg I.V., I.M., or subcutaneously up to maximum dose of 0.4 mg 30 to 60 minutes before anesthesia. May repeat every 4 to 6 hours p.r.n.
Infants weighing more than 5 kg: 0.03 mg/kg I.V. or I.M. every 4 to 6 hours p.r.n.
Infants weighing 5 kg or less: 0.04 mg/kg I.V. or I.M. every 4 to 6 hours p.r.n.
➤ **Antimuscarinic**
Adults and children weighing more than 41 kg: 0.4 to 0.6 mg I.V., I.M., or subcutaneously.
Children weighing 29.5 kg to 41 kg: 0.4 mg I.V., I.M., or subcutaneously.
Children weighing 18 kg to less than 29.5 kg: 0.3 mg I.V., I.M., or subcutaneously.
Children weighing 11 kg to less than 18 kg: 0.2 mg I.V., I.M., or subcutaneously.
Children weighing 7 kg to less than 11 kg: 0.15 mg I.V., I.M., or subcutaneously.
Children weighing 3 kg to less than 7 kg: 0.1 mg I.V., I.M., or subcutaneously.
➤ **Hypotonic radiography**
Adults: 1 mg I.M.
➤ **Stress echocardiography (adjunct chronotropic agent)** ◆

Reactions in bold italics are *life-threatening*. Interactions may have a *rapid onset* or a *delayed onset*.

Adults: 0.25 to 0.5 mg I.V. up to a total dose of 1 to 2 mg until 85% of target HR is achieved.

ADMINISTRATION

I.V.
▼ Give into a large vein or into I.V. tubing over at least 1 minute.
▼ Slow delivery may cause slowing of the HR.
▼ **Incompatibilities:** Pantoprazole, pentobarbital sodium, sodium bicarbonate. Consult detailed reference.

Subcutaneous
● Document administration site.

I.M.
● Auto-injection may be given through clothing.
● Firmly jab tip into outer thigh at 90-degree angle.
● Hold auto-injector in place for at least 10 seconds to allow time for complete administration.
● Make sure needle is visible after removing auto-injector. If needle didn't engage, repeat injection, jabbing more firmly.
● Massage injection site for several seconds after removing auto-injector.
● In very thin or young patients, pinch the skin on the thigh together before injection.

ACTION

Inhibits acetylcholine at parasympathetic neuroeffector junction, blocking vagal effects on SA and AV nodes, enhancing conduction through AV node and increasing HR.

Route	Onset	Peak	Duration
I.V.	Immediate	Unknown	Unknown
I.M.	Rapid	3 min	4 hr
Subcut.	Unknown	Unknown	Unknown

Half-life: I.M.: adults, 2 to 4 hours; children older than age 2, 1½ to 3½ hours; children younger than age 2, 4 to 10 hours.

ADVERSE REACTIONS

CNS: headache, restlessness, insomnia, dizziness, ataxia, disorientation, hallucinations, delirium, excitement, agitation, confusion.
CV: *bradycardia,* palpitations, tachycardia.

EENT: blurred vision, mydriasis, photophobia, cycloplegia, increased IOP.
GI: dry mouth, constipation, thirst, nausea, vomiting.
GU: urine retention, erectile dysfunction.
Other: *anaphylaxis.*

INTERACTIONS

Drug-drug. *Anticholinergics, drugs with anticholinergic effects (amantadine, antiarrhythmics, antiparkinsonians, glutethimide, meperidine, phenothiazines, TCAs):* May increase anticholinergic effects. Use together cautiously.
Potassium chloride wax-matrix tablets: May increase risk of mucosal lesions. Avoid combination.

EFFECTS ON LAB TEST RESULTS

None reported.

CONTRAINDICATIONS & CAUTIONS

● Contraindicated in patients hypersensitive to drug and in patients with hyperthermia.
● Contraindicated in patients with acute angle-closure glaucoma, obstructive uropathy, obstructive disease of GI tract, paralytic ileus, toxic megacolon, intestinal atony, unstable CV status in acute hemorrhage, tachycardia, myocardial ischemia, asthma, or myasthenia gravis.
● Use cautiously in patients with hyperthyroidism, hiatal hernia with reflux esophagitis, or renal or hepatic impairment, and in elderly patients.
● Use cautiously in patients with Down syndrome because they may be more sensitive to drug.
● Drug will be ineffective treatment of bradycardia in heart transplant patients due to lack of vagal nerve innervation.
Dialyzable drug: No.
⚠ **Overdose S&S:** Delirium, seizures, coma, tachycardia, fever, mydriasis, decreased salivation and sweating, urine retention, hypertension, vasodilation, hyperthermia.

PREGNANCY-LACTATION-REPRODUCTION

● Use in pregnant women only if clearly needed.
● Safe use in breast-feeding women hasn't been established. Use cautiously in breast-feeding women.

NURSING CONSIDERATIONS

• In adults, avoid doses less than 0.5 mg because of risk of paradoxical bradycardia.

🔔 **Alert:** Watch for tachycardia in cardiac patients because it may lead to ventricular fibrillation.

• Many adverse reactions (such as dry mouth and constipation) vary with dose.

• Monitor fluid intake and urine output. Drug causes urine retention and urinary hesitancy.

PATIENT TEACHING

• Instruct patient to report all adverse reactions and to immediately report urine retention, abnormal heartbeat, dizziness, passing out, difficulty breathing, weakness, tremors, and abdominal edema.

• Tell patient to protect the AtroPen from light and not to freeze it.

avanafil
a-VAN-ah-fill

Stendra

Therapeutic class: Erectile dysfunction drugs
Pharmacologic class: PDE5 inhibitors

AVAILABLE FORMS
Tablets: 50 mg, 100 mg, 200 mg

INDICATIONS & DOSAGES
➤ **Erectile dysfunction**
Adult men: 100 mg P.O. daily as needed 15 minutes before sexual activity. May increase to a maximum of 200 mg daily or decrease to 50 mg daily. Use lowest effective dosage.
Adjust-a-dose: In patients taking moderate CYP3A4 inhibitors, maximum dosage is 50 mg P.O. daily. In patients taking a stable dose of alpha blocker, initially give 50 mg P.O. daily; adjust as needed and tolerated.

ADMINISTRATION
P.O.
• May give without regard for food.
• Store at controlled room temperature; protect from light.

ACTION
Increases cyclic guanosine monophosphate level, prolongs smooth-muscle relaxation, and promotes blood flow into the corpus cavernosum.

Route	Onset	Peak	Duration
P.O.	Rapid	30–45 min	Unknown

Half-life: 5 hours.

ADVERSE REACTIONS
CNS: headache, dizziness.
CV: hypertension, flushing.
EENT: nasal congestion, nasopharyngitis, sinusitis, sinus congestion.
GI: dyspepsia, nausea, constipation, diarrhea.
Musculoskeletal: back pain, arthralgia.
Respiratory: URI, bronchitis.
Skin: rash.
Other: influenza.

INTERACTIONS
Drug-drug. *Alpha blockers, antihypertensives:* May cause additive hypotensive effect. Use cautiously together.
CYP450 inducers: Use together hasn't been evaluated and isn't recommended.
Moderate CYP3A4 inhibitors (amprenavir, aprepitant, diltiazem, erythromycin, fluconazole, fosamprenavir, verapamil): May increase avanafil concentration. Use cautiously together at maximum avanafil daily dosage of 50 mg.
Nitrates: May increase hypotensive effects. Use together is contraindicated. If nitrate administration is deemed medically necessary in a life-threatening situation, at least 12 hours should elapse after last dose of avanafil before nitrate administration.
PDE5 inhibitors (sildenafil, tadalafil): May cause additive hypotensive effects. Use together is contraindicated.
Strong CYP3A4 inhibitors (atazanavir, clarithromycin, indinavir, itraconazole, ketoconazole, nefazodone, nelfinavir, ritonavir, saquinavir, telithromycin): May increase avanafil concentration. Use together is contraindicated.
Drug-food. *Grapefruit juice:* May increase avanafil serum level. Don't use together.
Drug-lifestyle. *Alcohol use:* May increase risk of hypotension, including orthostatic

---

hypotension (increased HR, dizziness, headache). Discourage use together.
Street drug "poppers" (amyl nitrate, butyl nitrate): May increase risk of severe hypotensive effects. Discourage use together.

EFFECTS ON LAB TEST RESULTS
None reported.

CONTRAINDICATIONS & CAUTIONS
• Contraindicated in patients hypersensitive to drug or its components and in patients taking nitrates.
• Drug hasn't been studied in patients with severe renal disease, those on dialysis, or patients with severe hepatic disease. Don't use in these patients.
• Not recommended for use in patients with MI, stroke, life-threatening arrhythmia, or coronary revascularization within the past 6 months; resting hypotension or hypertension; unstable angina; angina with sexual intercourse; New York Heart Association Class 2 or greater HF; or conditions in which sexual activity isn't advised.
• Use cautiously in patients with anatomic deformities of the penis, including angulation, cavernosal fibrosis, and Peyronie disease, and in patients with conditions that may predispose them to priapism (such as sickle cell anemia, multiple myeloma, and leukemia).
Dialyzable drug: Unknown.

PREGNANCY-LACTATION-REPRODUCTION
• Not indicated for use in women.

NURSING CONSIDERATIONS
• Drug isn't for use in women.
• Assess patients with preexisting CV disease to determine if they're healthy enough for sexual activity.
• Monitor patients for loss of color discrimination and other visual changes.
• Monitor patients for sudden decrease in or loss of hearing, which is rare.

PATIENT TEACHING
• Teach patient that drug is only to be taken once daily.
• Caution patient to take drug only as prescribed.

• Advise patient that drug shouldn't be used with nitrates under any circumstances. Instruct patient who experiences chest pain after taking avanafil to seek immediate medical attention.
• Discuss with patient who has preexisting heart disease the potential cardiac risk of sexual activity; advise patient to seek immediate medical help if cardiac signs and symptoms occur upon initiation of sexual activity.
• Counsel patient to stop drug and seek prompt medical assistance if sudden loss of vision in one or both eyes or sudden decrease in or loss of hearing occurs.
• Advise patient to seek emergency medical attention for an erection lasting longer than 4 hours, whether painful or not.
• Tell patient that drug doesn't protect against sexually transmitted diseases, including HIV.
• Instruct patient to take drug approximately 30 minutes before sexual activity and that sexual stimulation is required for an erection to occur.

SAFETY ALERT!

axitinib
ax-I-ti-nib

Inlyta

Therapeutic class: Antineoplastics
Pharmacologic class: Kinase inhibitors

AVAILABLE FORMS
Tablets: 1 mg, 5 mg

INDICATIONS & DOSAGES
➤ **Advanced renal cell carcinoma after failure of one prior systemic therapy**
Adults: 5 mg P.O. b.i.d. approximately 12 hours apart. If patient tolerates drug for at least 2 consecutive weeks with adverse reactions no greater than grade 2 CTCAE guidelines, is normotensive, and isn't receiving antihypertensives, may increase dosage to 7 mg b.i.d., then 10 mg b.i.d.
Adjust-a-dose: Base dosage adjustment on individual safety and tolerability. Management of adverse reactions may require temporary interruption or permanent

discontinuation. If dosage reduction from 5 mg b.i.d. is needed, recommended dosage is 2 or 3 mg b.i.d. If a strong CYP3A4/5 inhibitor must be coadministered, decrease axitinib dosage by approximately half; may increase or decrease subsequent doses based on individual safety and tolerability. If strong CYP3A4/5 inhibitor is discontinued, return axitinib dosage to that used before initiation after inhibitor is out of system (3 to 5 half-life periods of the strong inhibitor). Reduce axitinib starting dose by approximately half in patients with baseline moderate hepatic impairment (Child-Pugh class B); may increase or decrease subsequent doses based on individual safety and tolerability.

ADMINISTRATION
P.O.
● Drug is considered hazardous: use safe handling and disposal precautions according to facility policy.
● May give without regard for food.
● Have patient swallow tablets whole with a glass of water.
● If a dose is missed or patient vomits, don't give an additional dose; give next prescribed dose at usual time.
● Store at room temperature.

ACTION
Inhibits receptor tyrosine kinase, which decreases cell proliferation, tumor growth, angiogenesis, and cancer progression.

Route	Onset	Peak	Duration
P.O.	Unknown	2½–4 hr	Unknown

Half-life: 2.5 to 6.1 hours.

ADVERSE REACTIONS
CNS: asthenia, fatigue, headache, dizziness, TIA.
CV: hypertension, *DVT.*
EENT: dysphonia, mucosal inflammation, stomatitis, dysgeusia, epistaxis, tinnitus, retinal-vein occlusion thrombosis, glossodynia.
GI: diarrhea, nausea, vomiting, constipation, abdominal pain, upper abdominal pain, dyspepsia, hemorrhoids, *rectal hemorrhage, hemoptysis.*
GU: hematuria, proteinuria.

Hematologic: anemia, *polycythemia.*
Metabolic: decreased appetite, decreased weight, hypothyroidism, dehydration.
Musculoskeletal: arthralgia, extremity pain, myalgia.
Respiratory: cough, dyspnea, *PE.*
Skin: alopecia, hand-foot syndrome, rash, dry skin, pruritus, erythema.

INTERACTIONS
Drug-drug. *Moderate CYP3A4/5 inducers (bosentan, efavirenz, etravirine, modafinil, nafcillin), strong CYP3A4/5 inducers (carbamazepine, dexamethasone, phenobarbital, phenytoin, rifabutin, rifampin, rifapentine):* May reduce axitinib level. Avoid concurrent use.
Strong CYP3A4/5 inhibitors (atazanavir, clarithromycin, indinavir, itraconazole, ketoconazole, nefazodone, nelfinavir, ritonavir, saquinavir, telithromycin, voriconazole): May increase axitinib level. Avoid concurrent use; if strong CYP3A4/5 inhibitor is absolutely necessary, reduce axitinib dosage.
Drug-herb. *St. John's wort:* May decrease axitinib plasma concentration. Discourage concurrent use.
Drug-food. *Grapefruit, grapefruit juice:* May increase axitinib plasma concentration. Discourage concurrent use.

EFFECTS ON LAB TEST RESULTS
● May increase potassium, amylase, lipase, alkaline phosphatase, ALT, AST, bilirubin, and creatinine levels. May decrease bicarbonate, calcium, albumin, phosphate, and thyroid hormone levels.
● May decrease Hb level and lymphocyte, neutrophil, and platelet counts.
● May increase or decrease glucose, sodium, and TSH levels.

CONTRAINDICATIONS & CAUTIONS
● Use isn't recommended in patients with recent GI bleeding or untreated brain metastases.
● Drug may be associated with impaired wound healing.
● Use cautiously in patients with hypertension; in those at risk for GI perforation, HF, fistula formation, thyroid dysfunction, or arterial or venous thromboembolic events;

Reactions in bold italics are *life-threatening*. Interactions may have a *rapid onset* or a ***delayed onset***.

and in patients with moderate hepatic impairment (Child-Pugh class B) or ESRD (CrCl less than 15 mL/minute). Drug hasn't been studied in patients with Child-Pugh class C hepatic impairment.

• Drug is associated with proteinuria.
• Drug may cause reversible posterior leukoencephalopathy syndrome (RPLS).
Dialyzable drug: Unknown.

⚠ *Overdose S&S:* Dizziness, hypertension, seizures, possible fatal hemoptysis.

PREGNANCY-LACTATION-REPRODUCTION
• Drug can cause fetal harm. Women of childbearing potential should be advised of potential hazard to the fetus and to avoid becoming pregnant during therapy.
• It isn't known if drug appears in breast milk. Patient should discontinue breast-feeding or discontinue drug.

NURSING CONSIDERATIONS
• Hypertension should be well controlled before start of therapy. Monitor patient for increased BP; treat as indicated. If hypertension persists despite antihypertensive use, decrease axitinib dosage, as ordered.
• Watch for hypotension if drug is withheld for any reason and patient continues antihypertensive use.
• Monitor patient for signs and symptoms of hematologic or neurologic disease, thromboembolic events, and GI disorders.
• Monitor patient for bleeding or hemorrhagic event. Temporarily interrupt treatment if bleeding occurs.
• Monitor use of all prescription drugs, OTC medications, grapefruit or grapefruit juice, and supplements.
• Obtain LFTs and renal function tests before and periodically during therapy.
• Stop drug at least 24 hours before surgery; resume based on clinical judgment of wound healing. Monitor wound healing carefully.
• Monitor patient for signs and symptoms of RPLS (headache, seizures, lethargy, confusion, blindness, and other visual disturbances) and other neurologic signs and symptoms. Discontinue drug if these occur.
• Monitor patient for proteinuria before and during therapy. For moderate or severe proteinuria, reduce dosage or withhold

drug. Monitor thyroid function before and periodically during therapy.

PATIENT TEACHING
• Counsel female patient to use effective birth control during treatment.
• Instruct patient that drug may be taken without regard to meals and that patient should swallow capsules whole with a glass of water.
• Tell patient to avoid grapefruit and grapefruit juice while taking this drug.
• Caution patient that if a dose is missed, to wait until next scheduled dose and never to take two doses at the same time to make up for a missed dose.
• Advise patient to alert prescriber if stomach pain, bruising, bleeding, delayed wound healing, fatigue, high BP, or neurologic signs and symptoms (headache, seizures, lethargy, confusion, blindness, other visual changes) occur.
• Teach patient to consult prescriber before starting new drugs or supplements.
• Instruct patient to keep lab test appointments as requested by prescriber to monitor drug's safety and effectiveness.

SAFETY ALERT!

azacitidine
ay-za-SYE-ti deen

Vidaza

Therapeutic class: Antineoplastics
Pharmacologic class: Pyrimidine nucleoside analogues

AVAILABLE FORMS
Powder for injection: 100-mg vials

INDICATIONS & DOSAGES
➤ **Myelodysplastic syndrome, including refractory anemia, refractory anemia with ringed sideroblasts (if patient has neutropenia or thrombocytopenia, or needs transfusions), refractory anemia with excess blasts, refractory anemia with excess blasts in transformation, or chronic myelomonocytic leukemia**
Adults: Initially, 75 mg/m² subcutaneously or I.V. daily for 7 days; repeat cycle every

4 weeks. May increase to 100 mg/m^2 if no response after two treatment cycles and nausea and vomiting are the only toxic reactions. Four to six treatment cycles are recommended.

Adjust-a-dose: If bicarbonate level is less than 20 mEq/L, reduce next dose by 50%. If BUN or creatinine levels rise during treatment, delay the next cycle until they are normal; then give 50% of previous dose.

For patients with baseline WBC count greater than or equal to 3 × 10^9/L, ANC greater than or equal to 1.5 × 10^9/L, and platelet count greater than or equal to 75 × 10^9/L, adjust the dose based on nadir counts as follows: If ANC is less than 0.5 × 10^9/L and platelet count is less than 25 × 10^9/L, give 50% of dose. If ANC is 0.5 to 1.5 × 10^9/L and platelet count is 25 to 50 × 10^9/L, give 67% of dose.

For patients with baseline WBC count less than 3 × 10^9/L, ANC less than 1.5 × 10^9/L, or platelet count less than 75 × 10^9/L, adjust dosage as shown in the table below.

If a nadir, as defined in the table, has occurred, the next course of treatment should be given 28 days after the start of the preceding course, provided that both the WBC and platelet counts are greater than 25% above the nadir and rising. If an increase greater than 25% above nadir isn't seen by day 28, counts should be reassessed every 7 days. If a 25% increase isn't seen by day 42, patient should be treated with 50% of scheduled dose. Adjust further dosages during therapy based on hematologic or renal toxicities.

➤ **Acute myeloid leukemia ◆**
Adults: 75 mg/m^2/day subcutaneously for 7 days every 4 weeks for at least six cycles. May continue treatment as long as patient continues to benefit or until disease progression or unacceptable toxicity.

ADMINISTRATION
I.V.
▼ Reconstitute drug with 10 mL of sterile water for injection.
▼ Vigorously shake or roll the vial until powder is dissolved. The resulting solution will be 10 mg/mL.
▼ Use only clear solution.
▼ Withdraw proper dose and mix in a total volume of 50 to 100 mL of NSS or lactated Ringer solution.
▼ Give the infusion over 10 to 40 minutes. Infusion must be completed within 1 hour of reconstitution.
▼ **Incompatibilities:** Dextrose 5%, hespan, bicarbonate.

Subcutaneous
● Dilute using aseptic and hazardous substances techniques.
● Reconstitute with 4 mL sterile water for injection. Vigorously shake or roll the vial until a uniform suspension forms. The resulting cloudy suspension will be 25 mg/mL.
● Draw up suspension into syringes for injection (no more than 4 mL per syringe).
● Just before giving drug, resuspend drug by vigorously rolling the syringe between the palms for 30 seconds. Divide doses greater than 4 mL into two syringes and inject into two separate sites.
● Give new injections at least 1 inch (2.5 cm) from previous site, and never into tender, bruised, red, or hardened skin.
● Reconstituted drug is stable for 1 hour at room temperature and 8 hours refrigerated at 36° to 46° F (2° to 8° C). After refrigeration, suspension may be allowed to warm for 30 minutes at room temperature.

ACTION
Causes hypomethylation of DNA and is toxic to abnormal hematopoietic cells in bone marrow. Hypomethylation may restore normal function to genes needed for

Azacitidine dosage adjustments based on nadir counts and bone marrow biopsy cellularity

| WBC or platelet nadir % decrease in counts from baseline | Bone marrow biopsy cellularity at time of nadir | | |
| | 30%–60% | 15%–30% | <15% |
		% dose in the next course	
50%–75%	100%	50%	33%
>75%	75%	50%	33%

Reactions in bold italics are *life-threatening*. Interactions may have a *rapid onset* or a *delayed onset*.

proliferation and differentiation. Drug has little effect on nonproliferating cells.

Route	Onset	Peak	Duration
I.V.	Unknown	Unknown	Unknown
Subcut.	Unknown	30 min	Unknown

Half-life: About 4 hours.

ADVERSE REACTIONS

CNS: anxiety, dizziness, fatigue, headache, insomnia, malaise, pain, weakness, lethargy, pyrexia.
CV: chest pain, edema, hypotension, hypertension, peripheral swelling.
EENT: nasopharyngitis, pharyngitis, rhinitis, nasal congestion.
GI: abdominal pain and tenderness, anorexia, constipation, diarrhea, nausea, vomiting, abdominal distention, dyspepsia, gingival bleeding, loose stools, stomatitis.
GU: UTI.
Hematologic: anemia, *febrile neutropenia, leukopenia, neutropenia, thrombocytopenia,* hematoma, postprocedural hemorrhage.
Metabolic: decreased weight, *hypokalemia.*
Musculoskeletal: arthralgia, bone pain, limb pain, myalgia, chest wall pain.
Respiratory: dyspnea, pneumonia, URI.
Skin: ecchymosis, erythema (including erythema at injection site), pallor, petechiae, pitting edema, rash, cellulitis, dry skin, granuloma, pigmentation, pruritus at injection site, skin nodules, swelling at injection site, urticaria.
Other: rigors.

INTERACTIONS
None reported.

EFFECTS ON LAB TEST RESULTS
• May increase BUN and creatinine levels. May decrease bicarbonate and potassium levels.
• May decrease neutrophil, platelet, and WBC counts.

CONTRAINDICATIONS & CAUTIONS
• Contraindicated in patients hypersensitive to azacitidine or mannitol and in patients with advanced malignant hepatic tumors.
• Use cautiously in patients with hepatic and renal disease.
Dialyzable drug: Unknown.

⚠ *Overdose S&S:* Diarrhea, nausea, vomiting.

PREGNANCY-LACTATION-REPRODUCTION
• Drug may cause fetal harm. Women of childbearing potential should be advised to avoid pregnancy during treatment.
• Men should be advised not to father a child during therapy.
• It isn't known if drug appears in breast milk. Patient should discontinue breast-feeding or discontinue drug.

NURSING CONSIDERATIONS
• Check LFT results and creatinine level before therapy starts.
• Obtain CBC before each cycle or more often. Bone marrow suppression is common.
• Premedicate patient for nausea and vomiting.
• Monitor renal function at baseline, before each cycle, and more frequently if indicated. Monitor renal function closely in elderly patients and in renally impaired patients receiving drug because renal impairment may increase toxicity.
• *Look alike–sound alike:* Don't confuse azacitidine with azathioprine.

PATIENT TEACHING
• Advise patient to report all adverse reactions and to immediately report signs and symptoms of infection (fever, cough, malaise), liver problems (dark urine, abdominal pain, yellowing of skin or eyes), or renal problems (urine retention, change in amount of urine, edema); abnormal bleeding; chest pain; dizziness; or severe GI signs and symptoms.
• Inform patient that blood counts may decrease with febrile neutropenia, thrombocytopenia, and anemia.
• Advise male and female patient to use birth control during therapy.

azathioprine

ay-za-THYE-oh-preen

Azasan, Imuran✤

azathioprine sodium

Therapeutic class: Immunosuppressants
Pharmacologic class: Purine antagonists

AVAILABLE FORMS
Powder for injection✤: 50 mg/vial
Tablets: 25 mg, 50 mg, 75 mg, 100 mg

INDICATIONS & DOSAGES
➤ **Immunosuppression in kidney transplantation**
Adults: Initially, 3 to 5 mg/kg P.O. or I.V. daily, usually beginning on day of transplantation. Maintained at 1 to 3 mg/kg daily based on patient response and tolerance.
Adjust-a-dose: Give drug in lower doses to patients with oliguria in the posttransplant period and in those with impaired renal function. In patients receiving allopurinol, decrease azathioprine dose to ⅓ to ¼ of the usual dose.
➤ **RA**
Adults: Initially, 1 mg/kg P.O. as single dose or divided into two doses. Usual dose is 50 to 100 mg. If patient response isn't satisfactory after 6 to 8 weeks, dosage may be increased by 0.5 mg/kg daily to maximum of 2.5 mg/kg daily at 4-week intervals. Maintenance therapy should be at lowest effective dose. Attempt gradual dose reduction once the patient is stable. Reduce dosage by 0.5 mg/kg (about 25 mg daily) every 4 weeks.

ADMINISTRATION
P.O.
● Give drug after meals to minimize adverse GI effects.
● Drug is a potential teratogen and mutagen. Use safe-handling procedures.
I.V.
▼ Drug is a potential teratogen and mutagen. Use safe handling procedures.
▼ Use only in patients who can't tolerate oral drugs.

▼ Reconstitute drug in 50-mg vial with 5 mL of sterile water for injection.
▼ Inspect for particles before use.
▼ Give by direct I.V. injection, or further dilute in NSS for injection or D₅W solution and infuse over 30 to 60 minutes.
▼ **Incompatibilities:** None reported.

ACTION
May alter antibody production and suppress T-cell effects.

Route	Onset	Peak	Duration
P.O., I.V.	Unknown	1–2 hr	Unknown

Half-life: About 2 hours.

ADVERSE REACTIONS
CNS: fever.
GI: nausea, vomiting, anorexia, *pancreatitis,* abdominal pain.
Hematologic: *leukopenia, myelosuppression, pancytopenia, thrombocytopenia, immunosuppression.*
Hepatic: *hepatotoxicity.*
Musculoskeletal: myalgia.
Other: infections, *increased risk of neoplasia.*

INTERACTIONS
Drug-drug. *ACE inhibitors:* May cause severe leukopenia and increase risk of anemia. Monitor patient closely.
Allopurinol: May impair inactivation of azathioprine. Avoid using if possible; decrease azathioprine to ⅓ to ¼ usual dose.
Cyclosporine: May decrease cyclosporine level. Monitor cyclosporine level closely.
Febuxostat: May increase risk of toxicity. Concomitant use is contraindicated.
DMARDs (abatacept, adalimumab, etanercept, hydroxychloroquine, leflunomide, methotrexate, minocycline, sulfasalazine, tocilizumab): Concomitant use hasn't been studied. Use together isn't recommended.
Live-virus vaccines: May reduce effectiveness of live-virus vaccines. Immunocompromised patients may be at increased risk for vaccine-induced infection. Defer live-virus vaccines until immune function improves.
Mercaptopurine: May increase risk of myelosuppression, including pancytopenia. Avoid concomitant use.

Nondepolarizing neuromuscular blockers:
May decrease or reverse pharmacologic
action of neuromuscular blockers. Monitor
respiratory function; dosage requirements
for nondepolarizing muscle relaxants may
need to be increased.
Ribavirin: May increase risk of severe
pancytopenia and azathioprine-related
myelotoxicity. Monitor CBC, including
platelet count.
*Sulfamethoxazole–trimethoprim and other
drugs that interfere with myelopoiesis:* May
cause severe leukopenia, especially in renal
transplant patients. Use together cautiously.
Tacrolimus (topical): May increase risk of
adverse effects of immunosuppressants.
Avoid use together.
Warfarin: May inhibit warfarin's anticoagulant effect. Monitor patient. Adjust warfarin
dosage as needed.
Drug-herb. *Cat's claw, echinacea:* May
reduce drug's therapeutic effects. Avoid
using together.

EFFECTS ON LAB TEST RESULTS
• May increase alkaline phosphatase, ALT,
AST, and bilirubin levels. May decrease Hb
and uric acid levels.
• May decrease platelet, RBC, and WBC
counts.

CONTRAINDICATIONS & CAUTIONS
• Contraindicated in patients hypersensitive
to drug or its components and in pregnant
women.
Black Box Warning Long-term immunosuppression with this drug increases risk
of neoplasia, including posttransplant lymphoma and hepatosplenic T-cell lymphoma
in patients with inflammatory bowel disease.
Prescribers using this drug should be very
familiar with its risks, the mutagenic potential to both men and women, and possible
hematologic toxicities. ■
• Use cautiously in patients with hepatic or
renal dysfunction.
• Benefits must be weighed against risk
when giving to patient with systemic viral
infection, such as chickenpox or herpes
zoster.
• Rare but life-threatening hepatic veno-
occlusive disease has been reported in

transplant patients. If this is suspected,
permanently discontinue drug.
• Patients with RA previously treated
with alkylating drugs, such as cyclophosphamide, chlorambucil, or melphalan, may
be at increased risk for tumor development
if treated with this drug. Use together is
contraindicated.
Dialyzable drug: 45% in an 8-hour dialysis
session.
⚠ **Overdose S&S:** Nausea, vomiting, diarrhea, abnormal liver function, leukopenia.

PREGNANCY-LACTATION-REPRODUCTION
• There are no adequate and well-controlled
studies in pregnant women. Drug can cause
fetal harm. Avoid use in pregnant women
when possible. Don't use to treat RA in
pregnant women. Women of childbearing
potential should be advised to avoid becoming pregnant.
• Drug appears in breast milk. Not recommended in breast-feeding women.

NURSING CONSIDERATIONS
• Consider genotype or phenotype testing
for thiopurine S-methyltransferase. Patients
with low or absent levels are at increased
risk for hematologic effects of drug.
• To prevent bleeding, avoid all I.M. injections when platelet count is below
$100,000/mm^3$.
• Monitor CBC and platelet counts weekly
for 1 month, twice monthly for 2 months,
then monthly unless more frequent monitoring is clinically indicated. Also monitor
counts at dosage changes. Notify prescriber
if counts drop suddenly or become danger-
ously low. Drug may need to be temporarily
withheld.
• Watch for early signs and symptoms of
hepatotoxicity (such as clay-colored stools,
dark urine, pruritus, and yellow skin and
sclera) and for increased alkaline phosphatase, bilirubin, AST, and ALT levels.
• Monitor patient for bacterial, viral, fungal,
protozoal, and opportunistic infections,
including reactivation of latent infections
such as tuberculosis.
• Watch for new-onset neurologic symptoms. Patients on immunosuppressive
therapy may be at increased risk for

JC virus–associated infection resulting in multifocal leukoencephalopathy.
- Aspirin, NSAIDs, and low-dose glucocorticoids may be continued during azathioprine therapy.
- Therapeutic response usually occurs within 8 weeks. Patients not improved after 12 weeks can be considered refractory to treatment.
- Consider obtaining genotype or phenotype for intermediate thiopurine S-methyltransferase activity. Patients with deficiency are at greater risk for severe bone marrow toxicity from azathioprine therapy.
- *Look alike–sound alike:* Don't confuse azathioprine with Azulfidine. Don't confuse Imuran with Inderal.

PATIENT TEACHING
Black Box Warning Warn patient of the risk of malignancy. ∎
- Warn patient to report even mild infections (colds, fever, sore throat, malaise), because drug is a potent immunosuppressant.
- Instruct patient to avoid conception during therapy and for 4 months after therapy stops.
- Warn patient that some hair thinning is possible.
- Tell patient taking drug for refractory RA that it may take up to 12 weeks to be effective.
- Advise patient to report unusual bleeding or bruising.
- Tell patient that drug may be taken with food to decrease nausea.
- Advise patient to use soft toothbrush and perform oral care cautiously.

---

azelastine hydrochloride
a-ZEL-as-teen

Astepro, Optivar

Therapeutic class: Antihistamines
Pharmacologic class: H_1-receptor antagonists

AVAILABLE FORMS
Intranasal: 0.1%, 0.15%
Ophthalmic solution: 0.05%

INDICATIONS & DOSAGES
➤ **Pruritus from allergic conjunctivitis**
Adults and children age 3 and older: Instill 1 drop into affected eye b.i.d.
➤ **Perennial allergic rhinitis**
Adults and children age 12 and older: Instill 2 sprays (0.15%) per nostril b.i.d.
Children ages 6 to 11: Instill 1 spray (0.1% or 0.15%) per nostril b.i.d.
Children age 6 months to 5 years: Instill 1 spray (0.1%) per nostril b.i.d.
➤ **Seasonal allergic rhinitis**
Adults and children age 12 and older: Instill 1 to 2 sprays (0.1% and 0.15%) per nostril b.i.d. or 2 sprays (0.15%) per nostril once daily.
Children ages 6 to 11: Instill 1 spray (0.1% or 0.15%) per nostril b.i.d.
Children ages 2 to 5: Instill 1 spray (0.1%) per nostril b.i.d.

ADMINISTRATION
Ophthalmic
- Keep bottle tightly closed when not in use.
- Don't touch tip of dropper to any surface.
Intranasal
- Before initial use of nasal spray, prime the delivery system with 4 sprays (0.1%) or 6 sprays (0.15%), or until a fine mist appears.
- If 3 or more days have elapsed since last use, reprime the delivery system with 2 sprays or until a fine mist appears.
- After each use, wipe spray tip with a clean tissue or cloth.

ACTION
Inhibits the release of histamine and other mediators from cells involved in the allergic response.

Route	Onset	Peak	Duration
Ophthalmic	3 min	Unknown	8 hr
Intranasal	Unknown	3–4 hr	Unknown

Half-life: 22 to 25 hours.

ADVERSE REACTIONS
CNS: anxiety, depression, dizziness, drowsiness, headache, fatigue, malaise, nervousness, sleep disorder, vertigo.
CV: flushing, hypertension, tachycardia.
EENT: transient eye burning or stinging, conjunctivitis, eye pain, temporary blurring,

---

Reactions in bold italics are *life-threatening*. Interactions may have a *rapid onset* or a *delayed onset*.

pharyngitis, rhinitis, nasal discomfort, nasal congestion, sinusitis, postnasal drip, sneezing, epistaxis, bitter taste.
GI: abdominal pain, constipation, diarrhea, nausea, vomiting, gastroenteritis, increased appetite.
GU: hematuria.
Respiratory: *asthma,* dyspnea, cough, URI.
Skin: pruritus.
Other: flulike syndrome, weight gain.

INTERACTIONS
Drug-drug. *Cimetidine:* May interfere with plasma concentrations of azelastine. Avoid use together.
CNS depressants: May enhance CNS depressant effect of azelastine. Avoid combination.
Drug-lifestyle. *Alcohol use:* May increase CNS depressant effect of azelastine. Avoid use together.

EFFECTS ON LAB TEST RESULTS
None reported.

CONTRAINDICATIONS & CAUTIONS
• Contraindicated in patients hypersensitive to drug or its components.
Dialyzable drug: Unknown.

PREGNANCY-LACTATION-REPRODUCTION
• Use cautiously in pregnant women and only if potential benefit justifies potential risk to fetus.
• It isn't known if drug appears in breast milk. Use cautiously in breast-feeding women.

NURSING CONSIDERATIONS
• Drug is for ophthalmic or intranasal use only. Don't inject or give orally.
• Don't use ophthalmic form for irritation caused by contact lenses.

PATIENT TEACHING
• Instruct patient not to touch any surface, eyelid, or surrounding areas with tip of dropper.
• Tell patient to keep bottle tightly closed when not in use.
• Advise patient not to wear contact lens if eye is red.

• Warn patient that soft contact lenses may absorb the preservative benzalkonium.
• Instruct patient who wears soft contact lenses and whose eyes aren't red to wait at least 10 minutes after instilling drug before inserting contact lenses.
• Tell patient to report all adverse reactions and to immediately report shortness of breath or severe nose irritation if taking intranasal form.
• Because drug may cause CNS depression, advise patient using intranasal form to avoid hazardous activities requiring complete mental alertness, such as driving or operating machinery.

azelastine hydrochloride–fluticasone propionate
a-ZEL-as-teen/floo-TIK-a-sone

Dymista

Therapeutic class: Antihistamines–corticosteroids
Pharmacologic class: H_1-receptor antagonists–corticosteroids

AVAILABLE FORMS
Nasal spray: 137 mcg azelastine hydrochloride and 50 mcg fluticasone propionate/spray

INDICATIONS & DOSAGES
➤ **Symptoms of seasonal allergic rhinitis**
Adults and children age 6 and older:
1 spray/nostril b.i.d.

ADMINISTRATION
Intranasal
• Shake gently before each use.
• Prime the spray before initial use; spray six times or until a fine mist appears. If the spray hasn't been used within the past 14 days, prime the spray again with 1 spray or until a fine mist appears.
• Store upright at room temperature with dust cap in place. Don't freeze or refrigerate.
• Protect from light.

ACTION
Azelastine inhibits release of histamine and other mediators from cells involved

in the allergic response. Fluticasone may decrease inflammation by inhibiting mast cells, macrophages, and mediators such as leukotrienes.

Route	Onset	Peak	Duration
Intranasal	Rapid	½ hr (azelastine), 1 hr (fluticasone)	Unknown

Half-life: Azelastine, 25 hours; fluticasone, unknown.

ADVERSE REACTIONS
CNS: headache, fever, pain.
EENT: epistaxis, nasal congestion, rhinitis, pharyngitis, oropharyngeal pain, otitis media, otitis externa.
GI: diarrhea, dysgeusia, nausea, vomiting, upper abdominal pain.
Respiratory: cough, URI.
Skin: urticaria.
Other: viral infection.

INTERACTIONS
Drug-drug. *CNS depressants:* May increase risk of drowsiness. Use together cautiously.
CYP3A4 inhibitors (fluconazole, ketoconazole): May increase fluticasone plasma level. Use together cautiously.
Ritonavir: May increase fluticasone plasma level and risk of systemic corticosteroid effects, including Cushing syndrome and adrenal suppression. Avoid use together.
Drug-lifestyle. *Alcohol use:* May increase risk of somnolence and CNS impairment. Discourage use together.

EFFECTS ON LAB TEST RESULTS
None reported.

CONTRAINDICATIONS & CAUTIONS
• Contraindicated in patients hypersensitive to either drug or its components.
• Avoid use in patients with current nasal ulcers, nasal trauma, or nasal surgery until healing occurs.
• Use cautiously in patients with glaucoma, cataracts, ongoing infection, or history of adrenal suppression.
Dialyzable drug: Unknown.

PREGNANCY-LACTATION-REPRODUCTION
• Use cautiously in pregnant and breast-feeding women and only if benefits outweigh risks.

NURSING CONSIDERATIONS
• Monitor patient for fungal, bacterial, or viral infections.
• Monitor patient for localized nasopharyngeal *Candida albicans* infection with prolonged use.
• Ensure patient receives regular eye exams to screen for cataracts and glaucoma with long-term use.
• Monitor growth rate in children using the spray long-term.
• Monitor patient for adrenal insufficiency (tiredness, weakness, nausea, vomiting, hypotension).

PATIENT TEACHING
• Instruct patient to shake bottle gently before each use and to prime the spray until a fine mist appears before initial use or if the spray hasn't been used in the past 14 days. Advise patient to follow full package directions for use.
• Caution patient to avoid spraying into eyes and, if exposure occurs, to flush eyes with water for 10 minutes.
• Warn patient to watch for changes in vision, which can indicate serious eye problems, such as glaucoma or cataracts. Advise patient to have regular eye exams while taking drug.
• Tell patient to watch for nasal problems, such as nosebleeds and nasal septal perforation.
• Advise patient that drug can decrease the body's ability to heal or fight infection. Tell patient to report fever, aches or pains, chills, fatigue, or exposure to chickenpox or measles. Caution patient to avoid exposure to communicable diseases.
• Warn patient that drug can cause drowsiness. Instruct patient to avoid alcohol and other drugs that cause drowsiness while taking this medication.
• Advise patient to avoid driving or tasks that require alertness until drug's effects are known.
• Instruct female patient to notify prescriber if she is pregnant, planning to become pregnant, or is breast-feeding.

azilsartan medoxomil

ay-zil-SAR-tan

Edarbi

Therapeutic class: Antihypertensives
Pharmacologic class: ARBs

AVAILABLE FORMS
Tablets: 40 mg, 80 mg

INDICATIONS & DOSAGES
➤ **Hypertension (alone or in combination with other antihypertensives)**
Adults: 80 mg P.O. once daily.
Adjust-a-dose: For patients treated with high doses of diuretics, consider initiating therapy at 40 mg P.O. daily.

ADMINISTRATION
P.O.
● Give drug with or without food.
● Store at room temperature in original container.
● Protect from moisture and light.

ACTION
Blocks vasoconstricting and aldosterone-secreting effects of angiotensin II by preventing angiotensin II from binding to angiotensin I receptors on vascular smooth muscle and the adrenal glands.

Route	Onset	Peak	Duration
P.O.	Rapid	1½–3 hr	Unknown

Half-life: 11 hours.

ADVERSE REACTIONS
CNS: asthenia, dizziness, fatigue.
CV: hypotension, orthostatic hypotension.
GI: diarrhea, nausea.
Musculoskeletal: muscle spasm, weakness.
Respiratory: cough.

INTERACTIONS
Drug-drug. *Aliskiren:* May increase risk of renal impairment, hypotension, and hyperkalemia in diabetic patients and those with moderate to severe renal impairment (GFR less than 60 mL/minute). Concomitant use is contraindicated in diabetic patients. Avoid concomitant use in those with moderate to severe renal impairment.
Lithium: May increase lithium serum concentration. Lithium dosage reduction may be needed.
NSAIDs: May decrease renal function and azilsartan effectiveness. Monitor renal function and BP periodically.

EFFECTS ON LAB TEST RESULTS
● May increase serum creatinine level.
● May increase or decrease platelet and WBC counts.
● May decrease Hb level, hematocrit, and RBC count.

CONTRAINDICATIONS & CAUTIONS
● Contraindicated in patients hypersensitive to drug or its components and when administered with aliskiren in diabetic patients.
● Use cautiously in patients with volume or salt depletion (such as those taking high-dose diuretics) because of the risk of symptomatic hypotension. Correct the cause before start of therapy or initiate drug at 40 mg P.O. daily.
Dialyzable drug: Unknown.

PREGNANCY-LACTATION-REPRODUCTION
Black Box Warning Use during pregnancy can cause injury and death to the developing fetus. When pregnancy is detected, stop drug as soon as possible. ■
● It isn't known if drug appears in breast milk. Patient should discontinue breast-feeding or discontinue drug.

NURSING CONSIDERATIONS
● Monitor BP closely. If BP isn't controlled with azilsartan alone, consider adding additional antihypertensives.
● If hypotension occurs, place patient in the supine position, and administer volume expanders if necessary.
● Monitor renal function periodically. Drug may cause oliguria or progressive azotemia and (rarely) acute renal failure or death in patients whose renal function may depend on the activity of the RAAS (such as those with HF).

PATIENT TEACHING

🜊 *Alert:* Advise female patient of childbearing potential of possible hazards to the fetus if drug is taken during pregnancy. Tell female patient who plans to become pregnant to notify provider so other treatment options can be considered.

🜊 *Alert:* Instruct female patient to report suspected pregnancy to prescriber immediately to prevent potential fetal harm.

🜊 *Alert:* Advise female patient who is breast-feeding to stop either drug or breast-feeding because of possible harm to the infant.

• Tell patient to notify provider if dizziness occurs, especially upon standing. If dizziness occurs, advise patient to lie down, rise slowly from a lying to standing position, and to climb stairs slowly.

• Teach patient that azilsartan may be prescribed alone or with other antihypertensives to control BP.

• Inform patient that azilsartan may be taken with or without food.

• Warn patient to store drug in its original container and to protect it from light and moisture.

• Advise patient that laboratory blood work will be needed to monitor renal function and drug tolerance.

---

azithromycin
ay-zi-thro-MY-sin

AzaSite, Zithromax✦, Zmax

Therapeutic class: Antibiotics
Pharmacologic class: Macrolides

AVAILABLE FORMS
Injection: 500 mg
Ophthalmic solution: 1%
Oral suspension (extended-release): 2 g
Powder for oral suspension: 100 mg/5 mL, 200 mg/5 mL; 1,000 mg/single-dose packet
Tablets: 250 mg, 500 mg, 600 mg

INDICATIONS & DOSAGES
➤ **Acute bacterial worsening of COPD caused by *Haemophilus influenzae*, *Moraxella catarrhalis*, or *Streptococcus pneumoniae*; uncomplicated skin and skin-structure infections caused by *Staphylococcus aureus*, *Streptococcus pyogenes*, or *Streptococcus agalactiae*; second-line therapy for pharyngitis or tonsillitis caused by *S. pyogenes***
Adults and adolescents age 16 and older: Initially, 500 mg P.O. as a single dose on day 1, followed by 250 mg daily on days 2 through 5. Total cumulative dose is 1.5 g. Or, for worsening COPD, 500 mg P.O. daily for 3 days.

➤ **Community-acquired pneumonia caused by *Chlamydia pneumoniae*, *H. influenzae*, *Mycoplasma pneumoniae*, *S. pneumoniae*, *Legionella pneumophila*, *M. catarrhalis*, or *S. aureus***
Adults and adolescents age 16 and older: For mild infections, give 500 mg P.O. as a single dose on day 1; then 250 mg P.O. daily on days 2 through 5. Total dose is 1.5 g. For more severe infections or those caused by *S. aureus*, give 500 mg I.V. as a single daily dose for 2 days; then 500 mg P.O. as a single daily dose to complete a 7- to 10-day course of therapy. Switch from I.V. to oral therapy based on patient response.

➤ **Community-acquired pneumonia caused by *C. pneumoniae*, *H. influenzae*, *M. pneumoniae*, or *S. pneumoniae***
Children age 6 months and older: 10 mg/kg oral suspension P.O. (maximum of 500 mg) as a single dose on day 1, followed by 5 mg/kg (maximum of 250 mg) daily on days 2 through 5. Or, a single dose of Zmax 60 mg/kg.

➤ **Single-dose treatment for mild to moderate acute bacterial sinusitis caused by *H. influenzae*, *M. catarrhalis*, or *S. pneumoniae* or for community-acquired pneumonia caused by *C. pneumoniae*, *H. influenzae*, *M. pneumoniae*, or *S. pneumoniae***
Adults: 2 g Zmax P.O. as a single dose taken 1 hour before or 2 hours after a meal.

➤ **Acute bacterial sinusitis caused by *H. influenzae*, *M. catarrhalis*, or *S. pneumoniae***
Adults: 500 mg P.O. daily for 3 days.
Children age 6 months and older: 10 mg/kg oral suspension P.O. once daily for 3 days.

➤ **Chancroid**
Adults: 1 g P.O. as a single dose.

➤ **Nongonococcal urethritis or cervicitis caused by *Chlamydia trachomatis***
Adults and adolescents age 16 and older:
1 g P.O. as a single dose.

➤ **To prevent disseminated *Mycobacterium avium* complex in patients with advanced HIV infection**
Adults and adolescents: 1.2 g P.O. once weekly alone or with rifabutin.

➤ ***M. avium* complex in patients with advanced HIV infection**
Adults: 600 mg P.O. daily with ethambutol 15 mg/kg daily.

➤ **Urethritis and cervicitis caused by *Neisseria gonorrhoeae***
Adults: 2 g P.O. as a single dose.

➤ **Pelvic inflammatory disease caused by *C. trachomatis*, *N. gonorrhoeae*, or *Mycoplasma hominis* in patients who need initial I.V. therapy**
Adults and adolescents age 16 and older:
500 mg I.V. as a single daily dose for 1 to 2 days; then 250 mg P.O. daily to complete a 7-day course of therapy. Switch from I.V. to oral therapy based on patient response.

➤ **Otitis media**
Children older than age 6 months: 30 mg/kg oral suspension P.O. as a single dose; or 10 mg/kg P.O. once daily for 3 days; or 10 mg/kg P.O. on day 1 and then 5 mg/kg once daily on days 2 to 5.

➤ **Pharyngitis, tonsillitis**
Children age 2 and older: 12 mg/kg oral suspension (maximum, 500 mg) P.O. daily for 5 days.

➤ **Bacterial conjunctivitis caused by coryneform group G, *H. influenzae*, *Staphylococcus aureus*, *Streptococcus mitis* group, and *S. pneumoniae***
Adults and children age 1 and older: Instill 1 drop in affected eye(s) b.i.d., 8 to 12 hours apart for first 2 days; then instill 1 drop in affected eye(s) once daily for next 5 days.

➤ **Babesiosis ◆**
Adults: 500 to 1,000 mg P.O. on day 1, then 250 mg P.O. daily thereafter for 7 to 10 days; higher dosages may be needed in immunocompromised patients (600 to 1,000 mg daily). Infectious Disease Society of America guidelines recommend the combination of azithromycin and atovaquone for 7 to 10 days as initial therapy for treatment of active babesiosis.

➤ **Cat scratch disease ◆**
Adults and children weighing 45.5 kg or more: 500 mg P.O. on day 1, then 250 mg P.O. daily on days 2 to 5.
Children weighing less than 45.5 kg:
10 mg/kg on day 1, then 5 mg/kg P.O. daily on days 2 to 5.

ADMINISTRATION
P.O.
● Obtain specimen for culture and sensitivity tests before giving first dose. Begin therapy while awaiting results.
● Reconstitute Zmax extended-release suspension with 60 mL of water. Shake well. Patient should consume within 12 hours of reconstitution.
● Give Zmax 1 hour before or 2 hours after a meal. Tablets and single-dose packets for oral suspension can be taken with or without food. Don't give with antacids.
● Reconstitute suspension packet with 2 ounces (60 mL) water. After taking, rinse glass with additional 2 ounces water and have patient drink it to ensure he has taken entire dose. Packets aren't for children.

I.V.
▼ Reconstitute drug in 500-mg vial with 4.8 mL of sterile water for injection to yield 100 mg/mL.
▼ Shake well until all drug is dissolved.
▼ Further dilute in 250- or 500-mL NSS solution, half-NSS, D$_5$W, or lactated Ringer solution to yield a final concentration of 1 or 2 mg/mL, respectively.
▼ Infuse a 500-mg dose of azithromycin I.V. over 1 hour or longer. Never give it as a bolus or I.M. injection.
▼ Reconstituted solution and diluted solution are stable for 24 hours when stored below 86° F (30° C). Diluted solution is stable for 7 days when refrigerated at 41° F (5° C).
▼ **Incompatibilities:** Amikacin sulfate, aztreonam, cefotaxime, ceftazidime, ceftriaxone sodium, cefuroxime, ciprofloxacin, clindamycin phosphate, famotidine, fentanyl citrate, furosemide, gentamicin sulfate, imipenem–cilastatin sodium, ketorolac tromethamine, levofloxacin, morphine sulfate, piperacillin–tazobactam sodium, potassium chloride, ticarcillin disodium–clavulanate potassium, tobramycin sulfate.

Ophthalmic
- Avoid contaminating applicator tip. Don't allow it to touch eye, fingers, or other surfaces.
- Invert closed bottle and shake once before each use. Remove cap with bottle still in the inverted position. Tilt head back, and with bottle inverted, gently squeeze bottle to instill 1 drop into affected eye(s).
- Store unopened bottle under refrigeration at 36° to 46° F (2° to 8° C). Once bottle has been opened, store at 36° to 77° F (2° to 25° C) for up to 14 days. Discard after 14 days.

ACTION

Binds to the 50S subunit of bacterial ribosomes, blocking protein synthesis; bacteriostatic or bactericidal, depending on concentration.

Route	Onset	Peak	Duration
P.O.	Unknown	2–5 hr	Unknown
I.V.	Unknown	Unknown	Unknown
Ophthalmic	Unknown	Unknown	Unknown

Half-life: About 3 days.

ADVERSE REACTIONS

CNS: fatigue, headache, somnolence, dizziness.
CV: chest pain, palpitations.
EENT: eye irritation (ophthalmic).
GI: abdominal pain, anorexia, diarrhea, nausea, vomiting, ***pseudomembranous colitis,*** dyspepsia, flatulence, melena.
GU: candidiasis, nephritis, vaginitis.
Hepatic: cholestatic jaundice.
Skin: photosensitivity reactions, rash, pain at injection site, pruritus.
Other: ***angioedema.***

INTERACTIONS

Drug-drug. *Antacids containing aluminum and magnesium:* May lower peak azithromycin level (immediate-release form). Separate doses by at least 2 hours.
Antiarrhythmics (amiodarone, quinidine): May increase risk of life-threatening arrhythmias, including torsades de pointes. Monitor ECG rhythm carefully.
Carbamazepine, phenytoin: May increase levels of these drugs. Monitor drug levels.

Cyclosporine: May elevate cyclosporine concentrations, with increased risk of nephrotoxicity and neurotoxicity. Monitor cyclosporine levels and renal function.
Digoxin: May increase digoxin level. Monitor digoxin level.
Drugs that prolong QT interval (fluoroquinolones, lithium, methadone, paliperidone, perflutren): May prolong QT interval. Use together with caution and monitor patient.
Ergotamine: May cause acute ergotamine toxicity. Monitor patient closely.
HMG-CoA reductase inhibitors (atorvastatin, lovastatin): May increase HMG-CoA reductase inhibitor levels, resulting in severe myopathy or rhabdomyolysis. Consider alternative therapy.
Nelfinavir: May increase azithromycin level. Monitor for liver enzyme abnormalities and hearing impairment.
Pimozide: May prolong QT interval and cause ventricular tachycardia. Concurrent use is contraindicated.
Theophylline: May increase theophylline level. Monitor theophylline level carefully.
Triazolam: May decrease triazolam clearance. Monitor patient closely.
Warfarin: May increase INR. Monitor INR carefully.
Drug-food. *Any food:* May decrease absorption of multidose oral suspension form. Advise patient to take drug on empty stomach.
Drug-lifestyle. *Sun exposure:* May cause photosensitivity reactions. Advise patient to avoid excessive sunlight exposure.

EFFECTS ON LAB TEST RESULTS
- May increase ALT, AST, creatinine, LDH, and bilirubin levels.

CONTRAINDICATIONS & CAUTIONS
- Contraindicated in patients hypersensitive to azithromycin, erythromycin, or other macrolide or ketolide antibiotics and in those with history of cholestatic jaundice or hepatic dysfunction from prior use of azithromycin.
- Don't use oral drug in patients with pneumonia or in those with moderate to severe illness or risk factors (such as cystic fibrosis, nosocomially acquired infections, known

or suspected bacteremia; hospitalized, elderly, or debilitated patients; or patients with immunodeficiency or functional asplenia).

• Use cautiously in patients with impaired hepatic function or myasthenia gravis.

⚠️ **Alert:** Use cautiously in patients at increased risk for torsades de pointes and fatal arrhythmias, including those with known prolonged QT interval, history of torsades de pointes, congenital long QT syndrome, bradyarrhythmias, uncompensated HF, uncorrected hypokalemia or hypomagnesemia, clinically significant bradycardia, or concomitant use of drugs known to prolong the QT interval or class IA (procainamide, quinidine) or class III (amiodarone, dofetilide, sotalol) antiarrhythmics.

⚠️ **Alert:** Elderly patients may be at increased risk for drug-associated QT-interval effects.

• Drug may cause CDAD ranging in severity from mild diarrhea to fatal colitis, which may occur over 2 months after administration. If CDAD is suspected or confirmed, drug may need to be discontinued and appropriate treatment begun.

• Prolonged use of ophthalmic solution may result in overgrowth of nonsusceptible organisms, including fungi. If superinfection occurs, discontinue drug and institute alternative therapy.

Dialyzable drug: Unknown.

PREGNANCY-LACTATION-REPRODUCTION
• There are no adequate and well-controlled studies in pregnant women. Use during pregnancy only if clearly needed.

• Drug appears in breast milk. Use cautiously in breast-feeding women.

NURSING CONSIDERATIONS
• Monitor patient for superinfection. Drug may cause overgrowth of nonsusceptible bacteria or fungi.

• If patient vomits within 60 minutes of taking Zmax, notify prescriber; additional or different therapy may be needed.

⚠️ **Alert:** Monitor patient for CDAD, which may range in severity from mild diarrhea to fatal colitis.

⚠️ **Alert:** Consider full risk profile when choosing appropriate antibiotic therapy. Alternative macrolide or fluoroquinolone class drugs also have the potential to cause

QT-interval prolongation and other significant adverse effects.

• Monitor patient for allergic and skin reactions. Discontinue drug if reaction occurs.

• Monitor patient for jaundice, hepatotoxicity, and hepatitis. Discontinue drug immediately if signs and symptoms (yellowing of skin or sclera, abdominal pain, nausea, vomiting, dark urine) occur.

⚠️ **Alert:** Exacerbation and new onset of myasthenia gravis have occurred with azithromycin use.

PATIENT TEACHING
• Tell patient to take drug as prescribed, even after he feels better.

• Advise patient to avoid excessive sunlight and to wear protective clothing and use sunscreen when outside.

• Tell patient to report adverse reactions promptly.

⚠️ **Alert:** Warn patient to seek immediate medical care for irregular heartbeat, shortness of breath, dizziness, or fainting.

• Advise patient not to stop taking drug without first contacting health care provider.

• Tell patient to take Zmax at least 1 hour before or 2 hours after a meal.

• Teach patient to reconstitute Zmax and to shake well before use.

• Tell patient that immediate-release tablets and suspension can be taken with or without food. Food may reduce GI upset.

• Instruct patient to thoroughly wash hands before instilling ophthalmic solution.

• Tell patient to avoid contaminating ophthalmic applicator tip and not to let tip touch eye, fingers, or other surfaces.

• Instruct patient how to instill ophthalmic solution.

• Advise patient to avoid contact lenses when diagnosed with bacterial conjunctivitis.

aztreonam
AZ-tree-oh-nam

Azactam, Cayston

Therapeutic class: Antibiotics
Pharmacologic class: Monobactams

AVAILABLE FORMS
Inhalation: 75-mg ampule
Injection: 1-g vials, 2-g vials

INDICATIONS & DOSAGES
➤ **UTI; septicemia; infections of lower respiratory tract, skin, and skin structures; intra-abdominal infections, surgical infections, and gynecologic infections caused by susceptible *Escherichia coli, Klebsiella pneumoniae, Proteus mirabilis, Pseudomonas aeruginosa, Enterobacter cloacae, Klebsiella oxytoca, Citrobacter* species, and *Serratia marcescens;* respiratory infections caused by *Haemophilus influenzae***
Adults: 500 mg to 2 g I.V. or I.M. every 8 to 12 hours. For severe systemic or life-threatening infections, 2 g every 6 to 8 hours. Maximum dose is 8 g daily.
Children ages 9 months and older: 30 mg/kg I.V. every 6 to 8 hours. Maximum dose is 120 mg/kg/day.
Adjust-a-dose: For adults with CrCl of 10 to 30 mL/minute, give 1 to 2 g; then give 50% of the usual dose at usual interval. If CrCl is less than 10 mL/minute, give 500 mg to 2 g; then give 25% of the usual dose at usual interval. For serious infections, add ⅛ of the initial dose to maintenance doses after each hemodialysis session.
➤ **To improve respiratory symptoms in cystic fibrosis patients with *P. aeruginosa* infection**
Adults and children age 7 and older: 75 mg inhalation t.i.d. for 28 days, followed by 28 days off.

ADMINISTRATION
Inhalational
● Give bronchodilator before administering aztreonam.
● Give short-acting bronchodilators 15 minutes to 4 hours before each dose or long-acting bronchodilators 30 minutes to 12 hours before each dose.
● Space doses at least 4 hours apart.
● Treatment order for patients on multiple therapies is bronchodilator, mucolytics, then aztreonam.
● Don't reconstitute until ready to give dose.
● Add one ampule of diluent to one amber glass vial of aztreonam. Replace rubber stopper on vial and gently swirl until contents have completely dissolved. Administer immediately.
● Don't use diluent or reconstituted drug if it's cloudy or if there are particles in the solution.
● Use only Altera Nebulizer System to administer drug.
● Never mix with other drugs in nebulizer.
● Administration usually takes 2 to 3 minutes.

I.V.
▼ Obtain specimen for culture and sensitivity tests before giving first dose. Begin therapy while awaiting results.
▼ For direct injection, reconstitute with 6 to 10 mL of sterile water for injection and immediately shake vial vigorously. Constituted solutions aren't for multiple-dose use. Discard unused solution.
▼ To give a bolus, inject drug over 3 to 5 minutes, directly into I.V. tubing.
▼ For infusion, reconstitute with a compatible I.V. solution to yield 20 mg/mL or less.
▼ Give infusions over 20 minutes to 1 hour.
▼ Give thawed solutions only by I.V. infusion.
▼ **Incompatibilities:** Acyclovir, amphotericin B, ampicillin sodium, azithromycin, chlorpromazine, daunorubicin, ganciclovir, lorazepam, metronidazole, mitomycin, mitoxantrone, nafcillin, prochlorperazine, streptozocin, vancomycin.

I.M.
● To prepare I.M. injection, add at least 3 mL of one of the following solutions per gram of aztreonam: sterile water for injection, bacteriostatic water for injection, NSS, or bacteriostatic NSS.
● Give I.M. injections deep into a large muscle, such as the upper outer quadrant of the gluteus maximus or the side of the thigh.
● Give doses larger than 1 g by I.V. route.

◑ Alert: Don't give I.M. injection to children.
● Pain and swelling may occur at injection site.

ACTION
Inhibits bacterial cell-wall synthesis, ultimately causing cell-wall destruction; bactericidal.

Route	Onset	Peak	Duration
I.V.	Unknown	Immediate	Unknown
I.M.	Unknown	<1 hr	Unknown
Inhalation	Unknown	1 hr	Unknown

Half-life: 1½ to 2 hours.

ADVERSE REACTIONS
CNS: *seizures,* confusion, headache, insomnia, pyrexia.
CV: hypotension, thrombophlebitis, chest discomfort.
EENT: nasal congestion, sore throat.
GI: *pseudomembranous colitis,* diarrhea, abdominal pain, nausea, vomiting.
Hematologic: *neutropenia, pancytopenia, thrombocytopenia,* anemia, leukocytosis, thrombocytosis.
Respiratory: bronchospasm, cough.
Skin: discomfort and swelling at I.M. injection site, rash, erythema multiforme.
Other: hypersensitivity reactions.

INTERACTIONS
Drug-drug. *Aminoglycosides:* May have synergistic nephrotoxic effects. Monitor renal function.
Cefoxitin, imipenem: May have antagonistic effect. Avoid using together.
Furosemide: May increase aztreonam level. Avoid using together.
Probenecid: May increase aztreonam level. Avoid using together.

EFFECTS ON LAB TEST RESULTS
● May increase ALT, AST, BUN, creatinine, and LDH levels. May decrease Hb level.
● May prolong PT and PTT, and increase INR.
● May decrease neutrophil and RBC counts. May increase or decrease platelet and WBC counts.
● May cause false-positive Coombs test result. May alter urine glucose determinations using cupric sulfate (Clinitest or Benedict reagent).

CONTRAINDICATIONS & CAUTIONS
● Contraindicated in patients hypersensitive to drug or its components and in those taking other beta-lactam antibiotics.
● Use cautiously in elderly patients and in those with impaired renal or hepatic function. Dosage adjustment may be needed. Monitor renal function test results.
● Drug may cause CDAD ranging in severity from mild diarrhea to fatal colitis occurring up to 2 months after administration. If CDAD is suspected or confirmed, drug may need to be discontinued and appropriate treatment begun.
● Rare cases of toxic epidermal necrolysis have been reported in patients undergoing bone marrow transplant with multiple risk factors, including sepsis, radiation therapy, and concomitantly administered drugs associated with toxic epidermal necrolysis.
Dialyzable drug: Yes.

PREGNANCY-LACTATION-REPRODUCTION
● There are no adequate and well-controlled studies in pregnant women. Use during pregnancy only if clearly needed.
● Drug appears in breast milk. Breast-feeding women should temporarily discontinue breast-feeding.

NURSING CONSIDERATIONS
● Observe patient for signs and symptoms of superinfection.
◑ Alert: Because drug is ineffective against gram-positive and anaerobic organisms, combine it with other antibiotics for immediate treatment of life-threatening illnesses.
◑ Alert: Patients allergic to penicillins or cephalosporins may not be allergic to this drug. Monitor closely those who have had an immediate hypersensitivity reaction to these antibiotics, especially to ceftazidime.
● Antibiotics may promote overgrowth of nonsusceptible organisms. Monitor patient for signs of superinfection.
● Dosage of Cayston isn't based on weight or adjusted for age.

PATIENT TEACHING

• Warn patient receiving I.M. drug that pain and swelling may occur at injection site.

• Tell patient to report discomfort at I.V. insertion site.

• Instruct patient to report adverse reactions and signs and symptoms of superinfection promptly.

• Instruct patient or caregiver in proper administration of drug by nebulizer.

• Teach patient or caregiver to use bronchodilator before using Cayston.

baclofen
BAK-loe-fen

Gablofen, Lioresal Intrathecal

Therapeutic class: Skeletal muscle relaxants
Pharmacologic class: Gamma-aminobutyric acid derivatives

AVAILABLE FORMS

Intrathecal injection: 50 mcg/mL, 500 mcg/mL, 1,000 mcg/mL, 2,000 mcg/mL
Tablets: 10 mg, 20 mg

INDICATIONS & DOSAGES

Adjust-a-dose (for all indications): For patients with impaired renal function, decrease oral and intrathecal doses.

➤ **Spasticity in MS; spinal cord injury**
Adults and children age 12 and older: Initially, 5 mg P.O. t.i.d. for 3 days; then 10 mg t.i.d. for 3 days, 15 mg t.i.d. for 3 days, 20 mg t.i.d. for 3 days. Increase daily dosage, based on response, to maximum of 80 mg (given as 20 mg q.i.d.).
Adjust-a-dose: For patients with psychiatric or brain disorders and for elderly patients, increase dose gradually.

➤ **To manage severe spasticity in patients who don't respond to or can't tolerate oral baclofen therapy**
Adults: For screening phase, after test dose to check responsiveness, give drug via implantable infusion pump. Give test dose of 1 mL of 50-mcg/mL dilution into intrathecal space by barbotage over 1 minute or longer. Significantly decreased severity or frequency of muscle spasm or reduced muscle tone should appear within 4 to 8 hours. If response is inadequate, give second test dose of 75 mcg/1.5 mL 24 hours after the first. If response is still inadequate, give final test dose of 100 mcg/2 mL after 24 hours. Patients unresponsive to the 100-mcg dose shouldn't be considered candidates for implantable pump.
Children: Initial test dose is the same as that for adults (50 mcg); for very small children, initial dose is 25 mcg.
For maintenance therapy: Adjust first dose based on screening dose that elicited an adequate response. Double this effective dose and give over 24 hours. However, if screening dose effectiveness was maintained for 8 hours or longer, don't double dose. After first 24 hours, increase dose slowly as needed and tolerated by 10% to 30% increments at 24-hour intervals in spasticity of spinal cord origin. In children with spasticity of spinal cord origin and adults and children with spasticity of cerebral origin, increase by 5% to 15% increments at 24-hour intervals. During prolonged maintenance therapy, increase daily dose by 10% to 40% in spasticity of spinal cord origin, or increase daily dose by 5% to 15% in spasticity of cerebral origin, if needed; if patient experiences adverse effects, decrease dose by 10% to 20%. Maintenance dosages range from 12 to 2,003 mcg daily, but experience with dosages of more than 1,000 mcg daily is limited. Most patients need 300 to 800 mcg daily.

ADMINISTRATION
P.O.

• Give drug with meals or milk to prevent GI distress.
Intrathecal
Black Box Warning Don't discontinue abruptly. This can result in high fever, altered mental status, exaggerated rebound spasticity, and muscle rigidity, which in rare cases, has led to rhabdomyolysis, multiple organ-system failure, and death. ■

• Don't give intrathecal injection by I.V., I.M., subcutaneous, or epidural route.
• If patient suddenly requires a large intrathecal dose increase, check for a catheter complication, such as kinking or dislodgment.

Reactions in bold italics are *life-threatening*. Interactions may have a *rapid onset* or a *delayed onset*.

• With long-term intrathecal use, about 5% of patients may develop tolerance to drug. In some cases, this may be treated by hospitalizing patient and slowly withdrawing drug over a 2- to 4-week period. After the "drug holiday," drug may be restarted at the initial continuous infusion dose.

ACTION

Hyperpolarizes fibers to reduce impulse transmission. Appears to reduce transmission of impulses from the spinal cord to skeletal muscle, thus decreasing the frequency and amplitude of muscle spasms in patients with spinal cord lesions.

Route	Onset	Peak	Duration
P.O.	Unknown	2–3 hr	Unknown
Intrathecal	30 min–1 hr	4 hr	4–8 hr

Half-life: 2½ to 4 hours.

ADVERSE REACTIONS

CNS: agitation, drowsiness, dizziness, headache, weakness, fatigue, hypotonia, confusion, insomnia, *seizures with intrathecal use,* paresthesia, asthenia, pain, speech disorder, depression.
CV: hypotension, peripheral edema.
EENT: nasal congestion.
GI: nausea, constipation, dry mouth.
GU: urinary frequency, urine retention, erectile dysfunction, incontinence.
Metabolic: hyperglycemia, weight gain.
Musculoskeletal: muscle rigidity or spasticity, muscle weakness.
Respiratory: dyspnea, pneumonia.
Skin: rash, pruritus, urticaria, excessive sweating.
Other: chills, accidental injury.

INTERACTIONS

Drug-drug. *CNS depressants:* May increase CNS depression. Avoid using together.
Drug-lifestyle. *Alcohol use:* May increase CNS depression. Discourage use together.

EFFECTS ON LAB TEST RESULTS

• May increase alkaline phosphatase, AST, CK, and glucose levels.
• May increase leukocyte count.

CONTRAINDICATIONS & CAUTIONS

• Contraindicated in patients hypersensitive to drug.
• Use cautiously in patients with impaired renal function, respiratory disease, or seizure disorder or when spasticity is used to maintain motor function.
• Use cautiously in patients with psychotic disorders, schizophrenia, or confusional states. Exacerbations of these conditions have occurred.
Dialyzable drug: Unknown.
⚠ *Overdose S&S:* Coma, dizziness, lightheadedness, diminished reflexes, vomiting, hypotonia, increased salivation, drowsiness, vision changes, respiratory depression, seizures.

PREGNANCY-LACTATION-REPRODUCTION

• Use in pregnant women only when potential benefits justify possible risks to the fetus.
• Oral drug appears in breast milk. It isn't known if drug appears in breast milk after intrathecal administration. Patient should avoid breast-feeding during therapy.

NURSING CONSIDERATIONS

🔔 *Alert:* Don't use oral drug to treat muscle spasm caused by rheumatic disorders, cerebral palsy, Parkinson disease, or stroke because drug's effectiveness for these indications hasn't been established.
🔔 *Alert:* Life-threatening CNS depression, CV collapse, and respiratory failure may occur with intrathecal use. Have trained staff and resuscitation equipment available during screening, dosage titration, and pump refill.
• Watch for sensitivity reactions, such as fever, skin eruptions, and respiratory distress.
• Expect an increased risk of seizures in patients with seizure disorder.
• The amount of relief determines whether dosage (and drowsiness) can be reduced.
• Some degree of muscle tone and spasticity may be necessary to sustain upright posture and balance with movement or to obtain optimal function, help support circulatory function, and prevent formation of DVT.
• When switching to intrathecal baclofen, attempt to discontinue concomitant oral

antispasmodics to avoid overdose or increased adverse effects. Reduce oral antispasmodic dosage slowly while monitoring patient closely.

Black Box Warning Don't withdraw intrathecal drug abruptly after long-term use unless severe adverse reactions demand it; doing so may precipitate seizures, high fever, hallucinations, or rebound spasticity. ∎

● *Look alike–sound alike:* Don't confuse baclofen with Bactroban.

PATIENT TEACHING

Black Box Warning Advise patient and caregivers, especially patients with spinal cord injuries at T6 or above, communication difficulties, or history of withdrawal symptoms from oral or intrathecal baclofen, of risks associated with abrupt discontinuation of intrathecal form. Tell them to keep scheduled refill visits and teach them the signs and symptoms of baclofen withdrawal. ∎

● Instruct patient to take oral form with meals or milk.

● Tell patient to avoid activities that require alertness until CNS effects of drug are known. Drowsiness usually is transient.

● Tell patient to avoid alcohol and OTC antihistamines while taking drug.

● Advise patient to follow prescriber's orders regarding rest and physical therapy.

● Teach patient and caregivers about the signs and symptoms of overdose and what to do if an overdose occurs.

● Teach patient and caregivers proper home care of pump and insertion site.

beclomethasone dipropionate (inhalation)
be-kloe-METH-a-sone

QVAR 40, QVAR 80

Therapeutic class: Antiasthmatics
Pharmacologic class: Corticosteroids

AVAILABLE FORMS

Oral inhalation aerosol: 40 mcg/metered spray, 80 mcg/metered spray

INDICATIONS & DOSAGES
➤ **Chronic asthma**

Adults and children age 12 and older: Starting dose, 40 to 80 mcg b.i.d. when patient previously used bronchodilators alone, or 40 to 160 mcg b.i.d. when patient previously used inhaled corticosteroids. Maximum, 320 mcg b.i.d.

Children ages 5 to 11: 40 mcg b.i.d., up to 80 mcg b.i.d.

ADMINISTRATION
Inhalational

● Prime the inhaler before first use or if it hasn't been used for more than 10 days by depressing canister twice into the air.

● Allow 1 minute to elapse between inhalations.

● Have patient rinse mouth and throat and spit after use.

ACTION

May decrease inflammation by decreasing the number and activity of inflammatory cells, inhibiting bronchoconstrictor mechanisms, producing direct smooth-muscle relaxation, and decreasing airway hyperresponsiveness.

Route	Onset	Peak	Duration
Inhalation	1–4 wk	½ hr	Unknown

Half-life: 2.8 hours.

ADVERSE REACTIONS

CNS: headache.
EENT: hoarseness, throat irritation, fungal infection of throat, pharyngitis, rhinitis, sinusitis.
GI: fungal infection of mouth, dry mouth.
Musculoskeletal: back pain.
Respiratory: cough, URI, exacerbation of asthma, wheezing.
Other: *angioedema,* facial edema, hypersensitivity reactions, *adrenal insufficiency,* suppression of HPA function.

INTERACTIONS
None significant.

EFFECTS ON LAB TEST RESULTS
None reported.

Reactions in bold italics are *life-threatening*. Interactions may have a *rapid onset* or a *delayed onset*.

CONTRAINDICATIONS & CAUTIONS
● Contraindicated in patients hypersensitive to drug or its ingredients and in those with status asthmaticus, nonasthmatic bronchial diseases, or asthma controlled by bronchodilators or other noncorticosteroids alone.
● Use cautiously, if at all, in patients with TB, fungal or bacterial infections, ocular HSV, or systemic viral infections.
● Use cautiously in patients receiving systemic corticosteroid therapy.
Dialyzable drug: No.

PREGNANCY-LACTATION-REPRODUCTION
● Use during pregnancy only when potential benefits justify possible risks to the fetus. After delivery, evaluate neonates for adrenal suppression if mother received substantial doses during pregnancy.
● Serious adverse reactions may occur in breast-feeding infants. A decision should be made to discontinue breast-feeding or discontinue drug, taking into account importance of drug to the mother.

NURSING CONSIDERATIONS
● Check mucous membranes frequently for signs and symptoms of fungal infection.
● During times of stress (trauma, surgery, or infection), systemic corticosteroids may be needed to prevent adrenal insufficiency in previously corticosteroid-dependent patients.
● Periodic measurement of growth and development may be needed during high-dose or prolonged therapy in children. Cataracts can occur. Closely monitor patients for vision changes.
● **Alert:** Taper oral corticosteroid therapy slowly. Acute adrenal insufficiency and death may occur in patients with asthma who change abruptly from oral corticosteroids to beclomethasone.
● **Alert:** Bronchospasm may occur after dosing and should be treated immediately with a short-acting inhaled bronchodilator.

PATIENT TEACHING
● Tell patient to prime inhaler before first use, or after 10 days of not using it, by depressing canister twice into the air.

● Inform patient that drug doesn't relieve acute asthma attacks.
● Tell patient who needs a bronchodilator to use it several minutes before beclomethasone.
● Instruct patient to carry or wear medical identification indicating his need for supplemental systemic corticosteroids during stress.
● Advise patient to allow 1 minute to elapse between inhalations of drug and to hold his breath for a few seconds to enhance drug action.
● Tell patient it may take up to 4 weeks to feel the full benefit of the drug.
● Tell patient to keep inhaler clean by wiping it weekly with a dry tissue or cloth; don't get it wet.
● Advise patient to prevent oral fungal infections by gargling or rinsing his mouth with water after each use. Caution him not to swallow the water.
● Tell patient to report evidence of corticosteroid withdrawal, including fatigue, weakness, arthralgia, orthostatic hypotension, and dyspnea.
● Instruct patient to store drug at 77° F (25° C). Advise patient to ensure delivery of proper dose by gently warming canister to room temperature before using.

beclomethasone dipropionate (intranasal)
be-kloe-METH-a-sone

Beconase AQ, Qnasl, Rivanase AQ✦

Therapeutic class: Corticosteroids
Pharmacologic class: Corticosteroids

AVAILABLE FORMS
Nasal aerosol solution: 40 mcg/actuation, 80 mcg/actuation
Nasal spray: 42 mcg/metered spray, 50 mcg/metered spray✦

INDICATIONS & DOSAGES
➤ **To relieve symptoms of seasonal or perennial rhinitis and nonallergic (vasomotor) rhinitis; to prevent nasal**

polyp recurrence after surgical removal (Beconase AQ)

Adults and children age 12 and older:
2 sprays (160 mcg total) QNasl in each nostril once daily. Or, 1 or 2 sprays (42 to 84 mcg Beconase AQ or 50 to 100 mcg Rivanase AQ) in each nostril b.i.d.

Children ages 6 to 12: Initially, 1 spray (42 mcg) in each nostril b.i.d. May increase to 2 sprays in each nostril b.i.d. Once adequate control is achieved, decrease to 1 spray in each nostril b.i.d. (Beconase AQ).

➤ **To relieve symptoms of seasonal or perennial rhinitis (Qnasl)**

Adults and children age 12 and older:
320 mcg/day administered as 2 nasal aerosol sprays in each nostril once daily.

Children ages 4 to 11: 1 spray (40 mcg) in each nostril once daily.

ADMINISTRATION
Intranasal

● Pump nasal spray six times or until a fine mist is produced before first use; repeat priming if nasal spray hasn't been used for 7 days (Beconase AQ). For Qnasl, prime four times before first use and two times if not used for 7 days or more.

● Shake before use.

ACTION

May reduce nasal inflammation by inhibiting mediators of inflammation.

Route	Onset	Peak	Duration
Intranasal	5–7 days	3 wk	Unknown

Half-life: About 4½ hours (major active metabolite).

ADVERSE REACTIONS

CNS: headache, light-headedness.
EENT: mild, transient nasal burning and stinging; dryness, epistaxis, nasal congestion, nasopharyngeal fungal infections, rhinorrhea, sneezing, watery eyes.
GI: nausea.
Metabolic: growth velocity reduction in children and adolescents.
Skin: rash, urticaria.

INTERACTIONS

None significant.

EFFECTS ON LAB TEST RESULTS
None reported.

CONTRAINDICATIONS & CAUTIONS

● Contraindicated in patients hypersensitive to drug and in those with untreated localized infection involving the nasal mucosa.
● Not recommended for children younger than age 6.
● Use cautiously, if at all, in patients with active or quiescent respiratory tract tuberculous infections or untreated fungal, bacterial, or systemic viral or ocular HSV infections.
● Use cautiously in patients who have recently had nasal septal ulcers, nasal surgery, or trauma until wound healing occurs.
Dialyzable drug: No.
⚠ *Overdose S&S:* Hypercorticism, adrenal suppression.

PREGNANCY-LACTATION-REPRODUCTION

● Use during pregnancy only when potential benefits justify possible risks to the fetus.
● It isn't known if drug appears in breast milk. Use cautiously in breast-feeding women.

NURSING CONSIDERATIONS

● Observe patient for fungal infections.
● Drug isn't effective for acute exacerbations of rhinitis. Decongestants or antihistamines may be needed.
● Stop drug if no significant symptom improvement occurs after 3 weeks.
● Monitor growth routinely in pediatric patients; reduction in growth rate may occur.
● Watch for hypercorticism and adrenal suppression with very high doses, or with standard doses in susceptible patients. If signs and symptoms occur, taper and discontinue drug.

PATIENT TEACHING

● Advise patient or parent to read package insert for instructions on drug use.
● Advise patient to pump nasal spray four to six times (based on individual product) until a fine mist is produced before first use. If nasal spray pump hasn't been used for 7 or more days in a row, it should be reprimed.
● To instill, instruct patient to blow nose to clear nasal passages, shake container, tilt

---

Reactions in bold italics are *life-threatening*. Interactions may have a *rapid onset* or a *delayed onset*.

B

head slightly forward, and insert nozzle into nostril, pointing away from septum. Tell him to hold other nostril closed and inhale gently while spraying, hold breath for a few seconds, and exhale through the mouth. Next, have him shake container and repeat in other nostril.

• Tell patient to clean the cap and nosepiece of the activator in warm water every day, and then allow them to air-dry.

• Advise patient to use drug regularly, as prescribed, because its effectiveness depends on regular use.

• Explain that unlike decongestants, drug doesn't work right away. Most patients notice improvement within a few days, but some may need 2 to 3 weeks.

• Warn patient not to exceed recommended dosage because of risk of HPA axis suppression.

• Tell patient to notify prescriber if signs and symptoms don't improve within 3 weeks or if nasal irritation persists.

• Teach patient good nasal and oral hygiene.

bedaquiline fumarate
bed-AK-wi-leen

Sirturo

Therapeutic class: Antituberculotics
Pharmacologic class: Diarylquinolines

AVAILABLE FORMS
Tablets ⊙*:* 100 mg

INDICATIONS & DOSAGES
Black Box Warning Drug should be reserved for use when an effective treatment regimen can't otherwise be provided. ■
➤ **Pulmonary multidrug-resistant TB as part of combination therapy**
Adults: Weeks 1 and 2, 400 mg P.O. once daily. Weeks 3 to 24, 200 mg P.O. three times a week (48 hours between doses) for a total of 600 mg/week.
Adjust-a-dose: In first 2 weeks, if a dose is missed, don't make it up but continue the dosing schedule. From 3 weeks on, if a dose is missed, have patient take dose as soon as possible, then resume the three-times-a-week schedule.

ADMINISTRATION
P.O.
• Administer by directly observed therapy (DOT).
• Give with food.
• Give tablets whole with water. Don't crush, split, or allow patient to chew tablets.
• Allow a minimum of 48 hours between doses after initial 2 weeks of therapy.
• Store tablets at room temperature in a light-resistant container with an expiration of not more than 3 months if transferred from the original container.

ACTION
Inhibits mycobacterial adenosine 5-triphosphate synthase, an enzyme essential for the generation of energy in *Mycobacterium tuberculosis.*

Route	Onset	Peak	Duration
P.O.	Unknown	5 hr	Unknown

Half-life: 5½ months.

ADVERSE REACTIONS
CNS: headache.
CV: chest pain, *QTc-interval prolongation.*
GI: nausea, anorexia.
Musculoskeletal: arthralgia.
Respiratory: hemoptysis.
Skin: rash.

INTERACTIONS
Drug-drug. **Black Box Warning** *Drugs that prolong QT interval (antiarrhythmics, clofazimine, dolasetron, fluoroquinolones, macrolides, mefloquine, pentamidine):* May increase risk of prolonged QT interval. Monitor ECG frequently. ■
Lopinavir–ritonavir: May increase bedaquiline level and risk of adverse reactions. Use together only if benefits outweigh risk.
Strong CYP3A4 inducers (rifabutin, rifampin, rifapentine): May decrease bedaquiline level. Avoid use together.
Strong CYP3A4 inhibitors (ketoconazole): May increase bedaquiline level. Avoid concomitant use for more than 14 consecutive days. Monitor patient for adverse reactions.
Drug-herb. *St. John's wort:* May decrease bedaquiline level. Avoid concurrent use.
Drug-lifestyle. *Alcohol use:* May increase risk of liver injury. Discourage use together.

✚Canada   ◇OTC   ◆ Off-label use   𝒫 Photoguide   ⊙ Do not crush   *Liquid contains alcohol.

EFFECTS ON LAB TEST RESULTS
• May increase transaminase and amylase levels.

CONTRAINDICATIONS & CAUTIONS
Black Box Warning Drug's use increased risk of death compared to placebo. Only use when an effective treatment regimen can't otherwise be provided. ∎

Black Box Warning QT-interval prolongation can occur. Use of bedaquiline with drugs that prolong QT interval may cause additive QT-interval prolongation. ∎

• Contraindicated in patients hypersensitive to drug or its components.

• Don't use drug for latent, extrapulmonary, or drug-sensitive TB.

• Use cautiously in patients with severe renal impairment, history of torsades de pointes, congenital long QT syndrome, hypothyroidism, bradyarrhythmia, uncompensated HF, hypocalcemia, hypomagnesemia, or hypokalemia.

• Use in severe hepatic dysfunction hasn't been studied. Avoid use.

Dialyzable drug: No.

PREGNANCY-LACTATION-REPRODUCTION
• Use in pregnant women hasn't been studied. Use only if clearly needed and if benefits outweigh risk.

• It isn't known if drug appears in breast milk. Patient should discontinue breastfeeding or discontinue drug.

NURSING CONSIDERATIONS
• There is a risk of treatment failure if patient is noncompliant. Drug must be given by DOT.

• Monitor LFTs at baseline and monthly as needed. Repeat within 48 hours if elevation of more than 3 × ULN occurs. Test for viral hepatitis and discontinue all hepatotoxic drugs.

• Discontinue drug if transaminase levels are elevated and are accompanied by total bilirubin level greater than 2 × ULN, or aminotransferase levels are more than 8 × ULN, or aminotransferase elevations are greater than 5 × ULN and remain elevated for more than 2 weeks.

• Monitor patient for hepatic dysfunction (fatigue, anorexia, nausea, jaundice, dark urine, liver tenderness, hepatomegaly).

• Monitor ECG before therapy and at 2, 12, and 24 weeks after start of therapy.

Black Box Warning Discontinue drug if clinically significant ventricular arrhythmia occurs or QTc interval is more than 500 msec. ∎

• Assess ECG for QT-interval prolongation with syncopal episode.

• Monitor potassium, calcium, and magnesium levels before therapy and correct if abnormal. Assess electrolyte levels if QT-interval prolongation is detected.

PATIENT TEACHING
• Inform patient that drug will be given as part of DOT.

• Advise patient to take drug with food, to swallow tablet whole, and not to dissolve, crush, or chew it.

• Caution patient to take bedaquiline with other medications prescribed for TB.

• Advise patient not to miss doses and to complete full course of therapy for treatment to be effective and to decrease risk of untreatable TB.

• Instruct patient to keep all follow-up appointments to monitor for drug's side effects.

• Warn patient to avoid alcohol and hepatotoxic drugs or herbal supplements while taking bedaquiline, to decrease risk of liver complications.

• Advise patient to consult practitioner if there is a personal or family history of congenital QT-interval prolongation or HF.

belimumab
beh-LIH-moo-mab

Benlysta

Therapeutic class: Immunosuppressants
Pharmacologic class: Human monoclonal antibodies

AVAILABLE FORMS
Injection: 120-mg, 400-mg single-use vials

INDICATIONS & DOSAGES

➤ **Active, autoantibody-positive systemic lupus erythematosus**

Adults: 10 mg/kg I.V. infusion every 2 weeks for first three doses, then every 4 weeks thereafter.

ADMINISTRATION

I.V.

▼ Consider premedicating with an antihistamine and antipyretic for prophylaxis against infusion or hypersensitivity reactions.

▼ Store unopened vials in refrigerator.

▼ Once vial has been at room temperature for 10 to 15 minutes, reconstitute with sterile water: 1.5 mL for 120-mg vial and 4.8 mL for 400-mg vial.

▼ Direct stream of sterile water toward side of vial to minimize foaming. Gently swirl for 60 seconds every 5 minutes until dissolved. Don't shake. Protect solution from light while dissolving. Usual reconstitution time is 10 to 15 minutes but may take up to 30 minutes.

▼ Solution should be opalescent and colorless to pale yellow.

▼ Dilute in 250 mL NSS only.

▼ From the 250-mL NSS bag, withdraw a volume of NSS equal to the amount of medication to be added so total volume remains at 250 mL. Add the medication to the 250-mL NSS bag and discard any unused drug solution.

▼ Protect unused reconstituted solution from light and store in refrigerator. Solutions in NSS may be stored in refrigerator or at room temperature.

▼ Administer as an I.V. infusion over 1 hour. Don't give as an I.V. push or bolus.

▼ Complete infusion within 8 hours of reconstitution.

▼ **Incompatibilities:** Dextrose solution, other I.V. drugs.

ACTION

Inhibits survival of B cells, including autoreactive B cells, and reduces their differentiation into immunoglobulin-producing plasma cells.

Route	Onset	Peak	Duration
I.V.	Unknown	Unknown	Unknown

Half-life: 19.4 days.

ADVERSE REACTIONS

CNS: anxiety, headache, insomnia, migraine, depression, fever.
EENT: nasopharyngitis, pharyngitis, sinusitis.
GI: nausea, diarrhea, viral gastroenteritis.
GU: cystitis, UTI.
Hematologic: *leukopenia.*
Musculoskeletal: extremity pain.
Respiratory: bronchitis, URI.
Other: infection, antibody detection, hypersensitivity reactions, infusion reactions.

INTERACTIONS

Drug-drug. *I.V. cyclophosphamide, other biological agents:* Use together hasn't been studied. Don't use together.
Live-virus vaccines: May impair response to vaccines. Don't give live-virus vaccines for 30 days before or concurrently with belimumab.
Drug-herb. *Echinacea:* May decrease drug's therapeutic effects. Consider therapy modification.

EFFECTS ON LAB TEST RESULTS

● May decrease leukocyte count.

CONTRAINDICATIONS & CAUTIONS

● Contraindicated in patients with a history of anaphylaxis to belimumab.

● Use cautiously in patients with a history of chronic infection, hypersensitivity reactions, infusion reactions, depression, or malignancies.

● Use cautiously in black patients because response rate may be lower.

● More deaths occurred with belimumab than with placebo during the controlled period of the main clinical trials. No single cause of death predominated, but possible causes included infection, CV disease, and suicide.

● Safety and effectiveness in children haven't been established.
Dialyzable drug: Unknown.

PREGNANCY-LACTATION-REPRODUCTION

- There are no adequate well-controlled studies in pregnant women. Use cautiously during pregnancy and only if potential benefit outweighs risk to the fetus. Pregnant women should enroll in a pregnancy registry that monitors maternal-fetal outcomes of exposure to belimumab by calling 1-877-681-6296.
- Women of childbearing potential should use adequate contraception during treatment and for at least 4 months after final dose.
- It isn't known if drug appears in breast milk. A decision should be made to discontinue breast-feeding or discontinue drug, taking into account importance of drug to the mother.

NURSING CONSIDERATIONS

- Patient shouldn't receive live-virus vaccines for 30 days before or concurrently with drug.
- Premedication is recommended to avoid or minimize allergic reactions.
- Drug should be administered only by a health care professional prepared to manage anaphylaxis.
- Watch for hypersensitivity reactions, even in patients who previously tolerated infusions.
- Monitor patient for infection. Serious and sometimes fatal infections have occurred in patients receiving immunosuppressants.
- Monitor patient for depression, suicidal ideation, malignancies, allergic reactions, and infusion reactions.
- Assess patients with new-onset or deteriorating neurologic signs and symptoms for JC virus–associated progressive multifocal leukoencephalopathy (PML). If PML is confirmed, therapy may have to be discontinued.

PATIENT TEACHING

- Inform patient that drug will be given in the doctor's office or hospital.
- Warn patient not to skip appointments to ensure drug is given on schedule to improve effectiveness of treatment.
- Tell patient to immediately report signs and symptoms of an allergic reaction (such as itching, hives, shortness of breath, swelling of the face, and throat closure).

- Teach patient infection-prevention measures.
- Instruct patient to immediately report signs and symptoms of infection (such as fever, body aches, cough, and sore throat).
- Tell patient to report history of cancer to health care provider.
- Instruct patient not to receive live-virus vaccines while taking drug.
- Counsel female patient of childbearing potential to use adequate contraception during treatment and for at least 4 months after final dose.
- Advise female patient to tell health care provider if she is pregnant or breast-feeding.

SAFETY ALERT!

belinostat
be-LIN-oh-stat

Beleodaq

Therapeutic class: Antineoplastics
Pharmacologic class: Histone deacetylase inhibitors

AVAILABLE FORMS
Injection: 500-mg single-use vial

INDICATIONS & DOSAGES
➤ **Relapsed or refractory peripheral T-cell lymphoma**
Adults: 1,000 mg/m^2 I.V. once daily on days 1 through 5 of a 21-day cycle over 30 minutes. Repeat cycles until disease progression or unacceptable toxicity occurs.
Adjust-a-dose: Before start of each cycle, and before resuming therapy after toxicity, ANC should be 1×10^9/L or higher and platelet count should be 50×10^9/L or higher. Nonhematologic adverse reactions must be grade 2 or less before retreatment.

For nadir ANC less than 0.5×10^9/L (with any platelet count), decrease dosage by 25% (to 750 mg/m^2). For platelet count less than 25×10^9/L (with any nadir ANC), decrease dosage by 25% (to 750 mg/m^2). For any grade 3 or 4 nonhematologic adverse reaction (except nausea, vomiting, or diarrhea), decrease dosage by 25% (to 750 mg/m^2). For grade 3 or 4 nausea, vomiting, or diarrhea, adjust dosage only if the duration is greater than 7 days with supportive therapy. For recurrent ANC nadirs less than 0.5×10^9/L or recurrent platelet count nadirs less than 25×10^9/L after two dosage reductions, discontinue drug. For recurrence of grade 3 or 4 non-hematologic adverse reactions after two dosage reductions, discontinue drug.

For patients homozygous for the UGT1A1*28 allele, reduce starting dose to 750 mg/m². (This may affect 20% of the black population, 10% of the white population, and 2% of the Asian population.)

For obese patients, use patient's actual body weight for calculating BSA or weight-based dosing.

ADMINISTRATION

I.V.

▼ Store vial at room temperature. Retain in original package until use.

▼ Follow safe handling and disposal procedures for cytotoxic drugs.

▼ Reconstitute each vial with 9 mL sterile water for injection to yield a concentration of 50 mg/mL. Swirl vial until there are no visible particles.

▼ May store reconstituted vial for up to 12 hours at ambient temperature (59° to 77° F [15° to 25° C]).

▼ Withdraw volume needed for required dose and transfer to infusion bag containing 250 mL NSS injection. The infusion bag with drug solution may be stored at ambient room temperature for up to 36 hours, including infusion time.

▼ Inspect solution for particulate matter. Don't use if solution is cloudy or contains particulates.

▼ Infuse drug over 30 minutes using 0.22-micron in-line filter. Infusion time may be extended to 45 minutes if infusion-site pain or other symptoms associated with the infusion occur.

▼ **Incompatibilities:** None known.

ACTION

Induces cell-cycle arrest or apoptosis of some transformed cells. Shows preferential cytotoxicity toward tumor cells compared to normal cells.

Route	Onset	Peak	Duration
I.V.	Rapid	Unknown	Unknown

Half-life: 1.1 hours.

ADVERSE REACTIONS

CNS: fatigue, pyrexia, chills, headache, dizziness.
CV: peripheral edema, *prolonged QT interval,* hypotension, phlebitis.
GI: nausea, vomiting, constipation, diarrhea, decreased appetite, abdominal pain.
GU: increased creatinine level.
Hematologic: anemia, *thrombocytopenia, leukopenia.*
Hepatic: *hepatic impairment,* increased blood LDH level.
Metabolic: *hypokalemia.*
Respiratory: dyspnea, cough, *pneumonia.*
Skin: rash, pruritus, injection-site pain.
Other: infection, *sepsis, multiorgan failure.*

INTERACTIONS

Drug-drug. *Strong inhibitors of UGT1A1 allele (atazanavir, indinavir):* May increase belinostat blood level. Monitor patient closely. Avoid use together if possible.

EFFECTS ON LAB TEST RESULTS

• May increase creatinine and blood LDH levels. May decrease potassium level.
• May decrease RBC, platelet, neutrophil, and lymphocyte counts.

CONTRAINDICATIONS & CAUTIONS

• Contraindicated in patients hypersensitive to drug or its components.
• Serious, sometimes fatal infections, including pneumonia and sepsis, can occur. Avoid giving to patients with an active infection. Those with history of extensive or intensive chemotherapy may be at increased risk for life-threatening infection.
• May cause hepatotoxicity, which may be fatal. Not recommended in patients with moderate to severe hepatic impairment or CrCl of 39 mL/minute or less; drug hasn't been studied in these populations.
• May cause tumor lysis syndrome, especially in patients with advanced disease or high tumor burden. Monitor patient closely;

if tumor lysis syndrome occurs, begin appropriate treatment.
● Use cautiously in patients with renal insufficiency.
● Safety and effectiveness in children haven't been established.
Dialyzable drug: Unknown.

PREGNANCY-LACTATION-REPRODUCTION
● Avoid use in pregnant women because of potential for teratogenicity or embryo-fetal death.
● May impair male fertility.
● Breast-feeding patients should discontinue breast-feeding or discontinue drug.

NURSING CONSIDERATIONS
● Monitor CBC at baseline and weekly, and adjust dosage as necessary.
● Monitor patients for infection.
● Before first dose of each cycle, obtain serum chemistry tests, including renal and hepatic function. Adjust dosage or interrupt or discontinue therapy as necessary.
● Monitor patients for signs and symptoms of tumor lysis syndrome (lethargy, arrhythmia, edema, renal failure, metabolic acidosis, hyperkalemia, hyperuricemia, hypocalcemia). Report signs or symptoms immediately.
● Monitor patient for nausea, diarrhea, and vomiting. Treat symptomatically.
● *Look alike–sound alike:* Don't confuse belinostat with beractant.

PATIENT TEACHING
● Advise patient to immediately report GI signs or symptoms, such as diarrhea, vomiting, or nausea.
● Explain importance of obtaining laboratory studies as instructed.
● Tell patient to report signs and symptoms of hepatic injury (yellowing of skin or eyes, dark urine, itching, pain in right upper quadrant of abdomen).
● Caution patient to report signs and symptoms of infection (fever, flulike symptoms, cough, shortness of breath, burning on urination, muscle aches, worsening of skin problems).
● Instruct patient to report unusual bleeding or bruising, weakness, tiredness, pallor, dyspnea, or infection.

● Teach patient to immediately report signs and symptoms of tumor lysis syndrome (lethargy, confusion, fatigue, rapid irregular heartbeat, rapid breathing, edema, low urine output, dark urine, nausea, tingling of arms or legs, aching joints, muscle weakness).
● Warn patient to avoid becoming pregnant and not to use drug while breast-feeding. Inform patient of potential hazard to fetus.
● Warn male patient taking belinostat that drug may impair fertility.

benazepril hydrochloride
ben-A-za-pril

Lotensin⬧

Therapeutic class: Antihypertensives
Pharmacologic class: ACE inhibitors

AVAILABLE FORMS
Tablets: 5 mg, 10 mg, 20 mg, 40 mg

INDICATIONS & DOSAGES
Adjust-a-dose (for all indications): If CrCl is below 30 mL/minute/1.73m^2 or serum creatinine level is greater than 3 mg/dL, give 5 mg P.O. daily. Daily dose may be adjusted up to 40 mg.
➤ **Hypertension**
Adults: For patients not receiving a diuretic, 10 mg P.O. daily initially. Adjust dosage as needed and tolerated; usually 20 to 40 mg daily in one or two divided doses. For patients receiving a diuretic, 5 mg P.O. daily initially.
Children age 6 and older: 0.2 mg/kg (between 0.1 and 0.6 mg/kg) P.O. daily. Adjust as needed up to 0.6 mg/kg (maximum 40 mg) P.O. daily.
➤ **Nephropathy (nondiabetic)** ◆
Adults: 10 to 20 mg P.O. daily.

ADMINISTRATION
P.O.
● Protect tablets from moisture.

ACTION
Inhibits ACE, preventing conversion of angiotensin I to angiotensin II, a potent vasoconstrictor. Less angiotensin II decreases peripheral arterial resistance, decreasing

aldosterone secretion, which reduces sodium and water retention and lowers BP. Drug also acts as antihypertensive in patients with low-renin hypertension.

Route	Onset	Peak	Duration
P.O.	1 hr	1–2 hr	24 hr

Half-life: 10 to 11 hours.

ADVERSE REACTIONS
CNS: headache, dizziness, somnolence.
CV: symptomatic hypotension.

INTERACTIONS
Drug-drug. *Aliskiren:* May increase risk of renal impairment, hypotension, and hyperkalemia in diabetic patients and those with moderate to severe renal impairment (GFR less than 60 mL/minute). Concomitant use is contraindicated in diabetic patients. Avoid concomitant use in those with moderate to severe renal impairment.
Angiotensin II receptor antagonists (telmisartan): May increase risk of renal dysfunction. Avoid concurrent use.
Antidiabetics, insulin: May increase risk of hypoglycemia. Monitor patient carefully.
Azathioprine: May increase risk of anemia or leukopenia. Monitor hematologic study results if used together.
Diuretics, other antihypertensives: May cause excessive hypotension. Stop diuretic or lower dosage of benazepril, as needed.
Everolimus: May increase risk of angioedema. Discontinue one or both agents if an interaction is suspected.
Gold salts: May increase risk of nitritoid reaction. Carefully monitor patients.
Iron salts (parenteral): May increase risk of adverse reactions to iron salts. Monitor patient closely.
Lithium: May increase lithium level and toxicity. Use together cautiously; monitor lithium level.
Nesiritide: May increase risk of hypotension. Monitor BP.
NSAIDs: May decrease antihypertensive effects. Monitor BP.
Pergolide, phenothiazines (chlorpromazine): May cause profound hypotension. Use with caution and monitor BP.

Potassium-sparing diuretics, potassium supplements: May cause hyperkalemia. Monitor potassium level and renal function.
Salicylates: May decrease hypotensive effects of benazepril. Consider increasing benazepril dosage or decreasing or stopping salicylate.
Thiazide diuretics: May attenuate potassium loss. Also may increase risk of renal failure. Monitor serum potassium level and renal function.
Trimethoprim: May increase risk of hyperkalemia. Monitor serum potassium level and clinical response.
Drug-herb. *Capsaicin:* May cause cough. Discourage use together.
Ma huang: May decrease antihypertensive effects. Discourage use together.
Drug-food. *Salt substitutes containing potassium:* May cause hyperkalemia. Monitor potassium level and renal function.

EFFECTS ON LAB TEST RESULTS
• May increase BUN, creatinine, and potassium levels.

CONTRAINDICATIONS & CAUTIONS
• Contraindicated in patients hypersensitive to ACE inhibitors and in those with a history of angioedema regardless of prior ACE inhibitor use.
• Use cautiously in patients with impaired hepatic or renal function. If jaundice develops or liver enzyme levels are markedly elevated, discontinue drug.
Dialyzable drug: Slightly.
⚠ **Overdose S&S:** Hypotension.

PREGNANCY-LACTATION-REPRODUCTION
Black Box Warning Drugs that act on the renin-angiotensin system can cause injury and death to a developing fetus. Discontinue drug as soon as possible once pregnancy is detected. ■
• Small amounts of drug appear in breast milk. Patient should discontinue breastfeeding or discontinue drug.

NURSING CONSIDERATIONS
• Monitor patient for hypotension. Excessive hypotension can occur when drug is given with diuretics. If possible, diuretic therapy should be stopped 2 to 3 days before

starting benazepril to decrease potential for excessive hypotensive response. If drug doesn't adequately control BP, diuretic may be cautiously reinstituted.

• Although ACE inhibitors reduce BP in all races, they reduce it less in blacks taking ACE inhibitors alone. Black patients should take drug with a thiazide diuretic for a more favorable response.

• Drug may increase risk of angioedema in black patients.

• Measure BP when drug level is at peak (2 to 6 hours after administration) and at trough (just before a dose) to verify adequate BP control.

• Assess renal and hepatic function before and periodically during therapy. Monitor potassium level.

• Monitor patient for excessive cough. Therapy may need to be changed if cough is intolerable.

• *Look alike–sound alike:* Don't confuse benazepril with Benadryl. Don't confuse Lotensin with lovastatin.

PATIENT TEACHING

• Instruct patient to avoid salt substitutes because they may contain potassium, which can cause high potassium level in patients taking drug.

• Inform patient that light-headedness can occur, especially during first few days of therapy. Tell him to rise slowly to minimize this effect and to report dizziness to prescriber. If fainting occurs, he should stop drug and call prescriber immediately.

• Warn patient to use caution in hot weather and during exercise. Inadequate fluid intake, vomiting, diarrhea, and excessive perspiration can lead to light-headedness and fainting.

• Advise patient to report signs of infection, such as fever and sore throat. Tell him to call prescriber if he develops easy bruising or bleeding; swelling of tongue, lips, face, eyes, mucous membranes, or extremities; difficulty swallowing or breathing; or hoarseness.

• *Alert:* Tell woman of childbearing potential to notify prescriber if she becomes pregnant. Drug will need to be stopped.

• Tell patient to contact physician if intolerable cough develops.

benztropine mesylate
BENZ-troe-peen

Cogentin

Therapeutic class: Antiparkinsonian drugs
Pharmacologic class: Anticholinergics

AVAILABLE FORMS
Injection: 1 mg/mL in 2-mL ampules
Tablets: 0.5 mg, 1 mg, 2 mg

INDICATIONS & DOSAGES
➤ **Drug-induced extrapyramidal disorders (except tardive dyskinesia)**
Adults: 1 to 4 mg P.O., I.V., or I.M. once daily or b.i.d.
➤ **Transient extrapyramidal disorders**
Adults: 1 to 2 mg P.O., I.V., or I.M. b.i.d. or t.i.d. After 1 or 2 weeks, withdraw drug to determine continued need.
➤ **Acute dystonic reaction**
Adults: 1 to 2 mg I.V. or I.M.; then 1 to 2 mg P.O. b.i.d. to prevent recurrence.
➤ **Parkinsonism**
Adults: 0.5 to 6 mg P.O., I.V., or I.M. daily. First dosage is 0.5 to 1 mg, increased by 0.5 mg every 5 to 6 days. Adjust dosage to meet individual requirements. Maximum, 6 mg daily.
➤ **Postencephalitic parkinsonism**
Adults: 2 mg P.O., I.V., or I.M. daily in one or more doses. In highly sensitive patients, therapy may be initiated with 0.5 mg P.O. or I.M. at bedtime, and increased as needed. Maximum, 6 mg daily.

ADMINISTRATION
P.O.
• Drug may be given before or after meals depending on patient reaction. If patient is prone to excessive salivation, give drug after meals. If his mouth dries excessively, give drug before meals unless it causes nausea.
I.V.
▼ Reserve I.V. delivery for emergencies, such as acute dystonic reactions.
▼ The I.V. form is seldom used because no significant difference in onset exists between it and the I.M. form.
▼ Use filtered needle to draw up solution from ampule.
▼ **Incompatibilities:** Haloperidol lactate.

I.M.
● Use filtered needle to draw up solution from ampule.

ACTION
Unknown. May block central cholinergic receptors, helping to balance cholinergic activity in the basal ganglia.

Route	Onset	Peak	Duration
P.O.	1–2 hr	7 hr	24 hr
I.V., I.M.	15 min	Unknown	24 hr

Half-life: Unknown.

ADVERSE REACTIONS
CNS: confusion, memory impairment, nervousness, depression, disorientation, hallucinations, toxic psychosis, fever.
CV: tachycardia.
EENT: dilated pupils, blurred vision.
GI: dry mouth, constipation, nausea, vomiting, paralytic ileus.
GU: urine retention, dysuria.
Musculoskeletal: muscle weakness.
Skin: decreased sweating.
Other: heat stroke.

INTERACTIONS
Drug-drug. *Amantadine, phenothiazines, TCAs:* May cause additive anticholinergic adverse reactions, such as confusion and hallucinations. Reduce dosage before giving.
Cholinergics (donepezil, galantamine, rivastigmine, tacrine): May antagonize the therapeutic effects of these drugs. If used together, monitor patient for therapeutic effect.

EFFECTS ON LAB TEST RESULTS
None reported.

CONTRAINDICATIONS & CAUTIONS
● Contraindicated in patients hypersensitive to drug or its components, in those with angle-closure glaucoma, and in children younger than age 3.
● Drug isn't recommended for use in patients with tardive dyskinesia.
● Drug may produce anhidrosis. Use cautiously in hot weather, in patients with mental disorders, in elderly patients, and in children age 3 and older.

● Use cautiously in patients with prostatic hyperplasia, arrhythmias, or seizure disorders.
Dialyzable drug: Unknown.
⚠ **Overdose S&S:** CNS depression preceded or followed by stimulation; confusion, nervousness, listlessness, intensification of mental symptoms or toxic psychosis (in patients with mental illness being treated with neuroleptic drugs), hallucinations, dizziness, muscle weakness, ataxia, dry mouth, mydriasis, blurred vision, palpitations, tachycardia, hypertension, nausea, vomiting, dysuria, numbness of fingers, dysphagia, allergic reactions, headache, delirium, coma, shock, seizures, respiratory arrest, anhidrosis, hyperthermia, glaucoma, constipation; hot, dry, flushed skin.

PREGNANCY-LACTATION-REPRODUCTION
● Safe use during pregnancy hasn't been established.
● It isn't known if drug appears in breast milk. Anticholinergic agents may suppress lactation.

NURSING CONSIDERATIONS
● Monitor vital signs carefully. Watch closely for adverse reactions, especially in elderly or debilitated patients. Call prescriber promptly if adverse reactions occur.
● At certain doses, drug produces atropine-like toxicity, which may aggravate tardive dyskinesia.
● Watch for intermittent constipation and abdominal distention and pain, which may indicate onset of paralytic ileus.
● Monitor elderly patients closely as they are more prone to severe adverse effects.
● **Alert:** Never stop drug abruptly. Reduce dosage gradually.
● **Look alike–sound alike:** Don't confuse benztropine with bromocriptine.

PATIENT TEACHING
● Warn patient to avoid activities that require alertness until CNS effects of drug are known.
● If patient takes a single daily dose, tell him to do so at bedtime.
● Advise patient to report signs and symptoms of urinary hesitancy or urine retention.

• Tell patient to relieve dry mouth with cool drinks, ice chips, sugarless gum, or hard candy.
• Advise patient to limit hot weather activities because drug-induced lack of sweating may cause overheating.

besifloxacin hydrochloride
beh-sih-FLOX-ah-sin

Besivance

Therapeutic class: Antibiotics
Pharmacologic class: Fluoroquinolones

AVAILABLE FORMS
Ophthalmic suspension: 0.6%

INDICATIONS & DOSAGES
➤ **Conjunctivitis caused by CDC coryne-form group G,** *Aerococcus viridans, Corynebacterium pseudodiphtheriticum, Corynebacterium striatum, Haemophilus influenzae, Moraxella catarrhalis, Moraxella lacunata, Pseudomonas aeruginosa, Staphylococcus aureus, Staphylococcus epidermidis, Staphylococcus hominis, Staphylococcus lugdunensis, Staphylococcus warneri, Streptococcus mitis* **group,** *Streptococcus oralis, Streptococcus pneumoniae,* **or** *Streptococcus salivarius*
Adults and children age 1 and older: Instill 1 drop into affected eye t.i.d., 4 to 12 hours apart, for 7 days.

ADMINISTRATION
Ophthalmic
• Invert bottle and shake once before use. Remove cap with bottle in inverted position.
🚫 *Alert:* Don't inject into eye or introduce into anterior chamber of eye.
🚫 *Alert:* Make sure patient doesn't wear contact lenses during treatment.

ACTION
Inhibits DNA gyrase and topoisomerase, preventing cell replication and division.

Route	Onset	Peak	Duration
Ophthalmic	Unknown	Unknown	Unknown

Half-life: 7 hours.

ADVERSE REACTIONS
CNS: headache.
EENT: blurred vision, conjunctival erythema, eye irritation, eye pain, eye pruritus.

INTERACTIONS
None reported.

EFFECTS ON LAB TEST RESULTS
None reported.

CONTRAINDICATIONS & CAUTIONS
• Although drug isn't intended for systemic administration, hypersensitivity reactions have been reported with systemic administration of quinolones. Discontinue drug at first sign of allergic reaction or rash.
• Prolonged use can result in superinfection.
• Safety and effectiveness in infants younger than age 1 haven't been established.
Dialyzable drug: Unknown.

PREGNANCY-LACTATION-REPRODUCTION
• Use during pregnancy only if potential benefit justifies risk to the fetus.
• Drug probably appears in breast milk. Use cautiously in breast-feeding women.

NURSING CONSIDERATIONS
• Be aware that prolonged use may lead to growth of resistant organisms.

PATIENT TEACHING
• Instruct patient to wash his hands before and after instilling the drug.
• Teach patient how to instill drug correctly. Remind him not to touch the tip of the bottle with his hands and not to let the tip touch the eye or surrounding tissue.
• Advise patient to avoid wearing contact lenses if he has signs and symptoms of conjunctivitis while taking the drug.
• Remind patient not to share washcloths or towels with other family members to avoid spreading infection.
• Tell patient to take drug exactly as prescribed for as long as prescribed, even if he's feeling better.
• Instruct patient to stop the drug and notify his prescriber if rash or allergic reaction occurs.

betamethasone dipropionate
bay-ta-METH-a-sone

Diprolene, Diprolene AF

betamethasone valerate
Beta-Val, Dermabet, Luxiq, Valnac

Therapeutic class: Corticosteroids
Pharmacologic class: Corticosteroids

AVAILABLE FORMS
betamethasone dipropionate
Cream: 0.05%
Gel: 0.05%
Lotion: 0.05%
Ointment: 0.05%
betamethasone valerate
Cream: 0.1%
Foam: 0.12%
Lotion: 0.1%
Ointment: 0.1%

INDICATIONS & DOSAGES
➤ **Inflammation and pruritus from corticosteroid-responsive dermatoses**
Adults and children older than age 12:
Clean area; apply cream, ointment, lotion, or gel sparingly. Give dipropionate products once daily to b.i.d.; give valerate 0.1% solution b.i.d., or valerate 0.1% cream or ointment once daily to t.i.d. Maximum dosage of augmented betamethasone dipropionate 0.05% ointment, cream, gel, or lotion is 45 g, 45 g, 50 g, or 50 mL per week, respectively. Therapy with augmented formulations shouldn't exceed 2 weeks.
➤ **Inflammation and pruritus from corticosteroid-responsive dermatoses of scalp (valerate only)**
Adults: Gently massage small amounts of foam into affected scalp areas b.i.d., morning and evening, until control is achieved. If no improvement is seen in 2 weeks, reassess diagnosis.

ADMINISTRATION
Topical
• Apply sparingly to affected areas. To prevent skin damage, rub in gently, leaving a thin coat.

• Decrease dosing frequency to once daily if clinical improvement is seen.
• Avoid applying near eyes or mucous membranes or in ear canal, groin area, or armpit.
• Don't dispense foam directly into warm hands because foam will begin to melt on contact.
• For patients with eczematous dermatitis whose skin may be irritated by adhesive material, hold dressing in place with gauze, elastic bandages, stockings, or stockinette.
🛈 *Alert:* Foam product is flammable. Avoid fire, flame, or smoking during use. Don't expose to heat.
🛈 *Alert:* Don't use occlusive dressings.
• Continue drug for a few days after lesions clear.

ACTION
Unclear. Is diffused across cell membranes to form complexes with receptors. Has anti-inflammatory, antipruritic, vasoconstrictive, and antiproliferative activity. Considered a medium-potency to very-high-potency drug (depending on product), according to vasoconstrictive properties.

Route	Onset	Peak	Duration
Topical	Unknown	Unknown	Unknown

Half-life: Unknown.

ADVERSE REACTIONS
GU: glycosuria (with dipropionate).
Metabolic: hyperglycemia.
Skin: burning, pruritus, irritation, dryness, erythema, folliculitis, striae, acneiform eruptions, perioral dermatitis, hypopigmentation, hypertrichosis, allergic contact dermatitis, secondary infection, maceration, atrophy, miliaria with occlusive dressings.
Other: *HPA axis suppression,* Cushing syndrome.

INTERACTIONS
None significant.

EFFECTS ON LAB TEST RESULTS
• May increase glucose level.

CONTRAINDICATIONS & CAUTIONS
• Contraindicated in patients hypersensitive to corticosteroids.

🍁Canada ◇OTC ◆Off-label use 🔎Photoguide ⓓDo not crush *Liquid contains alcohol.

• Don't use as monotherapy in primary bacterial infections (impetigo, paronychia, erysipelas, cellulitis, angular cheilitis), rosacea, perioral dermatitis, or acne.
• Don't use augmented betamethasone dipropionate 0.05% ointment; betamethasone dipropionate 0.05% gel, cream, and ointment; or betamethasone valerate 0.1% ointment on the face, groin, or axilla.
Dialyzable drug: No.
⚠ *Overdose S&S:* Systemic effects.

PREGNANCY-LACTATION-REPRODUCTION
• There are no adequate and well-controlled studies in pregnant women. Use during pregnancy only if potential benefit justifies potential risk to the fetus.
• Use cautiously in breast-feeding women.

NURSING CONSIDERATIONS
• Drug isn't for ophthalmic use.
• Because of alcohol content of vehicle, gel products may cause mild, transient stinging, especially when used on or near excoriated skin.
• If antifungal or antibiotic combined with corticosteroid fails to provide prompt improvement, stop corticosteroid until infection is controlled.
• Systemic absorption is likely with prolonged or extensive body surface treatment. Watch for symptoms of HPA axis suppression, manifestations of Cushing syndrome, hyperglycemia, and glycosuria. If HPA axis suppression occurs, attempt to withdraw drug or substitute a less potent steroid. Withdraw gradually.
• Evaluate patient for HPA axis suppression by using the urinary free cortisol and corticotropin stimulation tests.
🔊 *Alert:* Children may demonstrate greater susceptibility to HPA axis suppression and Cushing syndrome.
• Avoid using plastic pants or tight-fitting diapers on treated areas in young children. Children may absorb larger amounts of drug and be more susceptible to systemic toxicity.
🔊 *Alert:* Diprolene and Diprolene AF may not be replaced with generics because other products have different potencies.

PATIENT TEACHING
• Teach patient how to apply drug.

• Emphasize that drug is for external use only.
• Tell patient to wash hands after application.
• Tell patient to stop drug and report signs of systemic absorption, skin irritation or ulceration, hypersensitivity, or infection.
• Instruct patient not to use occlusive dressings.
• Discuss personal hygiene measures to reduce chance of infection.

bethanechol chloride
be-THAN-e-kole

Duvoid, Urecholine❧

Therapeutic class: Urinary stimulants
Pharmacologic class: Cholinergic agonists

AVAILABLE FORMS
Tablets: 5 mg, 10 mg, 25 mg, 50 mg

INDICATIONS & DOSAGES
➤ **Acute postoperative and postpartum nonobstructive (functional) urine retention, neurogenic atony of urinary bladder with urine retention**
Adults: 10 to 50 mg P.O. t.i.d. to q.i.d. Determine minimum effective dose by giving 5 or 10 mg and repeating same amount at hourly intervals until satisfactory response or maximum of 50 mg has been given.

ADMINISTRATION
P.O.
• Give drug 1 hour before or 2 hours after meals because drug may cause nausea and vomiting if taken soon after eating.

ACTION
Directly stimulates muscarinic cholinergic receptors, mimicking acetylcholine action, increasing GI tract tone and peristalsis and contraction of the detrusor muscle of the urinary bladder.

Route	Onset	Peak	Duration
P.O.	30–90 min	1 hr	6 hr

Half-life: Unknown.

Reactions in bold italics are *life-threatening*. Interactions may have a *rapid onset* or a *delayed onset*.

ADVERSE REACTIONS
CNS: headache, malaise, seizures.
CV: *bradycardia,* profound hypotension with reflexive tachycardia, flushing.
EENT: lacrimation, miosis.
GI: abdominal cramps, diarrhea, excessive salivation, nausea, belching, borborygmus.
GU: urinary urgency.
Respiratory: *bronchoconstriction, asthma attack.*
Skin: diaphoresis.

INTERACTIONS
Drug-drug. *Anticholinergics, atropine, belladonna alkaloids, procainamide, quinidine:* May reverse cholinergic effects. Observe patient for lack of drug effect.
Cholinesterase inhibitors (donepezil), cholinergic agonists: May cause additive effects or increase toxicity. Avoid using together.
Ganglionic blockers: May cause critical drop in BP, usually preceded by severe abdominal pain. Avoid using together.

EFFECTS ON LAB TEST RESULTS
• May increase amylase, lipase, and liver enzyme levels.

CONTRAINDICATIONS & CAUTIONS
• Contraindicated in patients hypersensitive to drug or its components and in those with uncertain strength or integrity of bladder wall, mechanical obstruction of GI or urinary tract, hyperthyroidism, peptic ulceration, latent or active bronchial asthma, obstructive pulmonary disease, pronounced bradycardia or hypotension, vasomotor instability, cardiac disease or CAD, AV conduction defects, hypertension, seizure disorder, Parkinson disease, spastic GI disturbances, acute inflammatory lesions of the GI tract, peritonitis, or marked vagotonia.
• Safe use in children hasn't been established.
Dialyzable drug: Unknown.
⚠ Overdose S&S: Abdominal discomfort, excessive salivation, flushing, hot feeling, sweating, nausea, vomiting.

PREGNANCY-LACTATION-REPRODUCTION
• It isn't known if drug affects reproduction. Use during pregnancy only if clearly needed.

• It isn't known if drug appears in breast milk. Patient should discontinue breast-feeding or discontinue drug.

NURSING CONSIDERATIONS
• Adverse effects are rare with oral use.
• Monitor vital signs frequently, especially respirations. Always have atropine injection available, and be prepared to give 0.6 mg subcutaneously or by slow I.V. push. Provide respiratory support, if needed.
• Monitor patient for orthostatic hypotension.
• Watch closely for adverse reactions that may indicate drug toxicity.

PATIENT TEACHING
• Tell patient to take drug on an empty stomach and at regular intervals.
• Inform patient that drug is usually effective 30 to 90 minutes after use.

SAFETY ALERT!

bevacizumab
beh-vah-SIZZ-yoo-mab

Avastin

Therapeutic class: Antineoplastics
Pharmacologic class: Monoclonal antibodies

AVAILABLE FORMS
Solution: 25 mg/mL in 4-mL and 16-mL vials

INDICATIONS & DOSAGES
Adjust-a-dose (for all indications): Although there are no recommended dosage reductions, temporarily suspend or stop drug in patients with severe infusion reactions, severe hypertension that isn't controlled with medical management, or moderate to severe proteinuria.
➤ **Platinum-resistant recurrent epithelial ovarian, fallopian tube, or primary peritoneal cancer**
Adults: 10 mg/kg I.V. every 2 weeks in combination with paclitaxel, pegylated liposomal doxorubicin, or weekly topotecan; or 15 mg/kg I.V. every 3 weeks in combination with topotecan.

➤ **Metastatic colorectal cancer with fluoropyrimidine-irinotecan–based or fluoropyrimidine-oxaliplatin–based chemotherapy for second-line treatment after progression on a first-line bevacizumab-containing regimen**
Adults: 5 mg/kg I.V. every 2 weeks or 7.5 mg/kg I.V. every 3 weeks.

➤ **Persistent, recurrent, or metastatic cervical cancer with paclitaxel and cisplatin or paclitaxel and topotecan**
Adults: 15 mg/kg I.V. infusion once every 3 weeks.

➤ **First- or second-line treatment, with 5-FU–based chemotherapy, for metastatic colon or rectal cancer**
Adults: If used with bolus irinotecan, 5-FU, and leucovorin (IFL) regimen, give 5 mg/kg I.V. every 14 days. If used with oxaliplatin, 5-FU, and leucovorin (known as FOLFOX 4) regimen, give 10 mg/kg I.V. every 14 days. Infusion rate varies by patient tolerance and number of infusions.

➤ **With carboplatin and paclitaxel as first-line treatment of unresectable, locally advanced, recurrent, or metastatic nonsquamous, non–small-cell lung cancer**
Adults: 15 mg/kg I.V. infusion once every 3 weeks.

➤ **With interferon alfa for metastatic renal cell carcinoma; as single agent for progressive glioblastoma following prior therapy**
Adults: 10 mg/kg I.V. every 14 days.

➤ **Glioblastoma as single agent for progressive disease following prior therapy**
Adults: 10 mg/kg I.V. every 14 days.

ADMINISTRATION

I.V.
▼ Don't freeze or shake vials.
▼ Dilute drug using aseptic technique. Withdraw proper dose and mix in a total volume of 100 mL NSS in an I.V. bag.
▼ Don't give by I.V. push or bolus.
▼ Give first infusion over 90 minutes and, if tolerated, second infusion over 60 minutes. Later infusions can be given over 30 minutes if previous infusions were tolerated.
▼ Discard unused portion; drug is preservative-free.

▼ Diluted drug is stable 8 hours if refrigerated at 36° to 46° F (2° to 8° C).
▼ Protect from light.
▼ **Incompatibilities:** Dextrose solutions.

ACTION

A recombinant humanized vascular endothelial growth factor inhibitor.

Route	Onset	Peak	Duration
I.V.	Unknown	Unknown	Unknown

Half-life: About 20 days.

ADVERSE REACTIONS

CNS: asthenia, dizziness, headache, abnormal gait, confusion, pain, syncope.
CV: *intra-abdominal thrombosis,* hypertension, *thromboembolism, DVT,* HF, hypotension.
EENT: epistaxis, excess lacrimation, gum bleeding, taste disorder, voice alteration.
GI: anorexia, constipation, diarrhea, dyspepsia, flatulence, stomatitis, vomiting, *GI hemorrhage,* abdominal pain, colitis, dry mouth, nausea.
GU: *vaginal hemorrhage,* proteinuria.
Hematologic: *leukopenia, neutropenia, thrombocytopenia.*
Metabolic: hypokalemia, weight loss, bilirubinemia.
Musculoskeletal: back pain, myalgia.
Respiratory: *hemoptysis,* dyspnea, URI.
Skin: alopecia, dry skin, exfoliative dermatitis, nail disorder, palmar-plantar erythrodysesthesia, skin ulcer.
Other: decreased wound healing, hypersensitivity.

INTERACTIONS

Drug-drug. *Antineoplastics (anthracyclines, systemic):* May increase cardiotoxic effects of antineoplastics. Monitor therapy.
Bisphosphonate derivatives: May increase risk of osteonecrosis of the jaw. Monitor therapy.
Live-virus vaccines: May reduce immune response. Avoid use together.
Sunitinib: May increase bevacizumab toxicities, including microangiopathic hemolytic anemia and hypertension. Avoid combination.

Reactions in bold italics are *life-threatening*. Interactions may have a *rapid onset* or a *delayed onset*.

EFFECTS ON LAB TEST RESULTS
• May increase bilirubin and urine protein levels. May decrease potassium level.
• May decrease neutrophil, platelet, and WBC counts.

CONTRAINDICATIONS & CAUTIONS
• Contraindicated in patients with recent hemoptysis or within 28 days after major surgery.
• Use cautiously in patients hypersensitive to drug or its components, in those who need surgery, are taking anticoagulants, or have significant CV disease.
Dialyzable drug: Unknown.
⚠ *Overdose S&S:* Headache.

PREGNANCY-LACTATION-REPRODUCTION
• Drug has shown teratogenic effects in animal studies. Avoid use in pregnant women.
• Because of bevicizumab's long half-life, patients should use adequate contraception during therapy and for 6 months or more after last dose.
🔵 *Alert:* May increase risk of ovarian failure and may impair fertility. Long-term effects on fertility are unknown.
• It isn't known if drug appears in breast milk. Women shouldn't breast-feed during therapy and for about 3 weeks after therapy ends.

NURSING CONSIDERATIONS
🔵 *Alert:* Posterior reversible leukoencephalopathy syndrome (PRLS)–associated symptoms (hypertension, headache, visual disturbances, altered mental function, seizures) may occur 16 hours to 1 year after starting the drug. Monitor patient closely. If syndrome occurs, stop drug and provide supportive care.
🔵 *Alert:* Monitor patient for arterial thromboembolic events and venous thromboembolic events (VTEs). Patients treated for cervical cancer may be at increased risk for VTEs. Permanently discontinue drug for grade 4 VTE, including PE.
🔵 *Alert:* Drug may increase risk of developing fistula, including non-GI fistulae (tracheoesophageal, bronchopleural, biliary, vaginal, renal, or bladder), which can be fatal.

• Permanently stop drug if patient develops any fistula of an internal organ.
• PRLS can be confirmed only by MRI.
• Hypersensitivity reactions can occur during infusion. Monitor the patient closely.
• If patient develops nephrotic syndrome, severe hypertension, hypertensive crisis, serious hemorrhage, or GI perforation that needs intervention, stop drug.
🔵 *Alert:* Drug may increase risk of serious arterial thromboembolic events, including MI, TIAs, stroke, and angina. Those patients at highest risk are age 65 or older, have a history of arterial thromboembolism, and have taken the drug before. If patient has an arterial thrombotic event, permanently stop drug.
Black Box Warning Drug may cause fatal GI perforation. Monitor patient closely. ∎
Black Box Warning Bevacizumab can result in life-threatening wound dehiscence. Permanently discontinue bevacizumab therapy in patients who experience wound dehiscence that requires medical intervention. Discontinue drug at least 28 days before elective surgery and don't restart drug for at least 28 days after surgery and until the surgical wound is fully healed. ∎
Black Box Warning Drug increases risk of severe or fatal hemorrhage, hemoptysis, GI bleeding, CNS hemorrhage, and vaginal bleeding. Don't give to patients with serious hemorrhage or recent hemoptysis. ∎
• Monitor urinalysis for worsening proteinuria. Patients with 2+ or greater urine dipstick test should undergo 24-hour urine collection. Discontinue use in patients with nephrotic syndrome.
• Monitor patient's BP every 2 to 3 weeks.
• Adverse reactions occur more often in older patients.

PATIENT TEACHING
• Inform patient about potential adverse reactions.
• Tell patient to report adverse reactions immediately, especially abdominal pain, constipation, and vomiting.
• Advise patient that BP and urinalysis will be monitored during treatment.
• Caution women of childbearing potential to avoid pregnancy during treatment.

◑ *Alert:* Inform women of the potential for ovarian failure and impaired fertility before starting treatment.

● Urge patient to alert other health care providers about treatment and to avoid elective surgery during treatment.

bimatoprost
by-MAT-oh-prost

Latisse, Lumigan

Therapeutic class: Antiglaucoma drugs
Pharmacologic class: Prostaglandin analogues

AVAILABLE FORMS
Ophthalmic solution: 0.01%, 0.03%
Topical solution: 0.03%

INDICATIONS & DOSAGES
➤ **Increased IOP in patients with open-angle glaucoma or ocular hypertension**
Adults: Instill 1 drop in conjunctival sac of affected eye(s) once daily in the evening.
➤ **Hypotrichosis of the eyelashes**
Adults: Apply 1 drop nightly directly to skin of upper eyelid margin at base of eyelashes with single-use applicator, using a second applicator for a second eye (if needed).

ADMINISTRATION
Ophthalmic
● Don't touch tip of dropper to eye or surrounding tissue.
● If more than one ophthalmic drug is being used, give drugs at least 5 minutes apart.
● Store drug in original container between 59° and 77° F (15° and 25° C).
Topical
● Before application, ensure face is clean and makeup and contact lenses are removed.
● Use new applicator for each eye; never reuse. Don't use any other brush or applicator.
● Blot excess solution from beyond eyelid margin.

ACTION
Has ocular hypotensive activity, which selectively mimics the effects of naturally occurring prostaglandins. Drug may also increase outflow of aqueous humor. Mechanism in treating hypotrichosis is unknown.

Route	Onset	Peak	Duration
Ophthalmic	4 hr	10 min	Unknown
Topical	Unknown	Unknown	Unknown

Half-life: 45 minutes.

ADVERSE REACTIONS
CNS: headache, asthenia.
EENT: conjunctival hyperemia, growth of eyelashes, ocular pruritus, allergic conjunctivitis, asthenopia, blepharitis, cataract, conjunctival edema; eye discharge, tearing, and pain; eyelash darkening, eyelid erythema, foreign body sensation, increase in iris pigmentation; ocular burning, dryness, and irritation; photophobia, superficial punctate keratitis, visual disturbance.
Respiratory: URI.
Skin: hirsutism, hyperpigmentation of periocular skin.
Other: infection.

INTERACTIONS
Drug-drug. *Latanoprost:* May increase IOP. Modify therapy.

EFFECTS ON LAB TEST RESULTS
● May cause abnormal LFT values.

CONTRAINDICATIONS & CAUTIONS
● Contraindicated in patients hypersensitive to bimatoprost, benzalkonium chloride, or other ingredients in product.
● Drug hasn't been approved for use in patients with angle-closure glaucoma or inflammatory or neovascular glaucoma.
● Use cautiously in patients with renal or hepatic impairment.
● Use cautiously in patients with active intraocular inflammation (iritis, uveitis), aphakic patients, pseudophakic patients with torn posterior lens capsule, and patients at risk for macular edema.
Dialyzable drug: No.

PREGNANCY-LACTATION-REPRODUCTION
● Adverse events have been observed in animal reproduction studies. Use only if benefit outweighs fetal risk.

Reactions in bold italics are *life-threatening*. Interactions may have a *rapid onset* or a ***delayed onset***.

• It isn't known if drug appears in breast milk. Use cautiously in breast-feeding women.

NURSING CONSIDERATIONS
• Temporary or permanent increased pigmentation of iris and eyelid, as well as increased pigmentation and growth of eyelashes, may occur.
• Patient should remove contact lenses before using solution. Lenses may be reinserted 15 minutes after administration.

PATIENT TEACHING
• Tell patient receiving treatment in only one eye about potential for increased brown pigmentation of iris, eyelid skin darkening, and increased length, thickness, pigmentation, or number of lashes in treated eye.
• Teach patient how to instill drops, and advise him to wash hands before and after instilling solution. Warn him not to touch tip of dropper to eye or surrounding tissue.
• If eye trauma or infection occurs or if eye surgery is needed, tell patient to seek medical advice before continuing to use multidose container.
• Advise patient to immediately report eye inflammation or lid reactions.
• Advise patient to apply light pressure on lacrimal sac for 1 minute after instillation of drops to minimize systemic absorption of drug.
• Tell patient to remove contact lenses before using solution and that lenses may be reinserted 15 minutes after administration.
• Teach patient that Latisse applicators are for single use only. Instruct patient to wash face and remove makeup and contact lenses before applicator use.
• Tell patient that effects of Latisse are gradual in onset and may not be significant for 2 months. Results last only as long as treatment is continued.
• Instruct patient to blot excess solution from beyond eyelid margin.
• If patient is using more than one ophthalmic drug, tell him to apply them at least 5 minutes apart.
• Stress importance of compliance with recommended therapy.

bisoprolol fumarate
BIS-oh-PROE-lol

Zebeta

Therapeutic class: Antihypertensives
Pharmacologic class: Selective beta blockers

AVAILABLE FORMS
Tablets: 5 mg, 10 mg

INDICATIONS & DOSAGES
➤ **Hypertension**
Adults: Initially, 2.5 to 5 mg P.O. daily alone or with other antihypertensives. May increase to 10 mg daily, then to 20 mg once daily if needed.
Adjust-a-dose: In patients with bronchospastic disease or hepatic or renal insufficiency (CrCl less than 40 mL/minute), initially give 2.5 mg; then titrate with caution.

ADMINISTRATION
P.O.
• May give without regard to meals.
• Store at room temperature. Protect from moisture.

ACTION
Selectively blocks cardiac adrenoceptors, reducing resting and exercise HR, decreasing cardiac output, depressing renin secretion, and decreasing tonic sympathetic outflow from the vasomotor centers in the brain.

Route	Onset	Peak	Duration
P.O.	Unknown	2–4 hr	Unknown

Half-life: 9 to 12 hours.

ADVERSE REACTIONS
CNS: headache, dizziness, hypoesthesia, insomnia, asthenia, fatigue.
CV: chest pain, peripheral edema, bradycardia.
EENT: dry mouth, pharyngitis, rhinitis, sinusitis.
GI: diarrhea, nausea, vomiting.
Musculoskeletal: arthralgia.
Respiratory: cough, dyspnea, URI.
Skin: sweating.

INTERACTIONS

Drug-drug. *Antiarrhythmics (disopyramide), calcium channel blockers (diltiazem, verapamil):* May increase myocardial depression or conduction delay. Use cautiously together.

Beta blockers: May increase beta blocker effects to unsafe level. Use together is contraindicated.

Catecholamine-depleting drugs (guanethidine, reserpine): May cause hypotension or bradycardia. Monitor patient closely.

Clonidine: May cause rebound hypertension if clonidine is discontinued. Stop bisoprolol for several days before discontinuing clonidine.

Digoxin: May increase risk of slow AV conduction and bradycardia. Use together cautiously.

Insulin, oral antidiabetics: May mask signs and symptoms of hypoglycemia, particularly tachycardia. Use together cautiously.

Rifampin: May increase bisoprolol metabolism. Monitor patient for decreased bisoprolol effects.

EFFECTS ON LAB TEST RESULTS

● May increase serum triglyceride, AST, ALT, uric acid, creatinine, BUN, potassium, glucose, and phosphorus levels.
● May decrease WBC and platelet counts.
● May cause ANA conversion.

CONTRAINDICATIONS & CAUTIONS

● Contraindicated in patients hypersensitive to drug and in those with cardiogenic shock, overt cardiac failure, second- or third-degree AV block, or marked sinus bradycardia.
● Use cautiously in patients with hepatic or renal insufficiency, hyperthyroidism, HF, arterial insufficiency, peripheral vascular disease (PVD), or diabetes.
● Use cautiously in patients with a history of severe anaphylactic reaction to a variety of allergens. Patients may be more sensitive if allergen is reintroduced; usual epinephrine doses may not be effective.
● Use cautiously in patients with bronchospastic disease who don't tolerate or respond to other antihypertensive treatment. Patients should have a bronchodilator on hand in the event of an episode.
Dialyzable drug: No.

PREGNANCY-LACTATION-REPRODUCTION

● There are no adequate and well-controlled studies in pregnant women. Use during pregnancy only if potential benefit justifies potential risk to the fetus.
● It isn't known if drug appears in breast milk. Use cautiously in breast-feeding women.

NURSING CONSIDERATIONS

● Monitor BP closely.
● Avoid use in patients with acute HF because of worsening of disease. If bisoprolol administration is necessary, monitor patient closely.
● Use cautiously in patients with known compensated HF. In patients without a history of HF, drug may precipitate signs and symptoms of new HF. Consider stopping drug at first indication of new HF. Drug may be continued while HF is being treated with other drugs.
● Drug interruption or abrupt discontinuation may exacerbate angina pectoris, MI, or ventricular arrhythmia and may exacerbate the signs and symptoms of hyperthyroidism, possibly leading to thyroid storm. If drug is to be discontinued, taper over approximately 1 week while monitoring patient. If withdrawal signs and symptoms occur, restart drug at least temporarily.
● A long-term bisoprolol regimen shouldn't be discontinued before major surgery. However, the impaired ability of the heart to respond to reflex adrenergic stimuli may increase risks of general anesthesia and surgical procedures.
● Drug may mask tachycardia caused by hyperthyroidism. In patients with suspected thyrotoxicosis, withdraw drug gradually to avoid thyroid storm.
● Drug may mask signs and symptoms of hypoglycemia in diabetic patients.
● Drug may cause or aggravate signs and symptoms of arterial insufficiency in patients with PVD.

PATIENT TEACHING

● Tell patient to report slowed heartbeat, difficulty breathing, or other signs of HF.
● Caution patient not to discontinue bisoprolol without first consulting health care provider.

Reactions in bold italics are *life-threatening*. Interactions may have a *rapid onset* or a *delayed onset*.

• Warn diabetic patient that bisoprolol may mask signs and symptoms of hypoglycemia (such as tachycardia, dizziness, and weakness).

• Urge patient to use caution when operating automobiles and machinery or performing activities requiring alertness.

SAFETY ALERT!

bivalirudin
bye-VAL-ih-roo-din

Angiomax

Therapeutic class: Anticoagulants
Pharmacologic class: Direct thrombin inhibitors

AVAILABLE FORMS
Injection: 250-mg vial

INDICATIONS & DOSAGES
Adjust-a-dose (for all indications): For patients with CrCl of 30 mL/minute or less, decrease infusion rate to 1 mg/kg/hour. For patients on hemodialysis, reduce infusion rate to 0.25 mg/kg/hour. No reduction of bolus dose is needed.

➤ **Anticoagulation in patients with unstable angina undergoing percutaneous transluminal coronary angioplasty (PTCA); anticoagulation in patients with unstable angina undergoing PCI, with provisional use of a platelet glycoprotein (Gp) IIb/IIIa inhibitor**
Adults: 0.75 mg/kg I.V. bolus followed by a continuous infusion of 1.75 mg/kg/hour during the procedure. Check activated clotting time 5 minutes after bolus dose is given. May give additional 0.3 mg/kg bolus dose if needed. Infusion may continue for up to 4 hours after procedure. After 4-hour infusion, may give an additional infusion of 0.2 mg/kg/hour for up to 20 hours, if needed. Use with 300 to 325 mg aspirin.

➤ **Patients undergoing PCI who have or are at risk for heparin-induced thrombocytopenia (HIT) or heparin-induced thrombocytopenia–thrombosis syndrome (HITTS)**
Adults: 0.75 mg/kg I.V. bolus, followed by a continuous infusion of 1.75 mg/kg/hour throughout the procedure. Infusion up to 4 hours after procedure is optional. After 4 hours, may give an additional infusion of 0.2 mg/kg/hour for up to 20 hours. Use with 300 to 325 mg aspirin.

➤ **ST-elevation MI in patients undergoing primary PCI ◆**
Adults: 0.75 mg/kg I.V. bolus, followed by 1.75 mg/kg/hour I.V. infusion for duration of procedure. May continue after procedure at reduced dosage if clinically indicated.

ADMINISTRATION
I.V.
▼ Reconstitute each 250-mg vial with 5 mL of sterile water for injection. Gently swirl until all material is dissolved.
▼ Reconstituted material will be a clear to slightly opalescent, colorless to slightly yellow solution.
▼ Dilute each reconstituted vial in 50 mL D_5W or NSS to yield a final concentration of 5 mg/mL.
▼ To prepare low-rate infusion, dilute each reconstituted vial in 500 mL D_5W or NSS to yield a final concentration of 0.5 mg/mL.
▼ Solutions with concentrations of 0.5 to 5 mg/mL are stable at room temperature for 24 hours.
▼ **Incompatibilities:** Alteplase, amiodarone, amphotericin B, chlorpromazine, diazepam, prochlorperazine, reteplase, streptokinase, vancomycin. *Note:* Compatible with dobutamine at concentrations up to 4 mg/mL, but incompatible at concentration of 12.5 mg/mL.

ACTION
Binds specifically and rapidly to thrombin, inhibiting its effects, thereby producing an anticoagulant effect.

Route	Onset	Peak	Duration
I.V.	Rapid	Immediate	1–2 hr

Half-life: 25 minutes in patients with normal renal function.

ADVERSE REACTIONS
CNS: anxiety, headache, insomnia, nervousness, fever, pain.
CV: *bradycardia,* hypertension, hypotension.

GI: abdominal pain, dyspepsia, nausea, vomiting.
GU: urine retention.
Hematologic: *severe, spontaneous bleeding (cerebral, retroperitoneal, GU, GI).*
Musculoskeletal: back pain, pelvic pain.
Skin: pain at injection site.

INTERACTIONS
Drug-drug. *Gp IIb/IIIa inhibitors (abciximab, eptifibatide, tirofiban), heparin, thrombolytics, warfarin:* May increase risk of hemorrhage. Use together cautiously.
Drug-herb. *Angelica (dong quai), boldo, bromelains, capsicum, chamomile, dandelion, danshen, devil's claw, fenugreek, feverfew, garlic, ginger, ginkgo, ginseng, horse chestnut, licorice, meadowsweet, onion, passion flower, red clover, willow:* May increase risk of bleeding. Discourage use together.

EFFECTS ON LAB TEST RESULTS
None reported.

CONTRAINDICATIONS & CAUTIONS
• Contraindicated in patients hypersensitive to drug or its components; in those with history of thrombocytopenia after tirofiban administration, major surgical procedure, or severe physical trauma within previous month; and in those with active major bleeding. Avoid using in patients with unstable angina who aren't undergoing PTCA or PCI or in patients with other acute coronary syndromes.
• Use cautiously in patients undergoing brachytherapy, in those with HIT or HITTS, in those with diseases linked to increased risk of bleeding, and in elderly patients.
Dialyzable drug: 25%.

PREGNANCY-LACTATION-REPRODUCTION
• Use cautiously in pregnant women and only if clearly indicated.
• It's unknown if drug appears in breast milk. Use cautiously in breast-feeding women.

NURSING CONSIDERATIONS
• There is no antidote for drug.
• Monitor coagulation test results, Hb level, and hematocrit before starting therapy and periodically thereafter.

• Circumstances for provisional use of a Gp inhibitor during PCI include decreased Thrombolysis in Myocardial Infarction (TIMI) flow (0–2) or slow reflow, dissection with decreased flow, new or suspected thrombus, persistent residual stenosis, distal embolization, an unplanned stent, suboptimal stenting, side-branch closure, abrupt closure, clinical instability, and prolonged ischemia.
• Obtain a complete list of patient's prescription and OTC drugs and supplements, including herbs.
♦ **Alert:** Hemorrhage can occur at any site in the body. If patient has unexplained decrease in hematocrit, decrease in BP, or other unexplained symptoms, suspect hemorrhage.
• Monitor venipuncture sites for bleeding, hematoma, or inflammation.
• Puncture-site hemorrhage and catheterization-site hematoma may occur in patients age 65 and older more often than in younger patients.
• Don't give drug I.M.

PATIENT TEACHING
• Advise patient that drug can cause bleeding, and tell him to report unusual bruising or bleeding (nosebleeds, bleeding gums) or tarry stools immediately.
• Counsel patient that drug is given with aspirin, and caution him to avoid other aspirin-containing drugs or NSAIDs while receiving this drug.
• Advise patient to consult with prescriber before initiating any herbal therapy; many herbs have anticoagulant, antiplatelet, and fibrinolytic properties.
• Advise patient to avoid activities that carry a risk of injury, and instruct him to use a soft toothbrush and electric razor while on drug.

Reactions in bold italics are *life-threatening*. Interactions may have a *rapid onset* or a ***delayed onset***.

bleomycin sulfate
blee-oh-MYE-sin

Therapeutic class: Antineoplastics
Pharmacologic class: Cytotoxic
glycopeptide antibiotics

AVAILABLE FORMS
Injection: 15-unit vials, 30-unit vials

INDICATIONS & DOSAGES
Adjust-a-dose (for all indications): For patients with CrCl of 40 to 50 mL/minute,
give 70% of dose; for CrCl of 30 to
39 mL/minute, give 60% of dose; for CrCl
of 20 to 29 mL/minute, give 55% of dose;
for CrCl of 10 to 19 mL/minute, give 45%
of dose; and for CrCl of 5 to 9 mL/minute,
give 40% of dose.
➤ **Squamous cell carcinoma (head,
neck, skin, penis, cervix, and vulva),
non-Hodgkin lymphoma, testicular
carcinoma**
Adults: Because an anaphylactoid reaction
is possible, treat lymphoma patients with
2 units or less for first two doses. If no acute
reaction occurs, then may follow regular
dosage schedule: 0.25 to 0.5 units/kg (10 to
20 units/m^2) I.V., I.M., or subcutaneously
once or twice weekly to total of 400 units.
➤ **Hodgkin lymphoma**
Adults: Because an anaphylactoid reaction
is possible, treat lymphoma patients with
2 units or less for first two doses. If no acute
reaction occurs, then may follow regular
dosage schedule: 0.25 to 0.5 units/kg (10 to
20 units/m^2) I.V., I.M., or subcutaneously
one or two times weekly. After 50% response, maintenance dose is 1 unit I.V. or
I.M. daily or 5 units I.V. or I.M. weekly.
Total cumulative dose is 400 units.
➤ **Malignant pleural effusion**
Adults: 60 units given as single-dose bolus
intrapleural injection.

ADMINISTRATION
I.V.
▼ Preparing and giving parenteral form
of drug may be mutagenic, teratogenic,
and carcinogenic. Follow facility policy to
reduce risks.

▼ Drug may adsorb to plastic I.V. bags. For
prolonged infusions, use glass containers.
▼ Reconstitute drug with 5 or 10 mL of
NSS for injection to equal 3 units/mL
solution.
▼ Administer slowly over 10 minutes.
▼ Use reconstituted solution within
24 hours.
▼ Refrigerate unopened vials containing
dry powder.
▼ Drug is an irritant and may cause
phlebitis. It isn't known to cause tissue
damage with extravasation. If signs or
symptoms of extravasation occur, stop
infusion immediately and institute appropriate care according to facility policy.
▼ **Incompatibilities:** Amino acids; aminophylline; ascorbic acid injection; cefazolin;
diazepam; drugs containing sulfhydryl
groups; fluids containing dextrose;
furosemide; hydrocortisone; methotrexate; mitomycin; nafcillin; penicillin G;
riboflavin; solutions containing divalent
and trivalent cations, especially calcium
salts and copper; terbutaline sulfate.
I.M.
● Dilute 15-unit vial in 1 to 5 mL or
30-unit vial in 2 to 10 mL of sterile water
for injection, bacteriostatic water for injection, or NSS for injection.
● Monitor injection site for irritation.
Subcutaneous
● Dilute 15-unit vial in 1 to 5 mL or
30-unit vial in 2 to 10 mL of sterile water
for injection, bacteriostatic water for injection, or NSS for injection.
● Monitor injection site for irritation.
Intrapleural
● For intrapleural use, dilute 60 units of
drug in 50 to 100 mL NSS for injection; give
drug through a thoracotomy tube.
● If patient's condition requires sclerosis, instill drug when chest tube drainage is 100 to
300 mL/24 hours; ideally, drainage should
be less than 100 mL. After instillation,
clamp thoracotomy tube and move patient
from his back to his left then right side
several times for the next 4 hours. Remove
clamp and reestablish suction. Length of
time chest tube is left in place after sclerosis
depends on patient's condition.

ACTION
May inhibit DNA synthesis and cause scission of single- and double-stranded DNA; also inhibits RNA and protein synthesis.

Route	Onset	Peak	Duration
I.V., subcut.	Unknown	30–60 min	Unknown
I.M.	Unknown	30–60 min	Unknown

Half-life: 2 hours.

ADVERSE REACTIONS
CNS: fever.
GI: stomatitis, anorexia, nausea, vomiting, diarrhea.
Metabolic: weight loss, hyperuricemia.
Respiratory: *pneumonitis, pulmonary fibrosis.*
Skin: erythema, hyperpigmentation, acne, rash, striae, skin tenderness, pruritus, reversible alopecia, hyperkeratosis, nail changes.
Other: chills, *anaphylactoid reactions.*

INTERACTIONS
Drug-drug. *Anesthesia:* May increase oxygen requirements. Monitor patient closely.
Brentuximab: May increase risk of pulmonary toxicity. Use together is contraindicated.
Cisplatin: May decrease bleomycin elimination. Monitor renal function and adjust bleomycin dosage as needed.
Fosphenytoin, phenytoin: May decrease phenytoin and fosphenytoin levels. Monitor drug levels closely.
Live-virus vaccines: May increase risk of vaccine-induced adverse reactions. Avoid concomitant use.
Oxygen: May increase risk of pulmonary toxicity due to increased sensitization of lung tissue from bleomycin. Use together cautiously.

EFFECTS ON LAB TEST RESULTS
• May increase uric acid level.

CONTRAINDICATIONS & CAUTIONS
• Contraindicated in patients hypersensitive to drug.
• Severe idiosyncratic reactions can occur (hypotension, mental confusion, fever, chills, wheezing), usually after first or second dose. Monitor patient carefully.
• Use cautiously in patients with renal or pulmonary impairment.
Dialyzable drug: Unknown.

PREGNANCY-LACTATION-REPRODUCTION
• Drug can cause fetal harm when administered to pregnant women. If used during pregnancy, or if patient becomes pregnant while receiving drug, apprise patient of the potential hazard to the fetus.
• Women of childbearing potential should avoid becoming pregnant during therapy.
• It isn't known if drug appears in breast milk. Patient should discontinue breastfeeding during therapy.

NURSING CONSIDERATIONS
Black Box Warning Drug should be administered under the supervision of a physician experienced in the use of cancer chemotherapeutic agents. ∎
• Pulmonary toxicities are common. Obtain pulmonary function tests. If tests show a marked decline, stop drug.
Black Box Warning Fatal pulmonary fibrosis may occur, especially when cumulative dose exceeds 400 units. ∎
Black Box Warning Monitor lymphoma patient for idiosyncratic reaction (hypotension, confusion, fever, chills, wheezing) after receiving drug. ∎
⚡ *Alert:* Adverse pulmonary reactions are more common in patients older than age 70. Also, in patients receiving radiation therapy, patients with lung disease, and patients who need oxygen therapy, pulmonary toxic adverse effects may be increased.
• Monitor chest X-ray and listen to lungs regularly.
• Watch for fever, which may be treated with antipyretics. Fever usually occurs within 3 to 6 hours of administration.
⚡ *Alert:* Watch for hypersensitivity reactions, which may be delayed for several hours, especially in patients with lymphoma. (Give test dose of 1 to 2 units before first two doses in patients with lymphoma. If no reaction occurs, follow regular dosage schedule.)

Reactions in bold italics are *life-threatening*. Interactions may have a *rapid onset* or a *delayed onset*.

PATIENT TEACHING

• Warn patient that hair loss may occur but is usually reversible.

• Tell patient to report adverse reactions promptly and to take infection-control and bleeding precautions.

• For patient who is to receive anesthesia, tell him to inform anesthesiologist that he has taken this drug. High oxygen levels inhaled during surgery may enhance pulmonary toxicity of drug.

SAFETY ALERT!

bortezomib
bore-TEZ-uh-mib

Velcade

Therapeutic class: Antineoplastics
Pharmacologic class: Proteasome inhibitors

AVAILABLE FORMS
Powder for injection: 3.5 mg

INDICATIONS & DOSAGES

Adjust-a-dose (for all indications): If patient has moderate to severe hepatic dysfunction with bilirubin level greater than 1.5 to $3 \times$ ULN, reduce dosage of first cycle to 0.7 mg/m^2. If patient tolerates this dosage, may increase to 1 mg/m^2 in subsequent cycles. Based on tolerability, dosage may be reduced to 0.5 mg/m^2.

➤ **Previously untreated multiple myeloma**

Adults: 1.3 mg/m^2 I.V. over 3 to 5 seconds or subcutaneously in combination with oral melphalan and oral prednisone for nine 6-week treatment cycles. In cycles 1 to 4, bortezomib is given twice weekly (days 1, 4, 8, 11, 22, 25, 29, and 32). In cycles 5 to 9, bortezomib is given once weekly (days 1, 8, 22, and 29). Separate consecutive doses of drug by at least 72 hours. Prior to initiating any cycle, platelet count should be $70 \times 10^9/L$ or greater, ANC should be $1 \times 10^9/L$ or greater, and nonhematologic toxicities should have resolved to grade 1 or baseline.

Adjust-a-dose: If prolonged grade 4 neutropenia or thrombocytopenia, or thrombocytopenia with bleeding in previous cycle, consider reducing melphalan dose by 25% for next cycle. If platelet count is less than or equal to $30 \times 10^9/L$ or ANC is $0.75 \times 10^9/L$ or less on a day other than day 1, withhold bortezomib dose. If several bortezomib doses in consecutive cycles are withheld due to toxicity, reduce dose by one dose level (from 1.3 mg/m^2 to 1 mg/m^2, or from 1 mg/m^2 to 0.7 mg/m^2). For grade 3 nonhematologic toxicities, withhold drug until symptoms are grade 1 or baseline, then restart with one dose level reduction. If patient has neuropathic pain, peripheral neuropathy, or both, see the table that follows.

➤ **Previously untreated mantle cell lymphoma**

Adults: 1.3 mg/m^2 I.V. over 3 to 5 seconds in combination with I.V. rituximab, cyclophosphamide, doxorubicin, and oral prednisone for six 3-week treatment cycles. Bortezomib is administered followed by rituximab. In cycles 1 and 2, bortezomib is given twice weekly (days 1, 4, 8, 11) followed by 10-day rest period on days 12 to 21. Patients who respond at cycle 6 should receive two additional cycles for a total of 8 cycles. Separate consecutive doses of drug by at least 72 hours. Before initiating any cycle other than cycle 1, platelet count should be $100 \times 10^9/L$ or greater, ANC should be $1.5 \times 10^9/L$ or greater, Hb level should be at least 8 g/dL or greater, and nonhematologic toxicities should have resolved to grade 1 or baseline.

Adjust-a-dose: For grade 3 neutropenia or platelet count less than $25 \times 10^9/L$, withhold bortezomib for up to 2 weeks until ANC is $0.75 \times 10^9/L$ or greater and platelet count is $25 \times 10^9/L$ or greater. If the toxicity doesn't resolve, discontinue bortezomib. If ANC is $0.75 \times 10^9/L$ or greater and platelet count is $25 \times 10^9/L$ or greater, decrease bortezomib dose by one dose level (from 1.3 mg/m^2 to 1 mg/m^2, or from 1 mg/m^2 to 0.7 mg/m^2). For grade 3 or greater nonhematologic toxicities, withhold drug until symptoms are grade 2 or better, then restart with one dose level reduction. If patient has neuropathic pain, peripheral neuropathy, or both, see table.

➤ **Multiple myeloma or mantle cell lymphoma that still progresses after at least one therapy**

Adults: 1.3 mg/m^2 by I.V. bolus or subcutaneously twice weekly for 2 weeks (days 1, 4, 8, and 11), followed by a 10-day rest period (days 12 through 21). This 3-week period is a treatment cycle. For therapy longer than eight cycles, may adjust dosage schedule to once weekly for 4 weeks on days 1, 8, 15, and 22, followed by a rest period on days 23 through 35. Separate consecutive doses of drug by at least 72 hours.

Adjust-a-dose: If grade 3 nonhematologic or grade 4 hematologic toxicity (excluding neuropathy) develops, withhold drug. When toxicity has resolved, restart at a 25% reduced dose. If patient has neuropathic pain, peripheral neuropathy, or both, see table.

Severity of neuropathy	Dosage
Grade 1 (asymptomatic; paresthesia, loss of reflexes, or both) without pain or loss of function	No change.
Grade 1 with pain or grade 2 (moderate symptoms limiting activities of daily living [ADLs])	Reduce to 1 mg/m^2.
Grade 2 with pain or grade 3 (severe symptoms with interference with ADLs)	Hold drug until toxicity resolves; then start at 0.7 mg/m^2 once weekly.
Grade 4 (life-threatening consequences; urgent intervention indicated)	Stop drug.

ADMINISTRATION

I.V.

▼ Use caution and aseptic technique when preparing and handling drug. Wear gloves and protective clothing to prevent skin contact.

▼ Reconstitute with 3.5 mL of NSS and give by I.V. bolus over 3 to 5 seconds.

▼ Inspect solution before administration. Don't give if discolored or if particles are seen.

▼ Reconstituted drug may be stored in a syringe at 59° to 86° F (15° to 30° C); total storage time must not exceed 8 hours.

▼ Store unopened vial at a controlled room temperature, in original packaging, protected from light.

▼ Drug is considered a hazardous agent. Use appropriate precautions for handling and disposal.

▼ **Incompatibilities:** None reported.

Subcutaneous

● Give at concentration of 2.5 mg/mL.

● Rotate injection sites. New injections should be given at least 1 inch (2.54 cm) from an old site and never in areas that are tender, bruised, reddened, or hard.

● If injection-site reactions occur, a less concentrated solution (1 mg/mL) may be used.

ACTION

Disrupts intracellular homeostatic mechanisms by inhibiting the 26S proteasome, which regulates intracellular levels of certain proteins, causing cells to die.

Route	Onset	Peak	Duration
I.V.	Unknown	Unknown	Unknown
Subcut.	Unknown	Unknown	Unknown

Half-life: 40 to 193 hours (1-mg/m^2 dose); 76 to 108 hours (1.3-mg/m^2 dose).

ADVERSE REACTIONS

CNS: anxiety, asthenia, dizziness, dysesthesia, fatigue, fever, headache, insomnia, paresthesia, peripheral neuropathy, rigors, pyrexia.
CV: edema, hypotension.
EENT: blurred vision.
GI: abdominal pain, constipation, decreased appetite, diarrhea, dysgeusia, dyspepsia, nausea, vomiting.
Hematologic: *neutropenia, thrombocytopenia,* anemia, leukopenia, lymphopenia.
Hepatic: *acute liver failure, hepatitis,* hyperbilirubinemia, increased liver enzyme levels.
Metabolic: anorexia.
Musculoskeletal: arthralgia, back pain, bone pain, limb pain, muscle cramps, myalgia.
Respiratory: cough, dyspnea, pneumonia, URI.
Skin: pruritus, rash.
Other: dehydration, herpes zoster.

INTERACTIONS

Drug-drug. *Antihypertensives:* May cause hypotension. Monitor patient's BP closely.

Reactions in bold italics are *life-threatening*. Interactions may have a *rapid onset* or a *delayed onset*.

Drugs linked to peripheral neuropathy, such as amiodarone, antivirals, isoniazid, nitrofurantoin, statins: May worsen neuropathy. Use together cautiously.

Drugs that prolong QT interval (antiarrhythmics [bretylium, disopyramide, dofetilide, procainamide, quinidine, sotalol], chlorpromazine, dolasetron, droperidol, mefloquine, mesoridazine, moxifloxacin, pentamidine, pimozide, tacrolimus, thioridazine, ziprasidone): May prolong QT interval and increase risk of life-threatening ventricular arrhythmias. Use together with caution.

Inhibitors or inducers of CYP3A4: May increase risk of toxicity or may reduce drug's effects. Monitor patient closely.

Oral antidiabetics: May cause hypoglycemia or hyperglycemia. Monitor glucose level closely.

Drug-herb. *St. John's wort:* May decrease bortezomib exposure. Avoid concomitant use.

EFFECTS ON LAB TEST RESULTS
- May decrease Hb level.
- May increase liver enzyme levels.
- May increase or decrease glucose level.
- May decrease neutrophil and platelet counts.

CONTRAINDICATIONS & CAUTIONS
- Contraindicated in patients hypersensitive to bortezomib, boron, or mannitol.
- Intrathecal administration is contraindicated.
- Use cautiously in patients with hepatic or renal impairment or with a history of syncope and in those who are dehydrated or receiving other drugs known to cause hypotension.

Dialyzable drug: Yes.

⚠ *Overdose S&S:* Symptomatic hypotension, thrombocytopenia.

PREGNANCY-LACTATION-REPRODUCTION
- There are no adequate and well-controlled studies in pregnant women. Drug may cause fetal harm. Use during pregnancy isn't recommended.
- Women of childbearing potential should avoid becoming pregnant and should use effective contraception during treatment.

- It isn't known if drug appears in breast milk. A decision should be made to discontinue breast-feeding or discontinue drug, taking into account importance of drug to the mother and risk to the infant.

NURSING CONSIDERATIONS
- Monitor for evidence of neuropathy, such as a burning sensation, hyperesthesia, hypoesthesia, paresthesia, discomfort, or neuropathic pain.
- Consider subcutaneous administration for patients at high risk for or with preexisting peripheral neuropathy.
- Monitor for signs and symptoms of tumor lysis syndrome (hyperuricemia, hyperkalemia, hyperphosphatemia, hypocalcemia, and acute renal failure).
- Watch carefully for adverse effects, especially in elderly patients.
- Be sure patient has an order for an antiemetic, antidiarrheal, or both to treat drug-induced nausea, vomiting, or diarrhea.
- Provide fluid and electrolyte replacement to prevent dehydration.
- To manage orthostatic hypotension, adjust antihypertensive dosage, maintain hydration status, and give mineralocorticoids and/or sympathomimetics.
- Dialysis may reduce drug level; give after dialysis.

🔆 *Alert:* Because thrombocytopenia is common, monitor patient's CBC and platelet counts carefully during treatment, before each dose, and especially on day 11.

PATIENT TEACHING
- Tell patient to notify prescriber about new or worsening peripheral neuropathy.
- Urge women to use effective contraception and not to breast-feed during treatment.
- Teach patient how to avoid dehydration, and stress the need to tell prescriber about dizziness, light-headedness, or fainting spells.
- Tell patient to use caution when driving or performing other hazardous activities because drug may cause fatigue, dizziness, faintness, light-headedness, and doubled or blurred vision.

bosentan
bow-SEN-tan

Tracleer

Therapeutic class: Vasodilators
Pharmacologic class: Endothelin-receptor antagonists

AVAILABLE FORMS
Tablets: 62.5 mg, 125 mg

INDICATIONS & DOSAGES
Black Box Warning Only prescribers and pharmacies registered with the Tracleer REMS Program (call 1-866-228-3546, option 1) may prescribe and distribute bosentan. ∎
➤ **Pulmonary arterial hypertension in patients with World Health Organization class III (with mild exertion) or IV (at rest) symptoms, to improve exercise ability and decrease rate of clinical worsening**
Adults: 62.5 mg P.O. b.i.d., in the morning and evening, for 4 weeks. If patient weighs 40 kg or more, increase to maintenance dosage of 125 mg P.O. b.i.d. in the morning and evening. If patient weighs less than 40 kg, maintenance dosage is 62.5 mg P.O. b.i.d.
Adjust-a-dose: For patients who develop ALT and AST abnormalities, dosage may need to be decreased or therapy stopped until ALT and AST levels return to normal. If therapy is resumed, begin with initial dose. Test levels within 3 days; then give using the following table. If liver function abnormalities are accompanied by symptoms of liver injury or if bilirubin level is at least 2 × ULN, stop treatment and don't restart. In patients who weigh less than 40 kg, the initial and maintenance dosage is 62.5 mg b.i.d.

ALT and AST levels	Treatment and monitoring recommendations
>3 and ≤5 × ULN	Confirm with repeat test; if confirmed, reduce dose to 62.5 mg b.i.d. or interrupt treatment and retest every 2 weeks. Once ALT and AST levels return to pretreatment levels, continue or reintroduce treatment at starting dose. If bosentan is reintroduced, it should be at the starting dose. Check aminotransferase levels within 3 days and thereafter at least every 2 weeks.
>5 and ≤8 × ULN	Confirm with repeat test; if confirmed, stop treatment and retest at least every 2 weeks. Once levels return to pretreatment levels, consider reintroduction of treatment.
>8 × ULN	Stop treatment; don't restart drug.

Discontinue bosentan at least 36 hours before starting ritonavir. After at least 10 days following the initiation of ritonavir, resume bosentan at 62.5 mg P.O. once daily or every other day.

ADMINISTRATION
P.O.
● Give drug in morning and evening without regard for meals.

ACTION
Specific and competitive antagonist for endothelin-1 (ET-1). ET-1 levels are elevated in patients with pulmonary arterial hypertension, suggesting a pathogenic role for ET-1 in this disease.

Route	Onset	Peak	Duration
P.O.	Unknown	3–5 hr	Unknown

Half-life: About 5 hours.

ADVERSE REACTIONS
CNS: headache, fatigue, syncope.
CV: edema, flushing, hypotension, palpitations, chest pain.
EENT: sinusitis.
Hematologic: anemia.
Hepatic: *hepatotoxicity.*
Musculoskeletal: arthralgia.
Respiratory: respiratory tract infection.

Reactions in bold italics are *life-threatening*. Interactions may have a *rapid onset* or a *delayed onset*.

B

INTERACTIONS
Drug-drug. *Clarithromycin:* May increase risk of bosentan hepatotoxicity. Monitor patient closely. Stop one or both drugs if an interaction is suspected.

Cyclosporine: May increase bosentan level and decrease cyclosporine level. Use together is contraindicated.

Glyburide: May increase risk of elevated LFT values and decrease levels of both drugs. Use together is contraindicated.

Hormonal contraceptives: May cause contraceptive failure. Patient should use two reliable methods of birth control.

Ketoconazole: May increase bosentan effect. Watch for adverse effects.

PDE5 inhibitors (sildenafil): May increase bosentan level and decrease sildenafil level. Use together with caution.

Rifampin: May alter bosentan level. Monitor hepatic function weekly for 4 weeks followed by routine monitoring.

Ritonavir: May increase risk of bosentan toxicity. Dosage adjustment may be needed. Discontinue bosentan at least 36 hours before start of ritonavir; at least 10 days after ritonavir start, resume bosentan at 62.5 mg once daily or every other day based on tolerability. If receiving ritonavir for at least 10 days, start bosentan at 62.5 mg once daily or every other day based on tolerability.

Simvastatin, other statins: May decrease levels of these drugs. Monitor cholesterol levels to assess need to adjust statin dose.

Tacrolimus: May increase bosentan levels. Use together cautiously.

Warfarin: May decrease warfarin level. Monitor coagulation tests and adjust warfarin dosage as needed.

EFFECTS ON LAB TEST RESULTS
Black Box Warning May increase AST, ALT, and bilirubin levels. ∎
• May decrease Hb level and hematocrit.

CONTRAINDICATIONS & CAUTIONS
• Contraindicated in patients hypersensitive to drug and in those taking cyclosporine or glyburide.

Black Box Warning Generally avoid using in patients with moderate to severe hepatic impairment or in those with elevated aminotransferase levels greater than 3 × ULN. ∎

• Use cautiously in patients with mild hepatic impairment.

• Safety and effectiveness in children haven't been established.

Dialyzable drug: Unlikely.

⚠ **Overdose S&S:** Headache, nausea, vomiting, hypotension, dizziness, blurred vision.

PREGNANCY-LACTATION-REPRODUCTION
Black Box Warning Drug is likely to cause major birth defects. Contraindicated in pregnant women. Exclude pregnancy before giving drug. Monthly pregnancy test must be obtained. ∎

Black Box Warning Females of childbearing potential must use two reliable methods of contraception during treatment unless they have a tubal sterilization, a Copper T 380A intrauterine device (IUD), or levonorgestrel 20 mcg/day intrauterine system (IUS); in these instances, no additional contraception is needed. Ensure contraception is continued until 1 month after completion of bosentan therapy. ∎

Black Box Warning There is a possibility of contraception failure when bosentan is administered with hormonal contraceptives; patient shouldn't use hormonal contraceptives alone when taking bosentan. ∎

• Decreased sperm counts have been observed in patients receiving drug.

• It isn't known if drug appears in breast milk. Use isn't recommended in breast-feeding women.

NURSING CONSIDERATIONS
Black Box Warning Use of this drug can cause serious liver injury. AST and ALT level elevations may be dose dependent and reversible, so measure these levels before treatment and monthly thereafter, adjusting dosage accordingly. If elevations are accompanied by symptoms of liver injury (nausea, vomiting, fever, abdominal pain, jaundice, or unusual lethargy or fatigue) or if bilirubin level increases by greater than 2 × ULN, discontinue drug and notify prescriber immediately. ∎

• Fluid retention and HF may occur. Patient may require diuretics, fluid management, or hospitalization for decompensating HF.

• Monitor Hb level after 1 and 3 months of therapy; then every 3 months.
• Gradually reduce dosage before stopping drug.

PATIENT TEACHING
• Advise patient to take doses in the morning and evening, with or without food.
Black Box Warning Warn patient to avoid becoming pregnant while taking this drug. Hormonal contraceptives, including oral, implantable, and injectable methods, may not be effective when used with this drug. Advise patient to use two acceptable methods of contraception during and for 1 month after treatment with bosentan. A monthly pregnancy test must be performed. ∎
• Tell women who have had tubal ligation or have Copper T 380A IUD or levonorgestrel 20 IUS that they can use those contraceptive methods alone.
• Inform male patients of risk of low sperm count.
• Advise patient to have LFTs and blood counts performed regularly.

SAFETY ALERT!

brentuximab vedotin
bren-TUX-eh-mab

Adcetris

Therapeutic class: Antineoplastics
Pharmacologic class: Antibodies

AVAILABLE FORMS
Powder for injection: 50-mg single-use vial

INDICATIONS & DOSAGES
Adjust-a-dose (for all indications): For severe renal impairment (CrCl less than 30 mL/minute), avoid use. For mild hepatic impairment (Child-Pugh class A), decrease starting dose to 1.2 mg/kg with a maximum dose of 120 mg. For moderate or severe hepatic impairment (Child-Pugh class B or C), avoid use. In patients with new or worsening grade 2 or 3 neuropathy, withhold dose until neuropathy improves to grade 1 or baseline; then restart at 1.2 mg/kg. For patients with grade 4 neuropathy, discontinue drug. For patients with grade 3 or 4 neutropenia,

withhold dose until resolution to baseline or grade 2 or lower. Consider the use of granulocyte-colony factor stimulating factor (G-CSF) for subsequent cycles in patients with grade 3 or 4 neutropenia. For recurrent grade 4 neutropenia despite the use of G-CSF, discontinue drug or reduce dosage to 1.2 mg/kg.

➤ **Classic Hodgkin lymphoma in patients at high risk for relapse or progression after autologous hematopoietic stem cell transplantation (auto-HSCT) consolidation**
Adults: 1.8 mg/kg I.V. infusion over 30 minutes every 3 weeks in 4 to 6 weeks after auto-HSCT or upon recovery from auto-HSCT for a maximum of 16 cycles or until patient exhibits signs of disease progression or toxicities. Maximum dose is 180 mg.

➤ **Hodgkin lymphoma after failure of auto-HSCT or after failure of at least two multiagent chemotherapy regimens in patients who aren't auto-HSCT candidates; systemic anaplastic large cell lymphoma after failure of at least one multiagent chemotherapy regimen**
Adults: 1.8 mg/kg I.V. infusion over 30 minutes every 3 weeks, or until patient exhibits signs of disease progression or toxicities. Maximum dose is 180 mg.

ADMINISTRATION
I.V.
▼ Drug is considered hazardous; use safe handling and disposal precautions.
▼ Reconstitute each 50-mg vial with 10.5 mL sterile water for injection to yield a single-use solution containing 5 mg/mL.
▼ Gently swirl contents; don't shake vial. Inspect for particulates and discoloration.
▼ Dilute further to yield 0.4 to 1.8 mg/mL in infusion bag of NSS injection, 5% dextrose injection, or lactated Ringer injection. Gently mix by inverting bag.
▼ After reconstitution, infuse immediately or store at 36° to 46° F (2° to 8° C) and use within 24 hours of reconstitution. Don't freeze. Discard unused portion left in vial.
▼ Administer drug only by I.V. infusion over 30 minutes; don't give by I.V. push or bolus.

Reactions in bold italics are *life-threatening*. Interactions may have a *rapid onset* or a ***delayed onset***.

▼ **Incompatibilities:** Don't mix or administer drug with other medications or fluids.

ACTION

Disrupts microtubule network of the cancer cell, which induces cell-cycle arrest and apoptotic death of the cells.

Route	Onset	Peak	Duration
I.V.	Rapid	1–3 days	Unknown

Half-life: 4 to 6 days.

ADVERSE REACTIONS

CNS: peripheral neuropathy (sensory, motor), headache, dizziness, fatigue, pyrexia, chills, insomnia, anxiety, pain, fever.
CV: peripheral edema, *PE, supraventricular arrhythmia,* lymphadenopathy.
EENT: oropharyngeal pain.
GI: nausea, diarrhea, abdominal pain, vomiting, constipation, decreased appetite.
GU: pyelonephritis, UTI.
Hematologic: *neutropenia,* anemia, *thrombocytopenia.*
Metabolic: decreased weight.
Musculoskeletal: arthralgia, myalgia, back pain, extremity pain, muscle spasms.
Respiratory: URI, cough, dyspnea, pneumonitis, pneumothorax.
Skin: rash, pruritus, alopecia, night sweats, dry skin, xeroderma.
Other: *septic shock, anaphylaxis,* immunogenicity.

INTERACTIONS

Drug-drug. *Bleomycin:* May increase risk of pulmonary toxicity. Concomitant use is contraindicated.
Inactivated-virus vaccines: Drug may diminish the therapeutic effect of vaccines. Complete all age-appropriate vaccinations at least 2 weeks before drug initiation. If patient is vaccinated during therapy, revaccinate at least 3 months after immunosuppressant is discontinued. Consider therapy modification.
Live-virus vaccines: Drug may enhance the adverse or toxic effects of vaccines. Avoid combination.

Strong CYP3A4 inducers (rifampin): May decrease brentuximab level. Monitor patient for brentuximab effectiveness.
Strong CYP3A4 inhibitors (ketoconazole): May increase brentuximab level. Monitor patient for increased adverse effects.

EFFECTS ON LAB TEST RESULTS

• May decrease RBC, WBC, platelet, and neutrophil counts.

CONTRAINDICATIONS & CAUTIONS

• Contraindicated in patients hypersensitive to drug.
Black Box Warning John Cunningham (JC) virus infection resulting in progressive multifocal leukoencephalopathy (PML) and death can occur in patients receiving brentuximab. ◼
◐ **Alert:** Infusion-related reactions, including anaphylaxis, have occurred. If anaphylaxis occurs, discontinue drug immediately and permanently and initiate appropriate therapy. Interrupt infusion for other infusion-related reactions and treat appropriately. Patients with prior infusion-related reactions should be premedicated (acetaminophen, antihistamine, corticosteroid) for subsequent infusions.
• Avoid use in patients with severe renal impairment or moderate or severe hepatic impairment due to increased risk of grade 3 or greater adverse events.
• Serious infections (pneumonia, bacteremia, sepsis, fatal septic shock) have been reported.
Dialyzable drug: Unknown.

PREGNANCY-LACTATION-REPRODUCTION

• Drug may cause fetal harm if administered during pregnancy. Women of childbearing potential should avoid pregnancy during and for 6 months after therapy ends.
• Drug may damage spermatozoa and testicular tissue, resulting in possible genetic abnormalities. Males with female sexual partners of childbearing potential should use effective contraception during therapy and for 6 months after therapy ends.
• It isn't known if drug appears in breast milk. Breast-feeding isn't recommended during treatment.

NURSING CONSIDERATIONS
• Drug may cause severe peripheral neuropathy. Monitor patient for new or worsening signs and symptoms.
• Drug may cause hepatotoxicity, which can be fatal, especially in patients with preexisting liver disease or elevated baseline liver enzymes and in those taking concomitant medications. Monitor liver enzymes and bilirubin. Delay or reduce dose, or discontinue drug as clinically indicated for new, worsening, or recurrent hepatotoxicity.
• Monitor patient closely for infusion-related adverse effects; interrupt therapy and treat as necessary.
• Monitor patient for signs and symptoms of neutropenia. Monitor CBC before each dose, and more frequently if patient exhibits grade 3 or 4 neutropenia. Delay or reduce dose, or discontinue drug as required.
• Monitor patient for tumor lysis syndrome, characterized by changes in electrolytes and kidney damage.
• Monitor patient for skin reactions, especially Stevens-Johnson syndrome. Discontinue drug if reactions occur.
• Monitor patient for vision loss, impaired speech, muscle weakness or paralysis, and cognitive deterioration, which may indicate PML. Hold drug for suspected PML and discontinue if diagnosis is confirmed.
• Monitor patient for noninfectious pulmonary toxicity (pneumonitis, interstitial lung disease, acute respiratory distress syndrome). Hold drug during evaluation of new or worsening pulmonary symptoms and until symptoms improve.
• Monitor patient for infection (bacterial, fungal, or viral) during treatment.

PATIENT TEACHING
• Tell patient to report muscle weakness or numbness or tingling of the hands or feet.
• Advise patient to report signs or symptoms of possible infection, including temperature of 100.5° F (38° C) or greater, chills, cough, or pain on urination.
• Warn patient to report signs or symptoms of possible infusion-related reactions, including fever, chills, rash, or breathing problems (wheezing, cough, chest tightness), blue skin color, and swelling of the face, lips, tongue or throat.

• Caution female patient to avoid becoming pregnant and not to breast-feed during and for 6 months after therapy ends. Tell her to report possible pregnancy immediately.
• Caution male patient with female partner of childbearing potential to use effective contraception during and for 6 months after therapy ends.

brexpiprazole
brex-PIP-ra-zole

Rexulti

Therapeutic class: Antipsychotics
Pharmacologic class: Atypical antipsychotics

AVAILABLE FORMS
Tablets: 0.25 mg, 0.5 mg, 1 mg, 2 mg, 3 mg, 4 mg

INDICATIONS & DOSAGES
Adjust-a-dose (for all indications): If patient is also taking a strong or moderate CYP2D6 inhibitor and a strong CYP3A4 inhibitor, give one-quarter usual dose. If patient is also taking a strong CYP3A4 inducer, double usual dose over 1 to 2 weeks. For patient who is a poor CYP2D6 metabolizer, decrease dose by one-half. If the CYP2D6 poor metabolizer patient is also taking a strong or moderate CYP3A4 inhibitor, give one-quarter of usual dose. If discontinuing a coadministered CYP2D6 or CYP3A4 inhibitor, adjust brexpiprazole to original dosage. If a CYP3A4 inducer is being discontinued, reduce brexpiprazole to original dosage over 1 to 2 weeks.
➤ **Adjunctive treatment of major depressive disorder**
Adults: Initially, 0.5 or 1 mg P.O. once daily. If starting at 0.5 mg, increase to 1 mg P.O. once daily after 1 week based on patient's response and tolerability. Then, increase to target dose of 2 mg P.O. once daily after 1 week. Maximum daily dose is 3 mg.
Adjust-a-dose: For patients also taking strong CYP3A4 inhibitors, give one-half usual dose. For patients with moderate to severe hepatic impairment (Child-Pugh score 7 or greater), maximum recommended

---

Reactions in bold italics are *life-threatening*. Interactions may have a *rapid onset* or a *delayed onset*.

dose is 2 mg P.O. once daily. For patients with moderate, severe, or end-stage renal impairment (CrCl less than 60 mL/minute), recommended maximum dose is 2 mg P.O. once daily.

➤ Schizophrenia

Adults: Initially, 1 mg P.O. once daily on days 1 through 4; then titrate to 2 mg P.O. once daily on days 5 through 7; then increase to 4 mg P.O. once daily on day 8 based on patient's response and tolerability. Recommended target dose is 2 to 4 mg daily. Maximum daily dose is 4 mg.

Adjust-a-dose: For patients also taking strong CYP2D6 inhibitors or strong CYP3A4 inhibitors, give one-half usual dose. For patients with moderate to severe hepatic impairment (Child-Pugh score 7 or more), maximum recommended dose is 3 mg P.O. once daily. For patients with moderate, severe, or end-stage renal impairment (CrCl less than 60 mL/minute), recommended maximum dose is 3 mg P.O. once daily.

ADMINISTRATION
P.O.
● Give without regard for food.
● If a dose is missed, give as soon as possible. If it's close to the time for next dose, skip missed dose and give next dose at the regular time. Don't double-dose.
● Store at 68° to 77° F (20° to 25° C).

ACTION
Exact mechanism unknown. Its effect may occur through partial agonist activity at serotonin 5-HT$_{1A}$ and dopamine D$_2$ receptors, as well as antagonist activity at serotonin 5-HT$_{2A}$ receptors.

Route	Onset	Peak	Duration
P.O.	Unknown	4 hr	Unknown

Half-life: 91 hours.

ADVERSE REACTIONS
CNS: fatigue, drowsiness, akathisia, headache, tremor, dizziness, anxiety, restlessness, somnolence, sedation, abnormal dreams, insomnia, extrapyramidal reactions.
EENT: blurred vision, nasopharyngitis, dry mouth, sialorrhea.

GI: constipation, dyspepsia, diarrhea, nausea, abdominal pain, flatulence.
GU: UTI.
Metabolic: weight gain, increased appetite.
Musculoskeletal: myalgia.

INTERACTIONS
Drug-drug. *Anticholinergics (diphenhydramine, meclizine, scopolamine):* May increase risk of body temperature dysregulation. Use together cautiously.
CNS depressants: May increase CNS depressant effects. Monitor therapy.
Strong CYP2D6 inhibitors (bupropion, fluoxetine, paroxetine, quinidine), strong CYP3A4 inhibitors (clarithromycin, itraconazole, ketoconazole, ritonavir): May increase brexpiprazole concentration. Reduce brexpiprazole dosage.
Strong CYP3A4 inducers (carbamazepine, phenytoin, rifampin): May decrease brexpiprazole concentration. Increase brexpiprazole dosage.
Drug-herb. *St. John's wort:* May decrease brexpiprazole concentration. Increase brexpiprazole dosage.
Drug-food. *Grapefruit juice:* May increase brexpiprazole concentration. Avoid use together.

EFFECTS ON LAB TEST RESULTS
● May increase CK, cortisol, triglyceride, and prolactin levels.
● May decrease WBC count.

CONTRAINDICATIONS & CAUTIONS
● Contraindicated in patients hypersensitive to drug or its components.
Black Box Warning Elderly patients with dementia-related psychosis treated with antipsychotics are at increased risk for death. Drug isn't approved for treatment of patients with dementia-related psychosis. ■
Black Box Warning Antidepressants have increased the risk of suicidal thoughts and behaviors in patients younger than age 24. Safety and effectiveness in children haven't been studied. ■
● Antipsychotics can cause neuroleptic malignant syndrome (NMS), which can be fatal.
● Antipsychotics can cause tardive dyskinesia, especially in elderly patients, most

notably elderly women, and may be irreversible.

• Atypical antipsychotics are associated with metabolic changes, such as weight gain, dyslipidemia, hyperglycemia, and diabetes.

• Antipsychotics may increase the risk of seizures. Use cautiously in patients with a history of seizures or conditions that could lower the seizure threshold.

• Drug may alter the body's ability to lower the core temperature.

• Use cautiously in patients who are poor metabolizers of CYP2D6, in patients with moderate to severe hepatic impairment (Child-Pugh score of 7 or more), and in those with moderate, severe, or end-stage renal impairment (CrCl less than 60 mL/minute); adjust dosage appropriately.

• Use cautiously in patients with preexisting hypotension or who are taking other antihypertensives; drug can cause orthostatic hypotension or syncope.

• Use cautiously in patients at risk for aspiration pneumonia. Esophageal dysmotility and aspiration have been associated with antipsychotic use.

• Antipsychotics can impair thinking, judgment, and motor skills.

• Tablets may contain lactose; avoid use in patients with lactose-intolerant conditions.

• Use cautiously in elderly patients because of the increased risk of adverse events.

Dialyzable drug: Unlikely.

PREGNANCY-LACTATION-REPRODUCTION

• There are no adequate studies in pregnant women. Neonates exposed to antipsychotics during the third trimester are at risk for extrapyramidal or withdrawal signs and symptoms, which can vary in severity but may require prolonged hospitalization. Routine use during pregnancy isn't recommended; risk and benefits should be considered.

• Women exposed to drug during pregnancy should be enrolled in the National Pregnancy Registry for Atypical Antipsychotics (1-866-961-2388).

• It's unknown if drug appears in breast milk. Consider risks and benefits before using in breast-feeding women.

NURSING CONSIDERATIONS

• Monitor patients for suicidal thoughts or behaviors, especially during the first few months of treatment and after dosage changes. Consider discontinuing drug in patients whose depression worsens or who experience suicidal thoughts or behaviors.

• Monitor patients for signs and symptoms of NMS (hyperpyrexia, muscle rigidity, change in mental status, tachycardia, change in BP or pulse, diaphoresis, arrhythmias, elevated CK level, rhabdomyolysis, acute renal failure). Discontinue drug if reactions appear, and treat appropriately.

• Monitor blood glucose, triglyceride, and lipid levels; observe for weight changes.

• Monitor patients for seizures, difficulty swallowing, and aspiration.

• Monitor patients with diabetes regularly for worsening of glucose control.

• Monitor patients at risk for diabetes (obesity, family history) before and periodically during treatment.

• Avoid exposing patients to extreme heat; make sure they are well hydrated.

• Monitor patients for tardive dyskinesia (involuntary, dyskinetic movements). Reassess need for continued treatment periodically. If tardive dyskinesia develops, consider discontinuing drug.

• Monitor patients with a history of significantly low WBC count or ANC or drug-induced neutropenia frequently during first few months of therapy. Consider discontinuing drug at first sign of significant decline in WBC count; monitor patients for fever or other signs or symptoms of infection. Discontinue drug in patients with severe neutropenia (ANC less than $1,000/mm^3$).

• Monitor patients for orthostatic hypotension and syncope. Patients at increased risk include those with dehydration, hypovolemia, history of CV disease (HF, MI, ischemia, conduction abnormalities), or history of cerebrovascular disease, those taking antihypertensives, and patients who are antipsychotic-naive. Lower starting dose and slower titration may be needed in these patients.

• Check with pharmacist regarding potential interactions with other drugs that are metabolized via the CYP450 enzyme system in the liver.

Reactions in bold italics are *life-threatening*. Interactions may have a *rapid onset* or a *delayed onset*.

• *Look alike–sound alike:* Don't confuse Rexulti with Maxalt.

PATIENT TEACHING

🕄 *Alert:* Counsel family members or caregivers to monitor for changes in behavior and to immediately report suicidal thoughts or behaviors to prescriber.

• Explain the potential for dystonic or extrapyramidal symptoms (involuntary, abnormal movements). Instruct patient to immediately report symptoms to prescriber.

• Teach diabetic patient to monitor blood glucose level closely and to report changes in glucose level.

• Advise patient to report lactose intolerance before starting therapy.

• Educate patient about the risk of metabolic changes, how to recognize hyperglycemia, and the need for blood tests for glucose and lipid levels. Encourage patient to report weight gain.

• Caution patient about risk of orthostatic hypotension and syncope, especially at start of therapy and with dosage changes.

• Advise female patient to contact prescriber immediately if she is or plans to become pregnant or is breast-feeding.

• Remind patient to avoid strenuous exercise, dehydration, or exposure to extreme heat. Encourage patient to drink plenty of water while taking drug.

• Instruct patient to report muscle rigidity, increased sweating, changes in BP, or irregular heartbeats.

• Warn patient about potential for drug interactions; advise him to report to prescriber all OTC drugs, prescription medications, and supplements being taken before start of therapy.

• Caution patient about risk of impaired judgment, thinking, or motor skills. Advise patient not to perform activities that require mental alertness, such as operating hazardous machinery, including motor vehicles, until drug's effects are known.

---

brimonidine tartrate
bri-MOE-ni-deen

Alphagan P, Mirvaso, Qoliana

Therapeutic class: Antiglaucoma drugs–dermatologic agents
Pharmacologic class: Selective alpha$_2$ agonists

AVAILABLE FORMS
Ophthalmic solution: 0.1%, 0.15%, 0.2%
Topical gel: 0.33%

INDICATIONS & DOSAGES
➤ **To reduce IOP in open-angle glaucoma or ocular hypertension**
Adults and children age 2 and older: 1 drop in affected eye t.i.d., about 8 hours apart.
➤ **Persistent erythema of rosacea**
Adults: Apply a pea-size amount to five areas of the face (central forehead, chin, nose, and each cheek) once daily.

ADMINISTRATION
Ophthalmic
• Don't touch tip of dropper to eye or surrounding tissue.
• If more than one ophthalmic product is being used, give them at least 5 minutes apart.
Topical
• Apply a thin layer across the entire face, avoiding the lips and eyes.
• Don't apply to open wounds or irritated skin.
• Wash hands after applying.

ACTION
Reduces aqueous humor production and increases uveoscleral outflow.

Route	Onset	Peak	Duration
Ophthalmic	Unknown	30 min–2½ hr	Unknown
Topical	Unknown	15 days	Unknown

Half-life: Ophthalmic, 2 hours; topical, unknown.

ADVERSE REACTIONS
CNS: asthenia, dizziness, headache, fatigue, somnolence.
CV: hypertension, hypotension.

EENT: allergic conjunctivitis, ocular hyperemia, pruritus, abnormal vision, allergic reaction, blepharitis, burning; conjunctival edema, hemorrhage, or inflammation; dryness, eyelid edema or erythema, follicular conjunctivitis, foreign body sensation, increased tearing, pain, pharyngitis, photophobia, rhinitis, sinus infection or inflammation, stinging, superficial punctate keratopathy, visual disturbances, visual field defect, vitreous floaters, worsened visual acuity, increased IOP (topical only).
GI: dyspepsia, oral dryness.
Metabolic: diabetes mellitus.
Musculoskeletal: arthralgia, arthritis, joint disorder, osteoporosis.
Respiratory: bronchitis, cough, dyspnea.
Skin: rash; acne rosacea, acne vulgaris, allergic contact dermatitis, dermatitis, erythema (topical only).
Other: flulike syndrome.

INTERACTIONS

Drug-drug. *Antihypertensives, beta blockers, cardiac glycosides:* May further decrease BP or pulse rate. Monitor vital signs.
Apraclonidine, dorzolamide, pilocarpine, timolol: May have additive IOP-lowering effects. Use cautiously together.
CNS depressants: May increase effects. Use cautiously together.
Linezolid, MAO inhibitors: May increase effects. Avoid using together.
TCAs: May interfere with brimonidine's effect. Use cautiously together.
Drug-lifestyle. *Alcohol use:* May increase CNS-depressant effect. Avoid alcohol.

EFFECTS ON LAB TEST RESULTS

• May increase cholesterol level.

CONTRAINDICATIONS & CAUTIONS

• Ophthalmic form is contraindicated in patients hypersensitive to drug or its components and in those taking MAO inhibitors.
• Use cautiously in patients with CV disease, cerebral or coronary insufficiency, hepatic or renal impairment, depression, Raynaud phenomenon, Sjögren syndrome, orthostatic hypotension, or thromboangiitis obliterans.
Dialyzable drug: Unknown.
⚠ **Overdose S&S:** Hypotension.

PREGNANCY-LACTATION-REPRODUCTION

• Use during pregnancy only if potential benefit justifies potential risk to the fetus.
• It isn't known if drug appears in breast milk. Consider discontinuing breast-feeding or discontinuing drug.

NURSING CONSIDERATIONS

• Monitor IOP because drug effect may reverse after first month of therapy.
• Intermittent flushing may occur after topical application and may resolve when therapy is discontinued.

PATIENT TEACHING

• Tell patient to wait at least 15 minutes after instilling ophthalmic drug before wearing soft contact lenses.
• Caution patient to avoid hazardous activities because of risk of decreased mental alertness, fatigue, or drowsiness.
• Advise patient to avoid alcohol.
• If patient is using more than one ophthalmic drug, tell him to apply them at least 5 minutes apart.
• Instruct patient how to apply topical form. Caution patient that topical form is for external use only and shouldn't be used orally, intravaginally, or in the eyes.

brivaracetam
See NEW DRUGS for information.

bromfenac sodium
BROM-fen-ak

Bromsite, Prolensa

Therapeutic class: Anti-inflammatory drugs (ophthalmic)
Pharmacologic class: NSAIDs

AVAILABLE FORMS
Ophthalmic solution: 0.07%, 0.075%, 0.09%

INDICATIONS & DOSAGES

➤ **Inflammation and pain after cataract surgery**
Adults: For generic solution, 1 drop in affected eye(s) b.i.d., starting 24 hours after surgery and continuing for 2 weeks. Or for Bromsite or Prolensa, 1 drop in affected

---

eye(s) once daily beginning 1 day before surgery, continued on the day of surgery and for the first 14 days after surgery.

ADMINISTRATION
Ophthalmic
• May give in conjunction with other topical ophthalmic medications. Give at least 5 minutes apart.
• After giving drop, have patient close his eyes and apply gentle pressure to lacrimal sac for 1 to 2 minutes.
• Don't touch tip of dropper to eye or surrounding tissue.

ACTION
Blocks prostaglandin synthesis by inhibiting cyclooxygenase 1 and 2.

Route	Onset	Peak	Duration
Ophthalmic	Unknown	Unknown	Unknown

Half-life: Unknown.

ADVERSE REACTIONS
EENT: abnormal sensation in the eye, burning, conjunctival hyperemia, eye irritation, eye pain, eye pruritus, eye redness, iritis, keratitis; anterior chamber inflammation, foreign body sensation, eye pain, photophobia, blurred vision.

INTERACTIONS
Topical corticosteroids: May delay wound healing. Monitor therapy.

EFFECTS ON LAB TEST RESULTS
• May prolong bleeding time.

CONTRAINDICATIONS & CAUTIONS
• Contraindicated in patients hypersensitive to drug or its components. Drug contains sulfite, which may cause allergic-type reactions, including anaphylaxis and life-threatening or less severe asthmatic episodes, in patients sensitive to sulfites.
• Use cautiously in patients with bleeding tendencies, those taking anticoagulants, and those sensitive to aspirin products, phenylacetic acid derivatives, and other NSAIDs.
• Use cautiously in patients who have had complicated or repeat ocular surgeries or those with corneal denervation, corneal epithelial defects, diabetes mellitus, oc-

ular surface diseases (such as dry-eye syndrome), or RA because of the increased risk of corneal adverse effects, which may threaten sight.
Dialyzable drug: Unknown.

PREGNANCY-LACTATION-REPRODUCTION
• Use in pregnant women only if potential benefit justifies risk to the fetus.
• Avoid use late in pregnancy because NSAIDs may cause premature closure of the ductus arteriosus.
• Use cautiously in breast-feeding women.

NURSING CONSIDERATIONS
• Ask patient if he's sensitive to sulfites, aspirin, or other NSAIDs before treatment. Drug contains sulfite, which may cause allergic-type reactions, including anaphylaxis and life-threatening or less severe asthmatic episodes, in patients sensitive to sulfites.
• Sulfite sensitivity is more common in patients with asthma than in those without asthma. If patient has asthma, monitor closely.
• If patient takes an anticoagulant or has known bleeding tendencies, watch closely for increased bleeding.
• Use for more than 24 hours before surgery and for longer than 2 weeks after surgery may increase risk of corneal adverse reactions.

PATIENT TEACHING
• Teach patient how to instill the drops.
• Instruct patient to take medication as prescribed.
• Tell patient not to use for longer than 2 weeks after surgery and not to save unused amount for other conditions.
• Tell patient the signs and symptoms of adverse effects. If bothersome or serious adverse effects occur, advise patient to stop therapy and contact prescriber.
• Tell patient to store drug at room temperature.
• Advise patient to remove contact lenses before instillation. Lenses may be reinserted after 10 minutes.

bromocriptine mesylate
broe-moe-KRIP-teen

Cycloset, Parlodel

Therapeutic class: Antiparkinsonian drugs
Pharmacologic class: Dopamine receptor agonists

AVAILABLE FORMS
Capsules: 5 mg
Tablets: 0.8 mg (Cycloset), 2.5 mg (Parlodel)

INDICATIONS & DOSAGES
➤ **Parkinson disease (not Cycloset)**
Adults: 1.25 mg P.O. b.i.d. with meals. Increase dosage by 2.5 mg/day every 14 to 28 days, up to 100 mg daily. Usual dose is 20 to 30 mg daily.
➤ **Amenorrhea and galactorrhea from hyperprolactinemia; hypogonadism, infertility (not Cycloset)**
Adults and adolescents age 16 and older: 1.25 to 2.5 mg P.O. daily, increased by 2.5 mg daily at 2- to 7-day intervals until desired effect occurs. Therapeutic daily dose is 2.5 to 15 mg.
Children ages 11 to 15: 1.25 to 2.5 mg P.O. daily. May increase as tolerated until therapeutic response is achieved. Range, 2.5 to 10 mg daily in children with prolactin-secreting pituitary adenomas.
➤ **Acromegaly (not Cycloset)**
Adults: 1.25 to 2.5 mg P.O. with bedtime snack for 3 days. Another 1.25 to 2.5 mg may be added every 3 to 7 days until therapeutic benefit occurs. Maximum, 100 mg daily.
➤ **Type 2 diabetes mellitus (Cycloset only)**
Adults: Initially, 0.8 mg P.O. daily within 2 hours after waking in the morning. May increase by 0.8 mg weekly until maximum tolerated dosage of 1.6 to 4.8 mg daily is achieved.
➤ **Traumatic brain injury ◆**
Adults: 2.5 mg P.O. daily. Continue long-term if response is adequate.

ADMINISTRATION
P.O.
● Give drug in the evening with food to minimize adverse reactions (except Cycloset).
● For treatment of type 2 diabetes mellitus, give Cycloset within 2 hours of patient's waking in the morning.

ACTION
Inhibits secretion of prolactin and acts as a dopamine receptor agonist by activating postsynaptic dopamine receptors; improves glycemic control.

Route	Onset	Peak	Duration
P.O.	2 hr	53–120 min	24 hr

Half-life: 5 hours (Parlodel); 6 hours (Cycloset).

ADVERSE REACTIONS
CNS: dizziness, headache, fatigue, *seizures,* **stroke,** mania, light-headedness, drowsiness, delusions, hallucinations, nervousness, insomnia, depression.
CV: orthostatic hypotension, *acute MI.*
EENT: nasal congestion, rhinitis, blurred vision.
GI: nausea, abdominal cramps, constipation, diarrhea, vomiting, anorexia.
GU: urine retention, urinary frequency.
Skin: coolness and pallor of fingers and toes.

INTERACTIONS
Drug-drug. *Amitriptyline, haloperidol, imipramine, loxapine, MAO inhibitors, methyldopa, phenothiazines, reserpine:* May interfere with bromocriptine's effects. Bromocriptine dosage may need to be increased.
Antihypertensives: May increase hypotensive effects. Adjust dosage of antihypertensive.
Chloramphenicol, probenecid, salicylates, sulfonamides: May increase unbound fraction of other highly protein-bound drugs. Monitor patient for increased adverse reactions.
CYP3A4 inhibitors or inducers: May increase or decrease circulating levels of Cycloset, respectively. Use together with caution. Limit Cycloset dose to 1.6 mg/day during concomitant use of moderate CYP3A4 inhibitors. Avoid

concomitant use with strong CYP3A4 inhibitors and ensure washout of the strong CYP3A4 inhibitor before initiating Cycloset.

Dopamine receptor antagonists (butyrophenones, phenothiazines, thioxanthenes): May diminish effects of Cycloset. Concurrent use isn't recommended.

Ergot-related drugs: May increase occurrence of ergot-related adverse effects and reduce effectiveness of these therapies. Avoid concomitant use.

Estrogens, hormonal contraceptives, progestins: May interfere with effects of bromocriptine. Avoid using together.

Levodopa: May have additive effects. Adjust dosage of levodopa, if needed.

Macrolides (erythromycin): May increase bromocriptine level and risk of adverse reactions. Use together cautiously.

Triptans (sumatriptan): May have additive vasoconstrictive effects. Concomitant use is contraindicated; don't use within 24 hours of one another.

Drug-lifestyle. *Alcohol use:* May enhance toxic or adverse effects of alcohol. Discourage use together.

EFFECTS ON LAB TEST RESULTS

● May increase alkaline phosphatase, ALT, AST, BUN, CK, and uric acid levels.

CONTRAINDICATIONS & CAUTIONS

● Contraindicated in patients hypersensitive to ergot derivatives and in those with uncontrolled hypertension, toxemia of pregnancy, severe ischemic heart disease, hereditary galactose intolerance, lactase deficiency, glucose-galactose malabsorption, or peripheral vascular disease.

● Cycloset is contraindicated in patients with syncopal migraines or severe psychotic disorders.

● Use cautiously in patients with impaired renal or hepatic function and in those with a history of MI with residual arrhythmias.

● Use cautiously in patients taking antihypertensives.

Dialyzable drug: Unknown.

⚠ **Overdose S&S:** Nausea, vomiting, constipation, diaphoresis, dizziness, pallor, severe hypotension, malaise, confusion, lethargy, drowsiness, delusions, hallucinations, repetitive yawning.

PREGNANCY-LACTATION-REPRODUCTION

● Drug should be discontinued immediately if pregnancy occurs and patient should be carefully observed throughout the pregnancy, including regular visual field checks, to monitor possible pituitary tumor expansion.

● If hypertensive disorder of pregnancy occurs, weigh benefit of Parolodel against risk. A decision should be made whether therapy continues to be medically necessary or can be withdrawn.

● Patient should use contraceptive methods other than oral contraceptives or subdermal implants during treatment.

● Drug may lead to early postpartum conception. After menses resumes, patient should be tested for pregnancy every 4 weeks or as soon as a period is missed.

● Drug shouldn't be used in breast-feeding women. Product labeling for Cycloset specifically contraindicates use in breast-feeding women.

NURSING CONSIDERATIONS

● For Parkinson disease, bromocriptine usually is given with levodopa or levodopa–carbidopa. The levodopa–carbidopa dosage may need to be reduced.

⊙ **Alert:** Monitor patient for adverse reactions, which occur in 68% of patients, particularly at start of therapy. Most reactions are mild to moderate; nausea is most common. Minimize adverse reactions by gradually adjusting dosages to effective levels. Adverse reactions are more common when drug is used for Parkinson disease.

● Baseline and periodic evaluations of cardiac, hepatic, renal, and hematopoietic function are recommended during prolonged therapy.

⊙ **Alert:** Prolactin-secreting adenomas in pregnant women may expand and compress the optic or other cranial nerves; emergency pituitary surgery may be necessary. Watch for signs and symptoms of cranial nerve compression.

● Drug can cause orthostatic hypotension and syncope, particularly at start of therapy or when dosage is increased. Assess

---

orthostatic vital signs before initiation of therapy and periodically thereafter.
● *Look alike–sound alike:* Don't confuse bromocriptine with benztropine or brimonidine. Don't confuse Parlodel with pindolol.

PATIENT TEACHING
● Instruct patient to take drug with meals.
● Tell patient to take Cycloset within 2 hours of waking in the morning.
● Advise patient to use contraceptive methods other than oral contraceptives or subdermal implants during treatment.
● Instruct patient to avoid dizziness and fainting by rising slowly to an upright position and avoiding sudden position changes.
● Inform patient that it may take 8 weeks or longer for menses to resume and excess production of milk to slow down.
● Advise patient to avoid alcohol while taking drug.
● Advise patients not to operate heavy machinery if somnolence occurs while taking Cycloset.

budesonide (inhalation; intranasal)
byoo-DES-oh-nide

Pulmicort Flexhaler, Pulmicort Respules, Pulmicort Turbuhaler❦, Rhinocort Allergy ◇, Rhinocort Aqua

Therapeutic class: Corticosteroids
Pharmacologic class: Corticosteroids

AVAILABLE FORMS
Dry powder inhaler: 90 mcg/dose, 100 mcg/dose❦, 180 mcg/dose, 200 mcg/dose❦, 400 mcg/dose❦
Inhalation suspension (Respules): 0.25 mg, 0.5 mg, 1 mg
Nasal spray: 32 mcg/metered spray

INDICATIONS & DOSAGES
➤ **As a preventative in maintenance of asthma**
All patients: Use lowest effective dose after stabilizing asthma.
Respules
Children ages 1 to 8 previously taking bronchodilator alone: 0.5 mg daily or 0.25 mg

b.i.d. suspension via jet nebulizer. Maximum dose is 0.5 mg daily.
Children ages 1 to 8 previously taking inhaled corticosteroid: 0.5 mg daily or 0.25 mg b.i.d. suspension via jet nebulizer to maximum dose of 1 mg/day.
Children ages 1 to 8 previously taking oral corticosteroid: 1 mg daily or 0.5 mg b.i.d. via jet nebulizer. Maximum dose is 0.5 mg/day.
Adjust-a-dose: Symptomatic children not responding to nonsteroidal therapy may require starting dose of 0.25 mg daily.
Flexhaler
Adults: Initially, inhaled dose of 360 mcg b.i.d. to maximum of 720 mcg b.i.d.
Children ages 6 to 17: Initially, inhaled dose of 180 mcg b.i.d. to maximum of 360 mcg b.i.d.
Turbuhaler❦
Adults and children age 12 and older when treatment with inhaled glucocorticosteroids is started, during periods of severe asthma, and while oral glucocorticosteroids are being reduced or discontinued: Initially, inhaled dose of 400 to 2,400 mcg daily divided into two to four administrations. Maintenance dose is usually 200 to 400 mcg b.i.d. Individualize dose to the lowest possible to meet therapeutic objective.
Children ages 6 to 12 when beginning budesonide, during periods of severe asthma, and while oral corticosteroids are being reduced or discontinued: Initially, inhaled dose of 100 to 200 mcg b.i.d. For maintenance, use lowest dose necessary to control symptoms.
➤ **Symptoms of seasonal or perennial allergic rhinitis**
Adults and children age 6 and older: 1 spray in each nostril once daily. Maximum dose is 4 sprays per nostril once daily (256 mcg/day) for adults and children older than age 12 and 2 sprays per nostril once daily (128 mcg/day) for children age 6 to less than age 12.

ADMINISTRATION
Inhalational
● Give inhalation suspension at regular intervals once or twice a day, as directed.
● Give suspension with a jet nebulizer connected to a compressor with adequate

airflow. Make sure that it's equipped with a mouthpiece or suitable face mask.

• Total daily dose may be increased or given as a divided dose to improve control if needed. Titrate dosage downward again after asthma is stabilized.

• When aluminum foil envelope has been opened, the shelf-life of unused ampules is 2 weeks when protected from light.

• Refer to manufacturer's instructions before use. Prime inhaler before first use. Have patient inhale deeply and forcefully each time unit is used and rinse mouth with water after inhalation.

Intranasal
• Prime pump by actuating eight times before first use. Reprime pump if not used for 2 or more days. Discard bottle after 120 sprays.

• Shake before each actuation.

ACTION
Exhibits potent glucocorticoid activity and weak mineralocorticoid activity. Drug inhibits mast cells, macrophages, and mediators (such as leukotrienes) involved in inflammation.

Route	Onset	Peak	Duration
Inhalation, powder	24 hr	1–2 wk	Unknown
Inhalation, Respules	2–8 days	4–6 wk	Unknown
Intranasal	10 hr	2 wk	Unknown

Half-life: Inhalation and intranasal, 2 to 3 hours.

ADVERSE REACTIONS
CNS: headache, asthenia, fever, hypertonia, insomnia, pain, syncope.
EENT: sinusitis, pharyngitis, rhinitis, otitis media, voice alteration; epistaxis and nasal irritation (intranasal).
GI: abdominal pain, dry mouth, dyspepsia, diarrhea, gastroenteritis, nausea, oral candidiasis, taste perversion, vomiting.
Metabolic: weight gain.
Musculoskeletal: back pain, fractures, myalgia.
Respiratory: respiratory tract infection, *bronchospasm,* increased cough.
Skin: ecchymoses.
Other: flulike symptoms, hypersensitivity reactions, viral infection.

INTERACTIONS
Drug-drug. *Ketoconazole, other strong CYP3A4 inhibitors (atazanavir, clarithromycin, indinavir, itraconazole, nefazodone, nelfinavir, ritonavir, saquinavir, telithromycin):* May inhibit metabolism and increase level of budesonide. Monitor patient for adverse reactions and adjust dosage as needed.

EFFECTS ON LAB TEST RESULTS
None reported.

CONTRAINDICATIONS & CAUTIONS
• Contraindicated in patients hypersensitive to drug, in those with severe hypersensitivity to milk proteins (powder for inhalation), and in those with status asthmaticus or other acute asthma episodes.

• Use nasal formulation cautiously in patients with septal ulcers, nasal surgery, nasal trauma, or untreated localized nasal mucosa infections.

• Use cautiously, if at all, in patients with active or inactive TB, ocular HSV infections, or untreated systemic fungal, bacterial, viral, or parasitic infections.
Dialyzable drug: No.
⚠ Overdose S&S: Hyperadrenocorticism.

PREGNANCY-LACTATION-REPRODUCTION
• Hypoadrenalism may occur in infants of women who received corticosteroids during pregnancy. These infants should be carefully monitored.

• Studies of pregnant women using inhaled or intranasal form haven't demonstrated an increased risk of abnormalities. Inhaled corticosteroids are recommended for the treatment of asthma during pregnancy.

• Drug appears in breast milk. Patient should use lowest possible dose immediately after breast-feeding to maximize time between dose and breast-feeding.

NURSING CONSIDERATIONS
⊘ Alert: When transferring from systemic corticosteroid to inhalation drug, use caution and gradually decrease corticosteroid dose to prevent adrenal insufficiency.

• Inhalation drug doesn't remove the need for systemic corticosteroid therapy in some situations.

- Systemic effects of corticosteroid therapy may occur if recommended daily dosage is exceeded.
- If bronchospasm occurs after inhalation use, stop therapy and treat with a bronchodilator.
- Lung function may improve within 24 hours of starting therapy, but maximum benefit may not be achieved for 1 to 2 weeks or longer.
- For Pulmicort Respules, lung function improves in 2 to 8 days, but maximum benefit may not be seen for 4 to 6 weeks.
- Watch for *Candida* infections of the mouth or pharynx.
- ⚠ *Alert:* Corticosteroids may increase risk of developing serious or fatal infections in patients exposed to viral illnesses, such as chickenpox or measles.
- In rare cases, inhaled corticosteroids have been linked to increased IOP and cataract development. Stop drug if local irritation occurs.
- Monitor bone mineral density in patients at risk for decreased bone mineral content (prolonged immobilization, family history of osteoporosis, postmenopausal status).
- Monitor children for reduction in growth velocity. Use lowest effective dose.
- Monitor patients for hypercorticism and adrenal suppression and if they occur, reduce dosage slowly.
- Rare cases of eosinophilic conditions and Churg-Strauss syndrome have occurred when systemic corticosteroids have been reduced or withdrawn. Monitor patients for eosinophilia, vasculitic rash, worsening pulmonary symptoms, cardiac symptoms, and neuropathy.

PATIENT TEACHING

- Tell patient that budesonide inhaler isn't a bronchodilator and isn't intended to treat acute episodes of asthma.
- Instruct patient to use the inhaler according to manufacturer's instructions at regular intervals because effectiveness depends on twice-daily use on a regular basis.
- Tell patient that improvement in asthma control may be seen within 24 hours, although maximum benefit may not appear for 1 to 2 weeks. If signs or symptoms worsen

during this time, instruct patient to contact prescriber.
- Advise patient to avoid exposure to chickenpox or measles and to contact prescriber if exposure occurs.
- Instruct patient using inhaler to carry or wear medical identification indicating need for supplementary corticosteroids during periods of stress or an asthma attack.
- Advise patient that unused Respules are good for 2 weeks after the foil envelope has been opened; however, unused Respules should be returned to envelope to protect them from light.
- Tell patient to read and follow patient information leaflet contained in package.
- To instill intranasal drug, instruct patient to shake container before use, blow nose to clear nasal passages, tilt head slightly forward, and insert nozzle into nostril, pointing away from septum. Tell him to hold other nostril closed and inhale gently while spraying. Next, have him shake container and repeat in other nostril. Advise patient to avoid blowing nose for 15 minutes after use and to wipe spray tip clean with a tissue.
- Advise patient to store nasal canister with valve upward and away from extreme heat or cold. Caution him not to incinerate or break canister because contents are under pressure.
- Advise patient using nasal formula to notify prescriber if signs or symptoms don't improve or if they worsen in 3 weeks.
- Teach patient good nasal and oral hygiene and not to share drug because this could spread infection.

budesonide (oral, rectal)
byoo-DES-oh-nide

Entocort EC, Uceris

Therapeutic class: Corticosteroids
Pharmacologic class: Glucocorticoids

AVAILABLE FORMS
Capsules ⒪: 3 mg
Foam: 2 mg/actuation
Tablets (extended-release) ⒪: 9 mg

INDICATIONS & DOSAGES

Adjust-a-dose (for all indications): In patients with moderate to severe liver disease who have increased signs or symptoms of hypercorticism, reduce dose.

➤ **Mild to moderate active Crohn disease involving the ileum, ascending colon, or both (capsules)**
Adults: 9 mg P.O. once daily in morning for up to 8 weeks. For recurrent episodes of active Crohn disease, a repeat 8-week course may be given.

➤ **To maintain remission in mild to moderate Crohn disease that involves the ileum or ascending colon (capsules)**
Adults: 6 mg P.O. daily for up to 3 months. If symptom control is maintained at 3 months, taper dose to stop therapy. Therapy for longer than 3 months doesn't have added benefit.

➤ **Induction of remission in active mild to moderate ulcerative colitis (tablets)**
Adults: 9 mg P.O. once daily in the morning for up to 8 weeks.

➤ **Induction of remission in mild to moderate distal ulcerative colitis (rectal foam)**
Adults: 2 mg (1 metered dose) P.R. b.i.d. for 2 weeks then 2 mg P.R. once daily for 4 weeks.

ADMINISTRATION
P.O.
● Give drug whole; don't break or crush capsule or tablet.
Rectal
● Wash hands before and after use.
● Attach applicator to canister nozzle. Warm canister in the hands while shaking it for 10 to 15 seconds.
● Unlock canister top; then turn it upside down and insert applicator tip into rectum.
● Push down on pump dome for 2 seconds and hold applicator in place for 10 to 15 seconds.
● Withdraw and discard used applicator.

ACTION
Significant glucocorticoid effects caused by drug's high affinity for glucocorticoid receptors.

Route	Onset	Peak	Duration
P.O.	Unknown	½–10 hr	Unknown
P.O. (extended-release)	Unknown	7.4–9.2 hr	Unknown
Rectal	Unknown	Unknown	Unknown

Half-life: About 2 hours.

ADVERSE REACTIONS
CNS: headache, dizziness, asthenia, hyperkinesia, paresthesia, tremor, vertigo, fatigue, malaise, agitation, confusion, insomnia, nervousness, somnolence, pain, sleep disorder.
CV: chest pain, hypertension, palpitations, tachycardia, flushing.
EENT: facial edema, ear infection, eye abnormality, abnormal vision, sinusitis.
GI: nausea, diarrhea, dyspepsia, abdominal pain, flatulence, vomiting, anal disorder, aggravated Crohn disease, enteritis, epigastric pain, fistula, glossitis, hemorrhoids, intestinal obstruction, tongue edema, tooth disorder, increased appetite.
GU: dysuria, micturition frequency, nocturia, intermenstrual bleeding, menstrual disorder, hematuria, pyuria, UTI.
Hematologic: leukocytosis, anemia.
Metabolic: hypercorticism, dependent edema, hypokalemia, increased weight.
Musculoskeletal: back pain, aggravated arthritis, cramps, arthralgia, myalgia.
Respiratory: respiratory tract infection, bronchitis, dyspnea.
Skin: acne, alopecia, dermatitis, eczema, skin disorder, increased sweating, purpura.
Other: flulike disorder, candidiasis, viral infection.

INTERACTIONS
Drug-drug. *Barbiturates (phenobarbital), rifamycins (rifampin):* May decrease budesonide effects. Adjust budesonide dosage as clinically indicated.
CYP inhibitors (erythromycin, indinavir, itraconazole, ketoconazole, ritonavir, saquinavir): May increase effects of budesonide. If use together is unavoidable, reduce budesonide dosage.
Gastric acid secretion inhibitors (antacids, H₂ blockers, PPIs): May affect dissolution of extended-release budesonide. Avoid use together or separate administration times by as much as possible and monitor clinical response to budesonide.

Quinolones (levofloxacin): May increase risk of tendon rupture when taken concomitantly with corticosteroids. Avoid use together.

Salicylates (aspirin): May decrease salicylate level and effectiveness and increase risk of GI bleeding. Monitor patient response and adjust salicylate dosage as needed.

Drug-food. *Grapefruit juice:* May increase drug effects. Discourage use together.

EFFECTS ON LAB TEST RESULTS
● May increase alkaline phosphatase and C-reactive protein levels. May decrease potassium and Hb levels.
● May increase erythrocyte sedimentation rate and WBC count.

CONTRAINDICATIONS & CAUTIONS
● Contraindicated in patients hypersensitive to drug.
● Use cautiously in patients with TB, hypertension, diabetes mellitus, osteoporosis, hepatic impairment, peptic ulcer disease, glaucoma, or cataracts; those with a family history of diabetes or glaucoma; and those with any other condition in which glucocorticoids may have unwanted effects.
Dialyzable drug: Unknown.
⚠ *Overdose S&S:* Hypercorticism, adrenal suppression.

PREGNANCY-LACTATION-REPRODUCTION
● Drug may be used cautiously for the induction of remission in pregnant women with inflammatory bowel disease. Use only if potential benefit justifies potential fetal risk.
● Glucocorticoids appear in breast milk, and infants may have adverse reactions. Use cautiously in breast-feeding women and only if benefits outweigh risks.

NURSING CONSIDERATIONS
● Reduced liver function affects elimination of this drug; systemic availability of drug may increase in patients with liver cirrhosis.
● Patients undergoing surgery or other stressful situations may need systemic glucocorticoid supplementation in addition to budesonide therapy.
● Carefully monitor patients transferred from systemic glucocorticoid therapy to budesonide for signs and symptoms of corticosteroid withdrawal. Watch for immunosuppression, especially in patients who haven't had diseases such as chickenpox or measles; these can be fatal in patients who are immunosuppressed or receiving glucocorticoids.
● Replacement of systemic glucocorticoids with this drug may unmask allergies, such as eczema and rhinitis, which were previously controlled by systemic drug.
● Long-term use of drug may cause hypercorticism and adrenal suppression.

PATIENT TEACHING
● Tell patient to swallow capsules whole and not to chew or break them.
● Advise patient to avoid grapefruit juice while taking drug.
● Tell patient to notify prescriber immediately if he is exposed to or develops chickenpox or measles.
● Tell patient to keep container tightly closed.
● Teach patient how to administer rectal formulation and to keep it away from flame.

---

bumetanide
byoo-MET-a-nide

Bumex, Burinex ✦

Therapeutic class: Diuretics
Pharmacologic class: Loop diuretics

AVAILABLE FORMS
Injection: 0.25 mg/mL
Tablets: 0.5 mg, 1 mg, 2 mg, 5 mg ✦

INDICATIONS & DOSAGES
➤ **Edema caused by HF or hepatic or renal disease**
Adults: 0.5 to 2 mg P.O. once daily. If diuretic response isn't adequate, a second or third dose may be given at 4- to 5-hour intervals. Maximum dose is 10 mg daily. May be given parenterally if oral route isn't possible. Usual first dose is 0.5 to 1 mg given I.V. or I.M. If response isn't adequate, a second or third dose may be given at 2- to 3-hour intervals. Maximum, 10 mg daily.

B

ADMINISTRATION
P.O.
● Give drug with food to minimize GI upset.
● To prevent nocturia, give drug in morning. If second dose is needed, give in early afternoon.
I.V.
▼ For direct injection, give drug over 1 to 2 minutes.
▼ For intermittent infusion, give diluted drug through an intermittent infusion device or piggyback into an I.V. line containing a free-flowing, compatible solution.
▼ Solutions should be freshly prepared and used within 24 hours.
▼ **Incompatibilities:** Dobutamine, fenoldopam, midazolam.
I.M.
● Document injection site.

ACTION
Inhibits sodium and chloride reabsorption in the ascending loop of Henle.

Route	Onset	Peak	Duration
P.O.	30–60 min	1–2 hr	4–6 hr
I.V.	Within min	15–30 min	30–60 min
I.M.	40 min	Unknown	5–6 hr

Half-life: 1 to 1½ hours.

ADVERSE REACTIONS
CNS: dizziness, headache, vertigo.
CV: orthostatic hypotension.
EENT: deafness, tinnitus.
GU: oliguria.
Metabolic: volume depletion and dehydration, hypokalemia, hypochloremic alkalosis, *hypomagnesemia,* asymptomatic hyperuricemia, hyponatremia, elevated blood glucose level.
Skin: rash, pruritus.

INTERACTIONS
Drug-drug. *Aminoglycoside antibiotics:* May increase ototoxicity. Avoid using together if possible.
Antidiabetics: May decrease hypoglycemic effects. Monitor glucose level.
Antihypertensives: May increase hypotensive effects. Consider dosage adjustment.
Cardiac glycosides: May increase risk of digoxin toxicity from bumetanide-induced

hypokalemia. Monitor potassium and digoxin levels.
Chlorothiazide, chlorthalidone, furosemide, hydrochlorothiazide, indapamide, metolazone: May cause excessive diuretic response, causing serious electrolyte abnormalities or dehydration. Adjust doses carefully, and monitor patient closely for signs and symptoms of excessive diuretic response.
Cisplatin: May increase risk of ototoxicity. Monitor patient closely.
Lithium: May decrease lithium clearance, increasing risk of lithium toxicity. Monitor lithium level.
Neuromuscular blockers: May prolong neuromuscular blockade. Monitor patient closely.
NSAIDs, probenecid: May inhibit diuretic response. Use together cautiously.
Other potassium-wasting drugs (such as amphotericin B, corticosteroids): May increase risk of hypokalemia. Use together cautiously.
Drug-herb. *Dandelion:* May interfere with drug activity. Discourage use together.
Licorice: May cause unexpected, rapid potassium loss. Discourage use together.

EFFECTS ON LAB TEST RESULTS
● May increase alkaline phosphatase, ALT, AST, bilirubin, cholesterol, creatinine, glucose, LDH, BUN, and urine urea levels.
● May decrease calcium, magnesium, potassium, sodium, and chloride levels.
● May decrease platelet count.

CONTRAINDICATIONS & CAUTIONS
● Contraindicated in patients hypersensitive to drug or sulfonamides (possible cross-sensitivity) and in patients with anuria, hepatic coma, or severe electrolyte depletion.
● Use cautiously in patients with hepatic cirrhosis and ascites, in elderly patients, and in those with decreased renal function.
Dialyzable drug: Unknown.
⚠ *Overdose S&S:* Electrolyte depletion, weakness, dizziness, confusion, anorexia, lethargy, vomiting, cramps, dehydration, circulatory collapse, vascular thrombosis, and embolism.

PREGNANCY-LACTATION-REPRODUCTION

● There are no adequate well-controlled studies in pregnant women. Use during pregnancy only if potential benefits justify potential risk to the fetus.
● Use in breast-feeding women isn't recommended.

NURSING CONSIDERATIONS

● Safest and most effective dosage schedule is alternate days or 3 or 4 consecutive days with 1 or 2 days off between cycles.
Black Box Warning Monitor BP and pulse rate during rapid diuresis. Profound water and electrolyte depletion may occur. ∎
● Monitor fluid intake and output, weight, and electrolyte, BUN, creatinine, and carbon dioxide levels frequently, especially in elderly patients.
● Watch for evidence of hypokalemia, such as muscle weakness and cramps. Instruct patient to report these symptoms.
● Consult prescriber and dietitian about a high-potassium diet. Foods rich in potassium include citrus fruits, tomatoes, bananas, dates, and apricots.
● Monitor glucose level in diabetic patients.
● Monitor uric acid level, especially in patients with history of gout.
● If oliguria or azotemia develops or increases, prescriber may stop drug.
● Drug can be safely used in patients allergic to furosemide; 1 mg of bumetanide equals about 40 mg of furosemide.
● Monitor patient for ototoxicity, especially when drug is given I.V. and at high doses.

PATIENT TEACHING

● Instruct patient to take drug with food to minimize GI upset.
● Advise patient to take drug in morning to avoid need to urinate at night; if patient needs second dose, have him take it in early afternoon.
● Advise patient to avoid sudden posture changes and to rise slowly to avoid dizziness upon standing quickly.
● Instruct patient to notify prescriber about extreme thirst, muscle weakness, cramps, nausea, or dizziness.
● Instruct patient to weigh himself daily to monitor fluid status.

SAFETY ALERT!

buprenorphine
byoo-pre-NOR-feen

Butrans

buprenorphine hydrochloride
Buprenex, Probuphine

Therapeutic class: Opioid analgesics
Pharmacologic class: Opioid agonist-antagonists–opioid partial agonists
Controlled substance schedule: III

AVAILABLE FORMS

Injection: 0.324 mg (equivalent to 0.3 mg base/mL)
Subdermal implant: 74.2 mg buprenorphine (equivalent to 80 mg of buprenorphine hydrochloride)
Sublingual tablets: 2 mg, 8 mg (as base)
Transdermal patch: 5 mcg/hour, 7.5 mcg/hour, 10 mcg/hour, 15 mcg/hour, 20 mcg/hour

INDICATIONS & DOSAGES

✸ *NEW INDICATION:* **Maintenance treatment of opioid dependence in patients who have achieved and sustained prolonged clinical stability on low to moderate doses (doses of no more than 8 mg/day of Subutex or Suboxone S.L. tablet equivalent or generic equivalent) of a transmucosal buprenorphine-containing product**
Adults: 1 dose (4 implants) inserted subdermally in the inner side of the upper arm and kept in place for 6 months.
➤ **Moderate to severe pain**
Adults and children age 13 and older: 0.3 mg I.M. or slow I.V. (over at least 2 minutes) every 6 hours p.r.n., or around the clock; repeat dose (up to 0.3 mg), as needed, 30 to 60 minutes after first dose. May increase I.M. dosing to 0.6 mg/dose.
Children ages 2 to 12: 2 to 6 mcg/kg I.M. or slow I.V. (over at least 2 minutes) every 4 to 6 hours.
Adjust-a-dose: In high-risk patients, such as debilitated or elderly patients, reduce dose by one-half.
➤ **Moderate to severe chronic pain in patients requiring continuous opioid analgesia for an extended period of time**

Reactions in bold italics are *life-threatening*. Interactions may have a *rapid onset* or a *delayed onset*.

B

Adults (opioid-naive): 5 mcg/hour transdermal patch once every 7 days. To achieve adequate analgesia and minimize adverse effects, consider patient's tolerance, condition, and other medications and titrate dosage to maximum of 20 mcg/hour. Allow minimum of 72 hours between dosage increases.

Adults (non–opioid-naive): Buprenorphine may precipitate withdrawal in patients already on opioids. For conversion from other opioids to buprenorphine, taper patient's current around-the-clock opioids for up to 7 days to no more than morphine 30 mg or equivalent per day before beginning treatment with buprenorphine. Patients may use short-acting analgesics as needed until analgesic efficacy with buprenorphine is attained. For patients whose daily dose was less than morphine 30 mg P.O. or equivalent, initiate treatment with buprenorphine transdermal patch 5 mcg/hour. For patients whose daily dose was between 30 and 80 mg of morphine equivalents, initiate treatment with buprenorphine transdermal patch 10 mcg/hour. To achieve adequate analgesia with tolerable adverse effects, consider patient's tolerance, condition, and other medications and titrate dose to maximum of 20 mcg/hour transdermal patch once every 7 days. Allow minimum of 72 hours between dosage increases. If patch must be discontinued, taper dosage gradually every 7 days to prevent withdrawal in the physically dependent patient; consider initiating immediate-release opioids, if needed.

Adjust-a-dose: For patients with mild to moderate hepatic impairment, start with buprenorphine dosage of 5 mcg/hour. Thereafter, individually titrate dosage to level that provides adequate analgesia and tolerable adverse effects, under close supervision of prescriber.

➤ **Opioid dependence**
Adults: 8 mg S.L. on day 1 and 16 mg S.L. on day 2. Maintenance dose is 12 to 16 mg S.L. as a single daily dose.

ADMINISTRATION

I.V.
▼ When mixed in a 1:1 volume ratio, drug is compatible with atropine sulfate, diphenhydramine hydrochloride, droperidol, glycopyrrolate, haloperidol lactate, hydroxyzine hydrochloride, promethazine hydrochloride, scopolamine hydrochloride, D_5W, 5% dextrose in NSS, NSS, lactated Ringer solution, and NSS injections.
▼ For direct injection, give slowly over at least 2 minutes into a vein or through tubing of a free-flowing, compatible I.V. solution.
▼ **Incompatibilities:** Diazepam, furosemide, lorazepam.
I.M.
● Give drug as deep I.M. injection.
S.L.
● Place all the tablets of the dose under the tongue until dissolved; if uncomfortable, patient should take at least two at the same time.
Subdermal
Black Box Warning Subdermal implant is only available through a restricted program called the Probuphine Risk Evaluation and Mitigations Strategies (REMS) program. All health care providers must become certified before performing insertions or prescribing implants. Patients must be monitored to ensure that implant is removed by a health care provider certified to perform insertions. ▊
● Each dose (4 implants) is inserted subdermally under local anesthesia in the inner side of the upper arm, remains in place for 6 months, then is removed at the end of the sixth month.
● At the time of implant removal, new implants may be inserted subdermally in an area of the inner side of either upper arm that hasn't been previously used, if continued treatment is desired. If new implants aren't inserted on the same day as implant removal, maintain patients on their previous dosage of transmucosal buprenorphine.
● After one insertion in each arm, most patients should be transitioned back to a transmucosal buprenorphine-containing product for continued treatment.
Transdermal
🜂 *Alert:* Avoid exposing patch or surrounding area to direct external heat source or direct sunlight. Increased temperature may increase amount of drug released, which can result in overdose and death.

🍁Canada　◇OTC　◆Off-label use　✐Photoguide　⊛Do not crush　*Liquid contains alcohol.

◑ Alert: Transdermal patch is indicated only for moderate to severe chronic pain that requires around-the-clock analgesia for an extended period of time.

● Each patch is intended to be worn for 7 days. If patch falls off during 7-day dosing interval, apply new patch to different site.

● Don't use if pouch seal is broken or patch is cut, damaged, or changed in any way. Apply patch to intact skin immediately after opening.

● Appropriate application sites are upper outer arm, upper chest, upper back, or side of the chest (eight total available sites).

● Application site should be hairless; clip hair if needed but don't shave site. If needed, clean selected site with water only and allow to dry completely before applying patch.

● Edges of patch may be taped to the skin if needed.

● After removing patch, fold it in half, seal it in patch-disposal unit, and place it in trash.

● Wait minimum of 3 weeks before applying new patch to same application site.

ACTION

Unknown. Binds with opioid receptors in the CNS, altering perception of and emotional response to pain.

Route	Onset	Peak	Duration
I.V.	Immediate	2 min	6 hr
I.M.	15 min	1 hr	6 hr
S.L.	Unknown	Unknown	Unknown
Subdermal	12 hr	Unknown	24 wk
Transdermal	17 hr	3–6 days	7 days

Half-life: 1 to 7 hours; subdermal, 24 to 48 hours; transdermal, 26 hours.

ADVERSE REACTIONS

CNS: dizziness, sedation, vertigo, *increased ICP,* asthenia (tablets only), confusion, depression, dreaming, euphoria, fatigue, headache, insomnia, nervousness, pain, paresthesia, psychosis, slurred speech, weakness, somnolence.
CV: *bradycardia,* cyanosis, flushing, hypertension, hypotension, tachycardia, peripheral edema.
EENT: blurred vision, conjunctivitis, diplopia, visual abnormalities, miosis, tinnitus, rhinitis (tablets only), dry mouth (patch), toothache, oropharyngeal pain.

GI: nausea, abdominal pain (tablets only), constipation, diarrhea (tablets only), vomiting, anorexia, dry mouth, dyspepsia.
GU: urine retention, UTI.
Musculoskeletal: arthralgia, back pain (tablets only), joint swelling, extremity pain.
Respiratory: *respiratory depression,* dyspnea, hypoventilation.
Skin: application-site rash or erythema (patch), diaphoresis, injection-site reactions, pruritus, sweating; implant-site pain, pruritus, erythema (Probuphine).
Other: chills, infection (tablets only), withdrawal syndrome.

INTERACTIONS
Drug-drug. **Black Box Warning** *Benzodiazepines, CNS depressants:* May cause slow or difficult breathing, sedation, and death. Avoid use together. If use together is necessary, limit dosage and duration of each drug to the minimum necessary for desired effect. ■
Class IA or III antiarrhythmics: May increase risk of prolonged QT syndrome. Avoid use with transdermal patch.
CYP3A4 inducers (carbamazepine, phenobarbital, phenytoin, rifampin): May increase clearance of buprenorphine. Monitor patient for clinical effects of drug.
CYP3A4 inhibitors (erythromycin, indinavir, ketoconazole, ritonavir, saquinavir): May decrease clearance of buprenorphine. Monitor patient for increased adverse effects.
MAO inhibitors: May cause additive effects. Use together cautiously.
◑ Alert: *Serotonergic drugs (amoxapine, antiemetics [dolasetron, granisetron, ondansetron, palonsetron], antimigraine drugs, buspirone, cyclobenzaprine, dextromethorphan, linezolid, lithium, MAO inhibitors, maprotiline, methylene blue, mirtazapine, nefazodone, SNRIs, SSRIs, TCAs, trazodone, tryptophan, vilazodone):* Can increase risk of serotonin syndrome. Use together cautiously; monitor patient for serotonin syndrome.
Skeletal muscle relaxants: May enhance neuromuscular blocking action and increase respiratory depression. Use together cautiously.
Drug-lifestyle. *Alcohol or illicit drug use:* May cause additive effects. Discourage use together.

Reactions in bold italics are *life-threatening.* Interactions may have a *rapid onset* or a *delayed onset.*

EFFECTS ON LAB TEST RESULTS
• May increase amylase level.

CONTRAINDICATIONS & CAUTIONS
• Contraindicated in patients hypersensitive to drug and in those with paralytic ileus or GI obstruction.

Black Box Warning Serious, life-threatening, or fatal respiratory depression may occur, especially during drug initiation or after a dosage increase. Misuse or abuse of drug by chewing, swallowing, snorting, or injecting buprenorphine extracted from the transdermal system will result in the uncontrolled delivery of buprenorphine and will pose a significant risk of overdose and death. ■

Black Box Warning Opioid drugs should only be prescribed with benzodiazepines or other CNS depressants to patients for whom alternative treatment options are inadequate. ■

Black Box Warning Insertion and removal of subdermal implants are associated with risk of implant migration, protrusion, and expulsion resulting from the procedure. Rare but serious complications, including nerve damage and migration resulting in embolism and death, may result from improper insertion of implants inserted in the upper arm. Additional complications may include local migration, protrusion, and expulsion. Incomplete insertions or infections may lead to protrusion or expulsion. ■

◑ *Alert:* Don't exceed dose of one 20-mcg/hour transdermal patch every 7 days due to risk of prolonging QTc interval.

◑ *Alert:* Patients are at increased risk for oversedation and respiratory depression if they snore or have a history of sleep apnea, haven't used opioids recently or are first-time opioid users, have increased opioid dosage requirements or opioid habituation, received general anesthesia for longer lengths of time, received other sedating drugs, have thoracic or other surgical incisions that may impair breathing, or have preexisting pulmonary or cardiac disease. Monitor these patients carefully.

◑ *Alert:* Drug may lead to rare but serious decrease in adrenal gland cortisol production.

◑ *Alert:* Drug may cause decreased sex hormone levels with long-term use.

• Use cautiously in elderly or debilitated patients; patients who are opioid dependent; in those undergoing biliary tract surgery and those with biliary tract disease or pancreatitis; in those with head injury, intracranial lesions, and increased ICP; severe respiratory, liver, or kidney impairment; CNS depression or coma; those at risk for hypotension and circulatory shock; and in those with thyroid irregularities, adrenal insufficiency, prostatic hypertrophy, urethral stricture, acute alcoholism, delirium tremens, or kyphoscoliosis.

• The transdermal patch is included in the REMS program for extended-release and long-acting opioids. Prescribers are encouraged to undergo REMS training and counsel patients on safe drug use.

Dialyzable drug: Unknown.

⚠ *Overdose S&S:* Respiratory depression, pinpoint pupils, sedation, hypotension, death, snoring, bradycardia, cool and clammy skin, partial or complete airway obstruction, skeletal muscle flaccidity, somnolence.

PREGNANCY-LACTATION-REPRODUCTION
• There are no adequate and controlled studies in pregnant women. Prolonged use can result in neonatal opioid withdrawal syndrome, which can be life-threatening. Use during pregnancy only if potential benefits justify risk to the fetus.

• Drug appears in breast milk. Use in breast-feeding women isn't recommended.

• Breast-feeding infants exposed to large doses of opioids should be monitored for apnea and sedation.

NURSING CONSIDERATIONS
Black Box Warning Buprenorphine has potential for abuse similar to other opioids and is a controlled substance. Patients at risk for opioid abuse include those with personal or family history of substance abuse or mental illness. Assess for risk of abuse before prescribing, and monitor patients regularly. ■

Black Box Warning Accidental exposure to drug, especially in children, can cause a fatal overdose. ■

◆ *Alert:* Carefully monitor vital signs, pain level, respiratory status, and sedation level in patients receiving opioids, especially those receiving I.V. opioid drugs postoperatively.

◆ *Alert:* If patient is taking opioids with serotonergic drugs, watch for signs and symptoms of serotonin syndrome (agitation, hallucinations, rapid HR, fever, excessive sweating, shivering or shaking, muscle twitching or stiffness, trouble with coordination, nausea, vomiting, diarrhea), especially when starting treatment or increasing dosages. Signs and symptoms may occur within several hours of coadministration but may also occur later, especially after dosage increase. Discontinue the opioid, serotonergic drug, or both if serotonin syndrome is suspected.

◆ *Alert:* Monitor patient for signs and symptoms of adrenal insufficiency (nausea, vomiting, loss of appetite, fatigue, weakness, dizziness, low BP). Perform diagnostic testing if adrenal insufficiency is suspected. If adrenal insufficiency is confirmed, treat with corticosteroids and wean patient off opioids if appropriate. Discontinue corticosteroids when clinically appropriate.

◆ *Alert:* Monitor patient for signs and symptoms of decreased sex hormone levels (low libido, erectile dysfunction, amenorrhea, infertility). If symptoms occur, evaluate patient and obtain laboratory testing.

◆ *Alert:* Monitor patient with subdermal implant for nerve damage; implant migration, protrusion, or expulsion; and infection.

● Taper dosage before discontinuing transdermal patch.

● Drug may worsen increased ICP and mask its signs and symptoms. Carefully monitor patient's pupillary reflexes and level of consciousness.

● Monitor patients with history of seizure disorders for worsening of condition.

● Monitor patients for signs and symptoms of hypotension after initiating therapy or increasing dosage.

● Monitor patients with fever or increased core body temperature after exertion; adjust dosage if signs or symptoms of respiratory or CNS depression occur.

● Watch for worsening of symptoms in patients with biliary tract disease, including acute pancreatitis; drug may cause spasm of sphincter of Oddi.

● Reassess patient's level of pain 15 and 30 minutes after parenteral administration.

● Buprenorphine 0.3 mg is equal to 10 mg of morphine and 75 mg of meperidine in analgesic potency. It has longer duration of action than morphine or meperidine.

◆ *Alert:* Naloxone won't completely reverse the respiratory depression caused by buprenorphine overdose; an overdose may require mechanical ventilation. Larger-than-usual doses of naloxone (more than 0.4 mg) and doxapram also may be indicated.

● Treat accidental skin exposure by removing exposed clothing and rinsing skin with water.

● Drug may cause constipation. Assess bowel function and need for stool softeners and stimulant laxatives.

◆ *Alert:* Drug's opioid antagonist properties may cause withdrawal syndrome in opioid-dependent patients.

● If dependence occurs, withdrawal symptoms may appear up to 14 days after drug is stopped.

● *Look alike–sound alike:* Don't confuse Buprenex with Bumex. Don't confuse buprenorphine with bupropion.

PATIENT TEACHING

◆ *Alert:* Encourage patient to report all medications being taken, including prescription and OTC drugs and supplements.

Black Box Warning Caution the patient or the caregiver of a patient taking an opioid drug with a benzodiazepine, CNS depressant, or alcohol to seek immediate medical attention if the patient has symptoms of dizziness, light-headedness, extreme sleepiness, slowed or difficult breathing, or unresponsiveness. ■

◆ *Alert:* Caution patient to immediately report signs and symptoms of serotonin syndrome, adrenal insufficiency, and decreased sex hormone levels.

● Caution ambulatory patient about getting out of bed or walking.

● When drug is used after surgery, encourage patient to turn, cough, and breathe deeply to prevent breathing problems.

● Explain assessment and monitoring process to patient and family. Instruct them to immediately report difficulty breathing

---

or other signs or symptoms of potential adverse opioid-related reaction.
• Tell patient to place all the tablets of dose under the tongue until dissolved; if this is uncomfortable, tell him to take at least two at the same time.
• Instruct patient in proper disposal of transdermal system.
• Teach patient proper patch application and advise him to read package instructions.
• Warn patient not to apply heat to patch application site or to cut patch.
• Tell patient and family to report adverse reactions to prescriber immediately.
• Warn patient not to take other long-acting opioids while using transdermal system.
• Advise patient with subdermal implant to report signs and symptoms of infection or delayed wound healing, including evidence of implant extrusion from the skin.
• Tell patient that evaluation by the health care provider will be needed at least 1 week after implant insertion and monthly thereafter.

buPROPion hydrobromide
byoo-PROE-pee-on

Aplenzin

buPROPion hydrochloride
Forfivo XL, Wellbutrin✒, Wellbutrin SR✒, Wellbutrin XL, Zyban✒

Therapeutic class: Antidepressants
Pharmacologic class: Aminoketones

AVAILABLE FORMS
bupropion hydrobromide
Tablets (extended-release) ⓒ: 174 mg, 348 mg, 522 mg
bupropion hydrochloride
Tablets (extended-release 12-hour) ⓒ: 100 mg, 150 mg, 200 mg
Tablets (extended-release 24-hour) ⓒ: 150 mg, 300 mg, 450 mg
Tablets (immediate-release) ⓒ: 75 mg, 100 mg

INDICATIONS & DOSAGES
➤ **Major depressive disorder (Aplenzin only)**
Adults: Initially, 174 mg P.O. (equivalent to 150 mg/day bupropion HCl) given as

a single daily dose in the morning. If the 174-mg initial dose is adequately tolerated, increase to the 348-mg/day target dose as early as day 4 of dosing. There should be an interval of at least 24 hours between successive doses. The full antidepressant effect may not be evident until after 4 weeks of treatment or longer. Consider increasing dosage to the maximum of 522 mg P.O. daily, given as a single dose, for patients in whom no clinical improvement is noted after several weeks of treatment at 348 mg/day. When switching patients from Wellbutrin, Wellbutrin SR, or Wellbutrin XL to Aplenzin, give the equivalent total daily dose when possible (522 mg bupropion HBr is equivalent to 450 mg bupropion HCl; 348 mg bupropion HBr is equivalent to 300 mg bupropion HCl; 174 mg bupropion HBr is equivalent to 150 mg bupropion HCl).
Adjust-a-dose: In patients with renal impairment or mild to moderate hepatic impairment, including hepatic cirrhosis, reduced frequency or dose should be considered. In patients with severe hepatic cirrhosis, don't exceed 174 mg every other day.
➤ **Seasonal affective disorder**
Adults: Start treatment in autumn before depressive symptoms appear. Wellbutrin XL: Initially, 150 mg extended-release P.O. once daily in the morning. After 1 week, increase to 300 mg once daily, if tolerated. Continue 300 mg daily during the autumn and winter and taper to 150 mg daily for 2 weeks before stopping the drug in the early spring. Aplenzin: 174 mg P.O. daily. May increase to 348 mg P.O. once daily after 7 days. Taper and discontinue drug in early spring.
➤ **Depression**
Adults: For immediate-release, initially, 100 mg P.O. b.i.d.; increase after 3 days to 100 mg P.O. t.i.d., if needed. If patient doesn't improve after several weeks of therapy, increase dosage to 150 mg t.i.d. No single dose should exceed 150 mg. Allow at least 6 hours between successive doses. Maximum dose is 450 mg daily. For sustained-release, initially, 150 mg P.O. every morning; increase to target dose of 150 mg P.O. b.i.d., as tolerated, as early as day 4 of dosing. Allow at least 8 hours between successive doses. Maximum dose is

400 mg daily. For extended-release, initially, 150 mg P.O. every morning; increase to target dosage of 300 mg P.O. daily, as tolerated, as early as day 4 of dosing. Allow at least 24 hours between successive doses. Maximum is 450 mg daily. Don't initiate treatment with Forfivo XL.

➤ **Aid to smoking-cessation treatment**
Adults: 150 mg Zyban P.O. daily for 3 days; increased to maximum of 300 mg daily in two divided doses at least 8 hours apart. Continue therapy for 7 to 12 weeks. Some patients may need continuous treatment.

Adjust-a-dose: In patients with mild to moderate hepatic cirrhosis or renal impairment, reduce frequency and dose. In patients with severe hepatic cirrhosis, don't exceed 75 mg immediate-release P.O. daily, 150 mg sustained-release P.O. every other day, or 150 mg extended-release P.O. every other day.

ADMINISTRATION
P.O.
- Don't crush, split, or allow patients to chew tablets.
- When switching patients from immediate-release or sustained-release tablets to extended-release tablets, give the same total daily dose (when possible) as the once-daily dosage provided.

ACTION
Unknown. Drug doesn't inhibit MAO, but it weakly inhibits norepinephrine, dopamine, and serotonin reuptake. Noradrenergic or dopaminergic mechanisms, or both, may cause drug's effect.

Route	Onset	Peak	Duration
P.O. (extended-release)	Unknown	5 hr	Unknown
P.O. (immediate-release)	Unknown	2 hr	Unknown
P.O. (sustained-release)	Unknown	3 hr	Unknown

Half-life: 8 to 24 hours.

ADVERSE REACTIONS
CNS: abnormal dreams, insomnia, headache, sedation, tremor, agitation, dizziness, *seizures, suicidal behavior,* anxiety, confusion, delusions, euphoria, fever, hostility, impaired concentration, impaired sleep quality, akinesia, akathisia, fatigue, syncope, somnolence.
CV: tachycardia, *arrhythmias,* hypertension, hypotension, palpitations, chest pain.
EENT: blurred vision, rhinitis, auditory disturbances, epistaxis, pharyngitis, sinusitis, dry mouth.
GI: constipation, nausea, vomiting, anorexia, taste disturbance, dyspepsia, diarrhea, abdominal pain, flatulence.
GU: erectile dysfunction, menstrual complaints, urinary frequency, urine retention.
Metabolic: increased appetite, weight loss, weight gain.
Musculoskeletal: arthritis, myalgia, arthralgia, muscle spasm or twitch.
Respiratory: upper respiratory complaints, increase in coughing.
Skin: excessive sweating, pruritus, rash, cutaneous temperature disturbance, urticaria.
Other: chills, decreased libido, accidental injury, hot flashes.

INTERACTIONS
Drug-drug. *Amantadine, levodopa:* May increase risk of adverse reactions. If used together, give small first doses of bupropion and increase dosage gradually.
Antidepressants (desipramine, fluoxetine, imipramine, nortriptyline, sertraline), antipsychotics (haloperidol, risperidone, thioridazine), systemic corticosteroids, theophylline: May lower seizure threshold. Use cautiously together.
Beta blockers, class IC antiarrhythmics: May increase levels of these drugs and adverse reactions. Use a reduced dose if used with bupropion.
Carbamazepine, phenobarbital, phenytoin: May enhance metabolism of bupropion and decrease its effect. Monitor patient closely.
CYP2B6 substrates or inhibitors (cyclophosphamide, orphenadrine, thiotepa), efavirenz, fluvoxamine, nelfinavir, norfluoxetine, paroxetine, ritonavir, sertraline: May increase bupropion activity. Monitor patient for expected therapeutic effects and adverse effects.
Linezolid, methylene blue, SSRIs: May cause serotonin syndrome. Use extreme caution and monitor closely.
MAO inhibitors (linezolid, methylene blue): May increase risk of bupropion toxicity.

Reactions in bold italics are *life-threatening*. Interactions may have a *rapid onset* or a *delayed onset*.

Don't use drugs within 14 days of each other.

Nicotine replacement agents: May cause hypertension. Monitor BP.

Drug-lifestyle. *Alcohol use:* May alter seizure threshold. Discourage use together.

Sun exposure: May increase risk of photosensitivity reactions. Advise patient to avoid excessive sunlight exposure.

EFFECTS ON LAB TEST RESULTS
• May increase LFT values.

CONTRAINDICATIONS & CAUTIONS
• Contraindicated in patients hypersensitive to drug, in those who have taken MAO inhibitors within previous 14 days, and in those with seizure disorders or history of bulimia or anorexia nervosa because of a higher risk of seizures.

❸ *Alert:* Concomitant use with SSRIs, linezolid, or methylene blue can cause serotonin syndrome (fever, mental status changes, muscle twitching, excessive sweating, shivering or shaking, diarrhea, loss of coordination). Use drug with SSRIs, linezolid, or methylene blue only for life-threatening or urgent conditions when the potential benefits outweigh the risks of toxicity.

• Hypersensitivity reactions, including anaphylaxis, pruritus, urticaria, angioedema, dyspnea, erythema multiforme, and Stevens-Johnson syndrome, have occurred.

• Contraindicated in patients abruptly stopping use of alcohol or sedatives (including benzodiazepines).

• Don't use with other drugs containing bupropion.

• Forfivo XL isn't recommended in patients with renal or hepatic impairment.

Black Box Warning Bupropion hydrobromide (Aplenzin) isn't approved for smoking cessation treatment. ■

Black Box Warning Bupropion isn't approved for use in children. ■

• Use cautiously in patients with recent history of MI; unstable heart disease; renal or hepatic impairment; a history of seizures, head trauma, or other predisposition to seizures; and in those being treated with drugs that lower seizure threshold.

Dialyzable drug: Unknown.

⚠ *Overdose S&S:* Seizures, ECG changes, hallucinations, loss of consciousness, sinus tachycardia, coma, fever, hypotension, muscle rigidity, rhabdomyolysis, respiratory failure, stupor.

PREGNANCY-LACTATION-REPRODUCTION
• Use during pregnancy only when potential benefits justify potential risks to the fetus.

• Prescriber should be notified if patient plans to or becomes pregnant.

• Drug and its metabolites appear in breast milk. Recommendations for breast-feeding vary by individual product; refer to manufacturer's labeling for recommendations.

NURSING CONSIDERATIONS
• Many patients experience a period of increased restlessness, including agitation, insomnia, and anxiety, especially at start of therapy.

❸ *Alert:* To minimize the risk of seizures, don't exceed maximum recommended dose.

❸ *Alert:* Patient with major depressive disorder may experience a worsening of depression and suicidal thoughts. Carefully monitor patient for worsening depression or suicidal thoughts, especially at the beginning of therapy and during dosage changes.

Black Box Warning Drug may increase the risk of suicidal thinking and behavior in children, adolescents, and young adults with major depressive disorder or other psychiatric disorder. ■

Black Box Warning Drug may cause hostility, agitation, psychosis, hallucinations, paranoia, delusions, homicidal ideation, anxiety, panic, and depressed mood in patients taking bupropion for smoking cessation. Monitor patients for neuropsychiatric reactions. ■

❸ *Alert:* If SSRIs, linezolid, or methylene blue must be given, bupropion must be stopped and the patient should be monitored for serotonin toxicity for 2 weeks or until 24 hours after the last dose of SSRIs, methylene blue, or linezolid, whichever comes first. Treatment with bupropion may be resumed 24 hours after last dose of SSRIs, methylene blue, or linezolid.

• Closely monitor patient with history of bipolar disorder. Antidepressants can cause manic episodes during the depressed phase of bipolar disorder. This may be less likely to occur with bupropion than with other antidepressants.

• Begin smoking-cessation treatment while patient is still smoking; about 1 week is needed to achieve steady-state drug levels.

• Stop smoking-cessation treatment if patient hasn't progressed toward abstinence by week 7. Treatment usually lasts up to 12 weeks. Patient can stop taking drug without tapering off.

• Monitor patients without iridectomy for narrow-angle glaucoma.

• Monitor BP for hypertension before and periodically during treatment.

Black Box Warning Zyban isn't indicated for treatment of depression. ∎

• *Look alike–sound alike:* Don't confuse bupropion with buspirone. Don't confuse Zyban with Diovan. Don't confuse Wellbutrin SR with Wellbutrin XL.

PATIENT TEACHING

Black Box Warning Advise families and caregivers to closely observe patient for increased suicidal thinking and behavior, as well as hostility, agitation, and depressed mood, and to contact health care provider immediately should these occur. ∎

🕔 *Alert:* Explain that excessive use of alcohol, abrupt withdrawal from alcohol or other sedatives, and addiction to cocaine, opiates, or stimulants during therapy may increase risk of seizures. Seizure risk is also increased in those using OTC stimulants, in anorectics, and in diabetic patients using oral antidiabetics or insulin.

🕔 *Alert:* Teach patient to recognize and immediately report symptoms of serotonin toxicity (fever, mental status changes, muscle twitching, excessive sweating, shivering or shaking, diarrhea, loss of coordination).

• Tell patient not to chew, crush, or divide tablets.

• Advise patient to consult prescriber before taking other prescription or OTC drugs.

• Advise patient to avoid hazardous activities that require alertness and good psychomotor coordination until effects of drug are known.

🕔 *Alert:* Advise patient that Zyban and Wellbutrin contain the same active ingredient and shouldn't be used together.

• Tell patient that it may take 4 weeks to reach full antidepressant effect.

🕔 *Alert:* Advise patient to report mood swings or suicidal thoughts immediately.

• Inform patient that tablets may have an odor.

• Tell patient taking extended-release form that the empty shell may appear in stool.

busPIRone hydrochloride
byoo-SPYE-rone

Therapeutic class: Anxiolytics
Pharmacologic class: Azaspirodecane-dione derivatives

AVAILABLE FORMS
Tablets: 5 mg, 7.5 mg, 10 mg, 15 mg, 30 mg

INDICATIONS & DOSAGES
➤ **Anxiety disorders**
Adults: Initially, 7.5 mg P.O. b.i.d. Increase dosage by 5 mg daily at 2- to 3-day intervals. Usual maintenance dosage is 20 to 30 mg daily in divided doses. Don't exceed 60 mg daily.

ADMINISTRATION
P.O.
• Don't give drug with grapefruit juice.
• Give drug at the same times each day, and always with or always without food.

ACTION
May inhibit neuronal firing and reduce serotonin turnover in cortical, amygdaloid, and septohippocampal tissue.

Route	Onset	Peak	Duration
P.O.	Unknown	40–90 min	Unknown

Half-life: 2 to 3 hours.

ADVERSE REACTIONS
CNS: dizziness, drowsiness, headache, nervousness, insomnia, light-headedness, fatigue, numbness, excitement, confusion, depression, anger, decreased concentration, paresthesia, incoordination, tremor, anger, hostility.
CV: tachycardia, nonspecific chest pain.
EENT: blurred vision.

Reactions in bold italics are *life-threatening*. Interactions may have a *rapid onset* or a *delayed onset*.

GI: dry mouth, nausea, diarrhea, abdominal distress, constipation, vomiting.
Musculoskeletal: aches and pains.
Skin: rash, sweating or clamminess.

INTERACTIONS
Drug-drug. *Azole antifungals:* May inhibit first-pass metabolism of buspirone. Monitor patient closely for adverse effects; adjust dosage as needed.
CNS depressants: May increase CNS depression. Use together cautiously.
CYP3A4 inducers (such as carbamazepine, dexamethasone, phenobarbital, phenytoin, rifabutin, rifampin): May decrease buspirone level. Adjust dosage as needed.
Drugs metabolized by CYP3A4 (clarithromycin, diltiazem, erythromycin, fluvoxamine, itraconazole, ketoconazole, nefazodone, ritonavir, verapamil): May increase buspirone level. Monitor patient; decrease buspirone dosage and adjust carefully.
Linezolid, methylene blue: May cause serotonin syndrome. Use extreme caution and monitor closely.
MAO inhibitors: May elevate BP. Avoid using together.
Nefazodone: May increase levels of both drugs. Use lower buspirone dosage if used together.
Sodium oxybate: May increase sleep duration and CNS depression. Use together is contraindicated.
Drug-food. *Grapefruit juice:* May increase drug level, increasing adverse effects. Give with liquid other than grapefruit juice.
Drug-lifestyle. *Alcohol use:* May increase CNS depression. Discourage use together.

EFFECTS ON LAB TEST RESULTS
None reported.

CONTRAINDICATIONS & CAUTIONS
• Contraindicated in patients hypersensitive to drug and within 14 days of MAO inhibitor therapy.
🕒 *Alert:* Concomitant use with linezolid or methylene blue can cause serotonin syndrome (fever, mental status changes, muscle twitching, excessive sweating, shivering or shaking, diarrhea, loss of coordination). Use drug with linezolid or methylene blue only for life-threatening or urgent conditions

when the potential benefits outweigh the risks of toxicity.
• Drug isn't recommended for patients with severe hepatic or renal impairment.
Dialyzable drug: No.
⚠ *Overdose S&S:* Nausea, vomiting, dizziness, drowsiness, miosis, gastric distress.

PREGNANCY-LACTATION-REPRODUCTION
• Use in pregnant and breast-feeding women isn't recommended. Use during pregnancy only if clearly needed.

NURSING CONSIDERATIONS
• Monitor patient closely for adverse CNS reactions. Drug is less sedating than other anxiolytics, but CNS effects may be unpredictable.
🕒 *Alert:* Before starting therapy, don't stop a previous benzodiazepine regimen abruptly because a withdrawal reaction may occur.
🕒 *Alert:* If linezolid or methylene blue must be given, buspirone must be stopped and the patient should be monitored for serotonin toxicity for 2 weeks or until 24 hours after the last dose of methylene blue or linezolid, whichever comes first. Treatment with buspirone may be resumed 24 hours after last dose of methylene blue or linezolid.
• Drug shows no potential for abuse and isn't classified as a controlled substance.
• *Look alike–sound alike:* Don't confuse buspirone with bupropion or risperidone.

PATIENT TEACHING
🕒 *Alert:* Teach patient to recognize and immediately report symptoms of serotonin toxicity (fever, mental status changes, muscle twitching, excessive sweating, shivering or shaking, diarrhea, loss of coordination).
• Warn patient to avoid hazardous activities that require alertness and good coordination until effects of drug are known.
• Remind patient that drug effects may not be noticeable for several weeks.
• Warn patient not to abruptly stop a benzodiazepine because of risk of withdrawal symptoms.
• Tell patient to avoid use of alcohol during therapy.
• Advise patient to take consistently; that is, always with or always without food.

butorphanol tartrate
byoo-TOR-fa-nole

Therapeutic class: Opioid analgesics
Pharmacologic class: Opioid agonist-antagonists–opioid partial agonists
Controlled substance schedule: IV

AVAILABLE FORMS
Injection: 1 mg/mL, 2 mg/mL
Nasal spray: 10 mg/mL (1 mg/spray)

INDICATIONS & DOSAGES
➤ **Moderate to severe pain**
Adults: 1 to 4 mg I.M. every 3 to 4 hours p.r.n., or around the clock. Not to exceed 4 mg per dose. Or, 0.5 to 2 mg I.V. every 3 to 4 hours p.r.n., or around the clock. Or, 1 mg by nasal spray every 3 to 4 hours (1 spray in one nostril); repeat in 60 to 90 minutes if pain relief is inadequate. For severe pain, 2 mg (1 spray in each nostril) every 3 to 4 hours.
Adjust-a-dose: For patients with renal or hepatic impairment, increase dosage interval to 6 to 8 hours and give 50% of the normal dose. For elderly patients, give 1 mg I.M. or 0.5 mg I.V.; wait 6 hours before repeating dose. For nasal use, 1 mg (1 spray in one nostril). May give another 1 mg in 1.5 to 2 hours. Wait 6 hours before repeating sequence.
➤ **Labor for patients at full term; early labor (without signs of fetal distress)**
Adults: 1 or 2 mg I.V. or I.M.; repeat after 4 hours as needed. Don't give dose less than 4 hours before anticipated delivery.
➤ **Preoperative anesthesia or preanesthesia**
Adults: 2 mg I.M. 60 to 90 minutes before surgery.
➤ **Adjunct to balanced anesthesia**
Adults: 2 mg I.V. shortly before induction, or 0.5 to 1 mg I.V. in increments during anesthesia.
Elderly patients: One-half usual dose, with repeat doses determined by patient's response.

ADMINISTRATION
I.V.
▼ Compatible solutions include D$_5$W and NSS.
▼ Give by direct injection into a vein or into the tubing of a free-flowing I.V. solution.
▼ **Incompatibilities:** Refer to detailed drug reference.
I.M.
● Give drug I.M.; don't give subcutaneously.
Intranasal
● Watch for nasal congestion with nasal spray use.

ACTION
May bind with opioid receptors in the CNS, altering perception of and emotional response to pain.

Route	Onset	Peak	Duration
I.V.	1 min	4–5 min	2–4 hr
I.M.	10–30 min	30–60 min	3–4 hr
Nasal	15 min	1–2 hr	2½–5 hr

Half-life: About 2 to 9 hours.

ADVERSE REACTIONS
CNS: dizziness, insomnia, somnolence, anxiety, asthenia, confusion, euphoria, headache, lethargy, nervousness, paresthesia, tremor.
CV: flushing, palpitations, vasodilation.
EENT: nasal congestion, blurred vision, nasal irritation, pharyngitis, sinus congestion, sinusitis, rhinitis, tinnitus.
GI: nausea, unpleasant taste, vomiting, anorexia, constipation, dry mouth, stomach pain.
Respiratory: bronchitis, cough, dyspnea, URI.
Skin: clamminess, excessive diaphoresis, pruritus.
Other: sensation of heat.

INTERACTIONS
Drug-drug. `Black Box Warning` *Benzodiazepines, CNS depressants:* May cause slow or difficult breathing, sedation, and death. Avoid use together. If use together is necessary, limit dosage and duration of each drug to the minimum necessary for desired effect. ∎
CNS depressants: May cause additive effects. Use together cautiously.
❸ *Alert:* Serotonergic drugs (amoxapine, antiemetics [dolasetron, granisetron, ondansetron, palonosetron], antimigraine drugs, buspirone, cyclobenzaprine,

---

dextromethorphan, linezolid, lithium, MAO inhibitors, maprotiline, methylene blue, mirtazapine, nefazodone, SNRIs, SSRIs, TCAs, trazodone, tryptophan, vilazodone): May increase risk of serotonin syndrome. Use together cautiously; monitor patient for serotonin syndrome.

Drug-herb. ❸ Alert: *St. John's wort:* May increase risk of serotonin syndrome. Use together cautiously; monitor patient for serotonin syndrome.

Drug-lifestyle. *Alcohol use:* May cause additive effects. Discourage use together.

EFFECTS ON LAB TEST RESULTS
None reported.

CONTRAINDICATIONS & CAUTIONS
• Contraindicated in patients hypersensitive to drug or to preservative, benzethonium chloride, and in those with opioid addiction; may cause withdrawal syndrome.

Black Box Warning Drug exposes patients and other users to risks of opioid addiction, abuse, and misuse, which can lead to overdose and death. Assess each patient's risk before prescribing butorphanol tartrate injection, and monitor all patients regularly for development of these behaviors or conditions. ∎

Black Box Warning Serious, life-threatening, or fatal respiratory depression may occur with use of butorphanol tartrate injection. Monitor patients for respiratory depression, especially during drug initiation and after dosage increase. ∎

Black Box Warning Opioid drugs should only be prescribed with benzodiazepines or other CNS depressants to patients for whom alternative treatment options are inadequate. ∎

❸ **Alert:** Drug may lead to rare but serious decrease in adrenal gland cortisol production.

❸ **Alert:** Drug may cause decreased sex hormone levels with long-term use.

• Use cautiously in patients with head injury, increased ICP, acute MI, ventricular dysfunction, coronary insufficiency, respiratory disease or depression, and renal or hepatic dysfunction.

• Use cautiously in patients who have recently received repeated doses of opioid analgesic.

• For patients who have been taking drug regularly, gradually titrate dosage downward to prevent signs and symptoms of withdrawal. *Dialyzable drug:* Unknown.

⚠ **Overdose S&S:** Respiratory depression, CNS depression, CV insufficiency, coma, death.

PREGNANCY-LACTATION-REPRODUCTION
• There are no adequate and well-controlled studies in pregnant women before 37 weeks' gestation. Use during pregnancy only if potential benefit justifies potential risk to the fetus.

• There have been rare reports of infant respiratory distress/apnea after butorphanol administration during labor. These reports have been associated with administration of a dose within 2 hours of delivery, use of multiple doses, use with additional analgesics or sedatives, or use in preterm pregnancies.

• If fetal HR pattern is abnormal, use butorphanol injection cautiously.

❸ **Alert:** Monitor breast-feeding women and infants for psychomimetic reactions. Monitor breast-feeding infants for apnea and sedation.

Black Box Warning Closely monitor neonates with prolonged opioid exposure during pregnancy for signs and symptoms of withdrawal (fever, diarrhea, vomiting, poor feeding, high-pitched crying, increased muscle tone, irritability, seizures), which may be life-threatening and may require management according to protocols developed by neonatology experts. ∎

NURSING CONSIDERATIONS
• Butorphanol nasal solution isn't recommended during labor or delivery; there is no clinical experience with its use in this setting.

❸ **Alert:** If patient is taking opioids with serotonergic drugs, monitor for signs and symptoms of serotonin syndrome (agitation, hallucinations, rapid HR, fever, excessive sweating, shivering or shaking, muscle twitching or stiffness, trouble with coordination, nausea, vomiting, diarrhea), especially when starting treatment or increasing dosages. Signs and symptoms may occur within several hours of coadministration but may also occur later, especially after dosage increase. Discontinue the opioid, serotonergic drug, or both if serotonin syndrome is suspected.

❸ *Alert:* Monitor patient for signs and symptoms of adrenal insufficiency (nausea, vomiting, loss of appetite, fatigue, weakness, dizziness, low BP). Perform diagnostic testing if adrenal insufficiency is suspected. If adrenal insufficiency is confirmed, treat with corticosteroids and wean patient off opioids if appropriate. Discontinue corticosteroids when clinically appropriate.

❸ *Alert:* Monitor patient for signs and symptoms of decreased sex hormone levels (low libido, erectile dysfunction, amenorrhea, infertility). If signs and symptoms occur, evaluate patient and obtain laboratory testing.

• Reassess patient's level of pain 15 and 30 minutes after administration.

• Respiratory depression apparently doesn't increase with larger dosage.

• Drug may cause constipation. Assess bowel function and need for stool softener and stimulant laxatives.

• Psychological and physical addiction may occur.

• Periodically monitor postoperative vital signs and bladder function. Because drug decreases both rate and depth of respirations, monitor arterial oxygen saturation to help assess respiratory depression.

PATIENT TEACHING

❸ *Alert:* Encourage patient to report all medications being taken, including prescription and OTC drugs and supplements.

Black Box Warning Caution the patient or the caregiver of a patient taking an opioid drug with a benzodiazepine, CNS depressant, or alcohol to seek immediate medical attention if the patient has symptoms of dizziness, light-headedness, extreme sleepiness, slowed or difficult breathing, or unresponsiveness. ∎

❸ *Alert:* Caution patient to immediately report signs and symptoms of serotonin syndrome, adrenal insufficiency, and decreased sex hormone levels.

• Caution ambulatory patient about getting out of bed or walking. Warn outpatient to avoid driving and other hazardous activities that require mental alertness until it's clear how the drug affects the CNS.

❸ *Alert:* Accidental ingestion of even one dose of nasal solution, especially by children, can result in a fatal overdose.

• Teach patient how to take nasal spray and how to store in child-resistant container.

• Instruct patient to avoid alcohol during therapy.

calcitonin salmon
kal-si-TOE-nin

Fortical, Miacalcin

Therapeutic class: Antiosteoporotics
Pharmacologic class: Polypeptide hormones

AVAILABLE FORMS
Injection: 200 units/mL in 2-mL ampules
Nasal spray: 200 units/activation

INDICATIONS & DOSAGES
➤ **Paget disease of bone (osteitis deformans)**
Adults: 100 units daily I.M. or subcutaneously.
➤ **Hypercalcemia**
Adults: 4 units/kg every 12 hours I.M. or subcutaneously. If response is inadequate after 1 or 2 days, increase dosage to 8 units/kg every 12 hours. If response remains unsatisfactory after 2 additional days, increase dosage to maximum of 8 units/kg every 6 hours.
➤ **Postmenopausal osteoporosis in women more than 5 years after menopause**
Adults: 200 units (one activation) daily intranasally, alternating nostrils daily. Or, 100 units I.M. or subcutaneously daily. Patient should receive adequate vitamin D and calcium supplements (at least 1,000 mg elemental calcium and 400 units of vitamin D) daily.

ADMINISTRATION
I.M.
• I.M. route is preferred if volume of dose exceeds 2 mL; use multiple injection sites.
• Store in refrigerator between 36° and 46° F (2° and 8° C).
Intranasal
• Alternate nostrils daily.

• Allow bottle to reach room temperature and prime pump before first use by releasing at least 5 sprays until full spray is produced. Don't prime pump every day.
• Discard spray container after 30 doses.
• Keep bottle refrigerated while unopened; store in an upright position at room temperature after opening.

Subcutaneous

• Alternate injection sites.
• Store in refrigerator between 36° and 46° F (2° and 8° C).

ACTION

Decreases osteoclastic activity by inhibiting osteocytic osteolysis; decreases mineral release and matrix or collagen breakdown in bone.

Route	Onset	Peak	Duration
I.M., subcut.	2 hr	23 min	6–8 hr
Intranasal	Rapid	10–13 min	Unknown

Half-life: I.M. and subcutaneous, 58 to 64 minutes; intranasal, 23 minutes.

ADVERSE REACTIONS

CNS: depression, headache, weakness, dizziness, paresthesia, fatigue.
CV: angina, chest pressure, facial flushing, edema of feet, hypertension.
EENT: eye pain, nasal congestion, rhinitis, abnormal tearing, sinusitis, conjunctivitis.
GI: constipation, transient nausea, unusual taste, diarrhea, anorexia, nausea, vomiting, epigastric discomfort, abdominal pain.
GU: cystitis, increased urinary frequency, nocturia.
Hematologic: infection, lymphadenopathy.
Musculoskeletal: arthrosis, myalgia.
Respiratory: ***bronchospasm,*** URI, shortness of breath, sinusitis.
Skin: rash, pruritus of ear lobes, inflammation at injection site, flushing of face and hands.
Other: hypersensitivity reactions, ***anaphylaxis,*** chills, tender palms and soles, flulike symptoms.

INTERACTIONS

Drug-drug. *Lithium:* May reduce plasma lithium concentration due to increased urinary clearance of lithium. Monitor level and adjust lithium dosage as needed.

EFFECTS ON LAB TEST RESULTS

None reported.

CONTRAINDICATIONS & CAUTIONS

• Contraindicated in patients hypersensitive to drug.

Dialyzable drug: Unknown.

⚠ ***Overdose S&S:*** Hypocalcemic tetany (increased neuromuscular irritability, repetitive neuromuscular movements after a single stimulus).

PREGNANCY-LACTATION-REPRODUCTION

• Use during pregnancy only if potential benefits justify possible risks to patient and fetus.
• It isn't known if drug appears in breast milk, but it has been shown to decrease milk production in animals. Use in breast-feeding women isn't recommended.

NURSING CONSIDERATIONS

• Skin test is usually done in patients with suspected drug sensitivity before therapy.
Alert: Systemic allergic reactions are possible because hormone is protein. Keep epinephrine nearby.
Alert: Observe patient for signs of hypocalcemic tetany during therapy (muscle twitching, tetanic spasms, and seizures when hypocalcemia is severe).
Alert: Periodically reevaluate need for continued therapy because of the possible association between malignancy and long-term calcitonin salmon use.
• Monitor calcium level closely. Watch for symptoms of hypercalcemia relapse: bone pain, renal calculi, polyuria, anorexia, nausea, vomiting, thirst, constipation, lethargy, bradycardia, muscle hypotonicity, pathologic fracture, psychosis, and coma.
• Periodic examinations of urine sediment are recommended.
• Periodic nasal examination with visualization of nasal mucosa, turbinates, septum, and mucosal blood vessel status is recommended to assess for ulceration in patients using intranasal form.
• Monitor periodic alkaline phosphatase and 24-hour urine hydroxyproline levels to evaluate drug effect.

• In Paget disease, maximum reductions of alkaline phosphatase and urinary hydroxyproline excretion may take 6 to 24 months of continuous treatment.

• In patients with good first response to drug who have a relapse, expect to evaluate antibody response to the hormone protein.

• If symptoms have been relieved after 6 months, treatment may be stopped until symptoms or radiologic signs recur.

• Nasal reactions occur more commonly in elderly patients.

• **Look alike–sound alike:** Don't confuse calcitonin with calcifediol or calcitriol.

PATIENT TEACHING

• When drug is given for postmenopausal osteoporosis, remind patient to take adequate calcium and vitamin D supplements.

• Prime pump of nasal spray bottle before first dose by holding bottle upright and depressing the two white side arms of pump toward bottle at least five times until a full spray is produced. Don't prime pump before each daily dose.

• Show home care patient and family member how to give drug. If nasal spray is prescribed, tell patient to alternate nostrils daily.

• Advise patient to notify prescriber if significant nasal irritation or evidence of an allergic response occurs.

• Inform patient that local inflammatory reactions have been reported at subcutaneous or I.M. injection sites in about 10% of patients and that facial flushing and warmth occur in 2% to 5% of patients within minutes of injection and usually last about 1 hour.

• Tell patient that nausea and vomiting may occur at the onset of therapy.

• Tell patient to inform prescriber promptly if signs and symptoms of hypercalcemia occur. Inform patient that, if drug loses its hypocalcemic activity, other drugs or increased dosages won't help.

• Advise patient not to breast-feed while taking drug.

calcitriol (1,25-dihydroxycholecalciferol)
kal-SIH-trye-ol

Rocaltrol, Vectical

Therapeutic class: Antihypocalcemics
Pharmacologic class: Vitamin D analogues

AVAILABLE FORMS
Capsules: 0.25 mcg, 0.5 mcg
Injection: 1 mcg/mL
Oral solution: 1 mcg/mL
Topical: 3 mcg/g

INDICATIONS & DOSAGES
➤ **Hypocalcemia in patients undergoing long-term dialysis (P.O.)**
Adults: Initially, 0.25 mcg P.O. daily. Increase by 0.25 mcg daily at 4- to 8-week intervals. Maintenance oral dosage is 0.25 mcg every other day up to 1 mcg daily (most patients respond to doses between 0.5 and 1 mcg/day).
➤ **Hypocalcemia in patients undergoing long-term dialysis (I.V.)**
Adults and children age 13 and older: Usual I.V. dosage is 1 to 2 mcg I.V. three times weekly (approximately every other day). Increase dose by 0.5 to 1 mcg at 2- to 4-week intervals.
➤ **Hypoparathyroidism, pseudohypoparathyroidism**
Adults and children age 6 and older: Initially, 0.25 mcg P.O. daily in the morning. Dosage may be increased at 2- to 4-week intervals. Maintenance dosage is 0.25 to 2 mcg P.O. daily.
➤ **Hypoparathyroidism**
Children ages 1 to 5: Give 0.25 to 0.75 mcg P.O. daily.
➤ **To manage secondary hyperparathyroidism and resulting metabolic bone disease in predialysis patients (with CrCl of 15 to 55 mL/minute)**
Adults and children age 3 and older: Initially, 0.25 mcg P.O. daily. Dosage may be increased to 0.5 mcg/day if needed.
Children younger than age 3: Initially, 0.01 to 0.015 mcg/kg P.O. daily.

➤ **Mild to moderate plaque psoriasis**
Adults: Apply topically to affected area
b.i.d. Maximum weekly dosage is 200 g.
➤ **Psoriasis (plaque-type)** ◆
Children and adolescents: Apply topically
to affected area b.i.d.

ADMINISTRATION
P.O.
● Give drug without regard for food.
● Don't give with magnesium-containing
antacids.
I.V.
▼ For hypocalcemia in patient undergoing
hemodialysis, give drug by rapid injection
through catheter at end of hemodialysis
session.
▼ **Incompatibilities:** None reported.
Topical
● Topical form isn't for oral, ophthalmic, or
intravaginal use.
● Gently rub into skin until no longer
visible.

ACTION
Stimulates calcium absorption from the GI
tract and promotes movement of calcium
from bone to blood.

Route	Onset	Peak	Duration
P.O.	2–6 hr	3–6 hr	3–5 days
I.V.	Immediate	Unknown	3–5 days
Topical	Unknown	Unknown	Unknown

Half-life: 5 to 8 hours.

ADVERSE REACTIONS
CNS: headache, somnolence, weakness,
irritability.
CV: hypertension, *arrhythmias.*
EENT: conjunctivitis, photophobia,
rhinorrhea.
GI: nausea, vomiting, constipation, polydip-
sia, *pancreatitis,* metallic taste, dry mouth,
anorexia.
GU: polyuria, nocturia, nephrocalcinosis,
hypercalciuria.
Metabolic: weight loss.
Musculoskeletal: bone and muscle pain.
Skin: pruritus, skin discomfort at applica-
tion area, psoriasis.
Other: hyperthermia, decreased libido.

INTERACTIONS
Drug-drug. *Cardiac glycosides:* May
increase risk of arrhythmias. Use together
cautiously.
*Cholestyramine, colestipol, excessive use of
mineral oil:* May decrease absorption of oral
vitamin D analogues. Avoid using together.
Corticosteroids: May counteract vitamin D
analogue effects. Avoid using together.
Magnesium-containing antacids: May cause
hypermagnesemia, especially in patients
with chronic renal failure. Avoid using
together.
Phenobarbital, phenytoin: May inhibit
calcitriol synthesis. Dose may need to be
increased.
Thiazides: May cause hypercalcemia. Use
together cautiously.

EFFECTS ON LAB TEST RESULTS
● May increase AST, ALT, BUN, creatinine,
cholesterol, urine albumin, and calcium
levels.

CONTRAINDICATIONS & CAUTIONS
● Contraindicated in patients with hypercalcemia or vitamin D toxicity. Withhold all
preparations containing vitamin D.
● Use cautiously in patients receiving cardiac glycosides and in those with sarcoidosis or hyperparathyroidism.
Dialyzable drug: Unknown.
⚠ **Overdose S&S:** Hypercalcemia, hyperphosphatemia, weakness, headache,
anorexia, nausea, vomiting, stomach
cramps, dizziness.

PREGNANCY-LACTATION-REPRODUCTION
● There are no adequate well-controlled
studies in pregnant women. Use during
pregnancy only if potential benefit justifies
risk to the fetus.
● Ingested calcitriol may appear in breast
milk. Women shouldn't breast-feed while
taking drug.

NURSING CONSIDERATIONS
● Effective therapy is dependent on adequate calcium intake.
● Monitor calcium level; this level times
the phosphate level shouldn't exceed 70.
During dose adjustment, determine calcium
level twice weekly. If hypercalcemia occurs,

stop drug and notify prescriber but resume after calcium level returns to normal. Patient should receive adequate daily intake of calcium. Observe for hypocalcemia, bone pain, and weakness before and during therapy.

• Monitor phosphorus level, especially in hypoparathyroid patients and dialysis patients.

• Reduce dose as parathyroid hormone levels decrease in response to therapy.

• Make sure patient taking calcitriol maintains adequate fluid status.

• The symptoms of vitamin D intoxication include headache, somnolence, weakness, irritability, hypertension, arrhythmias, conjunctivitis, photophobia, rhinorrhea, nausea, vomiting, constipation, polydipsia, pancreatitis, metallic taste, dry mouth, anorexia, nephrocalcinosis, polyuria, nocturia, weight loss, bone and muscle pain, pruritus, hyperthermia, and decreased libido.

• Protect drug from heat and light.

• *Look alike–sound alike:* Don't confuse calcitriol with calcifediol or calcitonin.

PATIENT TEACHING

• Tell patient to immediately report early symptoms of vitamin D intoxication: weakness, nausea, vomiting, dry mouth, constipation, muscle or bone pain, or metallic taste.

• Instruct patient to adhere to diet and calcium supplementation and to avoid unapproved OTC drugs and antacids that contain magnesium.

• Warn patient to avoid excessive exposure of topically treated areas to either artificial or natural sunlight, including phototherapy.

🔵 *Alert:* Tell patient that drug is the most potent form of vitamin D available and shouldn't be taken by anyone else.

calcium acetate
Calphron ◇, Eliphos, PhosLo Gelcaps, Phoslyra

calcium chloride

calcium citrate ◇
Citracal ◇, Citracal Liquitab ◇

calcium glubionate
Calcionate ◇

calcium gluconate

calcium lactate

calcium phosphate (tribasic)

Therapeutic class: Calcium supplements
Pharmacologic class: Calcium salts

AVAILABLE FORMS
calcium acetate
Contains 253 mg or 12.7 mEq of elemental calcium/g
Capsules: 667 mg
Gelcaps: 667 mg
Solution: 667 mg/5 mL
Tablets 🆗*:* 667 mg, 668 mg
calcium chloride
Contains 273 mg or 13.6 mEq of elemental calcium/g
Injection: 10% solution in 10-mL ampules, vials, and syringes
calcium citrate
Contains 211 mg or 10.6 mEq of elemental calcium/g
Capsules: 150 mg ◇
Granules for oral solution: 760 mg/3.5 g
Tablets: 200 mg ◇, 250 mg ◇
calcium glubionate
Contains 64 mg or 3.2 mEq elemental calcium/g
Syrup: 1.8 g/5 mL ◇
calcium gluconate
Contains 90 mg or 4.5 mEq of elemental calcium/g
Capsules: 500 mg
Injection: 10% solution in 10-mL ampules and vials, 10-mL or 50-mL vials
Tablets: 50 mg, 500 mg ◇, 650 mg ◇
calcium lactate
Contains 130 mg or 6.5 mEq of elemental calcium/g
Capsules: 500 mg (96 mg elemental calcium)
Tablets: 600 mg, 648 mg, 750 mg
calcium phosphate (tribasic)
Contains 400 mg or 20 mEq of elemental calcium/g
Tablets: 600 mg ◇

INDICATIONS & DOSAGES

➤ **Hypocalcemic emergency**
Adults: 7 to 14 mEq calcium I.V. May give
as a 10% calcium gluconate solution or
2% to 10% calcium chloride solution.
Children: 1 to 7 mEq calcium I.V.
Infants: Up to 1 mEq calcium I.V.

➤ **Hypocalcemic tetany**
Adults: 4.5 to 16 mEq calcium I.V. Repeat
until tetany is controlled.
Children: 0.5 to 0.7 mEq/kg calcium I.V.
t.i.d. to q.i.d. until tetany is controlled.
Neonates: 2.4 mEq/kg calcium I.V. daily in
divided doses.

➤ **Adjunctive treatment of magnesium
intoxication**
Adults: Initially, 7 mEq I.V. Base subsequent
doses on patient's response.

➤ **During exchange transfusions**
Adults: 1.35 mEq I.V. with each 100 mL
citrated blood.
Neonates: 0.45 mEq I.V. after each 100 mL
citrated blood.

➤ **Hyperphosphatemia**
Adults: 1,334 to 2,000 mg calcium acetate
P.O. t.i.d. with meals. Titrate dose every
2 to 3 weeks until an acceptable serum
phosphorus level is reached and watch for
hypercalcemia. Most dialysis patients need
3 to 4 tablets with each meal.

➤ **Dietary supplement**
Adults: 500 mg to 2 g P.O. daily.

➤ **Hyperkalemia with secondary cardiac
toxicity**
Adults: 2.25 to 14 mEq I.V. Repeat dose
after 1 to 2 minutes, if needed.

ADMINISTRATION

P.O.
● Give drug with a full glass of water.
● Give 1 to 1½ hours after meals if GI upset
occurs.

I.V.
▼ Calcium salts are not interchangeable;
verify preparation before use.
▼ Give calcium chloride only by I.V. route.
When adding to parenteral solutions that
contain other additives (especially phosphorus or phosphate), watch for precipitate. Use an in-line filter.
▼ When giving calcium gluconate as
injection, give only by I.V. route.

▼ Monitor ECG when giving calcium I.V.
Stop drug and notify prescriber if patient
complains of discomfort.
▼ Extravasation may cause severe necrosis
and tissue sloughing. Calcium gluconate
is less irritating to veins and tissues than
calcium chloride.

Direct injection
▼ Don't use scalp veins in children.
▼ Warm solution to body temperature
before giving it.
▼ For calcium chloride, give at
1 mL/minute (1.5 mEq/minute); for calcium gluconate, 2 mL/minute.
▼ Give slowly through a small needle
into a large vein or through an I.V. line
containing a free-flowing, compatible
solution.
▼ After injection, keep patient recumbent
for 15 minutes.

Intermittent infusion
▼ Infuse diluted solution through an I.V.
line containing a compatible solution.
▼ For calcium gluconate, don't exceed
200 mg/minute.
▼ **Incompatibilities:** Drug will precipitate
if given with sodium bicarbonate or other
alkaline drugs. Calcium chloride: amphotericin B, chlorpheniramine, dobutamine.
Calcium gluconate: amphotericin B, dobutamine, fluconazole, indomethacin sodium
trihydrate, methylprednisolone sodium
succinate, prochlorperazine edisylate.

ACTION

Replaces calcium and maintains calcium
level.

Route	Onset	Peak	Duration
P.O.	Unknown	Unknown	Unknown
I.V., I.M.	Immediate	Immediate	30 min–2 hr

Half-life: Unknown.

ADVERSE REACTIONS

CNS: tingling sensations, sense of oppres-
sion or heat waves with I.V. use, syncope
with rapid I.V. use.
CV: *bradycardia, arrhythmias, cardiac
arrest with rapid I.V. use,* mild drop in BP,
vasodilation.
GI: constipation, irritation, chalky taste,
hemorrhage, nausea, vomiting, thirst,
abdominal pain.

GU: polyuria, renal calculi.
Metabolic: hypercalcemia.
Skin: local reactions, including burning, necrosis, tissue sloughing, cellulitis, soft-tissue calcification with I.M. use.

INTERACTIONS

Drug-drug. *Bisphosphonates:* May reduce absorption of bisphosphonate from GI tract. Give calcium salts at least 30 minutes after alendronate or risedronate, at least 60 minutes after ibandronate, and not within 2 hours of etidronate.
Cardiac glycosides: May increase digoxin toxicity. Give calcium cautiously, if at all, to digitalized patients.
Fluoroquinolones: Oral calcium may decrease absorption of oral quinolones. Consider therapy modification.
Fosphenytoin, phenytoin: Use together may decrease absorption of both drugs. Avoid using together, or monitor levels carefully.
Iron supplements: May reduce iron absorption. Separate drug administration by 2 hours.
Sodium polystyrene sulfonate: May cause metabolic acidosis in patients with renal disease and a reduction of the resin's binding of potassium. Separate drugs by several hours.
Tetracyclines: May decrease serum concentration of tetracyclines. Avoid use together or, if concurrent use is absolutely necessary, consider separating administration of each agent by several hours.
Thiazide diuretics: May cause hypercalcemia. Avoid using together.
Verapamil: May reduce effects and toxicity of verapamil. Monitor patient closely.
Drug-food. *Foods containing oxalic acid (rhubarb, spinach), phytic acid (bran, whole-grain cereals), or phosphorus (dairy products, milk):* May interfere with calcium absorption. Discourage use together.

EFFECTS ON LAB TEST RESULTS

• May increase calcium level.

CONTRAINDICATIONS & CAUTIONS

• Contraindicated in cancer patients with bone metastases and in those with ventricular fibrillation, hypercalcemia, hypophosphatemia, or renal calculi.
Dialyzable drug: Yes.

⚠ *Overdose S&S:* Hypercalcemia, confusion, delirium, stupor, coma.

PREGNANCY-LACTATION-REPRODUCTION

• It isn't known if drug can cause fetal harm when used during pregnancy or if it can affect reproductive capacity. Use in pregnant women only if clearly needed.
• Calcium appears in breast milk, but is thought to be compatible with breast-feeding. Monitor maternal serum calcium levels.

NURSING CONSIDERATIONS

• Use all calcium products with extreme caution in digitalized patients and patients with sarcoidosis and renal or cardiac disease. Use calcium chloride cautiously in patients with cor pulmonale, respiratory acidosis, or respiratory failure.
◑ *Alert:* Double-check that you are giving the correct form of calcium; resuscitation cart may contain both calcium gluconate and calcium chloride.
• Monitor calcium levels frequently. Maintain calcium level of 9 to 10.4 mg/dL. Don't allow level to exceed 12 mg/dL. Hypercalcemia may result after large doses in chronic renal failure. Report abnormalities.
• Signs and symptoms of severe hypercalcemia may include stupor, confusion, delirium, and coma. Signs and symptoms of mild hypercalcemia may include anorexia, nausea, and vomiting.
• When calcium is given by the I.V. route, calcium gluconate is generally preferred over calcium chloride as it's less irritating to the veins.
• *Look alike–sound alike:* Don't confuse calcium with calcitriol, calcium gluconate with calcium glubionate, or calcium chloride with calcium gluconate.

PATIENT TEACHING

• Tell patient to take oral calcium 1 to 1½ hours after meals if GI upset occurs.
• Tell patient to take oral calcium with a full glass of water.
• Tell patient to report anorexia, nausea, vomiting, constipation, abdominal pain, dry mouth, thirst, or polyuria.
• Advise patient to notify prescriber if taking OTC products such as iron.

Reactions in bold italics are *life-threatening*. Interactions may have a *rapid onset* or a *delayed onset*.

● Warn patient that he shouldn't eat rhubarb, spinach, bran and whole-grain cereals, or dairy products in the meal before he takes calcium; these foods may interfere with calcium absorption.

● Inform patient that some products may contain phenylalanine or tartrazine.

canagliflozin
KAN-a-gli-FLOE-zin

Invokana

Therapeutic class: Antidiabetics
Pharmacologic class: Sodium-glucose cotransporter 2 inhibitors

AVAILABLE FORMS
Tablets: 100 mg, 300 mg

INDICATIONS & DOSAGES
➤ **Adjunct to diet and exercise to improve glycemic control in patients with type 2 diabetes**
Adults: 100 mg P.O. once daily before first meal of the day. May increase to 300 mg/day.
Adjust-a-dose: In patients tolerating 100 mg once daily who have an estimated GFR of 60 mL/minute/1.73 m^2 or greater and require additional glycemic control, may increase dosage to 300 mg once daily.

In those with moderate renal impairment (estimated GFR of 45 to <60 mL/minute/1.73 m^2), maximum dosage is 100 mg once daily. Don't initiate therapy in patients with an estimated GFR of less than 45 mL/minute/1.73 m^2. Discontinue drug in patients with an estimated GFR persistently less than 45 mL/minute/1.73 m^2.

If patient is also taking UDP-glucuronosyltransferase (UGT) inducers (phenobarbital, phenytoin, rifampin, ritonavir), may increase canagliflozin dosage to 300 mg once daily if patient is currently tolerating canagliflozin 100 mg once daily, has an estimated GFR greater than 60 mL/minute/1.73 m^2, and requires additional glycemic control; if estimated GFR is 45 to less than 60 mL/minute/1.73 m^2,

consider changing to another antidiabetic drug if need for concurrent UGTs exists.

ADMINISTRATION
P.O.
● Give before first meal of the day.
● Store tablets at room temperature.

ACTION
Inhibits sodium-glucose cotransporter 2, which reabsorbs glucose filtered by the kidneys, increasing amount of urinary glucose that is excreted.

Route	Onset	Peak	Duration
P.O.	Unknown	1–2 hr	Unknown

Half-life: 10.6 hours for 100-mg dose; 13.1 hours for 300-mg dose.

ADVERSE REACTIONS
CNS: fatigue, asthenia, syncope, postural dizziness.
CV: hypotension, orthostatic hypotension.
GI: thirst, constipation, nausea, abdominal pain, dehydration, *pancreatitis.*
GU: genital fungal infection, UTI, increased urination, vulvovaginal pruritus, renal impairment.
Hematologic: increased Hb level.
Metabolic: *hypoglycemia, hyperkalemia,* hypercholesterolemia, hypermagnesemia, hyperphosphatemia.
Musculoskeletal: bone fracture.
Other: hypersensitivity reactions.

INTERACTIONS
Drug-drug. *ACE inhibitors (enalapril, lisinopril, moexipril, quinapril), ARBs (candesartan, losartan, olmesartan, valsartan), eplerenone, potassium-sparing diuretics (amiloride, spironolactone):* May increase risk of hyperkalemia. Monitor potassium level closely.
Antihypertensives: May increase hypotension. Monitor patient closely.
Carbamazepine: May decrease canagliflozin serum concentration. Consider increasing canagliflozin dosage based on GFR.
Digoxin: May increase digoxin level. Monitor digoxin level periodically.
Insulin and insulin secretagogues (glipizide, repaglinide): May increase risk of

hypoglycemia. Consider lower dosage of insulin or insulin secretagogue.

Lomitapide: May increase lomitapide level. Limit maximum adult dosage of lomitapide to 30 mg daily.

Loop diuretics: May cause hypotension and intravascular volume depletion. Consider alternative therapy.

Salicylates: May increase hypoglycemic effects. Monitor patient closely.

SSRIs (citalopram, fluoxetine, sertraline): May increase canagliflozin level. Monitor patient closely. Canagliflozin dosage may need adjustment if SSRI is discontinued.

UGT inducers (phenobarbital, phenytoin, rifampin, ritonavir): May decrease canagliflozin level. Adjust canagliflozin dosage based on estimated GFR.

Drug-herb. *St. John's wort:* May decrease canagliflozin serum concentration. Consider increasing canagliflozin dosage based on GFR.

EFFECTS ON LAB TEST RESULTS
● May increase serum creatinine, potassium, magnesium, phosphate, Hb, LDL cholesterol, non-HDL cholesterol, and urine glucose levels.
● May decrease GFR and serum glucose level.

CONTRAINDICATIONS & CAUTIONS
● Contraindicated in patients hypersensitive to drug or its components, in those with type 1 diabetes, diabetic ketoacidosis, severe renal impairment (estimated GFR of <30 mL/minute/1.73 m^2), or ESRD, and in patients on dialysis.
◑ *Alert:* Drug may cause acidosis, which may require emergency department care or hospitalization.
◑ *Alert:* Drug may increase risk of bone fracture as early as 12 weeks after start of treatment and has been linked to decreased bone mineral density. Consider factors that may contribute to bone fracture risk prior to prescribing.
◑ *Alert:* Drug may increase risk of severe UTI, including urosepsis and pyelonephritis. Monitor patient and treat promptly if indicated.
● Drug isn't recommended for patients with severe hepatic disease (Child-Pugh class C).
● Drug increases serum creatinine level and decreases estimated GFR; patients with hypovolemia may be more susceptible to these

changes. Renal function abnormalities can occur after drug initiation. More frequent renal function monitoring is recommended in patients with an estimated GFR of less than 60 mL/minute/1.73 m^2.
● Use cautiously in elderly patients and in those with volume depletion, impaired renal function, chronic low systolic BP, or hypotension.
Dialyzable drug: No.

PREGNANCY-LACTATION-REPRODUCTION
● There are no adequate well-controlled studies in pregnant women. Use during pregnancy only if potential benefit justifies potential risk to the fetus.
● It isn't known if drug appears in breast milk. Patient should discontinue breast-feeding or discontinue drug, taking into account importance of drug to the mother.

NURSING CONSIDERATIONS
◑ *Alert:* Drug can increase risk of acute kidney injury. Before start of therapy, assess patient for factors that may predispose patient to acute kidney injury (decreased blood volume, chronic renal insufficiency, HF, concurrent use of other medications, such as diuretics, ACE inhibitors, ARBs, NSAIDs). Assess renal function before starting drug and monitor patient periodically. If acute kidney injury occurs, drug should be discontinued and the kidney impairment treated.
● Correct volume depletion before initiating drug. Observe for hypotension during therapy.
◑ *Alert:* Monitor patients for ketoacidosis, especially those with major illness, reduced food or fluid intake, or reduced insulin dose. Elevated urine or serum ketone levels without associated very high glucose levels have occurred with sodium-glucose cotransporter-2 inhibitor use.
● Monitor blood glucose level. Assess for signs and symptoms of hypoglycemia.
● Be aware that because of the drug's mechanism of action, urine test will be positive for glucose.
● Monitor electrolytes, such as potassium and magnesium. Correct levels as clinically indicated.
● Drug may increase lipid levels. Assess LDL cholesterol level periodically and treat as clinically indicated.

Reactions in bold italics are *life-threatening*. Interactions may have a *rapid onset* or a ***delayed onset***.

- Assess for genital mycotic (fungal) infections, especially in patients with a history of infection and in uncircumcised males. Treat appropriately.
- Monitor patient for hypersensitivity reaction (urticaria); reaction may occur hours to days after start of therapy. Discontinue drug and treat appropriately if hypersensitivity reaction occurs.

PATIENT TEACHING
- Advise patient to discontinue drug and immediately report hypersensitivity reaction (generalized urticarial rash).
- **❸ Alert:** Instruct patient to seek medical attention immediately for signs and symptoms of ketoacidosis (difficulty breathing, hyperventilation, anorexia, nausea, vomiting, abdominal pain, confusion, unusual fatigue or sleepiness).
- **❸ Alert:** Instruct patient to seek medical attention for signs and symptoms of UTI (dysuria, frequency, pelvic pain, hematuria, urgency, fever, back pain, nausea, vomiting).
- **❸ Alert:** Advise patient to seek immediate medical attention for signs and symptoms of acute kidney injury (decreased urine, swelling in legs or feet). Warn patient not to stop drug without first discussing with prescriber.
- Warn female patient of possible risks to fetus and infant during pregnancy or breast-feeding. Instruct breast-feeding woman that she should discontinue drug or discontinue breast-feeding.
- Caution patient to avoid dehydration, which can cause hypotension. Instruct patient regarding adequate fluid intake and to report signs and symptoms of hypotension (postural dizziness, weakness, syncope).
- Instruct patient on general diabetes care, including importance of diet and exercise and monitoring blood glucose and HbA_{1c} levels; signs and management of hypoglycemia and hyperglycemia; and assessing for diabetes complications.
- Advise patient to seek medical advice promptly during periods of stress (such as fever, trauma, infection, or surgery) because medication requirements may change.
- Instruct patient that if a dose is missed, to take it as soon as it's remembered unless it's almost time for the next dose, in which

case patient should skip missed dose and take drug at next regularly scheduled time. Advise patient not to take two doses of drug at the same time.

C

candesartan cilexetil
kan-dah-SAR-tan

Atacand

Therapeutic class: Antihypertensives
Pharmacologic class: Angiotensin II receptor antagonists

AVAILABLE FORMS
Tablets: 4 mg, 8 mg, 16 mg, 32 mg

INDICATIONS & DOSAGES
Adjust-a-dose (for all indications): If patient is taking a diuretic, especially a patient with impaired renal function, administer under close medical supervision and consider a lower starting dose.
➤ **Hypertension (used alone or with other antihypertensives)**
Adults: Initially, 16 mg P.O. once daily when used alone; usual range is 8 to 32 mg P.O. daily as a single dose or in two divided doses. Double the dose about every 2 weeks, as tolerated, to target dose of 32 mg once daily.
Adjust-a-dose: In patients with moderate hepatic impairment, initially give 8 mg P.O. once daily.
➤ **Pediatric hypertension (used alone or with other antihypertensives)**
Children ages 6 to younger than 17: Initially for patients weighing more than 50 kg, 8 to 16 mg P.O. once daily. May increase to 32 mg P.O. as single dose or divided doses as needed. Initially for patients weighing less than 50 kg, 4 to 8 mg P.O. once daily. May increase to 16 mg P.O. as single dose or divided doses as needed.
Children ages 1 to younger than 6: Initially, 0.2 mg/kg P.O. once daily. Dosage range is 0.05 to 0.4 mg/kg P.O. as single dose or divided doses.
➤ **HF (New York Heart Association class II to IV)**
Adults: Initially, 4 mg P.O. once daily. Double the dose about every 2 weeks as tolerated to a target dose of 32 mg once daily.

🍁 Canada   ◇ OTC   ◆ Off-label use   🖋 Photoguide   🚫 Do not crush   *Liquid contains alcohol.

ADMINISTRATION
P.O.
- Give drug without regard for food.
- Tablets may be made into suspension by pharmacist for patients unable to swallow pills.
- Suspension may be stored unopened at room temperature for 100 days.
- Shake suspension well before each use.
- Use suspension within 30 days of opening bottle.

ACTION
Inhibits vasoconstrictive action of angiotensin II by blocking angiotensin II receptor on the surface of vascular smooth muscle and other tissue cells.

Route	Onset	Peak	Duration
P.O.	Unknown	3–4 hr	24 hr

Half-life: 9 hours.

ADVERSE REACTIONS
CNS: dizziness, fatigue, headache.
CV: chest pain, peripheral edema.
EENT: pharyngitis, rhinitis, sinusitis.
GI: abdominal pain, diarrhea, nausea, vomiting.
GU: albuminuria.
Musculoskeletal: arthralgia, back pain.
Respiratory: coughing, bronchitis, URI.
Other: *angioedema.*

INTERACTIONS
Drug-drug. *ACE inhibitors, ARBs:* May increase risk of hypotension, hyperkalemia, and changes in renal function (including acute renal failure) when used with other drugs that cause blockade of the RAAS. Closely monitor BP, renal function, and electrolyte levels when administering with other agents that affect the RAS.
Aliskiren: May increase risk of renal impairment, hypotension, and hyperkalemia in diabetic patients and those with moderate to severe renal impairment (GFR <60 mL/minute). Concomitant use is contraindicated in diabetic patients. Avoid concomitant use in those with moderate to severe renal impairment.
Canagliflozin: May enhance hyperkalemic and hypotensive effects. Monitor potassium level and BP closely.

Lithium: May increase lithium concentration. Monitor lithium levels closely.
NSAIDs (celecoxib, ibuprofen): May decrease antihypertensive effect of candesartan. Coadministration in patients who are elderly, volume-depleted (including those taking diuretics), or with decreased renal function may result in deteriorating renal function. Monitor BP and renal function.
Potassium-sparing diuretics, potassium supplements: May cause hyperkalemia. Monitor patient closely.
Drug-herb. *Ma huang:* May decrease antihypertensive effects. Discourage use together.
Drug-food. *Salt substitutes containing potassium:* May cause hyperkalemia. Monitor patient closely.

EFFECTS ON LAB TEST RESULTS
- May increase potassium, BUN, and serum creatinine levels.

CONTRAINDICATIONS & CAUTIONS
- Contraindicated in patients hypersensitive to drug or its components, in children with GFR of less than 30 mL/min/1.73 m^2, and in children younger than age 1.
- Use cautiously in patients whose renal function depends on the RAAS (such as patients with HF) because of risk of oliguria and progressive azotemia with acute renal failure or death.
- Use cautiously in patients who are volume or salt depleted; may cause symptoms of hypotension. Start therapy with a lower dosage range, and monitor BP carefully.
- Don't use for hypertension in children younger than age 1 because of potential effects on the developing immature kidneys.
Dialyzable drug: No.
⚠ *Overdose S&S:* Hypotension, dizziness, tachycardia; possible bradycardia from parasympathetic stimulation.

PREGNANCY-LACTATION-REPRODUCTION
Black Box Warning Drugs such as candesartan that act directly on the RAAS can cause fetal and neonatal illness and death when given to pregnant women. If pregnancy is detected, discontinue candesartan as soon as possible. ■

Reactions in bold italics are *life-threatening*. Interactions may have a *rapid onset* or a *delayed onset*.

• It isn't known if drug appears in breast milk. Consider discontinuing breast-feeding or drug, taking into account importance of drug to the mother.

NURSING CONSIDERATIONS
• If hypotension occurs after a dose of cand-esartan, place patient in the supine position and, if needed, give an I.V. infusion of NSS.
• Most of drug's antihypertensive effect occurs within 2 weeks. Maximal effect may take 4 to 6 weeks. Diuretic may be added if BP isn't controlled by drug alone.
• Carefully monitor elderly patients and those with renal disease for therapeutic response and adverse reactions.

PATIENT TEACHING
• Inform women of childbearing potential of the consequences of exposure to drug during pregnancy. Prescriber should be noti-fied immediately if pregnancy is suspected.
• Advise breast-feeding women of the risk of adverse effects on the infant and the need to stop either breast-feeding or drug.
• Instruct patient to store drug at room temperature in tightly sealed container.
• Inform patient to report adverse reactions without delay.
• Tell patient that drug may be taken with-out regard to meals.

SAFETY ALERT!

cangrelor tetrasodium
KAN-grel-or

Kengreal

Therapeutic class: Antiplatelet drugs
Pharmacologic class: Platelet aggrega-tion inhibitors

AVAILABLE FORMS
Injection: 50 mg/10 mL in single-use vial

INDICATIONS & DOSAGES
➤ **As an adjunct to PCI for reducing risk of periprocedural MI, repeat coronary revascularization, and stent thrombosis in patients who haven't been treated with a P2Y12 platelet inhibitor and aren't receiving a glycoprotein IIb/IIIa inhibitor**

Adults: 30 mcg/kg I.V. bolus before PCI followed immediately by a 4-mcg/kg/minute I.V. infusion continued for at least 2 hours or for duration of PCI, whichever is longer. Transition patient to oral P2Y12 platelet inhibitor to maintain platelet inhibition. Recommended inhibitors include ticagrelor 180 mg P.O. at any time during infusion or immediately after discontinuation, or prasugrel 60 mg or clopidogrel 600 mg im-mediately after discontinuation of infusion, but not before.

ADMINISTRATION
I.V.
▼ For each 50-mg vial, reconstitute by adding 5 mL sterile water for injection. Swirl gently until all material is dissolved; avoid vigorous mixing. Ensure contents are fully dissolved, clear, colorless to pale yellow, and free from particulate matter.
▼ Dilute reconstituted drug immediately. Don't use without dilution.
▼ Further dilute each reconstituted vial by withdrawing contents from one reconsti-tuted vial and adding to one 250-mL NSS or dextrose 5% bag. Mix bag thoroughly. This dilution will result in a concentration of 200 mcg/mL and should be sufficient for at least 2 hours of dosing. Patients weigh-ing 100 kg or more will require a minimum of two bags.
▼ Discard any unused portion of reconsti-tuted solution remaining in vial.
▼ Administer via a dedicated I.V. line.
▼ Administer bolus volume rapidly (less than 1 minute) from the diluted bag via manual I.V. push or pump. Ensure bolus is completely administered before start of PCI. Start infusion immediately after administration of bolus.
▼ Diluted drug is stable for up to 12 hours in 5% dextrose injection and 24 hours in NSS at room temperature.

ACTION
A direct P2Y12 platelet receptor inhibitor that blocks adenosine diphosphate–induced platelet activation and aggregation. Binds selectively and reversibly to the P2Y12 receptor to prevent further signaling and platelet activation.

Route	Onset	Peak	Duration
I.V.	2 min	2 min	1 hr after discontinuation of infusion

Half-life: 3 to 6 minutes.

ADVERSE REACTIONS
CNS: *intracranial hemorrhage.*
GU: worsening renal function in patients with severe renal impairment.
Hematologic: *bleeding.*
Respiratory: dyspnea.

INTERACTIONS
Drug-drug. *Agents with antiplatelet properties (NSAIDs, P2Y12 inhibitors, SSRIs):* May enhance antiplatelet effects. Monitor therapy.
Anticoagulants: May increase anticoagulant effects. Monitor therapy.
Thienopyridines (clopidogrel, prasugrel): Negate antiplatelet effect. Don't give clopidogrel or prasugrel with cangrelor.
Drug-herb. *Alfalfa, anise, bilberry:* May increase risk of bleeding. Modify therapy.

EFFECTS ON LAB TEST RESULTS
None reported.

CONTRAINDICATIONS & CAUTIONS
• Contraindicated in patients hypersensitive to drug or its components and in those with significant active bleeding.
• Although rare, drug can cause serious hypersensitivity reactions, including anaphylaxis, bronchospasm, angioedema, and stridor.
• Safety and effectiveness in children haven't been established.
Dialyzable drug: Unknown.

PREGNANCY-LACTATION-REPRODUCTION
• There are no adequate studies in pregnant women. Some adverse effects were noted in animal studies.
• It isn't known if drug appears in breast milk.

NURSING CONSIDERATIONS
• Monitor patients for hypersensitivity reactions, including anaphylactic reactions, anaphylactic shock, bronchospasm, angioedema, and stridor. Discontinue drug immediately and treat emergently.

• Monitor patients for signs of overt bleeding and symptoms of active bleeding, such as reduction in Hb level of 3 g/dL or more or an absolute reduction in hematocrit of 9% or more.
• Platelet function will resume 1 hour after discontinuation of infusion.

PATIENT TEACHING
• Explain to patient that drug is used to inhibit platelet function during PCI and that platelet function and ability for clot formation will resume 1 hour after discontinuation of the infusion.
• Warn patient of the risk of bleeding; advise patient to immediately report signs and symptoms of bleeding (mental status changes, light-headedness, low BP, blood in stool or urine, bleeding from gums, joint pain and swelling, abnormal bruising, abdominal or chest pain).
• Caution patient that hypersensitivity reactions may occur; tell him to immediately report difficulty breathing, swelling of throat and lips, feeling faint, hives, or rash.

SAFETY ALERT!

capecitabine
kap-ah-SEAT-ah-been

Xeloda

Therapeutic class: Antineoplastics
Pharmacologic class: Pyrimidine analogues

AVAILABLE FORMS
Tablets ⓞⓝⓒ: 150 mg, 500 mg

INDICATIONS & DOSAGES
Adjust-a-dose (for all indications): Round to nearest dose that gives a whole tablet; don't cut tablets in half.
➤ **With docetaxel or alone, metastatic breast cancer resistant to both paclitaxel and an anthracycline-containing chemotherapy regimen or resistant to paclitaxel in patients for whom further anthracycline therapy isn't indicated; first-line treatment of metastatic colorectal cancer when fluoropyrimidine therapy**

Reactions in bold italics are *life-threatening*. Interactions may have a *rapid onset* or a *delayed onset*.

alone is preferred; Dukes stage C colon cancer after complete resection of primary tumor when fluoropyrimidine alone is preferred

Adults: 2,500 mg/m^2 daily P.O., in two divided doses, about 12 hours apart and after a meal, for 2 weeks, followed by a 1-week rest period; repeat every 3 weeks. Adjuvant treatment in patients with Dukes C colon cancer is recommended for a total of eight cycles (24 weeks).

Adjust-a-dose: Follow National Cancer Institute of Canada (NCIC) common toxicity criteria when adjusting dosage. Toxicity criteria relate to degrees of severity of diarrhea, nausea, vomiting, stomatitis, and hand-foot syndrome. Refer to drug package insert for specific toxicity definitions.

NCIC grade 1: Maintain dose level.

NCIC grade 2: At first appearance, stop treatment until resolved to grade 0 to 1; then restart at 100% of starting dose for next cycle. At second appearance, stop treatment until resolved to grade 0 to 1 and use 75% of starting dose for next cycle. At third appearance, stop treatment until resolved to grade 0 to 1 and use 50% of starting dose for next cycle. At fourth appearance, stop treatment permanently.

NCIC grade 3: At first appearance, stop treatment until resolved to grade 0 to 1 and use 75% of starting dose for next cycle. At second appearance, stop treatment until resolved to grade 0 to 1 and use 50% of starting dose for next cycle. At third appearance, stop treatment permanently.

NCIC grade 4: At first appearance, stop treatment permanently or until resolved to grade 0 to 1, and use 50% of starting dose for next cycle. Reduce starting dose for patients with CrCl of 30 to 50 mL/minute to 75% of the starting dose (from 1,250 to 950 mg/m^2 P.O. b.i.d.).

Consider reducing initial dose by 25% (1,900 mg/m^2 daily in two divided doses) in patients age 60 and older with breast cancer when used in combination with docetaxel, to minimize drug toxicity. In patients who develop grade 3 or 4 hyperbilirubinemia, interrupt treatment until bilirubin level is 3 × ULN or less; refer to dosage modification guidelines for dosage recommendations.

ADMINISTRATION

P.O.

- Give drug whole with water within 30 minutes after breakfast and dinner.
- Don't cut or crush tablets.
- Use gloves and safety glasses to avoid exposure if tablets break.

ACTION

Converted to active 5-FU, which causes cellular injury by interfering with DNA synthesis to inhibit cell division and with RNA processing and protein synthesis.

Route	Onset	Peak	Duration
P.O.	Unknown	90–120 min	Unknown

Half-life: About 45 minutes.

ADVERSE REACTIONS

CNS: dizziness, fatigue, headache, insomnia, paresthesia, pyrexia, lethargy, peripheral neuropathy, asthenia.
CV: edema, chest pain, *venous thrombosis.*
EENT: eye irritation, epistaxis, increased lacrimation, rhinorrhea.
GI: diarrhea, nausea, vomiting, stomatitis, abdominal pain, constipation, anorexia, dyspepsia, taste perversion.
Hematologic: *neutropenia, thrombocytopenia,* anemia, *lymphopenia.*
Metabolic: dehydration.
Musculoskeletal: myalgia, limb pain, back pain.
Respiratory: dyspnea.
Skin: hand-foot syndrome, dermatitis, nail disorder, alopecia, rash.
Other: neutropenic fever.

INTERACTIONS

Drug-drug. *Antacids containing aluminum hydroxide and magnesium hydroxide:* May increase exposure to capecitabine and its metabolites. Monitor patient.
Fosphenytoin, phenytoin: May increase toxicity or fosphenytoin/phenytoin effect. Consider therapy modification or monitor phenytoin level.
Leucovorin: May increase cytotoxic effects of 5-FU with enhanced toxicity. Monitor patient carefully.
Black Box Warning *Warfarin:* May decrease clearance of warfarin and increase risk of bleeding. Monitor PT and INR frequently. ∎

EFFECTS ON LAB TEST RESULTS

• May increase ALT and bilirubin levels. May decrease Hb level. May increase or decrease calcium level.

• May decrease neutrophil, platelet, and WBC counts.

Black Box Warning May prolong PT and increase INR (in patients taking warfarin concomitantly). ■

CONTRAINDICATIONS & CAUTIONS

• Contraindicated in patients hypersensitive to 5-FU, patients with known dihydropyrimidine dehydrogenase deficiency, and in those with severe renal impairment.

• Severe bone marrow suppression can occur and is more common when drug is used in combination therapy. Dosage adjustment may be needed.

• Use cautiously in elderly patients and those with history of CAD, mild to moderate hepatic dysfunction from liver metastases, hyperbilirubinemia, and renal insufficiency. Use cautiously in patients also taking warfarin.

Dialyzable drug: Unknown.

⚠ Overdose S&S: Nausea, vomiting, diarrhea, GI irritation and bleeding, bone marrow depression.

PREGNANCY-LACTATION-REPRODUCTION

• Fetal harm may occur if drug is administered during pregnancy. Women of childbearing potential should use effective contraception during treatment.

• It isn't known if drug appears in breast milk. Patient should discontinue breastfeeding or discontinue drug, taking into account importance of drug to the mother.

NURSING CONSIDERATIONS

• Patients older than age 80 may have a greater risk of adverse GI effects.

• Assess patient for severe diarrhea, and notify prescriber if it occurs. Give fluid and electrolyte replacement if patient becomes dehydrated. Drug may need to be immediately interrupted until diarrhea resolves or becomes less intense.

• Severe mucocutaneous reactions, such as Stevens-Johnson syndrome and toxic epidermal necrolysis, can occur. Drug will be permanently discontinued in patients who experience a severe mucocutaneous reaction.

• Monitor patient for hand-foot syndrome (numbness, paresthesia, painless or painful swelling, erythema, desquamation, blistering, and severe pain of hands or feet), hyperbilirubinemia, and severe nausea. Drug therapy must be immediately adjusted. Hand-foot syndrome is staged from 1 to 4; drug may be stopped if severe or recurrent episodes occur.

• Hyperbilirubinemia may require stopping drug.

Black Box Warning Frequently monitor INR and PT of patients taking capecitabine and oral coumarin-derivative anticoagulant therapy; adjust anticoagulant dose accordingly. ■

Black Box Warning Patients older than age 60 and those with a diagnosis of cancer are at increased risk of coagulopathy. ■

❸ Alert: Monitor patient carefully for toxicity, which may be managed by symptomatic treatment, dose interruptions, and dosage adjustments.

• *Look alike–sound alike:* Don't confuse Xeloda with Xenical.

PATIENT TEACHING

• Tell patient how to take drug. Drug is usually taken for 14 days, followed by 7-day rest period (no drug), as a 21-day cycle. Prescriber determines number of treatment cycles. Instruct patent to swallow tablets whole and not to cut or crush them.

❸ Alert: Tell patient who also takes warfarin to report significant bleeding or bruising.

• Instruct patient to take drug with water within 30 minutes after breakfast and dinner.

• If a combination of tablets is prescribed, teach patient importance of correctly identifying the tablets to avoid possible dosing error.

• For missed doses, instruct patient not to take the missed dose and not to double the next one. Instead, he should continue with regular dosing schedule and check with prescriber.

• Instruct patient to inform prescriber if he's taking folic acid.

• Inform patient and caregiver about expected adverse effects of drug, especially nausea, vomiting, diarrhea, and hand-foot syndrome (pain, swelling, or redness of hands or feet). Tell him that patient-specific dosage adaptations during therapy are expected and needed.

🚫 *Alert:* Instruct patient to stop taking drug and contact prescriber immediately if he develops diarrhea (more than four bowel movements daily or diarrhea at night), vomiting (two to five episodes in 24 hours), nausea, appetite loss or decrease in amount of food eaten each day, stomatitis (pain, redness, swelling, or sores in mouth), hand-foot syndrome, temperature of 100.5° F (38° C) or higher, or other evidence of infection.

• Tell patient that most adverse effects improve within 2 to 3 days after stopping drug. If patient doesn't improve, tell him to contact prescriber.

• Advise women of childbearing potential to avoid becoming pregnant during therapy.

• Advise breast-feeding women to stop breast-feeding during therapy.

captopril
KAP-toe-pril

Therapeutic class: Antihypertensives
Pharmacologic class: ACE inhibitors

AVAILABLE FORMS
Tablets: 12.5 mg, 25 mg, 50 mg, 100 mg

INDICATIONS & DOSAGES
Adjust-a-dose (for all indications): Patients with impaired renal function may respond to smaller or less frequent doses. In patients with significant renal impairment, reduce initial daily dosage, and use smaller increments for a slow titration (1- to 2-week intervals). Slowly back-titrate dosage after desired therapeutic effect has been achieved to determine the minimal effective dose. A loop diuretic such as furosemide, rather than a thiazide diuretic, is preferred in patients with severe renal impairment when concomitant diuretic therapy is required.

➤ **Hypertension (alone or in combination with other antihypertensives)**
Adults: Initially, 25 mg P.O. b.i.d. or t.i.d. If dosage doesn't control BP satisfactorily in 1 or 2 weeks, increase it to 50 mg b.i.d. or t.i.d. If that dosage doesn't control BP satisfactorily after another 1 or 2 weeks,

expect to add a diuretic. If patient needs further BP reduction, may increase dosage to 100 mg b.i.d. or t.i.d., then if necessary, to 150 mg b.i.d. or t.i.d. while continuing diuretic. Usual dosage range is 25 to 150 mg b.i.d. or t.i.d. Maximum daily dosage is 450 mg.

➤ **Diabetic nephropathy**
Adults: 25 mg P.O. t.i.d.

➤ **HF**
Adults: Initially, 25 mg P.O. t.i.d. Patients with normal or low BP who have been vigorously treated with diuretics and who may be hyponatremic or hypovolemic may start with 6.25 or 12.5 mg P.O. t.i.d.; starting dosage may be adjusted over several days. Gradually increase dosage to 50 mg P.O. t.i.d.; once patient reaches this dosage, delay further dosage increases for at least 2 weeks. Usual dosage is 50 to 100 mg P.O. t.i.d.; maximum dosage is 450 mg daily. Generally used in conjunction with a diuretic and a cardiac glycoside.

➤ **Left ventricular dysfunction after acute MI**
Adults: Start therapy as early as 3 days after MI with 6.25 mg P.O. for one dose, followed by 12.5 mg P.O. t.i.d. Increase over several days to 25 mg P.O. t.i.d.; then increase to 50 mg P.O. t.i.d. over several weeks.

ADMINISTRATION
P.O.
• Give 1 hour before meals to enhance drug absorption.

• Drug may be compounded into a suspension if patient can't swallow tablets.

• Refrigerate suspension and shake well before use. Suspension is stable for 56 days if refrigerated.

ACTION
Inhibits ACE, preventing conversion of angiotensin I to angiotensin II, a potent vasoconstrictor. Less angiotensin II decreases peripheral arterial resistance, decreasing aldosterone secretion, which reduces sodium and water retention and lowers BP.

Route	Onset	Peak	Duration
P.O.	Within 15 min	60–90 min	Unknown

Half-life: Less than 2 hours.

ADVERSE REACTIONS
CNS: dizziness, fainting, headache, malaise, fatigue, fever.
CV: tachycardia, hypotension, angina pectoris, palpitations.
GI: abdominal pain, anorexia, constipation, diarrhea, dry mouth, dysgeusia, nausea, vomiting.
Hematologic: *leukopenia, agranulocytosis, thrombocytopenia, pancytopenia,* anemia.
Metabolic: hyperkalemia.
Respiratory: dry, persistent, nonproductive cough; dyspnea.
Skin: urticarial rash, maculopapular rash, pruritus, alopecia.
Other: *angioedema.*

INTERACTIONS
Drug-drug. *Aliskiren:* May increase risk of renal impairment, hypotension, and hyperkalemia in diabetic patients and those with moderate to severe renal impairment (GFR <60 mL/minute). Concomitant use is contraindicated in diabetic patients. Avoid concomitant use in those with moderate to severe renal impairment.
Antacids: May decrease captopril effect. Separate dosage times.
Canagliflozin: May enhance hyperkalemic and hypotensive effects. Monitor potassium level and BP.
Diuretics, other antihypertensives: May cause excessive hypotension. May need to stop diuretic or reduce captopril dosage.
Insulin, oral antidiabetics: May cause hypoglycemia when captopril therapy is started. Monitor patient closely.
Lithium: May increase lithium level; symptoms of toxicity possible. Monitor lithium level and patient closely.
NSAIDs: May reduce antihypertensive effect. Monitor BP.
Potassium-sparing diuretics, potassium supplements: May cause hyperkalemia. Avoid using together unless hypokalemia is confirmed.
Drug-herb. *Black catechu:* May cause additional hypotensive effect. Discourage use together.
Capsaicin: May worsen cough. Discourage use together.

Drug-food. *Salt substitutes containing potassium:* May cause hyperkalemia. Monitor patient closely.

EFFECTS ON LAB TEST RESULTS
● May increase alkaline phosphatase, bilirubin, BUN, serum creatinine, and potassium levels. May decrease sodium, glucose, and Hb levels and hematocrit.
● May decrease granulocyte, platelet, RBC, and WBC counts.
● May cause false-positive urine acetone test results.

CONTRAINDICATIONS & CAUTIONS
● Contraindicated in patients hypersensitive to drug or other ACE inhibitors.
● Use cautiously in patients with impaired renal function or serious autoimmune disease, especially systemic lupus erythematosus, and in those who have been exposed to other drugs that affect WBC counts or immune response.
Dialyzable drug: Yes (hemodialysis in adults only).
⚠ *Overdose S&S:* Hypotension.

PREGNANCY-LACTATION-REPRODUCTION
Black Box Warning Use during pregnancy can cause injury and death to the developing fetus. When pregnancy is detected, stop drug as soon as possible. ∎
● Drug appears in breast milk. Patient should discontinue breast-feeding or discontinue drug, taking into account importance of drug to the mother.

NURSING CONSIDERATIONS
⟁ *Alert:* Black patients who take ACE inhibitors as monotherapy for hypertension have a smaller reduction in BP than nonblacks.
⟁ *Alert:* Black patients taking ACE inhibitors have a higher incidence of angioedema than nonblacks.
● Monitor patient's BP and pulse rate frequently.
⟁ *Alert:* Elderly patients may be more sensitive to drug's hypotensive effects.
● Assess patient for signs of angioedema.
● Drug causes cough, most frequently of all ACE inhibitors.

• In patients with impaired renal function or collagen vascular disease, monitor WBC and differential counts before starting treatment, every 2 weeks for the first 3 months of therapy, and periodically thereafter.

• *Look alike–sound alike:* Don't confuse captopril with Capitrol or carvedilol.

PATIENT TEACHING

• Instruct patient to take drug 1 hour before meals; food in the GI tract may reduce absorption.

• Inform patient that light-headedness is possible, especially during first few days of therapy. Tell him to rise slowly to minimize this effect and to report occurrence to prescriber. If fainting occurs, he should stop drug and call prescriber immediately.

• Tell patient to use caution in hot weather and during exercise. Lack of fluids, vomiting, diarrhea, and excessive perspiration can lead to light-headedness and syncope.

• Advise patient to report signs and symptoms of infection, such as fever and sore throat.

• Tell women to notify prescriber if pregnancy occurs. Drug will need to be stopped.

• Urge patient to promptly report swelling of the face, lips, or mouth or difficulty breathing.

• Advise patient not to use potassium-sparing diuretics, potassium supplements, or potassium-containing salt substitutes without first consulting prescriber.

---

carbamazepine
kar-ba-MAZ-e-peen

Carbatrol, Epitol, Equetro, Mazepine ♣, Tegretol, Tegretol-XR, Teril

Therapeutic class: Anticonvulsants
Pharmacologic class: Iminostilbene derivatives

AVAILABLE FORMS

Capsules (extended-release) ⓪: 100 mg, 200 mg, 300 mg
Oral suspension: 100 mg/5 mL
Tablets ⓪: 200 mg
Tablets (chewable): 100 mg

Tablets (extended-release) ⓪: 100 mg, 200 mg, 400 mg

INDICATIONS & DOSAGES

➤ **Generalized tonic-clonic and complex partial seizures, mixed seizure patterns (except Carbatrol and Equetro)**
Adults and children older than age 12: Initially, 200 mg P.O. b.i.d. (conventional or extended-release tablets), or 100 mg suspension P.O. q.i.d. with meals. May be increased weekly by 200 mg P.O. daily in divided doses at 12-hour intervals for extended-release tablets or 6- to 8-hour intervals for conventional tablets or suspension, adjusted to minimum effective level. Maximum, 1,000 mg daily in children ages 12 to 15 and 1,200 mg daily in patients older than age 15. Doses up to 1,600 mg daily have been used in adults in rare instances. Usual maintenance dosage is 800 to 1,200 mg daily.
Children ages 6 to 12: Initially, 100 mg P.O. b.i.d. (conventional or extended-release tablets) or 50 mg suspension P.O. q.i.d. with meals, increased at weekly intervals by up to 100 mg P.O. in three to four divided doses daily (in two divided doses for extended-release form). Maximum, 1,000 mg daily. Usual maintenance dosage is 400 to 800 mg daily or 20 to 30 mg/kg in three or four divided doses.
Children younger than age 6: 10 to 20 mg/kg in two to three divided doses (conventional tablets) or four divided doses (suspension). Maximum dosage is 35 mg/kg in 24 hours.
➤ **Epilepsy (Carbatrol only)**
Adults and children older than age 12: 200 mg P.O. b.i.d. Increase at weekly intervals by adding up to 200 mg daily until optimal response is obtained. Dosage shouldn't exceed 1,000 mg daily in children ages 12 to 15 and 1,200 mg daily in patients older than age 15. Usual effective maintenance level is 800 to 1,200 mg daily.
➤ **Acute manic and mixed episodes associated with bipolar I disorder (Equetro only)**
Adults: Initially, 200 mg Equetro P.O. b.i.d. Increase by 200 mg daily to achieve therapeutic response. Doses higher than 1,600 mg daily haven't been studied.

➤ **Trigeminal neuralgia (except Carbatrol and Equetro)**

Adults: Initially, 100 mg P.O. b.i.d. (conventional or extended-release tablets) or 50 mg suspension P.O. q.i.d. with meals, increased by 100 mg every 12 hours for tablets or 50 mg q.i.d. for suspension until pain is relieved. Maximum, 1,200 mg daily. Maintenance dosage is usually 200 to 400 mg P.O. b.i.d.

➤ **Trigeminal neuralgia (Carbatrol only)**

Adults: Initially, 200-mg capsule P.O. daily. Daily dosage may be increased by up to 200 mg/day every 12 hours, only as needed to achieve freedom from pain. Don't exceed 1,200 mg daily.

ADMINISTRATION
P.O.
● Shake oral suspension well before measuring dose.
● When converting from tablets to suspension, administer the same number of mg/day in smaller, more frequent doses.
● Give tablets with meals.
● Contents of extended-release capsules may be sprinkled over applesauce if patient has difficulty swallowing capsules. Capsules and tablets shouldn't be crushed or chewed, unless labeled as chewable form.
● When giving by NG tube, mix dose with an equal volume of water, NSS, or D_5W. Flush tube with 100 mL of diluent after giving dose.
● Don't crush or split extended-release form or give broken or chipped tablets.
● Patients converting from immediate-release to extended-release form should receive the same total daily dosage.

ACTION
Thought to stabilize neuronal membranes and limit seizure activity by either increasing efflux or decreasing influx of sodium ions across cell membranes in the motor cortex during generation of nerve impulses.

Route	Onset	Peak	Duration
P.O.	Unknown	1½–12 hr	Unknown
P.O. (extended-release)	Unknown	4–8 hr	Unknown

Half-life: 25 to 65 hours with single dose; 8 to 29 hours with long-term use.

ADVERSE REACTIONS
CNS: ataxia, dizziness, drowsiness, somnolence, vertigo, ***worsening of seizures,*** confusion, fatigue, fever, headache, syncope, pain, depression including ***suicidal ideation,*** speech disorder.
CV: ***arrhythmias, AV block, HF,*** aggravation of CAD, hypertension, hypotension.
EENT: blurred vision, conjunctivitis, diplopia, nystagmus, dry pharynx.
GI: nausea, vomiting, abdominal pain, anorexia, diarrhea, dry mouth, dyspepsia, glossitis, stomatitis.
GU: albuminuria, glycosuria, erectile dysfunction, urinary frequency, urine retention.
Hematologic: ***agranulocytosis, aplastic anemia, thrombocytopenia,*** eosinophilia, leukocytosis.
Hepatic: ***hepatitis.***
Metabolic: hyponatremia.
Respiratory: pulmonary hypersensitivity.
Skin: ***erythema multiforme, Stevens-Johnson syndrome,*** excessive diaphoresis, rash, urticaria, pruritus.
Other: SIADH, chills.

INTERACTIONS
Drug-drug. *Anticoagulants:* May reduce anticoagulant effect. Monitor PT when starting or stopping carbamazepine.
Aripiprazole: May decrease aripiprazole serum concentration. Double aripiprazole dose when carbamazepine is added, then base additional dosage increases on clinical evaluation. If carbamazepine is later withdrawn, reduce aripiprazole dose.
Atracurium, cisatracurium, pancuronium, rocuronium, vecuronium: May decrease the effects of nondepolarizing muscle relaxant, causing it to be less effective. May need to increase the dose of the nondepolarizing muscle relaxant.
Azole antifungals (itraconazole, ketoconazole): May increase carbamazepine level and decrease antifungal level. Monitor levels and effectiveness of drugs.
Cimetidine, danazol, diltiazem, fluoxetine, fluvoxamine, isoniazid, valproic acid, verapamil: May increase carbamazepine level. Use together cautiously.
Clarithromycin, erythromycin, troleandomycin: May inhibit metabolism of

carbamazepine, increasing carbamazepine level and risk of toxicity. Avoid using together.

Doxycycline, felbamate, haloperidol, hormonal contraceptives, phenytoin, theophylline, tiagabine, topiramate, valproate: May decrease levels of these drugs. Watch for decreased effect.

Lamotrigine: May decrease lamotrigine level and increase carbamazepine level. Monitor patient for clinical effects and toxicity.

Lithium: May increase CNS toxicity of lithium. Avoid using together.

MAO inhibitors: May increase depressant and anticholinergic effects. Avoid using together. Discontinue MAO inhibitors at least 14 days before starting carbamazepine.

Nefazodone: May increase carbamazepine levels and toxicity while reducing nefazodone levels and therapeutic benefits. Use together is contraindicated.

Oral and other hormonal contraceptives: May cause breakthrough bleeding and reduced contraceptive effectiveness. Consider back-up method of birth control.

Phenobarbital, phenytoin, primidone: May decrease carbamazepine level. Watch for decreased effect.

SSRIs, TCAs: May increase carbamazepine level and decrease levels of antidepressant. Closely monitor patient and adjust dosage as needed.

Drug-food. *Grapefruit juice:* May increase carbamazepine level. Avoid use together.

Drug-herb. *Plantains (psyllium seed):* May inhibit GI absorption of drug. Discourage use together.

EFFECTS ON LAB TEST RESULTS

• May increase BUN level. May decrease sodium and Hb levels and hematocrit.
• May increase LFT values and eosinophil and WBC counts. May decrease thyroid function test values and granulocyte and platelet counts.
• May cause false pregnancy test results.

CONTRAINDICATIONS & CAUTIONS

• Contraindicated in patients hypersensitive to this drug or TCAs and in those with a history of bone marrow suppression; also contraindicated in those who have taken an MAO inhibitor within 14 days. Concomitant use with delavirdine or other NNRTIs or nefazodone is also contraindicated.

• Use cautiously in patients with mixed seizure disorders because they may experience an increased risk of seizures. Also, use with caution in patients with hepatic dysfunction.

• Safety and effectiveness of Equetro in children and adolescents haven't been established.

Dialyzable drug: Yes.

⚠ Overdose S&S: Conduction disorders, hypotension or hypertension, impairment of consciousness, irregular breathing, respiratory depression, tachycardia, shock, seizures, adiadochokinesia, ataxia, athetoid movements, ballism, dizziness, drowsiness, dysmetria, motor restlessness, muscular twitching, mydriasis, nystagmus, opisthotonos, psychomotor disturbances, tremor; hyperreflexia followed by anuria or oliguria, hyporeflexia, nausea and vomiting, urine retention.

PREGNANCY-LACTATION-REPRODUCTION

• Drug can cause fetal harm, including major congenital malformations, when administered during pregnancy. Weigh benefits against the risks. If used in pregnant women, monotherapy, rather than use in combination with other anticonvulsants, is recommended to possibly reduce risk of teratogenic effects.

• Consider tests to detect defects using currently accepted procedures as part of routine prenatal care in pregnant women receiving drug.

• Pregnant women taking carbamazepine should enroll themselves in the North American Antiepileptic Drug Pregnancy Registry by calling 1-888-233-2334 or by visiting www.aedpregnancyregistry.org.

• Drug and its metabolite appear in breast milk. Patient should discontinue breastfeeding or discontinue drug, taking into account importance of drug to the mother.

NURSING CONSIDERATIONS

Black Box Warning Patients of Asian ancestry should be screened with blood tests to identify their genetic risk of rare, but serious skin reactions (toxic epidermal necrolysis, Stevens-Johnson syndrome).

Screen for HLA-B*1502 allele before starting treatment with carbamazepine. ∎

• Watch for worsening of seizures, especially in patients with mixed seizure disorders, including atypical absence seizures.

⊕ *Alert:* Closely monitor all patients taking or starting AEDs for changes in behavior indicating worsening of suicidal thoughts or behavior or depression. Symptoms such as anxiety, agitation, hostility, mania, and hypomania may be precursors to emerging suicidality.

• Obtain baseline determinations of urinalysis, BUN and iron levels, liver function, CBC, and platelet and reticulocyte counts. Monitor these values periodically thereafter.

Black Box Warning Aplastic anemia and agranulocytosis have been reported in association with carbamazepine therapy. Obtain complete pretreatment hematologic testing as a baseline. If patient in the course of treatment exhibits low or decreased WBC or platelet counts, monitor patient closely. Consider discontinuing drug if evidence of significant bone marrow depression develops. ∎

• Never stop drug suddenly when treating seizures. Notify prescriber immediately if adverse reactions occur.

• Adverse reactions may be minimized by increasing dosages gradually.

• Therapeutic level is 4 to 12 mcg/mL. Monitor level and effects closely. Ask patient when last dose was taken to better evaluate drug level.

• When managing seizures, take appropriate precautions.

⊕ *Alert:* Watch for signs of anorexia or subtle appetite changes, which may indicate excessive drug level.

• *Look alike–sound alike:* Don't confuse carbamazepine with oxcarbazepine. Don't confuse Tegretol or Tegretol-XR with Trental, Topamax, Toprol-XL, or Toradol. Don't confuse Carbatrol with carvedilol.

PATIENT TEACHING

• Instruct patient to take drug with food to minimize GI distress. Tell patient taking suspension form to shake container well before measuring dose.

• Tell patient not to crush or chew tablets or capsules and not to take broken or chipped tablets.

• Tell patient that Tegretol-XR tablet coating may appear in stool because it isn't absorbed.

• Advise patient to keep tablets in the original container and to keep the container tightly closed and away from moisture. Some formulations may harden when exposed to excessive moisture, so that less is available in the body, decreasing seizure control.

• Inform patient that when drug is used for trigeminal neuralgia, an attempt to decrease dosage or withdraw drug is usually made every 3 months.

• Advise patient to notify prescriber immediately if fever, sore throat, mouth ulcers, or easy bruising or bleeding occurs.

• Tell patient that drug may cause mild to moderate dizziness and drowsiness when first taken. Advise him to avoid hazardous activities until effects disappear, usually within 3 to 4 days.

• Advise patient that periodic eye examinations are recommended.

• Inform female patient of risks to fetus if pregnancy occurs while taking carbamazepine; advise her to enroll in the North American Antiepileptic Drug Pregnancy Registry.

• Advise women that breast-feeding isn't recommended during therapy.

SAFETY ALERT!

carboplatin
KAR-bo-pla-tin

Therapeutic class: Antineoplastics
Pharmacologic class: Platinum-containing compounds

AVAILABLE FORMS

Aqueous solution for injection: 50 mg/5 mL, 150 mg/15 mL, 450 mg/45 mL, 600 mg/60 mL, 1 g/100 mL

INDICATIONS & DOSAGES

➤ **Advanced ovarian cancer**
Adults: 360 mg/m² I.V. on day 1 every 4 weeks. Or, 300 mg/m² on day 1 every

4 weeks for six cycles when used with other chemotherapy drugs. Or, use the Calvert formula to calculate initial dosage:

$$\text{Total dose (mg)} = (\text{target AUC}) \times (\text{GFR} + 25)$$

where *target AUC* (area under the curve) is usually 4 to 6 mg/mL and *GFR* is measured in mL/minute. Doses shouldn't be repeated until platelet count exceeds 100,000/mm³ and neutrophil count exceeds 2,000/mm³. Subsequent doses are based on blood counts: If platelet count is greater than 100,000/mm³ and neutrophil count is greater than 2,000/mm³, give 125% of prior dose. If platelet count is 50,000/mm³ to 100,000/mm³ and neutrophil count is 500/mm³ to 2,000/mm³, keep same dose. If platelet count is less than 50,000/mm³ and neutrophil count is less than 500/mm³, give 75% of dose.

Adjust-a-dose: If CrCl is 41 to 59 mL/minute, first dose is 250 mg/m². If CrCl is 16 to 40 mL/minute, first dose is 200 mg/m². Drug isn't recommended for patients with CrCl of 15 mL/minute or less.

ADMINISTRATION
I.V.

Black Box Warning Anaphylaxis may occur within minutes of administration. Keep epinephrine, corticosteroids, and antihistamines available when giving carboplatin. ▪

▼ Preparing and giving parenteral form of drug may be mutagenic, teratogenic, or carcinogenic. Follow facility policy to reduce risks.

▼ Don't use aluminum needles or I.V. administration sets because drug may precipitate or lose potency.

▼ For premixed aqueous solution of 10 mg/mL, dilute for infusion with NSS or D₅W to a concentration as low as 0.5 mg/mL.

▼ Give drug by continuous or intermittent infusion over at least 15 minutes.

▼ Store unopened vials at room temperature. Protect from light.

▼ Once diluted as directed, drug is stable at room temperature for 8 hours.

▼ Because drug contains no preservatives, discard after 8 hours.

▼ **Incompatibilities:** Amphotericin B cholesteryl sulfate complex, 5-FU, mesna, sodium bicarbonate.

ACTION
May cross-link strands of cellular DNA and interfere with RNA transcription, causing an imbalance of growth that leads to cell death. Not specific to cell cycle.

Route	Onset	Peak	Duration
I.V.	Unknown	Unknown	Unknown

Half-life: Carboplatin, about 2½ to 6 hours; platinum, 5 or more days.

ADVERSE REACTIONS
CNS: dizziness, confusion, *stroke,* peripheral neuropathy, *central neurotoxicity,* pain, asthenia.
CV: *HF, embolism.*
EENT: ototoxicity.
GI: abdominal pain, constipation, diarrhea, nausea, vomiting, mucositis, change in taste, stomatitis.
GU: renal toxicity.
Hematologic: *thrombocytopenia, leukopenia, neutropenia,* anemia, *bone marrow suppression, bleeding.*
Skin: alopecia.
Other: hypersensitivity reactions.

INTERACTIONS
Drug-drug. *Bone marrow suppressants, including radiation therapy:* May increase hematologic toxicity. Monitor CBC with differential closely.
Nephrotoxic drugs, especially aminoglycosides and amphotericin B: May enhance nephrotoxicity of carboplatin. Use together cautiously.
Phenytoin: May decrease phenytoin level. Monitor serum level and patient for decreased effectiveness.
Vaccines (live): May diminish vaccine's effect. Don't give live vaccines for 3 months after carboplatin.

EFFECTS ON LAB TEST RESULTS
● May increase alkaline phosphatase, AST, BUN, and creatinine levels. May decrease electrolyte and Hb levels and hematocrit.
● May decrease neutrophil, platelet, RBC, and WBC counts.

CONTRAINDICATIONS & CAUTIONS
• Contraindicated in patients with severe bone marrow suppression or bleeding and in patients with history of hypersensitivity to cisplatin, platinum-containing compounds, or mannitol.
Dialyzable drug: Yes.
⚠ *Overdose S&S:* Bone marrow suppression, hepatotoxicity.

PREGNANCY-LACTATION-REPRODUCTION
• There are no adequate well-controlled studies in pregnant women. Drug may cause fetal harm when administered to a pregnant woman. Avoid use in women of childbearing potential. Women shouldn't become pregnant during therapy.
• It's unknown if drug appears in breast milk. Patient should discontinue breast-feeding during therapy.

NURSING CONSIDERATIONS
Black Box Warning Carboplatin should be administered under the supervision of a physician experienced in the use of chemotherapeutic agents. ■
• Determine electrolyte, creatinine, and BUN levels; CBC with differential; platelet count; and CrCl before first infusion and before each course of treatment.
◑ *Alert:* When using the Calvert formula, the total dose is calculated in mg, not mg/m^2.
• Monitor CBC with differential and platelet count frequently during therapy and, when indicated, until recovery. Lowest WBC and platelet counts usually occur by day 21. Levels usually return to baseline by day 28. Don't repeat unless platelet count exceeds $100,000/mm^3$.
Black Box Warning Bone marrow suppression is dose related and may be severe, resulting in infection or bleeding. ■
Black Box Warning Vomiting is another frequent drug-related side effect. ■
• Bone marrow suppression may be more severe in patients with CrCl below 60 mL/minute; adjust dosage.
◑ *Alert:* Carefully check ordered dose against laboratory test results. Only one increase in dosage is recommended. Subsequent doses shouldn't exceed 125% of starting dose.

• Therapeutic effects are commonly accompanied by toxicity.
• Drug has less nephrotoxicity and neurotoxicity than cisplatin, but it causes more severe myelosuppression.
• To prevent bleeding, avoid all I.M. injections when platelet count is below $50,000/mm^3$.
• Monitor vital signs during infusion.
• Give antiemetic to reduce nausea and vomiting.
Black Box Warning Anemia may be cumulative and may require transfusion support. ■
• Patients older than age 65 are at greater risk for neurotoxicity.
• *Look alike–sound alike:* Don't confuse carboplatin with cisplatin.

PATIENT TEACHING
• Advise patient of most common adverse reactions: nausea, vomiting, bone marrow suppression, anemia, and reduction in blood platelets.
• Advise patient to watch for signs of infection (fever, sore throat, fatigue) and bleeding (easy bruising, nosebleeds, bleeding gums, tarry stools). Tell patient to take temperature daily.
• Instruct patient to avoid OTC products containing aspirin and NSAIDs.
• Advise women to stop breast-feeding during therapy because of risk of toxicity to infant.
• Because of risk of sterility and menstruation cessation, counsel both men and women of childbearing potential before starting therapy. Also recommend that women consult prescriber before becoming pregnant.

cariprazine hydrochloride
kar-IP-ra-zeen

Vraylar

Therapeutic class: Antipsychotics
Pharmacologic class: Atypical antipsychotics

AVAILABLE FORMS
Capsules: 1.5 mg, 3 mg, 4.5 mg, 6 mg

INDICATIONS & DOSAGES

Adjust-a-dose (for all indications): If a strong CYP3A4 inhibitor is initiated while patient is on a stable dose of cariprazine, reduce cariprazine dosage by half; if patient is taking 4.5 mg daily, reduce to 1.5 or 3 mg daily; if patient is taking 1.5 mg daily, give every other day. Adjust cariprazine dosage when CYP3A4 inhibitor is discontinued. If initiating cariprazine while patient is on a strong CYP3A4 inhibitor, give 1.5 mg on days 1 and 3 (with no dose on day 2); from day 4 onward, give 1.5 mg daily, and increase to a maximum dose of 3 mg daily. Adjust cariprazine dosage when CYP3A4 inhibitor is discontinued. Concomitant use of cariprazine and CYP3A4 inducers hasn't been studied and isn't recommended.

➤ **Schizophrenia**
Adults: Initially, 1.5 mg P.O. once daily on day 1. May increase to 3 mg P.O. once daily on day 2. Based on patient's response and tolerability, may make further dosage adjustments in 1.5- or 3-mg increments. Recommended dosage range is 1.5 to 6 mg once daily. Maximum dose is 6 mg daily.

➤ **Manic or mixed episodes associated with bipolar I disorder**
Adults: Initially, 1.5 mg P.O. once daily on day 1; increase dose to 3 mg P.O. once daily on day 2. Based on patient's response and tolerability, may make further dosage adjustments in 1.5- or 3-mg increments. Recommended dosage range is 3 to 6 mg P.O. once daily.

ADMINISTRATION
P.O.
- May give with or without food.
- Store at room temperature.
- Protect 3- and 4.5-mg capsules from light to prevent potential color fading.

ACTION
Exact mechanism unknown. Action thought to occur through partial agonist activity at central dopamine D_2 and serotonin $5-HT_{1A}$ receptors as well as antagonist activity at serotonin $5-HT_{2A}$ receptors.

Route	Onset	Peak	Duration
P.O.	Unknown	3–6 hr	Unknown

Half-life: 48 to 96 hours (parent compound); 1 to 3 weeks (major metabolite).

C

ADVERSE REACTIONS
CNS: fatigue, pyrexia, extrapyramidal symptoms, akathisia, headache, somnolence, dizziness, agitation, insomnia, restlessness, anxiety.
CV: tachycardia, hypertension.
EENT: blurred vision, nasopharyngitis, dry mouth, toothache, oropharyngeal pain.
GI: abdominal pain, constipation, diarrhea, dyspepsia, nausea, vomiting.
GU: UTI.
Metabolic: weight gain, decreased appetite.
Musculoskeletal: arthralgia, back pain, extremity pain.
Respiratory: cough.
Skin: rash.

INTERACTIONS
Drug-drug. *CNS depressants:* May increase CNS depression. Monitor therapy.
CYP3A4 inducers (carbamazepine, rifampin): May increase or decrease cariprazine concentration. Use together isn't recommended.
Black Box Warning *Opioids:* May cause slow or difficult breathing, sedation, and death. Avoid use together. If use together is necessary, limit dosage and duration of each drug to the minimum necessary for desired effect. ∎
Strong CYP3A4 inhibitors (itraconazole, ketoconazole): May increase cariprazine concentration. Reduce cariprazine dosage.
Drug-food. *Grapefruit juice (CYP3A4 inhibitor):* May increase cariprazine concentration. Discourage use together.

EFFECTS ON LAB TEST RESULTS
- May increase CK and liver enzyme levels.
- May decrease WBC count.

CONTRAINDICATIONS & CAUTIONS
- Contraindicated in patients hypersensitive to drug or its components.
Black Box Warning Antipsychotics increase the risk of death in elderly patients with dementia-related psychosis. Drug isn't

approved to treat patients with dementia-related psychosis. ∎

Black Box Warning Opioid drugs should only be prescribed with benzodiazepines or other CNS depressants to patients for whom alternative treatment options are inadequate. ∎

🔴 *Alert:* Antipsychotics can cause leukopenia and neutropenia, which can be fatal. Use cautiously in patients with preexisting low WBC count or ANC or history of drug-induced leukopenia or neutropenia.

● Antipsychotics can cause orthostatic hypotension and syncope. Drug hasn't been evaluated in patients with a recent history of MI or unstable CV disease.

● Antipsychotics can cause neuroleptic malignant syndrome (NMS), which can be fatal.

● Drug may cause irreversible tardive dyskinesia, especially in elderly patients, most notably elderly women.

● Antipsychotics can disrupt the body's ability to reduce core body temperature; impair judgment, thinking, or motor skills; and increase risk of metabolic changes (hyperglycemia, diabetes mellitus, dyslipidemia, and weight gain), esophageal dysmotility, aspiration, and aspiration pneumonia.

● Antipsychotics increase risk of seizures, especially in patients with a history of seizures or with conditions that lower the seizure threshold.

● Drug is associated with dystonia, especially in males and younger age-groups, most commonly during first few days of treatment.

● Use isn't recommended in patients with severe hepatic or renal impairment.

● Safety and effectiveness in children haven't been established.

Dialyzable drug: Unlikely.

⚠ *Overdose S&S:* Orthostasis, sedation.

PREGNANCY-LACTATION-REPRODUCTION

● Drug may cause fetal harm. Neonates exposed to antipsychotics during the third trimester are at risk for extrapyramidal and withdrawal signs and symptoms, which can vary in severity and require prolonged hospitalization.

● Encourage women exposed to drug during pregnancy to enroll in the National

Pregnancy Registry for Atypical Antipsychotics (1-866-961-2388).

● It isn't known if drug appears in breast milk. Consider risks and benefits before using in breast-feeding women.

NURSING CONSIDERATIONS

● Monitor patients for hypersensitivity reactions (rash, pruritus, urticaria, swollen tongue or lips, facial edema, pharyngeal edema).

● Monitor patients closely for adverse reactions and treatment response for several weeks after drug initiation and after each dosage change.

● Monitor patients for signs and symptoms of NMS (hyperpyrexia, muscle rigidity, delirium, autonomic instability, elevated CK level, rhabdomyolysis, acute renal failure); discontinue drug immediately if reactions appear. Provide intensive symptomatic treatment and monitoring.

● Monitor patients for signs and symptoms of tardive dyskinesia (potentially irreversible, involuntary, dyskinetic movements). Drug may need to be discontinued.

● Monitor patients for signs and symptoms of dystonia (throat tightness, difficulty swallowing or breathing, tongue protrusion).

● Monitor blood glucose, triglyceride, and lipid levels and for changes in weight, waist circumference, and BMI.

● Monitor patients for clinically significant neutropenia, fever, or other signs and symptoms of infection; treat promptly. Discontinue drug for ANC less than $1,000/mm^3$ and monitor WBC count until abnormalities resolve.

● Monitor patients for orthostatic hypotension, especially in elderly patients and those with dehydration, hypovolemia, concomitant treatment with antihypertensives, and known CV or cerebrovascular disease.

● Ask patients about a history of seizures and review patients' medications for those that might lower the seizure threshold, as drug may increase the risk of seizures.

● Monitor patients who are exposed to strenuous exercise or extreme heat, are dehydrated, or are taking anticholinergics for elevated core body temperature.

● Watch for abnormal, involuntary movements, which may indicate extrapyramidal reactions; drug may need to be stopped.

● **Look alike–sound alike:** Don't confuse Vraylar with Valchlor.

PATIENT TEACHING

Black Box Warning Caution the patient or the caregiver of a patient taking an opioid drug with a benzodiazepine, CNS depressant, or alcohol to seek immediate medical attention if the patient has symptoms of dizziness, light-headedness, extreme sleepiness, slowed or difficult breathing, or unresponsiveness. ■

● Counsel patient on importance of following dosage escalation instructions.

● Explain potential for dystonic or extrapyramidal signs and symptoms (involuntary, abnormal movements). Advise patient to immediately report signs and symptoms to prescriber, as drug may need to be discontinued.

● Instruct patient to report signs and symptoms of NMS (excessive muscle rigidity, increased sweating, changes in BP, or irregular heartbeat).

● Educate patient about risk of metabolic changes and how to recognize signs and symptoms of hyperglycemia and diabetes mellitus. Instruct patient that laboratory monitoring of blood glucose and lipid levels and monitoring weight for changes may be necessary.

● Remind patient to avoid strenuous exercise or exposure to extreme heat and to drink plenty of water, as drug may impair body temperature–regulating ability.

● Counsel patient on risk of orthostatic hypotension and syncope, especially during treatment initiation and dosage increases.

● Warn patient about potential for drug interactions and to report to prescriber all OTC and prescription drugs and natural supplements being taken.

● Caution patient about operating hazardous machinery, including motor vehicles, until drug's effects on cognitive and motor skills are known.

● Advise female patient who is pregnant, considering pregnancy, or is breast-feeding to discuss risks and benefits with prescriber.

carisoprodol
kar-eye-soe-PROE-dol

Soma🖋

Therapeutic class: Skeletal muscle relaxants
Pharmacologic class: Carbamate derivatives
Controlled substance schedule: IV

AVAILABLE FORMS
Tablets: 250 mg, 350 mg

INDICATIONS & DOSAGES
➤ **Adjunctive treatment for acute, painful musculoskeletal conditions**
Adults: 250 to 350 mg P.O. t.i.d. and at bedtime for a maximum of 2 to 3 weeks.

ADMINISTRATION
P.O.
● Give drug with food or milk if GI upset occurs.

ACTION
May modify central perception of pain without modifying pain reflexes. Muscle relaxant effects may be related to sedative properties.

Route	Onset	Peak	Duration
P.O.	½ hr	1½–2 hr	4–6 hr

Half-life: 2 hours for carisoprodol, 10 hours for active metabolite.

ADVERSE REACTIONS
CNS: drowsiness, dizziness, headache.
Respiratory: *asthmatic episodes.*
Skin: *erythema multiforme,* pruritus, rash.
Other: *angioedema, anaphylaxis.*

INTERACTIONS
Drug-drug. *CNS depressants:* May increase CNS depression. Avoid using together.
CYP2C19 inducers (rifampin): May increase active metabolite (meprobamate) exposure and decrease available carisoprodol. Use cautiously together.
CYP2C19 inhibitors (fluvoxamine, omeprazole): May decrease metabolism of carisoprodol to meprobamate, increasing exposure to carisoprodol. Use cautiously together.

Meprobamate: May increase meprobamate level. Avoid use together.

Black Box Warning *Opioids:* May cause slow or difficult breathing, sedation, and death. Avoid use together. If use together is necessary, limit dosage and duration of each drug to the minimum necessary for desired effect. ∎

Drug-herb. *Kava kava:* May enhance CNS adverse or toxic effects. Monitor therapy.
St. John's wort: May increase active metabolite (meprobamate) exposure and decrease available carisoprodol. Use cautiously together.

Drug-lifestyle. *Alcohol use:* May increase CNS depression. Discourage use together.

EFFECTS ON LAB TEST RESULTS
● May increase eosinophil count.

CONTRAINDICATIONS & CAUTIONS
● Contraindicated in patients hypersensitive to related compounds (such as meprobamate) and in those with intermittent porphyria.
Black Box Warning Opioid drugs should only be prescribed with benzodiazepines or other CNS depressants to patients for whom alternative treatment options are inadequate. ∎
◑ **Alert:** Drug is Schedule IV controlled substance; cases of dependence, withdrawal, and abuse have occurred.
● Use cautiously in patients with impaired hepatic or renal function.
● Safety and effectiveness in adults older than age 65 and children younger than age 16 haven't been established.
Dialyzable drug: Yes.
⚠ **Overdose S&S:** Stupor, coma, seizures, shock, respiratory depression, drowsiness, dizziness, headache, diplopia, nystagmus, delirium, dystonia, muscular incoordination.

PREGNANCY-LACTATION-REPRODUCTION
● Safe use during pregnancy hasn't been established. Use in pregnant women only if potential benefit justifies risk to the fetus.
● Drug appears in breast milk. Use cautiously in breast-feeding women.

NURSING CONSIDERATIONS
◑ **Alert:** Watch for idiosyncratic reactions after first to fourth doses (weakness, ataxia,

visual and speech difficulties, fever, skin eruptions, and mental status changes) and for severe reactions, including bronchospasm, hypotension, and anaphylactic shock. After unusual reactions, withhold dose and notify prescriber immediately.
● Record amount of relief to help prescriber determine whether dosage can be reduced.
● Don't stop drug abruptly, which may cause mild withdrawal effects, such as insomnia, headache, nausea, or abdominal cramps.
● Monitor patient for dependence and signs and symptoms of abuse and overdose.

PATIENT TEACHING
Black Box Warning Caution the patient or the caregiver of a patient taking an opioid drug with a benzodiazepine, CNS depressant, or alcohol to seek immediate medical attention if the patient has symptoms of dizziness, light-headedness, extreme sleepiness, slowed or difficult breathing, or unresponsiveness. ∎
● Warn patient to avoid activities that require alertness until CNS effects of drug are known. Drowsiness is transient.
● Advise patient to avoid combining drug with alcohol or other CNS depressants.
● Tell patient to ask prescriber before using OTC cold or hay fever remedies.
● Instruct patient and family that drug can cause dependence.
● Advise patient to avoid sudden changes in posture if dizziness occurs.
● Tell patient to take drug with food or milk if GI upset occurs.

SAFETY ALERT!

carmustine (BCNU)
kar-MUS-teen

BiCNU, Gliadel Wafer

Therapeutic class: Antineoplastics
Pharmacologic class: Nitrosoureas

AVAILABLE FORMS
Injection: 100-mg vial (lyophilized), with a 3-mL vial of absolute alcohol supplied as a diluent
Wafer: 7.7 mg, for intracavitary use

INDICATIONS & DOSAGES
➤ **Brain tumor, Hodgkin lymphoma, malignant lymphoma, multiple myeloma**
Adults: 150 to 200 mg/m^2 I.V. by slow infusion every 6 weeks; may be divided into daily injections of 75 to 100 mg/m^2 on 2 successive days; repeat dose every 6 weeks if platelet count is greater than 100,000/mm^3 and WBC count is greater than 4,000/mm^3.

Adjust-a-dose: Dosage is reduced by 30% when WBC nadir is 2,000 to 2,999/mm^3 and platelet nadir is 25,000 to 74,999/mm^3. Dosage is reduced by 50% when WBC nadir is less than 2,000/mm^3 and platelet nadir is less than 25,000/mm^3.

➤ **Adjunct to surgery to prolong survival in patients with recurrent glioblastoma multiforme for whom surgical resection is indicated; adjunct to surgery and radiation in patients with newly diagnosed high-grade malignant glioma**
Adults: 8 wafers placed in the resection cavity if size and shape of cavity allow. If 8 wafers can't be accommodated, use maximum number of wafers allowed.

ADMINISTRATION
I.V.
▼ Preparing and giving parenteral form of drug may be mutagenic, teratogenic, or carcinogenic. Follow facility policy to reduce risks. Wear gloves when handling any form of drug.
▼ Prepare drug only in glass containers. Solution is unstable in plastic I.V. bags.
▼ If powder liquefies or appears oily, discard because decomposition has occurred.
▼ To reconstitute, dissolve 100 mg of drug in 3 mL of absolute alcohol provided by manufacturer.
▼ Dilute solution with 27 mL of sterile water for injection. Resulting solution should be clear and colorless to yellowish and contains 3.3 mg of carmustine/mL in 10% alcohol.
▼ For infusion, may further dilute in D$_5$W in glass container.
▼ Don't use polyvinyl chloride I.V. tubing. May use polyethylene I.V. tubing.
▼ Don't mix with other drugs during administration.

▼ Give at least 250 mL over at least 2 hours.
▼ To reduce pain on infusion, dilute further or slow infusion rate.
▼ Reconstituted solution may be stored in refrigerator for 24 hours. Once further diluted in D$_5$W, store at room temperature and give within 8 hours. It may decompose at temperatures above 80° F (27° C). Protect from light.
▼ **Incompatibilities:** Sodium bicarbonate.
Intracavitary
● Unopened foil pouches of wafer may be kept at room temperature for a maximum of 6 hours. Open only in the operating room immediately before implantation.
● Wafers broken in half may be used; however, discard wafers as hazardous waste if broken into more than two pieces.
● Use double gloves when handling wafers. Discard outer gloves into a biohazard waste container after use.

ACTION
Inhibits enzymatic reactions involved with DNA synthesis, cross-links strands of cellular DNA, and interferes with RNA transcription, causing an imbalance of growth that leads to cell death. Not specific to cell cycle.

Route	Onset	Peak	Duration
I.V., intra-cavitary	Unknown	Unknown	Unknown

Half-life: I.V.: Biphasic: initial, 1.4 minutes; secondary, 22 minutes (active metabolites: plasma half-life of 67 hours).

ADVERSE REACTIONS
(I.V. and intracavitary wafer)
CNS: ataxia, *brain edema, seizures.*
CV: *hemorrhage.*
EENT: visual disturbances.
GI: nausea, vomiting, anorexia, diarrhea, dysphagia, *GI hemorrhage.*
GU: *nephrotoxicity,* renal impairment.
Hematologic: *cumulative bone marrow suppression, leukopenia, thrombocytopenia, acute leukemia or bone marrow dysplasia,* anemia.
Hepatic: *hepatotoxicity.*
Metabolic: hyperglycemia, *hypokalemia,* hyponatremia.
Respiratory: *pulmonary fibrosis.*

Other: intense pain at infusion site from venous spasm.

(Intracavitary wafer only)
CNS: headache, hemiplegia, confusion, aphasia, depression, somnolence, speech disorder, amnesia, *intracranial hypertension,* personality disorder, anxiety, facial paralysis, neuropathy, hypoesthesia, abnormal thinking, abnormal gait, hallucinations, insomnia, incoordination, hypokinesia, pain. **CV:** deep vein thrombophlebitis, *hemorrhage,* chest pain, *PE.*
GI: constipation, abdominal pain.
GU: UTI, urinary incontinence.
Musculoskeletal: back pain, myasthenia.
Respiratory: dyspnea, pneumonia.
Skin: rash, facial edema, abscess.
Other: fever, allergic reaction, accidental injury, abnormal healing.

INTERACTIONS
Drug-drug. *Cimetidine:* May increase carmustine's bone marrow toxicity. Avoid using together.
Digoxin, phenytoin: May decrease levels of these drugs. Monitor patient.
Live-virus vaccines: May increase risk of infection in immunocompromised patients. Don't use together; don't give for at least 3 months after carmustine.
Myelosuppressants: May increase myelosuppression. Monitor patient.

EFFECTS ON LAB TEST RESULTS
• May increase alkaline phosphatase, AST, bilirubin, Hb, and urine urea levels.
• May decrease platelet and WBC counts.

CONTRAINDICATIONS & CAUTIONS
• Contraindicated in patients hypersensitive to drug.
• Drug may increase risk of secondary malignancies.
Dialyzable drug: No.

PREGNANCY-LACTATION-REPRODUCTION
• Drug may cause fetal harm if used during pregnancy. Women of childbearing potential should use effective contraception during treatment.
• Drug may impair fertility.

• It isn't known if drug appears in breast milk. Patient should discontinue breast-feeding during treatment.

NURSING CONSIDERATIONS
Black Box Warning Carmustine for injection should be administered under the supervision of a physician experienced in the use of cancer chemotherapeutic agents. ■
Black Box Warning Bone marrow suppression, notably thrombocytopenia and leukopenia, is the most common and severe of the toxic effects. It may contribute to bleeding and overwhelming infections in an already compromised patient. ■
Black Box Warning Pulmonary toxicity appears to be dose related. Patients receiving greater than 1,400 mg/m^2 cumulative dose are at higher risk. Pulmonary toxicity can occur years after treatment and can result in death, particularly in patients treated in childhood. ■
• Obtain pulmonary function tests before and during therapy.
Black Box Warning Bone marrow suppression is delayed with carmustine. Blood counts should be monitored weekly for at least 6 weeks after a dose and drug shouldn't be given more often than every 6 weeks. ■
Black Box Warning Bone marrow toxicity of carmustine for injection is cumulative; dosage adjustment must be considered on the basis of nadir blood cell counts from prior dose. ■
• Give antiemetic before drug to reduce nausea.
• If drug touches skin, wash off thoroughly. Avoid contact with skin because drug will stain skin brown.
• Perform liver, renal, and pulmonary function tests periodically.
• Monitor CBC with differential. The ANC may be used to better calculate patient's immunosuppressive state.
• Monitor uric acid level. To prevent hyperuricemia with resulting uric acid nephropathy, allopurinol may be used with adequate hydration.
• Therapeutic levels are commonly toxic.
• Acute leukemia or bone marrow dysplasia may occur after long-term use.
• To prevent bleeding, avoid using I.M. when platelet count is less than 50,000/mm^3.

Reactions in bold italics are *life-threatening*. Interactions may have a *rapid onset* or a *delayed onset*.

- Anticipate blood transfusions during treatment because of cumulative anemia.
- Monitor patient for secondary malignancies.

PATIENT TEACHING
- Advise patient about common adverse reactions to drug.
- Tell patient to watch for signs and symptoms of infection (fever, sore throat, fatigue) and bleeding (easy bruising, nosebleeds, bleeding gums, tarry stools). Tell him to take temperature daily.
- Instruct patient to avoid OTC products containing aspirin and NSAIDs unless prescribed by health care provider.
- Advise women to stop breast-feeding during therapy because of possible risk of toxicity to infant.
- Caution woman of childbearing potential to avoid becoming pregnant during therapy. Recommend that she consult prescriber before becoming pregnant.

carteolol hydrochloride
KAR-tee-oh-lol

Ocupress

Therapeutic class: Antiglaucoma drugs
Pharmacologic class: Nonselective beta blockers

AVAILABLE FORMS
Ophthalmic solution: 1%

INDICATIONS & DOSAGES
➤ **Chronic open-angle glaucoma, intraocular hypertension**
Adults: One drop into conjunctival sac of each affected eye b.i.d.

ADMINISTRATION
Ophthalmic
- Don't touch tip of dropper to eye or surrounding tissue.
- Apply light finger pressure on lacrimal sac for 1 minute after instilling to minimize systemic absorption.
- If more than one ophthalmic drug is being used, give at least 5 minutes apart.

ACTION
Exact mechanism unknown. Reduces IOP by decreasing aqueous humor production.

Route	Onset	Peak	Duration
Ophthalmic	Unknown	Unknown	Unknown

Half-life: Unknown.

ADVERSE REACTIONS
CNS: asthenia, dizziness, headache, insomnia.
CV: *arrhythmias, bradycardia,* hypotension, palpitations.
EENT: burning, conjunctival hyperemia, edema, ocular tearing, transient eye irritation, abnormal corneal staining, blepharoconjunctivitis, blurred and cloudy vision, corneal sensitivity, decreased night vision, photophobia, ptosis, sinusitis.
GI: constipation, diarrhea, nausea, taste perversion, vomiting.
Respiratory: *bronchospasm,* dyspnea.

INTERACTIONS
Drug-drug. *Catecholamine-depleting drugs such as reserpine, oral beta blockers:* May cause additive effects and development of hypotension or bradycardia. Monitor patient closely; monitor vital signs.
Insulin: May mask symptoms of hypoglycemia (such as tachycardia) as a result of beta blockade. Use together cautiously in patients with diabetes.
Drug-lifestyle. *Sun exposure:* May cause photophobia. Advise patient to wear sunglasses.

EFFECTS ON LAB TEST RESULTS
None reported.

CONTRAINDICATIONS & CAUTIONS
- Contraindicated in patients hypersensitive to drug or its components and in those with bronchial asthma, severe COPD, sinus bradycardia, second- or third-degree AV block, overt cardiac failure, or cardiogenic shock.
- Use cautiously in patients hypersensitive to other beta blockers; in those with nonallergic bronchospastic disease, diabetes mellitus, hyperthyroidism, or decreased pulmonary function; and in breast-feeding women.

Dialyzable drug: No.
⚠ *Overdose S&S:* Bradycardia, bronchospasm, HF, hypotension.

PREGNANCY-LACTATION-REPRODUCTION
• There are no adequate well-controlled studies in pregnant women. Use during pregnancy only if potential benefit justifies potential risk to the fetus.
• It's unknown if drug appears in breast milk. Use cautiously in breast-feeding women.

NURSING CONSIDERATIONS
• Monitor vital signs.
🌢 *Alert:* Stop drug at first sign of cardiac failure, and notify prescriber.

PATIENT TEACHING
• If patient is using more than one topical ophthalmic drug, tell him to apply them at least 5 minutes apart.
• Teach patient how to instill drops. Advise him to wash hands before and after instillation, and warn him not to touch tip of dropper to eye or surrounding tissue.
• Advise patient to apply light finger pressure on lacrimal sac for 1 minute after drug instillation to minimize systemic absorption.
• Tell patient to remove contact lenses before instilling drug.
• Instruct patient to keep bottle tightly closed when not in use and to protect it from light.
• Tell patient that drug is a beta blocker and, although given topically, may be absorbed systemically, causing adverse effects. Advise patient to monitor HR and BP closely, to report slow HR to prescriber and, if signs or symptoms of serious adverse reactions or hypersensitivity occur, to stop drug and notify prescriber immediately.
• Stress importance of compliance with recommended therapy.
• Advise patient to ease sun sensitivity by wearing sunglasses.

carvedilol
kar-VAH-da-lol

Coreg

carvedilol phosphate
Coreg CR

Therapeutic class: Antihypertensives
Pharmacologic class: Alpha-nonselective beta blockers

AVAILABLE FORMS
Capsules (extended-release) ⓞⓝⓒ: 10 mg, 20 mg, 40 mg, 80 mg
Tablets: 3.125 mg, 6.25 mg, 12.5 mg, 25 mg

INDICATIONS & DOSAGES
Adjust-a-dose (for all indications): In patients with pulse rate below 55 beats/minute, reduce dosage.
➤ **Hypertension**
Adults: Dosage highly individualized. For immediate-release tablets, initially, 6.25 mg P.O. b.i.d. Measure standing BP 1 hour after first dose. If tolerated, continue dosage for 7 to 14 days. May increase to 12.5 mg P.O. b.i.d. for 7 to 14 days, following same BP monitoring protocol as before. Maximum dose is 25 mg P.O. b.i.d. as tolerated. May be switched to extended-release capsule after controlled on immediate-release tablets. Or, for extended-release capsule, initially 20 mg P.O. once daily. Measure standing BP 1 hour after dose. May increase by 20 mg every 7 to 14 days to maximum of 80 mg P.O. once daily if needed and tolerated, using standing systolic pressure 1 hour after dosing as a guide for tolerance.
➤ **Left ventricular dysfunction after MI**
Adults: Dosage individualized. Start therapy after patient is hemodynamically stable and fluid retention has been minimized. For immediate-release tablets, initially, 6.25 mg P.O. b.i.d. Increase after 3 to 10 days to 12.5 mg b.i.d., then again after 3 to 10 days to a target dose of 25 mg b.i.d. Or start with 3.125 mg b.i.d., or adjust dosage more slowly if indicated. May be switched to extended-release capsule after controlled on immediate-release tablets. Or, 10 to 20 mg extended-release capsules P.O. once daily.

May increase after 3 to 10 days to 20 to 40 mg P.O. once daily; continue increasing dose every 3 to 10 days until target dose of 80 mg P.O. once daily based on tolerability is reached.

➤ **Mild to severe HF**
Adults: Dosage highly individualized. For immediate-release tablets, initially, 3.125 mg P.O. b.i.d. for 2 weeks; if tolerated, may increase to 6.25 mg P.O. b.i.d. Dosage may be doubled every 2 weeks, as tolerated. Maximum dose for patients in severe HF or who weigh less than 85 kg is 25 mg P.O. b.i.d.; for those weighing more than 85 kg, dose is 50 mg P.O. b.i.d. May be switched to extended-release capsule after controlled on immediate-release tablets. Or, 10-mg extended-release capsule P.O. once daily for 2 weeks. May increase to 20, 40, and 80 mg over successive intervals of at least 2 weeks if tolerated.

ADMINISTRATION
P.O.
● Give drug with food.
● Make sure patient doesn't crush, chew, or take capsules in divided doses.
● Capsules may be opened, mixed in cool applesauce, and taken immediately; don't store.
● Give capsules in the morning.
● Extended-release equivalent of 3.125 mg immediate-release b.i.d. is 10 mg, 6.25 mg immediate-release b.i.d. is 20 mg, 12.5 mg immediate-release b.i.d. is 40 mg, and 25 mg immediate-release b.i.d. is 80 mg. Dosage may be further titrated based on clinical response.
● Administer extended-release form and drugs that contain alcohol 2 hours apart.

ACTION
Nonselective beta blocker with alpha-blocking activity.

Route	Onset	Peak	Duration
P.O.	Rapid	1–2 hr	7–10 hr
P.O. (extended-release)	30 min	5 hr	Unknown

Half-life: Immediate-release, 7 to 10 hours; extended-release, unknown.

ADVERSE REACTIONS
CNS: asthenia, dizziness, fatigue, *stroke,* pain, headache, malaise, fever, hypesthesia, vertigo, somnolence, depression, insomnia, syncope, paresthesia.
CV: hypotension, orthostatic hypotension, *AV block, bradycardia,* edema, syncope, angina pectoris, peripheral edema, hypovolemia, fluid overload, hypertension, palpitations, chest pain.
EENT: abnormal vision, blurred vision.
GI: diarrhea, vomiting, nausea, melena, periodontitis, abdominal pain, dyspepsia.
GU: erectile dysfunction, abnormal renal function, albuminuria, hematuria, UTI.
Hematologic: *thrombocytopenia,* purpura.
Metabolic: hyperglycemia, weight gain, *hyperkalemia, hypoglycemia,* weight loss, hypercholesterolemia, hyperuricemia, hyponatremia, glycosuria, diabetes mellitus, gout.
Musculoskeletal: arthralgia, muscle cramps.
Respiratory: *lung edema,* cough, rales.
Other: hypersensitivity reactions.

INTERACTIONS
Drug-drug. *Amiodarone:* May increase risk of bradycardia, AV block, and myocardial depression. Monitor patient's ECG and vital signs.
Catecholamine-depleting drugs such as MAO inhibitors, reserpine: May cause bradycardia or severe hypotension. Monitor patient closely.
Cimetidine: May increase bioavailability of carvedilol. Monitor vital signs closely.
Clonidine: May increase BP-lowering and HR-lowering effects. Monitor vital signs closely.
Cyclosporine: May increase cyclosporine level. Monitor cyclosporine level.
CYP4502D6 inhibitors (fluoxetine, paroxetine, propafenone, quinidine): May increase level of carvedilol. Monitor patient for hypotension and dizziness.
Digoxin: May increase digoxin level by about 15% when given together. Monitor digoxin level.
Diltiazem, verapamil: May cause isolated conduction disturbances. Monitor patient's heart rhythm and BP.

Insulin, oral antidiabetics: May enhance hypoglycemic properties. Monitor glucose level.

NSAIDs, salicylates: May decrease antihypertensive effects. Monitor BP.

Rifampin: May reduce carvedilol level by 70%. Monitor vital signs closely.

Drug-herb. *Ma huang:* May decrease antihypertensive effects. Discourage use together.

EFFECTS ON LAB TEST RESULTS

● May increase alkaline phosphatase, ALT, AST, BUN, cholesterol, creatinine, GGT, nonprotein nitrogen, potassium, triglyceride, sodium, and uric acid levels. May increase or decrease glucose level.

● May shorten PT and decrease platelet count.

CONTRAINDICATIONS & CAUTIONS

● Contraindicated in patients hypersensitive to drug and in those with New York Heart Association class IV decompensated cardiac failure requiring I.V. inotropic therapy.

● Contraindicated in patients with bronchial asthma or related bronchospastic conditions, second- or third-degree AV block, sick sinus syndrome (unless a pacemaker is in place), cardiogenic shock, severe bradycardia, or severe hepatic impairment.

● Use cautiously in hypertensive patients with left-sided HF, perioperative patients who receive anesthetics that depress myocardial function (such as cyclopropane and trichloroethylene), and diabetic patients receiving insulin or oral antidiabetics, and in those subject to spontaneous hypoglycemia.

● Use cautiously in patients with thyroid disease (may mask hyperthyroidism; withdrawal may precipitate thyroid storm or exacerbation of hyperthyroidism), myasthenia gravis, pheochromocytoma, Prinzmetal or variant angina, bronchospastic disease (in those who can't tolerate other antihypertensives), or peripheral vascular disease (may precipitate or aggravate symptoms of arterial insufficiency).

● Safety and effectiveness in children younger than age 18 haven't been established.

Dialyzable drug: No.

⚠ *Overdose S&S:* Hypotension, bradycardia, cardiac insufficiency, cardiogenic shock, cardiac arrest, respiratory problems, bronchospasm, vomiting, lapses of consciousness, generalized seizures.

PREGNANCY-LACTATION-REPRODUCTION

● There are no adequate well-controlled studies in pregnant women. Use during pregnancy only if potential benefit outweighs potential risk to the fetus.

● It's unknown if drug appears in breast milk. Patient should discontinue breastfeeding or discontinue drug, taking into account importance of drug to the mother.

NURSING CONSIDERATIONS

⚠ *Alert:* Patients who have a history of severe anaphylactic reaction to several allergens may be more reactive to repeated challenge (accidental, diagnostic, or therapeutic). They may be unresponsive to dosages of epinephrine typically used to treat allergic reactions.

● Mild hepatocellular injury may occur during therapy. At first sign of hepatic dysfunction, perform tests for hepatic injury or jaundice; if present, stop drug.

● If drug must be stopped, do so gradually over 1 to 2 weeks, if possible.

● Monitor patient with HF for worsened condition, renal dysfunction, or fluid retention; diuretics may need to be increased.

● Monitor diabetic patient closely; drug may mask signs of hypoglycemia, or hyperglycemia may be worsened.

● Observe patient for dizziness or lightheadedness for 1 hour after giving each new dose.

● Monitor elderly patients carefully; drug levels are about 50% higher in elderly patients than in younger patients.

● *Look alike–sound alike:* Don't confuse carvedilol with carteolol or captopril.

PATIENT TEACHING

● Tell patient not to interrupt or stop drug without medical approval.

● Inform patient that improvement of HF symptoms might take several weeks of drug therapy.

● Advise patient with HF to call prescriber if weight gain or shortness of breath occurs.

Reactions in bold italics are *life-threatening*. Interactions may have a *rapid onset* or a *delayed onset*.

• Inform patient that he may experience low BP when standing. If dizziness or fainting occurs (rare), advise him to sit or lie down and to notify prescriber if symptoms persist.
• Caution patient against performing hazardous tasks during start of therapy.
• Advise diabetic patient to promptly report changes in glucose level.
• Inform patient who wears contact lenses that his eyes may feel dry.
• Tell patient to take drug with food. Extended-release capsule may be opened and contents mixed with cool applesauce and taken immediately; don't store.
• Advise patient that capsules shouldn't be crushed or chewed, or their contents divided.

---

caspofungin acetate
KAS-po-fun-gin

Cancidas

Therapeutic class: Antifungals
Pharmacologic class: Echinocandins

AVAILABLE FORMS
Lyophilized powder for injection: 50 mg, 70 mg in single-use vials

INDICATIONS & DOSAGES
Adjust-a-dose (for all indications): For adults receiving rifampin, give 70 mg I.V. once daily. Adults receiving nevirapine, efavirenz, carbamazepine, dexamethasone, or phenytoin may also require 70 mg I.V. once daily. For children receiving rifampin, give 70 mg/m² I.V. once daily (not to exceed an actual daily dose of 70 mg). Also consider giving 70 mg/m² I.V. once daily (not to exceed 70 mg) for children receiving nevirapine, efavirenz, carbamazepine, dexamethasone, or phenytoin. For patients with Child-Pugh score of 7 to 9, after initial 70-mg loading dose (when indicated), give 35 mg/day. Dosage adjustment in patients with Child-Pugh score of more than 9 is unknown.

➤ **Invasive aspergillosis in patients who are refractory to or intolerant of other therapies (amphotericin B, lipid forms of amphotericin B, or itraconazole); candidemia and *Candida*-caused intra-abdominal abscesses, peritonitis, and pleural space infections**
Adults: Single 70-mg I.V. loading dose on day 1, followed by 50 mg I.V. over about 1 hour once daily. Base treatment duration on severity of patient's underlying disease, recovery from immunosuppression, and clinical response.
Children age 3 months to 17 years: Single 70 mg/m² I.V. loading dose on day 1, followed by 50 mg/m² daily thereafter. May increase daily maintenance dose to 70 mg/m². Maximum loading dose and daily maintenance dose shouldn't exceed 70 mg.

➤ **Empirical treatment of presumed fungal infections in febrile, neutropenic patients**
Adults: Single 70-mg I.V. loading dose on day 1, followed by 50 mg I.V. over 1 hour once daily thereafter. Continue empirical therapy until neutropenia resolves. If fungal infection is confirmed, treat for a minimum of 14 days and continue therapy for at least 7 days after neutropenia and symptoms resolve. May increase daily dose to 70 mg if the 50-mg dose is well tolerated but clinical response is suboptimal.
Children age 3 months to 17 years: Single 70 mg/m² I.V. loading dose on day 1, followed by 50 mg/m² daily thereafter. May increase daily maintenance dose to 70 mg/m². Maximum loading dose and daily maintenance dose shouldn't exceed 70 mg.

➤ **Esophageal candidiasis**
Adults: 50 mg I.V. daily over 1 hour for 7 to 14 days after symptoms resolve. Don't administer a loading dose.
Children age 3 months to 17 years: Single 70-mg/m² I.V. loading dose on day 1, followed by 50 mg/m² daily thereafter. May increase daily maintenance dose to 70 mg/m². Maximum loading dose and daily maintenance dose shouldn't exceed 70 mg.

ADMINISTRATION
I.V.
▼ Let refrigerated vial warm to room temperature.
▼ Reconstitute drug by adding 10.8 mL of NSS, sterile water for injection, bacteriostatic water for injection with methylparaben and propylparaben, or bacteriostatic water for injection with benzyl

---

alcohol 0.9% to the vial. Resulting solution will be clear.

▼ Reconstitution will lead to a concentration of 5 mg/mL for 50-mg vial and 7 mg/mL for 70-mg vial.

▼ Use reconstituted vials within 1 hour of reconstitution or discard.

▼ For patients on fluid restriction, dilute the 35-mg and 50-mg doses in 100 mL NSS or lactated Ringer solution. For other patients, dilute 35-mg, 50-mg, and 70-mg doses in 250 mL NSS or lactated Ringer solution.

▼ Give drug by slow infusion over about 1 hour.

▼ Monitor site carefully for phlebitis.

▼ The final product for infusion (solution in I.V. bag or bottle) can be stored at room temperature for 24 hours or at 36° to 46° F (2° to 8° C) for 48 hours.

▼ **Incompatibilities:** Don't mix or infuse with other drugs or dextrose solutions.

ACTION
Inhibits synthesis of $1,3-\beta$-D-glucan, an essential component of the cell wall, in susceptible *Aspergillus* and *Candida* species. Drug is extensively distributed and has a prolonged half-life.

Route	Onset	Peak	Duration
I.V.	Unknown	Unknown	Unknown

Half-life: 9 to 11 hours; terminal, 40 to 50 hours.

ADVERSE REACTIONS
CNS: paresthesia, fever, headache.
CV: tachycardia, phlebitis, infused vein complications, hypotension.
GI: anorexia, nausea, vomiting, diarrhea, abdominal pain.
GU: proteinuria, hematuria.
Hematologic: anemia, eosinophilia.
Metabolic: hypokalemia.
Musculoskeletal: pain, myalgia.
Respiratory: dyspnea, crackles, cough, pneumonia, tachypnea.
Skin: histamine-mediated symptoms, including rash, facial swelling, pruritus, sensation of warmth.
Other: chills, sweating, mucosal inflammation.

INTERACTIONS
Drug-drug. *Cyclosporine:* May increase caspofungin level. May increase risk of elevated ALT level; avoid using together unless benefit outweighs risk.
Inducers of drug clearance or mixed inducer-inhibitors (carbamazepine, dexamethasone, efavirenz, nelfinavir, nevirapine, phenytoin, rifampin): May reduce caspofungin level. May need to adjust dosage upward to 70 mg in patients who are clinically unresponsive.
Tacrolimus: May reduce tacrolimus level. Monitor tacrolimus level; expect to adjust dosage.

EFFECTS ON LAB TEST RESULTS
● May increase glucose, alkaline phosphatase, and liver enzyme levels. May decrease albumin, calcium, Hb, potassium, magnesium, and protein levels.
● May increase eosinophil count.

CONTRAINDICATIONS & CAUTIONS
● Contraindicated in patients hypersensitive to drug or its components.
● Safety and effectiveness in neonates and infants younger than age 3 months aren't known.
Dialyzable drug: No.

PREGNANCY-LACTATION-REPRODUCTION
● There are no adequate studies in pregnant women. Use during pregnancy only if potential benefit justifies potential risk to the fetus.
● It's unknown if drug appears in breast milk. Use cautiously in breast-feeding women. Monitor infants for signs and symptoms of histamine release, such as facial swelling, rash, and GI symptoms.

NURSING CONSIDERATIONS
● Safety information is limited, but drug is well tolerated for therapy lasting longer than 2 weeks.
● Observe patients for histamine-mediated reactions, including rash, facial swelling, pruritus, and a sensation of warmth.

PATIENT TEACHING
● Instruct patient to report signs and symptoms of phlebitis.

Reactions in bold italics are *life-threatening*. Interactions may have a *rapid onset* or a *delayed onset*.

• Instruct patient to immediately report any signs of a hypersensitivity reaction.

cefadroxil
sef-a-DROX-ill

Therapeutic class: Antibiotics
Pharmacologic class: First-generation cephalosporins

AVAILABLE FORMS
Capsules: 500 mg
Oral suspension: 250 mg/5 mL, 500 mg/5 mL
Tablets: 1 g

INDICATIONS & DOSAGES
➤ **UTIs caused by** *Escherichia coli*, *Proteus mirabilis*, **and** *Klebsiella* **species; skin and soft-tissue infections caused by staphylococci and streptococci; pharyngitis or tonsillitis caused by group A beta-hemolytic streptococci**
Adults: 1 to 2 g P.O. daily, depending on infection being treated. Usually given once daily or in two divided doses.
Children: 30 mg/kg P.O. daily in a single dose or in two divided doses every 12 hours for tonsillitis, pharyngitis, and impetigo, and in two divided doses every 12 hours for other skin infections and UTIs. For beta-hemolytic strep infection, treat for 10 days.
Adjust-a-dose: In adult patient with renal impairment, give first dose of 1 g. Reduce additional doses based on CrCl. If CrCl is 25 to 50 mL/minute, give 500 mg P.O. every 12 hours. If CrCl is 10 to 25 mL/minute, give 500 mg P.O. every 24 hours; if CrCl is less than 10 mL/minute, give 500 mg P.O. every 36 hours.

ADMINISTRATION
P.O.
• Before administration, ensure patient isn't allergic to penicillins or cephalosporins.
• Obtain specimen for culture and sensitivity tests before giving first dose. Begin therapy while awaiting results.
• Administer without regard to meals but give drug with food or milk to lessen GI discomfort.

• Keep oral suspension refrigerated and discard unused portion after 14 days. Shake well before using.

ACTION
Inhibits cell-wall synthesis, promoting osmotic instability; usually bactericidal.

Route	Onset	Peak	Duration
P.O.	Unknown	70–90 min	Unknown

Half-life: About 1 to 2 hours.

ADVERSE REACTIONS
CNS: *seizures,* fever.
GI: *pseudomembranous colitis,* glossitis, abdominal cramps.
GU: genital pruritus, candidiasis, vaginitis, renal dysfunction.
Hematologic: *transient neutropenia, leukopenia, agranulocytosis, thrombocytopenia,* anemia, eosinophilia.
Skin: maculopapular and erythematous rashes, urticaria.
Other: *anaphylaxis, angioedema,* hypersensitivity reactions.

INTERACTIONS
Drug-drug. *Aminoglycosides:* May increase risk of nephrotoxicity. Avoid using together.
Live-virus vaccines: May decrease vaccine effectiveness. Don't give together.
Probenecid: May inhibit excretion and increase cefadroxil level. Use together cautiously.
Warfarin: May enhance anticoagulant effects. Monitor therapy.

EFFECTS ON LAB TEST RESULTS
• May increase alkaline phosphatase, ALT, AST, bilirubin, GGT, and LDH levels. May decrease Hb level.
• May increase eosinophil count. May decrease granulocyte, neutrophil, platelet, and WBC counts.
• May falsely increase serum or urine creatinine level in tests using Jaffe reaction. May cause false-positive results of Coombs test and urine glucose tests that use cupric sulfate, such as Benedict reagent and Clinitest.

CONTRAINDICATIONS & CAUTIONS
• Contraindicated in patients hypersensitive to drug or other cephalosporins.

♣ Canada   ◇ OTC   ♦ Off-label use   ✐ Photoguide   ⊗ Do not crush   *Liquid contains alcohol.

• Use cautiously in patients with a history of sensitivity to penicillin or GI diseases (colitis).

• Use cautiously in patients with impaired renal function; adjust dosage as needed.

❖ *Alert:* Seizures have occurred, particularly in patients with renal impairment when the dosage wasn't reduced. If seizures occur, discontinue drug and treat if clinically indicated.

❖ *Alert:* Drug can cause pseudomembranous colitis ranging from mild to life-threatening that can occur more than 2 months after treatment. Monitor patient for diarrhea and treat appropriately.

Dialyzable drug: Yes.

PREGNANCY-LACTATION-REPRODUCTION

• There are no adequate studies in pregnant women. Use during pregnancy only if potential benefit justifies potential risk to the fetus.

• It isn't known if drug appears in breast milk. Use cautiously in breast-feeding women.

NURSING CONSIDERATIONS

• If CrCl is less than 50 mL/minute, lengthen dosage interval so drug doesn't accumulate. Monitor renal function in patients with renal dysfunction.

• If large doses are given, therapy is prolonged, or patient is high risk, monitor patient for superinfection.

• *Look alike–sound alike:* Don't confuse drug with other cephalosporins that sound alike.

PATIENT TEACHING

• Instruct patient to take drug with food or milk to lessen GI discomfort.

• Tell patient to take entire amount of drug exactly as prescribed, even after he feels better.

• Advise patient to notify prescriber if rash develops or if signs and symptoms of superinfection appear, such as recurring fever, chills, and malaise.

cefazolin sodium
sef-AH-zoe-lin

Ancef, Kefzol

Therapeutic class: Antibiotics
Pharmacologic class: First-generation cephalosporins

AVAILABLE FORMS
Infusion: 1 g/50-mL bag, 2 g/50-mL bag
Injection (parenteral): 500 mg, 1 g

INDICATIONS & DOSAGES
Adjust-a-dose (for all indications): For adults with CrCl of 55 mL/minute or greater, give full dose every 6 to 8 hours; if CrCl is 35 to 54 mL/minute, give full dose every 8 hours or longer; if CrCl is 11 to 34 mL/minute, give 50% of usual dose every 12 hours; if CrCl is below 10 mL/minute, give 50% of usual dose every 18 to 24 hours.

➤ **Perioperative prevention in contaminated surgery**
Adults: 1 g I.M. or I.V. 30 to 60 minutes before surgery; then 0.5 to 1 g I.M. or I.V. every 6 to 8 hours for 24 hours. In operations lasting longer than 2 hours, give another 0.5- to 1-g dose I.M. or I.V. intraoperatively. Continue treatment for 3 to 5 days if life-threatening infection is likely.

➤ **Infections of respiratory, biliary, and GU tracts; skin, soft-tissue, bone, and joint infections; septicemia; endocarditis caused by** *Escherichia coli, Enterobacteriaceae,* **gonococci,** *Haemophilus influenzae, Klebsiella* **species,** *Proteus mirabilis, Staphylococcus aureus, Streptococcus pneumoniae,* **and group A beta-hemolytic streptococci**
Adults: 250 to 500 mg I.M. or I.V. every 8 hours for mild infections or 500 mg to 1.5 g I.M. or I.V. every 6 to 8 hours for moderate to severe or life-threatening infections. Maximum, 12 g/day in life-threatening situations.
Children older than age 1 month: 25 to 50 mg/kg/day I.M. or I.V. in three or four divided doses. In severe infections, dose may be increased to 100 mg/kg/day.
Adjust-a-dose: For children with CrCl of 40 to 70 mL/minute, give 60% of normal

daily dose divided every 12 hours; if CrCl is 20 to 40 mL/minute, give 25% of usual daily dose divided every 12 hours; if CrCl is 5 to 20 mL/minute, give 10% of usual dose every 24 hours.

ADMINISTRATION

I.V.

▼ Before giving first dose, obtain specimen for culture and sensitivity tests. Begin therapy while awaiting results.

▼ Before giving drug, ensure patient isn't allergic to penicillins or cephalosporins.

▼ Give commercially available frozen solutions in D_5W only by intermittent or continuous I.V. infusion.

▼ Reconstitute drug with sterile water, bacteriostatic water, or NSS as follows: Add 2 mL to 500-mg vial or 2.5 mL to 1-g vial, yielding 225 mg/mL or 330 mg/mL, respectively.

▼ Shake well until dissolved.

▼ For direct injection, further dilute with 5 mL of sterile water for injection.

▼ Inject into a large vein or into the tubing of a free-flowing I.V. solution over 3 to 5 minutes or as an intermittent infusion over 30 to 60 minutes.

▼ For intermittent infusion, add reconstituted drug to 50 to 100 mL of compatible solution or use premixed solution.

▼ If I.V. therapy lasts longer than 3 days, alternate injection sites. Use of small I.V. needles in larger available veins may be preferable.

▼ Reconstituted drug is stable 24 hours at room temperature or 10 days refrigerated.

▼ **Incompatibilities:** Amphotericin B cholesteryl sulfate complex, amiodarone, anakinra, caspofungin, cisatracurium, doxapram, hetastarch in NSS, hydromorphone, idarubicin, lidocaine, norepinephrine, pantoprazole, pemetrexed, pentamidine, promethazine, vancomycin, vinorelbine. Consult detailed drug reference.

I.M.

● Before giving first dose, obtain specimen for culture and sensitivity tests. Begin therapy while awaiting results.

● After reconstitution, inject drug I.M. without further dilution. This drug isn't as painful as other cephalosporins. Give injection deep into a large muscle.

ACTION

Inhibits cell-wall synthesis, promoting osmotic instability; usually bactericidal.

Route	Onset	Peak	Duration
I.V.	Immediate	Immediate	Unknown
I.M.	Unknown	½–2 hr	Unknown

Half-life: About 2 hours.

ADVERSE REACTIONS

CV: phlebitis, thrombophlebitis with I.V. injection.

GI: diarrhea, *pseudomembranous colitis,* anorexia, glossitis, dyspepsia, abdominal cramps, anal pruritus, oral candidiasis.

GU: genital pruritus, candidiasis, vaginitis.

Hematologic: *neutropenia, leukopenia, thrombocytopenia,* eosinophilia.

Skin: maculopapular and erythematous rashes, urticaria, pruritus, pain, induration, sterile abscesses, tissue sloughing at injection site, *Stevens-Johnson syndrome.*

Other: *anaphylaxis,* hypersensitivity reactions, drug fever.

INTERACTIONS

Drug-drug. *Aminoglycosides:* May increase risk of nephrotoxicity. Avoid using together.

Anticoagulants: May increase anticoagulant effects. Monitor PT and INR.

Live-virus vaccines: May decrease effectiveness of live-virus vaccines. Concurrent use isn't recommended.

Probenecid: May inhibit excretion and increase cefazolin level. Use together cautiously.

Warfarin: May enhance anticoagulant effects. Monitor therapy.

EFFECTS ON LAB TEST RESULTS

● May increase alkaline phosphatase, ALT, AST, bilirubin, GGT, and LDH levels and prolong INR.

● May increase eosinophil count. May decrease neutrophil, platelet, and WBC counts.

● May falsely increase serum or urine creatinine level in tests using Jaffe reaction. May cause false-positive results of Coombs test and urine glucose tests that use cupric sulfate, such as Benedict reagent and Clinitest.

CONTRAINDICATIONS & CAUTIONS
• Contraindicated in patients hypersensitive to drug or other cephalosporins.
• Use cautiously in patients hypersensitive to penicillin because of the possibility of cross-sensitivity with other beta-lactam antibiotics.
• Use cautiously in patients with a history of colitis, seizure disorders, or renal insufficiency.
• Prolonged use may result in fungal or bacterial superinfection, including CDAD, which can occur more than 2 months after treatment ends.
Dialyzable drug: Yes.
⚠ ***Overdose S&S:*** Pain, inflammation, and phlebitis at injection site; dizziness, paresthesia, headache, seizures; elevated creatinine, BUN, liver enzymes, and bilirubin levels; positive Coombs test; thrombocytosis, thrombocytopenia, eosinophilia, leukopenia; prolonged PT.

PREGNANCY-LACTATION-REPRODUCTION
• There are no adequate studies in pregnant women. Use during pregnancy only if clearly needed and potential benefit justifies potential risk to the fetus.
• Drug appears in very low concentrations in breast milk. Use cautiously in breastfeeding women.

NURSING CONSIDERATIONS
• If CrCl falls below 55 mL/minute in adults or 70 mL/minute in children, adjust dosage.
• If large doses are given, therapy is prolonged, or patient is at high risk, monitor patient for signs and symptoms of superinfection.
• ***Look alike–sound alike:*** Don't confuse drug with other cephalosporins that sound alike.

PATIENT TEACHING
• Instruct patient to report adverse reactions promptly.
• Tell patient to report discomfort at I.V. injection site.
• Advise patient to notify prescriber if a rash develops or if signs and symptoms

of superinfection, such as recurring fever, chills, and malaise, appear.

cefdinir
sef-DIN-er

Therapeutic class: Antibiotics
Pharmacologic class: Third-generation cephalosporins

AVAILABLE FORMS
Capsules: 300 mg
Suspension: 125 mg/5 mL, 250 mg/5 mL

INDICATIONS & DOSAGES
Adjust-a-dose (for all indications): If CrCl is less than 30 mL/minute, reduce dosage to 300 mg P.O. once daily for adults and 7 mg/kg (up to 300 mg) P.O. once daily for children. In patients receiving long-term hemodialysis, give 300 mg or 7 mg/kg P.O. at end of each dialysis session and then every other day.
➤ **Mild to moderate infections caused by susceptible strains of microorganisms in community-acquired pneumonia, acute worsening of chronic bronchitis, acute maxillary sinusitis, acute bacterial otitis media, and uncomplicated skin and skin-structure infections**
Adults and children age 13 and older: 300 mg P.O. every 12 hours or 600 mg P.O. every 24 hours for 10 days. Give every 12 hours for pneumonia and skin infections.
Children ages 6 months to 12 years: 7 mg/kg P.O. every 12 hours or 14 mg/kg P.O. every 24 hours for 10 days, up to maximum dose of 600 mg daily. Give every 12 hours for skin infections.
➤ **Pharyngitis, tonsillitis**
Adults and children age 13 and older: 300 mg P.O. every 12 hours for 5 to 10 days or 600 mg P.O. every 24 hours for 10 days.
Children ages 6 months to 12 years: 7 mg/kg P.O. every 12 hours for 5 to 10 days; or 14 mg/kg P.O. every 24 hours for 10 days.

ADMINISTRATION
P.O.
• Before administration, ensure patient isn't allergic to penicillins or cephalosporins.

- Give antacids and iron supplements 2 hours before or after a dose of cefdinir.
- Give drug without regard for meals.
- Give twice-daily doses every 12 hours.
- Shake suspension well before use.

ACTION

Inhibits cell-wall synthesis, promoting osmotic instability; usually bactericidal.

Route	Onset	Peak	Duration
P.O.	Unknown	2–4 hr	Unknown

Half-life: 1¾ hours.

ADVERSE REACTIONS

CNS: headache.
GI: diarrhea, *pseudomembranous colitis,* abdominal pain, nausea.
GU: vaginitis, increased urine proteins.
Hematologic: increased WBC and RBC counts.
Other: hypersensitivity reactions, *anaphylaxis.*

INTERACTIONS

Drug-drug. *Aminoglycosides:* May increase risk of nephrotoxicity. Avoid using together.
Antacids containing aluminum and magnesium, iron supplements, multivitamins containing iron: May decrease rate of absorption and bioavailability of cefdinir. Give such preparations 2 hours before or after cefdinir.
Live-virus vaccines: May decrease effectiveness of live-virus vaccines. Concurrent use isn't recommended.
Probenecid: May inhibit renal excretion of cefdinir. Monitor patient for adverse reactions.
Warfarin: May enhance anticoagulant effects. Monitor therapy.

EFFECTS ON LAB TEST RESULTS

- May increase alkaline phosphatase, GGT, and LDH levels. May decrease bicarbonate levels.
- May increase WBC, RBC, eosinophil, lymphocyte, and platelet counts.
- May falsely increase serum or urine creatinine level in tests using Jaffe reaction. May cause false-positive results of Coombs test and urine glucose tests that use cupric sulfate, such as Benedict reagent and Clinitest.

CONTRAINDICATIONS & CAUTIONS

- Contraindicated in patients hypersensitive to drug or other cephalosporins.
- Use cautiously in patients hypersensitive to penicillin because of the possibility of cross-sensitivity with other beta-lactam antibiotics.
- Use cautiously in patients with history of colitis or renal insufficiency.
Dialyzable drug: 63%.

PREGNANCY-LACTATION-REPRODUCTION

- There are no adequate studies in pregnant women. Use during pregnancy only if clearly needed and if potential benefit justifies potential risk to the fetus.
- It isn't known if drug appears in breast milk. Use cautiously in breast-feeding women.

NURSING CONSIDERATIONS

- Prolonged drug treatment may result in emergence and overgrowth of resistant organisms. Monitor patient for signs and symptoms of superinfection.
- Pseudomembranous colitis has been reported with cefdinir and can occur more than 2 months after therapy. Watch for diarrhea in patients after antibiotic therapy and in those with history of colitis.
- *Look alike–sound alike:* Don't confuse drug with other cephalosporins that sound alike.

PATIENT TEACHING

- Instruct patient to take antacids and iron supplements 2 hours before or after a dose of cefdinir.
- Inform diabetic patient that each teaspoon of suspension contains 2.86 g of sucrose.
- Tell patient that drug may be taken without regard to meals.
- Tell patient to take drug as prescribed, even after he feels better.
- Advise patient to report severe diarrhea or diarrhea with abdominal pain.
- Tell patient to report all adverse reactions or signs and symptoms of superinfection promptly.

cefepime hydrochloride
SEF-ah-peem

Maxipime

Therapeutic class: Antibiotics
Pharmacologic class: Fourth-generation cephalosporins

AVAILABLE FORMS
Injection: 500-mg vial, 1-g vial, 2-g vial, 1 g/50-mL Galaxy container, 2 g/100-mL Galaxy container, 1-g ADD-Vantage vial, 2-g ADD-Vantage vial, 1 g/50-mL duplex container, 2 g/50-mL duplex container

INDICATIONS & DOSAGES
Adjust-a-dose (for all indications): Adjust adult dosage based on CrCl, as shown in the table below. For patients receiving hemodialysis, about 68% of drug is removed after a 3-hour dialysis session. Cefepime dosage for patients receiving hemodialysis is 1 g on day 1, followed by 500 mg every 24 hours for treatment of all infections except febrile neutropenia. For patients with febrile neutropenia, give 1 g every 24 hours. Give cefepime after hemodialysis and at the same time each day. For patients receiving continuous ambulatory peritoneal dialysis, give normal dose every 48 hours. Because pediatric and adult cefepime pharmacokinetics are similar, change the pediatric dosing regimen proportional to the adult regimen.
➤ **Mild to moderate UTI caused by** *Escherichia coli, Klebsiella pneumoniae,* **or** *Proteus mirabilis,* **including concurrent bacteremia with these microorganisms**
Adults and children age 16 and older: 0.5 to 1 g I.M. or I.V. over 30 minutes every 12 hours for 7 to 10 days. Use I.M. only for *E. coli* infection when I.M. route

is considered more appropriate route of administration.
➤ **Severe UTI, including pyelonephritis, caused by** *E. coli* **or** *K. pneumoniae*
Adults and children age 16 and older: 2 g I.V. over 30 minutes every 12 hours for 10 days.
➤ **Moderate to severe pneumonia caused by** *Streptococcus pneumoniae, Pseudomonas aeruginosa, K. pneumoniae,* **or** *Enterobacter* **species**
Adults and children age 16 and older: 1 to 2 g I.V. over 30 minutes every 8 to 12 hours for 10 days.
➤ **Moderate to severe skin infection, uncomplicated skin infection, and skin-structure infection caused by** *Streptococcus pyogenes* **or methicillin-susceptible strains of** *Staphylococcus aureus*
Adults and children age 16 and older: 2 g I.V. over 30 minutes every 12 hours for 10 days.
➤ **Complicated intra-abdominal infection caused by** *E. coli,* **viridans group streptococci,** *P. aeruginosa, K. pneumoniae, Enterobacter* **species, or** *Bacteroides fragilis*
Adults and children age 16 and older: 2 g I.V. over 30 minutes every 8 to 12 hours for 7 to 10 days. Give with metronidazole.
➤ **Empirical therapy for febrile neutropenia**
Adults and children age 16 and older: 2 g I.V. every 8 hours for 7 days or until neutropenia resolves.
➤ **Uncomplicated and complicated UTI (including pyelonephritis), uncomplicated skin and skin-structure infection, pneumonia, empirical therapy for febrile neutropenic children**
Children ages 2 months to 16 years weighing up to 40 kg: 50 mg/kg/dose I.V. over 30 minutes every 12 hours for 10 days. For febrile neutropenia, 50 mg/kg every 8 hours

Adult dosage adjustments for renal impairment (cefepime hydrochloride)				
	If normal dosage would be			
CrCl (mL/min)	**500 mg every 12 hr**	**1 g every 12 hr**	**2 g every 12 hr**	**2 g every 8 hr**
30–60	500 mg every 24 hr	1 g every 24 hr	2 g every 24 hr	2 g every 12 hr
11–29	500 mg every 24 hr	500 mg every 24 hr	1 g every 24 hr	2 g every 24 hr
<11	250 mg every 24 hr	250 mg every 24 hr	500 mg every 24 hr	1 g every 24 hr

Reactions in bold italics are *life-threatening*. Interactions may have a *rapid onset* or a *delayed onset*.

for 7 days or until neutropenia resolves. For UTI, treat for 7 to 10 days. Don't exceed 2 g/dose.

ADMINISTRATION

I.V.
▼ Before giving drug, ensure patient isn't allergic to penicillins or cephalosporins.
▼ Obtain specimen for culture and sensitivity tests before giving. Begin therapy while awaiting results.
▼ Follow manufacturer's guidelines closely when reconstituting drug. They vary with concentration of drug ordered and how drug is packaged (duplex container, ADD-Vantage vial, or regular vial).
▼ The type of diluent varies with the product used. Use only solutions recommended by the manufacturer.
▼ Give intermittent I.V. infusion with a Y-type administration set and compatible solutions over 30 minutes.
▼ Interrupt flow of primary I.V. solution while drug is infusing.
▼ May also give by direct I.V. after vial reconstitution over 5 minutes.
▼ **Incompatibilities:** Aminophylline, amphotericin B, amphotericin B cholesteryl sulfate complex, ciprofloxacin, gentamicin, metronidazole, tobramycin, vancomycin.

I.M.
● Before giving drug, ensure patient isn't allergic to penicillins or cephalosporins.
● Obtain specimen for culture and sensitivity tests before giving. Begin therapy while awaiting results.
● Reconstitute drug using sterile water for injection, NSS for injection, D_5W injection, 0.5% or 1% lidocaine hydrochloride, or bacteriostatic water for injection with parabens or benzyl alcohol. Follow manufacturer's guidelines for quantity of diluent to use.
● Inspect solution for particulate matter before use. The powder and its solutions tend to darken, depending on storage conditions. If stored as recommended, potency isn't adversely affected.
● Pain may occur at injection site.

ACTION
Inhibits bacterial cell-wall synthesis, promotes osmotic instability, and destroys bacteria.

Route	Onset	Peak	Duration
I.V.	Unknown	30 min	Unknown
I.M.	Unknown	1–2 hr	Unknown

Half-life: Adults, 2 to 2½ hours.

ADVERSE REACTIONS
CNS: fever, headache.
CV: phlebitis.
GI: diarrhea, nausea, vomiting.
Skin: rash, pruritus.
Other: *anaphylaxis,* pain, inflammation, hypersensitivity reactions.

INTERACTIONS
Drug-drug. *Aminoglycosides:* May increase risk of nephrotoxicity. Monitor renal function closely.
Live-virus vaccines: May decrease effectiveness of live-virus vaccines. Concurrent use isn't recommended.
Potent diuretics: May increase risk of nephrotoxicity. Monitor renal function closely.
Probenecid: May inhibit renal excretion of cefepime. Monitor patient for adverse reactions.
Warfarin: May enhance anticoagulant effects. Monitor therapy.

EFFECTS ON LAB TEST RESULTS
● May increase ALT and AST levels. May decrease phosphorus level.
● May increase eosinophil count. May alter PT and PTT.
● May falsely increase serum or urine creatinine level in tests using Jaffe reaction. May cause false-positive results of Coombs test and urine glucose tests that use cupric sulfate, such as Benedict reagent and Clinitest.

CONTRAINDICATIONS & CAUTIONS
● Contraindicated in patients hypersensitive to drug, cephalosporins, beta-lactam antibiotics, or penicillins.
۞ Alert: Drug may increase risk of nonconvulsive status epilepticus (altered mental status, confusion, decreased responsiveness), especially in patients with renal

impairment. To decrease risk, follow dosage adjustment guidelines for patients with CrCl of 60 mL/minute or less. Discontinue drug in patients with seizures associated with drug.

• Use cautiously in patients hypersensitive to penicillin because of possibility of cross-sensitivity with other beta-lactam antibiotics.

• Use cautiously in patients with history of colitis or renal insufficiency.

Dialyzable drug: 68%.

⚠ *Overdose S&S:* Encephalopathy, myoclonus, seizures, neuromuscular excitability.

PREGNANCY-LACTATION-REPRODUCTION

• There are no adequate studies in pregnant women. Use during pregnancy only if clearly needed and potential benefit justifies potential risk to the fetus.

• Drug appears in breast milk in very low concentrations (0.5 mcg/mL). Use cautiously in breast-feeding women.

NURSING CONSIDERATIONS

• Monitor patient for superinfection, including CDAD and pseudomembranous colitis. Drug may cause overgrowth of nonsusceptible bacteria or fungi.

• Drug may reduce PT activity and increase bleeding risk. Patients at risk include those with renal or hepatic impairment or poor nutrition and those receiving prolonged therapy. Monitor PT and INR in these patients. Give vitamin K, as indicated.

• *Look alike–sound alike:* Don't confuse drug with other cephalosporins that sound alike.

PATIENT TEACHING

• Warn patient receiving drug I.M. that pain may occur at injection site.

• Advise patient to notify prescriber if a rash develops or if signs and symptoms of superinfection appear, such as recurring fever, chills, malaise, and diarrhea.

• Instruct patient to report adverse reactions promptly.

cefotaxime sodium
sef-oh-TAKS-eem

Claforan

Therapeutic class: Antibiotics
Pharmacologic class: Third-generation cephalosporins

AVAILABLE FORMS
Infusion: 1-g, 2-g premixed package
Injection: 500-mg, 1-g, 2-g

INDICATIONS & DOSAGES
Adjust-a-dose (for all indications): For patients with CrCl less than 20 mL/minute/ $1.73 m^2$, give half of usual dose at regular time interval. For patients receiving hemodialysis, give 0.5 to 2 g supplement after dialysis. For patients receiving continuous ambulatory peritoneal dialysis, give 1 g every 24 hours.

➤ **Perioperative prophylaxis in contaminated surgery**
Adults: 1 g I.M. or I.V. 30 to 90 minutes before surgery. In patients undergoing bowel surgery, provide preoperative mechanical bowel cleansing and give a nonabsorbable anti-infective, such as neomycin. In patients undergoing cesarean delivery, give 1 g I.M. or I.V. as soon as the umbilical cord is clamped; then 1 g I.M. or I.V. 6 and 12 hours later.

➤ **Uncomplicated gonorrhea caused by penicillinase-producing strains or non–penicillinase-producing strains of** *Neisseria gonorrhoeae*
Adults and adolescents: 500 mg I.M. as a single dose.

➤ **Rectal gonorrhea**
Men: 1 g I.M. as a single dose.
Women: 500 mg I.M. as a single dose.

➤ **Serious infection of the lower respiratory and urinary tract, CNS, skin, bone, and joints; gynecologic and intra-abdominal infection; bacteremia; septicemia caused by susceptible microorganisms, such as streptococci (including** *Streptococcus pneumoniae* **and** *S. pyogenes, Staphylococcus aureus* **[penicillinase- and non–penicillinase-producing], and** *S. epidermidis*),

---

Escherichia coli, Klebsiella, Haemophilus influenzae, Serratia marcescens, **and species of** *Pseudomonas* **(including** *P. aeruginosa***),** *Enterobacter, Proteus,* **and** *Peptostreptococcus*

Adults and children weighing 50 kg or more: 1 to 2 g I.V. or I.M. every 6 to 8 hours. Up to 12 g daily can be given for life-threatening infections.

Children ages 1 month to 12 years weighing less than 50 kg: 50 to 180 mg/kg/day I.M. or I.V. in four to six divided doses.

Neonates ages 1 to 4 weeks: 50 mg/kg I.V. every 8 hours.

Neonates to age 1 week: 50 mg/kg I.V. every 12 hours.

ADMINISTRATION

I.V.

▼ Before giving drug, ensure patient isn't allergic to penicillins or cephalosporins.

▼ Obtain specimen for culture and sensitivity tests before giving. Begin therapy while awaiting results.

▼ For direct injection, reconstitute drug in 500-mg, 1-g, or 2-g vials with 10 mL of sterile water for injection. Solutions containing 1 g/14 mL are isotonic.

▼ Inject drug over 3 to 5 minutes into a large vein or into the tubing of a free-flowing I.V. solution.

▼ For infusion, reconstitute drug in infusion vials with 50 to 100 mL of D₅W or NSS.

▼ Interrupt flow of primary I.V. solution, and infuse this drug over 20 to 30 minutes.

▼ **Incompatibilities:** Allopurinol, aminoglycosides, aminophylline, azithromycin, doxapram, filgrastim, fluconazole, hetastarch, pentamidine isethionate, sodium bicarbonate injection, vancomycin.

I.M.

● Before giving drug, ensure patient isn't allergic to penicillins or cephalosporins.

● Obtain specimen for culture and sensitivity tests before giving. Begin therapy while awaiting results.

● Reconstitute 500-mg vial with 2 mL, 1-g vial with 3 mL, and 2-g vial with 5 mL sterile water for injection.

● For doses of 2 g, divide the dose and give at different sites.

● Inject deep into a large muscle, such as the gluteus maximus or the side of the thigh.

ACTION

Inhibits cell-wall synthesis, promoting osmotic instability; usually bactericidal.

Route	Onset	Peak	Duration
I.V.	Immediate	Immediate	Unknown
I.M.	Unknown	30 min	Unknown

Half-life: 1 to 2 hours.

ADVERSE REACTIONS

CNS: fever, headache.

CV: phlebitis, thrombophlebitis.

GI: diarrhea, *pseudomembranous colitis,* nausea, vomiting.

Hematologic: *agranulocytosis, thrombocytopenia, transient neutropenia,* eosinophilia, hemolytic anemia.

Skin: maculopapular and erythematous rashes, urticaria, pain, induration, sterile abscesses, temperature elevation, tissue sloughing at I.M. injection site.

Other: *anaphylaxis,* hypersensitivity reactions, serum sickness.

INTERACTIONS

Drug-drug. *Aminoglycosides:* May increase risk of nephrotoxicity. Monitor patient's renal function tests.

Live-virus vaccines: May decrease effectiveness of live-virus vaccines. Concurrent use isn't recommended.

Probenecid: May inhibit excretion and increase cefotaxime level. Use together cautiously.

Warfarin: May enhance anticoagulant effects. Monitor therapy.

EFFECTS ON LAB TEST RESULTS

● May increase alkaline phosphatase, ALT, AST, bilirubin, GGT, and LDH levels. May decrease Hb level.

● May increase eosinophil count. May decrease granulocyte, neutrophil, and platelet counts.

● May cause positive Coombs test results.

CONTRAINDICATIONS & CAUTIONS

● Contraindicated in patients hypersensitive to drug or other cephalosporins.

- Use cautiously in patients hypersensitive to penicillin because of possibility of cross-sensitivity with other beta-lactam antibiotics.
- Prolonged use may result in fungal or bacterial superinfection, including CDAD and pseudomembranous colitis, which can occur more than 2 months after treatment ends.
- Use cautiously in patients with history of colitis or renal insufficiency.

Dialyzable drug: Yes.

⚠ *Overdose S&S:* Elevated BUN and creatinine levels.

PREGNANCY-LACTATION-REPRODUCTION
- There are no adequate studies in pregnant women. Use during pregnancy only if clearly needed.
- Low concentrations of drug appear in breast milk. Use cautiously in breastfeeding women.

NURSING CONSIDERATIONS
- If large doses are given, therapy is prolonged, or patient is at high risk, monitor patient for superinfection.
- *Look alike–sound alike:* Don't confuse drug with other cephalosporins that sound alike.

PATIENT TEACHING
- Tell patient to promptly report adverse reactions and signs and symptoms of superinfection, including diarrhea.
- Instruct patient to report discomfort at I.V. insertion site.

---

cefoxitin sodium
se-FOX-i-tin

Therapeutic class: Antibiotics
Pharmacologic class: Second-generation cephalosporins

AVAILABLE FORMS
Infusion: 1 g, 2 g in 50-mL duplex containers
Injection: 1 g, 2 g

INDICATIONS & DOSAGES
Adjust-a-dose (for all indications): For adults with renal insufficiency, give loading dose of 1 to 2 g. For adults with CrCl of 30 to 50 mL/minute, give 1 to 2 g every 8 to 12 hours; if CrCl is 10 to 29 mL/minute, 1 to 2 g every 12 to 24 hours; if CrCl is 5 to 9 mL/minute, 0.5 to 1 g every 12 to 24 hours; and if CrCl is less than 5 mL/minute, 0.5 to 1 g every 24 to 48 hours. For patients receiving hemodialysis, give a loading dose of 1 to 2 g after each hemodialysis session; then give the maintenance dose based on creatinine level. For patients receiving continuous ambulatory peritoneal dialysis, give 1 g every 24 hours.
➤ **Serious infection of the respiratory or GU tracts; skin, soft-tissue, bone, or joint infection; bloodstream or intra-abdominal infection caused by susceptible organisms (such as *Escherichia coli* and other coliform bacteria, penicillinase- and non–penicillinase-producing *Staphylococcus aureus, S. epidermidis*, streptococci, *Klebsiella, Haemophilus influenzae*, and *Bacteroides*, including *B. fragilis*)**
Adults: 1 to 2 g I.V. every 6 to 8 hours for uncomplicated infections. Up to 12 g daily may be used in life-threatening infections.
Children older than age 3 months: 80 to 160 mg/kg daily I.V., given in four to six equally divided doses. Maximum daily dose is 12 g.
➤ **Perioperative prophylaxis**
Adults: 2 g I.V. 30 to 60 minutes before surgery; then 2 g I.V. every 6 hours for up to 24 hours. For patients undergoing cesarean section, give 2 g I.V. as soon as the umbilical cord is clamped; may give additional 2-g doses 4 and 8 hours after initial dose.
Children age 3 months and older: 30 to 40 mg/kg I.V. 30 to 60 minutes before surgery; then 30 to 40 mg/kg every 6 hours for up to 24 hours.

ADMINISTRATION
I.V.
▼ Before giving drug, ensure patient isn't allergic to penicillins or cephalosporins.
▼ Obtain specimen for culture and sensitivity tests before giving. Begin therapy while awaiting results.
▼ Reconstitute 1 g with at least 10 mL of sterile water for injection and 2 g with 10 to 20 mL of sterile water for injection.

Solutions of D_5W and NSS for injection also may be used.

▼ After reconstitution, drug may be stored for 6 hours at room temperature or 1 week under refrigeration.

▼ For direct injection, give drug over 3 to 5 minutes into a large vein or into the tubing of a free-flowing I.V. solution.

▼ For intermittent infusion, add reconstituted drug to 50 or 100 mL of D_5W or NSS for injection and administer over 10 to 60 minutes.

▼ Interrupt flow of primary solution during cefoxitin infusion.

▼ Assess site often to detect evidence of thrombophlebitis.

▼ **Incompatibilities:** Aminoglycosides, filgrastim, hetastarch, pantoprazole, pentamidine.

ACTION

Inhibits cell-wall synthesis, promoting osmotic instability; usually bactericidal.

Route	Onset	Peak	Duration
I.V.	Immediate	Immediate	Unknown

Half-life: About ½ to 1 hour.

ADVERSE REACTIONS

CNS: fever.

CV: phlebitis, thrombophlebitis, hypotension.

GI: diarrhea, *pseudomembranous colitis,* nausea, vomiting.

GU: *acute renal failure.*

Hematologic: *thrombocytopenia, transient neutropenia,* eosinophilia, hemolytic anemia, anemia.

Respiratory: dyspnea.

Skin: maculopapular and erythematous rashes, urticaria, pain, induration, sterile abscesses, tissue sloughing at injection site, exfoliative dermatitis.

Other: *anaphylaxis,* hypersensitivity reactions, serum sickness.

INTERACTIONS

Drug-drug. *Aminoglycosides:* May increase risk of nephrotoxicity. Monitor patient's renal function tests.

Live-virus vaccines: May decrease effectiveness of live-virus vaccines. Concurrent use isn't recommended.

Probenecid: May inhibit excretion and increase cefoxitin level. Probenecid may be used for this effect.

Warfarin: May increase anticoagulation. Monitor PT, and adjust warfarin dosage as needed.

EFFECTS ON LAB TEST RESULTS

● May increase alkaline phosphatase, ALT, AST, bilirubin, and LDH levels. May decrease Hb level.

● May increase eosinophil count. May decrease neutrophil and platelet counts.

● May prolong PT.

● May falsely increase serum or urine creatinine level in tests using Jaffe reaction. May cause false-positive results of Coombs test and urine glucose tests that use cupric sulfate, such as Benedict reagent and Clinitest.

CONTRAINDICATIONS & CAUTIONS

● Contraindicated in patients hypersensitive to drug or other cephalosporins.

● Use cautiously in patients hypersensitive to penicillin because of possibility of cross-sensitivity with other beta-lactam antibiotics.

● Use cautiously in patients with history of colitis, renal insufficiency, or seizures.

● Drug can cause overgrowth of nonsusceptible organisms, including CDAD and pseudomembranous colitis, which can occur more than 2 months after treatment ends. Monitor patient for superinfection and treat appropriately.

● Higher doses have been associated with risk of eosinophilia and elevated AST levels in children age 3 months and older.

Dialyzable drug: Yes.

PREGNANCY-LACTATION-REPRODUCTION

● There are no adequate studies in pregnant women. Use during pregnancy only if potential benefit justifies potential risk to the fetus.

● Drug appears in breast milk in low concentrations. Use cautiously in breast-feeding women.

NURSING CONSIDERATIONS

🛈 *Alert:* The premixed frozen product is for I.V. use only.

• If large doses are given, therapy is prolonged, or patient is at high risk, monitor patient for signs and symptoms of superinfection.

• **Look alike–sound alike:** Don't confuse drug with other cephalosporins that sound alike.

PATIENT TEACHING

• Tell patient to report adverse reactions and signs and symptoms of superinfection promptly.

• Instruct patient to report discomfort at I.V. site.

• Advise patient to notify prescriber about loose stools or diarrhea.

cefpodoxime proxetil
SEF-pod-OX-eem

Therapeutic class: Antibiotics
Pharmacologic class: Third-generation cephalosporins

AVAILABLE FORMS
Oral suspension: 50 mg/5 mL or 100 mg/ 5 mL in 50-, 75-, or 100-mL bottles
Tablets (film-coated): 100 mg, 200 mg

INDICATIONS & DOSAGES
Adjust-a-dose (for all indications): For patients with CrCl less than 30 mL/minute, increase dosage interval to every 24 hours. Give to hemodialysis patients three times weekly after hemodialysis.

➤ **Acute community-acquired pneumonia caused by strains of *Haemophilus influenzae* or *Streptococcus pneumoniae***
Adults and children age 12 and older:
200 mg P.O. every 12 hours for 14 days.

➤ **Acute bacterial worsening of chronic bronchitis caused by *S. pneumoniae* or *H. influenzae* (strains that don't produce beta-lactamase only), or *Moraxella catarrhalis* (tablets only)**
Adults and children age 12 and older:
200 mg P.O. every 12 hours for 10 days.

➤ **Uncomplicated gonorrhea in men and women; rectal gonococcal infections in women**
Adults and children age 12 and older:
200 mg P.O. as a single dose.

➤ **Uncomplicated skin and skin-structure infections caused by *Staphylococcus aureus* or *Streptococcus pyogenes***
Adults and children age 12 and older:
400 mg P.O. every 12 hours for 7 to 14 days.

➤ **Acute otitis media caused by *S. pneumoniae* (penicillin-susceptible strains only), *S. pyogenes*, *H. influenzae*, or *M. catarrhalis***
Children ages 2 months to 12 years:
5 mg/kg oral suspension P.O. every 12 hours for 5 days. Don't exceed 200 mg per dose.

➤ **Pharyngitis or tonsillitis caused by *S. pyogenes***
Adults: 100 mg P.O. every 12 hours for 5 to 10 days.
Children ages 2 months to 12 years:
5 mg/kg oral suspension P.O. every 12 hours for 5 to 10 days. Don't exceed 100 mg per dose.

➤ **Uncomplicated UTIs caused by *Escherichia coli*, *Klebsiella pneumoniae*, *Proteus mirabilis*, or *Staphylococcus saprophyticus***
Adults: 100 mg P.O. every 12 hours for 7 days.

➤ **Mild to moderate acute maxillary sinusitis caused by *H. influenzae*, *S. pneumoniae*, or *M. catarrhalis***
Adults and adolescents age 12 and older:
200 mg P.O. every 12 hours for 10 days.
Children ages 2 months to 12 years:
5 mg/kg oral suspension P.O. every 12 hours for 10 to 14 days; maximum, 200 mg/dose.

ADMINISTRATION
P.O.
• Before administration, ensure patient isn't allergic to penicillins or cephalosporins.

• Obtain specimen for culture and sensitivity tests before giving. Begin therapy while awaiting results.

• Give tablets with food to enhance absorption. May give oral suspension without regard to food. Shake suspension well before using.

• Store suspension in the refrigerator (36° to 46° F [2° to 8° C]). Discard unused portion after 14 days.

ACTION
Inhibits cell-wall synthesis, promoting osmotic instability; usually bactericidal.

Route	Onset	Peak	Duration
P.O.	Unknown	2–3 hr	Unknown

Half-life: 2 to 3 hours.

ADVERSE REACTIONS
CNS: headache.
GI: diarrhea, *pseudomembranous colitis,* nausea, vomiting, abdominal pain.
GU: vaginal fungal infections.
Skin: rash.
Other: *anaphylaxis,* hypersensitivity reactions.

INTERACTIONS
Drug-drug. *Aminoglycosides:* May increase risk of nephrotoxicity. Monitor renal function tests closely.
Antacids, H_2-receptor antagonists: May decrease absorption of cefpodoxime. Separate H_2-receptor antagonist and cefpodoxime doses by at least 2 hours. Monitor therapy.
Live-virus vaccines: May decrease effectiveness of live-virus vaccines. Concurrent use isn't recommended.
Probenecid: May decrease excretion of cefpodoxime. Monitor patient for toxicity.
Warfarin: May prolong PT and INR. Monitor levels closely, and adjust warfarin dosage.

EFFECTS ON LAB TEST RESULTS
• May falsely increase serum or urine creatinine level in tests using Jaffe reaction.
• May decrease WBC, absolute neutrophil, platelet, and lymphocyte counts.
• May cause false-positive results of Coombs test and urine glucose tests that use cupric sulfate, such as Benedict reagent and Clinitest.

CONTRAINDICATIONS & CAUTIONS
• Contraindicated in patients hypersensitive to drug or other cephalosporins.
⚠ *Alert:* Drug can cause pseudomembranous colitis ranging from mild to life-threatening. Monitor patient for diarrhea and treat appropriately.
• Use cautiously in patients with a history of penicillin hypersensitivity because of risk of cross-sensitivity.
• Use cautiously in patients receiving nephrotoxic drugs because other

cephalosporins have been shown to have nephrotoxic potential.
⚠ *Alert:* Some dosage forms may contain benzoate, which is a metabolite of benzyl alcohol. Benzyl alcohol in large amounts has been linked to potentially fatal gasping syndrome in neonates. Avoid dosage forms with benzyl alcohol derivatives in neonates. Refer to manufacturer's labeling.
Dialyzable drug: 23%.

PREGNANCY-LACTATION-REPRODUCTION
• There are no adequate studies in pregnant women. Use during pregnancy only if clearly needed.
• Drug appears in breast milk. Patient should discontinue breast-feeding or discontinue drug, taking into account importance of drug to the mother.

NURSING CONSIDERATIONS
• Monitor renal function and compare with baseline.
• Monitor patient for superinfection. Drug may cause overgrowth of nonsusceptible bacteria or fungi.
• *Look alike–sound alike:* Don't confuse drug with other cephalosporins that sound alike.

PATIENT TEACHING
• Tell patient to take drug as prescribed, even after he feels better.
• Instruct patient to take tablets with food. If patient is using suspension, tell him to shake container before measuring dose and to keep container refrigerated.
• Tell patient to report all adverse reactions, especially rash or signs and symptoms of superinfection.
• Instruct patient to report loose stools or diarrhea.

cefprozil
sef-PRO-zil

Therapeutic class: Antibiotics
Pharmacologic class: Second-generation cephalosporins

AVAILABLE FORMS
Oral suspension: 125 mg/5 mL, 250 mg/5 mL
Tablets: 250 mg, 500 mg

INDICATIONS & DOSAGES
Adjust-a-dose (for all indications): If CrCl is less than 30 mL/minute, give 50% of standard dose at standard intervals. If patient is receiving dialysis, give dose after hemodialysis is completed; drug is removed by hemodialysis.

➤ **Pharyngitis or tonsillitis caused by** *Streptococcus pyogenes*
Adults and children age 13 and older: 500 mg P.O. daily for at least 10 days.
Children ages 2 to 12: 7.5 mg/kg P.O. every 12 hours for 10 days. Don't exceed adult dose.

➤ **Otitis media caused by** *Streptococcus pneumoniae, Haemophilus influenzae,* **or** *Moraxella catarrhalis*
Infants and children ages 6 months to 12 years: 15 mg/kg P.O. every 12 hours for 10 days. Don't exceed adult dosage.

➤ **Secondary bacterial infections of acute bronchitis and acute bacterial worsening of chronic bronchitis caused by** *S. pneumoniae, H. influenzae,* **or** *M. catarrhalis*
Adults and children age 13 and older: 500 mg P.O. every 12 hours for 10 days.

➤ **Uncomplicated skin and skin-structure infections caused by** *Staphylococcus aureus* **or** *S. pyogenes*
Adults and children age 13 and older: 250 or 500 mg P.O. every 12 hours or 500 mg P.O. daily for 10 days.
Children ages 2 to 12: 20 mg/kg P.O. every 24 hours for 10 days. Don't exceed adult dose.

➤ **Acute sinusitis caused by** *S. pneumoniae, H. influenzae* **(beta-lactamase–positive and beta-lactamase–negative strains), or** *M. catarrhalis* **(including strains that produce beta-lactamase)**
🛈 *Alert:* Because of variable rates of resistance among *S. pneumoniae,* clinical practice guidelines don't recommend drug as initial empirical treatment of acute bacterial rhinosinusitis.
Adults and children age 13 and older: 250 mg P.O. every 12 hours for 10 days; for moderate to severe infection, 500 mg P.O. every 12 hours for 10 days.
Children ages 6 months to 12 years: 7.5 mg/kg P.O. every 12 hours for 10 days; for moderate to severe infections, 15 mg/kg

P.O. every 12 hours for 10 days. Don't exceed adult dosage.

ADMINISTRATION
P.O.
● Obtain specimen for culture and sensitivity tests before giving first dose. Start therapy while awaiting results.
● Before giving, ensure patient isn't allergic to penicillins or cephalosporins.
● Administer without regard to meals.
● Shake suspension well before using.

ACTION
Inhibits cell-wall synthesis, promoting osmotic instability; usually bactericidal.

Route	Onset	Peak	Duration
P.O.	Unknown	1½ hr	Unknown

Half-life: 1¼ hours in adults with normal renal function; 1½ hours in children; 2 hours in patients with impaired hepatic function; 6 hours in patients with ESRD.

ADVERSE REACTIONS
CNS: dizziness.
GI: diarrhea, nausea, vomiting, abdominal pain.
GU: genital pruritus, vaginitis.
Hematologic: eosinophilia.
Skin: diaper rash.
Other: *anaphylaxis,* superinfection, hypersensitivity reactions, serum sickness.

INTERACTIONS
Drug-drug. *Aminoglycosides:* May increase risk of nephrotoxicity. Monitor renal function tests closely.
Live-virus vaccines: May decrease effectiveness of live-virus vaccines. Concurrent use isn't recommended.
Probenecid: May inhibit excretion and increase cefprozil level. Use together cautiously.
Warfarin: May enhance anticoagulant effects. Monitor therapy.

EFFECTS ON LAB TEST RESULTS
● May increase alkaline phosphatase, ALT, AST, bilirubin, BUN, creatinine, and LDH levels.
● May increase eosinophil count. May decrease platelet and WBC counts.

Reactions in bold italics are *life-threatening.* Interactions may have a *rapid onset* or a **delayed onset.**

- May prolong PT and PTT.
- May falsely increase serum or urine creatinine level in tests using Jaffe reaction. May cause false-positive results of Coombs test and urine glucose tests that use cupric sulfate, such as Benedict reagent and Clinitest.

CONTRAINDICATIONS & CAUTIONS
- Contraindicated in patients hypersensitive to drug or other cephalosporins.
- Use cautiously in patients hypersensitive to penicillin because of possibility of cross-sensitivity with other beta-lactam antibiotics.
- **❸ Alert:** May cause mild to life-threatening CDAD and pseudomembranous colitis, which can occur even more than 2 months after therapy; drug may need to be discontinued and other treatment initiated. Use cautiously in patients with a history of GI disease, especially colitis.
- Use cautiously in patients with history of colitis and renal insufficiency.
Dialyzable drug: Yes.

PREGNANCY-LACTATION-REPRODUCTION
- There are no adequate studies in pregnant women. Use during pregnancy only if clearly needed and potential benefit justifies potential risk to the fetus.
- Small amounts of drug appear in breast milk. Use cautiously in breast-feeding women.

NURSING CONSIDERATIONS
- Monitor renal function test and LFT results.
- Drug may cause overgrowth of nonsusceptible bacteria or fungi. Monitor patient for superinfection.
- Monitor patient for diarrhea.
- *Look alike–sound alike:* Don't confuse drug with other cephalosporins that sound alike.

PATIENT TEACHING
- Advise patient to take drug as prescribed, even after he feels better.
- Tell patient to shake suspension well before measuring dose.
- Inform patient or parent that oral suspension is bubble gum–flavored to improve palatability and promote compliance in children. Tell him to refrigerate reconstituted

suspension and to discard unused drug after 14 days.
- Instruct patient to report all adverse reactions and to immediately report rash or signs and symptoms of superinfection, including diarrhea.

ceftaroline fosamil
sef-TAR-oh-leen

Teflaro

Therapeutic class: Antibiotics
Pharmacologic class: Fifth-generation cephalosporins

AVAILABLE FORMS
Injection: 400-mg, 600-mg in single-use vials

INDICATIONS & DOSAGES
➤ **Acute bacterial skin and skin-structure infections caused by susceptible isolates of *Staphylococcus aureus, Streptococcus pyogenes, Streptococcus agalactiae, Escherichia coli, Klebsiella pneumoniae,* or *Klebsiella oxytoca;* community-acquired bacterial pneumonia (CABP) caused by susceptible isolates of *Streptococcus pneumoniae, S. aureus, Haemophilus influenzae, K. pneumoniae, K. oxytoca,* or *E. coli***
Adults: 600 mg I.V. over 5 to 60 minutes every 12 hours. For skin and skin-structure infections, continue treatment for 5 to 14 days; for CABP, continue treatment for 5 to 7 days.
Adjust-a-dose: For patients with CrCl of 31 to 50 mL/minute, give 400 mg I.V. every 12 hours. If CrCl is 15 to 30 mL/minute, give 300 mg I.V. every 12 hours. For patients with ESRD, including those on hemodialysis, give 200 mg I.V. every 12 hours. Administer after dialysis treatment.

ADMINISTRATION
I.V.
▼ Obtain specimen for culture before administration.
▼ Before administration, ensure patient isn't allergic to penicillins or cephalosporins.

▼ Reconstitute drug with 20 mL sterile water for injection, NSS, D5W, or lactated Ringer solution. Mix gently.

▼ Inspect solution for particulate matter. Color of solution ranges from clear to light to dark yellow.

▼ Further dilute in 50 to 250 mL I.V. fluid for infusion using the same diluent used for reconstitution or NSS injection, 5% dextrose injection, 2.5% dextrose in half-NSS injection, or lactated Ringer injection if sterile water was used earlier.

▼ A 600-mg dose in 50-mL infusion bag results in 12-mg/mL dose; a 400-mg dose in 50-mL infusion bag results in 8-mg/mL dose.

▼ Administer by I.V. infusion over 5 to 60 minutes.

▼ Final solution of ceftaroline is stable for 6 hours at room temperature or for 24 hours if refrigerated at 36° to 46° F (2° to 8° C).

▼ **Incompatibilities:** Other drugs, I.V. solutions not listed above.

ACTION

Bactericidal by binding to penicillin-binding proteins.

Route	Onset	Peak	Duration
I.V.	Unknown	1 hr	Unknown

Half-life: 1.6 to 2.7 hours.

ADVERSE REACTIONS

CNS: dizziness, *seizures,* pyrexia.
CV: *bradycardia,* palpitations, phlebitis.
GI: diarrhea, nausea, constipation, vomiting, abdominal pain, *CDAD.*
GU: *renal failure.*
Hematologic: anemia, eosinophilia, *neutropenia, thrombocytopenia.*
Hepatic: hepatitis.
Metabolic: *hypokalemia, hyperkalemia,* hyperglycemia.
Skin: rash, urticaria.
Other: hypersensitivity, *anaphylaxis.*

INTERACTIONS

Drug-drug. *Live-virus vaccines:* May decrease effectiveness of live-virus vaccines. Concurrent use isn't recommended.
Probenecid: May inhibit excretion and increase ceftaroline level. Monitor therapy.

Warfarin: May enhance anticoagulant effects. Monitor therapy.

EFFECTS ON LAB TEST RESULTS

● May increase serum glucose and transaminase levels.
● May decrease eosinophil, neutrophil, platelet, and RBC counts.
● May increase or decrease potassium level.
● May cause seroconversion of direct Coombs test from negative to positive.

CONTRAINDICATIONS & CAUTIONS

● Contraindicated in patients hypersensitive to drug or other cephalosporins, penicillins, or carbapenem drugs.
● Use cautiously in patients with history of beta-lactam allergy, renal failure, or drug-resistant infections.
● May cause mild to severe CDAD, which can occur more than 2 months after therapy ends and may be fatal.
● Safety and effectiveness in children haven't been established.
Dialyzable drug: Yes.

PREGNANCY-LACTATION-REPRODUCTION

● There are no adequate studies in pregnant women. Use during pregnancy only if potential benefit justifies potential risk to the fetus.
● It isn't known if drug appears in breast milk. Use cautiously if breast-feeding.

NURSING CONSIDERATIONS

● Prescribing drug without proven or strongly suspected bacterial infection is unlikely to provide benefit and increases the risk of drug resistance.
● Obtain a list of patient's known allergies before beginning treatment.
● Monitor for signs and symptoms of CDAD (frequent watery or bloody diarrhea).
● Monitor for anemia during and after therapy. Consider a diagnostic workup, including direct Coombs test for drug-induced hemolytic anemia.
● Monitor renal function periodically during therapy, especially in elderly patients and in those with decreased renal function.
● *Look alike–sound alike:* Don't confuse ceftaroline with ceftazidime or ceftriaxone.

Reactions in bold italics are *life-threatening*. Interactions may have a *rapid onset* or a *delayed onset*.

PATIENT TEACHING

● Instruct patient to inform prescriber if he's allergic to penicillin or cephalosporins before beginning treatment.

● Tell patient to report itching, hives, throat swelling, or shortness of breath.

● Tell patient that blood tests may be required to assess his tolerance to treatment.

● Warn patient that diarrhea may occur and to immediately report watery or bloody diarrhea.

● Advise female patient to tell prescriber if she's pregnant or is breast-feeding.

ceftazidime
sef-TAZ-i-deem

Fortaz, Tazicef

Therapeutic class: Antibiotics
Pharmacologic class: Third-generation cephalosporins

AVAILABLE FORMS

Infusion: 1 g, 2 g in 50-mL and 100-mL vials (premixed)
Injection (with sodium carbonate): 500 mg, 1 g, 2 g

INDICATIONS & DOSAGES

Adjust-a-dose (for all indications): If CrCl is 31 to 50 mL/minute, give 1 g every 12 hours; if CrCl is 16 to 30 mL/minute, give 1 g every 24 hours; if CrCl is 6 to 15 mL/minute, give 500 mg every 24 hours; if CrCl is less than 5 mL/minute, give 500 mg every 48 hours. Ceftazidime is removed by hemodialysis; give a loading dose of 1 g, followed by 1 g after each hemodialysis period. If patient is receiving continuous ambulatory peritoneal dialysis, give a loading dose of 1 g, followed by 500 mg every 24 hours. Or, add 250 mg per 2 L of dialysis fluid.

➤ **Serious UTI and lower respiratory tract infection; skin, gynecologic, intra-abdominal, bone and joint, and CNS infection; bacteremia; and septicemia caused by susceptible microorganisms, such as streptococci (including *Strep-tococcus pneumoniae* and *S. pyogenes*), penicillinase- and non–penicillinase-** producing *Staphylococcus aureus, Escherichia coli, Klebsiella, Proteus, Enterobacter, Haemophilus influenzae, Pseudomonas*, and some strains of *Bac-teroides*

Adults and children age 12 and older: 1 to 2 g I.V. or I.M. every 8 to 12 hours; up to 6 g daily in life-threatening infections.

Children ages 1 month to 12 years: 30 to 50 mg/kg I.V. every 8 hours. Maximum dose is 6 g/day. Use sodium carbonate formulation.

Neonates up to age 4 weeks: 30 mg/kg I.V. every 12 hours. Use sodium carbonate formulation.

➤ **Uncomplicated UTI**
Adults: 250 mg I.V. or I.M. every 12 hours.

➤ **Complicated UTI**
Adults and children age 12 and older: 500 mg to 1 g I.V. or I.M. every 8 to 12 hours.

➤ **Uncomplicated pneumonia**
Adults and children age 12 and older: 500 mg to 1 g I.V. or I.M. every 8 hours.

➤ **Lung infections caused by *Pseu-domonas* in patients with cystic fibrosis with healthy renal function**
Adults and children age 12 and older: 30 to 50 mg/kg I.V. every 8 hours. Maximum dose is 6 g/day.

➤ **Very severe life-threatening infections, especially in immunocompromised patients**
Adults and children older than age 12: 2 g I.V. every 8 hours.

ADMINISTRATION

I.V.

▼ Before administration, ensure patient isn't allergic to penicillins or cephalosporins.

▼ Obtain specimen for culture and sensitivity tests before giving. Begin therapy while awaiting results.

▼ Each brand of drug includes specific instructions for reconstitution. Read and follow them carefully.

▼ To reconstitute solution that contains sodium carbonate, add 5 mL sterile water for injection to a 500-mg vial, or add 10 mL to a 1-g or 2-g vial. Shake well to dissolve drug. Because carbon dioxide

---

is released during dissolution, positive pressure will develop in vial.

▼ Infuse drug over 15 to 30 minutes.

▼ **Incompatibilities:** Aminoglycosides, aminophylline, amiodarone, amphotericin B cholesteryl sulfate complex, azithromycin, clarithromycin, fluconazole, idarubicin, midazolam, pentamidine isethionate, ranitidine hydrochloride, sargramostim, sodium bicarbonate solutions, vancomycin.

I.M.

● Before administration, ensure patient isn't allergic to penicillins or cephalosporins.

● Obtain specimen for culture and sensitivity tests before giving. Begin therapy while awaiting results.

● Inject deep into a large muscle, such as the gluteus maximus or the side of the thigh.

ACTION

Inhibits cell-wall synthesis, promoting osmotic instability; usually bactericidal.

Route	Onset	Peak	Duration
I.V.	Immediate	Immediate	Unknown
I.M.	Unknown	1 hr	Unknown

Half-life: 2 hours.

ADVERSE REACTIONS

CNS: *seizures.*

CV: phlebitis, thrombophlebitis.

GI: *pseudomembranous colitis,* nausea, vomiting, diarrhea, abdominal cramps.

Hematologic: *agranulocytosis, leukopenia, thrombocytopenia,* eosinophilia, thrombocytosis, hemolytic anemia.

Skin: maculopapular and erythematous rashes, urticaria, pain, induration, sterile abscesses, tissue sloughing at injection site.

Other: *anaphylaxis,* hypersensitivity reactions, serum sickness.

INTERACTIONS

Drug-drug. *Aminoglycosides:* May cause additive or synergistic effect against some strains of *Pseudomonas aeruginosa* and *Enterobacteriaceae;* may increase risk of nephrotoxicity. Monitor patient for effects and monitor renal function.

Chloramphenicol: May cause antagonistic effect. Avoid using together.

Live-virus vaccines: May decrease effectiveness of live-virus vaccines. Concurrent use isn't recommended.

Probenecid: May increase serum concentrations of cephalosporins. Monitor therapy.

Warfarin: May increase anticoagulation effect. Monitor PT and INR closely.

EFFECTS ON LAB TEST RESULTS

● May increase alkaline phosphatase, ALT, AST, bilirubin, and LDH levels. May decrease Hb level.

● May increase eosinophil count. May decrease granulocyte and WBC counts. May increase or decrease platelet count.

● May prolong PTT and PT, and increase INR.

● May falsely increase serum or urine creatinine level in tests using Jaffe reaction. May cause false-positive results of Coombs test and urine glucose tests that use cupric sulfate, such as Benedict reagent and Clinitest.

CONTRAINDICATIONS & CAUTIONS

● Contraindicated in patients hypersensitive to drug or other cephalosporins.

● Use cautiously in patients hypersensitive to penicillin; may cause cross-sensitivity with other beta-lactam antibiotics.

● Prolonged use can result in superinfection, including CDAD and pseudomembranous colitis, which can occur even more than 2 months after treatment ends.

● Use cautiously in patients with history of colitis, renal insufficiency, or seizures.

Dialyzable drug: Yes.

⚠ *Overdose S&S:* Seizures, encephalopathy, asterixis, neuromuscular excitability, coma (in patients with renal failure).

PREGNANCY-LACTATION-REPRODUCTION

● There are no adequate studies in pregnant women. Use during pregnancy only if clearly needed.

● Drug appears in breast milk in low concentrations. Use caution in breast-feeding.

NURSING CONSIDERATIONS

● If large doses are given, therapy is prolonged, or patient is at high risk, monitor patient for superinfection.

● *Look alike–sound alike:* Don't confuse drug with other cephalosporins that sound alike.

Reactions in bold italics are *life-threatening*. Interactions may have a *rapid onset* or a *delayed onset*.

PATIENT TEACHING

- Tell patient to report adverse reactions or signs of superinfection promptly.
- Instruct patient to report discomfort at I.V. insertion site.
- Advise patient to notify prescriber about loose stools or diarrhea.

ceftazidime–avibactam
sef-TAZ-i-deem/A-vi-BAK-tam sodium

Avycaz

Therapeutic class: Antibiotics
Pharmacologic class: Cephalosporins–beta-lactamase inhibitors

AVAILABLE FORMS
Injection (single-use vials): 2 g ceftazidime and 0.5 g avibactam per vial

INDICATIONS & DOSAGES
Alert: Dosage recommendations are expressed as total grams of the ceftazidime–avibactam combination.
Adjust-a-dose (for all indications): If CrCl is 31 to 50 mL/minute, give 1.25 g (1 g ceftazidime and 0.25 g avibactam) every 8 hours. If CrCl is 16 to 30 mL/minute, give 0.94 g (0.75 g ceftazidime and 0.19 g avibactam) every 12 hours. If CrCl is 6 to 15 mL/minute, give 0.94 g (0.75 g ceftazidime and 0.19 g avibactam) every 24 hours. If CrCl is 5 mL/minute or less, give 0.94 g (0.75 g ceftazidime and 0.19 g avibactam) every 48 hours. If patient is on hemodialysis, administer after hemodialysis on hemodialysis days.
➤ **Complicated intra-abdominal infections caused by susceptible microorganisms (*Escherichia coli, Klebsiella pneumoniae, Proteus mirabilis, Providencia stuartii, Enterobacter cloacae, Klebsiella oxytoca,* or *Pseudomonas aeruginosa*) in combination with metronidazole**
Adults: 2.5 g (2 g ceftazidime and 0.5 g avibactam) I.V. every 8 hours for 5 to 14 days.
➤ **Complicated UTI, including pyelonephritis, caused by susceptible microorganisms (*E. coli, K. pneumoniae, Citrobacter koseri, Enterobacter aerogenes, E. cloacae, Citrobacter freundii, Proteus* spp., or *P. aeruginosa*)**
Adults: 2.5 g (2 g ceftazidime and 0.5 g avibactam) I.V. every 8 hours for 7 to 14 days.

ADMINISTRATION
I.V.
▼ Store unconstituted vials at 77° F (25° C); excursions permitted between 59° and 86° F (15° and 30° C). Protect from light.
▼ Reconstitute vial with 10 mL sterile water for injection, NSS, 5% dextrose, lactated Ringer solution, or all combinations of dextrose injection and sodium chloride injection containing up to 2.5% dextrose and 0.45% sodium chloride. Mix gently.
▼ Refer to package insert for specific information regarding volume to withdraw from vial to dilute further to 50 or 250 mL to administer renal doses of drug.
▼ Further dilute constituted solution with the same diluent used for constitution to achieve a total volume between 50 mL (40 and 10 mg/mL of ceftazidime and avibactam, respectively) and 250 mL (8 and 2 mg/mL of ceftazidime and avibactam, respectively). Mix gently. Inspect for particulate matter and discoloration (the color of solution ranges from clear to light yellow).
▼ Final solution is stable for 12 hours at room temperature and for 24 hours if refrigerated at 36° to 46° F (2° to 8° C). Use final solution within 12 hours of subsequent storage at room temperature.
▼ Infuse final solution over 2 hours.
▼ **Incompatibilities:** Solutions other than those listed above and all medications.

ACTION
Ceftazidime is a bactericidal agent that inhibits cell-wall synthesis, promoting osmotic instability. Avibactam increases ceftazidime's effectiveness by inactivating certain beta-lactamases, which destroy ceftazidime.

Route	Onset	Peak	Duration
I.V.	Rapid	Unknown	Unknown

Half-life: Ceftazidime, about 3 hours; avibactam, about 2½ hours.

ADVERSE REACTIONS
CNS: dizziness, anxiety.
GI: nausea, vomiting, constipation, abdominal pain, *CDAD.*
GU: *acute renal failure,* renal impairment.
Hematologic: eosinophilia, *thrombocytopenia.*
Hepatic: increased alkaline phosphatase, ALT, and GGT levels.
Metabolic: hypokalemia.
Skin: rash.
Other: hypersensitivity reaction, *drug-resistant bacterial infection.*

INTERACTIONS
Drug-drug. *Probenecid:* May decrease ceftazidime–avibactam excretion. Avoid use together.
Vitamin K antagonists (warfarin): May enhance anticoagulation effects. Monitor therapy.

EFFECTS ON LAB TEST RESULTS
● May increase alkaline phosphatase, GGT, and ALT levels. May decrease potassium level.
● May prolong PT.
● May cause false-positive reaction for glucose in the urine with certain methods.
● May result in seroconversion from a negative to a positive direct Coombs test.

CONTRAINDICATIONS & CAUTIONS
● Contraindicated in patients hypersensitive to cephalosporins and avibactam.
◑ *Alert:* Reserve use for patients who have limited or no alternative treatment options because of limited clinical safety and efficacy data.
● Use cautiously in patients with penicillin or other beta-lactam allergy because of cross-sensitivity.
◑ *Alert:* Drug may cause severe neurologic reactions, including encephalopathy, myoclonus, seizures, and nonconvulsive status epilepticus. Risk may increase in patients with renal impairment; ensure dosage adjustment for renal function. Discontinue drug if neurotoxicity occurs.
◑ *Alert:* Serious and fatal hypersensitivity reactions and anaphylaxis can occur.
● Use cautiously in patients with renal impairment. Decreased clinical response

may occur in patients with baseline CrCl of 30 to 50 mL/minute.
● CDAD has been reported with the use of nearly all systemic antibacterial drugs, and may range in severity from mild diarrhea to fatal colitis. CDAD may occur more than 2 months after use of antibacterial drugs.
● Safety and effectiveness in children haven't been established.
● Use cautiously in elderly patients, who are more likely to have renal dysfunction.
Dialyzable drug: Yes.

PREGNANCY-LACTATION-REPRODUCTION
● Use cautiously in pregnant women and only if benefits outweigh risk to the fetus.
● Ceftazidime appears in breast milk in low concentrations; it isn't known if avibactam appears in breast milk. Use cautiously in breast-feeding women.

NURSING CONSIDERATIONS
● To reduce the development of drug-resistant bacteria and maintain the effectiveness of antibacterial drugs, ceftazidime–avibactam should be used only to treat infections that are proven or strongly suspected to be caused by susceptible bacteria.
◑ *Alert:* Monitor renal function at baseline and at least daily in patients with renal impairment.
◑ *Alert:* Monitor patients for CNS reactions (including seizures, nonconvulsive status epilepticus, encephalopathy, coma, asterixis, neuromuscular excitability, and myoclonia), particularly in those with renal impairment. Adjust dosage based on CrCl level or discontinue therapy as clinically indicated.
◑ *Alert:* Watch for CDAD in patients who develop diarrhea. If CDAD is suspected or confirmed, antibacterial drugs not directed against CDAD may need to be discontinued. Manage fluid and electrolyte levels as appropriate, supplement protein intake, monitor antibacterial treatment of CDAD, and institute surgical evaluation as clinically indicated.
● Assess carefully for previous hypersensitivity reactions to cephalosporins, penicillins, or carbapenems.
● Monitor patient closely for hypersensitivity reaction. Discontinue drug if allergic reactions occur.

Reactions in bold italics are *life-threatening*. Interactions may have a *rapid onset* or a *delayed onset.*

- For patients with renal failure, give after hemodialysis on hemodialysis days.
- Urine glucose tests based on enzymatic glucose oxidase reactions are recommended. False-positive reactions may occur with other methods.
- *Look alike–sound alike:* Don't confuse Avycaz with Fortaz or Avelox. Don't confuse avibactam with aztreonam.

PATIENT TEACHING

- Instruct patient to immediately report changes in CNS status (disturbance of consciousness, including confusion, hallucinations, stupor, and coma; myoclonus, seizures).
- Advise patient that diarrhea, including frequent watery or bloody diarrhea, may occur even months after antibacterial treatment ends and to consult health care provider for evaluation.
- Teach patient to report signs and symptoms of hypersensitivity reactions.
- Inform patient that blood tests to assess renal function will be needed during treatment.
- Counsel patient, family, or caregivers that antibacterial drugs should be used to treat bacterial infections only and aren't effective in treating viral infections (such as the common cold).
- Advise patient that it's common to feel better early in the course of therapy but to take the full course of the drug as prescribed. Skipping doses or not completing the full course of therapy may decrease the effectiveness of treatment and increase the likelihood that bacteria will develop resistance and won't be treatable in the future.
- Instruct female patient to inform prescriber if she is pregnant, plans to become pregnant, or is breast-feeding.

ceftolozane–tazobactam
sef-TOL-oh-zane/TAZ-oh-BAK-tam

Zerbaxa

Therapeutic class: Antibiotics
Pharmacologic class: Cephalosporins–beta-lactamase inhibitors

AVAILABLE FORMS
Powder for injection: 1 g ceftolozane and 0.5 g tazobactam

INDICATIONS & DOSAGES

ℹ️ *Alert:* Dosage recommendations are expressed as total grams of the ceftazidime–avibactam combination.

Adjust-a-dose (for all indications): If CrCl is 30 to 50 mL/minute, give 750 mg (500 mg ceftolozane and 250 mg tazobactam) I.V. every 8 hours; if CrCl is 15 to 29 mL/minute, give 375 mg (250 mg ceftolozane and 125 mg tazobactam) I.V. every 8 hours; if on hemodialysis or with ESRD, give single loading dose of 750 mg (500 mg ceftolozane and 250 mg tazobactam) I.V. followed by maintenance dose of 150 mg (100 mg ceftolozane and 50 mg tazobactam) I.V. every 8 hours for remainder of treatment period. On hemodialysis days, give maintenance dose immediately after completion of dialysis. For patients with changing renal function, monitor CrCl at least daily and adjust dosage accordingly.

➤ **Complicated intra-abdominal infections caused by** *Enterobacter cloacae, Escherichia coli, Klebsiella oxytoca, Klebsiella pneumoniae, Proteus mirabilis, Pseudomonas aeruginosa, Bacteroides fragilis, Streptococcus anginosus, Streptococcus constellatus,* **and** *Streptococcus salivarius*
Adults: 1.5 g (1 g ceftolozane and 0.5 g tazobactam) I.V. every 8 hours for 4 to 14 days based on infection severity and clinical response. Give with metronidazole 500 mg I.V. every 8 hours.

➤ **Complicated UTIs, including pyelonephritis, caused by** *E. coli, K. pneumoniae, P. mirabilis,* **and** *P. aeruginosa*
Adults: 1.5 g (1 g ceftolozane and 0.5 g tazobactam) I.V. every 8 hours for 7 days.

ADMINISTRATION
I.V.
▼ Reconstitute vial with 10 mL sterile water for injection or NSS; gently shake to dissolve. The final volume is approximately 11.4 mL and must be added to a larger volume for infusion.
▼ To prepare required dose, withdraw appropriate volume from vial: for 1.5-g dose (1 g ceftolozane and 0.5 g tazobactam), withdraw entire contents of vial; for 750-mg dose (500 mg ceftolozane and 250 mg tazobactam), withdraw 5.7 mL;

for 375-mg dose (250 mg ceftolozane and 125 mg tazobactam), withdraw 2.9 mL; for 150-mg dose (100 mg ceftolozane and 50 mg tazobactam), withdraw 1.2 mL. Add withdrawn volume to infusion bag containing 100 mL NSS or D_5W.

▼ Administer by infusion over 60 minutes.

▼ Once reconstituted, vials are stable for 1 hour; once placed in infusion bag, drug is stable for 24 hours at room temperature or 7 days under refrigeration. Don't freeze vials or infusion bags that contain drug.

▼ Infusions range from clear, colorless solutions to solutions that are clear and slightly yellow. Variations in color within this range don't affect product's potency.

▼ Vial doesn't contain a bacteriostatic preservative.

▼ **Incompatibilities:** Don't mix with other drugs or solutions except D_5W or NSS.

ACTION

Ceftolozane inhibits cell-wall synthesis by binding to penicillin-binding proteins. Tazobactam is an irreversible inhibitor of some beta-lactamases.

Route	Onset	Peak	Duration
I.V.	Unknown	1 hr	Unknown

Half-life: Ceftolozane, 3 hours; tazobactam, 1 hour.

ADVERSE REACTIONS

CNS: headache, insomnia, anxiety, dizziness, fever.
CV: hypotension, atrial fibrillation.
GI: nausea, diarrhea, CDAD, constipation, vomiting, abdominal pain.
GU: renal impairment, including *renal failure.*
Hematologic: anemia, *thrombocytosis.*
Hepatic: increased AST and ALT levels.
Metabolic: *hypokalemia.*
Skin: rash.
Other: *hypersensitivity reaction.*

INTERACTIONS

Drug-drug. *Probenecid:* May increase ceftolozane–tazobactam serum concentration. Monitor therapy.
Vitamin K antagonists (warfarin): May enhance anticoagulant effects. Monitor PT and INR.

EFFECTS ON LAB TEST RESULTS

● May increase ALT and AST levels. May decrease potassium level.
● May increase platelet count. May decrease Hb level, hematocrit, and RBC count.

CONTRAINDICATIONS & CAUTIONS

● Contraindicated in patients with serious hypersensitivity to ceftolozane–tazobactam, piperacillin–tazobactam, or other members of the beta-lactam class.
● Use cautiously in patients hypersensitive to cephalosporins or tazobactam.
● Don't use unless proven or strongly suspected bacterial infection exists.
● May cause fungal or bacterial superinfection, including CDAD and pseudomembranous colitis. Stop drug and take appropriate measures if diarrhea develops. CDAD has occurred more than 2 months after antibacterial treatment.
● Safety and effectiveness in children haven't been established.
● Use cautiously in elderly patients. Risk of adverse effects may be increased.
Dialyzable drug: Ceftolozane, 66%; tazobactam, 56%.

PREGNANCY-LACTATION-REPRODUCTION

● Use in pregnant women hasn't been studied. Use cautiously and only if benefits outweigh potential risk to the fetus.
● It isn't known if drug appears in breast milk. Use cautiously in breast-feeding women.

NURSING CONSIDERATIONS

● Ensure a suspected or confirmed serious bacterial infection exists before giving drug.
● Obtain daily renal function tests, because drug's efficacy decreases in patients with baseline CrCl of 30 to 50 mL/minute. Adjust dosage as necessary based on CrCl.
● Before beginning treatment, obtain patient's history of allergy or hypersensitivity reactions to assess for cephalosporin or penicillin hypersensitivity.
● Monitor patient for signs and symptoms of hypersensitivity; institute appropriate therapy if needed.
● Monitor patient for development of superinfection, including diarrhea.
● *Look alike–sound alike:* Don't confuse Zerbaxa with Pradaxa.

PATIENT TEACHING
• Explain to patient that drug is used for presumed or actual serious bacterial infections.
• Teach patient that drug is given intravenously and to immediately report signs or symptoms of allergic reactions (wheezing, chest tightness, itching, or swelling of the face, lips, tongue, or throat).
• Advise patient not to skip doses, as this may decrease effectiveness of treatment.
• Counsel patient to report GI adverse effects such as diarrhea; GI effects commonly occur and may be serious. Tell patient to contact prescriber immediately if severe watery or bloody diarrhea occurs.
• Warn female patient to alert prescriber if she is pregnant or breast-feeding.

ceftriaxone sodium
sef-try-AX-ohn

Rocephin

Therapeutic class: Antibiotics
Pharmacologic class: Third-generation cephalosporins

AVAILABLE FORMS
Infusion: 1 g, 2 g, 1 g/50 mL, 2 g/50 mL premixed
Injection: 250 mg, 500 mg, 1 g, 2 g

INDICATIONS & DOSAGES
Adjust-a-dose (for all indications): In patients with significant renal disease and hepatic dysfunction, maximum dose is 2 g/day. In patients receiving intermittent hemodialysis, give 1 to 2 g I.V. every 24 hours after dialysis session. This recommendation assumes patient is receiving standard intermittent hemodialysis three times a week and completes the full dialysis sessions.
➤ **Uncomplicated gonococcal vulvo-vaginitis**
Adults: 250 mg I.M. as a single dose, plus azithromycin 1 g P.O. as a single dose or doxycycline 100 mg P.O. b.i.d. for 7 days.
➤ **UTI; lower respiratory tract, gynecologic, bone or joint, intra-abdominal, skin, or skin-structure infection; septicemia**
Adults and children older than age 12: 1 to 2 g I.M. or I.V. daily or in equally divided doses every 12 hours. Total daily dose shouldn't exceed 4 g. Treat for 4 to 14 days. Complicated infections may require longer treatment.
Children age 12 and younger: 50 to 75 mg/kg I.M. or I.V., not to exceed 2 g/day, given in divided doses every 12 hours or given once daily.
➤ **Meningitis**
Adults: 1 to 2 g I.M. or I.V. once daily or in two equally divided doses daily for 4 to 14 days.
Children: Initially, 100 mg/kg I.M. or I.V.; then 100 mg/kg/day as a single dose or in divided doses every 12 hours for 7 to 14 days. Maximum dose is 4 g/day.
➤ **Perioperative prophylaxis**
Adults: 1 g I.V. as a single dose 30 minutes to 2 hours before surgery.
➤ **Acute bacterial otitis media**
Adults: 1 to 2 g I.M. or I.V. once daily or in two equally divided doses daily for 4 to 14 days.
Children: 50 mg/kg I.M. as a single dose. Don't exceed 1 g.
➤ **Acute otitis media ♦**
Children: 50 mg/kg/day I.V. or I.M. for 1 to 3 consecutive days in patients unresponsive to initial antibiotic therapy and in penicillin-allergic patients.

ADMINISTRATION
I.V.
▼ Before giving drug, ensure patient isn't allergic to penicillins or cephalosporins.
▼ Obtain specimen for culture and sensitivity tests before giving first dose. Begin therapy while awaiting results.
▼ Reconstitute drug with sterile water for injection, NSS for injection, D_5W, or a combination of NSS and dextrose injection and other compatible solutions.
▼ Add 2.4 mL of diluent to the 250-mg vial, 4.8 mL to the 500-mg vial, 9.6 mL to the 1-g vial, and 19.2 mL to the 2-g vial. All reconstituted solutions average 100 mg/mL. For intermittent infusion, dilute further to achieve desired concentration, and give over 30 minutes.
▼ Diluted I.V. preparation is stable for 48 hours at room temperature or 10 days if refrigerated.

❸ Alert: Don't mix or administer ceftriaxone with calcium-containing I.V. solutions, including parenteral nutrition. This includes the use of different infusion lines at different sites. Don't administer within 48 hours of each other in any patient.

▼ **Incompatibilities:** Aminoglycosides, aminophylline, amphotericin B cholesteryl sulfate complex, azithromycin, calcium, clindamycin phosphate, filgrastim, fluconazole, gentamicin, labetalol, linezolid, metronidazole, pentamidine isethionate, theophylline, vancomycin, vinorelbine tartrate.

I.M.
● Before giving drug, ensure patient isn't allergic to penicillins or cephalosporins.
● Obtain specimen for culture and sensitivity tests before giving first dose. Begin therapy while awaiting results.
● Inject deep into a large muscle, such as the gluteus maximus or the lateral aspect of the thigh.

ACTION
Inhibits cell-wall synthesis, promoting osmotic instability; usually bactericidal.

Route	Onset	Peak	Duration
I.V.	Immediate	Immediate	Unknown
I.M.	Unknown	2–3 hr	Unknown

Half-life: Adults with normal renal and hepatic function, 5 to 9 hours.

ADVERSE REACTIONS
GI: *pseudomembranous colitis,* diarrhea.
Hematologic: eosinophilia, thrombocytosis, *leukopenia.*
Skin: pain, induration, tenderness at injection site, rash.
Other: hypersensitivity reactions, serum sickness, *anaphylaxis.*

INTERACTIONS
Drug-drug. *Aminoglycosides:* May increase nephrotoxicity and cause synergistic effect against some strains of *Pseudomonas aeruginosa* and *Enterobacteriaceae* species. Monitor patient.
Live-virus vaccines: May decrease effectiveness of live-virus vaccines. Concurrent use isn't recommended.

Probenecid: High doses (1 or 2 g daily) may enhance hepatic clearance of ceftriaxone and shorten its half-life. Avoid using together.
Warfarin: May increase anticoagulation effect. Monitor PT and INR closely.

EFFECTS ON LAB TEST RESULTS
● May increase alkaline phosphatase, ALT, AST, bilirubin, BUN, and LDH levels.
● May increase eosinophil and platelet counts. May decrease WBC count.
● May prolong PTT and PT, and increase INR.
● May falsely increase serum or urine creatinine level in tests using Jaffe reaction. May cause false-positive results of Coombs test and urine glucose tests that use cupric sulfate, such as Benedict reagent and Clinitest.

CONTRAINDICATIONS & CAUTIONS
● Contraindicated in patients hypersensitive to drug or other cephalosporins.
● Use cautiously in patients hypersensitive to penicillin because of possibility of cross-sensitivity with other beta-lactam antibiotics.
❸ Alert: May cause superinfection and mild to fatal CDAD. If suspected, manage appropriately; discontinue drug if needed.
❸ Alert: May cause hemolytic anemia, which can be fatal. If anemia develops during therapy, stop drug until cause is determined.
● Use cautiously in patients with history of colitis, renal insufficiency, or GI or gallbladder disease.
Dialyzable drug: No.

PREGNANCY-LACTATION-REPRODUCTION
● There are no adequate studies in pregnant women. Use during pregnancy only if clearly needed and potential benefit justifies potential risk to the fetus.
● Drug appears in breast milk in low concentrations. Use cautiously in breast-feeding women.

NURSING CONSIDERATIONS
● If large doses are given, therapy is prolonged, or patient is at high risk, monitor patient for signs and symptoms of superinfection.

Reactions in bold italics are *life-threatening*. Interactions may have a *rapid onset* or a *delayed onset*.

C

• Monitor PT and INR in patients with impaired vitamin K synthesis or low vitamin K stores. Vitamin K therapy may be needed.
• Drug is commonly used in home antibiotic programs for outpatient treatment of serious infections, such as osteomyelitis and community-acquired pneumonia.
• Monitor patients for superinfection, diarrhea, and anemia and treat appropriately.
• *Look alike–sound alike:* Don't confuse drug with other cephalosporins that sound alike.

PATIENT TEACHING
• Tell patient to report adverse reactions promptly.
• Instruct patient to report discomfort at I.V. insertion site.
• Teach patient and family receiving home care how to prepare and give drug.
• If home care patient is diabetic and is testing his urine for glucose, tell him drug may affect results of cupric sulfate tests; he should use an enzymatic test instead.
• Tell patient to notify prescriber about loose stools or diarrhea.

---

cefuroxime axetil
se-fyoor-OX-eem

Ceftin

cefuroxime sodium
Zinacef

Therapeutic class: Antibiotics
Pharmacologic class: Second-generation cephalosporins

AVAILABLE FORMS
cefuroxime axetil
Suspension: 125 mg/5 mL, 250 mg/5 mL
Tablets: 125 mg, 250 mg, 500 mg
cefuroxime sodium
Infusion: 750-mg, 1.5-g vials, infusion packs, and ADD-Vantage vials
Injection: 750 mg, 1.5 g

INDICATIONS & DOSAGES
Adjust-a-dose (for all indications): For injectable form in adults with CrCl of 10 to 20 mL/minute, give 750 mg I.V. or I.M. every 12 hours; if CrCl is less than 10 mL/minute, give 750 mg I.V. or I.M.

every 24 hours. Give patients on hemodialysis an additional dose after hemodialysis.
➤ **Serious lower respiratory tract infection, UTI, skin or skin-structure infections, bone or joint infection, septicemia, meningitis, and gonorrhea**
Adults and children age 13 and older:
750 mg to 1.5 g cefuroxime sodium I.V. or I.M. every 8 hours for 5 to 10 days. For life-threatening infections and infections caused by less susceptible organisms, 1.5 g I.V. or I.M. every 6 hours; for bacterial meningitis, up to 3 g I.V. every 8 hours.
Children ages 3 months to 12 years: 50 to 100 mg/kg/day cefuroxime sodium I.V. or I.M. in equally divided doses every 6 or 8 hours. Use higher dosage of 100 mg/kg/day, not to exceed maximum adult dosage, for more severe or serious infections. For bacterial meningitis, 200 to 240 mg/kg/day cefuroxime sodium I.V. in divided doses every 6 to 8 hours.
➤ **Perioperative prophylaxis**
Adults: 1.5 g I.V. 30 to 60 minutes before surgery; in lengthy operations, 750 mg I.V. or I.M. every 8 hours. For open-heart surgery, 1.5 g I.V. at induction of anesthesia and then every 12 hours for a total dose of 6 g.
➤ **Bacterial exacerbations of chronic bronchitis or secondary bacterial infection of acute bronchitis**
Adults and children age 13 and older:
250 or 500 mg P.O. b.i.d. for 10 days (chronic bronchitis) or 5 to 10 days (acute bronchitis).
➤ **Acute bacterial maxillary sinusitis**
Adults and children age 13 and older:
250 mg P.O. b.i.d. for 10 days.
Children ages 3 months to 12 years:
250 mg b.i.d. for 10 days. For children who can't swallow tablets whole, 30 mg/kg/day oral suspension in two divided doses for 10 days. Maximum daily dose for suspension is 1,000 mg.
➤ **Pharyngitis and tonsillitis**
Adults and children age 13 and older:
250 mg P.O. b.i.d. for 10 days.
Children ages 3 months to 12 years:
125 mg P.O. b.i.d. for 10 days. For children who can't swallow tablets whole, give 20 mg/kg daily of oral suspension in two divided doses for 10 days. Maximum daily dose for suspension is 500 mg.

➤ **Otitis media**
Children ages 3 months to 12 years:
250 mg P.O. b.i.d. for 10 days. For children who can't swallow tablets whole, give 30 mg/kg/day of oral suspension in two divided doses for 10 days. Maximum daily dose for suspension is 1,000 mg.

➤ **Uncomplicated skin and skin-structure infection**
Adults and children age 13 and older:
250 or 500 mg P.O. b.i.d. for 10 days.

➤ **Uncomplicated UTI**
Adults: 250 mg P.O. b.i.d. for 7 to 10 days.

➤ **Uncomplicated gonorrhea**
Adults: 1,000 mg P.O. as a single dose. Or, 1.5 g I.M. with 1 g probenecid P.O. for one dose.

➤ **Early Lyme disease**
Adults and children age 13 and older:
500 mg P.O. b.i.d. for 20 days.

➤ **Impetigo**
Children ages 3 months to 12 years:
30 mg/kg/day of oral suspension in two divided doses for 10 days. Maximum daily dose, 1,000 mg.

ADMINISTRATION
P.O.
• Before giving drug, ensure patient isn't allergic to penicillins or cephalosporins.
• Tablets and oral suspension aren't bioequivalent and aren't substitutable on a milligram-per-milligram basis.
• Obtain specimen for culture and sensitivity tests before giving first dose. Therapy may begin while awaiting results.
• Shake suspension well before each use.
• Give tablets without regard for meals; give oral suspension with food.
• Crush tablets, if absolutely necessary, for patients who can't swallow tablets. Tablets may be dissolved in small amounts of apple, orange, or grape juice or chocolate milk. However, the drug has a bitter taste that is difficult to mask, even with food.
• Store suspension at room temperature before reconstitution or under refrigeration after reconstitution. Discard reconstituted suspension after 10 days.

I.V.
▼ Before giving drug, ensure patient isn't allergic to penicillins or cephalosporins.

▼ Obtain specimen for culture and sensitivity tests before giving first dose. Therapy may begin while awaiting results.
▼ Reconstitute each 750-mg vial with 8 mL and each 1.5-g vial with 16 mL of sterile water for injection.
▼ Withdraw entire contents of vial for a dose.
▼ For direct injection, inject over 3 to 5 minutes into a large vein or into the tubing of a free-flowing I.V. solution.
▼ For intermittent infusion, add reconstituted drug to 100 mL D_5W, NSS for injection, or other compatible I.V. solution.
▼ Infuse over 15 to 60 minutes.
▼ **Incompatibilities:** Aminoglycosides, azithromycin, ciprofloxacin, cisatracurium, clarithromycin, cyclophosphamide, doxapram, filgrastim, fluconazole, gentamicin, midazolam, ranitidine, sodium bicarbonate injection, vancomycin, vinorelbine tartrate.

I.M.
• Before giving drug, ensure patient isn't allergic to penicillins or cephalosporins.
• Obtain specimen for culture and sensitivity tests before giving first dose. Therapy may begin while awaiting results.
• Reconstitute 750-mg vial with 3 mL sterile water for injection.
• Inject deep into a large muscle, such as the gluteus maximus or the side of the thigh.

ACTION
Inhibits cell-wall synthesis, promoting osmotic instability; usually bactericidal.

Route	Onset	Peak	Duration
P.O.	Unknown	2–4 hr	Unknown
I.V.	Immediate	2–3 min	Unknown
I.M.	Unknown	15–60 min	Unknown

Half-life: 1 to 2 hours.

ADVERSE REACTIONS
CV: phlebitis, thrombophlebitis.
GI: diarrhea, *pseudomembranous colitis,* nausea, anorexia, vomiting.
Hematologic: hemolytic anemia, *thrombocytopenia, transient neutropenia,* eosinophilia.
Skin: maculopapular and erythematous rashes, urticaria, pain, induration, sterile abscesses, temperature elevation, tissue sloughing at I.M. injection site.

Other: *anaphylaxis,* hypersensitivity reactions, serum sickness.

INTERACTIONS

Drug-drug. *Aminoglycosides:* May cause synergistic activity against some organisms; may increase nephrotoxicity. Monitor patient's renal function closely.
Live-virus vaccines: May decrease effectiveness of live-virus vaccines. Concurrent use isn't recommended.
Loop diuretics: May increase risk of adverse renal reactions. Monitor renal function test results closely.
Probenecid: May inhibit excretion and increase cefuroxime level. Probenecid may be used for this effect.
Warfarin: May increase anticoagulation effects. Monitor PT and INR closely.

EFFECTS ON LAB TEST RESULTS

● May increase alkaline phosphatase, ALT, AST, bilirubin, and LDH levels. May decrease Hb level and hematocrit.
● May prolong PT and may increase INR and eosinophil count. May decrease neutrophil and platelet counts.
● May falsely increase serum or urine creatinine level in tests using Jaffe reaction. May cause false-positive results of Coombs test and urine glucose tests that use cupric sulfate, such as Benedict reagent and Clinitest.

CONTRAINDICATIONS & CAUTIONS

● Contraindicated in patients hypersensitive to drug or other cephalosporins.
● Use cautiously in patients hypersensitive to penicillin because of possibility of cross-sensitivity with other beta-lactam antibiotics.
● According to the CDC, oral cephalosporins aren't recommended to treat gonococcal infections.
● According to clinical practice guidelines, cefotaxime or ceftriaxone should be used to treat childhood bacterial meningitis and pneumococcal and meningococcal meningitis caused by penicillin-resistant strains and *Haemophilus influenzae* type b meningitis.
● Use cautiously in patients with history of colitis and in those with renal insufficiency.

● **Alert:** Drug may cause pseudomembranous colitis ranging from mild to life-threatening, which can occur even 2 months after therapy. Monitor patient for diarrhea and treat appropriately.
● Some cephalosporins have been associated with seizures in patients with renal impairment when the dosage wasn't reduced. If drug-associated seizures occur, discontinue drug and treat with anticonvulsant therapy if indicated.
Dialyzable drug: Yes.

PREGNANCY-LACTATION-REPRODUCTION

● There are no adequate studies in pregnant women. Use during pregnancy only if clearly needed and potential benefit justifies potential risk to the fetus.
● Drug appears in breast milk. Patient should consider temporarily discontinuing breast-feeding during treatment.

NURSING CONSIDERATIONS

● Monitor patient for signs and symptoms of superinfection and diarrhea.
● Drug may increase INR and risk of bleeding. Monitor patient.
● **Look alike–sound alike:** Don't confuse drug with other cephalosporins that sound alike.

PATIENT TEACHING

● Tell patient to take drug as prescribed, even after he feels better.
● If patient has difficulty swallowing tablets, show him how to dissolve or crush tablets, but warn him that the bitter taste is hard to mask, even with food.
● Tell parent to shake suspension well before measuring dose. Suspension may be stored at room temperature or refrigerated, but must be discarded after 10 days.
● Instruct caregiver to give oral suspension with food.
● Instruct patient to notify prescriber about rash, loose stools, diarrhea, or evidence of superinfection.
● Advise patient receiving drug I.V. to report discomfort at I.V. insertion site.

celecoxib
sell-ah-COCKS-ib

Celebrex⬦

Therapeutic class: NSAIDs
Pharmacologic class: Cyclooxygenase-2 inhibitors

AVAILABLE FORMS
Capsules: 50 mg, 100 mg, 200 mg, 400 mg

INDICATIONS & DOSAGES
Adjust-a-dose (for all indications): For elderly patients and those weighing less than 50 kg, start at lowest dosage. For patients with Child-Pugh class B hepatic impairment, reduce dosage by about 50%. Don't use in patients with severe renal or severe hepatic impairment. For patients who are poor metabolizers of CYP2C9, start treatment at half the lowest recommended dose.

➤ **To relieve signs and symptoms of osteoarthritis**
Adults: 200 mg P.O. daily as a single dose or in two equally divided doses.

➤ **To relieve signs and symptoms of RA**
Adults: 100 to 200 mg P.O. b.i.d.

➤ **To relieve signs and symptoms of ankylosing spondylitis**
Adults: 200 mg P.O. once daily or in two divided doses. If no response after 6 weeks, may increase dose to 400 mg daily. If no response after 6 more weeks, consider other treatment.

➤ **To relieve signs and symptoms of juvenile RA**
Children age 2 and older weighing 10 to 25 kg: 50 mg P.O. b.i.d.
Children age 2 and older weighing more than 25 kg: 100 mg P.O. b.i.d.

➤ **Acute pain and primary dysmenorrhea**
Adults: 400 mg P.O., initially, followed by another 200-mg dose if needed. On subsequent days, 200 mg P.O. b.i.d. as needed.

➤ **Acute gout ♦**
Adults: 800 mg P.O. once, followed by 400 mg P.O. on day 1; then 400 mg P.O. b.i.d. for 1 week.

ADMINISTRATION
P.O.
● May give dosages up to 200 mg b.i.d. without regard to food.
● For patients who have difficulty swallowing capsules, capsule contents can be added to applesauce. Carefully empty entire contents of capsule onto a level teaspoon of cool or room-temperature applesauce and give immediately with water.

ACTION
Thought to inhibit prostaglandin synthesis, impeding cyclooxygenase-2, to produce anti-inflammatory, analgesic, and antipyretic effects.

Route	Onset	Peak	Duration
P.O.	Unknown	3 hr	Unknown

Half-life: 11 hours.

ADVERSE REACTIONS
CNS: headache, dizziness, insomnia.
CV: hypertension, peripheral edema.
EENT: pharyngitis, rhinitis, sinusitis.
GI: abdominal pain, diarrhea, dyspepsia, flatulence, GI reflux, nausea.
Metabolic: hyperchloremia.
Musculoskeletal: back pain.
Respiratory: dyspnea, URI.
Skin: *erythema multiforme, exfoliative dermatitis, Stevens-Johnson syndrome, toxic epidermal necrolysis,* rash.
Other: accidental injury.

INTERACTIONS
Drug-drug. *ACE inhibitors, ARBs:* May decrease antihypertensive effects. Monitor BP.
Antacids containing aluminum or magnesium: May decrease celecoxib level. Separate doses.
Anticoagulants, antiplatelets (clopidogrel, prasugrel): May increase bleeding risk. Use cautiously.
Aspirin: May increase risk of ulcers; low aspirin dosages can be used safely to reduce the risk of CV events. Monitor patient for signs and symptoms of GI bleeding.
Corticosteroids, SSRIs: May increase risk of GI bleeding. Use together cautiously.
CYP2C9 inhibitors (amiodarone, metronidazole, ritonavir, zafirlukast): May affect

celecoxib metabolism. Use together cautiously.

Digoxin: May increase digoxin serum concentration. Monitor concurrent therapy.

Fluconazole, voriconazole: May increase celecoxib level. Reduce dosage of celecoxib to minimal effective dose.

Furosemide, thiazides: May reduce sodium excretion caused by diuretics, leading to sodium retention. Monitor patient for swelling and increased BP.

Lithium: May increase lithium level. Monitor lithium level closely during treatment.

Warfarin: May prolong PT and cause bleeding complications. Monitor PT and INR, and check for signs and symptoms of bleeding.

Drug-herb. *Dong quai, feverfew, garlic, ginger, horse chestnut, red clover:* May increase risk of bleeding. Discourage use together.

White willow: Herb and drug contain similar components. Discourage use together.

Drug-lifestyle. *Long-term alcohol use, smoking:* May cause GI irritation or bleeding. Check for signs and symptoms of bleeding.

EFFECTS ON LAB TEST RESULTS

• May increase ALT, AST, BUN, creatinine, and chloride levels.

• May decrease phosphate level.

CONTRAINDICATIONS & CAUTIONS

Black Box Warning Contraindicated for the treatment of perioperative pain after CABG. ■

• Contraindicated in patients hypersensitive to drug, sulfonamides, aspirin, or other NSAIDs.

• Contraindicated in patients who experienced asthma, urticaria, or allergic-type reactions after taking aspirin or other NSAIDs and in those who have demonstrated allergic-type reactions to sulfonamides.

• Drug isn't recommended with any dose of a nonaspirin NSAID.

❸ Alert: NSAIDs can increase the risk of heart attack or stroke in patients with or without heart disease or risk factors for heart disease.

❸ Alert: The risk of heart attack or stroke can occur as early as the first weeks of NSAID use. Risk appears greater at higher doses. Use lowest effective dose for shortest duration possible.

❸ Alert: NSAIDs increase the risk of HF.

• Use cautiously in patients with history of ulcers or GI bleeding, advanced renal disease, dehydration, anemia, symptomatic liver disease, hypertension, edema, HF, or asthma, and in poor CYP2C9 metabolizers.

• Consider alternative therapies for treatment of juvenile RA in patients identified to be poor CYP2C9 metabolizers.

• Use cautiously in elderly or debilitated patients.

Dialyzable drug: Unlikely.

⚠ Overdose S&S: Lethargy, drowsiness, nausea, vomiting, epigastric pain, GI bleeding, hypertension, acute renal failure, respiratory depression, coma, anaphylaxis.

PREGNANCY-LACTATION-REPRODUCTION

• There are no adequate studies in pregnant women. Use during pregnancy isn't recommended because NSAID use close to conception may be associated with an increased risk of miscarriage, and use at 30 weeks' gestation and later may cause premature closure of the ductus arteriosus and other life-threatening fetal conditions.

• A registry is available for pregnant women exposed to autoimmune medications, including celecoxib. Contact the Organization of Teratology Information Specialists Autoimmune Diseases in Pregnancy Study at 1-877-311-8972.

• Drug appears in breast milk. Use cautiously in breast-feeding women. Patient should consider temporarily discontinuing breast-feeding during treatment.

• Long-term use of NSAIDs in women of reproductive age may be associated with infertility that's reversible upon discontinuation of NSAID.

NURSING CONSIDERATIONS

❸ Alert: Patients allergic to or with a history of anaphylactic reactions to sulfonamides, aspirin, or other NSAIDs may be allergic to this drug.

Black Box Warning NSAIDs cause an increased risk of serious GI adverse events, including bleeding, ulceration, and perforation of the stomach or intestines, which can be fatal. Elderly patients are at greater risk. ■

• Patient with history of ulcers or GI bleeding is at higher risk for GI bleeding while taking NSAIDs such as celecoxib. Other risk factors for GI bleeding include treatment with corticosteroids or anticoagulants, longer duration of NSAID treatment, smoking, alcoholism, older age, and poor overall health.

• Although drug may be used with low aspirin dosages, the combination may increase risk of GI bleeding.

• Watch for signs and symptoms of overt and occult bleeding.

Black Box Warning NSAIDs may increase the risk of serious thrombotic events, MI, or stroke. The risk may be greater with longer use or in patients with CV disease or risk factors for CV disease. ■

◑ Alert: Watch for and immediately evaluate signs and symptoms of heart attack (chest pain, shortness of breath, trouble breathing) or stroke (weakness in one part or side of the body, slurred speech).

• Drug can cause fluid retention; monitor patient with hypertension, edema, or HF.

• Assess patient for CV risk factors before therapy.

• Drug may be hepatotoxic; watch for signs and symptoms of liver toxicity.

• Before starting drug therapy, rehydrate dehydrated patient.

• Monitor patient's renal function; renal insufficiency is possible in patients with preexisting renal disease. Long-term administration may cause renal papillary necrosis and other renal injury.

• **Look alike–sound alike:** Don't confuse Celebrex with Cerebyx or Celexa.

PATIENT TEACHING

• Tell patient to report history of allergic reactions to sulfonamides, aspirin, or other NSAIDs before therapy.

• Instruct patient to promptly report signs of GI bleeding, such as blood in vomit, urine, or stool; or black, tarry stools.

◑ Alert: Advise patient to immediately report rash, unexplained weight gain, or swelling.

◑ Alert: Advise patient to seek medical attention immediately if chest pain, shortness of breath or trouble breathing, weakness in one part or side of the body, or slurred speech occurs.

• Tell woman to notify prescriber if she becomes pregnant or is planning to become pregnant during drug therapy.

• Instruct patient to take drug with food if stomach upset occurs.

• Tell patient who has trouble swallowing capsule whole that contents of capsule may be taken with applesauce.

• Tell patient that drug may harm the liver. Advise patient to stop therapy and notify prescriber immediately if he experiences signs and symptoms of hepatotoxicity, including nausea, fatigue, lethargy, itching, yellowing of skin or eyes, right upper quadrant tenderness, and flulike syndrome.

• Inform patient that it may take several days before he feels consistent pain relief.

• Advise patient that using OTC NSAIDs with celecoxib may increase the risk of GI toxicity.

cephalexin
sef-a-LEX-in

Apo-Cephalex✣, Keflex

Therapeutic class: Antibiotics
Pharmacologic class: First-generation cephalosporins

AVAILABLE FORMS
Capsules: 250 mg, 500 mg, 750 mg
Oral suspension: 125 mg/5 mL, 250 mg/5 mL
Tablets: 250 mg, 500 mg

INDICATIONS & DOSAGES
Adjust-a-dose (for all indications): Dosage adjustments may be required for patients with impaired renal function. For CrCl of 30 to 59 mL/minute, no dosage adjustment is needed but maximum daily dose shouldn't exceed 1 g; for CrCl of 15 to 29 mL/minute, reduce dose to 250 mg every 8 or 12 hours; for CrCl of 5 to 14 mL/minute in patients not yet on dialysis, reduce dose to 250 mg every 24 hours; and for CrCl of 1 to

4 mL/minute in patients not yet on dialysis, reduce dose to 250 mg every 48 or 60 hours.

➤ Respiratory tract infections caused by susceptible isolates of *Streptococcus pneumoniae* and *Streptococcus pyogenes;* GU tract infections caused by susceptible isolates of *Escherichia coli, Proteus mirabilis,* and *Klebsiella pneumoniae;* skin and skin-structure infections caused by susceptible isolates of *Staphylococcus aureus* or *S. pyogenes;* bone infections caused by susceptible isolates of *S. aureus* and *P. mirabilis;* and otitis media caused by susceptible isolates of *S. pneumoniae, Haemophilus influenzae, S. aureus, S. pyogenes,* and *Moraxella catarrhalis*

Adults and children age 15 and older: 250 mg to 1 g P.O. every 6 hours or 500 mg every 12 hours for 7 to 14 days. Maximum, 4 g daily.

Children older than age 1: 25 to 50 mg/kg/day P.O. in two to four equally divided doses for 7 to 14 days. For otitis media, 75 to 100 mg/kg P.O. in equally divided doses every 6 hours. For severe infections, 50 to 100 mg/kg P.O. in equally divided doses. Don't exceed recommended adult dosage.

ADMINISTRATION
P.O.
● Before giving, ensure patient isn't allergic to penicillins or cephalosporins.
● Obtain specimen for culture and sensitivity tests before giving. Begin therapy while awaiting results.
● To prepare oral suspension, add required amount of water to powder in two portions. Shake well after each addition. After mixing, store in refrigerator. Mixture will remain stable for 14 days. Keep tightly closed and shake well before using.
● May give without regard to meals but give drug with food or milk to lessen GI discomfort.

ACTION
Inhibits cell-wall synthesis, promoting osmotic instability; usually bactericidal.

Route	Onset	Peak	Duration
P.O.	Unknown	1 hr	Unknown

Half-life: Adults, 30 minutes to 1¼ hours; children ages 3 to 12 months, 2½ hours; neonates, 5 hours.

ADVERSE REACTIONS
CNS: dizziness, headache, fatigue, agitation, confusion, hallucinations.
GI: anorexia, diarrhea, *pseudomembranous colitis,* gastritis, glossitis, dyspepsia, abdominal pain, anal pruritus, tenesmus, oral candidiasis.
GU: genital pruritus, candidiasis, vaginitis, interstitial nephritis.
Hematologic: *neutropenia, thrombocytopenia,* eosinophilia, anemia.
Musculoskeletal: arthritis, arthralgia, joint pain.
Skin: maculopapular and erythematous rashes, urticaria.
Other: *anaphylaxis,* hypersensitivity reactions, serum sickness.

INTERACTIONS
Drug-drug. *Aminoglycosides:* May increase risk of nephrotoxicity. Avoid using together.
Live-virus vaccines: May decrease effectiveness of live-virus vaccines. Concurrent use isn't recommended.
Metformin: May increase metformin level. Monitor blood glucose level closely.
Multivitamins containing zinc, zinc: May decrease cephalexin absorption. Consider administering at least 3 hours after cephalexin. Consider therapy modification when used with zinc chloride.
Probenecid: May increase cephalosporin level. Use together isn't recommended.

EFFECTS ON LAB TEST RESULTS
● May increase alkaline phosphatase, ALT, AST, bilirubin, and LDH levels. May decrease Hb level and prolong PT.
● May increase eosinophil count. May decrease neutrophil and platelet counts.
● May falsely increase serum or urine creatinine level in tests using Jaffe reaction. May cause false-positive results of Coombs test and urine glucose tests that use cupric sulfate, such as Benedict reagent and Clinitest.

CONTRAINDICATIONS & CAUTIONS
● Contraindicated in patients hypersensitive to cephalosporins.
● Use cautiously in patients hypersensitive to penicillin because of possibility of cross-sensitivity with other beta-lactam antibiotics.

• Severe hypersensitivity reactions can occur. If an allergic reaction occurs, discontinue drug immediately and treat appropriately.

• Drug may increase risk of seizures. Use cautiously in patients with history of seizures.

• Use cautiously in patients with history of colitis and in those with renal insufficiency.

🕦 **Alert:** Drug can cause superinfection and CDAD and pseudomembranous colitis ranging from mild to life-threatening, which can occur even 2 months after therapy. Monitor patient for diarrhea and treat appropriately. *Dialyzable drug:* Unknown.

⚠ **Overdose S&S:** Nausea, vomiting, epigastric distress, diarrhea, hematuria.

PREGNANCY-LACTATION-REPRODUCTION

• There are no adequate studies in pregnant women. Use during pregnancy only if clearly needed and potential benefit justifies potential risk to the fetus.

• Drug appears in breast milk. Use cautiously in breast-feeding women.

NURSING CONSIDERATIONS

• If large doses are given or if therapy is prolonged, monitor patient for superinfection, especially if patient is high risk.

• Treat group A beta-hemolytic streptococcal infections for a minimum of 10 days.

• *Look alike–sound alike:* Don't confuse Keflex with Keppra. Don't confuse drug with other cephalosporins that sound alike.

PATIENT TEACHING

• Tell patient to take drug exactly as prescribed, even if feeling better.

• Instruct patient to take drug with food or milk to lessen GI discomfort. If patient is taking suspension form, instruct him to shake container well before measuring dose and to store in refrigerator.

• Tell patient to report all adverse reactions and to immediately report rash and signs and symptoms of superinfection or diarrhea.

certolizumab pegol
SERT-oh-LIZ-u-mahb PEGH-ol

Cimzia

Therapeutic class: Immunomodulators
Pharmacologic class: TNF blockers

AVAILABLE FORMS
Lyophilized powder for injection: 200 mg
Prefilled syringe: 200 mg/mL

INDICATIONS & DOSAGES
➤ **Crohn disease when response to conventional therapy is inadequate**
Adults: Initially and at weeks 2 and 4, 400 mg subcutaneously (given as two injections of 200 mg each), followed by a maintenance dose of 400 mg every 4 weeks, if adequate response.
➤ **RA**
Adults: Initially and at weeks 2 and 4, 400 mg subcutaneously (given as two injections of 200 mg each), followed by maintenance dose of 200 mg every other week or 400 mg every 4 weeks.
➤ **Psoriatic arthritis; active ankylosing spondylitis**
Adults: 400 mg subcutaneously (given as two injections of 200 mg each) initially; repeat dose at week 2 and then again at week 4. Maintenance dosage is 200 mg every other week, or 400 mg every 4 weeks.

ADMINISTRATION
Subcutaneous

• Bring drug to room temperature before reconstituting.

• Each 400-mg dose requires two vials. Reconstitute each vial with 1 mL of sterile water for injection, using a 20G needle. Gently swirl the vial without shaking. May take up to 30 minutes to fully reconstitute. Inspect vial for particulate matter and discoloration, and discard if present.

• Draw up each vial in its own syringe, switching each 20G needle to a 23G needle. Inject prepared or prefilled syringes into separate sites in the abdomen or thigh. Don't inject in areas where skin is tender, bruised, red, or hard. Discard unused portion of vial or syringe.

C

• Reconstituted drug is stable for 2 hours at room temperature or for up to 24 hours if refrigerated. Don't freeze.
• Give at room temperature.

ACTION
Selectively neutralizes TNFα, a proinflammatory cytokine responsible for stimulating the production of inflammatory mediators.

Route	Onset	Peak	Duration
Subcut.	Unknown	54–171 hr	Unknown

Half-life: 14 days.

ADVERSE REACTIONS
CNS: anxiety, bipolar disorder, *suicide attempt.*
CV: angina pectoris, *arrhythmias, HF,* hypertensive heart disease, *MI,* pericardial effusion and pericarditis, vasculitis.
EENT: optic neuritis, retinal hemorrhage, uveitis.
GI: abdominal pain.
GU: UTI.
Hematologic: anemia, *leukopenia,* lymphadenopathy, *pancytopenia,* thrombophilia.
Hepatic: elevated liver enzymes, *hepatitis.*
Musculoskeletal: arthralgia, extremity pain.
Respiratory: URI, TB.
Skin: alopecia, dermatitis, peripheral edema, erythema nodosum, urticaria, injection-site pain and erythema, *Stevens-Johnson syndrome, toxic epidermal necrolysis, erythema multiforme.*
Other: *anaphylaxis, opportunistic infection.*

INTERACTIONS
Drug-drug. *Abatacept, anakinra, canakinumab, natalizumab, rituximab:* May increase risk of serious infection and neutropenia. Avoid using together.
Live-virus vaccines: May cause infection. Avoid using together.
Drug-herb. *Echinacea:* May diminish therapeutic effects. Consider therapy modification.

EFFECTS ON LAB TEST RESULTS
• May falsely prolong PTT.

CONTRAINDICATIONS & CAUTIONS
• Use cautiously in patients hypersensitive to drug or its components; anaphylaxis or serious allergic reactions may occur.
• Use cautiously in patients with known hypersensitivity to other TNF blockers and those with underlying conditions that may increase the risk of infections.
• Use cautiously in patients with underlying hematologic disorders because significant hematologic abnormalities have occurred.
• Don't use in combination with biological DMARDs or other TNF-blocker therapy.
Black Box Warning Patients treated with certolizumab are at increased risk for serious infections that may lead to hospitalization or death. Most patients who developed these infections were taking concomitant immunosuppressants, such as methotrexate or corticosteroids. ∎
Black Box Warning Prophylactic antifungal therapy should be considered for patients at risk for invasive fungal infections who develop severe systemic illness. ∎
• Use cautiously in patients with a history of recurrent infections or concomitant immunosuppressive therapy and in those who have resided in regions where TB and histoplasmosis are endemic. Don't begin drug in patients with active infections.
• Use cautiously in patients with a history of CNS demyelinating disorder, hematologic disorders, or HF.
• Rare reactivation of HBV infection can occur, usually in chronic carriers who are also receiving immunosuppressants. Evaluate patient for HBV infection before initiating treatment. Monitor HBV carriers for clinical signs and symptoms of active infection and altered laboratory values during and for several months after therapy ends.
Black Box Warning Certolizumab isn't indicated for use in children or adolescents because of the risk of lymphoma and other malignancies reported with the use of TNF blockers. ∎
• Use cautiously in elderly patients because of increased risk of infection.
Dialyzable drug: Unknown.

PREGNANCY-LACTATION-REPRODUCTION
• Use during pregnancy only when clearly needed and benefits outweigh risks to the

---

fetus. Enroll women exposed to certolizumab pegol during pregnancy in the Mother-ToBaby Autoimmune Diseases Study by contacting the Organization of Teratology Information Specialists (1-877-311-8972).

• It isn't known if drug appears in breast milk. Patient should discontinue breast-feeding or discontinue drug, taking into account importance of drug to the mother.

NURSING CONSIDERATIONS

Black Box Warning Carefully consider risks and benefits of treatment before initiating therapy in patients with chronic or recurrent infection. ■

Black Box Warning Monitor patient for signs and symptoms of invasive fungal infection and other opportunistic infections during and after treatment. Discontinue treatment if serious infection or sepsis develops. Fatal infections have occurred. ■

Black Box Warning Invasive fungal infections, including histoplasmosis, coccidioidomycosis, candidiasis, aspergillosis, blastomycosis, and pneumocystis, may present with disseminated, rather than localized disease. Antigen and antibody testing for histoplasmosis may be negative in some patients with active infection. Consider empirical antifungal therapy in patients at risk for invasive fungal infections who develop severe systemic illness. ■

Black Box Warning Bacterial, viral, and other infections due to opportunistic pathogens, including *Legionella* and *Listeria*, have occurred. ■

• Before therapy, evaluate patient for TB risk factors and consider antituberculosis therapy in patients with history of latent or active TB when adequate treatment can't be confirmed.

Black Box Warning Test patient for latent TB before and during therapy; active TB, including reactivation of latent TB, has occurred. Initiate treatment for latent infection before starting therapy. ■

Black Box Warning Closely monitor patient for signs and symptoms of infection during and after treatment, including the possible development of TB in patients who tested negative for latent TB before starting therapy. ■

• Before therapy, evaluate patients at risk for HBV infection and test for previous HBV infection.

PATIENT TEACHING

Black Box Warning Teach patient to seek prompt medical attention if persistent fever, cough, shortness of breath, or fatigue develops. ■

• Advise patient to seek immediate medical attention for signs and symptoms of infection or for unusual bruising or bleeding.

• Instruct patient to seek immediate medical attention if any symptoms of severe allergic reaction develop.

• Tell patient to report signs and symptoms of HF.

• Show patient how to self-administer pre-filled syringes and how to properly dispose of needles and syringes.

SAFETY ALERT!

cetuximab
seh-TUX-eh-mab

Erbitux

Therapeutic class: Antineoplastics
Pharmacologic class: Monoclonal antibodies

AVAILABLE FORMS
Injection: 2 mg/mL

INDICATIONS & DOSAGES
Adjust-a-dose (for all indications): If patient develops a grade 1 or 2 CTCAE infusion reaction or a nonserious grade 3 CTCAE infusion reaction, permanently reduce infusion rate by 50%. If patient develops a serious infusion reaction requiring medical intervention or hospitalization, stop drug immediately and permanently. If patient develops a severe acneiform rash, follow these guidelines:

• After first occurrence, delay infusion 1 to 2 weeks. If patient improves, continue at 250 mg/m^2. If patient doesn't improve, stop drug.

• After second occurrence, delay infusion 1 to 2 weeks. If patient improves, reduce dose to 200 mg/m^2. If patient doesn't improve, stop drug.

• After third occurrence, delay infusion 1 to 2 weeks. If patient improves, reduce dose to 150 mg/m^2. If patient doesn't improve, stop drug.

• After fourth occurrence, stop drug.

➤ **Squamous cell carcinoma of the head and neck**

Adults: A loading dose of 400 mg/m^2 I.V. over 2 hours (maximum rate, 10 mg/minute) followed by weekly maintenance dose of 250 mg/m^2 I.V. over 1 hour. If used with radiation therapy, begin drug 1 week before radiation course or on day of initiation of platinum-based therapy with 5-FU. Complete administration 1 hour before radiation or platinum-based therapy with 5-FU. Continue for the duration (6 or 7 weeks) of radiation therapy or until disease progression or unacceptable toxicity occurs. If used as monotherapy for recurrent or metastatic disease after failure of platinum-based therapy, continue until disease progresses or unacceptable toxicity occurs.

➤ ***KRAS* mutation-negative (wild type), epidermal growth factor receptor–expressing, metastatic colorectal cancer as determined by FDA-approved tests in combination with FOLFIRI (irinotecan, 5-FU, leucovorin) chemotherapy regimen for first-line treatment, or in combination with irinotecan in patients refractory to irinotecan-based chemotherapy, or as a single agent in patients who have failed oxaliplatin- and irinotecan-based chemotherapy or who are intolerant to irinotecan**

Adults: Loading dose, 400 mg/m^2 I.V. over 2 hours (maximum, 10 mg/minute). Complete drug administration 1 hour before initiating FOLFIRI regimen. Maintenance dosage, 250 mg/m^2 I.V. weekly over 1 hour (maximum, 10 mg/minute) until disease progression or unacceptable toxicity occurs.

ADMINISTRATION

I.V.

▼ Drug is a potential teratogen. Follow safe handling procedures when preparing or administering.

▼ Premedicate with an H$_1$-antagonist such as diphenhydramine 50 mg I.V. 30 to 60 minutes before first dose. Premedication before subsequent doses should be based on clinical judgment and severity of prior infusion reactions.

▼ Solution should be clear and colorless and may contain a small amount of particulates.

▼ Don't shake or dilute.

▼ Drug can be given by infusion pump or syringe pump, piggybacked into patient's infusion line. Don't give drug by I.V. push or bolus.

▼ Give initial loading dose over 120 minutes and subsequent infusions over 60 minutes. Don't exceed infusion rate of 10 mg/minute.

▼ Give drug through a low–protein-binding 0.22-micrometer in-line filter.

▼ Flush line with NSS at the end of the infusion.

▼ Observe patient for 1 hour after administration.

▼ Store vials at 36° to 46° F (2° to 8° C). Don't freeze.

▼ Solution in infusion container is stable up to 12 hours at 36° to 46° F (2° to 8° C) and up to 8 hours at 68° to 77° F (20° to 25° C).

▼ **Incompatibilities:** Don't dilute with other solutions.

ACTION

An epidermal growth factor receptor (EGFR) antagonist that binds to the EGFR on normal and tumor cells.

Route	Onset	Peak	Duration
I.V.	Unknown	Unknown	Unknown

Half-life: 4.6 days.

ADVERSE REACTIONS

CNS: asthenia, depression, fever, headache, insomnia, pain.
CV: edema, *cardiopulmonary arrest, PE.*
EENT: conjunctivitis.
GI: abdominal pain, anorexia, constipation, diarrhea, dyspepsia, dysphagia, mucositis, nausea, stomatitis, vomiting, xerostomia.
GU: *acute renal failure.*
Hematologic: anemia, *leukopenia.*
Metabolic: dehydration, *hypomagnesemia,* weight loss.
Musculoskeletal: back pain.

Respiratory: cough, dyspnea.
Skin: alopecia, maculopapular rash, nail disorder, pruritus, radiation dermatitis, acneiform rash.
Other: *anaphylactoid reaction,* chills, infection, infusion reaction, *sepsis.*

INTERACTIONS
Drug-drug. *Live-virus vaccines:* May decrease immune response. Avoid using together.
Drug-lifestyle. *Sun exposure:* May worsen skin reactions. Advise patient to avoid excessive sun exposure.

EFFECTS ON LAB TEST RESULTS
• May decrease magnesium, calcium, and potassium levels.

CONTRAINDICATIONS & CAUTIONS
• Use cautiously in patients hypersensitive to drug, its components, or murine proteins. If used with radiation, use cautiously in patients with a history of CAD, arrhythmias, and HF.
• Determine *RAS* mutation and EGFR-negative expression status using FDA-approved tests before initiating treatment for colorectal cancer. Drug isn't indicated for treatment of *RAS*-mutant colorectal cancer or when results of *RAS* mutation tests are unknown; increased tumor progression, increased mortality, or lack of benefit may occur in patients with *RAS*-mutant metastatic colorectal cancer.
• Acneiform rash has been reported in up to 88% of patients. Rash usually develops in first 2 weeks of therapy and may require dosage modification and treatment with topical or oral antibiotics.
• Life-threatening and fatal bullous muco-cutaneous disease with blisters, erosions, and skin sloughing has been observed in patients treated with cetuximab. It couldn't be determined if these mucocutaneous adverse reactions were directly related to EGFR inhibition or to idiosyncratic immune-related effects (such as Stevens-Johnson syndrome or toxic epidermal necrolysis).
Dialyzable drug: No.

PREGNANCY-LACTATION-REPRODUCTION
• There are no adequate studies in pregnant women. Drug has the potential to cause fetal harm and isn't recommended for use during pregnancy. Use only if potential benefit justifies potential risk to the fetus.
• Women shouldn't breast-feed during therapy and for at least 60 days after last dose.
• All males and females of childbearing potential should use adequate contraception during therapy and for 6 months after last dose.

NURSING CONSIDERATIONS
Black Box Warning Severe infusion reactions, including acute airway obstruction, urticaria, and hypotension, may occur, usually with the first infusion. If a severe infusion reaction occurs, stop drug immediately and give symptomatic treatment. ■
• Keep epinephrine, corticosteroids, I.V. antihistamines, bronchodilators, and oxygen available for severe infusion reactions.
• Manage mild to moderate infusion reactions by decreasing infusion rate and premedicating with an antihistamine for subsequent infusions.
• Monitor patient for infusion reactions for 1 hour after infusion ends.
• Assess patient for acute onset or worsening of pulmonary symptoms. If interstitial lung disease is confirmed, stop drug.
• Monitor patient for skin toxicity, which starts most often during first 2 weeks of therapy. Treat with topical and oral antibiotics.
• Periodically monitor serum electrolyte levels during and for at least 8 weeks after therapy ends.
Black Box Warning In patients also receiving radiation therapy or platinum-based therapy with 5-FU, closely monitor electrolytes, especially magnesium, potassium, and calcium, during and after therapy. Cardiopulmonary arrest or sudden death has occurred. ■

PATIENT TEACHING
• Tell patient to promptly report adverse reactions, including dyspnea, chills, and fever.
• Inform patient that skin reactions may occur, typically during the first 2 weeks of treatment.
• Advise patient to avoid prolonged or unprotected sun exposure during and 2 months after treatment.

Reactions in bold italics are *life-threatening.* Interactions may have a *rapid onset* or a *delayed onset.*

• Instruct female patient not to breast-feed during therapy and for at least 60 days after last dose.
• Advise male and female patient of child-bearing potential to use adequate contraception during therapy and for 6 months after last dose.

chloroquine phosphate
KLO-ro-kwin

Aralen

Therapeutic class: Antimalarials
Pharmacologic class: Aminoquinolines

AVAILABLE FORMS
Tablets: 250 mg (equivalent to 150 mg base), 500 mg (equivalent to 300 mg base)

INDICATIONS & DOSAGES
❂ *Alert:* Prescribers should be completely familiar with this drug before prescribing.
➤ **Acute malarial attacks caused by *Plasmodium vivax, Plasmodium malariae, Plasmodium ovale*, and susceptible strains of *Plasmodium falciparum***
Adults: Initially, 1 g (600 mg base) P.O.; then 500 mg (300 mg base) at 6, 24, and 48 hours.
Children: Initially, 16.6 mg/kg (10 mg/kg base) P.O.; then 8.3 mg/kg (5 mg/kg base) at 6, 24, and 48 hours. Don't exceed adult dose.
➤ **To prevent malaria**
Adults: 500 mg (300 mg base) P.O. once weekly on the same day each week, for 1 to 2 weeks before entering a malaria-endemic area and continued for 4 weeks after leaving the area. If treatment begins after exposure, give 1 g (600 mg base) P.O. initially, in two divided doses 6 hours apart, followed by the usual dosing regimen.
Children: 8.3 mg/kg (5 mg/kg base) P.O. once weekly on the same day each week, for 1 to 2 weeks before entering a malaria-endemic area and continued for 4 to 8 weeks after leaving the area. Don't exceed 500 mg (300 mg base). If treatment begins after exposure, give 16.6 mg/kg (10 mg/kg base) P.O. initially, in two divided doses 6 hours apart, followed by the usual dosing regimen.

➤ **Extraintestinal amebiasis**
Adults: 1 g (600 mg base) P.O. once daily for 2 days; then 500 mg (300 mg base) daily for 2 to 3 weeks. Treatment is usually combined with an intestinal amebicide.

ADMINISTRATION
P.O.
❂ *Alert:* Drug dosage may be discussed in "mg" or "mg base"; be aware of the difference.
• To improve compliance when drug is used for prevention, advise patient to take drug immediately before or after a meal on the same day each week.
• An oral suspension can be prepared by pharmacist if patient can't swallow pills.

ACTION
May bind to and alter the properties of DNA in susceptible parasites.

Route	Onset	Peak	Duration
P.O.	Unknown	1–2 hr	Unknown

Half-life: 3 to 5 days.

ADVERSE REACTIONS
CNS: *seizures,* mild and transient headache, psychic stimulation, neuropathy, acute extrapyramidal reactions.
CV: hypotension, ECG changes, *cardiomyopathy.*
EENT: blurred vision, difficulty in focusing, reversible corneal changes; typically irreversible, sometimes progressive or delayed retinal changes (such as narrowing of arterioles, macular lesions, pallor of optic disk, optic atrophy, and patchy retinal pigmentation, typically leading to blindness); ototoxicity, nerve deafness, vertigo, tinnitus.
GI: anorexia, abdominal cramps, diarrhea, nausea, vomiting.
Hematologic: *agranulocytosis, aplastic anemia, thrombocytopenia.*
Hepatic: *hepatitis.*
Musculoskeletal: myopathy or neuromyopathy leading to progressive weakness and atrophy of proximal muscle groups.
Skin: pruritus, lichen planus eruptions, skin and mucosal pigmentary changes, pleomorphic skin eruptions, *erythema multiforme, Stevens-Johnson syndrome, toxic epidermal necrolysis,* exfoliative

dermatitis, urticaria, DRESS syndrome (drug rash with eosinophilia and systemic symptoms), hair loss and bleaching of hair pigment.
Other: *anaphylaxis, angioedema.*

INTERACTIONS
Drug-drug. *Aluminum salts (kaolin), magnesium:* May decrease GI absorption. Separate dose times by 4 hours.
Ampicillin: May significantly reduce bioavailability of ampicillin. Separate dose times by 2 hours.
Cimetidine: May decrease hepatic metabolism of chloroquine. Monitor patient for toxicity.
Cyclosporine: May cause a sudden increase in serum cyclosporine level. Monitor patient closely. If necessary, discontinue chloroquine.
Drugs that prolong QT interval: May have additive effects on QT interval. Avoid concurrent use if possible.
Mefloquine: May increase seizure risk. Avoid concurrent use, and delay administration of mefloquine until at least 12 hours after the last dose of chloroquine when possible.
Drug-lifestyle. *Sun exposure:* May worsen drug-induced dermatoses. Advise patient to avoid excessive sun exposure.

EFFECTS ON LAB TEST RESULTS
- May increase liver enzyme levels.
- May decrease Hb level and granulocyte and platelet counts.

CONTRAINDICATIONS & CAUTIONS
- Contraindicated in patients hypersensitive to drug and in those with retinal or visual field changes or porphyria.
- Use cautiously in patients with severe GI, neurologic, or blood disorders; hepatic disease or alcoholism; or G6PD deficiency or psoriasis.
- Don't use to treat *P. falciparum* acquired in an area of known chloroquine resistance or when chloroquine prophylaxis has failed. Use other antimalarials if patient has a resistant strain of plasmodia.
- Risk of toxic reactions may be greater in elderly patients and in those with impaired renal function because drug is substantially excreted by the kidneys. Monitor renal function closely.

Dialyzable drug: Unknown.
⚠ *Overdose S&S:* Headache, drowsiness, visual disturbances, nausea, vomiting, CV collapse, seizures, sudden and early respiratory and cardiac arrest; atrial standstill, nodal rhythm, prolonged intraventricular conduction time, progressive bradycardia leading to ventricular fibrillation or arrest.

PREGNANCY-LACTATION-REPRODUCTION
- Safety and effectiveness of chloroquine in pregnant women aren't known. Avoid use during pregnancy except in the suppression or treatment of malaria when benefit outweighs potential risk to the fetus.
- Serious adverse reactions may occur in breast-fed infants. Patient should discontinue breast-feeding or discontinue drug, taking into account importance of drug to the mother.

NURSING CONSIDERATIONS
- Ensure that baseline and periodic ophthalmic examinations are performed. Check periodically for ocular muscle weakness after long-term use.
- Make sure patient is tested with an audiometer before, during, and after therapy, especially if therapy is long-term.
- Monitor CBC and LFTs periodically during long-term therapy. If a severe blood disorder—not caused by the disease—develops, drug may need to be stopped.
- ⚠ *Alert:* Monitor patient for overdose, which can quickly lead to toxic symptoms. Children are extremely susceptible to toxicity; avoid long-term treatment.

PATIENT TEACHING
- To improve compliance when using drug for prevention, advise patient to take drug immediately before or after a meal on the same day each week.
- Instruct patient to avoid excessive sun exposure to prevent worsening of drug-induced dermatoses.
- Tell patient to report adverse reactions promptly, especially blurred vision, increased sensitivity to light, tinnitus, hearing loss, or muscle weakness.
- Instruct patient to keep drug out of reach of children. Overdose may be fatal.

cholestyramine
koe-LESS-tir-a-meen

Prevalite

Therapeutic class: Antilipemics
Pharmacologic class: Bile acid
sequestrants

AVAILABLE FORMS
Powder: 378-g cans, 9-g single-dose packets; each scoop of powder or single-dose packet contains 4 g of cholestyramine resin

INDICATIONS & DOSAGES
➤ **Primary hyperlipidemia or pruritus caused by partial bile obstruction, adjunct for reduction of increased cholesterol level in patients with primary hypercholesterolemia**
Adults: 4 g P.O. once daily or b.i.d. Maintenance dose is 8 to 16 g daily divided into two doses. Maximum daily dose is 24 g.
Children: 240 mg/kg P.O. daily in two to three divided doses, not to exceed 8 g/day.

ADMINISTRATION
P.O.
- Mix thoroughly with 60 to 180 mL of water, other noncarbonated beverage, highly fluid soup, or pulpy fruit with high moisture content, such as applesauce or crushed pineapple.
- Give drug with a meal.
- Give other drugs 1 hour before or at least 4 hours after cholestyramine to avoid impeding absorption.

ACTION
Binds bile acids in the intestinal tract, impeding their absorption and causing their elimination in feces. In response to this bile acid depletion, LDL cholesterol levels decrease as the liver uses LDL cholesterol to replenish reduced bile acid stores.

Route	Onset	Peak	Duration
P.O.	Unknown	Unknown	2–4 wk

Half-life: Unknown.

ADVERSE REACTIONS
CNS: dizziness, headache, vertigo, anxiety, fatigue, insomnia, syncope, tinnitus.

GI: abdominal discomfort, constipation, fecal impaction, nausea, anorexia, diarrhea, flatulence, *GI bleeding,* hemorrhoids, steatorrhea, vomiting.
GU: dysuria, hematuria.
Hematologic: anemia, bleeding tendencies, ecchymoses.
Metabolic: hyperchloremic acidosis.
Musculoskeletal: backache, muscle and joint pains, osteoporosis.
Skin: rash; irritation of skin, tongue, and perianal area.
Other: vitamin A, D, E, and K deficiencies from decreased absorption.

INTERACTIONS
Drug-drug. *Acetaminophen, beta blockers, cardiac glycosides, corticosteroids, estrogens, ezetimibe, fat-soluble vitamins (A, D, E, and K), iron preparations, niacin, penicillin G, phenobarbital, progestins, tetracycline, thiazide diuretics, thyroid hormones, warfarin and other coumarin derivatives:* May decrease absorption of these drugs. Give other drugs 1 to 2 hours before or 4 to 6 hours after cholestyramine.

EFFECTS ON LAB TEST RESULTS
- May increase alkaline phosphatase and triglyceride levels. May decrease Hb level and hematocrit.
- May prolong PT.
- May cause abnormal results in cholecystography that uses iopanoic acid because iopanoic acid is also bound by cholestyramine.

CONTRAINDICATIONS & CAUTIONS
- Contraindicated in patients hypersensitive to bile-acid sequestering resins and in those with complete biliary obstruction.
- Use cautiously in patients predisposed to constipation and in those with conditions aggravated by constipation, such as severe, symptomatic CAD.
Dialyzable drug: Unknown.
⚠ *Overdose S&S:* GI tract obstruction.

PREGNANCY-LACTATION-REPRODUCTION
- There are no adequate well-controlled studies in pregnant women. Drug may interfere with absorption of fat-soluble vitamins, causing fetal harm. Weigh potential benefit against potential risk to the fetus.

• Use cautiously in breast-feeding women. The possible lack of proper vitamin absorption may have an effect on breast-fed infants.

NURSING CONSIDERATIONS
• Monitor cholesterol and triglyceride levels regularly during therapy.
• Monitor levels of cardiac glycosides in patients receiving cardiac glycosides and cholestyramine together. If cholestyramine therapy is stopped, adjust dosage of cardiac glycosides, if necessary, to avoid toxicity.
• Monitor bowel habits. Encourage a diet high in fiber and fluids. If severe constipation develops, decrease dosage, add a stool softener, or stop drug.
• Watch for hyperchloremic acidosis with long-term use or very high doses.
• Long-term use may lead to deficiencies of vitamins A, D, E, and K and folic acid.
• For patients with phenylketonuria, light form contains 28.1 mg of phenylalanine per 6.4-g dose.

PATIENT TEACHING
◑ *Alert:* Tell patient never to take drug in its dry form because it may irritate the esophagus or cause severe constipation.
• Tell patient to prepare drug in a large glass containing water, milk, or juice (especially pulpy fruit juice). Tell him to sprinkle powder on the surface of the beverage, let the mixture stand for a few minutes, and then stir thoroughly. Discourage mixing with carbonated beverages because of excessive foaming. After drinking preparation, patient should swirl a small additional amount of liquid in the same glass and then drink again to make sure he has taken the entire dose.
• Tell patient to avoid sipping or holding the suspension in the mouth because drug may damage tooth surfaces. Advise patient to maintain good oral hygiene.
• Advise patient to take at mealtime, if possible.
• Advise patient to take all other drugs at least 1 to 2 hours before or 4 to 6 hours after cholestyramine to avoid blocking their absorption.
• Teach patient about proper dietary management of fats. When appropriate, recommend weight control, exercise, and smoking cessation programs.

• Tell patient that drug may deplete body stores of vitamins A, D, E, and K and folic acid. Patient should discuss need for supplements with prescriber.

ciclesonide (inhalation, intranasal)
si-CLEH-son-ide

Alvesco, Omnaris, Zetonna

Therapeutic class: Corticosteroids
Pharmacologic class: Corticosteroids

AVAILABLE FORMS
Nasal aerosol solution: 37 mcg/metered spray
Nasal spray: 50 mcg/metered spray
Oral inhalation aerosol: 80 mcg, 160 mcg

INDICATIONS & DOSAGES
➤ **Preventative during asthma maintenance (Alvesco)**
Adults and children age 12 and older who were previously taking bronchodilators alone: Initially, inhaled dose of 80 mcg b.i.d. to maximum of 160 mcg b.i.d.
Adults and children age 12 and older who were previously taking inhaled corticosteroids: Initially, 80 mcg b.i.d. to maximum of 320 mcg b.i.d.
Adults and children age 12 and older who were previously taking oral corticosteroids: 320 mcg b.i.d.
➤ **Signs and symptoms of perennial allergic rhinitis**
Adults and children age 12 and older: 2 sprays of Omnaris in each nostril once daily (200 mcg/day). Or, 1 actuation of Zetonna per nostril once daily.
➤ **Signs and symptoms of seasonal allergic rhinitis**
Adults and children age 12 and older: 1 actuation of Zetonna per nostril once daily.
Adults and children age 6 and older: 2 sprays of Omnaris in each nostril once daily (200 mcg/day).

ADMINISTRATION
Inhalational
• Patient should rinse mouth after inhalation.

Reactions in bold italics are *life-threatening*. Interactions may have a *rapid onset* or a *delayed onset*.

Intranasal

- Before first use of Omnaris, gently shake container, then prime by spraying eight times. If not used for 4 consecutive days, gently shake and reprime with 1 spray or until a fine mist appears.
- Before first use of Zetonna, prime by actuating three times. If not used for 10 consecutive days, prime by actuating three times. If the product is dropped, the canister and actuator may become separated; if this happens, instruct patients to reassemble product and test spray once into the air before using.

ACTION

May decrease inflammation by inhibiting macrophages, eosinophils, and mediators such as leukotrienes involved in the asthmatic response.

Route	Onset	Peak	Duration
Inhalation	>4 wk	1 hr	Unknown
Intranasal	1–2 days	1–5 wk	Unknown

Half-life: Inhalation drug, less than 1 hour; inhalation drug's active metabolite, 6 to 7 hours; intranasal drug, unknown.

ADVERSE REACTIONS

CNS: headache, back pain.
EENT: ear pain, nasopharyngitis, sinusitis, pharyngolaryngeal pain, nasal congestion or discomfort, epistaxis, URI.
Metabolic: growth retardation.
Musculoskeletal: arthralgia, pain in the extremities or back.

INTERACTIONS

Drug-drug. *Delavirdine:* May increase serum ciclesonide level. Use together cautiously.
Ketoconazole, other inhibitors of CYP450: May increase ciclesonide level and adverse effects. Use together cautiously; adjust ciclesonide dosage as needed.
Protease inhibitors (such as ritonavir): May increase serum level and effects of ciclesonide. Use lowest effective ciclesonide dosage and monitor patient closely for Cushing syndrome.

EFFECTS ON LAB TEST RESULTS

None reported.

CONTRAINDICATIONS & CAUTIONS

- Contraindicated as primary treatment of status asthmaticus or other acute asthmatic episodes, and in patients hypersensitive to drug or its components.
- Intranasal form is contraindicated in patients who have had recent nasal septal ulcers, nasal surgery, or nasal trauma until healing has occurred.
- Use cautiously in patients who have changed from systemic to inhaled corticosteroids because renal insufficiency, steroid withdrawal (pain, lassitude, depression), or acute worsening of symptoms may occur.
- Use cautiously in immunosuppressed patients and in those with wounds; corticosteroids suppress the immune system.
- Use cautiously in children; may cause a decline in growth rate.
- Use cautiously, if at all, in patients with active or quiescent respiratory TB infection; untreated systemic fungal, bacterial, viral, or parasitic infections; or ocular HSV infection.

Dialyzable drug: Unknown.
⚠ **Overdose S&S:** Hyperadrenocorticism.

PREGNANCY-LACTATION-REPRODUCTION

- There are no adequate well-controlled studies in pregnant women. Use during pregnancy only if potential benefit justifies potential risk to the fetus.
- If a woman takes a corticosteroid during pregnancy, monitor neonate for hypoadrenalism.
- It isn't known if drug appears in breast milk. Use cautiously in breast-feeding women.

NURSING CONSIDERATIONS

- **Alert:** Don't use for acute bronchospasm or acute asthma.
- Assess patient for bone loss during long-term use.
- Watch for evidence of localized mouth infections, glaucoma, cataracts, and immunosuppression.
- Monitor infants born to mothers using drug during pregnancy for hypoadrenalism.
- Monitor patients who are switched from systemic to inhaled corticosteroids for worsening of signs and symptoms and other adverse effects of withdrawal.

● Monitor children for decline in growth rate; the potential to regain growth after drug is stopped hasn't been studied.

● Monitor patients for nasal adverse effects.

● For patients who don't respond adequately to starting dose after 4 weeks of therapy, higher doses may provide additional asthma control.

● After asthma stability has been achieved, titrate to lowest effective dosage to minimize systemic effects.

PATIENT TEACHING

● Teach patient how to use drug properly. Refer patient to manufacturer's instructions.

● Tell patient to discard Omnaris bottle after 120 actuations following initial priming or 4 months after removal from foil pouch, whichever occurs first.

● Tell patient to replace Zetonna nasal aerosol when indicator shows zero.

● Inform patient that drug isn't indicated for the relief of acute bronchospasm.

● Instruct patient to rinse his mouth with water and spit out after inhalation.

● Advise patient to use drug at regular intervals or about the same time every day, as directed.

● Instruct patient using intranasal form to contact prescriber if there is no relief from symptoms after 1 week.

● Warn patient to avoid exposure to chickenpox, measles, or other infections and, if exposed, to consult prescriber immediately.

● Inform patient that asthma-related therapeutic results may take several weeks and to contact prescriber if symptoms don't improve after 4 weeks of treatment or if condition worsens.

● Advise parents of child receiving long-term therapy that child should have periodic growth measurements.

SAFETY ALERT!

cidofovir
sye-DOE-fo-veer

Therapeutic class: Antivirals
Pharmacologic class: Nucleosides–nucleotides

AVAILABLE FORMS
Injection: 75 mg/mL in 5-mL vial

INDICATIONS & DOSAGES

Black Box Warning Cidofovir is indicated only for the treatment of CMV retinitis in patients with AIDS. ▪

➤ **CMV retinitis in patients with AIDS**
Adults: Initially, 5 mg/kg I.V. infused over 1 hour once weekly for 2 consecutive weeks; then maintenance dose of 5 mg/kg I.V. infused over 1 hour once every 2 weeks. Give probenecid and prehydration with I.V. NSS simultaneously to reduce risk of nephrotoxicity.

Adjust-a-dose: For patients with creatinine level of 0.3 to 0.4 mg/dL above baseline, reduce dosage to 3 mg/kg at same rate and frequency. If creatinine level reaches 0.5 mg/dL or more above baseline, or patient develops 3+ or higher proteinuria, stop drug.

ADMINISTRATION
I.V.

▼ Drug has mutagenic effects; prepare it in a class II laminar flow biological safety cabinet and wear surgical gloves and a closed-front surgical gown with knit cuffs.

▼ If drug contacts skin, wash and flush thoroughly with water.

▼ Place excess drug and all materials used to prepare and give it in a leak-proof, puncture-proof container.

▼ Let drug reach room temperature before use.

▼ Using a syringe, withdraw prescribed dose and add to an I.V. bag containing 100 mL of NSS.

▼ Infuse over 1 hour using an infusion pump.

▼ Because of the risk of nephrotoxicity, don't exceed recommended dosages or frequency or rate of infusion.

▼ Discard any partially used vials.

▼ Give within 24 hours of preparing. Admixture may be refrigerated at 36° to 46° F (2° to 8° C) for up to 24 hours.

Black Box Warning Because of increased risk of nephrotoxicity, give 1 L NSS I.V. over 1 to 2 hours, immediately before giving drug. Also give probenecid with each cidofovir infusion. ▪

❸ *Alert:* If tolerated, a second liter of NSS may be administered over a 1- to 3-hour

---

period at the start of or immediately after cidofovir infusion.

▼ Compatibility of admixture with Ringer, lactated Ringer, and bacteriostatic solutions hasn't been evaluated.

▼ **Incompatibilities:** Other drugs or supplements.

ACTION
Suppresses CMV replication by selective inhibition of viral DNA synthesis.

Route	Onset	Peak	Duration
I.V.	Unknown	Unknown	Unknown

Half-life: Unknown.

ADVERSE REACTIONS
CNS: asthenia, fever, headache, *seizures,* abnormal gait, amnesia, anxiety, confusion, depression, dizziness, hallucinations, insomnia, neuropathy, paresthesia, somnolence, malaise.
CV: hypotension, orthostatic hypotension, pallor, syncope, tachycardia, vasodilation.
EENT: ocular hypotony, abnormal vision, amblyopia, conjunctivitis, eye disorders, iritis, pharyngitis, retinal detachment, rhinitis, sinusitis, uveitis.
GI: abdominal pain, anorexia, diarrhea, nausea, vomiting, aphthous stomatitis, colitis, constipation, dry mouth, dyspepsia, dysphagia, flatulence, gastritis, melena, mouth ulcers, oral candidiasis, rectal disorders, stomatitis, taste perversion, tongue discoloration.
GU: proteinuria, *nephrotoxicity,* glycosuria, hematuria, urinary incontinence, UTI.
Hematologic: anemia, *neutropenia, thrombocytopenia.*
Hepatic: hepatomegaly.
Metabolic: fluid imbalance, hyperglycemia, hyperlipidemia, hypocalcemia, hypokalemia, weight loss.
Musculoskeletal: arthralgia, myalgia, myasthenia; pain in back, chest, or neck.
Respiratory: dyspnea, asthma, bronchitis, coughing, hiccups, increased sputum, lung disorders, pneumonia.
Skin: alopecia, rash, acne, dry skin, pruritus, skin discoloration, sweating, urticaria.
Other: chills, infections, *sarcoma, sepsis,* allergic reactions, facial edema, HSV infection.

INTERACTIONS
Drug-drug. **Black Box Warning** *Nephrotoxic drugs (such as aminoglycosides, amphotericin B, foscarnet, I.V. pentamidine):* May increase nephrotoxicity. Don't use together. ■
Zidovudine: Stop zidovudine or reduce dosage by 50% on the days cidofovir is given; probenecid reduces metabolic clearance of zidovudine.

EFFECTS ON LAB TEST RESULTS
● May increase alkaline phosphatase, ALT, AST, BUN, creatinine, glucose, cholesterol, LDH, and urine protein levels.
● May decrease bicarbonate, calcium, potassium, and Hb levels.
● May decrease neutrophil and platelet counts.

CONTRAINDICATIONS & CAUTIONS
● Contraindicated in patients hypersensitive to drug, probenecid, and other sulfa drugs.
● Contraindicated in patients with creatinine level more than 1.5 mg/dL, CrCl of 55 mL/minute or less, or urine protein level of 100 mg/dL or more (equivalent to 2+ proteinuria or more).
Black Box Warning Renal failure has occurred with as few as one or two doses of cidofovir. Monitor renal function within 48 hours before each dose and modify dosage as needed. Contraindicated in patients receiving other drugs with nephrotoxic potential (stop such drugs at least 7 days before starting cidofovir therapy). ■
● Use within 1 month of placement of a ganciclovir ocular implant may cause profound hypotony.
● Direct intraocular injection is contraindicated and is associated with iritis, ocular hypotony, and permanent vision impairment.
● Use cautiously in patients with renal impairment. Monitor renal function tests and patient's fluid balance.
● Safety and effectiveness in children haven't been established.
Dialyzable drug: 75% (high-flux hemodialysis only).

PREGNANCY-LACTATION-REPRODUCTION
• There are no adequate studies in pregnant women. Use during pregnancy only if potential benefit justifies potential risk to the fetus.

Black Box Warning In animal studies, cidofovir was carcinogenic and teratogenic and caused hypospermia. ■

• It isn't known if drug appears in breast milk. Because of potential for adverse reactions and potential for tumorigenicity as shown in animal studies, drug shouldn't be used in breast-feeding women.

NURSING CONSIDERATIONS
Black Box Warning Due to increased risk of nephrotoxicity and bone marrow suppression, monitor creatinine and urine protein levels and WBC counts with differential before each dose. ■

Black Box Warning Neutropenia has been observed in association with treatment. Monitor neutrophil count during therapy. ■

• Drug may cause Fanconi syndrome and decreased bicarbonate level with renal tubular damage. Monitor patient closely.

• Drug may cause granulocytopenia.

PATIENT TEACHING
• Inform patient that drug doesn't cure CMV retinitis and that regular ophthalmologic examinations are needed.

• Alert patient taking zidovudine that he'll need to obtain dosage guidelines on days cidofovir is given.

• Tell patient that close monitoring of kidney function will be needed and that abnormalities may require a change in therapy.

• Stress importance of completing a full course of probenecid with each cidofovir dose. Tell patient to take probenecid after a meal to decrease nausea.

• Advise women of childbearing potential to use effective contraception, especially during and for 1 month after treatment.

• Advise male patient to practice barrier contraception during and for 3 months after treatment.

cilostazol
sill-AHS-tah-zoll

Pletal

Therapeutic class: Antiplatelet drugs
Pharmacologic class: cAMP phosphodiesterase inhibitors

AVAILABLE FORMS
Tablets: 50 mg, 100 mg

INDICATIONS & DOSAGES
➤ **To reduce symptoms of intermittent claudication**
Adults: 100 mg P.O. b.i.d., at least 30 minutes before or 2 hours after breakfast and dinner.

Adjust-a-dose: Decrease dose to 50 mg P.O. b.i.d. when giving with drugs that may interact to cause an increase in cilostazol level.

ADMINISTRATION
P.O.
• Give drug at least 30 minutes before or 2 hours after breakfast and dinner.

• Don't give with grapefruit juice.

ACTION
Thought to inhibit the enzyme phosphodiesterase III, thus inhibiting platelet aggregation and causing vasodilation.

Route	Onset	Peak	Duration
P.O.	Unknown	Unknown	Unknown

Half-life: 11 to 13 hours.

ADVERSE REACTIONS
CNS: dizziness, headache, vertigo.
CV: palpitations, peripheral edema, tachycardia.
EENT: pharyngitis, rhinitis.
GI: abnormal stools, diarrhea, abdominal pain, dyspepsia, flatulence, nausea.
Hematologic: bleeding.
Musculoskeletal: back pain, myalgia.
Respiratory: increased cough.
Other: infection.

Reactions in bold italics are *life-threatening*. Interactions may have a *rapid onset* or a ***delayed onset***.

INTERACTIONS
Drug-drug. *Diltiazem, omeprazole, ticlopidine:* May increase cilostazol level. Reduce cilostazol dosage to 50 mg b.i.d.
Erythromycin, other macrolides, strong or moderate CYP3A4 inhibitors (diltiazem, itraconazole, ketoconazole): May increase level of cilostazol and its metabolites. Reduce cilostazol dosage to 50 mg b.i.d.
Drug-food. *Grapefruit juice:* May increase drug level. Discourage use together.
Drug-herb. *Ginkgo biloba:* May prolong bleeding time. Discourage use together.
Drug-lifestyle. *Smoking:* May decrease drug exposure. Discourage smoking.

EFFECTS ON LAB TEST RESULTS
• May reduce triglyceride levels. May increase HDL level.

CONTRAINDICATIONS & CAUTIONS
• Contraindicated in patients hypersensitive to drug or its components.
Black Box Warning Contraindicated in patients with HF of any severity. ■
• Contraindicated in patients with hemostatic disorders or active bleeding, such as bleeding peptic ulcer and intracranial bleeding.
• Use cautiously in patients with severe underlying heart disease; also use cautiously with other drugs having antiplatelet activity.
• Use cautiously in patients with severe renal impairment (CrCl <25 mL/minute) and in those with moderate to severe hepatic impairment.
Dialyzable drug: No.
⚠ *Overdose S&S:* Severe headache, diarrhea, hypotension, tachycardia, cardiac arrhythmias.

PREGNANCY-LACTATION-REPRODUCTION
• There are no adequate studies in pregnant women. Therefore, assessment of fetal risk isn't possible.
• Drug may appear in breast milk. Patient should discontinue breast-feeding or discontinue drug, taking into account importance of drug to the mother.

NURSING CONSIDERATIONS
• Beneficial effects may not be seen for up to 12 weeks after therapy starts.

Black Box Warning Cilostazol and similar drugs that inhibit the enzyme phosphodiesterase decrease the likelihood of survival in patients with class III and IV HF. ■
🔔 *Alert:* CV risk is unknown in patients who use drug on long-term basis and in those with severe underlying heart disease.
• Dosage can be reduced or stopped without such rebound effects as platelet hyperaggregation.
• If aspirin is added to drug therapy, monitor patient for aspirin-related adverse reactions.

PATIENT TEACHING
• Instruct patient to take drug on an empty stomach, at least 30 minutes before or 2 hours after breakfast and dinner.
• Tell patient that beneficial effect of drug on cramping pain isn't likely to be noticed for 2 to 4 weeks and that it may take as long as 12 weeks.
• Advise patient to avoid drinking grapefruit juice during drug therapy.
• Inform patient that CV risk is unknown in patients who use drug on a long-term basis and in those with severe underlying heart disease.
• Tell patient that drug may cause dizziness. Caution patient not to drive or perform other activities that require alertness until response to drug is known.

cimetidine
sye-MET-i-deen

Tagamet HB ◊

cimetidine hydrochloride
Tagamet

Therapeutic class: Antiulcer drugs
Pharmacologic class: H_2 receptor antagonists

AVAILABLE FORMS
Oral liquid: 300 mg/5 mL*
Tablets: 200 mg ◊, 300 mg, 400 mg, 800 mg

INDICATIONS & DOSAGES
Adjust-a-dose (for all indications): In patients with renal impairment, decrease dosage to 300 mg P.O. every 12 hours, increasing

frequency to every 8 hours with caution. A renally impaired patient who also has liver dysfunction may require even further dosage reduction. Schedule dose at the end of hemodialysis.

➤ **Short-term treatment of duodenal ulcer; maintenance therapy**
Adults and children age 16 and older:
800 mg P.O. at bedtime. Or, 400 mg P.O. b.i.d. or 300 mg q.i.d. (with meals and at bedtime). Or, 200 mg P.O. t.i.d. with a 400-mg bedtime dose. Treatment lasts 4 to 6 weeks unless endoscopy shows healing. For maintenance therapy, 400 mg at bedtime.

➤ **Active benign gastric ulceration**
Adults: 800 mg P.O. at bedtime or 300 mg P.O. q.i.d. (with meals and at bedtime) for up to 8 weeks.

➤ **Pathologic hypersecretory conditions, such as Zollinger-Ellison syndrome, systemic mastocytosis, and multiple endocrine adenomas**
Adults and children age 16 and older:
300 mg P.O. q.i.d. with meals and at bedtime, adjusted to patient needs. Maximum oral amount, 2,400 mg daily.

➤ **GERD with erosive esophagitis**
Adults: 800 mg P.O. b.i.d. or 400 mg P.O. q.i.d. before meals and at bedtime for up to 12 weeks.

➤ **Heartburn**
Adults and children age 12 and older:
200 mg Tagamet HB P.O. with water as symptoms occur, or as directed, up to b.i.d. For prevention, 200 mg P.O. right before or up to 30 minutes before eating food or drinking beverages that cause heartburn. Maximum, 400 mg daily. Drug shouldn't be taken daily for longer than 2 weeks.

ADMINISTRATION
P.O.
● Give dose at end of hemodialysis.

ACTION
Competitively inhibits action of histamine on the H_2 receptor sites of parietal cells, decreasing gastric acid secretion.

Route	Onset	Peak	Duration
P.O.	1 hr	45–90 min	4–5 hr

Half-life: 2 hours.

ADVERSE REACTIONS
CNS: confusion, dizziness, hallucinations, headache, peripheral neuropathy, somnolence.
GI: mild and transient diarrhea.
GU: erectile dysfunction.
Musculoskeletal: arthralgia, muscle pain.
Other: mild gynecomastia if used longer than 1 month, hypersensitivity reactions.

INTERACTIONS
Drug-drug. *Amiodarone:* May increase amiodarone level. Avoid combination if possible. Monitor for increased amiodarone concentrations and effects. Consider therapy modification.
Antacids: May interfere with cimetidine absorption. Separate doses by at least 1 hour, if possible.
Carmustine: May enhance the bone marrow suppressant effects of carmustine. Avoid use together.
Digoxin, fluconazole, indomethacin, iron salts, ketoconazole, tetracycline: May decrease drug absorption. Separate doses by at least 2 hours.
Fosphenytoin, phenytoin, some benzodiazepines, theophylline: May inhibit hepatic microsomal enzyme metabolism of these drugs. Monitor drug level.
I.V. lidocaine: May decrease clearance of lidocaine, increasing the risk of toxicity. Consider using a different H_2 antagonist, if possible. Monitor lidocaine level closely.
Metoprolol, propranolol, timolol: May increase the effects of beta blocker. Consider another H_2 antagonist or decrease the dose of beta blocker.
Procainamide: May increase procainamide level. Avoid this combination, if possible. Monitor procainamide level closely and adjust the dose as necessary.
Warfarin-type anticoagulants: May increase blood levels of these drugs. Closely monitor PT and adjust anticoagulant dosage if necessary.
Drug-lifestyle. *Alcohol use:* May increase blood alcohol level. Discourage use together.
Smoking: May decrease drug's ability to inhibit nocturnal gastric secretion. Urge patient to quit smoking.

Reactions in bold italics are *life-threatening*. Interactions may have a *rapid onset* or a ***delayed onset***.

EFFECTS ON LAB TEST RESULTS

- May increase ALT, AST, and creatinine levels.
- May antagonize pentagastrin's effect during gastric acid secretion tests. May cause false-negative results in skin tests using allergen extracts. May impair interpretation of Hemoccult and Gastroccult test results on gastric content aspirate because of FD&C blue dye number 2 used in tablets.

CONTRAINDICATIONS & CAUTIONS

- Contraindicated in patients hypersensitive to drug.
- Use cautiously in elderly or debilitated patients because they may be more susceptible to drug-induced confusion.
- Use cautiously in patients with renal or hepatic impairment.
- Prolonged treatment (2 years or more) increases risk of vitamin B_{12} malabsorption and deficiency, especially in women and patients younger than age 30.
- Drug may increase risk of acute gastroenteritis and community-acquired pneumonia in children.

Dialyzable drug: Yes.

⚠ **Overdose S&S:** Mental deterioration, unresponsiveness, death.

PREGNANCY-LACTATION-REPRODUCTION

- There are no adequate studies in pregnant women. Use during pregnancy only if clearly needed and potential benefit justifies potential risk to the fetus.
- Drug appears in breast milk. As a general rule, women shouldn't breast-feed while taking drug.

NURSING CONSIDERATIONS

- Assess patient for abdominal pain. Note blood in emesis, stool, or gastric aspirate.
- Identify tablet strength when obtaining a drug history.
- Schedule dose at end of hemodialysis treatment because hemodialysis reduces drug levels.
- Wait at least 15 minutes after giving tablet before drawing sample for Hemoccult or Gastroccult test, and follow test manufacturer's instructions closely.
- Treatment of gastric ulcer isn't as effective as treatment of duodenal ulcer.

- **Look alike–sound alike:** Don't confuse cimetidine with simethicone.

PATIENT TEACHING

- Remind patient taking drug once daily to take it at bedtime and to take multiple daily doses with meals.
- Instruct patient taking Tagamet HB not to exceed recommended dosage and not to take daily for longer than 14 days.
- Urge patient to avoid cigarette smoking because it may increase gastric acid secretion and worsen disease.
- Advise patient to report all adverse reactions, including abdominal pain, blood in stools or emesis, black tarry stools, and coffee-ground emesis.
- Tell patient to check with prescriber or pharmacist before taking other drugs.

cinacalcet hydrochloride

sin-ah-KAL-set

Sensipar

Therapeutic class: Hyperparathyroidism drugs
Pharmacologic class: Calcimimetics

AVAILABLE FORMS

Tablets ⓓ: 30 mg, 60 mg, 90 mg

INDICATIONS & DOSAGES

Adjust-a-dose (for all indications): Patients with moderate to severe hepatic impairment (Child-Pugh class B or C) may experience increased exposure to cinacalcet and increased half-life. Dosage adjustments may be necessary based on serum calcium, serum phosphorus, or intact parathyroid hormone (iPTH) level.

➤ **Primary hyperparathyroidism**
Adults: Initially, 30 mg P.O. b.i.d. Titrate every 2 to 4 weeks through sequential doses of 30 mg b.i.d., 60 mg b.i.d., 90 mg b.i.d., and 90 mg t.i.d. or q.i.d. to normalize calcium levels.

➤ **Secondary hyperparathyroidism in patients with chronic kidney disease undergoing dialysis**
Adults: Initially, 30 mg P.O. once daily; adjust no more than every 2 to 4 weeks

---

through sequential doses of 60 mg, 90 mg, 120 mg, and 180 mg P.O. once daily to reach target range of 150 to 300 picograms (pg)/mL for iPTH level.

➤ **Hypercalcemia in patients with parathyroid carcinoma**

Adults: Initially, 30 mg P.O. b.i.d.; adjust every 2 to 4 weeks through sequential doses of 30 mg, 60 mg, and 90 mg P.O. b.i.d., and 90 mg P.O. t.i.d. or q.i.d. daily if needed to normalize calcium level.

ADMINISTRATION

P.O.

● Don't break or crush tablets; give them whole, with food or shortly after a meal.

ACTION

Increases sensitivity of calcium-sensing receptor to extracellular calcium, letting calcium be absorbed despite decreased PTH.

Route	Onset	Peak	Duration
P.O.	Unknown	2–6 hr	Unknown

Half-life: Terminal half-life, 30 to 40 hours.

ADVERSE REACTIONS

CNS: dizziness, asthenia, *seizures,* depression, fatigue, headache, paresthesia.
CV: chest pain, hypertension.
GI: diarrhea, nausea, vomiting, anorexia, constipation.
Hematologic: anemia.
Metabolic: hypocalcemia, dehydration, hypercalcemia.
Musculoskeletal: myalgia, arthralgia, fracture, limb pain.
Respiratory: URI.
Other: dialysis access infection.

INTERACTIONS

Drug-drug. *Amitriptyline:* Amitriptyline and nortriptyline exposure increases by 20% in patients who are CYP2D6 extensive metabolizers. Avoid using together, if possible.
Drugs metabolized mainly by CYP2D6 with a narrow therapeutic index (flecainide, thioridazine, most TCAs, vinblastine): May strongly inhibit CYP2D6, decreasing metabolism and increasing levels of these drugs. Adjust dosage of other drugs, as needed.

Drugs that strongly inhibit CYP3A4 (erythromycin, itraconazole, ketoconazole): May increase cinacalcet level. Use together cautiously, monitoring PTH and calcium level closely and adjusting cinacalcet dosage, as needed.

EFFECTS ON LAB TEST RESULTS

● May decrease calcium, phosphorus, and testosterone levels.

CONTRAINDICATIONS & CAUTIONS

● Contraindicated in patients hypersensitive to drug or its components and in patients with calcium level less than 8.4 mg/dL.
● Use cautiously in patients with history of seizures and in those with moderate to severe hepatic impairment.
● If iPTH level is less than 150 pg/mL, reduce dosage of cinacalcet and/or vitamin D sterols or discontinue therapy.
Dialyzable drug: No.
⚠ *Overdose S&S:* Hypocalcemia.

PREGNANCY-LACTATION-REPRODUCTION

● There are no adequate studies in pregnant women. Use during pregnancy only if potential benefit justifies potential risk to the fetus.
● Women who become pregnant during treatment are encouraged to enroll in Amgen's Pregnancy Surveillance Program by calling 1-800-772-6436.
● It isn't known if drug appears in breast milk. Patient should discontinue breastfeeding or discontinue drug, taking into account importance of drug to the mother.

NURSING CONSIDERATIONS

● *Alert:* Monitor calcium level closely, especially if patient has a history of seizures, because decreased calcium level lowers seizure threshold.
● Patients with moderate to severe hepatic impairment may need dosage adjustment based on PTH and calcium levels. Monitor these patients closely.
● Give drug alone or with vitamin D sterols, phosphate binders, or both.
● Measure calcium level within 1 week after starting therapy or adjusting dosage. After maintenance dose is established, measure calcium level monthly for patients with

chronic kidney disease receiving dialysis and every 2 months for those with parathyroid carcinoma.

• Watch carefully for evidence of hypocalcemia: paresthesia, myalgias, cramping, tetany, and seizures.

• If calcium level is 7.5 to 8.4 mg/dL or patient develops symptoms of hypocalcemia, give calcium-containing phosphate binders, vitamin D sterols, or both, to raise calcium level. If calcium level is below 7.5 mg/dL or hypocalcemia symptoms persist and the vitamin D dose can't be increased, withhold drug until calcium level reaches 8.0 mg/dL, hypocalcemia symptoms resolve, or both. Resume therapy with the next lowest dose.

• Measure iPTH level 1 to 4 weeks after therapy starts or dosage changes. After the maintenance dose is established, monitor PTH level every 1 to 3 months. Levels in patients with chronic kidney disease receiving dialysis should be 150 to 300 pg/mL.

• Adynamic bone disease may develop if iPTH levels are suppressed below 100 pg/mL. If this occurs, notify prescriber.

❸ **Alert:** Don't use drug in patients with chronic kidney disease who aren't receiving dialysis because they have an increased risk of hypocalcemia.

PATIENT TEACHING

• Tell patient not to divide tablets but to take them whole, with food or shortly after a meal.

• Advise patient to report to prescriber adverse reactions and signs of hypocalcemia, which include paresthesia, muscle weakness, muscle cramping, and muscle spasm.

---

ciprofloxacin
si-proe-FLOX-a-sin

Cipro✔, Cipro I.V., Cipro XR

Therapeutic class: Antibiotics
Pharmacologic class: Fluoroquinolones

AVAILABLE FORMS
Infusion (premixed): 200 mg in 100 mL D₅W, 400 mg in 200 mL D₅W
Injection: 200 mg, 400 mg

Suspension (oral): 250 mg/5 mL (5%), 500 mg/5 mL (10%)
Tablets (extended-release, film-coated) ⓓ: 500 mg, 1,000 mg
Tablets (film-coated): 100 mg, 250 mg, 500 mg, 750 mg

INDICATIONS & DOSAGES
Black Box Warning Use in patients with sinusitis, bronchitis, and uncomplicated UTI isn't recommended because of risk of serious adverse effects. Use in these patients only when there are no other treatment options. ∎

Adjust-a-dose (for all indications): For patients with a CrCl of 30 to 50 mL/minute, give 250 to 500 mg P.O. every 12 hours or the usual I.V. dose; if CrCl is 5 to 29 mL/minute, give 250 to 500 mg P.O. every 18 hours or 200 to 400 mg I.V. every 18 to 24 hours. If patient is receiving hemodialysis or peritoneal dialysis, give 250 to 500 mg P.O. every 24 hours after dialysis.

➤ **Complicated intra-abdominal infection**
Adults: 500 mg P.O. or 400 mg I.V. every 12 hours for 7 to 14 days. Give with metronidazole.

➤ **Severe or complicated bone or joint infection, severe respiratory tract infection, severe skin or skin-structure infection**
Adults: 750 mg P.O. every 12 hours or 400 mg I.V. every 8 hours.

➤ **Severe or complicated UTI; mild to moderate bone or joint infection; mild to moderate respiratory infection; mild to moderate skin or skin-structure infection; infectious diarrhea; typhoid fever**
Adults: 500 mg P.O. or 400 mg I.V. every 12 hours. Or, 1,000 mg extended-release tablets P.O. every 24 hours.

➤ **Complicated UTI or pyelonephritis**
Adults: 500 mg P.O. every 12 hours for 7 to 14 days. Or 1,000 mg extended-release tablets P.O. every 24 hours for 7 to 14 days.
Children ages 1 to 17: 6 to 10 mg/kg I.V. every 8 hours for 10 to 21 days. Maximum I.V. dose, 400 mg. Or, 10 to 20 mg/kg P.O. every 12 hours. Maximum P.O. dose, 750 mg. Don't exceed maximum dose, even in patients who weigh more than 51 kg.

Adjust-a-dose: If CrCl is less than 30 mL/minute, reduce the dosage of extended-release form from 1,000 to 500 mg daily. Administer extended-release form after hemodialysis or peritoneal dialysis is completed.

➤ **Nosocomial pneumonia**
Adults: 400 mg I.V. every 8 hours for 10 to 14 days.

➤ **Mild to moderate UTI**
Adults: 250 mg P.O. or 200 mg I.V. every 12 hours for 7 to 14 days.

➤ **Uncomplicated UTI**
Adults: 500 mg extended-release tablet P.O. once daily for 3 days, or 250 mg P.O. every 12 hours for 3 days.

➤ **Chronic bacterial prostatitis**
Adults: 500 mg P.O. every 12 hours or 400 mg I.V. every 12 hours for 28 days.

➤ **Mild to moderate acute sinusitis**
Adults: 500 mg P.O. or 400 mg I.V. every 12 hours for 10 days.

➤ **Empirical therapy in febrile neutropenic patients**
Adults: 400 mg I.V. every 8 hours used with piperacillin 50 mg/kg I.V. every 4 hours (not to exceed 24 g/day of piperacillin).

➤ **Inhalation anthrax (postexposure)**
Adults: 400 mg I.V. every 12 hours initially until susceptibility test results are known; then 500 mg P.O. b.i.d. Give drug with one or two additional antimicrobials. Switch to oral therapy when appropriate. Treat for 60 days (I.V. and P.O. combined).
Children: 10 mg/kg I.V. every 12 hours; then 15 mg/kg P.O. every 12 hours. Don't exceed 800 mg/day I.V. or 1,000 mg/day P.O. Give drug with one or two additional antimicrobials. Switch to oral therapy when appropriate. Treat for 60 days (I.V. and P.O. combined).

➤ **Plague due to *Yersinia pestis;* plague prophylaxis as soon as possible after suspected or confirmed exposure**
Adults: 400 mg I.V. every 8 to 12 hours or 500 to 750 mg P.O. every 12 hours for 14 days.
Children: 10 mg/kg I.V. or 15 mg/kg P.O. every 8 to 12 hours for 10 to 21 days. Maximum dosage, 500 mg/dose P.O. and 400 mg/dose I.V.

➤ **Surgical prophylaxis ◆**
Adults: 400 mg I.V. infused over 60 minutes and repeated every 4 to 10 hours. Or, 500 mg P.O. every 12 hours or a one-time dose of 1,500 mg.

ADMINISTRATION
P.O.
● Cipro XR and immediate-release oral forms aren't interchangeable.
● Obtain specimen for culture and sensitivity tests before giving first dose. Begin therapy while awaiting results.
● To avoid decreasing the effects of ciprofloxacin, give at least 2 hours before or 6 hours after certain drugs and vitamins. Food doesn't affect absorption but may delay peak levels.
● Caffeine should be avoided during therapy with this drug because of potential for increased caffeine effects.
● Give drug with plenty of fluids to reduce risk of urine crystals.
● Don't crush or split extended-release tablets.
● Shake oral suspension vigorously each time before use for approximately 15 seconds; don't give through feeding tube.

I.V.
▼ Obtain specimen for culture and sensitivity tests before giving first dose. Begin therapy while awaiting results.
▼ Dilute drug to 1 to 2 mg/mL using D_5W or NSS for injection.
▼ If giving drug through a Y-type set, stop the other I.V. solution while infusing.
▼ Infuse over 1 hour into a large vein to minimize discomfort and vein irritation.
▼ **Incompatibilities:** Aminophylline, ampicillin–sulbactam, azithromycin, cefepime, clindamycin phosphate, dexamethasone sodium phosphate, furosemide, heparin sodium, methylprednisolone sodium succinate, phenytoin sodium.

ACTION
Inhibits bacterial DNA synthesis, mainly by blocking DNA gyrase; bactericidal.

Route	Onset	Peak	Duration
P.O.	Unknown	30–120 min	Unknown
P.O. (extended-release)	Unknown	1–4 hr	Unknown
I.V.	Unknown	Immediate	Unknown

Half-life: 4 hours; Cipro XR, 6 hours in adults with normal renal function.

ADVERSE REACTIONS

CNS: *seizures,* confusion, headache, restlessness.
GI: *pseudomembranous colitis,* diarrhea, nausea, vomiting.
GU: crystalluria, interstitial nephritis.
Hematologic: *leukopenia, neutropenia, thrombocytopenia,* eosinophilia.
Musculoskeletal: tendon rupture.
Skin: rash, *Stevens-Johnson syndrome, toxic epidermal necrolysis.*
Other: hypersensitivity reactions.

INTERACTIONS
Drug-drug. *Aluminum hydroxide, aluminum-magnesium hydroxide, calcium carbonate, didanosine (chewable tablets, buffered tablets, or pediatric powder for oral solution), magnesium hydroxide, products containing zinc:* May decrease ciprofloxacin absorption and effects. Give ciprofloxacin 2 hours before or 6 hours after these drugs.
Cyclosporine: May increase risk for cyclosporine toxicity. Monitor cyclosporine level.
Drugs that prolong QT interval: May additionally increase QT interval and risk of life-threatening cardiac arrhythmias. Use together cautiously.
Iron salts: May decrease absorption of ciprofloxacin, reducing anti-infective response. Give at least 2 hours apart.
NSAIDs: May increase risk of CNS stimulation. Monitor patient closely.
Probenecid: May elevate level of ciprofloxacin. Monitor patient for toxicity.
Black Box Warning *Steroids:* May increase risk of tendinitis and tendon rupture. ∎
Sucralfate: May decrease ciprofloxacin absorption, reducing anti-infective response. If use together can't be avoided, give at least 6 hours apart.
Theophylline: May increase theophylline level and prolong theophylline half-life.

Monitor level of theophylline and watch for adverse effects.
Tizanidine: Increases tizanidine levels, causing low BP, somnolence, dizziness, and slowed psychomotor skills. Use together is contraindicated.
Warfarin: May increase anticoagulant effects. Monitor PT and INR closely.
Drug-herb. *Dong quai, St. John's wort:* May cause photosensitivity. Advise patient to avoid excessive sunlight exposure.
Yerba maté: May decrease clearance of herb's methylxanthines and cause toxicity. Discourage use together.
Drug-food. *Caffeine:* May increase effect of caffeine. Monitor patient closely.
Dairy products, other foods: May delay peak drug levels. Advise patient to take drug on an empty stomach.
Orange juice fortified with calcium: May decrease GI absorption of drug, reducing its effects. Discourage use together.
Drug-lifestyle. *Sun exposure:* May cause photosensitivity reactions. Advise patient to avoid excessive sunlight exposure.

EFFECTS ON LAB TEST RESULTS
• May increase alkaline phosphatase, ALT, AST, bilirubin, BUN, creatinine, LDH, and GGT levels.
• May increase eosinophil count. May decrease WBC, neutrophil, and platelet counts.

CONTRAINDICATIONS & CAUTIONS
• Contraindicated in patients sensitive to fluoroquinolones.
⊕ *Alert:* Serious and occasionally fatal hypersensitivity reactions, some after first dose, have been reported. Emergency treatment for anaphylaxis may be necessary. Immediately discontinue drug at first appearance of rash, jaundice, or other signs and symptoms of hypersensitivity.
⊕ *Alert:* Cases of severe hepatotoxicity, including fatal events, have been reported. Acute liver injury can be rapid and is frequently associated with hypersensitivity. If signs and symptoms of hepatitis occur, discontinue drug immediately.
• Use cautiously in patients with CNS disorders, such as severe cerebral arteriosclerosis or seizure disorders, and in

those at risk for seizures. Drug may cause CNS stimulation.

Black Box Warning Drug is associated with increased risk of tendinitis and tendon rupture, especially in patients older than age 60 and those with heart, kidney, or lung transplants. ∎

Black Box Warning Drug may exacerbate muscle weakness in patients with myasthenia gravis. Avoid use of fluoroquinolones in patients with a known history of myasthenia gravis. ∎

🔔 *Alert:* Oral or parenteral fluoroquinolones may increase the risk of peripheral neuropathy of the arms or legs. Symptoms can occur anytime during treatment and can last for months to years or be permanent. Stop drug immediately if patient develops symptoms and switch to a non-fluoroquinolone antibacterial drug unless the benefits of continued treatment outweigh the risks.

Black Box Warning Fluoroquinolones have been associated with disabling and potentially irreversible serious adverse reactions that have occurred together, including tendinitis and tendon rupture, peripheral neuropathy, and CNS effects. Drug is associated with increased risk of serious adverse CNS reactions (convulsions, toxic psychoses, increased ICP, pseudotumor cerebri, tremors, restlessness, anxiety, light-headedness, confusion, hallucinations, paranoia, depression, nightmares, insomnia and, rarely, suicidal thoughts or acts). If any of these serious adverse reactions occur, discontinue drug immediately. ∎

• Drug may cause CDAD ranging in severity from mild diarrhea to fatal colitis and possibly occurring more than 2 months after therapy ends. Drug may need to be discontinued if CDAD develops during therapy.
Dialyzable drug: Less than 10%.

PREGNANCY-LACTATION-REPRODUCTION

• There are no adequate studies in pregnant women. Use during pregnancy only if potential benefit justifies potential risk to the fetus.

• Pregnant women and immunocompromised patients should receive the usual doses and regimens for anthrax postexposure prophylaxis.

• Drug appears in breast milk, and the amount absorbed by a breast-feeding infant is unknown. Because of the risk of serious adverse reactions (including articular damage), a decision should be made to discontinue breast-feeding or discontinue drug, taking into account importance of drug to the mother.

NURSING CONSIDERATIONS

• Monitor patient's intake and output, and observe patient for signs of crystalluria.

Black Box Warning Tendon rupture may occur in patients receiving quinolones. If pain or inflammation occurs or if patient ruptures a tendon, stop drug. ∎

🔔 *Alert:* Monitor patient for symptoms of peripheral neuropathy (pain, burning, tingling, numbness, weakness, or a change in sensation to light touch, pain, temperature, or sense of body position), and report them immediately to the practitioner.

🔔 *Alert:* Immediately report signs and symptoms of hepatitis (anorexia, jaundice, dark urine, pruritus, abdominal tenderness) and discontinue drug.

• Long-term therapy may result in overgrowth of organisms resistant to drug.

• Cutaneous anthrax patients with signs of systemic involvement, extensive edema, or lesions on the head or neck need I.V. therapy and a multidrug approach.

• Additional antimicrobials for anthrax multidrug regimens can include rifampin, vancomycin, penicillin, ampicillin, chloramphenicol, imipenem, clindamycin, and clarithromycin.

• Steroids may be used as adjunctive therapy for anthrax patients with severe edema and for meningitis.

• Follow current CDC recommendations for anthrax.

PATIENT TEACHING

• Tell patient to take drug as prescribed, even after feeling better.

• Advise patient to drink plenty of fluids to reduce risk of urine crystals.

• Advise patient not to crush, split, or chew the extended-release tablets.

🔔 *Alert:* Warn patient to immediately notify his health care provider for signs and symptoms of serious adverse reactions including

---

unusual joint or tendon pain, muscle weakness, "pins and needles" tingling or pricking sensation, numbness in the arms or legs, confusion or hallucinations.

• Warn patient to avoid hazardous tasks that require alertness, such as driving, until effects of drug are known.

• Instruct patient to avoid caffeine while taking drug because of potential for increased caffeine effects.

• Advise patient that hypersensitivity reactions may occur even after first dose. If a rash or other allergic reaction occurs, tell patient to stop drug immediately and notify prescriber.

• Tell patient that tendon rupture can occur with drug and to notify prescriber if pain or inflammation occurs.

• Tell patient to avoid excessive sunlight or artificial ultraviolet light during therapy.

ciprofloxacin hydrochloride (ophthalmic, otic)
si-proe-FLOX-a-sin

Cetraxal, Ciloxan

Therapeutic class: Antibiotics
Pharmacologic class: Fluoroquinolones

AVAILABLE FORMS
Ophthalmic ointment: 0.3% (base)
Ophthalmic solution: 0.3% (base)
Otic solution: 0.2% (0.25 mL single-use container)

INDICATIONS & DOSAGES
➤ **Corneal ulcers caused by** *Pseudomonas aeruginosa, Staphylococcus aureus, Staphylococcus epidermidis, Streptococcus pneumoniae,* **or possibly** *Serratia marcescens* **or** *Streptococcus viridans*
Adults and children older than age 1: Give 2 drops in affected eye every 15 minutes for first 6 hours; then 2 drops every 30 minutes for remainder of first day. On the second day, 2 drops hourly. On days 3 to 14, 2 drops every 4 hours. Treatment may be continued after day 14 if reepithelialization hasn't occurred.

➤ **Bacterial conjunctivitis caused by** *Haemophilus influenzae, S. aureus, S. epidermidis,* **or possibly** *S. pneumoniae*
Adults and children older than age 1: Give 1 or 2 drops into conjunctival sac of affected eye every 2 hours while awake for first 2 days. Then, 1 or 2 drops every 4 hours while awake for next 5 days.
Adults and children older than age 2:
½-inch (1.27-cm) ribbon of ointment into conjunctival sac t.i.d. for the first 2 days, then ½-inch ribbon b.i.d. for next 5 days.
➤ **Acute otitis externa caused by susceptible isolates of** *P. aeruginosa* **or** *S. aureus*
Adults and children age 1 and older: Instill 0.5 mg (contents of one single-dose container) into affected ear b.i.d. for 7 days.

ADMINISTRATION
Ophthalmic
• Apply light finger pressure on lacrimal sac for 1 minute after drops are instilled.
Otic
• Containers are for single use only.
• Warm solution by holding container in hands for 1 minute.
• Patient should lie down with affected ear upward.
• Instill into affected ear; patient should remain lying down for 1 minute after drug is instilled.

ACTION
Inhibits bacterial DNA gyrase, an enzyme needed for bacterial replication.

Route	Onset	Peak	Duration
Ophthalmic, otic	Unknown	Unknown	Unknown

Half-life: 3 to 5 hours.

ADVERSE REACTIONS
EENT: headache, local burning or discomfort, white crystalline precipitate in superficial portion of corneal defect in patients with corneal ulcers (ophthalmic), allergic reactions, conjunctival hyperemia (ophthalmic), foreign body sensation (ophthalmic), itching.
GI: bad or bitter taste in mouth (ophthalmic).
Other: fungal superinfection of ear.

INTERACTIONS
None significant.

EFFECTS ON LAB TEST RESULTS
None reported.

CONTRAINDICATIONS & CAUTIONS
• Contraindicated in patients hypersensitive to drug or other fluoroquinolones.
• Serious and occasionally fatal hypersensitivity (anaphylactic) reactions, some after first dose, have been reported in patients receiving systemic quinolone therapy. Serious anaphylactic reactions require immediate emergency treatment with epinephrine and other resuscitation measures.
• Discontinue drug at first appearance of rash or other signs and symptoms of hypersensitivity reaction.
• Prolonged use can lead to superinfection (overgrowth of nonsusceptible organisms). If superinfection occurs, initiate appropriate therapy.
Dialyzable drug: Not applicable.

PREGNANCY-LACTATION-REPRODUCTION
• There are no adequate studies in pregnant women. Use during pregnancy only if potential benefit justifies potential risk to the fetus.
• It isn't known if drug appears in breast milk after application; however, drug given systemically appears in breast milk. Use cautiously in breast-feeding women using ophthalmic form. Patient using otic form should either discontinue breast-feeding or discontinue drug.

NURSING CONSIDERATIONS
❸ *Alert:* Stop drug at first sign of hypersensitivity, such as rash, and notify prescriber. Serious hypersensitivity reactions, including anaphylaxis, may occur in patients receiving systemic drug.
• A topical overdose may be flushed from eyes with warm tap water.
• If corneal epithelium is still compromised after 14 days of treatment, continue therapy.
• Institute appropriate therapy if superinfection occurs. Prolonged use may result in overgrowth of nonsusceptible organisms, including fungi.

• *Look alike–sound alike:* Don't confuse Ciloxan with Cytoxan.

PATIENT TEACHING
• Tell patient to clean eye area of excessive discharge before instilling.
• Teach patient how to instill drops or apply ointment, to wash hands before and after using drug, and not to touch tip of dropper to eye or surrounding tissues.
• Instruct patient to apply light finger pressure on lacrimal sac for 1 minute after drops are instilled.
• Teach patient how to correctly instill otic solution.
• Advise patient that ophthalmic drug may cause temporary blurring of vision or stinging after administration. If these symptoms become pronounced or worsen, tell patient to contact prescriber.
• Tell patient to avoid wearing contact lenses while treating bacterial conjunctivitis. If approved by prescriber, tell patient to wait at least 15 minutes after instilling drops before inserting contact lenses.
• Tell patient not to share drug, washcloths, or towels with family members and to notify prescriber if anyone develops same signs or symptoms.
• Stress importance of compliance with recommended therapy and of reporting adverse reactions promptly.

SAFETY ALERT!

cisatracurium besylate
sis-ah-trah-KYOO-ee-hum

Nimbex

Therapeutic class: Skeletal muscle relaxants
Pharmacologic class: Nondepolarizing neuromuscular blockers

AVAILABLE FORMS
Injection: 2 mg/mL, 10 mg/mL*

INDICATIONS & DOSAGES
➤ **Adjunct to general anesthesia to facilitate endotracheal intubation and relax skeletal muscles during surgery**

Adults: First dose of 0.15 mg/kg I.V.; then maintenance dosages of 0.03 mg/kg I.V. every 40 to 50 minutes p.r.n. Or, first dose of 0.2 mg/kg I.V.; then maintenance dosages of 0.03 mg/kg I.V. every 50 to 60 minutes p.r.n. Or, as a continuous infusion in operating room, after initial bolus dose, give a maintenance infusion at 3 mcg/kg/minute and reduce to 1 to 2 mcg/kg/minute as needed.

Children ages 2 to 12: 0.1 to 0.15 mg/kg I.V. over 5 to 10 seconds. After first dose, give a maintenance infusion of 3 mcg/kg/minute, then reduce to 1 to 2 mcg/kg/minute as needed.

Children ages 1 to 23 months: 0.15 mg/kg over 5 to 10 seconds. No information is available for continuous infusion.

Adjust-a-dose: During coronary artery bypass surgery (adults) with induced hypothermia, reduce infusion rate by 50%.

➤ **To maintain neuromuscular blockade during mechanical ventilation in ICU**
Adults: Principles for infusion in operating room apply to use in ICU. After first dose, give 3 mcg/kg/minute by I.V. infusion. Range, 0.5 to 10.2 mcg/kg/minute.

Adjust-a-dose: In patients with neuromuscular disease, such as myasthenia gravis, don't exceed 0.02 mg/kg. Patients with burns may need increased amount.

ADMINISTRATION

I.V.

▼ Drug is colorless to slightly yellow or green-yellow. Inspect vials for particulates and discoloration before use. Don't use unclear solutions or those with visible particulates.

▼ The 20-mL vial is intended for use only in the ICU.

▼ Use only under direct supervision of medical staff skilled in using neuromuscular blockers and maintaining airway patency. Don't give drug unless resources for intubation, mechanical ventilation, and oxygen therapy are within reach.

▼ Keep refrigerated; don't freeze. After removal from refrigeration to room temperature (77° F [25° C]), use within 21 days, even if rerefrigerated.

▼ Use drug within 24 hours when diluted to a concentration of 0.1 mg/mL in D$_5$W, NSS, or 5% dextrose and NSS.

▼ **Incompatibilities:** Acyclovir, alkaline solutions with pH higher than 8.5, aminophylline, amphotericin B, amphotericin B cholesteryl sulfate complex, ampicillin, ampicillin sodium–sulbactam sodium, cefazolin, cefotaxime, cefoxitin, ceftazidime, cefuroxime, diazepam, furosemide, ganciclovir, heparin sodium, ketorolac, lactated Ringer injection, methylprednisolone sodium succinate, piperacillin, piperacillin sodium–tazobactam sodium, propofol, sodium bicarbonate, sodium nitroprusside, thiopental sodium, ticarcillin disodium–clavulanate potassium, sulfamethoxazole–trimethoprim.

ACTION

Binds to cholinergic receptors on the motor end plate, antagonizing acetylcholine and blocking neuromuscular transmission.

Route	Onset	Peak	Duration
I.V.	2–3 min	3–5 min	35–45 min

Half-life: 22 to 29 minutes; about 3 hours for laudanosine.

ADVERSE REACTIONS

CV: *bradycardia,* hypotension, flushing.
Respiratory: *bronchospasm, prolonged apnea.*
Skin: rash.

INTERACTIONS

Drug-drug. *Aminoglycosides, bacitracin, clindamycin, colistimethate sodium, colistin, lithium, local anesthetics, magnesium salts, polymyxins, procainamide, quinidine, quinine, tetracyclines, vancomycin:* May enhance neuromuscular blocking action of cisatracurium. Use together cautiously.
Carbamazepine, phenytoin: May decrease the effects of cisatracurium. May need to increase cisatracurium dose.
Enflurane or isoflurane given with nitrous oxide or oxygen: May prolong cisatracurium duration of action. Patient may need less frequent maintenance doses, lower maintenance doses, or reduced infusion rate of cisatracurium. Effects are dependent on duration of volatile agent administration.
Succinylcholine: May shorten time to onset of maximal neuromuscular block. Monitor patient.

EFFECTS ON LAB TEST RESULTS
None reported.

CONTRAINDICATIONS & CAUTIONS
• Contraindicated in patients who are hypersensitive to drug, to other bis-benzylisoquinolinium drugs, or to benzyl alcohol (found in 10-mg/mL vial).
Dialyzable drug: Unknown.
⚠ *Overdose S&S:* Prolonged neuromuscular blockade.

PREGNANCY-LACTATION-REPRODUCTION
• There are no adequate studies in pregnant women. Use during pregnancy only if clearly needed and potential benefit justifies potential risk to the fetus.
• It isn't known if drug appears in breast milk. Use cautiously in breast-feeding women.

NURSING CONSIDERATIONS
• Drug isn't recommended for rapid-sequence endotracheal intubation because of its intermediate onset.
• Dosage requirements vary widely among patients.
◔ *Alert:* Drug has no known effect on consciousness, pain threshold, or cerebration. To avoid patient distress, don't induce neuromuscular block before unconsciousness.
◔ *Alert:* Never give by I.M. injection.
• Monitor neuromuscular function with nerve stimulator during drug administration. If stimulation doesn't elicit a response, stop infusion until response returns.
◔ *Alert:* Drug should only be given by clinicians experienced in its use. Don't give drug unless personnel and facilities for resuscitation, life-support, and drug antagonist are immediately available.
• To avoid inaccurate dosing, perform neuromuscular monitoring on a nonparetic arm or leg in patients with hemiparesis or paraparesis.
• Monitor acid-base balance and electrolyte levels. Abnormalities may potentiate or antagonize the action of cisatracurium.
• Monitor patient for malignant hyperthermia.
• Give analgesics, if indicated. Patient can feel pain but can't indicate its presence.

◔ *Alert:* Careful dosage calculation is essential. Always verify dosage with another health care professional.

PATIENT TEACHING
• Explain purpose of drug.
• Assure patient that monitoring will be continuous.
• Explain all procedures and events because patient can still hear.

SAFETY ALERT!

cisplatin (CDDP)
SIS-pla-tin

Therapeutic class: Antineoplastics
Pharmacologic class: Platinum-containing compounds

AVAILABLE FORMS
Injection: 1 mg/mL

INDICATIONS & DOSAGES
Adjust-a-dose (for all indications): If CrCl is 10 to 50 mL/minute, give 75% of normal dose; if CrCl is less than 10 mL/minute, give 50% of normal dose but consider avoiding use. For hemodialysis patients, give 50% of usual dose; give after dialysis on dialysis days. For peritoneal dialysis patients, give 50% of usual dose. For patients receiving continuous renal replacement therapy, give 75% of usual dose.
Black Box Warning Confirm dosages greater than 100 mg/m^2/cycle once every 3 to 4 weeks with prescriber. ∎
➤ **Adjunctive therapy in metastatic testicular cancer**
Adults: 20 mg/m^2 I.V. daily for 5 days. Repeat every 3 weeks for three cycles.
➤ **Adjunctive therapy in metastatic ovarian cancer**
Adults: 100 mg/m^2 I.V.; repeat every 4 weeks. Or, 75 to 100 mg/m^2 I.V. once every 4 weeks with cyclophosphamide.
➤ **Advanced bladder cancer**
Adults: 50 to 70 mg/m^2 I.V. every 3 to 4 weeks. Give 50 mg/m^2 every 4 weeks in patients who have received other antineoplastics or radiation therapy.

ADMINISTRATION

I.V.

▼ Preparing and giving parenteral form of drug may be mutagenic, teratogenic, or carcinogenic. Follow facility policy to reduce risks.

▼ Hydrate patient with NSS for 8 to 12 hours before giving drug and for 24 hours after administration. Maintain urine output of at least 100 mL/hour for 4 consecutive hours before therapy and for 24 hours after therapy.

Black Box Warning Anaphylactic-type reactions may occur within minutes of administration. Have emergency equipment available. ■

▼ Infusions are most stable in solutions containing chloride (such as NSS or half-NSS and 0.22% sodium chloride). Don't use D₅W alone.

▼ Further dilute with dextrose 5% in 0.3% sodium chloride injection or dextrose 5% in half-NSS for injection with 37.5 g mannitol added.

▼ Administer over 6 to 8 hours.

▼ Reconstituted solutions are stable for 20 hours at room temperature. Protect from light or use within 6 hours after removal from amber vial. Don't refrigerate.

▼ Don't use needles or I.V. sets containing aluminum parts for preparation or administration.

▼ **Incompatibilities:** Aluminum administration sets, amifostine, amphotericin B cholesteryl sulfate complex, cefepime, D₅W, etoposide–mannitol–potassium chloride, 5-FU, mesna, 0.1% sodium chloride solution, paclitaxel, piperacillin sodium–tazobactam sodium, sodium bicarbonate, sodium bisulfate, sodium thiosulfate, solutions with a chloride content less than 2%, thiotepa.

ACTION

May cross-link strands of cellular DNA and interfere with RNA transcription, causing an imbalance of growth that leads to cell death. Not specific to cell cycle.

Route	Onset	Peak	Duration
I.V.	Rapid	Unknown	Several days

Half-life: Initial phase, 14 to 49 minutes; beta, 0.7 to 4.6 hours; gamma, 24 to 127 hours.

ADVERSE REACTIONS

CNS: peripheral neuritis, *seizures.*
EENT: tinnitus, hearing loss.
GI: anorexia, diarrhea, loss of taste, nausea, vomiting.
GU: *prolonged renal toxicity with repeated courses of therapy.*
Hematologic: *myelosuppression, leukopenia, thrombocytopenia,* anemia.
Metabolic: *hypomagnesemia, hypokalemia, hypocalcemia.*
Other: *anaphylactoid reaction.*

INTERACTIONS

Drug-drug. *Aminoglycosides:* May increase nephrotoxicity. Carefully monitor renal function study results.
Aminoglycosides, bumetanide, ethacrynic acid, furosemide, torsemide: May increase ototoxicity. Avoid using together, if possible.
Aspirin, NSAIDs: May increase risk of bleeding. Avoid using together.
Fosphenytoin, phenytoin: May decrease phenytoin and fosphenytoin levels. Monitor levels.
Myelosuppressants: May increase myelosuppression. Monitor patient.

EFFECTS ON LAB TEST RESULTS

● May increase uric acid level. May decrease calcium, Hb, magnesium, phosphate, potassium, and sodium levels.
● May decrease platelet and WBC counts.

CONTRAINDICATIONS & CAUTIONS

Black Box Warning Anaphylaxis-like hypersensitivity reactions requiring emergency treatment have been reported. Facial edema, bronchoconstriction, tachycardia, and hypotension may occur within minutes of administration. Epinephrine, corticosteroids, and antihistamines have been used effectively to alleviate symptoms. ■

● Contraindicated in patients hypersensitive to drug or other platinum-containing compounds and in those with preexisting severe renal disease, hearing impairment, or myelosuppression.

● Use cautiously in patients previously treated with radiation or cytotoxic drugs and in those with peripheral neuropathies; also use cautiously with other ototoxic and nephrotoxic drugs.

• Secondary malignancies have been reported.
• Drug can cause hyperuricemia requiring antihyperuricemia therapy to reduce uric acid levels, especially with dosages higher than 50 mg/m².
Dialyzable drug: No.
⚠ *Overdose S&S:* Renal failure, liver failure, deafness, ocular toxicity, significant myelosuppression, intractable nausea and vomiting, neuritis, death.

PREGNANCY-LACTATION-REPRODUCTION
• Drug can cause fetal harm when used during pregnancy. Women of childbearing potential should be advised to avoid pregnancy during treatment.
• Drug appears in breast milk. Women shouldn't breast-feed during therapy.

NURSING CONSIDERATIONS
Black Box Warning Drug should be administered under the supervision of a physician experienced in the use of cancer chemotherapeutic agents. ■
Black Box Warning Be careful to avoid overdose. Doses greater than 100 mg/m² per cycle every 3 to 4 weeks are rare. Confirm that dose is total dose per cycle, not daily dose. ■
🜂 *Alert:* Myelosuppression is a major toxicity and occurs in approximately 30% of patients. Other dose-related toxicities include nausea and vomiting.
🜂 *Alert:* Cisplatin is considered a vesicant if more than 20 mL is administered or if it's given at a concentration of 0.5 mg/mL or more. Stop infusion immediately if extravasation occurs. Don't flush the line; drug must be aspirated out before extravasation treatment. Prepare for the provider to infiltrate the area with sodium thiosulfate and to institute other treatments.
• Monitor CBC, electrolyte levels (especially potassium and magnesium), platelet count, and renal function studies before initial and subsequent doses.
Black Box Warning Ototoxicity, which may be more pronounced in children, is manifested by tinnitus or loss of high-frequency hearing and, occasionally, deafness. ■
• To detect hearing loss, obtain audiometry tests before initial and subsequent doses.

• Prehydration and mannitol diuresis may significantly reduce renal toxicity and ototoxicity.
• Therapeutic effects are frequently accompanied by toxicity.
• Drug is highly emetogenic. Nausea and vomiting may occur immediately or may be delayed. Antiemetics are recommended. Monitor intake and output. Continue I.V. hydration until patient can tolerate adequate oral intake.
Black Box Warning Renal toxicity is cumulative; don't give next dose until renal function returns to normal. ■
• Don't repeat dose unless platelet count exceeds 100,000/mm³, WBC count exceeds 4,000/mm³, creatinine level is below 1.5 mg/dL, BUN level is below 25 mg/dL, and auditory acuity is within normal limits.
• To prevent bleeding, avoid all I.M. injections when platelet count is less than 50,000/mm³.
• Anticipate need for blood transfusions during treatment because of cumulative anemia.
Black Box Warning Immediately give epinephrine, corticosteroids, or antihistamines for anaphylactoid reactions. ■
• Safe use in children hasn't been established.
• *Look alike–sound alike:* Don't confuse cisplatin with carboplatin; they aren't interchangeable.

PATIENT TEACHING
• Teach patient to report all adverse reactions, including nausea and vomiting.
• Advise patient to watch for signs and symptoms of infection (fever, sore throat, fatigue) and bleeding (easy bruising, nosebleeds, bleeding gums, tarry stools). Tell patient to take temperature daily.
• Tell patient to immediately report ringing in the ears or numbness in hands or feet.
• Instruct patient to avoid OTC products containing aspirin.
• Advise female patient to stop breast-feeding during therapy because of risk of toxicity to infant.
• Advise female patient of childbearing potential to avoid becoming pregnant during therapy because drug may cause fetal harm.

---

citalopram hydrobromide
si-TAL-oh-pram

Celexa◊

Therapeutic class: Antidepressants
Pharmacologic class: SSRIs

AVAILABLE FORMS
Capsules: 10 mg, 20 mg, 40 mg
Solution: 10 mg/5 mL
Tablets: 10 mg, 20 mg, 40 mg

INDICATIONS & DOSAGES
Adjust-a-dose (for all indications): For patients with hepatic impairment and for those who are CYP2C19 poor metabolizers, are taking cimetidine or another CYP2C19 inhibitor, or are older than age 60, the maximum dosage is 20 mg/day.
➤ **Depression**
Adults: Initially, 20 mg P.O. once daily, increasing to 40 mg daily after no less than 1 week. Maximum recommended dose is 40 mg daily.
Elderly patients: 20 mg P.O. daily.
➤ **Obsessive-compulsive disorder** ◆
Adults: Initially, 20 mg P.O. daily, titrated to a target dose of 40 mg P.O. daily. Maximum dosage is 40 mg/day. Significant improvement is generally seen 4 to 6 weeks after start of therapy.

ADMINISTRATION
P.O.
● Give drug without regard for food.

ACTION
Probably linked to potentiation of serotonergic activity in the CNS resulting from inhibition of neuronal reuptake of serotonin.

Route	Onset	Peak	Duration
P.O.	1–4 wk	4 hr	1–2 days

Half-life: 35 hours.

ADVERSE REACTIONS
CNS: somnolence, insomnia, *suicide attempt,* anxiety, agitation, dizziness, paresthesia, migraine, impaired concentration, amnesia, depression, apathy, tremor, confusion, fatigue, fever.

CV: tachycardia, orthostatic hypotension, hypotension.
EENT: rhinitis, sinusitis, abnormal accommodation.
GI: dry mouth, nausea, diarrhea, anorexia, dyspepsia, vomiting, abdominal pain, taste perversion, increased saliva, flatulence, increased appetite.
GU: dysmenorrhea, amenorrhea, ejaculation disorder, erectile dysfunction, anorgasmia, polyuria.
Metabolic: decreased or increased weight.
Musculoskeletal: arthralgia, myalgia.
Respiratory: URI, coughing.
Skin: rash, pruritus.
Other: increased sweating, yawning, decreased libido.

INTERACTIONS
Drug-drug. *Amphetamines, buspirone, dextromethorphan, dihydroergotamine, meperidine, other SSRIs or SSNRIs (duloxetine, venlafaxine), TCAs,* **tramadol,** *trazodone, tryptophan:* May increase risk of serotonin syndrome. Avoid other drugs that increase the availability of serotonin in the CNS; monitor patient closely if used together.
Antiarrhythmics (Class IA [procainamide, quinidine], Class III [amiodarone, sotalol]), antibiotics (clarithromycin, erythromycin, levofloxacin, moxifloxacin), antipsychotics (chlorpromazine, thioridazine), drugs that prolong QTc interval (dolasetron, methadone, ondansetron, pentamidine): May cause QTc prolongation and increase risk of torsades de pointes. Use together isn't recommended.
Carbamazepine: May increase citalopram clearance. Monitor patient for effects.
CNS drugs: May cause additive effects. Use together cautiously.
Drugs that affect coagulation (aspirin, NSAIDs): May increase bleeding risk. Monitor patient closely.
Drugs that inhibit CYP3A4 and CYP2C19: May cause decreased clearance of citalopram. Monitor patient for increased adverse effects.
Imipramine, other TCAs: May increase level of imipramine metabolite desipramine by about 50%. Use together cautiously.

Linezolid, methylene blue: May cause serotonin syndrome. Use with extreme caution and monitor closely.
Lithium: May enhance serotonergic effect of citalopram. Use together cautiously, and monitor lithium level.
MAO inhibitors (phenelzine, selegiline, tranylcypromine): May cause serotonin syndrome or signs and symptoms resembling neuroleptic malignant syndrome. Avoid using within 14 days of MAO inhibitor therapy.
Sumatriptan: May cause weakness, hyperreflexia, and incoordination. Monitor patient closely.
Drug-herb. *St. John's wort:* May increase the risk of serotonin syndrome. Discourage use together.
Drug-lifestyle. *Alcohol use:* May increase CNS effects. Discourage use together.

EFFECTS ON LAB TEST RESULTS

None reported.

CONTRAINDICATIONS & CAUTIONS

• Contraindicated in patients hypersensitive to drug or its inactive components, within 14 days of MAO inhibitor therapy, and in patients taking pimozide.
Alert: Drug isn't recommended for patients with congenital long QT syndrome, bradycardia, hypokalemia, hypomagnesemia, recent acute MI, or uncompensated HF.
Alert: High doses can prolong the QT interval and cause torsades de pointes, a potentially fatal heart rhythm. Maximum dose is 40 mg/day.
Alert: Discontinue drug in patients with persistent QTc interval measurement longer than 500 msec.
Alert: Concomitant use with linezolid or methylene blue can cause serotonin syndrome (fever, mental status changes, muscle twitching, excessive sweating, shivering or shaking, diarrhea, loss of coordination). Use together is contraindicated.
• Use cautiously in patients with history of mania, seizures, suicidal thoughts, or hepatic or renal impairment.
Dialyzable drug: No.
Overdose S&S: Dizziness, sweating, nausea, vomiting, tremor, somnolence, sinus tachycardia, amnesia, confusion, coma, seizures, hyperventilation, cyanosis, rhabdomyolysis, ECG changes.

PREGNANCY-LACTATION-REPRODUCTION

• There are no adequate well-controlled studies in pregnant women. Use during pregnancy only if potential benefit justifies potential risk to the fetus.
• Use in third trimester may be linked to neonatal complications at birth. Consider risk versus benefit of treatment during this time.
• Drug appears in breast milk. Patient should discontinue breast-feeding or discontinue drug, taking into account importance of drug to the mother.

NURSING CONSIDERATIONS

• Correct electrolyte disturbances before starting drug; monitor patients at high risk for electrolyte disturbances periodically during therapy.
• Don't use at doses greater than 40 mg/day because of a dose-related association with QT-interval prolongation.
• Although drug hasn't been shown to impair psychomotor performance, any psychoactive drug has the potential to impair judgment, thinking, or motor skills.
• The possibility of a suicide attempt is inherent in depression and may persist until significant remission occurs. Closely supervise high-risk patients at start of drug therapy. Reduce risk of overdose by limiting amount of drug available per refill.
Black Box Warning Drug may increase the risk of suicidal thinking and behavior in children, adolescents, and young adults with major depressive disorder or other psychiatric disorders. Drug isn't approved for use in children. ■
• At least 14 days should elapse between MAO inhibitor therapy and citalopram therapy.
Alert: Combining triptans with an SSRI or an SSNRI may cause serotonin syndrome or neuroleptic malignant syndrome–like reactions. Signs and symptoms of serotonin syndrome may include restlessness, hallucinations, loss of coordination, fast heartbeat, rapid changes in BP, increased body temperature, overactive reflexes, nausea, vomiting,

and diarrhea. Serotonin syndrome may be more likely to occur when starting or increasing the dose of the triptan, SSRI, or SSNRI.

🌢 *Alert:* If linezolid or methylene blue must be given, stop drug and monitor patient for serotonin toxicity for 2 weeks, or until 24 hours after the last dose of methylene blue or linezolid, whichever comes first. Treatment may be resumed 24 hours after last dose of methylene blue or linezolid.

• Don't discontinue drug abruptly as a discontinuation syndrome can develop, with varying symptoms.

• *Look alike–sound alike:* Don't confuse Celexa with Zyprexa, Celebrex, or Cerebyx.

PATIENT TEACHING

Black Box Warning Advise families and caregivers to closely observe patient for increased suicidal thinking and behavior. ■

🌢 *Alert:* Teach patient to recognize and immediately report symptoms of serotonin toxicity (fever, mental status changes, muscle twitching, excessive sweating, shivering or shaking, diarrhea, loss of coordination).

• Caution patient against use of MAO inhibitors while taking citalopram.

• Inform patient that, although improvement may take 1 to 4 weeks, he should continue therapy as prescribed.

• Advise patient not to stop drug abruptly.

• Tell patient that drug may be taken in the morning or evening without regard to meals. If drowsiness occurs, he should take drug in evening.

• Instruct patient to exercise caution when driving or operating hazardous machinery; drug may impair judgment, thinking, and motor skills.

• Advise patient to consult prescriber before taking other prescription or OTC drugs.

• Advise women of childbearing potential to consult prescriber before breast-feeding.

• Warn patient to avoid alcohol during drug therapy.

• Instruct women of childbearing potential to use contraceptives during drug therapy and to notify prescriber immediately if pregnancy is suspected.

clarithromycin
klar-ITH-ro-my-sin

Biaxin🌢

Therapeutic class: Antibiotics
Pharmacologic class: Macrolides

AVAILABLE FORMS
Suspension: 125 mg/5 mL, 250 mg/5 mL
Tablets (extended-release) ⊙⊙⊙*:* 500 mg
Tablets (film-coated): 250 mg, 500 mg

INDICATIONS & DOSAGES
Adjust-a-dose (for all indications): In patients with CrCl of less than 30 mL/minute, reduce dosage by 50% or double frequency interval. For concomitant use with atazanavir or ritonavir in patients with CrCl of 30 to 60 mL/minute, reduce dosage by 50%; if CrCl is less than 30 mL/minute, reduce dosage by 75%.

➤ **Pharyngitis or tonsillitis caused by *Streptococcus pyogenes***
Adults: 250 mg P.O. every 12 hours for 10 days.
Children age 6 and older: 7.5 mg/kg P.O. every 12 hours for 10 days.

➤ **Acute maxillary sinusitis caused by *Streptococcus pneumoniae, Haemophilus influenzae*, or *Moraxella catarrhalis***
Adults: 500 mg P.O. every 12 hours for 14 days. Or, if using extended-release form, give two 500-mg tablets P.O. daily for 14 days.
Children age 6 and older: 7.5 mg/kg P.O. every 12 hours for 10 days.

➤ **Acute worsening of chronic bronchitis caused by *M. catarrhalis* or *S. pneumoniae;* community-acquired pneumonia caused by *H. influenzae, S. pneumoniae, Mycoplasma pneumoniae*, or *Chlamydia pneumoniae***
Adults: 250 mg P.O. every 12 hours for 7 days *(H. influenzae)* or 7 to 14 days (other bacteria).

➤ **Acute worsening of chronic bronchitis caused by *H. influenzae* or *Haemophilus parainfluenzae***
Adults: 500 mg P.O. every 12 hours for 7 days *(H. parainfluenzae)* or 7 to 14 days *(H. influenzae).*

➤ **Acute worsening of chronic bronchitis caused by *M. catarrhalis, S. pneumoniae, H. parainfluenzae*, or *H. influenzae***
Adults: Two 500-mg extended-release tablets P.O. daily for 7 days.

➤ **Mild to moderate community-acquired pneumonia caused by *H. influenzae, S. pneumoniae, C. pneumoniae*, or *M. pneumoniae***
Adults: 250 mg P.O. b.i.d. for 7 to 14 days.

➤ **Mild to moderate community-acquired pneumonia caused by *H. influenzae, H. parainfluenzae, M. catarrhalis, S. pneumoniae, C. pneumoniae*, or *M. pneumoniae***
Adults: Two 500-mg extended-release tablets P.O. once daily for 7 days.

➤ **Community-acquired pneumonia caused by *S. pneumoniae, C. pneumoniae*, or *M. pneumoniae***
Children age 6 and older: 7.5 mg/kg P.O. every 12 hours for 10 days.

➤ **Uncomplicated skin and skin-structure infections caused by *Staphylococcus aureus* or *S. pyogenes***
Adults: 250 mg P.O. every 12 hours for 7 to 14 days.
Children: 7.5 mg/kg P.O. every 12 hours for 10 days.

➤ **Acute otitis media**
Children age 6 and older: 7.5 mg/kg P.O. every 12 hours for 10 days.

➤ **To prevent and treat disseminated infection caused by *Mycobacterium avium* complex**
Adults: 500 mg P.O. b.i.d.
Children age 20 months and older: 7.5 mg/kg P.O. b.i.d., up to 500 mg b.i.d.

➤ **To reduce risk of duodenal ulcer recurrence in *H. pylori* infection**
Adults: 500 mg clarithromycin with 30 mg lansoprazole and 1 g amoxicillin, all given P.O. every 12 hours for 10 to 14 days. Or, 500 mg clarithromycin with 20 mg omeprazole and 1 g amoxicillin, all given P.O. every 12 hours for 10 days. Or, two-drug regimen with 500 mg clarithromycin P.O. every 8 hours and 40 mg omeprazole P.O. once daily for 14 days. Continue omeprazole for 14 additional days.

ADMINISTRATION
P.O.
- Obtain specimen for culture and sensitivity tests before giving. Begin therapy while awaiting results.
- Give drug with or without food.
- Don't refrigerate the suspension form; discard unused portion after 14 days.

ACTION
Binds to the 50S subunit of bacterial ribosomes, blocking protein synthesis; bacteriostatic or bactericidal, depending on concentration.

Route	Onset	Peak	Duration
P.O.	Unknown	2–3 hr	Unknown
P.O. (extended release)	Unknown	5–8 hr	Unknown

Half-life: 3 to 7 hours.

ADVERSE REACTIONS
CNS: headache.
GI: *pseudomembranous colitis,* abdominal pain or discomfort, diarrhea, nausea, taste perversion, vomiting (in children).
Hematologic: coagulation abnormalities.
Skin: rash (in children).

INTERACTIONS
Drug-drug. *Alprazolam, midazolam, triazolam:* May decrease clearance of these drugs, causing adverse reactions. Use together cautiously.
Apixaban, dabigatran: May increase apixaban and dabigatran concentrations. Apixaban or dabigatran dosage reductions or avoidance of combination may be necessary. Consider therapy modification.
Atazanavir, ritonavir: May increase clarithromycin level. Reduce clarithromycin dosage in renally impaired patients.
Carbamazepine, phenytoin: May inhibit metabolism of these drugs, increasing serum levels and risk of toxicity. Avoid using together.
Colchicine: May increase colchicine level. Concomitant use is contraindicated in patients with renal or hepatic impairment. In those with normal renal and hepatic function, reduce colchicine dose.
Cyclosporine: May increase cyclosporine levels. Monitor cyclosporine level.

CYP3A4 substrates (colchicine): May increase substrate concentration. Avoid use together or reduce substrate dosage.

Digoxin: May increase digoxin level. Monitor patient for digoxin toxicity.

Dihydroergotamine, ergotamine: May cause acute ergot toxicity. Avoid using together.

Fluconazole: May increase clarithromycin level. Monitor patient closely.

HMG-CoA reductase inhibitors: May increase levels of these drugs; may rarely cause rhabdomyolysis. Use together cautiously.

Other drugs that prolong QTc interval (amiodarone, antipsychotics, disopyramide, fluoroquinolones, fluoxetine, procainamide, quinidine, sotalol, TCAs): May have additive effects. Monitor ECG for QTc interval prolongation. Avoid using together if possible.

Pimozide: May cause torsades de pointes. Use together is contraindicated.

Rifamycin: May decrease therapeutic effects of clarithromycin while increasing adverse effects of rifamycin. Monitor patient.

Sildenafil: May prolong absorption of sildenafil. May need to reduce sildenafil dosage.

Theophylline: May increase theophylline level. Monitor drug level.

Warfarin: May prolong PT and increase INR. Monitor PT and INR carefully.

Zidovudine: May alter zidovudine level. Monitor patient closely.

Drug-herb. *St. John's wort:* May decrease clarithromycin level. Avoid use during clarithromycin therapy.

Drug-food. *Grapefruit juice:* May inhibit metabolism, increasing adverse effects. Don't take with grapefruit juice.

EFFECTS ON LAB TEST RESULTS
- May increase BUN level.
- May prolong PT and increase INR.

CONTRAINDICATIONS & CAUTIONS
- Severe acute hypersensitivity reactions, including anaphylaxis, Stevens-Johnson syndrome, toxic epidermal necrolysis, drug rash with eosinophilia, and Henoch-Schönlein purpura, have been reported. Discontinue drug and begin immediate treatment if these occur.
- Contraindicated in patients hypersensitive to clarithromycin, erythromycin, or other macrolides and in those receiving pimozide or other drugs that prolong QT interval or cause cardiac arrhythmias.
- Contraindicated in patients with a history of cholestatic jaundice or hepatic impairment associated with prior use of clarithromycin.
- Use cautiously in patients with hepatic or renal impairment or myasthenia gravis.
- May cause exacerbation of or new signs and symptoms in patients with myasthenia gravis. Use cautiously in these patients.
- Drug may cause CDAD and pseudomembranous colitis, which can occur more than 2 months after therapy ends.
- Safety and effectiveness in children younger than age 6 months haven't been established.

Dialyzable drug: No.

PREGNANCY-LACTATION-REPRODUCTION
- There are no adequate well-controlled studies in pregnant women; animal studies show adverse pregnancy outcome and embryo-fetal risk. Use during pregnancy only if potential benefit justifies potential risk to the fetus and when no alternative therapy is appropriate.
- Drug appears in breast milk. Use cautiously in breast-feeding women and weigh benefits against risks.

NURSING CONSIDERATIONS
- **Alert:** Be sure to use extended-release form to only treat infections for which it is approved.
- Monitor patient for superinfection. Drug may cause overgrowth of nonsusceptible bacteria or fungi.

PATIENT TEACHING
- Tell patient to take drug as prescribed, even after he feels better.
- Advise patient to report all adverse reactions.
- Inform patient that drug may be taken with or without food.
- Tell patient not to refrigerate the suspension form, but to discard unused portion after 14 days.

clevidipine
cle-VIH-deh-peen

Cleviprex

Therapeutic class: Antihypertensives
Pharmacologic class: Dihydropyridine
calcium channel blockers

AVAILABLE FORMS
Injection: 0.5 mg/mL in 50-, 100-, and
250-mL single-use vials

INDICATIONS & DOSAGES
➤ **To lower BP when oral therapy isn't
feasible or desirable**
Adults: Begin infusion at 1 to 2 mg/hour
and titrate by doubling the dose every
90 seconds. When BP approaches goal,
titrate every 5 to 10 minutes at less than
double the dose. Maintenance dose is usually 4 to 6 mg/hour. Maximum dose is
1,000 mL (average of 21 mg/hour) per
24-hour period. Drug isn't recommended for
use beyond 72 hours.

ADMINISTRATION
I.V.
▼ Store vials in cartons in refrigerator
because drug is photosensitive. May store
at controlled room temperature (77° F
[25° C]) for up to 2 months.
▼ Maintain aseptic technique when handling solution. Drug can support growth
of microorganisms; don't use if solution
might be contaminated.
▼ Invert vial several times to mix emulsion
before use.
▼ Inspect solution and discard if particulate matter or discoloration is present
before use. Don't dilute.
▼ Use a continuous infusion pump to
regulate flow.
▼ Discard unused portion within 12 hours.
▼ **Incompatibilities:** Don't administer drug in same I.V. line with other
medications.

ACTION
Inhibits calcium ion influx across cardiac
and smooth-muscle cells, decreasing
contractility and oxygen demand. Dilates
coronary arteries and arterioles, decreasing
systemic vascular resistance.

Route	Onset	Peak	Duration
I.V.	2–4 min	Unknown	5–15 min

Half-life: 15 minutes; metabolite, 9 hours.

ADVERSE REACTIONS
CNS: headache.
CV: atrial fibrillation.
GI: nausea, vomiting.
GU: *acute renal failure.*

INTERACTIONS
None reported.

EFFECTS ON LAB TEST RESULTS
● May increase bilirubin, AST, and ALT
levels.

CONTRAINDICATIONS & CAUTIONS
● Contraindicated in patients hypersensitive
to soy beans, soy products, eggs, or egg
products.
● Contraindicated in those with defective
lipid metabolism or severe aortic stenosis.
● Use cautiously in patients with HF, and
monitor for exacerbations.
● Safety and effectiveness in children
younger than age 18 haven't been established.
Dialyzable drug: Unknown.
⚠ *Overdose S&S:* Hypotension, reflex
tachycardia.

PREGNANCY-LACTATION-REPRODUCTION
● There are no adequate well-controlled
studies in pregnant women. Use during
pregnancy only if potential benefit justifies
potential risk to the fetus.
● It isn't known if drug appears in breast
milk. Consider the possibility of infant
exposure during breast-feeding, and monitor
infant for adverse effects.

NURSING CONSIDERATIONS
● Monitor BP and HR continuously, especially when starting drug and during dosage
adjustments.
● Drug may exacerbate HF; monitor patient
closely.
● Titrate dose slowly; rapid titration may
cause hypotension and reflex tachycardia. If
either occurs, decrease clevidipine dosage.

Reactions in bold italics are *life-threatening*. Interactions may have a *rapid onset* or a *delayed onset*.

● Monitor patient who received prolonged infusion for rebound hypertension for at least 8 hours after infusion is stopped if no other antihypertensive is prescribed.

● To convert to oral therapy, discontinue or titrate drug downward while appropriate oral therapy is established. When an oral antihypertensive is started, consider the lag time of onset of the oral agent's effect and continue BP monitoring until desired effect is achieved.

● Because drug contains lipids, restrict lipid intake in those with lipid metabolism disorders.

● Drug isn't a beta-adrenergic blocker; if given with beta-adrenergic blocker, gradually reduce beta-adrenergic blocker dosage to avoid withdrawal symptoms.

● Discard unopened vials that have been stored at room temperature for longer than 2 months.

PATIENT TEACHING

● Tell patient to report adverse reactions promptly.

● Advise patient to seek medical attention immediately if signs and symptoms of hypertensive emergency occur (visual changes, neurologic symptoms, HF).

clindamycin hydrochloride
klin-da-MYE-sin

Cleocin Hydrochloride, Dalacin C✤

clindamycin palmitate hydrochloride
Cleocin Pediatric, Dalacin C Flavored Granules✤

clindamycin phosphate (injection)
Cleocin Phosphate, Dalacin C Phosphate✤

Therapeutic class: Antibiotics
Pharmacologic class: Lincomycin derivatives

AVAILABLE FORMS
clindamycin hydrochloride
Capsules: 75 mg, 150 mg, 300 mg

clindamycin palmitate hydrochloride
Granules for oral solution: 75 mg/5 mL
clindamycin phosphate (injection)
Injectable infusion (in D$_5$W): 300 mg (50 mL), 600 mg (50 mL), 900 mg (50 mL)
Injection: 150 mg base/mL, 300 mg base/ 2 mL, 600 mg base/4 mL, 900 mg base/ 6 mL

INDICATIONS & DOSAGES
➤ **Infections caused by sensitive staphylococci, streptococci, pneumococci, *Bacteroides, Fusobacterium, Clostridium perfringens*, or other sensitive aerobic and anaerobic organisms**
Adults: 150 to 450 mg P.O. every 6 hours; or 300 to 600 mg I.M. or I.V. every 6, 8, or 12 hours. In more severe infections, dosage may be increased to 1,200 to 2,700 mg/day I.M. or I.V. in two, three, or four divided doses. In life-threatening infections, dosages as high as 4,800 mg daily can be given.
Children ages 1 month to 16 years: 20 to 40 mg/kg/day I.M. or I.V. in three or four equal doses. In beta-hemolytic streptococcal infections, treatment should continue for at least 10 days.
Neonates younger than age 1 month: 15 to 20 mg/kg/day I.M. or I.V. in three or four equal doses.

ADMINISTRATION
P.O.
● Obtain specimen for culture and sensitivity tests before giving first dose. Begin therapy while awaiting results.

● Give capsule form with a full glass of water to prevent esophageal irritation.

● Don't refrigerate reconstituted oral solution because it will thicken. Drug is stable for 2 weeks at room temperature.

I.V.
▼ Obtain specimen for culture and sensitivity tests before giving first dose. Begin therapy while awaiting results.

▼ Never give undiluted as a bolus.

▼ For infusion, dilute each 300 mg in 50 mL solution and give over 10 to 60 minutes at no more than 30 mg/minute.

▼ Check site daily for phlebitis and irritation.

▼ Drug may contain benzyl alcohol. Benzyl alcohol has been associated with a fatal gasping syndrome in premature infants.

▼ **Incompatibilities:** Allopurinol, aminophylline, ampicillin, azithromycin, barbiturates, calcium gluconate, cefazolin, ceftriaxone, ciprofloxacin hydrochloride, doxapram, filgrastim, fluconazole, gentamicin sulfate, idarubicin, magnesium sulfate, phenytoin sodium, ranitidine, rubber closures such as those on I.V. tubing, tobramycin sulfate.

I.M.
• Obtain specimen for culture and sensitivity tests before giving first dose. Begin therapy while awaiting results.
• Inject deep into muscle. Rotate sites. Don't exceed 600 mg per injection.

ACTION
Inhibits bacterial protein synthesis by binding to the 50S subunit of the ribosome.

Route	Onset	Peak	Duration
P.O.	Unknown	45–60 min	Unknown
I.V.	Immediate	Immediate	Unknown
I.M.	Unknown	3 hr	Unknown

Half-life: 2½ to 3 hours.

ADVERSE REACTIONS
CV: thrombophlebitis.
GI: nausea, *pseudomembranous colitis,* abdominal pain, diarrhea, vomiting.
Hematologic: *thrombocytopenia, transient leukopenia,* eosinophilia.
Hepatic: jaundice.
Skin: maculopapular rash, urticaria.
Other: *anaphylaxis.*

INTERACTIONS
Drug-drug. *Erythromycin:* May block access of clindamycin to its site of action. Avoid using together.
Neuromuscular blockers: May increase neuromuscular blockade. Monitor patient closely.
Paclitaxel: May increase paclitaxel effects. Observe patient for toxicity.
Drug-food. *Diet foods with sodium cyclamate:* May decrease drug level. Discourage patient from eating these foods.

EFFECTS ON LAB TEST RESULTS
• May increase alkaline phosphatase, AST, and bilirubin levels.
• May increase eosinophil count. May decrease platelet and WBC counts.

CONTRAINDICATIONS & CAUTIONS
• Contraindicated in patients hypersensitive to drug or lincomycin. Severe hypersensitivity reactions requiring emergency treatment have been reported.
• Clindamycin use may result in overgrowth of nonsusceptible organisms, particularly yeasts. Monitor patient for sign of superinfection.
⚠ *Alert:* Some oral products may contain tartrazine, which can cause allergic reactions that are frequently see in patients with aspirin hypersensitivity. Refer to manufacturer's instructions.
• Use cautiously in neonates and patients with renal or hepatic disease, asthma, history of GI disease, or significant allergies.
• Severe or fatal reactions such as toxic epidermal necrolysis have been reported. Discontinue drug if severe skin reaction occurs.
Black Box Warning Clindamycin has been associated with development of CDAD, which may evolve into severe, possibly fatal, colitis; its use should be reserved for serious infections. If CDAD is suspected or confirmed, drug may need to be discontinued and appropriate treatment initiated. ∎
Dialyzable drug: No.

PREGNANCY-LACTATION-REPRODUCTION
• There are no adequate studies in pregnant women. Use during pregnancy only if clearly needed and potential benefit justifies potential risk to the fetus.
• Drug appears in breast milk. Use in breast-feeding women isn't recommended.

NURSING CONSIDERATIONS
• I.M. injection may raise CK level in response to muscle irritation.
• Monitor renal, hepatic, and hematopoietic functions during prolonged therapy.
• Observe patient for signs and symptoms of superinfection.
⚠ *Alert:* Don't give opioid antidiarrheals to treat drug-induced diarrhea; they may prolong and worsen this condition.

Black Box Warning Diarrhea, colitis, and pseudomembranous colitis have developed up to 2 months after cessation of drug therapy. ■
● Drug doesn't penetrate blood-brain barrier.

PATIENT TEACHING
● Advise patient to take capsule form with a full glass of water to prevent esophageal irritation.
● Warn patient that I.M. injection may be painful.
● Tell patient to report discomfort at I.V. insertion site.
● Instruct patient to report adverse reactions (especially diarrhea). Warn patient not to self-treat diarrhea because drug may cause life-threatening colitis.

clindamycin phosphate (topical)
klin-da-MYE-sin

Cleocin, Cleocin T, Clinda-Derm, Clindagel, Clinda-T✤, Clindesse, Clindets, Dalacin T✤, Evoclin

Therapeutic class: Antibiotics
Pharmacologic class: Lincomycin derivatives

AVAILABLE FORMS
Foam: 1%
Gel: 1%
Lotion: 1%
Pledget: 1%*
Topical cream: 1%, 2%
Topical solution: 1%*
Vaginal cream: 2%
Vaginal suppositories: 100 mg

INDICATIONS & DOSAGES
➤ **Inflammatory acne vulgaris**
Adults and children age 12 and older: Apply to skin b.i.d., morning and evening, or once daily if using Clindagel or Evoclin.
➤ **Bacterial vaginosis**
Adults: 1 applicatorful vaginally at bedtime for 3 to 7 days in nonpregnant women or 7 days in pregnant women, or 1 suppository vaginally at bedtime for 3 days, or 1 applicatorful of Clindesse vaginally as a single dose.

ADMINISTRATION
Topical
● Wash area with warm water and soap, rinse, pat dry, and wait 30 minutes after washing or shaving to apply.
● Avoid excessive washing of affected area.
● Apply to entire area, but avoid contact with eyes, nose, mouth, and other mucous membranes.
● Remove pledgets from foil just before use.
● Use pledgets only once and then discard; more than 1 pledget may be used per application.
● If using foam or Clindagel, discontinue use if there has been no improvement after 6 to 8 weeks, or if condition worsens.
Vaginal
● Make sure patient knows how to use applicators that come with drug.

ACTION
Bacteriostatic or bactericidal based on drug level and susceptibility of organism; suppresses growth of susceptible organisms in sebaceous glands by blocking protein synthesis.

Route	Onset	Peak	Duration
Topical, vaginal	Unknown	Unknown	Unknown

Half-life: Topical and vaginal cream, 1½ to 2½ hours; vaginal suppositories, 11 hours.

ADVERSE REACTIONS
CNS: headache.
EENT: pharyngitis.
GI: abdominal pain, bloody diarrhea, colitis including *pseudomembranous colitis*, constipation, diarrhea, GI upset.
GU: *Candida albicans* overgrowth, cervicitis, vaginitis, vulvar irritation, UTI, vaginal discharge, vaginal candidiasis.
Skin: dryness, redness, burning, contact dermatitis, irritation, rash, pruritus, swelling.

INTERACTIONS
Drug-drug. *Erythromycin:* May antagonize clindamycin's effect. Separate doses.

Isotretinoin: May cause cumulative dryness, resulting in excessive skin irritation. Use together cautiously.

Neuromuscular blockers: May increase action of neuromuscular blocker. Use together cautiously.

Drug-lifestyle. *Abrasive or medicated soaps or cleansers, acne products, or other preparations containing peeling drugs (benzoyl peroxide, resorcinol, salicylic acid, sulfur, tretinoin), alcohol-containing products (aftershave, cosmetics, perfumed toiletries, shaving creams or lotions), astringent soaps or cosmetics, medicated cosmetics or cover-ups:* May cause cumulative dryness, resulting in excessive skin irritation. Urge caution.

EFFECTS ON LAB TEST RESULTS
• May increase liver enzyme levels.

CONTRAINDICATIONS & CAUTIONS
• Contraindicated in patients hypersensitive to clindamycin or lincomycin and in those with history of ulcerative colitis, regional enteritis, or antibiotic-related colitis.

Dialyzable drug: No.

⚠ *Overdose S&S:* Systemic effects.

PREGNANCY-LACTATION-REPRODUCTION
• There are no adequate studies in pregnant women. Use during pregnancy only if clearly needed and potential benefit justifies potential risk to the fetus.
• Drug appears in breast milk. Patient should discontinue breast-feeding or discontinue drug, taking into account importance of drug to the mother.

NURSING CONSIDERATIONS
• For treating acne, drug may be used with tretinoin or benzoyl peroxide, as well as systemic antibiotics.
• Drug can cause excessive dryness.
• Topical solution and pledgets contain alcohol base, which may irritate eyes.
• Monitor elderly patients for systemic effects.

PATIENT TEACHING
• Tell patient to wash area with warm water and soap, rinse, pat dry, and wait 30 minutes after washing or shaving to apply.

• Warn patient to avoid excessive washing of area. Tell patient to cover entire affected area but to avoid contact with eyes, nose, mouth, and other mucous membranes.
• Instruct patient to use other prescribed acne medicines at a different time.
• Tell patient to use only as prescribed.
• Instruct patient to dab, not roll, applicator-tipped bottle. If tip becomes dry, patient should invert bottle and depress tip several times to moisten.
• Warn patient not to smoke while applying topical solution.
• For vaginal treatment, instruct patient how to use vaginal applicators.
• Advise patient that the vaginal form contains mineral oil, which can weaken latex or rubber products, such as condoms and diaphragms, and that she should use another form of birth control during and within 3 days of therapy.
• Advise patient to avoid sexual intercourse during vaginal treatment.
• Advise patient to avoid use of tampons or douches during vaginal treatment.
• Instruct patient to notify prescriber immediately if abdominal pain or diarrhea occurs. Inform patient that an antidiarrheal may worsen condition and should only be used as directed by prescriber.
• Tell patient to remove pledgets from foil before use.
• Advise patient to use pledgets only once and then discard. Also, more than 1 pledget may be used per application.
• Advise patient to complete entire course of therapy.

clobazam
KLOE-ba-zam

Onfi

Therapeutic class: Anticonvulsants
Pharmacologic class: Benzodiazepines
Controlled substance schedule: IV

AVAILABLE FORMS
Oral suspension: 2.5 mg/mL
Tablets: 10 mg, 20 mg

INDICATIONS & DOSAGES
➤ **Adjunctive treatment of seizures associated with Lennox-Gastaut syndrome**
Adults and children age 2 and older weighing more than 30 kg: Initially, 5 mg P.O. b.i.d. for 6 days. On day 7, increase to 10 mg P.O. b.i.d.; on day 14, titrate to 20 mg P.O. b.i.d. as tolerated. Maximum dose is 40 mg/day.
Adults and children age 2 and older weighing 30 kg or less: Initially, 5 mg P.O. once daily for 6 days. On day 7, increase to 5 mg P.O. b.i.d.; on day 14, titrate to 10 mg P.O. b.i.d. as tolerated. Maximum dose is 20 mg/day.
Adjust-a-dose: For elderly patients, those with mild to moderate hepatic impairment (Child-Pugh score 5 to 9), and those who are poor CYP2C19 metabolizers, initially 5 mg P.O. daily. Then titrate according to weight but at half the recommended dose. If necessary, may start an additional titration to the maximum dosage (20 or 40 mg/day depending on weight) on day 21. There are no dosage recommendations for patients with severe hepatic or renal impairment.

ADMINISTRATION
P.O.
• May give tablets whole or crushed and mixed in applesauce.
• May give with or without food.
• Shake oral suspension well before every dose and use only oral dosing syringe supplied with product.
• Use oral suspension within 90 days of first opening; discard any remaining product.
• To discontinue drug, taper gradually by 5 to 10 mg/day on a weekly basis.

ACTION
Thought to involve potentiating GABA neurotransmission, which results from binding at the benzodiazepine site of the GABA$_A$ receptor.

Route	Onset	Peak	Duration
P.O.	Rapid	½–4 hr	Unknown

Half-life: 36 to 42 hours.

ADVERSE REACTIONS
CNS: somnolence, lethargy, pyrexia, irritability, fatigue, sedation, ataxia, psychomotor hyperactivity, insomnia, aggression.
EENT: drooling.
GI: vomiting, constipation, dysphagia.
GU: UTI.
Metabolic: increased or decreased appetite.
Musculoskeletal: dysarthria.
Respiratory: URI, pneumonia, cough, bronchitis.
Skin: *Stevens-Johnson syndrome, toxic epidermal necrolysis.*

INTERACTIONS
Drug-drug. *CNS depressants (opioids, TCAs):* May increase sedation. Avoid use together.
CYP2C19 inhibitors (fluconazole, fluvoxamine, ketoconazole, omeprazole, ticlopidine): May increase levels of clobazam or its metabolite. Decrease clobazam dosage if needed.
Drugs metabolized by CYP2D6 inhibitors (dextromethorphan): May increase levels of drugs metabolized by CYP2D6 inhibitors. Decreased dosages of these drugs may be needed.
Hormonal contraceptives: May diminish contraceptive effectiveness. Patient should use nonhormonal contraceptives as needed.
Black Box Warning *Opioids:* May cause slow or difficult breathing, sedation, and death. Avoid use together. If use together is necessary, limit dosage and duration of each drug to the minimum necessary for desired effect. ∎
Drug-lifestyle. *Alcohol use:* May increase clobazam level by up to 50% and increase CNS depression. Discourage alcohol use.

EFFECTS ON LAB TEST RESULTS
None reported.

CONTRAINDICATIONS & CAUTIONS
• Contraindicated in patients hypersensitive to drug or its components.
• Withdraw clobazam gradually to minimize risk of precipitating seizures, seizure exacerbation, status epilepticus, or withdrawal signs and symptoms (seizures, psychosis, hallucinations, behavioral disorder, tremor, anxiety).

Black Box Warning Opioid drugs should only be prescribed with benzodiazepines or other CNS depressants to patients for whom alternative treatment options are inadequate. ∎

• Use cautiously in patients with history of dependence.

• Drug may increase risk of suicidal thoughts or behavior.

Dialyzable drug: Unknown.

⚠ *Overdose S&S:* Drowsiness, confusion, lethargy, respiratory depression, hypotension, ataxia, coma.

PREGNANCY-LACTATION-REPRODUCTION

• There are no adequate well-controlled studies in pregnant women. Use during pregnancy only if benefit to mother outweighs risk to the fetus.

• Neonatal flaccidity, respiratory and feeding difficulties, hypothermia, and withdrawal signs and symptoms have occurred in infants born to women who received benzodiazepines, including clobazam, late in pregnancy.

• Advise pregnant women to enroll in the North American Antiepileptic Drug Pregnancy Registry by calling 1-888-233-2334 or visiting www.aedpregnancyregistry.org.

• Drug appears in breast milk. Patient should discontinue breast-feeding or discontinue drug, taking into account importance of drug to the mother.

NURSING CONSIDERATIONS

⚠ *Alert:* Monitor patients for skin reactions (rash, blistering or peeling skin, mouth sores, hives). Rare but serious skin reactions, including Stevens-Johnson syndrome and toxic epidermal necrolysis, have occurred with drug use, especially during first 8 weeks of treatment or when reintroducing therapy. Discontinue drug at first sign of reaction unless reaction is obviously not drug-related. Don't resume drug if rash is suggestive of Stevens-Johnson syndrome or toxic epidermal necrolysis.

⚠ *Alert:* Drug may increase risk of suicidal thoughts or behavior. Monitor patients treated with AEDs for indications of emergence or worsening of depression, suicidal thoughts or behavior, or unusual changes in mood or behavior.

• Monitor patients for signs and symptoms of abuse or physical dependence.

• Monitor patients for somnolence. This can occur at all dosage ranges, is usually seen within the first month, and then may subside with continued therapy.

• Monitor patients for dependence. Dependence may occur at the recommended dosage range over only a few weeks. Risk increases with increasing dosage and duration of treatment. Risk is increased in those with a history of alcohol or drug abuse.

PATIENT TEACHING

Black Box Warning Caution the patient or the caregiver of a patient taking an opioid drug with a benzodiazepine, CNS depressant, or alcohol to seek immediate medical attention if the patient has symptoms of dizziness, light-headedness, extreme sleepiness, slowed or difficult breathing, or unresponsiveness. ∎

• Advise patient and caregivers to notify health care providers before taking or giving clobazam with other CNS depressants (other benzodiazepines, opioids, TCAs, sedating antihistamines, alcohol).

• Inform patient to use caution if operating heavy machinery, including cars, when taking drug until its effects are known.

• Caution patient and caregivers not to stop drug or change dosage without first discussing with prescriber.

• Advise women using hormonal contraceptives to use nonhormonal methods during therapy and to continue these methods for 28 days after stopping drug.

• Caution patient and caregivers that drug may increase risk of suicidal thoughts. Tell them to report signs and symptoms of depression or changes in mood or behavior.

• Instruct female patient to inform health care provider if she is pregnant, plans to become pregnant, or plans to breast-feed during therapy.

• Instruct patient or caregiver to discard any remaining oral suspension within 90 days of first opening the bottle.

• Teach patient or caregiver how to use the dosing syringe for the oral suspension.

---

clobetasol propionate
kloe-BAY-ta-sol

Clobex, Cormax, Embeline,
Embeline E, Olux, Olux-E

Therapeutic class: Corticosteroids
Pharmacologic class: Corticosteroids

AVAILABLE FORMS
Cream: 0.05%
Foam: 0.05%*
Gel: 0.05%
Lotion: 0.05%
Ointment: 0.05%
Scalp application: 0.05%*
Shampoo: 0.05%*
Solution: 0.05%*
Spray: 0.05%*

INDICATIONS & DOSAGES
➤ **Short-term topical treatment for moderate to severe plaque-type psoriasis of nonscalp regions, excluding the face and intertriginous areas**
Adults: Apply thin layer of lotion or cream to affected areas b.i.d., morning and evening, for up to 14 days. Or, apply spray directly onto affected areas b.i.d. and rub in gently and completely. For localized lesions (less than 10% of BSA) that haven't improved sufficiently, continue treatment for up to 2 more weeks. Total dose shouldn't exceed 50 g (50 mL) weekly.
Adolescents age 16 and older: Apply thin layer of emollient cream to affected areas b.i.d. and rub in gently and completely. If applied to 5% to 10% of BSA, can be used for up to 4 consecutive weeks. Total dosage shouldn't exceed 50 g (50 mL) weekly.
➤ **Inflammation and pruritus from corticosteroid-responsive dermatoses**
Adults: Apply thin layer of cream, emollient cream, foam, gel, lotion, or ointment to affected areas b.i.d., morning and evening, for maximum of 14 days. Total dose shouldn't exceed 50 g (50 mL) weekly.
Children age 12 and older: Apply thin layer of cream, emollient cream, foam, gel, or ointment to affected areas b.i.d., morning and evening, for maximum of 14 days. Total dose shouldn't exceed 50 g (50 mL) weekly.

➤ **Short-term topical treatment of mild to moderate plaque-type psoriasis of nonscalp regions, excluding the face and intertriginous areas**
Adults and children age 12 and older: Apply thin layer of foam to affected areas b.i.d., morning and evening, for maximum of 14 days. Total dose shouldn't exceed 50 g (21 capfuls) weekly.
➤ **Inflammation and pruritus of moderate to severe corticosteroid-responsive dermatoses of the scalp**
Adults and children age 12 and older: Apply thin layer of solution to the affected scalp area b.i.d., morning and evening. Massage into affected scalp area gently and completely. Limit treatment to 14 days, with no more than 50 g (50 mL) weekly.
➤ **Moderate to severe scalp psoriasis**
Adults: Apply thin film of shampoo to affected areas of dry scalp once daily. Leave in place for 15 minutes before lathering and rinsing. Limit treatment to 4 consecutive weeks. If complete disease control isn't achieved after 4 weeks, substitute treatment with a less potent topical steroid. Maximum dose is 50 g (50 mL) weekly. Or, apply thin layer of foam to scalp b.i.d. for up to 2 weeks. Maximum dose is 50 g (21 capfuls) weekly.
Children age 12 and older: Apply thin layer of foam to scalp b.i.d. for up to 2 weeks. Maximum dose is 50 g (21 capfuls) weekly.

ADMINISTRATION
Topical
● Apply the smallest amount that will cover affected area.
● Gently wash skin before applying. To prevent skin damage, rub medication in gently and completely. When treating hairy sites, part hair and apply directly to lesions.
● To dispense foam, hold the can upside down and depress the actuator.
● Avoid applying near eyes or mucous membranes or in ear canal.
🛈 *Alert:* Don't use occlusive dressings or bandages. Don't cover or wrap treated areas unless directed by prescriber.

ACTION
Unclear. Diffuses across cell membranes to form complexes with receptors, showing

---

♣ Canada   ◇ OTC   ◆ Off-label use   ✔ Photoguide   ⊚ Do not crush   *Liquid contains alcohol.

anti-inflammatory, antipruritic, vasoconstrictive, and antiproliferative activity. Considered a very-high-potency to high-potency drug, according to vasoconstrictive properties.

Route	Onset	Peak	Duration
Topical	Unknown	Unknown	Unknown

Half-life: Unknown.

ADVERSE REACTIONS

GU: glycosuria.
Metabolic: hyperglycemia.
Skin: burning, pruritus, irritation, dryness, erythema, folliculitis, perioral dermatitis, allergic contact dermatitis, hypopigmentation, hypertrichosis, acneiform eruptions, skin atrophy, telangiectasia.
Other: *HPA axis suppression,* Cushing syndrome, finger numbness.

INTERACTIONS
None significant.

EFFECTS ON LAB TEST RESULTS
• May increase glucose level.

CONTRAINDICATIONS & CAUTIONS
• Contraindicated in patients hypersensitive to corticosteroids and in those with primary scalp infections (scalp solution only).
• Topical corticosteroids may be absorbed and cause hyperadrenocorticism or suppression of the HPA axis, particularly in younger children and in patients receiving high doses for prolonged periods.
• Rarely, prolonged treatment with corticosteroids is associated with development of Kaposi sarcoma.
• Don't use as monotherapy for primary bacterial infections (impetigo, paronychia, erysipelas, cellulitis, angular cheilitis, erythrasma), rosacea, perioral dermatitis, or acne.
• Don't use very-high-potency or high-potency agents on the face, groin, or axilla areas.
• Drug isn't for ophthalmic use.
• Use cautiously in children
Dialyzable drug: Unknown.
⚠ *Overdose S&S:* Systemic effects.

PREGNANCY-LACTATION-REPRODUCTION
• There are no adequate studies in pregnant women. Use during pregnancy only if potential benefit justifies potential risk to the fetus. Extensive use during pregnancy isn't recommended.
• It isn't known if drug appears in breast milk. Use cautiously in breast-feeding women.

NURSING CONSIDERATIONS
• If antifungal or antibiotic combined with corticosteroid fails to provide prompt improvement, stop corticosteroid until infection is controlled.
• Stop drug and notify prescriber if skin infection, striae, or atrophy occurs.
• HPA axis suppression occurs at doses as low as 2 g daily.

PATIENT TEACHING
• Teach patient how to apply drug and to avoid contact with eyes.
• Tell patient to wash hands after application.
• Tell patient to stop drug and report signs of systemic absorption, skin irritation or ulceration, hypersensitivity, or infection.
• Warn patient to use drug for no longer than 14 consecutive days, except shampoo, which can be used for 4 consecutive weeks.
• Tell patient using the foam to invert can and dispense a small amount of Olux foam (up to a golf ball-size dollop) into the cap of the can, onto a saucer or other cool surface, or directly on the lesion, taking care to avoid contact with the eyes. Dispensing directly onto hands isn't recommended because the foam will melt immediately on contact with warm skin. Tell him to move hair away from affected area of scalp so that foam can be applied to each affected area.
• Tell patient using foam that contents are flammable and under pressure, so he should avoid smoking during and immediately after application and should keep can away from flames. Also tell him not to puncture or incinerate container.

---

clonazepam
kloe-NAZ-e-pam

Klonopin🖉

Therapeutic class: Anticonvulsants
Pharmacologic class: Benzodiazepines
Controlled substance schedule: IV

AVAILABLE FORMS
ODTs: 0.125 mg, 0.25 mg, 0.5 mg, 1 mg, 2 mg
Tablets: 0.5 mg, 1 mg, 2 mg

INDICATIONS & DOSAGES
➤ **Lennox-Gastaut syndrome, atypical absence seizures, akinetic and myoclonic seizures**
Adults and children older than age 10 or weighing more than 30 kg: Initially, no more than 1.5 mg P.O. daily in three divided doses. May be increased by 0.5 to 1 mg every 3 days until seizures are controlled or adverse effects prevent further increases. If given in unequal doses, give largest dose at bedtime. Maximum recommended daily dose is 20 mg.
Children age 10 and younger or weighing 30 kg or less: Initially, 0.01 to 0.03 mg/kg P.O. daily (not to exceed 0.05 mg/kg daily) in two or three divided doses. Increase by 0.25 to 0.5 mg every third day to maximum maintenance dose of 0.1 to 0.2 mg/kg P.O. daily divided into three equal doses, as needed.
➤ **Panic disorder**
Adults: Initially, 0.25 mg P.O. b.i.d.; increase to target dose of 1 mg daily after 3 days. Some patients may benefit from dosages up to maximum of 4 mg daily. To achieve 4 mg daily, increase dosage in increments of 0.125 to 0.25 mg b.i.d. every 3 days, as tolerated, until panic disorder is controlled. Taper drug with decrease of 0.125 mg b.i.d. every 3 days until drug is stopped.

ADMINISTRATION
P.O.
● Have patient swallow tablets whole with water. Give ODT to patient with or without water.

● Peel back the foil of the ODT pouch carefully. Don't push ODT through foil.
● Pharmacist can prepare oral suspension from tablets if necessary for younger patients.

ACTION
Unknown. Probably acts by facilitating the effects of the inhibitory neurotransmitter GABA.

Route	Onset	Peak	Duration
P.O.	20–40 min	1–4 hr	6–12 hr

Half-life: Adults, 17 to 60 hours; children, 22 to 33 hours.

ADVERSE REACTIONS
CNS: amnesia, aphonia, choreiform movements, coma, confusion, depression, dysarthria, dysdiadochokinesis, "glassy-eyed" appearance, hallucinations, headache, hemiparesis, hypotonia, hysteria, increased libido, insomnia, psychosis, slurred speech, tremor, vertigo, paradoxical reactions (aggressive behavior, agitation, anxiety, excitability, hostility, irritability, nervousness, nightmares and vivid dreams, sleep disturbances), fever, ataxia, abnormal coordination, somnolence, dizziness, nervousness, reduced intellectual ability.
CV: palpitations.
EENT: abnormal eye movements, diplopia, nystagmus, blurred vision, pharyngitis, rhinitis, sinusitis.
GI: anorexia, coated tongue, constipation, diarrhea, dry mouth, encopresis, gastritis, increased or decreased appetite, nausea, sore gums, abdominal pain.
GU: dysuria, enuresis, nocturia, urine retention, colpitis, dysmenorrhea, delayed ejaculation, erectile dysfunction, urinary frequency, UTI.
Hematologic: anemia, eosinophilia, *leukopenia, thrombocytopenia.*
Hepatic: hepatomegaly, transient elevations of serum transaminases and alkaline phosphatase.
Metabolic: dehydration, weight loss or gain.
Musculoskeletal: muscle weakness, muscle pains.
Respiratory: chest congestion, hypersecretion in upper respiratory tract passages,

respiratory depression, rhinorrhea, shortness of breath, bronchitis, URI, cough.
Skin: hair loss, hirsutism, rash.
Other: ankle and facial edema, general deterioration, lymphadenopathy, allergic reaction, influenza.

INTERACTIONS
Drug-drug. *Carbamazepine, phenobarbital, phenytoin:* May lower clonazepam levels. Monitor patient closely.
Cimetidine: May increase effects of clonazepam. Adjust clonazepam dosage as needed.
Clozapine: May cause delirium, sedation, sialorrhea, ataxia, severe orthostatic hypotension, and respiratory depression. Don't start drugs simultaneously. Adding clonazepam to an established clozapine regimen may carry less risk than adding clozapine to clonazepam. Monitor patient carefully, especially during the first 48 hours of coadministration.
CNS depressants: May increase CNS depression. Avoid using together.
Digoxin: May increase digoxin level and toxicity. Monitor digoxin level.
Disulfiram: May increase toxic effects of clonazepam. Reduce clonazepam dosage as needed.
Fluconazole, itraconazole, ketoconazole, miconazole: May increase and prolong drug levels, CNS depression, and psychomotor impairment. Avoid using together.
Methadone: May increase potential for fatal respiratory depression. Use cautiously.
Omeprazole: May increase effects and toxicities of clonazepam. Adjust clonazepam dosage as needed or discontinue one or both drugs.
Black Box Warning *Opioids:* May cause slow or difficult breathing, sedation, and death. Avoid use together. If use together is necessary, limit dosage and duration of each drug to the minimum necessary for desired effect. ■
Protease inhibitors (nelfinavir, ritonavir): May cause severe respiratory depression. Monitor patient carefully.
Theophylline: May decrease clonazepam effects. Monitor patient closely.
Valproic acid: May increase clonazepam toxicity and increase seizure risk and teratogenic effects of both drugs in first trimester. Use cautiously.
Drug-herb. *St. John's wort:* May increase hepatic metabolism, resulting in decreased drug effects. Adjust clonazepam dosage as needed.
Drug-lifestyle. *Alcohol use:* May cause additive CNS effects. Discourage use together.
Smoking: May increase clearance of clonazepam. Monitor patient for decreased drug effects.

EFFECTS ON LAB TEST RESULTS
● May increase LFT values and eosinophil count. May decrease platelet and WBC counts.

CONTRAINDICATIONS & CAUTIONS
Black Box Warning Opioid drugs should only be prescribed with benzodiazepines or other CNS depressants to patients for whom alternative treatment options are inadequate. ■
● Contraindicated in patients hypersensitive to benzodiazepines and in those with significant hepatic disease or acute angle-closure glaucoma.
● Use cautiously in patients with mixed-type seizures because drug may cause generalized tonic-clonic seizures.
● Use cautiously in children and in patients with chronic respiratory disease, open-angle glaucoma, porphyria, or a history of drug or alcohol addiction.
● Use cautiously in elderly patients. Drug may accumulate due to potential decrease in hepatic and renal function.
Dialyzable drug: No.
⚠ *Overdose S&S:* Somnolence, confusion, coma, diminished reflexes.

PREGNANCY-LACTATION-REPRODUCTION
● Drug may cause fetal harm. Use during pregnancy only if clearly needed and potential benefit justifies potential risk to the fetus.
● Drug may cause neonatal flaccidity, respiratory and feeding difficulties, and hypothermia in infants born to women who received benzodiazepines late in pregnancy. In addition, neonates born to women who received benzodiazepines late in pregnancy may be at some risk for experiencing

---

Reactions in bold italics are *life-threatening*. Interactions may have a *rapid onset* or a *delayed onset*.

withdrawal symptoms during the postnatal period.

• Encourage women who are taking drug during pregnancy to register in the North American Antiepileptic Drug Pregnancy Registry by calling 1-888-233-2334 or visiting www.aedpregnancyregistry.org; registration must be done by patients themselves.

• Drug appears in breast milk. Patient should discontinue breast-feeding or discontinue drug, taking into account importance of drug to the mother.

NURSING CONSIDERATIONS

🔔 *Alert:* Closely monitor all patients for changes in behavior that may indicate worsening of suicidal thoughts or behavior or depression.

• Don't stop drug abruptly because this may worsen seizures. Call prescriber at once if adverse reactions develop.

• Assess elderly patient's response closely. Elderly patients are more sensitive to drug's CNS effects.

• Monitor patient for oversedation.

• Monitor CBC and LFTs.

• Withdrawal symptoms are similar to those of barbiturates.

• To reduce inconvenience of somnolence when drug is used for panic disorder, giving one dose at bedtime may be desirable.

• *Look alike–sound alike:* Don't confuse clonazepam with clonidine, clozapine, or lorazepam. Don't confuse Klonopin with clonidine.

PATIENT TEACHING

Black Box Warning Caution the patient or the caregiver of a patient taking an opioid drug with a benzodiazepine, CNS depressant, or alcohol to seek immediate medical attention if the patient has symptoms of dizziness, light-headedness, extreme sleepiness, slowed or difficult breathing, or unresponsiveness. ■

• Advise patient to avoid driving and other hazardous activities that require mental alertness until drug's CNS effects are known.

• Instruct parent to monitor child's school performance because drug may interfere with attentiveness.

• Warn patient and parents not to stop drug abruptly because seizures may occur.

• Advise patient that drug isn't for use during pregnancy or breast-feeding.

• Tell patient to open pouch of ODTs and peel back the foil. He shouldn't push the tablet *through* the foil.

• Tell patient to use dry hands when removing the ODT.

• Tell patient that ODTs can be taken with or without water but that regular tablets should be swallowed whole with water.

clonidine
KLOE-ni-deen

clonidine hydrochloride
Catapres, Catapres-TTS, Dixarit✿, Duraclon, Kapvay

Therapeutic class: Antihypertensives
Pharmacologic class: Centrally acting alpha agonists

AVAILABLE FORMS
Injection for epidural use: 100 mcg/mL
Injection for epidural use, concentrate: 500 mcg/mL
Tablets: 0.025 mg✿, 0.1 mg, 0.2 mg, 0.3 mg
Tablets (extended-release) 🚫: 0.1 mg, 0.2 mg
Transdermal: 0.1 mg/24 hours, 0.2 mg/24 hours, 0.3 mg/24 hours

INDICATIONS & DOSAGES
➤ **Essential and renal hypertension**
Adults and children age 12 and older: Initially, 0.1 mg P.O. b.i.d.; then increased by 0.1 mg daily on a weekly basis. Usual range is 0.2 to 0.6 mg daily in divided doses; infrequently, dosages as high as 2.4 mg daily are used.

Or, apply transdermal patch once every 7 days, starting with 0.1-mg system and adjusted with another 0.1-mg or larger system after 1 or 2 weeks if desired BP reduction isn't achieved.
➤ **Severe cancer pain that is unresponsive to epidural or spinal opiate analgesia or other more conventional methods of analgesia**

Adults: Initially, 30 mcg/hour by continuous epidural infusion. Experience with rates greater than 40 mcg/hour is limited.

Children: Initially, 0.5 mcg/kg/hour by epidural infusion. Dosage should be cautiously adjusted, based on response.

➤ **ADHD as monotherapy or as adjunctive therapy to stimulant medications**
Children ages 6 to 17: Initially, 0.1 mg extended-release tablet (Kapvay) P.O. at bedtime. Adjust by 0.1 mg/day at weekly intervals to desired response. With first dosage increase, give tablets b.i.d., with equal or higher dose given at bedtime. Maximum dose is 0.4 mg/day.

ADMINISTRATION
P.O.
● Don't crush, break, or allow patient to chew extended-release tablets.
● Immediate-release and extended-release forms can't be substituted on a milligram-per-milligram basis.
● Give last dose immediately before bedtime.
● Reduce dosage gradually over 2 to 4 days before discontinuing. Decrease dosage of extended-release form by no more than 0.1 mg every 3 to 7 days.

Transdermal
● Apply patch to nonhairy area of intact skin on upper arm or torso.
● When converting from oral to patch form, place patch on patient and gradually decrease oral dose over several days. Antihypertensive effect of patch takes 2 to 3 days to appear.

Epidural
Black Box Warning The injection form concentrate, containing 500 mcg/mL, must be diluted in NSS injection before use to yield 100 mcg/mL. ■

ACTION
Unknown. Thought to stimulate alpha$_2$ receptors and inhibit the central vasomotor centers, decreasing sympathetic outflow to the heart, kidneys, and peripheral vasculature, and lowering peripheral vascular resistance, BP, and HR.

Route	Onset	Peak	Duration
P.O. (immediate release)	30–60 min	1–3 hr	6–10 hr
P.O. (extended release)	1–2 wk	7–8 hr	Unknown
Transdermal	2–3 days	3 days	7 days
Epidural	Unknown	30–60 min	Unknown

Half-life: Immediate- and extended-release, 12 to 16 hours; transdermal, 20 hours; epidural, 1 to 2 hours.

ADVERSE REACTIONS
CNS: drowsiness, dizziness, sedation, weakness, fatigue, malaise, agitation, depression.
CV: *bradycardia, severe rebound hypertension,* orthostatic hypotension.
GI: constipation, dry mouth, nausea, vomiting, anorexia.
GU: urine retention, erectile dysfunction.
Metabolic: weight gain.
Skin: pruritus, dermatitis with transdermal patch, rash.
Other: loss of libido.

INTERACTIONS
Drug-drug. *Amitriptyline, amoxapine, clomipramine, desipramine, doxepin, imipramine, mirtazapine, nortriptyline, protriptyline, trimipramine:* May cause loss of BP control with life-threatening elevations in BP. Avoid using together.
Beta blockers: May cause life-threatening hypertension. Closely monitor BP.
CNS depressants: May increase CNS depression. Use together cautiously.
Digoxin, verapamil: May cause AV block and severe hypotension. Monitor BP and ECG.
Diuretics, other antihypertensives: May increase hypotensive effect. Monitor patient closely.
Levodopa: May reduce effectiveness of levodopa. Monitor patient.
MAO inhibitors, prazosin: May decrease antihypertensive effect. Use together cautiously.
Propranolol, other beta blockers: May cause paradoxical hypertensive response. Monitor patient carefully.

Reactions in bold italics are *life-threatening*. Interactions may have a *rapid onset* or a *delayed onset*.

Drug-herb. *Capsicum:* May reduce antihypertensive effectiveness. Discourage use together.

Ma huang: May decrease antihypertensive effects. Discourage use together.

EFFECTS ON LAB TEST RESULTS

● May decrease urinary excretion of vanillylmandelic acid and catecholamines. May cause a weakly positive Coombs test result.

CONTRAINDICATIONS & CAUTIONS

● Contraindicated in patients hypersensitive to drug.

● Transdermal form is contraindicated in patients hypersensitive to any component of the adhesive layer of transdermal system.

● Epidural form is contraindicated in patients receiving anticoagulant therapy, in those with bleeding diathesis, in those with an injection-site infection, and in those who are hemodynamically unstable or have severe CV disease.

● Use cautiously in patients with severe coronary insufficiency, conduction disturbances, recent MI, cerebrovascular disease, chronic renal failure, or impaired liver function.

Dialyzable drug: No.

⚠ *Overdose S&S:* Early hypertension, then hypotension; bradycardia; respiratory and CNS depression; hypothermia; drowsiness; decreased or absent reflexes; weakness; irritability; miosis. With large overdoses: Reversible cardiac conduction defects or arrhythmias, apnea, coma, seizures.

PREGNANCY-LACTATION-REPRODUCTION

● There are no adequate well-controlled studies in pregnant women. Use during pregnancy only if clearly needed and potential benefit justifies potential risk to the fetus.

Black Box Warning Epidural clonidine isn't recommended for obstetric, postpartum, or perioperative pain management due to the risk of hemodynamic instability, except in rare cases in which the potential benefits outweigh the risks. ■

● Drug appears in breast milk. Patient should discontinue breast-feeding or discontinue drug, taking into account importance of drug to the mother.

NURSING CONSIDERATIONS

● Drug may be given to lower BP rapidly in some hypertensive emergencies.

● Monitor BP and pulse rate frequently. Dosage is usually adjusted to patient's BP and tolerance.

● Elderly patients may be more sensitive than younger ones to drug's hypotensive effects.

● Observe patient for tolerance to drug's therapeutic effects, which may require increased dosage.

● Noticeable antihypertensive effects of transdermal clonidine may take 2 to 3 days. Oral antihypertensive therapy may have to be continued in the interim.

🔆 *Alert:* Remove transdermal patch before defibrillation or cardioversion to prevent arcing.

● Stop drug gradually by reducing dosage over 2 to 4 days to avoid rapid rise in BP, agitation, headache, and tremor. When stopping therapy in patients receiving both clonidine and a beta blocker, gradually withdraw the beta blocker several days before gradually stopping clonidine to minimize adverse reactions.

● Don't stop drug before surgery.

● When drug is given epidurally, carefully monitor infusion pump, and inspect catheter tubing for obstruction or dislodgment.

● *Look alike–sound alike:* Don't confuse clonidine with clonazepam, clozapine, Klonopin, quinidine, or clomiphene.

PATIENT TEACHING

● Instruct patient to take drug exactly as prescribed.

● Advise patient that stopping drug abruptly may cause severe high rebound BP. Tell him dosage must be reduced gradually over 2 to 4 days, as instructed by prescriber.

● Tell patient to take the last dose immediately before bedtime.

● Reassure patient that the transdermal patch usually remains attached despite showering and other routine daily activities. Instruct him on the use of the adhesive overlay to provide additional skin adherence, if needed. Also tell him to place patch at a different site each week.

● Caution patient that drug may cause drowsiness but that this adverse effect usually diminishes over 4 to 6 weeks.

• Inform patient that dizziness upon standing can be minimized by rising slowly from a sitting or lying position and avoiding sudden position changes.

• Advise patient that, if he is scheduled for an MRI, he should alert the facility that he is wearing a transdermal patch.

clopidogrel bisulfate
cloe-PID-oh-grel

Plavix◆

Therapeutic class: Antiplatelet drugs
Pharmacologic class: Platelet aggregation inhibitors

AVAILABLE FORMS
Tablets: 75 mg, 300 mg

INDICATIONS & DOSAGES
➤ **To reduce thrombotic events in patients with atherosclerosis documented by recent stroke, MI, or peripheral arterial disease**
Adults: 75 mg P.O. daily.
➤ **To reduce thrombotic events in patients with acute coronary syndrome (unstable angina/non-ST-elevation MI), including those receiving drugs and those undergoing PCI (with or without stent) or CABG**
Adults: Initially, a single 300-mg P.O. loading dose; then 75 mg P.O. once daily. Start and continue aspirin (75 to 325 mg once daily) with clopidogrel.
➤ **Acute ST-segment elevation MI**
Adults: 75 mg P.O. once daily, with aspirin, with or without thrombolytics. A 300-mg loading dose is optional.

ADMINISTRATION
P.O.
• Give drug without regard to meals.
• Patient shouldn't consume grapefruit or grapefruit juice.

ACTION
Inhibits the binding of adenosine diphosphate (ADP) to its platelet receptor, impeding ADP-mediated activation and subsequent platelet aggregation, and irreversibly modifies the platelet ADP receptor.

Route	Onset	Peak	Duration
P.O.	2 hr	45 min	5 days

Half-life: 6 hours.

ADVERSE REACTIONS
CNS: confusion, ***fatal intracranial bleeding,*** hallucinations.
CV: hypotension.
EENT: epistaxis, rhinitis, taste disorder.
GI: ***hemorrhage,*** abdominal pain, constipation, diarrhea, dyspepsia, gastritis, ulcers.
GU: UTI, hematuria.
Hematologic: ***thrombotic thrombocytopenic purpura.***
Musculoskeletal: arthralgia, myalgia, arthritis.
Respiratory: ***bronchospasm,*** interstitial pneumonitis, respiratory tract bleeding.
Skin: rash, pruritus, bruising, eczema, ***erythema multiforme,*** urticaria, ***Stevens-Johnson syndrome, toxic epidermal necrolysis.***
Other: flulike syndrome, ***angioedema, anaphylaxis,*** serum sickness.

INTERACTIONS
Drug-drug. *Aspirin, NSAIDs:* May increase risk of GI bleeding. Monitor patient.
Bupropion: May elevate bupropion plasma concentration. Closely monitor patient and adjust bupropion dosage as needed when clopidogrel is started or stopped.
Macrolides: May inhibit antiplatelet effect. Adjust clopidogrel dosage as needed. Consider using azithromycin if a macrolide is necessary.
Rifamycins: May increase antiplatelet effect. Carefully monitor platelet function when starting, stopping, or changing rifamycin dosage. Adjust clopidogrel dosage as needed.
Salicylates: May increase the risk of serious bleeding in patients with TIA or ischemic stroke. Avoid use together.
Strong or moderate CYP2C19 inhibitors (cimetidine, esomeprazole, etravirine, felbamate, fluconazole, fluoxetine, fluvoxamine, ketoconazole, omeprazole, PPIs, ticlopidine, voriconazole): May decrease effects of clopidogrel. Avoid use together.

Reactions in bold italics are ***life-threatening.*** Interactions may have a *rapid onset* or a ***delayed onset.***

Warfarin: May increase risk of bleeding. Use together cautiously.

Drug-herb. *Herbs with antiplatelet activity (anise, bilberry, cat's claw, chamomile, dong quai, evening primrose, fenugreek, garlic, ginger, ginkgo biloba, ginseng, green tea, horseradish, licorice, red clover, turmeric, and many others):* May increase risk of bleeding. Discourage use together.

Drug-food. *Grapefruit, grapefruit juice:* May reduce drug's antiplatelet effects. Avoid use together.

EFFECTS ON LAB TEST RESULTS
• May decrease platelet count.

CONTRAINDICATIONS & CAUTIONS
• Contraindicated in patients hypersensitive to drug or its components, in those with a history of hypersensitivity or hematologic reaction to other thienopyridines, and in those with pathologic bleeding (such as peptic ulcer or intracranial hemorrhage).
• Hypersensitivity reactions, including rash, angioedema, and hematologic reactions, have been reported.
• Consider discontinuing drug 5 days before elective surgery, including elective CABG. Platelet aggregation won't return to normal for at least 5 days after drug has been stopped.
• Premature interruption of therapy may result in stent thrombosis with subsequent fatal or nonfatal MI. Duration of therapy, in general, is determined by type of stent placed (bare metal or drug eluting) and whether an acute coronary syndrome event was ongoing at the time of placement.
• Use cautiously in patients at risk for increased bleeding from trauma, surgery, or other pathologic conditions and in those with renal or hepatic impairment.
Dialyzable drug: Unknown.
⚠ *Overdose S&S:* Prolonged bleeding time, bleeding complications.

PREGNANCY-LACTATION-REPRODUCTION
• Information related to use during pregnancy is limited. Use cautiously in pregnant women and only if clearly needed.
• It isn't known if drug appears in breast milk. Patient should discontinue breast-feeding or discontinue drug, taking into account importance of drug to the mother.

NURSING CONSIDERATIONS
Black Box Warning Drug effectiveness depends on the drug's activation to an active metabolite by the cytochrome P450 system, principally CYP2C19. Patients who are poor metabolizers exhibit higher CV event rates after acute coronary syndrome or PCI than patients with normal CYP2C19 function. Tests are available to assess a patient's CYP2C19 genotype. Consider alternative treatment for patients identified as poor metabolizers. ■
• Consider discontinuing drug 5 days before elective surgery, including elective CABG. Platelet aggregation won't return to normal for at least 5 days after drug has been stopped.
• *Alert:* Drug may cause fatal thrombotic thrombocytopenic purpura (thrombocytopenia, hemolytic anemia, neurologic findings, renal dysfunction, and fever) that requires urgent treatment, including plasmapheresis.
• *Look alike–sound alike:* Don't confuse Plavix with Paxil.

PATIENT TEACHING
• Advise patient that it may take longer than usual to stop bleeding. Tell him to refrain from activities in which trauma and bleeding may occur, and encourage him to wear a seat belt when in a car.
• Instruct patient to notify prescriber if unusual bleeding or bruising occurs.
• Tell patient to inform all health care providers, including dentists, before undergoing procedures or starting new drug therapy, that he is taking drug.
• Inform patient that drug may be taken without regard to meals.

clotrimazole
kloe-TRIM-a-zole

Canesten❖, Clotrimaderm❖, Cruex ◊, Desenex ◊, FungiCure Intensive NailGuard ◊, Gyne-Lotrimin ◊, Gyne-Lotrimin 3 ◊, Lotrimin AF ◊, Mycelex ◊, Mycelex-7 ◊, Trivagizole 3 ◊

Therapeutic class: Antifungals
Pharmacologic class: Imidazole derivatives

AVAILABLE FORMS
Combination pack: Vaginal tablets 100 mg and vulvar cream 1% ◊, vaginal tablets 200 mg and vulvar cream 1% ◊
Topical cream: 1%
Topical lotion: 1%
Topical solution: 1%
Troches (lozenges) ⓞⓉⓒ*:* 10 mg
Vaginal cream: 1% ◊, 2% ◊, 10%❖ ◊
Vaginal suppositories: 100 mg ◊, 200 mg ◊
Vaginal tablets: 100 mg ◊, 200 mg❖ ◊, 500 mg❖ ◊

INDICATIONS & DOSAGES
➤ **Superficial fungal infections (tinea corporis, tinea cruris, tinea pedis, tinea versicolor, candidiasis)**
Adults and children age 2 and older: Apply thin film and massage into affected and surrounding area, morning and evening, for 2 to 4 weeks. If improvement doesn't occur after 4 weeks, reevaluate patient.
➤ **Vulvovaginal candidiasis**
Adults and children age 12 and older: One 100-mg vaginal suppository inserted daily at bedtime for 7 consecutive days. Or, one 200-mg vaginal suppository at bedtime for 3 days. Or, 1 applicatorful of vaginal cream daily at bedtime for 3 days (2%) or 7 days (1%).
➤ **Oropharyngeal candidiasis**
Adults and children age 3 and older: Patient should dissolve lozenge in mouth over 15 to 30 minutes five times daily for 14 consecutive days. When drug is used for initial treatment in patients with HIV-1 infection, duration of therapy is 7 to 14 days.
➤ **To prevent oropharyngeal candidiasis in patients immunocompromised** by chemotherapy, radiotherapy, or corticosteroid therapy in the treatment of leukemia, solid tumors, or renal transplantation
Adults: Patient should dissolve lozenge in mouth over 15 to 30 minutes t.i.d. for duration of chemotherapy or until corticosteroid is reduced to maintenance levels.

ADMINISTRATION
P.O.
● Lozenges should dissolve in mouth and not be chewed, for full benefit.
Topical
● Clean and dry area before applying drug.
● Don't use occlusive wrappings or dressings.
Vaginal
● Insert suppository high into vagina.
● Applicators for cream and some suppositories are disposable. If not disposable, wash applicator with soap and warm water immediately after use. Rinse thoroughly and dry.

ACTION
Fungistatic or fungicidal, depending on level. Alters fungal cell-wall permeability and produces osmotic instability.

Route	Onset	Peak	Duration
P.O.	Unknown	Unknown	3 hr
Topical, vaginal	Unknown	Unknown	Unknown

Half-life: Unknown.

ADVERSE REACTIONS
GI: lower abdominal cramps, nausea and vomiting with lozenges.
GU: mild vaginal burning or irritation, urinary frequency.
Skin: erythema, blistering, burning, edema, general irritation, peeling, pruritus, skin fissures, stinging, urticaria.

INTERACTIONS
None significant.

EFFECTS ON LAB TEST RESULTS
● May increase liver enzyme levels.

CONTRAINDICATIONS & CAUTIONS
● Contraindicated in patients hypersensitive to drug.

Reactions in bold italics are *life-threatening*. Interactions may have a *rapid onset* or a *delayed onset*.

• Contraindicated for ophthalmic use.
Dialyzable drug: Unknown.

PREGNANCY-LACTATION-REPRODUCTION
• There are no adequate studies in pregnant women. Use lozenges during pregnancy only if potential benefit justifies potential risk to the fetus.
• Use topical clotrimazole during first trimester only if clearly indicated.
• Manual insertion of vaginal tablets may be preferred over use of vaginal applicator. Use only on advice of physician.
• It's unknown if drug appears in breast milk. Use cautiously in breast-feeding women. Patient should consider discontinuing breast-feeding.

NURSING CONSIDERATIONS
• Consult prescriber before using topical preparations in children younger than age 2. Don't use troches in children younger than age 3; don't use vaginal preparations in children younger than age 12.
• Watch for irritation or sensitivity; stop if irritation occurs, and notify prescriber.
• Improvement usually occurs within 1 week; if no improvement is seen within 4 weeks, review diagnosis.

PATIENT TEACHING
• Reassure patient that hypopigmentation from tinea versicolor will resolve gradually.
• Warn patient not to use occlusive wrappings or dressings.
• Warn patient to avoid contact with eyes.
• Caution patient that frequent or persistent yeast infections may suggest a more serious medical problem.
• Tell patient to refrain from sexual intercourse during vaginal treatment.
• Warn patient that topical preparation may stain clothing.
• Tell patient that using a sanitary napkin protects clothing when using vaginal preparation.
• Stress need to continue use of vaginal preparations, as prescribed, even if menstruation begins.
• Tell patient with athlete's foot to change shoes and cotton socks daily and to dry between the toes after bathing.

• Tell patient to allow lozenges to dissolve in mouth and not to chew, for full benefit.
• Stress need to continue treatment for full course and to notify prescriber if no improvement occurs after 4 weeks.

SAFETY ALERT!

clozapine
KLOE-za-peen

Clozaril🖋, FazaClo ODT, Versacloz

Therapeutic class: Antipsychotics
Pharmacologic class: Dibenzapine derivatives

AVAILABLE FORMS
ODTs: 12.5 mg, 25 mg, 100 mg, 150 mg, 200 mg
Oral suspension: 50 mg/mL
Tablets: 12.5 mg, 25 mg, 50 mg, 100 mg, 200 mg

INDICATIONS & DOSAGES
➤ **Schizophrenia in severely ill patients unresponsive to other therapies; to reduce risk of recurrent suicidal behavior in schizophrenia or schizoaffective disorders**
Adults: Initially, 12.5 mg P.O. once daily or b.i.d. Adjust dose upward by 25 to 50 mg daily (if tolerated) to 300 to 450 mg daily by end of 2 weeks. Individual dosage is based on clinical response, patient tolerance, and adverse reactions. Subsequent dosage shouldn't be increased more than once or twice weekly and shouldn't exceed 100-mg increments. Don't exceed 900 mg daily. For the general population, if ANC is 1,500/mm^3 or greater (normal baseline range), treatment may be initiated. Confirm all initial reports of ANC less than 1,500/mm^3 with a repeat ANC within 24 hours. For patients with benign ethnic neutropenia (BEN), obtain two baseline ANC levels before initiating treatment (normal ANC range for those with BEN is 1,000/mm^3 or greater). For patients with BEN, if ANC is 1,000/mm^3 or greater, treatment may be initiated. When restarting drug in those who have discontinued clozapine for 2 days or more, re-initiate at 12.5 mg once or twice daily to minimize the risk of hypotension, bradycardia, and syncope. If

that dose is well tolerated, the dose may be increased to the previously therapeutic dose more quickly than recommended for initial treatment.

Adjust-a-dose: Refer to manufacturer's instructions for ANC monitoring and dosage interruption for neutropenia, and for concurrent use with CYP1A2, CYP2D6, or CYP3A4 inhibitors or CYP1A2 or CYP3A4 inducers. Reduce dosages in those with significant renal or hepatic impairment and in those who are poor metabolizers of CYP2D6.

Discontinue drug in those with QT interval greater than 500 msec, those with symptoms of ventricular arrhythmias, or those with cardiomyopathy/myocarditis or neuroleptic malignant syndrome.

ADMINISTRATION
P.O.
- Give with or without food.
- Peel the foil from the ODT blister and gently remove the tablet immediately before giving.
- Give ODT with or without water.
- Shake bottle for 10 seconds before withdrawing suspension using provided oral syringe and syringe adaptor.

ACTION
Unknown. Binds selectively to dopaminergic receptors in the CNS and may interfere with adrenergic, cholinergic, histaminergic, and serotonergic receptors.

Route	Onset	Peak	Duration
P.O.	Unknown	1–6 hr	4–12 hr

Half-life: Proportional to dose; may range from 4 to 66 hours.

ADVERSE REACTIONS
CNS: drowsiness, sedation, dizziness, vertigo, headache, *seizures,* syncope, tremor, disturbed sleep or nightmares, restlessness, hypokinesia or akinesia, agitation, rigidity, akathisia, confusion, fatigue, insomnia, hyperkinesia, weakness, lethargy, ataxia, slurred speech, depression, myoclonus, anxiety, fever.
CV: tachycardia, hypotension, hypertension, chest pain, ECG changes, orthostatic hypotension.

EENT: visual disturbances.
GI: constipation, excessive salivation, dry, mouth, nausea, vomiting, heartburn, diarrhea.
GU: urinary frequency or urgency, urine retention, incontinence, abnormal ejaculation.
Hematologic: *leukopenia, neutropenia,* eosinophilia.
Metabolic: hyperglycemia, weight gain, hypercholesterolemia, hypertriglyceridemia.
Musculoskeletal: muscle pain or spasm, muscle weakness.
Respiratory: *respiratory arrest.*
Skin: rash, diaphoresis.

INTERACTIONS
Drug-drug. *Anticholinergics:* May potentiate anticholinergic effects of clozapine. Use together cautiously.
Antihypertensives: May potentiate hypotensive effects. Monitor BP.
🚫 *Alert: Benzodiazepines, other psychotropic drugs:* May increase risk of sedation and CV and respiratory arrest. Use together cautiously.
Bone marrow suppressants: May increase bone marrow toxicity. Avoid using together.
Citalopram, *fluoroquinolones,* **fluoxetine, fluvoxamine,** *paroxetine,* **sertraline:** May increase clozapine levels and toxicity. Adjust clozapine dose as needed.
CYP1A2 inducers (tobacco smoking): May decrease clozapine (oral suspension) effectiveness. Increase clozapine dosage as necessary.
CYP2D6 or CYP3A4 inhibitors (bupropion, cimetidine, duloxetine, erythromycin, escitalopram, fluoxetine, paroxetine, quinidine, sertraline, terbinafine); moderate or weak CYP1A2 inhibitors (caffeine, oral contraceptives): Monitor patient for adverse reactions. Reduce clozapine oral dosage if necessary.
Digoxin, other highly protein-bound drugs, warfarin: May increase levels of these drugs. Monitor patient closely for adverse reactions.
Black Box Warning *Opioids:* May cause slow or difficult breathing, sedation, and death. Avoid use together. If use together is necessary, limit dosage and duration of each drug to the minimum necessary for desired effect. ■

---

*Reactions in bold italics are **life-threatening.** Interactions may have a **rapid onset** or a **delayed onset.***

Phenytoin: May decrease clozapine level and cause breakthrough psychosis. Monitor patient for psychosis and adjust clozapine dosage.

Psychoactive drugs: May cause additive effects. Use together cautiously.

Ritonavir: May increase clozapine levels and toxicity. Avoid using together.

Strong CYP3A4 inducers (carbamazepine, phenytoin, rifampin): May decrease clozapine effectiveness. Use together isn't recommended. If coadministration is necessary, consider increasing clozapine dosage.

Strong CYP1A2 inhibitors (ciprofloxacin, fluvoxamine): May increase clozapine level. Reduce clozapine (oral suspension) dosage to one-third during coadministration.

Drug-herb. *St. John's wort:* May decrease drug level. Discourage use together.

Drug-lifestyle. *Alcohol use:* May increase CNS depression. Discourage use together.

Smoking: May decrease drug level. Urge patient to quit smoking. Monitor patient for effectiveness and adjust dosage.

EFFECTS ON LAB TEST RESULTS

● May increase glucose, cholesterol, and triglyceride levels.

● May increase eosinophil count. May decrease granulocyte, WBC counts, and ANC.

CONTRAINDICATIONS & CAUTIONS

Black Box Warning Because of risk of severe neutropenia, which can lead to fatal infections, drug is available only through the Clozapine REMS Program. Prescribers, patients, and dispensing pharmacists must enroll in the program and be certified. ■

Black Box Warning Obtain CBC with differential before initiating treatment: ANC must be at least 1,500/mm^3 for the general population and must be at least 1,000/mm^3 for patients with documented BEN. Monitor ANC regularly during treatment. ■

Black Box Warning Opioid drugs should only be prescribed with benzodiazepines or other CNS depressants to patients for whom alternative treatment options are inadequate. ■

● Contraindicated in patients with a history of serious hypersensitivity to drug or its components, in patients who experienced clozapine-induced agranulocytosis or severe granulocytopenia, and in patients with uncontrolled epilepsy.

● Closely monitor patients taking other drugs that suppress bone marrow function.

● Use cautiously in patients with prostatic hyperplasia or angle-closure glaucoma because drug has potent anticholinergic effects. Severe GI reactions (constipation, intestinal obstruction, fecal impaction, paralytic ileus) can also occur.

Black Box Warning Fatal myocarditis and cardiomyopathy may occur at any time during treatment. If signs or symptoms (chest pain, tachycardia, palpitations, dyspnea, fever, flulike symptoms, hypotension, ECG changes) occur, obtain a cardiac evaluation, and discontinue drug. Generally, patients with clozapine-related myocarditis or cardiomyopathy shouldn't be re-challenged with the drug. ■

● Drug is associated with development of eosinophilia, which usually occurs during the first month of treatment. Eosinophilia has been associated with organ involvement (myocarditis, pancreatitis, hepatitis, colitis, nephritis) and could be consistent with a drug-induced hypersensitivity syndrome. If eosinophilia develops, evaluate for signs and symptoms of systemic reactions and, if clozapine-related disease is suspected, discontinue drug immediately. If a cause for eosinophilia unrelated to clozapine is identified, the underlying cause should be treated and clozapine may be continued.

● Drug is associated with QT-interval prolongation and life-threatening ventricular arrhythmias. Use caution in those with risk factors for QT-interval prolongation or serious CV reactions and in those taking drugs known to prolong the QT interval. Consider obtaining a baseline ECG and serum chemistry panel, and correct electrolyte abnormalities before starting treatment. Discontinue clozapine if QTc interval is greater than 500 msec. Obtain a cardiac evaluation and discontinue drug if patient has symptoms of torsades de pointes or other arrhythmias (syncope, pre-syncope, dizziness, palpitations).

• Drug can cause neuroleptic malignant syndrome (NMS), which can be fatal. If signs and symptoms of NMS (hyperpyrexia, muscle rigidity, altered mental status, irregular pulse, fluctuating blood pressure, tachycardia, diaphoresis, cardiac arrhythmias, elevated creatinine phosphokinase, myoglobinuria, rhabdomyolysis, acute renal failure) occur, discontinue drug and begin appropriate treatment and monitoring.

• Tardive dyskinesia (TD), a syndrome of potentially irreversible, involuntary dyskinetic movements, has occurred in patients taking antipsychotics. Use the lowest effective dosage for the shortest duration possible. Consider discontinuing drug if TD occurs (*Note:* Some patients may require treatment despite TD syndrome).

• Safe and effective use in children hasn't been established.

Dialyzable drug: No.

⚠ *Overdose S&S:* Altered state of consciousness, drowsiness, delirium, coma, tachycardia, hypotension, respiratory depression or failure, hypersalivation, aspiration pneumonia, cardiac arrhythmias, seizures.

PREGNANCY-LACTATION-REPRODUCTION

• There are no adequate studies in pregnant women. Use during pregnancy only if clearly needed and potential benefit justifies potential risk to the fetus.

🜉 *Alert:* Neonates exposed to antipsychotics during the third trimester of pregnancy are at risk for developing extrapyramidal signs and symptoms (repetitive muscle movements of the face and body) and withdrawal symptoms (agitation, abnormally increased or decreased muscle tone, tremors, sleepiness, severe difficulty breathing, and difficulty feeding) after delivery.

• Drug appears in breast milk. Women receiving drug shouldn't breast-feed.

NURSING CONSIDERATIONS

Black Box Warning Drug increases the risk of fatal myocarditis and cardiomyopathy, especially during, but not limited to, the first month of therapy. In patients in whom myocarditis is suspected (unexplained fatigue, dyspnea, tachypnea, chest pain, tachycardia, fever, flulike symptoms, palpitations, and other signs or symptoms

of HF or ECG abnormalities, such as ST-T wave abnormalities or arrhythmias), stop therapy immediately and don't restart. ∎

🜉 *Alert:* Drug may cause hyperglycemia. Monitor patients with diabetes regularly. In patients with risk factors for diabetes, obtain fasting blood glucose test results at baseline and periodically.

🜉 *Alert:* Monitor patient for metabolic syndrome, including significant weight gain and increased BMI, hypertension, hyperglycemia, hypercholesterolemia, and hypertriglyceridemia.

• Monitor patient for signs and symptoms of myocarditis, and cardiomyopathy.

Black Box Warning Orthostatic hypotension, with or without syncope and bradycardia, can occur. Rarely, collapse can be profound and be accompanied by respiratory or cardiac arrest. Orthostatic hypotension is more likely to occur during initial titration with rapid dose escalation and can occur with the first dose and with doses as low as 12.5 mg. Start treatment with 12.5 mg once daily or b.i.d. and titrate slowly. Use caution in patients with CV or cerebrovascular disease or conditions that may cause hypotension. ∎

Black Box Warning Seizures may occur, especially in patients receiving high doses. Begin treatment at 12.5 mg, titrate gradually, and use divided dosing. Use caution with patients with a history of seizures or risk factors for seizures (CNS pathology, drugs that lower the seizure threshold, alcohol abuse). ∎

• Some patients experience transient fever with temperature higher than 100.4° F (38° C), especially in the first 3 weeks of therapy. Monitor these patients closely.

Black Box Warning Drug isn't indicated for use in elderly patients with dementia-related psychoses because of an increased risk of death from CV disease or infection. ∎

🜉 *Alert:* Fever may be the first sign of neutropenic infection. Interrupt therapy and obtain ANC level in any patient who develops fever (temperature 101.3° F [38.5° C]). If fever occurs in any patient with ANC less than 1,000/mm^3, initiate appropriate workup and treatment and monitor/manage patient appropriately.

- If drug is to be discontinued and patient doesn't have moderate to severe neutropenia, reduce dose gradually over 1 to 2 weeks. To discontinue the drug abruptly for a reason unrelated to neutropenia, continue to monitor ANC until it is 1,500/mm³ or greater (for the general population), or until ANC is 1,000/mm³ or greater or above patient's baseline (for those with BEN).
- If patient reports onset of fever (temperature 101.3° F or greater) while discontinuing drug, continue to monitor ANC for an additional 2 weeks after drug is discontinued.
- When discontinuing drug, monitor patients carefully for recurrence of psychotic symptoms and symptoms related to cholinergic rebound (profuse sweating, headache, nausea, vomiting, diarrhea).
- PE and DVT have occurred in patients taking clozapine. It isn't known whether these can be attributed to the drug or to some other patient characteristic. Monitor for PE if patient develops DVT, acute dyspnea, chest pain, or other respiratory signs and symptoms.
- Drug can cause sedation and impair cognitive and motor performance. Monitor patient carefully for CNS changes.
- *Look alike–sound alike:* Don't confuse clozapine with clonidine, clofazimine, clonazepam, or Klonopin. Don't confuse Clozaril with Colazal.

PATIENT TEACHING
Black Box Warning Tell patient about need for regular blood tests to check for low ANC. Advise patient to report flulike symptoms, fever, sore throat, lethargy, weakness malaise, or other signs of neutropenia or infection. ∎
Black Box Warning Warn patient to avoid hazardous activities that require alertness and good coordination and where sudden loss of consciousness could cause serious risk to himself or others, while taking drug. ∎
- Tell patient to check with prescriber before taking alcohol or OTC drugs.
- Advise patient that smoking may decrease drug effectiveness.
- Tell patient to rise slowly to avoid dizziness and to immediately report feeling faint,

loss of consciousness, or irregular or slow heartbeat.
- Tell patient to keep ODTs in the blister package until he is ready to take them.
- Inform patient about risk for metabolic changes, seizures, and TD.
- Caution patient not to restart drug if he misses more than 2 days of treatment and to notify his prescriber.

cobimetinib fumarate
See NEW DRUGS for information.

SAFETY ALERT!

codeine phosphate
koe-DEEN
codeine sulfate

Therapeutic class: Opioid analgesics
Pharmacologic class: Opioids
Controlled substance schedule: II

AVAILABLE FORMS
codeine phosphate
Injection: 30 mg/mL ♣, 60 mg/mL ♣
Syrup: 5 mg/mL ♣
Tablets: 15 mg ♣, 30 mg ♣
codeine sulfate
Tablets: 15 mg, 30 mg, 60 mg

INDICATIONS & DOSAGES
➤ **Mild to moderately severe pain**
Adults: 15 to 60 mg P.O. or 30 to 60 mg (phosphate) subcutaneously or I.M. every 4 to 6 hours p.r.n. Maximum 24-hour P.O. dose is 360 mg.
Children age 12 and older: 0.5 to 1 mg/kg (phosphate) subcutaneously or I.M. every 4 to 6 hours p.r.n.
Adjust-a-dose: Adjust codeine phosphate dosages in patients with renal failure. For CrCl of 10 to 50 mL/minute, decrease dosage by 25% and titrate. If CrCl is less than 10 mL/minute, decrease dosage by 50% and titrate.

ADMINISTRATION
P.O.
- Give drug with milk or meals to avoid GI upset.
I.M.
- Document injection site.

Subcutaneous

- Assess injection site for local irritation, pain, and induration.

ACTION

May bind with opioid receptors in the CNS, altering perception of and emotional response to pain. Also suppresses the cough reflex by direct action on the cough center in the medulla.

Route	Onset	Peak	Duration
P.O.	30–60 min	1–2 hr	4–6 hr
I.M.	10–30 min	30–60 min	4–6 hr
Subcut.	10–30 min	30–60 min	4–6 hr

Half-life: 2½ to hours.

ADVERSE REACTIONS

CNS: clouded sensorium, sedation, dizziness, euphoria, light-headedness, physical dependence.
CV: *bradycardia,* flushing, hypotension.
GI: constipation, dry mouth, ileus, nausea, vomiting.
GU: urine retention.
Respiratory: *respiratory depression.*
Skin: diaphoresis, pruritus.

INTERACTIONS

Drug-drug. Black Box Warning *Benzodiazepines, CNS depressants:* May cause slow or difficult breathing, sedation, and death. Avoid use together. If use together is necessary, limit dosage and duration of each drug to the minimum necessary for desired effect. ■
Cimetidine: May lead to increased effect or toxicity. Monitor patient response.
CNS depressants, general anesthetics, hypnotics, MAO inhibitors, other opioid analgesics, sedatives, TCAs, tranquilizers: May cause additive effects. Use together cautiously; monitor patient response.
Opioid antagonists: May reduce analgesic effect or precipitate withdrawal symptoms. Consider therapy modification.
ⱺ Alert: *Serotonergic drugs (amoxapine, antiemetics [dolasetron, granisetron, ondansetron, palonosetron], antimigraine drugs, buspirone, cyclobenzaprine, dextromethorphan, linezolid, lithium, MAO inhibitors, maprotiline, methylene blue, mirtazapine, nefazodone, SNRIs, SSRIs, TCAs, trazodone, tryptophan, vilazodone):* May

increase risk of serotonin syndrome. Use together cautiously and monitor patient for serotonin syndrome.
Drug-herb. **ⱺ Alert:** *St. John's wort:* May increase risk of serotonin syndrome. Use together cautiously and monitor patient for serotonin syndrome.
Drug-lifestyle. *Alcohol use:* May cause additive effects. Discourage use together.

EFFECTS ON LAB TEST RESULTS

- May increase amylase and lipase levels.

CONTRAINDICATIONS & CAUTIONS

- Contraindicated in patients hypersensitive to drug.

Black Box Warning Opioid drugs should only be prescribed with benzodiazepines or other CNS depressants to patients for whom alternative treatment options are inadequate. ■
ⱺ Alert: Safety and effectiveness and pharmacokinetics of codeine sulfate in children younger than age 18 haven't been established.
ⱺ Alert: Drug may lead to a rare but serious decrease in adrenal gland cortisol production.
ⱺ Alert: Drug may decrease sex hormone levels with long-term use.

Black Box Warning Children who receive codeine for pain relief after a tonsillectomy or adenoidectomy and are ultrarapid metabolizers have an increased risk of death. Codeine is contraindicated for pain management after these surgeries. ■
ⱺ Alert: For managing pain (not associated with tonsillectomy or adenoidectomy), codeine should be used in children only if benefits outweigh risks.
ⱺ Alert: Patients are at increased risk of oversedation and respiratory depression if they have snoring or history of sleep apnea, no recent opioid use or are first-time opioid users, increased opioid dose requirements or opioid habituation, received general anesthesia for longer lengths of time, received other sedating drugs, preexisting pulmonary or cardiac disease, or have thoracic or other surgical incisions that may impair breathing. Monitor patients carefully.
- Use cautiously in elderly or debilitated patients and in those with head injury,

increased ICP, increased CSF pressure, hepatic or renal disease, hypothyroidism, Addison disease, acute alcoholism, seizures, severe CNS depression, bronchial asthma, COPD, respiratory depression, and shock.
Dialyzable drug: Unknown.
⚠ *Overdose S&S:* CNS depression, respiratory depression, apnea, flaccid skeletal muscles, bradycardia, hypotension, circulatory collapse, death.

PREGNANCY-LACTATION-REPRODUCTION

❸ *Alert:* There are no adequate well-controlled studies in pregnant women. Use during pregnancy only if potential benefit justifies potential risk to the fetus. Neonatal codeine withdrawal has occurred in infants born to addicted and nonaddicted mothers who had been taking codeine-containing medications in the days before delivery. Codeine phosphate injection is contraindicated in pregnant women.

• Don't administer drug during labor when delivery of a premature infant is anticipated.
❸ *Alert:* Drug and metabolites (morphine) appear in breast milk. Breast-feeding women may put their infants at increased risk for morphine overdose if the mothers are ultrarapid codeine metabolizers. Weigh risk of infant exposure against benefits of breast-feeding for both mother and infant.

NURSING CONSIDERATIONS

❸ *Alert:* Carefully monitor vital signs, pain level, respiratory status, and sedation level in all patients receiving opioids, especially those receiving I.V. drugs, even those given postoperatively.
❸ *Alert:* If patient is taking opioids with serotonergic drugs, watch for signs and symptoms of serotonin syndrome (agitation, hallucinations, rapid HR, fever, excessive sweating, shivering or shaking, muscle twitching or stiffness, trouble with coordination, nausea, vomiting, diarrhea), especially at start of treatment or after dosage increases. Signs and symptoms may occur within several hours of coadministration but may occur later, especially after dosage increase. Discontinue opioid, serotonergic drug, or both if serotonin syndrome is suspected.

❸ *Alert:* Monitor patient for signs and symptoms of adrenal insufficiency (nausea, vomiting, loss of appetite, fatigue, weakness, dizziness, low BP). Perform diagnostic testing if adrenal insufficiency is suspected. If adrenal insufficiency is confirmed, treat with corticosteroids and wean patient off opioids if appropriate. Discontinue corticosteroids when clinically appropriate.
❸ *Alert:* Monitor patient for signs and symptoms of decreased sex hormone levels (low libido, erectile dysfunction, amenorrhea, infertility). If signs and symptoms occur, evaluate patient and obtain laboratory testing.

• Reassess patient's level of pain at least 15 and 30 minutes after use.
• Codeine and aspirin or acetaminophen are commonly prescribed together to provide enhanced pain relief.
• For full analgesic effect, give drug before patient has intense pain.
• Drug is an antitussive and shouldn't be used when cough is a valuable diagnostic sign or is beneficial (as after thoracic surgery).
• Monitor cough type and frequency.
• Monitor respiratory and circulatory status.
• Opioids may cause constipation. Assess bowel function and need for stool softeners and stimulant laxatives.
• Codeine may delay gastric emptying, increase biliary tract pressure from contraction of the sphincter of Oddi, and interfere with hepatobiliary imaging studies.
• *Look alike–sound alike:* Don't confuse codeine with Cardene or Cordran.

PATIENT TEACHING

Black Box Warning Caution the patient or the caregiver of a patient taking an opioid drug with a benzodiazepine, CNS depressant, or alcohol to seek immediate medical attention if the patient has symptoms of dizziness, light-headedness, extreme sleepiness, slowed or difficult breathing, or unresponsiveness. ∎
❸ *Alert:* Caution parents and caregivers to observe children for signs of toxicity (unusual sleepiness, confusion, or difficult or noisy breathing). If signs occur, stop drug and seek medical attention immediately.

---

❸ *Alert:* Encourage patient to report all medications being taken, including prescriptions and OTC medications and supplements.

❸ *Alert:* Caution patient to immediately report signs and symptoms of serotonin syndrome, adrenal insufficiency, and decreased sex hormone levels to health care provider.

• Explain the assessment and monitoring process to patient and family. Instruct them to immediately report if patient has any difficulty breathing or any other signs of a potential adverse opioid-related reaction.

• Advise patient that GI distress caused by taking drug orally can be eased by taking drug with milk or meals.

• Instruct patient to ask for or to take drug before pain is intense.

• Caution ambulatory patient about getting out of bed or walking. Warn outpatient to avoid driving and other hazardous activities that require mental alertness until drug's effects on the CNS are known.

• Advise patient to avoid alcohol during therapy.

• Warn breast-feeding woman to watch for increased sleepiness, difficulty breast-feeding or breathing, or limpness of infant. Tell her to immediately seek medical attention if this occurs.

SAFETY ALERT!

codeine phosphate–acetaminophen
koe-DEEN/a-seet-a-MIN-a-fen

Capital and Codeine, Tylenol with Codeine #3✐, Tylenol with Codeine #4

Therapeutic class: Opioid analgesics
Pharmacologic class: Opioids–para-aminophenol derivatives
Controlled substance schedule: III (tablets); V (liquid)

AVAILABLE FORMS
Oral solution or suspension: 12 mg codeine and 120 mg acetaminophen/5 mL*
Tablets: 15 mg codeine and 300 mg acetaminophen, 30 mg codeine and 300 mg acetaminophen, 60 mg codeine and 300 mg acetaminophen

INDICATIONS & DOSAGES
Adjust-a-dose (for all indications): Consider decreased dosage in patients with renal impairment, elderly patients, and patients overly sensitive to effects of opioids. For patients with hepatic impairment, maximum total daily acetaminophen dose is 2,000 mg.

➤ **Mild to moderately severe pain**
Adults and children older than age 12: Codeine 15 to 60 mg and acetaminophen 300 to 1,000 mg P.O. every 4 hours as needed for pain; adjust dosage based on pain severity and patient response. Maximum total daily dosage: acetaminophen 4,000 mg and codeine 360 mg.
Children ages 7 to 12: Codeine 0.5 to 1 mg/kg/dose every 4 to 6 hours; acetaminophen 10 to 15 mg/kg/dose every 4 hours as needed.
Children ages 3 up to 7: 5 mL oral solution or suspension P.O. t.i.d. or q.i.d. as needed.

ADMINISTRATION
P.O.
• Store tablets at room temperature.
• Give with milk or meals to avoid GI upset.

ACTION
Codeine may bind with opioid receptors in the CNS, altering perception and emotional response to pain. Acetaminophen is thought to produce analgesia by inhibiting prostaglandin and other substances that sensitize pain receptors.

Route	Onset	Peak	Duration
P.O. (codeine)	30–45 min	1–2 hr	4–6 hr
P.O. (acetaminophen)	Rapid	½–2 hr	3–4 hr

Half-life: Codeine, 2.9 hours; acetaminophen, 1.25 to 3 hours.

ADVERSE REACTIONS
CNS: drowsiness, light-headedness, dizziness, sedation, euphoria, dysphoria.
GI: nausea, vomiting, constipation, abdominal pain.
Hematologic: *thrombocytopenia, agranulocytosis.*
Respiratory: shortness of breath.
Skin: pruritus, rash.
Other: allergic reactions.

INTERACTIONS

Drug-drug. *Antipsychotics, general anesthetics, opioid analgesics, sedative-hypnotics, tranquilizers, other CNS depressants:* May increase CNS depression. Use together cautiously.

Black Box Warning *Benzodiazepines, CNS depressants:* May cause slow or difficult breathing, sedation, and death. Avoid use together. If use together is necessary, limit dosage and duration of each drug to the minimum necessary for desired effect. ■

Cimetidine: May enhance effects of codeine, increasing toxicity. Monitor patient carefully.

❸ *Alert: Serotonergic drugs (amoxapine, antiemetics [dolasetron, granisetron, ondansetron, palonosetron], antimigraine drugs, buspirone, cyclobenzaprine, dextromethorphan, linezolid, lithium, MAO inhibitors, maprotiline, methylene blue, mirtazapine, nefazodone, SNRIs, SSRIs, TCAs, trazodone, tryptophan, vilazodone):* May increase risk of serotonin syndrome. Use together cautiously and monitor patient for serotonin syndrome.

Drug-herb. ❸ *Alert: St. John's wort:* May increase risk of serotonin syndrome. Use together cautiously and monitor patient for serotonin syndrome.

Drug-lifestyle. *Alcohol use:* May increase CNS depression. Discourage use together.

EFFECTS ON LAB TEST RESULTS

• May increase serum amylase level.
• May cause false-positive results for urinary 5-hydroxyindoleacetic acid.

CONTRAINDICATIONS & CAUTIONS

• Contraindicated in patients hypersensitive to codeine or acetaminophen.

Black Box Warning Opioid drugs should only be prescribed with benzodiazepines or other CNS depressants to patients for whom alternative treatment options are inadequate. ■

Black Box Warning Children who receive codeine for pain relief after a tonsillectomy or adenoidectomy and are ultrarapid metabolizers have an increased risk of death. Codeine is contraindicated for pain management after these surgeries. ■

❸ *Alert:* For managing pain (not associated with tonsillectomy or adenoidectomy),

codeine should be used in children only if benefits outweigh risks.

❸ *Alert:* Drug may lead to a rare but serious decrease in adrenal gland cortisol production.

❸ *Alert:* Drug may decrease sex hormone levels with long-term use.

❸ *Alert:* Patients are at increased risk for oversedation and respiratory depression if they snore or have a history of sleep apnea, no recent history of opioid use or are first-time opioid users, have increased opioid dose requirements or opioid habituation, received general anesthesia for longer lengths of time, received other sedating drugs, have preexisting pulmonary or cardiac disease, or have thoracic or other surgical incisions that may impair breathing. Monitor patients carefully.

• Tablets aren't approved for use in children.
• Use cautiously in patients with head injury, intracranial lesions, increased ICP, or acute abdominal conditions.

Black Box Warning Acetaminophen has been associated with acute liver failure, usually at doses greater than 4,000 mg/day and often when more than one acetaminophen-containing product is used. Liver failure may result in liver transplant or death. ■

❸ *Alert:* May cause serious, potentially fatal skin reactions, including Stevens-Johnson syndrome, toxic epidermal necrolysis, and acute generalized exanthematous pustulosis. Reaction may occur with first or subsequent use when acetaminophen is used as monotherapy or when it is one component of combination drug therapy. Monitor for reddening of the skin, rash, blisters, and detachment of the upper surface of the skin. Stop drug immediately if skin reaction is suspected.

• Use cautiously in patients with asthma or sulfite sensitivity because allergy-type reactions, anaphylaxis, and asthmatic episodes may occur.
• Use cautiously in elderly or debilitated patients; in those with severe renal or hepatic impairment, hypothyroidism, urethral stricture, Addison disease, or prostatic hypertrophy; in patients identified as ultrarapid metabolizers of codeine; and in those with identified polymorphism of CYP2D6 genotype.

Dialyzable drug: Unknown.

⚠ *Overdose S&S:* Extreme sleepiness, confusion, shallow breathing. Codeine: Pinpoint pupils, respiratory depression, loss of consciousness, seizures. Acetaminophen: Hepatic necrosis, nausea, vomiting, diaphoresis, malaise, renal tubular necrosis, hypoglycemia, coma, coagulation defects.

PREGNANCY-LACTATION-REPRODUCTION

• There are no adequate studies in pregnant women. Use during pregnancy only if potential benefit justifies potential risk to the fetus; dependence and withdrawal in newborns may occur.

• Codeine and its metabolites and acetaminophen appear in breast milk. Use cautiously in breast-feeding women if benefits outweigh risks; closely monitor effects of codeine in infant.

NURSING CONSIDERATIONS

• Prescribe lowest effective dosage for shortest period of time and inform patients of risks and signs and symptoms of acetaminophen and codeine toxicity.

☯ *Alert:* If patient is taking opioids with serotonergic drugs, watch for signs and symptoms of serotonin syndrome (agitation, hallucinations, rapid HR, fever, excessive sweating, shivering or shaking, muscle twitching or stiffness, trouble with coordination, nausea, vomiting, diarrhea), especially when at start of treatment or after dosage increases. Signs and symptoms may occur within several hours of coadministration but may occur later, especially after dosage increase. Discontinue opioid, serotonergic drug, or both if serotonin syndrome is suspected.

☯ *Alert:* Monitor patient for signs and symptoms of adrenal insufficiency (nausea, vomiting, loss of appetite, fatigue, weakness, dizziness, low BP). Perform diagnostic testing if adrenal insufficiency is suspected. If adrenal insufficiency is confirmed, treat with corticosteroids and wean patient off opioids if appropriate. Discontinue corticosteroids when clinically appropriate.

☯ *Alert:* Monitor patient for signs and symptoms of decreased sex hormone levels (low libido, erectile dysfunction, amenorrhea, infertility). If signs and symptoms occur, evaluate patient and obtain laboratory testing.

☯ *Alert:* Carefully monitor vital signs, pain level, respiratory status, and sedation level in all patients receiving opioids, especially those receiving I.V. drugs, even those given postoperatively.

• Carefully monitor patients identified as ultrarapid metabolizers of codeine and those with identified polymorphism of CYP2D6 genotype. Overdose signs and symptoms and exaggerated adverse effects may occur at normal doses in these patients.

• Monitor serial renal function tests or LFTs in patients with severe hepatic or renal disease.

PATIENT TEACHING

Black Box Warning Caution the patient or the caregiver of a patient taking an opioid drug with a benzodiazepine, CNS depressant, or alcohol to seek immediate medical attention if the patient has symptoms of dizziness, light-headedness, extreme sleepiness, slowed or difficult breathing, or unresponsiveness. ■

☯ *Alert:* Caution parents and caregivers to observe children for signs of toxicity (unusual sleepiness, confusion, or difficult or noisy breathing). If signs occur, stop drug and seek medical attention immediately.

☯ *Alert:* Warn patient to stop drug and seek medical attention immediately if skin rash or reaction occurs while using acetaminophen.

☯ *Alert:* Encourage patient to report all medications being taken, including prescriptions and OTC medications and supplements.

☯ *Alert:* Caution patient to immediately report signs and symptoms of serotonin syndrome, adrenal insufficiency, and decreased sex hormone levels to health care provider.

• Explain the assessment and monitoring process to patient and family. Instruct them to immediately report if patient has any difficulty breathing or any other signs of a potential adverse opioid-related reaction.

• Inform patient with severe hepatic or renal disease that serial renal function tests or LFTs will be needed.

• Caution patient not to drive a car or operate heavy machinery while taking this drug.

• Discourage alcohol use during therapy.

C

• Warn patient that codeine may be habit-forming and to take only as long as it's prescribed and in the amounts prescribed.
• Advise breast-feeding women who are ultrarapid metabolizers to consult prescriber immediately, call 911, or go to the nearest emergency department if the infant shows signs and symptoms of codeine toxicity (sleepiness, difficulty breast-feeding, breathing difficulties, limpness).

colchicine
KOL-chih-seen

Colcrys✔, Mitigare

Therapeutic class: Antigout drugs
Pharmacologic class: Colchicum autumnale alkaloids

AVAILABLE FORMS
Capsules: 0.6 mg
Tablets: 0.6 mg

INDICATIONS & DOSAGES
➤ **Prevention of gout flares**
Adults: 0.6 mg P.O. once daily or b.i.d. Maximum daily dose is 1.2 mg.
Adjust-a-dose: For patients taking Colcrys with CrCl of less than 30 mL/minute, give 0.3 mg/day. Closely monitor patient after dosage increases. For patients on dialysis, starting doses should be 0.3 mg twice a week with close monitoring. Closely monitor patients with mild to moderate hepatic impairment; no dosage adjustment is required. Consider dosage reduction in patients with severe hepatic impairment.

For patients taking Mitigare, consider dosage reduction or alternative drug in patients with severe renal impairment; closely monitor patients undergoing hemodialysis for toxicity. Consider dosage reduction or alternative drug in patients with severe hepatic impairment.
➤ **Gout flares (Colcrys)**
Adults: 1.2 mg P.O. at first sign of a flare, followed by 0.6 mg 1 hour later; maximum dosage is 1.8 mg over a 1-hour period.
Adjust-a-dose: For patients with CrCl of less than 30 mL/minute or severe hepatic impairment, no dosage adjustment is needed

but treatment course should be repeated no more than once every 2 weeks. For patients with severe renal or hepatic impairment requiring repeated courses for the treatment of gout flares, consider alternative therapy. For patients on dialysis, reduce total recommended dose for treatment of gout flares to a single dose of 0.6 mg (one tablet). For these patients, treatment course shouldn't be repeated more than once every 2 weeks.
➤ **Familial Mediterranean fever (FMF) (Colcrys)**
Adults: 1.2 to 2.4 mg P.O. daily; may increase by 0.3 mg/day to maximum daily dosage given once daily or in two divided doses.
Adolescents age 13 and older: 1.2 to 2.4 mg P.O. once daily or in two divided doses.
Children ages 6 to 12: 0.9 to 1.8 mg P.O. once daily or in two divided doses.
Children ages 4 to 6: 0.3 to 1.8 mg P.O. once daily or in two divided doses.
Adjust-a-dose: For patients with CrCl of less than 30 mL/minute or ESRD requiring dialysis, initially 0.3 mg/day, carefully increasing dosage as needed. In patients with severe hepatic disease, consider dosage reduction with careful monitoring.

ADMINISTRATION
P.O.
• Give drug with or without food.

ACTION
Exact mechanism of action is not fully known; thought to involve a reduction in lactic acid produced by leukocytes, reducing uric acid deposits and phagocytosis, thereby decreasing the inflammatory process.

Route	Onset	Peak	Duration
P.O.	Unknown	30–180 min	Unknown

Half-life: 27 to 31 hours.

ADVERSE REACTIONS
CNS: fatigue, headache.
EENT: pharyngolaryngeal pain.
GI: diarrhea, nausea, vomiting.
Hematologic: *aplastic anemia, granulocytopenia, leukopenia, pancytopenia, thrombocytopenia.*
Other: gout.

INTERACTIONS

Drug-drug. *Acidifying agents:* May inhibit action of colchicine. Avoid use together.

Alkalinizing agents: May increase action of colchicine. Avoid use together.

CNS depressants, sympathomimetics (such as phenylephrine): May increase sensitivity to these drugs. Monitor patient closely and adjust dosage as needed.

Digoxin, HMG-CoA reductase inhibitors (atorvastatin, simvastatin): May increase risk of myopathy or rhabdomyolysis. Avoid use together. If coadministration can't be avoided, monitor patient carefully. Discontinue colchicine if signs or symptoms occur.

Moderate CYP3A4 inhibitors (amprenavir, aprepitant, diltiazem, erythromycin, fluconazole, fosamprenavir, verapamil), P-glycoprotein inhibitors (cyclosporine, ranolazine), strong CYP3A4 inhibitors (atazanavir, clarithromycin, indinavir, itraconazole, ketoconazole, lopinavir/ritonavir, nefazodone, nelfinavir, ritonavir, ritonavir-boosted darunavir, ritonavir-boosted fosamprenavir, ritonavir-boosted tipranavir, saquinavir, telithromycin; the fixed combination of elvitegravir–cobicistat–emtricitabine–tenofovir): May increase colchicine level, increasing the risk of toxic effects. Reduce colchicine dosage if alternative treatment isn't available. Concurrent use in patients with renal or hepatic impairment is contraindicated.

Drug-food. *Grapefruit, grapefruit juice:* May increase drug level. Discourage use together.

EFFECTS ON LAB TEST RESULTS

- May increase AST, ALT, and CK levels.
- May decrease Hb level and hematocrit.
- May decrease leukocyte, granulocyte, and platelet counts.
- May cause false-positive results when urine is tested for RBCs or Hb.

CONTRAINDICATIONS & CAUTIONS

- Contraindicated in patients with serious CV, renal, hepatic, or GI impairment and in those taking P-glycoprotein inhibitors or strong CYP3A4 inhibitors.
- Myelosuppression has been reported. Use cautiously in patients with hematologic disorders.

Dialyzable drug: No.

⚠ **Overdose S&S:** Abdominal pain, nausea, vomiting, diarrhea, hypovolemia, multiorgan failure, death.

PREGNANCY-LACTATION-REPRODUCTION

- There are no adequate studies in pregnant women. Use during pregnancy only if potential benefit justifies potential risk to the fetus.
- Drug isn't expected to appear in breast milk. Use cautiously in breast-feeding women and observe breast-fed infants for adverse effects related to vitamin absorption.

NURSING CONSIDERATIONS

- Safety and effectiveness of repeat treatment for gout flares haven't been established.
- ⊕ **Alert:** Colcrys and Mitigare are the only FDA-approved single-ingredient colchicine products.
- Drug isn't an analgesic and shouldn't be used to treat pain from other causes.
- Obtain baseline laboratory studies, including CBC, before starting therapy and periodically thereafter; watch for myelosuppression, leukopenia, granulocytopenia, thrombocytopenia, pancytopenia, and aplastic anemia.
- Monitor patient who has used drug for a prolonged period for neuromuscular toxicity and rhabdomyolysis.
- If nausea, vomiting, or diarrhea occurs, discontinue drug.
- Drug may increase risk of malignancy.
- When used for gout prophylaxis, colchicine must be given with allopurinol or a uricosuric drug (such as probenecid) to decrease serum uric acid level. However, colchicine should be started before the other agent because a sudden change in uric acid level may cause a gout attack.
- **Look alike–sound alike:** Don't confuse colchicine with Cortrosyn.

PATIENT TEACHING

- Tell patient that drug can be taken without regard to food but to avoid grapefruit and grapefruit juice.
- Advise patient to report muscle pain or weakness, tingling or numbness in fingers or

toes, unusual bleeding or bruising, increased infections, weakness, tiredness, cyanosis, nausea, vomiting, or diarrhea; advise patient to discontinue drug.

colesevelam hydrochloride
koe-leh-SEVE-eh-lam

Welchol⚘

Therapeutic class: Antilipemics
Pharmacologic class: Bile acid sequestrants

AVAILABLE FORMS
Oral suspension: 1.875-g, 3.75-g packets
Tablets: 625 mg

INDICATIONS & DOSAGES
➤ **Adjunct to diet and exercise, either alone or with an HMG-CoA reductase inhibitor, to reduce elevated LDL cholesterol (LDL-C) in patients with primary hypercholesterolemia (Fredrickson type IIa); in boys and postmenarchal girls, ages 10 to 17, with heterozygous familial hypercholesterolemia if, after an adequate trial of diet therapy, LDL-C is 190 mg/dL or higher or LDL-C is 160 mg/dL or higher and patient has a positive family history of premature CV disease or two or more other CV disease risk factors**
Adults: 3 tablets (1,875 mg) P.O. b.i.d. or 6 tablets (3,750 mg) once daily. Or, one 1.875-g packet P.O. b.i.d. or one 3.75-g packet P.O. once daily.
Children ages 10 to 17: One 1.875-g packet P.O. b.i.d. with meals or one 3.75-g packet P.O. once daily with a meal.
➤ **Adjunct to diet and exercise to improve glycemic control in type 2 diabetes mellitus**
Adults: 3 tablets (1,875 mg) P.O. b.i.d. or 6 tablets (3,750 mg) P.O. once daily. Or, one 1.875-g packet P.O. b.i.d. or one 3.75-g packet P.O. once daily.

ADMINISTRATION
P.O.
• Give drug with a meal and plenty of fluids.
• Store tablets at room temperature and protect them from moisture.

• Empty entire contents of one packet into glass and add 4 to 8 oz of water, fruit juice, or diet soft drink. Stir well and give immediately.

ACTION
Binds bile acids in the intestinal tract, impeding their absorption and causing their elimination in feces. In response to this bile acid depletion, LDL-C levels decrease as the liver uses LDL-C to replenish reduced bile acid stores.

Route	Onset	Peak	Duration
P.O.	Unknown	2 wk	Unknown

Half-life: Unknown.

ADVERSE REACTIONS
CNS: headache, asthenia, pain.
EENT: pharyngitis, rhinitis, sinusitis.
GI: constipation, flatulence, abdominal pain, diarrhea, dyspepsia, nausea.
Musculoskeletal: back pain, myalgia.
Respiratory: increased cough.
Other: infection, accidental injury, flulike syndrome.

INTERACTIONS
Drug-drug. *Amiodarone:* May decrease amiodarone bioavailability. Consider therapy modification.
Glyburide: May decrease glyburide level. Administer glyburide at least 4 hours before colesevelam dose.
Hormonal contraceptives (estrogens, progestins): May decrease levels of these contraceptives. Administer hormonal contraceptive at least 4 hours before or 4 to 6 hours after colesevelam dose.
Phenytoin: May decrease phenytoin level and increase seizure activity. Administer phenytoin 4 hours before colesevelam dose and monitor phenytoin level.
Thyroid hormones: Coadministration may increase TSH level. Administer thyroid hormone replacement 4 hours before colesevelam dose.
Warfarin: May decrease INR. Monitor INR and patient closely.

EFFECTS ON LAB TEST RESULTS
• May increase triglyceride levels.

CONTRAINDICATIONS & CAUTIONS

• Contraindicated in patients hypersensitive to drug or any of its components, in patients with triglyceride levels greater than 500 mg/dL, and in patients with bowel obstruction.

• Contraindicated for glycemic control in patients with type 1 diabetes and for the treatment of diabetic ketoacidosis.

• Use cautiously in patients susceptible to vitamin K or fat-soluble vitamin deficiencies and in patients with swallowing disorders, severe GI motility disorders, or major GI tract surgery.

• Use cautiously in patients with triglyceride levels greater than 300 mg/dL.

• Oral suspension contains 13.5 mg phenylalanine/1.875-g packet and 27 mg phenylalanine/3.75-g packet.

Dialyzable drug: Unknown.

⚠ *Overdose S&S:* Severe local GI reactions, especially constipation.

PREGNANCY-LACTATION-REPRODUCTION

• There are no adequate studies in pregnant women. Use during pregnancy may interfere with vitamin absorption. Use only if clearly needed.

• Drug doesn't appear in breast milk but may interfere with vitamin absorption and affect breast-feeding infants. Use cautiously in breast-feeding women and only when clearly needed.

NURSING CONSIDERATIONS

• Before starting drug, assess patient for underlying causes of hypercholesterolemia, such as poorly controlled diabetes, hypothyroidism, nephrotic syndrome, dysproteinemias, obstructive liver disease, other drug therapy, and alcoholism.

• Monitor patient's bowel habits. If severe constipation develops, decrease dosage, add a stool softener, or stop drug.

• Monitor the effects of patient's other drugs to identify drug interactions.

• Monitor INR, total cholesterol, and LDL-C and triglyceride levels periodically during therapy.

PATIENT TEACHING

• Instruct patient to take drug with a meal and plenty of fluids.

• Teach patient to monitor bowel habits. Encourage a diet high in fiber and fluids. Instruct patient to notify prescriber promptly if severe constipation develops.

• Encourage patient to follow prescribed diet, exercise, and monitoring of cholesterol and triglyceride levels.

• Tell patient to notify prescriber if she's pregnant or breast-feeding.

conivaptan hydrochloride
kah-nih-VAP-tan

Vaprisol

Therapeutic class: Vasopressin antagonists
Pharmacologic class: Arginine vasopressin receptor antagonists

AVAILABLE FORMS

Injection (premixed): 0.2 mg/mL in 100 mL D_5W

INDICATIONS & DOSAGES

➤ **Euvolemic hyponatremia (as from SIADH, hypothyroidism, adrenal insufficiency, pulmonary disorders) and hypervolemic hyponatremia in hospitalized patients**

Adults: Loading dose of 20 mg I.V. over 30 minutes; then 20 mg I.V. by continuous infusion over 24 hours for 1 to 3 days. If sodium level isn't rising at desired rate, increase to maximum dose of 40 mg/day by continuous infusion. Don't give for more than 4 days after loading dose.

Adjust-a-dose: If sodium level rises more than 12 mEq/L in 24 hours, stop infusion. If hyponatremia persists or recurs and patient has had no adverse neurologic effects from the rapid rise in sodium level, restart infusion at a reduced dose. If patient develops hypotension or hypovolemia, stop infusion. Monitor vital signs and volume status often. If hyponatremia persists once patient is no longer hypotensive and volume returns to normal, restart infusion at a reduced dose. In patients with moderate hepatic impairment, give a loading dose of 10 mg followed by a continuous infusion of 10 mg over 24 hours for 2 to 4 days. If serum sodium level isn't rising at desired rate, drug may be titrated upward to 20 mg over 24 hours. Don't use if CrCl is less than 30 mL/minute.

ADMINISTRATION
I.V.

▼ Give via a large vein, and change infusion site every 24 hours.

▼ Protect premixed solution from light until ready to use.

▼ **Incompatibilities:** Lactated Ringer solution, NSS. Don't mix or infuse with other I.V. drugs.

ACTION
Increases free water eliminated by kidneys, inhibiting inappropriate or excessive arginine vasopressin (ADH) secretion. Typically, this causes increased net fluid loss, increased urine output, and decreased urine osmolality.

Route	Onset	Peak	Duration
I.V.	Unknown	Unknown	12 hr

Half-life: 5 hours.

ADVERSE REACTIONS
CNS: headache, confusion, fever, insomnia.
CV: atrial fibrillation, hypertension, hypotension, orthostatic hypotension.
EENT: pharyngolaryngeal pain.
GI: constipation, diarrhea, dry mouth, nausea, oral candidiasis, vomiting.
GU: frequency, hematuria, polyuria, UTI.
Hematologic: anemia.
Metabolic: *hypoglycemia,* hypokalemia, dehydration, hyperglycemia, *hypomagnesemia,* hyponatremia.
Respiratory: pneumonia.
Skin: erythema.
Other: infusion-site reactions, thirst.

INTERACTIONS
Drug-drug. *Amlodipine:* May increase amlodipine level and half-life. Monitor BP.
Digoxin: May increase digoxin level. Monitor patient, and adjust digoxin dose, as needed.
Midazolam: May increase midazolam level. Monitor patient for respiratory depression and hypotension.
Potent CYP3A4 inhibitors (clarithromycin, indinavir, itraconazole, ketoconazole, ritonavir): May seriously increase levels and toxic effects. Use together is contraindicated.

Simvastatin: May increase simvastatin level. Monitor patient for signs of rhabdomyolysis, including muscle pain, weakness, and tenderness.

EFFECTS ON LAB TEST RESULTS
● May decrease potassium, magnesium, sodium, and Hb levels and hematocrit. May increase or decrease blood glucose level.

CONTRAINDICATIONS & CAUTIONS
● Contraindicated in patients with hypovolemic hyponatremia or anuria; patients hypersensitive to drug or its components, corn, or corn products; and those taking potent CYP3A4 inhibitors, such as clarithromycin, indinavir, itraconazole, ketoconazole, or ritonavir.
● Use cautiously in hyponatremic patients with underlying HF and patients with hepatic or renal impairment.
Dialyzable drug: Unknown.
⚠ *Overdose S&S:* Hypotension, thirst.

PREGNANCY-LACTATION-REPRODUCTION
● Although there are no adequate well-controlled studies in pregnant women, drug may cause fetal harm. Use during pregnancy only if potential benefit justifies potential risk to the fetus.
● It isn't known if drug appears in breast milk. Patient should discontinue breast-feeding or discontinue drug, taking into account importance of drug to the mother.

NURSING CONSIDERATIONS
● Monitor sodium level and neurologic status regularly during therapy.
⚡ *Alert:* Rapid correction of sodium level may cause osmotic demyelination syndrome. Monitor sodium level and volume status. Don't exceed a rise in serum sodium level greater than 12 mEq/L/24 hours.
● Drug may cause significant infusion-site reactions, even with proper dilution and administration. Rotate infusion site every 24 hours to reduce risk of reaction.

PATIENT TEACHING
● Inform patient that he may experience low BP when standing. If he feels dizzy or faint, advise him to sit or lie down.

- Advise patient to promptly report signs and symptoms of hypoglycemia, such as feeling shaky, nervous, tired, sweaty, cold, hungry, confused, irritable, or impatient.
- Emphasize the importance of reporting an unusually fast heartbeat or weakness.
- Tell patient that analgesics and moist heating pads can be used to treat pain and inflammation at the infusion site.
- Inform patient that the infusion will be given for a maximum of 4 days after the loading dose.

SAFETY ALERT!

crizotinib
kriz-OH-ti-nib

Xalkori

Therapeutic class: Antineoplastics
Pharmacologic class: Tyrosine kinase inhibitors

AVAILABLE FORMS
Capsules ⓄTC: 200 mg, 250 mg

INDICATIONS & DOSAGES
➤ **Metastatic non–small-cell lung cancer (NSCLC) that is anaplastic lymphoma kinase (ALK)–positive as detected by an FDA-approved test; metastatic NSCLC tumors that are ROS1-positive**
Adults: 250 mg P.O. b.i.d.
Adjust-a-dose: For patients with CrCl less than 30 mL/minute (not requiring dialysis), give 250 mg once daily.

For patients with grade 3 hematologic toxicity, withhold drug until recovery to grade 2 or lower; then resume at same dosing schedule. For patients with grade 4 hematologic toxicity, withhold drug until recovery to grade 2 or lower; then reduce dosage to 200 mg P.O. b.i.d. If recurrence occurs, withhold drug until recovery to grade 2 or lower; then resume at 250 mg P.O. once daily. Permanently discontinue drug for patients with grade 4 recurrence.

For patients with QTc interval greater than 500 msec on at least two separate ECGs, withhold drug until recovery to baseline or to QTc interval less than 481 msec; then resume at 200 mg P.O. b.i.d.

If QTc interval is greater than 500 msec or greater than or equal to a 60-msec change from baseline with torsades de pointes or polymorphic ventricular tachycardia or signs or symptoms of serious arrhythmia, permanently discontinue drug.

For patients with AST or ALT elevations greater than 5 × ULN and total bilirubin elevation 1.5 × ULN or less, withhold drug until recovery to baseline or to 3 × ULN or less; then resume at 200 mg P.O. b.i.d. For patients with AST or ALT elevations greater than 3 × ULN and concurrent total bilirubin elevation greater than 1.5 × ULN, in the absence of cholestasis or hemolysis, permanently discontinue drug.

Permanently discontinue drug if any grade drug-related interstitial lung disease or pneumonitis occurs or if bradycardia occurs with no concurrent contributing medication identified. If a contributory medication is identified and discontinued (or its dosage is adjusted), resume at 250 mg once daily upon recovery to asymptomatic bradycardia or to a HR of 60 beats/minute (bpm) or above, with frequent monitoring. Withhold drug until recovery to asymptomatic bradycardia or to a HR of 60 bpm or above.

ADMINISTRATION
P.O.
- Drug may only be prescribed to patients diagnosed by FDA-approved test to detect ALK-positive NSCLC. An approved test isn't currently available to detect *ROS1* rearrangements. Refer to manufacturer's instructions for clinical trials experience.
- Give capsules whole; don't crush, open, or dissolve them.
- Don't touch or handle crushed or broken capsules.
- May give drug with or without food.
- Don't give a missed dose if next dose is due within 6 hours; if patient vomits a dose, give next dose at the regular time.

ACTION
Inhibits tyrosine kinase receptors, including ALK and other growth factors, decreasing tumor-cell proliferation.

Reactions in bold italics are *life-threatening*. Interactions may have a *rapid onset* or a *delayed onset*.

Route	Onset	Peak	Duration
P.O.	Unknown	4–6 hr	Unknown

Half-life: 42 hours.

ADVERSE REACTIONS
CNS: dizziness, neuropathy, headache, insomnia, fatigue, fever.
CV: chest pain, edema, bradycardia.
EENT: visual disorders.
GI: nausea, diarrhea, vomiting, constipation, esophageal disorder, abdominal pain, stomatitis, decreased appetite, dysgeusia.
Musculoskeletal: arthralgia, back pain.
Respiratory: cough, pneumonia, dyspnea, *PE,* URI, *pneumonitis.*
Skin: rash.

INTERACTIONS
Drug-drug. *CYP3A substrates (alfentanil, cyclosporine, dihydroergotamine, ergotamine, fentanyl, pimozide, quinidine, sirolimus, tacrolimus):* May increase levels of these drugs. Avoid use together.
Moderate CYP3A inhibitors (aprepitant, diltiazem, erythromycin, fluconazole, verapamil): May increase crizotinib level. Use together cautiously.
P-glycoprotein substrates (daunorubicin, saquinavir, vinca alkaloids): May increase levels of these drugs. Avoid use together.
Strong CYP3A inducers (carbamazepine, phenobarbital, phenytoin, rifabutin, rifampin): May decrease crizotinib level. Avoid use together.
Strong CYP3A inhibitors (atazanavir, clarithromycin, indinavir, itraconazole, ketoconazole, nefazodone, nelfinavir, ritonavir, saquinavir, telithromycin, troleandomycin, voriconazole): May increase crizotinib level. Avoid use together.
Drug-herb. *St. John's wort:* May decrease crizotinib level. Avoid use together.
Drug-food. *Grapefruit, grapefruit juice:* May increase crizotinib level. Avoid use together.

EFFECTS ON LAB TEST RESULTS
- May increase ALT and AST levels.
- May decrease neutrophil, platelet, and lymphocyte counts.

CONTRAINDICATIONS & CAUTIONS
- Contraindicated in patients hypersensitive to drug or its components.
- Avoid use with other agents known to cause bradycardia (beta blockers, non-dihydropyridine calcium channel blockers, clonidine, digoxin) when possible. Monitor HR and BP regularly.
- Use cautiously in patients with hepatic disease, HF, bradyarrhythmias, or electrolyte abnormalities; in patients at risk for pneumonitis; and in patients taking medications that prolong QTc interval.
- Use cautiously in patients with moderate hepatic impairment, severe renal impairment (CrCl of less than 30 mL/minute), or ESRD.
- Use cautiously in Asian patients; drug levels at standard doses may be higher in this population.
Dialyzable drug: Unknown.

PREGNANCY-LACTATION-REPRODUCTION
- Although there are no adequate well-controlled studies in pregnant women, drug can cause fetal harm. Women of childbearing potential should avoid becoming pregnant during therapy.
- Women of childbearing potential who are receiving this drug should use adequate contraception during therapy and for at least 45 days after therapy ends; male patients receiving this drug who have partners of childbearing potential should use adequate contraception during therapy and for at least 90 days after therapy ends.
- It isn't known if drug appears in breast milk. Women shouldn't breast-feed during therapy and for 45 days after final dose.

NURSING CONSIDERATIONS
- An FDA-approved test for the detection of ROS1 positivity isn't currently available. Refer to product information for the tests used in the clinical study to identify patients with ROS1 positivity in NSCLC.
- Monitor patient for signs and symptoms of long QTc interval (such as dizziness or syncope).
- Monitor ECG in patients with HF, bradyarrhythmias, or electrolyte abnormalities and in patients taking medications that prolong QTc interval.

● Monitor electrolyte levels; correct levels as needed.

● Monitor patient for pulmonary signs and symptoms; discontinue drug if treatment-related pneumonitis occurs.

● Monitor LFTs and CBC at least monthly or as clinically indicated.

🔔 *Alert:* Monitor patient for new-onset vision loss. Discontinue drug for severe vision loss and obtain ophthalmologic evaluation.

● Drug is associated with moderate emetic potential. Consider antiemetic use.

PATIENT TEACHING

Black Box Warning Caution the patient or the caregiver of a patient taking an opioid drug with a benzodiazepine, CNS depressant, or alcohol to seek immediate medical attention if the patient has symptoms of dizziness, light-headedness, extreme sleepiness, slowed or difficult breathing, or unresponsiveness. ■

● Warn patient to swallow capsules whole and to avoid touching crushed or broken tablets.

● Advise patient to avoid grapefruit and grapefruit juice while taking drug.

● Instruct patient in the use of standard antiemetics, antidiarrheals, and laxatives to treat most frequent GI adverse effects.

● Tell patient to report visual disturbances, such as flashes of light, blurred vision, light sensitivity, or floaters.

● Teach patient that if he misses a dose, to take missed dose as soon as he remembers unless it's less than 6 hours until next dose; in that case, patient shouldn't take missed dose. Instruct patient to never take two doses at the same time to make up for a missed dose.

● Caution patient not to change dosage or stop drug without discussing with health care provider.

● Advise female patient of childbearing potential who is receiving drug to use adequate contraception during therapy and for at least 45 days after therapy ends; tell male patient receiving drug who has a partner of childbearing potential to use adequate contraception during therapy and for at least 90 days after therapy ends. Inform patient of potential risk to fetus.

cyclobenzaprine hydrochloride
sye-kloe-BEN-za-preen

Amrix

Therapeutic class: Skeletal muscle relaxants
Pharmacologic class: TCA derivatives

AVAILABLE FORMS
Capsules (extended-release) 🆕: 15 mg, 30 mg
Tablets: 5 mg, 7.5 mg, 10 mg

INDICATIONS & DOSAGES
➤ **Adjunct to rest and physical therapy to relieve muscle spasm from acute, painful musculoskeletal conditions**
Adults and children age 15 and older: 5 mg P.O. t.i.d. Based on response, dose may be increased to 10 mg t.i.d. Don't exceed 30 mg/day. Or, 15 to 30 mg extended-release capsule P.O. once daily (adults only). Use for longer than 2 or 3 weeks isn't recommended.

Adjust-a-dose: In elderly patients and in those with mild hepatic impairment, start with 5-mg conventional tablets and adjust slowly upward. Drug isn't recommended in patients with moderate to severe hepatic impairment. Don't use extended-release capsules in children, elderly patients, or those with impaired hepatic function.

ADMINISTRATION
P.O.
● Don't split the generic 10-mg tablets because of the high risk of inconsistent doses.
● Give extended-release capsules whole; don't crush or break.

ACTION
Unknown. Relieves skeletal muscle spasm of local origin without disrupting muscle function.

Route	Onset	Peak	Duration
P.O.	1 hr	4 hr	12–24 hr
P.O. (extended-release)	1.5 hr	7–8 hr	Unknown

Half-life: Tablets, 18 hours; extended-release capsules, 32 hours.

Reactions in bold italics are *life-threatening*. Interactions may have a *rapid onset* or a ***delayed onset***.

ADVERSE REACTIONS

CNS: dizziness, drowsiness, *seizures,* headache, tremor, insomnia, fatigue, asthenia, nervousness, confusion, paresthesia, depression, attention disturbances, dysarthria, ataxia, syncope.
CV: *arrhythmias,* palpitations, hypotension, tachycardia.
EENT: visual disturbances, blurred vision.
GI: dry mouth, dyspepsia, abnormal taste, constipation, nausea.
Skin: rash, pruritus, acne.

INTERACTIONS

Drug-drug. *CNS depressants:* May increase CNS depression. Avoid using together.
Guanethidine: May block guanethidine's antihypertensive effect. Monitor BP.
MAO inhibitors: May cause hyperpyretic crisis, seizures, and death when MAO inhibitors are used with TCAs; may also occur with cyclobenzaprine. Avoid using within 2 weeks of MAO inhibitor therapy.
Black Box Warning *Opioids:* May cause slow or difficult breathing, sedation, and death. Avoid use together. If use together is necessary, limit dosage and duration of each drug to the minimum necessary for desired effect. ▪
Naproxen: May increase drowsiness. Make patient aware of this interaction.
Tramadol: May increase risk of seizures. Use together cautiously.
Drug-lifestyle. *Alcohol use:* May increase CNS depression. Discourage use together.

EFFECTS ON LAB TEST RESULTS

• May cause false-positive serum TCA screen.

CONTRAINDICATIONS & CAUTIONS

• Contraindicated in patients hypersensitive to drug; in those with hyperthyroidism, heart block, arrhythmias, conduction disturbances, or HF; in those who have received MAO inhibitors within 14 days; and in those in the acute recovery phase of an MI.
• There is increased risk of potentially life-threatening serotonin syndrome when drug is used in combination with SSRIs, SNRIs, other TCAs, tramadol, bupropion, meperidine, or verapamil.
• Use cautiously in elderly or debilitated patients and in those with a history of urine

retention, acute angle-closure glaucoma, or increased IOP.
• Safety and effectiveness in children younger than age 15 haven't been established.
Dialyzable drug: Unknown.
⚠ Overdose S&S: Drowsiness, tachycardia, tremor, agitation, coma, ataxia, hypertension, slurred speech, confusion, dizziness, nausea, vomiting, hallucinations, cardiac arrest, chest pain, cardiac arrhythmias, ECG changes (changes in QRS axis or width).

PREGNANCY-LACTATION-REPRODUCTION

• There are no adequate well-controlled studies in pregnant women. Use during pregnancy only if clearly needed.
• It isn't known if drug appears in breast milk. Use cautiously in breast-feeding women.

NURSING CONSIDERATIONS

• Drug may cause toxic reactions similar to those caused by TCAs. Observe same precautions as when giving TCAs.
• Monitor patient for nausea, headache, and malaise, which may occur if drug is stopped abruptly after long-term use.
⟲ Alert: Notify prescriber immediately of signs and symptoms of overdose, including cardiac toxicity.

PATIENT TEACHING

Black Box Warning Caution the patient or the caregiver of a patient taking an opioid drug with a benzodiazepine, CNS depressant, or alcohol to seek immediate medical attention if the patient has symptoms of dizziness, light-headedness, extreme sleepiness, slowed or difficult breathing, or unresponsiveness. ▪
• Advise patient to report urinary hesitancy or urine retention. If constipation is a problem, suggest that patient increase fluid intake and use a stool softener.
• Warn patient to avoid activities that require alertness until CNS effects of drug are known.
• Warn patient not to combine with alcohol or other CNS depressants, including OTC cold or allergy remedies.
• Instruct patient not to split the generic 10-mg tablets because of the high risk of

C

inconsistent doses and not to crush or break capsules.

• Advise patient that using drug for longer than 2 to 3 weeks isn't recommended.

SAFETY ALERT!

cyclophosphamide
sye-kloe-FOSS-fa-mide

Procytox ✦

Therapeutic class: Antineoplastics
Pharmacologic class: Nitrogen mustards

AVAILABLE FORMS
Capsules ⚫: 25 mg, 50 mg
Injection: 200-mg✦, 500-mg, 1-g, 2-g vials
Tablets ⚫: 25 mg, 50 mg

INDICATIONS & DOSAGES
Adjust-a-dose (for all indications): Consider dosage reduction to 75% of usual dosage in patients with severe renal failure (CrCl of 0 to 10 mL/minute). Adjust dosage for patients with hepatic dysfunction as follows: If bilirubin level is 3.1 to 5 mg/dL or AST level is greater than 180 units/L, give 75% of dose. Don't give if bilirubin level is greater than 5 mg/dL.

➤ **Breast or ovarian cancer, Hodgkin lymphoma, chronic lymphocytic leukemia, chronic myelocytic leukemia, acute lymphoblastic leukemia, acute myelocytic and monocytic leukemia, neuroblastoma, retinoblastoma, malignant lymphoma, multiple myeloma, mycosis fungoides**
Adults and children: Initially for induction, 40 to 50 mg/kg I.V. in divided doses over 2 to 5 days. Or, 10 to 15 mg/kg I.V. every 7 to 10 days, 3 to 5 mg/kg I.V. twice weekly, or 1 to 5 mg/kg P.O. daily, based on patient tolerance. Adjust subsequent doses according to evidence of antitumor activity or leukopenia.

➤ **Minimal-change nephrotic syndrome in patients who failed to adequately respond to or are unable to tolerate adrenocorticosteroid therapy**
Children: 2 mg/kg P.O. daily for 8 to 12 weeks. Maximum cumulative dose, 168 mg/kg.

ADMINISTRATION
P.O.
• Don't give oral form at bedtime; infrequent urination during the night may increase possibility of cystitis.
• Make sure patient receives adequate fluids or is infused to force diuresis to reduce risk of urinary tract toxicity.
• Don't open, cut, crush, or allow patient to chew capsules or tablets.
• Drug is considered a hazardous agent. Follow appropriate precautions for safe handling and disposal.

I.V.
▼ Preparing and giving parenteral form of drug may be mutagenic, teratogenic, or carcinogenic. Follow facility policy to reduce risks.
▼ Reconstitute powder using sterile water for injection or bacteriostatic water for injection containing only parabens.
▼ Add 25 mL to 500-mg vial, 50 mL to 1-g vial, or 100 mL to 2-g vial to produce a solution containing 20 mg/mL. Shake vigorously to dissolve. If powder doesn't dissolve completely, let vial stand for a few minutes.
▼ Check reconstituted solution for small particles. Filter solution, if needed.
▼ Give by direct I.V. injection or infusion.
▼ For infusion, further dilute with D₅W, dextrose 5% in NSS for injection, dextrose 5% in Ringer injection, lactated Ringer injection, sodium lactate injection, or half-NSS for injection.
▼ Reconstituted solution is stable 6 days if refrigerated or 24 hours at room temperature. Use stored solutions cautiously because drug contains no preservatives.
▼ **Incompatibilities:** Amphotericin B cholesteryl sulfate complex.

ACTION
Cross-links strands of cellular DNA and interferes with RNA transcription, causing an imbalance of growth that leads to cell death. Not specific to cell cycle.

Route	Onset	Peak	Duration
P.O.	Unknown	Unknown	Unknown
I.V.	Unknown	2–3 hr	Unknown

Half-life: 3 to 12 hours.

Reactions in bold italics are *life-threatening*. Interactions may have a *rapid onset* or a **delayed onset**.

ADVERSE REACTIONS

CV: *cardiotoxicity with very high doses and with doxorubicin.*
GI: nausea and vomiting, anorexia, stomatitis.
GU: *hemorrhagic cystitis,* impaired fertility.
Hematologic: *leukopenia, thrombocytopenia,* anemia.
Hepatic: *hepatotoxicity.*
Metabolic: hyperuricemia, SIADH.
Respiratory: *pulmonary fibrosis with high doses.*
Skin: alopecia.
Other: *secondary malignant disease, anaphylaxis,* hypersensitivity reactions.

INTERACTIONS

Drug-drug. *Allopurinol, myelosuppressants:* May increase myelosuppression. Monitor patient for toxicity.
Amiodarone: May increase risk of pulmonary toxicity. Monitor therapy.
Anticoagulants: May increase anticoagulant effect. Monitor patient for bleeding.
Aspirin, NSAIDs: May increase risk of bleeding. Avoid using together.
Azole antifungals (itraconazole): May increase exposure to cyclophosphamide and its metabolites. Closely monitor patient for cyclophosphamide adverse reactions.
Barbiturates: May enhance cyclophosphamide toxicity. Monitor patient closely.
Carbamazepine: May increase cyclophosphamide level. Monitor patient carefully and adjust cyclophosphamide dosage as needed.
Cardiotoxic drugs: May increase adverse cardiac effects. Monitor patient for toxicity.
Chloramphenicol, corticosteroids: May reduce activity of cyclophosphamide. Use together cautiously.
Ciprofloxacin: May decrease antimicrobial effect. Monitor patient for effect.
Clozapine: May increase risk of neutropenia. Monitor therapy.
Digoxin: May decrease digoxin level. Monitor level closely.
Live-virus vaccines: May increase vaccine-induced adverse reactions. Don't give together.
Pentostatin: May cause respiratory distress, hypotension, hypothermia, and death. Avoid use together if possible.

Phenytoin: May increase risk of cyclophosphamide toxicity. If coadministration can't be avoided, monitor patient carefully and consider reducing initial dose of cyclophosphamide.
Quinolones: May decrease the antimicrobial effects of quinolones. Monitor patient.
Succinylcholine: May prolong neuromuscular blockade. Avoid using together.
Thiazide diuretics: May prolong antineoplastic-induced leukopenia. Monitor patient closely.
TNF blockers: May increase the incidence of noncutaneous solid malignancies. Use together isn't recommended.

EFFECTS ON LAB TEST RESULTS

• May increase uric acid level. May decrease Hb and pseudocholinesterase levels.
• May decrease platelet, RBC, and WBC counts.
• May suppress positive reaction to *Candida,* mumps, *Trichophyton,* and tuberculin skin test results. May cause a false-positive Papanicolaou test result.

CONTRAINDICATIONS & CAUTIONS

• Contraindicated in patients hypersensitive to drug and in those with severe bone marrow suppression or urinary outflow obstruction.
• Use cautiously in patients with leukopenia, thrombocytopenia, malignant cell infiltration of bone marrow, or hepatic or renal disease and in those who have recently undergone radiation therapy or chemotherapy.
Dialyzable drug: Yes.
⚠ **Overdose S&S:** Infection, myelosuppression, cardiotoxicity.

PREGNANCY-LACTATION-REPRODUCTION

• Drug may cause fetal harm if used during pregnancy. Women of childbearing potential should avoid pregnancy while receiving cyclophosphamide and for up to 1 year after completion of treatment. Male patients who are sexually active with female partners who are or may become pregnant should use a condom during and for at least 4 months after treatment.
• Amenorrhea, transient or permanent, develops in a proportion of women treated

with drug. The risk of premature menopause increases with age.

• Men treated with drug may develop oligospermia or azoospermia. Development of sterility appears to depend on dose, duration of therapy, and state of gonadal function at time of treatment. Sterility may be irreversible in some patients. Treatment for nephrotic syndrome beyond 90 days in boys increases the probability of sterility.

• Drug appears in breast milk. Patient should discontinue breast-feeding or discontinue drug, taking into account importance of drug to the mother.

NURSING CONSIDERATIONS

• If cystitis occurs, stop drug and notify prescriber. Cystitis can occur months after therapy ends. Mesna may be given to reduce frequency and severity of bladder toxicity. Test urine for blood.

• Adequately hydrate patients before and after dose to decrease risk of cystitis.

• Use caution to ensure correct dose to decrease risk of cardiac toxicity.

• Monitor CBC and renal function tests and LFT results.

• Monitor patient closely for leukopenia (nadir between days 8 and 15, recovery in 17 to 28 days).

• Monitor uric acid level. To prevent hyperuricemia with resulting uric acid nephropathy, allopurinol may be used with adequate hydration.

• To prevent bleeding, avoid all I.M. injections when platelet count is less than 50,000/mm^3.

• Anticipate blood transfusions because of cumulative anemia.

• Therapeutic effects are often accompanied by toxicity.

PATIENT TEACHING

• Warn patient that hair loss is likely to occur but is reversible.

• Advise patient to watch for signs and symptoms of infection (fever, sore throat, fatigue) and bleeding (easy bruising, nosebleeds, bleeding gums, tarry stools). Tell patient to take temperature daily.

• Instruct patient to avoid OTC products that contain aspirin.

• To minimize risk of hemorrhagic cystitis, encourage patient to urinate every 1 to 2 hours while awake and to drink at least 3 L of fluid daily.

• If patient is taking tablets or capsules, tell him not to take them at bedtime because infrequent urination during night increases risk of cystitis.

• Advise both men and women to practice contraception during therapy and for 4 months afterward for men and 12 months for women; drug may cause birth defects.

• Advise women to stop breast-feeding during therapy because of risk of toxicity to infant.

• Drug can cause irreversible sterility in both males and females. Before therapy, counsel patient who is considering parenthood. Also recommend that women consult prescriber before becoming pregnant.

cycloSPORINE
sye-kloe-SPOR-een

Sandimmune

cycloSPORINE (modified)
Gengraf, Neoral

Therapeutic class: Immunosuppressants
Pharmacologic class:
Immunosuppressants

AVAILABLE FORMS
Capsules for microemulsion (modified)*:
25 mg, 50 mg, 100 mg
Capsules (nonmodified): 25 mg, 50 mg, 100 mg
Injection: 50 mg/mL
Oral solution (modified and nonmodified):
100 mg/mL*

INDICATIONS & DOSAGES
➤ **To prevent organ rejection in renal, hepatic, or cardiac transplantation**
Adults and children: 15 mg/kg P.O. 4 to 12 hours before transplantation, continued daily for 1 to 2 weeks postoperatively. Then reduce dosage by 5% each week to maintenance level of 5 to 10 mg/kg daily. Or, 5 to 6 mg/kg I.V. concentrate 4 to 12 hours before transplantation as a slow I.V. infusion

---

Reactions in bold italics are *life-threatening*. Interactions may have a *rapid onset* or a *delayed onset*.

over 2 to 6 hours. Postoperatively, repeat dose daily until patient can tolerate oral forms.

For conversion from Sandimmune to Gengraf or Neoral, use same daily dose as previously used for Sandimmune. Monitor blood levels every 4 to 7 days after conversion, and monitor BP and creatinine level every 2 weeks during the first 2 months.

➤ **Severe, active RA that hasn't adequately responded to methotrexate**
Adults: 1.25 mg/kg P.O. b.i.d. Gengraf or Neoral. Dosage may be increased by 0.5 to 0.75 mg/kg daily after 8 weeks and again after 12 weeks to a maximum of 4 mg/kg daily. If no response is seen after 16 weeks, stop therapy.

Adjust-a-dose: If hypertension, serum creatinine elevations (30% above patient's pretreatment level), or clinically significant laboratory abnormalities occur, decrease dosage by 25% to 50% to control adverse reactions. If dosage reduction doesn't control abnormalities, or if the adverse reaction or abnormality is severe, discontinue drug.

➤ **Psoriasis**
Adults: 1.25 mg/kg Gengraf or Neoral daily P.O. b.i.d. for at least 4 weeks. Increase dosage by 0.5 mg/kg daily once every 2 weeks as needed to a maximum of 4 mg/kg daily.

Adjust-a-dose: If clinically significant laboratory abnormalities occur, decrease dosage by 25% to 50% to control adverse reactions. If the serum creatinine level is 25% or more above patient's pretreatment level, serum creatinine measurement should be repeated within 2 weeks. If the serum creatinine level remains at 25% or more above baseline, reduce dosage by 25% to 50%. If at any time the serum creatinine level increases by 50% or more above pretreatment level, reduce dosage by 25% to 50%. If reversibility (within 25% of baseline) of the serum creatinine level isn't achievable after two dosage modifications, discontinue drug.

If patient with no history of hypertension before initiation of therapy develops hypertension, reduce dosage by 25% to 50%. If patient continues to be hypertensive despite multiple dosage reductions, discontinue drug. For patients with previously treated hypertension, adjust their antihypertensive

medication. Discontinue cyclosporine if a change in hypertension management isn't effective or tolerable.

ADMINISTRATION
P.O.
● Drug is considered a potential teratogen and mutagen. Follow safe-handling procedures when preparing, administering, or dispensing.
● Give Neoral or Gengraf on an empty stomach.
● Measure oral solution doses carefully in an oral syringe. Don't rinse dosing syringe with water. If syringe is cleaned, it must be completely dry before reuse.
● To improve the taste of Sandimmune oral solution, mix it with milk, chocolate milk, or orange juice. Gengraf or Neoral oral solution may be mixed with orange or apple juice (not grapefruit juice); it's less palatable when mixed with milk.
● Use a glass container to mix, and have patient drink at once.

I.V.
▼ This form is usually reserved for patients who can't tolerate oral drugs.
▼ Immediately before use, dilute each milliliter of concentrate in 20 to 100 mL of D_5W or NSS for injection. Give at $\frac{1}{3}$ the oral dose.
▼ Infuse over 2 to 6 hours.
▼ Protect diluted drug from light.
▼ **Incompatibilities:** Amphotericin B cholesteryl sulfate complex, magnesium sulfate.

ACTION
May inhibit proliferation and function of T lymphocytes and inhibit production and release of lymphokines.

Route	Onset	Peak	Duration
P.O.	Unknown	90 min–3 hr	Unknown
I.V.	Unknown	Unknown	Unknown

Half-life: Initial phase, about 1 hour; terminal phase, 8½ to 27 hours.

ADVERSE REACTIONS
CNS: tremor, headache, confusion, paresthesia, *seizures.*
CV: hypertension, flushing.
EENT: gum hyperplasia, sinusitis.

GI: nausea, vomiting, diarrhea, abdominal discomfort.
GU: *nephrotoxicity.*
Hematologic: anemia, *leukopenia, thrombocytopenia.*
Hepatic: *hepatotoxicity.*
Metabolic: hyperglycemia.
Skin: hirsutism, acne.
Other: infections, *anaphylaxis.*

INTERACTIONS

Drug-drug. *Acyclovir, aminoglycosides, amphotericin B, cimetidine, diclofenac, gentamicin, ketoconazole, melphalan, NSAIDs, ranitidine, sulfamethoxazole–trimethoprim, tacrolimus, tobramycin, vancomycin:* May increase risk of nephrotoxicity. Avoid using together.
Allopurinol, **azole antifungals,** *bromocriptine,* **caspofungin,** *cimetidine, clarithromycin, danazol, diltiazem, erythromycin, imipenem–cilastatin, methylprednisolone, metoclopramide,* **micafungin,** *nicardipine, prednisolone, verapamil:* May increase cyclosporine level. Monitor patient for increased toxicity.
Azathioprine, corticosteroids, cyclophosphamide, verapamil: May increase immunosuppression. Monitor patient closely.
Carbamazepine, isoniazid, nafcillin, octreotide, **orlistat,** *phenobarbital,* **phenytoin, rifabutin, rifampin,** *ticlopidine:* May decrease immunosuppressant effect from low cyclosporine level. Cyclosporine dosage may need to be increased.
Digoxin, HMG-CoA reductase inhibitors (lovastatin), prednisolone: May decrease clearance of these drugs. Use together cautiously.
Mycophenolate mofetil: May decrease mycophenolate level. Monitor patient closely when cyclosporine is added to or removed from therapy.
Potassium-sparing diuretics: May induce hyperkalemia. Monitor patient closely.
Sirolimus: May increase sirolimus level. Take sirolimus at least 4 hours after cyclosporine dose. If separating doses isn't possible, monitor patient for increased adverse effects.
Vaccines: May decrease immune response. Delay routine immunization.

Drug-herb. *Astragalus, echinacea, licorice:* May interfere with drug's effect. Discourage use together.
St. John's wort: May reduce drug level, resulting in transplant failure. Discourage use together.
Drug-food. *Alfalfa sprouts:* May interfere with drug's effect. Discourage use together.
Grapefruit and grapefruit juice: May increase drug level and cause toxicity. Advise patient to avoid use together.
Drug-lifestyle. *Sun exposure:* May increase risk of sensitivity to sunlight. Advise patient to avoid excessive sun exposure.

EFFECTS ON LAB TEST RESULTS

• May increase ALT, AST, bilirubin, BUN, creatinine, glucose, and LDL levels.
• May decrease Hb and magnesium levels.
• May decrease platelet and WBC counts.

CONTRAINDICATIONS & CAUTIONS

• Contraindicated in patients hypersensitive to drug or polyoxyethylated castor oil (found in injectable form).
• Contraindicated in patients with RA or psoriasis with abnormal renal function, uncontrolled hypertension, or malignancies (Neoral or Gengraf).
• Contraindicated with psoralen and ultraviolet A light (PUVA), methotrexate or other immunosuppressive agents, ultraviolet B light (UVB), coal tar, or radiation therapy in psoriasis patients (Neoral or Gengraf).
Black Box Warning Manage patients receiving drug in facilities equipped and staffed with adequate laboratory and supportive medical resources. ∎
Dialyzable drug: No.

PREGNANCY-LACTATION-REPRODUCTION

• There are no adequate studies in pregnant women; use during pregnancy isn't recommended. If drug is needed during pregnancy, use only if potential benefit justifies potential risk to the fetus.
• Alcohol is present in cyclosporine preparations; this fact should be considered when using drug in pregnant women.
• Drug and ethanol present in cyclosporine preparations appear in breast milk. Patient should discontinue breast-feeding or

discontinue drug, taking into account importance of drug to the mother.

NURSING CONSIDERATIONS

Black Box Warning Only experienced physicians should prescribe this drug. ■

Black Box Warning Psoriasis patients previously treated with PUVA, methotrexate or other immunosuppressive agents, UVB, coal tar, or radiation therapy are at an increased risk for skin malignancies when taking Neoral or Gengraf. ■

• Drug can cause hepatotoxicity.

Black Box Warning Neoral and Gengraf may increase the susceptibility to infection and the development of neoplasia. ■

🜂 *Alert:* Drugs causing immunosuppression increase the risk of opportunistic infections, including activation of latent viral infections such as BK virus–associated neuropathy, which may lead to serious outcomes, including kidney graft loss.

Black Box Warning Monitor patient's renal function. ■

Black Box Warning Monitor cyclosporine level at regular intervals with prolonged Sandimmune use. Absorption of capsules and oral solution can be erratic during long-term use. ■

Black Box Warning Neoral and Gengraf have greater bioavailability than Sandimmune. A lower dose of Neoral or Gengraf may be needed to provide blood level similar to that achieved with Sandimmune. Monitor blood level when switching patients between these two brands. ■

Black Box Warning Gengraf is bioequivalent to and interchangeable with Neoral capsules, but neither is interchangeable with Sandimmune. ■

Black Box Warning Always give with corticosteroids; however, don't give Sandimmune with other immunosuppressants. ■

Black Box Warning Drug can cause systemic hypertension and nephrotoxicity; risk increases with increasing dosage and duration of therapy. ■

• Use Neoral or Gengraf to treat RA or psoriasis.

RA

• Before starting treatment, measure BP at least twice and obtain two creatinine levels to estimate baseline.

• Evaluate BP and creatinine level every 2 weeks during first 3 months and then monthly if patient is stable.

• Monitor BP and creatinine level after an increase in NSAID dosage or introduction of a new NSAID. Monitor CBC and LFTs monthly if patient also receives methotrexate.

Psoriasis

• Measure BP at least twice to determine a baseline. Monitor BP after dosage changes.

• Evaluate patient for occult infection and tumors initially and throughout treatment.

• Obtain baseline creatinine level (on two occasions), CBC, and BUN, magnesium, uric acid, potassium, and lipid levels.

• Evaluate BP, CBC, and uric acid, potassium, lipid, magnesium, creatinine, and BUN levels every 2 weeks during first 3 months and then monthly thereafter if patient is stable.

• Monitor creatinine level after increasing NSAID dose or starting a new NSAID.

• Improvement in psoriasis takes 12 to 16 weeks of therapy.

• *Look alike–sound alike:* Don't confuse cyclosporine with cyclophosphamide or cycloserine. Don't confuse Sandimmune with Sandostatin.

PATIENT TEACHING

• Encourage patient to take drug at same time each day and to be consistent with relation to meals.

• Teach patient how to measure dosage and mask taste of oral solution. Tell him not to take drug with grapefruit juice.

• Instruct patient to fill glass with water after dose and drink it to make sure he consumes all of drug.

• Advise patient to take drug with meals if nausea occurs.

• Advise patient to take Neoral or Gengraf on an empty stomach.

• Tell patient being treated for psoriasis that improvement may not occur until after 12 to 16 weeks of therapy.

• Stress that drug shouldn't be stopped without prescriber's approval.

• Explain to patient the importance of frequent laboratory monitoring while receiving therapy.

• Tell patient to avoid people with infections because drug lowers resistance to infection.

• Advise patient to perform careful oral care and to see a dentist regularly because drug can cause gum disease.

• Advise female patient to use barrier contraception, not hormonal contraceptives, during therapy. Advise patient of the potential risk during pregnancy and the increased risk of tumors, high BP, and renal problems.

• Warn patient to wear protection in the sun and to avoid excessive sun exposure.

SAFETY ALERT!

cytarabine (ara-C, cytosine arabinoside)
sye-TARE-a-been

Cytosar✶, DepoCyt

Therapeutic class: Antineoplastics
Pharmacologic class: Pyrimidine analogues

AVAILABLE FORMS
Injection: 20 mg/mL, 100 mg/mL
Liposomal intrathecal injection: 10 mg/mL

INDICATIONS & DOSAGES
Adjust-a-dose (for all indications): For conventional form, consider dosage reduction in patients with poor renal function.

➤ **Acute nonlymphocytic leukemia**
Adults and children: 100 mg/m² I.V. daily by continuous I.V. infusion or 100 mg/m² I.V. every 12 hours by rapid I.V. injection or I.V. infusion on days 1 to 7 in a course of therapy or daily until remission is attained.

➤ **Acute lymphocytic leukemia**
Consult literature for current recommendations.

➤ **Meningeal leukemia**
Adults and children: Varies from 5 to 75 mg/m² intrathecally. Frequency varies from once daily for 4 days to once every 4 days. The most frequently used dose is 30 mg/m² every 4 days until CSF is normal; then one additional dose.

➤ **Lymphomatous meningitis (liposomal)**
Adults: For induction, give 50 mg liposomal injection intrathecally every 14 days for two doses (weeks 1 and 3); then, for consolida-

tion therapy, give 50 mg liposomal injection intrathecally every 14 days for three doses (weeks 5, 7, and 9) followed by one additional dose at week 13. Maintenance dose, 50 mg liposomal injection intrathecally every 28 days for four doses (weeks 17, 21, 25, and 29).

Adjust-a-dose: For patients with neurotoxicity, reduce dose to 25 mg. If neurotoxicity persists, stop therapy.

➤ **Acute promyelocytic leukemia (induction)** ◆
Adults: 200 mg/m² I.V. daily by continuous I.V. infusion for 7 days beginning on day 3 of treatment (in combination with tretinoin and daunorubicin).

ADMINISTRATION
I.V.
▼ Preparing and giving parenteral drug may be mutagenic, teratogenic, or carcinogenic. Follow facility policy to reduce risks.

▼ To reduce nausea, give antiemetic before drug. Nausea and vomiting are more likely with large doses given by I.V. push. Dizziness may occur with rapid infusion.

▼ For I.V. infusion, dilute solution in vial using NSS for injection or D₅W.

▼ **Incompatibilities:** Allopurinol sodium, amphotericin B cholesteryl sulfate complex, 5-FU, ganciclovir sodium, heparin sodium, hydrocortisone sodium succinate, insulin, methylprednisolone sodium succinate, nafcillin, oxacillin, penicillin.

Intrathecal
• Drug is considered hazardous; use safe handling and disposal precautions.

Black Box Warning Give liposomal form with dexamethasone to help decrease symptoms of chemical arachnoiditis, which may be life-threatening. ∎

• Withdraw intrathecal cytarabine liposomal injection from the vial immediately before administration. It is a single-use vial, doesn't contain any preservative, and should be used within 4 hours of withdrawal from the vial. Discard unused portions of each vial properly.

• Don't use in-line filters when giving intrathecal cytarabine liposomal injection.

- After drug administration by lumbar puncture, instruct patient to lie flat for 1 hour.
- Patients should be observed by the physician for immediate toxic reactions.
- Refrigerate liposomal form at 36° to 46° F (2° to 8° C).

ACTION
Inhibits DNA synthesis.

Route	Onset	Peak	Duration
I.V., intrathecal	Unknown	Unknown	Unknown

Half-life: Initial, 8 minutes; terminal, 1 to 3 hours; in CSF, 2 hours.

ADVERSE REACTIONS
CNS: *neurotoxicity,* malaise, dizziness, headache, cerebellar syndrome, fever.
CV: thrombophlebitis, edema.
EENT: conjunctivitis.
GI: nausea, vomiting, diarrhea, anorexia, anal ulceration, abdominal pain, oral ulcers in 5 to 10 days, projectile vomiting, *bowel necrosis with high doses given by rapid I.V.*
GU: urine retention, renal dysfunction.
Hematologic: *leukopenia,* anemia, reticulocytopenia, *thrombocytopenia,* megaloblastosis.
Hepatic: *hepatotoxicity,* jaundice.
Metabolic: hyperuricemia.
Musculoskeletal: myalgia, bone pain.
Respiratory: *pulmonary edema,* shortness of breath, pulmonary hypersensitivity.
Skin: rash, pruritus, alopecia, freckling.
Other: flulike syndrome, infection, *anaphylaxis.*

INTERACTIONS
Drug-drug. *Digoxin, except oral liquid:* May decrease oral digoxin absorption. Monitor digoxin level closely.
Flucytosine: May decrease flucytosine activity. Avoid using together.
Gentamicin: May decrease activity against *Klebsiella pneumoniae.* Avoid using together.

EFFECTS ON LAB TEST RESULTS
- May increase bilirubin, phosphorus, potassium, and uric acid levels. May decrease Hb level.

- May increase megaloblast count. May decrease platelet, RBC, reticulocyte, and WBC counts.

CONTRAINDICATIONS & CAUTIONS
- Contraindicated in patients hypersensitive to drug and in those with active meningeal infection (liposomal cytarabine). Anaphylaxis has been reported (rare).
- Use cautiously in patients with hepatic or renal impairment, gout, or myelosuppression.
- Tumor lysis syndrome may occur. Consider antihyperuricemic therapy and ensure adequate hydration.
Alert: With high-dose therapy, drug is associated with sudden respiratory distress syndrome, which can be fatal.
Dialyzable drug: Yes.
Overdose S&S: Irreversible CNS toxicity, death (conventional form); severe chemical arachnoiditis (liposomal form).

PREGNANCY-LACTATION-REPRODUCTION
- Drug can cause fetal harm if a pregnant woman is exposed to drug systemically. Advise women of childbearing potential to avoid becoming pregnant during therapy. If drug is used during pregnancy or if patient becomes pregnant while taking drug, patient should be apprised of the potential harm to the fetus.
- It isn't known if drug appears in breast milk. Patient should discontinue breastfeeding or discontinue drug, taking into account importance of drug to the mother.

NURSING CONSIDERATIONS
Black Box Warning Cytarabine should be administered by physicians experienced in cancer chemotherapy. For induction therapy, patients should be treated in a facility with laboratory and supportive resources sufficient to monitor drug tolerance and protect and maintain a patient compromised by drug toxicity. The physician must judge possible benefit to patient against known toxic effects of cytarabine.
Black Box Warning Ensure that dexamethasone is given concurrently with liposomal form of drug.

- Drug is an irritant. If extravasation occurs, stop the infusion immediately and follow facility policy for monitoring and treatment.
- Monitor fluid intake and output carefully. Maintain high fluid intake and give allopurinol to avoid urate nephropathy in leukemia-induction therapy. Monitor uric acid level.
- Monitor renal function studies, LFTs, and CBC with differential.
- Therapy may be modified or stopped if granulocyte count is below 1,000/mm^3 or platelet count is below 50,000/mm^3.
- Corticosteroid eye drops help prevent drug-induced conjunctivitis.
- Provide diligent mouth care to help minimize stomatitis.

🔵 *Alert:* Assess patient receiving high doses for neurotoxicity, which may first appear as nystagmus but can progress to ataxia and cerebellar dysfunction.

- To prevent bleeding, avoid all I.M. injections when platelet count is below 50,000/mm^3.
- Anticipate blood transfusions because of cumulative anemia. Patient may receive RBC colony-stimulating factors to promote RBC production and decrease need for blood transfusions.

Black Box Warning Monitor patient for toxic effects, including bone marrow suppression, nausea, vomiting, diarrhea, oral ulceration, and hepatic dysfunction. ∎

- In leukopenia, initial WBC count nadir occurs 7 to 9 days after drug is stopped. A second, more severe nadir occurs 15 to 24 days after drug is stopped. In thrombocytopenia, platelet count nadir occurs on days 12 to 15.

🔵 *Alert:* A cytarabine syndrome has been described and is characterized by fever, myalgia, bone pain, occasionally chest pain, maculopapular rash, conjunctivitis, and malaise. It usually occurs 6 to 12 hours after drug administration. Corticosteroids have been shown to be beneficial in the treatment or prevention of this syndrome.

- *Look alike–sound alike:* Don't confuse conventional cytarabine with liposomal cytarabine.

PATIENT TEACHING
- Instruct patient to watch for signs and symptoms of infection (fever, sore throat, fatigue) and bleeding (easy bruising, nosebleeds, bleeding gums, tarry stools). Tell patient to take temperature daily.
- Advise patient to report visual changes, blurred vision, or eye pain to prescriber.
- Advise breast-feeding patient to stop breast-feeding during therapy because of risk of toxicity in infant.
- Caution female patient of childbearing potential to consult prescriber before becoming pregnant because drug may harm fetus.

SAFETY ALERT!

dabigatran etexilate mesylate
da-BIG-a-tran

Pradaxa🍂

Therapeutic class: Anticoagulants
Pharmacologic class: Direct thrombin inhibitors

AVAILABLE FORMS
Capsules 🆔*:* 75 mg, 110 mg, 150 mg

INDICATIONS & DOSAGES
➤ **To reduce risk of stroke and systemic embolism in patients with nonvalvular atrial fibrillation**
Adults: 150 mg P.O. b.i.d. if CrCl is greater than 30 mL/minute. When converting from warfarin to dabigatran, stop warfarin and start dabigatran when INR is below 2. When converting from dabigatran to warfarin and CrCl is 50 mL/minute or greater, start warfarin 3 days before stopping dabigatran; if CrCl is 31 to 50 mL/minute, start warfarin 2 days before stopping dabigatran; if CrCl is 15 to 30 mL/minute, start warfarin 1 day before stopping dabigatran; if CrCl is less than 15 mL/minute, no recommendations can be made. When converting from parenteral anticoagulants to dabigatran, start dabigatran 0 to 2 hours before the next scheduled dose of the parenteral anticoagulant, or at the time of discontinuing a continuously

administered parenteral drug (such as unfractionated heparin). When converting from dabigatran to parenteral anticoagulation and CrCl is 30 mL/minute or more, wait 12 hours or, if CrCl is less than 30 mL/minute, wait 24 hours after the last dose of dabigatran before beginning parenteral treatment.

Adjust-a-dose: For patients with CrCl of 15 to 30 mL/minute or for those with CrCl of 30 to 50 mL/minute who are taking dronedarone or oral ketoconazole concurrently, give 75 mg P.O. b.i.d. Don't use in patients on dialysis or in those with CrCl of less than 15 mL/minute.

➤ **To treat DVT and PE in patients with CrCl greater than 30 mL/minute who have been treated with a parenteral anticoagulant for 5 to 10 days; to reduce risk of recurrence of DVT and PE in patients with CrCl greater than 30 mL/minute who have been previously treated**
Adults: 150 mg P.O. b.i.d.
Adjust-a-dose: There are no dosing recommendations for patients with CrCl of 30 mL/minute or less or for those on dialysis. Avoid use in patients with CrCl of less than 50 mL/minute also taking P-glycoprotein inhibitors.

✷ **NEW INDICATION: Prophylaxis of DVT and PE after hip replacement surgery**
Adults: 110 mg P.O. 1 to 4 hours after surgery and after hemostasis has been achieved, then 220 mg once daily for 28 to 35 days. If drug isn't started on day of surgery, after hemostasis has been achieved, start treatment with 220 mg once daily.
Adjust-a-dose: There are no dosing recommendations for patients with CrCl of less than 30 mL/minute or for those on dialysis. Avoid use in patients with CrCl of less than 50 mL/minute also taking P-glycoprotein inhibitors.

ADMINISTRATION
P.O.
● Give without regard to food.
● Don't crush capsule, empty its contents, or allow patient to chew capsule. Capsule must be swallowed whole.
● Temporarily discontinue drug before invasive or surgical procedures. Restart drug promptly after procedure.

ACTION
Inhibits thrombin formation, preventing development of a thrombus.

Route	Onset	Peak	Duration
P.O.	Unknown	1–2 hr	Unknown

Half-life: 12 to 17 hours.

ADVERSE REACTIONS
GI: dyspepsia, abdominal pain, abdominal discomfort, gastritis-like symptoms, GERD, esophagitis, erosive gastritis, *gastric hemorrhage, hemorrhagic erosive gastritis,* GI ulcer, diarrhea, nausea, *GI bleeding.*
Hematologic: *life-threatening bleeding,* major bleeding, any bleeding.

INTERACTIONS
Drug-drug. *Antiplatelet drugs, aspirin, dronedarone, fibrinolytic therapy, heparin, ketoconazole:* May increase effectiveness of dabigatran. Consider reducing dabigatran dosage to 75 mg b.i.d. when giving concomitantly to patients with moderate renal impairment (CrCl of 30 to 50 mL/minute).
NSAIDs: May increase risk of bleeding. Avoid use together.
Rifampin: May reduce dabigatran level. Avoid use together.
Drug-herb. *St. John's wort:* May decrease dabigatran pharmacologic effects and plasma concentration. Avoid concurrent use.

EFFECTS ON LAB TEST RESULTS
● May increase aPTT, ecarin clotting time (ECT), and thrombin time.

CONTRAINDICATIONS & CAUTIONS
Black Box Warning Consider potential risk of epidural or spinal hematoma versus potential benefit in patients scheduled for spinal procedures, such as spinal or epidural anesthesia or spinal puncture. Hematomas may result in long-term or permanent paralysis. Increased risk may occur with use of indwelling epidural catheters, concomitant use of drugs that affect hemostasis (NSAIDs, platelet inhibitors, anticoagulants), history of traumatic or repeated epidural or spinal punctures, or history of spinal deformity or surgery. Optimal timing

between administration of drug and spinal or epidural procedure isn't known. ∎

• Contraindicated in patients hypersensitive to drug and in those with active pathologic bleeding.

• Contraindicated in patients with mechanical prosthetic valves. Use in patients with atrial fibrillation in the setting of other forms of valvular heart disease, including the presence of a bioprosthetic heart valve, isn't recommended.

• Use cautiously in elderly patients and in patients with history of bleeding.

• Because of risk of clot formation and stroke, avoid lapses in therapy when possible. Restart therapy as soon as possible.

Black Box Warning Discontinuing drug prematurely increases risk of thrombotic events. If drug must be discontinued for a reason other than pathologic bleeding, consider coverage with another anticoagulant. ∎

Dialyzable drug: Approximately 57%.

⚠ *Overdose S&S:* Hemorrhagic complications.

PREGNANCY-LACTATION-REPRODUCTION

• There are no adequate well-controlled studies in pregnant women. Consider risks of bleeding and stroke if drug is used during pregnancy.

• It isn't known if drug appears in breast milk. Patient should discontinue breast-feeding or discontinue drug, taking into account importance of drug to the mother.

NURSING CONSIDERATIONS

• Monitor patient for signs of bleeding. If bleeding occurs, stop drug, investigate cause, and provide supportive measures.

• Monitor ECT or aPPT to assess treatment effectiveness.

Black Box Warning Monitor patient for neurologic impairment (midline back pain, sensory or motor deficits such as numbness or weakness in lower limbs, bowel or bladder dysfunction). Treat impairment urgently. ∎

• Discontinue dabigatran 1 to 2 days before invasive or surgical procedures in patients with CrCl of 50 mL/minute or more and 3 to 5 days in patients with CrCl of less than 50 mL/minute. Consider longer times for patients undergoing major surgery, spinal puncture, or placement of a spinal or epidural catheter or port, in whom complete hemostasis may be required.

PATIENT TEACHING

🕯 *Alert:* Advise patient to keep drug in original bottle to protect from moisture, to remove only one capsule from the opened bottle at the time of use, to tightly close the bottle immediately after removing drug, and not to put drug in pill boxes or pill organizers.

• Tell patient that drug may be taken without regard to food.

• Advise patient to take dabigatran at approximately the same times each day. A missed dose may be skipped only if it can't be taken at least 6 hours before the next scheduled dose.

• Teach patient to swallow the capsule whole and not to open, crush, or chew it.

• Caution patient to take drug as prescribed and not to stop or change dosage without first consulting health care provider.

• Advise patient to tell all of his health care providers that he's taking this drug.

• Tell patient to inform health care provider about use of other drugs, including OTCs, vitamins, and herbs.

• Warn patient he may bruise more easily and bleed longer while taking this drug.

• Instruct patient to report bleeding when brushing teeth or shaving; blood in vomit, urine, or stool; heavier menstrual bleeding; or nosebleeds.

• Tell patient he will need to have regular blood tests to monitor drug's effects.

• Instruct patient to inform his health care provider of scheduled invasive procedures, including dental work. Drug may need to be stopped temporarily.

SAFETY ALERT!

dacarbazine (DTIC)
da-KAR-ba-zeen

Therapeutic class: Antineoplastics
Pharmacologic class: Triazenes

AVAILABLE FORMS
Injection: 100 mg, 200 mg

INDICATIONS & DOSAGES

➤ **Metastatic malignant melanoma**
Adults: 2 to 4.5 mg/kg I.V. daily for 10 days; repeat every 4 weeks as tolerated. Or, 250 mg/m^2 I.V. daily for 5 days; repeat every 3 weeks.

➤ **Hodgkin lymphoma**
Adults: 150 mg/m^2 I.V. daily (with other drugs) for 5 days; repeat every 4 weeks. Or, 375 mg/m^2 on first day of combination regimen; repeat every 15 days.

➤ **Advanced soft-tissue sarcomas** ◆
Adults: 250 mg/m^2 daily by continuous I.V. infusion for 4 days every 3 weeks (total dacarbazine dose is 1,000 mg/m^2 over 96 hours) (MAID regimen; in combination with mesna, doxorubicin, and ifosfamide).

ADMINISTRATION

I.V.

▼ Preparing and giving parenteral drug may be mutagenic, teratogenic, or carcinogenic. Follow facility policy to reduce risks.

▼ Reconstitute drug using sterile water for injection. Add 9.9 mL to 100-mg vial or 19.7 mL to 200-mg vial to yield a concentration of 10 mg/mL.

▼ For infusion, dilute further with NSS or D$_5$W.

▼ To decrease pain at insertion site, dilute drug further or decrease infusion rate.

▼ Watch for irritation and infiltration during infusion; extravasation can cause severe pain, tissue damage, and necrosis. If solution infiltrates, stop immediately, apply ice to area for 24 to 48 hours, and notify prescriber.

▼ Reconstituted solutions in the vial are stable 8 hours at room temperature and with normal lighting conditions, or up to 3 days if refrigerated.

▼ Solution should be colorless to clear yellow. If solution turns pink, it has decomposed. Discard it.

▼ Diluted solutions are stable 8 hours at room temperature and with normal lighting, or up to 24 hours if refrigerated.

▼ **Incompatibilities:** Allopurinol sodium, cefepime, hydrocortisone sodium succinate, piperacillin–tazobactam.

ACTION

May cross-link strands of cellular DNA and interfere with RNA and protein synthesis. Not specific to cell cycle.

Route	Onset	Peak	Duration
I.V.	Unknown	Unknown	Unknown

Half-life: Initial phase, 19 minutes; terminal phase, 5 hours.

ADVERSE REACTIONS

GI: anorexia, severe nausea and vomiting, stomatitis.
Hematologic: *leukopenia, thrombocytopenia.*
Skin: alopecia.
Other: *anaphylaxis,* severe pain with infiltration or a too-concentrated solution, tissue damage.

INTERACTIONS

Drug-lifestyle. *Sun exposure:* May cause photosensitivity reaction, especially during first 2 days of therapy. Advise patient to avoid excessive sunlight exposure.

EFFECTS ON LAB TEST RESULTS

● May increase BUN and liver enzyme levels.
● May decrease platelet, RBC, and WBC counts.

CONTRAINDICATIONS & CAUTIONS

● Contraindicated in hypersensitivity to drug.
● Use cautiously in patients with impaired bone marrow function and those with severe renal or hepatic dysfunction.
Dialyzable drug: Unknown.

PREGNANCY-LACTATION-REPRODUCTION

Black Box Warning Studies have demonstrated this agent to have a carcinogenic and teratogenic effect when used in animals. ■

● There are no adequate well-controlled studies in pregnant women. Use during pregnancy only if potential benefit justifies potential risk to the fetus.

● It isn't known if drug appears in breast milk. Patient should discontinue breast-feeding or discontinue drug, taking into account importance of drug to the mother.

NURSING CONSIDERATIONS

Black Box Warning Dacarbazine should be administered under the supervision of a physician experienced in the use of cancer chemotherapeutic agents. ∎

Black Box Warning The physician must carefully weigh the possibility of therapeutic benefit against the risk of toxicity for each patient. ∎

• Give antiemetics before giving this drug. Nausea and vomiting may subside after several doses.

• To prevent bleeding, avoid all I.M. injections when platelet count is below 50,000/mm^3.

Black Box Warning Hematopoietic depression is the most common toxicity. ∎

• Anticipate need for blood transfusions to combat anemia.

• Therapeutic effects commonly occur with toxicity. Monitor CBC and platelet count.

Black Box Warning Hepatic necrosis may occur. Monitor LFTs. ∎

• For Hodgkin lymphoma, drug is usually given with bleomycin, vinblastine, and doxorubicin.

• *Look alike–sound alike:* Don't confuse dacarbazine with procarbazine.

PATIENT TEACHING

• Tell patient to watch for signs of infection (fever, sore throat, fatigue) and bleeding (easy bruising, nosebleeds, bleeding gums, tarry stools) and to take temperature daily.

• Tell patient to avoid people with URIs.

• Advise patient to avoid sunlight and sunlamps for first 2 days after treatment.

• Reassure patient that fever, malaise, and muscle pain, beginning 7 days after treatment ends and possibly lasting 7 to 21 days, may be treated with mild fever reducers such as acetaminophen.

• Tell patient that restricting food intake for 4 to 6 hours before dose may help to decrease adverse GI effects.

• Reassure patient that hair loss is reversible.

• Advise female patient to avoid pregnancy and breast-feeding during therapy.

daclatasvir dihydrochloride
dak-LAT-as-vir

Daklinza

Therapeutic class: Antivirals
Pharmacologic class: Hepatitis C virus NS5A replication complex inhibitors

AVAILABLE FORMS
Tablets: 30 mg, 60 mg

INDICATIONS & DOSAGES
➤ **Treatment of chronic HCV genotype 1 or 3 infection in combination with sofosbuvir and with or without ribavirin**
Adults: 60 mg P.O. once daily for 12 weeks in combination with sofosbuvir.
Adjust-a-dose: When given with strong CYP3A inhibitors, reduce dosage to 30 mg once daily. When given with moderate CYP3A inducers, increase dosage to 90 mg once daily.

For patients with HCV genotype 1 or 3 infection with Child-Pugh class B or C decompensated cirrhosis and posttransplantation patients, give drug with sofosbuvir and ribavirin for 12 weeks. Starting dose of ribavirin is 600 mg P.O. daily, increasing up to 1,000 mg P.O. daily as tolerated. May decrease starting dose and on-treatment dose of ribavirin based on Hb level and CrCl.

For patients with HCV genotype 3 infection with compensated cirrhosis (Child-Pugh class A), give drug with sofosbuvir and ribavirin for 12 weeks. Recommended ribavirin dosage is based on weight (1,000 mg P.O. for patients weighing less than 75 kg and 1,200 mg P.O. for those weighing at least 75 kg administered in two divided doses with food).

ADMINISTRATION
P.O.
• May give with or without food.
• If a dose is missed, give as soon as possible within the same day. If missed dose isn't within the same day, give next scheduled dose at the appropriate time.
• Store at room temperature.

ACTION
Inhibits both viral RNA replication and virion assembly.

Route	Onset	Peak	Duration
P.O.	Unknown	2 hr	Unknown

Half-life: 12 to 15 hours.

ADVERSE REACTIONS
CNS: fatigue, headache.
GI: diarrhea, nausea.
Metabolic: elevated lipase level.

INTERACTIONS
Drug-drug. *Alert: Amiodarone:* May cause serious symptomatic bradycardia. Use together isn't recommended. If use together is required, use cardiac monitoring. ■
Dabigatran: May increase dabigatran level. Use together isn't recommended in specific patients with renal impairment. Refer to dabigatran manufacturer's instructions for specific recommendations.
Digoxin: May increase digoxin level. For patients already taking daclatasvir, initiate digoxin using lowest appropriate dosage; monitor and adjust digoxin dosage as needed. For those already taking digoxin, measure serum digoxin level before initiating daclatasvir. Reduce digoxin concentration by decreasing digoxin dosage by approximately 15% to 30% or by modifying dosing frequency; continue monitoring.
HMG-CoA reductase inhibitors (atorvastatin, fluvastatin, pitavastatin, pravastatin, rosuvastatin, simvastatin): May increase HMG-CoA reductase inhibitor level. Monitor for HMG-CoA reductase inhibitor–related adverse events such as myopathy.
Moderate CYP3A inducers (bosentan, dexamethasone, efavirenz, etravirine, modafinil, nafcillin, rifapentine): May reduce daclatasvir level. Increase daclatasvir dose to 90 mg once daily.
Moderate CYP3A inhibitors (atazanavir, ciprofloxacin, darunavir/ritonavir, diltiazem, erythromycin, fluconazole, fosamprenavir, verapamil): May increase daclatasvir level. Monitor patient for daclatasvir-related adverse events.
Strong CYP3A inducers (carbamazepine, phenytoin, rifampin): May reduce daclatasvir level. Use together is contraindicated.
Strong CYP3A inhibitors (atazanavir/ritonavir, clarithromycin, indinavir, itraconazole, ketoconazole, nefazodone, nelfinavir, posaconazole, ritonavir, saquinavir, telithromycin, voriconazole): May increase daclatasvir level. Reduce daclatasvir dosage to 30 mg once daily.
Drug-herb. *St. John's wort:* May diminish daclatasvir effectiveness. Use together is contraindicated.

EFFECTS ON LAB TEST RESULTS
● May increase lipase level.

CONTRAINDICATIONS & CAUTIONS
● Contraindicated in combination with drugs or herbs that strongly induce CYP3A (such as carbamazepine, phenytoin, rifampin, St. John's wort) because of loss of efficacy of daclatasvir.
● *Alert:* May cause serious symptomatic bradycardia when given with amiodarone. Bradycardia can occur hours after administration or up to 2 weeks after treatment initiation. Inpatient cardiac monitoring is recommended for first 48 hours if daclatasvir is used with amiodarone. Outpatient or self-monitoring of HR should occur on a daily basis for at least first 2 weeks of treatment.
● Patients who have recently discontinued amiodarone should undergo cardiac monitoring when beginning daclatasvir because of amiodarone's long half-life.
● Patients receiving beta blockers or with underlying cardiac comorbidities or advanced liver disease may be at increased risk for symptomatic bradycardia. Bradycardia usually resolves after daclatasvir is discontinued.
● Safe use in children hasn't been established.
Dialyzable drug: Unlikely.

PREGNANCY-LACTATION-REPRODUCTION
● There are no adequate studies in pregnant women. Consider risks and benefits before use during pregnancy.
● It isn't known if drug appears in breast milk. Use cautiously and consider risks and benefits to mother and infant.

NURSING CONSIDERATIONS

● Before treatment initiation in patients with genotype 1a, consider screening for the presence of NS5A polymorphisms at amino acid positions M28, Q30, L31, and Y93 in patients with cirrhosis.

● Drug must be taken in combination with sofosbuvir. If sofosbuvir is permanently discontinued, daclatasvir should be discontinued.

● Dosage reduction for adverse reactions isn't recommended. Lower dosage may cause loss of therapeutic effect and possible development of resistance.

● Review concomitant medications during therapy and monitor patients for adverse reactions associated with those drugs.

● Monitor patients for bradycardia (HR less than 60 beats/minute [bpm], syncope, near-syncope, dizziness, light-headedness, malaise, weakness, tiredness, dyspnea, chest pain, confusion, memory problems). Report signs and symptoms immediately.

● *Look alike–sound alike:* Don't confuse daclatasvir with ledipasvir or entecavir.

PATIENT TEACHING

● Counsel patient on importance of reporting to prescriber all other drugs and supplements being taken before beginning treatment, as some are contraindicated during daclatasvir therapy.

● Teach patient to self-monitor HR daily, especially if patient is also taking amiodarone, and to immediately report HR less than 60 bpm. Advise patient to immediately report signs and symptoms of serious bradycardia.

● Instruct patient that if a dose is missed to take dose as soon as possible if it's within the same day. If missed dose isn't remembered within the same day, patient should skip missed dose and should take next dose at the appropriate time.

● Teach patient appropriate precautions to prevent transmission of HCV during therapy.

---

daclizumab
See NEW DRUGS for information.

---

dalbavancin hydrochloride
dal-ba-VAN-sin

Dalvance

Therapeutic class: Antibiotics
Pharmacologic class: Lipoglycopeptides

AVAILABLE FORMS
Injection: 500-mg single-use vial

INDICATIONS & DOSAGES
➤ **Acute bacterial skin and skin-structure infections caused by susceptible strains of gram-positive microorganisms (*Staphylococcus aureus* [including MRSA], *Streptococcus pyogenes, Streptococcus agalactiae*, and *Streptococcus anginosus* group [*S. anginosus, S. intermedius, S. constellatus*])**
Adults: 1,500 mg I.V. infusion over 30 minutes as a single dose, or 1,000 mg I.V. infusion over 30 minutes followed by a second dose of 500 mg I.V. infusion over 30 minutes 1 week later.

Adjust-a-dose: For patients with CrCl of less than 30 mL/minute who aren't receiving hemodialysis, give 1,125 mg I.V. infusion over 30 minutes as a single dose, or 750 mg I.V. infusion over 30 minutes followed by a second dose of 375 mg I.V. infusion over 30 minutes 1 week later. No dosage adjustment is recommended for patients on regularly scheduled hemodialysis.

ADMINISTRATION
I.V.

▼ Reconstitute each vial with 25 mL sterile water for injection. Swirl gently, and invert vial until vial contents are completely dissolved. Don't shake. Reconstituted vial contains a concentration of 20 mg/mL. Dilute further with dextrose 5% to a final concentration of 1 to 5 mg/mL.

▼ Inspect for particulate matter before infusion. Don't infuse if particulate matter is identified.

▼ To reduce risk of infusion-related reactions, infuse drug over 30 minutes.

▼ Flush I.V. line before and after each dalbavancin infusion with 5% dextrose

---

Reactions in bold italics are *life-threatening*. Interactions may have a *rapid onset* or a *delayed onset*.

injection if line is used to administer other drugs in addition to dalbavancin.

▼ Store reconstituted vials or final I.V. bags or bottles in refrigerator or at room temperature. Use within 48 hours.

▼ **Incompatibilities:** Other medications, electrolytes, saline-based solutions.

ACTION

Bactericidal; interferes with cell-wall synthesis within the bacteria.

Route	Onset	Peak	Duration
I.V.	Unknown	Unknown	7 days

Half-life: 8½ days.

ADVERSE REACTIONS

CNS: headache, dizziness.
CV: flushing, phlebitis, spontaneous hematoma.
EENT: oral candidiasis.
GI: nausea, vomiting, diarrhea, *GI hemorrhage,* melena, hematochezia, abdominal pain, *Clostridium difficile colitis.*
GU: vulvovaginal mycotic infection.
Hematologic: anemia, *hemorrhagic anemia, leukopenia, neutropenia, thrombocytopenia,* eosinophilia, *thrombocytosis.*
Hepatic: *hepatotoxicity.*
Metabolic: *hypoglycemia.*
Respiratory: *bronchospasm.*
Skin: rash, pruritus, urticaria, petechiae.
Other: infusion-site reactions, *anaphylactoid reaction, wound hemorrhage.*

INTERACTIONS

None reported.

EFFECTS ON LAB TEST RESULTS

• May increase INR and ALT, AST, and alkaline phosphatase levels.
• May decrease Hb level and platelet and WBC counts.

CONTRAINDICATIONS & CAUTIONS

• Contraindicated in patients hypersensitive to drug or its components.
• Don't use unless proven or strongly suspected bacterial infection exists.
• Use cautiously in patients with known hypersensitivity to glycopeptides.

• Use cautiously in patients with moderate to severe hepatic impairment (Child-Pugh class B or C).
• Safety and effectiveness in children haven't been established.
• Use cautiously in elderly patients. Drug is substantially excreted by the kidneys.
Dialyzable drug: No.

PREGNANCY-LACTATION-REPRODUCTION

• There are no adequate well-controlled studies in pregnant women. Use during pregnancy only if clearly needed and potential benefit justifies potential risk to the fetus.
• It isn't known if drug appears in breast milk. Use cautiously in breast-feeding women.

NURSING CONSIDERATIONS

🛈 *Alert:* Monitor patient for development of CDAD, which can range from mild to fatal colitis. Stop drug and take appropriate measures if diarrhea develops. Signs and symptoms may occur up to 2 months after drug administration.
• Ensure a suspected or confirmed serious bacterial infection exists before administering drug.
• Monitor patient for infusion reactions or hypersensitivity. Discontinue drug if reaction occurs.
• Rapid infusion may result in "red man syndrome" (upper body flushing, urticaria, pruritus, rash). Stopping or slowing infusion may stop this reaction.

PATIENT TEACHING

• Instruct patient to notify prescriber of allergy or hypersensitivity to other glycopeptides such as vancomycin before treatment.
• Explain to patient that drug is used only for presumed or actual serious bacterial infections.
• Teach patient that drug will be given intravenously, and to immediately report signs or symptoms of reactions.
• Advise patient not to skip any doses of antibacterial drugs as this may decrease effectiveness of treatment.
• Tell patient to report GI side effects such as diarrhea, which is common and may be

---

serious. Tell patient to contact prescriber if severe watery or bloody diarrhea occurs.

• Warn female patient to alert prescriber if she is pregnant or breast-feeding.

SAFETY ALERT!

dalteparin sodium
DAHL-tep-ah-rin

Fragmin

Therapeutic class: Anticoagulants
Pharmacologic class: Low–molecular-weight heparins

AVAILABLE FORMS
Injection: 2,500 antifactor Xa international units/0.2-mL syringe, 5,000 antifactor Xa international units/0.2-mL syringe, 7,500 antifactor Xa international units/0.3-mL syringe, 10,000 antifactor Xa international units/1-mL syringe, 12,500 antifactor Xa international units/0.5-mL syringe, 15,000 antifactor Xa international units/0.6-mL syringe, 18,000 antifactor Xa international units/0.72-mL syringe, 95,000 antifactor Xa international units/3.8-mL vial*

INDICATIONS & DOSAGES
➤ **To prevent DVT in patients undergoing abdominal surgery who are at moderate to high risk for thromboembolic complications**
Adults: 2,500 international units subcutaneously daily, starting 1 to 2 hours before surgery and repeated once daily for 5 to 10 days postoperatively. Or, for patients at high risk, give 5,000 international units subcutaneously the evening before surgery, then once daily postoperatively for 5 to 10 days. Or, in patients with malignancy, give 2,500 international units subcutaneously 1 to 2 hours before surgery followed by 2,500 international units subcutaneously 12 hours later, then 5,000 international units subcutaneously once daily for 5 to 10 days postoperatively.
➤ **To prevent DVT in patients undergoing hip replacement surgery**
Adults: 2,500 international units subcutaneously within 2 hours before surgery and second dose of 2,500 international

units subcutaneously in the evening after surgery (4 to 8 hours after surgery or later if hemostasis hasn't been achieved). Starting on first postoperative day, allowing a minimum of 6 hours after postoperative dose, give 5,000 international units subcutaneously once daily for 5 to 10 days. Or, give 5,000 international units subcutaneously 10 to 14 hours before surgery; then 5,000 international units subcutaneously once daily starting 4 to 8 hours after surgery for 5 to 10 days postoperatively. Allow approximately 24 hours between preoperative and first postoperative doses.

If starting postoperatively, give 2,500 international units subcutaneously in the evening after surgery (4 to 8 hours after surgery, or later if hemostasis hasn't been achieved). Starting on first postoperative day, allowing a minimum of 6 hours after postoperative dose, give 5,000 international units subcutaneously once daily for 5 to 10 days.
➤ **Unstable angina; non-Q-wave MI**
Adults: 120 international units/kg subcutaneously every 12 hours with aspirin (75 to 165 mg daily) P.O., unless contraindicated. Maximum dose, 10,000 international units. Treatment usually lasts 5 to 8 days.
➤ **To prevent DVT in patients at risk for thromboembolic complications because of severely restricted mobility during acute illness**
Adults: 5,000 international units subcutaneously once daily for 12 to 14 days.
➤ **Symptomatic venous thromboembolism in cancer patients**
Adults: Initially, 200 international units/kg (maximum, 18,000 international units) subcutaneously daily for 30 days; then 150 international units/kg (maximum, 18,000 international units) subcutaneously daily months 2 through 6.
Adjust-a-dose: In patients with platelet count 50,000 to 100,000/mm^3, reduce dose by 2,500 international units until platelet count exceeds 100,000/mm^3. In patients with platelet count less than 50,000/mm^3, stop drug until platelet count exceeds 50,000/mm^3. In patients with CrCl of 30 mL/minute or less, monitor anti-Xa levels to determine appropriate dose.

Reactions in bold italics are *life-threatening*. Interactions may have a *rapid onset* or a *delayed onset*.

Target anti-Xa range is 0.5 to 1.5 international units/mL. Draw anti-Xa 4 to 6 hours after dose and only after patient has received three to four doses.

➤ **Venous thromboembolism prophylaxis in general surgery** ◆

Adults: 2,500 units subcutaneously once daily, starting 1 to 2 hours before surgery and repeated once daily postoperatively until hospital discharge.

Adjust-a-dose: In patients with other risk factors (such as cancer) that place them at high risk for venous thromboembolism, recommended dose is 5,000 units subcutaneously the evening before surgery, then once daily postoperatively at least until hospital discharge. Or, in patients with malignancy, give 2,500 units subcutaneously 1 to 2 hours before surgery followed by 2,500 units 12 hours later, then 5,000 units once daily postoperatively at least until hospital discharge. For selected high-risk general surgery patients, including some who have undergone major cancer surgery or have previously experienced venous thromboembolism, consider continuing dalteparin for up to 28 days after hospital discharge.

➤ **Venous thromboembolism prophylaxis in gynecologic surgery** ◆

Adults: 2,500 units subcutaneously once daily, starting 1 to 2 hours before surgery and repeated once daily postoperatively.

Adjust-a-dose: In patients with other risk factors (such as cancer) that place them at high risk for venous thromboembolism, recommended dose is 5,000 units subcutaneously the evening before surgery, then once daily postoperatively. Or, in patients with malignancy, give 2,500 units subcutaneously 1 to 2 hours before surgery followed by 2,500 units subcutaneously 12 hours later, then 5,000 units once daily postoperatively. All patients who have major gynecologic surgery should receive thromboprophylaxis at least until hospital discharge. For patients undergoing major gynecologic surgery who are at high risk for venous thromboembolism, including patients with a history of venous thromboembolism or patients who had surgery for cancer, consider continuing dalteparin for up to 28 days after hospital discharge.

ADMINISTRATION

Subcutaneous

● Before giving injection, obtain complete list of all prescribed and OTC medications and supplements, including herbs.

● Have patient sit or lie supine when giving drug.

● Injection sites include a U-shaped area around the navel, upper outer side of thigh, and upper outer quadrangle of buttock. Rotate sites daily.

● When area around the navel or thigh is used, use thumb and forefinger to lift up a fold of skin while giving injection.

● Give subcutaneous injection deeply, inserting entire length of needle at a 45- to 90-degree angle.

ACTION

Enhances inhibition of factor Xa and thrombin by antithrombin.

Route	Onset	Peak	Duration
Subcut.	1–2 hr	4 hr	>12 hr

Half-life: 2 to 5 hours.

ADVERSE REACTIONS

CNS: fever.

GU: hematuria.

Hematologic: *thrombocytopenia, hemorrhage,* ecchymoses, bleeding complications.

Skin: pruritus, rash, hematoma at injection site, injection-site pain.

Other: *anaphylaxis.*

INTERACTIONS

Drug-drug. *Antiplatelet drugs (aspirin, NSAIDs, clopidogrel, dipyridamole, ticlopidine), oral anticoagulants, SSRIs (fluoxetine), thrombolytics:* May increase risk of bleeding. Use together cautiously.

Drug-herb. *Angelica (dong quai), boldo, bromelains, capsicum, chamomile, dandelion, danshen, devil's claw, fenugreek, feverfew, garlic, ginger, ginkgo, ginseng, horse chestnut, licorice, meadowsweet, onion, passion flower, red clover, willow:* May increase risk of bleeding. Discourage use together.

EFFECTS ON LAB TEST RESULTS

● May increase ALT and AST levels.
● May decrease platelet count.

CONTRAINDICATIONS & CAUTIONS

• Contraindicated in patients hypersensitive to drug, heparin, or pork products; in those with active major bleeding; and in those with thrombocytopenia and antiplatelet antibodies in the presence of the drug.

• Contraindicated in patients with unstable angina or non-Q-wave MI who are undergoing regional anesthesia because of an increased risk of bleeding associated with the dose of dalteparin recommended for these indications.

• Use cautiously in patients with history of heparin-induced thrombocytopenia and in patients at increased risk for hemorrhage, such as those with severe uncontrolled hypertension, bacterial endocarditis, congenital or acquired bleeding disorders, active ulceration, angiodysplastic GI disease, or hemorrhagic stroke; also use with caution shortly after brain, spinal, or ophthalmic surgery. Monitor vital signs.

• Use cautiously in patients with bleeding diathesis, thrombocytopenia, platelet defects, severe hepatic or renal insufficiency, hypertensive or diabetic retinopathy, or recent GI bleeding.

Dialyzable drug: Unknown.

⚠ *Overdose S&S:* Hemorrhagic complications.

PREGNANCY-LACTATION-REPRODUCTION

• There are no adequate well-controlled studies in pregnant women. Use during pregnancy only if clearly needed.

• Use preservative-free formulations without benzyl alcohol (not multidose vial) when possible during pregnancy and only if clearly needed. Benzyl alcohol has been associated with fatal "gasping syndrome" in premature neonates.

• Small amounts of anti-Xa activity have been detected in breast milk; clinical implications, if any, on a breast-feeding infant are unknown. Use cautiously in breast-feeding women.

NURSING CONSIDERATIONS

Black Box Warning Patients who have received epidural or spinal anesthesia or spinal puncture are at increased risk for developing an epidural or spinal hematoma, which may result in long-term or permanent paralysis. Increased risk may occur with use of indwelling epidural catheters, concomitant use of drugs that affect hemostasis (NSAIDs, platelet inhibitors, anticoagulants), history of traumatic or repeated epidural or spinal punctures, or history of spinal deformity or surgery. Monitor these patients closely for neurologic impairment and treat urgently. ∎

Black Box Warning Monitor patients for neurologic impairment (midline back pain, sensory or motor deficits such as numbness or weakness in lower limbs, bowel or bladder dysfunction). Treat impairment urgently. ∎

Black Box Warning Optimal timing between administration of drug and neuraxial procedures isn't known. Consider benefits and risks before neuraxial intervention in patients anticoagulated or to be anticoagulated for thromboprophylaxis. ∎

• DVT is a risk factor in patients who are candidates for therapy, including those older than age 40, those who are obese, those undergoing surgery under general anesthesia lasting longer than 30 minutes, and those who have additional risk factors (such as malignancy or history of DVT or PE).

• Never give drug I.M.

• Don't mix with other injections or infusions unless specific compatibility data support such mixing.

⚠ *Alert:* Drug isn't interchangeable (unit for unit) with unfractionated heparin or other low–molecular-weight heparin.

• Periodic, routine CBC and fecal occult blood tests are recommended during therapy. Patients don't need regular monitoring of PT or aPTT.

• Monitor patient closely for thrombocytopenia and hyperkalemia.

• Stop drug if a thromboembolic event occurs despite dalteparin prophylaxis.

• Obtain a complete list of patient's prescription and OTC drugs and supplements, including herbs.

PATIENT TEACHING

• Instruct patient and family to watch for and report signs of bleeding (bruising and blood in stools) and to report all adverse reactions promptly.

Reactions in bold italics are *life-threatening*. Interactions may have a *rapid onset* or a *delayed onset*.

• Tell patient to avoid OTC drugs containing aspirin or other salicylates unless ordered by prescriber.
• Advise patient to consult with prescriber before initiating any herbal therapy; many herbs have anticoagulant, antiplatelet, and fibrinolytic properties.
• Tell patient to use a soft toothbrush and electric razor during treatment.

SAFETY ALERT!

dapagliflozin propanediol
DAP-a-gli-FLOE-zin PROE-pane-di-ol

Farxiga

Therapeutic class: Antidiabetics
Pharmacologic class: Sodium-glucose cotransporter 2 inhibitors

AVAILABLE FORMS
Tablets: 5 mg, 10 mg

INDICATIONS & DOSAGES
➤ **Adjunct to diet and exercise to improve glycemic control in patients with type 2 diabetes**
Adults: Initially, 5 mg P.O. once daily; may increase to 10 mg daily for patients who required additional glycemic control.
Adjust-a-dose: Discontinue in patients with persistently impaired real function (estimated GFR [eGFR] less than 60 mL/minute/1.73 m^2). Drug hasn't been studied in severe hepatic impairment.

ADMINISTRATION
P.O.
• Give dose in the morning.
• May give without regard for food.
• Store at room temperature.

ACTION
Reduces reabsorption of filtered glucose from the proximal renal tubule and lowers the renal threshold for glucose, resulting in increased glucose excretion.

Route	Onset	Peak	Duration
P.O.	Unknown	2 hr	Unknown

Half-life: 12.9 hours.

ADVERSE REACTIONS
CV: volume depletion (dehydration, hypovolemia, orthostatic hypotension, hypotension).
EENT: nasopharyngitis.
GI: nausea, constipation.
GU: genital mycotic infection, UTI, increased urination, dysuria.
Metabolic: dyslipidemia, *hypoglycemia.*
Musculoskeletal: back pain, extremity pain.
Other: influenza.

INTERACTIONS
Drug-drug. *Insulin, insulin secretagogues:* May increase risk of hypoglycemia. Monitor patient closely and adjust insulin and secretagogue dosages as necessary.
Loop diuretics: May increase risk of hypotension. Monitor patient closely.

EFFECTS ON LAB TEST RESULTS
• May increase hematocrit and serum phosphorus, creatinine, and LDL cholesterol levels. May decrease eGFR level.
• May cause positive urinary glucose.

CONTRAINDICATIONS & CAUTIONS
• Contraindicated in patients with active bladder cancer, moderate or severe renal impairment (eGFR less than 60 mL/minute/1.73 m^2), or ESRD; patients on dialysis; and patients with history of serious hypersensitivity reactions (anaphylaxis, angioedema, or severe cutaneous reactions) to dapagliflozin-containing products.
• Contraindicated in patients with type 1 diabetes or diabetic ketoacidosis.
• Use cautiously in elderly patients because of increased risk of adverse events.
• Use cautiously in patients with history of bladder cancer. Drug may increase risk of cancer reactivation.
⚠ *Alert:* Drug may cause acidosis, which may require emergency department care or hospitalization. Monitor patients for ketoacidosis, especially those with major illness, reduced food or fluid intake, or reduced insulin dosage. Elevated urine or serum ketone levels without associated very high glucose levels have occurred with sodium-glucose cotransporter 2 inhibitor use.
Dialyzable drug: Unknown.

PREGNANCY-LACTATION-REPRODUCTION

● There are no adequate studies in pregnant women. Use during pregnancy, especially during the second and third trimesters, isn't recommended. If needed during pregnancy, use only if potential benefit justifies potential risk to the fetus.

● It isn't known if drug appears in breast milk. Patient should discontinue breastfeeding or discontinue drug.

NURSING CONSIDERATIONS

◑ *Alert:* Drug can increase risk of acute kidney injury. Before starting therapy, assess patient for factors that may predispose to acute kidney injury (decreased blood volume, chronic renal insufficiency, HF, concurrent use of other medications such as diuretics, ACE inhibitors, ARBs, and NSAIDs). Assess renal function before start of therapy and monitor periodically. If acute kidney injury occurs, drug should be discontinued and the kidney impairment treated.

◑ *Alert:* Drug may increase risk of severe UTI, including urosepsis and pyelonephritis. Monitor patient and treat promptly if indicated.

● Monitor glucose levels closely, especially if patient is taking antidiabetic agents concurrently. Adjust hypoglycemic dosages if needed.

● Monitor patient for mycotic infections.

● Stop drug immediately if hypersensitivity, reduced renal function, or bladder cancer is suspected.

● Monitor volume status and watch for signs and symptoms of hypotension, particularly in patients with impaired renal function (eGFR less than 60 mL/minute/1.73 m^2), elderly patients, and patients taking loop diuretics. Increased urinary glucose excretion also results in increased urine volume.

PATIENT TEACHING

● Warn patient to use drug only as directed. If a dose is missed, patient should take the missed dose as soon as it's remembered unless it is almost time for the next dose. Caution patient not to double a dose.

◑ *Alert:* Advise patient to seek immediate medical attention for signs and symptoms of acute kidney injury (decreased urine output, swelling in legs or feet). Warn patient not to stop taking drug without first discussing with prescriber.

● Inform patient of increased risk of UTI. Teach patient to report painful urination or discolored urine.

● Instruct patient to report signs and symptoms of yeast infections (itching, burning, discharge) promptly. Counsel patient on importance of diet and exercise in addition to medication for diabetes control.

● Teach patient to obtain periodic blood testing as requested by prescriber.

◑ *Alert:* Instruct patient to seek medical attention immediately for signs and symptoms of ketoacidosis (difficulty breathing, hyperventilation, anorexia, nausea, vomiting, abdominal pain, confusion, and unusual fatigue or sleepiness).

◑ *Alert:* Instruct patient to seek medical attention for signs and symptoms of UTI (painful urination, urinary frequency, blood in urine, urgency, pelvic pain, fever, back pain, nausea, vomiting).

● Advise patient to watch for signs and symptoms of hypoglycemia (fatigue, weakness, confusion, headache, pallor, or profuse sweating).

● Caution patient to maintain adequate fluid intake to decrease risk of hypotension.

● Warn patient to contact prescriber for signs and symptoms of hypotension, such as light-headedness (especially with position change) and weakness.

● Advise patient to seek medical attention promptly for fever, trauma, infection, or when surgery is needed; dosage adjustment may be needed owing to stress.

daptomycin
dap-toe-MYE-sin

Cubicin

Therapeutic class: Antibiotics
Pharmacologic class: Cyclic lipopeptides

AVAILABLE FORMS
Powder for injection: 500-mg vial

INDICATIONS & DOSAGES

➤ **Bacteremia caused by *Staphylococcus aureus* (including right-sided endocarditis caused by methicillin-susceptible and methicillin-resistant strains)**

Adults: 6 mg/kg I.V. infusion over 30 minutes or I.V. injection over 2 minutes every 24 hours for at least 2 to 6 weeks based on patient response.

Adjust-a-dose: For bacteremic patients with CrCl of less than 30 mL/minute, give 6 mg/kg I.V. every 48 hours. When possible, give drug after hemodialysis on hemodialysis days.

➤ **Complicated skin or skin-structure infection (SSSI) caused by susceptible strains of *S. aureus* (including MRSA), *Streptococcus pyogenes*, *Streptococcus agalactiae*, *Streptococcus dysgalactiae*, and *Enterococcus faecalis* (vancomycin-susceptible strains only)**

Adults: 4 mg/kg I.V. infusion over 30 minutes or I.V. injection over 2 minutes every 24 hours for 7 to 14 days.

Adjust-a-dose: In patients with SSSI and CrCl of less than 30 mL/minute, including those receiving hemodialysis or continuous ambulatory peritoneal dialysis, give 4 mg/kg I.V. every 48 hours after dialysis.

ADMINISTRATION

I.V.

▼ Obtain specimen for culture and sensitivity tests before giving first dose. Begin therapy while awaiting results.

▼ Reconstitute 500-mg vial with 10 mL of NSS.

▼ Further dilute with NSS for I.V. infusion and infuse over 30 minutes.

▼ For I.V. injection over 2 minutes, give at a concentration of 50 mg/mL.

▼ Refrigerate vials at 36° to 46° F (2° to 8° C).

▼ Vials are for single use; discard excess.

▼ Reconstituted and diluted solutions are stable for 12 hours at room temperature or for 48 hours at 36° to 46° F.

▼ Don't use drug with ReadyMED elastomeric infusion pumps (Cardinal Health); an impurity may leach from the pump into the solution.

▼ **Incompatibilities:** Dextrose-containing solutions and other I.V. drugs. If an I.V. line is used for several drugs, flush the line with NSS or lactated Ringer solution injection between drugs.

ACTION

Binds to and depolarizes bacterial membranes to inhibit protein, DNA, and RNA synthesis, thus causing bacterial cell death.

Route	Onset	Peak	Duration
I.V.	Rapid	<1 hr	Unknown

Half-life: About 8 hours.

ADVERSE REACTIONS

CNS: anxiety, confusion, dizziness, fever, headache, insomnia.

CV: *cardiac failure,* chest pain, edema, hypertension, hypotension.

EENT: sore throat.

GI: *pseudomembranous colitis,* abdominal pain, constipation, decreased appetite, diarrhea, nausea, vomiting.

GU: *renal failure,* UTI.

Hematologic: anemia.

Metabolic: *hypoglycemia,* hyperglycemia, *hypokalemia.*

Musculoskeletal: limb and back pain, myopathy.

Respiratory: cough, dyspnea, eosinophilic pneumonia.

Skin: cellulitis, injection-site reactions, pruritus, rash.

Other: fungal infections.

INTERACTIONS

Drug-drug. *HMG-CoA reductase inhibitors:* May increase risk of myopathy. Consider stopping these drugs while giving daptomycin.

Tobramycin: May affect levels of both drugs. Use together cautiously.

Warfarin: May alter anticoagulant activity. Monitor PT and INR for the first several days of daptomycin therapy.

EFFECTS ON LAB TEST RESULTS

● May increase alkaline phosphatase and CK levels. May decrease potassium and Hb levels and hematocrit. May increase or decrease glucose level.

● May increase LFT values.

● May cause false elevation of INR and false prolongation of PT.

CONTRAINDICATIONS & CAUTIONS

• Contraindicated in patients hypersensitive to drug.
• Use cautiously in those with renal insufficiency and those older than age 65.
• Safety and effectiveness haven't been established in children younger than age 18. Avoid use in children younger than age 12 months because of risk of potential effects on muscular, neuromuscular, or nervous systems (either peripheral or central).
Dialyzable drug: Yes.

PREGNANCY-LACTATION-REPRODUCTION

• There are no adequate well-controlled studies in pregnant women. Use during pregnancy only if potential benefit justifies potential risk to the fetus.
• Drug appears in breast milk in low amounts. Use cautiously if breast-feeding.

NURSING CONSIDERATIONS

• Monitor CBC, renal function tests, and LFTs periodically.
❶ *Alert:* Because drug may increase the risk of myopathy, monitor CK level weekly. If CK level rises, monitor it more often. In patients with myopathy and CK elevation over 1,000 units/L or more than 10 × ULN, stop drug. Consider stopping all other drugs linked with myopathy (such as HMG-CoA reductase inhibitors) during therapy.
• Monitor patient for superinfection because drug may cause overgrowth of nonsusceptible organisms.
❶ *Alert:* Drug may cause eosinophilic pneumonia, a rare type of pneumonia in which eosinophil-type WBCs fill the lungs, causing fever, cough, shortness of breath, and difficulty breathing. Monitor patient closely.
• Watch for evidence of CDAD, which can occur more than 2 months after therapy.
• Monitor patient for muscle pain or weakness, particularly of the distal extremities.
• *Look alike–sound alike:* Don't confuse daptomycin with dactinomycin.

PATIENT TEACHING

• Advise patient to immediately report muscle weakness and infusion-site irritation.
• Tell patient to report all adverse reactions, especially severe diarrhea, rash, and infection.

• Inform patient about possible adverse reactions.

daratumumab
See NEW DRUGS for information.

SAFETY ALERT!

darbepoetin alfa
dar-bah-poe-E-tin

Aranesp

Therapeutic class: Colony stimulating factors
Pharmacologic class: Recombinant human erythropoietins

AVAILABLE FORMS

Injection (with albumin or polysorbate solution): 25 mcg/mL, 40 mcg/mL, 60 mcg/mL, 100 mcg/mL, 150 mcg/ 0.75 mL, 200 mcg/mL, 300 mcg/mL, 500 mcg/mL in single-dose vials
Prefilled syringe or autoinjector (with albumin or polysorbate solution): 10 mcg/ 0.4 mL, 25 mcg/0.42 mL, 40 mcg/0.4 mL, 60 mcg/0.3 mL, 100 mcg/0.5 mL, 150 mcg/ 0.3 mL, 200 mcg/0.4 mL, 300 mcg/0.6 mL, 500 mcg/mL

INDICATIONS & DOSAGES

➤ **Anemia from chronic renal failure**
Adults: The I.V. route is preferred for patients on dialysis. For patients on dialysis, give 0.45 mcg/kg I.V. or subcutaneously once weekly. Or, give 0.75 mcg/kg I.V. or subcutaneously once every 2 weeks. For patients not on dialysis, give 0.45 mcg/kg I.V. or subcutaneously at 4-week intervals. Give the lowest effective dose to gradually increase Hb to a level at which blood transfusion isn't necessary. Refer to manufacturer's instructions for specific dosing. Don't increase dose more often than once a month.
Children younger than age 18: For patients on dialysis, give 0.45 mcg/kg I.V. or subcutaneously once weekly. For patients not on dialysis, give 0.75 mcg/kg I.V. or subcutaneously once every 2 weeks.

Reactions in bold italics are *life-threatening*. Interactions may have a *rapid onset* or a *delayed onset*.

Adults and children older than age 1 who are on dialysis and converting from epoetin alfa: Base starting dose on the previous epoetin alfa dose (see table below). Don't use as initial treatment of anemia in children with chronic renal failure.

Previous epoetin alfa dose (units/wk)	Darbepoetin alfa dose (mcg/wk): Adults	Darbepoetin alfa dose (mcg/wk): Children
<1,500	6.25	Unknown
1,500–2,499	6.25	6.25
2,500–4,999	12.5	10
5,000–10,999	25	20
11,000–17,999	40	40
18,000–33,999	60	60
34,000–89,999	100	100
≥90,000	200	200

Give darbepoetin alfa less often than epoetin alfa. If patient was receiving epoetin alfa two to three times weekly, give darbepoetin alfa once weekly. If patient was receiving epoetin alfa once weekly, give darbepoetin alfa once every 2 weeks.

Adjust-a-dose: For patients with chronic renal disease who aren't on dialysis, if the Hb level exceeds 10 g/dL, reduce dosage or interrupt therapy; use the lowest dosage sufficient to reduce the need for RBC transfusions. For patients with chronic renal disease who are on dialysis, if the Hb level approaches or exceeds 11 g/dL, reduce dosage or interrupt therapy.

➤ **Anemia from chemotherapy in patients with nonmyeloid malignancies**
Adults: Initiate drug only if Hb level is less than 10 g/dL and if there is a minimum of 2 additional months of planned chemotherapy; 2.25 mcg/kg subcutaneously once weekly or 500 mcg subcutaneously once every 3 weeks.

Adjust-a-dose: For either dosing schedule, adjust dose to maintain a target Hb level necessary to avoid RBC transfusions. Give the lowest effective dose to gradually increase Hb to a level at which blood transfusion isn't necessary. If Hb exceeds a level needed to avoid RBC transfusion, withhold drug until Hb approaches a level at which RBC transfusion may be needed, then resume at 40% of previous dose. If Hb increases more than 1 g/dL in a 2-week

period, or when Hb reaches a level needed to avoid RBC transfusion, reduce dose by 40%. For patients receiving the drug on a once-a-week schedule, if Hb level increases less than 1 g/dL and remains below 10 g/dL after 6 weeks of therapy, increase dose up to 4.5 mcg/kg.

If after 8 weeks of therapy there is no response as measured by Hb levels or if transfusions are still required, discontinue drug. Discontinue drug after completion of chemotherapy course.

ADMINISTRATION

I.V.

⚠ *Alert:* The needle cover of the prefilled syringe contains dry natural rubber (a derivative of latex). Assess patient for a history of latex allergy.

▼ Don't shake. Shaking can denature drug.

▼ If drug contains particles or is discolored, don't use.

▼ Give undiluted by I.V. injection.

▼ Single-dose vials contain no preservatives; don't pool unused portions.

▼ Store drug in refrigerator; don't freeze. Don't use if drug has been frozen. Protect drug from light.

▼ **Incompatibilities:** Other I.V. drugs or solutions.

Subcutaneous

⚠ *Alert:* The needle cover of the prefilled syringe contains dry natural rubber (a derivative of latex). Assess patient for a history of latex allergy.

● Don't give subcutaneously in patients with chronic renal failure on dialysis.

● Don't shake. Shaking can denature drug.

● Store drug in refrigerator; don't freeze. Protect drug from light.

ACTION

Mimics effects of erythropoietin. Functions as a growth factor and as a differentiating factor, enhancing RBC production.

Route	Onset	Peak	Duration
I.V.	Unknown	Unknown	Unknown
Subcut.	Slow	48 hr	Unknown

Half-life: I.V., 21 hours; subcutaneous, 74 hours.

ADVERSE REACTIONS

CNS: *seizures,* dizziness, fatigue, fever, headache, asthenia, TIA, *stroke.*
CV: *cardiac arrest, cardiac arrhythmia,* edema, hypertension, hypotension, peripheral edema, *PE, acute MI, HF, thrombosis,* angina, chest pain, vascular access thrombosis.
GI: abdominal pain, constipation, diarrhea, nausea, vomiting, *peritonitis, GI hemorrhage.*
Metabolic: dehydration.
Musculoskeletal: arthralgia, limb pain, myalgia, back pain.
Respiratory: cough, dyspnea, URI, bronchitis, pneumonia.
Skin: pruritus, rash.
Other: infection, *sepsis,* abscess, access infection, fluid overload, flulike symptoms, injection-site pain.

INTERACTIONS
None reported.

EFFECTS ON LAB TEST RESULTS
None reported.

CONTRAINDICATIONS & CAUTIONS
• Contraindicated in patients hypersensitive to drug or its components and in those with uncontrolled hypertension.
• Safety and effectiveness haven't been established in patients with underlying hematologic disease, such as hemolytic anemia, sickle cell anemia, thalassemia, or porphyria. Use with caution.
Dialyzable drug: No.
⚠ *Overdose S&S:* CV and thrombotic reactions, polycythemia.

PREGNANCY-LACTATION-REPRODUCTION
• There are no adequate well-controlled studies in pregnant women; animal studies show that drug may cause fetal harm. Use during pregnancy only if potential benefit justifies potential risk to the fetus.
• Women who become pregnant during therapy are encouraged to enroll in Amgen's Pregnancy Surveillance Program by calling 1-800-772-6436 (1-800-77-AMGEN).
• It isn't known if drug appears in breast milk. Use cautiously in breast-feeding women.

NURSING CONSIDERATIONS

Black Box Warning Erythropoiesis-stimulating agents increase risk of death, MI, stroke, venous thromboembolism, vascular access thrombosis, and tumor progression or recurrence. No trial has identified an Hb target level, drug dose, or dosing strategy that doesn't increase these risks. ■
Black Box Warning Patients with chronic renal disease have an increased risk of death and serious CV events, including stroke, when erythropoiesis-stimulating agents are used to increase Hb level to greater than 11 g/dL. Therapy should be individualized for each patient; the lowest possible dose sufficient to reduce the need for RBC transfusions should be used. ■
Black Box Warning In patients with non–small-cell lung cancer and breast, head and neck, lymphoid, and cervical cancers, there is a risk of tumor growth and shortened survival when Hb levels exceed the lowest dose needed to avoid RBC transfusion. Target for the lowest dosage needed to avoid RBC transfusions. Use only for treatment of anemia due to concomitant myelosuppressive chemotherapy, and discontinue drug after chemotherapy course. ■
Black Box Warning Health care providers and hospitals must enroll in and comply with the ESA APPRISE Oncology Program to prescribe or dispense darbepoetin alfa to patients with cancer. Go to www.esa-apprise.com or call 1-866-284-8089 for more information. ■
Black Box Warning Drug isn't indicated for patients receiving myelosuppressive therapy when the anticipated outcome is cure. ■
• When initiating therapy or adjusting dosage, monitor Hb level at least weekly until stable; then, at least monthly.
• Hb level may not increase until 2 to 6 weeks after starting therapy.
• If patient has a minimal response or lack of response at recommended dose, check for deficiencies in folic acid, iron, or vitamin B_{12}. Other contributing factors include infection, malignancy, and occult blood loss.
🔵 *Alert:* If patient develops a sudden loss of response with severe anemia and low reticulocyte count, withhold drug and test patient for antierythropoietin antibodies. If antibodies are present, stop treatment. Don't

switch to another erythropoietic protein because a cross-reaction is possible.
• Control BP and monitor it carefully.
• Monitor renal function and electrolytes in predialysis patients.
• Monitor patency of vascular and dialysis access and report problems immediately.
• Patients who are marginally dialyzed may need adjustments in dialysis prescriptions.
• Serious allergic reactions, including skin rash and urticaria, may occur. If an anaphylactic reaction occurs, stop the drug and give appropriate therapy.

PATIENT TEACHING
• Instruct patients on proper administration and on proper use and disposal of needles.
• Advise patient of possible side effects and allergic reactions.
• Inform patient of the need for frequent monitoring of BP and Hb level; stress compliance with his treatment for high BP.
• Instruct patient how to take drug correctly at home, including how to store drug and dispose of supplies properly.

darifenacin hydrobromide
da-ree-FEN-ah-sin

Enablex🔗

Therapeutic class: Antispasmodics
Pharmacologic class: Anticholinergics

AVAILABLE FORMS
Tablets (extended-release) ⓓⓝⓒ*:* 7.5 mg, 15 mg

INDICATIONS & DOSAGES
➤ **Urge incontinence, urgency, and frequency from an overactive bladder**
Adults: Initially, 7.5 mg P.O. once daily. After 2 weeks, may increase to 15 mg P.O. once daily if needed.
Adjust-a-dose: If patient has hepatic impairment (Child-Pugh class B), don't exceed 7.5 mg P.O. once daily. Drug isn't recommended for use in patients with severe hepatic impairment (Child-Pugh class C).

ADMINISTRATION
P.O.
• Don't crush tablet; patient should swallow whole.
• Give drug without regard for food.

ACTION
Relaxes smooth muscle of bladder by antagonizing muscarinic receptors.

Route	Onset	Peak	Duration
P.O.	Unknown	7 hr	Unknown

Half-life: 13 to 19 hours.

ADVERSE REACTIONS
CNS: asthenia, dizziness, pain, headache, somnolence.
CV: hypertension, peripheral edema.
EENT: abnormal vision, dry eyes, pharyngitis, rhinitis, sinusitis.
GI: dry mouth, constipation, abdominal pain, diarrhea, dyspepsia, nausea, vomiting.
GU: urinary tract disorder, UTI, vaginitis, urine retention.
Metabolic: weight gain.
Musculoskeletal: arthralgia, back pain.
Respiratory: bronchitis.
Skin: dry skin, pruritus, rash.
Other: accidental injury, flulike syndrome.

INTERACTIONS
Drug-drug. *Anticholinergics:* May increase anticholinergic effects, such as dry mouth, blurred vision, and constipation. Monitor patient closely.
Digoxin: May increase digoxin level. Monitor digoxin level.
Drugs metabolized by CYP2D6 (flecainide, TCAs, thioridazine): May increase levels of these drugs. Use together cautiously.
Midazolam: May increase midazolam level. Monitor patient carefully.
Potent CYP3A4 inhibitors (clarithromycin, itraconazole, ketoconazole, nefazodone, nelfinavir, ritonavir): May increase darifenacin level. Maintain dosage no higher than 7.5 mg P.O. daily.
Drug-lifestyle. *Hot weather:* May cause heat prostration from decreased sweating. Urge caution.

EFFECTS ON LAB TEST RESULTS
None reported.

CONTRAINDICATIONS & CAUTIONS
• Contraindicated in patients hypersensitive to drug or its components. Angioedema can be life-threatening and has been reported after the first dose. If angioedema occurs, discontinue drug, start appropriate therapy, and ensure patent airway.
• Contraindicated in those with or at risk for urine retention, gastric retention, or uncontrolled angle-closure glaucoma.
• Avoid use in patients with severe hepatic impairment (Child-Pugh class C).
• Use cautiously in patients with bladder outflow or GI obstruction, ulcerative colitis, myasthenia gravis, severe constipation, controlled angle-closure glaucoma, decreased GI motility, or Child-Pugh class B hepatic impairment.
Dialyzable drug: Unknown.
⚠ *Overdose S&S:* Severe antimuscarinic effects (mydriasis, decreased secretions, ileus, urine retention, tachycardia, altered mental status).

PREGNANCY-LACTATION-REPRODUCTION
• There are no studies in pregnant women. Use only if potential benefit justifies potential risk to the fetus.
• It isn't known if drug appears in breast milk. Use cautiously if breast-feeding.

NURSING CONSIDERATIONS
• Assess bladder function, and monitor drug effects.
• If patient has bladder outlet obstruction, watch for urine retention.
• Assess patient for decreased gastric motility and constipation.

PATIENT TEACHING
• Tell patient to swallow tablet whole with plenty of liquid; caution against crushing or chewing tablet.
• Inform patient that drug may be taken with or without food.
• Tell patient to use caution, especially when performing hazardous tasks, until drug effects are known.
• Tell patient to report blurred vision, constipation, and urine retention and to immediately report swelling of the face, lips, or tongue or difficulty speaking.

• Discourage use of other drugs that may cause dry mouth, constipation, urine retention, or blurred vision.
• Tell patient that drug decreases sweating, and advise cautious use in hot environments and during strenuous activity.

defibrotide sodium
See NEW DRUGS for information.

SAFETY ALERT!

degarelix acetate
day-gah-REL-ix

Firmagon

Therapeutic class: Antineoplastics
Pharmacologic class: Gonadotropin-releasing hormone receptor antagonists

AVAILABLE FORMS
Injection: 80-mg, 120-mg vial

INDICATIONS & DOSAGES
➤ **Advanced prostate cancer**
Adult men: Initially, 240 mg Subcut., administered as two 120-mg injections at a concentration of 40 mg/mL. Maintenance dose is 80 mg Subcut. given as one injection at a concentration of 20 mg/mL every 28 days starting 28 days after first dose.

ADMINISTRATION
Subcutaneous
• Drug is considered hazardous; use safe handling and disposal precautions.
• Give drug within 1 hour of reconstitution.
• For 120-mg initial dose, draw up 3 mL sterile water for injection with a reconstitution needle (21G/2″). For 80-mg maintenance dose, draw up 4.2 mL sterile water for injection.
• Inject sterile water for injection slowly into degarelix 80-mg or 120-mg vial. To keep product and syringe sterile, don't remove syringe and needle.
• Keeping vial in an upright position, swirl it very gently until liquid looks clear and has no undissolved powder or particles. If powder adheres to vial over the liquid surface, vial can be tilted slightly to dissolve powder. Avoid shaking, to prevent foam formation.

Reactions in bold italics are *life-threatening*. Interactions may have a *rapid onset* or a ***delayed onset***.

A ring of small air bubbles on surface of liquid is acceptable. The reconstitution procedure may take up to 15 minutes.
• Turn vial upside down and withdraw 3 mL of degarelix 120 mg or 4.2 mL of degarelix 80 mg. Make sure to withdraw the precise volume and expel any air bubbles.
• Exchange reconstitution needle with administration needle for deep subcutaneous injection (27G/1¼″).
• Inject 3 mL degarelix 120 mg or 4.2 mL degarelix 80 mg subcutaneously immediately after reconstitution. Grasp skin of abdomen, and elevate subcutaneous tissue. Insert needle deeply at angle of not less than 45 degrees. Gently pull back plunger to check if blood is aspirated. If blood appears in syringe, reconstituted product can no longer be used. Discontinue procedure and discard syringe and needle. Reconstitute new dose.
• Repeat reconstitution procedure for second 120-mg initial dose. Choose different injection site and inject 3 mL.

ACTION
Reversibly binds to the pituitary GnRH receptors, reducing the release of gonadotropins, and consequently testosterone.

Route	Onset	Peak	Duration
Subcut.	Unknown	2 days	Unknown

Half-life: Loading dose, about 53 days; maintenance dose, about 31 days.

ADVERSE REACTIONS
CNS: asthenia, dizziness, fatigue, fever, headache, insomnia.
CV: hypertension, hot flashes.
GI: constipation, diarrhea, nausea.
GU: erectile dysfunction, UTI, testicular atrophy.
Metabolic: weight gain, increased GGT.
Musculoskeletal: arthralgia, back pain, decrease in bone density.
Skin: injection-site reactions (including pain, erythema, swelling, induration, and nodule formation), night sweats, hyperhidrosis.
Other: chills, gynecomastia.

INTERACTIONS
Drug-drug. *Class IA, Class III antiarrhythmics (amiodarone, procainamide, quinidine, sotalol):* May prolong QT interval. Avoid use together.

EFFECTS ON LAB TEST RESULTS
• May increase PSA, AST, ALT, and GGT levels.

CONTRAINDICATIONS & CAUTIONS
• Contraindicated in patients hypersensitive to drug or its components. Discontinue drug for serious hypersensitivity reactions and don't rechallenge.
• Drug may increase risk of CV disease, anemia, and diabetes.
• Androgen deprivation therapy may prolong the QT interval. Prescribers should consider whether benefits of therapy outweigh potential risks. Use cautiously in patients with congenital long QT syndrome, electrolyte abnormalities, or HF and in those taking Class IA or Class III antiarrhythmics.
• Use cautiously in patients with CrCl of less than 50 mL/minute or severe hepatic impairment.
Dialyzable drug: Unknown.

PREGNANCY-LACTATION-REPRODUCTION
• Drug isn't indicated for use in women and is contraindicated in women who are or may become pregnant or are breast-feeding.

NURSING CONSIDERATIONS
• Monitor QT interval and electrolyte levels in patients with congenital long QT syndrome, electrolyte abnormalities, or HF, and in those taking Class IA or Class III antiarrhythmics.
• Monitor PSA level; if level is elevated, monitor testosterone level.
• Monitor bone density tests periodically.
• Monitor LFT values, CBC, and glucose levels.

PATIENT TEACHING
• Teach injection technique and methods of record-keeping to patient or family if they will be giving drug.
• Emphasize to patient the importance of notifying health care provider of heart problems, such as HF, irregular heart

rhythm, or salt imbalance, before taking drug.
● Advise patient to inform all health care providers that he or she is taking drug.

delavirdine mesylate
dell-ah-VUR-den

Rescriptor

Therapeutic class: Antiretrovirals
Pharmacologic class: Nonnucleoside reverse transcriptase inhibitors

AVAILABLE FORMS
Tablets: 100 mg, 200 mg

INDICATIONS & DOSAGES
➤ **HIV-1 infection in combination with two other active antiretrovirals**
Adults and adolescents age 16 and older: 400 mg P.O. t.i.d.

Resistant virus emerges rapidly when delavirdine is administered as monotherapy. Always administer with appropriate antiretroviral therapy.

ADMINISTRATION
P.O.
● Patient may take drug with or without food.
● For patient with achlorhydria (absence of gastric acid in the stomach), drug should be taken with an acidic beverage, such as orange juice or cranberry juice.
● Patient should separate doses of delavirdine and antacid by at least 1 hour.
● Drug may be dispersed in water before ingestion. Add four 100-mg tablets to at least 3 oz (90 mL) of water, allow to stand for a few minutes, and stir until a uniform dispersion occurs. Tell patient to drink dispersion promptly, rinse glass, and swallow the rinse to ensure that entire dose is consumed. Don't try to disperse 200-mg tablets because they don't disperse well; take 200-mg tablets intact.

ACTION
A nonnucleoside reverse transcriptase inhibitor of HIV-1 that binds directly to reverse transcriptase and blocks RNA-

and DNA-dependent DNA polymerase activities.

Route	Onset	Peak	Duration
P.O.	Unknown	1 hr	Unknown

Half-life: 2 to 11 hours.

ADVERSE REACTIONS
CNS: anxiety, asthenia, fatigue, headache, depression, fever, insomnia, pain.
EENT: pharyngitis, sinusitis.
GI: nausea, abdominal cramps, diarrhea, distention or pain, vomiting.
Respiratory: bronchitis, cough, URI.
Skin: rash.
Other: flulike syndrome.

INTERACTIONS
Drug-drug. *Amphetamines, nonsedating antihistamines, benzodiazepines, calcium channel blockers, clarithromycin, dapsone, ergot alkaloid preparations, indinavir, rifabutin, sedative-hypnotics, warfarin:* May increase or prolong therapeutic and adverse effects of these drugs. Avoid using together or, if use together is unavoidable, reduce doses of indinavir and clarithromycin. Monitor INR for warfarin dosing.
Antacids: May reduce absorption of delavirdine. Separate doses by at least 1 hour.
Antiarrhythmics (amiodarone, bepridil, flecainide, lidocaine [systemic], quinidine, propafenone): May increase risk of arrhythmias. Use cautiously and monitor drug levels if possible.
Carbamazepine, phenobarbital, phenytoin: May decrease delavirdine level. Use together cautiously.
Didanosine: May decrease absorption of both drugs by 20%. Separate doses by at least 1 hour.
Fluoxetine, ketoconazole: May cause a 50% increase in delavirdine bioavailability. Monitor patient and reduce dose of clarithromycin.
H$_2$-receptor antagonists, PPIs: May increase gastric pH and reduce absorption of delavirdine. Long-term use together isn't recommended.
HMG-CoA reductase inhibitors (atorvastatin, lovastatin, simvastatin): May increase levels of these drugs, which increases risk of

myopathy, including rhabdomyolysis. Avoid using together.

Rifabutin, rifampin: May decrease delavirdine level. May increase rifabutin level by 100%. Avoid using together.

Saquinavir: May increase bioavailability of saquinavir fivefold. Monitor AST and ALT levels frequently when used together.

Sildenafil: May increase sildenafil level and may increase sildenafil adverse events, including hypotension, visual changes, and priapism. Tell patient not to exceed 25 mg of sildenafil in 48 hours.

Drug-herb. *St. John's wort:* May decrease drug level. Discourage use together.

EFFECTS ON LAB TEST RESULTS

● May increase alkaline phosphatase, ALT, amylase, AST, bilirubin level, CK, creatinine, GGT, and lipase levels. May decrease glucose and Hb levels and hematocrit.

● May increase eosinophil count; may prolong PT and PTT. May decrease granulocyte, neutrophil, platelet, RBC, and WBC counts.

CONTRAINDICATIONS & CAUTIONS

● Contraindicated in patients hypersensitive to drug or its components and in those taking drugs that are highly dependent on CYP3A metabolism (antihistamines, ergot derivatives, sedative-hypnotics).

● Use cautiously in elderly patients and in patients with impaired hepatic function.

Dialyzable drug: Unlikely.

PREGNANCY-LACTATION-REPRODUCTION

● There are no adequate well-controlled studies in pregnant women. Use during pregnancy only if potential benefit justifies potential risk to the fetus.

● HIV-positive women shouldn't breastfeed, to avid postnatal HIV transmission and possible adverse reactions in breast-fed infants.

● Encourage pregnant patients to enroll in the Antiretroviral Pregnancy Registry by calling 1-800-258-4263.

NURSING CONSIDERATIONS

● Because drug's effects in patients with hepatic or renal impairment haven't been

studied, monitor renal function test results and LFTs carefully.

● Drug-induced diffuse, maculopapular, erythematous, pruritic rash occurs most commonly on upper body and arms of patients with lower CD4 cell counts, usually within first 3 weeks of treatment. Dosage adjustment doesn't seem to affect rash. Treat symptoms with diphenhydramine, hydroxyzine, or topical corticosteroids.

● Drug doesn't reduce risk of transmission of HIV-1.

● Monitor patient's fluid balance and weight.

PATIENT TEACHING

● Tell patient to stop drug and call prescriber if severe rash or such symptoms as fever, fatigue, headache, nausea, abdominal pain, or cough occur.

● Inform patient that drug doesn't cure HIV-1 infection and that he may continue to acquire illnesses, including opportunistic infections related to HIV-1 infection. Therapy hasn't been shown to reduce the risk or frequency of such illnesses. Drug hasn't been shown to reduce transmission of HIV.

● Advise patient to remain under medical supervision when taking drug because the long-term effects aren't known.

● Tell patient to take drug as prescribed and not to alter doses without prescriber's approval. If a dose is missed, tell patient to take the next dose as soon as possible; he shouldn't double the next dose.

● Inform patient that drug may be dispersed in water before ingestion. Add four 100-mg tablets to at least 3 oz (90 mL) of water, allow to stand for a few minutes, and stir until a uniform dispersion occurs. Tell patient to drink dispersion promptly, rinse glass, and swallow the rinse to ensure that entire dose is consumed.

● Instruct patient to take 200-mg tablets whole; 200-mg tablets don't disperse well in water.

● Tell patient that drug may be taken with or without food.

● Tell patient with achlorhydria to take drug with an acidic beverage, such as orange or cranberry juice.

● Instruct patient to take drug and antacids at least 1 hour apart.

• Advise patient to report use of other prescription or nonprescription drugs, including herbal remedies.

• Advise patient taking sildenafil about an increased risk of sildenafil-related adverse events, including low BP, visual changes, and painful penile erection. Tell him to promptly report any symptoms to his prescriber. Tell patient not to exceed 25 mg of sildenafil in 48 hours.

denosumab
deh-KNOW-sue-mab

Prolia, Xgeva

Therapeutic class: Antiosteoporotics–antiresorptives
Pharmacologic class: Monoclonal antibodies

AVAILABLE FORMS
Injection: 60 mg/mL in prefilled syringe; 60 mg/mL, 70 mg/mL in single-use vial

INDICATIONS & DOSAGES
➤ **Osteoporosis in men and postmenopausal women at risk for fracture (Prolia only)**
Adults: 60 mg subcutaneously every 6 months. All patients should receive 1,000 mg of calcium daily and at least 400 international units of vitamin D daily.
➤ **Bone metastases from solid tumors (Xgeva only)**
Adults: 120 mg subcutaneously every 4 weeks with calcium and vitamin D as necessary to prevent or treat hypocalcemia.
➤ **To increase bone mass in men at high risk for fracture who are receiving androgen deprivation therapy for non-metastatic prostate cancer and in women who are receiving adjuvant aromatase inhibitor therapy for breast cancer (Prolia only)**
Adults: 60 mg subcutaneously once every 6 months. All patients should receive calcium 1,000 mg daily and at least 400 international units of vitamin D daily.
➤ **Giant cell tumor of bone (Xgeva only)**
Adults and skeletally mature adolescents age 13 and older: 120 mg subcutaneously every 4 weeks with additional 120-mg doses on days 8 and 15 of first month of therapy. Administer calcium and vitamin D as necessary to prevent or treat hypocalcemia.
➤ **Hypercalcemia of malignancy refractory to bisphosphonate therapy (Xgeva only)**
Adults: 120 mg subcutaneously every 4 weeks with additional 120-mg doses on days 8 and 15 of first month of therapy.

ADMINISTRATION
Subcutaneous
• Don't use if solution is discolored or cloudy or contains many particles or foreign particulate matter.
• Before administration, drug may be removed from refrigerator and brought to room temperature (up to 77° F [25° C]) by letting stand in original container. This generally takes 15 to 30 minutes. Don't warm drug in any other way. Avoid vigorous shaking of drug. Once removed from refrigerator, maintain at 77° F or lower and use within 14 days. Discard after 14 days if not used.
• Use 27G needle to withdraw drug from single-use vial, and inject entire contents of vial. Don't reenter vial.
• Administer via subcutaneous injection in upper arm, upper thigh, or abdomen.
• Drug is intended for subcutaneous route only and shouldn't be administered I.V., I.M., or intradermally.

ACTION
Inhibits osteoclast activity, thereby decreasing bone resorption and increasing bone mass and strength.

Route	Onset	Peak	Duration
Subcut.	Unknown	10 days	4–5 mo

Half-life: About 25 to 28 days.

ADVERSE REACTIONS
CNS: asthenia, insomnia, sciatica, vertigo, headache, fatigue.
CV: angina, atrial fibrillation, peripheral edema.
EENT: pharyngitis.
GI: flatulence, GERD, upper abdominal pain, nausea, decreased appetite, vomiting, constipation, diarrhea.

Reactions in bold italics are *life-threatening*. Interactions may have a *rapid onset* or a *delayed onset*.

GU: cystitis.
Hematologic: anemia.
Metabolic: hypercholesterolemia, *hypocalcemia,* hypophosphatemia.
Musculoskeletal: back pain, bone pain, extremity pain, musculoskeletal pain, myalgia, spinal osteoarthritis.
Respiratory: pneumonia, URI, dyspnea.
Skin: pruritus, rash, dermatitis.
Other: *anaphylaxis,* facial swelling, herpes zoster, *osteonecrosis of the jaw.*

INTERACTIONS

Drug-drug. *Immunosuppressants (except cytarabine [liposomal]):* May enhance adverse/toxic effect of immunosuppressants and increase risk of serious infections. Monitor patient closely.
Drug-lifestyle. *Alcohol use:* May increase risk of osteoporosis. Avoid use together.

EFFECTS ON LAB TEST RESULTS

• May increase cholesterol level. May decrease calcium and phosphate levels.

CONTRAINDICATIONS & CAUTIONS

• Contraindicated in patients with a history of systemic hypersensitivity to components of the product. Reactions have included anaphylaxis, facial swelling, and urticaria.
• Contraindicated in patients with hypocalcemia.
• Discontinue use if severe bone, joint, or muscle pain occurs.
• Xgeva isn't for use in prevention of skeletal-related events in patients with multiple myeloma.
• Use cautiously in patients with history of hypoparathyroidism, thyroid surgery, parathyroid surgery, malabsorption syndromes, excision of small intestine, or severe renal impairment.
• Use cautiously in patients taking immunosuppressants and in those with an impaired immune system.
Dialyzable drug: Unknown.

PREGNANCY-LACTATION-REPRODUCTION

• Drug may cause fetal harm and is contraindicated in pregnant women. If drug is used during pregnancy, or if patient becomes pregnant while taking drug, inform patient of potential hazard to a fetus.

• Women who become pregnant during treatment are encouraged to enroll in Amgen's Pregnancy Surveillance Program by calling 1-800-77-AMGEN (1-800-772-6436).
• Caution women of childbearing potential to use highly effective contraception during therapy and for at least 5 months after last dose.
• Advise male patient taking drug who has a pregnant partner that drug may appear in seminal fluid and that fetal exposure to drug may occur during unprotected sexual intercourse.
• It isn't known if drug appears in breast milk. Patient should discontinue breast-feeding or discontinue drug, taking into account importance of drug to the mother.

NURSING CONSIDERATIONS

• Make sure patient has adequate intake of calcium and vitamin D.
• Monitor calcium (especially in first weeks of therapy), vitamin D, magnesium, and phosphorus levels before and during therapy. Administer calcium, magnesium, and vitamin D as needed.
• Drug can cause severe symptomatic hypocalcemia; fatal cases have been reported. Correct hypocalcemia before starting drug.
• Drug may cause osteonecrosis of the jaw, which can occur spontaneously and is commonly associated with tooth extraction, local infection with delayed healing, or both.
• Consider stopping drug if severe skin reactions occur.
• Hypercalcemia may occur in patients with growing skeletons when treatment is discontinued. Monitor patients for signs and symptoms of hypercalcemia (nausea, vomiting, headache, decreased alertness) and treat appropriately.
• A REMS (risk evaluation and mitigation strategy) program is associated with Prolia. An FDA-approved patient medication guide must be dispensed with drug.
🔾 *Alert:* Needle cap on single-use syringe contains latex; keep away from those with latex allergy.
🔾 *Alert:* Prolia and Xgeva contain the same active ingredient, denosumab. Patients receiving Prolia should not receive Xgeva.

PATIENT TEACHING

- Caution patient to read medication guide that comes with prescription before starting treatment and at every prescription refill.
- Warn patient to immediately report signs and symptoms of low calcium (spasms, twitching or muscle cramps, and numbness or tingling of fingers or toes or around mouth); emphasize the importance of maintaining normal calcium levels.
- Advise patient to have a dental exam before treatment and to follow good oral hygiene practices during therapy.
- Instruct patient to tell dentist before dental procedures that he is taking drug, and to inform dentist or prescriber if persistent pain or slow healing of mouth or jaw occurs after dental surgery.
- Tell patient to report jaw pain, swelling, or numbness; loose teeth; or dramatic gum loss.
- Advise patient to seek prompt medical care if signs and symptoms of severe infection occur, including cellulitis or skin reactions (such as dermatitis, rash, or eczema).
- Advise patient to contact health care provider if severe bone, joint, or muscle pain occurs.
- Instruct patient with severe renal impairment about signs and symptoms of hypocalcemia and the importance of maintaining normal calcium levels.
- Tell patient to take calcium and vitamin D supplement, as directed by prescriber.

---

desipramine hydrochloride
dess-IP-ra-meen

Norpramin

Therapeutic class: Antidepressants
Pharmacologic class: TCAs

AVAILABLE FORMS
Tablets: 10 mg, 25 mg, 50 mg, 75 mg, 100 mg, 150 mg

INDICATIONS & DOSAGES
➤ **Depression**
Adults: 100 to 200 mg P.O. daily in divided doses; increase to maximum of 300 mg daily. Or, give entire dose at bedtime.

Adolescents and elderly patients: 25 to 100 mg P.O. daily in divided doses; increase gradually to maximum of 150 mg daily, if needed.

ADMINISTRATION
P.O.
- Give drug without regard for food.

ACTION
Unknown. Increases the amount of norepinephrine, serotonin, or both in the CNS by blocking their reuptake by the presynaptic neurons.

Route	Onset	Peak	Duration
P.O.	Unknown	About 6 hr	Unknown

Half-life: 15 to 24 hours.

ADVERSE REACTIONS
CNS: drowsiness, dizziness, *seizures,* excitation, tremor, weakness, confusion, anxiety, restlessness, agitation, headache, nervousness, EEG changes, extrapyramidal reactions, ataxia, delusions, insomnia, fatigue, peripheral neuropathy.
CV: tachycardia, orthostatic hypotension, ECG changes, hypertension.
EENT: blurred vision, tinnitus, mydriasis.
GI: dry mouth, constipation, nausea, vomiting, anorexia, paralytic ileus.
GU: urine retention, erectile dysfunction, nocturia, decreased libido, painful ejaculation, testicular swelling, urinary hesitancy.
Hematologic: *agranulocytosis, thrombocytopenia,* eosinophilia, purpura.
Metabolic: *hypoglycemia,* hyperglycemia, weight loss or gain.
Skin: rash, urticaria, photosensitivity reactions, diaphoresis, alopecia.
Other: *sudden death in children,* hypersensitivity reactions.

INTERACTIONS
Drug-drug. *Barbiturates, CNS depressants:* May enhance CNS depression. Avoid using together.
Cimetidine, **fluoxetine, fluvoxamine, paroxetine, sertraline:** May increase desipramine level. Monitor drug levels and patient for signs of toxicity.
Clonidine: May cause life-threatening BP elevations. Avoid using together.

Reactions in bold italics are *life-threatening*. Interactions may have a *rapid onset* or a *delayed onset*.

Drugs that prolong QT interval (antiarrhythmics, clarithromycin, droperidol, fluoroquinolones, pimozide, ziprasidone): May increase QT-interval prolongation and risk of ventricular arrhythmias. Avoid combination if possible.

Epinephrine, norepinephrine: May increase hypertensive effect. Use together cautiously.

Linezolid, methylene blue: May cause serotonin syndrome. Use with extreme caution and monitor closely.

MAO inhibitors: May cause severe excitation, hyperpyrexia, or seizures, usually with high doses. Avoid using within 14 days of MAO inhibitor therapy.

Quinolones: May increase the risk of life-threatening arrhythmias. Avoid using together.

Serotonergic drugs (buspirone, fentanyl, lithium, tramadol, triptans, tryptophan): Increase risk of serotonin syndrome. Monitor closely if use together is clinically warranted. Discontinue desipramine and other serotonergic drugs if syndrome occurs, and initiate supportive treatment.

Drug-herb. *Evening primrose oil:* May cause additive or synergistic effect, resulting in lower seizure threshold and increasing the risk of seizure. Discourage use together.

St. John's wort, *SAM-e, yohimbe:* May cause serotonin syndrome. Discourage use together.

Drug-food. *Grapefruit juice:* May increase desipramine level, increasing pharmacologic effects and risk of adverse reactions. Avoid use together.

Drug-lifestyle. *Alcohol use:* May enhance CNS depression. Discourage use together.

Smoking: May lower drug level. Monitor patient for lack of effect.

Sun exposure: May increase risk of photosensitivity reactions. Advise patient to avoid excessive sunlight exposure.

EFFECTS ON LAB TEST RESULTS
● May increase or decrease glucose level.
● May increase LFT values.
● May cause false-positive urine detection of amphetamines or methamphetamines.

CONTRAINDICATIONS & CAUTIONS
● Contraindicated in patients hypersensitive to drug and in those who have taken MAO inhibitors within previous 14 days.

● *Alert:* Concomitant use with linezolid or methylene blue can cause serotonin syndrome (fever, mental status changes, muscle twitching, excessive sweating, shivering or shaking, diarrhea, loss of coordination) and is contraindicated.

● Contraindicated during acute recovery phase after MI.

Black Box Warning Drug isn't approved for use in children. ■

● Use with extreme caution in patients with CV disease; in those with a family history of sudden death, cardiac arrhythmias, or cardiac conduction disturbances; in those with history of urine retention, glaucoma, seizure disorders, or thyroid disease; and in those taking thyroid drug.

● *Alert:* Treatment of patients who require as much as 300 mg desipramine should be initiated in hospitals where access to skilled health care providers and frequent ECGs is available. High doses may cause prolongation of the QRS or QT interval.

Dialyzable drug: No.

⚠ Overdose S&S: Cardiac arrhythmias, severe hypotension, seizures, CNS depression, coma, ECG changes, confusion, disturbed concentration, transient visual hallucinations, dilated pupils, agitation, hyperactive reflexes, stupor, drowsiness, muscle rigidity, vomiting, hypothermia, hyperpyrexia.

PREGNANCY-LACTATION-REPRODUCTION
● Safe use in pregnant women hasn't been established. Use during pregnancy only if clearly needed and potential benefit justifies potential risk to the fetus.

● Drug appears in breast milk. Patient should discontinue breast-feeding or discontinue drug, taking into account importance of drug to the mother.

NURSING CONSIDERATIONS
● *Alert:* Drug has been shown to lower the seizure threshold. Seizures precede cardiac arrhythmias and death in some patients.

● Monitor patient for nausea, headache, and malaise after abrupt withdrawal of long-term therapy; these symptoms don't indicate addiction.

• Don't withdraw drug abruptly.

• Because patients may experience hypertensive episodes, cardiac arrhythmias, or drug interactions with anesthesia during surgery, stop drug gradually several days before elective surgery.

◑ Alert: If linezolid or methylene blue must be given, stop drug and monitor the patient for serotonin toxicity for 2 weeks or until 24 hours after the last dose of methylene blue or linezolid, whichever comes first. Treatment may be resumed 24 hours after last dose of methylene blue or linezolid.

• If signs or symptoms of psychosis occur or increase, notify prescriber. Record mood changes. Monitor patient for suicidal tendencies.

Black Box Warning Drug may increase risk of suicidal thinking and behavior in children, adolescents, and young adults ages 18 to 24, especially during the first few months of treatment, especially in those with major depressive disorder or other psychiatric disorder. ∎

• Recommend sugarless hard candy or gum to relieve dry mouth. Saliva substitutes may be needed.

◑ Alert: Norpramin may contain tartrazine.

• **Look alike–sound alike:** Don't confuse desipramine with disopyramide or imipramine.

PATIENT TEACHING

Black Box Warning Advise families and caregivers to observe patient closely for increased suicidal thinking and behavior. ∎

• Advise patient to take full dose at bedtime to avoid daytime sedation; if insomnia occurs, tell patient to take drug in the morning.

• Warn patient to avoid hazardous activities that require alertness and good coordination until effects of drug are known. Drowsiness and dizziness usually subside after a few weeks.

◑ Alert: Teach patient to recognize and immediately report symptoms of serotonin toxicity (fever, mental status changes, muscle twitching, excessive sweating, shivering or shaking, diarrhea, loss of coordination).

• Advise patient to call prescriber if fever and sore throat occur. Blood counts may need to be obtained.

• Tell patient to avoid alcohol during therapy because it may antagonize effects of drug.

• Tell patient to consult prescriber before taking other prescription or OTC drugs.

• Warn patient not to stop drug suddenly.

• To prevent sensitivity to the sun, advise patient to use sunblock, wear protective clothing, and avoid prolonged exposure to strong sunlight.

desloratadine
dess-lor-AT-a-deen

Clarinex◆, Clarinex RediTabs

Therapeutic class: Antihistamines
Pharmacologic class: Piperidines

AVAILABLE FORMS
ODTs: 2.5 mg, 5 mg
Syrup: 0.5 mg/mL
Tablets: 5 mg

INDICATIONS & DOSAGES
➤ **Seasonal allergic rhinitis (patients age 2 and older); perennial allergic rhinitis and chronic idiopathic urticaria (patients age 6 months and older)**
Adults and children age 12 and older: 5 mg P.O. tablets or syrup once daily.
Children ages 6 to 11: 2.5 mg ODT or syrup P.O. once daily.
Children ages 12 months to 5 years: 1.25 mg P.O. once daily.
Infants ages 6 to 11 months: 1 mg P.O. once daily.
Adjust-a-dose: In adults with hepatic or renal impairment, start dosage at 5 mg P.O. every other day.

ADMINISTRATION
P.O.
• Give drug without regard for meals.
• Place ODTs on tongue immediately after opening blister pack.
• Give ODTs with or without water.

ACTION
Long-acting tricyclic antihistamine with selective H_1-receptor antagonist activity. It inhibits histamine release from human mast cells in vitro.

Route	Onset	Peak	Duration
P.O.	<1 hr	3 hr	Up to 24 hr

Half-life: 27 hours.

ADVERSE REACTIONS
CNS: headache, somnolence, fatigue, dizziness, irritability, fever.
EENT: pharyngitis, dry throat, rhinorrhea, epistaxis.
GI: nausea, diarrhea, dry mouth, dyspepsia.
GU: dysmenorrhea.
Musculoskeletal: myalgia.
Respiratory: bronchitis, cough, URI.

INTERACTIONS
Drug-drug. *CNS depressants:* May increase CNS depression. Monitor therapy.
Drug-lifestyle. *Alcohol use:* May increase CNS depression. Avoid use together.

EFFECTS ON LAB TEST RESULTS
• May prevent, reduce, or mask positive result in diagnostic skin test.

CONTRAINDICATIONS & CAUTIONS
• Contraindicated in patients hypersensitive to drug or its components, or to loratadine.
• Hypersensitivity reactions, including rash, pruritus, urticaria, edema, dyspnea, and anaphylaxis, have been reported. If these occur, stop drug immediately and consider alternative treatments.
• Use cautiously in elderly patients because of the greater likelihood of decreased hepatic, renal, or cardiac function and concomitant disease or other drug therapy.
Dialyzable drug: No.
⚠ **Overdose S&S:** Somnolence, increased QTc interval.

PREGNANCY-LACTATION-REPRODUCTION
• There are no adequate well-controlled studies in pregnant women. Use during pregnancy only if clearly needed and potential benefit justifies potential risk to the fetus.

• Drug appears in breast milk. Patient should discontinue breast-feeding or discontinue drug, taking into account importance of drug to the mother.

NURSING CONSIDERATIONS
• Stop drug 4 days before diagnostic skin testing because antihistamines can prevent, reduce, or mask positive skin test response.

PATIENT TEACHING
• Advise patient not to exceed recommended dosage. Higher doses don't increase effectiveness and may cause somnolence.
• Tell patient that drug can be taken without regard to meals.
• Instruct patient to remove ODTs from blister pack and place on tongue immediately to dissolve.
• ODTs may be taken with or without water.
• Tell patient to report adverse effects.
• Advise patient with phenylketonuria that each ODT contains 1.75 mg phenylalanine.

desmopressin acetate
des-moe-PRESS-in

DDAVP, Minirin, Stimate

Therapeutic class: Hemostatics
Pharmacologic class: Posterior pituitary hormones

AVAILABLE FORMS
Injection: 4 mcg/mL
Metered nasal spray: 10 mcg/spray, 150 mcg/spray
Nasal solution: 0.1 mg/mL, 1.5 mg/mL
Tablets: 0.1 mg, 0.2 mg

INDICATIONS & DOSAGES
➤ **Nonnephrogenic diabetes insipidus, temporary polyuria, and polydipsia related to pituitary trauma**
Intranasal, I.V., or subcutaneous
Adults and children older than age 12:
0.1 to 0.4 mL (10 to 40 mcg) intranasally daily in one to three doses. Most adults need 0.2 mL (20 mcg) daily in two divided doses. Or, give 0.5 to 1 mL (2 to 4 mcg) I.V. or subcutaneously daily, usually in two divided doses.

P.O.

Adults and children older than age 4: Initially, 0.05 mg (half of the 0.1-mg tablet) P.O. b.i.d.; adjust dosage to patient response. If patient previously received the drug intranasally, begin oral therapy 12 hours after last intranasal dose. Maximum dose is 1.2 mg/day (divided into 2 or 3 doses) for patients with diabetes insipidus.

Intranasal

Children ages 3 months to 12 years: 0.05 to 0.3 mL (5 to 30 mcg) intranasally daily in one or two doses.

➤ Hemophilia A and von Willebrand disease

Adults and children age 3 months and older: 0.3 mcg/kg diluted in NSS and infused I.V. over 15 to 30 minutes. Repeat dose, if needed, as indicated by laboratory response and patient's condition. If used preoperatively, give 30 minutes before the scheduled procedure.

Adults and children age 11 months and older: A total dose of 300 mcg (one spray [150 mcg] of solution containing 1.5 mg/mL in each nostril). Dose of 150 mcg (one spray of solution containing 1.5 mg/mL into a single nostril) may be adequate for patients weighing less than 50 kg. Give drug 2 hours before surgery.

➤ Primary nocturnal enuresis

Adults and children age 6 and older: Initially, 0.2 mg P.O. at bedtime; adjust dose up to 0.6 mg to achieve desired response.

➤ Prevention of surgical bleeding in patients with uremia ◆

Adults: 0.3 mcg/kg I.V. over 30 minutes.

ADMINISTRATION

P.O.

● Discontinue in patient with acute illness that may result in fluid or electrolyte imbalance.

● Store at controlled room temperature.

I.V.

▼ Don't give injection to patients with hemophilia A with factor VIII of up to 5% or with severe von Willebrand disease.

▼ For adults and children weighing more than 10 kg, dilute with 50 mL sterile physiologic saline solution. For children weighing 10 kg or less, 10 mL of diluent is recommended.

▼ Inspect drug for particulates and discoloration before infusing.

▼ Monitor BP and pulse rate during infusion.

▼ The comparable antidiuretic dose of the injection is about one-tenth of the intranasal dose.

▼ **Incompatibilities:** None reported.

Intranasal

● Ensure nasal passages are intact, clean, and free of obstruction before giving intranasally.

● Nasal spray pump delivers only doses of 10 mcg DDAVP (per 0.1-mL dose) or 150 mcg Stimate (per 0.1-mL dose). If doses other than these are required, use the nasal tube delivery system or injection.

Subcutaneous

● Teach patient to rotate injection sites to prevent tissue damage.

ACTION

Increases the permeability of renal tubular epithelium to adenosine monophosphate and water, enabling the epithelium to promote reabsorption of water and produce a concentrated urine. Also increases factor VIII activity by releasing endogenous factor VIII from plasma storage sites.

Route	Onset	Peak	Duration
P.O.	1 hr	1–1½ hr	6–14 hr
I.V.	30 min	1½–2 hr	6–14 hr
Intranasal	15–30 min	1–1½ hr	6–14 hr
Subcut.	Unknown	Unknown	Unknown

Half-life: P.O., 1½ to 2½ hours; I.V., 3 hours; intranasal, 7.8 minutes (initial phase) and 75.5 minutes (terminal phase).

ADVERSE REACTIONS

CNS: headache, *seizures.*
CV: flushing, slight rise in BP.
EENT: rhinitis, epistaxis, sore throat.
GI: nausea, abdominal cramps.
GU: vulvar pain.
Metabolic: hyponatremia.
Respiratory: cough.
Skin: local erythema, swelling, or burning after injection.

INTERACTIONS

Drug-drug. *Carbamazepine, chlorpropamide:* May increase ADH; may

---

Reactions in bold italics are *life-threatening*. Interactions may have a *rapid onset* or a *delayed onset*.

increase desmopressin effect. Avoid using together.

Clofibrate: May enhance and prolong effects of desmopressin. Monitor patient closely.

Demeclocycline, epinephrine, heparin, lithium, NSAIDs, SSRIs, TCAs: May increase risk of adverse effects. Monitor patient closely.

Pressor agents: May enhance pressor effects with large doses of desmopressin. Monitor patient closely.

Drug-lifestyle. *Alcohol use:* May increase risk of adverse effects. Discourage use together.

EFFECTS ON LAB TEST RESULTS
● May decrease sodium level.

CONTRAINDICATIONS & CAUTIONS
● Contraindicated in patients hypersensitive to drug and in those with type IIB von Willebrand disease, moderate to severe renal impairment, or hyponatremia.
● Use cautiously in patients with coronary artery insufficiency, hypertensive CV disease, and conditions linked to fluid and electrolyte imbalances, such as cystic fibrosis, because these patients are susceptible to hyponatremia.
● Use cautiously in patients at risk for water intoxication with hyponatremia.
Dialyzable drug: Unknown.
⚠ *Overdose S&S:* Confusion, drowsiness, continuing headache, problems passing urine, rapid weight gain due to fluid retention.

PREGNANCY-LACTATION-REPRODUCTION
● There are no adequate well-controlled studies in pregnant women. Use during pregnancy only if clearly needed and potential benefit justifies potential risk to the fetus.
● It isn't known if drug appears in breast milk. Use cautiously in breast-feeding women.

NURSING CONSIDERATIONS
● Morning and evening doses are adjusted separately for adequate diurnal rhythm of water turnover.

● Intranasal use can cause changes in the nasal mucosa, resulting in erratic, unreliable absorption. Report worsening condition to prescriber, who may recommend injectable DDAVP.
● Restrict fluid intake to reduce risk of water intoxication and sodium depletion, especially in children or elderly patients.
🔔 *Alert:* Overdose may cause oxytocic or vasopressor activity. Withhold drug and notify prescriber. If fluid retention is excessive, give furosemide.
● *Look alike–sound alike:* Don't confuse desmopressin with vasopressin.

PATIENT TEACHING
● Some patients may have trouble measuring and inhaling drug into nostrils. Teach patient and caregivers correct administration method.
● Instruct patient to clear nasal passages before giving drug.
● Instruct patient to press down four times to prime pump. Tell him to discard the bottle after 25 (150 mcg/spray) or 50 doses (10 mcg/spray), depending on the strength, because the amount left may be less than desired dose.
● Advise patient to report nasal congestion, allergic rhinitis, or URI to prescriber; dosage adjustment may be needed.
● Teach patient using subcutaneous drug to rotate injection sites to prevent tissue damage.
● Warn patient to drink only enough water to satisfy thirst.
● Inform patient with hemophilia A or von Willebrand disease that taking desmopressin may prevent hazards of using blood products.
● Advise patient to carry medical identification indicating use of drug.

desoximetasone
dess-OX-ee-MET-ah-sone

Topicort

Therapeutic class: Corticosteroids
Pharmacologic class: Corticosteroids

AVAILABLE FORMS
Cream: 0.05%, 0.25%
Gel: 0.05%*

Ointment: 0.05%, 0.25%
Spray: 0.25%

INDICATIONS & DOSAGES
➤ **Inflammation from corticosteroid-responsive dermatoses (except spray)**
Adults and children: Clean area; apply a thin film and rub in gently b.i.d. Don't use 0.25% ointment on children younger than age 10.
➤ **Plaque psoriasis (spray only)**
Adults: Apply a thin film to affected areas and rub in gently b.i.d. Treatment beyond 4 weeks isn't recommended.

ADMINISTRATION
Topical
• Gently wash skin before applying. To prevent skin damage, rub in gently, leaving thin coat. When treating hairy sites, part hair and apply directly to lesions.
• Avoid applying near eyes, mucous membranes, or in ear canal.
🖐 *Alert:* Don't bandage, cover, or wrap the treated skin area unless ordered.
• Stop drug and notify prescriber if skin infection, striae, or atrophy occur.
• Continue drug for a few days after lesions clear.
• Avoid using spray on face, axilla, or groin or if atrophy is present.

ACTION
Unclear. Diffuses across cell membranes to form complexes with receptors, showing anti-inflammatory, antipruritic, vasoconstrictive, and antiproliferative activity.

Route	Onset	Peak	Duration
Topical	Unknown	Unknown	Unknown

Half-life: 13 to 17 hours (urine).

ADVERSE REACTIONS
GU: glycosuria.
Metabolic: hyperglycemia.
Skin: burning, pruritus, irritation, dryness, erythema, folliculitis, hypertrichosis, acneiform eruptions, perioral dermatitis, hypopigmentation, allergic contact dermatitis, maceration, secondary infection, atrophy, striae, miliaria with occlusive dressings.
Other: *HPA axis suppression,* Cushing syndrome.

INTERACTIONS
None significant.

EFFECTS ON LAB TEST RESULTS
• May increase glucose level.

CONTRAINDICATIONS & CAUTIONS
• Contraindicated in patients hypersensitive to drug or its components.
• Don't use as monotherapy in primary bacterial infections (impetigo, paronychia, erysipelas, cellulitis, angular cheilitis), treatment of rosacea, perioral dermatitis, or acne.
• Don't use very-high-potency or high-potency agents on the face, groin, or axillae.
• Don't use spray if atrophy is present at treatment site.
• Drug isn't for ophthalmic use.
• Use cautiously in children. Spray isn't recommended for use in children.
Dialyzable drug: Unknown.
⚠ *Overdose S&S:* Systemic effects.

PREGNANCY-LACTATION-REPRODUCTION
• There are no adequate well-controlled studies in pregnant women. Use during pregnancy only if potential benefit justifies potential risk to the fetus.
• Don't use extensively, in large amounts, or for prolonged periods in pregnant patients.
• It isn't known if topical corticosteroids are sufficiently absorbed systemically to produce detectable quantities in breast milk. Use cautiously in breast-feeding women. If used during breast-feeding, don't apply on the chest, to avoid accidental ingestion by the infant.

NURSING CONSIDERATIONS
• If fever develops and occlusive dressing is in place, notify prescriber and remove occlusive dressing.
• If antifungal or antibiotic combined with corticosteroid fails to provide prompt improvement, stop corticosteroid until infection is controlled.
• Systemic absorption is likely with use of occlusive dressings, prolonged treatment, or extensive body surface treatment. Watch for symptoms of HPA axis suppression, Cushing syndrome, hyperglycemia, and glycosuria.

- Avoid using plastic pants or tight-fitting diapers on treated areas in young children. Children may absorb larger amounts of drug and be more susceptible to systemic toxicity.
- Gel contains alcohol and may cause burning or irritation in open lesions.
- *Look alike–sound alike:* Don't confuse desoximetasone with dexamethasone.

PATIENT TEACHING
- Teach patient how to apply drug and to report all adverse reactions.
- Tell patient this drug is for external use only and to avoid contact with the eyes.
- If an occlusive dressing is ordered, advise patient to leave it in place for no longer than 12 hours each day and not to use the dressing on infected or weeping lesions.
- Tell patient to stop drug and report signs of systemic absorption, skin irritation or ulceration, hypersensitivity, or infection.

---

desvenlafaxine
des-ven-lah-FAX-in

Khedezla

desvenlafaxine fumarate

desvenlafaxine succinate
Pristiq✒

Therapeutic class: Antidepressants
Pharmacologic class: SSNRIs

AVAILABLE FORMS
desvenlafaxine
Tablets (extended-release) ⓓⓝⓒ: 50 mg, 100 mg
desvenlafaxine fumarate
Tablets (extended-release) ⓓⓝⓒ: 50 mg, 100 mg
desvenlafaxine succinate
Tablets (extended-release) ⓓⓝⓒ: 25 mg, 50 mg, 100 mg

INDICATIONS & DOSAGES
Adjust-a-dose (for all indications): For patients with CrCl of 30 to 50 mL/minute, give 50 mg P.O. once daily. For patients with CrCl of less than 30 mL/minute or ESRD, give 25 mg P.O. daily or 50 mg P.O. every

other day. Don't give supplemental doses after dialysis. For patients with moderate to severe hepatic impairment, give 50 mg P.O. daily; dosage escalation above 100 mg/day isn't recommended for these patients.
➤ **Major depressive disorder**
Adults: 50 mg P.O. once daily.
➤ **Reduction of hot flash frequency or severity in women with natural or medically induced menopause** ◆
Adults: 100 to 150 mg P.O. once daily (maximum, 200 mg/day); titration during first 1 to 2 weeks of therapy may help manage adverse effects at therapy initiation.

ADMINISTRATION
P.O.
- Administer at approximately the same time each day with or without food.
- Patient must swallow tablets whole with fluid and not divide, crush, chew, or dissolve them.

ACTION
Thought to stimulate receptors, increasing the release of serotonin and norepinephrine.

Route	Onset	Peak	Duration
P.O.	Unknown	7½ hr	Unknown

Half-life: About 11 hours.

ADVERSE REACTIONS
CNS: abnormal dreams, anxiety, asthenia, chills, dizziness, fatigue, jittery feeling, headache, insomnia, irritability, paresthesia, somnolence, tremor.
CV: hot flashes, hypertension, palpitations, tachycardia.
EENT: blurred vision, mydriasis, tinnitus.
GI: constipation, diarrhea, dry mouth, dysgeusia, *GI bleeding,* nausea, vomiting.
GU: proteinuria.
Metabolic: decreased appetite, weight loss.
Skin: hyperhidrosis, rash.
Other: sexual dysfunction, yawning.

INTERACTIONS
Drug-drug. *Aspirin, NSAIDs, warfarin, other drugs that affect coagulation:* May increase risk of bleeding. Use together cautiously.
CNS drugs: Drug may cause additive CNS effects. Avoid using together.

CYP3A4 inhibitors (ketoconazole): May increase desvenlafaxine levels. Use together cautiously.

Desipramine, other drugs metabolized by CYP2D6: May increase levels of these drugs. Use together cautiously.

Linezolid, methylene blue: Increases risk of serotonin syndrome. Use together is contraindicated. If urgent treatment with either of these drugs is needed, stop desvenlafaxine immediately; then administer linezolid or methylene blue. Watch for signs and symptoms of serotonin syndrome for 7 days or until 24 hours after last dose of linezolid or methylene blue. Restart desvenlafaxine 24 hours after last dose of linezolid or methylene blue.

MAO inhibitors: May cause serotonin syndrome or signs and symptoms resembling neuroleptic malignant syndrome. Avoid using within 7 days of MAO inhibitor therapy.

Midazolam, other drugs metabolized by CYP3A4: May decrease levels of these drugs. Use together cautiously.

SSNRIs, SSRIs: May increase risk of serotonin syndrome. Monitor patient closely if used together.

Venlafaxine: Drug is a major active metabolite of venlafaxine. Avoid using together.

Drug-lifestyle. *Alcohol use:* May enhance CNS depression. Discourage use together.

EFFECTS ON LAB TEST RESULTS

• May increase total cholesterol, LDL, triglyceride, and sodium levels.
• May cause false-positive test for phencyclidine (PCP) and amphetamines.

CONTRAINDICATIONS & CAUTIONS

• Contraindicated in patients hypersensitive to drug or within 14 days of MAO inhibitor therapy.

❶ **Alert:** Concomitant use with linezolid or methylene blue can cause serotonin syndrome (fever, mental status changes, muscle twitching, excessive sweating, shivering or shaking, diarrhea, loss of coordination). Use with linezolid or methylene blue is contraindicated. Stop drug when linezolid or methylene blue is started and restart 24 hours after last dose of linezolid or methylene blue.

• Use cautiously in elderly patients and in patients with renal impairment, diseases or conditions that could affect hemodynamic responses or metabolism, and in those with a history of mania or seizures.

• Potentially life-threatening serotonin syndrome has been reported with desvenlafaxine alone, but particularly with concomitant use of other serotonergic drugs and with drugs that impair serotonin metabolism.

• Angle-closure glaucoma has occurred in patients with untreated anatomically narrow angles who have taken antidepressants.

• Drug may increase bleeding risk. Use with aspirin, NSAIDs, warfarin, or other anticoagulants may increase risk.

Black Box Warning Desvenlafaxine isn't approved for use in children. ∎

Dialyzable drug: No.

⚠ **Overdose S&S:** Headache, vomiting, agitation, dizziness, nausea, constipation, diarrhea, dry mouth, paresthesia, tachycardia, change in level of consciousness, mydriasis, seizures, ECG changes.

PREGNANCY-LACTATION-REPRODUCTION

• There are no adequate well-controlled studies in pregnant women. Use during pregnancy only if clearly needed and potential benefit justifies potential risk to the fetus.

• Drug appears in breast milk. Patient should discontinue breast-feeding or discontinue drug, taking into account importance of drug to the mother.

NURSING CONSIDERATIONS

Black Box Warning Closely monitor patient being treated for depression for signs and symptoms of clinical worsening and suicidal ideation, especially at the beginning of therapy and with dosage adjustments. Symptoms may include agitation, insomnia, anxiety, aggressiveness, or panic attacks. ∎

❶ **Alert:** If linezolid or methylene blue must be given, stop drug and monitor the patient for serotonin toxicity for 7 days, or until 24 hours after the last dose of methylene blue or linezolid, whichever comes first. Treatment may be resumed 24 hours after last dose of methylene blue or linezolid.

• Carefully monitor BP. Drug may cause dose-related increases in BP.

Reactions in bold italics are *life-threatening*. Interactions may have a *rapid onset* or a *delayed onset*.

- Monitor IOP in patients at risk for angle-closure glaucoma.
- Record mood changes. Monitor patient for suicidal tendencies and allow patient only a minimum supply of the drug.
- Monitor patient for signs and symptoms of bleeding.
- Monitor lipid and sodium levels before and during therapy.
- **Alert:** Don't stop drug abruptly. Withdrawal or discontinuation syndrome may occur if drug is stopped abruptly. Signs and symptoms of withdrawal syndrome include dizziness, nausea, headache, irritability, insomnia, diarrhea, anxiety, fatigue, abnormal dreams, and hyperhidrosis. Taper drug slowly.
- Monitor respiratory status. Drug may cause interstitial lung disease or eosinophilic pneumonia. If patient develops dyspnea, cough, or chest discomfort, discontinue drug.
- Monitor patient for signs and symptoms of serotonin syndrome, including mental status changes, autonomic instability, neuromuscular symptoms, seizures, and GI symptoms.

PATIENT TEACHING
- Advise a woman of childbearing potential to contact prescriber if she becomes pregnant, intends to become pregnant during therapy, or is breast-feeding.
- **Black Box Warning** Warn family members to closely monitor patient for signs and symptoms of worsening condition or suicidal ideation. ▪
- **Alert:** Teach patient to recognize and immediately report symptoms of serotonin toxicity (fever, mental status changes, muscle twitching, excessive sweating, shivering or shaking, diarrhea, loss of coordination).
- Tell patient to avoid alcohol and to consult prescriber before taking other prescription or OTC drugs.
- Teach patient to report all adverse reactions, including abnormal bleeding.
- Warn patient to avoid hazardous activities that require alertness and good coordination until effects of drug are known.
- If medication is to be stopped, tell patient to stop drug gradually by tapering the dosage as instructed by prescriber and not to abruptly stop taking drug.
- Tell patient not to divide, crush, chew, or dissolve tablets.

dexamethasone (ophthalmic)
dex-a-METH-a-sone

Maxidex, Ozurdex

dexamethasone sodium phosphate

Therapeutic class: Anti-inflammatory drugs (ophthalmic)
Pharmacologic class: Corticosteroids

AVAILABLE FORMS
dexamethasone
Intraocular implant: 0.7 mg
Ophthalmic suspension: 0.1%
dexamethasone sodium phosphate
Ophthalmic solution: 0.1%

INDICATIONS & DOSAGES
➤ **Uveitis; iridocyclitis; inflammatory conditions of eyelids, conjunctiva, cornea, and anterior segment of globe; corneal injury from chemical or thermal burns or penetration of foreign bodies; allergic conjunctivitis; suppression of graft rejection after keratoplasty; acne rosacea**
Adults and children: Initially, 1 or 2 drops of solution into conjunctival sac every hour during the day and every 2 hours during the night. Decrease to 1 drop every 4 hours when favorable response is noted. As condition improves, taper to 1 drop t.i.d. or q.i.d. to control symptoms, then to b.i.d., then once daily. Treatment may extend from a few days to several weeks. Or, give 1 or 2 drops of suspension in the conjunctival sac up to six times daily. In severe disease, drops may be used hourly, being tapered to discontinuation as inflammation subsides.
➤ **Macular edema; posterior-segment uveitis; diabetic macular edema**
Adults: 1 implant (0.7 mg) injected intravitreally into each affected eye.

ADMINISTRATION
Ophthalmic
• Shake suspension well before use.
• Apply light finger pressure on lacrimal sac for 1 minute after instillation.
• Implant should be injected under controlled aseptic conditions, with adequate anesthesia and administration of a broad-spectrum microbicide.

ACTION
Suppresses edema, fibrin deposition, capillary dilation, leukocyte migration, capillary proliferation, and collagen deposition.

Route	Onset	Peak	Duration
Ophthalmic	Unknown	Unknown	Unknown

Half-life: Unknown.

ADVERSE REACTIONS
(Implant)
CNS: headache.
CV: hypertension.
EENT: burning, stinging, or red eyes; cataracts, vitreous detachment, vitreous opacity, corneal erosion, conjunctival hemorrhage, defects in visual acuity and visual field, retinal aneurysm, retinal tear, eyelid ptosis, dry eyes, foreign body sensation, increased IOP, keratitis, ocular pain.
Respiratory: bronchitis.
(Solution)
EENT: burning eye sensation, decreased visual acuity, visual field defect, eye perforation, filtering blebs, glaucoma, secondary ocular infection.

INTERACTIONS
Drug-drug. *NSAIDs (ophthalmic):* May increase toxic effects of ophthalmic corticosteroids. Monitor therapy.

EFFECTS ON LAB TEST RESULTS
None reported.

CONTRAINDICATIONS & CAUTIONS
• Contraindicated in patients hypersensitive to drug or its components. Some products contain sulfite.
• Contraindicated in patients with ocular TB or acute superficial HSV infection (dendritic keratitis), vaccinia, varicella, or other fungal or viral diseases of cornea and conjunctiva; in patients with acute, purulent, untreated infections of eye; and in those who have had uncomplicated removal of superficial corneal foreign body. Ocular implant is also contraindicated in patients with advanced glaucoma.
• Use cautiously in patients with corneal abrasions that may be infected (especially with herpes).
• Use cautiously in patients with glaucoma (any form) because IOP may increase. Dosage of glaucoma drugs may need to be increased to compensate.
❸ *Alert:* Intravitreal implant is contraindicated in patients with glaucoma who have cup-to-disc ratios greater than 0.8 and in patients with torn or ruptured posterior lens capsule, except pseudophakic patients after laser posterior capsulotomy.
❸ *Alert:* Corticosteroids aren't recommended in patients with a history of ocular HSV infection because of the potential risk of reactivation of the viral infection.
Dialyzable drug: Unknown.

PREGNANCY-LACTATION-REPRODUCTION
• There are no adequate well-controlled studies in pregnant women. Use during pregnancy only if potential benefit justifies potential risk to the fetus.
• It isn't known if topical administration of corticosteroids results in systemic absorption sufficient to produce detectable quantities in breast milk. Patient should discontinue breast-feeding or discontinue drug, taking into account importance of drug to the mother.

NURSING CONSIDERATIONS
• Drug isn't for long-term use.
• Watch for corneal ulceration, which may require stopping drug.
• Corneal viral and fungal infections may be worsened by corticosteroid application.
• After injection of implant, monitor patient for elevated IOP and endophthalmitis.
• *Look alike–sound alike:* Don't confuse dexamethasone with desoximetasone. Don't confuse Maxidex with Maxzide.

PATIENT TEACHING
• Tell patient to shake suspension well before use.

Reactions in bold italics are *life-threatening*. Interactions may have a *rapid onset* or a *delayed onset*.

• Teach patient how to instill drops. Advise him to wash hands before and after applying solution, and warn him not to touch tip of dropper to eye or surrounding tissue.
• Tell patient to apply light finger pressure on lacrimal sac for 1 minute after instillation.
• Warn patient not to use leftover drug for new eye inflammation; doing so may cause serious problems.
🕄 *Alert:* Warn patient to call prescriber immediately and to stop drug if visual acuity changes or visual field diminishes.
• Tell patient not to share drug, washcloths, or towels with family members and to notify prescriber if anyone develops same signs or symptoms.
• Stress importance of compliance with recommended therapy.
• Tell patient who wears soft contact lenses to remove them before instillation and to wait at least 15 minutes after instillation to reapply them.
• Advise patient who wears hard contact lenses to check with prescriber before using the same lenses again.

dexamethasone (oral)
dex-a-METH-a-sone

Dexamethasone Intensol*

dexamethasone sodium phosphate injection

Therapeutic class: Corticosteroids
Pharmacologic class: Glucocorticoids

AVAILABLE FORMS
dexamethasone
Elixir: 0.5 mg/5 mL*
Oral concentrate: 1 mg/mL
Oral solution: 0.5 mg/5 mL
Tablets: 0.5 mg, 0.75 mg, 1 mg, 1.5 mg, 2 mg, 4 mg, 6 mg
dexamethasone sodium phosphate
Injection: 4 mg/mL, 10 mg/mL

INDICATIONS & DOSAGES
➤ **Cerebral edema**
Adults: Initially, 10 mg phosphate I.V.; then 4 mg I.M. every 6 hours until symptoms

subside (usually 2 to 4 days); then taper over 5 to 7 days. Oral therapy (1 to 3 mg t.i.d.) should replace I.M. dosing as soon as possible.
➤ **Palliative management of recurrent or inoperable brain tumors**
Adults: 2 mg I.M. or I.V. b.i.d. to t.i.d. for maintenance therapy.
➤ **Inflammatory conditions, neoplasias**
Adults: 0.75 to 9 mg/day P.O. or 0.5 to 9 mg/day phosphate I.M., depending on size and location of affected area.
➤ **Acute, self-limited allergic disorders; acute exacerbations of chronic allergic disorders**
Adults: On day one, give 4 or 8 mg I.M. (using 4 mg/mL preparation). On days two and three, give four 0.75-mg tablets P.O. in two divided doses. On day four, give two 0.75-mg tablets P.O. in two divided doses. On days five and six, give one 0.75-mg tablet P.O. A follow-up visit should take place on day eight.
➤ **Shock**
Adults: 20 mg phosphate I.V. as single first dose; then 3 mg/kg/24 hours via continuous I.V. infusion. Or, 1 to 6 mg/kg phosphate I.V. as single dose. Or, 40 mg phosphate I.V. every 2 to 6 hours, as needed, continued only until patient is stabilized (usually not longer than 48 to 72 hours).
➤ **Dexamethasone suppression test for Cushing syndrome**
Adults: Determine baseline 24-hour urine levels of 17-hydroxycorticosteroids; then, give 0.5 mg P.O. every 6 hours for 48 hours. Repeat 24-hour urine collection to determine 17-hydroxycorticosteroid excretion during second 24 hours of dexamethasone administration. Or, 1 mg P.O. as single dose at 11:00 p.m. with determination of plasma cortisol at 8 a.m. the next morning.
➤ **Adrenocortical insufficiency**
Children: 0.02 to 0.3 mg/kg or 0.6 to 9 mg/m^2 P.O. daily, in three or four divided doses.
➤ **Tuberculous meningitis**
Adults: 8 to 12 mg phosphate I.M. daily; taper over 6 to 8 weeks.
➤ **Acute exacerbation of MS**
Adults: 30 mg P.O. daily for 1 week, followed by 4 to 12 mg every other day for 1 month.

➤ **Adjunctive therapy for short-term administration in synovitis of osteoarthritis, RA, bursitis, acute gouty arthritis, epicondylitis, acute nonspecific tenosynovitis, posttraumatic osteoarthritis; lesions (keloids; localized, hypertrophic, infiltrated, inflammatory lesions of lichen planus, psoriatic plaques, granuloma annulare, or lichen simplex chronicus; discoid lupus erythematosus; necrobiosis lipoidica diabeticorum; alopecia areata; cystic tumors of an aponeurosis or tendon [ganglia])**

Adults: 0.2 to 6 mg intra-articular or intralesional injection ranging from one single injection to injection every 3 to 5 days to once every 2 to 3 weeks. Dosage and frequency of injection vary depending on condition and site of injection.

ADMINISTRATION
P.O.
● Give oral dose with food when possible. Patient may need measures to prevent GI irritation.

I.V.
▼ For direct injection, inject undiluted over at least 1 minute (doses 10 mg or less).
▼ For intermittent or continuous infusion, dilute solution according to manufacturer's instructions and give over prescribed duration.
▼ During continuous infusion, change solution every 24 hours.
▼ **Incompatibilities:** Ciprofloxacin, daunorubicin, diphenhydramine, doxapram, doxorubicin, glycopyrrolate, idarubicin, midazolam, vancomycin.

I.M.
● Give I.M. injection deep into gluteal muscle. Rotate injection sites to prevent muscle atrophy. Avoid subcutaneous injection because atrophy and sterile abscesses may occur.

Intra-articular, intralesional
● Frequent intra-articular injection may damage joint tissues.

ACTION
Unclear. Decreases inflammation, mainly by stabilizing leukocyte lysosomal membranes; suppresses immune response; stimulates bone marrow; and influences protein, fat, and carbohydrate metabolism.

Route	Onset	Peak	Duration
P.O.	1–2 hr	1–2 hr	2½ days
I.V.	1 hr	1 hr	Variable
I.M.	1 hr	1 hr	6 days
Intra-articular, intralesional	Unknown	Unknown	Unknown

Half-life: About 1 to 2 days.

ADVERSE REACTIONS
CNS: euphoria, insomnia, psychotic behavior, *pseudotumor cerebri,* vertigo, headache, paresthesia, *seizures,* depression.
CV: *HF,* hypertension, edema, *arrhythmias,* thrombophlebitis, *thromboembolism.*
EENT: cataracts, glaucoma.
GI: peptic ulceration, GI irritation, increased appetite, *pancreatitis,* nausea, vomiting.
GU: menstrual irregularities, increased urine glucose and calcium levels.
Metabolic: *hypokalemia,* hyperglycemia, carbohydrate intolerance, hypercholesterolemia, *hypocalcemia,* sodium retention, weight gain.
Musculoskeletal: growth suppression in children, muscle weakness, osteoporosis, tendon rupture, myopathy.
Skin: hirsutism, delayed wound healing, acne, various skin eruptions, atrophy at I.M. injection site, thin fragile skin.
Other: cushingoid state, susceptibility to infections, acute adrenal insufficiency after increased stress or abrupt withdrawal after long-term therapy, *angioedema.*
After abrupt withdrawal: rebound inflammation, fatigue, weakness, arthralgia, fever, dizziness, lethargy, fainting, orthostatic hypotension, dyspnea, anorexia, *hypoglycemia. After prolonged use, sudden withdrawal may be fatal.*

INTERACTIONS
Drug-drug. *Aminoglutethimide:* May cause loss of dexamethasone-induced adrenal suppression. Use together cautiously.
Antidiabetics, including insulin: May decrease response. May need dosage adjustment.

Reactions in bold italics are *life-threatening.* Interactions may have a *rapid onset* or a *delayed onset.*

Aspirin, indomethacin, other NSAIDs: May increase risk of GI distress and bleeding. Use together cautiously.

Barbiturates, carbamazepine, phenytoin, rifampin: May decrease corticosteroid effect. Increase corticosteroid dosage.

Cardiac glycosides: May increase risk of arrhythmia resulting from hypokalemia. May need dosage adjustment.

Cyclosporine: May increase toxicity. Monitor patient closely.

Oral anticoagulants: May alter dosage requirements. Monitor PT and INR closely.

Potassium-depleting drugs such as thiazide diuretics: May enhance potassium-wasting effects of dexamethasone. Monitor potassium level.

Salicylates: May decrease salicylate level. Monitor patient for lack of salicylate effectiveness.

Skin-test antigens: May decrease response. Postpone skin testing until therapy is completed.

Toxoids, vaccines: May decrease antibody response and may increase risk of neurologic complications. Avoid using together.

Drug-lifestyle. *Alcohol use:* May increase risk of gastric irritation and GI ulceration. Discourage use together.

EFFECTS ON LAB TEST RESULTS

• May increase cholesterol and glucose levels. May decrease calcium, potassium, T_3 and T_4 levels.

• May decrease ^{131}I uptake and protein-bound iodine levels in thyroid function tests.

• May cause false-negative results in nitro blue tetrazolium test for systemic bacterial infections. May alter reactions to skin tests.

CONTRAINDICATIONS & CAUTIONS

• Contraindicated in patients hypersensitive to drug or its ingredients, in those with systemic fungal infections, and in those receiving immunosuppressive doses together with live-virus vaccines. I.M. administration is contraindicated in patients with ITP.

• Use with caution in patient with recent MI.

• Use cautiously in patients with GI ulcer, renal disease, hypertension, osteoporosis, diabetes mellitus, hypothyroidism, cirrhosis, diverticulitis, nonspecific ulcerative colitis, recent intestinal anastomoses, thromboembolic disorders, seizures, myasthenia gravis, HF, TB, active hepatitis, ocular HSV infection, emotional instability, or psychotic tendencies.

• Because some forms contain sulfite preservatives, also use cautiously in patients sensitive to sulfites.

D

Dialyzable drug: No.

PREGNANCY-LACTATION-REPRODUCTION

• Use in pregnant women only if potential benefit justifies potential risk to the fetus. When systemic corticosteroids are needed during pregnancy, it's generally recommended to use lowest effective dose for shortest duration of time, avoiding high doses during first trimester.

• Drug appears in breast milk. Patient should discontinue breast-feeding or discontinue drug, taking into account importance of drug to the mother.

• Advise patient exposed to dexamethasone during pregnancy for autoimmune disease treatment to contact the OTIS Autoimmune Diseases in Pregnancy Study at 1-877-311-8972.

NURSING CONSIDERATIONS

⚠ *Alert:* Epidural corticosteroid injections to treat neck and back pain and radiating pain in the arms and legs may result in rare but serious adverse events (vision loss, stroke, paralysis, death). The use of epidural corticosteroid injections isn't approved by the FDA.

• Most adverse reactions to corticosteroids are dose- or duration-dependent.

• For better results and less toxicity, give once-daily dose in morning.

• Always adjust to lowest effective dose.

• Monitor patient's weight, BP, and electrolyte levels.

• Monitor patient for cushingoid effects, including moon face, buffalo hump, central obesity, thinning hair, hypertension, and increased susceptibility to infection.

• Watch for depression or psychotic episodes, especially in high-dose therapy.

• Diabetic patient may need increased insulin; monitor glucose levels.

• Drug may mask or worsen infections, including latent amebiasis.

- Elderly patients may be more susceptible to osteoporosis with long-term use.
- Inspect patient's skin for petechiae.
- Gradually reduce dosage after long-term therapy.
- *Look alike–sound alike:* Don't confuse dexamethasone with desoximetasone.

PATIENT TEACHING
- Instruct patient to take drug with food or milk.

🌓 *Alert:* Counsel patient receiving epidural corticosteroid injections to seek immediate medical attention for loss of vision or vision changes; tingling in the arms or legs; sudden weakness or numbness of the face, arm, or leg on one or both sides of the body; dizziness; severe headache; or seizures.

- Tell patient not to stop drug abruptly or without prescriber's consent.
- Teach patient signs and symptoms of early adrenal insufficiency: fatigue, muscle weakness, joint pain, fever, anorexia, nausea, shortness of breath, dizziness, and fainting.
- Instruct patient to carry medical identification indicating his need for supplemental systemic glucocorticoids during stress, especially when dosage is decreased. This card should contain prescriber's name, drug name, and dosage of drug.
- Warn patient on long-term therapy about cushingoid effects (moon face, buffalo hump) and the need to notify prescriber about sudden weight gain or swelling.
- Warn patient about easy bruising.
- Advise patient receiving long-term therapy to consider exercise or physical therapy. Tell him to ask prescriber about vitamin D or calcium supplement.
- Instruct patient receiving long-term therapy to have periodic eye examinations.
- Advise patient to avoid exposure to infections (such as measles and chickenpox) and to notify prescriber if such exposure occurs.
- Tell patient to avoid alcohol.

🌓 *Alert:* Counsel patient that, before undergoing epidural corticosteroid injection, to discuss benefits and risks along with other possible treatments with health care provider.

dexlansoprazole
decks-lan-SOH-prah-zole

Dexilant✎, Dexilant Solutab

Therapeutic class: Antiulcer drugs
Pharmacologic class: PPIs

AVAILABLE FORMS
Capsules ⬛: 30 mg, 60 mg
Delayed-release ODTs ⬛: 30 mg

INDICATIONS & DOSAGES
➤ **Healing of erosive esophagitis**
Adults: Initially, 60-mg capsule P.O. once daily for up to 8 weeks.
Adjust-a-dose: For patients with moderate hepatic impairment (Child-Pugh class B), maximum dose is 30-mg capsule or ODT P.O. daily for up to 8 weeks.
➤ **Maintenance of healed erosive esophagitis; heartburn relief**
Adults: One 30-mg capsule or ODT P.O. once daily for up to 6 months.
➤ **Symptomatic nonerosive GERD**
Adults: 30-mg capsule or ODT P.O. once daily for 4 weeks.

ADMINISTRATION
P.O.
🌓 *Alert:* Two 30-mg ODTs aren't interchangeable with one 60-mg capsule.
- Give capsule with or without food.
- Patient should swallow capsules whole. Or, capsules can be opened and the intact granules sprinkled on 1 tablespoon of applesauce and swallowed immediately. Or, give capsules or ODTs with water via oral syringe or NG tube.
- If a dose is missed, give as soon as possible. Don't give missed dose if next scheduled dose is due; give the next dose on time. Don't give two doses at one time.
- Make sure patient takes the ODT at least 30 minutes before a meal.
- Have patient place the ODT on the tongue, allow it to disintegrate, and swallow the microgranules without water; make sure patient doesn't chew the microgranules. Or, have patient swallow the ODT whole with water.

ACTION
Inhibits proton pump activity by binding to hydrogen–potassium adenosine triphosphatase, located at the secretory surface of the gastric parietal cells, to suppress gastric acid secretion.

Route	Onset	Peak	Duration
P.O.	Unknown	4 hr	Unknown

Half-life: 1 to 2 hours.

ADVERSE REACTIONS
GI: abdominal discomfort, abdominal tenderness, diarrhea, flatulence, nausea, vomiting.
Respiratory: URI.

INTERACTIONS
Drug-drug. *Atazanavir, nelfinavir:* May decrease antiviral effect and promote development of drug resistance. Don't use together.
Azole antifungals (itraconazole, ketoconazole): May decrease antifungal level. Avoid concomitant use if possible. If concomitant use is necessary, have patient take antifungal with an acidic beverage (cola) to increase absorption.
Clopidogrel: May reduce clopidogrel's plasma concentration and clinical effect. Avoid use together.
Drugs with pH-dependent absorption (ampicillin, digoxin, ketoconazole, iron): May decrease absorption of these drugs. Use together cautiously.
Fluvoxamine: May increase dexlansoprazole level. Monitor patient for dexlansoprazole-related adverse reactions.
Methotrexate: May increase methotrexate toxicity, especially with high doses. Consider discontinuing dexlansoprazole.
Rifampin: May decrease dexlansoprazole exposure. Avoid concomitant use.
Saquinavir: May increase saquinavir toxicity. Monitor for potential toxicity.
Warfarin: May increase INR and the risk of bleeding. Monitor patient closely.
Drug-herb. *St. John's wort:* May decrease dexlansoprazole exposure. Avoid concomitant use.
Drug-lifestyle. *Alcohol use:* May alter release rate of drug from ODT, possibly leading to decreased efficacy. Avoid use together.

EFFECTS ON LAB TEST RESULTS
● May increase alkaline phosphatase, ALT, and AST levels. May increase creatinine, gastrin, protein, glucose, and potassium levels.
● May increase or decrease bilirubin level. May decrease magnesium level.
● May decrease platelet count.
● May alter secretin stimulation test result.
● May cause false-positive urine drug screen for tetrahydrocannabinol (THC).

CONTRAINDICATIONS & CAUTIONS
● Contraindicated in patients hypersensitive to drug or its components and with rilpivirine-containing products.
❸ Alert: There may be an increased risk of hip, wrist, and spine fractures associated with PPIs.
● Use cautiously in patients with suspected gastric malignancy. Response to treatment doesn't eliminate the possibility of malignancy.
● Prolonged treatment (2 years or more) can lead to vitamin B_{12} malabsorption and deficiency, especially in women and those younger than age 30.
● May increase risk of GI infections.
● Acute interstitial nephritis has been observed in patients taking PPIs, may occur at any point during therapy, and is generally attributed to an idiopathic hypersensitivity reaction. Discontinue drug if acute interstitial nephritis develops.
● Drug isn't recommended in patients with severe hepatic impairment (Child-Pugh class C).
● Safety and effectiveness in children haven't been established.
Dialyzable drug: No.

PREGNANCY-LACTATION-REPRODUCTION
● There are no adequate well-controlled studies in pregnant women. Use during pregnancy only if clearly needed.
● It isn't known if drug appears in breast milk. Patient should discontinue breastfeeding or discontinue drug, taking into account importance of drug to the mother.

NURSING CONSIDERATIONS

● Monitor patient periodically for improvement in the signs and symptoms of GERD and erosive esophagitis to assess success of therapy.

● Monitor LFT results and glucose and electrolyte levels periodically during therapy.

● Monitor patient for bleeding during therapy.

● May cause false-positive results in diagnostic investigations for neuroendocrine tumors. Temporarily stop drug at least 14 days before assessing serum chromogranin A (CgA) levels and consider repeating test if initial CgA levels are high. If serial tests are performed (for example, for monitoring), use the same commercial laboratory for testing, as reference ranges among tests may vary.

◐ **Alert:** Prolonged use of PPIs may cause low magnesium levels. Monitor magnesium levels before starting treatment and periodically thereafter.

◐ **Alert:** Monitor patient for symptoms of low magnesium, such as abnormal HR or rhythm, palpitations, muscle spasms, tremor, or seizures. In children, abnormal HR may present as fatigue, upset stomach, dizziness, and light-headedness. Magnesium supplementation or drug discontinuation may be required.

◐ **Alert:** Drug may cause CDAD. Evaluate for CDAD in patients who develop diarrhea that doesn't improve.

PATIENT TEACHING

● Tell patient to report hypersensitivity reactions immediately.

● Tell patient to swallow capsule whole and not to crush, split, or chew it. Capsule may also be opened and its contents sprinkled on applesauce if desired.

● Advise patient that drug can be taken without regard to meals.

● Advise female patient to notify prescriber if she is pregnant, plans to become pregnant, or is breast-feeding.

● Tell patient to report all adverse reactions, including diarrhea.

● Teach patient to recognize and report signs and symptoms of low magnesium level.

● Advise patient to avoid alcohol use when taking ODT.

dexmethylphenidate hydrochloride
decks-meth-ill-FEN-i-date

Focalin, Focalin XR✦

Therapeutic class: CNS stimulants
Pharmacologic class: Methylphenidate derivatives
Controlled substance schedule: II

AVAILABLE FORMS

Capsules (extended-release) ⓞⓝⓖ: 5 mg, 10 mg, 15 mg, 20 mg, 25 mg, 30 mg, 35 mg, 40 mg
Tablets: 2.5 mg, 5 mg, 10 mg

INDICATIONS & DOSAGES

➤ **ADHD**

Immediate-release tablets
Adults and children age 6 and older:
For patients who aren't now taking methylphenidate, initially, 2.5 mg P.O. b.i.d., given at least 4 hours apart. Increase weekly by 2.5 to 5 mg daily, up to a maximum of 20 mg daily in divided doses.

For patients who are now taking methylphenidate, initially give half the current methylphenidate dosage, up to a maximum of 20 mg P.O. daily in divided doses.

Extended-release capsules
Adults: For patients who aren't now taking dexmethylphenidate or methylphenidate, or who are on stimulants other than methylphenidate, give 10 mg P.O. once daily in the morning. May adjust in weekly increments of 10 mg to a maximum dose of 40 mg daily.

For patients who are now taking methylphenidate, initially give half the total daily dose of methylphenidate. Patients who are now taking the immediate-release form of dexmethylphenidate may be switched to the same daily dose of extended-release form. Maximum daily dose is 40 mg.

Children age 6 and older: For patients who aren't now taking dexmethylphenidate or methylphenidate, or who are on stimulants

other than methylphenidate, give 2.5 mg
P.O. b.i.d. May adjust in weekly increments
of 5 mg to a maximum daily dose of 30 mg.

For patients who are now taking
methylphenidate, initially give half the total
daily dose of methylphenidate. Patients who
are now taking the immediate-release form
of dexmethylphenidate may be switched
to the same daily dose of extended-release
form. Maximum daily dose is 30 mg.

ADMINISTRATION
P.O.
● Capsules may be swallowed whole with
or without food or the contents sprinkled
on a small amount of applesauce and eaten
immediately.
● Don't crush or divide the capsule or its
contents.

ACTION
Blocks presynaptic reuptake of norepinephrine and dopamine and increases their
release, increasing concentration in the
synapse.

Route	Onset	Peak	Duration
P.O. (immediate-release)	Unknown	1–1½ hr	Unknown
P.O. (extended-release)	Unknown	1–4 hr; 4½–7 hr	Unknown

Half-life: 2 to 3 hours.

ADVERSE REACTIONS
CNS: headache, anxiety, feeling jittery,
nervousness, insomnia, fever, dizziness.
CV: tachycardia.
GI: anorexia, abdominal pain, nausea,
dyspepsia, dry mouth, decreased appetite,
vomiting.
Musculoskeletal: twitching (motor or
vocal tics).
Other: hypersensitivity reactions.

INTERACTIONS
Drug-drug. *Antacids, acid suppressants:*
May alter the release of extended-release
form. Avoid using together.
*Anticoagulants, phenobarbital, phenytoin,
primidone, TCAs:* May inhibit metabolism
of these drugs. May need to decrease dosage
of these drugs; monitor drug levels.

Antihypertensives: May decrease effectiveness of these drugs. Use together cautiously;
monitor BP.
*Clonidine, other centrally acting alpha
agonists:* May cause serious adverse effects.
Use together cautiously.
MAO inhibitors: May increase risk of hypertensive crisis. Using together within
14 days of MAO inhibitor therapy is contraindicated.

EFFECTS ON LAB TEST RESULTS
None reported.

CONTRAINDICATIONS & CAUTIONS
● Contraindicated in patients hypersensitive
to methylphenidate or other components.
● Contraindicated in patients with severe
anxiety, tension, or agitation; glaucoma;
motor tics; a family history or diagnosis of
Tourette syndrome; or within 14 days of
MAO inhibitor therapy.
🔆 **Alert:** Contraindicated in patients with
serious heart problems.
Black Box Warning Use cautiously in patients with a history of substance abuse,
including alcoholism. Chronic abuse can
lead to marked tolerance and psychological
dependence. Psychotic episodes can occur.
Withdraw patient carefully from abusive
use because severe depression can occur.
Withdrawal after long-term use may unmask signs and symptoms of an underlying
disorder that may require follow-up. ■
● Use cautiously in patients with a psychiatric illness, bipolar disorder, depression,
or family history of suicide, and in patients
with seizures, hypertension, hyperthyroidism, HF, stroke, or recent MI.
Dialyzable drug: Unknown.
⚠ **Overdose S&S:** Agitation, cardiac arrhythmias, confusion, seizures, delirium,
dryness of mucous membranes, euphoria,
flushing, hallucinations, headache, hyperpyrexia, hyperreflexia, hypertension, muscle
twitching, mydriasis, palpitations, sweating,
tachycardia, tremors, vomiting.

PREGNANCY-LACTATION-REPRODUCTION
● There are no adequate well-controlled
studies in pregnant women. Use during
pregnancy only if clearly needed and

potential benefit justifies potential risk to the fetus.

• It isn't known if drug appears in breast milk. Use cautiously in breast-feeding women.

NURSING CONSIDERATIONS

• Diagnosis of ADHD must be based on complete history and evaluation of the patient by psychological and educational experts.

• Obtain a detailed patient history, including a family history for mental disorders, family suicide, ventricular arrhythmias, or sudden death.

• Refer patient for psychological, educational, and social support.

• Periodically reevaluate the long-term usefulness of the drug.

• Monitor CBC and differential and platelet counts during prolonged therapy.

• Don't use for severe depression or normal fatigue states.

• Stop treatment or reduce dosage if symptoms worsen or adverse reactions occur.

• Long-term stimulant use may temporarily suppress growth. Monitor children for growth and weight gain. If growth slows or weight gain is lower than expected, stop drug.

⟐ Alert: Periodically monitor patient for changes in HR or BP. Promptly evaluate patients with chest pain, unexplained syncope, or other signs or symptoms of cardiac disease.

• Monitor patient for signs of drug dependence or abuse.

• If seizures occur, stop drug.

• **Look alike–sound alike:** Don't confuse dexmethylphenidate with methadone.

PATIENT TEACHING

• Stress the importance of taking the correct dose of drug at the same time every day. Report accidental overdose immediately.

⟐ Alert: Warn patient that the misuse of amphetamines can have serious effects, including sudden death.

• Advise patient unable to swallow capsules to empty the contents of the capsule onto a spoonful of applesauce and eat immediately.

⟐ Alert: Tell patient not to cut, crush, or chew the contents of the extended-release beaded capsule.

• Advise parents to monitor child for medication abuse or sharing. Also inform parents to watch for increased aggression or hostility and to report worsening behavior.

⟐ Alert: Instruct patient to immediately report chest pain, shortness of breath, or fainting.

• Advise parents to monitor child's height and weight and to tell the prescriber if they suspect growth is slowing.

• Caution patient to expect blurred vision or difficulty with accommodation and to exercise caution while performing activities that require a clear visual field. Advise patient to report blurred vision to the prescriber.

dextroamphetamine sulfate
dex-troe-am-FET-a-meen

Dexedrine, Procentra, Zenzedi

Therapeutic class: CNS stimulants
Pharmacologic class: Amphetamines
Controlled substance schedule: II

AVAILABLE FORMS
Capsules (extended-release) **ONC***:* 5 mg, 10 mg, 15 mg
Oral solution: 5 mg/5 mL
Tablets: 2.5 mg, 5 mg, 7.5 mg, 10 mg, 15 mg, 20 mg, 30 mg

INDICATIONS & DOSAGES
➤ **Narcolepsy**
Adults: 5 to 60 mg P.O. daily in divided doses.
Children age 12 and older: 10 mg P.O. daily. Increase by 10 mg at weekly intervals, as needed. Give first dose on awakening; give additional doses (one or two) at intervals of 4 to 6 hours.
Children ages 6 to 12: 5 mg P.O. daily. Increase by 5 mg at weekly intervals as needed.
➤ **ADHD**
Children age 6 and older: 5 mg P.O. once daily or b.i.d. Increase by 5 mg at weekly intervals, as needed. It's rarely necessary to exceed 40 mg/day.

ADMINISTRATION
P.O.
• Avoid late-evening doses, particularly with extended-release capsules, due to resulting insomnia.
• Certain formulations may contain tartrazine (immediate-release tablets) or benzoic acid, which is a derivative of benzyl alcohol (oral solution). Derivatives of benzyl alcohol are associated with potentially fatal "gasping syndrome" in neonates.
• Make sure patient doesn't chew or crush extended-release capsules.

ACTION
Unknown. Probably promotes nerve impulse transmission by releasing stored dopamine and norepinephrine from nerve terminals in the brain. Main sites of activity appear to be the cerebral cortex and the reticular activating system.

Route	Onset	Peak	Duration
P.O.	Unknown	3 hr	4–6 hr
P.O. (extended-release)	Unknown	8 hr	8 hr

Half-life: 10 to 12 hours.

ADVERSE REACTIONS
CNS: insomnia, nervousness, restlessness, tremor, dizziness, headache, chills, overstimulation, dysphoria, euphoria, dyskinesia.
CV: tachycardia, palpitations, *arrhythmias,* hypertension.
GI: dry mouth, taste perversion, diarrhea, constipation, anorexia, other GI disturbances.
GU: erectile dysfunction.
Metabolic: weight loss.
Musculoskeletal: *rhabdomyolysis.*
Skin: urticaria.
Other: increased libido.

INTERACTIONS
Drug-drug. *Acetazolamide, alkalizing drugs, antacids, sodium bicarbonate:* May increase renal reabsorption. Monitor patient for enhanced amphetamine effects.
Acidifying drugs, ammonium chloride, ascorbic acid: May decrease level and increase renal clearance of dextroam-

phetamine. Monitor patient for decreased amphetamine effects.
Adrenergic blockers: May inhibit adrenergic blocking effects. Avoid using together.
Antihypertensives: May diminish antihypertensive effects. Monitor BP.
Chlorpromazine, lithium: May inhibit central stimulant effects of amphetamines. Chlorpromazine may be used to treat amphetamine poisoning.
Insulin, oral antidiabetics: May decrease antidiabetic requirements. Monitor glucose level.
MAO inhibitors: May cause severe hypertension or hypertensive crisis. Avoid using within 14 days of MAO inhibitor therapy.
Meperidine: May potentiate analgesic effect. Use together cautiously.
Methenamine: May increase urinary excretion of amphetamines and reduce effectiveness. Monitor drug effects.
Norepinephrine: May enhance adrenergic effect of norepinephrine. Monitor patient.
Phenobarbital, phenytoin: May delay absorption of these drugs. Monitor patient closely.
Drug-food. *Acidic foods, fruit juice:* Decreases amphetamine absorption. May decrease effectiveness of oral solution. Avoid giving together.
Caffeine: May increase amphetamine and related amine effects. Urge caution.

EFFECTS ON LAB TEST RESULTS
• May increase corticosteroid level.

CONTRAINDICATIONS & CAUTIONS
• Contraindicated in patients hypersensitive to or with idiosyncratic reactions to sympathomimetic amines and in those with hyperthyroidism, moderate to severe hypertension, symptomatic CV disease, glaucoma, advanced arteriosclerosis, and history of drug abuse. Also contraindicated during or within 14 days after MAO inhibitor therapy.
⚠ *Alert:* Use cautiously in agitated patients and patients with motor tics, phonic tics, or Tourette syndrome. Also use cautiously in patients whose underlying condition may be worsened by an increase in BP or HR (preexisting hypertension, HF, recent MI); patients with a psychiatric illness, bipolar

disorder, depression, or family history of suicide; and those with a seizure disorder.
• Don't use in children or adolescents with structural cardiac abnormalities or other serious heart problems.
Dialyzable drug: Unknown.
⚠ *Overdose S&S:* Assaultiveness, confusion, hallucinations, hyperreflexia, rapid respiration, restlessness, rhabdomyolysis, tremor, hyperpyrexia, panic states, fatigue, depression, arrhythmias, hypertension, hypotension, circulatory collapse, nausea, vomiting, diarrhea, abdominal cramps, seizures, coma.

PREGNANCY-LACTATION-REPRODUCTION
• There are no adequate well-controlled studies in pregnant women. Use during pregnancy only if potential benefit justifies potential risk to the fetus.
• Drug appears in breast milk. Use in breast-feeding women isn't recommended.

NURSING CONSIDERATIONS
• Obtain a detailed patient history, including a family history for mental disorders, family suicide, ventricular arrhythmias, or sudden death.
• Monitor patients beginning treatment for ADHD for aggressive behavior or hostility.
• Drug shouldn't be used to prevent fatigue.
Black Box Warning Drug has a high abuse potential and may cause dependence. Monitor patient closely. Pay particular attention to the possibility of patients obtaining amphetamines for nontherapeutic use or distribution to others. ∎
◑ *Alert:* Periodically monitor patient for changes in HR or BP.
• Monitor for growth retardation in children.
• Don't crush extended-release capsules.
• *Look alike–sound alike:* Don't confuse Dexedrine with dextran or Excedrin.

PATIENT TEACHING
Black Box Warning Warn patient that the misuse of amphetamines can cause serious CV adverse events, including sudden death. ∎
• Tell patient not to chew or crush extended-release capsules.

◑ *Alert:* Instruct patient to immediately report chest pain, shortness of breath, or fainting.
• Warn patient to avoid activities that require alertness, a clear visual field, or good coordination until CNS effects of drug are known.
• Tell patient he may get tired as drug effects wear off.
• Ask patient to report signs and symptoms of excessive stimulation.
• Inform parents that children may show increased aggression or hostility and to report worsening of behavior.
• Advise patient to consume caffeine-containing products cautiously.
• Tell patient not to drink fruit juice at same time as oral solution.
• Warn patient with a seizure disorder that drug may decrease seizure threshold. Instruct him to notify prescriber if seizures occur.

dextroamphetamine sulfate–dextroamphetamine saccharate–amphetamine aspartate–amphetamine sulfate
dex-tro-am-PHET-ta-meen/
am-PHET-ta-meen

Adderall XR

Therapeutic class: CNS stimulants
Pharmacologic class: Amphetamines
Controlled substance schedule: II

AVAILABLE FORMS
Capsules (extended-release) ⓞⓝⓒ: 5 mg: 1.25 mg dextroamphetamine sulfate, 1.25 mg dextroamphetamine saccharate, 1.25 mg amphetamine aspartate, and 1.25 mg amphetamine sulfate; 10 mg: 2.5 mg dextroamphetamine sulfate, 2.5 mg dextroamphetamine saccharate, 2.5 mg amphetamine aspartate, and 2.5 mg amphetamine sulfate; 15 mg: 3.75 mg dextroamphetamine sulfate, 3.75 mg dextroamphetamine saccharate, 3.75 mg amphetamine aspartate, and 3.75 mg amphetamine sulfate; 20 mg: 5 mg dextroamphetamine sulfate, 5 mg

dextroamphetamine saccharate, 5 mg amphetamine aspartate, and 5 mg amphetamine sulfate; 25 mg: 6.25 mg dextroamphetamine sulfate, 6.25 mg dextroamphetamine saccharate, 6.25 mg amphetamine aspartate, and 6.25 mg amphetamine sulfate; 30 mg: 7.5 mg dextroamphetamine sulfate, 7.5 mg dextroamphetamine saccharate, 7.5 mg amphetamine aspartate, and 7.5 mg amphetamine sulfate.

Tablets: 5 mg: 1.25 mg dextroamphetamine sulfate, 1.25 mg dextroamphetamine saccharate, 1.25 mg amphetamine aspartate, and 1.25 mg amphetamine sulfate; 7.5 mg: 1.875 mg dextroamphetamine sulfate, 1.875 mg dextroamphetamine saccharate, 1.875 mg amphetamine aspartate, and 1.875 mg amphetamine sulfate; 10 mg: 2.5 mg dextroamphetamine sulfate, 2.5 mg dextroamphetamine saccharate, 2.5 mg amphetamine aspartate, and 2.5 mg amphetamine sulfate; 12.5 mg: 3.125 mg dextroamphetamine sulfate, 3.125 mg dextroamphetamine saccharate, 3.125 mg amphetamine aspartate, and 3.125 mg amphetamine sulfate; 15 mg: 3.75 mg dextroamphetamine sulfate, 3.75 mg dextroamphetamine saccharate, 3.75 mg amphetamine aspartate, and 3.75 mg amphetamine sulfate; 20 mg: 5 mg dextroamphetamine sulfate, 5 mg dextroamphetamine saccharate, 5 mg amphetamine aspartate, and 5 mg amphetamine sulfate; 30 mg: 7.5 mg dextroamphetamine sulfate, 7.5 mg dextroamphetamine saccharate, 7.5 mg amphetamine aspartate, and 7.5 mg amphetamine sulfate.

INDICATIONS & DOSAGES
➤ **Narcolepsy**

Adults and children age 12 and older: Initially, 10 mg (immediate-release) tablet P.O. daily. May increase daily dose by 10 mg at weekly intervals to maximum of 60 mg/day. Give first dose on awakening, then one or two additional doses at intervals of 4 to 6 hours.

Children ages 6 to younger than 12: Initially, 5 mg (immediate-release) tablet P.O. daily. May increase daily dose by 5 mg at weekly intervals until optimal response is achieved. Give first dose on awakening,

then one or two additional doses at intervals of 4 to 6 hours.

Adjust-a-dose: For adverse reactions (insomnia or anorexia), reduce dosage.

➤ **ADHD**

Adults: Initially, 5 mg (immediate-release) tablet P.O. once daily or b.i.d. May increase daily dose by 5 mg at weekly intervals until optimal response achieved; maximum dose, 40 mg/day. Or, 20-mg extended-release capsule P.O. once daily in morning. Maximum dose, 30 mg/day.

Adolescents ages 13 to 17 (extended-release): Initially, 10 mg P.O. daily in morning. May increase to 20 mg/day after 1 week if symptoms aren't controlled.

Children age 6 and older (immediate-release): Initially, 5 mg P.O. once daily or b.i.d. May increase daily dose by 5 mg at weekly intervals until optimal response is achieved. Rarely necessary to exceed a total of 40 mg/day.

Children ages 6 to 12 (extended-release): Initially, 5 to 10 mg P.O. once daily in morning. May increase daily dose by 5 or 10 mg at weekly intervals. Maximum dose, 30 mg/day.

Children ages 3 to 5 (immediate-release): Initially, 2.5 mg P.O. daily. May increase daily dose by 2.5 mg at weekly intervals until optimal response is achieved.

ADMINISTRATION
P.O.
● May give with or without food.
● Give first dose upon awakening to avoid insomnia.
● Make sure patient takes extended-release capsules whole, or open the capsules and sprinkle entire contents on applesauce and have patient consume immediately without chewing.

ACTION
Unknown. Thought to block reuptake of norepinephrine and dopamine into presynaptic neuron and increase release of same neurotransmitters into extraneuronal space.

Route	Onset	Peak	Duration
P.O. (immediate-release)	Unknown	3 hr	Unknown
P.O. (extended-release)	Unknown	7 hr	Unknown

Half-life: Immediate release, 9 to 14 hours; extended release, 10 to 14 hours.

ADVERSE REACTIONS

CNS: headache, insomnia, agitation, anxiety, dizziness, drowsiness, emotional lability, fatigue, speech disturbance, twitching, fever.
CV: systolic hypertension, palpitations, tachycardia.
EENT: dry mouth, teeth clenching, tooth infection.
GI: abdominal pain, decreased appetite, anorexia, constipation, diarrhea, dyspepsia, nausea, vomiting.
GU: decreased libido, erectile dysfunction, UTI.
Metabolic: weight loss.
Respiratory: dyspnea.
Skin: diaphoresis, skin photosensitivity.
Other: infection.

INTERACTIONS

Drug-drug. *Acetazolamide, thiazides:* May increase amphetamine concentration through decreased urine excretion. Monitor patient response.
Adrenergic blockers, antihistamines, antihypertensives, ethosuximide, phenobarbital, phenytoin: Amphetamines may reduce therapeutic effects of these drugs. Monitor patient response.
Antacids, MAO inhibitors, sodium bicarbonate: May increase amphetamine concentrations and risk of adverse reactions. Avoid concurrent use, and don't give drug within 14 days of MAO inhibitors.
Chlorpromazine, lithium carbonate: May reduce therapeutic effects of amphetamines. Monitor patient response.
Ammonium chloride, ascorbic acid, glutamic acid, guanethidine, methenamine, reserpine, sodium acid phosphate: May lower amphetamine blood level and absorption. Don't use together.
Meperidine, norepinephrine, TCAs: Amphetamines may increase effects of these drugs and risk of adverse reactions related to these drugs. Monitor patient response.
PPIs: May increase amphetamine absorption rate. Monitor therapy.
Drug-herb. *Ephedra:* May cause hypertension or arrhythmias. Don't use together.
Drug-lifestyle. *Alcohol use:* May increase risk of drug dependency. Avoid use together. Concurrent use is contraindicated in patients with a history of ethanol or drug dependency.
Caffeine: May alter amphetamine level. Avoid concurrent use.

EFFECTS ON LAB TEST RESULTS
• May increase plasma corticosteroid level.
• May interfere with urinary steroid testing.

CONTRAINDICATIONS & CAUTIONS
Black Box Warning Amphetamines have a high potential for abuse. Administration of amphetamines for prolonged periods of time may lead to drug dependence and must be avoided. Particular attention should be paid to the possibility of persons obtaining amphetamines for nontherapeutic use or distribution to others, and the drugs should be prescribed or dispensed sparingly. ■
Black Box Warning Misuse of amphetamines may cause sudden death and serious CV adverse events. ■
• Contraindicated in patients with advanced arteriosclerosis, symptomatic CV disease, moderate to severe hypertension, hyperthyroidism, known hypersensitivity or idiosyncrasy to sympathomimetic amines, glaucoma, agitated states, or history of drug abuse. Also contraindicated during or within 14 days after administration of MAO inhibitors.
❶ **Alert:** Sudden death has been reported at usual doses in patients with structural cardiac abnormalities and other serious heart problems. Stimulants generally should not be used in adults, children, or adolescents with structural cardiac abnormalities, cardiomyopathy, serious heart rhythm abnormalities, or other serious cardiac problems.
• Drug can increase BP. Use cautiously in patients with underlying medical conditions (preexisting hypertension, HF, recent MI, ventricular arrhythmia) that might be compromised by increases in BP or HR.

● Use cautiously in patients with a history of seizures, tics or Tourette syndrome, or mental problems, including psychosis, bipolar illness, mania, or depression.

● Drug may cause peripheral vasculopathy, including Raynaud phenomenon, which may improve after dosage reduction or drug discontinuation.

● Drug hasn't been studied in elderly patients.

● Immediate-release tablets aren't recommended for children with ADHD younger than age 3 or for children with narcolepsy younger than age 6. Use of extended-release capsules in children younger than age 6 hasn't been studied.

Dialyzable drug: Unknown.

⚠ **Overdose S&S:** Restlessness, tremor, hyperreflexia, rapid respiration, confusion, assaultiveness, hallucinations, panic states, hyperpyrexia, rhabdomyolysis; fatigue, depression (usually follow the central stimulation); arrhythmias, hypertension or hypotension, circulatory collapse; nausea, vomiting, diarrhea, abdominal cramps; seizures, coma (usually precede fatal poisoning).

PREGNANCY-LACTATION-REPRODUCTION

● There are no adequate well-controlled studies in pregnant women. Infants born to mothers dependent on amphetamines have an increased risk of premature delivery and low birth weight. These infants may also experience signs and symptoms of withdrawal, such as dysphoria, including agitation, and significant lassitude. Use during pregnancy only if potential benefit justifies potential risk to the fetus.

● Drug appears in breast milk. Breast-feeding women shouldn't use drug.

NURSING CONSIDERATIONS

● Administer drug upon awakening to prevent insomnia.

● Interrupt therapy occasionally to assess if behavioral symptoms warrant continued therapy.

● Perform a careful history and physical examination in all patients to assess for the presence of cardiac disease. Further cardiac evaluation may be needed. All patients who develop cardiac signs and symptoms (chest pain, syncope) during therapy should have a prompt cardiac evaluation.

● Evaluate patient for dependence on other prescription drugs, illicit drugs, or alcohol before start of therapy.

● Monitor BP during therapy.

● Screen patient for a family history of suicide, bipolar disorder, and depression before use. Monitor patient for increased aggression, worsening of existing psychiatric signs and symptoms, or psychosis.

● When used long term, drug may slow growth rate in children. Monitor growth rate; interrupt treatment for children not growing or gaining weight as expected.

● Monitor patient for risk of vasculopathies, including Raynaud phenomenon, and evaluate unexplained wounds on fingers and toes.

● Single doses of 20 mg extended-release capsules and 10 mg immediate-release tablets given b.i.d. (4 hours apart) have been shown to produce comparable plasma amphetamine concentrations.

● **Look alike–sound alike:** Don't confuse Adderall XR with Inderal.

PATIENT TEACHING

● Tell patient to report all drugs and supplements being taken before start of therapy, especially if patient has taken an MAO inhibitor within the past 2 weeks.

● Explain that serious cardiac effects are possible during therapy. Advise patient to immediately report chest pain, shortness of breath, or fainting.

● Advise patient to report development of such conditions as glaucoma, high BP, or hyperthyroidism.

● Advise patient to keep regular follow-up appointments for monitoring of HR and BP, and for growth checks in children.

● Advise patient to report worsening of psychiatric signs and symptoms or behavioral changes during therapy.

● Explain that drug may cause circulatory problems. Advise patient to immediately report unexplained wounds on fingers or toes.

● Instruct patient to take drug in early part of day (preferably upon awakening) to avoid insomnia.

● Advise patient to swallow capsules and tablets whole, but that extended-release capsules can be opened, the contents sprinkled on applesauce, and then the applesauce swallowed immediately without chewing.

diazepam
dye-AZ-e-pam

Diastat*, Diastat Acudial, Diazepam Intensol*, Valium✔

Therapeutic class: Anxiolytics
Pharmacologic class: Benzodiazepines
Controlled substance schedule: IV

AVAILABLE FORMS
Injection: 5 mg/mL
Oral solution: 5 mg/5 mL, 5 mg/mL*
Rectal gel twin packs:* 2.5 mg (pediatric); 10 mg, 20 mg (adult)
Tablets: 2 mg, 5 mg, 10 mg

INDICATIONS & DOSAGES
Adjust-a-dose (for all indications): For elderly or debilitated patients, give 2 to 2.5 mg P.O. daily or b.i.d. initially; increase gradually as needed and tolerated. Or, when using injection, use lower doses (2 to 5 mg) and increase dosage more gradually.
➤ **Anxiety**
Adults: Depending on severity, 2 to 10 mg P.O. b.i.d. to q.i.d. Or, 2 to 10 mg I.M. or I.V. May repeat in 3 to 4 hours if needed.
Children age 6 months and older: 1 to 2.5 mg P.O. t.i.d. or q.i.d., increased gradually, as needed and tolerated.
Elderly patients: Initially, 2 to 2.5 mg P.O. once daily or b.i.d.; increase gradually.
➤ **Acute alcohol withdrawal**
Adults: 10 mg P.O. t.i.d. or q.i.d. during first 24 hours; reduce to 5 mg P.O. t.i.d. or q.i.d., p.r.n. Or, 10 mg I.V. or I.M. initially; then 5 to 10 mg I.V. or I.M. again in 3 to 4 hours if needed.
➤ **Before endoscopic procedures**
Adults: Adjust I.V. dose to desired sedative response (up to 20 mg). Or, 5 to 10 mg I.M. 30 minutes before procedure.
➤ **Muscle spasm**
Adults: 2 to 10 mg P.O. b.i.d. to q.i.d. as an adjunct. Or, 5 to 10 mg I.V. or I.M. initially; then 5 to 10 mg I.V. or I.M. again in 3 to 4 hours if needed.

Children: 0.04 to 0.2 mg/kg/dose I.V. slowly every 2 to 4 hours; don't exceed 0.6 mg/kg within an 8-hour period.
➤ **Preoperative sedation**
Adults: 10 mg I.M. or I.V. before surgery.
➤ **Cardioversion**
Adults: 5 to 15 mg I.V. within 5 to 10 minutes before procedure.
➤ **Adjunctive treatment for seizure disorders**
Adults: 2 to 10 mg P.O. b.i.d. to q.i.d.
Children age 6 months and older: 1 to 2.5 mg P.O. t.i.d. or q.i.d. initially; increase as needed and as tolerated.
➤ **Status epilepticus, severe recurrent seizures**
Adults: 5 to 10 mg I.V. or I.M. initially. Use I.M. route only if I.V. access is unavailable. Repeat every 10 to 15 minutes, p.r.n., up to maximum dose of 30 mg. Repeat every 2 to 4 hours, if needed.
Children age 5 and older: 1 mg I.V. every 2 to 5 minutes up to maximum of 10 mg. Repeat in 2 to 4 hours if needed.
Children ages 1 month to 5 years: 0.2 to 0.5 mg I.V. slowly every 2 to 5 minutes up to maximum of 5 mg.
➤ **Patients on stable regimens of antiepileptic drugs who need diazepam intermittently to control bouts of increased seizure activity**
Adults and children age 12 and older: 0.2 mg/kg P.R., rounding up to the nearest available dose form. A second dose may be given 4 to 12 hours later.
Children ages 6 to 11: 0.3 mg/kg P.R., rounding up to the nearest available dose form. A second dose may be given 4 to 12 hours later.
Children ages 2 to 5: 0.5 mg/kg P.R., rounding up to the nearest available dose form. A second dose may be given 4 to 12 hours later.
➤ **Tetanus**
Adults: Initially, 5 to 10 mg I.V. or I.M. then 5 to 10 mg in 3 to 4 hours if needed. Larger doses may be required.
Children age 5 and older: 5 to 10 mg I.M. or I.V. repeated every 3 to 4 hours, p.r.n.
Children ages 1 month to younger than 5 years: 1 to 2 mg I.M. or I.V. slowly repeated every 3 to 4 hours, p.r.n.

Reactions in bold italics are *life-threatening*. Interactions may have a *rapid onset* or a *delayed onset*.

ADMINISTRATION
P.O.
● When using oral solution, dilute dose just before giving with liquid or semisolid food, such as water, juices, soda or sodalike beverages, applesauce, or pudding.

I.V.
▼ Keep emergency resuscitation equipment and oxygen at bedside.

▼ For adults, give at no more than 5 mg/minute.

▼ For children, administer slowly over 3 minutes. Don't exceed 0.25 mg/kg.

▼ Avoid infusion sets or containers made from polyvinyl chloride.

▼ If possible, inject directly into a large vein. If not, inject slowly through infusion tubing as near to the insertion site as possible. Watch closely for phlebitis at injection site.

▼ Monitor respirations every 5 to 15 minutes and before each dose.

▼ Don't store parenteral solution in plastic syringes.

▼ **Incompatibilities:** All other I.V. drugs, most I.V. solutions.

I.M.
● Use the I.M. route if I.V. administration is impossible.

● Use Diastat rectal gel to treat no more than five episodes per month and no more than one episode every 5 days because tolerance may develop.

🕲 *Alert:* Only caregivers who can distinguish the distinct cluster of seizures or events from the patient's ordinary seizure activity, who have been instructed and can give the treatment competently, who understand which seizures may be treated with Diastat, and who can monitor the clinical response and recognize when immediate professional medical evaluation is needed should give Diastat rectal gel.

ACTION
A benzodiazepine that probably potentiates the effects of GABA, depresses the CNS, and suppresses the spread of seizure activity.

Route	Onset	Peak	Duration
P.O.	30 min	¼–2½ hr	20–80 hr
I.V.	1–5 min	1–5 min	15–60 min
I.M.	Unknown	1 hr	Unknown
P.R.	Unknown	90 min	Unknown

Half-life: About 1 to 12 days. Varies with route and patient age.

ADVERSE REACTIONS
CNS: drowsiness, dysarthria, slurred speech, tremor, transient amnesia, fatigue, ataxia, headache, insomnia, paradoxical anxiety, hallucinations, minor changes in EEG patterns, pain, vertigo, confusion, depression.
CV: *CV collapse, bradycardia,* hypotension.
EENT: diplopia, blurred vision, nystagmus.
GI: nausea, constipation, diarrhea with rectal form, dry mouth.
GU: incontinence, urine retention.
Hematologic: *neutropenia.*
Hepatic: jaundice.
Respiratory: *respiratory depression, apnea,* hiccups.
Skin: rash, phlebitis at injection site.
Other: altered libido, physical or psychological dependence.

INTERACTIONS
Drug-drug. *Cimetidine, disulfiram, fluoxetine, fluvoxamine, hormonal contraceptives, isoniazid, metoprolol, propranolol, valproic acid:* May decrease clearance of diazepam and increase risk of adverse effects. Monitor patient for excessive sedation and impaired psychomotor function.
CNS depressants: May increase CNS depression. Use together cautiously.
Digoxin: May increase digoxin level and risk of toxicity. Monitor patient and digoxin level closely.
Diltiazem: May increase CNS depression and prolong effects of diazepam. Reduce dose of diazepam.
Fluconazole, itraconazole, ketoconazole, miconazole: May increase and prolong diazepam level, CNS depression, and psychomotor impairment. Avoid using together.
Levodopa: May decrease levodopa effectiveness. Monitor patient.
Black Box Warning *Opioids:* May cause slow or difficult breathing, sedation, and death. Avoid use together. If use together is

necessary, limit dosage and duration of each drug to the minium necessary for desired effect. ∎

Phenobarbital: May increase effects of both drugs. Use together cautiously.

Drug-herb. *Kava:* May increase sedation. Discourage use together.

Drug-lifestyle. *Alcohol use:* May cause additive CNS effects. Discourage use together. *Smoking:* May decrease effectiveness of drug. Monitor patient closely.

EFFECTS ON LAB TEST RESULTS
• May increase LFT values.
• May decrease neutrophil count.

CONTRAINDICATIONS & CAUTIONS
Black Box Warning Opioid drugs should only be prescribed with benzodiazepines or other CNS depressants to patients for whom alternative treatment options are inadequate. ∎
• Contraindicated in patients hypersensitive to drug and in infants younger than age 6 months (oral form).
• Diazepam (oral form) is contraindicated in patients with myasthenia gravis, severe respiratory insufficiency, severe hepatic insufficiency, or sleep apnea syndrome.
• Diazepam is contraindicated in patients with acute angle-closure glaucoma.
• Use cautiously in patients experiencing shock, coma, or acute alcohol intoxication (parenteral form).
• Use cautiously in elderly and debilitated patients and in patients with hepatic or renal impairment, depression, history of substance abuse, impaired gag reflex, or chronic open-angle glaucoma (who are receiving appropriate therapy) and in those at risk for falls.
• Some injectable forms may contain propylene glycol; large amounts are potentially toxic and have been associated with hyperosmolality, lactic acidosis, seizures, and respiratory depression.

Dialyzable drug: No.

⚠ Overdose S&S: Somnolence, confusion, coma, diminished reflexes.

PREGNANCY-LACTATION-REPRODUCTION
• Use during pregnancy isn't recommended, especially during first and third trimesters. If drug is needed during pregnancy, use only if potential benefit justifies potential risk to the fetus.
• Neonatal flaccidity, respiratory and feeding difficulties, hypothermia, and withdrawal symptoms have been reported in infants born to mothers who received benzodiazepines late in pregnancy.
• Drug appears in breast milk. Use in breast-feeding women isn't recommended.

NURSING CONSIDERATIONS
• Monitor periodic LFTs and renal and hematopoietic function studies in patients receiving repeated or prolonged therapy.
• Monitor elderly patients for dizziness, ataxia, and mental status changes. Patients are at an increased risk for falls.
◑ Alert: Use of drug may lead to abuse and addiction. Don't withdraw drug abruptly after long-term use; withdrawal symptoms may occur.
• **Look alike–sound alike:** Don't confuse diazepam with diazoxide or Ditropan. Don't confuse Valium with Valcyte.

PATIENT TEACHING
Black Box Warning Caution the patient or the caregiver of a patient taking an opioid drug with a benzodiazepine, CNS depressant, or alcohol to seek immediate medical attention if the patient has symptoms of dizziness, light-headedness, extreme sleepiness, slowed or difficult breathing, or unresponsiveness. ∎
• Warn patient to report all adverse reactions and to avoid activities that require alertness and good coordination until effects of drug are known.
• Tell patient to avoid alcohol while taking drug.
• Notify patient that smoking may decrease drug's effectiveness.
• Warn patient not to abruptly stop drug because withdrawal symptoms may occur.
• Advise female patient to avoid use during pregnancy; inform her of the potential hazard to the fetus if drug is used during pregnancy or if patient becomes pregnant while taking drug.
• Instruct patient's caregiver on the proper use of Diastat rectal gel.

Reactions in bold italics are *life-threatening*. Interactions may have a *rapid onset* or a *delayed onset*.

D

diclofenac (oral)
dye-KLOE-fen-ak

Zorvolex

diclofenac potassium
Apo-Diclo Rapide✦, Cambia, Cataflam, Voltaren Rapide✦, Zipsor

diclofenac sodium (oral)
Apo-Diclo✦, Voltaren SR✦

Therapeutic class: NSAIDs
Pharmacologic class: NSAIDs

AVAILABLE FORMS
diclofenac
Capsules: 18 mg, 35 mg
diclofenac potassium
Capsules: 25 mg*
Powder for solution: 50 mg/packet
Tablets: 50 mg
diclofenac sodium
Tablets (delayed-release) ⓞⓝⓒ*:* 25 mg, 50 mg, 75 mg
Tablets (extended-release) ⓞⓝⓒ*:* 100 mg

INDICATIONS & DOSAGES
Adjust-a-dose (for all indications): Patients with hepatic impairment may require lower initial dosages. Discontinue immediately if hepatic impairment occurs during therapy, including persistent or worsening abnormal LFT values, clinical signs or symptoms consistent with liver disease, or systemic manifestations of liver disease. Use Cambia in patients with hepatic impairment only if benefits outweigh risks. Initiate treatment with Zorvolex at the lowest dosage; if efficacy isn't achieved with the lowest dosage, discontinue drug.

➤ **Ankylosing spondylitis**
Adults: 25 mg delayed-release diclofenac sodium P.O. q.i.d.; may add another 25-mg dose at bedtime.
➤ **Osteoarthritis**
Adults: 50 mg P.O. b.i.d. or t.i.d., or 75 mg diclofenac potassium or delayed-release diclofenac sodium P.O. b.i.d. Or 35 mg Zorvolex P.O. t.i.d. Or, 100 mg extended-release diclofenac sodium P.O. daily.

➤ **RA**
Adults: 50 mg P.O. t.i.d. or q.i.d., or 75 mg diclofenac potassium or delayed-release diclofenac sodium P.O. b.i.d. Or, 100 mg extended-release diclofenac sodium P.O. daily or b.i.d.
➤ **Analgesia**
Adults: 50 mg diclofenac potassium P.O. t.i.d. For some patients, the first dose on the first day may be 100 mg, followed by 50 mg for the second and third doses; maximum dose for first day is 200 mg. Don't exceed 150 mg daily after the first day. Or, 25 mg Zipsor P.O. q.i.d. or 18 or 35 mg Zorvolex P.O. t.i.d.
➤ **Primary dysmenorrhea**
Adults: 50 mg diclofenac potassium P.O. t.i.d. For some patients, the first dose on the first day may be 100 mg, followed by 50 mg for the second and third doses; maximum dose for first day is 200 mg. Don't exceed 150 mg daily after the first day.
➤ **Migraine**
Adults: 50 mg (1 packet) P.O. as a single dose.

ADMINISTRATION
P.O.
● Give drug with milk, meals, or antacids.
● Don't crush or break delayed- or extended-release tablets.
● Mix powder in 30 to 60 mL water only. Use no other liquid.
● Mix solution well and have patient drink immediately.
● Powder (Cambia) and Zorvolex may be less effective if taken with food.
● Zorvolex capsules aren't interchangeable with other formulations of oral diclofenac even if the milligram strength is the same.

ACTION
May inhibit prostaglandin synthesis, to produce anti-inflammatory, analgesic, and antipyretic effects.

Route	Onset	Peak	Duration
P.O. (delayed-release)	30 min	2–3 hr	8 hr
P.O. (extended-release)	Unknown	5–6 hr	Unknown
P.O.	10 min	1 hr	8 hr

Half-life: 1 to 2 hours.

ADVERSE REACTIONS
CNS: anxiety, dizziness, drowsiness, headache, irritability.
CV: *HF,* edema, fluid retention, hypertension.
EENT: blurred vision, epistaxis, eye pain, night blindness, reversible hearing loss, swelling of the lips and tongue, tinnitus.
GI: abdominal distention, abdominal pain or cramps, *bleeding,* constipation, diarrhea, flatulence, indigestion, melena, nausea, peptic ulceration, taste disorder, bloody diarrhea, appetite change, colitis, vomiting.
GU: nephrotic syndrome, *acute renal failure,* fluid retention, interstitial nephritis, oliguria, papillary necrosis, proteinuria.
Hepatic: jaundice, *hepatitis, hepatotoxicity.*
Metabolic: *hypoglycemia,* hyperglycemia.
Musculoskeletal: back, leg, or joint pain.
Respiratory: *asthma, laryngeal edema.*
Skin: *Stevens-Johnson syndrome,* allergic purpura, alopecia, bullous eruption, dermatitis, eczema, photosensitivity reactions, pruritus, rash, urticaria.
Other: *anaphylactoid reactions, anaphylaxis, angioedema.*

INTERACTIONS
Drug-drug. *ACE inhibitors:* May enhance adverse or toxic effect of NSAIDs and result in a significant decrease in renal function. May diminish antihypertensive effect of ACE inhibitors. Monitor therapy.
Anticoagulants, antiplatelet agents, SNRIs, SSRIs, warfarin: May cause bleeding. Monitor patient closely.
Aspirin: May decrease effectiveness of diclofenac and increase GI toxicity. Avoid using together.
Beta blockers: May decrease antihypertensive effects. Monitor patient closely.
Cyclosporine, digoxin, lithium, methotrexate: May reduce renal clearance of these drugs and increase risk of toxicity. Monitor patient closely.
Diuretics: May decrease effectiveness of diuretics. Avoid using together.
Insulin, oral antidiabetics: May alter requirements for antidiabetics. Monitor patient closely.

Potassium-sparing diuretics: May enhance retention and increase level of potassium. Monitor potassium level.
Drug-herb. *Alfalfa, anise, bilberry:* May cause bleeding based on the known effects or components. Discourage use together.
White willow: May increase bleeding risk. Discourage use together.
Drug-lifestyle. *Sun exposure:* May cause photosensitivity reactions. Advise patient to avoid excessive sunlight exposure.

EFFECTS ON LAB TEST RESULTS
• May increase ALT, AST, bilirubin, BUN, and creatinine levels.
• May increase or decrease glucose level.

CONTRAINDICATIONS & CAUTIONS
Black Box Warning Contraindicated for the treatment of perioperative pain after CABG surgery. ■
• Contraindicated in patients hypersensitive to drug and in those with hepatic porphyria or history of asthma, urticaria, or other allergic reactions after taking aspirin or other NSAIDs. Zipsor is contraindicated in patients hypersensitive to bovine protein.
❸ Alert: NSAIDs can increase the risk of heart attack or stroke in patients with or without heart disease or risk factors for heart disease.
❸ Alert: The risk of heart attack or stroke can occur as early as the first weeks of NSAID use. Risk appears greater at higher doses. Use lowest effective dose for shortest duration possible.
❸ Alert: NSAIDs increase the risk of HF.
• Use cautiously in patients with history of peptic ulcer disease, hepatic dysfunction, cardiac disease, hypertension, fluid retention, or impaired renal function.
• Drug may cause photosensitivity as well as serious skin adverse events, including exfoliative dermatitis, Stevens-Johnson syndrome, and toxic epidermal necrolysis, which can be fatal. Discontinue at first sign of rash or hypersensitivity.
Dialyzable drug: Unknown.
⚠ Overdose S&S: Drowsiness, confusion, hypotonia, loss of consciousness, vomiting, aspiration, pneumonitis, increased ICP.

Reactions in bold italics are *life-threatening*. Interactions may have a *rapid onset* or a *delayed onset*.

PREGNANCY-LACTATION-REPRODUCTION

⊘ Alert: Drug can cause fetal harm when administered at 30 weeks' gestation or later. Use during pregnancy before 30 weeks' gestation only if potential benefit justifies potential risk to the fetus.

⊘ Alert: NSAIDs can cause premature closure of the ductus arteriosus. Avoid use during pregnancy, particularly late pregnancy.

● Drug may appear in breast milk. Patient should discontinue breast-feeding or discontinue drug, taking into account importance of drug to the mother.

NURSING CONSIDERATIONS

⊘ Alert: Monitor patient and immediately evaluate signs and symptoms of heart attack (chest pain, shortness of breath, trouble breathing) or stroke (weakness in one part or side of the body, slurred speech).

● Because NSAIDs impair the synthesis of renal prostaglandins, they can decrease renal blood flow and lead to reversible renal impairment, especially in patients with renal failure, HF, or liver dysfunction, in elderly patients, and in those taking diuretics. Monitor these patients closely.

● LFT values may increase during therapy. Monitor transaminase, especially ALT, levels periodically in patients undergoing long-term therapy. Make first transaminase measurement no later than 8 weeks after therapy begins.

Black Box Warning NSAIDs cause an increased risk of serious GI adverse events, including bleeding, ulceration, and perforation of the stomach or intestines, which can be fatal. Elderly patients are at greater risk. ∎

Black Box Warning NSAIDs may increase the risk of serious thrombotic events, MI, or stroke, which can be fatal. The risk may be greater with longer use or in patients with CV disease or risk factors for CV disease. ∎

⊘ Alert: Different formulations of oral diclofenac are not bioequivalent even if the milligram strength is the same.

● Because of their antipyretic and antiinflammatory actions, NSAIDs may mask the signs and symptoms of infection.

● Consider periodic CBC and chemistry profile monitoring with long-term NSAID treatment because serious GI bleeding, hepatotoxicity, and renal injury can occur without warning.

● **Look alike–sound alike:** Don't confuse diclofenac with Diflucan.

PATIENT TEACHING

● Tell patient to take tablets or capsules with milk, meals, or antacids to minimize GI distress; however, taking Cambia or Zorvolex with food may reduce its effectiveness.

● Instruct patient not to crush, break, or chew delayed- or extended-release tablets.

⊘ Alert: Advise patient to seek medical attention immediately if chest pain, shortness of breath or trouble breathing, weakness in one part or side of the body, or slurred speech occurs.

● Tell patient to mix powder form well in 30 to 60 mL of water only and to drink immediately.

● Advise patient not to take this drug with any other diclofenac-containing products (such as Arthrotec).

● Teach patient signs and symptoms of GI bleeding (blood in vomit, urine, or stool; coffee-ground vomit; black, tarry stools) and to notify prescriber immediately if any of these occur.

● Teach patient the signs and symptoms of damage to the liver, including nausea, fatigue, lethargy, itching, yellowed skin or eyes, right upper quadrant tenderness, and flulike symptoms. Tell patient to contact prescriber immediately if these symptoms occur.

● Advise patient to avoid drinking alcohol or taking aspirin during drug therapy.

● Tell patient to wear sunscreen or protective clothing because drug may cause sensitivity to sunlight.

● Warn patient to avoid hazardous activities that require alertness until it is known whether the drug causes CNS symptoms.

● Tell female patient who is pregnant to avoid use of drug during last trimester.

● Advise patient that use of OTC NSAIDs and diclofenac may increase risk of GI toxicity.

diclofenac epolamine
dye-KLOE-fen-ak

Flector

diclofenac sodium (topical)
Pennsaid, Solaraze, Voltaren

Therapeutic class: NSAIDs
Pharmacologic class: NSAIDs

AVAILABLE FORMS
Topical gel: 1%, 3%
Topical solution: 1.5%, 2%
Transdermal patch: 1.3%

INDICATIONS & DOSAGES
➤ **Actinic keratosis (Solaraze only)**
Adults: Apply gently to lesion b.i.d. for 60 to 90 days.
➤ **Osteoarthritis (Voltaren only)**
Adults: Apply 4 g of gel to affected foot, knee, or ankle q.i.d. Maximum dose of 16 g to any single joint of the lower extremities. Or apply 2 g of gel to affected hand, elbow, or wrist q.i.d. Maximum dose of 8 g to any single joint of the upper extremities. Total dose shouldn't exceed 32 g daily for all affected joints.
➤ **Acute pain due to minor strains, sprains, and contusions**
Adults: Apply 1 patch to most painful area b.i.d.
➤ **Osteoarthritis of the knee**
Adults: Count 10 drops at a time of 1.5% topical solution onto hand or directly onto knee. Apply to each side, front and back, spreading evenly, using a total of 40 drops q.i.d. Or, 2 pump actuations (40 mg) of 2% topical solution on each painful knee b.i.d. Dispense solution directly onto the knee or first into the hand and then onto the knee. Spread evenly around front, back, and sides of the knee.

ADMINISTRATION
Topical
• Apply to clean, dry skin.
• Don't apply to open wounds or broken skin.
• Avoid contact with eyes.

• Use enough gel to cover the lesion; for example, use 0.5 g of gel on a 5 × 5-cm lesion.
• Don't apply Flector patch to nonintact or damaged skin, including from exudative dermatitis, eczema, infected lesions, burns, or wounds.
• Patient shouldn't wear patch while bathing or showering.
• Measure gel using supplied dosing cards in package.
• Wear gloves to gently massage Voltaren into skin of entire joint.
• Wash hands after applying.
• Pump for 2% topical solution must be primed before first use. Depress pump four times while holding bottle upright; discard solution obtained during priming.

ACTION
Unknown. May produce anti-inflammatory and analgesic effects by ability to inhibit prostaglandin synthesis.

Route	Onset	Peak	Duration
Topical	Unknown	4–12 hr	Unknown
Transdermal	Unknown	10–20 hr	Unknown

Half-life: 1 to 3 hours; 12 hours for patch.

ADVERSE REACTIONS
CNS: paresthesia, headache, pain, asthenia, migraine, hypokinesia.
CV: chest pain, hypertension.
EENT: sinusitis, pharyngitis, rhinitis, conjunctivitis, eye pain.
GI: diarrhea, dyspepsia, abdominal pain.
GU: hematuria, renal impairment.
Hepatic: liver impairment.
Metabolic: hypercholesterolemia, hyperglycemia.
Musculoskeletal: arthralgia, arthrosis, back pain, myalgia, neck pain.
Respiratory: *asthma,* dyspnea, pneumonia.
Skin: reaction at application site, contact dermatitis, dry skin, exfoliation, localized pain, pruritus, rash, localized edema, acne, alopecia, photosensitivity reactions, skin ulcer.
Other: *anaphylaxis,* flulike syndrome, infection, allergic reaction.

INTERACTIONS
Drug-drug. *ACE inhibitors:* May enhance adverse or toxic effect of NSAIDs and result in a significant decrease in renal function. May diminish antihypertensive effect of ACE inhibitors. Monitor therapy.
Anticoagulants, antiplatelet agents, SNRIs, SSRIs, warfarin: May cause bleeding. Monitor patient closely.
Aspirin: May decrease effectiveness of diclofenac and increase GI toxicity. Avoid using together.
Beta blockers: May decrease antihypertensive effects. Monitor patient closely.
Cyclosporine, digoxin, lithium, methotrexate: May reduce renal clearance of these drugs and increase risk of toxicity. Monitor patient closely.
Diuretics: May decrease effectiveness of diuretics. Avoid using together.
Insulin, oral antidiabetics: May alter requirements for antidiabetics. Monitor patient closely.
Oral NSAIDs: May increase diclofenac effects. Minimize use together.
Potassium-sparing diuretics: May enhance retention and increase potassium level. Monitor potassium level.
Drug-lifestyle. *Sun exposure:* May increase risk of photosensitivity reactions. Advise patient to avoid excessive sun exposure.

EFFECTS ON LAB TEST RESULTS
• May increase ALT, AST, cholesterol, creatinine, glucose, and transaminase levels.

CONTRAINDICATIONS & CAUTIONS
• Contraindicated in patients hypersensitive to diclofenac, benzyl alcohol, polyethylene glycol monomethyl ether 350, or hyaluronic acid.
Black Box Warning Contraindicated for perioperative pain for CABG surgery. ∎
⊕ Alert: NSAIDs can increase risk of heart attack or stroke in patients with or without heart disease or risk factors for heart disease.
⊕ Alert: Risk of heart attack or stroke can occur as early as the first weeks of NSAID use. Risk appears greater at higher doses. Use lowest effective dose for shortest duration possible.
⊕ Alert: NSAIDs increase risk of HF.

• Use cautiously in patients with the aspirin triad; these patients are usually asthmatics who develop rhinitis, with or without nasal polyps, after taking aspirin or other NSAIDs.
• Use cautiously in patients with active GI bleeding or ulceration and in those with severe renal or hepatic impairment.
• May cause serious adverse skin events, including exfoliative dermatitis, Stevens-Johnson syndrome, and toxic epidermal necrolysis, which can be fatal. Discontinue use at first sign of rash or hypersensitivity.
Dialyzable drug: Unknown.

PREGNANCY-LACTATION-REPRODUCTION
⊕ Alert: Drug can cause fetal harm when administered at 30 weeks' gestation or later. Use during pregnancy before 30 weeks' gestation only if potential benefit justifies potential risk to the fetus.
• Drug may cause constriction of ductus arteriosus. Avoid use in late pregnancy.
• Drug may appear in breast milk. Patient should discontinue breast-feeding or discontinue drug, taking into account importance of drug to the mother.

NURSING CONSIDERATIONS
Black Box Warning NSAIDs may increase the risk of serious CV thrombotic events. The risk may increase with duration of use. Patients with CV disease or risk factors for CV disease may be at greater risk. ∎
Black Box Warning NSAIDs increase the risk of serious GI adverse reactions, including bleeding, ulceration, and perforation of the stomach or intestines, which can be fatal. These reactions can occur at any time and without warning. Elderly patients are at greater risk. ∎
⊕ Alert: Monitor patient and immediately evaluate signs and symptoms of heart attack (chest pain, shortness of breath, trouble breathing) or stroke (weakness in one part or side of the body, slurred speech).
• Avoid use in patients with recent MI unless benefits are expected to outweigh risk of recurrent CV thrombotic events. If used in patients with recent MI, watch for signs and symptoms of cardiac ischemia.
• Avoid use in patients with severe HF unless benefits are expected to outweigh risk

of worsening HF. If used in patients with severe HF, watch for signs and symptoms of worsening HF.

• Evaluate patient with signs or symptoms of liver dysfunction or with abnormal LFT results for development of more severe hepatic reaction while taking drug.

• If clinical signs or symptoms of liver disease develop, or if systemic manifestation (eosinophilia, rash) occurs, discontinue drug.

• Safety and effectiveness of sunscreens, cosmetics, or other topical medications used with drug are unknown.

• Complete healing or optimal therapeutic effect may not be seen until 30 days after therapy is complete.

• Reevaluate lesions that don't respond to therapy.

PATIENT TEACHING

• Inform patient about risk of skin reactions (rash, itchiness, pain, irritation) at the application site. Urge patient to seek medical attention if adverse reactions occur.

❸ *Alert:* Advise patient to seek medical attention immediately if chest pain, shortness of breath or trouble breathing, weakness in one part or side of the body, or slurred speech occurs.

• Instruct patient that pump solution must be primed (four pumps) before first use.

• Encourage patient to minimize sun exposure during therapy. Explain that sunscreen may be helpful but that the safety of using sunscreen with drug is unknown.

• Advise patient needing an MRI to inform the facility that he's wearing a transdermal patch.

• Tell patient using Solaraze that complete healing or optimal therapeutic effect may not occur for up to 30 days after stopping therapy.

• Caution patient not to apply gel to open wounds or broken skin.

• Instruct patient to avoid contact with eyes.

• Instruct patient not to apply other topical drugs or cosmetics to affected area while using drug, unless directed.

• Advise patient to use only on intact skin unless otherwise directed.

• Inform patient that if Flector patch begins to peel off, the edges may be taped

down. Instruct patient not to wear Flector patch during bathing or showering. Bathing should take place in between scheduled patch removal and application.

• Tell patient to wash his hands after applying gel unless the hands are the treated area and to wait at least 1 hour after application before washing hands.

• Instruct patient not to cover area with clothing for at least 10 minutes after applying gel and to wait at least 1 hour before showering or bathing.

• Tell female patient to notify prescriber if she is pregnant or breast-feeding.

---

dicyclomine hydrochloride
dye-SYE-kloe-meen

Bentyl, Bentylol✤, Protylol✤

Therapeutic class: Antispasmodics
Pharmacologic class: Anticholinergics–antimuscarinics

AVAILABLE FORMS
Capsules: 10 mg
Injection: 10 mg/mL
Syrup: 10 mg/5 mL
Tablets: 10 mg✤, 20 mg

INDICATIONS & DOSAGES
➤ **Irritable bowel syndrome, other functional GI disorders**
Adults: Initially, 20 mg P.O. q.i.d.; may increase to 40 mg P.O. q.i.d. after 1 week unless adverse effects limit dosage escalation. Or, 10 to 20 mg I.M. q.i.d. Don't use I.M. form for longer than 1 to 2 days.

ADMINISTRATION
P.O.
• Store in light-resistant container.
• Protect from excessive heat.
I.M.
❸ *Alert:* Don't give subcutaneously or I.V.
• Aspirate syringe before injecting to avoid I.V. injection; thrombosis and injection-site reaction may occur if drug is inadvertently injected I.V.
❸ *Alert:* Injection concentration is 10 mg/mL. Carefully calculate appropriate amount of solution for administering correct dose.

Reactions in bold italics are *life-threatening*. Interactions may have a *rapid onset* or a *delayed onset*.

ACTION

Inhibits action of acetylcholine on post-ganglionic, parasympathetic muscarinic receptors, decreasing GI motility. Drug possesses local anesthetic properties that may be partly responsible for spasmolysis.

Route	Onset	Peak	Duration
P.O., I.M.	Unknown	1–1½ hr	Unknown

Half-life: Initial, about 2 hours; secondary, 9 to 10 hours.

ADVERSE REACTIONS

CNS: asthenia, headache, dizziness, fever, insomnia, light-headedness, drowsiness, nervousness, confusion, excitement (in elderly patients), somnolence, tingling, dyskinesia, lethargy, weakness, numbness.
CV: palpitations, tachycardia.
EENT: blurred vision, increased IOP, mydriasis, photophobia, diplopia.
GI: constipation, dry mouth, thirst, vomiting, nausea, abdominal distention, heartburn, paralytic ileus.
GU: urinary hesitancy, urine retention, erectile dysfunction.
Skin: urticaria, decreased sweating or inability to sweat, local irritation, rash.
Other: allergic reactions, heat prostration.

INTERACTIONS

Drug-drug. *Amantadine, antihistamines, antiparkinsonians, disopyramide, glutethimide, meperidine, phenothiazines, procainamide, quinidine, TCAs:* May have additive adverse effects. Avoid using together.
Antacids: May interfere with dicyclomine absorption. Give dicyclomine at least 1 hour before antacid.
GI motility agents (metoclopramide): May decrease efficacy of motility agents. Monitor therapy.
Drug-lifestyle. *Alcohol use:* May cause additive sedative effects. Avoid use together.

EFFECTS ON LAB TEST RESULTS

None reported.

CONTRAINDICATIONS & CAUTIONS

• Contraindicated in patients hypersensitive to anticholinergics and in those with obstructive uropathy, obstructive disease of the GI tract, reflux esophagitis, severe ulcerative colitis, toxic megacolon, myasthenia gravis, unstable CV status in acute hemorrhage, tachycardia secondary to cardiac insufficiency or thyrotoxicosis, or glaucoma.
• Don't use in patients with myasthenia gravis except to reduce adverse muscarinic effects of an anticholinesterase.
• Use cautiously in patients with autonomic neuropathy, hyperthyroidism, CAD, arrhythmias, HF, hypertension, hiatal hernia, hepatic or renal disease, prostatic hyperplasia, known or suspected GI infection, and ulcerative colitis.
• Use cautiously in patients in hot or humid environments; drug can cause heatstroke.
• May affect GI absorption of various drugs by affecting GI motility (such as slowly dissolving dosage forms of digoxin), which may increase serum concentrations.
❶ *Alert:* Use cautiously in patients sensitive to anticholinergic drugs, especially elderly patients and those with mental illness, because of the risk of psychosis and delirium. When present, these signs and symptoms usually resolve within 12 to 24 hours after discontinuation of drug.
• Safety and effectiveness in children haven't been established. Contraindicated in children younger than age 6 months.
Dialyzable drug: Unknown.
⚠ *Overdose S&S:* Headache; nausea; vomiting; blurred vision; dilated pupils; hot, dry skin; dry mouth; dysphagia; CNS stimulation; muscle weakness; paralysis.

PREGNANCY-LACTATION-REPRODUCTION

• There are no adequate well-controlled studies in pregnant women. Use during pregnancy only if clearly needed.
• Drug appears in breast milk. Contraindicated in breast-feeding women.

NURSING CONSIDERATIONS

• Adjust dosage based on patient's needs and response. Dosages up to 40 mg P.O. q.i.d. have been used in adults, but safety and effectiveness for longer than 2 weeks haven't been established.
• Dicyclomine may have atropine-like adverse reactions.

◆ Alert: Overdose may cause curare-like effects, such as respiratory paralysis. Keep emergency equipment available.
• Monitor patient's vital signs and urine output carefully.
• **Look alike–sound alike:** Don't confuse dicyclomine with dyclonine or doxycycline. Don't confuse Bentyl with Benadryl.

PATIENT TEACHING
• Tell patient when to take drug, and stress importance of doing so on time and at evenly spaced intervals and to report all adverse reactions.
• Advise patient to avoid driving and other hazardous activities if drowsiness, dizziness, or blurred vision occurs; to drink plenty of fluids to help prevent constipation; and to report rash or other skin eruption.
• Warn patient that heat prostration may occur during therapy when environmental temperatures are high. If symptoms (fever, decreased sweating) occur, instruct patient to stop drug and contact his physician.
• Advise female patient not to breast-feed during therapy.

---

didanosine (ddI, dideoxyinosine)
dye-DAN-oh-seen

Videx, Videx EC

Therapeutic class: Antiretrovirals
Pharmacologic class: Nucleoside–nucleotide reverse transcriptase inhibitors

AVAILABLE FORMS
Capsules (delayed-release): 125 mg, 200 mg, 250 mg, 400 mg
Powder for oral solution (pediatric): 2 g/4-ounce glass bottle, 4 g/8-ounce glass bottle

INDICATIONS & DOSAGES
➤ **HIV infection**
Adults and children age 6 and older weighing 60 kg or more: 400-mg capsule P.O. daily. Or, 200 mg P.O. b.i.d. (preferred dosing).

Adults and children age 6 and older weighing 25 kg to less than 60 kg: 250-mg capsule P.O. daily. Or, 125 mg P.O. b.i.d. (preferred dosing).
Adults and children age 6 and older weighing 20 kg to less than 25 kg: 200-mg capsule P.O. daily. Or, 125 mg P.O. b.i.d. (preferred dosing).
Children older than age 8 months: 120 mg/m^2 of the pediatric powder for oral solution P.O. b.i.d. Maximum dose is 200 mg P.O. b.i.d.
Children ages 2 weeks to 8 months: 100 mg/m^2 of the pediatric powder for oral solution P.O. b.i.d. Maximum dose is 200 mg P.O. b.i.d.
Adjust-a-dose: For dialysis patients (with CrCl of less than 10 mL/minute) weighing 60 kg or more, 125 mg delayed-release capsule P.O. once daily or 100 mg of the pediatric powder for oral solution once daily. For dialysis patients weighing less than 60 kg, 75 mg of the pediatric powder for oral solution once daily. Don't use delayed-release capsules in dialysis patients who weigh less than 60 kg. If CrCl is less than 10 mL/minute, don't give a supplemental dose after hemodialysis for either drug.

In adults weighing 60 kg or more with CrCl of 30 to 59 mL/minute, 200-mg capsule P.O. once daily, or 200 mg P.O. once daily or 100 mg of the pediatric powder for oral solution b.i.d. If CrCl is 10 to 29 mL/minute, 125-mg capsule or 150 mg of the pediatric powder for oral solution once daily. If CrCl is less than 10 mL/minute, 125-mg capsule or 100 mg of the pediatric powder for oral solution once daily.

In adults weighing less than 60 kg with a CrCl of 30 to 59 mL/minute, 125-mg capsule P.O. once daily, or 150 mg once daily or 75 mg of the pediatric powder for oral solution b.i.d. If CrCl is 10 to 29 mL/minute, 125-mg capsule or 100 mg of the pediatric powder for oral solution once daily. For CrCl less than 10 mL/minute, 75 mg of the pediatric powder for oral solution once daily; capsule not indicated for these patients.

For adult patients taking tenofovir who weigh 60 kg or more with a CrCl of 60 mL/minute or more, reduce didanosine dose to 250 mg once daily. Avoid concomitant

---

Reactions in bold italics are *life-threatening*. Interactions may have a *rapid onset* or a *delayed onset*.

therapy in patients with CrCl less than 60 mL/minute. For adult patients taking tenofovir who weigh less than 60 kg with a CrCl of 60 mL/minute or more, reduce didanosine dose to 200 mg once daily. Avoid concomitant therapy in patients with CrCl less than 60 mL/minute.

D

ADMINISTRATION
P.O.

• Give drug on an empty stomach, at least 30 minutes before or 2 hours after eating; giving drug with meals can decrease absorption by 50%.

⊕ *Alert:* The pediatric powder for oral solution must be prepared by a pharmacist before dispensing. It must be constituted with purified USP water to an initial concentration of 20 mg/mL, then immediately diluted with an antacid to a final concentration of 10 mg/mL. The admixture is stable for 30 days at 36° to 46° F (2° to 8° C). Shake solution well before measuring dose. Discard unused portion after 30 days.

ACTION

Inhibits the enzyme HIV-RNA–dependent DNA polymerase (reverse transcriptase) and terminates DNA chain growth.

Route	Onset	Peak	Duration
P.O.	Unknown	15–90 min	Unknown
P.O. (delayed-release)	Unknown	2 hr	Unknown

Half-life: Adults, 1½ hours; children, about 1 hour.

ADVERSE REACTIONS

CNS: dizziness, fever, headache, peripheral neuropathy.
EENT: optic neuritis, retinal changes.
GI: abdominal pain, diarrhea, nausea, vomiting, *pancreatitis,* anorexia, dry mouth.
Hepatic: *hepatic failure.*
Metabolic: hyperuricemia.
Skin: alopecia, pruritus, rash.

INTERACTIONS

Drug-drug. *Allopurinol:* Increases didanosine level. Don't administer together.
Amprenavir, atazanavir, darunavir, delavirdine, indinavir, lopinavir, nelfinavir, rilpivirine, ritonavir, saquinavir, tipranavir: May alter pharmacokinetics of didanosine

or these drugs. Give didanosine at least 1 hour after these drugs.
Antacids containing magnesium or aluminum hydroxides: May enhance adverse effects of the antacid component (including diarrhea or constipation) when given with didanosine tablets or pediatric suspension. Avoid using together.
Dapsone, drugs that require gastric acid for adequate absorption, ketoconazole: May decrease absorption from buffering action. Give these drugs 2 hours before didanosine.
Fluoroquinolones, tetracyclines: May decrease absorption from buffering products in didanosine tablets or antacids in pediatric suspension. Separate dosage times by at least 2 hours.
Hydroxyurea: Enhances toxic effects of didanosine. Avoid combination.
Itraconazole: May decrease itraconazole level. Avoid using together.
Methadone: Increases didanosine concentration (with pediatric powder for oral solution). Give delayed-release capsule if methadone is required. Monitor clinical response closely, including changes in HIV-RNA viral load.
Ribavirin: Increases risk of fatal hepatic failure, peripheral neuropathy, pancreatitis, and systematic hyperlactemia/lactic acidosis. Don't use together.
Black Box Warning *Stavudine, other antiretrovirals:* Fatal lactic acidosis has been reported in pregnant women. Use only if potential benefits clearly outweigh potential risks. ∎
Sulfamethoxazole–trimethoprim, pentamidine, other drugs linked to pancreatitis: May increase risk of pancreatic toxicity. Use together cautiously; consider temporarily stopping didanosine during administration of these drugs.
Tenofovir: May increase didanosine levels and risk of life-threatening adverse effects, including lactic acidosis and pancreatitis. Adjust didanosine dosage.
Drug-herb. *St. John's wort:* May decrease drug level, decreasing therapeutic effects. Discourage use together.
Drug-food. *Any food:* May decrease rate of absorption. Advise patient to take drug on an empty stomach at least 30 minutes before a meal or 2 hours after eating.

Drug-lifestyle. *Alcohol use:* Increases risk of pancreatitis. Avoid use together.

EFFECTS ON LAB TEST RESULTS
• May increase alkaline phosphatase, ALT, AST, bilirubin, and uric acid levels. May decrease Hb level.
• May decrease granulocyte, platelet, and WBC counts.

CONTRAINDICATIONS & CAUTIONS
• Contraindicated in patients hypersensitive to drug or its components.
❸ **Alert:** Administration with allopurinol or ribavirin is contraindicated.
Black Box Warning Contraindicated in patients with confirmed pancreatitis. ■
Black Box Warning Use cautiously in patients with history of pancreatitis; deaths have occurred. ■
Black Box Warning Lactic acidosis and severe hepatomegaly with steatosis, including fatal cases, have been reported. ■
• Use cautiously in patients with peripheral neuropathy, renal or hepatic impairment, or hyperuricemia. Monitor LFTs and renal function tests.
Dializable drug: 7% or less.
⚠ **Overdose S&S:** Pancreatitis, peripheral neuropathy, diarrhea, hyperuricemia, hepatic dysfunction.

PREGNANCY-LACTATION-REPRODUCTION
• There are no adequate well-controlled studies in pregnant women. Use during pregnancy only in special circumstances and only if potential benefit justifies potential risk to the fetus.
• Not recommended for initial therapy in antiretroviral-naive pregnant women due to toxicity.
• It isn't known if drug appears in breast milk. Because of the potential for HIV transmission and for serious adverse reactions in breast-feeding infants, women shouldn't breast-feed during therapy.
• Enroll pregnant women exposed to antiretrovirals in the Antiretroviral Pregnancy Registry (1-800-258-4263 or www.apregistry.com).

NURSING CONSIDERATIONS
• Using drug in patients with advanced HIV disease or history of peripheral neuropathy or use with neurotoxic drugs may cause numbness, tingling, or pain in the hands and feet. Discontinue drug if neuropathy occurs.
• Patients may tolerate a reduced dose of Videx after symptoms of peripheral neuropathy resolve; if symptoms recur, consider permanently stopping drug.
• Because of a high rate of early virologic failure and emergence of resistance, using tenofovir with didanosine and lamivudine isn't recommended as a new treatment regimen for therapy-naive or therapy-experienced patients with HIV infection. Patients on this regimen should be considered for treatment modification.
• **Look alike–sound alike:** Don't confuse drug with other antiretrovirals that use abbreviations for identification.

PATIENT TEACHING
• Instruct patient to take drug on an empty stomach, 30 minutes before or 2 hours after eating.
• Inform patient that drug doesn't cure HIV infection, that opportunistic infections and other complications of HIV infection may continue to occur, and that transmission of HIV to others through sexual contact or blood contamination is still possible.
• Tell patient to report all adverse reactions and to immediately report signs and symptoms of inflammation of the pancreas (abdominal pain, nausea, vomiting, diarrhea) and signs and symptoms of peripheral neuropathy (numbness, tingling, or pain in hands or feet).

difluprednate
die-FLU-pred-nate

Durezol

Therapeutic class: Anti-inflammatory drugs (ophthalmic)
Pharmacologic class: Corticosteroids

AVAILABLE FORMS
Ophthalmic emulsion: 0.05%

INDICATIONS & DOSAGES
➤ **Inflammation and pain associated with ocular surgery**
Adults: 1 drop into the conjunctival sac of the affected eye q.i.d. beginning 24 hours after surgery for 2 weeks, then decrease to b.i.d. for 1 week, and then taper according to response.
➤ **Endogenous anterior uveitis**
Adults: 1 drop into the conjunctival sac of the affected eye q.i.d. for 14 days, then taper as clinically indicated.

ADMINISTRATION
Ophthalmic
● Shake well before each use.
● Don't touch tip of dropper to any surface, including eye.

ACTION
May inhibit the release of arachidonic acid, a precursor of inflammatory mediators, such as prostaglandins and leukotrienes.

Route	Onset	Peak	Duration
Ophthalmic	Rapid	Unknown	Unknown

Half-life: Unknown.

ADVERSE REACTIONS
EENT: anterior chamber cells, anterior chamber flare, blepharitis, ciliary and conjunctival hyperemia, conjunctival edema, corneal edema, eye inflammation, eye pain, iritis, photophobia, posterior capsule opacification, punctate keratitis, reduced visual acuity.

INTERACTIONS
None reported.

EFFECTS ON LAB TEST RESULTS
None reported.

CONTRAINDICATIONS & CAUTIONS
● Contraindicated in patients with ocular TB, epithelial HSV infection (dendritic keratitis), vaccinia, varicella, or other fungal or viral diseases of ocular structures.
● Use cautiously in patients with glaucoma (any form) because IOP may increase.
● Use can result in posterior subcapsular cataract formation.

● Use cautiously in patients with a history of HSV infection; drug may prolong or worsen the condition.
Dialyzable drug: Unknown.

PREGNANCY-LACTATION-REPRODUCTION
● Use in pregnant women hasn't been evaluated, and potential fetal harm can't be ruled out. Use during pregnancy only if potential benefit justifies potential risk to the fetus.
● It isn't known if drug appears in breast milk. Use cautiously in breast-feeding women.

NURSING CONSIDERATIONS
● Drug isn't intended for long-term use; if used for 10 days or more, monitor IOP. Watch for ocular bacterial, fungal, or viral infections.
● Drug may delay healing after cataract surgery; examine with slit-lamp biomicroscopy and, if appropriate, fluorescein staining if used for more than 28 days.
● Safety and effectiveness in children haven't been established.

PATIENT TEACHING
● Teach patient how to instill drops. Advise him to wash his hands before and after applying the drug, and warn him not to touch tip of dropper to eye or surrounding tissue.
● Advise patient to contact prescriber if pain develops or redness, itching, or inflammation worsens.
● Tell patient to remove contact lenses before instilling drug; preservative in drug may be absorbed by soft contact lenses. Lenses may be reinserted 10 minutes after administration.
● Tell patient who wears hard contact lenses to check with prescriber before using lenses again.
● Advise patient to store drug at room temperature in protective carton away from light, and to keep unused vials in foil pouch.

digoxin
di-JOX-in

Apo-Digoxin✽, Lanoxin*, Lanoxin
Pediatric, Toloxin✽

Therapeutic class: Inotropes
Pharmacologic class: Cardiac
glycosides

AVAILABLE FORMS
Elixir: 0.05 mg/mL (pediatric)
Injection: 0.05 mg/mL✽, 0.1 mg/mL
(pediatric), 0.25 mg/mL
Tablets: 0.0625 mg, 0.125 mg, 0.1875 mg,
0.25 mg

INDICATIONS & DOSAGES
◆ Alert: Factors to consider when a digoxin
dosing regimen is selected include body
weight, age, renal function, concomitant
drugs, and disease. Toxic levels of digoxin
are only slightly higher than therapeutic
levels.

Adjust-a-dose (for all indications): Refer
to manufacturer's information for recommended dosage adjustments based on renal
function and weight.

➤ **HF, rapid digitalization**
Tablets
Adults and children older than age 10:
Total loading dose is 10 to 15 mcg/kg P.O.
Initially, give half the total loading dose
followed by one-quarter of the loading dose
every 6 to 8 hours twice. Carefully assess
clinical response and toxicity before each
dose. Recommended starting maintenance
dose for patients with normal renal function is 3.4 to 5.1 mcg/kg/day P.O. once
daily. May increase every 2 weeks based on
clinical response, serum drug levels, and
toxicity. Refer to manufacturer's instructions
for once-daily maintenance dose recommendations based on renal function and lean
body weight.
Children ages 5 to 10: Total loading dose is
20 to 45 mcg/kg P.O. Initially, give half the
total loading dose followed by one-quarter
of the loading dose every 6 to 8 hours twice.
Carefully assess clinical response and toxic-

ity before each dose. Recommended starting
maintenance dosage for patients with normal renal function is 3.2 to 6.4 mcg/kg
P.O. twice daily. Refer to manufacturer's
instructions for daily maintenance dose recommendations based on renal function and
lean body weight.
Elixir
In pediatric patients, if a loading dose is
needed, it can be administered with roughly
half the total given as the first dose. Additional fractions of this planned total dose
may be given at 4- to 8-hour intervals, with
careful assessment of clinical response before each additional dose. If the patient's
clinical response necessitates a change from
the calculated loading dose of digoxin, base
the calculation of the maintenance dose on
the amount actually given as the loading
dose.
Children older than age 10: Loading dose
is 10 to 15 mcg/kg P.O. given in divided
doses, followed by maintenance dose of 3 to
4.5 mcg/kg P.O. once daily.
Children ages 5 to 10: Loading dose is
20 to 35 mcg/kg P.O. given in divided doses,
followed by maintenance dose of 2.8 to
5.6 mcg/kg/dose P.O. b.i.d.
Children ages 2 to 5: Loading dose is
30 to 45 mcg/kg P.O. given in divided doses,
followed by maintenance dose of 4.7 to
6.6 mcg/kg/dose P.O. b.i.d.
Infants ages 1 to 24 months: Loading dose is
35 to 60 mcg/kg P.O. given in divided doses,
followed by maintenance dose of 5.6 to
9.4 mcg/kg/dose P.O. b.i.d.
Full-term infants: Loading dose is 25 to
35 mcg/kg P.O. in divided doses, followed
by maintenance dose of 3.8 to 5.6 mcg/kg
P.O. b.i.d.
Preterm infants: Loading dose is 20 to
30 mcg/kg P.O. given in divided doses,
followed by maintenance dose of 2.3 to
3.9 mcg/kg/dose P.O. b.i.d.
I.V.
Initially for all patients, give half the total
loading dose followed by one-quarter of the
loading dose every 6 to 8 hours twice. Carefully assess clinical response and toxicity
before each dose. Recommended starting
maintenance doses assume the presence of
normal renal function. May increase every

---

2 weeks based on clinical response, serum drug levels, and toxicity. Refer to manufacturer's instructions for maintenance dose recommendations based on renal function and lean body weight.

Adults and children older than age 10: Total loading dose is 8 to 12 mcg/kg I.V. in divided doses, followed by a starting maintenance dose of 2.4 to 3.6 mcg/kg I.V. once daily.

Children ages 5 to 10: Total loading dose is 15 to 30 mcg/kg I.V. in divided doses, followed by a starting maintenance dose of 2.3 to 4.5 mcg/kg/dose I.V. b.i.d.

Children ages 2 to 5: Total loading dose is 25 to 35 mcg/kg I.V. in divided doses, followed by a starting maintenance dose of 3.8 to 5.3 mcg/kg/dose I.V. b.i.d.

Infants ages 1 to 24 months: Total loading dose is 30 to 50 mcg/kg I.V. in divided doses, followed by a starting maintenance dose of 4.5 to 7.5 mcg/kg/dose I.V. b.i.d.

Full-term infants: Total loading dose is 20 to 30 mcg/kg I.V. in divided doses, followed by a starting maintenance dose of 3 to 4.5 mcg/kg/dose I.V. b.i.d.

Preterm infants: Total loading dose is 15 to 25 mcg/kg I.V. in divided doses, followed by a starting maintenance dose of 1.9 to 3.1 mcg/kg/dose I.V. b.i.d.

➤ **HF, gradual digitalization**
Tablets
More gradual attainment of digoxin levels can also be accomplished by beginning an appropriate maintenance dosage without a loading dose in patients with normal renal function.

Adults and children older than age 10: Give starting maintenance dose of 3.4 to 5.1 mcg/kg P.O. once daily.

Children ages 5 to 10: Give starting maintenance dose of 3.2 to 6.4 mcg/kg/dose P.O. b.i.d.

Adjust-a-dose: Refer to manufacturer's instructions for dosage adjustment based on renal function and lean body weight.

Elixir
More gradual attainment of digoxin levels can also be accomplished by beginning an appropriate maintenance dosage without a loading dose in patients with normal renal function. In general, divided daily dosing is recommended for infants and children younger than age 10. In newborns, renal clearance of digoxin is diminished and suitable dosage adjustments must be observed, especially in preterm infants. Beyond the immediate newborn period, children generally require proportionally larger doses than adults on the basis of body weight or surface area. Children older than age 10 require adult dosages in proportion to their body weight.

Adults and children older than age 10: 3 to 4.5 mcg/kg P.O. once daily.

Children ages 5 to 10: 2.8 to 5.6 mcg/kg/dose P.O. b.i.d.

Children ages 2 to 5: 4.7 to 6.6 mcg/kg/dose P.O. b.i.d.

Infants ages 1 to 24 months: 5.6 to 9.4 mcg/kg/dose P.O. b.i.d.

Full-term infants: 3.8 to 5.6 mcg/kg/dose P.O. b.i.d.

Preterm infants: 2.3 to 3.9 mcg/kg/dose P.O. b.i.d.

Adjust-a-dose: Refer to manufacturer's instructions for dosage adjustment based on renal function and lean body weight.

I.V.
Gradual digitalization can be accomplished by beginning an appropriate maintenance dose. Recommended starting doses assume the presence of normal renal function. May increase every 2 weeks based on clinical response, serum drug levels, and toxicity. Refer to manufacturer's instructions for dose recommendations based on renal function and lean body weight.

Adults and children older than age 10: Give a starting dose of 2.4 to 3.6 mcg/kg I.V. once daily.

Children ages 5 to 10: Give a starting dose of 2.3 to 4.5 mcg/kg/dose I.V. b.i.d.

Children ages 2 to 5: Give a starting dose of 3.8 to 5.3 mcg/kg/dose I.V. b.i.d.

Infants ages 1 to 24 months: Give a starting dose of 4.5 to 7.5 mcg/kg/dose I.V. b.i.d.

Full-term infants: Give a starting dose of 3 to 4.5 mcg/kg/dose I.V. b.i.d.

Preterm infants: Give a starting dose of 1.9 to 3.1 mcg/kg/dose I.V. b.i.d.

➤ **Atrial fibrillation (chronic)**
P.O., I.V.
Adults: If a loading dose is used, total loading dose is 10 to 15 mcg/kg P.O. (tablets, elixir). Initially, give half the total loading

dose followed by one-quarter of the loading dose every 6 to 8 hours twice. Carefully assess clinical response and toxicity before each dose. Recommended starting maintenance dosage for patients with normal renal function is 3.4 to 5.1 mcg/kg (tablets) P.O. once daily or 3 to 4.5 mcg/kg (elixir) P.O. once daily.

Or, for more gradual P.O. digitalization in patients with normal renal function, begin with the starting maintenance dosage of 3.4 to 5.1 mcg/kg (tablets) P.O. once daily or 3 to 4.5 mcg/kg (elixir) P.O. once daily. May increase every 2 weeks based on clinical response, serum drug levels, and toxicity. Refer to manufacturer's instructions for once-daily maintenance dose recommendations based on renal function and lean body weight.

Or, if using an I.V. loading dose, give a total loading dose of 8 to 12 mcg/kg I.V. by initially giving half the total loading dose followed by one-quarter of the loading dose every 6 to 8 hours twice. Carefully assess clinical response and toxicity before each dose. Recommended starting maintenance dosage for patients with normal renal function is 2.4 to 3.6 mcg/kg I.V. once daily.

Or, for more gradual I.V. digitalization in patients with normal renal function, begin with the starting maintenance dosage of 2.4 to 3.6 mcg/kg I.V. once daily. Increase every 2 weeks according to clinical response, serum drug levels, and toxicity. Refer to manufacturer's instructions for dosage recommendations based on renal function and lean body weight.

ADMINISTRATION
P.O.
● Before giving loading dose, obtain baseline data (HR and rhythm, BP, and electrolyte levels) and ask patient about use of cardiac glycosides within the previous 2 to 3 weeks.
● Before giving drug, take apical-radial pulse for 1 minute. Record and notify prescriber of significant changes (sudden increase or decrease in pulse rate, pulse deficit, irregular beats and, particularly, regularization of a previously irregular rhythm). If these occur, check BP and obtain a 12-lead ECG.

I.V.
▼ Before giving loading dose, obtain baseline data (HR and rhythm, BP, and electrolyte levels) and ask patient about use of cardiac glycosides within the previous 2 to 3 weeks.
▼ Before giving drug, take apical-radial pulse for 1 minute. Record and notify prescriber of significant changes (sudden increase or decrease in pulse rate, pulse deficit, irregular beats and, particularly, regularization of a previously irregular rhythm). If these occur, check BP and obtain a 12-lead ECG.
▼ Dilute fourfold with D_5W, NSS, or sterile water for injection to reduce the chance of precipitation.
▼ Infuse drug slowly over at least 5 minutes.
▼ Protect solution from light.
▼ **Incompatibilities:** Amiodarone, amphotericin B cholesteryl sulfate complex, dobutamine, doxapram, fluconazole, foscarnet, propofol, remifentanil. Mixing with other drugs isn't recommended.

ACTION
Inhibits sodium-potassium–activated adenosine triphosphatase, promoting movement of calcium from extracellular to intracellular cytoplasm and strengthening myocardial contraction. Also acts on CNS to enhance vagal tone, slowing conduction through the SA and AV nodes.

Route	Onset	Peak	Duration
P.O.	30–120 min	2–6 hr	3–4 days
I.V.	5–30 min	1–4 hr	3–4 days

Half-life: With normal renal function: adults, 36 to 48 hours; children, 18 to 36 hours.

ADVERSE REACTIONS
CNS: agitation, fatigue, generalized muscle weakness, hallucinations, dizziness, headache, malaise, paresthesia, stupor, vertigo.
CV: *arrhythmias, heart block.*
EENT: blurred vision, diplopia, light flashes, photophobia, yellow-green halos around visual images.
GI: anorexia, nausea, diarrhea, vomiting.

Reactions in bold italics are *life-threatening*. Interactions may have a *rapid onset* or a *delayed onset*.

INTERACTIONS

Drug-drug. *Amiloride:* May decrease digoxin effect and increase renal clearance of digoxin. Monitor patient for altered digoxin effect.

Amiodarone, *diltiazem,* **dronedarone,** *in-domethacin, nifedipine,* **protease inhibitors, quinidine, verapamil:** May increase digoxin level. Monitor patient for toxicity.

Amphotericin B, carbenicillin, cortico-steroids, **diuretics (chlorthalidone, loop diuretics, metolazone),** *ticarcillin:* May cause hypokalemia and hypomagnesemia, predisposing patient to cardiac glycoside toxicity. Monitor electrolyte levels.

Antacids: May decrease absorption of oral digoxin. Separate doses as much as possible.

Antibiotics (azole antifungals, macrolides, telithromycin, tetracyclines), propafenone, ritonavir: May increase risk of cardiac gly-coside toxicity. Monitor patient for toxicity.

Anticholinergics: May increase absorption of oral digoxin tablets. Monitor drug level and observe for toxicity.

Beta blockers, calcium channel blockers: May have additive effects on AV node con-duction, causing advanced or complete heart block. Use cautiously.

Cholestyramine, colestipol, metoclo-pramide: May decrease absorption of oral digoxin. Monitor patient for decreased digoxin level and effect. Give digoxin 1½ hours before or 2 hours after other drugs.

Parenteral calcium, thiazides: May cause hypercalcemia and hypomagnesemia, predisposing patient to digitalis toxicity. Monitor calcium and magnesium levels.

Drug-herb. *Betel palm, foxglove, fumitory, goldenseal, hawthorn, lily of the valley, motherwort, rue, shepherd's purse:* May increase cardiac effects. Discourage use together.

Danshen, licorice, Siberian ginseng: May increase toxicity. Monitor patient closely.

St. John's wort: May decrease digoxin serum concentration. Monitor therapy.

EFFECTS ON LAB TEST RESULTS

● May prolong PR interval or depress ST segment.

CONTRAINDICATIONS & CAUTIONS

● Contraindicated in patients hypersensitive to drug and in those with digitalis-induced toxicity, ventricular fibrillation, or ventricu-lar tachycardia unless caused by HF.

● Don't use in patients with Wolff-Parkinson-White syndrome unless the conduction accessory pathway has been pharmacologically or surgically disabled.

● Use with extreme caution in elderly pa-tients and in those with acute MI, incom-plete AV block, sinus bradycardia, PVCs, chronic constrictive pericarditis, hyper-trophic cardiomyopathy, renal insufficiency, severe pulmonary disease, or hypothy-roidism.

Dialyzable drug: No.

⚠ *Overdose S&S:* Ventricular tachycardia, ventricular fibrillation, bradycardia, heart block, cardiac arrest, hyperkalemia.

PREGNANCY-LACTATION-REPRODUCTION

● It isn't known if drug can cause fetal harm when used during pregnancy or if drug can affect reproductive capacity. Use during pregnancy only if clearly needed.

● Drug appears in breast milk; however, a breast-feeding infant is exposed to an amount estimated to be far below the usual infant maintenance dose. Use cautiously, but the amount should have no pharmacologic effect on a breast-feeding infant.

NURSING CONSIDERATIONS

● Drug-induced arrhythmias may increase the severity of HF and hypotension.

● In children, cardiac arrhythmias, includ-ing sinus bradycardia, are usually early signs of toxicity.

● Patients with hypothyroidism are ex-tremely sensitive to cardiac glycosides and may need lower doses.

● According to the 2013 guideline for the management of HF (American College of Cardiology Foundation/American Heart Association), there is no reason to use load-ing doses to initiate digoxin therapy in patients with HF. The guideline indicates that digoxin therapy is usually initiated and maintained at 0.125 to 0.25 mg P.O. once daily; higher daily doses (up to 0.5 mg/day) are rarely necessary. If patient is older than age 70, has impaired renal function, or has a

low lean body mass, initially use low doses (0.125 mg daily or every other day).
• Monitor patient for toxicity. Toxic effects on the heart may be life-threatening and require immediate attention. Signs and symptoms of toxicity include anorexia, nausea, vomiting, visual changes, and cardiac arrhythmias. Patients with low body weight, advanced age, renal impairment, and electrolyte disturbances are at increased risk.
• Monitor digoxin level. Therapeutic level ranges from 0.8 to 2 nanograms/mL. Obtain blood for digoxin level at least 6 to 8 hours after last oral dose, preferably just before next scheduled dose.
◑ *Alert:* Excessively slow pulse rate (60 beats/minute or less) may be a sign of digitalis toxicity. Withhold drug and notify prescriber.
• Monitor potassium level carefully. Take corrective action before hypokalemia occurs. Hyperkalemia may result from digoxin toxicity.
• Reduce drug dose for 1 or 2 days before elective cardioversion. Adjust dosage after cardioversion.
• *Look alike–sound alike:* Don't confuse digoxin with doxepin.

PATIENT TEACHING
• Teach patient and a responsible family member about drug action, dosage regimen, how to take pulse, reportable signs, and follow-up care.
• Tell patient to report pulse rate less than 60 beats/minute (bpm) or more than 110 bpm, or skipped beats or other rhythm changes.
• Instruct patient to report all adverse reactions promptly. Nausea, vomiting, diarrhea, appetite loss, and visual disturbances may indicate toxicity.
• Encourage patient to eat a consistent amount of potassium-rich foods.
• Tell patient not to substitute one brand for another.
• Advise patient to avoid using herbal supplements and to consult prescriber before taking one.

diltiazem hydrochloride
dil-TYE-a-zem

Apo-Diltiaz❈, Cardizem✿,
Cardizem CD✿, Cardizem LA✿,
Cartia XT, Dilt XR, Diltzac, Matzim
LA, Taztia XT, Tiazac, Tiazac XC❈

Therapeutic class: Antihypertensives
Pharmacologic class: Calcium channel blockers

AVAILABLE FORMS
Capsules (extended-release) ⓞⓣⓒ: 60 mg, 90 mg, 120 mg, 180 mg, 240 mg, 300 mg, 360 mg, 420 mg
Injection: 5 mg/mL in 5-, 10-, 25-mL vials
Powder for injection: 100 mg
Tablets: 30 mg, 60 mg, 90 mg, 120 mg
Tablets (extended-release) ⓞⓣⓒ: 120 mg, 180 mg, 240 mg, 300 mg, 360 mg, 420 mg

INDICATIONS & DOSAGES
➤ **To manage Prinzmetal or variant angina or chronic stable angina pectoris**
Adults: 30 mg P.O. q.i.d. (immediate-release tablets) before meals and at bedtime. Increase dose gradually to maximum of 360 mg/day divided into three or four doses, as indicated. Or, give 120- or 180-mg extended-release capsule or 180-mg extended-release tablet P.O. once daily. Adjust over a 7- to 14-day period as needed and tolerated up to a maximum dose of 360 mg/day (Cardizem LA, Matzim LA), 480 mg/day (Cardizem CD, Cartia XT), or 540 mg/day (Tiazac, Taztia XT).
➤ **Hypertension, alone or as combination therapy**
Adults: Initially 180 to 240 mg P.O. once daily as monotherapy or 120 to 480 mg extended-release capsule P.O. once daily. Adjust dosage based on patient response to a maximum dose of 480 mg/day. Or, 120 to 540 mg extended-release tablet P.O. once daily. Dosage can be adjusted about every 2 weeks to a maximum of 540 mg daily.
➤ **Atrial fibrillation or flutter; paroxysmal supraventricular tachycardia**
Adults: 0.25 mg/kg I.V. as a bolus injection over 2 minutes. Repeat after 15 minutes if response isn't adequate with a dose of

0.35 mg/kg I.V. over 2 minutes. Follow bolus with continuous I.V. infusion at 5 to 15 mg/hour (for up to 24 hours).

➤ **Improvement of exercise tolerance in patients with chronic stable angina (Cardizem LA)**

Adults: Initially, 180 mg extended-release tablets P.O. once daily; increase dose at intervals of 7 to 14 days until adequate response is obtained. Maximum dosage is 360 mg.

ADMINISTRATION

P.O.
● Don't crush or allow patient to chew extended-release tablets or capsules; they should be swallowed whole.

● Tiazac and Taztia extended-release capsules can be opened and the contents sprinkled onto a spoonful of applesauce. The applesauce must be eaten immediately and without chewing, followed by a glass of cool water.

I.V.
▼ For direct injection, you need not dilute the 5 mg/mL injection.

▼ For continuous infusion, add 25 mL of drug to 100 mL solution, 50 mL of drug to 250 mL solution, or 50 mL of drug to 500 mL solution of 5 mg/mL injection to yield 1 mg/mL, 0.83 mg/mL, or 0.45 mg/mL, respectively. Compatible solutions include NSS, D$_5$W, or 5% dextrose and half-NSS.

▼ For direct injection or continuous infusion, give slowly while monitoring ECG and BP continuously.

▼ Don't infuse for longer than 24 hours.

▼ **Incompatibilities:** Acetazolamide, acyclovir, aminophylline, ampicillin, ampicillin sodium–sulbactam sodium, diazepam, furosemide, heparin, hydrocortisone, insulin, methylprednisolone, nafcillin, phenytoin, rifampin, sodium bicarbonate, thiopental.

ACTION
A calcium channel blocker that inhibits calcium ion influx across cardiac and smooth-muscle cells, decreasing myocardial contractility and oxygen demand. Drug also dilates coronary arteries and arterioles.

Route	Onset	Peak	Duration
P.O.	30–60 min	2–3 hr	6–8 hr
P.O. (extended-release capsule)	2–3 hr	10–14 hr	12–24 hr
P.O. (Cardizem LA, Matzim LA)	3–4 hr	11–18 hr	6–9 hr
I.V.	<3 min	2–7 min	1–10 hr

Half-life: 3 to 9 hours.

ADVERSE REACTIONS
CNS: headache, dizziness, asthenia, somnolence.
CV: edema, *arrhythmias, AV block, bradycardia, HF,* flushing, hypotension, conduction abnormalities, abnormal ECG.
GI: nausea, constipation, abdominal discomfort.
Hepatic: *acute hepatic injury.*
Skin: rash.

INTERACTIONS
Drug-drug. *Anesthetics:* May increase effects of anesthetics. Monitor patient.
Atazanavir, cimetidine: May inhibit diltiazem metabolism, increasing additive AV node conduction slowing. Monitor patient for toxicity.
Buspirone, quinidine, sirolimus, tacrolimus: May increase level of these drugs. Monitor drug levels and patient for toxicity.
Carbamazepine: May increase level of carbamazepine. Monitor carbamazepine level, and watch for signs and symptoms of toxicity.
Cyclosporine: May increase cyclosporine level. Monitor cyclosporine level with each dosage change.
Diazepam, midazolam, triazolam: May increase CNS depression and prolonged effects of these drugs. Use lower dose of these benzodiazepines.
Digoxin: May increase digoxin level. Monitor patient for digoxin toxicity.
Furosemide: May form a precipitate when mixed with diltiazem injection. Give through separate I.V. lines.
HMG-CoA reductase inhibitors (lovastatin, simvastatin): May increase risk of myopathy, rhabdomyolysis, and kidney failure. Use lower starting and maintenance doses of both agents.
Lithium: May reduce lithium level, causing loss of mania control. May also enhance

lithium's neurotoxic effects. Monitor therapy.

Propranolol, other beta blockers: May precipitate HF or prolong conduction time. Use together cautiously.

Rifampin: May lower diltiazem level significantly. Avoid use together.

Theophylline: May enhance action of theophylline, causing intoxication. Monitor theophylline levels.

EFFECTS ON LAB TEST RESULTS
None reported.

CONTRAINDICATIONS & CAUTIONS
• Contraindicated in patients hypersensitive to drug and in those with sick sinus syndrome or second- or third-degree AV block in the absence of an artificial pacemaker, cardiogenic shock, ventricular tachycardia, systolic BP below 90 mm Hg, acute MI, or pulmonary congestion (documented by X-ray).

• Contraindicated in I.V. form for patients who have atrial fibrillation or flutter with an accessory bypass tract, as in Wolff-Parkinson-White syndrome or short PR interval syndrome.

• Use cautiously in elderly patients and in those with HF, hypertrophic obstructive cardiomyopathy, or impaired hepatic or renal function.

Dialyzable drug: No.

⚠ *Overdose S&S:* Bradycardia, hypotension, heart block, cardiac failure.

PREGNANCY-LACTATION-REPRODUCTION
• There are no adequate well-controlled studies in pregnant women. Use during pregnancy only if clearly needed and potential benefit justifies potential risk to the fetus.

• Drug appears in breast milk. Patient should discontinue breast-feeding or discontinue drug, taking into account importance of drug to the mother.

NURSING CONSIDERATIONS
• Patients controlled on drug alone or with other drugs may be switched to Cardizem LA tablets once a day at the nearest equivalent total daily dose.

• Monitor BP and HR when starting therapy and during dosage adjustments.

• Maximal antihypertensive effect may not be seen for 14 days.

• If systolic BP is below 90 mm Hg or HR is below 60 beats/minute, withhold dose and notify prescriber.

• *Look alike–sound alike:* Don't confuse Tiazac with Ziac.

PATIENT TEACHING
• Instruct patient to take drug as prescribed, even when feeling better, and to report all adverse reactions.

• Advise patient to avoid hazardous activities during start of therapy.

• If nitrate therapy is prescribed during dosage adjustment, stress patient compliance. Tell patient that S.L. nitroglycerin may be taken with drug, as needed, when angina symptoms are acute.

⚠ *Alert:* Tell patient to swallow extended-release tablets whole, and not to crush or chew them.

• Inform patient taking Tiazac extended-release capsules that these capsules can be opened and the contents sprinkled on a spoonful of applesauce. Advise patient to eat the applesauce immediately and without chewing, and then drink a glass of cool water.

dimethyl fumarate
dye-METH-il

Tecfidera

Therapeutic class: Immunomodulators
Pharmacologic class: Nuclear factor–like 2 pathway activators

AVAILABLE FORMS
Capsules (delayed-release) ⬛: 120 mg, 240 mg

INDICATIONS & DOSAGES
➤ **Relapsing MS**
Adults: Initially, 120 mg P.O. b.i.d. for 7 days; then increase to maintenance dosage of 240 mg b.i.d.

Adjust-a-dose: Consider temporary dosage reduction to 120 mg b.i.d. for patient who can't tolerate maintenance dose. Resume recommended dose of 240 mg b.i.d. within

4 weeks; then consider discontinuing drug if patient is unable to tolerate return to maintenance dose.

Consider interrupting or discontinuing therapy in patients with lymphocyte counts less than 0.5×10^9/L persisting for more than 6 months. Consider withholding drug in patients with serious infections until resolution. Individualize decisions about restarting therapy based on clinical circumstances.

ADMINISTRATION
P.O.

● Make sure patient swallows capsules whole and intact. Don't allow patient to chew capsules, and don't crush or open capsule and sprinkle on food.

● Give without regard to meals; however, food may reduce incidence of flushing. Giving non-enteric-coated aspirin (up to a 325-mg dose) 30 minutes before may reduce incidence or severity of flushing.

● Store capsules in their original container to prevent exposure to light; once bottle has been opened, discard medication after 90 days. Store at room temperature.

ACTION

Unknown. The drug and its metabolite, monomethyl fumarate, have been shown to activate the nuclear factor–like 2 pathway, which reduces oxidative stress that contributes to myelin damage.

Route	Onset	Peak	Duration
P.O.	Unknown	2–2½ hr	Unknown

Half-life: 1 hour.

ADVERSE REACTIONS

CV: flushing.
GI: abdominal pain, diarrhea, nausea, vomiting, dyspepsia.
GU: albuminuria.
Hematologic: *lymphopenia.*
Skin: pruritus, rash, erythema.

INTERACTIONS
None reported.

EFFECTS ON LAB TEST RESULTS
● May increase AST and ALT levels.
● May decrease lymphocyte count.

CONTRAINDICATIONS & CAUTIONS
● Contraindicated in patients hypersensitive to drug or its components. Reactions have included anaphylaxis and angioedema and can occur after first dose or at any time during treatment. Discontinue drug if hypersensitivity signs or symptoms occur.
● Use cautiously in patients with lymphopenia and in those with increased risk of acquiring serious infections.
● **Alert:** Drug may increase risk of rare but serious brain infection, progressive multifocal leukoencephalopathy (PML), caused by John Cunningham virus.
Dialyzable drug: Unknown.

PREGNANCY-LACTATION-REPRODUCTION
● There are no adequate well-controlled studies in pregnant women. Use during pregnancy only if potential benefit justifies the potential risk to the fetus.
● It isn't known if drug appears in breast milk. Use cautiously in breastfeeding women. Women exposed to drug during pregnancy are encouraged to enroll in the pregnancy registry by calling 1-866-810-1462 or visiting www.tecfiderapregnancyregistry.com.

NURSING CONSIDERATIONS
● Obtain CBC, including lymphocyte count, before start of treatment, 6 months after starting treatment, then every 6 to 12 months thereafter and as clinically indicated.
● **Alert:** Watch for signs and symptoms of PML (new or worsening weakness; trouble using arms or legs; changes in orientation leading to confusion and personality changes; changes to thinking, memory, eyesight, strength, or balance).
● Monitor patient for signs and symptoms of hypersensitivity reactions, including anaphylaxis and angioedema (difficulty breathing, urticaria, and swelling of the throat and tongue).
● Transient increase in eosinophil count may occur during the first 2 months of therapy.
● If patient has a serious infection, consider withholding treatment until the infection is resolved.

• If patient experiences flushing during therapy, giving drug with food or non-enteric-coated aspirin (up to a 325-mg dose) 30 minutes before dose may decrease severity.

PATIENT TEACHING

• Instruct patients to swallow capsule whole and intact.
• Reassure patient that GI side effects usually decrease after the first month of therapy.
• Inform patient that flushing may occur after starting the medication and that taking it with food or non-enteric-coated aspirin (up to a 325-mg dose) 30 minutes before dose may help.
• Advise patient that a blood test will be needed before starting drug and then every 6 to 12 months to check for a low lymphocyte count.
• Instruct female patient that if she is pregnant or plans to become pregnant during therapy to inform her prescriber.
• Advise female patient who is pregnant to enroll in the pregnancy registry.

diphenhydrAMINE hydrochloride
dye-fen-HYE-drah-meen

Aler-Cap ◊, Banophen ◊, Benadryl ◊, Benadryl Allergy Childrens ◊, Diphenhist ◊, PediaCare Childrens Allergy ◊, Silphen Cough ◊, Simply Allergy ◊, Sominex ◊, TH Allergy Relief ◊, TH Childrens Allergy ◊, TheraFlu Multi-Symptom ◊, Total Allergy ◊, Triaminic MultiSymptom ◊*, Unisom SleepMelts ◊

Therapeutic class: Antihistamines
Pharmacologic class: Ethanolamines

AVAILABLE FORMS
Capsules: 25 mg ◊, 50 mg ◊
Elixir: 12.5 mg/5 mL ◊*
Injection: 50 mg/mL
ODTs: 12.5 mg ◊
Strips (orally disintegrating): 12.5 mg ◊*, 25 mg ◊*

Syrup: 12.5 mg/5 mL ◊*
Tablets: 25 mg ◊, 50 mg ◊
Tablets (chewable): 12.5 mg ◊, 25 mg

INDICATIONS & DOSAGES
➤ **Rhinitis, allergy symptoms, motion sickness, Parkinson disease**
Adults and children age 12 and older: 25 to 50 mg P.O. every 4 to 6 hours. Maximum, 300 mg P.O. daily. Or, 10 to 50 mg I.V. or deep I.M. Maximum I.V. or I.M. dosage, 400 mg daily. Don't exceed 25 mg/minute when giving I.V.
Children ages 6 to 11: 12.5 to 25 mg P.O. every 4 to 6 hours. Maximum dose is 150 mg daily. Or, 5 mg/kg deep I.M. or I.V. divided into four doses. Don't exceed 25 mg/minute when giving I.V. Maximum dose is 300 mg daily.
Children younger than age 6 and weighing more than 9 kg (prescription products only): 5 mg/kg P.O. daily or 150 mg/m^2 P.O. daily; maximum, 300 mg daily. Or, 5 mg/kg daily deep I.M. or I.V. divided into four doses. Don't exceed 25 mg/minute when giving I.V. Maximum dose is 300 mg daily. Don't use in neonates and premature infants.
➤ **Nighttime sleep aid**
Adults: 50 mg P.O. at bedtime.
➤ **Nonproductive cough**
Adults and children age 12 and older: 25 mg (syrup) P.O. every 4 hours. Don't exceed 150 mg daily. Or, 25 to 50 mg (liquid) P.O. every 4 hours. Don't exceed 300 mg daily.
Children ages 6 to 11: 12.5 mg syrup P.O. every 4 hours. Don't exceed 75 mg daily. Or, 12.5 to 25 mg liquid P.O. every 4 hours. Don't exceed 150 mg daily.

ADMINISTRATION
P.O.
• Give drug with food or milk to reduce GI distress.
I.V.
▼ For injection, don't exceed 25 mg/minute.
▼ **Incompatibilities:** Allopurinol, amobarbital, amphotericin B, cefepime, dexamethasone, foscarnet, haloperidol lactate, pentobarbital, phenobarbital, phenytoin, thiopental.

Reactions in bold italics are *life-threatening*. Interactions may have a *rapid onset* or a ***delayed onset***.

I.M.
• Give I.M. injection deep into large muscle; alternate injection sites to prevent irritation.

ACTION
Competes with histamine for H_1-receptor sites. Prevents, but doesn't reverse, histamine-mediated responses, particularly those of the bronchial tubes, GI tract, uterus, and blood vessels.

Route	Onset	Peak	Duration
P.O.	15 min	1–4 hr	6–8 hr
I.V.	Immediate	1–4 hr	6–8 hr
I.M.	Unknown	1–4 hr	6–8 hr

Half-life: About 2½ to 9½ hours.

ADVERSE REACTIONS
CNS: drowsiness, sedation, sleepiness, dizziness, incoordination, *seizures,* confusion, insomnia, headache, vertigo, fatigue, restlessness, tremor, nervousness.
CV: palpitations, hypotension, tachycardia.
EENT: diplopia, blurred vision, nasal congestion, tinnitus.
GI: dry mouth, nausea, epigastric distress, vomiting, diarrhea, constipation, anorexia.
GU: dysuria, urine retention, urinary frequency, early menses.
Hematologic: *thrombocytopenia, agranulocytosis,* hemolytic anemia.
Respiratory: thickening of bronchial secretions.
Skin: urticaria, photosensitivity, rash.
Other: *anaphylactic shock.*

INTERACTIONS
Drug-drug. *CNS depressants:* May increase sedation. Use together cautiously.
MAO inhibitors: May increase anticholinergic effects. Avoid using together.
Other products that contain diphenhydramine (including topical therapy): May increase risk of adverse reactions. Avoid using together.
Drug-lifestyle. *Alcohol use:* May increase CNS depression. Discourage use together.
Sun exposure: May cause photosensitivity reactions. Advise patient to avoid extensive sunlight exposure.

EFFECTS ON LAB TEST RESULTS
• May decrease Hb level and hematocrit.
• May decrease granulocyte and platelet counts.
• May prevent, reduce, or mask positive result in diagnostic skin test.
• May produce false-positives in urine detection of methadone and phencyclidine (PCP) and in serum TCA screens.

CONTRAINDICATIONS & CAUTIONS
• Contraindicated in patients hypersensitive to drug and other similar antihistamines; newborns; premature neonates; patients with angle-closure glaucoma, stenosing peptic ulcer, symptomatic prostatic hyperplasia, bladder neck obstruction, or pyloroduodenal obstruction; and those having an acute asthmatic attack.
• Avoid use in patients taking MAO inhibitors.
• Use with caution in patients with prostatic hyperplasia, asthma, COPD, increased IOP, hyperthyroidism, CV disease, and hypertension.
• Children younger than age 12 should use drug only as directed by prescriber.
Dialyzable drug: Unlikely.
⚠ *Overdose S&S:* Dry mouth, fixed or dilated pupils, flushing, GI symptoms.

PREGNANCY-LACTATION-REPRODUCTION
• There are no adequate well-controlled studies in pregnant women. Use during pregnancy only if clearly needed.
• Drug appears in breast milk. Contraindicated in breast-feeding women.

NURSING CONSIDERATIONS
• Stop drug 4 days before diagnostic skin testing.
• Injection form is for I.V. or I.M. administration only.
• Dizziness, excessive sedation, syncope, toxicity, paradoxical stimulation, and hypotension are more likely to occur in elderly patients.
• *Look alike–sound alike:* Don't confuse diphenhydramine with dimenhydrinate. Don't confuse Benadryl with Bentyl or benazepril.

PATIENT TEACHING

- Warn patient not to take this drug with any other products that contain diphenhydramine (including topical therapy) because of increased adverse reactions.
- Instruct patient to take drug 30 minutes before travel to prevent motion sickness.
- Tell patient to take diphenhydramine with food or milk to reduce GI distress.
- Warn patient to avoid alcohol and hazardous activities that require alertness until CNS effects of drug are known.
- Inform patient that sugarless gum, hard candy, or ice chips may relieve dry mouth.
- Tell patient to notify prescriber if tolerance develops because a different antihistamine may need to be prescribed.
- Drug is in many OTC sleep and cold products. Advise patient to consult prescriber before using these products.
- Warn patient of possible photosensitivity reactions. Advise use of a sunblock.

dipyridamole
dye-peer-IH-duh-mohl

Persantine

Therapeutic class: Antiplatelet drugs
Pharmacologic class: Pyrimidine analogues

AVAILABLE FORMS
Injection: 5 mg/mL in 2-mL, 10-mL vials
Tablets: 25 mg, 50 mg, 75 mg

INDICATIONS & DOSAGES
➤ **To inhibit platelet adhesion in prosthetic heart valves (given together with warfarin)**
Adults and children older than age 12: 75 to 100 mg P.O. q.i.d.
➤ **Alternative to exercise in evaluation of CAD during thallium myocardial perfusion scintigraphy**
Adults: 0.57 mg/kg (total dose) as an I.V. infusion at a constant rate over 4 minutes (0.142 mg/kg/minute).

ADMINISTRATION
P.O.
- If GI distress develops, give drug 1 hour before meals or with meals.

I.V.
▼ For use as a diagnostic drug, dilute in half-NSS, NSS, or D₅W in at least a 1:2 ratio for a total volume of 20 to 50 mL.
▼ Inject thallium-201 within 5 minutes after completing the 4-minute dipyridamole infusion.
▼ Don't mix in same syringe or infusion container with other drugs.
▼ **Incompatibilities:** Other drugs.

ACTION
May involve drug's ability to increase adenosine, which is a coronary vasodilator and platelet aggregation inhibitor.

Route	Onset	Peak	Duration
P.O.	Unknown	75 min	Unknown
I.V.	Unknown	2 min	Unknown

Half-life: 1 to 12 hours; alpha half-life of oral form, 40 minutes; beta half-life of oral form, 10 hours.

ADVERSE REACTIONS
CNS: dizziness, headache, fatigue.
CV: angina pectoris, chest pain, *ECG abnormalities,* flushing, hypotension, hypertension.
GI: nausea, abdominal distress, diarrhea, vomiting.
Skin: rash, pruritus.

INTERACTIONS
Drug-drug. *Adenosine:* May increase levels and cardiac effects of adenosine. Adjust adenosine dose as needed.
Cholinesterase inhibitors: May counteract anticholinesterase effects and aggravate myasthenia gravis. Monitor patient.
Heparin: May increase risk of bleeding. Monitor patient closely.
Theophylline, other xanthine derivatives: May prevent coronary vasodilation by I.V. dipyridamole, causing a false-negative thallium-imaging result. Avoid using together.

EFFECTS ON LAB TEST RESULTS
- May increase liver enzyme levels.

CONTRAINDICATIONS & CAUTIONS
- Contraindicated in patients hypersensitive to drug.

Reactions in bold italics are *life-threatening*. Interactions may have a *rapid onset* or a ***delayed onset***.

- Use cautiously in patients with hypotension or severe CAD.
- **Alert:** I.V. drug is associated with cardiac death, fatal and nonfatal MI, ventricular fibrillation, symptomatic ventricular tachycardia, stroke, transient cerebral ischemia, seizures, anaphylactoid reaction, and bronchospasm.
- Patients with myasthenia gravis who are receiving cholinesterase inhibitors may experience worsening of their disease when exposed to the I.V. drug.

Dialyzable drug: Unlikely.

Overdose S&S: Hypotension, warm feeling, flushes, sweating, restlessness, weakness, dizziness, tachycardia.

PREGNANCY-LACTATION-REPRODUCTION
- There are no adequate well-controlled studies in pregnant women. Use during pregnancy only if clearly needed.
- Drug appears in breast milk. Use cautiously in breast-feeding women.

NURSING CONSIDERATIONS
- Observe for adverse reactions, especially with large doses. Monitor BP.
- Observe for signs and symptoms of bleeding; note prolonged bleeding time (especially with large doses or long-term therapy).
- The value of drug as part of an antithrombotic regimen is controversial; its use may not provide significantly better results than aspirin alone.
- Dipyridamole injection may contain tartrazine, which may cause allergic reactions in some patients.
- **Look alike–sound alike:** Don't confuse dipyridamole with disopyramide. Don't confuse Persantine with Periactin or bosentan.

PATIENT TEACHING
- Instruct patient to take drug exactly as prescribed.
- Tell patient to report adverse reactions promptly.
- Tell patient receiving drug I.V. to report discomfort at insertion site.

SAFETY ALERT!

DOBUTamine hydrochloride
DOE-byoo-ta-meen

Therapeutic class: Inotropes
Pharmacologic class: Adrenergics–beta₁ agonists

AVAILABLE FORMS
Dobutamine in 5% dextrose: 1 mg/mL (250 or 500 mg); 2 mg/mL (500 mg); 4 mg/mL (1,000 mg)
Injection: 12.5 mg/mL in 20-mL and 40-mL vials (parenteral)

INDICATIONS & DOSAGES
➤ **Increased cardiac output in short-term treatment of cardiac decompensation caused by depressed contractility, such as during refractory HF; adjunctive therapy in cardiac surgery**
Adults and children: 0.5 to 1 mcg/kg/minute I.V. infusion, titrating to optimum dosage of 2 to 20 mcg/kg/minute. Usual effective range to increase cardiac output is 2.5 to 10 mcg/kg/minute. Usual maximum dosage is 20 mcg/minute and, rarely, rates up to 40 mcg/kg/minute may be needed.

ADMINISTRATION
I.V.
▼ Before starting therapy, give a plasma volume expander to correct hypovolemia and a cardiac glycoside.
▼ Dilute concentrate before injecting. Compatible solutions include D_5W, $D_{10}W$, half-NSS or NSS for injection, lactated Ringer solution for injection, Isolyte-M with D_5W, Normosol-M in D_5W, and 20% Osmitrol.
▼ Diluting one vial (250 mg) with 1,000 mL of solution yields 250 mcg/mL. Diluting with 500 mL yields 500 mcg/mL. Diluting with 250 mL yields 1,000 mcg/mL.
▼ Oxidation may slightly discolor admixture. This doesn't indicate a significant loss of potency, provided drug is used within 24 hours of reconstitution.
▼ Don't administer unless solution is clear and container is undamaged.

▼ Give through a central venous catheter or large peripheral vein using an infusion pump.

▼ Titrate rate according to patient's condition.

▼ Infusions lasting up to 72 hours produce no more adverse effects than shorter infusions.

▼ Watch for irritation and infiltration; extravasation can cause tissue damage and necrosis. Change I.V. sites regularly to avoid phlebitis.

▼ Solution remains stable for 24 hours. Don't freeze.

▼ **Incompatibilities:** Acyclovir, alkaline solutions, alteplase, aminophylline, bretylium, bumetanide, calcium chloride, calcium gluconate, cefazolin, cefepime, diazepam, digoxin, ethacrynate, furosemide, heparin, hydrocortisone sodium succinate, indomethacin, insulin, magnesium sulfate, midazolam, penicillin, phenytoin, phytonadione, piperacillin–tazobactam, potassium chloride, sodium bicarbonate, thiopental, verapamil, warfarin. Don't give through same line with other drugs.

ACTION

Stimulates heart's $beta_1$ receptors to increase myocardial contractility and stroke volume. At therapeutic dosages, drug increases cardiac output by decreasing peripheral vascular resistance, reducing ventricular filling pressure, and facilitating AV node conduction.

Route	Onset	Peak	Duration
I.V.	1–2 min	10 min	<5 min after infusion

Half-life: 2 minutes.

ADVERSE REACTIONS

CNS: headache.

CV: hypertension, increased HR, angina, PVCs, phlebitis, nonspecific chest pain, palpitations, ventricular ectopy, hypotension.

GI: nausea, vomiting.

Respiratory: *asthma attack,* shortness of breath.

Other: *anaphylaxis,* hypersensitivity reactions.

INTERACTIONS

Drug-drug. *Beta blockers:* May antagonize dobutamine effects. Avoid using together.

Bretylium: May increase risk of arrhythmias. Monitor ECG.

General anesthetics: May have greater risk of ventricular arrhythmias. Monitor ECG closely.

Guanethidine, oxytocic drugs: May increase pressor response, causing severe hypertension. Monitor BP closely.

Linezolid: May increase hypertensive effect of sympathomimetics. May need to decrease initial doses of dobutamine and titrate to effect.

TCAs: May potentiate pressor response and cause arrhythmias. Use together cautiously.

Drug-herb. *Rue:* May increase inotropic potential. Discourage use together.

EFFECTS ON LAB TEST RESULTS

● May decrease potassium level.
● May decrease platelet count.

CONTRAINDICATIONS & CAUTIONS

● Contraindicated in patients hypersensitive to drug or its components and in those with idiopathic hypertrophic subaortic stenosis.

● Use cautiously in patients with history of hypertension because drug may increase pressor response.

● Use cautiously after acute MI.

● Use cautiously in patients with history of sulfite sensitivity. Anaphylaxis or asthmatic episodes can occur.

Dialyzable drug: Unknown.

⚠ **Overdose S&S:** Anorexia, nausea, vomiting, tremor, anxiety, palpitations, headache, shortness of breath, anginal and nonspecific chest pain, hypertension, tachyarrhythmias, myocardial ischemia, ventricular fibrillation, hypotension.

PREGNANCY-LACTATION-REPRODUCTION

● There are no adequate well-controlled studies in pregnant women. Use during pregnancy only if clearly needed and potential benefit justifies potential risk to the fetus.

● It isn't known if drug appears in breast milk. Use cautiously in breast-feeding women or breast-feeding could be discontinued during therapy.

NURSING CONSIDERATIONS

🔔 *Alert:* Because drug increases AV node conduction, patients with atrial fibrillation may develop a rapid ventricular rate.

• Continuously monitor ECG, BP, pulmonary artery wedge pressure, cardiac output, and urine output.

• Correct hypovolemia before therapy.

• Monitor electrolyte levels. Drug may lower potassium level.

• *Look alike–sound alike:* Don't confuse dobutamine with dopamine.

PATIENT TEACHING

• Tell patient to report all adverse reactions promptly, especially labored breathing, angina, palpitations, dizziness, and drug-induced headache.

• Instruct patient to report discomfort at I.V. insertion site.

SAFETY ALERT!

docetaxel
dohs-eh-TAX-ell

Docefrez*, Taxotere*

Therapeutic class: Antineoplastics
Pharmacologic class: Taxoids

AVAILABLE FORMS
Injection: 20 mg*, 80 mg*, 140 mg*, 160 mg*, 200 mg* in single-dose vials

INDICATIONS & DOSAGES
➤ **Locally advanced or metastatic breast cancer after failure of previous chemotherapy**
Adults: 60 to 100 mg/m^2 I.V. over 1 hour every 3 weeks.
Adjust-a-dose: In patients receiving 100 mg/m^2 who experience febrile neutropenia, neutrophil count of less than 500/mm^3 for longer than 1 week, severe or cumulative cutaneous reactions, or severe peripheral neuropathy, reduce subsequent dose by 25%, to 75 mg/m^2. In patients who continue to experience reactions with decreased dose, either decrease it further to 55 mg/m^2 or stop drug.

➤ **Adjuvant postsurgery treatment of operable, node-positive breast cancer (excluding Docefrez)**
Adults: 75 mg/m^2 I.V. as a 1-hour infusion given 1 hour after doxorubicin 50 mg/m^2 and cyclophosphamide 500 mg/m^2 every 3 weeks for six cycles.
Adjust-a-dose: Patients who experience febrile neutropenia should receive granulocyte colony-stimulating factor (G-CSF) in all subsequent cycles. If febrile neutropenia doesn't resolve, continue G-CSF and reduce docetaxel dose to 60 mg/m^2. For patients who experience severe or cumulative cutaneous reactions or moderate neurosensory signs and symptoms, reduce dose to 60 mg/m^2. If these reactions persist at the reduced dosage, stop treatment.

➤ **Locally advanced or metastatic non–small-cell lung cancer (NSCLC) after failure of previous cisplatin-based chemotherapy**
Adults: 75 mg/m^2 I.V. over 1 hour every 3 weeks.
Adjust-a-dose: In patients who experience febrile neutropenia, neutrophil count of less than 500/mm^3 for longer than 1 week, severe or cumulative cutaneous reactions, or other grade 3 or 4 nonhematologic toxicities, withhold drug until toxicity resolves; then restart at 55 mg/m^2. In patients in whom peripheral neuropathy of grade 3 or above develops, stop drug.

➤ **With cisplatin, unresectable, locally advanced, or metastatic NSCLC not previously treated with chemotherapy (excluding Docefrez)**
Adults: 75 mg/m^2 docetaxel I.V. over 1 hour, immediately followed by cisplatin 75 mg/m^2 I.V. over 30 to 60 minutes every 3 weeks.
Adjust-a-dose: In patients whose lowest platelet count during the previous course of therapy was less than 25,000/mm^3, and those with febrile neutropenia or serious nonhematologic toxicities, decrease docetaxel dosage to 65 mg/m^2. For patients who require a further dosage reduction, a dosage of 50 mg/m^2 is recommended. For cisplatin dosage adjustments, see manufacturers' prescribing information.

➤ **Androgen-independent metastatic prostate cancer, with prednisone**

Adults: 75 mg/m² I.V., as a 1-hour infusion every 3 weeks, given with 5 mg prednisone P.O. b.i.d. continuously. Premedicate with dexamethasone 8 mg P.O. at 12 hours, 3 hours, and 1 hour before docetaxel infusion.

Adjust-a-dose: In patients who experience febrile neutropenia, neutrophil count less than 500/mm³ for more than 1 week, severe or cumulative cutaneous reactions, or moderate neurosensory signs or symptoms, reduce subsequent dose to 60 mg/m². In patients who continue to experience reactions with the decreased dose, stop treatment.

➤ **Advanced gastric adenocarcinoma, in combination with cisplatin and 5-FU (excluding Docefrez)**

Adults: Premedicate with antiemetics and hydration per cisplatin recommendations. Give 75 mg/m² docetaxel I.V. over 1 hour, followed by cisplatin 75 mg/m² I.V. over 1 to 3 hours both on day 1 only, then 5-FU 750 mg/m² I.V. daily as a 24-hour continuous infusion for 5 days beginning at the end of cisplatin infusion. Repeat cycle every 3 weeks.

Adjust-a-dose: Patients who experience febrile neutropenia should receive G-CSF in subsequent cycles. If episode recurs, reduce dose to 60 mg/m². If subsequent episodes of complicated neutropenia occur, reduce dose to 45 mg/m². In patients who experience grade 4 thrombocytopenia, reduce dosage to 60 mg/m². Don't re-treat until neutrophil count is greater than 1,500/mm³ and platelet count is greater than 100,000/mm³. Stop treatment if toxicity persists.

For patients who experience diarrhea, adjust dosage as follows: for first episode of grade 3 diarrhea, reduce 5-FU dose by 20%; for second episode, reduce docetaxel dose by 20%; for first episode of grade 4 diarrhea, reduce docetaxel and 5-FU doses by 20%; for second episode, stop drug.

For patients who experience stomatitis, adjust dosage as follows: for first episode of grade 3 stomatitis, reduce 5-FU dose by 20%; for second episode, stop 5-FU in subsequent cycles; for third episode, reduce docetaxel dose by 20%. For first episode of grade 4 stomatitis, stop 5-FU in subsequent cycles; for second episode, reduce docetaxel dose by 20%.

For patients who experience liver dysfunction, reduce docetaxel dose by 20%. If AST or ALT is greater than 5 × ULN or alkaline phosphatase is greater than 5 × ULN, stop treatment.

➤ **Induction treatment of inoperable locally advanced squamous cell cancer of the head and neck (SCCHN), with cisplatin and 5-FU (excluding Docefrez)**

Adults: 75 mg/m² I.V. infusion over 1 hour, followed by cisplatin 75 mg/m² I.V. infusion over 1 hour, on day 1, followed by 5-FU 750 mg/m² daily as a continuous I.V. infusion for 5 days. Repeat this regimen every 3 weeks for four cycles. After chemotherapy, patients should receive radiotherapy. Premedicate with antiemetics and appropriate hydration before and after giving cisplatin.

Adjust-a-dose: Use the same dosage adjustment schedule as for advanced gastric adenocarcinoma.

➤ **Induction treatment for locally advanced SCCHN with cisplatin and 5-FU before chemoradiotherapy (excluding Docefrez)**

Adults: 75 mg/m² I.V. infusion over 1 hour, followed by cisplatin 100 mg/m² I.V. infusion over 30 minutes to 3 hours on day 1, followed by 5-FU 1,000 mg/m² daily as a continuous I.V. infusion from day 1 to day 4. Repeat this regimen every 3 weeks for three cycles. After chemotherapy, patients should receive chemoradiotherapy. Premedicate with antiemetics and oral corticosteroids.

Adjust-a-dose: Use the same dosage adjustment schedule as for advanced gastric adenocarcinoma.

ADMINISTRATION

I.V.

▼ Wear gloves to prepare and give drug. If solution contacts skin, wash immediately and thoroughly with soap and water. If solution contacts mucous membranes, flush thoroughly with water.

▼ Dilute using supplied diluent. Let drug and diluent stand at room temperature for 5 minutes before mixing. After adding all the diluent to drug vial, gently rotate vial for about 45 seconds. Let solution stand for a few minutes so foam dissipates. All

---

Reactions in bold italics are *life-threatening*. Interactions may have a *rapid onset* or a *delayed onset*.

foam need not dissipate before preparing infusion solution.

▼ Prepare infusion solution by withdrawing needed amount of premixed solution from vial and injecting it into 250 mL NSS or D_5W to yield 0.3 to 0.74 mg/mL. Doses of more than 200 mg need a larger volume to stay below 0.74 mg/mL of drug. Mix infusion thoroughly by manual rotation.

▼ Prepare and store infusion solution in bottles (glass, polyolefin, or polypropylene) or plastic bags, and give through polyethylene-lined administration sets.

▼ Contact between undiluted concentrate and polyvinyl chloride equipment or devices isn't recommended.

▼ If solution isn't clear or if it contains precipitate, discard.

▼ The first dilution is stable for 8 hours. Use infusion solution within 4 hours.

▼ Infuse over 1 hour.

▼ Store unopened vials between 36° and 77° F (2° and 25° C).

▼ Mark all waste materials with CHEMOTHERAPY HAZARD labels.

▼ **Incompatibilities:** None reported.

ACTION

Promotes formation and stabilization of nonfunctional microtubules. This prevents mitosis and leads to cell death.

Route	Onset	Peak	Duration
I.V.	Rapid	Unknown	Unknown

Half-life: Alpha phase, 4 minutes; beta phase, 36 minutes; terminal phase, 11 hours.

ADVERSE REACTIONS

CNS: asthenia, paresthesia, peripheral neuropathy, weakness.
CV: fluid retention, peripheral edema, *arrhythmias,* chest tightness, flushing, hypotension.
EENT: altered hearing, tearing.
GI: anorexia, diarrhea, dysphagia, esophagitis, nausea, stomatitis, vomiting, dysgeusia.
Hematologic: *febrile neutropenia, leukopenia, myelosuppression, neutropenia, thrombocytopenia,* anemia.
Hepatic: *hepatotoxicity.*
Musculoskeletal: myalgia, arthralgia, back pain.

Respiratory: dyspnea, *pulmonary edema.*
Skin: alopecia, desquamation, skin eruptions, nail pigmentation alterations, nail pain, rash, reaction at injection site.
Other: infection, chills, drug fever, hypersensitivity reactions.

INTERACTIONS

Drug-drug. *Compounds that induce, inhibit, or are metabolized by CYP3A4 (cyclosporine, erythromycin, ketoconazole, troleandomycin):* May modify metabolism of docetaxel. Use together cautiously.
Ketoconazole or other CYP3A4 inhibitors: May increase docetaxel level and toxicity, including neutropenia: Monitor patient closely.

EFFECTS ON LAB TEST RESULTS

● May increase alkaline phosphatase, ALT, AST, and bilirubin levels. May decrease Hb level.
● May decrease platelet and WBC counts.

CONTRAINDICATIONS & CAUTIONS

● Contraindicated in patients severely hypersensitive to drug or to other forms containing polysorbate 80 and in those with neutrophil count below 1,500/mm³.
Black Box Warning Don't administer drug to patients with neutrophil counts less than 1,500/mm³. Perform frequent blood cell counts during therapy. ∎
Black Box Warning Treatment-related mortality increases in patients with abnormal liver function, those receiving higher doses, and patients with NSCLC and a history of prior treatment with platinum-based chemotherapy who receive docetaxel as a single agent at a dose of 100 mg/m². ∎
Black Box Warning Patients with severe hepatic impairment shouldn't receive this drug. Don't give drug to patients with bilirubin levels exceeding the ULN, or those with ALT or AST levels above $1\frac{1}{2} \times$ ULN and alkaline phosphatase levels above $2\frac{1}{2} \times$ ULN. Obtain bilirubin, AST or ALT, and alkaline phosphatase levels before each therapy cycle. ∎
Black Box Warning Contraindicated in patients with a history of hypersensitivity to polysorbate 80. Some dosage forms may contain polysorbate 80. ∎

❀Canada ◇OTC ◆Off-label use ✐Photoguide ⓓⓞDo not crush *Liquid contains alcohol.

- Safety and effectiveness in children haven't been established.
- Discontinue treatment if cystoid macular edema develops.

⊛ *Alert:* Some drug formulations may contain alcohol. Use cautiously in patients with hepatic impairment and in those in whom ethanol intake should be avoided or minimized. Some medications, such as pain relievers and sleep aids, may interact with the alcohol in the docetaxel infusion and worsen the intoxicating effects. A generic, nonalcoholic form of docetaxel is available.

Dialyzable drug: No.

⚠ *Overdose S&S:* Severe neutropenia, mild asthenia, cutaneous reactions, mild paresthesia, bone marrow suppression, peripheral neurotoxicity, mucositis.

PREGNANCY-LACTATION-REPRODUCTION

- Drug can cause fetal harm when used during pregnancy. Advise women of childbearing potential to avoid becoming pregnant during therapy.
- It isn't known if drug appears in breast milk. Patient should discontinue breastfeeding or discontinue drug, taking into account importance of drug to the mother.

NURSING CONSIDERATIONS

⊛ *Alert:* Drug should be administered only under the supervision of a physician experienced with antineoplastics and in a facility equipped to handle anaphylaxis.

- Give oral corticosteroid such as dexamethasone 16 mg P.O. (8 mg b.i.d.) daily for 3 days, starting 1 day before docetaxel administration, to reduce risk or severity of fluid retention and hypersensitivity reactions.
- Bone marrow toxicity is the most frequent and dose-limiting toxicity. Frequent blood count monitoring is needed during therapy.

Black Box Warning Monitor patient closely for hypersensitivity reactions, especially during first and second infusions. Severe and even fatal reactions have occurred in patients who have received recommended 3-day dexamethasone premedication. ∎

Black Box Warning Fluid retention is dose related and may be severe. Monitor patient closely. ∎

⊛ *Alert:* Evaluate patients for history of problems with alcohol or drinking, liver disease, or other conditions that may be affected by alcohol intake.

⊛ *Alert:* Monitor patients for signs and symptoms of alcohol intoxication during and after treatment (appearance of being drunk, confusion, stumbling, somnolence). Consider using formulation with lowest alcohol content for patients who experience adverse reactions. Slowing infusion rate during administration may help resolve signs and symptoms of alcohol intoxication.

⊛ *Alert:* When indicated, cisplatin dose should follow docetaxel dose.

- Monitor patient for vision changes. If they occur, patient should have a prompt, comprehensive eye examination.
- *Look alike–sound alike:* Don't confuse docetaxel with paclitaxel. Don't confuse Taxotere with Taxol.

PATIENT TEACHING

⊛ *Alert:* Caution patient to avoid driving, operating machinery, or performing other hazardous activities for 1 to 2 hours after treatment.

⊛ *Alert:* Instruct patient to immediately report signs and symptoms of alcohol intoxication that may occur during or 1 to 2 hours after treatment.

- Caution female patient of childbearing potential to avoid pregnancy or breastfeeding during therapy.
- Inform female patient of potential hazard to the fetus if drug is used during pregnancy, or if patient becomes pregnant during therapy.
- Remind patient that premedication with dexamethasone will be needed.
- Advise patient to report any pain or burning at injection site during or after administration.
- Warn patient that hair loss occurs in almost 80% of patients and reverses when treatment stops.
- Tell patient to promptly report sore throat, fever, or unusual bruising or bleeding, as well as signs and symptoms of fluid retention, such as swelling or shortness of breath.

D

dofetilide
doe-FE-ti-lyed

Tikosyn

Therapeutic class: Antiarrhythmics
Pharmacologic class: Antiarrhythmics

AVAILABLE FORMS
Capsules: 125 mcg, 250 mcg, 500 mcg

INDICATIONS & DOSAGES
➤ **To maintain normal sinus rhythm in patients with symptomatic atrial fibrillation or atrial flutter lasting longer than 1 week who have been converted to normal sinus rhythm; to convert atrial fibrillation and atrial flutter to normal sinus rhythm**
Adults: Individualized dosage based on CrCl and baseline QTc interval (or QT interval if HR is below 60 beats/minute), determined before first dose; usually 500 mcg P.O. b.i.d. for patients with CrCl greater than 60 mL/minute.
Adjust-a-dose: If CrCl is 40 to 60 mL/minute, starting dose is 250 mcg P.O. b.i.d.; if CrCl is 20 to 39 mL/minute, starting dose is 125 mcg P.O. b.i.d. Don't use drug at all if CrCl is less than 20 mL/minute.

Determine QTc interval 2 to 3 hours after first dose. If QTc interval has increased by more than 15% above baseline or if it's more than 500 msec (550 msec in patients with ventricular conduction abnormalities), adjust dosage as follows: If starting dose based on CrCl was 500 mcg P.O. b.i.d., give 250 mcg P.O. b.i.d. If starting dose based on CrCl was 250 mcg b.i.d., give 125 mcg b.i.d. If starting dose based on CrCl was 125 mcg b.i.d., give 125 mcg once a day.

Determine QTc interval 2 to 3 hours after each subsequent dose while patient is in hospital. If at any time after second dose the QTc interval exceeds 500 msec (550 msec in patients with ventricular conduction abnormalities), stop drug.

ADMINISTRATION
P.O.
• Give drug without regard for food or antacid administration.
• Don't give drug with grapefruit juice.

ACTION
Prolongs repolarization without affecting conduction velocity. Drug doesn't affect sodium channels, alpha-adrenergic receptors, or beta-adrenergic receptors.

Route	Onset	Peak	Duration
P.O.	Unknown	2–3 hr	Unknown

Half-life: 10 hours.

ADVERSE REACTIONS
CNS: headache, *stroke,* dizziness, insomnia, anxiety, migraine, cerebral ischemia, asthenia, paresthesia, syncope.
CV: chest pain, *ventricular fibrillation, ventricular tachycardia, torsades de pointes, AV block, heart block, bradycardia, cardiac arrest, MI,* bundle-branch block, angina, atrial fibrillation, hypertension, palpitations, edema.
GI: nausea, diarrhea, abdominal pain.
GU: UTI.
Hepatic: liver damage.
Musculoskeletal: back pain, arthralgia, facial paralysis.
Respiratory: respiratory tract infection, dyspnea, increased cough.
Skin: rash, sweating.
Other: *angioedema,* flulike syndrome, peripheral edema.

INTERACTIONS
Drug-drug. *Antiarrhythmics (classes I and III):* May increase dofetilide level. Withhold other antiarrhythmics for at least three plasma half-lives before giving dofetilide.
CYP3A4 inhibitors (amiodarone, **azole antifungals,** *cannabinoids, diltiazem,* **macrolides,** *nefazodone, norfloxacin, protease inhibitors, quinine, SSRIs, zafirlukast):* May decrease metabolism and increase dofetilide level. Use together cautiously.
Drugs secreted by renal tubular cationic transport (amiloride, metformin, triamterene): May increase dofetilide level. Use together cautiously; monitor patient for adverse effects.
Drugs that prolong QT interval: May increase risk of QT interval prolongation. Avoid using together.

Inhibitors of renal cationic secretion (cimetidine, ketoconazole, megestrol, prochlorperazine, sulfamethoxazole–trimethoprim), trimethoprim, verapamil: May increase dofetilide level. Use together is contraindicated.

Potassium-depleting diuretics: May increase risk of hypokalemia or hypomagnesemia. Monitor potassium and magnesium levels.

Thiazide diuretics: May cause hypokalemia and arrhythmias. Use together is contraindicated.

Drug-food. *Grapefruit juice:* May decrease hepatic metabolism and increase drug level. Discourage use together.

EFFECTS ON LAB TEST RESULTS
None reported.

CONTRAINDICATIONS & CAUTIONS
• Contraindicated in patients hypersensitive to drug, in those with congenital or acquired long QT interval syndromes or with baseline QTc interval greater than 440 msec (500 msec in patients with ventricular conduction abnormalities), and in those with CrCl less than 20 mL/minute.
• Use cautiously in patients with severe hepatic impairment.

Dialyzable drug: Unknown.

⚠ **Overdose S&S:** Prolonged QT interval, ventricular fibrillation, torsades de pointes, cardiac arrest.

PREGNANCY-LACTATION-REPRODUCTION
• There are no adequate well-controlled studies in pregnant women. Use during pregnancy only if clearly needed and potential benefit justifies potential risk to the fetus.
• It isn't known if drug appears in breast milk. Women shouldn't breast-feed while taking drug.

NURSING CONSIDERATIONS
Black Box Warning When dofetilide is initiated or reinitiated, patients should be hospitalized for a minimum of 3 days in a facility that can provide calculations of CrCl, continuous ECG monitoring, and cardiac resuscitation. Dofetilide is available only to hospitals and prescribers who have received appropriate education on dofetilide dosing and treatment initiation. ∎
• Don't discharge patient within 12 hours of conversion to normal sinus rhythm.
• Monitor patient for prolonged diarrhea, sweating, and vomiting. Report these signs to prescriber because electrolyte imbalance may increase potential for arrhythmia development.
• Monitor renal function and QTc interval every 3 months. Drug can cause torsades de pointes ventricular arrhythmia.
• Use of potassium-depleting diuretics may cause hypokalemia and hypomagnesemia, increasing the risk of torsades de pointes. Give dofetilide after potassium level reaches and stays in normal range.
• If patient doesn't convert to normal sinus rhythm within 24 hours of starting dofetilide, consider electrical conversion.
• Before starting dofetilide, stop previous antiarrhythmics while carefully monitoring patient for a minimum of three plasma half-lives. Don't give drug after amiodarone therapy until amiodarone level falls below 0.3 mcg/mL or until amiodarone has been stopped for at least 3 months.
• If dofetilide must be stopped to allow dosing with interacting drugs, allow at least 2 days before starting other drug therapy.

PATIENT TEACHING
• Tell patient to report any change in OTC drug, prescription drug, supplement, or herb use.
• Inform patient that drug can be taken without regard to meals or antacid administration.
• Tell patient to immediately report excessive or prolonged diarrhea, sweating, vomiting, or loss of appetite or thirst.
• Advise patient not to take drug with grapefruit juice.
• Advise patient to use antacids (aluminum and magnesium hydroxides) or acid suppressants, such as Zantac 75 mg, Pepcid, Prilosec, Axid, or Prevacid, instead of Tagamet HB if needed for ulcers or heartburn.
• Instruct patient to tell prescriber if she becomes pregnant.

• Advise patient not to breast-feed while taking dofetilide.
• If a dose is missed, tell patient not to double a dose but to skip that dose and take the next regularly scheduled dose.

dolasetron mesylate
doe-LAZ-e-tron

Anzemet

Therapeutic class: Antiemetics
Pharmacologic class: Selective serotonin receptor antagonists

AVAILABLE FORMS
Injection: 20 mg/mL
Tablets: 50 mg, 100 mg

INDICATIONS & DOSAGES
➤ **To prevent nausea and vomiting from cancer chemotherapy (P.O. only)**
Adults: 100 mg P.O. given as a single dose 1 hour before chemotherapy.
Children ages 2 to 16: 1.8 mg/kg P.O. given 1 hour before chemotherapy. Injectable formulation can be mixed with apple or apple-grape juice and given P.O. Maximum dose is 100 mg.
➤ **To prevent postoperative nausea and vomiting**
Adults: 12.5 mg as a single I.V. dose about 15 minutes before cessation of anesthesia.
Children ages 2 to 16: 1.2 mg/kg P.O. given within 2 hours before surgery, to maximum of 100 mg. I.V. form can be mixed with apple juice and given orally. Or 0.35 mg/kg, up to 12.5 mg, given as a single I.V. dose about 15 minutes before stopping anesthesia or as soon as nausea or vomiting starts.
➤ **Postoperative nausea and vomiting**
Adults: 12.5 mg as a single I.V. dose as soon as nausea or vomiting occurs.
Children ages 2 to 16: 0.35 mg/kg, to maximum dosage of 12.5 mg, given as a single I.V. dose as soon as nausea or vomiting occurs.

ADMINISTRATION
P.O.
• Mix injection for oral use in apple or apple-grape juice immediately before giving.
• Injection for oral use is stable in juice for 2 hours at room temperature.
I.V.
▼ Drug can be injected as rapidly as 100 mg over 30 seconds or diluted in 50 mL of compatible solution and infused over 15 minutes.
▼ Flush infusion line before and after administration.
▼ **Incompatibilities:** Other I.V. drugs.

ACTION
Blocks the action of serotonin and prevents serotonin from stimulating the vomiting reflex.

Route	Onset	Peak	Duration
P.O.	Rapid	1 hr	8 hr
I.V.	Rapid	36 min	7 hr

Half-life: 8 hours.

ADVERSE REACTIONS
CNS: headache, dizziness, drowsiness, fatigue, fever.
CV: *arrhythmias, bradycardia,* ECG changes, edema, hypertension, hypotension, tachycardia.
GI: diarrhea, abdominal pain, anorexia, constipation, dyspepsia.
GU: hematuria, polyuria, urine retention.
Skin: pruritus, rash, urticaria.
Other: chills, pain at injection site.

INTERACTIONS
Drug-drug. *Drugs that prolong ECG intervals (antiarrhythmics):* May increase risk of arrhythmia. Monitor patient closely.
Drugs that inhibit CYP enzymes (cimetidine): May increase level of hydrodolasetron, an active metabolite of dolasetron. Monitor patient for adverse effects.
Drugs that induce CYP enzymes (rifampin): May decrease level of hydrodolasetron, an active metabolite of dolasetron. Monitor patient for decreased effectiveness of antiemetic.

Serotonin antagonists (SNRIs, SSRIs): May cause serotonin syndrome. Monitor patient for signs and symptoms, including tremors, agitation, nausea, vomiting, incoordination, and seizures.

EFFECTS ON LAB TEST RESULTS
● May increase ALT and AST levels.
● May prolong PTT.

CONTRAINDICATIONS & CAUTIONS
● Contraindicated in patients hypersensitive to drug and in those with congenital long-QT syndrome.
⊕ *Alert:* Give with caution in patients who have or may develop prolonged cardiac conduction intervals, such as those with electrolyte abnormalities, history of arrhythmia, and history of cumulative high-dose anthracycline therapy.
⊕ *Alert:* Don't use injectable form in children and adults for the prevention of nausea and vomiting associated with cancer chemotherapy because of the increased risk of developing abnormal and sometimes fatal arrhythmias, including torsades de pointes. The tablet form, however, may be used for this indication.
● Drug isn't recommended for use in children younger than age 2.
Dialyzable drug: Unknown.
⚠ *Overdose S&S:* Hypotension; dizziness; prolonged PR, QRS, and QTc intervals.

PREGNANCY-LACTATION-REPRODUCTION
● There are no adequate well-controlled studies in pregnant women. Use during pregnancy only if clearly needed.
● It isn't known if drug appears in breast milk. Use cautiously in breast-feeding women.

NURSING CONSIDERATIONS
● Correct hypovolemia and hypomagnesemia before giving drug, and closely monitor electrolyte levels.
● Use ECG monitoring in elderly patients and in patients with HF, underlying heart disease, bradycardia, or renal impairment.
● Monitor patient for CV complications, such as heart block and tachyarrhythmias.
● *Look alike–sound alike:* Don't confuse Anzemet with Avandamet.

PATIENT TEACHING
● Tell patient about possible adverse effects, such as heart rhythm abnormalities and serotonin syndrome.
● Instruct patient to mix injection in juice for oral use immediately before giving.
● Tell patient to report nausea or vomiting.
● Tell patient to report a racing heartbeat, shortness of breath, dizziness, or fainting.

donepezil hydrochloride
doe-NEP-ah-zill

Aricept⌀, Aricept ODT

Therapeutic class: Anti-Alzheimer drugs
Pharmacologic class: Acetyl-cholinesterase inhibitors

AVAILABLE FORMS
ODTs ⓘ*:* 5 mg, 10 mg
Tablets ⓘ*:* 5 mg, 10 mg, 23 mg

INDICATIONS & DOSAGES
➤ **Mild to moderate Alzheimer dementia**
Adults: 5 or 10 mg P.O. once daily.
➤ **Moderate to severe Alzheimer disease**
Adults: Initially, 5 mg P.O. once daily for 4 to 6 weeks; dose may then be increased to 10 mg P.O. once daily. The dose may be increased to 23 mg P.O. once daily after patient has been taking 10 mg daily for 3 months.

ADMINISTRATION
P.O.
● Allow ODT to dissolve on tongue; then follow with water.
● Give drug at bedtime, without regard for food.
● Don't split or crush tablets.

ACTION
Thought to increase acetylcholine level by inhibiting cholinesterase enzyme, which causes acetylcholine hydrolysis.

Route	Onset	Peak	Duration
P.O.	Unknown	3–8 hr	Unknown

Half-life: 70 hours.

ADVERSE REACTIONS
CNS: headache, insomnia, *seizures,* dizziness, fatigue, depression, somnolence, syncope, pain, hallucinations.
CV: chest pain, hypertension, atrial fibrillation, hypotension, *bradycardia, heart block.*
EENT: cataract, blurred vision, eye irritation, sore throat.
GI: nausea, diarrhea, vomiting, anorexia, fecal incontinence, *GI bleeding,* weight loss.
GU: urinary incontinence, urinary frequency.
Metabolic: weight loss, dehydration.
Musculoskeletal: muscle cramps, arthritis, bone fracture.
Respiratory: dyspnea, bronchitis.
Skin: pruritus, urticaria, diaphoresis, ecchymoses.
Other: toothache, influenza, increased libido.

INTERACTIONS
Drug-drug. *Anticholinergics:* May decrease donepezil effects. Avoid using together.
Anticholinesterases, cholinomimetics: May have synergistic effect. Monitor patient closely.
Bethanechol, succinylcholine: May have additive effects. Monitor patient closely.
Carbamazepine, dexamethasone, phenobarbital, phenytoin, rifampin: May increase rate of donepezil elimination. Monitor patient.
Drugs that prolong QT interval: May increase risk of QT-interval prolongation. Monitor patient; consider therapy modification.
NSAIDs: May increase gastric acid secretions. Monitor for active or occult GI bleeding.

EFFECTS ON LAB TEST RESULTS
• May increase CK level.

CONTRAINDICATIONS & CAUTIONS
• Contraindicated in patients hypersensitive to drug or piperidine derivatives.
• Use cautiously in patients who take NSAIDs or have CV disease, are at risk for rhabdomyolysis and renal failure, or have asthma, obstructive pulmonary

disease, seizure disorders, urinary outflow impairment, GI bleeding, or history of ulcer disease.
Dialyzable drug: Unknown.
⚠ **Overdose S&S:** Severe nausea, vomiting, salivation, sweating, bradycardia, hypotension, respiratory depression, collapse, seizures, increasing muscle weakness.

PREGNANCY-LACTATION-REPRODUCTION
• There are no adequate well-controlled studies in pregnant women. Use during pregnancy only if clearly needed and potential benefit justifies potential risk to the fetus.
• It isn't known if drug appears in breast milk. Use cautiously in breast-feeding women.

NURSING CONSIDERATIONS
• Monitor patient for evidence of active or occult GI bleeding.
• Monitor patient for bradycardia because of potential for vagotonic effects.
• **Look alike–sound alike:** Don't confuse Aricept with Ascriptin.

PATIENT TEACHING
• Stress that drug doesn't alter underlying degenerative disease but can temporarily stabilize or relieve symptoms. Effectiveness depends on taking drug at regular intervals.
• Tell caregiver to give drug just before patient's bedtime.
• Tell patient and caregiver not to break or crush tablets.
• ODTs may be taken with or without food. Have patient allow tablet to dissolve on his tongue, then swallow with a sip of water.
• Advise patient and caregiver to report significant adverse effects or changes in overall health status immediately and to inform health care team that patient is taking drug before he receives anesthesia.
• Tell patient to avoid OTC cold or sleep remedies because of risk of increased anticholinergic effects.

DOPamine hydrochloride
DOE-pa-meen

Therapeutic class: Vasopressors
Pharmacologic class: Adrenergics

AVAILABLE FORMS
Injection: 40 mg/mL, 80 mg/mL,
160 mg/mL parenteral concentrate for
injection for I.V. infusion; 0.8 mg/mL
(200 or 400 mg) in D_5W; 1.6 mg/mL
(400 or 800 mg) in D_5W; 3.2 mg/mL
(800 mg) in D_5W parenteral injection for
I.V. infusion

INDICATIONS & DOSAGES
➤ **To treat shock and correct hemodynamic imbalances; to improve perfusion
to vital organs; to increase cardiac output; to correct hypotension**
Adults and children: Initially, 2 to
5 mcg/kg/minute by I.V. infusion. Titrate
dosage to desired hemodynamic or renal
response. Increase by 1 to 4 mcg/kg/minute
at 10- to 30-minute intervals. In seriously
ill patients, start with 5 mcg/kg/minute
and increase gradually in increments of
5 to 10 mcg/kg/minute to a rate of 20 to
50 mcg/kg/minute, as needed.
Adjust-a-dose: In patients with occlusive vascular disease, initial dose is
1 mcg/kg/minute or less. Initial dopamine
dosages shouldn't exceed one-tenth of the
usual dosage in patients who have received
MAO inhibitors within the prior 2 to
3 weeks.

ADMINISTRATION
I.V.
▼ Dilute with D_5W, NSS, D_5W in NSS
or half-NSS, lactated Ringer solution, or
D_5W in lactated Ringer solution. Mix just
before use.
▼ Use a central line or large vein, as in
the antecubital fossa, to minimize risk of
extravasation.
▼ Use a continuous infusion pump to
regulate flow rate. Avoid inadvertent administration of a bolus of the drug.
Black Box Warning Watch infusion site
carefully for extravasation; if it occurs,

stop infusion immediately and call prescriber. To prevent sloughing and necrosis
in ischemic areas, infiltrate the area with
5 to 10 mg phentolamine in 10 to 15 mL
NSS as soon as possible. ■
▼ Because solution will deteriorate rapidly,
discard after 24 hours or earlier if it's
discolored.
▼ **Incompatibilities:** Acyclovir sodium,
additives with dopamine and dextrose solution, alteplase, amphotericin B, cefepime,
furosemide, gentamicin, indomethacin
sodium trihydrate, iron salts, insulin, oxidizing agents, penicillin G potassium,
sodium bicarbonate or other alkaline solutions, thiopental. Don't mix other drugs in
I.V. container with dopamine.

ACTION
Stimulates dopaminergic and alpha and
beta receptors of the sympathetic nervous
system, resulting in a positive inotropic
effect and increased cardiac output. Action
is dose-related; large doses cause mainly
alpha stimulation.

Route	Onset	Peak	Duration
I.V.	5 min	Unknown	<10 min after infusion

Half-life: 2 minutes.

ADVERSE REACTIONS
CNS: headache, anxiety.
CV: hypotension, *ventricular arrhythmias
(high doses),* ectopic beats, tachycardia,
angina, palpitations, vasoconstriction.
GI: nausea, vomiting.
Metabolic: azotemia, hyperglycemia.
Respiratory: *asthmatic episodes,* dyspnea.
Skin: necrosis and tissue sloughing with
extravasation, piloerection.
Other: *anaphylactic reactions.*

INTERACTIONS
Drug-drug. *Alpha and beta blockers:* May
antagonize dopamine effects. Monitor
patient closely.
Diuretics (furosemide): May potentiate diuresis. Use together cautiously and monitor
fluid volume closely.
Ergot alkaloids: May cause extremely high
BP. Avoid using together.

Reactions in bold italics are *life-threatening*. Interactions may have a *rapid onset* or a ***delayed onset***.

Inhaled anesthetics: May increase risk of arrhythmias or hypertension. Monitor patient closely.

🕭 *Alert: MAO inhibitors (phenelzine, tranyl-cypromine):* May cause fever, hypertensive crisis, or severe headache. Avoid using to-gether; if patient received an MAO inhibitor in the past 2 to 3 weeks, initial dopamine dose is less than or equal to 10% of the usual dose.

Oxytocics: May cause severe, persistent hypertension. Use together cautiously.

Phenytoin: May cause severe hypotension, bradycardia, and cardiac arrest. Monitor patient carefully.

TCAs: May decrease pressor response. Monitor patient closely.

EFFECTS ON LAB TEST RESULTS
● May increase catecholamine, glucose, and urine urea levels.

CONTRAINDICATIONS & CAUTIONS
● Contraindicated in patients with uncor-rected tachyarrhythmias, pheochromocy-toma, or ventricular fibrillation.
● Use cautiously in patients with occlusive vascular disease, cold injuries, diabetic endarteritis, and arterial embolism; in those with a history of sulfite sensitivity; and in those taking MAO inhibitors.

Dialyzable drug: Unknown.

⚠ *Overdose S&S:* Excessive BP elevation.

PREGNANCY-LACTATION-REPRODUCTION
● There are no adequate well-controlled studies in pregnant women. Use during pregnancy only if potential benefit justifies potential risk to the fetus.
● If vasopressors are used to correct hy-potension or are added to a local anesthetic solution during labor or delivery, some oxytocics may cause severe persistent hy-pertension and may even cause rupture of a cerebral blood vessel during the postpartum period.
● It isn't known if drug appears in breast milk. Use cautiously in breast-feeding women.

NURSING CONSIDERATIONS
● Most patients receive less than 20 mcg/kg/minute. Doses of 0.5 to

2 mcg/kg/minute mainly stimulate dopamine receptors and dilate the renal vasculature. Doses of 2 to 10 mcg/kg/minute stimulate beta receptors for a positive in-otropic effect. Higher doses also stimulate alpha receptors, constricting blood vessels and increasing BP.
● Drug isn't a substitute for blood or fluid volume deficit. If deficit exists, replace fluid before giving vasopressors.
● During infusion, frequently monitor ECG, BP, cardiac output, central venous pressure, pulmonary artery wedge pressure, pulse rate, urine output, and color and temperature of limbs.
● If diastolic pressure rises disproportion-ately with a significant decrease in pulse pressure, decrease infusion rate and watch carefully for further evidence of predomi-nant vasoconstrictor activity, unless such an effect is desired.
● Observe patient closely for adverse re-actions; dosage may need to be adjusted or drug stopped.
● Check urine output often. If urine flow decreases without hypotension, notify pre-scriber because dosage may need to be reduced.

🕭 *Alert:* After drug is stopped, watch closely for sudden drop in BP. Taper dosage slowly to evaluate stability of BP.
● Acidosis decreases effectiveness of drug.
● *Look alike–sound alike:* Don't confuse dopamine with dobutamine.

PATIENT TEACHING
● Tell patient to report adverse reactions promptly.
● Instruct patient to immediately report discomfort at I.V. insertion site.

dorzolamide hydrochloride
dor-ZOLE-ah-mide

Trusopt

Therapeutic class: Antiglaucoma drugs
Pharmacologic class: Carbonic anhy-drase inhibitors–sulfonamides

AVAILABLE FORMS
Ophthalmic solution: 2%

INDICATIONS & DOSAGES
➤ **Increased IOP in patients with ocular hypertension or open-angle glaucoma**
Adults and children: One drop into conjunctival sac of each affected eye t.i.d.

ADMINISTRATION
Ophthalmic
• Don't touch tip of dropper to eye or surrounding tissue.
• Apply light finger pressure on lacrimal sac for 1 minute after instilling to minimize systemic absorption.
• If more than one ophthalmic drug is being used, give at least 5 minutes apart.
• Have patient remove contact lenses before administering drops; advise him to wait 15 minutes before reinserting.

ACTION
Decreases aqueous humor secretion, presumably by slowing the formation of bicarbonate ions. This reduces sodium and fluid transport, reducing IOP.

Route	Onset	Peak	Duration
Ophthalmic	Unknown	Unknown	8–12 hr

Half-life: 4 months.

ADVERSE REACTIONS
CNS: asthenia, fatigue, headache.
EENT: blurred vision; dryness; lacrimation; ocular allergic reaction; ocular burning, stinging, and discomfort; photophobia; superficial punctate keratitis; iridocyclitis.
GI: bitter taste, nausea.
GU: urolithiasis.
Skin: rash.

INTERACTIONS
Drug-drug. *Oral carbonic anhydrase inhibitors, salicylates:* May cause additive effects. Avoid using together.

EFFECTS ON LAB TEST RESULTS
None reported.

CONTRAINDICATIONS & CAUTIONS
• Contraindicated in patients hypersensitive to drug or its components.
• Use cautiously in patients hypersensitive to sulfonamides and in those with hepatic or renal impairment.

Dialyzable drug: Unknown.
⚠ **Overdose S&S:** Electrolyte imbalance, acidosis, CNS effects.

PREGNANCY-LACTATION-REPRODUCTION
• There are no adequate well-controlled studies in pregnant women. Use during pregnancy only if potential benefit justifies potential risk to the fetus.
• It isn't known if drug appears in breast milk. Patient should discontinue breastfeeding or discontinue drug, taking into account importance of drug to the mother.

NURSING CONSIDERATIONS
• Normal IOP is 10 to 21 mm Hg.
• Monitor patient who is hypersensitive to sulfonamides carefully. Drug may cause reactions similar to those seen with oral sulfonamides.
• Drug may be used with other topical ophthalmic drugs to lower IOP; separate drops by 5 minutes.

PATIENT TEACHING
• Teach patient how to instill drops. Advise him to wash hands before and after instillation, and warn him not to touch tip of dropper to eye or surrounding tissue.
• Tell patient that drug is a sulfonamide and, although it's given topically, it can be absorbed systemically. Advise patient to apply light finger pressure on lacrimal sac for 1 minute after drug instillation to minimize systemic absorption.
• Tell patient to stop drug and notify prescriber immediately if signs or symptoms of serious adverse reactions or hypersensitivity occur, including eye inflammation and eyelid reactions.
• Tell patient not to wear soft contact lenses during therapy. Contact lenses should be removed before instillation and may be reinserted 15 minutes after instillation.
• Stress importance of compliance with recommended therapy.
• Tell patient using more than one ophthalmic drug to allow at least 5 minutes between doses.

Reactions in bold italics are *life-threatening*. Interactions may have a *rapid onset* or a *delayed onset*.

doxazosin mesylate
dox-AY-zo-sin

Cardura⌀, Cardura XL

Therapeutic class: Antihypertensives
Pharmacologic class: Alpha blockers

AVAILABLE FORMS
Tablets (immediate-release): 1 mg, 2 mg, 4 mg, 8 mg
Tablets (extended-release) ⓓ*:* 4 mg, 8 mg

INDICATIONS & DOSAGES
➤ **Essential hypertension**
Adults: Initially, 1 mg immediate-release tablet P.O. daily; determine effect on standing and supine BP at 2 to 6 hours and 24 hours after dose. May increase to 2 mg and, thereafter, 4 mg and 8 mg once daily, if needed. Maximum daily dose is 16 mg, but doses over 4 mg daily increase the risk of adverse reactions. Don't use extended-release formulation to treat hypertension.
➤ **BPH**
Adults: Initially, 1 mg immediate-release tablet P.O. once daily in the morning or evening; may increase at 1- or 2-week intervals to 2 mg and, thereafter, 4 mg and 8 mg once daily, if needed. Or, one 4-mg extended-release tablet once daily with breakfast. May increase to 8 mg at 3- to 4-week intervals.

ADMINISTRATION
P.O.
• Patient should swallow extended-release tablets whole and not chew, divide, cut, or crush them.
• Give extended-release tablet with breakfast.
• Don't give evening dose the night before switching to extended-release tablets from immediate-release formula.

ACTION
An alpha blocker that acts on the peripheral vasculature to reduce peripheral vascular resistance and produce vasodilation. Drug also decreases smooth muscle tone in the prostate and bladder neck.

Route	Onset	Peak	Duration
P.O.	1–2 hr	2–3 hr	24 hr

Half-life: 19 to 22 hours.

ADVERSE REACTIONS
CNS: dizziness, asthenia, headache, vertigo, somnolence, drowsiness, pain.
CV: orthostatic hypotension, *arrhythmias,* hypotension, edema, palpitations, tachycardia.
EENT: rhinitis, pharyngitis, abnormal vision, dry mouth.
GI: nausea, vomiting, diarrhea, constipation.
GU: erectile dysfunction.
Hematologic: *leukopenia, neutropenia.*
Musculoskeletal: arthralgia, myalgia, back pain.
Respiratory: dyspnea.
Skin: rash, pruritus.

INTERACTIONS
Drug-drug. *Antihypertensives, diuretics:* May increase hypotensive effects. Adjust dosages as necessary.
Midodrine: May decrease the effectiveness of midodrine. Monitor patient for therapeutic effect.
PDE5 inhibitors (sildenafil, tadalafil, vardenafil): May cause additive hypotensive effects and symptomatic hypotension. Initiate PDE5 therapy at lowest possible dosage.
Drug-herb. *Butcher's broom:* May decrease effect of doxazosin. Discourage use together.
Ma huang: May decrease antihypertensive effects. Discourage use together.

EFFECTS ON LAB TEST RESULTS
• May decrease WBC and neutrophil counts.

CONTRAINDICATIONS & CAUTIONS
• Contraindicated in patients hypersensitive to drug and quinazoline derivatives (including prazosin and terazosin).
• Use cautiously in patients with impaired hepatic function.
• The 2014 guideline for the management of high BP in adults (Eighth Joint National Committee) doesn't recommend the use of doxazosin for the treatment of hypertension.

♣Canada   ◊OTC   ◆Off-label use   ⌀Photoguide   ⓓDo not crush   *Liquid contains alcohol.

However, according to the AHA/ACC/ASH 2015 scientific statement for the treatment of hypertension in patients with CAD, doxazosin should only be used if other drugs for hypertension and HF management don't achieve BP control at maximum tolerated doses.

● Rarely, drug has been associated with priapism (painful penile erection, sustained for hours and unrelieved by sexual intercourse or masturbation), which can lead to permanent erectile dysfunction if not promptly treated.

Dialyzable drug: No.

⚠ *Overdose S&S:* Hypotension.

PREGNANCY-LACTATION-REPRODUCTION
● There are no adequate well-controlled studies in pregnant women. Use during pregnancy only if clearly needed.
● Drug appears in breast milk. Use of extended-release form in breast-feeding women isn't recommended. Use immediate-release form cautiously.

NURSING CONSIDERATIONS
● Monitor BP closely.
● If syncope occurs, place patient in a recumbent position and treat supportively. A transient hypotensive response isn't considered a contraindication to continued therapy.
● Initial extended-release dose is 4 mg. If patient stops medication briefly, he should resume at 4-mg dose and titrate back to 8 mg if appropriate.
● Wait 3 to 4 weeks before increasing extended-release dose.
● *Look alike–sound alike:* Don't confuse doxazosin with doxapram, doxorubicin, or doxepin. Don't confuse Cardura with Coumadin, K-Dur, Cardene, or Cordarone.

PATIENT TEACHING
● Instruct patient to take drug exactly as prescribed.
◐ *Alert:* Advise patient that he is susceptible to a first-dose effect (marked low BP on standing up with dizziness or fainting). This is most common after first dose but also can occur during dosage adjustment or interruption of therapy.
● Advise patient to consult prescriber if dizziness or palpitations are bothersome.

● Advise patient to rise slowly from sitting or lying position.
● Advise patient to avoid driving and other hazardous activities until drug's effects are known.
● Inform male patient that drug has been associated with rare, but serious, priapism. Tell him to seek immediate medical treatment for a painful penile erection that's sustained for hours and unrelieved by sexual intercourse or masturbation because it can lead to permanent erectile dysfunction.

---

doxepin hydrochloride
DOKS-eh-pin

Silenor

Therapeutic class: Antidepressants
Pharmacologic class: TCAs

AVAILABLE FORMS
Capsules: 10 mg, 25 mg, 50 mg, 75 mg, 100 mg, 150 mg
Oral concentrate: 10 mg/mL
Tablets: 3 mg, 6 mg

INDICATIONS & DOSAGES
➤ **Depression; anxiety**
Adults: Initially, 75 mg P.O. daily. Usual dosage range is 75 to 150 mg daily to maximum of 300 mg daily in divided doses. Mild symptoms may require only 25 to 50 mg/day. Or, entire maintenance dose may be given once daily. Maximum dosage is 300 mg/day.
➤ **Insomnia (Silenor only)**
Adults: 3 to 6 mg P.O. once daily within 30 minutes of bedtime.
Adjust-a-dose: For elderly patients, give 3 mg P.O. once daily within 30 minutes of bedtime. May increase daily dose to 6 mg if indicated. For patients with hepatic impairment, initial dose is 3 mg P.O. once daily.

ADMINISTRATION
P.O.
● Dilute oral concentrate with 4 ounces (120 mL) of water, milk, or juice (orange, grapefruit, tomato, prune, or pineapple,

but not grape); don't mix preparation with carbonated beverages.
● Give at bedtime, if possible, because it may cause drowsiness and dizziness.
● Don't give Silenor within 3 hours of a meal.

ACTION

Unknown. Increases amount of norepinephrine, serotonin, or both in the CNS by blocking their reuptake by the presynaptic neurons.

Route	Onset	Peak	Duration
P.O.	Unknown	3½ hr	Unknown

Half-life: About 15 hours.

ADVERSE REACTIONS

CNS: drowsiness, dizziness, *seizures,* confusion, numbness, hallucinations, paresthesia, ataxia, weakness, headache, extrapyramidal reactions.
CV: orthostatic hypotension, tachycardia, ECG changes.
EENT: blurred vision, tinnitus.
GI: dry mouth, constipation, nausea, vomiting, anorexia.
GU: urine retention, change in libido.
Metabolic: *hypoglycemia,* hyperglycemia.
Skin: diaphoresis, rash, urticaria, photosensitivity reactions.
Other: hypersensitivity reactions, breast enlargement.

INTERACTIONS

Drug-drug. *Barbiturates, CNS depressants:* May enhance CNS depression. Avoid using together.
Cimetidine, **fluoxetine, fluvoxamine, paroxetine, sertraline:** May increase doxepin level. Monitor drug levels and patient for signs of toxicity.
Clonidine: May cause life-threatening hypertension. Avoid using together.
Drugs metabolized by CYP2D6 (cimetidine, flecainide, phenothiazines, propafenone, quinidine, sertraline, SSRIs): May increase doxepin level. Watch for signs and symptoms of toxicity.
Drugs that prolong QT interval (antiarrhythmics, clarithromycin, erythromycin, fluoroquinolones, ziprasidone): May

increase risk of arrhythmias. Avoid use together if possible.
Epinephrine, norepinephrine: May increase hypertensive effect. Use together cautiously.
Linezolid, methylene blue: May cause serotonin syndrome. Use with extreme caution and monitor closely.
MAO inhibitors: May cause severe excitation, hyperpyrexia, or seizures. Avoid using within 14 days of MAO inhibitor therapy.
Quinolones: May increase risk of life-threatening arrhythmias. Avoid use together.
Drug-herb. *Evening primrose oil:* May cause additive or synergistic effect, resulting in lower seizure threshold and increasing the risk of seizure. Discourage use together.
St. John's wort, SAM-e, yohimbe: May cause serotonin syndrome. Discourage use together.
Drug-lifestyle. *Alcohol use:* May enhance CNS depression. Discourage use together.
Sun exposure: May increase risk of photosensitivity reactions. Advise patient to avoid excessive sunlight exposure.

EFFECTS ON LAB TEST RESULTS

● May increase or decrease glucose level.
● May increase LFT values.

CONTRAINDICATIONS & CAUTIONS

● Contraindicated in patients hypersensitive to drug and in those with glaucoma or tendency toward urine retention; also contraindicated in those who have received an MAO inhibitor within past 14 days and during acute recovery phase of an MI.
Black Box Warning Doxepin isn't approved for use in children. Clinicians considering the use of doxepin in a child, adolescent, or young adult must balance risk with clinical need. ■
◔ Alert: Concomitant use with linezolid or methylene blue can cause serotonin syndrome (fever, mental status changes, muscle twitching, excessive sweating, shivering or shaking, diarrhea, loss of coordination). Use with linezolid or methylene blue only for life-threatening or urgent conditions when the potential benefits outweigh the risks of toxicity.
Dialyzable drug: No.
⚠ Overdose S&S: Cardiac arrhythmias, severe hypotension, seizures, CNS depression,

coma, confusion, disturbed concentration, transient visual hallucinations, dilated pupils, agitation, hyperactive reflexes, stupor, drowsiness, muscle rigidity, vomiting, hypothermia, hyperpyrexia.

PREGNANCY-LACTATION-REPRODUCTION

• There are no adequate well-controlled studies in pregnant women. Use during pregnancy only if clearly needed and potential benefit justifies potential risk to the fetus.
• Drug appears in breast milk. Use cautiously in breast-feeding women.

NURSING CONSIDERATIONS

• Don't withdraw drug abruptly; gradually taper dosage to minimize withdrawal symptoms.
• Monitor patient for nausea, headache, and malaise after abrupt withdrawal of long-term therapy; these symptoms don't indicate addiction.
• **Alert:** Because hypertensive episodes may occur during surgery in patients receiving drug, stop it gradually several days before surgery.
• **Alert:** If linezolid or methylene blue must be given, stop drug and monitor the patient for serotonin toxicity for 2 weeks, or until 24 hours after the last dose of methylene blue or linezolid, whichever comes first. Treatment may be resumed 24 hours after last dose of methylene blue or linezolid.
• If signs or symptoms of psychosis occur or increase, expect prescriber to reduce dosage. Record mood changes. Monitor patient for suicidal tendencies, and allow only a minimum supply of drug.
Black Box Warning Drug may increase risk of suicidal thinking and behavior in children, adolescents, and young adults ages 18 to 24, especially during the first few months of treatment, especially in those with major depressive disorder or other psychiatric disorder. ■
• Drug has strong anticholinergic effects and is one of the most sedating TCAs. Adverse anticholinergic effects can occur rapidly.
• Recommend use of sugarless hard candy or gum to relieve dry mouth.

• **Look alike–sound alike:** Don't confuse doxepin with doxazosin, digoxin, doxapram, or Doxidan.

PATIENT TEACHING

• **Alert:** Teach patient to recognize and immediately report symptoms of serotonin toxicity (fever, mental status changes, muscle twitching, excessive sweating, shivering or shaking, diarrhea, loss of coordination).
• Tell patient to dilute oral concentrate with 4 oz (120 mL) of water, milk, or juice (orange, grapefruit, tomato, prune, or pineapple, but not grape); preparation shouldn't be mixed with carbonated beverages.
Black Box Warning Advise families and caregivers to closely observe patient for increased suicidal thinking and behavior. ■
• Tell patient to take full dose at bedtime whenever he can, but warn him of possible morning dizziness on standing up quickly.
• Tell patient that, to minimize the potential for next-day effect, he should not take Silenor within 3 hours of a meal.
• Advise patient to consult prescriber before taking other prescription or OTC drugs.
• Warn patient to avoid hazardous activities that require alertness and good psychomotor coordination until effects of drug are known. Drowsiness and dizziness usually subside after a few weeks.
• Tell patient to avoid alcohol during drug therapy.
• Tell patient that maximal effect may not be evident for 2 to 3 weeks.
• Warn patient not to stop drug suddenly.
• To prevent sensitivity to the sun, advise patient to use sunblock, wear protective clothing, and avoid prolonged exposure to strong sunlight.

SAFETY ALERT!

DOXOrubicin hydrochloride
dox-oh-ROO-bi-sin

Therapeutic class: Antineoplastics
Pharmacologic class: Anthracycline glycoside antibiotics

AVAILABLE FORMS

Injection (preservative-free): 2 mg/mL
Powder for injection: 10 mg, 20 mg, 50 mg

INDICATIONS & DOSAGES

➤ **Bladder, breast, lung, ovarian, stomach, and thyroid cancers; non-Hodgkin lymphoma; Hodgkin lymphoma; acute lymphoblastic and myeloblastic leukemia; Wilms tumor; neuroblastoma; lymphoma; soft-tissue and bone sarcomas**
Adults and children: 60 to 75 mg/m^2 I.V. as single dose every 21 days, or when used in combination with other chemotherapy drugs, 40 to 75 mg/m^2 I.V. every 21 to 28 days.

Adjust-a-dose: Reduce dosage for patients with myelosuppression or impaired liver function. Lifetime cumulative dose shouldn't exceed 550 mg/m^2 (400 mg/m^2 for patients with chest irradiation) due to increased risk of cardiomyopathy. Elderly patients may need reduced dosages. Be prepared to decrease dosage if bilirubin level rises: Give 50% of dose when bilirubin level is 1.2 to 3 mg/dL; 25% when it's 3.1 to 5 mg/dL. Use is contraindicated in patients with severe hepatic impairment (Child-Pugh class C or bilirubin level above 5 mg/dL). Additional recommendations: Administer 75% of dose if transaminase levels are 2 to 3 × ULN and 50% of dose if transaminase levels are more than 3 × ULN.

ADMINISTRATION

I.V.

Black Box Warning Never give drug I.M. or subcutaneously. ∎

▼ Preparing and giving parenteral drug may be mutagenic, teratogenic, or carcinogenic. Follow facility policy to reduce risks.

▼ Reconstitute with preservative-free NSS for injection to yield 2 mg/mL; add 5 mL to 10-mg vial, 10 mL to 20-mg vial, or 25 mL to 50-mg vial. Shake vial to dissolve drug.

▼ Don't place I.V. catheter over joints or in limbs with poor venous or lymphatic drainage.

▼ Give by direct injection over 3 to 10 minutes into the tubing of a free-flowing I.V. solution containing D$_5$W or NSS for injection.

▼ Some protocols give doxorubicin as a prolonged infusion, which requires central venous access.

▼ If vein streaking proximal to the site of infusion or facial flushing occurs, slow administration rate. If welts appear, stop drug and notify prescriber.

Black Box Warning If extravasation occurs, stop infusion immediately, apply ice to the affected area, and notify prescriber. Extravasation can result in severe local tissue injury and necrosis requiring wide excision and skin grafting. ∎

▼ Refrigerated, reconstituted solution is stable 15 days; at room temperature, it's stable 7 days.

▼ **Incompatibilities:** Allopurinol, aluminum, aminophylline, bacteriostatic diluents, cefepime, dexamethasone sodium phosphate, diazepam, 5-FU, furosemide, ganciclovir, heparin sodium, hydrocortisone sodium succinate, piperacillin–tazobactam.

ACTION

May interfere with DNA-dependent RNA synthesis by intercalation.

Route	Onset	Peak	Duration
I.V.	Unknown	Unknown	Unknown

Half-life: Initial, 5 minutes; terminal, 20 to 48 hours.

ADVERSE REACTIONS

CV: cardiac depression, *arrhythmias, acute left ventricular failure, irreversible cardiomyopathy.*

GI: nausea, vomiting, diarrhea, stomatitis, esophagitis, anorexia.

GU: transient red urine.

Hematologic: *leukopenia, thrombocytopenia, myelosuppression.*

Metabolic: hyperuricemia.

Skin: severe cellulitis and tissue sloughing with drug extravasation, urticaria, facial flushing, complete alopecia within 3 to 4 weeks, hyperpigmentation of nail beds and dermal creases, radiation recall effect.

Other: chills, *anaphylaxis, secondary malignancy (acute myelogenous leukemia [AML], myelodysplastic syndrome).*

INTERACTIONS

Drug-drug. *Calcium channel blockers:* May increase cardiotoxic effects. Monitor patient's ECG closely.

Cyclosporine: May increase doxorubicin concentration. Monitor patient for toxicity.

Digoxin: May decrease digoxin level. Monitor digoxin level closely.

Fosphenytoin, phenytoin: May decrease level of phenytoin or fosphenytoin. Monitor drug level.

Paclitaxel: May decrease doxorubicin clearance. Monitor patient for toxicity.

Phenobarbital: May increase doxorubicin clearance. Monitor patient closely.

Progesterone: May enhance neutropenia and thrombocytopenia. Monitor patient and laboratory values closely.

Streptozocin: May increase and prolong doxorubicin level. Doxorubicin dosage may have to be adjusted.

Traztuzumab: May increase risk of cardiac abnormalities. Consider therapy modification.

Vaccines (inactivated): May diminish therapeutic effect of vaccines. If patient is vaccinated during therapy, revaccinate 3 months after stopping immunosuppressant.

Vaccines (live): May increase vaccine-related toxicities and decrease vaccine's therapeutic effects. Avoid use of live vaccines with immunosuppressants.

Drug-herb. *St. John's wort:* May decrease doxorubicin serum concentration. Avoid combination.

EFFECTS ON LAB TEST RESULTS
- May increase transaminase, bilirubin, and uric acid levels.
- May decrease platelet and WBC counts.

CONTRAINDICATIONS & CAUTIONS
- Contraindicated in patients with a history of sensitivity reactions to drug or its components.
- Contraindicated in patients with severe myocardial insufficiency, recent (past 4 to 6 weeks) MI, severe persistent drug-induced myelosuppression, or severe hepatic impairment (Child-Pugh class C or serum bilirubin level above 5 mg/dL).

Dialyzable drug: No.

PREGNANCY-LACTATION-REPRODUCTION
- May cause fetal harm if used during pregnancy. Female patients of reproductive potential and male patients with female

partners of reproductive potential should avoid pregnancy.
- Advise female patients of reproductive potential and male patients with female partners of reproductive potential to use effective nonhormonal contraception during and for 6 months after therapy ends.
- Drug appears in breast milk. Women shouldn't breast-feed during therapy.

NURSING CONSIDERATIONS
Black Box Warning Drug should be administered under the supervision of a physician experienced with cancer chemotherapeutic agents. ∎
- Perform cardiac function studies, including ECG and LVEF, before treatment and then periodically throughout therapy.
- Take preventive measures, including adequate hydration of the patient, before starting treatment. Rapid lysis of leukemic cells may cause hyperuricemia. Allopurinol may be ordered.
- Premedicate with antiemetic to reduce nausea.
- If skin or mucosal contact occurs, immediately wash with soap and water.

Black Box Warning Reduce dosage in patients with hepatic impairment. ∎
Black Box Warning Severe myelosuppression may occur, possibly resulting in hospitalization or death. ∎
Black Box Warning Risk of secondary AML or myelodysplastic syndrome increases with doxorubicin use, especially when given with DNA-damaging antineoplastics or radiotherapy, when patients have been heavily pretreated with cytotoxic drugs, when doses have been escalated, or when patients age 50 and older had an existing increased risk of secondary AML or myelodysplastic syndrome. Pediatric patients are also at risk for developing secondary AML. ∎
- Monitor CBC with differential and LFTs; monitor ECG monthly during therapy. If WBC count falls below 2,000/mm^3 or granulocyte count falls below 1,000/mm^3, follow institutional policy for infection control in immunocompromised patients.
- Monitor ECG for changes, such as sinus tachycardia, T-wave flattening, ST-segment depression, and voltage reduction.

• Leukopenia may occur during days 10 to 15, with recovery by day 21.

Black Box Warning Cardiomyopathy risk is proportional to the cumulative exposure, with incidence rates of 1% to 20% for cumulative doses ranging from 300 to 500 mg/m^2 when drug is given every 3 weeks. Cardiomyopathy risk is further increased with concomitant cardiotoxic therapy. Assess LVEF before, regularly during, and after doxorubicin treatment. ■

• If tachycardia develops, stop drug or slow rate of infusion, and notify prescriber.

Black Box Warning Myocardial toxicity, including acute left ventricular failure, may occur during therapy or months to years after termination of therapy. Assess LVEF regularly, during, and after treatment with doxorubicin. Pediatric patients are at increased risk for developing delayed cardiotoxicity. ■

⊎ Alert: If signs of HF develop, stop drug and notify prescriber. HF can often be prevented by increasing frequency of ECG assessments or multigated radionuclide angiography as the cumulative dose exceeds 300 mg/m^2 when patient is also receiving or has received cyclophosphamide, trastuzumab, or radiation therapy to cardiac area.

⊎ Alert: Reddish color of drug is similar to that of daunorubicin; don't confuse the two drugs.

• Esophagitis is common in patients who also have received radiation therapy.

⊎ Alert: If patient has previously received radiation therapy, he's susceptible to radiation recall effect.

• **Look alike–sound alike:** Don't confuse doxorubicin with doxorubicin liposomal, daunorubicin, or idarubicin.

PATIENT TEACHING

• Advise patient to report pain or burning at injection site during or after administration.

• Advise patient to watch for signs and symptoms of infection (fever, sore throat, fatigue) and bleeding (easy bruising, nosebleeds, bleeding gums, tarry stools) and to take temperature daily.

• Advise patient that orange to red urine for 1 to 2 days is normal and doesn't indicate presence of blood.

• Inform patient that hair loss may occur but that it's usually reversible. Hair may regrow 2 to 5 months after drug is stopped.

• Advise patient to take antiemetics on a regular basis to avoid nausea and vomiting.

SAFETY ALERT!

DOXOrubicin hydrochloride liposomal
dox-oh-ROO-bi-sin

Doxil

Therapeutic class: Antineoplastics
Pharmacologic class: Anthracycline glycoside antibiotics

AVAILABLE FORMS
Injection: 20 mg/10 mL, 50 mg/25 mL

INDICATIONS & DOSAGES
Adjust-a-dose (for all indications): Dosage modifications may be needed for stomatitis, myelosuppression, hand-foot syndrome, and other toxicities, based on toxicity grade (refer to manufacturer's instructions). Don't increase dosage after a dosage reduction for toxicity. Refer to manufacturer's directions.

Black Box Warning Don't exceed lifetime maximum cumulative dose of 550 mg/m^2 (400 mg/m^2 for adults having received mediastinal radiation or other cardiotoxic drugs). Prior use of other anthracyclines or anthracenediones should be included in calculations of total cumulative dosage. ■

➤ **Metastatic ovarian carcinoma refractory to both paclitaxel- and platinum-based chemotherapy regimens**
Women: 50 mg/m^2 I.V. initially at 1 mg/minute. If no infusion-related adverse reactions are observed, increase infusion rate to complete administration of the drug over 1 hour. Repeat treatment once every 28 days. Continue as long as condition doesn't progress, patient shows no evidence of cardiotoxicity, and patient continues to tolerate treatment.

➤ **AIDS-related Kaposi sarcoma refractory to previous combination chemotherapy and in patients intolerant of such therapy**

Adults: 20 mg/m^2 I.V. over 60 minutes once every 21 days. Initial rate should be 1 mg/minute to minimize infusion-related reactions. Continue as long as patient responds satisfactorily and tolerates treatment.

➤ **Multiple myeloma**
Adults: 30 mg/m^2 I.V. on day 4 following bortezomib, which is given at 1.3 mg/m^2 bolus on days 1, 4, 8, and 11 of each 21-day cycle. Initial rate of first dose of doxorubicin hydrochloride liposomal should be 1 mg/minute to minimize infusion-related reactions. If no infusion-related adverse reactions occur, increase infusion rate to complete administration over 1 hour. Treatment may continue for up to eight cycles, until disease progression or occurrence of unacceptable toxicity.

Adjust-a-dose: Dosage modifications may be necessary for toxicity when given in combination with bortezomib. Refer to manufacturer's directions.

➤ **Refractory metastatic breast cancer** ♦
Adults: 50 mg/m^2 I.V. over 1 hour every 4 weeks.

ADMINISTRATION

I.V.
▼ Don't give as an undiluted suspension or as an I.V. bolus. Don't give I.M. or subcutaneously.

▼ Follow procedures for proper handling and disposal of antineoplastics.

▼ Dilute doses up to 90 mg in 250 mL D$_5$W using aseptic technique. Dilute doses exceeding 90 mg in 500 mL D$_5$W.

❸ *Alert:* Carefully check label on I.V. bag before giving drug. Accidentally substituting doxorubicin hydrochloride liposomal for conventional doxorubicin hydrochloride may cause severe adverse reactions. The two products can't be substituted on a milligram-per-milligram basis.

▼ Don't use an in-line filter.

▼ Inspect product visually for particulate matter and discoloration before administration; don't use if a precipitate or foreign matter is present.

▼ Initiate infusion at 1 mg/minute and infuse over 60 minutes. Monitor patient carefully during infusion.

Black Box Warning Serious, sometimes fatal, allergic infusion reactions can

occur. Make sure emergency equipment and medications are available. Acute infusion-related reactions include flushing, shortness of breath, facial swelling, headache, chills, back pain, tightness in chest or throat, and hypotension. ■

▼ If extravasation occurs, stop infusion immediately and attempt to aspirate extravasated fluid before removing needle. Don't flush line or apply pressure to the site. Apply ice to the site intermittently for 15 minutes four times a day for 3 days. If extravasation is in an extremity, elevate the extremity. Restart infusion in another vein.

▼ Refrigerate diluted solution at 36° to 46° F (2° to 8° C) and give within 24 hours.

▼ **Incompatibilities:** Other I.V. drugs.

ACTION

Consists of doxorubicin hydrochloride encapsulated in liposomes. Action may involve drug's ability to bind DNA and inhibit nucleic acid synthesis.

Route	Onset	Peak	Duration
I.V.	Unknown	Unknown	Unknown

Half-life: 3.6 to 6.6 hours in first phase; 46.7 to 59.8 hours in second phase with doses of 10 to 20 mg/m^2.

ADVERSE REACTIONS

CNS: asthenia, paresthesia, headache, somnolence, dizziness, depression, insomnia, anxiety, malaise, emotional lability, fatigue, fever.
CV: chest pain, hypotension, tachycardia, peripheral edema, *cardiomyopathy, HF, arrhythmias,* pericardial effusion.
EENT: pharyngitis, rhinitis, conjunctivitis, retinitis, optic neuritis.
GI: nausea, vomiting, constipation, anorexia, diarrhea, abdominal pain, dyspepsia, oral candidiasis, enlarged abdomen, esophagitis, dysphagia, stomatitis, taste perversion, glossitis, secondary oral cancers.
Hematologic: *leukopenia, neutropenia, thrombocytopenia,* anemia.
Hepatic: hyperbilirubinemia.
Metabolic: dehydration, weight loss, *hypocalcemia,* hyperglycemia.
Musculoskeletal: myalgia, back pain.

Reactions in bold italics are *life-threatening*. Interactions may have a *rapid onset* or a *delayed onset*.

Respiratory: dyspnea, increased cough, pneumonia.

Skin: rash, alopecia, dry skin, pruritus, skin discoloration, skin disorder, exfoliative dermatitis, sweating, palmar–plantar erythrodysesthesia.

Other: allergic reaction, chills, herpes zoster, infection, infusion-related reactions.

INTERACTIONS

No formal drug interaction studies have been conducted. However, doxorubicin hydrochloride liposomal may interact with drugs that interact with conventional form of doxorubicin hydrochloride.

EFFECTS ON LAB TEST RESULTS

• May increase bilirubin and glucose levels. May decrease calcium and Hb levels.
• May prolong PT and increase INR. May decrease neutrophil, platelet, and WBC counts.

CONTRAINDICATIONS & CAUTIONS

• Contraindicated in patients hypersensitive to conventional formulation of doxorubicin hydrochloride or any component of the liposomal form.

Black Box Warning May cause myocardial damage, including HF, as the total cumulative doxorubicin dose approaches 550 mg/m^2. Risk of cardiomyopathy may be increased at lower cumulative doses in patients with prior mediastinal irradiation. ■

Black Box Warning Prior use of other anthracyclines or anthracenediones should be included in calculations of total cumulative dosage. ■

• Risk of cardiomyopathy with doxorubicin is generally proportional to the cumulative exposure, although the relationship between cumulative doxorubicin liposomal dose and risk of cardiotoxicity isn't known. Anthracycline-induced cardiotoxicity may be delayed (after discontinuation of anthracycline treatment).

Dialyzable drug: Unknown.

⚠ **Overdose S&S:** Leukopenia, mucositis, thrombocytopenia.

PREGNANCY-LACTATION-REPRODUCTION

• Drug may cause fetal harm if used during pregnancy. Female patients of reproductive potential and male patients with female partners of reproductive potential should use effective contraception during therapy and for 6 months after therapy ends.

• Drug appears in breast milk. Women should discontinue breast-feeding during treatment.

• Drug may damage spermatozoa and testicular tissue in males and may result in oligospermia, azoospermia, and permanent loss of fertility. May cause amenorrhea, infertility, and premature menopause in females. Recovery of menses and ovulation is related to age at time of treatment.

NURSING CONSIDERATIONS

• Consider previous or current therapy with related compounds such as daunorubicin when calculating total dose of drug to be given. HF and cardiomyopathy may occur after therapy ends.

• Assess left ventricular cardiac function (multigated radionuclide angiogram scan or echocardiogram) before drug initiation, during treatment to detect acute changes, and after treatment to detect delayed cardiotoxicity.

• Give drug to patient with history of CV disease only when benefit outweighs risk to patient.

⊛ **Alert:** Monitor patient for signs and symptoms of hand-foot syndrome, hematologic toxicity, and stomatitis. These adverse reactions may be managed with dosage delays and adjustments.

⊛ **Alert:** If an infusion-related reaction occurs, temporarily stop drug until resolution, then resume at a reduced infusion rate. Discontinue infusion for serious or life-threatening reactions.

• Evaluate patient's hepatic function before therapy, and reduce dosage for serum bilirubin level of 1.2 mg/dL or higher.

• Drug may increase toxicity of other antineoplastics.

• Closely monitor cardiac function by endomyocardial biopsy, echocardiography, or gated radionuclide scans. If results indicate possible cardiac injury, the benefit of continued therapy must be weighed against the risk of myocardial injury.

• Severe myelosuppression may occur.

• Monitor CBC, including platelets, before each dose and frequently throughout therapy. Leukopenia is usually transient. Persistent severe myelosuppression may result in superinfection or hemorrhage. Patient may need granulocyte colony-stimulating factor (or granulocyte-macrophage colony-stimulating factor) to support blood counts.

• Secondary oral cancers, primarily squamous cell carcinoma, have been reported during treatment and for up to 6 years after last dose in patients with long-term (more than 1 year) exposure to drug. Assess patients at regular intervals for the presence of oral ulceration or any oral discomfort that may indicate secondary oral cancer.

• Drug is cytotoxic. Follow applicable special handling and disposal procedures. Immediately wash thoroughly with soap and water if drug contacts skin or mucosa.

• **Look alike–sound alike:** Don't confuse doxorubicin with daunorubicin. Don't confuse Doxil with Paxil. Don't confuse regular formulation of doxorubicin with liposomal formulation.

PATIENT TEACHING

• Tell patient to notify prescriber if he experiences signs and symptoms of hand-foot syndrome (such as tingling or burning, redness, flaking, bothersome swelling, small blisters, or small sores on palms of hands or soles of feet).

• To reduce the risk of hand-foot syndrome, advise the patient to follow these guidelines at least 1 day before and for 3 to 5 days after treatment:

– Avoid direct sunlight and use sunblock SPF 15 or higher on all exposed skin.

– Wear loose clothing and comfortable, well-ventilated, low-heeled shoes.

– Avoid contact with hot water and take cool, short showers or baths.

– Don't put pressure on your skin. (Avoid kneeling, leaning on your elbows, wearing tight jewelry or undergarments, and chopping hard foods.)

• Advise patient to report signs and symptoms of mouth inflammation (such as painful redness, swelling, or sores in mouth).

• Warn patient to avoid exposure to people with infections. Tell patient to report temperature of 100.5° F (38° C) or higher.

• Tell patient to report nausea, vomiting, tiredness, weakness, rash, or mild hair loss.

• Advise female patient of childbearing potential to avoid pregnancy during therapy.

doxycycline
dox-i-SYE-kleen

Oracea

doxycycline calcium
Vibramycin

doxycycline hyclate
Acticlate, Acticlate Cap, Doryx, Doxy 100, Doxy 200, Periostat✦, Vibramycin

doxycycline monohydrate
Monodox, Vibramycin

Therapeutic class: Antibiotics
Pharmacologic class: Tetracyclines

AVAILABLE FORMS
doxycycline
Capsules: 40 mg, 50 mg, 75 mg, 100 mg, 150 mg
Injection: 100 mg/vial
Oral suspension: 25 mg/5 mL
Tablets: 50 mg, 75 mg, 100 mg, 150 mg
doxycycline calcium
Syrup: 50 mg/5 mL
doxycycline hyclate
Capsules: 50 mg, 100 mg
Capsules (coated pellets): 100 mg
Injection: 100 mg, 200 mg
Tablets: 20 mg, 100 mg
Tablets (delayed-release) ⊙**ℂ**: 50 mg, 75 mg, 100 mg, 150 mg, 200 mg
doxycycline monohydrate
Capsules: 50 mg, 75 mg, 100 mg
Oral suspension: 25 mg/5 mL
Tablets: 50 mg, 75 mg, 100 mg, 150 mg

INDICATIONS & DOSAGES
➤ **Infections caused by susceptible gram-positive and gram-negative organisms (including *Haemophilus ducreyi*,**

Yersinia pestis, and *Campylobacter fetus),*
Rickettsiae species, *Mycoplasma pneumo-*
niae, Chlamydia trachomatis, or *Borrelia*
burgdorferi (Lyme disease); psittacosis;
granuloma inguinale
Adults and children older than age 8 weigh-
ing at least 45 kg: 100 mg P.O. every
12 hours on first day; then 100 mg P.O. daily
as a single dose or in two divided doses. Or,
200 mg I.V. on first day in one or two infusions; then 100 to 200 mg I.V. daily. Daily
doses of 200 mg I.V. can be given as a single
dose or in two divided doses.
Children older than age 8 weighing less
than 45 kg: 4.4 mg/kg P.O. or I.V. daily, in
divided doses every 12 hours on first day;
then 2.2 to 4.4 mg/kg daily given as a single
dose or in two divided doses.

Give I.V. infusion slowly (minimum
1 hour). Infusion must be completed within
12 hours (within 6 hours in lactated Ringer
solution or dextrose 5% in lactated Ringer
solution).
➤ **Gonorrhea in patients allergic to**
penicillin
Adults: 100 mg P.O. b.i.d. for 7 days. Or,
300 mg P.O. once, followed in 1 hour with a
second 300-mg P.O. dose.
➤ **Syphilis in patients allergic to**
penicillin (except)
Adults: 100 mg P.O. b.i.d. for 14 days
(early). If more than 1-year duration,
100 mg P.O. b.i.d. for 4 weeks.
➤ **Primary or secondary syphilis in**
patients allergic to penicillin
Adults: 300 mg P.O. daily in divided doses
for 14 days.
➤ **Uncomplicated urethral, endocer-**
vical, or rectal infections caused by
C. trachomatis* or *Ureaplasma urealyticum
Adults: 100 mg P.O. b.i.d. for at least 7 days.
For acute epididymitis, use for 10 days.
➤ **To prevent malaria**
Adults: 100 mg P.O. daily beginning 1 to
2 days before travel to endemic area and
continued for 4 weeks after travel.
Children older than age 8: Give 2 mg/kg
P.O. once daily beginning 1 to 2 days before
travel to endemic area and continued for
4 weeks after travel. Don't exceed daily dose
of 100 mg.
➤ **Adjunct to other antibiotics for inhala-**
tion, GI, and oropharyngeal anthrax

Adults: 100 mg every 12 hours I.V. initially
until susceptibility test results are known.
Switch to 100 mg P.O. b.i.d. when appropriate. Treat for 60 days total.
Children older than age 8 weighing more
than 45 kg: 100 mg every 12 hours I.V.;
then switch to 100 mg P.O. b.i.d. when
appropriate. Treat for 60 days total.
Children older than age 8 weighing 45 kg
or less: 2.2 mg/kg every 12 hours I.V.; then
switch to 2.2 mg/kg (up to 100 mg) P.O.
b.i.d. when appropriate. Treat for 60 days
total.
Children age 8 and younger: 2.2 mg/kg I.V.
every 12 hours; then switch to 2.2 mg/kg
(up to 100 mg) P.O. b.i.d. when appropriate.
Treat for 60 days total.
➤ **Cutaneous anthrax**
Adults: 100 mg P.O. every 12 hours for
60 days.
Children older than age 8 weighing more
than 45 kg: 100 mg P.O. every 12 hours for
60 days.
Children older than age 8 weighing 45 kg
or less: 2.2 mg/kg (up to 100 mg) P.O. every
12 hours for 60 days.
Children age 8 and younger: 2.2 mg/kg (up
to 100 mg) P.O. every 12 hours for 60 days.
➤ **Adjunct to scaling and root planing to**
improve attachment and reduce pocket
depth in periodontitis
Adults: 20 mg Periostat P.O. b.i.d., more
than 1 hour before or 2 hours after the morning and evening meals and after scaling and
root planing. Effective for 9 months.
➤ **Inflammatory lesions of rosacea**
Adults: 40 mg Oracea P.O. once daily in
the morning, 1 hour before or 2 hours after
a meal. Give with a full glass of water.
Reevaluate treatment after 16 weeks.
➤ **Cervicitis** ◆
Adults: 100 mg P.O. b.i.d. for 7 days.

ADMINISTRATION
P.O.
● Obtain specimen for culture and sensitivity tests before giving. Begin therapy while
awaiting results.
🔆 *Alert:* Check expiration date. Outdated
or deteriorated tetracyclines may cause reversible nephrotoxicity (Fanconi syndrome).
● Give drug with food or milk if stomach
upset occurs.

• Increase fluid intake and don't administer tablets or capsules within 1 hour of bedtime because of possible esophageal irritation or ulceration.

• Give Oracea with a full glass of water.

• Don't crush delayed-release tablets or capsules. Delayed-released tablets and capsules can be carefully broken apart and their contents sprinkled onto a spoonful of applesauce and swallowed without chewing.

• Immediate-release tablets may be crushed and mixed with low-fat or chocolate milk, chocolate pudding, or apple juice mixed equally with sugar. Store mixtures in refrigerator (except apple juice mixture, which can be stored at room temperature) and discard after 24 hours.

I.V.

▼ Obtain specimen for culture and sensitivity tests before giving. Begin therapy while awaiting results.

▼ Reconstitute powder for injection with sterile water for injection. Use 10 mL in 100-mg vial and 20 mL in 200-mg vial. Further dilute solution to a concentration of 0.1 mg/mL to 1 mg/mL; don't infuse solution that contains more than 1 mg/mL. Refer to manufacturer's instructions for compatible solutions.

▼ Don't expose drug to light or heat. Protect it from sunlight during infusion.

▼ Infusion time varies with dose but usually ranges from 1 to 4 hours. Infusion must be completed within 12 hours.

▼ Monitor infusion site for evidence of thrombophlebitis.

▼ Reconstituted injectable solution is stable 72 hours if refrigerated and protected from light.

▼ **Incompatibilities:** Allopurinol, drugs that are unstable in acidic solutions (such as barbiturates), erythromycin lactobionate, heparin, meropenem, nafcillin, penicillin G potassium, piperacillin–tazobactam, riboflavin, sulfonamides.

ACTION

May exert bacteriostatic effect by binding to the 30S and possibly 50S ribosomal subunits of microorganisms and inhibiting protein synthesis. May also alter the cytoplasmic membrane of susceptible microorganisms.

Route	Onset	Peak	Duration
P.O.	Unknown	1½–4 hr	Unknown
P.O. (delayed-release)	Unknown	2–4 hr	Unknown
I.V.	Immediate	Unknown	Unknown

Half-life: About 1 day after multiple dosing.

ADVERSE REACTIONS

CNS: *intracranial hypertension,* headache.

CV: pericarditis, thrombophlebitis.

GI: diarrhea, epigastric distress, nausea, anorexia, glossitis, dysphagia, vomiting, oral candidiasis, enterocolitis, anogenital inflammation.

GU: vaginitis.

Hematologic: *neutropenia, thrombocytopenia,* eosinophilia, hemolytic anemia.

Musculoskeletal: bone growth retardation in children younger than age 8.

Skin: maculopapular and erythematous rashes, photosensitivity reactions, increased pigmentation, urticaria.

Other: *anaphylaxis,* hypersensitivity reactions, superinfection, permanent discoloration of teeth, enamel defects.

INTERACTIONS

Drug-drug. *Antacids and laxatives containing aluminum, magnesium, or calcium; antidiarrheals:* May decrease antibiotic absorption. Give antibiotic 1 hour before or 2 hours after these drugs.

Barbiturates, carbamazepine, phenobarbital, phenytoin, rifamycins: May decrease antibiotic effect. Consider therapy modification.

Ferrous sulfate and other iron products, zinc: May decrease antibiotic absorption. Give drug 2 hours before or 3 hours after iron.

Hormonal contraceptives: May decrease contraceptive effectiveness and increase risk of breakthrough bleeding. Advise use of a nonhormonal contraceptive.

Isotretinoin: May increase risk of pseudotumor cerebri. Avoid using together.

Methoxyflurane: May cause nephrotoxicity with tetracyclines. Avoid using together.

Oral anticoagulants: May increase anticoagulant effect. Monitor PT and INR, and adjust dosage.

Penicillins: May interfere with bactericidal action of penicillins. Avoid using together.

Reactions in bold italics are *life-threatening*. Interactions may have a *rapid onset* or a *delayed onset*.

Drug-lifestyle. *Alcohol use:* May decrease drug's effect. Discourage use together.
Sun exposure: May cause photosensitivity reactions. Advise patient to avoid excessive sunlight exposure.

EFFECTS ON LAB TEST RESULTS

- May increase BUN and liver enzyme levels. May decrease Hb level.
- May increase eosinophil count. May decrease platelet, neutrophil, and WBC counts.
- May falsely elevate fluorometric tests for urine catecholamines. May cause false-negative results in urine glucose tests using glucose oxidase reagent (Diastix or Chemstrip uG). Parenteral form may cause false-positive Clinitest results.

CONTRAINDICATIONS & CAUTIONS

- Contraindicated in patients hypersensitive to drug or other tetracyclines.
- Use cautiously in patients with impaired renal or hepatic function.
- CDAD has been reported and may range in severity from mild diarrhea to fatal colitis. If CDAD is suspected or confirmed, ongoing antibiotic use not directed against *Clostridium difficile* may need to be discontinued. Institute appropriate treatment.
- In a fetus in the last half of gestation or a child younger than age 8, drug may cause permanently discolored teeth, enamel defects, and bone growth retardation. Drug shouldn't be used in this age-group except for treatment of anthrax, unless other drugs aren't likely to be effective or are contraindicated.
Dialyzable drug: No.
⚠ **Overdose S&S:** Dizziness, nausea, vomiting.

PREGNANCY-LACTATION-REPRODUCTION

- Drug is generally considered a second-line antibiotic in pregnant women and use should be avoided. Use during pregnancy only when other drugs are contraindicated or ineffective. Contraindicated in second and third trimesters.
- In pregnant women and immunocompromised patients, use the usual dosage schedule for anthrax.

- Drug appears in breast milk. Patient should continue or discontinue breast-feeding, taking into account benefits versus risk of exposure to the infant.

NURSING CONSIDERATIONS

- If patient receives large doses or prolonged therapy or if patient is at high risk, watch for signs and symptoms of superinfection. If superinfection occurs, drug should be discontinued and appropriate therapy instituted.
- Cutaneous anthrax with signs of systemic involvement, extensive edema, or lesions on the head or neck requires I.V. therapy and a multidrug approach.
- Ciprofloxacin and doxycycline are first-line therapies for anthrax. If anthrax patient also has meningitis, ciprofloxacin is preferred because of better distribution to the CNS.
- Check patient's tongue for signs of fungal infection. Emphasize good oral hygiene.
- Photosensitivity reactions may occur within a few minutes to several hours after exposure and may last after therapy ends.
- ***Look alike–sound alike:*** Don't confuse doxycycline with doxylamine or dicyclomine. Don't confuse Oracea with Orencia.

PATIENT TEACHING

- Tell patient to take entire amount of drug exactly as prescribed, even after he feels better.
- Instruct patient to report adverse reactions promptly. If drug is being given I.V., tell him to report discomfort at I.V. site.
- Advise patient to take oral form of drug with food or milk if stomach upset occurs.
- Advise patient to increase fluid intake and not to take oral tablets or capsules within 1 hour of bedtime because of possible esophageal irritation or ulceration.
- Advise parent giving drug to a child that delayed-release tablets may not be crushed; however, immediate-release tablets may be crushed and mixed with low-fat or chocolate milk, chocolate pudding, or apple juice mixed equally with sugar. Tell parent to store mixtures in refrigerator (except apple juice mixture, which can be stored at room temperature) and to discard after 24 hours.

● Warn patient to avoid direct sunlight and ultraviolet light, wear protective clothing, and use sunscreen.
● Tell patient to report signs and symptoms of superinfection to prescriber.
● Tell patient taking Oracea to take drug with a full glass of water.

doxylamine succinate–pyridoxine hydrochloride
docks-ILL-ah-meen/peer-reh-DOCK-seen

Diclegis

Therapeutic class: Antiemetics
Pharmacologic class: Antihistamines–vitamin B$_6$ analogs

AVAILABLE FORMS
Tablets (delayed-release) ⒹⓄⒼ*:* doxylamine succinate 10 mg and pyridoxine hydrochloride 10 mg

INDICATIONS & DOSAGES
➤ **Nausea and vomiting of pregnancy in women who don't respond to conservative management**
Adults: Initially, doxylamine 20 mg and pyridoxine 20 mg at bedtime on day 1. If that dosage adequately controls symptoms the next day, continue taking at bedtime. If symptoms persist into the afternoon of day 2, patients should take doxylamine 20 mg and pyridoxine 20 mg at bedtime that night, then take doxylamine 10 mg and pyridoxine 10 mg in the morning and doxylamine 20 mg and pyridoxine 20 mg at bedtime on day 3. If that dosage adequately controls symptoms on day 4, patients should continue taking doxylamine 10 mg and pyridoxine 10 mg in the morning and doxylamine 20 mg and pyridoxine 20 mg at bedtime. Otherwise, they should take doxylamine 10 mg and pyridoxine 10 mg in the morning, doxylamine 10 mg and pyridoxine 10 mg midafternoon, and doxylamine 20 mg and pyridoxine 20 mg at bedtime on day 4.

ADMINISTRATION
P.O.
● Give tablets whole on an empty stomach with a glass of water. Don't crush, split, or allow patient to chew tablets.

● Patient should take tablets daily and not p.r.n.
● Store bottle at room temperature. Keep bottle tightly closed and protect from moisture. Don't remove desiccant canister from bottle.

ACTION
Unknown. The combination of antihistamine and vitamin B$_6$ may cause anticholinergic effects, decreasing nausea.

Route	Onset	Peak	Duration
P.O. (doxylamine)	Unknown	7½ hr	Unknown
P.O. (pyridoxine)	Unknown	5½ hr	Unknown

Half-life: Doxylamine, 12½ hours; pyridoxine, ½ hour.

ADVERSE REACTIONS
CNS: somnolence.

INTERACTIONS
Drug-drug. *CNS depressants (hypnotic sedatives and tranquilizers):* May have additive effects. Don't use together.
MAO inhibitors (selegiline, tranylcypromine): May prolong and intensify CNS anticholinergic effects. Use together is contraindicated.
Other ethanolamine derivative antihistamines (diphenhydramine): May have additive effects. Avoid use together.
Drug-food. *Any food:* May delay onset and reduce absorption if taken with food. Patient should take on an empty stomach with a glass of water.
Drug-lifestyle. *Alcohol use:* May cause additive CNS depression. Alcohol isn't recommended during pregnancy.

EFFECTS ON LAB TEST RESULTS
None reported.

CONTRAINDICATIONS & CAUTIONS
● Contraindicated in women hypersensitive to drug or its components.
● Contraindicated with MAO inhibitors.
● Use cautiously in patients with asthma, increased IOP, angle-closure glaucoma, stenosing peptic ulcer, or pyloroduodenal or urinary bladder neck obstruction because of anticholinergic effects.
Dialyzable drug: Unknown.

Reactions in bold italics are *life-threatening*. Interactions may have a *rapid onset* or a *delayed onset*.

⚠ **Overdose S&S:** Restlessness, dry mouth, dilated pupils, sleepiness, vertigo, mental confusion, tachycardia, seizures, rhabdomyolysis, acute renal failure, death.

PREGNANCY-LACTATION-REPRODUCTION
• Drug is intended for use in pregnant women. Drug hasn't been studied in women with hyperemesis gravidarum.
• Drug appears in breast milk. Women shouldn't breast-feed while taking drug.

NURSING CONSIDERATIONS
• Reassess for continued need for drug as the pregnancy progresses.
• Drug hasn't been studied in women with hyperemesis gravidarum.
• Monitor patient for anticholinergic effects (dry mouth, tachycardia, urine retention, constipation, ataxia).
• Monitor patient for somnolence, increased falls, and other CNS depressant effects.

PATIENT TEACHING
• Warn patient about side effects, including somnolence, increased falls, and other CNS depressant effects.
• Advise patient to avoid alcohol and sedating medications, including antihistamine cough and cold products, opioids, and sleep aids, while taking this drug because of increased risk of additive effects.
• Caution patient to avoid driving and operating heavy equipment or other activities that require complete mental alertness.

---

dronabinol (delta-9-tetrahydrocannabinol)
droe-NAB-i-nol

Marinol

Therapeutic class: Antiemetics
Pharmacologic class: Cannabinoids
Controlled substance schedule: III

AVAILABLE FORMS
Capsules: 2.5 mg, 5 mg, 10 mg

INDICATIONS & DOSAGES
➤ **Nausea and vomiting from cancer chemotherapy**

Adults and children: 5 mg/m^2 P.O. 1 to 3 hours before chemotherapy session. Then, 5 mg/m^2 every 2 to 4 hours after chemotherapy, for total of four to six doses/day. If needed, increase dosage in 2.5-mg/m^2 increments to maximum of 15 mg/m^2 per dose.

➤ **Anorexia and weight loss in patients with AIDS**
Adults: 2.5 mg P.O. b.i.d. before lunch and dinner. If patient can't tolerate twice-daily dosing, decrease to 2.5 mg P.O. given as a single dose daily in evening or at bedtime. May gradually increase to maximum of 20 mg daily given in divided doses.

ADMINISTRATION
P.O.
• Give 1 to 3 hours before chemotherapy.
• Store in cool environment, but protect from freezing.

ACTION
Unknown. A derivative of marijuana.

Route	Onset	Peak	Duration
P.O.	30–60 min	½–4 hr	4–6 hr (psychoactive effect); >24 hr (appetite stimulation)

Half-life: 1 to 1½ days.

ADVERSE REACTIONS
CNS: ataxia, dizziness, drowsiness, euphoria, paranoia, amnesia, asthenia, confusion, depersonalization, hallucinations, muddled thinking, somnolence.
CV: orthostatic hypotension, palpitations, tachycardia, vasodilation.
EENT: visual disturbances.
GI: abdominal pain, dry mouth, nausea, vomiting, diarrhea.

INTERACTIONS
Drug-drug. *CNS depressants, psychomimetic substances, sedatives:* May cause additive CNS depression. Avoid using together.
Drug-lifestyle. *Alcohol use:* May cause additive CNS depression. Discourage use together.

EFFECTS ON LAB TEST RESULTS
None reported.

CONTRAINDICATIONS & CAUTIONS
• Contraindicated in patients hypersensitive to sesame oil or cannabinoids.
• Use cautiously in children, elderly patients, and in those with heart disease, seizure disorders, psychiatric illness, or history of drug abuse.
Dialyzable drug: Unknown.
⚠ *Overdose S&S:* Mild—drowsiness, euphoria, heightened sensory awareness, altered time perception, reddened conjunctiva, dry mouth, tachycardia; moderate—memory impairment, depersonalization, mood alteration, urine retention, decreased bowel motility; severe—decreased motor coordination, lethargy, slurred speech, orthostatic hypotension.

PREGNANCY-LACTATION-REPRODUCTION
• There are no adequate well-controlled studies in pregnant women. Use during pregnancy only if potential benefit justifies potential risk to the fetus.
• Drug appears in breast milk. Use in breast-feeding women isn't recommended.

NURSING CONSIDERATIONS
• Expect drug to be prescribed only for patients who haven't responded satisfactorily to other antiemetics.
🖢 *Alert:* Drug is the principal active substance in *Cannabis sativa* (marijuana), which can produce both physiologic and psychological dependence and has a high risk of abuse. Use cautiously in patients receiving sedatives, hypnotics, or other psychoactive drugs.
• Monitor patient for hypotension, hypertension, syncope, and tachycardia.
• Monitor patient for worsening signs and symptoms of psychiatric illness.
• CNS effects are intensified at higher dosages.
• Drug effects may persist for days after treatment ends.
• *Look alike–sound alike:* Don't confuse dronabinol with droperidol.

PATIENT TEACHING
• Tell patient that drug may induce unusual changes in mood or other adverse behavioral effects.
• Advise patient against performing activities that require alertness until CNS effects of drug are known.
• Warn caregivers to supervise patient during and immediately after treatment.
• Advise patient to take drug 1 to 3 hours before chemotherapy.

dronedarone
dro-neh-DAR-rone

Multaq

Therapeutic class: Antiarrhythmics
Pharmacologic class: Benzofuran derivatives

AVAILABLE FORMS
Tablets: 400 mg

INDICATIONS & DOSAGES
➤ **To reduce risk of hospitalization in patients with recent episode of paroxysmal or persistent atrial fibrillation or flutter who have CV risk factors, such as age older than 70, diabetes, hypertension, stroke, left atrial diameter greater than 50 mm, or LVEF less than 40%, who are in normal sinus rhythm or who will be cardioverted**
Adults: 400 mg P.O. b.i.d.

ADMINISTRATION
P.O.
• Give drug with morning and evening meals.
• Don't give grapefruit juice to patient taking this drug.

ACTION
Unknown. Exhibits properties of all four Vaughan-Williams antiarrhythmic classes; it's unclear which of these is important in producing drug's clinical effects.

Route	Onset	Peak	Duration
P.O.	Unknown	3–6 hr	Unknown

Half-life: 13 to 19 hours.

ADVERSE REACTIONS
CNS: asthenia.
CV: *bradycardia, HF, QT interval prolongation.*

Reactions in bold italics are *life-threatening*. Interactions may have a *rapid onset* or a *delayed onset*.

GI: abdominal pain, diarrhea, dyspepsia, nausea, vomiting.
GU: prerenal azotemia, *acute renal failure,* elevated creatinine level.
Metabolic: hypovolemia.
Skin: allergic dermatitis, dermatitis, eczema, pruritus, rash.

INTERACTIONS
Drug-drug. *Beta blockers:* May cause bradycardia. Initially, give low dose of beta blocker and increase dosage only after monitoring ECG for tolerance.
Calcium channel blockers: May cause additive AV-blocking effects. Reduce initial dosage of calcium channel blocker; increase dosage only after monitoring ECG for tolerance.
CYP2C9 substrates (losartan, warfarin): May increase metabolite levels. Monitor patient closely; monitor INR in patient taking warfarin.
CYP3A inducers (carbamazepine, phenobarbital, phenytoin, rifampin): May decrease dronedarone level. Use together is contraindicated.
CYP3A inhibitors (clarithromycin, erythromycin, itraconazole, ketoconazole, ritonavir, voriconazole): May increase dronedarone level. Use together is contraindicated.
CYP3A substrates (sirolimus, tacrolimus): May increase levels of these drugs. Monitor drug levels.
Digoxin: May increase digoxin level and electrophysiologic effects of dronedarone. Avoid use together; if necessary to use together, decrease digoxin dosage by 50%.
Drugs that prolong QT interval (class I and III antiarrhythmics, macrolide antibiotics, phenothiazines, TCAs): May further increase QT interval, leading to torsades de pointes. Use together is contraindicated.
Statins: May increase statin level. Use together cautiously.
Drug-herb. *St John's wort:* May decrease drug level. Discourage use together.
Drug-lifestyle. *Grapefruit juice:* May increase drug level. Discourage use together.

EFFECTS ON LAB TEST RESULTS
• May increase serum creatinine level.

• May decrease potassium and magnesium levels (in patients taking potassium-depleting diuretics).

CONTRAINDICATIONS & CAUTIONS
Black Box Warning Contraindicated in patients with New York Heart Association class IV HF or class II to III HF with recent decompensation requiring hospitalization or referral to an HF clinic. ■
Black Box Warning Contraindicated in patients with atrial fibrillation who won't or can't be restored to normal sinus rhythm. Drug doubles risk of death, stroke, and hospitalization for HF in patients with permanent atrial fibrillation. ■
• Contraindicated in patients with second- or third-degree AV block or sick sinus syndrome (unless a functioning pacemaker is in place), bradycardia (less than 50 beats/minute), severe hepatic impairment, QTc interval of 500 msec or greater, or PR interval greater than 280 msec.
• Contraindicated with concomitant use of strong CYP3A inhibitors and drugs or herbal preparations that prolong QT interval.
❸ *Alert:* Discontinue class I or III antiarrhythmics, such as amiodarone, flecainide, propafenone, quinidine, disopyramide, dofetilide, and sotalol, and strong CYP3A inhibitors before starting drug.
❸ *Alert:* Drug may increase risk of severe hepatic injury or failure.
• Use cautiously in patients with new or worsening HF.
• Marked increase in serum creatinine level, prerenal azotemia, and acute renal failure, frequently in the setting of HF or hypovolemia, have been reported. Effects appear to be reversible upon drug discontinuation and with appropriate medical treatment. Monitor renal function periodically.
Dializable drug: Unknown.
⚠ *Overdose S&S:* QTc-interval prolongation.

PREGNANCY-LACTATION-REPRODUCTION
• Drug may cause fetal harm, and use in pregnant women is contraindicated. Women of childbearing potential should use effective birth control during therapy.

• It isn't known if drug appears in breast milk. Women should stop breast-feeding before using drug.

NURSING CONSIDERATIONS

• Potassium-depleting diuretics may cause hypokalemia and hypomagnesemia, increasing the risk of torsades de pointes. Initiate dronedarone therapy after potassium and magnesium levels reach and stay within normal range.
• Monitor CV status, ECG, and QTc interval routinely.
• Monitor renal function and electrolyte levels regularly.
• Monitor hepatic serum enzyme levels, especially during the first 6 months of therapy. Discontinue drug if hepatic injury is suspected.

PATIENT TEACHING

• Instruct patient to take drug with morning and evening meals.
• Tell patient to avoid grapefruit juice.
• Advise patient to report weight gain, dyspnea, fatigue, and peripheral edema, which may indicate worsening HF.
• Tell patient to report changes in OTC or prescription drug use, or in supplement or herb use.
• If patient misses a dose, tell patient not to double the dose but to skip that dose and take the next regularly scheduled dose.
• Instruct patient to report slowed heartbeat, diarrhea, nausea, vomiting, abdominal pain, indigestion, fatigue, or rash.
• Advise female patient of childbearing potential to use an effective method of birth control while taking drug and to notify prescriber if becoming pregnant or thinking of becoming pregnant.
• Advise female patient not to breast-feed while taking dronedarone because drug may appear in breast milk.

drospirenone–ethinyl estradiol
droh-SPYE-re-none/ETH-i-nill
es-tra-DYE-ole

Loryna, Mya✤, Nikki, Syeda, Yasmin, YAZ, Zamine 21✤, Zamine 28✤

Therapeutic class: Contraceptives
Pharmacologic class: Estrogen–progestin combinations

AVAILABLE FORMS
Tablets: 3 mg drospirenone and 0.03 mg ethinyl estradiol as 21 active (yellow) tablets and 7 inert (white) tablets (Syeda, Yasmin, Zamine 28); 3 mg drospirenone and 0.02 mg ethinyl estradiol as 24 active (light pink or peach) tablets and 4 inert (white) tablets (Loryna, Mya, Nikki, YAZ)

INDICATIONS & DOSAGES
➤ **Contraception**
Women: 1 active yellow tablet P.O. daily for 21 days beginning on day 1 of menstrual cycle or first Sunday after onset of menstruation. Then 1 white inert tablet P.O. daily on days 22 through 28. Or 1 light pink or peach active tablet P.O. daily for 24 days beginning on day 1 of menstrual cycle or first Sunday after onset of menstruation. Then 1 white inert tablet P.O. daily on days 25 through 28. Begin next and all subsequent 28-day regimens on same day of week that first regimen began, following same schedule. Restart yellow, light pink, or peach tablets on next day after last white tablet.
➤ **Premenstrual dysphoric disorder (YAZ)**
Women: 1 light pink tablet P.O. daily for 24 days beginning on day 1 of menstrual cycle or first Sunday after menstruation begins. Then 1 white inert tablet P.O. daily on days 25 through 28. Begin next and all subsequent 28-day regimens on same day of week that first regimen began, following same schedule. Restart light pink tablets on next day after last white tablet.
➤ **Acne in women at least age 14 and only if patient desires an oral contraceptive for birth control (Loryna, Nikki, YAZ)**

Women: Follow guidelines of use for contraception. The 28-day dosing regimen consists of 1 light peach or pink active tablet P.O. for 24 consecutive days followed by 1 inert tablet P.O. daily for 4 days. After 28 tablets are taken, new course is started next day.

ADMINISTRATION
P.O.
● Give pill at same time each day.

ACTION
Reduces chance of conception by inhibiting ovulation, inhibiting sperm progression, and reducing chance of implantation.

Route	Onset	Peak	Duration
P.O.	Unknown	1–3 hr	Unknown

Half-life: drospirenone, 30 hours; ethinyl estradiol, 24 hours.

ADVERSE REACTIONS
CNS: *cerebral hemorrhage, cerebral thrombosis,* asthenia, depression, dizziness, emotional lability, headache, migraine, nervousness.
CV: *arterial thromboembolism, mesenteric thrombosis, MI, PE,* hypertension, thrombophlebitis, fluid retention, edema.
EENT: cataracts, steepening of corneal curvature, intolerance to contact lenses, pharyngitis, retinal thrombosis, sinusitis.
GI: abdominal pain, abdominal cramping, bloating, changes in appetite, colitis, diarrhea, gastroenteritis, nausea, vomiting, gallbladder disease.
GU: amenorrhea, breakthrough bleeding, change in cervical erosion and secretion, change in menstrual flow, cystitis, cystitis-like syndrome, dysmenorrhea, impaired renal function, leukorrhea, menstrual disorder, premenstrual syndrome, spotting, temporary infertility after discontinuing treatment, UTI, vaginal candidiasis, vaginitis.
Hepatic: *Budd-Chiari syndrome, hepatic adenomas,* cholestatic jaundice, benign liver tumors.
Metabolic: reduced glucose tolerance, porphyria, weight change, *hyperkalemia.*
Musculoskeletal: back pain.
Respiratory: bronchitis, URI.

Skin: *erythema multiforme,* acne, erythema nodosum, hemorrhagic eruption, hirsutism, loss of scalp hair, melasma, pruritus, rash.
Other: changes in libido, breast tenderness.

INTERACTIONS
Drug-drug. *ACE inhibitors, aldosterone antagonists, ARBs, NSAIDs, potassium-sparing diuretics:* May increase risk of hyperkalemia. Monitor potassium level.
Acetaminophen: May increase level of contraceptive and decrease effectiveness of acetaminophen. Monitor patient for adverse effects. Adjust acetaminophen dose as needed.
Antibiotics, griseofulvin, penicillins, tetracycline: May decrease contraceptive effect. Advise patient to use additional method of birth control while taking the antibiotic.
Ascorbic acid, atorvastatin: May increase level of contraceptive. Monitor patient for adverse effects.
Carbamazepine, modafinil, oxcarbazepine, phenobarbital, phenytoin, protease inhibitors: May increase metabolism of ethinyl estradiol and decrease contraceptive effectiveness. Advise patient to use another method of birth control.
Clofibrate, morphine, salicylic acid, temazepam: May decrease levels and increase clearance of these drugs. Monitor patient for effectiveness.
Cyclosporine, prednisolone, theophylline: May increase levels of these drugs. Monitor patient for adverse effects and toxicity.
Rifampin: May decrease contraceptive effectiveness and increase menstrual irregularities. Advise patient to use another method of birth control.
Troleandomycin: May increase risk of intrahepatic cholestasis and decrease contraceptive effect. Advise patient to use an alternative method of birth control.
Warfarin, other anticoagulants: May increase or decrease anticoagulation effect. Monitor INR or consider therapy modification.
Drug-herb. *St. John's wort:* May decrease contraceptive effectiveness and increase breakthrough bleeding. Discourage use together, or advise use of additional method of birth control.

D

Drug-lifestyle. *Smoking:* May increase risk of adverse CV effects. Advise patient to avoid smoking.

EFFECTS ON LAB TEST RESULTS
• May increase potassium, corticoid, prothrombin, thyroid-binding globulin, total circulating sex steroid, total thyroid hormone, triglyceride, amylase, GGT, transferrin, prolactin, renin activity, vitamin A, and factor VII, VIII, IX, and X levels, as well as iron-binding capacity. May decrease antithrombin III level, folate, albumin, zinc, and vitamin B_{12}.
• May increase norepinephrine-induced platelet aggregation. May decrease glucose tolerance and free T_3 resin uptake.

CONTRAINDICATIONS & CAUTIONS
• Contraindicated in women with hepatic dysfunction, tumor, or disease; renal or adrenal insufficiency; thrombophlebitis, thromboembolic disorders, or history of DVT or thromboembolic disorders; cerebrovascular disease or CAD; headaches with focal neurologic symptoms; known or suspected breast cancer, endometrial cancer, or other estrogen-dependent neoplasia; abnormal genital bleeding; or cholestatic jaundice of pregnancy or jaundice with other hormonal contraceptive use; and in patients older than age 35 who smoke and in those who smoke 15 or more cigarettes daily.
• Contraindicated in women age 65 or older.
• Use cautiously in patients with CV risk factors such as hypertension, hyperlipidemias, obesity, and diabetes.
• Don't use in patients predisposed to hyperkalemia; drug may increase potassium level.
• Use cautiously in patients with conditions aggravated by fluid retention.
Dialyzable drug: Unknown.
⚠ *Overdose S&S:* Nausea, withdrawal uterine bleeding.

PREGNANCY-LACTATION-REPRODUCTION
• Contraindicated in women who are or may become pregnant. There is little or no increased risk of birth defects in women who inadvertently use combined oral contraceptives during early pregnancy.

• Small amounts of hormonal contraceptives appear in breast milk. Use of drug in breast-feeding women isn't recommended.

NURSING CONSIDERATIONS
🔔 *Alert:* The use of contraceptives causes increased risk of MI, thromboembolism, stroke, hepatic neoplasia, gallbladder disease, and hypertension. Risk increases in patients with hypertension, diabetes, hyperlipidemia, and obesity.
■ Black Box Warning Smoking increases the risk of serious CV adverse effects. The risk increases with age (especially age older than 35) and in patients who smoke 15 or more cigarettes daily. ■
• The relationship between the use of hormonal contraceptives and breast and cervical cancers is unclear. Encourage women to schedule a complete gynecologic examination at least yearly and to perform breast self-examinations monthly.
• In patients scheduled to have elective surgery that may increase the risk of thromboembolism, stop contraceptive use from at least 4 weeks before until 2 weeks after surgery. Also stop use during and after prolonged immobilization.
• Because of increased risk of thromboembolism in the postpartum period, don't start contraceptive earlier than 4 to 6 weeks after delivery.
• Stop use and evaluate patient if loss of vision, proptosis, diplopia, papilledema, or retinal vascular lesions occur. Recommend that contact lens wearers be evaluated by an ophthalmologist if visual changes or lens intolerance occurs.
• If patient misses two consecutive periods, she should obtain a negative pregnancy test result before continuing use of contraceptive.
• Immediately stop use if pregnancy is confirmed.
• Closely monitor patient with diabetes. Glucose intolerance may occur.
• Closely monitor patient with hypertension or a history of depression. Stop drug if these events occur.
• In patient at high risk for hyperkalemia and patient taking medications that may increase potassium, check potassium level during the first treatment cycle.

● Stop drug and evaluate patient if persistent, severe headaches occur or if migraines occur or are worsened.

● Evaluate patient for malignancy or pregnancy if she experiences breakthrough bleeding or spotting.

● Closely monitor patient with hyperlipidemias.

● Stop use if jaundice occurs.

● *Look alike–sound alike:* Don't confuse YAZ with Yasmin.

PATIENT TEACHING

● Advise patient to use additional method of birth control during the first 7 days of the first cycle of hormonal contraceptive.

● Inform patient that pills don't protect against sexually transmitted diseases such as HIV.

● Advise patient of the dangers of smoking while taking hormonal contraceptives. Suggest smokers choose a different form of birth control.

● Tell patient to schedule gynecologic examinations yearly and to perform breast self-examination monthly.

● Inform patient that spotting, light bleeding, or stomach upset may occur while she is taking the first one to three packs of pills. Tell her to continue taking the pills and to notify her health care provider if these symptoms persist.

● Tell patient to take the pill at the same time each day.

● Tell patient to immediately report sharp chest pain, coughing of blood or sudden shortness of breath, calf pain, crushing chest pain or chest heaviness, sudden severe headache or vomiting, dizziness or fainting, visual or speech disturbances, weakness or numbness in an arm or leg, vision loss, breast lumps, severe stomach pain or tenderness, difficulty sleeping, lack of energy, fatigue, change in mood, or jaundice with fever, fatigue, loss of appetite, dark urine, or light-colored bowel movements.

● Tell patient to notify health care provider if she wears contact lenses and notices a change in vision or has trouble wearing the lenses.

● Tell patient that risk of pregnancy increases with each active yellow, light pink,

or peach tablet she forgets to take. Inform patient what to do if she misses pills.

● Tell patient to use an additional method of birth control and to notify health care provider if she isn't sure what to do about missed pills.

● Advise patient who is breast-feeding to use an alternative method of birth control until infant is completely weaned. Quality and quantity of breast milk may be decreased. Yellowing of skin and eyes (jaundice) and breast enlargement may occur in breast-fed neonates.

droxidopa
droks-eye-DOE-pa

Northera

Therapeutic class: Vasopressors
Pharmacologic class: Norepinephrine precursors

AVAILABLE FORMS
Capsules ⓞⓣⓒ: 100 mg, 200 mg, 300 mg

INDICATIONS & DOSAGES
➤ **Symptomatic neurogenic orthostatic hypotension caused by primary autonomic failure (Parkinson disease, multiple system atrophy, and pure autonomic failure), dopamine beta-hydroxylase deficiency, nondiabetic autonomic neuropathy**
Adults: Initially, 100 mg P.O. t.i.d. Titrate to symptomatic response in increments of 100 mg t.i.d. every 24 to 48 hours. Maximum dose is 600 mg t.i.d.

ADMINISTRATION
P.O.

● Give on arising in morning, at midday, and in late afternoon at least 3 hours before bedtime.

● Monitor supine BP before initiating drug and after dosage increase.

● Give consistently with or without food.

● Ensure patient swallows capsule whole.

● Store capsules at room temperature.

ACTION

Metabolized to norepinephrine, which induces peripheral arterial and venous vasoconstriction, causing increased BP.

Route	Onset	Peak	Duration
P.O.	Rapid	1–4 hr	Unknown

Half-life: 2½ hours.

ADVERSE REACTIONS

CNS: headache, dizziness, syncope, fatigue.
CV: hypertension.
GI: nausea.
GU: UTI.
Other: falls.

INTERACTIONS

Drug-drug. *Carbidopa, dopa-decarboxylase inhibitors:* May decrease clearance of droxidopa. Monitor clinical effectiveness of droxidopa and adjust dosage as needed.
Drugs that increase BP (ephedrine, midodrine, norepinephrine, triptans [migraine indications]): May increase risk of supine hypertension. Monitor BP closely.
Serotonin 5-HT$_{1D}$ receptor agonists: May enhance hypertensive effects. Monitor therapy.
Drug-herb. *Ephedra, ma huang:* May increase BP. Don't use together.

EFFECTS ON LAB TEST RESULTS

None reported.

CONTRAINDICATIONS & CAUTIONS

• Contraindicated in patients hypersensitive to drug or its components.
Black Box Warning Droxidopa may cause or exacerbate supine hypertension, increasing risk of stroke, MI, or death if not well managed. ■
• Use cautiously in patients with ischemic heart disease, arrhythmias, or HF.
• Use cautiously in patients with hypersensitivity to FD + C Yellow No. 5 (tartrazine) or aspirin. Risk of allergic reaction to droxidopa may be increased in these patients.
• Safe use in children hasn't been established.
Dialyzable drug: Unknown.
⚠ *Overdose S&S:* Hypertensive crisis.

PREGNANCY-LACTATION-REPRODUCTION

• There are no adequate well-controlled studies in pregnant women.
• Drug may appear in breast milk. Consider discontinuing breast-feeding or drug.

NURSING CONSIDERATIONS

• Periodically assess patient for continued effectiveness of drug. Effectiveness beyond 2 weeks hasn't been established.
Black Box Warning Monitor supine BP before starting drug, periodically during treatment, and after dosage increases. Have patient elevate the head of the bed to reduce risk of supine hypertension when resting or sleeping. If elevating head of bed doesn't manage supine hypertension, reduce dosage or discontinue drug. ■
• Monitor BP in both supine and head-elevated sleeping positions.
• Monitor patient for worsening of existing ischemic heart disease, arrhythmias, or HF.
• Monitor patient when droxidopa dosage is changed or when concomitant levodopa dosage is reduced abruptly or when levodopa is discontinued for a symptom complex resembling neuroleptic malignant syndrome (fever, hyperthermia, muscle rigidity, involuntary movements, altered consciousness, mental status changes).

PATIENT TEACHING

• Tell patient to take droxidopa consistently, either with food or without food.
• Instruct patient to take last dose each day at least 3 hours before bedtime to reduce risk of supine hypertension.
Black Box Warning Educate patient to monitor supine BP regularly. ■
Black Box Warning Advise patient to elevate the head of the bed to reduce risk of supine hypertension. ■
• Caution patient to wait to take next scheduled dose if a dose is missed and never to double a dose to make up for missed dose.

Reactions in bold italics are *life-threatening*. Interactions may have a *rapid onset* or a *delayed onset*.

dulaglutide
DOO-la-gloo-tide

Trulicity

Therapeutic class: Antidiabetics
Pharmacologic class: Glucagon-like
peptide-1 receptor agonists

AVAILABLE FORMS
Injection: 0.75 mg/0.5 mL, 1.5 mg/0.5mL in
single-dose pens or prefilled syringes

INDICATIONS & DOSAGES
➤ **Adjunct to diet and exercise to improve glycemic control in patients with type 2 diabetes mellitus**
Adults: 0.75 mg subcutaneously once
weekly. May titrate to a maximum of
1.5 mg weekly.

ADMINISTRATION
Subcutaneous
● Inject into abdomen, thigh, or upper arm
once weekly any time of day. Use a different
injection site each week.
● May give without regard to meals.
● **Alert:** Don't mix dulaglutide with insulin.
Give as separate injections in nonadjacent
areas.
● Don't give I.M. or I.V.
● Inspect for particulate matter and discol-
oration before administration. Don't give if
present.
● Refrigerate at 36° to 46° F (2° to 8° C).
May store at room temperature for a total of
14 days if temperature doesn't exceed 86° F
(30° C).
● Don't freeze. Don't use drug if it has been
frozen.
● Protect from light by storing in original
carton until time of administration.
● Discard injection device after each use in
puncture-resistant container.
● If a dose is missed, give within 3 days of
missed dose; then resume prior schedule. If
less than 3 days remain until next scheduled
dose, skip the missed dose and give the next
dose on schedule.

● The day of weekly administration may be
changed if necessary as long as the last dose
was 3 or more days before the new day.

ACTION
A human glucagon-like peptide-1 (GLP-1)
receptor agonist that, like endogenous
GLP-1, binds to and activates the GLP-1
receptor in the pancreatic beta cells, leading
to glucose-dependent insulin release. Also
decreases glucagon secretion and slows
gastric emptying.

Route	Onset	Peak	Duration
Subcut.	Unknown	24–72 hr	Unknown

Half-life: About 5 days.

ADVERSE REACTIONS
CNS: fatigue, asthenia, malaise.
CV: tachycardia, increased PR interval,
first-degree AV block.
GI: *pancreatitis,* nausea, diarrhea, vom-
iting, decreased appetite, dyspepsia, con-
stipation, flatulence, GERD, eructation;
abdominal pain, tenderness, or distention.
GU: renal impairment.
Hepatic: elevated lipase and amylase levels.
Metabolic: *hypoglycemia.*
Other: *hypersensitivity reactions, thyroid
C-cell tumors (adenomas and carcinomas),*
antidrug antibody formation.

INTERACTIONS
Drug-drug. *Insulin, insulin secretagogues
(meglitinides, sulfonylureas):* May increase
risk of hypoglycemia. Consider reducing
insulin or insulin secretagogue dosage;
monitor blood glucose level closely.
Oral medications: May affect absorption of
oral medications since dulaglutide delays
gastric emptying. Monitor effects, especially when given with other drugs with a
narrow therapeutic index.

EFFECTS ON LAB TEST RESULTS
● May increase lipase and amylase levels.
May decrease glucose level.

CONTRAINDICATIONS & CAUTIONS
Black Box Warning Contraindicated in
patients with a personal or family history of
medullary thyroid carcinoma (MTC) and in

patients with multiple endocrine neoplasia syndrome type 2. ■

Black Box Warning Thyroid C-cell adenomas and carcinomas occurred in animal studies. It isn't known if dulaglutide causes thyroid C-cell tumors, including MTC, in humans. ■

• Contraindicated in patients with a serious hypersensitivity reaction to drug or its components.

• Drug hasn't been studied in patients with a history of pancreatitis. Consider alternatives.

• Drug isn't recommended as first-line therapy in patients who have inadequate response to diet and exercise.

• Drug shouldn't be used in patients with type 1 diabetes mellitus or for treatment of diabetic ketoacidosis. Drug isn't a substitute for insulin.

• To reduce risk of hypoglycemia, consider dosage reduction of concomitantly administered secretagogues or insulin when initiating dulaglutide.

• Avoid use in patients with severe GI disease, including severe gastroparesis; drug slows gastric emptying and hasn't been studied in this population.

• Concurrent use of dulaglutide and basal insulin hasn't been studied.

• Use cautiously in patients with hepatic or renal insufficiency or heart disease.

• Safety and effectiveness in children haven't been established.

Dialyzable drug: Unknown.

⚠ *Overdose S&S:* Mild or moderate GI symptoms, nonsevere hypoglycemia.

PREGNANCY-LACTATION-REPRODUCTION

• There are no adequate studies in pregnant women. Use cautiously during pregnancy and only if potential benefit justifies potential risk to the fetus.

• It isn't known if drug appears in breast milk. Patient should discontinue breastfeeding or discontinue drug.

NURSING CONSIDERATIONS

• Use caution when initiating dulaglutide therapy or escalating dosage in patients with renal insufficiency. Monitor renal function, especially in patients who report severe

GI adverse reactions (nausea, vomiting, diarrhea, dehydration).

• Monitor patients for signs and symptoms of pancreatitis (including persistent severe abdominal pain, sometimes radiating to the back, which may or may not be accompanied by vomiting). Discontinue drug if pancreatitis is suspected. Don't restart drug if pancreatitis is confirmed.

• Monitor patient for tachycardia; monitor ECG for PR-interval prolongation.

• Refer patients with elevated serum calcitonin level or thyroid nodules on examination or neck imaging to an endocrinologist.

• *Look alike–sound alike:* Don't confuse dulaglutide with duloxetine or dutasteride.

PATIENT TEACHING

• Explain to patient that dulaglutide isn't a substitute for insulin. Educate patient on general diabetes care, including the need to monitor glucose and HbA_{1c} levels, how to recognize the signs and symptoms of hypoglycemia or hyperglycemia, the importance of diet and exercise, and the impact stress or trauma may have on glucose levels.

• Warn patient to immediately discontinue drug and inform prescriber if hypersensitivity reactions occur.

• Advise patient to report heart palpitations or feelings of a racing heartbeat while at rest.

• Teach patient of risk of dehydration due to GI adverse reactions, including the associated risk of worsening renal function. Counsel patient to take precautions to avoid fluid depletion.

• Teach patient signs and symptoms of acute pancreatitis (persistent severe abdominal pain, sometimes radiating to the back, which may or may not be accompanied by vomiting) and to discontinue drug promptly and contact prescriber if any of these signs and symptoms occur.

Black Box Warning Inform patient of risk of MTC. Teach the signs and symptoms of thyroid tumors (a mass in the neck, dysphagia, dyspnea, persistent hoarseness). ■

• Instruct patient on the proper use of drug (rotating sites, inspecting solution for particles, discarding needles, storing pens and syringes, handling a missed dose).

D

• Caution patient never to mix insulin and dulaglutide but to give as separate injections. Although dulaglutide and insulin may be injected in the same region, they should never be injected adjacent to each other.
• Instruct female patient to tell prescriber if she is or plans to become pregnant or is breast-feeding.

duloxetine hydrochloride
do-LOCKS-ah-teen

Cymbalta♦

Therapeutic class: Antidepressants
Pharmacologic class: SSNRIs

AVAILABLE FORMS
Capsules (delayed-release) ⓓ: 20 mg, 30 mg, 40 mg, 60 mg

INDICATIONS & DOSAGES
Adjust-a-dose (for all indications): Duloxetine isn't recommended for patients with ESRD, severe renal dysfunction (CrCl of less than 30 mL/minute), or hepatic dysfunction.
➤ **Major depressive disorder**
Adults: Initially, 20 mg P.O. b.i.d.; then, 60 mg P.O. once daily or divided in two equal doses. May also start at 30 mg/day for 1 week to allow patients to adjust to medication. Maximum, 60 mg daily.
➤ **Generalized anxiety disorder**
Adults: 60 mg P.O. daily. Or, 30 mg P.O. daily for 1 week; then increase to 60 mg P.O. daily. May increase in increments of 30 mg daily to 120 mg P.O. once daily.
Children ages 7 to 17: 30 mg P.O. once daily for 2 weeks; may increase to 60 mg once daily. For doses greater than 60 mg/day, increase dosage in increments of 30 mg/day. Maximum, 120 mg daily.
Adjust-a-dose: In elderly patients, initially, 30 mg P.O. once daily for 2 weeks before considering an increase to target dose of 60 mg once daily. If needed, increase dosage further in increments of 30 mg once daily. Maximum, 120 mg daily.
➤ **Fibromyalgia**
Adults: Initially, 30 mg P.O. once daily for 1 week; increase to 60 mg P.O. once daily

after a week. Some patients may respond to the starting dose. Maximum dose is 60 mg/day. Base continued treatment on individual patient response.
➤ **Neuropathic pain related to diabetic peripheral neuropathy**
Adults: 60 mg P.O. once daily.
➤ **Chronic musculoskeletal pain**
Adults: Initially, 30 mg P.O. once daily for 1 week; then increase to 60 mg P.O. once daily.

ADMINISTRATION
P.O.
• Give whole; don't crush or open capsules.
• Give without regard to meals.

ACTION
May inhibit serotonin and norepinephrine reuptake in the CNS.

Route	Onset	Peak	Duration
P.O.	Unknown	6 hr	Unknown

Half-life: 12 hours.

ADVERSE REACTIONS
CNS: dizziness, fatigue, headache, insomnia, somnolence, ***suicidal thoughts,*** fever, hypoesthesia, irritability, lethargy, nervousness, nightmares, restlessness, sleep disorder, anxiety, asthenia, tremor.
CV: hot flashes, hypertension, increased HR.
EENT: blurred vision, nasopharyngitis, pharyngolaryngeal pain.
GI: constipation, diarrhea, dry mouth, nausea, dyspepsia, gastritis, vomiting.
GU: abnormal orgasm, abnormally increased frequency of urinating, delayed or dysfunctional ejaculation, dysuria, erectile dysfunction, urinary hesitation.
Metabolic: decreased appetite, ***hypoglycemia,*** increased appetite, weight gain or loss, hyponatremia.
Musculoskeletal: muscle cramps, myalgia.
Respiratory: cough.
Skin: increased sweating, night sweats, pruritus, rash.
Other: decreased libido, rigors.

INTERACTIONS

Drug-drug. *Anticoagulants (aspirin, NSAIDs, warfarin):* May increase bleeding risk. Monitor patient closely.

Class IC antiarrhythmics (flecainide, propafenone), phenothiazines: May increase levels of these drugs. Use together cautiously.

CNS drugs: May increase adverse effects. Use together cautiously.

CYP1A2 inhibitors (cimetidine, fluvoxamine, certain quinolones): May increase duloxetine level. Avoid using together.

CYP2D6 inhibitors (fluoxetine, paroxetine, quinidine): May increase duloxetine level. Use together cautiously.

Drugs that reduce gastric acidity: May cause premature breakdown of duloxetine's protective coating and early release of the drug. Monitor patient for effects.

Linezolid, methylene blue: May cause serotonin syndrome. Use with extreme caution and monitor closely.

Lithium, SSNRIs, SSRIs, tramadol: May increase risk of serotonin syndrome. Avoid use together.

🔆 *Alert:* *MAO inhibitors (phenelzine, rasagiline, selegiline):* May cause hyperthermia, rigidity, myoclonus, autonomic instability, rapid fluctuations of vital signs, agitation, delirium, and coma. Avoid use within 2 weeks after MAO inhibitor therapy; wait at least 5 days after stopping duloxetine before starting MAO inhibitor.

TCAs (amitriptyline, imipramine, nortriptyline): May increase levels of these drugs. Reduce TCA dose, and monitor drug levels closely.

Thioridazine: May prolong the QT interval and increase risk of serious ventricular arrhythmias and sudden death. Avoid using together.

Triptans: May cause serotonin syndrome (restlessness, hallucinations, loss of coordination, fast heartbeat, rapid changes in BP, increased body temperature, hyperreflexia, nausea, vomiting, and diarrhea) or neuroleptic malignant syndrome. Use cautiously and with increased monitoring, especially when starting or increasing dosages.

Drug-herb. *St. John's wort:* May increase sedative-hypnotic effects and risk of serotonin syndrome. Discourage use together.

Drug-lifestyle. *Alcohol use:* May increase risk of liver damage. Discourage use together.

EFFECTS ON LAB TEST RESULTS

● May increase alkaline phosphatase, ALT, AST, bilirubin, and CK levels.

CONTRAINDICATIONS & CAUTIONS

● Contraindicated in patients hypersensitive to drug or its ingredients, patients taking MAO inhibitors, and patients with a CrCl less than 30 mL/minute. Drug isn't recommended for patients with hepatic dysfunction or ESRD.

🔆 *Alert:* Before using duloxetine in a child or adolescent, balance potential risks with clinical need.

● Safety and effectiveness in children younger than age 7 haven't been established.

🔆 *Alert:* Concomitant use with linezolid or methylene blue can cause serotonin syndrome (fever, mental status changes, muscle twitching, excessive sweating, shivering or shaking, diarrhea, loss of coordination). Use with linezolid or methylene blue only for life-threatening or urgent conditions when the potential benefits outweigh the risks of toxicity.

● Use cautiously in patients with a history of mania or seizures, patients who drink substantial amounts of alcohol, patients with hypertension, patients with controlled angle-closure glaucoma, and those with conditions that slow gastric emptying.

● Pupil dilation that occurs after duloxetine use may trigger an angle-closure attack in a patient with anatomically narrow angles who doesn't have a patent iridectomy.

● Orthostatic hypotension, falls, and syncope have been reported with therapeutic doses and tend to occur within first week of therapy but can occur at any time during treatment, particularly after dosage increases. Fall risk appears to increase steadily with age and be related to degree of orthostatic decrease in BP as well as other factors that may increase the underlying risk of falls. Consider dosage reduction or discontinuing drug if falls occur.

Dialyzable drug: Unlikely.

⚠ *Overdose S&S:* Coma, hypotension, hypertension, seizures, serotonin syndrome, somnolence, syncope, tachycardia, vomiting.

PREGNANCY-LACTATION-REPRODUCTION

• There are no adequate well-controlled studies in pregnant women. Use during pregnancy only if potential benefit justifies potential risk to the fetus.

• Use during the third trimester may cause neonatal complications, including respiratory distress, cyanosis, apnea, seizures, vomiting, hypoglycemia, hypotonia, and hyperreflexia, which may require prolonged hospitalization, respiratory support, and tube feeding.

• Drug appears in breast milk. Use cautiously in breast-feeding women and only when benefits outweigh potential risks.

NURSING CONSIDERATIONS

Black Box Warning Drug may increase risk of suicidal thinking and behavior in children, adolescents, and young adults ages 18 to 24, especially during the first few months of treatment, and in those with major depressive disorder or other psychiatric disorder. ■

Black Box Warning Monitor all patients for worsening of depression or emergence of suicidal thoughts or behavior, especially when therapy starts or dosage changes. ■

⟳ *Alert:* If linezolid or methylene blue must be given, stop drug and monitor the patient for serotonin toxicity for 2 weeks, or until 24 hours after the last dose of methylene blue or linezolid, whichever comes first. Treatment may be resumed 24 hours after last dose of methylene blue or linezolid.

• Treatment of overdose is symptomatic. Don't induce emesis; gastric lavage or activated charcoal may be performed soon after ingestion or if patient is still symptomatic. Because drug undergoes extensive distribution, forced diuresis, dialysis, hemoperfusion, and exchange transfusion aren't useful. Contact a poison control center for information.

• If taken with TCAs, duloxetine metabolism will be prolonged, and patient will need extended monitoring.

• Periodically reassess patient to determine the need for continued therapy.

• Don't stop drug abruptly. Decrease dosage gradually, and watch for symptoms that may arise when drug is stopped, such as dizziness, nausea, headache, paresthesia, vomiting, irritability, and nightmares.

• If intolerable symptoms arise when decreasing or stopping drug, restart at previous dose and decrease even more gradually.

• Monitor BP periodically during treatment.

• Older patients may be more sensitive to drug effects than younger adults.

⟳ *Alert:* Combining triptans with an SSRI or an SSNRI may cause serotonin syndrome or neuroleptic malignant syndrome–like reactions. Signs and symptoms of serotonin syndrome may include restlessness, hallucinations, loss of coordination, fast heartbeat, rapid changes in BP, increased body temperature, overactive reflexes, nausea, vomiting, and diarrhea. Serotonin syndrome may be more likely to occur when starting or increasing the dose of triptan, SSRI, or SSNRI.

• *Look alike–sound alike:* Don't confuse duloxetine with fluoxetine or paroxetine. Don't confuse Cymbalta with Symbyax.

PATIENT TEACHING

Black Box Warning Warn families or caregivers to report signs of worsening depression (such as agitation, irritability, insomnia, hostility, impulsivity) and signs of suicidal behavior to prescriber immediately. ■

⟳ *Alert:* Teach patient to recognize and immediately report signs and symptoms of serotonin toxicity (fever, mental status changes, muscle twitching, excessive sweating, shivering or shaking, diarrhea, loss of coordination).

• Tell patient to not stop drug abruptly; dosage must be gradually reduced to avoid adverse effects.

• Tell patient to consult prescriber or pharmacist before taking other prescription or OTC drugs or herbal or other dietary supplements.

• Instruct patient to swallow capsules whole and not to chew, crush, or open them because they have an enteric coating.

• Urge patient to avoid activities that are hazardous or require mental alertness until he knows how the drug affects him.

• Warn against drinking alcohol during therapy.
• If patient takes drug for depression, explain that it may take 1 to 4 weeks to notice an effect.

dutasteride
doo-TAS-teh-ride

Avodart⊘

Therapeutic class: BPH drugs
Pharmacologic class: 5-alpha-reductase enzyme inhibitors

AVAILABLE FORMS
Capsules ⒪ⓃⒼ: 0.5 mg

INDICATIONS & DOSAGES
➤ **To treat and improve the symptoms of BPH, reduce the risk of acute urine retention, and reduce the need for BPH-related surgery**
Men: 0.5 mg P.O. once daily as monotherapy. May be given with tamsulosin 0.4 mg P.O. once daily as combination therapy.

ADMINISTRATION
P.O.
🜲 *Alert:* Drug is considered a teratogen. Follow safe handling and disposal procedures.
• Don't crush or break capsules.
• Give drug without regard for food.

ACTION
Inhibits conversion of testosterone to dihydrotestosterone, the androgen primarily responsible for the initial development and subsequent enlargement of the prostate gland.

Route	Onset	Peak	Duration
P.O.	Unknown	2–3 hr	Unknown

Half-life: About 5 weeks.

ADVERSE REACTIONS
GU: erectile dysfunction, decreased libido, ejaculation disorder.
Other: gynecomastia.

INTERACTIONS
Drug-drug. *CYP3A4 inhibitors (cimetidine, ciprofloxacin, diltiazem, ketoconazole, ritonavir, verapamil):* May increase dutasteride level. Use together cautiously and monitor therapy.

EFFECTS ON LAB TEST RESULTS
• May lower PSA level.

CONTRAINDICATIONS & CAUTIONS
• Contraindicated in women and children and in patients hypersensitive to dutasteride or its ingredients or to other 5-alpha-reductase inhibitors.
🜲 *Alert:* 5-Alpha-reductase inhibitors may increase the risk of high-grade prostate cancer. Before start of therapy, patients should be evaluated to rule out other urologic conditions, including prostate cancer, that might mimic BPH. Any increase in PSA level in patient receiving dutasteride should be considered significant, and the patient should be evaluated for prostate cancer.
• Use cautiously in patients with hepatic disease and in those taking long-term potent CYP450 inhibitors.
Dialyzable drug: Unknown.

PREGNANCY-LACTATION-REPRODUCTION
• Contraindicated in women of childbearing potential and during pregnancy.
🜲 *Alert:* Because drug may be absorbed through the skin, women who are or may become pregnant shouldn't handle drug, especially avoiding contact with crushed or broken tablets. If contact occurs, wash contact area immediately with soap and water.
• It isn't known if drug appears in breast milk. Contraindicated for use in breast-feeding women.
• Drug appears in semen.

NURSING CONSIDERATIONS
• If contact is made with a leaking capsule, wash the contact area immediately with soap and water.
• Carefully monitor patients with a large residual urine volume or severely diminished urine flow, or both, for obstructive uropathy.

Reactions in bold italics are *life-threatening*. Interactions may have a *rapid onset* or a *delayed onset*.

• Patients should wait at least 6 months after their last dose before donating blood.

• Establish a new baseline PSA level in men treated for 3 to 6 months, and use it to assess potentially cancer-related changes in PSA level.

• To interpret PSA values in men treated for 6 months or more, double the PSA value for comparison with normal values in untreated men.

• Evaluate patients for prostate cancer and other urologic conditions that may cause similar signs and symptoms before initiating therapy and periodically thereafter.

PATIENT TEACHING

• Tell patient to swallow the capsule whole.

• Inform patient that ejaculate volume may decrease but that sexual function should remain normal.

• Teach women who are pregnant or may become pregnant not to handle drug. A male fetus exposed to drug by the mother's swallowing or absorbing the drug through her skin may be born with abnormal sex organs.

✪ *Alert:* Tell patient not to donate blood for at least 6 months after final dose to prevent drug administration to a pregnant female transfusion recipient.

• Tell patient he'll need periodic blood tests to monitor therapeutic effects.

SAFETY ALERT!

edoxaban tosylate
e-DOX-a-ban

Savaysa

Therapeutic class: Factor Xa inhibitors
Pharmacologic class: Anticoagulants

AVAILABLE FORMS
Tablets: 15 mg, 30 mg, 60 mg

INDICATIONS & DOSAGES
Adjust-a-dose (for all indications): If CrCl is 15 to 50 mL/minute, decrease dosage to 30 mg P.O. once daily. For patients converting to edoxaban from warfarin or vitamin K antagonists, discontinue warfarin and start edoxaban when INR is 2.5 or less. For patients converting to edoxaban from oral anticoagulants other than warfarin, discontinue current oral anticoagulant and start edoxaban at the time of the next scheduled dose of the other oral anticoagulant. For patients converting to edoxaban from low-molecular-weight heparin (LMWH), discontinue LMWH and start edoxaban at the time of the next scheduled administration of LMWH. For patients converting to edoxaban from unfractionated heparin, discontinue infusion and start edoxaban 4 hours later.

For patients converting to oral warfarin and taking 60 mg of edoxaban, reduce edoxaban to 30 mg and begin concomitant warfarin; if patient is receiving 30 mg of edoxaban, reduce edoxaban to 15 mg and begin warfarin. Measure INR at least weekly and just before daily edoxaban dose to limit its influence on INR. Once INR is stable at 2.0 or greater, stop edoxaban and continue warfarin.

For patients converting to warfarin and a parenteral anticoagulant as a bridge, discontinue edoxaban and administer parenteral anticoagulant and warfarin at next scheduled edoxaban dose time. Once INR is stable at 2.0 or greater, stop parenteral anticoagulant and continue warfarin. For patients converting to non–vitamin K oral anticoagulants or other parenteral anticoagulants without concomitant warfarin, discontinue edoxaban and administer parenteral anticoagulant at next scheduled edoxaban dose time.

➤ **To reduce risk of stroke and systemic embolism in patients with nonvalvular atrial fibrillation (NVAF)**
Adults: 60 mg P.O. once daily.

Black Box Warning Don't use for treatment of NVAF in patients with CrCl greater than 95 mL/minute. ∎

➤ **Treatment of DVT and PE**
Adults: 60 mg P.O. once daily after 5 to 10 days of therapy with a parenteral anticoagulant.

Adjust-a-dose: If patient weighs 60 kg or less or is taking concomitant P-glycoprotein (P-gp) inhibitors, decrease dosage to 30 mg P.O. once daily.

ADMINISTRATION
P.O.
• Give without regard to meals.
• If a dose is missed, give as soon as possible on the same day. Resume normal schedule the following day. Don't double the dose to make up for missed dose.

ACTION
Inhibits free Factor Xa, prothrombinase activity, and thrombin-induced platelet aggregation. Inhibition of Factor Xa in the coagulation cascade reduces thrombin generation and thrombus formation.

Route	Onset	Peak	Duration
P.O.	Unknown	1–2 hr	Unknown

Half-life: 10 to 14 hours.

ADVERSE REACTIONS
CNS: *intracranial hemorrhage, hemorrhagic stroke, epidural or spinal hematoma.*
EENT: epistaxis, *oral hemorrhage.*
GI: *GI hemorrhage.*
GU: *vaginal hemorrhage,* hematuria.
Hematologic: *hemorrhage,* anemia, bruising.
Hepatic: abnormal LFT values.
Skin: rash, puncture-site bleeding.

INTERACTIONS
Drug-drug. *Anticoagulants, antiplatelet drugs (aspirin), NSAIDs, omega-3-fatty acids, thrombolytics, vitamin E, vorapaxar:* May increase risk of bleeding. Avoid concomitant use.
Digoxin: May increase digoxin level. Monitor digoxin level closely to determine if dosage adjustments are needed.
P-gp inducers (rifampin): May increase P-gp inducer exposure. Avoid concomitant use.
Verapamil: May decrease verapamil level. Monitor effects of verapamil and titrate dosage as necessary.
Drug-herb. *Alfalfa, anise, bilberry:* May increase bleeding risk. Don't use together.

EFFECTS ON LAB TEST RESULTS
• May increase LFT values.
• May decrease RBC count.

CONTRAINDICATIONS & CAUTIONS
• Contraindicated in patients hypersensitive to drug or its components and in those with active pathological bleeding.
Black Box Warning Contraindicated in patients with CrCl greater than 95 mL/minute. Efficacy is reduced in patients with NVAF with CrCl greater than 95 mL/minute, increasing the risk of stroke. There is an increased risk of ischemic stroke in patients with NVAF if their renal function improves and edoxaban blood level decreases. ∎
• Drug hasn't been studied in patients with mechanical heart valves or moderate to severe mitral stenosis or when CrCl is less than 15 mL/minute. Use isn't recommended in these patients.
• Use isn't recommended in patients with moderate to severe hepatic impairment (Child-Pugh classes B and C) because of possible intrinsic coagulation abnormalities.
Black Box Warning Epidural or spinal hematomas may occur in patients treated with edoxaban who are receiving neuraxial anesthesia or undergoing spinal puncture. Risk increases with indwelling epidural catheters, concomitant drugs that affect hemostasis (NSAIDs, platelet inhibitors, anticoagulants), spinal surgery or deformity, or a history of traumatic or repeated epidural or spinal punctures. The optimal timing between edoxaban administration and neuraxial procedures isn't known. Weigh risks and benefits before neuraxial intervention in patients who are or will be anticoagulated. ∎
• Safety and effectiveness in children haven't been established.
Dialyzable drug: 7%.
⚠ *Overdose S&S:* Bleeding.

PREGNANCY-LACTATION-REPRODUCTION
• There are no adequate studies in pregnant women. It isn't known if drug causes fetal harm. Use during pregnancy only if benefit outweighs risk to the fetus.
• It isn't known if drug appears in breast milk. Patient should discontinue breastfeeding or discontinue drug.

NURSING CONSIDERATIONS
Black Box Warning Premature discontinuation of drug increases risk of ischemic events. If drug is stopped for a reason other

than pathological bleeding or completion of treatment, consider transitioning to an alternative anticoagulant. ∎
• Monitor patient for bleeding. Immediately evaluate signs or symptoms of blood loss; discontinue drug if acute pathological bleeding occurs. Drug can cause serious and potentially fatal bleeding.
• Discontinue edoxaban at least 24 hours before invasive or surgical procedures. If surgery can't be delayed, weigh risk of bleeding against urgency of intervention.
• After surgery or other procedure, may restart edoxaban as soon as hemostasis has been achieved and patient can take oral medication.
⚠ **Alert:** Don't remove indwelling epidural or intrathecal catheters earlier than 12 hours after last dose of edoxaban. Don't give next dose earlier than 2 hours after removal of the catheter.
Black Box Warning Monitor patients frequently after spinal or epidural anesthesia or puncture for signs and symptoms of neurologic impairment (numbness or weakness of the legs, bowel or bladder dysfunction). Evaluate impairment urgently. ∎
• Be aware that vitamin K, protamine, tranexamic acid, and dialysis aren't expected to reverse the effects of edoxaban.

PATIENT TEACHING
• Warn patient that he or she may bleed more easily, bleed longer, or bruise more easily while taking drug.
• Instruct patient to immediately report unusual bleeding to prescriber.
• Instruct patient to take drug exactly as prescribed and, if a dose is missed, to take the next dose as soon as possible the same day and resume the normal dosing schedule the following day. Caution patient not to double a dose to make up for a missed dose.
• Advise patient not to discontinue drug without first consulting prescriber.
• Instruct patient that before scheduling surgery, medical, or dental procedures he should inform health care providers about taking edoxaban.
• Instruct patient to inform health care providers and dentists about prescription medications, OTC drugs, or herbal products he or she is taking or plans to take.

• Advise female patient to immediately report if she is pregnant, plans to become pregnant, is breast-feeding, or intends to breast-feed during treatment.
• Warn patient having neuraxial anesthesia or spinal puncture to watch for signs and symptoms of spinal or epidural hematoma, such as back pain, tingling, numbness (especially in the lower limbs), muscle weakness, and stool or urine incontinence. If any of these symptoms occur, advise patient to immediately contact health care provider.
• Warn patient to immediately report signs and symptoms of hemorrhage or adverse reactions, such as one-sided weakness, problems thinking or speaking, dizziness, balance changes, blurred vision, severe headache, and pale skin.

efavirenz
eff-ah-VYE-renz

Sustiva

Therapeutic class: Antiretrovirals
Pharmacologic class: NNRTIs

AVAILABLE FORMS
Capsules ⊚*:* 50 mg, 200 mg
Tablets ⊚*:* 600 mg

INDICATIONS & DOSAGES
➤ **HIV-1 infection, with a protease inhibitor with or without nucleoside analogue reverse transcriptase inhibitors**
Adults and children age 3 months and older weighing 40 kg or more: 600 mg (three 200-mg capsules or one 600-mg tablet) P.O. once daily on an empty stomach, preferably at bedtime.
Children age 3 months and older weighing 32.5 kg to less than 40 kg: 400 mg P.O. once daily on an empty stomach, preferably at bedtime.
Children age 3 months and older weighing 25 kg to less than 32.5 kg: 350 mg P.O. once daily on an empty stomach, preferably at bedtime.
Children age 3 months and older weighing 20 kg to less than 25 kg: 300 mg P.O. once daily on an empty stomach, preferably at bedtime.

Children age 3 months and older weighing 15 kg to less than 20 kg: 250 mg P.O. once daily on an empty stomach, preferably at bedtime.
Children age 3 months and older weighing 7.5 kg to less than 15 kg: 200 mg P.O. once daily on an empty stomach, preferably at bedtime.
Children age 3 months and older weighing 5 kg to less than 7.5 kg: 150 mg P.O. once daily on an empty stomach, preferably at bedtime.
Children age 3 months and older weighing 3.5 kg to less than 5 kg: 100 mg P.O. once daily on an empty stomach, preferably at bedtime.
Adjust-a-dose: For adults also taking voriconazole, increase voriconazole maintenance dose to 400 mg every 12 hours and decrease efavirenz dose to 300 mg once daily using capsule formulation. For adults and children weighing 50 kg or more who are also taking rifampin, recommended efavirenz dosage is 800 mg once daily.

ADMINISTRATION
P.O.
● Give drug at bedtime to decrease CNS adverse effects.
● In children, consider prophylaxis with antihistamines before initiating therapy, to prevent rash.
● Don't break or crush tablets. Don't crush capsules.
● Give on an empty stomach.
● For patients who can't swallow capsules or tablets, capsule contents may be sprinkled over a small amount (5 to 10 mL) of food and mixed gently. For patients who can tolerate solid foods, mix with soft food, such as applesauce, grape jelly, or yogurt.
● For young infants, dose can be gently mixed into 10 mL of reconstituted room-temperature infant formula in a medicine cup. Draw up dose mixture into a 10-mL dosing syringe to administer; then add an additional 10 mL to mixing cup and stir to disperse any remaining residue. Administer to infant.
● Give efavirenz mixture within 30 minutes of mixing. Patient shouldn't consume any additional food or additional formula for 2 hours after administration.

ACTION
Inhibits the transcription of HIV-1 RNA to DNA, a critical step in the viral replication process, suppressing viral replication.

Route	Onset	Peak	Duration
P.O.	Unknown	3–5 hr	Unknown

Half-life: Single dose, 52 to 76 hours; multiple doses, 40 to 55 hours.

ADVERSE REACTIONS
CNS: dizziness, abnormal dreams or thinking, agitation, amnesia, confusion, depersonalization, depression, euphoria, fever, fatigue, hallucinations, headache, hypoesthesia, impaired concentration, insomnia, nervousness, somnolence.
GI: diarrhea, nausea, abdominal pain, anorexia, dyspepsia, vomiting.
Skin: rash, *erythema multiforme, Stevens-Johnson syndrome, toxic epidermal necrolysis,* increased sweating, pruritus.

INTERACTIONS
Drug-drug. *Amprenavir, clarithromycin, indinavir, lopinavir:* May decrease levels of these drugs. Consider alternative therapy or dosage adjustment.
Atorvastatin, calcium channel blockers, itraconazole, pravastatin, rifampin, simvastatin: May decrease levels of these drugs. Dosage adjustments may be necessary.
Axitinib, bortezomib, bosutinib, cabazitaxel: May decrease pharmacologic effects of these drugs. Avoid concurrent use.
Bepridil, ergot derivatives, midazolam, pimozide, triazolam: May inhibit metabolism of these drugs and cause serious or life-threatening adverse events (such as arrhythmias, prolonged sedation, or respiratory depression). Avoid using together.
Bupropion: May decrease plasma concentrations and clinical effects of bupropion. Guide bupropion dosage by clinical response.
CYP2B6 inducers (strong): May increase metabolism of CYP2B6 substrates. Consider an alternative for one of the interacting drugs. Some combinations may be specifically contraindicated. Consult appropriate manufacturer labeling. Consider therapy modification.

Reactions in bold italics are *life-threatening*. Interactions may have a *rapid onset* or a *delayed onset*.

CYP2B6 inhibitors (moderate): May decrease metabolism of CYP2B6 substrates. Monitor therapy.

CYP2B6 inhibitors (strong): May decrease metabolism of CYP2B6 substrates. Consider therapy modification.

CYP2C19 substrates: CYP2C19 moderate inhibitors may decrease metabolism of CYP2C19 substrates. Monitor therapy.

CYP3A4 inducers (strong): May increase metabolism of CYP3A4 substrates. Consider an alternative for one of the interacting drugs. Some combinations may be specifically contraindicated. Consult appropriate manufacturer labeling. Consider therapy modification.

CYP3A4 substrates: CYP3A4 moderate inhibitors may decrease metabolism of CYP3A4 substrates. Monitor therapy.

Drugs that induce the CYP3A enzyme system (such as phenobarbital, phenytoin, rifampin): May decrease efavirenz level. Avoid using together. Refer to manufacturer's instructions for contraindications.

Estrogens, ritonavir: May increase drug levels. Monitor patient.

Hormonal contraceptives: May increase ethinyl estradiol level. Advise use of a reliable method of barrier contraception in addition to use of hormonal contraceptives.

Nevirapine: May decrease clinical effectiveness and increase risk of adverse reactions. Avoid using together.

Psychoactive drugs: May cause additive CNS effects. Avoid using together.

Rifabutin: May decrease rifabutin level. Increase daily rifabutin dosage by 50%. Consider doubling rifabutin dosage when rifabutin is given two to three times per week.

Ritonavir: May increase levels of both drugs. Monitor patient and liver function closely.

Saquinavir: May decrease saquinavir level and efavirenz exposure to the body. Don't use with saquinavir as sole protease inhibitor.

Voriconazole (in standard doses): Decreases voriconazole levels significantly, while efavirenz levels significantly increase. Avoid using together unless doses of each are adjusted.

Warfarin: May increase or decrease level and effects of warfarin. Monitor INR.

Drug-herb. *St. John's wort:* May decrease response and lead to possible resistance to efavirenz or all same-class drugs. Don't use together.

Drug-food. *High-fat meals:* May increase absorption of drug. Instruct patient to maintain a proper low-fat diet.

Drug-lifestyle. *Alcohol use:* May enhance CNS effects. Discourage use together.

EFFECTS ON LAB TEST RESULTS
● May increase ALT, AST, triglyceride, and cholesterol levels.
● May cause false-positive urine cannabinoid test results.

CONTRAINDICATIONS & CAUTIONS
● Contraindicated in patients hypersensitive to drug or its components and in those with moderate or severe hepatic impairment.
● Use cautiously in patients with mild hepatic impairment and in those receiving hepatotoxic drugs. Monitor LFTs in patients with history of hepatitis B or C and in those taking ritonavir.
● Serious psychiatric adverse reactions have been reported, including aggressive behavior, severe depression, suicidal ideation, nonfatal suicide attempts, paranoia, and mania. Use cautiously in patients with a history of mental illness or drug abuse.
● Use cautiously in patients with a history of seizures.
Dialyzable drug: No.
⚠ **Overdose S&S:** Increased nervous system symptoms, involuntary muscle contractions.

PREGNANCY-LACTATION-REPRODUCTION
● Because of the risk of neural tube defects, drug shouldn't be used in the first trimester. Advise pregnant women of the risk to a fetus. Other antiretrovirals should strongly be considered.
● Register pregnant women in the Antiretroviral Pregnancy Registry at 1-800-258-4263.
● Advise women not to breast-feed because of the risk of HIV transmission.
● Women of reproductive potential should undergo pregnancy testing before therapy starts and should use barrier contraception

in combination with other (hormonal) contraceptive methods during therapy and for 12 weeks after therapy ends.

NURSING CONSIDERATIONS

⚠ Alert: Drug shouldn't be used as monotherapy or added on as a single drug to a regimen failing because of viral resistance.

• Using drug with ritonavir may increase liver enzyme levels and adverse effects (such as dizziness, nausea, paresthesia).

• Rule out pregnancy before starting therapy in women of childbearing potential.

• Children may be more prone to adverse reactions, especially diarrhea, nausea, vomiting, and rash. Consider prophylaxis with antihistamines before initiating therapy, to prevent rash in this population.

• Discontinue if patient develops severe rash associated with blistering, desquamation, mucosal involvement, or fever.

• Monitor patients for elevated triglyceride and cholesterol levels before therapy and periodically during treatment.

PATIENT TEACHING

• Tell patient to immediately report signs and symptoms of serious psychiatric adverse effects.

• Instruct patient to take drug with water, preferably at bedtime and on an empty stomach. Tell patient not to break tablets.

• Inform patient about need for blood tests to monitor LFTs and cholesterol level.

• Tell patient to use a barrier contraceptive with a hormonal contraceptive during therapy and for 12 weeks after therapy ends and to notify prescriber immediately if pregnancy is suspected; drug is a known risk to the fetus.

• Inform patient that drug doesn't cure HIV infection, that opportunistic infections and other complications of HIV infection may continue to occur, and that transmission of HIV to others through sexual contact or blood contamination is still possible.

• Instruct patient to take drug at the same time every day and always with other antiretrovirals.

• Tell patient to take drug exactly as prescribed and not to stop it without medical approval. Also instruct patient to report adverse reactions.

• Inform patient that rash is the most common adverse effect. Tell patient to report rash immediately because it may be serious in rare cases.

• Advise patient to report use of other drugs, including OTC drugs and herbal supplements.

• Advise patient that dizziness, difficulty sleeping or concentrating, drowsiness, or unusual dreams may occur during the first few days of therapy. Reassure him that these symptoms typically resolve after 2 to 4 weeks and may be less problematic if drug is taken at bedtime.

• Tell patient to avoid alcohol, driving, or operating machinery until the drug's effects are known.

elbasvir–grazoprevir
See NEW DRUGS for information.

eletriptan hydrobromide
ell-ah-TRIP-tan

Relpax◆

Therapeutic class: Antimigraine drugs
Pharmacologic class: Serotonin 5-HT$_1$ receptor agonists

AVAILABLE FORMS
Tablets ⓐ: 20 mg, 40 mg

INDICATIONS & DOSAGES
➤ **Acute migraine with or without aura**
Adults: 20 to 40 mg P.O. at first migraine symptom. If headache recurs, dose may be repeated at least 2 hours later to a maximum of 80 mg daily.

ADMINISTRATION
P.O.
• Give drug without regard for food.
• Give drug whole; don't crush or break tablet.
• Give drug with a full glass of water.

ACTION
Binds to 5-HT$_1$ receptors and may constrict intracranial blood vessels and inhibit proinflammatory neuropeptide release.

Route	Onset	Peak	Duration
P.O.	½ hr	1½–2 hr	Unknown

Half-life: About 4 hours.

ADVERSE REACTIONS

CNS: asthenia, dizziness, headache, hypertonia, hypesthesia, pain, paresthesia, somnolence, vertigo.
CV: chest tightness, pain, and pressure; flushing, palpitations.
EENT: pharyngitis.
GI: abdominal pain, discomfort, or cramps; dry mouth, dyspepsia, dysphagia, nausea.
Musculoskeletal: back pain.
Skin: increased sweating.
Other: chills.

INTERACTIONS

Drug-drug. *CYP3A4 inhibitors (such as clarithromycin, itraconazole, ketoconazole, nefazodone, nelfinavir, ritonavir, troleandomycin):* May decrease eletriptan metabolism. Avoid use within 72 hours of these drugs.
Ergotamine-containing or ergot-type drugs (such as dihydroergotamine or methysergide), other triptans: May prolong vasospastic reactions. Avoid use within 24 hours of these drugs.
Linezolid: May enhance serotonergic effect of eletriptan, possibly resulting in serotonin syndrome. Discontinue eletriptan 2 weeks before starting linezolid, but if urgent initiation of linezolid is needed, discontinue eletriptan immediately and monitor patient.
MAO inhibitors, SNRIs, SSRIs, TCAs: May increase the risk of serotonin syndrome (weakness, hyperreflexia, and incoordination). Monitor patient closely.

EFFECTS ON LAB TEST RESULTS
None known.

CONTRAINDICATIONS & CAUTIONS

• Contraindicated in patients hypersensitive to drug or its components and in those with severe hepatic impairment, ischemic heart disease, history of MI, or silent ischemia; coronary artery vasospasm, including Prinzmetal variant angina; Wolff-Parkinson-White syndrome or arrhythmias associated with other cardiac accessory conduction pathway disorders; and other significant CV conditions.
• Contraindicated within 24 hours of treatment with another 5-HT$_1$ agonist or ergot-containing drug or within 72 hours of ketoconazole, itraconazole, nefazodone, clarithromycin, ritonavir, or nelfinavir.
• Contraindicated in patients with cerebrovascular syndromes, such as stroke or TIA; peripheral vascular disease, including ischemic bowel disease; uncontrolled hypertension; or hemiplegic or basilar migraine.
• Contraindicated in patients with risk factors for CAD, such as hypertension, hypercholesterolemia, smoking, obesity, diabetes, strong family history of CAD, postmenopausal women, or men older than age 40, unless patient is free from cardiac disease. Monitor patient closely after first dose.
• Safety of treating more than three migraine headaches in 30 days hasn't been established.
Dialyzable drug: Unknown.
⚠ Overdose S&S: Hypertension, more serious CV reactions.

PREGNANCY-LACTATION-REPRODUCTION

• Use cautiously in pregnant women and only if benefit outweighs possible risk to the fetus.
• Drug appears in breast milk. Use cautiously in breast-feeding women.

NURSING CONSIDERATIONS

• Drug isn't intended for migraine prevention.
❶ Alert: Combining a triptan with an SSRI or an SSNRI may cause serotonin syndrome. Signs and symptoms may include restlessness, hallucinations, loss of coordination, fast heartbeat, rapid changes in BP, increased body temperature, hyperreflexia, nausea, vomiting, and diarrhea. Serotonin syndrome may be more likely to occur when starting or increasing the dose of a triptan, SSRI, or SSNRI.
• Use drug only when patient has a clear diagnosis of migraine. If the first use produces no response, reconsider the migraine diagnosis.
❶ Alert: Serious cardiac events, including acute MI, arrhythmias, and death, occur rarely within a few hours after use of 5-HT$_1$ agonists.

- Ophthalmologic effects may occur with long-term use.
- Older patients may develop higher BP than younger patients after taking drug.

PATIENT TEACHING
- Instruct patient to take dose at first sign of a migraine headache. If the headache comes back after the first dose, patient may take a second dose after 2 hours. Caution patient not to take more than 80 mg in 24 hours.
- Warn patient to avoid driving and operating machinery if dizziness or fatigue occurs.
- Tell patient to immediately report pain, tightness, heaviness, or pressure in the chest, throat, neck, or jaw.
- Tell patient to swallow tablet whole with a full glass of water and not to split, crush, or chew it.

elotuzumab
See NEW DRUGS for information.

SAFETY ALERT!

eluxadoline
el-ux-AD-oh-leen

Viberzi

Therapeutic class: Anti–IBS drugs
Pharmacologic class: Mu-opioid receptor agonist
Controlled substance schedule: IV

AVAILABLE FORMS
Tablets: 75 mg, 100 mg

INDICATIONS & DOSAGES
➤ **Irritable bowel syndrome with diarrhea (IBS-D)**
Adults: 100 mg P.O. b.i.d.
Adjust-a-dose: Reduce dosage to 75 mg b.i.d. in patients who don't have a gallbladder, are unable to tolerate the 100-mg dose, are receiving concomitant OATP1B1 inhibitors (cyclosporine, gemfibrozil, atazanavir, lopinavir, ritonavir, saquinavir, tipranavir, rifampin, eltrombopag), or have mild to moderate (Child-Pugh class A or class B) hepatic impairment.

ADMINISTRATION
P.O.
- Give with food.
- If a dose is missed, give next dose at the regular time. Don't give two doses at the same time to make up for a missed dose.
- Store at room temperature.

ACTION
Mu-opioid receptor agonist, delta-opioid receptor antagonist, and kappa-opioid receptor agonist that decreases peristaltic action of the intestines. Acts locally to reduce abdominal pain and IBS-D without constipating adverse effects.

Route	Onset	Peak	Duration
P.O. (with food)	Unknown	1½ hr (range, 1–8 hr)	Unknown

Half-life: 3.7 to 6 hours.

ADVERSE REACTIONS
CNS: dizziness, fatigue, drowsiness, euphoria, intoxicated feeling, sedation.
EENT: nasopharyngitis.
GI: constipation, nausea, vomiting, abdominal pain, abdominal distention, flatulence, viral gastroenteritis.
Hepatic: elevated ALT and AST levels.
Respiratory: URI, bronchitis.
Skin: rash.

INTERACTIONS
Drug-drug. *CYP3A substrates with narrow therapeutic index (alfentanil, ergotamine, fentanyl, pimozide, quinidine, sirolimus, tacrolimus):* May increase concentration of CYP3A substrates. Monitor drug concentrations or other pharmacodynamic markers of drug effect when use with eluxadoline is initiated or discontinued.
Drugs that cause constipation (alosetron, anticholinergics, opioids): May increase risk of constipation-related adverse reactions. Avoid use together.
OATP1B1 inhibitors (atazanavir, cyclosporine, eltrombopag, gemfibrozil, lopinavir, rifampin, ritonavir, saquinavir, tipranavir): May increase eluxadoline concentration. Give eluxadoline at a dose of 75 mg b.i.d.; monitor patient for eluxadoline-related adverse reactions.

Reactions in bold italics are *life-threatening*. Interactions may have a *rapid onset* or a *delayed onset*.

Rosuvastatin: May increase rosuvastatin concentration and risk of myopathy/rhabdomyolysis. Use lowest effective rosuvastatin dose.

Strong CYP inhibitors (ciprofloxacin [CYP1A2], clarithromycin [CYP3A4], fluconazole [CYP2C19], gemfibrozil [CYP2C8], paroxetine and bupropion [CYP2D6]): May increase eluxadoline concentration. Monitor patient for eluxadoline-related adverse reactions.

Drug-lifestyle. *Alcohol use:* May increase risk of acute pancreatitis. Patient should avoid prolonged or acute excessive alcohol use while taking drug. Monitor patient closely.

EFFECTS ON LAB TEST RESULTS
● May increase ALT and AST levels.

CONTRAINDICATIONS & CAUTIONS
● Contraindicated in patients hypersensitive to drug or its components.
● Contraindicated in patients with known or suspected biliary duct obstruction or sphincter of Oddi disease or dysfunction. Permanently discontinue drug in patients who develop biliary duct obstruction or sphincter of Oddi spasm while taking eluxadoline.
● Contraindicated in patients with alcohol abuse, alcohol addiction, alcoholism, or consumption of more than three alcoholic beverages each day; history of pancreatitis or structural diseases of the pancreas or suspected pancreatic duct obstruction with severe hepatic impairment (Child-Pugh class C); history of chronic or severe constipation or sequelae from constipation; or known or suspected mechanical GI obstruction.
● Use cautiously in patients without a gallbladder because of increased risk of adverse reactions such as sphincter of Oddi spasm. Consider alternative therapies.
● Drug has potential for abuse and psychological dependence. Consider naloxone in the event of overdose.
● Safety and effectiveness in children haven't been established.
● Use cautiously in elderly patients, for whom the same effectiveness was observed but with a higher incidence of adverse reactions.
Dialyzable drug: Unlikely.

PREGNANCY-LACTATION-REPRODUCTION
● Use cautiously in pregnant women. Risk to fetus is unknown.
● It isn't known if drug appears in breast milk. Use cautiously in breast-feeding women, taking into account maternal benefits and risk to the fetus.

NURSING CONSIDERATIONS
● Monitor patients with hepatic impairment for impaired mental or physical abilities needed to perform potentially hazardous activities, such as driving or operating machinery.
● Monitor patients, especially those without a gallbladder, for sphincter of Oddi spasm (unusual or severe epigastric or upper right quadrant abdominal pain that may radiate to the back or shoulder, with or without nausea and vomiting, and with liver or pancreatic enzyme elevations). Discontinue drug if signs or symptoms develop.
● Monitor patients, especially those with excessive alcohol intake, for pancreatitis (new or worsening abdominal or epigastric pain that may radiate to the back, associated with elevated pancreatic enzyme levels). Discontinue drug if signs and symptoms occur.
● Monitor patients for constipation. Discontinue drug if severe constipation lasting more than 4 days develops.
● Watch for signs and symptoms of abuse of drug, including psychological dependence.

PATIENT TEACHING
● Advise patient to read the FDA-approved medication guide.
● Warn patient to stop drug and seek medical attention if unusual or severe abdominal pain occurs, especially if patient doesn't have a gallbladder.
● Advise patient to avoid prolonged and acute excessive alcohol use while taking drug.
● Advise patient to discontinue drug and contact prescriber for constipation lasting more than 4 days.
● Instruct patient to avoid taking drug with other medications that may cause constipation and to ask prescriber for a list of these medications.

E

• Inform patient that loperamide may occasionally be used with eluxadoline but must be stopped if constipation develops.
• Caution patient with hepatic impairment not to drive, operate machinery, or perform other dangerous activities until effects of drug are known.
• Advise patient that if a dose is missed to take the next dose at the regular time and not to take two doses at the same time to make up for the missed dose.

elvitegravir–cobicistat–emtricitabine–tenofovir disoproxil fumarate
el-vye-TEG-gra-veer/koe-BIK-i-stat/em-tra-SYE-tah-ben/te-NOE-fo-veer

Stribild

Therapeutic class: Antiretrovirals
Pharmacologic class: Antivirals–cytochrome P450 inhibitors–nucleoside and nucleotide reverse transcriptase inhibitors

AVAILABLE FORMS
Tablets: 150 mg elvitegravir, 150 mg cobicistat, 200 mg emtricitabine, and 300 mg tenofovir disoproxil fumarate

INDICATIONS & DOSAGES
➤ **HIV-1 infection in adults who are antiretroviral treatment–naive; to replace current antiretroviral regimen in adults who are virologically suppressed (HIV-1 RNA <50 copies/mL) on a stable regimen for at least 6 months with no history of treatment failure and no known substitutions associated with resistance to individual components**
Adults: 1 tablet P.O. once daily.
Adjust-a-dose: Discontinue drug in patients with estimated CrCl of less than 50 mL/minute and patients with Child-Pugh class C hepatic impairment.

ADMINISTRATION
P.O.
• Give with food.
• Drug is used as a complete treatment; don't give with other antiretrovirals.

ACTION
Combination of agents with differing mechanisms of action (integrase strand transfer inhibition, pharmacokinetic enhancement, nucleoside and nucleotide analogue HIV-1 reverse transcriptase inhibition) working together via differing mechanisms to inhibit HIV replication.

Route	Onset	Peak	Duration
P.O. (elvitegravir)	Unknown	4 hr	Unknown
P.O. (cobicistat, emtricitabine)	Unknown	3 hr	Unknown
P.O. (tenofovir)	Unknown	2 hr	Unknown

Half-life: Elvitegravir, 13 hours; cobicistat, 4 hours; emtricitabine, 10 hours; tenofovir, 17 hours.

ADVERSE REACTIONS
CNS: anxiety, headache, dizziness, insomnia, abnormal dreams, fatigue, somnolence, depression, fever, pain.
GI: diarrhea, nausea, flatulence.
GU: proteinuria, hematuria.
Musculoskeletal: arthralgia, back pain, bone fracture, myalgia.
Respiratory: cough, pneumonia.
Skin: rash.

INTERACTIONS
Drug-drug. *Acyclovir, cidofovir, ganciclovir, valacyclovir, valganciclovir:* May increase concentrations of these drugs, emtricitabine, and tenofovir due to competition for renal excretion. Use together carefully.
Additional antiretrovirals: May increase risk of drug interactions and altered pharmacokinetics of drug components. Use together is contraindicated.
Alfuzosin: May increase alfuzosin level and risk of severe hypotension. Use together is contraindicated.
Antacids: May decrease elvitegravir concentration. Separate administration times by 2 hours.
Antiarrhythmics, digoxin: May increase levels of these drugs. Use together cautiously and monitor drug levels if possible.
Antidepressants (SSRIs, TCAs, trazodone): May increase levels of these drugs. Use together cautiously and titrate antidepressant according to response.
Antifungals (itraconazole, ketoconazole, voriconazole): May increase levels of these

---

Reactions in bold italics are *life-threatening*. Interactions may have a *rapid onset* or a **delayed onset**.

drugs, elvitegravir, and cobicistat. Use together cautiously. Don't exceed 200 mg/day of ketoconazole or itraconazole.

Beta blockers (metoprolol, timolol): May increase beta blocker concentration. Monitor patient carefully and decrease beta blocker dosage as necessary.

Bosentan: May increase bosentan level. Give bosentan dose based on manufacturer's instructions and adjust according to patient tolerance.

Calcium channel blockers (amlodipine, diltiazem, felodipine, nicardipine, nifedipine, verapamil): May increase level of calcium channel blocker. Use together cautiously and monitor patient closely.

Carbamazepine, oxcarbazepine, phenobarbital, phenytoin: May significantly decrease elvitegravir and cobicistat levels; may increase carbamazepine level. Use together isn't recommended. Consider alternative anticonvulsants.

Clarithromycin, telithromycin: May increase level of clarithromycin, telithromycin, and cobicistat. Use together cautiously. Decrease clarithromycin dosage by 50% if CrCl is between 50 and 60 mL/minute.

Clonazepam, ethosuximide: May increase levels of these drugs. Use together cautiously.

Colchicine: May increase colchicine concentration. Adjust dosage according to manufacturer's instructions. Use together is contraindicated in patients with renal or hepatic impairment.

CYP2D6, CYP3A, P-glycoprotein substrates: May alter plasma concentrations of the four drug components (elvitegravir, cobicistat, emtricitabine, and tenofovir). Use together cautiously.

Dexamethasone: May significantly decrease cobicistat and elvitegravir levels. Monitor patient carefully for loss of therapeutic effect (elvitegravir, cobicistat) and development of resistance.

Ergot derivatives (dihydroergotamine, ergotamine): May increase levels of these drugs. Use together is contraindicated.

Fluticasone: May increase fluticasone level. Choose an alternative corticosteroid.

HMG-CoA reductase inhibitors (atorvastatin, lovastatin, simvastatin): May increase

statin drug level and risk of myopathy. Start statin at lowest dosage and titrate carefully.

Hormonal contraceptives: May alter levels of these drugs. Consider nonhormonal forms of birth control.

Immunosuppressants (cyclosporine, sirolimus, tacrolimus): May increase immunosuppressant level. Use together cautiously.

Midazolam: May increase midazolam level. Use with oral midazolam is contraindicated. Use parenteral form cautiously and monitor patient closely.

Neuroleptics (perphenazine, risperidone, thioridazine): May increase neuroleptic level. Decrease neuroleptic dosage as needed.

PDE5 inhibitors (sildenafil, tadalafil, vardenafil): May increase effects of PDE5 inhibitors. Adjust dosage according to manufacturer's instructions. Use with sildenafil for pulmonary arterial hypertension is contraindicated.

Pimozide: May increase risk of cardiac adverse effects. Use together is contraindicated.

Rifabutin, rifapentine: May decrease cobicistat and elvitegravir levels. Avoid use together.

Rifampin: May increase elvitegravir and cobicistat concentrations. Use together is contraindicated.

Salmeterol: May increase risk of CV effects of salmeterol, including QT-interval prolongation, palpitations, and tachycardia. Avoid use together.

Sedative/hypnotics (buspirone, clorazepate, diazepam, estazolam, flurazepam, triazolam, zolpidem): May increase concentrations of sedative/hypnotics. Use cautiously together and monitor patient carefully.

Warfarin: May increase warfarin concentration. Monitor INR carefully.

Drug-herb. *St. John's wort:* May reduce concentrations of drug components and decrease therapeutic effect. Discourage use together.

EFFECTS ON LAB TEST RESULTS
- May increase AST, amylase, CK, total cholesterol, HDL, LDL, and triglyceride levels.
- May increase urine RBC count.

CONTRAINDICATIONS & CAUTIONS

• Contraindicated in patients hypersensitive to drugs or their components and in those with CrCl of less than 70 mL/minute or severe hepatic impairment (Child-Pugh class C).

• Contraindicated with alfuzosin, rifampin, dihydroergotamine, ergotamine, methylergonovine, cisapride, St. John's wort, lovastatin, simvastatin, pimozide, sildenafil (for pulmonary arterial hypertension), triazolam, and oral midazolam.

• Use cautiously in new-onset or worsening renal impairment and in Fanconi syndrome.

• Use cautiously in patients with a history of pathologic fracture or other risk factors for osteoporosis or bone loss. Consider calcium and vitamin D supplementation.

Black Box Warning Drug isn't approved for the treatment of chronic HBV infection; safety and efficacy of drug haven't been established in patients infected with both HBV and HIV-1. Severe acute exacerbations of hepatitis B have been reported in patients who are infected with both HBV and HIV-1 and have discontinued emtricitabine (Emtriva) or tenofovir (Viread), which are components of this drug. Monitor hepatic function closely with both clinical and laboratory follow-up for at least several months in patients who are infected with both HIV-1 and HBV and discontinue this drug. If appropriate, initiation of anti–hepatitis B therapy may be warranted. ■

Black Box Warning Lactic acidosis and severe hepatomegaly with steatosis, including fatal cases, have been reported with use of nucleoside analogues, including tenofovir, in combination with other antiretrovirals. ■

• Drug may increase risk of pancreatitis. Use cautiously in patients at risk for or with a history of pancreatitis.

Dialyzable drug: Elvitegravir, unknown; cobicistat, unknown; emtricitabine, 30% hemodialysis; tenofovir, 10% hemodialysis.

PREGNANCY-LACTATION-REPRODUCTION

• Register pregnant women in the Antiretroviral Pregnancy Registry at 1-800-258-4263.

• Use cautiously in pregnant women and only if benefit outweighs possible risk to the fetus.

• Drug appears in breast milk. Because of risk of HIV transmission, women shouldn't breast-feed.

NURSING CONSIDERATIONS

• Suspend treatment in patients who develop signs and symptoms suggestive of lactic acidosis or pronounced hepatotoxicity (including nausea, vomiting, unusual or unexpected stomach discomfort, and weakness).

• Test for HBV before starting therapy; severe acute exacerbations of hepatitis B have been reported in patients infected with both HBV and HIV-1.

• Avoid concurrent or recent use of a nephrotoxic agent because renal impairment is possible.

• Assess CrCl, urine glucose, and urine protein before initiating and periodically during treatment.

• Monitor serum phosphorus level in patients at risk for renal impairment.

• Closely monitor patients with a confirmed increase in serum creatinine level of greater than 0.4 mg/dL from baseline for renal safety.

• Consider assessing bone mineral density (BMD) in patients with a history of pathologic bone fracture or other risk factors for osteoporosis or bone loss because of risk of drug-related decreased BMD.

• Redistribution or accumulation of body fat may occur in patients receiving antiretrovirals. The cause and long-term health effects of these conditions aren't known.

• Monitor patients for infection and development of immune reconstitution syndrome (inflammatory response to indolent or residual opportunistic infections, such as *Mycobacterium avium* infection, CMV, *Pneumocystis jiroveci* pneumonia, or TB), which may necessitate further evaluation and treatment.

• Autoimmune disorders (such as Graves disease, polymyositis, and Guillain-Barré syndrome) have also been reported in the setting of immune reconstitution; however, the time to onset is more variable, and the disorder can occur many months after initiation of treatment.

PATIENT TEACHING

- Caution patient to remain under the care of a health care provider and to comply with routine monitoring to decrease risk of adverse events.
- Inform patient that this drug isn't a cure for HIV-1 infection; patient must stay on continuous HIV therapy to control HIV-1 infection and decrease HIV-related illnesses.
- Instruct patient to avoid behaviors that can spread HIV-1 infection to others (such as sharing needles or other injection equipment; sharing personal items that may have blood or body fluids on them, such as toothbrushes and razor blades; or having sex without the protection of a latex or polyurethane condom).
- Warn female patient not to breast-feed because HIV-1 can be passed to the infant in breast milk.
- Teach patient to take drug on a regular dosing schedule with food and not to miss doses.
- Advise patient to immediately report nausea, vomiting, unusual or unexpected stomach discomfort, and weakness.
- Instruct patient not to change dose or stop drug without first consulting health care provider.
- Inform patient that redistribution or accumulation of body fat may occur.
- Caution patient to report signs and symptoms of infection.
- Teach patient to report yellowing of skin or sclera, dark urine, light-colored stools, loss of appetite, or nausea.

SAFETY ALERT!

empagliflozin
EM-pa-gli-FLOE-zin

Jardiance

Therapeutic class: Antidiabetics
Pharmacologic class: Sodium-glucose cotransporter 2 inhibitors

AVAILABLE FORMS
Tablets: 10 mg, 25 mg

INDICATIONS & DOSAGES
➤ **As adjunct to diet and exercise to improve glycemic control in patients with type 2 diabetes mellitus**
Adults: 10 mg P.O. daily in the morning. May increase to 25 mg daily.
Adjust-a-dose: Discontinue drug if GFR is less than 45 mL/minute.

ADMINISTRATION
P.O.
- May give without regard for food.
- Store at room temperature.

ACTION
Inhibits renal reabsorption of glucose and lowers renal threshold for glucose, resulting in increased urinary excretion of glucose.

Route	Onset	Peak	Duration
P.O.	Unknown	1½ hr	Unknown

Half-life: 12.4 hours.

ADVERSE REACTIONS
GI: nausea, thirst.
GU: genital mycotic infections, UTI, renal impairment, increased urination.
Metabolic: dyslipidemia, *hypoglycemia.*
Musculoskeletal: arthralgia.
Respiratory: URI.

INTERACTIONS
Drug-drug. *Diuretics:* May enhance diuretic effect. Closely monitor patient for volume depletion.
Insulin, insulin secretagogues, sulfonylureas, other antidiabetic agents: May increase hypoglycemic risk. Monitor patient closely.

EFFECTS ON LAB TEST RESULTS
- May increase hematocrit and LDL and serum creatinine levels. May decrease glucose level.
- May decrease GFR.
- May cause false-positive urine glucose tests.
- Interferes with 1,5-anhydroglucitol assay.

CONTRAINDICATIONS & CAUTIONS
- Contraindicated in patients with history of serious hypersensitivity reaction to drug or its components.

• Contraindicated in patients with GFR of less than 45 mL/minute.

❂ *Alert:* Drug may cause acidosis, which may require emergency department care or hospitalization for treatment. Monitor for ketoacidosis, especially in patients with major illness, reduced food or fluid intake, or reduced insulin dose. Elevated urine or serum ketone level without associated very high glucose levels has occurred with sodium-glucose cotransporter 2 inhibitor use.

• Drug isn't recommended for type 1 diabetes or for the treatment of diabetic ketoacidosis.

• Use cautiously in patients with low BP or moderate renal impairment and in those taking diuretics; drug may increase risk of hypotension.

• Drug may increase risk of adverse events related to volume depletion and reduced renal function, including UTI, especially in elderly patients and those with renal impairment.

• Drug may increase incidence of bone fractures. Per American Diabetes Association guidelines, sodium-glucose cotransporter 2 inhibitors should be avoided in patients with fracture risk factors.

• Use cautiously in patients with elevated hematocrit at baseline, as value may increase.

• Safety and effectiveness in children haven't been established.

Dialyzable drug: Unknown.

PREGNANCY-LACTATION-REPRODUCTION

• Drug hasn't been studied in pregnant women. Use in pregnant women only if benefit justifies risk to the fetus.

• It isn't known if drug appears in breast milk. Patient should discontinue breast-feeding or discontinue drug.

NURSING CONSIDERATIONS

• Assess renal function before initiating therapy and periodically during treatment. Don't start therapy if GFR is less than 45 mL/minute. Closely monitor patients with GFR of less than 60 mL/minute.

• Assess fluid status. Correct volume depletion before starting therapy.

• Monitor patients for signs and symptoms of hypotension (fatigue, dizziness, blurred vision, clammy skin) during therapy. Drug may increase risk of hypotension due to intravascular volume contraction.

• Monitor glucose level closely during drug initiation. Concomitant use of insulin and other antidiabetic agents may increase risk of hypoglycemia.

• Watch for genital mycotic infections and treat appropriately.

❂ *Alert:* Drug may increase risk of severe UTI, including urosepsis and pyelonephritis. Monitor patient and treat promptly if indicated.

• Monitor LDL cholesterol periodically; treat appropriately.

• Drug causes positive urine glucose tests. Avoid urine glucose testing for glycemic control monitoring.

• *Look alike–sound alike:* Don't confuse empagliflozin with canagliflozin or dapagliflozin. Don't confuse Jardiance with Januvia, Jantoven, or Janumet.

PATIENT TEACHING

• Instruct patient to take drug in the morning, with or without food.

• If a dose is missed, advise patient to take missed dose as soon as he remembers and not to double a dose.

• Stress importance of adhering to diet, weight reduction, exercise, personal hygiene, and blood glucose monitoring while on therapy.

• Teach patient to report all adverse reactions and how to identify and manage signs and symptoms of hypoglycemia (dizziness, weakness, shaking, fast heartbeat).

• Teach patient how to identify and manage signs and symptoms of hypotension (fatigue, dizziness, blurred vision, clammy skin). Encourage patient to maintain adequate fluid intake.

❂ *Alert:* Instruct patient to seek medical attention immediately for signs and symptoms of ketoacidosis (difficulty breathing, hyperventilation, anorexia, nausea, vomiting, abdominal pain, confusion, unusual fatigue or sleepiness).

• Instruct patient to seek medical advice during periods of stress or illness because medication requirements may change.

❯ Alert: Instruct patient to seek medical attention for signs and symptoms of UTI (difficulty urinating, frequency, urgency, pelvic pain, blood in urine, fever, back pain, nausea, vomiting).

● Inform patient that periodic monitoring of blood glucose and HbA_{1c} levels and renal function will be needed.

● Advise patient that urine glucose tests will be falsely positive because drug increases glucose excretion and recommend alternative methods to monitor glycemic control.

● Counsel patient to consult prescriber before starting new prescription or OTC medications or supplements.

● Advise patient to inform prescriber if she becomes pregnant, intends to become pregnant, or is breast-feeding.

emtricitabine
em-tra-SYE-tah-ben

Emtriva

Therapeutic class: Antiretrovirals
Pharmacologic class: Nucleoside reverse transcriptase inhibitors

AVAILABLE FORMS
Capsules: 200 mg
Oral solution: 10 mg/mL

INDICATIONS & DOSAGES
➤ HIV-1 infection, with other antiretrovirals
Adults: One 200-mg capsule or 240 mg (24 mL) oral solution P.O. once daily.
Children ages 3 months to 17 years: For children weighing more than 33 kg who can swallow intact capsules, give one 200-mg capsule P.O. once daily. Otherwise, give 6 mg/kg, up to a maximum dose of 240 mg (24 mL) oral solution P.O. once daily.
Children younger than age 3 months: 3 mg/kg oral solution P.O. once daily.
Adjust-a-dose: In adults with CrCl of 30 to 49 mL/minute, give one 200-mg capsule every 48 hours or 120 mg oral solution every 24 hours; if CrCl is 15 to 29 mL/minute, give one 200-mg capsule every 72 hours or 80 mg oral solution every 24 hours; if CrCl is less than 15 mL/minute or patient is receiving hemodialysis, give one 200-mg capsule every 96 hours or 60 mg oral solution every 24 hours. Give dose after hemodialysis session. In children with renal insufficiency, consider a dose reduction or increased dosing interval.

ADMINISTRATION
P.O.
● Give drug with or without food.
● Refrigerate oral solution; if stored at room temperature, use within 3 months.

ACTION
Inhibits replication of HIV by blocking viral DNA synthesis and inhibits reverse transcriptase by acting as an alternative for the enzyme's substrate, deoxycytidine triphosphate.

Route	Onset	Peak	Duration
P.O.	Unknown	1–2 hr	Unknown

Half-life: About 10 hours.

ADVERSE REACTIONS
CNS: abnormal dreams, asthenia, dizziness, headache, insomnia, depression, fatigue, neuritis, paresthesia, peripheral neuropathy.
EENT: rhinitis.
GI: abdominal pain, diarrhea, nausea, dyspepsia, vomiting.
Hepatic: *hepatotoxicity.*
Musculoskeletal: arthralgia, myalgia.
Respiratory: increased cough.
Skin: allergic skin reaction, discoloration, maculopapular rash, pruritus, urticarial and purpuric lesions, vesiculobullous rash.

INTERACTIONS
None reported.

EFFECTS ON LAB TEST RESULTS
● May increase ALT, amylase, AST, bilirubin, CK, lipase, glucose, and triglyceride levels.
● May decrease neutrophil count.

CONTRAINDICATIONS & CAUTIONS
● Contraindicated in patients hypersensitive to drug or its ingredients.
● In elderly patients, use cautiously because of the potential for other diseases and drug therapies and for decreased hepatic, renal, or cardiac function.

E

• Use cautiously in patients with impaired renal function.

Black Box Warning Drug isn't approved for treatment of chronic HBV infection; safety and efficacy haven't been established in patients infected with both HBV and HIV-1. Severe acute exacerbations of HBV infection have been reported in patients infected with both HBV and HIV-1 who have discontinued emtricitabine or tenofovir, which are components of this drug. Monitor hepatic function closely with both clinical and laboratory follow-up for at least several months in patients infected with both HIV-1 and HBV who discontinue this drug. If appropriate, initiation of anti–HBV therapy may be warranted. ■

Black Box Warning Lactic acidosis and severe hepatomegaly with steatosis, including fatal cases, have been reported with use of nucleoside analogues, alone or in combination with other antiretrovirals. ■

• Don't give drug with other emtricitabine-containing drugs or lamivudine.

Dialyzable drug: 30% hemodialysis.

PREGNANCY-LACTATION-REPRODUCTION

• Use drug during pregnancy only if clearly needed.

• Register pregnant women in the Antiretroviral Pregnancy Registry at 1-800-258-4263.

• Avoid breast-feeding because of potential for HIV-1 transmission and serious adverse reactions in breast-fed infants.

NURSING CONSIDERATIONS

• Test all patients for HBV before starting drug.

• Monitor hepatic function closely with both clinical and laboratory follow-up for at least several months in patients infected with both HIV-1 and HBV who discontinue this drug.

• Like other antiretrovirals, emtricitabine may cause changes or increases in body fat, including central obesity, buffalo hump, peripheral wasting, facial wasting, breast enlargement, and a cushingoid appearance.

PATIENT TEACHING

• Remind patient that anti-HIV medicine must be taken for life.

• Inform patient that drug doesn't cure HIV infection, that opportunistic infections and other complications of HIV infection may continue to occur, and that transmission of HIV to others through sexual contact or blood contamination is still possible.

• Explain possible adverse reactions, including lactic acidosis, hepatotoxicity, and changes or increases in body fat; advise patient to report all adverse reactions.

• Tell woman to notify prescriber immediately if she is or could be pregnant.

• Warn women against breast-feeding.

• Inform patient that the drug may be taken with or without food.

• Tell patient to refrigerate oral solution and, if stored at room temperature, to use solution within 3 months.

emtricitabine–rilpivirine–tenofovir alafenamide fumarate
See NEW DRUGS for information.

emtricitabine–tenofovir alafenamide fumarate
See NEW DRUGS for information.

enalaprilat
eh-NAH-leh-prel-at

enalapril maleate
Epaned Kit, Vasotec⬦

Therapeutic class: Antihypertensives
Pharmacologic class: ACE inhibitors

AVAILABLE FORMS
enalaprilat
Injection: 1.25 mg/mL
enalapril maleate
Oral solution: 1 mg/mL
Tablets: 2.5 mg, 5 mg, 10 mg, 20 mg

INDICATIONS & DOSAGES
➤ **Hypertension**
Adults: In patients not taking diuretics, initially, 5 mg P.O. once daily; then adjusted based on response. Usual dosage range is 10 to 40 mg daily as a single dose or two divided doses. Or, 1.25 mg I.V. infusion over 5 minutes every 6 hours.

Children ages 1 month to 16 years:
0.08 mg/kg (up to 5 mg) P.O. once daily; dosage should be adjusted as needed up to 0.58 mg/kg (maximum 40 mg). Don't use if CrCl is less than 30 mL/minute.

Adjust-a-dose: If patient is taking diuretics or CrCl is 30 mL/minute or less, initially, 2.5 mg P.O. once daily. Or, 0.625 mg I.V. over 5 minutes, and repeat in 1 hour, if needed; then 1.25 mg I.V. every 6 hours. For dialysis patients, give 2.5 mg P.O. on dialysis days; adjust dosage on dialysis days based on BP response.

➤ **To convert from I.V. therapy to oral therapy in patients receiving diuretics**
Adults: Initially, 2.5 mg P.O. once daily; if patient was receiving 0.625 mg I.V. every 6 hours, then 2.5 mg P.O. once daily. Adjust dosage based on response.

➤ **To convert from oral therapy to I.V. therapy**
Adults: 1.25 mg I.V. over 5 minutes every 6 hours.

➤ **To convert from I.V. therapy to oral therapy**
Adults: 5 mg P.O. once daily.

Adjust-a-dose: For patients with CrCl of 30 mL/minute or less, give 2.5 mg P.O. once daily.

➤ **To manage symptomatic HF**
Adults: Initially, 2.5 mg P.O. daily or b.i.d., increased gradually over several weeks. Maintenance is 5 to 20 mg daily in two divided doses. Maximum daily dose is 40 mg in two divided doses.

➤ **Asymptomatic left ventricular dysfunction**
Adults: Initially, 2.5 mg P.O. b.i.d. Increase as tolerated to target daily dose of 20 mg P.O. in divided doses.

ADMINISTRATION
P.O.
• Give drug without regard for food.
• Request oral suspension for patient who has difficulty swallowing.

I.V.
▼ Inspect solution for particulate matter and discoloration before administration.
▼ Compatible solutions include D₅W, NSS for injection, dextrose 5% in lactated Ringer injection, dextrose 5% in NSS for injection, and Isolyte E.
▼ Inject drug slowly over at least 5 minutes, or dilute in 50 mL of a compatible solution and infuse over 15 minutes.
▼ **Incompatibilities:** Amphotericin B, cefepime hydrochloride, phenytoin sodium.

ACTION
May inhibit ACE, preventing conversion of angiotensin I to angiotensin II, a potent vasoconstrictor. Less angiotensin II decreases peripheral arterial resistance, decreasing aldosterone secretion, reducing sodium and water retention, and lowering BP.

Route	Onset	Peak	Duration
P.O.	1 hr	3–4 hr	24 hr
I.V.	15 min	1–4 hr	6 hr

Half-life: 11 hours.

ADVERSE REACTIONS
CNS: asthenia, headache, dizziness, fatigue, vertigo, syncope, weakness.
CV: hypotension, chest pain, angina.
GI: anorexia, diarrhea, nausea, abdominal pain, vomiting.
GU: decreased renal function (in patients with bilateral renal artery stenosis or HF).
Hematologic: bone marrow depression.
Respiratory: bronchitis; dry, persistent, tickling, nonproductive cough; dyspnea.
Skin: rash.

INTERACTIONS
Drug-drug. *Aldosterone blockers (eplerenone), aliskiren, ARBs (candesartan, telmisartan), trimethoprim:* May increase risk of hyperkalemia. Monitor potassium level and clinical response.
Azathioprine: May increase risk of anemia or leukopenia. Monitor hematologic study results if used together.
Diuretics: May excessively reduce BP. Use together cautiously.
Insulin, oral antidiabetics: May cause hypoglycemia, especially at start of enalapril therapy. Monitor patient closely.
Lithium: May cause lithium toxicity. Monitor lithium level.

E

NSAIDs: May reduce antihypertensive effect. Monitor BP.

Potassium-sparing diuretics, potassium supplements: May cause hyperkalemia. Avoid using together unless hypokalemia is confirmed.

Drug-herb. *Capsaicin:* May cause cough. Discourage use together.

Ma huang: May decrease antihypertensive effects. Discourage use together.

Drug-food. *Salt substitutes containing potassium:* May cause hyperkalemia. Monitor patient closely.

EFFECTS ON LAB TEST RESULTS
- May increase bilirubin, BUN, creatinine, and potassium levels. May decrease sodium and Hb levels and hematocrit.
- May increase LFT values.

CONTRAINDICATIONS & CAUTIONS
- Contraindicated in patients hypersensitive to drug and in those with a history of angioedema related to previous treatment with an ACE inhibitor.
- Use cautiously in renally impaired patients or those with aortic stenosis or hypertrophic cardiomyopathy.
- According to the 2014 Evidence-Based Guideline for the Management of High Blood Pressure in Adults, ACE inhibitors are recommended as one of several preferred drugs for the initial treatment of hypertension; other options include ARBs, calcium channel blockers, and thiazide diuretics.

Dialyzable drug: Yes.

⚠ *Overdose S&S:* Hypotension.

PREGNANCY-LACTATION-REPRODUCTION
Black Box Warning Use during pregnancy can cause injury and death to the developing fetus. If pregnancy is detected, stop drug as soon as possible. ■
- Drug appears in breast milk. Breast-feeding isn't recommended.

NURSING CONSIDERATIONS
- Closely monitor BP response to drug.
- Monitor CBC with differential counts before and during therapy.
- Diabetic patients, those with impaired renal function or HF, and those receiving drugs that can increase potassium level may develop hyperkalemia. Monitor potassium intake and potassium level.
- Black patients who take ACE inhibitors as monotherapy for hypertension have a smaller reduction in BP than non-Black patients. Black patients taking ACE inhibitors have a higher incidence of angioedema than non-Blacks.
- *Look alike–sound alike:* Don't confuse enalapril with Anafranil or Eldepryl.
- *Look alike–sound alike:* Similar packaging and labeling of enalaprilat injection and pancuronium, a neuromuscular blocker, could result in a fatal medication error. Check all labels carefully.

PATIENT TEACHING
- Instruct patient to report breathing difficulty or swelling of face, eyes, lips, or tongue. Swelling of the face and throat (including swelling of the larynx) may occur, especially after first dose.
- Advise patient to report signs of infection, such as fever and sore throat.
- Inform patient that light-headedness can occur, especially during first few days of therapy. Tell him to rise slowly to minimize this effect and to notify prescriber if symptoms develop. If he faints, he should stop taking drug and call prescriber immediately.
- Tell patient to use caution in hot weather and during exercise. Inadequate fluid intake, vomiting, diarrhea, and excessive perspiration can lead to light-headedness and fainting.
- Advise patient to avoid salt substitutes; these products may contain potassium, which can cause high potassium levels in patients taking this drug.
- Tell female patient of childbearing potential to notify prescriber if pregnancy occurs. Drug will need to be stopped.

enfuvirtide
en-foo-VEER-tide

Fuzeon

Therapeutic class: Antiretrovirals
Pharmacologic class: Fusion inhibitors

AVAILABLE FORMS
Powder for injection: 108-mg single-use
vials (90 mg/mL after reconstitution)

INDICATIONS & DOSAGES
➤ **To help control HIV-1 infection, with
other antiretrovirals, in patients who
have continued HIV-1 replication despite
antiretroviral therapy**
Adults: 90 mg subcutaneously b.i.d.
Children ages 6 to 16: 2 mg/kg subcutaneously b.i.d. Maximum, 90 mg/dose.

ADMINISTRATION
Subcutaneous
● Reconstitute vial with 1 mL sterile water
for injection. Tap vial for 10 seconds and
then gently roll to prevent foaming. Let
drug stand for up to 45 minutes to ensure
reconstitution. Or, gently roll vial between
hands until product is completely dissolved.
Then draw up correct dose and inject drug.
● If you won't be using drug immediately
after reconstitution, refrigerate in original
vial and use within 24 hours. Don't inject
drug until it's at room temperature.
● Vial is for single use; discard unused
portion.
● Inject into upper arm, anterior thigh, or
abdomen. Rotate injection sites. Don't inject
into same site for two consecutive doses,
and don't inject into moles, scar tissue,
bruises, tattoos, or the navel, where large
nerves course close to the skin.
● Store unreconstituted vials at room
temperature.

ACTION
Interferes with entry of HIV-1 into cells
by inhibiting fusion of HIV-1 to cell
membranes.

Route	Onset	Peak	Duration
Subcut.	Unknown	4–8 hr	Unknown

Half-life: 3.8 hours.

ADVERSE REACTIONS
CNS: fatigue, insomnia, anxiety, asthenia,
depression, peripheral neuropathy.
EENT: conjunctivitis, sinusitis, taste distur-
bance.
GI: diarrhea, nausea, *pancreatitis,* abdomi-
nal pain, constipation, dry mouth.
Metabolic: anorexia, weight decrease.
Musculoskeletal: myalgia.
Respiratory: *bacterial pneumonia,* cough.
Skin: injection-site reactions, pruritus, skin
papilloma.
Other: herpes simplex, influenza,
influenza-like illness, lymphadenopathy.

INTERACTIONS
Drug-drug. *Protease inhibitors:* May
increase concentrations of either drug.
Monitor therapy.

EFFECTS ON LAB TEST RESULTS
● May increase ALT, amylase, AST, CK,
GGT, lipase, and triglyceride levels. May
decrease Hb level.
● May decrease eosinophil count.

CONTRAINDICATIONS & CAUTIONS
● Contraindicated in patients hypersensitive
to drug and in those not infected with HIV.
● Safety and effectiveness haven't been
established in children younger than age 6.
Dialyzable drug: Unlikely.

PREGNANCY-LACTATION-REPRODUCTION
● There are no well-controlled studies in
pregnant women. Use during pregnancy
only if clearly needed.
● Register pregnant women in the Antiretroviral Pregnancy Registry at 1-800-258-
4263.
● Because of the potential for HIV transmission, women shouldn't breast-feed.

NURSING CONSIDERATIONS
● Injection-site reactions (pain, discomfort,
induration, erythema, pruritus, nodules,
cysts, ecchymosis) are common and may
require analgesics or rest.

E

♣Canada   ◇OTC   ◆Off-label use   ✔Photoguide   ⊚Do not crush   *Liquid contains alcohol.

• Nerve pain (neuralgia or paresthesia) lasting up to 6 months and associated with administration at sites where large nerves course close to the skin, bruising, and hematomas have occurred. Patients receiving anticoagulants and those with hemophilia or other coagulation disorders may have a higher risk of postinjection bleeding.

◑ *Alert:* Monitor patient closely for evidence of bacterial pneumonia. Patients at high risk include those with a low initial CD4 count or high initial viral load, those who use I.V. drugs or smoke, and those with history of lung disease.

• Hypersensitivity may occur with first dose or later doses. If systemic symptoms occur, stop drug and don't rechallenge.

PATIENT TEACHING

• Teach patient how to prepare and give drug and how to safely dispose of used needles and syringes.

• Tell patient to rotate injection sites and to watch for cellulitis or local infection.

• Urge patient to immediately report evidence of pneumonia, such as cough with fever, rapid breathing, or shortness of breath.

• Tell patient to stop taking drug and seek medical attention if evidence of hypersensitivity develops, such as rash, fever, nausea, vomiting, chills, rigors, and hypotension.

• Teach patient that drug doesn't cure HIV infection and that it must be taken with other antiretrovirals.

• Tell patient to inform prescriber if she's pregnant, plans to become pregnant, or is breast-feeding while taking this drug. Because HIV could be transmitted to the infant, HIV-infected mothers shouldn't breast-feed.

• Tell patient that drug may affect the ability to drive or operate machinery.

• Tell patient that information on self-administration is available (1-877-4FUZEON [1-877-438-9366]).

SAFETY ALERT!

enoxaparin sodium
en-OCKS-a-par-in

Lovenox

Therapeutic class: Anticoagulants
Pharmacologic class: Low–molecular-weight heparins

AVAILABLE FORMS
Syringes (graduated prefilled): 60 mg/ 0.6 mL, 80 mg/0.8 mL, 100 mg/mL, 120 mg/0.8 mL, 150 mg/mL
Syringes (prefilled): 30 mg/0.3 mL, 40 mg/0.4 mL

INDICATIONS & DOSAGES
➤ **To prevent PE and DVT after hip or knee replacement surgery**
Adults: 30 mg subcutaneously every 12 hours for 7 to 10 days. Treatment for up to 14 days has been well tolerated. Give initial dose between 12 and 24 hours postoperatively, as long as hemostasis has been established. Continue treatment during postoperative period until risk of DVT has diminished. Hip replacement patients may receive 40 mg subcutaneously given 12 hours (range, 9 to 15 hours) preoperatively. After initial phase of therapy, hip replacement patients should continue with 40 mg subcutaneously daily for 3 weeks.
Adjust-a-dose: In patients with CrCl of less than 30 mL/minute, give 30 mg subcutaneously once daily.
➤ **To prevent PE and DVT after abdominal surgery**
Adults: 40 mg subcutaneously daily with initial dose 2 hours before surgery. Give subsequent dose, as long as hemostasis has been established, 24 hours after initial preoperative dose, and continue once daily for 7 to 10 days. Treatment for up to 12 days has been well tolerated. Continue treatment during postoperative period until risk of DVT has diminished.
Adjust-a-dose: In patients with CrCl of less than 30 mL/minute, give 30 mg subcutaneously once daily.

Reactions in bold italics are *life-threatening*. Interactions may have a *rapid onset* or a *delayed onset*.

enoxaparin sodium 529

➤ **To prevent PE and DVT in patients with acute illness who are at increased risk because of decreased mobility**
Adults: 40 mg subcutaneously once daily for 6 to 11 days. Treatment for up to 14 days has been well tolerated.
Adjust-a-dose: In patients with CrCl of less than 30 mL/minute, give 30 mg subcutaneously once daily.

➤ **To prevent ischemic complications of unstable angina and non–Q-wave MI with oral aspirin therapy**
Adults: 1 mg/kg subcutaneously every 12 hours until clinical stabilization (minimum 2 days) with aspirin 100 to 325 mg P.O. once daily. Usual duration of treatment is 2 to 8 days.
Adjust-a-dose: In patients with CrCl of less than 30 mL/minute, give 1 mg/kg subcutaneously once daily.

➤ **Acute ST-segment elevation MI**
Adults younger than age 75: 30 mg single I.V. bolus plus 1 mg/kg subcutaneously followed by 1 mg/kg subcutaneously every 12 hours (maximum of 100 mg for the first two doses only) with aspirin 75 to 325 mg P.O. once daily. When given with a thrombolytic, give enoxaparin from 15 minutes before to 30 minutes after the start of fibrinolytic therapy. For patients undergoing PCI, if the last subcutaneous dose was given less than 8 hours before balloon inflation, no additional dose is needed. If the last dose was given more than 8 hours before balloon inflation, give 0.3 mg/kg I.V. bolus.
Adults age 75 and older: Don't use an initial I.V. bolus. Give 0.75 mg/kg subcutaneously every 12 hours (maximum 75 mg for the first two doses only).
Adjust-a-dose: In adults younger than age 75 with severe renal impairment (CrCl of less than 30 mL/minute), 30 mg single I.V. bolus plus 1 mg/kg subcutaneously followed by 1 mg/kg subcutaneously once daily. In adults age 75 and older with severe renal impairment, 1 mg/kg subcutaneously once daily with no initial bolus. Give with aspirin.

➤ **Inpatient treatment of acute DVT with and without PE when given with warfarin sodium**
Adults: 1 mg/kg subcutaneously every 12 hours. Or, 1.5 mg/kg subcutaneously once daily (at same time daily) for 5 to 7 days until therapeutic oral anticoagulant effect (INR 2 to 3) is achieved. Warfarin sodium therapy is usually started within 72 hours of enoxaparin injection.
Adjust-a-dose: In patients with CrCl of less than 30 mL/minute, give 1 mg/kg subcutaneously once daily.

➤ **Outpatient treatment of acute DVT without PE when given with warfarin sodium**
Adults: 1 mg/kg subcutaneously every 12 hours for 5 to 7 days until therapeutic oral anticoagulant effect (INR 2 to 3) is achieved. Warfarin sodium therapy usually is started within 72 hours of enoxaparin injection.
Adjust-a-dose: In patients with CrCl of less than 30 mL/minute, give 1 mg/kg subcutaneously once daily.

➤ **To prevent PE and DVT in general surgery patients ◆**
Adults: 40 mg subcutaneously once daily, with initial dose given 2 hours before surgery. Usual duration of administration is until hospital discharge or up to 7 to 10 days; for selected high-risk general surgery patients, including those who have undergone major cancer surgery or have previously experienced a venous thrombotic event, consider continuation for up to 28 days after hospital discharge.
Adjust-a-dose: In patients with CrCl of less than 30 mL/minute, give 30 mg subcutaneously once daily.

ADMINISTRATION
I.V.
▼ If using multidose vial, use a tuberculin syringe to withdraw appropriate volume of drug.
▼ Flush I.V. access with sufficient amount of saline or dextrose solution before and after I.V. bolus administration.
▼ **Incompatibilities:** Don't mix or administer with other I.V. drugs.
Subcutaneous
• With patient lying down, give by deep subcutaneous injection, alternating doses between left and right anterolateral and posterolateral abdominal walls.
• Don't massage after subcutaneous injection. Watch for signs of bleeding at site. Rotate sites and keep record.

ACTION
Accelerates formation of antithrombin III–thrombin complex and deactivates thrombin, preventing conversion of fibrinogen to fibrin. Drug has a higher antifactor-Xa-to-antifactor-IIa activity ratio than heparin.

Route	Onset	Peak	Duration
I.V.	Unknown	Unknown	Unknown
Subcut.	Unknown	4 hr	Unknown

Half-life: 4½ hours after a single dose; 7 hours after repeated dosing.

ADVERSE REACTIONS
CNS: confusion, fever, pain.
CV: edema, peripheral edema.
GI: nausea, diarrhea.
Hematologic: *thrombocytopenia, hemorrhage,* ecchymoses, bleeding complications, hypochromic anemia.
Respiratory: dyspnea.
Skin: irritation, pain, hematoma, and erythema at injection site; rash; urticaria.
Other: *angioedema, anaphylaxis.*

INTERACTIONS
Drug-drug. *Anticoagulants, antiplatelet drugs, NSAIDs:* May increase risk of bleeding. Use together cautiously. Monitor PT and INR.
SSRIs: May increase risk of severe bleeding. Monitor PT, INR, and patient. Adjust therapy as needed.
Drug-herb. *Angelica (dong quai), boldo, bromelains, capsicum, chamomile, dandelion, danshen, devil's claw, fenugreek, feverfew, garlic, ginger, ginkgo, ginseng, horse chestnut, licorice, meadowsweet, onion, passion flower, red clover, willow:* May increase risk of bleeding. Discourage use together.

EFFECTS ON LAB TEST RESULTS
• May increase ALT and AST levels. May decrease Hb level.
• May decrease platelet count.

CONTRAINDICATIONS & CAUTIONS
• Contraindicated in patients hypersensitive to drug, heparin, or pork products; in those with active major bleeding; and in those with thrombocytopenia and antiplatelet antibodies in presence of drug.

• Use cautiously in patients with history of heparin-induced thrombocytopenia, aneurysms, cerebrovascular hemorrhage, spinal or epidural punctures (as with anesthesia), uncontrolled hypertension, or threatened abortion.
• Use cautiously in elderly patients and in those with conditions that place them at increased risk for hemorrhage, such as bacterial endocarditis, congenital or acquired bleeding disorders, ulcer disease, angiodysplastic GI disease, hemorrhagic stroke, or recent spinal, eye, or brain surgery.
• Use cautiously in patients with prosthetic heart valves, with regional or lumbar block anesthesia, blood dyscrasias, recent childbirth, pericarditis or pericardial effusion, renal insufficiency, or severe CNS trauma.
Dialyzable drug: Unknown.
⚠ *Overdose S&S:* Hemorrhagic complications.

PREGNANCY-LACTATION-REPRODUCTION
• There are no well-controlled studies in pregnant women. Monitor pregnant women closely for evidence of bleeding or excessive coagulation. Warn pregnant women and women of childbearing potential about potential risk of therapy.
• Consider using a shorter-acting anticoagulant as delivery approaches.
• Multidose vial shouldn't be used in pregnant women because of benzyl alcohol content.
• It isn't known if drug appears in breast milk. Patient should discontinue breast-feeding or discontinue drug.

NURSING CONSIDERATIONS
• It's important to achieve hemostasis at the puncture site after PCI. The vascular access sheath for instrumentation should remain in place for 6 hours after a dose if manual compression method is used; give next dose no sooner than 6 to 8 hours after sheath removal. Monitor vital signs and site for hematoma and bleeding.
• Monitor anti-Xa levels in pregnant women with mechanical heart valves and in patients with significant renal impairment.
Black Box Warning Patients who receive epidural or spinal anesthesia or spinal puncture during therapy are at increased risk for

---

developing an epidural or spinal hematoma, which may result in long-term or permanent paralysis. Factors that can increase these risks include use of indwelling epidural catheters, concurrent use of other drugs that affect hemostasis, history of traumatic or repeated epidural or spinal puncture, and history of spinal deformity or spinal surgery. Monitor these patients closely for neurologic impairment, as urgent treatment is necessary. ■

Black Box Warning Optimal timing between administration of enoxaparin and spinal procedures isn't known. ■

Alert: For spinal procedures, consider both dose and elimination half-life of drug. Delay placement or removal of a spinal catheter for at least 12 hours after prophylactic doses or for 24 hours for higher therapeutic doses of 1 mg/kg b.i.d. or 1.5 mg/kg daily. Give postprocedure doses no sooner than 4 hours after catheter removal.

- Draw blood to establish baseline coagulation parameters before therapy.
- Never give drug I.M.

Alert: Don't try to expel the air bubble from the 30- or 40-mg prefilled syringes. This may lead to loss of drug and an incorrect dose.

- Avoid I.M. injections of other drugs to prevent or minimize hematoma.
- Monitor platelet counts regularly. Patients with normal coagulation won't need close monitoring of PT or PTT.
- Regularly inspect patient for bleeding gums, bruises on arms or legs, petechiae, nosebleeds, melena, tarry stools, hematuria, and hematemesis.
- To treat severe overdose, give protamine sulfate (a heparin antagonist) by slow I.V. infusion at concentration of 1% to equal dose of drug injected.

Alert: Drug isn't interchangeable with heparin or other low-molecular-weight heparins.

PATIENT TEACHING

- Instruct patient and family to watch for signs of bleeding or abnormal bruising and to notify prescriber immediately.

Black Box Warning Tell patient to immediately report signs and symptoms of spinal or epidural hematoma, such as numbness (especially of the lower limbs) and muscle weakness. ■

- Tell patient to avoid OTC drugs containing aspirin or other salicylates unless ordered by prescriber.
- Advise patient to consult prescriber before initiating herbal therapy; many herbs have anticoagulant, antiplatelet, or fibrinolytic properties.

E

entecavir

en-TEK-ah-veer

Baraclude

Therapeutic class: Antivirals
Pharmacologic class: Nucleosides–nucleotides

AVAILABLE FORMS

Oral solution: 0.05 mg/mL
Tablets: 0.5 mg, 1 mg

INDICATIONS & DOSAGES

➤ **Chronic HBV infection in patients with active viral replication and either persistently increased aminotransferase levels or histologically active disease**

Adults and adolescents age 16 and older who have had no previous nucleoside treatment: 0.5 mg P.O. once daily at least 2 hours before or after a meal.

Adjust-a-dose: If CrCl is 30 to less than 50 mL/minute, give 0.25 mg P.O. once daily or 0.5 mg P.O. every 48 hours. If CrCl is 10 to less than 30 mL/minute, give 0.15 mg P.O. once daily or 0.5 mg P.O. every 72 hours. If CrCl is less than 10 mL/minute or patient is undergoing hemodialysis or continuous ambulatory peritoneal dialysis (CAPD), give 0.05 mg P.O. once daily or 0.5 mg P.O. every 7 days.

Children age 2 to younger than age 16 and weighing at least 10 kg who have had no previous nucleoside treatment: For children weighing more than 30 kg, 10 mL (0.5 mg) oral solution or one 0.5-mg tablet P.O. once daily. For children weighing more than 26 to 30 kg, 9 mL (0.45 mg) oral solution P.O. once daily. For children weighing more than 23 to 26 kg, 8 mL (0.4 mg) oral solution P.O.

once daily. For children weighing more than 20 to 23 kg, 7 mL (0.35 mg) oral solution P.O. once daily. For children weighing more than 17 to 20 kg, 6 mL (0.3 mg) oral solution P.O. once daily. For children weighing more than 14 to 17 kg, 5 mL (0.25 mg) oral solution P.O. once daily. For children weighing more than 11 to 14 kg, 4 mL (0.2 mg) oral solution P.O. once daily. For children weighing more than 10 to 11 kg, 3 mL (0.15 mg) oral solution P.O. once daily.

Adjust-a-dose: Insufficient data are available for specific dosage adjustments in children with renal impairment. Consider reducing dosage or increasing dosing interval similar to adjustments for adults.

Adults and adolescents age 16 and older who have a history of viremia and are taking lamivudine or telbivudine or have resistance mutations, or patients with decompensated liver disease: 1 mg P.O. once daily at least 2 hours before or after a meal.

Adjust-a-dose: If CrCl is 30 to less than 50 mL/minute, give 0.5 mg P.O. once daily or 1 mg P.O. every 48 hours. If CrCl is 10 to less than 30 mL/minute, give 0.3 mg P.O. once daily or 1 mg P.O. every 72 hours. If CrCl is less than 10 mL/minute or patient is undergoing hemodialysis or CAPD, give 0.1 mg P.O. once daily or 1 mg P.O. every 7 days.

Children age 2 to younger than age 16 and weighing at least 10 kg who are lamivudine-experienced: For children weighing more than 30 kg, 20 mL (1 mg) oral solution or one 1-mg tablet P.O. once daily. For children weighing more than 26 to 30 kg, 18 mL (0.9 mg) oral solution P.O. once daily. For children weighing more than 23 to 26 kg, 16 mL (0.8 mg) oral solution P.O. once daily. For children weighing more than 20 to 23 kg, 14 mL (0.7 mg) oral solution P.O. once daily. For children weighing more than 17 to 20 kg, 12 mL (0.6 mg) oral solution P.O. once daily. For children weighing more than 14 to 17 kg, 10 mL (0.5 mg) oral solution P.O. once daily. For children weighing more than 11 to 14 kg, 8 mL (0.4 mg) oral solution P.O. once daily. For children weighing more than 10 to 11 kg, 6 mL (0.3 mg) oral solution P.O. once daily.

Adjust-a-dose: Insufficient data are available for specific dosage adjustments in children

with renal impairment. Consider reducing dosage or increasing dosing interval similar to adjustments for adults.

ADMINISTRATION
P.O.
- Drug is considered hazardous; follow safe handling and disposal procedures.
- Drug should be taken on an empty stomach at least 2 hours before or after a meal to increase absorption.
- After oral solution has been opened, it can be used up to expiration date on the bottle.

ACTION
Inhibits HBV polymerase and reduces viral DNA levels.

Route	Onset	Peak	Duration
P.O.	Unknown	½–1½ hr	Unknown

Half-life: About 5 or 6 days.

ADVERSE REACTIONS
CNS: dizziness, fatigue, headache.
GI: diarrhea, dyspepsia, nausea.
GU: glycosuria, hematuria.
Hepatic: hepatomegaly.
Metabolic: *lactic acidosis.*

INTERACTIONS
Drug-drug. *Cyclosporine, tacrolimus:* May further decrease renal function. Monitor renal function carefully.
Drugs that reduce renal function or compete for active tubular secretion: May increase level of either drug. Monitor renal function, and watch for adverse effects.
Ganciclovir, valganciclovir: May increase entecavir serum concentration. Monitor patient for entecavir toxicity.
Ribavirin: May enhance hepatotoxic effect of entecavir. Monitor therapy.
Drug-food. *All foods:* Delays absorption and decreases drug level. Give drug at least 2 hours before or after a meal.

EFFECTS ON LAB TEST RESULTS
- May increase ALT, amylase, AST, blood glucose, creatinine, lipase, and total bilirubin levels.
- May decrease platelet count.

CONTRAINDICATIONS & CAUTIONS

• Contraindicated in patients hypersensitive to drug or its components.

Black Box Warning Don't use in patients infected with both HIV and HBV who aren't also receiving highly active antiretroviral therapy. ∎

• Use cautiously in patients with renal impairment and in patients who have had a liver transplant.

Dialyzable drug: 13%.

PREGNANCY-LACTATION-REPRODUCTION

• Use cautiously in pregnant women and only if benefit outweighs risk to the fetus.

• Register pregnant women in the Antiretro- viral Pregnancy Registry at 1-800-258- 4263.

• It isn't known if drug appears in breast milk. Patient should discontinue breast- feeding or discontinue drug.

NURSING CONSIDERATIONS

Black Box Warning Drug may cause life- threatening lactic acidosis and severe hepat- omegaly with steatosis when is used alone or in combination with antiretrovirals. ∎

Black Box Warning HBV infection may worsen severely after therapy stops. Monitor hepatic function for several months in pa- tients who stop therapy. If appropriate, start therapy for HBV infection. ∎

• Closely monitor patients with renal im- pairment and patients who have had a liver transplant.

• Oral solution should be used for patients weighing up to 30 kg and for doses less than 0.5 mg.

• In elderly patients, adjust dosage for age- related decrease in renal function.

PATIENT TEACHING

• Tell patient to take drug on an empty stomach at least 2 hours before or after a meal.

• Caution against mixing or diluting oral solution with any other substance. Teach proper use of dosing spoon.

• Tell patient to report all adverse effects of this drug and any new drugs being taken.

• Explain that drug doesn't reduce the risk of HBV transmission to others.

• Teach patient the signs and symptoms of lactic acidosis, such as muscle pain, weak- ness, dyspnea, GI distress, cold hands and feet, dizziness, or fast or irregular heartbeat.

• Teach patient the signs and symptoms of hepatotoxicity, such as jaundice, dark urine, light-colored stool, loss of appetite, nausea, and stomach pain.

• Warn patient not to stop drug abruptly.

epinastine hydrochloride
ep-ih-NAS-teen

Elestat

Therapeutic class: Antihistamines
Pharmacologic class: H_1-receptor antagonists–mast cell stabilizers

AVAILABLE FORMS

Ophthalmic solution: 0.05%

INDICATIONS & DOSAGES

➤ **To prevent pruritus from allergic conjunctivitis**

Adults and children age 3 and older: Instill 1 drop into each eye b.i.d. Continue treat- ment as long as allergen is present, even if symptoms resolve.

ADMINISTRATION

Ophthalmic

• Drug is for ophthalmic use only. Don't inject or give orally.

• Keep bottle tightly closed when not in use.

• Don't touch tip of dropper to any surface.

ACTION

Inhibits release of mediators from cells involved in hypersensitivity reactions, temporarily preventing pruritus.

Route	Onset	Peak	Duration
Ophthalmic	Immediate	Unknown	8 hr

Half-life: About 12 hours.

ADVERSE REACTIONS

CNS: headache.
EENT: cold symptoms, burning eyes, hyperemia, increased lymph nodes near eyes, pharyngitis, pruritus, rhinitis, sinusitis.
Respiratory: increased cough, URI.

INTERACTIONS
None reported.

EFFECTS ON LAB TEST RESULTS
None reported.

CONTRAINDICATIONS & CAUTIONS
• Contraindicated in patients hypersensitive to drug or its components.
• Contraindicated for irritation related to contact lenses.
• Safety and effectiveness haven't been established in children younger than age 3.
Dialyzable drug: Unknown.

PREGNANCY-LACTATION-REPRODUCTION
• Use cautiously in pregnant women and only if benefit outweighs possible risk to the fetus.
• It isn't known if drug appears in breast milk. Use cautiously in breast-feeding women.

NURSING CONSIDERATIONS
• Monitor patient for signs and symptoms of infection.
• Soft contact lenses may absorb the preservative benzalkonium.

PATIENT TEACHING
• Teach patient proper instillation technique. Instruct him not to touch any surface, eyelid, or surrounding areas with tip of dropper.
• Caution patient not to use drops to treat contact lens–related eye irritation and not to wear contact lenses if eyes are red.
• Tell patient to remove contact lenses before instillation and to wait at least 10 minutes after instilling drug before reinserting lenses.
• Warn patient that soft contact lenses may absorb the preservative benzalkonium.
• Advise patient to report adverse reactions to drug.
• Tell patient to keep bottle tightly closed when not in use.

SAFETY ALERT!

epinephrine (adrenaline)
ep-i-NEF-rin

epinephrine hydrochloride
Adrenaclick, Adrenalin, Auvi-Q, EpiPen, EpiPen Jr

Therapeutic class: Vasopressors
Pharmacologic class: Adrenergics

AVAILABLE FORMS
Injection: 0.1 mg/mL (1:10,000), 1 mg/mL (1:1,000) parenteral
Injection device: 0.15 mg/0.15 mL, 0.3 mg/0.3 mL

INDICATIONS & DOSAGES
➤ **Anaphylaxis**
Adults: 0.3 to 0.5 mg Adrenalin I.M. or subcutaneously, repeated every 5 to 10 minutes as needed. Or, 0.2 to 1 mg of generic 1:1,000 solution I.M. or subcutaneously. Repeat every 10 to 15 minutes as needed. Or, 0.1 to 0.25 mg of 1:10,000 solution I.V. slowly over 5 to 10 minutes. May repeat every 5 to 15 minutes as needed, or follow with a continuous I.V. infusion, starting at 1 mcg/minute and increasing to 4 mcg/minute, as needed. Or, 0.3 mg I.M. or subcutaneously with autoinjector into outer aspect of thigh, through clothing if necessary. Repeat as needed.
Children weighing 30 kg or more: 0.3 to 0.5 mg Adrenalin I.M. or subcutaneously, repeated every 5 to 10 minutes as needed.
Children weighing less than 30 kg: 0.01 mg/kg Adrenalin I.M. or subcutaneously, repeated every 5 to 10 minutes as needed.
Children: 0.01 mg/kg (10 mcg) of generic 1:1,000 solution subcutaneously. Repeat every 15 minutes for two doses, then every 4 hours as needed. Maximum single dose shouldn't exceed 0.5 mg. Or, 0.3 mg of 1:10,000 solution I.V. Repeat every 15 minutes for three or four doses p.r.n. Or, 0.15 mg by autoinjector if patient weighs 15 to 29 kg or 0.3 mg by autoinjector if patient weighs 30 kg or more, I.M. or subcutaneously, into outer aspect of thigh, through clothing if necessary. Repeat p.r.n.

➤ **Asthma (not Adrenalin)**
Adults: 0.2 to 1 mg of 1:1,000 solution subcutaneously. Start with small dose and increase if needed. Or, 0.1 to 0.25 mg of 1:10,000 solution given slowly I.V.
Children: 0.01 mg/kg (or 0.3 mg/m^2) of 1:1,000 solution subcutaneously to a maximum of 0.5 mg, repeated every 4 hours as needed.
Infants: 0.05 mg solution subcutaneously. May be repeated at 20- to 30-minute intervals.
Neonates: 0.01 mg/kg of 1:1,000 solution subcutaneously.

➤ **Cardiac stimulation (not Adrenalin)**
Adults: 0.1 mg/mL of 1:10,000 solution I.V. May follow with 0.3 mg of 1:1,000 solution subcutaneously. Or, 0.1 to 1 mg of 1:10,000 solution I.V., repeated every 5 minutes, if needed.
Children: 0.005 to 0.01 mg/kg of 1:10,000 solution I.V., repeated every 5 minutes, if needed.

➤ **Induction and maintenance of mydriasis during intraocular surgery (Adrenalin only)**
Adults and children: Dilute 1 mL of epinephrine 1:1,000 (1 mg/mL) in 100 to 1,000 mL of an ophthalmic irrigation fluid to create a concentration of 1:100,000 to 1:1,000,000. Irrigate eye as needed for surgical procedure. Or, dilute to 1:1,000,000 to 1:4,000,000 (10 to 2.5 mcg/mL) for injection intracamerally as a bolus dose.

ADMINISTRATION
I.V.
▼ Keep solution in light-resistant container, and don't remove before use.
▼ Just before use, mix with D$_5$W, NSS for injection, lactated Ringer injection, or combinations of dextrose in saline solution.
▼ Monitor BP, HR, and ECG when therapy starts and frequently thereafter.
▼ Discard solution if it's discolored or contains precipitate or after 24 hours.
▼ When giving as a continuous infusion, use a central line with an infusion pump.
▼ Don't give autoinjectors I.V.
▼ **Incompatibilities:** Aminophylline; ampicillin sodium; furosemide; hyaluronidase; Ionosol D-CM, PSL, and

T solutions with D$_5$W; mephentermine; thiopental sodium. Compatible with most other I.V. solutions. Rapidly destroyed by alkalies or oxidizing drugs, including halogens, nitrates, nitrites, permanganates, sodium bicarbonate, and salts of easily reducible metals, such as iron, copper, and zinc. Don't mix with alkaline solutions.
I.M.
● Avoid I.M. use of parenteral suspension into buttocks. Gas gangrene may occur because drug reduces oxygen tension of the tissues, encouraging growth of contaminating organisms.
● Massage site after I.M. injection to counteract vasoconstriction. Repeated local injection can cause necrosis at injection site.
● Don't give if solution is discolored or contains precipitate.
● Don't give autoinjectors I.V.
Subcutaneous
● Don't refrigerate; protect from light.
● Don't give if solution is discolored or contains precipitate.
● Don't give autoinjectors I.V.
● Don't inject too deeply and enter muscle.
● Protect from light and freezing; store between 59° and 77° F (15° and 25° C).
Intraocular
● Must dilute before administration.

ACTION
Relaxes bronchial smooth muscle by stimulating beta$_2$ receptors and alpha and beta receptors in the sympathetic nervous system.

Route	Onset	Peak	Duration
I.V.	Immediate	5 min	Short
I.M.	Variable	Unknown	1–4 hr
Subcut.	5–15 min	30 min	1–4 hr
Intraocular	Unknown	Unknown	Unknown

Half-life: Unknown.

ADVERSE REACTIONS
CNS: drowsiness, headache, nervousness, tremor, *cerebral hemorrhage, stroke,* vertigo, pain, disorientation, agitation, fear, restlessness, dizziness, weakness, *subarachnoid hemorrhage.*
CV: palpitations, *ventricular fibrillation, shock,* widened pulse pressure, hypertension, tachycardia, anginal pain, cardiac

E

arrhythmias, altered ECG (including decreased T-wave amplitude).
GI: nausea, vomiting.
Respiratory: dyspnea.
Skin: urticaria, hemorrhage at injection site, pallor, sweating.
Other: tissue necrosis.

INTERACTIONS

Drug-drug. *Alpha blockers:* May cause hypotension from unopposed beta-adrenergic effects. Avoid using together.

Antihistamines, thyroid hormones: When given with sympathomimetics, may cause severe adverse cardiac effects. Avoid using together.

Cardiac glycosides, general anesthetics (halogenated hydrocarbons): May increase risk of ventricular arrhythmias. Monitor ECG closely.

Carteolol, nadolol, penbutolol, pindolol, propranolol, timolol: May cause hypertension followed by bradycardia. Stop beta blocker 3 days before starting epinephrine.

Doxapram, methylphenidate: May enhance CNS stimulation or pressor effects. Monitor patient closely.

Ergot alkaloids: May decrease vasoconstrictor activity. Monitor patient closely.

Levodopa: May enhance risk of arrhythmias. Monitor ECG closely.

MAO inhibitors: May increase risk of hypertensive crisis. Monitor BP closely.

TCAs: May potentiate the pressor response and cause arrhythmias. Use together cautiously.

EFFECTS ON LAB TEST RESULTS

● May increase BUN, glucose, and lactic acid levels.

CONTRAINDICATIONS & CAUTIONS

● Contraindicated in patients with angle-closure glaucoma, shock (other than anaphylactic shock), organic brain damage, HF, cardiac dilation, arrhythmias, coronary insufficiency, or cerebral arteriosclerosis.

● Contraindicated in patients receiving general anesthesia with halogenated hydrocarbons or cyclopropane and in patients in labor (may delay second stage).

● Commercial products containing sulfites contraindicated in patients with sulfite

allergies, except when epinephrine is being used to treat serious allergic reactions or other emergency situations.

● Contraindicated for use in fingers, toes, ears, nose, or genitalia when used with local anesthetic.

● Use cautiously in patients with longstanding bronchial asthma or emphysema who have developed degenerative heart disease.

● Use cautiously in elderly patients and in those with hyperthyroidism, CV disease, hypertension, psychoneurosis, and diabetes.
Dialyzable drug: Unknown.

⚠ **Overdose S&S:** Precordial distress, vomiting, headache, dyspnea, hypertension, peripheral vascular constriction, pulmonary edema, cerebral hemorrhage, arrhythmias, extreme pallor and coldness of the skin, metabolic acidosis, kidney failure.

PREGNANCY-LACTATION-REPRODUCTION

● Use during pregnancy only if potential benefit justifies potential risk to the fetus.

● Parenteral administration of epinephrine, if used to support BP during low or other spinal anesthesia for delivery, can cause accelerated fetal HR and shouldn't be used in obstetrics when maternal BP exceeds 130/80 mm Hg.

● It isn't known if drug appears in breast milk. Patient should discontinue breastfeeding or discontinue drug.

NURSING CONSIDERATIONS

● In patients with Parkinson disease, drug increases rigidity and tremor.

● Drug interferes with tests for urinary catecholamines.

🟢 **Alert:** Be aware of ratio expressions on some drug labels. Note that 1 mg equals 1 mL of 1:1,000 solution or 10 mL of 1:10,000 solution.

● Epinephrine is drug of choice in emergency treatment of acute anaphylactic reactions.

● Observe patient closely for adverse reactions. Notify prescriber if adverse reactions develop; adjusting dosage or stopping drug may be necessary.

● If BP increases sharply, give rapid-acting vasodilators, such as nitrates and alpha blockers, to counteract the marked pressor effect of large doses.

- Drug is rapidly destroyed by oxidizing products, such as iodine, chromates, nitrites, oxygen, and salts of easily reducible metals (such as iron).
- When treating patient with reactions caused by other drugs given I.M. or subcutaneously, inject this drug into the site where the other drug was given to minimize further absorption.
- *Look alike–sound alike:* Don't confuse epinephrine with ephedrine or norepinephrine.

PATIENT TEACHING
- If patient has acute hypersensitivity reactions (such as to bee stings), you may need to teach him to self-inject drug.
- Instruct patient in autoinjector use.
- Tell patient to give autoinjector in outer thigh and not into buttock.
- Caution patient or caregiver to only give two sequential doses unless under direct medical supervision. Patient should seek immediate medical care for acute hypersensitivity reactions.

SAFETY ALERT!

epirubicin hydrochloride
ep-uh-ROO-bi-sin

Ellence

Therapeutic class: Antineoplastics
Pharmacologic class: Anthracycline glycoside antibiotics

AVAILABLE FORMS
Injection: 2 mg/mL, 50 mg/25 mL, 200 mg/100 mL

INDICATIONS & DOSAGES
➤ **Adjuvant therapy in patients with evidence of axillary node tumor involvement after resection of primary breast cancer**
Adults: 100 to 120 mg/m^2 I.V. infusion over 3 to 20 minutes, depending on dosage and infusion volume, through a free-flowing I.V. solution on day 1 of each cycle, or divided equally in two doses on days 1 and 8 of each cycle; cycle repeated every 3 to 4 weeks for six cycles; used with regimens containing

cyclophosphamide and 5-FU. Don't exceed cumulative dose of 900 mg/m^2.

Dosage modification after first cycle is based on toxicity. For patients with platelet count nadir below 50,000/mm^3, ANC below 250/mm^3, neutropenic fever, or grade 3 or 4 nonhematologic toxicity, reduce day 1 dose in subsequent cycles to 75% of day 1 dose given in current cycle. Delay day 1 therapy in subsequent cycles until platelet count is at least 100,000/mm^3, ANC is at least 1,500/mm^3, and nonhematologic toxicities recover to grade 1 or less.

For patients receiving divided doses (days 1 and 8), day 8 dose should be 75% of day 1 dose if platelet count is 75,000 to 100,000/mm^3 and ANC is 1,000 to 1,499/mm^3. If day 8 platelet count is below 75,000/mm^3, ANC is below 1,000/mm^3, or grade 3 or 4 nonhematologic toxicity has occurred, omit day 8 dose.

Adjust-a-dose: For patients with bone marrow dysfunction (heavily pretreated patients, patients with bone marrow depression, or those with neoplastic bone marrow infiltration), start at lower doses of 75 to 90 mg/m^2.

For patients with hepatic dysfunction, if bilirubin is 1.2 to 3 mg/dL or AST is 2 to 4 × ULN, give half recommended starting dose. If bilirubin level is above 3 mg/dL or AST is more than 4 × ULN, give ¼ recommended starting dose.

For patients with severe renal dysfunction (creatinine level over 5 mg/dL), consider lower doses.

ADMINISTRATION
I.V.
▼ Wear protective clothing (goggles, gown, disposable gloves) when handling drug, which is a vesicant.
Black Box Warning Never give drug I.M. or subcutaneously; severe tissue necrosis may result. Always give I.V. in free-flowing NSS or D$_5$W over 3 to 20 minutes depending on dosage and volume of infusion solution. ■
Black Box Warning Avoid veins over joints or in limbs with compromised venous or lymphatic drainage. ■
▼ Avoid repeated injection into the same vein.

▼ Facial flushing and erythematous streaking along vein may indicate overly rapid delivery.

Black Box Warning If burning or stinging occurs, stop infusion immediately and restart in another vein. ∎

▼ After vial has been penetrated, discard unused solution after 24 hours.

▼ Store refrigerated solution between 36° and 46° F (2° and 8° C). Don't freeze. Protect from light.

▼ **Incompatibilities:** 5-FU, heparin, ifosfamide with mesna, any alkaline pH solutions, other I.V. drugs.

ACTION

May form a complex with DNA by getting between nucleotide base pairs, inhibiting DNA, RNA, and protein synthesis; DNA cleavage occurs, resulting in cytocidal activity. Drug may also interfere with replication and transcription of DNA and may generate cytotoxic free radicals.

Route	Onset	Peak	Duration
I.V.	Unknown	Unknown	Unknown

Half-life: 31 to 35 hours.

ADVERSE REACTIONS

CNS: lethargy, fever.
CV: *cardiomyopathy, HF.*
EENT: conjunctivitis, keratitis.
GI: nausea, vomiting, diarrhea, anorexia, mucositis.
GU: amenorrhea, red urine.
Hematologic: *leukopenia, neutropenia, febrile neutropenia,* anemia, *thrombocytopenia.*
Skin: alopecia, rash, pruritus, skin changes, local toxicity.
Other: infection, hot flashes.

INTERACTIONS

Drug-drug. *Calcium channel blockers, other cardioactive compounds:* May increase risk of HF. Monitor cardiac function closely.
Cimetidine: May increase epirubicin level by 50%. Avoid using together.
Cytotoxic drugs: May cause additive toxicities (especially hematologic and GI). Monitor patient closely.

Live-virus vaccines: May increase risk of vaccine-induced adverse reactions. Avoid concomitant use; don't give for at least 3 months after drug.

EFFECTS ON LAB TEST RESULTS

● May decrease Hb level.
● May decrease neutrophil, platelet, and WBC counts.

CONTRAINDICATIONS & CAUTIONS

● Contraindicated in patients hypersensitive to drug, other anthracyclines, or anthracenediones, and in patients with baseline neutrophil counts below 1,500/mm^3, severe myocardial insufficiency, recent MI, serious arrhythmias, or severe hepatic dysfunction.
● Contraindicated in patients who have had previous treatment with anthracyclines to the maximum total cumulative doses.
● Use cautiously in patients with active or dormant cardiac disease, previous or current radiotherapy to mediastinal and pericardial areas, or previous therapy with other anthracyclines or anthracenediones.
● Use cautiously in patients receiving other cardiotoxic drugs.
Dialyzable drug: Unknown.
⚠ *Overdose S&S:* Bone marrow aplasia, grade 4 mucositis, GI bleeding, hyperthermia, multiple organ failure, lactic acidosis, increased LDH level, anuria, death.

PREGNANCY-LACTATION-REPRODUCTION

● Drug can cause fetal harm. If drug is used during pregnancy, or if patient becomes pregnant during therapy, apprise patient of potential fetal hazard. Women of childbearing potential should be advised to avoid becoming pregnant; men taking drug should use effective contraception.
● It isn't known if drug appears in breast milk. Patient should discontinue breastfeeding or discontinue drug.

NURSING CONSIDERATIONS

Black Box Warning Give drug under supervision of prescriber experienced in cancer chemotherapy. ∎
● Don't handle drug if you are pregnant.
● For patients taking 120 mg/m^2 regimen, give prophylactic antibiotic therapy.

Reactions in bold italics are *life-threatening*. Interactions may have a *rapid onset* or a *delayed onset*.

• Give antiemetic before drug to reduce nausea and vomiting.
• Before therapy, obtain total bilirubin, AST, and creatinine levels; CBC including ANC; and LVEF.
• Monitor LVEF regularly during therapy. Stop drug at first sign of impaired cardiac function. Early signs of cardiac toxicity include sinus tachycardia, ECG abnormalities, tachyarrhythmias, bradycardia, AV block, and bundle-branch block.

Black Box Warning Cardiac toxicity may occur during therapy or months to years after treatment ends; indications include reduced LVEF and signs and symptoms of HF (tachycardia, dyspnea, pulmonary edema, dependent edema, hepatomegaly, ascites, pleural effusion, and gallop rhythm). Delayed cardiac toxicity depends on cumulative dose of epirubicin. Don't exceed cumulative dose of 900 mg/m^2. ∎

Black Box Warning Severe myelosuppression may occur. ∎

• Obtain total and differential WBC, CBC, platelet count, and LFTs before and during each cycle of therapy.
• WBC nadir is usually reached 10 to 14 days after drug administration, and WBC count returns to normal by day 21.
• Monitor uric acid, potassium, calcium, phosphate, and creatinine levels immediately after initial chemotherapy administration in patients susceptible to tumor lysis syndrome. Hydration, urine alkalinization, and prophylaxis with allopurinol may prevent hyperuricemia and minimize potential complications of tumor lysis syndrome.
• Drug may enhance the effects of radiation therapy or cause an inflammatory cell reaction at irradiation site. Monitor patient closely.

Black Box Warning Secondary acute myeloid leukemia has been reported in patients with breast cancer treated with anthracyclines, including epirubicin. ∎

PATIENT TEACHING
• Advise patient to report any pain or burning at injection site during or after administration.
• Advise patient to report nausea, vomiting, mouth inflammation, dehydration, fever, evidence of infection, or symptoms of HF (rapid heartbeat, labored breathing, swelling).
• Tell patient that urine will be reddish pink for 1 to 2 days after treatment.
• Inform patient of risk of heart damage and treatment-related leukemia with use of drug.
• Advise men to use effective contraception during treatment.
• Advise women that irreversible, premature menopause may occur.
• Tell patient that hair usually regrows within 2 to 3 months after therapy stops.

eplerenone
ep-LER-eh-nown

Inspra

Therapeutic class: Antihypertensives
Pharmacologic class: Selective aldosterone receptor antagonists

AVAILABLE FORMS
Tablets: 25 mg, 50 mg

INDICATIONS & DOSAGES
➤ **Hypertension**
Adults: 50 mg P.O. once daily. If response is inadequate after 4 weeks, increase dosage to 50 mg P.O. b.i.d. Maximum daily dose, 100 mg/day.
Adjust-a-dose: In patients taking weak CYP3A4 inhibitors (erythromycin, fluconazole, saquinavir, verapamil), reduce eplerenone starting dose to 25 mg P.O. once daily.
➤ **HF after an MI**
Adults: Initially, 25 mg P.O. once daily. Increase within 4 weeks, as tolerated and according to potassium level, to 50 mg P.O. once daily.
Adjust-a-dose: If potassium level is less than 5 mEq/L, increase dosage from 25 mg every other day to 25 mg daily; or increase dosage from 25 mg daily to 50 mg daily. If potassium level is 5 to 5.4 mEq/L, don't adjust dosage. If potassium level is 5.5 to 5.9 mEq/L, decrease dosage from 50 mg daily to 25 mg daily; or decrease dosage from 25 mg daily to 25 mg every other day; or if dosage was 25 mg every other day, withhold drug. If potassium level is

greater than 6 mEq/L, withhold drug. May restart drug at 25 mg every other day when potassium level is less than 5.5 mEq/L.

ADMINISTRATION

P.O.
- Give drug without regard for meals.
- Don't give with grapefruit juice.

ACTION

Binds to mineralocorticoid receptors and blocks aldosterone, which increases BP through induction of sodium reabsorption and possibly other mechanisms.

Route	Onset	Peak	Duration
P.O.	Unknown	90 min	Unknown

Half-life: 4 to 6 hours.

ADVERSE REACTIONS

CNS: dizziness, fatigue.
GI: diarrhea, abdominal pain.
GU: albuminuria, abnormal vaginal bleeding.
Metabolic: *hyperkalemia.*
Respiratory: cough.
Other: flulike syndrome, gynecomastia.

INTERACTIONS

Drug-drug. *ACE inhibitors, ARBs:* May increase risk of hyperkalemia. Use together cautiously.
Azole antifungals (itraconazole, ketoconazole), macrolides (clarithromycin), nefazodone, protease inhibitors (nelfinavir, ritonavir): Inhibits the CYP3A4 metabolism of eplerenone. Use together is contraindicated.
Canagliflozin: May increase risk of hyperkalemia. Monitor therapy.
Lithium: May increase risk of lithium toxicity. Monitor lithium level.
NSAIDs: May reduce the antihypertensive effect and cause severe hyperkalemia in patients with impaired renal function. Monitor BP and potassium level.
Potassium supplements, potassium-sparing diuretics (amiloride, spironolactone, triamterene): May increase risk of hyperkalemia and sometimes-fatal arrhythmias. Use together is contraindicated.
Weak CYP3A4 inhibitors (erythromycin, fluconazole, saquinavir, verapamil): May increase eplerenone level. Reduce eplerenone starting dose to 25 mg P.O. once daily.
Drug-herb. *St. John's wort:* May decrease eplerenone level over time. Discourage use together.
Drug-food. *Grapefruit juice:* May increase eplerenone level by about 25%.

EFFECTS ON LAB TEST RESULTS

- May increase ALT, BUN, cholesterol, creatinine, GGT, potassium, triglyceride, and uric acid levels. May decrease sodium level.

CONTRAINDICATIONS & CAUTIONS

- When used for hypertension, contraindicated in patients with type 2 diabetes with microalbuminuria, creatinine level greater than 2 mg/dL in men or greater than 1.8 mg/dL in women, or CrCl less than 50 mL/minute and in patients taking potassium supplements or potassium-sparing diuretics (amiloride, spironolactone, triamterene).
- Contraindicated in patients with potassium level greater than 5.5 mEq/mL at initiation or CrCl of 30 mL/minute or less and in patients taking strong CYP3A4 inhibitors, such as ketoconazole, clarithromycin, ritonavir, nelfinavir, nefazodone, and itraconazole.
- Use cautiously in patients with mild to moderate hepatic impairment.
Dialyzable drug: No.
⚠ *Overdose S&S:* Hypotension, hyperkalemia.

PREGNANCY-LACTATION-REPRODUCTION

- Use in pregnant women only if potential benefits justify potential risk to the fetus.
- It isn't known if drug appears in breast milk. Patient should discontinue breastfeeding or discontinue drug.

NURSING CONSIDERATIONS

- Drug may be used alone or with other antihypertensives.
- Full therapeutic effect of the drug occurs in 4 weeks.
- In patients with HF, measure potassium level at baseline, within first week or after

---

dosage adjustment, at 1 month after starting therapy, and periodically thereafter.
• Monitor patient for signs and symptoms of hyperkalemia.
• *Look alike–sound alike:* Don't confuse Inspra with Spiriva.

PATIENT TEACHING
• Inform patient that drug may be taken with or without food.
• Advise patient to avoid potassium supplements and salt substitutes during treatment.
• Tell patient to report adverse reactions.

SAFETY ALERT!

epoetin alfa (erythropoietin)
i-POE-i-tin

Epogen, Eprex ♣, Procrit

Therapeutic class: Colony stimulating factors
Pharmacologic class: Recombinant human erythropoietins

AVAILABLE FORMS
Injection (single-use vial): 2,000 units/mL, 3,000 units/mL, 4,000 units/mL, 10,000 units/mL, 40,000 units/mL
Injection (multidose vial)*: 20,000 units/1 mL, 20,000 units/2 mL

INDICATIONS & DOSAGES
➤ **Anemia caused by chronic renal disease**
Adults: Dosage is individualized. For patients on hemodialysis, start treatment only if Hb level is less than 10 g/dL. For patients not on hemodialysis, start treatment only if Hb level is less than 10 g/dL, the decline of Hb level indicates that patient will require an RBC transfusion, and reducing the risk of alloimmunization and other RBC transfusion–related risks is a treatment goal. Starting dose is 50 to 100 units/kg subcutaneously or I.V. three times weekly. I.V. route is preferred for patients receiving hemodialysis. Maintenance dosage is highly individualized. Give the lowest effective dose to gradually increase Hb to a level at which blood transfusion isn't necessary.

Children age 1 month and older who are on dialysis: Initially, 50 units/kg I.V. or subcutaneously three times weekly. I.V. route is preferred for patients receiving hemodialysis. Maintenance dosage is highly individualized to keep Hb level within target range. Give the lowest effective dose to gradually increase Hb to a level at which blood transfusion isn't necessary.
Adjust-a-dose: Don't increase dosage more frequently than every 4 weeks. Reduce dosage by 25% when target Hb level approaches 12 g/dL or if it rises more than 1 g/dL in any 2-week period. If Hb level continues to increase, hold dose until Hb level begins to decrease; then restart at 25% below previous dose. Increase dosage by 25% if Hb level is less than 10 g/dL and hasn't increased by 1 g/dL after 4 weeks or if Hb level falls below 10 g/dL. For patients on dialysis, if Hb level approaches or exceeds 11 g/dL, reduce dosage or interrupt therapy. For patients not on dialysis, if Hb level exceeds 10 g/dL, reduce dosage or interrupt therapy.
➤ **Anemia from zidovudine therapy (4,200 mg/week or less) in HIV-infected patients**
Adults: Initially, 100 units/kg I.V. or subcutaneously three times weekly for 8 weeks or until target Hb level is reached. If response isn't satisfactory after 8 weeks, increase dosage by 50 to 100 units/kg I.V. or subcutaneously three times weekly. Evaluate response every 4 to 8 weeks thereafter; further increase dosage in increments of 50 to 100 units/kg three times weekly, up to maximum of 300 units/kg I.V. or subcutaneously. Give the lowest effective dose to gradually increase Hb to a level where blood transfusion isn't necessary. Withhold drug if Hb level exceeds 12 g/dL. Restart drug at 25% below the previous dosage if Hb level declines to less than 11 g/dL. Discontinue if an increase in Hb isn't achieved at 300 units/kg for 8 weeks.
➤ **Anemia from chemotherapy**
Adults: Start therapy if Hb level is less than 10 g/dL and a minimum of 2 additional months of chemotherapy is planned. Initially, 150 units/kg subcutaneously three times weekly. Or, 40,000 units subcutaneously weekly until completion of a

chemotherapy course. If Hb level hasn't increased by at least 1 g/dL (in the absence of RBC transfusion) and remains below 10 g/dL after initial 4 weeks of therapy, increase dosage up to 300 units/kg subcutaneously three times weekly or 60,000 units weekly. Give the lowest effective dose to gradually increase Hb to a level at which blood transfusion isn't necessary. Discontinue drug after 8 weeks if no response, as measured by Hb level or if transfusions are still required.

Children ages 5 to 18: 600 units/kg I.V. once weekly until completion of a chemotherapy course. If Hb level hasn't increased by at least 1 g/dL (in the absence of RBC transfusion) and remains below 10 g/dL after initial 4 weeks of therapy, increase dosage to 900 units/kg I.V. (maximum, 60,000 units). Discontinue drug after 8 weeks if no response, as measured by Hb level or if transfusions are still required.

Adjust-a-dose: Withhold drug if Hb level exceeds level needed to avoid an RBC transfusion. Restart drug at dosage 25% below previous dosage when Hb level approaches a level at which an RBC transfusion may be required. Reduce dosage by 25% if Hb level increases more than 1 g/dL in a 2-week period or reaches a level needed to avoid an RBC transfusion.

➤ **To reduce need for allogenic blood transfusion in anemic patients scheduled to have elective, noncardiac, nonvascular surgery**

Adults: 300 units/kg subcutaneously daily for 10 days before surgery, on day of surgery, and for 4 days after surgery. Or, 600 units/kg subcutaneously in once-weekly doses (21, 14, and 7 days before surgery), plus a fourth dose on day of surgery. DVT prophylaxis is recommended for surgery patients during epoetin therapy.

ADMINISTRATION

I.V.

▼ Store solution in refrigerator; don't freeze.

▼ Protect from light.

▼ Don't shake.

▼ Give by direct injection without dilution.

▼ If patient is having dialysis, drug may be given into venous return line after dialysis session. To keep drug from adhering to tubing, inject drug with blood still in the line. Then flush with NSS.

▼ Single-dose vials contain no preservatives. Discard unused portion. Don't reenter preservative-free vials.

▼ Store unused portions of multidose vials at 36° to 46° F (2° to 8° C). Discard 21 days after initial entry.

⊕ *Alert:* Multidose vials contain benzyl alcohol, which has been associated with sometimes fatal neurologic and other complications in premature infants.

▼ **Incompatibilities:** Other I.V. drugs.

Subcutaneous

● Store solution in refrigerator; don't freeze.

● Protect from light.

● Don't shake.

● Don't use if solution is discolored or has particulate matter.

● Give in upper arm, abdomen, mid-thigh, or outer buttocks.

● Single-use vial without preservative may be admixed in a syringe with bacteriostatic NSS for injection with benzyl alcohol 0.9% (bacteriostatic saline) at a 1:1 ratio to provide local anesthetic.

● Rotate injection sites and document.

ACTION

Mimics effects of erythropoietin. Functions as a growth factor and as a differentiating factor, enhancing RBC production.

Route	Onset	Peak	Duration
I.V.	Immediate	Immediate	Unknown
Subcut.	Unknown	5–24 hr	Unknown

Half-life: 4 to 13 hours.

ADVERSE REACTIONS

CNS: asthenia, dizziness, depression, fatigue, headache, insomnia, paresthesia, pyrexia, *seizures.*

CV: edema, hypertension, increased clotting of arteriovenous grafts.

EENT: pharyngitis.

GI: abdominal pain and constipation (in children), diarrhea, nausea, vomiting, stomatitis.

Metabolic: hyperglycemia, *hypokalemia,* hyperphosphatemia, hyperuricemia.

Musculoskeletal: arthralgia, myalgia, bone pain, muscle spasm.

Reactions in bold italics are *life-threatening.* Interactions may have a *rapid onset* or a *delayed onset.*

Respiratory: cough, shortness of breath, URI.
Skin: injection-site reactions, rash, urticaria.

INTERACTIONS
None significant.

EFFECTS ON LAB TEST RESULTS
● May increase BUN, creatinine, phosphate, potassium, and uric acid levels.

CONTRAINDICATIONS & CAUTIONS
● Contraindicated in patients hypersensitive to products derived from mammal cells or albumin (human), in those with uncontrolled hypertension or pure RBC aplasia that begins after treatment with epoetin, and in patients receiving myelosuppressive chemotherapy when the anticipated outcome is cure.
Dialyzable drug: Unknown.
⚠ Overdose S&S: Severe hypertension.

PREGNANCY-LACTATION-REPRODUCTION
● Use single-dose formulations during pregnancy only if potential benefit justifies potential risk to the fetus.
● Use of multidose vials (which contain benzyl alcohol) is contraindicated in pregnant women, neonates, infants, and breast-feeding women.
● It isn't known if drug appears in breast milk. Use single-dose vials cautiously in breast-feeding women.

NURSING CONSIDERATIONS
Black Box Warning Patients with chronic renal disease have an increased risk of death, serious adverse CV events, and stroke when erythropoiesis-stimulating agents are used to increase Hb level to more than 11 g/dL. Individualize therapy and use the lowest dosage needed to reduce the need for RBC transfusion. ■
● Before starting therapy, evaluate patient's iron status. Patient should receive adequate iron supplementation beginning no later than when epoetin alfa treatment starts and continuing throughout therapy. Patient also may need vitamin B_{12} and folic acid.
● Monitor BP before therapy. Most patients with chronic renal failure have hypertension. BP may increase, especially when hematocrit increases in the early part of therapy.
Black Box Warning In patients with non-small-cell lung cancer and breast, head and neck, lymphoid, and cervical cancers, there is a risk of tumor growth and shortened survival. Use the lowest dosage needed to avoid RBC transfusions. Use only for treatment of anemia due to concomitant myelosuppressive chemotherapy and discontinue drug following chemotherapy course. Erythropoiesis-stimulating agents (ESAs) aren't indicated for patients receiving myelosuppressive therapy when the anticipated outcome is cure. Patients and providers must be enrolled in the ESA APPRISE Oncology Program (www.esa-apprise.com). ■
● Institute diet restrictions or drug therapy to control BP.
● Monitor Hb level twice weekly until it stabilizes in the target range and maintenance dose is established, then continue to monitor at regular intervals. Resume twice-weekly testing after any dosage adjustments.
● When used in HIV-infected adults, dosage recommendations are for those with endogenous erythropoietin levels of 500 units/L or less and cumulative zidovudine doses of 4.2 g/week or less.
● Monitor blood counts; elevated hematocrit may cause excessive clotting. For patients with chronic renal disease, monitor Hb level weekly until stable and then at least monthly.
● Patient may need additional heparin to prevent clotting during dialysis treatments.
● Drug increases risk of seizures in patients with chronic kidney disease. Monitor patients closely for neurologic signs and symptoms.
Black Box Warning Due to increased risk of DVT, consider prophylaxis. ■
⚠ Alert: Evaluate patient who experiences a lack or loss of effect for pure red cell aplasia.
● **Look alike–sound alike:** Don't confuse Epogen with Neupogen.

PATIENT TEACHING
● Inform patient that pain or discomfort in limbs (long bones) and pelvis, feelings of cold, and sweating may occur after injection

(usually within 2 hours). Symptoms may last for 12 hours and then disappear.

● Advise patient to avoid driving or operating heavy machinery at start of therapy. There may be a relationship between too-rapid increase in hematocrit and seizures.

● Tell patient to monitor BP at home and to adhere to dietary restrictions.

● Advise female patient that she may resume menstruating after therapy and to consider the need for contraception.

SAFETY ALERT!

eptifibatide
ep-tiff-IB-ah-tide

Integrilin

Therapeutic class: Antiplatelet drugs
Pharmacologic class: Glycoprotein IIb/IIIa inhibitors

AVAILABLE FORMS
Injection: 10-mL (2 mg/mL), 100-mL (0.75 mg/mL), 100-mL (2 mg/mL) vials

INDICATIONS & DOSAGES
➤ **Acute coronary syndrome (unstable angina or non–ST-segment elevation MI) in patients receiving drug therapy and in those undergoing a PCI**
Adults: 180 mcg/kg I.V. bolus as soon as possible after diagnosis, followed by a continuous I.V. infusion at a rate of 2 mcg/kg/minute until hospital discharge or start of CABG surgery, for up to 72 hours. If patient is having a PCI, continue infusion until hospital discharge or for 18 to 24 hours after the procedure, whichever comes first, for up to 96 hours. Give aspirin (160 to 325 mg) and heparin (target aPTT, 50 to 70 seconds) daily.
Adjust-a-dose: If CrCl is less than 50 mL/minute, give 180 mcg/kg I.V. bolus as soon as possible after diagnosis, followed by a continuous I.V. infusion at 1 mcg/kg/minute.
➤ **PCI**
Adults: 180 mcg/kg I.V. bolus given just before the procedure, immediately followed by an infusion of 2 mcg/kg/minute and a second I.V. bolus of 180 mcg/kg given

10 minutes after the first bolus. Continue infusion until hospital discharge or for 18 to 24 hours, whichever comes first; the minimum duration of infusion is 12 hours. Give aspirin 160 to 325 mg 1 to 24 hours before PCI and daily thereafter; give heparin before PCI (but not after).
Adjust-a-dose: If CrCl is less than 50 mL/minute, give 180 mcg/kg I.V. bolus just before the procedure, immediately followed by a continuous I.V. infusion at 1 mcg/kg/minute and a second bolus of 180 mcg/kg given 10 minutes after the first bolus.

ADMINISTRATION
I.V.
▼ Inspect solution for particles before use; if they appear, drug may not be sterile. Discard it.
▼ Protect drug from light before giving.
▼ Drug may be given in same line with NSS, D_5W, alteplase, atropine, dobutamine, heparin, lidocaine, meperidine, metoprolol, midazolam, morphine, nitroglycerin, or verapamil. Main infusion may also contain up to 60 mEq/L of potassium chloride.
▼ For I.V. push, withdraw bolus dose from 10-mL vial into a syringe and give over 1 or 2 minutes.
▼ For infusion, give undiluted drug directly from 100-mL vial using an infusion pump.
▼ Administer drug with heparin titrated to dosing parameters.
▼ If patient needs thrombolytics, stop infusion.
▼ Refrigerate vials at 36° to 46° F (2° to 8° C). Store vials at room temperature for no longer than 2 months; afterward, discard them.
▼ **Incompatibilities:** Furosemide.

ACTION
Reversibly binds to the glycoprotein IIb/IIIa (GPIIb/IIIa) receptor on human platelets and inhibits platelet aggregation.

Route	Onset	Peak	Duration
I.V.	Immediate	Immediate	4–8 hr

Half-life: 2½ hours.

ADVERSE REACTIONS

CV: hypotension.
GU: hematuria.
Hematologic: *thrombocytopenia, major bleeding,* minor bleeding.
Other: bleeding at femoral artery access site.

INTERACTIONS

Drug-drug. *Apixaban, clopidogrel, dabigatran, dipyridamole, edoxaban, NSAIDs, oral anticoagulants (warfarin), rivaroxaban, SSRIs, thrombolytics, ticlopidine:* May increase risk of bleeding. Monitor patient closely for signs of bleeding.
Other inhibitors of GPIIb/IIIa: May cause serious bleeding. Avoid using together.

EFFECTS ON LAB TEST RESULTS

● May decrease platelet count.

CONTRAINDICATIONS & CAUTIONS

● Contraindicated in patients hypersensitive to drug or its ingredients and in those with history of bleeding diathesis or evidence of active abnormal bleeding within previous 30 days; severe hypertension (systolic BP higher than 200 mm Hg or diastolic BP higher than 110 mm Hg) not adequately controlled with antihypertensives; major surgery within previous 6 weeks; history of stroke within 30 days or history of hemorrhagic stroke; current or planned use of another parenteral GPIIb/IIIa inhibitor; or platelet count less than 100,000/mm³.
● Contraindicated in patients with creatinine level of 4 mg/dL or higher and in patients dependent on hemodialysis.
● Use cautiously in patients at increased risk for bleeding, in those with platelet count less than 150,000/mm³, in those with hemorrhagic retinopathy, and in those weighing more than 143 kg.
Dialyzable drug: Yes.

PREGNANCY-LACTATION-REPRODUCTION

● Use during pregnancy only if clearly needed.
● It isn't known if drug appears in breast milk. Use cautiously in breast-feeding women.

NURSING CONSIDERATIONS

● Drug is intended for use with heparin and aspirin.
● At least 4 hours before hospital discharge, stop this drug and heparin and achieve sheath hemostasis by standard compressive techniques.
● Remove sheath during infusion only after heparin has been stopped and its effects largely reversed.
● If patient is to undergo CABG, stop infusion at least 2 to 4 hours before surgery.
● Minimize use of arterial and venous punctures, I.M. injections, urinary catheters, and nasotracheal and NG tubes.
● When obtaining I.V. access, avoid use of noncompressible sites (such as subclavian or jugular veins).
● Monitor patient for bleeding.
⚠ *Alert:* If platelet count is less than 100,000/mm³, stop this drug and heparin.
● Perform baseline laboratory tests before start of drug therapy; also determine Hb level, hematocrit, PT, INR, aPTT, platelet count, and creatinine level.

PATIENT TEACHING

● Advise patient to inform health care provider of all drugs and supplements he takes.
● Explain that drug inhibits blood clotting and is used to prevent chest pain and heart attack.
● Explain that benefits of drug far outweigh risk of serious bleeding.
● Tell patient to report to prescriber chest discomfort or other adverse effects immediately.
● Tell patient to report unusual bleeding, bruising, or blood in stools.

SAFETY ALERT!

eribulin mesylate
er-ih-BYOO-lin

Halaven

Therapeutic class: Antineoplastics
Pharmacologic class: Microtubule inhibitors

AVAILABLE FORMS

Injection: 1 mg/2-mL vial

INDICATIONS & DOSAGES
➤ **To treat metastatic breast cancer in patients who have received at least two chemotherapeutic regimens for the treatment of metastatic disease, and whose treatments have included an anthracycline and a taxane in either the adjuvant or metastatic setting; unresectable or metastatic liposarcoma in patients who have received a prior anthracycline-containing regimen**

Adults: 1.4 mg/m^2 I.V. over 2 to 5 minutes on days 1 and 8 of a 21-day cycle. Assess for peripheral neuropathy and obtain CBCs before each dose. Don't administer drug on day 1 or 8 if ANC is less than 1,000/mm^3, platelet count is less than 75,000/mm^3, or grade 3 or 4 nonhematologic toxicities exist. May delay day-8 dose for a maximum of 1 week.

If toxicities don't resolve or improve to grade 2 or less by day 15, omit dose. If toxicities resolve or improve to grade 2 or less by day 15, give eribulin at a reduced dose and initiate next cycle no sooner than 2 weeks later.

Adjust-a-dose: In mild hepatic impairment (Child-Pugh class A) and in patients with moderate or severe renal impairment (CrCl of 15 to 49 mL/minute), give 1.1 mg/m^2 I.V. over 2 to 5 minutes on days 1 and 8 of a 21-day cycle. In moderate hepatic impairment (Child-Pugh class B), give 0.7 mg/m^2 I.V. over 2 to 5 minutes on days 1 and 8 of a 21-day cycle. If toxicities occur, refer to package insert for dosage adjustments. Don't reescalate dose after it has been reduced. Discontinue drug for any event requiring permanent dosage reduction while patient is receiving 0.7 mg/m^2.

ADMINISTRATION
I.V.

▼ Drug is considered hazardous; use safe handling and disposal precautions.

▼ Draw up required amount from vial and administer undiluted, or dilute in 100 mL NSS. Don't use dextrose.

▼ May store undiluted drug in a syringe or diluted solutions for 4 hours at room temperature or 24 hours if refrigerated.

▼ Discard unused portion of vial.

▼ **Incompatibilities:** Dextrose, other I.V. drugs.

ACTION
Causes cell death by inhibiting cell division.

Route	Onset	Peak	Duration
I.V.	Unknown	Unknown	Unknown

Half-life: About 40 hours.

ADVERSE REACTIONS
CNS: dizziness, depression, peripheral neuropathy, headache, insomnia, asthenia, fatigue, pyrexia.
CV: *QT-interval prolongation,* peripheral edema.
EENT: increased lacrimation, mucosal inflammation.
GI: anorexia, dysgeusia, dyspepsia, abdominal pain, stomatitis, dry mouth, constipation, diarrhea, nausea, vomiting.
GU: UTI.
Hematologic: *neutropenia,* anemia, *thrombocytopenia.*
Metabolic: weight loss, *hypokalemia.*
Musculoskeletal: muscle spasms, muscle weakness, arthralgia, myalgia, back pain, bone pain, pain in extremity.
Respiratory: URI, cough, dyspnea.
Skin: rash, alopecia.

INTERACTIONS
Drug-drug. *Class IA and III antiarrhythmics, other drugs known to prolong QT interval:* May further prolong QT interval. Use together cautiously and monitor patient carefully.
Live-virus vaccines: May increase risk of live-virus vaccine–induced adverse reactions. Concurrent use isn't recommended.

EFFECTS ON LAB TEST RESULTS
● May increase ALT and bilirubin levels. May decrease potassium level.
● May decrease Hb level and neutrophil and platelet counts.

CONTRAINDICATIONS & CAUTIONS
● Contraindicated in patients hypersensitive to drug or its components.
● Avoid use in patients with existing congenital long QT syndrome.

Reactions in bold italics are *life-threatening*. Interactions may have a *rapid onset* or a *delayed onset*.

• Use cautiously in patients with liver or renal insufficiency and in those at risk for neutropenia or peripheral motor or sensory neuropathy.

• Use cautiously in patients with HF, bradyarrhythmias, or electrolyte imbalance and in those taking drugs known to prolong QT interval or with a history of prolonged QT interval.

• Safety and effectiveness in children haven't been established.

Dialyzable drug: Unknown.

⚠ *Overdose S&S:* Neutropenia, hypersensitivity reaction.

PREGNANCY-LACTATION-REPRODUCTION

• There are no well-controlled studies in pregnant women, but drug is expected to cause fetal harm. Use during pregnancy only if benefits outweigh risk and patient is aware of potential fetal hazard.

• It isn't known if drug appears in breast milk. Patient should discontinue breast-feeding or discontinue drug.

NURSING CONSIDERATIONS

• Assess patient for peripheral neuropathy.

• Monitor patient for hypokalemia and hypomagnesemia before and periodically during therapy.

• Monitor patient for signs and symptoms of infection.

• Monitor blood counts and obtain CBC before each dose.

• Monitor LFTs and renal function tests during therapy.

• Monitor ECG for changes, especially QT-interval prolongation.

• Consider prophylactic antiemetics for nausea and vomiting.

PATIENT TEACHING

• Tell patient to report a temperature of 100.4° F (38° C) or greater and other signs or symptoms of infection, such as chills, cough, or burning or pain on urination.

• Advise patient that drug may cause nerve damage and to contact prescriber if burning, tingling, or radiating pain occurs in any extremity.

• Caution patient to immediately report irregular heartbeat.

• Warn patient to avoid pregnancy and to use effective contraception during treatment.

• Tell patient to consult prescriber before breast-feeding.

SAFETY ALERT!

erlotinib
ur-LOE-tih-nib

Tarceva

Therapeutic class: Antineoplastics
Pharmacologic class: Epidermal growth factor receptor inhibitors

AVAILABLE FORMS
Tablets ⓓ: 25 mg, 100 mg, 150 mg

INDICATIONS & DOSAGES
Adjust-a-dose (for all indications): In patients with severe skin reactions or severe diarrhea refractory to loperamide, reduce dose in 50-mg decrements or stop therapy.

In patients with severe hepatic impairment (AST level greater than 3 × ULN), reduce initial dose to 75 mg/day and gradually increase as tolerated. Interrupt therapy or discontinue drug if total bilirubin level increases to greater than 3 × ULN and/or transaminase levels are greater than 5 × ULN in patients with normal baseline hepatic function, or if bilirubin level doubles or transaminase levels triple in patients with preexisting hepatic impairment or biliary obstruction.

In patients with acute or worsening ocular disorders such as eye pain, consider discontinuing drug; if therapy is resumed, reinitiate with a 50-mg dosage reduction after toxicity has resolved to baseline or grade 1 or less and discontinue for corneal perforation or severe ulceration.

In patients with severe (grade 3 to 4) renal toxicity or in patients at risk for renal failure due to dehydration, consider discontinuing drug. May resume at previous dose after euvolemia has been reestablished. If treatment is withheld due to toxicity and therapy is resumed, reinitiate with a 50-mg dosage reduction after toxicity has resolved to baseline or grade 1 or less.

In patients who currently smoke cigarettes, increase by 50-mg increments at 2-week intervals to a maximum of 300 mg. Immediately reduce dosage to the recommended dosage (150 mg or 100 mg daily) upon cessation of smoking.

➤ **With gemcitabine, first-line treatment of locally advanced, unresectable, or metastatic pancreatic cancer**

Adults: 100 mg P.O. once daily taken at least 1 hour before or 2 hours after meals. Continue until disease progresses or intolerable toxicity occurs.

➤ **Maintenance therapy for locally advanced or metastatic non–small-cell lung cancer (NSCLC) in patients whose disease hasn't progressed after four cycles of platinum-based, first-line chemotherapy; locally advanced or metastatic NSCLC after failure of at least one chemotherapy regimen**

Adults: 150 mg P.O. once daily at least 1 hour before or 2 hours after meals. Continue until disease progresses or intolerable toxicity occurs.

➤ **Metastatic NSCLC in patients with tumors with epidermal growth factor receptor (*EGFR*) exon 19 deletions or exon 21 (L858R) substitution mutations as detected by an FDA-approved test**

Adults: 150 mg P.O. once daily at least 1 hour before or 2 hours after a meal. Continue until disease progresses or intolerable toxicity occurs.

ADMINISTRATION

P.O.

● Give drug 1 hour before or 2 hours after a meal.

● For patients unable to swallow tablets whole, tablets may be dissolved in 100 mL water and given orally or via feeding tube (silicone-based). To ensure full dose is received, rinse container with 40 mL water, administer residue, and repeat rinse.

● Drug is a hazardous agent. Use appropriate precautions for handling and disposal.

ACTION

Probably inhibits tyrosine kinase activity in EGFRs, which are expressed on the surface of normal and cancer cells. Is particularly selective for human EGFR1.

Route	Onset	Peak	Duration
P.O.	Unknown	4 hr	Unknown

Half-life: About 36 hours.

ADVERSE REACTIONS

CNS: fatigue, syncope, *stroke,* anxiety, depression, dizziness, headache, insomnia, neuropathies, pyrexia, rigors.

CV: chest pain, arrhythmias, edema, *MI, DVT.*

EENT: conjunctivitis, keratoconjunctivitis sicca, decreased tear production, abnormal eyelash growth.

GI: abdominal pain, anorexia, diarrhea, decreased appetite, nausea, stomatitis, vomiting, constipation, dyspepsia, flatulence, *pancreatitis.*

GU: renal insufficiency.

Hematologic: hemolytic anemia.

Metabolic: decreased weight.

Musculoskeletal: bone pain, myalgia.

Respiratory: cough, dyspnea, *pulmonary toxicity.*

Skin: acne, dry skin, pruritus, rash, alopecia, paronychia.

Other: infection.

INTERACTIONS

Drug-drug. *Antacids, H_2-receptor antagonists, PPIs:* May reduce bioavailability of drug. Separate doses by several hours.

Anticoagulants, such as warfarin: May increase risk of bleeding. Monitor PT and INR.

Ciprofloxacin: May increase erlotinib plasma concentration. Consider reducing erlotinib dosage if severe adverse reactions occur.

CYP3A4 inducers (carbamazepine, phenobarbital, phenytoin, rifabutin, rifampin): May increase erlotinib metabolism. Avoid use if possible and increase erlotinib dosage, as needed.

Strong CYP3A4 inhibitors (atazanavir, clarithromycin, indinavir, itraconazole, ketoconazole, nefazodone, nelfinavir, ritonavir, saquinavir, telithromycin, troleandomycin, voriconazole): May decrease erlotinib metabolism. Avoid use if possible; consider reducing erlotinib dosage.

Drug-herb. *St. John's wort:* May increase drug metabolism. Drug dosage may need to be increased. Discourage use together.

Drug-food. *Any food:* May increase bioavailability of drug. Give drug 1 hour before or 2 hours after meals.

Grapefruit or grapefruit juice: May increase drug level. Avoid use together.

Drug-lifestyle. *Cigarette smoking:* May decrease drug level. Encourage smoking cessation.

EFFECTS ON LAB TEST RESULTS

• May increase ALT, AST, and bilirubin levels.

• May increase INR and prolong PT.

CONTRAINDICATIONS & CAUTIONS

• Use cautiously in patients with pulmonary disease or liver impairment. Also use cautiously in patients who have received or are receiving chemotherapy because it may worsen adverse pulmonary effects.

• Withhold drug for acute onset of new or progressive unexplained pulmonary signs and symptoms, such as dyspnea, cough, and fever (pending diagnostic evaluation), and for grade 3 or 4 keratitis lasting more than 2 weeks. Withhold drug for acute or worsening ocular disorders such as eye pain, and consider discontinuation.

• Use cautiously in patients receiving other antiangiogenic agents, corticosteroids, NSAIDs, or taxane-based chemotherapy, and in those with a history of peptic ulcer disease because of increased risk of GI perforation.

• Interrupt therapy or discontinue drug in patients with dehydration at risk for renal failure.

• Discontinue if severe bullous, blistering, or exfoliating conditions develop.

Dialyzable drug: Unknown.

⚠ Overdose S&S: Severe adverse reactions (such as diarrhea, ALT or AST elevation, rash).

PREGNANCY-LACTATION-REPRODUCTION

• Drug may cause fetal harm. If drug is used during pregnancy, or if patient becomes pregnant during therapy, apprise patient of potential hazard to fetus.

• It isn't known if drug appears in breast milk. Patient should discontinue breast-feeding or discontinue drug.

NURSING CONSIDERATIONS

• Monitor renal function tests and LFTs periodically during therapy.

☉ Alert: GI perforation with fatalities has been reported. Permanently discontinue drug if GI perforation occurs.

☉ Alert: Rarely, serious interstitial lung disease may occur. If patient develops dyspnea, cough, and fever, notify prescriber. Therapy may need to be interrupted or stopped.

• Monitor patient for severe diarrhea, and give loperamide if needed.

• Monitor patient for eye ulcers, bullous blistering, and exfoliative skin conditions.

PATIENT TEACHING

☉ Alert: Tell patient to immediately report new or worsened cough, shortness of breath, eye irritation or pain, or severe or persistent diarrhea, nausea, anorexia, or vomiting.

• Instruct patient to take drug 1 hour before or 2 hours after food.

• Explain the likelihood of serious interactions with other drugs and herbal supplements and the need to tell prescriber about any change in drugs and supplements taken.

• Counsel patient about smoking cessation, as smoking may decrease drug level and effectiveness.

ertapenem sodium
er-tah-PEN-em

Invanz

Therapeutic class: Antibiotics
Pharmacologic class: Carbapenems

AVAILABLE FORMS

Injection: 1 g

INDICATIONS & DOSAGES

Adjust-a-dose (for all indications): In adult patients with CrCl of 30 mL/minute or less, give 500 mg/day. In hemodialysis patients receiving daily 500-mg dose less than 6 hours before hemodialysis, give supplementary 150-mg dose afterward.

In hemodialysis patients receiving dose 6 hours or more before hemodialysis, no supplementary dose is needed.

➤ **Complicated intra-abdominal infection caused by** *Escherichia coli, Clostridium clostridioforme, Eubacterium lentum, Peptostreptococcus* **species,** *Bacteroides fragilis, Bacteroides distasonis, Bacteroides ovatus, Bacteroides thetaiotaomicron,* **or** *Bacteroides uniformis*
Adults and children age 13 and older: 1 g I.V. or I.M. once daily for 5 to 14 days.
Infants and children ages 3 months to 12 years: 15 mg/kg I.V. or I.M. every 12 hours for 5 to 14 days. Don't exceed 1 g daily.

➤ **Complicated skin or skin-structure infection, including diabetic foot infections without osteomyelitis, caused by** *Staphylococcus aureus* **(methicillin-susceptible strains),** *Streptococcus agalactiae, Streptococcus pyogenes, E. coli, Klebsiella pneumoniae, Proteus mirabilis, B. fragilis, Peptostreptococcus* **species,** *Porphyromonas asaccharolytica,* **or** *Prevotella bivia*
Adults and children age 13 and older: 1 g I.V. or I.M. once daily for 7 to 14 days. Diabetic foot infections may need up to 28 days of treatment.
Infants and children ages 3 months to 12 years: 15 mg/kg I.V. or I.M. every 12 hours for 7 to 14 days. Don't exceed 1 g daily.

➤ **Community-acquired pneumonia from** *S. pneumoniae* **(penicillin-susceptible strains),** *Haemophilus influenzae* **(beta-lactamase–negative strains), or** *Moraxella catarrhalis;* **complicated UTI, including pyelonephritis caused by** *E. coli* **or** *K. pneumoniae*
Adults and children age 13 and older: 1 g I.V. or I.M. once daily for 10 to 14 days. If patient improves after at least 3 days of treatment, use appropriate oral therapy to complete the full course of therapy.
Infants and children ages 3 months to 12 years: 15 mg/kg I.V. or I.M. every 12 hours for 10 to 14 days. Don't exceed 1 g daily. If patient improves after at least 3 days of treatment, use appropriate oral therapy to complete the full course of therapy.

➤ **Acute pelvic infection, including postpartum endomyometritis, septic abortion, and postsurgical gynecologic infection caused by** *S. agalactiae, E. coli, B. fragilis, P. asaccharolytica, Peptostreptococcus* **species, or** *P. bivia*
Adults and children age 13 and older: 1 g I.V. or I.M. once daily for 3 to 10 days.
Infants and children ages 3 months to 12 years: 15 mg/kg I.V. or I.M. every 12 hours for 3 to 10 days. Don't exceed 1 g daily.

➤ **Prevention of surgical site infection after elective colorectal surgery**
Adults: 1 g I.V. 1 hour before surgical incision.

ADMINISTRATION

I.V.

▼ Obtain specimens for culture and sensitivity testing before giving. Begin therapy while awaiting results.

▼ Before giving first dose, check for previous hypersensitivity to penicillin, cephalosporin, beta-lactam, or local amide-type anesthetics.

▼ Reconstitute 1-g vial with 10 mL of sterile water for injection, NSS for injection, or bacteriostatic water for injection.

▼ Shake well to dissolve, and then immediately transfer contents to 50 mL of NSS.

▼ Infuse over 30 minutes.

▼ Complete the infusion within 6 hours of reconstitution or refrigerate for up to 24 hours. Infuse within 4 hours once removed from refrigeration. Don't freeze.

▼ **Incompatibilities:** Diluents containing dextrose (alpha-D-glucose), other I.V. drugs.

I.M.

● Obtain specimens for culture and sensitivity testing before giving. Begin therapy while awaiting results.

● Before giving first dose, check for previous hypersensitivity to penicillin, cephalosporin, beta-lactam, or local amide-type anesthetics.

● Reconstitute 1-g vial with 3.2 mL of 1% lidocaine hydrochloride injection (without epinephrine). Shake vial thoroughly to form solution. Immediately withdraw the contents of the vial and give by deep I.M. injection

---

into a large muscle, such as the gluteal muscles or lateral part of the thigh. Use the reconstituted I.M. solution within 1 hour after preparation. Don't give reconstituted solution I.V.

ACTION

Inhibits cell-wall synthesis through penicillin-binding proteins.

Route	Onset	Peak	Duration
I.V.	Immediate	30 min	24 hr
I.M.	Unknown	2 hr	24 hr

Half-life: 4 hours.

ADVERSE REACTIONS

CNS: altered mental status, anxiety, asthenia, dizziness, fatigue, fever, headache, insomnia.
CV: chest pain, edema, hypertension, hypotension, infused vein complication, phlebitis, swelling, tachycardia, thrombophlebitis.
EENT: pharyngitis.
GI: diarrhea, abdominal pain, acid regurgitation, constipation, dyspepsia, nausea, oral candidiasis, vomiting.
GU: renal dysfunction, vaginitis.
Hematologic: *leukopenia, neutropenia, thrombocytopenia,* anemia, coagulation abnormalities, eosinophilia, *thrombocytosis.*
Hepatic: jaundice.
Metabolic: *hyperkalemia, hypokalemia,* hyperglycemia.
Musculoskeletal: leg pain.
Respiratory: cough, dyspnea, rales, *respiratory distress,* rhonchi.
Skin: erythema, extravasation, infusion-site pain and redness, pruritus, rash.
Other: hypersensitivity reactions.

INTERACTIONS

Drug-drug. *Probenecid:* May reduce renal clearance and may increase half-life. Don't give together with probenecid to extend half-life.
Valproic acid: May decrease valproic acid levels, leading to loss of seizure control. Monitor valproic acid levels, and observe patient for signs of seizure activity.

EFFECTS ON LAB TEST RESULTS

● May increase albumin, ALT, alkaline phosphatase, AST, bilirubin, creatinine, glucose, and potassium levels. May decrease Hb level and hematocrit.
● May increase eosinophil count, urine RBC count, or urine WBC count. May prolong PT. May decrease segmented neutrophil and serum WBC counts. May increase or decrease platelet count.

CONTRAINDICATIONS & CAUTIONS

● Contraindicated in patients hypersensitive to any component of the drug or to other drugs in the same class and in patients who have had anaphylactic reactions to beta-lactams.
● I.M. use is contraindicated in patients hypersensitive to local anesthetics of the amide type (because of drug's diluent, lidocaine hydrochloride).
● Drug may cause CDAD, ranging in severity from mild to fatal colitis, that may occur during treatment or more than 2 months after treatment. Drug may need to be discontinued if CDAD is suspected.
● Use cautiously in patients with CNS disorders, elderly patients, and those with compromised renal function, as toxic reactions may occur in these patients.
Dialyzable drug: Yes.
⚠ *Overdose S&S:* Nausea, diarrhea, dizziness.

PREGNANCY-LACTATION-REPRODUCTION

● There are no well-controlled studies in pregnant women. Use during pregnancy only if clearly needed.
● Drug appears in breast milk. Use cautiously and only when expected benefit outweighs risk.

NURSING CONSIDERATIONS

● If patient has diarrhea during therapy, notify prescriber and collect stool specimen for culture to rule out CDAD.
● Vomiting occurs more frequently in children than adults. Monitor children closely for signs and symptoms of dehydration and electrolyte imbalance.
● If allergic reaction occurs, stop drug immediately.

• Anaphylactic reactions require immediate emergency treatment with epinephrine, oxygen, I.V. steroids, and airway management.
• Anticonvulsants may continue in patients with seizure disorders. If focal tremors, myoclonus, or seizures occur, notify prescriber. Drug may need to be decreased or stopped.
• Monitor renal, hepatic, and hematopoietic function during prolonged therapy.
• MRSA and *Enterococcus* species are resistant to drug.
• **Look alike–sound alike:** Don't confuse Invanz with Avinza.

PATIENT TEACHING
• Tell patient to report all adverse reactions.
• Tell patient to alert nurse if discomfort occurs at injection site.
• Tell patient to report diarrhea as soon as possible.

---

erythromycin (ophthalmic, topical)
er-ith-roe-MYE-sin

Erygel

Therapeutic class: Antibiotics
Pharmacologic class: Macrolides

AVAILABLE FORMS
Ointment: 2%
Ophthalmic ointment: 0.5%
Topical gel: 2%
Topical solution: 2%*

INDICATIONS & DOSAGES
➤ **Acute and chronic conjunctivitis, other eye infections (ophthalmic ointment)**
Adults and children: Apply a ribbon of ointment about 1 cm long directly to infected eye up to six times daily, depending on severity of infection.
➤ **To prevent ophthalmia neonatorum caused by *Neisseria gonorrhoeae* or *Chlamydia trachomatis* (ophthalmic ointment)**
Neonates: Apply a ribbon of ointment about 1 cm long in lower conjunctival sac of each eye shortly after birth.
➤ **Inflammatory acne vulgaris (topical gel, topical solution)**

Adults and children: Apply to affected areas b.i.d., morning and evening. If no improvement in 6 to 8 weeks, discontinue drug; prescriber should reevaluate treatment.

ADMINISTRATION
Ophthalmic
• Don't use for infection unless causative organism has been identified.
• To prevent ophthalmia neonatorum, apply ointment no later than 1 hour after birth. Use drug in neonates born either vaginally or by cesarean birth. Gently massage eyelids for 1 minute to spread ointment. Use new tube for each neonate.
Topical
• Wash, rinse, and pat affected areas dry before application.
• Wash hands after each application.
• Avoid contact with eyes, nose, mouth, other mucous membranes, and broken skin.

ACTION
Inhibits protein synthesis; usually bacteriostatic, but may be bactericidal in high concentrations or against highly susceptible organisms.

Route	Onset	Peak	Duration
Ophthalmic, topical	Unknown	Unknown	Unknown

Half-life: Unknown.

ADVERSE REACTIONS
EENT: minor ocular irritations, redness.
Skin: burning, dryness, pruritus, erythema, irritation, oily skin, peeling, sensitivity reactions.
Other: hypersensitivity reactions.

INTERACTIONS
Drug-drug. *Clindamycin (topical):* Topical erythromycin may antagonize clindamycin's effect. Avoid using together.
Drug-lifestyle. *Abrasive or medicated soaps or cleansers, acne products or other preparations containing peeling drugs (benzoyl peroxide, resorcinol, salicylic acid, sulfur, tretinoin), alcohol-containing products (aftershave, cosmetics, perfumed toiletries, shaving creams or lotions), astringent soaps or cosmetics, medicated cosmetics or cover-ups:* May cause

---

Reactions in bold italics are *life-threatening*. Interactions may have a *rapid onset* or a *delayed onset*.

cumulative dryness, resulting in excessive skin irritation. Urge caution.

EFFECTS ON LAB TEST RESULTS
None reported.

CONTRAINDICATIONS & CAUTIONS
• Contraindicated in patients hypersensitive to drug.
• Safety and effectiveness of topical drug in children haven't been established.
Dialyzable drug: Unknown.

PREGNANCY-LACTATION-REPRODUCTION
• Use during pregnancy only if clearly needed. Topical drug may be used to treat acne during pregnancy.
• It isn't known if drug appears in breast milk. Use cautiously in breast-feeding women.

NURSING CONSIDERATIONS
• For treating infants born to mothers with clinically apparent gonorrhea, give I.V. or I.M. injections of aqueous crystalline penicillin G; a single dose of 50,000 units for term infants or 20,000 units for infants of low birth weight.
• Store ophthalmic drug at room temperature in tightly closed, light-resistant container.
🕭 Alert: Prolonged topical use may result in fungal or bacterial superinfection, including pseudomembranous colitis and CDAD, during and even 2 months after treatment. Consider these diagnoses in patients who present with diarrhea; stop drug for significant diarrhea, abdominal cramps, or passage of blood or mucus.
• Topical drug may be flammable; keep away from heat and flame.

PATIENT TEACHING
• Tell patient to clean eye area of excessive discharge before ophthalmic application.
• Teach patient how to apply drug. Advise him to wash hands before and after applying ointment, and warn him not to touch tip of applicator to eye or surrounding tissue.
• Tell patient that vision may be blurred for a few minutes after applying ophthalmic ointment. Instruct patient to keep eyes

closed for 1 to 2 minutes after applying drug.
• Advise patient to watch for and report signs and symptoms of sensitivity (itching lids, redness, swelling, or constant burning).
• Tell patient not to share drug, washcloths, or towels with family members and to notify prescriber if anyone develops same signs or symptoms.
• Tell patient to wash hands after each application.
• Stress importance of compliance with recommended therapy.
• Advise patient to wash, rinse, and dry face thoroughly before each topical use.
• Advise patient to avoid topical use near eyes, nose, mouth, or other mucous membranes.
• Tell patient to stop using drug and notify prescriber if condition worsens, or if there is no improvement.
• Caution patient to keep topical drug away from heat and open flame.
• Advise patient to report diarrhea immediately.

---

erythromycin base
er-ith-roe-MYE-sin

Erythro Base🍁, Erybid🍁, Eryc✐, Ery-Tab✐, PCE

erythromycin ethylsuccinate
E.E.S. Granules, EryPed, Erythro-ES🍁

erythromycin lactobionate
Erythrocin

erythromycin stearate
Erythrocin Stearate, Erythro-S🍁

Therapeutic class: Antibiotics
Pharmacologic class: Macrolides

AVAILABLE FORMS
erythromycin base
Capsules (delayed-release): 250 mg
Tablets (enteric-coated): 250 mg, 333 mg, 500 mg
erythromycin ethylsuccinate
Oral suspension: 200 mg/5 mL, 400 mg/5 mL

Powder for oral suspension: 200 mg/5 mL, 400 mg/5 mL

Tablets: 400 mg, 600 mg✤

erythromycin lactobionate

Injection: 500-mg, 1-g vials

erythromycin stearate

Tablets (film-coated): 250 mg, 500 mg✤

INDICATIONS & DOSAGES

➤ **Acute pelvic inflammatory disease caused by** *Neisseria gonorrhoeae*

Adults: 500 mg I.V. every 6 hours for 3 days; then 500 mg P.O. every 12 hours or 333 mg P.O. every 8 hours for 7 days or 250 mg P.O. every 6 hours for 7 days.

➤ **Intestinal amebiasis caused by** *Entamoeba histolytica*

Adults: 500 mg P.O. every 12 hours, 333 mg P.O. every 8 hours, or 250 mg P.O. every 6 hours for 10 to 14 days.

Children: 30 to 50 mg/kg P.O. daily, in divided doses, for 10 to 14 days.

➤ **To prevent rheumatic fever recurrence in patients allergic to penicillin and sulfonamides**

Adults: 250 mg base or stearate P.O. b.i.d., or 400 mg ethylsuccinate P.O. b.i.d.

➤ **Mild to moderately severe respiratory tract, skin, or soft-tissue infection from sensitive group A beta-hemolytic streptococci,** *Streptococcus pneumoniae,* *Mycoplasma pneumoniae, Corynebacterium diphtheriae,* **or** *Bordetella pertussis;* *Listeria monocytogenes* **infection**

Adults: 250 mg P.O. every 6 hours, 333 mg P.O. every 8 hours, or 500 mg P.O. every 12 hours. Maximum dose is 4 g daily. Or 15 to 20 mg/kg I.V. daily, as continuous infusion or in divided doses every 6 hours for 10 days (3 weeks for *Mycoplasma* species infection). Maximum dosage is 4 g/day.

Children: 30 to 50 mg/kg P.O. daily, in divided doses every 6 hours; or 15 to 20 mg/kg I.V. daily, in divided doses every 4 to 6 hours for 10 days (3 weeks for *Mycoplasma* species infection).

➤ **Nongonococcal urethritis caused by** *Ureaplasma urealyticum*

Adults: 500 mg P.O. every 6 hours or 666 mg P.O. every 8 hours for at least 7 days.

➤ **Legionnaires disease**

Adults: 1 to 4 g P.O. daily in divided doses for 10 to 14 days alone or with rifampin. I.V. route may be used initially in severe cases.

➤ **Uncomplicated urethral, endocervical, or rectal infection caused by** *Chlamydia trachomatis,* **when tetracyclines are contraindicated**

Adults: 500 mg base P.O. q.i.d. for at least 7 days, or 666 mg P.O. every 8 hours for at least 7 days, or 250 mg P.O. q.i.d. for 14 days if patient can't tolerate higher doses.

➤ **Urogenital** *C. trachomatis* **infection during pregnancy**

Adults: 500 mg base or stearate P.O. q.i.d. for at least 7 days or 250 mg base or stearate or 400 mg ethylsuccinate P.O. q.i.d. for at least 14 days.

➤ **Conjunctivitis of the newborn caused by** *C. trachomatis*

Neonates: 50 mg/kg/day P.O. in divided doses for at least 2 weeks.

➤ **Pneumonia in infants caused by** *C. trachomatis*

Infants: 50 mg/kg/day base or stearate P.O. in four divided doses for 21 days, or 15 to 20 mg/kg/day lactobionate I.V. as a continuous infusion or in four divided doses.

➤ **Pertussis**

Adults: 40 to 50 mg/kg/day P.O. in divided doses for 5 to 14 days.

➤ **Preoperative prophylaxis for elective colorectal surgery**

Adults: Two 500-mg tablets, three 333-mg tablets, or four 250-mg tablets P.O. at 1 p.m., 2 p.m., and 11 p.m. on preoperative day 1 before 8 a.m. surgery.

➤ **Primary syphilis**

Adults: 30 to 40 g base or stearate P.O. or 48 to 64 g ethylsuccinate P.O. in divided doses for 10 to 15 days.

ADMINISTRATION

P.O.

• Obtain specimen for culture and sensitivity tests before giving. Begin therapy while awaiting results.

• When giving suspension, note the concentration.

• Give drug with full glass of water 2 hours before or 2 hours after meals for best absorption.

Reactions in bold italics are *life-threatening*. Interactions may have a *rapid onset* or a *delayed onset*.

E

• Give drug with food if GI upset occurs. Don't give drug with fruit juice. Make sure patient doesn't swallow chewable tablets whole.

• Coated tablets or encapsulated pellets cause less GI upset, so they may be better tolerated by patients who have trouble tolerating drug.

• Protect capsules from moisture and excessive heat.

I.V.

▼ Obtain specimen for culture and sensitivity tests before giving. Begin therapy while awaiting results.

▼ Reconstitute drug according to manufacturer's directions.

▼ Dilute each 250 mg in at least 100 mL of NSS.

▼ Infuse over 1 hour.

▼ **Incompatibilities:** Ascorbic acid injection, colistimethate, dextrose 2.5% in half-strength lactated Ringer solution, dextrose 5% in lactated Ringer solution, dextrose 5% in NSS, dextrose 5% in Normosol-M, dextrose 10% in water, D_5W, furosemide, heparin sodium, linezolid, metoclopramide, Normosol-R, Ringer injection, vitamin B complex with C.

ACTION

Inhibits bacterial protein synthesis by binding to the 50S subunit of the ribosome. Bacteriostatic or bactericidal, depending on concentration.

Route	Onset	Peak	Duration
P.O.	Unknown	1½ hr	Unknown
I.V.	Immediate	1½ hr	Unknown

Half-life: 1½ hours.

ADVERSE REACTIONS

CNS: fever.

CV: vein irritation or thrombophlebitis after I.V. injection, *ventricular arrhythmias.*

GI: *pseudomembranous colitis,* abdominal pain and cramping, diarrhea, nausea, vomiting.

Hepatic: hepatic dysfunction.

Skin: eczema, rash, urticaria.

Other: *anaphylaxis,* overgrowth of nonsusceptible bacteria or fungi.

INTERACTIONS

Drug-drug. *Azole antifungals (ketoconazole):* May increase erythromycin concentrations, leading to increased risk of adverse reactions, including sudden death from cardiac causes. Avoid use together.

Carbamazepine: May inhibit metabolism of carbamazepine, increasing blood level and risk of toxicity. Avoid using together.

Clindamycin, lincomycin: May be antagonistic. Avoid using together.

Clopidogrel: May inhibit antiplatelet effect of clopidogrel. Monitor platelet function when starting or stopping erythromycin. Adjust clopidogrel dosage as needed.

Colchicine: May increase colchicine level and risk of colchicine-related adverse reactions. Use cautiously and monitor patient for colchicine-related toxicity.

Cyclosporine: May increase cyclosporine level. Monitor drug level.

Digoxin: May increase digoxin level. Monitor patient for digoxin toxicity.

Dihydroergotamine, ergotamine, pimozide: May increase QTc interval and risk of ventricular arrhythmias. Use together is contraindicated.

Disopyramide: May increase disopyramide level, which may cause arrhythmias and prolonged QT intervals. Monitor ECG.

Fluoroquinolones, *other drugs that prolong the QTc interval (amiodarone, antipsychotics, procainamide, quinidine, sotalol, TCAs):* May have additive effects. Monitor ECG for QTc interval prolongation. Avoid using together, if possible.

HMG-CoA reductase inhibitors (lovastatin, simvastatin): May increase concentrations of HMG-CoA reductase inhibitors; rhabdomyolysis has occurred rarely. Monitor CK and serum transaminase levels.

Midazolam, triazolam: May increase effects of these drugs. Monitor patient closely.

Oral anticoagulants: May increase anticoagulant effect. Monitor PT and INR closely.

Rifamycins (rifabutin, rifampin, rifapentine): May decrease therapeutic effects of erythromycin while increasing adverse effects of rifamycin. Monitor patient.

Strong CYP3A inhibitors (diltiazem, verapamil): May increase the risk of sudden death from cardiac causes. Don't use together.

Theophylline: May decrease erythromycin level and increase theophylline toxicity. Use together cautiously.

Drug-food. *Grapefruit juice:* May inhibit drug's metabolism; caution patient to avoid grapefruit juice during therapy.

EFFECTS ON LAB TEST RESULTS
• May increase alkaline phosphatase, ALT, AST, and bilirubin levels.
• May interfere with fluorometric determination of urine catecholamines and with colorimetric assays.

CONTRAINDICATIONS & CAUTIONS
• Contraindicated in patients hypersensitive to drug or other macrolides.
⚠ **Alert:** Drug has been associated with prolonged QT interval and infrequent cases of arrhythmia, including torsades de pointes. Avoid drug in patients with known prolonged QT interval, proarrhythmic conditions, or clinically significant bradycardia, and in those receiving class IA (quinidine, procainamide) or class III (dofetilide, amiodarone, sotalol) antiarrhythmics.
• Use erythromycin salts cautiously in patients with impaired hepatic function.
• May cause infantile hypertrophic pyloric stenosis (HPS) requiring surgery. Benefit of therapy needs to be weighed against risk of developing HPS.
• Prolonged or repeated use may result in superinfection. If superinfection occurs, discontinue drug.
• Drug may cause CDAD, ranging in severity from mild to life-threatening colitis, during treatment and for up to 2 months after treatment. Drug may need to be discontinued if CDAD is suspected or confirmed.
• Don't use drug to treat neurosyphilis.
Dialyzable drug: No.

PREGNANCY-LACTATION-REPRODUCTION
• Use drug during pregnancy only if clearly needed.
• Drug appears in breast milk. Use cautiously in breast-feeding women.

NURSING CONSIDERATIONS
• Monitor patient for superinfection and diarrhea. Drug may cause overgrowth of nonsusceptible bacteria or fungi.

• Monitor hepatic function. Drug may cause hepatotoxicity.
• Elderly patients may be more at risk for developing drug-induced hearing loss. Monitor patient for new hearing loss.

PATIENT TEACHING
• Tell patient to take drug as prescribed, even after he feels better.
• Instruct patient to take oral form of drug with full glass of water 2 hours before or 2 hours after meals for best absorption.
• Drug may be taken with food if GI upset occurs. Tell patient not to take drug with fruit juice or to swallow the chewable tablets whole.
• Instruct patient to report adverse reactions, especially diarrhea, nausea, abdominal pain, vomiting, and fever.
• Instruct parents or caregivers to report vomiting or irritability immediately.

---

escitalopram oxalate
ess-si-TAL-oh-pram

Lexapro⬦

Therapeutic class: Antidepressants
Pharmacologic class: SSRIs

AVAILABLE FORMS
Oral solution: 5 mg/5 mL
Tablets: 5 mg, 10 mg, 20 mg

INDICATIONS & DOSAGES
Adjust-a-dose (for all indications): For elderly patients and those with hepatic impairment, 10 mg P.O. daily, initially and as maintenance dosages.
➤ **Treatment and maintenance therapy for patients with major depressive disorder**
Adults and adolescents: Initially, 10 mg P.O. once daily, increasing to 20 mg if needed after at least 1 week in adults and 3 weeks in adolescents.
➤ **Generalized anxiety disorder**
Adults: Initially, 10 mg P.O. once daily, increasing to 20 mg if needed after at least 1 week.
➤ **Hot flashes (flushes) related to natural or surgically induced menopause ♦**

Adult women: 10 to 20 mg P.O. once daily for 8 weeks.

ADMINISTRATION
P.O.
● Give drug without regard for food.
● Give once daily in the morning or evening.

ACTION
Action may be linked to increase of serotonergic activity in the CNS from inhibition of neuronal reuptake of serotonin. Drug is closely related to citalopram, which may be the active component.

Route	Onset	Peak	Duration
P.O.	Unknown	5 hr	Unknown

Half-life: 27 to 32 hours.

ADVERSE REACTIONS
CNS: *suicidal behavior,* fever, insomnia, dizziness, somnolence, paresthesia, lightheadedness, migraine, tremor, vertigo, abnormal dreams, irritability, impaired concentration, fatigue, lethargy.
CV: palpitations, hypertension, flushing, chest pain.
EENT: rhinitis, sinusitis, blurred vision, tinnitus, earache.
GI: nausea, diarrhea, constipation, indigestion, abdominal pain, vomiting, increased or decreased appetite, dry mouth, flatulence, heartburn, cramps, gastroesophageal reflux.
GU: ejaculation disorder, erectile dysfunction, anorgasmia, menstrual cramps, UTI, urinary frequency.
Metabolic: weight gain or loss, hyponatremia.
Musculoskeletal: arthralgia, myalgia, muscle cramps, pain in arms or legs.
Respiratory: bronchitis, cough.
Skin: rash, increased sweating.
Other: decreased libido, yawning, flulike symptoms.

INTERACTIONS
Drug-drug. *Antiparkinsonians (rasagiline, selegiline):* May cause serotonin syndrome. Avoid use together.
Aspirin, NSAIDs, other drugs known to affect coagulation: May increase the risk of bleeding. Use together cautiously.

Beta blockers: May cause bradycardia and increase risk of CNS toxicity. Monitor patient closely.
Buspirone, methylphenidate: May increase risk of serotonin syndrome. Monitor patient closely.
Carbamazepine: May increase escitalopram clearance. Monitor patient for expected antidepressant effect and adjust dose as needed.
Cimetidine: May increase escitalopram level. Monitor patient for increased adverse reactions to escitalopram.
Citalopram: May cause additive effects. Using together is contraindicated.
CNS drugs: May cause additive effects. Use together cautiously.
Desipramine, other drugs metabolized by CYP2D6: May increase levels of these drugs. Use together cautiously.
Linezolid, methylene blue: May cause serotonin syndrome. Use extreme caution and monitor closely.
Lithium: May enhance serotonergic effect of escitalopram. Use together cautiously, and monitor lithium level.
MAO inhibitors: May cause fatal serotonin syndrome or signs and symptoms resembling neuroleptic malignant syndrome. Avoid using within 14 days of MAO inhibitor therapy.
Triptans: May increase serotonergic effects, leading to weakness, hyperreflexia, incoordination, rapid changes in BP, nausea, and diarrhea. Use together cautiously, especially at the start of therapy or at dosage increases.
Tramadol: May cause serotonin syndrome. Monitor patient closely.
Drug-herb. *St. John's wort:* May cause serotonin syndrome. Use with caution.
Drug-lifestyle. *Alcohol use:* May increase CNS effects. Discourage use together.

EFFECTS ON LAB TEST RESULTS
None reported.

CONTRAINDICATIONS & CAUTIONS
● Contraindicated in patients taking pimozide, MAO inhibitors, or within 14 days of MAO inhibitor therapy and in those hypersensitive to escitalopram, citalopram, or any of its inactive ingredients.

Black Box Warning Escitalopram isn't approved for use in children age 11 and younger. ■

Alert: Concomitant use with methylene blue or linezolid can cause serotonin syndrome (fever, mental status changes, muscle twitching, sweating, shivering, shaking, diarrhea, loss of coordination). Use drug with methylene blue or linezolid only for life-threatening or urgent conditions when the potential benefits outweigh the risks of toxicity.

Alert: If linezolid or methylene blue must be given, the serotonergic drug must be stopped and patient should be monitored for serotonin toxicity for 2 weeks or until 24 hours after the last dose of methylene blue or linezolid, whichever comes first. Treatment with serotonergic drugs may be resumed 24 hours after the last dose of methylene blue or linezolid.

• Use cautiously in patients with a history of mania, seizure disorders, suicidal thoughts, or renal or hepatic impairment.

• Use cautiously in patients with diseases that produce altered metabolism or hemodynamic responses.

• Use with caution in elderly patients because they may have greater sensitivity to drug.

Dialyzable drug: Unknown.

⚠ *Overdose S&S:* Seizures, coma, dizziness, ECG changes, hypotension, insomnia, nausea, sinus tachycardia, somnolence, vomiting, acute renal failure.

PREGNANCY-LACTATION-REPRODUCTION

• Use in pregnant women only if potential benefit justifies potential risk to the fetus.

• Prescriber should consider tapering dosage in the third trimester by carefully weighing established benefit of treating depression with an antidepressant against potential risks; decision can only be made on a case-by-case basis.

• Drug appears in breast milk. Use cautiously in breast-feeding women; monitor infants for adverse reactions.

NURSING CONSIDERATIONS

Black Box Warning Drug may increase risk of suicidal thinking and behavior in children, adolescents, and young adults

ages 18 to 24, especially during the first few months of treatment, especially in those with major depressive disorder or other psychiatric disorder. ■

• Closely monitor patients at high risk of suicide.

• Evaluate patient for history of drug abuse, and observe for signs of misuse or abuse.

• When discontinuing drug, taper gradually and monitor patient for reemerging signs and symptoms.

• Periodically reassess patient to determine need for maintenance treatment and appropriate dosing.

Alert: Combining triptans with an SSRI or an SSNRI may cause serotonin syndrome or neuroleptic malignant syndrome-like reactions. Serotonin syndrome may be more likely to occur when starting or increasing the dose of triptan, SSRI, or SSNRI.

• *Look alike–sound alike:* Don't confuse escitalopram with estazolam.

PATIENT TEACHING

• Inform patient that symptoms should improve gradually over several weeks, rather than immediately.

• Tell patient that although improvement may occur within 1 to 4 weeks, he should continue drug as prescribed.

Black Box Warning Caution patient and patient's family to report signs of worsening depression (such as agitation, irritability, insomnia, hostility, impulsivity) and signs of suicidal behavior to prescriber immediately. ■

Alert: Teach patient to recognize and immediately report symptoms of serotonin toxicity (fever, mental status changes, muscle twitching, excessive sweating, shivering or shaking, diarrhea, loss of coordination).

• Tell patient to use caution while driving or operating hazardous machinery because of drug's potential to impair judgment, thinking, and motor skills.

• Advise patient to consult health care provider before taking other prescription or OTC drugs.

• Tell patient that drug may be taken in the morning or evening without regard to meals

• Encourage patient to avoid alcohol while taking drug.

Reactions in bold italics are *life-threatening*. Interactions may have a *rapid onset* or a *delayed onset*.

• Advise female patient to notify health care provider if she is pregnant or breast-feeding before starting therapy.

eslicarbazepine acetate
ES-lye-kar-BAY-ze-peen

Aptiom

Therapeutic class: Anticonvulsants
Pharmacologic class: Carboxamide derivatives

AVAILABLE FORMS
Tablets: 200 mg, 400 mg, 600 mg, 800 mg

INDICATIONS & DOSAGES
➤ **Monotherapy or adjunctive treatment for partial-onset seizures**
Adults: Initially, 400 mg P.O. once daily; may initiate treatment at 800 mg daily if need for additional seizure reduction outweighs an increased risk of adverse reactions. After 1 week at 400-mg daily dose, increase to recommended maintenance dosage of 800 mg P.O. once daily. May increase in weekly increments of 400 to 600 mg once daily to a recommended maintenance dose of 800 to 1,600 mg once daily. For monotherapy, consider the 800-mg once-daily maintenance dose in patients unable to tolerate 1,200-mg daily dose. For adjunctive therapy, consider the 1,600-mg daily dose in patients who didn't achieve a satisfactory response with a 1,200-mg daily dose.
Adjust-a-dose: For patients with moderate to severe renal impairment (CrCl of less than 50 mL/minute), the initial, titration, and maintenance doses should generally be reduced by 50%. Maintenance doses may be adjusted according to clinical response. Consider adjusting dosages of both eslicarbazepine and carbamazepine if given concurrently. Consider increasing eslicarbazepine dosage if given with enzyme-inducing antiepileptics, such as phenobarbital, primidone, or phenytoin.

ADMINISTRATION
P.O.
• Give drug without regard for food.

• Patient may swallow tablet whole or crushed.
• Store at room temperature.

ACTION
Unknown. Thought to inhibit voltage-gated sodium channels, resulting in decreased seizure activity.

Route	Onset	Peak	Duration
P.O.	Rapid	1–4 hr	Unknown

Half-life: 13 to 20 hours.

ADVERSE REACTIONS
CNS: asthenia, gait disturbance, dizziness, drowsiness, somnolence, headache, ataxia, balance disorder, tremor, dysarthria, memory impairment, depression, insomnia, fatigue, vertigo.
CV: hypertension, peripheral edema.
EENT: diplopia, blurred vision, visual impairment, nystagmus.
GI: nausea, vomiting, diarrhea, constipation, abdominal pain, gastritis.
GU: UTI.
Metabolic: hyponatremia.
Respiratory: cough.
Skin: rash.
Other: falls.

INTERACTIONS
Drug-drug. *Carbamazepine, phenobarbital, phenytoin, primidone:* May decrease eslicarbazepine concentration. Consider higher eslicarbazepine dosage.
Clobazam, omeprazole: May increase concentrations of these drugs. Monitor patient accordingly.
Ethinyl estradiol, levonorgestrel: May decrease hormone concentrations. Patient should use additional or alternative nonhormonal contraception.
Phenytoin: May increase phenytoin concentration. Monitor phenytoin level and adjust dosage accordingly.
Rosuvastatin, simvastatin: May lower statin level. Adjust statin dosage if significant change in lipids occur.
Warfarin: May decrease warfarin effect. Monitor INR and adjust dosage accordingly.
Drug-herb. *Evening primrose:* May decrease seizure threshold. Don't use together.

Drug-lifestyle. *Alcohol use:* May increase CNS depression. Avoid use together.

EFFECTS ON LAB TEST RESULTS
● May increase bilirubin, AST, ALT, total cholesterol, triglyceride, LDL, and CK levels.
● May decrease sodium, chloride, T_3, T_4, and Hb levels and hematocrit.

CONTRAINDICATIONS & CAUTIONS
● **Alert:** Contraindicated in patients hypersensitive to drug or its components. Rare cases of anaphylaxis and angioedema have been reported. Anaphylaxis and angioedema associated with laryngeal edema can be fatal. If patient develops any of these reactions after treatment, discontinue drug.
● **Alert:** Contraindicated in patients who have experienced dermatologic reaction, DRESS (drug rash with eosinophilia and systemic symptoms) syndrome, anaphylactic reactions, or angioedema while taking oxcarbazepine.
● Don't give oxcarbazepine to patients also taking eslicarbazepine. Drugs are chemically related.
● Use in patients with severe hepatic impairment hasn't been evaluated and isn't recommended.
● Use cautiously in patients at risk for suicidal thoughts and behavior.
Dialyzable drug: Yes.
⚠ **Overdose S&S:** Hyponatremia, dizziness, nausea, vomiting, somnolence, euphoria, oral paresthesia, ataxia, walking difficulty, diplopia.

PREGNANCY-LACTATION-REPRODUCTION
● Use in pregnancy only if potential benefit justifies potential risk to the fetus. Recommend that pregnant patients enroll in the North American Antiepileptic Drug Pregnancy Registry at 1-888-233-2334.
● Women of childbearing potential who use hormonal contraceptives should also use additional or alternative forms of nonhormonal contraceptives.
● Drug appears in breast milk. Patient should discontinue breast-feeding or discontinue drug.

NURSING CONSIDERATIONS
● To discontinue drug, reduce dosage gradually; avoid abrupt discontinuation.
● **Alert:** Anticonvulsants can increase risk of suicidal thoughts or behavior in patients taking these drugs for any indication. Monitor patients for new or worsening depression, development of suicidal thoughts and behavior, or unusual change in mood or behavior.
● Monitor sodium and chloride levels initially and periodically during treatment, especially in patients taking drugs known to decrease serum sodium level. Reduce dosage or discontinue drug as clinically indicated.
● Monitor patients for hyponatremia (nausea, vomiting, malaise, headache, lethargy, confusion, irritability, muscle weakness, spasms, obtundation, and increased seizure frequency or severity).
● Obtain thyroid function tests at baseline and periodically during treatment.
● Obtain LFTs at baseline and periodically during therapy. Discontinue drug if jaundice, liver injury, or laboratory results suggestive of liver injury occur.
● Monitor patient for dermatologic conditions, such as Stevens-Johnson syndrome and toxic epidermal necrolysis; discontinue drug if serious dermatologic changes occur.
● **Alert:** Monitor patients for DRESS syndrome or multiorgan hypersensitivity (fever, rash, lymphadenopathy, hepatitis, nephritis, hematologic abnormalities, myocarditis, or myositis). Discontinue drug if DRESS syndrome occurs.
● Monitor patients for development of dizziness or disturbances in gait and coordination (ataxia, vertigo, balance disorder, nystagmus), especially during dosage titration and in patients age 60 and older. Consider dosage modification.
● Monitor patients for dose-dependent somnolence or fatigue, cognitive dysfunction (memory impairment, disturbance in attention, amnesia, confusion, aphasia, speech disorder, slowness of thought, disorientation, or psychomotor retardation), or visual changes (diplopia, blurred vision, impaired vision).

PATIENT TEACHING

• Advise patient not to operate motor vehicles or hazardous machinery while taking drug until drug's effects are known.
• Tell patient to report CNS signs and symptoms, such as dizziness or disturbances in gait and coordination (ataxia, vertigo, balance disorder, nystagmus).
• Advise patient that laboratory monitoring will be needed during therapy.
• Inform patient and caregivers of increased risk of suicidal thoughts and behavior. Advise them to immediately report new or worsening depression, unusual changes in mood or behavior, thoughts of suicide, or thoughts about self-harm.
• Counsel patient to report rash or other skin reactions.
• Advise patient to report signs and symptoms of hyponatremia (nausea, vomiting, malaise, headache, lethargy, confusion, irritability, muscle weakness, spasms, obtundation, increased seizure frequency or severity).
• Caution patient not to stop drug without first discussing with prescriber. If drug needs to be stopped, it must be tapered gradually.

SAFETY ALERT!

esmolol hydrochloride
ESS-moe-lol

Brevibloc

Therapeutic class: Antiarrhythmics
Pharmacologic class: Selective beta blockers

AVAILABLE FORMS

Injection: 10 mg/mL vial
Premixed bags in sodium chloride: 10 mg/mL in 250-mL bags; 20 mg/mL in 100-mL bags

INDICATIONS & DOSAGES

➤ **Supraventricular tachycardia; noncompensatory sinus tachycardias**
Adults: 500 mcg/kg/minute as loading dose by I.V. infusion over 1 minute; then 4-minute maintenance infusion of 50 mcg/kg/minute. If adequate response doesn't occur within 5 minutes, may repeat loading dose and follow with maintenance infusion of 100 mcg/kg/minute for 4 minutes. May repeat loading dose and increase maintenance infusion by increments of 50 mcg/kg/minute. Range of maintenance dose is generally 50 to 200 mcg/kg/minute. Maximum maintenance infusion for tachycardia is 200 mcg/kg/minute. May continue maintenance infusions for up to 48 hours.

➤ **Intraoperative and postoperative tachycardia or hypertension**
Adults: For immediate control: 1 mg/kg as a bolus dose over 30 seconds, followed by 150 mcg/kg/minute I.V. infusion, if needed. Maximum dose for tachycardia is 200 mcg/kg/minute; maximum dose for hypertension is 300 mcg/kg/minute. For gradual control (stepwise dosing): Loading dose is 500 mcg/kg over 1 minute, then 50 mcg/kg/minute for 4 minutes. Optional loading dose if needed, then 100 mcg/kg/minute for 4 minutes. Optional loading dose if needed, then 150 mcg/kg/minute for 4 minutes. If necessary, may increase to 200 mcg/kg/minute. Maximum doses are 200 mcg/kg/minute for tachycardia and 300 mcg/kg/minute for hypertension.

ADMINISTRATION

I.V.
▼ Don't dilute in 10-mg/mL single-dose vials or premixed containers.
▼ Give with an infusion-control device rather than by I.V. push. Administer by continuous I.V. infusion with or without a loading dose and titrate using ventricular rate or BP at 4-minute or more intervals. Avoid infusing into small veins or through a butterfly catheter.
▼ If concentration exceeds 10 mg/mL, give drug through a central line.
▼ Don't use for longer than 48 hours. Watch infusion site carefully for signs of extravasation; if they occur, stop infusion immediately and call prescriber.
▼ **Incompatibilities:** Amphotericin B cholesteryl sulfate complex, diazepam, furosemide, procainamide, sodium bicarbonate 5%, thiopental sodium, warfarin sodium.

🍁Canada   ◊OTC   ◆Off-label use   ✿Photoguide   ⓓDo not crush   *Liquid contains alcohol.

ACTION
A class II antiarrhythmic and ultra-short-acting selective beta blocker that decreases HR, contractility, and BP.

Route	Onset	Peak	Duration
I.V.	Immediate	30 min	30 min after infusion

Half-life: About 9 minutes.

ADVERSE REACTIONS
CNS: dizziness, somnolence, headache, agitation, confusion.
CV: hypotension, peripheral ischemia.
GI: nausea, vomiting.
Skin: inflammation or induration at infusion site.

INTERACTIONS
Drug-drug. *Antidiabetic agents:* May increase blood glucose-lowering effect of antidiabetic agent. Closely monitor blood glucose concentration.
Calcium channel blockers (diltiazem, nicardipine, nifedipine, verapamil), flecainide: May potentiate pharmacologic effects of both drugs. I.V. administration in close proximity is contraindicated. Monitor cardiac function closely and adjust therapy as needed.
Clonidine: May cause life-threatening BP increases. Closely monitor BP. Discontinue either agent gradually, preferably esmolol first.
Digoxin: May increase digoxin level by 10% to 20%. Monitor digoxin level.
Lidocaine: May increase lidocaine concentration. Monitor patient closely and adjust dosage as needed.
MAO inhibitors: May worsen bradycardia or hypertension. Discontinue esmolol or reduce esmolol dosage if needed.
Morphine: May increase esmolol level. Adjust esmolol dosage carefully.
NSAIDs: May impair antihypertensive effect of esmolol. Monitor BP and adjust esmolol dosage as needed.
Prazosin: May increase risk of orthostatic hypertension. Help patient to stand slowly until effects are known.
Reserpine, other catecholamine-depleting drugs: May increase bradycardia and hypertension. Adjust esmolol dosage carefully.

Salicylates (aspirin): May impair antihypertensive effect of esmolol. Monitor patient and consider alternative therapy as needed.
Succinylcholine: May prolong neuromuscular blockade. Monitor patient closely.
Vasoconstrictive and positive inotropic agents (dopamine, epinephrine, norepinephrine): May increase risk of reduced cardiac contractility in presence of high systemic vascular resistance. Don't use together.
Verapamil: May increase effects of both drugs. Monitor cardiac function closely and decrease dosages as necessary.

EFFECTS ON LAB TEST RESULTS
None reported.

CONTRAINDICATIONS & CAUTIONS
● Contraindicated in patients hypersensitive to drug or its components and in those with severe sinus bradycardia, second- or third-degree heart block, sick sinus syndrome, cardiogenic shock, decompensated HF, pulmonary hypertension.
● Use cautiously in patients with renal impairment, diabetes, or bronchospasm.
◔ **Alert:** Don't withdraw drug abruptly, as angina, MI, and ventricular arrhythmias can occur.
Dialyzable drug: Unknown.
⚠ **Overdose S&S:** Bradycardia, hypotension, loss of consciousness, cardiac arrest, pulseless electrical activity.

PREGNANCY-LACTATION-REPRODUCTION
● Use during the third trimester can cause fetal bradycardia. Use in pregnant women only if potential benefit justifies potential risk to the fetus.
● It isn't known if drug appears in breast milk. Patient should discontinue breastfeeding or discontinue drug.

NURSING CONSIDERATIONS
● Dosage for postoperative treatment of tachycardia and hypertension is same as for supraventricular tachycardia.
◔ **Alert:** Monitor ECG and BP continuously during infusion. Nearly half of patients will develop hypotension. Diaphoresis and dizziness may accompany hypotension.

Reactions in bold italics are *life-threatening*. Interactions may have a *rapid onset* or a *delayed onset*.

Monitor patient closely, especially if he had low BP before treatment.

• Hypotension can usually be reversed within 30 minutes by decreasing the dose or, if needed, by stopping the infusion. Notify prescriber if this becomes necessary.

• If a local reaction develops at the infusion site, change to another site.

• When patient's HR becomes stable, replace drug with an alternative antiarrhythmic, such as propranolol, digoxin, or verapamil. Reduce infusion rate by half 30 minutes after the first dose of the new drug. Monitor patient response and, if HR is controlled for 1 hour after administration of the second dose of the replacement drug, stop esmolol infusion.

• Monitor serum electrolyte levels, as hyperkalemia can occur, especially in patients with renal impairment.

• Drug can mask signs and symptoms of hyperthyroidism. Monitor patient for thyrotoxicosis when withdrawing drug.

PATIENT TEACHING

• Instruct patient to report all adverse reactions promptly.

• Tell patient to report discomfort at I.V. site.

esomeprazole magnesium
ess-oh-ME-pray-zol

Nexium⬧

esomeprazole sodium
Nexium I.V.

Therapeutic class: Antiulcer drugs
Pharmacologic class: Proton pump inhibitors

AVAILABLE FORMS
esomeprazole magnesium
Capsules (delayed-release) ⬤*:* 20 mg, 40 mg
Powder for suspension (delayed-release): 2.5 mg, 5 mg, 10 mg, 20 mg, 40 mg
esomeprazole sodium
Powder for injection: 20-mg, 40-mg single-use vials

INDICATIONS & DOSAGES
Adjust-a-dose (for all indications): For patients with severe hepatic failure (Child-Pugh class C), maximum daily dose is 20 mg.

➤ **GERD; to heal erosive esophagitis**
Adults: 20 or 40 mg P.O. daily for 4 to 8 weeks. Maintenance dose for healing erosive esophagitis is 20 mg P.O. for up to 6 months.
Children ages 1 to 11 weighing less than 20 kg: 10 mg P.O. once daily for up to 8 weeks.
Children ages 1 to 11 weighing 20 kg or more: 10 or 20 mg P.O. once daily for up to 8 weeks.

➤ **Symptomatic GERD**
Adults: 20 mg P.O. daily for 4 weeks. If symptoms are unresolved, may continue treatment for 4 more weeks.
Children and adolescents ages 12 to 17: 20 mg P.O. once daily for up to 4 weeks.
Children ages 1 to 11: 10 mg P.O. once daily for up to 8 weeks.

➤ **Short-term therapy (up to 10 days) of GERD in patients with a history of erosive esophagitis who are unable to take drug orally**
Adult: Reconstitute 20 or 40 mg with 5 mL of D_5W, NSS, or lactated Ringer injection and give by I.V. bolus over 3 minutes. Or, further dilute to a total volume of 50 mL and give I.V. over 10 to 30 minutes. Switch patient to oral therapy as soon as he can tolerate it.
Children ages 1 to 17 weighing 55 kg or more: 20 mg I.V. infusion once daily over 10 to 30 minutes.
Children ages 1 to 17 weighing less than 55 kg: 10 mg I.V. infusion once daily over 10 to 30 minutes.
Children ages 1 month to younger than 1 year: 0.5 mg/kg I.V. infusion once daily over 10 to 30 minutes.

➤ **Erosive esophagitis due to acid-mediated GERD only**
Infants ages 1 to 11 months weighing more than 7.5 to 12 kg: 10 mg P.O. once daily for up to 6 weeks.
Infants ages 1 to 11 months weighing more than 5 to 7.5 kg: 5 mg P.O. once daily for up to 6 weeks.

E

Infants ages 1 to 11 months weighing 3 to 5 kg: 2.5 mg P.O. once daily for up to 6 weeks.

➤ **To reduce the risk of gastric ulcers in patients receiving continuous NSAID therapy**
Adults: 20 or 40 mg P.O. once daily for up to 6 months.

➤ **Long-term treatment of pathologic hypersecretory conditions, including Zollinger-Ellison syndrome**
Adults: 40 mg P.O. b.i.d. Adjust dosage based on patient response.

➤ **To eliminate** *Helicobacter pylori*
Adults: 40 mg esomeprazole magnesium P.O. daily, 1,000 mg amoxicillin P.O. b.i.d., and 500 mg clarithromycin P.O. b.i.d., given together for 10 days to reduce duodenal ulcer recurrence.

➤ **Reduction of risk of rebleeding of gastric or duodenal ulcers after therapeutic endoscopy**
Adults: 80 mg I.V. over 30 minutes, followed by continuous infusion of 8 mg/hour for a total I.V. treatment duration of 72 hours, followed by oral acid-suppressive therapy.

Adjust-a-dose: In patients with mild to moderate hepatic impairment (Child-Pugh classes A and B), maximum continuous infusion rate is 6 mg/hour. In patients with severe hepatic impairment (Child-Pugh class C), maximum continuous infusion rate is 4 mg/hour.

ADMINISTRATION
P.O.
● Give drug at least 1 hour before meals. If patient has difficulty swallowing the capsule, contents of the capsule can be emptied and mixed with 1 tablespoon of applesauce and swallowed (without chewing the enteric-coated pellets).
● If giving capsule via NG tube, open capsule and empty the granules into a 60-mL syringe. Mix with 50 mL of water. Replace the plunger and shake vigorously for 15 seconds. Flush NG tube with additional water after use. Don't give if pellets have dissolved or disintegrated.
● For oral suspension, mix contents of a 2.5- or 5-mg packet with 5 mL of water; mix contents of a 10-, 20-, or 40-mg packet with 15 mL of water. Then let it sit for 2 to

3 minutes to thicken. Stir the suspension and drink within 30 minutes.
● To give oral suspension via NG tube, add 5 mL of water to a syringe, then add contents of 2.5- or 5-mg packet; or add 15 mL of water to a syringe, then add contents of 10-, 20-, or 40-mg packet. Shake syringe and leave for 2 to 3 minutes to thicken. Shake syringe again and inject through NG or gastric tube within 30 minutes. Flush any remaining contents into the stomach with additional water.

I.V.
▼ Flush I.V. line with D_5W, NSS, or lactated Ringer injection before and after administration.
▼ Use reconstituted solution within 12 hours.
▼ Use admixture diluted with D_5W within 6 hours.
▼ If diluted with NSS or lactated Ringer injection, use within 12 hours.
▼ Store reconstituted solution and admixture at room temperature.
▼ **Incompatibilities:** Other I.V. drugs.

ACTION
Reduces gastric acid secretion and decreases gastric acidity.

Route	Onset	Peak	Duration
P.O.	Unknown	1½ hr	13–17 hr
I.V.	Unknown	Unknown	Unknown

Half-life: 1 to 1½ hours.

ADVERSE REACTIONS
CNS: headache, dizziness.
GI: abdominal pain, constipation, diarrhea, dry mouth, flatulence, nausea, vomiting.
Skin: pruritus.

INTERACTIONS
Drug-drug. *Calcium salts (calcium carbonate):* May interfere with GI absorption of calcium salts. Closely monitor clinical response to calcium; larger dosages of calcium may be needed.
Cilostazol: May increase concentrations of cilostazol and its active metabolite. Consider a cilostazol dose reduction when esomeprazole is given concurrently.
Clopidogrel: May decrease antiplatelet activity. Use esomeprazole magnesium

---

Reactions in bold italics are *life-threatening*. Interactions may have a *rapid onset* or a *delayed onset*.

or esomeprazole sodium cautiously with clopidogrel.

Clozapine: May increase clozapine plasma concentration and risk of toxicity. Closely monitor clinical status and laboratory values.

Dabigatran: May decrease concentration of active metabolite of dabigatran. Monitor patient closely.

Diazepam: May decrease clearance of diazepam. Monitor patient for diazepam toxicity.

Digoxin: May increase serum digoxin level. Monitor digoxin concentration and clinical response. If an interaction is suspected, adjust digoxin dosage as needed.

Drugs metabolized by CYP2C19: May alter clearance of esomeprazole, especially in elderly patients or patients with hepatic insufficiency. Monitor patient for toxicity.

Fluvoxamine: May increase risk of adverse reactions. Use cautiously.

Iron salts (ferrous sulfate): May interfere with absorption of iron salts. Temporary cessation of esomeprazole may be required to achieve appropriate clinical response to oral iron. If stopping esomeprazole isn't an option, parenteral iron may be a suitable alternative.

Ketoconazole, voriconazole: May increase esomeprazole concentration. Monitor therapy.

Macrolide antibiotics (clarithromycin): May increase esomeprazole level. Monitor patient for toxicity.

Methotrexate: May increase methotrexate concentration and risk of toxicity. Monitor patient closely.

Mycophenolate: May decrease mycophenolate plasma concentration and pharmacologic effects. Monitor clinical response and adjust mycophenolate dosage as needed.

Protease inhibitors (atazanavir, nelfinavir, saquinavir): May reduce plasma levels of atazanavir or nelfinavir. Use together isn't recommended. May increase saquinavir levels. Monitor carefully and reduce dosage if needed.

Rifampin: May decrease esomeprazole levels. Avoid using together.

Rilpivirine: May cause loss of virologic response or resistance. Use together is contraindicated.

Tacrolimus: May increase pharmacologic effects of tacrolimus and risk of adverse reactions. Closely monitor tacrolimus trough concentration when starting or stopping esomeprazole. Adjust tacrolimus dosage as needed.

Warfarin: May prolong PT and increase INR, causing abnormal bleeding. Monitor patient and his PT and INR.

Drug-herb. *St. John's wort:* May decrease esomeprazole level. Avoid use together.

Drug-food. *Any food:* May reduce drug level. Advise patient to take drug 1 hour before food.

EFFECTS ON LAB TEST RESULTS
● May decrease magnesium level.

CONTRAINDICATIONS & CAUTIONS
● Contraindicated in patients hypersensitive to drug or components of esomeprazole or omeprazole (a drug similar to this one).

⚠ **Alert:** There may be an increased risk of osteoporosis-related hip, wrist, and spine fractures associated with PPIs. Risk is increased in patients who received high-dose and long-term (greater than 1 year) therapy. The lowest dosage for the shortest duration should be used.

● Use cautiously in patients receiving continuous NSAID therapy who are at increased risk for gastric ulcers (those age 60 and older and those with a history of gastric ulcers).

● Drug-induced decreases in gastric acidity may increase serum chromogranin A (CgA) level, possibly causing false-positive results in diagnostic investigations for neuroendocrine tumors. Temporarily stop esomeprazole at least 14 days before assessing CgA level; consider repeating the test if initial CgA level is high.

Dialyzable drug: Unlikely.

⚠ **Overdose S&S:** Blurred vision, confusion, tremor, ataxia, intermittent clonic seizures, diaphoresis, drowsiness, flushing, headache, nausea, tachycardia.

PREGNANCY-LACTATION-REPRODUCTION
● Use during pregnancy only if potential benefit justifies potential risk to the fetus.

✤Canada   ◇OTC   ◆Off-label use   ✔Photoguide   ⓓ Do not crush   *Liquid contains alcohol.

• It isn't known if drug appears in breast milk, but omeprazole does. Use cautiously in breast-feeding women.

NURSING CONSIDERATIONS
• Antacids can be used while taking drug, unless otherwise directed by prescriber.
• Monitor patient for rash or signs and symptoms of hypersensitivity. Monitor GI symptoms for improvement or worsening. Monitor LFTs, especially in patients with preexisting hepatic disease.
❶ Alert: Prolonged use may cause low magnesium levels that require magnesium supplementation and possibly discontinuation of drug. Monitor magnesium level before treatment and periodically during treatment. Monitor patient for signs and symptoms of low magnesium level, such as abnormal HR or heart rhythm, palpitations, muscle spasms, tremor, and seizures. In children, abnormal HR may present as fatigue, upset stomach, dizziness, and light-headedness.
❶ Alert: May increase risk of CDAD. Evaluate for CDAD in patients who develop diarrhea that doesn't improve.
❶ Alert: Prolonged treatment (at least 2 years or more) may lead to vitamin B_{12} malabsorption and subsequent vitamin B_{12} deficiency, which is dose-related and stronger in women and those younger than age 30; prevalence decreases after discontinuation of therapy.
• Long-term therapy may cause atrophic gastritis.
• **Look alike–sound alike:** Don't confuse Nexium with Nexavar.

PATIENT TEACHING
• Instruct patient to take drug exactly as prescribed.
• Tell patient to take drug at least 1 hour before a meal.
• Advise patient that antacids can be used while taking drug unless otherwise directed by prescriber.
• Warn patient not to chew or crush drug pellets because this inactivates the drug.
• If patient has difficulty swallowing capsule, tell him to mix contents of capsule with 1 tablespoon of soft applesauce and swallow immediately.

• Advise patient to store capsules at room temperature in a tight container.
• Tell patient to inform prescriber of worsening signs and symptoms, pain, or diarrhea that doesn't improve.
• Instruct patient to alert prescriber if rash or other signs and symptoms of allergy occur.
• Warn patient to immediately report symptoms of low magnesium level.

esterified estrogens
ESS-tehr-eh-fide ESS-troe-jenz

Estragyn✸, Menest

Therapeutic class: Estrogens
Pharmacologic class: Estrogens

AVAILABLE FORMS
Tablets (film-coated): 0.3 mg, 0.625 mg, 1.25 mg, 2.5 mg

INDICATIONS & DOSAGES
➤ **Inoperable progressing prostate cancer**
Men: 1.25 to 2.5 mg P.O. t.i.d.
➤ **Palliative treatment for metastatic breast cancer**
Men and postmenopausal women: 10 mg P.O. t.i.d. for 3 or more months.
➤ **Hypogonadism**
Women: 2.5 to 7.5 mg P.O. daily in divided doses in cycles of 20 days on, 10 days off.
➤ **Castration, primary ovarian failure**
Women: 1.25 mg P.O. daily in cycles of 3 weeks on, 1 week off. Adjust for symptoms. Can be given continuously.
➤ **Vasomotor menopausal symptoms**
Women: 1.25 mg P.O. daily in cycles of 3 weeks on, 1 week off. Dosage may be increased to 2.5 to 3.75 mg P.O. daily, if needed. If patient is menstruating, cyclical administration is started on day 5 of bleeding.
➤ **Moderate to severe menopausal vulvar and vaginal atrophy**
Women: 0.3 to 1.25 mg or more P.O. daily, depending on tissue response of individual patient, in cycles of 3 weeks on, 1 week off.

ADMINISTRATION
P.O.
● Use lowest effective dose needed for specific indication.
● Reevaluate at 3- to 6-month intervals for tapering or discontinuation of therapy.
● Give without regard to food.

ACTION
Mimics the actions of endogenous estrogens; increases synthesis of DNA, RNA, and protein in responsive tissues; reduces release of FSH and luteinizing hormone from pituitary gland.

Route	Onset	Peak	Duration
P.O.	Unknown	Unknown	Unknown

Half-life: Unknown.

ADVERSE REACTIONS
CNS: headache, dizziness, chorea, depression, *stroke, seizures.*
CV: thrombophlebitis, *thromboembolism,* hypertension, edema, *PE, MI.*
EENT: worsening myopia or astigmatism, intolerance of contact lenses.
GI: nausea, vomiting, abdominal cramps, bloating, anorexia, increased appetite, *pancreatitis,* increased risk of gallbladder disease.
GU: breakthrough bleeding, altered menstrual flow, dysmenorrhea, amenorrhea, *increased risk of endometrial cancer,* cervical erosion, altered cervical secretions, enlargement of uterine fibromas, vaginal candidiasis, testicular atrophy, impotence.
Hepatic: cholestatic jaundice, *hepatic adenoma.*
Metabolic: hypercalcemia, weight changes, hypertriglyceridemia.
Skin: melasma, rash, hirsutism or hair loss, erythema nodosum, *erythema multiforme,* dermatitis.
Other: breast tenderness, enlargement or secretion; gynecomastia; *increased risk of breast cancer.*

INTERACTIONS
Drug-drug. *Anastrozole:* May interfere with anastrozole effectiveness. Avoid use together.
Carbamazepine, fosphenytoin, phenobarbital, phenytoin, rifampin: May decrease effectiveness of estrogen therapy. Monitor patient closely.
Clarithromycin, erythromycin, itraconazole, ketoconazole, ritonavir: May increase estrogen plasma levels and side effects. Monitor patient.
Corticosteroids: May increase corticosteroid effects. Monitor patient closely.
Cyclosporine: May increase risk of toxicity. Use together with caution, and monitor cyclosporine level frequently.
Dantrolene, hepatotoxic drugs: May increase risk of hepatotoxicity. Monitor liver function closely.
Oral anticoagulants: May decrease anticoagulant effects. Adjust dosage if needed. Monitor PT and INR.
Tamoxifen: May interfere with tamoxifen effectiveness. Avoid using together.
Drug-herb. *St. John's wort:* May decrease effects of drug. Discourage use together.
Drug-food. *Caffeine:* May increase caffeine level. Urge caution.
Grapefruit, grapefruit juice: May increase risk of adverse effects. Discourage use together.
Drug-lifestyle. *Smoking:* May increase risk of CV effects. If smoking continues, may need another form of therapy.

EFFECTS ON LAB TEST RESULTS
● May increase calcium, thyroid-binding globulin, serum triglyceride, serum phospholipid, and clotting factor VII, VIII, IX, and X levels.
● May increase norepinephrine-induced platelet aggregation and may prolong PT.
● May reduce metyrapone test results and cause impaired glucose tolerance.

CONTRAINDICATIONS & CAUTIONS
● Contraindicated in patients hypersensitive to drug and in patients with breast cancer (except metastatic disease), estrogen-dependent neoplasia, active thrombophlebitis, thromboembolic disorders, undiagnosed abnormal genital bleeding, or history of thromboembolic disease.
● Use cautiously in patients with history of hypertension, mental depression, cardiac or renal dysfunction, liver impairment, gallbladder disease, bone disease, migraine, seizures, or diabetes.

Black Box Warning Drug shouldn't be used for prevention of CV disease. Drug is associated with development of dementia in postmenopausal women age 65 and older. Estrogens with or without progestins should be prescribed at the lowest effective doses for the shortest duration consistent with treatment goals. ■

Dialyzable drug: Unknown.

⚠ *Overdose S&S:* Nausea, withdrawal bleeding in females.

PREGNANCY-LACTATION-REPRODUCTION

● Estrogens shouldn't be used during pregnancy.

● There is no indication for use in pregnancy. There appears to be little or no increased risk of birth defects in children born to women who have used estrogens and progestins from oral contraceptives inadvertently during early pregnancy.

● Estrogens have been shown to decrease the quantity and quality of breast milk. Use only if clearly needed; monitor infant's growth closely.

NURSING CONSIDERATIONS

☀ *Alert:* Drug is considered a high-risk medication for elderly patients.

● When used for vasomotor symptoms in menstruating women, cyclic administration is started on day 5 of bleeding.

● When given cyclically for short-term use, administration should be cyclic and attempts to discontinue or taper the medication should be made at 3- to 6-month intervals.

● Make sure patient has thorough physical examination before starting estrogen therapy. Patients receiving long-term therapy should have annual examinations. Periodically monitor body weight, BP, lipid levels, and hepatic function.

● Notify pathologist about patient's estrogen therapy when sending specimens to laboratory for evaluation.

☀ *Alert:* Because of risk of thromboembolism, stop therapy at least 4 to 6 weeks before procedures that cause prolonged immobilization or increased risk of thromboembolism, such as knee or hip surgery.

Black Box Warning Estrogens have been reported to increase the risk of endometrial carcinoma. ■

● Glucose tolerance may be impaired. Monitor glucose level closely in patients with diabetes.

PATIENT TEACHING

● Advise patient to report all adverse reactions promptly.

● Emphasize importance of regular physical examinations. Postmenopausal women who use estrogen replacement for longer than 5 years to treat menopausal symptoms may be at increased risk for endometrial cancer. This risk is reduced by using cyclic rather than continuous therapy and the lowest possible estrogen dosage. Adding progestins to the regimen decreases risk of endometrial hyperplasia, but it's unknown whether progestins affect risk of endometrial cancer.

☀ *Alert:* Warn patient to immediately report abdominal pain; pain, numbness, or stiffness in legs or buttocks; pressure or pain in chest or shortness of breath; severe headaches; visual disturbances, such as blind spots, flashing lights, or blurriness; vaginal bleeding or discharge; breast lumps; swelling of hands or feet; yellow skin or sclera; dark urine; or light-colored stools.

● Tell diabetic patient to report elevated glucose level so that antidiabetic dosage can be adjusted.

● Explain to woman receiving cyclic therapy for postmenopausal symptoms that she may experience withdrawal bleeding during week off drug. Tell her to report unusual vaginal bleeding.

● Teach woman to perform routine breast self-examination.

● Advise woman of childbearing potential to consult prescriber before taking drug and to advise prescriber immediately if she becomes pregnant.

● Teach patient methods to decrease risk of blood clots.

● Encourage patient to stop smoking or reduce number of cigarettes smoked because of the risk of CV complications.

estradiol (oestradiol)
ess-tra-DYE-ole

Alora, Climara, Estrace Vaginal
Cream, Estraderm, Estring Vaginal
Ring, Evamist, Menostar, Minivelle,
Vivelle, Vivelle-Dot

estradiol acetate
Femring

estradiol cypionate
Depo-Estradiol

estradiol gel
Divigel, Elestrin, EstroGel

estradiol hemihydrate
Vagifem

estradiol valerate (oestradiol valerate)
Delestrogen

Therapeutic class: Estrogens
Pharmacologic class: Estrogens

AVAILABLE FORMS
estradiol
Spray, topical solution: 1.53 mg/spray
Tablets (micronized): 0.5 mg, 1 mg, 2 mg
Transdermal: 0.014 mg/24 hours,
0.025 mg/24 hours, 0.0375 mg/24 hours,
0.05 mg/24 hours, 0.06 mg/24 hours,
0.075 mg/24 hours, 0.1 mg/24 hours
Vaginal cream (in nonliquefying base):
0.1 mg/g
Vaginal ring (extended-release): 2 mg
(0.0075 mg/24 hours
estradiol acetate
Vaginal ring: 0.05 mg/24 hours; 0.1 mg/
24 hours
estradiol cypionate
Injection (in oil): 5 mg/mL
estradiol gel
Transdermal gel: 0.06% (1.25 g/metered
dose), 0.06% (0.87 g/activation), 0.1% (in
0.25-, 0.5-, and 1-g single-dose packets)
estradiol hemihydrate
Vaginal tablets: 10 mcg

estradiol valerate
Injection (in oil): 10 mg/mL, 20 mg/mL,
40 mg/mL

INDICATIONS & DOSAGES
➤ **Vasomotor menopausal symptoms,
female hypogonadism, female castration,
primary ovarian failure**
Women: 1 to 2 mg P.O. estradiol daily. Or,
for vasomotor symptoms, 1 to 5 mg cypionate I.M. once every 3 to 4 weeks; for
female hypogonadism, 1.5 to 2 mg cypionate I.M. once every month.
Transdermal patch
Women: Apply patch according to manufacturer's instructions. Alora, Estraderm,
Vivelle, and Vivelle-Dot are applied twice
weekly. Climara and Menostar are applied
once a week. Apply to clean, dry area of the
trunk. Adjust dose, if necessary, after the
first 2 or 3 weeks of therapy; then every 3 to
6 months as needed. Rotate application sites
weekly with an interval of at least 1 week
between particular sites used. Adjust dosage
as needed.
➤ **Postmenopausal urogenital symptoms**
Women: One ring inserted into the upper
third of the vagina. Ring is kept in place for
3 months.
➤ **Vulvar and vaginal atrophy**
Women: 0.05 mg/24 hours Estraderm applied twice weekly in a cyclic regimen. Or,
0.05 mg/24 hours Climara applied weekly
in a cyclic regimen. Or, 2 to 4 g vaginal applications of cream daily for 1 to 2 weeks.
When vaginal mucosa is restored, maintenance dose is 1 g one to three times weekly
in a cyclic regimen. If using Vagifem for
atrophic vaginitis, give 1 tablet vaginally
once daily for 2 weeks. Maintenance dose is
1 tablet inserted vaginally twice weekly. Or,
10 to 20 mg valerate I.M. every 4 weeks as
needed. Or, 1 to 5 mg cypionate I.M. once
every 3 to 4 weeks. Or, 0.05 to 0.1 mg daily
by vaginal ring. Replace vaginal ring every
3 months. Or, 1.25 g EstroGel applied once
daily to skin.
➤ **Palliative treatment of advanced,
inoperable breast cancer**
Men and postmenopausal women: 10 mg
P.O. estradiol t.i.d. for 3 months.
➤ **Palliative treatment of advanced,
inoperable prostate cancer**

Men: 30 mg valerate I.M. every 1 to 2 weeks, or 1 to 2 mg estradiol P.O. t.i.d.

➤ **To prevent postmenopausal osteoporosis**

Women: Place a 6.5-cm² (0.025 mg/24 hours) Climara patch once weekly on clean, dry skin of lower abdomen or upper quadrant of buttock. Or, place a 3.25-cm² (0.014 mg/24 hours) Menostar patch once weekly to clean, dry area of the lower abdomen. Or, place a 0.5 mg/24 hours Estraderm patch twice weekly in a cyclic regimen in women with an intact uterus. In women with a hysterectomy, apply one Estraderm patch twice weekly in a continuous regimen. For each system, press firmly in place for about 10 seconds; ensure complete contact, especially around edges. Or, 0.025-mg/24 hours Vivelle, Vivelle-Dot, or Alora system applied to a clean, dry area of the trunk twice weekly. Or, 0.5 mg P.O. daily for 23 days, followed by 5 days without drug.

➤ **Moderate to severe vasomotor symptoms from menopause**

Women: Divigel 0.1% at dose of 0.25, 0.5, or 1 g/day. Start with Divigel 0.25 g daily and adjust dose based on individual patient response. Or, 1 pump per day of Elestrin applied to the upper arm. Or, Evamist 1 spray per day initially; may adjust dose based on clinical response. Or, 0.05 to 0.1 mg daily by vaginal ring. Replace vaginal ring every 3 months. Or, 1.25 g EstroGel applied once daily to skin.

ADMINISTRATION

P.O.

● Give without regard for food. If stomach upset occurs, give with food.
● Don't give drug with grapefruit juice.
● Store at controlled room temperature.

I.M.

● To give I.M. injection, make sure drug is well dispersed by rolling vial between palms. Inject deep into large muscle. Rotate injection sites to prevent muscle atrophy. Never give drug I.V.

Transdermal

● Apply Elestrin once daily to the upper arm.
● Apply EstroGel over the entire area of one arm on the inside and outside from wrist to shoulder. Don't massage or rub EstroGel.

Patient should allow gel to dry for 5 minutes before getting dressed.

● Apply Evamist each morning to adjacent, nonoverlapping areas on the inner surface of the forearm, starting near the elbow. Allow to dry for 2 minutes and do not wash the site for 30 minutes.

● Apply Divigel once daily on skin of either right or left upper thigh. Application surface area should be about 5 by 7 inches (about 12.5 by 18 cm; about the size of two palm prints). Apply entire contents of a unit-dose packet each day. To avoid potential skin irritation, apply Divigel to right or left upper thigh on alternating days. Don't apply Divigel on face, breasts, or irritated skin, or in or around the vagina. After application, allow gel to dry before dressing. Don't wash application site within 1 hour after applying Divigel. Avoid contact of gel with eyes. Wash hands after application.

● Apply transdermal patch to clean, dry, hairless, intact skin on abdomen or buttock. Don't apply to breasts, waistline, or other areas where clothing can loosen patch. When applying, ensure thorough contact between patch and skin, especially around edges, and hold in place for about 10 seconds. Apply patch immediately after opening and removing protective cover. Rotate application sites.

Vaginal

● Using the applicator, insert Vagifem as far into vagina as it can comfortably go, without using force.
● Remove vaginal ring from its pouch. Squeeze sides together and insert ring into vagina where comfortable.

ACTION

Increases synthesis of DNA, RNA, and protein in responsive tissues; reduces release of FSH and luteinizing hormone from the pituitary gland.

Route	Onset	Peak	Duration
P.O., I.M., vaginal	Unknown	Unknown	Unknown
Transdermal gel (EstroGel)	Immediate	1 hr	24–36 hr

Half-life: Alora transdermal patch, 1.75 ± 2.87 hours; Vivelle transdermal patch, 4.4 ± 2.3 hours; Vivelle-Dot transdermal patch, 5.9 to 7.7 hours; other forms, unknown.

Reactions in bold italics are *life-threatening*. Interactions may have a *rapid onset* or a **delayed onset**.

ADVERSE REACTIONS

CNS: *stroke,* headache, dizziness, chorea, depression, *seizures,* insomnia (Vagifem).
CV: thrombophlebitis, *thromboembolism,* hypertension, edema, *PE, MI.*
EENT: worsening myopia or astigmatism, intolerance of contact lenses, sinusitis (Vagifem).
GI: nausea, vomiting, abdominal cramps, bloating, increased appetite, *pancreatitis,* anorexia, gallbladder disease, dyspepsia (Vagifem).
GU: breakthrough bleeding, altered menstrual flow, dysmenorrhea, amenorrhea, *increased risk of endometrial cancer,* cervical erosion, abnormal Pap smear, altered cervical secretions, enlargement of uterine fibromas, vaginal candidiasis in women, testicular atrophy, erectile dysfunction, genital pruritus, hematuria, vaginal discomfort, vaginitis (Vagifem).
Hepatic: cholestatic jaundice, *hepatic adenoma.*
Metabolic: weight changes, hypothyroidism, hypercalcemia (in patients with breast cancer and bone metastases).
Respiratory: URI, allergy, bronchitis (Vagifem).
Skin: melasma, urticaria, erythema nodosum, dermatitis, hair loss, pruritus.
Other: gynecomastia; *increased risk of breast cancer;* hot flashes; pain (Vagifem); breast tenderness, enlargement, or secretion; flulike syndrome.

INTERACTIONS

Drug-drug. *Anastrozole:* May interfere with anastrozole effectiveness. Avoid use together.
Carbamazepine, fosphenytoin, phenobarbital, phenytoin, rifampin: May decrease effectiveness of estrogen therapy. Monitor patient closely.
Clarithromycin, erythromycin, itraconazole, ketoconazole, ritonavir: May increase estrogen plasma levels and side effects. Monitor patient.
Corticosteroids: May enhance effects of corticosteroids. Monitor patient closely.
Cyclosporine: May increase risk of toxicity. Use together with caution, and monitor cyclosporine level frequently.

Dantrolene, other hepatotoxic drugs: May increase risk of hepatotoxicity. Monitor liver function closely.
Oral anticoagulants: May decrease anticoagulant effect. Dosage adjustments may be needed. Monitor PT and INR.
Tamoxifen: May interfere with tamoxifen effectiveness. Avoid using together.
Thyroid hormones: May change thyroid hormone concentrations. May increase thyroid hormone requirements.
Drug-herb. *Black cohosh:* May increase drug's adverse effects. Discourage use together.
Saw palmetto: May negate drug's effects. Discourage use together.
St. John's wort: May decrease effects of drug. Discourage use together.
Drug-food. *Caffeine:* May increase caffeine level. Advise patient to avoid or minimize use of caffeine.
Grapefruit juice: May elevate drug level. Tell patient to take drug with liquid other than grapefruit juice.
Drug-lifestyle. *Smoking:* May increase risk of adverse CV effects. If smoking continues, may need another therapy.

EFFECTS ON LAB TEST RESULTS

● May increase clotting factor VII, VIII, IX, and X; total T_4; thyroid-binding globulin; and triglyceride levels; may increase LFT results.
● May increase norepinephrine-induced platelet aggregation and prolong PT.
● May decrease metyrapone test results.

CONTRAINDICATIONS & CAUTIONS

● Contraindicated in patients with thrombophlebitis or thromboembolic disorders, estrogen-dependent neoplasia, breast or reproductive organ cancer (except for palliative treatment), undiagnosed abnormal genital bleeding, or history of thrombophlebitis or thromboembolic disorders linked to previous estrogen use (except for palliative treatment of breast and prostate cancer).
● Contraindicated in patients with liver dysfunction or disease.
● Contraindicated in patients with known anaphylactic reaction or angioedema caused by drug. Exogenous estrogens may

exacerbate signs and symptoms of angioedema in women with hereditary angioedema.

• Use cautiously in patients with cerebrovascular disease or CAD, asthma, bone disease, migraine, seizures, or cardiac or renal dysfunction.

• Use cautiously in women who have a strong family history (grandmother, mother, sister) of breast cancer, breast nodules, fibrocystic breasts, or abnormal mammogram findings.

⚠ Alert: Postmenopausal women ages 50 to 79 who are taking estrogen and progestin have an increased risk of MI, stroke, invasive breast cancer, PE, and thrombosis. Postmenopausal women age 65 or older also have an increased risk of dementia.

Dialyzable drug: Unknown.

⚠ Overdose S&S: Nausea, vomiting, withdrawal uterine bleeding.

PREGNANCY-LACTATION-REPRODUCTION

• Drug is contraindicated in pregnancy.

• Use of estrogen and progestin as in combination hormonal contraceptives hasn't been associated with teratogenic effects when inadvertently taken early in pregnancy.

• Estrogens have been shown to decrease the quantity and quality of breast milk. Use only if clearly needed; monitor infant's growth closely.

NURSING CONSIDERATIONS

• Ensure that patient has physical examination before starting therapy. Patients receiving long-term therapy should have yearly examinations. Monitor lipid levels, BP, body weight, and hepatic function.

• Ask patient about allergies, especially to foods and plants. Estradiol is available as an aqueous solution or as a solution in peanut oil; estradiol cypionate, as a solution in cottonseed oil; estradiol valerate, as a solution in castor oil or sesame oil.

Black Box Warning Estrogen increases the risk of endometrial cancer. Use adequate diagnostic measures, including endometrial sampling when indicated, to rule out malignancy in all cases of undiagnosed persistent or recurring abnormal vaginal bleeding. ∎

Black Box Warning Don't use estrogens with or without progestins to prevent CV

disease or dementia. Use the lowest effective doses and for the shortest duration consistent with treatment goals. ∎

• When estrogen is prescribed for a postmenopausal woman with a uterus, also initiate a progestin to reduce the risk of endometrial cancer.

⚠ Alert: EstroGel contains alcohol. Avoid fire, flame, or smoking until area dries in 2 to 5 minutes.

• In women also taking oral estrogen, treatment with the Estraderm transdermal patch can begin 1 week after withdrawal of oral therapy, or sooner if menopausal symptoms appear before the end of the week.

• Transdermal systems may be used continually rather than cyclically. Other alternative regimens are 1 to 5 mg cypionate I.M. every 3 to 4 weeks and 10 to 20 mg valerate I.M. every 4 weeks, as needed.

• Instruct patients using Vagifem who have severely atrophic vaginal mucosa to be careful when inserting the applicator. After gynecologic surgery, tell patient to use any vaginal applicator cautiously and only if clearly indicated.

• The prescriber should assess patient's need to continue estradiol therapy. Make attempts to stop or taper at 3- to 6-month intervals.

• Because of risk of thromboembolism, stop therapy at least 1 month before high-risk procedures or those that cause prolonged immobilization, such as knee or hip surgery.

• Glucose tolerance may be impaired. Monitor glucose level closely in patients with diabetes.

• Notify pathologist about estrogen therapy when sending specimens to laboratory for evaluation.

PATIENT TEACHING

• Tell patient to read package insert describing estrogen's adverse effects and give her a verbal explanation of those effects.

Black Box Warning Advise patient not to allow contact between children and Evamist application site. Accidental exposure may cause breast budding and breast masses in prepubertal females and gynecomastia and breast masses in prepubertal males. Ensure children don't come in contact with application site. ∎

• Emphasize importance of regular physical examinations. Postmenopausal women who use estrogen replacement for longer than 5 years may be at increased risk for endometrial cancer. Risk is reduced by using cyclic rather than continuous therapy and the lowest possible dosages of estrogen. Adding progestins to the regimen decreases risk of endometrial hyperplasia; however, it isn't known whether progestins affect risk of endometrial cancer. No increased risk of breast cancer has been reported.

• Teach woman how to use cream. She should wash vaginal area with soap and water before applying and should insert cream high into the vagina (about two-thirds the length of the applicator). She should take drug at bedtime, or lie flat for 30 minutes after instillation to minimize drug loss.

• Tell patient using topical emulsion not to apply it with sunscreen.

• Tell patient to use transdermal system correctly, to rotate sites, to avoid breasts and waistline, and to reapply patch if it falls off.

• Teach patient using transdermal gel (EstroGel) to apply in a thin layer on one arm and allow to dry before smoking, getting near flames, dressing, or touching the arm. Recommend bathing before application to maintain full dosage.

• Tell patient that estradiol gel should never be applied directly to the breast.

• Tell patient to insert Vagifem by the applicator as far into vagina as it can comfortably go, without using force.

🛈 **Alert:** Warn patient to immediately report abdominal pain, pressure or pain in chest, shortness of breath, severe headaches, visual disturbances, vaginal bleeding or discharge, breast lumps, swelling of hands or feet, yellow skin or sclera, dark urine, light-colored stools, and pain, numbness, or stiffness in legs or buttocks.

• Explain to patient receiving cyclic therapy for postmenopausal symptoms that withdrawal bleeding may occur during week off drug. Tell her to report unusual vaginal bleeding.

• Tell diabetic patient to report elevated glucose level so that antidiabetic dosage can be adjusted.

• Teach woman how to perform routine breast self-examination.

• Teach patient methods to decrease risk of blood clots.

• Advise woman not to become pregnant during estrogen therapy.

• Encourage patient to stop or reduce smoking because of the risk of CV complications.

• Advise patient not to allow pets to lick or touch Evamist application site. If signs of illness occur, patient should contact pet's veterinarian.

estradiol–norethindrone acetate transdermal system
ess-tra-DYE-ole/nor-ETH-in-drone

CombiPatch

Therapeutic class: Estrogens
Pharmacologic class: Estrogen–progestin combinations

AVAILABLE FORMS
Transdermal: 9-cm^2 system releasing 0.05 mg estradiol and 0.14 mg norethindrone acetate daily; 16-cm^2 system releasing 0.05 mg estradiol and 0.25 mg norethindrone acetate daily

INDICATIONS & DOSAGES
➤ **Moderate to severe vasomotor symptoms from menopause; vulval and vaginal atrophy; hypoestrogenemia from hypogonadism, castration, or primary ovarian failure in woman with intact uterus**
Continuous combined regimen
Women: Wear 9-cm^2 patch system continuously on lower abdomen. Replace system twice weekly during 28-day cycle. May increase to 16-cm^2 patch.
Continuous sequential regimen
Women: For use in sequential regimen with an estradiol transdermal system (such as Alora, Estraderm, Vivelle), wear 0.05-mg estradiol transdermal patch for first 14 days of 28-day cycle; replace system twice weekly. Wear 9-cm^2 patch system on lower abdomen for rest of 28-day cycle; replace system twice weekly. May increase to 16-cm^2 patch.

ADMINISTRATION
Transdermal
- Apply patch system to a smooth (fold-free), clean, dry, nonirritated area of skin on lower abdomen, avoiding the waistline. Rotate application sites, with an interval of at least 1 week between applications to same site.
- Don't apply patch on or near breasts.
- Avoid applying to areas that may get prolonged sun exposure.
- Reapply patch, if needed, to another area of lower abdomen. If patch fails to adhere, replace with a new one.

ACTION
A matrix transdermal system in which estradiol and norethindrone are released continuously. Estrogen replacement therapy can reduce menopausal symptoms and release of FSH and luteinizing hormone in postmenopausal women.

Route	Onset	Peak	Duration
Transdermal	12–24 hr	Unknown	3–4 days

Half-life: Estradiol, 2 to 23 hours; norethindrone, 6 to 8 hours.

ADVERSE REACTIONS
CNS: asthenia, *stroke,* depression, insomnia, nervousness, dizziness, headache, pain.
CV: *thromboembolism,* thrombophlebitis, hypertension, edema, *PE, MI.*
EENT: pharyngitis, rhinitis, sinusitis, retinal vascular thrombosis, intolerance to contact lenses.
GI: abdominal pain, diarrhea, dyspepsia, changes in appetite, flatulence, nausea, constipation, gallbladder disease.
GU: dysmenorrhea, leukorrhea, menstrual disorder, suspicious Papanicolaou smears, vaginitis, menorrhagia, *vaginal hemorrhage.*
Hepatic: cholestatic jaundice.
Metabolic: weight changes, hypercalcemia, hypertriglyceridemia.
Musculoskeletal: arthralgia, back pain.
Respiratory: respiratory disorder, bronchitis.
Skin: application-site reactions, acne, melasma, chloasma.
Other: accidental injury, flulike syndrome, breast pain, tooth disorder, peripheral edema, breast enlargement, infection, changes in libido.

INTERACTIONS
Drug-drug. *Anastrozole:* May interfere with anastrozole effectiveness. Avoid using together.
Carbamazepine, fosphenytoin, phenobarbital, phenytoin, rifampin: May decrease estrogen therapy effectiveness. Monitor patient closely.
Clarithromycin, erythromycin, itraconazole, ketoconazole, ritonavir: May increase estrogen plasma levels and side effects. Monitor patient.
Corticosteroids: May enhance effects of corticosteroids. Monitor patient closely.
Cyclosporine: May increase risk of toxicity. Use together with caution; monitor cyclosporine level frequently.
Dantrolene, hepatotoxic drugs: May increase risk of hepatotoxicity. Monitor liver function closely.
Oral anticoagulants: May decrease effect of anticoagulant. May need to adjust dose. Monitor PT and INR.
Tamoxifen: May interfere with tamoxifen effectiveness. Avoid using together.
Drug-herb. *Black cohosh:* May increase adverse effects of drug. Discourage use together.
Saw palmetto: May cause antiestrogenic effects. Discourage use together.
St. John's wort: May decrease effects of drug. Discourage use together.
Drug-food. *Caffeine:* May increase caffeine level. Advise patient to avoid or minimize use of caffeine.
Grapefruit juice: May elevate estrogen level. Advise patient to take with liquid other than grapefruit juice.
Drug-lifestyle. *Smoking:* May increase risk of adverse CV effects. If smoking continues, may need alternative therapy.

EFFECTS ON LAB TEST RESULTS
- May increase T_3 and T_4, HDL, and triglyceride levels. May decrease LDL levels.
- May increase fibrinogen activity and platelet count. May decrease T_3 resin uptake. May alter aPTT, INR, and platelet aggregation times.

• May reduce metyrapone test values. May alter glucose tolerance test results.

CONTRAINDICATIONS & CAUTIONS
• Contraindicated in women hypersensitive to estrogen, progestin, or any component of the patch and in patients with known or suspected breast cancer, known or suspected estrogen-dependent neoplasia, known anaphylactic reaction or angioedema, known hepatic impairment or disease, thrombophilic disorders, known or suspected pregnancy, undiagnosed abnormal genital bleeding, active thrombophlebitis, thromboembolic disorders, or stroke.
• Exogenous estrogens may exacerbate signs and symptoms of angioedema in women with hereditary angioedema.
• Use cautiously in patients with impaired liver function, asthma, epilepsy, migraine, or cardiac or renal dysfunction.
Dialyzable drug: Unknown.
⚠ *Overdose S&S:* Nausea, withdrawal bleeding.

PREGNANCY-LACTATION-REPRODUCTION
• Don't give to pregnant women.
• Estrogen has been shown to decrease the quantity and quality of breast milk. Use cautiously in breast-feeding women.

NURSING CONSIDERATIONS
Black Box Warning Don't use estrogens, with or without progestins, to prevent CV disease or dementia. Use drug with or without progestins at the lowest effective doses and for the shortest duration consistent with treatment goals. ∎
Black Box Warning Postmenopausal women treated for 5 years have an increased risk of MI, stroke, invasive breast cancer, PE, and DVT. ∎
• Women not receiving continuous estrogen or combined estrogen–progestin therapy may start therapy at any time.
• Women receiving continuous hormone replacement therapy should complete the current cycle before starting therapy. Women commonly have withdrawal bleeding at completion of cycle; first day of withdrawal bleeding is an appropriate time to start therapy.

• Store patches in refrigerator before dispensing. Patient may then store patches at room temperature for up to 6 months, or the expiration date, whichever comes first.
• Reevaluate therapy at 3- to 6-month intervals.
• A combined estrogen–progestin regimen is indicated for a woman with an intact uterus. Progestins taken with estrogen significantly reduce, but don't eliminate, risk of endometrial cancer linked to use of estrogen alone.
• Because of risk of thromboembolism, stop therapy at least 4 to 6 weeks before surgery associated with an increased risk of thromboembolism, or during periods of prolonged immobilization.
• BP increases have been linked to estrogen use. Monitor patient's BP regularly.
• Treatment of postmenopausal symptoms usually starts during menopausal stage when vasomotor symptoms occur.
• Monitor glucose level closely in patients with diabetes.
⚠ *Alert:* Don't interchange CombiPatch with other estrogen patches. Verify therapy before application.

PATIENT TEACHING
• Teach woman how to apply patch properly. She should wear only one patch at any time during therapy. Tell her to apply patch immediately after opening protective cover.
• Tell patient that an oil-based cream or lotion may help remove adhesive from the skin after patch has been removed and the area allowed to dry for 15 minutes.
• Advise woman not to use patch if she's pregnant or plans to become pregnant.
• Urge woman of childbearing potential to consult prescriber before applying patch and to advise prescriber immediately if she becomes pregnant.
• Instruct patient that the continuous combined regimen may lead to irregular bleeding, particularly in the first 6 months, but that it usually decreases with time and often stops completely.
• Tell patient that, for the continuous sequential regimen, monthly withdrawal bleeding is common.
• Advise patient to alert prescriber and remove patch at first sign of clotting

disorders (thrombophlebitis, cerebrovascular disorders, and PE).
• Instruct patient to stop using patch and call prescriber about any loss of vision, sudden onset of protrusion of the eyeball (proptosis), double vision, or migraine.
• Encourage patient to stop or reduce smoking because of the risk of CV complications.
• Tell patient to perform monthly breast self-examinations and to have annual gynecologic and breast examinations by a health care provider.
• Advise patient not to store patches where extreme temperatures can occur.
• Tell patient undergoing an MRI to alert facility that she's using a transdermal patch.

estradiol valerate–estradiol valerate with dienogest
ess-tra-DYE-ole VAL-er-ate/
dye-EN-oh-jest

Natazia

Therapeutic class: Estrogens
Pharmacologic class: Estrogen–progestin combinations

AVAILABLE FORMS
Tablets: 28-day blister pack containing two 3-mg estradiol valerate, five 2-mg estradiol valerate with 2-mg dienogest, seventeen 2-mg estradiol valerate with 3-mg dienogest, two 1-mg estradiol valerate, and two inert tablets

INDICATIONS & DOSAGES
➤ Contraception; treatment of heavy menstrual bleeding in women without organic pathology who choose to use an oral contraceptive as their method of contraception
Women: 1 tablet P.O. daily beginning on first day of menstrual cycle as directed on blister pack at same time each day. When changing from another combination hormonal contraceptive, begin on first day of withdrawal bleeding. When changing from combination hormonal vaginal ring or transdermal patch, begin on day vaginal ring or transdermal patch is removed. When changing from progestin-only contraceptive, begin

next day. When changing from implant contraceptive or intrauterine system, begin day of implant or intrauterine system removal. When changing from injection contraceptive, begin day next injection is due.

ADMINISTRATION
P.O.
• Give at same time each day; don't delay by more than 12 hours.
• Tablets must be given in order indicated on blister pack.

ACTION
Prevents pregnancy by suppressing ovulation. May also cause changes in endometrium and cervical mucus, inhibiting sperm penetration and reducing likelihood of implantation.

Route	Onset	Peak	Duration
P.O.	Unknown	3 hr (estradiol); 1½ hr (dienogest)	Unknown

Half-life: Estradiol, 14 hours; dienogest, 11 hours.

ADVERSE REACTIONS
CNS: depression, headache.
CV: *MI, DVT,* hypertension.
GI: nausea, vomiting.
GU: amenorrhea, irregular uterine bleeding, metrorrhagia, oligomenorrhea, *uterine leiomyoma, ruptured ovarian cyst.*
Metabolic: weight gain, hyperglycemia.
Skin: acne.
Other: breast pain, tenderness, or discomfort.

INTERACTIONS
Drug-drug. *Antibiotics:* May reduce contraceptive effectiveness. Advise use of backup contraception during therapy.
HIV protease inhibitors: May either increase or decrease estrogen and progesterone levels. Use together cautiously and monitor patient for effectiveness of hormone treatment.
Lamotrigine: May decrease lamotrigine serum level, reducing seizure control. Adjust lamotrigine dosage as necessary.
Strong CYP3A4 inducers (such as barbiturates, carbamazepine, felbamate, griseofulvin, oxcarbazepine, phenytoin, rifampin, topiramate): May reduce contraceptive

---

Reactions in bold italics are *life-threatening*. Interactions may have a *rapid onset* or a *delayed onset*.

effectiveness or increase breakthrough bleeding. An alternative method of birth control should be used.

Strong and moderate inhibitors of CYP3A4 (such as cimetidine, erythromycin, ketoconazole, SSRIs, verapamil): May increase levels of hormones. Avoid use together. If drugs must be used together, monitor patient for adverse effects.

Thyroid hormone: May increase serum concentration of thyroid-binding globulin, leading to decreased effectiveness of thyroid replacement therapy. Monitor patient; thyroid hormone dosage may need adjustment.

Drug-herb. *St John's wort:* May reduce contraceptive effectiveness or increase breakthrough bleeding. Recommend alternative method of birth control.

Drug-food. *Grapefruit juice:* May increase levels of hormones. Avoid use together.

Drug-lifestyle. `Black Box Warning` *Smoking:* Increases risk of medical problems, such as stroke, emboli, or heart disease. Recommend smoking cessation. ∎

EFFECTS ON LAB TEST RESULTS

● May increase thyroid-binding globulin, glucose, cholesterol, and lipid levels.
● May increase levels of coagulation factors.

CONTRAINDICATIONS & CAUTIONS

● Contraindicated in patients with benign or malignant liver tumors; liver disease; breast cancer or history of breast cancer; undiagnosed abnormal genital bleeding; headaches with focal neurologic symptoms or migraine headaches with or without aura if older than age 35; diabetes with vascular disease; uncontrolled hypertension; hypertension with vascular disease; inherited or acquired hypercoagulopathies; thrombogenic valvular or thrombogenic rhythm disease of heart, such as endocarditis or atrial fibrillation; CAD; cerebrovascular disease; DVT; or current or past PE.

`Black Box Warning` Contraindicated in women who smoke and who are older than age 35. ∎

● Use cautiously in women with CV disease risk factors, history of cholestasis, history of well-controlled hypertension, prediabetes or well-controlled diabetes, history of hyperlipidemia, new-onset headaches, history of bleeding irregularities, history of emotional disorders, angioedema, or chloasma.

● Exogenous estrogens may exacerbate signs and symptoms of angioedema in women with hereditary angioedema.
● Safety and effectiveness in women with BMI greater than 30 kg/m^2 haven't been evaluated.
● Drug hasn't been studied in postmenopausal women and isn't indicated in this population.

Dialyzable drug: Unknown.

⚠ *Overdose S&S:* Nausea, withdrawal bleeding.

PREGNANCY-LACTATION-REPRODUCTION

● Don't give to pregnant women.
● There is little or no increased risk of birth defects in women who inadvertently use combined oral contraceptives during early pregnancy.
● Estrogen has been shown to decrease the quantity and quality of breast milk. Drug shouldn't be used in breast-feeding women.
● Use before menarche isn't indicated.

NURSING CONSIDERATIONS

● Start drug no earlier than 4 weeks after delivery in women who aren't breast-feeding. Risk of postpartum venous thrombotic event (VTE) decreases and ovulation risk increases after third postpartum week.
● Monitor BP; elevations are possible in nonhypertensive women.
● Monitor coagulation factors as appropriate.
● Monitor glucose and cholesterol levels regularly, especially in women who are prediabetic and in those with history of elevated lipid levels.
● Monitor women for headache. New-onset headaches may require discontinuing oral contraceptives.
● Carefully monitor women with history of depression for recurrence or exacerbation.
● Stop drug if arterial or deep VTE occurs. Highest risk of VTE is during first year of contraceptive use. If feasible, stop tablets at least 4 weeks before and for 2 weeks after major surgery.
● Oral contraceptives are associated with increased risk of thrombotic and hemorrhagic

strokes, especially in women older than age 35, in those with hypertension, and in smokers. Stop drug if unexplained vision loss, proptosis, diplopia, papilledema, or retinal vascular changes occur. Evaluate retinal vein thrombosis immediately.

• Risk of drug causing breast cancer or cervical or endometrial cancer is controversial and uncertain. As a precaution, women should have regular Papanicolaou tests, breast examinations, and mammograms.

• Discontinue drug if jaundice develops. Women who take oral contraceptives are at slightly higher risk for developing liver tumors and gallstones. Monitor patient for skin color changes and pain in right upper quadrant.

• Ensure that patient uses a nonhormonal contraceptive method, such as a condom or spermicide, for the first 9 days.

PATIENT TEACHING

• Teach patient to take tablet once daily and not to skip doses or delay taking tablet by more than 12 hours. Advise patient that tablets should be taken in the order marked on each pack.

• Instruct patient to read package insert for information on missed tablets or to contact her pharmacist or prescriber; tell her that backup contraception must be used.

• Tell patient starting drug for first time to begin taking tablets on day 1 of her period and to use backup contraceptive method for first 9 days.

• Instruct patient that spotting or light bleeding is normal at first.

• Advise patient that she may feel nauseous, especially during first few months, but that this symptom usually disappears and she shouldn't stop taking tablets. Tell patient to report to prescriber if nausea doesn't resolve.

• Warn patient to start drug no earlier than 4 weeks after giving birth.

• Advise patient to notify prescriber if she is pregnant before taking drug.

• Tell patient that breast-feeding while taking tablets isn't recommended because milk production may be reduced and small amounts of drug appear in breast milk.

• Inform patient taking tablets that blood tests may be needed to check blood glucose and cholesterol levels, as well as how her blood is clotting, and that her BP may also be checked.

• Tell patient to inform prescriber of all prescription, over-the-counter, and herbal supplements she is taking.

• Advise patient, if appropriate, to quit smoking before taking drug.

Black Box Warning Advise patient who smokes that she is at increased risk for serious CV events from combination oral contraceptive use. Risk increases with age, especially after age 35, and with number of cigarettes smoked. ■

• Warn patient that contraceptive use doesn't protect against HIV infection or other sexually transmitted diseases.

• Tell patient that a missed period may occur but that pregnancy should be ruled out if she misses two or more consecutive menstrual cycles.

• Warn patient to call prescriber immediately if she experiences persistent leg pain; sudden shortness of breath; sudden blindness (partial or complete); severe chest pain; sudden, severe headache; weakness or numbness in an arm or leg; trouble speaking; or yellowing of skin or eyes.

• Advise patient with tendency to chloasma to avoid sun exposure and ultraviolet radiation.

• Advise patient to stop smoking while taking oral contraceptive because of increased risk of stroke and other thromboembolic events.

---

estrogens (conjugated) (estrogenic substances, conjugated; oestrogens, conjugated)
ESS-troe-jenz

Cenestin, C.E.S.✤, Enjuvia, Premarin✒

Therapeutic class: Estrogens
Pharmacologic class: Estrogens

AVAILABLE FORMS
Injection: 25 mg/5 mL
Tablets: 0.3 mg, 0.45 mg, 0.625 mg, 0.9 mg, 1.25 mg
Vaginal cream: 0.625 mg/g

INDICATIONS & DOSAGES

➤ **Abnormal uterine bleeding (hormonal imbalance)**
Adults: 25 mg I.V. (preferred) or I.M. Repeat dose in 6 to 12 hours, if necessary.

➤ **Vulvar or vaginal atrophy; kraurosis vulvae**
Adults: 0.5 to 2 g cream intravaginally once daily in cycles of 21 days on, 7 days off.

➤ **Moderate to severe dyspareunia due to menopause-related vulvar and vaginal atrophy**
Adults: 0.5 g cream intravaginally twice weekly as a continuous regimen. Or, 0.5 g intravaginally once daily for 21 days followed by 7 days off.

➤ **Castration and primary ovarian failure**
Adults: Initially, 1.25 mg Premarin P.O. daily in cycles of 3 weeks on, 1 week off. Adjust dose as needed.

➤ **Female hypogonadism**
Adults: 0.3 to 0.625 mg Premarin P.O. daily, given cyclically 3 weeks on, 1 week off. Adjust dose depending on symptom severity and responsiveness of the endometrium.

➤ **Moderate to severe vasomotor symptoms with or without moderate to severe symptoms of vulvar and vaginal atrophy associated with menopause**
Adults: Initially, 0.3 mg Premarin or Enjuvia P.O. daily. Premarin may also be given cyclically 25 days on, 5 days off. Adjust dosage based on patient response.

➤ **Moderate to severe vasomotor symptoms from menopause**
Adults: 0.45 mg Cenestin P.O. daily. Adjust dose based on patient response.

➤ **Moderate to severe symptoms of vulvar and vaginal atrophy from menopause**
Adults: 0.3 mg Cenestin P.O. daily.

➤ **To prevent osteoporosis**
Adults: 0.3 mg Premarin P.O. daily, or cyclically 25 days on, 5 days off. Adjust dose based on response of bone mineral density testing.

➤ **Palliative treatment of inoperable prostatic cancer**
Adults: 1.25 to 2.5 mg Premarin P.O. t.i.d.

➤ **Palliative treatment of breast cancer**
Adults: 10 mg Premarin P.O. t.i.d. for at least 3 months.

ADMINISTRATION

P.O.
● Give drug at same time each day.

I.V.
▼ I.V. use is preferred because a more rapid response can be expected.
▼ Refrigerate before reconstituting.
▼ Reconstitute only with diluent provided. Agitate gently after adding diluent.
▼ Drug is compatible with NSS and dextrose or invert sugar solutions.
▼ Use reconstituted solution within a few hours, if possible. Reconstituted solution is stable under refrigeration for 60 days. Don't use if solution darkens or precipitates.
▼ Give direct injection slowly to avoid flushing reaction.
▼ **Incompatibilities:** Acidic solutions, ascorbic acid, protein hydrolysate.

I.M.
● Reconstitute only with diluent provided. Agitate gently after adding diluent.
● Inject deep into large muscle. Rotate injection sites to prevent muscle atrophy.

Vaginal
● Wash the vaginal area with soap and water, insert about two-thirds the length of the applicator into the vagina, and release drug. Give drug at bedtime or when patient will lie flat for 30 minutes after use to minimize drug loss.

ACTION

Increases synthesis of DNA, RNA, and protein in responsive tissues. Also reduces release of FSH and luteinizing hormone from the pituitary gland.

Route	Onset	Peak	Duration
P.O., I.V., I.M., vaginal	Unknown	Unknown	Unknown

Half-life: Unknown.

ADVERSE REACTIONS

CNS: headache, dizziness, chorea, depression, ***stroke, seizures.***
CV: flushing with rapid I.V. administration; thrombophlebitis, ***thromboembolism,*** hypertension, edema, ***PE, MI.***
EENT: worsening myopia or astigmatism, intolerance of contact lenses.

GI: nausea, vomiting, abdominal cramps, bloating, anorexia, increased appetite, *pancreatitis,* gallbladder disease.

GU: breakthrough bleeding, altered menstrual flow, dysmenorrhea, amenorrhea, *increased risk of endometrial cancer,* cervical erosion, altered cervical secretions, enlargement of uterine fibromas, vaginal candidiasis, testicular atrophy, impotence.

Hepatic: cholestatic jaundice, *hepatic adenoma.*

Metabolic: weight changes, hypercalcemia, hypertriglyceridemia.

Skin: melasma, chloasma, urticaria, hirsutism or hair loss, erythema nodosum, dermatitis.

Other: breast tenderness, enlargement, or secretion; gynecomastia; *increased risk of breast cancer;* changes in libido.

INTERACTIONS

Drug-drug. *Anastrozole:* May interfere with anastrozole effectiveness. Avoid use together.

Carbamazepine, fosphenytoin, phenobarbital, phenytoin, rifampin: May decrease effectiveness of estrogen therapy. Monitor patient closely.

Corticosteroids: May enhance corticosteroid effects. Monitor patient closely.

Cyclosporine: May increase risk of toxicity. Use together with caution, and monitor cyclosporine level frequently.

Dantrolene, other hepatotoxic drugs: May increase risk of hepatotoxicity. Monitor liver function closely.

Itraconazole, ketoconazole, macrolide antibiotics, ritonavir: May increase estrogen plasma levels and risk of adverse effects. Monitor patient.

Oral anticoagulants: May decrease anticoagulant effects. May need to adjust dosage. Monitor PT and INR.

Tamoxifen: May interfere with tamoxifen effectiveness. Avoid using together.

Thyroid hormones: May increase serum thyroxine-binding globulin levels, which may increase thyroid hormone requirements.

Drug-herb. *Black cohosh:* May increase adverse effects of drug. Discourage use together.

Saw palmetto: May have antiestrogenic effects. Discourage use together.

St. John's wort: May decrease effects of drug. Discourage use together.

Drug-food. *Caffeine:* May increase caffeine level. Advise caution.

Grapefruit juice: May increase concentration of estrogen. Avoid using together.

Drug-lifestyle. *Smoking:* May increase risk of adverse CV effects. If smoking continues, recommend nonhormonal contraception.

EFFECTS ON LAB TEST RESULTS

● May increase clotting factor VII, VIII, IX, and X; total T_4; phospholipid; thyroid-binding globulin; and triglyceride levels.

● May increase norepinephrine-induced platelet aggregation and PT.

● May cause a false-positive metyrapone test result.

CONTRAINDICATIONS & CAUTIONS

● Contraindicated in patients with liver dysfunction; thrombophlebitis, thromboembolic disorders; known protein C, protein S, or antithrombin deficiency or other thrombophilic disorders; estrogen-dependent neoplasia; breast or reproductive cancer (except for palliative treatment); undiagnosed abnormal genital bleeding; and known anaphylactic reaction or angioedema to conjugated estrogens.

● Use cautiously in patients with cerebrovascular disease or CAD, asthma, bone disease, migraine, seizures, or cardiac, hepatic, or renal dysfunction.

● Use cautiously in women who have a strong family history (mother, grandmother, sister) of breast or genital tract cancer, breast nodules, fibrocystic breasts, or abnormal mammogram findings.

● Exogenous estrogens may exacerbate signs and symptoms of angioedema in women with hereditary angioedema.

Dialyzable drug: Unknown.

⚠ **Overdose S&S:** Nausea, vomiting, breast tenderness, abdominal pain, drowsiness or fatigue, withdrawal uterine bleeding.

PREGNANCY-LACTATION-REPRODUCTION

● Don't use during pregnancy.

● Drug shouldn't be used during breast-feeding. Estrogen has been shown to

---

Reactions in bold italics are *life-threatening*. Interactions may have a *rapid onset* or a *delayed onset*.

decrease the quantity and quality of breast milk.

NURSING CONSIDERATIONS

● Make sure patient has thorough physical examination before starting therapy; patients receiving long-term therapy should have yearly examinations. Periodically monitor lipid levels, BP, body weight, and hepatic function.

● Rapid treatment of dysfunctional uterine bleeding or reduction of surgical bleeding usually requires delivery by I.V. or I.M. route.

Black Box Warning Don't use to prevent CV disease. In postmenopausal women receiving therapy for more than 5 years, drug may increase risks of MI, stroke, invasive breast cancer, PE, and DVT. Use the lowest effective doses for the shortest time, considering the benefits and risks. ■

Black Box Warning In postmenopausal women receiving therapy for more than 5 years, drug may increase risk of endometrial cancer. Cyclic therapy and the lowest possible dose reduces risk. Adding progestins decreases risk of endometrial hyperplasia, but it's unknown whether they affect risk of endometrial cancer. ■

Black Box Warning In postmenopausal women age 65 or older receiving 4 years of treatment with conjugated estrogens plus medroxyprogesterone acetate, drug may increase the risk of dementia. ■

● When used solely for the treatment of vulval and vaginal atrophy, consider topical products.

● Notify pathologist about estrogen therapy when sending specimens to laboratory for evaluation.

● Because of thromboembolism risk, stop therapy at least 4 to 6 weeks before procedures that prolong immobilization or raise the risk of thromboembolism, such as knee or hip surgery.

● Glucose tolerance may be impaired. Monitor glucose level closely in patients with diabetes.

● Reevaluate need for therapy at 3- to 6-month intervals.

● *Look alike–sound alike:* Don't confuse Premarin with Primaxin, Provera, or Remeron.

PATIENT TEACHING

● Teach patient about adverse effects and advise her to report them promptly.

● Emphasize importance of regular physical examinations.

● Teach woman how to use vaginal cream. Tell patient to wash the vaginal area with soap and water, insert about two-thirds the length of the applicator into the vagina, and release drug. Tell her to use drug at bedtime or to lie flat for 30 minutes after use to minimize drug loss.

● Explain to patient that cyclic therapy for postmenopausal symptoms may cause withdrawal bleeding during week off drug. Tell her to report unusual vaginal bleeding.

● *Alert:* Warn patient to immediately report abdominal pain; pain, numbness, or stiffness in legs or buttocks; pressure or pain in chest; shortness of breath; severe headaches; visual disturbances, such as blind spots, flashing lights, or blurriness; vaginal bleeding or discharge; breast lumps; swelling of hands or feet; yellow skin or sclera; dark urine; and light-colored stools.

● Tell diabetic patient to report elevated glucose level so that antidiabetic dosage can be adjusted.

● Teach woman how to perform routine breast self-examination.

● Advise woman not to become pregnant during estrogen therapy.

● Advise woman of childbearing potential to consult prescriber before taking drug and to advise prescriber immediately if she becomes pregnant.

● Encourage patient to stop smoking or reduce number of cigarettes smoked because of the risk of CV complications.

● Tell patient using drug for osteoporosis prevention to ensure adequate intake of calcium and vitamin D.

● Inform patient that vaginal cream has been reported to weaken latex condoms and to use an alternative method of birth control.

estropipate (piperazine estrone sulfate)
ess-troe-PIH-pate

Ogen .625, Ogen 1.25, Ogen 2.5, Ogen 5

Therapeutic class: Estrogens
Pharmacologic class: Estrogens

AVAILABLE FORMS
Tablets: 0.75 mg, 1.5 mg, 3 mg, 6 mg

INDICATIONS & DOSAGES
➤ **Vulval and vaginal atrophy**
Women: 0.75 to 6 mg P.O. daily, 3 weeks on and 1 week off. If patient is menstruating, start cyclic administration on day 5 of bleeding.
➤ **Primary ovarian failure, female castration, female hypogonadism**
Women: 1.5 to 9 mg P.O. daily for first 3 weeks; then a rest period of 8 to 10 days. If bleeding doesn't occur by end of rest period, cycle is repeated.
➤ **Moderate to severe vasomotor menopausal symptoms**
Women: 0.75 to 6 mg P.O. daily in cyclic method, 3 weeks on and 1 week off. Can be given continuously. If patient is menstruating, start cyclic administration on day 5 of bleeding.
➤ **To prevent osteoporosis**
Women: 0.75 mg P.O. daily for 25 consecutive days of a 31-day cycle, followed by 6 days without drug. Repeat regimen as indicated.

ADMINISTRATION
P.O.
● Give with or without food.
● Drug is hazardous. Use appropriate precautions for handling and disposal.

ACTION
Increases synthesis of DNA, RNA, and proteins in responsive tissues; reduces FSH and luteinizing hormone levels.

Route	Onset	Peak	Duration
P.O.	Unknown	Unknown	Unknown

Half-life: Unknown.

ADVERSE REACTIONS
CNS: depression, headache, dizziness, migraine, *seizures, stroke.*
CV: edema, thrombophlebitis, hypertension, *PE, MI, thromboembolism.*
EENT: steepening of corneal curvature, intolerance to contact lenses.
GI: nausea, vomiting, gallbladder disease, abdominal cramps, bloating.
GU: increased size of uterine fibromas, *endometrial cancer,* vaginal candidiasis, cystitis-like syndrome, dysmenorrhea, amenorrhea, breakthrough bleeding, condition resembling premenstrual syndrome.
Hepatic: cholestatic jaundice, *hepatic adenoma.*
Metabolic: weight changes, hypocalcemia, hypertriglyceridemia.
Skin: hemorrhagic eruption, erythema nodosum, *erythema multiforme,* hirsutism or hair loss, melasma.
Other: breast engorgement or enlargement, *breast cancer,* breast tenderness, changes in libido, leg cramps.

INTERACTIONS
Drug-drug. *Anastrozole:* May interfere with anastrozole effectiveness. Avoid use together.
Carbamazepine, fosphenytoin, phenobarbital, phenytoin, rifampin: May decrease estrogen effect. Monitor patient closely.
Clarithromycin, erythromycin, itraconazole, ketoconazole, ritonavir: May increase estrogen plasma levels and side effects. Monitor patient.
Corticosteroids: May enhance corticosteroid effect. Monitor patient closely.
Cyclosporine: May increase risk of toxicity. Use together with caution; frequently monitor cyclosporine level.
Dantrolene, other hepatotoxic drugs: May increase risk of hepatotoxicity. Monitor liver function closely.
Oral anticoagulants: May decrease anticoagulant effect. Dosage adjustments may be needed. Monitor PT and INR.
Tamoxifen: May interfere with tamoxifen effect. Avoid using together.
Drug-herb. *Black cohosh:* May increase adverse effects of estrogen. Discourage use together.

Reactions in bold italics are *life-threatening*. Interactions may have a *rapid onset* or a *delayed onset*.

Red clover: May interfere with hormonal therapies. Discourage use together.
St. John's wort: May decrease estrogen effect. Discourage use together.
Drug-food. *Caffeine:* May increase caffeine level. Advise caution.
Grapefruit juice: May increase concentration of drug and risk of adverse effects. Avoid use together.
Drug-lifestyle. *Smoking:* May increase risk of adverse CV effects. If smoking continues, may need alternative therapy.

EFFECTS ON LAB TEST RESULTS
● May increase clotting factor VII, VIII, IX, and X; total T_4; phospholipid; thyroid-binding globulin; and triglyceride levels.
● May increase norepinephrine-induced platelet aggregation and prolong PT.
● May reduce metyrapone test results.

CONTRAINDICATIONS & CAUTIONS
● Contraindicated in patients with known hypersensitivity to drug and in those with liver dysfunction, active thrombophlebitis, arterial thromboembolic disorders, estrogen-dependent neoplasia, undiagnosed genital bleeding, and breast, reproductive organ, or genital cancer.
● Use cautiously in patients with cerebrovascular disease or CAD; asthma; mental depression; bone disease; migraine; seizures; or cardiac, hepatic, or renal dysfunction.
● Use cautiously in women who have a family history (mother, grandmother, sister) of breast or genital tract cancer, breast nodules, fibrocystic breasts, or abnormal mammogram findings.
Dialyzable drug: Unknown.
⚠ Overdose S&S: Nausea, vomiting, withdrawal uterine bleeding.

PREGNANCY-LACTATION-REPRODUCTION
● There is no indication for use during pregnancy. Use is contraindicated.
● Estrogens can be detected in breast milk and have been shown to decrease the quantity and quality of milk. Use cautiously in breast-feeding women.

NURSING CONSIDERATIONS
● Make sure patient has thorough physical examination before starting estrogen therapy. Patients receiving long-term therapy should have examinations yearly. Periodically monitor lipid levels, BP, body weight, and hepatic function.
Black Box Warning Estrogens and progestins shouldn't be used to prevent CV disease. The Women's Health Initiative study reported increased risks of MI, stroke, invasive breast cancer, PE, and DVT in postmenopausal women during 5 years of combination therapy. Because of these risks, estrogens and progestins should be prescribed at the lowest effective doses and for the shortest duration consistent with treatment goals and risks for the individual woman. The Women's Health Initiative study also reported increased risk of the development of dementia in postmenopausal women age 65 and older during 4 years of treatment with oral conjugated estrogens plus medroxyprogesterone. It isn't known if this finding also applies to younger postmenopausal women or to women taking estrogen alone. ■
Black Box Warning Estrogens may increase the risk of endometrial cancer in postmenopausal women. ■
● When used to treat hypogonadism, duration of therapy needed to produce withdrawal bleeding depends on patient's endometrial response to drug. If satisfactory withdrawal bleeding doesn't occur, an oral progestin is added to the regimen. Explain to patient that, despite return of withdrawal bleeding, pregnancy can't occur because she doesn't ovulate.
● Because of risk of thromboembolism, stop therapy at least 4 to 6 weeks before procedures that prolong immobilization or raise the risk of thromboembolism, such as knee or hip surgery.
● Glucose tolerance may be impaired. Monitor glucose level closely in patients with diabetes.

PATIENT TEACHING
● Tell patient to read package insert describing estrogen's adverse effects; also, explain effects verbally.

🍁Canada   ◇OTC   ◆Off-label use   🖉Photoguide   ⓓDo not crush   *Liquid contains alcohol.

• Tell diabetic patient to report elevated glucose level to prescriber.
• Stress importance of regular physical examinations. Postmenopausal women who use estrogen replacement for longer than 5 years may have increased risk of endometrial cancer. Using cyclic therapy and lowest possible estrogen dosage reduces risk. Adding progestins to regimen decreases risk of endometrial hyperplasia; however, it isn't known whether progestins affect risk of endometrial cancer.

🕒 **Alert:** Warn patient to immediately report abdominal pain; pain, stiffness, or numbness in legs or buttocks; pressure or pain in chest; shortness of breath; severe headaches; visual disturbances, such as blind spots or flashing lights; vaginal bleeding or discharge; breast lumps; swelling of hands or feet; yellow skin or sclera; dark urine; and light-colored stools.

• Teach woman how to perform routine breast self-examination.
• Advise woman not to become pregnant while on estrogen therapy.
• Encourage patient to stop or reduce smoking because of the risk of CV complications.
• Advise woman of childbearing potential to consult prescriber before taking drug and to tell prescriber immediately if she becomes pregnant.
• Teach patient at risk for osteoporosis about the importance of adequate calcium and vitamin D intake.

SAFETY ALERT!

eszopiclone
ess-ZOP-ah-klone

Lunesta✐

Therapeutic class: Hypnotics
Pharmacologic class: Pyrrolopyrazine derivatives
Controlled substance schedule: IV

AVAILABLE FORMS
Tablets: 1 mg, 2 mg, 3 mg

INDICATIONS & DOSAGES
➤ **Insomnia**
Adults: 1 mg P.O. immediately before bedtime. Increase to 2 or 3 mg as needed.
Elderly and debilitated patients: 1 mg P.O. immediately before bedtime. Increase to 2 mg as needed. Maximum dose is 2 mg.
Adjust-a-dose: In patients with severe hepatic impairment and in those also taking a potent CYP3A4 inhibitor, start with 1 mg P.O. and increase to 2 mg as needed. Maximum dose is 2 mg.

ADMINISTRATION
P.O.
• Avoid giving drug after a high-fat meal.
• Give drug immediately before bedtime because drug may cause dizziness or lightheadedness.

ACTION
Probably interacts with GABA receptors at binding sites close or connected to benzodiazepine receptors.

Route	Onset	Peak	Duration
P.O.	Rapid	1 hr	Unknown

Half-life: 6 hours.

ADVERSE REACTIONS
CNS: abnormal dreams, anxiety, complex sleep-related behavior, confusion, depression, dizziness, hallucinations, headache, nervousness, pain, somnolence, neuralgia.
GI: diarrhea, dry mouth, dyspepsia, nausea, vomiting, unpleasant taste, gynecomastia.
GU: dysmenorrhea, UTI, decreased libido.
Skin: pruritus, rash.
Other: accidental injury, viral infection.

INTERACTIONS
Drug-drug. *CNS depressants:* May have additive CNS effects. Adjust dosage of either drug as needed.
CYP3A4 inhibitors (clarithromycin, itraconazole, ketoconazole, nefazodone, nelfinavir, ritonavir, troleandomycin): May decrease eszopiclone elimination, increasing the risk of toxicity. Use together cautiously. Limit eszopiclone dose to maximum of 2 mg.
Olanzapine: May impair cognitive function or memory. Use together cautiously.

Reactions in bold italics are *life-threatening*. Interactions may have a *rapid onset* or a *delayed onset*.

Rifampin: May decrease eszopiclone activity. Don't use together.

Drug-food. *High-fat meals:* May decrease drug absorption and effects. Discourage high-fat meals with or just before taking drug.

Drug-lifestyle. *Alcohol use:* May decrease psychomotor ability. Discourage use together.

EFFECTS ON LAB TEST RESULTS

None reported.

CONTRAINDICATIONS & CAUTIONS

• Rarely, drug may cause angioedema and anaphylaxis that require emergency treatment and can be fatal. Don't rechallenge patients who develop angioedema after treatment with drug.

• Use cautiously in elderly and debilitated patients, in patients with diseases or conditions that could affect metabolism or hemodynamic responses, and in patients with compromised respiratory function or severe hepatic impairment. Also use cautiously in patients with signs and symptoms of depression because of the increased risk of suicide.

• Dosage adjustments may be needed when drug is combined with other CNS depressants because of potentially additive effects.

⚠ **Overdose S&S:** CNS depression.

PREGNANCY-LACTATION-REPRODUCTION

• Use during pregnancy only if potential benefit justifies potential risk to the fetus.

• It isn't known if drug appears in breast milk. Breast-feeding isn't recommended.

NURSING CONSIDERATIONS

❸ **Alert:** Anaphylaxis and angioedema may occur as early as the first dose; monitor patient closely.

❸ **Alert:** Drug may increase risk of next-day impairment of driving and other activities that require full alertness. Recommended starting dose for all patients is 1 mg.

• Evaluate patient for physical and psychiatric disorders before treatment.

• Use the lowest effective dose.

❸ **Alert:** Give drug immediately before patient goes to bed or after patient has gone to bed and has trouble falling asleep.

• Use only for short periods (for example, 7 to 10 days). If patient still has trouble sleeping, check for other psychological disorders.

• Risk of abuse and dependence increases with the dose and duration of treatment and the concurrent use of other psychoactive drugs.

• Monitor patient for changes in behavior, such as decreased inhibition, aggression, and agitation, and including those that suggest depression or suicidal thinking. Amnesia and other neuropsychiatric symptoms may occur unpredictably.

PATIENT TEACHING

❸ **Alert:** Warn patient that drug may cause allergic reactions, facial swelling, and complex sleep-related behaviors, such as driving, eating, and making phone calls while asleep. Advise patient to report these adverse effects.

❸ **Alert:** Caution patient taking 3 mg of eszopiclone not to drive or engage in activities that are hazardous or require complete mental alertness the day after use.

• Urge patient to take drug immediately before going to bed because drug may cause dizziness or light-headedness.

• Caution patient not to take drug unless he can't get a full night's sleep.

• Advise patient to avoid taking drug after a high-fat meal.

• Tell patient to avoid activities that require mental alertness until the drug's effects are known.

• Advise patient to avoid alcohol while taking drug.

• Urge patient to immediately report changes in behavior and thinking.

• Warn patient not to stop drug abruptly or change dose without consulting the prescriber.

• Inform patient that tolerance or dependence may develop if drug is taken for a prolonged period.

etanercept
ee-tan-ER-sept

Enbrel, Enbrel SureClick

Therapeutic class: Antiarthritics
Pharmacologic class: TNF blockers

AVAILABLE FORMS
Injection: 25-mg multiuse vial
Prefilled autoinjector: 50 mg/mL
Prefilled syringe: 25 mg/0.5 mL, 50 mg/mL

INDICATIONS & DOSAGES
➤ **To reduce signs and symptoms of moderately to severely active polyarticular juvenile idiopathic arthritis in patients whose response to one or more DMARDs has been inadequate**
Children ages 2 to 17: For children weighing 63 kg or more, 50 mg subcutaneously weekly using the prefilled syringe or prefilled autoinjector. For children weighing less than 63 kg, 0.8 mg/kg subcutaneously weekly as two injections, either on the same day or 3 or 4 days apart using the multiuse vial. Maximum dosage is 50 mg/week. Glucocorticoids, NSAIDs, or analgesics may be continued during treatment. Use with methotrexate hasn't been studied in pediatric patients.
➤ **RA, psoriatic arthritis, ankylosing spondylitis**
Adults: 50 mg subcutaneously once weekly using the 50-mg/mL single-use prefilled syringe or prefilled autoinjector. Methotrexate, glucocorticoids, salicylates, NSAIDs, or analgesics may be continued during treatment.
➤ **Chronic moderate to severe plaque psoriasis in patients who are candidates for systemic therapy or phototherapy**
Adults: 50 mg subcutaneously twice weekly, 3 to 4 days apart, for 3 months. Then, reduce dose to 50 mg subcutaneously once weekly. Give dose using 50-mg/mL single-use prefilled syringes or prefilled autoinjector.

ADMINISTRATION
Subcutaneous
• Give 50-mg dose as one subcutaneous injection using a 50-mg/mL single-use prefilled syringe or prefilled autoinjector or as two 25-mg subcutaneous injections using multiuse vial. Give the two 25-mg injections on the same day or 3 to 4 days apart.
• Store prefilled syringe at 36° to 46° F (2° to 8° C), but let it reach room temperature (15 to 30 minutes) before use. Don't remove the needle cover while allowing syringe to reach room temperature.
• Store prefilled autoinjector at 36° to 46° F (2° to 8° C) but let it reach room temperature before use. Don't remove the needle cover while allowing syringe to reach room temperature.
• Reconstitute multiple-use vial aseptically with 1 mL of supplied sterile bacteriostatic water for injection (0.9% benzyl alcohol). Use a 25G needle rather than the supplied vial adapter if the vial will be used for multiple doses. Don't filter reconstituted solution when preparing or giving drug. Inject diluent slowly into vial. Refrigerate reconstituted vial for up to 14 days at 36° to 46° F (2° to 8° C) and discard 14 days after reconstitution.
• Minimize foaming by gently swirling during dissolution rather than shaking. Dissolution takes less than 10 minutes.
• Don't use solution if it's discolored or cloudy, or if it contains particulate matter.
• Separate injection sites by at least 1 inch (2.5 cm), rotate regularly, and never use areas where skin is tender, bruised, red, or hard. Use sites on the thigh, abdomen, and upper arm.
❸ *Alert:* Needle covers of diluent syringe and prefilled syringe contain latex and shouldn't be handled by persons sensitive to latex.
• **Incompatibilities:** Don't add other drugs or diluents to solution.

ACTION
Binds specifically to TNF and blocks its action with cell-surface TNF receptors, reducing inflammatory and immune responses found in RA.

Route	Onset	Peak	Duration
Subcut.	Unknown	72 hr	Unknown

Half-life: About 5 days.

ADVERSE REACTIONS
CNS: headache, asthenia, dizziness.
CV: peripheral edema.
EENT: rhinitis, pharyngitis, sinusitis, mouth ulcers.
GI: abdominal pain, dyspepsia, nausea, vomiting, diarrhea.
Respiratory: URI, cough, respiratory disorder.
Skin: injection-site reaction, rash, alopecia, urticaria, pruritus.
Other: infections, *malignancies.*

INTERACTIONS
Drug-drug. *Abatacept, anakinra, canakinumab, certolizumab pegol, natalizumab, velolizumab:* Increases rate of serious infection when used together. Use together cautiously.
Cyclophosphamide: May increase risk of solid malignancies. Concurrent use not recommended.
Leflunomide: May increase risk of hematologic toxicity (pancytopenia, agranulocytosis, or thrombocytopenia). Monitor patient closely for bone marrow suppression at least monthly; consider therapy modification.
Sulfasalazine: May cause decreased neutrophil count. Monitor patient carefully.
Vaccines (inactivated): May reduce vaccine efficacy. Complete all age-appropriate vaccinations at least 2 weeks before start of immunosuppressive therapy. If patient is vaccinated during immunosuppressive therapy, revaccinate at least 3 months after immunosuppressant discontinuation.
Vaccines (live-virus): May affect normal immune response. Postpone live-virus vaccination until 3 months after etanercept discontinuation.

EFFECTS ON LAB TEST RESULTS
None reported.

CONTRAINDICATIONS & CAUTIONS
• Contraindicated in patients hypersensitive to drug or its components, in those with sepsis, and in those receiving a live-virus vaccine.
• Drug isn't indicated for use in children younger than age 2.
• Use cautiously in patients age 65 and older and in patients with underlying diseases that predispose them to infection, such as diabetes, HF, or history of active or chronic infections.
• Use cautiously in RA patients with preexisting or recent onset of demyelinating disorders (MS, myelitis, and optic neuritis).
Dialyzable drug: Unknown.

PREGNANCY-LACTATION-REPRODUCTION
• Use during pregnancy only if clearly needed.
• Drug is present in low levels in breast milk and is minimally absorbed by a breast-fed infant. Use cautiously if breast-feeding.
• The Pregnancy Surveillance Program monitors outcomes in women exposed during pregnancy and the Lactation Surveillance Program monitors outcomes during breast-feeding. Patients or their physicians should call 1-800-77-AMGEN (1-800-772-6436) to enroll.

NURSING CONSIDERATIONS
• Methotrexate, glucocorticoids, salicylates, NSAIDs, or analgesics may be continued during treatment in adults.
Black Box Warning Patients treated with anti-TNF therapies are at increased risk for developing serious, sometimes fatal, infections (TB; invasive fungal infections; bacterial, viral, and other infections). Most patients who developed serious infections were also receiving immunosuppressants, such as methotrexate or corticosteroids. Monitor patient carefully; if serious infection occurs, stop therapy and notify prescriber. ■
Black Box Warning Infections, including bacterial sepsis and TB, have been reported. Evaluate patient's risk factors and test for latent TB. Begin treatment for latent TB before therapy with etanercept. ■
◕ *Alert:* Don't give live-virus vaccines during therapy.
• If possible, bring patients with juvenile RA up to date with all immunizations before starting treatment.
Black Box Warning Histoplasmosis, coccidioidomycosis, blastomycosis, and other opportunistic infections may develop with use of this drug. Consider empirical antifungal therapy in patients at risk for invasive fungal infections who develop severe systemic illness. ■

Black Box Warning Lymphoma and other malignancies, sometimes fatal, have been reported in children and adolescents. ∎

PATIENT TEACHING
• If patient is self-administering drug, advise him about mixing and injection techniques, including rotating injection sites.
• Tell patient that injection-site reactions generally occur within first month of therapy and decrease thereafter.
• Inform patient about avoiding live-virus vaccine administration during therapy.
• Stress importance of alerting other health care providers of etanercept use.
• Instruct patient to promptly report signs of infection, including persistent fever, cough, shortness of breath, or fatigue.
• Advise women to stop breast-feeding.

etanercept-szzs
See NEW DRUGS for information.

eteplirsen
See NEW DRUGS for information.

ethacrynate sodium
eth-uh-KRIH-nayt

Edecrin

ethacrynic acid
Edecrin

Therapeutic class: Diuretics
Pharmacologic class: Loop diuretics

AVAILABLE FORMS
ethacrynate sodium
Injection: 50 mg/vial
ethacrynic acid
Tablets: 25 mg

INDICATIONS & DOSAGES
➤ **Edema (rapid diuresis)**
Adults: 50 mg or 0.5 to 1 mg/kg I.V. Usually only one dose is needed, although a second dose may be needed.
➤ **Edema**
Adults: 50 to 200 mg P.O. daily. May increase to 200 mg b.i.d. for desired effect in 25- to 50-mg increments.

Children age 13 months and older: First dose is 25 mg P.O., increased cautiously by 25 mg daily until desired effect is achieved.
Adjust-a-dose: If added to an existing diuretic regimen, first dose is 25 mg and dosage adjustments are made in 25-mg increments.

ADMINISTRATION
P.O.
• Give in morning to prevent nocturia.
• Give after meals.
I.V.
▼ Add 50 mL of D₅W or NSS to vial.
▼ Don't use cloudy or opalescent solution.
▼ Give over several minutes through tubing of running infusion.
▼ If more than one I.V. dose is needed, use a new injection site to avoid thrombophlebitis.
▼ Discard unused solution after 24 hours.
▼ **Incompatibilities:** Hydralazine, Normosol-M, procainamide, ranitidine, reserpine, solutions or drugs with pH below 5, triflupromazine, whole blood and its derivatives.

ACTION
Potent loop diuretic; inhibits sodium and chloride reabsorption at the proximal and distal tubules and the ascending loop of Henle.

Route	Onset	Peak	Duration
P.O.	30 min	2 hr	6–8 hr
I.V.	5 min	15–30 min	2 hr

Half-life: 1 hour.

ADVERSE REACTIONS
CNS: malaise, confusion, fatigue, apprehension, vertigo, headache, fever.
CV: orthostatic hypotension.
EENT: transient or permanent deafness with over-rapid I.V. injection, blurred vision, tinnitus, hearing loss.
GI: cramping, diarrhea, anorexia, nausea, vomiting, *GI bleeding, pancreatitis.*
GU: oliguria, hematuria, nocturia, polyuria, frequent urination.
Hematologic: *agranulocytosis, neutropenia, thrombocytopenia,* azotemia.
Metabolic: asymptomatic hyperuricemia; hypokalemia; hypochloremic alkalosis; fluid

---

Reactions in bold italics are *life-threatening*. Interactions may have a *rapid onset* or a *delayed onset*.

and electrolyte imbalances, including dilutional hyponatremia, hypocalcemia, and hypomagnesemia; hyperglycemia and impaired glucose tolerance; volume depletion and dehydration.
Skin: rash.
Other: chills.

INTERACTIONS
Drug-drug. *Aminoglycoside antibiotics:* May increase ototoxic adverse reactions to both drugs. Use together cautiously.
Antidiabetics: May decrease hypoglycemic effects. Monitor glucose level.
Antihypertensives: May increase risk of hypotension. Use together cautiously.
Cardiac glycosides: May increase risk of digoxin toxicity from ethacrynate-induced hypokalemia. Monitor potassium and digoxin levels.
Chlorothiazide, chlorthalidone, hydrochlorothiazide, indapamide, metolazone: May cause excessive diuretic response, causing serious electrolyte abnormalities or dehydration. Adjust doses carefully, and monitor patient closely for signs and symptoms of excessive diuretic response.
Cisplatin: May increase risk of ototoxicity. Avoid using together.
Lithium: May decrease lithium clearance, increasing risk of lithium toxicity. Monitor lithium level.
Neuromuscular blockers: May enhance neuromuscular blockade. Monitor patient closely.
NSAIDs: May decrease diuretic effect. Use together cautiously.
Other potassium-wasting drugs (amphotericin B, corticosteroids): May increase risk of hypocalcemia. Use cautiously.
Probenecid: May decrease diuretic effect. Avoid using together.
Risperidone: May enhance adverse or toxic effect of risperidone. Consider therapy modification and maintain adequate hydration.
Warfarin: May increase anticoagulant effect. Use together cautiously.
Drug-herb. *Dandelion:* May interfere with diuretic activity. Discourage use together.
Licorice: May cause unexpected rapid potassium loss. Discourage use together.

EFFECTS ON LAB TEST RESULTS
● May increase glucose and uric acid levels. May decrease calcium, magnesium, potassium, and sodium levels.
● May decrease granulocyte, neutrophil, and platelet counts.

CONTRAINDICATIONS & CAUTIONS
● Contraindicated in infants, patients hypersensitive to drug, and patients with anuria.
🚯 *Alert:* Drug is potent diuretic and can cause severe diuresis with water and electrolyte depletion. Monitor patient closely.
● Use cautiously in patients with electrolyte abnormalities or hepatic impairment.
● Ototoxicity has been reported, most often with I.V. use and with excessive doses.
Dializyable drug: Unknown.
⚠ *Overdose S&S:* Dehydration, electrolyte depletion.

PREGNANCY-LACTATION-REPRODUCTION
● Use in pregnancy only if clearly needed.
● It isn't known if drug appears in breast milk. Patient should discontinue breastfeeding or discontinue drug.

NURSING CONSIDERATIONS
● Monitor fluid intake and output, weight, BP, and electrolyte levels.
● Watch for signs and symptoms of orthostatic hypotension (dizziness, vertigo, syncope) and hypokalemia (muscle weakness and cramps).
● Monitor glucose level in diabetic patients.
● Consult prescriber and dietitian about providing a high-potassium diet. Foods rich in potassium include citrus fruits, tomatoes, bananas, dates, and apricots. Potassium chloride and sodium supplements may be needed.
● Dosage may be on an alternate-day schedule, or more prolonged periods of diuretic therapy may be interspersed with rest periods. Intermittent dosage schedule allows time to correct electrolyte imbalance and may provide a more efficient diuretic response.
● Drug may increase risk of gastric hemorrhage caused by steroid treatment.
● Monitor elderly patients, who are especially susceptible to hypotension and other effects of excessive diuresis.

E

• Monitor uric acid level, especially in patients with history of gout.

🌙 **Alert:** If patient develops severe diarrhea, stop drug. Patient shouldn't receive drug again after diarrhea has resolved.

PATIENT TEACHING
• Instruct patient to take drug with food to minimize GI upset.
• Advise patient to take drug in morning to avoid need to urinate at night; if patient needs second dose, have him take it in early afternoon.
• Advise patient to avoid sudden posture changes and to rise slowly to avoid dizziness upon standing quickly.
• Tell patient to notify prescriber about muscle weakness, cramps, nausea, diarrhea, or dizziness.
• Caution patient not to perform hazardous activities if drug causes drowsiness.
• Advise diabetic patient to closely monitor glucose level.

ethambutol hydrochloride
e-THAM-byoo-tole

Etibi✤, Myambutol

Therapeutic class: Antituberculotics
Pharmacologic class: Synthetic antituberculotics

AVAILABLE FORMS
Tablets: 100 mg, 400 mg

INDICATIONS & DOSAGES
➤ **Adjunctive treatment for pulmonary TB**
Adults and children age 13 and older: In patients who haven't received prior antitubercular therapy, 15 mg/kg P.O. daily as a single dose once every 24 hours, combined with other antituberculotics. For retreatment, 25 mg/kg P.O. every 24 hours as a single dose for 60 days (or until bacteriologic smears and cultures become negative) with at least one other antituberculotic; after 60 days, decrease to 15 mg/kg/day as a single dose every 24 hours.
Adjust-a-dose: Reduce dosage in patients with impaired renal function according to serum drug levels.

ADMINISTRATION
P.O.
• Always give with other antituberculotics to prevent development of resistant organisms.
• Giving with food doesn't significantly alter absorption.
• Give on a once-every-24-hour basis only.

ACTION
May inhibit synthesis of one or more metabolites of susceptible bacteria, changing cell metabolism during cell division; bacteriostatic.

Route	Onset	Peak	Duration
P.O.	Unknown	2–4 hr	Unknown

Half-life: About 3½ hours.

ADVERSE REACTIONS
CNS: dizziness, fever, hallucinations, headache, malaise, mental confusion, peripheral neuritis.
EENT: optic neuritis, irreversible blindness.
GI: abdominal pain, anorexia, GI upset, nausea, vomiting.
Hematologic: *thrombocytopenia, leukopenia, neutropenia.*
Metabolic: hyperuricemia.
Musculoskeletal: joint pain.
Skin: *toxic epidermal necrolysis,* dermatitis, pruritus.
Other: *anaphylactoid reactions,* precipitation of acute gout.

INTERACTIONS
Drug-drug. *Aluminum salts:* May delay and reduce ethambutol absorption. Separate doses by at least 4 hours.

EFFECTS ON LAB TEST RESULTS
• May increase ALT, AST, bilirubin, and uric acid levels. May decrease glucose level.
• May decrease platelet count.

CONTRAINDICATIONS & CAUTIONS
• Contraindicated in children younger than age 13, patients hypersensitive to drug, and patients with optic neuritis.
• Use cautiously in patients with impaired renal function, cataracts, recurrent eye inflammation, gout, or diabetic retinopathy. Irreversible blindness has occurred.
Dialyzable drug: Unknown.

Reactions in bold italics are *life-threatening*. Interactions may have a *rapid onset* or a *delayed onset*.

PREGNANCY-LACTATION-REPRODUCTION
- Use during pregnancy only if benefit justifies potential risk to the fetus.
- Drug appears in breast milk. Use only if expected benefit to the mother outweighs potential risk to the infant.

NURSING CONSIDERATIONS
- Perform visual acuity and color discrimination tests before and during therapy. Patients taking more than 15 mg/kg/day should have monthly eye examinations.
- Ensure that any changes in vision don't result from an underlying condition.
- Obtain AST and ALT levels before therapy, and monitor these levels every 3 to 4 weeks.
- In patients with impaired renal function, base dosage on drug level.
- Monitor uric acid level; observe patient for signs and symptoms of gout.

PATIENT TEACHING
- Tell patient to report all vision changes immediately; explain that eye examinations will be necessary. Advise patient that visual disturbances usually disappear several weeks to months after drug is stopped. Inflammation of the optic nerve is related to dosage and duration of treatment.
- Inform patient that drug is given with other antituberculotics.
- Stress importance of compliance with drug therapy.
- Advise patient to report adverse reactions to prescriber.

ethinyl estradiol–desogestrel
ETH-i-nill/DAY-so-jest-rul

Monophasic
Desogen, Emoquette

Biphasic
Kariva, Viorele

Triphasic
Cyclessa, Velivet

ethinyl estradiol–ethynodiol diacetate
Monophasic
Kelnor 1/35, Zovia 1/35E-28, Zovia 1/50E-28

ethinyl estradiol–levonorgestrel
Monophasic
Altavera, Aviane-28, Falmina, Introvale, Lessina-28, Levora 0.15/30-28, Marlissa, Orsythia, Portia-28, Quasense, Seasonale

Biphasic
Lo Seasonique, Seasonique

Triphasic
Enpresse-28, Levonest, Myzilra, Trivora-28

ethinyl estradiol–norethindrone
Monophasic
Alyacen 1/35, Alyacen 777, Aranelle, Balziva-28, Brevicon 28-Day, Briellyn, Cyclafem 1/35, Dasetta 1/35, Modicon-28, Norinyl 1 + 35, Nortrel 0.5/35-28, Nortrel 1/35, Ortho-Novum 1/35-28, Philith, Wera

Triphasic
Alyacen 7/7/7, Aranelle, Cyclafem 7/7/7, Dasetta 7/7/7, Nortrel 7/7/7, Ortho-Novum 7/7/7-28, Tri-Norinyl 28-day

ethinyl estradiol–norethindrone acetate
Monophasic
Activella, Femhrt, Junel 1/20, Junel 1.5/30, Junel Fe 1/20, Junel Fe 1.5/30, Larin 1/20, Larin 1.5/30, Loestrin 21 1/20, Loestrin 21 1.5/30, Microgestin 1/20, Microgestin 1.5/30

ethinyl estradiol–norgestimate
Monophasic
Mono-Linyah, Ortho-Cyclen-28, Previfem, Sprintec

Triphasic
Ortho Tri-Cyclen, Ortho Tri-Cyclen Lo, Tri-Linyah, Tri-Previfem, Tri-Sprintec

ethinyl estradiol–norgestrel
Monophasic
Cryselle, Elinest, Lo/Ovral-28, Ogestrel 0.5/50-28

ethinyl estradiol–norethindrone acetate–ferrous fumarate
Monophasic
Femcon Fe, Gildess Fe 1/20, Gildess Fe 1.5/30, Junel Fe 1/20, Junel Fe 1.5/30, Larin 24 Fe, Larin Fe 1/20, Larin Fe 1.5/30, Loestrin 24 Fe, Loestrin Fe 1/20, Loestrin Fe 1.5/30, Lo Loestrin Fe, Microgestin Fe 1/20, Microgestin Fe 1.5/30

Triphasic
Estrostep Fe, Tri-Legest Fe

mestranol–norethindrone
Monophasic
Norinyl 1 + 50 28 Day

Therapeutic class: Contraceptives
Pharmacologic class: Estrogen–progestin combinations

AVAILABLE FORMS
Monophasic hormonal contraceptives
ethinyl estradiol–desogestrel
Tablets: ethinyl estradiol 30 mcg and desogestrel 0.15 mg (Desogen, Emoquette)
ethinyl estradiol–ethynodiol diacetate
Tablets: ethinyl estradiol 35 mcg and ethynodiol diacetate 1 mg (Kelnor 1/35, Zovia 1/35E-28); ethinyl estradiol 50 mcg and ethynodiol diacetate 1 mg (Zovia 1/50E-28)
ethinyl estradiol–levonorgestrel
Tablets: ethinyl estradiol 20 mcg and levonorgestrel 0.1 mg (Aviane-28, Falmina, Lessina-28, Orsythia); ethinyl estradiol 30 mcg and levonorgestrel 0.15 mg (Altavera, Introvale, Levora 0.15/30-28, Marlissa, Portia-28, Quasense, Seasonale); ethinyl estradiol 30 mcg and 0.15 mg levonorgestrel (84 tablets), and 10 mcg ethinyl estradiol (7 tablets) (Seasonale)

ethinyl estradiol–norethindrone
Tablets: ethinyl estradiol 35 mcg and norethindrone 0.4 mg (Balziva-28, Briellyn, Philith); ethinyl estradiol 35 mcg and norethindrone 0.5 mg (Brevicon 28-Day, Modicon-28, Nortrel 0.5/35-28, Wera); ethinyl estradiol 35 mcg and norethindrone 0.75 mg (Alyacen 777); ethinyl estradiol 35 mcg and norethindrone 1 mg (Alyacen 1/35, Alyacen 777, Cyclafem 1/35, Dasetta 1/35, Norinyl 1 + 35, Nortrel 1/35, Ortho-Novum 1/35-28)
ethinyl estradiol–norethindrone acetate
Tablets: ethinyl estradiol 2.5 mcg and norethindrone acetate 0.5 mg; ethinyl estradiol 5 mcg and norethindrone acetate 1 mg; ethinyl estradiol 20 mcg and norethindrone acetate 1 mg (Junel 1/20, Larin 1/20, Loestrin 21 1/20, Microgestin 1/20); ethinyl estradiol 30 mcg and norethindrone acetate 1.5 mg (Junel 1.5/30, Larin 1.5/30, Loestrin 21 1.5/30, Microgestin 1.5/30); ethinyl estradiol 0.5 mg and norethindrone acetate 0.1 mg; ethinyl estradiol 1 mg and norethindrone acetate 0.5 mg
ethinyl estradiol–norgestimate
Tablets: ethinyl estradiol 35 mcg and norgestimate 0.25 mg (Mono-Linyah, Ortho-Cyclen-28, Previfem, Sprintec)
ethinyl estradiol–norgestrel
Tablets: ethinyl estradiol 30 mcg and norgestrel 0.3 mg (Cryselle, Elinest, Lo/Ovral-28); ethinyl estradiol 50 mcg and norgestrel 0.5 mg (Ogestrel 0.5/50-28)
ethinyl estradiol–norethindrone acetate–ferrous fumarate
Chewable tablets: norethindrone 0.4 mg and ethinyl estradiol 35 mcg; inactive tablets contain ferrous fumarate 75 mg
Tablets: ethinyl estradiol 10 mcg, norethindrone acetate 1 mg, and ferrous fumarate 75 mg (Lo Loestrin Fe); ethinyl estradiol 20 mcg, norethindrone acetate 1 mg, and ferrous fumarate 75 mg (Gildess Fe 1/20, Junel Fe 1/20, Larin 24 Fe, Larin Fe 1/20, Loestrin Fe 1/20, Loestrin 24 Fe, Microgestin Fe 1/20); ethinyl estradiol 30 mcg, norethindrone acetate 1.5 mg, and ferrous fumarate 75 mg (Gildess Fe 1.5/30, Junel Fe 1.5/30, Larin Fe 1.5/30, Loestrin Fe 1.5/30, Microgestin Fe 1.5/30)

mestranol–norethindrone
Tablets: mestranol 50 mcg and norethindrone 1 mg (Norinyl 1 + 50 28 Day)
Biphasic hormonal contraceptives
ethinyl estradiol–desogestrel
Tablets: ethinyl estradiol 20 mcg and desogestrel 0.15 mg (21 days), then inert tablets (2 days), then ethinyl estradiol 10 mcg (5 days) (Kariva, Viorele)
ethinyl estradiol–levonorgestrel
Tablets: ethinyl estradiol 0.02 mg and levonorgestrel 0.1 mg (84 days), then ethinyl estradiol 0.01 mg (7 days) (Lo Seasonique); ethinyl estradiol 30 mcg and levonorgestrel 0.15 mg (84 days), then ethinyl estradiol 10 mcg (7 days) (Seasonique)
Triphasic hormonal contraceptives
ethinyl estradiol–desogestrel
Tablets: 0.1 mg desogestrel and 25 mcg ethinyl estradiol (7 tablets); 0.125 mg desogestrel and 25 mcg ethinyl estradiol (7 tablets); 0.15 mg desogestrel and 25 mcg ethinyl estradiol (7 tablets) (Cyclessa, Velivet)
ethinyl estradiol–levonorgestrel
Tablets: ethinyl estradiol 30 mcg and levonorgestrel 0.05 mg (6 days); ethinyl estradiol 40 mcg and levonorgestrel 0.075 mg (5 days); ethinyl estradiol 30 mcg and levonorgestrel 0.125 mg (10 days) (Enpresse-28, Levonest, Myzilra, Trivora-28)
ethinyl estradiol–norethindrone
Tablets: ethinyl estradiol 30 mcg and norethindrone 0.5 mg (7 days); ethinyl estradiol 35 mcg and norethindrone 1 mg (9 days); ethinyl estradiol 35 mcg and norethindrone 0.5 mg (5 days) (Aranelle, Tri-Norinyl 28-day); ethinyl estradiol 35 mcg and norethindrone 0.5 mg (7 days); ethinyl estradiol 35 mcg and norethindrone 0.75 mg (7 days); ethinyl estradiol 35 mcg and norethindrone 1 mg (7 days) (Alyacen 7/7/7, Cyclafem 7/7/7, Dasetta 7/7/7, Nortrel 7/7/7, Ortho-Novum 7/7/7-28)
ethinyl estradiol–norgestimate
Tablets: ethinyl estradiol 25 mcg and norgestimate 0.18 mg (7 days); ethinyl estradiol 25 mcg and norgestimate 0.215 mg (7 days); ethinyl estradiol 25 mcg and norgestimate 0.25 mg (7 days) (Ortho Tri-Cyclen Lo); ethinyl estradiol 35 mcg and norgestimate 0.18 mg (7 days); ethinyl estradiol 35 mcg and norgestimate

0.215 mg (7 days); ethinyl estradiol 35 mcg and norgestimate 0.25 mg (7 days) (Ortho Tri-Cyclen, Tri-Linyah, Tri-Previfem, Tri-Sprintec)
ethinyl estradiol–norethindrone acetate–ferrous fumarate
Tablets: ethinyl estradiol 20 mcg and norethindrone acetate 1 mg (5 days); ethinyl estradiol 30 mcg and norethindrone acetate 1 mg (7 days); ethinyl estradiol 35 mcg and norethindrone acetate 1 mg (9 days); 75-mg ferrous fumarate tablets (7 days) (Estrostep Fe, Tri-Legest Fe)

INDICATIONS & DOSAGES
➤ **Contraception**
Monophasic hormonal contraceptives
Women: 1 tablet P.O. daily beginning on first day of menstrual cycle or first Sunday after menstrual cycle begins. With 20- and 21-tablet package, new cycle begins 7 days after last tablet taken. With 28-tablet package, dosage is 1 tablet daily without interruption; extra tablets taken on days 22 to 28 are placebos or contain iron. Or, for Seasonale, 1 pink tablet P.O. daily beginning on first Sunday after menstrual cycle begins, for 84 consecutive days, followed by 7 days of white (inert) tablets. When changing from 21-day or 28-day combination oral contraceptive, begin on first day of withdrawal bleeding, at the latest 7 days after last active tablet. When changing from progestin-only pill, begin the next day. When changing from implant contraceptive, begin the day of implant removal. When changing from injection contraceptive, begin the day when next injection is due.
Biphasic hormonal contraceptives
Women: 1 color tablet P.O. daily for 10 days; then next color tablet for 11 days. With 21-tablet packages, new cycle begins 7 days after last tablet taken. With 28-tablet packages, dosage is 1 tablet daily without interruption. Or, for Seasonique, 1 light blue-green tablet P.O. once daily for 84 consecutive days followed by 1 yellow tablet for 7 consecutive days; then repeat cycle.
Triphasic hormonal contraceptives
Women: 1 tablet P.O. daily in the sequence specified by the brand. With 21-tablet packages, new dosing cycle begins 7 days after

E

last tablet taken. With 28-tablet packages, dosage is 1 tablet daily without interruption.
➤ **Moderate acne vulgaris in women age 15 and older who have no known contraindications to hormonal contraceptive therapy, who want oral contraception for at least 6 months, who have reached menarche, and who are unresponsive to topical antiacne drugs**
Women age 15 and older: 1 tablet Ortho Tri-Cyclen or Estrostep Fe P.O. daily (21 tablets contain active ingredients and 7 are inert).
➤ **Menopausal signs and symptoms; to prevent osteoporosis (Activella, Femhrt)**
Women with intact uterus: 1 tablet P.O. daily.

ADMINISTRATION
P.O.
● Give drug at the same time each day; give at night to reduce nausea and headaches.
● Chewable tablet may be swallowed whole or chewed and followed with a full glass of liquid.

ACTION
Inhibits ovulation and may prevent transport of the ovum (if ovulation should occur) through the fallopian tubes.
 Estrogen suppresses FSH, blocking follicular development and ovulation.
 Progestin suppresses luteinizing hormone so that ovulation can't occur even if the follicle develops; it also thickens cervical mucus, interfering with sperm migration, and prevents implantation of the fertilized ovum.

Route	Onset	Peak	Duration
P.O.	Unknown	2 hr (ethinyl estradiol), 0.5–4 hr (varies by progestin)	Unknown

Half-life: 6 to 20 hours (ethinyl estradiol); 5 to 45 hours (varies by progestin).

ADVERSE REACTIONS
CNS: headache, dizziness, depression, lethargy, migraine, *stroke, cerebral hemorrhage.*
CV: *thromboembolism,* hypertension, edema, *PE, MI.*
EENT: worsening myopia or astigmatism, intolerance of contact lenses, exophthalmos, diplopia.

GI: nausea, vomiting, abdominal cramps, bloating, anorexia, changes in appetite, gallbladder disease, *pancreatitis.*
GU: breakthrough bleeding, spotting, granulomatous colitis, dysmenorrhea, amenorrhea, cervical erosion or abnormal secretions, enlargement of uterine fibromas, vaginal candidiasis.
Hepatic: cholestatic jaundice, *liver tumors,* gallbladder disease.
Metabolic: weight change, additive insulin resistance in diabetics.
Skin: rash, acne, *erythema multiforme,* melasma, hirsutism.
Other: breast tenderness, enlargement, or secretion; *anaphylaxis; hemolytic-uremic syndrome.*

INTERACTIONS
Drug-drug. *Anastrozole:* May inhibit anastrozole effect. Avoid use together.
Anti-infectives (chloramphenicol, fluconazole, griseofulvin, neomycin, nitrofurantoin, penicillins, sulfonamides, tetracyclines): May decrease contraceptive effect. Advise patient to use another method of contraception.
Atorvastatin: May increase norethindrone and ethinyl estradiol levels. Monitor patient for adverse effects.
Benzodiazepines: May decrease or increase benzodiazepine levels. Adjust dosage, if necessary.
Beta blockers: May increase beta blocker level. Dosage adjustment may be necessary.
Carbamazepine, fosphenytoin, phenobarbital, phenytoin, rifampin: May decrease estrogen effect. Use together cautiously.
Corticosteroids: May enhance corticosteroid effect. Monitor patient closely.
Insulin, sulfonylureas: Glucose intolerance may decrease antidiabetic effects. Monitor these effects.
Iron supplements: Increase risk of iron-related toxicity if drug contains iron. Don't use together.
NNRTIs, protease inhibitors: May decrease hormonal contraceptive effect. Avoid using together, if possible.
Oral anticoagulants: May decrease anticoagulant effect. Dosage adjustments may be needed. Monitor PT and INR.

Reactions in bold italics are *life-threatening*. Interactions may have a *rapid onset* or a *delayed onset*.

Tamoxifen: May inhibit tamoxifen effect. Avoid using together.

Drug-herb. *Black cohosh:* May increase adverse effects of estrogen. Discourage use together.

Red clover: May interfere with drug. Discourage use together.

St. John's wort: May decrease drug effect because of increased hepatic metabolism. Discourage use together, or advise patient to use an additional method of contraception.

Drug-food. *Caffeine:* May increase caffeine level. Urge caution.

Grapefruit juice: May increase estrogen level. Advise patient to take with liquid other than grapefruit juice.

Drug-lifestyle. *Smoking:* May increase risk of adverse CV effects. If smoking continues, may need alternative therapy.

EFFECTS ON LAB TEST RESULTS

● May increase clotting factors II, VII, VIII, IX, and X; fibrinogen; phospholipid; plasminogen; thyroid-binding globulin; total T_4; and triglyceride levels.

● May increase norepinephrine-induced platelet aggregation and prolong PT.

● May reduce metyrapone test results. May cause false-positive result in nitroblue tetrazolium test.

CONTRAINDICATIONS & CAUTIONS

● Contraindicated in patients with thromboembolic disorders, cerebrovascular disease or CAD, diplopia or ocular lesions arising from ophthalmic vascular disease, classic migraine, MI, known or suspected breast cancer, known or suspected estrogen-dependent neoplasia, benign or malignant liver tumors, active liver disease or history of cholestatic jaundice with pregnancy or previous use of hormonal contraceptives, and undiagnosed abnormal vaginal bleeding.

● Use cautiously in patients with hyperlipidemia, hypertension, migraines, seizure disorders, asthma, bleeding irregularities, gallbladder disease, ocular disease, diabetes, emotional disorders, and cardiac, renal, or hepatic insufficiency.

Dialyzable drug: Unknown.

⚠ Overdose S&S: Nausea, withdrawal uterine bleeding.

PREGNANCY-LACTATION-REPRODUCTION

● Use during pregnancy isn't indicated. Discontinue if pregnancy is confirmed. There is little or no increased risk of birth defects in women who accidently use drug during early pregnancy.

● Estrogens can reduce the quantity and quality of breast milk. Breast-feeding women should use other forms of contraception while breast-feeding. Those not breast-feeding may start oral contraceptives 4 to 6 weeks postpartum.

NURSING CONSIDERATIONS

Black Box Warning Cigarette smoking increases the risk of serious CV adverse effects from oral contraceptives. Women who use oral contraceptives shouldn't smoke. ∎

● Triphasic hormonal contraceptives may cause fewer adverse reactions, such as breakthrough bleeding and spotting.

● The CDC reports that use of hormonal contraceptives may decrease risk of ovarian and endometrial cancers and doesn't seem to increase risk of breast cancer. However, the FDA reports that some studies suggest that hormonal contraceptives may be linked to an increase in cervical cancer.

● Monitor lipid levels, BP, body weight, and hepatic function.

🖲 Alert: Many hormonal contraceptives share similar names. Make sure to check the hormone strength for verification.

● Estrogens and progestins may alter glucose tolerance, thus changing dosage requirements for antidiabetics. Monitor glucose level.

● Stop hormonal contraceptives for a few weeks before adrenal function tests.

● Stop hormonal contraceptive and notify prescriber if patient develops granulomatous colitis.

● Stop drug at least 1 week before surgery to decrease risk of thromboembolism. Tell patient to use an alternative method of birth control.

● Women who are nonlactating mothers or those who have had second-trimester abortion must wait 28 days before starting oral contraception.

PATIENT TEACHING

• Tell patient to take tablets at same time each day; nighttime doses may reduce nausea and headaches.

• Advise patient to use additional method of birth control, such as condom or diaphragm with spermicide, for first week of first cycle.

• Tell patient that missing doses in midcycle greatly increases likelihood of pregnancy.

• Tell patient that missing a dose may cause spotting or light bleeding.

• Tell patient that hormonal contraceptives don't protect against HIV or other sexually transmitted diseases.

• Tell patient using Seasonale that there will be four planned menses per year, but spotting or bleeding between menses may occur.

• If 1 pill is missed, tell patient to take it as soon as possible (2 pills if remembered on the next day) and then to continue regular schedule. Advise an additional method of contraception for remainder of cycle. If 2 consecutive pills are missed, tell patient to take 2 pills a day for next 2 days and then resume regular schedule. Advise an additional method of contraception for the next 7 days or preferably for the remainder of cycle. If 2 consecutive pills are missed in the 3rd or 4th week or if patient misses 3 consecutive pills, tell patient to contact prescriber for instructions.

• Warn patient of common adverse effects, such as headache, nausea, dizziness, breast tenderness, spotting, and breakthrough bleeding, which usually diminish after 3 to 6 months.

• Instruct patient to weigh herself at least twice a week and to report any sudden weight gain or swelling to prescriber.

• Warn patient to avoid exposure to ultraviolet light or prolonged exposure to sunlight.

🔆 *Alert:* Warn patient to immediately report abdominal pain; numbness, stiffness, or pain in legs or buttocks; pressure or pain in chest; shortness of breath; severe headache; visual disturbances, such as blind spots, blurriness, or flashing lights; undiagnosed vaginal bleeding or discharge; two consecutive missed menstrual periods; lumps in the breast; swelling of hands or feet; or severe pain in the abdomen (tumor rupture in liver).

• Advise patient of increased risks created by simultaneous use of cigarettes and hormonal contraceptives.

• If one menstrual period is missed and tablets have been taken on schedule, tell patient to continue taking them. If two consecutive menstrual periods are missed, tell patient to stop drug and have pregnancy test. Progestins may cause birth defects if taken early in pregnancy.

• Tell patient to chew chewable tablet and follow with a full glass of liquid or swallow whole.

• Advise patient not to take same drug for longer than 12 months without consulting prescriber. Stress importance of Papanicolaou tests and annual gynecologic examinations.

• Advise patient to check with prescriber about how soon pregnancy may be attempted after hormonal therapy is stopped. Many prescribers recommend that women not become pregnant within 2 months after stopping drug.

• Warn patient of possible delay in achieving pregnancy when drug is stopped.

• Teach women how to perform routine breast self-examination.

• Teach patient methods to decrease risk of thromboembolism.

• Advise patient taking hormonal contraceptives to use additional form of birth control during concurrent treatment with certain antibiotics.

• Advise patient that hormonal contraceptives may change the fit of contact lenses.

---

etodolac
ee-toe-DOE-lak

Therapeutic class: NSAIDs
Pharmacologic class: NSAIDs

AVAILABLE FORMS
Capsules: 200 mg, 300 mg
Tablets: 400 mg, 500 mg
Tablets (extended-release): 400 mg, 500 mg, 600 mg

Reactions in bold italics are *life-threatening*. Interactions may have a *rapid onset* or a *delayed onset*.

INDICATIONS & DOSAGES

➤ **Acute pain**
Adults: 200 to 400 mg (immediate-release) P.O. every 6 to 8 hours p.m., not to exceed 1,000 mg daily.

➤ **Short- and long-term management of osteoarthritis and RA**
Adults: 600 to 1,000 mg (immediate-release) P.O. daily, divided into two or three doses. Maximum daily dose is 1,200 mg. For extended-release tablets, 400 to 1,000 mg P.O. daily. Maximum daily dose is 1,200 mg.

➤ **Juvenile RA**
Children ages 6 to 16 weighing 20 to 30 kg: 400 mg (extended-release) P.O. once daily.
Children ages 6 to 16 weighing 31 to 45 kg: 600 mg (extended-release) P.O. once daily.
Children ages 6 to 16 weighing 46 to 60 kg: 800 mg (extended-release) P.O. once daily.
Children ages 6 to 16 weighing more than 60 kg) or more: 1,000 mg (extended-release) P.O. once daily.

ADMINISTRATION

P.O.
● Give drug with milk or meals to minimize GI discomfort.

ACTION

Unknown. Produces anti-inflammatory, analgesic, and antipyretic effects, possibly by inhibiting prostaglandin synthesis.

Route	Onset	Peak	Duration
P.O.	30 min	1–2 hr	4–12 hr
P.O. (extended-release)	Unknown	3–12 hr	6–12 hr

Half-life: 7¼ hours.

ADVERSE REACTIONS

CNS: asthenia, malaise, dizziness, depression, drowsiness, nervousness, syncope, fever.
CV: fluid retention.
EENT: blurred vision, tinnitus.
GI: dyspepsia, flatulence, abdominal pain, diarrhea, nausea, constipation, gastritis, melena, vomiting.
GU: dysuria, urinary frequency.
Hepatic: *hepatitis.*
Skin: pruritus, rash.
Other: chills.

INTERACTIONS

Drug-drug. *Antacids:* May decrease peak level of etodolac. Watch for decreased effect of etodolac.
Anticoagulants, antiplatelet drugs, SSRIs: May enhance anticoagulant or antiplatelet effects. Monitor patient.
Aspirin: May decrease protein-binding of etodolac without altering its clearance. May increase GI toxicity. Avoid using together.
Beta blockers, diuretics: May blunt effects of these drugs. Monitor patient closely.
Cyclosporine: May increase risk of nephrotoxicity. Avoid using together.
Digoxin, lithium, methotrexate: May impair elimination of these drugs, increasing risk of toxicity. Monitor drug levels.
Diuretics: May increase risk of renal insufficiency with prolonged use. Monitor patient for evidence of kidney injury.
Phenytoin: May increase phenytoin level. Monitor patient for toxicity.
Warfarin: May decrease the protein binding of warfarin but doesn't change its clearance. Although no dosage adjustment is needed, monitor INR closely and watch for bleeding.
Drug-herb. *Dong quai, feverfew, garlic, ginger, horse chestnut, red clover:* May increase risk of bleeding. Discourage use together.
White willow: Herb and drug contain similar components. Discourage use together.
Drug-lifestyle. *Alcohol use:* May increase risk of adverse effects. Discourage use together.
Sun exposure: May cause photosensitivity reactions. Advise patient to avoid excessive sunlight exposure.

EFFECTS ON LAB TEST RESULTS

● May increase BUN and creatinine. May decrease uric acid and Hb levels and hematocrit.
● May decrease WBC count.
● May cause a false-positive test result for urine bilirubin, possibly from phenolic metabolites and ketone bodies.

CONTRAINDICATIONS & CAUTIONS

Black Box Warning Contraindicated for the treatment of perioperative pain after CABG surgery. ∎

• Contraindicated in patients hypersensitive to drug and in those with history of aspirin- or NSAID-induced asthma, rhinitis, urticaria, or other allergic reactions.

🌙 *Alert:* NSAIDs may increase the risk of heart attack or stroke in patients with or without heart disease or risk factors for heart disease.

🌙 *Alert:* Risk of heart attack or stroke may occur as early as the first weeks of NSAID use. Risk appears greater at higher doses. Use the lowest effective dose for the shortest duration possible.

• Use cautiously in elderly patients and in patients with history of renal or hepatic impairment, preexisting asthma, or GI bleeding, ulceration, and perforation.

Dialyzable drug: No.

⚠ *Overdose S&S:* Lethargy, drowsiness, nausea, vomiting, epigastric pain, GI bleeding, coma, hypertension, acute renal failure, respiratory depression, anaphylaxis.

PREGNANCY-LACTATION-REPRODUCTION

• Use in pregnancy only if potential benefit justifies potential risk to the fetus.

• Avoid use in third trimester because drug may cause premature closure of the ductus arteriosus.

• It isn't known if drug appears in breast milk. Patient should discontinue breast-feeding or discontinue drug.

NURSING CONSIDERATIONS

• Because NSAIDs impair the synthesis of renal prostaglandins, they can decrease renal blood flow and lead to reversible renal impairment, especially in patients with renal or heart failure or liver dysfunction, in elderly patients, and in those taking diuretics. Monitor these patients closely.

Black Box Warning NSAIDs cause an increased risk of serious GI adverse events, including bleeding, ulceration, and perforation of the stomach or intestines, which can be fatal. Elderly patients are at greater risk. ∎

Black Box Warning NSAIDs may increase the risk of serious thrombotic events, MI, or stroke, which can be fatal. The risk may be greater with longer use or in patients with CV disease or risk factors for CV disease. ∎

🌙 *Alert:* Watch for and immediately evaluate signs and symptoms of heart attack (chest pain, shortness of breath or trouble breathing) or stroke (weakness in one part or side of the body, slurred speech).

• May cause serious skin reactions (exfoliative dermatitis, Stevens-Johnson syndrome, toxic epidermal necrolysis). Discontinue drug at first sign of hypersensitivity or rash.

PATIENT TEACHING

• Tell patient to take drug with milk or meals to minimize GI discomfort.

• Teach patient signs and symptoms of GI bleeding, including blood in vomit, urine, or stool; coffee-ground vomit; and black, tarry stool. Tell him to notify prescriber immediately if any of these occurs.

🌙 *Alert:* Advise patient to seek medical attention immediately if chest pain, shortness of breath or trouble breathing, weakness in one part or side of the body, or slurred speech occurs.

• Advise patient to avoid consuming alcohol or aspirin while taking drug.

• Warn patient to avoid hazardous activities that require alertness until harmful CNS effects of drug are known.

• Teach patient signs and symptoms of liver damage, including nausea, fatigue, lethargy, itching, yellowed skin or eyes, right upper quadrant tenderness, and flulike symptoms. Tell him to contact prescriber immediately if any of these symptoms occurs.

• Advise patient to use a sunblock, wear protective clothing, and avoid prolonged exposure to sunlight because of possible sensitivity to sunlight.

• Advise patient that use of OTC NSAIDs and etodolac may increase the risk of GI toxicity.

---

etonogestrel–ethinyl estradiol vaginal ring
e-toe-noe-JES-trel/ETH-i-nill

NuvaRing

Therapeutic class: Contraceptives
Pharmacologic class: Estrogen–
progestin combinations

AVAILABLE FORMS
Vaginal ring: Delivers 0.12 mg etonogestrel
and 0.015 mg ethinyl estradiol daily

INDICATIONS & DOSAGES
➤ **Contraception**
Women: Insert 1 ring into the vagina and
leave in place for 3 weeks. Insert new ring
1 week after the previous ring is removed.

ADMINISTRATION
Vaginal
● In women who did not use hormonal
contraception during the previous month,
therapy should be initiated on the first day
of the menstrual cycle. A woman using a
combination oral contraceptive may switch
to NuvaRing on any day, but at the latest on
the day following the usual hormone-free
interval.
● Leave ring in place continuously for a full
3 weeks to maintain effect. It's then removed
for 1 week. During this time, withdrawal
bleeding occurs (usually starting 2 or 3 days
after removal). Insert a new ring 1 week
after removal of the previous one, regardless
of whether patient is still menstruating.

ACTION
Suppresses gonadotropins, which inhibits
ovulation, increases the viscosity of cervical
mucus (decreasing the ability of sperm to
enter the uterus), and alters the endometrial
lining (reducing potential for implantation).

Route	Onset	Peak	Duration
Vaginal	Immediate (etonogestrel), 60 hr (ethinyl estradiol)	200 hr	Unknown

Half-life: Etonogestrel, 29 hours; ethinyl estradiol, 45 hours.

ADVERSE REACTIONS
CNS: headache, emotional lability, migraine, *cerebral thrombosis, cerebral hemorrhage.*
CV: hypertension, edema, *thromboembolic
events, MI.*
EENT: sinusitis, changes in corneal curva-
ture, intolerance to contact lenses.
GI: nausea, vomiting.
GU: vaginitis, leukorrhea, device-related
events (for example, foreign body sensation,
coital difficulties, device expulsion), vaginal
discomfort, breakthrough bleeding.
Hematologic: *coagulation abnormalities.*
Hepatic: *hepatic adenomas,* benign liver
tumors, cholestatic jaundice.
Metabolic: weight gain.
Respiratory: URI.
Skin: melasma.

INTERACTIONS
Drug-drug. *Acetaminophen:* May decrease
acetaminophen level and increase ethinyl
estradiol level. Monitor patient for effects.
*Ampicillin, barbiturates, carbamazepine,
felbamate, griseofulvin, oxcarbazepine,
phenylbutazone, phenytoin, rifampin,
tetracyclines, topiramate:* May decrease
contraceptive effect and increase risk of
pregnancy, breakthrough bleeding, or both.
Tell patient to use an additional form of
contraception while taking these drugs.
Anastrozole: May diminish therapeutic
effect of anastrozole. Avoid use together.
Ascorbic acid, atorvastatin, itraconazole:
May increase ethinyl estradiol level. Monitor patient for adverse effects.
*Clofibrate, morphine, salicylic acid,
temazepam:* May increase clearance of these
drugs. Monitor patient for effectiveness.
Cyclosporine, prednisolone, theophylline:
May increase levels of these drugs. Monitor
levels if appropriate and adjust dosage.
HIV protease inhibitors: May affect contraceptive effect. Refer to the specific protease
inhibitor drug literature. May need to use a
backup method of contraception.
Miconazole (oil-based vaginal capsule):
May increase serum concentrations of
etonogestrel and ethinyl estradiol. Monitor
patient for adverse effects.
Drug-herb. *St. John's wort:* May reduce
drug effectiveness and increase the risk

of breakthrough bleeding and pregnancy. Discourage use together.

Drug-lifestyle. Black Box Warning
Smoking: May increase risk of serious CV adverse effects, especially in patients older than age 35 who smoke 15 or more cigarettes daily. Drug shouldn't be used in those older than age 35 and who smoke. Urge patient to avoid smoking. ■

EFFECTS ON LAB TEST RESULTS

● May increase coagulation factors; thyroid-binding globulin (leading to increased circulating total thyroid hormone levels); sex hormone-binding globulin (and other binding proteins); and triglyceride levels. May decrease antithrombin III and folate levels.

● May increase norepinephrine-induced platelet aggregation. May decrease T_3 resin uptake and glucose tolerance.

CONTRAINDICATIONS & CAUTIONS

● Contraindicated in patients hypersensitive to components of drug; patients older than age 35 who smoke 15 or more cigarettes daily; patients with thrombophlebitis, thromboembolic disorder, history of deep vein thrombophlebitis, cerebrovascular disease or CAD (current or previous), valvular heart disease with complications, severe hypertension, diabetes with vascular complications, headache with focal neurologic symptoms or migraine headaches with aura; women older than age 35 with migraine headaches; major surgery with prolonged immobilization; known or suspected cancer of the endometrium or breast; estrogen-dependent neoplasia; abnormal undiagnosed genital bleeding; jaundice related to pregnancy or previous use of hormonal contraceptives; active liver disease; or benign or malignant hepatic tumors.

● Use cautiously in patients with hypertension, hyperlipidemias, obesity, or diabetes.

● Use cautiously in patients with conditions that could be aggravated by fluid retention, and in patients with a history of depression.

Dialyzable drug: Unknown.

PREGNANCY-LACTATION-REPRODUCTION

● Not indicated for use in pregnancy; drug is contraindicated. Discontinue drug if pregnancy is confirmed.

● There is little or no increased risk of birth defects in women who accidently use combined hormonal contraceptives during early pregnancy.

● Drug may appear in breast milk and may decrease the quantity and quality of milk. Breast-feeding women should use other forms of contraception while breast-feeding.

NURSING CONSIDERATIONS

❸ *Alert:* Drug may increase the risk of MI, thromboembolism, stroke, hepatic neoplasia, and gallbladder disease.

Black Box Warning Cigarette smoking increases the risk of serious adverse cardiac effects. The risk increases with age and in patients who smoke 15 or more cigarettes daily. ■

● Stop drug at least 4 weeks before and for 2 weeks after procedures that may increase the risk of thromboembolism, and during and after prolonged immobilization.

● Stop drug and notify prescriber if patient develops unexplained partial or complete loss of vision, proptosis, diplopia, papilledema, retinal vascular lesions, migraines, depression, or jaundice.

● Monitor BP closely if patient has hypertension or renal disease.

● Rule out pregnancy if woman hasn't adhered to the prescribed regimen and a period is missed, if prescribed regimen has been adhered to and two periods are missed, or if patient has retained the ring for longer than 4 weeks.

PATIENT TEACHING

● Stress importance of having regular annual physical examinations to check for adverse effects or developing contraindications.

● Tell patient that drug doesn't protect against HIV and other sexually transmitted diseases.

● Advise patient not to smoke while using contraceptive.

● Tell patient to use backup method of contraception until ring has been used continuously for 7 days. Tell patient not to use diaphragm if backup method is needed.

• Tell patient who wears contact lenses to contact an ophthalmologist if vision or lens tolerance changes.

• Advise patient to follow manufacturer's instructions for use if switching from different form of hormonal contraceptive.

• Tell patient to insert ring into vagina (using fingers) and keep it in place continuously for 3 weeks to maintain effect, saving foil package for later disposal. Explain that it is then removed for 1 full week and that, during this time, withdrawal bleeding occurs (usually starting 2 or 3 days after removal). Tell patient to insert new ring 1 week after removing previous one, regardless of menstrual bleeding. Tell patient to reseal ring in the package after removing it from vagina.

• Advise patient that, if the ring is removed or expelled (such as while removing a tampon, straining, or moving bowels), it should be washed with cool to lukewarm (not hot) water and reinserted immediately. Stress that contraceptive effect may be compromised if the ring stays out for longer than 3 hours and that she should use a backup method of contraception until the newly reinserted ring has been used continuously for 7 days.

• Tell patient that there's no danger of the vaginal ring being pushed too far up in the vagina or getting lost.

SAFETY ALERT!

etoposide (VP-16-213)
e-toe-POE-side

etoposide phosphate
Etopophos

Therapeutic class: Antineoplastics
Pharmacologic class: Podophyllotoxin derivatives

AVAILABLE FORMS
etoposide
Capsules: 50 mg
Injection: 20 mg/mL in 5-mL, 25-mL, and 50-mL vials

etoposide phosphate
Injection: 119.3-mg vials equivalent to 100 mg etoposide

INDICATIONS & DOSAGES
Adjust-a-dose (for all indications): For patients with CrCl of 15 to 50 mL/minute, reduce dose by 25%. For patients with CrCl of less than 10 mL/minute, consider dosage reduction.

➤ **Refractory testicular cancer in combination with other chemotherapeutic agents**
Adults: 50 to 100 mg/m^2 daily I.V. on 5 consecutive days every 3 to 4 weeks. Or, 100 mg/m^2 daily I.V. on days 1, 3, and 5 every 3 to 4 weeks for three or four courses of therapy.

➤ **Small-cell carcinoma of the lung in combination with other chemotherapeutic agents**
Adults: 35 mg/m^2 daily I.V. for 4 days. Or, 50 mg/m^2 daily I.V. for 5 days. Repeat cycles every 3 to 4 weeks. Oral dose is two times I.V. dose (two times 35 mg/m^2 for 4 days to 50 mg/m^2 for 5 days), rounded to nearest 50 mg.

ADMINISTRATION
P.O.
• Give drug without regard for food.
• Don't give drug with grapefruit juice.
• Drug is hazardous. Use appropriate precautions for handling and disposal.
• Refrigerate capsules at 36° to 46° F (2° to 8° C). Don't freeze. Capsules are stable for 24 months under refrigeration.

I.V.
▼ Preparing and giving parenteral drug may be mutagenic, teratogenic, or carcinogenic. Follow facility policy to reduce risks. Use gloves.
▼ For etoposide infusion, dilute to 0.2 or 0.4 mg/mL in either D$_5$W or NSS. Higher concentrations may crystallize.
▼ Give etoposide by slow infusion over at least 30 to 60 minutes to prevent severe hypotension. Never give by rapid injection.
▼ For etoposide phosphate, reconstitute each vial with sterile water for injection, D$_5$W, NSS, bacteriostatic water for injection with benzyl alcohol, or bacteriostatic sodium chloride for injection with benzyl

alcohol to a concentration of 20 mg/mL or 10 mg/mL. After reconstitution, give without further dilution or dilute to as low as 0.1 mg/mL in either D_5W or NSS.

▼ Give etoposide phosphate over 5 to 210 minutes.

▼ Check BP every 15 minutes during infusion. Hypotension may occur if infusion is too rapid. If systolic pressure falls below 90 mm Hg, stop infusion and notify prescriber.

▼ Etoposide diluted to 0.2 mg/mL is stable for 96 hours at room temperature in plastic or glass, unprotected from light; at 0.4 mg/mL, it's stable for 24 hours under same conditions. Diluted etoposide phosphate solution stored in glass or plastic containers is stable under refrigeration for 7 days or for 24 to 48 hours at room temperature, depending on diluent. Further diluted solutions are stable under refrigeration or at room temperature for 24 hours.

▼ **Incompatibilities:** Cefepime hydrochloride, filgrastim, gallium nitrate, idarubicin.

ACTION
Inhibits topoisomerase II enzyme, causing inability to repair DNA strand breaks, which leads to cell death. Cell-cycle specific to G_2 portion of cell cycle.

Route	Onset	Peak	Duration
P.O., I.V.	Unknown	Unknown	Unknown

Half-life: Initial phase, ½ to 2 hours; terminal phase, 4 to 11 hours.

ADVERSE REACTIONS
CNS: peripheral neuropathy.
CV: hypotension.
GI: anorexia, diarrhea, nausea, vomiting, abdominal pain, stomatitis, mucositis.
Hematologic: *leukopenia, neutropenia, thrombocytopenia,* anemia, *myelosuppression.*
Hepatic: *hepatotoxicity.*
Skin: reversible alopecia, rash.
Other: *anaphylaxis,* hypersensitivity reactions.

INTERACTIONS
Drug-drug. *Cyclosporine:* May increase etoposide level and toxicity. Monitor CBC and adjust etoposide dose.

Live-virus vaccines: May increase risk of live-virus vaccine–induced adverse reactions. Concurrent use isn't recommended.
Phosphatase inhibitors: May decrease etoposide effectiveness. Monitor drug effects.
Warfarin: May further prolong PT. Monitor PT and INR closely.
Drug-food. *Grapefruit juice:* May reduce etoposide concentrations. Avoid using together.

EFFECTS ON LAB TEST RESULTS
● May decrease Hb level.
● May decrease neutrophil, platelet, RBC, and WBC counts.

CONTRAINDICATIONS & CAUTIONS
● Contraindicated in patients hypersensitive to drug.
● Use cautiously in patients who have had cytotoxic or radiation therapy and in those with hepatic impairment.
Dialyzable drug: No.

PREGNANCY-LACTATION-REPRODUCTION
● Drug can cause fetal harm if used during pregnancy. Advise women of childbearing potential to avoid becoming pregnant. If drug is used during pregnancy, or if patient becomes pregnant during therapy, patient should be apprised of potential fetal hazard.
● Drug appears in breast milk. Patient should discontinue breast-feeding or discontinue drug.

NURSING CONSIDERATIONS
Black Box Warning Give drug under the supervision of a physician experienced in the use of cancer chemotherapy. Severe myelosuppression with infection or bleeding may occur. ■
● Obtain baseline BP before starting therapy.
● Anticipate need for antiemetics.
● Have diphenhydramine, hydrocortisone, epinephrine, and emergency equipment available to establish an airway in case anaphylaxis occurs.
● Store capsules in refrigerator.
Black Box Warning Monitor CBC. Watch for evidence of bone marrow suppression, which could lead to infection or bleeding. ■

- Observe patient's mouth for signs of ulceration.
- To prevent bleeding, avoid all I.M. injections when platelet count is below 50,000/mm^3.
- Etoposide phosphate dose is expressed as etoposide equivalents; 119.3 mg of etoposide phosphate is equivalent to 100 mg of etoposide.

PATIENT TEACHING

- Tell patient to watch for signs and symptoms of infection (fever, sore throat, fatigue) and bleeding (easy bruising, nosebleeds, bleeding gums, tarry stools). Tell patient to take temperature daily.
- Inform patient of need for frequent BP readings during I.V. administration.
- Caution women of childbearing potential to avoid pregnancy and breast-feeding during therapy.

etravirine
eh-trah-VIGH-reen

Intelence

Therapeutic class: Antiretrovirals
Pharmacologic class: NNRTIs

AVAILABLE FORMS
Tablets ⓓⓝⓒ: 25 mg, 100 mg, 200 mg

INDICATIONS & DOSAGES
➤ **HIV-1 in treatment-experienced patients with evidence of viral replication and HIV-1 strains resistant to an NNRTI and other antiretrovirals**
Adults: 200 mg P.O. b.i.d. after meals. Given with other antiretrovirals.
Children age 6 and older weighing 30 kg or more: 200 mg P.O. b.i.d.
Children age 6 and older weighing 25 to less than 30 kg: 150 mg P.O. b.i.d.
Children age 6 and older weighing 20 to less than 25 kg: 125 mg P.O. b.i.d.
Children age 6 and older weighing 16 to less than 20 kg: 100 mg P.O. b.i.d.

ADMINISTRATION
P.O.
- Give drug after meals.

- Have patient swallow tablets whole with a liquid such as water.
- If patient can't swallow whole tablets, place tablets in a glass with 5 mL of water. Stir water well until it looks milky. May add more water, orange juice, or milk to glass (avoid grapefruit juice, fluids warmer than 104° F [40° C], or carbonated beverages) and have patient drink immediately. Rinse glass with water several times and have patient swallow each rinse completely.

ACTION
Binds to reverse transcriptase, an enzyme that replicates HIV.

Route	Onset	Peak	Duration
P.O.	Unknown	2½–4 hr	Unknown

Half-life: About 41 hours.

ADVERSE REACTIONS
CNS: abnormal dreams, amnesia, anxiety, confusion, disorientation, fatigue, headache, hypoesthesia, insomnia, paresthesia, peripheral neuropathy, *seizures,* sluggishness, syncope, tremors.
CV: angina, *atrial fibrillation,* hypertension, *MI.*
EENT: blurred vision, vertigo.
GI: abdominal distension, abdominal pain, anorexia, constipation, diarrhea, dry mouth, flatulence, gastritis, GERD, hematemesis, nausea, *pancreatitis,* retching, stomatitis, vomiting.
GU: *renal failure.*
Hepatic: *hepatitis,* hepatomegaly, increased liver enzyme levels.
Hematologic: anemia, hemolytic anemia.
Metabolic: *diabetes,* dyslipidemia.
Respiratory: *bronchospasm,* dyspnea.
Skin: rash.

INTERACTIONS
Drug-drug. *Amiodarone, bepridil, disopyramide, flecainide, lidocaine, mexiletine, propafenone, quinidine:* May decrease levels of these drugs. Use caution, and monitor patient closely.
Amprenavir and ritonavir: May increase amprenavir level. Avoid use together.
Atazanavir and ritonavir: May decrease atazanavir level and increase etravirine level. Avoid use together.

Atorvastatin, lovastatin, simvastatin: May decrease levels of these drugs. Adjust dosage, if needed.

Clarithromycin: May decrease clarithromycin level and increase etravirine level. Consider using azithromycin for treating *Mycobacterium avium* complex.

CYP3A4 inhibitors (itraconazole, ketoconazole): May decrease levels of these drugs. Adjust dosage, if needed.

CYP450 inducers (carbamazepine, phenobarbital, phenytoin): May decrease etravirine level. Avoid use together.

Delavirdine: May increase etravirine level. Avoid use together.

Dexamethasone: May decrease etravirine level. Avoid use together.

Diazepam: May increase diazepam level. Reduce diazepam dose, as needed.

Efavirenz, nevirapine: May decrease etravirine level. Avoid use together.

Fluconazole, posaconazole: May increase etravirine level. Use together cautiously.

Fluvastatin: May increase fluvastatin level. Adjust dosage, if needed.

Immunosuppressants (cyclosporine, sirolimus, tacrolimus): May decrease levels of these drugs. Use together cautiously, and monitor patient closely.

Lopinavir–ritonavir: May increase etravirine level. Use together cautiously.

Methadone: May cause withdrawal symptoms. Monitor patient, and consider increasing methadone dosage.

PDE5 inhibitors (sildenafil, tadalafil, vardenafil): May decrease effectiveness of these drugs. Adjust dosage, as needed.

Protease inhibitors (atazanavir, fosamprenavir, indinavir, nelfinavir): May alter protease inhibitor level if given without ritonavir. Avoid use together unless given with low-dose ritonavir.

Rifabutin: May decrease etravirine and rifabutin levels. If etravirine isn't given with a protease inhibitor and ritonavir, give rifabutin 300 mg daily. If etravirine is given with darunavir and ritonavir or with saquinavir and ritonavir, avoid rifabutin.

Rifampin, rifapentine: May decrease etravirine level. Avoid use together.

Ritonavir: May decrease etravirine level. Avoid use together.

Ritonavir and tipranavir: May decrease etravirine level. Avoid use together.

Warfarin: May increase warfarin level. Monitor INR closely, and adjust warfarin dosage if needed.

Drug-herb. *St. John's wort:* May decrease etravirine level. Avoid use together.

EFFECTS ON LAB TEST RESULTS

● May increase amylase, lipase, creatinine, total cholesterol, LDL, triglyceride, AST, ALT, and glucose levels.

● May decrease Hb level and WBC, neutrophil, and platelet counts.

CONTRAINDICATIONS & CAUTIONS

● Contraindicated in patients hypersensitive to etravirine or its components.

● Hypersensitivity reactions, including DRESS syndrome (drug rash with eosinophilia and systemic symptoms), ranging from rash to organ dysfunction, and severe, potentially life-threatening and fatal skin reactions (Stevens-Johnson syndrome, toxic epidermal necrolysis, erythema multiforme) have been reported. Discontinue drug immediately if signs or symptoms of hypersensitivity reactions or severe skin reactions develop.

● Use cautiously in elderly patients and patients with hepatic impairment or HBV or HCV infection.

● For children, don't exceed adult dosage or give to children younger than age 6.

Dialyzable drug: Unlikely.

PREGNANCY-LACTATION-REPRODUCTION

● Use only if potential benefit outweighs fetal risk.

● Register pregnant patients in the Antiretroviral Pregnancy Registry at 1-800-258-4263.

● It isn't known if drug appears in breast milk. Women with HIV infection shouldn't breast-feed.

NURSING CONSIDERATIONS

❸ *Alert:* Etravirine may interact with many drugs. Review patient's complete drug regimen.

● If patient can't swallow the tablet whole, dissolve it in water and have patient drink it immediately. To make sure patient receives

E

entire dose, refill the glass several times and have patient drink.

☉ Alert: Monitor patient closely for skin reactions. Fatalities have occurred due to toxic epidermal necrolysis, Stevens-Johnson syndrome, or erythema multiforme, and hypersensitivity reactions that may be accompanied by hepatic failure. Discontinue drug if severe skin or hypersensitivity reactions develop.

• Monitor patient for signs of fat redistribution (central obesity, buffalo hump, peripheral wasting, breast enlargement, cushingoid appearance).

• Immune reconstitution syndrome can occur. Monitor patient for inflammatory response to indolent or residual infections or autoimmune disorders.

• Notify prescriber if signs, symptoms, or laboratory abnormalities suggest pancreatitis. Monitor amylase and lipase levels.

• Monitor patient's CBC, platelet count, LFTs, and renal function studies. Report abnormalities.

PATIENT TEACHING

• Advise patient to take etravirine after a meal.

• Warn patient to tell prescriber about any other prescription drugs, OTC drugs, and herbal supplements he takes.

• Advise patient to report adverse effects to prescriber.

• Inform patient that drug doesn't cure HIV infection, that opportunistic infections and other complications of HIV infection may still occur, and that HIV may still be transmitted to others through sexual contact or blood contamination.

• Advise patient to take drug as prescribed and not to alter dose or stop drug without medical approval.

• If patient misses a dose, tell him to take it as soon as possible and then return to his normal schedule. Advise patient not to double the dose.

• Tell patient that routine blood tests will be needed to assess how he is tolerating drug therapy.

SAFETY ALERT!

everolimus
eh-ver-OH-lih-mus

Afinitor, Afinitor Disperz, Zortress

Therapeutic class: Antineoplastics
Pharmacologic class: Kinase inhibitors

AVAILABLE FORMS
Tablets (Afinitor) ⓝⓒ: 2.5 mg, 5 mg, 7.5 mg, 10 mg
Tablets (Afinitor Disperz) ⓝⓒ: 2 mg, 3 mg, 5 mg
Tablets (Zortress) ⓝⓒ: 0.25 mg, 0.5 mg, 0.75 mg

INDICATIONS & DOSAGES
➤ **Advanced renal cell carcinoma after treatment with sunitinib or sorafenib fails; renal angiomyolipoma with tuberous sclerosis complex; advanced hormone-receptor positive, HER2-negative breast cancer in postmenopausal women in combination with exemestane for recurrence or progression after treatment with letrozole or anastrozole; progressive neuroendocrine tumors of pancreatic origin (unresectable, locally advanced, or metastatic); progressive, well-differentiated, nonfunctional neuroendocrine tumors of GI or lung origin (locally advanced or metastatic) (Afinitor)**
Adults: 10 mg P.O. once daily. Continue until disease progression or unacceptable toxicity occurs.

Adjust-a-dose: For severe or intolerable adverse effects, reduce dosage to 5 mg P.O. daily or interrupt therapy. For mild hepatic impairment (Child-Pugh class A), reduce dosage to 7.5 mg P.O. daily; may decrease to 5 mg if not well tolerated. For moderate hepatic impairment (Child-Pugh class B), reduce dosage to 5 mg P.O. daily; may decrease to 2.5 mg if not well tolerated. For severe hepatic impairment (Child-Pugh class C), reduce dosage to 2.5 mg P.O. daily and use only if benefit outweighs risk; don't exceed 2.5 mg. If concomitant use of drugs that are moderate inhibitors of CYP3A4 or P-glycoprotein (P-gp) are required, decrease dosage to 2.5 mg P.O. daily; if tolerated, may increase to 5 mg daily. If concomitant use of drugs that are strong inducers of CYP3A4 can't be avoided, increase dosage in 5-mg increments to a maximum dosage of 20 mg P.O. daily.

➤ **Prevention of organ rejection in liver transplantation (Zortress only)**
Adults: 1 mg P.O. b.i.d. starting at least 30 days after transplant in combination with reduced-dose tacrolimus and corticosteroids. Adjust dosage based on trough concentrations obtained 4 to 5 days after previous dosing change to a target therapeutic range of 3 to 8 ng/mL.
Adjust-a-dose: In patients with mild hepatic impairment, reduce initial dose by a third. In patients with moderate to severe hepatic impairment, reduce initial dose by half and monitor blood concentrations.

➤ **Prevention of kidney transplant rejection in patients at low to moderate immunologic risk (Zortress only)**
Adults: Initially, 0.75 mg P.O. b.i.d. in combination with basiliximab induction and a reduced dose of cyclosporine and corticosteroids as soon as possible after transplantation. Dosage adjustments may be made at 4- to 5-day intervals based on patient response and clinical situation.
Adjust-a-dose: In patients with mild hepatic impairment, reduce initial dose by a third. In patients with moderate to severe hepatic impairment, reduce initial dose by half and monitor blood concentrations.

➤ **Subependymal giant cell astrocytoma with tuberous sclerosis in patients who aren't surgical candidates (Afinitor or Afinitor Disperz)**
Adults and children age 1 and older: Initially, 4.5 mg/m^2 P.O. once daily; round dose to nearest strength. Adjust dosage in 2-week intervals to trough concentration of 5 to 15 ng/mL. Don't combine the two dosage forms (Afinitor tablets and Afinitor Disperz tablets) to achieve the desired dose. Use one dosage form or the other. Once a stable dose is attained, monitor trough concentrations every 3 to 6 months in patients with changing BSA or every 6 to 12 months in patients with stable BSA for duration of treatment.
Adjust-a-dose: The recommended starting dose for patients with severe hepatic impairment (Child-Pugh class C) or requiring

moderate CYP3A4 or P-gp inhibitors is 2.5 mg/m^2, once daily. The recommended starting dose for patients requiring a concomitant strong CYP3A4 inducer is 9 mg/m^2 once daily. Assess trough concentrations approximately 2 weeks after initiation of treatment, a change in dose, a change in coadministration of CYP3A4 or P-gp inducers or inhibitors, a change in hepatic function, or a change in dosage form between Afinitor tablets and Afinitor Disperz. For severe or intolerable adverse reactions, reduce dose by approximately 50%. If dose reduction falls below lowest available strength, give every other day.

ADMINISTRATION
P.O.
Afinitor, Zortress
● Give drug at same time each day, consistently with or consistently without food.
● Have patient swallow tablets whole with a glass of water. Tablets shouldn't be chewed or crushed.
● Patient should avoid grapefruit or grapefruit juice while taking drug.

Afinitor Disperz
● Wear gloves to avoid possible contact with everolimus when preparing suspension.
● Give as a suspension only.
● Give drug orally once daily at the same time every day, either consistently with food or consistently without food.
● Administer suspension immediately after preparation. Discard suspension if not administered within 60 minutes after preparation. Prepare suspension in water only.
● To administer drug using an oral syringe, place the prescribed dose into a 10-mL syringe. Do not exceed a total of 10 mg per syringe. If higher doses are required, prepare an additional syringe. Do not break or crush tablets. Draw approximately 5 mL of water and 4 mL of air into the syringe. Place the filled syringe into a container (tip up) for 3 minutes, until the tablets are in suspension. Gently invert the syringe 5 times immediately prior to administration. After administration of the prepared suspension, draw approximately 5 mL of water and 4 mL of air into the same syringe, and swirl the contents to suspend remaining

particles. Administer the entire contents of the syringe.

• To administer using a small drinking glass, place the prescribed dose into a small drinking glass (maximum size 100 mL) containing approximately 25 mL of water. Do not exceed a total of 10 mg per glass. If higher doses are required, prepare an additional glass. Do not break or crush tablets. Allow 3 minutes for suspension to occur. Stir the contents gently with a spoon, immediately prior to drinking. After administration of the prepared suspension, add 25 mL of water and stir with the same spoon to re-suspend remaining particles. Administer the entire contents of the glass.

ACTION
Binds to an intracellular protein, thereby inhibiting mammalian target rapamycin (mTOR), a kinase. Inhibiting mTOR reduces cancer cell proliferation, angiogenesis, and glucose uptake.

Route	Onset	Peak	Duration
P.O.	Unknown	1–2 hr	Unknown

Half-life: 30 hours.

ADVERSE REACTIONS
CNS: asthenia, dizziness, dysgeusia, headache, insomnia, paresthesia, fever, fatigue, *seizures.*
CV: chest pain, *HF,* hypertension, tachycardia, *hemorrhage.*
EENT: conjunctivitis, eyelid edema, epistaxis, mucosal inflammation, nasopharyngitis, pharyngolaryngeal pain, rhinorrhea, sinusitis.
GI: abdominal pain, anorexia, diarrhea, dry mouth, dysphagia, hemorrhoids, nausea, stomatitis, vomiting, mouth ulcers, oral mucositis.
GU: renal failure, UTI, menstrual irregularities.
Hematologic: anemia, *leukopenia, neutropenia, thrombocytopenia.*
Hepatic: elevated alkaline phosphatase, AST, ALT levels.
Metabolic: exacerbation of diabetes mellitus, weight loss, fasting hyperglycemia, hypercholesterolemia, hypertriglyceridemia, hypophosphatemia.

Musculoskeletal: extremity pain, jaw pain, arthralgia.
Respiratory: bronchitis, cough, dyspnea, pleural effusion, pneumonia, *pneumonitis, bronchospasm.*
Skin: acneiform dermatitis, dry skin, erythema, hand-foot syndrome, nail disorder, pruritus, onychoclasis, rash, skin lesion.
Other: chills, peripheral edema, infection, hypersensitivity reactions, *angioedema.*

INTERACTIONS
Drug-drug. **Black Box Warning** *Cyclosporine:* Increased nephrotoxicity can occur with standard cyclosporine dosing in combination with everolimus. Decrease cyclosporine dosage, and monitor serum cyclosporine and everolimus levels. ■
Strong CYP3A4 inducers (carbamazepine, dexamethasone, phenobarbital, phenytoin, rifabutin, rifampin): May decrease everolimus level. Avoid using together; if drugs must be used together, increase everolimus dosage at 5 mg-increments up to 20 mg daily.
Strong or moderate CYP3A4 inhibitors (amprenavir, aprepitant, atazanavir, clarithromycin, delavirdine, diltiazem, erythromycin, fluconazole, fosamprenavir, indinavir, itraconazole, ketoconazole, nefazodone, nelfinavir, ritonavir, saquinavir, telithromycin, verapamil, voriconazole) and P-gp inhibitors (amiodarone, atorvastatin, spironolactone): May increase everolimus level. Avoid using together.
Vaccines (live-virus): Toxic effects of vaccines may increase and drug's therapeutic effects diminish. Avoid use together.
Drug-herb. *St. John's wort:* May alter drug level. Discourage use together.
Drug-food. *Grapefruit, grapefruit juice:* May increase drug level. Don't use together.

EFFECTS ON LAB TEST RESULTS
• May increase urinary protein and creatinine, cholesterol, triglyceride, and glucose levels.
• May decrease Hb level and lymphocyte, neutrophil, and platelet counts.

CONTRAINDICATIONS & CAUTIONS
Black Box Warning Use of Zortress has been shown to increase mortality in a heart

transplant clinical trial. Use in heart transplant patients isn't recommended. ∎

• Contraindicated in patients hypersensitive to drug, its components, other rapamycin derivatives, or sirolimus (Zortress only).

• Afinitor isn't indicated to treat functional carcinoid tumors.

• Avoid use in patients with severe hepatic impairment or severe infection.

Dialyzable drug: No.

PREGNANCY-LACTATION-REPRODUCTION

• Avoid use during pregnancy because of potential hazards to fetus.

• Women of reproductive potential should avoid pregnancy and use highly effective contraception during treatment and for up to 8 weeks after last dose.

• The National Transplantation Pregnancy Registry (NTPR) at Temple University is a registry for pregnant women taking immunosuppressants after any solid organ transplant. The NTPR encourages reporting all immunosuppressant exposures during pregnancy in transplant recipients at 1-877-955-6877.

• Drug may cause male and female infertility.

• It isn't known if drug appears in breast milk.

NURSING CONSIDERATIONS

Black Box Warning Zortress should only be prescribed by providers experienced in immunosuppressive therapy and management of transplant patients. ∎

• Don't crush tablets. Avoid direct contact with skin or mucous membranes. If contact occurs, wash area thoroughly.

Black Box Warning Zortress increases risk of infection and malignancies, such as lymphoma and skin cancer, due to immunosuppression. ∎

♻ Alert: Drug may cause immunosuppression, predisposing patients to bacterial, fungal, viral, or protozoal infections, including reactivation of hepatitis B virus. Infections may be severe or even fatal. Complete treatment of preexisting invasive fungal infections before starting therapy. Consider holding or stopping everolimus if infection occurs. Discontinue drug if invasive systemic fungal infection is diagnosed, and treat infection appropriately.

• Monitor patient for signs of infection (fever, chills, sore throat, fatigue).

Black Box Warning There is an increased risk of arterial and venous renal thrombosis leading to graft loss in patients taking Zortress, usually in first 30 days after transplant. ∎

Black Box Warning When drug is used with cyclosporine, increased nephrotoxicity can occur and reduced dosages of everolimus are needed. Monitor cyclosporine and everolimus whole blood trough concentrations. ∎

• Monitor renal function studies, glucose and lipid levels, and CBC before and during therapy.

• Avoid mouthwash containing alcohol or peroxide in patients who develop mouth ulcers, stomatitis, or oral mucositis.

• Monitor respiratory status for signs and symptoms of noninfectious pneumonitis (hypoxia, pleural effusion, cough, dyspnea). For severe cases, discontinue therapy and administer corticosteroids.

PATIENT TEACHING

• Advise female patient of childbearing potential to use an effective method of contraception during therapy and for 8 weeks afterward.

• Advise male and female patient that use may impair fertility.

• Tell patient to swallow the Afinitor or Zortress tablets whole with a glass of water.

• Tell patient to take drug at the same time each day, consistently with or without food.

• Instruct caregiver how to prepare and administer Afinitor Disperz.

• Instruct patient that if he misses a dose of Afinitor, he may still take it up to 6 hours after the normal time. If more than 6 hours have elapsed, tell him to skip that day's and take it at the usual time the next day.

• Advise patient to notify health care provider if mouth ulcers, fever, shortness of breath, cough, rash, headache, loss of appetite, nausea, vomiting, diarrhea, swelling of the extremities or face, weakness, tiredness, or nosebleeds occur.

● Tell patient not to receive live-virus vaccines and to avoid close contact with anyone who has received a live-virus vaccine.

evolocumab
E-voe-lok-ue-mab

Repatha

Therapeutic class: Antilipemics
Pharmacologic class: Proprotein convertase subtilisin kexin type 9 (PCSK9) antibody inhibitors

AVAILABLE FORMS
Injection: 140-mg/mL solution in single-dose prefilled syringe or autoinjector

INDICATIONS & DOSAGES
➤ **Adjunct to diet and maximally tolerated statin therapy for treatment of heterozygous familial hypercholesterolemia (HeFH) or primary hyperlipidemia in patients with established clinical atherosclerotic CV disease who require additional lowering of LDL cholesterol (LDL-C)**
Adults: 140 mg subcutaneously every 2 weeks or 420 mg subcutaneously once monthly. When switching dosage regimens, give first dose of new regimen on next scheduled date of prior regimen.
➤ **Adjunct to diet and other LDL-lowering therapies (statins, ezetimibe, LDL apheresis) for treatment of homozygous familial hypercholesterolemia (HoFH) in patients who require additional lowering of LDL-C**
Adults and adolescents age 13 and older: 420 mg subcutaneously once monthly.

ADMINISTRATION
Subcutaneous
🚫 *Alert:* Needle cover of glass prefilled syringe and autoinjector contains a latex derivative and may cause allergic reactions in patients sensitive to latex.
● Allow drug to warm to room temperature for at least 30 minutes before injecting. Don't warm in any other way.
● Don't use if solution is discolored or contains particulate matter.
● Don't shake.

● Administer into abdomen, thigh, or upper arm. Don't administer if areas are tender, bruised, red, or indurated.
● Rotate injection site with each injection.
● Don't administer with other injectable drugs at same injection site.
● To administer monthly 420-mg dose, use three different syringes or autoinjectors for each injection. Give all injections within 30 minutes.
● If dose is missed, give as soon as possible if there are more than 7 days until next scheduled dose. If there are less than 7 days until next scheduled dose, omit missed dose and give next dose according to original schedule.
● Store in refrigerator in original carton. Protect from direct light.
● If kept at room temperature in original carton, drug must be used within 30 days. Don't expose to temperatures above 77° F (25° C). Don't freeze.

ACTION
A human monoclonal antibody (IgG2) that targets PCSK9. By blocking PCSK9's ability to bind LDL receptors in the liver, more receptors are available to remove LDL-C from the blood, thereby lowering LDL levels.

Route	Onset	Peak	Duration
Subcut.	4 hr	3–4 days	Unknown

Half-life: 11 to 17 days.

ADVERSE REACTIONS
CNS: headache, dizziness, fatigue.
CV: hypertension.
EENT: nasopharyngitis, sinusitis.
GI: diarrhea, gastroenteritis, nausea.
GU: UTI.
Hematologic: contusion.
Musculoskeletal: back pain, myalgia, musculoskeletal pain, arthralgia, muscle spasms.
Respiratory: URI, cough.
Skin: rash.
Other: flulike symptoms, injection-site reactions (erythema, pain, bruising), hypersensitivity reactions.

E

INTERACTIONS
None reported.

EFFECTS ON LAB TEST RESULTS
• May decrease LDL, non-HDL, apo B, and total cholesterol to very low levels.

CONTRAINDICATIONS & CAUTIONS
• Contraindicated in patients with a history of serious hypersensitivity to drug or its components.
• Safety and effectiveness of drug haven't been established in children of any age with primary hyperlipidemia or HeFH or in children younger than age 13 with HoFH.
• Effect of drug on CV morbidity and mortality hasn't been determined.
Dialyzable drug: Unknown.

PREGNANCY-LACTATION-REPRODUCTION
• There are no adequate studies in pregnant women. Use cautiously during pregnancy and consider possible risk to the fetus.
• It isn't known if drug appears in breast milk. Use cautiously and consider risks and benefits of breast-feeding.

NURSING CONSIDERATIONS
• Measure LDL levels periodically. In patients with HoFH, measure LDL levels 4 to 8 weeks after start of therapy because response to therapy will depend on degree of LDL receptor function.
• Adverse consequences of long-term very low LDL-C levels (less than 25 mg/dL) aren't known.
• Monitor patients for hypersensitivity reactions (rash, urticaria). If serious allergic reaction occurs, discontinue drug.
• Long-term consequences of continuing evolocumab in the presence of anti–drug binding antibodies are unknown.
• *Look alike–sound alike:* Don't confuse evolocumab with ezetimibe.

PATIENT TEACHING
🡇 *Alert:* Before drug initiation, advise patient to report latex sensitivity because needle cover of the glass prefilled syringe and autoinjector contains a latex derivative that may cause allergic reactions.
• Explain that periodic blood tests to monitor treatment are necessary.

• Teach patient and caregivers how to store, prepare, administer, and dispose of drug.
• Advise patient to immediately report signs or symptoms of serious allergic reaction and any adverse reactions.

SAFETY ALERT!

exenatide
eks-EHN-uh-tyde

Bydureon, Byetta

Therapeutic class: Antidiabetics
Pharmacologic class: Incretin mimetics

AVAILABLE FORMS
Injection: 5 mcg/dose in 1.2-mL prefilled pen (60 doses); 10 mcg/dose in 2.4-mL prefilled pen (60 doses)
Injection (extended-release): 2 mg/dose in single-use vial, 2 mg/dose in single-dose pen

INDICATIONS & DOSAGES
➤ **Adjunct to diet and exercise to improve glycemic control in patients with type 2 diabetes**
Adults: 5 mcg subcutaneously b.i.d. within 60 minutes before morning and evening meals. If needed, increase to 10 mcg b.i.d. after 1 month. Or, 2 mg (extended-release) subcutaneously every 7 days.
Adjust-a-dose: Use caution when escalating doses of Byetta (injection) from 5 to 10 mcg in patients with moderate renal impairment (CrCl of 50 to 80 mL/minute). Bydureon and Byetta aren't recommended for patients with ESRD or severe renal impairment (CrCl of less than 30 mL/minute).

When converting from Byetta immediate-release to Bydureon extended-release formulation, initiate weekly administration of exenatide ER the day after discontinuing exenatide immediate-release. Patient may experience increased blood glucose levels for approximately 2 weeks after conversion. Pretreatment with exenatide immediate-release isn't required when initiating exenatide ER.

ADMINISTRATION
Subcutaneous
🕘 *Alert:* Multidose pens are for single patient use only. Pens should never be shared even if the needle is changed. Clearly label with patient identifying information where it will not obstruct the dosing window, warning, or other product information.
Bydureon
• Give Bydureon at any time during the day and without regard to meals.
• To administer: Attach vial connector to vial.
— Connect prefilled diluent syringe to vial.
— Push on syringe's plunger to inject diluent into vial. Continue to push on plunger while shaking vial to thoroughly mix powder and diluent. Solution will be cloudy.
— Invert vial and withdraw solution to the black-dashed dose line on syringe.
— Remove vial connector and attach needle.
— Give immediately as a subcutaneous injection in the thigh, abdomen, or back of upper arm. Rotate injection sites each week.
• Store in refrigerator at 36° to 46° F (2° to 8° C). May store at room temperature (68° to 77° F [20° to 25° C]) for up to 4 weeks. Don't freeze, and don't use drug if it has been frozen. Protect from light.
Byetta
• Drug comes in two strengths; check cartridge carefully before use.
• Don't give after a meal.
• Give as a subcutaneous injection in the thigh, abdomen, or upper arm.
• Before first use, store drug in refrigerator at 36° to 46° F (2° to 8° C). After first use, drug can be kept at room temperature up to 77° F (25° C). Don't freeze, and don't use drug if it has been frozen. Protect drug from light. Discard pen 30 days after first use, even if some drug remains.
• Don't mix with insulin.

ACTION
Reduces fasting and postprandial glucose levels in type 2 diabetes by stimulating insulin production in response to elevated glucose levels, inhibiting glucagon release after meals, and slowing gastric emptying.

Route	Onset	Peak	Duration
Subcut.	Unknown	2 hr	Unknown
Subcut. (extended-release)	Unknown	2 wk, 6–7 wk	10 wk

Half-life: 2½ hours; extended-release, unknown.

ADVERSE REACTIONS
CNS: dizziness, headache, fatigue, jittery feeling, nervousness, weakness.
GI: anorexia, constipation, decreased appetite, diarrhea, dyspepsia, nausea, *pancreatitis,* vomiting, GERD.
Metabolic: *hypoglycemia.*
Skin: excessive sweating.

INTERACTIONS
Drug-drug. *Acetaminophen:* May decrease acetaminophen concentration. Give acetaminophen at least 1 hour before or 4 hours after exenatide injection.
Digoxin, lisinopril, lovastatin: May decrease concentrations of these drugs. Monitor patient.
Drugs that are rapidly absorbed: May slow gastric emptying and reduce absorption of some oral drugs. Separate administration by 1 hour.
Oral drugs that need to maintain a threshold concentration to maintain effectiveness (antibiotics, hormonal contraceptives): May reduce rate and extent of absorption of these drugs. Give these drugs at least 1 hour before giving exenatide.
Other antidiabetic agents (insulin, meglitinides [repaglinide]): May increase risk of hypoglycemia. Closely monitor blood glucose concentrations when exenatide is started or stopped, and reinforce patient instructions for hypoglycemia management, especially in patients receiving insulin.
Sulfonylureas: May increase the risk of hypoglycemia. Reduce sulfonylurea dose as needed, and monitor patient closely.
Warfarin: May increase INR and increase bleeding risk when administered together. Monitor INR frequently, especially when starting drug or changing dosage.

EFFECTS ON LAB TEST RESULTS
• May increase INR.

CONTRAINDICATIONS & CAUTIONS

Black Box Warning Extended-release form is contraindicated in patients with personal or family history of medullary thyroid carcinoma and in patients with multiple endocrine neoplasia syndrome type 2. ∎

● Contraindicated in patients hypersensitive to drug or its components. Serious reactions (anaphylaxis, angioedema) have been reported. If hypersensitivity occurs, discontinue drug.

● Drug has been associated with acute pancreatitis, including fatal and nonfatal hemorrhagic or necrotizing pancreatitis. Discontinue immediately if pancreatitis is suspected. Don't restart if pancreatitis is confirmed.

● Don't use in patients with type 1 diabetes or diabetic ketoacidosis.

● Don't use in patients with ESRD, CrCl less than 30 mL/minute, or severe GI disease (including gastroparesis).

● Use cautiously in patients with renal transplant.

Dialyzable drug: Unknown.

⚠ *Overdose S&S:* Severe nausea, severe vomiting, hypoglycemia.

PREGNANCY-LACTATION-REPRODUCTION

● Use only if potential benefit justifies potential risk to the fetus.

● Prescribers are encouraged to register patients in the Exenatide Pregnancy Registry by calling 1-800-633-9081.

● It isn't known if drug appears in breast milk. Patient should discontinue breastfeeding or discontinue drug.

NURSING CONSIDERATIONS

● Assess GI and renal function before and during treatment.

⊙ *Alert:* Drug-related nausea, vomiting, and diarrhea resulting in dehydration have led to increased serum creatinine levels and acute renal failure.

● Monitor patient receiving Bydureon for serious injection-site reactions, such as abscess, cellulitis, and necrosis, with or without subcutaneous nodules.

● Monitor glucose level regularly and HbA_{1c} level periodically.

⊙ *Alert:* Stop drug if pancreatitis is suspected. Initiate appropriate treatment and

monitor patient carefully. Drug shouldn't be readministered.

● *Look alike–sound alike:* Don't confuse exenatide with ezetimibe.

PATIENT TEACHING

Black Box Warning Explain to patient taking Bydureon the risk and signs and symptoms of thyroid tumors. ∎

● Explain the risks of drug.

● Review proper use and storage of medication, particularly the one-time setup for each new pen or reconstitution procedure for powder.

● Inform patient that prefilled pen doesn't include a needle; the prescriber will indicate which needle length and gauge is appropriate.

● Instruct patient to inject Byetta in the thigh, abdomen, or upper arm within 60 minutes before morning and evening meals. Caution against injecting drug after a meal.

● Instruct patient to inject Bydureon in the thigh, abdomen, or back of upper arm immediately after mixing with diluent.

⊙ *Alert:* Warn patient not to share the multidose pen device with other people, even if the needle is changed due to the risk of transmission of blood-borne pathogens, including HIV and hepatitis viruses.

● Advise patient that drug may decrease appetite, food intake, and body weight, and that these changes don't warrant a change in dosage.

● Advise patient to seek immediate medical care if unexplained, persistent, severe abdominal pain, with or without vomiting, occurs.

● Inform patient receiving Bydureon about risk of serious injection-site reactions and to report signs and symptoms (erythema, pain, drainage, skin color changes) immediately.

● Review steps for managing hypoglycemia, especially if patient takes a sulfonylurea or insulin.

● Inform patient of potential risk of worsening renal function and signs and symptoms of renal dysfunction.

● Tell patient changing from Byetta to Bydureon that transient blood glucose elevations are possible during the first 2 weeks of therapy.

• Stress importance of proper storage (refrigeration), infection prevention, and timing of exenatide dose in relation to other oral drugs.

• Tell patient that if a dose of Byetta is missed to resume treatment as prescribed with the next scheduled dose.

• Tell patient that if a dose of Bydureon is missed to administer it as soon as noticed, provided the next regularly scheduled dose is due at least 3 days later, and then to resume once-every-7-days dosing schedule. If a dose is missed and the next regularly scheduled dose is due in 1 to 2 days, tell patient not to administer the missed dose and instead to resume therapy with next regularly scheduled dose.

ezetimibe
ee-ZET-ah-mibe

Zetia✔

Therapeutic class: Antilipemics
Pharmacologic class: Selective cholesterol absorption inhibitors

AVAILABLE FORMS
Tablets: 10 mg

INDICATIONS & DOSAGES
➤ **Adjunct to diet and exercise to reduce total cholesterol, LDL cholesterol (LDL-C), and apolipoprotein B (apo B) levels in patients with primary hypercholesterolemia, alone or combined with HMG-CoA reductase inhibitors (statins); adjunct to other lipid-lowering drugs (combined with atorvastatin or simvastatin) to reduce total cholesterol, and LDL-C levels in patients with homozygous familial hypercholesterolemia; adjunct to diet in patients with homozygous sitosterolemia to reduce sitosterol and campesterol levels; adjunct to fenofibrate and diet to reduce total cholesterol, LDL-C, apo B, and non-HDL-C levels in patients with mixed hyperlipidemia**
Adults and children age 10 and older: 10 mg P.O. daily.

ADMINISTRATION
P.O.
• Give drug without regard for meals.
• May give dose at same time as an HMG-CoA reductase inhibitor or fenofibrate.
• Give at least 2 hours before or at least 4 hours after administration of a bile acid sequestrant.

ACTION
Inhibits absorption of cholesterol by the small intestine, unlike other drugs used for cholesterol reduction; causes reduced hepatic cholesterol stores and increased cholesterol clearance from the blood.

Route	Onset	Peak	Duration
P.O.	Unknown	4–12 hr	Unknown

Half-life: 22 hours.

ADVERSE REACTIONS
CNS: dizziness, fatigue.
EENT: nasopharyngitis, sinusitis.
GI: diarrhea.
Musculoskeletal: arthralgia, back pain, pain in extremity, myalgia.
Respiratory: URI.
Other: viral infection.

INTERACTIONS
Drug-drug. *Bile acid sequestrant (cholestyramine):* May decrease ezetimibe level. Give ezetimibe at least 2 hours before or 4 hours after cholestyramine.
Cyclosporine, fenofibrate: May increase ezetimibe level. Monitor patient for adverse reactions.
Fibrates: May increase excretion of cholesterol into the gallbladder bile. Avoid using together.
Gemfibrozil: May increase risk of myopathy and cholelithiasis. Avoid use together.

EFFECTS ON LAB TEST RESULTS
• May increase LFT values.

CONTRAINDICATIONS & CAUTIONS
• Contraindicated in patients hypersensitive to components of drug.
• Contraindicated in combination with HMG-CoA reductase inhibitors in patients with active liver disease or unexplained increased transaminase levels.

• Rarely, myopathy, including rhabdomyolysis, has been reported. Risk may increase with concurrent use of statin or fibrate drugs. Discontinue ezetimibe and statin or fibrate immediately if myopathy is suspected or confirmed.

Dialyzable drug: Unknown.

PREGNANCY-LACTATION-REPRODUCTION
• Use only if potential benefit justifies potential risk to the fetus.
• When drug is used with a statin in a woman of childbearing potential, refer to pregnancy information and product labeling for the statin. All statins are contraindicated in pregnant and breast-feeding women.
• It isn't known if drug appears in breast milk. Use drug only if potential benefit justifies potential risk to the infant.

NURSING CONSIDERATIONS
• Before starting treatment, assess patient for underlying causes of dyslipidemia.
• Obtain baseline triglyceride and total cholesterol, LDL-C, and HDL-C levels.
• Using drug with an HMG-CoA reductase inhibitor significantly decreases total cholesterol and LDL-C, apo B, and triglyceride levels and (except with pravastatin) increases HDL-C level more than use of an HMG-CoA reductase inhibitor alone. Check LFT values when therapy starts and thereafter according to the HMG-CoA reductase inhibitor manufacturer's recommendations.
• Patient should maintain a cholesterol-lowering diet during treatment.
• Monitor patient for muscle pain, weakness, or tenderness. Discontinue drug if signs or symptoms of myopathy occur with CK more than $10 \times$ ULN.

PATIENT TEACHING
• Emphasize importance of following a cholesterol-lowering diet during drug therapy.
• Tell patient he may take drug without regard for meals.
• Advise patient to notify prescriber of unexplained muscle pain, weakness, or tenderness.
• Urge patient to tell prescriber about any herbal or dietary supplements he's taking.
• Advise patient to visit prescriber for routine follow-ups and blood tests.
• Tell woman to notify prescriber if she becomes pregnant.

ezogabine
e-ZOG-a-been

Potiga

Therapeutic class: Anticonvulsants
Pharmacologic class: Potassium channel activators
Controlled substance schedule: V

AVAILABLE FORMS
Tablets ⊙: 50 mg, 200 mg, 300 mg, 400 mg

INDICATIONS & DOSAGES
➤ **Adjunctive treatment of partial-onset seizures in patients who have responded inadequately to several alternative treatments and for whom benefits outweigh risk of retinal abnormalities and potential decline in visual acuity**
Adults: 100 mg P.O. t.i.d. in equally divided doses. Increase at weekly intervals by no more than 50 mg t.i.d. Maximum dosage is 400 mg P.O. t.i.d.

Adjust-a-dose: For patients older than age 65 and those with hepatic impairment (Child-Pugh score between 7 and 9), initially give 50 mg P.O. t.i.d.; may increase dosage at weekly intervals by no more than 50 mg P.O. t.i.d. to a maximum of 250 mg P.O. t.i.d. For patients with CrCl of less than 50 mL/minute, ESRD requiring hemodialysis, or severe hepatic impairment (Child-Pugh score greater than 9), initially give 50 mg P.O. t.i.d. May increase dosage at weekly intervals by no more than 50 mg P.O. t.i.d. to a maximum of 200 mg P.O. t.i.d.

ADMINISTRATION
P.O.
• May give with or without food.
• Patient should swallow tablets whole. Don't crush, dissolve, or allow patient to chew them.

Reactions in bold italics are *life-threatening*. Interactions may have a *rapid onset* or a *delayed onset*.

ACTION

Unknown. Thought to activate potassium channels, which stabilize the resting membrane potential and reduce brain excitability.

Route	Onset	Peak	Duration
P.O.	Rapid	½-2 hr	Unknown

Half-life: 7 to 11 hours.

ADVERSE REACTIONS

CNS: fatigue, dizziness, somnolence, tremor, abnormal coordination, confusion, aphasia, dysarthria, vertigo, asthenia, impaired memory, paresthesia, amnesia, anxiety, disorientation, psychosis, hallucinations, *suicidal thoughts or behaviors,* worsening depression, *withdrawal seizures;* disturbance in attention, gait, or balance.
CV: *QT-interval prolongation.*
EENT: diplopia, blurred vision.
GI: nausea, constipation, dyspepsia, dysphagia.
GU: dysuria, urinary hesitation, urine retention, hematuria, chromaturia.
Metabolic: weight gain.
Other: influenza.

INTERACTIONS

Drug-drug. *Antiarrhythmics (disopyramide, dofetilide, procainamide, quinidine, sotalol), arsenic trioxide, chlorpromazine, citalopram, clarithromycin, dolasetron, droperidol, erythromycin, fluoxetine, levofloxacin, mesoridazine, moxifloxacin, pentamidine, pimozide, QT-interval prolonging agents, thioridazine, ziprasidone:* May additively increase risk of QT-interval prolongation. Coadminister with caution. *Carbamazepine, phenytoin:* May decrease ezogabine level. Consider increasing ezogabine dosage.
Digoxin: May inhibit renal clearance of digoxin, increasing digoxin level. Monitor digoxin level closely.
Drug-lifestyle. *Alcohol use:* May increase ezogabine level and risk of adverse effects. Use together cautiously, if at all.

EFFECTS ON LAB TEST RESULTS

● May cause falsely elevated serum and urine bilirubin levels.

CONTRAINDICATIONS & CAUTIONS

● Contraindicated in patients hypersensitive to drug.
Black Box Warning Drug may cause retinal abnormalities that result in damage to photoreceptors and vision loss. Rate of progression of these abnormalities and their reversibility are unknown. Some patients have developed abnormal visual acuity; however, it isn't possible to determine whether ezogabine was responsible for the changes. Discontinue drug if retinal pigmentary abnormalities or vision changes are detected unless no other suitable treatment options are available and benefits of treatment outweigh potential risk of vision loss. Discontinue drug if patient fails to show substantial clinical benefit after adequate titration. ■
● If drug is discontinued, gradually reduce dosage over at least 3 weeks unless safety concerns require abrupt withdrawal.
● Use cautiously in patients with increased risk of urine retention, such as those with BPH, those unable to communicate symptoms, and those who use medications such as anticholinergics that affect voiding.
● Use cautiously in patients with prolonged QT interval, HF, ventricular hypertrophy, hypokalemia, or hypomagnesemia, and in those who are taking other drugs known to prolong QT interval.
● Use cautiously in patients with hepatic or renal insufficiency.
Dialyzable drug: Unknown.
⚠ Overdose S&S: Agitation, aggressive behavior, irritability, cardiac arrhythmia.

PREGNANCY-LACTATION-REPRODUCTION

● Use in pregnant women only if benefits outweigh potential risk to the fetus.
● Encourage patients to enroll in the North American Antiepileptic Drug Pregnancy Registry (1-888-233-2334 or www.aedpregnancyregistry.org).
● Because of the potential for serious adverse reactions in breast-feeding infants, patient should discontinue breast-feeding or discontinue drug.

E

NURSING CONSIDERATIONS

- Avoid stopping drug abruptly. Gradually reduce dosage over at least 3 weeks, unless safety concerns require abrupt withdrawal.
- May cause blue skin discoloration, which should prompt consideration of alternative treatment.

Black Box Warning Obtain eye examination by ophthalmic professional at baseline and periodically (every 6 months) during therapy that includes visual acuity and dilated fundus photography. ■

- Monitor patient for urine retention, weak urine stream, or pain on urination.
- Monitor patient for confusion, psychosis, hallucinations, dizziness, and somnolence.
- Monitor QT interval in patients with known prolonged QT interval, HF, ventricular hypertrophy, hypokalemia, or hypomagnesemia, or when patient is taking other drugs known to prolong the QT interval.
- Monitor patient for warning signs and symptoms of suicidal thoughts or behaviors, such as worsening depression or unusual changes in mood or behavior.

PATIENT TEACHING

Black Box Warning Warn patient to contact health care provider immediately if changes in vision occur. ■

- Tell patient to report discoloration of the skin, including lips and nail beds.
- Warn patient not to stop drug without first consulting health care provider, because seizures may worsen. Patient should contact prescriber if more than one dose is missed.
- Advise patient to report signs and symptoms of urine retention (bloating, bladder discomfort), weakening of urine stream, or painful urination.
- Warn patient not to drive, operate machinery, or perform other dangerous activities until the effects of ezogabine are known.
- **⊙ Alert:** Inform patient, caregivers, and family about the risk of confusion, psychosis, hallucinations, and suicidal thoughts and behavior. Caution them to immediately report changes in behavior to prescriber.
- Caution patient that drug can lead to abuse or dependence. Discuss careful follow-up with prescriber and need to protect drug from theft; discourage patient from giving drug to anyone else.

famciclovir
fam-SYE-kloe-vir

Famvir✷

Therapeutic class: Antivirals
Pharmacologic class: Nucleosides–nucleotides

AVAILABLE FORMS
Tablets: 125 mg, 250 mg, 500 mg

INDICATIONS & DOSAGES

➤ **Acute herpes zoster infection (shingles)**
Adults: 500 mg P.O. every 8 hours for 7 days.
Adjust-a-dose: For patients with CrCl of 40 to 59 mL/minute, give 500 mg P.O. every 12 hours; if CrCl is 20 to 39 mL/minute, give 500 mg P.O. every 24 hours; if CrCl is less than 20 mL/minute, give 250 mg P.O. every 24 hours. For hemodialysis patients, give 250 mg P.O. after each hemodialysis session.

➤ **Recurrent genital herpes**
Adults: 1,000 mg P.O. b.i.d. for a single day. Begin therapy at the first sign or symptom.
Adjust-a-dose: For patients with CrCl of 40 to 59 mL/minute, give 500 mg every 12 hours for 1 day; for CrCl of 20 to 39 mL/minute, give 500 mg P.O. as a single dose; if CrCl is less than 20 mL/minute, give 250 mg as a single dose. For hemodialysis patient, give 250 mg single dose after hemodialysis session.

➤ **Suppression of recurrent genital herpes**
Adults: 250 mg P.O. b.i.d. for up to 1 year.
Adjust-a-dose: For patients with CrCl of 20 to 39 mL/minute, give 125 mg P.O. every 12 hours; if CrCl is less than 20 mL/minute, give 125 mg P.O. every 24 hours. For hemodialysis patients, give 125 mg P.O. after each hemodialysis session.

➤ **Recurrent mucocutaneous herpes simplex infections in HIV-infected patients**
Adults: 500 mg P.O. b.i.d. for 7 days.
Adjust-a-dose: For patients with CrCl of 20 to 39 mL/minute, give 500 mg P.O.

every 24 hours; if CrCl is less than
20 mL/minute, give 250 mg P.O. every
24 hours. For hemodialysis patients, give
250 mg P.O. after each hemodialysis
session.
➤ **Recurrent herpes labialis (cold sores)**
Adults: 1,500 mg P.O. for one dose. Give at
the first sign or symptom of cold sore.
Adjust-a-dose: For patients with CrCl of
40 to 59 mL/minute, give 750 mg as a single
dose; for CrCl of 20 to 39 mL/minute, give
500 mg P.O. as a single dose; if CrCl is less
than 20 mL/minute, give 250 mg as a single
dose. For hemodialysis patient, give 250 mg
single dose after hemodialysis session.

ADMINISTRATION
P.O.
● Give drug without regard for meals.

ACTION
A guanosine nucleoside that is converted
to penciclovir, which enters viral cells and
inhibits DNA polymerase and viral DNA
synthesis.

Route	Onset	Peak	Duration
P.O.	Unknown	1 hr	Unknown

Half-life: 2 to 3 hours.

ADVERSE REACTIONS
CNS: headache, fatigue, dizziness, pares-
thesia, somnolence.
GI: nausea, abdominal pain, diarrhea,
vomiting, flatulence.
GU: dysmenorrhea.
Skin: pruritus, rash.
Other: zoster-related signs, symptoms, and
complications.

INTERACTIONS
Drug-drug. *Probenecid:* May increase
level of penciclovir, the active metabolite of
famciclovir. Monitor patient for increased
adverse reactions.
*Varicella virus vaccine, zoster vaccine
(live, attenuated):* May diminish effect
of vaccines. When possible, discontinue
famciclovir for at least 24 hours before and
14 days after vaccinations.

EFFECTS ON LAB TEST RESULTS
None reported.

CONTRAINDICATIONS & CAUTIONS
● Contraindicated in patients hypersensitive
to drug.
● Use cautiously in patients with renal or
hepatic impairment and in elderly patients.
Dialyzable drug: Yes.

PREGNANCY-LACTATION-REPRODUCTION
● Use drug during pregnancy only if benefit
clearly outweighs potential risk to the fetus.
● Women exposed to drug during pregnancy
should be enrolled in the Famvir Pregnancy
Reporting system (1-888-669-6682).
● It isn't known if drug appears in breast
milk. Use only if benefits outweigh risk to
the infant.

NURSING CONSIDERATIONS
● In patients with renal or hepatic impair-
ment, adjust dosage as needed.
● Monitor LFTs and renal function tests.

PATIENT TEACHING
● Inform patient that drug doesn't cure
genital herpes but can decrease the duration
and severity of symptoms.
● Teach patient how to avoid spreading
infection to others.
● Urge patient to recognize the early signs
and symptoms of herpes infection, such
as tingling, itching, and pain, and to report
them. Therapy is more effective if started
within 48 hours of rash onset.
● Drug may contain lactose. If patient is
lactose-intolerant, advise patient to notify
prescriber before taking drug.

famotidine
fa-MOE-ti-deen

Pepcid✿, Pepcid AC ◇

Therapeutic class: Antiulcer drugs
Pharmacologic class: H_2-receptor
antagonists

AVAILABLE FORMS
Injection: 0.4 mg/mL in NSS (premixed),
10 mg/mL
Powder for oral suspension: 40 mg/5 mL
after reconstitution
Tablets: 10 mg ◇, 20 mg ◇, 40 mg
Tablets (chewable): 10 mg ◇, 20 mg ◇

INDICATIONS & DOSAGES
Adjust-a-dose (for all indications): For patients with CrCl below 50 mL/minute, give half the dose, or increase dosing interval to every 36 to 48 hours.

➤ **Short-term treatment for duodenal ulcer**
Adults: For acute therapy, 40 mg P.O. once daily at bedtime or 20 mg P.O. b.i.d. Healing usually occurs within 4 weeks. For maintenance therapy, 20 mg P.O. once daily at bedtime.

➤ **Short-term treatment for benign gastric ulcer**
Adults: 40 mg P.O. daily at bedtime or 20 mg P.O. b.i.d. for 8 weeks.
Children ages 1 to 16: 0.5 mg/kg/day P.O. at bedtime or in two divided doses, up to 40 mg daily.

➤ **Pathologic hypersecretory conditions (such as Zollinger-Ellison syndrome)**
Adults: 20 mg P.O. every 6 hours, up to 160 mg every 6 hours. Maximum, 640 mg/day.

➤ **Hospitalized patients who can't take oral drug or who have intractable ulcers or hypersecretory conditions**
Adults: 20 mg I.V. every 12 hours.

➤ **GERD**
Adults: 20 mg P.O. b.i.d. for up to 6 weeks. For esophagitis caused by GERD, 20 to 40 mg b.i.d. for up to 12 weeks.
Children ages 1 to 16: 1 mg/kg/day P.O. in two divided doses up to 40 mg b.i.d.
Children ages 3 months to younger than 1 year: 0.5 mg/kg/dose oral suspension b.i.d. for up to 8 weeks.
Children younger than age 3 months: 0.5 mg/kg/dose oral suspension once daily for up to 8 weeks.

➤ **To prevent or treat heartburn**
Adults: 10 mg Pepcid AC P.O. 1 hour before meals to prevent symptoms, or 10 mg Pepcid AC P.O. with water when symptoms occur. Maximum daily dose is 20 mg. Drug shouldn't be taken daily for longer than 2 weeks.

➤ **Stress ulcer prevention in certain populations (such as general intensive-care patients and head and thermal injury patients)** ◆
Adults: 20 mg P.O. b.i.d. via NG tube. Or, 20 mg I.V. b.i.d. or 1.7 mg/hour by continuous I.V. infusion.

Adjust-a-dose: For patients with CrCl of less than 30 mL/minute, give 20 mg P.O. once daily via NG tube. Or, 20 mg I.V. b.i.d. or 0.85 mg/hour by continuous I.V. infusion.

ADMINISTRATION
P.O.
● Reconstitute and shake oral suspension before use.
● Store reconstituted oral suspension below 86° F (30° C). Discard after 30 days.
I.V.
▼ Compatible solutions include sterile water for injection, NSS for injection, D_5W or dextrose 10% in water for injection, 5% sodium bicarbonate injection, and lactated Ringer injection. Drug also can be added to total parenteral nutrition solutions.
▼ For direct injection, dilute 2 mL (20 mg) with compatible solution to a total volume of either 5 or 10 mL. Inject over at least 2 minutes.
▼ For intermittent infusion, dilute 20 mg (2 mL) in 100-mL compatible solution. The premixed 50-mL solution doesn't need further dilution. Infuse over 15 to 30 minutes.
▼ After dilution, solution is stable 48 hours at 36° to 46° F (2° to 8° C).
▼ **Incompatibilities:** Amphotericin B cholesteryl sulfate complex, azithromycin, cefepime, lansoprazole, pantoprazole, piperacillin–tazobactam, trimethoprim–sulfamethoxazole.

ACTION
Competitively inhibits action of histamine on the H_2-receptor sites of parietal cells, decreasing gastric acid secretion.

Route	Onset	Peak	Duration
P.O.	1 hr	1–3 hr	10–20 hr
I.V.	1 hr	1–4 hr	10–20 hr

Half-life: 2½ to 3½ hours.

ADVERSE REACTIONS
CNS: headache, dizziness.
GI: constipation, diarrhea.

INTERACTIONS
None significant.

EFFECTS ON LAB TEST RESULTS
• May increase BUN, creatinine, and liver enzyme levels.
• May cause false-negative results in skin tests using allergen extracts. May antagonize pentagastrin in gastric acid secretion tests.

CONTRAINDICATIONS & CAUTIONS
• Contraindicated in patients hypersensitive to drug or its components.
• Drug may cause reversible confusional states that clear within 3 to 4 days after discontinuation. Patients older than age 50 and those with renal or hepatic impairment may be more at risk.
• **Alert:** QT-interval prolongation and torsades de pointes have been reported in patients with renal dysfunction.
• Treatment lasting 2 years can cause vitamin B_{12} deficiency, which is dose-related and more likely to occur in women and those younger than age 30.
• **Alert:** Some forms may contain benzyl alcohol, which is linked to "gasping syndrome" (metabolic acidosis, respiratory distress, CNS dysfunction, hypotension, CV collapse) in neonates.
Dializable drug: No.

PREGNANCY-LACTATION-REPRODUCTION
• Drug crosses placental barrier and appears in breast milk. Use cautiously in pregnant and breast-feeding women.

NURSING CONSIDERATIONS
• Assess patient for abdominal pain.
• Look for blood in emesis, stool, or gastric aspirate.
• Monitor patients with renal dysfunction for QT-interval prolongation.

PATIENT TEACHING
• Instruct patient in proper use of OTC product, if appropriate.
• Warn patient with phenylketonuria that Pepcid AC chewable tablets contain phenylalanine.
• Tell patient to take prescription drug with snack, if desired.
  Advise patient to limit use of prescription drug to no longer than 8 weeks, unless ordered by prescriber, and OTC drug to no longer than 2 weeks.

• With prescriber's knowledge, let patient take antacids together, especially at beginning of therapy when pain is severe.
• Urge patient to avoid cigarette smoking because it may increase gastric acid secretion and worsen disease.
• Advise patient to report abdominal pain, blood in stools or vomit, black tarry stools, or coffee-ground emesis.

F

febuxostat
feb-UX-oh-stat

Uloric

Therapeutic class: Antigout drugs
Pharmacologic class: Xanthine oxidase inhibitors

AVAILABLE FORMS
Tablets: 40 mg, 80 mg

INDICATIONS & DOSAGES
➤ **Hyperuricemia associated with gout**
Adults: 40 mg P.O. daily. May increase dosage to 80 mg after 2 weeks if uric acid level remains above 6 mg/dL.

ADMINISTRATION
P.O.
• Give drug without regard to food or antacid use.

ACTION
Reduces uric acid production by inhibiting xanthine oxidase.

Route	Onset	Peak	Duration
P.O.	Rapid	1–1½ hr	Unknown

Half-life: 5 to 8 hours.

ADVERSE REACTIONS
CNS: dizziness.
GI: nausea.
Hepatic: liver function abnormalities.
Musculoskeletal: arthralgia.
Skin: rash.

INTERACTIONS
Drug-drug. *Azathioprine, didanosine, mercaptopurine:* May increase levels of these drugs, leading to toxicity. Use together is contraindicated.

Pegloticase: May increase toxic effects of pegloticase. Avoid use together.
Theophylline: May increase theophylline level. Use cautiously together.

EFFECTS ON LAB TEST RESULTS
● May increase alkaline phosphatase, AST, and ALT levels.

CONTRAINDICATIONS & CAUTIONS
● Contraindicated in patients hypersensitive to drug or its components and in those taking azathioprine, mercaptopurine, or didanosine.
● Use cautiously in patients with severe hepatic impairment (Child-Pugh class C) or renal impairment (CrCl of less than 30 mL/minute).
● Safety and effectiveness in children haven't been established.
Dialyzable drug: Unknown.

PREGNANCY-LACTATION-REPRODUCTION
● It isn't known if drug crosses the placental barrier. Use during pregnancy only if potential benefit justifies potential risk to the fetus.
● It isn't known if drug appears in breast milk. Use cautiously in breast-feeding women.

NURSING CONSIDERATIONS
● Acute gout flares may occur during first 6 weeks of therapy; colchicine or another anti-inflammatory may be added prophylactically and drug should be continued.
● Monitor hepatic function at baseline, 2 months and 4 months after starting therapy, and periodically thereafter.
❸ Alert: Patients with unexplained serum ALT level greater than 3 × ULN with total bilirubin level greater than 2 × ULN are at risk for severe drug-induced liver injury. Stop drug in these patients and don't restart.
● Monitor uric acid level.
● Patient taking drug may be at risk for thromboembolic events, such as MI and stroke. Monitor patient closely.

PATIENT TEACHING
● Warn patient about the risk of gout flares and the importance of taking an NSAID or colchicine during the first 6 weeks of treatment.

● Inform patient that drug may increase risk of MI or stroke. Advise patient to report all adverse reactions, including abnormal bleeding, nausea, malaise, light-colored stools, yellowing of eyes or skin, rash, chest pain, dyspnea, or neurologic symptoms of a stroke.

felodipine
fe-LOE-di-peen

Plendil✦

Therapeutic class: Antihypertensives
Pharmacologic class: Calcium channel blockers

AVAILABLE FORMS
Tablets (extended-release) **OTC**: 2.5 mg, 5 mg, 10 mg

INDICATIONS & DOSAGES
➤ **Hypertension**
Adults: Initially, 5 mg P.O. daily. Adjust dosage based on patient response, usually at intervals of not less than 2 weeks. Usual dosage is 2.5 to 10 mg daily; maximum dosage is 10 mg daily.
Elderly patients: 2.5 mg P.O. daily; adjust dosage as for adults. Maximum dosage is 10 mg daily.
Adjust-a-dose: Patients with impaired hepatic function may respond to lower doses. Monitor BP during dosage adjustments.

ADMINISTRATION
P.O.
● Give drug whole; don't crush or cut tablets.
● Give drug without food or with a light meal.
● Don't give drug with grapefruit juice.

ACTION
A dihydropyridine-derivative calcium channel blocker that prevents entry of calcium ions into vascular smooth muscle and cardiac cells; shows some selectivity for smooth muscle compared with cardiac muscle.

Route	Onset	Peak	Duration
P.O.	2–5 hr	2½–5 hr	24 hr

Half-life: 11 to 16 hours.

Reactions in bold italics are *life-threatening*. Interactions may have a *rapid onset* or a ***delayed onset***.

ADVERSE REACTIONS
CNS: headache, dizziness, paresthesia, asthenia.
CV: peripheral edema, chest pain, palpitations, flushing.
EENT: rhinorrhea, pharyngitis.
GI: abdominal pain, nausea, constipation, diarrhea, dyspepsia.
Musculoskeletal: muscle cramps, back pain.
Respiratory: URI, cough, sneezing.
Skin: rash.

INTERACTIONS
Drug-drug. *Anticonvulsants:* May decrease felodipine level. Avoid using together.
Antipsychotics (atypical): May enhance hypotensive effects. Monitor therapy.
CYP3A4 inhibitors (such as azole antifungals, cimetidine, erythromycin): May decrease clearance of felodipine. Reduce doses of felodipine; monitor patient for toxicity.
Metoprolol: May alter pharmacokinetics of metoprolol. Monitor patient for adverse reactions.
NSAIDs: May decrease antihypertensive effects. Monitor BP.
Tacrolimus: May increase tacrolimus level. Monitor patient closely.
Drug-herb. *Ma huang:* May decrease antihypertensive effects. Discourage use together.
Drug-food. *Grapefruit, lime:* May increase drug level and adverse effects. Discourage use together.

EFFECTS ON LAB TEST RESULTS
None reported.

CONTRAINDICATIONS & CAUTIONS
● Contraindicated in patients hypersensitive to drug.
● Drug may cause significant hypotension and rarely syncope.
● Safe use in patients with HF hasn't been established.
Dialyzable drug: Unknown.
⚠ *Overdose S&S:* Peripheral vasodilation, hypotension, bradycardia.

PREGNANCY-LACTATION-REPRODUCTION
● There are no well-controlled studies in pregnant women, but animal studies show potential fetal hazards.
● It isn't known if drug appears in breast milk. Patient should discontinue breast-feeding or discontinue drug.

NURSING CONSIDERATIONS
● Monitor BP for response.
● Monitor patient for peripheral edema, which appears to be both dose- and age-related. It's more common in patients taking higher doses, especially those older than age 60.

PATIENT TEACHING
● Tell patient to swallow tablets whole and not to crush or chew them.
● Tell patient to take drug without food or with a light meal.
● Advise patient not to take drug with grapefruit juice.
● Advise patient to continue taking drug even when he feels better, to watch his diet, and to check with prescriber or pharmacist before taking other drugs, including OTC drugs, nutritional supplements, or herbal remedies.
● Teach patient to report all adverse reactions.
● Advise patient to observe good oral hygiene and to see a dentist regularly; use of drug may cause mild gum problems.

---

fenofibrate
fee-no-FYE-brate

Antara, Fenoglide, Lipofen, TriCor✐, Triglide

fenofibrate (choline)
Trilipix

fenofibric acid
Fibricor

Therapeutic class: Antilipemics
Pharmacologic class: Fibric acid derivatives

AVAILABLE FORMS
fenofibrate
Capsules ⓓⓝⓒ: 50 mg, 150 mg

Capsules (micronized) ⓄⒸ: 30 mg, 43 mg, 67 mg, 90 mg, 130 mg, 134 mg, 200 mg
Tablets ⓄⒸ: 40 mg, 48 mg, 54 mg, 107 mg, 120 mg, 145 mg, 160 mg
fenofibrate (choline)
Capsules (delayed-release) ⓄⒸ: 45 mg, 135 mg
fenofibric acid
Tablets: 35 mg, 105 mg

INDICATIONS & DOSAGES
Adjust-a-dose (for all indications): In patients with CrCl less than 50 mL/minute or in elderly patients, initially 30 mg daily for Antara or Fibricor, 40 mg/day for Fenoglide, 50 mg daily for Lipofen, 48 mg daily for TriCor, or 45 mg once daily for Trilipix. Increase only after evaluating effects on renal function and triglyceride level at this dose.

➤ **Hypertriglyceridemia (Fredrickson types IV and V hyperlipidemia) in patients who don't respond adequately to diet alone**
Adults: For Antara, initial dose is 30 to 90 mg P.O. daily, with maximum dose of 90 mg daily. For Fibricor, initial dose is 35 to 105 mg daily, with maximum dose of 105 mg daily. For Fenoglide, initial dose is 40 to 120 mg/day, with maximum dose of 120 mg daily. For Lipofen, initial dose is 50 to 150 mg daily, with maximum dose of 150 mg daily. For TriCor, initial dose is 48 to 145 mg daily, with maximum dose of 145 mg daily. For Triglide, initial dose is 160 mg daily, with maximum dose of 160 mg daily. For Trilipix, initial dose is 45 to 135 mg once daily, with maximum dose of 135 mg once daily. For all forms, adjust dose based on patient response and repeat lipid determinations every 4 to 8 weeks.

➤ **Primary hypercholesterolemia or mixed dyslipidemia (Fredrickson types IIa and IIb) in patients who don't respond adequately to diet alone**
Adults: For Antara, initial dose is 90 mg P.O. daily. For Fenoglide, initial dose is 120 mg/day. For Fibricor, the dose is 105 mg P.O. daily. For Lipofen, initial dose is 150 mg daily. For TriCor, initial dose is 145 mg daily. For Triglide, initial dose is 160 mg daily. For Trilipix, initial dose is 135 mg once daily. May reduce dose if lipid levels fall significantly below the target range.

➤ **Mixed dyslipidemia in combination with HMG-CoA reductase inhibitors (Trilipix)**
Adults: 135 mg P.O. once daily with a statin. May give daily dose at the same time as the statin, following the dosing recommendations for each medication. Avoid administering with maximum dose of a statin unless the benefits are expected to outweigh the risks.

ADMINISTRATION
P.O.
● Administer Fenoglide and Lipofen with meals.
● Administer Antara, Tricor, Triglide, and Trilipix with or without food.
● Ensure patient swallows capsules and tablets whole. Don't open capsules or crush, dissolve, or allow patient to chew capsules or tablets.
● Protect Fibricor, Lipofen, and Triglide from light.

ACTION
May lower triglyceride levels by inhibiting triglyceride synthesis with less VLDL released into circulation. Drug may also stimulate breakdown of triglyceride-rich protein.

Route	Onset	Peak	Duration
P.O.	Unknown	2–8 hr	Unknown

Half-life: 20 hours.

ADVERSE REACTIONS
CNS: dizziness, headache, asthenia, fatigue, insomnia, localized pain, paresthesia.
CV: hypertension.
EENT: blurred vision, conjunctivitis, eye discomfort, eye floaters, earache, rhinitis, sinusitis, nasopharyngitis.
GI: abdominal pain, constipation, diarrhea, dyspepsia, eructation, flatulence, increased appetite, nausea, vomiting.
GU: polyuria, vaginitis, UTI.
Musculoskeletal: arthralgia, back pain, myalgia.
Respiratory: cough, bronchitis, URI.
Skin: pruritus, rash.

INTERACTIONS

Drug-drug. *Bile acid sequestrants:* May bind and inhibit absorption of fenofibrate. Give drug 1 hour before or 4 to 6 hours after bile acid sequestrants.

Coumarin-type anticoagulants: May potentiate anticoagulant effect, prolonging PT and INR. Monitor PT and INR closely. May need to reduce anticoagulant dosage.

Cyclosporine, immunosuppressants, nephrotoxic drugs: May induce renal dysfunction that may affect fenofibrate elimination. Use together cautiously.

HMG-CoA reductase inhibitors: May increase risk of adverse musculoskeletal effects. Avoid using together, unless potential benefit outweighs risk.

Drug-food. *Any food:* May increase capsule absorption. Advise patient to take capsule with meals.

Drug-lifestyle. *Alcohol use:* May increase triglyceride levels. Discourage use together.

EFFECTS ON LAB TEST RESULTS

● May increase ALT, AST, BUN, CK, and creatinine levels. May decrease uric acid and Hb levels and hematocrit.
● May decrease WBC count.

CONTRAINDICATIONS & CAUTIONS

● Contraindicated in patients hypersensitive to drug and in those with gallbladder disease, hepatic dysfunction, primary biliary cirrhosis, severe renal dysfunction or ESRD (including those receiving hemodialysis), or unexplained persistent liver function abnormalities.
● Use cautiously in patients with a history of pancreatitis.
● Select Trilipix dosage cautiously for elderly patients and those with renal impairment because of the increased risk of adverse reactions.
Dialyzable drug: No.

PREGNANCY-LACTATION-REPRODUCTION

● Safe use in pregnant women hasn't been established for all products. Refer to individual manufacturer's instructions for use during pregnancy.
● Contraindicated in breast-feeding women.

NURSING CONSIDERATIONS

● Obtain baseline lipid levels and LFT results before therapy, and monitor liver function periodically during therapy. Stop drug if enzyme levels persist above 3 × ULN.
● *Alert:* Watch for signs and symptoms of pancreatitis, myositis, rhabdomyolysis, hepatic impairment, cholelithiasis, and renal failure. Monitor patient for muscle pain, tenderness, or weakness, especially with malaise or fever.
● Monitor LFT values at baseline and during therapy. Discontinue drug in patients with persistent LFT values greater than 3 × ULN.
● If an adequate response isn't obtained after 2 months of treatment with maximum daily dose, stop therapy.
● Drug lowers uric acid level by increasing uric acid excretion in patients with or without hyperuricemia.
● Beta blockers, estrogens, and thiazide diuretics may increase triglyceride levels; evaluate need for continued use of these drugs.
● Hb level, hematocrit, and WBC count may decrease when therapy starts but will stabilize with long-term administration.

PATIENT TEACHING

● Inform patient that drug therapy doesn't reduce need for following a triglyceride-lowering diet.
● Advise patient to promptly report all adverse reactions, especially unexplained muscle weakness, pain, or tenderness, abdominal pain, and yellowing of skin or eyes, particularly with malaise or fever.
● Tell patient to take capsules with meals for best drug absorption.
● Advise patient to swallow capsules and tablets whole and not to open capsules or crush, dissolve, or chew capsules or tablets.
● Advise patient to continue weight control measures, including diet and exercise, and to limit alcohol before therapy.
● Instruct patient who is also taking a bile acid sequestrant to take fenofibrate 1 hour before or 4 to 6 hours after the bile acid sequestrant.
● Advise patient about risk of tumor growth.

fentanyl citrate
FEN-ta-nil

Sublimaze

fentanyl nasal spray
Lazanda

fentanyl sublingual spray
SUBSYS

fentanyl transdermal system
Duragesic-12, Duragesic-25,
Duragesic-50, Duragesic-75,
Duragesic-100, Ionsys

fentanyl transmucosal
Abstral, Actiq, Fentora

Therapeutic class: Opioid analgesics
Pharmacologic class: Opioid agonists
Controlled substance schedule: II

AVAILABLE FORMS
Injection: 50 mcg/mL
Nasal spray: 100 mcg, 300 mcg, 400 mcg
Transdermal device: 40 mcg/activation
Transdermal system: Patches that release
12 mcg, 25 mcg, 37.5 mcg, 50 mcg,
62.5 mcg, 75 mcg, 87.5 mcg, or 100 mcg
of drug per hour
Transmucosal (buccal tablet): 100 mcg,
200 mcg, 400 mcg, 600 mcg, 800 mcg
Transmucosal (lozenge): 200 mcg, 400 mcg,
600 mcg, 800 mcg, 1,200 mcg, 1,600 mcg
Transmucosal (sublingual spray): 100 mcg,
200 mcg, 400 mcg, 600 mcg, 800 mcg,
1,200 mcg, 1,600 mcg
Transmucosal (sublingual tablet): 100 mcg,
200 mcg, 300 mcg, 400 mcg, 600 mcg,
800 mcg

INDICATIONS & DOSAGES
➤ **Adjunct to general anesthetic**
Adults: For low-dose therapy, 1 to 2 mcg/kg
I.V. For moderate-dose therapy, 2 to
20 mcg/kg I.V.; then 25 to 100 mcg I.V.
or I.M. p.r.n. For high-dose therapy, 20 to
50 mcg/kg I.V.; then 25 mcg to one-half
initial loading dose I.V. p.r.n.

➤ **Adjunct to regional anesthesia**
Adults: 50 to 100 mcg I.M. or slowly I.V.
over 1 to 2 minutes p.r.n.
➤ **To induce and maintain anesthesia**
Children ages 2 and older: 2 to 3 mcg/kg
I.V. every 1 to 2 hours as needed.
➤ **Postoperative pain, restlessness,
tachypnea, and emergence delirium**
Adults: 50 to 100 mcg I.M. or I.V. every 1 to
2 hours p.r.n.
➤ **Preoperative medication**
Adults: 50 to 100 mcg I.M. 30 to 60 minutes
before surgery.
➤ **To manage persistent, moderate to
severe chronic pain in opioid-tolerant
patients who require around-the-clock
opioid analgesics for an extended time**
Adults and children age 2 and older: When
converting to transdermal system, base the
first dose on the daily dose, potency, and
characteristics of the current opioid therapy; the reliability of the relative potency
estimates used to calculate the needed dose;
the degree of opioid tolerance; and patient's
condition. Each patch may be worn for
72 hours, although some adult patients may
need a patch to be applied every 48 hours
during the first dosage period. May increase
dose 3 days after the first dose, then every
6 days thereafter.
Adjust-a-dose: For elderly, cachectic, or debilitated patients, start transdermal system
doses at no higher than 25 mcg/hr unless
these patients are already tolerating around-
the-clock opioid at a dose and potency comparable to fentanyl 25 mcg/hr transdermal
system.
➤ **To manage breakthrough cancer pain
in patients already receiving and tolerating an opioid**
Adults: 200 mcg Actiq initially; may give
second dose 15 minutes after completing the
first (30 minutes after first lozenge is placed
in mouth). Maximum dose is 2 lozenges per
breakthrough episode. If several episodes
of breakthrough pain requiring 2 lozenges
occur, dose may be increased to the next
available strength. After a successful dosage
has been reached, patient should limit use to
no more than 4 lozenges daily.

Or, initially 100 mcg buccal tablet between the upper cheek and gum. May repeat
same dose once per breakthrough episode

after at least 30 minutes. Adjust in 100-mcg increments. Doses above 400 mcg can be increased by 200 mcg. Generally, dosage should be increased when patient requires more than one dose per breakthrough episode. Once a successful maintenance dose has been established, reevaluate if patient experiences more than four breakthrough episodes per day.

Or, initially 100 mcg sublingual tablet. If adequate analgesia is obtained within 30 minutes, continue to treat subsequent episodes with this dose. If adequate analgesia isn't obtained, may give a second sublingual tablet after 30 minutes. Use no more than two doses per episode of breakthrough pain; it's essential to wait at least 2 hours before treating another episode. Dosage escalation may be performed in a stepwise manner over consecutive breakthrough episodes until adequate analgesia with tolerable adverse effects is achieved. Limit drug consumption to treat four or fewer breakthrough pain episodes per day once a successful dose is found.

Or, initially 100 mcg nasal spray. Titrate as needed to an effective dosage (from 100 to 200, to 300, to 400 mcg, to 600 mcg, up to maximum of 800 mcg) that gives adequate analgesia with tolerable adverse effects. Dose is a single spray into one nostril or single spray into each nostril per episode. Don't give more than four doses per 24 hours. Wait at least 2 hours before treating another episode. During an episode, if analgesia isn't achieved within 30 minutes, patient may use a rescue medication as directed by the health care provider.

Or, initially 100 mcg sublingual spray. If pain isn't relieved after 30 minutes during each breakthrough pain episode treated, one additional dose of the same strength may be given for that episode. May use a maximum of two doses for any breakthrough pain episode, and 4 hours must elapse before treating another episode of breakthrough pain with a higher dose. Titrate dosage level as needed to an effective dosage (from 100 to 200, to 400, to 600, to 800, to 1,200, to 1,600 mcg) that gives adequate analgesia with tolerable adverse effects using a single dose per breakthrough cancer pain episode.

When drug has been titrated to an effective dosage, patients should generally use only one dose of the appropriate strength per breakthrough pain episode.

➤ **Switching from Actiq to Fentora to manage breakthrough cancer pain in opioid-tolerant patients**
Adults: If current Actiq dose is 200 to 400 mcg, start with 100 mcg Fentora; if current Actiq dose is 600 to 800 mcg, use 200 mcg Fentora; if current Actiq dose is 1,200 to 1,600 mcg, use 400 mcg Fentora. Actiq and Fentora aren't bioequivalent.
Adjust-a-dose: For patients with renal or hepatic impairment, use lowest possible dose.

➤ **Acute postoperative pain (Ionsys only)**
Adults: Only patient may activate device (40-mcg dose). Maximum is six doses/hour or 80 doses in 24 hours for a maximum of 72 hours.

ADMINISTRATION
I.V.
▼ Only those trained to give I.V. anesthetics and manage adverse effects should give this form.
▼ Keep opioid antagonist (naloxone) and resuscitation equipment available.
▼ I.V. form often used with droperidol to produce neuroleptanalgesia.
▼ Inject slowly over 1 to 2 minutes.
▼ **Incompatibilities:** Azithromycin, fluorouracil, lidocaine, methohexital, pentobarbital sodium, phenytoin, thiopental.
I.M.
● Document administration site.
Intranasal
● Prime the device by spraying into the pouch (4 sprays in total).
● Insert the nozzle about ½ inch (1.25 cm) into the nose and point toward the bridge of the nose, tilting the bottle slightly.
● Press down firmly until a click is heard and the number in the counting window advances by one.
Transdermal
● Dosage equivalent charts are available to calculate the fentanyl transdermal dose based on the daily morphine intake; for example, for every 90 mg of oral morphine or 15 mg of I.M. morphine per 24 hours, 25 mcg/hour of transdermal fentanyl is needed.

F

● Clip hair at application site but don't use a razor, which may irritate skin. Wash area with clear water, if needed, but not with soaps, oils, lotions, alcohol, or other substances that may irritate skin or prevent adhesion. Dry area completely before application.

● Remove transdermal system from package just before applying, hold in place for 30 seconds, and be sure edges of patch stick to skin.

● Don't cut or otherwise alter transdermal patch before applying.

● Place transdermal patch on the upper back for a child or patient who's cognitively impaired to reduce the chance the patch will be removed and placed in the mouth.

Black Box Warning Heat from fever or heating pads, electric blankets, heat lamps, hot tubs, or water beds may increase transdermal delivery and cause toxicity. ∎

● Always wear gloves when handling Ionsys system.

● Make sure patient knows to avoid exposing Ionsys device to electronic security systems.

● Patient should apply one Ionsys device to healthy, unbroken/intact, nonirritated, nonirradiated skin on chest or upper outer arm only.

● Allow only patient to administer Ionsys doses. Each on-demand dose is delivered over a 10-minute period. Each device operates for up to 24 hours or 80 doses, whichever comes first.

● Refer to manufacturer's instructions for information on complete device activation, administration, and removal.

Transmucosal

● Remove foil just before giving.

● For Actiq: Place lozenge between patient's cheek and gum and allow to dissolve over about 15 to 20 minutes; it must not be bitten, sucked, or chewed. Lozenge may be moved from one side to the other using the stick. Discard stick in the trash after use or, if any drug matrix remains on the stick, place under hot running tap water until dissolved. Or, place in child-resistant container provided and discard as for schedule II drugs.

● For buccal tablet: Place tablet between patient's cheek and gum and leave there until disintegrated, usually 14 to 25 minutes. Tablet shouldn't be sucked, chewed, or

swallowed; this results in lower plasma concentrations. After 30 minutes, if remnants from tablet remain, they may be swallowed with a glass of water.

● For sublingual tablet: Place on the floor of the mouth directly under the tongue. Patient should let tablet completely dissolve and shouldn't chew, suck, or swallow it. Water may be used to moisten buccal mucosa before administration.

● For sublingual spray: Open blister package with scissors immediately before use. Carefully spray contents of unit into the mouth under the tongue. Advise patients and caregivers to properly dispose of used unit-dose systems immediately after use.

ACTION

Binds with opioid receptors in the CNS, altering perception of and emotional response to pain.

Route	Onset	Peak	Duration
I.V.	1–2 min	3–5 min	30–60 min
I.M.	7–15 min	20–30 min	1–2 hr
Intranasal	15–21 min	25–35 min	Unknown
Transdermal	12–24 hr	1–3 days	Variable
Transmucosal	5–15 min	20–30 min	Unknown

Half-life: Parenteral, 3½ hours; intranasal, 15 to 24.9 hours; transmucosal, 5 to 15 hours; transdermal, 18 hours.

ADVERSE REACTIONS

CNS: asthenia, clouded sensorium, confusion, euphoria, sedation, somnolence, *seizures,* anxiety, depression, dizziness, hallucinations, headache, nervousness.

CV: *arrhythmias,* chest pain, hypertension, hypotension, *DVT, PE.*

EENT: pharyngitis, dry eyes, swelling, strabismus, ptosis, epistaxis, nasal discomfort, rhinorrhea, nasal congestion, postnasal drip, rhinitis (intranasal).

GI: constipation, abdominal pain, anorexia, diarrhea, dyspepsia, dry mouth, ileus, nausea, vomiting.

GU: urine retention.

Musculoskeletal: skeletal muscle rigidity (dose-related).

Respiratory: *apnea, hypoventilation, respiratory depression,* dyspnea, cough, URI, bronchitis.

Reactions in bold italics are *life-threatening*. Interactions may have a *rapid onset* or a *delayed onset*.

Skin: diaphoresis, pruritus, erythema at application site (transdermal).
Other: physical dependence.

INTERACTIONS

Drug-drug. *Amiodarone:* May cause hypotension, bradycardia, and decreased cardiac output. Monitor patient closely.

Black Box Warning *Benzodiazepines, CNS depressants:* May cause slow or difficult breathing, sedation, and death. Avoid use together. If use together is necessary, limit dosage and duration of each drug to the minimum necessary for desired effect. ∎

CYP3A4 inducers (carbamazepine, phenytoin, rifampin): May decrease analgesic effects. Monitor patient for adequate pain relief.

Black Box Warning *CYP3A4 inhibitors (cyclosporine, itraconazole, ketoconazole):* May increase fentanyl level and cause fatal respiratory depression. Carefully monitor patient and adjust fentanyl dosage as needed. ∎

Diazepam: May cause CV depression when given with high doses of fentanyl. Monitor patient closely.

Droperidol: May cause hypotension and decrease pulmonary arterial pressure. Use together cautiously.

General anesthetics, hypnotics, MAO inhibitors, other opioid analgesics, sedatives, TCAs: May cause additive effects. Use together cautiously. Reduce dosages of these drugs and reduce fentanyl dose by ¼ to ⅓.

Protease inhibitors: May increase fentanyl levels and adverse effects. Monitor patient closely for respiratory depression.

❸ Alert: *Serotonergic drugs (antiemetics [dolasetron, granisetron, ondansetron, palonosetron], amoxapine, antimigraine drugs, buspirone, cyclobenzaprine, dextromethorphan, linezolid, lithium, MAO inhibitors, maprotiline, methylene blue, mirtazapine, nefazodone, SNRIs, SSRIs, TCAs, trazodone, tryptophan, vilazodone):* May increase risk of serotonin syndrome. Use together cautiously; monitor for serotonin syndrome.

Drug-herb. ❸ Alert: *St. John's wort:* May increase risk of serotonin syndrome. Use together cautiously; monitor for serotonin syndrome.

Drug-lifestyle. *Alcohol use:* May cause additive effects. Discourage use together.

EFFECTS ON LAB TEST RESULTS

● May increase amylase and lipase levels.

CONTRAINDICATIONS & CAUTIONS

● Contraindicated in patients intolerant to drug.

Black Box Warning Opioid drugs should only be prescribed with benzodiazepines or other CNS depressants to patients for whom alternative treatment options are inadequate. ∎

Black Box Warning Transdermal form contraindicated in patients hypersensitive to adhesives, those who are opioid-naive, those who need postoperative pain management, and those with acute, mild, or intermittent pain that can be managed with nonopioids. Don't use in patients with increased intracranial pressure, head injury, impaired consciousness, or coma. ∎

Black Box Warning Transmucosal forms contraindicated in those who need acute or postoperative pain management. ∎

Black Box Warning Nasal spray is contraindicated in opioid-nontolerant patients and in those who need acute or postoperative pain management. ∎

● Transdermal form is contraindicated in patients with acute or severe bronchial asthma, known or suspected paralytic ileus, and GI obstruction.

❸ Alert: Drug may lead to rare but serious decrease in adrenal gland cortisol production.

❸ Alert: Drug may cause decreased sex hormone levels with long-term use.

● Fentora contraindicated in patients with mucositis more severe than grade 1.

● Use with caution in patients with brain tumors, COPD, decreased respiratory reserve, potentially compromised respirations, hepatic or renal disease, or cardiac bradyarrhythmias.

● Use with caution in elderly or debilitated patients.

Dialyzable drug: Unknown.

⚠ Overdose S&S: CNS depression, respiratory depression, apnea, flaccid skeletal muscles, bradycardia, hypotension, circulatory collapse.

PREGNANCY-LACTATION-REPRODUCTION

● There are no well-controlled studies in pregnant women. Use during pregnancy only if potential benefit justifies potential risk to the fetus.

Black Box Warning Prolonged maternal use of opioids during pregnancy can cause neonatal withdrawal syndrome, which may be life-threatening and requires management by neonatology experts. Advise patient of the risk of neonatal withdrawal syndrome. ■

● Drug appears in breast milk. Refer to individual manufacturer's instructions for use in breast-feeding women.

NURSING CONSIDERATIONS

Black Box Warning Respiratory depression or death can occur even when transdermal drug has been used as recommended and has not been misused or abused. Drug should only be prescribed by health care providers knowledgeable in the use of potent opioids for management of long-term pain. Drug is contraindicated for use in conditions in which the risk of life-threatening respiratory depression is significantly increased. Ionsys transdermal patch is for hospital use only. ■

⊗ *Alert:* If patient is taking opioids with serotonergic drugs, monitor for signs and symptoms of serotonin syndrome (agitation, hallucinations, rapid HR, fever, excessive sweating, shivering or shaking, muscle twitching or stiffness, trouble with coordination, nausea, vomiting, diarrhea), especially when starting treatment or increasing dosage. Symptoms may occur within several hours of coadministration but may also occur later, especially after dosage increase. Discontinue the opioid, serotonergic drug, or both if serotonin syndrome is suspected.

⊗ *Alert:* Monitor patient for signs and symptoms of adrenal insufficiency (nausea, vomiting, loss of appetite, fatigue, weakness, dizziness, low BP). Perform diagnostic testing if adrenal insufficiency is suspected. If adrenal insufficiency is confirmed, treat with corticosteroids and wean patient off opioids if appropriate. Discontinue corticosteroids when clinically appropriate.

⊗ *Alert:* Monitor patient for signs and symptoms of decreased sex hormone levels (low libido, erectile dysfunction, amenorrhea,

infertility). If signs and symptoms occur, evaluate patient and obtain laboratory testing.

● For better analgesic effect, give drug before patient has intense pain.

⊗ *Alert:* High doses can produce muscle rigidity, which can be reversed with neuromuscular blockers; however, patient must be artificially ventilated.

● Monitor circulatory and respiratory status and urinary function carefully. Drug may cause respiratory depression, hypotension, urine retention, nausea, vomiting, ileus, or altered level of consciousness, no matter how it's given.

● Periodically monitor postoperative vital signs and bladder function. Because drug decreases both rate and depth of respirations, monitoring of arterial oxygen saturation (SaO_2) may help assess respiratory depression. Immediately report respiratory rate below 12 breaths/minute, decreased respiratory volume, or decreased SaO_2.

● Drug may cause constipation. Assess bowel function and need for stool softeners and stimulant laxatives.

Black Box Warning Fentanyl is an opioid agonist and schedule II controlled substance with potential for abuse. Be alert for signs of misuse, abuse, or diversion. ■

Transdermal form

Black Box Warning Transdermal drug levels peak between 24 and 72 hours after initial application and dose increases. Monitor patients for life-threatening hypoventilation, especially during these times. ■

● Fentanyl patches should be used only in patients age 2 or older who are opioid tolerant, who have chronic moderate to severe pain poorly controlled by other drugs, and who need a total daily opioid dose at least equivalent to the 25-mcg/hour fentanyl patch.

● When converting a patient from another opioid, determine the initial fentanyl dosage with great care; overestimating the dosage could be dangerous or fatal.

● Identify all daily drugs, particularly CYP3A4 inhibitors, which may increase fentanyl levels.

● Monitor patients closely, and provide immediate care for evidence of overdose, such as slow or shallow breathing, a slow heartbeat, severe sleepiness, cold and clammy skin, trouble walking and talking, and feeling faint, dizzy, or confused.

• Give patients detailed instructions for using fentanyl patches correctly and safely.

• Make dosage adjustments gradually in patient using the transdermal system. Reaching steady-state level of a new dosage may take up to 6 days; delay dosage adjustment until after at least two applications.

• Monitor patient who develops adverse reactions to the transdermal system for at least 12 hours after removal. Drug level drops gradually; it may take as long as 17 hours to decline by 50%.

• Most patients experience good control of pain for 3 days while wearing the transdermal system, but a few may need a new application after 48 hours.

• Because the drug level rises for the first 24 hours after application, analgesic effect can't be evaluated on the first day. Make sure patient has adequate supplemental analgesic to prevent breakthrough pain.

• When reducing opioid therapy or switching to a different analgesic, withdraw the transdermal system gradually. Because the drug level drops gradually after removal, give half the equianalgesic dose of the new analgesic 12 to 18 hours after removal.

⚠ *Alert:* Transdermal patches must be stored, used, and disposed of properly to prevent poisonings or other harm, especially to children and pets. A patch that has been worn for 3 days may still contain enough fentanyl to cause harm, or even kill a child or pet. Patches should only be handled by patient or patient's caregivers.

Intranasal and transmucosal forms

Black Box Warning Intranasal and transmucosal forms are used only to manage breakthrough cancer pain in patients who are already receiving and tolerating opioids. ■

Black Box Warning Intranasal and transmucosal forms aren't bioequivalent and can't be substituted on a microgram-per-microgram basis. ■

• *Look alike–sound alike:* Don't confuse fentanyl with alfentanil.

PATIENT TEACHING

Black Box Warning Caution the patient or the caregiver of a patient taking an opioid drug with a benzodiazepine, CNS depressant, or alcohol to seek immediate medical attention if the patient has symptoms of dizziness, light-headedness, extreme sleepiness, slowed or difficult breathing, or unresponsiveness. ■

• When drug is used for pain control, instruct patient to request drug before pain becomes intense.

⚠ *Alert:* Encourage patient to report all medications being taken, including prescription and OTC medications and supplements.

⚠ *Alert:* Caution patient to immediately report signs and symptoms of serotonin syndrome, adrenal insufficiency, and decreased sex hormone levels to health care provider.

• When drug is used after surgery, encourage patient to turn, cough, and breathe deeply to prevent lung problems.

• Instruct patient to avoid hazardous activities until CNS effects subside.

• Tell home care patient to avoid drinking alcohol or taking other CNS-type drugs because additive effects can occur.

• Advise patient not to stop drug abruptly.

• Teach patient about proper application of transdermal patch. Tell patient to clip hair at application site but not to use a razor, which may irritate skin. Wash area with clear water, if needed, but not with soaps, oils, lotions, alcohol, or other substances that may irritate skin or prevent adhesion. Dry area completely before application.

• Tell patient to remove transdermal system from package just before applying, hold in place for 30 seconds, and be sure the edges of patch stick to skin.

⚠ *Alert:* Teach patient not to alter the transdermal patch (such as by cutting it) before applying.

• Advise parent or caregiver to place transdermal patch on the upper back for a child or a patient who's cognitively impaired, to reduce the chance the patch will be removed and placed in the mouth.

• Teach patient to dispose of the transdermal patch by folding it so the adhesive side adheres to itself and then flushing it down the toilet.

• Tell patient that, if another patch is needed after 48 to 72 hours, he should apply it to a different skin site.

• Tell patient that pain relief with the patch may not occur for several hours after the patch is applied. Oral, immediate-release opioids may be needed for initial pain relief. **Black Box Warning** Inform patient that heat from fever or environment, such as from heating pads, electric blankets, heat lamps, hot tubs, or water beds, may increase transdermal delivery and cause toxicity requiring dosage adjustment. Instruct patient to notify prescriber if fever occurs or if he'll be spending time in a hot climate. ∎

⊙ *Alert:* Instruct patient that if an MRI is required, to inform the facility that patient is wearing a transdermal patch.

• Teach patient proper administration of transmucosal forms.

• Teach patient proper administration of the nasal spray. Tell him that a fine mist is not always felt and to rely on the audible click and advancement of the dose counter.

Black Box Warning Warn patient and patient's family that the amount of drug in transmucosal and intranasal forms can be fatal to a child. Advise patient to keep medicine well secured and out of children's reach. ∎

ferric carboxymaltose
FER-ik car-box-ee-MAL-tose

Injectafer

Therapeutic class: Iron supplements
Pharmacologic class: Hematinics

AVAILABLE FORMS
Injection: 750 mg of elemental iron in 15-mL single-dose vial

INDICATIONS & DOSAGES
➤ **Iron deficiency anemia in patients intolerant to or who have had unsatisfactory response to oral iron and in those with non-dialysis-dependent chronic kidney disease**
Adults: For patients weighing at least 50 kg, 750 mg I.V. on day 1; repeat dose after at least 7 days. May repeat course of therapy if anemia recurs. For patients weighing less than 50 kg, give 15 mg/kg body weight on day 1; repeat dose after at least 7 days. May repeat course of therapy if anemia recurs.

Maximum cumulative dose is 1,500 mg per treatment course.

ADMINISTRATION
I.V.
▼ Inspect vial for particulate matter and discoloration before administration.
▼ Give either as an undiluted slow I.V. push (at 100 mg [2 mL]/minute) or as an infusion. To administer by infusion, dilute up to 750 mg iron in maximum of 250 mL sterile NSS injection. Infusion concentration must be not less than 2 mg iron/mL.
▼ Give infusion over at least 15 minutes.
▼ Infusion is stable for 72 hours at room temperature at 2- to 4-mg/mL concentrations.
▼ Store vials at 68° to 77° F (20° to 25° C), with excursions permitted to 59° to 86° F (15° to 30° C). Don't freeze vials.
▼ Vials are single-use and have no preservative.
▼ Discard any excess drug remaining in vial.

ACTION
Colloidal iron (III) hydroxide acts in complex with carboxymaltose, a carbohydrate polymer that releases iron, an essential component in the formulation of Hb.

Route	Onset	Peak	Duration
I.V.	Unknown	15 min–1.21 hr	Unknown

Half-life: 7 to 12 hours.

ADVERSE REACTIONS
CNS: dizziness, headache, pyrexia, chills, syncope.
CV: hypertension, hypotension, flushing, tachycardia, chest discomfort.
GI: nausea, vomiting, constipation, dysgeusia.
Skin: injection-site discoloration, urticaria, pruritus, erythema.

INTERACTIONS
Drug-drug. *Dimercaprol:* May enhance nephrotoxic effect of iron salts. Avoid combination.

Reactions in bold italics are *life-threatening*. Interactions may have a *rapid onset* or a ***delayed onset***.

EFFECTS ON LAB TEST RESULTS
- May increase ALT and GGT levels.
- May decrease phosphorus level.
- May falsely elevate serum iron and transferrin-bound iron levels in the 24 hours after administration.

CONTRAINDICATIONS & CAUTIONS
- Contraindicated in patients hypersensitive to drug or its components, in patients with evidence of iron overload, and in those with anemia not caused by iron deficiency.
- Serious hypersensitivity reactions, including anaphylaxis, have been reported.
- Safety and effectiveness in children haven't been established.

Dialyzable drug: No.

⚠ *Overdose S&S:* Hemosiderosis, hypophosphatemic osteomalacia.

PREGNANCY-LACTATION-REPRODUCTION
- Use during pregnancy only if potential benefit justifies potential risk to the fetus.
- Drug appears in breast milk.

NURSING CONSIDERATIONS
- Before administering, assess patient for prior history of reactions to parenteral iron products.
- Monitor patient for extravasation during administration. Extravasation may cause persistent discoloration. If extravasation occurs, discontinue infusion at that site.
- Monitor vital signs before and after each dose. Monitor patient for hypertension after each dose.
- Monitor patient for hypersensitivity reactions during infusion and for at least 30 minutes after infusion or until patient is clinically stable. Only administer drug when personnel and therapies are immediately available for treatment of serious hypersensitivity reactions.
- Monitor iron status (Hb level and hematocrit, serum ferritin level, iron saturation) frequently during therapy.

PATIENT TEACHING
- Advise patient to report signs and symptoms of hypersensitivity reactions, such as rash, itching, dizziness, light-headedness, swelling, and breathing problems.
- Caution patient not to take oral iron supplements while receiving iron by infusion.
- Advise female patient to report pregnancy or intent to become pregnant to her practitioner.

fesoterodine fumarate
fezz-oh-TER-ah-deen

Toviaz

F

Therapeutic class: Antispasmodics
Pharmacologic class: Muscarinic receptor antagonists

AVAILABLE FORMS
Tablets (extended-release) ⓓ: 4 mg, 8 mg

INDICATIONS & DOSAGES
➤ **Urge incontinence, urinary urgency, and urinary frequency from overactive bladder**
Adults: 4 mg P.O. once daily; increase to 8 mg once daily if needed.

Adjust-a-dose: Don't exceed 4 mg in patients with CrCl of less than 30 mL/minute and in those taking CYP3A4 inhibitors.

ADMINISTRATION
P.O.
- Give drug with or without food.
- Don't divide or crush tablets. Give with liquid and have patient swallow whole.

ACTION
Antagonizes muscarinic (M3) receptors, increasing bladder capacity and decreasing unstable detrusor contractions.

Route	Onset	Peak	Duration
P.O.	Unknown	5 hr	Unknown

Half-life: 7 hours.

ADVERSE REACTIONS
CNS: headache, dizziness, insomnia.
CV: peripheral edema.
EENT: dry eyes.
GI: dry mouth, constipation, dyspepsia, nausea, abdominal pain.
GU: UTI, dysuria, urine retention.
Musculoskeletal: back pain.

Respiratory: URI, dry throat, cough.
Skin: rash.

INTERACTIONS
Drug-drug. *Anticholinergics, antimuscarinics:* May increase risk of anticholinergic effects (such as constipation, blurred vision, urine retention). Use together cautiously.
Potassium preparations: May slow GI motility, arresting or delaying transport of solid dosage forms of potassium. Use together is contraindicated.
Strong CYP3A4 inhibitors (such as clarithromycin, itraconazole, ketoconazole): May increase fesoterodine concentration. Fesoterodine doses of more than 4 mg aren't recommended when fesoterodine is used with strong CYP3A4 inhibitors.
Drug-lifestyle. *Alcohol use:* May cause additive CNS depression. Discourage use together.

EFFECTS ON LAB TEST RESULTS
● May increase ALT and GGT levels.

CONTRAINDICATIONS & CAUTIONS
● Contraindicated in patients with hypersensitivity to drug or its components and in those with urine retention, gastric retention, or uncontrolled angle-closure glaucoma.
● Life-threatening angioedema with upper airway swelling can occur after first dose. Ensure a patent airway and discontinue drug if this occurs.
● Avoid use in patients with severe hepatic impairment.
● Use cautiously in patients with bladder outlet obstruction, decreased GI motility, myasthenia gravis, or controlled angle-closure glaucoma.
Dialyzable drug: Unknown.
⚠ **Overdose S&S:** Confusion, blurred vision, tachycardia, constipation, dry mouth, light-headedness, difficulty starting and continuing urination, urinary incontinence.

PREGNANCY-LACTATION-REPRODUCTION
● Use during pregnancy and breast-feeding only if potential benefits outweigh potential fetal/neonatal risk.

NURSING CONSIDERATIONS
● Give drug without regard to food.
● Monitor patient for urinary symptoms and adverse reactions.

PATIENT TEACHING
● Warn patient to avoid hot environments because drug may decrease sweating, causing severe heat illness.
● Advise patient to avoid driving, operating machinery, and other dangerous activities until drug's effects are known.
● Tell patient to avoid alcohol as it may cause drowsiness.
● Tell patient to report all adverse reactions (especially swelling of the face, lips, or tongue), stomach or intestinal problems, constipation, difficulty emptying the bladder, weak urine stream, glaucoma, kidney or liver problems, or myasthenia gravis.
● Tell patient to take drug with water and to swallow tablet whole. Tell him not to chew, crush, or divide tablet.

fidaxomicin
fye-DAX-oh-MYE sin

Dificid

Therapeutic class: Antibiotics
Pharmacologic class: Macrolides

AVAILABLE FORMS
Tablets: 200 mg

INDICATIONS & DOSAGES
➤ **CDAD**
Adults: 200 mg P.O. b.i.d. for 10 days.

ADMINISTRATION
P.O.
● May give without regard for food.
● Store at room temperature.

ACTION
Acts on *Clostridium difficile* locally in the GI tract by inhibiting RNA synthesis through RNA polymerases.

Route	Onset	Peak	Duration
P.O.	<1 hr	1–5 hr	Unknown

Half-life: About 12 hours.

ADVERSE REACTIONS
GI: nausea, vomiting, abdominal pain or discomfort, *GI bleeding,* dyspepsia, flatulence, intestinal obstruction.
Hematologic: anemia, *neutropenia.*
Metabolic: hyperglycemia, *metabolic acidosis.*
Skin: drug eruption, rash, pruritus.

INTERACTIONS
None reported.

EFFECTS ON LAB TEST RESULTS
● May increase alkaline phosphatase, liver enzyme, and blood glucose levels.
● May decrease serum bicarbonate level and platelet count.

CONTRAINDICATIONS & CAUTIONS
● Contraindicated in patients hypersensitive to drug.
● Acute hypersensitivity reactions have been reported. Discontinue drug and treat appropriately. Patients with known macrolide allergies may have increased risk.
● Drug isn't an effective treatment for systemic *Clostridium* infections. Don't prescribe fidaxomicin unless a *C. difficile* infection has been proven or is strongly suspected because this may lead to the development of drug-resistant bacteria.
Dialyzable drug: Unknown.

PREGNANCY-LACTATION-REPRODUCTION
● Use drug in pregnant women only if clearly needed.
● It isn't known if drug appears in breast milk. Use cautiously if breast-feeding.

NURSING CONSIDERATIONS
● Obtain specimen for culture before start of treatment. Monitor response to treatment.
● Monitor glucose level, especially in diabetic patients.
● Monitor patient for abdominal pain or bleeding.
● Monitor patient for acute hypersensitivity.

PATIENT TEACHING
● Inform patient that drug can be taken with or without food.

● Advise patient that drug is used to treat CDAD only and shouldn't be used to treat other infections.
● Counsel patient to take the drug exactly as directed. Missing or skipping doses, or not completing the full course of therapy, may lead to reinfection, continued infection, or bacterial resistance.

filgrastim (G-CSF; granulocyte colony-stimulating factor)
fill-GRASS-tim

Neupogen

Therapeutic class: Colony-stimulating factors
Pharmacologic class: Hematopoietics

AVAILABLE FORMS
Injection: 300-mcg/mL, 480-mcg/1.6 mL vials; 300-mcg/0.5 mL, 480-mcg/0.8 mL prefilled syringes

INDICATIONS & DOSAGES
➤ **Acute exposure to myelosuppressive doses of radiation (hematopoietic syndrome of acute radiation syndrome)**
Adults and children: 10 mcg/kg subcutaneously as soon as possible after suspected or confirmed exposure to radiation doses greater than 2 gray (Gy). Continue daily administration until ANC remains greater than 1,000/mm^3 for three consecutive CBCs or exceeds 10,000/mm^3 after a radiation-induced nadir.
➤ **To decrease risk of infection in patients with nonmyeloid malignant disease receiving myelosuppressive antineoplastics**
Adults and children: 5 mcg/kg daily I.V. (as continuous or intermittent infusion), subcutaneous infusion, or subcutaneously as a single dose given no sooner than 24 hours after cytotoxic chemotherapy. Doses may be increased in increments of 5 mcg/kg for each chemotherapy cycle, depending on duration and severity of the nadir of ANC. Administer daily for up to 2 weeks.
➤ **To decrease risk of infection in patients with nonmyeloid malignant disease**

receiving myelosuppressive antineoplastics followed by bone marrow transplantation
Adults and children: 10 mcg/kg daily I.V. infusion for no longer than 24 hours or as continuous 24-hour subcutaneous infusion at least 24 hours after cytotoxic chemotherapy and bone marrow infusion. Adjust subsequent dosages based on neutrophil response.
Adjust-a-dose: For patients with ANC above 1,000/mm³ for 3 consecutive days, reduce dosage to 5 mcg/kg daily; if ANC remains above 1,000/mm³ for 3 more consecutive days, stop drug. If ANC decreases to below 1,000/mm³, resume therapy at 5 mcg/kg daily.

➤ **Congenital neutropenia**
Adults: 6 mcg/kg subcutaneously b.i.d. Adjust dosage based on patient response.
Adjust-a-dose: For patients with an ANC persistently above 10,000/mm³, reduce dosage, as directed.

➤ **Idiopathic or cyclic neutropenia**
Adults: 5 mcg/kg subcutaneously daily. Adjust dosage based on patient response.

➤ **Peripheral blood progenitor cell collection and therapy in cancer patients**
Adults: 10 mcg/kg subcutaneously (as bolus or continuous infusion) daily. Give 4 days before leukapheresis and continue until last leukapheresis.
Adjust-a-dose: Patients with WBC count over 100,000/mm³ may need dosage adjustment.

➤ **To reduce time to neutrophil recovery and fever duration after induction or consolidation chemotherapy treatment of adults with acute myeloid leukemia**
Adults: 5 mcg/kg/day subcutaneously beginning 24 hours after last dose of chemotherapy until neutrophil recovery (ANC 1,000/mm³ for 3 consecutive days or 10,000/mm³ for 1 day) or for a maximum of 35 days.

➤ **Hematopoietic stem cell mobilization in autologous transplantation in patients with non-Hodgkin lymphoma or multiple myeloma (in combination with plerixafor)** ◆
Adults: 10 mcg/kg subcutaneously once daily. Begin 4 days before initiation of

plerixafor; continue G-CSF on each day before apheresis for up to 8 days.

ADMINISTRATION
I.V.
▼ Dilute in 50 to 100 mL of D_5W. Dilution to less than 5 mcg/mL isn't recommended.
▼ Don't dilute with NSS.
▼ If drug yield is 5 to 15 mcg/mL, add albumin at 2 mg/mL (0.2%) to minimize binding of drug to plastic containers or tubing.
▼ Give by intermittent infusion over 15 to 60 minutes or by continuous infusion over 24 hours.
▼ **Incompatibilities:** Amphotericin B, cefepime, cefonicid, cefotaxime, cefoxitin, ceftizoxime, ceftriaxone, cefuroxime, clindamycin, dactinomycin, etoposide, fluorouracil, furosemide, heparin sodium, mannitol, methylprednisolone sodium succinate, metronidazole, mitomycin, piperacillin, prochlorperazine edisylate, sodium solutions, thiotepa.

Subcutaneous
● Rotate administration sites and record.
◑ *Alert:* Needle cover of Neupogen prefilled syringe may contain dry natural rubber (a derivative of latex).

ACTION
Binds cell receptors to stimulate proliferation, differentiation, commitment, and end-cell function of neutrophils.

Route	Onset	Peak	Duration
I.V.	5–60 min	24 hr	1–7 days
Subcut.	5–60 min	2–8 hr	1–7 days

Half-life: 3½ hours.

ADVERSE REACTIONS
CNS: fever, headache, weakness, fatigue, dizziness.
CV: *MI, arrhythmias,* chest pain, hypertension.
EENT: epistaxis, sore throat.
GI: nausea, vomiting, diarrhea, mucositis, stomatitis, constipation.
Hematologic: *thrombocytopenia,* anemia, leukocytosis, *neutropenic fever.*
Metabolic: hyperuricemia.
Musculoskeletal: bone pain.
Respiratory: dyspnea, cough, URI.

Skin: alopecia, rash, cutaneous vasculitis.
Other: hypersensitivity reactions.

INTERACTIONS
Drug-drug. *Bleomycin, cyclophosphamide:*
May increase pulmonary toxicity. Monitor
therapy.
Chemotherapeutic drugs: Rapidly dividing
myeloid cells may be sensitive to cytotoxic
drugs. Don't use within 24 hours before or
after a dose of one of these drugs.

EFFECTS ON LAB TEST RESULTS
• May increase alkaline phosphatase, creatinine, LDH, and uric acid levels.
• May increase WBC count. May decrease
platelet count.

CONTRAINDICATIONS & CAUTIONS
• Contraindicated in patients hypersensitive
to drug or its components or to proteins
derived from *Escherichia coli.*
• Severe allergic reactions, including anaphylaxis, can occur. Permanently discontinue drug for serious allergic reactions.
• Sickle cell crisis and fatalities have been
reported in patients with sickle cell trait or
sickle cell disease.
Dialyzable drug: Unknown.
⚠ **Overdose S&S:** Excessive leukocytosis.

PREGNANCY-LACTATION-REPRODUCTION
• Adverse effects have been seen in animal studies. Use with extreme caution in
pregnant and breast-feeding women.
• If used, consider enrolling patients in
Amgen's surveillance programs (1-800-
772-6436).

NURSING CONSIDERATIONS
🕦 **Alert:** Obtain baseline CBC after exposure to myelosuppressive doses of radiation;
don't delay administration if CBC isn't readily available. Monitor CBC every third day
until ANC remains greater than 1,000/mm^3
for 3 consecutive CBCs.
• Obtain baseline CBC and platelet count
before therapy.
• Once a dose is withdrawn, don't reuse
vial. Discard unused portion. Vials are for
single-dose use only.
• Obtain CBC and platelet count two to
three times weekly during therapy. Patients

who receive drug also may receive high
doses of chemotherapy, which may increase
risk of toxicities.
• A transiently increased neutrophil count
is common 1 or 2 days after therapy starts.
Give daily for up to 2 weeks or until ANC
has returned to 10,000/mm^3 after the expected chemotherapy-induced neutrophil
nadir.
• Glomerulonephritis can occur; dosage
reduction or drug discontinuation may be
necessary.
• Monitor patients with left upper abdominal or shoulder pain for enlarged spleen or
splenic rupture.
• Monitor patients for capillary lead syndrome (hypotension, hypoalbuminemia,
edema, hemoconcentration), which can be
life-threatening. Monitor patients closely;
intensive care may be needed.
• *Look alike–sound alike:* Don't confuse
Neupogen with Epogen or Neumega.

PATIENT TEACHING
• If patient will give drug, teach him how
to do so and how to dispose of used needles, syringes, drug containers, and unused
medicine.
🕦 **Alert:** Rarely, splenic rupture may occur.
Advise patient to immediately report left
upper abdominal or shoulder tip pain.
• Instruct patient to report all adverse reactions promptly.

filgrastim-sndz
fill-GRASS-tim

Zarxio

Therapeutic class: Colony-stimulating
factors
Pharmacologic class: Hematopoietics

AVAILABLE FORMS
Injection: 300 mcg/0.5 mL, 480 mcg/0.8 mL
prefilled syringes

INDICATIONS & DOSAGES
➤ **To decrease incidence of infection in
patients with nonmyeloid malignancies
receiving myelosuppressive chemotherapy associated with risk of severe febrile**

neutropenia; to reduce time to neutrophil recovery and duration of fever after induction or consolidation chemotherapy for acute myeloid leukemia

Adults and children: 5 mcg/kg by a single subcutaneous injection or short I.V. infusion (15 to 30 minutes), or continuous I.V. infusion once daily at least 24 hours after chemotherapy. Give daily for up to 2 weeks, until ANC reaches 10,000/mm³.

Adjust-a-dose: May increase dose by increments of 5 mcg/kg for each chemotherapy cycle, depending on duration and severity of ANC nadir.

➤ **To reduce duration of neutropenia and neutropenia-related clinical sequelae in patients with nonmyeloid malignancies undergoing myeloablative chemotherapy followed by bone marrow transplantation**

Adults and children: 10 mcg/kg/day as an I.V. infusion over no longer than 24 hours. Administer at least 24 hours after cytotoxic chemotherapy and at least 24 hours after bone marrow infusion. Titrate daily dosage during neutrophil recovery based on ANC.

Adjust-a-dose: For ANC greater than1,000/mm³ for 3 consecutive days, reduce dose to 5 mcg/kg/day. If ANC decreases to less than 1,000/mm³ with 5-mcg/kg/day dose, increase dose to 10 mcg/kg/day. If ANC remains greater than 1,000/mm³ for 3 more consecutive days, discontinue drug; if ANC decreases to less than 1,000/mm³, resume drug at 5 mcg/kg/day.

➤ **Mobilization of autologous peripheral blood progenitor cells (PBPC) before leukapheresis**

Adults and children: 10 mcg/kg/day subcutaneously. Begin treatment at least 4 days before first leukapheresis procedure and continue until last leukapheresis procedure.

Adjust-a-dose: Monitor daily neutrophil count after 4 days of treatment; discontinue drug for WBC count above 100,000/mm³.

➤ **Chronic severe neutropenia**

Adults and children: For patients with congenital neutropenia, starting dose is 6 mcg/kg subcutaneously b.i.d. For patients with idiopathic or cyclic neutropenia, starting dose is 5 mcg/kg as a single daily subcutaneous injection. Adjust dosage based on patient response.

ADMINISTRATION
General

● Give at least 24 hours after cytotoxic chemotherapy.

🚯 *Alert:* Direct administration of less than 0.3 mL isn't recommended because of potential for dosing errors.

🚯 *Alert:* Removable needle cap contains natural rubber latex. Safe use in latex-sensitive patients hasn't been studied.

● Store in refrigerator at 36° to 46° F (2° to 8° C) in original pack to protect from light. Don't shake.

● Before use, allow drug to reach room temperature for at least 30 minutes to a maximum of 24 hours (if beyond 24 hours, discard drug).

● Solution should be clear and colorless to slightly yellow. Discard if solution is discolored or contains particulate matter.

● Avoid freezing; if frozen, thaw in refrigerator before administering. Discard drug if frozen more than once.

● Discard unused portion of prefilled syringes.

I.V.

▼ Dilute in 5% dextrose to concentration between 5 and 15 mcg/mL and add albumin (human) to yield a final concentration of 2 mg/mL to minimize adsorption to plastic materials.

▼ When diluted in 5% dextrose or 5% dextrose plus albumin (human), drug is compatible with glass, polyvinylchloride, polyolefin, and polypropylene.

▼ Administer as a short I.V. infusion over 15 to 30 minutes or by continuous infusion over 24 hours.

▼ Diluted solution can be stored at room temperature for up to 24 hours, which includes the time during room-temperature storage of the infusion solution and the duration of the infusion.

▼ **Incompatibilities:** Amphotericin B, cefepime, cefotaxime, cefoxitin, ceftriaxone, cefuroxime, clindamycin, etoposide, 5-FU, furosemide, heparin, mannitol, methylprednisolone, metronidazole, mitomycin, NSS, piperacillin, prochlorperazine edisylate, sodium succinate, thiotepa.

Subcutaneous
• Administer in outer upper arms, abdomen, thighs, or upper outer areas of the buttock.
• Rotate injection sites.

ACTION
Binds to specific cell-surface receptors to stimulate proliferation, differentiation commitment, and some end-cell function activation of neutrophils.

Route	Onset	Peak	Duration
I.V.	Immediate	Unknown	Unknown
Subcut.	Rapid	2–8 hr	Unknown

Half-life: 3½ hours.

ADVERSE REACTIONS
CNS: fever, fatigue, dizziness, headache, asthenia, malaise, insomnia, hypoesthesia, pain.
CV: peripheral edema, hypertension, chest pain, arrhythmia.
EENT: epistaxis, oropharyngeal pain.
GI: nausea, constipation, diarrhea, vomiting, decreased appetite.
GU: UTI.
Hematologic: *thrombocytopenia,* anemia, *leukocytosis.*
Hepatic: increased alkaline phosphatase level.
Musculoskeletal: back pain, bone pain, extremity pain, arthralgia, muscle spasms.
Respiratory: cough, dyspnea, bronchitis, URI.
Skin: erythema, maculopapular rash, alopecia.
Other: *hypersensitivity reactions (anaphylaxis), transfusion reaction,* increased LDH level, *sepsis,* splenomegaly.

INTERACTIONS
None reported.

EFFECTS ON LAB TEST RESULTS
• May increase LDH and alkaline phosphatase levels.
• May increase WBC count. May decrease Hb level and platelet count.

CONTRAINDICATIONS & CAUTIONS
• Contraindicated in patients hypersensitive to human granulocyte colony-stimulating factors (G-CSF; filgrastim, pegfilgrastim).

• Serious allergic reactions, including anaphylaxis, have been reported. Most events occurred with initial exposure but can occur within days of discontinuing initial antiallergic treatment. Permanently discontinue drug in patients with serious allergic reactions.
• Safe use with simultaneous chemotherapy or radiation therapy hasn't been established.
• Drug isn't approved for use in healthy donors undergoing PBPC collection. Alveolar hemorrhage (pulmonary infiltrates, hemoptysis) has been reported.
• Splenic rupture (including fatal cases), sickle cell crisis (including fatal cases), ARDS, cutaneous vasculitis, and capillary leak syndrome, which may be life-threatening, have been reported.
• Use cautiously in severe chronic neutropenia; confirm diagnosis before initiating drug. Drug may increase risk of myelodysplastic syndrome and acute myelogenous leukemia.
• G-CSF drugs may act as a growth factor on any type of tumor. Transmission of tumor cells by PBPC therapy infusion may occur and hasn't been well studied.
• Use cautiously in children as studies regarding safety and effectiveness in children are limited.
Dialyzable drug: Unknown.

PREGNANCY-LACTATION-REPRODUCTION
• There are no adequate studies in pregnant women. Use during pregnancy only if benefits outweigh risks to the fetus.
• It isn't known if drug appears in breast milk. Use cautiously in breast-feeding women.

NURSING CONSIDERATIONS
• Filgrastim-sndz is biosimilar to the FDA-approved reference product filgrastim (Neupogen).
• Monitor platelet count during treatment.
• Monitor CBC routinely to adjust and determine length of treatment.
• Obtain CBC and platelet count at baseline then twice weekly during cytotoxic chemotherapy.
• For severe chronic neutropenia, monitor CBC with differential and platelet count during initial 4 weeks of treatment and during the 2 weeks after dosage adjustments.

Once patient is clinically stable, monitor monthly during first year of treatment, then as clinically indicated. Consider risks and benefits of continued treatment if abnormal cytogenetics or myelodysplasia occurs.

• Monitor patient for splenic enlargement and rupture (left upper abdominal or shoulder pain).

• Assess patients with fever, lung infiltrates, or respiratory distress for ARDS. Discontinue drug if ARDS is confirmed.

• Monitor patients for capillary leak syndrome (hypotension, hypoalbuminemia, edema, hemoconcentration). Treat as clinically indicated.

• Monitor patients for anaphylaxis or other serious hypersensitivity to drug. Permanently discontinue drug in those with serious allergic reactions.

• Watch for sickle cell crisis in patients with sickle cell trait or sickle cell disease.

• Monitor patients for signs and symptoms of cutaneous vasculitis (purpura, erythema), especially patients on long-term therapy. Withhold drug if cutaneous vasculitis develops. Consider restarting drug at a reduced dosage when signs and symptoms have resolved and ANC has decreased.

• Drug may cause transient positive bone-imaging changes because of increased hematopoietic activity.

• For patients on long-term therapy, assess patients and caregivers for ability to self-administer drug subcutaneously.

• **Look alike–sound alike:** Don't confuse filgrastim-sndz with filgrastim.

PATIENT TEACHING

• Instruct patient and caregivers on proper timing, administration, and disposal of subcutaneous self-administered drug.

• Patient with latex allergy shouldn't administer or receive drug.

• Teach patient signs and symptoms of allergic reaction (rash, facial edema, wheezing, dyspnea, hypotension, rapid HR); advise patient to seek immediate medical attention if they occur.

• Educate patient about signs and symptoms of splenic enlargement or rupture (left upper abdominal pain, left shoulder pain); advise patient to seek medical attention immediately if this type of pain occurs.

• Advise patient to immediately report difficulty breathing, fever, lung infiltrates, or respiratory distress.

• Discuss potential risks and benefits of drug for patient with sickle cell trait.

• Advise patient to immediately report purpura or erythema.

• Warn patient to seek immediate medical attention if swelling, decreased urination, shortness of breath, abdominal swelling or feeling of fullness, dizziness, or fatigue occurs.

• Caution patient not to inject a dose of 0.3 mL or less. Prefilled syringes aren't designed for lower doses.

• Tell patient that routine blood tests will be needed before and during treatment to monitor for effectiveness and safe use.

• Warn female patient who is pregnant or breast-feeding about drug's risks.

finasteride
fin-AS-teh-ride

Propecia, Proscar♦

Therapeutic class: BPH drugs
Pharmacologic class: 5-alpha reductase inhibitors

AVAILABLE FORMS
Tablets: 1 mg, 5 mg

INDICATIONS & DOSAGES
➤ **To improve symptoms of BPH and reduce risk of acute urine retention and need for surgery, including transurethral resection of prostate and prostatectomy (Proscar)**
Men: 5 mg P.O. daily.
➤ **With doxazosin, to reduce risk of BPH symptom progression (Proscar)**
Men: 5 mg P.O. daily.
➤ **Male pattern hair loss (androgenetic alopecia) in men only (Propecia)**
Men: 1 mg P.O. daily.

ADMINISTRATION
P.O.
• Give drug without regard for food.
🕲 **Alert:** Drug is a potential teratogen. Follow safe handling procedures.

ACTION
Inhibits 5-alpha reductase, resulting in inhibition of the conversion of testosterone to dihydrotestosterone (DHT), the androgen primarily responsible for the initial development and subsequent enlargement of the prostate gland. In male pattern baldness, the scalp contains miniaturized hair follicles and increased DHT level; drug decreases scalp DHT level in such cases.

Route	Onset	Peak	Duration
P.O.	Unknown	1–2 hr	24 hr

Half-life: 6 hours; 8 hours in elderly patients.

ADVERSE REACTIONS
CNS: dizziness, drowsiness, asthenia, headache, weakness.
EENT: rhinitis.
CV: hypotension, orthostatic hypotension.
GU: erectile dysfunction, decreased volume of ejaculate, decreased libido, erectile dysfunction, breast tenderness.
Respiratory: dyspnea.
Other: gynecomastia, rash.

INTERACTIONS
None reported.

EFFECTS ON LAB TEST RESULTS
• May decrease PSA level.

CONTRAINDICATIONS & CAUTIONS
• Contraindicated in patients hypersensitive to drug or to other 5-alpha reductase inhibitors, such as dutasteride.
⚠ *Alert:* Drug may increase the risk of high-grade prostate cancer. Before starting drug, patient should be evaluated to rule out other urologic conditions, including prostate cancer, that might mimic BPH. An increase in PSA level during therapy should be considered significant and patient should be evaluated for prostate cancer.
• Use cautiously in patients with liver dysfunction.
Dialyzable drug: Unknown.

PREGNANCY-LACTATION-REPRODUCTION
• Use isn't indicated in women. Contraindicated in pregnant women and women of childbearing potential.

• Pregnant women should avoid contact with drug and with semen from a male partner taking drug.
• It isn't known if drug appears in breast milk.

NURSING CONSIDERATIONS
• Before therapy, evaluate patient for conditions that mimic BPH, including hypotonic bladder, prostate cancer, infection, or stricture.
• Carefully monitor patients who have a large residual urine volume or severely diminished urine flow.
• Sustained increase in PSA level could indicate noncompliance with therapy.
• A minimum of 6 months of therapy may be needed for treatment of BPH.

PATIENT TEACHING
• Tell patient that drug may be taken with or without meals.
• Warn female patient who is or may become pregnant not to handle crushed or broken tablets because of risk of adverse effects on male fetus and to avoid contact with semen from a male partner exposed to finasteride.
• Inform patient that signs of improvement may require at least 3 months of daily use when drug is used to treat hair loss or at least 6 months when taken for BPH.
• Reassure patient that drug may decrease volume of ejaculate without impairing normal sexual function.
• Instruct patient to report breast changes, such as lumps, pain, or nipple discharge.

fingolimod
fin-GOL-ih-mod

Gilenya

Therapeutic class: Immunosuppressants
Pharmacologic class: Sphingosine 1-phosphate receptor modulators

AVAILABLE FORMS
Capsules: 0.5 mg

INDICATIONS & DOSAGES
➤ **To reduce frequency of clinical exacerbations and to delay accumulation of physical disability in relapsing forms of MS**
Adults: 0.5 mg P.O. once daily.

ADMINISTRATION
P.O.
● May give drug without regard for food.

ACTION
Unclear. May reduce migration of lymphocytes into CNS. Blocks activity of lymphocytes leaving lymph nodes, which reduces number of lymphocytes in the peripheral blood.

Route	Onset	Peak	Duration
P.O.	Unknown	12–16 hr	Unknown

Half-life: 6 to 9 days.

ADVERSE REACTIONS
CNS: asthenia, depression, dizziness, paresthesia, headache, migraine.
CV: *bradycardia,* hypertension.
EENT: sinusitis, blurred vision, eye pain.
GI: abdominal pain, gastroenteritis, diarrhea, nausea.
Hematologic: *lymphopenia, leukopenia.*
Hepatic: *hepatotoxicity.*
Metabolic: hypertriglyceridemia, weight loss.
Musculoskeletal: back pain.
Respiratory: bronchitis, cough, dyspnea.
Skin: tinea infections, alopecia, eczema, pruritus.
Other: flulike symptoms, herpes viral infections.

INTERACTIONS
Drug-drug. *Antineoplastics, immunomodulators, immunosuppressants:* May increase risk of immunosuppression. Use cautiously together.
❸ Alert: *Beta blockers, HR-lowering calcium channel blockers (diltiazem, verapamil), digoxin:* May increase risk of severe bradycardia or heart block. If possible, switch patient to cardiac drug that doesn't cause bradycardia before starting fingolimod. If change isn't possible, monitor patient with continuous ECG overnight after first dose to determine effects.
Class IA or III antiarrhythmics (amiodarone, procainamide, quinidine, sotalol): May increase risk of bradycardia or torsades de pointes. Contraindicated together.
Ketoconazole: May increase fingolimod level and risk of adverse effects. Use cautiously and monitor patient closely.
Live attenuated virus vaccines: May decrease vaccination effects or increase infection risk. Don't use together or give vaccine within 60 days of prior fingolimod use.

EFFECTS ON LAB TEST RESULTS
● May increase ALT, AST, GGT, and triglyceride levels.
● May decrease lymphocyte and neutrophil counts.

CONTRAINDICATIONS & CAUTIONS
● Contraindicated in patients hypersensitive to drug and in those with active acute or chronic infection.
❸ Alert: Contraindicated in patients with MI, unstable angina, stroke, TIA, decompensated HF requiring hospitalization, or Class III/IV HF within the past 6 months; in those with history or presence of Mobitz Type II second- or third-degree AV block or sick sinus syndrome unless patient has a functioning pacemaker; and in those with baseline QTc interval of 500 msec or greater.
❸ Alert: Use cautiously after cardiac evaluation in patients with ischemic heart disease, history of MI, HF, history of cardiac arrest, cerebrovascular disease, history of symptomatic bradycardia, recurrent syncope, severe untreated sleep apnea, AV block, or SA heart block. Monitor patient with continuous ECG overnight in medical facility after first dose.
● Use cautiously in patients with history of bradycardia, syncope, sick sinus syndrome, ischemic heart disease, or HF and in patients taking class IA or III antiarrhythmics, beta blockers, or calcium channel blockers.
● Use cautiously in patients with history of infection, macular edema, decreased pulmonary function test results, or liver disease.

- Use cautiously in patients older than age 65 who have concomitant disease or are taking other drugs.
- Safety and effectiveness in children haven't been established.

Dialyzable drug: No.

⚠ *Overdose S&S:* Chest tightness or discomfort.

PREGNANCY-LACTATION-REPRODUCTION

- Drug may cause fetal harm. Use in pregnant women only if benefit justifies risk to the fetus.
- Pregnant women should enroll in the Gilenya Pregnancy Registry at 1-877-598-7237.
- Women of childbearing potential should use effective contraception during therapy and for 2 months after last dose.
- It isn't known if drug appears in breast milk. Patient should discontinue breastfeeding or discontinue drug.

NURSING CONSIDERATIONS

🔔 *Alert:* Monitor HR and BP hourly for at least 6 hours after first dose in all patients. Obtain ECG before first dose and at the end of the observation period. Monitor BP routinely during treatment.

🔔 *Alert:* Monitor high-risk patients and those who may not tolerate bradycardia with continuous ECG overnight. High-risk patients include those who develop severe bradycardia after receiving the first dose, those with preexisting conditions who may not tolerate bradycardia, those receiving other drugs that slow the HR or AV conduction, those with QT-interval prolongation before taking fingolimod or prolonged QT interval that occurs during monitoring period, those receiving other drugs that prolong QT interval, and those at risk for QT-interval prolongation due to hypokalemia, hypomagnesemia, or congenital long-QT syndrome.

🔔 *Alert:* If CV symptoms occur (HR less than 45 beats/minute or at its lowest value 6 hours after dose, or new-onset second-degree or higher AV block 6 hours after dose), continue monitoring until symptoms resolve.

🔔 *Alert:* Repeat first-dose monitoring guidelines after second dose in patients who required pharmacologic intervention for symptomatic bradycardia after first dose.

- Obtain baseline ECG if one wasn't done within 6 months before start of therapy, especially in patients receiving antiarrhythmics, beta blockers, or calcium channel blockers and in those with cardiac risk factors or slow or irregular HR on physical examination.

🔔 *Alert:* Drug may cause progressive multifocal leukoencephalopathy (PML), which can cause severe disability or death. Monitor patient for progressive and diverse symptoms of PML (progressive weakness on one side of the body, clumsiness, vision problems, confusion, and changes in thinking, personality, memory, and orientation). Stop drug and perform diagnostic evaluation, including MRI, if PML is suspected.

- Test for varicella antibodies before treatment initiation, especially if patient has no history of chickenpox or immunization; consider vaccination against varicella zoster 1 month before start of fingolimod therapy.
- Obtain baseline ophthalmic examination and monitor patient for macular edema at 3 to 4 months after treatment initiation and if patient complains of visual disturbances. Although macular edema is a rare adverse reaction, patients with uveitis and diabetes are at increased risk.
- Monitor patient for signs and symptoms of infection during treatment and for 2 months after discontinuation of therapy. Obtain baseline CBC with differential within 6 months of beginning therapy. Consider suspending treatment if patient has active infection.
- Monitor patient for hepatic impairment (unexplained nausea, vomiting, abdominal pain, fatigue, anorexia, jaundice, dark urine). Obtain LFTs at baseline and as needed during therapy. Most enzyme elevations occur within 3 to 4 months of treatment initiation. Drug may need to be discontinued if severe liver injury occurs.
- Monitor patient for respiratory changes. Obtain spirometry and diffusion lung capacity tests if clinically indicated.
- Drug is associated with basal cell carcinoma. Monitor patient for suspicious skin lesions and evaluate promptly.
- Restart therapy as at initiation if patient discontinues treatment for more than 2 weeks.

PATIENT TEACHING
🌑 *Alert:* Teach patient to immediately contact the health care provider if signs and symptoms of a slowing HR, such as dizziness, tiredness, irregular heartbeat, or palpitations, occur.

🌑 *Alert:* Advise patient to immediately report symptoms of PML (new or worsening weakness; trouble using arms or legs; changes in thinking, eyesight, strength, or balance). Tell patient not to stop drug without first discussing with prescriber.

• Instruct patient to report visual disturbances, trouble breathing, changes in HR (low HR, dizziness, fatigue, chest pain) or rhythm (palpitations), infection (pain, fever, malaise), or suspicious skin lesions.

• Tell patient to immediately report unexplained nausea, vomiting, abdominal pain, fatigue, anorexia, jaundice, or dark urine.

• Advise patient to notify prescriber of any medication changes.

• Warn female patient of childbearing potential about possible risk to fetus; advise her to use effective contraception during treatment and for 2 months after treatment ends.

• Advise female patient to notify prescriber immediately if she is or plans to become pregnant.

---

flecainide acetate
FLEH-kay-nide

Tambocor ✢

Therapeutic class: Antiarrhythmics
Pharmacologic class: Benzamide derivatives

AVAILABLE FORMS
Tablets: 50 mg, 100 mg, 150 mg

INDICATIONS & DOSAGES
➤ **Prevention of paroxysmal supraventricular tachycardia, including AV nodal reentrant tachycardia and AV reentrant tachycardia or paroxysmal atrial fibrillation or flutter in patients without structural heart disease; life-threatening ventricular arrhythmias such as sustained ventricular tachycardia**

Adults: For paroxysmal supraventricular tachycardia or paroxysmal atrial fibrillation or flutter, 50 mg P.O. every 12 hours. Increase in increments of 50 mg b.i.d. every 4 days. Maximum dose is 300 mg/day. For life-threatening ventricular arrhythmias, 100 mg P.O. every 12 hours. Increase in increments of 50 mg b.i.d. every 4 days until desired effect occurs. Maximum dose for most patients is 400 mg/day.

Adjust-a-dose: If CrCl is 35 mL/minute or less, first dose is 100 mg P.O. once daily or 50 mg P.O. b.i.d.

ADMINISTRATION
P.O.
• Give drug without regard for food.

ACTION
A class IC antiarrhythmic that decreases excitability, conduction velocity, and automaticity by slowing atrial, AV node, His-Purkinje system, and intraventricular conduction; prolongs refractory periods in these tissues.

Route	Onset	Peak	Duration
P.O.	Unknown	1–6 hr	Unknown

Half-life: 12 to 27 hours.

ADVERSE REACTIONS
CNS: dizziness, headache, light-headedness, syncope, fatigue, fever, tremor, anxiety, insomnia, depression, malaise, paresthesia, ataxia, vertigo, asthenia, somnolence.
CV: *new or worsened arrhythmias, HF, cardiac arrest,* chest pain, palpitations, edema, flushing.
EENT: blurred vision and other visual disturbances, eye pain, eye irritation, dry mouth.
GI: nausea, constipation, abdominal pain, dyspepsia, vomiting, diarrhea, anorexia.
Respiratory: dyspnea.
Skin: rash.

INTERACTIONS
Drug-drug. *Amiodarone, cimetidine, CYP2D6 inhibitors (clozapine, quinidine):* May increase level of flecainide. Watch for toxicity. In the presence of amiodarone, reduce usual flecainide dose by 50% and

---

Reactions in bold italics are *life-threatening*. Interactions may have a *rapid onset* or a *delayed onset*.

monitor patient for adverse effects.

Digoxin: May increase digoxin level. Monitor digoxin level.

Disopyramide, verapamil: May increase negative inotropic properties. Avoid using together.

Propranolol, other beta blockers: May increase flecainide and propranolol levels. Watch for propranolol and flecainide toxicity.

Ritonavir: May significantly increase flecainide levels and toxicity. Use together is contraindicated.

Toremifene: May increase risk of life-threatening cardiac arrhythmias, including torsades de pointes, due to possibly additive prolongation of QT interval. Use together is contraindicated.

Urine-acidifying and urine-alkalizing drugs: May cause extremes of urine pH, which may alter flecainide excretion. Monitor patient for flecainide toxicity or decreased effectiveness.

Drug-food. *Milk:* May interfere with drug absorption. Monitor trough drug levels during major changes in dietary milk intake.

EFFECTS ON LAB TEST RESULTS
None reported.

CONTRAINDICATIONS & CAUTIONS
• Contraindicated in hypersensitivity to drug and in those with second- or third-degree AV block or right bundle-branch block with left hemiblock (in the absence of an artificial pacemaker), recent MI, or cardiogenic shock, and in those taking ritonavir.

Black Box Warning Patients who received flecainide for atrial fibrillation or flutter were at increased risk for ventricular tachycardia and ventricular fibrillation. Its use for these conditions isn't recommended. ∎

• Use cautiously in patients with structural heart disease, severe renal disease, prolonged QT interval, sick sinus syndrome, or blood dyscrasia. Avoid use in HF.

• In patients with hepatic disease, use drug only if potential benefits outweigh risk, and use frequent and early drug-level monitoring to guide dosage.

• When transferring patient from another antiarrhythmic to flecainide, allow two to four plasma half-lives to elapse for the drug being discontinued before starting flecainide at the usual dosage. Consider hospitalizing patients in whom withdrawal of a previous antiarrhythmic produced life-threatening arrhythmias.

Dialyzable drug: No.

PREGNANCY-LACTATION-REPRODUCTION
• Use during pregnancy only if potential benefit justifies potential risk to the fetus.
• Drug appears in breast milk. Consider discontinuing breast-feeding or drug.

NURSING CONSIDERATIONS
Black Box Warning When used to prevent ventricular arrhythmias, reserve drug for patients with documented life-threatening arrhythmias. For patients with sustained ventricular tachycardia, initiate therapy in the hospital and monitor rhythm. ∎

Black Box Warning Patients treated with flecainide for atrial flutter have a 1:1 AV conduction due to slowing of the atrial rate. A paradoxical increase in the ventricular rate may occur. Concomitant negative chronotropic therapy with digoxin or beta blockers may lower the risk of this complication. ∎

• Check that pacing threshold was determined 1 week before and after starting therapy in a patient with a pacemaker; flecainide can alter endocardial pacing thresholds.

• Correct hypokalemia or hyperkalemia before giving flecainide; these electrolyte disturbances may alter drug's effect.

• Monitor ECG for proarrhythmic effects.

• Most patients can be maintained on an every-12-hours dosing schedule; some need to receive flecainide every 8 hours.

• Monitor flecainide level, especially if patient has renal failure or HF. Therapeutic flecainide levels range from 0.2 to 1 mcg/mL. Risk of adverse effects increases when trough blood level exceeds 1 mcg/mL.

PATIENT TEACHING
• Stress importance of taking drug exactly as prescribed.

• Instruct patient to report adverse reactions promptly and to limit fluid and sodium intake to minimize fluid retention.

flibanserin

FLY-bann-ser-rin

Addyi

Therapeutic class: Miscellaneous sexual dysfunction aids
Pharmacologic class: Serotonin agonist/antagonist agents

AVAILABLE FORMS
Tablets: 100 mg

INDICATIONS & DOSAGES
➤ **Acquired, generalized hypoactive sexual desire disorder (HSDD) in premenopausal women, as characterized by low sexual desire that causes marked distress or interpersonal difficulty and isn't due to a coexisting medical or psychiatric condition, problems within the relationship, or effects of a drug or other drug substance**
Adults: 100 mg P.O. once daily at bedtime. If no improvement after 8 weeks, discontinue drug.

ADMINISTRATION
P.O.
• Give at bedtime to prevent hypotension, syncope, accidental injury, and CNS depression.
• If a dose is missed at bedtime, give next dose at bedtime the next day. Don't double next dose.
• Store at room temperature.

ACTION
Unknown. Drug demonstrates agonist activity at $5\text{-}HT_{1A}$ and antagonist activity at $5\text{-}HT_{2A}$ receptors. Moderate antagonist activity is seen at the $5\text{-}HT_{2B}$, $5\text{-}HT_{2C}$, and dopamine D_4 receptors.

Route	Onset	Peak	Duration
P.O.	Unknown	45 min–4 hr	Unknown

Half-life: About 11 hours.

ADVERSE REACTIONS
CNS: syncope, CNS depression, dizziness, insomnia, somnolence, sedation, vertigo, anxiety, fatigue.

CV: hypotension.
EENT: dry mouth.
GI: nausea, constipation, abdominal pain.
GU: metrorrhagia.
Skin: rash.
Other: accidental injury.

INTERACTIONS
Drug-drug. *CNS depressants (benzodiazepines, diphenhydramine, hypnotics, opioids):* May increase risk of somnolence and CNS depression. Monitor patient closely.
CYP3A4 inducers (carbamazepine, phenytoin, rifabutin, rifampin, rifapentine): May decrease flibanserin concentration. Use together isn't recommended.
Digoxin, sirolimus: May increase levels of these drugs, possibly leading to serious toxicity. Monitor drug levels closely.
Black Box Warning *Moderate or strong CYP3A4 inhibitors (amprenavir, atazanavir, ciprofloxacin, clarithromycin, conivaptan, diltiazem, erythromycin, fluconazole, fosamprenavir, indinavir, itraconazole, ketoconazole, nefazodone, nelfinavir, posaconazole, ritonavir, saquinavir, telithromycin, verapamil):* May increase flibanserin level and risk of hypotension and syncope. Use together is contraindicated. Discontinue flibanserin 2 days before starting moderate or strong CYP3A4 inhibitor; discontinue moderate or strong CYP3A4 inhibitor 2 weeks before starting flibanserin. ◼
Strong CYP2C19 inhibitors (antifungals, benzodiazepines, PPIs, SSRIs), weak CYP3A4 inhibitors (cimetidine, fluoxetine, oral contraceptives, ranitidine): May increase risk of hypotension, syncope, CNS depression. Monitor patient closely.
Drug-herb. *Ginkgo:* May increase flibanserin level and risk of hypotension, syncope, and CNS depression. Monitor patient closely.
St. John's wort: May decrease flibanserin level. Use together isn't recommended.
Drug-food. *Grapefruit juice:* May increase flibanserin level and risk of hypotension and syncope. Concurrent use is contraindicated.
Drug-lifestyle. **Black Box Warning** *Alcohol use:* May increase risk of hypotension, syncope, and CNS depression. Concurrent use is contraindicated. ◼

Reactions in bold italics are *life-threatening*. Interactions may have a *rapid onset* or a *delayed onset*.

EFFECTS ON LAB TEST RESULTS
None reported.

CONTRAINDICATIONS & CAUTIONS
Black Box Warning Drug is contraindicated in patients with hepatic impairment or concomitant alcohol use and in those taking concomitant strong or moderate CYP3A4 inhibitors because of risk of severe hypotension and syncope. ∎

Black Box Warning Because of the increased risk of hypotension and syncope due to an interaction with alcohol, drug is available only through a restricted program under a Risk Evaluation and Mitigation Strategy (REMS) called the ADDYI REMS Program. ∎

• Drug isn't indicated for treatment of HSDD in postmenopausal women or men, or to enhance sexual performance.

• Risk of hypotension and syncope increases if drug is taken during waking hours or at higher-than-recommended doses. Consider benefits of drug and risks of hypotension and syncope in patients with preexisting conditions that may cause hypotension.

• Use cautiously in poor metabolizers of CYP2C19.

• Drug isn't indicated for children or elderly patients.

Dialyzable drug: Unknown.

⚠ *Overdose S&S:* Hypotension, syncope, CNS depression.

PREGNANCY-LACTATION-REPRODUCTION

• There are no studies in pregnant women. Risk of using drug during pregnancy is unknown.

• It isn't known if drug appears in breast milk. Breast-feeding isn't recommended during therapy.

NURSING CONSIDERATIONS
Black Box Warning Prescribers and pharmacies must be certified with the ADDYI REMS Program in order to provide drug. Before drug is prescribed, patient's likelihood of abstaining from alcohol must be assessed. ∎

• Monitor patients for hypotension and syncope, especially with concurrent use

of herbal supplements or weak CYP3A4 inhibitors.

• Watch for signs and symptoms of hypotension and syncope in patients in whom the benefit of initiating a moderate or strong CYP3A4 inhibitor within 2 days of stopping the drug clearly outweighs the risk of flibanserin exposure–related hypotension and syncope.

• Drug may impair physical or mental abilities.

• *Look alike–sound alike:* Don't confuse Addyi with Adderall.

PATIENT TEACHING
Black Box Warning Warn patient about importance of not drinking alcohol while taking drug. ∎

• Caution patient to take drug at bedtime only. Explain that drug shouldn't be taken during waking hours because risk of hypotension and syncope increases.

• Advise patient to avoid activities that require full alertness (such as driving) for at least 6 hours after taking a dose and until drug's effects are known.

• Advise patient not to double a dose if she forgets to take it at bedtime and not to take more than the prescribed dose.

• Teach patient who experiences presyncopal signs and symptoms such as lightheadedness to immediately lie down and that it's important to promptly seek medical help if symptoms don't resolve.

• Discourage patient from taking other drugs that cause drowsiness or sedation and to report all drugs and supplements being taken before starting therapy.

• Advise patient not to take drug if she has liver damage.

• Inform patient not to drink grapefruit juice during therapy.

• Instruct patient that drug is only available through prescribers and pharmacies certified with the ADDYI REMS Program.

• Advise patient to inform prescriber if she becomes or is planning to become pregnant while taking flibanserin.

• Counsel patient not to breast-feed.

fluconazole
floo-KON-a-zole

Diflucan♦

Therapeutic class: Antifungals
Pharmacologic class: Bistriazole
derivatives

AVAILABLE FORMS
Injection: 100 mg/50 mL, 200 mg/100 mL,
400 mg/200 mL
Powder for oral suspension: 50 mg/5 mL,
200 mg/5 mL
Tablets: 50 mg, 100 mg, 150 mg, 200 mg

INDICATIONS & DOSAGES
*Adjust-a-dose (for all indications except
vulvovaginal candidiasis):* If CrCl is less than
50 mL/minute and patient isn't receiving
dialysis, give initial loading dose of 50 to
400 mg; then reduce dosage by 50%.
Patients receiving regular hemodialysis
treatment should receive usual dose after
each dialysis session.
➤ **Oropharyngeal candidiasis**
Adults: 200 mg P.O. or I.V. on first day, then
100 mg once daily for at least 2 weeks.
Children: 6 mg/kg P.O. or I.V. on first day,
then 3 mg/kg daily for 2 weeks.
*Adjust-a-dose for premature neonates
(gestational age, 26 to 29 weeks):* For first
2 weeks of life, give same dosage as for
older children every 72 hours. After first
2 weeks, give dose once daily.
➤ **Esophageal candidiasis**
Adults: 200 mg P.O. or I.V. on first day, then
100 mg once daily. Up to 400 mg daily has
been used, depending on patient's condition
and tolerance of treatment. Patients should
receive drug for at least 3 weeks and for
2 weeks after symptoms resolve.
Children: 6 mg/kg P.O. or I.V. on first day,
then 3 mg/kg daily for at least 3 weeks and
for at least 2 weeks after symptoms resolve.
Maximum daily dose 12 mg/kg.
*Adjust-a-dose for premature neonates
(gestational age, 26 to 29 weeks):* For first
2 weeks of life, give same dosage as for
older children every 72 hours. After first
2 weeks, give dose once daily.
➤ **Vulvovaginal candidiasis**
Adults: 150 mg P.O. for one dose only.

➤ **Systemic candidiasis**
Adults: Optimal therapeutic dosage and duration of therapy haven't been established;
doses of up to 400 mg P.O. or I.V. daily have
been used.
Children: 6 to 12 mg/kg/day P.O. or I.V.
*Adjust-a-dose for premature neonates
(gestational age, 26 to 29 weeks):* For first
2 weeks of life, give same dosage as for
older children every 72 hours. After first
2 weeks, give dose once daily.
➤ **Cryptococcal meningitis**
Adults: 400 mg P.O. or I.V. on first day, then
200 mg once daily for 10 to 12 weeks after
CSF culture result is negative. Doses up to
400 mg/day may be used.
Children: 12 mg/kg/day P.O. or I.V. on
first day, then 6 to 12 mg/kg/day for 10 to
12 weeks after CSF culture result is
negative.
*Adjust-a-dose for premature neonates
(gestational age, 26 to 29 weeks):* For the
first 2 weeks of life, administer the same
dosage as older children every 72 hours.
After the first 2 weeks, administer dose
once daily.
➤ **To prevent candidiasis in bone marrow
transplant and cancer patients**
Adults: 400 mg P.O. or I.V. once daily. Start
treatment several days before anticipated
agranulocytosis, and continue for 7 days
after neutrophil count exceeds 1,000/mm^3.
➤ **To suppress relapse of cryptococcal
meningitis in patients with AIDS**
Adults: 200 mg P.O. or I.V. daily.
Children: 6 mg/kg/day P.O. or I.V. once
daily.
*Adjust-a-dose for premature neonates
(gestational age, 26 to 29 weeks):* For first
2 weeks of life, give same dosage as for
older children every 72 hours. After first
2 weeks, give dose once daily.
➤ ***Candida*-related peritonitis; UTI**
Adults: 50 to 200 mg P.O. or I.V. once daily.

ADMINISTRATION
P.O.
● Drug is considered hazardous; use safe
handling and disposal precautions.
● Give drug without regard for food.
● Add 24 mL of distilled or purified water
to the bottle and shake oral suspension well
before giving.

I.V.

▼ Drug is considered hazardous; use safe handling and disposal precautions.

▼ To ensure product sterility, don't remove protective wrap from I.V. bag until just before use.

▼ The plastic container may show some opacity from moisture absorbed during sterilization. This doesn't affect drug and diminishes over time.

▼ To prevent air embolism, don't connect in series with other infusions.

▼ Use an infusion pump.

▼ Give by continuous infusion at no more than 200 mg/hour.

▼ Don't use if solution is cloudy or precipitated.

▼ **Incompatibilities:** Many other I.V. drugs. Infuse fluconazole separately. Don't add other drugs to I.V. bag.

ACTION

Inhibits fungal CYP450 (responsible for fungal sterol synthesis); weakens fungal cell walls.

Route	Onset	Peak	Duration
P.O.	Rapid	1–2 hr	30 hr
I.V.	Immediate	Immediate	Unknown

Half-life: 20 to 50 hours.

ADVERSE REACTIONS

CNS: headache, dizziness, seizures.
GI: nausea, vomiting, abdominal pain, diarrhea, dyspepsia, taste perversion.
Skin: rash.

INTERACTIONS

Drug-drug. *Alprazolam, chlordiazepoxide, clonazepam, clorazepate, diazepam, estazolam, flurazepam, midazolam, quazepam, triazolam:* Fluconazole may increase levels of these drugs and may cause increased CNS depression and psychomotor impairment. Avoid using together.
Cimetidine: May decrease fluconazole level. Monitor patient's response to fluconazole.
Cyclosporine, phenytoin, theophylline: May increase levels of these drugs. Monitor cyclosporine, phenytoin, and theophylline levels.
Erythromycin: May cause prolonged QT interval and sudden death. Don't use together.

HMG-CoA reductase inhibitors (atorvastatin, fluvastatin, lovastatin, pravastatin, simvastatin): May increase levels and adverse effects of these drugs. Avoid using together or reduce dosage of HMG-CoA reductase inhibitor.
Isoniazid, oral sulfonylureas, phenytoin, rifampin, valproic acid: May increase hepatic transaminase level. Monitor LFT results closely.
Oral sulfonylureas (glipizide, glyburide): May increase levels of these drugs. Monitor patient for enhanced hypoglycemic effect.
Rifampin: May enhance fluconazole metabolism. Monitor patient for lack of response to fluconazole.
Tacrolimus: May increase tacrolimus level and nephrotoxicity. Monitor patient carefully.
Warfarin: May increase risk of bleeding. Monitor PT and INR.
Zidovudine: May increase zidovudine-related toxicities. Monitor patient closely; zidovudine dosage decrease may be needed.
Zolpidem: May increase therapeutic effects of zolpidem. Monitor patient closely. A decrease in dosage may be needed.

EFFECTS ON LAB TEST RESULTS

● May increase alkaline phosphatase, ALT, AST, bilirubin, and GGT levels.
● May decrease platelet and WBC counts.

CONTRAINDICATIONS & CAUTIONS

● Rarely, anaphylaxis has been reported.
● Contraindicated in patients hypersensitive to drug.
● Contraindicated with CYP3A4 substrates that may lead to QT-interval prolongation (astemizole, erythromycin, pimozide, quinidine).
● Use cautiously in patients hypersensitive to other antifungal azole compounds.
● Oral suspension contains sucrose and shouldn't be used in patients with hereditary fructose, glucose, or galactose malabsorption or sucrase-isomaltase deficiency.
Dialyzable drug: 50%.
⚠ **Overdose S&S:** Hallucinations, paranoid behavior.

PREGNANCY-LACTATION-REPRODUCTION

● Contraindicated in pregnant women for most indications. Long-term treatment with high doses (400 to 800 mg/day) during the first trimester of pregnancy may be associated with birth defects.

- Drug appears in breast milk. Use cautiously in breast-feeding women.

NURSING CONSIDERATIONS

🜂 **Alert:** Serious hepatotoxicity has occurred in patients with underlying medical conditions. Monitor LFTs and discontinue drug if hepatic dysfunction develops.

- Rare cases of exfoliative skin disorders have been reported. Closely monitor patients who develop mild rash. Stop drug if lesions progress.
- Use cautiously in patients with renal impairment. Monitor renal function during treatment; dosage adjustment may be necessary.
- Likelihood of adverse reactions may be greater in HIV-infected patients.

PATIENT TEACHING

- Tell patient to take drug as directed, even after he feels better.
- Instruct patient to report all adverse reactions promptly.

SAFETY ALERT!

fludarabine phosphate
floo-DAR-a-been

Therapeutic class: Antineoplastics
Pharmacologic class: Purine antagonists

AVAILABLE FORMS

Liquid for injection: 50 mg/2 mL
Powder for injection: 50 mg

INDICATIONS & DOSAGES

➤ **B-cell chronic lymphocytic leukemia in patients with no or inadequate response to at least one standard alkylating drug regimen**
Adults: 25 mg/m² I.V. daily over 30 minutes for 5 consecutive days. Repeat cycle every 28 days. The optimal duration of treatment hasn't been established.
Adjust-a-dose: In patients with CrCl of 50 to 79 mL/minute, starting dose is 20 mg/m². In patients with CrCl of 30 to 49 mL/minute,

starting dose is 15 mg/m². If CrCl is less than 30 mL/minute, don't give drug.

ADMINISTRATION
I.V.

▼ Preparing and giving parenteral drug may be mutagenic, teratogenic, or carcinogenic. Follow facility policy to reduce risks.

▼ To prepare, add 2 mL of sterile water for injection to the vial. If using powder for injection, dissolution should occur within 15 seconds.

▼ Each milliliter contains 25 mg of drug.

▼ Dilute further in 100 or 125 mL of D₅W or NSS for injection.

▼ Use within 8 hours of reconstitution.

▼ Store drug in refrigerator at 36° to 46° F (2° to 8° C).

▼ **Incompatibilities:** Acyclovir sodium, amphotericin B, chlorpromazine, daunorubicin, ganciclovir, hydroxyzine hydrochloride, prochlorperazine edisylate.

ACTION

After conversion to its active metabolite, drug interferes with DNA synthesis by inhibiting DNA polymerase alpha, ribonucleotide reductase, and DNA primase, thus inhibiting DNA synthesis.

Route	Onset	Peak	Duration
I.V.	Unknown	Unknown	Unknown

Half-life: About 20 hours.

ADVERSE REACTIONS

CNS: fatigue, malaise, weakness, paresthesia, peripheral neuropathy, *stroke,* headache, sleep disorder, depression, cerebellar syndrome, *TIA, agitation, confusion, fever, coma, pain.*
CV: edema, angina, phlebitis, *arrhythmias, HF, MI,* supraventricular tachycardia, *DVT, aneurysm, hemorrhage.*
EENT: visual disturbances, delayed blindness, optic neuritis, optic neuropathy, hearing loss, epistaxis, sinusitis, pharyngitis.
GI: nausea, vomiting, diarrhea, constipation, anorexia, stomatitis, *GI bleeding,* esophagitis, mucositis.
GU: dysuria, UTI, urinary hesitancy, proteinuria, hematuria, *renal failure.*

Reactions in bold italics are *life-threatening*. Interactions may have a *rapid onset* or a *delayed onset*.

Hematologic: hemolytic anemia, *myelosuppression.*
Hepatic: *liver failure,* cholelithiasis.
Metabolic: hypocalcemia, hyperkalemia, hyperglycemia, dehydration, hyperuricemia, hyperphosphatemia.
Musculoskeletal: myalgia.
Respiratory: cough, pneumonia, dyspnea, URI, allergic pneumonitis, hemoptysis, hypoxia, bronchitis.
Skin: rash, pruritus, alopecia, seborrhea, diaphoresis.
Other: chills, *tumor lysis syndrome, infection, anaphylaxis.*

INTERACTIONS
Drug-drug. *Cytarabine:* May decrease metabolism of subsequently given fludarabine and inhibits fludarabine activity. Monitor patient closely.
Myelosuppressive agents: May increase toxicity. Avoid using together, if possible.
Black Box Warning *Pentostatin:* May increase risk of pulmonary toxicity, which can be fatal. Avoid using together. ■
Vaccines (live): May increase risk of vaccine-related reactions. Use together isn't recommended.

EFFECTS ON LAB TEST RESULTS
• May increase glucose, phosphate, potassium, and uric acid levels.
• May decrease calcium and Hb levels. May decrease platelet, RBC, and WBC counts.

CONTRAINDICATIONS & CAUTIONS
• Contraindicated in patients hypersensitive to drug or its components.
• Use cautiously in patients with renal insufficiency.
Black Box Warning May cause life-threatening and fatal autoimmune phenomena, such as acquired hemophilia, thrombocytopenia or thrombocytopenic purpura, Evans syndrome, and hemolytic anemia, after one or more cycles. ■
Dialyzable drug: Yes.
⚠ Overdose S&S: Delayed blindness, coma, thrombocytopenia, neutropenia, death.

PREGNANCY-LACTATION-REPRODUCTION
• May cause fetal harm. If used in pregnancy, apprise patient of potential fetal hazard.

• Women of childbearing potential and men with sexual partners of childbearing potential must use contraceptives during therapy and for at least for 6 months after therapy ends.
• Drug may damage testicular tissue and spermatozoa.
• It isn't known if drug appears in breast milk. Patient should discontinue breast-feeding or discontinue drug.

NURSING CONSIDERATIONS
Black Box Warning Administer under the supervision of a physician experienced in the use of antineoplastic therapy. ■
Black Box Warning Higher than recommended doses are associated with severe neurologic toxicity, including blindness, coma, and death. ■
☝ Alert: Monitor patient closely and expect modified dosage based on toxicity. Most toxic effects are dose dependent. Advanced age, renal insufficiency, and bone marrow impairment may predispose patients to increased or excessive toxicity.
Black Box Warning Careful hematologic monitoring is needed, especially of neutrophil and platelet counts. Bone marrow suppression can be severe. ■
Black Box Warning Instances of life-threatening and sometimes fatal autoimmune phenomena have been reported. Monitor patient for development of hemolysis. ■
• To prevent bleeding, avoid all I.M. injections when platelet count is below 50,000/mm³.
• Give blood transfusions because of cumulative anemia. Patients should be given irradiated blood only, to minimize transfusion-associated GFHD.
• Hyperuricemia, hypocalcemia, hyperkalemia, and renal failure may result from rapid lysis of tumor cells. Take preventive measures against tumor lysis syndrome, such as I.V. hydration, alkalinization of urine, and treatment with allopurinol as appropriate.
• *Look alike–sound alike:* Don't confuse fludarabine with floxuridine, fluorouracil, or flucytosine.

PATIENT TEACHING

● Instruct patient to watch for signs and symptoms of infection (fever, sore throat, fatigue) and bleeding (easy bruising, nosebleeds, bleeding gums, tarry stools). Tell patient to take temperature daily.

---

flunisolide (inhalation, intranasal)

floo-NISS-oh-lide

AeroSpan HFA

Therapeutic class: Corticosteroids
Pharmacologic class: Corticosteroids

AVAILABLE FORMS

Oral inhalant in a hydrofluoroalkane (HFA) inhaler: 80 mcg/metered dose (AeroSpan HFA)
Nasal spray: 25 mcg/spray, 29 mcg/spray

INDICATIONS & DOSAGES

➤ **Chronic asthma (inhalational)**
Adults and children age 12 and older:
2 inhalations (160 mcg) with AeroSpan HFA inhaler b.i.d. Titrate to lowest effective dose once asthma stability is achieved. Don't exceed 320 mcg b.i.d.
Children ages 6 to 11: 1 inhalation (80 mcg) with AeroSpan HFA inhaler b.i.d. Titrate to lowest effective dose once asthma stability is achieved. Don't exceed 160 mcg b.i.d.
➤ **Symptoms of seasonal or perennial allergic rhinitis (nasal spray)**
Adults and children age 15 and older: Starting dose is 2 sprays in each nostril b.i.d. If needed, may increase dosage to 2 sprays in each nostril t.i.d. Maximum total daily dose is 8 sprays in each nostril per day.
Children ages 6 to 14: Starting dose is 1 spray in each nostril t.i.d. or 2 sprays in each nostril b.i.d. Maximum total daily dose is 4 sprays in each nostril per day.

ADMINISTRATION

Inhalational
● For best results, the canister should be at room temperature before use.
● Allow 1 minute between doses.
● Prime before using for the first time by releasing two test sprays into the air away from the face. If the inhaler hasn't been used

for more than 2 weeks, prime the inhaler again by releasing two test sprays into the air away from the face.
Intranasal
● Shake well before each use.
● Before first use, prime nasal spray by pushing down on pump five or six times until a fine mist appears. If pump hasn't been used for 5 days or more, it must be primed again.

ACTION

A corticosteroid that may decrease inflammation by inhibiting macrophages, T cells, eosinophils, and mediators such as leukotrienes while reducing the number of mast cells within the airway.

Route	Onset	Peak	Duration
Inhalation	1–4 wk	Unknown	Unknown
Intranasal	Unknown	Unknown	Unknown

Half-life: Inhalation, about 1¾ hours; intranasal, 1 to 2 hours.

ADVERSE REACTIONS

CNS: headache, dizziness, insomnia, migraine.
CV: chest pain, edema.
EENT: conjunctivitis, ear pain, nasal dryness, nasal congestion, loss of smell, epistaxis, rhinitis, laryngitis, voice alteration, taste perversion, pharyngitis, sinusitis.
GI: dyspepsia, vomiting, diarrhea, gastroenteritis, nausea, oral moniliasis, abdominal pain.
GU: UTI, dysmenorrhea, vaginitis.
Musculoskeletal: neck pain, myalgia.
Respiratory: cough, bronchitis.
Skin: *erythema multiforme.*
Other: infection, allergic reaction.

INTERACTIONS

Inhalational
Drug-drug. *Aldesleukin:* May diminish antineoplastic effect of aldesleukin. Avoid using together.
Amphotericin B: May enhance hypokalemic effect of amphotericin B. Monitor patient.
Corticorelin: May diminish therapeutic effect of corticorelin. Monitor therapy.
CYP3A4 inhibitors (strong): May increase serum concentration of corticosteroids. Use together isn't recommended.

Reactions in bold italics are *life-threatening*. Interactions may have a *rapid onset* or a *delayed onset*.

Deferasirox: May enhance adverse effects of deferasirox. Monitor patient.

Loop diuretics, thiazide diuretics: May enhance hypokalemic effect of these drugs. Monitor patient.

Drug-herb. *Echinacea:* May diminish therapeutic effect of immunosuppressants. Consider therapy modification.

Intranasal

None significant.

EFFECTS ON LAB TEST RESULTS

None reported.

CONTRAINDICATIONS & CAUTIONS

• Contraindicated in patients hypersensitive to drug. Inhalational formulation is contraindicated in patients with status asthmaticus or acute asthma episodes.

• Inhalational drug isn't recommended in patients with nonasthmatic bronchial diseases or with asthma controlled by bronchodilator or other noncorticosteroid alone.

• Use cautiously, if at all, in patients with active or quiescent respiratory tract TB infections or untreated fungal, bacterial, or systemic viral or ocular herpes simplex infections.

❸ *Alert:* Drug is absorbed into the circulation, and excessive doses may suppress HPA axis function.

• Use intranasal form cautiously in patients who have recently had nasal septal ulcers, nasal surgery, or nasal trauma.

Dialyzable drug: Unknown.

PREGNANCY-LACTATION-REPRODUCTION

• Use during pregnancy only if potential benefit justifies potential risk to the fetus.

• Inhaled corticosteroids are likely acceptable to use in pregnant and breast-feeding women when weighed against patient's risk of asthma exacerbation(s).

• Use intranasal form cautiously during pregnancy and breast-feeding and at lowest effective dose.

NURSING CONSIDERATIONS

❸ *Alert:* All patients with asthma should have routine tests of adrenal cortical function, including measurement of early-morning resting cortisol levels to establish a baseline in the event of an emergency.

❸ *Alert:* There is an increased risk of death due to adrenal insufficiency in patients transferred from systematically active corticosteroids to flunisolide inhaler. Monitor patient carefully.

❸ *Alert:* Withdraw drug slowly in patients who have received long-term oral corticosteroid therapy.

❸ *Alert:* After withdrawing systemic corticosteroids, patient may need supplemental systemic corticosteroids if stress (trauma, surgery, or infection) causes adrenal insufficiency.

• If patient develops paradoxical bronchospasm immediately after using inhalational drug, treat immediately with a fast-acting bronchodilator and discontinue drug.

• Assess bone mineral density initially and periodically in patients at risk for osteoporosis who are using inhalational drug.

• Inhalational drug may increase risk of cataracts and increased IOP. Monitor patient closely.

• Intranasal drug isn't effective for acute exacerbations of rhinitis. Decongestants or antihistamines may be needed.

• Don't give intranasal drug for more than 3 weeks unless there is significant symptom improvement.

• *Look alike–sound alike:* Don't confuse flunisolide with fluocinonide.

PATIENT TEACHING

• Warn patient that drug doesn't relieve acute asthma attacks.

❸ *Alert:* Instruct patient to immediately contact prescriber if asthma episodes unresponsive to bronchodilators occur during treatment.

• Advise patient to ensure delivery of proper dose by gently warming the inhalation canister to room temperature before using. Some patients carry the canister in a pocket to keep it warm.

• Children should administer drug under adult supervision.

• Tell patient who also uses a bronchodilator to use it several minutes before beginning inhalational flunisolide treatment.

• Instruct patient to begin inhaling immediately before activating the canister to get the full dose.

• Instruct patient to allow 1 minute to elapse before repeating inhalations and to hold his breath for a few seconds to enhance drug action.

• Teach patient to keep inhaler clean and unobstructed. The HFA inhaler doesn't need cleaning during normal use.

• Advise patient to prevent oral fungal infections by gargling or rinsing mouth with water after each inhaler use. Caution patient not to swallow the water.

• Instruct patient to shake intranasal container before use, blow nose to clear nasal passages, tilt head slightly forward, and insert nozzle into nostril, pointing away from septum. Tell patient to hold other nostril closed and inhale gently while spraying and then to repeat procedure in other nostril. Advise patient to clean nosepiece with warm water daily.

• Explain that intranasal drug doesn't work right away. Most patients notice improvement within a few days, but some may need 2 to 3 weeks.

• Tell patient to stop intranasal drug and notify prescriber if signs and symptoms don't diminish in 3 weeks or if nasal irritation persists.

• Teach patient to check mucous membranes frequently for signs and symptoms of fungal infection.

• Warn patient to avoid exposure to chickenpox or measles. If exposed, contact prescriber immediately.

• Advise parents of a child receiving long-term therapy that the child should have periodic growth measurements and be checked for evidence of HPA axis suppression.

---

fluocinolone acetonide
floo-oh-SIN-oh-lone

Capex, Derma-Smoothe/FS, Dermotic, Synalar

Therapeutic class: Corticosteroids
Pharmacologic class: Corticosteroids

AVAILABLE FORMS
Cream: 0.01%, 0.025%
Oil: 0.01%
Oil/drops (otic): 0.01%
Ointment: 0.025%
Shampoo: 0.01%
Topical solution: 0.01%

INDICATIONS & DOSAGES
➤ **Inflammation from corticosteroid-responsive dermatoses**
Adults and children: Clean area; apply product sparingly t.i.d. to q.i.d.
➤ **Atopic dermatitis**
Adults: Apply thin film of topical oil t.i.d.
Children age 2 and older: Apply thin film of topical oil b.i.d. for maximum of 4 weeks. Avoid face and diaper area.
➤ **Scalp psoriasis**
Adults: Wet or dampen hair and scalp thoroughly. Apply a thin film of topical oil and massage into scalp. Cover with supplied shower cap overnight or for a minimum of 4 hours before washing thoroughly with regular shampoo and then rinsing thoroughly with water.
➤ **Seborrheic dermatitis of the scalp**
Adults: Apply no more than 30 mL of 0.01% shampoo to the scalp once daily, lather, and rinse thoroughly with water after 5 minutes.
➤ **Eczematous external otitis**
Adults and children age 2 and older: Apply 5 drops of oil (otic) into affected ear b.i.d. for 7 to 14 days.

ADMINISTRATION
Otic
• Tilt head to one side so the affected ear is facing up. Gently pull earlobe backward and upward and apply 5 drops of oil into the ear. Keep head tilted for at least 1 minute.
Topical
• Gently wash skin before applying. To prevent skin damage, rub in gently, leaving a thin coat. When treating hairy sites, part hair and apply directly to lesions.
• Avoid application near eyes or mucous membranes; in armpits, groin, or rectal area; or in ear canal if eardrum is perforated.
• Do not use occlusive dressing unless ordered.
• For patients with eczematous dermatitis whose skin may be irritated by adhesive material, hold dressing in place with gauze, elastic bandages, stockings, or stockinette.
• Change dressing as prescribed. Stop drug and notify prescriber if skin infection, striae, or atrophy occur.
• Shake shampoo well prior to use.

Reactions in bold italics are *life-threatening*. Interactions may have a *rapid onset* or a *delayed onset*.

ACTION

Unclear. Is diffused across cell membranes to form complexes with receptors. Shows anti-inflammatory, antipruritic, vasoconstrictive, and antiproliferative activity. Considered a medium-potency to low-potency drug, according to vasoconstrictive properties.

Route	Onset	Peak	Duration
Otic, topical	Unknown	Unknown	Unknown

Half-life: Unknown.

ADVERSE REACTIONS

GU: glycosuria.
Metabolic: hyperglycemia.
Skin: burning, pruritus, irritation, dryness, erythema, folliculitis, hypertrichosis, hypopigmentation, acneiform eruptions, perioral dermatitis, allergic contact dermatitis, maceration, secondary infection, atrophy, striae, miliaria with occlusive dressings.

INTERACTIONS

None significant.

EFFECTS ON LAB TEST RESULTS

● May increase glucose level.

CONTRAINDICATIONS & CAUTIONS

● Contraindicated in patients hypersensitive to drug or its components.
● Don't use as monotherapy in primary bacterial infections (impetigo, paronychia, erysipelas, cellulitis, angular cheilitis), treatment of rosacea, perioral dermatitis, or acne.
● Drug isn't for ophthalmic use.
● Use cautiously in patients with peanut sensitivity.
Dialyzable drug: Unknown.
⚠ *Overdose S&S:* Systemic effects.

PREGNANCY-LACTATION-REPRODUCTION

● Use cautiously in pregnant and breast-feeding women at lowest effective dose.

NURSING CONSIDERATIONS

● If an occlusive dressing has been applied and a fever develops, notify prescriber and remove dressing.
● If antifungal or antibiotic combined with corticosteroid fails to provide prompt improvement, stop corticosteroid until infection is controlled.
● Systemic absorption is likely with use of occlusive dressings, prolonged treatment, or extensive body surface treatment. Watch for symptoms, such as hyperglycemia, glycosuria, HPA axis suppression, or Cushing syndrome.
● Avoid using plastic pants or tight-fitting diapers on treated areas in young children. Children may absorb larger amounts of drug and be more susceptible to systemic toxicity.
🌢 *Alert:* Body oil and scalp oil formulations contain peanut oil.
● *Look alike–sound alike:* Don't confuse fluocinolone with fluocinonide or fluticasone.

PATIENT TEACHING

● Teach patient or family how to apply drug using gloves or sterile applicator.
● Tell patient to wash hands after application.
● If an occlusive dressing is used, advise patient to leave it in place for no longer than 12 hours each day and not to use dressing on infected or weeping lesions.
● Tell patient to stop using solution and notify prescriber if he develops signs of systemic absorption, skin irritation or ulceration, hypersensitivity, or infection.
● Advise patient using the shampoo not to bandage, cover, or wrap the treated scalp area unless directed.

fluocinonide
floo-oh-SIN-oh-nide

Vanos

Therapeutic class: Corticosteroids
Pharmacologic class: Corticosteroids

AVAILABLE FORMS

Cream: 0.05%, 0.1%
Gel: 0.05%
Ointment: 0.05%
Topical solution: 0.05%

INDICATIONS & DOSAGES

➤ **Inflammation from corticosteroid-responsive dermatoses**
Adults and children: Clean area; apply cream, gel, ointment, or topical solution

sparingly b.i.d. to q.i.d. In children, use lowest dosage that promotes healing. If using Vanos 0.1% cream in adults and children age 12 and older, apply a thin layer once daily or b.i.d. for up to 2 weeks.

ADMINISTRATION
Topical
- Gently wash skin before applying. To prevent skin damage, rub in gently, leaving a thin coat. When treating hairy sites, part hair and apply directly to lesion.
- Avoid applying near eyes or mucous membranes or in ear canal.
- Occlusive dressings may be used in severe or resistant dermatoses.
- For patients with eczematous dermatitis whose skin may be irritated by adhesive material, hold dressing in place with gauze, elastic bandages, stockings, or stockinette.
- Change dressing as prescribed. Stop drug and notify prescriber if skin infection, striae, or atrophy occur.
- Continue treatment for a few days after lesions clear.

ACTION
Diffuses across cell membranes to form complexes with cytoplasmic receptors, showing anti-inflammatory, antipruritic, vasoconstrictive, and antiproliferative activity. Considered a high-potency drug, according to vasoconstrictive properties.

Route	Onset	Peak	Duration
Topical	Unknown	Unknown	Unknown

Half-life: Unknown.

ADVERSE REACTIONS
GU: glycosuria.
Metabolic: hyperglycemia.
Skin: burning, pruritus, irritation, dryness, erythema, folliculitis, hypertrichosis, hypopigmentation, acneiform eruptions, perioral dermatitis, allergic contact dermatitis, maceration, secondary infection, atrophy, striae, miliaria with occlusive dressings.

INTERACTIONS
None significant.

EFFECTS ON LAB TEST RESULTS
- May increase glucose level.

CONTRAINDICATIONS & CAUTIONS
- Contraindicated in patients hypersensitive to drug or its components.
- Don't use as monotherapy in primary bacterial infections (impetigo, paronychia, erysipelas, cellulitis, angular cheilitis), treatment of rosacea, perioral dermatitis, or acne.
- Don't use very-high-potency or high-potency agents on the face, groin, or armpits.
- Drug isn't for ophthalmic use.
Dialyzable drug: Unknown.
⚠ *Overdose S&S:* Systemic effects.

PREGNANCY-LACTATION-REPRODUCTION
- Use cautiously in pregnant and breast-feeding women at lowest effective dose.

NURSING CONSIDERATIONS
- If an occlusive dressing has been applied and a fever develops, notify prescriber and remove dressing.
- If antifungal or antibiotic combined with corticosteroid fails to provide prompt improvement, stop corticosteroid until infection is controlled.
- Systemic absorption is likely with use of occlusive dressings, prolonged treatment, or extensive body surface treatment. Watch for such symptoms as hyperglycemia, glycosuria, and HPA axis suppression.
- Avoid using plastic pants or tight-fitting diapers on treated areas in young children. Children may absorb larger amounts of drug and be more susceptible to systemic toxicity.
- *Look alike–sound alike:* Don't confuse fluocinonide with fluocinolone or fluticasone.

PATIENT TEACHING
- Teach patient and family how to apply drug using careful hand washing and gloves or sterile applicator.
- If an occlusive dressing is ordered, advise patient to leave it in place no more than 12 hours each day and not to use the dressing on infected or weeping lesions.
- Tell patient to stop drug and report signs of systemic absorption, skin irritation or ulceration, hypersensitivity, or infection.

Reactions in bold italics are *life-threatening*. Interactions may have a *rapid onset* or a *delayed onset*.

SAFETY ALERT!

fluorouracil
(5-fluorouracil, 5-FU)
flure-oh-YOOR-a-sill

Carac, Efudex, Fluoroplex, Tolak

Therapeutic class: Antineoplastics
Pharmacologic class: Pyrimidine
analogues

AVAILABLE FORMS
Cream: 0.5%, 1%, 4%, 5%
Injection: 50 mg/mL
Topical solution: 2%, 5%

INDICATIONS & DOSAGES
➤ **Colon, rectal, breast, stomach, and
pancreatic cancers**
Adults: Initially, 12 mg/kg I.V. daily for
4 days (daily dose shouldn't exceed
800 mg); if no toxicity, give 6 mg/kg on
days 6, 8, 10, and 12; then give a single
weekly maintenance dose of 10 to 15 mg/kg
I.V. begun after toxicity (if any) from first
course has subsided. Don't exceed 1 g/week.
(Recommended dosages are based on actual body weight unless patient is obese or
retaining fluid.)
*Poor-risk patients and those not in an
adequate nutritional state:* Initially,
6 mg/kg/day for 3 days. If no toxicity is
observed, may give 3 mg/kg on the 5th,
7th, and 9th days unless toxicity occurs. No
therapy is given on the 4th, 6th, or 8th days.
Daily dose shouldn't exceed 400 mg.
➤ **Multiple actinic (solar) keratoses**
Adults: Apply Carac cream once daily for up
to 4 weeks. Or, apply Efudex or Fluoroplex
cream or topical solution b.i.d. for 2 to
6 weeks.
➤ **Superficial basal cell carcinoma**
Adults: Apply 5% Efudex cream or topical
solution b.i.d. usually for 3 to 6 weeks;
maximum, 12 weeks.

ADMINISTRATION
I.V.
▼ Preparing and giving parenteral drug
may be mutagenic, teratogenic, or carcinogenic. Follow facility policy to reduce
risks.

▼ To reduce nausea, give antiemetic before
5-FU.
▼ Don't use cloudy solution. If crystals
form, redissolve by warming.
▼ Drug may be given by direct injection
without dilution or infused over 2 to
24 hours to decrease toxicity.
▼ For infusion, dilute drug with D_5W,
sterile water for injection, or NSS for
injection.
▼ For continuous infusion, use plastic
I.V. containers. Solution is more stable in
plastic than in glass bottles.
▼ Don't refrigerate. Protect drug from
sunlight.
▼ Discard unused portion of vial after 1 hour.
▼ **Incompatibilities:** Aldesleukin, amphotericin B cholesteryl sulfate complex, carboplatin, cisplatin, cytarabine, diazepam,
doxorubicin, droperidol, epirubicin, fentanyl citrate, filgrastim, gallium nitrate,
leucovorin calcium, metoclopramide,
morphine sulfate, ondansetron, topotecan,
vinorelbine tartrate.
Topical
● Apply topical form cautiously near patient's eyes, nose, and mouth.
● Avoid occlusive dressings with topical
form because they increase risk of inflammatory reactions in adjacent normal skin.
● Apply topical form with nonmetal applicator or suitable gloves. Wash hands
immediately after handling topical form.
● The 1% topical strength is used on patient's face. Higher strengths, such as 5%,
are used for thicker skinned areas or resistant lesions, such as superficial basal cell
carcinoma.

ACTION
May interfere with DNA and RNA synthesis, leading to a thymine deficiency that
provokes unbalanced growth and death of
the cell.

Route	Onset	Peak	Duration
I.V., topical	Unknown	Unknown	Unknown

Half-life: 16 minutes (I.V.).

ADVERSE REACTIONS
CNS: malaise.
GI: stomatitis, GI ulcer, nausea, vomiting,
diarrhea, anorexia, *GI bleeding.*

Hematologic: *leukopenia, thrombocytopenia, agranulocytosis,* anemia.
Skin: dermatitis, erythema, scaling, pruritus, nail changes, pigmented palmar creases, erythematous contact dermatitis, desquamative rash of hands and feet, hand-foot syndrome with long-term use, photosensitivity reactions, reversible alopecia, pain, burning, soreness, suppuration, swelling, dryness, erosion with topical use.

INTERACTIONS
Drug-drug. *Leucovorin calcium:* May increase cytotoxicity and toxicity of fluorouracil. Monitor patient closely.
Live-virus vaccines: May increase risk of vaccine-induced adverse reactions. Concomitant use isn't recommended.
Drug-lifestyle. *Sun exposure:* May cause photosensitivity reactions. Advise patient to avoid excessive sunlight exposure.

EFFECTS ON LAB TEST RESULTS
• May increase alkaline phosphatase, AST, ALT, bilirubin, 5-hydroxyindoleacetic acid (in urine), and LDH levels. May decrease Hb and plasma albumin levels.
• May decrease granulocyte, platelet, RBC, and WBC counts.

CONTRAINDICATIONS & CAUTIONS
• Contraindicated in patients hypersensitive to drug and in those with bone marrow suppression (WBC counts of 3,500/mm³ or less or platelet counts of 100,000/mm³ or less) or potentially serious infections.
• Contraindicated in patients in a poor nutritional state.
◑ **Alert:** Discontinue I.V. drug at first sign of stomatitis or esophagopharyngitis, WBC count less than 3,500/mm³ or a rapidly falling WBC count, intractable vomiting, diarrhea, GI ulceration and bleeding, platelet count less than 100,000/mm³, or hemorrhage from any site.
• Use cautiously in patients who have received high-dose pelvic radiation or alkylating drugs and in those with impaired hepatic or renal function or widespread neoplastic infiltration of bone marrow.
Dialyzable drug: Yes.
⚠ **Overdose S&S:** Nausea, vomiting, diarrhea, GI ulceration and bleeding, bone

marrow depression (thrombocytopenia, leukopenia, agranulocytosis).

PREGNANCY-LACTATION-REPRODUCTION
• There are no well-controlled studies in pregnant women. Drug may cause fetal harm. Use during pregnancy only if potential benefit justifies potential risk to the fetus.
• Topical formulations contraindicated in women who are or may become pregnant during therapy.
• Women of childbearing potential should avoid becoming pregnant during therapy.
• Contraindicated in breast-feeding women.

NURSING CONSIDERATIONS
Black Box Warning I.V. drug should be administered under the supervision of a physician experienced in cancer chemotherapy. Patient should be hospitalized at least during the initial course of I.V. therapy. ■
• Ingestion and systemic absorption of topical form may cause leukopenia, thrombocytopenia, stomatitis, diarrhea, or GI ulceration, bleeding, and hemorrhage. Application to large ulcerated areas may cause systemic toxicity.
• Watch for stomatitis or diarrhea (signs of toxicity). Consider using topical oral anesthetic to soothe lesions. Stop drug and notify prescriber if diarrhea occurs.
• Encourage diligent oral hygiene to prevent superinfection of denuded mucosa.
• Monitor WBC and platelet counts. WBC counts with differential are recommended before each dose. Watch for ecchymoses, petechiae, easy bruising, and anemia.
• Monitor fluid intake and output, CBC, LFTs, and renal function tests.
• Long-term use may cause erythematous, desquamative rash of the hands and feet (hand-foot syndrome). Syndrome gradually resolves over 5 to 7 days after therapy interruption.
• Dermatologic adverse effects are reversible when drug is stopped.
• To prevent bleeding, avoid I.M. injections when platelet count is below 50,000/mm³.
• Anticipate blood transfusions because of cumulative anemia.
◑ **Alert:** Toxicity may be delayed for 1 to 3 weeks.

Reactions in bold italics are *life-threatening*. Interactions may have a *rapid onset* or a *delayed onset*.

* The WBC count nadir occurs 9 to 14 days after first dose; the platelet count nadir occurs in 7 to 14 days.
☼ Alert: Drug may be ordered as "5-fluorouracil" or "5-FU." The numeral "5" is part of the drug name and shouldn't be confused with dosage units.
* **Look alike–sound alike:** Don't confuse fluorouracil with floxuridine, fludarabine, or flucytosine.

PATIENT TEACHING
* Advise patient to immediately report all adverse reactions, especially infection, bleeding, severe nausea, vomiting, diarrhea, dark urine, yellowing of skin or eyes, malaise, or redness of hands or feet.
* Warn patient that hair loss may occur but is reversible.
* Caution patient to avoid prolonged exposure to sunlight or ultraviolet light when topical form is used.
* Tell patient to use highly protective sunblock to avoid inflammatory skin irritation.
* Warn patient that topically treated area may be unsightly during therapy and for several weeks afterward. Complete healing may take 1 or 2 months.

fluoxetine hydrochloride
floo-OX-e-teen

Prozac⚘, Prozac Weekly⚘, Sarafem⚘

Therapeutic class: Antidepressants
Pharmacologic class: SSRIs

AVAILABLE FORMS
Capsules (delayed-release) ⓓⓝⓒ*:* 90 mg
Capsules (pulvules): 10 mg, 20 mg, 40 mg
Oral solution: 20 mg/5 mL
Tablets: 10 mg, 15 mg, 20 mg, 60 mg

INDICATIONS & DOSAGES
Adjust-a-dose (for all indications): For patients with renal or hepatic impairment and those taking several drugs at the same time, reduce dose or increase dosing interval.
➤ **Depression, obsessive-compulsive disorder (OCD) (excluding Sarafem)**

Adults: Initially, 20 mg P.O. in the morning; increase dosage based on patient response. Maximum daily dose is 80 mg.
Children ages 7 to 17 (OCD): 10 mg P.O. daily. After 2 weeks, increase to 20 mg daily. Dosage is 20 to 60 mg daily.
Children ages 8 to 18 (depression): 10 mg P.O. once daily for 1 week; then increase to 20 mg daily.
➤ **Maintenance therapy for depression (excluding Sarafem) in stabilized patients (not for newly diagnosed depression)**
Adults: 90 mg Prozac Weekly P.O. once weekly. Start once-weekly doses 7 days after the last daily dose of Prozac 20 mg.
➤ **Short-term and long-term treatment of bulimia nervosa (excluding Sarafem)**
Adults: 60 mg P.O. daily in the morning.
➤ **Short-term treatment of panic disorder with or without agoraphobia (excluding Sarafem)**
Adults: 10 mg P.O. once daily for 1 week, then increase dose as needed to 20 mg daily. Maximum daily dose is 60 mg.
➤ **Depressive episodes associated with bipolar I disorder (with olanzapine)**
Adults: 20 mg P.O. with 5 mg P.O. olanzapine once daily in the evening. Dosage adjustments can be made based on efficacy and tolerability within ranges of fluoxetine 20 to 50 mg and olanzapine 5 to 12.5 mg.
Children ages 10 to 17: Initially, 20 mg P.O. with 2.5 mg olanzapine P.O. once daily in evening. Dosage adjustments can be made based on efficacy and tolerability within ranges of fluoxetine 20 to 50 mg and olanzapine 5 to 12 mg.
➤ **Premenstrual dysphoric disorder**
Adults: 20 mg Sarafem P.O. daily continuously (every day of the menstrual cycle) or intermittently (daily dose starting 14 days before the anticipated onset of menstruation through first full day of menses and repeating with each new cycle). Maximum daily dose, 80 mg P.O.
➤ **Treatment-resistant depression**
Adults: 20 mg P.O. with 5 mg P.O. olanzapine once daily in the evening. Dosage adjustments can be made based on efficacy and tolerability within ranges of fluoxetine 20 to 50 mg and olanzapine 5 to 20 mg.

F

ADMINISTRATION
P.O.
● Give drug without regard for food.
● Avoid giving drug in the afternoon, whenever possible, because doing so commonly causes nervousness and insomnia.
● Delayed-release capsules must be swallowed whole; don't crush or open.

ACTION
Thought to be linked to drug's inhibition of CNS neuronal uptake of serotonin.

Route	Onset	Peak	Duration
P.O.	Unknown	6–8 hr	Unknown

Half-life: Acute administration, 2 to 3 days; long-term administration, 4 to 6 days.

ADVERSE REACTIONS
CNS: nervousness, somnolence, anxiety, insomnia, headache, drowsiness, tremor, dizziness, asthenia, abnormal thinking, fatigue, fever.
CV: palpitations, hot flashes.
EENT: nasal congestion, pharyngitis, sinusitis.
GI: nausea, diarrhea, dry mouth, anorexia, dyspepsia, constipation, abdominal pain, vomiting, flatulence, increased appetite.
GU: sexual dysfunction, decreased libido.
Metabolic: weight loss, hyponatremia.
Musculoskeletal: muscle pain.
Respiratory: URI, cough.
Skin: rash, pruritus, diaphoresis.
Other: flulike syndrome.

INTERACTIONS
Drug-drug. *Amphetamines, buspirone, dextromethorphan, dihydroergotamine, lithium salts, meperidine, other SSRIs or SSNRIs (duloxetine, venlafaxine), TCAs,* **tramadol,** *trazodone, tryptophan:* May increase the risk of serotonin syndrome. Avoid combinations of drugs that increase the availability of serotonin in the CNS; monitor patient closely if used together.
Aspirin, NSAIDs: May increase risk of GI bleeding. Use together cautiously.
Benzodiazepines, lithium, TCAs: May increase CNS effects. Monitor patient closely.
Beta blockers, carbamazepine, flecainide, vinblastine: May increase levels of these drugs. Monitor drug levels and monitor patient for adverse reactions.
Cyclosporine: May increase renal toxicity of cyclosporine. Monitor patient carefully for cyclosporine toxicity.
Cyproheptadine: May reverse or decrease fluoxetine effect. Monitor patient closely.
Dextromethorphan: May cause unusual side effects such as visual hallucinations. Advise use of cough suppressant that doesn't contain dextromethorphan while taking fluoxetine.
Highly protein-bound drugs: May increase level of fluoxetine or other highly protein-bound drugs. Monitor patient closely.
Insulin, oral antidiabetics: May alter glucose level and antidiabetic requirements. Adjust dosage.
Linezolid, methylene blue: May cause serotonin syndrome. Use extreme caution and monitor closely.
MAO inhibitors (phenelzine, selegiline, tranylcypromine): May cause serotonin syndrome and signs and symptoms resembling neuroleptic malignant syndrome. Avoid using at the same time and for at least 5 weeks after stopping fluoxetine.
Phenytoin: May increase phenytoin level and risk of toxicity. Monitor phenytoin level and adjust dosage.
Pimozide, thioridazine: May increase levels of these drugs, increasing risk of serious ventricular arrhythmias and sudden death. Don't use together and don't use thioridazine for at least 5 weeks after stopping pimozide.
Tamoxifen: May decrease tamoxifen plasma level, leading to breast cancer recurrence. Monitor patient carefully.
Triptans: May cause weakness, hyperreflexia, incoordination, rapid changes in BP, nausea, and diarrhea. Monitor patient closely, especially at the start of treatment and when dosage increases.
Warfarin: May increase risk for bleeding. Monitor PT and INR.
Drug-herb. *Gotu kola, kava kava, St. John's wort, tryptophan, valerian:* May increase sedative and hypnotic effects; may cause serotonin syndrome. Discourage use together.
Drug-lifestyle. *Alcohol use:* May increase CNS depression. Discourage use together.

Reactions in bold italics are *life-threatening*. Interactions may have a *rapid onset* or a *delayed onset*.

EFFECTS ON LAB TEST RESULTS
• May decrease sodium level.

CONTRAINDICATIONS & CAUTIONS
• Contraindicated in patients hypersensitive to drug and within 14 days of stopping an MAO inhibitor intended to treat psychiatric disorders. MAO inhibitors shouldn't be started within 5 weeks of stopping fluoxetine. Avoid using thioridazine with fluoxetine or within 5 weeks after stopping fluoxetine.

Black Box Warning Drug may increase the risk of suicidal thinking and behavior in children, adolescents, and young adults with major depressive disorder or other psychiatric disorder. ■

Black Box Warning Fluoxetine is approved for use in children with major depressive disorder and OCD. Fluoxetine isn't approved for use in children younger than age 7. Sarafem isn't approved for use in children. ■

⊖ **Alert:** Concomitant use with linezolid or methylene blue can cause serotonin syndrome (fever, mental status changes, muscle twitching, excessive sweating, shivering or shaking, diarrhea, loss of coordination). Use drug with linezolid or methylene blue only for life-threatening or urgent conditions when the potential benefits outweigh the risks of toxicity.

• Use cautiously in patients at high risk for suicide and in those with history of diabetes mellitus, seizures, mania, or hepatic, renal, or CV disease.

Dialyzable drug: No.

⚠ *Overdose S&S:* Nausea, seizures, somnolence, tachycardia, vomiting, coma, delirium, ECG abnormalities, hypotension, mania, neuroleptic malignant syndrome-like reactions, pyrexia, stupor, syncope.

PREGNANCY-LACTATION-REPRODUCTION
• Use cautiously in pregnant women and only if benefit justifies possible risk to the fetus.
• Drug appears in breast milk. Use in breast-feeding women isn't recommended.

NURSING CONSIDERATIONS
⊖ *Alert:* If linezolid or methylene blue must be given, fluoxetine must be stopped and patient monitored for serotonin toxicity for 5 weeks or until 24 hours after the last dose of linezolid or methylene blue, whichever comes first. Treatment with fluoxetine may be resumed 24 hours after the last dose of linezolid or methylene blue.

• Use antihistamines or topical corticosteroids to treat rashes or pruritus.
• Watch for weight change during therapy, particularly in underweight or bulimic patients.
• Record mood changes. Watch for suicidal tendencies.
• Drug has a long half-life; monitor patient for adverse effects for up to 2 weeks after drug is stopped.

⊖ *Alert:* Combining triptans with an SSRI or an SSNRI may cause serotonin syndrome or neuroleptic malignant syndrome-like reactions. Serotonin syndrome may be more likely to occur when starting or increasing the dose of triptan, SSRI, or SSNRI.

• When discontinuing drug, taper dosage over 2 weeks to 1 month to avoid withdrawal syndrome.

• *Look alike–sound alike:* Don't confuse fluoxetine with fluvoxamine or fluvastatin. Don't confuse Prozac with Proscar or Prilosec.

PATIENT TEACHING
Black Box Warning Advise family and caregivers to carefully observe patient for worsening suicidal thinking or behavior. ■

⊖ *Alert:* Teach patient to recognize and immediately report symptoms of serotonin toxicity (fever, mental status changes, muscle twitching, excessive sweating, shivering or shaking, diarrhea, loss of coordination).

• Tell patient to avoid taking drug in the afternoon whenever possible because doing so commonly causes nervousness and insomnia.

• Drug may cause dizziness or drowsiness. Warn patient to avoid driving and other hazardous activities that require alertness and good psychomotor coordination until effects of drug are known.

• Tell patient to consult prescriber before taking other prescription or OTC drugs.

• Advise patient that full therapeutic effect may not be seen for 4 weeks or longer.

fluphenazine decanoate
floo-FEN-a-zeen

Modecate Concentrate ✦

fluphenazine hydrochloride

Therapeutic class: Antipsychotics
Pharmacologic class: Phenothiazines

AVAILABLE FORMS
fluphenazine decanoate
Depot injection: 25 mg/mL*, 100 mg/mL ✦
fluphenazine hydrochloride
Elixir: 2.5 mg/5 mL*
I.M. injection: 2.5 mg/mL
Oral concentrate: 5 mg/mL*
Tablets: 1 mg, 2.5 mg, 5 mg, 10 mg

INDICATIONS & DOSAGES
➤ **Psychotic disorders**
Adults: Initially, 2.5 to 10 mg/day
fluphenazine hydrochloride P.O. daily in
divided doses every 6 to 8 hours; may increase cautiously to 20 mg/day. Maximum
daily dose is 40 mg. Maintenance dose is
1 to 5 mg P.O. daily. I.M. doses are ⅓ to
½ of P.O. doses. Usual initial I.M. dose is
1.25 mg. Give more than 10 mg daily with
caution.

Or, 12.5 to 25 mg of fluphenazine decanoate I.M. or subcutaneously every 1 to
6 weeks; maintenance dose is 25 to 100 mg,
as needed.
Elderly patients: 1 to 2.5 mg fluphenazine
hydrochloride P.O. daily.

ADMINISTRATION
P.O.
• Oral liquid forms can cause contact dermatitis. Wear gloves when preparing solutions, and avoid contact with skin and
clothing.
• Protect drug from light. Slight yellowing
of concentrate is common and doesn't affect potency. Discard markedly discolored
solutions.
• Use calibrated device to measure desired
dose, and dilute liquid concentrate with
60 mL of tomato or fruit juice or milk just
before administration. Don't dilute in beverages containing caffeine (coffee, cola),

tannics (tea), or pectinates (apple juice).
I.M.
• Parenteral forms can cause contact dermatitis. Wear gloves when preparing solutions, and avoid contact with skin and
clothing.
• Protect drug from light. Slight yellowing
of injection is common and doesn't affect
potency. Discard markedly discolored solutions.
• For long-acting form (decanoate), which
is an oil preparation, use a dry needle of at
least 21G.
Subcutaneous
• Long-acting form (decanoate) is indicated
for subcutaneous administration.
• Use a dry syringe and needle of at least
21G.
• Don't use if solution is cloudy or contains
particulate matter.

ACTION
A piperazine phenothiazine that blocks
postsynaptic dopamine receptors in the
brain.

Route	Onset	Peak	Duration
P.O.	<1 hr	30 min	6–8 hr
I.M. (decanoate)	24–72 hr	Unknown	1–6 wk
I.M. (hydrochloride)	<1 hr	90–120 min	6–8 hr
Subcut.	Unknown	Unknown	Unknown

Half-life: Decanoate, 6 to 9 days; hydrochloride,
15 hours.

ADVERSE REACTIONS
CNS: extrapyramidal reactions, tardive
dyskinesia, pseudoparkinsonism, *seizures,*
neuroleptic malignant syndrome, sedation,
EEG changes, drowsiness, dizziness.
CV: orthostatic hypotension, tachycardia,
ECG changes.
EENT: blurred vision, ocular changes,
nasal congestion.
GI: dry mouth, constipation, increased
appetite.
GU: urine retention, dark urine, menstrual
irregularities, inhibited ejaculation.
Hematologic: *leukopenia, agranulocyto-*
sis, aplastic anemia, thrombocytopenia,
eosinophilia, hemolytic anemia.
Hepatic: cholestatic jaundice.

Metabolic: weight gain.
Skin: mild photosensitivity reactions, allergic reactions.
Other: gynecomastia, galactorrhea.

INTERACTIONS

Drug-drug. *Antacids:* May inhibit absorption of oral phenothiazines. Separate antacid and phenothiazine doses by at least 2 hours.
Anticholinergics: May increase anticholinergic effects. Use together cautiously.
Barbiturates, lithium: May decrease phenothiazine effect and increase neurologic adverse effects. Monitor patient.
Centrally acting antihypertensives: May decrease antihypertensive effect. Monitor BP.
CNS depressants: May increase CNS depression. Use together cautiously.
Black Box Warning *Opioids:* May cause slow or difficult breathing, sedation, and death. Avoid use together. If use together is necessary, limit dosage and duration of each drug to the minimum necessary for desired effect. ■
Drug-herb. *St. John's wort:* May increase risk of photosensitivity reactions. Advise patient to avoid excessive sunlight exposure.
Drug-lifestyle. *Alcohol use:* May increase CNS depression, especially that involving psychomotor skills. Strongly discourage alcohol use.
Sun exposure: May increase risk of photosensitivity reactions. Advise patient to avoid excessive sunlight exposure.

EFFECTS ON LAB TEST RESULTS

● May increase LFT values. May decrease Hb level and hematocrit.
● May increase eosinophil count. May decrease granulocyte, platelet, and WBC counts.
● May cause false-positive results for amylase, 5-hydroxyindoleacetic acid, urinary porphyrin, and urobilinogen tests and for urine pregnancy tests that use human chorionic gonadotropin.

CONTRAINDICATIONS & CAUTIONS

● Contraindicated in patients hypersensitive to drug and in those with coma, CNS depression, bone marrow suppression or other blood dyscrasia, subcortical damage, or liver damage.
Black Box Warning Opioid drugs should only be prescribed with benzodiazepines or other CNS depressants to patients for whom alternative treatment options are inadequate. ■
● Use cautiously in elderly or debilitated patients and in those with pheochromocytoma, severe CV disease (may cause sudden drop in BP), peptic ulcer, respiratory disorder, hypocalcemia, seizure disorder (drug may lower seizure threshold), severe reactions to insulin or electroconvulsive therapy, mitral insufficiency, glaucoma, or prostatic hyperplasia.
● Use cautiously in patients exposed to extreme heat or cold (including antipyretic therapy) or phosphorus insecticides.
● Use parenteral form cautiously in patients who have asthma or are allergic to sulfites.
Dialyzable drug: Unknown.
⚠ *Overdose S&S:* Stupor, coma, seizures in children.

PREGNANCY-LACTATION-REPRODUCTION

● Safe use during pregnancy hasn't been established. Use if only clearly needed and if benefit justifies risk.
🖐 *Alert:* Neonates exposed to antipsychotics during the third trimester are at risk for developing extrapyramidal signs and symptoms (repetitive muscle movements of the face and body) and withdrawal signs and symptoms (agitation, abnormally increased or decreased muscle tone, tremors, sleepiness, severe difficulty breathing, difficulty feeding) after delivery.
● Drug may appear in breast milk. Use cautiously in breast-feeding women.

NURSING CONSIDERATIONS

● Monitor patient for tardive dyskinesia, which may occur after prolonged use. It may not appear until months or years later and may disappear spontaneously or persist for life, despite ending drug.
🖐 *Alert:* Watch for signs and symptoms of neuroleptic malignant syndrome (extrapyramidal effects, hyperthermia, autonomic disturbance), which is rare but often fatal. It may not be related to length of drug use or type of neuroleptic.

• Withhold dose and notify prescriber if patient, especially child or pregnant woman, develops signs or symptoms of blood dyscrasia (fever, sore throat, infection, cellulitis, weakness) or extrapyramidal reactions persisting longer than a few hours. **Black Box Warning** Elderly patients with dementia-related psychosis treated with atypical or conventional antipsychotics are at increased risk for death. Antipsychotics aren't approved for the treatment of dementia-related psychosis. ■

• Don't withdraw drug abruptly unless serious adverse reactions occur.

• Abrupt withdrawal of long-term therapy may cause gastritis, nausea, vomiting, dizziness, tremor, feeling of warmth or cold, diaphoresis, tachycardia, headache, or insomnia.

PATIENT TEACHING
Black Box Warning Caution the patient or the caregiver of a patient taking an opioid drug with a benzodiazepine, CNS depressant, or alcohol to seek immediate medical attention if the patient has symptoms of dizziness, light-headedness, extreme sleepiness, slowed or difficult breathing, or unresponsiveness. ■

• Warn patient to avoid activities that require alertness and good coordination until effects of drug are known. Drowsiness and dizziness usually subside after first few weeks.

• Warn patient to avoid alcohol while taking drug.

• Tell patient to relieve dry mouth with sugarless gum or hard candy.

• Have patient report signs of urine retention or constipation.

• Advise patient to use sunblock and wear protective clothing to avoid sensitivity to the sun.

• Tell patient that drug may discolor urine.

SAFETY ALERT!

flutamide
FLOO-ta-mide

Therapeutic class: Antineoplastics
Pharmacologic class: Nonsteroidal antiandrogens

AVAILABLE FORMS
Capsules: 125 mg, 250 mg ✤

INDICATIONS & DOSAGES
➤ **Metastatic locally confined prostate cancer (stages B_2, C, D_2), combined with luteinizing hormone-releasing hormone analogues, such as leuprolide acetate or goserelin**
Men: 250 mg P.O. every 8 hours.

ADMINISTRATION
P.O.
• Drug is a hormonal agent and is considered a potential teratogen. Follow safe handling procedures.
• Give drug with a full glass of water.
• Give drug without regard for food.

ACTION
Inhibits androgen uptake or prevents binding of androgens in nucleus of cells in target tissues.

Route	Onset	Peak	Duration
P.O.	Unknown	2 hr	Unknown

Half-life: For steady-state metabolite, about 8 hours.

ADVERSE REACTIONS
CNS: drowsiness, confusion, depression, anxiety, nervousness, paresthesia.
CV: peripheral edema, hypertension, hot flashes.
GI: diarrhea, nausea, vomiting, anorexia.
GU: erectile dysfunction, urine discoloration.
Hematologic: anemia, *leukopenia, thrombocytopenia,* hemolytic anemia.
Skin: injection-site reaction, rash, photosensitivity reactions.
Other: loss of libido, gynecomastia.

Reactions in bold italics are *life-threatening*. Interactions may have a *rapid onset* or a *delayed onset*.

INTERACTIONS
Drug-drug. *Warfarin:* May prolong PT. Monitor PT and INR.
Drug-lifestyle. *Sun exposure:* May cause photosensitivity reactions. Advise patient to avoid excessive sunlight exposure.

EFFECTS ON LAB TEST RESULTS
• May increase BUN, creatinine, Hb, and liver enzyme levels.
• May decrease platelet and WBC counts.
• May alter pituitary-gonadal system tests during therapy and for 12 weeks after.

CONTRAINDICATIONS & CAUTIONS
• Contraindicated in patients hypersensitive to drug, in those with severe liver dysfunction, and in women.
Dialyzable drug: Unlikely.
⚠ **Overdose S&S:** Gynecomastia, breast tenderness, increased AST level.

PREGNANCY-LACTATION-REPRODUCTION
• Not indicated for use in women. May cause fetal harm.

NURSING CONSIDERATIONS
Black Box Warning Drug may cause liver failure. Obtain LFTs before the start of therapy, monthly for the first 4 months of therapy, periodically thereafter, and at the first signs and symptoms suggesting liver dysfunction (nausea, vomiting, anorexia, fatigue). Immediately stop drug if jaundice occurs or AST level rises above 2 × ULN. ■
• Monitor CBC periodically.
• Patients with hemoglobin M disease or G6PD deficiency and smokers are at risk for methemoglobinemia, hemolytic anemia, and cholestatic jaundice. Monitor methemoglobin level.
• Flutamide must be taken continuously with drug used for medical castration (such as leuprolide) to allow full therapeutic benefit. Leuprolide suppresses testosterone production, whereas flutamide inhibits testosterone action at cellular level; together, they can impair growth of androgen-responsive tumors.

PATIENT TEACHING
• Advise patient not to stop drug without consulting prescriber.

• Tell patient to take drug with a full glass of water.
• Tell patient drug may be taken without food, but if stomach irritation occurs, to take with food.
• Instruct patient to report adverse reactions promptly, especially dark yellow or brown urine, vomiting, or yellowing of the eyes or skin.

fluticasone furoate
floo-TIK-a-sone

Arnuity Ellipta, Veramyst

fluticasone propionate
Flonase, Flovent Diskus, Flovent HFA

Therapeutic class: Corticosteroids
Pharmacologic class: Corticosteroids

AVAILABLE FORMS
Nasal spray (furoate): 27.5 mcg/spray
Nasal spray (propionate): 50 mcg/metered spray
Oral inhalation aerosol: 44 mcg, 110 mcg, 220 mcg
Oral inhalation powder: 50 mcg, 100 mcg, 200 mcg, 250 mcg

INDICATIONS & DOSAGES
➤ **As preventative in maintenance of chronic asthma in patients requiring oral corticosteroid**
Flovent Diskus
Adults and children age 12 and older: In patients previously taking bronchodilators alone, initially, inhaled dose of 100 mcg b.i.d. to maximum of 500 mcg b.i.d.
Adults and children age 12 and older previously taking inhaled corticosteroids: Initially, inhaled dose of 100 to 250 mcg b.i.d. to maximum of 500 mcg b.i.d.
Adults and children age 12 and older previously taking oral corticosteroids: Inhaled dose of 500 to 1,000 mcg b.i.d. Maximum dose, 1,000 mcg b.i.d.
Children ages 4 to 11: For patients previously on bronchodilators alone or on inhaled corticosteroids, initially, inhaled dose of 50 mcg b.i.d. to maximum of 100 mcg b.i.d.

Flovent HFA
Adults and children age 12 and older: In those previously taking bronchodilators alone, initially, inhaled dose of 88 mcg b.i.d. to maximum of 440 mcg b.i.d.
Adults and children age 12 and older previously taking inhaled corticosteroids: Initially, inhaled dose of 88 to 220 mcg b.i.d. to maximum of 440 mcg b.i.d.
Adults and children age 12 and older previously taking oral corticosteroids: Initially, inhaled dose of 440 mcg b.i.d. to maximum of 880 mcg b.i.d.
Children ages 4 to 11 (Flovent only): 88 mcg inhaled b.i.d. regardless of prior therapy.

➤ **Nasal symptoms of seasonal and perennial allergic and nonallergic rhinitis**
Flonase
Adults: Initially, 2 sprays (100 mcg) in each nostril daily or 1 spray b.i.d. Once symptoms are controlled, decrease to 1 spray in each nostril daily. Or, for seasonal allergic rhinitis, 2 sprays in each nostril once daily, as needed, for symptom control.
Adolescents and children age 4 and older: Initially, 1 spray (50 mcg) in each nostril daily. If not responding, increase to 2 sprays in each nostril daily. Once symptoms are controlled, decrease to 1 spray in each nostril daily. Maximum dose is 2 sprays in each nostril daily.
Veramyst
Adults and children age 12 and older: 110 mcg once daily administered as 2 sprays (27.5 mcg/spray) in each nostril.
Children ages 2 to 11: 55 mcg once daily administered as 1 spray (27.5 mcg/spray) in each nostril.

ADMINISTRATION
Inhalational
• For best results, aerosol canister should be at room temperature.
• Prime and shake well before each use.
• Patients should rinse mouth after inhalation.
Intranasal
• Prime and shake well before use.

ACTION
Anti-inflammatory and vasoconstrictor that may decrease inflammation by inhibiting mast cells, macrophages, and mediators such as leukotrienes.

Route	Onset	Peak	Duration
Inhalation (nasal)	12 hr	Several days	1–2 wk
Inhalation (oral)	24 hr	Several days	1–2 wk

Half-life: 3 hours.

ADVERSE REACTIONS
CNS: headache, dizziness, fever, migraine, nervousness.
EENT: pharyngitis, blood in nasal mucus, cataracts, conjunctivitis, dry eye, dysphonia, epistaxis, eye irritation, hoarseness, laryngitis, nasal burning or irritation, nasal discharge, rhinitis, sinusitis.
GI: oral candidiasis, abdominal discomfort, abdominal pain, diarrhea, mouth irritation, nausea, viral gastroenteritis, vomiting.
GU: UTI.
Hematologic: eosinophilia.
Metabolic: cushingoid features, growth retardation in children, hyperglycemia, weight gain.
Musculoskeletal: aches and pains, symptoms of neck sprain or strain, joint pain, muscular soreness, osteoporosis.
Respiratory: URI, *bronchospasm,* asthma symptoms, bronchitis, chest congestion, cough, dyspnea.
Skin: dermatitis, urticaria.
Other: *angioedema,* influenza, viral infections.

INTERACTIONS
Drug-drug. *Cobicistat:* May increase serum concentration of oral inhalation drug. Avoid use together.
Ketoconazole, other CYP3A4 inhibitors: May increase mean fluticasone level. Use together cautiously.
Ritonavir: May cause systemic corticosteroid effects, such as Cushing syndrome and adrenal suppression. Avoid using together.

EFFECTS ON LAB TEST RESULTS
• Abnormal response to the 6-hour cosyntropin stimulation test may occur in patients taking high doses of fluticasone.

Reactions in bold italics are *life-threatening*. Interactions may have a *rapid onset* or a *delayed onset*.

CONTRAINDICATIONS & CAUTIONS

● Contraindicated in patients hypersensitive to ingredients in these preparations.
● Contraindicated as primary treatment of patients with status asthmaticus or other acute, intense episodes of asthma.
● Use cautiously in patients at risk for decreased bone mineralization.
● Drug can increase risk of vasculitis, Kaposi sarcoma, psychiatric disturbances, hypertension, fluid retention, GI perforation, and hyperglycemia.
Dialyzable drug: Unknown.
⚠ *Overdose S&S:* Hypercorticism.

PREGNANCY-LACTATION-REPRODUCTION

● Use during pregnancy only if potential benefit justifies potential risk to the fetus.
● Use cautiously in breast-feeding.

NURSING CONSIDERATIONS

● Because of risk of systemic absorption of inhaled corticosteroids, observe patient carefully for evidence of systemic corticosteroid effects.
● *Alert:* Monitor patient, especially postoperatively, during periods of stress or severe asthma attack for evidence of inadequate adrenal response.
● *Alert:* During withdrawal from oral corticosteroids, some patients may experience signs and symptoms of systemically active corticosteroid withdrawal, such as joint or muscle pain, lassitude, and depression, despite maintenance or even improvement of respiratory function. Deaths due to adrenal insufficiency have occurred with transfer from active corticosteroids to fluticasone propionate inhaler.
● For patients starting therapy who are currently receiving oral corticosteroid therapy, reduce dose of prednisone to no more than 2.5 mg/day on a weekly basis, beginning after at least 1 week of therapy with fluticasone.
● *Alert:* As with other inhaled asthma drugs, bronchospasm may occur with an immediate increase in wheezing after a dose. If bronchospasm occurs after a dose of inhalation aerosol, treat immediately with a fast-acting inhaled bronchodilator.
● Drug may increase risk of glaucoma and cataracts. Monitor patient.

PATIENT TEACHING

● Advise patient to report all adverse reactions.
● Tell patient that inhalation drug isn't indicated for the relief of acute bronchospasm.
● Advise patient to use drug at regular intervals, as directed.
● Instruct patient to contact prescriber if nasal spray doesn't improve condition after 4 days of treatment.
● Instruct patient to immediately contact prescriber if asthma episodes unresponsive to bronchodilators occur during treatment with fluticasone. During such episodes, patient may need therapy with oral corticosteroids.
● Warn patient to avoid exposure to chickenpox or measles and, if exposed, to consult prescriber immediately.
● Tell patient to carry or wear medical identification indicating that he may need supplementary corticosteroids during stress or a severe asthma attack.
● *Alert:* During periods of stress or a severe asthma attack, instruct patient who has been withdrawn from systemic corticosteroids to resume prescribed oral corticosteroids immediately and to contact prescriber for further instruction.
● Teach patient how to prime and use inhaler according to manufacturer's instructions.
● Advise patient to avoid spraying inhalation aerosol into eyes.
● Advise patient to store fluticasone powder in a dry place.

Flonase nasal spray
● Teach patient how to prime and use nasal inhaler according to manufacturer's instructions.
● Tell patient to contact provider if signs or symptoms don't improve within 4 days or if signs or symptoms worsen.

F

---

fluticasone furoate–vilanterol trifenatate
floo-TIK-a-sone/vye-LAN-ter-ol

Breo Ellipta

Therapeutic class: Corticosteroids–bronchodilators
Pharmacologic class: Corticosteroids–beta$_2$ adrenergic agonists

AVAILABLE FORMS
Powder for inhalation: Inhaler containing two double-foil blister strips of powder formulation: One strip contains fluticasone furoate 100 mcg/blister or 200 mcg/blister; the other contains vilanterol 25 mcg/blister

INDICATIONS & DOSAGES
➤ **Asthma; reducing exacerbations in patients with COPD**
Adults: 1 inhalation of 100 mcg fluticasone furoate–25 mcg vilanterol trifenatate or 200 mcg fluticasone furoate–25 mcg vilanterol trifenatate once daily.

ADMINISTRATION
Inhalational
• Patient shouldn't use more than 1 inhalation in 24 hours; may cause adverse effects.
• Have patient exhale fully before taking one long, steady, deep breath through the mouthpiece (patient shouldn't breathe through the nose), hold breath for 3 to 4 seconds, and exhale slowly and gently. After use, have patient rinse mouth with water without swallowing to help reduce the risk of oropharyngeal candidiasis.
• Give at the same time every day and not more than one time every 24 hours.
• Store at room temperature between 68° and 77° F (20° and 25° C).
• Keep drug stored inside the unopened moisture-protective foil tray; remove from tray immediately before initial use.
• Discard drug 6 weeks after opening foil tray or when the counter reads "0" (after all blisters have been used).
• Inhaler isn't reusable.
• Don't attempt to take the inhaler apart.

ACTION
Fluticasone is an anti-inflammatory and vasoconstrictor that may decrease inflammation by inhibiting mast cells, macrophages, and mediators such as leukotrienes. Vilanterol trifenatate relaxes bronchial smooth muscle and inhibits inflammatory mediators, especially mast cells.

Route	Onset	Peak	Duration
Inhalation (fluticasone)	Unknown	30–60 min	Unknown
Inhalation (vilanterol)	Unknown	10 min	Unknown

Half-life: Fluticasone, 24 hours; vilanterol, 21 hours.

ADVERSE REACTIONS
CNS: headache, pyrexia.
CV: hypertension, peripheral edema.
EENT: nasopharyngitis, oropharyngeal candidiasis, oropharyngeal pain, pharyngitis.
GI: diarrhea.
Musculoskeletal: back pain, arthralgia.
Respiratory: URI, COPD, pneumonia, bronchitis, sinusitis, cough.
Other: flulike symptoms.

INTERACTIONS
Drug-drug. *CYP3A4 inhibitors (clarithromycin, conivaptan, indinavir, itraconazole, ketoconazole, lopinavir, nefazodone, nelfinavir, ritonavir, saquinavir, telithromycin, troleandomycin, voriconazole):* May increase systemic effects of corticosteroids, and increased CV adverse effects may occur. Use together cautiously.
Loop or thiazide diuretics (furosemide, hydrochlorothiazide, torsemide): May increase risk of hypokalemia or ECG changes. Monitor patient closely with concurrent use.
MAO inhibitors, TCAs, other drugs known to prolong QTc interval: May increase adrenergic effects or risk of ventricular arrhythmias. Don't use together or within 2 weeks of discontinuation.
Nonselective beta blockers (carvedilol, propranolol, sotalol): May increase risk of bronchospasm. Use cardioselective agents only if absolutely needed.
Other long-acting beta-agonist drugs (arformoterol tartrate, formoterol fumarate,

---

Reactions in bold italics are *life-threatening*. Interactions may have a *rapid onset* or a *delayed onset*.

indacaterol, salmeterol): May increase risk of overdose. Don't use together.

EFFECTS ON LAB TEST RESULTS
• May increase glucose level. May decrease potassium level.

CONTRAINDICATIONS & CAUTIONS
• Contraindicated in patients with severe hypersensitivity to milk proteins and in those who have demonstrated hypersensitivity to fluticasone furoate, vilanterol, or their components.

Black Box Warning Use for asthma only when patient isn't adequately controlled on a long-term asthma control medication such as an inhaled corticosteroid (ICS) or if disease severity clearly warrants initiation of treatment with both an ICS and a long-acting beta$_2$-adrenergic agonist (LABA). LABAs such as vilanterol increase the risk of asthma-related death. Once asthma control is achieved and maintained, assess patient regularly and discontinue fluticasone–vilanterol if possible without loss of asthma control while maintaining patient on long-term medication such as an ICS. Don't use fluticasone–vilanterol in patients whose asthma is adequately controlled on a low- or medium-dose ICS. ■

❸ *Alert:* Contraindicated as primary treatment of status asthmaticus or other acute episodes of COPD or asthma where other intensive measures are required.

❸ *Alert:* Don't exceed recommended dosage; serious adverse events, including fatalities, have been associated with excessive use of inhaled sympathomimetics.

• Use cautiously in patients with existing TB; fungal, bacterial, viral, or parasitic infections; or ocular herpes simplex. Drug may suppress the immune system and infection may worsen.

• Use cautiously in patients with thyrotoxicosis, diabetes mellitus, ketoacidosis, or CV disorders (coronary insufficiency, arrhythmias, hypertension).

• Use cautiously in patients with increased IOP, cataracts, or glaucoma. Increased IOP, glaucoma, and cataracts have occurred with prolonged use.

• Use cautiously in patients with seizure disorders; beta agonists may cause CNS stimulation.
Dialyzable drug: Unknown.

PREGNANCY-LACTATION-REPRODUCTION
• Use cautiously in pregnant and breast-feeding women.
• Avoid use during labor as drug may interfere with uterine contractility.

NURSING CONSIDERATIONS
• If not already prescribed, initiate an inhaled, short-acting beta$_2$ agonist in patients taking this drug.
• Patients who have been taking oral or inhaled short-acting beta$_2$ agonists on a regular basis (q.i.d.) should discontinue regular use of these drugs and use them only for relief of acute respiratory symptoms.
• Monitor short-acting beta$_2$ agonist rescue use. Increased use signals disease deterioration.
• Slowly wean patients requiring oral corticosteroids from systemic corticosteroid use after switch to an inhaler. Reduce daily prednisone dosage by 2.5 mg on a weekly basis during therapy with inhaled drug.
• Patients may require supplemental corticosteroid during times of stress when weaning from systemic corticosteroids.
• Monitor lung function and watch for COPD signs and symptoms and adrenal insufficiency (fatigue, lassitude, weakness, nausea, vomiting, hypotension).
• Discontinue drug slowly if hypercortisolism or adrenal suppression is suspected.
• Monitor patient periodically for candidal infections of the mouth. Have patient rinse mouth after inhalation without swallowing to help reduce the risk.
• Monitor patient for signs and symptoms of pneumonia.
• If paradoxical bronchospasm occurs, discontinue drug and institute alternative therapy.
• Monitor patient for increased IOP and for development or worsening of glaucoma or cataracts.
• Monitor patient for hypokalemia and hyperglycemia.

F

- Serious or even fatal courses of chickenpox or measles can occur in susceptible patients.
- Monitor patient for CV effects (tachycardia, hypertension, supraventricular tachycardia, extrasystoles).
- Monitor patient for reduction in bone mineral density (BMD) initially and periodically with long-term use. Patients who use tobacco and those with prolonged immobilization, family history of osteoporosis, postmenopausal status, advanced age, poor nutrition, or long-term use of other drugs that can reduce BMD (anticonvulsants, oral corticosteroids) are at increased risk.

☼ Alert: Orally inhaled corticosteroids may slow growth rate when given to children and adolescents.

PATIENT TEACHING

- Teach patient to rinse mouth without swallowing after inhalation to help reduce the risk of candidal infections.
- Caution patient not to use drug for acute symptoms or asthma.
- Warn patient not to use drug with other LABAs.
- Instruct patient to immediately notify health care provider if adverse reactions occur, symptoms worsen, more inhalations than usual of rescue medication are needed, or a significant decrease in lung function occurs.
- Instruct patient not to discontinue drug without the guidance of health care provider.
- Advise patient to obtain regular eye examinations.
- Caution female patient to report pregnancy to health care provider as soon as possible.

fluticasone propionate (topical)
floo-TIK-a-sone

Cutivate

Therapeutic class: Corticosteroids
Pharmacologic class: Corticosteroids

AVAILABLE FORMS
Cream: 0.05%
Lotion: 0.05%
Ointment: 0.005%

INDICATIONS & DOSAGES

➤ **Inflammation and pruritus from dermatoses responsive to corticosteroids**
Adults: Apply sparingly to affected area b.i.d.; rub in gently and completely. If using lotion (0.05%) in adults and children age 1 year and older, apply once daily. Don't use for longer than 4 weeks.
Children age 3 months and older: Apply a thin film of cream (0.05%) to affected areas b.i.d. Rub in gently. Don't use for longer than 4 weeks.

➤ **Inflammation and pruritus from atopic dermatitis**
Children age 3 months and older: Apply thin film (0.05%) to affected areas once daily or b.i.d. Rub in gently. Don't use for longer than 4 weeks.

ADMINISTRATION
Topical
- Don't use drug with an occlusive dressing or in diaper area.

ACTION
Is diffused across cell membranes to form complexes with cytoplasmic receptors. Shows anti-inflammatory, antipruritic, vasoconstrictive, and antiproliferative activity. Considered a medium-potency drug, according to vasoconstrictive properties.

Route	Onset	Peak	Duration
Topical	Rapid	Unknown	10 hr

Half-life: About 7½ hours.

ADVERSE REACTIONS
CNS: light-headedness.
GU: glycosuria.
Metabolic: hyperglycemia.
Skin: urticaria, burning, hypertrichosis, pruritus, irritation, erythema, hives, dryness
Other: *HPA axis suppression,* Cushing syndrome.

INTERACTIONS
None significant.

EFFECTS ON LAB TEST RESULTS
- May increase glucose level.

Reactions in bold italics are *life-threatening*. Interactions may have a *rapid onset* or a **delayed onset.**

CONTRAINDICATIONS & CAUTIONS
• Contraindicated in patients hypersensitive to drug or its components.
• Don't use as monotherapy in primary bacterial, viral, fungal, herpetic, or tubercular skin infections or for treatment of rosacea, perioral dermatitis, or acne.
• Drug isn't for ophthalmic use.
Dialyzable drug: Unknown.
⚠ *Overdose S&S:* Systemic effects (including reversible HPA axis suppression, Cushing syndrome, hyperglycemia, glycosuria).

PREGNANCY-LACTATION-REPRODUCTION
• Use during pregnancy only if potential benefit justifies potential risk to the fetus.
• Use cautiously in breast-feeding women.

NURSING CONSIDERATIONS
• Don't mix drug with other bases or vehicles because doing so may affect potency.
• If adverse reactions occur, prescriber may order less potent drug.
• Stop drug if local irritation or systemic infection, absorption, or hypersensitivity occurs.
• May cause suppression of HPA axis in patients receiving high doses for prolonged periods, particularly in children.
• Absorption of corticosteroid is increased when drug is applied to inflamed or damaged skin, eyelids, or scrotal area; it's lowest when applied to intact normal skin, palms of hands, or soles of feet.
• *Look alike–sound alike:* Don't confuse fluticasone with fluconazole, fluocinolone, or fluocinonide.

PATIENT TEACHING
• Teach patient or family member how to apply drug using gloves, sterile applicator, or after careful hand washing.
• Tell patient to wash hands after application.
• Tell patient to avoid prolonged use and contact with eyes. Warn him not to apply to face, in skin creases, or around eyes, genitals, underarms, or rectum.
• Instruct patient to notify prescriber of all adverse reactions, if condition persists or worsens, or if burning or irritation develops.

fluticasone propionate–salmeterol inhalation powder
floo-TIK-a-sone/sal-MEE-ter-ol

Advair Diskus 100/50, Advair Diskus 250/50, Advair Diskus 500/50, Advair HFA 45/21, Advair HFA 115/21, Advair HFA 230/21

Therapeutic class: Antiasthmatics
Pharmacologic class: Corticosteroids–long-acting beta$_2$-adrenergic agonists

AVAILABLE FORMS
Inhalation powder: 100 mcg fluticasone propionate and 50 mcg salmeterol, 250 mcg fluticasone propionate and 50 mcg salmeterol, 500 mcg fluticasone propionate and 50 mcg salmeterol
Aerosol spray: 45 mcg fluticasone propionate and 21 mcg salmeterol, 115 mcg fluticasone propionate and 21 mcg salmeterol, 230 mcg fluticasone propionate and 21 mcg salmeterol

INDICATIONS & DOSAGES
➤ **Long-term maintenance of asthma**
Adults and children age 12 and older: 1 inhalation of Advair Diskus b.i.d., at least 12 hours apart; or 2 inhalations of Advair HFA b.i.d. at least 12 hours apart. Starting doses are dependent on patient's current asthma therapy. Maximum dose of Advair Diskus is 1 inhalation of fluticasone 500 mcg and salmeterol 50 mcg b.i.d. at least 12 hours apart. Maximum dose of Advair HFA is 2 inhalations of fluticasone 230 mcg and salmeterol 21 mcg b.i.d.
Children ages 4 to 11: 1 inhalation of Advair Diskus fluticasone 100 mcg and salmeterol 50 mcg b.i.d. about 12 hours apart.
➤ **Maintenance therapy for airflow obstruction in patients with COPD from chronic bronchitis; to reduce exacerbations of COPD in patients with a history of exacerbations**
Adults: 1 inhalation of Advair Diskus 250/50 only, b.i.d., about 12 hours apart.

ADMINISTRATION
Inhalational
• Prime Advair HFA before first use by releasing 4 test sprays into the air, away from the face, shaking well for 5 seconds before each spray. If inhaler hasn't been used for 4 weeks or has been dropped, prime inhaler again by shaking well before each spray and releasing 2 test sprays into the air.
• Discard Advair HFA canister when counter reads "000."
• After administration, have patient rinse his mouth without swallowing.

ACTION
Fluticasone is a synthetic corticosteroid with potent anti-inflammatory activity. Salmeterol xinafoate, a long-acting beta agonist, relaxes bronchial smooth muscle and inhibits release of mediators.

Route	Onset	Peak	Duration
Inhalation (fluticasone)	Unknown	1–2 hr	Unknown
Inhalation (salmeterol)	Unknown	5 min	Unknown

Half-life: Fluticasone, 8 hours; salmeterol, 5½ hours.

ADVERSE REACTIONS
CNS: headache, compressed nerve syndromes, hypnagogic effects, sleep disorders, tremors, pain.
CV: palpitations.
EENT: pharyngitis, blood in nasal mucosa, congestion, conjunctivitis, dental discomfort and pain, eye redness, hoarseness or dysphonia, keratitis, nasal irritation, rhinorrhea, rhinitis, sinusitis, sneezing, viral eye infections.
GI: abdominal pain and discomfort, appendicitis, constipation, diarrhea, gastroenteritis, nausea, oral candidiasis, oral discomfort and pain, oral erythema and rashes, oral ulcerations, unusual taste, vomiting.
Musculoskeletal: arthralgia, articular rheumatism, bone and cartilage disorders, muscle pain, muscle stiffness, rigidity, tightness.
Respiratory: URI, bronchitis, cough, lower respiratory tract infection, pneumonia.
Skin: disorders of sweat and sebum, infection, skin flakiness, sweating, urticaria.

Other: allergic reactions, chest symptoms, fluid retention, viral or bacterial infections.

INTERACTIONS
Drug-drug. *Beta blockers:* Blocked pulmonary effect of salmeterol may produce severe bronchospasm in patients with asthma. Avoid using together. If necessary, use a cardioselective beta blocker cautiously.
Ketoconazole, other inhibitors of CYP450: May increase fluticasone level and adverse effects. Use together cautiously.
Loop diuretics, thiazide diuretics: Potassium-wasting diuretics may cause or worsen ECG changes or hypokalemia. Use together cautiously.
MAO inhibitors, TCAs: May potentiate the action of salmeterol on the vascular system. Separate doses by 2 weeks.

EFFECTS ON LAB TEST RESULTS
• May increase liver enzyme levels.

CONTRAINDICATIONS & CAUTIONS
• Contraindicated in patients hypersensitive to drug or its components, to treat acute bronchospasm, and in those with severe hypersensitivity to milk proteins.
Black Box Warning When treating asthma, use only for patients not adequately controlled on a long-term asthma-controller medication such as an inhaled corticosteroid. ■
• Contraindicated as primary treatment of status asthmaticus or other acute asthmatic episodes.
❸ *Alert:* Don't use drug for transferring patients from systemic corticosteroid therapy. Deaths from adrenal insufficiency have occurred in patients with asthma during and after transfer from systemic corticosteroids to less systemically available inhaled corticosteroids.
• Use cautiously, if at all, in patients with active or quiescent respiratory TB infection; untreated systemic fungal, bacterial, viral, or parasitic infection; or ocular herpes simplex.
• Use cautiously in patients with CV disorders, seizure disorders, or thyrotoxicosis; in patients unusually responsive to sympathomimetic amines; and in patients with hepatic impairment.

Dialyzable drug: Unknown.

⚠ *Overdose S&S:* Hypercorticism, angina, arrhythmias, dizziness, dry mouth, fatigue, headache, hypertension, hypotension, insomnia, malaise, muscle cramps, nausea, nervousness, palpitations, seizures, tachycardia, prolonged QTc interval, hypokalemia, hyperglycemia, cardiac arrest, death.

PREGNANCY-LACTATION-REPRODUCTION

● Use during pregnancy only if potential benefit justifies potential risk to the fetus.
● Avoid use during labor as drug can interfere with uterine contractility.
● Use cautiously in breast-feeding women.

NURSING CONSIDERATIONS

Black Box Warning Rare, serious asthma episodes or asthma-related deaths have occurred in patients taking salmeterol. Don't use for patients whose asthma is adequately controlled on low- or medium-dose inhaled corticosteroids. ■
Black Box Warning When patient's asthma has been controlled and maintained, step down therapy, if possible, while assessing patient regularly. Ensure that asthma control is maintained; then maintain patient on long-term asthma control medication (corticosteroid). ■
🖐 *Alert:* Patient shouldn't be switched from systemic corticosteroids to Advair Diskus or Advair HFA because of HPA axis suppression. Death from adrenal insufficiency can occur. Several months are required for recovery of HPA function after withdrawal of systemic corticosteroids.
● Don't start therapy during rapidly deteriorating or potentially life-threatening episodes of asthma. Serious acute respiratory events, including fatality, can occur.
● The benefit of Advair 250/50 in treating patients with COPD for more than 6 months is unknown. If drug is used for longer than 6 months, periodically reevaluate patient to assess for benefits or risks of therapy.
● Monitor patient for urticaria, angioedema, rash, bronchospasm, or other signs of hypersensitivity.
● Don't use this drug to stop an asthma attack. Patients should carry an inhaled,

short-acting beta₂ agonist (such as albuterol) for acute symptoms.
● If drug causes paradoxical bronchospasm, treat immediately with a short-acting inhaled bronchodilator (such as albuterol), and notify prescriber.
● Monitor patient for increased use of inhaled short-acting beta₂ agonist. The dose of Advair may need to be increased.
● Closely monitor children for growth suppression.

PATIENT TEACHING

● Instruct patient on proper use of the prescribed inhaler to provide effective treatment.
● Tell patient to avoid exhaling into the dry-powder multidose inhaler; to activate and use the dry-powder multidose inhaler in a level, horizontal position; and not to use Advair Diskus with a spacer device.
● Instruct patient to keep the dry-powder multidose inhaler in a dry place, away from direct heat or sunlight, and to avoid washing the mouthpiece or other parts of the device. Patient should discard device 1 month after removal from the moisture-protective overwrap pouch or after every blister has been used, whichever comes first. He shouldn't attempt to take device apart.
● Instruct patient to rinse mouth after inhalation to prevent oral candidiasis.
● Inform patient that improvement may occur within 30 minutes after dose, but the full benefit may not occur for 1 week or more.
● Advise patient not to exceed recommended prescribing dose.
● Instruct patient not to relieve acute symptoms with Advair. Treat acute symptoms with an inhaled short-acting beta₂ agonist.
● Instruct patient to report decreasing effects or use of increasing doses of the short-acting inhaled beta₂ agonist.
● Tell patient to report all adverse reactions, especially palpitations, chest pain, rapid HR, tremor, or nervousness.
● Instruct patient to call immediately if exposed to chickenpox or measles.

F

fluvastatin sodium
flue-va-STA-tin

Lescol✏, Lescol XL

Therapeutic class: Antilipemics
Pharmacologic class: HMG-CoA
reductase inhibitors

AVAILABLE FORMS
Capsules ⊙: 20 mg, 40 mg
Tablets (extended-release) ⊙: 80 mg

INDICATIONS & DOSAGES
➤ **To reduce LDL cholesterol (LDL-C)
and total cholesterol levels in patients
with primary hypercholesterolemia
(types IIa and IIb); to slow progression
of coronary atherosclerosis in patients
with CAD; to reduce elevated triglyceride
and apolipoprotein B (apo B) levels in patients with primary hypercholesterolemia
and mixed dyslipidemia whose response
to dietary restriction and other nonphar-
macologic measures has been inadequate**
Adults: Initially, 20 to 40 mg P.O. at bedtime, increasing if needed to maximum
of 80 mg daily in divided doses or 80 mg
Lescol XL P.O. at bedtime.
➤ **Adjunct to diet to reduce LDL-C, total
cholesterol, and apo B levels in pediatric
patients with heterozygous familial hypercholesterolemia whose response to
dietary restriction hasn't been adequate
and for whom the following findings are
present: LDL-C remains at 190 mg/dL or
more, or LDL-C remains at 160 mg/dL or
more and there's a positive family history
of premature CV disease or two or more
other CV disease risk factors are present**
*Adolescent boys and girls (who are at least
1 year postmenarche) ages 10 to 16:* 20 mg
P.O. once daily at bedtime. Dosage adjustments may be made at 6-week intervals up
to maximum of 40 mg (capsule) P.O. b.i.d.
or 80 mg extended-release tablet P.O. once
daily.
➤ **To reduce the risk of undergoing coronary revascularization procedures**
Adults: In patients who must reduce LDL-C
level by at least 25%, initially 40 mg P.O.
once daily or b.i.d.; or one 80-mg extended-
release tablet as a single dose in the evening.
In patients who must reduce LDL-C level
by less than 25%, initially 20 mg P.O. daily.
Dosages range from 20 to 80 mg daily.

ADMINISTRATION
P.O.
• Give drug without regard for meals.
• For once-daily dosage, give immediate-
release capsules in the evening.
• Don't crush or break tablets; don't open or
crush capsules.
• Administer extended-release tablet as a
single dose at any time of the day.

ACTION
Inhibits HMG-CoA reductase, an early
(and rate-limiting) step in the cholesterol
synthesis pathway.

Route	Onset	Peak	Duration
P.O.	Unknown	1 hr	Unknown

Half-life: About 3 hours.

ADVERSE REACTIONS
CNS: dizziness, fatigue, headache,
insomnia.
EENT: pharyngitis, rhinitis, sinusitis.
GI: abdominal pain, constipation, diarrhea,
dyspepsia, flatulence, nausea, vomiting.
GU: UTI.
Hematologic: *leukopenia, thrombocytope-
nia,* hemolytic anemia.
Musculoskeletal: *rhabdomyolysis,* arthral-
gia, back pain, myalgia, arthropathy.
Respiratory: URI, bronchitis, cough.
Other: hypersensitivity reactions, acciden-
tal trauma, flulike illness.

INTERACTIONS
Drug-drug. *Cholestyramine, colestipol:*
May bind with fluvastatin in the GI tract and
decrease absorption. Separate doses by at
least 4 hours.
Cimetidine, omeprazole, ranitidine: May
decrease fluvastatin metabolism. Monitor
patient for enhanced effects.
*Cyclosporine and other immunosuppres-
sants, erythromycin, niacin:* May increase
risk of polymyositis and rhabdomyolysis.
Avoid using together.
Digoxin: May alter digoxin pharmacokinetics. Monitor digoxin level carefully.

Reactions in bold italics are *life-threatening*. Interactions may have a *rapid onset* or a *delayed onset*.

Erythromycin, nicotinic acid: May increase risk of myopathy and rhabdomyolysis. Don't use together.

Fibric acids (fenofibrate, gemfibrozil): May cause severe myopathy or rhabdomyolysis. If coadministration can't be avoided, monitor CK closely.

Fluconazole, itraconazole, ketoconazole: May increase fluvastatin level and adverse effects. Use cautiously together or, if given together, reduce dose of fluvastatin.

Glyburide: May increase levels of both drugs. Monitor serum glucose and signs and symptoms of toxicity.

Phenytoin: May increase phenytoin levels. Monitor phenytoin levels.

Protease inhibitors (atazanavir, darunavir, fosamprenavir, indinavir, nelfinavir, ritonavir, saquinavir, tipranavir): May increase fluvastatin level and risk of myopathy and rhabdomyolysis. Use together cautiously.

Rifampin: May enhance fluvastatin metabolism and decrease levels. Monitor patient for lack of effect.

Warfarin: May increase anticoagulant effect with bleeding. Monitor PT and INR.

Drug-herb. *Eucalyptus, jin bu huan, kava:* May increase risk of hepatotoxicity. Discourage use together.

Red yeast rice: May increase risk of adverse reactions because herb contains compounds similar to those in drug. Discourage use together.

Drug-lifestyle. *Alcohol use:* May increase risk of hepatotoxicity. Discourage use together.

EFFECTS ON LAB TEST RESULTS

● May increase ALT, AST, HbA₁c, fasting glucose, and CK levels. May decrease Hb level and hematocrit.
● May decrease platelet and WBC counts.

CONTRAINDICATIONS & CAUTIONS

● Contraindicated in patients hypersensitive to drug and in those with active liver disease or unexplained persistent elevations of transaminase levels; also contraindicated in women of childbearing potential.
● Drug may cause rhabdomyolysis in patients with renal function impairment.
● Use cautiously in patients with severe renal impairment or history of liver disease

or heavy alcohol use and in those age 65 or older.

Dialyzable drug: Unknown.

⚠ **Overdose S&S:** GI complaints, elevated AST and ALT levels.

PREGNANCY-LACTATION-REPRODUCTION

● Use contraindicated in pregnant and breast-feeding women.

NURSING CONSIDERATIONS

● Patient should follow a diet restricted in saturated fat and cholesterol during therapy.
● Exercise caution when giving to patients with a history of liver disease or heavy alcohol ingestion. Closely monitor these patients.
● Perform LFTs before initiating therapy and if signs and symptoms of liver injury occur.
● Monitor lipid levels before starting therapy, at 4 weeks, at times of dosage changes, and periodically thereafter.
● Watch for signs and symptoms of myopathy. Monitor patient for muscle pain or weakness with malaise and fever. Discontinue drug for markedly elevated CK levels or if myopathy is suspected or confirmed.
● *Look alike–sound alike:* Don't confuse fluvastatin with fluoxetine.

PATIENT TEACHING

● Tell patient that drug may be taken without regard for meals; if taken once daily, immediate-release capsules are taken in the evening.
● Advise patient who is also taking a bile acid sequestrant such as cholestyramine to take fluvastatin at bedtime, at least 4 hours after taking the sequestrant.
● Teach patient about proper dietary management, weight control, and exercise. Explain their importance in controlling elevated cholesterol and triglyceride levels.
● Warn patient to avoid alcohol.
● Tell patient to notify prescriber of adverse reactions, especially muscle aches and pains.
● Advise patient that it may take up to 4 weeks for the drug to be completely effective.

⭘ *Alert:* Tell female patient of childbearing potential to stop drug and notify prescriber immediately if she becomes pregnant.

fluvoxamine maleate
floo-VOX-a-meen

Luvox, Luvox CR

Therapeutic class: Antidepressants
Pharmacologic class: SSRIs

AVAILABLE FORMS
Capsules (extended-release) ⓞⓝⓒ: 100 mg, 150 mg
Tablets: 25 mg, 50 mg, 100 mg

INDICATIONS & DOSAGES
Adjust-a-dose (for all indications): In elderly patients and those with hepatic impairment, give lower first dose and adjust dose more slowly. When using extended-release capsules, titrate dosage more slowly after initial 100-mg dose.

➤ **Obsessive-compulsive disorder (OCD)**
Adults: Initially, 50 mg (tablet) P.O. daily at bedtime; increase by 50 mg every 4 to 7 days. Maximum, 300 mg daily. Give total daily amounts above 100 mg in two divided doses. Or, 100-mg extended-release capsule P.O. once per day as a single daily dose at bedtime. Increase in 50-mg increments every week, as tolerated, until maximum therapeutic benefit is achieved. Maximum dose is 300 mg/day.
Children ages 8 to 17: Initially, 25 mg P.O. daily at bedtime; increase by 25 mg every 4 to 7 days. Maximum, 200 mg daily for children ages 8 to less than 11 and 300 mg daily for children ages 11 to 17. Give total daily amounts over 50 mg in two divided doses.

ADMINISTRATION
P.O.
● Give drug without regard for food.
● Capsules shouldn't be crushed or chewed.
● Give extended-release capsules at bedtime.

ACTION
Unknown. Selectively inhibits the presynaptic neuronal uptake of serotonin, which may improve OCD.

Route	Onset	Peak	Duration
P.O. (capsules)	Unknown	Unknown	Unknown
P.O. (tablets)	Unknown	3–8 hr	Unknown

Half-life: 14 to 16 hours.

ADVERSE REACTIONS
CNS: agitation, headache, asthenia, somnolence, insomnia, nervousness, dizziness, tremor, anxiety, hypertonia, depression, CNS stimulation.
CV: palpitations, vasodilation.
EENT: amblyopia, rhinitis.
GI: nausea, diarrhea, constipation, dyspepsia, vomiting, dry mouth, anorexia, flatulence, dysphagia, taste perversion.
GU: abnormal ejaculation, urinary frequency, erectile dysfunction, anorgasmia, urine retention, dysmenorrhea.
Respiratory: URI, dyspnea.
Skin: rash, sweating.
Other: tooth disorder, flulike syndrome, chills, decreased libido, yawning.

INTERACTIONS
Drug-drug. *Antipsychotics, MAO inhibitors (phenelzine, selegiline, tranylcypromine):* May cause serotonin syndrome (CNS irritability, shivering, altered consciousness) or neuroleptic malignant syndrome. Avoid using within 2 weeks of MAO inhibitor.
Benzodiazepines, theophylline, warfarin: May reduce clearance of these drugs. Use together cautiously (except for diazepam, which shouldn't be used with fluvoxamine). Adjust dosage as needed.
Carbamazepine, clozapine, methadone, metoprolol, propranolol, TCAs, theophylline: May increase levels of these drugs. Use together cautiously, and monitor patient closely for adverse reactions. Dosage adjustments may be needed.
Diltiazem: May cause bradycardia. Monitor HR.
Linezolid, methylene blue: May cause serotonin syndrome. Use extreme caution and monitor closely.
Lithium, tryptophan: May enhance effects of fluvoxamine. Use together cautiously.

Reactions in bold italics are *life-threatening*. Interactions may have a *rapid onset* or a *delayed onset*.

Pimozide, thioridazine: May prolong QTc interval. Avoid using together.
Sumatriptan: May cause weakness, hyperreflexia, and incoordination. Monitor patient closely. May cause serotonin syndrome. Avoid using within 2 weeks of MAO inhibitor.
Tramadol: May cause serotonin syndrome. Monitor patient closely.
Drug-herb. *Alfalfa, anise, bilberry, bladderwrack, bromelain, dong quai, evening primrose, garlic, ginkgo biloba, ginseng (American, Panax, Siberian), white willow:* May increase antiplatelet activity. Avoid use together.
Kava kava, SAM-e, St. John's wort, tryptophan, valerian: May increase sedative-hypnotic effects and risk of serotonin syndrome. Avoid use together.
Melatonin: May increase melatonin bioavailability. Avoid use together.
Drug-lifestyle. *Alcohol use:* May increase CNS effects. Discourage use together.
Smoking: May decrease drug's effectiveness. Urge patient to stop smoking.

EFFECTS ON LAB TEST RESULTS
None reported.

CONTRAINDICATIONS & CAUTIONS
• Contraindicated in patients hypersensitive to drug or to other phenyl piperazine antidepressants; in those receiving pimozide, alosetron, tizanidine, or thioridazine therapy; and within 2 weeks of MAO inhibitor.
⊕ *Alert:* Concomitant use with linezolid or methylene blue can cause serotonin syndrome (fever, mental status changes, muscle twitching, excessive sweating, shivering or shaking, diarrhea, loss of coordination). Use drug with linezolid or methylene blue only for life-threatening or urgent conditions when the potential benefits outweigh the risks of toxicity.
• Use cautiously in patients with hepatic dysfunction, other conditions that may affect hemodynamic responses or metabolism, or history of mania or seizures.
Black Box Warning Fluvoxamine tablets aren't approved for use in children, except for those with OCD. Fluvoxamine extended-release capsules shouldn't be used in children. ∎

Dialyzable drug: Unlikely.
⚠ **Overdose S&S:** Nausea, vomiting, diarrhea, coma, hypokalemia, hypotension, respiratory difficulties, somnolence, tachycardia, ECG abnormalities, seizures, dizziness, liver function disturbances, tremor, increased reflexes.

PREGNANCY-LACTATION-REPRODUCTION
• Neonates exposed to drug late in the third trimester have developed complications requiring prolonged hospitalization, respiratory support, and tube feeding. Neonates exposed to SSRIs in late pregnancy may have an increased risk of persistent pulmonary hypertension of the newborn, which is associated with substantial neonatal morbidity and mortality. Risks and benefits of treatment should be carefully considered on a case-by-case basis.
• Drug appears in breast milk. Patient should discontinue breast-feeding or discontinue drug.

NURSING CONSIDERATIONS
Black Box Warning Drug may increase the risk of suicidal thinking and behavior in young adults ages 18 to 24, especially during first few months of treatment. Monitor patient closely for clinical worsening. ∎
• Record mood changes. Monitor patient for suicidal tendencies.
⊕ *Alert:* Combining an SSRI with a triptan may cause serotonin syndrome or neuroleptic malignant syndrome-like reactions. Serotonin syndrome is more likely to occur when starting or increasing the dose of a triptan.
⊕ *Alert:* If linezolid or methylene blue must be given, fluvoxamine must be stopped and patient should be monitored for serotonin toxicity for 2 weeks or until 24 hours after the last dose of linezolid or methylene blue, whichever comes first. Treatment with fluvoxamine may be resumed 24 hours after the last dose of linezolid or methylene blue.
• Patients shouldn't stop drug without first consulting prescriber; abruptly stopping drug may cause withdrawal syndrome, including headache, muscle ache, and flulike symptoms.
• *Look alike–sound alike:* Don't confuse fluvoxamine with fluoxetine.

PATIENT TEACHING

Black Box Warning Advise families and caregivers to closely observe patient for increased suicidal thinking or behavior. ■

☻ *Alert:* Teach patient to recognize and immediately report symptoms of serotonin toxicity (fever, mental status changes, muscle twitching, excessive sweating, shivering or shaking, diarrhea, loss of coordination).

• Warn patient to avoid hazardous activities until CNS effects of drug are known.

• Tell women to notify prescriber about planned, suspected, or known pregnancy.

• Tell patient who develops a rash, hives, or a related allergic reaction to notify prescriber.

• Inform patient that several weeks of therapy may be needed to obtain full therapeutic effect. Once improvement occurs, advise patient not to stop drug until directed by prescriber.

• Suggest that patient keep a diary of changes in mood or behavior. Tell patient to report suicidal thoughts immediately.

• Advise patient to check with prescriber before taking OTC drugs; drug interactions can occur.

• Tell patient drug can be taken with or without food.

SAFETY ALERT!

fondaparinux sodium
fon-da-PAR-i-nuks

Arixtra

Therapeutic class: Anticoagulants
Pharmacologic class: Activated factor X inhibitors

AVAILABLE FORMS
Injection: 2.5 mg/0.5 mL, 5 mg/0.4 mL, 7.5 mg/0.6 mL, 10 mg/0.8 mL in single-dose, prefilled syringe

INDICATIONS & DOSAGES
➤ **To prevent DVT, which may lead to PE, in patients undergoing surgery for hip fracture, hip replacement, knee replacement, or abdominal surgery**
Adults: 2.5 mg subcutaneously once daily for 5 to 9 days. Give first dose after hemostasis is established, 6 to 8 hours after surgery. Giving the dose earlier than 6 hours after surgery increases the risk of major bleeding. Patients undergoing hip fracture surgery should receive an extended prophylaxis course of up to 24 additional days; a total of 32 days (perioperative and extended prophylaxis) has been tolerated.

➤ **Acute DVT (with warfarin); acute PE (with warfarin) when treatment is started in the hospital**
Adults weighing more than 100 kg: 10 mg subcutaneously daily for 5 to 9 days (drug has been given for up to 26 days in clinical trials) and until INR is 2 to 3. Begin warfarin therapy as soon as possible, usually within 72 hours.

Adults weighing 50 to 100 kg: 7.5 mg subcutaneously daily for 5 to 9 days (drug has been given for up to 26 days in clinical trials) and until INR is 2 to 3. Begin warfarin therapy as soon as possible, usually within 72 hours.

Adults weighing less than 50 kg: 5 mg subcutaneously daily for 5 to 9 days (drug has been given for up to 26 days in clinical trials) and until INR is 2 to 3. Begin warfarin therapy as soon as possible, usually within 72 hours.

➤ **Acute symptomatic superficial vein thrombosis (at least 5 cm in length) of the legs**
Adults: 2.5 mg subcutaneously once daily for 45 days.

ADMINISTRATION
Subcutaneous

• Give subcutaneously only, never I.M. Inspect the single-dose, prefilled syringe for particulate matter and discoloration before giving.

☻ *Alert:* To avoid loss of drug, don't expel air bubble from the syringe.

• Give drug in fatty tissue, rotating injection sites. If drug has been properly injected, the needle will pull back into the syringe security sleeve and the white safety indicator will appear above the blue upper body. A soft click may be heard or felt when the syringe plunger is fully released. After injection of the syringe contents, the plunger automatically rises while the needle

---

Reactions in bold italics are *life-threatening*. Interactions may have a *rapid onset* or a *delayed onset*.

withdraws from the skin and retracts into the security sleeve. Don't recap the needle.
● **Incompatibilities:** Other injections or infusions.

ACTION

Binds to antithrombin III (AT-III) and potentiates the neutralization of factor Xa by AT-III, which interrupts coagulation and inhibits formation of thrombin and blood clots.

Route	Onset	Peak	Duration
Subcut.	Unknown	2–3 hr	Unknown

Half-life: 17 to 21 hours.

ADVERSE REACTIONS

CNS: insomnia, dizziness, confusion.
CV: hypotension.
EENT: epistaxis.
Hematologic: *hemorrhage,* anemia, hematoma, *postoperative hemorrhage, thrombocytopenia.*
Metabolic: hypokalemia.
Skin: mild local irritation (injection-site bleeding, rash, pruritus), bullous eruption, purpura, rash, increased wound drainage and infection.

INTERACTIONS

Drug-drug. *Drugs that increase risk of bleeding (anticoagulants, NSAIDs, platelet inhibitors):* May increase risk of hemorrhage. Stop these drugs before starting fondaparinux. If use together is unavoidable, monitor patient closely.
Drug-herb. *Angelica (dong quai), ginkgo, ginseng, willow:* May increase risk of bleeding. Discourage use together.

EFFECTS ON LAB TEST RESULTS

● May increase AST, ALT, and bilirubin levels. May decrease potassium and Hb levels and hematocrit.
● May decrease platelet count.

CONTRAINDICATIONS & CAUTIONS

● Contraindicated in patients with CrCl of less than 30 mL/minute and in those who are hypersensitive to drug.
● Contraindicated for venous thromboembolism prophylaxis in patients weighing less than 50 kg who are undergoing hip frac-

ture, hip replacement, knee replacement, or abdominal surgery.
● Contraindicated in patients with history of serious hypersensitivity reaction (angioedema, anaphylactoid/anaphylactic reactions) to fondaparinux.
● Contraindicated in patients with active major bleeding, bacterial endocarditis, or thrombocytopenia with a positive test result for antiplatelet antibody after taking fondaparinux.
● Use cautiously in patients being treated with platelet inhibitors; in those at increased risk for bleeding, such as those with congenital or acquired bleeding disorders; in those with active ulcerative and angiodysplastic GI disease; in those with hemorrhagic stroke; and in patients shortly after brain, spinal, or ophthalmologic surgery.
● Use cautiously in elderly patients, in patients with CrCl of 30 to 50 mL/minute, and in those with a history of heparin-induced thrombocytopenia, a bleeding diathesis, uncontrolled arterial hypertension, or a history of recent GI ulceration, diabetic retinopathy, or hemorrhage.
◑ Alert: Use cautiously in latex-sensitive patients; the packaging (needle guard) contains dry natural rubber.
Dialyzable drug: 20%.
⚠ Overdose S&S: Hemorrhagic complications.

PREGNANCY-LACTATION-REPRODUCTION

● Use cautiously in pregnant women and only if benefit justifies risk to the fetus.
● It isn't known if drug appears in breast milk. Use cautiously in breast-feeding women.

NURSING CONSIDERATIONS

● Don't use interchangeably with heparin, low-molecular-weight heparins, or heparinoids.
Black Box Warning Patients who receive epidural or spinal anesthesia, epidural catheters, or spinal puncture or have a history of spine deformity or surgery are at increased risk for developing an epidural or spinal hematoma, which may result in long-term or permanent paralysis. Other factors that increase risk include concurrent use of NSAIDs, platelet inhibitors, and other

anticoagulants, use of indwelling epidural catheters, and history of traumatic or repeated epidural or spinal surgery. Monitor these patients closely for neurologic impairment, and treat urgently. Consider the risk before neuraxial intervention in patients anticoagulated or to be anticoagulated for thromboprophylaxis. ■

• Monitor renal function periodically, and stop drug in patients who develop unstable renal function or severe renal impairment while receiving therapy.

• Routinely assess patient for signs and symptoms of bleeding, and regularly monitor CBC, platelet count, creatinine level, and stool occult blood test results. Stop use if platelet count is less than 100,000/mm³.

• Anticoagulant effects may last for 2 to 4 days after stopping drug in patients with normal renal function.

• PT and aPTT aren't suitable monitoring tests to measure drug activity. If coagulation parameters change unexpectedly or patient develops major bleeding, stop drug.

PATIENT TEACHING

• Tell patient to report signs and symptoms of bleeding or neurologic impairment.

• Instruct patient to avoid OTC products that contain aspirin or other salicylates.

• Advise patient to consult with prescriber before starting herbal therapy; many herbs have anticoagulant, antiplatelet, or fibrinolytic properties.

• Teach patient the correct technique for subcutaneous use, if needed.

formoterol fumarate
for-MOH-te-rol

Foradil Aerolizer, Perforomist

Therapeutic class: Bronchodilators
Pharmacologic class: Selective beta₂-adrenergic agonists

AVAILABLE FORMS
Capsules for inhalation: 12 mcg
Inhalation solution: 20 mcg/2-mL vial

INDICATIONS & DOSAGES
➤ **Maintenance treatment and prevention of bronchospasm in patients with reversible obstructive airway disease or nocturnal asthma, who usually require treatment with short-acting inhaled beta₂ agonists**
Adults and children age 5 and older:
One 12-mcg capsule by inhalation via Aerolizer inhaler every 12 hours. Total daily dosage shouldn't exceed 1 capsule b.i.d. (24 mcg/day). If symptoms occur between doses, use a short-acting beta₂ agonist for immediate relief.
➤ **To prevent exercise-induced bronchospasm**
Adults and children age 5 and older: One 12-mcg capsule by inhalation via Aerolizer inhaler at least 15 minutes before exercise p.r.n. Don't give additional doses within 12 hours of first dose.
➤ **Maintenance treatment of bronchoconstriction in patients with COPD (chronic bronchitis, emphysema)**
Adults: One 20 mcg/2-mL vial (Perforomist) by oral inhalation through a jet nebulizer every 12 hours. Maximum dose, 40 mcg/day. Or, one 12-mcg capsule (Foradil) by inhalation via Aerolizer inhaler every 12 hours; total daily dosage shouldn't exceed 24 mcg/day.

ADMINISTRATION
Inhalational Foradil
• Give Foradil capsules only by oral inhalation and only with the Aerolizer inhaler. They aren't for oral ingestion. Patient shouldn't exhale into the device. Capsules should remain in the unopened blister until administration time and be removed immediately before use.

• Pierce Foradil capsules only once. In rare instances, the gelatin capsule may break into small pieces and get delivered to the mouth or throat upon inhalation. The Aerolizer contains a screen that should catch any broken pieces before they leave the device. To minimize the possibility of shattering the capsule, strictly follow storage and use instructions.

Perforomist

● Give Perforomist inhalational solution through a standard jet nebulizer connected to an air compressor.

ACTION

Long-acting selective beta$_2$ agonist that causes bronchodilation. It ultimately increases cAMP, leading to relaxation of bronchial smooth muscle and inhibition of mediator release from mast cells.

Route	Onset	Peak	Duration
Inhalation powder	5 min	1–3 hr	12 hr
Inhalation solution	12 min	1–3 hr	12 hr

Half-life: Foradil, 10 hours; Perforomist, 7 hours.

ADVERSE REACTIONS

CNS: tremor, dizziness, insomnia, nervousness, headache, fatigue, malaise, anxiety.
CV: *arrhythmias,* chest pain, angina, hypertension, hypotension, tachycardia, palpitations.
EENT: dry mouth, tonsillitis, dysphonia, nasopharyngitis, sinusitis.
GI: nausea, vomiting, diarrhea.
Metabolic: *metabolic acidosis, hypokalemia,* hyperglycemia.
Musculoskeletal: muscle cramps.
Respiratory: bronchitis, chest infection, dyspnea.
Skin: rash, pruritus.
Other: viral infection.

INTERACTIONS

Drug-drug. *Adrenergics:* May potentiate sympathetic effects of formoterol. Use together cautiously.
Beta blockers: May antagonize effects of beta agonists, causing bronchospasm in asthmatic patients. Avoid use except when benefit outweighs risks. Use cardioselective beta blockers with caution to minimize risk of bronchospasm.
Diuretics, steroids, xanthine derivatives: May increase hypokalemic effect of formoterol. Use together cautiously.
MAO inhibitors, TCAs, other drugs that prolong QT interval: May increase risk of ventricular arrhythmias. Use together cautiously.

Non–potassium-sparing diuretics, such as loop or thiazide diuretics: May worsen ECG changes or hypokalemia. Use together cautiously, and monitor patient for toxicity.

EFFECTS ON LAB TEST RESULTS

● May increase glucose level. May decrease potassium level.

CONTRAINDICATIONS & CAUTIONS

● Contraindicated in patients hypersensitive to drug or its components, or with other long-acting beta$_2$ agonists.
● Use cautiously in patients with CV disease, especially coronary insufficiency, cardiac arrhythmias, and hypertension, and in those who are unusually responsive to sympathomimetic amines.
● Use cautiously in patients with diabetes mellitus because hyperglycemia and ketoacidosis have occurred rarely with the use of beta agonists.
● Use cautiously in patients with seizure disorders or thyrotoxicosis and in breast-feeding women.
Black Box Warning Use for asthma only as additional therapy for patients whose condition isn't adequately controlled with other long-term asthma-control medications. Once control is achieved and maintained, step down therapy while assessing patient regularly; discontinue drug, if possible, and maintain patient on a long-term asthma-control medication (corticosteroid). ▪
Dialyzable drug: Unknown.
⚠ *Overdose S&S:* Exaggeration of adverse reactions, hypotension, cardiac arrest.

PREGNANCY-LACTATION-REPRODUCTION

● Use cautiously in pregnant women and only if benefit outweighs risk to the fetus.
● Drug may interfere with uterine contractility if used during labor.
● Use cautiously in breast-feeding women.

NURSING CONSIDERATIONS

● Drug isn't indicated for patients who can control asthma symptoms with just occasional use of inhaled, short-acting beta$_2$ agonists or for treatment of acute bronchospasm requiring immediate reversal with short-acting beta$_2$ agonists or in patients with rapidly deteriorating or significantly worsening asthma.

• Drug may be used along with short-acting beta agonists, inhaled corticosteroids, and theophylline therapy for asthma management.

🌢 *Alert:* Drug isn't a substitute for short-acting beta₂ agonists for immediate relief of bronchospasm or as substitute for inhaled or oral corticosteroids.

• Patients using drug twice daily shouldn't take additional doses to prevent exercise-induced bronchospasm.

• For patients formerly using regularly scheduled short-acting beta₂ agonists, decrease use of the short-acting drug to an as-needed basis when starting long-acting formoterol.

Black Box Warning Drug may increase the risk of asthma-related death. Use only as additional therapy for patients not adequately controlled on low to medium dose of inhaled corticosteroids or in patients whose disease is severe and requires treatment with two maintenance therapies. ▪

Black Box Warning For children and adolescents with asthma who require the addition of a long-acting beta₂ agonist to an inhaled corticosteroid, a fixed-dose combination product containing an inhaled corticosteroid and long-acting beta₂ agonist should be considered to ensure adherence to both drugs. ▪

🌢 *Alert:* As with all beta₂ agonists, drug may produce life-threatening paradoxical bronchospasm. If bronchospasm occurs, treat immediately and notify prescriber promptly.

🌢 *Alert:* If patient develops tachycardia, hypertension, or other CV adverse effects, drug may need to be stopped.

• Watch for immediate hypersensitivity reactions, such as anaphylaxis, urticaria, angioedema, rash, and bronchospasm.

• *Look alike–sound alike:* Don't confuse Foradil with Toradol.

PATIENT TEACHING

• Tell patient not to increase the dosage or frequency of use without medical advice.

• Warn patient not to stop or reduce other medication taken for asthma.

• Advise patient that drug isn't to be used for acute asthmatic episodes. Prescriber should give a short-acting beta₂ agonist for this use.

• Advise patient to report worsening symptoms, treatment that becomes less effective, or increased use of short-acting beta agonists.

• Tell patient to report nausea, vomiting, shakiness, headache, fast or irregular heartbeat, or sleeplessness.

• Tell patient using drug for exercise-induced bronchospasm to take it at least 15 minutes before exercise and to wait 12 hours before taking additional doses.

• Tell patient not to use the Foradil Aerolizer with a spacer device or to exhale or blow into the Aerolizer.

• Advise patient to avoid washing the Aerolizer and to always keep it dry. Each refill contains a new device to replace the old one.

• Tell patient to avoid exposing capsules to moisture and to handle them only with dry hands.

• Advise female patient to notify prescriber if she becomes pregnant or is breast-feeding.

foscarnet sodium (PFA, phosphonoformic acid)
foss-CAR-net

Foscavir

Therapeutic class: Antivirals
Pharmacologic class: Pyrophosphate analogues

AVAILABLE FORMS
Injection: 2.4 g/100 mL

INDICATIONS & DOSAGES
Adjust-a-dose (for all indications):
Adjust dosage when CrCl is less than 1.4 mL/minute/kg. If CrCl falls below 0.4 mL/minute/kg, stop drug. Consult manufacturer's package insert for specific dosage adjustments.

Black Box Warning Drug is only indicated for use in immunocompromised patients with CMV retinitis and mucocutaneous acyclovir-resistant HSV infections. ▪

➤ **CMV retinitis in patients with AIDS**
Adults: Initially, for induction, 60 mg/kg
I.V. over a minimum of 1 hour every 8 hours
or 90 mg/kg I.V. over 1½ to 2 hours every
12 hours for 2 to 3 weeks, depending on
patient response. Follow with a maintenance
infusion of 90 to 120 mg/kg over 2 hours
daily. Maximum dosage, 180 mg/kg/day
(initial dosage) and 120 mg/kg/day (maintenance dosage).

➤ **Acyclovir-resistant HSV infections**
Adults: 40 mg/kg I.V. over 1 hour every
8 to 12 hours for 2 to 3 weeks or until
healed. Maximum dosage, 120 mg/kg/day.

ADMINISTRATION

I.V.

Black Box Warning To minimize renal
toxicity, make sure patient is adequately
hydrated before and during infusion. ∎

▼ Don't exceed the recommended dosage,
rate, or frequency of infusion. Doses must
be individualized according to patient's
renal function.

▼ Drug may be infused via a central or
peripheral vein with enough blood flow for
rapid distribution and dilution. If infusing
into a central vein, don't dilute the commercially available form (24 mg/mL). If
infusing into a peripheral vein, dilute to
12 mg/mL with D_5W or NSS to decrease
risk of local irritation. Use an infusion
pump.

▼ Give induction treatment over 1 to
2 hours, depending on dose, and maintenance infusions over 2 hours and at no
more than 1 mg/kg/minute.

▼ **Incompatibilities:** Acyclovir, amphotericin B, dextrose 30%, diazepam,
digoxin, ganciclovir, lactated Ringer solution, leucovorin, midazolam, pentamidine,
phenytoin, prochlorperazine, promethazine, solutions containing calcium (such
as total parenteral nutrition), trimetrexate,
sulfamethoxazole–trimethoprim, vancomycin.

ACTION

Inhibits herpes virus replication in vitro by
blocking the pyrophosphate-binding site on
DNA polymerases and reverse transcrip-
tases.

Route	Onset	Peak	Duration
I.V.	Unknown	Immediate	Unknown

Half-life: 3 hours.

ADVERSE REACTIONS

CNS: asthenia, dizziness, fatigue, fever,
headache, hypoesthesia, malaise, neuropathy, paresthesia, *seizures,* abnormal coordination, agitation, aggression, amnesia,
anxiety, aphasia, ataxia, cerebrovascular
disorder, confusion, dementia, depression,
EEG abnormalities, generalized spasms,
hallucinations, insomnia, meningitis, nervousness, pain, sensory disturbances, somnolence, stupor, tremor.

CV: ECG abnormalities, first-degree AV
block, flushing, hypertension, hypotension,
palpitations, sinus tachycardia, chest pain,
edema.

EENT: conjunctivitis, eye pain, pharyngitis,
rhinitis, sinusitis, visual disturbances.

GI: abdominal pain, anorexia, diarrhea,
nausea, vomiting, *pancreatitis,* constipation,
dysphagia, dry mouth, dyspepsia, flatulence,
melena, rectal hemorrhage, taste perversion,
ulcerative stomatitis.

GU: *acute renal failure,* abnormal renal
function, albuminuria, candidiasis, dysuria,
polyuria, urethral disorder, urine retention,
UTI.

Hematologic: anemia, *bone marrow suppression, granulocytopenia, leukopenia,
thrombocytopenia,* thrombocytosis.

Hepatic: abnormal hepatic function.

Metabolic: hyperphosphatemia, hypocalcemia, hypokalemia, *hypomagnesemia,*
hypophosphatemia, hyponatremia.

Musculoskeletal: arthralgia, back pain, leg
cramps, myalgia.

Respiratory: *bronchospasm,* cough, dyspnea, hemoptysis, pneumonitis, *pneumothorax,* pulmonary infiltration, *respiratory
insufficiency, stridor.*

Skin: diaphoresis, rash, erythematous rash,
facial edema, pruritus, seborrhea, skin
discoloration, skin ulceration.

Other: *sarcoma, sepsis,* abscess, bacterial
or fungal infections, flulike symptoms,
inflammation and pain at infusion site,
lymphadenopathy, lymphoma-like disorder,
rigors.

INTERACTIONS

Drug-drug. *Calcium:* May decrease serum level of ionized calcium. Avoid concurrent use.
Nephrotoxic drugs (such as aminoglycosides, amphotericin B): May increase risk of nephrotoxicity. Avoid using together.
Pentamidine: May increase risk of nephrotoxicity; severe hypocalcemia also has been reported. Monitor renal function tests and electrolytes.
Zidovudine: May increase risk or severity of anemia. Monitor blood counts.

EFFECTS ON LAB TEST RESULTS

- May increase alkaline phosphatase, ALT, AST, bilirubin, creatinine, and phosphate levels. May decrease calcium, Hb, magnesium, phosphate, potassium, and sodium levels.
- May increase platelet count. May decrease granulocyte, platelet, and WBC counts.

CONTRAINDICATIONS & CAUTIONS

- Contraindicated in patients hypersensitive to drug.

Black Box Warning In patients with abnormal renal function, use cautiously, maintain adequate hydration, and reduce dosage. Drug is nephrotoxic and can worsen renal impairment. Some degree of nephrotoxicity occurs in most patients. ■

Dialyzable drug: Yes.

⚠ ***Overdose S&S:*** Seizures, renal impairment, paresthesia (limb or perioral), calcium and phosphate electrolyte disturbances.

PREGNANCY-LACTATION-REPRODUCTION

- Use cautiously in pregnant women and only if clearly needed.
- Patient should discontinue breast-feeding or discontinue drug.

NURSING CONSIDERATIONS

Alert: Because drug is highly toxic, which is probably dose-related, always use the lowest effective maintenance dose.

Black Box Warning Frequent monitoring of serum creatinine, with dosage adjustment for changes in renal function, is imperative. ■

- Monitor CrCl frequently during therapy because of drug's adverse effects on renal function. Obtain a baseline 24-hour CrCl. Monitor level two to three times weekly during induction and at least once every 1 to 2 weeks during maintenance.

Black Box Warning Drug can cause seizures related to altered mineral and electrolyte levels; monitor levels using a schedule similar to that established for monitoring of CrCl. Assess patient for tetany and seizures, and treat with supplementation if necessary. ■

- Monitor patient's Hb level and hematocrit. Anemia occurs in about one-third of patients and may be severe enough to require transfusions.
- Drug may cause a dose-related transient decrease in ionized calcium, which may not always show up in patient's laboratory values.

PATIENT TEACHING

- Explain the importance of adequate hydration throughout therapy.
- Advise patient to report tingling around the mouth, numbness in the arms and legs, and pins-and-needles sensations.
- Tell patient to alert nurse about discomfort at I.V. insertion site.

fosinopril sodium

foe-SIN-oh-pril

Therapeutic class: Antihypertensives
Pharmacologic class: ACE inhibitors

AVAILABLE FORMS

Tablets: 10 mg, 20 mg, 40 mg

INDICATIONS & DOSAGES

➤ **Hypertension**

Adults: Initially, 10 mg P.O. daily; adjust dosage based on BP response at peak and trough levels. Usual dosage is 20 to 40 mg daily; maximum is 80 mg daily. Dosage may be divided.
Children weighing more than 50 kg: Initially, 5 to 10 mg P.O. once daily. Maximum dosage is 40 mg/day.

➤ **Adjunctive therapy for HF with diuretics or digoxin**

Adults: Initially, 10 mg P.O. once daily. Increase dosage over several weeks to a maximum of 40 mg P.O. daily, if needed.

ADMINISTRATION
P.O.
● Give drug without regard for meals.

ACTION
Inhibits ACE, preventing conversion of angiotensin I to angiotensin II, a potent vasoconstrictor. Less angiotensin II decreases peripheral arterial resistance, thus decreasing aldosterone secretion, which reduces sodium and water retention and lowers BP.

Route	Onset	Peak	Duration
P.O.	1 hr	3 hr	24 hr

Half-life: 11½ hours.

ADVERSE REACTIONS
CNS: dizziness, *stroke,* headache, fatigue, syncope, paresthesia, sleep disturbance, weakness.
CV: *MI,* chest pain, angina pectoris, rhythm disturbances, palpitations, hypotension, orthostatic hypotension, flushing.
EENT: tinnitus, sinusitis.
GI: *pancreatitis,* nausea, vomiting, diarrhea, dry mouth, abdominal distention, abdominal pain, constipation.
GU: sexual dysfunction, renal insufficiency, urinary frequency.
Hepatic: *hepatitis.*
Metabolic: *hyperkalemia.*
Musculoskeletal: arthralgia, musculoskeletal pain, myalgia.
Respiratory: dry, persistent, tickling, nonproductive cough; *bronchospasm.*
Skin: urticaria, rash, photosensitivity reactions, pruritus.
Other: *angioedema,* decreased libido, gout.

INTERACTIONS
Drug-drug. *Antacids:* May impair absorption. Separate dosage times by at least 2 hours.
Azathioprine: May increase risk of anemia or leukopenia. Monitor hematologic studies if used together.
Diuretics, other antihypertensives: May cause excessive hypotension. Stop diuretic or lower fosinopril dosage.
Lithium: May increase lithium level and lithium toxicity. Monitor lithium level.
Nesiritide: May increase hypotensive effects. Monitor BP.

NSAIDs: May decrease antihypertensive effects. Monitor BP.
Potassium-sparing diuretics, potassium supplements: May cause risk of hyperkalemia. Monitor patient closely.
Drug-herb. *Capsaicin:* May cause cough. Discourage use together.
Ma huang: May decrease antihypertensive effects. Discourage use together.
Drug-food. *Salt substitutes containing potassium:* May cause hyperkalemia. Discourage use together.

EFFECTS ON LAB TEST RESULTS
● May increase BUN, creatinine, potassium, and Hb levels and hematocrit.
● May increase LFT values.
● May cause falsely low digoxin level with the Digi-Tab radioimmunoassay kit for digoxin.

CONTRAINDICATIONS & CAUTIONS
● Contraindicated in patients hypersensitive to drug or other ACE inhibitors.
● Use cautiously in patients with impaired renal or hepatic function.
Dialyzable drug: 2% to 7%.
⚠ *Overdose S&S:* Hypotension.

PREGNANCY-LACTATION-REPRODUCTION
● Use in pregnant and breast-feeding women isn't recommended.
Black Box Warning Use during pregnancy can cause injury and death to the developing fetus. When pregnancy is detected, stop drug as soon as possible. ∎

NURSING CONSIDERATIONS
● Monitor BP for drug effect.
● Black patients who take ACE inhibitors as monotherapy for hypertension have a smaller reduction in BP than non-Black patients. Black patients taking ACE inhibitors have a higher incidence of angioedema than non-Blacks.
● Monitor potassium intake and potassium level. Diabetic patients, those with impaired renal function, and those receiving drugs that can increase potassium level may develop hyperkalemia.
● Other ACE inhibitors may cause agranulocytosis and neutropenia. Monitor CBC

with differential counts before therapy and periodically thereafter.

● Assess renal and hepatic function before and periodically throughout therapy.

● *Look alike–sound alike:* Don't confuse fosinopril with lisinopril. Don't confuse Monopril with Monurol.

PATIENT TEACHING

● Tell patient to avoid salt substitutes; these products may contain potassium, which can cause high potassium level in patients taking drug.

● Instruct patient to contact prescriber if light-headedness or fainting occurs.

● Advise patient to report evidence of infection, such as fever and sore throat.

● Instruct patient to call prescriber if he develops easy bruising or bleeding; swelling of tongue, lips, face, eyes, mucous membranes, arms, or legs; difficulty swallowing or breathing; cough; or hoarseness.

● Urge patient to use caution in hot weather and during exercise. Inadequate fluid intake, vomiting, diarrhea, and excessive perspiration can lead to light-headedness and fainting.

● Tell female patient of childbearing potential to notify prescriber if pregnancy occurs. Drug will need to be stopped.

fosphenytoin sodium
faws-FEN-i-toe-in

Cerebyx

Therapeutic class: Anticonvulsants
Pharmacologic class: Hydantoin derivatives

AVAILABLE FORMS
Injection: 100 mg phenytoin sodium equivalents/2 mL, 500 mg phenytoin sodium equivalents/10 mL vials

INDICATIONS & DOSAGES
Adjust-a-dose (for all indications): Phenytoin clearance is decreased slightly in elderly patients; lower or less frequent dosing may be required.

➤ **Status epilepticus**
Adults: 15 to 20 mg phenytoin sodium equivalent/kg I.V. at infusion rate of 100 to 150 mg phenytoin sodium equivalent/minute as loading dose; then 4 to 6 mg phenytoin sodium equivalent/kg daily I.V. or I.M. as maintenance dose.

➤ **To prevent and treat seizures during neurosurgery (nonemergent loading or maintenance dosing)**
Adults: Loading dose of 10 to 20 mg phenytoin sodium equivalent/kg I.M. or I.V. at infusion rate not exceeding 150 mg phenytoin sodium equivalent/minute. Maintenance dose is 4 to 6 mg phenytoin sodium equivalent/kg daily I.V. or I.M.

➤ **Short-term substitution for oral phenytoin therapy**
Adults: Same total daily dose equivalent as oral phenytoin sodium therapy given as a single daily dose I.M. or I.V. at infusion rate not exceeding 150 mg phenytoin sodium equivalent/minute. Some patients may need more frequent dosing.

ADMINISTRATION
I.V.
▼ If rapid phenytoin loading is a main goal, this form is preferred.

▼ For status epilepticus, give I.V. rather than I.M. because therapeutic phenytoin level occurs more rapidly.

▼ For infusion, dilute in D_5W or NSS for injection to yield 1.5 to 25 mg phenytoin sodium equivalent/mL.

Black Box Warning Don't give more than 150 mg phenytoin sodium equivalent/minute because of risk of severe hypotension and cardiac arrhythmias. For a 50-kg patient, infusion should take 5 to 7 minutes. (Infusion of identical molar dose of phenytoin takes at least 15 minutes, because giving phenytoin I.V. at more than 50 mg/minute causes adverse CV effects.) ■

▼ Patients receiving 20 mg phenytoin sodium equivalent/kg at 150 mg phenytoin sodium equivalent/minute typically feel discomfort, usually in the groin. To reduce discomfort, slow or temporarily stop infusion.

▼ Monitor patient's ECG, BP, and respirations continuously during maximum phenytoin level—about 10 to 20 minutes after end of fosphenytoin infusion. Severe CV complications are most common in elderly or gravely ill patients. If needed, decrease rate or stop infusion.

▼ Store drug under refrigeration. Don't store at room temperature longer than 48 hours. Discard vials that develop particulate matter.

▼ **Incompatibilities:** Other I.V. drugs.

I.M.

● Depending on dose ordered, may require two separate I.M. injections.

● I.M. administration generates systemic phenytoin levels similar enough to oral phenytoin sodium to allow essentially interchangeable use.

● Store drug under refrigeration. Don't store at room temperature longer than 48 hours. Discard vials that develop particulate matter.

ACTION

May stabilize neuronal membranes and limit seizure activity either by increasing efflux or decreasing influx of sodium ions across cell membranes in the motor cortex during generation of nerve impulses.

Route	Onset	Peak	Duration
I.V.	Unknown	End of infusion	Unknown
I.M.	Unknown	30 min	Unknown

Half-life: Fosphenytoin, 15 minutes; phenytoin, 12 to 29 hours.

ADVERSE REACTIONS

CNS: ataxia, dizziness, somnolence, ***brain edema, intracranial hypertension,*** agitation, asthenia, dysarthria, extrapyramidal syndrome, fever, headache, hypesthesia, incoordination, increased or decreased reflexes, nervousness, paresthesia, speech disorders, stupor, thinking abnormalities, tremor, vertigo.

CV: hypertension, hypotension, tachycardia, vasodilation.

EENT: nystagmus, amblyopia, deafness, diplopia, tinnitus.

GI: constipation, dry mouth, taste perversion, tongue disorder, vomiting.

GU: pelvic pain.

Metabolic: *hypokalemia.*

Musculoskeletal: back pain, myasthenia.

Respiratory: pneumonia.

Skin: pruritus, ecchymoses, injection-site reaction and pain, rash.

Other: accidental injury, chills, facial edema, infection.

INTERACTIONS

Drug-drug. *Amiodarone, chloramphenicol, chlordiazepoxide, cimetidine, diazepam, disulfiram, estrogens, ethosuximide, fluoxetine, H$_2$-receptor antagonists, halothane, isoniazid, methylphenidate, phenothiazines, phenylbutazone, salicylates, succinimides, sulfonamides, tolbutamide, trazodone:* May increase phenytoin level and effect. Use together cautiously.

Carbamazepine, reserpine: May decrease phenytoin level. Monitor patient.

Corticosteroids, doxycycline, estrogens, furosemide, hormonal contraceptives, quinidine, rifampin, theophylline, vitamin D, warfarin: May decrease effects of these drugs because of increased hepatic metabolism. Monitor patient closely.

Lithium: May increase lithium toxicity. Monitor patient's neurologic status closely. Marked neurologic symptoms have been reported despite normal lithium level.

Phenobarbital, valproate sodium, valproic acid: May increase or decrease phenytoin level. May increase or decrease levels of these drugs. Monitor patient.

TCAs: May lower seizure threshold and require adjustments in phenytoin dosage. Use together cautiously.

Drug-lifestyle. *Alcohol use:* Acute intoxication may increase phenytoin level and effect. Discourage use together.

Long-term alcohol use: May decrease phenytoin level. Monitor patient and strongly discourage use together.

EFFECTS ON LAB TEST RESULTS

● May increase alkaline phosphatase, GGT, and glucose levels. May decrease folate, potassium, and T$_4$ levels.

● May cause falsely low dexamethasone and metyrapone test results.

CONTRAINDICATIONS & CAUTIONS

● Contraindicated in patients hypersensitive to drug or its components, phenytoin, or other hydantoins.

● Contraindicated in patients with sinus bradycardia, SA block, second- or third-degree AV block, or Adams-Stokes syndrome.

● Contraindicated in patients taking delavirdine because of potential loss of virologic response and possible resistance to delavirdine or to NNRTIs.

Black Box Warning There is an increased risk of severe hypotension and cardiac arrhythmia (bradycardia, heart block, QT-interval prolongation, ventricular tachycardia, ventricular fibrillation) with I.V. infusion rate of greater than 150 mg phenytoin sodium equivalent/minute. CV effects can also occur at lower infusion rates; therefore, cardiac monitoring is needed during and after infusion. Reduce rate or discontinue drug as clinically necessary. ∎

● Use cautiously in patients with porphyria and in those with history of hypersensitivity to similarly structured drugs, such as barbiturates, oxazolidinediones, and succinimide.

● *Alert:* If patient develops acute hepatotoxicity, discontinue drug and don't readminister.

● *Alert:* Serious and sometimes fatal toxic epidermal necrolysis and Stevens-Johnson syndrome have been reported; usually onset of symptoms occurs within 28 days but sometimes later. Discontinue drug at first sign of rash unless rash is clearly not drug related. If rash occurs, evaluate patient for signs and symptoms of DRESS (drug reaction with eosinophilia and systemic symptoms).

Dialyzable drug: Unknown.

⚠ *Overdose S&S:* Asystole, bradycardia, cardiac arrest, hypocalcemia, hypotension, lethargy, metabolic acidosis, nausea, syncope, tachycardia, vomiting, death.

PREGNANCY-LACTATION-REPRODUCTION

● Drug is known to cause birth defects. Use with extreme caution in pregnant women after assessing maternal benefits and fetal risk.

● A potentially life-threatening bleeding disorder related to decreased levels of vitamin K–dependent clotting factors may occur in newborns exposed to phenytoin in utero. This drug-induced condition can be prevented with vitamin K administration to the mother before delivery and to the neonate after birth.

● Breast-feeding isn't recommended.

NURSING CONSIDERATIONS

● *Alert:* Because of risk of cardiac and local toxicity with I.V. fosphenytoin administration, use oral phenytoin whenever possible.

● Most significant drug interactions are those commonly seen with phenytoin.

● *Alert:* Drug should always be prescribed and dispensed in phenytoin sodium equivalent units. Don't make adjustments in the recommended doses when substituting fosphenytoin for phenytoin, and vice versa.

● In status epilepticus, phenytoin may be used as maintenance instead of fosphenytoin, using the appropriate dose.

● Phosphate load provided by fosphenytoin (0.0037 millimole phosphate/mg phenytoin sodium equivalent) must be taken into consideration when treating patients who need phosphate restriction, such as those with severe renal impairment. Monitor laboratory values.

● Asian patients who have tested positive for the allele HLA-B*1502 have a potentially increased risk of serious skin reactions, including Stevens-Johnson syndrome and toxic epidermal necrolysis. Monitor these patients carefully.

● If patient develops exfoliative, purpuric, or bullous rash or signs and symptoms of lupus erythematosus, Stevens-Johnson syndrome, or toxic epidermal necrolysis, stop drug and notify prescriber. If rash is mild (measles-like or scarlatiniform), therapy may resume after rash disappears. If rash recurs when therapy is resumed, further fosphenytoin or phenytoin administration is contraindicated. Document that patient is allergic to drug.

● Stop drug in patients with acute hepatotoxicity.

● After administration, phenytoin levels shouldn't be monitored until conversion to phenytoin is essentially complete—about 2 hours after the end of an I.V. infusion or 4 hours after I.M. administration.

● Interpret total phenytoin levels cautiously in patients with renal or hepatic disease or hypoalbuminemia caused by an increased fraction of unbound phenytoin. It may be more useful to monitor unbound phenytoin levels in these patients. When giving drug I.V., monitor patients with renal and hepatic

disease because they are at increased risk for more frequent and severe adverse reactions.
• Monitor glucose level closely in diabetic patients; drug may cause hyperglycemia.
• Abrupt withdrawal of drug may precipitate status epilepticus.
• *Look alike–sound alike:* Don't confuse Cerebyx with Cerezyme, Celexa, or Celebrex.

PATIENT TEACHING
• Warn patient that sensory disturbances may occur with I.V. administration.
• Instruct patient to immediately report adverse reactions, especially rash.
• Warn patient not to stop drug abruptly or adjust dosage without discussing with prescriber.
• Advise female patient of childbearing potential to discuss drug therapy with prescriber if considering pregnancy.
• Advise female patient of childbearing potential that breast-feeding isn't recommended during therapy.

frovatriptan succinate
frow-vah-TRIP-tan

Frova♥

Therapeutic class: Antimigraine drugs
Pharmacologic class: Serotonin 5-HT$_1$ receptor agonists

AVAILABLE FORMS
Tablets: 2.5 mg

INDICATIONS & DOSAGES
➤ **Acute treatment of migraine attacks with or without aura**
Adults: 2.5 mg P.O. taken at the first sign of migraine attack. If the headache recurs, a second tablet may be taken at least 2 hours after the first dose. The total daily dose shouldn't exceed 7.5 mg.

ADMINISTRATION
P.O.
• Give drug without regard for food.
• Give drug with a full glass of water.
• If headache returns after first dose, give a second dose after 2 hours. Don't give more than 3 tablets in 24 hours.

ACTION
May cause vasoconstriction in response to excessive dilation of extracerebral and intracranial arteries during migraine headaches.

Route	Onset	Peak	Duration
P.O.	Unknown	2–4 hr	Unknown

Half-life: 26 hours.

ADVERSE REACTIONS
CNS: dizziness, headache, fatigue, paresthesia, insomnia, anxiety, somnolence, dysesthesia, hypoesthesia, hot or cold sensation, pain, drowsiness.
CV: *coronary artery vasospasm, transient myocardial ischemia, MI, ventricular tachycardia, ventricular fibrillation,* chest pain, palpitations, flushing.
EENT: abnormal vision, tinnitus, sinusitis, rhinitis.
GI: dry mouth, dyspepsia, vomiting, abdominal pain, diarrhea, nausea.
Musculoskeletal: skeletal pain.
Skin: increased sweating.

INTERACTIONS
Drug-drug. *Ergotamine-containing or ergot-type drugs (such as dihydroergotamine or methysergide):* May cause prolonged vasospastic reactions. Separate doses by 24 hours.
5-HT$_1$ agonists: May cause additive effects. Separate doses by 24 hours.
SSRIs (such as citalopram, fluoxetine, fluvoxamine, paroxetine, sertraline): May cause weakness, hyperreflexia, and incoordination. Monitor patient closely.

EFFECTS ON LAB TEST RESULTS
None reported.

CONTRAINDICATIONS & CAUTIONS
• Contraindicated in patients hypersensitive to drug or its components.
• Contraindicated in patients with history or symptoms of ischemic heart disease or coronary artery vasospasm, including Prinzmetal variant angina, Wolff-Parkinson-White syndrome, or other cardiac accessory conduction pathway disorders; in those with cerebrovascular or peripheral vascular disease, including ischemic bowel disease;

in those with uncontrolled hypertension; and in those with hemiplegic or basilar migraine.

• Contraindicated within 24 hours of another triptan, drug containing ergotamine, or ergot-type drug.

• Contraindicated in patients with risk factors for CAD, such as hypertension, hypercholesterolemia, smoking, obesity, diabetes, strong family history of CAD, postmenopausal women, or men older than age 40, unless patient is free from cardiac disease. If drug is used in such a patient, monitor patient closely and consider obtaining an ECG after the first dose. Intermittent, long-term users of triptans or those with risk factors should undergo periodic cardiac evaluation while using drug.

• Safety of treating an average of more than four migraine headaches in a 30-day period hasn't been established.

Dialyzable drug: Unknown.

PREGNANCY-LACTATION-REPRODUCTION

• It isn't known if drug affects fetal development. Use during pregnancy only if potential benefit justifies potential fetal risk. Consider using a better-studied drug during pregnancy.

• It isn't known if drug appears in breast milk. Patient should discontinue breast-feeding or discontinue drug.

NURSING CONSIDERATIONS

◆ *Alert:* Serious cardiac events, including acute MI, life-threatening cardiac arrhythmias, and death, may occur within a few hours of taking a triptan.

• Use drug only when patient has a clear diagnosis of migraine. If a patient has no response for the first migraine attack treated with frovatriptan, reconsider the diagnosis of migraine.

◆ *Alert:* Combining a triptan with an SSRI or an SSNRI or agents that reduce frovatriptan's metabolism may cause serotonin syndrome. Symptoms may include restlessness, hallucinations, loss of coordination, fast heartbeat, rapid changes in BP, increased body temperature, hyperreflexia, nausea, vomiting, and diarrhea. Serotonin syndrome is more likely to occur when

starting or increasing the dose of a triptan, SSRI, or SSNRI.

PATIENT TEACHING

• Instruct patient to take dose at first sign of migraine headache. If headache comes back after first dose, he may take a second dose after 2 hours. Tell patient not to take more than 3 tablets in 24 hours.

• Caution patient to take extra care or avoid driving and operating machinery if dizziness or fatigue develops after taking drug.

• Stress importance of reporting all adverse reactions. Advise patient to immediately report pain, tightness, heaviness, or pressure in chest, throat, neck, or jaw; or rash or itching after taking drug.

• Instruct patient not to take drug within 24 hours of taking another serotonin-receptor agonist or ergot-type drug.

• Tell patient dose may be taken with or without food, but to take with a full glass of fluid.

SAFETY ALERT!

fulvestrant
full-VES-trant

Faslodex

Therapeutic class: Antineoplastics
Pharmacologic class: Estrogen antagonists

AVAILABLE FORMS
Injection: 50 mg/mL in 5-mL prefilled syringes*

INDICATIONS & DOSAGES
➤ **Hormone receptor–positive metastatic breast cancer with disease progression after antiestrogen therapy**
Postmenopausal women: 500 mg I.M. slowly into buttocks (over 1 to 2 minutes per injection) as two 5-mL injections, one in each buttock on days 1, 15, 29, and then once monthly thereafter.

Adjust-a-dose: For patients with moderate hepatic impairment (Child-Pugh class B), give 250 mg I.M. slowly into buttocks over 1 to 2 minutes as one 5-mL injection on days 1, 15, 29, and then monthly thereafter.

Reactions in bold italics are *life-threatening*. Interactions may have a *rapid onset* or a *delayed onset*.

✳ NEW INDICATION: Hormone receptor-positive, human epidermal growth factor receptor 2 (HER2)-negative advanced or metastatic breast cancer in combination with palbociclib in women with disease progression after endocrine therapy

Adults: 500 mg I.M. slowly into buttocks (1 to 2 minutes per injection) as two 5-mL injections, one in each buttock, on days 1, 15, 29, and then once monthly thereafter. Recommended palbociclib dose is a 125-mg capsule P.O. once daily for 21 consecutive days followed by 7 days off each 28-day cycle. Premenopausal and perimenopausal women treated with this combination should be treated with luteinizing hormone-releasing hormone (LHRH) agonists according to current clinical practice standards.

Adjust-a-dose: For patients with moderate hepatic impairment (Child-Pugh class B), give 250 mg I.M. as one 5-mL injection on days 1, 15, 29, and then once monthly thereafter. Refer to palbociclib prescribing information for dosage adjustments and management of toxicity related to palbociclib.

ADMINISTRATION
I.M.
● Drug is a potential teratogen. Follow safe handling procedures.
● Drug may be warmed before use by storing at room temperature for 1 hour or rolling injection gently in hands.
● Expel gas bubble from syringe before giving.
● Give slowly into buttocks.

ACTION
Competitively binds estrogen receptors and downregulates estrogen-receptor protein in human breast cancer cells. It's effective in treating estrogen receptor–positive breast tumors.

Route	Onset	Peak	Duration
I.M.	Unknown	7 days	1 mo

Half-life: About 40 days.

ADVERSE REACTIONS
CNS: asthenia, headache, pain, dizziness, insomnia, fever, paresthesia, depression, anxiety, fatigue.

CV: hot flashes, chest pain, peripheral edema, vasodilation.
EENT: pharyngitis.
GI: nausea, vomiting, constipation, abdominal pain, diarrhea, anorexia.
GU: UTI.
Hematologic: anemia.
Musculoskeletal: bone pain, back pain, pelvic pain, arthritis.
Respiratory: dyspnea, cough.
Skin: injection-site pain, rash, sweating.
Other: accidental injury, flulike syndrome.

INTERACTIONS
None reported.

EFFECTS ON LAB TEST RESULTS
● May decrease Hb level and hematocrit.

CONTRAINDICATIONS & CAUTIONS
● Contraindicated in patients allergic to drug or its components.
● Use cautiously in patients with moderate or severe hepatic impairment.
Dialyzable drug: Unknown.

PREGNANCY-LACTATION-REPRODUCTION
● Drug can cause fetal harm. Women of childbearing potential should be advised not to become pregnant during therapy. If drug is used during pregnancy, or if patient becomes pregnant during therapy, apprise patient of potential hazard to the fetus. Women should use effective contraception during therapy and for 1 year after last dose.
● It isn't known if drug appears in breast milk. Patient should discontinue breast-feeding or discontinue drug.

NURSING CONSIDERATIONS
● Because drug is given I.M., use cautiously in patients with bleeding diatheses or thrombocytopenia, and in those taking anticoagulants.
● Pregnancy testing is recommended within 7 days before initiating drug.

PATIENT TEACHING
● Caution female patient to avoid pregnancy during therapy and for 1 year after last dose and to report suspected pregnancy immediately.

● Inform patient of the most common adverse effects, including pain at injection site, headache, GI symptoms, back pain, hot flashes, and sore throat. Advise patient to report all adverse reactions.

furosemide
fur-OH-se-mide

Lasix◆, Lasix Special✦

Therapeutic class: Antihypertensives
Pharmacologic class: Loop diuretics

AVAILABLE FORMS
Injection: 10 mg/mL
Oral solution: 10 mg/mL, 40 mg/5 mL
Tablets: 20 mg, 40 mg, 80 mg, 500 mg✦

INDICATIONS & DOSAGES
➤ **Acute pulmonary edema**
Adults: 40 mg I.V. injected slowly over 1 to 2 minutes; then 80 mg I.V. in 60 to 90 minutes if needed. Maximum is 200 mg/dose.
➤ **Edema**
Adults: 20 to 80 mg P.O. daily in the morning. If response is inadequate, give a second dose, and each succeeding dose, every 6 to 8 hours. Carefully increase dose in 20- to 40-mg increments up to 600 mg daily. Once effective dose is attained, may give once daily or b.i.d. Or, 20 to 40 mg I.V. or I.M., increased by 20 mg 2 hours after previous dose until desired effect achieved.
Infants and children: 2 mg/kg P.O. daily, increased by 1 to 2 mg/kg in 6 to 8 hours if needed; carefully adjusted up to maximum of 6 mg/kg if needed. Or, 1 mg/kg slowly I.V. or I.M. May increase dosage by 1 mg/kg 2 hours after previous dose if needed up to 6 mg/kg. Maximum dose is 1 mg/kg/day for premature infants.
➤ **Hypertension**
Adults: 40 mg P.O. b.i.d. Dosage adjusted based on response. May be used as adjunct to other antihypertensives if needed.

ADMINISTRATION
P.O.
● To prevent nocturia, give in the morning. Give second dose if ordered in early afternoon, 6 to 8 hours after morning dose.

● Store tablets in light-resistant container to prevent discoloration (doesn't affect potency). Refrigerate oral solution to ensure drug stability.
I.V.
▼ If discolored yellow, don't use.
▼ For direct injection, give over 1 to 2 minutes.
▼ For infusion, dilute with D_5W, NSS, or lactated Ringer solution.
◑ *Alert:* To avoid ototoxicity, infuse no more than 4 mg/minute.
▼ Use prepared infusion solution within 24 hours.
▼ **Incompatibilities:** Acidic solutions, amrinone, ciprofloxacin, milrinone.
I.M.
● To prevent nocturia, give in the morning. Give second dose if ordered in early afternoon, 6 to 8 hours after morning dose.
● Record administration site.

ACTION
Inhibits sodium and chloride reabsorption at the proximal and distal tubules and the ascending loop of Henle.

Route	Onset	Peak	Duration
P.O.	20–60 min	1–2 hr	6–8 hr
I.V.	Within 5 min	30 min	2 hr
I.M.	Unknown	30 min	2 hr

Half-life: 2 hours.

ADVERSE REACTIONS
CNS: vertigo, headache, dizziness, paresthesia, weakness, restlessness, fever.
CV: orthostatic hypotension, thrombophlebitis with I.V. administration.
EENT: blurred or yellowed vision, transient deafness, tinnitus.
GI: abdominal discomfort and pain, diarrhea, anorexia, nausea, vomiting, constipation, *pancreatitis.*
GU: azotemia, nocturia, polyuria, frequent urination, oliguria.
Hematologic: *agranulocytosis, aplastic anemia, leukopenia, thrombocytopenia,* anemia.
Hepatic: hepatic dysfunction, jaundice.
Metabolic: volume depletion and dehydration, asymptomatic hyperuricemia, impaired glucose tolerance, *hypokalemia,* hypochloremic alkalosis, hyperglycemia,

---

*Reactions in bold italics are **life-threatening**. Interactions may have a rapid onset or a **delayed onset**.*

dilutional hyponatremia, *hypocalcemia, hypomagnesemia.*
Musculoskeletal: muscle spasm.
Skin: dermatitis, purpura, photosensitivity reactions, transient pain at I.M. injection site, *toxic epidermal necrolysis, Stevens-Johnson syndrome, erythema multiforme.*
Other: gout.

INTERACTIONS
Drug-drug. *Aminoglycoside antibiotics, cisplatin:* May increase ototoxicity. Use together cautiously.
Amphotericin B, corticosteroids, corticotropin, metolazone: May increase risk of hypokalemia. Monitor potassium level closely.
Antidiabetics: May decrease hypoglycemic effects. Monitor glucose level.
Antihypertensives: May increase risk of hypotension. Use together cautiously. Decrease antihypertensive dose if needed.
Cardiac glycosides, neuromuscular blockers: May increase toxicity of these drugs from furosemide-induced hypokalemia. Monitor potassium level.
Chlorothiazide, chlorthalidone, hydrochlorothiazide, indapamide, metolazone: May cause excessive diuretic response, causing serious electrolyte abnormalities or dehydration. Adjust doses carefully, and monitor patient closely for signs and symptoms of excessive diuretic response.
Ethacrynic acid: May increase risk of ototoxicity. Avoid using together.
Lithium: May decrease lithium excretion, resulting in lithium toxicity. Monitor lithium level.
NSAIDs: May inhibit diuretic response. Use together cautiously.
Phenytoin: May decrease diuretic effects of furosemide. Use together cautiously.
Propranolol: May increase propranolol level. Monitor patient closely.
Salicylates: May cause salicylate toxicity. Use together cautiously.
Sucralfate: May reduce diuretic and antihypertensive effect. Separate doses by 2 hours.
Drug-herb. *Aloe:* May increase drug effect. Discourage use together.
Bayberry, blue cohosh, cayenne, ephedra, ginger, ginseng (American), kola, licorice:
May worsen hypertension. Discourage use together.
Black cohosh, California poppy, coleus, golden seal, hawthorn, mistletoe, periwinkle, quinine, shepherd's purse: May increase antihypertensive effect. Discourage use together.
Dandelion: May interfere with drug activity. Discourage use together.
Licorice: May cause unexpected rapid potassium loss. Discourage use together.
Drug-food. *Any food:* May decrease furosemide serum level. Don't give with food.
Drug-lifestyle. *Sun exposure:* May increase risk of photosensitivity reactions. Advise patient to avoid excessive sunlight exposure.

EFFECTS ON LAB TEST RESULTS
● May increase cholesterol, glucose, BUN, creatinine, and uric acid levels. May decrease calcium, Hb, magnesium, potassium, and sodium levels.
● May decrease granulocyte, platelet, and WBC counts.

CONTRAINDICATIONS & CAUTIONS
● Contraindicated in patients hypersensitive to drug and in those with anuria.
● Use cautiously in patients with hepatic cirrhosis and in those allergic to sulfonamides. Use during pregnancy only if potential benefits to mother clearly outweigh risks to fetus.
● **Alert:** Drug may cause tinnitus and reversible or irreversible hearing loss. Ototoxicity is associated with rapid injection, severe renal impairment, use of higher-than-recommended doses, hypoproteinemia, or use with other ototoxic drugs.
● Drug may exacerbate or activate systemic lupus erythematosus.
● Premature infants may be at increased risk for persistent patent ductus arteriosus with furosemide treatment during first weeks of life.
Dialyzable drug: No.
▲ *Overdose S&S:* Dehydration, blood volume reduction, hypotension, electrolyte imbalance.

PREGNANCY-LACTATION-REPRODUCTION

• There are no well-controlled studies in pregnant women. Use during pregnancy only if potential benefit justifies potential risk to the fetus.

• Drug appears in breast milk. Use cautiously in breast-feeding women.

NURSING CONSIDERATIONS

❸ *Alert:* Monitor weight, BP, and pulse rate routinely with long-term use.

Black Box Warning Drug is potent diuretic and can cause severe diuresis with water and electrolyte depletion. Monitor patient closely and adjust dose carefully. ■

• If oliguria or azotemia develops or increases, drug may need to be stopped.

• Monitor fluid intake and output and electrolyte, BUN, and carbon dioxide levels frequently.

• Watch for signs of hypokalemia, such as muscle weakness and cramps.

• Consult prescriber and dietitian about a high-potassium diet or potassium supplements. Foods rich in potassium include citrus fruits, tomatoes, bananas, dates, and apricots.

• Monitor glucose level in diabetic patients.

• Drug may not be well absorbed orally in patient with severe HF. Drug may need to be given I.V. even if patient is taking other oral drugs.

• Monitor uric acid level, especially in patients with a history of gout.

• Monitor elderly patients, who are especially susceptible to excessive diuresis, because circulatory collapse and thromboembolic complications are possible.

• Monitor patients with severe symptoms of urine retention due to bladder emptying disorders, prostate enlargement, or urethral narrowing or worsening of symptoms, especially during initial treatment.

• Drug may increase fetal birth weight. Monitor fetal growth during pregnancy.

• Nephrocalcinosis and nephrolithiasis have occurred in premature infants and in children younger than age 4 on long-term furosemide therapy. Monitor renal function and renal ultrasounds.

• *Look alike–sound alike:* Don't confuse furosemide with torsemide. Don't confuse Lasix with Lonox, Lidex, or Luvox.

PATIENT TEACHING

• Advise patient to take drug in morning to prevent need to urinate at night. If patient needs second dose, tell him to take it in early afternoon, 6 to 8 hours after morning dose.

• Inform patient of possible need for potassium or magnesium supplements.

• Instruct patient to stand slowly to prevent dizziness and to limit alcohol intake and strenuous exercise in hot weather to avoid worsening dizziness upon standing quickly.

• Advise patient to report all adverse reactions and to immediately report ringing in ears, severe abdominal pain, or sore throat and fever; these symptoms may indicate toxicity.

❸ *Alert:* Discourage patient from storing different types of drugs in the same container, increasing risk of drug errors. (The most popular strengths of furosemide and digoxin are white tablets that are about equal in size.)

• Tell patient to consult prescriber or pharmacist before taking OTC drugs.

• Teach patient to avoid direct sunlight and to use protective clothing and sunblock because of risk of photosensitivity reactions.

---

gabapentin
gab-ah-PEN-tin

Gralise, Neurontin✐

gabapentin enacarbil
Horizant

Therapeutic class: Anticonvulsants
Pharmacologic class: GABA structural analogues

AVAILABLE FORMS

Capsules: 100 mg, 300 mg, 400 mg
Oral solution: 250 mg/5 mL
Tablets: 100 mg, 300 mg, 400 mg, 600 mg, 800 mg
Tablets (extended-release) ⓞⓡⓒ: 300 mg, 600 mg

INDICATIONS & DOSAGES

Adjust-a-dose (for all indications): For immediate-release formulation in patients age 12 and older with CrCl of 30 to 59 mL/minute, give 400 to 1,400 mg

---

daily divided into two doses. For CrCl of 15 to 29 mL/minute, give 200 to 700 mg daily in a single dose. For CrCl of less than 15 mL/minute, give 100 to 300 mg daily in a single dose. Reduce daily dosage in proportion to CrCl (patients with a CrCl of 7.5 mL/minute should receive half the daily dosage of those with a CrCl of 15 mL/minute). For patients receiving hemodialysis, maintenance dosage is based on estimates of CrCl. Give supplemental dose of 125 to 350 mg after each 4 hours of hemodialysis.

➤ **Adjunctive treatment of partial seizures with or without secondary generalization in patients with epilepsy (excluding Gralise)**

Adults and children age 12 and older: Initially, 300 mg P.O. t.i.d. Increase dosage as needed and tolerated to 1,800 mg daily in divided doses. Dosages up to 3,600 mg daily have been well tolerated.

➤ **Adjunctive treatment to control partial seizures in children (excluding Gralise)**

Starting dosage, children ages 3 to 11: 10 to 15 mg/kg daily P.O. in three divided doses, adjusting over 3 days to reach effective dosage.

Effective dosage, children ages 5 to 11: 25 to 35 mg/kg daily P.O. in three divided doses.

Effective dosage, children ages 3 to 4: 40 mg/kg daily P.O. in three divided doses.

➤ **Moderate to severe primary restless legs syndrome (Horizant)**

Adults: 600 mg extended-release tablet P.O. daily at about 5 p.m. If dose isn't taken at the recommended time, the next dose should be taken the following day as prescribed.

Adjust-a-dose: If CrCl is 30 to 59 mL/minute, give 300 mg daily (may increase to 600 mg if needed). If CrCl is 15 to 29 mL/minute, give 300 mg daily in the morning; increase to 300 mg b.i.d. if needed. If CrCl is less than 15 mL/minute, give 300 mg every other day in the morning; increase to 300 mg once daily in the morning if needed. Don't give to patients receiving hemodialysis.

➤ **Postherpetic neuralgia (immediate-release)**

Adults: 300 mg P.O. once daily on first day, 300 mg b.i.d. on day 2, and 300 mg t.i.d.

on day 3. Adjust as needed for pain to a maximum daily dose of 1,800 mg in three divided doses.

➤ **Postherpetic neuralgia (Gralise)**

Adults: Titrate dosage to 1,800 mg P.O. once daily with the evening meal. On day 1, give 300 mg; on day 2, 600 mg; on days 3 to 6, 900 mg; on days 7 to 10, 1,200 mg; on days 11 to 14, 1,500 mg; and on day 15 and thereafter, 1,800 mg.

Adjust-a-dose: For patients with reduced renal function, initiate Gralise at a daily dose of 300 mg. For patients with CrCl of 30 to 60 mL/minute, titrate dosage to 600 to 1,800 mg daily as tolerated. Don't give Gralise to patients with CrCl of less than 30 mL/minute or to those receiving hemodialysis.

➤ **Postherpetic neuralgia (Horizant)**

Adults: 600 mg P.O. in morning for 3 days; increase to 600 mg b.i.d. on day 4. If dose isn't taken at recommended time, skip dose, and take next dose at time of next scheduled dose.

Adjust-a-dose: If CrCl is 30 to 59 mL/minute, give 300 mg in the morning for 3 days; then increase to 300 mg b.i.d. (may increase to 600 mg b.i.d. as needed). If CrCl is 15 to 29 mL/minute, give 300 mg in the morning on days 1 and 3, then 300 mg daily in the morning (increase to 300 mg b.i.d. if needed). If CrCl is less than 15 mL/minute, give 300 mg in the morning every other day (increase to 300 mg daily in the morning if needed). If CrCl is less than 15 mL/minute and patient is on hemodialysis, give 300 mg after each dialysis treatment (increase to 600 mg after every dialysis treatment if needed).

ADMINISTRATION

P.O.

• Give immediate-release forms without regard for food.
• Give extended-release tablets with food.
• Give Gralise tablets with the evening meal.
• Give drug 2 hours after an antacid.
• Refrigerate oral solution.
• Patient should swallow extended-release tablets whole and shouldn't cut, crush, or chew them.

G

• Gralise, Horizant, and other gabapentin products aren't interchangeable.

ACTION
Unknown. Structurally related to GABA but doesn't interact with GABA receptors, isn't converted into GABA or GABA agonist, doesn't inhibit GABA reuptake, and doesn't prevent degradation.

Route	Onset	Peak	Duration
P.O. (immediate-release)	Unknown	2 hr	Unknown
P.O. (extended-release)	Unknown	8 hr	Unknown
P.O. (enacarbil)	Unknown	5–7 hr	Unknown

Half-life: Gabapentin, 5 to 7 hours; gabapentin enacarbil, 5 to 6 hours.

ADVERSE REACTIONS
CNS: ataxia, dizziness, fatigue, somnolence, abnormal thinking, amnesia, depression, dysarthria, incoordination, nervousness, tremor.
CV: peripheral edema, vasodilation.
EENT: amblyopia, diplopia, nystagmus, pharyngitis, rhinitis, dry throat.
GI: constipation, dry mouth, dyspepsia, increased appetite, flatulence, nausea, vomiting; diarrhea (Gralise).
GU: erectile dysfunction; UTI (Gralise).
Hematologic: *leukopenia.*
Metabolic: weight gain.
Musculoskeletal: back pain, fractures, myalgia.
Respiratory: coughing.
Skin: abrasion, pruritus.
Other: dental abnormalities.

INTERACTIONS
Drug-drug. *Antacids:* May decrease absorption of gabapentin. Separate dosage times by at least 2 hours.
CNS depressants: May increase risk of CNS depressant–related adverse effects. Monitor therapy.
Hydrocodone: May enhance CNS depressant effect of hydrocodone. Consider reducing hydrocodone dosage by 20% to 30% initially.

EFFECTS ON LAB TEST RESULTS
• May decrease WBC count.

• May cause false-positive results with the Ames N-Multistix SG dipstick test for urine protein when used with other anticonvulsants.

CONTRAINDICATIONS & CAUTIONS
• Contraindicated in patients hypersensitive to drug.
• In elderly patients, adjust dosage based on CrCl values due to potentially decreased renal function.
• Gabapentin enacarbil isn't recommended for patients who must sleep during the day and remain awake at night.
• Anaphylaxis and angioedema can occur any time during therapy and require emergency treatment and discontinuation of drug.
• DRESS syndrome (drug reaction with eosinophilia and systemic symptoms), with such symptoms as fever, rash, lymphadenopathy, and other organ system involvement, which can be life-threatening, can occur. Evaluate patient immediately if symptoms occur and discontinue drug.
Dialyzable drug: Yes.
⚠ *Overdose S&S:* Double vision, slurred speech, drowsiness, lethargy, diarrhea.

PREGNANCY-LACTATION-REPRODUCTION
• Use during pregnancy only if potential benefit justifies potential risk to the fetus.
• Use in breast-feeding women only if benefit to the mother outweighs potential risk to the infant.

NURSING CONSIDERATIONS
⤷ *Alert:* Closely monitor all patients taking or starting antiepileptic drugs for changes in behavior indicating worsening of suicidal thoughts or behavior or depression. Symptoms such as anxiety, agitation, hostility, mania, and hypomania may be precursors to emerging suicidality.
• If drug is to be stopped or an alternative drug substituted, do so gradually over at least 1 week to minimize risk of precipitating seizures.
⤷ *Alert:* Don't suddenly withdraw other anticonvulsants in patients starting gabapentin therapy.

G

- Routine monitoring of drug levels isn't necessary. Drug doesn't appear to alter levels of other anticonvulsants.

PATIENT TEACHING
- Advise patient that immediate-release form may be taken without regard for meals.
- Advise patient to take extended-release tablets with food.
- Instruct patient to take first dose at bedtime to minimize adverse reactions.
- Tell patient with seizures that the maximum time interval between doses shouldn't exceed 12 hours.
- Warn patient that extended-release formulas can cause significant dizziness and sleepiness.
- Warn patient to report all adverse reactions and to avoid driving and operating heavy machinery until drug's CNS effects are known.
- Advise patient not to take extended-release formulas with alcohol or other drugs that may cause sleepiness or dizziness.
- Advise patient not to stop drug abruptly.
- Advise female patient to discuss drug therapy with prescriber if considering pregnancy.
- Tell patient to keep oral solution refrigerated.

galantamine hydrobromide
gah-LAN-tah-meen

Razadyne, Razadyne ER,
Reminyl ER✤

Therapeutic class: Anti-Alzheimer drugs
Pharmacologic class: Cholinesterase inhibitors

AVAILABLE FORMS
Capsules (extended-release): 8 mg, 16 mg, 24 mg
Oral solution: 4 mg/mL
Tablets: 4 mg, 8 mg, 12 mg

INDICATIONS & DOSAGES
➤ **Mild to moderate Alzheimer dementia**
Adults: Initially, 4 mg b.i.d., preferably with morning and evening meals. If dose is well tolerated after minimum of 4 weeks

of therapy, increase dosage to 8 mg b.i.d. A further increase to 12 mg b.i.d. may be attempted, but only after at least 4 weeks of therapy at the previous dosage. Dosage range is 16 to 24 mg daily in two divided doses.

Or, 8 mg extended-release capsule P.O. once daily in the morning with food. Increase to 16 mg P.O. once daily after a minimum of 4 weeks. May further increase to 24 mg once daily after a minimum of 4 weeks, based on patient response and tolerability.
Adjust-a-dose: For patients with Child-Pugh score of 7 to 9, dosage usually shouldn't exceed 16 mg daily. Drug isn't recommended for patients with Child-Pugh score of 10 to 15. For patients with moderate renal impairment, dosage usually shouldn't exceed 16 mg daily. For patients with CrCl less than 9 mL/minute, drug isn't recommended.

ADMINISTRATION
P.O.
🛈 *Alert:* Give Razadyne tablets b.i.d.; give Razadyne ER capsules once daily. To avoid dosing errors, verify any prescription that suggests a different dosing schedule.
- Give drug with food and antiemetics, and ensure adequate fluid intake to decrease the risk of nausea and vomiting.
- Use proper technique when dispensing the oral solution with the pipette provided by the manufacturer. Dilute dose in 100 mL of a nonalcoholic beverage and give to patient right away.

ACTION
Thought to enhance cholinergic function by increasing acetylcholine level in brain.

Route	Onset	Peak	Duration
P.O.	Unknown	1 hr	Unknown
Extended-release	Unknown	4½–5 hr	Unknown

Half-life: About 7 hours.

ADVERSE REACTIONS
CNS: asthenia, depression, dizziness, headache, tremor, insomnia, somnolence, fatigue, syncope, tremor, lethargy, malaise.
CV: *bradycardia, AV block.*
EENT: rhinitis.

GI: diarrhea, nausea, vomiting, abdominal pain, dyspepsia, anorexia.
GU: UTI, hematuria, urinary incontinence.
Hematologic: anemia.
Metabolic: weight loss.

INTERACTIONS
Drug-drug. *Amitriptyline, fluoxetine, fluvoxamine, quinidine:* May decrease galantamine clearance. Monitor patient closely.
Anticholinergics: May antagonize anticholinergic activity. Monitor patient.
Antipsychotics: May enhance neurotoxic effects of antipsychotics; severe extrapyramidal symptoms have occurred. Monitor therapy.
Cholinergics (bethanechol, succinylcholine): May have synergistic effect. Monitor patient closely. May need to avoid use before procedures using general anesthesia with succinylcholine-type neuromuscular blockers.
Cimetidine, clarithromycin, erythromycin, ketoconazole, paroxetine: May increase galantamine bioavailability. Monitor patient closely.
Highest risk QTc-prolonging agents: May enhance QTc-prolonging effects. Monitor for QTc prolongation and arrhythmias; consider therapy modification.
NSAIDs: May increase risk of bleeding due to increased gastric acid secretion. Monitor patient for symptoms of active or occult GI bleeding.
Drug-lifestyle. *Alcohol use:* May increase CNS effects. Avoid use.

EFFECTS ON LAB TEST RESULTS
None reported.

CONTRAINDICATIONS & CAUTIONS
• Contraindicated in patients hypersensitive to drug or its components.
• Use cautiously in patients with supraventricular cardiac conduction disorders and in those taking other drugs that significantly slow HR.
• Use cautiously during or before procedures involving anesthesia using succinylcholine-type or similar neuromuscular blockers.
• Use cautiously in patients with history of peptic ulcer disease and in those taking NSAIDs. Because of the potential for cholinomimetic effects, use cautiously in patients with bladder outflow obstruction, seizures, asthma, or COPD.
Dialyzable drug: Unknown.
⚠ *Overdose S&S:* Muscle weakness, muscle fasciculations, nausea, vomiting, GI cramping, excessive salivation, excessive lacrimation, sweating, bradycardia, hypotension, respiratory depression, syncope, seizures, QT-interval prolongation, hallucinations.

PREGNANCY-LACTATION-REPRODUCTION
• There are no well-controlled studies in pregnant women. Use during pregnancy only if potential benefit justifies potential risk to the fetus.
• It isn't known if drug appears in breast milk. Use cautiously in breast-feeding women.

NURSING CONSIDERATIONS
⊕ *Alert:* Drug may cause bradycardia and heart block. Consider all patients at risk for adverse effects on cardiac conduction.
• If drug is stopped for 3 days or longer, restart at the lowest dose and gradually increase, at 4-week or longer intervals, to the previous dosage level.
• Because of the risk of increased gastric acid secretion, monitor patients closely for symptoms of active or occult GI bleeding, especially those with an increased risk of developing ulcers.
• Monitor patient's weight during therapy.
• Monitor patients closely for seizures.
• Serious skin reactions such as Stevens-Johnson syndrome have been reported. Monitor patient for serious rash and discontinue therapy if needed.

PATIENT TEACHING
• Advise caregiver to give drug with morning and evening meals (for the conventional form), or only in the morning (for the extended-release form) and with food.
• Inform patient that nausea and vomiting are common adverse effects.
• Teach caregiver the proper technique when measuring the oral solution with the pipette. Tell her to place measured amount in 100 mL of a nonalcoholic beverage and have patient drink right away.

Reactions in bold italics are *life-threatening*. Interactions may have a *rapid onset* or a *delayed onset*.

- Urge patient or caregiver to report slow heartbeat immediately.
- Advise patient and caregiver that although drug may improve cognitive function, it doesn't alter the underlying disease process.
- Instruct patient to watch for serious skin reactions and to stop drug at first appearance of a rash.

ganciclovir (DHPG)
gan-SYE-kloe-vir

Cytovene, Zirgan

Therapeutic class: Antivirals
Pharmacologic class: Nucleosides–nucleotides

AVAILABLE FORMS
Injection: 500 mg/vial
Ophthalmic gel: 0.15%

INDICATIONS & DOSAGES
Black Box Warning Ganciclovir I.V. is indicated only for the treatment of cytomegalovirus (CMV) retinitis in immunocompromised patients and for the prevention of CMV disease in transplant patients at risk for CMV disease. ■
Adjust-a-dose (for all indications): Adjust dosage in patient with renal impairment according to the table. If patient is receiving hemodialysis, give dose shortly after session is complete.

Initial I.V. therapy

CrCl (mL/min)	Dose (mg/kg)	Interval
50–69	2.5	12 hr
25–49	2.5	24 hr
10–24	1.25	24 hr
<10	1.25	3 times weekly after hemodialysis

Maintenance I.V. therapy

CrCl (mL/min)	Dose (mg/kg)	Interval
50–69	2.5	24 hr
25–49	1.25	24 hr
10–24	0.625	24 hr
<10	0.625	3 times weekly after hemodialysis

➤ **CMV retinitis in immunocompromised patients, including those with AIDS and normal renal function**
Adults: Induction treatment is 5 mg/kg I.V. (given at a constant rate over 1 hour) every 12 hours for 14 to 21 days. Maintenance treatment is 5 mg/kg I.V. daily 7 days per week or 6 mg/kg I.V. daily five times weekly.
➤ **To prevent CMV disease in transplant recipients with normal renal function**
Adults: 5 mg/kg I.V. (given at a constant rate over 1 hour) every 12 hours for 7 to 14 days; then 5 mg/kg daily 7 days per week or 6 mg/kg daily five times weekly. Duration of therapy depends on degree of immunosuppression.
➤ **Acute herpetic keratitis**
Adults and children age 2 and older: 1 drop in affected eye five times daily (approximately every 3 hours while awake) until the corneal ulcer heals; then 1 drop t.i.d. for 7 days.

ADMINISTRATION
I.V.
▼ Drug is hazardous. Use safe handling precautions. I.V. solutions are alkaline; avoid direct contact with skin or mucous membranes. If contact occurs, wash area thoroughly with soap and water; thoroughly rinse eyes with plain water.
▼ To reconstitute, add 10 mL sterile water for injection to 500-mg vial. Shake vial well to dissolve drug.
▼ Further dilute in 50 to 250 mL (usually 100 mL) of compatible I.V. solution.
▼ If fluids are being restricted, dilute to no more than 10 mg/mL.
▼ Don't give as bolus.
▼ Use an infusion pump.
▼ Infuse over at least 1 hour.
▼ Infusing drug too rapidly has toxic effects.
◑ *Alert:* Don't give subcutaneously or I.M.
▼ Discard vial if particulate matter or discoloration is observed.
▼ Reconstituted solution is stable at room temperature for 12 hours. Don't refrigerate. Use solution within 24 hours of dilution to reduce risk of bacterial contamination.
▼ **Incompatibilities:** Aldesleukin, amifostine, aztreonam, cefepime, cytarabine, doxorubicin hydrochloride, fludarabine,

foscarnet, ondansetron, other I.V. drugs, paraben (bacteriostatic agent), piperacillin sodium–tazobactam, sargramostim, vinorelbine.

Ophthalmic
● Store at 59° to 77° F (15° to 20° C). Don't freeze.

ACTION

Inhibits binding of deoxyguanosine triphosphate to DNA polymerase, resulting in inhibition of DNA synthesis.

Route	Onset	Peak	Duration
I.V.	Unknown	Immediate	Unknown
Ophthalmic	Unknown	Unknown	Unknown

Half-life: I.V., about 3 to 5 hours; ophthalmic, unknown.

ADVERSE REACTIONS

CNS: fever, *coma, seizures,* abnormal thinking, agitation, altered dreams, amnesia, anxiety, asthenia, ataxia, confusion, dizziness, headache, somnolence, tremor, neuropathy, paresthesia.
EENT: retinal detachment in CMV retinitis patients; blurred vision, eye irritation, punctate keratitis, conjunctival hyperemia (ophthalmic).
GI: abdominal pain, anorexia, diarrhea, nausea, vomiting, dry mouth, dyspepsia, flatulence.
Hematologic: anemia, *agranulocytosis, leukopenia, thrombocytopenia.*
Respiratory: pneumonia.
Skin: rash, sweating, inflammation, pruritus, pain and phlebitis at injection site.
Other: *sepsis,* chills, infection.

INTERACTIONS

Drug-drug. *Amphotericin B, cyclosporine, other nephrotoxic drugs:* May increase risk of nephrotoxicity. Monitor renal function.
Cytotoxic drugs: May increase toxic effects, especially hematologic effects and stomatitis. Use together only if benefits outweigh risks; monitor patient closely.
Imipenem–cilastatin: May increase seizure activity. Use together only if potential benefits outweigh risks.
Immunosuppressants (such as azathioprine, corticosteroids, cyclosporine): May enhance immune and bone marrow suppression. Use together cautiously.
Probenecid: May increase ganciclovir level. Monitor patient closely.
Zidovudine: May increase risk of agranulocytosis. Use together cautiously; monitor hematologic function closely.

EFFECTS ON LAB TEST RESULTS

● May increase alkaline phosphatase, ALT, AST, creatinine, and GGT levels. May decrease Hb level.
● May decrease granulocyte, neutrophil, platelet, and WBC counts.

CONTRAINDICATIONS & CAUTIONS

Black Box Warning Clinical toxicity of ganciclovir I.V. includes granulocytopenia, anemia, and thrombocytopenia. Animal studies indicate that drug is carcinogenic and teratogenic and causes aspermatogenesis. ∎
● Contraindicated in patients hypersensitive to drug or acyclovir and in those with an ANC below 500/mm^3 or a platelet count below 25,000/mm^3.
● Use cautiously and reduce dosage in patients with renal dysfunction. Monitor renal function tests.
Dialyzable drug: About 50%.
⚠ *Overdose S&S:* Persistent bone marrow suppression, reversible neutropenia or granulocytopenia, hepatitis, renal toxicity, seizures (all with I.V. form).

PREGNANCY-LACTATION-REPRODUCTION

● Ganciclovir I.V. may be teratogenic or embryotoxic at recommended doses. Use during pregnancy only if potential benefits justify risks to the fetus.
● Women of childbearing potential should use effective contraception during treatment. Men should practice barrier contraception during treatment and for at least 90 days after treatment ends.
● Women receiving ganciclovir I.V. shouldn't breast-feed. It isn't known when breast-feeding can be safely resumed after last dose.

NURSING CONSIDERATIONS

● Because of the frequency of agranulocytosis and thrombocytopenia, obtain neutrophil

and platelet counts every 2 days during twice-daily dosing and at least weekly thereafter.
• Carefully monitor renal function; adjust dosages in patients with renal impairment.

PATIENT TEACHING
• Explain importance of drinking plenty of fluids during therapy.
• Instruct patient to report adverse reactions promptly.
• Tell patient to report discomfort at I.V. insertion site.
• Advise patient using gel not to let dropper touch any surface because dropper is sterile.
• Advise patient not to wear contact lenses while undergoing ophthalmic treatment.
• Advise patient undergoing ophthalmic treatment to notify prescriber if eye pain, redness, itching, or inflammation becomes aggravated.

gatifloxacin
ga-ti-FLOKS-a-sin

Zymar♣, Zymaxid

Therapeutic class: Antibiotics
Pharmacologic class: Fluoroquinolones

AVAILABLE FORMS
Solution: 0.3%, 0.5%

INDICATIONS & DOSAGES
➤ **Bacterial conjunctivitis caused by** *Corynebacterium propinquum, Streptococcus mitis, Staphylococcus aureus, Staphylococcus epidermidis, Streptococcus pneumoniae,* **or** *Haemophilus influenzae*
Adults and children age 1 and older: Instill 1 drop of Zymar into affected eye every 2 hours while patient is awake, up to eight times daily for 2 days. Then instill 1 drop up to q.i.d. while patient is awake for 5 more days.
➤ **Bacterial conjunctivitis caused by** *S. mitis, S. aureus, S. epidermidis, S. pneumoniae,* **or** *H. influenzae*
Adults and children age 1 and older: Instill 1 drop Zymaxid into affected eye every 2 hours while patient is awake, up to eight times on Day 1. Then instill 1 drop b.i.d. to q.i.d. while patient is awake on Days 2 to 7.

ADMINISTRATION
Ophthalmic
• Apply gentle pressure to the inside corner of the eyelid for 1 to 2 minutes after instilling drop.

ACTION
Inhibits DNA gyrase and topoisomerase, preventing cell replication and division.

Route	Onset	Peak	Duration
Ophthalmic	Unknown	Unknown	Unknown

Half-life: Unknown.

ADVERSE REACTIONS
CNS: headache.
EENT: conjunctival irritation, increased lacrimation, keratitis, papillary conjunctivitis, chemosis, conjunctival hemorrhage, discharge, dry eyes, eye irritation, eyelid edema, pain, red eyes, reduced visual acuity.
GI: taste disturbance.

INTERACTIONS
None reported.

EFFECTS ON LAB TEST RESULTS
None reported.

CONTRAINDICATIONS & CAUTIONS
• Contraindicated in patients hypersensitive to drug or other quinolones.
• Safety and effectiveness in infants younger than age 1 year have not been established.
Dialyzable drug: Unknown.

PREGNANCY-LACTATION-REPRODUCTION
• Use cautiously in pregnant and breastfeeding women.

NURSING CONSIDERATIONS
• Solution isn't for injection subconjunctivally or into the anterior chamber of the eye.
• Systemic drug may cause serious hypersensitivity reactions. If allergic reaction occurs, stop drug and treat symptoms.
• Monitor patient for superinfection.
• Growth of resistant organisms, including fungi, may occur with prolonged use. Monitor patient carefully.

PATIENT TEACHING

• Urge patient to immediately stop drug and seek medical treatment if evidence of a serious allergic reaction, such as itching, rash, swelling of the face or throat, or difficulty breathing, develops.

• Instruct patient to apply gentle pressure to inside corner of eyelid for 1 to 2 minutes after instilling drop.

• Tell patient not to wear contact lenses during treatment.

• Warn patient to avoid touching the applicator tip to anything, including eyes and fingers.

• Teach patient that prolonged use may encourage infections with nonsusceptible bacteria.

SAFETY ALERT!

gemcitabine hydrochloride
jem-SITE-ah-been

Gemzar

Therapeutic class: Antineoplastics
Pharmacologic class: Pyrimidine analogues

AVAILABLE FORMS
Powder for injection: 200-mg, 1-g vials
Solution for injection: 200-mg, 1-g, 2-g vials

INDICATIONS & DOSAGES
Adjust-a-dose (for all indications): Permanently discontinue drug for any of the following nonhematologic adverse reactions: unexplained dyspnea or other evidence of severe pulmonary toxicity, severe hepatotoxicity, hemolytic-uremic syndrome, capillary leak syndrome, or posterior reversible encephalopathy syndrome. Withhold drug or reduce dosage by 50% for other severe (grade 3 or 4) nonhematologic toxicity until resolved. No dosage modifications are recommended for alopecia, nausea, or vomiting.

➤ **Locally advanced or metastatic adenocarcinoma of pancreas**
Adults: 1,000 mg/m^2 I.V. over 30 minutes once weekly for up to 7 weeks, unless toxi-

city occurs. Monitor CBC with differential and platelet count before giving each dose.
Adjust-a-dose: If bone marrow suppression is detected, adjust therapy. If absolute granulocyte count (AGC) is 1,000/mm^3 or more and platelet count is 100,000/mm^3 or more, give full dose. If AGC is 500 to 999/mm^3 or platelet count is 50,000 to 99,000/mm^3, give 75% of dose. If AGC is below 500/mm^3 or platelet count is below 50,000/mm^3, withhold dose. Course of 7 weeks is followed by 1 week of rest. Subsequent dosage cycles consist of one infusion weekly for 3 consecutive weeks out of every 4 weeks. Dosage adjustments for subsequent cycles are based on AGC and platelet count nadirs and degree of nonhematologic toxicity.

➤ **With cisplatin, first-line treatment of inoperable, locally advanced (stage IIIA or IIIB), or metastatic (stage IV) non–small-cell lung cancer**
Adults: For 4-week schedule, 1,000 mg/m^2 I.V. over 30 minutes on days 1, 8, and 15 of each 28-day cycle.

For 3-week schedule, 1,250 mg/m^2 I.V. over 30 minutes on days 1 and 8 of each 21-day cycle.
Adjust-a-dose: If bone marrow suppression is detected, adjust therapy. If AGC is 1,000/mm^3 or more and platelet count is 100,000/mm^3 or more, give full dose. If AGC is 500 to 999/mm^3 or platelet count is 50,000 to 99,000/mm^3, give 75% of dose. If AGC is below 500/mm^3 or platelet count is below 50,000/mm^3, withhold dose.

➤ **With carboplatin, for treatment of advanced ovarian cancer that relapsed at least 6 months after platinum-based therapy**
Adults: 1,000 mg/m^2 I.V. over 30 minutes on days 1 and 8 of each 21-day cycle. Check CBC with differential and platelet count before each dose. The AGC should be 1,500/mm^3 or higher and platelet count 100,000/mm^3 or higher before each cycle.
Adjust-a-dose: Base adjustment on AGC and platelet count results on day 8 of cycle. If AGC is 1,000 to 1,499/mm^3, give 50% of dose. If AGC is below 1,000/mm^3 or platelet count is below 75,000/mm^3, withhold dose. Adjustments for subsequent cycles based on observed toxicities.

Reactions in bold italics are *life-threatening*. Interactions may have a *rapid onset* or a *delayed onset*.

➤ **Metastatic breast cancer (first-line treatment after failure of adjuvant anthracycline chemotherapy) with paclitaxel**

Adults: 1,250 mg/m^2 I.V. over 30 minutes on days 1 and 8 of each 21-day cycle. Adjust dosage based on total AGC and platelet counts taken on days 1 and 8 of the cycle.

Adjust-a-dose: On day 1, if AGC is below 1,500/mm^3 or if platelet count is below 100,000/mm^3, withhold dose. On day 8, if AGC is 1,000 to 1,199/mm^3 or platelet count is 50,000 to 75,000/mm^3, give 75% of dose. If AGC is 700 to 999/mm^3 and platelet count is 50,000/mm^3 or above, give 50% of dose. If AGC is below 700/mm^3 or platelet count is below 50,000/mm^3, withhold dose.

ADMINISTRATION

I.V.

▼ Preparing and giving parenteral drug may be mutagenic, teratogenic, or carcinogenic. Follow safe handling precautions and use gloves.

▼ To prepare solution, add 5 mL of unpreserved NSS for injection to 200-mg vial or 25 mL to 1-g vial. Shake to dissolve.

▼ Resulting concentration is 38 mg/mL (accounting for the volume displaced by the powder); reconstitution at concentrations higher than 40 mg/mL isn't recommended.

▼ If needed, dilute to as little as 0.1 mg/mL by adding NSS for injection.

▼ Make sure solution is clear to light straw-colored and free of particles.

▼ Don't extend infusion time beyond 60 minutes or give drug more often than once weekly; doing so may increase toxicity.

▼ Drug is stable for 24 hours at room temperature.

▼ Don't refrigerate reconstituted drug because it may crystallize.

▼ **Incompatibilities:** Compatibility with other drugs hasn't been studied.

ACTION

Cytotoxic and specific to cell cycle; inhibits DNA synthesis and blocks progression of cells.

Route	Onset	Peak	Duration
I.V.	Unknown	Unknown	Unknown

Half-life: About 2½ to 19 hours (influenced by length of the infusion, age, and gender).

ADVERSE REACTIONS

CNS: drowsiness, paresthesia, pain, fever.
CV: edema, peripheral edema.
GI: stomatitis, nausea, vomiting, constipation, diarrhea.
GU: proteinuria, hematuria.
Hematologic: anemia, *leukopenia, neutropenia, thrombocytopenia, hemorrhage.*
Hepatic: *hepatotoxicity.*
Respiratory: dyspnea, *bronchospasm, pneumonitis.*
Skin: alopecia, rash, pain at injection site.
Other: flulike syndrome, infection, *anaphylactoid reactions,* injection-site reactions.

INTERACTIONS

Drug-drug. *Bleomycin:* May increase risk of pulmonary toxicity. Consider therapy modification.
Clozapine: May increase risk of neutropenia. Avoid combination.
Live-virus vaccines: May increase risk of vaccine-induced adverse reactions. Defer use of live-virus vaccines.
Warfarin: May increase the anticoagulant effect of warfarin. Monitor patient and INR.

EFFECTS ON LAB TEST RESULTS

● May increase ALT, AST, BUN, and creatinine levels. May decrease Hb level.
● May decrease neutrophil, platelet, and WBC counts.

CONTRAINDICATIONS & CAUTIONS

● Contraindicated in patients hypersensitive to drug.
● Use cautiously in patients with renal or hepatic impairment.
● Use cautiously when given within 7 days of radiation therapy.
● Prolonging infusion duration beyond 60 minutes or administering more frequently than weekly has resulted in an increased incidence of toxicities, including clinically significant hypotension, severe flulike symptoms, myelosuppression, and asthenia.

• Capillary leak syndrome with severe consequences has been reported when drug has been used alone or in combination with other chemotherapeutic agents. Discontinue if syndrome develops.

• Hemolytic-uremic syndrome that may lead to renal failure has been reported. Watch for evidence of anemia with microangiopathic hemolysis (elevated bilirubin or LDH level, reticulocytosis, severe thrombocytopenia, or renal failure), and monitor renal function at baseline and periodically during treatment. Permanently discontinue if hemolytic-uremic syndrome or severe renal impairment occurs; renal failure may not be reversible despite discontinuation.

• Myelosuppression, manifested by neutropenia, thrombocytopenia, and anemia, occurs with gemcitabine used alone; risk increases when drug is combined with other cytotoxic drugs.

• Pulmonary toxicity, including interstitial pneumonitis, pulmonary fibrosis, pulmonary edema, and ARDS, has been reported; it may lead to respiratory failure (some fatal) despite discontinuation of therapy. Onset of pulmonary symptoms may occur up to 2 weeks after last dose of gemcitabine. Discontinue for unexplained dyspnea, with or without bronchospasm, or other evidence of pulmonary toxicity.

• Serious hepatotoxicity, including liver failure and death, has been reported with gemcitabine alone or in combination with other potentially hepatotoxic drugs. Administration in patients with concurrent liver metastases or preexisting medical history of hepatitis, alcoholism, or liver cirrhosis can lead to exacerbation of the underlying hepatic insufficiency. Assess hepatic function before initiating gemcitabine and periodically during treatment. Discontinue if severe liver injury develops.

• Posterior reversible encephalopathy syndrome (PRES) has been reported in patients receiving gemcitabine alone or in combination with other chemotherapeutic agents. PRES can present with headache, seizure, lethargy, hypertension, confusion, blindness, and other visual and neurologic disturbances. Confirm PRES diagnosis with MRI; discontinue gemcitabine if PRES develops during therapy.

• Safety and effectiveness in children haven't been determined.

Dialyzable drug: Unknown.

⚠ ***Overdose S&S:*** Myelosuppression, paresthesia, severe rash.

PREGNANCY-LACTATION-REPRODUCTION

• There are no adequate studies in pregnant women. Based on drug's mechanism of action, its use is expected to result in adverse reproductive effects. If drug is used during pregnancy or if patient becomes pregnant during therapy, apprise her of potential fetal hazard.

• Patient should discontinue breast-feeding or discontinue drug.

NURSING CONSIDERATIONS

• Monitor patient closely. Expect dosage modification according to toxicity and degree of myelosuppression. Age, gender, and presence of renal impairment may predispose patient to toxicity.

• Monitor hematologic values carefully, especially neutrophil and platelet counts.

• Obtain baseline and periodic renal and hepatic laboratory tests.

PATIENT TEACHING

• Advise patient to report all adverse reactions and to immediately report evidence of infection (fever, sore throat, fatigue) and bleeding (easy bruising, nosebleeds, bleeding gums, tarry stools). Tell patient to take temperature daily.

• Advise patient to immediately report changes in color or volume of urine output.

• Advise patient to promptly report flulike symptoms, breathing problems, abdominal pain, or yellowing of skin.

• Tell patient that adverse effects may continue after treatment ends.

Reactions in bold italics are *life-threatening*. Interactions may have a *rapid onset* or a ***delayed onset***.

gemfibrozil
jem-FI-broe-zil

Lopid🖊

Therapeutic class: Antilipemics
Pharmacologic class: Fibric acid
derivatives

AVAILABLE FORMS
Tablets: 600 mg

INDICATIONS & DOSAGES
➤ **As adjunct to diet in adults with hyper-triglyceridemia (types IV and V hyper-lipidemia) unresponsive to diet and who are at risk for pancreatitis; to reduce risk of CAD in patients without CAD symptoms and with type IIb hyperlipidemia who are refractory to treatment with diet, exercise, and other drugs, and who have decreased HDL levels and increased LDL and triglyceride levels**
Adults: 1,200 mg P.O. daily in two divided doses, 30 minutes before morning and evening meals.

ADMINISTRATION
P.O.
● Give drug 30 minutes before breakfast and dinner.

ACTION
Inhibits peripheral lipolysis and reduces triglyceride synthesis in the liver; lowers triglyceride and VLDL levels and increases HDL levels.

Route	Onset	Peak	Duration
P.O.	2–5 days	1–2 hr	Unknown

Half-life: 1½ hours.

ADVERSE REACTIONS
CNS: fatigue, headache, vertigo.
GI: abdominal and epigastric pain, dyspepsia, acute appendicitis, constipation, diarrhea, nausea, vomiting.
Hematologic: *leukopenia, thrombocytopenia,* anemia, eosinophilia.
Hepatic: bile duct obstruction.
Metabolic: *hypokalemia.*
Skin: dermatitis, eczema, pruritus, rash.

INTERACTIONS
Drug-drug. *Colestipol:* May decrease colestipol effects. Separate administration times by 2 hours.
Cyclosporine: May decrease cyclosporine level; may increase risk of nephrotoxicity. Monitor renal function and cyclosporine level, and adjust dose as needed.
CYP2C8, CYP2C9, CYP2C19 substrates: May increase levels of substrates metabolized through these enzymes. Consider therapy modification.
Glyburide, pioglitazone: May increase hypoglycemic effects. Monitor glucose level, and watch for signs of hypoglycemia.
HMG-CoA reductase inhibitors: May cause myopathy with rhabdomyolysis. Avoid using together.
Montelukast: May increase montelukast level and effects. Monitor clinical response and adjust montelukast dosage.
Oral anticoagulants: May enhance effects of oral anticoagulants. Monitor patient closely.
Repaglinide: May increase repaglinide level. Concurrent use is contraindicated.

EFFECTS ON LAB TEST RESULTS
● May increase ALT, AST, and CK levels.
● May decrease potassium and Hb level and hematocrit.
● May decrease eosinophil, WBC, and platelet counts.

CONTRAINDICATIONS & CAUTIONS
● Contraindicated in patients hypersensitive to drug and in those with hepatic or severe renal dysfunction (including primary biliary cirrhosis) or gallbladder disease.
Dialyzable drug: Unknown.

PREGNANCY-LACTATION-REPRODUCTION
● Use in pregnancy only if potential benefit justifies potential risk to the fetus.
● Patient should discontinue breast-feeding or discontinue drug.

NURSING CONSIDERATIONS
● Check CBC and LFTs periodically during the first 12 months of therapy.
● If drug has no benefits after 3 months of therapy, stop drug.

G

PATIENT TEACHING
● Instruct patient to take drug 30 minutes before breakfast and dinner.
● Teach patient about proper dietary management of cholesterol and triglycerides. When appropriate, recommend weight control, exercise, and smoking cessation programs.
● Because of possible dizziness and blurred vision, advise patient to avoid driving and other hazardous activities until effects of drug are known.
● Tell patient to observe bowel movements and to report evidence of excess fat in feces or other signs of bile duct obstruction.
● Advise patient to report all adverse reactions and muscle pain to prescriber.

---

gemifloxacin mesylate
jem-ah-FLOX-a-sin

Factive

Therapeutic class: Antibiotics
Pharmacologic class: Fluoroquinolones

AVAILABLE FORMS
Tablets ⊙*:* 320 mg

INDICATIONS & DOSAGES
Black Box Warning Fluoroquinolone use in patients with acute bacterial sinusitis, acute bacterial exacerbation of bronchitis, and uncomplicated UTIs isn't recommended because of risk of serious adverse effects. Use drug in these patients only when there are no other treatment options. ■
Adjust-a-dose (for all indications): If CrCl is 40 mL/minute or less, or if patient receives routine hemodialysis or continuous ambulatory peritoneal dialysis, reduce dosage to 160 mg P.O. once daily.
➤ **Acute bacterial worsening of chronic bronchitis caused by** *Streptococcus pneumoniae, Haemophilus influenzae, H. parainfluenzae,* **or** *Moraxella catarrhalis*
Adults: 320 mg P.O. once daily for 5 days.
➤ **Mild to moderate community-acquired pneumonia caused by** *S. pneumoniae* **(including multidrug-resistant strains),** *H. influenzae, M. catarrhalis, Mycoplasma*

pneumoniae, Chlamydia pneumoniae, **or** *Klebsiella pneumoniae*
Adults: 320 mg P.O. once daily for 5 to 7 days.

ADMINISTRATION
P.O.
● Give drug with or without food; however, it must be given 2 hours before or 3 hours after an antacid or multivitamin.
● Give plenty of fluids during treatment.

ACTION
Prevents cell growth by inhibiting DNA gyrase and topoisomerase IV, which interferes with DNA synthesis.

Route	Onset	Peak	Duration
P.O.	Unknown	½–2 hr	Unknown

Half-life: 4 to 12 hours.

ADVERSE REACTIONS
CNS: headache, dizziness.
GI: diarrhea, nausea, abdominal pain, vomiting.
Hematologic: *neutropenia,* neutrophilia.
Musculoskeletal: ruptured tendons.
Skin: rash.

INTERACTIONS
Drug-drug. *Antacids (magnesium or aluminum), didanosine (chewable tablets, buffered tablets, or pediatric powder for oral solution), ferrous sulfate or multivitamins containing metal cations (such as iron, magnesium or zinc), sucralfate:* May decrease gemifloxacin level. Give these drugs at least 3 hours before or 2 hours after gemifloxacin.
Antiarrhythmics of class IA (procainamide, quinidine) or class III (amiodarone, sotalol): May increase risk of prolonged QTc interval. Avoid using together.
Antipsychotics, erythromycin, ivabradine, mifepristone, TCAs: May increase risk of prolonged QTc interval. Use together cautiously.
Black Box Warning *Corticosteroids:* May increase risk of tendinitis and tendon rupture. Monitor patient for tendon pain or inflammation. ■
Probenecid: May increase gemifloxacin level. May use with probenecid for this reason.

Reactions in bold italics are *life-threatening*. Interactions may have a *rapid onset* or a *delayed onset*.

Sevelamer: May decrease gemifloxacin level. Give drug at least 2 hours before or 6 hours after sevelamer; consider therapy modification.

Sucralfate: May decrease gemifloxacin level. Use together cautiously.

Warfarin: May increase anticoagulation effect. Monitor PT and INR.

Drug-lifestyle. *Sun exposure:* May increase risk of photosensitivity. Advise patient to avoid excessive sunlight exposure.

EFFECTS ON LAB TEST RESULTS

● May increase alkaline phosphatase, ALT, AST, bilirubin, BUN, CK, creatinine, GGT, and potassium levels. May decrease albumin, protein, and sodium levels.

● May increase or decrease calcium and Hb levels and hematocrit.

● May increase or decrease neutrophil, platelet, and RBC counts.

CONTRAINDICATIONS & CAUTIONS

Black Box Warning Drug is associated with increased risk of tendinitis and tendon rupture, especially in patients older than age 60 and those with heart, kidney, or lung transplants. ■

Black Box Warning Drug may exacerbate muscle weakness in patients with myasthenia gravis. Avoid using fluoroquinolones in patients with a known history of myasthenia gravis. ■

Black Box Warning Fluoroquinolones have been associated with disabling and potentially irreversible serious adverse reactions that have occurred together, including tendinitis and tendon rupture, peripheral neuropathy, and CNS effects (seizures, toxic psychoses, increased ICP, pseudotumor cerebri, tremors, restlessness, anxiety, light-headedness, confusion, hallucinations, paranoia, depression, nightmares, insomnia and, rarely, suicidal thoughts or acts). If any of these serious adverse reactions occur, discontinue drug immediately. ■

● Contraindicated in patients hypersensitive to fluoroquinolones, gemifloxacin, or their components.

● Contraindicated in patients with a history of prolonged QTc interval, those with uncorrected electrolyte disorders (such as hypokalemia or hypomagnesemia), and

those taking a drug that could prolong the QTc interval.

● Use cautiously in patients with a proarrhythmic condition, epilepsy, or a predisposition to seizures.

● Safety and effectiveness haven't been established in children younger than age 18.

Dialyzable drug: 20% to 30%.

PREGNANCY-LACTATION-REPRODUCTION

● Don't use in pregnant or breast-feeding women unless potential benefit justifies risk to the fetus or infant.

NURSING CONSIDERATIONS

● Use drug only for infections caused by susceptible bacteria.

🕓 **Alert:** Don't exceed recommended dosage because this increases the risk of prolonging the QTc interval.

Black Box Warning Monitor patient for symptoms of peripheral neuropathy (pain, burning, tingling, numbness, weakness, or a change in sensation to light touch, pain, temperature, or the sense of body position) and report them immediately to practitioner. ■

● Mild to moderate maculopapular rash may appear, usually 8 to 10 days after therapy starts. It's more likely in women younger than age 40 and postmenopausal women taking hormone therapy. Stop drug if rash appears.

🕓 **Alert:** Serious, occasionally fatal, hypersensitivity reactions may occur, even with first dose. Stop drug immediately if hypersensitivity reaction occurs, and treat severe reactions emergently.

Black Box Warning Fluoroquinolones may cause tendon rupture, arthropathy, or osteochondrosis; stop drug if patient reports pain or inflammation or ruptures a tendon. ■

● Stop drug if patient has a photosensitivity reaction.

● Fluoroquinolones may cause CNS effects, such as tremors and anxiety. Monitor patient carefully.

● CDAD, ranging in severity from mild to fatal colitis, may occur, even up to months after therapy ends. Drug may need to be stopped.

● Keep patient adequately hydrated to avoid concentration of urine.

G

PATIENT TEACHING

Black Box Warning Warn patient to immediately report signs and symptoms of serious adverse reactions, including unusual joint or tendon pain, muscle weakness, "pins and needles" tingling or pricking sensation, numbness in the arms or legs, confusion, or hallucinations. ∎

• Urge patient to finish full course of treatment, even if symptoms improve.

• Tell patient that drug may be taken with or without food, but that it shouldn't be taken within 3 hours after or 2 hours before an antacid or multivitamin.

• Tell patient to stop drug and seek medical care if evidence of hypersensitivity reaction develops.

• Instruct patient to drink fluids liberally.

• Warn patient against taking OTC drugs or dietary supplements without consulting prescriber.

• Tell patient to avoid excessive exposure to sunlight or ultraviolet light.

• Urge patient to report all adverse reactions.

• Warn patient to avoid driving or other hazardous activities until effects of drug are known.

gentamicin sulfate (injection)
jen-ta-MYE-sin

Therapeutic class: Antibiotics
Pharmacologic class: Aminoglycosides

AVAILABLE FORMS

Injection: 40 mg/mL (adults), 10 mg/mL (children)
I.V. infusion (premixed): 40 mg, 60 mg, 80 mg, 100 mg, 120 mg, mg, 160 mg, 200 mg in 100 mL NSS

INDICATIONS & DOSAGES

➤ **Serious infections caused by sensitive strains of *Pseudomonas aeruginosa, Escherichia coli, Proteus, Klebsiella, Serratia,* or *Staphylococcus***
Adults: 3 mg/kg I.M. or I.V. infusion daily in three divided doses every 8 hours. For life-threatening infections, may give up to 5 mg/kg daily in three or four divided doses;

reduce dosage to 3 mg/kg daily as soon as patient improves.
Children: 2 to 2.5 mg/kg I.M. or I.V. infusion every 8 hours.
Neonates older than 1 week and infants: 2.5 mg/kg I.M. or I.V. infusion every 8 hours.
Neonates younger than 1 week and preterm infants: 2.5 mg/kg I.M. or I.V. infusion every 12 hours.
Adjust-a-dose: For adults with impaired renal function, doses and frequency are determined by drug level and renal function. To maintain therapeutic levels, adults should receive 1 to 1.7 mg/kg I.M. or I.V. infusion after each dialysis session, and children should receive 2 to 2.5 mg/kg I.M. or I.V. infusion after each dialysis session.

ADMINISTRATION

I.V.
▼ Obtain specimen for culture and sensitivity tests before giving. Begin therapy while awaiting results.
▼ For intermittent infusion, dilute with 50 to 200 mL of D₅W or NSS for injection.
▼ Infuse over 30 minutes to 2 hours.
▼ After completing infusion, flush the line with NSS or D₅W.
▼ Premixed, single-dose, flexible containers should be administered I.V. only.
▼ **Incompatibilities:** Don't physically premix gentamicin with other drugs; administer separately according to the recommended route of administration and dosage schedule.

I.M.
• Obtain specimen for culture and sensitivity tests before giving. Begin therapy while awaiting results.
• Obtain blood for peak level 1 hour after I.M. injection or 30 minutes after I.V. infusion finishes; for trough levels, draw blood just before next dose. Don't collect blood in a heparinized tube; heparin is incompatible with aminoglycosides.

ACTION

Inhibits protein synthesis by binding directly to the 30S ribosomal subunit; bactericidal.

Route	Onset	Peak	Duration
I.V.	Immediate	30–60 min	Unknown
I.M.	Unknown	30–60 min	Unknown

Half-life: 2 to 3 hours; longer in patients with renal impairment and in infants.

ADVERSE REACTIONS
CNS: *encephalopathy, seizures,* fever, headache, lethargy, confusion, dizziness, numbness, peripheral neuropathy, vertigo, ataxia, tingling.
CV: hypotension.
EENT: ototoxicity, blurred vision, tinnitus.
GI: vomiting, nausea.
GU: *nephrotoxicity,* possible increase in urinary excretion of casts.
Hematologic: *agranulocytosis, leukopenia, thrombocytopenia,* anemia, eosinophilia.
Musculoskeletal: muscle twitching, myasthenia gravis–like syndrome.
Respiratory: *apnea.*
Skin: rash, urticaria, pruritus, injection-site pain.
Other: *anaphylaxis.*

INTERACTIONS
Drug-drug. **Black Box Warning** *Amikacin, cephaloridine, cidofovir, cisplatin, colistin, neomycin, paramycin, polymyxin B, streptomycin, tobramycin, vancomycin, viomycin, other aminoglycosides:* May increase ototoxicity and nephrotoxicity. Monitor hearing and renal function test results. Avoid concurrent or sequential use. ∎
Atracurium, pancuronium, rocuronium, vecuronium: May increase effects of nondepolarizing muscle relaxants, including prolonged respiratory depression. Use together only when necessary, and expect to reduce dosage of nondepolarizing muscle relaxant.
General anesthetics: May increase neuromuscular blockade. Monitor patient closely.
Indomethacin: May increase peak and trough levels of gentamicin. Monitor gentamicin level.
Black Box Warning *I.V. loop diuretics (ethacrynic acid, furosemide):* May increase risk of ototoxicity. Avoid use together. ∎
Nondepolarizing muscle relaxants (pancuronium, vecuronium): May increase neuromuscular-blocking effects of these

drugs and cause prolonged respiratory depression and apnea. Use together with caution.
Parenteral penicillins (ampicillin, ticarcillin): May inactivate gentamicin in vitro. Don't mix together.

EFFECTS ON LAB TEST RESULTS
• May increase ALT, AST, bilirubin, BUN, creatinine, LDH, and nonprotein nitrogen levels.
• May decrease Hb and serum calcium, magnesium, sodium, and potassium levels.
• May increase eosinophil count. May decrease platelet and WBC counts.

CONTRAINDICATIONS & CAUTIONS
• Contraindicated in patients hypersensitive to drug or other aminoglycosides.
• Use cautiously in neonates, infants, elderly patients, and patients with impaired renal function or neuromuscular disorders.
• Use drug for short-term treatment if possible.
Dialyzable drug: 50%.
⚠ *Overdose S&S:* Nephrotoxicity, neurotoxicity, ototoxicity.

PREGNANCY-LACTATION-REPRODUCTION
Black Box Warning Aminoglycosides can cause fetal harm when used during pregnancy. ∎
• If drug is used during pregnancy or if patient becomes pregnant during therapy, apprise patient of potential hazard (deafness) to the fetus.
• Drug appears in breast milk.

NURSING CONSIDERATIONS
Black Box Warning Evaluate patient's hearing before and during therapy. Notify prescriber if patient complains of tinnitus, vertigo, or hearing loss. ∎
• Weigh patient and review renal function studies before therapy begins.
🔆 *Alert:* Use preservative-free form when intrathecal or intraventricular route is used adjunctively for serious CNS infections, such as meningitis and ventriculitis.
Black Box Warning Maintain peak levels at 4 to 12 mcg/mL and trough levels at 1 to 2 mcg/mL. The maximum peak level is usually 8 mcg/mL, except in patients

with cystic fibrosis, who need increased lung penetration. Prolonged peak levels of 10 to 12 mcg/mL or prolonged trough levels greater than 2 mcg/mL may increase risk of toxicity. ▉

Black Box Warning Nephrotoxicity risk is greater in patients with renal impairment and in those who receive high-dosage or prolonged therapy. Monitor renal function: urine output, specific gravity, urinalysis, BUN and creatinine levels, and CrCl. Report to prescriber evidence of declining renal function. ▉

Black Box Warning High-risk patients should have serial audiograms, especially if they show signs and symptoms of ototoxicity (dizziness, vertigo, ataxia, tinnitus, hearing loss). ▉

• Watch for signs and symptoms of superinfection (especially of upper respiratory tract), such as continued fever, chills, and increased pulse rate.

• Therapy usually continues for 7 to 10 days. If no response occurs in 3 to 5 days, stop therapy and obtain new specimens for culture and sensitivity testing.

PATIENT TEACHING

• Instruct patient to promptly report adverse reactions, such as vision changes, dizziness, vertigo, unsteady gait, ringing in the ears, hearing loss, numbness, tingling, muscle twitching, seizures, changes in urine amount, edema.

• Encourage patient to drink plenty of fluids.

• Warn patient to avoid hazardous activities if adverse CNS reactions occur.

gentamicin sulfate (ophthalmic, topical)
jen-ta-MYE-sin

Genoptic, Gentak

Therapeutic class: Antibiotics
Pharmacologic class: Aminoglycosides

AVAILABLE FORMS

Cream: 0.1%
Ointment: 0.1%
Ophthalmic ointment: 0.3% (base)
Ophthalmic solution: 0.3% (base)

INDICATIONS & DOSAGES

➤ **External ocular infections (conjunctivitis, keratoconjunctivitis, corneal ulcers, blepharitis, blepharoconjunctivitis, acute meibomianitis, and dacryocystitis) caused by susceptible organisms (*Staphylococcus aureus, Staphylococcus epidermidis, Streptococcus pyogenes, Streptococcus pneumoniae, Enterobacter aerogenes, Escherichia coli, Haemophilus influenzae, Klebsiella pneumoniae, Neisseria gonorrhoeae, Pseudomonas aeruginosa, Serratia marcescens*)**

Adults and children: 1 to 2 drops in affected eye every 4 hours. In severe infections, up to 2 drops every hour. Or, apply ointment (approximately ½ inch [1.25 cm]) to lower conjunctival sac b.i.d. or t.i.d.

➤ **To treat or prevent superficial infections and superficial burns of the skin caused by susceptible bacteria**

Adults and children older than age 1: Rub in small amount gently t.i.d. or q.i.d., with or without gauze dressing.

ADMINISTRATION
Ophthalmic
• Store drug away from heat.
• Apply light finger pressure on lacrimal sac for 1 minute after drops are instilled.
• Wait at least 10 minutes before instilling other eyedrops.

Topical
• Topical forms are for dermatologic use only; not for ophthalmic use.
• Clean affected area and remove crusts of impetigo before applying to increase absorption. Be sure to avoid further contamination of the skin.
• Wash hands after each application.
• Store drug in cool place.

ACTION

Inhibits protein synthesis by binding directly to the 30S ribosomal subunit; bactericidal.

Route	Onset	Peak	Duration
Ophthalmic, topical	Unknown	Unknown	Unknown

Half-life: Unknown.

ADVERSE REACTIONS

EENT: burning, stinging, or blurred vision with ointment; conjunctival hyperemia, transient irritation from solution, bacterial and fungal corneal ulcers.

Skin: allergic contact dermatitis, erythema, minor skin irritation, photosensitivity.

Other: overgrowth of nonsusceptible organisms with long-term use.

INTERACTIONS

None significant.

EFFECTS ON LAB TEST RESULTS

None reported.

CONTRAINDICATIONS & CAUTIONS

• Contraindicated in patients hypersensitive to drug.
• Use cautiously in patients with history of sensitivity to aminoglycosides because cross-sensitivity may occur.

Dialyzable drug: Unknown.

PREGNANCY-LACTATION-REPRODUCTION

• Use in pregnancy only if potential benefit justifies potential risk to the fetus.
• Drug appears in breast milk in small amounts and is absorbed by breast-feeding infants.

NURSING CONSIDERATIONS

• Obtain culture before giving drug. Therapy may begin before culture results are known.
• Ophthalmic solution isn't for injection into conjunctiva or anterior chamber of eye.
• If ophthalmic gentamicin is given together with systemic gentamicin, monitor gentamicin level.
❸ Alert: Avoid excessive ophthalmic use and topical use on large skin lesions or over a wide area because of possible systemic toxic effects.
❸ Alert: The topical ointment helps retain moisture and has been useful in infections on dry, eczematous, or psoriatic skin. The topical cream is for wet, oozing primary infections and greasy secondary infections. It's water-washable.
• Prolonged use can cause superinfection; bacterial resistance can also develop.

Report worsening signs and symptoms to prescriber. Drug should be discontinued.

PATIENT TEACHING

• Tell patient to clean eye area of excessive discharge before instilling drug.
• Teach patient how to instill drops or apply ophthalmic ointment. Advise patient to wash hands before and after applying ointment or solution and not to touch tip of dropper or tube to eye or surrounding tissues.
• Instruct patient to apply light finger pressure on lacrimal sac for 1 minute after drops are instilled.
• Tell patient to wait at least 10 minutes before instilling other eyedrops.
• Instruct patient to stop drug and notify prescriber if signs and symptoms of sensitivity (itching lids, swelling, or constant burning) or worsening signs and symptoms occur.
• Tell patient that vision may be blurred for a few minutes after application of ophthalmic ointment.
❸ Alert: Stress importance of following recommended therapy. *Pseudomonas* infections can cause complete vision loss within 24 hours if infection isn't controlled.
• Tell patient using topical forms to clean affected area, avoiding further skin contamination, and to remove crusts of impetigo before applying, to increase absorption.
• Tell patient to wash hands after each application.
• Advise patient not to share drug, washcloths, or towels with family members and to notify prescriber if anyone develops same signs or symptoms.
• Tell patient to stop using drug and notify prescriber immediately if no improvement occurs or if condition worsens.

SAFETY ALERT!

glatiramer acetate
glah-TEER-ah-mer

Copaxone, Glatopa

Therapeutic class: MS drugs
Pharmacologic class: Biological
response modifiers

AVAILABLE FORMS
Injection: 20 mg glatiramer acetate and
40 mg mannitol (20 mg/mL), USP, in
a single-use prefilled syringe; 40 mg
glatiramer acetate and 40 mg mannitol
(40 mg/mL), USP, in a single-use prefilled
syringe

INDICATIONS & DOSAGES
➤ **For first clinical episode and to reduce
frequency of relapse in patients with
relapsing-remitting MS**
Adults: 20 mg subcutaneously daily, or
40 mg (Copaxone) subcutaneously three
times per week given at least 48 hours apart.

ADMINISTRATION
Subcutaneous
• Give drug only subcutaneously in arms,
abdomen, hips, or thighs; rotate injection
sites to prevent lipoatrophy.
• Administer 40-mg dose on same 3 days
each week (e.g., Monday, Wednesday,
Friday) at least 48 hours apart.
• Drug doesn't contain preservatives;
discard if solution is cloudy or contains
particulate matter.
• Don't try to expel the air bubble from the
prefilled syringe. This may lead to loss of
drug and an incorrect dose.
• Store drug in refrigerator (36° to 46° F
[2° to 8° C]); allow drug to warm to room
temperature for 20 minutes before use.
If refrigeration isn't available, may store
at room temperature for up to 1 month
(refrigeration is preferred).

ACTION
May modify immune processes responsible
for the pathogenesis of MS.

Route	Onset	Peak	Duration
Subcut.	Unknown	Unknown	Unknown

Half-life: Unknown.

ADVERSE REACTIONS
CNS: anxiety, asthenia, abnormal dreams,
agitation, confusion, emotional lability,
fever, migraine, nervousness, pain, speech
disorder, stupor, syncope, tremor, vertigo.
CV: chest pain, palpitations, vasodilation,
hypertension, tachycardia, edema.
EENT: eye disorder, diplopia, visual field
deficit, ear pain, rhinitis, laryngismus, nasopharyngitis.
GI: diarrhea, nausea, anorexia, bowel urgency, gastroenteritis, GI disorder, oral
candidiasis, salivary gland enlargement,
ulcerative stomatitis, vomiting.
GU: urinary urgency, *vaginal hemorrhage,*
abnormal Papanicolaou smear, amenorrhea,
dysmenorrhea, hematuria, erectile dysfunction, menorrhagia, vaginal candidiasis.
Hematologic: lymphadenopathy,
ecchymosis.
Metabolic: weight gain.
Musculoskeletal: arthralgia, back pain,
hypertonia, neck pain.
Respiratory: dyspnea, cough, bronchitis,
hyperventilation.
Skin: diaphoresis, injection-site reaction,
pruritus, rash, eczema, erythema or hemorrhage, residual mass at injection site, skin
atrophy, urticaria, warts.
Other: flulike syndrome, infection, bacterial infection, chills, cyst, herpes simplex
and zoster, peripheral and facial edema.

INTERACTIONS
Drug-drug. *Denosumab, natalizumab,
roflumilast:* May increase risk of serious
infection. Consider therapy modification.
Leflunomide: May increase risk of hematologic toxicity, such as pancytopenia, agranulocytosis, or thrombocytopenia. Consider
therapy modification.
Live-virus vaccines: Immunosuppressants
may enhance adverse or toxic effect of
live-virus vaccines. Avoid use for at least
3 months after immunosuppressive therapy.
Pimecrolimus, tacrolimus (topical): May
enhance adverse or toxic effect of immunosuppressants. Avoid this combination.

Reactions in bold italics are *life-threatening*. Interactions may have a *rapid onset* or a *delayed onset*.

Tofacitinib: May enhance immunosuppressive effect of tofacitinib. Avoid combination.
Trastuzumab: May enhance neutropenic effect of immunosuppressants. Monitor therapy.
Drug-herb. *Echinacea:* May diminish therapeutic effect of immunosuppressants. Consider therapy modification.

EFFECTS ON LAB TEST RESULTS
• May diminish diagnostic effect of coccidioidin skin test.

CONTRAINDICATIONS & CAUTIONS
• Contraindicated in patients hypersensitive to drug or mannitol.
Dialyzable drug: Unknown.

PREGNANCY-LACTATION-REPRODUCTION
• There are no well-controlled studies in pregnant women. Use in pregnancy only if clearly needed.
• Use cautiously in breast-feeding women.

NURSING CONSIDERATIONS
• Immediate postinjection reactions may occur; symptoms include flushing, chest pain, palpitations, anxiety, dyspnea, constriction of the throat, and urticaria. They typically are transient and self-limiting and don't need specific treatment. Onset of postinjection reaction may occur several months after treatment starts, and patients may have more than one episode.
• Patient may experience at least one episode of transient chest pain, which usually begins at least 1 month after treatment starts; it isn't accompanied by other signs or symptoms.

PATIENT TEACHING
• Instruct patient how to self-inject drug. Supervise first injection. Injection sites include arms, abdomen, hips, and thighs.
• Tell patient to rotate injection sites daily.
• Explain need for aseptic self-injection techniques, and warn patient against reuse of needles and syringes. Periodically review proper disposal of needles, syringes, drug containers, and unused drug.
• Tell patient to notify prescriber about planned, suspected, or known pregnancy.

• Tell women to notify prescriber if breast-feeding.
• Advise patient not to change drug or dosage schedule or to stop drug without medical approval.
• Tell patient to notify prescriber of all adverse reactions and to immediately report if dizziness, hives, profuse sweating, chest pain, difficulty breathing, or severe pain occurs after drug injection.

SAFETY ALERT!

G

glimepiride
glye-MEH-per-ide

Amaryl◆

Therapeutic class: Antidiabetics
Pharmacologic class: Sulfonylureas

AVAILABLE FORMS
Tablets: 1 mg, 2 mg, 3 mg, 4 mg, 6 mg, 8 mg

INDICATIONS & DOSAGES
Adjust-a-dose (for all indications): For patients with renal impairment, those at risk for hypoglycemia, and elderly patients, initially, 1 mg P.O. once daily; then adjust cautiously to appropriate dosage, if needed.
➤ **Adjunct to diet and exercise to lower glucose level in patients with type 2 diabetes**
Adults: Initially, 1 or 2 mg P.O. once daily; usual maintenance dose is 1 to 4 mg P.O. once daily. After reaching 2 mg, dosage is increased in increments not exceeding 2 mg every 1 to 2 weeks, based on patient's glucose level response. Maximum dose is 8 mg daily.

ADMINISTRATION
P.O.
• Give drug with first main meal of the day.

ACTION
Lowers glucose level, possibly by stimulating release of insulin from functioning pancreatic beta cells, and may lead to increased sensitivity of peripheral tissues to insulin.

Route	Onset	Peak	Duration
P.O.	1 hr	2–3 hr	>24 hr

Half-life: 9 hours.

ADVERSE REACTIONS

CNS: dizziness, asthenia, headache.
EENT: changes in accommodation.
GI: nausea.
Hematologic: *leukopenia,* hemolytic anemia, *agranulocytosis, thrombocytopenia, aplastic anemia, pancytopenia.*
Metabolic: *hypoglycemia,* dilutional hyponatremia.

INTERACTIONS

Drug-drug. *Beta blockers:* May mask symptoms of hypoglycemia. Monitor glucose level.
Drugs that tend to produce hyperglycemia (such as corticosteroids, estrogens, fosphenytoin, hormonal contraceptives, isoniazid, nicotinic acid, phenothiazines, phenytoin, thyroid products): May lead to loss of glucose control. Adjust dosage.
Insulin: May increase risk of hypoglycemia. Use together cautiously.
NSAIDs, other drugs that are highly protein-bound (such as beta blockers, chloramphenicol, coumarin, MAO inhibitors, probenecid, sulfonamides): May increase hypoglycemic action of sulfonylureas such as glimepiride. Monitor glucose level carefully.
Rifamycins, thiazide diuretics: May increase risk of hyperglycemia. Monitor glucose level.
Salicylates: May increase hypoglycemic effects of sulfonylurea. Monitor glucose level.
Drug-lifestyle. *Alcohol use:* May alter glycemic control, most commonly causing hypoglycemia. May also cause disulfiram-like reaction. Discourage use together.

EFFECTS ON LAB TEST RESULTS

● May increase alkaline phosphatase, AST, BUN, and creatinine levels.
● May decrease glucose, Hb, and sodium levels.
● May decrease granulocyte, platelet, RBC, and WBC counts.

CONTRAINDICATIONS & CAUTIONS

● Contraindicated in patients hypersensitive to drug and in those with diabetic ketoacidosis, which should be treated with insulin.
● Contraindicated as sole therapy for type 1 diabetes.
● Contraindicated in patients with sulfonamide allergy.
● Use cautiously in debilitated or malnourished patients and in those with adrenal, pituitary, or renal insufficiency; these patients are more susceptible to the hypoglycemic action of glucose-lowering drugs.
● Use cautiously with drugs that can cause hypoglycemia.
● Use cautiously in elderly patients and in patients allergic to sulfonamides.
● Patients with G6PD deficiency may be at increased risk for sulfonylurea-induced hemolytic anemia. Use cautiously and consider therapy modification.
● Safety and effectiveness in children haven't been established.
Dialyzable drug: Unknown.
⚠ *Overdose S&S:* Hypoglycemia.

PREGNANCY-LACTATION-REPRODUCTION

● Use drug in pregnancy only if potential benefit justifies potential risk to the fetus.
● May cause hypoglycemia in breast-fed infants. Patient should discontinue breast-feeding or discontinue drug.

NURSING CONSIDERATIONS

● Glimepiride and insulin may be used together in patients who lose glucose control after first responding to therapy.
● Monitor fasting glucose level periodically to determine therapeutic response. Also monitor HbA_{1c} level, usually every 3 to 6 months, to precisely assess long-term glycemic control.
⚠ *Alert:* Use of oral antidiabetics may carry higher risk of CV mortality than use of diet alone or of diet and insulin therapy.
● When changing patient from other sulfonylureas to glimepiride, a transition period isn't needed. Monitor patient carefully for 1 to 2 weeks when changing from longer half-life sulfonylureas, such as chlorpropamide.

• *Look alike–sound alike:* Don't confuse glimepiride with glyburide or glipizide. Don't confuse Amaryl with Altace.

PATIENT TEACHING
• Tell patient to take drug with first meal of the day.
• Make sure patient understands that therapy relieves symptoms but doesn't cure the disease. He should also understand potential risks and advantages of taking drug and of other treatment methods.
• Stress importance of adhering to diet, weight reduction, exercise, and personal hygiene programs. Explain to patient and family how and when to monitor glucose level, and teach recognition of and intervention for signs and symptoms of high and low glucose levels.
• Advise patient to wear or carry medical identification at all times.
• Advise patient to consult prescriber before taking any OTC products or supplements.
• Teach patient to carry candy or other simple sugars to treat mild episodes of low glucose level. Patient experiencing severe episode may need hospital treatment.
• Advise patient to avoid alcohol, which lowers glucose level.

SAFETY ALERT!

glipiZIDE
GLIP-i-zide

Glucotrol♦, Glucotrol XL♦

Therapeutic class: Antidiabetics
Pharmacologic class: Sulfonylureas

AVAILABLE FORMS
Tablets (extended-release) ⓝ: 2.5 mg, 5 mg, 10 mg
Tablets (immediate-release): 5 mg, 10 mg

INDICATIONS & DOSAGES
➤ **Adjunct to diet and exercise to lower glucose level in patients with type 2 diabetes**
Immediate-release tablets
Adults: Initially, 5 mg P.O. daily 30 minutes before breakfast. Titrate by 2.5- to 5-mg increments no less than every few days

based on blood glucose levels. Maximum once-daily dose is 15 mg. Divide doses of more than 15 mg. Maximum daily dose is 40 mg.
Adjust-a-dose: For patients with hepatic insufficiency or patients older than age 65, initially give 2.5 mg P.O. daily.
Extended-release tablets
Adults: Initially, 5 mg P.O. with breakfast daily. Increase by 5 mg every 3 months, depending on level of glycemic control. Maximum daily dose is 20 mg.
➤ **To replace insulin therapy**
Adults: If insulin dosage is 20 units or less daily, insulin may be stopped when glipizide starts. If insulin dosage is more than 20 units daily, start patient at usual dosage in addition to 50% of insulin dose. In some cases, especially if insulin dose is more than 40 units daily, it may be advisable to transition to glipizide in a hospital setting.

ADMINISTRATION
P.O.
• Give immediate-release tablet about 30 minutes before meals.
• Give extended-release tablet with breakfast.
• Don't split or crush extended-release tablets.

ACTION
Unknown. Probably stimulates insulin release from pancreatic beta cells, reduces glucose output by the liver, and increases peripheral sensitivity to insulin.

Route	Onset	Peak	Duration
P.O. (immediate-release)	15–30 min	1–3 hr	24 hr
P.O. (extended-release)	2–3 hr	6–12 hr	24 hr

Half-life: 2 to 5 hours.

ADVERSE REACTIONS
CNS: dizziness, headache, syncope, asthenia, nervousness, tremor, anxiety, depression, insomnia, pain.
EENT: blurred vision.
GI: nausea, dyspepsia, flatulence, constipation, diarrhea, vomiting.
GU: polyuria.

G

Hematologic: *leukopenia,* hemolytic anemia, *agranulocytosis, thrombocytopenia, aplastic anemia.*
Metabolic: *hypoglycemia.*
Musculoskeletal: arthralgia, leg cramps.
Respiratory: rhinitis.
Skin: pruritus, photosensitivity reactions.

INTERACTIONS

Drug-drug. *Amantadine, anabolic steroids, antifungals, chloramphenicol, clofibrate, guanethidine, MAO inhibitors, NSAIDs, probenecid, quinolones, **salicylates**, sulfonamides:* May increase hypoglycemic activity. Monitor glucose level.
Beta blockers: May prolong hypoglycemic effect and mask symptoms of hypoglycemia. Use together cautiously.
*Corticosteroids, glucagon, phenytoin, **rifamycins**, **thiazide diuretics**:* May decrease hypoglycemic response. Monitor glucose level.
Oral anticoagulants: May increase hypoglycemic activity or enhance anticoagulant effect. Monitor glucose level, PT, and INR.
Drug-lifestyle. *Alcohol use:* May alter glycemic control, most commonly causing hypoglycemia. May cause disulfiram-like reaction. Discourage use together.

EFFECTS ON LAB TEST RESULTS

• May increase alkaline phosphatase, AST, LDH, BUN, cholesterol, and creatinine levels.
• May decrease glucose and Hb levels.
• May decrease granulocyte, platelet, and WBC counts.

CONTRAINDICATIONS & CAUTIONS

• Contraindicated in patients hypersensitive to drug and in those with diabetic ketoacidosis with or without coma.
• Contraindicated in patients with sulfonamide allergy.
• Patients with G6PD deficiency may be at increased risk for sulfonylurea-induced hemolytic anemia. Use cautiously and consider therapy modification.
• Use cautiously in patients with severe GI narrowing, or renal or hepatic disease, and in debilitated, malnourished, or elderly patients.

Dialyzable drug: Unknown.
⚠ *Overdose S&S:* Hypoglycemia.

PREGNANCY-LACTATION-REPRODUCTION

• Insulin is drug of choice to control diabetes during pregnancy. If used during pregnancy, discontinue at least 1 month before expected delivery date.
• Drug may cause hypoglycemia in breast-fed infants. Patient should discontinue breast-feeding or discontinue drug.

NURSING CONSIDERATIONS

• Some patients may attain effective control on a once-daily regimen, whereas others respond better with divided dosing.
• Patient may switch from immediate-release to extended-release tablets at the nearest equivalent total daily dose.
• Glipizide is a second-generation sulfonylurea. The frequency of adverse reactions appears to be lower than with first-generation drugs such as chlorpropamide.
🔆 *Alert:* Use of oral antidiabetic drugs may carry a higher risk of CV mortality than use of diet alone or of diet and insulin therapy.
• During periods of increased stress, patient may need insulin therapy. Monitor patient closely for hyperglycemia in these situations.
• Patient switching from insulin therapy to an oral antidiabetic should check glucose level at least three times a day before meals. Patient may need hospitalization during transition.
• *Look alike–sound alike:* Don't confuse glipizide with glyburide or glimepiride.

PATIENT TEACHING

• Instruct patient about disease and importance of following therapeutic regimen, adhering to diet, losing weight, getting exercise, following personal hygiene programs, and avoiding infection. Explain how and when to monitor glucose level, and teach recognition of episodes of low and high glucose levels.
• Tell patient to carry candy or other simple sugars to treat mild low-glucose episodes. Patient experiencing severe episode may need hospital treatment.

Reactions in bold italics are *life-threatening*. Interactions may have a *rapid onset* or a *delayed onset*.

- Instruct patient not to change drug dosage without prescriber's consent and to report abnormal blood or urine glucose test results.
- Tell patient not to take other drugs, including OTC drugs, without first checking with prescriber.
- Advise patient to wear or carry medical identification at all times.
- Advise patient to avoid alcohol, which lowers glucose level.
- Tell patient that he may occasionally notice something in stool that looks like a tablet; assure him that it's the nonabsorbable shell of the extended-release tablet.

SAFETY ALERT!

glyBURIDE (glibenclamide)
GLYE-byoor-ide

DiaBeta✔, Euglucon✤, Glynase

Therapeutic class: Antidiabetics
Pharmacologic class: Sulfonylureas

AVAILABLE FORMS
Tablets: 1.25 mg, 2.5 mg, 5 mg
Tablets (micronized): 1.5 mg, 3 mg, 4.5 mg, 6 mg

INDICATIONS & DOSAGES
➤ **Adjunct to diet to lower glucose level in patients with type 2 diabetes**
Nonmicronized form
Adults: Initially, 2.5 to 5 mg P.O. once daily with breakfast or first main meal. Adjust to maintenance dose at no more than 2.5-mg increments at weekly intervals. Usual daily maintenance dose is 1.25 to 20 mg, in single dose or divided doses. Maximum daily dose is 20 mg P.O.
Micronized form
Adults: Initially, 1.5 to 3 mg P.O. daily with breakfast or first main meal. Adjust to maintenance dose at no more than 1.5-mg increments at weekly intervals. Usual daily maintenance dose is 0.75 to 12 mg. Dosages exceeding 6 mg daily may have better response with b.i.d. dosing. Maximum dose is 12 mg P.O. daily.
Adjust-a-dose: For elderly patients, patients who are more sensitive to antidiabetics, and for those with renal, hepatic, adrenal, or

pituitary insufficiency, start with 1.25 mg (nonmicronized) or 0.75 mg (micronized) daily.
➤ **To replace insulin therapy**
Adults: If insulin dose is less than 40 units/day, patient may be switched directly to glyburide when insulin is stopped. If insulin dose is less than 20 units/day, initial dose is 2.5 to 5 mg (1.5 to 3 mg micronized) P.O. daily. If insulin dose is 20 to 40 units/day, initial dose is 5 mg (3 mg micronized) P.O. daily. If insulin dose is 40 or more units/day, initially, 5 mg (3 mg micronized) P.O. once daily in addition to 50% of insulin dose. Gradually taper off insulin as the glyburide dose is increased.

ADMINISTRATION
P.O.
- Give drug with breakfast or first main meal.

ACTION
Unknown. Probably stimulates insulin release from pancreatic beta cells, reduces glucose output by the liver, and increases peripheral sensitivity to insulin.

Route	Onset	Peak	Duration
P.O. (micronized)	1 hr	2–3 hr	12–24 hr
P.O. (non-micronized)	2–4 hr	2–4 hr	16–24 hr

Half-life: DiaBeta, 10 hours; Euglucon, 1.9 to 16 hours; Glynase, 4 hours.

ADVERSE REACTIONS
EENT: changes in accommodation or blurred vision.
GI: nausea, epigastric fullness, heartburn.
Hematologic: *leukopenia,* hemolytic anemia, *agranulocytosis, thrombocytopenia, aplastic anemia.*
Hepatic: cholestatic jaundice, *hepatitis.*
Metabolic: *hypoglycemia, hyponatremia.*
Musculoskeletal: arthralgia, myalgia.
Skin: rash, pruritus, other allergic reactions.
Other: *angioedema.*

INTERACTIONS
Drug-drug. *Anabolic steroids, azole antifungals, chloramphenicol, clofibrate, fluoroquinolones, guanethidine, MAO inhibitors, NSAIDs, probenecid, phenylbutazone,*

salicylates, sulfonamides: May increase hypoglycemic activity. Monitor glucose level.

Beta blockers: May prolong hypoglycemic effect and mask symptoms of hypoglycemia. Use together cautiously.

Bosentan: Increases risk of elevated LFT values. Use together is contraindicated.

Carbamazepine, corticosteroids, glucagon, **rifamycins, thiazide diuretics:** May decrease hypoglycemic response. Monitor glucose level.

Oral anticoagulants: May increase hypoglycemic activity or enhance anticoagulant effect. Monitor glucose level, PT, and INR.

Drug-lifestyle. *Alcohol use:* May alter glycemic control, most commonly causing hypoglycemia. May cause disulfiram-like reaction. Discourage use together.

EFFECTS ON LAB TEST RESULTS

● May increase alkaline phosphatase, AST, ALT, bilirubin, BUN, and cholesterol levels.

● May decrease glucose, sodium, and Hb levels.

● May decrease granulocyte, platelet, and WBC counts.

CONTRAINDICATIONS & CAUTIONS

● Contraindicated in patients hypersensitive to drug and in those with type 1 diabetes or diabetic ketoacidosis with or without coma.

● Use cautiously in patients with hepatic or renal impairment; in debilitated, malnourished, or elderly patients; and in patients allergic to sulfonamides.

Dialyzable drug: Unknown.

⚠ *Overdose S&S:* Hypoglycemia.

PREGNANCY-LACTATION-REPRODUCTION

● Insulin is drug of choice to control diabetes during pregnancy. If used during pregnancy, discontinue at least 2 weeks before expected delivery date.

● Drug may cause hypoglycemia in breast-fed infants. Patient should discontinue breast-feeding or discontinue drug.

NURSING CONSIDERATIONS

🛈 *Alert:* Micronized glyburide (Glynase) contains drug in a smaller particle size and isn't bioequivalent to regular glyburide

tablets. In patients who have been taking DiaBeta, adjust dosage.

● Although most patients may take drug once daily, those taking more than 10 mg daily may achieve better results with twice-daily dosage.

● Drug is a second-generation sulfonylurea. Adverse effects are less common with second-generation drugs than with first-generation drugs such as chlorpropamide.

🛈 *Alert:* Use of oral antidiabetic drugs may carry a higher risk of CV mortality than use of diet alone or of diet and insulin therapy.

● During periods of increased stress, such as infection, fever, surgery, or trauma, patient may need insulin therapy. Monitor patient closely for hyperglycemia in these situations.

● Patient switching from insulin therapy to an oral antidiabetic should check glucose level at least three times a day before meals. Patient may need hospitalization during transition.

● *Look alike–sound alike:* Don't confuse glyburide with glimepiride or glipizide.

PATIENT TEACHING

● Teach patient about diabetes and the importance of following therapeutic regimen, adhering to specific diet, losing weight, getting exercise, following personal hygiene programs, and avoiding infection. Explain how and when to monitor glucose level, and teach recognition of and intervention for low and high glucose levels.

● Tell patient not to change drug dosage without prescriber's consent and to report abnormal blood or urine glucose test results.

● Teach patient to carry candy or other simple sugars for mild low glucose level. Patient experiencing severe episode may need hospital treatment.

● Advise patient not to take other drugs, including OTC drugs, without first checking with prescriber.

● Advise patient to wear or carry medical identification at all times.

🛈 *Alert:* Instruct patient to report episodes of low glucose to prescriber immediately; a severely low glucose level is sometimes fatal in patients receiving as little as 2.5 to 5 mg daily.

• Advise patient to avoid alcohol, which may lower glucose level.

golimumab
go-LIM-myoo-mab

Simponi, Simponi Aria

Therapeutic class: Antiarthritics
Pharmacologic class: TNF blockers

AVAILABLE FORMS
Injection (subcutaneous): 50 mg/0.5 mL, 100 mg/mL prefilled syringe; 50 mg/0.5 mL, 100 mg/mL prefilled autoinjector
Injection (I.V.): 50 mg/4 mL single-use vial

INDICATIONS & DOSAGES
➤ **Moderate to severe active RA in combination with methotrexate; active psoriatic arthritis alone or in combination with methotrexate; active ankylosing spondylitis**
Adults: 50 mg subcutaneously monthly.
➤ **Moderate to severe ulcerative colitis in patients who have demonstrated an inadequate response or intolerance to prior treatment or who require continuous steroid therapy**
Adults: Initially, 200 mg subcutaneously, followed by 100 mg subcutaneously at week 2, then 100 mg subcutaneously every 4 weeks.
➤ **Moderate to severe RA in combination with methotrexate (Simponi Aria)**
Adults: 2 mg/kg I.V. infusion at weeks 0 and 4, and then every 8 weeks thereafter.

ADMINISTRATION
I.V.
▼ Dilute with NSS to a final volume of 100 mL.
▼ Administer over 30 minutes. Use a 0.22-micron low protein-binding filter.
▼ Don't infuse with other drugs in the same I.V. line.
▼ Solutions diluted for infusion may be stored at room temperature for 4 hours.
Subcutaneous
• Remove drug from refrigerator 30 minutes before administration and allow it to reach room temperature.

• Inspect solution before administration. Don't use solution if discolored or cloudy or if foreign particles are present. Drug is normally colorless to slightly opalescent to light yellow.
• Prefilled syringe and prefilled autoinjector contain latex. Don't handle if sensitive to latex.
• Don't use any leftover product remaining in prefilled syringe or prefilled autoinjector.
• Rotate injection sites. Don't inject drug into areas where skin is tender, bruised, red, or hard.
• If multiple injections are required, administer injections at different sites on the body.

ACTION
Binds to human TNF-alpha to neutralize its activity and inhibit its binding with receptors, thereby reducing the infiltration of inflammatory cells.

Route	Onset	Peak	Duration
I.V.	Unknown	12 weeks	Unknown
Subcut.	Unknown	2–6 days	Unknown

Half-life: 2 weeks.

ADVERSE REACTIONS
CNS: dizziness, paresthesia, fever.
CV: hypertension.
EENT: nasopharyngitis, oral herpes, pharyngitis, rhinitis, sinusitis.
Respiratory: bronchitis, URI.
Skin: injection-site reactions, superficial fungal infections.
Other: flulike syndrome, infection, antibody development.

INTERACTIONS
Drug-drug. *Abatacept, anakinra, other immunosuppressants:* May increase risk of serious infection. Avoid using together.
CYP450 substrates (such as cyclosporine, theophylline, warfarin): May alter levels of these drugs. Monitor patient closely and adjust dosages as needed.
Live-virus vaccines: May increase risk of infection. Postpone live-virus vaccine until 3 months after therapy has ended.

G

EFFECTS ON LAB TEST RESULTS
- May increase LFT values.
- May decrease platelet, WBC, and neutrophil counts.
- May diminish diagnostic effect of coccidioidin skin test.
- May cause positive ANA titer.

CONTRAINDICATIONS & CAUTIONS
- Use cautiously in patients with malignancies; invasive fungal infection; chronic infection (HBV, TB); history of recurrent infection, hematologic abnormalities, or HF; or preexisting or recent onset of CNS demyelination.
- Safe use in children hasn't been established.

Dialyzable drug: Unknown.

PREGNANCY-LACTATION-REPRODUCTION
- Use in pregnant women only if benefit justifies fetal risk and only if clearly needed.
- It isn't known if drug appears in breast milk. Patient should discontinue breastfeeding or discontinue drug.

NURSING CONSIDERATIONS
Black Box Warning Monitor patient closely for signs and symptoms of infection before and after treatment. TB, invasive fungal infection, and other bacterial and viral opportunistic infections, which are sometimes fatal, may occur in patients receiving golimumab. Stop drug if serious infection or sepsis develops during treatment. ■
Black Box Warning Evaluate patient for latent TB with tuberculin skin test before initiating treatment. Treat latent TB before therapy with golimumab. Monitor all patients for active TB during treatment even if initial latent TB test is negative. ■
- Drug increases risk of reactivation of HBV infection, which can be fatal, in patients who are HBV carriers. Before starting therapy, patient should be tested for HBV infection.
- Monitor patient for new or worsening HF; stop drug if signs and symptoms occur.
Black Box Warning Lymphoma and other malignancies, some fatal, have been reported in children and adolescents treated with TNF blockers, including golimumab. ■

- Monitor patient for lymphomas and other malignancies.
- Monitor CBC regularly during therapy.

PATIENT TEACHING
- Teach patient how to give subcutaneous injection. First self-injection should be under supervision of qualified health care practitioner.
- Advise patient that prefilled syringes and prefilled autoinjectors contain latex or a latex derivative.
- Instruct patient to report all adverse reactions, especially signs and symptoms of infection, new or worsening HF, or liver or nervous system problems.
- Tell patient to avoid live-virus vaccines while taking drug.

granisetron
gran-IZ-e-tron

Sancuso, Sustol

granisetron hydrochloride

Therapeutic class: Antiemetics
Pharmacologic class: 5-HT$_3$ receptor antagonists

AVAILABLE FORMS
Injection: 0.1 mg/mL in 1-mL single-use vials; 1 mg/mL in 1-mL, single-dose, preservative-free vials and 4-mL multidose vials containing benzyl alcohol
Injection (extended-release): 10 mg/0.4 mL single-dose syringe
Tablets: 1 mg
Transdermal patch: 3.1 mg per 24 hours

INDICATIONS & DOSAGES
➤ **Prevention of nausea and vomiting from emetogenic cancer chemotherapy**
Adults and children age 2 and older:
10 mcg/kg I.V. undiluted and given by direct injection over 30 seconds, or diluted and infused over 5 minutes. Start giving at least 30 minutes before chemotherapy. Or, for adults, 1 mg P.O. up to 1 hour before chemotherapy and repeated 12 hours later. Or, for adults, 2 mg P.O. daily given up to 1 hour before chemotherapy. Or, for adults,

apply a single patch to the upper outer arm 24 to 48 hours before chemotherapy. Remove the patch a minimum of 24 hours after completion of chemotherapy or a maximum of 7 days.

Or, for adults, 10 mg extended-release form subcutaneously with dexamethasone at least 30 minutes before chemotherapy on day 1. Don't give extended-release form more frequently than once every 7 days. Refer to manufacturer's instructions for dexamethasone dosages.

Adjust-a-dose: In patients with moderate renal impairment (CrCl of 30 to 59 mL/minute), don't give extended-release form more frequently than once every 14 days. Don't give extended-release form to patients with severe renal impairment (CrCl of less than 30 mL/minute).

➤ **Prevention of nausea and vomiting from radiation, including total body irradiation and fractionated abdominal radiation**
Adults: 2 mg P.O. once daily within 1 hour of radiation.

ADMINISTRATION
P.O.
● Store tablets between 68° and 77° F (20° and 25° C). Protect from light.
I.V.
▼ For direct injection, give drug undiluted over 30 seconds.
▼ For intermittent infusion, dilute with NSS for injection or D_5W to a volume of 20 to 50 mL.
▼ Infuse over 5 minutes, starting within 30 minutes before chemotherapy and only on days chemotherapy is given.
▼ Diluted solutions are stable 24 hours at room temperature.
▼ Don't freeze vials.
▼ Once the multiuse vial is penetrated, use contents within 30 days.
▼ **Incompatibilities:** Other I.V. drugs.
Subcutaneous
● Extended-release form is for subcutaneous injection only.
● Drug should only be administered by a health care provider.
● Remove extended-release form kit from refrigerator 1 hour before administration.

● Refer to manufacturer's syringe preparation instructions for warming syringe to body temperature using syringe warming pouches included in kit.
● Don't give drug if discoloration or particulate matter is noted in syringe; be aware that syringe is amber-colored glass.
● Give drug by subcutaneous injection in the skin of the back of the upper arm or in the skin of the abdomen at least 1 inch (2.54 cm) from the umbilicus.
● Topical anesthetic may be used at injection site before giving drug.
● Avoid injecting into skin that's burned, hardened, inflamed, swollen, or otherwise compromised.
● Give drug as a slow, sustained subcutaneous injection over 20 to 30 seconds.
● Store in refrigerator at 36° to 46° F (2° to 8° C). Protect from light; don't freeze.
● Once drug has been removed from refrigerator, it can remain at room temperature for up to 7 days.
Transdermal
● Apply patch to clean, intact, healthy skin on the upper outer arm.
● Each patch is packed in a pouch and should be applied directly after the pouch has been opened.
● Don't cut patch into pieces.

ACTION
May block 5-HT$_3$ in the CNS in the chemoreceptor trigger zone and in the peripheral nervous system on nerve terminals of the vagus nerve.

Route	Onset	Peak	Duration
P.O., I.V.	Unknown	Unknown	Unknown
Subcut. (extended-release)	Unknown	11–12 hr	7 days
Transdermal	Unknown	48 hr	Unknown

Half-life: P.O., I.V., transdermal, 5 to 9 hours; extended-release, 24 hours.

ADVERSE REACTIONS
CNS: asthenia, headache, fever, agitation, anxiety, CNS stimulation, dizziness, insomnia, somnolence, pain, weakness, drowsiness, syncope.
CV: hypertension, hypotension, prolonged QT interval; atrial fibrillation (extended-release form).

GI: constipation, nausea, vomiting, abdominal pain, decreased appetite, diarrhea, dyspepsia, flatulence, taste disorder, GERD.
Hematologic: anemia, *leukocytosis, leukopenia, thrombocytopenia.*
Skin: alopecia, rash, dermatitis, injection-site reactions, *hypersensitivity reactions.*

INTERACTIONS
Drug-drug. *Apomorphine:* May increase risk of profound hypotension and loss of consciousness. Avoid use together.
Drug that prolong QT interval: May increase risk of life-threatening cardiac arrhythmias, including torsades de pointes. Use together cautiously and monitor patient.
Serotonin modulators (fentanyl, lithium, MAO inhibitors, methylene blue I.V., mirtazapine, SNRIs, SSRIs, tramadol): May increase risk of serotonin syndrome. Monitor therapy.

EFFECTS ON LAB TEST RESULTS
● May increase ALT and AST levels. May decrease Hb level and hematocrit. May alter fluid and electrolyte levels with prolonged use.
● May decrease platelet and WBC counts.

CONTRAINDICATIONS & CAUTIONS
● Contraindicated in patients hypersensitive to drug or other 5-HT$_3$ receptor antagonists.
● Hypersensitivity reactions, including anaphylaxis, may occur up to 7 days or longer after administration of extended-release form.
🕓 *Alert:* QT-interval prolongation has been reported, and drug may increase risk of ventricular arrhythmias. Use caution in patients with preexisting arrhythmias, cardiac conduction disorders, cardiac disease, or electrolyte abnormalities; in patients receiving cardiotoxic chemotherapy; and in those receiving medications that prolong QT interval.
● May increase risk of serotonin syndrome, which can be fatal, especially if drug is used with other serotonergic drugs.
● Use of extended-release form with successive emetogenic chemotherapy cycles for more than 6 months isn't recommended.
● Injection-site bruising and hematoma, which can be severe, may occur more than

5 days after administration of extended-release form. Patients receiving anticoagulants or antiplatelet drugs be at greater risk.
Dialyzable drug: Unknown.
⚠ *Overdose S&S:* Headache.

PREGNANCY-LACTATION-REPRODUCTION
● Use in pregnancy only if clearly needed.
● Use cautiously in breast-feeding women.

NURSING CONSIDERATIONS
● Drug regimen is given only on days when chemotherapy is given. Treatment at other times isn't useful.
● Monitor patient for signs and symptoms of serotonin syndrome (mental status changes, neuromuscular signs and symptoms, autonomic instability, seizures, GI symptoms). If signs or symptoms of serotonin syndrome occur, discontinue drug and initiate treatment.
● Monitor patients receiving extended-release form for injection-site infections, bruising, and hematoma.
● Monitor patients receiving extended-release form for signs and symptoms of hypersensitivity reactions (dyspnea, wheezing, rash, hives, fever, swelling).

PATIENT TEACHING
● Stress importance of taking second dose of oral drug 12 hours after the first for maximum effectiveness.
● Tell patient to report adverse reactions immediately.
● Teach patient receiving extended-release form that hypersensitivity reactions can occur up to 7 days or later after subcutaneous administration and to immediately report signs and symptoms.
● Teach patient signs and symptoms of serotonin syndrome and to report them immediately.
● Tell patient to report injection-site reactions (infection, bruising, hematoma, bleeding) to prescriber.

Reactions in bold italics are *life-threatening*. Interactions may have a *rapid onset* or a ***delayed onset***.

haloperidol
ha-loe-PER-i-dole

Novo-Peridol✣

haloperidol decanoate
Haldol Decanoate, Haloperidol LA✣

haloperidol lactate
Haldol

Therapeutic class: Antipsychotics
Pharmacologic class: Butyrophenone
derivatives

AVAILABLE FORMS
haloperidol
Tablets: 0.5 mg, 1 mg, 2 mg, 5 mg, 10 mg,
20 mg
haloperidol decanoate
Injection: 50 mg/mL, 100 mg/mL
haloperidol lactate
Injection: 5 mg/mL
Oral solution (concentrate): 2 mg/mL

INDICATIONS & DOSAGES
Adjust-a-dose (for all indications): For indications with oral dosing and for oral dosing
in elderly and debilitated patients, initially,
0.5 to 2 mg P.O. b.i.d. or t.i.d.; increase gradually, as needed.
➤ **Psychotic disorders**
Adults and children older than age 12:
Dosage varies for each patient. Initially,
0.5 to 5 mg P.O. b.i.d. or t.i.d. Maximum,
100 mg P.O. daily. Or, 2 to 5 mg lactate
I.M. every 4 to 8 hours, although hourly
administration may be needed until control
is obtained.
Children ages 3 to 12 weighing 15 to 40 kg:
Initially, 0.5 mg P.O. in two or three divided
doses daily. May increase dose by 0.5 mg
at 5- to 7-day intervals, depending on therapeutic response and patient tolerance.
Maintenance dose, 0.05 to 0.15 mg/kg P.O.
daily given in two or three divided doses.
Severely disturbed children may need higher
doses.
➤ **Chronic psychosis requiring prolonged
therapy**
Adults: 50 to 200 mg decanoate I.M. every
4 weeks.

Adjust-a-dose: For elderly or debilitated
patients, lower initial dose and gradual adjustments are recommended. Recommended
initial and maintenance dosage is 10 to
15 times the daily oral dose, administered
I.M. every 4 weeks.
➤ **Nonpsychotic behavior disorders**
Children ages 3 to 12: 0.05 to 0.075 mg/kg
P.O. daily, in two or three divided doses.
Maximum, 6 mg daily. Severely disturbed
nonpsychotic or hyperactive children with
conduct disorders may only require short-
term use.
➤ **Tourette syndrome**
Adults: Initially, 0.5 to 5 mg P.O. b.i.d., t.i.d.,
or as needed. Up to about 100 mg/day may
be needed.
Children ages 3 to 12: 0.05 to 0.075 mg/kg
P.O. daily, in two or three divided doses.
Elderly patients: 0.5 to 2 mg P.O. b.i.d. or
t.i.d.; increase gradually, as needed.

ADMINISTRATION
P.O.
❸ ***Alert:*** Haloperidol isn't approved for I.V.
use.
● Protect drug from light. Slight yellowing
of concentrate is common and doesn't affect
potency. Discard very discolored solutions.
I.M.
● Protect drug from light. Slight yellowing
of solution is common and doesn't affect
potency. Discard very discolored solutions.
● Use a 21G needle. Maximum volume
per injection site shouldn't exceed 3 mL.
Give in gluteal muscle by deep I.M. injection; Z-track techniques are recommended
(haloperidol decanoate).
● When switching from tablets to I.M.
decanoate injection, give 10 to 20 times
the oral dose once a month (maximum,
100 mg). If initial dose conversion requires
more than 100 mg, give in two injections
(100 mg maximum) separated by 3 to
7 days. If patient is elderly or debilitated
or if oral haloperidol dose is 10 mg/day or
less, initiate dose at 10 to 15 times the daily
oral dose. If patient is at high risk for relapse or oral haloperidol dose is greater than
10 mg/day, initiate dose at 20 times the oral
daily dose.

Subcutaneous
● Protect drug from light. Slight yellowing of solution is common and doesn't affect potency. Discard very discolored solutions.

ACTION
A butyrophenone that probably exerts antipsychotic effects by blocking postsynaptic dopamine receptors in the brain.

Route	Onset	Peak	Duration
P.O.	Unknown	2–6 hr	Unknown
I.M. (decanoate)	Unknown	3–9 days	Unknown
I.M. (lactate)	Unknown	10–20 min	Unknown
Subcut.	Unknown	Unknown	Unknown

Half-life: P.O., 14 to 37 hours; I.M. decanoate, 3 weeks; I.M. lactate, 20 hours.

ADVERSE REACTIONS
CNS: severe extrapyramidal reactions, dystonia, tardive dyskinesia, *neuroleptic malignant syndrome, seizures,* sedation, drowsiness, lethargy, headache, insomnia, confusion, vertigo, agitation, anxiety, depression, euphoria, restlessness, tonic-clonic seizures, hallucinations.
CV: tachycardia, hypotension, hypertension; *prolonged QT interval* and other ECG changes, *torsades de pointes* with high doses.
EENT: blurred vision, cataracts, retinopathy.
GI: dry mouth, anorexia, constipation, diarrhea, nausea, vomiting, dyspepsia.
GU: urine retention, menstrual irregularities, priapism.
Hematologic: *leukopenia,* leukocytosis.
Hepatic: jaundice.
Metabolic: hyperglycemia, hypoglycemia.
Skin: rash, other skin reactions, diaphoresis.
Other: gynecomastia.

INTERACTIONS
Drug-drug. *Anticholinergics:* May increase anticholinergic effects and glaucoma. Use together cautiously.
Azole antifungals, buspirone, macrolides: May increase haloperidol level. Monitor patient for increased adverse reactions; haloperidol dose may need to be adjusted.
Beta blockers: May cause an unexpected severe hypotensive reaction. If this occurs, provide supportive treatment.
Carbamazepine: May decrease haloperidol level. Monitor patient.

CNS depressants: May increase CNS depression. Use together cautiously.
Lithium: May cause lethargy and confusion after high doses. Monitor patient.
Methyldopa: May cause dementia. Monitor patient closely.
Black Box Warning *Opioids:* May cause slow or difficult breathing, sedation, and death. Avoid use together. If use together is necessary, limit dosage and duration of each drug to the minimum necessary for desired effect. ■
Rifampin: May decrease haloperidol level. Monitor patient for clinical effect.
Drug-lifestyle. *Alcohol use:* May increase CNS depression. Discourage use together.

EFFECTS ON LAB TEST RESULTS
● May increase LFT values. May increase or decrease glucose level.
● May increase or decrease WBC count.

CONTRAINDICATIONS & CAUTIONS
● Contraindicated in patients hypersensitive to drug and in those with Parkinson disease or CNS depression.
Black Box Warning Opioid drugs should only be prescribed with benzodiazepines or other CNS depressants to patients for whom alternative treatment options are inadequate. ■
● Use cautiously in elderly and debilitated patients; in patients with history of seizures or EEG abnormalities, prolonged QT interval and other severe CV disorders, allergies, glaucoma, or urine retention; and in those taking anticonvulsants, anticoagulants, antiparkinsonians, or lithium.
● Blood dyscrasias have been reported. Discontinue drug for ANC less than 1,000/mm³ or for leukopenia or agranulocytosis.
Dialyzable drug: Unknown.
⚠ *Overdose S&S:* Severe extrapyramidal reactions, hypotension, sedation.

PREGNANCY-LACTATION-REPRODUCTION
🜂 *Alert:* Antipsychotic use during the third trimester may result in abnormal muscle movements (extrapyramidal symptoms) and withdrawal symptoms in newborns. Use during pregnancy only if clearly needed. Use minimum effective maternal dose.
● Breast-feeding isn't recommended.

Reactions in bold italics are *life-threatening*. Interactions may have a *rapid onset* or a *delayed onset*.

NURSING CONSIDERATIONS

• Monitor patient for tardive dyskinesia, which may occur after prolonged use. It may not appear until months or years later and may disappear spontaneously or persist for life, despite ending drug.

🜂 *Alert:* Watch for signs and symptoms of neuroleptic malignant syndrome (extrapyramidal effects, hyperthermia, autonomic disturbance), which is rare but commonly fatal.

🜂 *Alert:* Monitor ECG when drug is given in high doses because of the increased risk of QT-interval prolongation and torsades de pointes.

Black Box Warning Elderly patients with dementia-related psychosis treated with atypical or conventional antipsychotics are at increased risk for death. Antipsychotics aren't approved for the treatment of dementia-related psychosis. ∎

• Don't withdraw drug abruptly unless required by severe adverse reactions.

• Esophageal dysmotility and aspiration can occur. Use cautiously in patients at risk for aspiration (those with pneumonia, Alzheimer disease).

• *Look alike–sound alike:* Don't confuse Haldol with Halcion or Halog.

PATIENT TEACHING

Black Box Warning Caution the patient or the caregiver of a patient taking an opioid drug with a benzodiazepine, CNS depressant, or alcohol to seek immediate medical attention if the patient has symptoms of dizziness, light-headedness, extreme sleepiness, slowed or difficult breathing, or unresponsiveness. ∎

• Advise patient to report all adverse reactions.

• Although drug is the least sedating of the antipsychotics, warn patient to avoid activities that require alertness and good coordination until effects of drug are known. Drowsiness and dizziness usually subside after a few weeks.

• Warn patient to avoid alcohol during therapy.

• Tell patient to relieve dry mouth with sugarless gum or hard candy.

heparin sodium
HEP-ah-rin

Heparin Lock Flush Solution (with Tubex), Heparin Sodium Injection

Therapeutic class: Anticoagulants
Pharmacologic class: Anticoagulants

AVAILABLE FORMS

Products are derived from beef lung or pork intestinal mucosa.

heparin sodium
Carpuject: 5,000 units/mL
Premixed I.V. solutions: 1,000 units in 500 mL (2 units/mL) of NSS; 2,000 units in 1,000 mL (2 units/mL) of NSS; 12,500 units in 250 mL (50 units/mL) of half-NSS; 25,000 units in 250 mL (100 units/mL) of half-NSS; 25,000 units in 500 mL (50 units/mL) of half-NSS; 10,000 units in 100 mL (100 units/mL) of D_5W; 12,500 units in 250 mL (50 units/mL) of D_5W; 20,000 units in 500 mL (40 units/mL) of D_5W; 25,000 units in 250 mL (100 units/mL) of D_5W; 25,000 units in 500 mL (50 units/mL) of D_5W
Single-dose ampules and vials: 1,000 units/mL, 5,000 units/mL, 10,000 units/mL, 20,000 units/mL
Syringes: 1,000 units/mL, 2,500 units/mL, 5,000 units/mL, 7,500 units/mL, 10,000 units/mL, 20,000 units/mL
Unit-dose vials: 1,000 units/mL, 2,500 units/mL, 5,000 units/mL, 7,500 units/mL, 10,000 units/mL, 20,000 units/mL
Vials (multidose): 1,000 units/mL, 2,000 units/mL, 2,500 units/mL, 5,000 units/mL, 10,000 units/mL, 20,000 units/mL
heparin sodium flush
Syringes: 1 unit/mL, 10 units/mL, 100 units/mL
Vials: 10 units/mL, 100 units/mL

INDICATIONS & DOSAGES

➤ **Thromboprophylaxis**
Adults: 5,000 units subcutaneously every 8 to 12 hours for a minimum of 7 days or for 10 to 14 days for patients undergoing total hip arthroplasty, total knee arthroplasty, or

hip fracture surgery according to American College of Chest Physicians guidelines.

➤ **Full-dose continuous I.V. infusion therapy for DVT, MI, or PE**
Adults: Initially, 5,000 units by I.V. bolus; then 20,000 to 40,000 units/day by I.V. infusion with pump. Titrate hourly rate based on PTT results (every 4 to 6 hours in the early stages of treatment).
Children: Initially, 50 units/kg I.V.; then 100 units/kg I.V. infusion every 4 hours or 20,000 units/m² daily by I.V. infusion pump. Titrate dosage based on PTT.

➤ **Full-dose subcutaneous therapy for DVT, MI, or PE**
Adults: Initially, 5,000 units I.V. bolus and 10,000 to 20,000 units in a concentrated solution subcutaneously; then 8,000 to 10,000 units subcutaneously every 8 hours or 15,000 to 20,000 units in a concentrated solution every 12 hours.

➤ **Full-dose intermittent I.V. therapy for DVT, MI, or PE**
Adults: Initially, 10,000 units by I.V. bolus; then titrated according to PTT, and 5,000 to 10,000 units I.V. every 4 to 6 hours.

➤ **Fixed low-dose therapy for prevention of venous thrombosis, PE, embolism associated with atrial fibrillation, and postoperative DVT**
Adults: 5,000 units subcutaneously every 12 hours. In surgical patients, give first dose 2 hours before procedure; then 5,000 units subcutaneously every 8 to 12 hours for 5 to 7 days or until patient can walk.

ADMINISTRATION
I.V.
▼ Draw blood to establish baseline coagulation parameters before therapy.
▼ Use an infusion pump to provide maximum safety. Check continuous infusions regularly, even when pumps are in good working order, to ensure correct dosing. Place notice above patient's bed to caution I.V. team or laboratory personnel to apply pressure dressings after taking blood.
▼ During intermittent infusion, always draw blood 30 minutes before next scheduled dose to avoid falsely prolonged PTT. Blood for PTT may be drawn 4 hours after continuous I.V. heparin therapy starts. Never draw blood for PTT from the tubing of the heparin infusion or from the infused vein, because falsely prolonged PTT will result. Always draw blood from the opposite arm.
▼ Don't skip a dose or try to "catch up" with a solution containing heparin. If solution runs out, restart it as soon as possible, and reschedule bolus dose immediately. Monitor PTT.
▼ Concentrated heparin solutions (more than 100 units/mL) can irritate blood vessels.
▼ Never piggyback other drugs into an infusion line while heparin infusion is running. Never mix another drug and heparin in same syringe when giving a bolus.
▼ **Incompatibilities:** Alteplase, amiodarone, amphotericin B cholesteryl sulfate complex, caspofungin, ciprofloxacin, doxorubicin, doxycycline hyclate, droperidol, ergotamine, filgrastim, haloperidol, idarubicin, levofloxacin, methotrimeprazine, mitoxantrone, nesiritide, phenytoin sodium, reteplase. For additional information, consult detailed drug reference.

Subcutaneous
● Give low-dose injections sequentially between iliac crests in lower abdomen deep into subcutaneous fat. Inject drug subcutaneously slowly into fat pad.
● Don't massage injection site; watch for signs of bleeding there.
● Alternate sites every 12 hours—right for morning, left for evening. Record location.

ACTION
Accelerates formation of antithrombin III–thrombin complex and deactivates thrombin, preventing conversion of fibrinogen to fibrin.

Route	Onset	Peak	Duration
I.V.	Immediate	Unknown	Variable
Subcut.	20–60 min	2–4 hr	Variable

Half-life: 1 to 2 hours. Half-life is dose-dependent and nonlinear and may be disproportionately prolonged at higher doses.

ADVERSE REACTIONS
CNS: fever.
EENT: rhinitis.

Hematologic: *hemorrhage, overly pro-longed clotting time, thrombocytopenia, white clot syndrome.*
Metabolic: *hyperkalemia,* hypoaldosteronism.
Musculoskeletal: osteoporosis.
Skin: irritation, mild pain, hematoma, ulcer-ation, cutaneous or subcutaneous necrosis, pruritus, urticaria, transient alopecia.
Other: hypersensitivity reactions, including chills; *anaphylactoid reactions.*

INTERACTIONS
Drug-drug. *Antihistamines, digoxin, ni-trates, tetracycline:* May decrease heparin effect. Monitor coagulation tests.
Antiplatelet drugs, salicylates: May increase anticoagulant effect. Use together cau-tiously. Monitor coagulation studies and patient closely.
Nitroglycerin: May decrease effects of heparin. Monitor patient closely.
Oral anticoagulants: May increase additive anticoagulation. Monitor PT, INR, and PTT.
Thrombolytics: May increase risk of hemor-rhage. Monitor patient closely.
Drug-herb. *Alfalfa, angelica (dong quai), anise, bilberry, devil's claw, feverfew, gar-lic, ginger, ginkgo, ginseng, licorice, mead-owsweet, passion flower, red clover, white willow:* May increase risk of bleeding. Dis-courage herb use.
Drug-lifestyle. *Smoking:* May interfere with anticoagulant effect of heparin. Dis-courage smoking.

EFFECTS ON LAB TEST RESULTS
• May increase ALT, AST, and potassium levels.
• May increase INR and prolong PT and PTT. May decrease platelet count.
• Drug may cause false elevations in some tests for thyroxine level.

CONTRAINDICATIONS & CAUTIONS
• Contraindicated in patients hypersensitive to drug. Conditionally contraindicated in pa-tients with active bleeding, blood dyscrasia, or bleeding tendencies, such as hemophilia, thrombocytopenia, history of heparin-induced thrombocytopenia (HIT), or hepatic disease with hypoprothrombinemia; sus-pected intracranial hemorrhage; suppurative thrombophlebitis; inaccessible ulcerative

lesions (especially of GI tract) and open ulcerative wounds; extensive denudation of skin; ascorbic acid deficiency; and other conditions that cause increased capillary permeability.
• Conditionally contraindicated during or after brain, eye, or spinal cord surgery; dur-ing spinal tap or spinal anesthesia; during continuous tube drainage of stomach or small intestine; and in subacute bacterial endocarditis, shock, advanced renal disease, threatened abortion, or severe hypertension.
• Use cautiously in women during menses or after childbirth and in patients with mild hepatic or renal disease, alcoholism, occu-pations with high risk of physical injury, or history of allergies, asthma, or GI ulcerations.
• May reduce bone mineral density with prolonged use (longer than 6 months).
• Use cautiously in women older than age 60 because of an increased risk of bleeding.
Dialyzable drug: Unknown.
⚠ Overdose S&S: Bleeding, nosebleeds, hematuria, tarry stools, easy bruising, pe-techial formations.

PREGNANCY-LACTATION-REPRODUCTION
• Drug doesn't cross placental barrier. Use during pregnancy only if potential benefit justifies potential risk to the fetus.
• Use cautiously in breast-feeding women.
• Use preservative-free formulations (with-out benzyl alcohol) in pregnant and breast-feeding women.

NURSING CONSIDERATIONS
• Although heparin use is clearly hazardous in certain conditions, its risks and benefits must be evaluated.
• If a woman needs anticoagulation during pregnancy, most prescribers use heparin.
❸ Alert: Some commercially available hep-arin injections contain benzyl alcohol. Avoid using these products in neonates and pregnant women if possible.
• Drug requirements are higher in early phases of thrombogenic diseases and febrile states; they are lower when patient's condi-tion stabilizes.
• Elderly patients should usually start at lower dosage.
❸ Alert: Check order and vial carefully; heparin comes in various concentrations. It's

now required that the label clearly state the strength of the entire container followed by how much medication is in 1 mL. Products with both the old and new labels will be available during a transition period.

☻ *Alert:* USP and international units aren't equivalent for heparin.

☻ *Alert:* Heparin, low-molecular-weight heparins, and danaparoid aren't interchangeable.

☻ *Alert:* Don't change concentrations of infusions unless absolutely necessary. This is a common source of dosage errors.

☻ *Alert:* There is the potential for delayed onset of HIT, a serious antibody-mediated reaction resulting from irreversible aggregation of platelets. HIT may progress to the development of venous and arterial thromboses, a condition referred to as heparin-induced thrombocytopenia and thrombosis (HITT). Thrombotic events may be the initial presentation for HITT, which can occur up to several weeks after stopping heparin therapy. Evaluate patients presenting with thrombocytopenia or thrombosis after stopping heparin for HIT and HITT.

• Draw blood for PTT 4 to 6 hours after dose given subcutaneously.

• Avoid I.M. injections of other drugs to prevent or minimize hematoma.

• Measure PTT carefully and regularly. Anticoagulation is present when PTT values are 1½ to 2 times the control values.

• Monitor platelet count regularly. When new thrombosis accompanies thrombocytopenia (white clot syndrome), stop heparin.

• Regularly inspect patient for bleeding gums, bruises on arms or legs, petechiae, nosebleeds, melena, tarry stools, hematuria, and hematemesis.

• Monitor vital signs.

☻ *Alert:* To treat severe overdose, use protamine sulfate (1% solution), a heparin antagonist. Dosage is based on the dose of heparin, its route of administration, and the time since it was given. Generally, 1 mg of protamine neutralizes 100 USP units of heparin. Don't give more than 50 mg protamine in a 10-minute period. Protamine can cause severe hypotension and anaphylactoid reactions. Ensure emergency treatment is available.

• Abrupt withdrawal may cause increased coagulability; warfarin therapy usually overlaps heparin therapy for continuation of prophylaxis or treatment.

• *Look alike–sound alike:* Don't confuse heparin with Hespan. Don't confuse heparin sodium injection 10,000 units/mL and Hep-Lock 10 units/mL.

PATIENT TEACHING

• Instruct patient and family to report all adverse reactions.

• Advise patient and family to watch for signs and symptoms of bleeding or bruising and to notify prescriber immediately if any occur.

• Tell patient to avoid OTC drugs containing aspirin, other salicylates, or drugs that may interact with heparin unless ordered by prescriber.

• Advise patient to consult with prescriber before starting herbal therapy; many herbs have anticoagulant, antiplatelet, or fibrinolytic properties.

hydrALAZINE hydrochloride
hye-DRAL-a-zeen

Apresoline ✤

Therapeutic class: Antihypertensives
Pharmacologic class: Peripheral dilators

AVAILABLE FORMS
Injection: 20 mg/mL in 1-mL vial
Tablets: 10 mg, 25 mg, 50 mg, 100 mg

INDICATIONS & DOSAGES
➤ **Essential hypertension**
Adults: Initially, 10 mg P.O. q.i.d. for the first 2 to 4 days, 25 mg q.i.d. for the balance of the first week; 50 mg q.i.d. from the second week on, based on patient tolerance and response.
Children age 1 and older: Initially, 0.75 mg/kg daily P.O. divided into four doses; gradually increase over 3 to 4 weeks to maximum of 7.5 mg/kg/day in four divided doses or 200 mg/day.
➤ **Severe essential hypertension**
Adults: 20 to 40 mg I.M. or I.V.; repeat as needed. Switch to oral form as soon as possible.

Reactions in bold italics are *life-threatening*. Interactions may have a *rapid onset* or a *delayed onset*.

Children: 1.7 to 3.5 mg/kg/day I.M. or I.V. divided into four to six doses.
➤ **HF ◆**
Adults: Initially, 25 to 50 mg P.O. t.i.d. or q.i.d. in combination with isosorbide dinitrate. Maximum dose is 300 mg daily in divided doses.

ADMINISTRATION
P.O.
● Give drug with food to increase absorption.
I.V.
▼ Give drug as a rapid bolus injection directly into the vein only when the drug can't be given orally. Repeat p.r.n., generally every 4 to 6 hours. It shouldn't be added to infusion solutions.
▼ Drug may discolor upon contact with metal; discolored solutions should be discarded. Use immediately after the vial is opened.
▼ Replace parenteral therapy with oral therapy as soon as possible.
▼ **Incompatibilities:** Aminophylline, ampicillin sodium, chlorothiazide, D$_5$W, dextrose 10% in lactated Ringer solution, dextrose 10% in NSS, diazoxide, doxapram, edetate calcium disodium, ethacrynate, fructose 10% in NSS, fructose 10% in water, furosemide, hydrocortisone sodium succinate, mephentermine, metaraminol bitartrate, methohexital, nitroglycerin, phenobarbital sodium, verapamil.
I.M.
● Switch to oral form as soon as possible.

ACTION
Unknown. A direct-acting peripheral vasodilator that relaxes arteriolar smooth muscle.

Route	Onset	Peak	Duration
P.O.	20–30 min	1–2 hr	2–4 hr
I.V.	5–20 min	10–80 min	2–6 hr
I.M.	10–30 min	1 hr	2–6 hr

Half-life: Oral, 3 to 7 hours; I.V. and I.M., unknown.

ADVERSE REACTIONS
CNS: headache, dizziness.
CV: angina pectoris, palpitations, tachycardia, orthostatic hypotension, edema, flushing.
EENT: nasal congestion, conjunctivitis.

GI: nausea, vomiting, diarrhea, anorexia, constipation, paralytic ileus.
GU: difficult urination.
Hematologic: *neutropenia, leukopenia, agranulocytosis,* eosinophilia, *thrombocytopenia with or without purpura.*
Respiratory: dyspnea.
Skin: rash.

INTERACTIONS
Drug-drug. *Diazoxide, MAO inhibitors:* May cause severe hypotension. Use together cautiously.
Diuretics, other hypotensive drugs: May cause excessive hypotension. Dosage adjustment may be needed.
Indomethacin: May decrease effects of hydralazine. Monitor BP.
Metoprolol, propranolol: May increase levels and effects of these beta blockers. Monitor patient closely. May need to adjust dosage of either drug.
Drug-food. *Any food:* Food may increase drug absorption. Encourage patient to take with food.

EFFECTS ON LAB TEST RESULTS
● May decrease Hb level.
● May decrease neutrophil, WBC, granulocyte, platelet, and RBC counts.
● May cause positive ANA titers.

CONTRAINDICATIONS & CAUTIONS
● Contraindicated in patients hypersensitive to drug.
● Drug may contain tartrazine and cause allergic reactions, especially in patients hypersensitive to aspirin.
● Contraindicated in those with CAD or mitral valvular rheumatic heart disease.
● Use cautiously in patients with suspected cardiac disease, stroke, or severe renal impairment and in those taking other antihypertensives.
● May cause blood dyscrasias. Discontinue drug if they occur..
Dialyzable drug: Unknown.
⚠ *Overdose S&S:* Hypotension, tachycardia, headache, flushing.

PREGNANCY-LACTATION-REPRODUCTION
● Drug crosses the placental barrier and is associated with fetal toxicity in the third

trimester. Use during pregnancy only if expected benefit justifies potential risk to the fetus.

• Use cautiously in breast-feeding women.

NURSING CONSIDERATIONS

• Monitor patient's BP, pulse rate, and body weight frequently. Drug may be given with diuretics and beta blockers to decrease sodium retention and tachycardia and to prevent angina attacks.

• Elderly patients may be more sensitive to drug's hypotensive effects.

• Obtain CBC, lupus erythematosus cell preparation, and ANA titer determination before therapy and periodically during long-term therapy.

🜨 **Alert:** Monitor patient closely for signs and symptoms of lupuslike syndrome (sore throat, fever, muscle and joint aches, rash), and notify prescriber immediately if they develop. Pyridoxine should be given.

• **Look alike–sound alike:** Don't confuse hydralazine with hydroxyzine.

PATIENT TEACHING

• Instruct patient to take oral form with meals to increase absorption.

• Inform patient that low BP and dizziness upon standing can be minimized by rising slowly and avoiding sudden position changes.

• Tell woman of childbearing potential to notify prescriber if she suspects pregnancy. Drug will need to be stopped.

• Tell patient to notify prescriber of all adverse reactions, including unexplained prolonged general tiredness or fever, muscle or joint aching, or chest pain.

---

hydrochlorothiazide
hye-droe-klor-oh-THYE-a-zide

Apo-Hydro🍁, Microzide, Oretic, Urozide🍁

Therapeutic class: Diuretics
Pharmacologic class: Thiazide diuretics

AVAILABLE FORMS
Capsules: 12.5 mg
Tablets: 12.5 mg, 25 mg, 50 mg, 100 mg🍁

INDICATIONS & DOSAGES
Adjust-a-dose (for all indications): In patients older than age 65, 12.5 mg daily initially. Adjust in increments of 12.5 mg, if needed.
➤ **Edema**
Adults: 25 to 100 mg P.O. daily or intermittently.
Children ages 6 months to 12 years: Initially, 1 to 2 mg/kg/day P.O. in a single dose or two divided doses. May increase to a maximum of 37.5 mg/day for children ages 6 months to 2 years and 100 mg/day for children ages 2 to 12 years.
Children younger than age 6 months: May give up to 3 mg/kg/day P.O. in two divided doses.
➤ **Hypertension**
Adults: 12.5 to 50 mg P.O. once daily. Increase or decrease daily dose based on BP.
Children ages 6 months to 12 years: Initially, 1 to 2 mg/kg/day P.O. in a single dose or two divided doses. May increase to a maximum of 37.5 mg/day for children ages 6 months to 2 years and 100 mg/day for children ages 2 to 12 years.
Children younger than age 6 months: May give up to 3 mg/kg/day P.O. in two divided doses.

ADMINISTRATION
P.O.
• To prevent nocturia, give drug in morning. If second dose is needed, give in early afternoon.

ACTION
Increases sodium and water excretion by inhibiting sodium and chloride reabsorption in distal segment of the nephron.

Route	Onset	Peak	Duration
P.O.	2 hr	1–5 hr	6–12 hr

Half-life: 6 to 15 hours.

ADVERSE REACTIONS
CNS: dizziness, vertigo, headache, paresthesia, weakness, restlessness.
CV: orthostatic hypotension, allergic myocarditis, vasculitis.
GI: *pancreatitis,* anorexia, nausea, epigastric distress, vomiting, abdominal pain, diarrhea, constipation.

Reactions in bold italics are *life-threatening*. Interactions may have a *rapid onset* or a *delayed onset*.

GU: *renal failure,* polyuria, frequent urination, interstitial nephritis, erectile dysfunction.

Hematologic: *aplastic anemia, agranulocytosis, leukopenia, thrombocytopenia,* hemolytic anemia.

Hepatic: jaundice.

Metabolic: asymptomatic hyperuricemia; *hypokalemia;* hyperglycemia and impaired glucose tolerance; fluid and electrolyte imbalances, including dilutional hyponatremia and hypochloremia; metabolic alkalosis; hypercalcemia; volume depletion and dehydration.

Musculoskeletal: muscle cramps.

Respiratory: *respiratory distress,* pneumonitis.

Skin: dermatitis, photosensitivity reactions, rash, purpura, alopecia, *erythema multiforme,* exfoliative dermatitis.

Other: *anaphylactic reactions,* hypersensitivity reactions, gout.

INTERACTIONS

Drug-drug. *Amphotericin B, corticosteroids:* May increase risk of hypokalemia. Monitor potassium level closely.

Antidiabetics: May decrease hypoglycemic effects. Adjust dosage if needed. Monitor glucose level.

Antihypertensives: May have additive antihypertensive effect. Use together cautiously.

Barbiturates, opioids: May increase orthostatic hypotensive effect. Monitor patient closely.

Bumetanide, ethacrynic acid, furosemide, torsemide: May cause excessive diuretic response, causing serious electrolyte abnormalities or dehydration. Adjust doses carefully, and monitor patient closely for signs and symptoms of excessive diuretic response.

Cardiac glycosides: May increase risk of digoxin toxicity from diuretic-induced hypokalemia. Monitor potassium and digoxin levels.

Cholestyramine, colestipol: May decrease intestinal absorption of thiazides. Separate doses by 2 hours.

Diazoxide: May increase antihypertensive, hyperglycemic, and hyperuricemic effects. Use together cautiously.

Lithium: May decrease lithium excretion, increasing risk of lithium toxicity. Consider therapy modification.

NSAIDs: May increase risk of renal failure. May decrease diuretic and antihypertensive effects. Monitor renal function and BP.

Drug-herb. *Licorice:* May cause unexpected rapid potassium loss. Discourage use together.

Drug-lifestyle. *Alcohol use:* May increase orthostatic hypotensive effect. Discourage use together.

EFFECTS ON LAB TEST RESULTS

• May increase glucose, cholesterol, triglyceride, calcium, and uric acid levels.

• May decrease potassium, sodium, chloride, serum protein-bound iodine, and Hb levels.

• May decrease granulocyte, WBC, and platelet counts.

CONTRAINDICATIONS & CAUTIONS

• Contraindicated in patients with anuria and patients hypersensitive to other thiazides or other sulfonamide derivatives.

• Drug can cause systemic lupus activation or exacerbation.

• Use cautiously in children and in patients with severe renal disease, impaired hepatic function, or progressive hepatic disease.

Dialyzable drug: Unknown.

⚠ *Overdose S&S:* Electrolyte imbalance, dehydration.

PREGNANCY-LACTATION-REPRODUCTION

• Drug crosses the placental barrier; maternal use may adversely affect fetus.

• Women using thiazide diuretics for treatment of hypertension before pregnancy may continue their use.

• Patient should discontinue breast-feeding or discontinue drug.

NURSING CONSIDERATIONS

• Monitor fluid intake and output, weight, BP, and electrolyte levels; correct electrolyte disturbances before start of therapy.

• Watch for signs and symptoms of hypokalemia, such as muscle weakness and cramps.

• Drug may be used with potassium-sparing diuretic to prevent potassium loss.

• Consult prescriber and dietitian about a high-potassium diet or potassium supplement.

• Monitor creatinine and BUN levels regularly. Cumulative effects of drug may occur with impaired renal function.

• Monitor uric acid level, especially in patients with history of gout.

• Monitor glucose level, especially in diabetic patients.

• Monitor elderly patients, who are especially susceptible to excessive diuresis.

• Stop thiazides and thiazide-like diuretics before parathyroid function tests.

• In patients with hypertension, therapeutic response may be delayed several weeks.

PATIENT TEACHING

• Instruct patient to take drug with food to minimize GI upset.

• Advise patient to take drug in morning to avoid need to urinate at night; if patient needs second dose, have him take it in early afternoon.

• Advise patient to avoid sudden posture changes and to rise slowly to avoid dizziness upon standing quickly.

• Encourage sunblock use to prevent photosensitivity reactions.

• Tell patient to check with prescriber or pharmacist before using OTC drugs.

SAFETY ALERT!

hydrocodone bitartrate
hye-droe-KOE-done

Hysingla ER, Zohydro ER

Therapeutic class: Opioid analgesics
Pharmacologic class: Opioid analgesics
Controlled substance schedule: II

AVAILABLE FORMS

Capsules (extended-release) ⑩: 10 mg, 15 mg, 20 mg, 30 mg, 40 mg, 50 mg
Tablets (extended-release) ⑩: 20 mg, 30 mg, 40 mg, 60 mg, 80 mg, 100 mg, 120 mg

INDICATIONS & DOSAGES

➤ **Management of pain severe enough to require daily, around-the-clock,**

long-term opioid treatment and for which alternative treatment options are inadequate

Adults who are opioid naive or who aren't opioid tolerant: Initially, 10 mg (Zohydro ER) P.O. every 12 hours. Gradually adjust dosage, preferably in increments of 10 mg every 12 hours every 3 to 7 days, until adequate pain relief and acceptable adverse reactions have been achieved. Or, 20 mg (Hysingla ER) P.O. once daily. Increase dosage in increments of 10 to 20 mg once daily every 3 to 5 days as needed to achieve adequate analgesia. Patients who experience breakthrough pain may require a dosage increase or may need a rescue medication.

Adults who are opioid tolerant: Discontinue all other around-the-clock opioids before initiating therapy. Refer to manufacturer's instructions when converting from other oral opioids to Zohydro ER or Hysingla ER; doses aren't equianalgesic.

Adjust-a-dose: In patients with moderate renal impairment to ESRD, start with 50% of the Hysingla ER initial dose or with low Zohydro ER dose and monitor closely. For severe hepatic impairment, start with 10 mg (Zohydro ER) P.O. every 12 hours or use 50% of initial dose of Hysingla ER. Monitor patient closely for adverse events such as respiratory depression. Decrease initial dose in elderly patients, who may be more sensitive to adverse effects.

ADMINISTRATION
P.O.

Black Box Warning Give capsules and tablets whole. Don't crush, dissolve, or allow patient to chew capsules or tablets because of the risk of rapid release and absorption of a potentially fatal dose of hydrocodone. ■

• Administer capsules or tablets one at a time with enough water to ensure complete swallowing immediately after placing in the mouth.

• Store at room temperature.

ACTION

Acts as a full agonist primarily at the mu opioid receptor, binding to and activating opioid receptors at various sites in the CNS to produce analgesia.

Route	Onset	Peak	Duration
P.O. (Hysingla ER)	Unknown	6–30 hr	Unknown
P.O. (Zohydro ER)	Unknown	5 hr	Unknown

Half-life: Hysingla ER, about 7 to 9 hours; Zohydro ER, about 8 hours.

ADVERSE REACTIONS

CNS: somnolence, tremor, lethargy, migraine, paresthesia, anxiety, depression, insomnia, fatigue, dizziness, drowsiness, pyrexia, migraine, pain, paresthesia, sedation.
CV: peripheral edema, hot flashes, hypertension.
EENT: tinnitus, nasopharyngitis, oropharyngeal pain, nasal congestion, sinusitis, dry mouth.
GI: constipation, nausea, vomiting, abdominal pain, GERD, decreased appetite, diarrhea, dyspepsia, viral gastroenteritis.
GU: UTI.
Metabolic: dehydration, *hypokalemia.*
Musculoskeletal: muscle spasms, back pain, foot fracture, joint injury, joint sprain, muscle strain, arthralgia, musculoskeletal pain, myalgia, neck pain, osteoarthritis, extremity pain, noncardiac chest pain, osteoarthritis.
Respiratory: URI, cough, dyspnea.
Skin: pruritus, contusion, skin laceration, hyperhidrosis, night sweats, rash.
Other: fall, flulike syndrome.

INTERACTIONS

Drug-drug. *Anticholinergics:* May increase risk of urine retention, severe constipation, or paralytic ileus. Monitor patient for signs and symptoms of urine retention and constipation in addition to respiratory and CNS depression. Use together cautiously.
Black Box Warning *Benzodiazepines, CNS depressants:* May cause slow or difficult breathing, sedation, and death. Avoid use together. If use together is necessary, limit dosage and duration of each drug to the minimum necessary for desired effect. ■
Black Box Warning *CYP2D6 inhibitors (bupropion, fluoxetine, paroxetine), CYP3A4 inhibitors (amiodarone, erythromycin, ketoconazole, nefazodone, protease inhibitors, ritonavir, telithromycin):* May increase hydrocodone plasma concentration and prolong opioid effects, especially use of CYP3A4 and CYP2D6 inhibitors is

concomitant. Monitor patient for respiratory depression and sedation; consider dosage adjustments until drug effects are stable. ■
Black Box Warning *CYP3A4 inducers (carbamazepine, phenytoin, rifampin):* May induce metabolism and decrease hydrocodone plasma concentration, decreasing efficacy and potentially causing withdrawal symptoms. Monitor patient for effectiveness of drug and for opioid withdrawal symptoms. Consider dosage adjustments until stable. If CYP3A4 inducer is stopped, monitor patient for increased therapeutic and adverse effects, especially respiratory depression. ■
MAO inhibitors: May potentiate effects of opioid analgesics. Don't use in patients who have received MAO inhibitors within past 14 days.
Mixed agonist/antagonists (butorphanol, nalbuphine, pentazocine), partial agonists (buprenorphine): May reduce analgesic effect of hydrocodone or precipitate withdrawal symptoms. Avoid concurrent use.
⊎ Alert: *Serotonergic drugs (amoxapine, antiemetics [dolasetron, granisetron, ondansetron, palonosetron], antimigraine drugs, buspirone, cyclobenzaprine, dextromethorphan, linezolid, lithium, MAO inhibitors, maprotiline, methylene blue, mirtazapine, nefazodone, SNRIs, SSRIs, TCAs, trazodone, tryptophan, vilazodone):* May increase risk of serotonin syndrome. Use together cautiously. Monitor patient for serotonin syndrome.
Drug-herb. **⊎ Alert:** *St. John's wort:* May increase risk of serotonin syndrome. Use together cautiously. Monitor patient for serotonin syndrome.
Drug-lifestyle. **Black Box Warning** *Alcohol use:* May increase hydrocodone plasma level and risk of fatal overdose. Patients shouldn't consume alcoholic beverages or use other drugs that contain alcohol. ■

EFFECTS ON LAB TEST RESULTS
• May increase cholesterol and GGT levels.
• May decrease potassium level.

CONTRAINDICATIONS & CAUTIONS
Black Box Warning Drug exposes patient to risks of addiction, abuse, and misuse even at recommended doses, which can lead to overdose and death. Assess each patient's

risk before prescribing and monitor patients for these behaviors or conditions. ■

Black Box Warning Accidental ingestion of even one dose of this drug, especially by children, can result in a fatal overdose of hydrocodone. ■

Black Box Warning Opioid drugs should only be prescribed with benzodiazepines or other CNS depressants to patients for whom alternative treatment options are inadequate. ■

۰ Alert: Drug should only be prescribed by health care professionals knowledgeable in the use of potent opioids for pain management. Drug should only be used when alternative treatment options are ineffective, not tolerated, or otherwise inadequate to provide sufficient pain management.

۰ Alert: Drug may lead to rare but serious decrease in adrenal gland cortisol production.

۰ Alert: Drug may reduce sex hormone levels with long-term use.

• Contraindicated for use as an as-needed analgesic. Drug should be prescribed in the smallest appropriate quantity.

• Use cautiously in patients with hypersensitivity to morphine, oxycodone, and codeine because cross-reactivity may occur.

• Contraindicated in patients with significant respiratory depression, acute or severe bronchial asthma, known or suspected paralytic ileus, or hypersensitivity to drug or its components.

• Use cautiously in cachectic or debilitated patients; there is potential for crucial respiratory depression even at therapeutic dosages.

• Use cautiously in patients with a history of seizures and adrenal insufficiency.

۰ Alert: When giving first dose, it's preferable to underestimate a patient's 24-hour oral hydrocodone requirements and provide rescue medication (immediate-release opioid) than to overestimate the 24-hour oral hydrocodone requirements, which could result in adverse reactions.

• Use cautiously in patients taking concomitant CNS depressants; in elderly, cachectic, or debilitated patients; and in those with chronic pulmonary disease, seizure disorder, hypotension or depleted blood volume, or hepatic or renal impairment.

۰ Alert: Avoid use in patients with head injuries, increased ICP, brain tumors, impaired consciousness, or coma. Drug reduces respiratory drive, increasing carbon dioxide retention and ICP.

• QTc interval may be prolonged when doses greater than 160 mg daily are used. Use cautiously in patients with HF, bradyarrhythmias, or electrolyte abnormalities, and when patients are using other drugs known to prolong the QTc interval. Don't use in those with congenital long QT syndrome. If QTc-interval prolongation occurs, consider dosage reduction of 33% to 50% or change to another analgesic.

• Esophageal obstruction, dysphagia, and choking have occurred with Hysingla ER use. Patients with underlying GI disorders or with a small GI lumen are at greater risk. Consider another analgesic in these patients.

• Safety and effectiveness in children younger than age 18 haven't been established.

Dialyzable drug: Unknown.

⚠ Overdose S&S: Respiratory depression, somnolence (can lead to stupor or coma), skeletal muscle flaccidity, cold clammy skin, constricted pupils (although mydriasis rather than miosis may occur due to severe hypoxia in overdose situations), pulmonary edema, bradycardia, hypotension, death.

PREGNANCY-LACTATION-REPRODUCTION

• Use in pregnant women only if benefit outweighs risk to the fetus.

Black Box Warning Prolonged use during pregnancy can result in neonatal opioid withdrawal syndrome, which may be life-threatening if not recognized and treated according to protocols developed by neonatology experts. ■

Black Box Warning If opioid use is required for a prolonged period during pregnancy, advise patient of risk of neonatal opioid withdrawal syndrome (poor feeding, diarrhea, irritability, tremor, rigidity, seizures) and assure her that appropriate treatment will be available. ■

• Don't use during labor and delivery; neonatal respiratory depression may occur.

• Opioids may appear in breast milk. Patient should discontinue breast-feeding or discontinue drug.

Reactions in bold italics are **life-threatening**. Interactions may have a *rapid onset* or a **delayed onset**.

• Monitor infants exposed to drug through breast milk for excess sedation and respiratory depression. Also watch for withdrawal symptoms in breast-feeding infants when maternal administration of an opioid analgesic is stopped, or when breast-feeding is stopped.

NURSING CONSIDERATIONS

• Drug may be targeted for theft, diversion, and misuse.

Black Box Warning Monitor patients for respiratory depression, especially within first 24 to 72 hours of drug initiation or after dosage increase. Serious, life-threatening, or fatal respiratory depression may occur. ■

Black Box Warning Monitor patients for abuse or misuse of drug, especially those with a personal or family history of substance abuse (drug or alcohol addiction or abuse, mental illness). Counsel patients about risks and proper use of drug. ■

❸ *Alert:* If patient is taking opioids with serotonergic drugs, watch for signs and symptoms of serotonin syndrome (agitation, hallucinations, rapid HR, fever, excessive sweating, shivering or shaking, muscle twitching or stiffness, trouble with coordination, nausea, vomiting, diarrhea), especially when starting treatment or increasing dosages. Signs and symptoms may occur within several hours of coadministration but may also occur later, especially after dosage increase. Discontinue the opioid, serotonergic drug, or both if serotonin syndrome is suspected.

❸ *Alert:* Monitor patient for signs and symptoms of adrenal insufficiency (nausea, vomiting, loss of appetite, fatigue, weakness, dizziness, low BP). Perform diagnostic testing if adrenal insufficiency is suspected. If adrenal insufficiency is confirmed, treat with corticosteroids and wean patient off opioids if appropriate. Discontinue corticosteroids when clinically appropriate.

❸ *Alert:* Monitor patient for signs and symptoms of decreased sex hormone levels (low libido, erectile dysfunction, amenorrhea, infertility). If signs and symptoms occur, evaluate patient and obtain laboratory testing.

Patients considered opioid tolerant are those receiving, for 1 week or longer, at least 60 mg morphine per day, 25 mcg/hour transdermal fentanyl, 30 mg oral oxycodone per day, 8 mg oral hydromorphone per day or more, 25 mg oral oxymorphone per day or more, or an equianalgesic dose of another opioid.

• Closely monitor patients converting from methadone because methadone has a long half-life and can accumulate in plasma, resulting in significant respiratory depression.

• Closely monitor patients converting from fentanyl patches because of risk of additive effects.

• Elderly patients receiving drug may become confused and oversedated, especially those with impaired hepatic or renal function. Start with low doses of hydrocodone and observe closely for adverse events such as respiratory depression.

• Watch for decreased bowel motility in postoperative patients and for biliary spasm in patients with biliary tract disease or acute pancreatitis.

• Monitor patients with history of seizure disorder for worsening seizure control.

• Use lowest initial dose in patients with renal impairment or severe hepatic impairment, and monitor patients closely for adverse events such as respiratory depression.

❸ *Alert:* Don't stop drug abruptly; withdraw slowly. Gradually titrate downward every 2 to 4 days to prevent signs and symptoms of withdrawal in physically dependent patients. When tapering Hysingla ER dosage, the next dose should be at least 50% of the prior dose. When Hysingla ER dosage has reached 20 mg daily for 2 to 4 days, it may be discontinued. Monitor patients closely for signs and symptoms of opioid withdrawal, such as restlessness, lacrimation, rhinorrhea, yawning, perspiration, chills, myalgia, and mydriasis. Such symptoms may indicate a need to taper more slowly.

• Periodically reevaluate patient's need for therapy.

• *Look alike–sound alike:* Don't confuse hydrocodone ER with hydrocodone standard release. Don't confuse hydrocodone with oxycodone or hydromorphone.

PATIENT TEACHING

Black Box Warning Caution the patient or the caregiver of a patient taking an opioid

---

drug with a benzodiazepine, CNS depressant, or alcohol to seek immediate medical attention if the patient has symptoms of dizziness, light-headedness, extreme sleepiness, slowed or difficult breathing, or unresponsiveness. ∎

Black Box Warning Instruct patient to avoid alcoholic beverages, prescription drugs, and OTC products that contain alcohol during treatment. ∎

Black Box Warning Instruct patient to swallow drug whole to avoid exposure to a potentially fatal dose of hydrocodone. Crushing, chewing, snorting, or injecting the dissolved product allows uncontrolled delivery of drug and may result in overdose and death. ∎

Black Box Warning Inform female patient that prolonged use of drug during pregnancy can result in neonatal opioid withdrawal syndrome, which may be life-threatening. ∎

⊙ *Alert:* Encourage patient to report all medications being taken, including prescription and OTC medications and supplements.

⊙ *Alert:* Caution patient to immediately report signs and symptoms of serotonin syndrome, adrenal insufficiency, and decreased sex hormone levels.

● Caution patient not to share drug and to protect it from theft or misuse.

● Inform patient that potentially serious additive effects may occur if drug is used with other CNS depressants and to avoid such drugs unless supervised by a health care provider.

● Advise patient to report signs and symptoms of respiratory depression (respiratory rate less than 12 breaths/minute, shortness of breath, confusion, excessive drowsiness, nausea, vomiting) and to seek immediate medical attention. Risk of respiratory depression is greatest at drug initiation and dosage increases.

● Warn patient that use of drug, even when taken as recommended, can result in addiction, abuse, and misuse, which can lead to overdose or death. Instruct patient not to discontinue drug without first discussing the need for a tapering regimen with prescriber.

● Caution patient not to drive or operate dangerous machinery unless he knows and is tolerant to drug's effects.

● Warn patient about potential for severe constipation; teach management instructions and when to seek medical attention.

● Inform patient that drug may cause orthostatic hypotension and fainting. Teach how to recognize signs and symptoms of low BP and how to reduce risk of serious consequences of hypotension (e.g., sit or lie down, carefully rise from a sitting or lying position).

● Caution patient to seek medical attention immediately if hypersensitivity reactions, including anaphylaxis, occur.

● Instruct patient to store drug securely and away from children, to dispose of drug properly when no longer needed, and not to throw in regular trash. Accidental ingestion, especially by children, may result in respiratory depression or death.

● Inform patient to dispose of unused capsules through a drug take-back program. If such a program isn't available in patient's area, instruct patient to flush unused capsules down the toilet.

SAFETY ALERT!

hydrocodone bitartrate–acetaminophen
hye-droe-KOE-done/a-seet-a-MIN-a fen

Norco

Therapeutic class: Opioid analgesics
Pharmacologic class: Opioid analgesics–para-aminophenol derivatives
Controlled substance schedule: II

AVAILABLE FORMS
Oral solution*: 7.5 mg hydrocodone/325 mg acetaminophen per 15 mL, 10 mg hydrocodone/300 mg acetaminophen per 15 mL, 10 mg hydrocodone/325 mg acetaminophen per 15 mL
Tablets: 2.5 mg hydrocodone/325 mg acetaminophen, 5 mg hydrocodone/300 mg acetaminophen, 5 mg hydrocodone/325 mg acetaminophen, 7.5 mg hydrocodone/300 mg acetaminophen, 7.5 mg hydrocodone/325 mg acetaminophen, 10 mg hydrocodone/300 mg acetaminophen, 10 mg hydrocodone/325 mg acetaminophen

---

INDICATIONS & DOSAGES

➤ **Moderate to moderately severe pain**
Adults and children age 14 and older: Adjust dosage according to severity of pain and patient response. Give 1 or 2 tablets (hydrocodone 2.5 to 10 mg/acetaminophen 300 to 750 mg) P.O. every 4 to 6 hours or 15 mL P.O. every 4 to 6 hours as needed. Maximum dosage is 60 mg hydrocodone/4,000 mg acetaminophen.
Children ages 2 to 13: 0.135 mg/kg (hydrocodone) P.O. every 4 to 6 hours as needed.
Adjust-a-dose: For patients with chronic alcoholism, limit acetaminophen to 2,000 mg daily. Acetaminophen intake shouldn't exceed 4,000 mg/day in adults and children age 13 and older; 3,200 mg/day for children age 12; 2,400 mg/day for children age 11; 2,000 mg/day for children ages 9 to 10; 1,600 mg/day for children ages 6 to 8; 1,200 mg/day for children ages 4 to 5; and 800 mg/day for children ages 2 to 3.

ADMINISTRATION

P.O.

• Give drug with food or milk.
• Administer oral solution by a calibrated device such as syringe or dropper.
• Only oral solution is approved for pediatric use.

ACTION

Inhibits synthesis of prostaglandins and binds to opiate receptors in CNS and peripherally blocks pain impulse generation; produces antipyresis by direct action on hypothalamic heat-regulating center; causes cough suppression by direct central action in medulla; may produce generalized CNS depression.

Route	Onset	Peak	Duration
P.O. (hydrocodone)	Unknown	1⅓ hr	Unknown
P.O. (acetaminophen)	Unknown	½–2 hr	3–4 hr

Half-life: Hydrocodone, 3.8 hours; acetaminophen, 2 to 3 hours.

ADVERSE REACTIONS

CNS: light-headedness, dizziness, sedation, drowsiness, mental clouding, lethargy, impairment of mental and physical performance, anxiety, fear, dysphoria, psycho-logical dependence, mood changes, *stupor, coma.*
CV: *bradycardia, cardiac arrest, circulatory collapse,* hypotension.
EENT: hearing impairment, permanent hearing loss.
GI: nausea, vomiting, constipation, abdominal pain, gastric distress, heartburn, peptic ulcer.
GU: urethral spasms, spasm of vesical sphincters, urine retention, *renal tubular necrosis,* renal toxicity.
Hematologic: *thrombocytopenia, agranulocytosis,* occult blood loss, hemolytic anemia, iron deficiency anemia, prolonged bleeding time.
Hepatic: *hepatic necrosis, hepatitis,* increased LFT values.
Metabolic: *hypoglycemia, hypoglycemic coma.*
Musculoskeletal: muscle flaccidity.
Respiratory: *respiratory depression, acute airway obstruction,* apnea, dyspnea.
Skin: rash, pruritus, cold clammy skin, diaphoresis.
Other: allergic reaction.

INTERACTIONS

Drug-drug. *Anticholinergics:* May increase risk of paralytic ileus. Avoid use together.
Antidepressants, antihistamines, antipsychotics, anxiolytics, barbiturates or other CNS depressants, other opioids: May produce additive effects. Avoid use together.
Barbiturates, metyrapone, mipomersen: May increase risk of hepatotoxicity from acetaminophen. Monitor therapy.
Carbamazepine, dasatinib, hydantoins, isoniazid: May increase risk of hepatotoxicity from acetaminophen. Use cautiously together. Consider alternative therapy.
MAO inhibitors: May decrease BP or cause additive effects. Avoid use together.
Phenothiazines, TCAs: May increase effect of either antidepressant or hydrocodone. Avoid use together.
 Alert: Serotonergic drugs (amoxapine, antiemetics [dolasetron, granisetron, ondansetron, palonosetron], antimigraine drugs, buspirone, cyclobenzaprine, dextromethorphan, linezolid, lithium, MAO inhibitors, maprotiline, methylene blue, mirtazapine, nefazodone, SNRIs, SSRIs,

H

TCAs, trazodone, tryptophan, vilazodone): May increase risk of serotonin syndrome. Use together cautiously. Monitor patient for serotonin syndrome.

Sodium oxybate: May increase sleep duration and CNS depression. Consider therapy modification.

Drug-herb. *Kava kava, valerian:* May increase risk of excessive sedation. Avoid use together.

↯ Alert: *St. John's wort:* May increase risk of serotonin syndrome. Use together cautiously. Monitor patient for serotonin syndrome.

Drug-lifestyle. *Alcohol use:* May produce additive CNS effects and increase risk of hepatotoxicity. Discourage use together.

EFFECTS ON LAB TEST RESULTS
• May increase amylase and lipase levels.
• Acetaminophen may produce false-positive results on urinary 5-hydroxyindoleacetic acid test.

CONTRAINDICATIONS & CAUTIONS
Black Box Warning Acetaminophen has been associated with acute liver failure, at times resulting in liver transplant and death. Most liver injury has been associated with the use of acetaminophen at doses exceeding 4,000 mg/day, and often involves more than one acetaminophen-containing product. ■

Black Box Warning Opioid drugs should only be prescribed with benzodiazepines or other CNS depressants to patients for whom alternative treatment options are inadequate. ■

↯ Alert: May cause serious, potentially fatal skin reactions, including Stevens-Johnson syndrome, toxic epidermal necrolysis, and acute generalized exanthematous pustulosis. Reaction may occur with first or subsequent use when acetaminophen is used as monotherapy or when it's one component of combination drug therapy. Monitor patient for reddening of the skin, rash, blisters, and detachment of the upper surface of the skin. Stop drug immediately if skin reaction is suspected.

↯ Alert: Patients with any of the following conditions are at increased risk for oversedation and respiratory depression and require

close monitoring: snoring or sleep apnea, first-time opioid use or previous (nonrecent) opioid use, opioid habituation or need for increased opioid doses, need for prolonged general anesthesia or other sedating drugs, preexisting pulmonary or cardiac disease, or thoracic or other surgical incisions that may impair breathing.

• Contraindicated in patients hypersensitive to drug or its components.

• Use cautiously in patients who are allergic to other opioids because cross-sensitivity may occur.

↯ Alert: Drug may lead to rare but serious decrease in adrenal gland cortisol production.

↯ Alert: Drug may reduce sex hormone levels with long-term use.

• Use cautiously in patients with a history of respiratory depression, drug abuse, head injury or increased ICP, acute abdominal conditions, liver disease, recent anesthesia, pulmonary disease, renal impairment, hypothyroidism, Addison disease, or BPH and urethral stricture, and in elderly or debilitated patients and those sensitive to CNS depressants.

• Use cautiously in patients with sulfite sensitivity; drug may contain sodium bisulfite.

Dialyzable drug: Unknown.

⚠ Overdose S&S: Hydrocodone: Loss of consciousness, pinpoint pupils, respiratory depression, stupor, coma, skeletal muscle flaccidity, cold clammy skin, bradycardia, hypotension, apnea, circulatory collapse, cardiac arrest, death. Acetaminophen: Fatal hepatic necrosis, renal tubular necrosis, hypoglycemic coma, thrombocytopenia, nausea, vomiting, diaphoresis, general malaise.

PREGNANCY-LACTATION-REPRODUCTION
↯ Alert: Carefully weigh risks and benefits of using drug during pregnancy. Use only if benefits outweigh risks. May increase risk of respiratory depression and physical dependence in neonates.

• Patient should discontinue breast-feeding or discontinue drug.

NURSING CONSIDERATIONS
• Monitor patients closely for an allergic reaction, particularly those who are allergic to other opioids.

Reactions in bold italics are *life-threatening*. Interactions may have a *rapid onset* or a *delayed onset*.

❗ *Alert:* Carefully monitor vital signs, pain level, respiratory status, and sedation level in all patients receiving opioids, especially those receiving I.V. drugs, even those given postoperatively.

❗ *Alert:* If patient is taking opioids with serotonergic drugs, watch for signs and symptoms of serotonin syndrome (agitation, hallucinations, rapid HR, fever, excessive sweating, shivering or shaking, muscle twitching or stiffness, trouble with coordination, nausea, vomiting, diarrhea), especially when starting treatment or increasing dosages. Signs and symptoms may occur within several hours of coadministration but may also occur later, especially after dosage increase. Discontinue the opioid, serotonergic drug, or both if serotonin syndrome is suspected.

❗ *Alert:* Monitor patient for signs and symptoms of adrenal insufficiency (nausea, vomiting, loss of appetite, fatigue, weakness, dizziness, low BP). Perform diagnostic testing if adrenal insufficiency is suspected. If adrenal insufficiency is confirmed, treat with corticosteroids and wean patient off opioids, if appropriate. Discontinue corticosteroids when clinically appropriate.

❗ *Alert:* Monitor patient for signs and symptoms of decreased sex hormone levels (low libido, erectile dysfunction, amenorrhea, infertility). If signs and symptoms occur, evaluate patient and obtain laboratory testing.

● Monitor patients for signs and symptoms of drug dependence or abuse.

● Monitor respiratory status.

● Monitor patients who have had a head injury.

● Use of opioids in patients with acute abdominal disorders may mask symptoms.

● Constipation is a very common adverse effect. Treat constipation aggressively.

● Monitor liver and kidney function. Acetaminophen elimination may be increased in patients with hepatic impairment.

● Monitor patient's ability to urinate; report urine retention.

● Monitor BP and pulse regularly.

● Make sure to use a calibrated measuring device to administer oral solution.

PATIENT TEACHING

Black Box Warning Caution the patient or the caregiver of a patient taking an opioid drug with a benzodiazepine, CNS depressant, or alcohol to seek immediate medical attention if the patient has symptoms of dizziness, light-headedness, extreme sleepiness, slowed or difficult breathing, or unresponsiveness. ■

● For best results, instruct patient to take drug before pain becomes severe.

● Explain the assessment and monitoring process to patient and family. Instruct them to immediately report if patient has any difficulty breathing or any other signs of a potential adverse opioid-related reaction.

● Inform patient that it's very important to take this medication only as prescribed and, if oral solution is prescribed, to make sure to measure doses accurately using a calibrated device, such as a dropper or a syringe.

● Caution patient that this medication can be habit forming and that a tolerance to the dose may develop. Explain that drug is for short-term use only.

● Advise patient that this medication may impair judgment and not to operate heavy machinery or drive until the drug's effects are known.

● Instruct patient to avoid alcohol while taking this medication.

Black Box Warning Warn patient that this medicine contains acetaminophen (or Tylenol). Caution patient not to take more than 4,000 mg of acetaminophen on a daily basis (including from all medications being taken). Instruct patient to contact health care provider if he has taken more than 4,000 mg in a day, even if he is feeling well. ■

❗ *Alert:* Encourage patient to report all medications being taken, including prescription and OTC medications and supplements.

❗ *Alert:* Caution patient to immediately report signs and symptoms of serotonin syndrome, adrenal insufficiency, and decreased sex hormone levels.

● Teach patient to eat a high-fiber diet, drink plenty of fluids, and use a stool softener or bulk laxative to prevent constipation.

● Tell patient to stop drug and immediately report blurred vision, rash, or yellowing of the skin.

❗ *Alert:* Warn patient to stop drug and seek medical attention immediately if rash or reaction occurs while using acetaminophen.

hydrocortisone (oral, injection, rectal)
hye-droe-KOR-ti-sone

Colocort, Cortef, Cortenema

hydrocortisone cypionate
Cortef

hydrocortisone sodium succinate
A-Hydrocort, Solu-Cortef

Therapeutic class: Corticosteroids
Pharmacologic class: Glucocorticoids

AVAILABLE FORMS
hydrocortisone
Enema: 100 mg/60 mL
Tablets: 5 mg, 10 mg, 20 mg
hydrocortisone cypionate
Tablets: 5 mg, 10 mg, 20 mg
hydrocortisone sodium succinate
Injection*: 100-mg vial, 250-mg vial, 500-mg vial, 1,000-mg vial

INDICATIONS & DOSAGES
➤ **Rheumatic disorders (adjunctive therapy for short-term administration in psoriatic arthritis, RA, including juvenile RA, ankylosing spondylitis, acute and subacute bursitis, acute nonspecific tenosynovitis, acute gouty arthritis, posttraumatic osteoarthritis, synovitis of osteoarthritis, epicondylitis)**
Adults: 20 to 240 mg P.O. daily. Or, initially, 100 to 500 mg succinate I.M. or I.V.; repeat every 2, 4, or 6 hours as needed.
➤ **Collagen diseases (systemic lupus erythematosus, acute rheumatic carditis, systemic dermatomyositis)**
Adults: 20 to 240 mg P.O. daily. Or, initially, 100 to 500 mg succinate I.M. or I.V.; repeat every 2, 4, or 6 hours as needed.
➤ **Dermatologic diseases (pemphigus, bullous dermatitis herpetiformis, severe erythema multiforme [Stevens-Johnson syndrome], exfoliative dermatitis, mycosis fungoides, severe psoriasis, severe seborrheic dermatitis)**
Adults: 20 to 240 mg P.O. daily. Or, initially, 100 to 500 mg succinate I.M. or I.V.; repeat every 2, 4, or 6 hours as needed.

➤ **Severe or intractable allergic states (seasonal or perennial allergic rhinitis, bronchial asthma, contact dermatitis, atopic dermatitis, serum sickness, drug hypersensitivity reactions, transfusion reactions)**
Adults: 20 to 240 mg P.O. daily. Or, initially, 100 to 500 mg succinate I.M. or I.V.; repeat every 2, 4, or 6 hours as needed.
➤ **Severe acute and chronic allergic and inflammatory processes involving the eye and its adnexa (allergic conjunctivitis, keratitis, allergic corneal marginal ulcers, herpes zoster ophthalmicus, iritis and iridocyclitis, chorioretinitis, anterior segment inflammation, diffuse posterior uveitis and choroiditis, optic neuritis, sympathetic ophthalmia)**
Adults: 20 to 240 mg P.O. daily. Or, initially, 100 to 500 mg succinate I.M. or I.V.; repeat every 2, 4, or 6 hours as needed.
➤ **Respiratory diseases (symptomatic sarcoidosis, Loeffler syndrome not manageable by other means, berylliosis, fulminating or disseminated pulmonary TB when used concurrently with appropriate antituberculous chemotherapy, aspiration pneumonitis)**
Adults: 20 to 240 mg P.O. daily. Or, initially, 100 to 500 mg succinate I.M. or I.V.; repeat every 2, 4, or 6 hours as needed.
➤ **Hematologic disorders (ITP in adults [I.M. form is contraindicated], secondary thrombocytopenia in adults, acquired [autoimmune] hemolytic anemia, erythroblastopenia, congenital [erythroid] hypoplastic anemia)**
Adults: 20 to 240 mg P.O. daily. Or, initially, 100 to 500 mg succinate I.M. or I.V.; repeat every 2, 4, or 6 hours as needed.
➤ **Neoplastic diseases (palliative management of leukemias and lymphomas in adults and acute leukemia of childhood)**
Adults: 20 to 240 mg P.O. daily. Or, initially, 100 to 500 mg succinate I.M. or I.V.; repeat every 2, 4, or 6 hours as needed.
Children: 0.56 to 8 mg/kg/day I.V. or I.M. in three or four divided doses.
➤ **Edematous states (to induce diuresis or remission of proteinuria in nephrotic syndrome, without uremia, of the idiopathic type or that is due to lupus erythematosus)**

Reactions in bold italics are *life-threatening*. Interactions may have a *rapid onset* or a *delayed onset*.

Adults: 20 to 240 mg P.O. daily. Or, initially, 100 to 500 mg succinate I.M. or I.V.; repeat every 2, 4, or 6 hours as needed.

➤ **Ulcerative colitis, regional enteritis**
Adults: 20 to 240 mg P.O. daily. Or, initially, 100 to 500 mg succinate I.M. or I.V.; repeat every 2, 4, or 6 hours as needed.

➤ **Nervous system disorders (acute exacerbations of MS, cerebral edema associated with brain tumors or craniotomy [I.V.], tuberculous meningitis with subarachnoid block or impending block when used concurrently with appropriate antituberculotics, trichinosis with neurologic or myocardial involvement)**
Adults: 20 to 240 mg P.O. daily. Or, initially, 100 to 500 mg succinate I.M. or I.V.; repeat every 2, 4, or 6 hours as needed.

➤ **Severe inflammation**
Adults: 20 to 240 mg P.O. daily. Or, initially, 100 to 500 mg succinate I.M. or I.V.; repeat every 2, 4, or 6 hours as needed.

➤ **Endocrine disorders (adrenal insufficiency, congenital adrenal hyperplasia, nonsuppurative thyroiditis, hypercalcemia associated with cancer)**
Adults: 20 to 240 mg P.O. daily. Or, initially, 100 to 500 mg succinate I.M. or I.V.; repeat every 2, 4, or 6 hours as needed.

➤ **Adjunctive treatment for ulcerative colitis and proctitis**
Adults: 1 enema (100 mg) P.R. nightly for 21 days. Or, 1 applicatorful (90-mg foam) P.R. daily or b.i.d. for 14 to 21 days.

ADMINISTRATION
P.O.
● Give drug with milk or food when possible. Patient may need another drug to prevent GI irritation.
I.V.
▼ Don't use acetate form for I.V. route.
▼ Reconstitute hydrocortisone sodium succinate with no more than 2 mL bacteriostatic water or bacteriostatic saline solution before adding to I.V. solutions. For direct injection, inject over 30 seconds to 10 minutes. For infusion, dilute with D_5W, NSS, or dextrose 5% in NSS to 1 mg/mL or less. Give intermittent I.V. infusion over 20 to 30 minutes.

▼ **Incompatibilities:** Solutions other than D_5W, NSS, or dextrose 5% in NSS, and other drugs.
I.M.
● Inject deep into gluteal muscle. Rotate injection sites to prevent muscle atrophy. Avoid subcutaneous injection because atrophy and sterile abscesses may occur.
● Injectable forms aren't used for alternate-day therapy.
Rectal
● Have patient lie on his left side during administration and for 30 minutes afterward to allow fluid to distribute throughout the left colon. Have patient try to retain the enema for at least 1 hour but preferably all night.

ACTION
Not clearly defined. Decreases inflammation, mainly by stabilizing leukocyte lysosomal membranes; suppresses immune response; stimulates bone marrow; and influences protein, fat, and carbohydrate metabolism.

Route	Onset	Peak	Duration
P.O.	Variable	1 hr	Variable
I.V., I.M., P.R.	Variable	Variable	Variable

Half-life: Oral, 100 minutes; I.V., I.M., and P.R., 8 to 12 hours.

ADVERSE REACTIONS
CNS: euphoria, insomnia, psychotic behavior, *pseudotumor cerebri,* vertigo, mood swings, headache, paresthesia, *seizures.*
CV: *HF,* hypertension, edema, *arrhythmias,* thrombophlebitis, *thromboembolism.*
EENT: cataracts, glaucoma.
GI: peptic ulceration, GI irritation, increased appetite, *pancreatitis,* nausea, vomiting.
GU: menstrual irregularities, increased urine calcium levels.
Hematologic: easy bruising.
Metabolic: *hypokalemia,* hyperglycemia, carbohydrate intolerance, hypercholesterolemia, *hypocalcemia.*
Musculoskeletal: growth suppression in children, muscle weakness, osteoporosis, tendon rupture.
Skin: hirsutism, delayed wound healing, acne, skin eruptions.

H

Other: cushingoid state, susceptibility to infections, *acute adrenal insufficiency after increased stress or abrupt withdrawal after long-term therapy.*

After abrupt withdrawal: rebound inflammation, fatigue, weakness, arthralgia, fever, dizziness, lethargy, depression, fainting, orthostatic hypotension, dyspnea, anorexia, *hypoglycemia. After prolonged use, sudden withdrawal may be fatal.*

INTERACTIONS

Drug-drug. *Antidiabetic agents:* May diminish antidiabetic therapeutic effects. Monitor therapy.

Aspirin, indomethacin, other NSAIDs: May increase risk of GI distress and bleeding. Use together cautiously.

Barbiturates, carbamazepine, fosphenytoin, phenytoin, rifampin: May decrease corticosteroid effect. Increase corticosteroid dosage.

Cyclosporine: May increase toxicity. Monitor patient closely.

Ketoconazole, troleandomycin: May decrease clearance of hydrocortisone. Titrate hydrocortisone dosage to avoid steroid toxicity.

Live attenuated virus vaccines, other toxoids and vaccines: May decrease antibody response and increase risk of neurologic complications. Avoid using together.

Oral anticoagulants: May alter dosage requirements. Monitor PT and INR closely.

Potassium-depleting drugs (thiazide diuretics): May enhance potassium-wasting effects of hydrocortisone. Monitor potassium level.

Skin-test antigens: May decrease response. Postpone skin testing until after therapy.

Drug-herb. *Echinacea, ginseng:* May increase immune-stimulating effects. Discourage use together.

EFFECTS ON LAB TEST RESULTS

● May increase glucose and cholesterol levels. May decrease T_3, T_4, potassium, and calcium levels.

● May cause decreased ^{131}I uptake and protein-bound iodine levels in thyroid function tests. May cause false-negative results in nitroblue tetrazolium test for systemic bacterial infections. May alter reactions to coccidioidin skin tests.

CONTRAINDICATIONS & CAUTIONS

● Contraindicated in patients hypersensitive to drug or its ingredients, in those with systemic fungal infections, and in those receiving immunosuppressive doses together with live-virus vaccines.

● Use with caution in patients with recent MI.

● Use cautiously in patients with GI ulcer, renal disease, hypertension, osteoporosis, diabetes mellitus, hypothyroidism, cirrhosis, diverticulitis, nonspecific ulcerative colitis, active hepatitis, recent intestinal anastomoses, thromboembolic disorders, seizures, myasthenia gravis, HF, TB, ocular herpes simplex, emotional instability, and psychotic tendencies.

● Kaposi sarcoma has been reported. Clinical remission is possible once corticosteroids are discontinued.

Dialyzable drug: Unknown.

PREGNANCY-LACTATION-REPRODUCTION

● Use cautiously in pregnant and breastfeeding women. When essential during pregnancy, use lowest possible dose for the shortest duration. Avoid high doses in first trimester.

● Steroids may alter the motility and number of sperm in some patients.

NURSING CONSIDERATIONS

● Determine whether patient is sensitive to other corticosteroids.

● Most adverse reactions to corticosteroids are dose- or duration-dependent.

● For better results and less toxicity, give a once-daily dose in morning.

❸ *Alert:* Salts aren't interchangeable.

❸ *Alert:* Only hydrocortisone sodium succinate can be given I.V.

❸ *Alert:* Epidural corticosteroid injections to treat neck and back pain and radiating pain in the arms and legs may result in rare but serious adverse events (vision loss, stroke, paralysis, death). The use of epidural corticosteroid injections isn't approved by the FDA.

● Enema may produce same systemic effects as other forms of hydrocortisone. If enema therapy must exceed 21 days, taper off by giving every other night for 2 to 3 weeks.

● High-dose therapy usually isn't continued beyond 48 hours.

Reactions in bold italics are *life-threatening*. Interactions may have a *rapid onset* or a *delayed onset*.

- Always adjust to lowest effective dose.
- Monitor patient's weight, BP, and electrolyte levels.
- Monitor patient for cushingoid effects, including moon face, buffalo hump, central obesity, thinning hair, hypertension, and increased susceptibility to infection.
- Unless contraindicated, give a low-sodium diet that's high in potassium and protein. Give potassium supplements.
- Drug may mask or worsen infections, including latent amebiasis.
- Stress (fever, trauma, surgery, and emotional problems) may increase adrenal insufficiency. Increase dosage.
- Watch for depression or psychotic episodes, especially during high-dose therapy.
- Inspect patient's skin for petechiae.
- Diabetic patient may need increased insulin; monitor glucose level.
- Periodic measurement of growth and development may be needed during high-dose or prolonged therapy in children.
- Elderly patients may be more susceptible to osteoporosis with prolonged use.
- Gradually reduce dosage after long-term therapy.
- *Look alike–sound alike:* Don't confuse Solu-Cortef with Solu-Medrol. Don't confuse hydrocortisone with hydroxychloroquine.

PATIENT TEACHING
- Tell patient not to stop drug abruptly or without prescriber's consent.
- Instruct patient to take oral form of drug with milk or food.
- Warn patient on long-term therapy about cushingoid effects (moon face, buffalo hump) and the need to notify prescriber about sudden weight gain or swelling.
- Teach patient signs and symptoms of early adrenal insufficiency: fatigue, muscle weakness, joint pain, fever, anorexia, nausea, shortness of breath, dizziness, and fainting.
- Instruct patient to carry a card with his prescriber's name and name and dosage of drug, indicating his need for supplemental systemic glucocorticoids during stress.
- Warn patient about easy bruising.
- Urge patient receiving long-term therapy to consider exercise or physical therapy. Also, tell him to ask prescriber about vitamin D or calcium supplement.

- Advise patient receiving long-term therapy to have periodic eye examinations.
- Caution patient to avoid exposure to infections (such as chickenpox or measles) and to notify prescriber if such exposure occurs.
- **Alert:** Counsel patient who receives epidural corticosteroid injections to seek immediate medical attention for vision loss or vision changes; tingling in the arms or legs; sudden weakness or numbness of the face, arm, or leg on one or both sides of the body; dizziness; severe headache; or seizures.
- **Alert:** Advise patient that before undergoing epidural corticosteroid injection, to discuss benefits and risks along with other possible treatments with health care provider.

H

hydrocortisone (topical)
hye-droe-KOR-ti-sone

Ala-Cort, Ala-Scalp, Anusol HC, Cortizone-5 ◊, Cortizone-10 ◊, Nutracort, Procort ◊, Scalpicin ◊, Synacort ◊, Texacort

hydrocortisone acetate (topical, rectal)
Anusol HC ◊, Cortaid ◊, Corticaine ◊, Cortifoam, Gynecort 10 ◊, Micort-HC, ProctoFoam-HC, U-cort

hydrocortisone butyrate
Locoid, Locoid Lipocream

hydrocortisone probutate
Pandel

hydrocortisone valerate

Therapeutic class: Corticosteroids
Pharmacologic class: Corticosteroids

AVAILABLE FORMS
hydrocortisone
Cream: 0.5% ◊, 1%, 2.5% ◊
Gel: 1%, 2%
Lotion: 0.25%, 0.5% ◊, 1% ◊, 1%, 2%, 2.5% ◊
Ointment: 0.5% ◊, 1%, 2.5% ◊
Rectal cream: 1%, 2.5% ◊
Rectal ointment: 1%
Topical solution: 1%, 2.5%

---

hydrocortisone acetate
Cream: 0.5% ◇, 1% ◇, 1%, 2%, 2.5% ◇
Lotion: 0.5%
Ointment: 0.5% ◇, 1% ◇
Rectal foam: 90 mg per application
Rectal suppositories: 25 mg
hydrocortisone butyrate
Cream: 0.1%
Ointment: 0.1%
Solution: 0.1%
hydrocortisone probutate
Cream: 0.1%
hydrocortisone valerate
Cream: 0.2%
Ointment: 0.2%

INDICATIONS & DOSAGES
➤ **Inflammation and pruritus from corticosteroid-responsive dermatoses, adjunctive topical management of seborrheic dermatitis of scalp**
Adults and children: Clean area; apply cream, gel, lotion, ointment, or topical solution sparingly daily to q.i.d. until acute phase is controlled; then reduce dosage to one to three times weekly as needed. Give children lowest dose that provides positive results.
➤ **Inflammation from proctitis; adjunctive treatment of chronic ulcerative colitis, cryptitis**
Adults: 1 applicatorful of rectal foam P.R. daily or b.i.d. for 2 to 3 weeks; then every other day as needed. Or, 1 suppository P.R. b.i.d. to t.i.d. or 2 suppositories P.R. b.i.d. for 2 weeks. In factitial proctitis, recommended duration of therapy is 6 to 8 weeks.

ADMINISTRATION
Rectal
● Refer to manufacturer's instructions to properly fill applicator barrel.
● Once applicator is properly filled, gently insert tip into anus. Once in place, push plunger to expel foam; then withdraw applicator.
● Thoroughly clean all applicator parts after each use.
● Avoid excessive handling of suppository, which is designed to melt at body temperature.
● Insert suppository, pointed end first, into rectum using gentle pressure.

Topical
● Gently wash skin before applying. To prevent skin damage, rub in gently, leaving a thin coat. When treating hairy sites, part hair and apply directly to lesions.
● Check individual products for frequency of administration.
● Avoid applying near eyes or mucous membranes or in ear canal; may be safely used on face, groin, armpits, and under breasts.
● Change dressing as prescribed. Stop drug and tell prescriber if skin infection, striae, or atrophy occurs.
● Continue treatment for a few days after lesions clear.

ACTION
Unclear. Diffuses across cell membranes to form complexes with cytoplasmic receptors, showing anti-inflammatory, antipruritic, vasoconstrictive, and antiproliferative activity. Considered a low-potency (hydrocortisone, hydrocortisone acetate) and a medium-potency (hydrocortisone butyrate, hydrocortisone probutate, hydrocortisone valerate) drug, according to vasoconstrictive properties.

Route	Onset	Peak	Duration
Topical, P.R.	Unknown	Unknown	Unknown

Half-life: Unknown.

ADVERSE REACTIONS
Topical
GU: glycosuria.
Metabolic: hyperglycemia.
Skin: burning, pruritus, irritation, dryness, erythema, folliculitis, hypertrichosis, hypopigmentation, acneiform eruptions, allergic contact dermatitis, atrophy, maceration, secondary infection, striae, miliaria with occlusive dressings.
Other: *HPA axis suppression,* Cushing syndrome.
Rectal
CNS: *seizures, increased ICP,* vertigo, headache.
CV: hypertension.
EENT: cataracts, glaucoma.
GI: peptic ulcer, *pancreatitis,* abdominal distention.
GU: menstrual irregularities.

Reactions in bold italics are *life-threatening*. Interactions may have a *rapid onset* or a *delayed onset*.

Metabolic: fluid or electrolyte disturbances, decreased carbohydrate tolerance.
Musculoskeletal: muscle weakness, osteoporosis, necrosis and fractures in bone.
Skin: impaired wound healing, fragile skin, petechiae, erythema, sweating.

INTERACTIONS
None significant.

EFFECTS ON LAB TEST RESULTS
● May increase glucose level.

CONTRAINDICATIONS & CAUTIONS
● Contraindicated in patients hypersensitive to drug or its components.
● Don't use as monotherapy in primary bacterial infections (impetigo, paronychia, erysipelas, cellulitis, angular cheilitis), treatment of rosacea, perioral dermatitis, or acne.
● Drug isn't for ophthalmic use.
Dialyzable drug: Unknown.
⚠ *Overdose S&S:* Systemic effects.

PREGNANCY-LACTATION-REPRODUCTION
● There are no well-controlled studies in pregnant women. Use during pregnancy only if potential benefit justifies potential risk to the fetus.
● Use cautiously in breast-feeding women.

NURSING CONSIDERATIONS
● If an occlusive dressing is applied and a fever develops, notify prescriber and remove dressing.
● If antifungal or antibiotic combined with corticosteroid fails to provide prompt improvement, stop corticosteroid until infection is controlled.
● Systemic absorption is likely with use of occlusive dressings, prolonged treatment, or extensive body surface treatment. Watch for symptoms, such as hyperglycemia, glycosuria, and HPA axis suppression.
● Avoid using plastic pants or tight-fitting diapers on treated areas in young children. Children may absorb larger amounts of drug and be more susceptible to systemic toxicity.
● Monitor patient for fluid or electrolyte disturbances (sodium and fluid retention, potassium loss, hypokalemic alkalosis,

negative nitrogen balance from catabolism of protein).
● Drug may suppress skin reaction testing.
● ***Look alike–sound alike:*** Don't confuse hydrocortisone with hydroxychloroquine.

PATIENT TEACHING
● Teach patient or family member how to apply drug.
● Tell patient to wash hands after application.
● If an occlusive dressing is ordered, advise patient to leave it in place for no longer than 12 hours each day and not to use the dressing on infected or weeping lesions.
● Teach patient how to use rectal foam applicator or suppository if needed.
● Tell patient to stop drug and report signs of systemic absorption, skin irritation or ulceration, hypersensitivity, infection, or lack of improvement.
● For perianal application, instruct patient to place small amount of drug on a tissue and gently rub in.
● Tell patient to disassemble applicator and clean with warm water after each use.
● Tell patient to stop using this product if condition worsens or if symptoms persist for more than 7 days.

SAFETY ALERT!

hydromorphone hydrochloride (dihydromorphinone hydrochloride)
hye-droe-MOR-fone

Dilaudid, Dilaudid-HP, Exalgo

Therapeutic class: Opioid analgesics
Pharmacologic class: Opioids
Controlled substance schedule: II

AVAILABLE FORMS
Injection: 1 mg/mL, 2 mg/mL, 4 mg/mL, 10 mg/mL
Lyophilized powder for injection: 10 mg/mL
Oral liquid: 5 mg/5 mL
Tablets: 2 mg, 4 mg, 8 mg ⊜
Tablets (extended-release) ⊜: 8 mg, 12 mg, 16 mg, 32 mg

INDICATIONS & DOSAGES

➤ **Moderate to severe pain**

Adults: For opioid-naive patients, 2 to 4 mg immediate-release tablets P.O. every 4 to 6 hours p.r.n. Or, 0.8 to 1 mg I.M. or subcutaneously every 3 to 4 hours or 0.2 to 0.6 mg I.V. (slowly over at least 2 to 5 minutes) every 2 to 3 hours p.r.n. Or, 2.5 to 10 mg oral liquid every 3 to 6 hours p.r.n. Or, for opioid-tolerant adults currently on immediate-release hydromorphone who require continuous analgesia for an extended period, starting dose of extended-release form is equivalent to total daily dose of immediate-release form. May increase every 3 to 4 days.

Adjust-a-dose: For elderly patients, use with caution and reduce initial oral starting dose. Initial I.V. starting dose for elderly or debilitated patients should be 0.2 mg. For those with moderate renal impairment, reduce dose to 50% of usual starting dose. For those with renal or hepatic impairment, reduce dose to 25% to 50% of usual starting dose. Use an alternative analgesic for those with severe hepatic impairment.

ADMINISTRATION

P.O.

● Give drug with food if GI upset occurs.

Black Box Warning Patient should swallow extended-release tablets whole; don't break, chew, dissolve, crush, or inject them. ∎

Black Box Warning Don't give extended-release tablets with other extended-release opioids. ∎

I.V.

▼ Reconstitute powder for solution immediately before use with 25 mL of sterile water for injection.

▼ Give by direct injection over no less than 2 minutes.

▼ Respiratory depression and hypotension can occur. Give slowly, and monitor patient constantly. Keep resuscitation equipment available.

▼ **Incompatibilities:** Alkalies, amphotericin B cholesteryl complex, ampicillin sodium, bromides, cefazolin, dexamethasone, diazepam, gallium nitrate, haloperidol, heparin sodium, iodides, minocycline, phenobarbital sodium, phenytoin sodium, prochlorperazine edisylate, sargramostim, sodium bicarbonate, sodium phosphate, thiopental.

I.M.

● Document administration site.

Subcutaneous

● Rotate injection sites to avoid induration with subcutaneous injection.

ACTION

Unknown. Binds with opioid receptors in the CNS, altering perception of and emotional response to pain. Also suppresses the cough reflex by direct action on the cough center in the medulla.

Route	Onset	Peak	Duration
P.O.	15–30 min	30–60 min	4–5 hr
P.O. (extended-release)	15–30 min	12–16 hr	18–24 hr
I.V.	10–15 min	15–30 min	2–3 hr
I.M.	15 min	30–60 min	4–5 hr
Subcut.	15 min	30–90 min	4 hr

Half-life: 2½ to 4 hours; P.O. (extended-release), 11 hours.

ADVERSE REACTIONS

CNS: sedation, somnolence, dizziness, euphoria, light-headedness, insomnia, drug withdrawal syndrome (extended-release form), headache, confusion.

CV: *cardiac arrest,* hypotension, flushing, *bradycardia,* chest discomfort, edema.

EENT: blurred vision, diplopia, nystagmus.

GI: nausea, vomiting, constipation, anorexia, weight loss, diarrhea, ileus, dry mouth, abdominal pain, biliary colic, taste alterations.

GU: urine retention.

Musculoskeletal: arthralgia, muscle contractions.

Respiratory: *apnea, respiratory depression, bronchospasm.*

Skin: diaphoresis, pruritus, hyperhidrosis.

Other: induration with repeated subcutaneous injections, physical dependence, pain.

INTERACTIONS

Drug-drug. *Anticholinergics:* May increase risk of urine retention or severe constipation. Use together cautiously.

Antipsychotics: May enhance opioid analgesic effects. Monitor therapy.

Reactions in bold italics are *life-threatening*. Interactions may have a *rapid onset* or a *delayed onset*.

Black Box Warning *Benzodiazepines, CNS depressants:* May cause slow or difficult breathing, sedation, and death. Avoid use together. If use together is necessary, limit dosage and duration of each drug to the minimum necessary for desired effect. ■

Droperidol, general anesthetics, minocycline, nabilone, neuromuscular blockers, other opioid analgesics, TCAs, tranquilizers: May cause additive effects. Monitor therapy carefully.

MAO inhibitors: May cause respiratory and CNS depression. Use together isn't recommended and use of extended-release tablets within 14 days of MAO inhibitors isn't recommended. If coadministration of extended-release form and MAO inhibitors is unavoidable, monitor patient carefully for respiratory and CNS depression.

✪ Alert: *Serotonergic drugs (amoxapine, antiemetics [dolasetron, granisetron, ondansetron, palonosetron], antimigraine drugs, buspirone, cyclobenzaprine, dextromethorphan, linezolid, lithium, MAO inhibitors, maprotiline, methylene blue, mirtazapine, nefazodone, SNRIs, SSRIs, TCAs, trazodone, tryptophan, vilazodone):* May increase risk of serotonin syndrome. Use together cautiously and monitor patient for serotonin syndrome.

Drug-herb. *Gotu kola, kava kava, valerian:* May increase CNS depression. Avoid use together.

✪ Alert: *St. John's wort:* May increase risk of serotonin syndrome. Use together cautiously and monitor patient for serotonin syndrome.

Drug-lifestyle. **Black Box Warning** *Alcohol use:* May cause additive effects. Discourage use together. ■

EFFECTS ON LAB TEST RESULTS

• May increase amylase and lipase levels.
• May interfere with hepatobiliary imaging studies because delayed gastric emptying and contraction of sphincter of Oddi may increase biliary tract pressure.

CONTRAINDICATIONS & CAUTIONS

Black Box Warning Opioid drugs should only be prescribed with benzodiazepines or other CNS depressants to patients for whom alternative treatment options are inadequate. ■

• Contraindicated in patients hypersensitive to drug; in those with intracranial lesions that cause increased ICP; in those with paralytic ileus or narrowed or obstructed GI tract; for obstetric analgesia; and in those with depressed ventilation, such as in status asthmaticus, COPD, cor pulmonale, emphysema, and kyphoscoliosis.

Black Box Warning Extended-release form is contraindicated in opioid-naive patients. It isn't indicated for acute pain or postoperative pain or as a p.r.n. analgesic. Fatal respiratory depression may occur in patients who aren't opioid-tolerant. Accidental intake, especially in children, can cause fatal hydromorphone overdose. ■

Black Box Warning Hydromorphone is an opioid agonist with an abuse liability similar to other opioid agonists, legal or illicit. Risk of abuse is increased in patients with a personal or family history of substance abuse or mental illness. Use with ethanol, other opioids, and other CNS depressants can increase risk of adverse events, including death. ■

✪ Alert: Patients with any of the following conditions are at increased risk for oversedation and respiratory depression and require close monitoring: snoring or sleep apnea; first-time opioid use or previous (nonrecent) opioid use; opioid habituation or need for increased opioid doses; need for prolonged general anesthesia or other sedating drugs; preexisting pulmonary or cardiac disease; or thoracic or other surgical incisions that may impair breathing.

✪ Alert: Drug may lead to rare but serious decrease in adrenal gland cortisol production.

✪ Alert: Drug may reduce sex hormone levels with long-term use.

• Use with caution in elderly or debilitated patients and in those with hepatic or renal disease, hypothyroidism, Addison disease, prostatic hyperplasia, or urethral stricture.

Dialyzable drug: Unknown.

⚠ Overdose S&S: Constricted pupils, cold clammy skin, extreme somnolence progressing to stupor or coma, respiratory depression, skeletal muscle flaccidity, bradycardia, hypotension, apnea, cardiac arrest, circulatory collapse, death.

PREGNANCY-LACTATION-REPRODUCTION

❸ *Alert:* Drug crosses placental barrier. Carefully weigh benefits and risks of using drug during pregnancy.

Black Box Warning Use in pregnancy can cause neonatal withdrawal syndrome, which can be life-threatening, and requires management by neonatology experts. Advise women of the risk and ensure appropriate treatment is available. ∎

● Drug appears in breast milk in low concentrations. Breast-feeding infants exposed to large doses of opioids should be monitored for apnea and sedation.

● Long-term use can cause hypogonadism and infertility.

NURSING CONSIDERATIONS

❸ *Alert:* Vial stopper may contain latex.

● Reassess patient's level of pain at least 15 and 30 minutes after administration.

● For better analgesic effect, give drug on a regular schedule, before patient has intense pain.

Black Box Warning Routinely monitor all patients for signs and symptoms of misuse, abuse, and addiction during treatment. ∎

Black Box Warning Dilaudid-HP, a highly concentrated form (10 mg/mL), may be given in smaller volumes to prevent the discomfort of large-volume I.M. or subcutaneous injections. Don't confuse Dilaudid-HP with standard parenteral formulations. Check dosage carefully. ∎

❸ *Alert:* Carefully monitor vital signs, pain level, respiratory status, and sedation level in all patients receiving opioids, especially those receiving I.V. drugs, even those given postoperatively.

❸ *Alert:* If patient is taking opioids with serotonergic drugs, watch for signs and symptoms of serotonin syndrome (agitation, hallucinations, rapid HR, fever, excessive sweating, shivering or shaking, muscle twitching or stiffness, trouble with coordination, nausea, vomiting, diarrhea), especially when starting treatment or increasing dosages. Signs and symptoms may occur within several hours of coadministration but may also occur later, especially after dosage increase. Discontinue the opioid, serotonergic drug, or both if serotonin syndrome is suspected.

❸ *Alert:* Monitor patient for signs and symptoms of adrenal insufficiency (nausea, vomiting, loss of appetite, fatigue, weakness, dizziness, low BP). Perform diagnostic testing if adrenal insufficiency is suspected. If adrenal insufficiency is confirmed, treat with corticosteroids and wean patient off opioids, if appropriate. Discontinue corticosteroids when clinically appropriate.

❸ *Alert:* Monitor patient for signs and symptoms of decreased sex hormone levels (low libido, erectile dysfunction, amenorrhea, infertility). If signs and symptoms occur, evaluate patient and obtain laboratory testing.

● Discontinue all other extended-release opioids before giving extended-release form of hydromorphone.

● Monitor respiratory and circulatory status and bowel function.

● Keep opioid antagonist (naloxone) available.

● Don't use extended-release form within 14 days of stopping MAO inhibitor.

● Discontinue use of extended-release form if stopped for more than 3 days.

● Drug may worsen or mask gallbladder pain.

● Drug is a commonly abused opioid.

● Drug may cause constipation. Assess bowel function and need for stool softeners and stimulant laxatives.

❸ *Alert:* Cough syrup may contain tartrazine.

● *Look alike–sound alike:* Don't confuse hydromorphone with morphine or oxymorphone. Don't confuse Dilaudid with Dilantin.

PATIENT TEACHING

● Instruct patient to request or take drug before pain becomes intense and to report all adverse reactions.

Black Box Warning Caution the patient or the caregiver of a patient taking an opioid drug with a benzodiazepine, CNS depressant, or alcohol to seek immediate medical attention if the patient has symptoms of dizziness, light-headedness, extreme sleepiness, slowed or difficult breathing, or unresponsiveness. ∎

Black Box Warning Warn patient that extended-release tablets must be taken whole. Caution patient not to cut, chew, crush, dissolve, or inject them. ∎

🕪 **Alert:** Encourage patient to report all medications being taken, including prescription and OTC medications and supplements.

🕪 **Alert:** Caution patient to immediately report signs and symptoms of serotonin syndrome, adrenal insufficiency, and decreased sex hormone levels.

• Explain the assessment and monitoring process to patient and family. Instruct them to immediately report if patient has any difficulty breathing or any other signs of a potential adverse opioid-related reaction.

• Advise patient to take drug with food if GI upset occurs.

• When drug is used after surgery, encourage patient to turn, cough, and breathe deeply to avoid lung problems.

• Caution patient about getting out of bed or walking. Warn outpatient to avoid hazardous activities that require mental alertness until drug's CNS effects are known.

• Advise patient to avoid alcohol during therapy.

hydroxychloroquine sulfate
hye-drox-ee-KLOR-oh-kwin

Plaquenil

Therapeutic class: Antimalarials
Pharmacologic class: Aminoquinolines

AVAILABLE FORMS
Tablets: 200 mg (equivalent to 155 mg base)

INDICATIONS & DOSAGES
Black Box Warning Prescribers should be completely familiar with this drug before prescribing. ∎

➤ **Suppressive prevention of malaria attacks caused by *Plasmodium vivax, P. malariae, P. ovale*, and susceptible strains of *P. falciparum***
Adults: 400 mg P.O. weekly on the same day each week, beginning 2 weeks before entering malaria-endemic area and continuing for 8 weeks after leaving area. If not started before exposure, double first dose to 800 mg in two divided doses 6 hours apart and continue for 8 weeks after leaving area.

Children: 6.5 mg/kg P.O. weekly on the same day each week, beginning 1 to 2 weeks before entering malaria-endemic area and continuing for 8 weeks after leaving area. Don't exceed adult dose. If not started before exposure, double first dose to 13 mg/kg in two divided doses 6 hours apart.

➤ **Acute malarial attacks**
Adults: Initially, 800 mg P.O., followed by 400 mg 6 to 8 hours after first dose; then 400 mg daily for 2 consecutive days.
Children: Initially, 13 mg/kg (up to 800 mg) P.O.; then 6.5 mg/kg (up to 400 mg) at 6 hours, 24 hours, and 48 hours after first dose.

➤ **Lupus erythematosus**
Adults: Initially, 400 mg P.O. daily or b.i.d., continued for several weeks or months, depending on response. For prolonged maintenance dose, 200 to 400 mg daily in one or two divided doses.

➤ **RA**
Adults: Initially, 400 to 600 mg P.O. daily. When good response occurs, usually in 4 to 12 weeks, cut dosage in half and continue at 200 to 400 mg daily in one or two divided doses. If objective improvement doesn't occur within 6 months, discontinue drug.

ADMINISTRATION
P.O.
🕪 **Alert:** Drug dosage may be discussed in "mg" or "mg base"; be aware of the difference.

• Give drug with food or milk to minimize GI upset.

• To improve compliance when drug is used for prevention, advise patient to take drug immediately before or after a meal on the same day each week.

ACTION
May bind to and alter the properties of DNA in susceptible organisms.

Route	Onset	Peak	Duration
P.O.	Unknown	2–4½ hr	Unknown

Half-life: 32 to 50 days.

ADVERSE REACTIONS
CNS: *seizures,* irritability, nightmares, ataxia, psychosis, vertigo, dizziness,

hypoactive deep tendon reflexes, lassitude, headache.

CV: *cardiomyopathy.*

EENT: blurred vision, difficulty in focusing, reversible corneal changes, typically irreversible nystagmus, sometimes progressive or delayed retinal changes such as narrowing of arterioles, macular lesions, pallor of optic disk, optic atrophy.

GI: anorexia, abdominal cramps, diarrhea, nausea, vomiting.

Hematologic: *agranulocytosis, leukopenia, thrombocytopenia, hemolysis in patients with G6PD deficiency, aplastic anemia.*

Metabolic: weight loss.

Musculoskeletal: skeletal muscle weakness.

Skin: pruritus, lichen planus eruptions, skin and mucosal pigmentary changes, pleomorphic skin eruptions, worsened psoriasis, alopecia, bleaching of hair.

INTERACTIONS

Drug-drug. *Aluminum salts (kaolin), magnesium:* May decrease GI absorption. Separate dose times by 2 to 4 hours.

Artemether: May increase toxic effects of hydroxychloroquine. Avoid use together.

Beta blockers: May increase CV effects of certain beta blockers (metoprolol). Carefully monitor patient. Consider using alternative beta blocker (atenolol).

Digoxin: May increase digoxin level. Monitor drug levels; monitor patient for toxicity.

Mefloquine: May increase QTc-interval prolongation and seizure risk when used concurrently. Avoid use together.

EFFECTS ON LAB TEST RESULTS

● May decrease Hb level.
● May decrease granulocyte, WBC, and platelet counts.

CONTRAINDICATIONS & CAUTIONS

● Contraindicated in patients hypersensitive to drug, in those with retinal or visual field changes or porphyria, and for long-term treatment in children.
● Use cautiously in patients with severe GI, neurologic, or blood disorders.
● Use cautiously in patients with hepatic disease or alcoholism or when used with hepatotoxic drugs.

● Use with caution in those with G6PD deficiency or psoriasis because drug may worsen these conditions.

🔆 *Alert:* Suicidal behavior has been reported in very rare cases.

Dialyzable drug: Unknown.

⚠ *Overdose S&S:* Headache, drowsiness, visual disturbances, CV collapse, seizures, sudden and early respiratory and cardiac arrest, atrial standstill, nodal rhythm, prolonged intraventricular conduction time, progressive bradycardia leading to ventricular fibrillation or arrest.

PREGNANCY-LACTATION-REPRODUCTION

● Drug doesn't appear to pose a significant risk to the fetus, especially with lower doses.
● Pregnant women exposed to drug for the treatment of RA or systemic lupus erythematosus may be enrolled in the Organization of Teratology Information Specialists Autoimmune Diseases in Pregnancy Study (1-877-311-8972).
● Considered compatible with breast-feeding.

NURSING CONSIDERATIONS

● Ensure that baseline and periodic ophthalmic examinations are performed at baseline and annually. Check periodically for ocular muscle weakness after long-term use. Retinal toxicity is largely dose-related.
● Monitor CBC and LFTs periodically during long-term therapy; if severe blood disorder not caused by disease develops, drug may need to be stopped.

🔆 *Alert:* Monitor patient for possible overdose, which can quickly lead to toxic signs or symptoms. Children are extremely susceptible to toxicity.

PATIENT TEACHING

● Advise patient taking drug for prevention to take drug immediately before or after a meal on the same day each week, to improve compliance.
● Instruct patient to report adverse reaction promptly.
● Tell patient that dizziness may occur and to use caution while driving or performing other tasks that require alertness, coordination, or physical dexterity.

---

hydroxyurea
hye-drox-ee-yoor-EE-a

Droxia, Hydrea

Therapeutic class: Antineoplastics
Pharmacologic class: Antimetabolites

AVAILABLE FORMS
Capsules: 200 mg, 300 mg, 400 mg, 500 mg

INDICATIONS & DOSAGES
Adjust-a-dose (for all indications): Base dosage on patient's actual or ideal weight, whichever is less. Dosage adjustment is recommended in renal impairment. According to manufacturer, if CrCl is less than 59 mL/minute, give 50% of the usual dose. If patient is on hemodialysis, give 50% of usual dose after dialysis on dialysis days.

➤ **Carcinoma of the head (excluding lip) and neck, with radiation; resistant chronic myelocytic leukemia (Hydrea)**
Adults: Initially, 15 mg/kg/day P.O. Individualize treatment based on tumor type, disease state, patient response, patient risk factors, and clinical practice standards. Prophylactic administration of folic acid is recommended. Evaluate hematologic status before and during treatment. Modify dosage or discontinue drug as needed.

➤ **To reduce frequency of painful crises and need for blood transfusions in adult patients with sickle cell anemia with recurrent moderate to severe painful crises (Droxia)**
Adults: 15 mg/kg Droxia P.O. once daily. If blood counts are in acceptable range, dose may be increased by 5 mg/kg daily every 12 weeks until maximum tolerated dose or 35 mg/kg daily has been reached. If blood counts are considered toxic, withhold drug until counts recover. Resume treatment after reducing dose by 2.5 mg/kg daily. Every 12 weeks, drug may then be adjusted up or down in 2.5-mg/kg daily increments until patient is at a stable, nontoxic dose for 24 weeks.

➤ **Thrombocytopenia** ◆
Adults: 15 to 20 mg/kg P.O. daily. Titrate to maintain platelet count of 400,000/mm³

or less and ANC of greater than 1,000 cells/mm³.

ADMINISTRATION
P.O.
• Wear gloves when handling drug or its container, and wash hands before and after contact with bottle or capsule. If powder from capsule is spilled, wipe up immediately with a damp towel. Dispose of towel in a closed container such as a plastic bag.

ACTION
May inhibit DNA synthesis.

Route	Onset	Peak	Duration
P.O.	Unknown	1–4 hr	24 hr

Half-life: 3 to 4 hours.

ADVERSE REACTIONS
CNS: malaise, fever, drowsiness.
GI: anorexia, nausea, vomiting, diarrhea, stomatitis, constipation.
Hematologic: *leukopenia, thrombocytopenia,* anemia, megaloblastosis, *bone marrow suppression.*
Metabolic: hyperuricemia, weight gain.
Skin: rash, itching, alopecia, cutaneous vasculitic toxicities (including vasculitic ulcerations and gangrene).
Other: chills.

INTERACTIONS
Drug-drug. ⊕ *Alert: Antiretrovirals (didanosine, stavudine):* May cause hepatotoxicity and hepatic failure, resulting in death. When given with didanosine to HIV-infected patients, severe peripheral neuropathy or fatal pancreatitis may occur. Avoid using with didanosine and stavudine.
Cytotoxic drugs, radiation therapy: May enhance toxicity of hydroxyurea. Use together cautiously.
Interferon: May increase the risk of cutaneous vasculitic toxicities, including vasculitic ulcerations and gangrene. Stop drug.
Live-virus vaccines: May increase risk of vaccine-related adverse reactions, viral replication, and severe infection. Avoid vaccinations during and for 3 months after therapy ends.

H

Uricosuric agents (probenecid): Increases uric acid levels. Adjust dosage of uricosuric agent as needed.

EFFECTS ON LAB TEST RESULTS
- May increase BUN, creatinine, hepatic enzyme, and uric acid levels. May decrease Hb level.
- May decrease WBC, RBC, and platelet counts.

CONTRAINDICATIONS & CAUTIONS
- Contraindicated in patients hypersensitive to drug and in those with WBC count less than 2,500/mm^3, platelet count less than 100,000/mm^3, or severe anemia.
- Use cautiously in patients with renal dysfunction and in the elderly.

Dialyzable drug: 50% to 74%.

⚠ *Overdose S&S:* Acute mucocutaneous toxicity; soreness, violet erythema on palms and soles followed by scaling of hands and feet; severe generalized hyperpigmentation of the skin; stomatitis.

PREGNANCY-LACTATION-REPRODUCTION
- Don't use during pregnancy; may be mutagenic. Advise women of childbearing potential who are taking drug to avoid pregnancy.
- Patient should discontinue breast-feeding or discontinue drug.

NURSING CONSIDERATIONS
- **Black Box Warning** Droxia may cause severe myelosuppression. Monitor blood counts at baseline and throughout therapy. Treatment interruption and dosage reductions may be needed. ∎
- **Black Box Warning** Droxia is carcinogenic. Monitor patient for malignancies. ∎
- Routinely measure BUN, uric acid, liver enzyme, and creatinine levels; monitor blood counts every 2 weeks.
- Acceptable blood counts during dosage adjustment for sickle cell anemia are neutrophil count of 2,500/mm^3 or more, platelet count of 95,000/mm^3 or more, Hb level more than 5.3 g/dL, and reticulocyte count (if Hb level is below 9 g/dL) at least 95,000/mm^3. Toxic levels are neutrophil count less than 2,000/mm^3, platelet count less than 80,000/mm^3, Hb level less than

4.5 g/dL, and reticulocyte count (if Hb level is below 9 g/dL) less than 80,000/mm^3.
- Hydroxyurea may dramatically lower WBC count in 24 to 48 hours.
- ⚠ *Alert:* Patients who have received or are currently receiving interferon may be at greater risk for developing cutaneous vasculitic toxicities. Monitor patients closely; discontinue drug if toxicities occur.
- ⚠ *Alert:* Patients with HIV infection who are also receiving didanosine may be at increased risk for severe peripheral neuropathy and fatal pancreatitis. Avoid this combination.
- Monitor patient for pancreatitis. If it occurs, discontinue drug permanently.
- Drug may increase risk of hyperuricemia. Monitor fluid intake and output; keep patient hydrated.
- To prevent bleeding, avoid all I.M. injections when platelet count is less than 50,000/mm^3.
- Blood transfusions may be necessary for cumulative anemia.
- Dosage change may be needed after chemotherapy or radiation therapy.
- Auditory and visual hallucinations and hematologic toxicity increase when renal function decreases.
- Drug crosses blood-brain barrier.
- Radiation therapy may increase risk or severity of GI distress or stomatitis.

PATIENT TEACHING
- Tell patient and caregiver to wear gloves when handling drug or its container and to wash their hands before and after contact with the bottle or capsule. If powder from capsule is spilled, wipe up immediately with a damp towel and dispose of the towel in a closed container such as a plastic bag.
- Advise patient to watch for signs and symptoms of infection (fever, sore throat, fatigue) and bleeding (easy bruising, nosebleeds, bleeding gums, tarry stools). He also should take his temperature daily.
- Caution women of childbearing potential to consult prescriber before becoming pregnant.
- **Black Box Warning** Advise patient to use sun protection and that monitoring for development of secondary malignancies will be needed. ∎

hydrOXYzine hydrochloride
hye-DROX-i-zeen

Atarax✤, Vistaril

hydrOXYzine pamoate
Vistaril

Therapeutic class: Antihistamines
Pharmacologic class: Piperazine
derivatives

AVAILABLE FORMS
hydroxyzine hydrochloride
Injection: 25 mg/mL, 50 mg/mL
Syrup: 2 mg/mL✤, 10 mg/5 mL
Tablets: 10 mg, 25 mg, 50 mg
hydroxyzine pamoate
Capsules: 25 mg, 50 mg

INDICATIONS & DOSAGES
Adjust-a-dose (for all indications): In elderly
patients, initiate drug at the lower end of
dosage range and observe closely.
➤ **Anxiety**
Adults: 50 to 100 mg P.O. q.i.d. Or, 50 to
100 mg I.M. t.i.d. or q.i.d.
Children age 6 and older: 50 to 100 mg P.O.
daily in divided doses.
Children younger than age 6: 50 mg P.O.
daily in divided doses.
➤ **Preoperative and postoperative
adjunctive therapy for sedation**
Adults: 25 to 100 mg P.O. or I.M.
Children: 0.6 mg/kg/dose P.O. or
1.1 mg/kg/dose I.M.
➤ **Pruritus**
Adults: 25 mg P.O. or I.M. t.i.d. or q.i.d.
Children age 6 and older: 50 to 100 mg P.O.
daily in divided doses.
Children younger than age 6: 50 mg P.O.
daily in divided doses.
➤ **Nausea and vomiting**
Adults: 25 to 100 mg/dose I.M.
Children: 1.1 mg/kg/dose I.M.

ADMINISTRATION
P.O.
● Give drug without regard for meals.
● Shake suspension well before giving.

I.M.
● Parenteral form (hydroxyzine hydrochloride) is for I.M. use only, preferably by
Z-track injection.
🔴 *Alert:* Never give drug I.V., subcutaneously, or intra-arterially.
● Aspirate I.M. injection carefully to prevent inadvertent I.V. injection. Inject deeply
into a large muscle (don't inject into lower
and mid-third of upper arm).

ACTION
Suppresses activity in certain essential
regions of the subcortical area of the CNS.

Route	Onset	Peak	Duration
P.O.	15–30 min	2 hr	4–6 hr
I.M.	Unknown	Unknown	4–6 hr

Half-life: 3 hours.

ADVERSE REACTIONS
CNS: drowsiness, dizziness, fatigue, invol-
untary motor activity.
EENT: blurred vision.
GI: dry mouth.
Respiratory: respiratory depression.
Skin: pain at I.M. injection site.

INTERACTIONS
Drug-drug. *Anticholinergics:* May cause
additive anticholinergic effects. Use together cautiously.
CNS depressants: May increase CNS depression. Use together cautiously; dosage
adjustments may be needed.
Epinephrine: May inhibit and reverse vasopressor effect of epinephrine. Avoid using
together.
Drug-lifestyle. *Alcohol use:* May increase
CNS depression. Discourage use together.

EFFECTS ON LAB TEST RESULTS
● May cause false increase in urinary 17-
hydroxycorticosteroid level.
● May cause false-negative skin allergen
tests by reducing or inhibiting the cutaneous
response to histamine.

CONTRAINDICATIONS & CAUTIONS
● Contraindicated in patients hypersensitive
to drug. Oral drug is contraindicated in
patients with prolonged QTc interval.

H

• Drug can prolong QTc interval. Use injectable formulation cautiously in patients with risk factors for QTc-interval prolongation and in patients with conditions that predispose to QTc-interval prolongation and ventricular arrhythmia.

• Use cautiously in patients with glaucoma, BPH, urinary stricture, asthma, or COPD and in elderly patients.

Dialyzable drug: Unknown.

⚠ Overdose S&S: Hypersedation.

PREGNANCY-LACTATION-REPRODUCTION

• Contraindicated in early pregnancy and in breast-feeding women.

NURSING CONSIDERATIONS

• If patient takes other CNS drugs, watch for oversedation.

• Elderly patients may be more sensitive to adverse anticholinergic effects; monitor these patients for dizziness, excessive sedation, confusion, hypotension, syncope, and dysuria.

• **Look alike–sound alike:** Don't confuse hydroxyzine with hydroxyurea, Hydrogesic, or hydralazine. Don't confuse Vistaril with Restoril.

PATIENT TEACHING

• Warn patient to avoid hazardous activities that require alertness and good coordination until effects of drug are known.

• Tell patient to report all adverse reactions, especially heart palpitations, dizziness, fainting, difficulty breathing, difficulty urinating, or vision changes.

• Tell patient to avoid use of alcohol while taking drug.

• Advise patient to use sugarless hard candy or gum to relieve dry mouth.

---

ibandronate sodium

eh-BAN-drow-nate

Boniva✿

Therapeutic class: Antiosteoporotics
Pharmacologic class: Bisphosphonates

AVAILABLE FORMS

Injection: 3 mg/3-mL prefilled syringe
Tablets ⓄⓉⒸ: 150 mg

INDICATIONS & DOSAGES

➤ **To treat or prevent postmenopausal osteoporosis**

Women: 150 mg P.O. once monthly on the same day each month, with a large glass of plain water. Or, for treatment, 3 mg I.V. bolus once every 3 months.

➤ **Hypercalcemia of malignancy ♦**

Adults: 2 to 6 mg as a single I.V. infusion over 15 minutes to 4 hours every 4 weeks. May give additional infusions up to 6 mg (including initial dose) if the albumin-corrected serum calcium level hasn't normalized by day 4 after the initial infusion.

➤ **Metastatic bone disease due to breast cancer ♦**

Adults: 6 mg I.V. every 3 to 4 weeks.

ADMINISTRATION

P.O.

• Give drug 1 hour before first food or drink and before any other drugs.

• Make sure patient doesn't lie down for at least 1 hour after receiving drug.

• Give drug with plain water only.

• Don't allow patient to chew or suck tablets as this may cause oropharyngeal ulceration.

I.V.

▼ Prefilled syringes are for single use only.

▼ Give undiluted using needle provided with the syringe.

▼ Give by I.V. bolus over 15 to 30 seconds.

▼ Don't use if drug is discolored or contains particulate matter.

▼ Store at room temperature.

▼ **Incompatibilities:** Calcium-containing solutions and other I.V. drugs.

ACTION

Inhibits bone breakdown and removal to reduce bone loss and increase bone mass.

Route	Onset	Peak	Duration
P.O.	Unknown	½–2 hr	Unknown
I.V.	Rapid	Unknown	Unknown

Half-life: P.O., 1½ to 6½ days for the 150-mg dose; I.V., approximately 5 to 25½ hours.

ADVERSE REACTIONS

CNS: asthenia, dizziness, depression, fatigue, headache, insomnia, vertigo.
CV: hypertension.
EENT: nasopharyngitis, pharyngitis.

Reactions in bold italics are *life-threatening*. Interactions may have a *rapid onset* or a *delayed onset*.

GI: dyspepsia, abdominal pain, constipation, diarrhea, gastritis, nausea, vomiting.
GU: cystitis, UTI.
Musculoskeletal: back pain, arthralgia, arthritis, joint disorder, limb pain, localized osteoarthritis, muscle cramps, myalgia.
Respiratory: bronchitis, URI, pneumonia.
Skin: rash.
Other: allergic reaction, infection, influenza, tooth disorder.

INTERACTIONS
Drug-drug. *Aspirin, NSAIDs:* May increase GI irritation. Use together cautiously.
Drugs that prolong QTc interval: May enhance QTc-prolonging effects. For high-risk QTc-prolonging agents, consider therapy modification. For moderate-risk QTc-prolonging drugs, monitor therapy.
PPIs: May decrease ibandronate therapeutic effects. Monitor therapy.
Products containing aluminum, calcium, magnesium, or iron: May decrease ibandronate absorption. Give oral ibandronate 1 hour before vitamins, minerals, or antacids.
Drug-food. *Food, milk, beverages (except water):* May decrease drug absorption. Give oral drug on an empty stomach with plain water.
Drug-lifestyle. *Alcohol use:* May decrease drug absorption and increase risk of esophageal irritation. Discourage use together.

EFFECTS ON LAB TEST RESULTS
• May decrease total alkaline phosphatase level. May interfere with bone-imaging agents.

CONTRAINDICATIONS & CAUTIONS
• Contraindicated in patients hypersensitive to drug and in those with uncorrected hypocalcemia. Oral form is contraindicated in those who can't stand or sit upright for 60 minutes.
⚠ **Alert:** There may be an increased risk of atypical fractures of the thigh in patients treated with bisphosphonates.
⚠ **Alert:** Drug may cause osteonecrosis, mainly in the jaw. Avoid invasive dental procedures if possible.
• Drug may cause hypocalcemia, especially if dietary intake of calcium or vitamin D is inadequate.

• Don't give to patients with severe renal impairment (CrCl less than 30 mL/minute).
• Use cautiously in patients with a history of GI disorders.
Dialyzable drug: Yes.
⚠ **Overdose S&S:** Hypocalcemia, hypophosphatemia, hypomagnesemia.

PREGNANCY-LACTATION-REPRODUCTION
• There are no adequate studies in pregnant women. Use during pregnancy only if potential benefit justifies potential risk to the fetus.
• It isn't known if drug appears in breast milk. Use cautiously in breast-feeding women.

NURSING CONSIDERATIONS
• Correct hypocalcemia or other disturbances of bone and mineral metabolism before therapy.
• Make sure patient has adequate intake of calcium and vitamin D.
• Obtain serum creatinine level and perform an oral examination before each dose in patients receiving I.V. ibandronate.
• Watch for signs of esophageal irritation (dysphagia, painful swallowing, retrosternal pain, heartburn).
• Monitor patient for bone, joint, and muscle pain, which may be severe and incapacitating and may occur within days, months, or years of start of therapy. When drug is stopped, symptoms may resolve.
• Watch for signs of uveitis and scleritis.

PATIENT TEACHING
• Tell patient receiving I.V. form that if she misses a dose to reschedule the missed dose as soon as possible. Subsequent injections should be rescheduled once every 3 months from that dose. She shouldn't receive more than one dose in a 3-month time frame.
• Tell patient taking monthly dose to take it on same date each month and to wait at least 7 days between doses if she misses a scheduled dose.
• Instruct patient to take oral drug 1 hour before any food or fluids and before any other drugs, including OTC drugs.
• Advise patient to swallow drug whole with a full glass of plain water while standing or sitting and to remain upright for at least 1 hour after taking drug.

• Advise patient to take calcium and vitamin D supplements as prescribed.
• Tell patient to report any bone, joint, or muscle pain.
• Advise patient to stop drug and immediately report signs and symptoms of esophageal irritation.
• Advise patient to have periodic dental exams to monitor for osteonecrosis of jaw.

SAFETY ALERT!

ibrutinib
eye-BROO-ti-nib

Imbruvica

Therapeutic class: Antineoplastics
Pharmacologic class: Kinase inhibitors

AVAILABLE FORMS
Capsules ⒹⒸ: 140 mg

INDICATIONS & DOSAGES
Adjust-a-dose (for all indications): Interrupt therapy for grade 3 or greater nonhematologic toxicities, grade 3 or greater neutropenia with infection or fever, or grade 4 hematologic toxicities. Once signs and symptoms of toxicity have resolved to grade 1 or baseline (recovery), may restart at the starting dose. If toxicity recurs, reduce dosage by one capsule (140 mg/day). May consider a second dosage reduction by 140 mg as needed. If toxicities persist or recur after two dosage reductions, discontinue drug. Recommended dosage for patients with mild hepatic impairment is 140 mg daily. Avoid use in patients with moderate or severe hepatic impairment.
➤ **Patients with mantle cell lymphoma who have received at least one prior therapy**
Adults: 560 mg (four 140-mg capsules) P.O. once daily.
➤ **Patients with chronic lymphocytic leukemia or small lymphocytic lymphoma who have received at least one prior therapy; patients with chronic lymphocytic leukemia or small lymphocytic lymphoma with 17p deletion**
Adults: 420 mg (three 140-mg capsules) P.O. once daily.

➤ **Patients with Waldenström macroglobulinemia**
Adults: 420 mg (three 140-mg capsules) P.O. once daily until disease progression or unacceptable toxicity occurs.

ADMINISTRATION
P.O.
• Give capsules whole with water at approximately same time each day.
• Patient should swallow capsules whole. Don't break, open, or crush capsules.
• If a dose is missed, administer as soon as missed dose is remembered on same day; return to normal scheduling the following day. Don't give extra capsules to make up for missed dose.
• Drug is hazardous; use safe handling precautions.
• Store at room temperature in original package.

ACTION
Inhibits Bruton tyrosine kinase activity, resulting in decreased malignant B-cell proliferation and survival.

Route	Onset	Peak	Duration
P.O.	Unknown	1–2 hr	Unknown

Half-life: 4 to 6 hours.

ADVERSE REACTIONS
CNS: dizziness, headache, fatigue, pyrexia, asthenia, subdural hematoma, insomnia, pain.
CV: atrial fibrillation, hypertension, peripheral edema.
EENT: blurred vision, decreased visual acuity, sinusitis, epistaxis.
GI: diarrhea, nausea, constipation, abdominal pain, vomiting, stomatitis, dyspepsia, decreased appetite, GERD, *GI bleeding.*
GU: UTI, *renal failure,* hematuria.
Hematologic: *neutropenia, thrombocytopenia,* anemia.
Metabolic: dehydration, hyperuricemia.
Musculoskeletal: musculoskeletal pain, muscle spasms, arthralgia, weakness.
Respiratory: URI, pneumonia, dyspnea, cough.
Skin: skin infections, bruising, rash, petechiae.
Other: chills, other malignancies, infection.

Reactions in bold italics are *life-threatening*. Interactions may have a *rapid onset* or a *delayed onset*.

INTERACTIONS

Afatinib, bosutinib, brentuximab, colchicine, dabigatran, doxorubicin (conventional), edoxaban, ledipasvir, naloxegol, pazopanib: May increase serum concentrations of these drugs. Refer to individual manufacturer's instructions regarding therapy modifications.

Anticoagulants, antiplatelet agents: May increase risk of bleeding. Monitor bleeding risk and patient closely.

Digoxin: May increase digoxin level. Monitor drug concentrations.

Moderate CYP3A inhibitors (amprenavir, aprepitant, atazanavir, ciprofloxacin, crizotinib, darunavir, diltiazem, erythromycin, fluconazole, fosamprenavir, imatinib, verapamil): May increase ibrutinib level. Avoid concurrent use. If ibrutinib must be used, reduce ibrutinib dosage to 140 mg P.O. daily and monitor patient for toxicities.

Strong CYP3A inducers (carbamazepine, phenytoin, rifampin): May decrease ibrutinib level. Avoid concurrent use and consider agents with less CYP3A induction.

Strong CYP3A inhibitors (clarithromycin, indinavir, itraconazole, ketoconazole, nefazodone, nelfinavir, posaconazole, ritonavir, saquinavir, telithromycin, voriconazole): May increase ibrutinib level. Avoid concurrent use or withhold ibrutinib for antibiotic or antifungal regimens lasting less than 7 days. Monitor patient closely for toxicities.

Drug-herb. *St. John's wort:* May decrease ibrutinib level. Discourage use together.

Drug-food. *Grapefruit products, Seville oranges:* May increase ibrutinib level. Discourage use together.

EFFECTS ON LAB TEST RESULTS

• May increase uric acid and creatinine levels. May decrease Hb level.
• May increase lymphocyte count. May decrease platelet and neutrophil counts.

CONTRAINDICATIONS & CAUTIONS

• Contraindicated in patients hypersensitive to drug or its components.
• Drug may increase risk of renal failure. Fatalities have been reported.
• Avoid use in patients with moderate or severe hepatic impairment (Child-Pugh class B or C).

• Drug may cause atrial fibrillation or atrial flutter, particularly in patients with cardiac risk factors, hypertension, acute infections, or a previous history of atrial fibrillation.
• Use cautiously in elderly patients because of increased risk of adverse effects.
Dialyzable drug: Unknown.

PREGNANCY-LACTATION-REPRODUCTION

• Drug may cause fetal harm; avoid use in pregnant women. Patient should avoid pregnancy for 1 month after therapy ends.
• It isn't known if drug appears in breast milk. Patient should discontinue breastfeeding or discontinue drug.

NURSING CONSIDERATIONS

• Monitor patients for signs and symptoms of hypersensitivity reactions (wheezing, chest tightness, fever, itching, heavy cough, blue-colored skin, seizures, or swelling of face, lips, tongue, or throat).
• Fatal bleeding events have occurred. Monitor patients for bleeding and evaluate risk-benefit of use in patients receiving anticoagulants or antiplatelet drugs.
• Consider interrupting therapy for 3 to 7 days before and after surgery, depending on procedure type and risk of bleeding.
• Monitor patients closely for fever and other signs of infection. Serious, sometimes fatal, infections have occurred.
• Monitor blood counts monthly, as indicated.
• Monitor for hyperuricemia and evaluate renal function; maintain hydration.
• Evaluate patients for new malignancy during treatment.
• Monitor patients for hypertension or cardiac abnormalities.

PATIENT TEACHING

• Caution patient to swallow capsules whole and not to open, break, or chew them.
• Caution patient to immediately report signs and symptoms of significant hypersensitivity reaction (wheezing, chest tightness, fever, itching, heavy cough, blue-colored skin, seizures, or swelling of face, lips, tongue, or throat).
• Instruct patient to contact prescriber if diarrhea, nausea, vomiting, abdominal pain, fever, infection, bleeding, or easy bruising occurs.

● Caution female patient to avoid becoming pregnant during therapy and for 1 month after therapy ends. Counsel patient to use effective birth control during treatment because drug may cause fetal harm.

ibuprofen
eye-byoo-PROH-fen

Advil ◇, Advil Gel Caplets ◇, Advil Infants' Concentrated Drops ◇, Caldolor, Children's Advil ◇, Children's Motrin Jr Strength ◇, ibuprofen ◇, Infant's Advil ◇, Junior Strength Advil ◇, Novo-Profen✢, Pamprin Ibuprofen Formula✢ ◇, pms-Ibuprofen✦

ibuprofen lysine
NeoProfen

Therapeutic class: NSAIDs
Pharmacologic class: NSAIDs

AVAILABLE FORMS
ibuprofen
Capsules: 200 mg ◇
Capsules (liqui-gel): 200 mg ◇
Injection: 800 mg/8-mL (100 mg/mL) single-dose vials
Oral drops: 40 mg/mL ◇, 50 mg/1.25 mL ◇
Oral suspension: 40 mg/mL ◇, 100 mg/ 5 mL ◇
Tablets: 100 mg ◇, 200 mg ◇, 300 mg✢ ◇, 400 mg, 600 mg, 800 mg
Tablets (chewable): 50 mg ◇, 100 mg ◇
ibuprofen lysine
Injection: EQ 20 mg base/2 mL (EQ 10 mg base/mL)

INDICATIONS & DOSAGES
➤ **RA, osteoarthritis, arthritis**
Adults: 300 to 800 mg P.O. t.i.d. or q.i.d. Maximum daily dose is 3.2 g.
➤ **Mild to moderate pain; moderate to severe pain as an adjunct to opioid analgesics; fever reduction in children**
Children ages 12 to 17: 400 mg I.V. every 4 to 6 hours p.r.n. Infusion time must be at least 10 minutes. Maximum daily dose is 2,400 mg.

Children ages 6 months to younger than 12 years: 10 mg/kg I.V. up to a maximum single dose of 400 mg every 4 to 6 hours p.r.n. Infusion time must be at least 10 minutes. Maximum daily dose is 40 mg/kg or 2,400 mg, whichever is less.
➤ **Mild to moderate pain, fever**
Adults: 200 to 400 mg P.O. every 4 to 6 hours p.r.n. Or, for pain, 400 to 800 mg I.V. every 6 hours p.r.n.; for fever, 400 mg I.V. followed by 400 mg I.V. every 4 to 6 hours or 100 to 200 mg I.V. every 4 hours p.r.n. Infuse over at least 30 minutes. Maximum dose, 3,200 mg/day. Use smallest effective dose.
Children age 12 and older: 200 to 400 mg P.O. every 4 to 6 hours. Maximum daily dose is 1.2 g. Use smallest effective dose.
Children age 11 weighing 33 to 43 kg: 300 mg chewable tablets or 15 mL (300 mg) oral suspension P.O. every 6 to 8 hours up to q.i.d.
Children ages 9 to 10 weighing 27 to 32 kg: 250 mg chewable tablets or 12.5 mL (250 mg) oral suspension P.O. every 6 to 8 hours up to q.i.d.
Children ages 6 to 8 weighing 22 to 27 kg: 200 mg chewable tablets or 10 mL (200 mg) oral suspension P.O. every 6 to 8 hours up to q.i.d.
Children ages 4 to 5 weighing 16 to 21 kg: 150 mg chewable tablets or 7.5 mL (150 mg) oral suspension P.O. every 6 to 8 hours up to q.i.d.
Children ages 2 to 3 weighing 11 to 16 kg: 100 mg (5 mL) oral suspension every 6 to 8 hours up to q.i.d.
Children ages 12 to 23 months weighing 8 to 10 kg: 75 mg (1.875 mL) oral drops every 6 to 8 hours up to q.i.d.
Children ages 6 to 11 months weighing 5 to 8 kg: 50 mg (1.25 mL) oral drops every 6 to 8 hours up to q.i.d.
Adjust-a-dose: For children ages 6 months to 11 years, use weight to determine dosage if possible; otherwise, use age. If needed, dose may be repeated every 6 to 8 hours but no more frequently than q.i.d. or a maximum of 30 mg/kg in 24 hours. Consult a health care provider before giving ibuprofen 100 mg chewable tablets to children younger than age 6 or those weighing less than 22 kg, 50 mg chewable tablets to children younger

than age 4 or those weighing less than 16 kg, 50 mg oral suspension to children younger than age 2 or those weighing less than 11 kg, or 50 mg oral drops to infants younger than age 6 months or those weighing less than 5 kg. Ibuprofen oral drops should be dosed at 7.5 mg/kg of body weight.

✳ *NEW INDICATION:* **Relief of signs and symptoms of juvenile arthritis**
Children: Recommended dose is 30 to 40 mg/kg/day of oral suspension divided into three to four doses; patients with milder disease may be adequately treated with 20 mg/kg/day. Doses above 50 mg/kg/day aren't recommended because they haven't been studied and may increase risk of serious adverse events. Lower dosage to the smallest dose needed to maintain adequate symptom control when clinical effect is obtained.

➤ **Migraine**
Adults: 400 mg (2 capsules) P.O. in 24 hours.

➤ **Clinically significant patent ductus arteriosus (ibuprofen lysine)**
Premature infants weighing between 500 and 1,500 g who are no more than 32 weeks' gestational age: 10 mg/kg I.V. followed by 5 mg/kg I.V. 24 hours later followed by a third dose of 5 mg/kg I.V. 24 hours after second dose.

Adjust-a-dose: If anuria or marked oliguria (urinary output less than 0.6 mL/kg/hour) is evident at the scheduled time of the second or third dose, don't give additional dose until renal function has returned to normal. If the ductus arteriosus closes or is significantly reduced in size after completion of the first course of ibuprofen lysine, no further doses are necessary.

ADMINISTRATION
P.O.
● Give drug with milk or meals.
● Shake oral suspension and drops well before using.

I.V.
▼ Dilute drug with NSS, 5% dextrose, or lactated Ringer solution. For 800-mg dose, use at least 200 mL of diluent. In adults, give over at least 30 minutes; in children, over at least 10 minutes; in neonates, over at least 15 minutes (lysine injection).

▼ For weight-based dosing at 10 mg/kg, ensure that drug concentration is 4 mg/mL or less.
▼ Diluted solutions are stable for 24 hours at room temperature.
▼ Correct dehydration before administering drug.
▼ **Incompatibilities:** TPN solutions.

ACTION
May inhibit prostaglandin synthesis, to produce anti-inflammatory, analgesic, and antipyretic effects.

Route	Onset	Peak	Duration
P.O.	Variable	1–2 hr	4–6 hr
I.V.	Unknown	Unknown	Unknown

Half-life: 2 to 4 hours.

ADVERSE REACTIONS
CNS: dizziness, headache, nervousness.
CV: edema, fluid retention.
EENT: tinnitus.
GI: abdominal pain, bloating, constipation, decreased appetite, diarrhea, dyspepsia, epigastric distress, flatulence, heartburn, nausea, nonnecrotizing enterocolitis, vomiting.
GU: *acute renal failure,* azotemia, cystitis, hematuria.
Hematologic: *agranulocytosis, aplastic anemia, leukopenia, neutropenia, pancytopenia, thrombocytopenia,* anemia, prolonged bleeding time.
Metabolic: *hypokalemia, hypoglycemia.*
Skin: pruritus, rash.

INTERACTIONS
Drug-drug. *Anticoagulants (warfarin):* May increase risk of serious GI bleeding. Use with extreme caution if concomitant use can't be avoided. Monitor patient closely.
Antihypertensives, furosemide, thiazide diuretics: May decrease the effectiveness of diuretics or antihypertensives. Monitor patient closely.
Apixaban, rivaroxaban: May increase bleeding risk. Coadminister with caution.
Aspirin: May negate the antiplatelet effect of low-dose aspirin therapy. Advise patient on the appropriate spacing of doses.
Aspirin, corticosteroids: May cause adverse GI reactions. Avoid using together.

Bisphosphonates: May increase risk of gastric ulceration. Monitor patient for signs of gastric irritation or bleeding.

Cyclosporine: May increase nephrotoxicity of both drugs. Avoid using together.

Digoxin, lithium: May increase levels or effects of these drugs. Monitor patient for toxicity.

Direct thrombin inhibitors (dabigatran, desirudin): May increase risk of bleeding. Coadminister with caution.

Methotrexate: May decrease methotrexate clearance and increase toxicity. Use together cautiously.

SSRIs (fluoxetine, venlafaxine): May increase risk of upper GI bleeding. If coadministration is unavoidable, closely watch for signs and symptoms of GI bleeding. Consider acid suppression therapy.

Triamterene: May increase risk of acute renal failure. Avoid coadministration; if unavoidable, closely monitor renal function.

Drug-herb. *Dong quai, feverfew, garlic, ginger, ginkgo biloba, horse chestnut, red clover:* May increase risk of bleeding, based on the known effects of components. Discourage use together.

White willow: Herb and drug contain similar components. Discourage use together.

Drug-lifestyle. *Alcohol use:* May cause adverse GI reactions. Discourage use together.

Sun exposure: May cause photosensitivity reactions. Advise patient to avoid excessive sunlight exposure.

EFFECTS ON LAB TEST RESULTS

- May increase BUN, creatinine, ALT, AST, and potassium levels.
- May decrease glucose and Hb levels and hematocrit.
- May decrease neutrophil, WBC, RBC, platelet, and granulocyte counts.

CONTRAINDICATIONS & CAUTIONS

- Contraindicated in patients hypersensitive to drug and in those with angioedema, syndrome of nasal polyps, or bronchospastic reaction to aspirin or other NSAIDs.

Black Box Warning Contraindicated for the treatment of perioperative pain after CABG surgery. ∎

Black Box Warning NSAIDs can increase risk of heart attack or stroke in patients with or without heart disease or risk factors for heart disease. ∎

Black Box Warning Risk of heart attack or stroke can occur as early as the first weeks of using an NSAID. Risk appears greater at higher doses. Use lowest effective dose for shortest duration possible. ∎

⟴ *Alert:* NSAIDs increase risk of HF.

- Use cautiously in elderly patients and in patients with GI disorders, history of peptic ulcer disease, hepatic or renal disease, cardiac decompensation, hypertension, asthma, or intrinsic coagulation defects.
- May increase risk of aseptic meningitis, with fever and coma, particularly in patients with systemic lupus erythematosus and related connective tissue disease. If signs or symptoms of meningitis occur, consider whether they're related to ibuprofen therapy.

Dialyzable drug: Unknown.

⚠ *Overdose S&S:* Abdominal pain, nausea, vomiting, lethargy, drowsiness, headache, tinnitus, nystagmus, CNS depression, seizures, hypotension, bradycardia, tachycardia, atrial fibrillation, metabolic acidosis, coma, acute renal failure, hyperkalemia, respiratory depression and failure.

PREGNANCY-LACTATION-REPRODUCTION

- There are no adequate studies in pregnant women. Drug can cause fetal harm and is contraindicated in pregnant women starting at 30 weeks' gestation. Before 30 weeks' gestation, use during pregnancy only if potential benefit justifies potential risk to the fetus.
- Drug appears into breast milk. Patient should discontinue breast-feeding or discontinue drug.

NURSING CONSIDERATIONS

- Check renal and hepatic function periodically in patients on long-term therapy. Stop drug if abnormalities occur and notify prescriber.
- Monitor BP because drug can lead to new-onset hypertension or worsening of preexisting hypertension, which may contribute to the increased incidence of CV events.
- Because of their antipyretic and anti-inflammatory actions, NSAIDs may mask signs and symptoms of infection.

Reactions in bold italics are *life-threatening*. Interactions may have a *rapid onset* or a *delayed onset*.

- Blurred or diminished vision and changes in color vision may occur.
- Full anti-inflammatory effects may take 1 or 2 weeks to develop.

❸ Alert: Watch for and immediately evaluate signs and symptoms of heart attack (chest pain, shortness of breath or trouble breathing) or stroke (weakness in one part or side of the body, slurred speech).

Black Box Warning NSAIDs cause an increased risk of serious GI adverse events, including bleeding, ulceration, and perforation of the stomach or intestines, which can be fatal. Elderly patients are at greater risk. ■

- Monitor patients for signs and symptoms of GI ulceration and bleeding.
- Monitor patient for signs or symptoms of aseptic meningitis (fever, headache, sensitivity to light, vomiting) and report immediately if they occur.

Black Box Warning NSAIDs may increase the risk of serious thrombotic events, MI, or stroke, which can be fatal. The risk may be greater with longer use or in patients with CV disease or risk factors for CV disease. ■

- If patient consumes three or more alcoholic drinks per day, drug may cause stomach bleeding.

PATIENT TEACHING

- Tell patient to take with meals or milk to reduce adverse GI reactions.

❸ Alert: Drug is available OTC. Instruct patient not to exceed 1.2 g daily for adults and children age 12 and older or 30 mg/kg for children ages 6 months to 11 years, not to give to children younger than age 6 months, and not to take for extended periods (longer than 3 days for fever or longer than 10 days for pain) without consulting prescriber.

- Tell patient that full therapeutic effect for arthritis may be delayed for 2 to 4 weeks. Although pain relief occurs at low dosage levels, inflammation doesn't improve at dosages less than 400 mg q.i.d.
- Caution patient that use with aspirin, anticoagulants, alcohol, or corticosteroids may increase risk of GI adverse reactions.
- Teach patient to watch for and immediately report to prescriber signs and symptoms of GI bleeding, including blood in

vomit, urine, or stool; coffee-ground vomit; and black, tarry stool.

❸ Alert: Advise patient to seek medical attention immediately if chest pain, shortness of breath or trouble breathing, weakness in one part or side of the body, or slurred speech occurs.

- Tell patient to contact prescriber before using this drug if fluid intake hasn't been adequate or if fluids have been lost as a result of vomiting or diarrhea.
- Warn patient to avoid hazardous activities that require mental alertness until effects on CNS are known.
- Advise patient to wear sunscreen to avoid hypersensitivity to sunlight.

SAFETY ALERT!

ibutilide fumarate
eye-BYOO-ti-lyed

Corvert

Therapeutic class: Antiarrhythmics
Pharmacologic class: Methanesulfonanilide derivatives

AVAILABLE FORMS

Injection: 0.1 mg/mL in 10-mL vials

INDICATIONS & DOSAGES

➤ **Rapid conversion of recent onset atrial fibrillation or atrial flutter to sinus rhythm**

Adults weighing 60 kg or more: 1 mg I.V. infusion over 10 minutes. May repeat dose if arrhythmia doesn't respond within 10 minutes after completing first dose.

Adults weighing less than 60 kg: 0.01 mg/kg I.V. infusion over 10 minutes. May repeat dose if arrhythmia doesn't respond within 10 minutes after completing first dose.

ADMINISTRATION

I.V.

▼ Give drug undiluted or diluted in 50 mL of diluent, and add to NSS for injection or D_5W before infusion. Add contents of 10-mL vial (0.1 mg/mL) to 50-mL infusion bag to form admixture of about 0.017 mg ibutilide/mL. Use drug with polyvinyl chloride plastic bags or polyolefin bags.

▼ Give drug over 10 to 30 minutes.

▼ Stop infusion if arrhythmia is terminated or patient develops ventricular tachycardia or marked prolongation of QT or QTc interval. If arrhythmia doesn't respond within 10 minutes after infusion ends, may repeat dose.

▼ Admixtures with approved diluents are stable for 24 hours at room temperature and for 48 hours if refrigerated.

▼ Don't infuse parenteral products that contain particulate matter or are discolored.

▼ **Incompatibilities:** None reported.

ACTION
Prolongs action potential in isolated cardiac myocyte and increases atrial and ventricular refractoriness, namely class III electrophysiologic effects.

Route	Onset	Peak	Duration
I.V.	Unknown	Unknown	Unknown

Half-life: Averages about 6 hours.

ADVERSE REACTIONS
CNS: headache.
CV: *sustained polymorphic ventricular tachycardia, AV block, bradycardia, HF,* ventricular extrasystoles, *nonsustained ventricular tachycardia,* hypotension, bundle-branch block, hypertension, *prolonged QT interval,* palpitations, tachycardia.
GI: nausea.

INTERACTIONS
Drug-drug. *Class IA antiarrhythmics (disopyramide, procainamide, quinidine), other class III antiarrhythmics (amiodarone, sotalol):* May increase potential for prolonged refractoriness. Don't give these drugs for at least five half-lives before and 4 hours after ibutilide dose.
Digoxin: Supraventricular arrhythmias may mask cardiotoxicity from excessive digoxin level. Use with caution in patients who may have an increased digoxin therapeutic range.
H_1-receptor antagonists, phenothiazines, TCAs, tetracyclic antidepressants, other drugs that prolong QT interval: May increase risk for proarrhythmia. Monitor patient closely.

EFFECTS ON LAB TEST RESULTS
None reported.

CONTRAINDICATIONS & CAUTIONS
Black Box Warning Administer drug only when the benefits of maintaining sinus rhythm outweigh the immediate risks of ibutilide administration and the risks of maintenance therapy. ■

● Contraindicated in patients hypersensitive to drug or its components.

● Contraindicated in patients with history of polymorphic ventricular tachycardia.

● Use cautiously in patients with hepatic or renal dysfunction.

● Safety and effectiveness of drug haven't been established in children.

● Drug's effectiveness hasn't been determined in patients with arrhythmias of more than 90 days' duration.

Dialyzable drug: Unknown.

⚠ *Overdose S&S:* Ventricular ectopy, ventricular tachycardia, third-degree AV block.

PREGNANCY-LACTATION-REPRODUCTION
● Drug causes fetal harm in animals. Use during pregnancy only if clearly needed and potential benefit justifies potential risk to the fetus.

● It isn't known if drug appears in breast milk. Use isn't recommended in breast-feeding women.

NURSING CONSIDERATIONS
Black Box Warning Drug can cause potentially fatal arrhythmias. Only skilled personnel trained in identification and treatment of acute ventricular arrhythmias, particularly polymorphic ventricular tachycardia, should give drug. ■

● Before therapy, correct hypokalemia and hypomagnesemia to reduce risk of proarrhythmia.

Black Box Warning Patients with atrial fibrillation lasting longer than 2 to 3 days must be adequately anticoagulated, generally over at least 2 weeks. ■

● Monitor ECG continuously during administration and for at least 4 hours afterward or until QTc interval returns to baseline; drug can induce or worsen ventricular arrhythmias. Longer monitoring is required if ECG shows arrhythmia or patient has hepatic insufficiency.

• Don't give class IA or other class III antiarrhythmics with infusion or for 4 hours afterward.

PATIENT TEACHING
• Tell patient to report adverse reactions promptly.
• Instruct patient to alert nurse of discomfort at injection site.

SAFETY ALERT!

idarubicin hydrochloride
eye-duh-ROO-bi-sin

Idamycin PFS

Therapeutic class: Antineoplastics
Pharmacologic class: Semisynthetic anthracyclines

AVAILABLE FORMS
Injection: 1 mg/mL in 5-, 10-, and 20-mL single-dose vials

INDICATIONS & DOSAGES
Dosages vary. Check treatment protocol with prescriber.
➤ **Acute myeloid leukemia, including French-American-British classifications M1 through M7, with other approved antileukemic drugs**
Adults: 12 mg/m^2 daily for 3 days by slow I.V. injection (over 10 to 15 minutes) with 100 mg/m^2 daily of cytarabine for 7 days by continuous I.V. infusion. Or, cytarabine may be given as 25-mg/m^2 bolus; then 200 mg/m^2 daily for 5 days by continuous I.V. infusion. A second course may be given, if needed.
Adjust-a-dose: If patient experiences severe mucositis, delay second course of therapy until recovery is complete; reduce dosage by 25%. Reduce dosage for renal impairment. If serum creatinine level is greater than 2 mg/dL, reduce dosage by 25%. If serum bilirubin level is 2.6 to 5 mg/dL, give 50% of usual dose. Don't give drug if bilirubin is greater than 5 mg/dL.
➤ **Acute myeloid leukemia (newly diagnosed)** ◆
Infants, children, adolescents: Per clinical trial CCG-2961, for induction and

consolidation, 5 mg/m^2/dose I.V. daily for 4 days on days 0 to 3 in combination with cytarabine, etoposide, thioguanine, and dexamethasone. Or, for consolidation only, 12 mg/m^2/dose I.V. daily for 3 days on days 0 to 2 in combination with fludarabine and cytarabine.
Adjust-a-dose: For patients with GFR of 50 mL/minute/1.73 m^2 or lower and those on intermittent hemodialysis, peritoneal dialysis, or continuous renal replacement therapy, give 75% of dose.
Black Box Warning Reduce dosage in patients with hepatic or renal impairment. Don't give idarubicin if bilirubin level exceeds 5 mg/dL. ■

ADMINISTRATION
I.V.
▼ Preparing and giving parenteral drug may be mutagenic, teratogenic, or carcinogenic. Follow facility policy to reduce risks.
▼ Reconstitute to final concentration of 1 mg/mL using NSS for injection without preservatives. Add 5 mL to 5-mg vial, 10 mL to 10-mg vial, or 20 mL to 20-mg vial. Don't use bacteriostatic water solution. Vial is under negative pressure.
Black Box Warning Give drug over 10 to 15 minutes into a free-flowing I.V. infusion. Don't give I.M. or subcutaneously. Drug is a vesicant; tissue necrosis may occur. ■
▼ If extravasation occurs, stop infusion immediately and notify prescriber. Treat with intermittent ice packs for ½ hour immediately and then for ½ hour q.i.d. for 3 days.
▼ Reconstituted solutions are stable for 72 hours at 59° to 86° F (15° to 30° C) and for 7 days if refrigerated and protected from light. Label unused solutions with chemotherapy hazard label.
▼ **Incompatibilities:** Many other drugs.

ACTION
Unknown. Probably inhibits nucleic acid synthesis and interacts with the enzyme topoisomerase II. Drug is highly lipophilic, which increases rate of cellular uptake.

Route	Onset	Peak	Duration
I.V.	Unknown	Few min	Unknown

Half-life: 20 to 22 hours.

ADVERSE REACTIONS

CNS: headache, changed mental status, peripheral neuropathy, *seizures,* fever.
CV: *hemorrhage, HF, MI, myocardial insufficiency, arrhythmias, myocardial toxicity,* atrial fibrillation, chest pain, asymptomatic decline in LVEF.
GI: nausea, vomiting, cramps, diarrhea, mucositis.
GU: renal dysfunction, red urine.
Hematologic: *myelosuppression.*
Hepatic: changes in hepatic function.
Metabolic: hyperuricemia.
Skin: alopecia, rash, urticaria, bullous erythrodermatous rash on palms and soles, erythema at previously irradiated sites, tissue necrosis if extravasation occurs.
Other: *infection,* hypersensitivity reactions.

INTERACTIONS

Drug-drug. *Alkaline solutions, heparin:* These combinations are incompatible. Don't mix idarubicin with other drugs unless specific compatibility data are known.
Live-virus vaccines: May increase risk of vaccine-induced adverse reactions. Avoid using together.

EFFECTS ON LAB TEST RESULTS

• May increase uric acid level. May decrease Hb level.
• May decrease WBC, neutrophil, and platelet counts.

CONTRAINDICATIONS & CAUTIONS

Black Box Warning Don't give idarubicin if serum bilirubin level exceeds 5 mg/dL. ■
• Use cautiously in patients with bone marrow suppression induced by previous drug therapy or radiotherapy, impaired hepatic or renal function, previous treatment with anthracyclines or cardiotoxic drugs, or a cardiac condition.
Dialyzable drug: Unlikely.
⚠ Overdose S&S: Severe and prolonged myelosuppression, increased severity of GI toxicity, severe arrhythmia, acute cardiac toxicity, increased incidence of delayed HF.

PREGNANCY-LACTATION-REPRODUCTION

• There are no adequate studies in pregnant women. If used during pregnancy, or if patient becomes pregnant during therapy, inform her of potential hazard to the fetus. Advise women of childbearing potential to avoid pregnancy.
• It isn't known if drug appears in breast milk. Patient should stop breast-feeding before using drug.

NURSING CONSIDERATIONS

Black Box Warning Drug should be given only under the supervision of a physician experienced in the use of cancer chemotherapeutic agents. ■
Black Box Warning Cardiotoxicity is the dose-limiting toxicity of drug. It is more common in those who have received prior anthracyclines or who have preexisting cardiac disease. No maximum cumulative lifetime dose for cardiotoxicity has been determined. ■
• CV adverse effects occur with greater frequency in older patients.
• Make sure patient is adequately hydrated before treatment. Hyperuricemia may result from rapid lysis of leukemic cells. Allopurinol may be ordered.
• Assess patient for systemic infection and ensure that it's controlled before therapy begins.
• Give antiemetics to prevent or treat nausea and vomiting.
• Monitor LFTs and renal function tests and CBC frequently.
• To prevent bleeding, avoid all I.M. injections when platelet count is below 50,000/mm^3.
Black Box Warning Severe myelosuppression may occur. ■
• Anticipate need for blood transfusions for anemia.
• Notify prescriber if signs or symptoms of HF occur.
• *Look alike–sound alike:* Don't confuse idarubicin with daunorubicin or doxorubicin.

PATIENT TEACHING

• Teach patient to recognize signs and symptoms of leakage of drug into surrounding tissue, and tell him to report them if they occur.

Reactions in bold italics are *life-threatening.* Interactions may have a *rapid onset* or a *delayed onset.*

• Warn patient to watch for signs and symptoms of infection (fever, sore throat, fatigue) and bleeding (easy bruising, nosebleeds, bleeding gums, tarry stools).

• Advise patient that red urine for several days is normal and doesn't indicate presence of blood.

• Caution woman of childbearing potential to avoid becoming pregnant during therapy. Recommend that she consult prescriber before becoming pregnant.

idarucizumab
EYE-da-roo-siz-ue-mab

Praxbind

Therapeutic class: Antidotes
Pharmacologic class: Humanized monoclonal antibody fragments

AVAILABLE FORMS
Injection: 2.5 g/50 mL in single-use vials

INDICATIONS & DOSAGES
➤ **To reverse anticoagulant effects of dabigatran etexilate mesylate (Pradaxa) for emergency surgery or urgent procedures; for life-threatening or uncontrolled bleeding**
Adults: 5 g (two 2.5-g vials) as two consecutive I.V. infusions or as two bolus injections, injecting contents of both vials consecutively, one after the other, using syringes.

ADMINISTRATION
I.V.

▼ Inspect for discoloration and particulate matter before giving. Solution is colorless to slightly yellow and clear to slightly opalescent.

▼ Give drug within 1 hour of removal from vial.

▼ A preexisting I.V. line may be used for administration but line must be flushed with NSS before infusion.

▼ Don't administer other infusions at the same time using the same I.V. access.

▼ Store vials in refrigerator at 36° to 46° F (2° to 8° C). Don't freeze or shake.

▼ Before use, unopened vial may be kept at room temperature (77° F [25° C]) for up to 48 hours if stored in the original package to protect from light, or up to 6 hours when exposed to light.

▼ **Incompatibilities:** Other I.V. drugs or infusions.

ACTION
A humanized monoclonal antibody fragment that binds specifically to dabigatran and its acylglucuronide metabolites with higher affinity than the binding affinity of dabigatran to thrombin, neutralizing dabigatran's anticoagulant effects within minutes.

Route	Onset	Peak	Duration
I.V.	Rapid	Unknown	24 hr

Half-life: 10.3 hours.

ADVERSE REACTIONS
CNS: headache, delirium, pyrexia.
GI: constipation.
Metabolic: *hypokalemia.*
Respiratory: pneumonia.
Other: *hypersensitivity.*

INTERACTIONS
None reported.

EFFECTS ON LAB TEST RESULTS
• May decrease potassium level.
• May prolong aPTT and ecarin clotting time.

CONTRAINDICATIONS & CAUTIONS
• Hypersensitivity and anaphylactoid reactions, such as pyrexia, bronchospasm, hyperventilation, rash, and pruritus, may occur. If reactions occur, discontinue drug.

• Reversing dabigatran therapy exposes patients to the thrombotic risk of their underlying disease. To reduce this risk, consider resumption of anticoagulant therapy as soon as medically appropriate. Dabigatran therapy can be started 24 hours after idarucizumab is given.

❸ *Alert:* Drug contains sorbitol. Use cautiously in patients with hereditary fructose intolerance, as serious and even fatal reactions, including hypoglycemia, hypophosphatemia, metabolic acidosis, increased uric acid level, and acute liver failure, have been reported. The minimum amount of

sorbitol at which serious adverse reactions may occur in these patients isn't known.
Dialyzable drug: Unknown.

PREGNANCY-LACTATION-REPRODUCTION

• There are no adequate studies in pregnant women. It isn't known if drug can cause fetal harm or affect reproductive capacity. Use during pregnancy only if clearly needed.
• It isn't known if drug appears in breast milk. Use cautiously in breast-feeding women.

NURSING CONSIDERATIONS

• For patients with elevated coagulation parameters and reappearance of clinically relevant bleeding, or who require a second emergency surgery or urgent procedure, an additional 5 g of drug may be considered. Safety and effectiveness of repeat treatment haven't been established.
• Assess patient for history of hereditary fructose intolerance before giving drug.
• Drug hasn't been studied in patients with hepatic impairment.
• Safety and effectiveness in children haven't been established.

PATIENT TEACHING

• Warn patient to immediately report signs and symptoms of hypersensitivity and anaphylactoid reactions (fever, bronchospasm, dyspnea, rash, itching), as drug will need to be discontinued.
• Instruct patient to seek immediate medical attention for signs or symptoms of bleeding.
• Warn patient that reversing dabigatran therapy exposes patient to the thromboembolic risk of the underlying disease. Advise patient that anticoagulant therapy may be resumed as soon as possible to reduce this risk.
• Teach patient with hereditary fructose intolerance to report this condition before receiving drug because drug contains sorbitol and may cause serious and even fatal reactions.

idelalisib
eye-DEL-a-lis-ib

Zydelig

Therapeutic class: Antineoplastics
Pharmacologic class: Kinase inhibitors

AVAILABLE FORMS

Tablets ⓞⓣⓒ: 100 mg, 150 mg

INDICATIONS & DOSAGES

➤ **Relapsed chronic lymphocytic leukemia, in combination with rituximab, in patients for whom rituximab alone would be considered appropriate therapy due to other comorbidities; relapsed follicular B-cell non-Hodgkin lymphoma or relapsed small lymphocytic lymphoma in patients who have received at least two prior systemic therapies**
Adults: 150 mg P.O. b.i.d. Continue treatment until disease progression or unacceptable toxicity.
Adjust-a-dose: Discontinue drug in patients with symptomatic pneumonitis of any severity. For AST/ALT level greater than 3 to 5 × ULN, maintain dosage and monitor at least weekly until AST/ALT level is 1 × ULN or less. If ALT/AST level is greater than 5 to 20 × ULN, withhold drug and monitor at least weekly until ALT/AST level is 1 × ULN or less; then resume at 100 mg b.i.d. If AST/ALT level is greater than 20 × ULN or hepatotoxicity recurs, discontinue drug permanently.
  If bilirubin level is greater than 1.5 to 3 × ULN, maintain dosage and monitor at least weekly until level is 1 × ULN or less. If bilirubin level is greater than 3 to 10 × ULN, withhold drug and monitor at least weekly until bilirubin level is 1 × ULN or less; then resume at 100 mg b.i.d. If bilirubin level is greater than 10 × ULN or hepatotoxicity recurs, discontinue drug permanently.
  If diarrhea occurs and is moderate (increase of four to six stools per day over baseline), maintain dosage and monitor at least weekly until resolved. If diarrhea is severe (seven or more stools per day over baseline) or requires hospitalization,

withhold drug and monitor at least weekly until resolved; then resume at 100 mg b.i.d. If diarrhea is life-threatening, discontinue drug permanently.

If ANC is 1,000 to less than 1,500 cells/mm^3, maintain dosage. If ANC is 500 to less than 1,000 cells/mm^3, maintain dosage and monitor ANC at least weekly. If ANC is less than 500 cells/mm^3, interrupt therapy and monitor ANC at least weekly until ANC is 500 cells/mm^3 or more; then resume at 100 mg b.i.d.

If thrombocytopenia occurs and platelet count is 50,000 to less than 75,000 cells/mm^3, maintain dosage. If platelet count is 25,000 to less than 50,000 cells/mm^3, maintain dosage and monitor platelet count at least weekly. If platelet count is less than 25,000 cells/mm^3, interrupt therapy and monitor platelet count at least weekly; may resume at 100 mg b.i.d. when platelet count recovers to greater than 25,000 cells/mm^3.

For other severe or life-threatening drug-related toxicities, withhold drug until toxicity is resolved. If resuming drug after interruption for other severe or life-threatening toxicities, reduce dosage to 100 mg b.i.d. Discontinue drug permanently for recurrence of other severe or life-threatening drug-related toxicities upon rechallenge.

ADMINISTRATION
P.O.
- Drug is considered hazardous; use safe-handling precautions.
- Give without regard for food.
- Patients should swallow tablets whole. Don't crush or split tablets.
- If a dose is missed by less than 6 hours, give missed dose right away and give next dose as usual. If a dose is missed by more than 6 hours, wait to give the next dose at the usual time.

ACTION
Induces apoptosis and inhibits proliferation in cell lines derived from malignant B cells and in primary tumor cell. Also inhibits several cell-signaling pathways to halt movement of B cells to lymph nodes and bone marrow.

Route	Onset	Peak	Duration
P.O.	Unknown	1½ hr	Unknown

Half-life: About 8 hours.

ADVERSE REACTIONS
CNS: headache, pain, night sweats, pyrexia, fatigue, asthenia, insomnia.
CV: peripheral edema.
EENT: nasal congestion, sinusitis.
GI: abdominal pain, nausea, vomiting, *diarrhea,* decreased appetite, GERD, stomatitis, *colitis.*
GU: UTI.
Hematologic: *neutropenia.*
Hepatic: *hepatotoxicity.*
Musculoskeletal: arthralgia.
Respiratory: pneumonia, cough, dyspnea, bronchitis, URI.
Skin: rash.
Other: chills, *sepsis.*

INTERACTIONS
Drug-drug. *CYP3A inducers (carbamazepine, phenytoin, rifampin):* May decrease idelalisib concentration. Avoid use together.
CYP3A inhibitors (ketoconazole, nefazodone, ritonavir, telithromycin): May increase idelalisib level. Monitor patient for toxicity; modify dosage if adverse reactions occur.
CYP3A substrates (alfentanil, cyclosporine, dihydroergotamine, ergotamine, fentanyl, pimozide, quinidine, sirolimus, tacrolimus): May increase substrate concentration. Avoid use together.
Hepatotoxic drugs: May increase risk of hepatotoxicity. Don't use together.
Other drugs that cause diarrhea: May increase risk of diarrhea and toxicity. Avoid use together.
Drug-herb. *St. John's wort:* May decrease idelalisib concentration. Don't use together.

EFFECTS ON LAB TEST RESULTS
- May increase ALT, AST, GGT, bilirubin, and triglyceride levels. May decrease sodium level.
- May increase or decrease glucose level.
- May decrease Hb level and neutrophil and platelet counts.
- May increase or decrease lymphocyte count.

CONTRAINDICATIONS & CAUTIONS

• Contraindicated in patients hypersensitive to drug or its components and in those with history of anaphylaxis or toxic epidermal necrolysis when exposed to drug.

• Severe or life-threatening cutaneous reactions can occur. Discontinue drug for any severe reaction.

Black Box Warning Drug may cause serious or fatal hepatotoxicity, severe diarrhea or colitis, pneumonitis, or intestinal perforation. ∎

• Safety and effectiveness in children younger than age 18 haven't been established.

Dialyzable drug: Unknown.

PREGNANCY-LACTATION-REPRODUCTION

• Women of childbearing potential should avoid becoming pregnant while taking drug. If drug is used during pregnancy, or if patient becomes pregnant while taking drug, she should be told of potential hazard to a fetus.

• Women of childbearing potential should use effective contraception during treatment and for at least 1 month after last dose.

• It isn't known if drug appears in breast milk. Patient should discontinue breastfeeding or discontinue drug.

NURSING CONSIDERATIONS

Black Box Warning Monitor AST, ALT, and bilirubin levels because hepatotoxicity may occur; monitor patient carefully and discontinue drug if necessary. Obtain baseline LFTs every 2 weeks for first 3 months of treatment, every 4 weeks for next 3 months, then every 1 to 3 months thereafter. Obtain LFTs weekly to monitor for hepatotoxicity if ALT or AST level rises above 3 × ULN; monitor levels until resolved. Withhold drug if ALT or AST level is greater than 5 × ULN; continue to monitor AST, ALT, and total bilirubin levels weekly until the abnormality is resolved. ∎

Black Box Warning Monitor patient carefully for diarrhea, colitis, and intestinal perforation (new or worsening abdominal pain, chills, fever, nausea, or vomiting); discontinue drug if necessary. ∎

Black Box Warning Monitor patient for respiratory signs and symptoms (cough,

dyspnea, hypoxia, bilateral interstitial infiltrates on X-ray, decrease in oxygen saturation level by more than 5%). If pneumonitis is suspected, interrupt therapy until cause of the pulmonary symptoms has been determined. If pneumonitis is secondary to drug, discontinue drug and treat with corticosteroids. ∎

Black Box Warning Serious infections (pneumonia, sepsis, febrile neutropenia), including fatal infections, have occurred. Monitor for signs and symptoms of infection and interrupt drug for Grade 3 or higher infection. ∎

❸ *Alert:* Consider Pneumocystis jirovecii pneumonia, (PJP) prophylaxis. Interrupt treatment in patient with suspected PJP infection of any grade and permanently discontinue drug if PJP infection is confirmed.

❸ *Alert:* Interrupt treatment for positive cytomegalovirus (CMV) infection until infection has resolved. Monitor for CMV reactivation at least monthly if drug is resumed.

• Monitor CBC, ANC, and platelet count at least every 2 weeks for first 3 months of therapy, and at least weekly in patients whose neutrophil count is less than 1,000 cells/mm^3.

• Drug responds poorly to antimotility agents given for diarrhea.

• Monitor patient for rash.

• Older patients may have increased risk of adverse effects. Monitor these patients carefully.

• Monitor patients for anaphylaxis; discontinue drug if anaphylaxis occurs.

• *Look alike–sound alike:* Don't confuse Zydelig with Zykadia.

PATIENT TEACHING

• Advise patient to take drug exactly as prescribed. If a dose is missed by less than 6 hours, tell patient to take missed dose right away and to take next dose as usual. If a dose is missed by more than 6 hours, advise patient to wait and take next dose at usual time.

Black Box Warning Instruct patient to report jaundice, bruising, abdominal pain, or bleeding. ∎

Black Box Warning Caution patient to immediately notify prescriber if the number

---

Reactions in bold italics are *life-threatening*. Interactions may have a *rapid onset* or a *delayed onset*.

of bowel movements in a day increases by six or more. ∎

Black Box Warning Warn patient to immediately notify prescriber if severe abdominal pain, chills, fever, nausea, or vomiting occurs, because of risk of colitis and intestinal perforation. ∎

• Advise patient to immediately notify prescriber if fever or signs or symptoms of infection occur.

Black Box Warning Advise patient to report new or worsening respiratory signs and symptoms, including cough or dyspnea. ∎

• Instruct patient that blood tests will be needed periodically, as ordered, to minimize risk of adverse reactions.

• Caution patient that drug may cause severe cutaneous reactions and to notify prescriber immediately if a severe skin reaction develops.

• Counsel female patient to avoid pregnancy and to use adequate contraception during therapy and for at least 1 month after therapy ends.

• Advise female patient to contact prescriber if she becomes pregnant or suspects she is pregnant.

• Caution patient not to breast-feed during therapy.

SAFETY ALERT!

ifosfamide
eye-FOSS-fa-mide

Ifex

Therapeutic class: Antineoplastics
Pharmacologic class: Nitrogen mustards

AVAILABLE FORMS
Powder for injection: 1-g, 3-g vials

INDICATIONS & DOSAGES
➤ **Germ cell testicular cancer**
Adults: 1.2 g/m^2 I.V. daily for 5 consecutive days. Repeat treatment every 3 weeks or after patient recovers from hematologic toxicity. Don't repeat doses until WBC count exceeds 4,000/mm^3 and platelet count exceeds 100,000/mm^3.
Adjust-a-dose: For patients with renal insufficiency, reduce dosage as follows: If GFR is 30 to 60 mL/minute, give 75% of usual dose; if GFR is 10 to 30 mL/minute, give 50% of usual dose. Don't give dose if GFR is less than 10 mL/minute. For patients with hepatic dysfunction, consider decreasing dosage to 25% of usual dose if serum AST level is greater than 300 units/L or if bilirubin level is greater than 3 mg/dL.

ADMINISTRATION
I.V.
▼ Preparing and giving drug may be mutagenic, teratogenic, or carcinogenic. Follow facility policy to reduce risks.
▼ Give a protective drug such as mesna to prevent hemorrhagic cystitis. Ifosfamide and mesna are physically compatible and may be mixed in the same I.V. solution.
▼ Obtain urinalysis before each dose. If microscopic hematuria occurs, notify prescriber. Adjust dosage of mesna, if needed. Adequate fluid intake (2 L daily, either P.O. or I.V.) is essential before, and 72 hours after, therapy.
▼ Reconstitute each gram of drug with 20 mL of diluent to yield a solution of 50 mg/mL. Use sterile water for injection or bacteriostatic water for injection. Solutions may then be further diluted with sterile water, dextrose 2.5% or 5% in water, half-NSS or NSS for injection, dextrose 5% and NSS for injection, or lactated Ringer injection.
▼ Infuse each dose over at least 30 minutes.
▼ Reconstituted solution is stable for 1 week at room temperature or 6 weeks if refrigerated. However, use solution within 6 hours if drug was reconstituted with sterile water without a preservative (such as benzyl alcohol or parabens).
▼ **Incompatibilities:** Cefepime, mesna with epirubicin, methotrexate sodium.

ACTION
Cross-links strands of cellular DNA and interferes with RNA transcription, causing an imbalance of growth that leads to cell death. Not specific to cell cycle.

Route	Onset	Peak	Duration
I.V.	Unknown	Unknown	Unknown

Half-life: Dose-dependent mean terminal, 7 to 15 hours.

ADVERSE REACTIONS

CNS: somnolence, confusion, hallucinations, depressive psychosis, fever, *seizures, coma.*
GI: nausea, vomiting.
GU: hemorrhagic cystitis, hematuria, dysuria, urinary frequency.
Hematologic: *leukopenia, thrombocytopenia, myelosuppression.*
Skin: alopecia.
Other: infection, phlebitis.

INTERACTIONS

Drug-drug. *Anticoagulants, aspirin, NSAIDs:* May increase risk of bleeding. Avoid using together.
Barbiturates, chloral hydrate, fosphenytoin, phenytoin: May increase ifosfamide toxicity. Monitor patient closely.
Corticosteroids: May inhibit hepatic enzymes, reducing ifosfamide's effect. Monitor patient for increased ifosfamide toxicity if corticosteroid dosage is suddenly reduced or stopped.
Cyclophosphamide: May increase risk of cardiac tamponade in patients with thalassemia. Monitor patient closely.
Live-virus vaccines: May increase risk of vaccine-induced adverse reactions. Avoid using together.
Myelosuppressive drugs: May enhance hematologic toxicity. Dosage adjustment may be needed.

EFFECTS ON LAB TEST RESULTS

• May increase liver enzyme levels.
• May decrease WBC and platelet counts.

CONTRAINDICATIONS & CAUTIONS

• Contraindicated in patients hypersensitive to drug and in those with severe bone marrow suppression or urinary outflow obstruction.
• Use cautiously in patients with renal impairment or compromised bone marrow reserve, as indicated by leukopenia, granulocytopenia, extensive bone marrow metastases, previous radiation therapy, or previous therapy with cytotoxic drugs.
• Don't give drug if CrCl is less than 10 mL/minute.

• Drug may suppress immune response and increase risk of serious infection, sepsis, or septic shock. Use cautiously.
Dialyzable drug: 75% to 100%.

PREGNANCY-LACTATION-REPRODUCTION

• Drug can cause fetal harm. Women shouldn't become pregnant and men shouldn't father a child during therapy and for up to 6 months after therapy ends.
• Drug appears in breast milk. Women mustn't breast-feed during therapy.
• Drug interferes with oogenesis and spermatogenesis. Amenorrhea, azoospermia, and sterility in both sexes have been reported and appear to depend on drug dosage, duration of therapy, and state of gonadal function at time of treatment. Sterility may be irreversible in some patients.

NURSING CONSIDERATIONS

Black Box Warning Urotoxic adverse effects, especially hemorrhagic cystitis, and CNS toxicities, such as confusion and coma, may require cessation of ifosfamide therapy. Hemorrhagic cystitis can be reduced by prophylactic use of mesna. ∎
Black Box Warning Myelosuppression can be severe and lead to fatal infections. Monitor blood counts before and at intervals after each treatment cycle. ∎
• Give antiemetic before drug, to reduce nausea.
• Ensure that patient is adequately hydrated during therapy.
• Patients are at increased risk for hemorrhagic cystitis. Obtain urinalysis before each dose. Withhold drug for microscopic hematuria (greater than 10 RBCs per high power field) until completely resolved.
• If cystitis develops, stop drug and notify prescriber.
• Bladder irrigation with NSS may be done to treat cystitis.
• Monitor CBC, renal function, and LFT values.
• To prevent bleeding, avoid all I.M. injections when platelet count is less than $50,000/mm^3$.
• Anticipate blood transfusions because of cumulative anemia.
• Assess patient for CNS toxicity, which may be severe and cause death; dosage

---

Reactions in bold italics are *life-threatening*. Interactions may have a *rapid onset* or a *delayed onset*.

reduction may be needed. Discontinue drug if encephalopathy occurs.

● *Look alike–sound alike:* Don't confuse ifosfamide with cyclophosphamide.

PATIENT TEACHING

● Remind patient to urinate frequently to minimize contact of drug and its metabolites with the lining of the bladder.

● Advise patient to watch for signs and symptoms of infection (fever, sore throat, fatigue) and bleeding (easy bruising, nosebleeds, bleeding gums, tarry stools). Tell patient to take temperature daily.

● Instruct patient to avoid OTC products that contain aspirin.

● Advise women to stop breast-feeding during therapy because of possible risk of toxicity to infant.

● Advise men to avoid fathering a child during therapy and for up to 6 months after therapy ends.

● Caution woman of childbearing potential to avoid becoming pregnant during therapy. Recommend that she consult prescriber before becoming pregnant.

iloperidone
ill-oh-PER-ih-done

Fanapt

Therapeutic class: Antipsychotics
Pharmacologic class: Dopamine–serotonin antagonists

AVAILABLE FORMS
Tablets: 1 mg, 2 mg, 4 mg, 6 mg, 8 mg, 10 mg, 12 mg

INDICATIONS & DOSAGES
➤ **Schizophrenia**
Adults: Initially, 1 mg P.O. b.i.d. Increase dosage daily as needed according to the following dosing schedule: 2 mg P.O. b.i.d. on day 2; 4 mg P.O. b.i.d. on day 3; 6 mg P.O. b.i.d. on day 4; 8 mg P.O. b.i.d. on day 5; 10 mg P.O. b.i.d. on day 6; 12 mg P.O. b.i.d. on day 7. Maximum dosage is 12 mg P.O. b.i.d.

Adjust-a-dose: For patients who are poor metabolizers of CYP2D6 and those taking CYP2D6 inhibitors (fluoxetine, paroxetine, quinidine) or CYP3A4 inhibitors (clarithromycin, ketoconazole), reduce dosage by half.

ADMINISTRATION
P.O.
● Give drug with or without food.

ACTION
May antagonize dopamine type 2 and serotonin type 2.

Route	Onset	Peak	Duration
P.O.	Unknown	2–4 hr	Unknown

Half-life: 18 to 37 hours.

ADVERSE REACTIONS
CNS: aggression, delusion, dizziness, extrapyramidal effects, fatigue, lethargy, restlessness, somnolence, tremor.
CV: hypotension, orthostatic hypotension, palpitations, tachycardia.
EENT: blurred vision, conjunctivitis, dry mouth, nasal congestion, nasopharyngitis.
GI: abdominal discomfort, diarrhea, nausea.
GU: ejaculation failure, erectile dysfunction, urinary incontinence.
Hematologic: hyperprolactinemia.
Metabolic: weight gain, weight loss.
Musculoskeletal: arthralgia, muscle spasm, musculoskeletal stiffness, myalgia.
Respiratory: dyspnea, URI.
Skin: rash.

INTERACTIONS
Drug-drug. *Alpha$_1$ blockers:* May enhance antihypertensive effects. Use together cautiously.
CYP3A4 or CYP2D6 inhibitors (clarithromycin, fluoxetine, ketoconazole, paroxetine, quinidine): May increase iloperidone level. Reduce dosage by half.
Dextromethorphan: May increase dextromethorphan level. Avoid use together.
Drugs that prolong QT interval: May cause lethal arrhythmias. Avoid use together.
Black Box Warning *Opioids:* May cause slow or difficult breathing, sedation, and death. Avoid use together. If use together is necessary, limit dosage and duration of each

drug to the minimum necessary for desired effect. ■

Drug-lifestyle. *Alcohol use:* May increase CNS effects. Discourage use together.

EFFECTS ON LAB TEST RESULTS

- May decrease hematocrit.

CONTRAINDICATIONS & CAUTIONS

- Contraindicated in patients hypersensitive to drug or its components; anaphylaxis, angioedema, and other hypersensitivity reactions have been reported.

Black Box Warning Opioid drugs should only be prescribed with benzodiazepines or other CNS depressants to patients for whom alternative treatment options are inadequate. ■

- Avoid use with other drugs known to prolong the QT interval, in patients with history of cardiac arrhythmias, and in elderly patients with dementia-related psychosis.
- Use cautiously in patients with history of stroke, TIA, QT-interval prolongation, diabetes, seizures, orthostatic hypotension, neuroleptic malignant syndrome, tardive dyskinesia, leukopenia, neutropenia, agranulocytosis, suicidal ideation, or priapism.
- Use cautiously in patients with moderate hepatic impairment. Use in patients with severe hepatic impairment isn't recommended.

Dialyzable drug: Unknown.

⚠ ***Overdose S&S:*** Prolonged QT interval, drowsiness, sedation, tachycardia, hypotension.

PREGNANCY-LACTATION-REPRODUCTION

- There are no adequate studies in pregnant women. Use during pregnancy only if potential benefit justifies potential risk to the fetus.

Alert: Neonates exposed to antipsychotics during the third trimester are at risk for developing extrapyramidal symptoms (repetitive muscle movements of face and body) and withdrawal symptoms (agitation, abnormally increased or decreased muscle tone, tremors, sleepiness, severe difficulty breathing, difficulty feeding) after delivery.

- It isn't known if drug appears in breast milk. Use in breast-feeding women isn't recommended.

NURSING CONSIDERATIONS

Black Box Warning Fatal CV events may occur in elderly patients with dementia. Drug isn't approved for use in patients with dementia-related psychosis. ■

- Symptom control may be delayed during the first 1 to 2 weeks of treatment compared to other antipsychotics that don't require similar titration.

Alert: Obtain baseline BP measurements before starting therapy, and monitor BP regularly. Watch for orthostatic hypotension, especially during first dosage adjustments.

Alert: Watch for evidence of neuroleptic malignant syndrome (hyperthermia, muscle rigidity, altered mental status, and autonomic instability), which is rare but can be fatal.

Alert: Life-threatening hyperglycemia may occur in patients taking atypical antipsychotics. Monitor patients with diabetes regularly. Monitor fasting blood glucose level at drug initiation and periodically during therapy in patients with risk factors for diabetes.

- Monitor patient for tardive dyskinesia, which may occur with prolonged use of drug. If tardive dyskinesia occurs, discontinue drug unless patient's condition warrants continued use.
- Monitor patient for suicidal thinking and behavior.
- Dispense lowest appropriate quantity of drug to reduce the risk of overdose.
- Monitor patient for weight gain.
- Periodically reassess patient to determine continued need for therapy.
- Monitor CBC frequently during the first few months of therapy and discontinue drug if WBC count drops with no other underlying cause.
- Monitor potassium and magnesium levels at baseline and periodically in patients at risk for electrolyte imbalance.
- Drug may lower seizure threshold in patients with a history of seizures; monitor these patients closely.

PATIENT TEACHING

Black Box Warning Caution the patient or the caregiver of a patient taking an opioid drug with a benzodiazepine, CNS depressant, or alcohol to seek immediate medical attention if the patient has symptoms of dizziness, light-headedness, extreme sleepiness, slowed or difficult breathing, or unresponsiveness. ■

• Warn patient to avoid driving and other hazardous activities that require mental alertness until the drug's effects are known.

• Tell patient drug can be taken with or without food.

• Warn patient to rise slowly, avoid hot showers, and use other precautions to avoid fainting when starting therapy.

• Advise patient to avoid becoming overheated or dehydrated.

• Tell female patient of childbearing potential to notify prescriber about planned, suspected, or known pregnancy.

• Advise breast-feeding women not to breast-feed during therapy.

• Instruct patient to report symptoms of dizziness, palpitations, or fainting to prescriber.

• Advise patient to avoid alcohol use while taking drug.

• Tell male patient to seek emergency medical care if an erection lasts more than 4 hours.

• Warn patient and caregiver about the risk of neuroleptic malignant syndrome, and advise them to seek emergency medical care if symptoms occur.

• Tell patient to notify prescriber about other prescription or OTC drugs he's taking or plans to take.

iloprost
EYE-loe-prost

Ventavis

Therapeutic class: Pulmonary vasodilators
Pharmacologic class: Prostacyclin analogues

AVAILABLE FORMS
Inhalation solution: 10 mcg/mL, 20 mcg/mL in single-dose ampules

INDICATIONS & DOSAGES
➤ **Pulmonary arterial hypertension (PAH) in patients with New York Heart Association (NYHA) Class III or IV symptoms**
Adults: Initially, 2.5 mcg inhaled using the I-neb Adaptive Aerosol Delivery (AAD) or Prodose AAD systems. As tolerated, increase to 5 mcg inhaled six to nine times daily while patient is awake, as needed, but to no more than every 2 hours. Maximum, 5 mcg nine times daily.

Adjust-a-dose: For patients with hepatic impairment (Child-Pugh class B or C), consider increasing dosing interval to every 3 to 4 hours depending on patient response.

ADMINISTRATION
Inhalational
• Use only I-neb AAD or Prodose AAD delivery devices, per manufacturer's instructions.

ACTION
Lowers pulmonary arterial pressure by dilating systemic and pulmonary arterial beds. Drug also affects platelet aggregation, although effect in pulmonary hypertension treatment isn't known.

Route	Onset	Peak	Duration
Inhalation	Unknown	Within 5 min	30–60 min

Half-life: 20 to 30 minutes.

ADVERSE REACTIONS
CNS: headache, insomnia, syncope.
CV: hypotension, vasodilation, chest pain, *HF, supraventricular tachycardia,* palpitations, peripheral edema.
GI: nausea, tongue pain, vomiting.
GU: *renal failure.*
Musculoskeletal: trismus, back pain, muscle cramps.
Respiratory: cough, dyspnea, hemoptysis, pneumonia.
Other: flulike syndrome.

INTERACTIONS
Drug-drug. *Anticoagulants, antiplatelet drugs:* May increase risk of bleeding. Monitor patient closely.
Antihypertensives, vasodilators: May increase effects of these drugs. Monitor BP.

EFFECTS ON LAB TEST RESULTS
● May increase alkaline phosphatase and GGT levels.

CONTRAINDICATIONS & CAUTIONS
● No known contraindications. Avoid using in patients whose systolic BP is less than 85 mm Hg.
● Use cautiously in elderly patients, patients with hepatic or renal impairment, and patients with COPD, severe asthma, or acute pulmonary infection.
● PAH may worsen if drug is withdrawn abruptly or dosages are reduced.
Dialyzable drug: Unknown.
⚠ *Overdose S&S:* Diarrhea, flushing, headache, hypotension, nausea, vomiting.

PREGNANCY-LACTATION-REPRODUCTION
● There are no adequate studies in pregnant women. Use during pregnancy only if potential benefit justifies potential risk to the fetus.
● It isn't known if drug appears in breast milk. Patient should discontinue breast-feeding or discontinue drug.

NURSING CONSIDERATIONS
● Keep drug away from skin and eyes; avoid inhaling while providing treatment.
● The 2-mL ampule must be used with the Prodose AAD and may be used with the I-neb AAD. The 1-mL ampule must be used only with the I-neb AAD.
● Monitor patient's vital signs carefully at start of treatment. Monitor patient for syncope.
● If patient develops evidence of pulmonary edema, stop treatment immediately.

PATIENT TEACHING
● Advise patient to take drug exactly as prescribed and using Prodose AAD or I-neb AAD.
● Advise patient to keep a backup Prodose AAD or I-neb AAD in case the original malfunctions.
● Tell patient to keep drug away from skin and eyes and to rinse the area immediately if contact occurs.
● Inform patient that drug may cause dizziness and fainting. Urge him to stand up slowly from a sitting or lying position and to report to prescriber worsening of symptoms.

● Tell patient to take drug before physical exertion, no more than every 2 hours.
● Tell patient not to expose others, especially pregnant women and infants, to drug.
● Teach patient how to clean equipment and safely dispose of used ampules after each treatment. Caution patient not to save or use leftover solution.

SAFETY ALERT!

imatinib mesylate
eh-MAT-eh-nib

ACT-Imatinib ✤, Apo-Imatinib ✤, Gleevec, Teva-Imatinib ✤

Therapeutic class: Antineoplastics
Pharmacologic class: Protein–tyrosine kinase inhibitors

AVAILABLE FORMS
Tablets ⓞ: 100 mg, 400 mg

INDICATIONS & DOSAGES
Adjust-a-dose (for all indications): For patients with CrCl of 40 to 59 mL/minute, don't exceed 600 mg daily; if CrCl is 20 to 39 mL/minute, decrease starting dose by 50% and don't exceed 400 mg daily; if CrCl is less than 20 mL/minute, don't exceed 100 mg daily. For patients with severe hepatic failure, reduce dosage by 25%. See manufacturer's package insert for full details on dosage adjustments for children; patients with neutropenia, thrombocytopenia, or hepatotoxicity; and those with adverse reactions.
➤ **Relapsed or refractory Philadelphia chromosome–positive (Ph+) acute lymphoblastic leukemia (ALL)**
Adults: 600 mg P.O. daily.
➤ **Newly diagnosed Ph+ ALL in pediatric patients in combination with chemotherapy**
Children age 1 and older: 340 mg/m^2 P.O. daily. Maximum dosage is 600 mg daily.
➤ **Aggressive systemic mastocytosis (ASM) without the D816V c-*Kit* mutation or with c-*Kit* mutational status unknown**
Adults: 400 mg P.O. daily.
Adjust-a-dose: For patients with ASM associated with eosinophilia, a clonal

hematologic disease related to the fusion kinase FIP1L1-PDGFRα, initial dose is 100 mg/day. Increase dose from 100 mg to 400 mg/day if no adverse drug reactions and if insufficient response to therapy.

➤ **Hypereosinophilic syndrome (HES) or chronic eosinophilic leukemia (CEL), or both**
Adults: 400 mg P.O. daily.

Adjust-a-dose: In HES/CEL patients with demonstrated FIP1L1-PDGFRα fusion kinase, initial dose is 100 mg/day. Increase dose from 100 mg to 400 mg/day if no adverse drug reactions and if insufficient response to therapy.

➤ **Myelodysplastic (MDS) or myeloprolif-erative (MPD) disease with *PDGFR* gene rearrangements**
Adults: 400 mg P.O. daily.

➤ **Unresectable, recurrent, or metastatic dermatofibrosarcoma protuberans (DFSP)**
Adults: 800 mg P.O. daily.

➤ **Chronic myeloid leukemia (CML) in blast crisis, in accelerated phase, or in chronic phase after failure of alfa interferon therapy; newly diagnosed Ph+ chronic-phase CML**
Adults: For chronic-phase CML, 400 mg P.O. daily as single dose with a meal and large glass of water. For accelerated-phase CML or blast crisis, 600 mg P.O. daily as single dose with a meal and large glass of water. Continue treatment as long as patient continues to benefit. May increase daily dose to 600 mg P.O. in chronic phase or to 800 mg P.O. (400 mg P.O. b.i.d.) in accelerated phase or blast crisis.
Children age 1 and older: For newly di-agnosed Ph+ chronic-phase CML only, give 340 mg/m² daily P.O. Don't exceed 600 mg/day.

➤ ***Kit* (CD117)-positive or GI stromal tumors (GISTs) after resection**
Adults: 400 mg P.O. daily.

➤ ***Kit*-positive unresectable or metastatic malignant GISTs**
Adults: 400 mg P.O. daily or b.i.d.

ADMINISTRATION
P.O.
• For daily dosing of 800 mg and above, use the 400-mg tablet to reduce exposure to iron.

• For patients unable to swallow tablets, disperse the tablets in water or apple juice (50 mL for 100-mg tablet and 200 mL for 400-mg tablet). Stir and have patient drink immediately.
• Drug is hazardous. Avoid exposure to crushed tablets. If necessary to manipulate tablets (e.g., to prepare an oral solution), double gloving, wearing a protective gown, and preparing in a controlled device is recommended.

ACTION
Inhibits the abnormal tyrosine kinase cre-ated by the Philadelphia chromosome ab-normality in CML; it inhibits tumor growth of murine myeloid cells and leukemia lines from CML patients in blast crisis.

Route	Onset	Peak	Duration
P.O.	Unknown	2–4 hr	Unknown

Half-life: Adults, 18 hours (parent drug), 40 hours (active metabolite); children, 15 hours (parent drug).

ADVERSE REACTIONS
CNS: *cerebral hemorrhage,* fatigue, headache, pyrexia, weakness, depression, dizziness, insomnia.
CV: edema.
EENT: epistaxis, nasopharyngitis.
GI: *GI hemorrhage,* abdominal pain, anorexia, constipation, diarrhea, dyspep-sia, nausea, vomiting.
Hematologic: *hemorrhage, neutropenia, thrombocytopenia,* anemia.
Metabolic: hypokalemia, weight increase.
Musculoskeletal: arthralgia, myalgia, mus-cle cramps, musculoskeletal pain, growth suppression in children.
Respiratory: cough, dyspnea, pneumonia.
Skin: petechiae, rash, pruritus.
Other: night sweats.

INTERACTIONS
Drug-drug. *CYP3A4 inducers (carba-mazepine, dexamethasone, phenobarbi-tal, phenytoin, rifampin):* May increase metabolism and decrease imatinib level. Use together cautiously.
CYP3A4 inhibitors (clarithromycin, eryth-romycin, itraconazole, ketoconazole): May decrease metabolism and increase imatinib level. Monitor patient for toxicity.

Dihydropyridine–calcium channel blockers, certain HMG-CoA reductase inhibitors (simvastatin), cyclosporine, pimozide, triazolo-benzodiazepines: May increase levels of these drugs. Monitor patient for toxicity, and obtain drug levels, if appropriate.

Levothyroxine: May increase levothyroxine clearance, causing increased TSH levels and symptoms of hypothyroidism. Monitor thyroid function.

Warfarin: May alter metabolism of warfarin. Avoid using together; use standard heparin or a low–molecular-weight heparin.

Drug-herb. *Ginseng:* May increase risk of hepatotoxicity. Avoid use together.

St. John's wort: May decrease drug effects. Discourage use together.

Drug-food. *Grapefruit juice:* May increase imatinib level. Patient should avoid grapefruit juice.

EFFECTS ON LAB TEST RESULTS

• May increase creatinine, bilirubin, alkaline phosphatase, AST, and ALT levels. May decrease potassium and Hb levels.

• May decrease neutrophil and platelet counts.

CONTRAINDICATIONS & CAUTIONS

• Contraindicated in patients hypersensitive to drug or its components.

• Use cautiously in elderly patients and in those with hepatic impairment.

• Severe HF and left ventricular dysfunction have occurred in patients taking imatinib. Use cautiously in patients with cardiac disease or risk factors for HF.

• Growth retardation has occurred in children and preadolescents receiving imatinib; long-term effects of prolonged treatment are unknown.

• Safety and effectiveness in children younger than age 1 haven't been established.

Dialyzable drug: Unknown.

⚠ **Overdose S&S:** Muscle cramps; ascites; vomiting; diarrhea; GI pain; elevated creatinine, AST, ALT, and bilirubin levels.

PREGNANCY-LACTATION-REPRODUCTION

• Drug can harm fetus. Sexually active women should use highly effective contraception during therapy.

• Drug appears in breast milk. Patient should discontinue breast-feeding or discontinue drug.

NURSING CONSIDERATIONS

• Monitor patient closely for possibly severe fluid retention. Elderly patients may have an increased risk of edema.

• There have been postmarketing reports of severe bullous skin reactions. Monitor patient for skin reactions. Drug may need to be withheld.

• Fatal tumor lysis syndrome can occur. Correct dehydration and treat high uric acid levels before starting therapy.

• Monitor weight daily. Report unexpected, rapid weight gain.

• Monitor CBC weekly for first month, every other week for second month, and periodically thereafter.

• Monitor LFTs carefully because hepatotoxicity (occasionally severe) may occur; decrease dosage as needed.

• Monitor growth of children being treated with imatinib.

• May increase dosage if no severe adverse reactions or severe non–leukemia-related neutropenia or thrombocytopenia occur in the following circumstances: disease progression, failure to achieve a satisfactory hematologic response after at least 3 months of treatment, or loss of a previously achieved hematologic response.

• In patients with HES and cardiac involvement, cases of cardiogenic shock/left ventricular dysfunction have been associated with the initiation of imatinib therapy. The condition is reversible with administration of systemic steroids and circulatory support measures, and by temporarily withholding imatinib. Monitor echocardiogram and serum troponin in patients with HES/CEL and in patients with MDS/MPD or ASM associated with high eosinophil levels.

• Grade 3/4 hemorrhage has been reported in patients with newly diagnosed CML and with GIST. GI tumor sites may be the source of GI bleeds in GIST.

• GI perforations, some fatal, have been reported.

PATIENT TEACHING

• Tell patient to take drug with food and a large glass of water.
• Advise patient unable to swallow tablets to mix them in water or apple juice (50 mL for 100-mg tablet and 200 mL for 400-mg tablet). Tell him to stir and drink immediately.
• Advise patient to report adverse effects, such as fluid retention and sudden weight gain.
• Advise patient that periodic laboratory tests will be needed to monitor therapy.
• Inform patient and caregivers that growth retardation has occurred in children and preadolescents receiving imatinib, and that long-term effects of prolonged treatment are unknown. Monitor growth closely.
• Advise patient of the risk of dizziness, blurred vision, or somnolence during treatment and to use caution when driving a car or operating machinery.
• Advise female patient to avoid pregnancy during therapy and to inform health care provider if she thinks she may be pregnant.
• Advise female patient not to breast-feed during therapy.

---

imipenem–cilastatin sodium
im-ih-PEN-em/sye-luh-STAT-in

Primaxin 500 ✤, Primaxin I.V.

Therapeutic class: Antibiotics
Pharmacologic class: Carbapenems–beta-lactams

AVAILABLE FORMS
Powder for injection: 250 mg, 500 mg

INDICATIONS & DOSAGES
Adjust-a-dose (for all indications): If CrCl is less than 70 mL/minute, adjust dosage and monitor renal function test results. Consult manufacturer's package insert for specific dosage adjustments. For patients on hemodialysis, administer dose after hemodialysis and at 12-hour intervals timed from the end of that dialysis session. Dosage regimen for adults with normal renal function is based on type and severity of infection. Consult manufacturer's package insert for dosing.

➤ **Serious lower respiratory tract, bone, intra-abdominal, gynecologic, joint, skin, and soft-tissue infections; UTIs; endocarditis; and bacterial septicemia, caused by** *Acinetobacter, Enterococcus, Staphylococcus aureus, Streptococcus, Escherichia coli, Haemophilus, Klebsiella, Morganella, Proteus, Enterobacter, Pseudomonas aeruginosa,* **or** *Bacteroides,* **including** *B. fragilis*
Adults weighing more than 70 kg: 250 to 1,000 mg by I.V. infusion every 6 to 8 hours. Maximum daily dose is 50 mg/kg/day or 4 g/day, whichever is less.
Adults weighing less than 70 kg: 125 to 1,000 mg by I.V. infusion every 6 to 8 hours. Maximum daily dosage is 50 mg/kg/day or 4 g/day, whichever is less.
Children age 3 months and older (except for CNS infections): 15 to 25 mg/kg I.V. every 6 hours. Maximum daily dose is 2 to 4 g.
Infants ages 4 weeks to 3 months weighing 1.5 kg or more (except for CNS infections): 25 mg/kg I.V. every 6 hours.
Neonates ages 1 to 4 weeks weighing 1.5 kg or more (except for CNS infections): 25 mg/kg I.V. every 8 hours.
Neonates younger than age 1 week weighing 1.5 kg or more (except for CNS infections): 25 mg/kg I.V. every 12 hours.

ADMINISTRATION
I.V.
▼ Obtain specimens for culture and sensitivity testing before giving first dose. Begin therapy while awaiting results.
▼ Reconstitute piggyback units with 100 mL of compatible I.V. solution to provide solution containing 2.5 to 5 mg/mL.
▼ When reconstituting powder, shake until the solution is clear. Solutions may be colorless to yellow; variations of color within this range don't affect drug's potency.
▼ After reconstitution, solution is stable for 4 hours at room temperature and for 24 hours when refrigerated.
▼ Don't give by direct I.V. bolus injection.
▼ For adults, give each 250- or 500-mg dose by I.V. infusion over 20 to 30 minutes. Infuse each 750-mg to 1-g dose over 40 to 60 minutes.

▼ For children, infuse doses of 500 mg or less over 15 to 30 minutes. Infuse doses greater than 500 mg over 40 to 60 minutes. If nausea occurs, the infusion may be slowed.

▼ **Incompatibilities:** Allopurinol, antibiotics, amiodarone, amphotericin B cholesteryl sulfate complex, azithromycin, dextrose 5% in lactated Ringer injection, etoposide, fluconazole, gemcitabine, lorazepam, meperidine, midazolam, milrinone, sargramostim, sodium bicarbonate.

ACTION
Inhibits bacterial cell-wall synthesis. Cilastatin prevents metabolism of imipenem, resulting in increased urinary recovery and decreased renal toxicity.

Route	Onset	Peak	Duration
I.V.	Immediate	Immediate	Unknown

Half-life: 1 hour after I.V. dose.

ADVERSE REACTIONS
CV: thrombophlebitis.
GI: diarrhea, nausea, vomiting.
GU: urine discoloration.
Skin: injection-site pain, rash.

INTERACTIONS
Drug-drug. *Cyclosporine:* May increase CNS adverse effects. Use together cautiously.
Ganciclovir: May cause seizures. Avoid using together.
Probenecid: May increase cilastatin level. Don't give concurrently.
Valproic acid: May decrease valproic acid level and increase risk of seizures. Monitor patient and valproic acid level carefully. Adjust valproic acid level or consider alternative antibiotic.

EFFECTS ON LAB TEST RESULTS
• May increase BUN, creatinine, ALT, AST, alkaline phosphatase, bilirubin, chloride, and LDH levels. May increase or decrease sodium level.
• May increase eosinophil count. May decrease Hb level, hematocrit, and WBC and platelet counts.

• May interfere with glucose determination by Benedict solution, Fehling's solution, or Clinitest.

CONTRAINDICATIONS & CAUTIONS
• Contraindicated in patients hypersensitive to drug or its components and in those with CrCl of 5 mL/minute/$1.73 m^2$ or less unless hemodialysis is begun within 48 hours.
• Use cautiously in patients allergic to penicillins or cephalosporins because drug has similar chemical structure. Also use cautiously in patients with a history of sensitivity to multiple allergens. Serious anaphylactic reactions require immediate emergency measures.
• Use cautiously in patients with history of seizure disorders, especially if they also have compromised renal function.
• Drug may cause CDAD, ranging in severity from mild to fatal colitis and occurring even 2 months after drug administration.
• Prolonged use may result in superinfection.
• Repeated evaluation of patient's condition is essential.
• Use cautiously in children younger than age 3 months. Drug isn't recommended for children with CNS infections because of increased risk of seizures or in children with impaired renal function who weigh less than 30 kg.
Dialyzable drug: Yes.

PREGNANCY-LACTATION-REPRODUCTION
• There are no adequate studies in pregnant women. Use during pregnancy only if potential benefit justifies potential hazards to the fetus.
• It isn't known if drug appears in breast milk. Use cautiously in breast-feeding women.

NURSING CONSIDERATIONS
◑ *Alert:* Don't use for CNS infections in children because of seizure risk.
◑ *Alert:* If seizures develop and persist despite anticonvulsant therapy, stop drug.
• For patients receiving hemodialysis, drug is recommended only when benefits outweigh possible risk of seizures.
• Monitor patient for superinfections during and after therapy.

Reactions in bold italics are *life-threatening*. Interactions may have a *rapid onset* or a *delayed onset*.

PATIENT TEACHING
• Instruct patient to report adverse reactions promptly.
• Tell patient to report discomfort at I.V. insertion site.
• Urge patient to notify prescriber as soon as possible about loose stools or diarrhea.
• Advise patient taking valproic acid or divalproex sodium that seizure therapy may need adjustment.

imipramine hydrochloride
im-IP-ra-meen

Novo-pramine ✤, PMS-Imipramine ✤, Tofranil

imipramine pamoate

Therapeutic class: Antidepressants
Pharmacologic class: TCAs

AVAILABLE FORMS
imipramine hydrochloride
Tablets: 10 mg, 25 mg, 50 mg
imipramine pamoate
Capsules: 75 mg, 100 mg, 125 mg, 150 mg

INDICATIONS & DOSAGES
➤ **Depression**
Adults: Initially, 75 mg (outpatients) to 100 mg (inpatients) P.O. daily in divided doses or (for outpatients) as a single bedtime dose. Maximum daily dose is 200 mg for outpatients and 300 mg for hospitalized patients.
Adolescents: 30 to 40 mg P.O. once daily, preferably at bedtime, or in divided doses if necessary. Dosage increases above 100 mg daily are generally unnecessary.
Elderly patients: Initially, 30 to 40 mg daily; maximum shouldn't exceed 100 mg daily.
➤ **Childhood enuresis**
Children age 6 and older: Initially, 25 mg imipramine hydrochloride P.O. 1 hour before bedtime. If patient doesn't improve within 1 week, increase dose to a maximum of 50 mg if child is younger than age 12; increase dose to a maximum of 75 mg for children age 12 and older.
➤ **Panic disorder** ◆
Adults: Initially, 10 mg P.O. daily titrated up to 300 mg daily.

ADMINISTRATION
P.O.
• Give drug without regard for food.
• Give full dose at bedtime if possible.

ACTION
Unknown. Increases norepinephrine, serotonin, or both in the CNS by blocking their reuptake by the presynaptic neurons.

Route	Onset	Peak	Duration
P.O.	Unknown	2–6 hr	Unknown

Half-life: 8 to 21 hours.

ADVERSE REACTIONS
CNS: drowsiness, dizziness, *seizures, stroke,* excitation, tremor, confusion, hallucinations, anxiety, ataxia, paresthesia, nervousness, EEG changes, extrapyramidal reactions, agitation.
CV: orthostatic hypotension, tachycardia, ECG changes, *MI, arrhythmias, heart block,* hypertension, *precipitation of HF,* palpitations.
EENT: blurred vision, tinnitus, mydriasis.
GI: dry mouth, constipation, nausea, vomiting, anorexia, paralytic ileus, abdominal cramps, black tongue, diarrhea.
GU: urine retention, urinary frequency.
Hematologic: *bone marrow depression, thrombocytopenia.*
Metabolic: *hypoglycemia,* hyperglycemia.
Skin: rash, urticaria, photosensitivity reactions, pruritus, diaphoresis.
Other: hypersensitivity reactions.

INTERACTIONS
Drug-drug. *Aclidinium:* May enhance anticholinergic effects. Avoid using together.
Barbiturates, CNS depressants: May enhance CNS depression. Avoid using together.
Cimetidine, **fluoxetine, fluvoxamine, paroxetine, sertraline:** May increase imipramine level. Monitor drug levels and patient for signs of toxicity.
Clonidine: May cause life-threatening hypertension. Avoid using together.
Epinephrine, norepinephrine: May increase hypertensive effect. Use together cautiously.
Linezolid, methylene blue: May cause serotonin syndrome. Use with extreme caution and monitor patient closely.

MAO inhibitors: May cause hyperpyretic crisis, severe seizures, and death. Don't use within 14 days of MAO inhibitor therapy.

QTc-prolonging drugs (quinidine, quinolones): May increase the risk of life-threatening arrhythmias. Avoid using together.

Drug-herb. *SAM-e, St. John's wort, yohimbe:* May cause serotonin syndrome. Discourage use together.

Drug-lifestyle. *Alcohol use:* May enhance CNS depression. Discourage use together.

Smoking: May lower level of drug. Monitor patient for lack of effect.

Sun exposure: May increase risk of photosensitivity reactions. Advise patient to avoid excessive sunlight exposure.

EFFECTS ON LAB TEST RESULTS

● May increase or decrease glucose level.
● May increase LFT values.

CONTRAINDICATIONS & CAUTIONS

Black Box Warning Antidepressants increase risk of suicidal thinking and behavior in children, adolescents, and young adults with major depressive disorder and other psychiatric disorders. Imipramine isn't approved for use in children except for those with nocturnal enuresis. ∎

● Contraindicated in patients hypersensitive to drug and in those receiving MAO inhibitors; also contraindicated during acute recovery phase of MI.

● **Alert:** Concomitant use with linezolid or methylene blue can cause serotonin syndrome (fever, mental status changes, muscle twitching, excessive sweating, shivering or shaking, diarrhea, and loss of coordination). Use imipramine with linezolid or methylene blue only for life-threatening or urgent conditions when the potential benefits outweigh the risks of toxicity.

● Use with extreme caution in patients at risk for suicide; in elderly patients and in patients with history of urine retention, angle-closure glaucoma, or seizure disorders; in patients with increased IOP, CV disease, impaired hepatic function, hyperthyroidism, or impaired renal function; and in patients receiving thyroid drugs.

● **Alert:** Imipramine pamoate shouldn't be used in children of any age because of increased risk of acute overdose.

Dialyzable drug: No.

⚠ **Overdose S&S:** Cardiac arrhythmias, severe hypotension, seizures, CNS depression, coma, ECG changes, drowsiness, stupor, ataxia, restlessness, agitation, hyperactive reflexes, muscle rigidity, athetoid and choreiform movements, tachycardia, HF, respiratory depression, cyanosis, shock, vomiting, hyperpyrexia, mydriasis, diaphoresis.

PREGNANCY-LACTATION-REPRODUCTION

● There are no adequate studies in pregnant women; however, fetal risk can't be excluded. Use during pregnancy only if potential benefit clearly justifies potential risk to the fetus.

● Drug appears in breast milk. Use in breast-feeding women isn't recommended.

NURSING CONSIDERATIONS

● **Alert:** If linezolid or methylene blue must be given, discontinue imipramine and monitor patient for serotonin toxicity for 2 weeks (5 weeks if fluoxetine was taken) or until 24 hours after the last dose of methylene blue or linezolid, whichever comes first. May resume imipramine 24 hours after last dose of methylene blue or linezolid.

● Monitor WBC count during therapy, and monitor patient for fever and sore throat. Discontinue drug if pathologic neutrophil depression occurs.

● Monitor patient for nausea, headache, and malaise after abrupt withdrawal of long-term therapy; these symptoms don't indicate addiction.

● Don't withdraw drug abruptly.

● Because of hypertensive episodes during surgery in patients receiving TCAs, stop drug gradually several days before surgery.

● If signs or symptoms of psychosis occur or increase, expect prescriber to reduce dosage. Monitor mood changes. Monitor patient for suicidal tendencies, and allow only a minimum supply of drug.

● To prevent relapse in children receiving drug for enuresis, withdraw drug gradually.

● Recommend sugarless hard candy or gum to relieve dry mouth. Saliva substitutes may be useful.

◑ Alert: Tofranil and Tofranil-PM may contain tartrazine.

● **Look alike–sound alike:** Don't confuse imipramine with desipramine.

PATIENT TEACHING

Black Box Warning Advise families and caregivers to closely observe patient for increased suicidal thinking and behavior. ■

◑ Alert: Teach patient to recognize and immediately report symptoms of serotonin toxicity (fever, mental status changes, muscle twitching, excessive sweating, shivering or shaking, diarrhea, and loss of coordination).

● Tell patient to take full dose at bedtime whenever possible, but warn him of possible morning dizziness upon standing up quickly.

● If child is an early-night bed-wetter, tell parents it may be more effective to divide dose and give the first dose earlier in day.

● Tell patient to avoid alcohol while taking this drug.

● Advise patient to consult prescriber before taking other prescription or OTC drugs.

● Warn patient to avoid hazardous activities that require alertness and good coordination until effects of the drug are known. Drowsiness and dizziness usually subside after a few weeks.

● Warn patient not to stop drug suddenly.

● To prevent oversensitivity to the sun, advise patient to use sunblock, wear protective clothing, and avoid prolonged exposure to strong sunlight.

indacaterol maleate
in-da-KAT-er-ol

Arcapta Neohaler

Therapeutic class: Bronchodilators
Pharmacologic class: Beta$_2$-adrenergic agonists

AVAILABLE FORMS
Capsules (powder for inhalation): 75 mcg

INDICATIONS & DOSAGES
➤ **Long-term maintenance therapy for COPD**
Adults: 75 mcg (1 capsule) daily by oral inhalation.

ADMINISTRATION
Inhalational
● Patient shouldn't swallow capsules.

● Use inhalation capsules with the Neohaler device only. Always use the new Neohaler device that comes with each prescription. Administer inhaled capsules using the Neohaler device according to the package instructions.

● Don't wash the Neohaler device. The inhaler may be wiped between uses with a clean, dry, lint-free cloth or a clean, dry, soft brush.

● Don't use other inhaler devices from other inhaled medications to administer indacaterol capsules.

● Always store capsules in the blister packaging and remove just before using. Don't keep or store capsules in the Neohaler device. Protect capsules from light and moisture.

● Administer indacaterol at the same time each day; patient shouldn't use more than once in 24 hours.

ACTION
Binds to beta$_2$ receptors in the lung and increases cAMP levels, resulting in relaxation of bronchial smooth muscle.

Route	Onset	Peak	Duration
Inhalation	5 min	15 min	24 hr

Half-life: 46 to 126 hours.

ADVERSE REACTIONS
CNS: headache, dizziness.
CV: peripheral edema, tachycardia, palpitations.
EENT: nasopharyngitis, sinusitis, oropharyngeal pain.
GI: nausea.
Metabolic: hyperglycemia.
Musculoskeletal: muscle spasm, musculoskeletal pain.
Respiratory: cough, URI, dyspnea.
Skin: pruritus, rash.

INTERACTIONS
Drug-drug. *Adrenergics (dobutamine, dopamine):* May increase risk of additive effects and adverse reactions. Use together cautiously.

Beta$_2$ agonists (formoterol): May result in overdose. Avoid use with other long-acting beta$_2$ agonists.

Beta blockers: May block therapeutic effects of beta-adrenergic agonists and cause severe bronchospasm. If beta blocker use can't be avoided, administer indacaterol with extreme caution.

Drugs that prolong QTc interval, MAO inhibitors, TCAs: May increase risk of ventricular arrhythmias. Monitor carefully.

Xanthine derivatives (caffeine, theophylline), non-potassium-sparing diuretics, steroids: May cause hypokalemia. Monitor electrolyte levels closely.

EFFECTS ON LAB TEST RESULTS
• May increase glucose level. May decrease potassium level.

CONTRAINDICATIONS & CAUTIONS
Black Box Warning Long-acting beta$_2$-adrenergic agonists increase risk of asthma-related death. The safety and effectiveness of indacaterol in patients with asthma haven't been established. Inhaled indacaterol isn't indicated to treat asthma. ∎

• Contraindicated in patients with acutely deteriorating COPD, when used more than once daily or at doses higher than prescribed, or in addition to drugs containing long-acting beta$_2$-adrenergic agonists.

• Use cautiously in patients with a history of CV disorders (coronary insufficiency, arrhythmias, hypertension), seizures, thyrotoxicosis, diabetes, or abnormal electrolyte levels and in patients abnormally responsive to sympathomimetic amines.

Dialyzable drug: Unknown.

⚠ *Overdose S&S:* Angina, hypertension or hypotension, tachycardia, cardiac arrest, arrhythmias, nervousness, headache, tremor, dry mouth, palpitations, muscle cramps, nausea, dizziness, fatigue, malaise, hypokalemia, hyperglycemia, metabolic acidosis, insomnia, death.

PREGNANCY-LACTATION-REPRODUCTION
• There are no adequate studies in pregnant women. Use during pregnancy only if potential benefit justifies potential risk to the fetus.

• Drug may interfere with uterine contractions. Use during labor only if benefit clearly outweighs risks.

• It isn't known if drug appears in breast milk. Use cautiously in breast-feeding.

NURSING CONSIDERATIONS
❸ *Alert:* Drug may produce paradoxical bronchospasm that may be life-threatening. If paradoxical bronchospasm occurs, discontinue drug immediately and institute alternative therapy.

• Discontinue routine use of short-acting beta$_2$-adrenergic agonists when indacaterol therapy is begun. Short-acting beta$_2$-adrenergic agonists should be used only for symptomatic relief of acute symptoms.

• As long as the capsule is empty after inhalation, the full dose of medication has been received even if patient coughs. Monitor patient for worsening of symptoms, decreased effectiveness, or increased need for short-acting rescue inhaler.

PATIENT TEACHING
Black Box Warning Inform patient that indacaterol isn't for use in asthma and can increase the risk of asthma-related death. ∎

• Instruct patient on the proper administration, use, and storage of the Neohaler device and capsules. Remind patient to use only the Neohaler device and no other inhaler to administer the medication.

• Warn patient that indacaterol isn't to be used for acute exacerbations of COPD and that acute symptoms should be treated with a short-acting inhaler such as albuterol.

• Advise patient not to use indacaterol with other long-acting beta-adrenergic agonists because of the risk of significant CV effects.

• Advise patient to notify prescriber of worsening symptoms, decreased effectiveness of drug, or the need for more frequent use of a short-acting inhaler.

• Warn patient not to stop therapy without first discussing with health care provider.

Reactions in bold italics are *life-threatening*. Interactions may have a *rapid onset* or a *delayed onset*.

indapamide
in-DAP-a-mide

Lozide ♣

Therapeutic class: Diuretics
Pharmacologic class: Thiazide-like diuretics

AVAILABLE FORMS
Tablets: 1.25 mg, 2.5 mg

INDICATIONS & DOSAGES
➤ **Edema of HF**
Adults: Initially, 2.5 mg P.O. daily in the morning, increased to 5 mg daily after 1 week, if needed.
➤ **Hypertension**
Adults: Initially, 1.25 mg P.O. daily in the morning, increased to 2.5 mg daily after 4 weeks, if needed. Increased to 5 mg daily after 4 more weeks, if needed. If response is inadequate, a second antihypertensive, given at 50% of the usual starting dose, may be needed.

ADMINISTRATION
P.O.
• Give drug with food or milk to minimize GI upset.
• To prevent nocturia, give drug in the morning.

ACTION
Enhances excretion of sodium chloride and water by interfering with sodium transport in the distal tubule.

Route	Onset	Peak	Duration
P.O.	Unknown	Within 2 hr	Unknown

Half-life: About 14 hours.

ADVERSE REACTIONS
CNS: headache, nervousness, dizziness, light-headedness, weakness, vertigo, restlessness, drowsiness, fatigue, anxiety, depression, numbness of limbs, irritability, agitation, lethargy, hypertonia.
CV: orthostatic hypotension, palpitations, PVCs, irregular heartbeat, vasculitis, flushing, chest pain, edema.

EENT: rhinorrhea, blurred vision, pharyngitis, sinusitis, conjunctivitis.
GI: anorexia, nausea, epigastric distress, vomiting, abdominal pain or cramps, diarrhea, constipation, dyspepsia.
GU: nocturia, polyuria, frequent urination, erectile dysfunction.
Metabolic: asymptomatic hyperuricemia; fluid and electrolyte imbalances, including dilutional hyponatremia, hypochloremia, metabolic alkalosis, and hypokalemia; weight loss; volume depletion and dehydration; hyperglycemia.
Musculoskeletal: muscle cramps and spasms.
Respiratory: cough.
Skin: rash, pruritus, urticaria.
Other: gout, infection.

INTERACTIONS
Drug-drug. *Amphotericin B, corticosteroids:* May increase risk of hypokalemia. Monitor potassium level closely.
Antidiabetics: May decrease hypoglycemic effect of sulfonylureas, causing elevated glucose levels. Adjust dosage, if needed. Monitor glucose level.
Barbiturates, opioids: May increase orthostasis. Monitor patient closely.
Bumetanide, ethacrynic acid, furosemide, torsemide: May cause excessive diuretic response, causing serious electrolyte abnormalities or dehydration. Adjust doses carefully, and monitor patient closely for signs and symptoms of excessive diuretic response.
Cardiac glycosides: May increase risk of digoxin toxicity from indapamide-induced hypokalemia. Monitor potassium and digoxin levels.
Cholestyramine, colestipol: May decrease absorption of thiazides. Separate doses by 2 hours.
Diazoxide: May increase antihypertensive, hyperglycemic, and hyperuricemic effects. Use together cautiously.
Lithium: May decrease lithium clearance, which may increase lithium toxicity. Avoid using together.
NSAIDs: May increase risk of NSAID-induced renal failure. Monitor patient for signs and symptoms of renal failure.

Drug-herb. *Licorice:* May cause unexpected rapid potassium loss and hypertension. Discourage use together.
Drug-lifestyle. *Alcohol use:* May increase orthostatic hypotensive effect. Discourage use together.

EFFECTS ON LAB TEST RESULTS
• May increase BUN, creatinine, glucose, cholesterol, triglyceride, calcium, and uric acid levels.
• May decrease potassium, sodium, phosphate, and chloride levels.

CONTRAINDICATIONS & CAUTIONS
• Contraindicated in patients hypersensitive to other sulfonamide-derived drugs and in those with anuria.
• Use cautiously in patients with severe renal disease, gout, impaired hepatic function, or progressive hepatic disease.
Dialyzable drug: Unknown.
⚠ *Overdose S&S:* Nausea, vomiting, GI disorders, weakness, electrolyte imbalance, hypotension, depressed respirations.

PREGNANCY-LACTATION-REPRODUCTION
• There are no adequate studies in pregnant women. Use during pregnancy only if clearly needed.
• It isn't known if drug appears in breast milk. Patient should discontinue breastfeeding or discontinue drug.

NURSING CONSIDERATIONS
• Monitor fluid intake and output, weight, BP, and electrolyte levels.
• Watch for signs of hypokalemia, such as muscle weakness and cramps. Drug may be used with potassium-sparing diuretic to prevent potassium loss.
• Consult prescriber and dietitian about a high-potassium diet or potassium supplement. Foods rich in potassium include citrus fruits, tomatoes, bananas, and dates.
• Monitor creatinine and BUN levels regularly. Cumulative effects of drug may occur in patients with impaired renal function.
• Monitor uric acid level, especially in patients with history of gout.
• Monitor glucose level, especially in diabetic patients.

• Monitor elderly patients, who are especially susceptible to excessive diuresis.
• Stop thiazides and thiazide-like diuretics before parathyroid function tests.
• Therapeutic response may be delayed several weeks in hypertensive patients.

PATIENT TEACHING
• Instruct patient to take drug in morning to prevent need to urinate at night.
• Tell patient to take drug with food to minimize GI upset.
• Advise patient to avoid sudden posture changes and to rise slowly to avoid dizziness upon standing quickly.

---

indinavir sulfate
in-DIN-ah-ver

Crixivan🍁

Therapeutic class: Antiretrovirals
Pharmacologic class: Protease inhibitors

AVAILABLE FORMS
Capsules: 200 mg, 400 mg

INDICATIONS & DOSAGES
➤ **HIV infection, with other antiretrovirals, when antiretrovirals are warranted**
Adults: 800 mg P.O. every 8 hours. Consider reducing indinavir to 600 mg every 8 hours when patient is taking delavirdine 400 mg t.i.d. Reduce indinavir to 600 mg every 8 hours when patient is taking itraconazole 200 mg b.i.d. or ketoconazole. When patient is taking indinavir and rifabutin, decrease rifabutin to one-half the standard dosage and increase indinavir to 1,000 mg every 8 hours.
Adjust-a-dose: For patients with mild to moderate hepatic insufficiency from cirrhosis, reduce dosage to 600 mg P.O. every 8 hours.

ADMINISTRATION
P.O.
• Give drug on an empty stomach with water 1 hour before or 2 hours after a meal. Or, give it with other liquids (such as skim milk, juice, coffee, or tea) or a light meal.

A meal high in fat, calories, and protein reduces drug absorption.

● Store capsules in the original container and keep desiccant in the bottle; capsules are sensitive to moisture.

ACTION

Inhibits HIV protease by binding to the protease-active site and inhibiting activity of the enzyme, preventing cleavage of the viral polyproteins and forming immature noninfectious viral particles.

Route	Onset	Peak	Duration
P.O.	Rapid	<1 hr	Unknown

Half-life: 1½ to 2 hours.

ADVERSE REACTIONS

CNS: asthenia, dizziness, fatigue, headache, insomnia, malaise, somnolence, fever.
GI: nausea, abdominal pain, acid regurgitation, anorexia, diarrhea, dry mouth, taste perversion, vomiting.
GU: hematuria, nephrolithiasis, dysuria.
Hematologic: *neutropenia, thrombocytopenia,* anemia.
Metabolic: hyperbilirubinemia, hyperglycemia.
Musculoskeletal: back pain.
Skin: pruritus, rash.
Other: flank pain.

INTERACTIONS

Drug-drug. *Alfuzosin, alprazolam, amiodarone, oral midazolam, pimozide, sildenafil (when used for pulmonary arterial hypertension), triazolam:* May increase plasma concentrations of these drugs and cause life-threatening reactions. Use together is contraindicated.
Atorvastatin, pitavastatin, rosuvastatin: May increase level of statin and risk of myopathy and rhabdomyolysis. Use together cautiously and use the lowest appropriate statin dose.
Carbamazepine, phenobarbital, phenytoin: May decrease indinavir concentration and effectiveness. Use with caution.
Clarithromycin: May alter clarithromycin level. Dosage adjustments not needed.
Delavirdine, itraconazole, ketoconazole: May increase indinavir level. Consider reducing indinavir to 600 mg every 8 hours.

Didanosine: May alter absorption of indinavir. Separate doses by 1 hour and give on an empty stomach.
Direct factor Xa inhibitors (rivaroxaban): May increase plasma concentrations and effects of direct factor Xa inhibitors. Avoid use together.
Efavirenz, nevirapine: May decrease indinavir level. Closely monitor clinical response.
Ergot derivatives (dihydroergotamine, ergonovine, ergotamine, methylergonovine): May cause acute ergot toxicity, characterized by peripheral vasospasm and ischemia of the extremities and other tissues. Use together is contraindicated.
Lopinavir–ritonavir: May increase indinavir level. Adjust indinavir dosage to 600 mg b.i.d.
Lovastatin, simvastatin: May increase levels of these drugs and increase risk of myopathy and rhabdomyolysis. Use together is contraindicated.
Nelfinavir: May increase indinavir level. Monitor patient closely.
Pantoprazole, rabeprazole: May reduce the antiviral activity of indinavir. Monitor clinical response and adjust indinavir dosage as needed.
Rifabutin: May increase rifabutin level and decrease indinavir level. Avoid using together or adjust dosages accordingly.
Rifampin: May decrease indinavir level. Avoid using together.
Ritonavir: May increase indinavir level twofold to fivefold. Monitor clinical response and adjust dosage if needed.
Sildenafil, tadalafil, vardenafil: May increase levels of these drugs and increase adverse effects (hypotension, visual changes, priapism). Tell patient not to exceed prescribed dosage. Sildenafil dosage shouldn't exceed 25 mg in a 48-hour period. Tadalafil dosage shouldn't exceed 10 mg in a 72-hour period. Vardenafil dosage shouldn't exceed 2.5 mg in a 24-hour period.
Drug-herb. *Garlic supplements:* May decrease indinavir level. Use together isn't recommended.
St. John's wort: May reduce drug level by more than half. Avoid use together.

Drug-food. *Grapefruit, grapefruit juice:*
May decrease drug level and therapeutic effect. Discourage use together.

EFFECTS ON LAB TEST RESULTS
• May increase ALT, AST, bilirubin, amylase, Hb, and glucose levels.
• May decrease neutrophil and platelet counts.

CONTRAINDICATIONS & CAUTIONS
• Contraindicated in patients hypersensitive to drug or its components.
• Contraindicated with alfuzosin, alprazolam, amiodarone, dihydroergotamine, ergonovine, ergotamine, lovastatin, methylergonovine, oral midazolam, pimozide, sildenafil (when used to treat pulmonary hypertension), simvastatin, and triazolam.
• Fatal cases of hemolytic anemia have occurred. If hemolytic anemia occurs, treat appropriately and discontinue drug.
• Use cautiously in patients with hepatic insufficiency from cirrhosis.
• Safety and effectiveness in children haven't been established.
Dialyzable drug: Unknown.
⚠ **Overdose S&S:** Nephrolithiasis/urolithiasis, flank pain, hematuria, nausea, vomiting, diarrhea.

PREGNANCY-LACTATION-REPRODUCTION
• There are no adequate studies in pregnant women. Use during pregnancy only if potential benefit justifies potential fetal risk.
• It isn't known if drug appears in breast milk. Women shouldn't breast-feed during therapy.

NURSING CONSIDERATIONS
• Drug must be taken at 8-hour intervals.
• Drug may cause nephrolithiasis. If signs and symptoms of nephrolithiasis occur, prescriber may stop drug for 1 to 3 days during acute phases.
• To prevent nephrolithiasis, patient should maintain adequate hydration (at least 48 oz or 1.5 L of fluids every 24 hours while taking indinavir).

PATIENT TEACHING
• Tell patient that drug doesn't cure HIV infection and that he may continue to develop opportunistic infections and other complications of HIV infection. Drug hasn't been shown to reduce the risk of HIV transmission.
• Advise patient to use barrier protection during sexual intercourse.
• Caution patient not to adjust dosage or stop therapy without first consulting prescriber.
• Advise patient that if a dose is missed, he should take the next dose at the regularly scheduled time and shouldn't double the dose.
• Instruct patient to take drug on an empty stomach with water 1 hour before or 2 hours after a meal. Or, he may take it with other liquids (such as skim milk, juice, coffee, or tea) or a light meal.
• Instruct patient to store capsules in the original container and to keep desiccant in the bottle; capsules are sensitive to moisture.
• Tell patient to drink at least 48 oz (1.5 L) of fluid daily.
• Advise women to avoid breast-feeding because drug may appear in breast milk. Also, to prevent transmitting virus to infant, advise HIV-positive women not to breast-feed.

indomethacin
in-doe-METH-a-sin

Indocin, Ratio-Indomethacin✦, Tivorbex

indomethacin sodium trihydrate
Indocin I.V.

Therapeutic class: NSAIDs
Pharmacologic class: NSAIDs

AVAILABLE FORMS
indomethacin
Capsules: 20 mg, 25 mg, 40 mg, 50 mg
Capsules (extended-release): 75 mg
Injection: 1 mg/vial
Oral suspension: 25 mg/5 mL*
Suppositories: 50 mg, 100 mg✦
indomethacin sodium trihydrate
Injection: 1-mg vials

INDICATIONS & DOSAGES

➤ **Moderate to severe RA or osteoarthritis, ankylosing spondylitis (excluding Tivorbex)**
Adults and children age 15 and older: 25 mg P.O. b.i.d. or t.i.d. with food or antacids or 25 mg P.R. b.i.d. or t.i.d.; increase daily dose by 25 or 50 mg every 7 days, up to 200 mg daily. Or, 75 mg extended-release capsules P.O. to start, in morning or at bedtime, followed by 75 mg extended-release capsules b.i.d. if needed.

➤ **Acute gouty arthritis (excluding Tivorbex)**
Adults and children age 15 and older: 50 mg P.O. or P.R. t.i.d. Reduce dose as soon as possible; then stop therapy. Don't use extended-release form.

➤ **Acute painful shoulders (bursitis or tendinitis) (excluding Tivorbex)**
Adults and children age 15 and older: 75 to 150 mg P.O. or P.R. daily in divided doses t.i.d. or q.i.d. for 7 to 14 days. Or, 75 mg (extended-release) P.O. daily or b.i.d. for 7 to 14 days.

➤ **Mild to moderate acute pain (Tivorbex)**
Adults: 20 mg P.O. t.i.d. or 40 mg P.O. t.i.d. or q.i.d.

➤ **To close a hemodynamically significant patent ductus arteriosus in premature neonates**
Neonates older than age 7 days: 0.2 mg/kg I.V.; then two doses of 0.25 mg/kg at 12- to 24-hour intervals.
Neonates ages 2 to 7 days: 0.2 mg/kg I.V.; then two doses of 0.2 mg/kg at 12- to 24-hour intervals.
Neonates younger than 48 hours: 0.2 mg/kg I.V.; then two doses of 0.1 mg/kg I.V. at 12- to 24-hour intervals.

ADMINISTRATION
P.O.
● Give drug with food, milk, or antacid.
I.V.
▼ Reconstitute powder for injection with sterile water or NSS. For each 1-mg vial, add 1 or 2 mL of diluent for a solution containing 1 mg/mL or 0.5 mg/mL, respectively. Give over 20 to 30 minutes.
▼ Use only preservative-free sterile saline solution or sterile water to prepare. Never use diluents containing benzyl alcohol because it has been linked to toxicity in newborns.
▼ Because injection contains no preservatives, reconstitute drug immediately before use and discard unused solution.
▼ If anuria or marked oliguria is evident, withhold administration of second or third scheduled I.V. dose and notify prescriber.
▼ Watch carefully for bleeding and for reduced urine output.
▼ **Incompatibilities:** Amino acid injection, calcium gluconate, cimetidine, dextrose injection, dobutamine, dopamine, gentamicin, levofloxacin, solutions with pH less than 6, tobramycin sulfate, tolazoline.
Rectal
● If suppository is too soft, place in refrigerator for 15 minutes or run under cold water in wrapper.

ACTION
May inhibit prostaglandin synthesis, to produce anti-inflammatory, analgesic, and antipyretic effects.

Route	Onset	Peak	Duration
P.O.	30 min	1–4 hr	4–6 hr
I.V.	Immediate	Immediate	4–6 hr
P.R.	Unknown	Unknown	4–6 hr

Half-life: 4¼ hours.

ADVERSE REACTIONS
P.O. and rectal
CNS: headache, dizziness, depression, fatigue, somnolence, syncope, vertigo.
CV: edema, hypertension.
EENT: hearing loss, tinnitus.
GI: *pancreatitis,* abdominal pain, anorexia, constipation, diarrhea, dyspepsia, *GI bleeding,* nausea, peptic ulceration.
Other: hypersensitivity reactions.
I.V.
GU: hematuria, interstitial nephritis, proteinuria.

INTERACTIONS
Drug-drug. *ACE inhibitors (benazepril, enalaprilat), angiotensin II receptor blockers (candesartan, valsartan):* May reduce antihypertensive effects; may worsen renal

function in those with impaired renal function. Monitor patient closely.

Aminoglycosides, cyclosporine, methotrexate: May enhance toxicity of these drugs. Avoid using together.

Anticoagulants: May cause bleeding. Monitor patient closely.

Antihypertensives: May decrease antihypertensive effect. Monitor patient closely.

Antihypertensives, furosemide, thiazide diuretics: May impair response to both drugs. Avoid using together, if possible.

Aspirin: May increase adverse reactions, including risk of GI toxicity. Avoid using together.

Bisphosphonates: May increase risk of gastric ulceration. Monitor patient for symptoms of gastric irritation or GI bleeding.

Corticosteroids: May increase risk of GI toxicity. Avoid using together.

Cyclosporine: May increase cyclosporine toxicity. Use cautiously and monitor renal function.

Diflunisal, probenecid: May decrease indomethacin excretion. Watch for increased indomethacin adverse effects.

Digoxin: May prolong half-life of digoxin. Use together cautiously.

Dipyridamole: May enhance fluid retention. Avoid using together.

Lithium: May increase lithium level. Monitor patient for toxicity.

Methotrexate: May increase methotrexate toxicity. Use together cautiously.

Penicillamine: May increase bioavailability of penicillamine. Monitor patient closely.

Phenytoin: May increase phenytoin level. Monitor patient closely.

SSRIs: May increase risk of GI bleeding. Adjust dosage as needed.

Triamterene: May cause nephrotoxicity. Avoid using together.

Drug-herb. *Alfalfa, anise, bilberry, dong quai, garlic:* May cause bleeding. Discourage use together.

Senna: May inhibit diarrheal effects. Discourage use together.

White willow: Herb and drug contain similar components. Don't use together.

Drug-lifestyle. *Alcohol use:* May cause GI toxicity. Discourage use together.

EFFECTS ON LAB TEST RESULTS

• May increase potassium level.
• May decrease Hb level and hematocrit.
• May increase LFT values.

CONTRAINDICATIONS & CAUTIONS

• Contraindicated in patients hypersensitive to drug and in those with a history of aspirin- or NSAID-induced asthma, rhinitis, or urticaria.

• Contraindicated in neonates with untreated infection, active bleeding, coagulation defects or thrombocytopenia, congenital heart disease needing patency of the ductus arteriosus, necrotizing enterocolitis, or significant renal impairment.

Black Box Warning NSAIDs can increase risk of heart attack or stroke in patients with or without heart disease or risk factors for heart disease. ■

Black Box Warning Risk of heart attack or stroke can occur as early as the first weeks of NSAID use. Risk appears greater at higher doses. Use lowest effective dose for shortest duration possible. ■

❸ *Alert:* Avoid use in patients with severe HF unless benefits are expected to outweigh risk of worsening HF.

• Suppositories are contraindicated in patients with history of proctitis or recent rectal bleeding.

Black Box Warning Contraindicated for the treatment of perioperative pain after CABG surgery. ■

• Use cautiously in elderly patients, those with history of GI disease, and those with epilepsy, parkinsonism, hepatic or renal disease, CV disease, infection, and mental illness or depression.

Dialyzable drug: Unknown.

⚠ *Overdose S&S:* Drowsiness, lethargy, confusion, nausea, vomiting, paresthesia, numbness, aggressive behavior, disorientation, seizures, headache, dizziness, GI bleeding.

PREGNANCY-LACTATION-REPRODUCTION

❸ *Alert:* Drug can cause fetal harm starting at 30 weeks' gestation; avoid use. Before 30 weeks' gestation, use during pregnancy only if potential benefit justifies potential fetal risk. Because NSAIDs may cause premature closure of the ductus arteriosus,

---

Reactions in bold italics are *life-threatening*. Interactions may have a *rapid onset* or a *delayed onset*.

NSAID use in late pregnancy should be avoided.

• Drug appears in breast milk. Use in breast-feeding women isn't recommended by most manufacturers.

• Long-term use of NSAIDs in women of reproductive age may be associated with infertility that's reversible upon discontinuation of drug.

NURSING CONSIDERATIONS

• Because of the high risk of adverse effects from long-term use, drug shouldn't be used routinely as an analgesic or antipyretic.

❸ *Alert:* Watch for and immediately evaluate signs and symptoms of heart attack (chest pain, shortness of breath or trouble breathing) or stroke (weakness in one part or side of the body, slurred speech).

• If ductus arteriosus reopens, a second course of one to three doses may be given. If ineffective, surgery may be needed.

• Watch for bleeding in patients receiving anticoagulants, patients with coagulation defects, and neonates.

• Because NSAIDs impair synthesis of renal prostaglandins, they can decrease renal blood flow and lead to reversible renal impairment, especially in patients with renal failure, HF, or hepatic dysfunction; in elderly patients; and in those taking diuretics. Monitor these patients closely.

• Drug causes sodium retention; watch for weight gain (especially in elderly patients) and increased BP in patients with hypertension.

• Monitor patient for rash and respiratory distress, which may indicate a hypersensitivity reaction.

• Because of their antipyretic and antiinflammatory actions, NSAIDs may mask signs and symptoms of infection.

Black Box Warning NSAIDs cause an increased risk of serious GI adverse events, including bleeding, ulceration, and perforation of the stomach or intestines, which can be fatal. Elderly patients are at greater risk. ∎

Black Box Warning NSAIDs may increase the risk of serious thrombotic events, MI, or stroke, which can be fatal. The risk may be greater with longer use or in patients with CV disease or risk factors for CV disease. ∎

• Monitor patient on long-term oral therapy for toxicity by conducting regular eye examinations, hearing tests, CBCs, and kidney function tests.

PATIENT TEACHING

• Tell patient to take oral dose with food, milk, or antacid to prevent GI upset.

❸ *Alert:* Advise patient to seek medical attention immediately if chest pain, shortness of breath or trouble breathing, weakness in one part or side of the body, or slurred speech occurs.

• Alert patient that using oral form with aspirin, alcohol, other NSAIDs, or corticosteroids may increase risk of adverse GI reactions.

• Teach patient signs and symptoms of GI bleeding, including blood in vomit, urine, or stool; coffee-ground vomit; and black, tarry stool. Tell him to notify prescriber immediately if any of these occurs.

• Tell patient to immediately report signs or symptoms of cardiac events, such as chest pain, shortness of breath, weakness, and slurred speech.

• Warn patient to avoid hazardous activities that require mental alertness until CNS effects are known.

• Tell patient to notify prescriber immediately if visual or hearing changes occur.

• Tell patient to notify prescriber if unexplained weight gain or edema occurs.

infliximab
in-FLICKS-ih-mab

Remicade

Therapeutic class: Anti-inflammatory drugs
Pharmacologic class: TNF blockers

AVAILABLE FORMS
Lyophilized powder for injection: 100-mg vial

INDICATIONS & DOSAGES
➤ **Moderately to severely active Crohn disease; reduction in the number of draining enterocutaneous and rectovaginal fistulas and maintenance of fistula**

closure in patients with fistulizing Crohn disease
Adults: 5 mg/kg I.V. infusion over at least 2 hours. Repeat at 2 and 6 weeks, then every 8 weeks thereafter. For patients who respond and then lose their response, consider 10 mg/kg. Patients who don't respond by week 14 are unlikely to respond with continued therapy. In those patients, consider stopping drug.
Children ages 6 to 17: For Crohn disease, 5 mg/kg I.V. infusion over at least 2 hours. Repeat at 2 and 6 weeks, then every 8 weeks thereafter.

➤ **Moderately to severely active RA**
Adults: 3 mg/kg I.V. infusion over at least 2 hours. Repeat at 2 and 6 weeks after first infusion and every 8 weeks thereafter. Dose may be increased up to 10 mg/kg, or doses may be given every 4 weeks if response is inadequate. Use with methotrexate.

➤ **Moderate to severe ulcerative colitis**
Adults: Induction dose, 5 mg/kg I.V. over at least 2 hours. Repeat at 2 and 6 weeks, then every 8 weeks thereafter.

➤ **Moderate to severe ulcerative colitis in children who have had an inadequate response to conventional therapy**
Children age 6 and older: Initially, 5 mg/kg I.V. infusion over at least 2 hours at 0, 2, and 6 weeks, followed by a maintenance regimen of 5 mg/kg I.V. infusion over at least 2 hours every 8 weeks.

➤ **Ankylosing spondylitis**
Adults: 5 mg/kg I.V. infusion over at least 2 hours. Repeat at 2 and 6 weeks, then every 6 weeks thereafter.

➤ **Psoriatic arthritis, with or without methotrexate**
Adults: 5 mg/kg I.V. infusion over at least 2 hours. Repeat at 2 and 6 weeks after first infusion, then every 8 weeks thereafter.

➤ **Chronic severe plaque psoriasis**
Adults: 5 mg/kg I.V. infusion over at least 2 hours. Repeat dose in 2 and 6 weeks, then give 5 mg/kg every 8 weeks thereafter.

ADMINISTRATION

I.V.
▼ Reconstitute with 10 mL sterile water for injection, using syringe with 21G or smaller needle. Don't shake; gently swirl to dissolve powder. Solution should be color-

less to light yellow and opalescent. It may also develop a few translucent particles; don't use if other types of particles develop or discoloration occurs.
▼ Dilute total volume of reconstituted drug to 250 mL with NSS for injection. Infusion concentration range is 0.4 to 4 mg/mL.
▼ Use an in-line, sterile, nonpyrogenic, low-protein-binding filter with a pore size less than 1.2 micrometer.
▼ Begin infusion within 3 hours of preparation and give over at least 2 hours.
▼ **Incompatibilities:** Other I.V. drugs. Don't infuse with other drugs.

ACTION

Binds to human TNF-alpha to neutralize its activity and inhibit its binding with receptors, thereby reducing the infiltration of inflammatory cells and TNF-alpha production in inflamed areas of the intestine.

Route	Onset	Peak	Duration
I.V.	Unknown	Unknown	Unknown

Half-life: 7½ to 9½ days.

ADVERSE REACTIONS

CNS: fatigue, fever, headache, dizziness, depression, insomnia, malaise, pain, systemic and cutaneous vasculitis.
CV: hypertension, chest pain, flushing, hypotension, pericardial effusion, tachycardia, bradycardia.
EENT: pharyngitis, rhinitis, sinusitis, conjunctivitis.
GI: abdominal pain, diarrhea, dyspepsia, nausea, *intestinal obstruction,* constipation, flatulence, oral pain, ulcerative stomatitis, vomiting.
GU: UTI, dysuria, increased urinary frequency.
Hematologic: *leukopenia, neutropenia, pancytopenia, thrombocytopenia,* anemia, hematoma.
Musculoskeletal: arthralgia, back pain, arthritis, myalgia.
Respiratory: coughing, URI, bronchitis, dyspnea, respiratory tract allergic reaction.
Skin: rash, acne, alopecia, candidiasis, dry skin, eczema, erythema, erythematous rash, increased sweating, maculopapular rash, papular rash, urticaria.

Reactions in bold italics are *life-threatening*. Interactions may have a *rapid onset* or a *delayed onset*.

Other: abscess, chills, ecchymosis, flulike syndrome, hot flashes, peripheral edema, toothache.

INTERACTIONS

Drug-drug. *Live-virus vaccines:* May affect normal immune response. Postpone live-virus vaccine until therapy stops. Use live-virus vaccines cautiously in infants born to female patients treated with infliximab.
TNF blockers (abatacept, anakinra, golimumab, rilonacept): May increase the risk of serious infections and neutropenia. Avoid using together.

EFFECTS ON LAB TEST RESULTS

● May increase liver enzyme levels. May decrease Hb level and hematocrit.
● May decrease WBC and platelet counts.
● May cause false-positive ANA test result.

CONTRAINDICATIONS & CAUTIONS

● Contraindicated in patients hypersensitive to murine proteins or other components of drug. Doses greater than 5 mg/kg are contraindicated in patients with moderate to severe HF.
Black Box Warning Lymphoma and other malignancies, some fatal, have occurred in children and adolescents treated with TNF blockers, including infliximab. ■
Black Box Warning Hepatosplenic T-cell lymphoma, a rare type of lymphoma, has occurred in adolescents and young adults with inflammatory bowel disease treated with TNF blockers, including infliximab. ■
Black Box Warning Histoplasmosis, coccidioidomycosis, blastomycosis, bacterial sepsis, *Listeria, Legionella,* and other opportunistic infections may develop with use of this drug. ■
Black Box Warning Carefully consider risks and benefits of treatment before initiating infliximab therapy in patients with long-term or recurrent infection. ■
● Use cautiously in elderly patients; in patients with active infection, history of chronic or recurrent infections, a history of hematologic abnormalities, or preexisting or recent-onset CNS demyelinating or seizure disorders; or in those who have lived in regions where histoplasmosis is endemic.
Dialyzable drug: Unknown.

PREGNANCY-LACTATION-REPRODUCTION

● It isn't known if drug can cause fetal harm or can affect reproductive capacity if used during pregnancy. Use in pregnant women only if clearly needed.
● It isn't known if drug appears in breast milk. Patient should discontinue breast-feeding or discontinue drug.

NURSING CONSIDERATIONS

♦ Alert: Watch for infusion-related reactions, including fever, chills, pruritus, urticaria, dyspnea, hypotension, hypertension, and chest pain during administration and for 2 hours afterward. If an infusion-related reaction occurs, stop drug, notify prescriber, and give acetaminophen, antihistamines, corticosteroids, and epinephrine.
● Give for Crohn disease and ulcerative colitis only after patient has an inadequate response to conventional therapy.
● Consider stopping treatment in patient who develops significant hematologic abnormalities or CNS adverse reactions.
● Notify prescriber for symptoms of new or worsening HF.
Black Box Warning Patients with histoplasmosis or other invasive fungal infections may present with disseminated rather than localized disease. Antigen and antibody testing for histoplasmosis may be negative in some patients with active infection. Consider empirical antifungal therapy in patients at risk for invasive fungal infections who develop severe systemic illness. ■
Black Box Warning Discontinue drug if serious infection or sepsis develops. ■
Black Box Warning Watch for development of lymphoma and infection. Patient with chronic Crohn disease and long-term exposure to immunosuppressants is more likely to develop lymphoma and infection. ■
● Drug may affect normal immune responses. Patient may develop autoimmune antibodies and lupus-like syndrome; stop drug if this happens. Symptoms should resolve.
Black Box Warning Drug may cause disseminated or extrapulmonary TB and fatal opportunistic infections. ■
Black Box Warning Evaluate patient for latent TB infection with a tuberculin skin test. Treat latent TB infection before therapy. ■

Black Box Warning Closely monitor patients for signs and symptoms of infection during and after infliximab treatment, including possible development of TB in patients who tested negative for latent TB infection before start of therapy. ■

● *Look alike–sound alike:* Don't confuse Remicade with Renacidin. Don't confuse infliximab with rituximab.

PATIENT TEACHING

● Tell patient about infusion-reaction symptoms and adverse effects and the need to report them promptly.

● Advise patient to reports all adverse reactions and to seek immediate medical attention for signs and symptoms of infection (persistent fever, cough, shortness of breath, fatigue, unusual bleeding or bruising).

● Tell female patient to stop breast-feeding.

● Tell patient alert prescriber to therapy before receiving vaccines.

● Advise parent to make sure child is up-to-date for all vaccines before therapy.

infliximab-dyyb
See NEW DRUGS for information.

ingenol mebutate
IN-je-nol

Picato

Therapeutic class: Immunomodulators
Pharmacologic class: Immune response modifiers

AVAILABLE FORMS
Topical gel: 0.015%, 0.05%

INDICATIONS & DOSAGES
➤ **Actinic keratosis on the face and scalp**
Adults: Apply 0.015% strength gel to affected area once daily for 3 days.
➤ **Actinic keratosis on the trunk and extremities**
Adults: Apply 0.05% strength gel to affected area once daily for 2 consecutive days.

ADMINISTRATION
Topical
● Store gel in refrigerator. Don't freeze.

● Spread evenly over treatment area using 1 unit-dose tube, and allow to dry.
● *Alert:* Don't apply to a treatment area of more than 25 cm².
● Wash hands after application to avoid transferring gel to other areas of the body, including periocular area, lips, and mouth.
● Avoid washing and touching treated area for 6 hours after application; after 6 hours, area may be washed with a mild soap.
● One unit-dose tube covers about a 2-inch × 2-inch (5 cm × 5 cm) area. Use each tube only once; throw away open tube after use even if it still contains gel.

ACTION
Unknown. Thought to induce cell death.

Route	Onset	Peak	Duration
Topical	Unknown	Unknown	Unknown

Half-life: Unknown.

ADVERSE REACTIONS
CNS: headache.
EENT: nasopharyngitis, periorbital edema.
Skin: erythema, flaking, scaling, crusting, swelling, vesiculation, pustulation, erosion, ulceration, pain, pruritus, infection at treatment site, irritation.

INTERACTIONS
None reported.

EFFECTS ON LAB TEST RESULTS
None reported.

CONTRAINDICATIONS & CAUTIONS
● *Alert:* Allergic reactions, including anaphylaxis, allergic contact dermatitis, and herpes zoster reactivation, have occurred in patients using drug. For severe allergic reactions, stop drug immediately.
● *Alert:* Severe eye injury (severe pain, chemical conjunctivitis, corneal burn, eyelid edema, ptosis, periorbital edema) may occur with eye exposure to drug.
● Drug can cause severe skin reactions in treated area. Don't administer until after skin has healed after previous treatments.
Dialyzable drug: Unknown.

Reactions in bold italics are *life-threatening*. Interactions may have a *rapid onset* or a *delayed onset*.

PREGNANCY-LACTATION-REPRODUCTION
● There are no adequate studies in pregnant women. Use during pregnancy only if potential benefit justifies potential risk to the fetus.
● No data are available concerning breast-feeding.

NURSING CONSIDERATIONS
● Monitor skin for serious adverse effects.
● Gel is for external use only; don't use via oral, ophthalmic, or intravaginal route.
● Don't use gel if skin hasn't healed from previous drug therapy, sunburn, or surgical treatment.
● Don't apply bandages or closed dressings to the treated area.

PATIENT TEACHING
● Warn patient that gel is for external use only and not to apply near mouth, eyes, or vagina.
● Teach patient proper application technique and to avoid drug transfer to nontreatment areas such as the periocular area.
● **Alert:** Caution patient not to use on an area of skin larger or for a period of time longer than prescribed.
● **Alert:** Advise patient not to apply makeup or insert contact lenses right after applying gel.
● Advise patient to wash hands well after applying drug to prevent transferring drug to eye or mouth area.
● **Alert:** If accidental eye exposure occurs, tell patient to flush eyes thoroughly with water and seek medical care.
● **Alert:** Warn patient not to mix gel with other topical drugs or lotions, or to cover treatment area with a bandage, dressing, or overlay.
● Instruct patient to keep drug out of the reach of children.
● Tell patient to store gel in refrigerator and not to freeze.
● Instruct patient to use gel only after skin has healed from previous drug therapy, sunburn, or surgical treatment.
● Caution patient not to use gel immediately after showering or less than 2 hours before bedtime, and not to perform activities that cause increased sweating for 6 hours after applying gel. Advise patient to allow treated area to dry for 15 minutes after application.

● Tell patient to report serious adverse skin effects.
● Instruct patient to use each tube only once and to throw away the open tube after use even if there is still gel in it.

Insulins (fixed combinations)
IN-su-lins

insulin degludec–insulin aspart
Ryzodeg 70/30

insulin lispro protamine– insulin lispro
Humalog Mix 75/25, Humalog Mix 50/50

isophane insulin suspension–insulin injection combinations
Humulin 70/30 ◇, Novolin 70/30 ◇

insulin aspart (rDNA origin) protamine suspension– insulin aspart (rDNA origin) injection
Novolog Mix 70/30

Therapeutic class: Antidiabetics
Pharmacologic class: Insulins

AVAILABLE FORMS
Injection: Humalog Mix 75/25 (75% insulin lispro protamine suspension and 25% insulin lispro) and 50/50 (50% insulin lispro protamine suspension and 50% insulin lispro) 100 units per mL (U-100) in 10-mL vial, 3-mL prefilled KwikPen syringe
Injection: Humulin 70/30 (70% isophane insulin suspension and 30% regular insulin) 100 units per mL (U-100) in 3-mL and 10-mL vials, 3-mL prefilled pens and KwikPen
Injection: Novolog Mix 70/30 (70% insulin aspart protamine suspension and 30% insulin aspart) 100 units per mL (U-100) in 10-mL vial, 3-mL prefilled FlexPen syringe
Injection: Novolin 70/30 (70% isophane insulin suspension and 30% regular insulin) 100 units per mL (U-100) in 10-mL vial

Injection: Ryzodeg 70/30 (210 units insulin degludec and 90 units insulin aspart) 100 units per mL (U-100) in 3-mL prefilled FlexTouch pen

INDICATIONS & DOSAGES
Adjust-a-dose (for all indications): Individualize dosage based on metabolic needs, blood glucose monitoring, and glycemic control goal. Insulin requirements may be altered during acute illness, emotional distress, or stress. Adjust as needed in patients who are elderly, have renal or hepatic dysfunction, or have changes in physical activity or meal patterns, and in patients concurrently taking drugs that lower blood glucose level. Refer to manufacturer's instructions for dosage adjustments when converting from other insulin regimens and formulations. Obese patients may need a maintenance dosage of up to 1.2 units/kg/day.
➤ **To improve glycemic control in patients with diabetes mellitus**
Adults: For Novolog Mix 70/30, usual dosage is 0.5 to 1 unit/kg/day subcutaneously in divided doses within 15 minutes before a meal or, in type 2 diabetes, given up to 15 minutes after start of a meal. Drug isn't intended for initial treatment, but may be transitioned to after basal insulin requirements are determined. Generally, 50% to 75% daily insulin dose is given as an intermediate- or long-acting form of insulin in one to two daily subcutaneous injections. The remaining portion of the 24-hour insulin requirement is divided and given as either regular insulin or a rapid-acting form of insulin at the same time before breakfast and dinner.
Adults: For Humalog Mix 50/50 and 75/25, dosage is individualized and given subcutaneously within 15 minutes before a meal.
Adults and children: For Humulin 70/30 and Novolin 70/30, usual dosage is 0.5 to 1 unit/kg/day subcutaneously divided into two doses given about 30 to 45 minutes before a meal. During puberty, insulin requirements may increase to 1.2 units/kg/day during growth spurts.
Adults: For Ryzodeg 70/30, individualize and titrate dose based on patient's metabolic needs, blood glucose monitoring results, and glycemic control goal. Adjust dosage

according to fasting blood glucose measurements before breakfast. Recommended time between dosage increases is 3 to 4 days.
   In insulin-naive patients with type 1 diabetes, recommended starting dose is approximately one-third to one-half of the total daily insulin dose. The remainder of the total daily insulin dose should be given as a short- or rapid-acting insulin divided among each daily meal.
   As a general rule, the initial total daily insulin dose for insulin-naive patients with type 1 diabetes is 0.2 to 0.4 unit/kg/day. In insulin-naive patients with type 2 diabetes, recommended starting dose is 10 units subcutaneously once daily.

ADMINISTRATION
Subcutaneous
• Inspect vials and syringes. Drug should appear uniformly white and cloudy. Don't use if it looks clear or contains solid particles.
• Administer all insulin mixtures at room temperature.
• Don't freeze vials or pens; discard if frozen.
• Drug is a suspension; administer only subcutaneously, never I.V.
• Don't use in insulin infusion pumps.
• Don't mix with other insulins.
• Keep away from direct heat and sunlight.
• Discard insulin exposed to temperatures above 98.6° F (37° C).
• Follow product-specific pen device directions for preparation and administration.
🕔 *Alert:* Multidose pens are for single patient use only. Pens should never be shared even if the needle is changed. Clearly label with patient identifying information where it won't obstruct dosing window, warning, or other product information.
Novolog Mix 70/30
• Keep all unopened Novolog Mix 70/30 refrigerated between 36° and 46° F (2° and 8° C).
• Once opened or unopened vial has been stored at room temperature, stability is 28 days.
• Once a Novolog Mix 70/30 FlexPen has been punctured, it should be kept at temperatures below 86° F (30° C) for up to

14 days. Don't store a Novolog Mix 70/30 FlexPen that's in use in refrigerator.

Humulin 70/30

• Discard opened or unopened vials stored at room temperature after 31 days.

• Store unopened pen or KwikPen in refrigerator at 36° to 46° F (2° to 8° C). Discard unopened pens stored at room temperature after 10 days.

• Store opened pen or KwikPen at room temperature; discard after 10 days even if syringe contains insulin.

Novolin 70/30

• Store unopened vials in refrigerator at 36° to 46° F (2° to 8° C).

• If refrigeration isn't possible, may keep unopened vials at room temperature for up to 6 weeks (42 days), as long as temperature is at or below 77° F (25° C). Keep unopened vials in carton to protect from light.

• If unopened vials are stored in refrigerator, follow expiration date on label.

• Keep open vials at room temperature.

• Throw away open vial after 6 weeks (42 days) of use, even if insulin remains in vial.

Humalog Mix 75/25 and Humalog Mix 50/50

• Refrigerate vials and pens at 36° to 46° F (2° to 8° C) until ready to use.

• Unrefrigerated (below 86° F [30° C]) vials must be used within 28 days or discarded.

• Unrefrigerated (below 86° F [30° C]) KwikPen and pen must be used within 10 days and then discarded, even if syringe contains insulin.

Ryzodeg 70/30

• Refrigerate unopened FlexTouch pens at 36° to 46° F (2° to 8° C) until ready to use; discard after expiration date.

• Unrefrigerated (below 86° F [30° C]) unopened pens must be used within 28 days or discarded.

• Don't refrigerate opened pens. Keep at room temperature (below 86° F [30° C]), away from direct heat and light for up to 28 days.

Don't dilute or mix with other insulin products or solutions.

ACTION

Regulates glucose metabolism by binding to insulin receptors on muscle, liver, and fat cells; facilitates cellular uptake of glucose; and promotes uptake and storage of glucose in the form of glycogen in the liver.

Route	Onset	Peak	Duration
Subcut. (Novolog Mix 70/30)	15 min	60 min	Up to 24 hr
Subcut. (Humulin 70/30)	30 min	2.2 hr	Up to 24 hr
Subcut. (Humalog Mix 75/25 and 50/50)	15 min	30–90 min	Up to 24 hr
Subcut. (Novolin 70/30)	30 min	2.2 hr	Up to 24 hr
Subcut. (Ryzodeg 70/30)	14 min (aspart)	72 min (aspart)	>24 hr

Half-life: Novolog Mix 70/30, 8 to 9 hours; Humulin 70/30, unknown; Humalog Mix 75/25 and 50/50, unknown; Ryzodeg 70/30, about 25 hours (insulin degludec).

ADVERSE REACTIONS

CNS: asthenia, headache, fever, pain.
CV: peripheral edema.
EENT: pharyngitis, rhinitis.
GI: abdominal pain, diarrhea, nausea.
GU: UTI, dysmenorrhea.
Metabolic: *hypoglycemia, hypokalemia,* weight gain.
Musculoskeletal: myalgia.
Respiratory: bronchitis, cough.
Skin: lipodystrophy, injection-site reactions.
Other: *allergic reactions,* insulin antibody production, flulike syndrome, infection.

INTERACTIONS

Drug-drug. *ACE inhibitors, antidiabetic agents (oral), ARBs, disopyramide, fibrates, fluoxetine,* **MAO inhibitors,** *octreotide, pentoxifylline, pramlintide, salicylates, sulfonamide antibiotics:* May increase risk of hypoglycemia. Monitor glucose level closely and adjust insulin dosage as needed. *Atypical antipsychotics, corticosteroids, danazol, diuretics, estrogens, glucagon, hormonal contraceptives, isoniazid, niacin, phenothiazines, protease inhibitors,* *sympathomimetics (albuterol, epinephrine, terbutaline), somatropin, thyroid hormones:* May decrease blood glucose–lowering effects. Monitor glucose level closely and adjust insulin dosage as needed.

Beta blockers, clonidine, guanethidine, reserpine: May mask signs and symptoms of hypoglycemia. Avoid concurrent use, if possible, or monitor patient closely.

Beta blockers, clonidine, lithium salts, pentamidine: May cause hypoglycemia or hyperglycemia. Monitor glucose level closely.

Thiazolidinediones (TZDs; pioglitazone, rosiglitazone): May cause fluid retention that can lead to HF. Monitor patient closely and adjust or stop TZDs as clinically indicated.

Drug-herb. *Ginseng:* May increase drug's effects. Discourage use together.

Drug-lifestyle. *Alcohol use:* May cause hyperglycemia or hypoglycemia. Monitor glucose level closely and discourage concurrent use.

EFFECTS ON LAB TEST RESULTS
• May decrease blood glucose and potassium levels.

CONTRAINDICATIONS & CAUTIONS
• Contraindicated during episodes of hypoglycemia or ketoacidosis.
• Contraindicated in patients with a history of hypersensitivity to drug or its components. Severe, life-threatening, generalized allergy, including anaphylaxis, can occur with insulin products.
• Changes in insulin or oral antidiabetic dosages may affect glycemic control and should be made only under medical supervision.
• Use cautiously in patients susceptible to hypokalemia, such as patients who are fasting, are taking potassium-lowering drugs, or are concurrently taking drugs that may affect potassium levels, including I.V. insulin. Untreated hypokalemia can cause respiratory paralysis, ventricular arrhythmias, and death.
• Hypoglycemia is the most common adverse reaction. Severe hypoglycemia can cause seizures, and may be life-threatening or fatal. Hypoglycemia can occur suddenly,

and signs and symptoms may differ. Risk increases with intensity of glycemic control and changes in glycemic treatment, meal patterns, physical activity, or concomitant medications, and in patients with renal or hepatic impairment.
• Use cautiously in elderly patients, who may be at increased risk for adverse effects; signs and symptoms of hypoglycemia may be more difficult to recognize in these patients.

Dialyzable drug: Unknown.

⚠ ***Overdose S&S:*** Hypoglycemia, hypokalemia.

PREGNANCY-LACTATION-REPRODUCTION
• Use cautiously in pregnant women and only if clearly needed.
• Monitor blood glucose levels closely in pregnant patients, in women who have recently given birth, and in breast-feeding women; insulin requirements may change.
• It isn't known if insulin appears in breast milk. Use cautiously in breast-feeding women.

NURSING CONSIDERATIONS
• Don't mix combination insulins with other insulins.
• Rotate injection sites to reduce risk of lipodystrophy.
• The time course of the action of insulin mixtures may vary among patients and in same patient depending on time of day, injection site, blood supply, temperature, and physical activity.
• Observe injection sites for reactions, such as redness, swelling, itching, or burning. These reactions should resolve within a few days or weeks.
• Assess patient and notify prescriber for signs and symptoms of hypoglycemia (sweating, shaking, trembling, confusion, headache, irritability, hunger, rapid, pulse, nausea) and hyperglycemia (drowsiness, fruity breath odor, frequent urination, thirst).
• Signs and symptoms of hypoglycemia may occur in patients with diabetes regardless of glucose value.
• Monitor blood glucose level and adjust insulin dosages as needed with medical supervision.

• Closely monitor patients also taking other medications because other drugs can mask signs and symptoms of hypoglycemia or cause an increase or decrease in blood glucose level.

• Increase frequency of glucose monitoring in patients who are acutely ill or under emotional stress, or if changes in diet, exercise, or medication regimen occur. These situations may affect rate of insulin absorption.

• Increase frequency of glucose monitoring when initiating therapy or when changes in insulin strength, dosage, manufacturer, or type or method of administration are made. Such changes may affect glycemic control and increase risk of hypoglycemia.

• Monitor patient carefully for signs and symptoms of hypoglycemia. Symptom awareness may be decreased in patients with long-standing diabetes, diabetic nerve disease, renal disease, or hepatic impairment and in patients who have experienced recurrent hypoglycemia. Treat according to individual facility policy and procedure if necessary.

• Mild episodes of hypoglycemia may be treated with oral glucose. More severe episodes of hypoglycemia, such as coma, seizure, or neurologic impairment, may be treated with I.M. or subcutaneous glucagon or concentrated I.V. glucose.

• Monitor potassium levels in patients at risk for hypokalemia (those receiving potassium-depleting drugs or I.V. insulin).

• Monitor patients for generalized allergic reactions, rash (including pruritus) over entire body, shortness of breath, wheezing, hypotension, rapid pulse, sweating, and anaphylaxis.

• Periodically measure HbA_{1c} levels.

Observe for signs and symptoms of HF when used with TZDs; consider dosage reduction or discontinuation of TZD if HF occurs.

Look alike–sound alike: Don't confuse NovoLog with Novolin; don't confuse Humalog with Humulin.

PATIENT TEACHING

Caution patient not to mix insulin combination products with other insulins.

• **Alert:** Warn patient not to share multidose pen with other people, even if the needle

is changed, because of risk of bloodborne pathogen transmission, including HIV and hepatitis.

• Advise patient that hypoglycemic episodes can impair the ability to concentrate and react; advise patient to use caution while driving and operating machinery.

• Instruct patient to keep hard candy or glucose tablets on hand to treat mild cases of hypoglycemia.

• Advise patient to keep a log of glucose levels.

• Instruct patient on long-term sequelae of diabetes if not managed properly.

• Instruct patient to carry identification or wear jewelry indicating that he has diabetes.

• Advise patient that allergic and hypersensitivity reactions can occur, including injection-site reactions (local pain, redness, or swelling), and to report symptoms to health care provider. Teach patient signs and symptoms of anaphylaxis and to seek emergency medical attention promptly if anaphylaxis occurs.

• Instruct patient on self-management procedures, including glucose monitoring, proper administration technique, and management of hypoglycemia and hyperglycemia.

• Warn patient about special situations, such as concurrent conditions (illness, stress, or emotional disturbances), inadequate or skipped insulin dose, inadvertent administration of an increased insulin dose, inadequate food intake, and skipped meals.

• Advise women with diabetes to inform their doctor if they are pregnant or plan to become pregnant.

• Advise pregnant women of the change in insulin requirements that may occur during pregnancy and after childbirth.

• Teach patient that alcohol and some other medications may increase or decrease glucose levels. Advise patient to inform health care provider of all medications and supplements being taken.

• Caution patient not to stop insulin abruptly or change amount taken without consulting prescriber.

• Advise patient that any insulin change should be made cautiously and only under medical supervision. Changes in insulin strength, manufacturer, type (regular, NPH,

or insulin analogs), species (animal, human), or method of manufacture (rDNA versus animal-source insulin) may result in the need for a dosage change. Dosage of concomitant oral antidiabetic agents may need adjustment.
• Teach patient to give insulin at appropriate time around a meal, depending on product.
• Instruct patient to rotate injection sites and of the importance of avoiding lipodystrophy.
• Teach patient to store insulin products properly, depending on individual products.
• Explain importance of checking insulin label before each injection as accidental mixups among insulin types have been reported.

SAFETY ALERT!

Insulins (intermediate-acting)

IN-su-lins

isophane insulin suspension (NPH)
Humulin N ◊, Humulin N KwikPen ◊, Novolin N ◊

Therapeutic class: Antidiabetics
Pharmacologic class: Insulins

AVAILABLE FORMS
Injection: 100 units/mL in 3-mL vial, 10-mL vial, 3-mL pen (Humulin N)

INDICATIONS & DOSAGES
Adjust-a-dose (for all indications): Individualize dosage based on metabolic needs, blood glucose monitoring, and glycemic control goal. Adjust dosage to achieve premeal plasma glucose level of 90 to 130 mg/dL and peak postprandial plasma and bedtime glucose level of less than 180 mg/dL. Insulin requirements may be altered during acute illness, emotional distress, or stress. Adjust as needed in patients who are elderly, have renal or hepatic dysfunction, or have changes in physical activity or meal patterns, and in patients concurrently taking drugs that lower blood glucose level. Refer to manufacturer's instructions for dosage adjustments when converting from other insulin regimens and formulations.

➤ **Patients with type 1 diabetes mellitus; patients with type 2 diabetes mellitus that can't be properly controlled by diet, exercise, and weight control**
Adults and children age 12 and older: Usual dosage is 0.5 to 1 unit/kg/day, often given in two divided doses to provide a more constant level of basal insulin.

ADMINISTRATION
Subcutaneous
• Give by subcutaneous injection only; not for I.M., I.V., or insulin pump administration.
• Give injection in abdominal region, buttocks, thigh, or upper arm. Subcutaneous injection into abdominal wall is generally associated with faster absorption than other injection sites.
• Rotate injection sites within same region to reduce risk of lipodystrophy. A general rule is to not administer within 1 inch (2.5 cm) of same site for 1 month.
• Injection into a lifted skin fold minimizes risk of I.M. injection.
• Roll vial gently between the hands before each dose to uniformly disperse NPH insulin. Avoid vigorous shaking that may cause air bubbles or foam.
• NPH insulin should be uniformly cloudy or milky after gentle mixing and shouldn't contain particulate matter.
• When mixing NPH insulin with regular insulin, always draw clear regular insulin into syringe first; then administer immediately.
• NPH insulin is typically given within 60 minutes of a meal. However, time of administration depends on patient-specific variables; NPH insulin may be given with meal-time regular or Humalog insulin if indicated.
❸ Alert: Multidose pens are for single patient use only. Pens should never be shared even if the needle is changed. Clearly label with patient identifying information where it won't obstruct dosing window, warning, or other product information.
• Store Humulin N at room temperature, below 86° F (30° C), if not exposed to direct sunlight for 31 days (vial) or 14 days (pen). May store opened vials and unopened vials and pens in refrigerator at 36° to 46° F

(2° to 8° C); don't refrigerate opened pens. Don't freeze vials or pens.

• Store opened or unopened Novolin N away from direct heat or light at room temperature, below 77° F (25° C), for up to 42 days. Unopened Novolin N can be stored in refrigerator at 36° to 46° F (2° to 8° C) and used until expiration date on label. Don't freeze.

ACTION

Lowers blood glucose level by stimulating peripheral glucose uptake by binding to insulin receptors on skeletal muscle and in fat cells and by inhibiting hepatic glucose production; also inhibits lipolysis and proteolysis, and enhances protein synthesis. Intermediate-acting insulin suspensions of human insulin with protamine and zinc provide a slower onset and a longer duration of activity.

Route	Onset	Peak	Duration
Subcut.	1–1½ hr	4–12 hr	Up to 24 hr

Half-life: About 4.4 hours.

ADVERSE REACTIONS

CV: peripheral edema.
Metabolic: hypoglycemia, hypokalemia, weight gain.
Skin: injection-site reaction, lipodystrophy, pruritus, rash.
Other: allergic reactions, immunogenicity.

INTERACTIONS

Drug-drug. *ACE inhibitors, antidiabetic agents (oral), ARBs, disopyramide, fibrates, fluoxetine, MAO inhibitors, octreotide, pentoxifylline, pramlintide, salicylates, sulfonamide antibiotics:* May increase risk of hypoglycemia. Monitor glucose level closely and adjust insulin dosage as needed.
Atypical antipsychotics, corticosteroids, danazol, diuretics, estrogens, glucagon, hormonal contraceptives, isoniazid, niacin, phenothiazines, protease inhibitors, sympathomimetics (albuterol, epinephrine, terbutaline), somatropin, thyroid hormones: May decrease blood glucose–lowering effects. Monitor glucose level closely and adjust insulin dosage as needed.
Beta blockers, clonidine, guanethidine, reserpine: May mask signs and symptoms of hypoglycemia. Avoid concurrent use, if possible, and monitor patient closely.
Beta blockers, clonidine, lithium salts, pentamidine: May cause hypoglycemia or hyperglycemia. Monitor glucose level closely.
Thiazolidinediones (TZDs; pioglitazone, rosiglitazone): May cause fluid retention that can lead to HF. Monitor patient closely and adjust or stop TZDs as clinically indicated.
Drug-lifestyle. *Alcohol use:* May cause hyperglycemia or hypoglycemia. Monitor glucose level closely, and discourage concurrent use.

EFFECTS ON LAB TEST RESULTS

• May decrease blood glucose and potassium levels.
• May develop antibodies that react with human insulin.

CONTRAINDICATIONS & CAUTIONS

• Contraindicated during episodes of hypoglycemia or ketoacidosis.
• Contraindicated in patients with a history of hypersensitivity to drug or its components. Severe, life-threatening, generalized allergy, including anaphylaxis, can occur with insulin products.
• Use cautiously in patients susceptible to hypokalemia, such as patients who are fasting, are taking potassium-lowering drugs, or are concurrently taking drugs that may affect potassium level. Untreated hypokalemia can cause respiratory paralysis, ventricular arrhythmias, and death.
• Hypoglycemia is the most common adverse reaction. Severe hypoglycemia can cause seizures, and may be life-threatening or fatal. Hypoglycemia can occur suddenly and symptoms may differ. Risk increases with intensity of glycemic control and changes in glycemic treatment, meal patterns, physical activity, and concomitant medications and in patients with renal or hepatic impairment.
• Use cautiously in elderly patients, who may at increased risk for adverse effects; signs and symptoms of hypoglycemia may be more difficult to recognize in these patients.
Dialyzable drug: Unknown.

⚠ *Overdose S&S:* Hypoglycemia, hypokalemia.

PREGNANCY-LACTATION-REPRODUCTION
• Use cautiously in pregnant women and monitor patients closely.
• Monitor blood glucose levels closely in pregnant patients, in women who have recently given birth, and in breast-feeding women; insulin requirements may change.
• It isn't known if insulin appears in breast milk. Use cautiously in breast-feeding women.

NURSING CONSIDERATIONS
• Monitor blood glucose levels and adjust insulin dosages as needed.
• Monitor patients taking other medications with insulin more closely because other drugs may mask signs and symptoms of hypoglycemia or may cause an increase or decrease in blood glucose level.
• Increase frequency of glucose monitoring in patients who are acutely ill or under emotional stress, or if changes in diet, exercise, or medication regimen occur, as these may affect rate of insulin absorption. Also closely monitor patients after changes to insulin dosage.
• Monitor patients carefully for signs and symptoms of hypoglycemia. Treat according to individual facility policy and procedure if necessary.
• Mild episodes of hypoglycemia may be treated with oral glucose. More severe episodes of hypoglycemia, such as coma, seizure, or neurologic impairment, may be treated with I.M. or subcutaneous glucagon or concentrated I.V. glucose.
• Monitor potassium levels in patients at risk for hypokalemia, especially those taking potassium-depleting drugs.
• Assess patient for signs and symptoms of hypoglycemia (seizures, sweating, shaking, trembling, confusion) and hyperglycemia (drowsiness, fruity breath odor, frequent urination, thirst). Notify prescriber if any of these signs or symptoms occur.
• Periodically measure HbA$_{1c}$ levels.
• Observe for signs and symptoms of HF with concomitant use of TZDs. Consider dosage reduction or discontinuation if HF occurs.

• Monitor patients for generalized allergic reactions, including anaphylaxis.
• *Look alike–sound alike:* Don't confuse Humulin with Humalog; don't confuse Novolin with Novolog.

PATIENT TEACHING
• Instruct patient in self-management, including glucose monitoring, injection technique, proper storage of insulin, and recognition and management of hypoglycemia and hyperglycemia.
• Explain to patient that insulin requirements may vary due to illness, stress or emotional disturbance, inadequate food intake, and skipped meals.
• Advise patient that hypoglycemic episodes can impair the ability to concentrate and react; advise patient to use caution while driving and operating machinery.
• Advise patient that allergic and hypersensitivity reactions can occur, including injection-site reactions (local pain, redness, or swelling), and to report signs and symptoms to health care provider. Teach patient signs and symptoms of anaphylaxis and to seek emergency medical attention promptly if anaphylaxis occurs.
• Instruct patient to rotate injection sites to avoid developing lipodystrophy.
• *Alert:* Warn patient not to share multidose pen with other people, even if the needle is changed, because of risk of bloodborne pathogen transmission, including HIV and hepatitis.
• Explain importance of checking insulin label before each injection as accidental mix-ups among insulin types have been reported.
• Explain that intermediate-acting insulins can be mixed with regular insulin.
• Instruct patient to visually inspect insulin before use to ensure that there's no particulate matter in vial and that the medication appears uniformly cloudy.
• Teach patient that alcohol and some other medications may increase or decrease glucose levels. Advise patient to inform health care provider of all medications and supplements he or she is taking.
• Instruct patient not to stop insulin abruptly or change amount injected without consulting prescriber.

Reactions in bold italics are *life-threatening*. Interactions may have a *rapid onset* or a *delayed onset*.

• Advise patient that any insulin changes should be made cautiously and only under medical supervision. Changes in insulin strength, manufacturer, type (regular, NPH, or insulin analogs), species (animal, human), or method of manufacture (rDNA versus animal-source insulin) may result in the need for a dosage change. Dosage of concomitant oral antidiabetic agents may need adjustment.

• Warn female patient to inform prescriber if she is pregnant or plans to become pregnant.

• Advise female patient of childbearing potential of importance of maintaining tight glucose control if she is pregnant or plans to become pregnant.

• Advise pregnant women of the change in insulin requirements that may occur during pregnancy and after childbirth.

• Instruct patient not to use insulin after the printed expiration date; inform him that vials are good for 31 days at room temperature and pens are good for 14 days at room temperature.

Insulins (long-acting)
IN-su-lins

insulin degludec
Tresiba

insulin detemir (rDNA) origin injection
Levemir, Levemir FlexTouch

insulin glargine (rDNA origin) injection
Lantus, Lantus SoloStar, Toujeo SoloStar

Therapeutic class: Antidiabetics
Pharmacologic class: Insulins

AVAILABLE FORMS
Injection: 100 units/mL in 10-mL vial, 100 and 200 units/mL in 3-mL pens, 300 units/mL in 1.5-mL pen

INDICATIONS & DOSAGES
Adjust-a-dose (for all indications): Individualize dosage based on metabolic needs, blood glucose monitoring, and glycemic control goal. Insulin requirements may be altered during acute illness, emotional distress, or stress. Adjust dosage as needed in patients who are elderly, in those who have renal or hepatic dysfunction or have changes in physical activity or meal patterns, and in patients who are concurrently taking drugs that lower blood glucose level. Refer to manufacturer's instructions for dosage adjustments when converting from other insulin regimens and formulations.

➤ **To improve glycemic control in patients with type 1 diabetes mellitus**
Adults (degludec, detemir, glargine) and children age 2 and older (detemir) or age 6 and older (glargine): Initial dosage is approximately one-third (Levemir, Lantus) or one-third to one-half (Toujeo, Tresiba) of total daily insulin requirements once daily at any time of day (Tresiba, Lantus) or with evening meal or at bedtime. Satisfy the remainder of the daily insulin requirements with rapid- or short-acting premeal insulin. Or, in patients who require twice-daily detemir dosing, give evening dose with evening meal, at bedtime, or 12 hours after morning dose.

➤ **To improve glycemic control in patients with type 2 diabetes mellitus**
Adults: Initial insulin degludec dosage is 10 units once daily at any time of day. Initial insulin detemir dosage is 10 units (0.1 to 0.2 unit/kg) once daily in evening or divided into two daily doses in patients inadequately controlled on oral antidiabetic agents, or once daily in the evening in patients inadequately controlled on a glucagon-like peptide 1 (GLP-1) receptor antagonist. Initial insulin glargine dosage is 0.2 unit/kg (up to 10 units) once daily. Adjust dosage as needed.

ADMINISTRATION
Subcutaneous
General
• Don't give long-acting insulins by insulin infusion pumps or by I.M. or I.V. injection.
• Administer by subcutaneous injection only in the thigh, abdominal wall, or upper

arm. Rotate sites within same region (abdomen, thigh, or deltoid) from one injection to the next to reduce risk of lipodystrophy.

● Don't mix or dilute long-acting insulins with other insulins or solutions because the pharmacokinetic and pharmacodynamic profile (onset of action, time to peak effect) of the insulin may be altered unpredictably.

● Inspect visually for particulate matter and discoloration before administration, whenever solution and container permit; use only if solution appears clear and colorless.

● Instructions for priming and using pens vary from one to another, are very detailed, and involve multiple steps. Refer to manufacturer's instructions for use.

🌙 **Alert:** Multidose pens are for single patient use only. Pens should never be shared even if the needle is changed. Clearly label with patient identifying information where it won't obstruct dosing window, warning, or other product information.

Insulin degludec

● Give insulin degludec once daily at any time of day.

● Individualize and titrate dosage every 3 to 4 days based on patient's metabolic needs, blood glucose monitoring results, and glycemic control goal.

● Don't perform dose conversion when using FlexTouch pen. The dose window for both 100-unit and 200-unit pens shows the number of insulin units to be delivered and no conversion is needed.

● In patients with type 1 or type 2 diabetes mellitus already on insulin therapy, start insulin degludec at the same unit dose as the total daily long- or intermediate-acting insulin unit dose.

● Always use a new needle for each injection to help ensure sterility and prevent blocked needles.

● Store unused pens in refrigerator at 36° to 46° F (2° to 8° C); may be used until expiration date on label. Don't freeze or use if pens have been frozen.

● Store open pen away from heat or light at room temperature, below 86° F (30° C). Discard after 56 days, even if pen still contains insulin and expiration date hasn't passed.

Insulin detemir

● Give insulin detemir once or twice daily. For patients treated with insulin detemir once daily, give dose with evening meal or at bedtime. For patients who require twice-daily dosing, administer evening dose with evening meal, at bedtime, or 12 hours after morning dose.

● When using insulin detemir with a GLP-1 receptor agonist, give as separate injections; never mix together. Insulin detemir and a GLP-1 receptor agonist may be injected in same body region, but the injections shouldn't be adjacent to each other.

● If converting from insulin glargine or NPH insulin to insulin detemir, maintain the same unit dose. Monitor glucose level closely during transition.

● Store unused (unopened) insulin detemir vials and pens between 36° and 46° F (2° and 8° C). Don't freeze and don't use if vials or pens have been frozen. Keep in carton so that vials or pens stay clean and protected from light.

● If refrigeration isn't possible, unused (unopened) insulin detemir can be kept unrefrigerated at room temperature, below 86° F (30° C), as long as it's kept as cool as possible and away from direct heat and light. Discard unrefrigerated insulin detemir 42 days after it's first kept out of the refrigerator, even if the pen or vial still contains insulin.

● After initial use, store vials in refrigerator; never freeze. If refrigeration isn't possible, the in-use vial can be kept unrefrigerated at room temperature, below 86° F (30° C), as long as it's kept as cool as possible and away from direct heat and light. Discard refrigerated insulin detemir vials 42 days after initial use.

● Pens (in use): After initial use, don't store insulin detemir pen in refrigerator and don't store with the needle in place; keep opened insulin detemir pen away from direct heat and light at room temperature, below 86° F (30° C). Discard unrefrigerated insulin detemir pens 42 days after they're first kept out of refrigerator.

Insulin glargine

● Give subcutaneously once daily at same time every day, at any time during the day.

• If converting from insulin detemir to insulin glargine, maintain the same unit dose. Monitor glucose level closely during transition.

• If changing from once-daily Toujeo 300 units/mL to once-daily Lantus, recommended initial Lantus dose is 80% of the Toujeo dose that's being discontinued.

• If switching from once-daily NPH insulin to once-daily Lantus, the recommended initial glargine dose is the same as the dose of NPH that is being discontinued.

• If switching from twice-daily NPH insulin to once-daily Lantus, the recommended initial insulin glargine dose is 80% of the total NPH insulin dose that is being discontinued.

• Store unopened insulin glargine vials and pens at 36° to 46° F (2° to 8° C); don't freeze, and discard if frozen. If refrigeration isn't possible, the open vial in use can be kept unrefrigerated for up to 28 days away from direct heat and light, as long as the room temperature isn't above 86° F (30° C).

• Opened vials, whether or not refrigerated, must be used within a 28-day period or they must be discarded.

• Opened pens shouldn't be refrigerated but should be kept at room temperature, below 86° F (30° C), away from direct heat and light; discard opened pens kept at room temperature after 28 days.

ACTION

Lowers blood glucose level by stimulating peripheral glucose uptake by binding to insulin receptors on skeletal muscle and in fat cells, and by inhibiting hepatic glucose production; also inhibits lipolysis and proteolysis, and enhances protein synthesis.

Route	Onset	Peak	Duration
Subcut. (degludec)	1 hr	9 hr	24 hr
Subcut. (detemir)	Unknown	Constant	24 hr
Subcut. (glargine)	3–6 hr	Constant	24 hr

Half-life: Degludec, 25 hours; detemir, 5 to 7 hours; glargine, unknown.

ADVERSE REACTIONS

CNS: headache, pyrexia.
CV: peripheral edema.
EENT: pharyngitis, rhinitis.
GI: abdominal pain, gastroenteritis, nausea, vomiting.

Metabolic: *hypoglycemia,* sodium retention, weight gain.
Musculoskeletal: back pain.
Respiratory: URI, bronchitis, cough.
Skin: injection-site reactions, lipodystrophy, pruritus, rash.
Other: allergic reactions, flulike symptoms.

INTERACTIONS

Drug-drug. *ACE inhibitors, antidiabetic agents (oral), ARBs, disopyramide, fibrates, fluoxetine,* **MAO inhibitors,** *octreotide, pentoxifylline, pramlintide, salicylates, sulfonamide antibiotics:* May increase blood glucose–lowering effect of insulin, increasing risk of hypoglycemia. Monitor glucose level and patient closely. Adjust insulin dosage as necessary.

Antiadrenergics (beta blockers, clonidine, guanethidine, reserpine): May mask signs and symptoms of hypoglycemia. Avoid concurrent use, if possible, and monitor patient closely.

Atypical antipsychotics, corticosteroids, danazol, diuretics, estrogens, glucagon, hormonal contraceptives, isoniazid, niacin, phenothiazines, protease inhibitors, somatropin, sympathomimetics (albuterol, epinephrine, terbutaline), thyroid hormones: May decrease blood glucose–lowering effect of insulin, increasing risk of hyperglycemia. Monitor glucose level and patient closely. Adjust insulin dosage as necessary.

Beta blockers, clonidine, lithium salts, pentamidine: May increase risk of either hypoglycemia or hyperglycemia. Monitor glucose level closely.

GLP-1 receptor agonists (albiglutide, exenatide, liraglutide): May increase risk of hypoglycemia. Monitor glucose level closely and decrease insulin dosage if necessary.

Thiazolidinediones (TZDs; pioglitazone, rosiglitazone): May cause fluid retention that can lead to HF. Monitor patient closely, and adjust or stop TZD as clinically necessary.

Drug-lifestyle. *Alcohol use:* May cause hyperglycemia or hypoglycemia. Monitor glucose level and discourage concurrent use.

EFFECTS ON LAB TEST RESULTS
● May decrease blood glucose level.

CONTRAINDICATIONS & CAUTIONS
● Contraindicated during episodes of hypoglycemia or diabetic ketoacidosis.
● Contraindicated in patients hypersensitive to drug or its components. Severe, life-threatening, generalized allergy, including anaphylaxis, can occur with insulin products.
◐ **Alert:** Adjust insulin regimen only with appropriate glucose monitoring under medical supervision.
● Use cautiously in patients susceptible to hypokalemia, such as patients who are fasting, are taking potassium-lowering drugs, or are concurrently taking drugs that may affect potassium level. Untreated hypokalemia can cause respiratory paralysis, ventricular arrhythmias, and death.
● Hypoglycemia is the most common adverse reaction. Severe hypoglycemia can cause seizures, and may be life-threatening or fatal. Hypoglycemia can occur suddenly, and symptoms may differ. Risk increases with intensity of glycemic control and changes in glycemic treatment, meal patterns, physical activity, and concomitant medications and in patients with renal or hepatic impairment.
● Use cautiously in elderly patients, who may be at risk for increased sensitivity to drug's effects. Signs and symptoms of hypoglycemia may be more difficult to recognize in these patients.
Dialyzable drug: Unknown.
⚠ *Overdose S&S:* Hypoglycemia.

PREGNANCY-LACTATION-REPRODUCTION
● Insulin detemir: Use cautiously in pregnant women. Carefully monitor glucose level.
● Insulin degludec, glargine: There are no well-controlled studies in pregnant women. Use during pregnancy only if potential benefit justifies potential risk to the fetus.
● Closely monitor blood glucose levels in pregnant patients, in women who have recently given birth, and in breast-feeding women; insulin requirements may change.

● It isn't known if insulin appears in breast milk. Use cautiously in breast-feeding women. Insulin doses may need adjustment.

NURSING CONSIDERATIONS
● Prolonged effect of long-acting insulin may delay recovery from hypoglycemia. Monitor patient carefully.
● Monitor patients taking other medications with insulin more closely because other drugs can mask signs and symptoms of hypoglycemia or cause an increase or a decrease in blood glucose level.
● Adjust dosages regularly, depending on patient-specific glucose measurements.
● Monitor patient carefully for signs and symptoms of hypoglycemia, especially in long-standing disease. Treat according to individual facility policy and procedure if necessary.
● Mild episodes of hypoglycemia may be treated with oral glucose. More severe episodes of hypoglycemia, such as coma, seizure, or neurologic impairment, may be treated with I.M. or subcutaneous glucagon or concentrated I.V. glucose.
● Assess patient for signs and symptoms of hypoglycemia (sweating, shaking, trembling, confusion) and hyperglycemia (drowsiness, fruity breath odor, frequent urination, thirst). Notify prescriber if any of these signs or symptoms occur.
● Periodically measure HbA_{1c} levels.
● Observe for signs and symptoms of HF with concomitant use of TZDs. Consider dosage reduction or discontinuation of TZD if HF occurs.
● Increase frequency of glucose monitoring in patients who are acutely ill or under emotional stress, or if changes in diet, exercise, or medication regimen occur, as these may affect the rate of insulin absorption. Also, closely monitor patient after changes to insulin dosage.
● *Look alike–sound alike:* Don't confuse insulin glargine with insulin glulisine.

PATIENT TEACHING
● Instruct patient in self-management, including glucose monitoring, injection technique, proper storage of insulin, and recognition and management of hypoglycemia and hyperglycemia.

• Explain to patient that insulin requirements may vary due to illness, stress or emotional disturbance, change in activity level, inadequate food intake, and skipped meals.

• Teach patient to watch for signs and symptoms of hypoglycemia (sweating, shaking, trembling, confusion) and hyperglycemia (drowsiness, frequent urination, thirst).

• Advise patient that hypoglycemic episodes may impair the ability to concentrate and react; advise patient to use caution while driving and operating machinery.

• Instruct patient to keep hard candy or glucose tablets on hand to treat mild cases of hypoglycemia.

• Advise patient that allergic and hypersensitivity reactions can occur, including injection-site reactions (local pain, redness, or swelling) and generalized reactions and to report signs or symptoms to health care provider. Teach patient signs and symptoms of anaphylaxis and to seek emergency medical attention promptly if anaphylaxis occurs.

• Instruct patient to rotate injection sites within same region to reduce risk of lipodystrophy.

• **Alert:** Warn patient not to share multidose pen with other people, even if the needle is changed, because of risk of bloodborne pathogen transmission, including HIV and hepatitis.

• Teach patient to store insulin products properly, depending on individual products, and to use only if solution appears clear and colorless.

• Explain importance of checking insulin label before each injection as accidental mix-ups among insulin types have been reported.

• Explain that long-acting insulins shouldn't be diluted or mixed with other insulins or drugs.

• Teach patient that alcohol may affect glucose levels and should be avoided.

• Inform patient that any insulin change should be made cautiously and only under medical supervision. Changes in insulin strength, manufacturer, type (regular, NPH, or insulin analogs), species (animal, human), or method of manufacture (rDNA versus animal-source insulin) may result

in the need for a dosage change. Dosage of concomitant oral antidiabetic agents may need adjustment.

• Instruct patient not to stop insulin abruptly or change amount injected without consulting prescriber.

• Warn female patient to contact prescriber if she is pregnant or plans to become pregnant.

• Advise pregnant patient of the change in insulin requirements that may occur during pregnancy and after childbirth.

SAFETY ALERT!

Insulins (rapid-acting)
IN-su-lins

insulin aspart (rDNA origin) injection
NovoLog, NovoRapid ✦

insulin glulisine (rDNA origin) injection
Apidra, Apidra SoloStar

insulin (human)
Afrezza

insulin (lispro)
Humalog

Therapeutic class: Antidiabetics
Pharmacologic class: Insulins

AVAILABLE FORMS
Inhalation powder (Afrezza): 4-unit, 8-unit, 12-unit single-use cartridges
Injection (aspart): 10-ml vials, 3-ml prefilled pens and cartridges
Injection (glulisine): 10-ml vials, 3-ml prefilled pens
Injection (lispro): 10-ml vials, 3-ml prefilled pens and cartridges

INDICATIONS & DOSAGES
Adjust-a-dose (for all indications): Individualize dosage based on metabolic needs, blood glucose monitoring, and glycemic control goal. Insulin requirements may be altered during acute illness, emotional distress, or stress. Adjust as needed in patients who are elderly, have renal or hepatic dysfunction,

or have changes in physical activity or meal patterns, and in those who are concurrently taking drugs that lower blood glucose level. Refer to manufacturer's instructions for dosage adjustments when converting from other insulin regimens or formulations. Obese patients may need a maintenance dose up to 1.2 units/kg/day. During puberty, insulin requirements may substantially increase to 1 to 2 units/kg/day.

➤ **To improve glycemic control in patients with diabetes mellitus (aspart, glulisine, lispro)**
Adults: For insulin aspart, initially, 0.2 to 0.6 unit/kg/day in divided doses subcutaneously immediately (5 to 10 minutes) before a meal. Usual maintenance dose is 0.5 to 1 unit/kg/day subcutaneously in divided doses. When continuous subcutaneous infusion pump is used, approximately 50% of total dose is given as meal-related boluses and the remainder as a basal infusion. Usual I.V. concentration is 0.05 to 1 unit/mL in NSS infused under close medical supervision.

For insulin glulisine, usual maintenance dose is 0.5 to 1 unit/kg/day subcutaneously in divided doses within 15 minutes before a meal or 20 minutes after starting a meal. When continuous subcutaneous infusion pump is used, base initial dosing on total daily insulin dose of the previous regimen. Usual I.V. concentration is 0.05 to 1 unit/mL in NSS infused under close medical supervision.

For lispro, usual maintenance dose is 0.5 to 1 unit/kg/day subcutaneously in divided doses within 15 minutes before a meal or immediately after a meal. When continuous subcutaneous infusion pump is used, approximately 50% of total dose is usually given as meal-related boluses and the remainder as a basal infusion. Usual I.V. concentration is 0.1 to 1 unit/mL in NSS infused under close medical supervision.
Children age 2 and older with type 1 diabetes mellitus (aspart): Initially, 0.2 to 0.4 unit/kg/day in divided doses subcutaneously 5 to 10 minutes before a meal. Usual maintenance dose is 0.5 to 1 unit/kg/day subcutaneously in divided doses.

Children age 4 and older with type 1 diabetes (glulisine): Usual maintenance dose is 0.5 to 1 unit/kg/day subcutaneously in divided doses within 15 minutes before a meal or 20 minutes after starting a meal.
Children age 3 and older with type 1 diabetes (lispro): Usual maintenance dose is 0.5 to 1 unit/kg/day subcutaneously in divided doses within 15 minutes before a meal or immediately after a meal.

➤ **To improve glycemic control in patients with diabetes mellitus (inhalation)**
Adults: For insulin-naive patients, initially 4 units inhaled at beginning of each meal. To convert to inhaled insulin from subcutaneous mealtime insulin, determine appropriate dose for each meal as follows: If using injected insulin up to 4 units, use 4 units of inhaled insulin; if injected insulin is 5 to 8 units, use 8 units of inhaled insulin; if injected insulin is 9 to 12 units, use 12 units inhaled insulin; if injected insulin is 13 to 16 units, use 16 units inhaled insulin; if injected insulin is 17 to 20 units, use 20 units inhaled insulin; if injected insulin is 21 to 24 units, use 24 units inhaled insulin. For patients using subcutaneous premixed insulin, estimate mealtime injected dose by dividing half of total daily injected premixed insulin dose equally among the three meals of the day; then convert each estimated injected mealtime dose to an appropriate inhaled dose as listed above. Administer half of total daily injected premixed dose as an injected basal insulin dose.

ADMINISTRATION
General
● Rapid-acting insulins are usually given in a regimen that includes an intermediate-acting or a long-acting insulin.
● Don't use if solution is viscous or cloudy; use only if clear and colorless.
♦ *Alert:* Multidose pens are for single patient use only. Pens should never be shared even if the needle is changed. Clearly label with patient identifying information where it won't obstruct dosing window, warning, or other product information.
● Store unopened insulin aspart vials, cartridges, and pens under refrigeration (36° to 46° F [2° to 8° C]) until expiration date or at room temperature of less than

---

Reactions in bold italics are *life-threatening*. Interactions may have a *rapid onset* or a ***delayed onset***.

86° F (30° C) for 28 days; don't freeze. Keep away from heat and sunlight. Once opened, vials may be stored under refrigeration or at room temperature of less than 86° F (30° C); use within 28 days. Cartridges and pens that have been opened should be stored at temperatures less than 86° F (30° C) and used within 28 days; don't freeze or refrigerate.

• Store insulin glulisine under refrigeration at 36° to 46° F (2° to 8° C) and protect from light. Don't store in freezer. Don't allow insulin glulisine to freeze; discard if it has been frozen. Unopened vials and cartridge systems not stored in refrigerator must be used within 28 days. Opened vials, whether or not refrigerated, must be used within 28 days. If refrigeration isn't possible, open vials can be kept at room temperature of less than 77° F (25° C) for up to 28 days away from direct heat and light. Don't refrigerate opened cartridge system, but keep below 77° F (25° C) and away from direct heat and light. Opened cartridge systems must be discarded after 28 days. Don't store pen, with or without cartridge system, in refrigerator at any time.

• Store lispro in refrigerator (36° to 46° F [2° to 8° C]), but not in freezer. Protect from direct heat and light. Don't use if frozen. Store unopened vials and pens in refrigerator until expiration date; if stored unopened at room temperature, discard after 28 days. If opened, vials can be stored for 28 days under refrigeration or at room temperature; opened pens and cartridges should be stored for 28 days at room temperature. Discard if exposed to temperatures greater than 98.6° F (37° C).

• **Incompatibilities:** Don't mix with any other insulin except NPH.

I.V.

▼ Rapid-acting insulin may be administered I.V. with close monitoring of blood glucose and serum potassium levels under appropriate medical supervision.

▼ Flush I.V. tubing with priming infusion of 20 mL from insulin infusion whenever new I.V. tubing set is added to insulin infusion container, to avoid adsorption to I.V. tubing.

▼ Use NSS and polyvinyl chloride or polypropylene infusion bags for I.V. infusions.

▼ Always administer I.V. infusions using an infusion pump.

Subcutaneous

• Administer by subcutaneous injection in abdominal region, buttocks, thigh, or upper arm. Subcutaneous injection into abdominal wall is generally associated with faster absorption than other injection sites.

• Rotate injection sites within same region to reduce risk of lipodystrophy.

• Injection into a lifted skin fold minimizes risk of I.M. injection.

• When used for continuous subcutaneous insulin infusion, insulin aspart contained within an external insulin pump reservoir should be replaced at least every 6 days and infusion sets and insertion sites should be changed at least every 3 days. Discard if exposed to temperatures greater than 98.6° F (37° C).

• NovoLog may be diluted with Insulin Diluting Medium for NovoLog for subcutaneous injection. Diluting one part NovoLog to nine parts diluent will yield a concentration one-tenth that of NovoLog (equivalent to U-10). Diluting one part NovoLog to one part diluent will yield a concentration one-half that of NovoLog (equivalent to U-50).

• When using for continuous subcutaneous insulin infusion, change insulin glulisine in reservoir and infusion set (reservoirs, tubing, and catheters) every 48 hours or after exposure to temperatures greater than 98.6° F (37° C).

• When using for continuous subcutaneous insulin infusion, change lispro in reservoir every 7 days, and change infusion sets every 3 days.

• Don't use mixed insulins in external insulin pumps.

Inhalational

• Administer using a single inhalation per cartridge using Afrezza inhaler only. Inhaler can be used for both 4-unit and 8-unit cartridges.

• Administer at beginning of a meal.

• Keep inhaler level, with white mouthpiece on top and purple base on bottom, after a cartridge has been inserted into inhaler.

- Loss of drug effect can occur if inhaler is turned upside down, held with mouthpiece pointing down, or shaken or dropped after the cartridge has been inserted but before dose has been administered. If any of these occur, replace cartridge before use.
- May mix and match between 4-unit (blue) and 8-unit (green) cartridges to obtain correct dose.
- Store unused foil packages of inhalation powder until expiration date under refrigeration (36° to 46° F [2° to 8° C]) or if at room temperature, use within 10 days. If in use, unopened blister cards and strips must be used within 10 days and opened strips must be used within 3 days.
- Inhaler can be refrigerated but should be at room temperature before use. Cartridges should be at room temperature for 10 minutes before use.
- Replace inhaler after 15 days of use.

ACTION

Lowers blood glucose level by stimulating peripheral glucose uptake by binding to insulin receptors on skeletal muscle and in fat cells and by inhibiting hepatic glucose production; also inhibits lipolysis and proteolysis, and enhances protein synthesis.

Route	Onset	Peak	Duration
Aspart (I.V.)	Immediate	Unknown	3–5 hr
Aspart (Subcut.)	15 min	1–3 hr	3–5 hr
Glulisine (I.V.)	Immediate	Unknown	5 hr
Glulisine (Subcut.)	15 min	1 hr	5 hr
Lispro (I.V.)	Immediate	Unknown	Unknown
Lispro (Subcut.)	15 min	30–90 min	3–5 hr
Inhalation	Unknown	12–15 min	180 min

Half-life: Aspart I.V., unknown; aspart subcut., 81 minutes; glulisine I.V., 13 minutes; glulisine subcut., 42 minutes; lispro I.V., 26 minutes; lispro subcut., 1 hour; inhalation, 28 to 39 minutes.

ADVERSE REACTIONS

CNS: headache, *seizures,* asthenia, fever, fatigue (inhalation), sensory disturbance.
CV: hypertension, peripheral edema.
EENT: nasopharyngitis.
GI: nausea, diarrhea.
GU: UTI, dysmenorrhea.

Metabolic: *hypoglycemia, hypokalemia,* weight gain.
Musculoskeletal: myalgia.
Respiratory: URI, cough; bronchospasm, throat pain or irritation, bronchitis, decreased pulmonary function (inhaled product).
Skin: injection- or infusion-site reactions, lipodystrophy, pruritus, rash.
Other: *allergic reactions, anaphylaxis,* insulin antibody production, flulike symptoms.

INTERACTIONS

Drug-drug. *ACE inhibitors, antidiabetic agents (oral), ARBs, disopyramide, fibrates, fluoxetine,* **MAO inhibitors,** *octreotide, pentoxifylline, pramlintide, salicylates, sulfonamide antibiotics:* May increase risk of hypoglycemia. Monitor glucose level closely and adjust insulin dosage as needed.
Atypical antipsychotics, corticosteroids, danazol, diuretics, estrogens, glucagon, hormonal contraceptives, isoniazid, niacin, phenothiazines, protease inhibitors, somatropin, sympathomimetics (albuterol, epinephrine, terbutaline), thyroid hormones: May decrease blood glucose–lowering effects. Monitor glucose level closely and adjust insulin dosage as needed.
Beta blockers, clonidine, guanethidine, reserpine: May mask signs and symptoms of hypoglycemia. Avoid concurrent use, if possible, or monitor patient closely.
Beta blockers, clonidine, lithium salts, pentamidine: May cause hypoglycemia or hyperglycemia. Monitor glucose level closely.
Thiazolidinediones (TZDs; pioglitazone, rosiglitazone): May cause fluid retention that can lead to HF. Monitor patient closely and adjust or stop TZDs as clinically indicated.
Drug-lifestyle. *Alcohol use:* May cause hyperglycemia or hypoglycemia. Monitor glucose level closely and discourage concurrent use.

EFFECTS ON LAB TEST RESULTS

- May decrease glucose and potassium levels.

Reactions in bold italics are *life-threatening.* Interactions may have a *rapid onset* or a *delayed onset.*

CONTRAINDICATIONS & CAUTIONS

Black Box Warning Inhaled insulin is contraindicated in patients with chronic lung disease, such as asthma or COPD, as acute bronchospasm has been observed in these patients. ■

• Contraindicated during episodes of hypoglycemia.

• Contraindicated in patients with a history of hypersensitivity to drug or its components. Severe, life-threatening, generalized allergic reaction, including anaphylaxis, can occur with insulin products.

• Inhaled insulin is contraindicated in patients with active lung cancer. Use cautiously in those with a history of lung cancer or who are at risk for lung cancer, considering risks and benefits of therapy.

• Inhaled insulin may increase risk of diabetic ketoacidosis (DKA). Closely monitor patients at risk for DKA. Change to an alternative route of insulin delivery if needed.

• Inhaled insulin isn't recommended in patients who smoke.

• Use cautiously in patients susceptible to hypokalemia, such as patients who are fasting, are taking potassium-lowering drugs, or are concurrently taking drugs that may affect potassium levels. Untreated hypokalemia can cause respiratory paralysis, ventricular arrhythmias, and death.

• Hypoglycemia is the most common adverse reaction. Severe hypoglycemia can cause seizures, and may be life-threatening or fatal. Hypoglycemia can occur suddenly, and symptoms may differ. Risk increases with intensity of glycemic control and changes in glycemic treatment, meal patterns, physical activity, and concomitant medications and in patients with renal or hepatic impairment.

• Use cautiously in elderly patients, who may be at increased risk for adverse effects. Signs and symptoms of hypoglycemia may be more difficult to recognize in these patients.

Dialyzable drug: Unknown.

⚠ *Overdose S&S:* Hypoglycemia, hypokalemia.

PREGNANCY-LACTATION-REPRODUCTION

• There are no adequate studies in pregnant women. Don't use during pregnancy unless potential benefit justifies risk to the fetus.

• Monitor blood glucose levels closely in pregnant patients, in women who have recently given birth, and in breast-feeding women; insulin requirements may change.

• It isn't known if insulin appears in breast milk. Refer to manufacturer's instructions for use in breast-feeding women.

NURSING CONSIDERATIONS

Black Box Warning Before initiating inhaled insulin, perform a detailed medical history, physical examination, and spirometry (forced expiratory volume in 1 second [FEV_1]) to identify potential lung disease in all patients. ■

• Assess pulmonary function (spirometry) before initiating inhalation product, after 6 months of therapy, and annually, even in the absence of pulmonary symptoms.

• Increase frequency of pulmonary assessment in patients with such symptoms as wheezing, bronchospasm, breathing difficulties, or persistent or recurring cough. Discontinue drug for persistent symptoms and consider stopping drug for decline of 20% or more in FEV_1 from baseline.

• Monitor blood glucose level and adjust insulin dosage as needed.

• Closely monitor patients also taking other medications as other drugs can mask signs and symptoms of hypoglycemia or cause an increase or decrease in blood glucose level.

• Increase frequency of glucose monitoring in patients who are acutely ill or under emotional stress, or if changes in diet, exercise, or medication regimen occur, because these may affect rate of insulin absorption.

• Closely monitor patients at risk for DKA from acute illness or infection; consider changing from inhaled product to alternative route of insulin delivery.

• Increase frequency of glucose monitoring when initiating therapy or when changes in insulin strength, dosage, manufacturer, or type or method of administration are made. Changes may affect glycemic control and increase risk of hypoglycemia.

• Monitor patient carefully for signs and symptoms of hypoglycemia. Symptom awareness may be decreased in patients with long-standing diabetes, diabetic nerve disease, renal disease, or hepatic impairment and in patients who have experienced recurrent hypoglycemia. Treat according to individual facility policy if necessary.

• Mild episodes of hypoglycemia may be treated with oral glucose. More severe episodes of hypoglycemia, such as coma, seizure, or neurologic impairment, may be treated with I.M. or subcutaneous glucagon or concentrated I.V. glucose.

• Monitor potassium levels in patients at risk for hypokalemia (those receiving potassium-depleting drugs or I.V. insulin).

• Monitor patients for generalized allergic reactions, including anaphylaxis.

• Assess patients and notify prescriber for signs or symptoms of hypoglycemia (sweating, shaking, trembling, confusion) and hyperglycemia (drowsiness, fruity breath odor, frequent urination, thirst).

• Periodically measure HbA_{1c} levels.

• Observe for signs and symptoms of HF with concomitant use of TZDs; consider dosage reduction or discontinuation of TZD if HF occurs.

• Monitor external pump for malfunction as this may cause a rapid decline in blood glucose level.

• *Look alike–sound alike:* Don't confuse NovoLog with Novolog 70/30. Don't confuse Humalog with Humalog 50/50 or 75/25. Don't confuse insulin glulisine with insulin glargine.

PATIENT TEACHING
General
• Advise patient that hypoglycemic episodes can impair the ability to concentrate and react; advise patient to use caution while driving and operating machinery.

• Instruct patient to keep hard candy or glucose tablets on hand to treat mild cases of hypoglycemia.

• Advise patient to keep a log of his glucose levels.

• Instruct patient on the long-term sequelae of diabetes if not managed properly.

• Instruct patient to carry identification or wear jewelry indicating that he has diabetes.

• Advise patient that allergic and hypersensitivity reactions can occur, including injection-site reactions (local pain, redness or swelling), and to report symptoms to health care provider. Teach patient signs and symptoms of anaphylaxis and to seek emergency medical attention promptly if anaphylaxis occurs.

• Instruct patient on self-management procedures, including glucose monitoring, proper administration technique, and management of hypoglycemia and hyperglycemia.

• Warn patient that insulin requirements may vary due to illness, stress, emotional disturbances, inadequate or skipped insulin dose, inadvertent administration of an increased insulin dose, inadequate food intake, or skipped meals.

❶ *Alert:* Warn patient not to share multidose pen with other people, even if the needle is changed, because of risk of bloodborne pathogen transmission, including HIV and hepatitis.

• Advise woman with diabetes to inform physician if she is pregnant or plans to become pregnant.

• Advise pregnant women of change in insulin requirements that may occur during pregnancy and after childbirth.

• Teach patient that alcohol and some other medications may increase or decrease glucose levels. Advise patient to inform health care provider of all medications and supplements he is taking.

• Caution patient not to stop insulin abruptly or change amount taken without consulting prescriber.

• Advise patient that any change of insulin should be made cautiously and only under medical supervision. Changes in insulin strength, manufacturer, type (regular, NPH, or insulin analogs), species (animal, human), or method of manufacture (rDNA versus animal-source insulin) may result in need for a dosage change. Dosage of concomitant oral antidiabetic agents may need adjustment.

Injection
• Teach patient to give insulin at appropriate time around a meal, depending on product.

• Instruct patient to rotate injection sites and of the importance of avoiding lipodystrophy.

• Instruct patient that when mixing two types of insulin, always draw up the shorter-acting insulin first, followed by NPH insulin, and inject immediately.

- Teach patient how to use external insulin pumps properly, to use the appropriate insulin in the pump, not to dilute it or mix it with other insulin formulations, to change the infusion set every 3 days, to rotate infusion sites, and to follow instructions for patient's specific type of pump.
- Teach patient to store insulin products properly, depending on individual products.
- Explain importance of checking insulin label before each injection as accidental mix-ups among insulin types have been reported.
- Instruct patient not to share pens with others, even if needles are changed.

Inhalation

- Instruct patient to read inhaler's medication guide before starting inhalation therapy and to reread it each time the prescription is renewed.
- Caution patient not to open cartridges, place cartridges in mouth, or swallow cartridges.
- Inform patient that inhaled insulin can cause a decline in lung function and that lung function will be evaluated by spirometry before initiation of treatment and periodically during treatment.
- Instruct patient to promptly report respiratory difficulty or signs or symptoms of lung cancer (hemoptysis, cough).
- Inform patient that if inhaled product isn't being used, it should be stored in refrigerator. If inhaler is being used, tell patient to leave it at room temperature and use unopened strips within 10 days and opened strips within 3 days.
- Instruct patient never to wash inhaler but to wipe it with a clean, dry cloth.
- Advise patient that inhalers should be discarded and replaced every 15 days.

SAFETY ALERT!

Insulins (short-acting)

IN-su-lins

insulin (regular)

Humulin R ◇, Humulin R U-500 (concentrated), Humulin R U-500 KwikPen, Novolin R ◇

Therapeutic class: Antidiabetics
Pharmacologic class: Insulins

AVAILABLE FORMS

Injection: 100 units/mL in 3- and 10-mL vials; 500 units/mL in 3-mL pen and 20-mL vial

INDICATIONS & DOSAGES

Adjust-a-dose (for all indications): Individualize dosage based on metabolic needs, blood glucose monitoring, and glycemic control. Insulin requirements may be altered during acute illness, emotional distress, or stress. Adjust dosage as needed in patients who are elderly, have renal or hepatic dysfunction, or have changes in physical activity or meal patterns, and in those who are concurrently taking drugs that lower blood glucose level. Dosage may also need adjustment when switching from another insulin formulation, manufacturer, or strength. I.V. administration of regular insulin is possible under medical supervision with close monitoring of blood glucose and potassium levels to avoid hypoglycemia and hypokalemia. I.V. administration of insulin is commonly used in the treatment of diabetic ketoacidosis, perioperative management of diabetes, and maintenance of glycemic control during labor in pregnant women with diabetes.

➤ **As adjunct to diet and exercise to improve glycemic control in patients with type 1 and type 2 diabetes mellitus**
Adults and children: Initially, 0.2 to 0.4 unit/kg/day subcutaneously divided into three or more doses. Dosage may be increased to maintenance dose of 0.5 to 1 unit/kg/day subcutaneously divided into three or more doses as needed. In patients with insulin resistance, daily insulin requirement may be more than 200 units daily.

❸ *Alert:* U-500 concentrate is used for the treatment of insulin-resistant patients with diabetes who require daily doses of more than 200 units because a large dose may be given subcutaneously in a reasonable volume. Don't give U-500 concentrated insulin I.V. or I.M.

ADMINISTRATION
General
● Store unopened vials and pens in refrigerator at 36° to 46° F (2° to 8° C). Don't freeze and don't use if vial has been frozen.
❸ *Alert:* Multidose pens are for single patient use only. Pens should never be shared even if the needle is changed. Clearly label with patient identifying information where it won't obstruct dosing window, warning, or other product information.
● Novolin R vials can be kept at room temperature (not greater than 77° F [25° C]), away from heat or light, for up to 42 days; don't refrigerate after first use. Discard after 42 days even if vial is unopened or isn't empty.
● Opened (in use) Humulin R vials can be kept at room temperature (not greater than 86° F [30° C]), away from heat or light, for up to 31 days. Discard after 31 days even if vial is unopened or isn't empty.
● Opened and unopened Humulin R U-500 vials can be kept at room temperature, below 86° F (30° C); discard after 40 days. Also discard opened refrigerated vials after 40 days.
● Opened and unopened Humulin R U-500 pens can be kept at room temperature, below 86° F (30° C); discard after 28 days. Don't store opened pens in refrigerator.

I.V.
▼ Don't use if solution is viscous or cloudy; use only if clear and colorless.
▼ I.V. administration requires close monitoring of blood glucose and serum potassium levels. Appropriate medical supervision is required.
▼ Onset of action when administered I.V. is more rapid in comparison to subcutaneous administration.
▼ Use of regular insulin in insulin pumps isn't recommended because of risk of precipitation.

▼ For I.V. use, Humulin R U-100 should be used at a concentration of 0.1 to 1 unit/mL in NSS using polyvinyl chloride infusion bags. Novolin R should be used at concentrations of 0.05 to 1 unit/mL in infusion systems using polypropylene infusion bags and one of the following infusion solutions: NSS, 5% dextrose, or 10% dextrose with potassium chloride 40 mmol/L.
▼ Always administer I.V. infusions using an infusion pump.
▼ Infusion bags prepared with Humulin R are stable when stored in refrigerator for 48 hours at 36° to 46° F (2° to 8° C) and may be used at room temperature for up to an additional 48 hours.
▼ Infusion bags prepared with Novolin R are stable at room temperature for 24 hours.
▼ **Incompatibilities:** Don't mix regular insulin with any other insulin except NPH; don't mix regular concentrated insulin with any other insulin.

Subcutaneous
● Regular insulin administered by subcutaneous injection should generally be used in regimens that include an intermediate- or long-acting insulin. It may also be used in combination with oral antidiabetic agents.
● Subcutaneous injection should be followed by a meal within 30 minutes of administration.
● Administer by subcutaneous injection in abdominal region, buttocks, thigh, or upper arm. Subcutaneous injection into abdominal wall is generally associated with faster absorption than other injection sites.
● Injection sites should be rotated within same region to reduce risk of lipodystrophy.
● Injection into a lifted skin fold minimizes risk of I.M. injection.
● Don't perform dose conversion when using the Humulin R U-500 KwikPen. The dose window of the pen shows the number of units of Humulin R U-500 to be injected and no dose conversion is required.
● Don't transfer Humulin R U-500 from the pen into a syringe for administration because overdose and severe hypoglycemia can occur.
● Don't use if solution is viscous or cloudy; use only if clear and colorless.

ACTION

Lowers blood glucose level by stimulating peripheral glucose uptake by binding to insulin receptors on skeletal muscle and in fat cells and by inhibiting hepatic glucose production; also inhibits lipolysis and proteolysis, and enhances protein synthesis.

Route	Onset	Peak	Duration
I.V.	10–15 min	Unknown	4 hr
U-100 (Subcut.)	30 min	1½–3½ hr	8 hr
U-500 (Subcut.)	30 min	3 hr	24 hr

Half-life: Unknown.

ADVERSE REACTIONS

CV: peripheral edema.
Metabolic: *hypoglycemia, hypokalemia,* weight gain.
Skin: injection-site reactions, lipodystrophy.
Other: allergic reactions, *anaphylaxis,* insulin antibody production.

INTERACTIONS

Drug-drug. *ACE inhibitors, antidiabetic agents (oral), ARBs, disopyramide, fibrates, fluoxetine,* **MAO inhibitors,** *salicylates, sulfonamide antibiotics, octreotide, pentoxifylline, pramlintide:* May cause hypoglycemia. Monitor glucose level and adjust insulin dosage as needed.
Atypical antipsychotics, corticosteroids, danazol, diuretics, estrogens, glucagon, hormonal contraceptives, isoniazid, niacin, phenothiazines, protease inhibitors, somatropin, sympathomimetics (albuterol, epinephrine, terbutaline), thyroid hormones: May cause hyperglycemia. Monitor glucose level and adjust insulin dosage as needed.
Beta blockers, clonidine, guanethidine, reserpine: May mask signs and symptoms of hypoglycemia. Avoid concurrent use, if possible, or monitor patient closely.
Beta blockers, clonidine, lithium salts, **pentamidine:** May cause hypoglycemia or hyperglycemia. Monitor glucose level.
Thiazolidinediones (TZDs; pioglitazone, rosiglitazone): May cause fluid retention that can lead to HF. Monitor patient closely, and adjust or stop TZD as clinically necessary.

Drug-lifestyle. *Alcohol use:* May cause hyperglycemia or hypoglycemia. Monitor glucose level closely and discourage concurrent use.

EFFECTS ON LAB TEST RESULTS

● May decrease glucose and potassium levels.
● May develop antibodies that react with human insulin.

CONTRAINDICATIONS & CAUTIONS

● Contraindicated during episodes of hypoglycemia.
● Contraindicated in patients with a history of hypersensitivity to drug or its components. Severe, life-threatening, generalized allergic reactions, including anaphylaxis, can occur with insulin products.
● Use cautiously in patients susceptible to hypokalemia, such as patients who are fasting, are taking potassium-lowering drugs, or are concurrently taking drugs that may affect potassium level. Untreated hypokalemia can cause respiratory paralysis, ventricular arrhythmias, and death.
● Hypoglycemia is the most common adverse reaction. Severe hypoglycemia can cause seizures, and may be life-threatening or fatal. Hypoglycemia can occur suddenly, and symptoms may differ. Risk increases with intensity of glycemic control and changes in glycemic treatment, meal patterns, physical activity, and concomitant medications and in patients with renal or hepatic impairment.
● Use cautiously in elderly patients, who may be at increased risk for adverse effects. Signs and symptoms of hypoglycemia may be more difficult to recognize in these patients.
Dialyzable drug: Unknown.
⚠ **Overdose S&S:** Hypoglycemia, hypokalemia.

PREGNANCY-LACTATION-REPRODUCTION

● Use cautiously in pregnant women.
● Monitor blood glucose levels closely in pregnant women, in women who have recently given birth, and in breast-feeding women; insulin requirements may change.

● It isn't known if insulin appears in breast milk. Use cautiously in breast-feeding women. Adjust insulin dose as needed.

NURSING CONSIDERATIONS

● Regular insulins are generally used in regimens that also include an intermediate- or long-acting insulin.

● Monitor blood glucose level and adjust insulin dosage as needed for patient-specific goals.

● Monitor patient carefully when initiating therapy. Time course of insulins varies with each patient.

● Monitor patient carefully for signs and symptoms of hypoglycemia, especially in long-standing disease. Treat according to individual facility policy if necessary.

● Mild episodes of hypoglycemia may be treated with oral glucose. More severe episodes of hypoglycemia, such as coma, seizure, or neurologic impairment, may be treated with I.M. or subcutaneous glucagon or concentrated I.V. glucose.

● Assess patient and notify prescriber for signs and symptoms of hypoglycemia (sweating, shaking, trembling, confusion) and hyperglycemia (drowsiness, fruity breath odor, frequent urination, thirst).

● Periodically measure HbA_{1c} levels.

● Monitor potassium levels in patients at risk for hypokalemia, including those taking potassium-depleting drugs.

● Increase frequency of glucose monitoring in patients who are acutely ill or under emotional stress, or if changes in diet, exercise, or medication regimen occur because these may affect the rate of insulin absorption. Also monitor patient closely after changes to insulin dosage.

● Observe for signs and symptoms of HF with concomitant use of TZDs. Consider dosage reduction or discontinuation of TZD if HF occurs.

● Monitor patients for generalized allergic reactions, including anaphylaxis.

● *Look alike–sound alike:* Don't confuse Humulin with Humalog. Don't confuse Novolin with NovoLog.

PATIENT TEACHING

● Instruct patient in self-management, including glucose management, injection technique, proper storage of insulin, and recognition and management of hypo-glycemia and hyperglycemia.

● Teach patient to eat within 30 minutes of injecting short-acting insulin.

● Instruct patient to only use syringes calibrated for their particular concentration of insulin.

🜚 *Alert:* Warn patient not to share multidose pen with other people, even if the needle is changed, because of risk of bloodborne pathogen transmission, including HIV and hepatitis.

● Teach patient to rotate injection sites and the importance of avoiding lipodystrophy.

● Instruct patient that when mixing two types of insulin, always draw up the shorter-acting insulin first, followed by NPH, and inject immediately.

● Explain importance of checking insulin label before each injection as accidental mix-ups among insulin types have been reported.

● Instruct patient to keep hard candy or glucose tablets on hand to treat mild cases of hypoglycemia.

● Caution patient that hypoglycemic episodes can impair the ability to concentrate and react; advise patient to use caution while driving and operating machinery.

● Advise patient to track his glucose levels.

● Instruct patient on long-term risks of diabetes if not managed properly.

● Instruct patient to carry identification or wear jewelry indicating that he has diabetes.

● Advise patient that allergic reactions, including injection-site reactions (local pain, redness or swelling) and generalized allergic reaction and anaphylaxis (whole-body rash, shortness of breath, wheezing, reduced BP, fast pulse, sweating), can occur. Teach patient to immediately seek emergency medical attention for generalized reactions.

● Warn patient that insulin requirements may vary due to illness, stress, emotional disturbances, inadequate or skipped insulin dose, inadvertent administration of an increased insulin dose, inadequate food intake, skipped meals or pregnancy.

● Caution patient not to stop insulin abruptly or to change amount injected without consulting prescriber.

Reactions in bold italics are *life-threatening*. Interactions may have a *rapid onset* or a *delayed onset*.

• Warn patient that any change in insulin should be made cautiously and only under medical supervision. Changes in insulin strength, manufacturer, type (regular, NPH, or insulin analogs), species (animal, human), or method of manufacture (rDNA, animal-source insulin) may result in the need for a dosage change.

• Caution patient to discuss adjustments to the administration schedule if travelling across more than two time zones.

SAFETY ALERT!

interferon alfa-2b (recombinant) (IFN-alpha 2b)
in-ter-FEER-on

Intron A

Therapeutic class: Antivirals
Pharmacologic class: Biological response modifiers

AVAILABLE FORMS
Powder for injection: 10, 18, and 50 million international units/vial with diluent
Solution for injection: 18 and 25 million international units/vial (6 and 10 million international units/mL)

INDICATIONS & DOSAGES
Adjust-a-dose (for all indications): (For all indications except condylomata acuminata, if adverse effects occur, stop drug until they abate; then resume drug at 50% of the previous dose. If intolerance persists, stop drug. See package insert for specific guidance.

➤ **Hairy cell leukemia**
Adults: 2 million international units/m² I.M. or subcutaneously three times weekly for 6 months or more if patient is responding to treatment. Give subcutaneously if platelet count is less than 50,000/mm³.

➤ **AIDS-related Kaposi sarcoma**
Adults: 30 million international units/m² subcutaneously or I.M. three times weekly. Maintain dose until disease progression or maximal response has been achieved after 16 weeks of treatment. Don't use solution for injection in vials for this indication.

➤ **Chronic HBV infection**
Adults: 30 to 35 million international units I.M. or subcutaneously weekly, given as 5 million international units daily or 10 million international units three times weekly for 16 weeks.
Children ages 1 to 17: 3 million international units/m² subcutaneously three times weekly for first week; then increase to 6 million international units/m² subcutaneously three times weekly (maximum is 10 million international units three times weekly) for total of 16 to 24 weeks.
Adjust-a-dose: If WBC count is less than 1.5×10^9/L, granulocyte count is less than 0.75×10^9/L, or platelet count is less than 50×10^9/L, reduce dose by 50%. Permanently discontinue drug if WBC count is less than 1×10^9/L, granulocyte count is less than 0.5×10^9/L, or platelet count is less than 25×10^9/L.

➤ **Chronic HCV infection**
Adults: 3 million international units I.M. or subcutaneously three times weekly. In patients tolerating therapy with normalization of ALT at 16 weeks of therapy, continue for 18 to 24 months. In patients who haven't normalized the ALT, consider stopping therapy.

➤ **Adjunct to surgical treatment in patients with malignant melanoma who are asymptomatic after surgery but at high risk for systemic recurrence for up to 8 weeks after surgery**
Adults: Initially, 20 million international units/m² by I.V. infusion over 20 minutes 5 consecutive days weekly for 4 weeks; then maintenance dose of 10 million international units/m² subcutaneously three times weekly for 48 weeks. Solution for injection in vials isn't recommended for I.V. administration and shouldn't be used for the induction phase.

➤ **First treatment of clinically aggressive follicular non-Hodgkin lymphoma with chemotherapy containing anthracycline**
Adults: 5 million international units subcutaneously three times weekly for up to 18 months.
Adjust-a-dose: For neutrophil count of more than 1,000/mm³ but less than 1,500/mm³, decrease dosage by 50%. May resume starting dose if neutrophil count returns to more

than 1,500/mm^3. Withhold drug if neutrophil count is less than 1,000/mm^3 or platelet count is less than 50,000/mm^3.

➤ **Condylomata acuminata (genital or venereal warts)**

Adults: 1 million international units for each lesion (maximum five lesions in a single course) intralesionally three times weekly for 3 weeks. Additional course may be given at 12 to 16 weeks. Don't use the 18-million or 50-million international units powder for injection or the 18-million international units multidose solution for injection for this indication.

ADMINISTRATION
I.V.
▼ Prepare infusion solution immediately before use.

▼ Based on desired dose, reconstitute appropriate vial strength of drug with diluent provided. Withdraw dose and inject into a 100-mL bag of NSS. Final yield of drug shouldn't be less than 10 million international units/100 mL.

▼ Infuse over 20 minutes.

▼ Store solution in refrigerator. Store powder before and after reconstitution in refrigerator. Use within 24 hours.

▼ **Incompatibilities:** Dextrose solutions.
I.M.
● Carefully monitor injection sites in patient with thrombocytopenia. Avoid I.M. injections if possible.

● In patients whose platelet count is below 50,000/mm^3, give subcutaneously.

● Give drug at bedtime to minimize daytime drowsiness.
Subcutaneous
● For condylomata acuminata intralesional injection, use only 10 million-international unit vial because dilution of other strengths for intralesional use results in a hypertonic solution.

● Don't reconstitute drug in 10 million-international unit vial with more than 1 mL of diluent.

● Use tuberculin or similar syringe and 25G to 30G needle.

● Don't inject too deep beneath lesion or too superficially. As many as five lesions can be treated at one time.

● To ease discomfort, give in evening with acetaminophen.

ACTION
Unknown. May inhibit tumor or viral cell replication and modulate host immune response by enhancing macrophage activity and improving specific lymphocytes' cytotoxicity for target cells.

Route	Onset	Peak	Duration
I.V.	Unknown	15–60 min	4 hr
I.M., subcut.	Unknown	3–12 hr	16 hr

Half-life: I.V., 2 hours; I.M., 2 to 3 hours.

ADVERSE REACTIONS
CNS: apathy, amnesia, asthenia, depression, difficulty in thinking or concentrating, dizziness, fatigue, insomnia, paresthesia, somnolence, anxiety, lethargy, nervousness, weakness, headache, rigors.

CV: chest pain, *cyanosis,* edema, hypotension.

EENT: conjunctivitis, earache, rhinorrhea, sinusitis, pharyngitis, rhinitis.

GI: anorexia, diarrhea, dry mouth, dyspepsia, nausea, vomiting, abdominal pain, constipation, esophagitis, flatulence, stomatitis.

GU: decreased libido, impotence, amenorrhea.

Hematologic: *leukopenia, thrombocytopenia, anemia, neutropenia.*

Hepatic: *hepatitis.*

Metabolic: weight loss.

Respiratory: coughing, dyspnea.

Skin: alopecia, dryness, increased diaphoresis, pruritus, rash, dermatitis.

Other: flulike syndrome, injection-site reaction.

INTERACTIONS
Drug-drug. *Aldesleukin, telbivudine:* May enhance adverse or toxic effects of these drugs. Avoid use together.

Aminophylline, theophylline: May reduce theophylline clearance. Monitor theophylline level.

CNS depressants: May increase CNS effects. Avoid using together.

Ribavirin: May enhance adverse effects, including hemolytic anemia. Monitor therapy.

Reactions in bold italics are *life-threatening*. Interactions may have a *rapid onset* or a *delayed onset*.

Zidovudine: May cause synergistic adverse effects (higher risk of neutropenia). Carefully monitor WBC count.

EFFECTS ON LAB TEST RESULTS
• May increase calcium, phosphate, AST, ALT, LDH, alkaline phosphatase, triglyceride, and fasting glucose levels. May decrease Hb level.
• May increase INR and prolong PT and PTT.
• May decrease WBC and platelet counts.
• May increase or decrease TSH level.

CONTRAINDICATIONS & CAUTIONS
• Contraindicated in patients hypersensitive to drug or its components and in those with autoimmune hepatitis or decompensated liver disease.
• Use cautiously in elderly patients and in those with history of CV disease, pulmonary disease, diabetes mellitus, coagulation disorders, renal impairment, and severe myelosuppression.
• Depression, psychosis, and suicidal behavior have been linked to drug use; patients with psychotic disorders, especially depression, shouldn't continue drug treatment.
❸ *Alert:* Neurotoxicity and cardiotoxicity are more common in elderly patients, especially those with underlying CNS or cardiac impairment.
Dialyzable drug: No.
⚠ *Overdose S&S:* Abnormal liver enzyme levels, renal failure, hemorrhage, MI.

PREGNANCY-LACTATION-REPRODUCTION
• There are no adequate studies in pregnant women. Use during pregnancy only if potential benefit justifies potential risk to the fetus.
❸ *Alert:* Combination therapy with ribavirin is contraindicated in pregnant women and in men whose female partners are pregnant.
❸ *Alert:* Because of fetal risk, warn women of childbearing potential and male patients with partners of childbearing potential who are receiving combination therapy with ribavirin to use two forms of contraception.
• It isn't known if drug appears in breast milk. Patient should discontinue breast-feeding or discontinue drug.

NURSING CONSIDERATIONS
Black Box Warning Alpha interferons cause or aggravate fatal or life-threatening neuropsychiatric, autoimmune, ischemic, and infectious disorders. Monitor patients closely with periodic clinical and laboratory evaluations. Withdraw patients with persistently severe or worsening signs or symptoms of these conditions from therapy. ∎
❸ *Alert:* Not all dosage forms are appropriate for all indications. Refer to manufacturer's instructions for approved indications before use.
• Powder for injection doesn't contain a preservative. Discard vial after reconstitution and withdrawal of a single dose; don't reenter vial.
• Ensure patient is well hydrated, especially at beginning of treatment.
• At start of treatment, monitor patient for flulike signs and symptoms, which tend to diminish with continued therapy. Premedicate patient with acetaminophen to minimize these symptoms.
• Periodically check for adverse CNS reactions, such as decreased mental status and dizziness, during therapy.
• Monitor CBC with differential, platelet count, blood chemistry and electrolyte studies, and LFTs. Monitor ECG before and during treatment if patient has cardiac disorder or advanced stages of cancer.
• For patients who develop thrombocytopenia, exercise extreme care in performing invasive procedures; inspect injection site and skin frequently for signs and symptoms of bruising; limit frequency of I.M. injections; test urine, emesis fluid, stool, and secretions for occult blood.
• Severe adverse reactions may need dosage reduction to one-half or withholding of drug until reactions subside.
• Use with blood dyscrasia-causing drugs, bone marrow suppressants, or radiation therapy may increase bone marrow suppression. Dosage reduction may be needed.
• For condylomata acuminata, maximum response usually occurs in 4 to 8 weeks. If results are not satisfactory after 12 to 16 weeks, a second course may be started. Patients with 6 to 10 condylomata may receive a second course of treatment; patients

with more than 10 condylomata may receive additional courses.

PATIENT TEACHING

• Advise patient to avoid contact with persons with viral illness; patient is at increased risk for infection during therapy.

• Advise patient that laboratory tests will be performed before and periodically during therapy.

• Teach patient proper oral hygiene during treatment because bone marrow suppressant effects of interferon may lead to microbial infection, delayed healing, and bleeding gums. Drug also may decrease saliva.

• Advise patient to check with prescriber for instructions after missing a dose.

• Stress need to follow prescriber's instructions about taking and recording temperature and how and when to take acetaminophen.

• If patient will give drug to himself, teach him how to prepare injection and to use disposable syringe. Give him information on drug stability.

• Tell patient that drug may cause temporary partial hair loss; hair should return after drug is stopped.

• Advise patient to report all adverse reactions and to immediately report neuropsychiatric symptoms (depression, mania, psychosis, suicidal ideation).

SAFETY ALERT!

interferon beta-1a
in-ter-FEER-on

Avonex, Rebif

Therapeutic class: Antivirals
Pharmacologic class: Biological response modifiers

AVAILABLE FORMS

Avonex
Lyophilized powder for injection: 30 mcg/single-use vial (6.6 million international units)
Prefilled syringe or autoinjector: 30 mcg (6 million international units)/0.5 mL

Rebif
Parenteral: 8.8 mcg (2.4 million international units)/0.2 mL, 22 mcg (6 million international units)/0.5mL, 44 mcg (12 million international units)/0.5mL in prefilled syringe or autoinjector

INDICATIONS & DOSAGES

Adjust-a-dose (for all indications): To decrease incidence and severity of flulike symptoms that may occur when initiating Avonex at a dose of 30 mcg, initiate once-weekly dosing with 7.5 mcg I.M. (week 1); then increase dose in increments of 7.5 mcg once weekly (weeks 2 to 4) up to recommended dose (30 mcg once weekly).

➤ **To slow accumulation of physical disability and decrease frequency of clinical worsening in patients with relapsing forms of MS**

Adults age 18 and older: 30 mcg Avonex I.M. once weekly. Or, initially, 4.4 or 8.8 mcg Rebif subcutaneously three times weekly for 2 weeks; then increase dose to 11 or 22 mcg three times weekly for another 2 weeks. Then increase to a maintenance dose of 22 or 44 mcg subcutaneously three times weekly.

Adjust-a-dose: For Rebif, in patients with leukopenia or elevated LFT values (ALT greater than 5 × ULN), reduce dosage until toxicity is resolved. Stop treatment if jaundice or other signs of hepatic injury occur.

➤ **First MS attack if brain MRI shows abnormalities consistent with MS**

Adults: 30 mcg Avonex I.M. once weekly.

ADMINISTRATION

Subcutaneous

• Visually inspect Rebif for particulate matter and discoloration before administration.

• Rotate sites of injection.

• Administer Rebif at same time on same 3 days at least 48 hours apart each week (late afternoon or evening on Monday, Wednesday, and Friday).

• Use only prefilled syringes for titration to 22 mcg prescribed dose of Rebif.

• Store Rebif in the refrigerator between 36° and 46° F (2° and 8° C). Don't freeze. Rebif may be stored at or below 77° F

(25° C) for up to 30 days if away from heat and light.

I.M.

• To reconstitute lyophilized Avonex, inject 1.1 mL of supplied diluent (sterile water for injection) into vial and gently swirl to dissolve drug. Don't shake.

• Use drug as soon as possible; may be used up to 6 hours after being reconstituted if stored at 36° to 46° F.

• Rotate sites of injection.

• The Avonex and diluent vials are for single use only; discard unused portions.

• Store Avonex prefilled syringes and autoinjectors in the refrigerator at 36° to 46° F. If refrigeration is unavailable, may store at 77° F for up to 7 days. Once refrigerated, syringes and autoinjectors must not be stored above 77° F. Once removed from refrigerator, warm to room temperature (about 30 minutes). Don't use external heat sources, such as hot water, to warm syringe, or expose to high temperatures. Don't freeze. Protect from light.

• After giving each dose, discard any remaining product in the syringe or autoinjector.

ACTION

Unknown. Interacts with specific cell receptors found on the surface of cells. Binding of these receptors causes the expression of a number of interferon-induced gene products believed to mediate the biological actions of interferon beta-1a.

Route	Onset	Peak	Duration
Subcut.	Unknown	16 hr	Unknown
I.M.	12 hr	6–36 hr	4 days

Half-life: Subcutaneous, 69 hours; I.M., 8 to 54 hours.

ADVERSE REACTIONS

CNS: asthenia, dizziness, fatigue, fever, headache, pain, sleep difficulty, depression, *seizures, suicidal ideation or attempt, suicidal tendency,* abnormal coordination, ataxia, hypertonia, malaise, speech disorder, syncope.

CV: chest pain, vasodilation.

EENT: abnormal vision, sinusitis, decreased hearing, otitis media.

GI: abdominal pain, diarrhea, dyspepsia, nausea, anorexia, dry mouth.

GU: increased urinary frequency, ovarian cyst, urinary incontinence, vaginitis, UTI.

Hematologic: lymphadenopathy, *leukopenia, pancytopenia, thrombocytopenia,* anemia.

Hepatic: abnormal hepatic function, *autoimmune hepatitis,* bilirubinemia, hepatic injury, *hepatitis.*

Metabolic: hyperthyroidism, hypothyroidism.

Musculoskeletal: back pain, muscle ache, skeletal pain, arthralgia, muscle spasm.

Respiratory: URI, dyspnea.

Skin: injection-site reaction, alopecia, ecchymosis at injection site, nevus, urticaria.

Other: chills, flulike syndrome, infection, hypersensitivity reactions, herpes simplex, herpes zoster, neutralizing antibodies.

INTERACTIONS

Drug-drug. *Myelosuppressive drugs:* May cause added hematologic toxicities; use cautiously together. Monitor CBC.

Theophylline derivatives (except dyphylline): Interferon beta-1a may decrease metabolism of theophylline derivative. Monitor therapy.

Drug-lifestyle. *Sun exposure:* May cause photosensitivity reactions. Advise patient to take precautions against sun exposure.

EFFECTS ON LAB TEST RESULTS

• May increase liver enzyme levels. May decrease Hb level and hematocrit. May increase or decrease thyroid function test levels.

• May increase eosinophil count. May decrease WBC and platelet counts.

CONTRAINDICATIONS & CAUTIONS

• Contraindicated in patients hypersensitive to natural or recombinant interferon beta, human albumin, or other components of drug.

• Use cautiously in patients with depression, seizure disorders, or severe cardiac conditions.

• Thrombotic microangiopathy (TMA), including thrombotic thrombocytopenic purpura and hemolytic-uremic syndrome, sometimes fatal, has been reported with

interferon beta products and may occur several weeks to years after start of therapy.
- Safety and effectiveness of drug in chronic progressive MS or in children younger than age 18 haven't been established.
Dialyzable drug: Unknown.

PREGNANCY-LACTATION-REPRODUCTION
- There are no adequate studies in pregnant women. Use during pregnancy only if potential benefit justifies potential risk to the fetus.
- It isn't known if drug appears in breast milk. Use cautiously in breast-feeding women.

NURSING CONSIDERATIONS
- Monitor patient closely for depression and suicidal ideation. It isn't known if these symptoms are related to the underlying neurologic basis of MS or to the drug.
- Monitor WBC count, platelet count, and blood chemistries, including LFTs. Rare but severe liver injury, including liver failure, may occur in patients taking Avonex.
- Monitor patient for TMA and discontinue drug if clinical signs and symptoms and laboratory findings consistent with TMA occur; manage as clinically indicated.
- Give analgesics or antipyretics to decrease flulike symptoms.

PATIENT TEACHING
- Advise patient to read medication guide that comes with drug.
- Teach patient and family member how to reconstitute drug and give Avonex I.M.
- Advise patient not to inject where skin is irritated, red, bruised, scarred, or infected.
- Caution patient not to change dosage or schedule of administration. If a dose is missed, tell him to take it as soon as he remembers. He may then resume his regular schedule. Tell patient not to take two injections within 48 hours of each other.
- Show patient how to store drug.
- Inform patient that flulike signs and symptoms (such as fever, fatigue, muscle aches, headache, chills, and joint pain) aren't uncommon at start of therapy and that analgesics/antipyretics may be prescribed on treatment days to lessen severity of flulike signs and symptoms.

- Advise patient to report depression, suicidal thoughts, or other adverse reactions.
- If pregnancy occurs, instruct patient to notify prescriber immediately.
- Instruct patient to keep syringes and needles away from children. Also, instruct him not to reuse needles or syringes and to discard them in a syringe-disposal unit.
- Advise patient to use sunscreen and avoid sun exposure while taking drug because photosensitivity may occur.
- Tell patient to store drug in the refrigerator between 36° and 46° F (2° and 8° C) and not to freeze. Drug may also be stored at or below 77° F (25° C) for up to 30 days and away from heat and light.

interferon beta-1b (recombinant)
in-ter-FEER-on

Betaseron, Extavia

Therapeutic class: Antivirals
Pharmacologic class: Biological response modifiers

AVAILABLE FORMS
Powder for injection: 9.6 million international units (0.3 mg)

INDICATIONS & DOSAGES
➤ **To reduce frequency of exacerbations in relapsing forms of MS, including patients who have experienced a first clinical episode and have MRI features consistent with MS**
Adults: 0.0625 mg subcutaneously every other day for weeks 1 and 2; then 0.125 mg subcutaneously every other day for weeks 3 and 4; then 0.1875 mg subcutaneously every other day for weeks 5 and 6; then 0.25 mg subcutaneously every other day thereafter.

ADMINISTRATION
Subcutaneous
⟳ *Alert:* The removable rubber cap of the Extavia diluent prefilled syringe contains natural rubber latex, which may cause

allergic reactions and shouldn't be handled by latex-sensitive individuals.

- To reconstitute, inject 1.2 mL of supplied diluent (half-NSS for injection) into vial and gently swirl to dissolve drug.
- Reconstituted solution contains 8 million international units (0.25 mg)/mL.
- Don't shake. Discard vial that contains particulates or discolored solution.
- Inject immediately after preparation.
- Rotate injection sites to minimize local reactions and observe site for necrosis.
- Store at room temperature. After reconstitution, if not used immediately, drug may be refrigerated for up to 3 hours.

ACTION

A naturally occurring antiviral and immunoregulatory drug derived from human fibroblasts. Drug attaches to membrane receptors and causes cellular changes, including increased protein synthesis.

Route	Onset	Peak	Duration
Subcut.	Unknown	1–8 hr	Unknown

Half-life: 8 minutes to 4¼ hours.

ADVERSE REACTIONS

CNS: depression, anxiety, emotional lability, depersonalization, *suicidal tendencies,* confusion, hypertonia, asthenia, migraine, *seizures,* headache, pain, dizziness, malaise, fever, chills, insomnia, ataxia.
CV: chest pain, peripheral edema, palpitations, hypertension, tachycardia, peripheral vascular disorder.
EENT: laryngitis, sinusitis, conjunctivitis, abnormal vision.
GI: diarrhea, constipation, abdominal pain, vomiting, dyspepsia, nausea.
GU: menstrual bleeding or spotting, early or delayed menses, fewer days of menstrual flow, menorrhagia, urgency, impotence, prostate disorder, frequency.
Hematologic: *leukopenia,* lymphadenopathy.
Musculoskeletal: myasthenia, arthralgia, myalgia, leg cramps.
Respiratory: dyspnea.
Skin: inflammation, pain, necrosis at injection site, diaphoresis, alopecia, rash, skin disorder.

Other: breast pain, flulike syndrome, pelvic pain, generalized edema.

INTERACTIONS

Theophylline derivatives (except dyphylline): May decrease metabolism of these drugs. Monitor therapy.
Zidovudine: May decrease zidovudine metabolism and enhance its adverse or toxic effects. Monitor therapy.

EFFECTS ON LAB TEST RESULTS

- May increase ALT and bilirubin levels.
- May decrease WBC and neutrophil counts.

CONTRAINDICATIONS & CAUTIONS

- Contraindicated in patients hypersensitive to interferon beta, human albumin, or components of drug.
- Drug-induced lupus erythematosus has been reported and has occurred with positive serologic testing (including positive antinuclear or anti-double-stranded DNA antibody testing).
- Thrombotic microangiopathy (TMA), including thrombotic thrombocytopenic purpura and hemolytic-uremic syndrome, sometimes fatal, has been reported with interferon beta products and may occur several weeks to years after start of therapy. *Dialyzable drug:* Unknown.

PREGNANCY-LACTATION-REPRODUCTION

- There are no adequate studies in pregnant women; however, spontaneous abortions have been reported in clinical trials. Use during pregnancy only if potential benefit justifies potential risk to the fetus.
- It isn't known if drug appears in breast milk. Patient should discontinue breast-feeding or discontinue drug.

NURSING CONSIDERATIONS

- **Alert:** Serious liver damage, including hepatic failure requiring transplant, can occur. Monitor liver function at 1, 3, and 6 months after therapy starts and periodically thereafter.
- Drug is intended for use under the guidance and supervision of a physician. If patients or caregivers are to administer

drug, train them in the proper technique for self-administering.

• Monitor patient for signs and symptoms of drug-induced lupus erythematosus (rash, serositis, polyarthritis, nephritis, Raynaud phenomenon); discontinue therapy if they occur.

• Monitor patient for TMA and discontinue drug if clinical signs and symptoms and laboratory findings consistent with TMA occur; manage as clinically indicated.

• Monitor patient for symptoms of depression and severe psychiatric effects (mania, suicidal behavior or ideation, psychosis).

• Monitor CBC at 1, 3, and 6 months after therapy starts and periodically thereafter.

• Monitor thyroid function tests every 6 months in patients being treated for thyroid disorder.

PATIENT TEACHING

• Warn woman about dangers to fetus. If pregnancy occurs during therapy, tell her to notify prescriber.

• Advise patient to read medication guide that comes with drug.

• Teach patient how to perform subcutaneous injections, including solution preparation, aseptic technique, injection-site rotation, and equipment disposal. Periodically reevaluate patient's technique.

• Tell patient to report sign and symptoms of drug-induced lupus erythematosus.

• Tell patient to take drug at bedtime to minimize mild flulike signs and symptoms that commonly occur.

• Advise patient to report suicidal thoughts or depression.

• Urge patient to immediately report signs or symptoms of tissue death at injection site.

• Advise patient of importance of obtaining routine blood tests.

ipilimumab
IP-ih-LIM-yoo-mab

Yervoy

Therapeutic class: Antineoplastics
Pharmacologic class: Monoclonal antibodies

AVAILABLE FORMS
Injection: 50 mg/10 mL (5 mg/mL), 200 mg/40 mL (5 mg/mL)

INDICATIONS & DOSAGES

Adjust-a-dose (for all indications): Withhold dose in patients with grade 2 immune-mediated adverse reactions or symptomatic endocrinopathy. Resume therapy with complete or partial resolution of adverse reactions or of symptomatic endocrinopathy to grade 0 to 1 in patients who are receiving less than 7.5 mg prednisone or equivalent per day. Permanently discontinue drug in patients with grade 2 reactions, symptomatic endocrinopathy lasting 6 weeks or longer, or the inability to reduce corticosteroid dosage to 7.5 mg prednisone or its equivalent daily. Permanently discontinue drug for grade 2 through 4 ophthalmologic reactions not improving to grade 1 within 2 weeks while patient is receiving topical therapy or if systemic therapy is required.
Black Box Warning For patients with severe immune-mediated reactions, initiate systemic corticosteroids (prednisone or equivalent) at 1 to 2 mg/kg/day and permanently discontinue ipilimumab. ∎

➤ **Treatment of unresectable or metastatic melanoma**
Adults: 3 mg/kg I.V. infusion over 90 minutes every 3 weeks for a total of four doses. All treatment must be administered within 16 weeks of first dose.

✳ *NEW INDICATION:* **Adjuvant treatment of cutaneous melanoma with pathologic involvement of regional lymph nodes of more than 1 mm after complete resection, including total lymphadenectomy**
Adults: 10 mg/kg I.V. over 90 minutes every 3 weeks for four doses, followed by 10 mg/kg every 12 weeks for up to 3 years

---

Reactions in bold italics are *life-threatening*. Interactions may have a *rapid onset* or a *delayed onset*.

or until documented disease recurrence or unacceptable toxicity. If toxicity occurs, omit, don't delay, doses.

ADMINISTRATION

I.V.

▼ Store vials in refrigerator at 36° to 46° F (2° to 8° C). Don't freeze or shake vials. Protect from light.

▼ Visually inspect solution. Solution may be clear to pale yellow. Discard if cloudy or discolored or if particles (other than translucent-to-white, amorphous particles) are present.

▼ Allow vials to come to room temperature for 5 minutes before preparing infusion.

▼ Withdraw required volume of drug and transfer into I.V. bag of NSS or D_5W. Final concentration should range from 1 to 2 mg/mL. Invert bag gently to mix.

▼ Store diluted solution up to 24 hours under refrigeration or at room temperature (68° to 77° F [20° to 25° C]).

▼ Administer diluted solution over 90 minutes through I.V. line containing a sterile, nonpyrogenic, low-protein-binding in-line filter.

▼ After each dose, flush I.V. line with NSS or D_5W.

▼ Discard unused portion of vial.

▼ **Incompatibilities:** Other I.V. drugs and solutions other than NSS or D_5W.

ACTION

Binds to the cytotoxic T-lymphocyte-associated antigen 4; this blockade has been shown to augment T-cell–mediated antitumor immune responses.

Route	Onset	Peak	Duration
I.V.	Rapid	Unknown	Unknown

Half-life: 15 days.

ADVERSE REACTIONS

CNS: fatigue, neuropathy.
GI: diarrhea, colitis, enterocolitis.
GU: nephritis.
Hepatic: *hepatotoxicity.*
Metabolic: endocrinopathy, hypopituitarism.
Skin: pruritus, rash, dermatitis, urticaria.
Other: *adrenal insufficiency.*

INTERACTIONS

Cardiac glycosides: May decrease oral absorption of these drugs. Monitor therapy.
Vitamin K antagonists: May enhance anticoagulant effects. Monitor therapy.

EFFECTS ON LAB TEST RESULTS

● May increase liver enzyme levels.
● May increase eosinophil count.
● May increase or decrease thyroid hormone levels.

CONTRAINDICATIONS & CAUTIONS

● Contraindicated in patients hypersensitive to drug or its components.

Black Box Warning Ipilimumab can cause severe and fatal immune-mediated adverse reactions involving any organ system, especially such reactions as enterocolitis, hepatitis, dermatitis (including toxic epidermal necrolysis), neuropathy, and endocrinopathy. Reactions usually occur during treatment, but may present weeks to months after therapy ends. If severe immune-mediated reactions occur, permanently discontinue ipilimumab and initiate systemic high-dose corticosteroid therapy. Assess patient for these reactions. ■

● Permanently discontinue drug for any of the following: persistent moderate adverse reactions or inability to reduce corticosteroid dose to 7.5 mg of prednisone or equivalent daily; failure to complete full treatment course for unresectable or metastatic melanoma within 16 weeks from administration of first dose; severe or life-threatening adverse reactions, including colitis with abdominal pain, fever, ileus, or peritoneal signs and symptoms; increase in stool frequency (seven or more over baseline); fecal incontinence; need for I.V. hydration for more than 24 hours; GI hemorrhage; GI perforation; AST or ALT level more than 5 × ULN or total bilirubin level more than 3 × ULN; Stevens-Johnson syndrome; toxic epidermal necrolysis; rash complicated by full-thickness dermal ulceration or necrotic, bullous, or hemorrhagic manifestations; severe motor or sensory neuropathy; Guillain-Barré syndrome; myasthenia gravis; severe immune-mediated reactions involving any organ system (nephritis, pneumonitis, pancreatitis,

noninfectious myocarditis); or immune-mediated ocular disease unresponsive to topical immunosuppressive therapy.
Dialyzable drug: Unknown.

PREGNANCY-LACTATION-REPRODUCTION
• Based on its mechanism of action and data from animal studies, drug can cause fetal harm when given to a pregnant woman.
• Advise women of childbearing potential to use effective contraception during treatment and for 3 months after last dose.
• Drug may appear in breast milk. Because of the risk of serious adverse reactions in breast-feeding infants, patient should discontinue breast-feeding or discontinue drug. Women shouldn't breast-feed for 3 months after final dose.

NURSING CONSIDERATIONS
Black Box Warning Assess patients for signs and symptoms of enterocolitis, dermatitis, neuropathy, and endocrinopathy, and evaluate clinical chemistry values, including ACTH level and LFT and thyroid function test results, at baseline and before each dose. ■
• Review LFT results and assess patient for signs and symptoms of hepatotoxicity (jaundice, dark urine, nausea, vomiting, right upper quadrant pain, abnormal bleeding or bruising) before each dose. For patients with hepatotoxicity (AST or ALT level more than 5 × ULN or total bilirubin level more than 3 × ULN), rule out infectious or malignant causes and increase frequency of LFT monitoring until resolution. When LFT results show sustained improvement or return to baseline, initiate corticosteroid tapering and continue to taper over 1 month. Withhold ipilimumab in patients with grade 2 hepatotoxicity.
• Monitor patients for signs and symptoms of enterocolitis and bowel perforation (abdominal pain, fever, ileus, or peritoneal signs and symptoms; increase in stool frequency to seven or more over patient's baseline; fecal incontinence; need for I.V. hydration for more than 24 hours; GI hemorrhage; GI perforation). Rule out infection and consider endoscopic evaluation for persistent or severe symptoms. With improvement to grade 1 or less, taper corticosteroid dosage

over at least 1 month. If moderate symptoms occur, administer antidiarrheal and, if persistent for more than 1 week, start systemic corticosteroids (prednisone or equivalent) at 0.5 mg/kg/day. May consider adding anti-TNF or other immunosuppressive therapy for management of immune-mediated enterocolitis unresponsive to 3 to 5 days of systemic corticosteroids or recurring after symptomatic improvement.
• Monitor patients for signs and symptoms of motor or sensory neuropathy. Withhold ipilimumab in patients with moderate neuropathy. Permanently discontinue drug in patients with severe neuropathy that interferes with daily activities, such as Guillain-Barré–like syndromes (unilateral or bilateral weakness, sensory changes, paresthesia). Consider systemic corticosteroids (1 to 2 mg/kg/day prednisone or equivalent) for severe neuropathies.
• Monitor patients for signs and symptoms of dermatitis (rash, pruritus) and consider these symptoms immune-mediated unless an alternative cause is identified. Permanently discontinue ipilimumab in patients with Stevens-Johnson syndrome, toxic epidermal necrolysis, or rash complicated by full-thickness dermal ulceration or necrotic, bullous, or hemorrhagic manifestations. When dermatitis is controlled, taper corticosteroids over at least 1 month. For patients with mild to moderate dermatitis, treat symptomatically; give topical or systemic corticosteroids if there is no improvement within 1 week. Withhold ipilimumab in patients with moderate to severe signs and symptoms.
• Monitor patients for signs and symptoms of hypophysitis, adrenal insufficiency (including adrenal crisis), and hyperthyroidism or hypothyroidism (headaches, fatigue, feeling cold, weight gain, changes in mood or behavior, dizziness, or fainting). Endocrinopathies should be considered immune-mediated unless an alternative cause is identified. Withhold drug in symptomatic patients. Give corticosteroids and hormone replacement as appropriate.
• Monitor patients for ocular symptoms (vision changes, eye pain or redness). Administer corticosteroid eyedrops to patients who develop uveitis, iritis, or episcleritis.

Permanently discontinue drug in patients with immune-mediated ocular disease unresponsive to local immunosuppressive therapy.

PATIENT TEACHING
● Instruct patient to report history of immune system disorders, such as ulcerative colitis, Crohn disease, lupus, or sarcoidosis; organ transplant; or liver damage.
● Teach patient the signs and symptoms of serious immune-mediated adverse reactions and to immediately report them to prescriber.
● Advise patient that blood chemistry studies will be needed before start of therapy and before each dose.
● Instruct patient to read the Yervoy Medication Guide before taking each dose.
● Warn female patient that ipilimumab can cause fetal harm and to report pregnancy immediately.
● Advise female patient of childbearing potential to use effective contraception during treatment and for 3 months after last dose.
● Tell breast-feeding patient not to breast-feed while taking drug.

ipratropium bromide
ih-pra-TROE-pee-um

Atrovent, Atrovent HFA

Therapeutic class: Bronchodilators
Pharmacologic class: Anticholinergics

AVAILABLE FORMS
Inhaler: 17 mcg/metered dose (Atrovent HFA)
Nasal spray: 0.03% (21 mcg/metered dose), 0.06% (42 mcg/metered dose)
Solution (for inhalation): 0.02% (500 mcg/vial)

INDICATIONS & DOSAGES
➤ **Bronchospasm in chronic bronchitis and emphysema**
Adults: Usually, 2 inhalations q.i.d.; patient may take additional inhalations as needed but shouldn't exceed 12 inhalations in 24 hours. Or, 250 to 500 mcg every 6 to 8 hours via oral nebulizer.

Children age 12 and older: 500 mcg every 6 to 8 hours (t.i.d. to q.i.d.) via oral nebulizer.
➤ **Rhinorrhea caused by allergic and nonallergic perennial rhinitis**
Adults and children age 6 and older: Two 0.03% nasal sprays (42 mcg) per nostril b.i.d. or t.i.d.
➤ **Rhinorrhea caused by the common cold**
Adults and children age 12 and older: Two 0.06% nasal sprays (84 mcg) per nostril t.i.d. or q.i.d.
Children ages 5 to 11: Two 0.06% nasal sprays (84 mcg) per nostril t.i.d.
➤ **Rhinorrhea caused by seasonal allergic rhinitis**
Adults and children age 5 and older: Two 0.06% nasal sprays (84 mcg) per nostril q.i.d. Total dose is 672 mcg/day.
➤ **Acute asthma exacerbations, in combination with a short-acting beta agonist ◆**
Adults and adolescents age 13 and older: 500 mcg via oral nebulizer every 20 minutes for three doses, then as needed; or 8 inhalations of inhalation aerosol every 20 minutes as needed for up to 3 hours.
Children ages 6 to 12: 250 to 500 mcg via oral nebulizer every 20 minutes for three doses, then as needed; or 4 to 8 inhalations of inhalation aerosol every 20 minutes as needed for up to 3 hours.
Children age 5 and younger: 250 mcg via oral nebulizer every 20 minutes for 1 hour; or 2 inhalations of inhalation aerosol every 20 minutes if needed for 1 hour.

ADMINISTRATION
Inhalation
● Shake canister before use, except for HFA aerosol.
● If more than 1 inhalation is ordered, wait at least 2 minutes between inhalations.
● Use spacer device to improve drug delivery, if appropriate.
● Inhalation solution is for use with oral nebulizer. Refer to manufacturer's instructions for use.
Intranasal
● Prime nasal spray with 7 sprays of pump before first use; prime with 2 sprays after pump hasn't been used for more than 24 hours.

• Tilt patient's head backward after dose to allow drug to spread to back of nose.

ACTION

Inhibits vagally mediated reflexes by antagonizing acetylcholine at muscarinic receptors on bronchial smooth muscle.

Route	Onset	Peak	Duration
Inhalation	5–15 min	1–2 hr	3–6 hr
Intranasal	Unknown	Unknown	Unknown

Half-life: Inhalation, about 2 hours; intranasal, 1.6 hours.

ADVERSE REACTIONS

CNS: dizziness, pain, headache.
CV: palpitations, chest pain, hypertension.
EENT: blurred vision, rhinitis, pharyngitis, sinusitis, epistaxis.
GI: nausea, GI distress, dry mouth, constipation, dyspepsia.
GU: UTI.
Musculoskeletal: back pain.
Respiratory: URI, bronchitis, ***bronchospasm***, cough, dyspnea, increased sputum.
Skin: rash.
Other: flulike symptoms, hypersensitivity reactions.

INTERACTIONS

Drug-drug. *Anticholinergics:* May increase anticholinergic effects. Avoid using together.

EFFECTS ON LAB TEST RESULTS

None reported.

CONTRAINDICATIONS & CAUTIONS

• Contraindicated in patients hypersensitive to drug, atropine, or its derivatives.
• Use cautiously in patients with angle-closure glaucoma, prostatic hyperplasia, or bladder-neck obstruction.
۞ Alert: Drug isn't indicated for initial treatment of acute episodes of bronchospasm, for which rescue therapy is required for rapid response.
• Safety and effectiveness of nebulization or inhaler in children younger than age 12 haven't been established.
Dialyzable drug: Unknown.

PREGNANCY-LACTATION-REPRODUCTION

• There are no adequate studies in pregnant women. Use during pregnancy only if clearly needed and if potential benefit justifies potential risk to the fetus.
• It isn't known if drug appears in breast milk. Use cautiously in breast-feeding women.

NURSING CONSIDERATIONS

• If patient uses a face mask for a nebulizer, take care to prevent leakage around the mask because eye pain or temporary blurring of vision may occur.
• Safety and effectiveness of intranasal use beyond 4 days in patients with a common cold haven't been established.

PATIENT TEACHING

• Warn patient that drug isn't effective for treating acute episodes of bronchospasm when rapid response is needed.
• Teach patient to use metered-dose inhaler (MDI) or oral nebulizer correctly. Refer to manufacturer's instructions for use.
• Inform patient that use of a spacer device with an MDI may improve drug delivery to lungs.
• Warn patient to avoid accidentally spraying drug into eyes. Temporary blurring of vision may result.
• If more than 1 inhalation is prescribed, tell patient to wait at least 2 minutes before repeating procedure.
• If patient is also using a corticosteroid inhaler, instruct him to use ipratropium first and then to wait about 5 minutes before using the corticosteroid. This lets the bronchodilator open air passages for maximal effectiveness of the corticosteroid.
• Instruct patient to prime nasal spray by pumping seven times before first use or after it has not been used for 1 week. Prime with two pumps after it has not been used for 1 day.
• Instruct patient to sniff deeply after each spray and to breathe out through mouth. Tell him to tilt head backward to allow drug to spread to back of nose.

Reactions in bold italics are *life-threatening*. Interactions may have a *rapid onset* or a ***delayed onset***.

irbesartan
er-bah-SAR-tan

Avapro✦

Therapeutic class: Antihypertensives
Pharmacologic class: Angiotensin II
receptor antagonists

AVAILABLE FORMS
Tablets: 75 mg, 150 mg, 300 mg

INDICATIONS & DOSAGES
Adjust-a-dose (for all indications): For
volume- and sodium-depleted patients,
initially, 75 mg P.O. daily.
➤ **Hypertension**
Adults: Initially, 150 mg P.O. daily, in-
creased to maximum of 300 mg daily, if
needed.
➤ **Nephropathy in patients with type 2
diabetes**
Adults: Target maintenance dose is 300 mg
P.O. once daily.

ADMINISTRATION
P.O.
● Give drug without regard for meals.

ACTION
Produces antihypertensive effect by competitive antagonist activity at the angiotensin II
receptor.

Route	Onset	Peak	Duration
P.O.	Unknown	1½–2 hr	>24 hr

Half-life: 11 to 15 hours.

ADVERSE REACTIONS
CNS: fatigue, anxiety, dizziness, headache.
CV: chest pain, edema, tachycardia.
EENT: pharyngitis, rhinitis, sinus abnor-
mality.
GI: diarrhea, dyspepsia, abdominal pain,
nausea, vomiting.
GU: UTI.
Musculoskeletal: musculoskeletal trauma
or pain.
Respiratory: URI, cough.
Skin: rash.
Other: flulike symptoms.

INTERACTIONS
ACE inhibitors: May increase risk of hypotension, renal dysfunction, and hyperkalemia. Use together cautiously; closely
monitor BP, renal function, and potassium
level.
⊕ *Alert: Aliskiren:* May increase risk of renal
impairment, hypotension, and hyperkalemia
in diabetic patients and those with moderate to severe renal impairment (GFR less
than 60 mL/minute). Concomitant use is
contraindicated in diabetic patients. Avoid
concomitant use in those with moderate to
severe renal impairment.
Lithium: May increase lithium concentration, possibly causing toxicity. Monitor
lithium serum concentration, and observe
patient's clinical response. Adjust lithium
dosage as needed.
*NSAIDs, selective cyclooxygenase-2 in-
hibitors (celecoxib):* May result in deterioration of renal function, including possible
acute renal failure, in patients who are elderly, volume-depleted (including those on
diuretic therapy), or who have compromised
renal function. May decrease antihypertensive effect of irbesartan. Periodically
monitor renal function during coadministration.
*Potassium-sparing diuretics, potassium
supplements, trimethoprim:* May increase
risk of hyperkalemia. Closely monitor
serum potassium concentration and adjust
treatment as needed.

EFFECTS ON LAB TEST RESULTS
None reported.

CONTRAINDICATIONS & CAUTIONS
● Contraindicated in patients hypersensitive
to drug or its components.
● Use cautiously in patients with impaired
renal function, HF, and renal artery stenosis.
Dialyzable drug: No.
⚠ *Overdose S&S:* Hypotension, tachycardia,
bradycardia.

PREGNANCY-LACTATION-REPRODUCTION
Black Box Warning Use during pregnancy
can cause injury and death to the developing
fetus. When pregnancy is detected, stop
drug as soon as possible. ∎

● It isn't known if drug appears in breast milk. Patient should discontinue breast-feeding or discontinue drug.

NURSING CONSIDERATIONS
● Drug may be given with a diuretic or other antihypertensive, if needed, for control of hypertension.
● Symptomatic hypotension may occur in volume- or sodium-depleted patients (vigorous diuretic use or dialysis). Correct the cause of volume depletion before administration or before a lower dose is used.
● If hypotension occurs, place patient in a supine position and give an I.V. infusion of NSS, if needed. Once BP has stabilized after a transient hypotensive episode, drug may be continued.
● Dizziness and orthostatic hypotension may occur more frequently in patients with type 2 diabetes and renal disease.

PATIENT TEACHING
● Warn woman of childbearing potential of consequences of drug exposure to fetus. Tell her to notify prescriber immediately if pregnancy is suspected.
● Tell patient that drug may be taken without regard for food.
● Tell patient to report all adverse reactions and to inform prescriber of other prescription and OTC drugs and supplements being taken.

SAFETY ALERT!

irinotecan hydrochloride
eh-rin-OH-te-kan

Camptosar

Therapeutic class: Antineoplastics
Pharmacologic class: DNA topoisomerase inhibitors

AVAILABLE FORMS
Injection: 20 mg/mL in 2-, 5-, and 15-mL vials

INDICATIONS & DOSAGES
➤ **Metastatic carcinoma of the colon or rectum that has recurred or progressed after 5-FU therapy**

Adults: Initially, 125 mg/m^2 by I.V. infusion over 90 minutes on days 1, 8, 15, and 22; then 2-week rest period. Thereafter, additional courses of treatment may be repeated every 6 weeks with 4 weeks on and 2 weeks off. Subsequent doses may be adjusted to low of 50 mg/m^2 or maximum of 150 mg/m^2 in 25- to 50-mg/m^2 increments based on patient's tolerance. Or, 350 mg/m^2 by I.V. infusion over 90 minutes once every 3 weeks. Additional courses may continue indefinitely in patients who respond favorably and in those whose disease remains stable, provided intolerable toxicity doesn't occur.

Adjust-a-dose: Consider reducing starting dose in patients age 65 and older, in those who have received pelvic or abdominal radiation, or in those who have a performance status of 2 or increased bilirubin level. Give 300 mg/m^2 by I.V. infusion over 90 minutes once every 3 weeks. Or, give 100 mg/m^2 by I.V. infusion over 90 minutes once weekly. See manufacturer's package insert for details on dosage adjustments due to toxicities.

➤ **First-line therapy for metastatic colorectal cancer with 5-FU and leucovorin**
Regimen 1
Adults: 125 mg/m^2 I.V. over 90 minutes on days 1, 8, 15, and 22; then leucovorin 20 mg/m^2 I.V. bolus on days 1, 8, 15, and 22 and 5-FU 500 mg/m^2 I.V. bolus on days 1, 8, 15, and 22. Courses are repeated every 6 weeks.
Regimen 2
Adults: 180 mg/m^2 I.V. over 90 minutes on days 1, 15, and 29; then leucovorin 200 mg/m^2 I.V. over 2 hours on days 1, 2, 15, 16, 29, and 30; then 5-FU 400 mg/m^2 I.V. bolus on days 1, 2, 15, 16, 29, and 30 and 5-FU 600 mg/m^2 I.V. infusion over 22 hours on days 1, 2, 15, 16, 29, and 30.
Adjust-a-dose: Consider reducing starting dose by one dose level for patients with any of the following conditions: prior pelvic or abdominal radiotherapy, performance status of 2, or increased bilirubin level. See manufacturer's package insert for details on all dosage adjustments.
➤ **Esophageal cancer, metastatic or locally advanced ◆**
Adults: 65 mg/m^2 I.V. over 90 minutes on days 1, 8, 15, and 22 of a 6-week

cycle (in combination with cisplatin), or 180 mg/m^2 I.V. over 90 minutes every 2 weeks (in combination with leucovorin and 5-FU), or 250 mg/m^2 I.V. every 3 weeks (in combination with capecitabine).

➤ **Gastric cancer, metastatic or locally advanced** ◆

Adults: 150 mg/m^2 I.V. (as a single agent) on days 1 and 15 of a 4-week cycle, or 65 mg/m^2 I.V. over 90 minutes on days 1, 8, 15, and 22 of a 6-week cycle (in combination with cisplatin), or 70 mg/m^2 I.V. over 90 minutes on days 1 and 15 of a 4-week cycle (in combination with cisplatin) for up to six cycles, or 180 mg/m^2 I.V. over 90 minutes every 2 weeks (in combination with leucovorin and 5-FU), or 250 mg/m^2 I.V. every 3 weeks (in combination with capecitabine).

➤ **Non-small-cell lung cancer, advanced** ◆

Adults: 60 mg/m^2 I.V. on days 1, 8, and 15 every 4 weeks (in combination with cisplatin).

➤ **Pancreatic cancer, advanced** ◆

Adults: 180 mg/m^2 I.V. over 90 minutes every 2 weeks (in combination with oxaliplatin, leucovorin, and 5-FU).

➤ **Small-cell lung cancer, extensive stage** ◆

Adults: 60 mg/m^2 I.V. on days 1, 8, and 15 every 4 weeks (in combination with cisplatin), or 65 mg/m^2 I.V. on days 1 and 8 every 3 weeks (in combination with cisplatin), or 175 mg/m^2 I.V. on day 1 every 3 weeks (in combination with carboplatin), or 50 mg/m^2 I.V. on days 1, 8, and 15 every 4 weeks (in combination with carboplatin).

ADMINISTRATION

I.V.

▼ Drug packaged in plastic blister to protect against inadvertent breakage and leakage. Inspect vial for damage and signs of leakage before removing blister.

▼ Wear gloves while handling and preparing infusion solutions. If drug contacts skin, wash thoroughly with soap and water. If drug contacts mucous membranes, flush thoroughly with water.

▼ Dilute drug in D$_5$W injection (preferred) or NSS for injection before infusion to yield 0.12 to 2.8 mg/mL.

▼ Solution is stable for up to 24 hours at 77° F (25° C) in ambient fluorescent lighting. Solutions diluted in D$_5$W, stored at 36° to 46° F (2° to 8° C), and protected from light are stable for 48 hours. However, because microbial contamination may occur during dilution, use admixture within 24 hours if refrigerated or 6 hours if kept at room temperature. Refrigerating admixtures using NSS isn't recommended because of low and sporadic risk of visible particulate. Don't freeze admixture because drug may precipitate.

▼ Premedicate patient with antiemetic drugs on day of treatment starting at least 30 minutes before giving irinotecan.

▼ Watch for irritation and infiltration; extravasation can cause tissue damage. If extravasation occurs, flush site with sterile water and apply ice. Notify prescriber.

▼ Store vial at 59° to 86° F (15° to 30° C). Protect from light.

▼ **Incompatibilities:** Gemcitabine, pemetrexed.

ACTION

Interacts with topoisomerase I, inducing reversible single-strand DNA breaks. Drug binds to the topoisomerase I–DNA complex and prevents religation of these single-strand breaks.

Route	Onset	Peak	Duration
I.V.	Unknown	1 hr	Unknown

Half-life: About 6 to 12 hours; active metabolite, 10 to 20 hours.

ADVERSE REACTIONS

CNS: asthenia, dizziness, fever, headache, insomnia, pain, akathisia, confusion, somnolence.

CV: edema, vasodilation, orthostatic hypotension.

EENT: rhinitis.

GI: *diarrhea,* abdominal cramping, abdominal pain and enlargement, anorexia, constipation, dyspepsia, flatulence, nausea, stomatitis, vomiting.

Hematologic: anemia, *leukopenia, neutropenia, thrombocytopenia.*

Metabolic: dehydration, weight loss.

Musculoskeletal: back pain.

Respiratory: dyspnea, increased cough, pneumonia.
Skin: alopecia, rash, sweating.
Other: chills, infection.

INTERACTIONS
Drug-drug. *CYP3A4 enzyme-inducing anticonvulsants (carbamazepine, phenobarbital, phenytoin), rifampin, rifabutin:* May significantly decrease irinotecan levels. For patients requiring anticonvulsant treatment, consider substituting non–enzyme-inducing anticonvulsants at least 2 weeks before start of irinotecan therapy.
CYP3A4 inhibitors (clarithromycin, indinavir, itraconazole, lopinavir, nefazodone, nelfinavir, ritonavir, saquinavir, voriconazole), UGT1A1 inhibitors (atazanavir, gemfibrozil, indinavir): May increase systemic exposure to irinotecan. Discontinue strong CYP3A4 inhibitors at least 1 week before starting irinotecan. Don't give strong CYP3A4 or UGT1A1 inhibitors with irinotecan unless there are no therapeutic alternatives.
Diuretics: May increase risk of dehydration and electrolyte imbalance. Consider stopping diuretic during active periods of nausea and vomiting.
Ketoconazole: May increase irinotecan levels, leading to drug toxicity. Stop ketoconazole at least 1 week before starting irinotecan therapy. Ketoconazole is contraindicated during irinotecan therapy.
Laxatives: May increase risk of diarrhea. Avoid using together.
Live-virus vaccines: May cause serious or fatal infection. Don't give together.
Neuromuscular blockers: May prolong the neuromuscular-blocking effects of succinylcholine, and the neuromuscular blockade of nondepolarizing drugs may be antagonized. Monitor patient for prolonged effects of succinylcholine if given together.
Other antineoplastics: May cause additive adverse effects, such as myelosuppression and diarrhea. Monitor patient closely.
Prochlorperazine: May increase risk of akathisia. Monitor patient closely.
Vaccines (killed or inactivated virus): May diminish response to vaccine. Avoid use together.

Drug-herb. *St. John's wort:* May decrease drug levels. Use together is contraindicated.
Drug-food. *Grapefruit juice:* May increase irinotecan serum concentration. Avoid combination.

EFFECTS ON LAB TEST RESULTS
● May increase alkaline phosphatase, AST, and bilirubin levels. May decrease Hb level.
● May decrease WBC and neutrophil counts.

CONTRAINDICATIONS & CAUTIONS
● Contraindicated in patients hypersensitive to drug.
● Fatal interstitial pulmonary disease (IPD) has been reported. Patients with preexisting lung disease, patients taking pulmonary toxic drugs or colony-stimulating factors, and patients receiving radiation therapy are at increased risk. If IPD is diagnosed, all chemotherapy will be discontinued.
● Safety and effectiveness in children haven't been established.
● Use cautiously in elderly patients.
Dialyzable drug: Unknown.
⚠ **Overdose S&S:** Severe neutropenia, severe diarrhea.

PREGNANCY-LACTATION-REPRODUCTION
● May cause fetal harm. Women of childbearing potential should avoid becoming pregnant during therapy.
● It isn't known if drug appears in breast milk. Patient should discontinue breastfeeding or discontinue drug.

NURSING CONSIDERATIONS
● Administer drug under the supervision of a physician experienced with cancer chemotherapy.
Black Box Warning Drug may cause severe myelosuppression. ▮
● Pelvic or abdominal irradiation may increase risk of severe myelosuppression. Avoid use of drug in patients undergoing irradiation.
● Patients with UGT1A1*28 allele or UGT1A1 7/7 genotype are at increased risk for neutropenia. Patient should be considered for initial minus 1 level dosage adjustment; monitor patient closely.

• If neutropenic fever occurs or if ANC drops below 500/mm^3, temporarily stop therapy. Reduce dosage, especially if WBC count is below 2,000/mm^3, neutrophil count is below 1,000/mm^3, Hb level is below 8 g/dL, or platelet count is below 100,000/mm^3.

• A colony-stimulating factor may be helpful in patients with significant neutropenia.

• Monitor WBC count with differential, Hb level, and platelet count before each dose.

Black Box Warning Drug can cause severe diarrhea. Treat diarrhea occurring within 24 hours of drug administration with 0.25 to 1 mg atropine I.V., unless contraindicated. Treat late diarrhea (more than 24 hours after irinotecan administration) promptly with loperamide. Monitor patient for dehydration, electrolyte imbalance, or sepsis, and treat appropriately. Institute antibiotic therapy if patient develops ileus, fever, or severe neutropenia. Interrupt therapy and reduce subsequent doses if severe diarrhea occurs. ■

• Delay subsequent doses until normal bowel function returns for at least 24 hours without antidiarrheal. If grade 2, 3, or 4 late diarrhea occurs, decrease subsequent doses within the current cycle.

• To decrease risk of dehydration, withhold diuretic during treatment and periods of active vomiting or diarrhea.

• Monitor patient for respiratory signs and symptoms (dyspnea, cough, fever) before and during treatment.

• **Look alike–sound alike:** Don't confuse irinotecan with topotecan.

PATIENT TEACHING

• Inform patient about risk of diarrhea and methods to treat it; tell him to avoid laxatives.

• Instruct patient to report all adverse reactions and to immediately contact prescriber if any of the following occur: diarrhea for the first time during treatment; black or bloody stools; symptoms of dehydration such as light-headedness, dizziness, or faintness; inability to drink fluids due to nausea or vomiting; inability to control diarrhea within 24 hours; fever or infection; dyspnea or cough.

• Warn patient that hair loss may occur.

• Caution female patient to avoid pregnancy and breast-feeding during therapy.

iron dextran
DexFerrum, DexIron✦, InFeD

Therapeutic class: Iron supplements
Pharmacologic class: Hematinics

AVAILABLE FORMS

1 mL iron dextran provides 50 mg elemental iron.
Injection: 50 mg elemental iron/mL in 1-mL and 2-mL single-dose vials

INDICATIONS & DOSAGES

➤ **Iron deficiency anemia**
Adults and children weighing more than 15 kg: I.V. or I.M. test dose is required. (See manufacturer's instructions.) Total dose may be calculated using dosage table in package insert or by using the following formula:

$$\text{Dose (mL)} = 0.0442 \, (\text{desired Hb} - \text{observed Hb}) \times \text{LBW} + (0.26 \times \text{LWB})$$

Note: LBW = lean body weight in kg. For males, LBW = 50 kg + 2.3 kg for each inch of patient's height over 5 feet. For females, LBW = 45.5 kg + 2.3 kg for each inch of patient's height over 5 feet.
Children weighing 5 to 15 kg: Use dosage table in package insert or calculate dose as follows:

$$\text{Dose (mL)} = 0.0442 \, (\text{desired Hb} - \text{observed Hb}) \times \text{weight in kg} + (0.26 \times \text{weight in kg})$$

I.V.
Adults and children: Inject 0.5-mL test dose over at least 5 minutes. If no reaction occurs in 1 hour, give remainder of therapeutic I.V. dose. Repeat therapeutic I.V. dose daily. Single daily dose shouldn't exceed 100 mg. Give slowly (1 mL/minute). Don't give drug in the first 4 months of life.
I.M. (by Z-track method)
Adults and children: Inject 0.5-mL test dose. If no reaction occurs in 1 hour, give remainder of dose. Daily dose ordinarily shouldn't exceed 0.5 mL (25 mg) for infants weighing less than 5 kg; 1 mL (50 mg) for

those weighing less than 10 kg; and 2 mL (100 mg) for heavier children and adults. Don't give drug in the first 4 months of life.

➤ **Iron replacement for blood loss**
Adults and children older than age 4 months: Replacement iron (in mg) = blood loss (in mL) × hematocrit.
Note: This formula is based on the approximation that 1 mL of normocytic, normochromic red cells contains 1 mg of elemental iron.

ADMINISTRATION
I.V.
▼ Check hospital policy before giving I.V.
▼ Give at slow gradual rate not to exceed 50 mg (1 mL)/minute.
▼ After completing I.V. dose, flush the vein with 10 mL of NSS.
▼ Patient should rest for 15 to 30 minutes after I.V. administration.
▼ **Incompatibilities:** Other I.V. drugs, parenteral nutrition solutions for I.V. infusion.
I.M.
● Inject I.M. deep into upper outer quadrant of buttock—never into the arm or other exposed area—with a 2″ to 3″19G or 20G needle.
● Use Z-track method to avoid leakage into subcutaneous tissue and staining of skin.
● After drawing up drug, use a new sterile needle to give injection.

ACTION
Provides elemental iron, an essential component in the formation of Hb.

Route	Onset	Peak	Duration
I.V.	Unknown	7–9 days	Unknown
I.M.	72 hr	Unknown	3–4 wk

Half-life: 5 to 20 hours. Half-life values don't represent iron clearance from the body. Iron isn't easily eliminated, and the accumulation of iron can be toxic.

ADVERSE REACTIONS
CNS: headache, transitory paresthesia, dizziness, malaise, fever, chills, *seizures,* disorientation.
CV: chest pain, tachycardia, *bradycardia,* hypotensive reaction, peripheral vascular flushing, arrhythmias, *cardiac arrest, shock,* hypertension.

GI: nausea, anorexia, abdominal pain, diarrhea, vomiting.
GU: hematuria.
Hematologic: leukocytosis, lymphadeno-pathy.
Musculoskeletal: arthralgia, myalgia.
Respiratory: *bronchospasm,* dyspnea, wheezing, *respiratory arrest.*
Skin: rash, urticaria, soreness, inflammation, brown skin discoloration at I.M. injection site, local phlebitis at I.V. injection site, sterile abscess, necrosis, atrophy.
Other: fibrosis, *anaphylaxis, delayed sensitivity reactions.*

INTERACTIONS
Drug-drug. *ACE inhibitors:* Increases risk of adverse systemic reactions. Stop one of the agents if interaction occurs.
Chloramphenicol: May increase iron level. Monitor patient closely.

EFFECTS ON LAB TEST RESULTS
● May cause false increase in bilirubin level and false decrease in calcium level. Use of more than 250 mg iron may color the serum brown. Drug may alter measurement of iron level and total iron-binding capacity for up to 3 weeks; I.M. injection may cause dense areas of activity for 1 to 6 days on bone scans using technetium-99m diphosphonate.

CONTRAINDICATIONS & CAUTIONS
Black Box Warning Fatal anaphylactic reactions have been reported. Fatal reactions have occurred when the test dose was tolerated. Patients with history of drug allergy may be at increased risk. Give only when indications have been clearly established and for iron deficiencies not amenable to oral iron therapy. Keep emergency equipment readily available. ■
● Contraindicated in patients hypersensitive to drug, in those with acute infectious renal disease, and in those with any anemia except iron deficiency anemia.
● Use cautiously in patients who have serious hepatic impairment, RA, or other inflammatory diseases.
● Use cautiously in patients with history of significant allergies or asthma.
Dialyzable drug: No.
⚠ *Overdose S&S:* Hemosiderosis.

Reactions in bold italics are *life-threatening*. Interactions may have a *rapid onset* or a *delayed onset*.

PREGNANCY-LACTATION-REPRODUCTION
• Use during pregnancy only if potential benefit justifies potential risk to the fetus.
• Traces of unmetabolized drug appear in breast milk. Use caution in breast-feeding.

NURSING CONSIDERATIONS
Black Box Warning Administer test dose of iron dextran before first therapeutic dose. If no signs or symptoms of anaphylactic-type reactions follow test dose, administer full therapeutic iron dextran dose. Fatal reactions have followed test dose. Observe for signs and symptoms of anaphylactic-type reactions with every dose given. Have emergency equipment immediately available. ■
• Don't give iron dextran with oral iron drug.
• I.V. or I.M. injections of iron are advisable only for patients in whom oral administration is impossible or ineffective.
• Monitor Hb level, hematocrit, and reticulocyte count.
• Maximum daily dose should not exceed 2 mL undiluted iron dextran.

PATIENT TEACHING
• Teach patient signs and symptoms of hypersensitivity and iron toxicity; tell patient to report all adverse reactions to prescriber.
• Inform patient that drug may stain skin.

---

iron sucrose injection
Venofer

Therapeutic class: Iron supplements
Pharmacologic class: Hematinics

AVAILABLE FORMS
Injection: 20 mg/mL of elemental iron in 2.5-mL, 5-mL, and 10-mL single-dose vials

INDICATIONS & DOSAGES
➤ **Iron deficiency anemia in patients who are hemodialysis dependent and are receiving erythropoietin therapy**
Adults: 100 mg (5 mL) of elemental iron I.V. directly in the dialysis line by slow injection over 2 to 5 minutes or by infusion of 100 mg diluted in a maximum of 100 mL NSS over 15 minutes during the dialysis session one to

three times a week to a total of 1,000 mg in 10 doses; repeat as needed.
➤ **Iron deficiency anemia in chronic kidney disease patients not on dialysis**
Adults: 200 mg by undiluted slow I.V. injection over 2 to 5 minutes, or as an infusion of 200 mg in a maximum of 100 mL NSS over 15 minutes, on five separate occasions in a 14-day period to a total cumulative dose of 1,000 mg.
➤ **Iron deficiency anemia in peritoneal dialysis-dependent chronic kidney disease patients**
Adults: 300 mg I.V. infusion over 90 minutes on two separate occasions 14 days apart, followed by one 400-mg infusion over 2½ hours 14 days later. Dilute in a maximum of 250 mL NSS.
➤ **Maintenance treatment in pediatric patients with hemodialysis-dependent chronic kidney disease, nondialysis-dependent chronic kidney disease who are receiving erythropoietin, or peritoneal dialysis-dependent chronic kidney disease who are receiving erythropoietin**
Children ages 2 and older: 0.5 mg/kg I.V. every 2 weeks for 12 weeks. Give undiluted by slow I.V. injection over 5 minutes or diluted in 25 mL NSS and administered over 5 to 60 minutes. May repeat treatment if necessary. Don't give more than 100 mg per dose.

ADMINISTRATION
I.V.
▼ Inspect drug for particulate matter and discoloration before giving.
▼ For infusion, dilute 100 mg elemental iron in a maximum of 100 mL NSS immediately before infusion, and infuse over at least 15 minutes. Dilute 300 mg or greater in a maximum of 250 mL NSS.
▼ **Incompatibilities:** Other I.V. drugs, parenteral nutrition solutions.

ACTION
Exogenous source of iron that replenishes depleted body iron stores and is essential for Hb synthesis.

Route	Onset	Peak	Duration
I.V.	Unknown	Unknown	Variable

Half-life: 6 hours.

ADVERSE REACTIONS

CNS: headache, asthenia, malaise, dizziness, fever.
CV: *HF,* hypotension, chest pain, hypertension, fluid retention.
GI: nausea, vomiting, diarrhea, abdominal pain, taste perversion.
Metabolic: gout, *hypoglycemia,* hyperglycemia.
Musculoskeletal: leg cramps, bone and muscle pain, arthralgia, back pain.
Respiratory: dyspnea, wheezing, pneumonia, cough.
Skin: rash, pruritus, injection-site reaction.
Other: accidental injury, pain, *sepsis, hypersensitivity reactions.*

INTERACTIONS

Drug-drug. *Oral iron preparations:* May reduce absorption of oral iron preparations. Avoid using together.

EFFECTS ON LAB TEST RESULTS

None reported.

CONTRAINDICATIONS & CAUTIONS

• Contraindicated in patients with hypersensitivity to drug or its components, evidence of iron overload, or anemia not caused by iron deficiency.
Dialyzable drug: No.
⚠ *Overdose S&S:* Accumulation of iron in storage sites, potentially leading to hemosiderosis.

PREGNANCY-LACTATION-REPRODUCTION

• There are no adequate studies in pregnant women. Use during pregnancy only if clearly needed.
• It isn't known if drug appears in breast milk. Use cautiously in breast-feeding women.

NURSING CONSIDERATIONS

⟳ *Alert:* Rare but fatal hypersensitivity reactions, characterized by anaphylactic shock, loss of consciousness, collapse, hypotension, dyspnea, or seizures, may occur. Have epinephrine readily available.
• Mild to moderate hypersensitivity reactions, with wheezing, dyspnea, hypotension, rash, or pruritus, may occur.

• Infusing drug may reduce hypotension risk.
• Transferrin saturation level increases rapidly after I.V. administration of drug. Obtain iron level 48 hours after I.V. use.
• Monitor ferritin level, transferrin saturation, Hb level, and hematocrit.
• Withhold dose in patient with signs and symptoms of iron overload.
• Keep dose selection in elderly patients conservative because of decreased hepatic, renal, or cardiac function; other disease; and other drug therapy.

PATIENT TEACHING

• Instruct patient to report all adverse reactions and notify prescriber immediately if symptoms of overdose or allergic reaction occur.

---

isavuconazonium sulfate
EYE-sa-vue-KOE-na-zoe-nee-um

Cresemba

Therapeutic class: Antifungals
Pharmacologic class: Triazole antifungals

AVAILABLE FORMS

Capsules ⓄⓉⒸ: 186 mg (equal to isavuconazole 100 mg)
Injection: 372 mg (equal to isavuconazole 200 mg)/vial

INDICATIONS & DOSAGES

➤ **Invasive aspergillosis; invasive mucormycosis fungal infection**
Adults: Give loading doses of 372 mg I.V. or P.O. every 8 hours for six doses (48 hours); then give maintenance dose of 372 mg I.V. or P.O. once daily. Initiate maintenance dose 12 to 24 hours after last loading dose. Switching between I.V. and P.O. formulations of isavuconazonium sulfate is acceptable for maintenance dosing. It isn't necessary to restart dosing with a loading dose when switching between formulations.

ADMINISTRATION
P.O.
• May give with or without food.

- Give capsules whole; capsules shouldn't be chewed, crushed, dissolved, or opened.
- Store in original packaging at 68° to 77° F (20° to 25° C).

I.V.

▼ Reconstitute one vial of isavuconazonium with 5 mL sterile water for injection; shake gently to dissolve.

▼ Inspect for particulate matter and discoloration.

▼ Reconstituted solution may be stored below 77° F (25° C) for a maximum of 1 hour before preparation of the admixed solution.

▼ Remove 5 mL of reconstituted solution from vial and add it to an infusion bag containing 250 mL NSS or D_5W.

▼ Diluted solution may show visible translucent to white particulates of isavuconazole (which will be removed by the in-line filter). Use gentle mixing or roll bag to minimize formation of particulates. Avoid unnecessary vibration or vigorous shaking of solution. Don't use a pneumatic transport system.

▼ Infuse through an in-line filter with a microporous membrane pore size of 0.2 to 1.2 microns to remove particulates.

▼ Infuse over a minimum of 1 hour. Don't give as an I.V. bolus injection.

▼ Complete I.V. administration within 6 hours of dilution. If this isn't possible, immediately refrigerate admixed solution at 36° to 46° F (2° to 8° C) and complete infusion within 24 hours. Don't freeze.

▼ Flush I.V. line with NSS or D_5W before and after infusion.

▼ **Incompatibilities:** I.V. medications and I.V. solutions other than NSS or D_5W.

ACTION

Isavuconazonium, a prodrug of isavuconazole, inhibits synthesis of ergosterol, a key component of the fungal cell membrane, weakening the membrane structure and function.

Route	Onset	Peak	Duration
P.O.	Unknown	2–3 hr	Unknown
I.V.	Rapid	Within 1 hr	Unknown

Half-life: 130 hours (I.V.).

ADVERSE REACTIONS

CNS: anxiety, fatigue, headache, insomnia, delirium, confusion, hallucination, depression, drowsiness, *seizures,* encephalopathy, hypoesthesia, migraine, peripheral neuropathy, paresthesia, somnolence, stupor, syncope, tremor, malaise, chills, vertigo.

CV: chest pain, hypotension, peripheral edema, thrombophlebitis, atrial fibrillation, atrial flutter, *bradycardia,* decreased QT interval, palpitations, supraventricular extrasystoles, supraventricular tachycardia, PVCs, *cardiac arrest,* catheter-site thrombosis.

EENT: optic neuropathy, tinnitus, gingivitis, stomatitis.

GI: abdominal pain, constipation, decreased appetite, diarrhea, nausea, vomiting, dyspepsia, dysgeusia, abdominal distention, gastritis, cholecystitis, cholelithiasis.

GU: hematuria, proteinuria, *acute renal failure.*

Hematologic: *agranulocytosis, leukopenia, pancytopenia.*

Hepatic: increased bilirubin level, elevated LFT values, *hepatitis,* hepatomegaly, *hepatic failure.*

Metabolic: hypoglycemia, *hypokalemia, hypomagnesemia,* hypoalbuminemia, hyponatremia.

Musculoskeletal: back pain, myositis, bone pain, neck pain.

Respiratory: cough, dyspnea, *bronchospasm,* tachypnea.

Skin: pruritus, rash, alopecia, dermatitis, exfoliative dermatitis, erythema, petechiae, urticaria.

Other: injection-site reactions, hypersensitivity reaction, falls.

INTERACTIONS

Drug-drug. *Atorvastatin:* May increase atorvastatin level. Monitor patient for atorvastatin-related adverse reactions.

Bupropion: May decrease bupropion level. Bupropion dosage increase may be needed but shouldn't exceed maximum recommended dose.

Cyclosporine, sirolimus, tacrolimus: May increase levels of concomitant drugs. Monitor concentrations of concomitant drugs; adjust their dosages as needed.

Digoxin: May increase digoxin level. Monitor digoxin level and titrate dose during concurrent use.

Lopinavir–ritonavir: May increase isavuconazonium level and decrease lopinavir and ritonavir levels, which may result in loss of antiviral efficacy. Use cautiously together, and monitor patient closely. Use with high-dose (400 mg) ritonavir is contraindicated.

Midazolam: May increase midazolam level. Consider midazolam dosage reduction.

Mycophenolate mofetil: May increase mycophenolate level. Monitor patient for mycophenolate–related toxicities.

Strong CYP3A4 inducers (carbamazepine, long-acting barbiturates, rifampin): May significantly decrease isavuconazonium level. Concomitant use is contraindicated.

Strong CYP3A4 inhibitors (ketoconazole, high-dose ritonavir): May significantly increase isavuconazonium level. Concomitant use is contraindicated.

Drug-herb. *St. John's wort:* May significantly decrease drug level. Concomitant use is contraindicated.

EFFECTS ON LAB TEST RESULTS

• May increase total bilirubin, AST, ALT, alkaline phosphatase, and GGT levels.
• May decrease potassium, magnesium, albumin, glucose, and sodium levels.
• May decrease WBC count.

CONTRAINDICATIONS & CAUTIONS

• Contraindicated in patients hypersensitive to drug or its components.
• Contraindicated with strong CYP3A4 inhibitors and inducers.
• **Alert:** Serious hypersensitivity reactions and severe skin reactions, such as anaphylaxis and Stevens-Johnson syndrome, have been reported. Discontinue drug for severe cutaneous reaction. Use cautiously in patients with serious underlying medical conditions and in patients hypersensitive to other azole drugs.
• Contraindicated in patients with familial short QT syndrome; drug shortens QTc interval in a concentration-related manner.
• Use cautiously in patients with severe hepatic impairment and only when benefits outweigh risks.

• Safety and effectiveness in children younger than age 18 haven't been established.

Dialyzable drug: No.

⚠ **Overdose S&S:** Headache, dizziness, paresthesia, somnolence, disturbance in attention, dysgeusia, dry mouth, diarrhea, oral hypoesthesia, vomiting, hot flushes, anxiety, restlessness, palpitations, tachycardia, photophobia, arthralgia.

PREGNANCY-LACTATION-REPRODUCTION

• There are no adequate studies in pregnant women. Drug may cause fetal harm. Use during pregnancy only if potential benefit outweighs risk to the fetus.
• Women shouldn't breast-feed during therapy.

NURSING CONSIDERATIONS

• Obtain specimens for fungal culture to isolate and identify causative organism before initiating antifungal therapy. May start therapy before results are available; however, adjust therapy accordingly when results are known.
• Infusion-related reactions can occur; monitor patients for dyspnea, hypotension, chills, dizziness, paresthesia, and hypotension. Discontinue infusion if reaction occurs.
• Monitor patients for hypersensitivity reactions and severe skin reactions, including anaphylaxis and Stevens-Johnson syndrome. Discontinue drug for exfoliative cutaneous reaction.
• Assess LFT values before and periodically during treatment.
• Monitor patients who develop abnormal LFT values during therapy for development of more severe hepatic injury. Discontinue drug if liver disease develops that may be attributed to drug.

PATIENT TEACHING

• Advise patient that routine blood tests will be needed to evaluate liver function.
• Instruct patient to report any adverse reactions, including infusion-related and skin-related reactions, to prescriber.
• Counsel patient to swallow capsules whole.

Reactions in bold italics are *life-threatening*. Interactions may have a *rapid onset* or a *delayed onset*.

• Instruct female patient to inform prescriber if she becomes pregnant during therapy. Inform her of fetal risks.
• Warn female patient not to breast-feed during therapy.

isoniazid (INH, isonicotinic acid hydrazide)
eye-soe-NYE-a-zid

Isotamine ✤, PDP-Isoniazid ✤

Therapeutic class: Antituberculotics
Pharmacologic class: Isonicotinic acid hydrazines

AVAILABLE FORMS
Injection: 100 mg/mL
Oral solution: 50 mg/5 mL
Tablets: 50 mg ✤, 100 mg, 300 mg

INDICATIONS & DOSAGES
Adjust-a-dose (for all indications): Give dose after hemodialysis.
➤ **Actively growing tubercle bacilli**
Adults and children age 15 and older: 5 mg/kg daily P.O. or I.M. in a single daily dose, up to 300 mg/day, with other drugs, continued for 6 months to 2 years. For intermittent multiple-drug regimen, 15 mg/kg (up to 900 mg) P.O. or I.M. up to 3 times/week.
Infants and children: 10 to 15 mg/kg P.O. or I.M. in a single daily dose, up to 300 mg/day, continued long enough to prevent relapse. Give with at least one other antituberculotic. For intermittent multidrug regimen, 20 to 40 mg/kg (up to 900 mg) P.O. or I.M. two or three times weekly.
➤ **To prevent tubercle bacilli in those exposed to TB or those with positive skin test results whose chest X-rays and bacteriologic study results indicate non-progressive TB**
Adults weighing more than 30 kg: 300 mg P.O. daily in a single dose, continued for 6 months to 1 year.
Infants and children: 10 mg/kg P.O. daily in a single dose, up to 300 mg/day, continued for up to 1 year. In situations in which adherence with daily preventative therapy can't be assured, 20 to 30 mg/kg (not to exceed

900 mg) twice weekly under the direct observation of a health care worker at the time of administration.

ADMINISTRATION
P.O.
• Always give drug with other antituberculotics to prevent development of resistant organisms.
• Don't give with food.
I.M.
• Solution may crystallize at a low temperature. Warm vial to room temperature before use to redissolve crystals.
• Inject deep I.M. into a large muscle mass.

ACTION
May inhibit cell-wall biosynthesis by interfering with lipid and DNA synthesis; bactericidal.

Route	Onset	Peak	Duration
P.O., I.M.	Unknown	1–2 hr	Unknown

Half-life: 1 to 4 hours.

ADVERSE REACTIONS
CNS: peripheral neuropathy, *seizures, toxic encephalopathy,* memory impairment, toxic psychosis.
EENT: optic neuritis and atrophy.
GI: epigastric distress, nausea, vomiting.
Hematologic: *agranulocytosis, aplastic anemia, thrombocytopenia,* eosinophilia, hemolytic anemia, sideroblastic anemia.
Hepatic: *hepatitis,* bilirubinemia, jaundice.
Metabolic: hyperglycemia, hypocalcemia, hypophosphatemia, *metabolic acidosis.*
Skin: irritation at injection site.
Other: gynecomastia, hypersensitivity reactions, pyridoxine deficiency, rheumatic and lupuslike syndromes.

INTERACTIONS
Drug-drug. *Acetaminophen:* May inhibit acetaminophen metabolism. Monitor patient closely for hepatotoxicity.
Antacids and laxatives containing aluminum: May decrease isoniazid absorption. Give isoniazid at least 1 hour before antacid or laxative.
Benzodiazepines (diazepam, triazolam): May inhibit metabolic clearance of benzodiazepines that undergo oxidative metabolism,

possibly increasing benzodiazepine activity. Monitor for adverse effects.

Carbamazepine: May increase carbamazepine levels. Monitor drug levels closely.

Cycloserine: May increase CNS adverse reactions. Use safety precautions.

Disulfiram: May cause neurologic symptoms, including changes in behavior and coordination. Avoid using together.

Enflurane: In rapid acetylators of isoniazid, may cause high-output renal failure because of nephrotoxic inorganic fluoride level. Monitor renal function.

Ketoconazole: May decrease ketoconazole level. Monitor for lack of effectiveness.

Meperidine: May increase CNS adverse reactions and hypotension. Use safety precautions.

Oral anticoagulants: May enhance anticoagulant activity. Monitor PT and INR.

Phenytoin: May inhibit phenytoin metabolism and increase phenytoin level. Monitor patient for phenytoin toxicity.

Rifampin: May increase the risk of hepatotoxicity. Monitor LFTs closely.

Drug-food. *Foods containing histamines (saury, skipjack, tuna, other tropical fish):* May cause headache, sweating, palpitations, flushing, diarrhea, itching, wheezing, dyspnea, or hypotension. Patients should avoid these foods during therapy.

Foods containing tyramine (aged cheese, beer, chocolate): May cause hypertensive crisis. Patients should avoid such foods.

Drug-lifestyle. *Alcohol use:* May increase risk of drug-related hepatitis. Discourage use of alcohol.

EFFECTS ON LAB TEST RESULTS

• May increase transaminase, glucose, and bilirubin levels. May decrease calcium, phosphate, and Hb levels.

• May increase eosinophil count. May decrease granulocyte and platelet counts.

• May alter result of urine glucose tests that use cupric sulfate method, such as Benedict reagent and Diastix.

CONTRAINDICATIONS & CAUTIONS

Black Box Warning Contraindicated in patients with acute hepatic disease or isoniazid-related liver damage. Severe

and sometimes fatal hepatitis associated with drug may occur even after months of treatment but usually occurs during first 3 months of treatment. Risk of developing hepatitis is age-related (increases with age), increases with daily alcohol use, and may be more common in black and Hispanic women, particularly during the postpartum period. If signs or symptoms suggest hepatic damage, discontinue isoniazid because a more severe form of liver damage can occur. ■

• Use cautiously in the elderly, those with chronic non–isoniazid-related liver disease or chronic alcoholism, those with seizure disorders (especially if taking phenytoin), and those with severe renal impairment.

Dialyzable drug: Yes.

⚠ **Overdose S&S:** Nausea, vomiting, dizziness, slurring of speech, blurring of vision, visual hallucinations, respiratory distress, CNS depression progressing from stupor to coma, seizures, severe metabolic acidosis, acetonuria, hyperglycemia.

PREGNANCY-LACTATION-REPRODUCTION

• There are no adequate studies in pregnant women; however, drug should be used as a treatment for active TB during pregnancy because benefit justifies potential risk to the fetus.

• Weigh benefit of preventive therapy against possible risk to the fetus. Preventive therapy generally should be started after delivery to prevent putting fetus at risk for exposure.

• Small amounts of drug in breast milk don't produce toxicity in breast-feeding infants. Breast-feeding shouldn't be discouraged.

NURSING CONSIDERATIONS

• Drug's pharmacokinetics vary among patients because drug is metabolized in the liver by genetically controlled acetylation. Fast acetylators metabolize drug up to 5 times faster than slow acetylators. About 50% of blacks and whites are fast acetylators; more than 80% of Chinese, Japanese, and Inuits are fast acetylators. A report suggests the risk of fatal hepatitis increases in black and Hispanic women and in the postpartum period. The risk of hepatitis

---

increases with daily alcohol use and with age.
• Peripheral neuropathy is more common in patients who are slow acetylators, malnourished, alcoholic, or diabetic. Give pyridoxine to prevent peripheral neuropathy.
Black Box Warning Monitor and interview patients monthly. For those patients older than age 35, also measure hepatic enzyme levels before and periodically throughout treatment. Elevated LFT results occur in about 15% of patients; most abnormalities are mild and transient, but some may persist throughout treatment, and progressive liver dysfunction may occur. If LFT values exceed 3 to 5 × ULN, strongly consider discontinuing treatment. ■

PATIENT TEACHING
• Instruct patient to take drug exactly as prescribed; warn against stopping drug without prescriber's consent.
• Advise patient that drug shouldn't be taken with food.
Black Box Warning Tell patient to notify prescriber immediately if signs and symptoms of liver impairment occur, such as appetite loss, fatigue, malaise, yellowing of skin or eyes, dark urine, fever of more than 3 days' duration, and abdominal tenderness, particularly of the right upper quadrant. ■
• Advise patient to avoid alcoholic beverages while taking drug. Also tell him to avoid certain foods: fish, such as skipjack tuna, and products containing tyramine, such as aged cheese, beer, and chocolate, because drug has some MAO inhibitor activity.
• Encourage patient to comply fully with treatment, which may take months or years.

isosorbide dinitrate
eye-soe-SOR-bide

ISDN✤, Dilatrate-SR, Isordil

isosorbide mononitrate
Apo-ISMN✤, Imdur✤, Monoket, PMS-ISMN✤, PRO-ISMN✤

Therapeutic class: Antianginals
Pharmacologic class: Nitrates

AVAILABLE FORMS
isosorbide dinitrate
Capsules (sustained-release) ⊕: 40 mg
Tablets: 5 mg, 10 mg, 20 mg, 30 mg, 40 mg
Tablets (sustained-release) ⊕: 40 mg
isosorbide mononitrate
Tablets: 10 mg, 20 mg
Tablets (extended-release) ⊕: 30 mg, 60 mg, 120 mg

INDICATIONS & DOSAGES
➤ **Treatment (Monoket only) and prevention of angina pectoris**
Adults (dinitrate): For immediate release, 5 to 20 mg P.O. b.i.d. to t.i.d., titrated to a maximum of 40 mg P.O. b.i.d. to t.i.d. For sustained release, usual dose is 40 to 160 mg P.O. daily. For Dilatrate-SR only, titrate to a maximum of 160 mg P.O. daily.
Adults (mononitrate): For immediate release, 5 to 20 mg P.O. b.i.d., with the two doses given 7 hours apart. For extended release, 30 to 60 mg P.O. daily; titrate every 3 days to 120 mg P.O. daily. Rarely, 240 mg may be required.
➤ **HF (isosorbide dinitrate)** ◆
Adults: 20 to 30 mg immediate-release P.O. t.i.d. to q.i.d. (in combination with hydralazine) according to American College of Cardiology Foundation/American Heart Association HF guidelines. Maximum dosage is 120 mg daily in divided doses.

ADMINISTRATION
P.O.
• Tell patient taking isosorbide dinitrate to swallow oral tablet whole on an empty stomach either 30 minutes before or 1 to 2 hours after meals.

- Store drug in a cool place, in a tightly closed container, and away from light.
- Don't crush or allow patient to chew extended- or sustained-release tablets or capsules.

ACTION

Thought to reduce cardiac oxygen demand by decreasing preload and afterload. Drug also may increase blood flow through the collateral coronary vessels.

Route	Onset	Peak	Duration
P.O.	15–40 min	Unknown	4–8 hr
P.O. (extended-release)	½–4 hr	Unknown	6–12 hr

Half-life: Dinitrate P.O., 5 to 6 hours; mononitrate, about 5 hours.

ADVERSE REACTIONS

CNS: headache, dizziness, weakness.
CV: orthostatic hypotension, tachycardia, palpitations, ankle edema, flushing, fainting.
EENT: sublingual burning.
GI: nausea, vomiting.
Skin: cutaneous vasodilation, rash.

INTERACTIONS

Drug-drug. *Antihypertensives:* May increase hypotensive effects. Monitor patient closely during initial therapy.
PDE5 inhibitors (avanafil, sildenafil, tadalafil, vardenafil), riociguat: May cause life-threatening hypotension. Use of nitrates in any form with these drugs is contraindicated.
Drug-lifestyle. *Alcohol use:* May increase hypotension. Discourage use together.

EFFECTS ON LAB TEST RESULTS

- May falsely reduce value in cholesterol tests using the Zlatkis-Zak color reaction.

CONTRAINDICATIONS & CAUTIONS

- Contraindicated in patients with hypersensitivity or idiosyncrasy to nitrates and in those with severe hypotension, angle-closure glaucoma, increased ICP, shock, or acute MI with low left ventricular filling pressure.
- Contraindicated in patients concurrently using PDE5 inhibitors or riociguat.

- Use cautiously in patients with blood volume depletion (such as from diuretic therapy), mild hypotension, or suspected right ventricular infarction.
Dialyzable drug: Mononitrate, yes; dinitrate, unknown.
⚠ **Overdose S&S:** Venous pooling, decreased cardiac output, hypotension, methemoglobinemia, headache, confusion, vertigo, fever, palpitations, nausea, vomiting (possibly with colic and bloody diarrhea), syncope, air hunger, dyspnea, slow breathing, diaphoresis, flushed skin, heart block, bradycardia, paralysis, coma.

PREGNANCY-LACTATION-REPRODUCTION

- There are no adequate studies in pregnant women. Use during pregnancy only if clearly needed.
- It isn't known if drug appears in breast milk. Use cautiously in breast-feeding women.

NURSING CONSIDERATIONS

- To prevent tolerance, a nitrate-free interval of 10 to 14 hours per day is recommended. The regimen for isosorbide mononitrate (1 tablet on awakening with the second dose in 7 hours, or 1 extended-release tablet daily) is intended to minimize nitrate tolerance by providing a substantial nitrate-free interval.
- Monitor BP, HR, and intensity and duration of drug response.
- Drug may cause headaches, especially at beginning of therapy. Dosage may be reduced temporarily, but tolerance usually develops. Treat headache with aspirin or acetaminophen.
- Methemoglobinemia has been seen with nitrates. Symptoms are those of impaired oxygen delivery despite adequate cardiac output and adequate arterial partial pressure of oxygen.
- *Look alike–sound alike:* Don't confuse Isordil with Plendil, Isuprel, or Inderal.

PATIENT TEACHING

- Caution patient to take drug as prescribed and to keep it accessible at all times.
⚠ *Alert:* Advise patient that stopping drug abruptly may cause increased angina symptoms and risk of heart attack.

Reactions in bold italics are *life-threatening*. Interactions may have a *rapid onset* or a *delayed onset*.

• Advise patient on isosorbide dinitrate to take oral tablet on an empty stomach either 30 minutes before or 1 to 2 hours after meals and to swallow oral tablets whole.

• Tell patient to stand up by changing to upright position slowly. Advise him to climb stairs carefully and to lie down at first sign of dizziness.

• Caution patient to avoid alcohol because it may worsen low BP effects.

• Advise patient that use of sildenafil, tadalafil, vardenafil, or avanafil with any nitrate may cause severe low BP. Patient should talk to his prescriber before using these drugs together.

• Tell patient to store drug in a cool dark place, in a tightly closed container.

isotretinoin
eye-so-TRET-i-noyn

Absorica, Claravis, Myorisan, Zenatane

Therapeutic class: Antiacne drugs
Pharmacologic class: Retinoic acid derivatives

AVAILABLE FORMS
Capsules: 10 mg, 20 mg, 25 mg, 30 mg, 35 mg, 40 mg

INDICATIONS & DOSAGES
➤ **Severe nodular acne that's unresponsive to conventional therapy**
Adults and adolescents older than age 12: 0.5 to 1 mg/kg P.O. daily in two divided doses with food for 15 to 20 weeks. Or, 2 mg/kg/day for adults whose disease is very severe with scarring or whose disease is primarily on the trunk.

ADMINISTRATION
P.O.
• Before use, have patient read patient information and sign consent form.
• Give drug with or shortly after meals to facilitate absorption.

ACTION
May normalize keratinization, reversibly decrease size of sebaceous glands, and make sebum less viscous and less likely to plug follicles.

Route	Onset	Peak	Duration
P.O.	Unknown	3–5 hr	Unknown

Half-life: 21 to 24 hours.

ADVERSE REACTIONS
CNS: pseudotumor cerebri, depression, *psychosis, suicidal ideation or attempts, suicide, aggressive and violent behavior,* emotional instability, headache, fatigue, dizziness, drowsiness, insomnia, weakness.
CV: palpitations, *stroke,* tachycardia.
EENT: conjunctivitis, epistaxis, drying of mucous membranes, dry nose, corneal deposits, dry eyes, hearing impairment (sometimes irreversible), decreased night vision, visual disturbances.
GI: nonspecific GI symptoms, nausea, vomiting, abdominal pain, dry mouth, anorexia, gum bleeding and inflammation, *acute pancreatitis,* inflammatory bowel disease.
GU: abnormal menses, hematuria.
Hematologic: increased erythrocyte sedimentation rate, anemia, *thrombocytosis.*
Hepatic: *hepatitis.*
Metabolic: hypertriglyceridemia, hyperglycemia.
Musculoskeletal: *rhabdomyolysis,* skeletal hyperostosis, tendon and ligament calcification, premature epiphyseal closure, decreased bone mineral density and other bone abnormalities, back pain, arthralgia, arthritis, tendinitis.
Respiratory: *bronchospasm,* respiratory tract infections.
Skin: cheilitis, cheilosis, fragility, rash, dry skin, facial skin desquamation, petechiae, pruritus, nail brittleness, thinning of hair, skin infection, peeling of palms and toes, photosensitivity reaction.

INTERACTIONS
Drug-drug. *Corticosteroids:* May increase risk of osteoporosis. Use together cautiously.
Medicated soaps, cleansers, and cover-ups; preparations containing alcohol; topical resorcinol peeling agents (benzoyl peroxide): May have cumulative drying effect. Use together cautiously.

Micro-dose progesterone hormonal contraceptives ("minipills") that don't contain estrogen: May decrease effectiveness of contraceptive. Advise patient to use different contraceptive method.

Phenytoin: May increase risk of osteomalacia. Use together cautiously.

Products containing vitamin A: May increase toxic effects of isotretinoin. Avoid using together.

Tetracyclines: May increase risk of pseudotumor cerebri. Avoid using together.

Drug-food. *Any high-fat food:* May increase absorption of drug. Advise patient to take drug with milk, a meal, or shortly after a meal.

Drug-lifestyle. *Alcohol use:* May increase risk of hypertriglyceridemia. Discourage use together.

Sun exposure: May increase photosensitivity reaction. Advise patient to avoid excessive sunlight exposure.

EFFECTS ON LAB TEST RESULTS

• May increase AST, ALT, alkaline phosphatase, triglyceride, glucose, and uric acid levels.

• May decrease serum HDL levels.

• May increase platelet count and erythrocyte sedimentation rate.

CONTRAINDICATIONS & CAUTIONS

• Contraindicated in patients hypersensitive to parabens (used as preservatives), vitamin A, or other retinoids.

• Use cautiously in patients with a history of mental illness or a family history of psychiatric disorders, asthma, liver disease, diabetes, heart disease, hypertriglyceridemia, hearing impairment, osteoporosis, genetic predisposition for age-related osteoporosis, history of childhood osteoporosis, weak bones, anorexia nervosa, osteomalacia, or other disorders of bone metabolism.

• Drug may cause erythema multiforme and severe skin reactions (such as Stevens-Johnson syndrome or toxic epidermal necrolysis), which may be serious and result in hospitalization, disability, life-threatening events, or death.

Dialyzable drug: Unknown.

⚠ *Overdose S&S:* Vomiting, facial flushing, abdominal pain, headache, dizziness, ataxia.

PREGNANCY-LACTATION-REPRODUCTION

Black Box Warning Women and adolescents who are pregnant or who may become pregnant must not use drug. There is an extremely high risk of severe birth defects if pregnancy occurs while patient is taking isotretinoin in any amount, even for short periods. Potentially, any fetus exposed during pregnancy can be affected; there are no accurate means of determining whether an exposed fetus has been affected. There is an increased risk of spontaneous abortion, and premature births have been reported. Cases of IQ scores less than 85 with or without other abnormalities have been reported. Documented external abnormalities include skull abnormalities, ear abnormalities (anotia, micropinna, small or absent external auditory canals), eye abnormalities (microphthalmia), facial dysmorphia, and cleft palate. Documented internal abnormalities include CNS abnormalities (cerebral abnormalities, cerebellar malformation, hydrocephalus, microcephaly, cranial nerve deficit), CV abnormalities, thymus gland abnormality, and parathyroid hormone deficiency. In some cases, these abnormalities have resulted in death. ■

Black Box Warning To minimize risk of fetal exposure, drug is only available through a restricted FDA-approved distribution program called iPLEDGE. ■

🖲 *Alert:* Patient must have negative results from two urine or serum pregnancy tests, one performed in the office when patient is qualified for therapy and the second performed during the first 5 days of the next normal menstrual period immediately preceding beginning of therapy. A pregnancy test must be repeated every month and must be negative before each course of therapy. For patients with amenorrhea, the second test should be done within 7 days after office visit and immediately preceding beginning of therapy. A pregnancy test must be repeated every month before patient receives the prescription. For patients with irregular cycles, or for those using a contraceptive method that precludes withdrawal bleeding, the second pregnancy test must be done within 7 days after office visit, immediately preceding beginning of therapy, and after

---

patient has used two forms of contraception for 1 month.

Black Box Warning If pregnancy does occur during treatment, discontinue drug immediately and refer patient to an obstetrician-gynecologist experienced in reproductive toxicity. ■

• It isn't known if drug appears in breast milk. Patient should discontinue breast-feeding or discontinue drug.

NURSING CONSIDERATIONS

• If total nodule count has been reduced by more than 70% before patient has completed 15 to 20 weeks of treatment, drug may be discontinued.

• Monitor baseline lipid studies, LFTs, and pregnancy tests before therapy and at monthly intervals.

• Regularly monitor glucose level and CK levels in patients who participate in vigorous physical activity.

• Closely watch for and report severe skin reactions. Drug may need to be discontinued.

• Most adverse reactions occur at doses exceeding 1 mg/kg daily. Reactions are generally reversible when therapy is stopped or dosage is reduced.

🕄 **Alert:** If patient experiences headache, nausea and vomiting, or visual disturbances, screen for papilledema. Signs and symptoms of pseudotumor cerebri require stopping the drug immediately and beginning neurologic interventions promptly.

🕄 **Alert:** Monitor patient for mood disturbance, psychosis, aggressive behavior, or suicidal ideation. Drug may need to be discontinued and patient evaluated.

• A second course of therapy may begin 8 weeks after completion of the first course, if necessary. Improvements may continue after first course is complete.

• Patients may be at increased risk of bone fractures or injury when participating in sports with repetitive impact.

• Spontaneous reports of osteoporosis, osteopenia, bone fractures, and delayed healing of bone fractures have occurred in patients taking drug. To decrease this risk, don't exceed recommended doses and duration.

PATIENT TEACHING

🕄 **Alert:** Warn woman of childbearing potential that, if this drug is used during pregnancy, severe fetal abnormalities may occur. Advise her to either abstain from sex or use two reliable forms of contraception simultaneously for 1 month before, during, and for 1 month after treatment. An isotretinoin medication guide must be given to patient each time isotretinoin is dispensed, as required by law.

• Advise patient to take drug with or shortly after meals to facilitate absorption.

• Tell patient to immediately report visual disturbances and bone, muscle, or joint pain.

• Warn patient that contact lenses may feel uncomfortable during therapy.

• Advise patient not to drive at night until effect on vision is known. Drug may decrease night vision.

• Warn patient against using abrasives, medicated soaps and cleansers, acne preparations containing peeling drugs, and topical products containing alcohol (including cosmetics, aftershave, cologne) because they may cause cumulative irritation or excessive drying of skin.

• Tell patient to avoid prolonged sun exposure and to use sunblock. Drug may have additive effect if used with other drugs that cause photosensitivity reaction.

• Warn patient that transient exacerbations may occur during therapy.

• Warn patient not to donate blood during therapy and for 1 month after stopping drug because drug could harm fetus of a pregnant recipient.

• Tell patient to report adverse reactions immediately, especially depression, suicidal thoughts, persistent headaches, visual disturbances, severe skin reactions, and persistent GI pain.

🕄 **Alert:** Advise patient to read iPLEDGE carefully and to fully understand all information before signing it.

itraconazole
eye-tra-KON-a-zole

Onmel, Sporanox

Therapeutic class: Antifungals
Pharmacologic class: Synthetic triazoles

AVAILABLE FORMS
Capsules: 100 mg
Oral solution: 10 mg/mL
Tablets: 200 mg

INDICATIONS & DOSAGES
➤ **Pulmonary and extrapulmonary blastomycosis, nonmeningeal histoplasmosis (capsules)**
Adults: 200 mg P.O. daily; increase as needed and tolerated by 100 mg to maximum of 400 mg daily. Give dosages exceeding 200 mg P.O. daily in two divided doses. Continue treatment for at least 3 months. In life-threatening illness, give a loading dose of 200 mg P.O. t.i.d. for 3 days.
➤ **Aspergillosis (capsules)**
Adults: 200 to 400 mg P.O. daily for at least 3 months. In life-threatening illness, give a loading dose of 200 mg P.O. t.i.d. for first 3 days of treatment.
➤ **Onychomycosis of the toenail (with or without fingernail involvement)**
Adults: 200 mg P.O. once daily for 12 consecutive weeks.
➤ **Onychomycosis of the fingernail**
Adults: 200 mg P.O. b.i.d. for 1 week, followed by 3 weeks drug-free. Repeat dosage.
➤ **Oropharyngeal candidiasis**
Adults: 200 mg oral solution swished in mouth vigorously and swallowed daily, for 1 to 2 weeks.
➤ **Oropharyngeal candidiasis in patients unresponsive to fluconazole tablets**
Adults: 100 mg oral solution swished in mouth vigorously and swallowed b.i.d., for 2 to 4 weeks.
➤ **Esophageal candidiasis**
Adults: 100 to 200 mg oral solution swished in mouth vigorously and swallowed daily, for at least 3 weeks. Treatment should continue for 2 weeks after symptoms resolve.

ADMINISTRATION
P.O.
● Before starting therapy, confirm diagnosis of onychomycosis by sending nail specimens for testing.
● Don't interchange capsules and oral solution.
● Give capsules and tablets with a full meal.
● Give oral solution on an empty stomach if possible.
● Have patient vigorously swish oral solution in mouth for several seconds and then swallow.

ACTION
Interferes with fungal cell-wall synthesis by inhibiting ergosterol formation and increasing cell-wall permeability, leading to osmotic instability.

Route	Onset	Peak	Duration
P.O.	Unknown	2–5 hr	Unknown

Half-life: 34 to 42 hours.

ADVERSE REACTIONS
CNS: headache, fever, dizziness, somnolence, fatigue, malaise, asthenia, pain, tremor, abnormal dreams, anxiety, depression.
CV: *HF,* hypertension, edema, orthostatic hypotension.
EENT: rhinitis, sinusitis, pharyngitis.
GI: nausea, vomiting, diarrhea, abdominal pain, anorexia, dyspepsia, flatulence, increased appetite, constipation, gastritis, gastroenteritis, ulcerative stomatitis, gingivitis.
GU: albuminuria.
Hematologic: *neutropenia.*
Hepatic: *hepatotoxicity, liver failure,* impaired hepatic function.
Metabolic: hypokalemia, hypertriglyceridemia.
Musculoskeletal: myalgia.
Respiratory: *pulmonary edema,* URI.
Skin: rash, pruritus.
Other: decreased libido, injury, herpes zoster, hypersensitivity reactions (urticaria, *angioedema, Stevens-Johnson syndrome*).

INTERACTIONS
Drug-drug. *Alprazolam:* May increase and prolong drug levels, CNS depression,

and psychomotor impairment. Avoid using together.

*Antacids, carbamazepine, H₂-receptor antagonists, isoniazid, phenobarbital, **phenytoin**, rifabutin, rifampin:* May decrease itraconazole level. Avoid using together.
Chlordiazepoxide, clonazepam, clorazepate, diazepam, estazolam, flurazepam, quazepam: May increase and prolong drug levels, CNS depression, and psychomotor impairment. Avoid using together.
Clarithromycin, erythromycin: May increase itraconazole levels. Monitor patient for signs of itraconazole toxicity.
*Cyclosporine, **digoxin**, tacrolimus:* May increase levels of these drugs. Monitor drug levels.
Black Box Warning *Dofetilide, ergometrine, ergot alkaloids, ergotamine, felodipine, levacetylmethadol, lovastatin, methadone, methylergotamine, midazolam (oral), nisoldipine, pimozide, quinidine, simvastatin, triazolam:* May increase levels of these drugs by CYP450 metabolism, causing serious CV events, including torsades de pointes, QT-interval prolongation, ventricular tachycardia, cardiac arrest, and sudden death. Use together is contraindicated. ■
HMG-CoA reductase inhibitors (atorvastatin, fluvastatin, pravastatin): May increase levels and adverse effects of these drugs. Avoid using together, or reduce dose of HMG-CoA reductase inhibitor.
NNRTIs (nevirapine): May decrease itraconazole level. Use together isn't recommended.
Oral anticoagulants: May enhance anticoagulant effect. Monitor PT and INR.
Oral antidiabetics: May cause hypoglycemia, similar to effect of other antifungals. Monitor glucose level. Avoid using together.
PDE5 inhibitors (avanafil, sildenafil, tadalafil, vardenafil): May increase levels of these drugs, increasing adverse effects. Give PDE5 inhibitors with caution and in reduced doses.
Protease inhibitors (indinavir, ritonavir, saquinavir): May increase levels of these drugs; indinavir and ritonavir may increase itraconazole levels. Monitor patient for toxicity.

EFFECTS ON LAB TEST RESULTS
● May increase alkaline phosphatase, ALT, AST, bilirubin, triglyceride, and GGT levels. May decrease potassium level.

CONTRAINDICATIONS & CAUTIONS
Black Box Warning Contraindicated in patients hypersensitive to drug; in those receiving methadone, disopyramide, dofetilide, dronedarone, quinidine, ergot alkaloids (dihydroergotamine, ergometrine [ergonovine], ergotamine, methylergometrine [methylergonovine]), irinotecan, lurasidone, oral midazolam, pimozide, triazolam, felodipine, nisoldipine, ranolazine, eplerenone, cisapride, lovastatin, simvastatin, ticagrelor, colchicine, fesoterodine, telithromycin, and solifenacin; and in patients with varying degrees of renal or hepatic impairment. Administration with itraconazole can cause elevated plasma concentrations and may increase or prolong pharmacologic effects and adverse reactions to these drugs. For example, increased plasma concentrations of some of these drugs can lead to QT prolongation and ventricular tachyarrhythmias, including torsades de pointes. ■
● Use cautiously in patients with hypochlorhydria; they may not absorb drug readily.
Black Box Warning Don't use drug to treat onychomycosis in patients with evidence of ventricular dysfunction, such as HF or history of HF. If signs or symptoms of HF occur while giving oral solution, reassess continued use. If signs or symptoms of HF occur while giving capsules or tablets, discontinue use. ■
● Use cautiously in HIV-infected patients because hypochlorhydria can accompany HIV infection.
● Use cautiously in patients receiving other highly bound drugs.
● Drug may cause transient or permanent hearing loss, particularly in elderly patients.
Dialyzable drug: No.

PREGNANCY-LACTATION-REPRODUCTION
● Don't use to treat onychomycosis in pregnant women, those contemplating pregnancy, or women of childbearing potential unless they are using effective contraceptive

measures and they begin therapy on the second or third day after onset of menses. Effective contraception should be continued throughout therapy and for 2 months after therapy ends.

• Drug may cause maternal or fetal harm. Use to treat systemic fungal infections in pregnant women only if benefit justifies potential risk.

• Drug appears in breast milk. Weigh expected benefits for mother against potential risk to infant.

NURSING CONSIDERATIONS

🕄 *Alert:* Oral solution isn't interchangeable with other forms.

• Perform baseline LFTs and monitor results periodically. In patients with baseline hepatic impairment, give drug only if patient's condition is life threatening. If liver dysfunction occurs during therapy, notify prescriber immediately.

• Monitor patient for hearing loss.

PATIENT TEACHING

• Teach patient to recognize and report signs and symptoms of liver disease (anorexia, dark urine, pale stools, unusual fatigue, and jaundice) or hearing loss.

• Instruct patient not to use oral solution interchangeably with capsules or tablets.

• For the oral solution, tell patient to take 10 mL at a time.

• Tell patient to take solution without food; capsules or tablets, with a full meal.

• Urge patient to list other drugs he's taking, to avoid drug interactions.

• Advise female patient of childbearing potential that an effective form of contraception must be used during therapy and for two menstrual cycles after stopping therapy with capsules or tablets.

ivabradine
eye-VAB-ra-deen

Corlanor

Therapeutic class: Antianginals
Pharmacologic class: Cyclic nucleotide-gated channel blockers

AVAILABLE FORMS
Tablets: 5 mg, 7.5 mg

INDICATIONS & DOSAGES

➤ **To reduce risk of hospitalization for worsening HF in patients with stable, symptomatic chronic HF with LVEF of 35% or more who are in sinus rhythm with resting HR of 70 beats/minute (bpm) or more and either are on maximally tolerated doses of beta blockers or have a contraindication to beta blocker use**

Adults: Initially, 5 mg P.O. b.i.d. with meals. After 2 weeks, adjust dosage to achieve resting HR of 50 to 60 bpm if necessary. Maximum dose is 7.5 mg b.i.d.

Adjust-a-dose: If HR is greater than 60 bpm, increase dosage by 2.5 mg b.i.d. up to a maximum of 7.5 mg b.i.d. If HR is less than 50 bpm or patient has signs and symptoms of bradycardia, decrease dosage by 2.5 mg b.i.d.; however, if current dosage is 2.5 mg b.i.d., discontinue therapy. In patients with a history of conduction defects and in those whose bradycardia could lead to hemodynamic compromise, initiate therapy at 2.5 mg b.i.d. before increasing dosage based on HR.

ADMINISTRATION
P.O.
• Give with meals.
• Store tablets at room temperature.

ACTION
Reduces HR by blocking hyperpolarization-activated cyclic nucleotide-gated channel responsible for the cardiac pacemaker I_f current.

Route	Onset	Peak	Duration
P.O.	Rapid	2 hr	Unknown

Half-life: 6 hours.

ADVERSE REACTIONS
CV: *bradycardia, conduction disturbances,* hypertension, atrial fibrillation.
EENT: phosphenes, visual brightness.

INTERACTIONS
Drug-drug. *CYP3A4 inducers (barbiturates, phenytoin, rifampin):* May decrease ivabradine level. Avoid use together.
Drugs that decrease HR (amiodarone, beta blockers, digoxin): May increase risk of bradycardia. Monitor HR.
Moderate CYP3A4 inhibitors (diltiazem, verapamil): May increase ivabradine level, causing bradycardia and conduction disturbances. Avoid use together.
Strong CYP3A4 inhibitors (clarithromycin, HIV protease inhibitors [nelfinavir], itraconazole, nefazodone, telithromycin): May significantly increase ivabradine level, leading to bradycardia and conduction disturbances. Use together is contraindicated.
Drug-herb. *St. John's wort:* May decrease ivabradine level. Discourage use together.
Drug-food. *Grapefruit juice:* May increase ivabradine level, causing bradycardia and conduction disturbances. Discourage use together.

EFFECTS ON LAB TEST RESULTS
None reported.

CONTRAINDICATIONS & CAUTIONS
• Contraindicated in patients hypersensitive to drug or its components and in those with acute decompensated HF or BP less than 90/50 mm Hg; sick sinus syndrome, SA block, or third-degree AV block unless a functioning demand pacemaker is present; resting HR less than 60 bpm before treatment; severe hepatic impairment; pacemaker dependence (HR maintained exclusively by the pacemaker); or concomitant use of strong CYP3A4 inhibitors.
• Avoid use in patients with second-degree AV block unless a functioning demand pacemaker is present and in those taking diltiazem or verapamil concomitantly.
• Use cautiously in patients with sinus node dysfunction, conduction defects (first- or second-degree AV block, bundle-branch block), or ventricular dyssynchrony and in those taking other negative chronotropes

(digoxin, amiodarone) concomitantly. Drug may increase risk of bradycardia, sinus arrest, and heart block.
• Not recommended in those with demand pacemakers set to rates of 60 bpm or greater.
• Use cautiously in patients with CrCl of less than 15 mL/minute.
• Safety and effectiveness in children haven't been established.
Dialyzable drug: Unknown.
⚠ **Overdose S&S:** Severe and prolonged bradycardia.

PREGNANCY-LACTATION-REPRODUCTION
• There are no adequate studies in pregnant women, but animal studies showed fetal harm. Avoid use during pregnancy because of risk of fetal harm; advise pregnant women of potential risk to the fetus. Women of childbearing potential should use effective contraception during treatment.
• If drug must be used during pregnancy, monitor patients, especially during first trimester, for destabilization of HF that could result from slowing HR. Monitor pregnant women with HF who are in the third trimester for signs and symptoms of preterm birth. Pregnant patients with LVEF less than 35% on maximally tolerated doses of beta blockers may be particularly HR-dependent for augmenting cardiac output.
• Drug may appear in breast milk. Women shouldn't breast-feed during therapy.

NURSING CONSIDERATIONS
• Regularly monitor cardiac rhythm. Drug may increase risk of atrial fibrillation. Discontinue drug if atrial fibrillation develops.
• Monitor patients for phosphenes (transient enhanced brightness in a limited area of the visual field, halos, image decomposition, colored bright lights, or multiple images), which may be triggered by sudden variations in light intensity. Onset is typically within first 2 months of treatment; phosphenes may resolve without discontinuing treatment.

PATIENT TEACHING
• Instruct patient to take tablets with meals.
• Warn female patient of childbearing potential that drug may cause fetal harm. Instruct her to use effective contraception

during treatment and to notify prescriber if she is pregnant or suspects she is pregnant.

● Advise breast-feeding patient to avoid breast-feeding during therapy because of potential risk of fetal harm.

● Advise patient to immediately seek medical attention for significant decreases in HR or such signs and symptoms as dizziness, fatigue, or hypotension.

● Advise patient to report all adverse reactions and to immediately report signs and symptoms of atrial fibrillation (heart palpitations or racing, chest pressure, worsened shortness of breath).

● Warn patient about possibility of developing luminous phenomena (phosphenes), resulting in transient visual brightness. Advise patient to use caution while driving or operating machinery in situations in which sudden changes in light intensity may occur, especially at night. Inform patient that phosphenes may subside during treatment.

● Warn patient to avoid grapefruit juice and St. John's wort and to report all drugs and supplements being taken before starting drug.

ixazomib citrate
See NEW DRUGS for information.

ixekizumab
See NEW DRUGS for information.

ketoconazole (oral)
kee-toe-KOE-na-zole

Therapeutic class: Antifungals
Pharmacologic class: Imidazole derivatives

AVAILABLE FORMS
Tablets: 200 mg

INDICATIONS & DOSAGES
Black Box Warning Drug should only be used when other effective antifungal therapy isn't available or tolerated and potential benefits outweigh potential risks. ∎

➤ **Fungal infections (coccidioidomycosis, blastomycosis, histoplasmosis, chromomycosis, and paracoccidioidomycosis)**
Adults: Initially, 200 mg P.O. daily in a single dose. May increase dosage to 400 mg

once daily in patients who don't respond. Maximum dosage is 400 mg once daily.
Children age 2 and older: 3.3 to 6.6 mg/kg P.O. daily in a single dose. Maximum dosage is 400 mg once daily.

➤ **Prostate cancer, advanced** ◆
Adults: 400 mg P.O. t.i.d. (in combination with oral hydrocortisone) until disease progression.

ADMINISTRATION
P.O.
● Patient should wait at least 2 hours after dose before taking antacids, anticholinergics, and H_2-receptor antagonists.

ACTION
Interferes with fungal cell-wall synthesis by inhibiting formation of ergosterol and increasing cell-wall permeability that makes the fungus susceptible to osmotic instability.

Route	Onset	Peak	Duration
P.O.	Unknown	1–2 hr	Unknown

Half-life: 8 hours.

ADVERSE REACTIONS
CNS: insomnia, nervousness, dizziness, asthenia, headache, fatigue, malaise, paresthesia, somnolence, fever, chills.
CV: orthostatic hypotension, peripheral edema, prolonged QT interval.
EENT: epistaxis, photophobia.
GI: nausea, vomiting, upper abdominal pain, diarrhea, constipation, dry mouth, dysgeusia, dyspepsia, flatulence, increased appetite, anorexia, tongue discoloration.
Hematologic: *leukopenia, thrombocytopenia.*
Hepatic: *hepatitis,* jaundice.
Skin: pruritus, rash, *erythema multiforme,* dermatitis, erythema, alopecia, xeroderma.
Other: *anaphylaxis,* gynecomastia, hot flush, adrenal insufficiency.

INTERACTIONS
Drug-drug. *Aliskiren:* May increase aliskiren level. Monitor therapy.
Alosetron: May increase alosetron serum concentration. Monitor therapy.
Amphotericin B: May decrease therapeutic effect of amphotericin B. Monitor therapeutic effect.

Antacids, anticholinergics, H₂-receptor antagonists: May decrease ketoconazole absorption. Wait at least 2 hours after ketoconazole dose before giving these drugs.

Bosentan: May increase risk of bosentan-related adverse effects. Monitor closely.

Buspirone: May increase buspirone level and risk of adverse effects. Reduce initial dosage of buspirone; adjust dosage as needed.

Calcium channel blockers metabolized by CYP3A4 pathway (amlodipine, felodipine, nicardipine, nifedipine): May increase plasma concentrations of calcium channel blockers and risk of adverse effects. Monitor plasma concentrations; reduce dosage of calcium channel blockers if needed.

Carbamazepine: May increase carbamazepine level. Closely monitor carbamazepine plasma level.

Chlordiazepoxide, clonazepam, clorazepate, diazepam, estazolam, flurazepam, midazolam, quazepam, triazolam: May increase and prolong levels of these drugs. May cause CNS depression and psychomotor impairment. Avoid using together.

Cilostazol: May increase cilostazol level and risk of cilostazol-related adverse effects such as headache. Consider reducing cilostazol dosage by 50%.

Cyclosporine, methylprednisolone, tacrolimus: May increase levels of these drugs. Monitor drug levels, if appropriate.

Digoxin: May increase digoxin level. Monitor digoxin level.

Black Box Warning *Disopyramide, dofetilide, dronedarone, methadone, pimozide, quinidine, ranolazine:* There is risk of elevated plasma concentrations of these drugs and QT-interval prolongation. Use together is contraindicated. ■

Docetaxel: May prolong clearance of docetaxel by 50%. Consider reducing docetaxel dosage.

Eplerenone: May cause hyperkalemia and hypotension. Use together is contraindicated.

Ergot alkaloids: May cause severe vasospasm and cerebral or extremity ischemia. Use together is contraindicated.

Fentanyl: May increase fentanyl level. Monitor fentanyl-related adverse effects and reduce fentanyl dosage if needed.

HMG-CoA reductase inhibitors (atorvastatin, fluvastatin, lovastatin, pravastatin, simvastatin): May increase levels and adverse effects of these drugs. Use together is contraindicated.

Indinavir: May increase indinavir plasma concentration. Reduce indinavir dosage if needed.

Isoniazid, rifampin, rifabutin: May decrease ketoconazole level. Use together isn't recommended.

Methylprednisolone: May alter methylprednisolone metabolism and methylprednisolone level. Adjust methylprednisolone dosage if needed.

Nevirapine: May decrease ketoconazole concentration. Use together isn't recommended.

Nisoldipine: May increase nisoldipine level. Use together is contraindicated.

Oral antidiabetics: May cause hypoglycemia. Monitor glucose level.

Paclitaxel: May increase paclitaxel level. Monitor patient carefully.

PDE5 inhibitors (sildenafil, tadalafil, vardenafil): May increase levels of these drugs. Use together cautiously and reduce dosage of PDE5 inhibitor.

Phenytoin: May alter metabolism of one or both drugs. Monitor patient for adverse effects.

Ritonavir: May increase bioavailability of ketoconazole. When used together, maximum dosage of ketoconazole is 200 mg/day.

Sirolimus: May increase sirolimus level. Use together isn't recommended.

Tacrolimus (topical): May increase tacrolimus level. Monitor tacrolimus level carefully; adjust dosage if needed.

Telithromycin: May alter telithromycin metabolism. Use cautiously and monitor patient for telithromycin-related adverse effects.

Theophylline: May decrease theophylline level. Monitor theophylline level.

Tolterodine: May increase tolterodine level. Consider reducing tolterodine dosage by 50%.

Verapamil: May increase verapamil serum concentration. Use together cautiously.

Vinca alkaloids (vinblastine, vincristine, vinorelbine): May inhibit metabolism of

K

vinca alkaloids. Monitor patient closely for vinca alkaloid–related toxicities.

Warfarin: May enhance effects of anticoagulant. Monitor PT and INR, and adjust dosage as needed.

Drug-herb. *St. John's wort:* May decrease ketoconazole level. Consider therapy modification.

Yew: May inhibit drug metabolism. Discourage use together.

Drug-lifestyle. *Alcohol use:* May cause disulfiram-like reaction (flushing, rash, peripheral edema, nausea, headache). Don't use together.

EFFECTS ON LAB TEST RESULTS
• May increase lipid, alkaline phosphatase, ALT, and AST levels.
• May decrease Hb level and platelet and WBC counts.

CONTRAINDICATIONS & CAUTIONS
• Contraindicated in patients hypersensitive to drug or its components.

Black Box Warning Administration with dofetilide, pimozide, quinidine, methadone, disopyramide, dronedarone, or ranolazine is contraindicated because ketoconazole can cause elevated levels of these drugs and prolong the QT interval, resulting in life-threatening ventricular arrhythmias. ∎

Black Box Warning Drug can cause serious hepatotoxicity that may be fatal or require liver transplantation, even in patients with no obvious risk factors for liver disease. Drug is contraindicated in patients with acute or chronic liver disease. ∎

• Drug decreases adrenal corticosteroid secretions at doses of 400 mg. Don't exceed recommended dose of 400 mg.

Dialyzable drug: No.

PREGNANCY-LACTATION-REPRODUCTION
• There are no adequate studies in pregnant women. Use during pregnancy only if potential benefit justifies potential risk to the fetus.
• Drug has been shown to lower serum testosterone level, which returns to baseline when therapy is discontinued. Testosterone levels are impaired with doses of 800 mg daily and abolished by 1,600 mg daily. Clinical manifestations may include gynecomastia, impotence, and oligospermia.

• Drug appears in breast milk. Women shouldn't breast-feed during therapy.

NURSING CONSIDERATIONS
⚠ *Alert:* Because of risk of hepatotoxicity, drug shouldn't be used for less serious conditions, such as fungal infections of the skin or nails.

Black Box Warning Because of increased risk of hepatotoxicity, monitor patient for signs and symptoms of hepatotoxicity, including elevated liver enzyme levels, nausea that doesn't subside, unusual fatigue, jaundice, dark urine, or pale stool. ∎

⚠ *Alert:* Drug is a potent inhibitor of the CYP450 enzyme system. Giving this drug with drugs metabolized by CYP3A4 may lead to increased drug levels, which could increase or prolong therapeutic and adverse effects.

• Monitor adrenal function in patients with adrenal insufficiency or borderline adrenal function and in those experiencing prolonged periods of stress (such as major surgery).
• Assess liver function status (AST, ALT, total bilirubin, alkaline phosphatase, PT, and INR) before starting drug.
• Measure ALT level weekly for duration of treatment. If ALT levels increase above the ULN or 30% above baseline, or if patient develops signs and symptoms of hepatotoxicity, obtain a full set of LFTs. Repeat LFTs to ensure normalization of values. If drug is restarted, monitor patient frequently.
• Review all medications patient is receiving for potential drug interactions with ketoconazole.

PATIENT TEACHING
• Instruct patient to wait at least 2 hours after dose before taking antacids, anticholinergics, or H2-receptor antagonists.
• Make sure patient understands that treatment should continue until all tests indicate that active fungal infection has subsided. If drug is stopped too soon, infection will recur. Treatment for systemic fungal infections may last 6 months.
• Reassure patient that nausea is common early in therapy but will subside. To minimize nausea, instruct patient to divide daily

---

amount into two doses or to take drug with meals.

• Review signs and symptoms of hepatotoxicity with patient; instruct him to stop drug and notify prescriber if they occur.

• Instruct patient to immediately report irregular heartbeats, palpitations, feeling faint, dizziness, or light-headedness.

• Advise patient to discuss any new drugs or herbal supplements he may be taking with prescriber.

• Caution patient to avoid alcohol consumption during treatment.

ketoconazole (topical)
kee-toe-KOE-na-zole

Extina, Ketoderm❧, Ketozole, Nizoral, Nizoral A-D ◊, Xolegel

Therapeutic class: Antifungals
Pharmacologic class: Imidazoles

AVAILABLE FORMS
Cream: 2%
Foam: 2%
Gel: 2%
Shampoo: 1% ◊, 2%

INDICATIONS & DOSAGES
➤ **Seborrheic dermatitis in immunocompetent patients**
Adults and children age 12 and older: Apply foam to affected area b.i.d. for 4 weeks. Apply gel to affected area once daily for 2 weeks. Apply cream to affected area b.i.d. for 4 weeks or until clearing.
➤ **Tinea corporis, tinea cruris, tinea pedis, tinea versicolor from susceptible organisms; seborrheic dermatitis; cutaneous candidiasis**
Adults: Cover affected and immediate surrounding areas daily for at least 2 weeks. For seborrheic dermatitis, apply b.i.d. for 4 weeks. Patients with tinea pedis need 6 weeks of treatment. For tinea (pityriasis) versicolor, apply 2% shampoo to affected area of damp skin, lather, leave on for 5 minutes, and rinse (one application is usually sufficient).

➤ **Scaling caused by dandruff**
Adults and children age 12 and older: Using 1% OTC shampoo, wet hair, lather, and rinse thoroughly; repeat. Use every 3 to 4 days for up to 8 weeks; then apply only as needed to control dandruff.

ADMINISTRATION
Topical
• Don't let drug come in contact with eyes.
• When using foam, dispense into cap of can or other cool surface; don't spray directly onto affected skin or the hands. If fingers are warm, rinse them in cold water and dry well; then, using fingertips, gently massage foam into affected areas until it disappears.
• Don't wash areas where gel was applied for at least 3 hours. Have patient wait at least 20 minutes after application before applying makeup or sunscreen to the affected areas.

ACTION
Probably inhibits yeast growth by altering the permeability of the cell membrane.

Route	Onset	Peak	Duration
Topical	Unknown	Unknown	Unknown

Half-life: Unknown.

ADVERSE REACTIONS
Skin: abnormal hair texture; increase in normal hair loss; irritation, pruritus, oiliness, or dryness of hair and scalp with shampoo use; scalp pustules; severe irritation, pruritus, and stinging or burning with cream, foam, and gel.

INTERACTIONS
None known.

EFFECTS ON LAB TEST RESULTS
None reported.

CONTRAINDICATIONS & CAUTIONS
• Contraindicated in patients hypersensitive to drug or its components.
• Ketoconazole cream contains sulfites that may cause allergic reactions, including anaphylaxis, in susceptible patients.
Dialyzable drug: No.

K

PREGNANCY-LACTATION-REPRODUCTION
• There are no adequate studies in pregnant women. Use during pregnancy only if potential benefit justifies potential fetal risk.
• It isn't known if appears in breast milk. Patient should discontinue breast-feeding or discontinue drug.

NURSING CONSIDERATIONS
• Most patients show improvement soon after treatment begins.
• Treatment of tinea corporis or tinea cruris should continue for at least 2 weeks to reduce possibility of recurrence.
❸ **Alert:** Product contains sodium sulfite anhydrous, which may cause severe or life-threatening allergic reactions, including anaphylaxis, in patients with asthma.

PATIENT TEACHING
• Tell patient to stop drug and notify prescriber if hypersensitivity reaction occurs.
• Advise patient to check with prescriber if condition worsens; drug may have to be stopped and diagnosis reevaluated.
• Tell patient to avoid using shampoo on scalp if skin is broken or inflamed.
• Advise patient that foam and gel are flammable and to avoid fire, flame, and smoking during and immediately after application.
• Instruct patient to dispense foam into cap of can or other cool surface and not to spray directly onto affected skin or the hands. If fingers are warm, tell patient to rinse them in cold water and dry well; then, using fingertips, to gently massage foam into affected areas until it disappears.
• Instruct patient to not wash areas where gel was applied for at least 3 hours and to wait at least 20 minutes after application before applying makeup or sunscreen to the affected areas.
• Warn patient that shampoo applied to permanent-waved hair removes curl.
• Warn patient to avoid drug contact with eyes.
• Tell patient to continue drug for intended duration of therapy, even if signs and symptoms improve soon after starting treatment.
• Tell patient not to store drug above room temperature (77° F [25° C]) and to protect from light.

ketoprofen
kee-toe-PROE-fen

Therapeutic class: NSAIDs
Pharmacologic class: NSAIDs

AVAILABLE FORMS
Capsules: 50 mg, 75 mg
Capsules (extended-release): 200 mg

INDICATIONS & DOSAGES
Adjust-a-dose (for all indications): For patients age 75 and older, reduce dosage. For patients with mildly impaired renal function, maximum daily dose is 150 mg. For patients with GFR of less than 25 mL/minute/1.73 m^2, ESRD, or impaired liver function and serum albumin level less than 3.5 g/dL, maximum daily dose is 100 mg.
➤ **RA, osteoarthritis**
Adults: 75 mg P.O. t.i.d. or 50 mg P.O. q.i.d., or 200 mg as an extended-release capsule once daily. Maximum dose is 300 mg daily, or 200 mg daily for extended-release capsules.
➤ **Mild to moderate pain, dysmenorrhea**
Adults: 25 to 50 mg P.O. every 6 to 8 hours p.r.n. Maximum dose is 300 mg daily.

ADMINISTRATION
P.O.
• Give drug 30 minutes before or 2 hours after meals with a full glass of water. If adverse GI reactions occur, drug may be given with milk or meals.
• Don't open extended-release capsules.

ACTION
Unknown. Produces anti-inflammatory, analgesic, and antipyretic effects, possibly by inhibiting prostaglandin synthesis.

Route	Onset	Peak	Duration
P.O.	1–2 hr	30–120 min	3–4 hr
P.O. (extended-release)	2–3 hr	6–7 hr	Unknown

Half-life: Immediate-release capsules, 2 to 4 hours; extended-release capsules, 3 to 7½ hours.

ADVERSE REACTIONS

CNS: headache, dizziness, CNS excitation (insomnia, nervousness, and dreams) or CNS depression (somnolence and malaise).
CV: peripheral edema.
EENT: tinnitus, visual disturbances.
GI: dyspepsia, abdominal pain, anorexia, constipation, diarrhea, flatulence, nausea, stomatitis, vomiting.
GU: *nephrotoxicity,* UTI signs and symptoms.
Skin: photosensitivity reactions, rash.

INTERACTIONS

Drug-drug. *Aspirin, corticosteroids:* May increase risk of adverse GI reactions. Avoid using together.
Aspirin, probenecid: May increase ketoprofen level. Avoid using together.
Cyclosporine: May increase nephrotoxicity. Avoid using together.
Hydrochlorothiazide, other diuretics: May decrease diuretic effectiveness. Monitor patient for lack of effect.
Lithium, methotrexate, phenytoin: May increase levels of these drugs, leading to toxicity. Monitor patient closely.
Warfarin: May increase risk of bleeding. Monitor patient closely.
Drug-herb. *Dong quai, feverfew, garlic, ginger, horse chestnut, red clover:* May cause bleeding based on the known effects of components. Discourage use together.
White willow: Herb and drug contain similar components. Discourage use together.
Drug-lifestyle. *Alcohol use:* May cause GI toxicity. Discourage use together.
Smoking: May increase risk of GI bleeding. Discourage use together.
Sun exposure: May cause photosensitivity reactions. Advise patient to avoid excessive sunlight exposure.

EFFECTS ON LAB TEST RESULTS

- May increase creatinine, BUN, ALT, and AST levels.
- May increase bleeding time.
- May increase or decrease iron test results.
- May falsely increase bilirubin level.

CONTRAINDICATIONS & CAUTIONS

- Contraindicated in patients hypersensitive to drug and in those with history of aspirin or NSAID-induced asthma, urticaria, or other allergic reactions.

Black Box Warning Contraindicated for the treatment of perioperative pain after CABG surgery. ■

Black Box Warning NSAIDs can increase risk of heart attack or stroke in patients with or without heart disease or risk factors for heart disease. Risk may increase with duration of use. ■

❸ *Alert:* Risk of heart attack or stroke can occur as early as the first weeks of NSAID use. Risk appears greater at higher doses. Use lowest effective dose for shortest duration possible.

❸ *Alert:* NSAIDs increase risk of HF.
- Drug isn't recommended for children.
- Use cautiously in patients with history of peptic ulcer disease, renal dysfunction, hypertension, HF, or fluid retention.
Dialyzable drug: Unlikely.
⚠ *Overdose S&S:* Lethargy, drowsiness, nausea, vomiting, epigastric pain, respiratory depression, coma, seizures, GI bleeding, hypotension, hypertension, acute renal failure.

PREGNANCY-LACTATION-REPRODUCTION

❸ *Alert:* Use during pregnancy only if potential benefit outweighs risk. Avoid use during last trimester because drug may cause premature closure of the ductus arteriosus.
- It isn't known if drug appears in breast milk. Women shouldn't breast-feed during therapy.

NURSING CONSIDERATIONS

- Don't use sustained-release form for patients in acute pain.
- Because NSAIDs impair synthesis of renal prostaglandins, they can decrease renal blood flow and lead to reversible renal impairment, especially in patients with renal or HF or liver dysfunction, in elderly patients, and in those taking diuretics. Monitor these patients closely.
- Check renal and hepatic function every 6 months or as indicated.
❸ *Alert:* Watch for and immediately evaluate signs and symptoms of heart attack (chest pain, shortness of breath or trouble breathing) or stroke (weakness in one part or side of the body, slurred speech).

K

● Drug decreases platelet adhesion and aggregation, and can prolong bleeding time about 3 to 4 minutes from baseline. **Black Box Warning** NSAIDs cause an increased risk of serious GI adverse events, including bleeding, ulceration, and perforation of the stomach or intestines, which can occur at any time during use and without warning signs and symptoms; it can be fatal. Elderly patients are at greater risk. ∎

Black Box Warning NSAIDs may increase the risk of serious thrombotic events, MI, or stroke, which can be fatal. The risk may be greater with longer use or in patients with CV disease or risk factors for CV disease. ∎

● NSAIDs may mask signs and symptoms of infection because of their antipyretic and anti-inflammatory actions.

PATIENT TEACHING

● Tell patient to take drug 30 minutes before or 2 hours after meals with a full glass of water. If adverse GI reactions occur, patient may take drug with milk or meals.

● Tell patient not to open extended-release capsules.

● **Alert:** Advise patient to seek medical attention immediately if chest pain, shortness of breath or trouble breathing, weakness in one part or side of the body, or slurred speech occurs.

● Tell patient that full therapeutic effect may be delayed for 2 to 4 weeks.

● Teach patient signs and symptoms of GI bleeding, including blood in vomit, urine, or stool; coffee-ground vomit; and black, tarry stools. Tell him to notify prescriber immediately if any of these occurs.

● Alert patient that using with aspirin, alcohol, other NSAIDs, or corticosteroids may increase risk of adverse GI reactions.

● Warn patient to avoid hazardous activities that require mental alertness until CNS effects are known.

● Because of possibility of sensitivity to the sun, advise patient to use a sunblock, wear protective clothing, and avoid prolonged exposure to sunlight.

● Instruct patient to report problems with vision or hearing immediately.

● Tell patient to protect drug from direct light and excessive heat and humidity.

ketorolac tromethamine (ophthalmic)
KEE-toe-role-ak

Acular, Acular LS, Acuvail

Therapeutic class: Anti-inflammatory drugs (ophthalmic)
Pharmacologic class: NSAIDs

AVAILABLE FORMS
Ophthalmic solution: 0.4%, 0.45%, 0.5%

INDICATIONS & DOSAGES
➤ **Relief from ocular itching caused by seasonal allergic conjunctivitis (Acular)**
Adults and children age 2 and older: 1 drop into conjunctival sac in each eye q.i.d.
➤ **Relief of postoperative inflammation in patients who have had cataract extraction (Acular)**
Adults and children age 2 and older: 1 drop to affected eye q.i.d. beginning 24 hours after cataract surgery and continuing through first 2 weeks of postoperative period.
➤ **Reduce ocular pain, burning, and stinging after corneal refractive surgery (Acular LS)**
Adults and children age 3 and older: 1 drop q.i.d. to affected eye, as needed, for up to 4 days after surgery.
➤ **Reduce pain and inflammation after cataract surgery (Acuvail)**
Adults: 1 drop b.i.d. to affected eye beginning 1 day before surgery, continuing on day of surgery, and through first 2 weeks after surgery.

ADMINISTRATION
Ophthalmic
● Apply light finger pressure on lacrimal sac for 1 minute after instillation.
● Store drug away from heat in a dark, tightly closed container and protect from freezing.
● Have patient remove contact lenses before administration.

ACTION
Thought to inhibit the action of cyclooxygenase, an enzyme responsible for prostaglandin synthesis. Prostaglandins

mediate the inflammatory response and cause miosis.

Route	Onset	Peak	Duration
Ophthalmic	Unknown	Unknown	Unknown

Half-life: 4 hours.

ADVERSE REACTIONS
CNS: headache (Acular LS).
EENT: transient stinging and burning on instillation, conjunctival hyperemia, corneal edema, corneal infiltrates, iritis, ocular edema and ocular pain (Acular LS), ocular inflammation (Acular), ocular irritation, superficial keratitis, superficial ocular infections.
Other: hypersensitivity reactions.

INTERACTIONS
None significant.

EFFECTS ON LAB TEST RESULTS
None reported.

CONTRAINDICATIONS & CAUTIONS
• Contraindicated in patients hypersensitive to components of drug and in those wearing soft contact lenses.
• Use cautiously in patients with bleeding disorders, in those receiving other drugs that may prolong bleeding time, and in those hypersensitive to other NSAIDs or aspirin.
• May slow or delay healing, especially when used with other topical NSAIDs or topical steroids.
Dialyzable drug: Unknown.

PREGNANCY-LACTATION-REPRODUCTION
🜂 *Alert:* Carefully weigh risks and benefits of using drug during pregnancy. Avoid use during late pregnancy because of risk of closure of the ductus arteriosus.
• Amount of drug available systemically after topical application is significantly less than that after oral doses. Use cautiously in breast-feeding women.

NURSING CONSIDERATIONS
• Acuvail may be used with other topical ophthalmics when given at least 5 minutes apart.

PATIENT TEACHING
• Teach patient how to instill drops. Advise him to wash hands before and after instilling solution, and warn him not to touch tip of dropper to eye or surrounding tissue.
• Advise patient to apply light finger pressure on lacrimal sac for 1 minute after instillation.
• Stress importance of compliance with recommended therapy.
• Tell patient not to instill drops while wearing contact lenses.
• Advise patient to report excessive bleeding or bruising to prescriber.
• Remind patient to discard drug when it's no longer needed.

ketorolac tromethamine (oral, nasal, injection)
KEE-toe-role-ak

Sprix, Toradol🍁

Therapeutic class: NSAIDs
Pharmacologic class: NSAIDs

AVAILABLE FORMS
Injection*: 10 mg/mL in 1-mL ampules🍁, 15 mg/mL in 1- and 2-mL vials and 1-mL Tubex syringes; 30 mg/mL in 1- and 2-mL single-dose vials, 1- and 2-mL Tubex syringes, and 10-mL multiple-dose vials
Nasal spray: 15.75 mg/spray
Tablets: 10 mg

INDICATIONS & DOSAGES
➤ **Short-term management of moderately severe, acute pain for single-dose treatment**
Adults younger than age 65 and adolescents age 17 and older: 60 mg I.M. or 30 mg I.V.
Adults age 65 and older: 30 mg I.M. or 15 mg I.V.
Adjust-a-dose: For renally impaired patients or those who weigh less than 50 kg, 30 mg I.M. or 15 mg I.V.
➤ **Short-term management of moderately severe, acute pain for multiple-dose treatment**
Adults younger than age 65 and adolescents age 17 and older: 30 mg I.M. or I.V. every 6 hours for maximum of 5 days. Maximum

daily dose is 120 mg. Or, 31.5 mg (one 15.75-mg spray in each nostril) every 6 to 8 hours; maximum daily dose is 126 mg. *Adults age 65 and older:* 15 mg I.M. or I.V. every 6 hours for maximum of 5 days. Maximum daily dose is 60 mg. Or, 15.75 mg (1 spray in only one nostril) every 6 to 8 hours; maximum daily dose is 63 mg.

Adjust-a-dose: For renally impaired patients or those who weigh less than 50 kg, 15 mg I.M. or I.V. every 6 hours. Maximum daily dose is 60 mg. Or, 15.75 mg (1 spray in only one nostril) every 6 to 8 hours; maximum daily dose is 63 mg.

➤ **Short-term management of moderately severe, acute pain when switching from parenteral to oral administration (oral therapy is indicated only as continuation of parenterally given drug and should never be given without patient first having received parenteral therapy)**
Adults younger than age 65 and adolescents age 17 and older: 20 mg P.O. as single dose; then 10 mg P.O. every 4 to 6 hours for maximum of 5 days. Maximum daily dose is 40 mg.
Adults age 65 and older: 10 mg P.O. as single dose; then 10 mg P.O. every 4 to 6 hours for maximum of 5 days. Maximum daily dose is 40 mg.

Adjust-a-dose: For renally impaired patients or those who weigh less than 50 kg, give 10 mg P.O. as single dose; then 10 mg P.O. every 4 to 6 hours. Maximum daily dose is 40 mg.

ADMINISTRATION
P.O.
● Give drug with food if GI upset occurs.
I.V.
▼ Dilute with NSS, D_5W, 5% dextrose and NSS, Ringer solution, lactated Ringer solution, or Plasma-Lyte A.
▼ Give injection over at least 15 seconds.
▼ Protect from light.
▼ **Incompatibilities:** Azithromycin; fenoldopam mesylate; haloperidol lactate; nalbuphine; solutions that result in a relatively low pH, such as hydroxyzine, meperidine, morphine sulfate, and prochlorperazine; thiethylperazine.
I.M.
● When appropriate, give by deep I.M. injection.

● Patient may feel pain at injection site.
● Put pressure on site for 15 to 30 seconds after injection to minimize local effects.
Intranasal
● Discard nasal spray within 24 hours of first dose, even if bottle still contains medication.
● Each 1.7-g bottle contains eight sprays.
● Activate pump before first use by pumping five times.
● Have patient blow his nose before use, sit upright or stand, and tilt his head slightly forward.
● Insert tip into the nostril, point away from the septum, and spray once.

ACTION
May inhibit prostaglandin synthesis to produce anti-inflammatory, analgesic, and antipyretic effects.

Route	Onset	Peak	Duration
P.O.	30–60 min	30–60 min	6–8 hr
I.V.	Immediate	1–3 min	6–8 hr
I.M.	10 min	30–60 min	6–8 hr
Intranasal	Unknown	½–2 hr	6–8 hr

Half-life: 4 to 6 hours.

ADVERSE REACTIONS
CNS: headache, dizziness, drowsiness, sedation.
CV: *arrhythmias,* edema, hypertension, palpitations.
EENT: (nasal spray only) increased lacrimation, nasal discomfort, rhinalgia, rhinitis, throat irritation.
GI: dyspepsia, GI pain, nausea, constipation, diarrhea, flatulence, peptic ulceration, stomatitis, vomiting.
GU: *renal failure.*
Hematologic: decreased platelet adhesion, prolonged bleeding time, purpura.
Skin: diaphoresis, pruritus, rash.
Other: pain at injection site.

INTERACTIONS
Drug-drug. *ACE inhibitors, angiotensin II receptor blockers:* May cause renal impairment, particularly in volume-depleted patients. Avoid using together in volume-depleted patients.

Anticoagulants: May increase anticoagulant levels in the blood. Use together with extreme caution and monitor patient closely.

Anticonvulsants (carbamazepine, phenytoin): May increase seizure activity. Use together cautiously.

Antihypertensives, diuretics: May decrease effectiveness. Monitor patient closely.

Disulfiram: May cause severe alcohol intolerance because injection form contains alcohol. Don't use together.

Lithium: May increase lithium level. Monitor patient closely for lithium toxicity.

Methotrexate: May decrease methotrexate clearance and increase toxicity. Avoid using together.

Pentoxifylline: May increase risk of bleeding. Use together is contraindicated.

Probenecid: May increase level and toxicity of ketorolac. Use together is contraindicated.

Salicylates: May increase risk of serious ketorolac adverse effects. Use together is contraindicated.

SSRIs: May increase risk of GI bleeding. Use together cautiously.

Drug-herb. *Dong quai, feverfew, garlic, ginger, horse chestnut, red clover:* May cause bleeding. Discourage use together.

White willow: Herb and drug contain similar components. Discourage use together.

Drug-lifestyle. *Alcohol use:* May increase risk of GI bleeding. Use with caution.

Smoking: May increase risk of GI bleeding. Discourage use together.

EFFECTS ON LAB TEST RESULTS

● May increase ALT and AST levels.
● May increase bleeding time.

CONTRAINDICATIONS & CAUTIONS

Black Box Warning Drug is contraindicated in patients who have previously demonstrated hypersensitivity to ketorolac or allergic manifestations to aspirin or other NSAIDs. Hypersensitivity reactions, ranging from bronchospasm to anaphylactic shock, have occurred and appropriate counteractive measures must be available when first dose of ketorolac injection is given. ■

Black Box Warning Contraindicated in children younger than age 17, as prophylactic analgesic before major surgery, and intraoperatively when hemostasis is critical; in patients with advanced renal impairment; and in those at risk for renal failure from volume depletion. ■

Black Box Warning Contraindicated in patients with suspected or confirmed cerebrovascular bleeding, hemorrhagic diathesis, or incomplete hemostasis, and in those at high risk for bleeding because drug inhibits platelet function. ■

Black Box Warning NSAIDs can cause peptic ulcers, GI bleeding, or perforation of the stomach or intestines, which can be fatal. These events can occur at any time during therapy and without warning. Contraindicated in patients with active peptic ulcer disease, recent GI bleeding or perforation, and a history of peptic ulcer disease or GI bleeding. Elderly patients are at greater risk for serious GI events. ■

Black Box Warning Contraindicated for treatment of perioperative pain in patients requiring CABG surgery. ■

Black Box Warning Contraindicated in patients currently receiving aspirin, probenecid, or other NSAIDs because of the cumulative risks of inducing serious NSAID-related adverse reactions. ■

Black Box Warning NSAIDs can increase risk of heart attack or stroke in patients with or without heart disease or risk factors for heart disease. Risk of heart attack or stroke can occur as early as the first weeks of NSAID use. Risk appears greater at higher doses. Use lowest effective dose for shortest duration possible. ■

⚙ *Alert:* NSAIDs increase risk of HF.

● Use cautiously in patients who are elderly or have hepatic or renal impairment or cardiac decompensation.

Dialyzable drug: Unlikely.

⚠ **Overdose S&S:** Abdominal pain, nausea, vomiting, peptic ulcers, GI bleeding, hyperventilation, renal dysfunction, metabolic acidosis, hypertension, lethargy, drowsiness, respiratory depression, coma, anaphylaxis.

PREGNANCY-LACTATION-REPRODUCTION

Black Box Warning Contraindicated in women during labor and delivery because drug may adversely affect fetal circulation and inhibit uterine contractions. ■

◑ *Alert:* Carefully weigh risks and benefits of use during pregnancy. Avoid use in late pregnancy.

• Prolonged use of NSAIDs in women of childbearing potential may be associated with infertility that's reversible upon drug discontinuation.

• Low concentrations of drug appear in breast milk. Use cautiously in breast-feeding women.

NURSING CONSIDERATIONS
• Correct hypovolemia before giving drug.

Black Box Warning Drug is indicated for short-term management (up to 5 days in adults) of moderately severe acute pain that requires analgesia at the opioid level and only as continuation treatment after I.V. or I.M. dosing, if necessary. Total combined duration of use of nasal spray, tablets, and injection shouldn't exceed 5 days because of increased risk of serious adverse events. Recommended total daily dose of ketorolac tablets (maximum, 40 mg) is significantly lower than for ketorolac injection (maximum, 120 mg). ∎

Black Box Warning Contraindicated for epidural or intrathecal administration because of its alcohol content. ∎

Black Box Warning Drug isn't indicated for minor or long-term painful conditions. ∎

◑ *Alert:* Watch for and immediately evaluate signs and symptoms of heart attack (chest pain, shortness of breath or trouble breathing) or stroke (weakness in one part or side of the body, slurred speech).

• Carefully observe patients with coagulopathies and those taking anticoagulants. Drug inhibits platelet aggregation and can prolong bleeding time. This effect disappears within 48 hours of stopping drug and doesn't alter platelet count, INR, PTT, or PT.

Black Box Warning NSAIDs may increase the risk of serious thrombotic events, MI, or stroke, which can be fatal. The risk may be greater with longer use or in patients with CV disease or risk factors for CV disease. ∎

Black Box Warning Adjust dosage for patients age 65 and older, weighing less than 50 kg, and with moderately elevated serum creatinine level. Doses of ketorolac injection aren't to exceed 60 mg (total dose per day) in these patients. ∎

• NSAIDs may mask signs and symptoms of infection because of their antipyretic and anti-inflammatory actions.

• *Look alike–sound alike:* Don't confuse ketorolac with Ketalar.

PATIENT TEACHING
• Tell patient to discard nasal spray within 24 hours of the first dose, even if medication remains in the bottle.

• Warn patient using nasal spray that transient, mild to moderate nasal irritation may occur that lasts for a few minutes and won't worsen with next dose.

• Advise patient to take a sip of water after using nasal spray to decrease throat sensation.

• Teach patient to read package insert and full directions for use of nasal spray bottle.

• Warn patient not to take ketorolac with other NSAIDs.

◑ *Alert:* Advise patient to seek medical attention immediately for chest pain, shortness of breath or trouble breathing, weakness in one part or side of the body, or slurred speech.

• Advise patient to maintain adequate fluid intake.

• Advise patient to be alert for signs and symptoms of CV events (chest pain, shortness of breath, weakness, slurred speech) and to seek medical attention immediately if they occur.

• Tell patient to promptly report edema and weight gain.

• Teach patient the warning signs and symptoms of hepatotoxicity (nausea, fatigue, lethargy, pruritus, jaundice, right upper quadrant abdominal tenderness, flulike symptoms), and advise him to stop drug and seek medical help immediately if they occur.

• Instruct female patient to notify prescriber immediately if she is pregnant.

• Warn patient receiving drug I.M. that pain may occur at injection site.

• Teach patient signs and symptoms of GI bleeding (including blood in vomit, urine, or stool; coffee-ground vomit; and black, tarry stools) and to notify prescriber immediately if any of these occurs.

• Tell patient not to take drug for more than 5 days in a row.

Reactions in bold italics are *life-threatening*. Interactions may have a *rapid onset* or a *delayed onset*.

labetalol hydrochloride
la-BET-ah-loll

Trandate

Therapeutic class: Antihypertensives
Pharmacologic class: Alpha–beta blockers

AVAILABLE FORMS
Injection: 5 mg/mL in 20- and 40-mL multiple-dose vials and 4-mL syringes
Tablets: 100 mg, 200 mg, 300 mg

INDICATIONS & DOSAGES
➤ **Hypertension**
Adults (inpatients): 200 mg P.O., followed by 200 to 400 mg P.O. in 6 to 12 hours depending on BP response. May increase by 200 mg P.O. b.i.d. at 1-day intervals. Usual dosage range is 100 to 300 mg P.O. b.i.d.
Adults (outpatients): 100 mg P.O. b.i.d. with or without a diuretic. If needed, dosage is increased to 200 mg b.i.d. after 2 days. Further increases may be made every 2 to 3 days until optimal response is reached. Usual maintenance dosage is 200 to 400 mg b.i.d. Maximum dose is 2.4 g daily in two divided doses given alone or with a diuretic.
➤ **Severe hypertension, hypertensive emergencies**
Adults (inpatients): 200 mg diluted in 160 mL of a commonly used I.V. fluid infused at 2 mg/minute I.V. or 200 mg diluted in 250 mL of a commonly used I.V. fluid and administered at 3 mL/minute I.V. until satisfactory response is obtained; then infusion is stopped. Maximum dose is 300 mg.

Or, give by repeated I.V. injection; initially, 20 mg I.V. slowly over 2 minutes. Repeat injections of 40 to 80 mg every 10 minutes until maximum dose of 300 mg is reached, as needed.

ADMINISTRATION
P.O.
● When switching from I.V. to P.O. form, begin P.O. regimen at 200 mg after BP begins to rise; repeat dose with 200 to 400 mg in 6 to 12 hours. Adjust dosage according to BP response.

● If dizziness occurs, give dose at bedtime or in smaller doses t.i.d.
I.V.
▼ Give by slow, direct I.V. injection over 2 minutes at 10-minute intervals.
▼ For I.V. infusion, prepare by diluting with D5W, NSS, or other compatible I.V. solution (refer to manufacturer's instructions for other compatible solutions) to yield 1 mg/mL or 2 mg/3 mL. Infuse at 2 mg/minute.
▼ Give labetalol infusion with an infusion-control device.
▼ Monitor BP during and after completion of infusion or I.V. injections.
▼ Patient should remain supine for 3 hours after infusion. When given I.V. for hypertensive emergencies, drug produces a rapid, predictable fall in BP within 5 to 10 minutes.
▼ Store at room temperature. Protect from light.
▼ **Incompatibilities:** Alkali solutions, amphotericin B, cefoperazone, ceftriaxone, furosemide, heparin, nafcillin, sodium bicarbonate, thiopental, warfarin.

ACTION
May be related to reduced peripheral vascular resistance, as a result of alpha and beta blockade.

Route	Onset	Peak	Duration
P.O.	20–120 min	1–2 hr	8–12 hr
I.V.	2–5 min	5–15 min	2–18 hr

Half-life: I.V., about 5½ hours; oral, 6 to 8 hours.

ADVERSE REACTIONS
CNS: dizziness, fatigue, headache, paresthesia, transient scalp tingling, syncope, vertigo, asthenia.
CV: orthostatic hypotension, *ventricular arrhythmias.*
EENT: nasal congestion.
GI: nausea, vomiting, dyspepsia.
GU: sexual dysfunction, urine retention.
Respiratory: *bronchospasm,* dyspnea.
Skin: rash.

INTERACTIONS
Drug-drug. *Beta agonists:* May blunt bronchodilator effect of these drugs in patients

with bronchospasm. May need to increase dosages of these drugs.

Cimetidine: May enhance labetalol's effect. Use together cautiously.

CV drugs, diuretics: May increase hypotensive effects. Monitor BP.

Halothane: May increase hypotensive effect. Monitor BP closely.

Insulin, oral antidiabetics: May alter dosage requirements in previously stabilized diabetic patient. Monitor patient closely.

Nitroglycerin: May blunt reflex tachycardia produced by nitroglycerin but not the hypotension. Monitor BP if used together.

NSAIDs: May decrease antihypertensive effects. Monitor BP.

TCAs: May increase incidence of tremor. Monitor patient for tremor.

Drug-herb. *Ma huang:* May decrease antihypertensive effects. Discourage use together.

EFFECTS ON LAB TEST RESULTS
• May increase transaminase and urea levels.
• May cause false-positive increase of urine free and total catecholamine levels when measured by a nonspecific trihydroxyindole fluorometric method. May cause false-positive test result for amphetamines when screening urine for drugs.

CONTRAINDICATIONS & CAUTIONS
• Contraindicated in patients hypersensitive to drug or its components and in those with bronchial asthma, overt cardiac failure, greater than first-degree heart block (except in patients with a functioning pacemaker), cardiogenic shock, severe bradycardia, and other conditions that may cause severe and prolonged hypotension.
• Use cautiously in patients with HF, hepatic failure, chronic bronchitis, emphysema, peripheral vascular disease, and pheochromocytoma.

Dialyzable drug: No.

⚠ *Overdose S&S:* Orthostatic hypotension, bradycardia, HF, bronchospasm, seizures.

PREGNANCY-LACTATION-REPRODUCTION
• There are no adequate studies in pregnant women. Use during pregnancy only if potential benefit justifies potential fetal risk.

• Low amounts of drug appear in breast milk and can be detected in the serum of breast-feeding infants. Use cautiously in breast-feeding women.

NURSING CONSIDERATIONS
• Monitor BP frequently. Drug masks common signs and symptoms of shock.
• In diabetic patients, monitor glucose level closely because beta blockers may mask certain signs and symptoms of hypoglycemia.
• Don't routinely withdraw long-term beta-blocker therapy before surgery.
• Rare occurrences of severe hepatic injury have been reported. Monitor LFTs.

PATIENT TEACHING
⟁ *Alert:* Tell patient that stopping drug abruptly can worsen chest pain and trigger a heart attack.
• Advise patient that dizziness is the most troublesome adverse reaction and tends to occur in the early stages of treatment, in patients taking diuretics, and with higher dosages. Inform patient that dizziness can be minimized by rising slowly and avoiding sudden position changes.
• Warn patient that occasional, harmless scalp tingling may occur, especially when therapy begins.

---

lacosamide
lah-COSS-ah-mide

Vimpat

Therapeutic class: Anticonvulsants
Pharmacologic class: Functionalized amino acids
Controlled substance schedule: V

AVAILABLE FORMS
Injection: 200 mg/20-mL vial
Oral solution: 10 mg/mL
Tablets: 50 mg, 100 mg, 150 mg, 200 mg

INDICATIONS & DOSAGES
Adjust-a-dose (for all indications): In patients with mild or moderate hepatic impairment or severe renal impairment (CrCl of 30 mL/minute or less), maximum recommended daily dosage is 300 mg. Withhold

---

drug in patients with severe hepatic impairment. Dosage supplementation of up to 50% should be considered following a 4-hour hemodialysis treatment. Reduce dosage as needed in patients with hepatic or renal impairment who are taking strong CYP3A4 and CYP2C9 inhibitors because of increased lacosamide exposure.

➤ **Adjunctive therapy for partial-onset seizures**
Adults and adolescents age 17 and older:
Initially, 50 mg P.O. b.i.d.; increase at weekly intervals to recommended daily dosage of 100 to 200 mg P.O. b.i.d. (200 to 400 mg daily). Or, initially 200 mg P.O. as a single loading dose followed approximately 12 hours later by 100 mg P.O. b.i.d. for 1 week. Then, increase by 50 mg b.i.d. as needed based on patient response and tolerance up to recommended maintenance dose of 200 mg b.i.d.

May administer I.V. at an equivalent daily dosage and frequency when oral administration is temporarily not feasible.

➤ **Monotherapy for partial-onset seizures**
Adults and adolescents age 17 and older: Initially, 100 mg P.O. b.i.d.; increase at weekly intervals by 50 mg b.i.d. (100 mg/day) to recommended daily dosage of 150 to 200 mg P.O. b.i.d. Or, initially 200 mg P.O. as a single loading dose followed approximately 12 hours later by 100 mg P.O. b.i.d. for 1 week. Then, increase by 50 mg b.i.d. as needed based on patient response and tolerance up to recommended maintenance dose of 150 to 200 mg P.O. b.i.d. When converting from another single antiepileptic, titrate lacosamide to therapeutic dose of 150 to 200 mg P.O. b.i.d. and maintain for at least 3 days before initiating withdrawal of concomitant drug. Gradually withdraw concomitant drug over at least 6 weeks. May administer drug I.V. at an equivalent daily dosage and frequency when oral administration is temporarily not feasible.

ADMINISTRATION
P.O.
● Give drug with or without food.
I.V.
▼ Reconstitute with NSS, D₅W, or lactated Ringer solution. Discard solution if dis-

colored or if particulate matter is present. Solution is stable for 4 hours at room temperature.
▼ Infuse over 15 to 60 minutes; 30 to 60 minutes is preferred.
▼ Discard unused solution in vial.
▼ Limit I.V. use to 5 days of consecutive treatment.
▼ **Incompatibilities:** None known.

ACTION
May selectively enhance slow inactivation of sodium channels, stabilizing hyperexcitable neuronal membranes and inhibiting repetitive neuronal firing.

Route	Onset	Peak	Duration
P.O.	Unknown	1–4 hr	Unknown
I.V.	Unknown	30–60 min	Unknown

Half-life: About 13 hours.

ADVERSE REACTIONS
CNS: asthenia, ataxia, balance disorder, depression, dizziness, fatigue, gait disturbance, headache, memory impairment, somnolence, tremor.
EENT: blurred vision, diplopia, nystagmus, vertigo.
GI: diarrhea, nausea, vomiting.
Skin: pruritus, skin laceration.
Other: contusion.

INTERACTIONS
Drug-drug. *Drugs that prolong PR interval (beta blockers, calcium channel blockers):* May increase risk of bradycardia or AV block. Monitor patient closely, especially with I.V. formulation.
Drug-lifestyle. *Alcohol use:* May cause additive drowsiness. Don't use together.

EFFECTS ON LAB TEST RESULTS
● May increase LFT values.

CONTRAINDICATIONS & CAUTIONS
● Lacosamide isn't recommended for patients with severe hepatic impairment.
● Use cautiously in patients with known cardiac conduction problems, depression, myocardial ischemia, or HF and in those with a history of suicidal thoughts.

- Use cautiously in patients with phenylketonuria because oral solution contains phenylalanine.
- Safety and effectiveness in children younger than age 17 haven't been established.

Dialyzable drug: 50%.

⚠ *Overdose S&S:* Coma.

PREGNANCY-LACTATION-REPRODUCTION

- There are no adequate studies in pregnant women. Use during pregnancy only if potential benefit justifies potential risk to the fetus.
- Encourage pregnant women taking drug to enroll in the Antiepileptic Drug Pregnancy Registry (1-888-233-2334 or www.aedpregnancyregistry.org/).
- It isn't known if drug appears in breast milk. Patient should discontinue breast-feeding or discontinue drug.

NURSING CONSIDERATIONS

⚫ *Alert:* Give loading dose under medical supervision because of increased risk of CNS adverse reactions.

⚫ *Alert:* Monitor patient for syncopal episodes; drug may increase risk of syncope, especially in patients with cardiac disease and in those receiving drugs that slow AV conduction.

⚫ *Alert:* Obtain ECG before starting therapy and after titrating to maintenance dose in patients with known conduction problems (marked first-degree AV block, second- or third-degree AV block, or sick sinus syndrome without pacemaker), sodium channelopathies (Brugada syndrome), concomitant use of drugs that prolong PR interval, or severe cardiac disease (MI, HF, structural heart disease). Also closely monitor this population when giving I.V. lacosamide.

- Monitor patient for signs and symptoms of multiorgan hypersensitivity reaction, including fever, rash, eosinophilia, hepatitis, nephritis, lymphadenopathy, and myocarditis. If reaction is suspected, discontinue drug and begin alternative treatment.
- Obtain an ECG in patients with severe cardiac disease or known conduction defects before starting drug.

⚫ *Alert:* Withdraw drug gradually over 1 week to minimize potential for increased seizure activity.

⚫ *Alert:* Drug may increase risk of suicidal thinking and behavior. Monitor patient closely for worsening depression, suicidal thoughts or behavior, and unusual changes in mood or behavior.

- Closely observe patients with mild to moderate hepatic impairment during dosage titration.

PATIENT TEACHING

- Inform patient that drug may be taken without regard to meals.
- Tell patient to report mood changes or suicidal thoughts immediately.
- Warn patient to avoid driving and operating heavy machinery until drug's CNS effects are known.
- Advise woman to notify prescriber if she suspects or is considering pregnancy or plans to breast-feed.
- Warn patient not to stop drug abruptly.
- Tell patient to avoid alcohol while taking drug.
- Advise patient to report blurred vision, dizziness, double vision, nausea, uncoordinated movement, or vertigo.

lamivudine (3TC)
lam-ah-VEW-den

Epivir, Epivir-HBV, Heptovir✦

Therapeutic class: Antiretrovirals
Pharmacologic class: Nucleoside–nucleotide reverse transcriptase inhibitors

AVAILABLE FORMS
Epivir
Oral solution: 10 mg/mL
Tablets: 150 mg, 300 mg
Epivir-HBV
Oral solution: 5 mg/mL
Tablets: 100 mg

INDICATIONS & DOSAGES
Black Box Warning Lamivudine tablets and oral solution used to treat HIV-1 infection contain a higher dose of the active ingredient

---

than do lamivudine tablets and oral solution used to treat chronic HBV infection. Patients with HIV-1 infection should receive only dosing forms appropriate for HIV-1 treatment. ∎

➤ **HIV infection, with other antiretrovirals**

Adults: 300 mg Epivir P.O. once daily or 150 mg P.O. b.i.d.

Children ages 3 months to 18 years: 4 mg/kg Epivir solution P.O. b.i.d. or 8 mg/kg P.O. once daily. Maximum dose is 300 mg daily.

Children weighing 14 kg or more who can reliably swallow tablets: For 14 to less than 20 kg, give 1 tablet (150 mg) P.O. once daily or ½ tablet (75 mg) P.O. b.i.d.; for 20 kg to less than 25 kg, give 1½ tablets (225 mg) P.O. once daily or ½ tablet (75 mg) P.O. in morning and 1 tablet (150 mg) P.O. in evening; for 25 kg or more, give 2 tablets (300 mg) P.O. once daily or 150 mg P.O. b.i.d.

Adjust-a-dose: For patients with HIV infection and CrCl of 30 to 49 mL/minute, give 150 mg Epivir P.O. daily. If CrCl is 15 to 29 mL/minute, give 150 mg P.O. on day 1 and then 100 mg daily; if CrCl is 5 to 14 mL/minute, give 150 mg on day 1 and then 50 mg daily; if CrCl is less than 5 mL/minute, give 50 mg on day 1 and then 25 mg daily.

➤ **Chronic HBV infection with evidence of HBV replication and active liver inflammation**

Adults: 100 mg Epivir-HBV P.O. once daily.

Children ages 2 to 17 years: 3 mg/kg Epivir-HBV P.O. once daily, up to a maximum dose of 100 mg daily. Optimum duration of treatment isn't known; safety and effectiveness of treatment beyond 1 year haven't been established.

Adjust-a-dose: For adult patients with chronic HBV infection and CrCl of 30 to 49 mL/minute, give first dose of 100 mg Epivir-HBV; then give 50 mg P.O. once daily. If CrCl is 15 to 29 mL/minute, give first dose of 100 mg; then give 25 mg P.O. once daily. If CrCl is 5 to 14 mL/minute, give first dose of 35 mg; then give 15 mg P.O. once daily. If CrCl is less than 5 mL/minute, give first dose of 35 mg; then give 10 mg P.O. once daily.

ADMINISTRATION

P.O.

● Give without regard for food.

ACTION

A synthetic nucleoside analogue that inhibits HIV and HBV reverse transcription via viral DNA chain termination. RNA- and DNA-dependent DNA polymerase activities.

Route	Onset	Peak	Duration
P.O.	Unknown	1–3 hr	Unknown

Half-life: Adults, 5 to 7 hours; children, 2 hours.

ADVERSE REACTIONS

Adverse reactions pertain to the combination therapy of lamivudine and zidovudine.

CNS: dizziness, fatigue, fever, headache, insomnia and other sleep disorders, malaise, neuropathy, depressive disorders.

EENT: nasal symptoms.

GI: anorexia, diarrhea, nausea, vomiting, abdominal cramps, abdominal pain, dyspepsia.

Hematologic: *neutropenia, thrombocytopenia,* anemia.

Hepatic: *hepatotoxicity.*

Metabolic: *lactic acidosis.*

Musculoskeletal: musculoskeletal pain, arthralgia, myalgia.

Respiratory: cough.

Skin: rash.

Other: chills.

INTERACTIONS

Drug-drug. *Emtricitabine:* May increase adverse or toxic effects of emtricitabine. Avoid combination.

Sulfamethoxazole–trimethoprim: May increase lamivudine level because of decreased clearance of drug. Monitor patient for toxicity.

EFFECTS ON LAB TEST RESULTS

● May increase ALT, bilirubin, and serum lipase and CK levels.

● May decrease Hb level and neutrophil and platelet counts.

CONTRAINDICATIONS & CAUTIONS

Black Box Warning Lactic acidosis and severe hepatomegaly with steatosis, including fatal cases, have been reported. ∎

• Contraindicated in patients hypersensitive to drug.
• Use cautiously in patients with renal impairment.
• Safety and efficacy of lamivudine haven't been established for treatment of chronic HBV infection in patients dually infected with HIV-1 and HBV. Emergence of HBV variants associated with resistance to lamivudine has also been reported in HIV-1-infected patients who have received lamivudine-containing antiretroviral regimens in the presence of concurrent HBV infection.
• Use Epivir-HBV only when an alternative antiviral with a higher genetic barrier to resistance isn't available or appropriate. Drug hasn't been evaluated in patients with HBV/HIV-1 coinfection, HCV infection, or hepatitis delta virus; in patients with chronic HBV infection with decompensated liver disease; or in liver transplant recipients.
❸ **Alert:** Use drug cautiously, if at all, in children with history of pancreatitis or other significant risk factors for development of pancreatitis.
Dialyzable drug: Unknown.

PREGNANCY-LACTATION-REPRODUCTION

• There are no adequate studies of Epivir-HBV use in pregnant women. Use during pregnancy only if potential benefit justifies potential risk to the fetus.
• Epivir is one of the preferred drugs used for the treatment of HIV infection in pregnant women.
• The Antiretroviral Pregnancy Registry monitors maternal-fetal outcomes of pregnant women exposed to lamivudine. To register, call the registry at 1-800-258-4263.
• Because of the potential for HIV transmission, women taking Epivir shouldn't breast-feed.
• Epivir-HBV appears in breast milk. Because of the potential for serious adverse reactions in breast-fed infants, a decision should be made whether to discontinue breast-feeding, taking into consideration

importance of continued HBV therapy to the mother and the benefits of breast-feeding.

NURSING CONSIDERATIONS

❸ **Alert:** Stop treatment immediately and notify prescriber if signs, symptoms, or laboratory abnormalities suggest pancreatitis. Monitor amylase level.
❸ **Alert:** Lactic acidosis and hepatotoxicity have been reported. Notify prescriber if signs of lactic acidosis or hepatotoxicity occur.
Black Box Warning Hepatitis may recur in some patients with chronic HBV infection when they stop taking drug. Monitor hepatic function closely. ∎
• Safety and effectiveness of Epivir-HBV for longer than 1 year haven't been established; optimum duration of treatment isn't known.
Black Box Warning Provide HIV counseling and test patients for HIV before starting treatment and during therapy because form and dosage of lamivudine in Epivir-HBV aren't appropriate for those infected with both HBV and HIV. If lamivudine is given to patients with HBV and HIV, use the higher dosage indicated for HIV therapy as part of an appropriate combination regimen. ∎
• Because of a high rate of early virologic resistance, don't use triple antiretroviral therapy with abacavir or didanosine, lamivudine, and tenofovir as new treatment for never-treated or pretreated patients. Monitor patients currently taking this therapy and those who take it with other antiretrovirals, and consider a different therapy.
• Monitor patient's CBC, platelet count, LFTs, and renal function studies. Report abnormalities.

PATIENT TEACHING

• Inform patient that long-term effects of drug aren't known.
• Stress importance of taking drug exactly as prescribed.
Black Box Warning Offer HIV counseling and testing to all patients before beginning treatment with Epivir-HBV and periodically during treatment because Epivir-HBV contains a lower dose of the same active ingredient as in lamivudine tablets and oral solution used to treat HIV. If treatment with

---

Reactions in bold italics are *life-threatening*. Interactions may have a *rapid onset* or a *delayed onset*.

Epivir-HBV is prescribed for chronic HBV infection in patient with unrecognized or untreated HIV infection, HIV resistance is likely because of the subtherapeutic dose and inappropriate monotherapy. ∎

• Inform patient that drug doesn't cure HIV infection, that opportunistic infections and other complications of HIV infection may still occur, and that transmission of HIV to others through sexual contact or blood contamination is still possible.

• Teach parents or guardians the signs and symptoms of pancreatitis. Advise them to report signs and symptoms immediately.

lamotrigine
la-MO-tri-geen

Lamictal, Lamictal CD, Lamictal ODT, Lamictal XR

Therapeutic class: Anticonvulsants
Pharmacologic class: Phenyltriazines

AVAILABLE FORMS
ODTs: 25 mg, 50 mg, 100 mg, 200 mg
Tablets: 25 mg, 100 mg, 150 mg, 200 mg
Tablets (chewable dispersible): 2 mg, 5 mg, 25 mg
Tablets (extended-release) ⓓⓝⓒ*:* 25 mg, 50 mg, 100 mg, 200 mg, 250 mg, 300 mg

INDICATIONS & DOSAGES
❸ *Alert:* Extended-release formula isn't for use as initial monotherapy or for conversion to monotherapy from two or more concomitant antiepileptic drugs (AEDs).

➤ **Conversion to monotherapy using extended-release formula in patients with partial seizures who are receiving treatment with a single enzyme-inducing AED**

Adults and children age 13 and older: Add 50 mg P.O. extended-release tablet daily to current drug regimen for 2 weeks, followed by 100 mg P.O. daily for 2 weeks. Then, increase by 100 mg every week until a dosage of 500 mg P.O. daily is reached. The concomitant enzyme-inducing AED can then be gradually reduced by 20% decrements each week over a 4-week period. Two weeks after completing withdrawal

of the enzyme-inducing AED, decrease lamotrigine (extended-release tablet) no faster than 100 mg/day each week to achieve the monotherapy maintenance dosage of 250 to 300 mg/day.

➤ **Conversion to monotherapy using extended-release formula in patients with partial seizures who are receiving adjunctive treatment with valproate**

Adults and children age 13 and older: Add 25 mg extended-release P.O. every other day for 2 weeks; then increase to 25 mg P.O. daily for weeks 3 and 4. Increase to 50 mg P.O. daily for week 5, 100 mg P.O. daily for week 6, and 150 mg P.O. daily for week 7. Maintain dosage at 150 mg P.O. daily while decreasing valproate dosage by no more than 500 mg/day each week until 500 mg/day is achieved; maintain for 1 week. Then, simultaneously increase extended-release tablet to 200 mg/day while decreasing valproate to 250 mg/day; maintain for 1 week. Increase to 250 or 300 mg P.O. daily as maintenance dosage and discontinue valproate.

➤ **Conversion to monotherapy using extended-release formula in patients with partial seizures who are receiving treatment with a single drug other than an enzyme-inducing AED or valproate**

Adults and children age 13 and older: Add 25 mg extended-release P.O. daily for 2 weeks; then increase to 50 mg P.O. daily for weeks 3 and 4. Increase to 100 mg P.O. daily for week 5. Starting with week 6, continue increasing dosage each week by 50 mg P.O. daily until a dosage of 250 to 300 mg P.O. daily is achieved; then withdraw concomitant AED therapy by 20% decrements each week over a 4-week period. No additional lamotrigine (extended-release tablet) adjustment is needed.

➤ **Adjunctive treatment of partial seizures or primary generalized tonic-clonic seizures caused by epilepsy or generalized seizures of Lennox-Gastaut syndrome**

Adults and children older than age 12 taking valproate: 25 mg immediate-release P.O. every other day for 2 weeks; then 25 mg P.O. daily for 2 weeks. Continue to increase, as needed, by 25 to 50 mg daily every 1 to 2 weeks until an effective maintenance dosage of 100 to 400 mg daily given in one or two divided doses is reached. When added to valproate alone, the usual daily maintenance dose is 100 to 200 mg. Or, 25 mg extended-release P.O. every other day for 2 weeks; then 25 mg P.O. daily for 2 weeks; then 50 mg P.O. daily for 1 week; then 100 mg P.O. daily for 1 week; then 150 mg P.O. daily for 1 week. Daily maintenance dose is 200 to 250 mg.

Adults and children older than age 12 not taking carbamazepine, phenytoin, phenobarbital, primidone, or valproate: 25 mg extended-release P.O. daily for 2 weeks; then 50 mg P.O. daily for 2 weeks; then 100 mg P.O. daily for 1 week; then 150 mg P.O. daily for 1 week; then 200 mg P.O. daily for 1 week. Daily maintenance dose is 300 to 400 mg.

Adults and children older than age 12 taking anticonvulsant drugs but not carbamazepine, phenytoin, phenobarbital, primidone, or valproate: 25 mg immediate-release P.O. daily for 1 to 2 weeks; then 50 mg P.O. daily for another 2 weeks. Continue to increase by 50 mg/day every 1 to 2 weeks until an effective maintenance dose is reached. Daily maintenance dose is 225 to 375 mg P.O. daily in two divided doses.

Adults and children older than age 12 taking carbamazepine, phenytoin, phenobarbital, or primidone but not valproate: 50 mg immediate-release P.O. daily for 2 weeks; then 100 mg P.O. daily in two divided doses for 2 weeks. Increase, as needed, by 100 mg daily every 1 to 2 weeks. Usual maintenance dosage is 300 to 500 mg P.O. daily in two divided doses. Or, 50 mg extended-release P.O. daily for 2 weeks; then 100 mg P.O. daily for 2 weeks; then 200 mg P.O. daily for 1 week; then 300 mg P.O. daily for 1 week; then 400 mg P.O. daily for 1 week. Daily maintenance dose is 400 to 600 mg.

Children ages 2 to 12 weighing 7 to 40 kg taking valproate: 0.15 mg/kg P.O. daily in one or two divided doses (rounded down to nearest whole tablet) for 2 weeks. Increase to 0.3 mg/kg daily in one or two divided doses for 2 weeks, followed by increasing the daily dose every 1 or 2 weeks with an additional 0.3 mg/kg daily in one or two divided doses. Thereafter, usual maintenance dosage is 1 to 5 mg/kg daily (maximum,

200 mg daily in one to two divided doses). In patients weighing less than 30 kg, maintenance dosage may need to be increased by as much as 50% based on clinical response.

Children ages 2 to 12 weighing 7 to 40 kg taking anticonvulsant drugs but not carbamazepine, phenytoin, phenobarbital, primidone, or valproate: 0.3 mg/kg immediate-release P.O. daily in one or two divided doses (rounded down to the nearest whole tablet) for 2 weeks; then 0.6 mg/kg P.O. daily in two divided doses for another 2 weeks; then increase the daily dose every 1 to 2 weeks with an additional 0.6 mg/kg P.O. daily in two divided doses. Thereafter, usual maintenance dose is 4.5 to 7.5 mg/kg P.O. daily. Maximum dose is 300 mg daily in two divided doses. In patients weighing less than 30 kg, maintenance dosage may need to be increased by as much as 50% based on clinical response.

Children ages 2 to 12 weighing 7 to 40 kg taking carbamazepine, phenytoin, phenobarbital, or primidone but not valproate: 0.6 mg/kg P.O. daily in two divided doses (rounded down to nearest whole tablet) for 2 weeks. Increase to 1.2 mg/kg P.O. daily in two divided doses for 2 weeks; then increase the daily dose every 1 to 2 weeks with an additional 1.2 mg/kg daily in two divided doses. Usual maintenance dosage is 5 to 15 mg/kg P.O. daily (maximum 400 mg daily in two divided doses). In patients weighing less than 30 kg, maintenance dosage may need to be increased by as much as 50% based on clinical response.

➤ **To convert patients from therapy with a hepatic enzyme-inducing AED alone to lamotrigine therapy**
Adults and children age 16 and older: Add 50 mg immediate-release P.O. once daily to current drug regimen for 2 weeks, followed by 100 mg P.O. daily in two divided doses for 2 weeks. Then increase daily dosage by 100 mg every 1 to 2 weeks until maintenance dose of 500 mg daily in two divided doses is reached. The concomitant hepatic enzyme-inducing AED can then be gradually reduced by 20% decrements weekly for 4 weeks.

Adjust-a-dose: For patients with severe renal impairment, use lower maintenance dosage.

➤ **To convert patients with partial seizures from adjunctive therapy with valproate to therapy with lamotrigine alone**

Adults and children age 16 and older:
Add immediate-release form until 200 mg daily is achieved; then gradually decrease valproate to 500 mg daily by decrements of no more than 500 mg daily per week. Maintain these dosages for 1 week, then increase lamotrigine to 300 mg daily while decreasing valproate to 250 mg daily. Maintain these dosages for 1 week, then stop valproate completely while increasing lamotrigine by 100 mg daily every week until a dose of 500 mg daily is reached.

➤ **Bipolar disorder for maintenance treatment to delay time to occurrence of mood episodes (depression, mania, hypomania, mixed episodes) in patients treated for acute mood episodes with standard therapy**

Adults: Initially, 25 mg immediate-release P.O. once daily for 2 weeks; then 50 mg P.O. once daily for 2 weeks. Dosage may then be doubled at weekly intervals, to maintenance dosage of 200 mg daily.

Adults taking carbamazepine or other hepatic enzyme-inducing drugs without valproate: Initially, 50 mg immediate-release P.O. once daily for 2 weeks; then 100 mg daily in two divided doses for 2 weeks. Dosage is then increased by 100 mg weekly to maintenance dosage of 400 mg daily, given in two divided doses.

Adults taking valproate: Initially, 25 mg immediate-release P.O. every other day for 2 weeks; then 25 mg P.O. once daily for 2 weeks. Dosage may then be doubled at weekly intervals to maintenance dosage of 100 mg daily.

ADMINISTRATION
P.O.
● Starter and titration kits are available to provide doses consistent with recommended titration schedule for the first 5 weeks of treatment.
● Chewable dispersible tablets may be swallowed whole, chewed, or dispersed in water or diluted fruit juice.

● If tablets are chewed, give a small amount of water or diluted fruit juice to aid in swallowing.
● ODTs should be placed on the tongue and moved around in the mouth.
● ODTs may be swallowed with or without water and without regard to food.
● Give extended-release tablets once daily with or without food. Patient must swallow tablets whole and must not chew, crush, or divide them.

ACTION
Unknown. May inhibit release of glutamate and aspartate (excitatory neurotransmitters) in the brain via action at voltage-sensitive sodium channels.

Route	Onset	Peak	Duration
P.O. (immediate-release)	Unknown	1–5 hr	Unknown
P.O. (extended-release)	Unknown	4–11 hr	Unknown

Half-life: 7 to 148 hours, depending on age, dosage schedule, use of other anticonvulsants, and other medical conditions.

ADVERSE REACTIONS
CNS: ataxia, dizziness, drowsiness, headache, somnolence, fatigue, anxiety, abnormal thinking, memory, depression, confusion, dysarthria, emotional lability, fever, incoordination, insomnia, irritability, malaise, *suicidal ideation.*
CV: palpitations, chest pain, edema.
EENT: blurred vision, diplopia, vision abnormality, rhinitis, nystagmus, pharyngitis.
GI: nausea, vomiting, abdominal pain, anorexia, constipation, diarrhea, dry mouth, dyspepsia.
GU: amenorrhea, dysmenorrhea, urinary frequency.
Musculoskeletal: arthralgia, back pain, muscle spasm, neck pain, weakness.
Respiratory: cough, dyspnea, bronchitis.
Skin: rash, dermatitis.

INTERACTIONS
Drug-drug. *Acetaminophen:* May decrease therapeutic effects of lamotrigine. Monitor patient.
Carbamazepine: May decrease effects of lamotrigine while increasing toxicity of

carbamazepine. Adjust doses and monitor patient.

Ethosuximide, oxcarbazepine, phenobarbital, phenytoin, primidone: May decrease lamotrigine level. Monitor patient closely.

Folate inhibitors (methotrexate, sulfamethoxazole–trimethoprim): May have additive effect because lamotrigine inhibits dihydrofolate reductase, an enzyme involved in folic acid synthesis. Monitor patient.

Hormonal contraceptives containing estrogen, rifampin: May decrease lamotrigine levels. Adjust dosage. By the end of the "pill-free" week, lamotrigine levels may double.

Valproate: May decrease clearance of lamotrigine, which increases lamotrigine level; also decreases valproate level. Monitor patient for toxicity.

Drug-lifestyle. *Sun exposure:* May cause photosensitivity reactions. Advise patient to avoid excessive sun exposure.

EFFECTS ON LAB TEST RESULTS

● May result in false-positive readings in rapid urine drug screens, particularly for phencyclidine.

CONTRAINDICATIONS & CAUTIONS

● Contraindicated in patients hypersensitive to drug or its components.

☼ Alert: Rare, multiorgan hypersensitivity reactions that can be fatal have occurred.

● Use cautiously in patients with renal, hepatic, or cardiac impairment.

● Drug isn't recommended for treatment of acute manic or mixed episodes of bipolar disorder because effectiveness hasn't been established.

Dialyzable drug: 20%.

⚠ Overdose S&S: Ataxia, nystagmus, increased seizures, decreased level of consciousness, coma, intraventricular conduction delay.

PREGNANCY-LACTATION-REPRODUCTION

● There are no adequate studies in pregnant women; in animal studies, lamotrigine was developmentally toxic. Use during pregnancy only if potential benefit justifies potential risk to the fetus.

● Pregnant patients are encouraged to register in the Antiepileptic Drug Pregnancy Registry (1-888-233-2334).

● Drug appears in breast milk. Closely monitor breast-feeding infants for adverse events resulting from drug use. Women should discontinue breast-feeding if infants develop drug toxicity. Use cautiously in breast-feeding women.

NURSING CONSIDERATIONS

☼ Alert: Closely monitor all patients taking or starting AEDs for changes in behavior indicating worsening of suicidal thoughts or behavior or depression. Symptoms such as anxiety, agitation, hostility, mania, and hypomania may be precursors to emerging suicidality.

● Don't stop drug abruptly because this may increase seizure frequency. Instead, taper drug over at least 2 weeks.

Black Box Warning Serious rashes, including Stevens-Johnson syndrome, requiring hospitalization and discontinuation of treatment have been reported. Most life-threatening rashes have been documented between 2 and 8 weeks of treatment initiation, but isolated cases have been reported with prolonged treatment (e.g., 6 months). Rate of serious rash is greater in children than in adults. Don't exceed initial dose or recommended dosage escalation, or maintain coadministration with valproate. Stop drug at first sign of rash, unless rash is clearly not drug-related. ∎

Black Box Warning Stopping treatment may not prevent a rash from becoming life-threatening or permanently disabling or disfiguring. ∎

Black Box Warning Extended-release form isn't approved for children younger than age 13. ∎

☼ Alert: Drug may cause aseptic meningitis. Monitor patient for symptoms such as headache, fever, neck stiffness, nausea, vomiting, rash, and photophobia. Discontinue drug if no other cause of meningitis is found.

● Reduce lamotrigine dose if drug is added to a multidrug regimen that includes valproic acid.

● Evaluate patients for changes in seizure activity. Check adjunct anticonvulsant level

● **Look alike–sound alike:** Don't confuse lamotrigine with lamivudine or levothyroxine. Don't confuse Lamictal with Lamisil, labetalol, or Lomotil.

PATIENT TEACHING

● Inform patient that drug may cause rash. Combination therapy of valproic acid and lamotrigine may cause a serious rash. Tell patient to report rash or signs or symptoms of hypersensitivity promptly to prescriber; drug may need to be stopped.

● Warn patient not to engage in hazardous activity until drug's CNS effects are known.

● Teach patient or caregiver to immediately report headache, fever, mouth ulcers, bruising or petechiae, signs of infection (fever, cough, dyspnea), neck stiffness, nausea, vomiting, rash, drowsiness, confusion, or light sensitivity.

● Warn patient that the drug may trigger sensitivity to the sun and to take precautions until tolerance is determined.

● Warn patient not to stop drug abruptly.

✪ **Alert:** Advise female patient of childbearing potential to discuss drug therapy with prescriber if considering pregnancy. Infants exposed to drug during the first trimester have a greater risk of cleft lip or palate.

● Advise women of childbearing potential that breast-feeding isn't recommended during therapy.

---

lansoprazole
lanz-AH-pray-zol

Prevacid✐, Prevacid SoluTab, Prevacid 24 Hour ◇

Therapeutic class: Antiulcer drugs
Pharmacologic class: PPIs

AVAILABLE FORMS

Capsules (delayed-release) ⓞⓝⓒ: 15 mg, 30 mg
ODTs (delayed-release): 15 mg, 30 mg

INDICATIONS & DOSAGES

➤ **Short-term treatment of active duodenal ulcer**
Adults: 15 mg P.O. daily before eating for 4 weeks.

➤ **Maintenance of healed duodenal ulcers**
Adults: 15 mg P.O. daily.

➤ **Short-term treatment of active benign gastric ulcer**
Adults: 30 mg P.O. once daily for up to 8 weeks.

➤ **Short-term treatment of erosive esophagitis**
Adults: 30 mg P.O. daily before eating for up to 8 weeks. If healing doesn't occur, 8 more weeks of therapy may be given. Maintenance dosage for healing is 15 mg P.O. daily.
Children ages 12 to 17: 30 mg P.O. once daily for up to 8 weeks.
Children ages 1 to 11 weighing more than 30 kg: 30 mg P.O. once daily for up to 12 weeks. Increase dosage up to 30 mg b.i.d. in patients who remain symptomatic after 2 weeks.
Children ages 1 to 11 weighing 30 kg or less: 15 mg P.O. once daily for up to 12 weeks. Increase dosage up to 30 mg b.i.d. in patients who remain symptomatic after 2 weeks.

➤ **Long-term treatment of pathologic hypersecretory conditions, including Zollinger-Ellison syndrome**
Adults: Initially, 60 mg P.O. once daily. Increase dosage, as needed. Give daily amounts above 120 mg in evenly divided doses.

➤ ***Helicobacter pylori* eradication to reduce risk of duodenal ulcer recurrence**
Adults: For patients receiving dual therapy, 30 mg P.O. lansoprazole with 1 g P.O. amoxicillin, each given t.i.d. for 14 days. For patients receiving triple therapy, 30 mg P.O. lansoprazole with 1 g P.O. amoxicillin and 500 mg P.O. clarithromycin, all given b.i.d. for 10 to 14 days.

➤ **Short-term treatment of symptomatic GERD**
Adults: 15 mg P.O. once daily for up to 8 weeks.
Children ages 12 to 17: 15 mg P.O. once daily for up to 8 weeks.
Children ages 1 to 11 weighing more than 30 kg: 30 mg P.O. once daily for up to 12 weeks. Dosage can be increased up to 30 mg b.i.d. in patients who remain symptomatic after 2 weeks.

L

Children ages 1 to 11 weighing 30 kg or less: 15 mg P.O. once daily for up to 12 weeks. Dosage can be increased up to 30 mg b.i.d. in patients who remain symptomatic after 2 weeks.
➤ **NSAID-related ulcer in patients who continue NSAID use**
Adults: 30 mg P.O. daily for 8 weeks.
➤ **To reduce risk of NSAID-related ulcer in patients with history of gastric ulcer who need NSAIDs**
Adults: 15 mg P.O. daily for up to 12 weeks.

ADMINISTRATION
P.O.
• Give 30 to 60 minutes before a meal.
• Don't crush or allow patient to chew capsules.
• For patients who have difficulty swallowing capsules, the capsules can be opened and the intact granules sprinkled on 1 tablespoon of applesauce, Ensure pudding, cottage cheese, yogurt, or strained pears and swallowed immediately. Or, capsule contents may be emptied into a small volume (60 mL) of apple, orange, or tomato juice and swallowed.
• Contents of capsule can be mixed with 40 mL of apple juice in a syringe and given within 3 to 5 minutes via an NG or nasojejunal tube. Flush with additional apple juice to give entire dose and maintain patency of the tube.
• Place ODT on patient's tongue and allow it to disintegrate with or without water until the particles can be swallowed.
• To give ODTs using an oral syringe, dissolve a 15-mg tablet in 4 mL water or a 30-mg tablet in 10 mL water and give within 15 minutes. Refill syringe with about 2 mL (15-mg tablet) or 5 mL (30-mg tablet) of water, shake gently, and give any remaining contents.
• To give ODTs through an 8 French or larger NG tube, dissolve a 15-mg tablet in 4 mL water or a 30-mg tablet in 10 mL water and give within 15 minutes. Refill syringe with about 5 mL of water, shake gently, and flush the NG tube.
• ODTs contain 2.5 mg phenylalanine/ 15-mg tablet and 5.1 mg phenylalanine/ 30-mg tablet.

ACTION
Inhibits proton pump activity by binding to hydrogen-potassium adenosine triphosphates, located at secretory surface of gastric parietal cells, to suppress gastric acid secretions.

Route	Onset	Peak	Duration
P.O.	1–3 hr	1.7 hr	24 hr

Half-life: Less than 2 hours.

ADVERSE REACTIONS
GI: abdominal pain, constipation, diarrhea, nausea.

INTERACTIONS
Drug-drug. *Ampicillin esters, digoxin, iron salts, ketoconazole:* May inhibit absorption of these drugs. Monitor patient closely.
Atazanavir: May reduce GI absorption of atazanavir, reducing antiviral activity. Don't use together.
Clarithromycin: May increase lansoprazole levels and adverse effects. Monitor patient.
Clopidogrel: May interfere with conversion of clopidogrel to its active metabolite. Avoid use together.
Digoxin: May cause hypomagnesemia. Monitor magnesium level before and during treatment.
Methotrexate: May increase methotrexate serum level. Monitor methotrexate concentration and adjust dosage as needed.
Rilpivirine: May decrease rilpivirine concentration. Avoid use together.
Sucralfate: May cause delayed lansoprazole absorption. Give lansoprazole at least 30 minutes before sucralfate.
Theophylline: May mildly increase theophylline clearance. Adjust theophylline dosage when lansoprazole is started or stopped. Use together cautiously.
Warfarin: May increase bleeding risk. Monitor INR and PT.
Drug-herb. *St. John's wort:* May increase risk of sun sensitivity. Advise patient to avoid excessive sunlight exposure.
Drug-food. *Any food:* May decrease rate and extent of GI absorption. Advise patient to take before meals.

Reactions in bold italics are *life-threatening*. Interactions may have a *rapid onset* or a ***delayed onset***.

EFFECTS ON LAB TEST RESULTS
• May increase LFT values and creatinine, serum potassium, and serum urea levels. May increase gastrin, globulin, and LDH levels.
• May increase or decrease electrolyte levels.
• May cause abnormal CBC. May increase or decrease WBC and platelet counts.

CONTRAINDICATIONS & CAUTIONS
• Contraindicated in patients hypersensitive to drug or its components. Reactions may include anaphylaxis, anaphylactic shock, angioedema, bronchospasm, acute interstitial nephritis, and urticaria.
🔄 **Alert:** Prolonged use of PPIs or use with medications such as digoxin or drugs that may cause hypomagnesemia (e.g., diuretics) may cause low magnesium levels that may require magnesium supplementation and possible discontinuation of drug. Monitor magnesium levels before starting treatment and periodically thereafter.
🔄 **Alert:** There may be an increased risk of hip, wrist, and spine fractures associated with PPIs.
• Acute interstitial nephritis has been observed in patients taking PPIs, including lansoprazole. It may occur at any point during therapy, and is generally attributed to an idiopathic hypersensitivity reaction. Discontinue drug if condition develops.
• Prolonged treatment (2 years or more) may cause cyanocobalamin (vitamin B_{12}) malabsorption caused by hypochlorhydria or achlorhydria. Observe for clinical signs and symptoms consistent with cyanocobalamin deficiency.
Dialyzable drug: No.

PREGNANCY-LACTATION-REPRODUCTION
• There are no adequate studies in pregnant women. Use during pregnancy only if clearly needed.
• It isn't known if drug appears in breast milk. Patient should discontinue breastfeeding or discontinue drug.

NURSING CONSIDERATIONS
🔄 **Alert:** Monitor patient for signs and symptoms of low magnesium level, such as abnormal HR or rhythm, palpitations, muscle spasms, tremor, or seizures. In children, abnormal HR may present as fatigue, upset stomach, dizziness, and light-headedness.
🔄 **Alert:** May increase risk of CDAD. Evaluate for CDAD in patients who develop diarrhea that doesn't improve.
• Patients with severe liver disease may need dosage adjustment, but don't adjust dosage for elderly patients or those with renal insufficiency.
• Just because symptoms respond to therapy, gastric malignancy shouldn't be ruled out.
• **Look alike–sound alike:** Don't confuse Prevacid with Pepcid, Prilosec, or Prevpac.

PATIENT TEACHING
• For best effect, instruct patient to take drug 30 to 60 minutes before eating.
• Teach patient how to take drug and alternative methods if needed.
• Teach patient to recognize and report all adverse reactions, especially signs and symptoms of low magnesium level.

latanoprost
lah-TAN-oh-prost

Xalatan

Therapeutic class: Antiglaucoma drugs
Pharmacologic class: Prostaglandin analogues

AVAILABLE FORMS
Ophthalmic solution: 0.005% (50 mcg/mL)

INDICATIONS & DOSAGES
➤ **Increased IOP in patients with ocular hypertension or open-angle glaucoma**
Adults: Instill 1 drop in conjunctival sac of each affected eye once daily in the evening.

ADMINISTRATION
Ophthalmic
• Don't allow tip of dispenser to contact eye or surrounding tissue. Serious damage to eye and subsequent vision loss may be caused by contaminated solutions.
• Apply light finger pressure on lacrimal sac for 1 minute after instilling drug to minimize systemic absorption.

● If more than one ophthalmic drug is being used, give at least 5 minutes apart.

ACTION
Thought to increase outflow of aqueous humor, thereby lowering IOP.

Route	Onset	Peak	Duration
Ophthalmic	3–4 hr	8–12 hr	Unknown

Half-life: 17 minutes.

ADVERSE REACTIONS
CV: angina pectoris.
EENT: blurred vision, burning, foreign body sensation, increased brown pigmentation of the iris, itching, stinging, conjunctival hyperemia, dry eye, excessive tearing, eye pain, eyelash changes, lid crusting or edema, lid discomfort, photophobia, punctate epithelial keratopathy.
Musculoskeletal: muscle, joint, or back pain.
Respiratory: URI.
Skin: allergic skin reaction, rash.
Other: cold, flulike syndrome.

INTERACTIONS
Drug-drug. *Eyedrops that contain thimerosal:* May cause precipitation of eyedrops. Give at least 5 minutes apart.

EFFECTS ON LAB TEST RESULTS
None reported.

CONTRAINDICATIONS & CAUTIONS
● Contraindicated in patients hypersensitive to drug, benzalkonium chloride, or other components of drug.
● Use cautiously in patients with impaired renal or hepatic function.
● Use cautiously in patients with a history of intraocular inflammation (iritis or uveitis).
● Don't use in patients with active intraocular inflammation.
● Drug may cause macular edema. Use cautiously in patients without an intact posterior capsule or who have risk factors for macular edema.
● Safety and effectiveness in children haven't been established.
Dialyzable drug: Unknown.
⚠ *Overdose S&S:* Ocular irritation, conjunctival or episcleral congestion.

PREGNANCY-LACTATION-REPRODUCTION
● There are no adequate studies in pregnant women. Use during pregnancy only if potential benefit justifies potential risk to the fetus.
● It isn't known if drug appears in breast milk. Use cautiously in breast-feeding women.

NURSING CONSIDERATIONS
● Don't give drug while patient is wearing contact lenses.
● Giving drug more frequently than recommended may decrease its IOP-lowering effects; don't exceed once-daily dosing.
● Drug may gradually change eye color, increasing amount of brown pigment in iris. This change in iris color occurs slowly and may not be noticeable for months or years. Increased pigmentation may be permanent.

PATIENT TEACHING
● Inform patient of risk that iris color may change in treated eye.
● Inform patient that darkening of eyelid may occur.
● Teach patient about potential changes to eyelashes (increased length, thickness, pigmentation, number of lashes).
● Teach patient how to instill drops, and advise him to wash hands before and after instilling solution. Warn him not to touch tip of dropper to eye or surrounding tissue.
● Advise patient to apply light finger pressure on lacrimal sac for 1 minute after instillation to minimize systemic absorption.
● Tell patient to report all adverse reactions and eye reactions, especially inflammation and lid reactions.
● Tell contact lens wearers to remove lenses before instilling solution and not to reinsert them for 15 minutes.
● If patient is using more than one topical ophthalmic drug, tell him to apply them at least 5 minutes apart.
● If patient develops another eye condition (such as trauma or infection) or needs eye surgery, advise him to contact prescriber about continued use of multidose container.
● Stress importance of compliance with recommended therapy.

Reactions in bold italics are *life-threatening*. Interactions may have a *rapid onset* or a *delayed onset*.

ledipasvir–sofosbuvir
LED-i-pas-vir/soe-FOS-bue-vir

Harvoni

Therapeutic class: Antivirals
Pharmacologic class: Antivirals

AVAILABLE FORMS
Tablets: 90 mg ledipasvir/400 mg sofosbuvir

INDICATIONS & DOSAGES
⚠ *Alert:* Sofosbuvir and its metabolite accumulate in patients with severe renal impairment (CrCl of less than 30 mL/minute). There are no dosing guidelines provided by the manufacturer.

➤ **Chronic HCV genotype 1 infection in treatment-naive patients with or without compensated cirrhosis or in treatment-experienced patients without cirrhosis**
Adults: One tablet P.O. once daily for 12 weeks. If pretreatment HCV-RNA is less than 6 million international units/mL in treatment-naive patients without cirrhosis, may consider treatment course of 8 weeks.

➤ **Chronic HCV genotype 1 infection in treatment-experienced patients with compensated cirrhosis**
Adults: One tablet P.O. once daily for 24 weeks.

➤ **Chronic HCV genotype 1 infection in treatment-naive and treatment-experienced patients with decompensated cirrhosis, in combination with ribavirin; chronic HCV genotype 1 or 4 infection in treatment-naive and treatment-experienced liver transplant patients without cirrhosis or with compensated cirrhosis, in combination with ribavirin**
Adults: One tablet P.O. once daily with ribavirin for 12 weeks.

➤ **Chronic HCV genotype 4,5,6 infection in treatment-naive patients without cirrhosis or with compensated cirrhosis**
Adults: One tablet P.O. once daily for 12 weeks.

ADMINISTRATION
P.O.
● May give without regard for food.

● Store at room temperature in original container.

ACTION
Ledipasvir and sofosbuvir are direct-acting antivirals against HCV. Ledipasvir inhibits the NS5A protein, and sofosbuvir inhibits the NS5B RNA polymerase, both of which are required for viral replication.

Route	Onset	Peak	Duration
P.O. (ledipasvir)	Unknown	4–4½ hr	Unknown
P.O. (sofosbuvir)	Unknown	0.8–1 hr	Unknown

Half-life: Ledipasvir, 47 hours; sofosbuvir, ½ hour.

ADVERSE REACTIONS
CNS: fatigue, headache, insomnia.
GI: nausea, diarrhea.
Hepatic: increased bilirubin and lipase levels.

INTERACTIONS
Drug-drug. ⚠ *Alert: Amiodarone:* May increase risk of symptomatic bradycardia, requiring pacemaker intervention, and cardiac arrest. Avoid use together. If use together can't be avoided, advise patient of risk and monitor patient carefully.
Antacids (aluminum hydroxide, magnesium hydroxide): May decrease ledipasvir level. Separate administration of antacids and ledipasvir–sofosbuvir by 4 hours.
Anticonvulsants (carbamazepine, oxcarbazepine, phenobarbital, phenytoin), antimycobacterials (rifabutin, rifampin, rifapentine), P-glycoprotein inducers (rifampin): May decrease ledipasvir–sofosbuvir concentrations. Use together isn't recommended.
Digoxin: May increase digoxin concentration. Monitor digoxin level.
H₂-receptor antagonists (famotidine): May decrease ledipasvir level. Separate administration by 12 hours or administer simultaneously if H₂-receptor antagonist dose doesn't exceed equivalent of famotidine 40 mg b.i.d.
HIV antiretroviral regimen containing tenofovir disoproxil fumarate, an HIV protease inhibitor (atazanavir, darunavir, lopinavir), and ritonavir: May increase tenofovir-associated adverse reactions. Safety of use together hasn't been established. Consider

alternative HCV or antiretroviral therapy or monitor patient closely for tenofovir-associated adverse reactions.

HIV antiretroviral regimen containing tenofovir disoproxil fumarate, cobicistat, elvitegravir, and emtricitabine: May increase tenofovir level. Safety of use together hasn't been established; use together isn't recommended.

HIV antiretroviral regimen containing tenofovir disoproxil fumarate, efavirenz, and emtricitabine: May increase tenofovir concentration and risk of toxicity. Monitor patient for tenofovir-associated adverse reactions.

HIV antiretroviral regimen containing tipranavir and ritonavir: May decrease ledipasvir–sofosbuvir concentrations and effectiveness. Use together isn't recommended.

HMG-CoA reductase inhibitors (rosuvastatin): May increase concentration of reductase inhibitor and increase risk of myopathy, including rhabdomyolysis. Use together isn't recommended.

Other products containing sofosbuvir: Duplicates therapy. Contraindicated for use together.

PPIs (omeprazole): May decrease ledipasvir level. May give PPI doses equivalent to 20 mg or less of omeprazole simultaneously with ledipasvir–sofosbuvir on an empty stomach.

Simeprevir: May increase ledipasvir–sofosbuvir concentrations. Use together isn't recommended.

Drug-herb. *St. John's wort:* May significantly decrease drug plasma level and reduce efficacy. Discourage use together.

EFFECTS ON LAB TEST RESULTS
• May increase bilirubin, lipase, and CK levels.

CONTRAINDICATIONS & CAUTIONS
• Contraindicated in patients hypersensitive to either drug or their components.

Black Box Warning Reactivation of hepatitis B virus (HBV) may occur in hepatitis C virus (HCV) co-infected patients, and result in fulminant hepatitis, hepatic failure and death. Screen all patients for current or prior HBV infection prior to treatment and if positive for HBV infection, assess baseline HBV DNA. ∎

• Use with other drugs containing sofosbuvir isn't recommended.

⊕ Alert: Symptomatic bradycardia, including fatal cardiac arrest and cases requiring pacemaker intervention, have been reported when drug is given with amiodarone. Patients taking amiodarone who are also taking beta blockers or have underlying cardiac comorbidities or advanced liver disease may be at increased risk. Symptoms may occur within hours to up to 2 weeks after start of treatment of HCV infection.

• Safety and effectiveness in children haven't been established.

Dialyzable drug: Ledipasvir, unlikely; sofosbuvir, 18%.

PREGNANCY-LACTATION-REPRODUCTION
• Use in pregnant women hasn't been well studied. Use cautiously and only if benefits outweigh potential risk to the fetus.
• It isn't known if drug appears in breast milk. Use cautiously in breast-feeding women and only if benefits outweigh potential risk to the fetus.

NURSING CONSIDERATIONS
Black Box Warning Monitor patient with current or prior HBV infection, for hepatitis flare or HBV reactivation with laboratory testing and watch for signs and symptoms of liver injury during active and post-treatment follow-up. ∎

⊕ Alert: Monitor patients taking amiodarone and those who must start amiodarone or who recently discontinued amiodarone for signs and symptoms of bradycardia (near-fainting or fainting, dizziness, lightheadedness, malaise, weakness, excessive fatigue, shortness of breath, chest pain, confusion, or memory problems). Utilize inpatient cardiac monitoring for first 48 hours; continue outpatient or self-monitoring of HR for bradycardia daily through at least first 2 weeks of treatment. Discontinue HCV treatment if signs or symptoms of bradycardia occur.

• Monitor bilirubin, liver enzyme, and serum creatinine levels at baseline and periodically when clinically indicated.

Reactions in bold italics are **life-threatening**. Interactions may have a *rapid onset* or a **delayed onset**.

• Monitor serum HCV-RNA level at baseline, during treatment, at end of treatment, during treatment follow-up, and when clinically indicated.
• Assess patient's concomitant medication use for potential drug interactions.

PATIENT TEACHING

Black Box Warning Warn patient to immediately report signs and symptoms of liver injury (fatigue, weakness, loss of appetite, nausea, vomiting, yellow skin or eyes, light-colored stool). ∎
• Instruct patient to take only one tablet at same time each day, with or without food. If a dose is missed within the calendar day it's usually taken, patient should take dose as soon as possible. If the calendar day when dose is usually taken has passed, patient shouldn't take missed dose and should resume usual dosing schedule.
• **Alert:** Caution patient to seek immediate medical attention for signs and symptoms of bradycardia.
• Inform patient that the effect of treatment on HCV transmission isn't known and to follow precautions to prevent transmission.
• Advise patient to report to prescriber all other prescription drugs, OTC medications, vitamins, and herbal supplements being taken because drug interactions are possible.
• Caution patient not to stop drug without first discussing with prescriber.
• Tell patient to report signs and symptoms of adverse reactions (fatigue, nausea, and headache).
• Advise patient to immediately report signs and symptoms of hypersensitivity reactions (wheezing, chest tightness, fever, itching, or swelling of the face, lips, tongue, or throat).

leflunomide
leh-FLEW-no-mide

Arava

Therapeutic class: Antiarthritics
Pharmacologic class: Pyrimidine synthesis inhibitors

AVAILABLE FORMS
Tablets: 10 mg, 20 mg, 100 mg

INDICATIONS & DOSAGES
➤ **To reduce signs and symptoms of active RA; to slow structural damage as shown by erosions and joint space narrowing seen on X-ray; to improve physical function**
Adults: 100 mg P.O. loading dose every 24 hours for 3 days; then 20 mg (maximum daily dose) P.O. every 24 hours. Eliminating loading dose may decrease risk of adverse reactions, especially in patients at risk for hematologic or hepatic toxicity. Dose may be decreased to 10 mg daily if higher dose isn't well tolerated.
Adjust-a-dose: If confirmed ALT elevations between 2 and 3 × ULN occur during treatment, stop drug and investigate cause; monitor LFTs.

ADMINISTRATION
P.O.
• Give drug without regard for food.

ACTION
An immunomodulatory drug that inhibits dihydroorotate dehydrogenase, an enzyme involved in pyrimidine synthesis that has antiproliferative activity and anti-inflammatory effects.

Route	Onset	Peak	Duration
P.O.	Unknown	6–12 hr	Unknown

Half-life: Teriflunomide (active metabolite), 18 to 19 days.

ADVERSE REACTIONS
CNS: anxiety, depression, dizziness, fever, headache, insomnia, malaise, migraine, neuralgia, neuritis, pain, paresthesia, sleep disorder, vertigo.
CV: hypertension, angina pectoris, chest pain, palpitations, peripheral edema, tachycardia, varicose veins, vasculitis, vasodilation, hematoma.
EENT: blurred vision, cataracts, conjunctivitis, epistaxis, eye disorder, pharyngitis, rhinitis, sinusitis.
GI: diarrhea, abdominal pain, anorexia, cholelithiasis, colitis, constipation, dry mouth, dyspepsia, enlarged salivary glands, esophagitis, flatulence, gastritis, gastroenteritis, gingivitis, melena, nausea, oral candidiasis, stomatitis, taste perversion, vomiting.

GU: cystitis, dysuria, hematuria, menstrual disorder, pelvic pain, prostate disorder, urinary frequency, UTI, vaginal candidiasis.
Hematologic: anemia.
Hepatic: *hepatotoxicity.*
Metabolic: *diabetes mellitus,* hyperglycemia, hyperlipidemia, hyperthyroidism, hypokalemia, weight loss.
Musculoskeletal: arthralgia, arthrosis, back pain, bone necrosis, bursitis, joint disorder, leg cramps, muscle cramps, myalgia, neck pain, synovitis, tendon rupture, tenosynovitis.
Respiratory: respiratory infection, *asthma,* bronchitis, dyspnea, cough, lung disorder.
Skin: alopecia, rash, acne, contact dermatitis, dry skin, eczema, fungal dermatitis, hair discoloration, maculopapular rash, nail disorder, pruritus, skin discoloration, skin disorder, skin nodule, skin ulcer, subcutaneous nodule.
Other: abscess, allergic reaction, cyst, ecchymoses, herpes simplex, herpes zoster, increased sweating, injury or accident.

INTERACTIONS
Drug-drug. *Charcoal, cholestyramine:* May decrease leflunomide level. Sometimes used for this effect in leflunomide toxicity.
Methotrexate, other hepatotoxic drugs: May increase risk of hepatotoxicity. Monitor liver enzyme levels.
NSAIDs (diclofenac, ibuprofen): May increase NSAID level. Monitor patient.
Rifampin: May increase active leflunomide metabolite level. Use together cautiously.
Tolbutamide: May increase tolbutamide level. Monitor patient.
Vaccines: May increase vaccine-related toxic effects. Modify therapy.
Vitamin K antagonists (warfarin): May enhance anticoagulant effect of these drugs. Monitor therapy.

EFFECTS ON LAB TEST RESULTS
• May increase AST, ALT, glucose, lipid, and CK levels.
• May decrease potassium level.

CONTRAINDICATIONS & CAUTIONS
• Contraindicated in patients hypersensitive to drug or its components.
• Drug isn't recommended for patients with evidence of HBV or HBC infection, severe immunodeficiency, bone marrow dysplasia, or severe uncontrolled infections; in women who are breast-feeding; in patients younger than age 18; or in men attempting to father a child.
Black Box Warning Drug isn't recommended for patients with preexisting liver disease or ALT more than 2 × ULN. ■
Black Box Warning Use cautiously in patients taking other drugs that can cause liver damage. ■
• Use cautiously in patients with renal insufficiency.
Dialyzable drug: No.
⚠ *Overdose S&S:* Diarrhea, abdominal pain, leukopenia, anemia, elevated LFT results.

PREGNANCY-LACTATION-REPRODUCTION
Black Box Warning Contraindicated in pregnant women and women of childbearing potential who aren't using reliable contraception because of the potential for fetal harm. Pregnancy must be excluded before start of therapy. ■
• To monitor fetal outcomes of pregnant women exposed to leflunomide, patients should be registered with the Leflunomide Pregnancy Registry (1-877-311-8972).
• It isn't known if drug appears in breast milk. Patient should discontinue breast-feeding or discontinue drug.
• Patients should avoid pregnancy after drug administration until undetectable serum concentrations (less than 0.02 mg/L) are verified, which may be accomplished by use of the recommended leflunomide removal protocol.
↻ *Alert:* Men planning to father a child should stop drug and follow recommended leflunomide removal protocol. In addition to cholestyramine use, verify that drug levels are less than 0.02 mg/L by two separate tests at least 14 days apart.

NURSING CONSIDERATIONS
• Vaccination with live-virus vaccines isn't recommended. Consider the long half-life of drug when contemplating giving a live-virus vaccine after stopping drug treatment.
• Risk of malignancy, particularly lymphoproliferative disorders, is increased with use of some immunosuppressants, including leflunomide.

Black Box Warning Liver enzyme levels
should be monitored at least monthly for
6 months after beginning therapy and every
6 to 8 weeks thereafter. If ALT level rises
to more than 3 × ULN, interrupt therapy.
If drug is determined to be the cause, start
cholestyramine washout (8 g P.O. t.i.d.
for 11 days) and monitor LFT values until
normalized. ■

❸ Alert: Monitor platelet and WBC counts
and Hb level or hematocrit at baseline and
monthly for 6 months after starting therapy
and every 6 to 8 weeks thereafter.

❸ Alert: Monitor AST, ALT, and serum albumin levels monthly if treatment includes
methotrexate or other potential immunosuppressants.

• Monitor patient for peripheral neuropathy
as drug may need to be stopped.

• Stop drug and start cholestyramine or
charcoal therapy if bone marrow suppression occurs.

• Watch for overlapping hematologic toxicity when switching to another antirheumatic.

Black Box Warning Rare cases of severe
liver injury, including cases with fatal outcome, have occurred during leflunomide
therapy. Most cases occur within 6 months
of therapy and in a setting of multiple risk
factors for hepatotoxicity (liver disease,
other hepatotoxins). ■

• Carefully monitor patient after dose reduction. Because the active metabolite of
leflunomide has a prolonged half-life, it may
take several weeks for levels to decline.

PATIENT TEACHING

• Explain need for and frequency of required blood tests and monitoring.

Black Box Warning Instruct patient to use
birth control during course of treatment and
until it's been determined that drug is no
longer active. ■

• Warn patient to notify prescriber if signs
or symptoms of pregnancy (such as late
menstrual periods or breast tenderness)
occur because of risk of fetal birth defects.

• Advise women to stop breast-feeding.

• Instruct patient to report all adverse reactions and to immediately report rash or
mucous membrane lesions, unusual tiredness, abdominal pain, jaundice, easy bruising, bleeding, fever, recurrent infections, or
pallor, which may be warnings of infrequent
but serious adverse reactions.

• Inform patient he may continue taking
aspirin, other NSAIDs, and low-dose corticosteroids during treatment.

• Inform patient that it may take 4 weeks to
begin to see improvement from therapy.

lesinurad
See NEW DRUGS for information.

SAFETY ALERT!

letrozole
LE-tro-zol

Femara

Therapeutic class: Antineoplastics
Pharmacologic class: Aromatase
inhibitors

AVAILABLE FORMS
Tablets: 2.5 mg

INDICATIONS & DOSAGES

Adjust-a-dose (for all indications): In patients
with cirrhosis and severe hepatic impairment, give 2.5 mg every other day.

➤ **Metastatic breast cancer with disease
progression after antiestrogen therapy
(such as tamoxifen)**

Postmenopausal women: 2.5 mg P.O. as
single daily dose.

➤ **First-line treatment of hormone
receptor–positive or hormone receptor–
unknown, locally advanced, or metastatic
breast cancer**

Postmenopausal women: 2.5 mg P.O. once
daily until tumor progression is evident.

➤ **Adjuvant treatment of hormone sensitive early breast cancer**

Postmenopausal women: 2.5 mg P.O. daily.

➤ **Extended adjuvant treatment of early
breast cancer following 5 years of adjuvant tamoxifen therapy**

Postmenopausal women: 2.5 mg P.O. once
daily for 5 years.

ADMINISTRATION
P.O.

• Drug is a hormonal agent and considered
a potential teratogen. Follow safe handling
procedures.

• Give drug without regard for meals.

♣Canada   ◇OTC   ◆Off-label use   *Photoguide   ⓓ Do not crush   *Liquid contains alcohol.

ACTION

Inhibits conversion of androgens to estrogens, which decreases tumor mass or delays progression of tumor growth in some women.

Route	Onset	Peak	Duration
P.O.	Unknown	2–6 wk (steady-state plasma)	Unknown

Half-life: About 2 days.

ADVERSE REACTIONS

CNS: headache, somnolence, dizziness, fatigue, asthenia, mood changes, depression.
CV: hot flashes or flushing, *MI, thromboembolism,* chest pain, edema, hypertension.
GI: nausea, vomiting, constipation, diarrhea, abdominal pain, anorexia.
Metabolic: hypercholesterolemia, weight gain.
Musculoskeletal: bone pain, limb pain, back pain, arthralgia, fractures.
Respiratory: dyspnea, cough.
Skin: rash, pruritus, alopecia, diaphoresis.
Other: viral infections, breast pain.

INTERACTIONS

Drug-drug. *Estrogens:* May produce antagonistic effects with letrozole. Use together isn't recommended.
Tamoxifen: May reduce plasma letrozole levels. Monitor therapy.

EFFECTS ON LAB TEST RESULTS

• May increase cholesterol level.
• May decrease lymphocyte count.

CONTRAINDICATIONS & CAUTIONS

• Contraindicated in patients hypersensitive to drug or its components.
• Use cautiously in patients with severe liver impairment; dosage adjustment isn't needed in those with mild to moderate liver dysfunction.
Dialyzable drug: Unknown.

PREGNANCY-LACTATION-REPRODUCTION

• May cause fetal harm. Contraindicated in women who are or may become pregnant.
• It isn't known if drug appears in breast milk. Patient should discontinue breastfeeding or discontinue drug.

NURSING CONSIDERATIONS

• Dosage adjustment isn't needed in patients with CrCl of 10 mL/minute or more.
• Use drug only in postmenopausal women. Rule out pregnancy before starting drug.
• *Look alike–sound alike:* Don't confuse Femara with FemHRT.

PATIENT TEACHING

• Instruct patient to take drug exactly as prescribed.
• Tell patient to take drug with a small glass of water, with or without food.
• Inform patient about potential adverse effects and to report them.
• Advise patient to use caution performing tasks that require alertness, coordination, or dexterity, such as driving, until effects are known.
• Advise patient of childbearing potential to use adequate contraceptive methods.

SAFETY ALERT!

leuprolide acetate
loo-PROE-lide

Eligard, Lupron, Lupron Depot, Lupron Depot-Ped

Therapeutic class: Antineoplastics
Pharmacologic class: Gonadotropin-releasing hormone analogues

AVAILABLE FORMS

Depot injection: 3.75 mg, 7.5 mg, 11.25 mg, 15 mg, 22.5 mg, 30 mg, 45 mg
Injection: 5 mg/mL in 2.8-mL multiple-dose vials

INDICATIONS & DOSAGES

➤ **Advanced prostate cancer**
Adults: 1 mg subcutaneously daily. Or, 7.5 mg I.M. depot injection monthly. Or, 7.5 mg subcutaneous Eligard once monthly. Or, 22.5 mg I.M. depot injection every 3 months. Or, 22.5 mg subcutaneous Eligard every 3 months. Or, 30 mg I.M. depot injection every 4 months. Or, 30 mg subcutaneous Eligard every 4 months. Or, 45 mg subcutaneous Eligard every 6 months. Or, 45 mg I.M. depot injection every 6 months.

➤ **Endometriosis (alone or in combination with norethindrone acetate)**
Adults: 3.75 mg I.M. depot injection as single injection once monthly for up to 6 months. Or, 11.25 mg I.M. every 3 months for up to 6 months.

➤ **Central precocious puberty**
Children: Initially, 50 mcg/kg/day subcutaneously. Titrate dosage upward by 10 mcg/kg/day until no progression of condition is noted. Discontinue drug at the appropriate age of puberty onset.
Children age 2 and older (Lupron Depot-Ped): Initially, for child weighing more than 37.5 kg, 15 mg I.M. once monthly. For child weighing more than 25 to 37.5 kg, 11.25 mg I.M. once monthly. For child weighing 25 kg or less, 7.5 mg I.M. once monthly. Or, for 3-month formulation, usual dosage is 11.25 or 30 mg I.M. once every 3 months. If clinical suppression isn't achieved with starting dose, increase dose to next available higher dose. Discontinue drug at the appropriate age of puberty onset.

➤ **Anemia related to uterine fibroids (with iron therapy)**
Adults: 3.75 mg I.M. depot injection once monthly for up to 3 consecutive months. Or 11.25 mg I.M. depot injection for 1 dose.

ADMINISTRATION

• Products have specific mixing and administration instructions. Read manufacturer's directions closely.
• Drug is considered hazardous; use safe-handling precautions.
I.M.
• Never give by I.V. injection.
• Give depot injections under medical supervision.
• Use supplied diluent to reconstitute drug (extra diluent is provided; discard remainder).
• Inject into vial; shake well. Suspension will appear milky. Use immediately.
• Draw appropriate amount into a syringe with a 22G needle.
• When using prefilled dual-chamber syringes, prepare for injection according to manufacturer's instructions.
• Gently shake syringe to form a uniform milky suspension. If particles adhere to stopper, tap syringe against your finger.

• Remove needle guard and advance plunger to expel air from syringe. Inject entire contents I.M. as with a normal injection.
Subcutaneous
• For the two-syringe mixing system, connect the syringes and inject the liquid contents according to manufacturer's instructions.
• Mix product by pushing contents back and forth between syringes for about 45 seconds; shaking the syringes won't mix the contents enough.
• Attach the needle provided in the kit and inject subcutaneously.
• Suspension settles very quickly. Remix if settling occurs. Must be given within 30 minutes.
• Never give by I.V. injection.

ACTION

Stimulates and then inhibits release of FSH and luteinizing hormone, which suppresses testosterone and estrogen levels.

Route	Onset	Peak	Duration
I.M., subcut.	Variable	1–2 mo	60–90 days

Half-life: Unknown.

ADVERSE REACTIONS

CNS: dizziness, depression, headache, pain, insomnia, paresthesia, asthenia.
CV: *arrhythmias,* angina, *MI,* peripheral edema, ECG changes, hypotension, hypertension, murmur, hot flashes.
GI: nausea, vomiting, anorexia, constipation.
GU: impotence, vaginitis, urinary frequency, hematuria, UTI, amenorrhea.
Hematologic: anemia.
Metabolic: weight gain or loss.
Musculoskeletal: transient bone pain during first week of treatment, joint disorder, myalgia, neuromuscular disorder, bone loss.
Respiratory: dyspnea, sinus congestion, *pulmonary fibrosis.*
Skin: injection-site reactions, dermatitis, acne.
Other: gynecomastia, androgen-like effects.

INTERACTIONS
None significant.

EFFECTS ON LAB TEST RESULTS

- May increase bilirubin, cholesterol, BUN, calcium, creatinine, glucose, LDH, phosphorus, AST, ALT, and uric acid levels.
- May decrease albumin, protein, and potassium levels.
- May increase WBC. May decrease Hb level and hematocrit.
- May prolong PT and PTT.
- May increase or decrease platelet count.
- May alter results of pituitary-gonadal system tests during therapy and for 12 weeks after.

CONTRAINDICATIONS & CAUTIONS

- Contraindicated in patients hypersensitive to drug or other gonadotropin-releasing hormone analogues and in women with undiagnosed vaginal bleeding.
- Androgen deprivation therapy may prolong QT/QTc interval. Consider if benefits of therapy outweigh potential risks in patients with congenital long QT syndrome, HF, or frequent electrolyte abnormalities, and in patients taking drugs known to prolong QT interval.
- Seizures have been reported in patients taking leuprolide, including those with a history of seizures, epilepsy, cerebrovascular disorders, or CNS anomalies or tumors; in patients taking concomitant medications associated with seizures, such as bupropion and SSRIs; and in patients with none of the conditions mentioned above.
- The 30- and 45-mg depot injections are contraindicated in women and children.
- Use cautiously in patients hypersensitive to benzyl alcohol.

Dialyzable drug: Unknown.

PREGNANCY-LACTATION-REPRODUCTION

- Contraindicated in women who are or may become pregnant during therapy.
- It isn't known if drug appears in breast milk. Use is contraindicated in breast-feeding women.

NURSING CONSIDERATIONS

- A fractional dose of drug formulated to give every 3, 4, or 6 months isn't equivalent to same dose of once-a-month formulation.
- Correct electrolyte abnormalities before starting drug; consider periodic monitoring of ECGs and electrolytes.

- After starting treatment for central precocious puberty, monitor patient response every 1 to 2 months with a gonadotropin-releasing hormone stimulation test and sex corticosteroid level determinations. Measure bone age for advancement every 6 to 12 months.

⚠ Alert: During first few weeks of treatment for prostate cancer, signs and symptoms of disease may temporarily worsen or additional signs and symptoms may occur (tumor flare).

- May increase risk of diabetes and CV events. Monitor patient closely.
- *Look alike–sound alike:* Don't confuse Lupron Depot with Lupron Depot-Ped.

PATIENT TEACHING

- Before starting child on treatment for central precocious puberty, make sure parents understand importance of continuous therapy.
- Carefully instruct patient who will give himself subcutaneous injection about the proper technique, and advise him to use only the syringes provided by manufacturer.
- Advise patient that, if another syringe must be substituted, a low-dose insulin syringe (U-100, 0.5 mL) may be an appropriate choice but that needle gauge should be no smaller than 22G.
- Instruct patient to store leuprolide acetate powder (depot) and diluent at room temperature, to refrigerate unopened vials of leuprolide acetate injection, and to protect leuprolide acetate injection from heat and light.
- Inform patient with history of undesirable effects from other endocrine therapies that leuprolide is easier to tolerate. Advise patient to report all adverse effects.
- Explain that symptoms of prostate cancer or central precocious puberty may worsen at first.
- Advise female patient of childbearing potential to use a nonhormonal form of contraception during treatment.

levalbuterol hydrochloride
lev-al-BYOO-ter-ol

Xopenex

levalbuterol tartrate
Xopenex HFA

Therapeutic class: Bronchodilators
Pharmacologic class: Beta₂ agonists

AVAILABLE FORMS
Inhalation aerosol: 45 mcg per actuation
Solution for inhalation: 0.31 mg, 0.63 mg, or 1.25 mg in 3-mL vials; 1.25 mg/0.5-mL vials (concentrate)

INDICATIONS & DOSAGES
➤ **To prevent or treat bronchospasm in patients with reversible obstructive airway disease**
Adults and adolescents age 12 and older: 0.63 mg t.i.d. every 6 to 8 hours, by oral inhalation via a nebulizer. Patients with more severe asthma who don't respond adequately to 0.63 mg t.i.d. may benefit from 1.25 mg t.i.d.
Children ages 6 to 11: 0.31 mg inhaled by nebulizer t.i.d. Routine dosage shouldn't exceed 0.63 mg t.i.d.
Adults and children age 4 and older: 2 inhalations Xopenex HFA (90 mcg) every 4 to 6 hours. In some patients, 1 inhalation (45 mcg) every 4 hours is sufficient.

ADMINISTRATION
Inhalation
● Keep unopened vial in foil pouch. After opened, vial must be used within 2 weeks and protected from light.
● Release four test sprays before first use of inhaler or after inhaler has not been used for more than 3 days.
● Shake canister well before use.
● Use a spacer device to improve inhalation, as appropriate.
   Dilute concentrated solution (1.25 mg/0.5 mL) with sterile NSS before administration by nebulization.

ACTION
Relaxes bronchial smooth muscle by stimulating beta₂ receptors; also inhibits release of mediators from mast cells in the airway.

Route	Onset	Peak	Duration
Inhalation	5–15 min	1 hr	3–4 hr

Half-life: 3¼ to 4 hours.

ADVERSE REACTIONS
CNS: dizziness, migraine, nervousness, pain, tremor, anxiety, asthenia, fever, headache.
CV: tachycardia.
EENT: rhinitis, sinusitis, turbinate edema, pharyngitis.
GI: dyspepsia, diarrhea.
Musculoskeletal: leg cramps.
Respiratory: increased cough, asthma.
Other: viral infection, flulike syndrome, accidental injury, lymphadenopathy.

INTERACTIONS
Drug-drug. *Beta blockers:* May block pulmonary effect of the drug and cause severe bronchospasm. Avoid using together, if possible. If use together is unavoidable, consider a cardioselective beta blocker, but use cautiously.
Digoxin: May decrease digoxin levels up to 22%. Monitor digoxin level.
Loop or thiazide diuretics: May cause ECG changes and hypokalemia. Use together cautiously.
MAO inhibitors, TCAs: May potentiate action of levalbuterol on the vascular system. Avoid using within 2 weeks of MAO inhibitor or TCA therapy.
Other short-acting sympathomimetic aerosol bronchodilators, epinephrine: May increase adrenergic adverse effects. Use together cautiously.

EFFECTS ON LAB TEST RESULTS
None reported.

CONTRAINDICATIONS & CAUTIONS
● Contraindicated in patients hypersensitive to drug or to racemic albuterol.
● Use cautiously in patients with CV disorders (especially coronary insufficiency, hypertension, and arrhythmias), seizure disorders, hyperthyroidism, or diabetes

L

mellitus, and in those who are unusually responsive to sympathomimetic amines.
Dialyzable drug: Unknown.

⚠ *Overdose S&S:* Exaggeration of adverse reactions, hypokalemia, seizures, angina, hypertension, hypotension, arrhythmias, muscle cramps, dry mouth, palpitations, nausea, insomnia, cardiac arrest, sudden death.

PREGNANCY-LACTATION-REPRODUCTION
● There are no adequate studies in pregnant women. Use during pregnancy only if potential benefit justifies potential risk to the fetus.
● It isn't known if drug appears in breast milk. Patient should discontinue breastfeeding or discontinue drug.

NURSING CONSIDERATIONS
❸ *Alert:* As with other inhaled beta agonists, drug can produce paradoxical bronchospasm or life-threatening CV effects. If this occurs, stop drug immediately and notify prescriber.
● Drug may worsen diabetes mellitus and ketoacidosis.
● Monitor potassium level, as drug may temporarily decrease potassium level.
● The compatibility of levalbuterol mixed with other drugs in a nebulizer hasn't been established.

PATIENT TEACHING
● Tell patient not to increase dosage without consulting prescriber.
● Advise patient not to use more frequently than recommended.
● Urge patient to seek medical attention immediately if levalbuterol becomes less effective, if signs and symptoms worsen, or if patient is using drug more frequently than usual.
● Tell patient that the effects of levalbuterol may last up to 8 hours.
● Tell patient not to double the next dose if a dose is missed and to take doses at least 6 hours apart.
● Advise patient to use other inhalational drugs and antiasthmatics only as directed while taking levalbuterol.
● Inform patient that common adverse reactions include palpitations, rapid HR,

headache, dizziness, tremor, and nervousness.
● Encourage female patient to contact prescriber if she becomes pregnant or is breastfeeding.
● Tell patient to keep unopened vials in foil pouch. After the foil pouch is opened, vials must be used within 2 weeks. Inform patient that vials removed from the pouch, if not used immediately, should be protected from light and excessive heat and used within 1 week.
● Teach patient to use drug correctly when inhaling by nebulizer.
● Instruct patient to shake inhaler well before using and to breathe as calmly, deeply, and evenly as possible until no more mist is formed in the nebulizer reservoir (5 to 15 minutes).
● Tell patient using the inhaler to release four test sprays into the air away from the face before the first use or if it hasn't been used for more than 3 days.
● Instruct patient to thoroughly wash and dry plastic actuator of inhaler at least once a week to prevent medication build-up and blockage. If actuator becomes blocked, washing actuator will remove blockage.

levetiracetam
lee-vah-tih-RACE-ah-tam

Keppra, Keppra XR, Spritam

Therapeutic class: Anticonvulsants
Pharmacologic class: Pyrrolidine derivatives

AVAILABLE FORMS
Injection: 500 mg/5 mL single-use vial
Injection (premixed in NSS): 500 mg/100 mL (5 mg/mL), 1,000 mg/100 mL (10 mg/mL), 1,500 mg/100 mL (15 mg/mL)
Oral solution: 100 mg/mL
Tablets 🔵*:* 250 mg, 500 mg, 750 mg, 1,000 mg
Tablets (extended-release) 🔵*:* 500 mg, 750 mg, 1,000 mg, 1,500 mg
Tablets for oral suspension: 250 mg, 500 mg, 750 mg, 1,000 mg

---

Reactions in bold italics are *life-threatening*. Interactions may have a *rapid onset* or a ***delayed onset***.

INDICATIONS & DOSAGES

Adjust-a-dose (for all indications): For immediate-release and oral solution, in adults with CrCl of 50 to 80 mL/minute, give 500 to 1,000 mg every 12 hours; if CrCl is 30 to 50 mL/minute, give 250 to 750 mg every 12 hours; if CrCl is less than 30 mL/minute, give 250 to 500 mg every 12 hours. For dialysis patients, give 500 to 1,000 mg every 24 hours. Give a 250- to 500-mg dose after dialysis.

For extended-release tablets, if CrCl is 50 to 80 mL/minute, give 1,000 to 2,000 mg every 24 hours. If CrCl is 30 to 50 mL/minute, give 500 to 1,500 mg every 24 hours. If CrCl is less than 30 mL/minute, give 500 to 1,000 mg every 24 hours.

➤ **Adjunctive therapy for myoclonic seizures of juvenile myoclonic epilepsy**
Adults and adolescents age 12 and older: Initially, 500 mg P.O. or I.V. b.i.d. Increase by 1,000 mg/day every 2 weeks to a dose of 1,500 mg P.O. or I.V. b.i.d. (3,000 mg/day).

➤ **Adjunctive therapy for primary generalized tonic-clonic seizures**
Adults and adolescents age 16 and older: Initially, 500 mg P.O. or I.V. b.i.d. Increase dose by 500 mg b.i.d. every 2 weeks to dose of 1,500 mg b.i.d.
Children ages 6 to younger than 16: Initially, 10 mg/kg P.O. or I.V. b.i.d. Increase dose by 10 mg/kg b.i.d. at 2-week intervals to dose of 30 mg/kg b.i.d. For children weighing more than 20 kg, use either tablets or oral solution. For children weighing 20 kg or less, use oral solution.

➤ **Adjunctive therapy for primary generalized tonic-clonic seizures (Spritam)**
Adults and children age 6 and older weighing more than 40 kg: 500 mg P.O. b.i.d.; increase as needed and tolerated by 500 mg P.O. b.i.d. every 2 weeks to a maximum recommended dose of 1,500 mg b.i.d.
Children age 6 and older weighing 20 to 40 kg: 250 mg P.O. b.i.d.; increase by 250 mg P.O. b.i.d. every 2 weeks to a maximum of 750 mg b.i.d.

➤ **Adjunctive treatment for partial-onset seizures in patients with epilepsy**
Adults and adolescents age 16 and older: Initially, 500 mg P.O. or I.V. b.i.d. Increase dosage by 500 mg b.i.d., as needed, for seizure control at 2-week intervals to maximum of 1,500 mg b.i.d.
Children ages 4 to younger than 16: Initially, 10 mg/kg b.i.d. Increase dose by 10 mg/kg b.i.d. at 2-week intervals to recommended dose of 30 mg/kg b.i.d. If patient can't tolerate this dose, reduce it. For children who weigh 20 kg or less, use the oral solution.
Children ages 6 months to younger than 4 years: Initially, 10 mg/kg P.O. or I.V. b.i.d. Increase by 10 mg/kg b.i.d. at 2-week intervals to recommended dosage of 25 mg/kg b.i.d. Reduce dosage if patient can't tolerate total daily dose of 50 mg/kg.
Children ages 1 month to 6 months: Initially, 7 mg/kg P.O. or I.V. b.i.d. Increase by 7 mg/kg b.i.d. at 2-week intervals to recommended dosage of 21 mg/kg b.i.d.

➤ **Adjunctive treatment for partial-onset seizures in patients with epilepsy (Spritam)**
Adults and children age 4 and older weighing more than 40 kg: 500 mg P.O. b.i.d.; increase as needed and tolerated by 500 mg P.O. b.i.d. every 2 weeks to a maximum recommended dose of 1,500 mg b.i.d.
Children age 4 and older weighing 20 to 40 kg: 250 mg P.O. b.i.d.; increase by 250 mg P.O. b.i.d. every 2 weeks to a maximum of 750 mg b.i.d.

➤ **Adjunctive treatment for partial-onset seizures in patients with epilepsy (extended-release)**
Adults and children age 12 and older: Initially, 1,000 mg P.O. once daily. May adjust once-daily dosage in increments of 1,000 mg every 2 weeks to maximum recommended once-daily dose of 3,000 mg.

ADMINISTRATION
P.O.

• Give drug without regard for food.
• Oral and I.V. forms are bioequivalent.
• Tablets should be swallowed whole and shouldn't be chewed, broken, or crushed.
• Tablets for oral solution are intended to disintegrate in the mouth. Place tablet on tongue with a dry hand. Follow with a sip of liquid and have patient swallow only after tablet disintegrates; patient shouldn't swallow tablet intact. Don't give partial tablets. Or, add whole tablet to a small

L

volume of liquid in a cup (1 tablespoon or enough to cover tablet); allow tablet to disperse, then have patient immediately consume entire contents.

• Don't push tablets for oral solution through the foil; peel foil from blister by bending up and lifting peel tab around the blister seal.

I.V.

▼ Dilute drug before giving.

▼ For adults and adolescents receiving adult dosages, dilute 500-mg, 1,000-mg, or 1,500-mg dose in 100 mL NSS, D₅W, or lactated Ringer injection and infuse within 4 hours over 15 minutes.

▼ For children, calculate the amount of diluent to not exceed a maximum levetiracetam concentration of 15 mg/mL of diluted solution; infuse within 4 hours over 15 minutes.

▼ Drug is compatible with diazepam, lorazepam, and valproate sodium for 4 hours at a controlled room temperature.

▼ Store premixed solution for infusion at 68° to 77° F (20° to 25° C); don't dilute.

▼ Store vials for injection at 77° F (25° C); excursions permitted to 59° to 86° F (15° to 30° C).

▼ **Incompatibilities:** Unknown with other antiepileptics besides diazepam, lorazepam, and valproate sodium.

ACTION

May act by inhibiting simultaneous neuronal firing that leads to seizure activity.

Route	Onset	Peak	Duration
P.O. (immediate-release), I.V.	1 hr	1 hr	12 hr
P.O. (extended-release)	Unknown	4 hr	Unknown

Half-life: About 6 to 8 hours in adult patients with normal renal function.

ADVERSE REACTIONS

CNS: asthenia, headache, somnolence, amnesia, anxiety, ataxia, depression, dizziness, emotional lability, hostility, nervousness, paresthesia, pain, vertigo.
EENT: diplopia, pharyngitis, rhinitis, sinusitis.

GI: anorexia.
Hematologic: *leukopenia, neutropenia.*
Respiratory: cough.
Other: infection.

INTERACTIONS

Drug-drug. *Antihistamines, benzodiazepines, opioids, other drugs that cause drowsiness, TCAs:* May lead to severe sedation. Avoid using together.
Drug-lifestyle. *Alcohol use:* May lead to severe sedation. Discourage use together.

EFFECTS ON LAB TEST RESULTS

• May alter LFT results. May decrease Hb and hematocrit.
• May decrease WBC, RBC, and neutrophil counts.
• May increase eosinophil count.

CONTRAINDICATIONS & CAUTIONS

• Contraindicated in patients hypersensitive to drug.
• Use cautiously in patients with history of psychiatric symptoms, especially psychotic symptoms and behaviors.
• Serious skin reactions, including toxic epidermal necrolysis and Stevens-Johnson syndrome, have been reported. Recurrence following rechallenge is possible. Discontinue drug for hypersensitivity reaction or unspecified rash.
• Don't abruptly discontinue drug because withdrawal seizures may occur.
• Drug may cause hematologic abnormalities, including decreased RBC, WBC, and neutrophil counts, Hb level, and hematocrit, and increased eosinophil count. Cases of agranulocytosis have been reported in the postmarketing setting.
Dialyzable drug: 50%.
⚠ **Overdose S&S:** Drowsiness, aggression, agitation, coma, depressed level of consciousness, respiratory depression, somnolence.

PREGNANCY-LACTATION-REPRODUCTION

• There are no adequate studies in pregnant women. Use during pregnancy only if potential benefit justifies potential risk to the fetus.
• Pregnant patients taking drug should enroll themselves in the North American

---

*Reactions in bold italics are **life-threatening**. Interactions may have a rapid onset or a **delayed onset**.*

Antiepileptic Drug Pregnancy Registry by calling 1-888-233-2334.
• Drug appears in breast milk. Patient should discontinue breast-feeding or discontinue drug.

NURSING CONSIDERATIONS

• Use drug only with other anticonvulsants; it's not recommended for monotherapy.
• Seizures can occur if drug is stopped abruptly. Tapering is recommended.
• Monitor patients for signs and symptoms of somnolence and fatigue. Somnolence and asthenia occurred most frequently within first 4 weeks of treatment.
• Monitor patients closely for such adverse reactions as dizziness, which may lead to falls.
• Monitor patients ages 1 month to younger than 4 years for increases in diastolic BP.
⚠ **Alert:** Closely monitor all patients taking or starting antiepileptic drugs for changes in behavior indicating psychosis or worsening of suicidal thoughts or behavior or depression. Symptoms such as anxiety, agitation, hostility, mania, and hypomania may be precursors to emerging suicidality.
• **Look alike–sound alike:** Don't confuse levetiracetam with levofloxacin. Don't confuse Keppra with Kaletra or Keflex.

PATIENT TEACHING

• Tell patient to seek medical attention for emerging or worsening depression, suicidal thoughts or behavior, or unusual changes in mood or behavior and to report such symptoms as anxiety, agitation, hostility, mania, and hypomania, which may be precursors to emerging suicidality.
• Warn patient to use extra care when sitting or standing to avoid falling.
• Advise patient to call prescriber and not to stop drug suddenly if adverse reactions occur.
• Tell patient to take with other prescribed seizure drugs.
• For the oral solution, tell patient or parent to use a calibrated measuring device, not a household spoon.
• Warn patient that drug may cause dizziness and somnolence and that he should avoid driving, operating heavy machinery,

bike riding, or other hazardous activities until he knows how the drug will affect him.
• Inform patient that drug can be taken with or without food.
• Tell patient not to chew, crush, or break tablets.
• Teach patient how to use tablets for oral solution correctly.
• Advise patient not to stop drug abruptly because doing so may increase seizure frequency.

levobunolol hydrochloride
LEE-voe-BYOO-no-lahl

Betagan

Therapeutic class: Antiglaucoma drugs
Pharmacologic class: Nonselective beta blockers

AVAILABLE FORMS
Ophthalmic solution: 0.5%

INDICATIONS & DOSAGES
➤ **Chronic open-angle glaucoma, ocular hypertension**
Adults: 1 or 2 drops once daily. May give 0.5% solution b.i.d. in patients with more severe or uncontrolled glaucoma.

ADMINISTRATION
Ophthalmic
• Don't let tip of dropper touch patient's eye or surrounding tissue.
• Apply light finger pressure on lacrimal sac for 1 minute after instilling drug to minimize systemic absorption.

ACTION
Thought to reduce formation, and possibly increase outflow, of aqueous humor.

Route	Onset	Peak	Duration
Ophthalmic	1 hr	2–6 hr	24 hr

Half-life: Unknown.

ADVERSE REACTIONS
CNS: syncope, depression, headache, insomnia.
CV: hypotension, *bradycardia, HF,* slight reduction in resting HR, heart block, stroke,

cerebral ischemia, palpitations, *cardiac arrest.*
EENT: transient eye stinging and burning, blepharoconjunctivitis, corneal punctate staining, decreased corneal sensitivity, erythema, itching, keratitis, photophobia, tearing, nasal congestion.
GI: nausea, diarrhea.
Respiratory: *bronchospasm,* dyspnea.
Skin: urticaria.

INTERACTIONS
Drug-drug. *Dipivefrin, epinephrine, systemically administered carbonic anhydrase inhibitors, topical miotics:* May further reduce IOP. Use together cautiously.
Metoprolol, propranolol, other oral beta blockers: May increase ocular and systemic effects. Avoid use together.
Reserpine, other catecholamine-depleting drugs: May increase hypotensive and brady-cardiac effects. Monitor BP and HR closely.
Drug-lifestyle. *Sun exposure:* May cause photophobia. Advise patient to wear sunglasses.

EFFECTS ON LAB TEST RESULTS
None reported.

CONTRAINDICATIONS & CAUTIONS
• May be absorbed systemically. Contraindicated in patients hypersensitive to drug and in those with bronchial asthma, sinus bradycardia, second- or third-degree AV block, cardiac failure, cardiogenic shock, or history of bronchial asthma or severe COPD.
• Use cautiously in patients taking oral beta blockers and in those with chronic bronchitis, emphysema, diabetes mellitus, hyperthyroidism, sulfite sensitivity, or myasthenia gravis.
Dialyzable drug: Unknown.
⚠ Overdose S&S: Bradycardia, hypotension, bronchospasm, acute HF.

PREGNANCY-LACTATION-REPRODUCTION
• There are no adequate studies in pregnant women. Use during pregnancy only if potential benefit justifies potential fetal risk.
• It isn't known if drug appears in breast milk. Use cautiously in breast-feeding women.

NURSING CONSIDERATIONS
• Normal IOP is 10 to 21 mm Hg.
• Don't use two or more topical ophthalmic beta-adrenergic blockers simultaneously.

PATIENT TEACHING
• Teach patient how to instill drug. Advise him to wash hands before and after instillation and to apply light finger pressure on lacrimal sac for 1 minute after drops are instilled.
• Warn patient not to touch tip of dropper to eye or surrounding tissue.
• Advise elderly patient to report shortness of breath, chest pain, or heart irregularities to prescriber. Drug may be absorbed systemically and produce signs and symptoms of beta blockade.
• Advise patient to carry medical identification at all times during therapy.

levocetirizine dihydrochloride
LEE-voe-se-TIR-a-zeen

Xyzal

Therapeutic class: Antihistamines
Pharmacologic class: H_1-receptor antagonists

AVAILABLE FORMS
Oral solution: 2.5 mg/5 mL
Tablets: 5 mg

INDICATIONS & DOSAGES
Adjust-a-dose (for all indications): For patients age 12 and older with CrCl of 50 to 80 mL/minute, give 2.5 mg P.O. once daily; with CrCl of 30 to 50 mL/minute, give 2.5 mg P.O. every other day; with CrCl of 10 to 30 mL/minute, give 2.5 mg P.O. twice weekly (once every 3 to 4 days).
➤ **Perennial allergic rhinitis; uncomplicated skin manifestations of chronic idiopathic urticaria**
Adults and children age 12 and older: 5 mg P.O. once daily in the evening; 2.5 mg P.O. once daily in the evening may be adequate for some patients.
Children ages 6 to 11: 2.5 mg P.O. once daily in the evening.

Children ages 6 months to 5 years: 1.25 mg
(2.5 mL) P.O. daily in the evening. Don't
exceed this dose.

➤ **Seasonal allergic rhinitis**
Adults and children age 12 and older: 5 mg
P.O. once daily in the evening; 2.5 mg P.O.
once daily in the evening may be adequate
for some patients.
Children ages 6 to 11: 2.5 mg P.O. once
daily in the evening.
Children ages 2 to 5: 1.25 mg (2.5 mL) P.O.
daily in the evening. Don't exceed this dose.

ADMINISTRATION
P.O.
• Give drug in the evening without regard
for food.

ACTION
H_1-receptor inhibition creates antihistamine
effect, relieving allergy symptoms.

Route	Onset	Peak	Duration
P.O.	Unknown	1 hr	24 hr

Half-life: Adults, 8 to 9 hours; children, 6 hours.

ADVERSE REACTIONS
CNS: fatigue, pyrexia, somnolence.
EENT: dry mouth, epistaxis, nasopharyngi-
tis, pharyngitis.
GI: diarrhea, vomiting, constipation.
Respiratory: cough.

INTERACTIONS
Drug-drug. *CNS depressants:* May have
additive effects when taken together. Avoid
using together.
Ritonavir: May increase serum concentra-
tion and increase half-life of levocetirizine.
Use cautiously together.
Theophylline: May decrease the clearance of
levocetirizine. Use cautiously together.
Drug-lifestyle. *Alcohol use:* May have ad-
ditive effect when taken with levocetirizine.
Discourage use together.

EFFECTS ON LAB TEST RESULTS
May prevent, reduce, or mask positive
result skin wheal in diagnostic skin test.

CONTRAINDICATIONS & CAUTIONS
• Contraindicated in patients hypersensitive
drug or to cetirizine.

• Contraindicated in patients with CrCl of
less than 10 mL/minute or those undergoing
hemodialysis.
• Contraindicated in patients ages 6 to 11
with impaired renal function, in those with
ESRD, and in those undergoing dialysis.
• Use cautiously in patients with predisposing factors for urine retention, such as
spinal cord lesion or prostatic hyperplasia.
Discontinue drug if urine retention occurs.
Dialyzable drug: Less than 10%.
⚠ **Overdose S&S:** Drowsiness; initial agitation and restlessness, then drowsiness
(in children).

PREGNANCY-LACTATION-REPRODUCTION
• There are no adequate studies in pregnant
women. Use only if clearly needed.
• Drug may appear in breast milk. Use in
breast-feeding women isn't recommended.

NURSING CONSIDERATIONS
• Monitor patient's renal function.
• Patient should avoid engaging in hazardous occupations requiring mental alertness and motor coordination, such as operating machinery or driving a motor vehicle.
• Safety and effectiveness in patients
younger than age 6 months haven't been
established.

PATIENT TEACHING
• Warn patient not to perform hazardous
tasks or those requiring alertness and coordination until CNS effects are known.
• Advise patient to avoid use of alcohol and
other CNS depressants while taking this
drug.
• Advise patient not to take more than the
recommended dose because of increased
risk of somnolence at higher doses.

L

---

levodopa–carbidopa
lee-voe-DOE-pa/kar-bih-DOE-pa

Duopa, Rytary, Sinemet◆,
Sinemet CR◆

Therapeutic class: Antiparkinsonians
Pharmacologic class: Decarboxylase
inhibitors–dopamine precursors

AVAILABLE FORMS
Capsules (extended-release) ⬛*:* 95 mg
levodopa with 23.75 mg carbidopa, 145 mg
levodopa with 36.25 mg carbidopa, 195 mg
levodopa with 48.75 mg carbidopa, 245 mg
levodopa with 61.25 mg carbidopa
Enteral suspension: levodopa 20 mg/mL
with 4.63 mg/mL carbidopa in single-use
cassettes
ODTs: 100 mg levodopa with 10 mg carbidopa, 100 mg levodopa with 25 mg
carbidopa, 250 mg levodopa with 25 mg
carbidopa
Tablets (extended-release) ⬛*:* 200 mg levodopa with 50 mg carbidopa (Sinemet CR),
100 mg levodopa with 25 mg carbidopa
(Sinemet CR)
Tablets (immediate-release): 100 mg levodopa with 10 mg carbidopa (Sinemet
10–100), 100 mg levodopa with 25 mg carbidopa (Sinemet 25–100), 250 mg levodopa
with 25 mg carbidopa (Sinemet 25–250)

INDICATIONS & DOSAGES
➤ **Idiopathic Parkinson disease, postencephalitic parkinsonism, and symptomatic parkinsonism resulting from
carbon monoxide or manganese intoxication**
Adults: 1 immediate-release tablet of
100 mg levodopa with 25 mg carbidopa
P.O. t.i.d.; then increased by 1 tablet daily
or every other day, as needed, to maximum
daily dose of 8 tablets. May use 250 mg
levodopa with 25 mg carbidopa or 100 mg
levodopa with 10 mg carbidopa tablets,
as directed, to obtain maximal response.
Optimum daily dose must be determined
by careful adjustment for each patient. Or,
1 extended-release capsule of 95 mg levodopa with 23.75 mg carbidopa t.i.d. for
3 days; on day 4, increase to 145 mg le-

vodopa with 36.25 mg carbidopa t.i.d. Adjust dose as needed; may increase dose up
to 390 mg levodopa with 97.5 mg t.i.d. May
increase frequency of dosing to maximum
of five times daily if needed and tolerated.
Maximum recommended daily dose is
2,450 mg levodopa with 612.5 mg carbidopa. Or, 1 extended-release tablet of levodopa 200 mg with 50 mg carbidopa b.i.d.
at intervals of 6 hours or more. Increase or
decrease doses and dosing intervals based
on response. Most patients have been adequately treated with a dose that provides
400 to 1,600 mg of levodopa per day (divided doses) at intervals of 4 to 8 hours
while awake. Allow at least a 3-day interval
between dosage adjustments.

Refer to manufacturer's instructions
to convert from immediate-release to
extended-release formulation. Patients given
conventional tablets may receive extended-
release tablets; dosage is calculated on
current levodopa intake. Extended-release
tablets should provide 10% more levodopa
daily, increased as needed and as tolerated
to 30% more levodopa daily. Give in divided
doses at intervals of 4 to 8 hours. Allow
at least a 3-day interval between dosage
adjustments.
➤ **Motor fluctuations in patients with
advanced Parkinson disease (Duopa)**
⊘ *Alert:* Before initiating enteral therapy,
convert patient from all other forms of levodopa to oral immediate-release levodopa-
carbidopa tablets (1:4 ratio).
Adults: Total daily dose (expressed in terms
of levodopa) consists of a morning dose,
a continuous dose, and extra doses, which
can be used to manage acute "off" symptoms not controlled by the morning and
continuous dose. Refer to manufacturer's
labeling for morning dose and continuous
dose calculations and titration instructions.
Maximum dose of morning and continuous
dose is 2,000 mg of the levodopa component over 16 hours. Maximum of extra
doses is one extra dose every 2 hours. Give
patient's routine nighttime dosage of oral
immediate-release levodopa–carbidopa aft
discontinuation of daily infusion.
Adjust-a-dose: For dyskinesias or levodopa
related adverse reactions within 1 hour of
morning dose on preceding day, decrease

morning dose by 1 mL. For dyskinesias or adverse reactions lasting 1 hour or more on preceding day, decrease continuous dose by 0.3 mL/hour. For dyskinesias or adverse reactions lasting for two or more periods of 1 hour or more on preceding day, decrease continuous dose by 0.6 mL/hour.

ADMINISTRATION
P.O.
- Give drug with food to decrease GI upset, but avoid giving with high-protein meals, which can impair absorption and reduce effectiveness.
- Don't crush or break extended-release form.
- Give ODT immediately after removing from bottle. Place tablet on patient's tongue, where it will dissolve in seconds and be swallowed with saliva. No additional fluid is needed.
- For patients who have difficulty swallowing, capsules may be opened and the entire contents sprinkled on a small amount of applesauce (1 to 2 tablespoons) and then consumed immediately (don't store for future use).
Enteral
- Before use, fully thaw in refrigerator. To ensure controlled thawing, take cartons containing the seven individual cassettes out of the transport box and separate cartons from each other.
- Assign a 12-week, use-by date based on the time the cartons are put into the refrigerator to thaw (may take up to 96 hours to thaw).
- Once thawed, individual cartons may be packed in a closer configuration within the refrigerator.
- Remove one cassette from refrigerator 20 minutes before administration (failure to use at room temperature may result in inaccurate dosage).
- Administer through either a nasojejunal tube (temporary administration) or a percutaneous endoscopic gastrostomy-jejunostomy tube (long-term administration) connected to the CADD-Legacy 1400 pump.
- Disconnect tube from the pump at end of infusion and flush tube with room temperature drinking water with a syringe.

- Cassettes are for single use only and should be discarded daily after infusion. Don't reuse opened cassettes.

ACTION
Levodopa, a dopamine precursor, relieves parkinsonian symptoms by being converted to dopamine in the brain. Carbidopa inhibits the decarboxylation of peripheral levodopa, which allows more intact levodopa to travel to the brain.

Route	Onset	Peak	Duration
P.O.	Unknown	30–120 min	Unknown
Enteral	Unknown	2½ hr	Unknown

Half-life: 1½ to 2 hours.

ADVERSE REACTIONS
CNS: syncope, agitation, bradykinetic episodes, confusion, dementia, *suicidal tendencies,* dizziness, dream abnormalities, headache, insomnia, *neuroleptic malignant syndrome,* paresthesia, psychotic episodes, somnolence.
CV: cardiac irregularities, hypertension, hypotension, orthostatic hypotension, palpitations, phlebitis, *MI.*
GI: anorexia, constipation, dark saliva, duodenal ulcer, diarrhea, dry mouth, dyspepsia, *GI bleeding,* taste alterations, vomiting.
GU: dark urine, urinary frequency, UTI.
Hematologic: *agranulocytosis,* hemolytic and nonhemolytic anemia, *leukopenia, thrombocytopenia.*
Musculoskeletal: back pain, muscle cramps, shoulder pain.
Respiratory: dyspnea, URI.
Skin: alopecia, rash, diaphoresis, dark sweat.
Other: increased libido, hypersensitivity.

INTERACTIONS
Drug-drug. *Antihypertensives:* May cause additive hypotensive effects. Use together cautiously.
Antipsychotics (butyrophenones, phenothiazines, risperidone): May decrease levodopa activity and increase risk of neuroleptic malignant syndrome. Monitor patient closely.
Benzodiazepines (chlordiazepoxide, diazepam): May reduce effects of levodopa. Use together cautiously.

Iron salts (oral): May reduce bioavailability of levodopa–carbidopa. Give iron 1 hour before or 2 hours after oral levodopa–carbidopa.

MAO inhibitors: May cause risk of severe hypertension. Avoid using together.

Methylphenidate: May increase risk of adverse effects related to levodopa–carbidopa. Monitor patient carefully.

Metoclopramide: May decrease therapeutic effects of levodopa–carbidopa. Monitor therapeutic effects.

Isoniazid: May antagonize antiparkinsonian actions. Use together cautiously. Therapy modification may be necessary.

Papaverine, phenytoin: May antagonize antiparkinsonian actions. Avoid using together.

Sapropterin: May increase risk of levodopa-related adverse effects. Monitor patient carefully.

TCAs: May cause increase in BP and dyskinesia. Use together cautiously.

Drug-herb. *Kava:* May decrease action of drug. Discourage kava use altogether.

Drug-food. *Foods high in protein:* May decrease levodopa absorption. Don't give levodopa with high-protein foods.

EFFECTS ON LAB TEST RESULTS

• May increase BUN, creatinine, uric acid, ALT, AST, alkaline phosphatase, LDH, and bilirubin levels.

• May decrease Hb level and hematocrit and WBC, granulocyte, and platelet counts.

• May falsely increase urinary catecholamine level and serum and urinary uric acid levels in colorimetric tests. May falsely decrease urinary vanillylmandelic acid level. May cause false-positive results in urine ketone tests using sodium nitroprusside reagent and in urine glucose tests using cupric sulfate reagent. May cause false-negative urine glucose or false-positive urine acetone results in tests using glucose oxidase. May alter results of urine screening tests for phenylketonuria.

• May cause positive Coombs test.

CONTRAINDICATIONS & CAUTIONS

• Contraindicated in patients hypersensitive to drug and in those with angle-closure glaucoma, melanoma, or undiagnosed skin lesions.

• Contraindicated within 14 days of MAO inhibitor therapy.

• Use cautiously in patients with severe CV, renal, hepatic, endocrine, or pulmonary disorders; orthostatic hypotension; history of peptic ulcer; psychiatric illness; MI with residual arrhythmias; bronchial asthma; emphysema; or well-controlled, chronic open-angle glaucoma.

• Potentially fatal GI complications, including bezoar, ileus, implant-site erosion or ulcer, intestinal hemorrhage, intestinal ischemia, intestinal obstruction, intestinal perforation, pancreatitis, peritonitis, pneumoperitoneum, and postoperative wound infection, may occur in patients receiving enteral therapy.

• May increase risk of impulse-control disorders, dyskinesia, melanoma, orthostatic hypotension, and sudden somnolence.

Dialyzable drug: Unknown.

⚠ **Overdose S&S:** Muscle twitching, blepharospasm.

PREGNANCY-LACTATION-REPRODUCTION

• There are no adequate studies in pregnant women. Use during pregnancy only if potential benefit justifies potential risk to the fetus.

• Drug appears in breast milk. Use cautiously in breast-feeding women.

NURSING CONSIDERATIONS

• Determine optimum daily dose by careful titration in each patient. Therapy should be individualized and adjusted according to the desired therapeutic response.

• Observe patient and monitor vital signs, especially changes in BP, when changing positions and while adjusting dosage. Report significant changes.

⚠ **Alert:** Because of risk of precipitating a symptom complex resembling neuroleptic malignant syndrome, observe patient closely if levodopa dosage is reduced abruptly or stopped.

• Hallucinations may require reduction or withdrawal of drug.

• Test patients receiving long-term therapy regularly for diabetes and acromegaly, and periodically for hepatic, renal, and hematopoietic function.

Reactions in bold italics are *life-threatening*. Interactions may have a *rapid onset* or a **delayed onset**.

PATIENT TEACHING

• Tell patient to take drug with food to minimize GI upset; however, high-protein meals can impair absorption and reduce effectiveness.
• Tell patient not to chew or crush extended-release form.
• Advise patient to have skin checks.
• Warn patient and caregivers not to increase or decrease dosage without prescriber's orders.
• Caution patient about possible dizziness when standing up quickly, especially at start of therapy. Tell patient to change positions slowly and dangle legs before getting out of bed.
• Instruct patient to report adverse reactions (such as somnolence, loss of impulse control) and therapeutic effects.
• Advise patient receiving enteral therapy to immediately report abdominal pain, prolonged constipation, nausea, vomiting, fever, or melanotic stool.
• Inform patient that pyridoxine (vitamin B_6) doesn't reverse beneficial effects of levodopa–carbidopa. Multivitamins can be taken without reversing levodopa's effects.
• Teach patient to take ODT immediately after taking from bottle and to place on top of tongue. Tablet will dissolve in seconds and will be swallowed with saliva. No additional fluid is needed.

---

levodopa–carbidopa–entacapone
lee-voe-DOE-pa/kar-bih-DOE-pa/en-ta-KAP-own

Stalevo✐

Therapeutic class: Antiparkinsonians
Pharmacologic class: Dopamine precursors–decarboxylase inhibitors–catecholamine-*O*-methyltransferase inhibitors

AVAILABLE FORMS

Tablets (film-coated) ⓜ: 50 mg levodopa, 12.5 mg carbidopa, and 200 mg entacapone; 75 mg levodopa, 18.75 mg carbidopa, and 200 mg entacapone; 100 mg levodopa, 25 mg carbidopa, and 200 mg entacapone; 125 mg levodopa, 31.25 mg carbidopa, and 200 mg entacapone; 150 mg levodopa, 37.5 mg carbidopa, and 200 mg entacapone; 200 mg levodopa, 50 mg carbidopa, and 200 mg entacapone

INDICATIONS & DOSAGES

➤ **Idiopathic Parkinson disease, to replace (with equivalent strengths) levodopa, carbidopa, and entacapone given individually or to replace immediate-release levodopa–carbidopa for patient who has end-of-dose "wearing off," who's taking a total daily levodopa dose of 600 mg or less, and who has no dyskinesia**
Adults: 1 tablet P.O.; determine dose and interval by therapeutic response. Maximum, 8 tablets daily for all strengths except levodopa 200 mg, carbidopa 50 mg, and entacapone 200 mg; for these strengths, give 6 tablets/day.

ADMINISTRATION
P.O.
• Don't cut tablets.
• Give only 1 tablet at each dosing interval.
• Give drug with food to decrease GI upset, but avoid giving with high-protein meal, which can decrease absorption.

ACTION
Levodopa, a dopamine precursor, relieves parkinsonian symptoms by converting to dopamine in the brain. Carbidopa inhibits the decarboxylation of peripheral levodopa, which allows more intact levodopa to travel to the brain. Entacapone is a reversible catecholamine-*O*-methyltransferase (COMT) inhibitor that increases levodopa level.

Route	Onset	Peak	Duration
P.O.	Unknown	1–3½ hr	Unknown

Half-life: Carbidopa, 1½ to 2 hours; levodopa, 1 to 3¼ hours; entacapone, ¾ to 1 hour.

ADVERSE REACTIONS
levodopa and carbidopa
CNS: syncope, agitation, bradykinetic episodes, confusion, dementia, *suicidal tendencies*, dizziness, dream abnormalities, headache, insomnia, *neuroleptic malignant*

syndrome, paresthesia, psychotic episodes, somnolence, hallucinations.
CV: cardiac irregularities, hypertension, hypotension, orthostatic hypotension, palpitations, phlebitis, *MI.*
GI: anorexia, constipation, dark saliva, duodenal ulcer, diarrhea, dry mouth, dyspepsia, *GI bleeding,* taste alterations, vomiting.
GU: dark urine, urinary frequency, UTI.
Hematologic: *agranulocytosis,* hemolytic and nonhemolytic anemia, *leukopenia, thrombocytopenia.*
Musculoskeletal: back pain, muscle cramps, shoulder pain.
Respiratory: dyspnea, URI.
Skin: alopecia, rash, diaphoresis, dark sweat.
Other: increased libido, hypersensitivity.
entacapone
CNS: dyskinesia, hyperkinesia, agitation, anxiety, asthenia, dizziness, fatigue, hypokinesia, somnolence.
GI: diarrhea, nausea, abdominal pain, constipation, dry mouth, dyspepsia, flatulence, gastritis, taste perversion, vomiting.
GU: urine discoloration.
Musculoskeletal: back pain.
Respiratory: dyspnea.
Skin: increased sweating, purpura.
Other: bacterial infection.

INTERACTIONS
Drug-drug. *Ampicillin, chloramphenicol, cholestyramine, erythromycin, probenecid, rifampin:* May interfere with entacapone excretion. Use together cautiously.
Antihypertensives: May cause orthostatic hypotension. Adjust antihypertensive dosage as needed.
CNS depressants: Additive effects. Use together cautiously.
Dopamine (D2) receptor antagonists such as butyrophenones, iron salts, isoniazid, metoclopramide, phenothiazines, phenytoin, risperidone: May decrease levodopa, carbidopa, and entacapone effects. Monitor patient for effectiveness.
Drugs metabolized by COMT, such as apomorphine, dobutamine, dopamine, epinephrine, isoetharine, isoproterenol, methyldopa, norepinephrine: May increase HR, arrhythmias, and excessive BP changes. Use together cautiously.
Metoclopramide: May increase availability of levodopa and carbidopa by increasing gastric emptying. Monitor patient for adverse effects.
Nonselective MAO inhibitors: May disrupt catecholamine metabolism. Avoid using together.
Selegiline: May cause severe hypotension. Use together cautiously, and monitor BP.
TCAs: May increase risk of hypertension and dyskinesia. Monitor patient closely.

EFFECTS ON LAB TEST RESULTS
• May increase alkaline phosphatase, AST, ALT, LDH, glucose, BUN, and bilirubin levels. May decrease Hb level and hematocrit.
• May decrease platelet and WBC counts.
• May cause false-positive reaction for urinary ketone bodies on a test tape. May cause false-negative result for glycosuria with glucose oxidase testing methods.
• May cause positive Coombs test.

CONTRAINDICATIONS & CAUTIONS
• Contraindicated in patients hypersensitive to drug or its ingredients.
⊘ Alert: Drug may increase risk of MI, stroke, and death. Monitor CV status closely.
• Contraindicated in patients with angle-closure glaucoma, suspicious undiagnosed skin lesions, or a history of melanoma.
• Contraindicated within 2 weeks of MAO inhibitor therapy.
• Use cautiously in patients with past or current psychosis and in patients with severe CV or pulmonary disease; bronchial asthma; biliary obstruction; peptic ulcer; or renal, hepatic, or endocrine disease.
• Use cautiously in patients with chronic open-angle glaucoma, hepatic impairment, or a history of MI and residual atrial, nodal, or ventricular arrhythmias.
Dialyzable drug: Unlikely.
⚠ Overdose S&S: CNS disturbances, hypotension, tachycardia, rhabdomyolysis, transient renal insufficiency, abdominal pain, loose stools.

PREGNANCY-LACTATION-REPRODUCTION
• There are no adequate studies in pregnant women. Use only if potential benefit justifies potential risk to the fetus.

• It isn't known if drug appears in breast milk. Use cautiously in breast-feeding women.

NURSING CONSIDERATIONS
• Certain CNS effects, such as dyskinesia, may occur at lower dosages and sooner with levodopa–carbidopa–entacapone than with levodopa alone. Dyskinesia may require a reduced dosage.
• Monitor patients for orthostatic hypotension, especially during dosage escalation.
• During the first adjustment period, monitor patient with CV disease carefully and in a facility equipped to provide intensive cardiac care.
• Neuroleptic malignant syndrome may develop when levodopa and carbidopa are reduced or stopped, especially in patients taking antipsychotic drugs. Watch patient carefully for fever, hyperthermia, muscle rigidity, involuntary movements, altered consciousness, mental status changes, and autonomic dysfunction.
• During extended therapy, periodically monitor hepatic, hematopoietic, CV, and renal function.
• Diarrhea is common; it usually develops 4 to 12 weeks after treatment starts but may appear as early as the first week or as late as many months after treatment starts.
◐ **Alert:** Monitor patient for hallucinations, depression, and suicidal tendencies.

PATIENT TEACHING
• Advise patient to take drug exactly as prescribed and not to split tablets.
• Tell patient to report a "wearing-off" effect, which may occur at the end of the dosing interval.
• Tell patient that urine, sweat, and saliva may turn dark (red, brown, or black) during treatment.
• Advise patient to notify the prescriber if problems making voluntary movements increase.
• Tell patient that diarrhea is common with this treatment.
• Inform patient that hallucinations may occur.
• Urge patient to immediately report depression, suicidal thoughts, or loss of impulse control.

• Explain that patient may become dizzy if rising quickly. Urge patient to use caution when rising.
• Tell patient that a high-protein diet, excessive acidity, and iron salts may reduce drug's effectiveness.
• Urge patient to avoid hazardous activities until CNS effects of drug are known.
• Advise female patient to notify prescriber if she becomes pregnant.

levofloxacin
lee-voe-FLOX-a-sin

Levaquin✔

Therapeutic class: Antibiotics
Pharmacologic class: Fluoroquinolones

AVAILABLE FORMS
Infusion (premixed): 250 mg in 50 mL D_5W, 500 mg in 100 mL D_5W, 750 mg in 150 mL D_5W
Ophthalmic solution: 0.5%
Oral solution: 25 mg/mL
Single-use vials: 500 mg, 750 mg
Tablets: 250 mg, 500 mg, 750 mg

INDICATIONS & DOSAGES
Black Box Warning Use in patients with acute bacterial sinusitis, acute bacterial exacerbation of bronchitis, and uncomplicated UTI isn't recommended because of risk of serious adverse effects. Use in these patients only when they have no other treatment options. ■
Adjust-a-dose (for all indications): For patients with CrCl of less than 50 mL/minute, adjust the oral or I.V. dosage regimen according to the manufacturer's instructions.
➤ **Acute bacterial sinusitis caused by susceptible strains of *Streptococcus pneumoniae*, *Moraxella catarrhalis*, or *Haemophilus influenzae***
Adults: 500 mg P.O. or I.V. infusion over 60 minutes every 24 hours for 10 to 14 days or 750 mg P.O. or I.V. every 24 hours for 5 days.

➤ **Mild to moderate skin and skin-structure infections caused by *Staphylococcus aureus* or *Streptococcus pyogenes***

Adults: 500 mg P.O. or I.V. infusion over 60 minutes every 24 hours for 7 to 10 days.

➤ **Acute bacterial worsening of chronic bronchitis caused by S. aureus, S. pneumoniae, M. catarrhalis, H. influenzae, or Haemophilus parainfluenzae**

Adults: 500 mg P.O. or I.V. infusion over 60 minutes every 24 hours for 7 days.

➤ **To prevent inhalation anthrax after confirmed or suspected exposure to Bacillus anthracis**

Adults: 500 mg I.V. infusion or P.O. every 24 hours for 60 days.

Children age 6 months and older weighing at least 50 kg: 500 mg P.O. or by slow I.V. infusion every 24 hours for 60 days.

Children age 6 months and older weighing less than 50 kg: 8 mg/kg (not to exceed 250 mg/dose) P.O. or by slow I.V. infusion every 12 hours for 60 days.

➤ **Chronic bacterial prostatitis caused by Escherichia coli, Enterococcus faecalis, or Staphylococcus epidermidis**

Adults: 500 mg P.O. or I.V. over 60 minutes every 24 hours for 28 days.

➤ **Community-acquired pneumonia from S. pneumoniae (excluding multidrug-resistant strains), H. influenzae, H. parainfluenzae, Mycoplasma pneumoniae, or Chlamydia pneumoniae**

Adults: 750 mg P.O. or I.V. over 90 minutes every 24 hours for 5 days.

➤ **Community-acquired pneumonia caused by methicillin-susceptible S. aureus, S. pneumoniae, H. influenzae, H. parainfluenzae, Klebsiella pneumoniae, M. catarrhalis, C. pneumoniae, Legionella pneumophila, or M. pneumoniae**

Adults: 500 mg P.O. or I.V. every 24 hours for 7 to 14 days.

➤ **Complicated skin and skin-structure infections caused by methicillin-sensitive S. aureus, E. faecalis, S. pyogenes, or Proteus mirabilis**

Adults: 750 mg P.O. or I.V. infusion over 90 minutes every 24 hours for 7 to 14 days.

➤ **Nosocomial pneumonia caused by methicillin-susceptible S. aureus, Pseudomonas aeruginosa, Serratia marcescens, E. coli, K. pneumoniae, H. influenzae, or S. pneumoniae**

Adults: 750 mg P.O. or I.V. infusion over 90 minutes every 24 hours for 7 to 14 days.

➤ **Complicated UTI caused by E. faecalis, Enterobacter cloacae, E. coli, K. pneumoniae, P. mirabilis, or P. aeruginosa; acute pyelonephritis caused by E. coli**

Adults: 250 mg P.O. or I.V. over 60 minutes every 24 hours for 10 days.

➤ **Complicated UTI caused by E. coli, K. pneumoniae, or P. mirabilis; acute pyelonephritis caused by E. coli**

Adults: 750 mg P.O. or I.V. over 90 minutes daily for 5 days.

➤ **Mild to moderate uncomplicated UTI caused by E. coli, K. pneumoniae, or Staphylococcus saprophyticus**

Adults: 250 mg P.O. daily for 3 days.

➤ **Prophylaxis or treatment of pneumonic and septicemic plague (Yersinia pestis)**

Adults: 500 mg P.O. or I.V. every 24 hours for 10 to 14 days.

Children age 6 months and older weighing 50 kg or more: 500 mg P.O. or by slow I.V. infusion every 24 hours for 10 to 14 days.

Children age 6 months and older weighing less than 50 kg: 8 mg/kg (not to exceed 250 mg/dose) P.O. or by slow I.V. infusion every 12 hours for 10 to 14 days.

➤ **Bacterial conjunctivitis**

Adults and children age 6 and older: On days 1 and 2, instill 1 to 2 drops in affected eye(s) every 2 hours while patient is awake up to eight times a day. On days 3 through 7, instill 1 to 2 drops in affected eye(s) every 4 hours while patient is awake up to four times a day.

ADMINISTRATION
P.O.

• Obtain specimen for culture and sensitivity tests before therapy and as needed to determine if bacterial resistance has occurred.

• Give drug with plenty of fluids.

• Give 2 hours before or 2 hours after antacids, sucralfate, and products containing iron or zinc.

• Give oral solution 1 hour before or 2 hours after a meal.

I.V.

▼ Obtain specimen for culture and sensitivity tests before therapy and as needed

---

Reactions in bold italics are *life-threatening*. Interactions may have a *rapid onset* or a ***delayed onset***.

to determine if bacterial resistance has occurred.

▼ Give this form only by infusion.

▼ Dilute drug in single-use vials, according to manufacturer's instructions, with D_5W or NSS for injection to a final concentration of 5 mg/mL.

▼ Infuse doses of 500 mg or less over 60 minutes and doses of 750 mg over 90 minutes.

▼ Reconstituted solution should be clear, slightly yellow, and free of particulate matter.

▼ Reconstituted drug is stable for 72 hours at room temperature, for 14 days when refrigerated in plastic containers, and for 6 months when frozen.

▼ Thaw at room temperature or in refrigerator.

▼ **Incompatibilities:** Acyclovir sodium, alprostadil, azithromycin, furosemide, heparin sodium, indomethacin sodium trihydrate, insulin, magnesium, mannitol 20%, nitroglycerin, propofol, sodium bicarbonate, sodium nitroprusside. The manufacturer recommends not mixing or infusing other drugs with levofloxacin.

Ophthalmic

● Avoid touching applicator tip to eye or other surfaces.

ACTION

Inhibits bacterial DNA gyrase and prevents DNA replication, transcription, repair, and recombination in susceptible bacteria.

Route	Onset	Peak	Duration
P.O., I.V.	Unknown	1–2 hr	Unknown
Ophthalmic	Unknown	Unknown	Unknown

Half-life: About 6 to 8 hours.

ADVERSE REACTIONS

CNS: *encephalopathy, seizures,* dizziness, headache, insomnia; headache (ophthalmic).

EENT: foreign body or burning sensation in eye, eye pain, vision loss, photophobia (ophthalmic).

GI: *pseudomembranous colitis,* abdominal pain, constipation, diarrhea, dyspepsia, nausea, vomiting.

GU: vaginitis.

Hematologic: *lymphopenia,* eosinophilia, hemolytic anemia.

Metabolic: *hypoglycemia.*

Musculoskeletal: back pain, tendon rupture.

Respiratory: allergic pneumonitis, dyspnea.

Skin: *erythema multiforme, Stevens-Johnson syndrome,* photosensitivity, pruritus, rash.

Other: *anaphylaxis, multisystem organ failure, hypersensitivity reactions.*

INTERACTIONS

Drug-drug. *Aluminum hydroxide, aluminum–magnesium hydroxide, calcium carbonate, didanosine, magnesium hydroxide, products containing zinc, sucralfate:* May interfere with GI absorption of levofloxacin. Give levofloxacin 2 hours before or 2 hours after these products.

Antiarrhythmics (Class IA [procainamide, quinidine] or Class III [amiodarone, dofetilide]), chlorpromazine, erythromycin, fluconazole, imipramine, ziprasidone: May increase risk of life-threatening cardiac arrhythmias. Avoid use together.

Antidiabetics: May alter glucose level. Monitor glucose level closely.

Iron salts: May decrease absorption of levofloxacin, reducing anti-infective response. Separate doses by at least 2 hours.

NSAIDs: May increase CNS stimulation. Monitor patient for seizure activity.

Black Box Warning *Steroids:* May increase risk of tendinitis and tendon rupture. Monitor patient for tendon pain or inflammation. ■

Theophylline: May decrease clearance of theophylline. Monitor theophylline level.

Warfarin and derivatives: May increase effect of oral anticoagulant. Monitor PT and INR.

Drug-herb. *Dong quai, St. John's wort:* May cause photosensitivity reactions. Advise patient to avoid excessive sunlight exposure.

Drug-lifestyle. *Sun exposure:* May cause photosensitivity reactions. Advise patient to avoid excessive sunlight exposure.

EFFECTS ON LAB TEST RESULTS

● May decrease glucose and Hb levels.

• May increase eosinophil count. May decrease WBC count.

• May produce false-positive opioid assay results.

CONTRAINDICATIONS & CAUTIONS

Black Box Warning Drug is associated with increased risk of tendinitis and tendon rupture, especially in patients older than age 60, in patients taking corticosteroids, and in those with heart, kidney, or lung transplants. ∎

Black Box Warning Drug may exacerbate muscle weakness in patients with myasthenia gravis. Avoid using fluoroquinolones in patients with a history of myasthenia gravis. ∎

⊍ *Alert:* Drug is associated with an increased incidence of musculoskeletal disorders (arthralgia, arthritis, tendinopathy, and gait abnormality) in pediatric patients. Testing of drug in immature animals has resulted in increased osteochondrosis, erosions in weight-bearing joints, and other signs and symptoms of arthropathy.

• Contraindicated in patients hypersensitive to drug, its components, or other fluoroquinolones.

• Use cautiously in patients with history of seizure disorders or other CNS diseases, such as cerebral arteriosclerosis.

• Use cautiously and with dosage adjustment in patients with renal impairment.

• Drug is indicated in children (age 6 months and older) only for postexposure inhalational anthrax prevention and for plague.

Dialyzable drug: No.

PREGNANCY-LACTATION-REPRODUCTION

• There are no adequate studies in pregnant women. Use during pregnancy only if potential benefit justifies potential fetal risk.

• Drug probably appears in breast milk. Patient should discontinue breast-feeding or discontinue drug.

NURSING CONSIDERATIONS

Black Box Warning Fluoroquinolones have been associated with disabling and potentially irreversible serious adverse reactions that have occurred together, including tendinitis and tendon rupture, peripheral neuropathy, and CNS effects (seizures, toxic psychoses, increased ICP, pseudotumor cerebri, tremors, restlessness, anxiety, light-headedness, confusion, hallucinations, paranoia, depression, nightmares, insomnia and, rarely, suicidal thoughts or acts). If any of these serious adverse reactions occur, discontinue drug immediately. ∎

• Patients with acute hypersensitivity reactions may need treatment with epinephrine, oxygen, I.V. fluids, antihistamines, corticosteroids, pressor amines, and airway management.

Black Box Warning Monitor patient for signs and symptoms of peripheral neuropathy (pain, burning, tingling, numbness, weakness, or a change in sensation to light touch, pain, temperature, or sense of body position), and report them immediately to health care provider. ∎

• Most antibacterials can cause pseudomembranous colitis. If diarrhea occurs, notify prescriber; drug may be stopped.

• Drug may cause an abnormal ECG.

⊍ *Alert:* If *P. aeruginosa* is a confirmed or suspected pathogen, use with a beta-lactam.

• Monitor glucose level and results of renal function tests, LFTs, and blood counts.

• *Look alike–sound alike:* Don't confuse levofloxacin with levetiracetam.

PATIENT TEACHING

Black Box Warning Warn patient to immediately notify prescriber for signs and symptoms of serious adverse reactions, including unusual joint or tendon pain, muscle weakness, "pins and needles" tingling or prickling sensation, numbness in the arms or legs, confusion, or hallucinations. ∎

• Tell patient to take drug as prescribed, even if signs and symptoms disappear.

• Advise patient to take drug with plenty of fluids and to space antacids, sucralfate, and products containing iron or zinc.

• Tell patient to take oral solution 1 hour before or 2 hours after eating.

• Warn patient to avoid hazardous tasks until adverse effects of drug are known.

• Advise patient to avoid excessive sunlight exposure.

• Instruct patient to stop drug and notify prescriber if rash or other signs or symptoms of hypersensitivity develop.

Reactions in bold italics are *life-threatening*. Interactions may have a *rapid onset* or a *delayed onset*.

• Instruct diabetic patient to monitor glucose level and notify prescriber about low-glucose reaction.

• Instruct patient to notify prescriber of all adverse reactions, including loose stools or diarrhea.

• Instruct patient not to use contact lenses during treatment for bacterial conjunctivitis.

levomilnacipran hydrochloride
lee-voe-mil-NAY-sih-pran

Fetzima

Therapeutic class: Antidepressants
Pharmacologic class: SSNRIs

AVAILABLE FORMS
Capsules (extended-release) ⓞⓝⓒ: 20 mg, 40 mg, 80 mg, 120 mg

INDICATIONS & DOSAGES
➤ **Major depressive disorder**
Adults: Initially, 20 mg P.O. once daily for 2 days; then increase to 40 mg once daily. May increase in increments of 40 mg at intervals of 2 or more days. Maximum dosage is 120 mg once daily.
Adjust-a-dose: For patients with CrCl of 30 to 59 mL/minute, maximum maintenance dosage is 80 mg once daily. If CrCl is 15 to 29 mL/minute, maximum maintenance dosage is 40 mg once daily. Don't use for patients with ESRD.

ADMINISTRATION
P.O.
• Give drug with or without food.
• Make sure patient swallows extended-release capsules whole and doesn't chew, crush, or open them.
• Give drug at approximately the same time each day.

ACTION
Unclear. Drug is a potent inhibitor of neuronal norepinephrine and serotonin reuptake.

Route	Onset	Peak	Duration
P.O.	Unknown	6–8 hr	Unknown

Half-life: 12 hours.

ADVERSE REACTIONS
CNS: syncope, agitation, extrapyramidal reaction, panic attack, migraine, paresthesia, tension, aggressive behavior, anger outburst, yawning.
CV: orthostatic hypotension, angina, chest pain, flushing, palpitations, tachycardia, premature atrial contractions, PVCs.
EENT: blurred vision, dry eye syndrome, conjunctival hemorrhage.
GI: abdominal pain, constipation, decreased appetite, dry mouth, flatulence, nausea, vomiting, thirst, teeth grinding.
GU: hematuria, proteinuria, urinary frequency; in men—dysuria, ejaculation disorder, erectile dysfunction, libido decrease, prostatitis, scrotal pain, testicular pain, testicular swelling, urethral pain, urinary hesitation, urine retention, urine flow decrease.
Metabolic: hypercholesterolemia.
Skin: hyperhidrosis, pruritus, urticaria, rash, dry skin.
Other: hot flashes.

INTERACTIONS
Drug-drug. *Antipsychotics (risperidone), cyclobenzaprine, dopamine antagonists (metoclopramide):* May increase risk of neuroleptic malignant syndrome and serotonin syndrome. If use together can't be avoided, closely monitor patient and if signs and symptoms occur, discontinue drug.
🟊 *Alert:Aspirin, NSAIDs, warfarin:* May increase risk of bleeding. Use together cautiously.
Lithium, other serotonergic drugs: May cause serotonin syndrome (diarrhea, dysreflexia, fever, hallucinations, loss of coordination, nausea, tachycardia). Avoid use together.
MAO inhibitors: May cause hyperthermia, rigidity, myoclonus, autonomic instability, rapid fluctuations of vital signs, agitation, delirium, and coma. Avoid using drug within 2 weeks after MAO inhibitor therapy; wait at least 7 days after stopping levomilnacipran before starting MAO inhibitor.

Methylene blue: May cause CNS toxicity and serotonin syndrome. Avoid use together.
Drug-herb. *Herbs with anticoagulant properties (alfalfa, anise, bilberry):* May increase bleeding risk. Discourage use together.
St. John's wort: Increases risk of serotonin syndrome. Don't use together.
Drug-lifestyle. *Alcohol use:* May cause more rapid release of levomilnacipran and enhance CNS depression.

EFFECTS ON LAB TEST RESULTS
● May increase LFT values.
● May decrease sodium level.

CONTRAINDICATIONS & CAUTIONS
● Contraindicated in patients hypersensitive to levomilnacipran, milnacipran hydrochloride, or components of the formulation.
● Contraindicated in patients being treated with MAO inhibitors (within 7 days of discontinuing drug or within 2 weeks of discontinuing MAO inhibitor), linezolid, or I.V. methylene blue.
● Drug isn't approved for treatment of fibromyalgia.
◑ *Alert:* Pupillary dilation that occurs after drug use may trigger an angle-closure attack in patients with anatomically narrow angles who don't have a patent iridectomy.
◑ *Alert:* Serotonin syndrome, a potentially life-threatening condition, may occur, particularly with concomitant use of serotonergic drugs (including triptans, TCAs, lithium, and tramadol) and drugs that impair serotonin metabolism (including MAO inhibitors). Discontinue drug for signs and symptoms of serotonin syndrome, including mental status changes (agitation, coma, hallucinations), autonomic instability (hyperthermia, labile BP, tachycardia), neuromuscular aberrations (hyperreflexia, incoordination), and diarrhea, nausea, and vomiting.
● Not recommended for use in patients with ESRD.
● Use cautiously in patients with a history of mania, seizures, hypertension, tachyarrhythmias, CV disease, glaucoma, or dysuria.
● Avoid use in patients with bipolar disorder.
Dialyzable drug: Unlikely.

PREGNANCY-LACTATION-REPRODUCTION
● There are no adequate studies in pregnant women. Use during pregnancy only if potential benefit justifies potential fetal risk. Neonates exposed to SSRIs/SNRIs late in the third trimester have developed complications requiring prolonged hospitalization, respiratory support, and tube feeding.
● It isn't known if Fetzima appears in breast milk. Patient should discontinue breastfeeding or discontinue drug, taking into account importance of drug to the mother.

NURSING CONSIDERATIONS
Black Box Warning Drug may increase the risk of suicidal thinking and behavior in children, adolescents, and young adults with major depressive disorder or other psychiatric disorder. Drug isn't approved for use in children. ■
● At least 14 days should elapse between discontinuation of an MAO inhibitor and initiation of levomilnacipran. Allow at least 7 days after stopping levomilnacipran before starting an MAO inhibitor.
● Monitor patient closely for worsening depression or suicidal behavior, especially during first few months of therapy and with dosage adjustments. Screen patients with depressive symptoms for bipolar disorder.
● To prevent withdrawal signs and symptoms, decrease dosage gradually, and watch for signs and symptoms that may arise when drug is stopped, such as dysphoria, irritability, agitation, dizziness, sensory disturbances, anxiety, confusion, headache, lethargy, emotional lability, insomnia, hypomania, tinnitus, and seizures.
● Carefully monitor HR and BP.
● Monitor patient for signs of hyponatremia (headache, difficulty concentrating, memory impairment, confusion, weakness, unsteadiness, hallucination, syncope, seizures, coma, respiratory arrest). Volume depletion, diuretic use, and increased age increase risk.
● Monitor LFT values and sodium level before and during therapy.

PATIENT TEACHING
Black Box Warning Warn families and caregivers to immediately report signs and symptoms of worsening depression (such as

---

agitation, irritability, insomnia, hostility, and impulsivity) and suicidal behavior. ∎

• Tell patient to consult prescriber before taking other prescription or OTC drugs and to avoid taking NSAIDs and aspirin to reduce risk of bleeding.

• Tell patient to avoid alcohol while taking drug.

• Instruct patient that frequent HR and BP monitoring will be needed and to report dizziness, passing out, or palpitations.

• Tell patient to report urinary hesitation or urine retention.

• Instruct woman of childbearing potential to notify prescriber if she becomes pregnant, is planning pregnancy during therapy, or is breast-feeding.

• Warn patient not to stop drug suddenly.

• Warn patient to avoid hazardous activities that require alertness and good coordination until drug's effects are known.

• Tell patient that drug may be taken with or without food but that food may increase tolerability.

• Instruct patient to swallow capsules whole and not to chew, crush, or open them.

---

levothyroxine sodium
(T_4, L-thyroxine sodium)
lee-voe-thye-ROX-een

Eltroxin✤, Euthyrox✤, Levo-T, Levoxyl✐, Synthroid✐, Tirosint, Unithroid

Therapeutic class: Thyroid hormone replacements
Pharmacologic class: Thyroid hormones

AVAILABLE FORMS
Capsules ⓓ: 13 mcg, 25 mcg, 50 mcg, 75 mcg, 88 mcg, 100 mcg, 112 mcg, 125 mcg, 137 mcg, 150 mcg
Powder for injection: 100 mcg, 200 mcg, 500 mcg
Tablets: 25 mcg, 50 mcg, 75 mcg, 88 mcg, 100 mcg, 112 mcg, 125 mcg, 137 mcg, 150 mcg, 175 mcg, 200 mcg, 300 mcg

INDICATIONS & DOSAGES
➤ **Thyroid hormone replacement**
Adults: For patients younger than age 50 or those older than age 50 who have been recently treated for hyperthyroidism or have been hypothyroid for a short time, 1.7 mcg/kg P.O. once daily. Monitor TSH levels every 6 to 8 weeks, making dosage adjustments in 12.5- to 25-mcg increments until patient is euthyroid and TSH level normalizes.
Adults: For patients age 50 or older or those younger than age 50 with underlying cardiac disease, 25 to 50 mcg P.O. daily. Adjust dose every 6 to 8 weeks, if needed, until patient is euthyroid and TSH level normalizes.
Children in whom growth and puberty are complete: 1.7 mcg/kg P.O. once daily.
Children older than age 12 in whom growth and puberty are incomplete: 2 to 3 mcg/kg P.O. daily.
Children ages 6 to 12: 4 to 5 mcg/kg P.O. daily.
Children ages 1 to 5: 5 to 6 mcg/kg P.O. daily.
Children ages 6 months to 1 year: 6 to 8 mcg/kg P.O. daily.
Children ages 3 to 6 months: 8 to 10 mcg/kg P.O. daily.
Infants and neonates birth to age 3 months: 10 to 15 mcg/kg P.O. daily. In neonates at risk for cardiac failure, use a lower initial dose (such as 25 mcg daily) and increase every 4 to 6 weeks as needed.
Elderly patients (older than age 50) with underlying CV disease: 12.5 to 25 mcg P.O. daily; increase by 12.5 to 25 mcg every 4 to 6 weeks, depending on response.
➤ **Severe, long-standing hypothyroidism**
Adults: 12.5 to 25 mcg P.O. daily. Increase in increments of 25 mcg every 2 to 4 weeks as needed.
Children: 25 mcg P.O. daily. Increase in increments of 25 mcg every 2 to 4 weeks as needed.
➤ **Subclinical hypothyroidism**
Adults: 1 mcg/kg P.O. daily.
➤ **Myxedema coma**
Adults: Initially, 300 to 500 mcg (0.3 to 0.5 mg) I.V. as solution followed by 50 to 100 mcg I.V. once daily until patient is able to tolerate oral administration. Consider smaller doses in patients with CV disease.

✦Canada   ◇OTC   ◆Off-label use   ✐Photoguide   ⓓ Do not crush   *Liquid contains alcohol.

ADMINISTRATION

P.O.

● Synthroid may contain tartrazine.
● Give drug at same time each day on an empty stomach, preferably ½ to 1 hour before breakfast.
● Give Levoxyl with a full glass of water to prevent difficulty swallowing.
● If necessary, crush tablet and suspend it in small amount of formula (except soy formula, which may decrease absorption), breast milk, or water, and give by spoon or dropper. Crushed tablet can also be sprinkled over food, except foods containing large amounts of soybean, fiber, or iron.

I.V.

▼ Reconstitute by adding 5 mL NSS injection only.
▼ Shake vial.
▼ Use immediately after reconstitution.
▼ Discard any unused portion.
▼ **Incompatibilities:** Don't mix or give with anything other than NSS injection.

ACTION

Not completely defined. Stimulates metabolism of all body tissues by accelerating rate of cellular oxidation.

Route	Onset	Peak	Duration
P.O.	3–5 days	2 hr	Unknown
I.V.	6–8 hr	Unknown	Unknown

Half-life: 6 to 8 days in euthyroidism; 3 to 4 days in hyperthyroidism; 9 to 10 days in hypothyroidism.

ADVERSE REACTIONS

CNS: insomnia, tremor, headache, fever, fatigue, anxiety, emotional lability.
CV: tachycardia, palpitations, *arrhythmias,* angina pectoris, *cardiac arrest,* hypertension, *HF, MI.*
GI: diarrhea, vomiting, abdominal cramps.
GU: menstrual irregularities.
Metabolic: weight loss, increased appetite.
Musculoskeletal: decreased bone density, muscle weakness, tremors.
Respiratory: dyspnea.
Skin: allergic skin reactions, diaphoresis, hair loss.
Other: heat intolerance, impaired fertility.

INTERACTIONS

Drug-drug. *Amiodarone, iodide (including iodine-containing radiographic contrast agents), lithium:* May reduce thyroid hormone secretion. Monitor thyroid function studies if used together.
Antacids, calcium carbonate, cholestyramine, colestipol, ferrous sulfate, sucralfate: May impair levothyroxine absorption. Separate doses by 4 to 5 hours.
Beta blockers: May reduce beta-blocker effects. Monitor patient.
Carbamazepine, hydantoins, phenobarbital, rifampin: May increase hepatic metabolism, resulting in hypothyroidism. Monitor patient.
Digoxin: May decrease cardiac glycoside effects. Monitor patient for clinical effect.
Estrogens: May decrease thyroid levels. Monitor levels after 12 weeks of therapy and adjust levothyroxine dosage as needed.
Fosphenytoin, phenytoin: May release free thyroid hormone. Monitor patient for tachycardia.
Insulin, oral antidiabetics: May alter glucose level. Monitor glucose level. Dosage adjustments may be needed.
Ketamine: May produce marked hypertension and tachycardia. Use together cautiously.
SSRIs: May increase levothyroxine requirements. Adjust dosage as needed.
Sympathomimetics such as epinephrine: May increase risk of coronary insufficiency. Monitor patient closely.
TCAs, tetracyclic antidepressants: May increase therapeutic effects and toxicity of both drugs. Monitor patient closely.
Theophylline: May decrease theophylline clearance in hypothyroidism; clearance may return to normal when euthyroid state is achieved. Monitor theophylline level.
Warfarin: May increase anticoagulant effects. Monitor patient for bleeding, and check PT and INR closely. Warfarin dosage adjustment may be needed.
Drug-herb. *Horseradish:* May cause abnormal thyroid function. Discourage use in patients undergoing thyroid function tests.
Lemon balm: May have antithyroid effects; may inhibit TSH. Discourage use together.
Drug-food. *Cottonseed meal, dietary fiber, soybean flour, walnuts:* May decrease

---

Reactions in bold italics are *life-threatening*. Interactions may have a *rapid onset* or a ***delayed onset***.

absorption of drug. Dosage adjustments may be needed.

EFFECTS ON LAB TEST RESULTS

• May decrease thyroid function test results. May alter results of liothyronine, protein-bound iodine, and radioactive ^{131}I uptake studies.

CONTRAINDICATIONS & CAUTIONS

• Contraindicated in patients hypersensitive to drug and in those with acute MI uncomplicated by hypothyroidism, untreated subclinical or overt thyrotoxicosis, or uncorrected adrenal insufficiency.

Black Box Warning Don't use either alone or with other therapeutic agents for treatment of obesity or for weight loss. ∎

Black Box Warning Doses beyond the range of daily hormonal requirements may produce serious or even life-threatening toxicities, especially if given with sympathomimetic amines. ∎

• Use cautiously in elderly patients and in those with angina pectoris, hypertension, other CV disorders, renal insufficiency, or ischemia.

• Use cautiously in patients with diabetes mellitus, diabetes insipidus, or myxedema and during rapid replacement in those with arteriosclerosis.

Dialyzable drug: No.

⚠ *Overdose S&S:* Signs and symptoms of hyperthyroidism, confusion, disorientation, cerebral embolism, shock, coma, seizures, death.

PREGNANCY-LACTATION-REPRODUCTION

• Drug is safe to use in pregnancy and shouldn't be discontinued during pregnancy. If hypothyroidism is diagnosed during pregnancy, patient should be promptly treated.

• Dosage may need to be increased in pregnant patients.

• Drug appears minimally in breast milk. Adequate replacement doses of levothyroxine are generally needed to maintain normal lactation and should be continued during breast-feeding.

NURSING CONSIDERATIONS

• Patients with diabetes mellitus may need increased antidiabetic doses when starting thyroid hormone replacement.

• Watch for angina, coronary occlusion, or stroke in patients with arteriosclerosis who are receiving rapid replacement.

• In patients with CAD who must receive thyroid hormone, observe carefully for possible coronary insufficiency.

• Patients with adult hypothyroidism are unusually sensitive to thyroid hormone. Start at lowest dosage, and adjust to higher dosages according to patient's symptoms and laboratory data until euthyroid state is reached.

• When changing from levothyroxine to liothyronine, stop levothyroxine and begin liothyronine. Increase dosage in small increments after residual effects of levothyroxine have disappeared. When changing from liothyronine to levothyroxine, start levothyroxine several days before withdrawing liothyronine to avoid relapse. Drugs aren't interchangeable.

• Long-term therapy causes bone loss in premenopausal and postmenopausal women. Consider a basal bone density measurement, and monitor patient closely for osteoporosis.

• Patients taking levothyroxine who need to have ^{131}I uptake studies performed must stop drug 4 weeks before test.

• Patients taking anticoagulants may need their dosage modified and require careful monitoring of coagulation status.

• Drug shouldn't be used for infertility (unless associated with hypothyroidism).

Black Box Warning Drug should not be used for the treatment of obesity or for weight loss. ∎

• *Look alike–sound alike:* Don't confuse levothyroxine with lamotrigine or Lanoxin.

PATIENT TEACHING

• Teach patient the importance of compliance. Tell him to take drug at same time each day, preferably ½ to 1 hour before breakfast, to maintain constant hormone levels and help prevent insomnia.

• Make sure patient understands that replacement therapy is usually for life. The drug should never be stopped unless directed by prescriber.

• Warn patient (especially elderly patient) to notify prescriber immediately about chest pain, palpitations, sweating, nervousness, shortness of breath, or other signals of overdose or aggravated CV disease.

• Tell caregiver of infant or child who can't swallow tablets to crush tablet and suspend in small amount of water and give by spoon or dropper. Crushed tablet can be sprinkled over food, except foods containing large amounts of soybean, fiber, or iron.

• Tell patient using Levoxyl to take pill with plenty of water to avoid choking, gagging, or getting the pill stuck in his throat.

• Advise patient who has achieved stable response not to change brands.

• Tell patient to report unusual bleeding and bruising or any other adverse reaction.

• Advise patient not to take OTC or other prescription drugs without first consulting prescriber.

• Advise patient to tell health care provider about all medications he or she is taking, both OTC and prescription.

• Tell patient who plans to have surgery to notify physician or dentist about taking levothyroxine.

• Advise patient to report pregnancy to prescriber because dosage may need adjustment.

• Advise patient to protect tablets from light and moisture.

SAFETY ALERT!

lidocaine hydrochloride
LYE-doe-kane

Xylocaine, Xylocard✦

Therapeutic class: Antiarrhythmics
Pharmacologic class: Amide derivatives

AVAILABLE FORMS
Infusion (premixed): 0.2% (2 mg/mL), 0.4% (4 mg/mL), 0.8% (8 mg/mL)
Injection (for direct I.V. use): 1% (10 mg/mL), 2% (20 mg/mL)
Injection (for I.V. admixtures): 4% (40 mg/mL), 10% (100 mg/mL), 20% (200 mg/mL)

INDICATIONS & DOSAGES
➤ **Ventricular arrhythmias caused by MI, cardiac manipulation, or cardiac glycosides**
Adults: 50 to 100 mg (1 to 1.5 mg/kg) by I.V. bolus at 25 to 50 mg/minute. Bolus dose is repeated every 5 minutes until arrhythmias subside or adverse reactions develop. Don't exceed 300-mg total bolus during a 1-hour period. Simultaneously, constant infusion of 20 to 50 mcg/kg/minute (1 to 4 mg/minute) is begun. If single bolus has been given, smaller bolus dose may be repeated 15 to 20 minutes after start of infusion to maintain therapeutic level.
Children: 1 mg/kg by I.V. or intraosseous bolus. Start infusion at 30 mcg/kg/minute.
Elderly patients: Reduce dosage and rate of infusion.
Adjust-a-dose: For patients with HF, with renal or liver disease, or who weigh less than 50 kg, reduce dosage.

ADMINISTRATION
I.V.
▼ Injections (additive syringes and single-use vials) containing 40, 100, or 200 mg/mL are for the preparation of I.V. infusion solutions only and must be diluted before use.
▼ Prepare I.V. infusion by adding 1 g (using 25 mL of 4% or 5 mL of 20% injection) to 1 L of D_5W injection to provide a solution containing 1 mg/mL.
▼ Use a more concentrated solution of up to 8 mg/mL in fluid-restricted patient.
▼ Patients receiving infusions must be on a cardiac monitor and must be attended at all times. Use an infusion control device for giving infusion precisely. Don't exceed 4 mg/minute; faster rate greatly increases risk of toxicity.
▼ Avoid giving injections containing preservatives.
▼ **Incompatibilities:** Amphotericin, ampicillin, cefazolin, ceftriaxone, fentanyl citrate (higher pH brands), methohexital sodium, phenytoin sodium, sodium bicarbonate, thiopental sodium.

ACTION
A class IB antiarrhythmic that decreases the depolarization, automaticity, and

---

excitability in the ventricles during the diastolic phase by direct action on the tissues, especially the Purkinje network.

Route	Onset	Peak	Duration
I.V.	Immediate	Immediate	10–20 min

Half-life: 1½ to 2 hours (may be prolonged in patients with HF or hepatic disease).

ADVERSE REACTIONS
CNS: confusion, tremor, stupor, restlessness, light-headedness, *seizures,* lethargy, somnolence, anxiety, hallucinations, nervousness, paresthesia, muscle twitching.
CV: hypotension, *bradycardia, new or worsened arrhythmias, cardiac arrest.*
EENT: tinnitus, blurred or double vision.
GI: vomiting.
Respiratory: *respiratory depression and arrest.*
Skin: soreness at injection site.
Other: *anaphylaxis,* sensation of cold.

INTERACTIONS
Drug-drug. *Atenolol, metoprolol, nadolol, pindolol, propranolol:* May reduce hepatic metabolism of lidocaine, increasing the risk of toxicity. Give bolus doses of lidocaine at a slower rate, and monitor lidocaine level and patient closely.
Cimetidine: May decrease clearance of lidocaine, increasing the risk of toxicity. Consider using a different H_2-receptor antagonist if possible. Monitor lidocaine level closely.
Ergot-type oxytocic drugs: May cause severe, persistent hypertension or stroke. Avoid using together.
Mexiletine: May increase pharmacologic effects. Avoid using together.
Phenytoin, procainamide, propranolol, quinidine: May increase cardiac depressant effects. Monitor patient closely.
Succinylcholine: May prolong neuromuscular blockade. Monitor patient closely.

EFFECTS ON LAB TEST RESULTS
None reported.

CONTRAINDICATIONS & CAUTIONS
• Contraindicated in patients hypersensitive to amide-type local anesthetics.

• Contraindicated in those with Adams-Stokes syndrome, Wolff-Parkinson-White syndrome, and severe degrees of SA, AV, or intraventricular block in the absence of an artificial pacemaker.
• Use cautiously and at reduced dosages in patients with complete or second-degree heart block or sinus bradycardia, in elderly patients, in those with HF or renal or hepatic disease, and in those weighing less than 50 kg.
Dialyzable drug: No.
⚠ **Overdose S&S:** Circulatory depression, change in level of consciousness, seizures, hypoventilation.

PREGNANCY-LACTATION-REPRODUCTION
• There are no adequate studies with I.V. lidocaine in pregnant women. Use cautiously if clearly needed, especially during early pregnancy.
• Drug appears in breast milk. Use cautiously in breast-feeding women.

NURSING CONSIDERATIONS
• Monitor drug level. Therapeutic levels are 2 to 5 mcg/mL.
⚕ **Alert:** Monitor patient for toxicity. In many severely ill patients, seizures may be the first sign of toxicity, but severe reactions are usually preceded by somnolence, confusion, tremors, and paresthesia. If signs of toxicity occur, stop drug at once and notify prescriber. Continuing could lead to seizures and coma. Give oxygen through a nasal cannula if not contraindicated. Keep oxygen and cardiopulmonary resuscitation equipment available.
• Monitor patient's response, especially BP and electrolytes, BUN, and creatinine levels. Notify prescriber promptly if abnormalities develop.
• If arrhythmias worsen or ECG changes occur (for example, QRS complex widens or PR interval substantially prolongs), stop infusion and notify prescriber.

PATIENT TEACHING
• Tell patient to report adverse reactions promptly because toxicity can occur.

lifitegrast
See NEW DRUGS for information.

SAFETY ALERT!

linagliptin
lin-a-GLIP-tin

Tradjenta

Therapeutic class: Antidiabetics
Pharmacologic class: DPP-4 inhibitors

AVAILABLE FORMS
Tablets: 5 mg

INDICATIONS & DOSAGES
➤ **Adjunct to diet and exercise to improve glycemic control in adults with type 2 diabetes as monotherapy or as combination therapy with an insulin secretagogue (such as a sulfonylurea) or insulin**
Adults: 5 mg P.O. daily.
Adjust-a-dose: When used in combination with an insulin secretagogue or insulin, use lower doses of those drugs to decrease the risk of hypoglycemia.

ADMINISTRATION
P.O.
● Give drug without regard for food.
● Store tablets at 77° F (25° C) with excursions permitted to between 59° and 86° F (15° to 30° C).
● Store tablets out of reach of children.

ACTION
Inhibits DPP-4, an enzyme that rapidly inactivates incretin hormones, which play a part in the body's regulation of glucose.

Route	Onset	Peak	Duration
P.O.	Rapid	1½ hr	Unknown

Half-life: About 12 hours (accumulation).

ADVERSE REACTIONS
CNS: headache.
EENT: nasopharyngitis.
GI: diarrhea.
Metabolic: *hypoglycemia.*
Musculoskeletal: arthralgia, back pain, myalgia.
Respiratory: cough, URI.

INTERACTIONS
Drug-drug. *CYP3A4 or P-glycoprotein inducers (such as rifampin):* May decrease linagliptin level. Avoid use together.
Ritonavir: May increase linagliptin effects and risk of adverse effects. Use with caution; monitor response, and adjust dosage as necessary.
Sulfonylureas (glyburide), insulin: May increase risk of hypoglycemia. Monitor glucose level carefully and adjust sulfonylurea or insulin dosage as necessary.

EFFECTS ON LAB TEST RESULTS
● May increase uric acid level.
● May decrease fasting glucose and HbA$_{1C}$ levels.

CONTRAINDICATIONS & CAUTIONS
● Contraindicated in patients hypersensitive to drug (with such signs and symptoms as urticaria, angioedema, and bronchial hyperactivity).
● Drug not for use in patients with type 1 diabetes or for treatment of diabetic ketoacidosis.
● Acute pancreatitis, including fatal pancreatitis, has occurred in patients taking linagliptin. It's unknown whether patients with a history of pancreatitis are at increased risk for development of pancreatitis while using linagliptin.
⚠ *Alert:* Drug may cause joint pain that can be severe and disabling. Report severe and persistent joint pain to prescriber; drug may need to be discontinued.
● Safety in children hasn't been established.
Dialyzable drug: Unlikely.

PREGNANCY-LACTATION-REPRODUCTION
● There are no adequate studies in pregnant women. Use during pregnancy only if clearly needed.
● It isn't known if drug appears in breast milk. Use cautiously in breast-feeding women.

NURSING CONSIDERATIONS
● Monitor HbA$_{1C}$ and fasting blood glucose levels periodically.
● Monitor patient for signs and symptoms of hypoglycemia (anxiety, confusion,

---

Nursing 2018

DRUG

HANDBOOK®

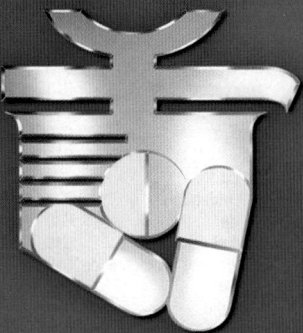

Photoguide to tablets and capsules

This photoguide includes 452 tablets and capsules, representing the most commonly prescribed generic and trade name drugs. These drugs, organized alphabetically by generic name, are shown in actual size and color with cross-references to drug information. Each product is labeled with its trade name and its strength.

INDEX OF TRADE NAMES IN PHOTOGUIDE TO TABLETS AND CAPSULES

Abilify	C3	Eryc	C10	Procardia XL	C21
Accupril	C24	Ery-Tab	C10	Proscar	C12
Aciphex	C24	Evista	C25	Protonix	C22
Actonel	C25	Famvir	C11	Provera	C18
Actos	C23	Flomax	C28	Provigil	C20
Aldactone	C27	Focalin XR	C8	Prozac	C12
Amaryl	C13	Fosamax	C3	Prozac Weekly	C12
Ambien	C32	Frova	C13	Ranexa	C25
Amitiza	C18	Geodon	C32	Relpax	C10
Aricept	C9	Glucophage	C18	Restoril	C29
Arimidex	C3	Glucophage XR	C18	Retrovir	C32
Ativan	C17	Glucotrol	C14	Reyataz	C4
Avandia	C26	Glucotrol XL	C14	Risperdal	C25
Avapro	C14	Imitrex	C28	Ritalin	C19
Avelox	C20	Inderal	C24	Ritalin-SR	C19
Avodart	C9	Inderal LA	C24	rivastigmine tartrate	C26
Azilect	C25	Januvia	C27	Sarafem	C12
Bactrim DS	C28	Kaletra	C17	Savella	C20
Benicar	C22	Klonopin	C6	Seroquel	C24
Benicar HCT	C22	Lasix	C13	Sinemet	C15
Biaxin	C6	Latuda	C18	Sinemet CR	C15
Boniva	C14	Lescol	C13	Singulair	C20
Bystolic	C20	Levaquin	C15	Soma	C5
Calan	C31	Levitra	C31	Stalevo	C15
Carafate	C28	Levoxyl	C16	Strattera	C4
Cardizem	C8	Lexapro	C10	Sutent	C28
Cardizem CD	C8	Lipitor	C4	Synthroid	C16
Cardizem LA	C8	Lopid	C13	Tenormin	C4
Cardura	C9	Lopressor	C19	Topamax	C29
Celebrex	C5	Lotensin	C5	Toprol-XL	C19
Celexa	C6	Lovaza	C22	TriCor	C22
Chantix	C31	Lunesta	C11	Tylenol with Codeine #3	C6
Cialis	C28	Lyrica	C23	Ultracet	C30
Cipro	C5	Macrodantin	C21	Uroxatral	C3
Clarinex	C7	Mavik	C30	Valium	C8
Clozaril	C6	Medrol	C19	Valtrex	C30
Colcrys	C7	methadone hydrochloride	C19	Vasotec	C10
Combivir	C15	Micardis	C29	Verelan	C31
Concerta	C19	Namenda	C18	VESIcare	C27
Coumadin	C32	Naprosyn	C20	Viagra	C27
Cozaar	C18	Neurontin	C13	Viibryd	C32
Crestor	C26	Nexium	C10	Viread	C29
Crixivan	C14	Nitrostat	C21	Vytorin	C11
Cymbalta	C9	Norvasc	C3	Vyvanse	C17
Demadex	C30	Nucynta	C29	Welchol	C7
Demerol	C18	Nucynta ER	C29	Wellbutrin	C5
Depakote	C9	Onglyza	C26	Wellbutrin SR	C5
Depakote Sprinkle	C9	OxyContin	C22	Xanax	C3
Detrol	C29	Pamelor	C21	Xarelto	C26
Dexilant	C7	Pepcid	C11	Zantac	C25
DiaBeta	C14	Plavix	C6	Zestril	C17
Diflucan	C12	Pradaxa	C7	Zetia	C11
Diovan	C30	Pravachol	C23	Zithromax	C4
Diovan HCT	C31	Premarin	C11	Zocor	C27
Effexor XR	C31	Prevacid	C15	Zoloft	C27
Effient	C23	Prinivil	C17	Zyban	C5
Enablex	C7	Pristiq	C7	Zyprexa	C21

ALENDRONATE SODIUM

Fosamax
(Page 87)

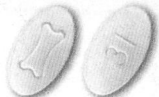

70 mg

ALFUZOSIN HYDROCHLORIDE

Uroxatral
(Page 89)

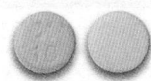

10 mg

ALPRAZOLAM

Xanax
(Page 98)

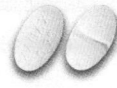
0.25 mg

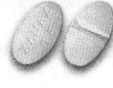
0.5 mg

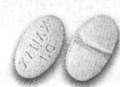
1 mg

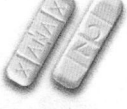

2 mg

AMLODIPINE BESYLATE

Norvasc
(Page 118)

2.5 mg

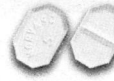
5 mg

ANASTROZOLE

Arimidex
(Page 134)

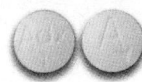

1 mg

ARIPIPRAZOLE

Abilify
(Page 145)

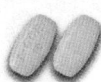
10 mg

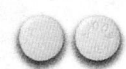
15 mg

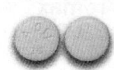
30 mg

ATAZANAVIR SULFATE

Reyataz
(Page 157)

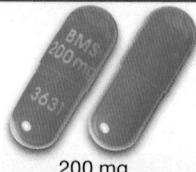

200 mg

ATENOLOL

Tenormin
(Page 163)

25 mg

50 mg

100 mg

ATOMOXETINE HYDROCHLORIDE

Strattera
(Page 165)

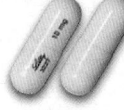

10 mg

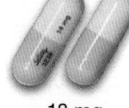

18 mg

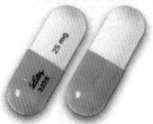

25 mg

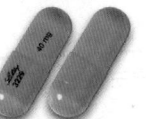

40 mg

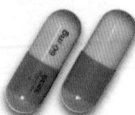

60 mg

ATORVASTATIN CALCIUM

Lipitor
(Page 167)

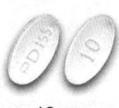

10 mg

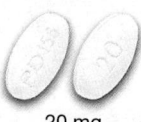

20 mg

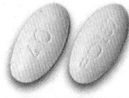

40 mg

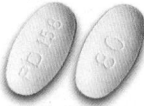

80 mg

AZITHROMYCIN

Zithromax
(Page 186)

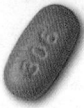

250 mg

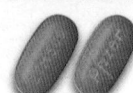

500 mg

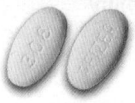

600 mg

BENAZEPRIL HYDROCHLORIDE

Lotensin
(Page 202)

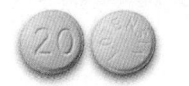 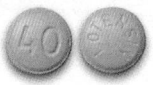

20 mg   40 mg

BUPROPION HYDROCHLORIDE

Wellbutrin
(Page 245)

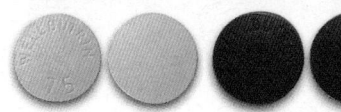

75 mg   100 mg

Wellbutrin SR
(Page 245)

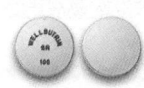  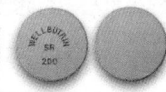

100 mg   150 mg   200 mg

Zyban
(Page 245)

150 mg

CARISOPRODOL

Soma
(Page 277)

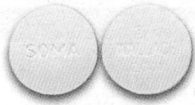

350 mg

CELECOXIB

Celebrex
(Page 314)

 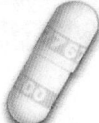

100 mg   200 mg

CIPROFLOXACIN

Cipro
(Page 335)

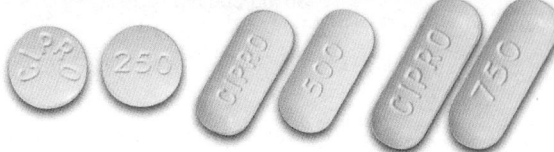

250 mg   500 mg   750 mg

CITALOPRAM HYDROBROMIDE

Celexa
(Page 345)

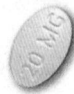

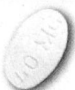

20 mg   40 mg

CLARITHROMYCIN

Biaxin
(Page 347)

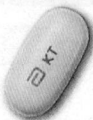

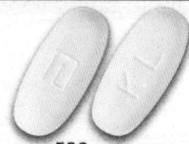

250 mg   500 mg

CLONAZEPAM

Klonopin
(Page 359)

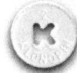

0.5 mg   1 mg   2 mg

CLOPIDOGREL BISULFATE

Plavix
(Page 364)

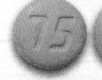

75 mg

CLOZAPINE

Clozaril
(Page 367)

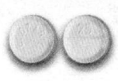

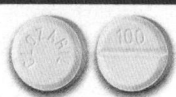

25 mg   100 mg

CODEINE PHOSPHATE—ACETAMINOPHEN

Tylenol with Codeine #3
(Page 374)

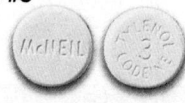

30 mg/300 mg

COLCHICINE

Colcrys
(Page 377)

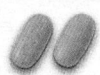

0.6 mg

COLESEVELAM HYDROCHLORIDE

Welchol
(Page 379)

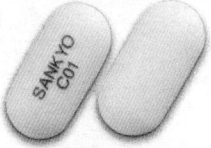

625 mg

DABIGATRAN ETEXILATE MESYLATE

Pradaxa
(Page 394)

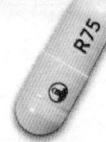 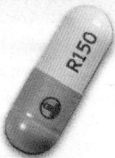

75 mg   150 mg

DARIFENACIN HYDROBROMIDE

Enablex
(Page 411)

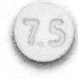

7.5 mg   15 mg

DESLORATADINE

Clarinex
(Page 420)

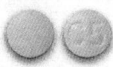

5 mg

DESVENLAFAXINE SUCCINATE

Pristiq
(Page 425)

50 mg   100 mg

DEXLANSOPRAZOLE

Dexilant
(Page 432)

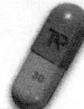 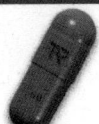

30 mg   60 mg

DEXMETHYLPHENIDATE HYDROCHLORIDE

Focalin XR
(Page 434)

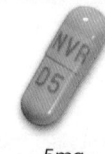

5mg

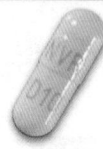

10 mg

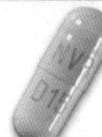

15 mg

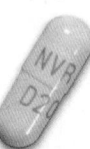

20 mg

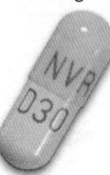

30 mg

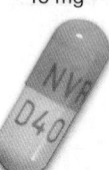

40 mg

DIAZEPAM

Valium
(Page 442)

2 mg

5 mg

10 mg

DILTIAZEM HYDROCHLORIDE

Cardizem
(Page 460)

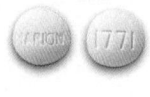

30 mg

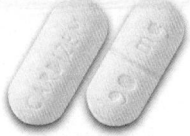

90 mg

Cardizem CD
(Page 460)

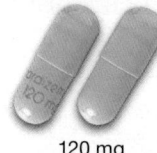

120 mg

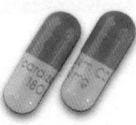

180 mg

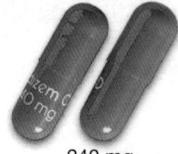

240 mg

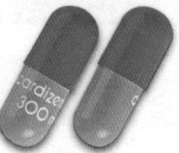

300 mg

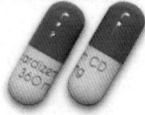

360 mg

Cardizem LA
(Page 460)

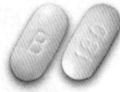

180 mg

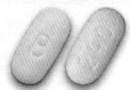

240 mg

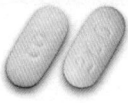

360 mg

DIVALPROEX SODIUM

Depakote
(Page 1519)

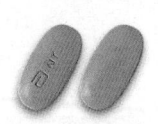 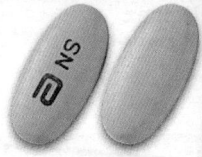

125 mg   250 mg   500 mg

Depakote Sprinkle
(Page 1519)

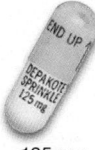

125 mg

DONEPEZIL HYDROCHLORIDE

Aricept
(Page 476)

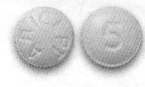   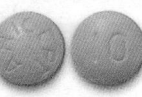

5 mg   10 mg

DOXAZOSIN MESYLATE

Cardura
(Page 481)

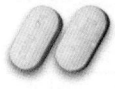   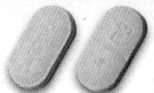

1 mg   2 mg   4 mg

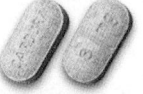

8 mg

DULOXETINE HYDROCHLORIDE

Cymbalta
(Page 505)

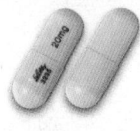   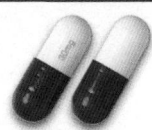   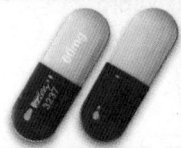

20 mg   30 mg   60 mg

DUTASTERIDE

Avodart
(Page 508)

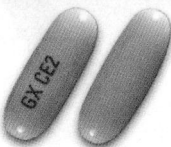

0.5 mg

ELETRIPTAN HYDROBROMIDE

Relpax
(Page 514)

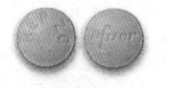

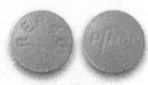

20 mg   40 mg

ENALAPRIL MALEATE

Vasotec
(Page 524)

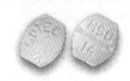

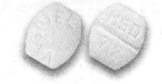

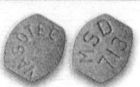

2.5 mg   5 mg   10 mg

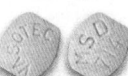

20 mg

ERYTHROMYCIN BASE

Eryc
(Page 553)

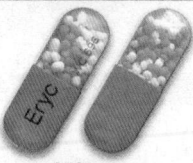

250 mg

Ery-Tab
(Page 553)

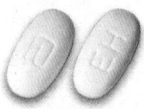

333 mg

ESCITALOPRAM OXALATE

Lexapro
(Page 556)

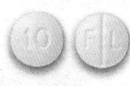

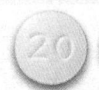

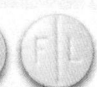

10 mg   20 mg

ESOMEPRAZOLE MAGNESIUM

Nexium
(Page 563)

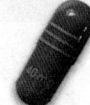

20 mg   40 mg

ESTROGENS (CONJUGATED)

Premarin
(Page 578)

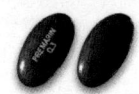

0.3 mg

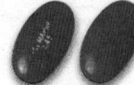

0.45 mg

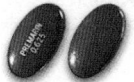

0.625 mg

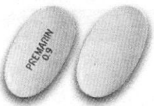

0.9 mg

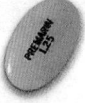

1.25 mg

ESZOPICLONE

Lunesta
(Page 584)

1 mg

2 mg

3 mg

EZETIMIBE

Zetia
(Page 613)

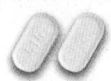

10 mg

EZETIMIBE—SIMVASTATIN

Vytorin
(Page 1662)

10 mg/10 mg

10 mg/20 mg

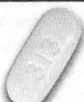

10 mg/40 mg

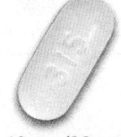

10 mg/80 mg

FAMCICLOVIR

Famvir
(Page 616)

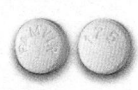

125 mg

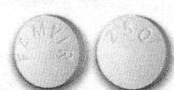

250 mg

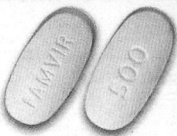

500 mg

FAMOTIDINE

Pepcid
(Page 617)

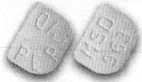

20 mg

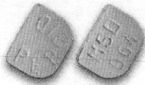

40 mg

FENOFIBRATE

TriCor
(Page 621)

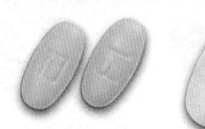 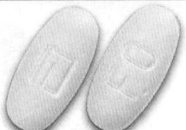

48 mg   145 mg

FINASTERIDE

Proscar
(Page 638)

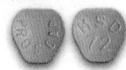

5 mg

FLUCONAZOLE

Diflucan
(Page 646)

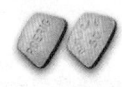   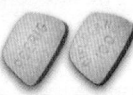   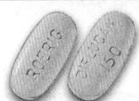

50 mg   100 mg   150 mg

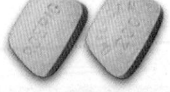

200 mg

FLUOXETINE HYDROCHLORIDE

Prozac
(Page 657)

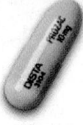   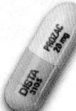   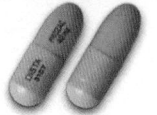

10 mg   20 mg   40 mg

Prozac Weekly
(Page 657)

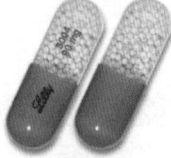

90 mg

Sarafem
(Page 657)

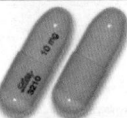   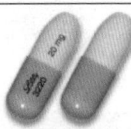

10 mg   20 mg

FLUVASTATIN SODIUM

Lescol
(Page 672)

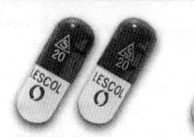

20 mg   40 mg

FROVATRIPTAN SUCCINATE

Frova
(Page 687)

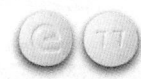

2.5 mg

FUROSEMIDE

Lasix
(Page 690)

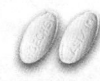   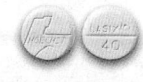   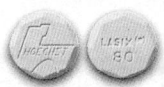

20 mg   40 mg   80 mg

GABAPENTIN

Neurontin
(Page 692)

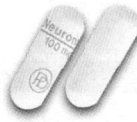   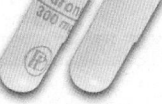   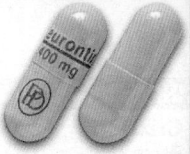

100 mg   300 mg   400 mg

GEMFIBROZIL

Lopid
(Page 703)

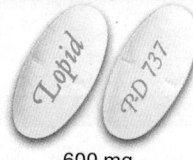

600 mg

GLIMEPIRIDE

Amaryl
(Page 711)

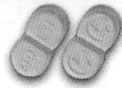   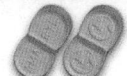   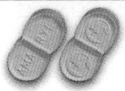

1 mg   2 mg   4 mg

GLIPIZIDE

Glucotrol
(Page 713)

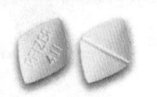

5 mg   10 mg

Glucotrol XL
(Page 713)

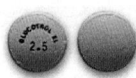 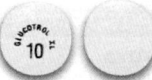

2.5 mg   5 mg   10 mg

GLYBURIDE

DiaBeta
(Page 715)

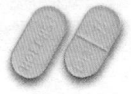   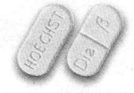

1.25 mg   2.5 mg   5 mg

IBANDRONATE SODIUM

Boniva
(Page 752)

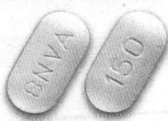

150 mg

INDINAVIR SULFATE

Crixivan
(Page 782)

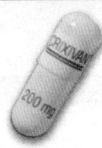   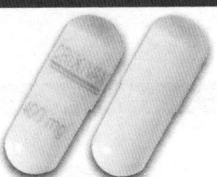

200 mg   400 mg

IRBESARTAN

Avapro
(Page 825)

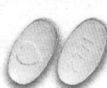   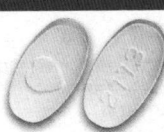

75 mg   150 mg   300 mg

LAMIVUDINE—ZIDOVUDINE

Combivir
(Page 1660)

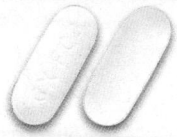

150 mg/300 mg

LANSOPRAZOLE

Prevacid
(Page 867)

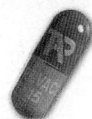 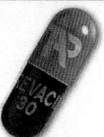

15 mg   30 mg

LEVODOPA— CARBIDOPA

Sinemet
(Page 886)

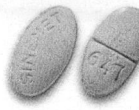 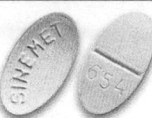

100 mg/10 mg   250 mg/25 mg

Sinemet CR
(Page 886)

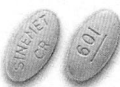

100 mg/25 mg

LEVODOPA—CARBIDOPA—ENTACAPONE

Stalevo
(Page 889)

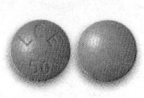 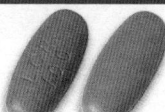 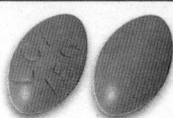

50 mg/12.5 mg/   100 mg/25 mg/   150 mg/37.5 mg/
200 mg   200 mg   200 mg

LEVOFLOXACIN

Levaquin
(Page 891)

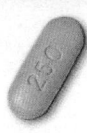 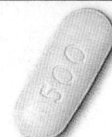

250 mg   500 mg

LEVOTHYROXINE SODIUM

Levoxyl
(Page 897)

 25 mcg

 50 mcg

75 mcg

 88 mcg

100 mcg

 112 mcg

125 mcg

 137 mcg

150 mcg

 175 mcg

 200 mcg

Synthroid
(Page 897)

 25 mcg

50 mcg

75 mcg

 88 mcg

100 mcg

112 mcg

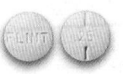 125 mcg

 150 mcg

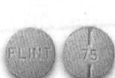 175 mcg

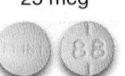 200 mcg

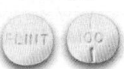 300 mcg

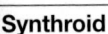
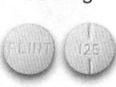
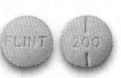
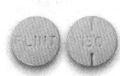
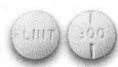
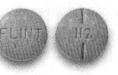
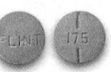

LISDEXAMFETAMINE DIMESYLATE

Vyvanse
(Page 908)

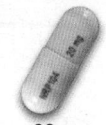 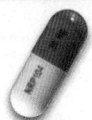 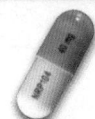

20 mg   30 mg   40 mg

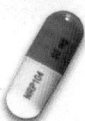 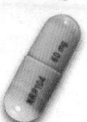 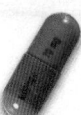

50 mg   60 mg   70 mg

LISINOPRIL

Prinivil
(Page 910)

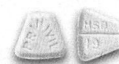 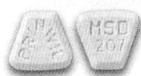

5 mg   10 mg   20 mg

40 mg

Zestril
(Page 910)

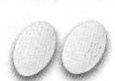 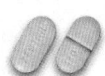

2.5 mg   5 mg   10 mg

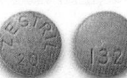 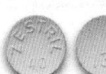

20 mg   40 mg

LOPINAVIR—RITONAVIR

Kaletra
(Page 920)

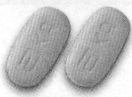

200 mg/50 mg

LORAZEPAM

Ativan
(Page 924)

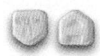 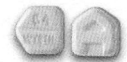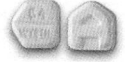 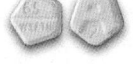

0.5 mg   1 mg   2 mg

LOSARTAN POTASSIUM

Cozaar
(Page 928)

25 mg   50 mg

LUBIPROSTONE

Amitiza
(Page 1683)

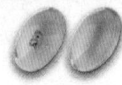

24 mcg

LURASIDONE HYDROCHLORIDE

Latuda
(Page 935)

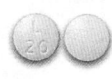 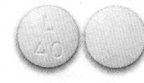 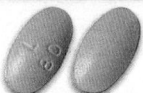

20 mg   40 mg   80 mg

MEDROXYPROGESTERONE ACETATE

Provera
(Page 943)

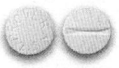 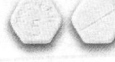 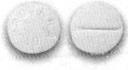

2.5 mg   5 mg   10 mg

MEMANTINE HYDROCHLORIDE

Namenda
(Page 952)

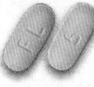 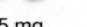 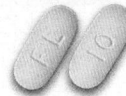

5 mg   10 mg

MEPERIDINE HYDROCHLORIDE

Demerol
(Page 954)

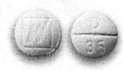 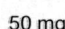

50 mg   100 mg

METFORMIN HYDROCHLORIDE

Glucophage
(Page 963)

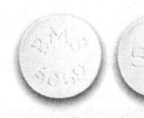 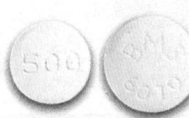 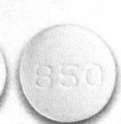 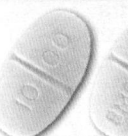

500 mg   850 mg   1,000 mg

Glucophage XR
(Page 963)

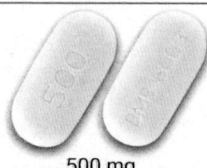

500 mg

METHADONE HYDROCHLORIDE
(Page 966)

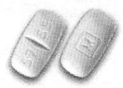

5 mg

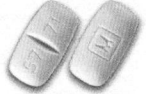

10 mg

METHYLPHENIDATE HYDROCHLORIDE

Concerta
(Page 979)

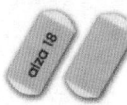

18 mg

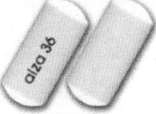

36 mg

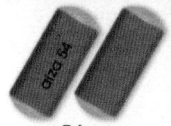

54 mg

Ritalin
(Page 979)

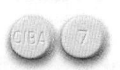

5 mg

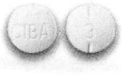

10 mg

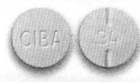

20 mg

Ritalin-SR
(Page 979)

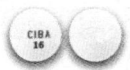

20 mg

METHYLPREDNISOLONE

Medrol
(Page 984)

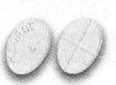

4 mg

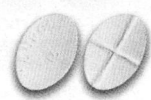

16 mg

METOPROLOL SUCCINATE

Toprol-XL
(Page 992)

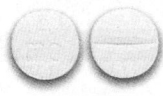

50 mg

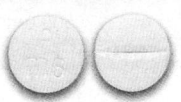

100 mg

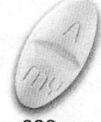

200 mg

METOPROLOL TARTRATE

Lopressor
(Page 992)

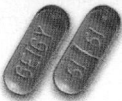

50 mg

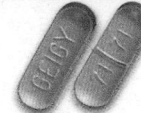

100 mg

MILNACIPRAN HYDROCHLORIDE

Savella
(Page 1006)

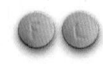

12.5 mg

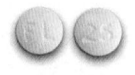

25 mg

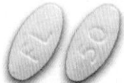

50 mg

MODAFINIL

Provigil
(Page 1022)

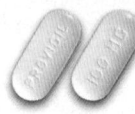

100 mg

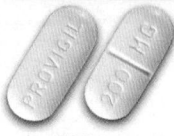

200 mg

MONTELUKAST SODIUM

Singulair
(Page 1027)

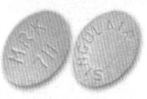

4 mg

5 mg

10 mg

MOXIFLOXACIN HYDROCHLORIDE

Avelox
(Page 1038)

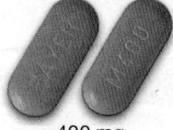

400 mg

NAPROXEN

Naprosyn
(Page 1054)

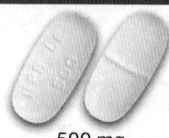

500 mg

NEBIVOLOL HYDROCHLORIDE

Bystolic
(Page 1061)

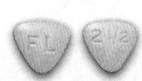

2.5 mg

5 mg

10 mg

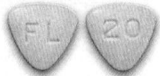

20 mg

NIFEDIPINE

Procardia XL
(Page 1072)

30 mg

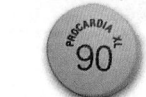

60 mg 90 mg

NITROFURANTOIN MACROCRYSTALS

Macrodantin
(Page 1075)

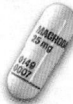 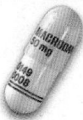 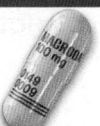

25 mg 50 mg 100 mg

NITROGLYCERIN

Nitrostat
(Page 1076)

0.4 mg

NORTRIPTYLINE HYDROCHLORIDE

Pamelor
(Page 1090)

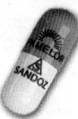 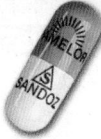 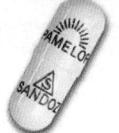

10 mg 25 mg 50 mg

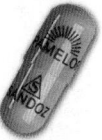

75 mg

OLANZAPINE

Zyprexa
(Page 1103)

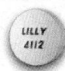 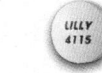 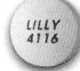

2.5 mg 5 mg 7.5 mg

  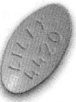

10 mg 15 mg 20 mg

OLMESARTAN MEDOXOMIL

Benicar
(Page 1106)

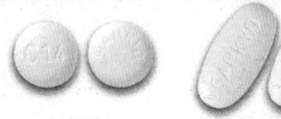

20 mg   40 mg

OLMESARTAN MEDOXOMIL—HYDROCHLOROTHIAZIDE

Benicar HCT
(Page 1656)

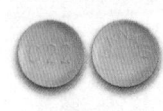   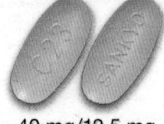   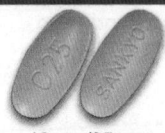

20 mg/12.5 mg   40 mg/12.5 mg   40 mg/25 mg

OMEGA-3-ACID ETHYL ESTERS

Lovaza
(Page 1116)

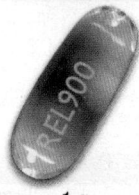

1 g

OXYCODONE HYDROCHLORIDE

OxyContin
(Page 1142)

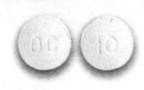   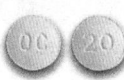   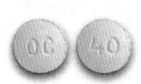

10 mg   20 mg   40 mg

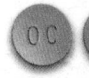

80 mg

PANTOPRAZOLE SODIUM

Protonix
(Page 1173)

          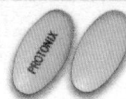

20 mg   40 mg

PIOGLITAZONE HYDROCHLORIDE

Actos
(Page 1223)

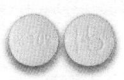 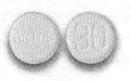 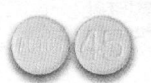

15 mg   30 mg   45 mg

PRASUGREL HYDROCHLORIDE

Effient
(Page 1240)

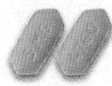 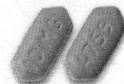

5 mg   10 mg

PRAVASTATIN SODIUM

Pravachol
(Page 1241)

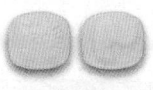 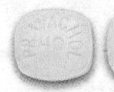

20 mg   40 mg

PREGABALIN

Lyrica
(Page 1250)

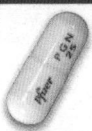 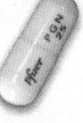 

25 mg   50 mg   75 mg

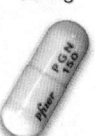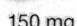

100 mg   150 mg   200 mg

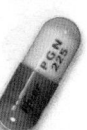 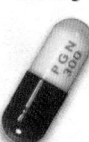

225 mg   300 mg

PROPRANOLOL HYDROCHLORIDE

Inderal
(Page 1267)

40 mg

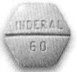
60 mg

80 mg

Inderal LA
(Page 1267)

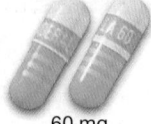
60 mg

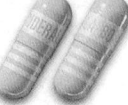
80 mg

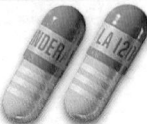
120 mg

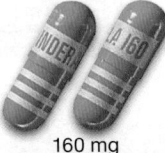
160 mg

QUETIAPINE FUMARATE

Seroquel
(Page 1272)

25 mg

50 mg

100 mg

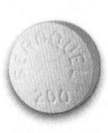
200 mg

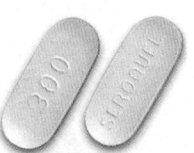
300 mg

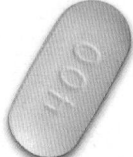
400 mg

QUINAPRIL HYDROCHLORIDE

Accupril
(Page 1276)

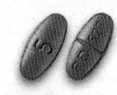
5 mg

10 mg

20 mg

40 mg

RABEPRAZOLE SODIUM

Aciphex
(Page 1280)

20 mg

RALOXIFENE HYDROCHLORIDE

Evista
(Page 1282)

60 mg

RANITIDINE HYDROCHLORIDE

Zantac
(Page 1294)

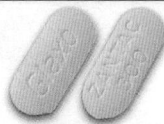

150 mg   300 mg

RANOLAZINE

Ranexa
(Page 1296)

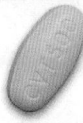

500 mg

RASAGILINE MESYLATE

Azilect
(Page 1297)

0.5 mg   1 mg

RISEDRONATE SODIUM

Actonel
(Page 1313)

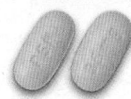

5 mg   35 mg

RISPERIDONE

Risperdal
(Page 1315)

                       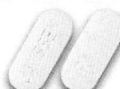

0.25 mg   0.5 mg   1 mg

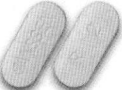   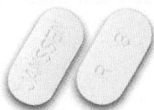   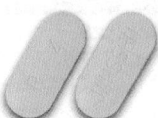

2 mg   3 mg   4 mg

RIVAROXABAN

Xarelto
(Page 1325)

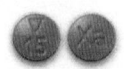

15 mg

20 mg

RIVASTIGMINE TARTRATE

(Page 1327)

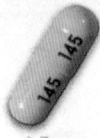

1.5 mg

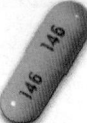

3 mg

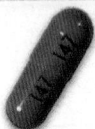

4.5 mg

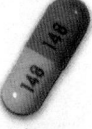

6 mg

ROSIGLITAZONE MALEATE

Avandia
(Page 1335)

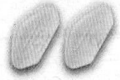

2 mg

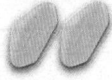

4 mg

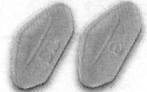

8 mg

ROSUVASTATIN CALCIUM

Crestor
(Page 1337)

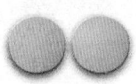

5 mg

10 mg

20 mg

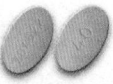

40 mg

SAXAGLIPTIN

Onglyza
(Page 1349)

2.5 mg

5 mg

SERTRALINE HYDROCHLORIDE

Zoloft
(Page 1354)

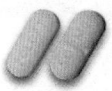 50 mg

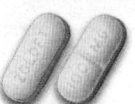 100 mg

SILDENAFIL CITRATE

Viagra
(Page 1358)

 25 mg

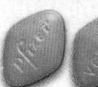 50 mg

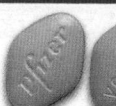 100 mg

SIMVASTATIN

Zocor
(Page 1365)

 5 mg

 10 mg

 20 mg

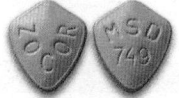 40 mg

SITAGLIPTIN PHOSPHATE

Januvia
(Page 1371)

 100 mg

SOLIFENACIN SUCCINATE

VESIcare
(Page 1376)

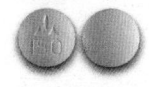 5 mg

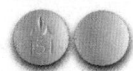 10 mg

SPIRONOLACTONE

Aldactone
(Page 1384)

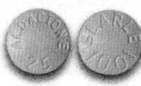 25 mg

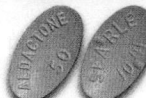 50 mg

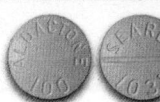 100 mg

SUCRALFATE

Carafate
(Page 1390)

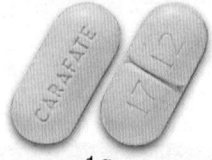

1 g

SULFAMETHOXAZOLE—TRIMETHOPRIM

Bactrim DS
(Page 1392)

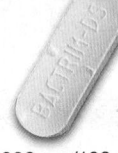

800 mg/160 mg

SUMATRIPTAN SUCCINATE

Imitrex
(Page 1397)

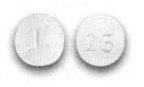 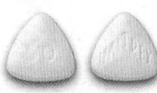

25 mg   50 mg

SUNITINIB MALATE

Sutent
(Page 1399)

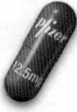 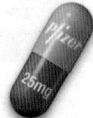 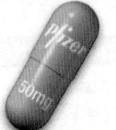

12.5 mg   25 mg   50 mg

TADALAFIL

Cialis
(Page 1409)

2.5 mg   5 mg   10 mg

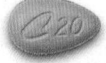

20 mg

TAMSULOSIN HYDROCHLORIDE

Flomax
(Page 1414)

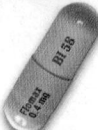

0.4 mg

TAPENTADOL HYDROCHLORIDE

Nucynta
(Page 1416)

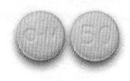

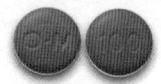

50 mg   100 mg

Nucynta ER
(Page 1416)

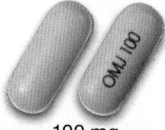

100 mg

TELMISARTAN

Micardis
(Page 1424)

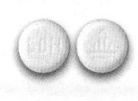   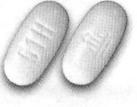   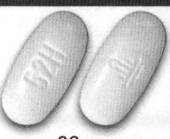

20 mg   40 mg   80 mg

TEMAZEPAM

Restoril
(Page 1425)

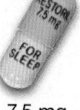   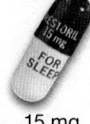   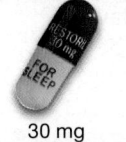

7.5 mg   15 mg   30 mg

TENOFOVIR DISOPROXIL FUMARATE

Viread
(Page 1430)

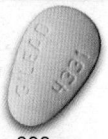

300 mg

TOLTERODINE TARTRATE

Detrol
(Page 1476)

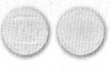   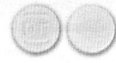

1 mg   2 mg

TOPIRAMATE

Topamax
(Page 1479)

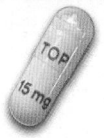   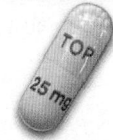   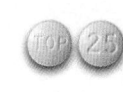

15 mg   25 mg   25 mg

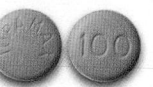   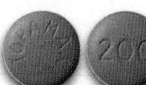   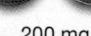

50 mg   100 mg   200 mg

TORSEMIDE

Demadex
(Page 1485)

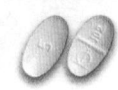 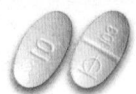 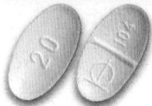

5 mg   10 mg   20 mg

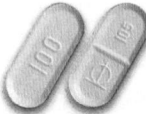

100 mg

TRAMADOL HYDROCHLORIDE—ACETAMINOPHEN

Ultracet
(Page 1651)

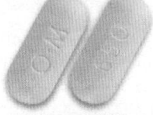

37.5 mg/325 mg

TRANDOLAPRIL

Mavik
(Page 1748)

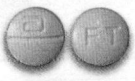   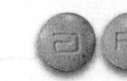

1 mg   2 mg   4 mg

VALACYCLOVIR HYDROCHLORIDE

Valtrex
(Page 1515)

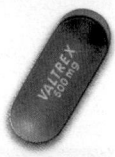   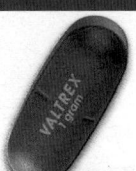

500 mg   1,000 mg

VALSARTAN

Diovan
(Page 1522)

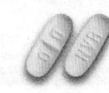 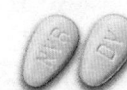 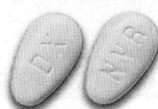

40 mg   80 mg   160 mg

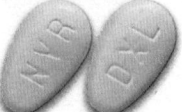

320 mg

VALSARTAN—HYDROCHLOROTHIAZIDE

Diovan HCT
(Page 1656)

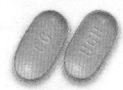

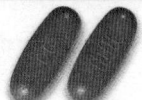

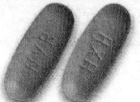

80 mg/12.5 mg   160 mg/12.5 mg   160 mg/25 mg

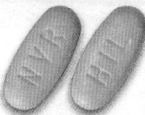

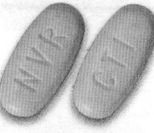

320 mg/12.5 mg   320 mg/25 mg

VARDENAFIL HYDROCHLORIDE

Levitra
(Page 1526)

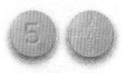

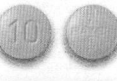

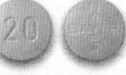

5 mg   10 mg   20 mg

VARENICLINE TARTRATE

Chantix
(Page 1527)

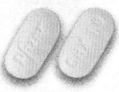

0.5 mg   1 mg

VENLAFAXINE HYDROCHLORIDE

Effexor XR
(Page 1529)

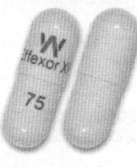

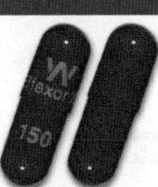

75 mg   150 mg

VERAPAMIL HYDROCHLORIDE

Calan
(Page 1532)

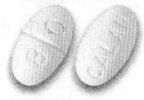

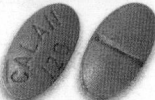

80 mg   120 mg

Verelan
(Page 1532)

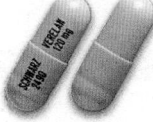

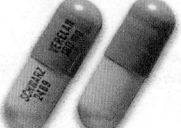

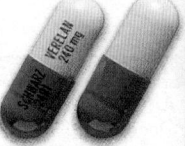

120 mg   180 mg   240 mg

VILAZODONE HYDROCHLORIDE

Viibryd
(Page 1537)

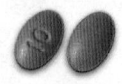
10 mg

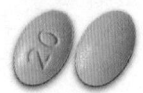
20 mg

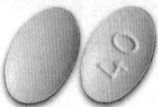
40 mg

WARFARIN SODIUM

Coumadin
(Page 1554)

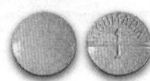
1 mg

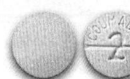
2 mg

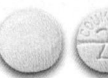
2.5 mg

3 mg

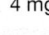
4 mg

5 mg

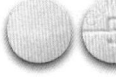

6 mg

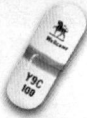
3 mg

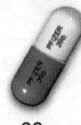
6 mg

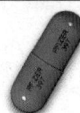
7.5 mg

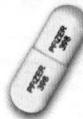
10 mg

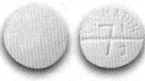
4 mg

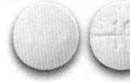
5 mg

ZIDOVUDINE

Retrovir
(Page 1559)

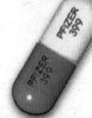
100 mg

ZIPRASIDONE HYDROCHLORIDE

Geodon
(Page 1562)

20 mg

40 mg

60 mg

80 mg

ZOLPIDEM TARTRATE

Ambien
(Page 1570)

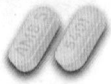
5 mg

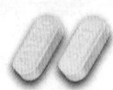
10 mg

diaphoresis, tachycardia, paresthesia) and hyperglycemia (excess thirst, urination).
• Monitor patient for signs and symptoms of pancreatitis (persistent, severe abdominal pain, which may radiate to the back, and vomiting). If pancreatitis is suspected, promptly discontinue linagliptin and initiate appropriate management.

PATIENT TEACHING

• Inform patient of the potential risks and benefits of linagliptin and of alternative modes of therapy.
• Instruct patient to take drug only as prescribed. If a dose is missed, advise patient not to double the next dose.
• Explain the importance of proper diet, regular physical activity, and periodic blood glucose monitoring.
• Teach patient to recognize and manage hypoglycemia and hyperglycemia.
• Advise patient to notify the health care provider promptly during periods of stress (such as fever, trauma, infection, or surgery) because medication requirements may change.
• Teach patient signs and symptoms of pancreatitis and to immediately contact prescriber if they occur.

linezolid
lih-NEH-zoe-lid

Zyvox

Therapeutic class: Antibiotics
Pharmacologic class: Oxazolidinones

AVAILABLE FORMS
Injection: 2 mg/mL
Powder for oral suspension: 100 mg/5 mL when reconstituted
Tablets: 600 mg

INDICATIONS & DOSAGES
Adjust-a-dose (for all indications): Administer after hemodialysis on dialysis days.
➤ **Vancomycin-resistant** *Enterococcus faecium* **infections, including those with concurrent bacteremia**
Adults and children age 12 and older: 600 mg I.V. or P.O. every 12 hours for 14 to 28 days.

Neonates age 7 days or older and infants and children through age 11: 10 mg/kg I.V. or P.O. every 8 hours for 14 to 28 days.
Neonates younger than age 7 days: 10 mg/kg I.V. or P.O. every 12 hours for 14 to 28 days. Increase to 10 mg/kg every 8 hours when patient is 7 days old. Consider this dosage increase if neonate has inadequate response.
➤ **Hospital-acquired pneumonia caused by** *Staphylococcus aureus* **(methicillin-susceptible [MSSA] and MRSA strains) or** *Streptococcus pneumoniae* **(including multidrug-resistant strains [MDRSP]); complicated skin and skin-structure infections, including diabetic foot infections without osteomyelitis caused by** *S. aureus* **(MSSA and MRSA),** *Streptococcus pyogenes,* **or** *Streptococcus agalactiae;* **community-acquired pneumonia caused by** *S. pneumoniae* **(including MDRSP), including those with concurrent bacteremia, or** *S. aureus* **(MSSA only)**
Adults and children age 12 and older: 600 mg I.V. or P.O. every 12 hours for 10 to 14 days.
Neonates age 7 days or older, infants, and children through age 11: 10 mg/kg I.V. or P.O. every 8 hours for 10 to 14 days.
Neonates younger than age 7 days: 10 mg/kg I.V. or P.O. every 12 hours for 10 to 14 days. Increase to 10 mg/kg every 8 hours when patient is 7 days old. Consider this dosage increase if neonate has inadequate response.
➤ **Uncomplicated skin and skin-structure infections caused by** *S. aureus* **(MSSA only) or** *S. pyogenes*
Adults: 400 mg P.O. every 12 hours for 10 to 14 days.
Children ages 12 to 18: 600 mg P.O. every 12 hours for 10 to 14 days.
Children ages 5 to 11: 10 mg/kg P.O. every 12 hours for 10 to 14 days.
Neonates age 7 days or older, infants, and children younger than age 5: 10 mg/kg P.O. every 8 hours for 10 to 14 days.
Neonates younger than age 7 days: 10 mg/kg P.O. every 12 hours for 10 to 14 days. Increase to 10 mg/kg every 8 hours when patient is 7 days old. Consider this dosage increase if neonate has inadequate response.

ADMINISTRATION
P.O.
- Give tablets and suspension with or without meals.
- Reconstitute suspension according to manufacturer's instructions.
- Store reconstituted suspension at room temperature and use within 21 days.

I.V.
▼ Inspect solution for particulate matter and leaks.
▼ Drug is compatible with D_5W injection, NSS for injection, and lactated Ringer injection.
▼ Don't inject additives into infusion bag. Give other I.V. drugs separately or via a separate I.V. line to avoid incompatibilities. If single I.V. line is used, flush line before and after infusion with a compatible solution.
▼ Infuse over 30 minutes to 2 hours. Don't infuse drug in a series connection.
▼ Store drug at room temperature in its protective overwrap. Solution may turn yellow over time, but this doesn't affect drug's potency.
▼ **Incompatibilities:** Amphotericin B, chlorpromazine hydrochloride, diazepam, pentamidine isethionate, phenytoin sodium.

ACTION
Prevents bacterial protein synthesis by interfering with DNA translation in the ribosomes. Also prevents formation of a functional 70S ribosomal subunit by binding to a site on the bacterial 50S ribosomal subunit.

Route	Onset	Peak	Duration
P.O.	Unknown	1–2 hr	Unknown
I.V.	Unknown	30 min	Unknown

Half-life: Adults, 4 to 5 hours; children age 1 week to 11 years, 1½ to 3 hours.

ADVERSE REACTIONS
CNS: headache, dizziness, fever, insomnia; vertigo (children).
GI: diarrhea, nausea, altered taste, constipation, oral candidiasis, tongue discoloration, vomiting, abdominal pain.
GU: vaginal candidiasis.

Hematologic: *leukopenia, myelosuppression, neutropenia, thrombocytopenia,* anemia.
Skin: rash.
Other: fungal infection.

INTERACTIONS
Drug-drug. *Adrenergic drugs (dopamine, epinephrine, pseudoephedrine):* May cause hypertension. Monitor BP and HR; start continuous infusions of dopamine and epinephrine at lower doses and titrate to response.
Insulin, oral antidiabetic agents: May cause symptomatic hypoglycemia. Monitor patient closely.
Serotonergic drugs: May cause serotonin syndrome, including confusion, delirium, restlessness, tremors, blushing, diaphoresis, and hyperpyrexia. Notify prescriber immediately of signs and symptoms of serotonin syndrome.
Drug-food. *Foods and beverages high in tyramine (aged cheeses, air-dried meats, red wines, sauerkraut, soy sauce, tap beers):* May increase BP. Provide a list of foods containing tyramine and advise patient that tyramine content of meals shouldn't exceed 100 mg.

EFFECTS ON LAB TEST RESULTS
- May increase ALT, AST, bilirubin, alkaline phosphatase, BUN, creatinine, amylase, lipase, LDH, and BUN levels. May decrease Hb level.
- May decrease glucose level and WBC, neutrophil, and platelet counts.

CONTRAINDICATIONS & CAUTIONS
- Contraindicated in patients hypersensitive to drug or its components.
- **⚠ Alert:** Concomitant use with psychiatric drugs or within 2 weeks of taking psychiatric drugs that work through the serotonin system of the brain (SSRIs, SSNRIs, TCAs, MAO inhibitors, and others) can cause serotonin syndrome (fever, mental status changes, muscle twitching, excessive sweating, shivering or shaking, diarrhea, and loss of coordination). Use linezolid with these drugs only for life-threatening or

urgent conditions when the potential benefits outweigh the risks of toxicity.
Dialyzable drug: 30%.

PREGNANCY-LACTATION-REPRODUCTION
• There are no adequate studies in pregnant women. Use during pregnancy only if potential benefit justifies potential risk to the fetus.
• Drug may appear in breast milk. Use cautiously in breast-feeding women.

NURSING CONSIDERATIONS
• No dosage adjustment is needed when switching from I.V. to oral forms.
◑ *Alert:* Before giving linezolid, stop any serotonergic drug and monitor patient for serotonin toxicity for 2 weeks (5 weeks if fluoxetine was taken) or until 24 hours after the last dose of linezolid, whichever comes first. May resume serotonergic psychiatric drugs 24 hours after last dose of linezolid.
◑ *Alert:* Nausea and vomiting may be symptoms of lactic acidosis. Monitor patient for unexplained acidosis or low bicarbonate level, and notify prescriber immediately if these occur.
◑ *Alert:* Drug may cause thrombocytopenia. In patients at increased risk for bleeding, those with existing thrombocytopenia, those taking other drugs that may cause thrombocytopenia, and those receiving this drug for longer than 14 days, monitor platelet count.
◑ *Alert:* Drug may lead to myelosuppression. Monitor CBC weekly.
◑ *Alert:* Prolonged use can cause superinfection, including CDAD, which can occur more than 2 months after treatment ends. Consider these diagnoses and take appropriate measures in patients with persistent diarrhea or secondary infections.
◑ *Alert:* Drug may cause symptomatic hypoglycemia in patients taking insulin or oral antidiabetic agents. Monitor patient closely.
• Inappropriate use of antibiotics may lead to development of resistant organisms; carefully consider other drugs before starting therapy, especially in outpatient setting.
• Use cautiously in patients with seizure disorder.

• *Look alike–sound alike:* Don't confuse Zyvox with Zovirax. Both come in a 400-mg strength.

PATIENT TEACHING
• Tell patient that tablets and oral suspension may be taken with or without meals.
• Stress importance of completing entire course of therapy, even if patient feels better.
• Tell patient to alert prescriber if he has high BP; is taking cough or cold preparations, insulin, or oral antidiabetic agents; or is being treated with SSRIs or other antidepressants.
◑ *Alert:* Teach patient to recognize and immediately report signs and symptoms of serotonin toxicity (fever, mental status changes, muscle twitching, excessive sweating, shivering or shaking, diarrhea, and loss of coordination).
• Advise patient that he may need to stop taking prescribed psychiatric drugs while taking linezolid but that he shouldn't stop them without first speaking to the prescriber.
• Teach patient to avoid eating large quantities of tyramine-containing foods (aged cheeses, soy sauce, tap beers, red wine) during therapy.
• Inform patient with phenylketonuria that each 5 mL of oral suspension contains 20 mg of phenylalanine. Tablets and injection don't contain phenylalanine.

SAFETY ALERT!

liraglutide
leer-ah-GLOO-tide

Saxenda, Victoza

Therapeutic class: Antidiabetics
Pharmacologic class: Glucagon-like peptide-1 receptor agonists

AVAILABLE FORMS
Injection: 0.6 mg, 1.2 mg, 1.8 mg, 2.4 mg, 3 mg in prefilled multidose pens

INDICATIONS & DOSAGES
➤ **As adjunct to diet and exercise to improve glycemic control in patients with type 2 diabetes mellitus (Victoza)**

L

Adults: Initially, 0.6 mg subcutaneously daily; after 1 week, increase dosage to 1.2 mg subcutaneously daily. May increase dosage to 1.8 mg subcutaneously daily if needed to achieve glycemic control.

➤ **As adjunct to diet and exercise for long-term weight management in adults with initial BMI of 30 kg/m² or greater (obese) or 27 kg/m² or greater (overweight) in the presence of at least one weight-related comorbid condition (hypertension, type 2 diabetes mellitus, or dyslipidemia) (Saxenda)**

Adults: Initially, 0.6 mg subcutaneously once daily for 1 week. Increase by 0.6 mg/day subcutaneously at weekly intervals to a target dose of 3 mg once daily. If patient can't tolerate an increased dose during titration period, consider delaying dose escalation for 1 week.

ADMINISTRATION
Subcutaneous

● Drug is considered hazardous; use safe handling precautions.

● Give drug once daily at any time of day, independently of meals. Inject into abdomen, thigh, or upper arm. Injection site and timing can be changed without dosage adjustment.

● Don't mix drug with insulin for injection or inject liraglutide and insulin in adjacent areas at the same time.

● If a dose is missed, don't double subsequent dose. Resume once-daily regimen.

● Inspect solution before each injection. Use solution only if it is clear, colorless, and contains no particles.

🜂 *Alert:* Multidose pens are for single patient use only. Pens should never be shared even if the needle is changed. Clearly label with patient identifying information where it won't obstruct dosing window, warning, or other product information.

● Before first use, store drug in refrigerator between 36° and 46° F (2° and 8° C). Discard if pen freezes.

● After initial use of liraglutide pen, pen can be stored for 30 days at room temperature (59° to 86° F [15° to 30° C]) or in refrigerator (36° to 46° F). Keep pen cap on when not in use. Discard pen after 30 days.

ACTION

Stimulates insulin release in the presence of elevated glucose levels by increasing intracellular cAMP.

Route	Onset	Peak	Duration
Subcut.	Unknown	8–12 hr	Unknown

Half-life: 13 hours.

ADVERSE REACTIONS

CNS: headache, dizziness, fatigue.
CV: increased HR, tachycardia.
GI: constipation, diarrhea, dyspepsia, nausea, vomiting, abdominal distention or pain, decreased appetite, flatulence, GERD.
GU: UTI.
Hepatic: cholelithiasis.
Metabolic: hypoglycemia.
Respiratory: URI.
Skin: injection-site reactions.
Other: flulike syndrome, *thyroid cancer,* anti-liraglutide antibody formation.

INTERACTIONS

Drug-drug. *Insulin secretagogues (sulfonylureas):* May increase risk of hypoglycemia. Reduce dosage of insulin secretagogue before beginning drug.
Oral medications: May impair absorption of oral drugs because of delayed gastric emptying. Use together cautiously.

EFFECTS ON LAB TEST RESULTS

● May increase serum bilirubin and lipase levels and serum calcitonin concentration.
● May decrease blood glucose level.

CONTRAINDICATIONS & CAUTIONS

Black Box Warning Drug causes dose-dependent and treatment duration–dependent thyroid C-cell tumors at clinically relevant exposures in both genders of rats and mice. It isn't known if drug causes thyroid C-cell tumors, including medullary thyroid carcinoma (MTC), in humans, as the human relevance of liraglutide-induced rodent thyroid C-cell tumors hasn't been determined. ■

Black Box Warning Contraindicated in patients with personal or family history of MTC and in patients with multiple endocrine neoplasia syndrome type 2. ■

Reactions in bold italics are *life-threatening*. Interactions may have a *rapid onset* or a *delayed onset*.

• Contraindicated in patients with a prior serious hypersensitivity reaction to liraglutide or its components.

• Use cautiously in patients with renal or hepatic impairment and in those with history of pancreatitis.

⚠ *Alert:* Acute pancreatitis, including fatal pancreatitis and nonfatal hemorrhagic or necrotizing pancreatitis, has occurred in patients taking liraglutide.

• Saxenda isn't indicated for treatment of type 2 diabetes mellitus.

• Saxenda and Victoza both contain the same active ingredient and shouldn't be used together.

• Saxenda shouldn't be used in combination with other GLP-1 receptor agonists.

• Safety and effectiveness of Saxenda in combination with other products intended for weight loss haven't been established.

• Elderly adults may be more sensitive to drug. Use cautiously.

Dialyzable drug: Unknown.

⚠ *Overdose S&S:* Nausea, vomiting, hypoglycemia.

PREGNANCY-LACTATION-REPRODUCTION

• There are no adequate studies of Victoza in pregnant women. Use during pregnancy only if potential benefit justifies potential risk to the fetus.

• Saxenda is contraindicated during pregnancy because weight loss offers no potential benefit to a pregnant woman and may result in fetal harm.

• It isn't known if drug appears in breast milk. Patient should either discontinue breast-feeding or discontinue drug.

NURSING CONSIDERATIONS

Black Box Warning Drug may cause thyroid C-cell tumors, including MTC. Monitor patient closely. ∎

• Discontinue Saxenda if dose of 3 mg once daily isn't tolerated because effectiveness hasn't been established at lower doses. Evaluate change in body weight 16 weeks after start of therapy; discontinue if body weight loss of at least 4% of baseline hasn't been achieved.

• Monitor patient closely for signs and symptoms of pancreatitis (persistent, severe abdominal pain, which may radiate to the

back, and vomiting). Discontinue drug promptly if pancreatitis is suspected. Don't restart if pancreatitis is confirmed.

⚠ *Alert:* Patients with thyroid nodules found on examination or neck imaging or with elevated serum calcitonin levels should be evaluated by an endocrinologist.

• Drug isn't recommended for first-line therapy in patients who have inadequate glycemic control with diet and exercise.

• Victoza isn't a substitute for insulin; it shouldn't be used for treatment of diabetic ketoacidosis or type 1 diabetes mellitus.

• Victoza hasn't been studied in combination with prandial insulin.

• Monitor blood glucose and HbA_{1C} levels. Consider decreasing insulin and insulin secretagogue (such as sulfonylurea) dosage when initiating liraglutide.

• Monitor patient for signs and symptoms of hypoglycemia (tachycardia, palpitations, anxiety, hunger, nausea, diaphoresis, tremors, pallor, restlessness, headache, and speech and motor dysfunction).

• Monitor GI status; drug slows gastric emptying.

PATIENT TEACHING

Black Box Warning Counsel patient regarding potential risk of MTC and describe signs and symptoms of thyroid tumors (neck mass, dysphagia, dyspnea, persistent hoarseness). Routine monitoring of serum calcitonin level or use of thyroid ultrasound is of uncertain value for early detection of MTC. ∎

• Warn patient that drug may increase risk of thyroid tumor; tell him to report such signs and symptoms as hoarseness, difficulty swallowing, difficulty breathing, or lump in the neck.

• Advise patient to stop taking drug and notify health care provider if he experiences persistent, severe abdominal pain that may radiate to the back and may or may not be accompanied by vomiting.

⚠ *Alert:* Warn patient not to share multidose pen with other people, even if needle is changed, because of risk of bloodborne pathogen transmission, including HIV and hepatitis.

• Tell patient that stress, such as fever, trauma, infection, or surgery, may change

drug requirements and to seek medical advice promptly if these occur.
- Emphasize to patient importance of adhering to a diet and exercise program and monitoring glucose and HbA_{1C} levels.
- Advise patient of risk of dehydration; encourage hydration.
- Warn patient of risk of hypersensitivity reactions and to report reactions should they occur.
- Teach patient how to give subcutaneous injection; instruct patient to rotate sites to prevent injection-site reactions.
- Instruct patient to discard pen after 30 days.

lisdexamfetamine dimesylate
lis-DEX-am-FET-a-meen

Vyvanse✷

Therapeutic class: CNS stimulants
Pharmacologic class: Amphetamines
Controlled substance schedule: II

AVAILABLE FORMS
Capsules ⓞⓝⓒ: 10 mg, 20 mg, 30 mg, 40 mg, 50 mg, 60 mg, 70 mg

INDICATIONS & DOSAGES
Adjust-a-dose (for all indications): For patients with severe renal impairment (GFR of 15 to 30 mL/minute/1.73 m²), maximum dose is 50 mg/day. For those with ESRD (GFR less than 15 mL/minute/1.73 m²), maximum dose is 30 mg/day.
➤ **ADHD**
Adults and children ages 6 to 17: Initially, 30 mg P.O. once daily in the morning. Increase by 10 or 20 mg at weekly intervals to a maximum of 70 mg daily.
➤ **Moderate to severe binge eating disorder**
Adults: Initially, 30 mg P.O. once daily in the morning. Increase by 20 mg at weekly intervals to target dose of 50 to 70 mg/day. Maximum dose is 70 mg/day.

ADMINISTRATION
P.O.
- Give drug in the morning to prevent insomnia.

- Give drug without regard for meals.
- Capsules may be swallowed whole or the contents dissolved in a glass of water and taken immediately.
- Don't divide the dose of a single capsule.

ACTION
May increase the release of norepinephrine and dopamine into extraneural spaces by blocking their reuptake into the presynaptic neuron.

Route	Onset	Peak	Duration
P.O.	Rapid	1 hr	Unknown

Half-life: Lisdexamfetamine, less than 1 hour; dextroamphetamine, 10 to 13 hours.

ADVERSE REACTIONS
CNS: anxiety, headache, insomnia, irritability, aggressive or hostile behavior, agitation, delusional thinking, dizziness, fever, hallucinations, labile affect, restlessness, seizures, somnolence, tic, tremor.
CV: *cardiomyopathy,* increased BP, increased HR, palpitations, peripheral vasculopathy, Raynaud phenomenon.
EENT: abnormal vision, blurred vision.
GI: abdominal pain, decreased appetite, dry mouth, nausea, vomiting, anorexia, diarrhea.
GU: frequent or prolonged erections.
Metabolic: slow growth, weight loss.
Respiratory: dyspnea.
Skin: hyperhidrosis, rash, *Stevens-Johnson syndrome.*

INTERACTIONS
Drug-drug. *Adrenergic blockers:* May inhibit adrenergic-blocking effects. Monitor BP and adjust adrenergic blocker dosage if necessary.
Antihistamines: May inhibit sedative effects of antihistamines. Monitor patient.
Antihypertensives, veratrum alkaloids: May inhibit antihypertensive effects of these drugs. If use together can't be avoided, closely monitor BP when lisdexamfetamine is started or stopped, and adjust antihypertensive dosage as needed.
Chlorpromazine, haloperidol: May decrease effectiveness of amphetamines. Monitor patient closely.

Reactions in bold italics are *life-threatening*. Interactions may have a *rapid onset* or a *delayed onset*.

Ethosuximide: May delay absorption of this drug. Monitor patient closely.

Lithium: May inhibit anorectic and CNS stimulant effects of amphetamine. Monitor patient closely.

MAO inhibitors: May cause severe hypertension or hypertensive crisis. Use is contraindicated within 14 days of MAO inhibitor therapy.

Meperidine: May increase the analgesic effect of meperidine. Use together cautiously.

Norepinephrine: May increase adrenergic effects of norepinephrine. Monitor patient closely.

Phenobarbital, phenytoin: May delay intestinal absorption of these drugs and enhance their anticonvulsant effects. Monitor patient closely.

TCAs: May cause adverse CV effects. Avoid using together.

Urine acidifiers (ammonium chloride, sodium acid phosphate), methenamine: May decrease serum level due to increased renal excretion of amphetamine. Monitor patient for decreased drug effects.

Urine alkalinizers (sodium bicarbonate): May increase lisdexamfetamine serum level because of decreased renal excretion of amphetamine. Monitor patient for increased drug effects and adjust dosage accordingly.

Drug-food. *Caffeine:* May increase CNS stimulation. Discourage use together.

Drug-lifestyle. *Alcohol use:* May increase CNS depression. Don't use together.

EFFECTS ON LAB TEST RESULTS
• May increase corticosteroid level.
• May interfere with urinary steroid test.

CONTRAINDICATIONS & CAUTIONS
Black Box Warning Drug has a high potential for abuse and dependence. ■
• Contraindicated in patients hypersensitive to sympathomimetic amines or in those with idiosyncratic reactions to them, in agitated patients, and in those with a history of drug abuse.
• Contraindicated within 14 days of MAO inhibitor therapy.
• Anaphylactic reactions, Stevens-Johnson syndrome, angioedema, and urticaria have been noted in postmarketing reports.

☉ Alert: Drug isn't indicated or recommended for weight loss.
• Contraindicated in patients with advanced arteriosclerosis, hyperthyroidism, symptomatic CV disease, structural cardiac abnormalities, cardiomyopathy, serious heart arrhythmia, moderate to severe hypertension, or glaucoma, and those intolerant of changes in HR or BP.
• Use cautiously in patients with a history of arrhythmias, MI, stroke, or seizures.
• Use cautiously in patients with preexisting psychosis, bipolar disorder, aggressive behavior, or Tourette syndrome.

Dializable drug: No.

⚠ Overdose S&S: Assaultiveness, confusion, hallucinations, hyperpyrexia, hyperreflexia, panic states, rapid respiration, restlessness, rhabdomyolysis, tremor, fatigue, depression, arrhythmias, circulatory collapse, hypertension, hypotension, abdominal cramps, diarrhea, nausea, vomiting, seizures, coma.

PREGNANCY-LACTATION-REPRODUCTION
• There are no adequate studies in pregnant women. Use during pregnancy only if potential benefit justifies potential fetal risk.
• Drug appears in breast milk. Patient should discontinue breast-feeding or discontinue drug.

NURSING CONSIDERATIONS
• Diagnosis of ADHD must be based on complete history and evaluation of the child with consultation of psychological, educational, and social resources.
• Evaluate for bipolar disorder before initiating therapy.
• Give the lowest effective dose in the morning. Afternoon doses may cause insomnia.
Black Box Warning Assess the risk of abuse before initiating therapy, and monitor patient for signs of drug dependence or abuse. Misuse may cause sudden death. ■
☉ Alert: Periodically monitor patients for changes in HR or BP.
• Abruptly stopping the drug can cause severe fatigue and depression.
• Monitor patient closely for adverse CV effects, new or worsening behavior (aggression, mania), vision problems, or seizures.
• Monitor BP and pulse routinely.

- Carefully observe patient for digital changes because stimulants used to treat ADHD are associated with peripheral vasculopathy, including Raynaud phenomenon.
- Effectiveness of this drug when taken longer than 4 weeks isn't known. Periodically interrupt therapy to determine whether continuation is necessary.
- Growth may be suppressed with long-term stimulant use. Monitor the child for growth and weight gain. Stop treatment if growth is suppressed or if weight gain is lower than expected.
- The drug may trigger Tourette syndrome. Monitor patient, especially at the start of therapy.
- Monitor patient for the appearance or worsening of aggressive behavior or hostility, especially when treatment is initiated.
- May cause psychotic or manic episodes in patients with no prior history or exacerbation of signs and symptoms in patients with preexisting psychosis.

PATIENT TEACHING
- Warn patient that the misuse of amphetamines can cause serious CV adverse events, including sudden death.
- ❸ **Alert:** Instruct patient to immediately report chest pain, shortness of breath, or fainting.
- Tell patient or caregiver that drug should be taken in the morning to prevent insomnia.
- Advise patient to swallow capsule whole. If he's unable to do so, the contents may be dissolved in a glass of water and taken immediately. Once dissolved, don't store for later use.
- Tell patient or caregiver that abruptly stopping drug can cause severe fatigue, depression, or general withdrawal reaction.
- Caution patient to avoid activities that require alertness or good psychomotor coordination until CNS effects of drug are known.
- Warn patient with seizure disorder that drug may decrease seizure threshold. Urge him to notify his prescriber if a seizure occurs.
- Instruct patient or caregiver to report palpitations or visual disturbances.

- Tell patient or caregiver to report worsening aggression, hallucinations, delusions, or mania.
- Advise patient or caregiver that drug may slow growth and cause weight loss.
- Instruct patient to immediately report unexplained wounds appearing on fingers or toes while taking drug.
- Advise patient to avoid caffeine and alcohol consumption while taking drug.

lisinopril
lye-SIN-oh-pril

Prinivil◆, Zestril◆

Therapeutic class: Antihypertensives
Pharmacologic class: ACE inhibitors

AVAILABLE FORMS
Tablets: 2.5 mg, 5 mg, 10 mg, 20 mg, 30 mg, 40 mg

INDICATIONS & DOSAGES
➤ **Hypertension**
Adults: Initially, 10 mg P.O. daily for patients not taking a diuretic. Most patients are well controlled on 20 to 40 mg daily as a single dose. For patients taking a diuretic, initially, 5 mg P.O. daily.
Children age 6 and older: Initially, 0.07 mg/kg (up to 5 mg) P.O. once daily. Increase dosage based on patient response and tolerance. Maximum dose, 0.61 mg/kg (don't exceed 40 mg). Don't use in children with a CrCl of less than 30 mL/minute.
Adjust-a-dose: In adults, if CrCl is 10 to 30 mL/minute, give 5 mg P.O. daily; if CrCl is less than 10 mL/minute, give 2.5 mg P.O. daily. May titrate dosage up to 40 mg/day.
➤ **Adjunctive treatment (with diuretics and cardiac glycosides) for HF**
Adults: Initially, 5 mg P.O. daily; increased as needed to maximum of 20 mg (40 mg for Zestril) P.O. daily.
Adjust-a-dose: If sodium level is less than 130 mEq/L, serum creatinine greater than 3 mg/dL, or CrCl less than 30 mL/minute, start treatment at 2.5 mg daily.
➤ **Hemodynamically stable patients within 24 hours of acute MI to improve survival**

Adults: Initially, 5 mg P.O.; then 5 mg after 24 hours, 10 mg after 48 hours, followed by 10 mg once daily for 6 weeks.

Adjust-a-dose: For patients with systolic BP 120 mm Hg or less when treatment is started or during first 3 days after an infarct, decrease dosage to 2.5 mg P.O. If systolic BP drops to 100 mm Hg or less, reduce daily maintenance dose of 5 mg to 2.5 mg, if needed. If prolonged systolic BP stays under 90 mm Hg for longer than 1 hour, withdraw drug.

ADMINISTRATION
P.O.
● Give drug without regard for food.
● If made into a suspension by pharmacist, shake before each use.

ACTION
Causes decreased production of angiotensin II and suppression of the RAAS.

Route	Onset	Peak	Duration
P.O.	1 hr	7 hr	24 hr

Half-life: 12 hours.

ADVERSE REACTIONS
CNS: dizziness, headache, fatigue, paresthesia.
CV: orthostatic hypotension, hypotension, chest pain.
EENT: nasal congestion.
GI: diarrhea, nausea, dyspepsia.
GU: impaired renal function, impotence.
Metabolic: *hyperkalemia.*
Respiratory: dyspnea; dry, persistent, tickling, nonproductive cough.
Skin: rash.
Other: *angioedema.*

INTERACTIONS
Drug-drug. *Aliskiren:* May increase risk of renal impairment, hypotension, and hyperkalemia in diabetic patients and those with moderate to severe renal impairment (GFR less than 60 mL/minute). Concomitant use is contraindicated in diabetic patients. Avoid concomitant use in those with moderate to severe renal impairment.
Allopurinol: May cause hypersensitivity reaction. Use together cautiously.

Azathioprine: May increase risk of anemia or leukopenia. Monitor hematologic studies if used together.
Diuretics, thiazide diuretics: May cause excessive hypotension with diuretics. Monitor BP closely.
Indomethacin, NSAIDs: May reduce hypotensive effects of drug. Adjust dose as needed.
Insulin, oral antidiabetics: May cause hypoglycemia, especially at start of lisinopril therapy. Monitor glucose level.
Lithium: May cause lithium toxicity. Monitor lithium levels.
Phenothiazines: May increase hypotensive effects. Monitor BP closely.
Potassium-sparing diuretics, potassium supplements: May cause hyperkalemia. Monitor laboratory values.
Tizanidine: May cause severe hypotension. Monitor patient.
Drug-herb. *Capsaicin:* May cause ACE inhibitor–induced cough. Discourage use together.
Ma huang: May decrease antihypertensive effects. Discourage use together.
Drug-food. *Potassium-containing salt substitutes:* May cause hyperkalemia. Monitor laboratory values.

EFFECTS ON LAB TEST RESULTS
● May increase BUN, creatinine, potassium, and bilirubin levels.
● May increase LFT values.

CONTRAINDICATIONS & CAUTIONS
● Contraindicated in patients hypersensitive to ACE inhibitors and in those with a history of angioedema related to previous treatment with ACE inhibitor.
● Use cautiously in patients with impaired renal function; adjust dosage.
● Use cautiously in patients at risk for hyperkalemia or hypotension and in those with aortic stenosis or hypertrophic cardiomyopathy. The safety and effectiveness of lisinopril on BP control in children younger than age 6 or in children with GFR less than 30 mL/minute hasn't been established.
۞ *Alert:* Although rare, angioedema, which can be fatal, may occur at any time during treatment, including after first dose; it may involve the head and neck (potentially

compromising the airway) or the intestine (presenting with abdominal pain). Black patients and patients with idiopathic or hereditary angioedema may be at increased risk. Patients concurrently receiving mammalian target of rapamycin (mTOR) inhibitor therapy (temsirolimus, sirolimus, everolimus) also may be at increased risk.

Dialyzable drug: Yes.

⚠ *Overdose S&S:* Hypotension.

PREGNANCY-LACTATION-REPRODUCTION
<u>Black Box Warning</u> Drug acts directly on the RAAS and can cause injury and death to a developing fetus. When pregnancy is detected, stop drug as soon as possible. ∎
• It isn't known if drug appears in breast milk. Patient should discontinue breast-feeding or discontinue drug.

NURSING CONSIDERATIONS
• When using drug in acute MI, give patient the appropriate and standard recommended treatment, such as thrombolytics, aspirin, and beta blockers.
• Although ACE inhibitors reduce BP in all races, BP reduction is less in blacks taking an ACE inhibitor alone. Black patients should take drug with a thiazide diuretic for a more favorable response.
• Monitor BP frequently. If drug doesn't adequately control BP, diuretics may be added.
• Monitor WBC with differential counts before therapy, every 2 weeks for first 3 months of therapy, and periodically thereafter.
• *Look alike–sound alike:* Don't confuse lisinopril with fosinopril or Lioresal. Don't confuse Zestril with Zostrix, Zetia, Zebeta, or Zyrtec. Don't confuse Prinivil with Proventil or Prilosec.

PATIENT TEACHING
☺ *Alert:* Rarely, facial and throat swelling (including swelling of the larynx) or intestinal swelling may occur, especially after first dose. Advise patient to report abdominal pain, breathing problems, or swelling of face, eyes, lips, or tongue.
• Tell patient that light-headedness can occur, especially during first few days of therapy, to rise slowly to minimize this

effect, and to report symptoms to prescriber. If fainting occurs, advise patient to stop drug and call prescriber immediately.
• If unpleasant adverse reactions occur, tell patient not to stop drug suddenly but to notify prescriber.
• Advise patient to report signs and symptoms of infection, such as fever and sore throat.
• Tell female patient of childbearing potential to notify prescriber if pregnancy occurs. Drug will need to be stopped.
• Instruct patient not to use salt substitutes that contain potassium without first consulting prescriber.
• Inform patient that a dry, nonproductive cough may develop during therapy.

lisinopril–hydrochlorothiazide
lye-SIN-oh-pril/hye-droe-klor-oh-THYE-a-zide

Zestoretic

Therapeutic class: Antihypertensives
Pharmacologic class: ACE inhibitors–thiazide diuretics

AVAILABLE FORMS
Tablets: 10 mg lisinopril and 12.5 mg hydrochlorothiazide, 20 mg lisinopril and 12.5 mg hydrochlorothiazide, 20 mg lisinopril and 25 mg hydrochlorothiazide

INDICATIONS & DOSAGES
➤ **Hypertension in patients not adequately controlled on lisinopril or hydrochlorothiazide monotherapy**
Adults: Initially, 10 mg lisinopril and 12.5 mg hydrochlorothiazide or 20 mg lisinopril and 12.5 mg hydrochlorothiazide P.O. once daily; titrate based on clinical response. Don't increase the hydrochlorothiazide component until 2 to 3 weeks have elapsed. In patients on adequate pressure control on single-agent hydrochlorothiazide 25 mg P.O. daily but with significant potassium loss, switch to 10 mg lisinopril and 12.5 mg hydrochlorothiazide tablets. Maximum dosage is 80 mg lisinopril and 50 mg hydrochlorothiazide P.O. once daily.

Adjust-a-dose: Not for use in patients with CrCl of less than 30 mL/minute/1.73 m². Dosage selection for elderly patients should be cautious, usually starting at low end of dosing range.

ADMINISTRATION
P.O.
● Store at controlled room temperature; protect from excessive light and humidity.
● May give without regard for food.

ACTION
Lisinopril inhibits ACE, leading to decreased angiotensin II production, decreased aldosterone secretion, and increased potassium level. Hydrochlorothiazide increases aldosterone secretion, increasing excretion of sodium, chloride, and water and decreasing excretion of potassium.

Route	Onset	Peak	Duration
P.O. (lisinopril)	1 hr	7 hr	Unknown
P.O. (hydro-chlorothiazide)	2 hr	4 hr	6–12 hr

Half-life: Lisinopril, 12 hours; hydrochlorothiazide, 5.6 to 14.8 hours.

ADVERSE REACTIONS
CNS: dizziness, headache, fatigue, asthenia, paresthesia.
CV: orthostatic effects, hypotension.
GI: diarrhea, nausea, vomiting, dyspepsia.
GU: erectile dysfunction.
Metabolic: *hypokalemia, hyperkalemia,* hyperglycemia.
Musculoskeletal: muscle cramps.
Respiratory: cough, URI.
Skin: rash.

INTERACTIONS
Drug-drug. *Aliskiren:* May increase risk of renal impairment, hypotension, and hyperkalemia in diabetic patients and in those with moderate to severe renal impairment (GFR less than 60 mL/minute). Concomitant use is contraindicated in diabetic patients. Avoid concomitant use in patients with moderate to severe renal impairment.
Antidiabetic agents, insulin: May increase blood glucose level. Monitor patient carefully; adjust dosage of antidiabetic as needed.

Barbiturates, opioids: May increase risk of orthostatic hypotension. Avoid use together.
Colestipol resins, cholestyramine: May impair absorption of hydrochlorothiazide. Separate administration times by at least 4 hours.
Corticosteroids, corticotropin: May worsen electrolyte depletion, particularly hypokalemia. Monitor patient carefully.
Diuretics, other antihypertensives: May increase hypotensive effects. Monitor patient carefully.
Gold injections: May increase risk of nitritoid effects (flushing, nausea, vomiting, hypotension). Avoid use together.
Lithium: May increase lithium level. Monitor patient carefully.
Nondepolarizing skeletal muscle relaxants (tubocurarine): May increase response to muscle relaxant. Avoid use together.
NSAIDs: May diminish antihypertensive effects. Use cautiously together.
Potassium-sparing diuretics, potassium supplements: May increase risk of hyperkalemia. Avoid use together.
Pressor amines (norepinephrine): May decrease response to pressor amines. Use together cautiously.
Drug-food. *Potassium-containing salt substitutes:* May increase risk of hyperkalemia. Discourage use together.
Drug-lifestyle. *Alcohol use:* May increase risk of orthostatic hypotension. Discourage use together.
Sun exposure: May increase risk of photosensitivity. Discourage sun exposure.

EFFECTS ON LAB TEST RESULTS
● May increase glucose, cholesterol, triglyceride, BUN, creatinine, potassium, and bilirubin levels and LFT values.
● May decrease calcium, potassium, and magnesium levels and WBC count.

CONTRAINDICATIONS & CAUTIONS
● Contraindicated in patients hypersensitive to either drug or sulfonamides and in those with history of angioedema related to previous treatment with an ACE inhibitor, hereditary or idiopathic angioedema, or anuria.
● Use cautiously in patients with a history or risk of angioedema, anaphylactoid

reactions, salt or volume depletion, collagen vascular disease, obstruction in the outflow tract of the left ventricle, HF, renal artery stenosis, renal disease, jaundice or hepatic disease, asthma, systemic lupus erythematosus, history of aortic stenosis, hypertrophic cardiomyopathy, existing hyperkalemia or other electrolyte imbalance, or hyperuricemia.

❸ *Alert:* Although rare, angioedema, which can be fatal, may occur at any time during treatment, including after first dose; it may involve the head and neck (potentially compromising the airway) or the intestine (presenting with abdominal pain). Black patients and patients with idiopathic or hereditary angioedema may be at increased risk. Patients concurrently receiving mammalian target of rapamycin (mTOR) inhibitor therapy (e.g., temsirolimus, sirolimus, everolimus) also may be at increased risk.

Dialyzable drug: Yes (lisinopril); unknown (hydrochlorothiazide).

⚠ *Overdose S&S:* Hypotension, dehydration, electrolyte imbalance.

PREGNANCY-LACTATION-REPRODUCTION

Black Box Warning Drugs that act directly on the RAAS can cause injury and death to a developing fetus. When pregnancy is detected, discontinue drug as soon as possible. ∎

• It isn't known if lisinopril appears in breast milk; hydrochlorothiazide does appear in breast milk. Patient should discontinue breast-feeding or discontinue drug.

NURSING CONSIDERATIONS

• Drug isn't to be used for initial therapy. Begin combination therapy only after patient has failed to achieve desired effect with monotherapy.

• Consider ACE inhibitor–induced cough if patient develops cough of unknown etiology.

• Correct lisinopril-induced hypotension before major surgery and anesthesia.

• If hypotension occurs, place patient in supine position and give I.V. NSS if appropriate. May resume drug once BP has increased.

• Monitor glucose, electrolyte, and lipid levels during therapy.

• Monitor WBC count in patients with collagen vascular disease or renal disease.

• Monitor patient for jaundice and elevated liver enzyme levels. Discontinue drug and treat appropriately if these occur.

• Drug may cause intestinal angioedema. Monitor patient for abdominal pain.

• Monitor patient for angioedema of the face, extremities, lips, tongue, glottis, or larynx, which may occur at any time during treatment. If symptoms occur, discontinue drug, treat appropriately, and monitor patient until symptoms have resolved.

• If airway obstruction is likely, give subcutaneous epinephrine solution 1:1,000 or other appropriate treatment as necessary to ensure patent airway.

• Black patients and patients with a history of angioedema unrelated to ACE inhibitors may be at increased risk for angioedema from ACE inhibitors.

• Black patients may have a more limited response to lisinopril than non-black patients.

PATIENT TEACHING

Black Box Warning Counsel female patient to report possible pregnancy to prescriber as soon as possible. ∎

• Instruct patient to stop drug and immediately report signs or symptoms suggesting angioedema (abdominal pain; swelling of the face, extremities, eyes, lips, or tongue; difficulty swallowing or breathing).

• Caution patient to report lightheadedness, especially during first few days of therapy, and if syncope occurs, to discontinue drug and notify prescriber.

• Tell patient to consult prescriber if fluid losses occur (excessive perspiration, dehydration, vomiting, or diarrhea).

• Advise patient to immediately report signs and symptoms of fluid and electrolyte imbalance (dry mouth, thirst, weakness, lethargy, drowsiness, restlessness, confusion, seizures, muscle pains or cramps, muscle fatigue, decreased urination, rapid heartbeat, nausea, vomiting).

• Instruct patient to promptly report signs and symptoms of infection (sore throat, fever).

• Warn patient to avoid salt substitutes containing potassium.

Reactions in bold italics are *life-threatening*. Interactions may have a *rapid onset* or a *delayed onset*.

● Inform patient that a dry, nonproductive cough may develop during therapy.

lithium carbonate
LITH-ee-um

Carbolith❋, Lithane❋, Lithobid

lithium citrate

Therapeutic class: Antimanics
Pharmacologic class: Alkali metals

AVAILABLE FORMS
lithium carbonate
Capsules: 150 mg, 300 mg, 600 mg
Tablets: 300 mg
Tablets (extended-release) ⓓ*ⓝⓒ:* 300 mg, 450 mg
lithium citrate
Syrup (sugarless): 8 mEq lithium/5 mL; 5 mL lithium citrate liquid contains 8 mEq lithium, equal to 300 mg lithium carbonate

INDICATIONS & DOSAGES
➤ **To prevent or control mania in bipolar disorder**
Adults and children age 12 and older: 600 mg immediate-release tablets P.O. t.i.d. Or, 900-mg extended-release tablets P.O. every 12 hours. Or, 10 mL (lithium 16 mEq) P.O. t.i.d. Increase dosage based on blood levels to achieve optimum dosage. Recommended therapeutic lithium levels are 1 to 1.5 mEq/L for acute mania and 0.6 to 1.2 mEq/L for maintenance therapy.
Adjust-a-dose: In elderly patients, start with lower doses. If CrCl is 10 to 50 mL/minute, give 50% to 75% of normal dose. If CrCl is less than 10 mL/minute, give 25% to 50% of normal dose. For patients with ESRD, give dose after dialysis.

ADMINISTRATION
P.O.
● Give drug after meals with plenty of water to minimize GI upset.
● Don't crush extended-release tablets.

ACTION
Probably alters chemical transmitters in the CNS, possibly by interfering with ionic pump mechanisms in brain cells, and may compete with or replace sodium ions.

Route	Onset	Peak	Duration
P.O. (immediate-release)	Unknown	30 min–3 hr	Unknown
P.O. (extended-release)	Unknown	2–6 hr	Unknown
P.O. (syrup)	Unknown	¼–1 hr	Unknown

Half-life: 18 to 36 hours.

ADVERSE REACTIONS
CNS: fatigue, lethargy, *coma, seizures,* tremors, drowsiness, headache, confusion, restlessness, dizziness, psychomotor retardation, blackouts, EEG changes, worsened organic mental syndrome, impaired speech, ataxia, incoordination.
CV: *arrhythmias, bradycardia,* reversible ECG changes, *severe bradycardia,* hypotension, Brugada syndrome.
EENT: blurred vision, exophthalmos, nystagmus, tinnitus.
GI: vomiting, anorexia, diarrhea, thirst, nausea, metallic taste, dry mouth, abdominal pain, flatulence, indigestion.
GU: polyuria, *renal toxicity with long-term use,* glycosuria, decreased CrCl, albuminuria, urinary incontinence, erectile dysfunction.
Hematologic: leukocytosis.
Metabolic: transient hyperglycemia, goiter, hypothyroidism, hyponatremia.
Musculoskeletal: muscle weakness.
Skin: pruritus, rash, diminished or absent sensation, drying and thinning of hair, psoriasis, acne, alopecia.
Other: ankle and wrist edema.

INTERACTIONS
Drug-drug. *ACE inhibitors:* May increase lithium level. Monitor lithium level; adjust lithium dosage, as needed.
Aminophylline, sodium bicarbonate, urine alkalinizers: May increase lithium excretion. Avoid excessive salt, and monitor lithium levels.
Antiarrhythmics and other drugs that prolong QT interval: May increase risk of life-threatening arrhythmias. Avoid use together.
Calcium channel blockers (verapamil): May decrease lithium levels and may

increase risk of neurotoxicity. Use together cautiously.

Carbamazepine, fluoxetine, methyldopa, NSAIDs, probenecid: May increase effect of lithium. Monitor patient for lithium toxicity.

Neuromuscular blockers: May cause prolonged paralysis or weakness. Monitor patient closely.

Thiazide diuretics: May increase reabsorption of lithium by kidneys, with possible toxic effect. Use with caution, and monitor lithium and electrolyte levels (especially sodium).

Drug-food. *Caffeine:* May decrease lithium level and drug effect. Advise patient who ingests large amounts of caffeine to tell prescriber before stopping caffeine. Adjust lithium dosage, as needed.

Sodium (salt): May change renal elimination of drug if sodium intake changes. Avoid major changes in sodium intake.

EFFECTS ON LAB TEST RESULTS

● May increase glucose and creatinine and TSH levels. May decrease sodium, T_3, T_4, and protein-bound iodine levels.

● May increase ^{131}I uptake and WBC and neutrophil counts.

CONTRAINDICATIONS & CAUTIONS

● Contraindicated if therapy can't be closely monitored.

● Use extreme caution in patients receiving neuromuscular blockers and diuretics; in elderly or debilitated patients; and in patients with thyroid disease, seizure disorder, infection, renal or CV disease, severe debilitation or dehydration, or sodium depletion.

● Patients with Brugada syndrome (abnormal ECG with increased risk of sudden death) or with risk factors for this condition shouldn't take lithium.

Dialyzable drug: Yes.

⚠ **Overdose S&S:** Diarrhea, vomiting, drowsiness, muscular weakness, lack of coordination, giddiness, ataxia, blurred vision, confusion, tinnitus, large output of dilute urine, slurred speech, loss of consciousness, myoclonic limb movements, agitation, urinary or fecal incontinence, seizures, arrhythmias, hypotension, peripheral vascular collapse, coma.

PREGNANCY-LACTATION-REPRODUCTION

● Drug may cause fetal harm if used during pregnancy; data from lithium birth registries suggest an increase in cardiac and other anomalies. If drug is used in women of childbearing potential or during pregnancy, or if patient becomes pregnant while taking drug, apprise patient of potential hazard to the fetus.

● Drug appears in breast milk. Use in breast-feeding women isn't recommended.

NURSING CONSIDERATIONS

Black Box Warning Lithium toxicity is closely related to serum lithium levels and can occur at doses close to therapeutic levels. Facilities for prompt and accurate serum lithium determinations should be available before initiation of therapy. ■

● Monitor patient and discontinue drug for signs and symptoms of lithium toxicity (ataxia, drowsiness, weakness, tremor, vomiting).

● When drug level is less than 1.5 mEq/L, adverse reactions are usually mild.

● Monitor baseline ECG, thyroid studies, renal studies, and electrolyte levels.

● Check fluid intake and output, especially when surgery is scheduled.

● Weigh patient daily; check for edema or sudden weight gain.

● Adjust fluid and salt ingestion to compensate if excessive loss occurs from protracted diaphoresis or diarrhea. Under normal conditions, patient fluid intake should be 2½ to 3 L daily, and he should follow a balanced diet with adequate salt intake.

● Check urine specific gravity and report level below 1.005, which may indicate diabetes insipidus.

● Drug alters glucose tolerance in diabetic patients. Monitor glucose level closely.

● Perform outpatient follow-up of thyroid and renal function every 2 to 3 months during 6 months of treatment, then as clinically indicated. Monitor CBC and ECG (patients older than age 40) before therapy and as needed. Monitor lithium level twice weekly until stable and levels are stable, then every 1 to 2 months or as needed.

● Palpate thyroid to check for enlargement. Monitor weight before and during therapy.

• *Look alike–sound alike:* Don't confuse lithium carbonate with lanthanum carbonate.

PATIENT TEACHING

• Tell patient to take drug with plenty of water and after meals to minimize GI upset.
• Explain the importance of having regular blood tests to determine drug levels and to monitor therapy; even slightly high values can be dangerous.
• Warn patient and caregivers to expect transient nausea, large amounts of urine, thirst, and discomfort during first few days and to watch for evidence of toxicity.
• Instruct patient to withhold one dose and call prescriber immediately if signs and symptoms of toxicity appear, but not to stop drug abruptly.
• Warn patient to avoid hazardous activities that require alertness and good psychomotor coordination until CNS effects are known.
• Tell patient not to switch brands or take other prescription or OTC drugs without prescriber's guidance.
• Advise patient to immediately seek emergency assistance if fainting, light-headedness, abnormal heartbeat, or shortness of breath occurs because these signs and symptoms are associated with a potentially life-threatening heart disorder known as Brugada syndrome.
• Tell patient to wear or carry medical identification at all times.

lixisenatide
See NEW DRUGS for information.

lomitapide mesylate
lom-i-TA-pide

Juxtapid

Therapeutic class: Antilipemics
Pharmacologic class: Microsomal triglyceride transfer protein inhibitors

AVAILABLE FORMS
Capsules ⓞⓤⓒ: 5 mg, 10 mg, 20 mg, 30 mg, 40 mg, 60 mg

INDICATIONS & DOSAGES
➤ As an adjunct to low-fat diet and other lipid-lowering treatments, including LDL apheresis where available, to reduce LDL, total cholesterol, apolipoprotein B, and non-HDL cholesterol levels in patients with homozygous familial hypercholesterolemia (HoFH)
Adults: 5 mg P.O. once daily. May increase to 10 mg daily after at least 2 weeks; may increase at least 4 weeks later to 20 mg, then at least 4 weeks later to 40 mg, then at least 4 weeks later to 60 mg. Measure ALT and AST levels before any dosage increase. Maximum daily dosage is 60 mg.
Adjust-a-dose: Decrease maximum daily dosage to 30 mg daily with concomitant use of weak CYP3A4 inhibitors, but to 40 mg daily with concomitant use of oral contraceptives. When initiating a weak CYP3A4 inhibitor in patient already taking 10 mg daily or more, decrease lomitapide dose by half.

In patients with ESRD receiving dialysis and in patients with mild hepatic impairment (Child-Pugh class A), don't exceed 40 mg P.O. daily. If ALT or AST level is 3 × to less than 5 × ULN, confirm result within 1 week; reduce dosage and monitor liver enzyme levels weekly. May resume drug at a reduced dosage when transaminase levels are less than 3 × ULN; monitor liver enzyme levels more frequently. If bilirubin level or INR increases, or transaminase levels rise above 5 × ULN or don't fall below 3 × ULN within 4 weeks, stop drug and obtain additional liver-related tests (alkaline phosphatase, total bilirubin, INR) and investigate for probable cause. If ALT or AST elevation is accompanied by signs and symptoms of liver injury (nausea, vomiting, abdominal pain, fever, jaundice, lethargy, flulike symptoms), increases in bilirubin level greater than 2 × ULN, or active liver disease, discontinue drug and investigate probable cause.

ADMINISTRATION
P.O.
• Give drug with a glass of water on an empty stomach at least 2 hours after evening meal.
• Don't crush or open capsules.

Black Box Warning Check LFTs (ALT, AST, alkaline phosphatase, and total bilirubin) before starting and periodically during treatment. ∎

• To reduce risk of developing a fat-soluble nutrient deficiency, patients should take drug with concurrent daily doses of vitamin E, 400 IU; linoleic acid, 200 mg; alpha linolenic acid, 210 mg; eicosapentaenoic acid, 110 mg; and docosahexaenoic acid, 80 mg.

ACTION

Inhibits microsomal triglyceride transfer protein, stopping synthesis of chylomicrons and VLDL, leading to reduced levels of plasma LDL cholesterol.

Route	Onset	Peak	Duration
P.O.	Unknown	6 hr	Unknown

Half-life: 39.7 hours.

ADVERSE REACTIONS

CNS: headache, dizziness, fever, fatigue.
CV: chest pain, angina pectoris, palpitations.
EENT: nasopharyngitis, pharyngolaryngeal pain, nasal congestion.
GI: diarrhea, nausea, dyspepsia, vomiting, abdominal pain, abdominal discomfort, abdominal distention, constipation, flatulence, GERD, defecation urgency, rectal tenesmus, gastroenteritis.
Hepatic: increased ALT level, hepatic steatosis, *hepatotoxicity.*
Metabolic: weight loss.
Musculoskeletal: back pain.
Other: flulike symptoms.

INTERACTIONS

Drug-drug. *Bile acid sequestrants (cholestyramine, colesevelam, colesevelam hydrochloride, colestipol, colestipol hydrochloride):* May interfere with absorption of lomitapide. Separate doses by 4 hours.
Hepatotoxins (acetaminophen [more than 4 g/day for 3 days/week or more], amiodarone, isotretinoin, methotrexate, tamoxifen, tetracyclines): May accelerate liver injury. Use together cautiously and monitor LFTs frequently.

Lovastatin: May increase risk of myopathy. Use together cautiously; consider lower lovastatin dosage.
Moderate CYP3A4 inhibitors (amprenavir, aprepitant, atazanavir, ciprofloxacin, crizotinib, darunavir/ritonavir, diltiazem, erythromycin, fluconazole, fosamprenavir, imatinib, verapamil): May increase lomitapide concentration. Use together is contraindicated.
P-glycoprotein substrates (aliskiren, ambrisentan, colchicine, dabigatran, digoxin, everolimus, fexofenadine, imatinib, lapatinib, maraviroc, nilotinib, posaconazole, ranolazine, saxagliptin, sirolimus, sitagliptin, talinolol, tolvaptan, topotecan): May increase level of substrate. Use together cautiously; consider substrate dosage reduction.
Simvastatin: May increase risk of myopathy. Decrease simvastatin dosage to 20 mg daily, or to 40 mg for patients previously taking 80 mg daily with no muscle toxicity in last year.
Strong CYP3A4 inhibitors (clarithromycin, conivaptan, indinavir, itraconazole, ketoconazole, lopinavir–ritonavir, mibefradil, nefazodone, nelfinavir, posaconazole, ritonavir, saquinavir, telithromycin, voriconazole): May increase lomitapide level. Use together is contraindicated.
Warfarin: May increase INR. Use together cautiously. Monitor INR carefully, especially after lomitapide dosage adjustments.
Weak CYP3A4 inhibitors (alprazolam, amiodarone, amlodipine, atorvastatin, bicalutamide, cilostazol, cimetidine, cyclosporine, fluoxetine, fluvoxamine, isoniazid, lapatinib, nilotinib, oral contraceptives, pazopanib, ranitidine, ranolazine, tipranavir/ritonavir, ticagrelor, zileuton): Use together cautiously, with maximum lomitapide dosage of 30 mg P.O. daily; maximum dosage is 40 mg P.O. daily with oral contraceptives.
Drug-herb. *Ginkgo biloba, goldenseal:* May increase lomitapide level. Use together cautiously, with maximum lomitapide dosage of 30 mg daily.
Drug-food. *Fat-soluble nutrients (alpha-linolenic acid, docosahexaenoic acid, eicosapentaenoic acid, linoleic acid, vitamin E):* May decrease absorption of

---

Reactions in bold italics are *life-threatening*. Interactions may have a *rapid onset* or a *delayed onset*.

these nutrients. Supplements should be given.

Grapefruit juice: May adversely affect absorption. Discourage use together.

Drug-lifestyle. *Alcohol use:* May exacerbate liver injury and increase hepatic fat levels. Discourage consumption of more than one alcoholic drink per day.

EFFECTS ON LAB TEST RESULTS

● May increase INR and transaminase, bilirubin, and alkaline phosphatase levels.

CONTRAINDICATIONS & CAUTIONS

Black Box Warning Because of risk of hepatotoxicity, lomitapide is available only through a restricted program under a Risk Evaluation and Mitigation Strategy (REMS) called the Juxtapid REMS program. Safety and effectiveness haven't been established in patients with hypercholesterolemia who don't have HoFH. ■

● Contraindicated in patients hypersensitive to drug or its components and in those with moderate or severe hepatic impairment (Child-Pugh class B or C) or active liver disease, including unexplained persistent elevations of serum transaminases.

● Contraindicated with concomitant administration of moderate or strong CYP3A4 inhibitors.

Black Box Warning Drug causes increased hepatic fat (steatosis), a risk factor for progressive liver disease, including steatohepatitis and cirrhosis. ■

● Drug hasn't been studied when given with other LDL-lowering agents that can also increase hepatic fat. Use together isn't recommended.

● Avoid use in patients with galactose intolerance, Lapp lactase deficiency, or glucose–galactose malabsorption; decreased absorption of concurrent drugs may result.

Dialyzable drug: Unlikely.

PREGNANCY-LACTATION-REPRODUCTION

◑ Alert: Rule out pregnancy in women of childbearing potential before starting treatment.

Drug may cause fetal harm and is contraindicated during pregnancy. Women of childbearing potential should have a nega-

tive pregnancy test before therapy and use effective contraception during therapy.

● Women who become pregnant during therapy should stop drug immediately and notify their prescriber.

◑ Alert: Discontinue drug immediately if pregnancy occurs during therapy and enroll patient in the Global Lomitapide Pregnancy Exposure Registry at 1-877-902-4099.

● It isn't known if drug appears in breast milk. Patient should discontinue breastfeeding or discontinue drug.

NURSING CONSIDERATIONS

Black Box Warning Drug may cause hepatic steatosis or transaminase elevations. Measure AST, ALT, alkaline phosphatase, and total bilirubin levels before treatment; then obtain AST and ALT levels periodically and with dosage changes. Adjust dosage if AST or ALT level is greater than $3 \times$ ULN. Discontinue drug for clinically significant liver toxicity. ■

● Assess liver-related tests (ALT and AST, at a minimum) monthly or before each dosage increase, whichever occurs first during the first year; then assess at least every 3 months and before any dosage increase.

● If transaminase elevations are accompanied by clinical signs and symptoms of liver injury (e.g., nausea, vomiting, abdominal pain, fever, jaundice, lethargy, or flulike symptoms), increase in bilirubin level $2 \times$ ULN or more, or active liver disease, discontinue treatment and investigate probable cause.

● Monitor patient for GI adverse effects. Absorption of oral medications, including oral contraceptives, may be affected in patients with diarrhea and vomiting.

● Monitor patients who are more susceptible to complications from diarrhea, such as older patients and patients taking drugs that can lead to volume depletion or hypotension, because of risk of severe diarrhea.

PATIENT TEACHING

● Inform patient about participation in drug's registry program. Information is available at www.juxtapid.com.

● Advise patient to limit alcohol to one drink daily.

- Instruct patient to report severe stomach upset or other GI signs and symptoms, fever, jaundice, lethargy, or flulike symptoms as these may be signs of liver injury.
- Instruct patient to stop drug and contact prescriber if severe diarrhea occurs or if patient experiences signs and symptoms of volume depletion, such as light-headedness, decreased urine output, or tiredness.
- Teach female patient that drug may harm a fetus and to use effective contraception during therapy and to discontinue drug and immediately notify prescriber if she becomes pregnant.
- Teach female patient of childbearing potential who is taking oral contraceptives to use additional contraceptive methods if vomiting and diarrhea occur.
- Remind patient to take vitamin E and other supplements as required.
- Caution patient to adhere to low-fat diet (less than 20% of calories from fat) and to take drug at least 2 hours after evening meal to minimize GI adverse effects.
- Warn patient to contact health care provider if drug has been stopped for more than a week.

lopinavir–ritonavir
low-PIN-ah-ver/ri-TON-ah-veer

Kaletra*✍

Therapeutic class: Antiretrovirals
Pharmacologic class: Protease inhibitors

AVAILABLE FORMS
Solution: lopinavir 400 mg and ritonavir 100 mg/5 mL (80 mg and 20 mg/mL)*
Tablets ⓘ: lopinavir 100 mg and ritonavir 25 mg; lopinavir 200 mg and ritonavir 50 mg

INDICATIONS & DOSAGES
➤ **HIV infection, with other antiretrovirals but not efavirenz, nevirapine, or nelfinavir**
Adults: 800 mg lopinavir and 200 mg ritonavir P.O. once daily (only in patients with less than three lopinavir resistance–associated substitutions) or in two evenly divided doses.

Children ages 6 months to 18 years: 230 mg lopinavir and 57.5 mg/m^2 ritonavir (oral solution) P.O. b.i.d. with food. Or, if patient weighs more than 35 kg, give four tablets of lopinavir 100 mg and ritonavir 25 mg P.O. b.i.d. If patient weighs between 25 and 35 kg, give three tablets of lopinavir 100 mg and ritonavir 25 mg P.O. b.i.d. If patient weighs 15 to 25 kg, give two tablets of lopinavir 100 mg and ritonavir 25 mg P.O. b.i.d. Maximum dosage is lopinavir 400 mg and ritonavir 100 mg P.O. b.i.d.
Children ages 14 days to 6 months: 16 mg lopinavir and 4 mg ritonavir/kg P.O. b.i.d. Or, lopinavir 300 mg and ritonavir 75 mg/m^2 P.O. b.i.d.
Adjust-a-dose: In pregnant women with no documented lopinavir resistance–associated substitutions, give 400 mg lopinavir and 100 mg ritonavir tablets b.i.d.; avoid oral solution. Once-daily dosing isn't recommended. There are insufficient data to recommend dosing in pregnant women with documented lopinavir resistance–associated substitutions. No dosage adjustment is required during the postpartum period.
➤ **HIV infection, in combination with other antiretrovirals (efavirenz, nevirapine, or nelfinavir)**
Adults: 500 mg lopinavir and 125 mg ritonavir (tablets) P.O. b.i.d., or 520 mg lopinavir and 130 mg ritonavir (oral solution) P.O. b.i.d. with food.
Children ages 6 months to 18 years: 300 mg lopinavir and 75 mg/m^2 ritonavir (oral solution) P.O. b.i.d. with food. Maximum dosage is lopinavir 533 mg and ritonavir 133 mg (oral solution) P.O. b.i.d. with food. Or, if patient weighs more than 45 kg, give five tablets of lopinavir 100 mg and ritonavir 25 mg P.O. b.i.d. If patient weighs between 30 and 45 kg, give four tablets of lopinavir 100 mg and ritonavir 25 mg P.O. b.i.d. If patient weighs 20 to 30 kg, give three tablets of lopinavir 100 mg and ritonavir 25 mg P.O. b.i.d. If patient weighs 15 to 20 kg, give two tablets of lopinavir 100 mg and ritonavir 25 mg P.O. b.i.d. Maximum dosage is lopinavir 500 mg and ritonavir 125 mg (tablets) P.O. b.i.d.

ADMINISTRATION
P.O.
❸ Alert: Many drug interactions are possible. Review all drugs patient is taking.
● Give oral solution with food. Give tablets without regard for food.
● Calculate children's doses based on either body weight or BSA.
● Tablets must be swallowed whole; don't crush or divide, and tell patient not to chew.
● Refrigerated solution remains stable until expiration date on package. If stored at room temperature, use drug within 2 months.

ACTION
Lopinavir is an HIV protease inhibitor, which produces immature, noninfectious viral particles. Ritonavir, also an HIV protease inhibitor, slows lopinavir metabolism, thereby increasing lopinavir level.

Route	Onset	Peak	Duration
P.O.	Unknown	4–6 hr	Unknown

Half-life: About 5 to 6 hours.

ADVERSE REACTIONS
CNS: *encephalopathy,* abnormal dreams, abnormal thinking, agitation, amnesia, anxiety, asthenia, ataxia, confusion, depression, dizziness, dyskinesia, emotional lability, fever, headache, hypertonia, insomnia, malaise, nervousness, neuropathy, pain, paresthesia, peripheral neuritis, somnolence, tremors.
CV: chest pain, *DVT,* edema, hypertension, palpitations, thrombophlebitis, vasculitis.
EENT: abnormal vision, eye disorder, otitis media, sinusitis, tinnitus.
GI: *hemorrhagic colitis, pancreatitis,* diarrhea, nausea, abdominal pain, abnormal stools, anorexia, cholecystitis, constipation, dry mouth, dyspepsia, dysphagia, enterocolitis, eructation, esophagitis, fecal incontinence, flatulence, gastritis, gastroenteritis, GI disorder, increased appetite, inflammation of the salivary glands, stomatitis, taste perversion, ulcerative stomatitis, vomiting.
GU: abnormal ejaculation, hypogonadism, renal calculus, urine abnormality.
Hematologic: *leukopenia, neutropenia, thrombocytopenia in children,* anemia.
Hepatic: hyperbilirubinemia in children.

Metabolic: Cushing syndrome, dehydration, decreased glucose tolerance, hyperglycemia, hyperuricemia, hyponatremia in children, hypothyroidism, *lactic acidosis,* weight loss.
Musculoskeletal: arthralgia, arthrosis, back pain, myalgia.
Respiratory: bronchitis, dyspnea, lung edema.
Skin: acne, alopecia, benign skin neoplasm, dry skin, exfoliative dermatitis, furunculosis, nail disorder, pruritus, rash, skin discoloration, sweating.
Other: chills, decreased libido, facial edema, flu syndrome, gynecomastia, immune reconstitution syndrome, lymphadenopathy, viral infection.

INTERACTIONS
Drug-drug. *Amiodarone, bepridil, lidocaine, quinidine:* May increase antiarrhythmic level. Use together cautiously. Monitor levels of these drugs, if possible.
Antiarrhythmics (flecainide, propafenone), pimozide: May increase risk of cardiac arrhythmias. Avoid using together.
Atorvastatin: May increase level of this drug and risk of myopathy and rhabdomyolysis. Use lowest possible dose and monitor patient carefully.
Atovaquone, methadone: May decrease levels of these drugs. Consider increasing doses of these drugs.
Bosentan: May increase bosentan level. Withhold bosentan for at least 36 hours before starting lopinavir–ritonavir, and decrease bosentan dosage and frequency.
Bupropion: May decrease bupropion level and antidepressant effect. Monitor patient for adequate clinical response and adjust bupropion dosage as needed.
Carbamazepine, phenobarbital, phenytoin: May decrease lopinavir level. Use together cautiously. Don't use once-daily lopinavir–ritonavir. Consider therapy modification.
Clarithromycin: May increase clarithromycin level in patients with renal impairment. Adjust clarithromycin dosage.
Cobicistat: May enhance therapeutic effects of ritonavir. Avoid use together.
Colchicine: May increase colchicine level. Don't use together in patient with renal or hepatic impairment. Decrease colchicine

dosage if used together in patient with normal renal and hepatic function.

Cyclosporine, rapamycin, tacrolimus: May increase levels of these drugs. Monitor therapeutic levels.

Dasatinib, nilotinib: May increase levels of these drugs and risk of adverse events. Adjust dasatinib and nilotinib dosages as needed.

Delavirdine: May increase lopinavir level. Avoid using together.

Didanosine: May decrease absorption of didanosine because lopinavir–ritonavir combination is taken with food. Give didanosine 1 hour before or 2 hours after lopinavir–ritonavir combination.

Disulfiram, metronidazole: May cause disulfiram-like reaction in patients using oral solution (contains alcohol). Avoid use together.

Drugs that prolong PR interval (atazanavir, beta blockers, calcium channel blockers, digoxin): May further prolong PR interval. Use cautiously together.

Drugs that prolong QT interval (amiodarone, flecainide, propafenone): May further prolong QT interval and increase risk of ventricular arrhythmias. Avoid use together.

Efavirenz, nelfinavir, nevirapine: May decrease lopinavir level. Consider increasing lopinavir–ritonavir combination dose. Don't use a once-daily regimen of lopinavir–ritonavir combination with these drugs.

Elvitegravir: May increase elvitegravir concentration. Reduce dosages of both drugs and consider modifying therapy.

Ergot derivatives (dihydroergotamine, ergonovine, ergotamine, methylergonovine): May increase risk of ergot toxicity characterized by peripheral vasospasm and ischemia. Avoid using together.

Felodipine, nicardipine, nifedipine: May increase levels of these drugs. Use together cautiously.

Fentanyl, triazolam: May increase or prolong sedation or cause respiratory depression. Monitor patient carefully.

Fluticasone: May increase fluticasone plasma concentration, leading to decreased serum cortisol level, Cushing syndrome, and adrenal suppression. Use together isn't

recommended unless benefits outweigh risks.

Fosamprenavir with ritonavir: May increase rate of adverse reactions. Appropriate doses of the combinations with respect to safety and efficacy haven't been established.

Hormonal contraceptives (ethinyl estradiol): May decrease effectiveness of contraceptives. Recommend nonhormonal contraceptives.

Indinavir, saquinavir: May increase levels of these drugs. Avoid using together.

Itraconazole, ketoconazole: May increase levels of these drugs. Don't give more than 200 mg/day of these drugs.

Lovastatin, simvastatin: May increase risk of adverse reactions, such as myopathy and rhabdomyolysis. Use together is contraindicated.

Methadone: May decrease methadone level. Monitor clinical response and increase methadone dosage as needed.

Midazolam (parenteral), triazolam: May cause prolonged or increased sedation or respiratory depression. Avoid using together. Don't give with oral midazolam.

Pitavastatin, pravastatin: May increase statin level and risk of myopathy and rhabdomyolysis. Use together cautiously.

Rifabutin: May increase rifabutin level. Decrease rifabutin dosage by at least 75% or a maximum of 150 mg every other day or three times a week. Monitor patient carefully and adjust dosage as needed.

Rifampin: May decrease effectiveness of Kaletra. Avoid using together.

Rosuvastatin: May increase statin level and risk of myopathy and rhabdomyolysis. Rosuvastatin dosage shouldn't exceed 10 mg daily.

Salmeterol: May increase salmeterol level and risk of CV adverse reactions. Use together isn't recommended.

Sildenafil, tadalafil, vardenafil: May increase level of these drugs and adverse effects, such as hypotension and prolonged erection. Warn patient not to take more than 25 mg of sildenafil in 48 hours, more than 10 mg of tadalafil in 72 hours, or more than 2.5 mg vardenafil in 72 hours.

Trazodone: May increase trazodone level and risk of adverse reactions. Consider lower dosage of trazodone.

Reactions in bold italics are *life-threatening*. Interactions may have a *rapid onset* or a ***delayed onset***.

Vinblastine, vincristine: May increase levels of these drugs and risk of adverse reactions. Temporarily withhold antiretroviral regimen for hematologic or GI adverse reactions. If cancer treatment is prolonged, consider other antivirals.

Warfarin: May affect warfarin level. Monitor PT and INR.

Drug-herb. *St. John's wort:* Loss of virologic response and possible resistance to drug. Discourage use together.

Drug-food. *Any food:* May increase absorption of oral solution. Tell patient to take with food.

EFFECTS ON LAB TEST RESULTS
● May increase glucose, amylase, lipase, cholesterol, uric acid, and triglyceride levels and LFT values. May decrease Hb level and hematocrit.

● May decrease RBC, WBC, neutrophil, and platelet counts.

CONTRAINDICATIONS & CAUTIONS
● Contraindicated in patients hypersensitive to drug or any of its components.

● Contraindicated with drugs metabolized by CYP3A, including dihydroergotamine, ergonovine, lovastatin, methylergonovine, midazolam, pimozide, rifampin, simvastatin, triazolam, and St. John's wort.

● Concomitant use with certain other drugs may result in known or potentially significant drug interactions. Consult full prescribing information before and during treatment for potential drug interactions.

● The number of baseline lopinavir resistance–associated substitutions affects drug's virologic response.

● Avoid use in patients with congenital long QT syndrome or hypokalemia and in those taking drugs that prolong QT interval. Correct potassium abnormalities before starting therapy.

● Use cautiously in patients with a history of pancreatitis, hepatic impairment, HBV or HCV infection, marked elevations in liver enzyme levels, or hemophilia.

● Use cautiously in patients with cardiac conduction abnormalities or underlying cardiac disease.

● Use cautiously in elderly patients.

● Oral solution contains 42.4% (volume/volume) alcohol and 15.3% (weight/volume) propylene glycol; use with care, especially in infants and young children. Consider total amounts of alcohol and propylene glycol from all drugs given to children ages 14 days to 6 months to avoid toxicity.

❸ **Alert:** Safety and effectiveness in neonates younger than age 14 days haven't been established. Use only if benefit outweighs risk. Monitor neonates for toxicity, such as hyperosmolality with or without lactic acidosis, renal toxicity, CNS depression (stupor, coma, apnea), seizures, hypotonia, cardiac arrhythmias, ECG changes, and hemolysis. Toxicity in preterm neonates can be severe or fatal.

Dialyzable drug: Unlikely.

⚠ **Overdose S&S:** Alcohol-related toxicity.

PREGNANCY-LACTATION-REPRODUCTION
● Drug is recommended with dosage adjustments for pregnant women with HIV infection.

● Avoid use of oral solution during pregnancy because it contains alcohol.

● Once-daily dosing isn't recommended in pregnant women with any documented lopinavir resistance–associated amino acid substitutions.

● The Antiretroviral Pregnancy Registry monitors maternal-fetal outcomes of pregnant women taking Kaletra. Health care providers are encouraged to enroll patients by calling 1-800-258-4263.

● Patients with HIV-1 infection shouldn't breast-feed, to avoid risk of postnatal transmission of HIV-1.

NURSING CONSIDERATIONS
● Don't administer tablets or oral solution as a once-daily dosing regimen when combined with efavirenz, nevirapine, or nelfinavir.

● Avoid once-daily dosing in children younger than age 18.

● Calculate appropriate dose of drug for each individual pediatric patient based on body weight or BSA to avoid underdosing or exceeding the recommended adult dose.

● Assess children for ability to swallow intact tablets before drug is prescribed; use oral solution in a calibrated dosing syringe if a child is unable to reliably swallow a tablet.

● During initial phase of treatment, patients responding to antiretroviral therapy may develop an inflammatory response to indolent or residual opportunistic infections (CMV, *Mycobacterium avium* complex, *Pneumocystis jiroveci* pneumonia, TB), which may necessitate further evaluation and treatment. Autoimmune disorders (such as Graves disease, polymyositis, and Guillain-Barré syndrome) have also been reported in the setting of immune reconstitution; however, time to onset is more variable, and onset can occur many months after initiation of antiretroviral treatment.

● Monitor patient for signs of fat redistribution, including central obesity, buffalo hump, peripheral wasting, breast enlargement, and cushingoid appearance.

● Monitor glucose, total cholesterol, and triglyceride levels before starting therapy and periodically thereafter.

● Monitor patient for signs and symptoms of pancreatitis (nausea, vomiting, abdominal pain, or increased lipase and amylase values).

● Monitor patient for signs and symptoms of bleeding (hypotension, rapid HR) and for adverse reactions associated with concomitant drugs.

● Consider potential for drug interactions before and during therapy. Review concomitant medications and monitor patient for adverse reactions associated with the concomitant medications.

● *Look alike–sound alike:* Don't confuse Kaletra with Keppra.

PATIENT TEACHING

● Tell patient to take oral solution with food. Tablets may be taken without regard to food.
🚺 *Alert:* Tablets must be swallowed whole; don't crush or divide, and tell patient not to chew.

● Tell patient also taking didanosine to take it 1 hour before or 2 hours after lopinavir–ritonavir combination.

● Advise patient to report all side effects to prescriber.

● Teach patient signs and symptoms of acute pancreatitis and to seek emergency medical treatment if signs and symptoms occur.

● Tell patient to immediately report severe nausea, vomiting, or abdominal pain.

● Inform patient that drug doesn't cure HIV infection, that opportunistic infections and other complications of HIV infection may still occur, and that transmission of HIV to others through sexual contact or blood contamination remains possible.

● Advise patient taking an erectile dysfunction drug of the increased risk of adverse effects, including low BP, visual changes, and painful erections, and to promptly report any symptoms to his prescriber. Tell him not to take more often than directed.

● Warn patient to tell prescriber about any other prescription or nonprescription medicine that he's taking, including herbal supplements.

SAFETY ALERT!

lorazepam
lor-AZ-e-pam

Ativan✦, Lorazepam Intensol, Lorazepam Preservative Free

Therapeutic class: Anxiolytics
Pharmacologic class: Benzodiazepines
Controlled substance schedule: IV

AVAILABLE FORMS
Injection: 2 mg/mL, 4 mg/mL
Oral solution: 2 mg/mL
Tablets: 0.5 mg, 1 mg, 2 mg

INDICATIONS & DOSAGES
➤ **Anxiety**
Adults: 2 to 6 mg P.O. daily in divided doses, with the largest dose taken before bedtime. Maximum, 10 mg daily.
Elderly patients: 1 to 2 mg P.O. daily in divided doses. Maximum, 10 mg daily.
➤ **Insomnia from anxiety or transient situational stress**
Adults: 2 to 4 mg P.O. at bedtime.
➤ **Preoperative sedation**
Adults: 2 mg I.V. total or 0.044 mg/kg I.V., whichever is smaller, 15 to 20 minutes before the anticipated operative procedure. Larger doses up to 0.05 mg/kg I.V., to total

of 4 mg, may be needed. Or, 0.05 mg/kg
I.M. 2 hours before procedure. Total dose
shouldn't exceed 4 mg.

➤ **Status epilepticus**
Adults: 4 mg I.V. at a rate of 2 mg/minute.
If seizures continue or recur after 10 to
15 minutes, an additional 4-mg dose may be
given. Drug may be given I.M. if I.V. access
isn't available.

ADMINISTRATION
P.O.
● Use only the calibrated dropper provided.
● Mix oral solution with liquid or semisolid
food, such as water, juices, carbonated
beverages, applesauce, or pudding. Gently
stir liquid or food for a few seconds and
have patient immediately consume entire
mixture.

I.V.
▼ Keep emergency resuscitation equipment and oxygen available.
▼ Dilute with an equal volume of sterile
water for injection, NSS for injection,
or D5W. Give slowly at no more than
2 mg/minute.
▼ Monitor respirations every 5 to 15 minutes and before each I.V. dose.
▼ Contains benzyl alcohol. Avoid use in
neonates.
▼ Refrigerate intact vials and protect from
light.
▼ **Incompatibilities:** Aldesleukin,
aztreonam, buprenorphine, caffeine citrate, floxacillin, foscarnet, idarubicin,
imipenem–cilastatin sodium, omeprazole,
ondansetron hydrochloride, sargramostim,
sufentanil citrate, thiopental.

I.M.
● For status epilepticus, drug may be given
I.M. if I.V. access isn't available.
● For I.M. use, inject deeply into a muscle.
Don't dilute.
● Refrigerate parenteral form to prolong
shelf life.

ACTION
May potentiate the effects of GABA, depress the CNS, and suppress the spread of
seizure activity.

Route	Onset	Peak	Duration
P.O.	1 hr	2 hr	12–24 hr
I.V.	5 min	60–90 min	6–8 hr
I.M.	15–30 min	60–90 min	6–8 hr

Half-life: 10 to 20 hours.

ADVERSE REACTIONS
CNS: drowsiness, sedation, amnesia,
insomnia, agitation, dizziness, weakness,
unsteadiness, disorientation, depression,
headache.
CV: hypotension.
EENT: visual disturbances, nasal congestion.
GI: abdominal discomfort, nausea, change
in appetite.

INTERACTIONS
Drug-drug. *Clozapine:* May cause delirium, sedation, sialorrhea, and ataxia. Don't
start simultaneously. Carefully monitor
patient, especially during first 48 hours of
coadministration.
Black Box Warning *Opioids:* May cause
slow or difficult breathing, sedation, and
death. Avoid use together. If use together is
necessary, limit dosage and duration of each
drug to the minimum necessary for desired
effect. ∎
Oral hormonal contraceptives: May decrease lorazepam level. Monitor closely;
lorazepam dosage may need to be increased.
Probenecid: May result in prolonged lorazepam half-life and a decrease in its total
clearance. Reduce lorazepam dosage by
50% when coadministered.
Sodium oxybate: May result in additive
effects, including increased sleep duration
and CNS depression. Use together is contraindicated.
Valproate: May increase lorazepam plasma
concentration. Reduce lorazepam dosage
to 50% of normal adult dose when used
together.
Drug-lifestyle. *Alcohol use:* May cause additive CNS effects. Discourage use together.

EFFECTS ON LAB TEST RESULTS
● May increase LDH and LFT values.

CONTRAINDICATIONS & CAUTIONS

• Contraindicated in patients hypersensitive to drug, other benzodiazepines, or the vehicle used in parenteral dosage form, and in patients with acute angle-closure glaucoma. I.V. administration is contraindicated in patients with sleep apnea and in patients with severe respiratory insufficiency, except those who are mechanically ventilated.

• Contraindicated for intra-arterial administration.

Black Box Warning Opioid drugs should only be prescribed with benzodiazepines or other CNS depressants to patients for whom alternative treatment options are inadequate. ■

• Use cautiously in patients with pulmonary, renal, or hepatic impairment, or history of substance abuse.

• Use cautiously in elderly, acutely ill, or debilitated patients.

Dialyzable drug: Unknown.

⚠ *Overdose S&S:* Drowsiness, confusion lethargy, ataxia, hypotonia, hypotension, hypnotic state, stage 1 to 3 coma, death.

PREGNANCY-LACTATION-REPRODUCTION

• May cause fetal harm, including neonatal withdrawal symptoms. Avoid use during pregnancy except in life-threatening situations (status epilepticus) when safer drugs can't be used.

• Drug appears in breast milk. Use in breast-feeding women isn't recommended.

NURSING CONSIDERATIONS

• Monitor hepatic, renal, and hematopoietic function periodically in patients receiving repeated or prolonged therapy.

🕙 *Alert:* Use of this drug may lead to abuse and addiction. Don't stop drug abruptly after long-term use because withdrawal symptoms may occur.

• *Look alike–sound alike:* Don't confuse lorazepam with alprazolam, clonazepam, or Lovaza. Don't confuse Ativan with Atgam.

PATIENT TEACHING

Black Box Warning Caution the patient or the caregiver of a patient taking an opioid drug with a benzodiazepine, CNS depressant, or alcohol to seek immediate medical attention if the patient has symptoms of dizziness, light-headedness, extreme sleepiness, slowed or difficult breathing, or unresponsiveness. ■

• When used before surgery, drug causes substantial preoperative amnesia. Patient teaching requires extra care to ensure adequate recall. Provide written materials or inform a family member, if possible.

• Warn patient to avoid hazardous activities that require alertness or good coordination until effects of drug are known.

• Tell patient to avoid use of alcohol while taking drug.

• Notify patient that smoking may decrease drug's effectiveness.

• Warn patient not to stop drug abruptly because withdrawal symptoms may occur.

• Advise women to avoid becoming pregnant while taking drug.

lorcaserin hydrochloride
lor-ca-SER-in

Belviq

Therapeutic class: Appetite suppressants
Pharmacologic class: Serotonin 2C receptor agonists

AVAILABLE FORMS
Tablets: 10 mg

INDICATIONS & DOSAGES
➤ **Weight management in patients with initial BMI of 30 kg/m² or greater (obese) or 27 kg/m² or greater (overweight) in the presence of at least one weight-related comorbid condition as adjunct to reduced-calorie diet and increased physical activity**
Adults: 10 mg P.O. b.i.d.
Adjust-a-dose: If patient hasn't lost at least 5% of baseline body weight by week 12, discontinue drug.

ADMINISTRATION
P.O.
• Store at room temperature.
• May give without regard for food.

ACTION

Exact mechanism of action unknown. May decrease food consumption and promote satiety by selectively activating 5-HT_{2C} receptors on anorexigenic pro-opiomelanocortin neurons located in the hypothalamus.

Route	Onset	Peak	Duration
P.O.	Unknown	1½–2 hr	Unknown

Half-life: 11 hours.

ADVERSE REACTIONS

CNS: headache, dizziness, fatigue, anxiety, insomnia, stress, depression, impaired memory and attention.
CV: hypertension, *valvulopathy,* peripheral edema.
EENT: eye disorder, nasopharyngitis, oropharyngeal pain, sinus congestion, toothache, dry mouth.
GI: nausea, vomiting, diarrhea, constipation, gastroenteritis.
GU: UTI.
Metabolic: *hypoglycemia,* worsening of diabetes mellitus, decreased appetite.
Musculoskeletal: back pain, musculoskeletal pain, muscle spasms.
Respiratory: URI, cough.
Skin: rash.

INTERACTIONS

Drug-drug. *Antipsychotics, bupropion, dextromethorphan, dopamine antagonists, linezolid, lithium, MAO inhibitors, SNRIs, SSRIs, tramadol, TCAs, triptans:* May increase risk of serotonin syndrome or neuroleptic malignant syndrome (NMS)–like reactions. Use together cautiously.
CYP2D6 substrates (antipsychotics, dextromethorphan, metoclopramide, SSNRIs, SSRIs, TCAs): May increase levels of CYP2D6 substrates. Use together cautiously.
Insulin, sulfonylureas: May increase risk of hypoglycemia in patients with type 2 diabetes. Monitor patient closely; adjust antidiabetic regimen as needed.
PDE5 inhibitors (sildenafil): May increase risk of priapism. Use together cautiously.
Potent 5-HT$_{2B}$ agonists (cabergoline): May increase risk of valvulopathy. Don't use together.

Drug-herb. *St. John's wort, tryptophan:* May increase risk of serotonin syndrome or NMS-like reactions. Discourage use together.

EFFECTS ON LAB TEST RESULTS

● May increase prolactin level. May decrease glucose level.
● May decrease Hb level and hematocrit and total WBC, lymphocyte, neutrophil, and total RBC counts.

CONTRAINDICATIONS & CAUTIONS

● Contraindicated in patients hypersensitive to drug or its components. Drug isn't recommended in patients with severe renal impairment or ESRD.
● Contraindicated for administration in combination with serotonergic and dopaminergic drugs that are potent 5-HT$_{2B}$ receptor agonists and are known to increase risk of heart valvulopathy.
● May increase risk of potentially life-threatening serotonin syndrome or NMS.
● Use cautiously in patients with moderate renal impairment, severe hepatic impairment, HF, hemodynamically significant valvular disease, bradycardia, or heart block greater than first degree.
● Use cautiously in patients with type 2 diabetes mellitus being treated with insulin or antidiabetic agents because weight loss may increase risk of hypoglycemia.
● Use cautiously in men who have conditions that might predispose them to priapism (sickle cell anemia, multiple myeloma, or leukemia) and in men with anatomic deformation of the penis (angulation, cavernosal fibrosis, or Peyronie disease).
Dialyzable drug: No.
⚠ Overdose S&S: Headache, nausea, abdominal discomfort, dizziness.

PREGNANCY-LACTATION-REPRODUCTION

● Contraindicated in pregnant women; drug may cause fetal harm. If used during pregnancy, or if patient becomes pregnant during therapy, apprise her of potential hazard to the fetus.
● It isn't known if drug appears in breast milk. Patient should discontinue breast-feeding or discontinue drug.

NURSING CONSIDERATIONS

- Safety and effectiveness of using drug with other products intended for weight loss, including prescription drugs, OTC drugs, and herbal preparations, haven't been established.
- Measure blood glucose levels before and during treatment in patients with type 2 diabetes.
- Monitor patient for dyspnea, dependent edema, HF, or new murmur. Effect on CV morbidity and mortality hasn't been established.
- Monitor CBC periodically.
- Measure prolactin level if gynecomastia or galactorrhea occurs.
- Monitor patient for serotonin syndrome (mental status changes, tachycardia, labile BP, hyperthermia, hyperreflexia, incoordination, nausea, vomiting, diarrhea).
- Monitor patient for confusion or impaired attention and memory.
- Monitor patient for new or worsening depression, suicidal thoughts or behaviors, or unusual changes in mood or behavior. Discontinue drug if symptoms occur.

PATIENT TEACHING

- Teach patient to use drug only in conjunction with a reduced-calorie diet and increased physical activity.
- Tell patient drug will be discontinued if 5% weight loss isn't achieved by 12 weeks of treatment.
- Warn patient to seek medical attention if signs or symptoms of valvular heart disease (dyspnea or dependent edema) occur.
- Advise patient to seek medical attention in the event of emerging or worsening depression, suicidal thoughts or behavior, or unusual changes in mood or behavior.
- Caution patient not to operate hazardous machinery, including automobiles, until drug's effects are known.
- Warn patient never to increase dosage.
- Advise men experiencing an erection lasting longer than 4 hours, whether painful or not, to immediately stop drug and seek emergency medical attention.
- Instruct patient to inform prescriber of all medications, nutritional supplements, and vitamins (including weight-loss products) they are using while taking this drug.

- Caution women to avoid pregnancy and not to breast-feed while taking this drug and to notify prescriber immediately if pregnancy occurs.

losartan potassium
low-SAR-tan

Cozaar♦

Therapeutic class: Antihypertensives
Pharmacologic class: Angiotensin II receptor antagonists

AVAILABLE FORMS
Tablets: 25 mg, 50 mg, 100 mg

INDICATIONS & DOSAGES
➤ **Hypertension**
Adults: Initially, 50 mg P.O. daily. Maximum daily dose is 100 mg in one or two divided doses.
Children age 6 and older: 0.7 mg/kg (up to 50 mg) P.O. daily, adjusted as needed up to 1.4 mg/kg/day (maximum 100 mg).
Adjust-a-dose: For adults with hepatic impairment or intravascular volume depletion (such as those taking diuretics), initially, 25 mg.
➤ **Nephropathy in patients with type 2 diabetes**
Adults: 50 mg P.O. once daily. Increase dosage to 100 mg once daily based on BP response.
➤ **To reduce risk of stroke in patients with hypertension and left ventricular hypertrophy**
Adults: Initially, 50 mg P.O. once daily. Adjust dosage based on BP response, adding hydrochlorothiazide 12.5 mg once daily, increasing losartan to 100 mg daily, or both. If further adjustments are required, may increase the daily dosage of hydrochlorothiazide to 25 mg.

ADMINISTRATION
P.O.
- Give drug without regard for meals.
- If made into suspension by pharmacist, store in refrigerator and shake well before each use.

ACTION

Inhibits vasoconstrictive and aldosterone-secreting action of angiotensin II by blocking angiotensin II receptor on the surface of vascular smooth muscle and other tissue cells.

Route	Onset	Peak	Duration
P.O.	6 hr	1–2 hr	Unknown

Half-life: Parent drug, about 1½ to 3 hours; active metabolite, about 4½ to 10 hours.

ADVERSE REACTIONS

Patients with hypertension or left ventricular hypertrophy
CNS: dizziness, asthenia, fatigue, headache, insomnia.
CV: edema, chest pain.
EENT: nasal congestion, sinusitis, pharyngitis, sinus disorder.
GI: abdominal pain, nausea, diarrhea, dyspepsia.
Musculoskeletal: muscle cramps, myalgia, back or leg pain.
Respiratory: cough, URI.
Other: *angioedema.*
Patients with nephropathy
CNS: asthenia, fatigue, fever, hypoesthesia.
CV: chest pain, hypotension, orthostatic hypotension.
EENT: sinusitis, cataract.
GI: diarrhea, dyspepsia, gastritis, nausea.
GU: UTI.
Hematologic: anemia.
Metabolic: *hyperkalemia, hypoglycemia,* hyponatremia, weight gain.
Musculoskeletal: back pain, leg or knee pain, muscle weakness.
Respiratory: cough, bronchitis.
Skin: cellulitis.
Other: flulike syndrome, *diabetic vascular disease, angioedema,* infection, trauma, diabetic neuropathy.

INTERACTIONS

Drug-drug. *Aliskiren:* May increase risk of renal impairment, hypotension, and hyperkalemia in diabetic patients and those with moderate to severe renal impairment (GFR less than 60 mL/minute). Concomitant use is contraindicated in diabetic patients. Avoid concomitant use in those with moderate to severe renal impairment.

Lithium: May increase lithium level. Monitor lithium level and patient for toxicity.
NSAIDs: May decrease antihypertensive effects. Monitor BP and renal function.
Potassium-sparing diuretics, potassium supplements: May cause hyperkalemia. Monitor patient closely.
Drug-herb. *Ma huang:* May decrease antihypertensive effects. Discourage use together.
Drug-food. *Salt substitutes containing potassium:* May cause hyperkalemia. Monitor patient closely.

EFFECTS ON LAB TEST RESULTS

• May increase liver enzyme or bilirubin levels.

CONTRAINDICATIONS & CAUTIONS

• Contraindicated in patients hypersensitive to drug.
• Concomitant use with aliskiren is contraindicated in diabetic patients.
• Use cautiously in patients with impaired renal or hepatic function.
Dialyzable drug: No.
⚠ **Overdose S&S:** Hypotension, tachycardia, bradycardia.

PREGNANCY-LACTATION-REPRODUCTION

Black Box Warning Drugs that act directly on the RAAS can cause fetal injury and death. If pregnancy is suspected, notify prescriber because drug should be stopped as soon as possible. ∎
• It isn't known if drug appears in breast milk. Patient should discontinue breastfeeding or discontinue drug, taking into account importance of drug to the mother.

NURSING CONSIDERATIONS

• Drug can be used alone or with other antihypertensives.
• If antihypertensive effect is inadequate using once-daily doses, a twice-daily regimen using the same or increased total daily dose may give a more satisfactory response.
• Monitor patient's BP closely to evaluate effectiveness of therapy. When used alone, drug has less of an effect on BP in black patients than in patients of other races.
• Monitor patients who are also taking diuretics for symptomatic hypotension.

• Regularly assess patient's renal function (via creatinine and BUN levels).
• Patients with severe HF whose renal function depends on the angiotensin-aldosterone system may develop acute renal failure during therapy. Closely monitor patient's BP, renal function, and potassium levels, especially during first few weeks of therapy and after dosage adjustments.
• *Look alike–sound alike:* Don't confuse Cozaar with Zocor or Colace.

PATIENT TEACHING
• Tell patient to avoid salt substitutes; these products may contain potassium, which can cause high potassium level in patients taking losartan.
• Inform woman of childbearing potential about consequences of taking drug while pregnant. Advise her to notify prescriber immediately if she suspects she is pregnant.
• Advise patient not to breast-feed while taking drug.
• Advise patient to report all adverse reactions and to immediately report swelling of face, eyes, lips, or tongue or breathing difficulty.

---

lovastatin (mevinolin)
loe-va-STA-tin

Altoprev, Mevacor

Therapeutic class: Antilipemics
Pharmacologic class: HMG-CoA reductase inhibitors

AVAILABLE FORMS
Tablets: 10 mg, 20 mg, 40 mg
Tablets (extended-release) ⬛: 20 mg, 40 mg, 60 mg

INDICATIONS & DOSAGES
Adjust-a-dose (for all indications): Avoid use of lovastatin with fibrates or niacin at doses greater than 1 g daily. For patients also taking danazol, diltiazem, dronedarone, or verapamil, start lovastatin at 10 mg (immediate-release) and don't exceed 20 mg daily. For patients also taking amiodarone, lovastatin dosage shouldn't exceed 40 mg daily unless clinical benefit is

likely to outweigh increased risk of myopathy or rhabdomyolysis. For elderly patients or patients with CrCl of less than 30 mL/minute, carefully consider dosage increase greater than 20 mg daily and implement cautiously if necessary. For patients requiring smaller reductions in cholesterol levels, use immediate-release lovastatin.

➤ **To prevent and treat CAD; hyperlipidemia**
Adults: Initially, 20 mg (immediate-release) P.O. once daily with evening meal. Recommended range is 10 to 80 mg as a single dose or in two divided doses; maximum daily recommended dose is 80 mg. Or, 20 to 60 mg extended-release tablets P.O. at bedtime.

Make dosage adjustments at intervals of 4 weeks or more.

➤ **Heterozygous familial hypercholesterolemia in adolescents**
Adolescents ages 10 to 17: Give 10 to 40 mg (immediate-release) daily P.O. with evening meal. Patients requiring reductions in LDL cholesterol level of 20% or more should start with 20 mg daily.

➤ **Primary prevention of CV disease**
Adults ages 40 to 75 with type 1 or type 2 diabetes (moderate-intensity therapy): 40 mg (immediate-release) P.O. once daily.
Adults ages 40 to 75 with an estimated 10-year atherosclerotic CV disease risk of 7.5% or more (moderate- to high-intensity therapy): 40 mg (immediate-release) P.O. once daily.

➤ **Secondary prevention of CV disease (moderate-intensity therapy)**
Adults older than age 75 or who aren't candidates for high-intensity therapy: 40 mg (immediate-release) P.O. once daily.

ADMINISTRATION
P.O.
• Give immediate-release drug with evening meal, which improves absorption and cholesterol biosynthesis. Give extended-release drug at bedtime.
• Don't crush, split, or allow patient to chew extended-release tablets.

ACTION
Inhibits HMG-CoA reductase, an early (and rate-limiting) step in cholesterol biosynthesis.

Route	Onset	Peak	Duration
P.O.	Unknown	2–4 hr	Unknown
P.O. (extended-release)	Unknown	12–14 hr	Unknown

Half-life: 1.1 to 1.7 hours.

ADVERSE REACTIONS
CNS: headache, dizziness, insomnia, peripheral neuropathy.
EENT: blurred vision.
GI: abdominal pain or cramps, constipation, diarrhea, dyspepsia, flatulence, heartburn, nausea, vomiting.
GU: UTI.
Musculoskeletal: muscle cramps, myalgia, myositis, *rhabdomyolysis.*
Skin: alopecia, rash, pruritus.
Other: flulike syndrome, pain, infection.

INTERACTIONS
Drug-drug. *Amiodarone:* May decrease the metabolism of lovastatin. Avoid combining lovastatin at doses exceeding 40 mg daily with amiodarone unless clinical benefit is likely to outweigh increased risk of myopathy.
Azole antifungals: May cause myopathy and rhabdomyolysis. Avoid using together.
Colchicine: May increase risk of myopathy or rhabdomyolysis. If coadministration can't be avoided, monitor patient for unexplained muscle pain, tenderness, or weakness.
Cyclosporine, gemfibrozil: May cause severe myopathy and rhabdomyolysis. Avoid this combination.
Danazol, diltiazem, dronedarone, verapamil: May cause myopathy and rhabdomyolysis. Don't exceed 20 mg lovastatin daily.
Dronedarone: May increase lovastatin serum concentration. Limit lovastatin to maximum of 20 mg/day (in adults). Increase monitoring for signs and symptoms of lovastatin toxicity (such as myopathy and rhabdomyolysis). Consider therapy modification.
Erythromycin, protease inhibitors (atazanavir, darunavir, fosamprenavir, indinavir, nefazodone, nelfinavir, riton-avir, saquinavir, tipranavir), strong CYP3A inhibitors (clarithromycin, itraconazole, ketoconazole, posaconazole, telithromycin, voriconazole): Increase risk of myopathy and rhabdomyolysis. Use together is contraindicated.
Macrolides (azithromycin, clarithromycin, telithromycin), nefazodone: May decrease metabolism of HMG-CoA reductase inhibitor, increasing toxicity. Monitor patient for adverse effects and report unexplained muscle pain.
Mifepristone (CYP3A4 inhibitor): May increase lovastatin plasma level, increasing risk of toxicity. Use together is contraindicated.
Niacin, other fibrates: May increase the risk for adverse and toxic effects of lovastatin. Avoid use of lovastatin with fibrates or niacin at doses greater than 1 g daily.
Oral anticoagulants: May increase anticoagulant effect. Monitor patient closely.
Phenytoin: May decrease serum concentration of HMG-CoA reductase inhibitors. Consider therapy modification.
Ranolazine: May increase risk of myopathy and rhabdomyolysis. Consider lovastatin dosage adjustment.
Drug-herb. *Eucalyptus, kava:* May increase risk of hepatotoxicity. Discourage use together.
Red yeast rice: May increase risk of adverse reactions because herb contains compounds similar to those in drug. Discourage use together.
Drug-food. *Grapefruit juice:* May increase drug level, increasing risk of adverse effects. Discourage use together.
Drug-lifestyle. *Alcohol use:* May increase risk of hepatotoxicity. Discourage use together.

EFFECTS ON LAB TEST RESULTS
• May increase ALT, AST, and CK levels.
• May cause thyroid function test abnormalities.

CONTRAINDICATIONS & CAUTIONS
• Contraindicated in patients hypersensitive to drug and in those with active liver disease or unexplained persistently increased transaminase level.

● Contraindicated in patients also taking erythromycin, protease inhibitors (atazanavir, darunavir, fosamprenavir, indinavir, nefazodone, nelfinavir, ritonavir, saquinavir, tipranavir), or strong CYP3A inhibitors (clarithromycin, itraconazole, ketoconazole, posaconazole, voriconazole, telithromycin) because of myopathy and rhabdomyolysis risk.

● Use cautiously in patients who consume substantial quantities of alcohol or have a history of liver disease.

Dialyzable drug: Unknown.

PREGNANCY-LACTATION-REPRODUCTION

● Drug may cause fetal harm and is contraindicated in women who are pregnant or may become pregnant. If patient becomes pregnant during therapy, apprise her of potential hazard to the fetus.

● It isn't known if drug appears in breast milk. Use in breast-feeding women is contraindicated.

NURSING CONSIDERATIONS

● Have patient follow a diet restricted in saturated fat and cholesterol during therapy.

● Obtain LFT results at the start of therapy; then monitor results periodically.

● Heterozygous familial hypercholesterolemia can be diagnosed in adolescent boys and in girls who are at least 1 year postmenarche and are 10 to 17 years old; if after an adequate trial of diet therapy LDL cholesterol level remains over 189 mg/dL or LDL cholesterol over 160 mg/dL and patient has a positive family history of premature CV disease or two or more other CV disease risk factors.

● Obtain CK level in patients with unexplained muscle pain.

● Discontinue lovastatin immediately if markedly elevated CK levels occur or myopathy is diagnosed or suspected.

● Predisposing factors for skeletal muscle effects include advanced age (65 and older), female gender, uncontrolled hypothyroidism, and renal impairment.

● *Look alike–sound alike:* Don't confuse lovastatin with Lotensin.

PATIENT TEACHING

● Instruct patient to take immediate-release drug with the evening meal and extended-release drug at bedtime.

● Teach patient about proper dietary management of cholesterol and triglycerides. When appropriate, recommend weight control, exercise, and smoking cessation programs.

● Instruct patient to store tablets at room temperature in a light-resistant container.

● Advise patient of the risk of myopathy and rhabdomyolysis and tell him to promptly report unexplained muscle pain, tenderness, or weakness, particularly when accompanied by malaise or fever.

● Teach patient about substances that shouldn't be taken with lovastatin and tell him to inform other health care providers that he's taking lovastatin, especially if a new medication is being prescribed.

● Caution patient to avoid grapefruit juice while taking drug.

⊙ *Alert:* Tell woman to stop drug and notify prescriber immediately if she is or may be pregnant or if she's breast-feeding.

⊙ *Alert:* Advise patient not to crush or chew extended-release tablets.

lumacaftor–ivacaftor
LOO-ma-kaf-tor/EYE-va-kaf-tor

Orkambi

Therapeutic class: Metabolic agents
Pharmacologic class: Cystic fibrosis transmembrane conductance regulator (CFTR) potentiators

AVAILABLE FORMS
Tablets: 200 mg lumacaftor/125 mg ivacaftor

INDICATIONS & DOSAGES
➤ **Treatment of cystic fibrosis (CF) in patients who are homozygous for the F508del mutation in the *CFTR* gene**
Adults and children age 12 and older: 400 mg lumacaftor/250 mg ivacaftor P.O. every 12 hours.

Adjust-a-dose: In patients with moderate hepatic impairment (Child-Pugh class B), reduce dose to 2 tablets in the morning and 1 tablet in the evening. In patients with severe hepatic impairment (Child-Pugh class C), use cautiously and give 1 tablet in the morning and 1 tablet in the evening or less if medically indicated, weighing risks and benefits of treatment. In patients currently taking strong CYP3A inhibitors (clarithromycin, itraconazole, ketoconazole, posaconazole, telithromycin, voriconazole), initiate drug at reduced dose of 1 tablet daily for first week of treatment, then continue with recommended daily dose. No dosage adjustment is needed when CYP3A inhibitors are initiated in patients already taking lumacaftor–ivacaftor. If drug is interrupted for more than 1 week and then reinitiated in patients taking strong CYP3A inhibitors, reduce dosage to 1 tablet daily for first week of treatment reinitiation, then continue with recommended daily dose. Withhold drug in patients with ALT or AST level greater than 5 × ULN when not associated with elevated bilirubin level and in those with ALT or AST elevations greater than 3 × ULN with bilirubin elevations greater than 2 × ULN. After resolution of transaminase elevations, consider benefits and risks of resuming drug.

ADMINISTRATION
P.O.
● If patient's genotype is unknown, use an FDA-cleared CF mutation test to detect the presence of the F508del mutation on both alleles of the *CFTR* gene before prescribing drug.
● Give drug with fat-containing foods (eggs, avocados, nuts, butter, peanut butter, cheese pizza, whole-milk dairy products).
● If a dose is missed, give missed dose within 6 hours. If more than 6 hours has elapsed after the usual dosing time, skip missed dose and resume normal schedule for the following dose. Don't double-dose.
● Store at room temperature (68° to 77° F [20° to 25° C]).

ACTION
Lumacaftor improves the conformational stability of F508del-*CFTR*, allowing for greater activity processing and trafficking mature protein to the cell surface. Ivacaftor

is a CFTR potentiator that facilitates increased chloride transport by potentiating the movement of CFTR protein at the cell surface. Increasing and potentiating CFTR help combat the pathophysiology of CF.

Route	Onset	Peak	Duration
P.O.	Unknown	4 hr	Unknown

Half-life: Lumacaftor, 26 hours; ivacaftor, 9 hours.

ADVERSE REACTIONS
CNS: fatigue.
EENT: nasopharyngitis, rhinorrhea.
GI: nausea, diarrhea, flatulence.
GU: menstrual abnormalities.
Respiratory: cough, dyspnea, URI, abnormal respirations, hemoptysis.
Skin: rash.
Other: flulike symptoms.

INTERACTIONS
Drug-drug. *Antacids (except calcium carbonate), H$_2$ blockers, PPIs (esomeprazole, lansoprazole, omeprazole):* May reduce effectiveness of these drugs. Adjust dosage as needed to achieve desired clinical effects.
Clarithromycin, erythromycin, telithromycin: May reduce effectiveness of anti-infective. Consider alternative agents, such as ciprofloxacin, azithromycin, or levofloxacin.
CYP2B6, CYP2C8, CYP2C9, CYP2C19 substrates: May alter concentrations of these substrates. Monitor patient carefully.
CYP3A substrates (cyclosporine, everolimus, midazolam, sirolimus, tacrolimus, triazolam): May decrease concentrations of CYP3A substrates. Don't use together.
Digoxin: May alter digoxin concentration. Monitor digoxin level and titrate dosage as needed.
Hormonal contraceptives (implantable, injectable, oral, transdermal): May reduce effectiveness of contraceptive and increase occurrence of abnormal menstrual events. Avoid concomitant use and consider nonhormonal contraceptive methods.
Ibuprofen, citalopram, escitalopram, methylprednisolone, montelukast, prednisone, sertraline: May reduce effectiveness of these drugs. Consider higher doses of these drugs to obtain desired effects.

Itraconazole, ketoconazole, posaconazole, voriconazole: May decrease effectiveness of antifungals. If these drugs are necessary, monitor patient for breakthrough fungal infections. Consider an alternative drug such as fluconazole.

Strong CYP3A inducers (carbamazepine, phenobarbital, phenytoin, rifabutin, rifampin): May decrease ivacaftor concentration. Concomitant use isn't recommended.

Strong CYP3A inhibitors (clarithromycin, itraconazole, ketoconazole, posaconazole, telithromycin, voriconazole): May increase ivacaftor concentration. When initiating in patients taking strong CYP3A inhibitors, reduce dose to 1 tablet daily for first week of treatment, then continue with recommended daily dose.

Sulfonylureas, repaglinide: May reduce effectiveness of these drugs. Adjust dosage of these drugs as needed to obtain desired clinical effect.

Warfarin: May affect warfarin concentration. Monitor INR.

Drug-herb. *St. John's wort:* May decrease ivacaftor concentration. Concomitant use isn't recommended.

EFFECTS ON LAB TEST RESULTS

● May increase blood CK, AST, ALT, and bilirubin levels.

CONTRAINDICATIONS & CAUTIONS

● Use cautiously in patients with advanced liver disease and only if benefits are expected to outweigh risks. Worsening of liver function, including hepatic encephalopathy, in patients with advanced liver disease has been reported.

● Use cautiously in patients with FEV_1 (forced expiratory volume in 1 second) less than 40%. Respiratory events (chest discomfort, dyspnea, abnormal respirations) have been reported.

● Use cautiously in patients with severe renal impairment (CrCl of less than 30 mL/minute) or ESRD.

● Drug may contribute to cataract development in children.

● Safety and effectiveness in children younger than age 12 haven't been established.

Dialyzable drug: Unlikely.

PREGNANCY-LACTATION-REPRODUCTION

● There are no adequate studies in pregnant women. Use cautiously during pregnancy and only if clearly needed.

● Both drug components may appear in breast milk. Use cautiously in breastfeeding women.

NURSING CONSIDERATIONS

● Assess ALT, AST, and bilirubin levels before therapy initiation, every 3 months during first year of treatment, and annually thereafter. For patients with a history of ALT, AST, or bilirubin elevation, consider more frequent monitoring. Monitor patients with ALT, AST, or bilirubin increases until abnormalities resolve.

● Closely monitor patients with advanced liver disease after initiation of treatment, and reduce dosage accordingly.

● Baseline and regular ophthalmologic examinations are recommended in children and adolescents because drug may contribute to cataract development.

● Interrupt therapy for ALT or AST elevation greater than 5 × ULN when not associated with elevated bilirubin level or for ALT or AST elevations greater than 3 × ULN with bilirubin elevations greater than 2 × ULN. Weigh risks and benefits before resuming drug.

● Monitor pulmonary function, especially if FEV_1 is less than 40%.

PATIENT TEACHING

● Teach patient to always take drug with high-fat foods.

● Explain to patient that a missed dose can be taken within 6 hours of dosing time but that if more than 6 hours have elapsed, the missed dose should be skipped and the normal schedule should be resumed for the following dose. Warn patient not to double-dose.

● Inform patient that chest discomfort, dyspnea, and abnormal respirations are more common at start of treatment.

● Teach patient to immediately report signs and symptoms of liver disease (pain or discomfort in upper right abdominal area, loss of appetite, dark amber-colored urine, yellowing of the skin or eyes, nausea or vomiting, confusion).

Reactions in bold italics are ***life-threatening***. Interactions may have a *rapid onset* or a ***delayed onset***.

- Instruct patient of need for regular blood work to monitor liver function.
- Advise patient and family that drug isn't a cure for CF.
- Inform patient taking hormonal contraceptives to switch to a nonhormonal contraceptive during therapy, because hormonal contraceptives may be less effective.
- Instruct patient to inform prescriber of all drugs, supplements, and OTC products being taken, because they may interfere with drug.
- Instruct parents of children and adolescents that these patients should undergo regular eye examinations during therapy.
- Caution patient that this drug combination may cause dizziness and to avoid driving, using machinery, or performing tasks that require alertness until drug's effects are known.

lurasidone hydrochloride
loo-RAS-i-dohne

Latuda✐

Therapeutic class: Antipsychotics
Pharmacologic class: Dopamine–serotonin receptor antagonists

AVAILABLE FORMS
Tablets: 20 mg, 40 mg, 60 mg, 80 mg, 120 mg

INDICATIONS & DOSAGES
Adjust-a-dose (for all indications): For patients with moderate (CrCl of 30 to less than 50 mL/minute) or severe (CrCl of less than 30 mL/minute) renal impairment or those concomitantly taking a moderate CYP3A4 inhibitor (such as diltiazem), the recommended starting dose is 20 mg and the maximum recommended dose is 80 mg. For patients with moderate (Child-Pugh score 7 to 9) or severe (Child-Pugh score 10 to 15) hepatic impairment, the recommended starting dose is 20 mg. The maximum recommended dose is 80 mg for patients with moderate hepatic impairment and 40 mg for those with severe hepatic impairment.

➤ **Schizophrenia**
Adults: Initially, 40 mg P.O. once daily. May increase to maximum dose of 160 mg daily.
➤ **Depressive episodes associated with bipolar I disorder as monotherapy or as adjunctive therapy with lithium or valproate**
Adults: Initially, 20 mg P.O. once daily. May increase to maximum of 120 mg daily.

ADMINISTRATION
P.O.
- Give with food (at least 350 calories).

ACTION
Exact mechanism is unknown. Drug's efficacy is mediated through antagonism at the dopamine type 2 and serotonin type 2 receptors.

Route	Onset	Peak	Duration
P.O.	Unknown	1–3 hr	Unknown

Half-life: 18 hours.

ADVERSE REACTIONS
CNS: somnolence, akathisia, parkinsonism (bradykinesia, cogwheel rigidity, drooling, extrapyramidal disorder, hypokinesia, muscle rigidity, psychomotor retardation, tremor), agitation, dystonia, dizziness, insomnia, anxiety, restlessness, seizures, fatigue.
CV: tachycardia.
EENT: blurred vision, nasopharyngitis.
GI: nausea, vomiting, dyspepsia, abdominal pain, diarrhea, dysphagia, increased appetite.
GU: UTI.
Metabolic: dyslipidemia, hyperglycemia, weight gain.
Musculoskeletal: back pain.
Skin: rash, pruritus.

INTERACTIONS
Drug-drug. *Antihypertensives:* May increase risk of hypotension. Monitor orthostatic vital signs and adjust antihypertensive dosage as needed.
Centrally acting drugs: May increase risk of adverse effects (increased cognitive impairment). Avoid use together.
Moderate inhibitors of CYP3A4 (atazanavir, diltiazem, erythromycin,

fluconazole, verapamil): May increase lurasidone level. Use together cautiously and reduce lurasidone dosage by 50%. Initial recommended lurasidone dose is 20 mg daily, with maximum dose of 80 mg daily.

Black Box Warning *Opioids:* May cause slow or difficult breathing, sedation, and death. Avoid use together. If use together is necessary, limit dosage and duration of each drug to the minimum necessary for desired effect. ■

Strong inducers of CYP3A4 (avasimibe, carbamazepine, phenytoin, rifampin): May significantly reduce lurasidone level. Don't use together.

Strong inhibitors of CYP3A4 (clarithromycin, ketoconazole, mibefradil, ritonavir, voriconazole): May significantly increase lurasidone level. Don't use together.

Drug-lifestyle. *Alcohol use:* May increase risk of adverse effects (such as increased cognitive impairment). Discourage use together.

Drug-food. *Grapefruit, grapefruit juice:* May increase lurasidone level. Patient should avoid grapefruit and grapefruit juice during therapy.

Drug-herb. *St. John's wort:* May significantly reduce lurasidone level. Don't use together.

EFFECTS ON LAB TEST RESULTS

● May increase prolactin, total cholesterol, triglyceride, glucose, serum creatinine, AST, ALT, and CK levels.
● May decrease WBC, neutrophil, and granulocyte counts.

CONTRAINDICATIONS & CAUTIONS

● Contraindicated in patients hypersensitive to drug or its components.
● Contraindicated for concomitant use with strong CYP3A4 inhibitors or inducers. If used concomitantly with a moderate CYP3A4 inducer, it may be necessary to increase lurasidone dosage after long-term treatment (7 days or more) with the CYP3A4 inducer.

Black Box Warning Opioid drugs should only be prescribed with benzodiazepines or other CNS depressants to patients for

whom alternative treatment options are inadequate. ■

Black Box Warning Elderly patients with dementia-related psychosis treated with atypical or conventional antipsychotics are at increased risk for death. Antipsychotics aren't approved for the treatment of dementia-related psychosis. ■

● Use cautiously in patients with hyperlipidemia, diabetes or risk factors for diabetes (family history, obesity), seizures or conditions that lower the seizure threshold (Alzheimer dementia), body temperature dysregulation, major depressive disorder, suicide attempts, dysphagia, or concomitant illness.
● Use cautiously in patients with known CV disease, cerebrovascular disease, and conditions that cause hypotension (dehydration, hypovolemia, antihypertensive use) and in antipsychotic-naive patients because of increased risk of dizziness, tachycardia or bradycardia, and syncope.
● Use cautiously in patients with preexisting low WBC count or a history of drug-induced neutropenia or leukopenia.
● Safety and effectiveness in children haven't been established.

Dialyzable drug: Unknown.

PREGNANCY-LACTATION-REPRODUCTION

● There are no adequate studies in pregnant women. Use during pregnancy only if clearly needed and potential benefit justifies potential risk to the fetus. Drug may cause abnormal muscle movements (extrapyramidal symptoms) or withdrawal symptoms in newborns.
● Enroll women ages 18 to 45 exposed to lurasidone during pregnancy in the National Pregnancy Registry for Atypical Antipsychotics (1-866-961-2388).
● It isn't known if drug appears in breast milk. Patient should discontinue breastfeeding or discontinue drug.

NURSING CONSIDERATIONS

Black Box Warning Antidepressants increase risk of suicidal thinking and behavior in children, adolescents, and young adults. Monitor all patients for worsening of depression or emergence of suicidal thoughts and behaviors. ■

• Monitor patients for tardive dyskinesia. Risk increases in elderly patients and women and with long-term administration. Use the lowest dose for the shortest time possible to minimize risk. Discontinue drug if symptoms occur.

• Monitor patients for orthostatic hypotension, syncope, and excessive sedation.

• Monitor patients for signs and symptoms of neuroleptic malignant syndrome (NMS), such as fever, diaphoresis, muscle rigidity, altered mental status, irregular pulse or BP, cardiac arrhythmias, increased CK level, rhabdomyolysis, and acute renal failure. Discontinue drug immediately if NMS occurs.

• Monitor CBC, renal function, and prolactin level periodically; discontinue drug if severe neutropenia develops.

• Monitor patients for metabolic changes (such as weight gain and elevated blood glucose, triglyceride, or cholesterol levels), and treat appropriately.

• Psychotic illness predisposes patients to suicide. Assess patients for suicidal thoughts and prescribe drug in small quantities to reduce risk of overdose.

PATIENT TEACHING
Black Box Warning Caution the patient or the caregiver of a patient taking an opioid drug with a benzodiazepine, CNS depressant, or alcohol to seek immediate medical attention if the patient has symptoms of dizziness, light-headedness, extreme sleepiness, slowed or difficult breathing, or unresponsiveness. ∎

Black Box Warning Advise family or caregivers to observe patient closely for worsening of depression or suicidal thoughts and behaviors. Encourage them to report such behaviors to health care provider immediately. ∎

• Advise patient to take drug on a regular basis and not to skip doses.

• Inform patient that periodic blood tests will be needed to monitor tolerance to the drug.

• Tell patient to avoid overheating and to maintain adequate hydration.

• Teach patient to monitor weight and maintain a healthy diet because drug may increase weight and blood glucose and cholesterol levels.

• Instruct patient to report all adverse reactions and to immediately report sudden changes in temperature or BP, irregular HR, or severe muscle rigidity.

• Counsel female patient to tell her prescriber if she is pregnant or breast-feeding before taking drug.

• Tell patient to avoid alcohol and grapefruit products during therapy.

• Warn patient to avoid driving or operating hazardous machinery until drug's effects are known.

SAFETY ALERT!

magnesium sulfate

Therapeutic class: Electrolyte replacements
Pharmacologic class: Minerals

AVAILABLE FORMS
Injectable: 4%, 8%, 50% in 2-, 10-, 20-, and 50-mL ampules, vials, and prefilled syringes
Injection solution: 1% in D_5W, 2% in D_5W, 4% in water for injection, 8% in water for injection

INDICATIONS & DOSAGES
Adjust-a-dose (for all indications): In severe renal impairment, reduce dosage and obtain frequent serum magnesium levels.
➤ **Mild hypomagnesemia**
Adults: 1 g I.M. every 6 hours for four doses, depending on magnesium level.
➤ **Symptomatic severe hypomagnesemia, with magnesium level of 0.8 mEq/L or less**
Adults: 5 g I.V. in 1 L of D_5W or NSS over 3 hours. Base subsequent doses on magnesium level.
➤ **Magnesium supplementation in total parenteral nutrition (TPN)**
Adults: 8 to 24 mEq I.V. daily added to TPN solution.
Infants: 2 to 10 mEq/day I.V. added to TPN solution.
➤ **Seizures in preeclampsia or eclampsia**
Adults: Total initial dose is 10 to 14 g I.V. To accomplish this, give 4 to 5 g I.V. in 250 mL of solution and simultaneously give up to

10 g I.M. (5 g or 10 mL of the undiluted 50% solution in each buttock). Base subsequent doses on magnesium level. Don't exceed 40 g in a 24-hour period. Maximum dose in patients with severe renal insufficiency is 20 g/48 hours.

ADMINISTRATION
P.O.
● Store between 68° and 77° F (20° and 25° C).
I.V.
▼ Concentration should be 200 mg/mL or less.
▼ Inject bolus dose slowly at a rate of 150 mg/minute or less, or use infusion pump for continuous infusion to avoid respiratory or cardiac arrest. Maximum infusion rate is 150 mg/minute. Rapid drip causes feeling of heat.
▼ For severe hypomagnesemia, watch for respiratory depression and evidence of heart block. Respirations should be better than 16 breaths/minute before giving dose.
▼ **Incompatibilities:** Alcohol (in high concentrations), alkali carbonates and bicarbonates, amiodarone, barium, calcium chloride, calcium gluconate, clindamycin, heavy metals, hydrocortisone, polymyxin B, procaine, salicylates, sodium bicarbonate, soluble phosphates, strontium, tartrates.
I.M.
● Undiluted 50% solutions may be given by deep I.M. injection to adults. Dilute solutions to 20% or less for use in children.

ACTION
Replaces magnesium and maintains magnesium level; as an anticonvulsant, reduces muscle contractions by interfering with release of acetylcholine at myoneural junction.

Route	Onset	Peak	Duration
P.O.	Unknown	4 hr	4–6 hr
I.V.	Immediate	Unknown	30 min
I.M.	1 hr	Unknown	3–4 hr

Half-life: Unknown.

ADVERSE REACTIONS
CNS: toxicity, weak or absent deep tendon reflexes, flaccid paralysis, drowsiness, stupor.
CV: slow, weak pulse; *arrhythmias;* hypotension; *circulatory collapse;* flushing.
GI: diarrhea.
Metabolic: hypocalcemia.
Respiratory: *respiratory paralysis.*
Skin: diaphoresis.
Other: hypothermia.

INTERACTIONS
Drug-drug. *Alendronate, fluoroquinolones, nitrofurantoin, penicillamine, sodium polystyrene sulfonate, tetracyclines:* May decrease bioavailability with oral magnesium supplements. Separate doses by 2 to 3 hours.
Cardiac glycosides: May cause serious cardiac conduction changes. Use together with caution.
CNS depressants: May have additive effect. Use together cautiously.
Neuromuscular blockers: May cause increased neuromuscular blockage. Use together cautiously.
Nifedipine: May increase risk of neuromuscular blockade and hypotension. Closely monitor clinical response.
Drug-lifestyle. *Alcohol use:* May decrease magnesium level. Discourage use together.

EFFECTS ON LAB TEST RESULTS
● May increase magnesium level. May decrease calcium level.

CONTRAINDICATIONS & CAUTIONS
● Contraindicated in patients with myocardial damage, heart block, or coma.
● Use cautiously in patients with impaired renal function.
�ును *Alert:* Using magnesium sulfate to stop preterm labor isn't an FDA-approved use of drug; safety and effectiveness of drug for this indication haven't been established.
Dialyzable drug: Yes.
⚠ *Overdose S&S:* Hypotension, facial flushing, feeling of warmth, thirst, nausea, vomiting, lethargy, dysarthria, drowsiness, diminished deep tendon reflexes, shallow respirations, apnea, coma, cardiac arrest,

---

Reactions in bold italics are *life-threatening*. Interactions may have a *rapid onset* or a *delayed onset*.

respiratory paralysis, disappearance of patellar reflex.

PREGNANCY-LACTATION-REPRODUCTION

🚯 *Alert:* Drug can cause fetal abnormalities (fetal hypocalcemia, bone abnormalities), especially when given beyond 5 to 7 days to pregnant women. Use during pregnancy only if clearly needed and inform patient of potential fetal harm.

• Contraindicated in pregnant women in actively progressing labor and in pregnant women with toxemia of pregnancy during the 2 hours preceding delivery.

• Drug appears in breast milk. Use cautiously in breast-feeding women.

NURSING CONSIDERATIONS

• Keep I.V. calcium available to reverse magnesium intoxication.

• Test knee-jerk and patellar reflexes before each additional dose. If absent, notify prescriber and give no more magnesium until reflexes return; otherwise, patient may develop temporary respiratory failure and need cardiopulmonary resuscitation or I.V. administration of calcium.

• Check magnesium level after repeated doses. Monitor levels hourly in patients with severe hypomagnesemia.

• Monitor fluid intake and output. Output should be 100 mL or more during 4-hour period before dose.

• Monitor renal function.

• Drug may contain aluminum. Premature neonates are at higher risk for aluminum toxicity due to immature renal function. Aluminum exposure of more than 4 to 5 mcg/kg/day is associated with CNS and bone toxicity.

• *Look alike–sound alike:* Don't confuse magnesium sulfate with manganese sulfate.

PATIENT TEACHING

• Explain use and administration of drug to patient and family.

• Tell patient to report all adverse effects.

mannitol
MAN-i-tole

Osmitrol

Therapeutic class: Diuretics
Pharmacologic class: Osmotic diuretics

AVAILABLE FORMS

Injection: 5%, 10%, 15%, 20%, 25%
Solution for irrigation: 5 g/100 mL

INDICATIONS & DOSAGES

➤ **Test dose for marked oliguria or suspected inadequate renal function**
Adults and children older than age 12: 200 mg/kg (about 75 mL of a 20% I.V. solution or 50 mL of a 25% solution) over 3 to 5 minutes. Response is adequate if 30 to 50 mL of urine/hour is excreted over 2 to 3 hours; if response is inadequate, a second test dose is given. If still no response after second dose, stop drug.

➤ **Oliguria**
Adults and children older than age 12: 50 to 100 g I.V. as a 20% solution over 90 minutes to several hours.

➤ **To prevent oliguria or acute renal failure**
Adults and children older than age 12: 50 to 100 g I.V. of a 5% to 25% solution. Determine exact concentration by fluid requirements.

➤ **To reduce intraocular or intracranial pressure or cerebral edema**
Adults and children older than age 12: 1.5 to 2 g/kg as a 15%, 20%, or 25% I.V. solution over 30 to 60 minutes. For maximum IOP reduction before surgery, give 60 to 90 minutes preoperatively.

➤ **Diuresis in drug intoxication**
Adults and children older than age 12: 5% to 25% solution continuously up to 200 g I.V., while maintaining 100 to 500 mL urine output/hour and a positive fluid balance.

➤ **Irrigating solution during transurethral surgical procedures**
Adults: 2.5% to 5% solution.

M

ADMINISTRATION
I.V.

▼ Change I.V. administration apparatus every 24 hours.

▼ To redissolve crystallized solution (crystallization occurs at low temperatures or in concentrations higher than 15%), warm bottle or bag by appropriate means to approximately 140° F (60° C) with occasional shaking. Cool to body temperature before giving. Don't use solution with undissolved crystals.

▼ Give as intermittent or continuous infusion at prescribed rate, using an inline filter and an infusion pump. Don't give as direct injection.

▼ Check patency at infusion site before and during administration.

▼ Monitor patient for signs and symptoms of infiltration; if it occurs, watch for inflammation, edema, and necrosis.

▼ **Incompatibilities:** Blood products and other drugs.

ACTION
Increases osmotic pressure of glomerular filtrate, thus inhibiting tubular reabsorption of water and electrolytes. Drug elevates plasma osmolality and increases urine output.

Route	Onset	Peak	Duration
I.V.	30–60 min	1 hr	6–8 hr

Half-life: About 1½ hours.

ADVERSE REACTIONS
CNS: *seizures,* dizziness, headache, fever.
CV: edema, thrombophlebitis, hypotension, hypertension, *HF,* tachycardia, angina-like chest pain, vascular overload.
EENT: blurred vision, rhinitis.
GI: thirst, dry mouth, nausea, vomiting, diarrhea.
GU: urine retention.
Metabolic: dehydration, fluid and electrolyte imbalance.
Respiratory: *pulmonary edema.*
Skin: local pain, urticaria.
Other: chills, thirst.

INTERACTIONS
Drug-drug. *Lithium:* May increase urinary excretion of lithium. Monitor lithium level closely.
Nephrotoxic drugs (aminoglycosides, cyclosporine): May increase risk of toxicity and renal failure. Avoid use together.
Opioid analgesics: May increase diuretic-related adverse effects and diminish therapeutic effects of diuretics. Monitor therapy.

EFFECTS ON LAB TEST RESULTS
● May increase or decrease electrolyte levels.
● May interfere with tests for inorganic phosphorus or ethylene glycol level.

CONTRAINDICATIONS & CAUTIONS
● Contraindicated in patients hypersensitive to drug.
● Contraindicated in patients with anuria; severe pulmonary congestion; frank pulmonary edema; active intracranial bleeding (except during craniotomy); severe dehydration; metabolic edema; previous progressive renal disease or dysfunction after starting drug, including increasing azotemia and oliguria; previous progressive HF or pulmonary congestion after treatment with drug; or failure to respond to test dose.
Dialyzable drug: Yes.
⚠ *Overdose S&S:* Increased electrolyte excretion, orthostatic tachycardia or hypotension, decreased central venous pressure, impaired neuromuscular function, intestinal dilation and ileus, pulmonary edema or water intoxication if urine output is inadequate.

PREGNANCY-LACTATION-REPRODUCTION
● There are no adequate studies in pregnant women. Use during pregnancy only if clearly needed and potential benefit justifies potential risk to the fetus.
● It isn't known if drug appears in breast milk. Use cautiously in breast-feeding women.

NURSING CONSIDERATIONS
● Monitor vital signs, including central venous pressure and fluid intake and output hourly. Report increasing oliguria. Check weight, renal function, fluid balance, and

---

serum and urine sodium and potassium levels daily.

• In comatose or incontinent patient, use urinary catheter because therapy is based on strict evaluation of fluid intake and output. If patient has urinary catheter, use an hourly urometer collection bag to evaluate output accurately and easily.

• To relieve thirst, give frequent mouth care or fluids.

• Drug is commonly used in chemotherapy regimens to enhance diuresis of renally toxic drugs.

• Don't give electrolyte-free solutions with blood. If blood is given simultaneously, add at least 20 mEq of sodium chloride to each liter of drug solution to avoid pseudoagglutination.

PATIENT TEACHING
• Tell patient that he may feel thirsty or have a dry mouth, and emphasize importance of drinking only the amount of fluids ordered.

• Instruct patient to promptly report adverse reactions and discomfort at I.V. site.

maraviroc
mahr-AY-vih-rok

Selzentry

Therapeutic class: Antiretrovirals
Pharmacologic class: CCR5 co-receptor antagonists

AVAILABLE FORMS
Tablets: 150 mg, 300 mg

INDICATIONS & DOSAGES
➤ **Combined with CYP3A4 inhibitors, including protease inhibitors (except tipranavir and ritonavir), to treat CCR5-tropic HIV-1 infection with evidence of viral replication or HIV-1 strains resistant to multiple antiretrovirals**
Adults and children age 16 and older: 150 mg P.O. b.i.d.

Adjust-a-dose: Use isn't recommended in patients with CrCl of less than 30 mL/minute or in those with ESRD on regular hemodialysis.

➤ **Combined with nucleoside reverse transcriptase inhibitors, tipranavir–ritonavir, nevirapine, raltegravir, or enfuvirtide to treat CCR5-tropic HIV-1 infection**
Adults and children age 16 and older: 300 mg P.O. b.i.d.

Adjust-a-dose: For patients with severe renal impairment (CrCl of less than 30 mL/minute) or ESRD on hemodialysis give 300 mg b.i.d.; if patient experiences orthostatic hypotension, reduce dosage to 150 mg P.O. b.i.d.

➤ **Combined with CYP3A inducers, including efavirenz, without strong CYP3A inhibitors, to treat CCR5-tropic HIV-1 infection**
Adults and children age 16 and older: 600 mg P.O. b.i.d.

Adjust-a-dose: Use isn't recommended in patients with CrCl of less than 30 mL/minute or in those with ESRD on regular hemodialysis.

ADMINISTRATION
P.O.
• Give drug without regard for food.

ACTION
Blocks viral entry into cells by binding to chemokine receptor type 5 co-receptor and preventing the initiation of HIV replication cycle.

Route	Onset	Peak	Duration
P.O.	Unknown	½–4 hr	Unknown

Half-life: 14 to 18 hours.

ADVERSE REACTIONS
CNS: anxiety, dizziness, paresthesia, sensory abnormalities, peripheral neuropathy, sleep disturbances, depressive disorders, pyrexia, pain, disturbances in consciousness, *stroke.*
CV: unstable angina, *acute cardiac failure,* CAD, endocarditis, *MI,* myocardial ischemia, vascular hypertensive disorders.
EENT: conjunctivitis, ocular infections, otitis media, nasal congestion, paranasal sinus disorders, sinusitis.
GI: abdominal pain, constipation, dyspepsia, stomatitis, appetite disorders.
GU: urinary tract signs and symptoms.

Hepatic: *cirrhosis, hepatic failure,* cholestatic jaundice.
Metabolic: lipodystrophies.
Musculoskeletal: muscle pains, joint pain, myositis, osteonecrosis, *rhabdomyolysis.*
Respiratory: URI, bronchitis, cough, pneumonia.
Skin: rash, pruritus, dermatitis, eczema, folliculitis, condyloma acuminata.
Other: herpes infection, immune reconstitution syndrome, influenza.

INTERACTIONS

Drug-drug. *Clarithromycin, CYP3A inhibitors (protease inhibitors except tipranavir–ritonavir), delavirdine, elvitegravir–ritonavir, itraconazole, ketoconazole, nefazodone, telithromycin:* May increase maraviroc level. Decrease maraviroc dosage.
CYP3A inducers (carbamazepine, efavirenz, etravirine, phenobarbital, phenytoin, rifampin): May decrease maraviroc level. Increase maraviroc dosage.
Drug-herb. *St. John's wort:* May decrease maraviroc level. Discourage use together.

EFFECTS ON LAB TEST RESULTS

● May increase AST, ALT, bilirubin, amylase, lipase, and CK levels.
● May decrease ANC.

CONTRAINDICATIONS & CAUTIONS

● Contraindicated in patients hypersensitive to drug or its components.
Black Box Warning Hepatotoxicity has been reported with maraviroc use. Severe rash or evidence of a systemic allergic reaction (fever, eosinophilia, or elevated immunoglobulin E level) before the development of hepatotoxicity may occur. Immediately evaluate patients with signs or symptoms of hepatitis or allergic reaction after drug use. ■
● Severe and potentially life-threatening skin and hypersensitivity reactions, including Stevens-Johnson syndrome, toxic epidermal necrolysis, and drug rash with eosinophilia with systemic symptoms (DRESS), have been reported. Discontinue drug if signs or symptoms of hypersensitivity occur.

● Contraindicated in patients with severe renal impairment or ESRD (CrCl of less than 30 mL/minute) who are taking potent CYP3A inhibitors or inducers.
● Use cautiously in patients with preexisting liver dysfunction or patients who are infected with HBV or HCV.
● Use cautiously in patients at risk for CV events, with a history of postural hypotension, or taking another medication known to lower BP.
● During initial phase of treatment, patients treated with combination antiretroviral therapy may develop an inflammatory response to indolent or residual opportunistic infections (CMV, *Mycobacterium avium* complex, *Pneumocystis jiroveci* pneumonia, TB), which may necessitate further evaluation and treatment. Autoimmune disorders (such as Graves disease, polymyositis, and Guillain-Barré syndrome) have also been reported in the setting of immune reconstitution; however, time to onset is more variable, and onset can occur many months after initiation of antiretroviral treatment.
● Safety and effectiveness haven't been established in children younger than age 16.
Dialyzable drug: No.

PREGNANCY-LACTATION-REPRODUCTION

● There are no adequate studies in pregnant women. Use during pregnancy only if potential benefit justifies potential fetal risk.
● Pregnant women exposed to drug should be registered in the Antiretroviral Pregnancy Registry (1-800-258-4263).
● Patient shouldn't breast-feed while taking drug because of potential for HIV transmission and serious adverse reactions in infants.

NURSING CONSIDERATIONS

● Effectiveness hasn't been established in patients with dual, mixed, or CXCR4-tropic HIV-1 infection.
● Monitor patient closely for signs and symptoms of infection.

PATIENT TEACHING

● Instruct patient to immediately report signs or symptoms of hepatitis or allergic reaction (rash, yellow eyes or skins, dark urine, vomiting, and abdominal pain).

Reactions in bold italics are *life-threatening*. Interactions may have a *rapid onset* or a *delayed onset*.

- Caution patient that drug doesn't cure HIV infection and that he may still develop HIV-related illness, including opportunistic infections.
- Caution patient that drug doesn't reduce risk of transmission of HIV to others.
- If patient feels dizzy while taking drug, advise him to avoid driving or operating machinery.
- Instruct woman to tell her prescriber if she's pregnant or planning to become pregnant while taking drug.
- Advise patient not to breast-feed during therapy.
- Advise patient to take drug every day as prescribed with other antiretrovirals. Tell patient not to change the dose or dosing schedule or stop any antiretroviral without consulting prescriber.

---

medroxyPROGESTERone acetate
me-DROX-ee-proe-JESS-te-rone

Depo-Provera, Depo-subQ
Provera 104, Provera✔

Therapeutic class: Estrogens
Pharmacologic class: Progestins

AVAILABLE FORMS
Injection (suspension): 104 mg/0.65 mL, 150 mg/mL, 400 mg/mL
Tablets: 2.5 mg, 5 mg, 10 mg

INDICATIONS & DOSAGES
➤ **Abnormal uterine bleeding caused by hormonal imbalance**
Women: 5 to 10 mg P.O. daily for 5 to 10 days beginning on day 16 or 21 of menstrual cycle. If patient also has received estrogen, give 10 mg P.O. daily for 10 days beginning on day 16 or 21 of cycle.
➤ **Secondary amenorrhea**
Women: 5 to 10 mg P.O. daily for 5 to 10 days. Start at any time during menstrual cycle (usually during latter half of cycle).
➤ **Endometrial hyperplasia**
Postmenopausal women (intact uterus) receiving conjugated estrogen 0.625 mg: 5 or 10 mg P.O. daily for 12 to 14 consecutive days per month, beginning day 1 or 16 of cycle.

➤ **Adjunctive therapy and palliative treatment of inoperable, recurrent, and metastatic endometrial or renal cancer**
Adults: 400 to 1,000 mg I.M. weekly. Dosage may be decreased to 400 mg/month when disease has stabilized.
➤ **Contraception**
Women: 150 mg (Depo-Provera) I.M. once every 3 months. Or, 104 mg Depo-subQ Provera subcutaneously once every 3 months. Give first dose during first 5 days of normal menstrual period; only within first 5 days postpartum if patient isn't breast-feeding; and, if patient is exclusively breast-feeding, only at sixth postpartum week.
➤ **Endometriosis-associated pain**
Women: 104 mg subcutaneously every 3 months (12 to 14 weeks).

ADMINISTRATION
P.O.
- Giving this drug immediately before or after a meal increases its bioavailability.
I.M.
- Shake vigorously before use.
- Give by deep I.M. injection in the gluteal or deltoid muscle.
- I.M. injection may be painful. Monitor sites for evidence of sterile abscess. Rotate injection sites to prevent muscle atrophy.
- For multidose vials, use a povidone-iodine solution or similar product to clean vial top before aspirating contents. Take special care to prevent contamination of vial's contents, especially when multidose vial is used for endometrial or renal carcinoma.
Subcutaneous
- Shake vigorously before use.
- Give subcutaneous injection into the anterior thigh or abdomen.

ACTION
Suppresses ovulation, possibly by inhibiting pituitary gonadotropin secretion, thus preventing follicular maturation and causing endometrial thinning.

Route	Onset	Peak	Duration
P.O.	Rapid	2–4 hr	3–5 days
I.M.	Slow	3 wk	3–4 mo
Subcut.	Unknown	1 wk	Unknown

Half-life: Oral, 12 to 17 hours; I.M., 50 days; subcutaneous, 43 days.

ADVERSE REACTIONS

CNS: anxiety, depression, fatigue, insomnia, somnolence, dementia, *stroke,* pain, dizziness, headache.
CV: thrombophlebitis, *PE,* edema, *thromboembolism,* syncope.
EENT: exophthalmos, diplopia, optic neuritis.
GI: bloating, abdominal pain, nausea.
GU: breakthrough bleeding, dysmenorrhea, amenorrhea, cervical erosion, abnormal secretions, changes in libido.
Hepatic: cholestatic jaundice.
Metabolic: weight changes.
Musculoskeletal: loss of bone mineral density.
Skin: rash, induration, sterile abscesses, acne, pruritus, melasma, alopecia, hirsutism.
Other: breast tenderness, enlargement, or secretion; hot flashes.

INTERACTIONS

Drug-drug. *Aminoglutethimide, carbamazepine, fosphenytoin, phenobarbital, phenytoin, rifampin, topiramate:* May decrease progestin effects. Monitor patient for diminished therapeutic response. Tell patient to use a nonhormonal contraceptive during therapy with these drugs.
Anticonvulsants, corticosteroids: These drugs can also reduce bone mass. Monitor patient.
NNRTIs, protease inhibitors: May cause significant changes (increase or decrease) in plasma levels of progestins. Monitor patients for diminished progestin response and advise using nonhormonal contraception during therapy.
Strong CYP3A inducers (carbamazepine, phenobarbital, phenytoin, rifabutin, rifampin, rifapentine): May decrease progestin effects. Avoid use together.
Strong CYP3A inhibitors (clarithromycin, indinavir, itraconazole, ketoconazole, nefazodone, ritonavir, telithromycin, voriconazole): May increase progestin effects. Monitor therapy.
Drug-herb. *St. John's wort:* May decrease progestin effects. Avoid use together.
Drug-food. *Caffeine:* May increase caffeine level. Advise caution.

Drug-lifestyle. *Smoking:* May increase risk of adverse CV effects. If smoking continues, may need alternative therapy.

EFFECTS ON LAB TEST RESULTS

● May increase LFT values, thyroid-binding globulin levels, HDL and triglyceride levels, coagulation tests, and prothrombin factors VII, VIII, IX, and X.
● May decrease plasma and urinary steroid levels, gonadotropin levels, and sex hormone–binding globulin concentrations.
● May reduce metyrapone test results. May alter glucose level.

CONTRAINDICATIONS & CAUTIONS

Black Box Warning Estrogens with progestins shouldn't be used for prevention of CV disease or dementia. ■
● Contraindicated in patients hypersensitive to drug and in those with active thromboembolic disorders or history of thromboembolic disorders, cerebrovascular disease, stroke, breast cancer, history of breast cancer, undiagnosed abnormal vaginal bleeding, missed abortion, or hepatic dysfunction. Tablets are contraindicated in patients with liver dysfunction or known or suspected malignant disease of genital organs.
Black Box Warning Injectable drug shouldn't be used for long-term birth control (more than 2 years) unless other forms of birth control are inadequate. ■
● Use cautiously in patients with diabetes, seizures, migraine, cardiac or renal disease, strong family history of breast cancer, asthma, depression, or breast nodules.
Black Box Warning The Women's Health Initiative (WHI) Estrogen Plus Progestin substudy reported increased risks of MI, stroke, invasive breast cancer, PE, and DVT in postmenopausal women (ages 50 to 79) during 5.6 years of treatment with daily oral conjugated estrogens 0.625 mg combined with medroxyprogesterone 2.5 mg relative to placebo. The WHI Memory Study, a substudy of the WHI study, reported increased risk of developing probable dementia in postmenopausal women age 65 and older during 4 years of treatment with daily conjugated estrogens 0.625 mg combined with medroxyprogesterone 2.5 mg relative to placebo. It's unknown whether this finding

---

Reactions in bold italics are *life-threatening*. Interactions may have a *rapid onset* or a *delayed onset*.

applies to younger postmenopausal women. In the absence of comparable data, these risks should be assumed to be similar for other doses of conjugated estrogens and medroxyprogesterone and other combinations and dosage forms of estrogens and progestins. Because of these risks, estrogens with or without progestins should be prescribed at lowest effective doses and for shortest durations consistent with treatment goals and risks for the individual woman. ■
Dialyzable drug: Unknown.

⚠ Overdose S&S: Nausea, vomiting, dizziness, breast tenderness, abdominal pain, drowsiness/fatigue, withdrawal bleeding.

PREGNANCY-LACTATION-REPRODUCTION

● Drug is contraindicated in women who are pregnant, suspected to be pregnant, or as a diagnostic test for pregnancy.

● Be alert to the possibility of an ectopic pregnancy in women using medroxyprogesterone contraceptive injection who become pregnant or complain of severe abdominal pain.

● Drug appears in breast milk. Tablets aren't recommended for use breast-feeding women. The manufacturer recommends that the injectable form be used with caution in breast-feeding women.

● High doses impair fertility.

NURSING CONSIDERATIONS

Black Box Warning Depo-Provera and Depo-subQ Provera may cause a significant loss of bone mineral density. Loss is greater with increasing duration of use and may not be reversible. In adolescents and young adults, drug may reduce peak bone mass and increase risk of osteoporotic fractures in later life. ■

● Monitor patient for pain, swelling, warmth, or redness in calves; sudden, severe headaches; visual disturbances; numbness in extremities; signs of depression; and signs of liver dysfunction (abdominal pain, dark urine, jaundice).

Black Box Warning Carefully monitor women with a strong family history of breast cancer. ■

PATIENT TEACHING

● According to FDA regulations, patient must read package insert explaining possible adverse effects of progestins before receiving first dose. Also, give patient verbal explanation.

Black Box Warning Teach patient that this product does not protect against HIV or other sexually transmitted diseases. ■

● Advise patient to take medication with food if GI upset occurs.

❸ Alert: Tell patient to report unusual symptoms immediately and to stop drug and notify prescriber about visual disturbances or migraine.

● Advise patient of the importance of an annual physical examination, including BP, breasts, abdomen, pelvic organs, and Papanicolaou test.

● Teach female patient how to perform routine breast self-examination.

● Advise patient to immediately report to prescriber any breast abnormalities, vaginal bleeding, swelling, yellowed skin or eyes, dark urine, clay-colored stools, shortness of breath, chest pain, or pregnancy.

● Advise patient that injection must be given every 3 months to maintain adequate contraceptive effects.

● Tell patient that because this is a long-acting method of birth control, it may take some time for fertility to return after the last injection.

● Tell female patient to immediately report a suspected pregnancy to prescriber.

● Advise patient that amenorrhea is possible with prolonged use.

● Encourage adequate intake of calcium and vitamin D.

mefloquine hydrochloride
MEH-flow-kwin

Therapeutic class: Antimalarials
Pharmacologic class: Quinine derivatives

AVAILABLE FORMS
Tablets: 250 mg

M

INDICATIONS & DOSAGES
➤ **Acute malaria infections caused by mefloquine-sensitive strains of *Plasmodium falciparum* or *P. vivax***
Adults: 1,250 mg (5 tablets) P.O. as a single dose with food and at least 8 oz of water. Patients with *P. vivax* infections should receive further therapy with primaquine or other 8-aminoquinolines to avoid relapse after treatment of the initial infection.
Children age 6 months and older: 20 to 25 mg/kg P.O. as a single dose with food and at least 8 oz of water. Maximum dose 1,250 mg. Dosage may be divided into two doses given 6 to 8 hours apart to reduce the incidence and severity of adverse effects. Patients with *P. vivax* infections should receive further therapy with primaquine or other 8-aminoquinolines to avoid relapse after treatment of the initial infection.
➤ **To prevent malaria**
Adults and children age 6 months and older weighing more than 45 kg: 250 mg P.O. once weekly. Preventive therapy should start 1 week before entering endemic area and continue for 4 weeks after returning. Give subsequent doses on same day of each week, preferably after main meal.
Children age 6 months and older weighing 30 to 45 kg: 187.5 mg (¾ of a 250-mg tablet) P.O. once weekly.
Children age 6 months and older weighing 20 to less than 30 kg: 125 mg (½ of a 250-mg tablet) P.O. once weekly.

ADMINISTRATION
P.O.
● Recommended prophylactic dose of mefloquine is approximately 5 mg/kg body weight once weekly.
● Because giving quinine and mefloquine together poses a health risk, give mefloquine no sooner than 12 hours after the last dose of quinine or quinidine.
● Patient should avoid taking drug on empty stomach and should always take it with at least 8 oz of water.
● May crush tablets and suspend in a small amount of water, milk, or other beverage when giving to small children and other patients unable to swallow tablets whole.

ACTION
May be caused by drug's ability to form complexes with hemin and to raise intravesicular pH in parasite acid vesicles.

Route	Onset	Peak	Duration
P.O.	Unknown	7–24 hr	Unknown

Half-life: About 21 days.

ADVERSE REACTIONS
CNS: *seizures, suicidal behavior,* fever, dizziness, syncope, headache, psychotic changes, hallucinations, confusion, anxiety, fatigue, vertigo, depression, abnormal dreams, insomnia, paresthesia, tremor, ataxia, mood changes, panic attacks, loss of balance.
CV: chest pain, edema.
EENT: tinnitus, visual disturbances.
GI: vomiting, nausea, loose stools, diarrhea, abdominal discomfort or pain, dyspepsia.
Hematologic: *leukopenia, thrombocytopenia.*
Musculoskeletal: myalgia.
Skin: rash.
Other: chills.

INTERACTIONS
Drug-drug. *Antiarrhythmics or beta-blockers, antihistamines or H₁-blockers, calcium channel blockers, phenothiazines, TCAs:* May prolong QTc interval and increase risk of life-threatening cardiac arrhythmias. Coadminister with caution.
Carbamazepine, phenytoin, valproic acid: May decrease drug levels and loss of seizure control at start of mefloquine therapy. Monitor anticonvulsant level.
Chloroquine, quinidine, quinine: May increase risk of seizures and ECG abnormalities. Give mefloquine at least 12 hours after last dose.
CYP3A4 inducers: May decrease mefloquine plasma concentration and reduce drug's effect. Use together cautiously.
CYP3A4 inhibitors: May increase mefloquine plasma concentration and risk of adverse reactions. Use together cautiously.
Halofantrine: May cause fatal prolongation of QTc interval if given with or within 15 weeks of last mefloquine dose. Don't use together.

Reactions in bold italics are *life-threatening*. Interactions may have a *rapid onset* or a *delayed onset*.

Ketoconazole: May increase mefloquine plasma concentration, leading to potentially fatal QT-interval prolongation. Don't use ketoconazole within 15 weeks of last dose of mefloquine.
Rifampin: May decrease mefloquine plasma concentration. Use together cautiously.
Vaccines (live): May decrease immunization result. Complete vaccination at least 3 days before start of mefloquine.

EFFECTS ON LAB TEST RESULTS
• May increase transaminase level.
• May decrease hematocrit.
• May decrease WBC and platelet counts.

CONTRAINDICATIONS & CAUTIONS
• Contraindicated in patients hypersensitive to mefloquine or related compounds, in those with a history of seizures, and in patients with active or recent history of depression, generalized anxiety disorder, psychosis, schizophrenia, or other major psychiatric disorders.
• Other I.V. antimalarials should be used to initially treat life-threatening or serious malarial infections. Mefloquine may be used after I.V. treatment is completed.
Black Box Warning Drug may cause neuropsychiatric adverse reactions that can persist after therapy ends. Drug shouldn't be prescribed for prophylaxis in patients with major psychiatric disorders. ∎
• If psychiatric symptoms occur with prophylactic treatment, discontinue drug.
• Use cautiously when treating patients with cardiac disease or seizure disorders.
• Cases of agranulocytosis and aplastic anemia have been reported in patients taking mefloquine.
• In certain cases, such as when a traveler is taking other medications, it may be desirable to start prophylaxis 2 to 3 weeks before departure, to ensure that the combination of drugs is well tolerated.
Dialyzable drug: No.
⚠ *Overdose S&S:* Possibly more pronounced adverse reactions.

PREGNANCY-LACTATION-REPRODUCTION
• Studies in pregnant women have shown no increase in the risk of teratogenic effects after mefloquine use; however, risk to a developing fetus can't be ruled out. Use only if clearly needed.
• Drug appears in breast milk in small amounts. Use cautiously in breast-feeding women.

NURSING CONSIDERATIONS
• Patients with *P. vivax* infections are at high risk for relapse because drug doesn't eliminate the hepatic-phase exoerythrocytic parasites. Give follow-up therapy with primaquine.
• Monitor LFT results periodically.
• If patient vomits within 30 minutes of receiving dose, repeat full dose; if within 30 to 60 minutes, give a half dose.
• If overdose is suspected, induce vomiting or perform gastric lavage because of risk of cardiotoxicity. Mefloquine has produced cardiac reactions similar to those caused by quinidine and quinine.
❸ *Alert:* Monitor patient for neurologic signs and symptoms (dizziness, vertigo, tinnitus, seizures, insomnia) or psychiatric signs and symptoms (anxiety, paranoia, hallucinations, depression, restlessness, confusion, behavior changes). Signs and symptoms may be more difficult to detect in children.
Black Box Warning During prophylactic use, if psychiatric or neurologic signs and symptoms occur, the drug should be discontinued and an alternative medication prescribed. ∎

PATIENT TEACHING
• Advise patient taking drug for prevention to take dose immediately before or after a meal on the same day each week, to improve compliance beginning 1 week before arrival at endemic area.
• Tell patient not to take drug on an empty stomach and always to take it with at least 8 oz of water.
• Instruct patient to read the medication guide and always to carry the information wallet card during therapy.
• Advise patient to use caution when performing activities that require alertness and coordination because dizziness, disturbed sense of balance, and neuropsychiatric reactions may occur.

M

◑ Alert: Inform patient that dizziness, vertigo, and tinnitus can occur during treatment, may continue for months or years after treatment, or may be permanent.

◑ Alert: Warn patient to contact prescriber immediately if neurologic or psychiatric signs or symptoms occur and not to stop drug until discussing with prescriber. Encourage patient to read the medication guide that comes with every prescription.

• Advise patient undergoing long-term therapy to have periodic ophthalmic exams because drug may cause ocular lesions.

• Advise patient that drug may cause insomnia.

• Advise women of childbearing potential to use reliable contraception during treatment.

SAFETY ALERT!

megestrol acetate
me-JESS-trole

Megace, Megace ES, Megace OS✤

Therapeutic class: Antineoplastics
Pharmacologic class: Progestins

AVAILABLE FORMS
Oral suspension: 40 mg/mL
Oral suspension (concentrated):
125 mg/mL
Tablets: 20 mg, 40 mg

INDICATIONS & DOSAGES
➤ **Breast cancer (palliative treatment)**
Adults: 40 mg P.O. q.i.d.
➤ **Endometrial cancer (palliative treatment)**
Adults: 40 to 320 mg P.O. daily in divided doses.
➤ **Anorexia, cachexia, or unexplained significant weight loss in patients with AIDS**
Adults: 800 mg P.O. (20 mL regular oral suspension) or 625 mg P.O. (5 mL concentrated oral suspension) once daily.
➤ **Hot flashes ◆**
Adults: 20 mg P.O. once daily.

ADMINISTRATION
P.O.
• Drug is a hormonal agent and is considered a teratogen. Follow safe handling procedures.
• Give drug without regard for meals.
• Shake suspension well before pouring.

ACTION
Inhibits hormone-dependent tumor growth by inhibiting pituitary and adrenal steroidogenesis. Drug may also have direct cytotoxicity; its appetite-stimulating mechanism is unknown.

Route	Onset	Peak	Duration
P.O.	Unknown	2–5 hr	Unknown

Half-life: Mean, 34.2 hours.

ADVERSE REACTIONS
CV: thrombophlebitis, *HF,* hypertension, *thromboembolism, cardiomyopathy,* palpitations, chest pain.
CNS: confusion, seizures, depression, headache, neuropathy, insomnia, abnormal thinking, mood changes, fever, asthenia.
EENT: pharyngitis.
GI: nausea, vomiting, diarrhea, flatulence, constipation, dry mouth, increased appetite, abdominal pain, dyspepsia.
GU: breakthrough menstrual bleeding, erectile dysfunction, UTI, urinary incontinence, urinary frequency.
Hematologic: *leukopenia.*
Metabolic: hyperglycemia, weight gain.
Musculoskeletal: carpal tunnel syndrome.
Respiratory: *PE,* dyspnea, pneumonia.
Skin: alopecia, rash.
Other: gynecomastia, tumor flare.

INTERACTIONS
Dofetilide: May increase dofetilide plasma level, increasing risk of life-threatening cardiac arrhythmias, including torsades de pointes. Avoid use together.
Indinavir: May decrease exposure of indinavir. Consider increasing indinavir dosage when coadministering.
Rifamycins (rifampin): May increase megestrol metabolism due to induction of CYP3A4 pathway, reducing pharmacologic effects. Consider increasing megestrol dosage.

Reactions in bold italics are *life-threatening*. Interactions may have a *rapid onset* or a *delayed onset*.

EFFECTS ON LAB TEST RESULTS
• May increase glucose level.

CONTRAINDICATIONS & CAUTIONS
• Contraindicated in patients hypersensitive to drug.
• Use cautiously in patients with history of thrombophlebitis or thromboembolism.
Dialyzable drug: Unlikely.

PREGNANCY-LACTATION-REPRODUCTION
• Drug may cause fetal harm. Oral solution is contraindicated in pregnancy. If tablets are used during pregnancy, or if patient becomes pregnant during therapy, apprise her of potential hazard to the fetus. Women of childbearing potential should avoid becoming pregnant.
• Drug appears in breast milk. Women shouldn't breast-feed during therapy.

NURSING CONSIDERATIONS
• May increase glucose level in diabetic patients.
• Drug isn't intended for prophylactic use to avoid weight loss. Start treatment with megestrol acetate oral suspension only after treatable causes of weight loss are sought and addressed.
• Two months is an adequate trial period in patients with cancer.

PATIENT TEACHING
• Inform patient that therapeutic response isn't immediate. Drug must be taken for at least 2 months to determine effectiveness.
• Tell patient drug may be taken without regard for food.
• **Alert:** Tell patient that the ES oral suspension is more concentrated than the regular oral suspension, so a smaller amount is needed if prescription is changed.
• Advise women to stop breast-feeding during therapy because of risk of toxicity to infant.
• Advise women of childbearing potential to use an effective form of contraception while receiving drug.

melphalan (L-PAM, phenylalanine mustard)
MEL-fa-lan

Alkeran

melphalan hydrochloride
Alkeran, Evomela

Therapeutic class: Antineoplastics
Pharmacologic class: Nitrogen mustards

AVAILABLE FORMS
Lyophilized powder for injection: 50 mg
Tablets: 2 mg

INDICATIONS & DOSAGES
➤ **Multiple myeloma (palliative treatment)**
Adults: Initially, 6 mg P.O. daily for 2 to 3 weeks; then stop drug for up to 4 weeks or until WBC and platelet counts stop dropping and begin to rise again; maintenance dose is 2 mg daily. Or, 10 mg/day for 7 to 10 days, followed by 2 mg/day when WBC is greater than 4,000 cells/mm^3 and platelet count is greater than 100,000 cells/mm^3; dosage is adjusted to between 1 and 3 mg/day depending on hematologic response. Or, 0.15 mg/kg P.O. daily for 7 days followed by a rest period of at least 14 days; maintenance dose is 0.05 mg/kg/day or less. Or 0.25 mg/kg/day for 4 consecutive days (or 0.2 mg/kg/day for 5 consecutive days) for a total dose of 1mg/kg/course; repeat every 4 to 6 weeks.

Or, give I.V. to patients who can't tolerate oral therapy, 16 mg/m^2 given by infusion over 15 to 20 minutes at 2-week intervals for four doses. After patient has recovered from toxicity, give drug at 4-week intervals.
Adjust-a-dose: Withhold drug until recovery for WBC count less than 3,000/mm^3 or platelet count less than 100,000/mm^3. For moderate to severe renal impairment, consider a reduced P.O. dose initially. For patients with renal insufficiency (BUN level of 30 mg/dL or more), consider reducing I.V. dose 50%.

M

➤ **Nonresectable advanced epithelial ovarian cancer (palliative treatment)**
Adults: 0.2 mg/kg P.O. daily for 5 days. Repeat every 4 to 5 weeks, depending on bone marrow recovery.
Adjust-a-dose: For moderate to severe renal impairment, consider a reduced dose initially.

✱ *NEW INDICATION:* **Multiple myeloma (conditioning treatment before hematopoietic stem cell transplantation; Evomela)**
Adults: 100 mg/m^2/day by I.V. infusion over 30 minutes for 2 consecutive days (day −3 and day −2) before autologous stem cell transplantation (day 0).
Adjust-a-dose: For patients weighing more than 130% of their ideal body weight, calculate BSA based on adjusted ideal body weight. For patients with renal insufficiency (BUN level of 30 mg/dL or more), consider reducing I.V. dose 50%.

➤ **Amyloidosis, light chain ◆**
Adults: 0.22 mg/kg/day P.O. for 4 days every 28 days (in combination with oral dexamethasone), or 10 mg/m^2/day P.O. for 4 days every month (in combination with oral dexamethasone) for 12 to 18 treatment cycles.

ADMINISTRATION
P.O.
● Give on an empty stomach; food decreases drug absorption.
● Store tablets in refrigerator. Protect from light.

I.V.
Black Box Warning Preparing and giving this form may be mutagenic, teratogenic, or carcinogenic. Follow facility safe handling policy to reduce risks. ∎
▼ Because drug isn't stable in solution, reconstitute immediately before giving with the 10 mL of sterile diluent supplied by manufacturer, using 20G or larger needle. Shake vigorously until solution is clear. The resulting solution will contain 5 mg/mL of melphalan. Immediately dilute required dose in NSS for injection to no more than 0.45 mg/mL. Give infusion over at least 15 minutes.
▼ Monitor infusion carefully; drug is considered a vesicant and extravasation

may cause local damage. If extravasation occurs, stop infusion immediately, notify prescriber, and follow facility protocol for treatment.
▼ Reconstituted product begins to degrade within 30 minutes. After final dilution, nearly 1% of drug degrades every 10 minutes. Administration must be finished within 60 minutes of reconstitution.
▼ Don't refrigerate reconstituted product because precipitate will form.

Evomela
▼ Use 8.6 mL NSS as directed to reconstitute and make a 50-mg/10 mL (5-mg/mL) nominal concentration of melphalan. The NSS should appear to be pulled into vial by the negative pressure in vial. Discard any vial (and replace with another) if there is no vacuum present when reconstituting vial.
▼ Reconstituted drug is stable for 24 hours when refrigerated (41° F [5° C]) without any precipitation because of the high solubility, and is stable for 1 hour at room temperature.
▼ Withdraw required volume needed for dose from vial and add to the appropriate volume of NSS to a final concentration of 0.45 mg/mL. Infuse over 30 minutes via injection port or central venous catheter.
▼ Admixture solution is stable for 4 hours at room temperature in addition to the 1 hour after reconstitution.
▼ Don't mix Evomela with other melphalan hydrochloride for injection products.
▼ Extravasation may cause local tissue damage. Don't administer by direct injection into a peripheral vein; inject slowly into a fast-running I.V. infusion via a central venous access line.
▼ **Incompatibilities:** Amphotericin B, chlorpromazine, D$_5$W, lactated Ringer injection. Compatibility with NSS injection depends on the concentration; don't prepare solutions with a concentration exceeding 0.45 mg/mL.

ACTION
Cross-links strands of cellular DNA and interferes with RNA transcription, causing an imbalance of growth that leads to cell death. Not specific to cell cycle.

Reactions in bold italics are *life-threatening*. Interactions may have a *rapid onset* or a *delayed onset*.

Route	Onset	Peak	Duration
P.O.	Unknown	About 1–2 hr	Unknown
I.V.	Unknown	Unknown	Unknown

Half-life: Oral, about ½ to 2¼ hours; I.V., about 75 minutes.

ADVERSE REACTIONS

CV: vasculitis.
GI: nausea, vomiting, diarrhea, oral ulceration, stomatitis.
Hematologic: *thrombocytopenia, leukopenia, bone marrow suppression,* hemolytic anemia.
Hepatic: *hepatotoxicity.*
Respiratory: *pneumonitis, pulmonary fibrosis.*
Skin: pruritus, alopecia, urticaria, ulceration at injection site.
Other: *anaphylaxis,* hypersensitivity reactions.

INTERACTIONS

Drug-drug (I.V. melphalan only). *Anticoagulants, aspirin, NSAIDs:* May increase risk of bleeding. Avoid using together.
Carmustine: May decrease threshold for pulmonary toxicity. Use together cautiously.
Cimetidine: May decrease melphalan level. Monitor patient closely.
Cisplatin: May increase renal impairment, decreasing melphalan clearance. Monitor patient closely.
Cyclosporine: May cause severe renal impairment. Monitor renal function closely.
Disulfiram: May cause acute alcohol intolerance. Don't use together.
Interferon alfa: May increase melphalan elimination. Monitor patient closely.
Live-virus vaccines: May increase risk of toxicity from live-virus vaccines. Postpone immunization with live-virus vaccines for at least 3 months after last dose of melphalan.
Nalidixic acid: May cause hemorrhagic ulcerative colitis or intestinal necrosis. Use together is contraindicated.
Drug-food. *Any food:* May decrease oral drug absorption. Advise patient to take drug on an empty stomach.

EFFECTS ON LAB TEST RESULTS

• May increase urine urea level. May decrease Hb level.

• May decrease RBC, WBC, and platelet counts.
• May cause a false-positive direct Coombs test.

CONTRAINDICATIONS & CAUTIONS

• Contraindicated in patients hypersensitive to drug and in those with disease resistant to drug.
• Contraindicated in patients with severe leukopenia, thrombocytopenia, or anemia and in those with chronic lymphocytic leukemia.
• Use cautiously in patients receiving radiation and chemotherapy.
• Drug is a vesicant and may cause local tissue damage if extravasation occurs. If signs or symptoms of extravasation develop, stop infusion immediately and notify prescriber.
Dialyzable drug: No.
⚠ Overdose S&S: Vomiting, ulceration of the mouth, diarrhea, GI hemorrhage, bone marrow suppression.

PREGNANCY-LACTATION-REPRODUCTION

• There are no adequate studies in pregnant women, but drug may cause fetal harm. Women of childbearing potential should avoid becoming pregnant.
• It isn't known if drug appears in breast milk; however, excretion into breast milk is likely. Don't give to breast-feeding women.
• Drug suppresses ovarian function in premenopausal women, resulting in amenorrhea in a significant number of patients.
• May damage spermatozoa and testicular tissue, resulting in possible genetic fetal abnormalities. Reversible and irreversible testicular suppression has also been reported.

NURSING CONSIDERATIONS

Black Box Warning Administer drug only under the supervision of a physician experienced in the use of cancer chemotherapeutic agents. ■
Black Box Warning Severe bone marrow suppression with resulting bleeding or infection may occur. ■
Black Box Warning Drug is leukemogenic. It produces chromosomal aberrations in vitro and in vivo and should be considered potentially mutagenic in humans. ■

M

Black Box Warning Controlled trials comparing I.V. to oral melphalan have shown more myelosuppression with the I.V. formulation. Hypersensitivity reactions, including anaphylaxis, have occurred in approximately 2% of patients who received the I.V. formulation. ■

• Dosage may need to be reduced in patients with renal impairment.

• Monitor uric acid level and CBC.

• To prevent bleeding, avoid all I.M. injections when platelet count is less than 50,000/mm³.

• Blood transfusions may be needed for cumulative anemia.

• Anaphylaxis may occur. Keep antihistamines and steroids readily available to give if needed.

• *Look alike–sound alike:* Don't confuse melphalan with Mephyton.

PATIENT TEACHING

• Advise patient to take tablets on empty stomach.

• Advise patient to report pain or redness at I.V. site.

• Advise patient to watch for signs and symptoms of infection (fever, sore throat, fatigue) and bleeding (easy bruising, nosebleeds, bleeding gums, tarry stools). Tell patient to take temperature daily.

• Advise women to stop breast-feeding during therapy because of risk of toxicity to infant.

• Advise women of childbearing potential to avoid becoming pregnant while taking the drug. Advise patient that the drug can interfere with menstrual cycle in women and stop sperm production in men.

• Advise male patient with female sexual partners of childbearing potential to use effective contraception during and after treatment.

• Advise female patient of childbearing potential to avoid pregnancy (which may include use of effective contraceptive methods) during and after treatment.

---

memantine hydrochloride
meh-MAN-teen

Ebixa❦, Namenda⬧, Namenda XR

Therapeutic class: Anti-Alzheimer drugs
Pharmacologic class: N-methyl-D-aspartate receptor antagonists

AVAILABLE FORMS
Capsules (extended-release) Ⓞ*:* 7 mg, 14 mg, 21 mg, 28 mg
Oral solution: 2 mg/mL
Tablets: 5 mg, 10 mg

INDICATIONS & DOSAGES
➤ **Moderate to severe Alzheimer dementia**
Adults: Initially, 5 mg P.O. once daily. Increase by 5 mg/day every week until target dose is reached. Maximum, 10 mg P.O. b.i.d. Doses greater than 5 mg should be given in two divided doses.

Or, for extended-release capsules, initial dose is 7 mg P.O. once daily. Increase as tolerated by 7-mg increments each week to target dosage of 28 mg P.O. once daily.
To convert from immediate-release to extended-release form: Patients taking immediate-release 10 mg b.i.d. may switch to extended-release 28 mg once daily the day following the last immediate-release tablet. Patients with severe renal failure taking immediate-release 5 mg b.i.d. may switch to extended-release 14 mg once daily the day following the last immediate-release tablet.

Adjust-a-dose: For immediate-release form, no dosage adjustment is recommended for patients with mild to moderate renal impairment; target dosage of 5 mg b.i.d. is recommended for patients with severe renal impairment (CrCl of 5 to 29 mL/minute). For extended-release form, no dosage adjustment is recommended for patients with mild to moderate renal impairment; a target dosage of 14 mg/day is recommended for patients with severe renal impairment (CrCl of 5 to 29 mL/minute).

ADMINISTRATION
P.O.
● Give drug without regard for food.
● Patients may take capsules intact or capsules may be opened, sprinkled on applesauce, then swallowed. Don't allow patients to divide, chew, or crush capsules.

ACTION
Antagonizes N-methyl-D-aspartate receptors, the persistent activation of which seems to increase Alzheimer symptoms.

Route	Onset	Peak	Duration
P.O. (tablets)	Unknown	3–7 hr	Unknown
P.O. (capsules)	Unknown	9–12 hr	Unknown

Half-life: 60 to 80 hours.

ADVERSE REACTIONS
CNS: *stroke,* aggressiveness, agitation, anxiety, ataxia, confusion, depression, dizziness, fatigue, hallucinations, headache, hypokinesia, insomnia, pain, somnolence, syncope, TIA, vertigo.
CV: *HF,* edema, hypertension.
EENT: cataracts, conjunctivitis.
GI: anorexia, constipation, diarrhea, nausea, vomiting.
GU: incontinence, urinary frequency, UTI.
Hematologic: anemia.
Metabolic: weight loss or gain.
Musculoskeletal: arthralgia, back pain.
Respiratory: bronchitis, coughing, dyspnea, flulike symptoms, pneumonia, URI.
Skin: rash.
Other: abnormal gait, falls, injury.

INTERACTIONS
Drug-drug. *Cimetidine, hydrochlorothiazide, quinidine, ranitidine, triamterene:* May alter levels of both drugs. Monitor patient.
NMDA antagonists (amantadine, dextromethorphan, ketamine): Effects of combined use unknown. Use together cautiously.
Urine alkalinizers (carbonic anhydrase inhibitors, sodium bicarbonate): May decrease memantine clearance. Monitor patient for adverse effects.
Drug-food. *Foods that alkalinize urine:* May increase drug level and adverse effects. Use together cautiously.

Drug-lifestyle. *Alcohol use:* May alter drug adherence, decrease its effectiveness, or increase adverse effects. Discourage use together.
Nicotine: May alter levels of drug and nicotine. Discourage use together.

EFFECTS ON LAB TEST RESULTS
● May increase alkaline phosphatase level.
● May decrease Hb level and hematocrit.

CONTRAINDICATIONS & CAUTIONS
● Contraindicated in patients allergic to drug or its components.
● Immediate-release form isn't recommended for patients with severe renal impairment.
● Use cautiously in patients with seizures, CV disease, or severe hepatic or renal impairment.
● Use cautiously in patients who may have an increased urine pH (from drugs, diet, renal tubular acidosis, or severe UTI, for example).
Dialyzable drug: Unknown.
⚠ **Overdose S&S:** Restlessness, psychosis, visual hallucinations, somnolence, stupor, loss of consciousness, agitation, asthenia, bradycardia, confusion, coma, dizziness, ECG changes, hypertension, lethargy, unsteady gait, vertigo, vomiting, weakness.

PREGNANCY-LACTATION-REPRODUCTION
● There are no adequate studies in pregnant women. Use during pregnancy only if potential benefit justifies potential risk to the fetus.
● It isn't known if drug appears in breast milk. Use cautiously in breast-feeding women.

NURSING CONSIDERATIONS
● In elderly patients, even those with a normal creatinine level, use of this drug may impair renal function. Estimate CrCl; reduce dosage in patients with moderate renal impairment. Don't give drug to patients with severe renal impairment.
● Monitor patient carefully for adverse reactions as he may not be able to recognize changes or communicate effectively.

M

PATIENT TEACHING
● Explain that drug doesn't cure Alzheimer disease but may aid patient to maintain function for a longer period of time.
● Tell patient or caregiver to report adverse effects.
● Urge patient to avoid alcohol during treatment.
● To avoid possible interactions, advise patient not to take herbal or OTC products without consulting prescriber.

SAFETY ALERT!

meperidine hydrochloride (pethidine hydrochloride)
me-PER-i-deen

Demerol⬦

Therapeutic class: Opioid analgesics
Pharmacologic class: Opioids
Controlled substance schedule: II

AVAILABLE FORMS
Injection: 10 mg/mL, 25 mg/mL, 50 mg/mL, 75 mg/mL, 100 mg/mL
Syrup: 50 mg/5 mL
Tablets: 50 mg, 100 mg

INDICATIONS & DOSAGES
➤ **Moderate to severe pain**
Adults: 50 to 150 mg P.O., I.M., or subcutaneously every 3 to 4 hours p.r.n. Or, 10 mg I.V. slowly by patient-controlled analgesia device, with range of 1 to 5 mg per dose; lockout interval is 6 to 10 minutes. Or, continuous I.V. infusion of 15 to 35 mg/hour.
Children: 1.1 to 1.8 mg/kg P.O., or 1.1 to 1.8 mg/kg I.M. or subcutaneously every 3 to 4 hours. Maximum, 50 to 150 mg every 4 hours p.r.n.
Adjust-a-dose: Reduce meperidine doses by 25% to 50% when administered with phenothiazines or other tranquilizers because they potentiate the action of meperidine. Reduce dosage in elderly patients and in those with hepatic and renal impairment. If CrCl is 10 to 50 mL/minute, give 75% of normal dose. If CrCl is less than 10 mL/minute, give 50% of normal dose. Avoid use in dialysis patients.

➤ **Preoperative analgesia**
Adults: 50 to 100 mg I.M. or subcutaneously 30 to 90 minutes before surgery.
Children: 1.1 to 2.2 mg/kg I.M. or subcutaneously up to the adult dose 30 to 90 minutes before anesthesia.
Adjust-a-dose: Reduce dosage in elderly patients and in those with hepatic or renal impairment. If CrCl is 10 to 50 mL/minute, give 75% of normal dose. If CrCl is less than 10 mL/minute, give 50% of normal dose. Avoid use in dialysis patients.

➤ **Adjunct to anesthesia**
Adults: Repeated slow I.V. injections of fractional doses (10 mg/mL). Or, continuous I.V. infusion of a more dilute solution (1 mg/mL) titrated to patient's needs.

➤ **Obstetric analgesia**
Adults: 50 to 100 mg I.M. or subcutaneously when pain becomes regular; may repeat at 1- to 3-hour intervals.

ADMINISTRATION
P.O.
● Syrup has local anesthetic effect on mucous membranes. Give with a half glass of water.
● Oral dose is less than half as effective as parenteral dose. Give I.M. if possible. When changing from parenteral to oral route, increase dosage.

I.V.
▼ Keep opioid antagonist (naloxone) available.
▼ Give drug slowly by direct injection.
▼ Drug may also be given by slow continuous infusion. Drug is compatible with most solutions, including D_5W, NSS, and Ringer or lactated Ringer solutions.
▼ Protect from light and store at room temperature.
▼ **Incompatibilities:** Barbiturates, allopurinol, aminophylline, amobarbital, amphotericin B, cefepime, cefoperazone, doxorubicin liposomal, ephedrine, furosemide, heparin, hydrocortisone sodium succinate, idarubicin, imipenem–cilastatin sodium, methicillin, methylprednisolone sodium succinate, morphine, pentobarbital, phenobarbital sodium, phenytoin, sodium bicarbonate, sodium iodide, sulfadiazine, sulfisoxazole, thiopental.

Reactions in bold italics are *life-threatening*. Interactions may have a *rapid onset* or a **delayed onset**.

I.M.

● Inject deep into large muscle mass, taking care to avoid nerve trunks.

Subcutaneous

● Subcutaneous injection isn't recommended because it's very painful, but it may be suitable for occasional use. Monitor patient for pain at injection site, local tissue irritation, and induration after subcutaneous injection.

ACTION

Unknown. Binds with opioid receptors in the CNS, altering perception of and emotional response to pain.

Route	Onset	Peak	Duration
P.O.	15 min	60–90 min	2–4 hr
I.V.	1 min	5–7 min	2–4 hr
I.M., subcut.	10–15 min	30–50 min	2–4 hr

Half-life: 2½ to 4 hours.

ADVERSE REACTIONS

CNS: agitation, incoordination, clouded sensorium, dizziness, euphoria, lightheadedness, sedation, somnolence, *seizures,* hallucinations, headache, paradoxical anxiety, physical dependence, syncope, tremor.
CV: *bradycardia, cardiac arrest, shock,* hypotension, tachycardia, palpitations.
GI: biliary tract spasms, constipation, dry mouth, ileus, nausea, vomiting.
GU: urine retention.
Musculoskeletal: muscle twitching.
Respiratory: *respiratory arrest, respiratory depression.*
Skin: diaphoresis, pruritus, urticaria.
Other: induration, local tissue irritation, pain at injection site, phlebitis after I.V. delivery.

INTERACTIONS

Drug-drug. *Acyclovir:* Increases meperidine plasma concentration and risk of adverse reactions. Use together cautiously.
Aminophylline, barbiturates, heparin, methicillin, morphine sulfate, phenytoin, sodium bicarbonate, sulfonamides: Incompatible when mixed in same I.V. container. Avoid using together.
Black Box Warning *Benzodiazepines, CNS depressants:* May cause slow or difficult breathing, sedation, and death. Avoid use

together. If use together is necessary, limit dosage and duration of each drug to the minimum necessary for desired effect. ■
Chlorpromazine: May cause excessive sedation and hypotension. Avoid using together.
Cimetidine: May increase respiratory and CNS depression. Monitor patient closely.
General anesthetics, phenothiazines, TCAs: May cause respiratory depression, hypotension, profound sedation, or coma. Use together with caution; reduce meperidine dosage.
MAO inhibitors: May increase CNS excitation or depression that can be severe or fatal. Use together is contraindicated.
Phenytoin: May decrease meperidine level. Watch for decreased analgesia.
Protease inhibitors: May increase respiratory and CNS depression. Avoid using together.
● *Alert:* Serotonergic drugs (amoxapine, antiemetics [dolasetron, granisetron, ondansetron, palonosetron], antimigraine drugs, buspirone, cyclobenzaprine, dextromethorphan, linezolid, lithium, MAO inhibitors, maprotiline, methylene blue, mirtazapine, nefazodone, SNRIs, SSRIs, TCAs, trazodone, tryptophan, vilazodone): May increase risk of serotonin syndrome. Use together cautiously and monitor patient for serotonin syndrome.
Sodium oxybate: May increase CNS depression and sleep duration. Use together is contraindicated.
Drug-herb. ● *Alert: St. John's wort:* May increase risk of serotonin syndrome. Use together cautiously and monitor patient for serotonin syndrome.
Drug-lifestyle. *Alcohol use:* May cause additive effects. Discourage use together.

EFFECTS ON LAB TEST RESULTS

● May increase amylase and lipase levels.

CONTRAINDICATIONS & CAUTIONS

● Contraindicated in patients hypersensitive to drug and in those who have received MAO inhibitors within past 14 days.
Black Box Warning Opioid drugs should only be prescribed with benzodiazepines or other CNS depressants to patients for

M

whom alternative treatment options are inadequate. ∎

◑ *Alert:* Drug may lead to a rare but serious decrease in adrenal gland cortisol production.

◑ *Alert:* Drug may cause decreased sex hormone levels with long-term use.

◑ *Alert:* Patients are at increased risk for oversedation and respiratory depression if they snore or have a history of sleep apnea, haven't used opioids recently or are first-time opioid users, have increased opioid dosage requirements or opioid habituation, have received general anesthesia for longer lengths of time or received other sedating drugs, have preexisting pulmonary or cardiac disease, or have thoracic or other surgical incisions that may impair breathing. Monitor patients carefully.

● Avoid use in patients with ESRD.

● Use cautiously in elderly or debilitated patients and in those with increased ICP, head injury, asthma and other respiratory conditions, supraventricular tachycardias, seizures, acute abdominal conditions, hepatic or renal disease, hypothyroidism, Addison disease, urethral stricture, and prostatic hyperplasia.

● Meperidine can produce drug dependence of the morphine type and, therefore, has the potential for abuse. Psychic dependence, physical dependence, and tolerance may develop upon repeated administration.

Dialyzable drug: Unknown.

⚠ *Overdose S&S:* Respiratory depression, somnolence progressing to stupor, coma, bradycardia, hypotension, hypothermia, delirium, skeletal muscle flaccidity, circulatory collapse, death.

PREGNANCY-LACTATION-REPRODUCTION

● Don't use in pregnant women before labor unless physician determines potential benefits outweigh possible risks; safe use in pregnancy before labor hasn't been established relative to possible adverse effects on fetal development.

● Drug appears in breast milk. Patient should discontinue breast-feeding or discontinue drug.

NURSING CONSIDERATIONS

● In elderly patients, patients using meperidine for longer than 48 hours, those with preexisting renal or CNS disease, and those taking more than 600 mg/day, the active metabolite may accumulate, causing increased adverse CNS reactions. Avoid prolonged use.

◑ *Alert:* Carefully monitor vital signs, pain level, respiratory status, and sedation level in all patients receiving opioids, especially those receiving I.V. drugs, even those given postoperatively.

◑ *Alert:* If patient is taking opioids with serotonergic drugs, watch for signs and symptoms of serotonin syndrome (agitation, hallucinations, rapid HR, fever, excessive sweating, shivering or shaking, muscle twitching or stiffness, trouble with coordination, nausea, vomiting, diarrhea), especially when starting treatment or increasing dosages. Signs and symptoms may occur within several hours of coadministration but may also occur later, especially after dosage increase. Discontinue the opioid, serotonergic drug, or both if serotonin syndrome is suspected.

◑ *Alert:* Monitor patient for signs and symptoms of adrenal insufficiency (nausea, vomiting, loss of appetite, fatigue, weakness, dizziness, low BP). Perform diagnostic testing if adrenal insufficiency is suspected. If adrenal insufficiency is confirmed, treat with corticosteroids and wean patient off opioids if appropriate. Discontinue corticosteroids when clinically appropriate.

◑ *Alert:* Monitor patient for signs and symptoms of decreased sex hormone levels (low libido, erectile dysfunction, amenorrhea, infertility). If signs and symptoms occur, evaluate patient and obtain laboratory testing.

● When giving drug parenterally, make sure patient is lying down.

● Drug may be used in some patients who are allergic to morphine.

● Reassess patient's level of pain at least 15 and 30 minutes after administration.

● Because drug toxicity frequently appears after several days of treatment, drug isn't recommended for treatment of chronic pain.

• In neonates exposed to drug during labor, monitor respirations. Have resuscitation equipment and naloxone available.

• Monitor respiratory and CV status carefully. Don't give if respirations are below 12 breaths/minute, if respiratory rate or depth is decreased, or if change in pupils is noted.

• If drug is stopped abruptly after long-term use, monitor patient for withdrawal symptoms.

• In postoperative patients, monitor bladder function.

• Monitor bowel function. Patient may need a stimulant laxative and stool softener.

• *Look alike–sound alike:* Don't confuse Demerol with Demulen.

PATIENT TEACHING

Black Box Warning Caution the patient or the caregiver of a patient taking an opioid drug with a benzodiazepine, CNS depressant, or alcohol to seek immediate medical attention if the patient has symptoms of dizziness, light-headedness, extreme sleepiness, slowed or difficult breathing, or unresponsiveness. ▪

❸ *Alert:* Explain assessment and monitoring process to patient and family. Instruct them to immediately report difficulty breathing or other signs or symptoms of an adverse opioid-related reaction.

❸ *Alert:* Encourage patient to report all medications being taken, including prescription and OTC medications and supplements.

❸ *Alert:* Caution patient to immediately report signs and symptoms of serotonin syndrome, adrenal insufficiency, and decreased sex hormone levels.

• Encourage postoperative patient to turn, cough, deep-breathe, and use an incentive spirometer to prevent lung problems.

• Caution ambulatory patient about getting out of bed or walking. Warn outpatient to avoid driving and other potentially hazardous activities that require mental alertness until drug's CNS effects are known.

• Advise patient to avoid alcohol and sleep aids during therapy.

• Caution patient that drug isn't intended for long-term use.

mercaptopurine (6-mercaptopurine, 6-MP)
mer-kap-toe-PYOOR-een

Purixan

Therapeutic class: Antineoplastics
Pharmacologic class: Purine antagonists

AVAILABLE FORMS
Oral suspension: 20 mg/mL
Tablets (scored): 50 mg

INDICATIONS & DOSAGES
➤ **Acute lymphatic leukemia**
Adults and children: 1.5 to 2.5 mg/kg P.O. once daily (rounded to nearest 25 mg). After remission is attained, usual maintenance dose for adults and children is 1.5 to 2.5 mg/kg once daily.
Adjust-a-dose: For patients with CrCl of less than 50 mL/minute, or patients receiving hemodialysis, continuous ambulatory peritoneal dialysis, or continuous renal replacement therapy, give dose every 48 hours. If given concurrently with allopurinol, reduce dosage to 25% to 33% of usual dose.
➤ **Acute promyelocytic leukemia, maintenance ◆**
Adults: 60 mg/m^2/day for 1 year (in combination with tretinoin and methotrexate).

ADMINISTRATION
P.O.
• Drugs is a hazardous agent; follow safe handling and disposal procedures.
• Give total daily dosage at one time, calculated to the nearest multiple of 25 mg.
• Give on an empty stomach.
• Give in the evening to reduce risk of relapse.
• Shake oral suspension vigorously for at least 30 seconds to ensure it's well mixed.
• Once opened, use oral suspension within 6 weeks.

ACTION
Inhibits RNA and DNA synthesis.

Route	Onset	Peak	Duration
P.O.	Unknown	<2 hr	Unknown

Half-life: Adults, 47 minutes; children, 21 minutes.

ADVERSE REACTIONS

GI: nausea, vomiting, anorexia, painful oral ulcers, diarrhea, *pancreatitis,* GI ulceration.
Hematologic: *leukopenia, thrombocytopenia,* anemia, myelosuppression.
Hepatic: jaundice, *hepatotoxicity, hepatic necrosis.*
Metabolic: hyperuricemia.
Skin: rash, hyperpigmentation.

INTERACTIONS

Drug-drug. *Allopurinol:* Slows inactivation of mercaptopurine. Decrease mercaptopurine to 25% or 33% of normal dose.
Azathioprine: Increased risk of severe myelosuppression. Avoid giving together.
Febuxostat: May increase risk of toxicity. Use together is contraindicated.
Hepatotoxic drugs: May enhance hepatotoxicity of mercaptopurine. Monitor patient for hepatotoxicity.
Live-virus vaccines: May increase risk of toxicity from vaccine and infection. Consider therapy modification.
Nondepolarizing neuromuscular blockers: May antagonize muscle relaxant effect. Notify anesthesiologist that patient is receiving mercaptopurine.
Sulfamethoxazole–trimethoprim: May enhance bone marrow suppression. Monitor CBC with differential carefully.
Warfarin: May decrease or increase anticoagulant effect. Monitor PT and INR.

EFFECTS ON LAB TEST RESULTS

• May increase uric acid, transaminase, alkaline phosphatase, and bilirubin levels.
• May decrease Hb level.
• May decrease WBC, RBC, and platelet counts.

CONTRAINDICATIONS & CAUTIONS

• Contraindicated in patients resistant or hypersensitive to drug.
• Drug can cause myelosuppression and hepatotoxicity.
• Drug may increase risk of neoplasia.
• Use cautiously in elderly patients.

Dialyzable drug: Unlikely.
⚠ *Overdose S&S:* Anorexia, nausea, vomiting, diarrhea, myelosuppression, hepatic dysfunction, gastroenteritis.

PREGNANCY-LACTATION-REPRODUCTION

• Drug may cause fetal harm. Women of childbearing potential should avoid becoming pregnant during therapy.
• Drug may appear in breast milk. Patient should discontinue breast-feeding or discontinue drug.

NURSING CONSIDERATIONS

⚠ *Alert:* A diagnosis of acute lymphatic leukemia must be established before starting therapy. The supervising physician must be knowledgeable in assessing response to chemotherapy.
• After start of therapy, initially monitor CBC weekly and when needed to monitor ANC and platelet count to ensure sufficient drug exposure and to adjust for excessive hematologic toxicity.
• Risk of relapse is lower with evening administration than with morning administration.
⚠ *Alert:* Patients with thiopurine S-methyltransferase (TPMT) deficiency are at increased risk for severe mercaptopurine toxicity and generally require substantial dosage reduction. Determine TPMT status before starting therapy.
• Consider modifying dosage after chemotherapy or radiation therapy in patients who have depressed neutrophil or platelet counts or impaired hepatic or renal function.
⚠ *Alert:* Drug may be ordered as "6-mercaptopurine" or as "6-MP." The numeral 6 is part of drug name and doesn't refer to dosage.
• Monitor CBC and transaminase, alkaline phosphatase, and bilirubin levels weekly during induction and monthly during maintenance.
• Leukopenia, thrombocytopenia, or anemia may persist for several days after drug is stopped.
• Watch for signs of bleeding and infection
• Monitor fluid intake and output. Encourage 3 L fluid intake daily.

Reactions in bold italics are *life-threatening*. Interactions may have a *rapid onset* or a *delayed onset*.

◑ Alert: Watch for jaundice, clay-colored stools, and frothy, dark urine. Hepatic dysfunction is reversible when drug is stopped. If right-sided abdominal tenderness occurs, stop drug and notify prescriber.

• Monitor uric acid level. Use allopurinol cautiously.

• To prevent bleeding, avoid all I.M. injections when platelet count is below 100,000/mm^3.

• Anticipate need for blood transfusions because of cumulative anemia.

• GI adverse reactions are less common in children than in adults.

PATIENT TEACHING

• Educate patient or caregivers on proper handling, storage, administration, and disposal of drug and how to clean up accidental spillage of the solution.

• Instruct patient to watch for signs and symptoms of infection (fever, sore throat, fatigue) and bleeding (easy bruising, nosebleeds, bleeding gums, tarry stools). Tell patient to take temperature daily.

• Tell patient to take drug on an empty stomach in the evening.

• Caution female patient of childbearing potential to consult prescriber before becoming pregnant.

• Advise female patient to stop breastfeeding during therapy because of risk of toxicity to infant.

---

meropenem
mare-oh-PEN-em

Merrem

Therapeutic class: Antibiotics
Pharmacologic class: Carbapenems

AVAILABLE FORMS
Powder for injection: 500 mg, 1 g

INDICATIONS & DOSAGES
Adjust-a-dose (for all indications): For adults with CrCl of 26 to 50 mL/minute, give usual dose every 12 hours. If CrCl is 10 to 25 mL/minute, give half usual dose every 12 hours; if CrCl is less than 10 mL/minute, give half usual dose every 24 hours.

➤ **Complicated skin and skin-structure infections from *Staphylococcus aureus* (methicillin-susceptible isolates only), *Streptococcus pyogenes*, *Streptococcus agalactiae*, viridans group streptococci, *Enterococcus faecalis* (excluding vancomycin-resistant isolates), *Escherichia coli*, *Proteus mirabilis*, *Bacteroides fragilis*, or *Peptostreptococcus* species**
Adults and children weighing more than 50 kg: 500 mg I.V. every 8 hours over 15 to 30 minutes as I.V. infusion.
Children age 3 months and older weighing 50 kg or less: 10 mg/kg I.V. every 8 hours over 15 to 30 minutes as I.V. infusion or over 3 to 5 minutes as I.V. bolus injection (5 to 20 mL); maximum dose is 500 mg I.V. every 8 hours.

➤ **Complicated skin and skin-structure infections caused by *Pseudomonas aeruginosa***
Adults and children weighing more than 50 kg: 1 g as I.V. infusion every 8 hours over 15 to 30 minutes.
Children age 3 months and older weighing 50 kg or less: 20 mg/kg I.V. every 8 hours over 15 to 30 minutes as I.V. infusion or over 3 to 5 minutes as I.V. bolus injection (5 to 20 mL); maximum dose is 1 g I.V. every 8 hours.

➤ **Complicated intra-abdominal infections caused by viridans group streptococci, *E. coli*, *Klebsiella pneumoniae*, *P. aeruginosa*, *Bacteroides fragilis*, *B. thetaiotaomicron*, or *Peptostreptococcus* species**
Adults and children weighing more than 50 kg: 1 g I.V. every 8 hours over 15 to 30 minutes as I.V. infusion or over 3 to 5 minutes as I.V. bolus injection (5 to 20 mL).
Children age 3 months and older weighing 50 kg or less: 20 mg/kg I.V. every 8 hours over 15 to 30 minutes as I.V. infusion or over 3 to 5 minutes as I.V. bolus injection (5 to 20 mL); maximum dose is 1 g I.V. every 8 hours.
Children 32 weeks' or more gestational age (GA) and 14 days or more postnatal age (PNA): 30 mg/kg I.V. infusion every 8 hours over 30 minutes.

M

Children 32 weeks' or more GA and less than 14 days PNA: 20 mg/kg I.V. infusion every 8 hours over 30 minutes.
Children less than 32 weeks' GA and 14 days or more PNA: 20 mg/kg I.V. infusion every 8 hours over 30 minutes.
Children less than 32 weeks' GA and less than 14 days PNA: 20 mg/kg I.V. infusion every 12 hours over 30 minutes.

➤ **Bacterial meningitis caused by *S. pneumoniae, Haemophilus influenzae,* or *Neisseria meningitidis***
Children weighing more than 50 kg: 2 g I.V. every 8 hours.
Children age 3 months and older weighing 50 kg or less: 40 mg/kg I.V. every 8 hours; maximum dose, 2 g I.V. every 8 hours.

ADMINISTRATION

I.V.

▼ Obtain specimen for culture and sensitivity tests before giving first dose. Begin therapy while awaiting results.

Alert: Serious hypersensitivity reactions may occur in patients receiving beta-lactams. Before therapy begins, determine if patient has had previous hypersensitivity reactions to penicillins, cephalosporins, beta-lactams, or other allergens. If an allergic reaction occurs, stop drug and notify prescriber. Serious anaphylactic reactions require emergency treatment.

▼ Use freshly prepared solutions of drug immediately whenever possible. Stability of drug varies with form of drug used (injection vial, infusion vial, or ADD-Vantage container).

▼ For bolus, add 10 mL of sterile water for injection to 500 mg/20-mL vial or 20 mL to 1 g/30-mL vial. Shake to dissolve, and let stand until clear. Give over 3 to 5 minutes. May be stored for up to 3 hours at up to 77° F (25° C) or for 13 hours at up to 41° F (5° C).

▼ For infusion, an infusion vial (500 mg/100 mL or 1 g/100 mL) may be directly reconstituted with a compatible infusion fluid. Or, an injection vial may be reconstituted and the resulting solution added to an I.V. container and further diluted with an appropriate infusion fluid. Don't use ADD-Vantage vials for this purpose. Give over 15 to 30 minutes.

▼ Solutions prepared with NSS at 1 to 20 mg/mL may be stored for 1 hour at up to 77° F (25° C) or 15 hours at up to 41° F (5° C); use solutions prepared with D_5W immediately.

▼ For ADD-Vantage vials, constitute only with half-NSS for injection, NSS for injection, or D_5W in 50-, 100-, or 250-mL Abbott ADD-Vantage flexible diluent containers. Follow manufacturer's guidelines closely when using ADD-Vantage vials.

▼ **Incompatibilities:** Amphotericin B, diazepam, metronidazole, pantoprazole. Other I.V. drugs are variable; consult a detailed reference.

ACTION

Inhibits cell-wall synthesis in bacteria. Readily penetrates cell wall of most gram-positive and gram-negative bacteria to reach penicillin-binding protein targets.

Route	Onset	Peak	Duration
I.V.	Unknown	1 hr	Unknown

Half-life: 1 to 1.5 hours.

ADVERSE REACTIONS

CNS: ***seizures,*** headache.
CV: phlebitis, thrombophlebitis, peripheral vascular disorder.
EENT: oral candidiasis, glossitis.
GI: ***CDAD,*** constipation, diarrhea, glossitis, nausea, vomiting.
GU: RBCs in urine.
Hematologic: anemia.
Respiratory: ***apnea,*** pneumonia.
Skin: injection-site inflammation, pruritus, rash.
Other: ***anaphylaxis, sepsis,*** hypersensitivity reactions, inflammation, pain.

INTERACTIONS

Drug-drug. *Probenecid:* May decrease renal excretion of meropenem; probenecid competes with meropenem for active tubular secretion, which significantly increases elimination half-life of meropenem and extent of systemic exposure. Avoid using together.
Valproic acid: May decrease valproic acid levels, increasing the risk of breakthrough seizures. Monitor levels frequently and

observe patient for seizure activity. Consider alternative antibiotic or supplemental anticonvulsant therapy.

EFFECTS ON LAB TEST RESULTS
• May increase ALT, AST, bilirubin, alkaline phosphatase, LDH, creatinine, and BUN levels.
• May decrease Hb level and hematocrit.
• May increase eosinophil count. May decrease WBC count. May increase or decrease INR and platelet count. May prolong or shorten PT and PTT.

CONTRAINDICATIONS & CAUTIONS
• Contraindicated in patients hypersensitive to components of drug or other drugs in same class and in patients who have had anaphylactic reactions to beta-lactams.
• Use cautiously in elderly patients and in those with a history of seizure disorders or impaired renal function.
Dialyzable drug: Yes.
⚠ *Overdose S&S:* Exaggerated adverse reactions.

PREGNANCY-LACTATION-REPRODUCTION
• There are no adequate studies in pregnant women. Use during pregnancy only if clearly needed.
• Drug appears in breast milk. Use cautiously in breast-feeding women.

NURSING CONSIDERATIONS
• In patients with CNS disorders, bacterial meningitis, and compromised renal function, drug may cause seizures and other CNS adverse reactions.
• If seizures occur during therapy, stop infusion and notify prescriber. Dosage adjustment may be needed.
• Monitor patient for signs and symptoms of superinfection. Drug may cause overgrowth of nonsusceptible bacteria or fungi.
• Periodic assessment of organ system functions, including renal, hepatic, and hematopoietic function, is recommended during prolonged therapy.
• Monitor patient's fluid balance and weight carefully.

PATIENT TEACHING
• Instruct patient to report adverse reactions or signs and symptoms of superinfection.
• Advise patient to report loose stools to prescriber.

---

mesalamine
me-SAL-a-meen

Apriso, Asacol HD, Canasa, Delzicol, Lialda, Mesasal❦, Mezavant❦, Pentasa, Rowasa, Salofalk❦, sfRowasa

Therapeutic class: Anti-inflammatory drugs
Pharmacologic class: Salicylates

AVAILABLE FORMS
Capsules (controlled-release) ⓓⓝⓒ: 250 mg, 375 mg, 500 mg
Rectal suspension: 2 g/60 mL❦, 4 g/60 mL, 1 g/100 mL❦, 4 g/100 mL❦
Suppositories: 1,000 mg
Tablets (delayed-release) ⓓⓝⓒ: 400 mg❦, 800 mg, 1.2 g
Capsules (delayed-release) ⓓⓝⓒ: 400 mg, 800 mg

INDICATIONS & DOSAGES
➤ **Active mild to moderate distal ulcerative colitis, proctitis, or proctosigmoiditis**
Adults: Two 400-mg tablets (800 mg) P.O. t.i.d. for total dose of 2.4 g daily for 6 weeks. Or 1 g capsules P.O. q.i.d. for total dose of 4 g up to 8 weeks. Or 1,000 mg suppository P.R., retained in the rectum for 1 to 3 hours or longer, once daily at bedtime. Or 4 g retention enema once daily (preferably at bedtime); retain approximately 8 hours.
➤ **Remission-induction of active, mild to moderate ulcerative colitis**
Lialda
Adults: Two to four 1.2-g tablets (2.4 to 4.8 g) P.O. once daily with a meal for up to 8 weeks.
Pentasa
Adults: Four 250-mg capsules or two 500-mg capsules (1 g) P.O. q.i.d. for a total dose of 4 g for up to 8 weeks.
Delzicol
Adults: 800 mg t.i.d. for 6 weeks.

M

➤ **Maintenance of remission of ulcerative colitis**

Adults: 1.5 g Apriso P.O. once daily in the morning. Or, 1.6 g Asacol daily in divided doses. Or, two 1.2-g tablets Lialda P.O. once daily. Or, 1 g Pentasa P.O. q.i.d. Or, 1.6 g Delzicol P.O. in two to four divided doses.

➤ **Treatment of ulcerative colitis (Delzicol)**

Children age 5 and older weighing 54 to 90 kg: 27 to 44 mg/kg/day P.O. in two divided doses daily for 6 weeks. Maximum dose is 2.4 g/day.

Children age 5 and older weighing 33 to less than 54 kg: 37 to 61 mg/kg/day P.O. in two divided doses daily for 6 weeks. Maximum dose is 2 g/day.

Children age 5 and older weighing 17 to less than 33 kg: 36 to 71 mg/kg/day P.O. in two divided doses daily for 6 weeks. Maximum dose 1.2 g/day.

ADMINISTRATION

P.O.
- Give Lialda with food.
- Don't administer drug with antacids.
- Don't crush or cut delayed-release or controlled-release forms.
- Intact or partially intact tablets may be seen in stool. Notify prescriber if this occurs repeatedly.
- Give Delzicol 1 hour before or 2 hours after a meal.
- If patient is unable to swallow Pentasa capsules whole, they may be opened and the contents sprinkled on applesauce or yogurt and consumed immediately.

Rectal
- Patient should retain rectal dosage form overnight (for about 8 hours). Usual course of therapy for rectal form is 3 to 6 weeks.
- Shake suspension well before each use and remove sheath before inserting into rectum.
- Patient should retain suppository for 1 to 3 hours or longer, if possible.

ACTION

An active metabolite of sulfasalazine, drug probably acts topically by inhibiting prostaglandin production in the colon.

Route	Onset	Peak	Duration
P.O., P.R.	Unknown	3–12 hr	Unknown

Half-life: About 5 to 10 hours.

ADVERSE REACTIONS

CNS: headache, dizziness, fever, fatigue, malaise, asthenia, insomnia.
CV: chest pain.
EENT: nasopharyngitis, pharyngitis, rhinitis, sinusitis.
GI: abdominal pain, cramps, discomfort, flatulence, diarrhea, rectal pain, bloating, nausea, pancolitis, vomiting, constipation, eructation, *hemorrhage.*
GU: interstitial nephritis, nephropathy, *nephrotoxicity.*
Musculoskeletal: arthralgia, myalgia, back pain, hypertonia.
Respiratory: wheezing, bronchitis, cough, dyspnea.
Skin: itching, rash, urticaria, hair loss.
Other: chills, acne.

INTERACTIONS

Drug-drug. *Antacids, H_2 antagonists, PPIs:* May cause premature release of delayed- or extended-release products. Avoid concurrent administration. Consider therapy modification.
Azathioprine, mercaptopurine: May cause blood disorders. Monitor blood cell counts and adjust therapy as needed.
Vaccines (varicella virus): May enhance adverse effect of varicella virus–containing vaccines, causing Reye syndrome. Consider therapy modification.
Warfarin: May decrease anticoagulation effect. Monitor effectiveness of therapy closely.

EFFECTS ON LAB TEST RESULTS

- May increase bilirubin, BUN, creatinine, AST, ALT, alkaline phosphatase, LDH, amylase, triglyceride, and lipase levels.
- May decrease Hb level and hematocrit and RBC and WBC counts.

CONTRAINDICATIONS & CAUTIONS

- Contraindicated in children and in patients allergic to mesalamine, sulfites (including sulfasalazine), any salicylates, or any component of the preparation.

• Use cautiously in elderly patients, in patients with renal or hepatic impairment, and in those taking nephrotoxic drugs.
Dialyzable drug: Unknown.
⚠ ***Overdose S&S:*** Confusion, diarrhea, headache, hyperventilation, diaphoresis, tinnitus, vertigo, vomiting.

PREGNANCY-LACTATION-REPRODUCTION

• There are no adequate studies in pregnant women. Use during pregnancy only if clearly needed.
• Drug appears in breast milk. Use cautiously in breast-feeding women.

NURSING CONSIDERATIONS

• Monitor periodic renal function studies and blood cell counts in patients on long-term therapy.
• Because the mesalamine rectal suspension contains potassium metabisulfite, it may cause hypersensitivity reactions in patients sensitive to sulfites.
• Absorption of drug may be nephrotoxic.
• Drug may be associated with an acute intolerance syndrome in which signs and symptoms (abdominal pain, cramping, bloody diarrhea, headache, fever, rash) may be similar to an ulcerative colitis exacerbation. If acute intolerance syndrome is suspected, discontinue drug.
• ***Look alike–sound alike:*** Don't confuse Asacol with Os-Cal.

PATIENT TEACHING

• Instruct patient to carefully follow instructions supplied with drug and to swallow tablets whole without crushing or chewing.
• Tell patient not to take drug with antacids.
• Advise patient to report all adverse reactions and to stop drug if fever or rash occurs. Patient intolerant of sulfasalazine may also be hypersensitive to mesalamine.
• Tell patient to remove foil wrapper from suppositories before inserting into rectum.
• Teach patient about proper use of retention enema.

SAFETY ALERT!

metformin hydrochloride

met-FORE-min

Fortamet, Glucophage✐, Glucophage XR✐, Glumetza, Glycon✱, Riomet

Therapeutic class: Antidiabetics
Pharmacologic class: Biguanides

AVAILABLE FORMS

Oral solution: 500 mg/5 mL
Tablets: 500 mg, 850 mg, 1,000 mg
Tablets (extended-release) (DNC): 500 mg, 750 mg, 1,000 mg

INDICATIONS & DOSAGES

Adjust-a-dose (for all indications): Obtain patient's estimated GFR (eGFR) before starting drug. Contraindicated in patients with eGFR below 30 mL/minute/1.73 m^2. Starting drug in patients with eGFR between 30 and 45 mL/minute/1.73 m^2 isn't recommended. If eGFR falls below 45 mL/minute/1.73 m^2 in patients taking drug, assess benefits and risks of continuing treatment. Discontinue if eGFR falls below 30 mL/minute/1.73 m^2. Obtain eGFR at least annually in all patients taking drug. In patients at increased risk for development of renal impairment such as the elderly, assess renal function more frequently.

For elderly or debilitated patients, use conservative initial and maintenance dosage because of potential decrease in renal function. Adjust dosage carefully. Don't adjust to maximum dosage.

➤ **Adjunct to diet to lower glucose level in patients with type 2 diabetes**
Adults: If using regular-release tablets or oral solution, initially 500 mg P.O. b.i.d. given with morning and evening meals, or 850 mg P.O. once daily given with morning meal. Titrate immediate-release forms in increments of 500 mg weekly or 850 mg every other week to maximum dose of 2,550 mg P.O. daily in divided doses. If using extended-release formulation, start therapy at 500 mg (500 to 1,000 mg for Fortamet) P.O. once daily with the evening meal. May increase dose as tolerated weekly

M

(every 1 to 2 weeks for Glumetza) in increments of 500 mg daily, up to a maximum dose of 2,000 mg once daily (2,500 mg for Fortamet). If higher doses are required, consider a trial of 1,000 mg b.i.d. or using the regular-release formulation up to its maximum dose.

Children ages 10 and older: 500 mg P.O. b.i.d. using the regular-release formulation only. Increase dosage in increments of 500 mg weekly up to a maximum of 2,000 mg daily in divided doses.

➤ **Adjunct to diet and exercise in type 2 diabetes as monotherapy or with a sulfonylurea or insulin (Fortamet)**
Adults age 17 and older: Initially, 500 mg P.O. with evening meal for patients on insulin therapy. Increase dosage based on glucose level in increments of 500 mg weekly to a maximum of 2,500 mg daily. Decrease insulin dose by 10% to 25% when fasting blood glucose level is less than 120 mg/dL.

If patient has not responded to 4 weeks of maximum-dose Fortamet monotherapy, consider gradual addition of an oral sulfonylurea.

ADMINISTRATION
P.O.
• Give drug with meals. Maximum doses may be better tolerated if total dose is divided and given in three doses with meals (immediate-release tablets only).
• Don't cut or crush extended-release tablets.
• Give Fortamet with full glass of water with the evening meal.

ACTION
Decreases hepatic glucose production and intestinal absorption of glucose and improves insulin sensitivity (increases peripheral glucose uptake and use).

Route	Onset	Peak	Duration
P.O. (conventional)	Unknown	2–4 hr	Unknown
P.O. (extended-release)	Unknown	4–8 hr	Unknown
P.O. (solution)	Unknown	2½ hr	Unknown

Half-life: About 6 hours.

ADVERSE REACTIONS
CNS: asthenia, headache, dizziness, chills, light-headedness.
CV: chest discomfort, palpitations, hypertension.
EENT: ear pain, rhinitis, seasonal allergy, toothache, tooth abscess, tonsillitis.
GI: diarrhea, nausea, vomiting, abdominal bloating, flatulence, anorexia, taste disorder, abnormal stools, constipation, dyspepsia.
Metabolic: *lactic acidosis, hypoglycemia.*
Musculoskeletal: myalgia, limb pain.
Respiratory: URI.
Skin: flushing, nail disorder.
Other: accidental injury, infection.

INTERACTIONS
Drug-drug. *Beta blockers:* Hypoglycemia may be difficult to recognize in patients using beta blockers. Monitor patient and blood glucose.
Calcium channel blockers, corticosteroids, estrogens, fosphenytoin, hormonal contraceptives, isoniazid, nicotinic acid, phenothiazines, phenytoin, sympathomimetics, thiazide and other diuretics, thyroid drugs: May produce hyperglycemia. Monitor patient's glycemic control. Metformin dosage may need to be increased.
Cationic drugs (such as amiloride, cimetidine, digoxin, morphine, procainamide, quinidine, quinine, ranitidine, triamterene, trimethoprim, vancomycin): May compete for common renal tubular transport systems, which may increase metformin level. Monitor glucose level.
Nifedipine: May increase metformin level. Monitor patient closely. Metformin dosage may need to be decreased.
Radiologic contrast dye: May cause acute renal failure. Withhold metformin at the time of or prior to the procedure and 48 hours after the procedure. Restart drug only after renal function is evaluated and found to be normal.
Drug-herb. *Guar gum:* May decrease hypoglycemic effect. Discourage use together.
Drug-lifestyle. *Alcohol use:* May increase drug effects. Discourage use together.

EFFECTS ON LAB TEST RESULTS
• May decrease vitamin B_{12} and Hb levels.

Reactions in bold italics are *life-threatening*. Interactions may have a *rapid onset* or a *delayed onset*.

CONTRAINDICATIONS & CAUTIONS

• Contraindicated in patients hypersensitive to drug and in those with hepatic disease or metabolic acidosis, including diabetic ketoacidosis with or without coma.

• Contraindicated in patients with eGFR below 30 mL/minute/1.73 m². Not recommended in patients with eGFR between 30 and 45 mL/minute/1.73 m².

• Contraindicated in patients with acute HF requiring pharmacologic intervention and in patients with conditions predisposing to renal dysfunction, CV collapse, MI, hypoxia, and septicemia.

• Discontinue drug at the time of or before an iodinated contrast imaging procedure in patients with eGFR between 30 and 60 mL/minute/1.73 m²; in patients with a history of liver disease, alcoholism, or HF; and in patients who will be receiving intra-arterial iodinated contrast. Reevaluate eGFR 48 hours after imaging procedure; restart drug if renal function is stable.

Black Box Warning Because of risk of lactic acidosis, drug is contraindicated in patients older than age 80, unless CrCl indicates normal renal function. Withhold drug for conditions associated with hypoxemia, dehydration, or sepsis. Caution patients that acute or chronic excessive alcohol intake may increase risk of lactic acidosis. ■

• Administration of Glumetza with an insulin secretagogue (e.g., sulfonylurea) or insulin may require lower doses of the insulin secretagogue or insulin to reduce risk of hypoglycemia.

• Use cautiously in elderly, debilitated, or malnourished patients and in those with adrenal or pituitary insufficiency because of increased risk of hypoglycemia.

Dialyzable drug: Yes.

⚠ *Overdose S&S:* Hypoglycemia, lactic acidosis.

PREGNANCY-LACTATION-REPRODUCTION

• Abnormal blood glucose levels during pregnancy may cause fetal harm. Most experts recommend that insulin be used during pregnancy to maintain blood glucose levels as close to normal as possible. Use metformin during pregnancy only if clearly needed.

• Drug appears in breast milk. Patient should discontinue breast-feeding or discontinue drug, taking into account importance of drug to the mother and risk of hypoglycemia in the infant. Consider insulin therapy.

NURSING CONSIDERATIONS

• Before therapy begins and at least annually thereafter, assess patient's renal function. If renal impairment is detected, a different antidiabetic may be indicated.

• When switching patients from chlorpropamide to metformin, take care during the first 2 weeks of metformin therapy because the prolonged retention of chlorpropamide increases the risk of hypoglycemia during this time.

• Monitor patient's glucose level regularly to evaluate effectiveness of therapy. Notify prescriber if glucose level increases despite therapy.

• If patient hasn't responded to 4 weeks of therapy with maximum dosage, an oral sulfonylurea can be added while keeping metformin at maximum dosage. If patient still doesn't respond after several months of therapy with both drugs at maximum dosage, prescriber may stop both and start insulin therapy.

• Monitor patient closely during times of increased stress, such as infection, fever, surgery, or trauma. Insulin therapy may be needed in these situations.

Black Box Warning Suspect lactic acidosis in diabetic patients with metabolic acidosis who don't have evidence of ketoacidosis. Lactic acidosis is a medical emergency and must be treated in a hospital setting. Risk of drug-induced lactic acidosis is very low; however, when it occurs, it is fatal in approximately 50% of cases. Reported cases have occurred primarily in diabetic patients with significant renal insufficiency; in those with other medical or surgical problems; and in those with other drug regimens. Risk increases with degree of renal impairment and patient age. Hemodialysis may be necessary. ■

Black Box Warning Stop drug temporarily for surgical procedures (except minor procedures that don't restrict intake of food and fluids) and for patients undergoing radiologic studies involving use of contrast media containing iodine. Don't restart drug until patient's oral intake has resumed and renal function has been deemed normal by prescriber and at least 48 hours after contrast media. ■

• Monitor patient's hematologic status for evidence of megaloblastic anemia. Patients with inadequate vitamin B_{12} or calcium intake or absorption appear to be predisposed to developing subnormal vitamin B_{12} level. These patients should have routine vitamin B_{12} level determinations every 2 to 3 years.

• **Look alike–sound alike:** Don't confuse Glucophage with Glucovance or Glucotrol.

PATIENT TEACHING

• Instruct patient about nature of diabetes and importance of following therapeutic regimen, adhering to specific diet, losing weight, getting exercise, following personal hygiene programs, and avoiding infection. Explain how and when to monitor glucose level. Teach evidence of low and high glucose levels. Explain emergency measures.
Black Box Warning Instruct patient to stop drug and immediately notify prescriber about unexplained hyperventilation, muscle pain, malaise, dizziness, light-headedness, unusual sleepiness, unexplained stomach pain, feeling of coldness, slow or irregular HR, or other nonspecific symptoms of early lactic acidosis. ■

• Warn patient not to consume excessive alcohol while taking drug.

• Tell patient not to change drug dosage without prescriber's knowledge. Encourage patient to report abnormal glucose level test results.

• **Alert:** Advise patient not to cut, crush, or chew extended-release tablets; instead, he should swallow them whole.

• Tell patient that inactive ingredients may be eliminated in the stool as a soft mass resembling the original tablet.

• Advise patient not to take other drugs, including OTC drugs, without first checking with prescriber.

• Instruct patient to carry medical identification at all times.

• Tell patient to report all adverse reactions and that diarrhea, nausea, and upset stomach generally subside over time.

SAFETY ALERT!

methadone hydrochloride⌀
METH-a-done

Dolophine, Methadose

Therapeutic class: Opioid analgesics
Pharmacologic class: Opioid agonists
Controlled substance schedule: II

AVAILABLE FORMS
Dispersible tablets and diskets (for methadone maintenance therapy): 40 mg
Injection: 10 mg/mL
Oral solution: 5 mg/5 mL, 10 mg/5 mL, 10 mg/mL (concentrate)
Tablets: 5 mg, 10 mg

INDICATIONS & DOSAGES
Adjust-a-dose (for all indications): For elderly patients and those with renal or hepatic impairment, reduce initial dose.
➤ **Severe pain in opioid nontolerant patients**
Adults: Initiate dosing regimen for each patient individually, taking into account patient's prior analgesic treatment experience and risk factors for addiction, abuse, and misuse. Initially, 2.5 mg P.O. every 8 to 12 hours, or 2.5 to 10 mg I.M., I.V., or subcutaneously every 8 to 12 hours p.r.n. Titrate slowly, no more frequently than every 3 to 5 days, and increase dosage as needed or use rescue drug as needed to maintain analgesia.
➤ **Opioid detoxification; maintenance treatment of opioid addiction**
Adults: Initially, 20 to 30 mg P.O. daily to suppress withdrawal symptoms (highly individualized; some patients may require a higher dose). Initial dose shouldn't exceed 30 mg. Maintenance dose is 20 to 120 mg P.O. daily. Dosage adjusted, as needed.

ADMINISTRATION
P.O.
• Oral form legally required in maintenance programs. Completely dissolve dispersible tablets, disket, or oral solution in ½ cup of orange juice or powdered citrus drink.
• Oral dose is half as potent as injected dose.

I.V.
▼ Store at controlled room temperature (59° to 86° F [15° to 30° C]).
▼ Protect from light.
▼ **Incompatibilities:** Unknown.

I.M.
● For parenteral use, I.M. injection is preferred. Rotate injection sites.
● Store at controlled room temperature (59° to 86° F [15° to 30° C]).
● Protect from light.

Subcutaneous
● Monitor patient for pain at injection site, tissue irritation, and induration after injection.
● Store at controlled room temperature (59° to 86° F [15° to 30° C]).
● Protect from light.

ACTION
Unknown. Binds with opioid receptors in the CNS, altering perception of and emotional response to pain.

Route	Onset	Peak	Duration
P.O.	30–60 min	1–7½ hr	4–8 hr
I.V.	Unknown	Unknown	Unknown
I.M., subcut.	10–20 min	1–2 hr	4–5 hr

Half-life: 8 to 59 hours.

ADVERSE REACTIONS
CNS: clouded sensorium, hallucinations, dizziness, light-headedness, sedation, somnolence, *seizures,* agitation, choreic movements, euphoria, headache, insomnia, syncope.
CV: *arrhythmias, bradycardia, prolonged QT interval, cardiac arrest, shock, cardiomyopathy, HF,* flushing, phlebitis, edema, hypotension, palpitations.
EENT: visual disturbances.
GI: nausea, vomiting, abdominal pain, anorexia, biliary tract spasm, constipation, dry mouth, glossitis, ileus.
GU: urine retention.
Metabolic: hypokalemia, *hypomagnesemia,* weight gain.
Respiratory: *respiratory arrest, respiratory depression, pulmonary edema.*
Skin: diaphoresis, pruritus, urticaria.
Other: decreased libido, induration, pain at injection site, physical dependence, tissue irritation.

INTERACTIONS
Drug-drug. *Ammonium chloride, other urine acidifiers:* May reduce methadone effect. Watch for decreased pain control.
General anesthetics, hypnotics, MAO inhibitors, TCAs: May cause respiratory depression, hypotension, profound sedation, or coma. Use together with caution. Monitor patient response.
CYP2C9 inhibitors (fluvoxamine), CYP3A4 inhibitors (clarithromycin, erythromycin, itraconazole, ketoconazole, telithromycin, voriconazole): May increase or prolong adverse drug effects and cause fatal respiratory depression. Monitor patient closely and reduce dosage if necessary.
CYP450 inducers (carbamazepine, phenytoin, rifampin): May decrease methadone effect and precipitate a withdrawal syndrome. Monitor patient closely.
NNRTIs (delavirdine, efavirenz, nevirapine), protease inhibitors (lopinavir and ritonavir, nelfinavir, ritonavir), rifamycins: May increase methadone metabolism, causing opioid withdrawal symptoms. Monitor patient and adjust dose as needed.
Black Box Warning *Opioids:* May cause slow or difficult breathing, sedation, and death. Avoid use together. If use together is necessary, limit dosage and duration of each drug to the minimum necessary for desired effect. ■
Protease inhibitors, cimetidine, fluvoxamine: May increase respiratory and CNS depression. Monitor patient closely.
✪ Alert: *Serotonergic drugs (amoxapine, antiemetics [dolasetron, granisetron, ondansetron, palonosetron], antimigraine drugs, buspirone, cyclobenzaprine, dextromethorphan, linezolid, lithium, MAO inhibitors, maprotiline, methylene blue, mirtazapine, nefazodone, SNRIs, SSRIs, TCAs, trazodone, tryptophan, vilazodone):* May increase risk of serotonin syndrome. Use together cautiously and monitor patient for serotonin syndrome.
Drug-herb. ✪ Alert: *St. John's wort:* May reduce methadone effect and precipitate a withdrawal syndrome. May increase risk of serotonin syndrome. Use together cautiously and monitor patient closely.
Drug-lifestyle. *Alcohol use:* May cause additive effects. Discourage use together.

M

EFFECTS ON LAB TEST RESULTS
• May increase amylase level.

CONTRAINDICATIONS & CAUTIONS
• Contraindicated in patients hypersensitive to drug.

Black Box Warning Accidental ingestion of methadone, especially in children, can result in a fatal overdose of methadone. ∎

Black Box Warning Prolonged QT interval and serious arrhythmia (torsades de pointes) have occurred during methadone treatment. Most cases involve patients being treated for pain with large, multiple daily doses, although cases have been reported in patients receiving doses commonly used for maintenance treatment of opioid addiction. ∎

Black Box Warning Opioid drugs should only be prescribed with benzodiazepines or other CNS depressants to patients for whom alternative treatment options are inadequate. ∎

☉ *Alert:* Drug may lead to a rare but serious decrease in adrenal gland cortisol production.

☉ *Alert:* Drug may cause decreased sex hormone levels with long-term use.

• Use with caution in elderly or debilitated patients and in those with acute abdominal conditions, severe hepatic or renal impairment, hypothyroidism, Addison disease, prostatic hyperplasia, urethral stricture, head injury, increased ICP, asthma, and other respiratory conditions.

☉ *Alert:* Patients are at increased risk for oversedation and respiratory depression if they snore or have a history of sleep apnea, haven't used opioids recently or are first-time opioid users, have increased opioid dosage requirements or opioid habituation, have received general anesthesia for longer lengths of time or received other sedating drugs, have preexisting pulmonary or cardiac disease, or have thoracic or other surgical incisions that may impair breathing. Monitor patients carefully.

☉ *Alert:* Deaths have been reported during initiation of methadone therapy for opioid dependence. Exercise extreme caution when initiating treatment.

☉ *Alert:* Drug isn't indicated as a p.r.n. analgesic.

Dialyzable drug: No.

⚠ *Overdose S&S:* Miosis, respiratory depression, somnolence, coma, cool clammy skin, skeletal muscle flaccidity, hypotension, apnea, bradycardia, noncardiac pulmonary edema, death.

PREGNANCY-LACTATION-REPRODUCTION
• Use drug during pregnancy only if potential benefit justifies fetal risk. Methadone clearance may increase during pregnancy, particularly during second and third trimesters. Dosage may need to be increased or dosing interval decreased. Use lowest possible dosage.

Black Box Warning Prolonged use during pregnancy can cause neonatal opioid withdrawal syndrome, which can be life-threatening and requires management by neonatology experts. If use is required for a prolonged period during pregnancy, apprise patient of the risk and ensure that appropriate treatment will be available. ∎

• Drug appears in breast milk. Sedation and respiratory depression in breast-feeding infants have been reported. Monitor infants for respiratory depression and sedation and slowly wean to prevent withdrawal symptoms.

• When methadone is used to treat opioid addiction in breast-feeding women, and if additional illicit substances are being abused, patient should pump and discard breast milk until sobriety is established.

• Long-term opioid use may cause secondary hypogonadism, which may lead to sexual dysfunction or infertility.

• Advise patients who developed amenorrhea secondary to substance abuse that pregnancy may occur after initiation of methadone maintenance treatment. Provide contraception counseling to prevent unplanned pregnancies.

NURSING CONSIDERATIONS
Black Box Warning Methadone is an opioid agonist and Schedule II controlled substance with an abuse liability similar to that of other opioid agonists, legal or illicit. Assess each patient's risk of opioid abuse or addiction before prescribing methadone. Risk of opioid abuse increases in patients with personal or family history of substance abuse (including drug or alcohol abuse or

---

Reactions in bold italics are *life-threatening*. Interactions may have a *rapid onset* or a *delayed onset*.

addiction) or mental illness (such as major depressive disorder). Routinely monitor all patients receiving methadone for signs and symptoms of misuse, abuse, and addiction during treatment. ∎

Black Box Warning Oral methadone can only be dispensed by certified treatment programs or during inpatient care for conditions other than concurrent opioid addiction. ∎

Black Box Warning Respiratory depression that can be life-threatening or fatal, QT-interval prolongation, and torsades de pointes have been observed during treatment. Be vigilant during treatment initiation and dosage titration. ∎

Black Box Warning Carefully monitor vital signs, pain level, respiratory status, and sedation level in all patients receiving opioids, especially those receiving I.V. drugs, even when given postoperatively. ∎

Black Box Warning Caution the patient or the caregiver of a patient taking an opioid drug with a benzodiazepine, CNS depressant, or alcohol to seek immediate medical attention if the patient has symptoms of dizziness, light-headedness, extreme sleepiness, slowed or difficult breathing, or unresponsiveness. ∎

⟁ *Alert:* If patient is taking opioids with serotonergic drugs, watch for signs and symptoms of serotonin syndrome (agitation, hallucinations, rapid HR, fever, excessive sweating, shivering or shaking, muscle twitching or stiffness, trouble with coordination, nausea, vomiting, diarrhea), especially when starting treatment or increasing dosages. Signs and symptoms may occur within several hours of coadministration but may also occur later, especially after dosage increase. Discontinue the opioid, serotonergic drug, or both if serotonin syndrome is suspected.

⟁ *Alert:* Monitor patient for signs and symptoms of adrenal insufficiency (nausea, vomiting, loss of appetite, fatigue, weakness, dizziness, low BP). Perform diagnostic testing if adrenal insufficiency is suspected. If adrenal insufficiency is confirmed, treat with corticosteroids and wean patient off opioids if appropriate. Discontinue corticosteroids when clinically appropriate.

⟁ *Alert:* Monitor patient for signs and symptoms of decreased sex hormone levels (low libido, erectile dysfunction, amenorrhea, infertility). If signs and symptoms occur, evaluate patient and obtain laboratory testing.

● Reassess patient's level of pain at least 15 and 30 minutes after parenteral administration and 30 minutes after oral administration.

Black Box Warning When used for detoxification and maintenance of opioid dependence, treatment products in oral form shall be dispensed only by opioid treatment programs. Administer in accordance with treatment standards cited in 42 CFR (Code of Federal Regulations) Section 8, including limitations on unsupervised administration. Dispensing hospitals and pharmacies are approved by the FDA and designated state authorities. ∎

● An around-the-clock regimen is needed to manage severe, chronic pain.

● Patient treated in methadone maintenance program usually needs an additional analgesic if pain control is needed.

● Monitor patient closely because drug has cumulative effect; marked sedation can occur after repeated doses.

● Monitor circulatory and respiratory status and bladder and bowel function. Patient may need a stool softener and stimulant laxative.

⟁ *Alert:* Respiratory depressant effects may last longer than analgesic effects. Monitor patient's respiratory status closely.

● When used as an adjunct in the treatment of opioid addiction (maintenance), withdrawal is usually delayed and mild.

⟁ *Alert:* Use caution when dosing. Confusion has occurred between milliliter and milligram doses.

● *Look alike–sound alike:* Don't confuse methadone with ketorolac, methylphenidate (Metadate CD, Metadate ER), dexmethylphenidate, and Mephyton.

PATIENT TEACHING

⟁ *Alert:* Explain assessment and monitoring process to patient and family. Instruct them to immediately report difficulty breathing or other signs or symptoms of a potential adverse opioid-related reaction.

M

⚠ *Alert:* Encourage patient to report all medications being taken, including prescription and OTC medications and supplements.

⚠ *Alert:* Caution patient to immediately report signs and symptoms of serotonin syndrome, adrenal insufficiency, and decreased sex hormone levels.

• Caution ambulatory patient about getting out of bed or walking. Warn outpatient to avoid hazardous activities that require mental alertness until drug's CNS effects are known.

• Instruct patient to increase fluid and fiber in diet, if not contraindicated, to combat constipation.

• Advise patient to avoid alcohol during therapy.

• Instruct breast-feeding women to monitor their infants for respiratory depression and sedation and when to contact health care provider for emergency care.

• Caution patients not to use CNS depressants during initiation of treatment with methadone.

methimazole
meth-IM-a-zole

Tapazole

Therapeutic class: Antihyperthyroid drugs
Pharmacologic class: Thyroid hormone antagonists

AVAILABLE FORMS
Tablets: 5 mg, 10 mg

INDICATIONS & DOSAGES
➤ **Hyperthyroidism**
Adults: If mild, 15 mg P.O. daily in three divided doses given at 8-hour intervals. If moderately severe, 30 to 40 mg daily in three divided doses given at 8-hour intervals. If severe, 60 mg daily in three divided doses given at 8-hour intervals. Maintenance dosage is 5 to 15 mg daily.
Children: 0.4 mg/kg P.O. in three divided doses daily given at 8-hour intervals. Maintenance dosage is 0.2 mg/kg in three divided doses daily.

ADMINISTRATION
P.O.
• Give drug with meals to minimize adverse GI effects.

ACTION
Inhibits synthesis of thyroid hormones.

Route	Onset	Peak	Duration
P.O.	Rapid	1–2 hr	36–72 hr

Half-life: 4 to 6 hours.

ADVERSE REACTIONS
CNS: headache, drowsiness, vertigo, paresthesia, neuritis, neuropathies, CNS stimulation, fever.
CV: edema.
GI: nausea, vomiting, salivary gland enlargement, loss of taste, epigastric distress.
Hematologic: *agranulocytosis, leukopenia, thrombocytopenia, aplastic anemia.*
Hepatic: jaundice, hepatic dysfunction, *hepatitis.*
Metabolic: hypothyroidism.
Musculoskeletal: arthralgia, myalgia.
Skin: rash, urticaria, discoloration, pruritus, erythema nodosum, exfoliative dermatitis, lupuslike syndrome, abnormal hair loss.
Other: lymphadenopathy.

INTERACTIONS
Drug-drug. *Aminophylline, theophylline:* May decrease clearance of these drugs. Dosage may need to be adjusted.
Anticoagulants: May increase anticoagulant effect due to anti–vitamin K activity. Monitor patient closely.
Beta blockers: Beta-blocker clearance may be enhanced by hyperthyroidism. Dosage of beta blocker may need to be reduced when patient becomes euthyroid.
Cardiac glycosides: May increase cardiac glycoside level. Cardiac glycoside dosage may need to be reduced.
Potassium iodide: May decrease response to drug. Methimazole dosage may need to be increased.
Warfarin: May alter dosage requirements. Monitor PT and INR, and adjust warfarin dosage as needed.

EFFECTS ON LAB TEST RESULTS
• May decrease Hb level.

Reactions in bold italics are *life-threatening*. Interactions may have a *rapid onset* or a *delayed onset*.

• May decrease granulocyte, WBC, and platelet counts.
• May alter thyroid uptake of ^{123}I or ^{131}I.

CONTRAINDICATIONS & CAUTIONS

• Contraindicated in patients hypersensitive to drug.
• Drug may cause hypoprothrombinemia and bleeding. Monitor patient for bleeding.
Dialyzable drug: No.
⚠ *Overdose S&S:* Nausea, vomiting, epigastric distress, headache, fever, joint pain, pruritus, edema, aplastic anemia, agranulocytosis, hepatitis, nephrotic syndrome, exfoliative dermatitis, neuropathies, CNS stimulation or depression.

PREGNANCY-LACTATION-REPRODUCTION

• Drug may cause fetal harm, particularly in first trimester; consider other agents during this time. If used during pregnancy or if patient becomes pregnant during therapy, apprise her of potential hazard to the fetus.
• Pregnant women may need lower doses as pregnancy progresses, and drug may be stopped during last few weeks of pregnancy. Monitor thyroid function studies closely.
• Drug appears in breast milk. Use cautiously and administer after breast-feeding and in divided doses.

NURSING CONSIDERATIONS

• Monitor CBC periodically to detect impending leukopenia, thrombocytopenia, and agranulocytosis; also monitor hepatic function. Stop drug if liver abnormality occurs.
🔔 *Alert:* Doses higher than 40 mg daily increase risk of agranulocytosis.
• Watch for evidence of hypothyroidism (mental depression, cold intolerance, and hard, nonpitting edema); notify prescriber because patient may need dosage adjustment.
🔔 *Alert:* Stop drug and notify prescriber if severe rash or enlarged cervical lymph nodes develop.
• *Look alike–sound alike:* Don't confuse methimazole with mebendazole, methazolamide, metolazone, or metronidazole.

PATIENT TEACHING

• Tell patient to take drug with meals to reduce adverse GI reactions.
• Warn patient to report fever, sore throat, mouth sores, skin eruptions, anorexia, itching, right upper quadrant pain, or yellow skin or eyes.
• Tell patient to ask prescriber about using iodized salt and eating shellfish because the iodine in these foods may make the drug less effective.
• Warn patient that drug may cause drowsiness; advise patient to use caution when operating machinery or a vehicle.
• Instruct patient to store drug in light-resistant container.
• Teach patient to watch for evidence of hypothyroidism (unexplained weight gain, fatigue, cold intolerance) and to notify prescriber if it arises.

SAFETY ALERT!

methotrexate (amethopterin)
meth-oh-TREX-ate

Otrexup, Rasuvo

methotrexate sodium
Trexall

Therapeutic class: Antineoplastics
Pharmacologic class: Folate antagonists

AVAILABLE FORMS

Autoinjector: 7.5 mg/0.15 mL, 7.5 mg/0.4 mL, 10 mg/0.2 mL, 10 mg/0.4 mL, 12.5 mg/0.25 mL, 15 mg/0.3 mL, 15 mg/0.4 mL, 17.5 mg/0.35 mL, 20 mg/0.4 mL, 22.5 mg/0.45 mL, 25 mg/0.4 mL, 25 mg/0.5 mL, 27.5 mg/0.55 mL, 30 mg/0.6 mL
Injection: 25 mg/mL in 2-mL, 4-mL, 8-mL, 10-mL, 20-mL, and 40-mL preservative-free single-use vials; 25 mg/mL in 2-mL and 10-mL vials containing benzyl alcohol
Lyophilized powder: 2.5 mg/mL, 25 mg/mL in 1,000-mg preservative-free vials
Tablets (scored): 2.5 mg, 5 mg, 7.5 mg, 10 mg, 15 mg

M

INDICATIONS & DOSAGES

Adjust-a-dose (for all indications): Reduce dosage in patients with impaired renal function.

➤ **Trophoblastic tumors (choriocarcinoma, hydatidiform mole) (except Otrexup, Rasuvo)**

Adults: 15 to 30 mg P.O. or I.M. daily for 5 days. Repeat after 1 or more weeks, based on response or toxicity. Number of courses is three to maximum of five.

➤ **Acute lymphocytic leukemia (except Otrexup, Rasuvo)**

Adults and children: 3.3 mg/m^2 daily P.O., I.V., or I.M. with 60 mg/m^2 prednisone daily for 4 to 6 weeks or until remission occurs; then 30 mg/m^2 P.O. or I.M. weekly in two divided doses or 2.5 mg/kg I.V. every 14 days.

➤ **Meningeal leukemia (except Otrexup, Rasuvo)**

Adults and children: 12 mg/m^2 or less (maximum 15 mg) intrathecally every 2 to 5 days until CSF is normal; then one additional dose. Or, for children, use dosages based on age.

Children age 3 and older: 12 mg intrathecally every 2 to 5 days.

Children ages 2 to younger than 3: 10 mg intrathecally every 2 to 5 days.

Children ages 1 to younger than 2: 8 mg intrathecally every 2 to 5 days.

Children younger than age 1: 6 mg intrathecally every 2 to 5 days.

➤ **Burkitt lymphoma (stage I, II) (except Otrexup, Rasuvo)**

Adults: 10 to 25 mg P.O. daily for 4 to 8 days, with 7- to 10-day rest intervals.

➤ **Lymphosarcoma (stage III) (except Otrexup, Rasuvo)**

Adults: 0.625 to 2.5 mg/kg daily P.O., I.M., or I.V.

➤ **Osteosarcoma (except Otrexup, Rasuvo)**

Adults: Initially, 12 g/m^2 I.V. (maximum dose, 20 g) as 4-hour infusion. If dose isn't sufficient to produce peak serum methotrexate concentration of 1,000 mcM (10^{-3} mol/L), may increase subsequent doses to 15 g/m^2 I.V., as 4-hour I.V. infusion at postoperative weeks 4, 5, 6, 7, 11, 12, 15, 16, 29, 30, 44, and 45. Give with leucovorin, 15 mg P.O. every 6 hours for 10 doses, be-

ginning 24 hours after start of methotrexate infusion.

➤ **Mycosis fungoides (except Otrexup, Rasuvo)**

Adults: 5 to 50 mg P.O. or I.M. once weekly; or 15 to 37.5 mg I.M. twice weekly.

➤ **Psoriasis**

Adults: 10 to 25 mg P.O., I.M., I.V., or subcutaneously as single weekly dose; or 2.5 to 5 mg P.O. every 12 hours for three doses weekly. Dosage shouldn't exceed 30 mg/week.

➤ **RA**

Adults: Initially, 7.5 mg P.O. I.M., or subcutaneously weekly, either in single dose or divided as 2.5 mg P.O. every 12 hours for three doses once weekly. Dosage may be gradually increased to maximum of 20 mg weekly.

➤ **Polyarticular course, juvenile RA**

Children and adolescents age 2 to 16: 10 mg/m^2 P.O., I.M., or subcutaneously once weekly. Or, 20 to 30 mg/m^2/week I.M. or subcutaneously.

ADMINISTRATION

P.O.

● Give drug when patient has an empty stomach.

I.V.

▼ Preparing and giving parenteral drug may be mutagenic, teratogenic, or carcinogenic. Follow facility policy to reduce risks.

▼ Dilution of drug depends on product, and infusion guidelines vary, depending on dose.

▼ Reconstitute 20-mg vial to a concentration no greater than 25 mg/mL. Reconstitute 1-g vial to a concentration of 50 mg/mL.

▼ If giving infusion, dilute total dose in D$_5$W.

▼ Reconstitute solutions without preservatives with NSS or D$_5$W immediately before use, and discard unused drug.

▼ **Incompatibilities:** Bleomycin, chlorpromazine, droperidol, gemcitabine, idarubicin, ifosfamide, midazolam, nalbuphine, promethazine, propofol.

I.M.

● Preparing and giving parenteral drug may be mutagenic, teratogenic, or carcinogenic. Follow facility policy to reduce risks.

Subcutaneous

● Administer subcutaneously in the abdomen or thigh only.

● Otrexup is a single-dose autoinjector for once-weekly subcutaneous use only and is available in specific dosage strengths. Use another formulation for dosing by other routes, doses less than 7.5 mg/week, doses more than 25 mg/week, high-dose regimens, or dosage adjustments between the available doses.

Intrathecal

● Preparing and giving parenteral drug may be mutagenic, teratogenic, or carcinogenic. Follow facility policy to reduce risks.

Black Box Warning Use preservative-free form for intrathecal or high-dose administration. ■

ACTION

Reversibly binds to dihydrofolate reductase, blocking reduction of folic acid to tetrahydrofolate, a cofactor necessary for purine, protein, and DNA synthesis.

Route	Onset	Peak	Duration
P.O.	Unknown	1–2 hr	Unknown
I.V.	Immediate	Immediate	Unknown
I.M.	Unknown	30 min–1 hr	Unknown
Subcut.	Unknown	1–2 hr	Unknown
Intrathecal	Unknown	Unknown	Unknown

Half-life: For doses below 30 mg/m² , about 3 to 10 hours; for doses of 30 mg/m² and above, 8 to 15 hours.

ADVERSE REACTIONS

CNS: *arachnoiditis within hours of intrathecal use,* subacute neurotoxicity possibly beginning a few weeks later, demyelination, malaise, fatigue, dizziness, aphasia, hemiparesis, fever.

EENT: pharyngitis, blurred vision.

GI: gingivitis, stomatitis, diarrhea, GI ulceration and *bleeding,* enteritis, nausea, vomiting.

GU: nephropathy, tubular necrosis, *renal failure,* menstrual dysfunction, abortion, cystitis.

Hematologic: *leukopenia, thrombocytopenia.*

Hepatic: *acute toxicity, chronic toxicity,* including cirrhosis and *hepatic fibrosis.*

Metabolic: *diabetes,* hyperuricemia.

Musculoskeletal: arthralgia, myalgia, osteoporosis in children on long-term therapy.

Respiratory: *pulmonary interstitial infiltrates,* pneumonitis.

Skin: urticaria, pruritus, hyperpigmentation, erythematous rashes, ecchymoses, rash, photosensitivity reactions, alopecia, acne, psoriatic lesions aggravated by exposure to sun.

Other: chills, reduced resistance to infection, *septicemia, sudden death.*

INTERACTIONS

Drug-drug. *Acitretin:* May increase the risk of hepatitis. Avoid using together.

Acyclovir: Use with intrathecal methotrexate may cause neurologic abnormalities. Monitor patient closely.

Digoxin: May decrease digoxin level. Monitor digoxin level closely.

Folic acid derivatives: Antagonizes methotrexate effect. Avoid using together, except for leucovorin rescue with high-dose methotrexate therapy.

Fosphenytoin, phenytoin: May decrease phenytoin and fosphenytoin levels. Monitor drug levels closely.

Hepatotoxic drugs: May increase risk of hepatotoxicity. Monitor patient closely.

NSAIDs, salicylates: May increase methotrexate toxicity. Avoid using together.

Oral antibiotics: May decrease absorption of methotrexate. Monitor patient closely.

Penicillins, sulfonamides, trimethoprim: May increase methotrexate level. Monitor patient for methotrexate toxicity.

Probenecid: May impair excretion of methotrexate, causing increased level, effect, and toxicity of methotrexate. Monitor methotrexate level closely and adjust dosage accordingly.

❸ *Alert: PPIs:* May cause methotrexate toxicity, especially when high doses of methotrexate are given. Use cautiously.

Procarbazine: May increase risk of nephrotoxicity. Monitor patient closely.

Theophylline: May increase theophylline level. Monitor theophylline level closely.

M

Thiopurines: May increase thiopurine level. Monitor patient closely.

Vaccines: May make immunizations ineffective; may cause risk of disseminated infection with live-virus vaccines. Postpone immunization, if possible.

Drug-food. *Any food:* May delay absorption and reduce peak level of methotrexate. Instruct patient to take drug on an empty stomach.

Drug-lifestyle. *Alcohol use:* May increase hepatotoxicity. Discourage use together.

Sun exposure: May cause photosensitivity reactions. Advise patient to avoid excessive sunlight exposure.

EFFECTS ON LAB TEST RESULTS

● May increase uric acid level. May decrease Hb level.

● May decrease WBC, RBC, and platelet counts.

● May alter results of laboratory assay for folate, which interferes with detection of folic acid deficiency.

CONTRAINDICATIONS & CAUTIONS

● Contraindicated in patients hypersensitive to drug and in those with psoriasis or RA who also have alcoholism, alcoholic liver, chronic liver disease, immunodeficiency syndromes, or blood dyscrasias.

Black Box Warning Use drug only in patients with life-threatening neoplastic diseases and in those with severe psoriasis or RA not adequately responsive to other therapy; deaths have occurred. Closely monitor patients for bone marrow, liver, lung, and kidney toxicities. ∎

Black Box Warning Methotrexate given with radiotherapy may increase the risk of soft-tissue necrosis and osteonecrosis. ∎

Black Box Warning Unexpectedly severe (sometimes fatal) bone marrow suppression, aplastic anemia, and GI toxicity have been reported with concomitant administration of methotrexate (usually in high dosage) with some NSAIDs. ∎

Black Box Warning Use cautiously and at modified dosage in patients with impaired hepatic or renal function, bone marrow suppression, aplasia, leukopenia, thrombocytopenia, or anemia. ∎

● Use cautiously in very young, elderly, or debilitated patients and in those with infection, peptic ulceration, or ulcerative colitis.

Dialyzable drug: Yes (using a high-flux dialyzer).

⚠ **Overdose S&S:** Leukopenia, thrombocytopenia, anemia, pancytopenia, bone marrow suppression, mucositis, stomatitis, oral ulceration, nausea, vomiting, GI ulceration, GI bleeding, sepsis or septic shock, renal failure, aplastic anemia, headache, seizures, acute toxic encephalopathy, cerebellar herniation associated with increased ICP, death.

PREGNANCY-LACTATION-REPRODUCTION

Black Box Warning Contraindicated during pregnancy. Don't use in women of childbearing potential unless benefits outweigh risks. ∎

● Contraindicated in breast-feeding women.

● If either partner is receiving methotrexate, they should avoid conception during and for a minimum of 3 months after therapy for males, and during and for at least one ovulatory cycle after therapy for females.

● Drug has been reported to cause impaired fertility, oligospermia, and menstrual dysfunction during and for a short period after therapy ends.

NURSING CONSIDERATIONS

Black Box Warning Methotrexate should be used only by health care providers whose knowledge and experience include the use of antimetabolite therapy. ∎

Black Box Warning Methotrexate-induced lung disease is a potentially dangerous lesion that may occur at any time during therapy. It isn't always fully reversible. Pulmonary symptoms (especially a dry, nonproductive cough) may require interruption of treatment and careful investigation. ∎

Black Box Warning Diarrhea and ulcerative stomatitis require interruption of therapy; hemorrhagic enteritis and death from intestinal perforation may occur. ∎

Black Box Warning Malignant lymphomas may occur in patients receiving low-dose methotrexate and may regress upon discontinuing drug. ∎

Black Box Warning Methotrexate may induce tumor lysis syndrome in patients with rapidly growing tumors. ∎

Black Box Warning Severe, occasionally fatal skin reactions have been reported following single or multiple doses of methotrexate. Reactions have occurred within days of methotrexate administration. Recovery has been reported with discontinuation of therapy. ∎

Black Box Warning Potentially fatal opportunistic infections, especially *Pneumocystis jiroveci* pneumonia, may occur with methotrexate therapy. ∎

Black Box Warning The high-dose regimens for osteosarcoma require meticulous care. ∎

❸ *Alert:* Drug may be given daily or once weekly, depending on the disease. To avoid administration errors, know your patient's dosing schedule.

• Monitor pulmonary function tests periodically and fluid intake and output daily. Encourage fluid intake of 2 to 3 L daily.

• Monitor uric acid level.

• Drug distributes readily into pleural effusions and other third-space compartments, such as ascites, leading to prolonged systemic level and risk of toxicity. Use drug cautiously in these patients.

❸ *Alert:* Alkalinize urine by giving sodium bicarbonate tablets or fluids to prevent precipitation of drug, especially at high doses. Maintain urine pH above 7. If BUN level is 20 to 30 mg/dL or creatinine level is 1.2 to 2 mg/dL, reduce dosage. If BUN level exceeds 30 mg/dL or creatinine level is higher than 2 mg/dL, stop drug and notify prescriber.

Black Box Warning It's essential to monitor CBC with differential, platelet count, and liver and renal function periodically. Watch for increases in AST, ALT, and alkaline phosphatase levels, which may signal hepatic dysfunction. Periodic liver biopsies are recommended for psoriatic patients who are receiving long-term treatment. Monitor patients at risk for impaired drug elimination (renal dysfunction, pleural effusions, ascites) more frequently. ∎

• Watch for signs and symptoms of bleeding (especially GI) and infection.

• To prevent bleeding, avoid all I.M. injections when platelet count is below 50,000/mm^3.

• Give blood transfusions for cumulative anemia. Patient may receive injections of RBC colony-stimulating factors to promote RBC production and decrease need for blood transfusions.

• Leucovorin rescue is needed with doses of more than 100 mg and starts 24 hours after therapy starts. Leucovorin is continued until methotrexate level falls below 5×10^{-8} M. Consult specialized references for specific recommendations for leucovorin dosage. Monitor methotrexate level and adjust leucovorin dose.

• The WBC and platelet count nadirs usually occur on day 7.

PATIENT TEACHING

• Advise patient to watch for signs and symptoms of infection (fever, sore throat, fatigue) and bleeding (easy bruising, nosebleeds, bleeding gums, tarry stools). Tell patient to take temperature daily.

Black Box Warning Fully inform patient of the risks involved with methotrexate therapy. ∎

• Teach and encourage diligent mouth care to reduce risk of superinfection in the mouth.

• Instruct patient how to take leucovorin. Stress the importance of taking as prescribed until instructed by prescriber to stop.

• Tell patient to use highly protective sunblock when exposed to sunlight.

• Advise women to stop breast-feeding during therapy.

M

methyldopa
meth-ill-DOE-pa

methyldopate hydrochloride

Therapeutic class: Antihypertensives
Pharmacologic class: Centrally acting
antiadrenergics

AVAILABLE FORMS
methyldopa
Tablets: 125 mg❖, 250 mg, 500 mg
methyldopate hydrochloride
Injection: 50 mg/mL

INDICATIONS & DOSAGES
➤ **Hypertension, hypertensive crisis**
Adults: Initially, 250 mg P.O. b.i.d. to t.i.d.
in first 48 hours. Increase if needed every
2 days. May give entire daily dose in
evening or at bedtime. Adjust dosages if
other antihypertensives are added to or
deleted from therapy. Adjust dosage at
48-hour intervals. Maintenance dosage is
500 mg to 2 g daily in two to four divided
doses. Maximum recommended P.O. daily
dose is 3 g. Or, 250 to 500 mg I.V. every
6 hours as required. Maximum I.V. dosage is
1 g every 6 hours. Switch to oral antihypertensives as soon as possible.
Children: Initially, 10 mg/kg P.O. daily
in two to four divided doses; or, 20 to
40 mg/kg/day I.V. in four divided doses.
Increase dose daily until desired response
occurs. Maximum daily dose is 65 mg/kg or
3 g, whichever is less.

ADMINISTRATION
P.O.
● If unpleasant adverse reactions occur,
patient shouldn't suddenly stop taking drug
but should notify the prescriber.
I.V.
▼ Dilute appropriate dose in 100 mL D₅W.
Infuse slowly over 30 to 60 minutes.
▼ **Incompatibilities:** Amphotericin B;
drugs with poor solubility in acidic media,
such as barbiturates and sulfonamides;
methohexital; some total parenteral nutrition solutions.

ACTION
May inhibit the central vasomotor centers,
decreasing sympathetic outflow to the heart,
kidneys, and peripheral vasculature.

Route	Onset	Peak	Duration
P.O.	4–6 hr	Unknown	12–48 hr
I.V.	4–6 hr	Unknown	10–16 hr

Half-life: About 2 hours.

ADVERSE REACTIONS
CNS: decreased mental acuity, sedation,
headache, weakness, dizziness, paresthesia,
parkinsonism, involuntary choreoathetoid
movements, psychic disturbances, depression, nightmares.
CV: orthostatic hypotension, edema, ***bradycardia, HF, myocarditis,*** aggravated angina,
paradoxical pressor response with I.V. use.
EENT: nasal congestion.
GI: dry mouth, ***pancreatitis,*** nausea, vomiting, diarrhea, constipation, flatus, sore or
"black" tongue.
GU: galactorrhea, dark urine.
Hematologic: ***thrombocytopenia, leukopenia, bone marrow depression,*** hemolytic
anemia.
Hepatic: ***hepatic necrosis, hepatitis,***
jaundice.
Musculoskeletal: arthralgia.
Skin: rash.
Other: drug-induced fever, gynecomastia,
hyperprolactinemia.

INTERACTIONS
Drug-drug. *Amphetamines, nonselective
beta blockers, norepinephrine, phenothiazines, TCAs:* May cause hypertensive
effects. Monitor patient closely.
Anesthetics: May need lower doses of anesthetics. Use together cautiously.
Barbiturates: May decrease actions of
methyldopa. Monitor patient closely.
Ferrous sulfate: May decrease bioavailability of methyldopa. Separate doses.
Haloperidol: May increase antipsychotic
effects of haloperidol or cause psychosis.
Use together cautiously.
Levodopa: May increase hypotensive effects, which may increase adverse CNS
reactions. Monitor patient closely.

Lithium: May increase lithium level. Watch for increased lithium level and signs and symptoms of toxicity.

MAO inhibitors: May cause excessive sympathetic stimulation. Avoid using together.

EFFECTS ON LAB TEST RESULTS

• May increase creatinine level. May decrease Hb level and hematocrit.

• May increase LFT values. May decrease platelet and WBC counts.

• May interfere with results of urinary uric acid testing, serum creatinine test, and AST test. May cause positive Coombs test result. May falsely increase urine catecholamine level, interfering with the diagnosis of pheochromocytoma.

CONTRAINDICATIONS & CAUTIONS

• Contraindicated in patients hypersensitive to drug and in those with active hepatic disease (such as acute hepatitis) or active cirrhosis.

• Contraindicated in those whose previous methyldopa therapy caused liver problems and in those taking MAO inhibitors.

• Use cautiously in patients with history of impaired hepatic function or sulfite sensitivity.

Dialyzable drug: Yes.

⚠ **Overdose S&S:** Sedation, acute hypotension, weakness, bradycardia, dizziness, constipation, abdominal distention, flatus, diarrhea, nausea, vomiting, light-headedness.

PREGNANCY-LACTATION-REPRODUCTION

• There are no well-controlled studies in pregnant women in the first trimester. Use only if clearly needed. Available data show use during pregnancy doesn't cause fetal harm and may improve fetal outcomes.

• Drug appears in breast milk. Use cautiously in breast-feeding women.

NURSING CONSIDERATIONS

• Monitor patient's BP regularly. Elderly patients are more likely to experience hypotension, syncope, and sedation.

• Occasionally, tolerance may occur, usually between the second and third months of therapy. Adding a diuretic or adjusting dosage may be needed. If patient's response changes significantly, notify prescriber.

• After dialysis, monitor patient for hypertension and notify prescriber, if needed. Patient may need an extra dose of drug.

• Monitor CBC with differential counts before therapy and periodically thereafter.

• Patients who need blood transfusions should have direct and indirect Coombs tests to prevent cross-matching problems.

• Monitor patient's Coombs test results. In patients who have received drug for several months, positive reaction to direct Coombs test may indicate hemolytic anemia.

• Report involuntary choreoathetoid movements. Drug may be stopped.

PATIENT TEACHING

• If unpleasant adverse reactions occur, advise patient not to suddenly stop taking drug but to notify prescriber.

• Instruct patient to report signs and symptoms of infection, yellowing of the skin, flulike symptoms, and muscle aches.

• Tell patient to check his weight daily and to notify prescriber if he gains 900 g in 1 day or 2.3 kg in 1 week. Sodium and water retention may occur but can be relieved with diuretics.

• Warn patient that, particularly at the start of therapy, drug may impair ability to perform tasks that require mental alertness. A once-daily dose at bedtime minimizes daytime drowsiness.

• Inform patient that low BP and dizziness upon rising can be minimized by rising slowly and avoiding sudden position changes and that dry mouth can be relieved by chewing gum or sucking on hard candy or ice chips.

• Tell patient that urine may turn dark if left sitting in toilet bowl or if toilet bowl has been treated with bleach.

M

methylnaltrexone bromide
meth-eel-NAHL-trek-zone

Relistor

Therapeutic class: GI drugs
Pharmacologic class: Peripherally acting
mu-opioid receptor antagonists

AVAILABLE FORMS
Injection: 8 mg/0.4 mL, 12 mg/0.6 mL
single-use vials
Tablets: 150 mg

INDICATIONS & DOSAGES
Adjust-a-dose (for all indications): If CrCl
is less than 30 mL/minute, reduce dose by
one-half.
➤ **Opioid-induced constipation (OIC)
in those receiving palliative care for advanced illness when response to laxatives
is insufficient**
Adults weighing more than 114 kg:
0.15 mg/kg subcutaneously every other
day, as needed.
Adults weighing 62 to 114 kg: 12 mg subcutaneously every other day, as needed.
Adults weighing 38 to less than 62 kg: 8 mg
subcutaneously every other day, as needed.
Adults weighing less than 38 kg: 0.15 mg/kg
subcutaneously every other day, as needed.
Adjust-a-dose: In patients with moderate or
severe renal impairment, give subcutaneous
dose every other day. If patient weighs more
than 114 kg, give 0.075 mg/kg; if weight is
62 to 114 kg, give 6 mg; if weight is 38 to
less than 62 kg, give 4 mg; if weight is less
than 38 kg, five 0.075 mg/kg.
➤ **OIC in patients with chronic noncancer pain**
Adults: 450 mg P.O. or 12 mg subcutaneously once daily. Discontinue maintenance laxative therapy before starting
methylnaltrexone. May resume laxative after patient has taken methylnaltrexone for
3 days if OIC symptoms persist. Reevaluate need for drug when opioid regimen is
changed.
Adjust-a-dose: For CrCl of less than
60 mL/minute, give 150 mg P.O. once daily
or 6 mg subcutaneously once daily. For
moderate or severe hepatic impairment, give

150 mg P.O. once daily. Or, for moderate or
severe hepatic impairment, if patient weighs
more than 114 kg, give 0.075 mg/kg subcutaneously; if weight is 62 to 114 kg, give
6 mg subcutaneously; if weight is 38 to less
than 62 kg, give 4 mg subcutaneously; if
weight is less than 38 kg, give 0.075 mg/kg
subcutaneously.

ADMINISTRATION
P.O.
● Give tablets with water on an empty stomach at least 30 minutes before first meal of
the day.
Subcutaneous
● Administer no more than one dose within
24 hours.
● To determine injection volume for the
0.15 mg/kg dose, multiply patient's weight
in pounds by 0.0034 and round up to the
nearest 0.1 mL, or multiply patient's weight
in kilograms by 0.0075 and round up to the
nearest 0.1 mL.
● Store drug at room temperature, away
from light.
● After drawn into a syringe as directed,
drug is stable at room temperature for
24 hours.
● Give injections subcutaneously into the
abdomen, thighs, or upper arms; rotate
injection sites. Don't inject into bruised,
tender, red, or hard areas.

ACTION
Antagonizes GI mu-opioid receptors, preventing opioid-induced slowing of GI motility and transit time.

Route	Onset	Peak	Duration
P.O.	Unknown	1½ hr	Unknown
Subcut.	Unknown	30 min	Unknown

Half-life: P.O., 15 hours; subcut., about 8 hours.

ADVERSE REACTIONS
CNS: dizziness, tremor, headache, anxiety.
EENT: rhinorrhea.
GI: abdominal pain, abdominal distention,
flatulence, nausea, diarrhea, vomiting.
Musculoskeletal: muscle spasms.
Other: chills, hot flushes, hyperhidrosis.

Reactions in bold italics are *life-threatening*. Interactions may have a *rapid onset* or a *delayed onset*.

INTERACTIONS
Drug-drug. *Opioid antagonists:* May increase risk of opioid withdrawal. Avoid combination.

EFFECTS ON LAB TEST RESULTS
None reported.

CONTRAINDICATIONS & CAUTIONS
❸ **Alert:** Contraindicated in patients with known or suspected GI obstruction and in those at increased risk for recurrent obstruction because of increased risk of GI perforation.
❸ **Alert:** Use cautiously in patients with peptic ulcer disease, Ogilvie syndrome, diverticular disease, infiltrative GI tract malignancies, or peritoneal metastases because of increased risk of GI perforation.
• Contraindicated in patients hypersensitive to drug.
❸ **Alert:** GI perforation has occurred rarely in patients with reduced GI tract integrity. Use cautiously.
• Use cautiously in patients with peritoneal catheters.
• Patients with disruptions to the blood-brain barrier may be at increased risk for opioid withdrawal or reduced analgesia. Consider overall risk-benefit profile.
• Drug hasn't been studied in patients with ESRD requiring dialysis.
• Safety and effectiveness in children haven't been established.
Dialyzable drug: Unknown.
⚠ **Overdose S&S:** Orthostatic hypotension, signs and symptoms of opioid withdrawal.

PREGNANCY-LACTATION-REPRODUCTION
• Don't use in pregnant women unless benefits outweigh fetal risks. Use in pregnancy may cause opioid withdrawal in a fetus.
• It isn't known if drug appears in breast milk. Patient should discontinue breast-feeding or discontinue drug.

NURSING CONSIDERATIONS
❸ **Alert:** Watch for symptoms of perforation (severe, persistent, or worsening abdominal pain). If symptoms occur, stop drug and evaluate patient.
• Discontinue drug if treatment with the opioid pain medication is also discontinued.

PATIENT TEACHING
• Inform patient that drug may be effective within a few minutes to a few hours after administration.
• Instruct patient to discontinue drug and notify prescriber if severe, persistent, or worsening abdominal pain or diarrhea or rash occurs.
• Tell patient to take tablets once daily with water at least 30 minutes before first meal of the day.
• Inform patient that vial is for single-use only; remaining drug should be discarded.
• Advise patient to avoid injecting the drug into areas where the skin is tender, bruised, red, or hard, to avoid areas with scars or stretch marks, and to rotate injection sites.
• Warn patient that no more than one dose should be taken within a 24-hour period.
• Advise patient to report loss of analgesia or signs and symptoms of opioid withdrawal (hyperhidrosis, chills, diarrhea, abdominal pain, anxiety, yawning).
• Warn patient to report all adverse reactions, to immediately report severe, worsening, or persistent abdominal pain, and to discontinue drug for severe or persistent diarrhea.

M

methylphenidate hydrochloride
meth-ill-FEN-i-date

Aptensio XR, Concerta✔, Metadate CD, Metadate ER, Methylin, QuilliChew ER, Quillivant XR, Ritalin✔, Ritalin LA, Ritalin-SR✔

methylphenidate transdermal system
Daytrana

Therapeutic class: CNS stimulants
Pharmacologic class: Piperidine derivatives
Controlled substance schedule: II

AVAILABLE FORMS
Oral solution (Methylin): 5 mg/5 mL, 10 mg/5 mL
Tablets (chewable): 2.5 mg, 5 mg, 10 mg
Tablets (Ritalin): 5 mg, 10 mg, 20 mg

Extended-release

Capsules (Aptensio XR) ⓞ: 10 mg, 15 mg, 20 mg, 30 mg, 40 mg, 50 mg, 60 mg
Capsules (Metadate CD) ⓞ: 10 mg, 20 mg, 30 mg, 40 mg, 50 mg, 60 mg
Capsules (Ritalin LA) ⓞ: 10 mg, 20 mg, 30 mg, 40 mg, 60 mg
Oral suspension: 25 mg/5 mL
Tablets (chewable; QuilliChew ER) ⓞ: 20 mg, 30 mg, 40 mg
Tablets (Concerta) ⓞ: 18 mg, 27 mg, 36 mg, 54 mg
Tablets (Metadate ER) ⓞ: 20 mg
Sustained-release
Tablets (Ritalin-SR) ⓞ: 20 mg
Transdermal system
Patch: 10 mg, 15 mg, 20 mg, 30 mg

INDICATIONS & DOSAGES
➤ **ADHD**

Adults: 10 mg (immediate-release) P.O. b.i.d. or t.i.d. Dosage varies; maximum dosage is 60 mg daily.
Children age 6 and older: Initially, 5 mg P.O. b.i.d. immediate-release form before breakfast and lunch, increasing by 5 to 10 mg at weekly intervals, as needed, until an optimum daily dose of 2 mg/kg is reached, not to exceed 60 mg/day.

To use Ritalin-SR and Metadate ER tablets in place of immediate-release methylphenidate tablets, calculate methylphenidate dosage in 8-hour intervals.

Concerta
Adults ages 18 to 65 not taking methylphenidate, or for patients taking other stimulants: Initially, 18 or 36 mg P.O. daily. May increase dosage in 18-mg increments at weekly intervals to maximum of 72 mg daily.
Adolescents ages 13 to 17 not currently taking methylphenidate, or for patients taking other stimulants: 18 mg P.O. extended-release Concerta once daily in the morning. Adjust dosage by 18 mg at weekly intervals to a maximum of 72 mg P.O. once daily in the morning.
Children ages 6 to 12 not currently taking methylphenidate, or for patients taking other stimulants: 18 mg extended-release P.O. once daily every morning. Adjust dosage by 18 mg at weekly intervals to a

maximum of 54 mg daily every morning.
Adolescents and children age 6 and older currently taking methylphenidate: If previous methylphenidate dosage was 5 mg b.i.d. or t.i.d., give 18 mg P.O. every morning. If previous dosage was 10 mg b.i.d. or t.i.d., give 36 mg P.O. every morning. If previous dosage was 15 mg b.i.d. or t.i.d., give 54 mg P.O. every morning. Maximum conversion daily dose is 54 mg. Once conversion is complete, adjust maximum dose in adolescents ages 13 to 17 to 72 mg once daily.
Metadate CD
Adults and children age 6 and older: Initially, 10 to 20 mg P.O. daily before breakfast, increasing by 10 to 20 mg at weekly intervals to a maximum of 60 mg daily.
Aptensio XR
Adults and children age 6 and older: Initially, 10 mg P.O. daily in the morning. Increase dosage weekly in increments of 10 mg to maximum of 60 mg daily.
Ritalin LA
Adults and children age 6 and older: Initially, 10 to 20 mg P.O. once daily. Increase by 10 mg at weekly intervals to a maximum of 60 mg daily. If previous methylphenidate dosage was 5 mg P.O. b.i.d., give 10 mg P.O. once daily. If previous methylphenidate dosage was 10 mg b.i.d., give 20 mg P.O. once daily. If previous methylphenidate dosage was 15 mg b.i.d., give 30 mg P.O. once daily. If previous methylphenidate dosage was 20 mg b.i.d., give 40 mg P.O. once daily. If previous methylphenidate dosage was 30 mg b.i.d., give 60 mg P.O. once daily.
Daytrana
Adults and children ages 6 to 17: Initially, apply one 10-mg patch to clean, dry, nonirritated skin on the hip, alternating sites daily. Apply 2 hours before desired effect and remove 9 hours later. Increase dose weekly as needed to a maximum of 30 mg daily. Base final dose and wear time on patient response.
Quillivant XR
Children age 6 and older: Initially, 10 to 20 mg P.O. once daily in a.m. May titrate weekly in dosages of 10 to 20 mg. Maximum dosage is 60 mg daily.

QuilliChew ER
Children age 6 and older: Initially, 20 mg P.O. once daily in the morning. Titrate dose up or down weekly in increments of 10 mg, 15 mg, or 20 mg. Maximum dosage is 60 mg daily.

➤ **Narcolepsy (except Aptensio XR, Concerta, Metadate CD, Ritalin LA, QuilliChew ER, and Quillivant XR)**
Adults: 10 mg immediate-release P.O. b.i.d. or t.i.d. 30 to 45 minutes before meals. Dosage varies; maximum dose is 60 mg/day.
Children age 6 and older: Initially, 5 mg immediate-release P.O. b.i.d. (before breakfast and lunch). Increase dosage, if needed, by 5 to 10 mg weekly. Maximum dose is 60 mg. To use Ritalin-SR or Metadate ER tablets in place of immediate-release methylphenidate tablets, calculate the dose of methylphenidate in 8-hour intervals.

ADMINISTRATION
P.O.
● Give chewable tablet with at least 8 oz (240 mL) of water or other liquid.
● Give immediate-release tablets, chewable tablets, and oral solution in divided doses b.i.d. or t.i.d., preferably 30 to 45 minutes before meals. Give last daily dose before 6 p.m. to prevent insomnia.
● Metadate CD, Aptensio XR, or Ritalin LA may be swallowed whole, or the contents of the capsule may be sprinkled onto a small amount of cool applesauce and taken immediately.
● Extended-release and sustained-release tablets (Metadate ER, Ritalin-SR) must be swallowed whole and never crushed, chewed, or divided.
● Concerta may be taken with or without food and must be swallowed whole. Don't crush, divide, or allow patient to chew Concerta tablets.
● Vigorously shake oral suspension bottle for 10 seconds before administering dose. Use oral dosing dispenser to measure dose. May give with or without food.
Transdermal
● Avoid placing the patch on the waistline or where tight clothing may rub it off. If possible, alternate sides of the body daily.

ACTION
Releases nerve terminal stores of norepinephrine, promoting nerve impulse transmission. At high doses, effects are mediated by dopamine.

Route	Onset	Peak	Duration
P.O. (Methylin, Ritalin)	Unknown	2 hr	Unknown
P.O. (Ritalin-SR)	Unknown	5 hr	8 hr
Aptensio XR	Unknown	2 hr; 8 hr	Unknown
P.O. (Metadate CD)	Unknown	1½ hr; 4½ hr	Unknown
P.O. (Ritalin LA)	Unknown	1–3 hr; 4–7 hr	Unknown
P.O. (Concerta)	Unknown	6–8 hr	Unknown
P.O. (Quillivant XR)	Unknown	5 hr	Unknown
P.O. (QuilliChew XR)	Unknown	5 hr	Unknown
Transdermal	2 hr	Variable	14 hr

Half-life: Conventional, 3 to 6 hours; extended-release (Metadate ER, Ritalin-SR), 3 to 8 hours; (Concerta, Metadate CD, Ritalin LA), 8 to 12 hours; (Aptensio XR), 5 hours; (Quillivant XR), 6 hours; (QuilliChew XR), 5 hours; transdermal, 3 to 4 hours.

M

ADVERSE REACTIONS
CNS: nervousness, headache, insomnia, *seizures,* tics, dizziness, akathisia, dyskinesia, drowsiness, mood swings, anxiety, irritability, depressed mood, tremor.
CV: palpitations, tachycardia, *arrhythmias,* hypertension.
EENT: blurred vision, pharyngitis, sinusitis, bruxism.
GI: nausea, abdominal pain, anorexia, decreased appetite, vomiting.
Hematologic: *thrombocytopenia, thrombocytopenic purpura, leukopenia,* anemia.
Metabolic: weight loss.
Respiratory: cough, URI.
Skin: exfoliative dermatitis, *erythema multiforme,* rash, urticaria, application-site irritation (redness, swelling, papules).
Other: viral infection, hyperhidrosis.

INTERACTIONS
Drug-drug. *Anticonvulsants (such as phenobarbital, phenytoin, primidone), SSRIs, TCAs (clomipramine, desipramine, imipramine), warfarin:* May increase levels of these drugs. Monitor patient for adverse reactions, and decrease dose of these drugs

as needed. Monitor drug levels (or coagulation times if patient is also taking warfarin).
Centrally acting alpha$_2$ agonists, clonidine: May cause serious adverse events. Avoid using together.
Centrally acting antihypertensives: May decrease antihypertensive effect. Monitor BP.
H$_2$ antagonists, PPIs: May interfere with normal release of Ritalin LA extended-release tablets. Monitor therapy.
MAO inhibitors: May cause severe hypertension or hypertensive crisis. Avoid using within 14 days of MAO inhibitor therapy.
Drug-food. *Caffeine:* May increase amphetamine and related amine effects. Discourage use together.
Drug-lifestyle. *Alcohol use:* May increase methylphenidate concentration, causing toxicity. Patient should avoid alcohol during therapy.

EFFECTS ON LAB TEST RESULTS
● May decrease Hb level and hematocrit.
● May decrease platelet and WBC counts.

CONTRAINDICATIONS & CAUTIONS
● Contraindicated in patients hypersensitive to drug and within 14 days of MAO inhibitor therapy. Some formulations are contraindicated in patients with glaucoma, motor tics, family history or diagnosis of Tourette syndrome, or history of marked anxiety, tension, or agitation. Refer to individual manufacturer's instructions.
● Avoid use in patients with structural cardiac abnormalities (Metadate CD is contraindicated).
◑ **Alert:** Drug may increase risk of prolonged, painful erection (priapism) in males of any age, with or without sexual stimulation. Incidence is rare, but if not treated immediately, priapism may lead to permanent damage to the penis.
● Because it doesn't dissolve, Concerta isn't recommended in patients with a history of peritonitis or with severe GI narrowing (such as small-bowel inflammatory disease, short-gut syndrome caused by adhesions or decreased transit time, cystic fibrosis, chronic intestinal pseudo-obstruction, or Meckel diverticulum).

● Use cautiously in patients with a history of emotional disorder, preexisting psychosis or bipolar disorder, seizures, EEG abnormalities, or hypertension, and in patients whose underlying medical conditions might be compromised by increases in BP or HR, such as those with preexisting hypertension, HF, recent MI, or hyperthyroidism.
Black Box Warning Drug has a high potential for abuse and dependence. Use cautiously in patients with a history of drug dependence or alcoholism. Long-term abusive use can lead to tolerance and psychological dependence. Psychotic episodes can occur. Monitor patient for severe depression and the effects of chronic overactivity during drug withdrawal. ■
◑ **Alert:** Chewable tablets contain phenylalanine.
◑ **Alert:** The transdermal patch may cause irreversible chemical leukoderma (loss of skin color) at patch application site and other areas of the body. Although not harmful, if hypopigmentation occurs, consider alternative treatments.
Dializable drug: Unknown.
⚠ *Overdose S&S:* Agitation, cardiac arrhythmias, confusion, seizures, coma, delirium, dryness of mucous membranes, euphoria, flushing, hallucinations, headache, hyperpyrexia, hyperreflexia, hypertension, muscle twitching, mydriasis, palpitations, sweating, tachycardia, tremors, vomiting.

PREGNANCY-LACTATION-REPRODUCTION
● There are no adequate studies in pregnant women. Use during pregnancy only if potential benefit justifies potential fetal risk.
● It isn't known if drug appears in breast milk. Use cautiously in breast-feeding women.

NURSING CONSIDERATIONS
● Don't use drug to prevent fatigue or treat severe depression.
● Drug may trigger Tourette syndrome in children. Monitor patient, especially at start of therapy.
● Observe patient for signs of excessive stimulation. Monitor BP.
● Check CBC, differential, and platelet counts with long-term use, particularly if patient shows signs or symptoms of

hematologic toxicity (fever, sore throat, easy bruising).

• Monitor height and weight in children on long-term therapy. Drug may delay growth spurt, but children will attain normal height when drug is stopped.

• Monitor patient for tolerance or psychological dependence.

• Carefully observe patient for digital changes because stimulants used to treat ADHD are associated with peripheral vasculopathy, including Raynaud phenomenon.

• If ADHD hasn't improved after a 1-month period at the appropriate dose, prescriber may discontinue drug.

❸ *Alert:* Monitor patients using patch for chemical leukoderma. Report skin changes to prescriber.

• *Look alike–sound alike:* Don't confuse methylphenidate with methadone. Don't confuse Ritalin with ritodrine or Rifadin. Don't confuse Ritalin SR with Ritalin LA.

PATIENT TEACHING

• Tell patient or caregiver to give drug 30 to 45 minutes before meals and to give last daily dose at 6 p.m. to prevent insomnia.

• Advise patient to avoid alcohol during therapy.

❸ *Alert:* Advise patient with phenylketonuria that the chewable tablets contain phenylalanine.

❸ *Alert:* Inform male patient of any age and caregivers of the rare but possible risk of priapism. Caution patient to seek medical attention if priapism or an erection lasting longer than 4 hours occurs.

• Warn patient against chewing sustained-release tablets.

• Metadate CD or Ritalin LA may be swallowed whole, or the contents of the capsule may be sprinkled onto a small amount of cool applesauce and taken immediately.

❸ *Alert:* Warn patient to take chewable tablet with at least 8 oz (240 mL) of water. Not using enough liquid to swallow tablet may cause the tablet to swell and block the throat, causing choking.

❸ *Alert:* Advise patient and caregiver to watch for signs of chemical leukoderma, especially under skin patch site, and to report any skin changes to prescriber. Caution

patient not to stop treatment without first consulting prescriber.

• Caution patient to avoid activities that require alertness or good psychomotor coordination until CNS effects of drug are known.

• Warn patient with seizure disorder that drug may decrease seizure threshold. Urge him to notify prescriber if seizure occurs.

• Advise patient to avoid beverages containing caffeine while taking drug.

• Teach parent to always use oral dosing dispenser to measure oral suspension dose.

• Tell parent to apply patch in morning immediately after opening; don't use if pouch seal is broken. Press firmly in place for about 30 seconds using the palm of your hand, being sure there is good contact with the skin, especially around the edges. Once the patch has been applied correctly, the child may shower, bathe, or swim as usual.

• Inform parent that, if patch comes off, a new one may be applied on a different site, but the total wear time for that day should be 9 hours. Upon removal, fold patch in half so the sticky sides adhere to each other, then flush down toilet or dispose of in a lidded container.

• If the applied patch is missing, have parent ask the child when or how the patch came off. Teach child that patch shouldn't be shared or removed except by parent or health care provider.

• Encourage parent to use the application chart provided with patch carton to keep track of application and removal.

• Tell parent to remove patch sooner than 9 hours if the child has decreased evening appetite or has difficulty sleeping.

• Tell parent the effects of the patch last for several hours after its removal.

• Warn parent and patient to avoid exposing patch to direct external heat sources, such as heating pads, electric blankets, and heated water beds.

• Tell parent to notify prescriber if the child develops bumps, swelling, or blistering at the patch application site or is experiencing blurred vision or other serious side effects.

M

methylPREDNISolone
meth-ill-pred-NISS-oh-lone

Medrol✐

methylPREDNISolone acetate
Depo-Medrol

methylPREDNISolone sodium succinate
Solu-Medrol

Therapeutic class: Corticosteroids
Pharmacologic class: Glucocorticoids

AVAILABLE FORMS
methylprednisolone
Tablets: 2 mg, 4 mg, 8 mg, 16 mg, 32 mg
methylprednisolone acetate
Injection (suspension): 20 mg/mL,
40 mg/mL, 80 mg/mL
methylprednisolone sodium succinate
Injection: 40-mg vial, 125-mg vial, 500-mg
vial, 1,000-mg vial, 2,000-mg vial

INDICATIONS & DOSAGES
➤ **Severe inflammation or immunosuppression**
Adults and children: 4 to 48 mg P.O. daily
depending on the disease treated. After
favorable response is noted, determine
maintenance dosage by decreasing until
lowest dosage that will maintain adequate
clinical response is achieved. Or, 10 to
80 mg acetate I.M. daily, or 10 to 40 mg
succinate I.M. or I.V., with subsequent doses
dictated by patient's clinical response and
condition. Or, 4 to 40 mg acetate into small
to medium joints or 20 to 80 mg acetate into
larger joints. Intralesional use is usually
20 to 60 mg acetate. Repeat intralesional
and intra-articular injections every 1 to
5 weeks.
Children: 0.11 to 1.6 mg/kg/day P.O., I.M.,
or I.V. (sodium succinate).

ADMINISTRATION
P.O.
● Give drug with milk or food when possible. Critically ill patients may need to
take drug with an antacid or H_2-receptor
antagonist.

I.V.
▼ Use only methylprednisolone sodium
succinate, never the acetate form.
▼ Reconstitute according to manufacturer's
directions using supplied diluent, or use
bacteriostatic water for injection with
benzyl alcohol.
▼ Compatible solutions include D_5W,
NSS, and dextrose 5% in NSS.
▼ For direct injection, inject diluted drug
into vein or free-flowing compatible I.V.
solution over at least 1 minute.
▼ For I.V. infusion, dilute solution according to manufacturer's instructions and give
over prescribed duration.
▼ For doses greater than 0.5 g, give I.V.
over at least 10 minutes to prevent arrhythmias and circulatory collapse. Recommended infusion rate is giving over at least
30 minutes.
▼ Discard reconstituted solution after
48 hours.
▼ **Incompatibilities:** Allopurinol,
aminophylline, calcium gluconate,
ciprofloxacin, cytarabine, diltiazem, docetaxel, doxapram, etoposide, filgrastim,
gemcitabine, glycopyrrolate, nafcillin,
ondansetron, paclitaxel, penicillin G
sodium, potassium chloride, propofol,
sargramostim, vinorelbine, vitamin B
complex with C.
I.M.
● Give injection deeply into gluteal muscle.
Avoid subcutaneous injection because
atrophy and sterile abscesses may occur.
● Dermal atrophy may occur with large
doses of acetate form. Use several small
injections rather than a single large dose,
and rotate injection sites.

ACTION
Not clearly defined. Decreases inflammation, mainly by stabilizing leukocyte
lysosomal membranes; suppresses immune
response; stimulates bone marrow; and
influences protein, fat, and carbohydrate
metabolism.

Reactions in bold italics are *life-threatening*. Interactions may have a *rapid onset* or a ***delayed onset***.

Route	Onset	Peak	Duration
P.O.	Rapid	2–3 hr	30–36 hr
I.V.	Rapid	Immediate	1 wk
I.M.	6–48 hr	4–8 days	4–8 days
Intra-articular	Rapid	7 days	1–5 wk

Half-life: 18 to 36 hours.

ADVERSE REACTIONS

CNS: euphoria, insomnia, psychotic be-havior, *pseudotumor cerebri,* vertigo, headache, depression, syncope, person-ality changes, paresthesia, *seizures,* malaise, emotional instability.
CV: *arrhythmias, HF, cardiomyopathy,* hypertension, tachycardia, syncope, my-ocardial rupture after MI, edema, throm-bophlebitis, *thromboembolism, cardiac arrest, circulatory collapse after rapid use of large I.V. dose.*
EENT: cataracts, glaucoma, IOP, exoph-thalmoses.
GI: peptic ulceration, GI irritation, in-creased appetite, *pancreatitis,* nausea, vomiting.
GU: menstrual irregularities.
Metabolic: hypokalemia, hyperglycemia, sodium and water retention, carbohydrate intolerance, hypercholesterolemia, hypocal-cemia.
Musculoskeletal: growth suppression in children, muscle weakness, osteoporosis.
Skin: hirsutism, delayed wound healing, acne, various skin eruptions.
Other: cushingoid state, susceptibility to infections, *acute adrenal insufficiency after increased stress or abrupt withdrawal after long-term therapy.*

INTERACTIONS

Drug-drug. *Aspirin, indomethacin, other NSAIDs:* May increase risk of GI distress and bleeding. Use together cautiously.
Barbiturates, carbamazepine, phenytoin, rifampin: May decrease corticosteroid effect. Increase corticosteroid dosage.
Cyclosporine: May increase toxicity. Monitor patient closely.
Ketoconazole and macrolide antibiotics: May decrease methylprednisolone clear-ance. Decreased dose may be required.
Oral anticoagulants: May alter dosage requirements. Monitor PT and INR closely.

Potassium-depleting drugs (thiazide di-uretics): May enhance potassium-wasting effects of methylprednisolone. Monitor potassium level.
Salicylates: May decrease salicylate lev-els. Monitor patient for lack of salicylate effectiveness.
Skin-test antigens: May decrease response. Postpone skin testing until after therapy.
Toxoids, vaccines: May decrease antibody response and may increase risk of neuro-logic complications. Avoid using together.
Drug-herb. *Echinacea:* May decrease therapeutic effects of immunosuppressants. Discourage use together.
Ginseng: May increase immune-regulating response. Discourage use together.

EFFECTS ON LAB TEST RESULTS

• May increase glucose and cholesterol levels and ALT, AST, alkaline phosphatase, and urine calcium levels.
• May decrease T_3, T_4, potassium, and calcium levels.
• May decrease ^{131}I uptake and protein-bound iodine levels in thyroid function tests. May cause false-negative results in nitroblue tetrazolium test for systemic bacterial infections. May alter reactions to skin tests.

CONTRAINDICATIONS & CAUTIONS

• Contraindicated in patients hypersensitive to drug or its ingredients, in those with sys-temic fungal infections, in premature infants (acetate and succinate), and in patients re-ceiving immunosuppressive doses together with live-virus vaccines.
• Use cautiously in patients with GI ul-ceration or renal disease, hypertension, osteoporosis, diabetes mellitus, hypothy-roidism, cirrhosis, diverticulitis, nonspecific ulcerative colitis, recent intestinal anasto-moses, thromboembolic disorders, seizures, active hepatitis, myasthenia gravis, HF, TB, ocular herpes simplex, emotional instability, and psychotic tendencies.
• Prolonged use may increase risk of infec-tion, mask signs of infection, and activate latent infections.
*Dialyzable drug:*Unknown.

M

PREGNANCY-LACTATION-REPRODUCTION

● There are no adequate studies in pregnant women. Use during pregnancy only if potential benefit justifies potential risk to the fetus. Use lowest effective dose for shortest duration.

● Drug appears in breast milk. Patient should discontinue breast-feeding or discontinue drug.

NURSING CONSIDERATIONS

◔ *Alert:* Epidural corticosteroid injections to treat neck and back pain and radiating pain in the arms and legs may result in rare but serious adverse events (loss of vision, stroke, paralysis, death). The use of epidural corticosteroid injections isn't approved by the FDA.

◔ *Alert:* Counsel patients who receive epidural corticosteroid injections to seek immediate medical attention if they experience loss of vision or vision changes; tingling in the arms or legs; sudden weakness or numbness of the face, arm, or leg on one or both sides of the body; dizziness; severe headache; or seizures.

◔ *Alert:* Drug may cause suppression of the HPA axis, which can lead to adrenal crisis. Younger children and patients receiving high doses are at increased risk. Withdrawal from corticosteroids should be done slowly and with careful patient monitoring.

● Medrol may contain tartrazine. Watch for allergic reaction to tartrazine in patients with sensitivity to aspirin.

● Drug may be used for alternate-day therapy.

● Most adverse reactions to corticosteroids are dose- or duration-dependent. For better results and less toxicity, give a once-daily dose in the morning.

◔ *Alert:* Different salts aren't interchangeable.

◔ *Alert:* Don't give Solu-Medrol intrathecally because severe adverse reactions may occur.

● If immediate onset of action is needed, don't use acetate form.

● Always adjust to lowest effective dose.

● Monitor patient's weight, BP, electrolyte level, and sleep patterns. Euphoria may initially interfere with sleep, but patients typically adjust to therapy in 1 to 3 weeks.

● Monitor patient for cushingoid effects, including moon face, buffalo hump, central obesity, thinning hair, hypertension, and increased susceptibility to infection.

● Measure growth and development periodically in children during high-dose or prolonged treatment.

● Watch for depression or psychotic episodes, especially in high-dose therapy.

● Diabetic patient may need increased insulin; monitor glucose level.

● Watch for an enhanced response to drug in patients with hypothyroidism or cirrhosis.

● Unless contraindicated, give low-sodium diet that's high in potassium and protein. Give potassium supplements as needed.

● Elderly patients may be more susceptible to osteoporosis with prolonged use.

● Taper off dosage after long-term therapy.

● *Look alike–sound alike:* Don't confuse Solu-Medrol with Solu-Cortef. Don't confuse methylprednisolone with medroxyprogesterone or methyltestosterone.

PATIENT TEACHING

◔ *Alert:* Counsel patient that before undergoing epidural corticosteroid injection, to discuss benefits and risks and other possible treatments with health care provider.

● Tell patient not to stop drug abruptly or without prescriber's consent.

● Instruct patient to take oral form of drug with milk or food.

● Teach patient signs and symptoms of early adrenal insufficiency: fatigue, muscle weakness, joint pain, fever, anorexia, nausea, shortness of breath, dizziness, and fainting.

● Instruct patient to carry or wear medical identification indicating his need for supplemental systemic glucocorticoids during stress. This card should contain prescriber's name, name of drug, and dosage taken.

● Warn patient on long-term therapy about cushingoid effects (moon face, buffalo hump) and the need to notify prescriber about sudden weight gain or swelling.

● Advise patient receiving long-term therapy to consider exercise or physical therapy. Also, tell patient to ask prescriber about vitamin D or calcium supplement.

● Instruct patient to avoid exposure to infections (such as chickenpox or measles) and to contact prescriber if such exposure occurs.

Reactions in bold italics are *life-threatening*. Interactions may have a *rapid onset* or a *delayed onset*.

methylTESTOSTERone
meth-ill-tes-TOSS-ter-own

Android, Testred

Therapeutic class: Androgens
Pharmacologic class: Androgens
Controlled substance schedule: III

AVAILABLE FORMS
Capsules: 10 mg
Tablets: 10 mg

INDICATIONS & DOSAGES
➤ **Metastatic breast cancer**
Women 1 to 5 years after menopause: 50 to 200 mg P.O. daily.
➤ **Hypogonadism; delayed puberty in carefully selected males**
Men and adolescents: 10 to 50 mg P.O. daily.

ADMINISTRATION
P.O.
● Drug is hazardous; use safe handling and disposal precautions.
● Give without regard for food.

ACTION
Stimulates target tissues to develop normally in androgen-deficient men. May have some antiestrogen properties, making it useful in treating certain estrogen-dependent breast cancers.

Route	Onset	Peak	Duration
P.O.	Unknown	2 hr	Unknown

Half-life: Varies from 10 to 100 minutes.

ADVERSE REACTIONS
CNS: headache, anxiety, depression, paresthesia, *stroke.*
CV: edema, venous thromboembolism, *MI.*
GI: irritation of oral mucosa with buccal administration, nausea.
GU: oligospermia, decreased ejaculatory volume, priapism, amenorrhea.
Hematologic: *suppression of clotting factors,* polycythemia.
Hepatic: reversible jaundice, *cholestatic hepatitis.*

Metabolic: hypernatremia, *hyperkalemia,* hyperphosphatemia, hypercholesterolemia, hypercalcemia.
Musculoskeletal: muscle cramps or spasms.
Skin: hypersensitivity reactions, acne.
Other: androgenic effects in women, altered libido, gynecomastia, hypoestrogenic effects in women, excessive hormonal effects in men, male-pattern baldness.

INTERACTIONS
Drug-drug. *Cyclosporine (systemic):* May increase cyclosporine hepatotoxicity. Consider therapy modification.
Hepatotoxic drugs: May increase risk of hepatotoxicity. Monitor liver function closely.
Insulin, oral antidiabetics: May decrease glucose level; may alter dosage requirements. Monitor glucose level in diabetic patients.
Oral anticoagulants: May increase sensitivity to oral anticoagulants; may alter dosage requirements. Monitor PT and INR.
Oxyphenbutazone: May increase methyltestosterone serum level. Monitor therapy.

EFFECTS ON LAB TEST RESULTS
● May increase sodium, potassium, phosphate, liver enzyme, lipid, and calcium levels. May decrease thyroxine-binding globulin and total T_4 levels.
● May increase RBC count and resin uptake of T_3 and T_4.

CONTRAINDICATIONS & CAUTIONS
● Contraindicated in men with breast or prostate cancer.
● Use cautiously in elderly patients; patients with cardiac, renal, or hepatic disease; and healthy males with delayed puberty.
Dialyzable drug: Unknown.
⚠ **Overdose S&S:** Nausea, edema.

PREGNANCY-LACTATION-REPRODUCTION
● Contraindicated in women who are or may become pregnant. Use during pregnancy may cause virilization of the female fetus. If patient becomes pregnant during therapy, apprise her of potential hazard to the fetus.

M

• It isn't known if drug appears in breast milk. Patient should discontinue breast-feeding or discontinue drug.

NURSING CONSIDERATIONS

• In children, obtain X-rays of wrist bones before therapy begins to establish bone maturation level. During treatment, bones may mature more rapidly than they grow in length. Periodically review X-rays to monitor bone maturation.

• Drug is typically used only for intermittent therapy. Because of potential hepatotoxicity, watch closely for jaundice.

• Promptly report evidence of virilization in women, such as deepening of the voice, increased hair growth, acne, or baldness.

• Watch for hypoestrogenic effects in women (flushing, diaphoresis, vaginal bleeding, nervousness, emotional lability, menstrual irregularities, and vaginitis, including itching, dryness, and burning).

• Watch for excessive hormonal effects in men. If patient is prepubertal, watch for premature epiphyseal closure, acne, priapism, growth of body and facial hair, and phallic enlargement. If he's postpubertal, watch for testicular atrophy, oligospermia, decreased ejaculatory volume, impotence, gynecomastia, and epididymitis.

• Unless contraindicated, use with high-calorie, high-protein diet. Give small, frequent meals.

• Periodically check cholesterol, calcium, and Hb levels, hematocrit, and cardiac and LFT results.

• Check weight regularly. Control edema with sodium restriction or diuretics.

🕄 *Alert:* In breast cancer, therapeutic response usually occurs within 3 months. If disease appears to progress, stop drug.

• Report signs of hypercalcemia. In metastatic breast cancer, hypercalcemia may indicate progression of bone metastases.

• Evaluate semen every 3 to 4 months, especially in adolescent boys.

🕄 *Alert:* Don't use to enhance athletic performance or physique.

• *Look alike–sound alike:* Testosterone and methyltestosterone aren't interchangeable. Don't confuse methyltestosterone with medroxyprogesterone.

PATIENT TEACHING

• Ensure patient understands importance of using effective contraception during therapy.

• Teach patient about potential adverse reactions and to report them.

• Tell female patient of childbearing potential to report menstrual irregularities and to stop drug while awaiting examination.

• Instruct patient to stop drug immediately and notify prescriber if pregnancy is suspected.

• Tell female patient to immediately report evidence of virilization, such as acne, swelling, weight gain, increased hair growth, hoarseness, clitoral enlargement, decreased breast size, deepening of voice, changes in libido, male pattern baldness, and oily skin or hair.

• Teach patient signs and symptoms of low glucose level (hypoglycemia) and method for checking glucose level; drug enhances hypoglycemia. Instruct patient to report signs or symptoms of hypoglycemia immediately.

• Advise adolescent and parents about the potential adverse effect on bone maturation before start of therapy.

---

metoclopramide hydrochloride
met-oh-KLOE-pra-mide

Apo-Metoclop✼, Metonia✼, Metozolv ODT, Reglan

Therapeutic class: GI stimulants
Pharmacologic class: Dopamine antagonists

AVAILABLE FORMS

Injection: 5 mg/mL
ODTs: 5 mg
Syrup: 1 mg/mL✼, 5 mg/5 mL
Tablets: 5 mg, 10 mg

INDICATIONS & DOSAGES

Adjust-a-dose (for all indications): For patients with CrCl below 40 mL/minute, decrease dosage by half.

➤ **To prevent or reduce nausea and vomiting from emetogenic cancer chemotherapy**

Adults: 1 to 2 mg/kg I.V. 30 minutes before chemotherapy; repeat every 2 hours for two doses, then every 3 hours for three doses.

➤ **To prevent or reduce postoperative nausea and vomiting**
Adults: 10 to 20 mg I.M. near end of surgical procedure; repeat every 4 to 6 hours, as needed.

➤ **To facilitate small-bowel intubation**
Adults and children older than age 14:
10 mg I.V. as a single dose over 1 to 2 minutes.
Children ages 6 to 14: 2.5 to 5 mg I.V. slowly over 1 to 2 minutes.
Children younger than age 6: 0.1 mg/kg I.V. slowly over 1 to 2 minutes.

➤ **To aid in radiologic examination**
Adults: 10 mg I.V. as a single dose over 1 to 2 minutes.

➤ **Delayed gastric emptying secondary to diabetic gastroparesis**
Adults: 10 mg P.O. 30 minutes before each meal and at bedtime for mild symptoms. Or, give 10 mg by slow I.V. infusion over 1 to 2 minutes 30 minutes before each meal and at bedtime for up to 10 days for severe symptoms; then P.O. dose may be started and continued for 2 to 8 weeks.

➤ **GERD**
Adults: 10 to 15 mg P.O. q.i.d., as needed, 30 minutes before meals and at bedtime.

ADMINISTRATION
P.O.
● Give drug 30 minutes before each meal and at bedtime when used for gastroparesis and GERD.

P.O. (ODT)
● Give drug at least 30 minutes before eating and at bedtime.
● Give immediately after opening sealed blister. If the tablet breaks or crumbles, throw it away and obtain a new one.
● Place tablet on patient's tongue. Tell him to let it melt for approximately 1 minute and then swallow.

I.V.
▼ Drug is compatible with D$_5$W, NSS for injection, dextrose 5% in half-NSS, Ringer injection, and lactated Ringer injection. NSS is the preferred diluent; drug is most stable in this solution.

▼ Give doses of 10 mg or less by direct injection over 1 to 2 minutes. Dilute doses larger than 10 mg in 50 mL of compatible diluent, and infuse over at least 15 minutes. Monitor BP closely.

▼ There is no need to protect drug from light if infusion mixture is given within 24 hours. If protected from light and refrigerated, it's stable for 48 hours.

▼ **Incompatibilities:** Allopurinol, ampicillin, amphotericin B cholesteryl sulfate complex, amsacrine, calcium gluconate, cefepime, chloramphenicol, doxorubicin liposomal, furosemide, pantoprazole, penicillin G potassium, sodium bicarbonate.

I.M.
● Inspect for particulate matter and discoloration. If either is present, don't use.

ACTION
Stimulates motility of upper GI tract, increases lower esophageal sphincter tone, and blocks dopamine receptors at the chemoreceptor trigger zone.

Route	Onset	Peak	Duration
P.O.	30–60 min	1–2 hr	1–2 hr
I.V.	1–3 min	Unknown	1–2 hr
I.M.	10–15 min	Unknown	1–2 hr

Half-life: 4 to 6 hours.

ADVERSE REACTIONS
CNS: anxiety, drowsiness, dystonic reactions, fatigue, lassitude, restlessness, *seizures, suicidal ideation,* akathisia, confusion, depression, dizziness, extrapyramidal symptoms, fever, hallucinations, headache, insomnia, tardive dyskinesia.
CV: *bradycardia, supraventricular tachycardia,* hypotension, transient hypertension.
GI: bowel disorders, diarrhea, nausea.
GU: incontinence, urinary frequency, erectile dysfunction.
Hematologic: *agranulocytosis, neutropenia.*
Skin: rash, urticaria.
Other: loss of libido, prolactin secretion, gynecomastia, amenorrhea.

INTERACTIONS
Drug-drug. *Anticholinergics, opioid analgesics:* May antagonize GI motility effects of metoclopramide. Use together cautiously.

M

CNS depressants: May cause additive CNS effects. Avoid using together.

Levodopa: Levodopa and metoclopramide have opposite effects on dopamine receptors. Avoid using together.

MAO inhibitors: May increase release of catecholamines in patients with hypertension. Use together cautiously.

Phenothiazines: May increase risk of extrapyramidal effects. Monitor patient closely.

Drug-lifestyle. *Alcohol use:* May cause additive CNS effects. Discourage use together.

EFFECTS ON LAB TEST RESULTS

● May increase LFT values, aldosterone levels, and prolactin levels.

● May decrease neutrophil and granulocyte counts.

CONTRAINDICATIONS & CAUTIONS

● Contraindicated in patients hypersensitive to drug and in those with pheochromocytoma, tardive dyskinesia, or seizure disorders.

● Contraindicated in patients for whom stimulation of GI motility might be dangerous (those with hemorrhage, obstruction, or perforation).

Black Box Warning Drug can cause irreversible tardive dyskinesia, even after drug is stopped. Risk increases with duration of therapy and total cumulative dose; there is no treatment. Discontinue drug if signs and symptoms occur. Except in rare cases, avoid treatment for longer than 12 weeks. ■

☯ Alert: Neuroleptic malignant syndrome has occurred rarely and may be fatal. If signs and symptoms develop (fever, CNS symptoms, irregular pulse, cardiac arrhythmias, or abnormal BP), discontinue drug.

● Use cautiously in patients with history of depression, Parkinson disease, or hypertension.

Dialyzable drug: No.

⚠ Overdose S&S: Drowsiness, disorientation, extrapyramidal reactions; seizures, lethargy (in infants and children).

PREGNANCY-LACTATION-REPRODUCTION

● There are no adequate studies in pregnant women. Use during pregnancy only if clearly needed.

● Drug appears in breast milk. Use cautiously in breast-feeding women.

NURSING CONSIDERATIONS

● Monitor bowel sounds.

● Safety and effectiveness of drug haven't been established for therapy lasting longer than 12 weeks.

● Metozolv ODT contains acesulfame K and mannitol.

● Monitor patient for involuntary movements of face, tongue, and extremities, which may indicate tardive dyskinesia.

● Monitor patient for fever, CNS symptoms, irregular pulse, cardiac arrhythmias, or abnormal BP, which may indicate neuroleptic malignant syndrome.

● Monitor patient for dizziness, headache, or nervousness after metoclopramide is stopped; these may indicate withdrawal.

● Diphenhydramine or benztropine may be used to counteract extrapyramidal adverse effects from high doses.

PATIENT TEACHING

● Instruct patient to take ODTs 30 minutes before food and at bedtime and not to repeat dose if inadvertently taken with food.

● Tell patient taking ODTs to open blister pack with dry hands and immediately place tablet on tongue, let it melt completely, and then swallow. (Taking it with water isn't necessary.) If tablet breaks or crumbles, advise patient to throw it away and take a new tablet out of the blister pack.

● Tell patient to avoid activities that require alertness for 2 hours after doses.

● Urge patient to report persistent or serious adverse reactions promptly.

● Advise patient not to drink alcohol during therapy.

● Teach patient signs and symptoms of tardive dyskinesia and neuroleptic malignant syndrome and to report any signs and symptoms that develop.

metolazone
me-TOLE-a-zone

Zaroxolyn

Therapeutic class: Diuretics
Pharmacologic class: Thiazide-like
diuretics

AVAILABLE FORMS
Tablets: 2.5 mg, 5 mg, 10 mg

INDICATIONS & DOSAGES
➤ **Edema in HF or renal disease**
Adults: 5 to 20 mg P.O. once daily.
➤ **Hypertension**
Adults: 2.5 to 5 mg P.O. once daily. Base
maintenance dosage on BP.

ADMINISTRATION
P.O.
● Give drug in the morning without regard
for meals.
🚫 *Alert:* Don't interchange Zaroxolyn tablets
and other formulations of metolazone that
share its slow and incomplete bioavailability.

ACTION
Increases sodium and water excretion by
inhibiting sodium reabsorption in ascending
loop of Henle.

Route	Onset	Peak	Duration
P.O.	1 hr	8 hr	≥24 hr

Half-life: 6 to 20 hours.

ADVERSE REACTIONS
CNS: dizziness, headache, fatigue, vertigo,
paresthesia, weakness, restlessness, drowsiness, anxiety, depression, nervousness,
blurred vision.
CV: orthostatic hypotension, palpitations,
chest pain, venous thrombosis.
GI: *pancreatitis,* anorexia, nausea, epigastric distress, vomiting, abdominal pain,
diarrhea, constipation, dry mouth.
GU: nocturia, polyuria, impotence.
Hematologic: *aplastic anemia, agranulocytosis, leukopenia,* purpura.
Hepatic: jaundice, *hepatitis.*

Metabolic: hyperglycemia and impaired
glucose tolerance; fluid and electrolyte
imbalances, including hypokalemia, hypomagnesemia, dilutional hyponatremia
and hypochloremia, metabolic alkalosis,
and hypercalcemia; volume depletion and
dehydration.
Musculoskeletal: muscle cramps.
Skin: dermatitis, photosensitivity reactions,
rash, pruritus, urticaria, skin necrosis, purpura, *Stevens-Johnson syndrome, toxic
epidermal necrolysis,* necrotizing angiitis.

INTERACTIONS
Drug-drug. *Amphotericin B, corticosteroids:* May increase risk of hypokalemia.
Monitor potassium level closely.
Anticoagulants: May decrease anticoagulant
response. Monitor PT and INR.
Antidiabetics: May alter glucose level and
require dosage adjustment of antidiabetics.
Monitor glucose level.
Barbiturates, opioids: May increase orthostatic hypotensive effect. Monitor patient
closely.
*Bumetanide, ethacrynic acid, furosemide,
torsemide:* May cause excessive diuretic
response, causing serious electrolyte abnormalities or dehydration. Adjust doses
carefully, and monitor patient closely for
signs and symptoms of excessive diuretic
response.
Cholestyramine, colestipol: May decrease
intestinal absorption of thiazides. Separate
doses.
Diazoxide: May increase antihypertensive,
hyperglycemic, and hyperuricemic effects.
Use together cautiously.
Lithium: May decrease lithium clearance,
increasing risk of lithium toxicity. Monitor
lithium level.
NSAIDs: May increase risk of renal failure.
May decrease diuretic and antihypertensive
effects. Monitor renal function and BP.
Other antihypertensives: May have additive
effects. Use together cautiously.
Drug-herb. *Licorice:* May cause hypokalemia. Discourage use together.
Drug-lifestyle. *Alcohol use:* May increase
orthostatic hypotensive effect. Discourage
use together.

M

Sun exposure: May cause photosensitivity reaction. Advise patient to avoid excessive sunlight exposure.

EFFECTS ON LAB TEST RESULTS
• May increase glucose, calcium, cholesterol, BUN, and triglyceride levels. May decrease potassium, sodium, magnesium, and chloride levels.
• May decrease Hb level and granulocyte and WBC counts.

CONTRAINDICATIONS & CAUTIONS
• Contraindicated in patients hypersensitive to thiazides, other sulfonamide-derived drugs, or metolazone and in those with anuria, hepatic coma, or precoma.
• Use cautiously in patients with impaired renal or hepatic function, systemic lupus erythematosus, diabetes, or gout.
Dialyzable drug: Unlikely.
⚠ *Overdose S&S:* Orthostatic hypotension, dizziness, drowsiness, lethargy, syncope, CNS depression, electrolyte abnormalities, hemoconcentration, depressed respirations, GI irritation and hypermotility.

PREGNANCY-LACTATION-REPRODUCTION
• There are no adequate studies in pregnant women. Use during pregnancy only if clearly needed. Drug isn't for routine use.
• Drug appears in breast milk. Patient should discontinue breast-feeding or discontinue drug.

NURSING CONSIDERATIONS
• Monitor fluid intake and output, weight, BP, and electrolyte levels.
• Watch for signs and symptoms of hypokalemia, such as muscle weakness and cramps. Drug may be used with potassium-sparing diuretic to prevent potassium loss.
• Consult dietitian about a high-potassium diet.
• Monitor glucose level, especially in diabetic patients.
• Monitor uric acid level, especially in patients with history of gout.
• Monitor elderly patients, who are especially susceptible to excessive diuresis.
• In hypertensive patients, therapeutic response may be delayed several weeks.

• Monitor BP. If response is inadequate, another antihypertensive may be added.
• Metolazone and furosemide may be used together to enhance diuretic effect.
• Unlike thiazide diuretics, metolazone is effective in patients with decreased renal function.
• Stop thiazides and thiazide-like diuretics before parathyroid function tests.
• *Look alike–sound alike:* Don't confuse Zaroxolyn with Zarontin.

PATIENT TEACHING
• Tell patient to take drug in morning to prevent need to urinate at night.
• Advise patient to avoid sudden posture changes and to rise slowly to avoid effects of dizziness upon standing quickly.
• Instruct patient to use a sunblock to prevent photosensitivity reactions.
• Instruct patient to increase dietary intake of potassium-containing foods.
• Teach patient about adverse reactions and to report them promptly.

metoprolol succinate
meh-TOH-pruh-lol

Toprol-XL⬗

metoprolol tartrate
Lopresor✽, Lopresor SR✽, Lopressor⬗

Therapeutic class: Antihypertensives
Pharmacologic class: Selective beta-adrenergic blockers

AVAILABLE FORMS
metoprolol succinate
Tablets (extended-release) ⓄⓃⒸ: 25 mg, 50 mg, 100 mg, 200 mg
metoprolol tartrate
Injection: 1 mg/mL in 5-mL ampules
Tablets: 25 mg, 37.5 mg, 50 mg, 75 mg, 100 mg
Tablets (extended-release) ⓄⓃⒸ: 100 mg✽, 200 mg✽

INDICATIONS & DOSAGES

➤ **Hypertension**

Adults: Initially, 50 mg P.O. b.i.d. or 100 mg P.O. once daily; then up to 100 to 450 mg daily in two or three divided doses. Or, 25 to 100 mg extended-release tablets (tartrate equivalent) P.O. once daily. Adjust dosage as needed and tolerated at intervals of not less than 1 week to maximum of 400 mg (extended-release) daily or 450 mg (immediate-release) daily.

Children ages 6 to 16 (metoprolol succinate): 1 mg/kg P.O. once daily, not to exceed 50 mg P.O. once daily.

➤ **Early intervention in acute MI**

Adults: 5 mg metoprolol tartrate I.V. bolus every 2 minutes for three doses. Then, starting 15 minutes after the last I.V. dose, 25 to 50 mg P.O. every 6 hours for 48 hours. Maintenance dosage is 100 mg P.O. b.i.d.

➤ **Angina pectoris**

Adults: Initially, 100 mg P.O. daily as a single dose or in two equally divided doses; increased at weekly intervals until an adequate response or a pronounced decrease in HR is seen. Effects of daily dose beyond 400 mg aren't known. Or, 100 mg extended-release tablets (tartrate equivalent) once daily. Adjust dosage as needed and tolerated at intervals of not less than 1 week to maximum of 400 mg daily.

➤ **Stable symptomatic HF (New York Heart Association class II) resulting from ischemia, hypertension, or cardiomyopathy**

Adults: 25 mg Toprol-XL P.O. once daily for 2 weeks. Double the dose every 2 weeks, as tolerated, to a maximum of 200 mg daily.

Adjust-a-dose: In patients with more severe HF, start with 12.5 mg Toprol-XL P.O. once daily for 2 weeks.

➤ **Episodic migraine prevention ◆**

Adults: 50 to 200 mg P.O. daily.

ADMINISTRATION

P.O.

● Give drug with or immediately after meal.
● Extended-release tablets may be cut in half on scored line, but never crushed or chewed.

I.V.

▼ Give drug undiluted by direct injection.

▼ Although best avoided, drug can be mixed with meperidine hydrochloride or morphine sulfate or given with an alteplase infusion at a Y-site connection.

▼ Store drug at room temperature and protect from light. Discard solution if it's discolored or contains particles.

▼ **Incompatibilities:** Amphotericin B.

ACTION

Unknown. A selective beta blocker that selectively blocks beta$_1$ receptors; decreases cardiac output, peripheral resistance, and cardiac oxygen consumption; and depresses renin secretion.

Route	Onset	Peak	Duration
P.O.	15 min	1 hr	6–12 hr
P.O. (extended-release)	15 min	6–12 hr	24 hr
I.V.	5 min	20 min	5–8 hr

Half-life: 3 to 7 hours.

ADVERSE REACTIONS

CNS: fatigue, dizziness, depression, headache, insomnia, mental confusion, nightmares, short-term memory loss.
CV: hypotension, *bradycardia, HF,* edema, palpitations.
GI: nausea, diarrhea, constipation, heartburn, dry mouth, flatulence, gastric pain.
Respiratory: dyspnea, wheezing, *bronchospasm.*
Skin: rash, pruritus.

INTERACTIONS

Drug-drug. *Amiodarone:* May increase bradycardic effects. Monitor therapy.
Barbiturates: May reduce metoprolol effect. Monitor therapy.
Calcium channel blockers: May increase hypotensive effects. Monitor therapy.
Cardiac glycosides: May cause excessive bradycardia and increased depressant effect on myocardium. Use together cautiously.
Catecholamine-depleting drugs (MAO inhibitors, reserpine): May have additive effect. Monitor patient for hypotension and bradycardia.
Fluoxetine, paroxetine, propafenone, quinidine: May increase metoprolol level. Monitor vital signs.

M

Hydralazine: May increase levels and effects of both drugs. Monitor patient closely. May need to adjust dosage.

Indomethacin, NSAIDs: May decrease antihypertensive effect. Monitor BP and adjust dosage.

Insulin, oral antidiabetics: May alter dosage requirements in previously stabilized diabetic patients. Monitor patient closely.

I.V. lidocaine: May reduce hepatic metabolism of lidocaine, increasing risk of toxicity. Give bolus doses of lidocaine at a slower rate, and monitor lidocaine level closely.

Terbutaline: May antagonize bronchodilatory effects of terbutaline. Monitor patient.

Verapamil: May increase effects of both drugs. Monitor cardiac function closely, and decrease dosages as needed.

Drug-herb. *Ma huang:* May decrease antihypertensive effects. Discourage use together.

Drug-food. *Any food:* May increase absorption. Encourage patient to take drug with food.

EFFECTS ON LAB TEST RESULTS
• May increase transaminase, alkaline phosphatase, LDH, and uric acid levels.

CONTRAINDICATIONS & CAUTIONS
• Contraindicated in patients hypersensitive to drug or other beta blockers.
• Contraindicated in patients with sinus bradycardia, greater than first-degree heart block, cardiogenic shock, sick sinus syndrome (unless a permanent pacemaker is in place), or overt cardiac failure when used to treat hypertension or angina. When used to treat MI, drug is contraindicated in patients with HR less than 45 beats/minute, greater than first-degree heart block, PR interval of 0.24 second or longer with first-degree heart block, systolic BP less than 100 mm Hg, or moderate to severe cardiac failure.
• Use cautiously in patients with HF, diabetes, or respiratory or hepatic disease.
• Avoid initiating high-dose, extended-release drug in patients undergoing non-cardiac surgery because drug has been associated with bradycardia, hypotension, stroke, and death.

• Don't routinely withdraw long-term beta-blocker therapy before surgery.

Dialyzable drug: Unknown.

⚠ **Overdose S&S:** Bradycardia, hypotension, bronchospasm, cardiac failure, cardiac arrest, coma, AV block, nausea, vomiting.

PREGNANCY-LACTATION-REPRODUCTION
• There are no adequate studies in pregnant women. Use during pregnancy only if clearly needed.
• Drug appears in breast milk in very small quantities; an infant consuming 1 L of breast milk daily would receive a metoprolol dose of less than 1 mg. Consider possible infant exposure when giving to breast-feeding women.

NURSING CONSIDERATIONS
• Always check patient's apical pulse rate before giving drug. If it's slower than 60 beats/minute, withhold drug and call prescriber immediately.
• In diabetic patients, monitor glucose level closely because drug masks common signs and symptoms of hypoglycemia.
• Monitor BP frequently; drug masks common signs and symptoms of shock.
• Beta blockers may mask tachycardia caused by hyperthyroidism. In patients with suspected thyrotoxicosis, taper off beta blocker to avoid thyroid storm.
Black Box Warning When stopping therapy, taper dosage over 1 to 2 weeks. Abrupt discontinuation may cause exacerbations of angina or MI. Don't discontinue therapy abruptly even in patients treated only for hypertension. ■
• Beta selectivity is lost at higher doses. Watch for peripheral side effects.
• **Look alike–sound alike:** Don't confuse metoprolol succinate with metoprolol tartrate. Don't confuse metoprolol with metaproterenol, misoprostol, or metolazone. Don't confuse Toprol-XL with Topamax, Tegretol, or Tegretol-XR.

PATIENT TEACHING
• Instruct patient to take drug exactly as prescribed and with meals.
• Caution patient to avoid driving and other tasks requiring mental alertness until response to therapy has been established.

Reactions in bold italics are *life-threatening*. Interactions may have a *rapid onset* or a *delayed onset*.

• Advise patient to inform dentist or prescriber about use of this drug before procedures or surgery.

• Tell patient to report all adverse reactions, especially shortness of breath.

Black Box Warning Instruct patient not to stop drug suddenly but to notify prescriber about unpleasant adverse reactions. Inform him that drug must be withdrawn gradually over 1 or 2 weeks. ∎

metronidazole (oral, injection)
me-troe-NI-da-zole

Flagyl, Flagyl ER, Novo-Nidazol✤, PMS-metronidazole✤

metronidazole hydrochloride
Flagyl IV RTU, Metro I.V. in Plastic Container

Therapeutic class: Antiprotozoals
Pharmacologic class: Nitroimidazoles

AVAILABLE FORMS
Capsules: 375 mg, 500 mg✤
Injection: 500 mg/100 mL in ready-to-use (RTU) minibags
Tablets: 250 mg, 500 mg
Tablets (extended-release) ⓞⓝⓒ: 750 mg

INDICATIONS & DOSAGES
Black Box Warning Use metronidazole only for the conditions for which it's indicated because it may be carcinogenic. Avoid unnecessary use. ∎

Adjust-a-dose (for all indications): For severe hepatic impairment (Child-Pugh class C), reduce dose of immediate-release tablets and I.V. infusion by 50%. Use of extended-release tablets isn't recommended.

➤ **Amebic liver abscess**
Adults: 500 to 750 mg P.O. t.i.d. for 5 to 10 days; or, 500 mg I.V. every 6 hours for 10 days if patient can't tolerate oral route.
Children: 35 to 50 mg/kg daily in three divided doses for 7 to 10 days.

➤ **Intestinal amebiasis (immediate-release)**
Adults: 750 mg P.O. t.i.d. for 5 to 10 days.

Children: 35 to 50 mg/kg P.O. daily in three divided doses for 7 to 10 days.
Adjust-a-dose: For severe hepatic impairment (Child-Pugh class C), reduce dose of immediate-release capsules to 375 mg P.O. every 8 hours.

➤ **Trichomoniasis (immediate-release)**
Adults: One 250-mg tablet P.O. b.i.d. for 7 days, or 2 g P.O. in single dose (may give the 2-g dose in two 1-g doses, both on the same day); wait 4 to 6 weeks before repeating course. Or, one 375-mg capsule P.O. b.i.d. for 7 days.
Adjust-a-dose: For severe hepatic impairment (Child-Pugh class C), reduce dose of immediate-release capsules to 375 mg P.O. once daily.

➤ **Refractory trichomoniasis**
Adults: 500 mg (immediate-release) P.O. b.i.d. for 7 days.

➤ **Bacterial infections caused by anaerobic microorganisms**
Adults: Loading dose is 15 mg/kg I.V. infused over 1 hour. Maintenance dose is 7.5 mg/kg I.V. or 500 mg (immediate-release) P.O. every 6 hours. Give first maintenance dose 6 hours after loading dose. Maximum dose shouldn't exceed 4 g daily.

➤ **To prevent postoperative infection in contaminated or potentially contaminated colorectal surgery**
Adults: Infuse 15 mg/kg I.V. over 30 to 60 minutes and complete about 1 hour before surgery. Then, infuse 7.5 mg/kg I.V. over 30 to 60 minutes at 6 and 12 hours after first dose.

➤ **Bacterial vaginosis (nonpregnant women)**
Adults: 750 mg Flagyl ER P.O. daily for 7 days. Or, 500 mg P.O. b.i.d. for 7 days.

➤ **CDAD (mild to moderate)** ◆
Adults: 500 mg P.O. t.i.d. for 10 to 14 days. Or, 500 mg I.V. every 8 hours for 10 to 14 days with vancomycin when P.O. route isn't practical.

➤ **Sinusitis (unimproved after 21 to 28 days of initial therapy)** ◆
Adults: 7.5 mg/kg P.O. q.i.d. for 7 to 10 days. Maximum dose is 4 g in 24 hours.

M

ADMINISTRATION

P.O.

● Give tablets and capsules with food if GI upset occurs.

● Give extended-release tablets (750 mg) at least 1 hour before or 2 hours after meals.

● Don't split, crush, or allow patient to chew extended-release tablets.

I.V.

▼ Flagyl IV RTU minibags need no preparation.

▼ Don't use aluminum needles or hubs to reconstitute the drug or to transfer reconstituted drug. Equipment that contains aluminum will turn the solution orange; the potency isn't affected.

▼ To reconstitute lyophilized vials, add 4.4 mL of sterile water for injection, bacteriostatic water for injection, sterile NSS for injection, or bacteriostatic NSS for injection. Reconstituted drug contains 100 mg/mL. Add contents of vial to 100 mL of D_5W, lactated Ringer injection, or NSS to yield 5 mg/mL. Neutralize this highly acidic solution by carefully adding 5 mEq sodium bicarbonate to each 500 mg; the carbon dioxide gas that forms may need to be vented.

▼ Don't give by I.V. push. Infuse over 30 to 60 minutes.

▼ Don't refrigerate the neutralized diluted solution; precipitation may occur. Refrigerated Flagyl IV RTU may form crystals, which disappear after the solution warms to room temperature.

▼ **Incompatibilities:** Aluminum, amphotericin B, aztreonam, filgrastim, pemetrexed, other I.V. drugs.

ACTION

Direct-acting trichomonicide and amebicide that works inside and outside the intestines. It's thought to enter the cells of microorganisms that contain nitroreductase, forming unstable compounds that bind to DNA and inhibit synthesis, causing cell death.

Route	Onset	Peak	Duration
P.O.	Unknown	2 hr	Unknown
I.V.	Immediate	1 hr	Unknown

Half-life: 6 to 8 hours.

ADVERSE REACTIONS

CNS: headache, *seizures,* fever, vertigo, ataxia, dizziness, syncope, incoordination, confusion, irritability, depression, weakness, insomnia, peripheral neuropathy.

CV: flattened T wave, edema, flushing, thrombophlebitis after I.V. infusion.

EENT: rhinitis, sinusitis, pharyngitis.

GI: nausea, abdominal cramping or pain, stomatitis, epigastric distress, vomiting, anorexia, diarrhea, constipation, proctitis, dry mouth, metallic taste.

GU: vaginitis, darkened urine, polyuria, dysuria, cystitis, dyspareunia, dryness of vagina and vulva, vaginal candidiasis, genital pruritus, *UTI,* dysmenorrhea.

Hematologic: *transient leukopenia, neutropenia.*

Musculoskeletal: transient joint pains.

Respiratory: URI.

Skin: rash, genital pruritus.

Other: decreased libido; overgrowth of nonsusceptible organisms, especially *Candida;* flulike symptoms.

INTERACTIONS

Drug-drug. *Busulfan:* May increase busulfan toxicity. Avoid using together.

Cimetidine: May increase risk of metronidazole toxicity because of inhibited hepatic metabolism. Monitor for toxicity.

CYP3A4 substrates: May increase concentration of aripiprazole, dofetilide, lomitapide, and pimozide. Monitor therapy.

Disulfiram: May cause acute psychosis and confusion. Avoid giving metronidazole within 2 weeks of disulfiram.

Lithium: May increase lithium level, which may cause toxicity. Monitor lithium level.

Mebendazole: May increase risk of Stevens-Johnson syndrome or toxic epidermal necrolysis. Consider therapy modification.

Phenobarbital, phenytoin: May decrease metronidazole effectiveness; may reduce total phenytoin clearance. Monitor patient.

Warfarin: May increase anticoagulant effects and risk of bleeding. Reduce warfarin as needed.

Drug-lifestyle. *Alcohol use:* May cause disulfiram-like reaction, including nausea, vomiting, headache, cramps, and flushing. Warn patient to avoid alcohol during and for 3 days after completing drug therapy.

Reactions in bold italics are *life-threatening*. Interactions may have a *rapid onset* or a *delayed onset*.

EFFECTS ON LAB TEST RESULTS
• May decrease WBC and neutrophil counts.
• May falsely decrease triglyceride and aminotransferase levels.
• May interfere with ALT, AST, glucose, and LDH testing.

CONTRAINDICATIONS & CAUTIONS
• Contraindicated in patients hypersensitive to drug or other nitroimidazole derivatives. Use disulfiram within 2 weeks or use with alcohol or propylene glycol products during treatment and for 3 days after.
• Use cautiously in patients with history of blood dyscrasia, CNS disorder, or retinal or visual field changes.
• Use cautiously in patients who take hepatotoxic drugs or have hepatic disease or alcoholism.
Dialyzable drug: Yes.
⚠ *Overdose S&S:* Nausea, vomiting, ataxia, neurotoxicity.

PREGNANCY-LACTATION-REPRODUCTION
• Contraindicated during first trimester. Consult current guidelines for appropriate use in pregnant women.
• Drug appears in breast milk. Patient should discontinue breast-feeding or discontinue drug.

NURSING CONSIDERATIONS
• Monitor LFT results carefully in elderly patients.
• Observe patient for edema, especially if he's receiving corticosteroids; Flagyl IV RTU may cause sodium retention.
• Record number and character of stools when drug is used to treat amebiasis. Give drug only after *Trichomonas vaginalis* infection is confirmed by wet smear or culture or *Entamoeba histolytica* is identified.
• Sexual partners of patients being treated for *T. vaginalis* infection, even if asymptomatic, must also be treated to avoid reinfection.
• *Look alike–sound alike:* Don't confuse metronidazole with metformin.

PATIENT TEACHING
• Instruct patient to take extended-release tablets at least 1 hour before or 2 hours after meals but to take all other oral forms with food to minimize GI upset.
• Inform patient with trichomoniasis of need for sexual partners to be treated simultaneously to avoid reinfection.
• Tell patient to avoid alcohol and alcohol-containing drugs during and for at least 3 days after treatment course.
• Tell patient he may experience a metallic taste and have dark or red-brown urine.
• Tell patient to report to prescriber symptoms of candidal overgrowth.
• Tell patient to report all adverse reactions to prescriber immediately, especially any neurologic symptoms (seizures, peripheral neuropathy).

metronidazole (topical, vaginal)
me-troe-NI-da-zole

MetroCream, MetroGel, MetroGel Vaginal, MetroLotion, Noritate, Nuvessa, Vandazole

Therapeutic class: Antibacterials (topical)
Pharmacologic class: Nitroimidazoles

M

AVAILABLE FORMS
Topical cream: 0.75%, 1%
Topical gel: 0.75%, 1%
Topical lotion: 0.75%
Vaginal gel: 0.75%, 1.3%

INDICATIONS & DOSAGES
➤ **Inflammatory papules and pustules of acne rosacea**
Adults: If using a 0.75% preparation, apply thin film to affected area b.i.d., morning and evening. If using a 1% preparation, apply thin film to affected area once daily. After response is seen (usually within 3 weeks), adjust frequency and duration of therapy.
➤ **Bacterial vaginosis**
Adults: One applicatorful of 0.75% (approximately 37.5 mg) vaginally daily or b.i.d. for 5 days. For once-daily use, give at bedtime. Or, one applicatorful (approximately 65 mg) of 1.3% vaginal gel intravaginally once as a single dose at bedtime.

ADMINISTRATION
Topical
● Clean area thoroughly before use, and then wait 15 to 20 minutes before applying drug to minimize risk of local irritation. Avoid contact with eyes.
Vaginal
● Screw the end of the applicator onto the tube and squeeze slowly. The plunger will stop when the applicator is full.
● Wash plunger and barrel in warm, soapy water and rinse thoroughly. Dry before reassembling.

ACTION
Unknown. May cause bactericidal effect by interacting with bacterial DNA. Drug is active against many anaerobic gram-negative bacilli, anaerobic gram-positive cocci, *Gardnerella vaginalis*, and *Campylobacter fetus*.

Route	Onset	Peak	Duration
Topical	Unknown	8–12 hr	Unknown
Vaginal	Unknown	6–12 hr	Unknown

Half-life: Unknown.

ADVERSE REACTIONS
Topical form
EENT: lacrimation if applied around eyes, eye irritation.
Skin: transient redness, dryness, mild burning, stinging, contact dermatitis, pruritus, rash.
Vaginal form
CNS: headache, dizziness, depression.
GI: cramps, nausea, loose stools, metallic or bad taste in mouth, pain, vomiting, diarrhea.
GU: cervicitis, vaginitis, perineal and vulvovaginal itching, vaginal burning, vaginal discharge, pelvic discomfort.
Skin: transient redness, dryness, mild burning, stinging.
Other: overgrowth of nonsusceptible organisms.

INTERACTIONS
Drug-drug. *Disulfiram:* May cause disulfiram-like reaction when used with vaginal form of metronidazole. Don't use together, and wait 2 weeks after stopping disulfiram before starting metronidazole vaginal therapy.

Lithium: May increase lithium level. Monitor lithium level.
Oral anticoagulants: May increase anticoagulant effect. Monitor patient for adverse reactions.
Drug-lifestyle. *Alcohol use:* May cause disulfiram-like reaction when used with vaginal form. Don't use together.

EFFECTS ON LAB TEST RESULTS
● May interfere with AST, ALT, LDH, triglyceride, and glucose levels.
● May increase or decrease WBC count.

CONTRAINDICATIONS & CAUTIONS
● Contraindicated in patients hypersensitive to drug or its ingredients, such as parabens, and other nitroimidazole derivatives.
● Use cautiously in patients with history or evidence of blood dyscrasia and in those with hepatic impairment.
● Use vaginal gel cautiously in patients with history of CNS diseases. Oral form may cause seizures and peripheral neuropathy.
● Prolonged use of vaginal form can lead to fungal or bacterial superinfection.
Dialyzable drug: Unknown.

PREGNANCY-LACTATION-REPRODUCTION
● There are no adequate studies in pregnant women. Use during pregnancy only if clearly needed and benefit justifies potential risk to the fetus.
● Drug may appear in breast milk after vaginal or topical use because some of drug is absorbed systemically. Patient should discontinue breast-feeding or discontinue drug.

NURSING CONSIDERATIONS
● Topical therapy hasn't been linked to the adverse effects observed with parenteral or oral therapy, but some drug may be absorbed after topical use.
● Don't use vaginal gel in patients who have taken disulfiram within past 2 weeks.
● Monitor patient for worsening symptoms.

PATIENT TEACHING
● Instruct patient to avoid use of topical gel around eyes.
● Advise patient to clean area thoroughly before use and to wait 15 to 20 minutes

---

after cleaning skin before applying drug to minimize risk of local irritation. Cosmetics may be used 5 minutes after medication has dried.

• If local reactions occur, advise patient to apply drug less frequently or stop using it and notify prescriber.

• Advise patient to avoid sexual intercourse while using vaginal preparation.

• Caution patient to avoid alcohol while being treated with vaginal preparation.

micafungin sodium
mick-a-FUN-gin

Mycamine

Therapeutic class: Antifungals
Pharmacologic class: Echinocandins

AVAILABLE FORMS
Lyophilized powder for injection: 50 mg, 100 mg single-use vial

INDICATIONS & DOSAGES
➤ **Candidemia, acute disseminated candidiasis, and *Candida* peritonitis and abscesses**
Adults: 100 mg I.V. daily for 10 to 47 days (mean duration, 15 days).
Children age 4 months and older: 2 mg/kg I.V. once daily. Maximum dosage is 100 mg daily.
➤ **Esophageal candidiasis**
Adults: 150 mg I.V. daily for 10 to 30 days (mean duration, 15 days).
Children age 4 months and older weighing more than 30 kg: 2.5 mg/kg I.V. once daily. Maximum dosage is 150 mg daily.
Children age 4 months and older weighing 30 kg or less: 3 mg/kg I.V. once daily.
➤ **To prevent candidal infection in hematopoietic stem cell transplant recipients**
Adults: 50 mg I.V. daily for 6 to 51 days (mean duration, 19 days).
Children age 4 months and older: 1 mg/kg I.V. once daily. Maximum dosage is 50 mg daily.

ADMINISTRATION
I.V.
▼ Use aseptic technique when preparing drug.
▼ Reconstitute each 50-mg or 100-mg vial with 5 mL of NSS without a bacteriostatic agent or D_5W for injection. To minimize foaming, dissolve powder by swirling the vial; don't shake it.
▼ For adult, dilute dose in 100 mL of NSS or D_5W for injection.
▼ For children's doses: Add reconstituted drug to NSS or D_5W I.V. infusion bag or syringe. Ensure that final concentration of solution is between 0.5 and 4 mg/mL. To minimize risk of infusion reactions, administer concentrations of greater than 1.5 mg/mL via central catheter.
▼ Flush line with NSS for injection before infusing drug.
▼ Infuse drug over 1 hour.
▼ Reconstituted product and diluted infusion may be stored for up to 24 hours at room temperature.
▼ Protect diluted solution from light.
▼ **Incompatibilities:** Drug may precipitate when mixed with commonly used drugs.

ACTION
Inhibits synthesis of an essential component of fungal cell walls. Drug is active against *Candida albicans, C. glabrata, C. krusei, C. parapsilosis*, and *C. tropicalis*.

Route	Onset	Peak	Duration
I.V.	Unknown	Unknown	Unknown

Half-life: 11 to 21 hours.

ADVERSE REACTIONS
CNS: headache, insomnia, anxiety, dizziness.
CV: atrial fibrillation, bradycardia, cardiac disorders, hypertension, hypotension, tachycardia, vascular disorders, edema, *cardiac arrest, MI, pericardial effusion.*
GI: abdominal pain, diarrhea, nausea, vomiting, anorexia, dyspepsia, mucositis, constipation.
Hematologic: *leukopenia, neutropenia, thrombocytopenia,* anemia.
Metabolic: hypocalcemia, hypokalemia, *hypomagnesemia,* hypophosphatemia,

M

hyperglycemia, hypoglycemia, hyper-kalemia, hypernatremia, *hypocalcemia.*
Respiratory: cough, dyspnea.
Skin: infusion-site inflammation, phlebitis, pruritus, rash.
Other: pyrexia, rigors.

INTERACTIONS
Drug-drug. *CYP3A4 substrates:* May increase concentration of aripiprazole, dofetilide, lomitapide, and pimozide. Monitor therapy.
Itraconazole: May increase itraconazole level. Monitor for itraconazole toxicity, and reduce itraconazole dose if needed.
Nifedipine: May increase nifedipine level. Monitor BP, and decrease nifedipine dose if needed.
Sirolimus: May increase sirolimus level. Monitor patient for evidence of toxicity, and decrease sirolimus dose if needed.

EFFECTS ON LAB TEST RESULTS
• May increase alkaline phosphatase, ALT, AST, bilirubin, BUN, creatinine, and LDH levels.
• May decrease calcium, magnesium, phosphorus, potassium, and Hb levels and hematocrit.
• May decrease neutrophil and platelet counts.

CONTRAINDICATIONS & CAUTIONS
• Contraindicated in patients hypersensitive to drug.
• Effects of micafungin are unknown in patients with severe hepatic disease.
Dialyzable drug: No.

PREGNANCY-LACTATION-REPRODUCTION
• There are no adequate studies in pregnant women. Use during pregnancy only if potential benefit justifies potential fetal risk.
• It isn't known if drug appears in breast milk. Use cautiously in breast-feeding women.

NURSING CONSIDERATIONS
• Injection-site reactions occur more often in patients receiving drug by peripheral I.V.
• To reduce the risk of histamine-mediated reactions, infuse drug over at least 1 hour.

⊎ Alert: If patient develops signs of serious hypersensitivity reaction, including shock, stop infusion and notify prescriber immediately.
• Monitor hepatic and renal function during therapy.
• Monitor patient for hemolysis and hemolytic anemia.

PATIENT TEACHING
• Advise patient to report pain or redness at infusion site.
• Teach patient about adverse reactions and to report them immediately.
• Tell patient he'll likely need laboratory tests to monitor his hematologic, renal, and hepatic function.

miconazole
my-KON-a-zole

Oravig

miconazole nitrate
Desenex ◇, Fungoid Tincture ◇, Lotrimin AF ◇, Micatin ◇, Micozole✤ ◇, Monistat 1 ◇, Monistat 3 ◇, Monistat 7 ◇, M-Zole 3 ◇, Tetterine ◇, Vagistat-3 ◇, Zeasorb-AF ◇

Therapeutic class: Antifungals
Pharmacologic class: Imidazoles

AVAILABLE FORMS
Aerosol powder: 2% ◇
Aerosol spray: 2% ◇
Buccal tablets ⓞⓝⓑ: 50 mg
Lotion: 2% ◇
Powder: 2% ◇
Topical cream: 2% ◇
Topical ointment: 2% ◇
Topical solution: 2% ◇
Vaginal cream: 2% ◇, 4% ◇
Vaginal suppositories: 100 mg ◇, 200 mg ◇, 1,200 mg ◇

INDICATIONS & DOSAGES
➤ **Tinea corporis, tinea cruris, tinea pedis, cutaneous candidiasis, common dermatophyte infections**

Adults and children older than age 2: Apply sparingly b.i.d. for 2 to 4 weeks. Powder or spray can be used liberally over affected area. In children younger than age 2, use only under the direction and supervision of a physician.

➤ **Vulvovaginal candidiasis**
Adults and children age 12 and older: One applicatorful 2% or 100-mg Monistat 7 suppository vaginally at bedtime for 7 days; repeat course, if needed. Or, one applicatorful 4% or 200-mg Monistat 3 suppository vaginally at bedtime for 3 days. Or, one 1,200-mg Monistat 1 suppository vaginally at bedtime for 1 day. May apply topical cream sparingly to affected area b.i.d. for 7 days or as needed for external symptoms.

➤ **Oropharyngeal candidiasis**
Adults and children age 16 and older: One 50-mg buccal tablet to the upper gum region once daily for 14 consecutive days.

ADMINISTRATION
P.O.
• Apply buccal tablet to the gum in the morning with dry hands after patient has brushed teeth.
• Place the rounded surface of the tablet against the gum just above the incisor. Apply slight pressure over the upper lip for 30 seconds to ensure adhesion.
• Alternate sides of the mouth for each dose.
• Instruct patient not to crush, chew, or swallow buccal tablets.
Topical
• Don't use occlusive dressings.
• Lotion is preferred in skin folds.
Vaginal
• Suppository is inserted high into vagina with applicator provided.
• Store between 59° and 86° F (15° and 30° C).

ACTION
Fungicidal; disrupts fungal cell membrane permeability.

Route	Onset	Peak	Duration
P.O.	Unknown	7 hr	15 hr
Topical, vaginal	Unknown	Unknown	Unknown

Half-life: Unknown.

ADVERSE REACTIONS
CNS: headache, fatigue, pain.
GI: diarrhea, nausea, dysgeusia, upper abdominal pain, vomiting (buccal tablets), oral discomfort, dry mouth, gastroenteritis.
GU: pelvic cramps, pruritus, and irritation with vaginal cream; vulvovaginal burning.
Hematologic: anemia, lymphopenia, neutropenia.
Skin: allergic contact dermatitis, burning, irritation, maceration, pain, edema, URI.

INTERACTIONS
Drug-drug. *Warfarin:* Buccal form of drug may enhance anticoagulant effect. Monitor PT and INR, and observe patient for bleeding.
Drug-herb. *Saccharomyces boulardii:* Antifungals may decrease therapeutic effect. Consider alternative therapy.

EFFECTS ON LAB TEST RESULTS
• May decrease WBC and RBC counts (oral form).

CONTRAINDICATIONS & CAUTIONS
• Contraindicated in patients hypersensitive to drug or its components. Cross-sensitivity to imidazole antifungals may occur.
• Safety and effectiveness of Oravig haven't been established for children younger than age 16.
• Don't use in children younger than age 2.
Dialyzable drug: Unknown.

PREGNANCY-LACTATION-REPRODUCTION
• There are no adequate studies in pregnant women. Use oral form during pregnancy only if potential benefit justifies potential risk to the fetus.
🔴 *Alert:* Vaginal preparation shouldn't be used during first trimester and should be used during pregnancy only if recommended by prescriber.
• Use cautiously in breast-feeding women.

NURSING CONSIDERATIONS
• Avoid using within 72 hours of certain vaginal and latex products, such as condoms or vaginal contraceptive diaphragms, because drug causes latex breakdown.

M

PATIENT TEACHING

• Advise patient that vaginal form of drug is for perineal or vaginal use only and to keep drug out of eyes.

• Caution patient that frequent or persistent yeast infections may suggest a more serious medical problem.

• Tell patient to cautiously insert vaginal form high into the vagina with applicator provided.

• Tell patient that drug may stain clothing.

• Warn patient to stop drug if sensitivity or chemical irritation occurs.

• Tell patient to use drug for full treatment period prescribed and to notify prescriber if symptoms persist or worsen despite therapy.

• Advise patient to avoid tampons and sexual intercourse during vaginal treatment.

• Instruct patient to apply sparingly in skin folds and rub in well to prevent skin breakdown.

• Tell patient to store vaginal product between 59° and 86° F (15° and 30° C).

• Tell patient not to crush, chew, or swallow buccal tablets.

• Advise patient that he can eat and drink with the buccal tablet in place but to avoid chewing gum.

• Instruct patient how to use buccal tablet.

• Tell patient that if the tablet falls off or is swallowed after it is in place for at least 6 hours, he shouldn't apply a new tablet until the next regularly scheduled dose.

SAFETY ALERT!

midazolam hydrochloride
mid-AY-zoh-lam

Therapeutic class: Anxiolytics
Pharmacologic class: Benzodiazepines
Controlled substance schedule: IV

AVAILABLE FORMS

Injection: 1 mg/mL, 5 mg/mL
Injection (preservative-free): 1 mg/mL, 5 mg/mL
Syrup: 2 mg/mL

INDICATIONS & DOSAGES

➤ **Preoperative sedation (to induce sleepiness or drowsiness and relieve apprehension)**

Adults: 0.07 to 0.08 mg/kg I.M. up to 1 hour before surgery.

➤ **Moderate sedation before short diagnostic or endoscopic procedures**

Adults younger than age 60: Initially, small dose not to exceed 2.5 mg I.V. given slowly over at least 2 minutes; wait at least 2 minutes to evaluate sedative effect. Then repeat in 2 minutes p.r.n., in small increments of first dose over at least 2 minutes each to achieve desired effect. Total dose of up to to 5 mg may be used. Additional doses to maintain desired level of sedation may be given by slow titration in increments of 25% of dose used to first reach the sedative end point.

Patients age 60 or older and debilitated patients: 0.5 to 1.5 mg I.V. over at least 2 minutes. Incremental doses shouldn't exceed 1 mg. A total dose of up to 3.5 mg is usually sufficient.

➤ **To induce sleepiness and amnesia and to relieve apprehension before anesthesia or before and during procedures**
P.O.

Children ages 6 to 16 who are cooperative: 0.25 to 0.5 mg/kg P.O. as a single dose, up to 20 mg.

Infants and children ages 6 months to 5 years or less cooperative, older children: 0.25 to 1 mg/kg P.O. as a single dose, up to 20 mg.

I.V.

Children ages 12 to 16: Initially, no more than 2.5 mg I.V. given slowly; repeat in 2 minutes, if needed, in small increments of first dose over at least 2 minutes to achieve desired effect. Total dose of up to 10 mg may be used. Additional doses to maintain desired level of sedation may be given by slow titration in increments of 25% of dose used to first reach the sedative end point. *Children ages 6 to 12:* 0.025 to 0.05 mg/kg I.V. over 2 to 3 minutes. Additional doses may be given in small increments after 2 to 3 minutes. Total dose of up to 0.4 mg/kg, not to exceed 10 mg, may be used. *Children ages 6 months to 5 years:* 0.05 to 0.1 mg/kg I.V. over 2 to 3 minutes. Additional doses may be given in small increments after 2 to 3 minutes. Total dose of up to 0.6 mg/kg, not to exceed 6 mg, may be used.

Reactions in bold italics are *life-threatening*. Interactions may have a *rapid onset* or a *delayed onset*.

I.M.

Children: 0.1 to 0.15 mg/kg I.M. Use up to 0.5 mg/kg in more anxious patients.

Adjust-a-dose: For obese children, base dose on ideal body weight; high-risk or debilitated children and children receiving other sedatives need lower doses.

➤ **To induce general anesthesia**

Adults older than age 55: 0.3 mg/kg I.V. infusion over 20 to 30 seconds if patient hasn't received premedication, or 0.2 mg/kg I.V. infusion over 20 to 30 seconds if patient has received a sedative or opioid premedication. Allow 2 minutes for effect. Additional increments of 25% of first dose may be needed to complete induction.

Adults younger than age 55: 0.3 to 0.35 mg/kg I.V. infusion over 20 to 30 seconds if patient hasn't received premedication, or 0.25 mg/kg I.V. infusion over 20 to 30 seconds if patient has received a sedative or opioid premedication. Allow 2 minutes for effect. Additional increments of 25% of first dose may be needed to complete induction.

Adjust-a-dose: For debilitated patients, initially, 0.2 to 0.25 mg/kg. As little as 0.15 mg/kg may be needed. Reduce doses in elderly patients.

➤ **As continuous infusion to sedate intubated patients in critical care unit**

Adults: Initially, 0.01 to 0.05 mg/kg may be given I.V. over several minutes, repeated at 10- to 15-minute intervals until adequate sedation is achieved. To maintain sedation, usual initial infusion rate is 0.02 to 0.1 mg/kg/hour. Higher loading dose or infusion rates may be needed in some patients. Use the lowest effective rate.

Children: Initially, 0.05 to 0.2 mg/kg may be given I.V. over 2 to 3 minutes or longer; then continuous infusion at rate of 0.06 to 0.12 mg/kg/hour. Increase or decrease infusion to maintain desired effect.

Neonates more than 32 weeks' gestational age: Initially, 0.06 mg/kg/hour I.V. Adjust rate, as needed, using lowest possible rate.

Neonates less than 32 weeks' gestational age: Initially, 0.03 mg/kg/hour I.V. Adjust rate, as needed, using lowest possible rate.

Black Box Warning Avoid rapid injection (less than 2 minutes) in neonates because rapid injection has been associated with severe hypotension, particularly when neonate has also received fentanyl. Severe hypotension has also been observed in neonates receiving a continuous infusion of midazolam who then receive a rapid I.V. injection of fentanyl. Seizures have been reported in several neonates after rapid I.V. administration. ■

➤ **Status epilepticus (seizures lasting longer than 5 minutes or occurring after patient has had intermittent seizures without regaining consciousness for longer than 5 minutes)** ◆

Adults: 10 mg I.M. once or 0.2 mg/kg I.M. once. Maximum dose is 10 mg I.M.

Children age 1 and older: For patients weighing more than 40 kg, give 10 mg I.M. once; for those weighing 13 to 40 kg, give 5 mg I.M. once. Or, give 0.2 mg/kg intranasally using 5-mg/mL injectable concentrated solution to deliver dose.

ADMINISTRATION

P.O.

Black Box Warning Midazolam syrup has been associated with respiratory depression and respiratory arrest, especially when used in noncritical-care settings. Midazolam syrup should only be used in hospital or ambulatory care settings that can provide continuous respiratory and cardiac function monitoring. Availability of appropriate resuscitative drugs and equipment and personnel trained in their use and skilled in airway management should be ensured. ■

• Give drug without regard for food. Dispense syrup directly into the mouth and don't mix with any liquid (such as grapefruit juice) before dispensing.

• Refer to manufacturer's instructions for use of oral dispenser and press-in bottle dispenser.

I.V.

Black Box Warning I.V. midazolam has been associated with respiratory depression and respiratory arrest, especially when used in noncritical setting. It should only be used in hospital or ambulatory care settings, including physicians' and dental offices that can provide continuous monitoring of cardiac and respiratory function. Availability of appropriate resuscitative drugs and equipment and personnel trained in their use and skilled in airway management should be ensured. ■

▼ Drug may be mixed in the same syringe with morphine sulfate, meperidine, atropine, or scopolamine.

▼ When mixing infusion, use 5-mg/mL vial and dilute to 0.5 mg/mL with D_5W or NSS.

Black Box Warning Give slowly over at least 2 minutes, and wait at least 2 minutes when initiating or titrating doses to fully evaluate therapeutic effect. Initial adult dose shouldn't exceed 2.5 mg. Lower initial doses are necessary for adults age 60 and older, for debilitated patients, and for those receiving concomitant opioids or other CNS depressants. ■

Black Box Warning Don't administer by rapid injection in the neonatal population. ■

▼ **Incompatibilities:** Acyclovir, azithromycin, cefazolin, cefepime, ceftazidime, dexamethasone, furosemide, hydrocortisone, lactated Ringer injection, micafungin, pantoprazole, piperacillin–tazobactam, sodium bicarbonate.

I.M.

● Inject deeply into a large muscle.

ACTION

May potentiate the effects of GABA, depress the CNS, and suppress the spread of seizure activity.

Route	Onset	Peak	Duration
P.O.	10–20 min	45–60 min	2–6 hr
I.V.	90 sec–5 min	Rapid	2–6 hr
I.M.	15 min	15–60 min	2–6 hr

Half-life: 2 to 6 hours.

ADVERSE REACTIONS

CNS: oversedation, drowsiness, amnesia, headache, seizures, involuntary movements, nystagmus, hiccups, paradoxical behavior or excitement.
CV: variations in BP and pulse rate.
EENT: nystagmus.
GI: nausea, vomiting.
Respiratory: *apnea,* decreased respiratory rate, oxygen desaturation, coughing.
Other: pain at injection site, redness.

INTERACTIONS

Drug-drug. *Cimetidine:* May increase and prolong sedation. Avoid use together.
CNS depressants: May cause apnea. Use together cautiously. Adjust dosage of midazolam if used with opiates or other CNS depressants.
Diltiazem: May increase CNS depression and prolong effects of midazolam. Use lower dose of midazolam.
Erythromycin: May alter metabolism of midazolam. Use together cautiously.
Fluconazole, itraconazole, ketoconazole, miconazole: May increase and prolong midazolam level, CNS depression, and psychomotor impairment. Avoid using together. If must be given together, monitor patient closely.
Hormonal contraceptives: May prolong half-life of midazolam. Use together cautiously.
Protease inhibitors (ritonavir, saquinavir): May increase midazolam level. Use together cautiously.
Theophylline: May antagonize sedative effect of midazolam. Use together cautiously.
Verapamil: May increase midazolam level. Monitor patient closely.
Drug-herb. *Ginkgo biloba, St. John's wort:* May decrease drug level. Discourage use together.
Drug-food. *Grapefruit juice:* May increase bioavailability of oral drug. Don't use together.
Drug-lifestyle. *Alcohol use:* May cause additive CNS effects. Don't use together.

EFFECTS ON LAB TEST RESULTS
None reported.

CONTRAINDICATIONS & CAUTIONS
● Contraindicated in patients hypersensitive to drug and in those with acute angle-closure glaucoma, shock, coma, or acute alcohol intoxication.
🕒 *Alert:* Drug should only be used with individualization of the dosage.
● Use cautiously in patients with uncompensated acute illness and in elderly or debilitated patients.
Black Box Warning Pediatric dosages must be calculated on a mg/kg basis, and all dosages should be titrated slowly. ■

Reactions in bold italics are *life-threatening*. Interactions may have a *rapid onset* or a *delayed onset*.

Black Box Warning Midazolam should only be administered by persons specifically trained in the use of anesthetics and the management of respiratory effects of anesthetics, including resuscitation of patients in the age-group being treated. The appropriate emergency equipment must always be immediately available. ■

● When overdose is suspected, flumazenil may be used as a reversal agent. It's used as an adjunct to proper benzodiazepine overdose management.

Dialyzable drug: Unknown.

⚠ *Overdose S&S:* Excessive sedation, somnolence, confusion, impaired coordination, diminished reflexes, coma, altered vital signs.

PREGNANCY-LACTATION-REPRODUCTION
● Several studies suggest an increased risk of congenital malformations associated with benzodiazepine use. Use in pregnancy isn't recommended.
● Drug appears in breast milk. Use cautiously in breast-feeding women.

NURSING CONSIDERATIONS
Black Box Warning A qualified individual, other than the practitioner performing the procedure, should monitor patient throughout procedure. Have oxygen and resuscitation equipment available in case of severe respiratory depression. Excessive amounts and rapid infusion have been linked to respiratory arrest. Continuously monitor patient, including children taking syrup form, for life-threatening respiratory depression. ■
● Monitor BP, HR and rhythm, respirations, airway integrity, and pulse oximetry during procedure.

PATIENT TEACHING
● Teach patient about drug's use and potential adverse reactions and to immediately report difficulty breathing.
● Because drug diminishes patient's recall of events around the time of surgery, provide written information, family member instructions, and follow-up contact.
● Warn patient to avoid hazardous activities that require alertness or good coordination until effects of drug are known.

SAFETY ALERT!

miglitol
MIG-lah-tall

Glyset

Therapeutic class: Antidiabetics
Pharmacologic class: Alpha-glucosidase inhibitors

AVAILABLE FORMS
Tablets: 25 mg, 50 mg, 100 mg

INDICATIONS & DOSAGES
➤ **Adjunct to diet in patients with type 2 diabetes, alone or with a sulfonylurea**
Adults: 25 mg P.O. t.i.d. May start with 25 mg P.O. daily and increase gradually to t.i.d. to minimize GI upset; dosage may be increased after 4 to 8 weeks to 50 mg P.O. t.i.d. Dosage may then be further increased after 3 months, based on HbA$_{1c}$ level, to maximum of 100 mg P.O. t.i.d.

ADMINISTRATION
P.O.
● Give drug with first bite of each main meal.

ACTION
Lowers glucose level by inhibiting enzymes in the small intestine, which delays the digestion of carbohydrates after a meal, resulting in a smaller increase in postprandial glucose level.

Route	Onset	Peak	Duration
P.O.	Unknown	2–3 hr	Unknown

Half-life: About 2 hours.

ADVERSE REACTIONS
GI: abdominal pain, diarrhea, flatulence.
Skin: rash.

INTERACTIONS
Drug-drug. *Digoxin, propranolol, ranitidine:* May decrease bioavailability of these drugs. Monitor clinical response and adjust dosage.
Insulin, sulfonylureas: May increase risk of hypoglycemia. Consider decreasing dosages of miglitol, insulin, and sulfonylureas.

Intestinal adsorbents (charcoal), digestive enzyme preparations (amylase, pancreatin): May reduce effect of miglitol. Avoid using together.

EFFECTS ON LAB TEST RESULTS
● May decrease iron level.

CONTRAINDICATIONS & CAUTIONS
● Contraindicated in patients hypersensitive to drug or its components and in those with diabetic ketoacidosis, inflammatory bowel disease, colonic ulceration, partial intestinal obstruction, chronic intestinal diseases with marked disorders of digestion or absorption, or conditions that may deteriorate because of increased gas formation in the intestine.
● Contraindicated in those predisposed to intestinal obstruction and in those with creatinine level greater than 2 mg/dL.
Dialyzable drug: Unknown.
⚠ Overdose S&S: Transient increases in flatulence, diarrhea, and abdominal discomfort.

PREGNANCY-LACTATION-REPRODUCTION
● Safe use in pregnancy hasn't been established. Abnormal blood glucose levels during pregnancy may cause fetal harm. Most experts recommend insulin be used during pregnancy to maintain blood glucose levels. Don't use miglitol during pregnancy unless clearly needed.
● Drug appears in breast milk. Use in breast-feeding women isn't recommended.

NURSING CONSIDERATIONS
● In patients also taking insulin or a sulfonylurea, dosage adjustment of these drugs may be needed. Monitor patient for hypoglycemia.
● Diabetes management should include diet control, an exercise program, and regular testing of urine and glucose level.
● Monitor glucose level regularly, especially during situations of increased stress, such as infection, fever, surgery, or trauma.
● Monitor HbA$_{1c}$ level every 3 months to evaluate long-term glycemic control.
● Treat mild to moderate hypoglycemia with a ready form of sugar, such as glucose tablets or gel. Severe hypoglycemia may necessitate I.V. glucose or glucagon.
● Monitor patient for adverse GI effects.

PATIENT TEACHING
● Stress importance of adhering to diet, weight reduction, and exercise instructions. Urge patient to have glucose and HbA$_{1c}$ levels tested regularly.
● Inform patient that drug treatment relieves symptoms but doesn't cure diabetes.
● Teach patient how to recognize high and low glucose levels.
● Instruct patient to have a source of glucose readily available to treat hypoglycemia.
● Advise patient that sucrose (table sugar, cane sugar) or fruit juices shouldn't be used to treat low-glucose reactions with this drug. Oral glucose (dextrose) or glucagon is necessary to increase glucose.
● Advise patient to seek medical advice promptly during periods of stress, such as fever, trauma, infection, or surgery, because dosage may have to be adjusted.
● Instruct patient to take drug three times daily with first bite of each main meal.
● Show patient how and when to monitor glucose level.
● Advise patient that adverse GI effects are most common during first few weeks of therapy and should improve over time.
● Urge patient to carry medical identification at all times.

milnacipran hydrochloride
Savella⬦

Therapeutic class: Antifibromyalgia drugs
Pharmacologic class: SSNRIs

AVAILABLE FORMS
Tablets: 12.5 mg, 25 mg, 50 mg, 100 mg

INDICATIONS & DOSAGES
➤ **Fibromyalgia**
Adults: Initially, 12.5 mg P.O. once daily; increase dosage to 12.5 mg b.i.d. on days 2 and 3, followed by 25 mg b.i.d. on days 4 to 7. Increase to 50 mg b.i.d. after day 7. May increase to 100 mg P.O. b.i.d. based on individual response.
Adjust-a-dose: For patients with CrCl of 5 to 29 mL/minute, give 25 mg b.i.d. May increase to 50 mg b.i.d. based on individual tolerance.

Reactions in bold italics are ***life-threatening***. Interactions may have a *rapid onset* or a ***delayed onset***.

ADMINISTRATION

P.O.

• Give drug with or without food.

ACTION

Unclear. Milnacipran is a potent inhibitor of neuronal norepinephrine and serotonin reuptake; however, it doesn't affect the uptake of dopamine or other transmitters.

Route	Onset	Peak	Duration
P.O.	Unknown	2–4 hr	36–48 hr

Half-life: 6 to 8 hours; active metabolite, 8 to 10 hours

ADVERSE REACTIONS

CNS: anxiety, depression, dizziness, falls, fatigue, fever, hypesthesia, irritability, insomnia, migraine, paresthesia, *seizures,* stress, somnolence, tension headache, tremors.
CV: chest discomfort, chest pain, flushing, hypertension, palpitations, peripheral edema, tachycardia, fever.
EENT: blurred vision.
GI: abdominal distention, abdominal pain, constipation, decreased appetite, diarrhea, dry mouth, flatulence, GERD, dyspepsia, dysgeusia, nausea, vomiting.
GU: cystitis, UTI; in men—dysuria, ejaculation disorder, ejaculation failure, erectile dysfunction, libido decrease, prostatitis, scrotal pain, testicular pain, testicular swelling, urethral pain, urinary hesitation, urine retention, urine flow decrease.
Metabolic: hypercholesterolemia, weight loss or gain.
Respiratory: dyspnea, URI.
Skin: hyperhidrosis, pruritus, rash.
Other: chills, contusion, hot flush, night sweats.

INTERACTIONS

Drug-drug. *Antipsychotics (risperidone), cyclobenzaprine, dopamine antagonists (metoclopramide):* May cause serotonin syndrome (diarrhea, dysreflexia, fever, hallucinations, loss of coordination, nausea, tachycardia). If use together can't be avoided, closely monitor patient for signs and symptoms of serotonin syndrome.
◑ *Alert: Aspirin, NSAIDs, warfarin:* May increase risk of bleeding. Use together cautiously.

Clomipramine: May cause euphoria and orthostatic hypotension when switching from clomipramine to milnacipran. Use together may also increase risk of serotonin syndrome. Monitor patient closely.
Digoxin: May cause orthostatic hypotension and tachycardia and digoxin-related adverse effects. Avoid use of digoxin I.V.; when using oral digoxin and drug together, monitor patient closely.
Lithium, other serotonergic drugs: May cause serotonin syndrome. Avoid use together.
MAO inhibitors: May cause serotonin syndrome. Avoid using drug within 2 weeks after MAO inhibitor therapy; wait at least 5 days after stopping milnacipran or before starting MAO inhibitor.
Methylene blue: May cause CNS toxicity and serotonin syndrome. Avoid use together.
Drug-herb. *Herbs with anticoagulant properties (alfalfa, anise, bilberry):* May increase risk of bleeding. Use together cautiously.
Drug-lifestyle. *Alcohol use:* May enhance psychomotor impairment and aggravate preexisting liver disease. Don't administer to patients using alcohol or with chronic liver disease.

EFFECTS ON LAB TEST RESULTS

• May increase LFT values.
• May decrease sodium level.

CONTRAINDICATIONS & CAUTIONS

• Contraindicated in patients hypersensitive to drug or its components.
• Contraindicated in patients being treated with MAO inhibitors, such as linezolid or I.V. methylene blue.
◑ *Alert:* Pupillary dilation that occurs after drug use may trigger an angle-closure attack in patients with anatomically narrow angles who don't have a patent iridectomy.
◑ *Alert:* Serotonin syndrome, a potentially life-threatening condition, may occur, particularly with concomitant use of serotonergic drugs (including triptans and tramadol) and drugs that impair serotonin metabolism (including MAO inhibitors). Signs and symptoms of serotonin syndrome include mental status changes (agitation, coma, hallucinations), autonomic instability

M

(hyperthermia, labile BP, tachycardia), neuromuscular aberrations (hyperreflexia, incoordination), and diarrhea, nausea, and vomiting.
• Use cautiously in patients with a history of mania, seizures, severe hepatic impairment, or dysuria; in patients who consume substantial amounts of alcohol; and in those with hypertension or controlled angle-closure glaucoma.
• Drug isn't approved for use in children.
Dialyzable drug: Unlikely.
⚠ *Overdose S&S:* Hypertension, cardiac arrest, decreased level of consciousness, confusion, dizziness, elevated LFT results.

PREGNANCY-LACTATION-REPRODUCTION
• There are no adequate studies in pregnant women. Use during pregnancy only if potential benefit justifies potential risk to the fetus. Neonates exposed to SSRIs/SNRIs late in the third trimester have developed complications requiring prolonged hospitalization, respiratory support, and tube feeding.
• Savella appears in breast milk. Use cautiously in breast-feeding women.

NURSING CONSIDERATIONS
Black Box Warning Drug may increase risk of suicidal thinking and behavior in children, adolescents, and young adults with major depressive disorder or other psychiatric disorder. Drug isn't approved for use in children. ∎
• At least 14 days should elapse between discontinuation of an MAO inhibitor and initiation of milnacipran. Allow at least 5 days after stopping milnacipran before starting an MAO inhibitor.
• Monitor patient closely for worsening depression or suicidal behavior, especially during the first few months of therapy and with dosage adjustments.
• To prevent withdrawal signs and symptoms, decrease dosage gradually, and watch for signs and symptoms that may arise when drug is stopped, such as dysphoria, irritability, agitation, dizziness, sensory disturbances, anxiety, confusion, headache, lethargy, emotional lability, insomnia, hypomania, tinnitus, and seizures.
• Carefully monitor HR and BP.

• Monitor patient for signs and symptoms of hyponatremia (headache, difficulty concentrating, memory impairment, confusion, weakness, unsteadiness, hallucination, syncope, seizures, coma, respiratory arrest).
• Monitor LFT values and sodium level before and during therapy.

PATIENT TEACHING
Black Box Warning Warn families and caregivers to immediately report signs and symptoms of worsening depression (such as agitation, irritability, insomnia, hostility, and impulsivity) and suicidal behavior. ∎
• Advise patient to avoid taking NSAIDs and aspirin while taking drug to reduce risk of bleeding.
• Tell patient to avoid alcohol while taking drug.
• Instruct patient to have frequent HR and BP monitoring.
• Tell patient to report urinary hesitation or urine retention.
• Instruct female patient of childbearing potential to notify prescriber if she becomes pregnant, is planning pregnancy during therapy, or is breast-feeding.
• Warn patient not to stop drug suddenly.
• Tell patient to consult prescriber before taking other prescription or OTC drugs.
• Warn patient to avoid hazardous activities that require alertness and good coordination until drug's effects are known.
• Tell patient that drug may be taken with or without food but that food may increase tolerability.

SAFETY ALERT!

milrinone lactate
MILL-ri-none

Therapeutic class: Inotropes
Pharmacologic class: Bipyridine phosphodiesterase inhibitors

AVAILABLE FORMS
Injection: 1 mg/mL
Injection (premixed): 200 mcg/mL in D$_5$W

INDICATIONS & DOSAGES
➤ **Short-term treatment of acutely decompensated HF**

Adults: Give first loading dose of 50 mcg/kg I.V. slowly over 10 minutes; then give continuous I.V. infusion of 0.375 to 0.75 mcg/kg/minute. Titrate infusion dose based on clinical and hemodynamic responses. Don't exceed 1.13 mg/kg/day.
Adjust-a-dose: If CrCl is 50 mL/minute, infusion rate is 0.43 mcg/kg/minute; if 40 mL/minute, infusion rate is 0.38 mcg/kg/minute; if 30 mL/minute, infusion rate is 0.33 mcg/kg/minute; if 20 mL/minute, infusion rate is 0.28 mcg/kg/minute; if 10 mL/minute, infusion rate is 0.23 mcg/kg/minute; and if 5 mL/minute, infusion rate is 0.2 mcg/kg/minute. Don't exceed 1.13 mg/kg/day.

ADMINISTRATION

I.V.
▼ Give loading dose undiluted as a direct injection over 10 minutes.
▼ Prepare I.V. infusion solution using half-NSS, NSS, or D₅W. Prepare the 100-mcg/mL solution by adding 180 mL of diluent per 20-mg (20-mL) vial, the 150-mcg/mL solution by adding 113 mL of diluent per 20-mg (20-mL) vial, and the 200-mcg/mL solution by adding 80 mL of diluent per 20-mg (20-mL) vial.
▼ **Incompatibilities:** Bumetanide, furosemide, imipenem–cilastatin sodium, procainamide, torsemide.

ACTION
Produces inotropic action by increasing cellular levels of cAMP and vasodilation by relaxing vascular smooth muscle.

Route	Onset	Peak	Duration
I.V.	5–15 min	1–2 hr	3–6 hr

Half-life: 2½ to 3¾ hours.

ADVERSE REACTIONS
CNS: headache.
CV: *ventricular arrhythmias,* ventricular ectopic activity, *sustained ventricular tachycardia,* hypotension, nonsustained ventricular tachycardia, chest pain.

INTERACTIONS
None significant.

EFFECTS ON LAB TEST RESULTS
● May cause abnormal LFT results.
● May cause electrolyte changes.

CONTRAINDICATIONS & CAUTIONS
● Contraindicated in patients hypersensitive to drug. Solutions containing dextrose may be contraindicated in patients with known allergy to corn or corn products.
⊗ *Alert:* Use of milrinone for more than 48 hours in patients with HF hasn't been shown to be safe or effective.
⊗ *Alert:* Drug has been associated with increased frequency of ventricular arrhythmias, including nonsustained ventricular tachycardia and supraventricular and ventricular arrhythmias in the high-risk population. Closely monitor patient.
● Contraindicated in patients with severe aortic or pulmonary valvular disease in place of surgery and during acute phase of MI.
● Use cautiously in patients with atrial flutter or fibrillation because drug may increase ventricular response rate.
Dialyzable drug: Unknown.
⚠ *Overdose S&S:* Hypotension.

PREGNANCY-LACTATION-REPRODUCTION
● There are no adequate studies in pregnant women. Use during pregnancy only if potential benefit justifies potential risk to the fetus.
● It isn't known if drug appears in breast milk. Use cautiously in breast-feeding women.

NURSING CONSIDERATIONS
● In patients with atrial flutter or fibrillation, drug is typically given with digoxin and diuretics.
● Improved cardiac output may increase urine output. Reduce diuretic dosage when HF improves. Potassium loss may cause digitalis toxicity.
● Monitor fluid and electrolyte status, BP, HR, and renal function during therapy. Excessive decrease in BP requires stopping or slowing rate of infusion.
● Correct hypoxemia and electrolyte imbalances, especially hypokalemia and hypomagnesemia, before use and throughout therapy.

PATIENT TEACHING
● Instruct patient to report adverse reactions promptly, especially angina or palpitations.
● Tell patient that drug may cause headache, which can be treated with analgesics.
● Tell patient to report discomfort at I.V. insertion site.

minocycline hydrochloride
mi-noe-SYE-kleen

Dynacin, Minocin, Solodyn

Therapeutic class: Antibiotics
Pharmacologic class: Tetracyclines

AVAILABLE FORMS
Capsules ⓞⓝⓒ: 50 mg, 75 mg, 100 mg
Injection: 100 mg
Tablets: 50 mg, 75 mg, 100 mg
Tablets (extended-release) ⓞⓝⓒ: 45 mg, 55 mg, 65 mg, 80 mg, 90 mg, 105 mg, 115 mg, 135 mg

INDICATIONS & DOSAGES
Adjust-a-dose (for all indications): Decrease dosage or increase dosing interval in patients with renal impairment. Don't exceed 200 mg Minocin in 24 hours.
➤ **Infections caused by susceptible gram-negative and gram-positive organisms (including *Haemophilus ducreyi, Yersinia pestis*, and *Campylobacter fetus*), *Rickettsiae* species, *Mycoplasma pneumoniae*, or *Chlamydia trachomatis;* psittacosis; granuloma inguinale**
Adults: 200 mg P.O. or I.V. initially; then 100 mg P.O. or I.V. every 12 hours. May use 100 or 200 mg P.O. initially; then 50 mg q.i.d.
Children older than age 8: Initially, 4 mg/kg P.O. or I.V.; then, 2 mg/kg P.O. or I.V. every 12 hours. Maximum dose is 100 mg/dose or 200 mg/dose for the loading dose.
➤ **Gonorrhea in patients allergic to penicillin**
Adults: Initially, 200 mg P.O.; then 100 mg every 12 hours for at least 4 days. Obtain samples for follow-up cultures within 2 to 3 days after treatment.
➤ **Syphilis in patients allergic to penicillin**

Adults: Initially, 200 mg P.O.; then 100 mg every 12 hours for 10 to 15 days.
➤ **Meningococcal carrier state**
Adults: 100 mg P.O. every 12 hours for 5 days.
➤ **Uncomplicated urethral, endocervical, or rectal infection caused by *C. trachomatis* or *Ureaplasma urealyticum***
Adults: 100 mg P.O. every 12 hours for at least 7 days.
➤ **Uncomplicated gonococcal urethritis**
Men: 100 mg P.O. every 12 hours for 5 days.
➤ **Treatment of inflammatory lesions of nonnodular moderate to severe acne vulgaris**
Adults and children age 12 and older: 1 mg/kg extended-release tablets P.O. once daily for 12 weeks.

ADMINISTRATION
P.O.
● Obtain specimen for culture and sensitivity tests before first dose. Begin therapy while awaiting results.
● Give pellet-filled capsules and tablets 1 hour before or 2 hours after a meal.
● Give drug with a full glass of water. Drug may be taken with food.
● Drug shouldn't be given within 1 hour of bedtime, to avoid esophageal irritation or ulceration.
● Give capsules and extended-release tablets at the same time each day, with or without food.
● Capsules and extended-release tablets must be swallowed whole and not crushed, chewed, or split.

I.V.
▼ Reconstitute powder with 5 mL sterile water for injection; further dilute to 500 to 1,000 mL with sodium chloride injection, dextrose injection, dextrose and sodium chloride injection, Ringer injection, or lactated Ringer injection. (Don't use solutions containing calcium except for lactated Ringer, because a precipitate may form.)
▼ Infuse over 60 minutes, avoid rapid administration, and don't administer with other drugs.
▼ Parenteral therapy is indicated only when oral therapy is inadequate or isn't tolerated. Institute oral therapy as soon as possible.

Reactions in bold italics are *life-threatening*. Interactions may have a *rapid onset* or a *delayed onset*.

ACTION

May be bacteriostatic by binding to microorganism's ribosomal subunits, inhibiting protein synthesis; may also alter the cytoplasmic membrane of susceptible microorganisms.

Route	Onset	Peak	Duration
P.O.	Unknown	1–4 hr	Unknown
P.O. (extended-release)	Unknown	3½–4 hr	Unknown
I.V.	Unknown	Unknown	Unknown

Half-life: P.O., 11 to 17 hours; I.V., 15 to 23 hours.

ADVERSE REACTIONS

CNS: *intracranial hypertension,* headache, light-headedness, dizziness, vertigo, fatigue, mood alterations, somnolence.
CV: thrombophlebitis, pericarditis.
EENT: tooth disorder, tinnitus.
GI: anorexia, diarrhea, nausea, dysphagia, glossitis, oral candidiasis, vomiting, dyspepsia, pancreatitis, dry mouth.
GU: *acute renal failure.*
Hematologic: *neutropenia, thrombocytopenia,* eosinophilia, hemolytic anemia.
Hepatic: *hepatotoxicity.*
Musculoskeletal: bone growth retardation in children younger than age 8, arthralgia, myalgia.
Respiratory: *bronchospasm,* cough, dyspnea, asthma exacerbation, pneumonitis.
Skin: increased pigmentation, maculopapular and erythematous rashes, photosensitivity reactions, pruritus, urticaria, alopecia.
Other: *anaphylaxis,* enamel defects, hypersensitivity reactions, permanent discoloration of teeth, superinfection, pain at injection site.

INTERACTIONS

Drug-drug. *Antacids (including sodium bicarbonate) and laxatives containing aluminum, magnesium, or calcium; antidiarrheals:* May decrease antibiotic absorption. Give antibiotic 1 hour before or 2 hours after these drugs.
Ferrous sulfate and other iron products, zinc: May decrease antibiotic absorption. Give drug 2 hours before or 3 hours after iron.

Hormonal contraceptives: May decrease contraceptive effectiveness and increase risk of breakthrough bleeding. Advise patient to use nonhormonal contraceptive.
Live-virus vaccines: May decrease vaccine effectiveness. Avoid administering together.
Methoxyflurane: May cause nephrotoxicity when given with tetracyclines. Avoid using together.
Oral anticoagulants: May increase anticoagulant effect. Monitor PT and INR, and adjust dosage.
Penicillins: May disrupt bactericidal action of penicillins. Avoid using together.
Retinoids: May increase risk of pseudotumor cerebri. Avoid administering together.
Drug-lifestyle. *Sun exposure:* May cause photosensitivity reactions. Advise patient to avoid excessive sunlight exposure.

EFFECTS ON LAB TEST RESULTS

● May increase BUN and liver enzyme levels. May decrease Hb level.
● May increase eosinophil count. May decrease platelet and neutrophil counts.
● May falsely elevate fluorometric test results for urine catecholamines. Parenteral form may cause false-positive results on copper sulfate test (Clinitest). May cause false-negative results on urine glucose tests using glucose oxidase reagent (Diastix or Chemstrip uG).

CONTRAINDICATIONS & CAUTIONS

● Contraindicated in patients hypersensitive to drug or other tetracyclines.
❸ *Alert:* Severe cases of anaphylaxis, serious skin reactions (Stevens-Johnson syndrome, erythema multiforme, drug reaction with eosinophilia and systemic symptoms [DRESS syndrome]), and death have been reported.
❸ *Alert:* Some products may contain tartrazine, which can cause allergy-type reactions (including bronchial asthma). Although incidence of this sensitivity is low, these reactions are frequently seen in patients who are also sensitive to aspirin.
● Use cautiously in patients with impaired renal or hepatic function. Use of these drugs during last half of pregnancy and in children younger than age 8 may cause permanent

M

discoloration of teeth, enamel defects, and bone growth retardation.

● Drug may cause superinfection. If overgrowth of nonsusceptible organisms occurs, discontinue drug and begin appropriate therapy.

Dialyzable drug: No.

⚠ *Overdose S&S:* Dizziness, nausea, vomiting.

PREGNANCY-LACTATION-REPRODUCTION

● There are no adequate studies in pregnant women. Drug may cause fetal harm. Avoid use in pregnancy.

● If patient becomes pregnant during therapy, stop drug immediately and apprise her of potential hazard to the fetus.

● Drug appears in breast milk. Patient should discontinue breast-feeding or discontinue drug.

● Drug shouldn't be used to treat acne in males or females attempting to conceive a child.

NURSING CONSIDERATIONS

● Monitor renal function and LFT results.

🔆 *Alert:* Check expiration date. Outdated or deteriorated drug may cause reversible nephrotoxicity (Fanconi syndrome).

● Don't expose drug to light or heat. Keep cap tightly closed.

● If large doses are given, therapy is prolonged, or patient is at high risk, monitor patient for signs and symptoms of superinfection.

● Drug may cause mild to severe CDAD, which can occur up to 2 months after therapy ends. If diarrhea occurs, evaluate patient for CDAD. Drug may need to be discontinued and appropriate therapy begun.

● Check patient's tongue for signs of candidal infection. Stress good oral hygiene.

● Drug may discolor teeth in older children and young adults, more commonly when used as long-term treatment. Watch for brown pigmentation, and notify prescriber if it occurs.

● Photosensitivity reactions may occur within a few minutes to several hours after exposure. Photosensitivity lasts after therapy ends.

● Monitor patient for DRESS syndrome. Discontinue drug immediately if syndrome occurs.

● *Look alike–sound alike:* Don't confuse Minocin with niacin or Minoxidil.

PATIENT TEACHING

● Tell patient to take entire amount of drug exactly as prescribed, even after he feels better.

● Instruct patient to take drug with a full glass of water. Drug may be taken with food. Tell patient not to take within 1 hour of bedtime to avoid esophageal irritation or ulceration.

● Teach patient about potential adverse reactions and tell him to report them promptly.

● Warn patient to avoid driving or other hazardous tasks because of possible adverse CNS effects.

● Caution patient to avoid direct sunlight and ultraviolet light, wear protective clothing, and use sunscreen.

● Tell patient to take extended-release tablets at the same time each day, with or without food.

● Tell patient to swallow extended-release tablet whole and not to crush, chew, or split tablet.

● Warn patient not to take more than one extended-release tablet each day.

● Warn patient that diarrhea may occur up to 2 months after last dose. Tell patient to report diarrhea to prescriber.

● Tell female patient not to take drug if pregnant or trying to become pregnant because of potential fetal hazard.

● Warn patient that drug can decrease hormonal contraceptive effectiveness. Advise the use of a nonhormonal method.

---

mipomersen sodium
MI-poe-MER-sen

Kynamro

Therapeutic class: Antilipemics
Pharmacologic class: Oligonucleotides

AVAILABLE FORMS
Injection: 200 mg/mL single-use vials or prefilled syringes

INDICATIONS & DOSAGES

➤ **Adjunctive treatment for homozygous familial hypercholesterolemia (HoFH) with lipid-lowering medications and diet to reduce LDL cholesterol, apolipoprotein B, total cholesterol, and non-HDL cholesterol**

Adults: 200 mg subcutaneously once weekly on same day each week.

Adjust-a-dose: If AST or ALT level is $3 \times$ ULN to less than $5 \times$ ULN, repeat measurement within 1 week; if elevations are confirmed, withhold drug. Perform additional LFTs if not already measured (such as total bilirubin, alkaline phosphatase, and INR) and investigate to identify probable cause of elevations.

Consider monitoring LFTs more frequently if resuming drug after transaminase levels resolve to less than $3 \times$ ULN. If AST or ALT is $5 \times$ ULN or greater, withhold drug. Perform additional liver-related tests to identify probable cause. If transaminase elevations are accompanied by clinical symptoms of liver injury (such as nausea, vomiting, abdominal pain, fever, jaundice, lethargy, and flulike symptoms), increases in bilirubin level at least $2 \times$ ULN, or active liver disease, discontinue treatment and identify probable cause.

ADMINISTRATION

Subcutaneous

● Store refrigerated at 36° to 46° F (2° to 8° C). Protect from light and keep in original carton until time of use. If refrigeration isn't possible, store at or below 86° F (30° C), away from heat sources, for up to 14 days.

● Remove from refrigeration at least 30 minutes before use.

● Inspect solution for clarity or particulate matter; if solution is cloudy or contains particles, return product to pharmacy.

● Administer first dose under supervision of health care provider.

● Administration sites include the abdomen, thigh region, and outer area of the upper arm. Alternate sites.

● Don't inject in areas of active skin disease or injury (such as sunburn, rash, inflammation, skin infection, or active areas of psoriasis). Avoid tattooed and scarred skin.

● Vials and syringes are for single use only. Discard excess solution; product contains no preservatives.

● Don't give I.V. or I.M.

● Don't mix or administer this drug with other products.

● If a dose is missed, give missed dose at least 3 days from the next scheduled weekly dose.

ACTION

Inhibits synthesis of apolipoprotein B-100, a primary component of LDL cholesterol and its metabolic precursor, VLDL.

Route	Onset	Peak	Duration
Subcut.	Unknown	3–4 hr	Unknown

Half-life: 1 to 2 months.

ADVERSE REACTIONS

CNS: fatigue, headache, pyrexia, chills, insomnia.

CV: angina pectoris, palpitations, peripheral edema, hypertension.

GI: nausea, vomiting, abdominal pain.

GU: proteinuria.

Hepatic: *hepatotoxicity,* hepatic steatosis, hepatic enzyme increase.

Musculoskeletal: extremity pain, musculoskeletal pain.

Skin: injection-site reactions (pain, hematoma, erythema, pruritus, swelling, discoloration).

Other: flulike symptoms, benign neoplasms, *malignant neoplasms.*

INTERACTIONS

Drug-drug. *Hepatotoxic drugs (acetaminophen, amiodarone, isotretinoin, methotrexate, tamoxifen, tetracyclines):* May increase risk of liver injury. Monitor LFTs frequently.

Drug-lifestyle. *Alcohol use:* May increase risk of hepatotoxicity. Limit alcohol intake to one drink per day.

EFFECTS ON LAB TEST RESULTS

● May increase AST, ALT, and urine protein levels.

CONTRAINDICATIONS & CAUTIONS

Black Box Warning Drug may cause elevated transaminase levels and may increase

M

hepatic fat, with or without concomitant increases in transaminase levels. Hepatic steatosis is a risk factor for advanced liver disease, including steatohepatitis and cirrhosis. Measure ALT, AST, alkaline phosphatase, and total bilirubin levels before initiating treatment, and monitor ALT and AST levels regularly as recommended. During treatment, withhold dose if ALT or AST level is 3 × ULN or more. Discontinue drug for clinically significant liver toxicity. ■

• Contraindicated in patients with known hypersensitivity to drug or its components and in those with moderate or severe hepatic impairment (Child-Pugh class B or C) or active liver disease, including unexplained, persistent serum transaminase elevations. **Black Box Warning** Only patients with a clinical or laboratory diagnosis of HoFH should use drug. Safety and effectiveness haven't been established in patients with hypercholesterolemia who don't have HoFH. ■

• Drug isn't recommended in patients with severe renal impairment or clinically significant proteinuria, or in patients on renal dialysis.

• Using drug as an adjunct to LDL apheresis isn't recommended.

Dialyzable drug: Unlikely.

PREGNANCY-LACTATION-REPRODUCTION

• Drug may cause fetal harm. Women of childbearing potential should use effective contraception during therapy. Use drug only if clearly needed.

• It isn't known if drug appears in breast milk. Patient should discontinue breastfeeding or discontinue drug.

NURSING CONSIDERATIONS

• If baseline LFT values are abnormal, consider treatment only after appropriate evaluation and resolution or explanation of any abnormalities.

• Obtain LFT values monthly for first year, then at least every 3 months thereafter. Discontinue drug if persistent or clinically significant increases occur.

• If transaminase elevations are accompanied by clinical signs and symptoms of liver injury (nausea, vomiting, abdominal pain, fever, jaundice, lethargy, flulike symptoms), increases in bilirubin to 2 × ULN or more,

or active liver disease, discontinue drug and identify probable cause.

• Measure lipid levels at least every 3 months for first year. Measure LDL levels after 6 months, since maximum LDL reduction occurs at that time. Assess whether drug is effective, taking into account possible hepatotoxicity.

Black Box Warning Because of hepatotoxicity, only providers and pharmacies certified through the Kynamro REMS (Risk Evaluation and Mitigation Strategy) program may prescribe and administer this medication. For more information, call 1-877-KYNAMRO (1-877-596-2676) or go to www.kynamrorems.com. ■

• Drug's effect on CV morbidity and mortality hasn't been determined.

• Proper injection technique may help decrease risk of injection-site reactions, which occur in the majority of patients and typically consist of one or more of the following: erythema, pain, tenderness, pruritus, and local swelling.

• Flulike symptoms, which typically develop within 2 days after an injection, may occur and include one or more of the following: flulike illness, pyrexia, chills, myalgia, arthralgia, malaise, and fatigue.

PATIENT TEACHING

• Caution patient that there must be at least 3 days between a missed dose and the next regularly scheduled weekly dose.

• Instruct patient or caregiver on the proper technique for administering this drug, including use of aseptic technique. Needles or syringes may only be used once, and should be properly disposed of in a suitable puncture-resistant container. Proper administration technique may decrease risk of injection-site reactions.

• Advise patient to avoid or limit alcohol to one drink per day because of additive liver toxicity.

• Tell patient to report signs and symptoms of liver damage, including nausea, vomiting, fever, anorexia, fatigue, jaundice, dark urine, pruritus, and abdominal pain. Encourage compliance with follow-up blood tests to monitor safe use of drug.

• Advise patient that injection-site reactions (erythema, pain, tenderness, pruritus, or local swelling) may occur.
• Advise patient that flulike symptoms, typically appearing within 2 days after an injection, may occur and include flulike illness, pyrexia, chills, myalgia, arthralgia, malaise, and fatigue.

mirabegron
MIR-a-BEG-ron

Myrbetriq

Therapeutic class: Bladder antispasmodics
Pharmacologic class: Beta-3 adrenergic agonists

AVAILABLE FORMS
Tablets (extended-release) ⊙: 25 mg, 50 mg

INDICATIONS & DOSAGES
➤ **Overactive bladder with symptoms of urge incontinence, urgency, and frequency**
Adults: Initially, 25 mg P.O. once daily. May increase to 50 mg after 8 weeks if necessary.
Adjust-a-dose: For patients with severe renal impairment (CrCl of 15 to 29 mL/minute) or moderate hepatic impairment (Child-Pugh class B), give no more than 25 mg daily. Drug isn't recommended for patients with ESRD (CrCl of less than 15 mL/minute) or for patients with severe hepatic impairment (Child-Pugh class C).

ADMINISTRATION
P.O.
• May give without regard to food.
• Patient should swallow tablets whole with water; don't crush or divide tablets.

ACTION
Relaxes the detrusor smooth muscle during storage phase of the urinary bladder fill-void cycle, increasing bladder capacity.

Route	Onset	Peak	Duration
P.O.	Unknown	3½ hr	Unknown

Half-life: 50 hours.

ADVERSE REACTIONS
CNS: headache, fatigue, dizziness.
CV: *hypertension,* tachycardia.
EENT: nasopharyngitis, dry mouth, sinusitis.
GI: constipation, diarrhea, abdominal pain.
GU: UTI, cystitis, urine retention.
Musculoskeletal: arthralgia, back pain.
Respiratory: URI.
Other: flulike symptoms.

INTERACTIONS
Drug-drug. *Antimuscarinics (pirenzepine):* May increase risk of urine retention. Use cautiously together.
Digoxin: May increase digoxin level. Monitor digoxin level and titrate mirabegron to lowest effective dosage.
Drugs metabolized by CYP2D6 (desipramine, flecainide, metoprolol, propafenone, thioridazine): May increase levels of these drugs. Monitor patient for adverse events; adjust dosage as needed.
Warfarin: May increase warfarin level. Monitor INR; adjust warfarin dosage as necessary.

EFFECTS ON LAB TEST RESULTS
• May increase ALT, AST, GGT, LDH, and digoxin levels.
• May increase INR.

CONTRAINDICATIONS & CAUTIONS
• Avoid use in patients hypersensitive to drug or its components and in those with severe, uncontrolled hypertension.
• Use cautiously in patients with hypertension, urine retention, or bladder outlet obstruction.
Dialyzable drug: Unknown.
⚠ *Overdose S&S:* Palpitations, increased HR, increased BP.

PREGNANCY-LACTATION-REPRODUCTION
• There are no adequate studies in pregnant women. Use during pregnancy only if potential benefit justifies potential risk to the fetus.
• It isn't known if drug appears in breast milk. Patient should discontinue breastfeeding or discontinue drug.

M

NURSING CONSIDERATIONS
● Monitor BP and pulse regularly, especially in patients with hypertension or atrial fibrillation.
● Monitor patient for angioedema of the face, lips, tongue, or larynx, which may be life threatening and can occur after first dose. Promptly discontinue drug if involvement of the tongue, hypopharynx, or larynx occurs, and ensure a patent airway.
● Monitor patients closely for urine retention and bladder obstruction, especially in those already taking bladder antispasmodics.
● Monitor LFT values periodically.
● Monitor patients for rash or pruritus.

PATIENT TEACHING
● Tell patient not to crush, chew, or cut tablets and that drug may be taken without regard to food.
● Warn patient that drug may cause an increase in BP or pulse. Teach patient to monitor BP and pulse at home and to report increases to the health care provider.
● Advise patient that he may experience difficulty in emptying his bladder and infrequent bladder infections and to report concerns to his health care provider.
● Tell patient to report rash or itching, which may indicate an allergy or a serious adverse reaction.
● Advise patient to immediately report signs and symptoms of a significant reaction (fast heartbeat, palpitations, back pain, bloody urine, chills, severe dizziness, passing out, severe headache, wheezing, chest tightness, fever, bad cough, blue skin, seizures, or swelling of face, lips, tongue, or throat).
● Teach female patient to report pregnancy to her health care provider as soon as possible.

mirtazapine
mer-TAH-zah-peen

Remeron, Remeron SolTab

Therapeutic class: Antidepressants
Pharmacologic class: Tetracyclic antidepressants

AVAILABLE FORMS
ODTs ⊕: 15 mg, 30 mg, 45 mg
Tablets: 7.5 mg, 15 mg, 30 mg, 45 mg

INDICATIONS & DOSAGES
➤ **Major depressive disorder**
Adults: Initially, 15 mg P.O. at bedtime. Maintenance dose is 15 to 45 mg daily. Adjust dosage at intervals of at least 1 week.

ADMINISTRATION
P.O.
● Give drug without regard for food.
● Remove ODT from blister pack and immediately place on patient's tongue.
● ODT may be given with or without water.
● Don't split or crush ODT.

ACTION
Thought to enhance central noradrenergic and serotonergic activity.

Route	Onset	Peak	Duration
P.O.	Unknown	2 hr	Unknown

Half-life: About 20 to 40 hours.

ADVERSE REACTIONS
CNS: somnolence, dizziness, asthenia, abnormal dreams, abnormal thinking, tremors, confusion.
CV: edema, peripheral edema, hypertension, vasodilatation.
EENT: dry mouth.
GI: increased appetite, dry mouth, constipation, nausea.
GU: urinary frequency.
Metabolic: weight gain.
Musculoskeletal: myalgia, weakness, back pain.
Respiratory: dyspnea.
Skin: pruritus, rash.
Other: flulike syndrome.

Reactions in bold italics are *life-threatening*. Interactions may have a *rapid onset* or a *delayed onset*.

INTERACTIONS

Drug-drug. *Diazepam, other CNS depressants:* May cause additive CNS effects. Avoid using together.

❸ **Alert:** *Linezolid, methylene blue, rasagiline:* May cause serotonin syndrome. Use extreme caution and monitor patient closely.

❸ **Alert:** *MAO inhibitors:* May sometimes cause fatal reactions. Avoid using within 14 days of MAO inhibitor therapy.

Warfarin: May increase anticoagulant effect. Closely monitor INR when mirtazapine is started or stopped, and adjust warfarin dosage as needed.

Drug-herb. *St. John's wort:* May increase risk of serotonin syndrome. Use together cautiously and monitor patient closely for adverse reactions.

Drug-lifestyle. *Alcohol use:* May cause additive CNS effects. Discourage use together.

EFFECTS ON LAB TEST RESULTS

• May increase ALT, cholesterol, and triglyceride levels.

CONTRAINDICATIONS & CAUTIONS

• Contraindicated in patients hypersensitive to drug and within 14 days of MAO inhibitor therapy.

❸ **Alert:** Concomitant use with linezolid or methylene blue can cause serotonin syndrome (fever, mental status changes, muscle twitching, excessive sweating, shivering or shaking, diarrhea, or loss of coordination). Use together is contraindicated.

Black Box Warning Drug may increase risk of suicidal thinking and behavior in children, adolescents, and young adults with major depressive or other psychiatric disorders. Drug isn't approved for use in children. ∎

• Use cautiously in patients with CV or cerebrovascular disease, seizure disorders, suicidal thoughts, hepatic or renal impairment, or history of mania or hypomania.

• Use cautiously in patients with conditions that predispose them to hypotension, such as dehydration, hypovolemia, or antihypertensive therapy.

• Give drug cautiously to elderly patients; decreased clearance has occurred in this age group.

Dialyzable drug: Unknown.

⚠ **Overdose S&S:** Disorientation, drowsiness, impaired memory, tachycardia.

PREGNANCY-LACTATION-REPRODUCTION

• There are no adequate studies in pregnant women. Use during pregnancy only if clearly needed.

• Drug may appear in breast milk. Use cautiously in breast-feeding women.

NURSING CONSIDERATIONS

❸ **Alert:** If linezolid or methylene blue must be given, mirtazapine must be stopped and patient should be monitored for serotonin toxicity for 2 weeks, or until 24 hours after the last dose of methylene blue or linezolid, whichever comes first. Treatment with mirtazapine may be resumed 24 hours after last dose of methylene blue or linezolid.

• Don't use within 14 days of MAO inhibitor therapy.

Black Box Warning Appropriately monitor and closely observe patients of all ages who are started on antidepressants for clinical worsening, mood changes, suicidality, or unusual changes in behavior. ∎

• Although agranulocytosis occurs rarely, stop drug and monitor patient closely if he develops a sore throat, fever, stomatitis, or other signs and symptoms of infection with a low WBC count.

• Lower dosages tend to be more sedating than higher dosages.

PATIENT TEACHING

Black Box Warning Advise families and caregivers to closely observe patient for increasing suicidal thinking and behavior. ∎

❸ **Alert:** Teach patient to recognize and immediately report signs and symptoms of serotonin toxicity.

• Instruct patient to take drug at bedtime. Caution patient not to perform hazardous activities if he gets too sleepy.

• Tell patient to report signs and symptoms of infection, such as fever, chills, sore throat, mucous membrane irritation, or flulike syndrome.

• Instruct patient not to use alcohol or other CNS depressants while taking drug.

• Instruct patient not to take other drugs without prescriber's approval.

M

• Tell women of childbearing potential to report suspected pregnancy immediately and to notify prescriber if breast-feeding.
• Instruct patient to remove ODTs from blister pack and place immediately on tongue. Tell patient to be sure his hands are clean and dry if he touches the tablet.
• Advise patient not to break or split tablet.

SAFETY ALERT!

mitomycin (mitomycin-C)
mye-toe-MYE-sin

Therapeutic class: Antineoplastics
Pharmacologic class: Antineoplastic antibiotics

AVAILABLE FORMS
Powder for injection: 5-mg, 20-mg, 40-mg vials

INDICATIONS & DOSAGES
Dosage and indications vary. Check treatment protocol with prescriber.
➤ **Disseminated adenocarcinoma of stomach or pancreas in combination with other chemotherapeutic agents**
Adults: 10 to 20 mg/m^2 I.V. as a single dose at 6- to 8-week intervals if patient has full hematologic recovery. Fully evaluate patient after each cycle and reduce dosage if toxicities occur. Discontinue drug if disease progresses after two courses of therapy.
Adjust-a-dose: For patients with myelosuppression, if WBC count is 3,000 to 3,999/mm^3 and platelet count is 75,000 to 99,000/mm^3, give 100% of prior dose. If WBC count is 2,000 to 2,999/mm^3 and platelet count is 25,000 to 74,999/mm^3, give 70% of prior dose. If WBC count is less than 2,000/mm^3 and platelet count is less than 25,000/mm^3, give 50% of prior dose. Don't repeat full dosage until WBC count has returned to 4,000/mm^3 and platelet count to 100,000/mm^3.

ADMINISTRATION
I.V.
▼ Hazardous drug; use safe handling and disposal precautions.
▼ Drug is a vesicant. Never give drug I.M. or subcutaneously.

▼ Preparing and giving drug may be mutagenic, teratogenic, or carcinogenic. Follow institutional policy to reduce risks.
▼ Using sterile water for injection, reconstitute drug in 5-mg vials with 10 mL, 20-mg vials with 40 mL, and 40-mg vials with 80 mL. Solution will appear clear to pale blue. Protect from light.
▼ Give drug by slow I.V. push or slow I.V. infusion over 15 to 30 minutes into the side arm of a free-flowing I.V. line.
▼ When reconstituted with sterile water, solution is stable for 14 days under refrigeration and for 7 days at room temperature, if protected from light. When diluted, drug is stable in D$_5$W for no more than 3 hours, in NSS for no more than 12 hours, and in sodium lactate for no more than 24 hours.
▼ The combination of mitomycin (5 to 15 mg) and heparin (1,000 to 10,000 units) in 30 mL NSS is stable for 48 hours at room temperature.
▼ Stop infusion immediately and notify prescriber if extravasation occurs because of potential for severe ulceration and necrosis.
▼ **Incompatibilities:** Aztreonam, bleomycin, cefepime, etoposide, filgrastim, gemcitabine, piperacillin sodium–tazobactam sodium, sargramostim, topotecan, vinorelbine.

ACTION
Similar to an alkylating drug, cross-linking strands of DNA and causing an imbalance of cell growth, leading to cell death.

Route	Onset	Peak	Duration
I.V.	Unknown	Unknown	Unknown

Half-life: About 50 minutes.

ADVERSE REACTIONS
CNS: headache, neurologic abnormalities, confusion, drowsiness, fatigue, fever, pain.
EENT: blurred vision.
GI: mucositis, nausea, vomiting, anorexia, diarrhea, stomatitis.
GU: *renal toxicity, hemolytic-uremic syndrome.*
Hematologic: *thrombocytopenia, leukopenia, microangiopathic hemolytic anemia.*

Reactions in bold italics are *life-threatening*. Interactions may have a *rapid onset* or a *delayed onset*.

Respiratory: *interstitial pneumonitis, pulmonary edema,* dyspnea, nonproductive cough.

Skin: cellulitis, induration, desquamation, pruritus, pain at injection site, reversible alopecia, purple bands on nails, rash, sloughing with extravasation, alopecia.

Other: *septicemia,* ulceration.

INTERACTIONS
None reported.

EFFECTS ON LAB TEST RESULTS
• May increase BUN and creatinine levels. May decrease Hb level.
• May decrease WBC and platelet counts.

CONTRAINDICATIONS & CAUTIONS
• Contraindicated in patients hypersensitive to drug and in those with thrombocytopenia, coagulation disorders, or an increased bleeding tendency from other causes.
• Don't give to patients with serum creatinine level greater than 1.7 mg/dL.
Dialyzable drug: 25% to 45%.

PREGNANCY-LACTATION-REPRODUCTION
• Drug can cause fetal harm. If used during pregnancy, or if patient becomes pregnant during therapy, apprise her of potential hazard to the fetus and potential risk of loss of the pregnancy.
• It isn't known if drug appears in breast milk. Patient should discontinue breast-feeding or discontinue drug.

NURSING CONSIDERATIONS
Black Box Warning Administer drug under the supervision of a physician experienced with cancer chemotherapeutic agents. ∎

Black Box Warning Bone marrow suppression (thrombocytopenia and leukopenia), which may contribute to overwhelming infections in an already compromised patient, is the most common and severe toxic effect. ∎

Reevaluate patient fully after each course of mitomycin, and reduce dosage if patient has experienced toxicities.

Alert: Pulmonary toxicity, which may be severe and life-threatening, has been reported infrequently. Signs and symptoms may include dyspnea with a nonproductive cough and pulmonary infiltrates on X-ray. Drug may need to be discontinued.

Alert: Extravasation may occur, causing cellulitis, ulceration, and tissue slough. If signs or symptoms of these conditions occur, stop infusion immediately and notify prescriber. Withdraw 3 to 5 mL of blood; then remove infusion needle. Treatment may include ice compresses, application of dimethyl sulfoxide, limb elevation, and protecting site from friction. If skin necrosis develops, skin grafting may be necessary.
• Continue CBC and blood studies at least 8 weeks after therapy stops. Leukopenia and thrombocytopenia are cumulative. If WBC count falls below 2,000/mm^3 or granulocyte count falls below 1,000/mm^3, follow institutional policy for infection control in immunocompromised patients.
• To prevent bleeding, avoid all I.M. injections when platelet count is less than 100,000/mm^3.
• If disease progresses after two courses of mitomycin, chances of response are minimal and drug should be discontinued.
• Anticipate need for blood transfusions to combat anemia.
• Monitor patient for dyspnea with nonproductive cough; chest X-ray may show infiltrates.
• Monitor renal function tests.
• Leukopenia may occur up to 8 weeks after therapy and may be cumulative with successive doses.

Black Box Warning Drug can cause hemolytic-uremic syndrome, which is characterized by microangiopathic hemolytic anemia, thrombocytopenia, and irreversible renal failure. The syndrome may occur at any time during systemic therapy with mitomycin as a single agent or in combination with other cytotoxic drugs; however, most cases occur at doses of 60 mg or more. Blood product transfusion may exacerbate symptoms associated with this syndrome. ∎

PATIENT TEACHING
• Advise patient to report all adverse reactions and to immediately report pain or burning at injection site during or after administration.
• Warn patient to watch for signs and symptoms of infection (fever, sore throat,

fatigue), bleeding (easy bruising, nose-bleeds, bleeding gums, tarry stools), and pulmonary toxicity (dyspnea with nonproductive cough). Tell patient to take temperature daily.

• Inform patient that hair loss may occur but that it's usually reversible.

• Inform patient of the potential for fetal harm if drug is used during pregnancy or if patient becomes pregnant during therapy.

SAFETY ALERT!

mitoxantrone hydrochloride
mye-toe-ZAN-trone

Therapeutic class: Antineoplastics
Pharmacologic class: DNA-reactive drugs–anthracenediones

AVAILABLE FORMS
Injection: 2 mg/mL

INDICATIONS & DOSAGES
➤ **Combination initial therapy for acute nonlymphocytic leukemia (ANLL)**
Adults: Induction begins with 12 mg/m^2 I.V. daily on days 1 to 3, with 100 mg/m^2 daily of cytarabine on days 1 to 7 as a continuous 24-hour infusion. A second induction with mitoxantrone for 2 days and cytarabine for 5 days may be given if response isn't adequate. Consolidation therapy: 12 mg/m^2 I.V. infusion daily on days 1 and 2 and cytarabine 100 mg/m^2 for 5 days given as a continuous 24-hour infusion on days 1 through 5. The first course is given approximately 6 weeks after the final induction course; the second is generally given 4 weeks after the first. Severe myelosuppression has occurred with this regimen.

➤ **To reduce neurologic disability and frequency of relapse in chronic progressive, progressive relapsing, or worsening relapsing-remitting MS**
Adults: 12 mg/m^2 I.V. over 5 to 15 minutes every 3 months. Maximum cumulative lifetime dose is 140 mg/m^2.

➤ **Advanced hormone-refractory prostate cancer**
Men: 12 to 14 mg/m^2 as a short I.V. infusion every 21 days. Drug is given as an adjunct to corticosteroid therapy.

ADMINISTRATION
I.V.
▼ Preparing and giving drug may be mutagenic, teratogenic, or carcinogenic. Follow facility policy to reduce risks.

▼ Dilute dose in at least 50 mL of NSS for injection or D$_5$W injection. Don't mix with other drugs.

Black Box Warning Give slowly into a free-flowing I.V. infusion of NSS or D$_5$W injection over at least 3 minutes. ∎

Black Box Warning Never give subcutaneously, intra-arterially, intramuscularly, or intrathecally. ∎

Black Box Warning Severe local tissue damage may result if extravasation occurs. ∎

▼ If extravasation occurs, stop infusion immediately and notify prescriber. Place ice packs over the area intermittently.

▼ Once vial is penetrated, undiluted solution may be stored for 7 days at room temperature or 14 days in refrigerator. Don't freeze.

▼ **Incompatibilities:** Amphotericin B, aztreonam, cefepime, doxorubicin liposomal, heparin sodium, hydrocortisone, other I.V. drugs, paclitaxel, piperacillin sodium–tazobactam sodium, propofol, sargramostim.

ACTION
Reacts with DNA, producing cytotoxic effect. Probably not specific to cell cycle.

Route	Onset	Peak	Duration
I.V.	Unknown	Unknown	Unknown

Half-life: Terminal half-life, 23 to 215 hours.

ADVERSE REACTIONS
CNS: fever, headache, *seizures.*
CV: *arrhythmias,* ECG abnormalities, *HF,* tachycardia.
EENT: conjunctivitis, sinusitis.
GI: abdominal pain, bleeding, constipation, diarrhea, mucositis, nausea, stomatitis, vomiting.
GU: amenorrhea, menstrual disorder, UTI, *renal failure.*
Hematologic: *myelosuppression,* anemia.
Hepatic: jaundice.
Metabolic: hyperuricemia.
Musculoskeletal: back pain.

Reactions in bold italics are *life-threatening*. Interactions may have a *rapid onset* or a *delayed onset*.

Respiratory: cough, dyspnea, URI, pneumonia.
Skin: alopecia, ecchymoses, local irritation or phlebitis, petechiae.
Other: fungal infections, *sepsis.*

INTERACTIONS
Cyclosporine: May increase effects of mitoxantrone. Monitor patient closely.
Digoxin: May decrease digoxin level. Monitor serum level and patient closely, and adjust digoxin dosage as needed.
Hydantoins (phenytoin): May decrease levels of these drugs, increasing risk of seizure. Monitor levels and adjust hydantoin dosage as needed.
Live-virus vaccines: May increase risk of vaccine-induced adverse reactions. Defer vaccination until mitoxantrone therapy has been completed.
Natalizumab: May increase risk of concurrent infection. Avoid use together.
Palifermin: May increase severity of oral mucositis. Don't give palifermin within 24 hours before or after mitoxantrone dose.
Tofacitinib: May increase immunosuppressive effect of tofacitinib. Avoid use together.
Trastuzumab: May increase risk of trastuzumab-induced cardiac dysfunction. Monitor patient closely for signs and symptoms of cardiac dysfunction.

EFFECTS ON LAB TEST RESULTS
• May increase ALT, AST, bilirubin, GGT, and uric acid levels. May decrease Hb level and hematocrit.
• May decrease leukocyte and granulocyte counts.

CONTRAINDICATIONS & CAUTIONS
• Contraindicated in patients hypersensitive to drug.
Black Box Warning Drug can cause potentially fatal HF during therapy or months to years after therapy. Evaluate LVEF before initiating treatment and before administering each dose of mitoxantrone to patients with MS. All patients with MS who have finished treatment should receive yearly, quantitative LVEF evaluation to detect late-occurring cardiotoxicity. Additional doses of mitoxantrone shouldn't be given to patients with MS who have experienced either

a drop in LVEF to below the lower limit of normal or a clinically significant reduction in LVEF during mitoxantrone therapy. ■
Black Box Warning Present or history of CV disease, radiotherapy to mediastinal/pericardial area, previous therapy with other anthracyclines or anthracenediones, or use of other cardiotoxic drugs may increase risk of cardiotoxicity. ■
• Significantly myelosuppressed patients shouldn't receive drug unless benefits outweigh risks.
Dialyzable drug: No.
⚠ **Overdose S&S:** Severe leukopenia.

PREGNANCY-LACTATION-REPRODUCTION
• Drug may cause fetal harm. Women of childbearing potential should avoid becoming pregnant during therapy. If used during pregnancy or if patient becomes pregnant during therapy, apprise her of potential risk to the fetus.
• There are no adequate studies in pregnant women. Women with MS who are biologically capable of becoming pregnant should have a pregnancy test before each dose, and results should be known before drug administration.
• Drug appears in breast milk. Patient should discontinue breast-feeding before starting drug.

NURSING CONSIDERATIONS
Black Box Warning Administer under the supervision of a physician experienced with cytotoxic chemotherapy. ■
Black Box Warning Except when used to treat ANLL, mitoxantrone should generally not be given to patients with baseline neutrophil counts less than 1,500 cells/mm^3. Frequently monitor peripheral blood cell counts for all patients using drug. ■
Black Box Warning Assess all patients for cardiac signs and symptoms by history, physical examination, and ECG before start of therapy. Assess patients with MS for cardiac signs and symptoms by history, physical examination and ECG before each dose. ■
Black Box Warning Patients with MS shouldn't receive a cumulative mitoxantrone dose greater than 140 mg/m^2. ■

- Closely monitor hematologic and laboratory chemistry parameters, including LFTs. Obtain CBC and platelet count before each course of treatment. Patient may require blood transfusion or RBC or WBC colony-stimulating factors.
- Avoid all I.M. injections if platelet count falls below 50,000/mm³.

Black Box Warning Use of drug has been associated with cardiotoxicity; all patients should have an ECG before initiation of therapy. Monitor LVEF before initiating therapy and prior to each dose; risk of cardiotoxicity increases with cumulative dose of 140 mg/m², although toxicities may occur at any dose. Continue ongoing cardiac monitoring to detect late occurring cardiotoxicity. ∎

- If severe nonhematologic toxicity occurs during first course, delay second course until patient recovers.

Black Box Warning Secondary acute myelocytic leukemia has been reported with mitoxantrone therapy. ∎

☻ *Alert:* Women of childbearing potential with MS should have a pregnancy test even if they are using contraception. Results should be known before administration of each dose.

PATIENT TEACHING

- Advise patient to immediately report injection-site discomfort.
- Tell patient that urine may appear blue-green within 24 hours after receiving drug and that the whites of his eyes may turn blue. These effects are not harmful but may persist during therapy.
- Teach patient about potential adverse reactions and to report them. Advise patient to watch for signs and symptoms of bleeding and infection.
- Advise female patient to use appropriate contraceptive method to avoid pregnancy while receiving drug.

modafinil
moe-DAFF-in-ill

Alertec✦, Provigil⌀

Therapeutic class: CNS stimulants
Pharmacologic class: Analeptics
Controlled substance schedule: IV

AVAILABLE FORMS
Tablets: 100 mg, 200 mg

INDICATIONS & DOSAGES

➤ **To improve wakefulness in patients with excessive daytime sleepiness caused by narcolepsy, obstructive sleep apnea-hypopnea syndrome, and shift-work sleep disorder**
Adults and adolescents age 16 and older: 200 mg P.O. daily, as a single dose in the morning. Patients with shift-work sleep disorder should take dose about 1 hour before the start of their shift. Maximum dose is 400 mg P.O. daily as a single dose.
Adjust-a-dose: In patients with severe hepatic impairment, give 100 mg P.O. daily, as a single dose in the morning.

ADMINISTRATION
P.O.
- Give drug without regard for food; however, food may delay effect of drug.

ACTION
Unknown. Similar to action of sympathomimetics, including amphetamines, but drug is structurally distinct from amphetamines and doesn't alter release of dopamine or norepinephrine.

Route	Onset	Peak	Duration
P.O.	Unknown	2–4 hr	Unknown

Half-life: 15 hours.

ADVERSE REACTIONS
CNS: headache, nervousness, dizziness, drowsiness, insomnia, depression, anxiety, paresthesia, hypertonia, confusion, emotional lability, vertigo, tremor, dyskinesia, agitation.
CV: hypertension, vasodilation, chest pain palpitations, tachycardia, edema.

Reactions in bold italics are *life-threatening*. Interactions may have a *rapid onset* or a *delayed onset*.

EENT: abnormal vision, epistaxis, rhinitis, dry mouth, mouth ulcer, pharyngitis.
GI: nausea, diarrhea, anorexia, gingivitis, thirst, dyspepsia, constipation, flatulence, taste perversion.
GU: abnormal urine.
Hematologic: eosinophilia.
Metabolic: weight loss.
Musculoskeletal: back or neck pain.
Respiratory: *asthma.*
Skin: sweating.
Other: chills.

INTERACTIONS
Drug-drug. *Carbamazepine, phenobarbital, rifampin, other inducers of CYP3A4:* May alter modafinil level. Monitor patient closely.
Cyclosporine, theophylline: May reduce levels of these drugs. Use together cautiously.
Dextroamphetamine, methylphenidate: May cause 1-hour delay in modafinil absorption. Separate dosing times.
Diazepam, phenytoin, propranolol, other drugs metabolized by CYP2C19: May inhibit CYP2C19 and lead to higher levels of drugs metabolized by this enzyme. Use together cautiously; adjust dosage as needed.
Hormonal contraceptives: May reduce contraceptive effectiveness. Advise patient to use alternative or additional method of contraception during modafinil therapy and for 1 month after drug is stopped.
Itraconazole, ketoconazole, other inhibitors of CYP3A4: May alter modafinil level. Monitor patient closely.
Phenytoin, warfarin: May inhibit CYP2C9 and increase phenytoin and warfarin levels. Monitor patient closely for toxicity.
TCAs: May increase TCA level. Reduce dosage of these drugs.
Drug-lifestyle. *Alcohol use:* Coadministration hasn't been studied. Avoid using together.

EFFECTS ON LAB TEST RESULTS
• May increase glucose, GGT, and AST levels.
• May increase eosinophil count.

CONTRAINDICATIONS & CAUTIONS
• Contraindicated in patients hypersensitive to drug and in those with a history of left ventricular hypertrophy or ischemic ECG changes, chest pain, arrhythmias, or other evidence of mitral valve prolapse linked to CNS stimulant use.
• Use cautiously in patients with recent MI or unstable angina and in those with history of psychosis.
• Use cautiously and give reduced dosage to patients with severe hepatic impairment, with or without cirrhosis.
• Use cautiously in patients taking MAO inhibitors.
• Safety and effectiveness in patients with severe renal impairment haven't been determined.
• Modafinil isn't approved for use in children younger than age 16 for any indication.
Dialyzable drug: Unknown.
⚠ **Overdose S&S:** Agitation or excitation, insomnia, slight or moderate elevations in hemodynamic parameters, aggressiveness, anxiety, confusion, shortened PT, diarrhea, irritability, nausea, nervousness, palpitations, sleep disturbances, tremor, bradycardia, chest pain, hypertension, tachycardia, hallucination, restlessness.

PREGNANCY-LACTATION-REPRODUCTION
• There are no adequate studies in pregnant women. Use during pregnancy only if potential benefit justifies potential fetal risk.
• A pregnancy registry has been established to collect information on pregnancy outcomes of women exposed to modafinil. Prescribers are encouraged to register pregnant patients, or pregnant women may self-enroll in the registry, by calling 1-866-404-4106.
• Caution patient that use of hormonal contraceptives (including depot or implantable contraceptives) with modafinil may reduce contraceptive effectiveness. Recommend an alternative method of contraception during therapy and for 1 month after therapy ends.
• It isn't known if drug appears in breast milk. Use cautiously in breast-feeding women.

NURSING CONSIDERATIONS
• Life-threatening angioedema and multiorgan hypersensitivity reactions can occur. Monitor patient for rash, dysphagia, bronchospasm, fever, and organ dysfunction. Stop drug and begin appropriate treatment.

● Monitor patient for emergence or exacerbation of psychiatric signs and symptoms and hypertension.

● *Look alike–sound alike:* Don't confuse Provigil with Nuvigil or Alertec with Arthrotec.

PATIENT TEACHING

🕩 *Alert:* Advise patient to stop drug and notify prescriber if rash, peeling skin, trouble swallowing or breathing, or other symptoms of allergic reaction occur. Rare cases of serious rash, including Stevens-Johnson syndrome, toxic epidermal necrolysis, and drug rash with eosinophilia and hypersensitivity, have been reported.

● Advise female patient to notify prescriber about planned, suspected, or known pregnancy, or if she's breast-feeding.

● Tell patient to avoid alcohol while taking drug.

● Warn patient to avoid activities that require alertness or good coordination until CNS effects of drug are known.

mometasone furoate
moe-MEH-tah-zone

Asmanex HFA, Asmanex Twisthaler, Elocon

mometasone furoate monohydrate
Nasonex

Therapeutic class: Anti-inflammatory drugs
Pharmacologic class: Glucocorticoids

AVAILABLE FORMS
Cream: 0.1%
Inhalation aerosol: 100 mcg/actuation, 200 mcg/actuation
Inhalation powder: 110 mcg/inhalation, 220 mcg/inhalation
Lotion: 0.1%
Nasal spray: 50 mcg/spray
Ointment: 0.1%

INDICATIONS & DOSAGES
➤ **Maintenance therapy for asthma; asthma in patients who take an oral corticosteroid**

Asmanex Twisthaler
Adults and children age 12 and older who previously used a bronchodilator or inhaled corticosteroid: Initially, 220 mcg by oral inhalation every day in the evening. Maximum, 440 mcg/day.
Adults and children age 12 and older who previously received an oral corticosteroid: 440 mcg by oral inhalation b.i.d. Maximum, 880 mcg/day.
Adjust-a-dose: For patients on long-term oral corticosteroid therapy, reduce oral corticosteroid dosage by no more than 2.5 mg/day at weekly intervals, beginning at least 1 week after starting mometasone. After stopping oral corticosteroid, reduce mometasone dosage to lowest effective amount. Carefully monitor patient for signs and symptoms of asthma instability and adrenal insufficiency.
Children ages 4 to 11: 110 mcg by oral inhalation once daily in the evening.
Asmanex HFA
Adults and children age 12 and older who previously used a medium-dose inhaled corticosteroid: Using a 100-mcg inhaler, 2 inhalations b.i.d. (morning and evening). Maximum, 800 mcg/day.
Adults and children age 12 and older who previously used a high-dose inhaled corticosteroid: Using a 200-mcg inhaler, 2 inhalations b.i.d. (morning and evening). Maximum, 800 mcg/day.
Adults and children age 12 and older who previously received an oral corticosteroid: 400 mcg by oral inhalation b.i.d. (morning and evening). Maximum, 800 mcg/day.
Adjust-a-dose: For patients currently receiving long-term oral corticosteroid therapy, wean prednisone slowly, beginning after at least 1 week of Asmanex HFA therapy. Carefully monitor patient for signs and symptoms of asthma instability and adrenal insufficiency.

If a dosage regimen fails to provide adequate asthma control, reevaluate the therapeutic regimen and consider additional therapeutic options, such as replacing the current strength of inhaler with a higher strength, initiating an inhaled corticosteroid and long-acting beta$_2$-agonist combination product, or initiating oral corticosteroids.

➤ **Allergic rhinitis**
Adults and children age 12 and older:
2 sprays (50 mcg/spray) in each nostril once daily.
Children ages 2 to 11: 1 spray
(50 mcg/spray) in each nostril once daily.
➤ **Prophylaxis of seasonal allergic rhinitis**
Adults and children age 12 and older:
2 sprays (50 mcg/spray) in each nostril once daily 2 to 4 weeks before anticipated start of pollen season.
➤ **Nasal polyps**
Adults: 2 sprays (50 mcg/spray) in each nostril once daily to b.i.d.
➤ **Dermatoses**
Adults: Apply thin film of cream or ointment to affected areas once daily. Or, apply a few drops of lotion to affected areas and massage lightly. Discontinue when control is achieved. If no improvement is seen within 2 weeks, reassess diagnosis.
Children age 12 and older: Apply a few drops of lotion to affected areas once daily and massage lightly. Discontinue when control is achieved. If no improvement is seen within 2 weeks, reassess diagnosis.
Children age 2 and older: Apply thin film of cream or ointment to affected areas once daily. Discontinue when control is achieved. If no improvement is seen within 2 weeks, reassess diagnosis.

ADMINISTRATION
Inhalational aerosol
• Shake well before each inhalation.
• Prime before first use by releasing four test sprays into the air, away from the face, shaking well before each spray.
• If the inhaler hasn't been used for more than 5 days, prime inhaler again with four test sprays.
• Have patient rinse mouth with water without swallowing after administration.
Inhalational powder
• Have patient exhale fully before bringing Twisthaler up to the mouth, placing between lips, and inhaling quickly and deeply.
• Patient shouldn't breathe out through inhaler but should remove inhaler and hold breath for 10 seconds if possible.

• Have patient rinse mouth after administration.
• Discard 45 days after opening foil pouch or when dose counter reads "00."
Intranasal
• Before initial use, prime nasal spray pump 10 times or until fine spray appears.
• Pump may be stored for 1 week without repriming. If unused for more than 1 week, reprime two times or until a fine spray appears.
• Shake well before each use.
Topical
• Drug is for topical use only; not for oral, ophthalmic, or intravaginal use. Avoid use on axillae, groin, or face.
• Don't use with occlusive dressings or in diaper area if child still requires diapers or plastic pants unless directed by prescriber.

ACTION
Unknown, although corticosteroids inhibit many cells and mediators involved in inflammation and the asthmatic response.

Route	Onset	Peak	Duration
Inhalation	Unknown	1–2½ hr	Unknown
Intranasal	Unknown	Unknown	Unknown
Topical	8 hr	Unknown	Unknown

Half-life: Oral, 5 hours; nasal, topical, 5.8 hours.

ADVERSE REACTIONS
CNS: headache, depression, fatigue, insomnia, pain, paresthesia.
EENT: allergic rhinitis, pharyngitis, dry throat, dysphonia, earache, epistaxis, nasal irritation, sinus congestion, sinusitis, oral candidiasis.
GI: abdominal pain, anorexia, dyspepsia, flatulence, gastroenteritis, nausea, vomiting.
GU: dysmenorrhea, menstrual disorder, UTI.
Metabolic: decreased glucocorticoid levels.
Musculoskeletal: arthralgia, back pain, myalgia.
Respiratory: URI, respiratory disorder.
Skin: burning, pruritus, skin atrophy, furunculosis, folliculitis, skin depigmentation, candidiasis, bacterial infection.
Other: flulike symptoms, infection.

INTERACTIONS
Drug-drug. *Ketoconazole:* May increase mometasone level. Use together cautiously.

EFFECTS ON LAB TEST RESULTS
None reported.

CONTRAINDICATIONS & CAUTIONS
• Contraindicated in patients hypersensitive to drug or its components, in those hypersensitive to milk proteins (Asmanex Twisthaler only), and in those with status asthmaticus or other acute forms of asthma or bronchospasm (as primary treatment).
• Use cautiously in patients at high risk for decreased bone mineral content (those with a family history of osteoporosis, prolonged immobilization, long-term use of drugs that reduce bone mass), patients switching from a systemic to an inhaled corticosteroid, and patients with active or dormant TB, untreated systemic infections, cataracts, glaucoma, ocular herpes simplex, diabetes, myasthenia, MI, thyroid disease, or immunosuppression.
• Topical drug may cause reversible HPA axis suppression with potential for glucocorticosteroid insufficiency during treatment or after treatment withdrawal. Evaluate patient periodically for HPA suppression.
🔸 *Alert:* Children treated with topical corticosteroids are at greater risk than adults for HPA axis suppression and Cushing syndrome. Don't use in treatment of diaper dermatitis.
• If patient develops allergic contact dermatitis, usually diagnosed by a failure to heal, drug should be discontinued.
• If skin infections are present or develop, topical drug may need to be discontinued until infection is controlled.
Dialyzable drug: Unknown.
⚠ *Overdose S&S:* Hypercorticism with long-term overdose.

PREGNANCY-LACTATION-REPRODUCTION
• There are no adequate studies in pregnant women. Use during pregnancy only if clearly needed and potential benefit justifies potential risk to the fetus.
• Systemically administered corticosteroids appear in breast milk and could suppress growth, interfere with endogenous cortico-steroid production, or cause other untoward effects. Use cautiously in breast-feeding women.

NURSING CONSIDERATIONS
🔸 *Alert:* Don't use inhalation form for acute bronchospasm. Life-threatening paradoxical bronchospasm can occur after inhalation. Stop drug and use a fast-acting bronchodilator.
• Wean patient slowly from a systemic corticosteroid after he switches to mometasone. Monitor pulmonary function tests, beta-agonist use, and asthma symptoms.
🔸 *Alert:* If patient is switching from an oral corticosteroid to an inhaled form, watch closely for evidence of adrenal insufficiency, such as fatigue, lethargy, weakness, nausea, vomiting, and hypotension.
• After an oral corticosteroid is withdrawn, HPA function may not recover for months. If patient has trauma, stress, infection, or surgery during this HPA recovery period, he is particularly vulnerable to adrenal insufficiency or adrenal crisis.
• Because inhaled and topical corticosteroids can be systemically absorbed, watch for cushingoid effects.
• Assess patient for bone loss during long-term use.
• Watch for evidence of localized mouth infections, vision changes, loss of glucose control, and immunosuppression.
• If female patient has taken a corticosteroid during pregnancy, monitor neonate for hypoadrenalism.
• Monitor elderly patients for increased sensitivity to drug effects.

PATIENT TEACHING
• Instruct patient on proper use and routine care of the inhaler or nasal spray pump.
• Tell patient to use drug regularly and at the same time each day. If he uses it only once daily, tell him to do so in the evening.
• Caution patient not to use drug for immediate relief of an asthma attack or bronchospasm.
• Inform patient that maximal benefits might not occur for 1 to 2 weeks or longer after therapy starts; instruct him to notify his prescriber if his condition fails to improve or worsens.

Reactions in bold italics are *life-threatening*. Interactions may have a *rapid onset* or a *delayed onset*.

• Tell patient that if he has bronchospasm after taking drug, he should immediately use a fast-acting bronchodilator. Urge him to contact prescriber immediately if bronchospasm doesn't respond to the fast-acting bronchodilator.

⚠ **Alert:** If patient has been weaned from an oral corticosteroid, urge him to contact prescriber immediately if an asthma attack occurs or if he is experiencing a period of stress. The oral corticosteroid may need to be resumed.

• Warn patient to avoid exposure to chickenpox or measles and to notify prescriber if such contact occurs.

• Long-term use of an inhaled corticosteroid may increase risk of cataracts or glaucoma; tell patient to report vision changes.

• Advise patient to write the date on a new inhaler on the day inhaler is opened and to discard the inhaler after 45 days or when the dose counter reads "00."

• Instruct patient not to use topical form with occlusive dressings or diapers unless instructed by prescriber.

montelukast sodium
mon-tell-OO-kast

Singulair⧓

Therapeutic class: Antiasthmatics
Pharmacologic class: Leukotriene-receptor antagonists

AVAILABLE FORMS
Oral granules: 4-mg packet
Tablets (chewable): 4 mg, 5 mg
Tablets (film-coated): 10 mg

INDICATIONS & DOSAGES
➤ **Asthma, seasonal allergic rhinitis, perennial allergic rhinitis**
Adults and children age 15 and older: 10 mg P.O. once daily in evening.
Children ages 6 to 14: 5 mg chewable tablet P.O. once daily in evening.
Children ages 2 to 5: 4 mg chewable tablet or 1 packet of 4-mg oral granules P.O. once daily in the evening.
Children ages 12 to 23 months (asthma only): 1 packet of 4-mg oral granules P.O. once daily in the evening.

Children ages 6 to 23 months (perennial allergic rhinitis only): 1 packet of 4-mg oral granules P.O. once daily in the evening.
➤ **Prevention of exercise-induced bronchoconstriction**
Adults and children age 15 and older: 10 mg P.O. at least 2 hours before exercise. Patients already taking a daily dose shouldn't take an additional dose. Also, an additional dose shouldn't be taken within 24 hours of a previous dose.
Children ages 6 to 14: 5 mg P.O. at least 2 hours before exercise (1 chewable tablet). An additional dose shouldn't be taken within 24 hours of a previous dose.

ADMINISTRATION
P.O.
• Give oral granules directly in the mouth, dissolved in 5 mL of cold or room-temperature baby formula or breast milk, or mixed with a spoonful of cold or room-temperature soft foods (use only applesauce, carrots, rice, or ice cream). Use within 15 minutes of opening the packet.
• May be taken without regard to food.

ACTION
Reduces early and late-phase bronchoconstriction from antigen challenge.

Route	Onset	Peak	Duration
P.O. (chewable, granules)	Unknown	2–2½ hr	24 hr
P.O. (film-coated)	Unknown	3–4 hr	24 hr

Half-life: 2¾ to 5½ hours.

ADVERSE REACTIONS
CNS: headache, asthenia, dizziness, fatigue, fever, somnolence, weakness.
EENT: conjunctivitis, otitis media, nasal congestion, nosebleed, laryngitis, sinusitis, pharyngitis, rhinitis, tonsillitis, dental pain.
GI: abdominal pain, dyspepsia, infectious gastroenteritis, nausea, diarrhea.
GU: pyuria.
Hematologic: systemic eosinophilia.
Respiratory: URI, cough, wheezing, pneumonia.
Skin: rash, dermatitis, urticaria, eczema.
Other: flulike symptoms, trauma, varicella, viral infection.

M

INTERACTIONS

Drug-drug. *Gemfibrozil:* May increase montelukast plasma concentration. Adjust montelukast dosage as needed.
Phenobarbital, rifampin: May decrease bioavailability of montelukast because of hepatic metabolism induction. Monitor patient for effectiveness.

EFFECTS ON LAB TEST RESULTS
● May increase ALT and AST levels.

CONTRAINDICATIONS & CAUTIONS
● Contraindicated in patients hypersensitive to drug or its ingredients.
● Patients with asthma may present with systemic eosinophilia that may manifest as clinical features of vasculitis consistent with Churg-Strauss syndrome. Churg-Strauss syndrome is often treated with systemic corticosteroid therapy. These reactions have sometimes been associated with reduction of oral corticosteroid dosage. Be alert to development of eosinophilia, vasculitic rash, worsening pulmonary symptoms, cardiac complications, or neuropathy.
● Use cautiously and with appropriate monitoring in patients whose dosages of systemic corticosteroids are reduced.
❸ Alert: Neuropsychiatric events have been reported in adults, adolescents, and children taking montelukast. Postmarketing reports include agitation, aggressive behavior or hostility, anxiousness, depression, disorientation, disturbance in attention, dream abnormalities, hallucinations, insomnia, irritability, memory impairment, restlessness, somnambulism, suicidal thinking and behavior (including suicide), and tremor.
Dialyzable drug: Unknown.
⚠ Overdose S&S: Headache, vomiting, psychomotor hyperactivity, thirst, somnolence, hyperkinesia, abdominal pain.

PREGNANCY-LACTATION-REPRODUCTION
● There are no adequate studies in pregnant women. Use during pregnancy only if clearly needed.
● It isn't known if drug appears in breast milk. Use cautiously in breast-feeding women.

NURSING CONSIDERATIONS
● Assess patient's underlying condition, and monitor him for effectiveness.
❸ Alert: Don't abruptly substitute drug for inhaled or oral corticosteroids. Dose of inhaled corticosteroids may be reduced gradually.
❸ Alert: Drug isn't indicated for use in patients with acute asthmatic attacks, status asthmaticus, or as monotherapy for management of exercise-induced bronchospasm. Continue appropriate rescue drug for acute worsening.
● Drug may cause behavior and mood changes. Monitor patient and consider discontinuing drug if neuropsychiatric symptoms develop.

PATIENT TEACHING
● Inform caregiver that the oral granules may be given directly into the child's mouth, dissolved in 1 teaspoon of cold or room-temperature baby formula or breast milk, or mixed in a spoonful of applesauce, carrots, rice, or ice cream.
● Tell caregiver not to open packet until ready to use and, after opening, to give the full dose within 15 minutes. Tell her that if she's mixing the drug with food, not to store excess for future use and to discard the unused portion.
● Advise patient to take drug daily, even if asymptomatic, and to contact his prescriber if asthma isn't well controlled.
● Warn patient not to reduce or stop taking other prescribed antiasthmatics without prescriber's approval.
● Advise patient to seek medical attention if short-acting inhaled bronchodilators are needed more often than usual during drug therapy.
● Warn patient that drug isn't beneficial in acute asthma attacks or in acute exercise-induced bronchospasm, and advise him to keep appropriate rescue drugs available.
● Warn patient that drug may cause behavior and mood changes, and to report development of these symptoms to prescriber.
● Advise patient with known aspirin sensitivity to continue to avoid using aspirin and NSAIDs during drug therapy.

Alert: Advise patient with phenylke-tonuria that chewable tablet contains phenyl-alanine.

SAFETY ALERT!

morphine hydrochloride
MOR-feen

Doloral✤, Ratio-Morphine✤

morphine sulfate
Astramorph PF, Duramorph PF, Infumorph, Kadian, M-Eslon✤, MorphaBond, Morphine LP Epidural✤, MS Contin, MS.IR✤, Statex✤, Statex DPS✤

Therapeutic class: Opioid analgesics
Pharmacologic class: Opioids
Controlled substance schedule: II

AVAILABLE FORMS
morphine hydrochloride
Syrup: 1 mg/mL✤*, 5 mg/mL✤*, 10 mg/mL✤*, 20 mg/mL✤*
Tablets (extended-release) ⓐ: 15 mg, 30 mg✤, 60 mg✤, 100 mg
morphine sulfate
Capsules (extended-release microgran-ules [M-Eslon]) ⓐ: 10 mg✤, 15 mg✤, 30 mg✤, 60 mg✤, 100 mg✤, 200 mg✤
Capsules (extended-release pellets) ⓐ: 30 mg, 45 mg, 60 mg, 75 mg, 90 mg, 120 mg
Capsules (extended-release pellets [Kadian]) ⓐ: 10 mg, 20 mg, 30 mg, 40 mg, 50 mg, 60 mg, 70 mg, 80 mg, 100 mg, 130 mg, 150 mg, 200 mg
Drops: 20 mg/mL✤, 50 mg/mL✤
Injection (epidural): 0.5 mg/mL, 1 mg/mL, 10 mg/mL, 25 mg/mL
Injection (with preservative): 0.5 mg/mL, 1 mg/mL, 2 mg/mL, 5 mg/mL, 10 mg/mL, 15 mg/mL, 25 mg/mL, 50 mg/mL
Injection (without preservative): 0.5 mg/mL, 1 mg/mL, 5 mg/mL, 10 mg/mL, 25 mg/mL
Injection (without preservative [Carpuject and prefilled syringes]): 2 mg/mL, 4 mg/mL, 8 mg/mL, 10 mg/mL, 15 mg/mL

Oral solution: 10 mg/5 mL, 20 mg/5 mL, 20 mg/mL (concentrate), 100 mg/5 mL (concentrate)
Suppositories: 5 mg, 10 mg, 20 mg, 30 mg
Syrup: 1 mg/mL✤, 5 mg/mL✤, 10 mg/mL
Tablets: 5 mg✤, 10 mg✤, 15 mg✤, 25 mg✤, 30 mg, 50 mg✤, 100 mg✤, 200 mg✤
Tablets (extended-release) ⓐ: 15 mg, 30 mg, 60 mg, 100 mg, 200 mg

INDICATIONS & DOSAGES
➤ **Moderate to severe pain**
Adults: 5 to 20 mg subcutaneously or I.M. or 5 to 15 mg I.V. every 4 hours p.r.n. Or, 5 to 30 mg (immediate-release tablets) P.O., or 10 to 20 mg (oral solution) P.O., or 10 to 20 mg P.R. every 4 hours p.r.n.

For extended-release tablet, give 15 or 30 mg P.O. every 8 to 12 hours.

For epidural injection, give 5 mg by epidural catheter; then, if pain isn't relieved adequately in 1 hour, give supplementary doses of 1 to 2 mg at intervals sufficient to assess effectiveness. Maximum total epidural dose shouldn't exceed 10 mg/24 hours.

For intrathecal injection, a single dose of 0.2 to 1 mg may provide pain relief for 24 hours (only in the lumbar area). Don't repeat injections.

➤ **Moderate to severe pain requiring continuous, around-the-clock oral opioid**
Adults: For patients receiving other oral morphine formulations, may convert to extended-release capsules by administer-ing patient's total daily oral morphine dose as extended-release capsules once daily or by administering one-half of patient's total daily oral morphine dose as Kadian b.i.d. Don't give Avinza more frequently than every 24 hours; don't give Kadian more fre-quently than every 12 hours. Supplemental pain medication may be required until re-sponse to patient's daily Avinza dosage has stabilized (up to 4 days).

For controlled-release tablets, patient may convert in one of two ways: by ad-ministering one-half of patient's 24-hour requirement as MS Contin on an every-12-hour schedule or by administering one-third of patient's daily requirement as MS Contin on an every-8-hour schedule.

M

✤ Canada   ◇ OTC   ◆ Off-label use   ⭮ Photoguide   ⓐ Do not crush   *Liquid contains alcohol.

➤ **Severe, chronic pain associated with terminal cancer**
Adults: Before initiating continuous morphine infusion, a loading dose of 15 mg by I.V. push may be necessary. Then give continuous infusion of 0.8 to 80 mg/hour via infusion pump.

ADMINISTRATION
P.O.
Black Box Warning Take care when administering morphine oral solution to avoid dosing errors because of confusion among different concentrations and between milligrams and milliliters, which could result in accidental overdose and death. Take care to ensure the proper dose is communicated and dispensed. ■
● Oral solutions of various concentrations and an intensified oral solution (20 mg/mL) are available. Carefully note the strength given.
Black Box Warning Oral solutions of various concentrations and an intensified oral solution (20 mg/mL) are available. Carefully note strength given. The 20-mg/mL concentration is indicated for use only in opioid-tolerant patients because of the risk of fatal respiratory depression in opioid-naive patients. It's packaged with a calibrated oral syringe for accurate dosing. ■
Black Box Warning Instruct patient to swallow extended-release or long-acting morphine sulfate oral formulations whole, without crushing, chewing, or dissolving, which may cause rapid, uncontrolled release and absorption of a potentially fatal dose of morphine. If necessary, capsules (Kadian) may be carefully opened and entire contents poured into cool, soft foods such as applesauce and swallowed immediately without chewing. ■
● Give morphine sulfate without regard to food.

I.V.
▼ For direct injection, dilute 2.5 to 15 mg in 4 or 5 mL of sterile water for injection and give slowly over 4 to 5 minutes.
▼ For continuous infusion, mix drug with D_5W to yield 0.1 to 1 mg/mL, and give by a continuous infusion device.

▼ In adults with severe, chronic pain, maintenance I.V. infusion is 0.8 to 80 mg/hour; sometimes higher doses are needed.
▼ Make sure an opioid antagonist is immediately available before administering I.V.
Black Box Warning Infumorph and Duramorph are supplied in sealed ampules. Treat accidental dermal exposure to these drugs by removing contaminated clothing and rinsing affected area with water. ■
Black Box Warning Inspect parenteral drug products for particulate matter before opening the amber ampule and again for color after removing contents from ampule. Don't use if solution in the unopened ampule contains a precipitate that doesn't disappear upon shaking. After removal, don't use unless solution is colorless or pale yellow. ■
▼ **Incompatibilities:** Aminophylline, amobarbital, cefepime, chlorothiazide, 5-FU, haloperidol, heparin sodium, meperidine, pentobarbital, phenobarbital sodium, phenytoin sodium, prochlorperazine, sodium bicarbonate, thiopental.

I.M.
● Document injection site.
● Store injection solution at room temperature and protect from light.
Black Box Warning Solution may darken with age. Don't use if injection is darker than pale yellow, discolored, or contains precipitate. ■

Subcutaneous
● Document injection site.
● Store injection solution at room temperature and protect from light.
Black Box Warning Solution may darken with age. Don't use if injection is darker than pale yellow, discolored, or contains precipitate. ■

Epidural
● Document injection site.
● Verify proper placement of needle or catheter in the epidural space before injecting drug.
Black Box Warning Inspect for particulate matter and discoloration before administration. Don't use if it's darker than pale yellow, discolored in any other way, or contains a precipitate. ■

Reactions in bold italics are *life-threatening*. Interactions may have a *rapid onset* or a *delayed onset*.

• Store injection solution at room temperature until ready to use; discard unused portion.
• Protect from light; don't freeze or heat sterilize.

Rectal
• Refrigeration of rectal suppository isn't needed.

ACTION

Unknown. Binds with opioid receptors in the CNS, altering perception of and emotional response to pain.

Route	Onset	Peak	Duration
P.O.	30 min	1–2 hr	4–12 hr
P.O. (extended-release)	1–2 hr	3–4 hr	12–24 hr
I.V.	5 min	20 min	4–5 hr
I.M.	10–30 min	30–60 min	4–5 hr
Subcut.	10–30 min	50–90 min	4–5 hr
P.R.	20–60 min	20–60 min	4–5 hr
Epidural	15–60 min	15–60 min	24 hr
Intrathecal	15–60 min	30–60 min	24 hr

Half-life: 2 to 3 hours.

ADVERSE REACTIONS

CNS: dizziness, euphoria, light-headedness, nightmares, sedation, somnolence, *seizures,* depression, hallucinations, nervousness, physical dependence, syncope, anxiety.
CV: *bradycardia, cardiac arrest, shock,* hypertension, hypotension, tachycardia, palpitations, peripheral circulatory collapse.
GI: constipation, nausea, vomiting, anorexia, biliary tract spasms, dry mouth, ileus.
GU: urine retention.
Hematologic: *thrombocytopenia.*
Respiratory: *apnea, respiratory arrest, respiratory depression.*
Skin: diaphoresis, edema, pruritus, skin flushing.
Other: decreased libido.

INTERACTIONS

Drug-drug. **Black Box Warning** *Benzodiazepines, CNS depressants:* May cause slow or difficult breathing, sedation, and death. Avoid use together. If use together is necessary, limit dosage and duration of each drug to the minimum necessary for desired effect. ■

Cimetidine: May increase respiratory and CNS depression when given with morphine sulfate. Monitor patient closely.
General anesthetics, hypnotics, MAO inhibitors, other opioid analgesics, TCAs: May cause respiratory depression, hypotension, profound sedation, or coma. Use together with caution, reduce morphine dose, and monitor patient response.
 ☻ *Alert:* Serotonergic drugs (amoxapine, antiemetics [dolasetron, granisetron, ondansetron, palonosetron], antimigraine drugs, buspirone, cyclobenzaprine, dextromethorphan, linezolid, lithium, MAO inhibitors, maprotiline, methylene blue, mirtazapine, nefazodone, SNRIs, SSRIs, TCAs, trazodone, tryptophan, vilazodone):* May increase risk of serotonin syndrome. Use together cautiously and monitor patient for serotonin syndrome.
Drug-herb. ☻ *Alert: St. John's wort:* May increase risk of serotonin syndrome. Use together cautiously and monitor patient for serotonin syndrome.
Drug-lifestyle. **Black Box Warning** *Alcohol use:* May cause additive CNS effects and fatal overdose. Warn patient to avoid alcohol and products containing alcohol. ■

EFFECTS ON LAB TEST RESULTS

• May increase amylase level. May decrease Hb level (morphine sulfate).
• May decrease platelet count.
• May cause abnormal LFT values (morphine sulfate).

CONTRAINDICATIONS & CAUTIONS

• Contraindicated in patients hypersensitive to drug and in those with conditions that would preclude I.V. administration of opioids (acute bronchial asthma or upper airway obstruction).
Black Box Warning Opioid drugs should only be prescribed with benzodiazepines or other CNS depressants to patients for whom alternative treatment options are inadequate. ■
Black Box Warning Use of extended-release or long-acting morphine sulfate forms may increase the risk of addiction, abuse, and misuse, even at recommended doses, and has a greater risk of overdose and death. Reserve their use for patients

for whom alternative treatment options are ineffective, not tolerated, or are otherwise insufficient to provide adequate pain management. ∎

Black Box Warning Accidental ingestion of even one dose of extended-release or long-acting forms of morphine sulfate, especially by children, can result in a fatal overdose. Keep out of reach of children. ∎

⦿ *Alert:* Drug may lead to a rare but serious decrease in adrenal gland cortisol production.

⦿ *Alert:* Drug may cause decreased sex hormone levels with long-term use.

⦿ *Alert:* Patients are at increased risk for oversedation and respiratory depression if they snore or have a history of sleep apnea, haven't used opioids recently or are first-time opioid users, have increased opioid dosage requirements or opioid habituation, have received general anesthesia for longer lengths of time or received other sedating drugs, have preexisting pulmonary or cardiac disease, or have thoracic or other surgical incisions that may impair breathing. Monitor patients carefully.

• Contraindicated in patients with GI obstruction.

• Use with caution in elderly or debilitated patients and in those with head injury, increased ICP, seizures, chronic pulmonary disease, prostatic hyperplasia, severe hepatic or renal disease, acute abdominal conditions, hypothyroidism, Addison disease, and urethral stricture.

• Use with caution in patients with circulatory shock, biliary tract disease, CNS depression, toxic psychosis, acute alcoholism, delirium tremens, and seizure disorders.

Dialyzable drug: Yes.

⚠ *Overdose S&S:* Miosis, CNS depression, respiratory depression, apnea, flaccid skeletal muscles, bradycardia, hypotension, circulatory collapse, cardiac arrest, respiratory arrest, death.

PREGNANCY-LACTATION-REPRODUCTION

⦿ *Alert:* Carefully weigh risks and benefits of using drug in pregnant women. Drug should be used in pregnancy only if need for opioid analgesia clearly outweighs potential fetal risks.

Black Box Warning Prolonged use of opioids during pregnancy can result in neonatal opioid withdrawal syndrome, which may be life-threatening if not recognized and treated, and requires management according to protocols developed by neonatology experts. If opioid use is required for a prolonged period, apprise pregnant patient of risk to the neonate and ensure appropriate treatment will be available. ∎

• Because of the potential for serious adverse reactions in breast-feeding infants, including respiratory depression, sedation, and possibly withdrawal symptoms upon cessation of morphine to the mother, patient should discontinue breast-feeding or discontinue drug, taking into account importance of drug to the mother.

• If morphine use is necessary in a breast-feeding patient, use cautiously. Limit use and supplement with nonopioid agents. Monitor infant for increased sleepiness, difficulty feeding or breathing, and limpness.

NURSING CONSIDERATIONS

Black Box Warning Assess each patient's risk of addiction, abuse, or misuse before prescribing extended-release or long-acting forms of morphine sulfate, and monitor all patients regularly for development of these behaviors. ∎

Black Box Warning Monitor patients for respiratory depression, especially during initiation of extended-release or long-acting morphine sulfate or after a dosage increase. Serious, life-threatening, or fatal respiratory depression may occur. ∎

⦿ *Alert:* If patient is taking opioids with serotonergic drugs, watch for signs and symptoms of serotonin syndrome (agitation, hallucinations, rapid HR, fever, excessive sweating, shivering or shaking, muscle twitching or stiffness, trouble with coordination, nausea, vomiting, diarrhea), especially at start of treatment and at dosage increases. Signs and symptoms may occur within several hours of coadministration but may also occur later, especially after dosage increase. Discontinue the opioid, serotonergic drug, or both if serotonin syndrome is suspected.

⦿ *Alert:* Monitor patient for signs and symptoms of adrenal insufficiency (nausea, vomiting, loss of appetite, fatigue, weakness,

---

dizziness, low BP). Perform diagnostic testing if adrenal insufficiency is suspected. If adrenal insufficiency is confirmed, treat with corticosteroids and wean patient off opioids if appropriate. Discontinue corticosteroids when clinically appropriate.

◑ Alert: Monitor patient for signs and symptoms of decreased sex hormone levels (low libido, erectile dysfunction, amenorrhea, infertility). If signs and symptoms occur, evaluate patient and obtain laboratory testing.

◑ Alert: Carefully monitor vital signs, pain level, respiratory status, and sedation level in all patients receiving opioids, especially those receiving I.V. drugs, even those given postoperatively.

• Reassess patient's level of pain at least 15 and 30 minutes after giving parenterally and 30 minutes after giving orally.

◑ Alert: Extended-release capsules aren't for use on an as-needed basis.

Black Box Warning Keep opioid antagonist (naloxone) and resuscitation equipment available. ■

• Monitor circulatory, respiratory, bladder, and bowel functions carefully. Drug may cause hypotension, urine retention, nausea, vomiting, ileus, or altered level of consciousness regardless of the route.

Black Box Warning Intrathecal dosage is usually one-tenth of epidural dosage. ■

Black Box Warning Life-threatening respiratory depression may occur with morphine use, even when drug has been used as recommended and not misused or abused. Proper dosing and titration are essential, and morphine should only be prescribed by health care providers knowledgeable in the use of potent opioids for management of long-term pain. Monitor patients for respiratory depression, especially during initiation of morphine or after a dosage increase. Instruct patients to swallow morphine capsule whole or to sprinkle contents of capsule on applesauce and swallow without chewing. Crushing, dissolving, or chewing pellets within the capsule can cause rapid release and absorption of a potentially fatal dose of morphine. ■

• If respirations drop below 12 breaths/minute, withhold dose and notify prescriber.

Black Box Warning Morphine has an abuse liability similar to other opioid analgesics and may be misused, abused, or diverted. ■

◑ Alert: Extended-release tablets and capsules aren't for use on an as-needed basis for mild or acute pain or for postoperative pain, unless patient has already been receiving long-term opioid therapy before surgery or if postoperative pain is expected to be moderate to severe and persist for an extended period.

• Preservative-free preparations are available for epidural and intrathecal use.

Black Box Warning When the epidural or intrathecal route is used, observe patients in a fully equipped and staffed environment for at least 24 hours after the initial dose. ■

Black Box Warning Infumorph isn't recommended for single-dose I.V., I.M., or subcutaneous administration. ■

Black Box Warning Improper or erroneous substitution of Infumorph 200 or 500 (10 or 25 mg/mL, respectively) for regular Duramorph (0.5 or 1 mg/mL) is likely to result in serious overdose, leading to seizures, respiratory depression, and possibly fatal outcome. ■

• When drug is given epidurally, monitor patient closely for respiratory depression up to 24 hours after the injection. Check respiratory rate and depth every 30 to 60 minutes for 24 hours. Watch for pruritus and skin flushing.

• Morphine is drug of choice in relieving MI pain; may cause transient decrease in BP.

• An around-the-clock regimen best manages severe, chronic pain.

• Morphine may worsen or mask gallbladder pain.

• Constipation is commonly severe with maintenance dose. Ensure that stool softener or stimulant laxative is ordered.

• Taper morphine sulfate therapy gradually when stopping therapy.

Black Box Warning Each ampule of Infumorph and Duramorph contains a large amount of a potent opioid that has been associated with abuse and dependence among health care providers. Due to the limited indications for this product, risk of overdose, and risk of its diversion and abuse, special measures should be taken to control this product within the hospital or clinic.

M

Infumorph and Duramorph should be subject to rigid accounting, rigorous control of wastage, and restricted access. ∎

Black Box Warning Accidental consumption of morphine, especially by children, can result in a fatal overdose of morphine. ∎

• *Look alike–sound alike:* Don't confuse morphine with hydromorphone. Don't confuse MS Contin with Oxycontin. Don't confuse Avinza with Invanz or Evista.

PATIENT TEACHING

Black Box Warning Caution the patient or the caregiver of a patient taking an opioid drug with a benzodiazepine, CNS depressant, or alcohol to seek immediate medical attention if the patient has symptoms of dizziness, light-headedness, extreme sleepiness, slowed or difficult breathing, or unresponsiveness. ∎

⊗ *Alert:* Explain assessment and monitoring process to patient and family. Instruct them to immediately report difficulty breathing or other signs or symptoms of a potential adverse opioid-related reaction.

⊗ *Alert:* Encourage patient to report all medications being taken, including prescription and OTC medications and supplements.

⊗ *Alert:* Caution patient to immediately report signs and symptoms of serotonin syndrome, adrenal insufficiency, and decreased sex hormone levels.

• When drug is used after surgery, encourage patient to turn, cough, deep-breathe, and use incentive spirometer to prevent lung problems.

• Caution ambulatory patient about getting out of bed or walking. Warn outpatient to avoid driving and other potentially hazardous activities that require mental alertness until drug's adverse CNS effects are known.

Black Box Warning Drinking alcohol or taking drugs containing alcohol while taking extended-release capsules may cause additive CNS effects and potentially fatal overdose. Warn patient to read labels on OTC drugs carefully for alcohol content and not to use alcohol in any form. ∎

• Tell patient to swallow morphine sulfate whole or to open capsule and sprinkle beads or pellets on a small amount of applesauce immediately before taking.

Black Box Warning Tell patient to keep morphine oral preparations out of the reach of children. In case of accidental ingestion, advise patient to seek emergency medical help immediately. ∎

⊗ *Alert:* Warn patient not to crush, break, or chew extended-release forms.

SAFETY ALERT!

morphine sulfate–naltrexone hydrochloride
MOR-feen/nal-TREX-own

Embeda

Therapeutic class: Opioid analgesics
Pharmacologic class: Opioid agonist–antagonists
Controlled substance schedule: II

AVAILABLE FORMS

Capsules ⬛*:* 20 mg morphine and 0.8 mg naltrexone, 30 mg morphine and 1.2 mg naltrexone, 50 mg morphine and 2 mg naltrexone, 60 mg morphine and 2.4 mg naltrexone, 80 mg morphine and 3.2 mg naltrexone, 100 mg morphine and 4 mg naltrexone

INDICATIONS & DOSAGES

➤ **Moderate to severe pain when a continuous, around-the-clock opioid analgesic is needed for an extended period of time**

Adults: Individualize dosage according to patient's previous analgesic treatment, general condition, concurrent medication, type and severity of pain, and degree of opioid tolerance. Initially, give lowest dose possible; titrate no more frequently than every other day to allow for stabilization before escalating dosage. If pain relief is inadequate, administer every 12 hours.

Initial treatment with Embeda as patient's first opioid analgesic or in patients who aren't opioid tolerant is one 20-mg morphine/0.8 mg naltrexone capsule P.O. every 24 hours. Use of higher starting doses in patients who aren't opioid tolerant may cause fatal respiratory depression. The 100-mg morphine/4-mg naltrexone capsules are for use only in opioid-tolerant patients. First dose of Embeda may be taken with last dose of any immediate-release (short-acting) opioid medication because of extended-release characteristics of Embeda.

Adjust-a-dose: For patients receiving other morphine preparations, convert by administering half of patient's daily morphine dose as Embeda every 12 hours or by administering total morphine dose as Embeda every 24 hours.

ADMINISTRATION
P.O.

Black Box Warning If patient has difficulty swallowing whole capsule, open capsule, sprinkle pellets onto small amount of applesauce, and administer immediately. Caution patient not to chew pellets. Have patient rinse mouth to make sure all pellets are swallowed. ■

Black Box Warning Crushing, chewing, cutting, or dissolving morphine–naltrexone capsules can cause rapid release and absorption of a potentially fatal dose of morphine. ■

• Don't administer pellets through an NG or gastric tube.

ACTION
Morphine is a selective mu agonist that produces analgesia and sedation by binding with the mu opioid receptor. Naltrexone is a centrally acting mu agonist that reverses subjective and analgesic effects of morphine by competing for mu receptor sites.

Route	Onset	Peak	Duration
P.O.	Unknown	7½ hr	Days

Half-life: 29 hours.

ADVERSE REACTIONS
CNS: anxiety, depression, dizziness, fatigue, headache, insomnia, irritability, lethargy, restlessness, sedation, somnolence, tremor.
CV: *cardiac arrest,* flushing, peripheral edema, *shock.*
GI: abdominal pain, anorexia, constipation, decreased appetite, diarrhea, dyspepsia, flatulence, nausea, stomach discomfort, vomiting, dry mouth.
Musculoskeletal: arthralgia, muscle spasms.

Respiratory: *apnea, respiratory arrest, respiratory depression.*
Skin: hyperhidrosis, pruritus.
Other: hot flush, chills.

INTERACTIONS
Drug-drug. *Anticholinergics:* May cause urine retention, severe constipation, or paralytic ileus. Use together cautiously and monitor patient closely.

Black Box Warning *Benzodiazepines, CNS depressants:* May cause slow or difficult breathing, sedation, and death. Avoid use together. If use together is necessary, limit dosage and duration of each drug to the minimum necessary for desired effect. ■
Cimetidine: May cause confusion and severe respiratory depression. Avoid use together.
General anesthetics: May cause respiratory depression, hypotension, profound sedation, or coma. Use together cautiously; reduce initial dosage of one or both agents by at least 50% and monitor patient closely.
Diuretics: May cause antidiuretic hormone release, rendering diuretics ineffective, and urine retention due to bladder sphincter spasm. Use together cautiously.
MAO inhibitors: May cause anxiety, confusion, significant respiratory depression, or coma. Avoid use together and within 14 days of stopping treatment with MAO inhibitors.
Mixed agonist–antagonist opioid analgesics (butorphanol, nalbuphine, pentazocine): May reduce analgesic effects and precipitate withdrawal symptoms. Consider therapy modification.
Muscle relaxants: May enhance neuromuscular blocking action of skeletal muscle relaxants, causing respiratory depression. Use together cautiously.
P-glycoprotein inhibitors (such as quinidine): May increase morphine level and risk of adverse effects. Use together cautiously.
Rifamycins (rifampin): May reduce morphine level and analgesic effect. Monitor response and increase morphine–naltrexone dosage if necessary.
☻ Alert: Serotonergic drugs (amoxapine, antiemetics [dolasetron, granisetron, ondansetron, palonosetron], antimigraine drugs, buspirone, cyclobenzaprine, dextromethorphan, linezolid, lithium, MAO

M

inhibitors, maprotiline, methylene blue, mirtazapine, nefazodone, SNRIs, SSRIs, TCAs, trazodone, tryptophan, vilazodone): May increase risk of serotonin syndrome. Use together cautiously and monitor patient for serotonin syndrome.

Drug-herb. ❸ Alert: *St. John's wort:* May increase risk of serotonin syndrome. Use together cautiously and monitor patient for serotonin syndrome.

Drug-lifestyle. *Alcohol use:* May cause additive CNS effects and fatal overdose. Warn patient to avoid alcohol.

EFFECTS ON LAB TEST RESULTS
• May interfere with tests that use enzymes to detect opioids.

CONTRAINDICATIONS & CAUTIONS
• Contraindicated in patients hypersensitive to drug or its components and in those with significant respiratory depression, acute or severe bronchial asthma, or hypercapnia in unmonitored settings without resuscitative equipment.

Black Box Warning Opioid drugs should only be prescribed with benzodiazepines or other CNS depressants to patients for whom alternative treatment options are inadequate. ∎

• Drug should be prescribed only by health care professionals knowledgeable in the use of potent opioids for management of chronic pain.

❸ Alert: Drug may lead to a rare but serious decrease in adrenal gland cortisol production.

❸ Alert: Drug may cause decreased sex hormone levels with long-term use.

❸ Alert: Patients are at increased risk for oversedation and respiratory depression if they snore or have a history of sleep apnea, haven't used opioids recently or are first-time opioid users, have increased opioid dosage requirements or opioid habituation, have received general anesthesia for longer lengths of time or received other sedating drugs, have preexisting pulmonary or cardiac disease, or have thoracic or other surgical incisions that may impair breathing. Monitor patients carefully.

• Contraindicated in patients with known or suspected paralytic ileus.

• Use cautiously in patients with mental health conditions, COPD, cor pulmonale, decreased respiratory reserve, hypoxia, hypercapnia, head injury, increased ICP, shock, seizures, biliary tract disease including pancreatitis, CNS depression, toxic psychosis, acute alcoholism, or delirium tremens.

• Use cautiously in elderly and debilitated patients and in those with severe renal or hepatic insufficiency, Addison disease, myxedema, hypothyroidism, prostatic hypertrophy, and urethral stricture.

• Individualize dosing regimen for each patient.

Dialyzable drug: Morphine, yes; naltrexone, no.

⚠ Overdose S&S: Respiratory depression, somnolence progressing to stupor or coma, skeletal muscle flaccidity, cold and clammy skin, constricted pupils, pulmonary edema, bradycardia, hypotension, death.

PREGNANCY-LACTATION-REPRODUCTION
• There are no adequate studies in pregnant women. Use during pregnancy only if clearly needed and potential benefit justifies potential risk to the fetus.

Black Box Warning Prolonged use during pregnancy can result in neonatal opioid withdrawal syndrome, which may be life-threatening if not recognized and treated, and requires management according to protocols developed by neonatology experts. If opioid use is required for a prolonged period, advise pregnant patient of risk to neonate and ensure that appropriate treatment will be available. ∎

• Morphine appears in breast milk. Because of potential for adverse reactions in breast-fed infants, patient should discontinue breast-feeding or discontinue drug, taking into account importance of drug to the mother.

• Closely monitor infants of breast-feeding women receiving drug. Withdrawal symptoms can occur in breast-fed infants when maternal administration of morphine is stopped.

• Long-term opioid use may cause secondary hypogonadism, which may lead to sexual dysfunction or infertility.

NURSING CONSIDERATIONS

Black Box Warning Capsules contain pellets of morphine sulfate. The pellets shouldn't be crushed, dissolved, or chewed because drug will be released and absorbed rapidly; resulting dose may be fatal, especially in opioid-naive patients. ∎

Black Box Warning Drug has an abuse liability similar to that of other opioid agonists, legal or illicit. Assess each patient's risk of opioid abuse or addiction before prescribing. Risk of opioid abuse increases in patients with personal or family history of substance abuse (including drug or alcohol abuse or addiction) or mental illness (such as major depressive disorder). Routinely monitor all patients receiving drug for signs and symptoms of misuse, abuse, and addiction during treatment. ∎

❍ *Alert:* If patient is taking opioids with serotonergic drugs, watch for signs and symptoms of serotonin syndrome (agitation, hallucinations, rapid HR, fever, excessive sweating, shivering or shaking, muscle twitching or stiffness, trouble with coordination, nausea, vomiting, diarrhea), especially when at start of treatment or at dosage increases. Signs and symptoms may occur within several hours of coadministration but may also occur later, especially after dosage increase. Discontinue the opioid, serotonergic drug, or both if serotonin syndrome is suspected.

❍ *Alert:* Monitor patient for signs and symptoms of adrenal insufficiency (nausea, vomiting, loss of appetite, fatigue, weakness, dizziness, low BP). Perform diagnostic testing if adrenal insufficiency is suspected. If adrenal insufficiency is confirmed, treat with corticosteroids and wean patient off opioids if appropriate. Discontinue corticosteroids when clinically appropriate.

❍ *Alert:* Monitor patient for signs and symptoms of decreased sex hormone levels (low libido, erectile dysfunction, amenorrhea, infertility). If signs and symptoms occur, evaluate patient and obtain laboratory testing.

● Monitor patients closely for respiratory depression, especially within first 24 to 72 hours of start of therapy.

❍ *Alert:* Don't use for mild or acute pain, on an as-needed basis, or for postoperative pain, unless patient has already been receiving long-term opioid therapy before surgery or if postoperative pain is expected to be moderate to severe and persist for an extended period.

● Morphine 100 mg/naltrexone 4 mg is for use in opioid-tolerant patients only.

Black Box Warning Respiratory depression, including fatal cases, may occur with morphine–naltrexone, even when drug has been used as recommended and not misused or abused. Proper dosing and titration are essential, and drug should only be prescribed by health care professionals knowledgeable in the use of potent opioids for management of chronic pain. Monitor patient for respiratory depression, especially during initiation of drug or after a dosage increase. ∎

❍ *Alert:* Carefully monitor vital signs, pain level, respiratory status, and sedation level in all patients receiving opioids, especially those receiving I.V. drugs, even those given postoperatively.

● Monitor circulatory, respiratory, bladder, and bowel functions carefully. Drug may cause hypotension, urine retention, nausea, vomiting, constipation, ileus, or altered level of consciousness.

● Taper drug gradually when stopping therapy to avoid withdrawal symptoms.

Black Box Warning Accidental ingestion of drug can result in fatal overdose of morphine, especially in children. ∎

● Keep opioid antagonist (naloxone) and resuscitation equipment available.

PATIENT TEACHING

Black Box Warning Caution the patient or the caregiver of a patient taking an opioid drug with a benzodiazepine, CNS depressant, or alcohol to seek immediate medical attention if the patient has symptoms of dizziness, light-headedness, extreme sleepiness, slowed or difficult breathing, or unresponsiveness. ∎

● Explain assessment and monitoring process to patient and family. Instruct them to immediately report difficulty breathing or other signs or symptoms of a potential adverse opioid-related reaction.

Black Box Warning Warn patient taking drug that consuming alcoholic beverages

---

or prescription or OTC drugs containing alcohol may cause dose to be fatal. ∎

Black Box Warning Tell patient to swallow capsules whole or open capsule and sprinkle pellets on small amount of applesauce immediately before taking; instruct patient that capsules shouldn't be crushed, cut, dissolved, or chewed. ∎

۞ Alert: Encourage patient to report all medications being taken, including prescription and OTC medications and supplements.

۞ Alert: Caution patient to immediately report signs and symptoms of serotonin syndrome, adrenal insufficiency, and decreased sex hormone levels.

• Caution patient that drug has potential for abuse and should be protected from theft.

Black Box Warning Tell patient to keep morphine oral preparations out of the reach of children. In case of accidental ingestion, advise patient to seek emergency medical help immediately. ∎

• Warn patient to avoid driving and other potentially hazardous activities that require mental alertness until drug's effects are known.

• Caution ambulatory patient about getting out of bed or walking because drug may cause a drop in BP with position change.

• Tell patient the importance of dietary changes, stool softeners, and laxatives to prevent constipation, a common adverse effect of drug.

moxifloxacin hydrochloride
mocks-ah-FLOX-a-sin

Avelox✐, Avelox I.V., Moxeza, Vigamox

Therapeutic class: Antibiotics
Pharmacologic class: Fluoroquinolones

AVAILABLE FORMS
Injection: 400 mg/250 mL
Ophthalmic solution: 0.5%
Tablets (film-coated): 400 mg

INDICATIONS & DOSAGES
Black Box Warning Use in patients with acute bacterial sinusitis, acute bacterial exacerbation of bronchitis, and uncompli-

cated UTI isn't recommended due to risk of serious adverse effects. Use drug in these patients only when they have no other treatment options. ∎

➤ **Acute bacterial sinusitis caused by** *Streptococcus pneumoniae, Haemophilus influenzae,* **or** *Moraxella catarrhalis*
Adults: 400 mg P.O. or I.V. every 24 hours for 10 days.

➤ **Complicated skin and skin-structure infections caused by methicillin-susceptible** *Staphylococcus aureus, Escherichia coli, Klebsiella pneumoniae,* **or** *Enterobacter cloacae*
Adults: 400 mg P.O. or I.V. every 24 hours for 7 to 21 days.

➤ **Complicated intra-abdominal infection caused by** *E. coli, Bacteroides fragilis, Streptococcus anginosus, Streptococcus constellatus, Enterococcus faecalis, Proteus mirabilis, Clostridium perfringens, Bacteroides thetaiotaomicron,* **or** *Peptostreptococcus* **species**
Adults: 400 mg P.O. or I.V. every 24 hours for 5 to 14 days. Start with the I.V. form; switch to P.O. when appropriate.

➤ **Community-acquired pneumonia from multidrug-resistant** *S. pneumoniae* **(resistance to two or more of the following antibiotics: penicillin, second-generation cephalosporins, macrolides, sulfamethoxazole–trimethoprim, tetracyclines),** *S. aureus, M. catarrhalis, H. influenzae, H. parainfluenzae, K. pneumoniae, Chlamydia pneumoniae, Legionella pneumophila,* **or** *Mycoplasma pneumoniae*
Adults: 400 mg P.O. or I.V. every 24 hours for 7 to 14 days.

➤ **Acute bacterial worsening of chronic bronchitis caused by** *S. pneumoniae, H. influenzae, H. parainfluenzae, K. pneumoniae, S. aureus,* **or** *M. catarrhalis*
Adults: 400 mg P.O. or I.V. every 24 hours for 5 days.

➤ **Uncomplicated skin-structure or skin infection caused by** *S. aureus* **or** *S. pyogenes*
Adults: 400 mg P.O. or I.V. every 24 hours for 7 days.

➤ **Plague (pneumonic and septicemic) caused by susceptible isolates of** *Yersinia pestis*

Reactions in bold italics are *life-threatening*. Interactions may have a *rapid onset* or a *delayed onset*.

Adults: For prophylaxis and treatment, 400 mg P.O. or I.V. every 24 hours for 10 to 14 days.
➤ **Bacterial conjunctivitis caused by susceptible strains of aerobic gram-positive and gram-negative organisms and *Chlamydia trachomatis***
Adults and children age 1 and older (Vigamox): 1 drop into affected eye(s) t.i.d. for 7 days.
Adults and children age 4 months and older (Moxeza): 1 drop into affected eye(s) b.i.d. for 7 days.

ADMINISTRATION
P.O.
- Give drug without regard for food. Give at same time each day.
- Give dose 4 hours before or 8 hours after antacids, sucralfate, multivitamins, didanosine buffered tablets for oral suspension or pediatric powder for oral solution, and other products containing aluminum, magnesium, iron, and zinc, to avoid decreasing drug's therapeutic effects.
- Store drug at controlled room temperature.

I.V.
▼ Don't refrigerate. Product precipitates if refrigerated.
▼ Don't use if particulate matter is visible.
▼ Flush I.V. line with a compatible solution such as D_5W, NSS, or lactated Ringer solution before and after use.
▼ Give only by infusion over 1 hour. Avoid rapid or bolus infusion.
▼ **Incompatibilities:** Other I.V. drugs.

Ophthalmic
- Place gentle pressure on lacrimal duct for 1 to 2 minutes after instilling drop.
- Solution isn't for injection subconjunctivally or into anterior chamber of the eye.

ACTION
Interferes with action of enzymes needed for bacterial replication. Inhibits topoisomerases I (DNA gyrase) and IV, impairing bacterial DNA replication, transcription, repair, and recombination.

Route	Onset	Peak	Duration
P.O., I.V.	Unknown	1–3 hr	Unknown
Ophthalmic	Unknown	Unknown	Unknown

Half-life: P.O., I.V., about 12 hours; ophthalmic, 13 hours.

ADVERSE REACTIONS
CNS: dizziness, headache, insomnia, fever.
EENT: with ophthalmic use: conjunctivitis; dry eyes; increased lacrimation; keratitis; ocular discomfort, pain, or pruritus; reduced visual acuity; subconjunctival hemorrhage; otitis media; pharyngitis; rhinitis.
GI: abdominal pain, anorexia, constipation, diarrhea, dyspepsia, nausea, vomiting.
Hematologic: anemia.
Hepatic: abnormal liver function.
Metabolic: hypokalemia.
Respiratory: *hypoxia.*

INTERACTIONS
Drug-drug. *Aluminum hydroxide, aluminum–magnesium hydroxide, calcium carbonate, didanosine, magnesium hydroxide, multivitamins, products containing zinc:* May interfere with GI absorption of moxifloxacin. Give moxifloxacin 4 hours before or 8 hours after these products.
Class IA antiarrhythmics (procainamide, quinidine), class III antiarrhythmics (amiodarone, sotalol): May increase risk of cardiac arrhythmias. Avoid using together.
Drugs that prolong QT interval (antipsychotics, erythromycin, TCAs): May have additive effect. Avoid using together.
Live-virus vaccines: May decrease effectiveness of live-virus vaccines. Don't give live-virus vaccines during therapy.
NSAIDs: May increase risk of CNS stimulation and seizures. Monitor patient and adjust treatment as needed.
Black Box Warning *Steroids:* May increase risk of tendinitis and tendon rupture. Monitor patient for tendon pain or inflammation. ■
Sucralfate: May decrease absorption of moxifloxacin, reducing anti-infective response. If use together can't be avoided, give at least 6 hours apart.
Warfarin: May increase anticoagulant effects. Monitor PT and INR closely.

M

Drug-lifestyle. *Sun exposure:* May cause moderate to severe photosensitivity reactions. Advise patient to avoid excessive sunlight exposure.

EFFECTS ON LAB TEST RESULTS

● May increase ALT, ionized calcium, chloride, globulin, and albumin levels and PT and INR.
● May decrease potassium, glucose, and amylase levels and oxygen partial pressure.
● May increase or decrease bilirubin and glucose levels.
● May increase WBC count. May decrease RBC, eosinophil, and basophil counts and Hb level and hematocrit. May increase or decrease neutrophil count.

CONTRAINDICATIONS & CAUTIONS

Black Box Warning Drug is associated with increased risk of tendinitis and tendon rupture, especially in patients older than age 60, patients taking corticosteroids, and those with heart, kidney, or lung transplants. ■

❸ **Alert:** Disturbances in blood glucose level, including hypoglycemia and hyperglycemia, have been reported. Elderly patients with diabetes receiving an oral hypoglycemic agent (e.g., sulfonylurea) or insulin concomitantly are at increased risk. If a hypoglycemic reaction occurs, discontinue drug and initiate appropriate therapy immediately. Carefully monitor glucose level.

● Contraindicated in patients hypersensitive to drug or other fluoroquinolones, in those with prolonged QT interval or uncorrected hypokalemia, and in those taking class 1A (procainamide) or class III (amiodarone) antiarrhythmics.

❸ **Alert:** Drug can prolong QT interval in some patients. Use cautiously in patients with ongoing proarrhythmic conditions, such as clinically significant bradycardia or acute myocardial ischemia.

● Discontinue drug at first sign of rash, jaundice, or other signs or symptoms of hypersensitivity.

● Seizures, increased ICP, and pseudotumor cerebri have been reported in patients taking fluoroquinolones. Drug may cause CNS events (including agitation, anxiety, confusion, depression, insomnia and, rarely, suicidal ideation), which may occur after

first dose. Use cautiously in patients who may have CNS disorders or risk factors for seizures. Drug may need to be discontinued.

Black Box Warning Drug may exacerbate muscle weakness in patients with myasthenia gravis. Avoid use of fluoroquinolones in patients with known history of myasthenia gravis. ■

● Drug may cause CDAD, ranging in severity from mild diarrhea to fatal colitis, and which can occur more than 2 months after therapy. If CDAD is suspected or confirmed, drug may need to be discontinued and appropriate therapy initiated.

● Safety and effectiveness in children and adolescents younger than age 18 haven't been established.

Dialyzable drug: No.

PREGNANCY-LACTATION-REPRODUCTION

● There are no adequate studies in pregnant women. Use during pregnancy only if potential benefit justifies potential fetal risk.

● Drug may appear in breast milk. Patient should discontinue breast-feeding or discontinue drug.

NURSING CONSIDERATIONS

Black Box Warning Fluoroquinolones have been associated with disabling and potentially irreversible serious adverse reactions that have occurred together, including tendinitis and tendon rupture, peripheral neuropathy, and CNS effects (seizures, toxic psychoses, increased ICP, pseudotumor cerebri, tremors, restlessness, anxiety, light-headedness, confusion, hallucinations, paranoia, depression, nightmares, insomnia and, rarely, suicidal thoughts or acts). If any of these serious adverse reactions occur, discontinue drug immediately. ■

Black Box Warning Monitor patient for signs and symptoms of peripheral neuropathy (pain, burning, tingling, numbness, weakness, or change in sensation to light touch, pain or temperature, or sense of body position) and immediately report them. ■

● Monitor patient for hypersensitivity reactions, including anaphylaxis.

● If diarrhea develops during therapy, send stool specimen for *Clostridium difficile* test.

● Rupture of the Achilles and other tendons is linked to fluoroquinolone use. If pain,

inflammation, or tendon rupture occurs, stop drug and notify prescriber.
● *Look alike–sound alike:* Don't confuse Avelox with Avonex.

PATIENT TEACHING
Black Box Warning Warn patient to immediately report signs and symptoms of serious adverse reactions, including unusual joint or tendon pain, muscle weakness, "pins and needles" tingling or prickling sensation, numbness in the arms or legs, confusion, or hallucinations. ■
● Instruct patient to take drug once daily, at the same time each day, without regard to meals.
● Tell patient to finish entire course of therapy, even if symptoms are relieved.
● Advise patient to drink plenty of fluids.
● Tell patient to space antacids, sucralfate, multivitamins, and products containing aluminum, magnesium, iron, and zinc to avoid decreasing drug's therapeutic effects.
☢ Alert: Warn patient to immediately report signs and symptoms of hypoglycemia.
● Instruct patient to contact prescriber and stop drug if allergic reaction, rash, heart palpitations, fainting, or persistent diarrhea occurs.
● Direct patient to contact prescriber, stop drug, rest, and refrain from exercise if pain, inflammation, or tendon rupture occurs.
● Warn patient that drug may cause dizziness and light-headedness. Tell patient to avoid hazardous activities, such as driving or operating machinery, until effects of drug are known.
● Instruct patient to avoid excessive sunlight exposure and ultraviolet light and to report photosensitivity reactions to prescriber.
● Tell patient not to wear contact lenses during ophthalmic treatment.
● Instruct patient not to touch ophthalmic dropper tip to anything, including eyes and fingers.

mupirocin
myoo-PIHR-oh-sin

Bactroban, Centany

Therapeutic class: Antibacterials (topical)
Pharmacologic class: Antibiotics

AVAILABLE FORMS
Intranasal ointment: 2%
Topical cream: 2%
Topical ointment: 2%

INDICATIONS & DOSAGES
➤ **Impetigo (topical ointment)**
Adults and children age 2 months and older: Apply to affected areas t.i.d. Reevaluate patient in 3 to 5 days; may cover affected area with dressing.
➤ **Traumatic skin lesions infected with *Staphylococcus aureus* or *Streptococcus pyogenes* (cream)**
Adults and children age 3 months and older: Apply thin film t.i.d. for 10 days; may cover with gauze dressing, if needed. Reevaluate patient if improvement doesn't occur in 3 to 5 days.
➤ **To eradicate nasal colonization by MRSA in adult patients and health care workers (intranasal ointment)**
Adults and children age 12 and older: Divide ointment in single-use tube between nostrils (½ tube per nostril) b.i.d. for 5 days. After application, close nostrils by pressing together and releasing sides of nose repeatedly for 1 minute to spread ointment throughout nares.

ADMINISTRATION
Topical
● Cosmetics and other skin products shouldn't be used on treated area.
Intranasal
● Other nasal products shouldn't be used with intranasal ointment.

ACTION
Inhibits bacterial protein synthesis by reversibly and specifically binding to bacterial isoleucyl transfer-RNA synthetase.

M

Route	Onset	Peak	Duration
Topical, intranasal	Unknown	Unknown	Unknown

Half-life: Unknown.

ADVERSE REACTIONS
CNS: headache.
EENT: rhinitis, pharyngitis, burning or stinging with intranasal use.
GI: taste perversion, nausea.
Respiratory: upper respiratory tract congestion, cough with intranasal use.
Skin: burning, erythema with topical use, pain, pruritus, rash, stinging.

INTERACTIONS
Drug-drug. *Bacillus Calmette-Guérin (BCG):* May diminish therapeutic effect of BCG. Avoid combination.
Other nasal products: May interfere with absorption of other nasal drugs. Don't use together.
Sodium picosulfate, typhoid vaccine: May diminish therapeutic effect of sodium picosulfate and typhoid vaccine. Consider therapy modification.

EFFECTS ON LAB TEST RESULTS
None reported.

CONTRAINDICATIONS & CAUTIONS
● Contraindicated in patients hypersensitive to drug or its components.
● Use cautiously in patients with burns or large open wounds and in those with impaired renal function because serious renal toxicity may occur.
Dialyzable drug: Unknown.

PREGNANCY-LACTATION-REPRODUCTION
● There are no adequate studies in pregnant women. Use during pregnancy only if clearly needed.
● It isn't known if drug appears in breast milk. Use cautiously in breast-feeding women.

NURSING CONSIDERATIONS
● Drug isn't for ophthalmic or internal use.
● Drug may cause CDAD, ranging in severity from mild diarrhea to fatal colitis and which can occur more than 2 months after therapy ends. If CDAD is suspected or con-

firmed, drug may need to be discontinued and appropriate therapy initiated.
● Discontinue drug if sensitization or severe local irritation occurs.
● Prolonged use may cause overgrowth of nonsusceptible bacteria and fungi.
● *Look alike–sound alike:* Don't confuse Bactroban with bacitracin, baclofen, or Bactrim.

PATIENT TEACHING
● Tell patient to notify prescriber immediately if condition doesn't improve or gets worse in 3 to 5 days.
● Advise patient to avoid contact with eyes and if accidental contact occurs, to rinse well with water.
● Urge patient to immediately report diarrhea.
● Tell patient not to use other nasal products with intranasal ointment.
● Warn patient about local adverse reactions related to drug use.
● Caution patient not to use cosmetics or other skin products on treated area.

---

mycophenolate mofetil
my-koe-FIN-oh-late

CellCept

mycophenolate mofetil hydrochloride
CellCept Intravenous

mycophenolic acid (mycophenolate sodium)
Myfortic

Therapeutic class: Immunosuppressants
Pharmacologic class: Mycophenolic acid derivatives

AVAILABLE FORMS
mycophenolate mofetil
Capsules ⊙: 250 mg
Powder for oral suspension: 200 mg/mL
Tablets: 500 mg
mycophenolate mofetil hydrochloride
Injection: 500 mg/vial

---

mycophenolic acid
Tablets (extended-release) 🔴*:* 180 mg, 360 mg

INDICATIONS & DOSAGES

➤ **To prevent organ rejection in patients receiving allogeneic renal transplants**
Adults: 1 g I.V. or P.O. (regular-release) b.i.d. with corticosteroids and cyclosporine. Or, 720 mg extended-release tablets P.O. b.i.d. 1 hour before or 2 hours after food.
Children ages 5 to 16 (extended-release): 400 mg/m^2 P.O. b.i.d. Maximum dose, 720 mg P.O. b.i.d. Or, for patients with body surface area (BSA) of 1.19 to 1.58 m^2, give 540 mg P.O. b.i.d. If BSA is greater than 1.58 m^2, give 720 mg P.O. b.i.d. Extended-release formulation isn't recommended for BSA of less than 1.19 m^2.
Children ages 3 months to 18 years: For oral suspension, give 600 mg/m^2 P.O. b.i.d.; maximum dose is 1 g b.i.d. Or, for patients with BSA of 1.25 to 1.5 m^2, give 750 mg (capsules) P.O. b.i.d. If BSA is greater than 1.5 m^2, give 1 g (tablets or capsules) P.O. b.i.d.
Adjust-a-dose: For patients with severe chronic renal impairment outside of immediate posttransplant period, avoid doses above 1 g b.i.d. If neutropenia develops, interrupt or reduce dosage.

➤ **To prevent organ rejection in patients receiving allogeneic cardiac transplant**
Adults: 1.5 g P.O. or I.V. b.i.d. with cyclosporine and corticosteroids.

➤ **To prevent organ rejection in patients receiving allogeneic hepatic transplants**
Adults: 1 g I.V. b.i.d. over no less than 2 hours or 1.5 g P.O. b.i.d. with cyclosporine and corticosteroids.
Adjust-a-dose: If neutropenia develops, stop or reduce dosage.

ADMINISTRATION
P.O.
🔵 *Alert:* Drug is considered a potential mutagen and teratogen. Follow safe-handling procedures when preparing, administering, or dispensing.
● Don't crush tablets; don't open or crush capsules.
● Avoid inhaling powder in capsule or having it contact skin or mucous membranes. If

contact occurs, wash skin thoroughly with soap and water, and rinse eyes with water.
● The extended-release tablets are not interchangeable with other forms.
● Suspension may be administered via NG tube with a minimum size 8 French catheter (at least 1.7-mm interior diameter).
I.V.
▼ Reconstitute and dilute to 6 mg/mL using 14 mL of D$_5$W.
▼ Never give by rapid or bolus I.V. injection. Infuse drug over at least 2 hours.
▼ Use within 4 hours of reconstitution and dilution.
▼ **Incompatibilities:** Other I.V. drugs or solutions.

ACTION
Inhibits proliferative response of T and B lymphocytes, suppresses antibody formation by B lymphocytes, and may inhibit recruitment of leukocytes into sites of inflammation and graft rejection.

Route	Onset	Peak	Duration
P.O.	Unknown	30–75 min	7–18 hr
P.O. (extended-release)	Unknown	1½–2¾ hr	8–17 hr
I.V.	Unknown	Unknown	10–17 hr

Half-life: About 18 hours.

ADVERSE REACTIONS
CNS: asthenia, fever, headache, pain, tremor, dizziness, insomnia, *progressive multifocal leukoencephalopathy,* depression, psychosis, anxiety.
CV: chest pain, edema, hypertension, hypotension, tachycardia, *hemorrhage.*
EENT: pharyngitis, ear pain, deafness.
GI: abdominal pain, constipation, diarrhea, dyspepsia, nausea, anorexia, oral candidiasis, vomiting, *hemorrhage.*
GU: hematuria, UTI, *renal tubular necrosis, acute renal failure.*
Hematologic: anemia, *leukopenia, thrombocytopenia,* hypochromic anemia, leukocytosis.
Metabolic: hypercholesterolemia, hyperglycemia, *hyperkalemia,* hypokalemia, hypophosphatemia.
Musculoskeletal: back pain.

M

Respiratory: cough, dyspnea, infection, bronchitis, pneumonia.
Skin: acne, rash, alopecia, skin carcinoma.
Other: infection, *sepsis.*

INTERACTIONS

Drug-drug. *Acyclovir, ganciclovir, other drugs that undergo renal tubular secretion:* May increase risk of toxicity for both drugs. Monitor patient closely.

Antacids with magnesium and aluminum hydroxides: May decrease mycophenolate absorption. Separate dosing times.

Azathioprine: May increase risk of bone marrow suppression. Don't use together.

Cholestyramine: May interfere with entero-hepatic recirculation, reducing mycophenolate bioavailability. Avoid using together.

Cyclosporine, drugs that alter normal GI flora, rifamycins (rifampin): May decrease mycophenolate level. Monitor response to therapy and increase dosage if necessary.

Hormonal contraceptives: May decrease effectiveness of contraceptive. Recommend addition of barrier form of contraception during treatment and for 6 weeks after treatment ends.

Immunosuppressants (sirolimus, tacrolimus): May increase mycophenolate level. Monitor patient closely.

Live-virus vaccines: May decrease vaccine effectiveness. Avoid using together.

Phenytoin, theophylline: May increase both drug levels. Monitor drug levels closely.

Probenecid, salicylates: May increase mycophenolate level. Monitor patient closely.

Drug-herb. *Cat's claw, echinacea:* May increase immunostimulation. Discourage use together.

Drug-food. *Any food:* May delay absorption of extended-release form. Advise patient to take on an empty stomach 1 hour before or 2 hours after a meal.

EFFECTS ON LAB TEST RESULTS

● May increase cholesterol and glucose levels. May decrease phosphorus and Hb levels. May increase or decrease potassium level.

● May decrease platelet count. May increase or decrease WBC count.

CONTRAINDICATIONS & CAUTIONS

● Contraindicated in patients hypersensitive to drug, its ingredients, or mycophenolic acid and in patients sensitive to polysorbate 80.

● Use cautiously in patients with GI disorders. Bleeding and perforation may occur.

● Oral suspension contains aspartame; use cautiously in patients with phenylketonuria.
Dialyzable drug: No.

⚠ **Overdose S&S:** Nausea, vomiting, diarrhea, neutropenia.

PREGNANCY-LACTATION-REPRODUCTION

`Black Box Warning` Use during pregnancy is associated with increased risk of first-trimester pregnancy loss and congenital malformations. Women of childbearing potential must be counseled regarding pregnancy prevention and planning. ∎

● For women using drug at any time during pregnancy and those becoming pregnant within 6 weeks of discontinuing therapy, prescriber should report pregnancy to the Mycophenolate Pregnancy Registry (1-800-617-8191).

● It isn't known if drug appears in breastmilk. Breast-feeding isn't recommended during therapy and for 6 weeks after therapy ends.

NURSING CONSIDERATIONS

`Black Box Warning` Increased risk of infection and lymphoma may result from immunosuppression. ∎

`Black Box Warning` Drug should only be used by health care providers experienced in immunosuppressive therapy and management of renal, cardiac, or hepatic transplant patients and in facilities equipped and staffed with adequate laboratory and supportive medical resources. ∎

● Start drug therapy within 24 hours after transplantation. Use I.V. form in patients unable to take oral forms.

● I.V. form can be given for up to 14 days; switch patient to capsules or tablets as soon as oral drugs can be tolerated.

🜂 *Alert:* Polyomavirus-associated nephropathy, progressive multifocal leukoencephalopathy, CMV infections, and reactivation of HBV or HCV infection have been reported in patients treated with

---

immunosuppressants. Consider reducing immunosuppressant dosage in patients who develop evidence of new or reactivated viral infections.

🔸 *Alert:* Drugs causing immunosuppression increase the risk of opportunistic infections, including activation of latent viral infections such as BK virus-associated neuropathy, which may lead to serious outcomes, including kidney graft loss.

🔸 *Alert:* Pure red cell aplasia (PRCA) has occurred in patients treated with this drug in combination with other immunosuppressants. Patients may experience fatigue, lethargy, or pallor. PRCA may be reversible with dose reduction or stopping drug. However, this may put graft at risk.

PATIENT TEACHING

• Warn patient not to open or crush capsules nor to cut, crush, or chew extended-release tablets, but to swallow them whole on an empty stomach 1 hour before or 2 hours after a meal.

• Stress importance of following treatment as prescribed.

• Inform patient of the importance of follow-up visits and ongoing laboratory tests during therapy.

• Tell female patient to have a pregnancy test 1 week before therapy begins and then again 8 to 10 days later. Inform her that repeat tests should be performed during routine follow-up visits.

• Instruct female patient to use two forms of contraception during therapy and for 6 weeks afterward, even if she has a history of infertility. Tell her to notify prescriber immediately if she suspects pregnancy.

• Instruct breast-feeding patient that she shouldn't breast-feed during therapy and for 6 weeks after therapy ends.

Black Box Warning Warn patient of the increased risk of infection and lymphoma and other malignancies. ∎

---

nadolol
nay-DOE-lol

Corgard

Therapeutic class: Antihypertensives
Pharmacologic class: Nonselective beta blockers

AVAILABLE FORMS
Tablets: 20 mg, 40 mg, 80 mg, 160 mg❧

INDICATIONS & DOSAGES

Adjust-a-dose (for all indications): If CrCl is 31 to 50 mL/minute, change dosing interval to every 24 to 36 hours; if CrCl is 10 to 30 mL/minute, every 24 to 48 hours; and if CrCl is less than 10 mL/minute, every 40 to 60 hours.

➤ **Angina pectoris**
Adults: 40 mg P.O. once daily. Increase in 40- to 80-mg increments at 3- to 7-day intervals until optimal response occurs. Usual maintenance dose is 40 to 80 mg once daily; up to 240 mg once daily may be needed.

➤ **Hypertension**
Adults: 40 mg P.O. once daily. Increase in 40- to 80-mg increments until optimal response occurs. Usual maintenance dose is 40 to 80 mg once daily. Doses of 320 mg daily may be needed.

ADMINISTRATION
P.O.

• Give drug without regard for food.

• Check apical pulse before giving drug. If slower than 60 beats/minute, withhold drug and call prescriber.

Black Box Warning Abruptly stopping drug may worsen angina and cause an MI. Reduce dosage gradually over 1 to 2 weeks. ∎

ACTION
Reduces cardiac oxygen demand by blocking catecholamine-induced increases in HR, BP, and force of myocardial contraction. Depresses renin secretion.

Route	Onset	Peak	Duration
P.O.	Unknown	3–4 hr	24 hr

Half-life: About 20 to 24 hours.

ADVERSE REACTIONS

CNS: fatigue, dizziness, fever.
CV: *bradycardia, HF,* hypotension, peripheral vascular disease, rhythm and conduction disturbances.

INTERACTIONS

Drug-drug. *Antihypertensives:* May increase antihypertensive effect. Monitor BP closely.
Cardiac glycosides: May cause excessive bradycardia and additive effects on AV conduction. Use together cautiously.
Epinephrine: May decrease patient response to epinephrine for treatment of an allergic reaction. Monitor patient closely for decreased clinical effect.
General anesthetics: May increase hypotensive effects. Consider stopping nadolol before surgery.
Insulin: May mask symptoms of hypoglycemia (such as tachycardia), as a result of beta blockade. Use with caution in patients with diabetes.
I.V. lidocaine: May reduce hepatic metabolism of lidocaine, increasing the risk of toxicity. Give bolus doses of lidocaine at a slower rate and monitor lidocaine level closely.
MAO inhibitors: May enhance orthostatic hypotensive effect. Monitor patient.
NSAIDs: May decrease antihypertensive effect. Monitor BP and adjust dosage.
Oral antidiabetics: May alter dosage requirements in previously stabilized diabetic patients. Monitor glucose closely.
Phenothiazines: May increase hypotensive effects. Monitor BP.
Prazosin: May increase risk of orthostatic hypotension in the early phases of use together. Assist patient to stand slowly until effects are known.
Reserpine: May increase hypotension or bradycardia. Monitor patient for adverse effects, such as dizziness, syncope, and postural hypotension.
Verapamil: May increase effects of both drugs. Monitor cardiac function closely and decrease dosages as necessary.
Drug-herb. *Dong quai, ephedra, garlic, ginseng, licorice, yohimbe:* May worsen hypertension or affect fluid and electrolytes. Avoid use.

EFFECTS ON LAB TEST RESULTS

None reported.

CONTRAINDICATIONS & CAUTIONS

● Contraindicated in patients with bronchial asthma, sinus bradycardia and greater than first-degree heart block, cardiogenic shock, and overt HF.
● Use cautiously in patients with HF, chronic bronchitis, emphysema, or renal or hepatic impairment and in patients undergoing major surgery involving general anesthesia. Drug shouldn't be routinely withdrawn before major surgery.
● Generally, patients with bronchospastic disease shouldn't receive beta blockers because they may block bronchodilation.
● Use cautiously in diabetic patients because beta blockers may mask certain signs and symptoms of hypoglycemia.
Black Box Warning Exacerbation of ischemic heart disease may occur following abrupt withdrawal of drug. Exacerbation of angina and, in some cases, MI have occurred after abrupt discontinuation of therapy. ■
Dialyzable drug: Yes.
⚠ *Overdose S&S:* Bradycardia, cardiac failure, hypotension, bronchospasm.

PREGNANCY-LACTATION-REPRODUCTION

● Use cautiously in pregnant women and only if benefit justifies possible fetal risk.
● Drug appears in breast milk. Patient should discontinue breast-feeding or discontinue drug.

NURSING CONSIDERATIONS

● Monitor BP frequently. If patient develops severe hypotension, give vasopressors, as prescribed.
● Drug masks signs and symptoms of shock and hyperthyroidism.
Black Box Warning If nadolol is to be discontinued after long-term administration, particularly in patients with ischemic heart disease, dosage should be gradually reduced over a period of 1 to 2 weeks and patient carefully monitored. If angina markedly worsens or acute coronary insufficiency develops after drug cessation, nadolol should be temporarily restarted and other measures taken to appropriately manage unstable angina. Because CAD is common and may

---

Reactions in bold italics are *life-threatening*. Interactions may have a *rapid onset* or a *delayed onset*.

be unrecognized, don't discontinue nadolol therapy abruptly, even in patients treated only for hypertension. ∎

PATIENT TEACHING
● Explain importance of taking drug as prescribed, with or without regard to food, even when patient feels well.
● Teach patient how to check pulse rate and tell him to check it before each dose. If pulse rate is below 60 beats/minute, tell patient to notify prescriber.
Black Box Warning Warn patient not to stop drug suddenly. ∎

nafcillin sodium
naf-SIL-in

Therapeutic class: Antibiotics
Pharmacologic class: Penicillinase-resistant penicillins

AVAILABLE FORMS
Infusion: 1-g, 2-g, 10-g premixed or Add-Vantage vials

INDICATIONS & DOSAGES
Adjust-a-dose (for all indications): In patients with renal failure and hepatic insufficiency, measure nafcillin serum levels and adjust dosage accordingly. Duration of therapy depends on type and severity of the infection and overall condition of patient. In severe infection, continue for at least 14 days. Continue for at least 48 hours after patient is afebrile and asymptomatic and cultures are negative. Treatment of endocarditis and osteomyelitis may require a longer duration of therapy.
➤ Systemic infection caused by susceptible organisms (methicillin-sensitive *Staphylococcus aureus*)
Adults: 500 mg to 1 g I.V. every 4 hours, or 500 mg to 1 g I.M. every 4 to 6 hours, depending on severity of infection.
Infants and children weighing less than 40 kg: 25 mg/kg I.M. b.i.d.
Neonates: 10 mg/kg I.M. b.i.d.

ADMINISTRATION
I.V.
▼ Before giving drug, ask patient about allergic reactions to penicillin.
▼ Obtain specimen for culture and sensitivity tests before giving. Begin therapy while awaiting results.
▼ Check container for leaks, cloudiness, or precipitate before use. Discard if present.
▼ Give drug over 30 to 60 minutes.
▼ Change site every 48 hours to prevent vein irritation.
▼ Reconstituted vials of 10 to 40 mg/mL are stable for 24 hours at room temperature.
▼ **Incompatibilities:** Other drugs.
I.M.
● Reconstitute with sterile water for injection, NSS for injection, or bacteriostatic water for injection. Add 6.6 mL to 2-g vial. Reconstituted vials contain 250 mg/mL.
● Administer clear solution by deep intragluteal I.M. injection immediately after reconstitution.

ACTION
Inhibits cell-wall synthesis during bacterial multiplication.

Route	Onset	Peak	Duration
I.V.	Immediate	Immediate	Unknown
I.M.	Unknown	30–60 min	Unknown

Half-life: About 30 to 60 minutes.

ADVERSE REACTIONS
CNS: *neurotoxicity.*
CV: thrombophlebitis, vein irritation.
GI: nausea, *pseudomembranous colitis,* diarrhea, vomiting.
Hematologic: *agranulocytosis, leukopenia, neutropenia, thrombocytopenia,* anemia, eosinophilia.
Skin: severe tissue necrosis (with subcutaneous extravasation).
Other: *anaphylaxis,* hypersensitivity reactions.

INTERACTIONS
Drug-drug. *Aminoglycosides:* May have synergistic effect; drugs are chemically and physically incompatible. Don't combine in same I.V. solution.

N

Cyclosporine: May cause subtherapeutic cyclosporine levels. Monitor cyclosporine levels.

Hormonal contraceptives: May decrease contraceptive effectiveness. Advise use of additional form of contraception during therapy.

Live-virus vaccines: May reduce effectiveness of live-virus vaccine. Don't use concurrently.

Methotrexate: May cause methotrexate toxicity. Monitor patient closely.

Probenecid: May increase nafcillin level. Probenecid may be used for this purpose.

Rifampin: May cause dose-dependent antagonism. Monitor patient closely.

Tetracycline: May decrease nafcillin's effectiveness. Avoid concurrent use.

Warfarin: May decrease effects of warfarin. Monitor PT and INR closely.

EFFECTS ON LAB TEST RESULTS
● May decrease Hb level and hematocrit.
● May cause false-positive Coombs test and false-positive urinary and serum protein levels.
● May decrease neutrophil, WBC, eosinophil, granulocyte, and platelet counts.

CONTRAINDICATIONS & CAUTIONS
● Contraindicated in patients hypersensitive to drug or other penicillins.
● Use cautiously in patients with GI distress and in those with other drug allergies (especially to cephalosporins) because of possible cross-sensitivity.
● Superinfection and CDAD can occur during therapy and up to 2 months after therapy ends. Drug may need to be discontinued and appropriate treatment initiated.
● Drug may infrequently cause renal tubular damage and interstitial nephritis.
● Skin sloughing from subcutaneous extravasation has been reported.

Dialyzable drug: No.

⚠ *Overdose S&S:* Neuromuscular hyperexcitability, seizures.

PREGNANCY-LACTATION-REPRODUCTION
● Use during pregnancy only if clearly needed.
● Penicillins appear in breast milk. Use cautiously in breast-feeding women.

NURSING CONSIDERATIONS
● If large doses are given or if therapy is prolonged, bacterial or fungal superinfection may occur, especially in elderly, debilitated, or immunosuppressed patients.
● Monitor sodium level because each gram of drug contains 2.9 mEq of sodium.
● Monitor WBC counts twice weekly in patients receiving drug for longer than 2 weeks. Neutropenia commonly occurs in the third week.
● Monitor patient for signs and symptoms of interstitial nephritis (abnormal urinalysis results, rash, fever, eosinophilia, hematuria, proteinuria, renal insufficiency).

PATIENT TEACHING
● Tell patient to report burning or irritation at the I.V. site.
● Advise patient to notify prescriber of all adverse reactions, especially rash or signs and symptoms of superinfection (recurring fever, chills, malaise) or CDAD (unexplained diarrhea).

SAFETY ALERT!

nalbuphine hydrochloride
NAL-byoo-feen

Nubain ✤

Therapeutic class: Opioid analgesics
Pharmacologic class: Opioid agonist-antagonists–opioid partial agonists

AVAILABLE FORMS
Injection: 10 mg/mL, 20 mg/mL

INDICATIONS & DOSAGES
Adjust-a-dose (for all indications): In patients with renal or hepatic impairment, decrease dosage.

➤ **Moderate to severe pain (non-opioid-tolerant patients); obstetric analgesia during labor and delivery**
Adults: For patient weighing about 70 kg, 10 to 20 mg subcutaneously, I.M., or I.V. every 3 to 6 hours p.r.n. Maximum, 160 mg daily. Adjust dosage according to the severity of pain, physical status, and other drugs patient is receiving.

Reactions in bold italics are ***life-threatening***. Interactions may have a *rapid onset* or a ***delayed onset***.

➤ **Adjunct to balanced anesthesia**
Adults: 0.3 to 3 mg/kg I.V. over 10 to
15 minutes; then maintenance dose of
0.25 to 0.5 mg/kg in single I.V. dose p.r.n.

ADMINISTRATION
I.V.
▼ Inject slowly over at least 2 to 3 minutes
into a vein or into an I.V. line containing a
compatible, free-flowing I.V. solution, such
as D5W, NSS, or lactated Ringer solution.
▼ Respiratory depression can be reversed
with naloxone. Keep resuscitation equip-
ment available, particularly when giving
I.V.
▼ **Incompatibilities:** Nafcillin, ketorolac.
I.M.
● Document injection site.
● Store vial in carton to protect from light.
Subcutaneous
● Document injection site.
● Store vial in carton to protect from light.

ACTION
Unknown. Binds with opioid receptors in
the CNS, altering perception of and emotional response to pain.

Route	Onset	Peak	Duration
I.V.	2–3 min	30 min	3–6 hr
I.M.	15 min	1 hr	3–6 hr
Subcut.	15 min	Unknown	3–6 hr

Half-life: 5 hours.

ADVERSE REACTIONS
CNS: dizziness, headache, sedation,
vertigo.
CV: *bradycardia.*
EENT: dry mouth.
GI: nausea, vomiting.
Respiratory: *respiratory depression.*
Skin: clamminess, diaphoresis.

INTERACTIONS
Drug-drug. *CNS depressants, general
anesthetics, hypnotics, MAO inhibitors,
sedatives, tranquilizers, TCAs:* May cause
respiratory depression, hypertension, profound sedation, or coma. Use together with
caution, and monitor patient response.
Opioid analgesics: May decrease analgesic
effect. Avoid using together.

🕑 *Alert:* Serotonergic drugs (amoxapine,
antiemetics [dolasetron, granisetron, ondansetron, palonosetron], antimigraine
drugs, buspirone, cyclobenzaprine, dextromethorphan, linezolid, lithium, MAO
inhibitors, maprotiline, methylene blue,
mirtazapine, nefazodone, SNRIs, SSRIs,
TCAs, trazodone, tryptophan, vilazodone):
May increase risk of serotonin syndrome.
Use together cautiously. Monitor patient for
serotonin syndrome.
Drug-lifestyle. *Alcohol use:* May cause
additive effects. Discourage use together.
🕑 *Alert:* St. John's wort: May increase
risk of serotonin syndrome. Use together
cautiously. Monitor patient for serotonin
syndrome. ∎

EFFECTS ON LAB TEST RESULTS
None reported.

CONTRAINDICATIONS & CAUTIONS
● Contraindicated in patients hypersensitive
to drug.
● Use cautiously and at low doses in patients
with preexisting respiratory compromise.
🕑 *Alert:* Drug should only be administered
as a supplement to general anesthesia by
those specifically trained in the use of I.V.
anesthetics and management of respiratory effects of potent opioids. Naloxone
hydrochloride and emergency resuscitative
equipment should be readily available.
🕑 *Alert:* Patients are at increased risk for
oversedation and respiratory depression if
they snore or have a history of sleep apnea,
haven't used opioids recently or are first-
time opioid users, have increased opioid
dosage requirements or opioid habituation,
have received general anesthesia for longer
lengths of time or received other sedating drugs, have preexisting pulmonary or
cardiac disease, or have thoracic or other
surgical incisions that may impair breathing.
Monitor patients carefully.
🕑 *Alert:* Drug may lead to a rare but serious
decrease in adrenal gland cortisol production.
🕑 *Alert:* Drug may cause decreased sex
hormone levels with long-term use.
● Use cautiously in patients with history of
drug abuse and in those with emotional
instability, head injury, increased ICP,

N

impaired ventilation, MI accompanied by nausea and vomiting, upcoming biliary surgery, or hepatic, renal, or adrenal insufficiency.

● Drug may cause mood disorders and osteoporosis.

❂ **Alert:** Certain commercial preparations contain sodium metabisulfite.

Dialyzable drug: Unknown.

⚠ **Overdose S&S:** Sleepiness, mild dysphoria.

PREGNANCY-LACTATION-REPRODUCTION

● There are no adequate studies in pregnant women. Use only if clearly needed.

Black Box Warning Prolonged use of drug during pregnancy can result in neonatal withdrawal syndrome, which may be life-threatening and which requires management according to neonatology expert protocols. ■

● Use cautiously in breast-feeding women.

● Long-term opioid use can cause secondary hypogonadism, infertility, and sexual dysfunction.

NURSING CONSIDERATIONS

● Reassess patient's level of pain at least 15 and 30 minutes after parenteral administration.

❂ **Alert:** Carefully monitor vital signs, pain level, respiratory status, and sedation level in all patients receiving opioids, especially those receiving I.V. drugs, even those given postoperatively.

Black Box Warning Drug can cause life-threatening or fatal respiratory depression. Monitor patient for respiratory depression, especially at start of therapy and after dosage increase. ■

Black Box Warning Before starting drug, assess patient's risk of opioid abuse, misuse, and addiction. Regularly monitor patients for development of these behaviors or conditions. ■

❂ **Alert:** If patient is taking opioids with serotonergic drugs, watch for signs and symptoms of serotonin syndrome (agitation, hallucinations, rapid HR, fever, excessive sweating, shivering or shaking, muscle twitching or stiffness, trouble with coordination, nausea, vomiting, diarrhea), especially at start of therapy and after dosage increase.

Signs and symptoms may occur within several hours of coadministration but may also occur later, especially after dosage increase. Discontinue opioid, serotonergic drug, or both if serotonin syndrome is suspected.

❂ **Alert:** Monitor patient for signs and symptoms of adrenal insufficiency (nausea, vomiting, loss of appetite, fatigue, weakness, dizziness, low BP). Perform diagnostic testing if adrenal insufficiency is suspected. If adrenal insufficiency is confirmed, treat with corticosteroids and wean patient off opioids if appropriate. Discontinue corticosteroids when clinically appropriate.

❂ **Alert:** Monitor patient for signs and symptoms of decreased sex hormone levels (low libido, erectile dysfunction, amenorrhea, infertility). If signs and symptoms occur, evaluate patient and obtain laboratory testing.

● Drug acts as an opioid antagonist and may cause withdrawal syndrome. For patients who have received long-term opioids, give 25% of the usual dose initially. Watch for signs of withdrawal.

❂ **Alert:** Drug causes respiratory depression, which at 10 mg is equal to respiratory depression produced by 10 mg of morphine.

● Monitor circulatory and respiratory status and bladder and bowel function. If respirations are shallow or rate is below 12 breaths/minute, withhold dose and notify prescriber.

● Constipation is commonly severe with maintenance therapy. Make sure stool softener or other stimulant laxative is ordered.

● Psychological and physical dependence may occur with prolonged use.

● **Look alike–sound alike:** Don't confuse Nubain with Navane.

PATIENT TEACHING

❂ **Alert:** Encourage patient to report all medications being taken, including prescription and OTC medications and supplements.

❂ **Alert:** Caution patient to immediately report signs and symptoms of serotonin syndrome, adrenal insufficiency, and decreased sex hormone levels.

● Explain assessment and monitoring process to patient and family. Instruct them to immediately report difficulty breathing or

---

other signs and symptoms of a potential adverse opioid-related reaction.
• Caution ambulatory patient about getting out of bed or walking. Warn outpatient to avoid driving and other hazardous activities that require mental alertness until drug's CNS effects are known.
• Teach patient how to manage troublesome adverse effects such as constipation.

naltrexone
nal-TREX-one

Vivitrol

naltrexone hydrochloride
ReVia

Therapeutic class: Opioid cessation drugs
Pharmacologic class: Opioid antagonists

AVAILABLE FORMS
naltrexone
Injection: 380-mg vial dose kit
naltrexone hydrochloride
Tablets: 25 mg, 50 mg, 100 mg

INDICATIONS & DOSAGES
➤ **Adjunct for maintaining opioid-free state in detoxified patients**
Adults: Initially, 25 mg P.O. If no withdrawal signs or symptoms occur within 1 hour, may start patient on 50 mg every 24 hours the following day. Or, 50 mg P.O. every weekday with a 100-mg dose on Saturday, 100 mg every other day, or 150 mg every third day. Or, 380 mg I.M. every 4 weeks or once a month.
➤ **Alcohol dependence**
Adults: 50 mg P.O. once daily for up to 12 weeks, or 380 mg I.M. in the gluteal muscle every 4 weeks or once monthly.

ADMINISTRATION
P.O.
• Keep container tightly closed and protect from light.
• Give without regard to meals; give with food if GI upset occurs.

I.M.
• Use only the diluent, needles, and other components supplied with the dose kit. Don't substitute.
• Allow drug to reach room temperature before administering.
• Administer I.M. into gluteal muscle. Avoid giving I.V., subcutaneously, or inadvertently into fatty tissue. Monitor the injection site.

ACTION
Probably reversibly blocks the effects of I.V. opioids by competitively occupying opiate receptors in the brain.

Route	Onset	Peak	Duration
P.O.	15–30 min	1 hr	24 hr
I.M.	Unknown	2–3 days	>30 days

Half-life: About 4 hours.

ADVERSE REACTIONS
CNS: insomnia, anxiety, nervousness, headache, depression, dizziness, fatigue, somnolence, syncope, low energy, irritability.
GI: nausea, diarrhea, vomiting, abdominal pain, anorexia, constipation, increased thirst.
GU: delayed ejaculation, decreased potency.
Musculoskeletal: muscle and joint pain.
Skin: injection-site reaction, rash.
Other: chills.

INTERACTIONS
Drug-drug. *Products that contain opioids:* May decrease effect of opioid. Avoid using together.
Thioridazine: May increase somnolence and lethargy. Monitor patient closely.

EFFECTS ON LAB TEST RESULTS
• May increase AST, ALT, and LDH levels.
• May increase lymphocyte count.

CONTRAINDICATIONS & CAUTIONS
• Contraindicated in patients hypersensitive to drug or dependent on opioids, those receiving opioid analgesics, those who fail the naloxone challenge test or who have a positive urine screen for opioids, or those in acute opioid withdrawal.
• Drug may precipitate opioid withdrawal.

N

• Dose-related hepatic injury is possible. Use cautiously in patients with mild hepatic disease or history of recent hepatic disease.
• Suicidal ideation and depression have been noted in postmarketing reports.
• Drug should be part of a comprehensive treatment plan that includes psychosocial support.
Dialyzable drug: Unknown.
⚠ *Overdose S&S:* Injection-site reaction, nausea, abdominal pain, somnolence, dizziness.

PREGNANCY-LACTATION-REPRODUCTION
• Use during pregnancy only if potential benefit justifies potential fetal risk.
• Drug appears in breast milk. Use cautiously in breast-feeding women.

NURSING CONSIDERATIONS
❸ *Alert:* Discontinue drug if patient develops signs or symptoms of acute hepatitis.
• Monitor patient for the development of depression or suicidal thinking.
• Don't begin treatment for opioid dependence until patient receives naloxone challenge, a test of opioid dependence. If signs and symptoms of opioid withdrawal persist after naloxone challenge, don't give drug.
• Patient must be completely free from opioids before taking naltrexone or severe withdrawal symptoms may occur. Patients who have been addicted to short-acting opioids, such as heroin and meperidine, must wait at least 7 days after last opioid dose before starting drug. Patients who have been addicted to longer-acting opioids such as methadone should wait at least 10 days.
• In an emergency, patient may be given an opioid analgesic, but dose must be higher than usual to overcome naltrexone's effect. Watch for respiratory depression from the opioid; it may be longer and deeper.
• For patients expected to be noncompliant because of history of opioid dependence, use a flexible maintenance-dose regimen of 100 mg on Monday and Wednesday and 150 mg on Friday.
• Monitor patient for an injection-site reaction, including pain, tenderness, swelling, erythema, bruising, or pruritus. In some cases, an injection-site reaction may be very severe, with induration, cellulitis, hematoma, abscess, sterile abscess, and necrosis.
• Use drug only as part of a comprehensive rehabilitation program.
• *Look alike–sound alike:* Don't confuse naltrexone with naloxone.

PATIENT TEACHING
• Advise patient to carry medical identification and to tell medical personnel that he takes naltrexone.
• Tell patient that drug can block the effects of opioids and opioid-like drugs, including heroin, pain medicine, antidiarrheals, or cough medicine.
❸ *Alert:* Warn patient if he uses large doses of heroin or any other opioid that serious injury, coma, or death can occur.
• Advise patient who previously used opioids that he may be more sensitive to lower doses of opioids once naltrexone therapy is stopped.
• Warn patient of risk of hepatic injury and tell him to seek medical attention if signs or symptoms of acute hepatitis occur.
❸ *Alert:* Tell caregiver of alcohol-dependent patient to monitor him closely for signs of depression or suicidal ideation and to report this immediately to prescriber.
• Give patient the names of nonopioid drugs that he can continue to take for pain, diarrhea, or cough.
• Tell patient to report pain, swelling, tenderness, induration, bruising, pruritus, or redness at the injection site.

naphazoline hydrochloride
naf-AZ-oh-leen

Albalon♣ ◇, All Clear ◇, Clear Eyes ◇, Naphcon-A ◇, Naphcon Forte♣ ◇

Therapeutic class: Vasoconstrictors
Pharmacologic class:
Sympathomimetics

AVAILABLE FORMS
Ophthalmic solution: 0.012% ◇, 0.03% ◇, 0.1%, 0.5%♣

INDICATIONS & DOSAGES
➤ **Ocular congestion, irritation, itching**
Adults: Instill 1 or 2 drops into the conjunctival sac of affected eye(s) every 3 to 4 hours as needed (0.1% solution), or up to q.i.d. (0.012%, 0.03% solution).

ADMINISTRATION
Ophthalmic
● Store drug in tightly closed container.

ACTION
Thought to cause vasoconstriction by local adrenergic action on blood vessels of conjunctiva.

Route	Onset	Peak	Duration
Ophthalmic	10 min	Unknown	2–6 hr

Half-life: Unknown.

ADVERSE REACTIONS
CNS: dizziness, headache, nervousness, weakness.
EENT: blurred vision, eye irritation, increased IOP, keratitis, lacrimation, photophobia, pupillary dilation, transient eye stinging.
GI: nausea.
Skin: diaphoresis.

INTERACTIONS
Drug-drug. *Anesthetics:* Cyclopropane and halothane may sensitize the myocardium to sympathomimetics; local anesthetics may increase the absorption of topical drugs. Monitor patient for increased adverse effects.
Beta blockers: May cause more systemic adverse effects. Monitor patient for adverse systemic effects.
MAO inhibitors, maprotiline, TCAs: May cause hypertensive crisis if naphazoline is systemically absorbed. Use together cautiously.

EFFECTS ON LAB TEST RESULTS
None reported.

CONTRAINDICATIONS & CAUTIONS
● Contraindicated in patients hypersensitive to drug's ingredients and in those with acute angle-closure glaucoma.

● Use cautiously in patients with hyperthyroidism, cardiac disease, hypertension, or diabetes mellitus.
● Safety and effectiveness in children haven't been established.
● Accidental ingestion by children of OTC imidazoline derivative eyedrops and nasal sprays, even in small amounts (1 to 2 mL), may cause serious harm.
Dialyzable drug: Unknown.

PREGNANCY-LACTATION-REPRODUCTION
● Use during pregnancy only if clearly needed.
● It isn't known if drug appears in breast milk. Use cautiously in breast-feeding women.

NURSING CONSIDERATIONS
● Drug is most widely used ocular decongestant.
● Rebound congestion and conjunctivitis may occur with frequent or prolonged use.

PATIENT TEACHING
● Teach patient how to instill drug. Advise him to wash hands before and after instillation and to apply light finger pressure on lacrimal sac for 1 minute after drops are instilled. Warn him not to touch tip of dropper to eye or surrounding tissue.
● Warn patient not to exceed recommended dosage to avoid rebound congestion and conjunctivitis.
● Tell patient to notify prescriber if sun sensitivity, blurred vision, pain, or lid swelling develops.
● Advise patient to keep drug out of the reach of children and to immediately contact a poison control center and seek emergency medical care if accidental ingestion occurs.
● Instruct patient not to use OTC preparations for longer than 72 hours without consulting prescriber.

N

naproxen
na-PROX-en

EC-Naprosyn, Naprosyn✒,
Naproxen-EC✤

naproxen sodium
Aleve ◊, Anaprox, Anaprox DS, Apo-
Napro-Na✤, Flanax Pain Relief ◊,
Maxidol✤, Mediproxen ◊, Motrimax,
Naprelan, Pamprin All Day Relief ◊

Therapeutic class: NSAIDs
Pharmacologic class: NSAIDs

AVAILABLE FORMS
naproxen
Oral suspension: 125 mg/5 mL
Tablets: 250 mg, 375 mg, 500 mg
Tablets (delayed-release) ⓒ: 375 mg,
500 mg
naproxen sodium
Capsules: 105 mg✤ ◊, 200 mg ◊,
220 mg✤ ◊
Tablets (extended-release) ⓒ: 375 mg,
500 mg, 750 mg
Tablets (film-coated) ⓒ: 220 mg ◊, 275 mg,
550 mg
Note: 275 mg of naproxen sodium contains
250 mg of naproxen

INDICATIONS & DOSAGES
Adjust-a-dose (for all indications): Consider
lower dosage in elderly patients and patients
with renal or hepatic impairment. Not recommended for patients with moderate to
severe renal impairment (CrCl less than
30 mL/minute).
➤ **Acute gout**
Adults: 750 mg naproxen P.O.; then
250 mg every 8 hours until attack subsides.
Or, 825 mg naproxen sodium P.O.; then
275 mg every 8 hours until attack subsides.
Or, 1,000 to 1,500 mg extended-release
tablets P.O. on day 1, followed by 1,000 mg
daily until attack subsides.
➤ **Acute tendinitis, bursitis, pain,
primary dysmenorrhea**
Adults: 550 mg naproxen sodium P.O., then
550 mg P.O. every 12 hours or 275 mg every
6 to 8 hours. Initial total daily dose shouldn't
exceed 1,375 mg; thereafter, total daily dose

shouldn't exceed 1,100 mg. Or, 500 mg
naproxen P.O. followed by 500 mg P.O.
every 12 hours or 250 mg P.O. every 6 to
8 hours. Or, 1,000 mg extended-release
tablets P.O. once daily for a limited time.
➤ **Ankylosing spondylitis, osteoarthritis,
RA**
Adults: 275 to 550 mg naproxen sodium
P.O. b.i.d. Or, 250 to 500 mg naproxen tablet
or suspension P.O. b.i.d. Or, 375 or 500 mg
naproxen delayed-release tablet P.O. b.i.d.
Or, 750 to 1,000 mg extended-release
tablets P.O. once daily. During long-term
administration, the dose of naproxen may
be adjusted up or down depending on patient's clinical response. In patients who
tolerate lower doses well, the dose may be
increased to 1,500 mg/day when a higher
level of anti-inflammatory/analgesic activity
is required.
➤ **Juvenile arthritis**
Children age 2 and older: 10 mg/kg
naproxen suspension P.O. daily given in two
divided doses. Don't exceed 15 mg/kg/day.

ADMINISTRATION
P.O.
• Give drug with food or milk to minimize
GI upset. Have patient drink a full glass of
water or other liquid with each dose.
• Shake suspension well.
• Make sure patient swallows delayed-
release, extended-release, and film-coated
tablets whole and doesn't break, crush, or
chew them.

ACTION
May inhibit prostaglandin synthesis to
produce anti-inflammatory, analgesic, and
antipyretic effects.

Route	Onset	Peak	Duration
P.O. (immediate-release)	1 hr	2–4 hr	7 hr
P.O. (delayed-release)	1 hr	4–24 hr	<21 hr
P.O. (suspension)	1 hr	1–4 hr	<12 hr

Half-life: 10 to 21 hours.

ADVERSE REACTIONS
CNS: dizziness, drowsiness, headache,
vertigo.
CV: edema, palpitations.

EENT: tinnitus, auditory disturbances, visual disturbances.
GI: abdominal pain, constipation, diarrhea, dyspepsia, epigastric pain, heartburn, nausea, occult blood loss, peptic ulceration, stomatitis, thirst.
Hematologic: ecchymoses, increased bleeding time.
Respiratory: dyspnea.
Skin: diaphoresis, pruritus, purpura.

INTERACTIONS

Drug-drug. *ACE inhibitors:* May cause renal impairment. Use together cautiously.
Antihypertensives, diuretics: May decrease effect of these drugs. Monitor patient closely.
Aspirin, corticosteroids: May cause adverse GI reactions. Avoid using together.
Digoxin: May increase serum digoxin level. Monitor levels.
Lithium: May increase lithium level. Observe patient for toxicity and monitor level. Adjustment of lithium dosage may be required.
Loop diuretics, thiazide diuretics: May reduce diuretic effects. Monitor patient and consider therapy modification.
Methotrexate: May cause toxicity. Monitor patient closely.
Oral anticoagulants, NSAIDs, SSRIs, other sulfonylureas, highly protein-bound drugs: May cause toxicity. Monitor patient closely.
Potassium-sparing diuretics: May reduce antihypertensive effects and enhance hyperkalemic effects. Monitor patient closely.
Probenecid: May decrease elimination of naproxen. Monitor patient for toxicity.
Drug-herb. *Alfalfa, anise, bilberry, dong quai, feverfew, garlic, ginger, ginkgo, horse chestnut, licorice, red clover:* May cause bleeding, based on the known effects of components. Discourage use together.
White willow: Herb and drug contain similar components. Discourage use together.
Drug-lifestyle. *Alcohol use:* May cause GI irritation. Discourage use together.

EFFECTS ON LAB TEST RESULTS

● May increase BUN, creatinine, ALT, AST, and potassium levels.
● May increase bleeding time.

● May interfere with urinary 5-hydroxy-indoleacetic acid and 17-hydroxycorticosteroid determinations.

CONTRAINDICATIONS & CAUTIONS

● Contraindicated in patients hypersensitive to drug and in those with the syndrome of aspirin-sensitive asthma, rhinitis, and nasal polyps.
● Drug can cause serious skin reactions (Stevens-Johnson syndrome, toxic epidermal necrolysis). Stop drug at first sign of rash or hypersensitivity.
Black Box Warning Naproxen is contraindicated for the treatment of perioperative pain after CABG surgery. ■
● Use cautiously in elderly patients and in patients with hypertension, hyperkalemia, renal disease, CV disease, GI disorders, hepatic disease, or history of peptic ulcer disease.
● Drug may increase risk of aseptic meningitis, especially in patients with lupus and mixed connective tissue disorders.
Dialyzable drug: No.
⚠ Overdose S&S: Drowsiness, heartburn, indigestion, nausea, vomiting, seizures.

PREGNANCY-LACTATION-REPRODUCTION

● Drug shouldn't be used in pregnant women, especially during last trimester, as closure of the ductus arteriosus can occur.
● Avoid use in breast-feeding women.

NURSING CONSIDERATIONS

● Because NSAIDs impair synthesis of renal prostaglandins, they can decrease renal blood flow and lead to reversible renal impairment, especially in patients with renal failure, HF, or liver dysfunction; in elderly patients; and in those taking diuretics. Monitor these patients closely.
● Monitor CBC and renal and hepatic function every 4 to 6 months during long-term therapy.
● Monitor patient for neurologic effects (drowsiness, dizziness, blurred vision), which may impair physical or mental abilities.
⚡ Alert: Watch for and immediately evaluate signs and symptoms of heart attack (chest pain, shortness of breath or trouble

breathing) or stroke (weakness in one part or side of the body, slurred speech).

Black Box Warning NSAIDs cause an increased risk of serious GI adverse events, including bleeding, ulceration, and perforation of the stomach or intestines, which can be fatal. Elderly patients are at greater risk. ■

Black Box Warning NSAIDs may increase the risk of serious thrombotic events, MI, or stroke, which can be fatal. The risk may be greater with longer use or in patients with CV disease or risk factors for CV disease. ■

• Because of their antipyretic and anti-inflammatory actions, NSAIDs may mask signs and symptoms of infection.

• Drug may prolong bleeding time and anemias can occur.

PATIENT TEACHING

◑ **Alert:** Drug is available without prescription (naproxen sodium, 220 mg). Instruct adult not to take more than 440 mg of naproxen sodium in any 8- to 12-hour period or 660 mg of naproxen sodium in a 24-hour period.

• Advise patient to take drug with food or milk to minimize GI upset. Tell him to drink a full glass of water or other liquid with each dose.

• Tell patient taking prescription doses for arthritis that full therapeutic effect may be delayed 2 to 4 weeks.

• Warn patient against taking naproxen and naproxen sodium at the same time.

◑ **Alert:** Advise patient to seek medical attention immediately if chest pain, shortness of breath or trouble breathing, weakness in one part or side of the body, or slurred speech occurs.

• Teach patient signs and symptoms of GI bleeding, including blood in vomit, urine, or stool; coffee-ground vomit; and black, tarry stools. Tell him to notify prescriber immediately if any of these occurs.

• Caution patient that use with aspirin, alcohol, other NSAIDs, or corticosteroids may increase risk of adverse GI reactions.

• Warn patient against hazardous activities that require mental alertness until CNS effects are known.

---

naratriptan hydrochloride
nar-ah-TRIP-tan

Amerge

Therapeutic class: Antimigraine drugs
Pharmacologic class: Serotonin 5-HT$_1$ receptor agonists

AVAILABLE FORMS
Tablets ⓞⓝⓔ: 1 mg, 2.5 mg

INDICATIONS & DOSAGES
➤ **Acute migraine attacks with or without aura**
Adults: 1 or 2.5 mg P.O. as a single dose. If headache returns or responds only partially, dose may be repeated after 4 hours. Maximum, 5 mg in 24 hours.
Adjust-a-dose: For patients with mild to moderate renal or hepatic impairment, reduce dosage. Maximum, 2.5 mg in 24 hours; a 1-mg starting dose is recommended.

ADMINISTRATION
P.O.
• Give drug with fluid without regard for food.
• Give drug whole; don't split or crush tablet.

ACTION
May act as an agonist at serotonin receptors on extracerebral intracranial blood vessels, which constricts the affected vessels, inhibits neuropeptide release, and reduces pain transmission in the trigeminal pathways.

Route	Onset	Peak	Duration
P.O.	Unknown	2–3 hr	Unknown

Half-life: 6 hours.

ADVERSE REACTIONS
CNS: paresthesia, dizziness, drowsiness, malaise, fatigue, vertigo, pain.
CV: *tachyarrhythmias,* abnormal ECG changes, palpitations, hypertension.
EENT: ear, nose, and throat infections; photophobia.
GI: nausea, hyposalivation, vomiting.

Reactions in bold italics are *life-threatening*. Interactions may have a *rapid onset* or a *delayed onset*.

Other: sensations of warmth, cold, pressure, tightness, or heaviness.

INTERACTIONS
Drug-drug. *Drugs that prolong QT interval (antiarrhythmics, arsenic trioxide, chlorpromazine, dolasetron, droperidol, mefloquine, mesoridazine, moxifloxacin, pentamidine, pimozide, tacrolimus, thioridazine, ziprasidone):* May cause an additive effect and prolong QT interval. Monitor patient closely.
Ergot-containing or ergot-type drugs (dihydroergotamine, methysergide), other 5-HT$_1$ agonists: May prolong vasospastic reactions. Avoid using within 24 hours of naratriptan.
Hormonal contraceptives: May slightly increase naratriptan level. Monitor patient.
MAO inhibitors: May decrease metabolic elimination of naratriptan. Don't use together.
SSRIs (fluoxetine, fluvoxamine, paroxetine, sertraline): May cause weakness, hyperreflexia, and incoordination. Monitor patient.
Drug-herb. *St. John's wort:* May increase serotonergic effect. Discourage use together.
Drug-lifestyle. *Smoking:* May increase naratriptan clearance. Discourage smoking.

EFFECTS ON LAB TEST RESULTS
None reported.

CONTRAINDICATIONS & CAUTIONS
• Contraindicated in patients hypersensitive to drug or its components and in those with prior or current cardiac ischemia, vasospastic CAD, arrhythmias associated with accessory conduction pathways, cerebrovascular (stroke, TIA) or peripheral vascular syndromes, hemiplegic or basilar migraines, ischemic bowel disease, or uncontrolled hypertension.
• Contraindicated in elderly patients, patients with severe renal impairment (CrCl less than 15 mL/minute), patients with severe hepatic impairment (Child-Pugh class C), and patients who have used ergot-containing, ergot-type, or other 5-HT$_1$ agonists within 24 hours.
⚠ *Alert:* Coronary artery spasm, transient ischemia, MI, ventricular tachycardia,

and ventricular fibrillation and death have been reported within a few hours of administration. Discontinue drug if these occur. If signs or symptoms of angina occur after dose, evaluate patient for CAD or Prinzmetal angina before additional doses are given and monitor ECG.
• Use cautiously in patients with risk factors for CAD, such as hypertension, hypercholesterolemia, obesity, diabetes, smoking, strong family history of CAD, and postmenopausal women, and men older than age 40, unless patient is free from cardiac disease. Monitor patient closely after first dose.
• Use cautiously in patients with renal or hepatic impairment.
• Safety and effectiveness when treating cluster headaches or more than four headaches in a 30-day period haven't been established.
Dialyzable drug: Unknown.
⚠ *Overdose S&S:* Chest pain, ischemic ECG changes.

PREGNANCY-LACTATION-REPRODUCTION
• There are no adequate studies in pregnant women. Use only if potential benefit justifies potential risk to the fetus.
• Patient should discontinue breast-feeding or discontinue drug.

NURSING CONSIDERATIONS
• Assess cardiac status in patients who develop risk factors for CAD.
⚠ *Alert:* Drug can cause coronary artery vasospasm and increased risk of cerebrovascular events.
• Drug isn't intended to prevent migraines or manage hemiplegic or basilar migraine.
• Use drug only when patient has a clear diagnosis of migraine.
⚠ *Alert:* Combining drug with an SSRI or an SSNRI may cause serotonin syndrome. Symptoms include restlessness, hallucinations, loss of coordination, fast heartbeat, rapid changes in BP, increased body temperature, hyperreflexia, nausea, vomiting, and diarrhea. Serotonin syndrome is more likely to occur when starting or increasing the dose of naratriptan, the SSRI, or the SSNRI.
• *Look alike–sound alike:* Don't confuse Amerge with Altace or Amaryl.

N

PATIENT TEACHING

• Instruct patient to take drug only as prescribed and to read the accompanying patient instruction leaflet before using drug.

• Tell patient that drug is intended to relieve, not prevent, migraines.

• Instruct patient to take dose soon after headache starts. If no response occurs with first tablet, tell him to seek medical approval before taking second tablet. Tell patient that if more relief is needed after first tablet (if a partial response occurs or headache returns), and prescriber has approved a second dose, he may take a second tablet (but not sooner than 4 hours after first tablet). Tell him not to exceed 2 tablets within 24 hours.

• Advise patient to increase fluid intake.

• Advise patient not to use drug if she suspects or knows that she's pregnant.

• Tell patient to alert prescriber about bothersome adverse effects.

• Tell patient to swallow tablet whole, and not to split, crush, or chew tablet.

---

natalizumab
nah-tah-LIZ-yoo-mab

Tysabri

Therapeutic class: Immunomodulators
Pharmacologic class: Monoclonal antibodies

AVAILABLE FORMS
Injection: 300 mg/15 mL single-use vials

INDICATIONS & DOSAGES
➤ **To slow the accumulation of physical disabilities and reduce the frequency of clinical exacerbations in relapsing forms of MS for patients who failed to respond or were unable to tolerate other therapies; moderate to severe Crohn disease in patients with inadequate response or intolerance to conventional therapy**
Adults: 300 mg I.V. over 1 hour every 4 weeks.

ADMINISTRATION
I.V.
▼ Dilute 300 mg in 100 mL NSS.
▼ Invert I.V. bag gently to mix solution; don't shake.

▼ Infuse over 1 hour; don't give by I.V. push or bolus.
▼ Flush I.V. line with NSS after infusion is complete.
▼ Refrigerate solution and use within 8 hours if not used immediately. Protect from light.
▼ **Incompatibilities:** Don't mix or infuse with other drugs. Don't use any diluent other than NSS.

ACTION
May block interaction between adhesion molecules on inflammatory cells and receptors on endothelial cells of vessel walls.

Route	Onset	Peak	Duration
I.V.	Unknown	Unknown	Unknown

Half-life: 3 to 17 days.

ADVERSE REACTIONS
CNS: *progressive multifocal leukoencephalopathy (PML),* depression, fatigue, headache, somnolence, vertigo.
CV: chest discomfort, peripheral edema.
EENT: tonsillitis.
GI: abdominal discomfort, diarrhea, gastroenteritis, nausea.
GU: UTI, vaginitis, amenorrhea, dysmenorrhea, irregular menstruation, urinary frequency, urinary urgency, ovarian cyst.
Metabolic: weight increase or decrease.
Musculoskeletal: arthralgia, extremity pain, muscle cramps, swollen joints.
Respiratory: upper and lower respiratory tract infection.
Skin: rash, dermatitis, pruritus, urticaria, night sweats.
Other: hypersensitivity reaction, infusion-related reaction, tooth infections, herpes infection, rigors, seasonal allergy, cholelithiasis.

INTERACTIONS
Drug-drug. *Corticosteroids, immunosuppressants, TNF inhibitors:* May increase risk of infection. Avoid using together.
Live-virus vaccines: May cause reduced effectiveness of the vaccine. Defer vaccine administration until immune function has returned.

Reactions in bold italics are *life-threatening*. Interactions may have a *rapid onset* or a **delayed onset**.

Drug-herb. *Echinacea:* May decrease effectiveness of natalizumab. Consider therapy modification.

EFFECTS ON LAB TEST RESULTS
• May increase LFT values and lymphocyte, monocyte, eosinophil, basophil, and nucleated RBC counts.
• May cause transient decrease in Hb level.

CONTRAINDICATIONS & CAUTIONS
• Contraindicated in patients hypersensitive to drug or its components or in those with current or history of PML. Use with other immunosuppressants or TNF-α inhibitors isn't recommended.

Black Box Warning Patients who test positively for anti-JC virus antibodies are at increased risk for developing PML. Consider testing for anti-JC virus antibodies before or during treatment if antibody status is unknown. Use drug cautiously in patients who are anti-JC virus antibody-positive and especially in those with one or more additional PML risk factors. ■

• Safety and effectiveness in patients with chronic progressive MS haven't been established.
Dialyzable drug: Unknown.

PREGNANCY-LACTATION-REPRODUCTION
• Use in pregnancy only if benefit justifies potential risk to the fetus.
• Drug appears in breast milk. Effects on infants are unknown.

NURSING CONSIDERATIONS
Black Box Warning Only prescribers registered in the TOUCH Prescribing Program may prescribe drug. Contact the TOUCH Prescribing Program at 1-800-456-2255. ■
• Report serious opportunistic and atypical infections to Biogen Idec at 1-800-456-2255 and to the FDA's MedWatch Program at 1-800-FDA-1088.
• The safety and effectiveness of natalizumab treatment beyond 2 years are unknown.
Black Box Warning Drug may cause PML. Withhold drug immediately at the first signs or symptoms suggestive of PML. Symptoms include clumsiness; progressive weakness;

and visual, speech, and sometimes personality changes. Gadolinium-enhanced MRI and CSF analysis for JC viral DNA are recommended for diagnosis. ■

Black Box Warning Risk of PML increases with duration of therapy, number of infusions, prior use of immunosuppressants, and presence of anti–JC virus antibodies. Consider these factors in the context of expected benefit when initiating and continuing treatment. ■

• Obtain a brain MRI scan before starting therapy.
🜚 *Alert:* Watch for evidence of hypersensitivity reaction during and for 1 hour after infusion, which may include dizziness, urticaria, fever, rash, rigors, pruritus, nausea, flushing, hypotension, dyspnea, and chest pain.
• If hypersensitivity reaction occurs, stop drug and notify prescriber.
🜚 *Alert:* Drug increases risk of developing encephalitis and meningitis caused by herpes simplex and varicella zoster viruses. Monitor patient for signs and symptoms of these conditions. Discontinue drug if either occurs and initiate appropriate treatment.
• Patients who develop antibodies to drug have an increased risk of infusion-related reaction.
• Discontinue drug in patients with jaundice or other evidence of significant liver injury. Elevated serum hepatic enzymes and elevated total bilirubin levels may occur as early as 6 days after the first dose.

PATIENT TEACHING
• Inform patient that he must be enrolled in and comply with the TOUCH program.
• Tell patient to read the "Medication Guide for Tysabri" before each infusion.
• Urge patient to immediately report progressively worsening symptoms persisting over several days, including changes in thinking, eyesight, balance, or strength.
• Advise patient to inform all health care providers caring for him that he's receiving this drug.
• Tell patient to schedule follow-up appointments with prescriber at 3 and 6 months after the first infusion, then at least every 6 months thereafter.

N

• Urge patient to immediately report rash, hives, dizziness, fever, shaking chills, or itching while drug is infusing or up to 1 hour afterward.
• Tell patient about the potential for liver injury.

SAFETY ALERT!

nateglinide
nah-TEG-lah-nyde

Starlix

Therapeutic class: Antidiabetics
Pharmacologic class: Meglitinide derivatives

AVAILABLE FORMS
Tablets: 60 mg, 120 mg

INDICATIONS & DOSAGES
➤ **Type 2 diabetes, as monotherapy, or with metformin or a thiazolidinedione**
Adults: 120 mg P.O. t.i.d. taken 1 to 30 minutes before meals. Patients near goal HbA$_{1c}$ level when treatment is started may receive 60 mg P.O. t.i.d.

ADMINISTRATION
P.O.
• Give drug 1 to 30 minutes before a meal.
• If a meal is skipped, dose should be skipped to reduce risk of hypoglycemia.

ACTION
Lowers glucose level by stimulating insulin secretion from pancreatic beta cells.

Route	Onset	Peak	Duration
P.O.	20 min	1 hr	4 hr

Half-life: About 1½ hours.

ADVERSE REACTIONS
CNS: dizziness.
GI: diarrhea.
Metabolic: *hypoglycemia.*
Musculoskeletal: back pain, arthropathy.
Respiratory: URI, bronchitis, coughing.
Other: flulike symptoms, accidental trauma.

INTERACTIONS
Drug-drug. *Corticosteroids, rifamycins, sympathomimetics, thiazides, thyroid products:* May reduce hypoglycemic action of nateglinide. Monitor glucose level closely.
MAO inhibitors, nonselective beta blockers, NSAIDs, salicylates: May increase hypoglycemic action of nateglinide. Monitor glucose level closely.

EFFECTS ON LAB TEST RESULTS
• May increase uric acid level.

CONTRAINDICATIONS & CAUTIONS
• Contraindicated in patients hypersensitive to drug and in those with type 1 diabetes or diabetic ketoacidosis.
• Use cautiously in patients with moderate to severe liver dysfunction or adrenal or pituitary insufficiency, and in elderly and malnourished patients.
• Safety and effectiveness in children haven't been established.
Dialyzable drug: Yes.
⚠ **Overdose S&S:** Hypoglycemic symptoms.

PREGNANCY-LACTATION-REPRODUCTION
• Drug shouldn't be used in pregnant or breast-feeding women.

NURSING CONSIDERATIONS
• Don't use with glyburide or other oral antidiabetics; may use with metformin or a thiazolidinedione.
• Monitor glucose level regularly to evaluate drug's effectiveness.
• Observe patient for signs and symptoms of hypoglycemia. To minimize risk of hypoglycemia, make sure that patient has a meal immediately after dose. If hypoglycemia occurs and patient remains conscious, give him an oral form of glucose. If he's unconscious, treat with I.V. glucose.
• Risk of hypoglycemia increases with strenuous exercise, alcohol ingestion, or insufficient caloric intake.
• Symptoms of hypoglycemia may be masked in patients with autonomic neuropathy and in those who use beta blockers.
• Insulin therapy may be needed for glycemic control in patients with fever, infection, or trauma and in those undergoing surgery.

Reactions in bold italics are *life-threatening*. Interactions may have a *rapid onset* or a *delayed onset*.

- Monitor glucose level closely when other drugs are started or stopped, to detect possible drug interactions.
- Periodically monitor HbA$_{1c}$ level.
- Drug's effectiveness may decrease over time.
- Usually, no special dosage adjustments are necessary in elderly patients, but some elderly patients may have greater sensitivity to glucose-lowering effect.

PATIENT TEACHING
- Tell patient to take drug 1 to 30 minutes before a meal.
- Advise patient to skip the scheduled dose if he skips a meal to reduce risk of hypoglycemia.
- Instruct patient on risk of hypoglycemia, its signs and symptoms (sweating, rapid pulse, trembling, confusion, headache, irritability, and nausea), and ways to treat these symptoms by eating or drinking something containing sugar.
- Teach patient how to monitor and log glucose levels to evaluate diabetes control.
- Advise patient to notify prescriber for persistent low or high glucose level.
- Instruct patient to adhere to prescribed diet and exercise regimen.
- Explain possible long-term complications of diabetes and importance of regular preventive therapy.
- Encourage patient to wear a medical identification bracelet.
- Inform patient of potential drug-drug interactions with nateglinide.

nebivolol hydrochloride
neh-BIH-voh-lawl

Bystolic✔

Therapeutic class: Antihypertensives
Pharmacologic class: Beta blockers

AVAILABLE FORMS
Tablets: 2.5 mg, 5 mg, 10 mg, 20 mg

INDICATIONS & DOSAGES
➤ **Hypertension**
Adults: Initially, 5 mg P.O. once daily. Increase at 2-week intervals to a maximum dose of 40 mg, if needed.

Adjust-a-dose: For patients with severe renal impairment (CrCl less than 30 mL/minute) or moderate hepatic impairment, start with 2.5 mg P.O. once daily. Increase dose cautiously, if needed.

ADMINISTRATION
P.O.
- May give drug without regard to food.

ACTION
Selectively blocks beta$_1$-adrenergic receptors, reducing HR, myocardial contractility, and sympathetic tone. Nebivolol also reduces BP by suppressing renin activity and decreasing peripheral vascular resistance.

Route	Onset	Peak	Duration
P.O.	Unknown	1½–4 hr	Unknown

Half-life: 12 to 19 hours.

ADVERSE REACTIONS
CNS: asthenia, dizziness, fatigue, headache, insomnia, paresthesia.
CV: *bradycardia,* chest pain, peripheral edema.
GI: abdominal pain, diarrhea, nausea.
Metabolic: hypercholesterolemia, hyperuricemia.
Respiratory: dyspnea.
Skin: rash.

INTERACTIONS
Drug-drug. *Alpha$_1$ blockers:* May enhance severity and duration of hypotension. A smaller starting dose of alpha$_1$ blocker may be necessary.
Antidiabetic agents (insulin, sulfonylureas): May mask signs of hypoglycemia. Monitor blood glucose level.
Beta agonists (dobutamine, isoproterenol): May reverse nebivolol effects or cause protracted, severe hypotension. Avoid concomitant use.
Beta blockers (atenolol, nadolol): May increase synergistic activity and bradycardia. Don't use together.
Catecholamine-depleting drugs (such as guanethidine, reserpine): May cause bradycardia or severe hypotension. Monitor patient closely.

N

Clonidine: May cause further decrease in BP. Simultaneous withdrawal may cause life-threatening rebound hypertension. Discontinue nebivolol for several days before gradual tapering of clonidine.

CYP2D6 inhibitors (fluoxetine, paroxetine, propafenone, quinidine): May increase nebivolol level. Monitor BP closely, and adjust nebivolol dose as needed.

Digoxin, diltiazem, disopyramide, verapamil: May increase the risk of bradycardia. Monitor patient's ECG and vital signs.

Fingolimod: May increase risk of bradycardia. Monitor patient closely.

Mefloquine: May cause CV toxicity. Consider an alternative drug.

NSAIDs: May decrease antihypertensive effect. Monitor BP; adjust nebivolol dosage as needed.

EFFECTS ON LAB TEST RESULTS
- May increase BUN, uric acid, and triglyceride levels. May decrease HDL and cholesterol levels.
- May decrease platelet count.

CONTRAINDICATIONS & CAUTIONS
- Contraindicated in patients hypersensitive to drug and in those with decompensated HF, severe bradycardia, second- or third-degree AV block, sick sinus syndrome (unless a permanent pacemaker is in place), cardiogenic shock, bronchial asthma or related bronchospastic conditions, or severe hepatic impairment (greater than Child-Pugh class B).
- Use cautiously in patients with compensated HF, in perioperative patients receiving anesthetics that depress myocardial function (such as cyclopropane and trichloroethylene), in diabetic patients receiving insulin or oral antidiabetics or subject to spontaneous hypoglycemia, in patients with severe renal impairment, and in patients with thyroid disease (use may mask hyperthyroidism and withdrawal may worsen it), pheochromocytoma, or peripheral vascular disease (may cause or worsen symptoms of arterial insufficiency).
- Don't stop drug abruptly in patients with CAD, angina, or MI as severe exacerbations and ventricular arrhythmias can occur.

- Don't withdraw drug routinely before major surgery; continue drug throughout perioperative period if possible.
- Safety and effectiveness in children haven't been established.

Dialyzable drug: Unknown.

⚠ *Overdose S&S:* Bradycardia, hypotension, cardiac failure, fatigue, dizziness, hypoglycemia, vomiting, bronchospasm, heart block.

PREGNANCY-LACTATION-REPRODUCTION
- Use drug during pregnancy only if benefit justifies potential risk to the fetus.
- Don't use drug in breast-feeding women.

NURSING CONSIDERATIONS
🔆 *Alert:* Patients with a history of severe anaphylactic reaction to several allergens may be more reactive to repeated exposure to nebivolol (accidental, diagnostic, or therapeutic), and they may not respond to amounts of epinephrine typically used to treat allergic reactions.
- Check patient's BP and HR often.
- Monitor LFTs and renal function test results.
- If nebivolol must be stopped, do so gradually over 1 to 2 weeks. If angina worsens or acute coronary syndrome occurs, restart drug promptly.
- Because beta blockers may mask tachycardia caused by hyperthyroidism, be sure to withdraw nebivolol gradually in patients with suspected thyrotoxicosis to avoid thyroid storm.
- Observe a diabetic patient closely because drug may mask evidence of hypoglycemia.
- If patient has a history of HF, watch for worsening symptoms, renal dysfunction, or fluid retention. Patient's diuretic dosage may need to be increased.
- Store drug at room temperature in a light-resistant container.

PATIENT TEACHING
- Instruct patient not to stop drug suddenly but to notify prescriber about unpleasant adverse reactions. Explain that drug must be withdrawn gradually over 1 or 2 weeks.
- Caution patient to avoid driving and other tasks requiring alertness until his response to therapy is known.

Reactions in bold italics are *life-threatening*. Interactions may have a *rapid onset* or a *delayed onset*.

- Tell patient to alert prescriber if shortness of breath occurs.
- Caution patient with diabetes or spontaneous hypoglycemia that drug may mask symptoms of low blood glucose level, especially increased HR.
- Urge female patient not to breast-feed.

necitumumab
See NEW DRUGS for information.

nelfinavir mesylate
nell-FIN-ah-veer

Viracept

Therapeutic class: Antiretrovirals
Pharmacologic class: Protease inhibitors

AVAILABLE FORMS
Tablets: 250 mg, 625 mg

INDICATIONS & DOSAGES
➤ **HIV infection**
Adults and children age 13 and older:
1,250 mg P.O. b.i.d. or 750 mg P.O. t.i.d. in combination with other antiretrovirals. Maximum dosage is 2,500 mg/day.
Children ages 2 to 12: 45 to 55 mg/kg P.O. b.i.d. or 25 to 35 mg/kg P.O. t.i.d. in combination with other antiretrovirals; don't exceed 2,500 mg/day (b.i.d. dosing) or 2,250 mg/day (t.i.d. dosing).

ADMINISTRATION
P.O.
- Give tablets with a meal.
- May dissolve tablets in a small amount of water. The cloudy liquid should then be given immediately and the glass rinsed and given to patient to ensure entire dose is consumed.

ACTION
An HIV-1 protease inhibitor, which prevents cleavage of the viral polyprotein, resulting in the production of immature, noninfectious virus.

Route	Onset	Peak	Duration
P.O.	Unknown	2–4 hr	Unknown

Half-life: 3½ to 5 hours.

ADVERSE REACTIONS
CNS: *seizures, suicidal ideation,* anxiety, asthenia, depression, dizziness, emotional lability, headache, hyperkinesia, insomnia, malaise, migraine, paresthesia, sleep disorder, somnolence.
CV: *QTc prolongation, torsades de pointes.*
GI: diarrhea, *pancreatitis,* flatulence, nausea, abdominal pain, anorexia, dyspepsia, epigastric pain, GI bleeding, mouth ulceration, pancreatitis, vomiting.
Hematologic: *leukopenia, thrombocytopenia, anemia.*
Hepatic: *hepatitis.*
Metabolic: *hypoglycemia,* dehydration, *diabetes mellitus,* hyperlipidemia, hyperuricemia.
Skin: rash, dermatitis, folliculitis, fungal dermatitis, pruritus, sweating, urticaria.
Other: redistribution or accumulation of body fat.

INTERACTIONS
Drug-drug. *Alfuzosin, amiodarone, ergot derivatives, oral midazolam, pimozide, quinidine, triazolam:* May increase levels of these drugs, causing increased risk of life-threatening adverse events. Avoid using together.
🛈 **Alert:** *Atorvastatin:* May increase statin level and risk of myopathy and rhabdomyolysis. Atorvastatin dosage shouldn't exceed 40 mg/day.
Azithromycin: May increase azithromycin level. Monitor patient for liver impairment.
Carbamazepine, phenobarbital: May reduce the effectiveness of nelfinavir. Use together cautiously.
Cyclosporine, sirolimus, tacrolimus: May increase levels of these immunosuppressants. Use together cautiously.
Delavirdine, HIV protease inhibitors (indinavir, saquinavir): May increase levels of protease inhibitors. Use together cautiously.
Didanosine: May decrease didanosine absorption. Take nelfinavir with food at least 2 hours before or 1 hour after didanosine.
Drugs that prolong QT interval: May increase risk of life-threatening cardiac arrhythmias such as torsades de pointes. Monitor patient and ECG closely.
Ethinyl estradiol: May decrease contraceptive level and effectiveness. Advise patient

N

to use alternative contraceptive measures during therapy.

✪ Alert: *Lovastatin, simvastatin:* May increase statin level and risk of myopathy and rhabdomyolysis. Use together is contraindicated.

Methadone, phenytoin: May decrease levels of these drugs. Adjust dosage of these drugs accordingly.

Rifabutin: May increase rifabutin level and decrease nelfinavir level. Reduce dosage of rifabutin to half the usual dose and increase nelfinavir to 1,250 mg b.i.d.

Rifampin: May decrease nelfinavir level. Use together is contraindicated.

Sildenafil: May increase adverse effects of sildenafil. Caution patient not to exceed 25 mg of sildenafil in a 48-hour period.

Drug-herb. *St. John's wort:* May decrease drug level. Discourage use together.

EFFECTS ON LAB TEST RESULTS

• May increase ALT, AST, alkaline phosphatase, bilirubin, GGT, amylase, CK, and lipid levels.

• May decrease Hb level. May increase or decrease glucose level.

• May decrease WBC and platelet counts.

CONTRAINDICATIONS & CAUTIONS

• Contraindicated in patients hypersensitive to drug or its components and in those with moderate or severe hepatic impairment.

• Contraindicated with drugs that are highly dependent on CYP3A for clearance (alfuzosin, amiodarone, ergot derivatives, rifampin, lovastatin, simvastatin, pimozide, quinidine, sildenafil used for pulmonary hypertension, oral midazolam, triazolam).

• Use cautiously in patients with hepatic dysfunction or hemophilia types A or B. Monitor LFT results.

Dialyzable drug: Unlikely.

PREGNANCY-LACTATION-REPRODUCTION

• Use in pregnant women only if potential benefit justifies potential risk to the fetus.

• Enroll pregnant women taking nelfinavir in the Antiretroviral Pregnancy Registry (1-800-258-4263).

• It isn't known if drug appears in breast milk. Women shouldn't breast-feed during therapy because of risk of transmitting HIV to infant.

NURSING CONSIDERATIONS

• Drug dosage is the same whether drug is used alone or with other antiretrovirals.

• Drug may cause hyperglycemia. Monitor glucose levels carefully.

• **Look alike–sound alike:** Don't confuse nelfinavir with nevirapine. Don't confuse Viracept with Viramune or Viramune XR.

PATIENT TEACHING

• Advise patient to take drug with food.

• Inform patient that drug doesn't cure HIV infection.

• Tell patient that long-term effects of drug are unknown and that there are no data stating that nelfinavir reduces risk of HIV transmission.

• Advise patient to take drug daily as prescribed and not to alter dose or stop drug without medical approval.

• If patient misses a dose, tell him to take it as soon as possible and then return to his normal schedule. Advise patient not to double the dose.

• Tell patient that diarrhea is the most common adverse effect and that it can be controlled with loperamide, if needed.

• Instruct patient taking hormonal contraceptives to use alternative or additional contraceptive measures while taking nelfinavir.

✪ Alert: Advise patient taking sildenafil about an increased risk of sildenafil-related adverse events, including low BP, visual changes, and painful erections. Tell him to promptly report any symptoms. Tell him not to exceed 25 mg of sildenafil in a 48-hour period.

• Advise patient to report use of other prescribed or OTC drugs because of possible drug interactions.

neomycin sulfate
nee-o-MYE-sin

Neo-Fradin

Therapeutic class: Antibiotics
Pharmacologic class: Aminoglycosides

AVAILABLE FORMS
Oral solution: 125 mg/5 mL
Tablets: 500 mg

INDICATIONS & DOSAGES
➤ **To suppress intestinal bacteria before surgery (tablets only)**
Adults: After saline cathartic, 1 g neomycin with 1 g erythromycin base P.O. at 1 p.m., 2 p.m., and 11 p.m., on day before 8 a.m. surgery.
➤ **Adjunctive treatment for hepatic coma**
Adults: 4 to 12 g P.O. daily in divided doses for 5 to 6 days.

ADMINISTRATION
P.O.
● For preoperative disinfection, provide a low-residue diet and a cathartic immediately before therapy.

ACTION
Inhibits protein synthesis by binding directly to the 30S ribosomal subunit; bactericidal.

Route	Onset	Peak	Duration
P.O.	Unknown	1–4 hr	8 hr

Half-life: 2 to 3 hours.

ADVERSE REACTIONS
CNS: *neuromuscular blockade.*
EENT: ototoxicity.
GI: nausea, vomiting, diarrhea, malabsorption syndrome, CDAD.
GU: *nephrotoxicity,* possible increase in urinary excretion of casts.

INTERACTIONS
Drug-drug. Black Box Warning *Acyclovir, amphotericin B, cephalosporins, cidofovir, cisplatin, methoxyflurane, vancomycin, other aminoglycosides:* May increase nephrotoxicity. Monitor renal function test results. ■
Black Box Warning *Anesthetics, neuromuscular blockers (e.g., decamethonium, succinylcholine, tubocurarine):* May increase effects of nondepolarizing muscle relaxants, including prolonged respiratory depression and respiratory paralysis. Use together only when necessary, and expect to reduce dosage of nondepolarizing muscle relaxants. Mechanical ventilation may be needed. ■
Digoxin: May decrease digoxin absorption. Monitor digoxin level.
Black Box Warning *I.V. loop diuretics (furosemide):* May increase ototoxicity. Monitor patient's hearing. ■
Oral anticoagulants: May inhibit vitamin K–producing bacteria; may increase anticoagulant effect. Monitor PT and INR.

EFFECTS ON LAB TEST RESULTS
● May increase BUN, creatinine, and nonprotein nitrogen levels.

CONTRAINDICATIONS & CAUTIONS
● Contraindicated in patients hypersensitive to other aminoglycosides, in those with intestinal obstruction or inflammatory or ulcerative GI disease, and in patients who are breast-feeding.
● Use cautiously in elderly patients and in those with impaired renal function or neuromuscular disorders.
● Prolonged use can cause superinfection including CDAD, which can occur 2 months after therapy ends.
● Safety and effectiveness of oral neomycin sulfate in patients younger than age 18 haven't been established.
Dialyzable drug: Yes.
⚠ *Overdose S&S:* Neurotoxicity, ototoxicity, nephrotoxicity.

PREGNANCY-LACTATION-REPRODUCTION
● Drug may cause fetal harm. Use only if clearly needed.
● Patient should discontinue breast-feeding or discontinue drug.

NURSING CONSIDERATIONS
Black Box Warning Due to increased risk of nephrotoxicity, monitor renal function: urine

output, specific gravity, urinalysis, BUN and creatinine levels, and creatinine clearance. Report evidence of declining renal function to prescriber. ▪

Black Box Warning Due to increased risk of neurotoxicity and ototoxicity, evaluate patient's hearing before and during prolonged therapy. Notify prescriber if patient has tinnitus, vertigo, or hearing loss. Deafness may start several weeks after drug is stopped. ▪

Black Box Warning Don't use with other aminoglycosides or neurotoxic or nephrotoxic drugs; risk of toxicities increase. ▪

• Watch for signs and symptoms of superinfection (chills, fever, diarrhea), including CDAD, which can occur more than 2 months after therapy ends.

Black Box Warning Neuromuscular blockade and respiratory paralysis have been reported after administration of aminoglycosides. Monitor patient closely. ▪

• For adjunctive treatment for hepatic coma, decrease patient's dietary protein and assess neurologic status frequently during therapy.

• The ototoxic and nephrotoxic properties of drug limit its usefulness.

PATIENT TEACHING

• Instruct patient to report all adverse reactions promptly, especially fever, chills, diarrhea, changes in hearing, changes in urine amount, or dark urine.

• Encourage patient to maintain adequate fluid intake.

SAFETY ALERT!

nesiritide
neh-SIR-ih-tide

Natrecor

Therapeutic class: Vasodilators
Pharmacologic class: Human B-type natriuretic peptides

AVAILABLE FORMS
Injection: Single-dose vials of 1.5 mg sterile, lyophilized powder

INDICATIONS & DOSAGES

➤ **Acutely decompensated HF in patients with dyspnea at rest or with minimal activity**

Adults: 2 mcg/kg by I.V. bolus over 60 seconds, followed by continuous infusion of 0.01 mcg/kg/minute. Maximum dosage is 0.03 mcg/kg/minute.

Adjust-a-dose: If hypotension develops during administration, reduce dosage or stop drug. Restart drug at dosage reduced by 30% with no bolus doses.

ADMINISTRATION

I.V.

▼ Reconstitute one 1.5-mg vial with 5 mL of diluent (such as D_5W, NSS, 5% dextrose and 0.2% saline solution injection, or 5% dextrose and half-NSS) from a prefilled 250-mL I.V. bag.

▼ Gently rock (don't shake) vial until solution becomes clear and colorless.

▼ Withdraw contents of vial and add back to the 250-mL I.V. bag to yield 6 mcg/mL. Invert the bag several times to ensure complete mixing, and use the solution within 24 hours.

▼ Use the formulas below to calculate bolus volume (2 mcg/kg) and infusion flow rate (0.01 mcg/kg/minute):

Bolus volume = patient weight ÷ 3
  (mL)   (kg)

Infusion flow rate = 0.1 × patient weight
  (mL/hr)   (kg)

▼ Before giving bolus dose, prime the I.V. tubing with 5 mL of solution. Withdraw the bolus and give over 60 seconds through an I.V. port in the tubing.

▼ Immediately after giving bolus, infuse drug at 0.1 mL/kg/hour to deliver 0.01 mcg/kg/minute.

▼ Store drug at 68° to 77° F (20° to 25° C). Protect from light. May store reconstituted vials at 36° to 77° F (2° to 25° C) for up to 24 hours.

▼ **Incompatibilities:** Bumetanide, enalaprilat, ethacrynate sodium, furosemide, heparin, hydralazine, insulin, sodium metabisulfite.

ACTION
Increases cyclic guanosine monophosphate level, relaxes smooth muscle, and dilates veins and arteries. Drug reduces pulmonary capillary wedge pressure and systemic arterial pressure in patients with HF.

Route	Onset	Peak	Duration
I.V.	15 min	1 hr	3 hr

Half-life: 18 minutes.

ADVERSE REACTIONS
CNS: anxiety, confusion, dizziness, fever, headache, insomnia, paresthesia, somnolence, tremor.
CV: hypotension, *bradycardia, ventricular tachycardia,* angina, atrial fibrillation, AV node conduction abnormalities, ventricular extrasystoles.
GI: abdominal pain, nausea, vomiting.
Hematologic: anemia.
Musculoskeletal: back pain, leg cramps.
Respiratory: *apnea,* cough, hemoptysis.
Skin: injection-site reactions, rash, pruritus, sweating.

INTERACTIONS
Drug-drug. *ACE inhibitors, ARBs:* May increase hypotension symptoms. Monitor BP closely.

EFFECTS ON LAB TEST RESULTS
• May increase creatinine level more than 0.5 mg/dL above baseline. May decrease Hb level and hematocrit.

CONTRAINDICATIONS & CAUTIONS
• Contraindicated in patients hypersensitive to drug or its components.
• Contraindicated in patients with cardiogenic shock, systolic BP below 100 mm Hg, low cardiac filling pressures, conditions in which cardiac output depends on venous return, or conditions that make vasodilators inappropriate (valvular stenosis, restrictive or obstructive cardiomyopathy, constrictive pericarditis, pericardial tamponade).
• Safety and effectiveness in children haven't been established.
Dialyzable drug: Unknown.
⚠ Overdose S&S: Excessive hypotension.

PREGNANCY-LACTATION-REPRODUCTION
• Use during pregnancy only if potential benefit justifies possible fetal risk.
• It isn't known if drug appears in breast milk. Use cautiously if breast-feeding.

NURSING CONSIDERATIONS
• Don't start drug at higher-than-recommended dosage; this may cause hypotension and increase creatinine level.
⊕ Alert: This drug may cause hypotension. Monitor patient's BP closely, particularly if patient is also taking an ACE inhibitor or ARB.
⊕ Alert: Drug binds to heparin, including the heparin lining of a coated catheter, decreasing the amount of nesiritide delivered. Don't give nesiritide through a central heparin-coated catheter.
• Drug may affect renal function. In patients with severe HF whose renal function depends on the RAAS, use may lead to azotemia.
• There is limited experience with giving this drug for longer than 96 hours.

PATIENT TEACHING
• Tell patient to report I.V. site discomfort.
• Urge patient to report to prescriber symptoms of hypotension, such as dizziness, lightheadedness, blurred vision, or sweating.
• Tell patient to report other adverse effects to prescriber promptly.

nevirapine
neh-VEER-ah-pine

Viramune, Viramune✸,
Viramune XR, Viramune XR✸

Therapeutic class: Antiretrovirals
Pharmacologic class: Nonnucleoside reverse transcriptase inhibitors

AVAILABLE FORMS
Oral suspension: 50 mg/5 mL
Tablets: 200 mg
Tablets (extended-release) ⓪: 100 mg, 400 mg

INDICATIONS & DOSAGES
➤ **Adjunctive treatment in HIV-infected adults who have experienced clinical or**

immunologic deterioration; used with nucleoside analogue antiretrovirals

Black Box Warning Adhere strictly to 14-day lead-in period with nevirapine 200-mg daily dosing. ■

Adults: 200 mg (immediate-release) P.O. daily for the first 14 days; then 200 mg P.O. b.i.d. Or, 400 mg (extended-release) P.O. once daily after 14-day lead-in period with 200-mg daily dosing.

Children age 6 to less than 18 years: Initially 150 mg/m² (immediate-release) P.O. once daily for 14 days. Maximum dose is 200 mg/day. Then if BSA is 0.58 to 0.83 m², increase to 200 mg (extended-release) once daily; if BSA is 0.84 to 1.16 m², increase to 300 mg (extended-release) once daily; if BSA is greater than or equal to 1.17 m², increase to 400 mg (extended-release) once daily.

Children age 15 days and older: 150 mg/m² (immediate-release) P.O. once daily for 14 days. Then, 150 mg/m² P.O. b.i.d. maintenance dosage. Maximum dosage is 400 mg daily.

Adjust-a-dose: For patients on dialysis, give an additional 200-mg (immediate-release) dose after each dialysis treatment. Patients with a CrCl equal to or greater than 20 mL/minute don't require dosage adjustment. Extended-release formula hasn't been studied in patients with renal impairment.

ADMINISTRATION
P.O.
● Use drug with at least one other antiretroviral.
● Administer with or without food.
● Extended-release tablets must be swallowed whole and shouldn't be crushed, chewed, or divided.
● Shake the suspension gently before administering. An oral dosing syringe is recommended.

ACTION
Binds directly to reverse transcriptase and blocks RNA-dependent and DNA-dependent DNA polymerase activities by disrupting the enzyme's catalytic site.

Route	Onset	Peak	Duration
P.O.	Unknown	4 hr	Unknown

Half-life: 25 to 30 hours.

ADVERSE REACTIONS
CNS: fever, headache, paresthesia, fatigue.
GI: nausea, abdominal pain, diarrhea.
Hematologic: *neutropenia.*
Hepatic: *hepatitis.*
Musculoskeletal: myalgia.
Skin: blistering, rash, *Stevens-Johnson syndrome.*

INTERACTIONS
Drug-drug. *Drugs extensively metabolized by CYP450:* May lower levels of these drugs. Dosage adjustment of these drugs may be needed.
Efavirenz: May decrease efavirenz concentration and increase adverse reactions. Concurrent use isn't recommended.
Ketoconazole: May decrease ketoconazole level. Avoid using together.
Protease inhibitors or hormonal contraceptives: May decrease levels of these drugs. Use together cautiously.
Rifabutin, rifampin: Dosage adjustment may be needed. Monitor patient closely.
Warfarin: May increase anticoagulant effect of warfarin. Monitor INR and adjust warfarin dose as needed.
Drug-herb. *St. John's wort:* May decrease drug level. Don't use together.

EFFECTS ON LAB TEST RESULTS
● May increase ALT, AST, GGT, and bilirubin levels. May decrease Hb level.
● May decrease neutrophil count.

CONTRAINDICATIONS & CAUTIONS
● Contraindicated in patients hypersensitive to drug.
Black Box Warning Use in patients with moderate or severe hepatic impairment or as part of occupational or nonoccupational postexposure prophylaxis regimens is contraindicated because of increased risk of hepatic failure. ■
Black Box Warning Severe, life-threatening and, in some cases, fatal hepatotoxicity, particularly in the first 18 weeks, has been reported in patients treated with nevirapine.

Reactions in bold italics are *life-threatening*. Interactions may have a *rapid onset* or a *delayed onset*.

In some cases, patients presented with nonspecific prodromal signs or symptoms of hepatitis and progressed to hepatic failure. These events are often associated with rash and fever. ■

Black Box Warning Women and patients with higher CD4$^+$ cell counts at start of therapy are at increased risk for life-threatening hepatotoxicity. Women with CD4$^+$ cell counts higher than 250/mm^3, including pregnant women receiving drug in combination with other antiretrovirals for treatment of HIV-1 infection, are at greatest risk. However, hepatotoxicity associated with nevirapine use can occur in both genders, at all CD4$^+$ cell counts, and at any time during treatment. ■

Black Box Warning Severe, life-threatening, sometimes fatal skin reactions have occurred, including Stevens-Johnson syndrome, toxic epidermal necrolysis, and hypersensitivity reactions characterized by rash, constitutional findings, and organ dysfunction. ■

• Use cautiously in patients with mild hepatic impairment; pharmacokinetics haven't been evaluated in these patients.

Dialyzable drug: Yes.

⚠ *Overdose S&S:* Edema, erythema nodosum, fatigue, fever, headache, insomnia, nausea, pulmonary infiltrates, rash, vertigo, vomiting, weight decrease.

PREGNANCY-LACTATION-REPRODUCTION

• Use cautiously in pregnant women. Advise women who are pregnant or may become pregnant to enroll in the Antiretroviral Pregnancy Registry (1-800-258-4263).

• Women with HIV infection shouldn't breast-feed.

NURSING CONSIDERATIONS

• Perform laboratory tests, including renal function tests, before therapy and regularly throughout.

Black Box Warning Monitor patient intensively during first 18 weeks of therapy to detect potentially life-threatening hepatotoxicity or skin reactions. Extra vigilance is warranted during first 6 weeks of therapy, which is the period of greatest risk of these reactions. ■

🖕 *Alert:* Monitor patient for blistering, oral lesions, conjunctivitis, muscle or joint aches, or general malaise. Especially look for severe rash or rash accompanied by fever. Immediately report these signs and symptoms to prescriber.

🖕 *Alert:* Be vigilant for signs or symptoms of hepatitis, such as fatigue, malaise, anorexia, nausea, jaundice, bilirubinuria, acholic stools, liver tenderness, or hepatomegaly. Consider diagnosis of hepatotoxicity in this setting, even if transaminase levels are initially normal or alternative diagnoses are possible.

Black Box Warning Check AST and ALT levels immediately if patient has signs or symptoms suggestive of hepatitis or hypersensitivity reaction. Check these levels for all patients who develop a rash in first 18 weeks of treatment. ■

Black Box Warning Patients with signs or symptoms of hepatitis or with increased ALT or AST levels combined with rash or other systemic symptoms, including hypersensitivity reactions, must stop drug and immediately seek medical evaluation. ■

Black Box Warning Don't restart drug after clinical hepatitis, elevated transaminase levels combined with rash or other systemic symptoms, or after severe rash or hypersensitivity reactions. In some cases, hepatic injury has progressed despite discontinuation of treatment. ■

🖕 *Alert:* If mild to moderate rash occurs during 14-day lead-in period with immediate-release nevirapine, don't increase dosage until the rash has resolved. Total duration of the once-daily lead-in dosing shouldn't exceed 28 days, at which point an alternative regimen should be sought.

🖕 *Alert:* If rash is present beyond 14-day lead-in period with immediate-release formulation, don't begin extended-release drug. The lead-in period before switching to extended-release formula isn't required if patient is already taking twice-daily immediate-release formulation in combination with other antiretrovirals.

🖕 *Alert:* Patients who have stopped therapy for more than 7 days should restart therapy as if receiving drug for the first time.

• Antiretroviral therapy may be changed if disease progresses during nevirapine

N

therapy. Drug shouldn't be used as monotherapy for HIV infection because of the rapid emergence of resistance.

● Drug may cause body-fat redistribution.

● ***Look alike–sound alike:*** Don't confuse nevirapine with nelfinavir. Don't confuse Viramune with Viracept.

PATIENT TEACHING

● Inform patient that drug doesn't cure HIV and that illnesses from advanced HIV infection still may occur. Explain that drug doesn't reduce risk of HIV transmission.

● Instruct patient to report rash immediately and to stop drug until told to resume.

● Tell patient with signs or symptoms of hepatitis (such as fatigue, malaise, anorexia, nausea, jaundice, liver tenderness or hepatomegaly, with or without initially abnormal transaminase levels) to stop drug and seek medical evaluation immediately.

● Stress importance of taking drug exactly as prescribed. If a dose is missed, tell patient to take the next dose as soon as possible and not to double next dose.

● Advise patient that if therapy is interrupted for more than 7 days, the 14-day lead-in dosages will be needed.

● Tell patient not to use other drugs unless approved by prescriber.

● Advise female patient of childbearing potential not to use hormonal contraceptives and other hormonal methods of birth control while taking nevirapine.

---

niCARdipine hydrochloride
nye-KAR-de-peen

Cardene, Cardene I.V.

Therapeutic class: Antihypertensives
Pharmacologic class: Calcium channel blockers

AVAILABLE FORMS
Capsules: 20 mg, 30 mg
Injection: 2.5-mg/mL vial; 20 mg/200-mL, 40 mg/200-mL premixed bag

INDICATIONS & DOSAGES
➤ **Chronic stable angina (used alone or with other antianginals)**

Adults: Initially, 20-mg capsule P.O. t.i.d. Adjust dosage no sooner than every 3 days based on patient response. Usual range, 20 to 40 mg t.i.d.

➤ **Hypertension**
Adults: Initially, 20 mg capsule P.O. t.i.d.; range, 20 to 40 mg t.i.d. Adjust dosage every 3 days based on patient response. Or, for patient who is starting on nicardipine and can't take oral form, 5 mg/hour I.V. infusion initially; then, increase by 2.5 mg/hour every 5 minutes for rapid control or every 15 minutes for gradual control to maximum of 15 mg/hour. After achieving BP goal, decrease infusion rate to 3 mg/hour. Or, as a substitute for oral nicardipine therapy, if patient is taking 20 mg P.O. every 8 hours, give 0.5 mg/hour I.V. infusion; if patient is taking 30 mg P.O. every 8 hours, give 1.2 mg/hour I.V. infusion; if patient is taking 40 mg P.O. every 8 hours, give 2.2 mg/hour I.V. infusion.

ADMINISTRATION
P.O.
● Give drug with or without food, but avoid giving with high-fat meal.
● Patient should avoid grapefruit juice during therapy.
I.V.
▼ Dilute to a concentration of 0.1 mg/mL with D_5W, dextrose 5% in NSS or half-NSS, or NSS or half-NSS.
▼ Check premixed bags for leaks, solution clarity, and intact seal. Don't add other drugs to bag.
▼ Give by slow infusion.
▼ Closely monitor BP during and after completion of infusion.
▼ If hypotension or tachycardia occurs, titrate infusion rate.
▼ Administer via central line or through a large peripheral vein. To minimize risk of peripheral venous irritation, change infusion site every 12 hours.
▼ Don't combine premixed or injection with any product in the same I.V. line or premixed container.
▼ When switching to oral form, give first dose of t.i.d. regimen 1 hour before stopping infusion. If using a different oral drug, start it when infusion ends.

▼ If solution is kept at room temperature, use within 24 hours.

▼ **Incompatibilities:** Ampicillin sodium, ampicillin–sulbactam sodium, cefepime, ceftazidime, furosemide, heparin sodium, lactated Ringer solution, sodium bicarbonate, thiopental.

ACTION

Inhibits calcium ion influx across cardiac and smooth muscle cells but is more selective to vascular smooth muscle than cardiac muscle. Drug also dilates coronary arteries and arterioles.

Route	Onset	Peak	Duration
P.O.	20 min	1–2 hr	Unknown
I.V.	Immediate	Immediate	Unknown

Half-life: 2 to 4 hours.

ADVERSE REACTIONS

CNS: headache, dizziness, lightheadedness, asthenia, drowsiness, paresthesia.
CV: angina, peripheral edema, palpitations, flushing, hypotension, tachycardia.
GI: nausea, vomiting, abdominal discomfort, dry mouth.
Musculoskeletal: myalgia and weakness (I.V. form).
Skin: rash, diaphoresis, injection-site reaction.

INTERACTIONS

Drug-drug. *Antihypertensives, protease inhibitors:* May increase antihypertensive effect. Monitor BP closely.
Cimetidine: May decrease metabolism of calcium channel blockers. Monitor patient for increased pharmacologic effect.
Cyclosporine: May increase plasma level of cyclosporine. Monitor patient for toxicity.
Digoxin: May increase digoxin level. Monitor digoxin level.
Drugs that prolong QT interval: May have an additive effect. Monitor patient and ECG.
Fentanyl: May cause severe hypotension. Closely monitor BP.
Drug-food. *Grapefruit and grapefruit juice:* May increase bioavailability of nicardipine. Discourage use together.
High-fat foods: May decrease absorption of nicardipine. Discourage use together.

EFFECTS ON LAB TEST RESULTS

● May decrease potassium level (I.V. form).

CONTRAINDICATIONS & CAUTIONS

● Contraindicated in patients hypersensitive to drug and in those with advanced aortic stenosis.
● Use cautiously in patients with hypotension or impaired hepatic or renal function and in elderly patients.
● Avoid systemic hypotension when administering drug to patients who have sustained an acute cerebral infarction or hemorrhage.
● Consider lower dosages and closely monitor responses in patients with hepatic impairment or reduced hepatic blood flow.
● Titrate gradually in patients with renal impairment.
● MI and increased angina have been noted when calcium channel blockers have been started or doses titrated. Abrupt withdrawal can cause rebound angina in patients with CAD.
● Avoid use of calcium channel blockers in patients with HF due to increased risk of worse outcomes.
● Safety and effectiveness in patients younger than age 18 haven't been established.
Dializable drug: No.
⚠ Overdose S&S: Hypotension, bradycardia, palpitations, flushing, drowsiness, confusion, slurred speech.

PREGNANCY-LACTATION-REPRODUCTION

● There are no adequate studies in pregnant women. Drug isn't recommended for use during pregnancy.
● Use cautiously in breast-feeding women, and monitor infant for adverse effects. Some manufacturers recommend that patient should avoid breast-feeding during therapy.

NURSING CONSIDERATIONS

● Closely monitor BP and HR. Drug can cause symptomatic hypotension or tachycardia. Measure BP frequently during initial therapy. Maximal response occurs in about 1 hour. Check for orthostatic hypotension. Because large swings in BP may occur based on drug level, assess antihypertensive effect 8 hours after dosing.

N

◑ Alert: Only immediate-release form is approved for treatment of angina.
● **Look alike–sound alike:** Don't confuse Cardene with Cardura or codeine.

PATIENT TEACHING
● Tell patient to take oral form exactly as prescribed.
● Tell patient to report injection-site pain.
● Advise patient to report chest pain immediately. Some patients may experience increased frequency, severity, or duration of chest pain at beginning of therapy or during dosage adjustments.
● Tell patient to get up from a sitting or lying position slowly to avoid dizziness caused by a decrease in BP.
● Tell patient drug may be taken with or without food but shouldn't be taken with high-fat foods or grapefruit products.

NIFEdipine
nye-FED-i-peen

Adalat CC, Adalat XL✤,
Afeditab CR, Apo-Nifed PA-SRT✤,
PMS-nifedipine✤, Procardia,
Procardia XL✐

Therapeutic class: Antihypertensives
Pharmacologic class: Calcium channel blockers

AVAILABLE FORMS
Capsules: 5 mg✤, 10 mg, 20 mg
Tablets (extended-release) ⓪: 20 mg✤, 30 mg, 60 mg, 90 mg

INDICATIONS & DOSAGES
Adjust-a-dose (for all indications): For elderly patients and patients with renal and hepatic impairment, initiate drug at the low end of the dosing range.
➤ **Vasospastic angina (Prinzmetal or variant angina), classic chronic stable angina pectoris**
Adults: Initially, 10 mg short-acting capsule P.O. t.i.d. Usual effective dosage range is 10 to 20 mg t.i.d. Some patients may require up to 30 mg q.i.d. Maximum daily dose is 180 mg. Adjust dosage over 7 to 14 days to evaluate response. Or, 30 to

60 mg (extended-release tablets, except Adalat CC or Afeditab CR) P.O. once daily. Maximum daily dose is 120 mg. Adjust dosage over 7 to 14 days to evaluate response. Use doses of more than 90 mg cautiously and only when clinically warranted.
➤ **Hypertension**
Adults: Initially, 30 mg extended-release tablet (Adalat CC or Afeditab CR) or 30 or 60 mg extended-release tablet (Procardia XL) P.O. once daily, adjusted over 7 to 14 days. Maximum dose is 90 mg (Adalat CC or Afeditab CR) or 120 mg/day (Procardia XL).
➤ **Ureteral calculi (distal)** ◆
Adults: 10 to 30 mg P.O. t.i.d. for up to 4 weeks or until expulsion of lower stones.

ADMINISTRATION
P.O.
● Don't give immediate-release capsules within 1 week of acute MI or in acute coronary syndrome.
◑ Alert: Don't use capsules S.L. to rapidly reduce severe high BP because the result may be fatal.
● Give extended-release tablets whole; don't break or crush tablet.
● Don't give drug with grapefruit juice.
● Protect capsules from direct light and moisture and store at room temperature.

ACTION
Thought to inhibit calcium ion influx across cardiac and smooth muscle cells, decreasing contractility and oxygen demand. Drug may also dilate coronary arteries and arterioles.

Route	Onset	Peak	Duration
P.O.	20 min	30–60 min	4–8 hr
P.O. (extended-release)	20 min	6 hr	24 hr

Half-life: 2 to 5 hours.

ADVERSE REACTIONS
Immediate-release
CNS: dizziness, light-headedness, giddiness, headache, weakness, nervousness, mood changes, shakiness, sleep disturbances, fever.
CV: flushing, heat sensation, peripheral edema, palpitations, transient hypotension.

EENT: nasal congestion, sore throat, blurred vision.
GI: nausea, heartburn, diarrhea, constipation, cramps, flatulence.
Musculoskeletal: muscle cramps, tremor, inflammation, joint stiffness.
Respiratory: dyspnea, cough, wheezing, chest congestion, shortness of breath.
Skin: dermatitis, pruritus, urticaria, sweating.
Other: difficulties in balance, chills, sexual difficulties.
Extended-release
CNS: dizziness, headache, fatigue, insomnia, nervousness, paresthesia, somnolence, asthenia, pain.
CV: palpitations, chest pain, flushing.
GI: nausea, constipation, abdominal pain, diarrhea, dry mouth, dyspepsia, flatulence.
GU: erectile dysfunction, polyuria.
Musculoskeletal: arthralgia, leg cramps.
Respiratory: dyspnea.
Skin: pruritus, rash.

INTERACTIONS
Drug-drug. *ACE inhibitors (benazepril):* May increase hypotensive effects. Monitor BP and adjust nifedipine dosage as needed.
Alpha₁ blockers (doxazosin): May increase nifedipine plasma concentration. Monitor BP and adjust nifedipine dosage as needed.
Antiretrovirals, cimetidine, verapamil: May decrease nifedipine metabolism. Monitor BP closely; adjust nifedipine dose as needed.
Azole antifungals, erythromycin, nefazodone, quinupristin–dalfopristin, valproic acid: May increase the effects of nifedipine. Monitor BP closely and decrease nifedipine dosage as needed.
Cyclosporine, tacrolimus: May increase serum levels of these drugs and increase risk of toxicity. Monitor serum levels and adjust dosage as needed.
Digoxin: May cause elevated digoxin level. Monitor digoxin level.
Diltiazem: May increase the effects of nifedipine. Monitor patient closely.
Diuretics, fentanyl: May increase hypotensive effects. Monitor BP.
PDE5 inhibitors (sildenafil): Increases risk of hypotension. Monitor BP and adjust nifedipine dosage if needed.

Phenytoin: May reduce nifedipine metabolism. Monitor patient and adjust nifedipine dosage as needed.
Propranolol, other beta blockers: May cause hypotension and HF. Use together cautiously.
Quinidine: May decrease levels and effects of quinidine while increasing effects of nifedipine. Monitor HR and adjust nifedipine dose as needed.
Strong CYP3A4 inducers (carbamazepine, dexamethasone, phenytoin, rifabutin, rifampin): May decrease nifedipine level. Use together is contraindicated.
Warfarin: May increase PT. Monitor coagulation parameters and adjust warfarin dosage as needed.
Drug-herb. *Ginkgo:* May increase effects of drug. Discourage use together.
Ginseng: May increase drug levels with possible toxicity. Discourage use together.
Melatonin, St. John's wort: May interfere with antihypertensive effect. Discourage use together.
Drug-food. *Grapefruit juice:* May increase bioavailability of drug. Discourage use together.

EFFECTS ON LAB TEST RESULTS
● May increase ALT, AST, alkaline phosphatase, and LDH levels.

CONTRAINDICATIONS & CAUTIONS
● Contraindicated in patients hypersensitive to drug, in those taking strong CYP450 inducers (rifampin), and in patients with cardiogenic shock or ST-segment elevation MI.
● Increased angina and MI have occurred at start of therapy or with dosage titration of dihydropyridine calcium channel blockers. Reflex tachycardia may occur, resulting in angina or MI in patients with obstructive coronary disease, especially in the absence of concurrent beta blockade.
● BP must be lowered at a rate appropriate for patient's clinical condition to avoid symptomatic hypotension with or without syncope. The use of immediate-release nifedipine in hypertensive emergencies and urgencies is neither safe nor effective. Serious adverse events (death, cerebrovascular ischemia, syncope, stroke, acute MI,

N

fetal distress) have been reported. Don't use immediate-release nifedipine for acute BP reduction or to manage primary hypertension.

● Avoid use in patients with HF; drug may worsen symptoms.

● Use with extreme caution in patients with severe aortic stenosis. Drug may reduce coronary perfusion, resulting in ischemia.

● Use cautiously in patients with hypertrophic cardiomyopathy and outflow tract obstruction because reduction in afterload may worsen symptoms.

● Use cautiously before major surgery. Cardiopulmonary bypass, intraoperative blood loss, or vasodilating anesthesia may result in severe hypotension or increased fluid requirements. Consider withdrawing nifedipine more than 36 hours before surgery if possible.

● Rare reversible elevations in BUN and serum creatinine levels have been reported in patients with preexisting chronic renal insufficiency.

● Use cautiously in patients with hepatic impairment. Clearance of nifedipine is reduced in cirrhotic patients, leading to increased systemic exposure and possibly increasing toxicities; monitor patient and consider dosage adjustments.

🛈 *Alert:* Immediate-release drug is considered a high-risk drug for elderly patients because of the potential for hypotension and increased risk of precipitating myocardial ischemia in this population. Avoid use.

🛈 *Alert:* Use extended-release form cautiously because of an increased risk of serious GI obstruction in patients both with and without risk factors. (Risk factors for GI obstruction include altered GI anatomy, GI hypomotility related to GERD, colon cancer, ileus, obesity, hypothyroidism, diabetes, and concomitant use of H_2 blockers, NSAIDs, laxatives, anticholinergic agents, and levothyroxine.)

● Safety and effectiveness in children haven't been established.

Dialyzable drug: Unlikely.

⚠ *Overdose S&S:* Hypotension, dizziness, palpitations, flushing, nervousness.

PREGNANCY-LACTATION-REPRODUCTION

● There are no adequate studies in pregnant women. Use only when potential benefit justifies possible risk to the fetus.

● Use cautiously in breast-feeding women. Monitor breast-fed infants for adverse effects.

NURSING CONSIDERATIONS

● Monitor BP and HR regularly, especially in patients who take beta blockers or antihypertensives.

● Watch for symptoms of HF.

● The most common adverse effect is peripheral edema, which occurs within 2 to 3 weeks of start of therapy.

● *Look alike–sound alike:* Don't confuse nifedipine with nimodipine or nicardipine.

PATIENT TEACHING

● If patient is kept on nitrate therapy while nifedipine dosage is being adjusted, urge continued compliance. Patient may take S.L. nitroglycerin, as needed, for acute chest pain.

● Tell patient that chest pain may worsen briefly as therapy starts or dosage increases.

● Instruct patient to swallow extended-release tablets without breaking, crushing, or chewing them.

● Advise patient to avoid taking drug with grapefruit juice.

● Tell patient not to abruptly stop drug unless directed by prescriber. Abrupt withdrawal may cause rebound angina in patients with CAD.

● Advise patient that Adalat CC tablets contain lactose and shouldn't be used by patients with galactose intolerance, Lapp lactase deficiency, or glucose-galactose malabsorption.

● Reassure patient taking the extended-release tablet that the wax mold may be passed in the stools. Assure him that drug has already been completely absorbed.

● Tell patient to protect capsules from direct light and moisture and to store at room temperature.

nitrofurantoin macrocrystals
nye-troh-fyoo-RAN-toyn

Macrobid, Macrodantin🖉

nitrofurantoin microcrystals
Furadantin

Therapeutic class: Antibiotics
Pharmacologic class: Nitrofurans

AVAILABLE FORMS
nitrofurantoin macrocrystals
Capsules: 25 mg, 50 mg, 100 mg
nitrofurantoin microcrystals
Oral suspension: 25 mg/5 mL

INDICATIONS & DOSAGES
➤ **UTIs caused by susceptible**
Escherichia coli, Staphylococcus
aureus, enterococci, or certain strains
of *Klebsiella* and *Enterobacter* species
Adults and children older than age 12:
50 to 100 mg P.O. q.i.d. with meals and at
bedtime. Continue for 1 week or for at least
3 days after sterility of urine is obtained. Or,
100 mg Macrobid P.O. every 12 hours for
7 days.
Children ages 1 month to 12 years: 5 to
7 mg/kg P.O. daily in four divided doses.
Continue for 1 week or for at least 3 days
after sterility of urine is obtained.
➤ **Long-term suppression therapy**
Adults: 50 to 100 mg P.O. daily at bedtime.
Children: 1 to 2 mg/kg P.O. daily in a single
dose at bedtime or divided into two doses
given every 12 hours.

ADMINISTRATION
P.O.
• Obtain urine specimen for culture and
sensitivity tests before giving. Repeat as
needed. Begin therapy while awaiting
results.
• Give drug with food or milk to minimize
GI distress and improve absorption.

ACTION
May interfere with bacterial enzyme systems and bacterial cell-wall formation.

Route	Onset	Peak	Duration
P.O.	Unknown	Unknown	Unknown

Half-life: 20 minutes to 1 hour.

ADVERSE REACTIONS
CNS: *ascending polyneuropathy with*
high doses or renal impairment, dizziness,
drowsiness, headache, peripheral neuropathy.
GI: anorexia, diarrhea, nausea, vomiting,
abdominal pain.
GU: overgrowth of nonsusceptible organisms in urinary tract.
Hematologic: *agranulocytosis, hemolysis*
in patients with G6PD deficiency, thrombo-
cytopenia.
Hepatic: *hepatic necrosis, hepatitis.*
Metabolic: *hypoglycemia.*
Respiratory: *asthmatic attacks,* pulmonary
sensitivity reactions.
Skin: *Stevens-Johnson syndrome;* exfoliative dermatitis; maculopapular, erythematous, or eczematous eruption; pruritus;
transient alopecia; urticaria.
Other: *anaphylaxis,* drug fever, hypersensitivity reactions.

INTERACTIONS
Drug-drug. *Antacids containing magne-*
sium: May decrease nitrofurantoin absorption. Separate dosage times by 1 hour.
Probenecid, sulfinpyrazone: May inhibit
excretion of nitrofurantoin, increasing drug
levels and risk of toxicity. The resulting
decreased urinary levels could lessen antibacterial effects. Avoid using together.
Drug-food. *Any food:* May increase absorption. Advise patient to take drug with food
or milk.

EFFECTS ON LAB TEST RESULTS
• May increase bilirubin and alkaline phosphatase levels. May decrease glucose level.
• May decrease granulocyte and platelet
counts.
• May cause false-positive results in urine
glucose tests using cupric sulfate (such
as Benedict reagent, Fehling solution, or
Chemstrip uG).

N

CONTRAINDICATIONS & CAUTIONS

• Contraindicated in infants age 1 month and younger; in patients with anuria, oliguria, or CrCl less than 60 mL/minute; and in patients with a history of cholestatic jaundice or hepatic dysfunction associated with nitrofurantoin use.

• Use cautiously in patients with renal impairment, asthma, anemia, diabetes mellitus, electrolyte abnormalities, vitamin B deficiency, debilitating disease, and G6PD deficiency.

Dialyzable drug: Yes.

⚠ *Overdose S&S:* Vomiting.

PREGNANCY-LACTATION-REPRODUCTION

• Contraindicated in pregnant women at 38 to 42 weeks' gestation, during labor and delivery, and when onset of labor is imminent due to possible hemolytic anemia in the neonate.

• Because of possible serious adverse reactions in infants younger than age 1 month, patient should discontinue breast-feeding or discontinue drug.

NURSING CONSIDERATIONS

• Drug may cause an asthma attack in patients with a history of asthma.

• Monitor fluid intake and output carefully. Treatment may turn urine brown or dark yellow.

• Monitor CBC, renal function, and pulmonary status regularly.

🕃 *Alert:* Monitor patient for signs and symptoms of superinfection, which can occur up to 2 months after therapy ends. Use of nitrofurantoin may result in growth of nonsusceptible organisms, especially *Pseudomonas* species, or cause fungal or bacterial superinfection, such as CDAD and pseudomembranous colitis.

• Monitor patient for pulmonary sensitivity reactions, including cough, chest pain, fever, chills, dyspnea, and pulmonary infiltration with consolidation or effusions.

🕃 *Alert:* Hypersensitivity may develop when drug is used for long-term therapy.

• Some patients may experience fewer adverse GI effects with nitrofurantoin macrocrystals.

• Dual-release capsules (25 mg nitrofurantoin macrocrystals combined with 75 mg

nitrofurantoin monohydrate) enable patients to take drug only twice daily.

• Continue treatment for 3 days after sterile urine specimens have been obtained.

• Store drug in amber container. Don't store in metals other than stainless steel or aluminum to avoid precipitation.

PATIENT TEACHING

• Instruct patient to take drug for as long as prescribed, exactly as directed, even after he feels better.

• Tell patient to take drug with food or milk to minimize stomach upset.

• Instruct patient to report adverse reactions, especially peripheral neuropathy, which can become severe or irreversible.

• Alert patient that drug may turn urine dark yellow or brown.

• Warn patient not to store drug in metals other than stainless steel or aluminum.

• Advise patient not to use antacid preparations containing magnesium trisilicate.

SAFETY ALERT!

nitroglycerin (glyceryl trinitrate)
nye-troe-GLIH-ser-in

Gonitro, Minitran, Nitro-Dur, Nitrolingual, NitroMist, Nitrostat♂, Rectiv, Trinipatch✤

Therapeutic class: Vasodilators
Pharmacologic class: Nitrates

AVAILABLE FORMS

Aerosol (translingual): 0.4 mg/metered spray
Injection: 5 mg/mL, 100 mcg/mL, 200 mcg/mL, 400 mcg/mL
Ointment: 0.4%, 2%
Powder (S.L.): 400 mcg
Tablets (S.L.): 0.3 mg ($\frac{1}{200}$ grain), 0.4 mg ($\frac{1}{150}$ grain), 0.6 mg ($\frac{1}{100}$ grain)
Transdermal patch: 0.1 mg/hour, 0.2 mg/hour, 0.3 mg/hour, 0.4 mg/hour, 0.6 mg/hour, 0.8 mg/hour release rate

INDICATIONS & DOSAGES

➤ **To prevent chronic anginal attacks**

Adults: For 2% ointment: Start dosage with ½ inch ointment, increasing by ½-inch increments until desired results are achieved. Range of dosage with ointment is ½ inch to 5 inches (1.25 to 12.7 cm). Usual dose is 1 to 2 inches (2.5 to 5.08 cm) every 6 to 8 hours. Or, transdermal patch 0.2 to 0.4 mg/hour once daily.

➤ **Acute angina pectoris; to prevent or minimize anginal attacks before stressful events**

Adults: 1 S.L. tablet ($\frac{1}{200}$ grain, $\frac{1}{150}$ grain, or $\frac{1}{100}$ grain) dissolved under the tongue or in the buccal pouch as soon as angina begins. Repeat every 5 minutes, if needed, for 15 minutes. Or, 1 or 2 metered-dose sprays Nitrolingual into mouth, preferably onto or under the tongue. Repeat every 3 to 5 minutes, if needed, to a maximum of three doses within a 15-minute period. Or, 1 or 2 packets of S.L. powder dissolved under the tongue at onset of angina or 5 to 10 minutes before activities that might precipitate an acute angina attack. Give 1 additional packet every 5 minutes as need but not more than 3 total packets (1,200 mcg) within a 15-minute period.

➤ **Hypertension from surgery, HF after MI, angina pectoris in acute situations; to produce controlled hypotension during surgery (by I.V. infusion)**

Adults: Initially, infuse at 5 mcg/minute, increasing as needed by 5 mcg/minute every 3 to 5 minutes until response occurs. If a 20-mcg/minute rate doesn't produce a response, increase dosage by as much as 20 mcg/minute every 3 to 5 minutes. Up to 100 mcg/minute may be needed.

➤ **Moderate to severe pain from chronic anal fissure**

Adults: 1 inch (2.5 cm) of ointment P.R. every 12 hours for up to 3 weeks.

ADMINISTRATION

P.O.

● Give 30 minutes before or 1 to 2 hours after meals.

● Drug must be swallowed whole and not chewed.

I.V.

▼ Dilute with D_5W or NSS for injection. Concentration shouldn't exceed 400 mcg/mL.

▼ Always give with an infusion control device and titrate to desired response.

▼ Regular polyvinyl chloride tubing can bind up to 80% of drug, making it necessary to infuse higher dosages. A special nonabsorbent polyvinyl chloride tubing is available from the manufacturer. Always mix in glass bottles and avoid using a filter.

▼ Use the same type of infusion set when changing lines.

▼ When changing the concentration of infusion, flush the administration set with 15 to 20 mL of the new concentration before use. This will clear the line of the old drug solution.

▼ **Incompatibilities:** Other drugs.

Topical

● To apply ointment, measure the prescribed amount on the application paper; then place the paper on any nonhairy area. Don't rub in. Cover with plastic film to aid absorption and to protect clothing. Remove all excess ointment from previous site before applying the next dose. Avoid getting ointment on fingers.

P.R.

● Cover a finger with plastic wrap, disposable surgical glove, or a finger cot.

● Apply 1 inch of ointment onto the covered finger.

● Gently insert the ointment into the anal canal using the covered finger no further than the first finger joint.

Transdermal

● Patch can be applied to any nonhairy part of the skin except distal parts of the arms or legs. (Absorption won't be maximal at distal sites.) Patch may cause contact dermatitis.

● A cardioverter-defibrillator shouldn't be discharged through a paddle electrode that overlies a nitroglycerin patch.

● Remove patch before defibrillation. Because of the aluminum backing on the patch, the electric current may cause arcing that can damage the paddles and burn patient.

● When stopping transdermal treatment of angina, gradually reduce the dosage and frequency of application over 4 to 6 weeks.

N

S.L.

● Give tablet at first sign of attack. Patient should wet the tablet with saliva and place it under tongue until absorbed. Dose may be repeated every 5 minutes for a maximum of three doses. If drug doesn't provide relief, obtain prompt medical attention.

● Give dose of 1 or 2 packets of S.L. powder as prescribed. Hold packet close to patient's mouth, tear packet at red line, and pour all of the powder under the tongue. Patient shouldn't swallow until all of the powder has dissolved.

Buccal

● The tablet should be placed between the lip and gum above the incisors or between the cheek and gum. Tablets shouldn't be swallowed or chewed.

Translingual

● Patient using translingual aerosol form shouldn't inhale the spray but should release it onto or under the tongue. He should wait about 10 seconds or so before swallowing.

ACTION

Reduces cardiac oxygen demand by decreasing left ventricular end-diastolic pressure (preload) and, to a lesser extent, systemic vascular resistance (afterload). Also increases blood flow through the collateral coronary vessels.

Route	Onset	Peak	Duration
P.O.	20–45 min	Unknown	3–8 hr
I.V.	Immediate	Immediate	3–5 min
Topical	30 min	Unknown	2–12 hr
Transdermal	30 min	Unknown	24 hr
S.L.	1–3 min	Unknown	30–60 min
Buccal	3 min	Unknown	3–5 hr
Translingual	2–4 min	Unknown	30–60 min
P.R.	Immediate	Unknown	Unknown

Half-life: About 1 to 4 minutes.

ADVERSE REACTIONS

CNS: headache, dizziness, syncope, weakness.
CV: orthostatic hypotension, tachycardia, flushing, palpitations.
EENT: S.L. burning.
GI: nausea, vomiting.
Skin: cutaneous vasodilation, contact dermatitis, rash.
Other: hypersensitivity reactions.

INTERACTIONS

Drug-drug. *Alteplase:* May decrease tissue plasminogen activator antigen level. Avoid using together; if unavoidable, use lowest effective dose of nitroglycerin.
Antihypertensives: May increase hypotensive effect. Monitor BP closely.
Heparin: I.V. nitroglycerin may interfere with anticoagulant effect of heparin. Monitor PTT.
Riociguat: May cause hypotension. Avoid use together.
Sildenafil, tadalafil, vardenafil: May cause severe hypotension. Use of nitrates in any form with these drugs is contraindicated.
Drug-lifestyle. *Alcohol use:* May increase hypotension. Discourage use together.

EFFECTS ON LAB TEST RESULTS

● May falsely decrease values in cholesterol determination tests using the Zlatkis-Zak color reaction.

CONTRAINDICATIONS & CAUTIONS

● Contraindicated in patients hypersensitive to drug.
● Contraindicated in patients with early MI (oral and sublingual), severe anemia, increased ICP, angle-closure glaucoma, orthostatic hypotension, allergy to adhesives (transdermal), or hypersensitivity to nitrates.
● I.V. nitroglycerin is contraindicated in patients hypersensitive to I.V. form, with cardiac tamponade, restrictive cardiomyopathy, or constrictive pericarditis.
● Use cautiously in patients with hypotension or volume depletion.
Dialyzable drug: Unknown.
⚠ *Overdose S&S:* Vasodilation, decreased cardiac output, venous pooling, hypotension, methemoglobinemia.

PREGNANCY-LACTATION-REPRODUCTION

● There are no adequate studies in pregnant women. Use only if clearly needed.
● It isn't known if drug appears in breast milk. Use cautiously in breast-feeding women.

NURSING CONSIDERATIONS

● Closely monitor vital signs, particularly BP, during infusion, especially in patient

---

Reactions in bold italics are *life-threatening*. Interactions may have a *rapid onset* or a *delayed onset*.

with an MI. Excessive hypotension can worsen ischemia.
• Monitor BP and intensity and duration of drug response.
• Drug may cause headaches, especially at beginning of therapy. Dosage may be reduced temporarily, but tolerance usually develops. Treat headache with aspirin or acetaminophen.
• Tolerance to drug can be minimized with a 10- to 12-hour nitrate-free interval. To achieve this, remove the transdermal system in the early evening and apply a new system the next morning or omit the last daily dose of a buccal, sustained-release, or ointment form. Check with the prescriber for alterations in dosage regimen if tolerance is suspected.
• Wipe off nitroglycerin paste or remove patch before defibrillation to avoid patient burns.
• *Look alike–sound alike:* Don't confuse nitroglycerin with nitroprusside.

PATIENT TEACHING
• Caution patient to take nitroglycerin regularly, as prescribed, and to have it accessible at all times.
⚠ Alert: Advise patient that stopping drug abruptly may cause coronary artery spasm.
• Teach patient how to give the prescribed form of nitroglycerin.
• Tell patient to take S.L. tablet at first sign of attack. Patient should wet the tablet with saliva, place it under tongue until absorbed, and then sit down and rest. Dose may be repeated every 5 minutes for a maximum of three doses. If drug doesn't provide relief, he should obtain medical help promptly.
• Advise patient who complains of a tingling sensation with S.L. drug to try holding tablet in cheek.
• Tell patient not to use more than 3 packets of S.L. powder in a 15-minute period and to obtain medical help promptly if drug doesn't provide relief. Advise patient not to swallow or spit for 5 minutes after taking each packet.
• Tell patient to take oral tablets on an empty stomach either 30 minutes before or 1 to 2 hours after meals, to swallow oral tablets whole, and not to chew tablets.

• Remind patient using translingual aerosol form that he shouldn't inhale the spray but should release it onto or under the tongue. Tell him to wait about 10 seconds or so before swallowing.
• Tell patient to place the buccal tablet between the lip and gum above the incisors or between the cheek and gum. Tablets shouldn't be swallowed or chewed.
• Tell patient to take an additional dose before anticipated stress or at bedtime if chest pain occurs at night.
• Urge patient using skin patches to dispose of them carefully because enough medication remains after normal use to be hazardous to children and pets.
• If patients using skin patches are scheduled for an MRI scan, advise them to notify the facility that they are wearing a patch.
• Advise patient to avoid alcohol.
• To minimize dizziness when standing up, tell patient to rise slowly. Advise him to go up and down stairs carefully and to lie down at the first sign of dizziness.
⚠ Alert: Advise patient that use of sildenafil, tadalafil, or vardenafil with any nitrate may cause life-threatening low BP. Use together is contraindicated.
• Tell patient to store drug in cool, dark place in a tightly closed container. Tell him to remove cotton from container because it absorbs drug.
• Tell patient to store S.L. tablets in original container or other container specifically approved for this use and to carry the container in a jacket pocket or purse, not in a pocket close to the body.

SAFETY ALERT!

nitroprusside sodium
nye-troe-PRUSS-ide

Nipride ✦, Nitropress

Therapeutic class: Antihypertensives
Pharmacologic class: Vasodilators

AVAILABLE FORMS
Injection: 25 mg/mL

INDICATIONS & DOSAGES
➤ **To lower BP quickly in hypertensive emergencies; to produce controlled hypotension to reduce bleeding during surgery; treatment of acute HF**
Adults and children: Begin infusion at 0.3 mcg/kg/minute I.V. and gradually titrate every few minutes until desired effect is achieved or until the maximum dose of 10 mcg/kg/minute.
Adjust-a-dose: Patients also taking other antihypertensives are extremely sensitive to nitroprusside. Titrate dosage accordingly. Use with caution in patients with severe renal impairment or hepatic insufficiency; use minimum effective dose.

ADMINISTRATION
I.V.
▼ Prepare solution by dissolving 50 mg in 2 to 3 mL of D₅W injection or according to manufacturer's instructions.
Black Box Warning Drug isn't for direct injection and must be further diluted before infusion. Further dilute concentration in 250, 500, or 1,000 mL of D₅W to provide solutions with 200, 100, or 50 mcg/mL, respectively. ■
Black Box Warning Immediately discontinue infusion if adequate BP reduction isn't obtained within 10 minutes at maximum dose. ■
▼ Reconstitute ADD-Vantage vials labeled as containing 50 mg of drug according to manufacturer's directions.
▼ Because drug is sensitive to light, wrap solution in foil or other opaque material; it's not necessary to wrap the tubing. Fresh solution has a faint brownish tint. Discard if highly discolored after 24 hours.
▼ Use an infusion pump. Drug is best given via piggyback through a peripheral line with no other drug. Don't titrate rate of main I.V. line while drug is being infused. Even a small bolus can cause severe hypotension.
Black Box Warning Use drug only when available equipment and personnel allow BP to be continuously monitored using either a continually reinflated sphygmomanometer or (preferably) an intra-arterial pressure sensor. ■

▼ When drug is used to treat HF, titration of infusion rate must be guided by results of invasive hemodynamic monitoring with simultaneous monitoring of urine output.
▼ Confirm drug's effect at any infusion rate after an additional 5 minutes before titrating to a higher dose to achieve desired BP.
▼ If severe hypotension occurs, stop infusion; effects of drug quickly reverse. Notify prescriber.
▼ If possible, start an arterial pressure line. Regulate drug flow to desired BP response.
▼ **Incompatibilities:** Amiodarone, atracurium besylate, bacteriostatic water for injection, cisatracurium, drotrecogin alfa, haloperidol lactate, levofloxacin, pantoprazole. Don't mix with other I.V. drugs or preservatives.

ACTION
Relaxes arteriolar and venous smooth muscle.

Route	Onset	Peak	Duration
I.V.	Immediate	1–2 min	10 min

Half-life: 2 minutes.

ADVERSE REACTIONS
CNS: headache, dizziness, *increased ICP,* loss of consciousness, apprehension, restlessness.
CV: *bradycardia,* hypotension, tachycardia, palpitations, ECG changes, flushing.
GI: nausea, abdominal pain, ileus.
Hematologic: *methemoglobinemia.*
Metabolic: acidosis, hypothyroidism.
Musculoskeletal: muscle twitching.
Skin: diaphoresis, pink color, rash.
Other: *thiocyanate toxicity, cyanide toxicity,* venous streaking, irritation at I.V. site.

INTERACTIONS
Drug-drug. *Antihypertensives:* May cause sensitivity to nitroprusside. Adjust dosage.
Ganglionic-blocking drugs, general anesthetics, negative inotropic drugs, other antihypertensives: May cause additive effects. Monitor BP closely.
Sildenafil, vardenafil: May increase hypotensive effects. Avoid use together.

EFFECTS ON LAB TEST RESULTS
• May increase creatinine level.
• May decrease RBC and WBC counts.

CONTRAINDICATIONS & CAUTIONS
• Contraindicated in patients hypersensitive to drug.
• Contraindicated in patients with compensatory hypertension (such as in arteriovenous shunt or coarctation of the aorta), inadequate cerebral circulation, acute HF with reduced peripheral vascular resistance (e.g., high-output HF in endotoxic sepsis), congenital optic atrophy, or tobacco-induced amblyopia.
• Use with extreme caution in patients with increased ICP.
• Use cautiously in patients with hypothyroidism, hepatic or renal disease, hyponatremia, or low vitamin B level and in those who are poor surgical risks.
Dialyzable drug: Yes.
⚠ Overdose S&S: Hypotension, acidosis, cyanide or thiocyanate toxicity.

PREGNANCY-LACTATION-REPRODUCTION
• There are no adequate studies in pregnant women. Use only if clearly needed.
• It isn't known if drug appears in breast milk. Patient should discontinue breastfeeding or discontinue drug.

NURSING CONSIDERATIONS
Black Box Warning Drug may cause rapid decrease in BP. Use drug only when available equipment and personnel allow BP to be continuously monitored. ∎
• Obtain baseline vital signs before giving drug; ascertain parameters prescriber wants to achieve. Monitor BP continuously. Patients receiving other antihypertensives may be more sensitive to drug.
• Keep patient in supine position when starting therapy or titrating drug.
Black Box Warning Giving excessive doses of 500 mcg/kg delivered faster than 2 mcg/kg/minute or using maximum infusion rate of 10 mcg/kg/minute for more than 10 minutes can cause cyanide toxicity. ∎
Black Box Warning Although acid-base balance and venous oxygen concentration should be monitored and may indicate

cyanide toxicity, these laboratory tests provide imperfect guidance. ∎
☉ Alert: If patient is at risk, check thiocyanate level every 72 hours. Level higher than 100 mcg/mL may be toxic. If profound hypotension, metabolic acidosis, dyspnea, headache, confusion, loss of consciousness, ataxia, or vomiting occurs, stop drug immediately and notify prescriber.
• **Look alike–sound alike:** Don't confuse nitroprusside with nitroglycerin.

PATIENT TEACHING
• Instruct patient to report all adverse reactions promptly, especially signs and symptoms of hypotension and cyanide toxicity.
• Tell patient to alert nurse if discomfort occurs at I.V. insertion site.

SAFETY ALERT!

nivolumab
neh-VOL-you-mab

Opdivo

Therapeutic class: Antineoplastics
Pharmacologic class: Monoclonal antibodies

N

AVAILABLE FORMS
Injection (single-use vials): 40 mg/4 mL, 100 mg/10 mL

INDICATIONS & DOSAGES
Adjust-a-dose (for all indications): Refer to manufacturer's instructions for dosage adjustments for adverse reactions and treatment-related toxicities.
➤ **Unresectable or metastatic melanoma with disease progression following ipilimumab and, if BRAF V600 mutation–positive, a BRAF inhibitor; metastatic squamous non-small-cell lung cancer with progression on or after platinum-based chemotherapy; patients with *EGFR* or *ALK* genomic tumor aberrations with disease progression on FDA-approved therapy**
Adults: 240 mg I.V. infusion every 2 weeks until disease progression or unacceptable toxicity occurs.

➤ **BRAF V600 wild-type unresectable or metastatic melanoma, in combination with ipilimumab**
Adults: 1 mg/kg I.V. infusion followed by ipilimumab on the same day, every 3 weeks for four doses, then nivolumab 240 mg I.V. every 2 weeks until disease progression or unacceptable toxicity occurs.

➤ **Advanced renal carcinoma in patients who have received prior anti-angiogenic therapy**
Adults: 240 mg I.V. infusion once every 2 weeks until disease progression or unacceptable toxicity.

✳ *NEW INDICATION:* **Classical Hodgkin lymphoma that has relapsed or progressed after autologous hematopoietic stem cell transplantation and posttransplantation brentuximab vedotin; recurrent or metastatic squamous cell carcinoma of the head and neck with disease progression on or after platinum-based therapy**
Adults: 3 mg/kg I.V. infusion every 2 weeks until disease progression or unacceptable toxicity.

ADMINISTRATION
I.V.
▼ Visually inspect for particulate matter and discoloration (solution should be clear to opalescent, colorless to pale yellow).
▼ Store vial refrigerated at 36° to 46° F (2° to 8° C). Don't freeze.
▼ Protect from light by storing in original package until time of use.
▼ To prepare: Withdraw required volume of nivolumab and dilute with NSS or 5% dextrose injection to yield a final concentration of 1 to 10 mg/mL. Mix by gentle inversion; don't shake.
▼ Discard all partially used or empty vials.
▼ Diluted solution is stable at room temperature for no more than 4 hours, including room temperature storage of infusion in the I.V. container and time for administration of infusion.
▼ Diluted solution is stable under refrigeration (36° to 46° F [2° to 8° C]) for no more than 24 hours from time of infusion preparation. Don't freeze.
▼ Give through I.V. line containing a sterile, nonpyrogenic, low protein-binding in-line filter (pore size, 0.2 to 1.2 micrometers) over 60 minutes.
▼ Flush I.V. line at end of infusion.
▼ **Incompatibilities:** Don't administer with other drugs through same I.V. line.

ACTION
A humanized monoclonal antibody that binds to the PD1 receptor found on the surface of T cells, reversing T-cell suppression and resulting in decreased tumor growth.

Route	Onset	Peak	Duration
I.V.	Unknown	Unknown	Unknown

Half-life: About 27 days.

ADVERSE REACTIONS
CNS: dizziness, peripheral and sensory neuropathy, fatigue, asthenia.
CV: peripheral edema, *ventricular arrhythmia,* chest pain.
EENT: iridocyclitis, stomatitis.
GI: abdominal pain, colitis, nausea, vomiting, constipation.
GU: renal dysfunction, nephritis.
Hepatic: increased AST, ALT, and alkaline phosphatase levels; *hepatitis.*
Metabolic: hyponatremia, *hyperkalemia,* weight loss, anemia, lymphopenia, thrombocytopenia.
Respiratory: cough, URI, dyspnea, pneumonitis or *interstitial lung disease,* pleural effusion, hemoptysis.
Skin: rash, pruritus, exfoliative dermatitis, *erythema multiforme,* psoriasis, skin depigmentation.
Musculoskeletal: pain.
Other: infusion-related reactions, fever.

INTERACTIONS
None reported.

EFFECTS ON LAB TEST RESULTS
● May increase creatinine, total bilirubin, potassium, amylase, lipase, ALT, AST, and thyroid function levels. May decrease sodium level.
● May decrease RBC, lymphocyte, and platelet counts.

CONTRAINDICATIONS & CAUTIONS
● Contraindicated in patients hypersensitive to drug or its components.

⟐ *Alert:* If nivolumab is withheld for an adverse reaction, also withhold ipilimumab.
⟐ *Alert:* Drug can cause severe immune-mediated pneumonitis or interstitial lung disease, which can be fatal.
• Drug can cause the following immune-mediated conditions: colitis, hepatitis, nephritis and renal dysfunction, hypothyroidism and hyperthyroidism, rash, encephalitis, and other serious adverse reactions.
• Drug can cause hypophysitis and adrenal insufficiency.
• Drug hasn't been studied in patients with moderate or severe hepatic impairment.
• Safety and effectiveness in children haven't been established.
Dialyzable drug: Unknown.

PREGNANCY-LACTATION-REPRODUCTION
⟐ *Alert:* Use cautiously in pregnant women. Drug may cause fetal harm and increase risk of abortion and premature infant death.
• Women of childbearing potential should use effective contraception during treatment and for at least 5 months after last dose.
• It isn't known if drug appears in breast milk. Patient should discontinue breast-feeding during treatment because of possible serious adverse effects in breast-feeding infants.

NURSING CONSIDERATIONS
• Infusion-related reactions, which can be severe or life-threatening, can occur. Discontinue drug for severe or life-threatening reactions. For mild to moderate reactions, either interrupt infusion or decrease infusion rate.
• Monitor patient for signs and symptoms of immune-mediated severe pneumonitis or interstitial lung disease (fever, cough, dyspnea, chest pain) or colitis (fever, abdominal pain, diarrhea, bloody stools). Adjust dosage or discontinue drug as needed. Refer to manufacturer's instructions for corticosteroid treatment if indicated.
• Obtain LFT values at baseline and monitor periodically during treatment because of risk of immune-mediated hepatitis. Adjust dosages or discontinue drug as needed. Refer to manufacturer's instructions for corticosteroid treatment if indicated.

• Obtain serum creatinine level at baseline and monitor periodically during treatment because of risk of immune-mediated nephritis and renal dysfunction. Adjust dosages or discontinue drug as needed. Refer to manufacturer's instructions for corticosteroid treatment if indicated.
• Monitor thyroid function at baseline and periodically during treatment because of risk of immune-mediated hypothyroidism and hyperthyroidism. Administer hormone replacement therapy for hypothyroidism, or initiate medical management for control of hyperthyroidism. There are no recommended nivolumab dosage adjustments for hypothyroidism or hyperthyroidism.
• Monitor patient for other immune-mediated adverse reactions, which may occur during or after nivolumab has been discontinued. Rule out other causes of reactions first. Based on severity of reaction, withhold drug, administer corticosteroids, or initiate hormone-replacement therapy, if appropriate.
• *Look alike–sound alike:* Don't confuse Opdivo with Optivite or Osphena. Don't confuse nivolumab with Nabilone, natalizumab, nebivolol, nepafenac, NephPlex, or nofetumomab.

PATIENT TEACHING
• Instruct patient to inform prescriber if patient has known disease that affects the immune system, lungs, liver, or kidney or has had an organ transplant.
• Educate patient and family to recognize and immediately report signs and symptoms of pneumonitis (new or worsening cough, chest pain, shortness of breath), colitis (diarrhea, bloody stools, dark tarry stools, severe abdominal pain or tenderness), hepatic dysfunction (dark urine, yellowing of eyes, nausea, vomiting, right-sided abdominal pain, lethargy, easy bruising or bleeding), renal dysfunction (decreased urine output, blood in urine, edema, loss of appetite), hormone gland problems (weight gain or loss, feeling hot or cold, constipation, persistent or unusual headaches, extreme fatigue, changes in mood or behavior, dizziness, hair loss, deepening voice), rash, vision changes, severe or persistent muscle or joint pains, or severe muscle weakness.

◑ *Alert:* Warn pregnant patient of the possibility of fetal harm. Advise female patient of childbearing potential to use effective contraception during and for at least 5 months after last dose.

• Advise female patient to report known or suspected pregnancy to prescriber.

• Caution female patient not to breast-feed while taking drug.

• Reinforce importance of laboratory tests and instruct patient to keep follow-up appointments to monitor drug's safety and effectiveness.

norelgestromin–ethinyl estradiol transdermal system
nor-el-JES-troe-min/ETH-i-nill

Xulane

Therapeutic class: Contraceptives
Pharmacologic class: Estrogen–progestin combinations

AVAILABLE FORMS
Transdermal patch: norelgestromin 6 mg and ethinyl estradiol 0.75 mg per patch, delivering 150 mcg norelgestromin and 35 mcg ethinyl estradiol daily

INDICATIONS & DOSAGES
➤ **Contraception**
Women of childbearing potential: Apply 1 patch weekly for 3 weeks (21 total days). Apply each new patch on the same day of the week. Week 4 is patch-free, and withdrawal bleeding is expected. On the day after week 4 ends, apply a new patch to start a new 4-week cycle. The patch-free interval between cycles should never be longer than 7 days.

ADMINISTRATION
Transdermal
• Apply patch to a clean, dry area of the skin on the buttocks, abdomen, upper outer arm, or upper torso. Don't apply to the breasts or to skin that is red, irritated, or cut.

ACTION
Combination hormonal contraceptives act by suppressing gonadotropins. The primary mechanism of this action is ovulation inhibition. However, changes in cervical mucus increase the difficulty of sperm entry into the uterus, and changes in the endometrium decrease the likelihood of implantation.

Route	Onset	Peak	Duration
Transdermal	Rapid	2 days	Unknown

Half-life: Ethinyl estradiol, 6 to 45 hours; norelgestromin, 28 hours.

ADVERSE REACTIONS
CNS: headache, emotional lability, dizziness, fatigue.
EENT: contact lens intolerance, changes in corneal curvature.
GI: nausea, diarrhea, abdominal pain, vomiting, gallbladder disease, cholestatic jaundice.
GU: dysmenorrhea, changes in menstrual flow, vaginal candidiasis.
Metabolic: weight changes.
Skin: application-site reaction, melasma, pruritus, acne.
Other: breast tenderness, enlargement, or secretion.

INTERACTIONS
Drug-drug. *Acetaminophen, clofibric acid, morphine, salicylic acid, temazepam:* May decrease levels or increase clearance of these drugs. Monitor for lack of effect.
Ampicillin, barbiturates, carbamazepine, felbamate, griseofulvin, oxcarbazepine, phenylbutazone, phenytoin, rifampin, tetracyclines, topiramate: May reduce contraceptive effectiveness, resulting in unintended pregnancy or breakthrough bleeding. Encourage backup method of contraception if used together.
Anticoagulants: May increase or decrease effect of anticoagulant. Monitor patient and laboratory values.
Ascorbic acid, atorvastatin, itraconazole, ketoconazole: May increase hormone levels Use together cautiously.
Cyclosporine, prednisolone, theophylline: May increase levels of these drugs. Monitor patient for adverse reactions.
HIV protease inhibitors: May affect contraceptive effectiveness and safety. Use together cautiously.

Reactions in bold italics are *life-threatening*. Interactions may have a *rapid onset* or a ***delayed onset***.

Drug-herb. *St. John's wort:* May reduce effectiveness of drug and cause breakthrough bleeding. Discourage use together.

Drug-lifestyle. `Black Box Warning` *Smoking:* May increase risk of CV adverse effects, related to age and smoking 15 or more cigarettes daily. Urge patient not to smoke. ∎

EFFECTS ON LAB TEST RESULTS

● May increase circulating total thyroid hormone, triglyceride, other binding protein, sex hormone–binding globulin, total circulating endogenous sex steroid, corticoid, and factor VII, VIII, IX, and X levels. May decrease antithrombin III and folate levels.
● May decrease free T_3 resin uptake and glucose tolerance.

CONTRAINDICATIONS & CAUTIONS

`Black Box Warning` Cigarette smoking increases the risk of serious adverse cardiac effects from hormonal contraceptive use. Risk increases with age, especially in women older than age 35, and with the number of cigarettes smoked. Hormonal contraceptives are contraindicated in women older than age 35 who smoke. ∎

`Black Box Warning` There is an increased risk of venous thromboembolism in women ages 15 to 44 using the norelgestromin–ethinyl estradiol transdermal system compared to women using oral contraceptives containing 30 to 35 mcg of ethinyl estradiol and either levonorgestrel or norgestimate. ∎

`Black Box Warning` The contraceptive patch has higher steady-state concentrations and lower peak concentrations than oral contraceptives. It's unknown whether there are changes in the risk of serious adverse events based on the differences in pharmacokinetic profiles of ethinyl estradiol in women using the contraceptive patch compared with women using oral contraceptives containing ethinyl estradiol 30 to 35 mcg. Increased estrogen exposure may increase the risk of adverse events, including venous thromboembolism. ∎

Contraindicated in patients hypersensitive to components of drug; in those with history of DVT or related disorder; in patients at high risk for arterial or venous thrombotic diseases or with current or past history of cerebrovascular disease or CAD; in those

with uncontrolled hypertension; and in patients with headaches with focal neurologic conditions, migraine headaches with aura, or migraine headaches if older than age 35.
● Contraindicated in patients with past or current known or suspected breast cancer, endometrial cancer, or other known or suspected estrogen-dependent neoplasia; or hepatic adenoma or cancer.
● Contraindicated in patients with thrombophlebitis, thromboembolic disorders, valvular heart disease with complications, diabetes with vascular involvement, major surgery with prolonged immobilization, undiagnosed abnormal genital bleeding, cholestatic jaundice of pregnancy or jaundice with previous hormonal contraceptive use, or acute or chronic hepatocellular disease with abnormal hepatic function.
● Use cautiously in patients with CV disease risk factors, conditions that might be aggravated by fluid retention, or history of depression.
Dialyzable drug: Unknown.
⚠ *Overdose S&S:* Nausea, vomiting, withdrawal uterine bleeding.

PREGNANCY-LACTATION-REPRODUCTION

● Contraindicated in women who are or may be pregnant. Studies haven't shown an increased risk of birth defects when drug was inadvertently taken during early pregnancy.
● Breast-feeding women should use alternative forms of contraception until infant is completely weaned.
● In women who choose not to breast-feed, don't begin drug until 4 weeks after childbirth.

NURSING CONSIDERATIONS

✵ *Alert:* Patients taking combination hormonal contraceptives may be at increased risk for thrombophlebitis, venous thrombosis with or without embolism, PE, MI, cerebral hemorrhage, cerebral thrombosis, hypertension, gallbladder disease, hepatic adenomas, benign liver tumors, mesenteric thrombosis, and retinal thrombosis.
● Increased risk of MI occurs primarily in smokers and women with hypertension, hypercholesterolemia, morbid obesity, and diabetes.

• Encourage women with a history of hypertension or renal disease to use a different contraceptive. If this drug is used, monitor BP closely and stop use if hypertension occurs.

• Drug may be less effective in women who weigh 90 kg or more.

• The risk of thromboembolic disease increases if therapy is used postpartum or postabortion.

• Rule out pregnancy if withdrawal bleeding fails to occur for two consecutive cycles.

• If skin becomes irritated, the patch may be removed and a new patch applied at a different site.

• Stop drug and notify prescriber at least 4 weeks before and for 2 weeks after an elective surgery that increases the risk of thromboembolism, and during and after prolonged immobilization. Teach patient about alternative methods of contraception during this time.

• Stop drug and notify prescriber if patient has headaches, vision loss, proptosis, diplopia, papilledema, retinal vascular lesions, jaundice, or depression.

PATIENT TEACHING

• Emphasize the importance of having regular annual physical examinations to check for adverse effects or developing contraindications.

• Tell patient that drug doesn't protect against HIV and other sexually transmitted diseases.

• Advise women to initiate and apply patch on the first day of menstrual cycle and then on the same day each week.

• Advise patient to use a backup method of contraception for the first 7 days.

• Tell patient switching from estrogen–progestin oral contraceptives to apply first patch on the first day of withdrawal bleeding. If no bleeding occurs within 5 days of last hormonally active pill, advise patient to obtain a pregnancy test.

• Advise patient to immediately apply a new patch once the used patch is removed, on the same day of the week every 7 days for 3 weeks. Week 4 is patch-free. Withdrawal bleeding is expected to occur during this time.

• Tell patient to apply each patch to a clean, dry area of the skin on the buttocks, abdomen, upper outer arm, or upper torso. Tell patient not to apply to the breasts or to skin that's red, irritated, or cut.

• Tell patient to carefully fold the used patch in half so that it sticks to itself before discarding.

• Tell women to immediately stop use if pregnancy is confirmed.

• Tell patient who wears contact lenses to report visual changes or changes in lens tolerance.

• Advise patient not to smoke while using the patch.

• Tell patient that if a patch becomes detached for less than 1 day, to reapply it or replace it immediately and continue the schedule. If the patch is detached for more than 1 day, a new cycle should be started and back-up contraception should be used for the first week.

• Stress that if patient isn't sure what to do about mistakes with patch use, she should use a backup method of birth control and contact her health care provider.

• Tell patient undergoing an MRI scan to alert facility that she's using a transdermal patch.

• Advise patient to report all drugs and supplements she is taking as some can decrease contraceptive effectiveness; a backup contraceptive method may be needed.

SAFETY ALERT!

norepinephrine bitartrate (levarterenol bitartrate, noradrenaline acid tartrate)
nor-ep-i-NEF-rin

Levophed

Therapeutic class: Vasopressors
Pharmacologic class: Direct-acting adrenergics

AVAILABLE FORMS
Injection: 1 mg/mL

INDICATIONS & DOSAGES
➤ **To restore BP in acute hypotension; severe hypotension during cardiac arrest**

Adults: Initially, 8 to 12 mcg/minute by I.V. infusion; then titrate to maintain systolic BP at 80 to 100 mm Hg in previously normotensive patients and 40 mm Hg below preexisting systolic BP in previously hypertensive patients. Average maintenance dose is 2 to 4 mcg/minute.

ADMINISTRATION

I.V.

▼ Use a central venous catheter (preferred) or large vein, such as the antecubital fossa, to minimize risk of extravasation. Give in D_5W alone or D_5W in NSS for injection. Use continuous infusion pump to regulate infusion flow rate and a piggyback setup so I.V. line stays open if norepinephrine is stopped.

▼ Never leave patient unattended during infusion. Check BP every 2 minutes until stabilized; then check every 5 minutes.

▼ During infusion, frequently monitor ECG, cardiac output, central venous pressure, pulmonary artery wedge pressure, pulse rate, urine output, and color and temperature of limbs. Titrate infusion rate based on findings and prescriber guidelines.

Black Box Warning Check site frequently for signs and symptoms of extravasation. If they appear, stop infusion immediately and call prescriber. To prevent sloughing and necrosis, use a fine hypodermic needle to infiltrate area with 5 to 10 mg phentolamine in 10 to 15 mL of NSS as soon as possible. Immediate local hyperemic changes will occur if area is infiltrated within 12 hours. Also, check for blanching along course of infused vein, which may progress to superficial sloughing. ∎

▼ Protect drug from light. Discard discolored solution or solution that contains precipitate. Solution will deteriorate after 24 hours.

▼ If prolonged therapy is needed, change injection site frequently.

▼ Avoid mixing with alkaline solutions, oxidizing drugs, or iron salts. The use of NSS alone isn't recommended because of the lack of oxidation protection.

▼ **Incompatibilities:** Alkalis, drotrecogin alfa, iron salts, oxidizers, regular insulin, thiopental.

ACTION

Stimulates alpha and beta$_1$ receptors in the sympathetic nervous system, causing vasoconstriction and cardiac stimulation.

Route	Onset	Peak	Duration
I.V.	Immediate	Immediate	1–2 min after infusion

Half-life: About 1 minute.

ADVERSE REACTIONS

CNS: headache, anxiety.
CV: *bradycardia, severe hypertension, arrhythmias.*
Respiratory: *asthma attacks,* respiratory difficulties.
Skin: irritation with extravasation, necrosis and gangrene secondary to extravasation.
Other: *anaphylaxis.*

INTERACTIONS

Drug-drug. *Alpha blockers:* May antagonize drug effects. Avoid using together.
Antihistamines, atropine, ergot alkaloids, guanethidine, MAO inhibitors, methyldopa, oxytocics: When given with sympathomimetics, may cause severe hypertension (hypertensive crisis). Avoid using together.
Inhaled anesthetics: May increase risk of arrhythmias. Monitor ECG.
TCAs: May potentiate the pressor response and cause arrhythmias. Use together cautiously.

EFFECTS ON LAB TEST RESULTS

None reported.

CONTRAINDICATIONS & CAUTIONS

● Contraindicated in patients with mesenteric or peripheral vascular thrombosis, profound hypoxia, hypercarbia, or hypotension resulting from blood volume deficit.
● Contraindicated during cyclopropane and halothane anesthesia due to risk of ventricular arrhythmias.
● Use cautiously in patients taking MAO inhibitors, TCAs, or imipramine-type antidepressants.
● Use cautiously in patients with sulfite sensitivity.
Dialyzable drug: Unknown.
⚠ *Overdose S&S:* Headache, severe hypertension, reflex bradycardia, increased

peripheral resistance, decreased cardiac output.

PREGNANCY-LACTATION-REPRODUCTION
• Safe use in pregnancy hasn't been established. Use in pregnant women only if clearly needed.
• It isn't known if drug appears in breast milk. Use cautiously in breast-feeding women.

NURSING CONSIDERATIONS
• Drug isn't a substitute for blood or fluid replacement therapy. If patient has volume deficit, replace fluids before giving vasopressors.
• Keep emergency drugs on hand to reverse effects of drug: atropine for reflex bradycardia, phentolamine to decrease vasopressor effects, and propranolol for arrhythmias.
• Notify prescriber immediately of decreased urine output.
• When stopping drug, gradually slow infusion rate. Continue monitoring vital signs, watching for possible severe drop in BP.
• **Alert:** Monitor infusion site carefully as extravasation can cause tissue necrosis.
• **Look alike–sound alike:** Don't confuse norepinephrine with epinephrine.

PATIENT TEACHING
• Tell patient to report adverse reactions promptly.
• Advise patient that vital signs will be monitored frequently and to immediately report discomfort at I.V. insertion site.

norethindrone
nor-ETH-in-drone

Camila, Errin, Heather, Jencycla, Micronor, Nor-QD

norethindrone acetate
Aygestin

Therapeutic class: Contraceptives
Pharmacologic class: Progestins

AVAILABLE FORMS
norethindrone
Tablets: 0.35 mg

norethindrone acetate
Tablets: 5 mg

INDICATIONS & DOSAGES
➤ **Amenorrhea, abnormal uterine bleeding**
Women: 2.5 to 10 mg norethindrone acetate P.O. daily for 5 to 10 days, beginning in the assumed latter half of the menstrual cycle.
➤ **Endometriosis**
Women: 5 mg norethindrone acetate P.O. daily for 14 days; then increased by 2.5 mg daily every 2 weeks, up to 15 mg daily. Therapy may continue for 6 to 9 months or until breakthrough bleeding warrants temporary termination.
➤ **Contraception**
Women of childbearing potential and menarchal girls: Initially, 0.35 mg norethindrone P.O. on first day of menstruation; then 0.35 mg daily.

ADMINISTRATION
P.O.
• When used for contraception, give drug at same time every day, continuously, with no interruption between pill packs.
• Give norethindrone acetate without regard to meals. May give with food if GI upset occurs.

ACTION
Suppresses ovulation, possibly by inhibiting pituitary gonadotropin secretion, and forms thick cervical mucus.

Route	Onset	Peak	Duration
P.O.	Unknown	Unknown	Unknown

Half-life: 5 to 14 hours.

ADVERSE REACTIONS
CNS: depression, *stroke,* headache, mood swings.
CV: thrombophlebitis, *PE,* edema, *thromboembolism.*
GI: bloating, abdominal pain or cramping.
GU: breakthrough bleeding, dysmenorrhea, amenorrhea, cervical erosion, abnormal secretions.
Hepatic: cholestatic jaundice.
Metabolic: weight changes.
Skin: melasma, rash, acne, pruritus, alopecia, hirsutism, hemorrhagic skin eruptions.

Reactions in bold italics are *life-threatening*. Interactions may have a *rapid onset* or a *delayed onset.*

Other: breast tenderness, enlargement, or secretion; premenstrual-like syndrome, *anaphylactic reactions.*

INTERACTIONS

Drug-drug. *Barbiturates, carbamazepine, fosphenytoin, phenytoin, rifampin:* May decrease progestin effects. Monitor patient for diminished therapeutic response.

Drug-food. *Caffeine:* May increase caffeine level. Urge caution.

Drug-lifestyle. *Smoking:* May increase risk of adverse CV effects. If smoking continues, may need alternative therapy.

EFFECTS ON LAB TEST RESULTS

● May increase LFT values. May alter coagulation factors and thyroid function tests.

● May decrease metyrapone test results and HDL levels. May increase LDL/HDL ratio.

CONTRAINDICATIONS & CAUTIONS

● Contraindicated in patients hypersensitive to drug and in those with breast cancer, undiagnosed abnormal vaginal bleeding, severe hepatic disease, missed abortion, or current or previous thromboembolic disorders.

● Use cautiously in patients with diabetes, seizures, migraines, cardiac or renal disease, asthma, and depression.

● *Alert:* Norethindrone acetate may cause papilledema or retinal vascular lesions. If these occur, discontinue drug.

Dialyzable drug: Unknown.

PREGNANCY-LACTATION-REPRODUCTION

● Contraindicated in pregnant women; may cause fetal harm.

● Use cautiously in breast-feeding women.

NURSING CONSIDERATIONS

● If switching from combined oral contraceptives to progestin-only pills (POPs), take the first POP the day after the last active combined pill.

● If switching from POPs to combined pills, take the first active combined pill on the first day of menstruation, even if the POP pack isn't finished.

● *Alert:* Norethindrone acetate is twice as potent as norethindrone. Norethindrone acetate shouldn't be used for contraception.

● Patients with menstrual disorders usually need preliminary estrogen treatment.

● Watch patient closely for signs of edema.

● Monitor BP.

● *Look alike–sound alike:* Don't confuse Micronor with Micro-K.

PATIENT TEACHING

● According to FDA regulations, patient must read package insert explaining possible adverse effects before receiving first dose. Also, give patient verbal explanation.

● Tell patient to take drug at the same time every day when used as a contraceptive. If she's more than 3 hours late taking the pill or if she has missed a pill, she should take the pill as soon as she remembers, and then continue the normal schedule. Also tell her to use a backup method of contraception for the next 48 hours.

● *Alert:* Tell patient to report unusual symptoms immediately and to stop drug and notify prescriber about visual disturbances or migraine, or pain or numbness in her arms or legs.

● Teach patient how to perform routine breast self-examination.

● Tell patient to report suspected pregnancy to prescriber.

● Encourage patient to stop or reduce smoking because of the risk of CV complications.

● Tell patient with diabetes that glucose levels may be affected and to closely monitor her levels.

● Advise patient to immediately report sudden partial or complete loss of vision, diplopia, migraine, or bulging of the eye.

● Tell patient that drug does not protect against HIV or other sexually transmitted diseases.

● Tell patient that if she vomits soon after taking a pill to use a back-up method of birth control for 48 hours.

N

nortriptyline hydrochloride
nor-TRIP-ti-leen

Pamelor⌀*

Therapeutic class: Antidepressants
Pharmacologic class: TCAs

AVAILABLE FORMS
Capsules: 10 mg, 25 mg, 50 mg, 75 mg
Oral solution: 10 mg/5 mL*

INDICATIONS & DOSAGES
➤ **Depression**
Adults: 25 mg P.O. t.i.d. or q.i.d., gradually increased to maximum of 150 mg daily. Or, give total daily dose at bedtime. Monitor level when doses above 100 mg daily are given.
Elderly patients and adolescents: 30 to 50 mg P.O. daily given once or in divided doses.

ADMINISTRATION
P.O.
● Give drug without regard for food.
● Whenever possible, give full dose at bedtime.

ACTION
Unknown. Increases the amount of norepinephrine, serotonin, or both in the CNS by blocking reuptake by the presynaptic neurons.

Route	Onset	Peak	Duration
P.O.	Unknown	7–8½ hr	Unknown

Half-life: 18 to 24 hours.

ADVERSE REACTIONS
CNS: *stroke,* numbness, tingling, paresthesia of extremities, incoordination, ataxia, tremors, peripheral neuropathy, extrapyramidal symptoms, *seizures,* alteration in EEG, confusional states, anxiety, restlessness, agitation, insomnia, nightmares, hypomania, exacerbation of psychosis, drowsiness, dizziness, weakness, fatigue, headache.
CV: edema, hypotension, hypertension, tachycardia, palpitations, *MI,* arrhythmias, *heart block,* flushing.

EENT: blurred vision, disturbance of accommodation, mydriasis, tinnitus.
GI: dry mouth, constipation, paralytic ileus, nausea and vomiting, anorexia, epigastric distress, diarrhea, peculiar taste, stomatitis, abdominal cramps, black tongue.
GU: urine retention, delayed micturition, dilation of the urinary tract, erectile dysfunction, testicular swelling, urinary frequency, nocturia.
Hematologic: bone marrow depression, eosinophilia, purpura, *thrombocytopenia.*
Hepatic: jaundice, altered liver function.
Metabolic: weight gain or loss.
Skin: rash, petechiae, urticaria, itching, photosensitivity, alopecia.
Other: drug fever, gynecomastia, breast enlargement and galactorrhea in women, increased or decreased libido, SIADH, diaphoresis.

INTERACTIONS
Drug-drug. *Barbiturates, CNS depressants:* May enhance CNS depression. Avoid using together.
Cimetidine, **fluoxetine, fluvoxamine, paroxetine, sertraline:** May increase nortriptyline level. Monitor drug levels and patient for signs of toxicity.
Clonidine: May cause life-threatening hypertension. Avoid using together.
Drugs that prolong QT interval: May increase risk of life-threatening cardiac arrhythmias, including torsades de pointes. Monitor patient and ECG.
Epinephrine, norepinephrine: May increase hypertensive effect. Use together cautiously.
Linezolid, methylene blue: May cause serotonin syndrome. Use extreme caution and monitor patient closely.
MAO inhibitors: May cause severe excitation, hyperpyrexia, or seizures, usually with high doses. Avoid using within 14 days of MAO inhibitor therapy.
Quinolones: May increase the risk of life-threatening arrhythmias. Avoid using together.
Drug-herb. *Evening primrose oil:* May cause additive or synergistic effect, lowering seizure threshold and increasing the risk of seizure. Discourage use together.

St. John's wort, SAM-e, yohimbe: May cause serotonin syndrome and reduced drug level. Discourage use together.
Drug-lifestyle. *Alcohol use:* May enhance CNS depression. Discourage use together.
Smoking: May decrease drug level. Monitor patient for lack of effect.
Sun exposure: May increase risk of photo-sensitivity reactions. Advise patient to avoid excessive sunlight exposure.

EFFECTS ON LAB TEST RESULTS
● May increase or decrease glucose level.
● May increase eosinophil count and LFT values. May decrease WBC, RBC, granulo-cyte, and platelet counts.

CONTRAINDICATIONS & CAUTIONS
● Contraindicated in patients hypersensitive to drug and during acute recovery phase of MI; also contraindicated within 14 days of MAO inhibitor therapy.
Black Box Warning Nortriptyline isn't approved for use in children. ■
Alert: Concomitant use with linezolid or methylene blue can cause serotonin syn-drome (fever, mental status changes, muscle twitching, excessive sweating, shivering or shaking, diarrhea, loss of coordination). Use drug with linezolid or methylene blue only for life-threatening or urgent conditions when the potential benefits outweigh the risks of toxicity.
● Drug isn't approved for use in patients with bipolar depression. Screen for bipolar depression before starting drug.
● Use with extreme caution in patients with glaucoma, suicidal tendency, history of urine retention or seizures, CV disease, or hyperthyroidism and in those receiving thyroid drugs.
Dialyzable drug: No.
⚠ Overdose S&S: Cardiac arrhythmias, severe hypotension, shock, HF, pulmonary edema, seizures, CNS depression, coma, ECG changes, confusion, restlessness, disturbed concentration, transient visual hallucinations, dilated pupils, agitation, hyperactive reflexes, stupor, drowsiness, muscle rigidity, vomiting, hypothermia, hyperpyrexia.

PREGNANCY-LACTATION-REPRODUCTION
● Safe use during pregnancy and breast-feeding hasn't been established. Weigh potential benefits against possible hazards.
● Monitor pregnant and breast-feeding infants for adverse reactions.

NURSING CONSIDERATIONS
Alert: If linezolid or methylene blue must be given, stop nortriptyline and monitor patient for serotonin toxicity for 2 weeks or until 24 hours after the last dose of methy-lene blue or linezolid, whichever comes first. Treatment with nortriptyline may resume 24 hours after the last dose of methylene blue or linezolid.
● To withdraw drug, gradually taper dosage and monitor for reemerging symptoms.
● Because patients using TCAs may suffer hypertensive episodes during surgery, stop drug gradually several days before surgery.
● If signs or symptoms of psychosis occur or increase, expect to reduce dosage. Record mood changes. Monitor patient for suicidal tendencies and allow him only a minimum supply of drug.
Black Box Warning Drug may increase the risk of suicidal thinking and behavior in children, adolescents, and young adults with major depressive disorder or other psychiatric disorder. ■
● *Look alike–sound alike:* Don't confuse nortriptyline with amitriptyline.

PATIENT TEACHING
Black Box Warning Advise families and caregivers to closely observe patient for increased suicidal thinking or behavior. ■
● Teach patient to recognize and imme-diately report signs and symptoms of serotonin syndrome (fever, mental status changes, muscle twitching, excessive sweat-ing, shivering or shaking, diarrhea, loss of coordination).
● Advise patient to take full dose at bed-time whenever possible to reduce risk of dizziness upon standing quickly.
● Warn patient to avoid activities that re-quire alertness and good coordination until effects of drug are known. Drowsiness and dizziness usually subside after a few weeks.

N

• Recommend use of sugarless hard candy or gum to relieve dry mouth. Saliva substitutes may be needed.
• Tell patient to consult prescriber before taking other prescription or OTC drugs.
• Warn patient not to stop drug suddenly.
• To prevent oversensitivity to the sun, advise patient to use sun block, wear protective clothing, and avoid prolonged exposure to strong sunlight.

nystatin
nye-STAT-in

Nystop

Therapeutic class: Antifungals
Pharmacologic class: Polyene macrolides

AVAILABLE FORMS
Cream: 100,000 units/g
Ointment: 100,000 units/g
Oral suspension: 100,000 units/mL
Powder: 100,000 units/g
Powder (bulk): 50, 150, or 500 million units; 1, 2, or 5 billion units
Tablets: 500,000 units

INDICATIONS & DOSAGES
➤ **Intestinal candidiasis**
Adults: 500,000 to 1 million units P.O. as tablets t.i.d.
➤ **Mycotic infections**
Adults and children: Apply cream or ointment liberally to affected areas b.i.d. Or, apply powder to lesions b.i.d. to t.i.d. until lesions have healed.
➤ **Oral candidiasis (thrush)**
Adults and children: 400,000 to 600,000 units P.O. as oral suspension q.i.d. for up to 14 days.
Infants: 200,000 units P.O. as oral suspension q.i.d.
Low-birth-weight and premature infants: 100,000 units P.O. oral suspension q.i.d.

ADMINISTRATION
P.O.
• To treat oral candidiasis, after patient's mouth is clean of food debris, have him hold suspension in mouth for several minutes

before swallowing. When treating infants, swab medication on oral mucosa.
• Suspension made with bulk powder contains no preservatives. Use immediately; don't store.
Topical
• Store at room temperature.

ACTION
Probably binds to sterols in fungal cell membrane, altering cell permeability and allowing leakage of intracellular components.

Route	Onset	Peak	Duration
P.O., topical	Unknown	Unknown	Unknown

Half-life: Unknown.

ADVERSE REACTIONS
GI: transient nausea, vomiting, diarrhea.
GU: irritation, sensitization, vulvovaginal burning (vaginal form).
Skin: rash.

INTERACTIONS
None significant.

EFFECTS ON LAB TEST RESULTS
None reported.

CONTRAINDICATIONS & CAUTIONS
• Contraindicated in patients hypersensitive to drug.
• Rarely, Stevens-Johnson syndrome has been reported.
Dialyzable drug: Unknown.
⚠ *Overdose S&S:* Nausea, GI upset.

PREGNANCY-LACTATION-REPRODUCTION
• Use cautiously in pregnant and breast-feeding women and only when needed.

NURSING CONSIDERATIONS
• Drug isn't effective against systemic infections.
• Monitor patient for rash.

PATIENT TEACHING
• Advise patient to continue taking drug for at least 2 days after symptoms resolve.
• Instruct patient to continue therapy during menstruation.
• Advise patient to report redness, swelling, or irritation.

Reactions in bold italics are *life-threatening*. Interactions may have a *rapid onset* or a *delayed onset*.

- Tell patient that overusing mouthwash or wearing poorly fitting dentures may promote infection.
- For fungal foot infections, teach patient to dust powder freely on the feet.

obeticholic acid
See NEW DRUGS for information.

obiltoxaximab
See NEW DRUGS for information.

SAFETY ALERT!

obinutuzumab
OH-bi-nue-TOOZ-ue-mab

Gazyva

Therapeutic class: Antineoplastics
Pharmacologic class: Monoclonal antibodies

AVAILABLE FORMS
Solution: 25 mg/mL

INDICATIONS & DOSAGES
➤ **Chronic lymphocytic leukemia previously untreated, in combination with chlorambucil**
Adults: Each cycle lasts 28 days. Cycle 1, day 1: 100 mg I.V. at 25 mg/hour over 4 hours; don't increase infusion rate. Cycle 1, day 2: 900 mg I.V. at 50 mg/hour; may increase infusion rate in increments of 50 mg/hour every 30 minutes to maximum rate of 400 mg/hour. Cycle 1, days 8 and 15: If no infusion reaction occurred during previous infusion and final infusion rate was 100 mg/hour or faster, give 1,000 mg I.V. at 100 mg/hour; may increase infusion rate by 100 mg/hour every 30 minutes to maximum rate of 400 mg/hour. For cycles 2 to 6 on day 1 only: If no infusion reaction occurred during previous infusion and final infusion rate was 100 mg/hour or faster, give 1,000 mg I.V. at 100 mg/hour; may increase infusion rate in increments of 100 mg/hour every 30 minutes to maximum of 400 mg/hour.

If a dose is missed, administer dose as soon as possible and adjust future doses accordingly. If appropriate, patients who don't complete the day-1, cycle-1 dose may proceed to the day-2, cycle-1 dose.

Adjust-a-dose: If grade 4 life-threatening reactions occur, stop infusion and permanently discontinue treatment. For grade 3 severe reactions, interrupt infusion and manage symptoms. Once symptoms resolve, may restart drug at no more than half the previous infusion rate. If patient doesn't experience further reaction symptoms, may increase dosage to prescribed rate for that treatment cycle. If grade 3 infusion reaction reappears, permanently discontinue treatment. The day-1 infusion rate may be increased back up to 25 mg/hour after 1 hour but not increased further. For grade 1 to 2 mild to moderate reactions, reduce rate or interrupt infusion and treat symptoms. Once symptoms resolve, continue or resume infusion. If patient tolerates infusion, may increase to prescribed infusion rate for that treatment cycle. The day-1 infusion rate may be increased back up to 25 mg/hour after 1 hour but not increased further.

If patient experiences an infection, grade 3 or 4 cytopenia, or a grade 2 or greater nonhematologic toxicity, consider treatment interruption.
➤ **Follicular lymphoma, in combination with bendamustine followed by obinutuzumab monotherapy in patients who relapsed after, or are refractory to, a rituximab-containing regimen**
Adults: Each cycle lasts 28 days. Cycle 1, day 1: 1,000 mg I.V. at 50 mg/hour; may increase infusion rate in increments of 50 mg/hour every 30 minutes to maximum rate of 400 mg/hour. Cycle 1, days 8 and 15: If no infusion reaction occurred during previous infusion and final infusion rate was 100 mg/hour or faster, give 1,000 mg I.V. at 100 mg/hour; may increase infusion rate by 100 mg/hour every 30 minutes to maximum rate of 400 mg/hour. For cycles 2 to 6 on day 1 only: If no infusion reaction occurred during previous infusion and final infusion rate was 100 mg/hour or faster, give 1,000 mg I.V. at 100 mg/hour; may increase infusion rate in increments of 100 mg/hour every 30 minutes to maximum of 400 mg/hour.

Give missed dose as soon as possible and adjust future doses accordingly. During monotherapy, maintain the original dosing schedule for subsequent doses.

♣ Canada   ◇ OTC   ◆ Off-label use   ✐ Photoguide   ⊜ Do not crush   *Liquid contains alcohol.

Patients who achieve stable disease, complete response, or partial response to the initial 6 cycles of obinutuzumab in combination with bendamustine should continue on obinutuzumab 1,000 mg as monotherapy for two years.

Adjust-a-dose: If grade 4 life-threatening reactions occur, stop infusion and permanently discontinue treatment. For grade 3 severe reactions, interrupt infusion and manage symptoms. Once symptoms resolve, may restart drug at no more than half the previous infusion rate. If patient doesn't experience further reaction symptoms, may increase dosage to prescribed rate for that treatment cycle. If grade 3 infusion reaction reappears, permanently discontinue treatment. For grade 1 to 2 mild to moderate reactions, reduce rate or interrupt infusion and treat symptoms. Once symptoms resolve, continue or resume infusion. If patient tolerates infusion, may increase to prescribed infusion rate for that treatment cycle. If patient experiences an infection, grade 3 or 4 cytopenia, or a grade 2 or greater nonhematologic toxicity, consider treatment interruption.

ADMINISTRATION
I.V.

⚠️ *Alert:* Premedicate all patients with acetaminophen and an antihistamine (such as diphenhydramine) at least 30 minutes before infusion and a glucocorticoid (dexamethasone or methylprednisolone) at least 1 hour before each infusion to reduce infusion-related reactions. Refer to manufacturer's instructions for premedication dosage instructions.

▼ Single-use vials contain preservative-free solution.

▼ Store vials in refrigerator at 36° to 46° F (2° to 8° C).

▼ Protect vials from light; don't freeze or shake vials.

▼ Administer through a dedicated I.V. line; don't administer as an I.V. push or bolus.

▼ Solution should be used immediately but is stable in refrigerator for up to 24 hours followed by 48 hours (including infusion time) at room temperature.

▼ **Incompatibilities:** Don't mix with other drugs or solutions, other than NS.

ACTION
Binds to CD20 antigen, mediating lysis of both normal and malignant B cells.

Route	Onset	Peak	Duration
I.V.	Rapid	Unknown	Unknown

Half-life: 26-37 days.

ADVERSE REACTIONS
CNS: pyrexia, asthenia.
CV: *worsening of cardiac conditions, causing death.*
EENT: sinusitis, nasopharyngitis.
GI: nausea, diarrhea, constipation.
GU: UTI.
Hematologic: *neutropenia, lymphopenia, leukopenia, thrombocytopenia,* anemia.
Hepatic: elevated ALT, AST, and alkaline phosphatase levels; *reactivation of HBV.*
Metabolic: *hypocalcemia, hypokalemia, hyperkalemia,* hyponatremia, hypoalbuminemia.
Musculoskeletal: bone and muscle pain.
Respiratory: cough, URI.
Other: *infusion-related reaction, tumor lysis syndrome.*

INTERACTIONS
Drug-drug. *Alfuzosin, amifostine, antipsychotics (second generation [atypical]), barbiturates, brimonidine (topical), diazoxide, duloxetine, nicorandil, PDE5 inhibitors, pentoxifylline, prostacyclin analogues:* May increase risk of hypotension. Monitor therapy closely.
Anticoagulants, antiplatelet drugs (aspirin, NSAIDs): May increase risk of bleeding. Monitor therapy closely.
Antihypertensives: May increase risk of hypotension. Consider withholding antihypertensives for 12 hours before, during, and for first hour after giving obinutuzumab.
Belimumab: May enhance adverse effects of belimumab. Avoid use together.
Deferiprone: May increase risk of neutropenia. Avoid use together.
Denosumab, natalizumab: May increase risk of serious infections. Monitor patient closely.
Fingolimod: May increase risk of immunosuppression. Avoid use together if possible or consider therapy modification.

Reactions in bold italics are ***life-threatening***. Interactions may have a *rapid onset* or a ***delayed onset***.

Inactivated vaccines: May diminish therapeutic effect of inactivated vaccines. Complete all appropriate vaccinations at least 2 weeks before starting drug. If patient is vaccinated during obinutuzumab therapy, revaccinate at least 3 months after drug is discontinued.

Leflunomide: May increase risk of hematologic toxicity. Monitor patient for bone marrow suppression at least monthly. Consider modifying leflunomide dosage.

Live-virus vaccines: May increase risk of infection. Live-virus vaccination isn't recommended during treatment and until B-cell recovery. Avoid use together.

Nivolumab: May diminish effect of nivolumab. Consider therapy modification.

Pimecrolimus, tacrolimus (topical): May enhance adverse effects of obinutuzumab. Avoid use together.

Roflumilast: May enhance immunosuppressive effect. Consider therapy modification.

Sipuleucel-T: May diminish effect of Sipuleucel-T. Monitor therapy closely.

Tofacitinib: May enhance immunosuppressive effect of tofacitinib. Avoid use together.

Trastuzumab: May enhance neutropenic effect of obinutuzumab. Monitor patient closely.

Drug-herb. *Echinacea:* May diminish therapeutic effect of obinutuzumab. Avoid use together.

EFFECTS ON LAB TEST RESULTS
• May decrease Hb and WBC, lymphocyte, and platelet counts.
• May decrease calcium, sodium, and albumin levels.
• May increase creatinine, alkaline phosphatase, AST, and ALT levels.
• May increase or decrease potassium level.
• May diminish diagnostic effect of coccidioidin skin test.

CONTRAINDICATIONS & CAUTIONS
• Contraindicated in patients hypersensitive to drug or its components.
Black Box Warning HBV reactivation, including fulminant hepatitis, hepatic failure, and death, may occur. Screen all patients for HBV infection before starting therapy and monitor carriers for active HBV infection for several months after therapy is complete.

Discontinue therapy and any concomitant chemotherapy if HBV reactivates and treat appropriately. The decision to restart therapy should be discussed with physician experienced in treating HBV infection. ■
Black Box Warning JC virus infection, resulting in progressive multifocal leukoencephalopathy (PML), has been reported. Monitor patients for new-onset neurologic symptoms or change in existing neurologic symptoms. Discontinue therapy and reduce or stop concomitant chemotherapy or immunosuppressive therapy in patients who develop PML. ■
• Use cautiously in patients with history of recurring or chronic infections.
• Patients with neutropenia should receive antimicrobial prophylaxis throughout treatment. Also consider antiviral and antifungal prophylaxis and granulocyte colony-stimulating factors (G-CSFs).
• Consider withholding other drugs that may increase bleeding risk.
• May cause severe infusion reactions, including bronchospasm, shortness of breath, tachycardia, hypotension, hypertension, nausea, vomiting, diarrhea, headache, and chills. Delayed reactions (up to 48 hours) may occur. Premedicate appropriately and consider infusion rate reduction, interruption of therapy, or discontinuation if reactions persist.
• Give in a facility with access to resuscitative emergency equipment.
• Use cautiously in patients with cardiac or pulmonary conditions; these patients may be at increased risk for serious infusion reactions.
• Consider temporarily withholding antihypertensives for 12 hours before, during, and for 1 hour after administration due to risk of hypotension.
Dialyzable drug: Unknown.

PREGNANCY-LACTATION-REPRODUCTION
• There are no adequate studies in pregnant women. Use only if potential benefit justifies potential risk to the fetus.
• Adverse effects were observed in animal reproduction studies
• It isn't known if drug appears in breast milk. Patient should discontinue breast-feeding or discontinue drug.

NURSING CONSIDERATIONS

⊕ *Alert:* Monitor patient for infusion reactions (hypotension, tachycardia, dyspnea, respiratory symptoms, nausea, vomiting, diarrhea, hypertension, flushing headache, pyrexia, chills), which can be fatal. Symptoms may occur up to 24 hours after infusion.

● Premedicate patient with acetaminophen, antihistamine, and I.V. glucocorticoid to reduce risk of infusion reactions.

● Cases of tumor lysis syndrome with fatalities have been reported. Acute renal failure, hyperkalemia, hypocalcemia, hyperuricemia, or hyperphosphatemia may occur. Administer prophylaxis (antihyperuricemic therapy [e.g., allopurinol] and hydration) in patients at high risk or with high tumor burden or renal impairment before therapy. Correct electrolyte abnormalities and monitor renal function and hydration.

● Patient may develop detectable antibodies to obinutuzumab.

● Regularly monitor blood counts. If neutropenia occurs, consider prophylaxis with antiviral and antifungal agents. Neutropenia may occur 28 days or more after end of treatment and last for more than 28 days.

● Monitor patient for clinical and laboratory signs and symptoms of hepatitis or HBV reactivation during and for several months after treatment.

● Monitor patient for bleeding and thrombocytopenia. Transfuse blood products if appropriate.

● Monitor BP before, during, and after infusion. Consider withholding antihypertensives for 12 hours before, during, and for 1 hour after infusion if appropriate.

PATIENT TEACHING

● Advise patient to seek immediate medical attention for infusion-related reactions, such as dizziness, nausea, chills, fever, vomiting, diarrhea, breathing problems, or chest pain.

● Advise patient to seek immediate medical attention for signs and symptoms of tumor lysis syndrome, such as nausea, vomiting, diarrhea, and lethargy.

● Tell patient to report signs and symptoms of infection, including fever and cough.

Black Box Warning Educate patient to report signs and symptoms of hepatitis, such as worsening fatigue or yellowing of skin or eyes. Inform patient that he or she will be monitored for hepatitis reactivation and will be treated appropriately. ∎

Black Box Warning Advise patient to immediately report new or changed neurologic signs and symptoms, such as confusion, dizziness or loss of balance, difficulty talking or walking, or vision problems. ∎

octreotide acetate
ok-TREE-oh-tide

Sandostatin, Sandostatin LAR Depot

Therapeutic class: Growth hormones
Pharmacologic class: Somatostatin analogues

AVAILABLE FORMS

Injection (ampules): 50 mcg/mL, 100 mcg/mL
Injection (single-dose vials): 50 mcg/mL, 100 mcg/mL, 500 mcg/mL
Injection (multidose vials): 200 mcg/mL, 1,000 mcg/mL
Injection for LAR (powder for suspension): 10 mg/5 mL, 20 mg/5 mL, 30 mg/5 mL

INDICATIONS & DOSAGES

➤ **Flushing and diarrhea from carcinoid tumors**

Adults: 100 to 600 mcg subcutaneously or I.V. daily in two to four divided doses for first 2 weeks of therapy. Usual daily dosage is 450 mcg but can range from 50 to 1,500 mcg/day. Base subsequent dosage on individual response. If Sandostatin LAR Depot is used, give 20 mg I.M. (intragluteally) at 4-week intervals for 2 months. Patients should continue to receive octreotide solution subcutaneously for 2 weeks at same dosage they were taking before the switch. After 2 months, adjust dosage based on symptoms.

➤ **Watery diarrhea from vasoactive intestinal polypeptide–secreting tumors (VIPomas)**

Adults: 200 to 300 mcg subcutaneously or I.V. daily in two to four divided doses for first 2 weeks of therapy. Base subsequent dosage on individual response, but usually shouldn't exceed 450 mcg daily. If Sandostatin LAR Depot is used, give 20 mg I.M. (intragluteally) at 4-week intervals for 2 months. Patients should continue to receive octreotide solution subcutaneously for 2 weeks at same dosage they were taking before the switch. After 2 months, adjust dosage based on symptoms.

➤ **Acromegaly**
Adults: Initially, 50 mcg subcutaneously or I.V. t.i.d.; then adjust based on IGF-1 (somatomedin C) levels every 2 weeks. Usual dosage is 100 mcg subcutaneously or I.V. t.i.d.; some patients require up to 500 mcg t.i.d. If Sandostatin LAR Depot is used, give 20 mg I.M. (intragluteally) at 4-week intervals for 3 months; then adjust dosage based on growth hormone and somatomedin C levels and symptoms. See manufacturer's instructions for a detailed dosing schedule.

Adjust-a-dose: In patients with cirrhosis of the liver or renal failure requiring dialysis, starting dose of Sandostatin LAR is 10 mg I.M. every 4 weeks.

ADMINISTRATION

I.V.
▼ For other uses, dilute in 50 to 200 mL D_5W or NSS and infuse over 15 to 30 minutes.
▼ May be given by I.V. push over 3 minutes.
▼ Solution is stable for 24 hours.
▼ **Incompatibilities:** Total parenteral nutrition.

I.M.
● Don't use if particulates or discoloration are observed.
● Follow the mixing instructions included in the packaging and give immediately after mixing.
● Rotate injection sites.
● Avoid deltoid muscle injections. May cause significant discomfort.
🕚 *Alert:* Never give the injectable suspension by I.V. or subcutaneous routes.

Subcutaneous
● Don't use if particulates or discoloration is observed.

ACTION
Mimics action of naturally occurring somatostatin.

Route	Onset	Peak	Duration
I.V.	Rapid	30 min	<12 hr
I.M.	Unknown	2–3 wk	Unknown
Subcut.	30 min	30 min	<12 hr

Half-life: About 1½ hours; long-acting, unknown.

ADVERSE REACTIONS
CNS: dizziness, fatigue, headache, lightheadedness, depression, weakness.
CV: *arrhythmias, bradycardia,* conduction abnormalities, edema.
EENT: blurred vision.
GI: abdominal pain or discomfort, diarrhea, gallbladder abnormalities, loose stools, nausea, *pancreatitis,* constipation, fat malabsorption, flatulence, vomiting.
GU: urinary frequency, UTI.
Metabolic: *hypoglycemia,* hyperglycemia, hypothyroidism, suppressed secretion of growth hormone and gastroenterohepatic peptides (gastrin, VIP, insulin, glucagon, secretin, motilin, and pancreatic polypeptide).
Musculoskeletal: backache, joint pain.
Skin: alopecia, erythema or pain at injection site, flushing, wheal, bruising, hair loss.
Other: cold symptoms, flulike symptoms, pain or burning at subcutaneous injection site.

INTERACTIONS
Drug-drug. *Androgens, MAO inhibitors, quinolone antibiotics, salicylates, SSRIs:* May increase risk of hypoglycemia. Monitor patient closely.
Beta blockers (propranolol) and other drugs that may cause bradycardia, ivabradine: May have additive effect and further lower HR. Decrease beta blocker dosage as needed.
Bromocriptine: May decrease bromocriptine availability. Monitor patient for effectiveness.
Cyclosporine: May decrease cyclosporine level. Monitor patient closely.
Drugs that prolong QT interval (antiarrhythmics, SSRIs, TCAs): May increase risk

of life-threatening cardiac arrhythmias, including torsades de pointes. Monitor patient and ECG.

Insulin, oral antidiabetics: May enhance hypoglycemic effects of antidiabetics and increase risk of hyperglycemia. Monitor patient and adjust dosage of antidiabetics as needed.

Lacosamide: May increase risk of AV-blocking effect of lacosamide. Monitor patient closely.

Quinidine, rifampin: May decrease excretion of these drugs. Use with caution and reduce dosage as needed.

Drug-food. *Any food:* May alter absorption of dietary fats. Administer injections between meals.

EFFECTS ON LAB TEST RESULTS
● May decrease vitamin B_{12} level. May increase or decrease glucose level.
● May alter LFT values.

CONTRAINDICATIONS & CAUTIONS
● Contraindicated in patients hypersensitive to drug or its components.
● Use cautiously in elderly patients, who may be more sensitive to drug.
● Use cautiously in patients with pancreatitis, gallbladder or bile disorders, cardiac abnormalities, diabetes, or nutritional disorders; octreotide may cause or exacerbate these conditions.
● Use cautiously in patients with renal impairment requiring dialysis or hepatic cirrhosis. Dosage adjustment may be needed.
Dialyzable drug: Unknown.
⚠ **Overdose S&S:** Hypoglycemia, flushing, dizziness, nausea.

PREGNANCY-LACTATION-REPRODUCTION
● Use cautiously in pregnant women and only if clearly needed and benefit justifies possible risks to the fetus.
● Drug appears in breast milk. Use cautiously breast-feeding women.

NURSING CONSIDERATIONS
● Monitor baseline thyroid function tests.
● Monitor somatomedin C levels every 2 weeks. Dosage adjustments are based on this level.

● Periodically monitor laboratory tests, such as thyroid function, glucose, urine 5-hydroxyindoleacetic acid, plasma serotonin, and plasma substance P (for carcinoid tumors).
● Monitor patient regularly for gallbladder disease. Therapy may be related to the development of cholelithiasis because of its effect on gallbladder motility or fat absorption.
● Monitor patient closely for signs and symptoms of glucose imbalance. Patients with type 1 diabetes mellitus and those receiving oral antidiabetics or oral diazoxide may need dosage adjustments during therapy. Monitor glucose level.
● Monitor patient closely for bradycardia, arrhythmias, conduction abnormalities, and other ECG changes (e.g., prolonged QT interval).
● Drug may alter fluid and electrolyte balance; other therapies may need adjusting.
● Half-life may be altered in patients with ESRD who are receiving dialysis.
● *Look alike–sound alike:* To avoid giving drug by the wrong route, don't confuse octreotide acetate injection with injectable depot suspension product.
● *Look alike–sound alike:* Don't confuse Sandostatin with Sandimmune or Sandoglobulin.

PATIENT TEACHING
● Urge patient to report signs and symptoms of abdominal discomfort immediately.
● Stress importance of the need for periodic laboratory testing during octreotide therapy.
● Advise patient that drug may restore fertility in some women with acromegaly and that she should use effective birth control if pregnancy isn't desired.
● Tell patient that drug may cause dizziness, drowsiness, or vision changes and that these symptoms may increase with alcohol use or certain other medications. Advise patient not to drive or perform hazardous tasks until drug's effects are known.
● Warn diabetic patient to monitor blood glucose level closely and to discuss results with prescriber before making dosage changes.

Reactions in bold italics are *life-threatening*. Interactions may have a *rapid onset* or a *delayed onset*.

ofloxacin (ophthalmic)
oh-FLOX-a-sin

Ocuflox

ofloxacin (otic)

Therapeutic class: Antibiotics
Pharmacologic class: Fluoroquinolones

AVAILABLE FORMS
Ophthalmic solution: 0.3%
Otic solution: 0.3%

INDICATIONS & DOSAGES
➤ **Conjunctivitis caused by** *Staphylococcus aureus, Staphylococcus epidermidis, Streptococcus pneumoniae, Enterobacter cloacae, Haemophilus influenzae, Proteus mirabilis,* **or** *Pseudomonas aeruginosa*
Adults and children older than age 1: Give 1 or 2 drops in conjunctival sac every 2 to 4 hours daily while patient is awake, for first 2 days; then q.i.d. for up to 5 additional days.
➤ **Bacterial corneal ulcer caused by** *S. aureus, S. epidermidis, S. pneumoniae, P. aeruginosa, Serratia marcescens,* **or** *Propionibacterium acnes*
Adults and children older than age 1: Give 1 or 2 drops every 30 minutes while patient is awake and 1 or 2 drops 4 and 6 hours after patient goes to bed on days 1 and 2. On day 3, 1 or 2 drops hourly while patient is awake; continue for 4 to 6 days. Then, 1 or 2 drops q.i.d. for an additional 3 days or until cured.
➤ **Chronic suppurative otitis media with perforated tympanic membrane**
Adults and children age 12 and older: 10 drops instilled into the affected ear b.i.d. for 14 days.
➤ **Otitis externa**
Adults and children age 13 and older: 10 drops instilled into the affected ear once daily for 7 days.
Children ages 6 months to 13 years: 5 drops into the affected ear once daily for 7 days.
➤ **Acute otitis media in children with tympanostomy tubes**
Children ages 1 to 12: 5 drops instilled into the affected ear b.i.d. for 10 days.

ADMINISTRATION
Ophthalmic
● Apply light finger pressure on lacrimal sac for 1 minute after drug instillation.
Otic
● Before instilling drops, warm the bottle by holding it in the hand for 1 to 2 minutes.
● Have patient lie with the affected ear upward, instill the drops, and have patient maintain this position for 5 minutes.

ACTION
Inhibits bacterial DNA gyrase, an enzyme needed for bacterial replication.

Route	Onset	Peak	Duration
Ophthalmic, otic	Unknown	Unknown	Unknown

Half-life: 4 to 8 hours.

ADVERSE REACTIONS
CNS: dizziness, vertigo.
EENT: transient ocular burning or discomfort, chemical conjunctivitis or keratitis, eye dryness, eye pain, itching, lacrimation, periocular or facial edema, photophobia, eye redness, stinging, earache, taste perversion.
Skin: rash.

INTERACTIONS
None significant.

EFFECTS ON LAB TEST RESULTS
None reported.

CONTRAINDICATIONS & CAUTIONS
● Contraindicated in patients hypersensitive to drug or other fluoroquinolones.
Dialyzable drug: Unknown.

PREGNANCY-LACTATION-REPRODUCTION
● There are no adequate studies in pregnant women. Use only if potential benefit justifies risks to the fetus.
● It isn't known if drug appears in breast milk after otic or ophthalmic administration. Patient should discontinue breast-feeding or discontinue drug.

NURSING CONSIDERATIONS
● Stop drug if improvement doesn't occur within 7 days, and obtain cultures.

Prolonged use may result in overgrowth of nonsusceptible organisms, including fungi.
• Ophthalmic solution isn't for injection into conjunctiva or anterior chamber of the eye.
• Otic solution isn't for ophthalmic use or injection.
• *Look alike–sound alike:* Don't confuse Ocuflox with Ocufen.

PATIENT TEACHING
• If an allergic reaction occurs, tell patient to stop drug and notify prescriber. Serious acute hypersensitivity reactions may need emergency treatment.
• Tell patient to clean excessive discharge from eye area before application.
• Teach patient how to instill drops. Advise him to wash hands before and after instilling solution, and warn him not to touch tip of ophthalmic dropper to eye or surrounding tissue.
• Advise patient to apply light finger pressure on lacrimal sac for 1 minute after drug instillation.
• Tell patient not to share drug, washcloths, or towels with family members and to notify prescriber if anyone develops same signs or symptoms.
• Stress importance of compliance with recommended therapy.
• Warn patient not to use leftover drug for new eye infection.
• Remind patient to discard drug when it's no longer needed.
• Warn patient not to touch the otic applicator.
• Teach patient to warm the bottle in his hand for 1 to 2 minutes to avoid dizziness from instilling cold eardrops, then to lie with the affected ear upward for instillation of the drops. This position should be maintained for 5 minutes.

ofloxacin (oral)
oh-FLOX-a-sin

Therapeutic class: Antibiotics
Pharmacologic class: Fluoroquinolones

AVAILABLE FORMS
Tablets: 200 mg, 300 mg, 400 mg

INDICATIONS & DOSAGES
Black Box Warning Use in patients with acute bacterial sinusitis, acute bacterial exacerbation of bronchitis, and uncomplicated UTIs isn't recommended because of risk of serious adverse effects. Use drug in these patients only when they have no other treatment options. ■
Adjust-a-dose (for all indications): For patients with CrCl of 20 to 50 mL/minute, give first dose as recommended; then give usual maintenance dose every 24 hours. For patients with CrCl less than 20 mL/minute, give 50% of recommended dose every 24 hours. For patients with hepatic impairment, don't exceed 400 mg/day.
➤ **Acute bacterial worsening of chronic bronchitis, uncomplicated skin and skin-structure infections, and community-acquired pneumonia**
Adults: 400 mg P.O. every 12 hours for 10 days.
➤ **Acute, uncomplicated urethral and cervical gonorrhea**
Adults: 400 mg P.O. as a single dose.
➤ **Mixed infection of the urethra and cervix due to** *Chlamydia trachomatis* **and** *Neisseria gonorrhoeae;* **nongonococcal cervicitis/urethritis due to** *C. trachomatis*
Adults: 300 mg P.O. every 12 hours for 7 days.
➤ **Uncomplicated cystitis caused by** *Escherichia coli, Klebsiella pneumoniae,* **or other organisms**
Adults: 200 mg P.O. every 12 hours for 3 days *(E. coli* or *K. pneumoniae)* or 200 mg P.O. every 12 hours for 7 days (other organisms).
➤ **Complicated UTI**
Adults: 200 mg P.O. every 12 hours for 10 days.
➤ **Prostatitis from** *E. coli*
Adults: 300 mg P.O. every 12 hours for 6 weeks.
➤ **Acute pelvic inflammatory disease**
Adults: 400 mg P.O. every 12 hours with metronidazole for 10 to 14 days.
➤ **Spontaneous bacterial peritonitis** ◆
Adults: 400 mg P.O. b.i.d.

Reactions in bold italics are *life-threatening.* Interactions may have a *rapid onset* or a *delayed onset.*

ADMINISTRATION
P.O.
- Give drug with or without food but not at the same time as antacids and vitamins.
- Give drug with plenty of fluids.

ACTION
Interferes with DNA gyrase, which is needed for synthesis of bacterial DNA. Spectrum of action includes many gram-positive and gram-negative aerobic bacteria, including *Enterobacteriaceae* and *Pseudomonas aeruginosa*.

Route	Onset	Peak	Duration
P.O.	Unknown	60–120 min	Unknown

Half-life: 4 to 7½ hours.

ADVERSE REACTIONS
CNS: *seizures, increased ICP,* dizziness, drowsiness, fatigue, fever, headache, insomnia, lethargy, malaise, nervousness, sleep disorders, visual disturbances.
CV: chest pain, phlebitis.
GI: nausea, *pseudomembranous colitis,* abdominal pain or discomfort, anorexia, constipation, diarrhea, dry mouth, dysgeusia, flatulence, vomiting.
GU: external genital pruritus in women, glycosuria, hematuria, proteinuria, vaginal discharge, vaginitis.
Hematologic: *leukopenia, neutropenia,* anemia, eosinophilia, leukocytosis.
Metabolic: *hypoglycemia,* hyperglycemia.
Musculoskeletal: body pain, tendon rupture, myalgia.
Skin: photosensitivity, pruritus, rash.
Other: *anaphylactoid reaction,* hypersensitivity reactions.

INTERACTIONS
Drug-drug. *Aluminum hydroxide, aluminum-magnesium hydroxide, calcium carbonate, magnesium hydroxide:* May decrease effects of ofloxacin. Give antacid at least 2 hours before or 2 hours after ofloxacin.
Antidiabetics: May affect glucose level, causing hypoglycemia or hyperglycemia. Monitor patient closely.
Didanosine (chewable or buffered tablets or pediatric powder for oral solution): May interfere with GI absorption of ofloxacin. Separate doses by 2 hours.

Drugs that prolong QT interval (antiarrhythmics, pimozide, ziprasidone): May increase risk of life-threatening ventricular arrhythmias. Avoid use together.
Iron salts: May decrease absorption of ofloxacin, reducing anti-infective response. Separate doses by at least 2 hours.
NSAIDs: May enhance seizure-potentiating effect of ofloxacin. Monitor therapy closely.
Black Box Warning *Steroids:* May increase risk of tendinitis and tendon rupture. Monitor patient for tendon pain or inflammation. ∎
Sucralfate: May decrease absorption of ofloxacin, reducing anti-infective response. If use together can't be avoided, give ofloxacin 2 hours before or 6 hours after sucralfate.
Theophylline: May increase theophylline level. Monitor patient closely and adjust theophylline dosage as needed.
Warfarin: May prolong PT and INR. Monitor PT and INR.
Drug-lifestyle. *Sun exposure:* May cause photosensitivity reactions. Advise patient to avoid excessive sunlight exposure.

EFFECTS ON LAB TEST RESULTS
- May increase BUN, creatinine, and liver enzyme levels. May decrease Hb level and hematocrit. May increase or decrease glucose level.
- May increase erythrocyte sedimentation rate and eosinophil count. May decrease neutrophil count. May increase or decrease WBC count.
- May produce false-positive urine screen results for opiates.

CONTRAINDICATIONS & CAUTIONS
Black Box Warning Drug is associated with increased risk of tendinitis and tendon rupture, especially in patients older than age 60 and those with heart, kidney, or lung transplants. ∎
Black Box Warning Drug may exacerbate muscle weakness in patients with myasthenia gravis. Avoid use in patients with a known history of myasthenia gravis. ∎
- Contraindicated in patients hypersensitive to drug or other fluoroquinolones.
- **Alert:** Serious, even fatal, hypersensitivity reactions can occur, even after first dose.

Discontinue drug at first sign of rash or hypersensitivity. Emergency treatment with epinephrine and resuscitative measures may be needed.

Black Box Warning Oral or parenteral fluoroquinolones may increase the risk of peripheral neuropathy of the arms or legs. Symptoms can occur at any time during treatment and can last for months or years or be permanent. Stop drug immediately if patient develops symptoms, and switch to a non-fluoroquinolone antibacterial drug. ■

• Use cautiously in patients with seizure disorders, CNS diseases such as cerebral arteriosclerosis, hepatic disorders, or renal impairment.

• Mild to life-threatening CDAD can occur during therapy and up to 2 months after therapy ends. Monitor patient for diarrhea as drug may need to be discontinued and other therapy begun.

• Safety and effectiveness in children younger than age 18 haven't been established.

Dialyzable drug: No.

⚠ *Overdose S&S:* Nausea, vomiting, seizures, vertigo, dysgeusia, psychosis, dizziness, drowsiness, hot and cold flushes, facial swelling and numbness, slurred speech, mild to moderate disorientation.

PREGNANCY-LACTATION-REPRODUCTION

• There are no adequate studies in pregnant women. Use only if potential benefit justifies risks to the fetus.

• Drug appears in breast milk in levels similar to those found in plasma. Patient should discontinue breast-feeding or discontinue drug.

NURSING CONSIDERATIONS

Black Box Warning Fluoroquinolones have been associated with disabling and potentially irreversible serious adverse reactions that have occurred together, including tendinitis and tendon rupture, peripheral neuropathy, and CNS effects (seizures, toxic psychoses, increased ICP, pseudotumor cerebri, tremors, restlessness, anxiety, light-headedness, confusion, hallucinations, paranoia, depression, nightmares, insomnia and, rarely, suicidal thoughts or acts). If any

of these serious adverse reactions occur, discontinue drug immediately. ■

Black Box Warning Monitor patient for symptoms of peripheral neuropathy (pain, burning, tingling, numbness, weakness, or a change in sensation to light touch, pain, temperature, or the sense of body position) and report them immediately. ■

❸ *Alert:* Patients treated for gonorrhea should be tested for syphilis. Drug isn't effective against syphilis, and treating gonorrhea may mask or delay syphilis symptoms.

• Periodically assess organ system functions during prolonged therapy.

• Monitor patient for overgrowth of nonsusceptible organisms.

• Monitor renal and hepatic studies and CBC in prolonged therapy.

• Monitor glucose level closely.

• Monitor patient for adverse CNS effects, including dizziness, headache, seizures, or depression. Stop drug and notify prescriber if these effects occur.

• Monitor patient for hypersensitivity reactions. Stop drug and initiate supportive therapy, as indicated.

PATIENT TEACHING

Black Box Warning Warn patient to immediately report signs and symptoms of serious adverse reactions, including unusual joint or tendon pain, muscle weakness, "pins and needles" tingling or prickling sensation, numbness in the arms or legs, confusion, or hallucinations. ■

• Tell patient to drink plenty of fluids during drug therapy and to finish the entire prescription, even after starting to feel better.

• Tell patient drug may be taken with or without food, but not to take antacids and vitamins at the same time as ofloxacin.

• Warn patient that dizziness and light-headedness may occur. Advise caution when driving or operating hazardous machinery until effects of drug are known.

• Warn patient that hypersensitivity reactions may follow first dose. Advise patient to stop drug at first sign of rash or other allergic reaction and call prescriber immediately.

• Advise patient to avoid prolonged exposure to direct sunlight and to use a sunscreen when outdoors.

Reactions in bold italics are *life-threatening*. Interactions may have a *rapid onset* or a *delayed onset*.

olanzapine
oh-LAN-za-peen

Zyprexa✐, Zyprexa Zydis

olanzapine pamoate
Zyprexa Relprevv

Therapeutic class: Antipsychotics
Pharmacologic class: Dibenzapine derivatives

AVAILABLE FORMS
Injection: 10 mg
Injection (extended-release): 210-mg base/vial, 300-mg base/vial, 405-mg base/vial
ODTs: 5 mg, 10 mg, 15 mg, 20 mg
Tablets: 2.5 mg, 5 mg, 7.5 mg, 10 mg, 15 mg, 20 mg

INDICATIONS & DOSAGES
➤ **Schizophrenia**
Adults: Initially, 5 to 10 mg P.O. once daily with the goal to be at 10 mg daily within several days of starting therapy. Adjust dose in 5-mg increments at intervals of 1 week or more. Most patients respond to 10 to 15 mg daily. Safety of dosages greater than 20 mg daily hasn't been established. Or, for maintenance dosing, 150 mg (extended-release) I.M. every 2 weeks, or 300 mg (extended-release) I.M. every 4 weeks, or 210 mg (extended-release) I.M. every 2 weeks, or 405 mg (extended-release) I.M. every 4 weeks.
Children age 13 and older: 2.5 or 5 mg P.O. once daily. Adjust dose as needed in increments of 2.5 or 5 mg. Maintenance dose is 10 mg/day.

➤ **Short-term treatment of acute manic episodes linked to bipolar I disorder**
Adults: Initially, 10 to 15 mg P.O. daily. Adjust dosage as needed in 5-mg daily increments at intervals of 24 hours or more. Maximum, 20 mg P.O. daily. Duration of treatment is 3 to 4 weeks.
Children age 13 and older: 2.5 or 5 mg P.O. once daily. Adjust dose as needed in increments of 2.5 or 5 mg. Maintenance dose is 10 mg/day.

➤ **Short-term treatment, with lithium or valproate, of acute mixed or manic episodes linked to bipolar I disorder**
Adults: 10 mg P.O. once daily. Dosage range is 5 to 20 mg daily. Duration of treatment is 6 weeks.

➤ **Long-term treatment of bipolar I disorder**
Adults: 5 to 20 mg P.O. daily.
Adjust-a-dose: In elderly or debilitated patients, those predisposed to hypotensive reactions, patients who may metabolize olanzapine more slowly than usual (nonsmoking women older than age 65) or may be more pharmacodynamically sensitive to olanzapine, initially, 5 mg P.O. Increase dose cautiously.

➤ **Agitation caused by schizophrenia and bipolar I mania**
Adults: 10 mg I.M. (short-acting) (range 2.5 to 10 mg). Subsequent doses of up to 10 mg may be given 2 hours after the first dose or 4 hours after the second dose, up to 30 mg I.M. daily. If maintenance therapy is required, convert patient to 5 to 20 mg P.O. daily.
Adjust-a-dose: In elderly patients, give 5 mg I.M. In debilitated patients, in those predisposed to hypotension, and in patients sensitive to effects of drug, give 2.5 mg I.M.

➤ **Depressive episodes associated with bipolar I disorder**
Adults: 5 mg P.O. with fluoxetine 20 mg P.O. once daily in the evening. Dosage adjustments can be made based on effectiveness and tolerability within ranges of olanzapine 5 to 12.5 mg and fluoxetine 20 to 50 mg.
Children age 10 and older: 2.5 mg P.O. with 20 mg fluoxetine P.O. once daily in the evening. Adjust dosage based on efficacy and tolerability. Doses above 12 mg (olanzapine) with fluoxetine 50 mg haven't been evaluated.

➤ **Treatment-resistant depression**
Adults: 5 mg P.O. with 20 mg fluoxetine P.O. once daily in the evening. Dosage adjustments can be made based on effectiveness and tolerability within ranges of olanzapine 5 to 20 mg and fluoxetine 20 to 50 mg.

ADMINISTRATION
P.O.
● Give drug without regard for food.

- Don't push tablet through foil backing; remove foil from package, then remove tablet.
- Place ODT on patient's tongue immediately after opening package.
- ODT may be given without water.

I.M.

- Inspect I.M. solution for particulate matter and discoloration before administration.
- To reconstitute I.M. injection, dissolve contents of one vial with 2.1 mL of sterile water for injection to yield a clear yellow 5 mg/mL solution. Store at room temperature and give within 1 hour of reconstitution. Discard any unused solution.
- For Zyprexa Relprevv extended-release injection, follow specific manufacturer's instructions for the appropriate diluent to add for each dosage.
- Olanzapine extended-release formula is intended for deep gluteal I.M. injection only.

ACTION

May block dopamine and 5-HT$_2$ receptors.

Route	Onset	Peak	Duration
P.O.	Unknown	6 hr	Unknown
I.M.	Rapid	15–45 min	Unknown
I.M. (extended-release)	Unknown	1 wk	Months

Half-life: 21 to 54 hours; extended release, 30 days.

ADVERSE REACTIONS

CNS: somnolence, insomnia, parkinsonism, dizziness, *neuroleptic malignant syndrome, suicide attempt,* abnormal gait, asthenia, personality disorder, akathisia, tremor, articulation impairment, tardive dyskinesia, fever, extrapyramidal events (I.M.).
CV: orthostatic hypotension, tachycardia, chest pain, hypertension, ecchymosis, peripheral edema, hypotension (I.M.).
EENT: amblyopia, rhinitis, pharyngitis, conjunctivitis.
GI: constipation, dry mouth, dyspepsia, increased appetite, increased salivation, vomiting, thirst.
GU: hematuria, metrorrhagia, urinary incontinence, UTI, amenorrhea, vaginitis.
Hematologic: *leukopenia.*
Metabolic: hyperglycemia, weight gain.

Musculoskeletal: joint pain, extremity pain, back pain, neck rigidity, twitching, hypertonia.
Respiratory: increased cough, dyspnea.
Skin: sweating, injection-site pain (I.M.).
Other: flulike syndrome, injury.

INTERACTIONS

Drug-drug. *Antihypertensives:* May potentiate hypotensive effects. Monitor BP closely.
Carbamazepine, omeprazole, rifampin: May increase clearance of olanzapine. Monitor patient.
Ciprofloxacin: May increase olanzapine level. Monitor patient for increased adverse effects.
Diazepam: May increase CNS effects. Monitor patient.
Dopamine agonists, levodopa: May antagonize activity of these drugs. Monitor patient.
Fluoxetine: May increase olanzapine level. Use together cautiously.
Fluvoxamine: May increase olanzapine level. May need to reduce olanzapine dose.
Lamotrigine: May increase sedative effect of olanzapine. Monitor patient.
Black Box Warning *Opioids:* May cause slow or difficult breathing, sedation, and death. Avoid use together. If use together is necessary, limit dosage and duration of each drug to minimum necessary for desired effect. ∎
Drug-herb. *Kava kava:* May increase adverse/toxic effect of olanzapine. Monitor patient.
St. John's wort: May decrease drug level. Discourage use together.
Drug-lifestyle. *Alcohol use:* May increase CNS effects. Discourage use together.
Smoking: May increase drug clearance. Urge patient to quit smoking.

EFFECTS ON LAB TEST RESULTS

- May increase AST, ALT, GGT, CK, glucose, triglyceride, and prolactin levels.
- May decrease bilirubin level.
- May increase eosinophil count. May decrease WBC count.

Reactions in bold italics are *life-threatening*. Interactions may have a *rapid onset* or a *delayed onset*.

CONTRAINDICATIONS & CAUTIONS

• Contraindicated in patients hypersensitive to drug.

Black Box Warning Sedation (including coma) or delirium have been reported following injections of olanzapine extended-release formula. This drug must be administered in a registered health care facility with ready access to emergency response services. After each injection, patient must be observed at the health care facility by a health care provider for at least 3 hours. Olanzapine extended-release is available only through the restricted Zyprexa Relprevv Patient Care Program (1-877-772-9390). ∎

Black Box Warning Drug may increase risk of CV or infection-related death in elderly patients with dementia. Olanzapine isn't approved to treat patients with dementia-related psychosis. ∎

Black Box Warning Opioids should only be prescribed with benzodiazepines or other CNS depressants to patients for whom alternative treatment options are inadequate. ∎

• Use cautiously in patients with heart disease, cerebrovascular disease, conditions that predispose patient to hypotension, history of seizures or conditions that might lower the seizure threshold, and hepatic impairment.

• Use cautiously in elderly patients, those with a history of paralytic ileus, and those at risk for aspiration pneumonia, prostatic hyperplasia, or angle-closure glaucoma.

Dialyzable drug: No.

⚠ Overdose S&S: Agitation, aggressiveness, dysarthria, tachycardia, extrapyramidal symptoms, reduced level of consciousness, aspiration, cardiopulmonary arrest, cardiac arrhythmias, delirium, neuroleptic malignant syndrome, respiratory depression or arrest, seizures, hypertension, hypotension.

PREGNANCY-LACTATION-REPRODUCTION

• There are no adequate studies in pregnant women. Use only if potential benefit justifies potential fetal risk. Use during pregnancy should be individualized.

❸ Alert: Neonates exposed to antipsychotics during the third trimester are at risk for developing extrapyramidal signs and symptoms (repetitive muscle movements of the face and body) and withdrawal signs and symptoms (agitation, abnormally increased or decreased muscle tone, tremors, sleepiness, severe difficulty breathing, difficulty feeding) after delivery and may require intensive care support.

• Prescribers should enroll women exposed to drug during pregnancy in the National Pregnancy Registry for Atypical Antipsychotics (1-866-961-2388).

• Drug appears in breast milk. Breastfeeding isn't recommended.

NURSING CONSIDERATIONS

❸ Alert: Watch for evidence of neuroleptic malignant syndrome (hyperpyrexia, muscle rigidity, altered mental status, autonomic instability), which is rare but commonly fatal. Stop drug immediately; monitor and treat patient as needed.

❸ Alert: Drug may cause hyperglycemia. Monitor patients with diabetes regularly. In patients with risk factors for diabetes, obtain fasting blood glucose test results at baseline and periodically.

❸ Alert: Monitor patient for symptoms of metabolic syndrome (significant weight gain and increased BMI, hypertension, hyperglycemia, hypercholesterolemia, and hypertriglyceridemia).

❸ Alert: Monitor patient for DRESS (drug reaction with eosinophilia and systemic symptoms), which can be fatal. DRESS consists of three or more of the following signs and symptoms: cutaneous reaction, eosinophilia, fever, and lymphadenopathy, plus one or more of the following systemic complications: hepatitis, myocarditis, pericarditis, nephritis, and pneumonia. Discontinue drug immediately if DRESS is suspected and provide supportive care.

• ODTs contain phenylalanine.

• Monitor patient for abnormal body temperature regulation, especially if patient exercises, is exposed to extreme heat, takes anticholinergics, or is dehydrated.

• Obtain baseline and periodic LFT results.

• Monitor patient for weight gain.

• Monitor patient for mental status changes, sedation, coma, or delirium.

• Monitor patient for tardive dyskinesia, which may occur after prolonged use. It may not appear until months or years later and

may disappear spontaneously or persist for life, despite stopping drug.
● Periodically reevaluate the long-term usefulness of olanzapine.
● Patient who feels dizzy or drowsy after an I.M. injection should remain recumbent until he can be assessed for orthostatic hypotension and bradycardia. Patient should rest until the feeling passes.
◐ *Alert:* Drug may increase risk of suicidal thinking and behavior in young adults ages 18 to 24 during first 2 months of treatment.
◐ *Alert:* Monitor patient receiving extended-release injection for postinjection delirium sedation syndrome (PDSS). Signs and symptoms that may be consistent with overdose and PDSS include sedation, coma, delirium, confusion, disorientation, agitation, anxiety, and other cognitive impairment. Other possible signs and symptoms of PDSS include dysarthria, ataxia, aggression, dizziness, weakness, hypertension, and seizures.
◐ *Alert:* After receiving extended-release injection and after postinjection observation period, patients must be alert, oriented, and absent of signs or symptoms of PDSS before release. Patients must be accompanied to their destination upon leaving the facility. If PDSS is suspected, patients must remain under medical supervision.
● *Look alike–sound alike:* Don't confuse olanzapine with olsalazine. Don't confuse Zyprexa with Zyrtec.

PATIENT TEACHING
Black Box Warning Caution patient or caregiver of patient taking an opioid with a benzodiazepine, CNS depressant, or alcohol to seek immediate medical attention if patient experiences dizziness, light-headedness, extreme sleepiness, slowed or difficult breathing, or unresponsiveness. ∎
◐ *Alert:* Inform patient of risk of DRESS and importance of reporting symptoms immediately.
● Warn patient to avoid hazardous tasks until full effects of drug are known.
● Warn patient against exposure to extreme heat; drug may impair body's ability to reduce temperature.
● Inform patient of potential for weight gain.

● Advise patient to avoid alcohol.
● Tell patient to rise slowly to avoid dizziness upon standing up quickly.
● Inform patient that ODTs contain phenylalanine.
● Tell patient to peel foil away from ODT, not to push tablet through. Have patient take tablet immediately, allowing tablet to dissolve on tongue and be swallowed with saliva; no additional fluid is needed.
● Tell patient to take drug with or without food.
● Urge female patient of childbearing potential to notify prescriber if she becomes pregnant or plans or suspects pregnancy. Tell her not to breast-feed during therapy.
◐ *Alert:* Warn patient not to drive or operate heavy machinery for rest of day after receiving extended-release injection and to seek medical attention if signs and symptoms of PDSS occur.

olmesartan medoxomil
ol-ma-SAR-tan

Benicar◆

Therapeutic class: Antihypertensives
Pharmacologic class: Angiotensin II receptor antagonists

AVAILABLE FORMS
Tablets: 5 mg, 20 mg, 40 mg

INDICATIONS & DOSAGES
➤ **Hypertension**
Adults: 20 mg P.O. once daily if patient has no volume depletion. May increase dosage to 40 mg P.O. once daily if BP isn't reduced after 2 weeks of therapy.
Children ages 6 to 16: For children weighing 35 kg or more, initially, 20 mg P.O. daily, with maintenance dosage of 20 to 40 mg daily. For children weighing 20 to less than 35 kg, initially, 10 mg P.O. daily, with maintenance dosage of 10 to 20 mg daily.
Adjust-a-dose: In patients with possible depletion of intravascular volume (those with impaired renal function who are taking diuretics), consider a lower starting dose.

ADMINISTRATION

P.O.

• Give drug without regard for food.

• Drug may be made into suspension by pharmacist if patient is unable to swallow pills.

• Refrigerate suspension, which may be stored for up to 28 days.

• Shake suspension well before use.

ACTION

Blocks vasoconstrictor and aldosterone-secreting effects of angiotensin II by selectively blocking the binding of angiotensin II to the angiotensin I, or AT_1, receptor in the vascular smooth muscle.

Route	Onset	Peak	Duration
P.O.	Rapid	1–2 hr	24 hr

Half-life: 13 hours.

ADVERSE REACTIONS

CNS: headache, dizziness.

EENT: pharyngitis, rhinitis, sinusitis.

GI: diarrhea.

GU: hematuria.

Metabolic: hyperglycemia, hypertriglyceridemia.

Musculoskeletal: back pain.

Respiratory: bronchitis, URI.

Other: flulike symptoms.

INTERACTIONS

Drug-drug. *ACE inhibitors:* May increase risk of hyperkalemia and decrease renal function. Consider monotherapy; if coadministration can't be avoided, monitor renal function and serum potassium level.

◑ *Alert: Aliskiren:* May increase risk of renal impairment, hypotension, and hyperkalemia in diabetic patients and those with moderate to severe renal impairment (GFR less than 60 mL/minute). Concomitant use is contraindicated in diabetic patients. Avoid concomitant use in those with moderate to severe renal impairment.

Colesevelam: Reduces olmesartan level. Give olmesartan at least 4 hours before colesevelam.

Cyclo-oxygenase-2 inhibitors, NSAIDs: May decrease antihypertensive effects of olmesartan. Coadministration in elderly or volume-depleted patients or in those with compromised renal function may result in deterioration of renal function, including possible acute renal failure. Monitor BP and renal function periodically.

Lithium: May increase serum lithium level and risk of toxicity. Closely monitor serum lithium level and adjust dosage as needed.

Potassium: May increase risk of hyperkalemia, possibly with cardiac arrhythmias or arrest. Closely monitor serum potassium level and renal function; adjust therapy as needed.

Potassium-sparing diuretics: May increase risk of hyperkalemia. Closely monitor serum potassium level.

Trimethoprim: May increase risk of hyperkalemia, especially in elderly patients. If use together can't be avoided, closely monitor potassium level.

EFFECTS ON LAB TEST RESULTS

• May increase glucose, triglyceride, uric acid, liver enzyme, bilirubin, and CK levels.

• May decrease Hb level and hematocrit.

CONTRAINDICATIONS & CAUTIONS

• Contraindicated in patients hypersensitive to drug or its components and in patients who experienced angioedema with ARBs.

• Use cautiously in patients who are volume- or sodium-depleted, those whose renal function depends on the RAAS (such as patients with severe HF), and those with unilateral or bilateral renal artery stenosis.

◑ *Alert:* Drug can cause spruelike enteropathy (severe chronic diarrhea with substantial weight loss).

Dialyzable drug: Unknown.

⚠ *Overdose S&S:* Hypotension, tachycardia, bradycardia.

PREGNANCY-LACTATION-REPRODUCTION

Black Box Warning Drug may cause fetal and neonatal complications and death. If patient becomes pregnant, stop drug immediately. ■

• It isn't known if drug appears in breast milk. Patient should discontinue breastfeeding or discontinue drug.

NURSING CONSIDERATIONS

• Symptomatic hypotension may occur in patients who are volume- or sodium-depleted, especially those being treated with high doses of a diuretic. If hypotension occurs, place patient supine and treat supportively. Treatment may continue once BP is stabilized.

• If BP isn't adequately controlled, a diuretic or other antihypertensive drugs also may be prescribed.

• Closely monitor patients with HF for oliguria, azotemia, and acute renal failure.

• Monitor BUN and creatinine level in patients with unilateral or bilateral renal artery stenosis.

• The antihypertensive effects of ACE inhibitors and ARBs are reduced in black patients; use of these drugs as initial antihypertensive therapy in these patients isn't recommended.

PATIENT TEACHING

• Tell patient to take drug exactly as prescribed and not to stop taking it, even if he feels better.

• Tell patient to take drug without regard to meals.

• Tell patient to promptly report all adverse reactions, especially light-headedness and fainting.

☼ **Alert:** Tell patient to contact prescriber if severe chronic diarrhea with substantial weight loss develops, even if months to years have elapsed before symptoms occur.

• Advise female patient of childbearing potential that drug can cause fetal harm and to immediately report pregnancy to health care provider.

• Inform diabetic patient that glucose readings may rise and that dosage of diabetes drugs may need adjustment.

• Warn patient that inadequate fluid intake, excessive perspiration, diarrhea, or vomiting may lead to an excessive drop in BP, light-headedness, and possibly fainting.

• Instruct patient that other antihypertensives can have additive effects. Patient should inform prescriber of all medications being taken, including OTC drugs.

olodaterol
OH-loe-DA-ter-ol

Striverdi Respimat

Therapeutic class: Bronchodilators
Pharmacologic class: Long-acting selective beta$_2$-adrenergic agonists

AVAILABLE FORMS
Inhalation aerosol: 2.5 mcg/actuation

INDICATIONS & DOSAGES
➤ **Long-term maintenance treatment of airway obstruction in patients with COPD, including chronic bronchitis and emphysema**
Adults: 2 inhalations once daily. Maximum dose is 2 inhalations in 24 hours.

ADMINISTRATION
Inhalation
• Prime inhaler by spraying toward ground until aerosol cloud is seen; then repeat spray three more times before first use or if inhaler hasn't been used for more than 21 days. If not used for more than 3 days, spray once toward ground to prime.

• To administer dose, have patient breathe in slowly through the mouth and press the dose release button. Patient should then continue to breathe in slowly as long as possible and then hold his breath for 10 seconds if possible. Repeat for the second inhalation.

• While patient is inhaling dose, have him hold inhaler flat and make sure he doesn't cover air vents on the mouthpiece.

• Give at same time each day.

ACTION
Binds and activates beta$_2$ adrenoceptors in the lungs, resulting in relaxation of smooth muscle cells and bronchodilation.

Route	Onset	Peak	Duration
Inhalation	5 min	10–20 min	24 hr

Half-life: 7½ hours.

ADVERSE REACTIONS
EENT: nasopharyngitis.
GI: diarrhea, constipation.

Reactions in bold italics are *life-threatening*. Interactions may have a *rapid onset* or a *delayed onset*.

GU: UTI.
Musculoskeletal: back pain, arthralgia.
Respiratory: bronchitis.

INTERACTIONS

Drug-drug. *Atomoxetine, linezolid, tedizolid:* May have additive tachycardic effect. Monitor patient carefully.
Atosiban: May increase risk of pulmonary edema or dyspnea. Monitor therapy.
Beta blockers: May diminish effect of both drugs and increase risk of bronchospasm. Avoid combination if possible.
Corticosteroids, non-potassium-sparing diuretics, xanthine derivatives (caffeine, theophylline): May increase risk of hypokalemia. Monitor potassium level.
Drugs that prolong QT interval (antiarrhythmics, droperidol, mifepristone, TCAs, thioridazine): May increase risk of life-threatening cardiac arrhythmias. Use together cautiously.
Linezolid: May cause additive hypertensive effect. Consider therapy modification.
MAO inhibitors, TCAs: May increase CV effects. Use together cautiously.
Other beta$_2$ agonists (long-acting): May have additive risk of toxic adverse effects. Use together is contraindicated.
Drug-food. *Caffeine:* May increase risk of hypokalemia. Discourage use together.

EFFECTS ON LAB TEST RESULTS

● May increase glucose level. May decrease potassium level.

CONTRAINDICATIONS & CAUTIONS

Black Box Warning Long-acting beta agonists such as olodaterol have been associated with increased risk of asthma-related death. Safety and effectiveness in patients with asthma haven't been established. Drug isn't indicated for use in asthma. ∎
● *Alert:* Rare, paradoxical, life-threatening bronchospasm has been reported. Discontinue drug immediately and treat emergently.
● Discontinue drug if hypersensitivity reactions such as angioedema occur.
● Don't initiate drug in patients with acute deterioration of COPD.
● Contraindicated as rescue therapy for acute symptoms.

● Use cautiously in patients with extreme sensitivity to other sympathomimetics, CV conditions (coronary insufficiency, cardiac arrhythmias, hypertrophic obstructive cardiomyopathy, hypertension), seizure disorders, diabetes, or thyrotoxicosis.
● Use cautiously in patients with known or suspected prolongation of QT interval.
● Safety and effectiveness in children haven't been established.
Dialyzable drug: Unknown.
⚠ **Overdose S&S:** CV toxicity, hypertension or hypotension, tachycardia, arrhythmias, palpitations, dizziness, nervousness, insomnia, anxiety, headache, tremor, dry mouth, muscle spasms, nausea, fatigue, malaise, hypokalemia, hyperglycemia, metabolic acidosis.

PREGNANCY-LACTATION-REPRODUCTION

● There are no adequate studies in pregnant women. Use during pregnancy only if potential benefit justifies potential risks to the fetus.
● It isn't known if drug appears in breast milk. Use cautiously in breast-feeding women.

NURSING CONSIDERATIONS

● Patient must also be prescribed a short-acting inhaled beta$_2$ agonist to provide symptomatic relief.
● Monitor patient for increased use of inhaled beta$_2$ agonist and decreased control of symptoms of bronchospasm. Evaluate for deterioration of disease.
● *Alert:* Excessive use of drug by using more frequently, increasing the number of inhalations, or using in combination with other medications containing long-acting beta$_2$ agonists may cause CV effects and death.
● Monitor patient for hypokalemia (which may increase risk of cardiac arrhythmias) and hyperglycemia.
● *Look alike–sound alike:* Don't confuse olodaterol with olopatadine. Don't confuse Striverdi Respimat with Combivent Respimat.

PATIENT TEACHING

Black Box Warning Warn patient that drug isn't approved for treatment of asthma.

People with asthma who take long-acting beta$_2$-adrenergic agonists have an increased risk of death from asthma complications. ■
- Teach patient how to use the Respimat device; then ask patient to demonstrate its use.
- Advise patient to take medication at same time each day.
- Explain that drug has a long-acting effect and should never be used as a "rescue medication" to relieve acute symptoms. Advise patient to always carry a rescue inhaler.
- Advise patient to report worsening signs or symptoms of COPD, increased frequency of rescue medication use, and decrease in effectiveness of rescue medication.
- Warn patient not to use drug with other long-acting beta$_2$ agonists and not to regularly use short-acting beta$_2$ agonists. Short-acting beta$_2$ agonists should only be used for acute symptoms.
- Instruct patient to report palpitations, chest pain, rapid heartbeat, muscle spasms, weakness, tremor or nervousness, URI, confusion, flushed dry skin, excessive thirst, urination, or hunger.
- Teach patient to seek emergency medical care for serious allergic reactions (breathing problems, rash, hives, or swelling of the face, mouth, or tongue).
- Caution patient not to stop drug without first discussing with prescriber.
- Instruct patient to consult prescriber before starting new prescription or OTC medications or herbal or nutritional supplements.
- Advise female patient to inform prescriber if she becomes pregnant, intends to become pregnant, or is breast-feeding.

olsalazine sodium
ol-SAL-uh-zeen

Dipentum

Therapeutic class: Anti-inflammatory drugs
Pharmacologic class: Salicylates

AVAILABLE FORMS
Capsules: 250 mg

INDICATIONS & DOSAGES
➤ **Maintenance of remission of ulcerative colitis in patients intolerant of sulfasalazine**
Adults: 500 mg P.O. b.i.d.

ADMINISTRATION
P.O.
- Give drug with food.

ACTION
Unknown. After oral use, converts to 5-aminosalicylic acid (5-ASA, or mesalamine) in the colon, where it has local anti-inflammatory effect.

Route	Onset	Peak	Duration
P.O.	Unknown	1 hr	Unknown

Half-life: About 1 hour.

ADVERSE REACTIONS
CNS: headache, depression, vertigo, dizziness, fatigue.
GI: diarrhea, nausea, abdominal pain, dyspepsia, bloating, anorexia, stomatitis, vomiting.
Musculoskeletal: arthralgia.
Respiratory: URI.
Skin: rash, itching.

INTERACTIONS
Drug-drug. *Anticoagulants:* May prolong PT and increase INR. Monitor bleeding study results.
Drug-food. *Any food:* May decrease GI irritation. Advise patient to take drug with food.

EFFECTS ON LAB TEST RESULTS
- May increase ALT and AST levels.

CONTRAINDICATIONS & CAUTIONS
- Contraindicated in patients hypersensitive to salicylates.
- Use cautiously in patients with severe allergies, asthma, hepatic impairment, and renal disease.
- Safety and effectiveness in children haven't been established.
Dializable drug: Unknown.

PREGNANCY-LACTATION-REPRODUCTION

• There are no adequate studies in pregnant women. Use only if potential benefit justifies risks to the fetus.
• Drug appears in breast milk. Use in breast-feeding women only if benefits outweigh risks.

NURSING CONSIDERATIONS

• Regularly monitor BUN and creatinine levels and urinalysis in patients with renal disease.
• Monitor liver enzyme levels in patients with hepatic impairment.
• Absorption of drug or its metabolites may cause renal tubular damage.
• Diarrhea sometimes occurs during therapy. Although diarrhea appears to be dose-related, it's difficult to distinguish from worsening of disease symptoms.
• Similar drugs have caused worsening of disease.
• *Look alike–sound alike:* Don't confuse olsalazine with olanzapine or sulfasalazine.

PATIENT TEACHING

• Teach patient to take drug in evenly divided doses and with food to minimize adverse GI reactions.
• Instruct patient to report persistent or severe adverse reactions promptly.

omalizumab
oh-mah-LIZ-uh-mab

Xolair

Therapeutic class: Antiasthmatics
Pharmacologic class: Monoclonal antibodies

AVAILABLE FORMS
Powder for injection: 150 mg in 5-mL vial

INDICATIONS & DOSAGES
➤ **Moderate to severe persistent asthma in patients with positive skin test or in vitro reactivity to a perennial aeroallergen and whose symptoms aren't adequately controlled by inhaled corticosteroids**

Adults and adolescents age 12 and older:
150 to 375 mg subcutaneously every 2 or 4 weeks. Dose and frequency vary with pretreatment immunoglobulin E (IgE) level (international units/mL) and patient weight. Divide doses larger than 150 mg among more than one injection site.
➤ **Chronic idiopathic urticaria in patients who are symptomatic despite antihistamine treatment**
Adults and adolescents age 12 and older:
150 to 300 mg subcutaneously every 4 weeks. Dosing isn't dependent on serum IgE level or body weight. Periodically reassess need for continued therapy; treatment duration hasn't been evaluated.

ADMINISTRATION
Subcutaneous
• Reconstitute with sterile water for injection only. Swirl gently, don't shake. Use 18G needle to draw medication into syringe, then replace with a 25G needle for administration.
• The lyophilized product takes 15 to 20 minutes to dissolve completely.
• The fully reconstituted product will appear clear or slightly opalescent and may have a few small bubbles or foam around the edge of the vial.
• Because the solution is slightly viscous, it may take 5 to 10 seconds to administer.
• Use reconstituted solution within 4 hours if at room temperature or within 8 hours if refrigerated.

ACTION
Inhibits binding of IgE to high-affinity receptor on surface of mast cells and basophils, which limits release of allergic response mediators.

Route	Onset	Peak	Duration
Subcut.	Unknown	7–8 days	Unknown

Half-life: About 24 to 26 days.

ADVERSE REACTIONS
CNS: anxiety, headache, dizziness, fatigue, pain, migraine.
CV: *MI, PE, thrombosis,* angina pectoris, peripheral edema.
EENT: pharyngitis, sinusitis, earache.

Musculoskeletal: arm pain, arthralgia, fracture, leg pain.
Respiratory: URI, cough, asthma.
Skin: injection-site reaction, dermatitis, pruritus.
Other: viral infections.

INTERACTIONS
None reported.

EFFECTS ON LAB TEST RESULTS
• May increase IgE level.

CONTRAINDICATIONS & CAUTIONS
• Contraindicated in patients severely hypersensitive to drug.
Black Box Warning Anaphylaxis presenting as bronchospasm, hypotension, syncope, urticaria, or angioedema of the throat or tongue has been reported after administration as early as the first dose and even after a year of treatment. ■
• Drug should be given only in a health care setting under direct medical supervision because of the risk of anaphylaxis.
❸ Alert: Drug isn't indicated for other allergic conditions or other forms of urticaria.
• Safety and effectiveness in children younger than age 12 haven't been established.
Dialyzable drug: Unknown.

PREGNANCY-LACTATION-REPRODUCTION
• There are no adequate studies in pregnant women. Use only if clearly needed.
• Encourage patients exposed to drug during pregnancy to call the EXPECT Pregnancy Registry (1-866-4XOLAIR).
• It isn't known if drug appears in breast milk. Use cautiously in breast-feeding women.

NURSING CONSIDERATIONS
❸ Alert: Don't use this drug to treat acute bronchospasm or status asthmaticus.
• Don't abruptly stop systemic or inhaled corticosteroid when omalizumab therapy starts; taper the dose gradually and under supervision.
• Injection-site reactions, such as bruising, redness, warmth, burning, stinging, itching, hives, pain, induration, and inflammation, may occur, usually within 1 hour after the

injection. These reactions last fewer than 8 days and decrease in frequency with subsequent injections.
Black Box Warning Observe patient for at least 2 hours after the injection, and keep drugs available to respond to anaphylactic reactions (such as bronchospasm, hypotension, syncope, urticaria, or angioedema of the throat or tongue). These reactions usually occur within 2 hours of subcutaneous injection; however, delayed reactions may occur up to 24 hours after administration. Anaphylaxis has also occurred beyond 1 year after beginning regularly administered treatment. If patient has a severe hypersensitivity reaction, stop treatment. ■
❸ Alert: Drug may slightly increase risk of CV and cerebrovascular events (TIA, MI, chest pain, pulmonary hypertension, DVT, PE). Periodically reassess the need for continued therapy based on disease severity and asthma control.
• Drug increases IgE level, so it can't be used to determine appropriate dosage during therapy or for 1 year after therapy ends.
• Patient medication guide must be given with each dose.

PATIENT TEACHING
• Tell patients not to stop or reduce the dosage of any other asthma drugs unless directed by the prescriber. Patient medication guide must be given with each dose.
• Explain that patient may not notice an immediate improvement in asthma after therapy starts.
Black Box Warning Teach patient the signs and symptoms of anaphylaxis and tell him to seek immediate medical care if symptoms occur. ■

Reactions in bold italics are *life-threatening*. Interactions may have a *rapid onset* or a *delayed onset*.

ombitasvir–paritaprevir–ritonavir–dasabuvir
om-BIT-as-vir/par-i-TA-pre-vir/
ri-TON-ah-veer/da-SA-bue-vir

Viekira Pak, Viekira XR

Therapeutic class: Antivirals
Pharmacologic class: Antivirals

AVAILABLE FORMS
Copackaged 28-day supply
Tablets: ombitasvir 12.5 mg/paritaprevir
75 mg/ritonavir 50 mg
Tablets: dasabuvir 250 mg
Tablets (24-hour extended-release) ⓝ:
ombitasvir 8.33 mg/paritaprevir 50 mg/
ritonavir 33.33 mg/ dasabuvir 200 mg

INDICATIONS & DOSAGES
➤ **Chronic HCV genotype 1 infection,
including patients with compensated
cirrhosis, with or without ribavirin**
Adults: For Viekira Pak, give two
ombitasvir–paritaprevir–ritonavir tablets
P.O. once daily (in morning) and one
dasabuvir tablet P.O. b.i.d. (morning and
evening), with a meal, or 3 tablets (Viekira
XR) P.O. once daily with a meal.
Adjust-a-dose: For patients with HCV
genotype 1a infection or unknown genotype without cirrhosis, give Viekira Pak
or Viekira XR plus ribavirin for 12 weeks.
For patients with genotype 1a infection
or unknown genotype with compensated
cirrhosis, give Viekira Pak or Viekira XR
plus ribavirin for 24 weeks. For patients
with genotype 1b infection with or without compensated cirrhosis, give Viekira
Pak or Viekira XR for 12 weeks. For liver
transplant patients with normal hepatic
function and mild fibrosis, regardless of
genotype 1 subtype, give Viekira Pak or
Viekira XR plus ribavirin for 24 weeks. For
ALT level greater than 10 × ULN, consider discontinuing antiviral therapy. If ALT
level is elevated and associated with liver
inflammation, increasing bilirubin or alkaline phosphatase level or INR, discontinue
treatment.

ADMINISTRATION
P.O.
● Must give with a meal but without regard
to fat or calorie content.
● Patient should swallow extended-release
tablets whole and not split, crush, or chew
them.
● Store at room temperature.

ACTION
Ombitasvir inhibits HCV NS5A, an enzyme
needed for viral RNA replication and assembly of virions. Paritaprevir inhibits HCV
NS3/4A protease, an enzyme essential for
viral replication and responsible for HCV
protein cleavage. Ritonavir doesn't have
activity against HCV but acts as a potent
inhibitor of CYP3A, thereby significantly
increasing paritaprevir exposure. Dasabuvir inhibits NS5B polymerase, an enzyme
essential for replication of the viral genome.

Route	Onset	Peak	Duration
P.O. (ombitasvir)	Unknown	4–5 hr	Unknown
P.O. (paritaprevir)	Unknown	4–5 hr	Unknown
P.O. (ritonavir)	Unknown	4–5 hr	Unknown
P.O. (dasabuvir)	Unknown	4–5 hr	Unknown

Half-life: Ombitasvir, 21 to 25 hours; paritaprevir,
5½ hours; ritonavir, 4 hours; dasabuvir, 5½ to
6 hours.

ADVERSE REACTIONS
CNS: insomnia, fatigue, asthenia, headache.
EENT: scleral icterus.
GI: nausea, diarrhea.
Hematologic: anemia.
Hepatic: ALT and serum bilirubin eleva-
tions.
Musculoskeletal: muscle spasms.
Respiratory: cough, dyspnea.
Skin: pruritus, rash, erythema, eczema,
dermatitis, exfoliation, psoriasis, ulcer,
urticaria, photosensitivity.

INTERACTIONS
Drug-drug. *Alpha$_1$-adrenoreceptor antagonists (alfuzosin):* May increase risk of
hypotension. Use together is contraindicated.
Alprazolam: May increase alprazolam
level. Monitor patient closely for clinical
effects of alprazolam and decrease dosage if
indicated.

Antiarrhythmics (amiodarone, bepridil, disopyramide, flecainide, lidocaine [systemic], mexiletine, propafenone, quinidine): May increase antiarrhythmic concentration. Use together cautiously and monitor drug levels, if available.

Atazanavir/ritonavir: May increase paritaprevir concentration. Give atazanavir 300 mg without ritonavir in morning.

Calcium channel blockers (e.g., amlodipine): May increase amlodipine level. Consider amlodipine dosage reduction and monitor patient closely.

Corticosteroids, fluticasone (inhaled/nasal): May increase fluticasone level and decrease cortisol concentration. Consider alternative corticosteroids, especially if using long term.

Cyclosporine: May increase cyclosporine level and risk of cyclosporine-related adverse reactions. When used together, decrease cyclosporine dosage and monitor renal function.

Darunavir/ritonavir: May decrease darunavir trough level. Use together isn't recommended.

Dihydroergotamine, ergonovine, ergotamine, methylergonovine: May increase risk of acute ergot toxicity (vasospasm, tissue ischemia) when given with ritonavir. Use together is contraindicated.

Diuretics (furosemide): May increase furosemide maximum concentration. Monitor patient and adjust furosemide dosage as clinically indicated.

Drugs highly dependent on CYP3A for clearance (oral midazolam, triazolam): May increase risk of high plasma levels of drugs dependent on CYP3A for clearance and serious or life-threatening adverse effects. Use together is contraindicated.

Efavirenz: Caused liver enzyme elevations in clinical trials. Use together is contraindicated.

Estrogen (conjugated estrogens for hormone replacement therapy, estradiol): May increase ALT level. Use cautiously together and monitor liver enzyme levels.

❸ Alert: *Ethinyl estradiol (combined oral contraceptives):* May significantly increase ALT level. Use together is contraindicated. Discontinue ethinyl estradiol–containing medication before starting antiviral treatment. Alternative methods of contraception (progestin only or nonhormonal) are recommended. Ethinyl estradiol may be restarted 2 weeks after completion of antiviral treatment.

Immunosuppressants (cyclosporine, tacrolimus): May increase cyclosporine and tacrolimus levels. Reduce cyclosporine dosage to one-fifth of patient's dose and closely monitor cyclosporine blood concentration. Reduce tacrolimus dosage to 0.5 mg every 7 days, monitor tacrolimus level frequently, and adjust dosage as needed. May resume higher doses after completion of antiviral therapy based on cyclosporine or tacrolimus level.

Ketoconazole: May increase ketoconazole level. Limit daily dose of ketoconazole to 200 mg.

Long-acting beta-adrenoceptor agonists (salmeterol): May increase salmeterol concentration and risk of QT-interval prolongation. Coadministration isn't recommended.

Lopinavir–ritonavir: May increase paritaprevir level. Use together isn't recommended.

Lovastatin, simvastatin: May significantly increase risk of myopathy, including rhabdomyolysis. Use together is contraindicated.

Opioid analgesics (buprenorphine/naloxone, hydrocodone): May increase concentrations of opioids. Monitor patient closely for sedative and cognitive effects and reduce hydrocodone dosage by 50%.

Pimozide: May increase risk of cardiac arrhythmias. Use together is contraindicated.

PPIs (omeprazole): May decrease omeprazole concentration. Monitor patient closely for omeprazole effectiveness and consider increasing omeprazole dosage if symptoms aren't well controlled; avoid using more than 40 mg/day of omeprazole.

Pravastatin, rosuvastatin: May increase pravastatin and rosuvastatin levels. Limit pravastatin to 40 mg/day and rosuvastatin to 10 mg/day.

Rilpivirine: May increase rilpivirine level and risk of QT-interval prolongation. Use together isn't recommended.

Sildenafil (at doses for treatment of pulmonary arterial hypertension): May increase risk of sildenafil-associated adverse effects (visual disturbances, hypotension, priapism, syncope). Use together is contraindicated.

Strong CYP2C8 and CYP3A inducers (carbamazepine, phenobarbital, phenytoin, rifampin): May reduce efficacy of ombitasvir, paritaprevir, ritonavir, and dasabuvir, and increase risk of resistance. Use together is contraindicated.

Strong CYP2C8 inhibitors (gemfibrozil): May increase dasabuvir level and risk of QT-interval prolongation. Use together is contraindicated.

Voriconazole: May decrease voriconazole level. Use together isn't recommended unless benefit outweighs risks.

Drug-herb. *St. John's wort:* May decrease ombitasvir, paritaprevir, ritonavir, and dasabuvir levels. Use together is contraindicated.

Drug-lifestyle. *Alcohol use:* May alter release of extended-release tablets. Avoid use 4 hours before or after taking drug.

EFFECTS ON LAB TEST RESULTS
- May increase ALT and bilirubin levels.
- May decrease Hb level.

CONTRAINDICATIONS & CAUTIONS
- If ombitasvir–paritaprevir–ritonavir and dasabuvir are administered with ribavirin, the contraindications for ribavirin also apply.
- Contraindicated in patients hypersensitive to any of the drugs or their components. Contraindicated in patients with known hypersensitivity (toxic epidermal necrolysis or Stevens-Johnson syndrome) to ritonavir.
- Contraindicated with drugs that are extensively metabolized by CYP3A, are strong inducers of CYP3A and CYP2C8, or are strong inhibitors of CYP2C8.
- **⊕ Alert:** Contraindicated in patients with moderate or severe hepatic impairment (Child-Pugh class B or C) because of potential toxicity.
- **⊕ Alert:** Patients with cirrhosis are at risk for hepatic decompensation and hepatic failure, including liver transplantation and death, during therapy.
- **Black Box Warning** Reactivation of HBV may occur in patients coinfected with HCV, and result in fulminant hepatitis, hepatic

failure, and death. Screen all patients for current or prior HBV infection before treatment and if positive for HBV infection, assess baseline HBV DNA. ■
- Use cautiously in patients with HIV infection. HIV-positive patients should also be on suppressive antiretroviral regimen to reduce risk of HIV-1 protease inhibitor drug resistance.
- Safety and effectiveness in children haven't been established.
Dialyzable drug: Unknown.

PREGNANCY-LACTATION-REPRODUCTION
- Use in pregnant women, without concomitant ribavirin, only if clearly needed.
- It isn't known if drug combination causes fetal harm. Drug combination, when taken with concomitant ribavirin, is contraindicated in pregnant women and in men whose female partners are pregnant.
- Encourage pregnant women with HCV/HIV-1 coinfection who are taking concomitant antiretrovirals to register with the Antiretroviral Pregnancy Registry (1-800-258-4263).
- It isn't known if ombitasvir, paritaprevir, ritonavir, dasabuvir, or their metabolites appear in breast milk. Use cautiously in breast-feeding women. HIV-infected women shouldn't breast-feed.

NURSING CONSIDERATIONS
Black Box Warning Use laboratory testing to monitor patient with current or prior HBV infection for hepatitis flare or HBV reactivation and watch for signs and symptoms of hepatic injury during active and posttreatment follow-up. ■
⊕ Alert: Perform LFTs at baseline, during first 4 weeks of therapy, then as clinically indicated. If ALT level, bilirubin level, or both are elevated above baseline, repeat tests and monitor patient closely. Drug may need to be discontinued if ALT level remains persistently greater than 10 × ULN.
⊕ Alert: Monitor patient for hepatic decompensation (elevated bilirubin level, ascites, hepatic encephalopathy, variceal hemorrhage). Discontinue drug if hepatic decompensation occurs.

O

• Monitor serum HCV-RNA level at baseline, end of treatment, during treatment follow-up, and when clinically indicated.
• Review patient's medication profile carefully before and periodically during therapy; many drug interactions are possible.
• Monitor patient for hepatotoxicity (fatigue, weakness, lack of appetite, nausea, vomiting, jaundice, discolored feces).

PATIENT TEACHING
• Explain to patient that this combination therapy is supplied as a monthly carton for a total of 28 days of treatment.
• Teach patient to take medication with a meal and not to crush, chew, or split extended-release tablets.
• **Alert:** Inform patient with cirrhosis of the increased risk of hepatic decompensation and failure with therapy, and the need for close monitoring.
Black Box Warning Warn patient to immediately report signs and symptoms of hepatic injury (fatigue, weakness, appetite loss, nausea, vomiting, yellowing of the skin or eyes, light-colored stool). ■
• Advise female patient to avoid becoming pregnant during therapy, especially if using drug combination concomitantly with ribavirin. Counsel her to notify prescriber immediately if she becomes pregnant.
• Inform female patient that contraceptives containing ethinyl estradiol are contraindicated during treatment and to use alternative contraceptive methods.
• Instruct patient to report all current or new medications to prescriber because of possible drug-drug interactions.
• Inform patient to take medication as prescribed, without missing any doses. If a dose of ombitasvir–paritaprevir–ritonavir is missed, it can be taken within 12 hours of missed dose. If a dose of dasabuvir is missed, it can be taken within 6 hours of missed dose. If more than 12 hours have passed since ombitasvir–paritaprevir–ritonavir is typically taken or more than 6 hours have passed since dasabuvir is typically taken, patient shouldn't take the missed dose but should take the next scheduled dose per the usual schedule.

• Caution patient to take medication as prescribed for full treatment period, to avoid virologic treatment failure and resistance.
• Explain to patient importance of obtaining laboratory tests as ordered.
• Advise patient to continue precautions to prevent HCV transmission during treatment.

omega-3–acid ethyl esters
oh-may-gah-three ASS-id

Epanova, Lovaza◆, Omtryg, Vascepa

Therapeutic class: Antilipemics
Pharmacologic class: Ethyl esters

AVAILABLE FORMS
Capsules ⬛: 1 g, 1.2 g

INDICATIONS & DOSAGES
➤ **Adjunct to diet to reduce triglyceride levels 500 mg/dL or higher**
Adults: 4 g (Epanova, Lovaza) P.O. once daily or divided as 2 g P.O. b.i.d. Or, 4.8 g (Omtryg) P.O. once daily or 2.4 g P.O. b.i.d. Or, 2 g (Vascepa) P.O. b.i.d.

ADMINISTRATION
P.O.
• May give Epanova and Lovaza with or without meals. Give Omtryg and Vascepa with meals.
• Make sure patient swallows capsules whole and doesn't chew, crush, dissolve, or extract contents of capsule.

ACTION
May reduce hepatic formation of triglycerides because two components of drug are poor substrates for the necessary enzymes. These components also block formation of other fatty acids.

Route	Onset	Peak	Duration
P.O.	Unknown	Unknown	Unknown

Half-life: Unknown.

ADVERSE REACTIONS
GI: altered taste, abdominal pain, belching, dyspepsia, diarrhea, nausea.

Reactions in bold italics are *life-threatening*. Interactions may have a *rapid onset* or a ***delayed onset***.

Musculoskeletal: arthralgia, back pain.
Skin: rash.

INTERACTIONS
Drug-drug. *Anticoagulants, antiplatelet drugs:* May prolong bleeding time. Monitor patient.

EFFECTS ON LAB TEST RESULTS
• May increase ALT, AST, and LDL cholesterol levels.

CONTRAINDICATIONS & CAUTIONS
• Contraindicated in patients hypersensitive to drug or its components.
• Use cautiously in patients sensitive to fish.
• Use cautiously in patients with coagulopathy and in those receiving therapeutic anticoagulation or antiplatelet therapy because of risk of prolonged bleeding time.
• Effect of drug on risk of pancreatitis and on CV mortality and morbidity hasn't been determined.
• Safety and effectiveness in children haven't been established.
Dialyzable drug: Unknown.

PREGNANCY-LACTATION-REPRODUCTION
• There are no adequate studies in pregnant women. Use cautiously and only if benefit justifies possible risks to the fetus.
• Drug may appear in breast milk. Use cautiously in breast-feeding women.

NURSING CONSIDERATIONS
• Assess patient for conditions that contribute to increased triglycerides, such as diabetes and hypothyroidism, before treatment.
• Monitor patient for changes in INR after drug initiation and after omega-3 fatty acid dosage changes in patients receiving warfarin.
• Evaluate patient's current drug regimen for any drugs known to sharply increase triglyceride levels, including estrogen therapy, thiazide diuretics, and beta blockers. Stopping these drugs, if appropriate, may negate the need for drug.
• Continue diet and lifestyle modifications during treatment.
• Obtain baseline triglyceride levels to confirm that they're consistently abnormal

before therapy; then recheck periodically during treatment. If patient has an inadequate response after 2 months, stop drug.
• Monitor LDL level to make sure it doesn't increase excessively during treatment.
• ***Look alike–sound alike:*** Don't confuse Lovaza with lorazepam or lovastatin.

PATIENT TEACHING
• Explain that taking drug doesn't reduce the importance of following the recommended diet and exercise plan.
• Remind patient of the need for follow-up blood work to evaluate progress.
• Advise patient to notify prescriber about bothersome side effects.
• Tell patient to report planned or suspected pregnancy.

omeprazole
oh-ME-pray-zole

Losec✤

omeprazole magnesium
Prilosec OTC ◇

Therapeutic class: Antiulcer drugs
Pharmacologic class: PPIs

AVAILABLE FORMS
Capsules (delayed-release) 🞕*:* 10 mg, 20 mg, 40 mg
Powder for delayed-release oral suspension: 2.5 mg/packet, 10 mg/packet
Tablets (delayed-release) 🞕*:* 20 mg ◇

INDICATIONS & DOSAGES
➤ **Symptomatic GERD without esophageal lesions**
Adults: 20 mg P.O., as delayed-release form or oral suspension, daily for 4 weeks for patients who respond poorly to customary medical treatment, usually including an adequate course of H_2-receptor antagonists.
Children ages 1 to 16 weighing 20 kg or more: 20 mg P.O. daily for up to 4 weeks.
Children ages 1 to 16 weighing 10 to less than 20 kg: 10 mg P.O. daily for up to 4 weeks.
Children ages 1 to 16 weighing 5 to less than 10 kg: 5 mg P.O. daily for up to 4 weeks.

➤ **Erosive esophagitis (EE)**
Adults: 20 mg P.O. daily. For recurrent EE or GERD signs and symptoms, treat for up to 12 months.
Adjust-a-dose: When drug is used for maintenance of healing of EE, dosage reduction to 10 mg once daily is recommended for patients with hepatic impairment (Child-Pugh class A, B, or C) and Asian patients.
Children ages 1 to 16 weighing 20 kg or more: 20 mg P.O. daily for 4 to 8 weeks.
Children ages 1 to 16 weighing 10 to less than 20 kg: 10 mg P.O. daily for 4 to 8 weeks.
Children ages 1 to 16 weighing 5 to less than 10 kg: 5 mg P.O. daily for 4 to 8 weeks.
➤ **Pathologic hypersecretory conditions (such as Zollinger-Ellison syndrome)**
Adults: Initially, 60 mg P.O. daily; adjust dosage based on patient response. If daily dose exceeds 80 mg, give in divided doses. Doses up to 120 mg t.i.d. have been given. Continue therapy as long as clinically indicated.
➤ **Duodenal ulcer (short-term treatment)**
Adults: 20 mg P.O., as delayed-release form or oral suspension, daily for 4 weeks.
➤ *Helicobacter pylori* **infection and duodenal ulcer disease, to eradicate** *H. pylori* **with clarithromycin (dual therapy)**
Adults: 40 mg P.O. every morning with clarithromycin 500 mg P.O. t.i.d. for 14 days. For patients with an ulcer at start of therapy, give another 14 days of omeprazole 20 mg P.O. once daily.
➤ *H. pylori* **infection and duodenal ulcer disease, to eradicate** *H. pylori* **with clarithromycin and amoxicillin (triple therapy)**
Adults: 20 mg P.O. with clarithromycin 500 mg P.O. and amoxicillin 1,000 mg P.O., each given b.i.d. for 10 days. For patients with an ulcer at start of therapy, give another 18 days of omeprazole 20 mg P.O. once daily.
➤ **Short-term treatment of active benign gastric ulcer**
Adults: 40 mg P.O. once daily for 4 to 8 weeks.
➤ **Frequent heartburn (2 or more days a week)**
Adults: 20 mg Prilosec OTC P.O. once daily before breakfast for 14 days. May repeat the 14-day course every 4 months.

ADMINISTRATION
P.O.
● Don't crush tablets or capsules. For patients who have difficulty swallowing, capsules may be opened and contents mixed with 15 mL of applesauce. Follow with water to ensure complete swallowing of pellets.
● Give drug at least 1 hour before meals.
● For oral suspension, empty contents of 2.5-mg packet into container containing 5 mL water; empty contents of 10-mg packet into container containing 15 mL water. Stir and leave for 2 to 3 minutes to thicken. Stir and administer within 30 minutes. If material remains after drinking, add more water, stir, and give immediately.
● For patients with an NG or gastric tube in place, add 5 mL water to catheter-tipped syringe; then add contents of 2.5-mg packet (or 15 mL water for 10-mg packet). Immediately shake syringe and leave for 2 to 3 minutes to thicken. Shake syringe and inject through NG or gastric tube, #6 French or larger, into stomach within 30 minutes. Refill syringe with an equal amount of water. Shake and flush any remaining contents from NG or gastric tube into stomach.

ACTION
Inhibits proton pump activity by binding to hydrogen–potassium adenosine triphosphatase, located at secretory surface of gastric parietal cells, to suppress gastric acid secretion.

Route	Onset	Peak	Duration
P.O.	1 hr	30 min–2 hr	<3 days

Half-life: 30 to 60 minutes.

ADVERSE REACTIONS
CNS: asthenia, dizziness, headache.
GI: abdominal pain, constipation, diarrhea, flatulence, nausea, vomiting, acid regurgitation.
Musculoskeletal: back pain.
Respiratory: cough, URI.
Skin: rash.

INTERACTIONS
Drug-drug. *Ampicillin esters, azole antifungals (such as ketoconazole), erlotinib, iron derivatives, nilotinib:* May cause poor bioavailability of these drugs because they

---

Reactions in bold italics are *life-threatening*. Interactions may have a *rapid onset* or a *delayed onset*.

need a low gastric pH for optimal absorption. Avoid using together.

Atazanavir, nelfinavir: May decrease plasma concentrations of these drugs, possibly resulting in loss of therapeutic effect. Avoid use together.

Benzodiazepines (metabolized by hepatic oxidation), fosphenytoin, phenytoin, warfarin: May decrease hepatic clearance, possibly leading to increased levels of these drugs. Monitor drug levels.

Calcium salts: May decrease GI absorption of calcium salts. Closely monitor clinical response and increase calcium dosage if needed.

Cilostazol: May increase cilostazol level. Reduce cilostazol dosage.

Clopidogrel: May decrease antiplatelet activity. Avoid use together.

Digoxin: May increase digoxin level, causing toxicity. Monitor digoxin level.

Fluvoxamine: May increase omeprazole level. Monitor patient for increased adverse reactions.

Iron salts: May interfere with iron absorption. Omeprazole may need to be temporarily stopped, or parenteral iron may be given as an alternative.

Mycophenolate: May decrease mycophenolate serum concentration; may reduce formation of active metabolite for mycophenolate. Monitor therapy.

Methotrexate: May increase methotrexate level, causing toxicity. Monitor patient closely.

Rifampin: May substantially decrease omeprazole concentration. Avoid concomitant use.

Salicylates: Enteric-coated forms may dissolve faster, increasing risk of gastric adverse effects. Use together cautiously.

Saquinavir: May increase saquinavir serum concentration, resulting in increased toxicity. Monitor therapy.

Tacrolimus: May increase tacrolimus level and risk of toxicity. Monitor tacrolimus trough concentration when omeprazole is started and stopped.

Voriconazole: May increase serum concentrations of both drugs. Consider reducing omeprazole dosage by 50%; monitor therapy.

EFFECTS ON LAB TEST RESULTS

• May increase LFT values and falsely elevate serum chromogranin A (CgA) level.
• May decrease magnesium, sodium, and glucose levels.

CONTRAINDICATIONS & CAUTIONS

• Contraindicated in patients hypersensitive to drug or its components.
🔆 **Alert:** High-dose, long-term PPI therapy may be associated with an increased risk of hip, wrist, and spine fractures.
• Use cautiously in patients with hypokalemia and respiratory alkalosis in patients on a low-sodium diet, and in breast-feeding women.
• Long-term administration of bicarbonate with calcium or milk can cause milk-alkali syndrome.
Dialyzable drug: Unlikely.
⚠ **Overdose S&S:** Confusion, drowsiness, blurred vision, tachycardia, nausea, vomiting, diaphoresis, flushing, headache, dry mouth.

PREGNANCY-LACTATION-REPRODUCTION

• Use during pregnancy only if potential benefit justifies fetal risks. When treating GERD in pregnant women, PPIs may be used when necessary.
• Drug appears in breast milk. Use cautiously in breast-feeding women.

NURSING CONSIDERATIONS

🔆 **Alert:** May increase risk of CDAD. Evaluate for CDAD in patients who develop diarrhea that doesn't improve.
• False-positive results in diagnostic investigations for neuroendocrine tumors may occur due to increased CgA level. Temporarily stop omeprazole treatment at least 14 days before assessing CgA level and consider repeating the test if initial CgA level is high. If serial tests are performed (e.g., for monitoring), the same commercial laboratory should be used for testing, as reference ranges between tests may vary.
• Long-term therapy may cause vitamin B_{12} absorption problems. Assess patient for signs and symptoms of cyanocobalamin deficiency (weakness, heart palpitations, dyspnea, paresthesia, pale skin, smooth tongue, CNS changes, loss of appetite).

• Dosage adjustments may be necessary in Asians and patients with hepatic impairment.

• Periodically assess patient for osteoporosis.

• Drug increases its own bioavailability with repeated doses. Drug is unstable in gastric acid; less drug is lost to hydrolysis because drug increases gastric pH.

• Gastrin level rises in most patients during the first 2 weeks of therapy.

◐ *Alert:* Prolonged use of PPIs may cause low magnesium levels. Monitor magnesium levels before starting treatment and periodically thereafter.

◐ *Alert:* Monitor patients for signs and symptoms of low magnesium level, such as abnormal HR or rhythm, palpitations, muscle spasms, tremors, or seizures. In children, an abnormal HR may present as fatigue, upset stomach, dizziness, and lightheadedness. Magnesium supplementation or drug discontinuation may be required.

• *Look alike–sound alike:* Don't confuse Prilosec OTC with Prozac, prilocaine, or Prinivil.

PATIENT TEACHING

• Tell patient to swallow tablets whole and not to open, crush, or chew them.

• Give patient instructions on how to take oral suspension.

• Instruct patient to take drug at least 1 hour before meals.

• Caution patient to avoid hazardous activities if he gets dizzy.

• Advise patient that Prilosec OTC isn't intended to treat infrequent heartburn (one episode of heartburn a week or less), or for those who want immediate relief of heartburn.

• Inform patient that Prilosec OTC may take 1 to 4 days for full effect, although some patients may get complete relief of symptoms within 24 hours.

• Teach patient to recognize and report signs and symptoms of low magnesium levels.

onabotulinumtoxinA
OH-na-BOT-ue-LYE-num-TOX-in A

Botox

onabotulinumtoxinA (cosmetic)
Botox Cosmetic

Therapeutic class: Neuromuscular transmission blockers
Pharmacologic class: Acetylcholine release inhibitors

AVAILABLE FORMS
onabotulinumtoxinA
Injection: 50 units/vial, 100 units/vial, 200 units/vial
onabotulinumtoxinA (cosmetic)
Injection: 50 units/vial, 100 units/vial

INDICATIONS & DOSAGES
Adjust-a-dose (for all indications): When adults are being treated for one or more indications, maximum cumulative dose generally shouldn't exceed 400 units in a 3-month interval (Botox) or 360 units in a 3-month interval (Botox Cosmetic).

➤ **Overactive bladder signs and symptoms (urge urinary incontinence, urgency, and frequency) in patients with inadequate response to or intolerant of anticholinergic medication (Botox)**
Adults: Recommended total dose is 100 units, given as 0.5 mL (5 units) I.M. across 20 sites into the detrusor muscle. Give prophylactic antibiotics (except aminoglycosides) 1 to 3 days before treatment, on treatment day, and 1 to 3 days after treatment to reduce likelihood of procedure-related UTI. Consider retreatment no sooner than 12 weeks from prior injection.

➤ **Urinary incontinence due to detrusor overactivity associated with a neurologic condition, such as spinal cord injury or MS, after inadequate response to or intolerance of anticholinergic medication (Botox)**
Adults: Recommended total dose is 200 units, given as 30 injections of 1 mL (6.7 units) each (total volume of 30 mL) I.M. across 30 sites into the detrusor muscle.

Give prophylactic antibiotics (except aminoglycosides) 1 to 3 days before treatment, on treatment day, and 1 to 3 days after treatment to reduce likelihood of procedure-related UTI. Consider retreatment no sooner than 12 weeks from prior injection.

➤ **Prophylaxis of headaches in patients with chronic migraine (15 days per month or more, with headache lasting 4 hours a day or longer) (Botox)**
Adults: Recommended total dose is 155 units, given as 0.1 mL (5 units) per site I.M. divided across seven head/neck muscles, every 12 weeks. Refer to manufacturer's instructions for injection-site diagrams.

➤ **Upper limb spasticity (Botox)**
Adults: 12.5 to 50 units per site I.M. The lowest recommended starting dose should be used. Tailor dosing in initial and sequential treatment sessions to the individual based on the size, number, and location of muscles involved; severity of spasticity; presence of local muscle weakness; and patient's response to previous treatment or adverse event history with onabotulinumtoxinA. Administer no more than 50 units per site. Refer to manufacturer's instructions for specific sites and dosages. Consider retreatment no sooner than 12 weeks from prior injection.

✷ *NEW INDICATION:* **Lower limb spasticity (Botox)**
Adults: 300 to 400 units I.M. divided among five muscles (gastrocnemius, soleus, tibialis posterior, flexor hallucis longus, and flexor digitorum longus). Use lowest recommended starting dose and administer no more than 50 units per site. Individualize dosing in initial and sequential treatment sessions based on size, number, and location of muscles involved; severity of spasticity; presence of local muscle weakness; and patient's response to previous treatment or adverse event history with onabotulinumtoxinA. Refer to manufacturer's instructions for specific sites and dosages.

➤ **Cervical dystonia to reduce severity of abnormal head position and neck pain (Botox)**
Adults and children age 16 and older: Adjust initial and subsequent dosing based on patient's head and neck position, localiza-

tion of pain, muscle hypertrophy, patient response, and adverse event history. Use lower initial dose in botulinum toxin–naive patients. Administer no more than 50 units per site.

➤ **Severe axillary hyperhidrosis inadequately managed by topical agents (Botox)**
Adults: 50 units (2 mL) injected intradermally in 0.1- to 0.2-mL aliquots to each axilla, evenly distributed in 10 to 15 sites approximately 1 to 2 cm apart. May administer repeat injections when clinical effect of a previous injection diminishes.

➤ **Blepharospasm associated with dystonia (Botox)**
Adults and children age 12 and older: 1.25 to 2.5 units (0.05 to 0.1 mL volume at each site) I.M. into medial and lateral pretarsal orbicularis oculi of upper lid and into lateral pretarsal orbicularis oculi of lower lid. Cumulative dose in a 30-day period shouldn't exceed 200 units.

➤ **Strabismus (Botox)**
Adults and children age 12 and older: For vertical muscles, and for horizontal strabismus of less than 20 prism diopters: 1.25 to 2.5 units in any one muscle. For horizontal strabismus of 20 to 50 prism diopters: 2.5 to 5 units in any one muscle. Maximum dose is 25 units for any one muscle.

➤ **Persistent cranial nerve VI palsy lasting 1 month or longer**
Adults and children age 12 and older: 1.25 to 2.5 units I.M. in medial rectus muscle.

➤ **Temporary improvement in appearance of moderate to severe glabellar lines associated with corrugator or procerus muscle activity (Botox Cosmetic)**
Adults: Inject 4 units (0.1 mL) I.M. into each of five sites, two in each corrugator muscle and one in the procerus muscle for a total dose of 20 units. An effective dose for facial lines is determined by gross observation of patient's ability to activate the superficial muscles injected.

➤ **Temporary improvement in appearance of moderate to severe lateral canthal lines associated with orbicularis oculi activity (Botox Cosmetic)**
Adults: Inject 4 units (0.1 mL) I.M. into each of three sites per side (six total

O

injection points) in the lateral orbicularis oculi muscle for a total of 24 units (0.6 mL) (12 units per side).

➤ **Anal fissures ♦**
Adults: 20 units (0.2 mL) I.M. on either the left or right side in the intersphincteric groove at the internal anal sphincter once monthly for 3 months. For posterior fissures, injecting dose anteriorly in the anal canal may provide better healing rates than posterior administration.

ADMINISTRATION
I.M., intradermal
● Reconstitute each vial with sterile, non-preserved NSS for injection by drawing up proper amount of diluent (see manufacturer's instructions) in appropriate-sized syringe (see manufacturer's instructions) and slowly injecting diluent into vial.
● Gently mix drug with the NSS by rotating vial.
● Administer within 24 hours after reconstitution; store in refrigerator until administration.

ACTION
Blocks neuromuscular transmission by inhibiting release of acetylcholine. I.M. doses chemically denervate muscle, reducing muscular activity either temporarily or permanently. Intradermal administration causes temporary chemical denervation of sweat glands, resulting in local reduction in sweating. Intradetrusor injection affects detrusor muscle activity via inhibition of acetylcholine release.

Route	Onset	Peak	Duration
I.M., intra-dermal	Varies by site	Unknown	Varies by site

Half-life: Unknown.

ADVERSE REACTIONS
Overactive bladder symptoms
GU: UTI, dysuria, urine retention, bacteriuria, residual urine volume, hematuria.
Other: injection-site soreness or ***hemorrhage.***
Urinary incontinence due to detrusor overactivity associated with a neurologic condition
GI: constipation.

GU: UTI, dysuria, urine retention, hematuria.
Musculoskeletal: weakness, muscle spasm, gait disturbance, falls.
Other: injection-site soreness or ***hemorrhage.***
Chronic migraine headache prophylaxis
CNS: headache, worsening migraine.
CV: hypertension.
EENT: ptosis, facial paresis.
Musculoskeletal: neck pain, weakness, stiffness, myalgia, muscle spasm.
Respiratory: bronchitis.
Other: injection-site pain.
Upper and lower limb spasticity
CNS: fatigue.
GI: nausea.
Musculoskeletal: extremity pain, weakness.
Respiratory: bronchitis.
Other: injection-site soreness or ***hemorrhage.***
Cervical dystonia
CNS: headache, dizziness, drowsiness, fever, speech disorder, numbness, asthenia, drowsiness.
EENT: rhinitis, oral dryness, ptosis, diplopia.
GI: nausea, dysphagia.
Musculoskeletal: neck pain, back pain, stiffness, hypertonia.
Respiratory: URI, increased cough, dyspnea.
Other: flulike syndrome, injection-site soreness.
Severe axillary hyperhidrosis
CNS: headache, fever, anxiety.
EENT: pharyngitis.
Metabolic: nonaxillary sweating.
Musculoskeletal: neck or back pain.
Skin: pruritus.
Other: flulike syndrome, injection-site pain or ***hemorrhage,*** infection.
Blepharospasm associated with dystonia
EENT: ptosis, superficial punctate keratitis, eye dryness, irritation, tearing, lagophthalmos, photophobia, ectropion, keratitis, diplopia, entropion, local swelling of eyelid skin.
Skin: diffuse rash.
Other: injection-site soreness or ***hemorrhage.***

Reactions in bold italics are *life-threatening*. Interactions may have a *rapid onset* or a ***delayed onset***.

Strabismus
EENT: vertical deviation due to effect on adjacent extraocular muscles, ptosis.
Other: injection-site soreness or **hemorrhage.**
Persistent cranial nerve VI palsy
Other: injection-site soreness or **hemorrhage.**
Glabellar lines
CNS: facial paresis.
EENT: eyelid ptosis.
Musculoskeletal: muscular weakness.
Other: facial pain.
Lateral canthal lines
EENT: eyelid edema.

INTERACTIONS

Drug-drug. *Aminoglycosides, neuromuscular blockers (curare or curare-like compounds):* May increase effect of toxin and risk of respiratory depression. Don't use together.
Anticholinergics: May increase systemic anticholinergic effects. Avoid use together.
Anticoagulants, antiplatelet drugs: May increase risk of bleeding. Discontinue antiplatelet therapy at least 3 days before injection procedure; monitor patients on anticoagulant therapy carefully.
Muscle relaxants, other botulinum neurotoxin products: May cause excessive neuromuscular weakness. Avoid use together.

EFFECTS ON LAB TEST RESULTS
None reported.

CONTRAINDICATIONS & CAUTIONS
Black Box Warning The effects of onabotulinumtoxinA and all botulinum toxin products may spread from the injection area to produce signs and symptoms consistent with botulinum toxin effects. These may include asthenia, generalized muscle weakness, diplopia, ptosis, dysphagia, dysphonia, dysarthria, urinary incontinence, and breathing difficulties, which have reportedly occurred hours to weeks after injection. Swallowing and breathing difficulties can be life-threatening; deaths have been reported. Risk of symptoms developing is probably greatest in children treated for spasticity, but symptoms can also occur in adults treated for spasticity and other conditions, particu-

larly in those with an underlying condition predisposing them to these symptoms. In unapproved uses (including spasticity in children) and in approved indications, cases of spread of effect have been reported at doses comparable to those used to treat cervical dystonia and at lower doses. ■
🔔 *Alert:* In the event of overdose, antitoxin against botulinum toxin is available from the CDC. However, the antitoxin will not reverse botulinum toxin-induced effects already apparent by the time of antitoxin administration. In the event of suspected or actual cases of botulinum toxin poisoning, contact your local or state health department to process a request for antitoxin through the CDC. If you don't receive a response within 30 minutes, contact the CDC directly at 1-770-488-7100.
• Contraindicated in known hypersensitivity to botulinum toxin and in patient with infection at injection sites.
• Contraindicated in patients being treated for overactive bladder with UTIs and in patients with overactive bladder or detrusor overactivity associated with a neurologic condition who have postvoid residual urine volume but don't catheterize routinely (patients with MS or diabetes mellitus).
• Use cautiously in patients with inflammation at the proposed injection site or when excessive weakness or atrophy is present in the target muscle.
• Use cautiously in patients with preexisting neuromuscular disorders, compromised respiratory function, or corneal exposure and ulceration due to reduced blinking.
Dialyzable drug: Unknown.
⚠ *Overdose S&S:* Neuromuscular weakness, aspiration pneumonia, respiratory muscle paralysis, respiratory failure, death.

PREGNANCY-LACTATION-REPRODUCTION
• There are no adequate studies in pregnant women. Use only if benefit justifies risks to the fetus.
• It isn't known if drug appears in breast milk. Use cautiously in breast-feeding women.

NURSING CONSIDERATIONS
🔔 *Alert:* Signs and symptoms of overdose usually don't occur immediately after

injection. Should accidental injection or oral ingestion occur or overdose be suspected, patient should be medically supervised for several weeks for signs and symptoms of systemic muscular weakness, which could be local or distant from the injection.

Black Box Warning Monitor patient for swallowing and breathing difficulties, which can lead to death. ■

• Prescribers administering the drug must understand the relevant neuromuscular or orbital anatomy and any alterations to that anatomy due to prior surgical procedures.

• Understanding of standard electromyographic techniques is required for treatment of strabismus and upper limb spasticity, and may be useful for the treatment of cervical dystonia.

• Botox and Botox Cosmetic contain the same active ingredient in the same formulation but aren't interchangeable.

• Drug isn't interchangeable with other preparations of botulinum toxin products and can't be converted into units of other botulinum toxin products.

• Start treatment at lowest recommended dosage.

• Watch for bronchitis and URI in patients being treated for upper limb spasticity.

• Discontinue antiplatelet therapy at least 3 days before the injection procedure; patients on anticoagulant therapy need to be managed appropriately to decrease bleeding risk.

• Repeat treatment may be administered when effect of previous injection has diminished, but generally no sooner than 12 weeks after previous injection.

• Follow indication-specific dosage and administration recommendations. Don't exceed a total dose of 360 units in a 3-month interval.

• Degree or pattern of muscle spasticity at the time of reinjection may necessitate alterations in dosage and of muscles to be injected.

• To prepare eye for injection, several drops of a local anesthetic and an ocular decongestant are instilled several minutes before injection.

• Monitor patient for retrobulbar hemorrhages and compromised retinal circulation after eye injections.

PATIENT TEACHING

Black Box Warning Caution patient to seek immediate medical attention if serious side effects occur, such as difficulty swallowing, speaking, or breathing. These side effects can occur hours, days, or even weeks after injection and can be fatal. ■

• Teach patient to report signs and symptoms of botulism toxicity, such as loss of strength or muscle weakness, double vision, blurred vision, drooping eyelids, hoarseness, change in or loss of voice, trouble speaking clearly, or loss of bladder control. Inform patient that, if these side effects occur, patient shouldn't drive a car, operate machinery, or perform other dangerous activities.

• Advise patient that onabotulinumtoxinA injections may cause reduced blinking or reduced effectiveness of blinking, and to seek immediate medical attention if eye pain or irritation occurs after treatment.

• Instruct patient to report voiding difficulties after bladder injections for urinary incontinence.

ondansetron
on-DAN-sah-tron

Zuplenz

ondansetron hydrochloride
Zofran, Zofran ODT

Therapeutic class: Antiemetics
Pharmacologic class: Selective serotonin (5-HT$_3$) receptor antagonists

AVAILABLE FORMS
Injection: 2 mg/mL, 4 mg/2 mL
ODTs: 4 mg, 8 mg
Oral soluble film: 4 mg, 8 mg
Oral solution: 4 mg/5 mL
Tablets: 4 mg, 8 mg, 16 mg, 24 mg

INDICATIONS & DOSAGES
Adjust-a-dose (for all indications): For patients with severe hepatic impairment, total daily dose shouldn't exceed 8 mg.
➤ **To prevent nausea and vomiting from highly emetogenic chemotherapy**

Reactions in bold italics are *life-threatening*. Interactions may have a *rapid onset* or a *delayed onset*.

Adults: 24 mg P.O. 30 minutes before chemotherapy. Or, three successive 8-mg P.O. doses (ODT/film) 30 minutes before start of single-day highly emetogenic chemotherapy.

If patient can't take oral form, give 0.15 mg/kg I.V. over 15 minutes beginning 30 minutes before chemotherapy. Give a second 0.15-mg/kg I.V. dose 4 hours later, then a third 0.15-mg/kg I.V. dose 8 hours after first dose. Don't exceed 16 mg/dose. *Children ages 6 months to 18 years:* 0.15 mg/kg I.V. over 15 minutes beginning 30 minutes before chemotherapy. Give second dose of 0.15 mg/kg I.V. over 15 minutes 4 hours after first dose. Give third 0.15-mg/kg I.V. dose 8 hours after first dose. No single I.V. dose should exceed 16 mg.

➤ **To prevent nausea and vomiting from moderately emetogenic chemotherapy**
Adults: 8 mg P.O. 30 minutes before chemotherapy. Then, 8 mg P.O. 8 hours after first dose. Then, 8 mg P.O. every 12 hours for 1 to 2 days after completion of chemotherapy. Or, three doses of 0.15 mg/kg I.V. For three-dose regimen, give first dose 30 minutes before chemotherapy and subsequent doses 4 and 8 hours after first dose. Infuse drug over 15 minutes. No single I.V. dose should exceed 16 mg. Or, 8 mg P.O. (film) 30 minutes before chemotherapy, followed by 8 mg P.O. (film) 8 hours after first dose. Then give 8 mg P.O. (film) every 12 hours for 1 to 2 days after completing chemotherapy.
Children ages 12 and older: 8 mg P.O. (ODT, tablet, solution) 30 minutes before chemotherapy, then 8 mg P.O. 8 hours after the first dose. Then, 8 mg every 12 hours for 1 to 2 days after completion of chemotherapy.
Children ages 4 to 11: 4 mg P.O. 30 minutes before chemotherapy. Then, 4 mg P.O. 4 and 8 hours after first dose. Then, 4 mg P.O. every 8 hours for 1 to 2 days after completion of chemotherapy.
Infants and children ages 6 months to 18 years: Three doses of 0.15 mg/kg I.V. Give first dose 30 minutes before chemotherapy; give subsequent doses 4 and 8 hours after first dose. Infuse drug

over 15 minutes. No single I.V. dose should exceed 16 mg.
➤ **To prevent postoperative nausea and vomiting**
Adults: 4 mg undiluted solution for injection I.M. or I.V. over 2 to 5 minutes immediately before induction of anesthesia. Or, 16 mg P.O. or two successive 8-mg oral soluble films or tablets 1 hour before induction of anesthesia.
Children ages 1 month to 12 years weighing more than 40 kg: 4 mg I.V. as a single dose.
Children ages 1 month to 12 years weighing 40 kg or less: 0.1 mg/kg I.V. as a single dose.
➤ **To prevent nausea and vomiting from radiation therapy in patients receiving total body irradiation, single high-dose fraction radiation therapy to abdomen, or daily fractionated radiation therapy to abdomen**
Adults: 8 mg P.O. t.i.d. For patients receiving total body irradiation, give 8 mg P.O. or oral soluble film 1 to 2 hours before each fraction of radiation therapy each day. For patients receiving single high-dose fraction radiation therapy to the abdomen, give 8 mg P.O. or oral soluble film 1 to 2 hours before therapy, then every 8 hours for 1 to 2 days after completion of therapy. For patients receiving daily fractionated radiation therapy, give 8 mg P.O. or oral soluble film 1 to 2 hours before therapy, then every 8 hours for each day therapy is given.

ADMINISTRATION
P.O.
● Open blister of ODT just before use by peeling backing off. Don't push ODT through foil blister.
● For Zuplenz, open film pouch with dry hands and immediately place film on top of the tongue, where it will dissolve in 4 to 20 seconds. Then have patient swallow with or without liquid. Wash hands after giving Zuplenz.
● Protect 4-mg tablets and oral solution from light.

I.V.
❶ *Alert:* No single I.V. dose should exceed 16 mg due to the risk of QT-interval prolongation.

▼ If precipitate is noted in vial, shake vigorously until dissolved.

▼ Dilute drug in 50 mL of D_5W injection or NSS for injection.

▼ Drug is stable for up to 48 hours after dilution in D_5W, 5% dextrose in half-NSS for injection, 5% dextrose in NSS, and 3% sodium chloride solution for injection.

▼ Infuse over 15 minutes.

▼ **Incompatibilities:** Alkaline solutions.

I.M.

● Document injection site.

● If precipitate is noted in vial, shake vigorously until dissolved.

● Give I.M. injection undiluted.

ACTION

May block 5-HT_3 in the CNS in the chemoreceptor trigger zone and in the peripheral nervous system on nerve terminals of the vagus nerve.

Route	Onset	Peak	Duration
P.O.	Unknown	Unknown	Unknown
I.V.	Immediate	10 min	Unknown
I.M.	Unknown	41 min	Unknown

Half-life: 4 hours.

ADVERSE REACTIONS

CNS: dizziness, fatigue, headache, malaise, sedation, extrapyramidal syndrome, fever, pain.

CV: *arrhythmias,* chest pain.

GI: constipation, diarrhea, abdominal pain, decreased appetite, xerostomia.

GU: gynecologic disorders, urine retention.

Respiratory: *hypoxia.*

Skin: pruritus, rash.

Other: chills, injection-site reaction.

INTERACTIONS

Drug-drug. ❸ *Alert: Apomorphine:* May cause profound hypotension and loss of consciousness. Use together is contraindicated.

Drugs (such as cimetidine) that alter hepatic drug-metabolizing enzymes, phenobarbital, rifampin: May change pharmacokinetics of ondansetron, but there is no need to adjust dosage based on clinical data.

Drugs that prolong QTc interval (antiarrhythmics, antipsychotics, antidepressants): May result in ventricular arrhythmias. Use cautiously and avoid combination with

drugs at highest risk for QTc-interval prolongation.

SNRIs, SSRIs: May result in serotonin syndrome. Use cautiously and monitor patient for mental status changes, tachycardia, sweating, flushing, nausea, vomiting, tremors, and muscle rigidity.

Drug-herb. *Horehound:* May enhance serotonergic effects. Discourage use together.

St. John's wort: May decrease ondansetron serum concentration. Consider therapy modification.

EFFECTS ON LAB TEST RESULTS

● May increase ALT and AST levels.

CONTRAINDICATIONS & CAUTIONS

● Contraindicated in patients hypersensitive to drug.

● ECG changes, including prolonged QT interval and torsades de pointes, have been reported. Avoid use in patients with congenital long QT syndrome. Monitor patient carefully.

● Use cautiously in patients with hepatic impairment.

Dialyzable drug: Unlikely.

⚠ *Overdose S&S:* Sudden transient blindness, severe constipation, hypotension.

PREGNANCY-LACTATION-REPRODUCTION

● There are no adequate studies in pregnant women. Drug crosses placental barrier during first trimester. Use only if clearly needed.

● It isn't known if drug appears in breast milk. Use cautiously in breast-feeding women.

NURSING CONSIDERATIONS

❸ *Alert:* Drug may increase the risk of prolonged QT interval and torsades de pointes (a potentially fatal heart rhythm). Monitor ECG in patients with congenital long QT syndrome, in those with HF or bradyarrhythmias, and in those taking other medications that can prolong the QT interval.

❸ *Alert:* Correct electrolyte abnormalities (hypokalemia or hypomagnesemia) before infusing drug.

Reactions in bold italics are *life-threatening*. Interactions may have a *rapid onset* or a *delayed onset*.

• Monitor LFT results. Don't exceed 8 mg in patients with hepatic impairment.
• *Look alike–sound alike:* Don't confuse Zofran with Zosyn, Zantac, or Zoloft.

PATIENT TEACHING

🕓 *Alert:* Caution patient to contact health care provider immediately if he experiences signs and symptoms of abnormal HR or rhythm, such as palpitations, dyspnea, or dizziness.
• Tell patient that an ECG may be necessary to monitor HR and rhythm.
• Instruct patient to immediately report difficulty breathing after drug administration.
• Tell patient receiving drug I.V. to report discomfort at insertion site.
• Tell patient taking ODTs to open blister just before use by peeling backing off and not by pushing through foil blister, and tell him that taking it with liquid isn't required.
• Teach patient to place ODTs or film on tongue, allow to dissolve, then swallow with saliva.

---

oritavancin diphosphate
or-it-a-VAN-sin

Orbactiv

Therapeutic class: Antibiotics
Pharmacologic class: Lipoglycopeptides

AVAILABLE FORMS
Powder for injection: 400-mg vial

INDICATIONS & DOSAGES
➤ **Acute bacterial skin and skin-structure infections caused or suspected to be caused by susceptible gram-positive bacteria, including *Staphylococcus aureus* (methicillin-sensitive and methicillin-resistant); *Streptococcus* species, including *S. pyogenes, S. agalactiae, S. dysgalactiae, S. anginosus, S. intermedius,* and *S. constellatus;* and vancomycin-susceptible *Enterococcus faecalis***
Adults: A single dose of 1,200 mg I.V. over 3 hours.

ADMINISTRATION
I.V.
▼ Obtain specimen for culture and sensitivity testing before giving.
▼ Prepare three 400-mg vials for a single 1,200-mg I.V. dose.
▼ Reconstitute each vial with 40 mL of sterile water for injection to provide a solution containing 10 mg/mL/vial. Inspect for particulate matter. Solution should be clear and colorless to pale yellow.
▼ For infusion, further dilute in 1,000 mL D₅W; withdraw 120 mL from 1,000-mL D₅W bag and add oritavancin reconstituted solution.
▼ Infuse drug over 3 hours. If I.V. line is also used to infuse other drugs, flush it with D₅W before and after each infusion.
▼ Refrigerate solution after reconstitution and use within 12 hours or within 6 hours when stored at room temperature, including 3-hour infusion time.
▼ **Incompatibilities:** NSS.

ACTION
Disrupts bacterial cell-wall synthesis and bacterial membrane integrity.

Route	Onset	Peak	Duration
I.V.	Unknown	Unknown	Unknown

Half-life: 245 hours.

ADVERSE REACTIONS
CNS: headache, dizziness.
CV: tachycardia, peripheral edema, injection-site phlebitis, *leukocytoclastic vasculitis.*
GI: nausea, vomiting, diarrhea.
Hematologic: anemia, eosinophilia.
Hepatic: elevated ALT and AST levels.
Metabolic: *hypoglycemia,* hyperuricemia.
Musculoskeletal: tenosynovitis, myalgia, osteomyelitis.
Respiratory: *bronchospasm,* wheezing.
Skin: limb and subcutaneous abscesses, rash, urticaria, *erythema multiforme,* cellulitis.
Other: infusion reaction, infusion-site erythema, extravasation, induration, pruritus, hypersensitivity, *angioedema.*

O

INTERACTIONS
Drug-drug. *Dextromethorphan, midazolam:* May decrease concentrations of these drugs. Monitor patient for efficacy.
Omeprazole: May increase omeprazole level. Monitor patient for omeprazole toxicity.
Unfractionated heparin sodium (I.V.): May falsely elevate aPTT test results for up to 120 hours (5 days). Heparin use is contraindicated for 120 hours after oritavancin administration.
Warfarin: May increase warfarin level and risk of bleeding. Monitor INR and patient for bleeding.

EFFECTS ON LAB TEST RESULTS
● May artificially prolong aPTT for up to 120 hours, prolong PT and increase INR for up to 12 hours, and prolong activated clotting time for up to 24 hours after dose is given.
● May increase AST, ALT, uric acid, and total bilirubin levels. May decrease glucose level.

CONTRAINDICATIONS & CAUTIONS
● Contraindicated in patients hypersensitive to drug or its components.
● Use cautiously in patients with history of hypersensitivity to glycopeptides (vancomycin, telavancin, dalbavancin); serious hypersensitivity reactions have been reported. If acute reaction occurs, discontinue drug and treat immediately.
● Unfractionated heparin I.V. is contraindicated for 120 hours after drug is given. Oritavancin falsely prolongs aPTT.
● Drug can cause superinfection, including CDAD and pseudomembranous colitis, which can occur more than 2 months after therapy ends.
● Drug may increase risk of osteomyelitis; an alternative antibacterial therapy may be needed.
● Drug hasn't been studied in patients with severe renal or hepatic impairment.
Dializable drug: No.

PREGNANCY-LACTATION-REPRODUCTION
● There are no adequate studies in pregnant women. Use only if potential benefit justifies potential fetal risks.

● It isn't known if drug appears in breast milk. Use cautiously in breast-feeding women.

NURSING CONSIDERATIONS
● Monitor patient for signs and symptoms of superinfection (frequent, watery stools) and osteomyelitis (fever, erythema, edema, pain).
● Infusion-related reactions (pruritus, urticaria, flushing) have been reported. Slow rate or interrupt infusion if reaction develops.
● If anticoagulation is needed, consider using anticoagulants that don't require PTT or INR monitoring.
● ***Look alike–sound alike:*** Don't confuse Orbactiv with Activase, Vibativ, or Factive. Don't confuse oritavancin with telavancin or dalbavancin.

PATIENT TEACHING
● Explain that antibiotics can change normal intestinal flora and that patient should report severe watery or bloody diarrhea as this may indicate a more serious intestinal infection.
● Instruct patient to report discomfort at I.V. insertion site.
● Warn patient that allergic reactions, including serious allergic reactions, can occur and require immediate treatment.

oseltamivir phosphate
oz-el-TAM-ah-ver

Tamiflu

Therapeutic class: Antivirals
Pharmacologic class: Selective neuraminidase inhibitors

AVAILABLE FORMS
Capsules: 30 mg, 45 mg, 75 mg
Oral suspension: 6 mg/mL after reconstitution

INDICATIONS & DOSAGES
➤ **To prevent influenza during a community outbreak or within 2 days after close contact with an infected person**

Adults and adolescents age 13 and older:
75 mg P.O. once daily for at least 10 days.
For a community outbreak, safety and effectiveness have been demonstrated for up to
6 weeks in immunocompetent patients.
*Children ages 1 to 12 weighing 40.1 kg or
more:* 75 mg (12.5 mL) P.O. once daily for
10 days.
*Children ages 1 to 12 weighing 23.1 to
40 kg:* 60 mg (10 mL) P.O. once daily for
10 days.
*Children ages 1 to 12 weighing 15.1 to
23 kg:* 45 mg (7.5 mL) P.O. once daily for
10 days.
*Children ages 1 to 12 weighing 15 kg or
less:* 30 mg (5 mL) P.O. once daily for
10 days.
Adjust-a-dose: For adults and adolescents
with CrCl of 30 to 60 mL/minute, reduce
dosage to 30 mg P.O. once daily. For CrCl
of 10 to 30 mL/minute, reduce dosage to
30 mg every other day. For patients on
hemodialysis (CrCl <10 mL/minute),
give 30 mg P.O. after alternate hemodialysis
sessions. May give an initial dose before
start of dialysis. For patients on continuous ambulatory peritoneal dialysis (CrCl
<10 mL/minute), give 30 mg P.O. once
weekly immediately after dialysis exchange.
➤ **To treat influenza**
Adults and adolescents age 13 and older:
75 mg P.O. b.i.d. for 5 days. Begin treatment within 2 days of onset of influenza
symptoms.
*Children ages 1 to 12 weighing 40.1 kg or
more:* 75 mg (12.5 mL) P.O. b.i.d. for 5 days.
*Children ages 1 to 12 weighing 23.1 to
40 kg:* 60 mg (10 mL) P.O. b.i.d. for 5 days.
*Children ages 1 to 12 weighing 15.1 to
23 kg:* 45 mg (7.5 mL) P.O. b.i.d. for 5 days.
*Children ages 1 to 12 weighing 15 kg or
less:* 30 mg (5 mL) P.O. b.i.d. for 5 days.
*Children ages 2 weeks to younger than
1 year:* 3 mg/kg P.O. b.i.d. for 5 days. Begin
treatment within 2 days of influenza onset.
Adjust-a-dose: For adults and adolescents
with CrCl of 30 to 60 mL/minute, reduce
dosage to 30 mg P.O. b.i.d. for 5 days.
For CrCl of 10 to 30 mL/minute, reduce
dosage to 30 mg P.O. once daily for 5 days.
For patients on hemodialysis (CrCl
<10 mL/minute), give 30 mg P.O. after
every hemodialysis session. Don't exceed

treatment duration of longer than 5 days.
For patients on continuous ambulatory peritoneal dialysis (CrCl <10 mL/minute), give
a single dose of 30 mg P.O. immediately
after dialysis exchange.

For children age 1 and older with ESRD
on hemodialysis: If child weighs more than
40 kg, give 30 mg after each dialysis session. If child weighs more than 23 but less
than 40 kg, give 15 mg after each dialysis
session. If child weighs more than 15 but
less than 23 kg, give 10 mg after each dialysis session. If child weighs 15 kg or less,
give 7.5 mg after each dialysis session.

ADMINISTRATION
P.O.
● Give drug with meals to decrease GI
adverse effects.
● Store at controlled room temperature
(59° to 86° F [15° to 30° C]).
● Capsules may be opened and mixed with
sweetened liquids such as chocolate syrup.
● Shake oral suspension well before use.
● For emergency (e.g., shortage) compounding of an oral suspension (6 mg/mL) from
capsules, refer to manufacturer's information instructions.
● May give via NG or orogastric tube. Dissolve powder from capsule in 20 mL sterile
water and inject in tube; follow with 10-mL
sterile water flush.

ACTION
Inhibits influenza A and B virus enzyme
neuraminidase, which is thought to play a
role in viral particle aggregation and release
from the host cell and appears to interfere
with viral replication.

Route	Onset	Peak	Duration
P.O.	Unknown	Unknown	Unknown

Half-life: 1 to 10 hours.

ADVERSE REACTIONS
CNS: dizziness, fatigue, headache, insomnia, vertigo.
EENT: epistaxis, sinusitis, conjunctivitis,
ear disorder, otitis media, tympanic membrane disorder (children).
GI: abdominal pain, diarrhea, nausea,
vomiting.

Respiratory: bronchitis, cough, asthma (children).
Skin: dermatitis (children).
Other: lymphadenopathy (children).

INTERACTIONS

Live/attenuated influenza virus vaccine:
May decrease effect of live/attenuated influenza virus vaccine. Avoid oseltamivir 48 hours before vaccination and 2 weeks after.
Probenecid: May increase active metabolite of oseltamivir. Consider alternative to probenecid, or reduced oseltamivir dosage may be needed.

EFFECTS ON LAB TEST RESULTS
None reported.

CONTRAINDICATIONS & CAUTIONS
● Contraindicated in patients hypersensitive to drug or its components.
● Use cautiously in patients with renal failure, chronic cardiac or respiratory diseases, or any medical condition that may require imminent hospitalization.
● Don't administer live/attenuated influenza vaccine within 2 weeks before or 48 hours after oseltamivir administration unless medically indicated.
Dialyzable drug: Yes.
⚠ *Overdose S&S:* Nausea, vomiting.

PREGNANCY-LACTATION-REPRODUCTION
● Drug is recommended for treatment or prophylaxis of influenza in pregnant women and in women up to 2 weeks postpartum. It shouldn't be used as a substitute for vaccination in pregnant women.
● Drug appears in breast milk in small amounts. According to the CDC, patient may continue oseltamivir while breastfeeding.

NURSING CONSIDERATIONS
● Drug must be given within 2 days of onset of symptoms.
● Safety and effectiveness of repeated treatment courses haven't been established.
� *Alert:* Closely monitor patients with influenza for neuropsychiatric symptoms, such as hallucinations, delirium, and ab-

normal behavior. Risks and benefits of continuing drug should be evaluated.

PATIENT TEACHING
● Instruct patient to begin treatment as soon as possible after appearance of flu symptoms.
● Inform patient that drug may be taken with or without meals. If nausea or vomiting occurs, he can take drug with food or milk.
● Tell patient to take a missed dose as soon as possible. However, if next dose is due within 2 hours, tell him to skip the missed dose and take the next dose on schedule.
● Advise patient to complete the full course of treatment, even if symptoms resolve.
● Alert patient that drug isn't a replacement for the annual influenza vaccination. Patients for whom vaccine is indicated should continue to receive the vaccine each fall.

osimertinib
See NEW DRUGS for information.

ospemifene
os-PEM-i-feen

Osphena

Therapeutic class: Selective estrogen receptor modulators
Pharmacologic class: Selective estrogen agonist–antagonists

AVAILABLE FORMS
Tablets: 60 mg

INDICATIONS & DOSAGES
➤ **Moderate to severe dyspareunia due to menopause**
Adults: 60 mg P.O. once daily.

ADMINISTRATION
P.O.
● Give with food.
● Store medication at room temperature.

ACTION
Binds to estrogen receptors, activating estrogenic pathways in some tissues (agonism) and blocking estrogenic pathways in others (antagonism).

Reactions in bold italics are *life-threatening*. Interactions may have a *rapid onset* or a ***delayed onset***.

Route	Onset	Peak	Duration
P.O.	Unknown	2 hr	Unknown

Half-life: 26 hours.

ADVERSE REACTIONS
CV: hot flush.
GU: vaginal or genital discharge.
Musculoskeletal: muscle spasms.
Skin: hyperhidrosis.

INTERACTIONS
Drug-drug. *CYP2C9, CYP2C19, CYP3A4 inducers (rifampin):* May decrease ospemifene level, decreasing therapeutic effect. Avoid use together.
CYP2C9, CYP2C19, CYP3A4 inhibitors (fluconazole, ketoconazole, omeprazole): May increase ospemifene level, increasing risk of ospemifene-related adverse effects. Avoid use together.
Estrogen agonists–antagonists, estrogens: Safety of concomitant use hasn't been established. Don't use together.
Highly protein-bound drugs (phenytoin, tolbutamide): May increase exposure of ospemifene or highly protein-bound drug, increasing adverse reactions. Monitor clinical response when either drug is started or stopped.
Drug-herb. *St. John's wort:* May decrease drug level and therapeutic effect. Avoid use together.

EFFECTS ON LAB TEST RESULTS
None reported.

CONTRAINDICATIONS & CAUTIONS
● Contraindicated in women hypersensitive to drug or its components; in those with severe hepatic impairment, undiagnosed abnormal genital bleeding, or known or suspected estrogen-dependent neoplasm; and in those with active or previous DVT or PE or active or previous arterial thromboembolic disease (stroke, MI).
   Don't use in women with known or suspected breast cancer or in those with a history of breast cancer. Drug hasn't been studied in this population.
   Use cautiously in women with an increased risk of CV disorders, arterial vascular disease, or venous thromboembolism (obesity, systemic lupus erythematosus, family history, personal history).
Dialyzable drug: Unknown.

PREGNANCY-LACTATION-REPRODUCTION
● Drug may cause fetal harm and is contraindicated in women who are or may become pregnant.
● It isn't known if drug appears in breast milk.

NURSING CONSIDERATIONS
Black Box Warning Risk of endometrial cancer is increased in women with a uterus who use unopposed estrogens; consider adding a progestin in these women. Women without a uterus don't need a progestin. Evaluate patient for uterine cancer if patient experiences persistent abnormal genital bleeding. ■
Black Box Warning Postmenopausal women who received daily oral conjugated estrogens as part of the Women's Health Initiative experienced an increased risk of stroke and DVT. To reduce these risks, this drug should be used for the shortest period of time necessary. Periodically reevaluate the need to continue therapy. ■
● Discontinue drug immediately if a venous thromboembolism or thromboembolic or hemorrhagic stroke is suspected or occurs.
● Discontinue drug at least 4 to 6 weeks before surgery that's associated with an increased risk of thromboembolism or during periods of extended immobilization.

PATIENT TEACHING
● Instruct patient to take drug with food for better absorption.
● Inform patient that drug may initiate or worsen hot flashes.
● Advise patient to immediately report all adverse reactions, especially unusual vaginal discharge or bleeding.

oxaliplatin
ox-ah-li-PLA-tin

Eloxatin

Therapeutic class: Antineoplastics
Pharmacologic class: Platinum-
containing compounds

AVAILABLE FORMS
Solution for injection: 5 mg/mL in 10-mL,
20-mL, and 40-mL single-use vials

INDICATIONS & DOSAGES
➤ **First-line treatment of advanced colorectal cancer with 5-FU and leucovorin
(5-FU/LV)**
Adults: On day 1, give 85 mg/m^2 oxaliplatin
I.V. in 250 to 500 mL D_5W and leucovorin
200 mg/m^2 I.V. in D_5W simultaneously over
120 minutes, in separate bags using a Y-line,
followed by 5-FU 400 mg/m^2 I.V. bolus
over 2 to 4 minutes, followed by 600 mg/m^2
5-FU I.V. infusion in 500 mL D_5W over
22 hours.

On day 2, give 200 mg/m^2 leucovorin
I.V. infusion over 120 minutes, followed by
400 mg/m^2 5-FU I.V. bolus over 2 to
4 minutes, followed by 600 mg/m^2 5-FU
I.V. infusion in 500 mL D_5W over 22 hours.

Repeat cycle every 2 weeks.
Adjust-a-dose: In patients with unresolved
and persistent grade 2 neurosensory events,
reduce oxaliplatin to 65 mg/m^2. In those
with persistent grade 3 neurosensory events,
consider stopping drug. In patients recovering from grade 3 or 4 GI or hematologic
events, reduce dose to 65 mg/m^2 and reduce
dose of 5-FU by 20%. Delay dose until neutrophil count is 1.5×10^9/L or more and
platelet count is 75×10^9/L or more.
➤ **With 5-FU/LV for the adjuvant treatment of stage III colon cancer in patients
who have had complete resection of the
primary tumor**
Adults: On day 1, give oxaliplatin,
85 mg/m^2 I.V. in 250 to 500 mL D_5W and
200 mg/m^2 leucovorin I.V. infusion in D_5W,
both over 120 minutes at the same time, in
separate bags, using a Y-line. Follow with
400 mg/m^2 5-FU I.V. bolus over 2 to 4 min-

utes, then 600 mg/m^2 5-FU in 500 mL D_5W
as a 22-hour continuous infusion.

On day 2, give leucovorin, 200 mg/m^2
I.V. infused over 120 minutes, followed by
400 mg/m^2 5-FU as an I.V. bolus over 2 to
4 minutes, then 600 mg/m^2 5-FU in 500 mL
D_5W as a 22-hour infusion.

Repeat cycle every 2 weeks for a total of
6 months. Premedicate with antiemetics,
with or without dexamethasone.
Adjust-a-dose: For patients with persistent
grade 2 neurotoxicity, consider an oxaliplatin dosage reduction to 75 mg/m^2. In
those with persistent grade 3 neurosensory events, consider stopping drug. For
patients who recovered from grade 4 neutropenia, grade 3 or 4 thrombocytopenia, or
a grade 3 or 4 GI event, reduce oxaliplatin to
75 mg/m^2 and 5-FU to a 300 mg/m^2 bolus
and 500 mg/m^2 22-hour infusion. Delay
dose until neutrophils are 1.5×10/L or
more and platelets are 75×10^9/L or more.

ADMINISTRATION
I.V.
▼ Preparing and giving drug may be mutagenic, teratogenic, or carcinogenic. Follow
facility policy to reduce risks.
▼ Reconstitute powder using sterile water
for injection or D_5W. Add 10 mL to a
50-mg vial or 20 mL to a 100-mg vial, for a
yield of 5 mg/mL. Never reconstitute with
sodium chloride solution or other solution
containing chloride.
▼ Reconstituted solutions must be further
diluted in an infusion solution of 250 to
500 mL of D_5W.
▼ Inspect bag for particulate matter and
discoloration before giving, and discard if
present.
▼ Don't use needles or I.V. administration
sets that contain aluminum because it
displaces the platinum, causing it to lose
potency and form a black precipitate.
▼ Give oxaliplatin and leucovorin over
2 hours at the same time in separate bags,
using a Y-line. Extend the infusion time to
6 hours to decrease acute toxicities.
▼ Store unopened vials at room temperature. Reconstituted solutions are stable
if refrigerated (36° to 46° F [2° to 8° C])
for up to 24 hours. After final dilution,
solutions are stable for 6 hours at room

Reactions in bold italics are *life-threatening*. Interactions may have a *rapid onset* or a ***delayed onset***.

temperature and up to 24 hours under refrigeration.

▼ **Incompatibilities:** Alkaline solutions or drugs such as 5-FU. Flush infusion line with D_5W before giving any other drugs simultaneously.

ACTION

Inhibits cell replication and transcription by forming platinum complexes that cross-link with DNA molecules. Not specific to cell cycle.

Route	Onset	Peak	Duration
I.V.	Unknown	Unknown	Unknown

Half-life: 391 hours (long, terminal phase).

ADVERSE REACTIONS

CNS: pain, peripheral neuropathy, fatigue, headache, dizziness, insomnia, fever, anxiety, depression.
CV: chest pain, *thromboembolism,* edema, flushing, peripheral edema, hypotension.
EENT: rhinitis, pharyngolaryngeal dysesthesias, pharyngitis, epistaxis, abnormal lacrimation.
GI: nausea, vomiting, diarrhea, stomatitis, abdominal pain, anorexia, constipation, dyspepsia, taste perversion, gastroesophageal reflux, flatulence, mucositis.
GU: dysuria, hematuria.
Hematologic: *febrile neutropenia,* anemia, *leukopenia, thrombocytopenia.*
Hepatic: venoocclusive disease.
Metabolic: *hypokalemia,* hypocalcemia, dehydration.
Musculoskeletal: back pain, arthralgia, myalgia.
Respiratory: dyspnea, cough, URI, hiccups, *pulmonary toxicity.*
Skin: injection-site reaction, rash, alopecia, dry skin, flushing, pruritus, sweating.
Other: *anaphylaxis,* hand-foot syndrome, allergic reaction, rigors.

INTERACTIONS

Drug-drug. *Clozapine:* May increase risk of agranulocytosis. Avoid use together.
Denosumab: May increase risk of serious infections. Monitor therapy.
Digoxin (oral): May decrease digoxin absorption. Monitor therapy.

Fosphenytoin, phenytoin: May decrease serum concentration of fosphenytoin and phenytoin. Monitor therapy.
Leflunomide: May increase risk of pancytopenia, agranulocytosis, or thrombocytopenia. Consider not using a leflunomide loading dose in patients receiving other immunosuppressants. Monitor patient for bone marrow suppression at least monthly. Consider therapy modification.
Live-virus vaccines, pimecrolimus, tacrolimus (topical): May enhance adverse or toxic effects of these drugs. Avoid combination.
Natalizumab: May enhance adverse or toxic effect of natalizumab; specifically, may increase risk of concurrent infection. Avoid combination.
Nephrotoxic drugs (such as gentamicin): May decrease elimination of these drugs and increase gentamicin level. Monitor patient for toxicity.
Roflumilast: May enhance immunosuppressive effect of roflumilast. Consider therapy modification.
Sipuleucel-T: May diminish sipuleucel-T therapeutic effect. Monitor therapy.
Taxane derivatives: May enhance myelosuppressive effect of taxane derivatives. Administer taxane derivative before platinum derivative when given as sequential infusions to limit toxicity. Consider therapy modification.
Tofacitinib: May enhance immunosuppressive effect of tofacitinib. Avoid combination.
Topotecan: May enhance adverse or toxic effect of topotecan. Consider therapy modification.
Trastuzumab: May increase neutropenia. Monitor therapy.
Vaccines (inactivated): May diminish therapeutic effect of inactivated vaccines. Monitor therapy.
Vitamin K antagonists (warfarin): May enhance anticoagulant effect of vitamin K antagonists. Monitor therapy and adjust vitamin K antagonist dosage as needed.

EFFECTS ON LAB TEST RESULTS

● May increase glucose, creatinine, bilirubin, AST, and ALT levels. May decrease potassium, albumin, calcium, sodium, and Hb levels.

• May decrease neutrophil, WBC, and platelet counts.

CONTRAINDICATIONS & CAUTIONS
• Contraindicated in patients allergic to drug or other platinum-containing compounds.
• Oxaliplatin may cause early-onset (occurs within hours or 1 to 2 days) or persistent (greater than 14 days) peripheral sensory neuropathy.
• Oxaliplatin has been associated with rare, sometimes fatal, pulmonary fibrosis.
• Extravasation of oxaliplatin can cause tissue necrosis. If extravasation occurs, stop infusion and notify health care provider immediately.
• Use cautiously in patients with renal impairment or peripheral sensory neuropathy.
Dialyzable drug: Unknown.
⚠ *Overdose S&S:* Thrombocytopenia, dyspnea, wheezing, paresthesia, vomiting, chest pain, respiratory failure, bradycardia, dysesthesia, laryngospasm, myelosuppression, nausea, diarrhea, neurotoxicity.

PREGNANCY-LACTATION-REPRODUCTION
• Drug may cause fetal harm. Use is contraindicated during first trimester. Advise women of childbearing potential to avoid becoming pregnant and to use effective contraception during therapy.
• It isn't known if drug appears in breast milk. Patient should discontinue breastfeeding or discontinue drug.

NURSING CONSIDERATIONS
• Administer drug under the supervision of a physician experienced in the use of cancer chemotherapeutic agents.
• Premedication with antiemetics, including 5-HT$_3$ receptor antagonists with or without dexamethasone, is recommended.
• Drug doesn't require patient prehydration.
• Give antiemetic with or without dexamethasone before drug to reduce nausea.
• Drug clearance is reduced in patients with renal impairment. Dosage adjustment for patients with renal impairment hasn't been established.
• Monitor CBC, platelet count, LFTs, and kidney function tests before each chemotherapy cycle.

Black Box Warning Monitor patient for anaphylactic reactions, which may occur within minutes of administration. Keep epinephrine, corticosteroids, and antihistamines available. ∎
• Monitor patient for injection-site reaction; extravasation may occur.
• Monitor patient for neuropathy and pulmonary toxicity. Peripheral neuropathy may be acute or persistent. Acute neuropathy is reversible; it occurs within 2 days of dosing and resolves within 14 days. Persistent peripheral neuropathy occurs more than 14 days after dosing and causes paresthesia, dysesthesia, hypoesthesia, and other neurologic impairment that can interfere with daily activities (such as walking or swallowing).
• Avoid ice and cold exposure during infusion of drug because cold temperatures can worsen acute neurologic symptoms. Cover patient with a blanket during infusion.
• Diarrhea, dehydration, hypokalemia, and fatigue may occur more frequently in elderly patients.

PATIENT TEACHING
• Inform patient of potential serious adverse reactions and to report them promptly.
• Tell patient to avoid exposure to cold or cold objects (such as cold drinks or ice cubes), which can bring on or worsen acute symptoms of peripheral neuropathy. Advise patient to drink warm drinks, wear warm clothing, and cover any exposed skin (hands, face, and head).
• Tell patient to immediately report trouble breathing or signs and symptoms of an allergic reaction, such as rash, hives, swelling of lips or tongue, or sudden cough.
• Tell patient to report fever, signs and symptoms of infection, persistent vomiting, diarrhea, or signs and symptoms of dehydration (thirst, dry mouth, light-headedness, and decreased urination).
• Caution female patient of childbearing potential not to becoming pregnant during therapy.

Reactions in bold italics are *life-threatening*. Interactions may have a *rapid onset* or a *delayed onset*.

SAFETY ALERT!

oxazepam
ox-AZ-e-pam

Novoxapam ✤, Oxpam ✤

Therapeutic class: Anxiolytics
Pharmacologic class: Benzodiazepines
Controlled substance schedule: IV

AVAILABLE FORMS
Capsules: 10 mg, 15 mg, 30 mg

INDICATIONS & DOSAGES
➤ **Alcohol withdrawal, severe anxiety**
Adults: 15 to 30 mg P.O. t.i.d. or q.i.d.
➤ **Mild to moderate anxiety**
Adults and children older than age 12: 10 to
15 mg P.O. t.i.d. or q.i.d.
Elderly patients: Initially, 10 mg P.O. t.i.d.;
cautiously increase to 15 mg t.i.d. to q.i.d.
➤ **Severe anxiety syndromes; agitation;
anxiety associated with depression**
Adults and children older than age 12: 15 to
30 mg P.O. t.i.d. or q.i.d.
➤ **Anxiety, tension, irritability, agitation**
Elderly patients: 10 mg P.O. t.i.d. May
increase cautiously to 15 mg t.i.d. or q.i.d.

ADMINISTRATION
P.O.
● Give drug without regard for meals.

ACTION
May stimulate GABA receptors in the ascending reticular activating system.

Route	Onset	Peak	Duration
P.O.	Unknown	3 hr	Unknown

Half-life: 5 to 13 hours.

ADVERSE REACTIONS
CNS: drowsiness, lethargy, dizziness,
vertigo, headache, syncope, tremor, slurred
speech, changes in EEG patterns.
CV: edema.
GI: nausea.
Hepatic: *hepatic dysfunction.*
Skin: rash.
Other: altered libido.

INTERACTIONS
Drug-drug. *CNS depressants:* May increase
CNS depression. Use together cautiously.
Black Box Warning *Opioids:* May cause
slow or difficult breathing, sedation, and
death. Avoid use together. If use together
is necessary, limit dosage and duration of
each drug to minimum necessary for desired
effect. ■
Drug-herb. *Kava kava:* May increase sedation. Discourage use together.
Drug-lifestyle. *Alcohol use:* May cause additive CNS effects. Discourage use together.

EFFECTS ON LAB TEST RESULTS
● May increase LFT values.

CONTRAINDICATIONS & CAUTIONS
● Contraindicated in patients hypersensitive
to drug and in those with psychoses.
Black Box Warning Opioids should only be
prescribed with benzodiazepines or other
CNS depressants to patients for whom alternative treatment options are inadequate. ■
● Use cautiously in elderly patients and in
those with history of substance abuse or
in whom a decrease in BP might lead to
cardiac problems.
● Safety and effectiveness in children
younger than age 6 haven't been established.
Dialyzable drug: No.
⚠ Overdose S&S: Drowsiness, confusion,
lethargy, ataxia, hypotonia, hypotension,
hypnotic state, stage 1 to 3 coma, death.

PREGNANCY-LACTATION-REPRODUCTION
● Drug crosses placental barrier and may
adversely affect the fetus (premature birth,
low birth weight, hypoglycemia, respiratory problems), especially in first and third
trimesters.
● Neonatal withdrawal signs and symptoms
may occur within days to weeks after birth.
Avoid use during pregnancy, especially in
first trimester.
● Drug appears in breast milk. Drowsiness, lethargy, or weight loss may occur
in breast-fed infants. Breast-feeding isn't
recommended.

O

NURSING CONSIDERATIONS

• Monitor hepatic, renal, and hematopoietic function periodically in patients receiving repeated or prolonged therapy.

☉ Alert: Use of this drug may lead to abuse and addiction. Don't stop drug abruptly because withdrawal symptoms may occur.

• **Look alike–sound alike:** Don't confuse oxazepam with oxaprozin.

PATIENT TEACHING

Black Box Warning Caution patient or caregiver of patient taking an opioid with a benzodiazepine, CNS depressant, or alcohol to seek immediate medical attention if patient experiences dizziness, light-headedness, extreme sleepiness, slowed or difficult breathing, or unresponsiveness. ▪

• Warn patient to avoid hazardous activities that require alertness or good coordination until effects of drug are known.

• Tell patient to avoid use of alcohol.

• Notify patient that smoking may decrease drug's effectiveness.

• Warn patient not to stop drug abruptly because withdrawal symptoms may occur.

• Warn female patient of childbearing potential to avoid use during pregnancy.

---

oxcarbazepine
oks-car-BAZ-e-peen

Oxtellar XR, Trileptal

Therapeutic class: Anticonvulsants
Pharmacologic class: Carboxamide derivatives

AVAILABLE FORMS

Oral suspension: 300 mg/5 mL (60 mg/mL)
Tablets (extended-release) **ONC:** 150 mg, 300 mg, 600 mg
Tablets (film-coated): 150 mg, 300 mg, 600 mg

INDICATIONS & DOSAGES

Adjust-a-dose (for all indications): If CrCl is less than 30 mL/minute, start therapy at 150 mg P.O. b.i.d. (one-half usual starting dose) and increase slowly to achieve desired response.

➤ **Adjunctive treatment of partial seizures in patients with epilepsy**
Adults: Initially, 300 mg immediate-release tablets/suspension P.O. b.i.d. Increase by a maximum of 600 mg daily (300 mg P.O. b.i.d.) at weekly intervals. Recommended daily dose is 1,200 mg P.O. in two divided doses. Or, 600 mg extended-release tablets P.O. daily. May increase at weekly intervals in 600-mg/day increments. Usual dosage is 1,200 to 2,400 mg daily.
Children ages 4 to 16 (immediate-release): Initially, 8 to 10 mg/kg P.O. daily in two divided doses, not to exceed 600 mg daily. The target maintenance dose depends on patient's weight and should be divided in two doses. If patient weighs between 20 and 29 kg, target maintenance dose is 900 mg daily. If patient weighs between 29.1 and 39 kg, target maintenance dose is 1,200 mg daily. If patient weighs more than 39 kg, target maintenance dose is 1,800 mg daily. Target doses should be achieved over 2 weeks.
Children ages 2 to 4 (immediate-release): Initially, 8 to 10 mg/kg P.O. daily in two divided doses, not to exceed 600 mg daily. If patient weighs less than 20 kg, a starting dose of 16 to 20 mg/kg may be considered. Maximum maintenance dosage should be achieved over 2 to 4 weeks and shouldn't exceed 60 mg/kg/day in a two-dose divided regimen.
Children ages 6 to 17 (extended-release): 8 to 10 mg/kg P.O. once daily, not to exceed 600 mg daily in first week. May increase at weekly intervals in 8- to 10-mg/kg increments once daily, not to exceed 600 mg. Target daily dose in patients weighing more than 39 kg is 1,800 mg/day; from 29.1 to 39 kg, 1,200 mg/day; and from 20 to 29 kg, 900 mg/day.
Elderly patients: When using extended-release tablets, consider a lower starting dose (300 or 450 mg/day). Dosage increases can be made at weekly intervals in increments of 300 to 450 mg/day.
➤ **To change from multidrug to single-drug treatment of partial seizures in patients with epilepsy**
Adults: Initially, 300 mg immediate-release tablets/suspension P.O. b.i.d., while reducing dose of concomitant anticonvulsant.

Reactions in bold italics are *life-threatening*. Interactions may have a *rapid onset* or a *delayed onset*.

Increase oxcarbazepine by a maximum of 600 mg daily at weekly intervals over 2 to 4 weeks. Recommended daily dose is 2,400 mg P.O. in two divided doses. Withdraw other anticonvulsant completely over 3 to 6 weeks.

Children ages 4 to 16: Initially, 8 to 10 mg/kg immediate-release tablets/suspension P.O. daily in two divided doses, while reducing dose of concomitant anticonvulsant. Increase oxcarbazepine by a maximum of 10 mg/kg daily at weekly intervals to achieve the recommended daily dose shown in the table. Withdraw other anticonvulsant completely over 3 to 6 weeks. See chart below for weight-based maintenance dosing with oxcarbazepine monotherapy.

➤ **To start single-drug treatment of partial seizures in patients with epilepsy**
Adults: Initially, 300 mg immediate-release tablets/suspension P.O. b.i.d. Increase dosage by 300 mg daily every third day to a daily dose of 1,200 mg in two divided doses.

Children ages 4 to 16: Initially, 8 to 10 mg/kg immediate-release tablets/suspension P.O. daily in two divided doses, increasing the dosage by 5 mg/kg daily every third day to the recommended daily dose range shown in the table.

Recommended maintenance doses for children during monotherapy

Weight (kg)	Dose (mg/day)
20	600–900
25	900–1,200
30	900–1,200
35	900–1,500
40	900–1,500
45	1,200–1,500
50	1,200–1,800
55	1,200–1,800
60	1,200–2,100
65	1,200–2,100
70	1,500–2,100

ADMINISTRATION
P.O.
- Shake suspension well.
- Mix suspension with water or give directly from syringe.
- Give immediate-release tablets without regard for food.

- Give extended-release tablets on an empty stomach (at least 1 hour before or 2 hours after a meal). Don't cut or crush tablets. For ease of swallowing, use multiple lower-strength tablets for appropriate dose.
- When converting from immediate-release to extended-release form, higher doses may be needed.
- Oral tablets and suspension may be interchanged at equal doses.

ACTION
Thought to prevent seizure spread in the brain by blocking voltage-sensitive sodium channels and to produce anticonvulsant effects by increasing potassium conduction and modulating high-voltage activated calcium channels.

Route	Onset	Peak	Duration
P.O.	Unknown	Variable	Unknown

Half-life: Immediate-release: About 2 hours for the drug; about 9 hours for the active metabolite. Children younger than age 8 have a 30% to 40% increase in clearance. Extended-release: 7 to 11 hours.

ADVERSE REACTIONS
CNS: abnormal gait, ataxia, dizziness, fatigue, headache, somnolence, tremor, vertigo, *aggravated seizures,* abnormal coordination, agitation, amnesia, anxiety, asthenia, confusion, emotional lability, feeling abnormal, fever, hypesthesia, impaired concentration, insomnia, nervousness, speech disorder.
CV: chest pain, edema, hypotension.
EENT: abnormal vision, diplopia, nystagmus, abnormal accommodation, ear pain, epistaxis, pharyngitis, rhinitis, sinusitis.
GI: abdominal pain, nausea, vomiting, rectal hemorrhage, anorexia, constipation, diarrhea, dry mouth, dyspepsia, gastritis, taste perversion, thirst.
GU: urinary frequency, UTI, vaginitis.
Metabolic: hyponatremia, weight gain.
Musculoskeletal: back pain, muscular weakness.
Respiratory: URI, bronchitis, pulmonary infection, coughing.
Skin: acne, bruising, hot flashes, increased sweating, purpura, rash.

O

Other: allergic reaction, infection, lymphadenopathy, toothache.

INTERACTIONS
Drug-drug. *Carbamazepine, valproic acid, verapamil:* May decrease level of active metabolite of oxcarbazepine. Monitor patient and level closely.
CYP3A4 substrates (cyclosporine, itraconazole, rivaroxaban): May decrease serum concentrations of substrates. Substrate dosage modifications may be needed.
Felodipine: May decrease felodipine level. Monitor patient closely.
Hormonal contraceptives: May decrease levels of ethinyl estradiol and levonorgestrel, reducing hormonal contraceptive effectiveness. Caution women of childbearing potential to use alternative forms of contraception.
Phenobarbital: May decrease level of active metabolite of oxcarbazepine; may increase phenobarbital level. Monitor patient closely.
Phenytoin: May decrease level of active metabolite of oxcarbazepine; may increase phenytoin level in adults receiving high doses of oxcarbazepine. Monitor phenytoin level closely when starting therapy in these patients.
Rifampin: May decrease serum concentrations of active metabolite(s) of oxcarbazepine. Monitor therapy.
Thiazide and thiazide-like diuretics: May enhance oxcarbazepine adverse effects, specifically hyponatremia. Monitor therapy.
Drug-lifestyle. *Alcohol use:* May increase CNS depression. Discourage use together.

EFFECTS ON LAB TEST RESULTS
• May decrease sodium and thyroxine levels.

CONTRAINDICATIONS & CAUTIONS
• Contraindicated in patients hypersensitive to drug or its components.
❸ *Alert:* Serious dermatologic reactions, including Stevens-Johnson syndrome and toxic epidermal necrolysis, have been reported in both children and adults in association with oxcarbazepine use. Such serious skin reactions may be life-threatening, and some patients have required hospitalization, with very rare reports of fatal outcome. The median time of onset for reported cases was 19 days after treatment initiation. Recurrence of serious skin reactions after rechallenge with oxcarbazepine has also been reported.
• Screen patients of Asian ancestry for the human leukocyte antigen allele B*1502 before therapy; these patients may be at increased risk for Stevens-Johnson syndrome or toxic epidermal necrolysis with oxcarbazepine therapy.
Dialyzable drug: Unknown.

PREGNANCY-LACTATION-REPRODUCTION
• There are no adequate studies in pregnant women; drug may cause fetal harm. Use cautiously in pregnant women and only if benefit justifies possible risk to the fetus.
• Patients exposed to drug during pregnancy are encouraged to enroll themselves in the Antiepileptic Drug Pregnancy Registry (1-888-233-2334).
• Drug and its active metabolite appear in breast milk in small amounts. Patient should discontinue breast-feeding or discontinue drug.

NURSING CONSIDERATIONS
❸ *Alert:* Between 25% and 30% of patients with history of hypersensitivity reaction to carbamazepine may develop hypersensitivities to oxcarbazepine. Ask patient about carbamazepine hypersensitivity and stop drug immediately if signs or symptoms of hypersensitivity occur.
❸ *Alert:* Closely monitor all patients taking or starting antiepileptic drugs for changes in behavior indicating worsening of suicidal thoughts or behavior or depression. Symptoms such as anxiety, agitation, hostility, mania, and hypomania may be precursors to emerging suicidality.
❸ *Alert:* Withdraw drug gradually to minimize potential for increased seizure frequency.
❸ *Alert:* Rare serious and sometimes fatal dermatologic reactions can occur. If skin reactions occur, discontinue drug.
• Watch for signs and symptoms of hyponatremia, including nausea, malaise, headache, lethargy, confusion, and decreased sensation.

Reactions in bold italics are *life-threatening*. Interactions may have a *rapid onset* or a *delayed onset*.

• Monitor sodium level in patients receiving oxcarbazepine for maintenance treatment, especially patients receiving other therapies that may decrease sodium levels.

• Oxcarbazepine use has been linked to several nervous system-related adverse reactions, including psychomotor slowing, difficulty with concentration, speech or language problems, somnolence, fatigue, and coordination abnormalities, such as ataxia and gait disturbances.

• **Look alike–sound alike:** Don't confuse oxcarbazepine with carbamazepine or oxaprozin.

PATIENT TEACHING

• Tell patient to take drug with or without food. For extended-release, tell patient to take on an empty stomach and not to cut, crush, or chew tablets.

• Tell patient to contact prescriber before interrupting or stopping drug.

• Advise patient to report signs and symptoms of low sodium in the blood, such as nausea, malaise, headache, lethargy, and confusion.

🔴 **Alert:** Multiorgan hypersensitivity reactions may occur. Tell patient to report fever and swollen lymph nodes to prescriber.

🔴 **Alert:** Serious skin reactions, including Stevens-Johnson syndrome and toxic epidermal necrolysis, can occur. Advise patient to immediately report rashes to prescriber.

• Caution patient to avoid driving and other potentially hazardous activities that require mental alertness until effects of drug are known.

• Instruct female patient using hormonal contraceptives to use alternative form of contraception while taking drug.

• Tell patient to avoid alcohol while taking drug.

• Advise patient to inform prescriber if he has ever experienced hypersensitivity reaction to carbamazepine.

oxybutynin
ox-i-BYOO-ti-nin

Gelnique 3%, Oxytrol, Oxytrol for Women ◇

oxybutynin chloride
Ditropan XL, Gelnique

Therapeutic class: Urinary antispasmodics
Pharmacologic class: Antimuscarinics

AVAILABLE FORMS
oxybutynin
Topical gel: 3%
Transdermal patch: 36-mg patch delivering 3.9 mg/day ◇
oxybutynin chloride
Syrup: 5 mg/5 mL
Tablets: 5 mg
Tablets (extended-release) 🚫: 5 mg, 10 mg, 15 mg
Topical gel: 10%

INDICATIONS & DOSAGES
➤ **Bladder instability associated with voiding**
Adults: 5 mg (immediate-release) P.O. b.i.d. to t.i.d., to maximum of 5 mg q.i.d.
Children age 5 and older: 5 mg (immediate-release) P.O. b.i.d., to maximum of 5 mg t.i.d.
Elderly patients: A lower initial starting dose of 2.5 mg (immediate-release) P.O. b.i.d. or t.i.d. is recommended.
➤ **Overactive bladder**
Adults: Initially, 5 mg Ditropan XL P.O. once daily. Dosage adjustments may be made weekly in 5-mg increments, as needed, to maximum of 30 mg P.O. daily. Or, apply one patch twice weekly (every 3 to 4 days) to dry, intact skin on the abdomen, hip, or buttock. Or, 1 g topical gel (10%) or 3 pumps (84 mg) of 3% topical gel once daily applied to dry, intact skin on the abdomen, upper arms or shoulders, or thighs.
Elderly patients: A lower initial starting dose of 2.5 mg (immediate-release) P.O. b.i.d. or t.i.d. is recommended.

> ➤ **Symptoms of detrusor overactivity associated with a neurologic condition (e.g., spina bifida)**
Children age 6 and older: 5 mg Ditropan XL P.O. once daily. May increase in 5-mg increments, as needed, to maximum of 20 mg P.O. daily.
Children age 5 and older (immediate-release): 5 mg P.O. b.i.d. or t.i.d.

ADMINISTRATION
P.O.
● Don't crush extended-release tablets.
● Give extended-release tablets without regard for food.
Topical (gel)
● Use immediately after sachets are opened.
● Apply to dry, intact skin on the abdomen, upper arms or shoulders, or thighs.
● Rotate application sites.
Transdermal
● Apply immediately after removing from protective pouch.
● Apply to dry, intact skin on the abdomen, hip, or buttock.
● Avoid reapplication to the same site within 7 days.
● Don't expose patch to sunlight.

ACTION
Relaxes smooth muscle of bladder by antagonizing muscarinic receptors, relieving symptoms of overactive bladder.

Route	Onset	Peak	Duration
P.O.	30–60 min	3–4 hr	6–10 hr
P.O. (extended-release)	Unknown	4–6 hr	24 hr
Topical (gel)	Unknown	Unknown	Unknown
Transdermal	24–48 hr	Varies	96 hr

Half-life: Tablets or oral solution, 2 to 3 hours; extended-release tablets, 12 to 13 hours; patch, 7 to 8 hours; gel, 64 hours.

ADVERSE REACTIONS
Oral
CNS: dizziness, insomnia, restlessness, hallucinations, asthenia, fever, headache, somnolence.
CV: palpitations, tachycardia, vasodilation.
EENT: mydriasis, cycloplegia, decreased lacrimation, amblyopia, blurred vision, dry eyes.

GI: constipation, dry mouth, nausea, vomiting, decreased GI motility, abdominal pain.
GU: urinary hesitancy, urine retention, impotence, UTI.
Skin: rash, decreased diaphoresis.
Other: suppression of lactation.
Topical (gel)
CNS: dizziness, fatigue.
EENT: dry mouth.
GI: viral gastroenteritis.
GU: UTI.
Respiratory: URI.
Skin: application-site reaction.
Transdermal patch
CNS: fatigue, somnolence, headache.
CV: flushing.
EENT: abnormal vision.
GI: dry mouth, diarrhea, abdominal pain, nausea, flatulence, constipation.
GU: dysuria.
Musculoskeletal: back pain.
Skin: pruritus, erythema, vesicles, macules, rash, burning at application site.

INTERACTIONS
Drug-drug. *Amantadine, anticholinergics:* May increase anticholinergic effects. Use together cautiously.
Beta blockers (atenolol), digoxin: May increase levels of these drugs. Monitor drug levels closely.
CNS depressants: May increase CNS effects. Use together cautiously.
CYP3A4 inhibitors (ketoconazole): May alter oxybutynin concentration. Use together cautiously.
Haloperidol: May decrease haloperidol level. Monitor drug level closely.
Drug-lifestyle. *Alcohol use:* May increase CNS effects. Discourage use together.
Exercise, hot weather: May cause heatstroke. Advise patient to use with caution in hot weather.

EFFECTS ON LAB TEST RESULTS
None reported.

CONTRAINDICATIONS & CAUTIONS
● Contraindicated in patients hypersensitive to drug or its components and in those with GI obstruction and conditions that decrease GI motility, uncontrolled narrow-angle

glaucoma, urine or gastric retention, or obstructive uropathy.
- Contraindicated in elderly or debilitated patients with intestinal atony and in hemorrhaging patients with unstable CV status.
- Use cautiously in elderly patients and in those with autonomic neuropathy, reflux esophagitis, myasthenia gravis, or hepatic or renal disease.
- Extended-release form isn't recommended for children who can't swallow the tablet whole without chewing, dividing, or crushing or for children younger than age 6.
- Use extended-release form cautiously in patients with bladder outflow obstruction, gastric obstruction, ulcerative colitis, intestinal atony, myasthenia gravis, or gastroesophageal reflux and in those taking drugs that worsen esophagitis (bisphosphonates).
Dialyzable drug: Unknown.

⚠ *Overdose S&S:* Restlessness, tremors, irritability, seizures, delirium, hallucinations, flushing, fever, dehydration, cardiac arrhythmias, vomiting, urine retention, hypotension or hypertension, respiratory failure, paralysis, coma.

PREGNANCY-LACTATION-REPRODUCTION
- Use cautiously in pregnant women and only if benefit justifies risk to the fetus.
- It isn't known if drug appears in breast milk. Use cautiously in breast-feeding women.
- Lactation suppression has been reported.

NURSING CONSIDERATIONS
- Before giving drug, get confirmation of neurogenic bladder by cystometry and rule out partial intestinal obstruction in patients with diarrhea, especially those with colostomy or ileostomy.
- If patient has UTI, treat with antibiotics.
- Drug may aggravate symptoms of hyperthyroidism, CAD, HF, arrhythmias, tachycardia, hypertension, or prostatic hyperplasia.
- Obtain periodic cystometry as directed to evaluate response to therapy.
- Monitor patient for residual urine after voiding.
- Oxytrol for Women has been FDA-approved as an OTC product. The

3.9-mg/day patch should be applied to the skin every 3 to 4 days.
- *Look alike–sound alike:* Don't confuse Ditropan with diazepam. Don't confuse oxybutynin with Oxycontin.

PATIENT TEACHING
- Warn patient to avoid hazardous activities, such as operating machinery or driving, until CNS effects of drug are known.
- Caution patient that using drug during very hot weather may cause fever or heatstroke because it suppresses sweating.
- Tell patient to swallow extended-release tablet whole and not to chew or crush it.
- Instruct patient to measure syrup with a teaspoon.
- Advise patient to store drug in tightly closed container at 59° to 86° F (15° to 30° C).
- Instruct patient using transdermal patch to change patch twice a week (every 3 to 4 days) and to choose a new application site with each new patch to avoid the same site within 7 days. Warn patient to only wear one patch at a time. Tell patient to dispose of old patches carefully in the trash in a manner that prevents accidental application or ingestion by children and pets.
- Tell patient using transdermal patch to keep patch in sealed pouch until immediately before application, not to expose patch to sunlight, and to wear patch under clothing.
- Tell patient to remove patch before undergoing an MRI scan.
- Advise patient using topical gel to rotate application sites.
- Advise patient to avoid alcohol while taking drug.
- Tell patient that drug may cause dry mouth.

O

SAFETY ALERT!

oxycodone hydrochloride
ox-i-KOE-done

Oxaydo, OxyContin*, Oxy IR*,
Roxicodone, Supeudol*

Therapeutic class: Opioid analgesics
Pharmacologic class: Opioids
Controlled substance schedule: II

AVAILABLE FORMS
Capsules: 5 mg
Oral solution: 5 mg/5 mL
Oral solution (concentrate): 20 mg/mL
Tablets (extended-release) ⓞⓝⓒ: 10 mg,
15 mg, 20 mg, 30 mg, 40 mg, 60 mg, 80 mg
Tablets (immediate-release): 5 mg, 10 mg,
15 mg, 20 mg, 30 mg
Tablets (immediate-release; abuse-deterrent): 5 mg, 7.5 mg

INDICATIONS & DOSAGES
➤ **Moderate to severe pain**
Adults: 5 to 15 mg immediate-release form
or oral solution P.O. every 4 to 6 hours.
Titrate dosage based on response. Usual
dosage is 10 to 30 mg every 4 hours p.r.n.
For control of severe, chronic pain, give on a
regularly scheduled basis every 4 to 6 hours.
➤ **Moderate to severe pain in patients not
currently receiving opioids, who need a
continuous, around-the-clock analgesic
for an extended period of time**
Adults: 10 mg extended-release tablets P.O.
every 12 hours. May increase dose every
1 to 2 days as needed.
Adjust-a-dose: For elderly or debilitated
patients and those with hepatic impairment,
decrease initial starting dose by one-third to
one-half.

ADMINISTRATION
P.O.
• To minimize GI upset, give drug after
meals or with milk.
Black Box Warning Patient must swallow
extended-release tablets whole. ■
Black Box Warning The 60- and 80-mg
extended-release tablets, or a single 40-mg
dose, or a total daily dose of more than

80 mg is limited to opioid-tolerant
patients. ■
Black Box Warning Oxycodone concentrated oral solution, available as a 20-mg/mL
concentration, is indicated for use in opioid-
tolerant patients only. ■
• Don't crush or dissolve extended-release
tablets.

ACTION
Unknown. Binds with opioid receptors in
the CNS, altering perception of and emotional response to pain.

Route	Onset	Peak	Duration
P.O. (immediate-release)	10–15 min	1 hr	3–6 hr
P.O. (extended-release)	Unknown	2½ hr	12 hr

Half-life: 2 to 3 hours; extended-release, 4.5 hours.

ADVERSE REACTIONS
CNS: clouded sensorium, dizziness, eupho-
ria, light-headedness, physical dependence,
sedation, somnolence, headache, asthenia.
CV: *bradycardia,* hypotension.
GI: constipation, nausea, vomiting, ileus.
GU: urine retention.
Respiratory: *respiratory depression.*
Skin: diaphoresis, pruritus.

INTERACTIONS
Drug-drug. *Anticoagulants:* Oxycodone
hydrochloride products containing aspirin
may increase anticoagulant effect. Monitor
clotting times. Use together cautiously.
Black Box Warning *Benzodiazepines, CNS
depressants:* May cause slow or difficult
breathing, sedation, and death. Avoid use
together. If use together is necessary, limit
dosage and duration of each drug to minimum necessary for desired effect. ■
*General anesthetics, hypnotics, MAO in-
hibitors, TCAs:* May cause additive adverse
effects (e.g., CNS or respiratory depression). Use together with caution. Reduce
oxycodone dose and monitor patient response.
Black Box Warning *CYP3A4 inhibitors
such as azole antifungals (ketoconazole),
macrolide antibiotics (erythromycin), protease inhibitors (ritonavir):* May increase
oxycodone level, increase or prolong adverse effects, and cause fatal respiratory

---

Reactions in bold italics are *life-threatening*. Interactions may have a *rapid onset* or a *delayed onset*.

depression. Carefully monitor patient over extended period of time and adjust oxycodone dosage as needed. ■

⊙ Alert: *Serotonergic drugs (amoxapine, antiemetics [dolasetron, granisetron, ondansetron, palonosetron], antimigraine drugs, buspirone, cyclobenzaprine, dextromethorphan, linezolid, lithium, MAO inhibitors, maprotiline, methylene blue, mirtazapine, nefazodone, SNRIs, SSRIs, TCAs, trazodone, tryptophan, vilazodone):* May increase risk of serotonin syndrome. Use together cautiously and monitor patient for serotonin syndrome.

Drug-herb. ⊙ Alert: *St. John's wort:* May increase risk of serotonin syndrome. Use together cautiously and monitor patient for serotonin syndrome.

Drug-lifestyle. *Alcohol use:* May cause additive effects. Don't use together.

EFFECTS ON LAB TEST RESULTS
● May increase amylase and lipase levels.

CONTRAINDICATIONS & CAUTIONS
● Drug should be prescribed only by health care professionals knowledgeable in the use of potent opioids for the management of chronic pain.

Black Box Warning Opioids should only be prescribed with benzodiazepines or other CNS depressants to patients for whom alternative treatment options are inadequate. ■

⊙ Alert: Patients are at increased risk for oversedation and respiratory depression if they snore or have a history of sleep apnea, haven't used opioids recently or are firsttime opioid users, have increased opioid dosage requirements or opioid habituation, have received general anesthesia for longer lengths of time or received other sedating drugs, have preexisting pulmonary or cardiac disease, or have thoracic or other surgical incisions that may impair breathing. Monitor patients carefully.

⊙ Alert: Drug may lead to rare but serious decrease in adrenal gland cortisol production.

⊙ Alert: Drug may cause decreased sex hormone levels with long-term use.

● Contraindicated in patients hypersensitive to drug.

● Contraindicated in known or suspected paralytic ileus, significant respiratory depression, and acute or severe bronchial asthma.

● Use with caution in elderly and debilitated patients and in those with head injury, increased ICP, seizures, asthma, COPD, prostatic hyperplasia, severe hepatic or renal disease, acute abdominal conditions, urethral stricture, hypothyroidism, Addison disease, and arrhythmias.

Black Box Warning Serious, lifethreatening, or fatal respiratory depression may occur with use of extended-release oxycodone. Monitor patient for respiratory depression, especially during initiation of therapy and after a dosage increase. Instruct patient to swallow extended-release oxycodone tablets whole; crushing, dissolving, or chewing the tablets can cause rapid release and absorption of a potentially fatal dose of oxycodone. ■

Black Box Warning Accidental ingestion of even one dose of extended-release oxycodone, especially by children, can result in a fatal oxycodone overdose. ■

Black Box Warning Patients must be screened for increased risk of opioid abuse (personal or family history of substance abuse or mental illness) before being prescribed opioids. ■

Black Box Warning Oxycodone extendedrelease tablets are indicated for the management of moderate to severe pain, when a continuous, around-the-clock opioid analgesic is needed for an extended period of time. They aren't intended for use as asneeded analgesics. ■

Dialyzable drug: Unknown.

⚠ Overdose S&S: CNS depression, respiratory depression, apnea, flaccid skeletal muscles, bradycardia, hypotension, circulatory collapse, cardiac arrest, respiratory arrest, death.

PREGNANCY-LACTATION-REPRODUCTION
⊙ Alert: Carefully weigh risks and benefits of using drug during pregnancy.

Black Box Warning Prolonged use of extended-release oxycodone during pregnancy can result in neonatal opioid withdrawal syndrome, which may be lifethreatening if not recognized and treated and requires management according to protocols developed by neonatology experts. ■

● There are no adequate studies in pregnant women. Use only if potential benefit justifies potential fetal risks.

● Drug isn't recommended for use during or immediately before labor as uterine contractions may be adversely affected.

● Prolonged opioid use during pregnancy may cause respiratory depression or withdrawal signs and symptoms in the neonate. Naloxone should be available to reverse opioid-induced respiratory depression in the neonate.

● Drug appears in breast milk. Breastfeeding isn't recommended.

● Long-term opioid use may cause secondary hypogonadism, which may lead to sexual dysfunction or infertility.

NURSING CONSIDERATIONS

Black Box Warning Use care when prescribing and administering oxycodone concentrated oral solution, to avoid dosing errors due to confusion between milligram and milliliter and among other oxycodone solutions with different concentrations, which could result in accidental overdose and death. Take care to ensure the proper dose is communicated and dispensed. ■

Black Box Warning Routinely monitor all patients on opioids for signs and symptoms of misuse, abuse, and addiction. ■

⊕ **Alert:** Carefully monitor vital signs, pain level, respiratory status, and sedation level in all patients receiving opioids, especially those receiving I.V. drugs, even when given postoperatively.

● Reassess patient's level of pain at least 15 and 30 minutes after administration.

● For full analgesic effect, give drug before patient has intense pain.

⊕ **Alert:** If patient is taking opioids with serotonergic drugs, watch for signs and symptoms of serotonin syndrome (agitation, hallucinations, rapid HR, fever, excessive sweating, shivering or shaking, muscle twitching or stiffness, trouble with coordination, nausea, vomiting, diarrhea), especially at start of treatment or with dosages increases. Signs and symptoms may occur within several hours of coadministration but may also occur later, especially after dosage

increase. Discontinue opioid, serotonergic drug, or both if serotonin syndrome is suspected.

⊕ **Alert:** Monitor patient for signs and symptoms of adrenal insufficiency (nausea, vomiting, loss of appetite, fatigue, weakness, dizziness, low BP). Perform diagnostic testing if adrenal insufficiency is suspected. If adrenal insufficiency is confirmed, treat with corticosteroids and wean patient off opioids if appropriate. Discontinue corticosteroids when clinically appropriate.

⊕ **Alert:** Monitor patient for signs and symptoms of decreased sex hormone levels (low libido, erectile dysfunction, amenorrhea, infertility). If signs and symptoms occur, evaluate patient and obtain laboratory testing.

● Patients taking extended-release form around-the-clock may need to take immediate-release form for worsening of pain or prevention of incident pain (e.g., breakthrough pain).

● Single-drug oxycodone solution or tablets are especially useful for patients who shouldn't take aspirin or acetaminophen.

● Monitor circulatory and respiratory status closely, especially within the first 24 to 72 hours of initiation of therapy. Withhold dose and notify prescriber if respirations are shallow or if respiratory rate falls below 12 breaths/minute.

● Monitor patient's bladder and bowel patterns. Patient may need a stimulant laxative because drug has a constipating effect.

● For patients who are taking more than 60 mg daily, stop drug gradually to prevent withdrawal symptoms.

● Extended-release formula isn't intended for as-needed use or for immediate postoperative pain. Drug is indicated only for postoperative use if patient was receiving it before surgery or if pain is expected to persist for an extended time.

⊕ **Alert:** Drug is potentially addictive, even at recommended doses, and if drug is misused. Chewing, crushing, snorting, or injecting it can lead to overdose and death.

● OxyContin has been formulated to prevent immediate access to full-dose oxycodone by cutting, chewing, or breaking the tablet. Attempts to dissolve tablets will result in a gummy substance that can't be drawn up into a syringe or injected.

PATIENT TEACHING

Black Box Warning Caution patient or caregiver of patient taking an opioid with a benzodiazepine, CNS depressant, or alcohol to seek immediate medical attention if patient experiences dizziness, light-headedness, extreme sleepiness, slowed or difficult breathing, or unresponsiveness. ■

• Instruct patient to take drug before pain is intense.

• Explain assessment and monitoring process to patient and family. Instruct them to immediately report difficulty breathing or other signs or symptoms of a potential adverse opioid-related reaction.

• Tell patient to take drug with milk or after eating.

Black Box Warning If a pregnant woman requires an opioid for a prolonged period, advise her of the risk of neonatal opioid withdrawal syndrome; ensure her that appropriate treatment will be available. ■

Black Box Warning Instruct patient or caregiver to keep drug out of the reach of children because accidental ingestion can result in a fatal oxycodone overdose. Advise patient or caregiver that if accidental ingestion occurs, to seek emergency medical help immediately. ■

Black Box Warning Tell patient to swallow extended-release tablets whole. ■

۞ Alert: Encourage patient to report all medications being taken, including prescription and OTC medications and supplements.

۞ Alert: Caution patient to immediately report symptoms of serotonin syndrome, adrenal insufficiency, and decreased sex hormone levels.

• Caution ambulatory patient about getting out of bed or walking. Warn outpatient to avoid driving and other hazardous activities that require mental alertness until drug's CNS effects are known.

• Advise patient to avoid alcohol use during therapy.

• Tell patient not to stop drug abruptly.

SAFETY ALERT!

oxycodone hydrochloride–acetaminophen
ox-i-KOE-done/a-seet-a-MIN-a-fen

Endocet✦, Oxycet, Percocet, Roxicet, Xartemis XR

Therapeutic class: Opioid analgesics
Pharmacologic class: Opioid agonists–para-aminophenol derivatives
Controlled substance schedule: II

AVAILABLE FORMS

Oral solution*: 325 mg acetaminophen and 5 mg oxycodone hydrochloride per 5 mL
Tablets: 5 mg oxycodone hydrochloride and 300 mg acetaminophen, 7.5 mg oxycodone hydrochloride and 300 mg acetaminophen, 10 mg oxycodone hydrochloride and 300 mg acetaminophen, 2.5 mg oxycodone hydrochloride and 325 mg acetaminophen, 5 mg oxycodone hydrochloride and 325 mg acetaminophen, 7.5 mg oxycodone hydrochloride and 325 mg acetaminophen, 10 mg oxycodone hydrochloride and 325 mg acetaminophen
Tablets (extended-release) ⓓⓝⓒ*:* 7.5 mg oxycodone hydrochloride and 325 mg acetaminophen

INDICATIONS & DOSAGES

➤ **Moderate to moderately severe pain (immediate-release)**
Adults: Oxycodone 2.5 to 10 mg and acetaminophen 325 mg P.O. every 6 hours as needed for pain. Adjust dosage based on pain severity and patient response. Maximum daily doses shouldn't exceed 60 mg oxycodone or 4 g acetaminophen.
Adjust-a-dose: Consider decreased dosage in patients with renal or hepatic impairment, chronic alcoholics, elderly patients, and patients overly sensitive to effects of opioids. Gradually taper dosage if therapy lasts for more than a few weeks.

➤ **Acute pain (extended-release)**
Adults: 2 tablets P.O. every 12 hours. May give second dose early (8 hours after first dose) if needed, with subsequent doses of 2 tablets every 12 hours.

Adjust-a-dose: For patients with renal or hepatic impairment, consider an initial dose of 1 tablet P.O. every 12 hours and adjust as needed.

ADMINISTRATION
P.O.
● Store drug at room temperature.
● Don't crush, split, dissolve, break, or allow patient to chew extended-release tablets.

ACTION
Oxycodone binds with opioid receptors in the CNS, altering perception of and emotional response to pain. Acetaminophen is thought to produce analgesia by inhibiting prostaglandin and other substances that sensitize pain receptors. The combination reduces pain more effectively than acetaminophen alone.

Route	Onset	Peak	Duration
P.O. (acetaminophen)	Unknown	½–2 hr	3–4 hr
P.O. (oxycodone)	10–15 min	1 hr	3–6 hr

Half-life: Acetaminophen, 1 to 4 hours; oxycodone, 3½ hours.

ADVERSE REACTIONS
CNS: paresthesia, hypoesthesia, dizziness, drowsiness, fatigue, headache, euphoria, dysphoria, insomnia.
CV: peripheral edema, circulatory depression, hypotension, *shock.*
EENT: dry mouth.
GI: constipation, dyspepsia, nausea, vomiting.
GU: dysuria.
Hematologic: *hemolytic anemia, neutropenia, pancytopenia, thrombocytopenia.*
Respiratory: cough, *apnea, respiratory arrest,* respiratory depression.
Skin: pruritus, erythema, erythematous dermatitis, excoriation, rash, flushing.
Other: *anaphylactoid reaction.*

INTERACTIONS
Drug-drug. *Anticholinergics (atropine, dicyclomine, scopolamine):* May increase risk of paralytic ileus. Monitor patient closely.

Black Box Warning *Benzodiazepines, CNS depressants:* May cause slow or difficult breathing, sedation, and death. Avoid use together. If use together is necessary, limit dosage and duration of each drug to minimum necessary for desired effect. ■
General anesthetics, neuromuscular blockers, opioid analgesics: May increase CNS depression. Use together cautiously, decreasing dosage of one or both agents.
Beta blockers (propranolol): May inhibit acetaminophen metabolism. Use together carefully.
CYP3A4 inhibitors (such as azole antifungals [ketoconazole]): May increase oxycodone level, increase or prolong adverse effects, and cause fatal respiratory depression. Carefully monitor patient over extended period and adjust oxycodone dosage as needed.
Lamotrigine, loop diuretics, zidovudine: May decrease effects of these drugs when used with acetaminophen. Use together cautiously.
Mixed opioid agonist–antagonist combinations: May decrease effects of oxycodone and precipitate withdrawal. Use together carefully.
Oral contraceptives: May decrease acetaminophen half-life. Use together cautiously.
Probenecid: May increase effectiveness of acetaminophen. Use together cautiously.
۞ Alert: *Serotonergic drugs (amoxapine, antiemetics [dolasetron, granisetron, ondansetron, palonosetron], antimigraine drugs, buspirone, cyclobenzaprine, dextromethorphan, linezolid, lithium, MAO inhibitors, maprotiline, methylene blue, mirtazapine, nefazodone, SNRIs, SSRIs, TCAs, trazodone, tryptophan, vilazodone):* May increase risk of serotonin syndrome. Use together cautiously and monitor patient for serotonin syndrome.
Drug-herb. *St. John's wort:* May increase risk of serotonin syndrome. Use together cautiously and monitor patient for serotonin syndrome.
Drug-lifestyle. *Alcohol use:* May increase risk of hepatotoxicity and CNS effects. Don't use together.

EFFECTS ON LAB TEST RESULTS
• May increase potassium, amylase, bilirubin, or liver enzyme levels. May increase or decrease blood glucose level.
• May decrease platelet count.
• Oxycodone may cause cross-reactivity with urinary assays used to detect cocaine and marijuana.
• Quinolones (levofloxacin, ofloxacin) may cause a false-positive urine screen result for opioids.
• Acetaminophen may cause false-positive result for urinary 5-hydroxyindoleacetic acid.

CONTRAINDICATIONS & CAUTIONS
• Contraindicated in patients hypersensitive to components of drug and in those with significant respiratory depression, acute or severe bronchial asthma, hypercarbia, or suspected or known paralytic ileus.

Black Box Warning Acetaminophen may increase risk of acute liver failure, liver transplant, and death. Liver injury is generally associated with use of acetaminophen at doses exceeding 4,000 mg/day and the use of more than one acetaminophen-containing product. ∎

Black Box Warning Serious, life-threatening, or fatal respiratory depression may occur with use of oxycodone–acetaminophen extended-release form. Monitor patient for respiratory depression, especially during initiation of therapy and after a dosage increase. Instruct patients to swallow oxycodone–acetaminophen extended-release tablets whole; crushing, dissolving, or chewing tablets can cause rapid release and absorption of a potentially fatal dose of oxycodone. ∎

Black Box Warning Accidental ingestion of even one dose of extended-release oxycodone–acetaminophen, especially by children, can result in a fatal overdose of oxycodone. ∎

Black Box Warning Patients must be screened for increased risk of opioid abuse (personal or family history of substance abuse or mental illness) before being prescribed opioids. ∎

Black Box Warning Opioids should only be prescribed with benzodiazepines or other CNS depressants to patients for whom alternative treatment options are inadequate. ∎

☻ **Alert:** Patients are at increased risk for oversedation and respiratory depression if they snore or have a history of sleep apnea, haven't used opioids recently or are first-time opioid users, have increased opioid dosage requirements or opioid habituation, have received general anesthesia for longer lengths of time or received other sedating drugs, have preexisting pulmonary or cardiac disease, or have thoracic or other surgical incisions that may impair breathing. Monitor patients carefully.

☻ **Alert:** May cause serious, potentially fatal skin reactions, including Stevens-Johnson syndrome, toxic epidermal necrolysis, and acute generalized exanthematous pustulosis. Reaction may occur with first or subsequent use when acetaminophen is used as monotherapy or when it is one component of combination drug therapy. Monitor for reddening of the skin, rash, blisters, and detachment of the upper surface of the skin. Stop drug immediately if skin reaction is suspected.

☻ **Alert:** Drug may lead to rare but serious decrease in adrenal gland cortisol production.

☻ **Alert:** Drug may cause decreased sex hormone levels with long-term use.

• Use cautiously in patients with increased sensitivity to codeine, head injury, increased ICP, intracranial lesions, seizures, alcoholism, delirium tremens, biliary disease including pancreatitis, liver disease, COPD, preexisting respiratory impairment, or cor pulmonale.
• Use cautiously in acute abdominal conditions because this drug may obscure diagnostic signs or markedly increase respiratory depression or CSF pressure.
• Use cautiously in hypotensive patients, elderly or debilitated patients, and in those with severe renal or hepatic impairment, hypothyroidism, urethral stricture, or Addison disease.

Dialyzable drug: Oxycodone, unknown; acetaminophen, unknown.

⚠ *Overdose S&S:* Oxycodone: Pinpoint pupils, respiratory depression, loss of consciousness, somnolence, stupor, coma, skeletal muscle flaccidity, cold and clammy

skin, bradycardia, hypotension, apnea, circulatory collapse, cardiac arrest, death.
Acetaminophen: *Nausea, vomiting, diaphoresis, general malaise, hepatic necrosis, renal tubular necrosis, hypoglycemic coma, coagulation defects.*

PREGNANCY-LACTATION-REPRODUCTION
❂ *Alert:* Carefully weigh risks and benefits of using drug during pregnancy.

Black Box Warning Prolonged use of extended-release oxycodone–acetaminophen during pregnancy can result in neonatal opioid withdrawal syndrome, which may be life-threatening if not recognized and treated and requires management according to protocols developed by neonatology experts. ■

• Don't use immediately before labor. Prolonged use of opioids during pregnancy can result in neonatal withdrawal syndrome. Use only if benefits outweigh fetal risks.

• Use during breast-feeding isn't recommended.

NURSING CONSIDERATIONS
• Monitor circulatory and respiratory status closely, especially within the first 24 to 72 hours of initiating therapy. Withhold dose and notify prescriber if respirations are shallow or if respiratory rate falls below 12 breaths/minute.

❂ *Alert:* Carefully monitor vital signs, pain level, respiratory status, and sedation level in all patients receiving opioids, especially those receiving I.V. drugs, even those given postoperatively.

• The lowest effective dosage should be prescribed for the shortest period of time. Inform patients of risks and signs and symptoms of morphine toxicity.

Black Box Warning Assess patients identified as potential abusers; drug should be prescribed with extreme care. Drug may cause physical dependence and tolerance with long-term therapy. ■

Black Box Warning Drug is potentially addictive. Chewing, crushing, dissolving, or injecting it can lead to overdose and death. ■

Black Box Warning All patients using opioids should be routinely monitored for signs and symptoms of misuse, abuse, and addiction. ■

❂ *Alert:* If patient is taking opioids with serotonergic drugs, watch for signs and symptoms of serotonin syndrome (agitation, hallucinations, rapid HR, fever, excessive sweating, shivering or shaking, muscle twitching or stiffness, trouble with coordination, nausea, vomiting, diarrhea), especially at start of treatment and at dosage increases. Signs and symptoms may occur within several hours of coadministration but may also occur later, especially after dosage increase. Discontinue opioid, serotonergic drug, or both if serotonin syndrome is suspected.

❂ *Alert:* Monitor patient for signs and symptoms of adrenal insufficiency (nausea, vomiting, loss of appetite, fatigue, weakness, dizziness, low BP). Perform diagnostic testing if adrenal insufficiency is suspected. If adrenal insufficiency is confirmed, treat with corticosteroids and wean patient off opioids if appropriate. Discontinue corticosteroids when clinically appropriate.

❂ *Alert:* Monitor patient for signs and symptoms of decreased sex hormone levels (low libido, erectile dysfunction, amenorrhea, infertility). If signs and symptoms occur, evaluate patient and obtain laboratory testing.

• Monitor patients for orthostatic hypotension.

• Monitor patients with head injury carefully. Oxycodone's effects on pupillary response and consciousness may mask worsening of neurologic status.

• Monitor patients with acute abdominal conditions closely. Drug may mask signs and symptoms in these patients.

• Observe for seizures in patients with convulsive disorders.

• Monitor bowel motility postoperatively, especially after intra-abdominal surgery.

PATIENT TEACHING
Black Box Warning Caution patient or caregiver of patient taking an opioid with a benzodiazepine, CNS depressant, or alcohol to seek immediate medical attention if patient experiences dizziness, light-headedness, extreme sleepiness, slowed or difficult breathing, or unresponsiveness. ■

Black Box Warning Teach patient to look for acetaminophen on labels of all prescriptions and OTC medications he takes and

---

to not use more than one product containing acetaminophen. Warn patient to seek medical attention if acetaminophen intake exceeds 4,000 mg/day even if feeling well. ■
• Explain assessment and monitoring process to patient and family. Instruct them to immediately report difficulty breathing or other signs or symptoms of a potential adverse opioid-related reaction.

Black Box Warning If a pregnant woman requires an opioid for a prolonged period, advise her of the risk of neonatal opioid withdrawal syndrome; assure her that appropriate treatment will be available. ■

Black Box Warning Instruct patient or caregiver to keep drug out of the reach of children because accidental ingestion can result in a fatal overdose of oxycodone. Advise patient or caregiver that if accidental ingestion occurs, to seek emergency medical help immediately. ■

Black Box Warning Tell patient to swallow oxycodone–acetaminophen extended-release tablets whole. ■

◑ *Alert:* Encourage patient to report all medications being taken, including prescription and OTC medications and supplements.

◑ *Alert:* Caution patient to immediately report signs and symptoms of serotonin syndrome, adrenal insufficiency, and decreased sex hormone levels.

◑ *Alert:* Warn patient to stop drug and seek medical attention immediately if rash or reaction occurs while using acetaminophen.
• Inform patient with severe hepatic or renal disease that serial blood tests will be needed.
• Advise patient not to drive a car or operate heavy machinery while taking this drug.
• Warn patient to avoid alcohol and other CNS depressants.

Black Box Warning Caution patient that oxycodone may be habit-forming and to take drug only as long as prescribed in the amounts prescribed. Advise patient that if drug is taken for more than a few weeks, it should be tapered off gradually. ■
• Caution breast-feeding patient not to use drug because it can cause morphine toxicity (sleepiness, difficulty breast-feeding, breathing difficulties, limpness) in infants.

oxymorphone hydrochloride
ox-i-MOR-fone

Opana, Opana ER

Therapeutic class: Opioid analgesics
Pharmacologic class: Opioids
Controlled substance schedule: II

AVAILABLE FORMS
Injection: 1 mg/mL
Tablets: 5 mg, 10 mg
Tablets (extended-release) ⓓⓝⓒ: 5 mg, 7.5 mg, 10 mg, 15 mg, 20 mg, 30 mg, 40 mg

INDICATIONS & DOSAGES
Adjust-a-dose (for all indications): For patients with mild hepatic impairment or CrCl less than 50 mL/minute, start with the lowest possible dose and slowly increase as tolerated.

➤ **Moderate to severe pain**
Adults: 1 to 1.5 mg I.M. or subcutaneously every 4 to 6 hours p.r.n. Or, 0.5 mg I.V. every 4 to 6 hours p.r.n. Or, in opioid-naive patients, 10 to 20 mg immediate-release tablets P.O. every 4 to 6 hours. If needed, begin dosing at 5 mg P.O. and adjust based on patient response.

➤ **Moderate to severe pain in patients requiring continuous, around-the-clock opioid treatment for an extended period of time**
Opioid-naive adults: Using extended-release (ER) form, give 5 mg P.O. every 12 hours. Increase 5 to 10 mg every 12 hours every 3 to 7 days as needed and tolerated.
Nonopioid-naive adults: Patients taking Opana immediate-release tablets can be switched to Opana ER tablets by giving one-half patient's total daily dose as Opana ER every 12 hours. Patients receiving oxymorphone I.V. can be switched to Opana ER by giving 10 times patient's total daily I.V. oxymorphone dose as Opana ER in two equally divided doses or Opana (immediate-release) in four or six equally divided doses.

➤ **Preoperative medication, anesthesia, analgesia; analgesia during labor; relief of anxiety in patients with dyspnea** associated with pulmonary edema secondary to acute left ventricular dysfunction

Adults: Initially, 0.5 mg I.V. or 1 to 1.5 mg subcutaneously or I.M. every 4 to 6 hours as needed.

ADMINISTRATION

P.O.

❸ *Alert:* Starting doses of more than 20 mg aren't recommended because of potential serious adverse reactions.

● Take tablets 1 hour before or 2 hours after a meal.

Black Box Warning Don't crush, break, allow patient to chew, or dissolve extended-release tablets. ■

Black Box Warning Extended-release tablets aren't for as-needed use. ■

I.V.

▼ Assess respiratory status before giving. Withhold dose and notify prescriber for signs or symptoms of respiratory depression (decrease in respiratory rate or tidal volume, Cheyne-Stokes respirations, cyanosis).

▼ If necessary, dilute drug in NSS.

▼ Give drug by direct I.V. injection.

▼ **Incompatibilities:** None reported.

I.M.

● Rotate administration sites and document.

● Assess respiratory status before giving. Withhold dose and notify prescriber for respiratory depression (decreased respiratory rate or tidal volume, Cheyne-Stokes respirations, cyanosis).

Subcutaneous

● Rotate administration sites and document.

● Assess respiratory status before giving. Withhold dose and notify prescriber if respirations are shallow or rate falls below 12 breaths/minute.

ACTION

May bind with opioid receptors in the CNS, altering perception of and emotional response to pain.

Route	Onset	Peak	Duration
P.O.	Varies	Varies	Varies
I.V.	5–10 min	15–30 min	3–4 hr
I.M.	10–15 min	30–90 min	3–6 hr
Subcut.	10–20 min	60–90 min	3–6 hr

Half-life: Parenteral, unknown; extended-release tablets, 7 to 12 hours; immediate-release tablets, 3 to 12 hours.

ADVERSE REACTIONS

CNS: clouded sensorium, dizziness, euphoria, headache, sedation, somnolence, *seizures,* dysphoria, light-headedness, hallucinations, physical dependence, fever, restlessness, confusion.

CV: hypotension, *bradycardia,* palpitations, tachycardia, flushing.

EENT: blurred vision, diplopia, miosis.

GI: constipation, nausea, vomiting, ileus.

GU: urine retention.

Respiratory: *respiratory depression, laryngeal edema, bronchospasm.*

Skin: increased sweating, pruritus.

INTERACTIONS

Drug-drug. *Agonist or antagonist analgesics (mixed or partial):* May reduce analgesic effect or precipitate withdrawal symptoms. Don't use together.

Anticholinergics: May increase risk of urine retention or severe constipation, leading to paralytic ileus. Monitor patient for abdominal pain or distention.

Black Box Warning *Benzodiazepines, CNS depressants:* May cause slow or difficult breathing, sedation, and death. Avoid use together. If use together is necessary, limit dosage and duration of each drug to minimum necessary for desired effect. ■

Cimetidine: May increase CNS reactions. Monitor patient closely.

CNS depressants, general anesthetics, phenothiazines, sedative-hypnotics, TCAs: May cause additive effects. Use together with caution and reduce opioid dosage.

MAO inhibitors: May cause severe opioid potentiation. Don't use opioids if patient has received MAO inhibitors within 14 days. Avoid combination.

Propofol: May increase bradycardia risk. Monitor ECG closely.

❸ *Alert: Serotonergic drugs (amoxapine, antiemetics [dolasetron, granisetron,*

Reactions in bold italics are *life-threatening*. Interactions may have a *rapid onset* or a *delayed onset*.

ondansetron, palonosetron], antimigraine drugs, buspirone, cyclobenzaprine, dextromethorphan, linezolid, lithium, MAO inhibitors, maprotiline, methylene blue, mirtazapine, nefazodone, SNRIs, SSRIs, TCAs, trazodone, tryptophan, vilazodone): May increase risk of serotonin syndrome. Use together cautiously and monitor patient for serotonin syndrome.

Drug-lifestyle. **Black Box Warning** *Alcohol use:* Alcoholic beverages or medications containing alcohol may cause additive effects and result in a potentially fatal overdose of oxymorphone. Don't use together. ■

❸ Alert: *St. John's wort:* May increase risk of serotonin syndrome. Use together cautiously and monitor patient for serotonin syndrome.

EFFECTS ON LAB TEST RESULTS
• May increase amylase and lipase levels.

CONTRAINDICATIONS & CAUTIONS
• Contraindicated in patients hypersensitive to drug; in those with acute asthma attacks, severe respiratory depression, upper airway obstruction, or paralytic ileus; or in those with moderate to severe hepatic impairment.
• Contraindicated in patients with pulmonary edema caused by a respiratory irritant.

Black Box Warning Serious, life-threatening, or fatal respiratory depression may occur with use of extended-release oxymorphone. Monitor patient for respiratory depression, especially during initiation of therapy and after a dosage increase. Instruct patients to swallow oxymorphone extended-release tablets whole; crushing, dissolving, or chewing the tablets can cause rapid release and absorption of a potentially fatal oxymorphone dose. ■

Black Box Warning Opioids should only be prescribed with benzodiazepines or other CNS depressants to patients for whom alternative treatment options are inadequate. ■

Black Box Warning Accidental ingestion of even one dose of extended-release oxymorphone, especially by children, can result in a fatal oxymorphone overdose. ■

Black Box Warning Patients must be screened for increased risk of opioid abuse (personal or family history of substance abuse or mental illness) before being prescribed opioids. ■

❸ Alert: Drug may lead to rare but serious decrease in adrenal gland cortisol production.

❸ Alert: Drug may cause decreased sex hormone levels with long-term use.

❸ Alert: Patients are at increased risk for oversedation and respiratory depression if they snore or have a history of sleep apnea, haven't used opioids recently or are first-time opioid users, have increased opioid dosage requirements or opioid habituation, have received general anesthesia for longer lengths of time or received other sedating drugs, have preexisting pulmonary or cardiac disease, or have thoracic or other surgical incisions that may impair breathing. Monitor patients carefully.

• Use with caution in elderly or debilitated patients and in those with head injury, increased ICP, seizures, asthma, COPD, acute abdominal conditions, biliary tract disease (including pancreatitis), acute alcoholism, delirium tremens, prostatic hyperplasia, renal or mild hepatic impairment, urethral stricture, respiratory depression, hypothyroidism, Addison disease, and arrhythmias.

Dialyzable drug: Unknown.

⚠ Overdose S&S: Miosis, CNS depression, respiratory depression, apnea, flaccid skeletal muscles, bradycardia, hypotension, circulatory collapse, cardiac arrest, respiratory arrest, death.

PREGNANCY-LACTATION-REPRODUCTION
• Opioids cross placental barrier. During pregnancy, use minimum effective dose and only if benefit justifies risks to the fetus.
• Use cautiously during labor as uterine contractions may be affected.

Black Box Warning Prolonged use of extended-release oxymorphone during pregnancy can result in neonatal opioid withdrawal syndrome, which may be life-threatening if not recognized and treated and requires management according to protocols developed by neonatology experts. ■

❸ Alert: Use cautiously in breast-feeding women. Monitor infants for apnea and sedation.

NURSING CONSIDERATIONS

• Keep opioid antagonist (naloxone) and resuscitation equipment available.

Black Box Warning Monitor circulatory and respiratory status closely, especially within the first 24 to 72 hours of initiation of therapy or after a dosage increase. Withhold dose and notify prescriber for signs or symptoms of respiratory depression. ∎

Black Box Warning Assess patients identified as potential abusers; drug should be prescribed with extreme care. Drug may cause physical dependence and tolerance with long-term use. ∎

Black Box Warning Drug is potentially addictive. Chewing, crushing, snorting, or injecting it can lead to overdose and death. ∎

Black Box Warning All patients using opioids should be routinely monitored for signs and symptoms of misuse, abuse, and addiction. ∎

❸ *Alert:* Carefully monitor vital signs, pain level, respiratory status, and sedation level in all patients receiving opioids, especially those receiving I.V. drugs, even those given postoperatively.

❸ *Alert:* If patient is taking opioids with serotonergic drugs, watch for signs and symptoms of serotonin syndrome (agitation, hallucinations, rapid HR, fever, excessive sweating, shivering or shaking, muscle twitching or stiffness, trouble with coordination, nausea, vomiting, diarrhea), especially at start of treatment or dosage increases. Signs and symptoms may occur within several hours of coadministration but may also occur later, especially after dosage increase. Discontinue opioid, serotonergic drug, or both if serotonin syndrome is suspected.

❸ *Alert:* Monitor patient for signs and symptoms of adrenal insufficiency (nausea, vomiting, loss of appetite, fatigue, weakness, dizziness, low BP). Perform diagnostic testing if adrenal insufficiency is suspected. If adrenal insufficiency is confirmed, treat with corticosteroids and wean patient off opioids if appropriate. Discontinue corticosteroids when clinically appropriate.

❸ *Alert:* Monitor patient for signs and symptoms of decreased sex hormone levels (low libido, erectile dysfunction, amenorrhea, infertility). If signs and symptoms occur, evaluate patient and obtain laboratory testing.

• Use of this drug may worsen gallbladder pain.

• Drug isn't for mild pain. For better effect, give drug before patient has intense pain.

• Monitor bladder and bowel function. Patient may need a stimulant laxative.

❸ *Alert:* Closely monitor neonate whose mother received opioid analgesics during labor for signs and symptoms of respiratory depression. A specific opioid antagonist, such as naloxone or nalmefene, should be available for reversal of opioid-induced respiratory depression in a neonate.

• *Look alike–sound alike:* Don't confuse oxymorphone with oxymetholone or oxycodone.

PATIENT TEACHING

❸ *Alert:* Encourage patient to report all medications being taken, including prescription and OTC medications and supplements.

❸ *Alert:* Caution patient to immediately report signs and symptoms of serotonin syndrome, adrenal insufficiency, and decreased sex hormone levels.

• Instruct patient to ask for drug before pain is intense. Inform patient that extended-release tablets must be taken around the clock.

• Explain the assessment and monitoring process to patient and family. Instruct them to immediately report difficulty breathing or other signs of a potential adverse opioid-related reaction.

Black Box Warning Caution patient or caregiver of patient taking an opioid with a benzodiazepine, CNS depressant, or alcohol to seek immediate medical attention if patient experiences dizziness, light-headedness, extreme sleepiness, slowed or difficult breathing, or unresponsiveness. ∎

Black Box Warning If a pregnant woman requires an opioid for a prolonged period, advise her of the risk of neonatal opioid withdrawal syndrome; assure her that appropriate treatment will be available. ∎

Black Box Warning Inform patient that the use of oxymorphone, even when taken as recommended, can result in addiction, abuse, and misuse, which can lead to overdose or death. ∎

Reactions in bold italics are *life-threatening*. Interactions may have a *rapid onset* or a *delayed onset*.

• Instruct patient not to share oxymorphone with others and to take steps to protect oxymorphone from theft or misuse.

• When drug is used I.M. or I.V. after surgery, encourage patient to turn, cough, and deep-breathe and to use incentive spirometer to avoid lung problems.

• Caution ambulatory patient about getting out of bed or walking. Warn outpatient to avoid driving and other hazardous activities that require mental alertness until drug's CNS effects are known.

Black Box Warning Caution patient not to consume alcohol or take any prescription or OTC drug containing alcohol with oral form as this can lead to an overdose. ■

Black Box Warning Warn patient not to crush, break, chew, or dissolve extended-release tablets; doing so may lead to a fatal overdose. ■

• Tell patient to take tablets 1 hour before or 2 hours after a meal.

Black Box Warning Instruct patient to keep tablets in a child-resistant container and in a safe place out of the reach of children. Accidental ingestion by a child can result in death. In case of accidental ingestion, seek emergency medical help immediately. ■

SAFETY ALERT!

oxytocin (synthetic injection)
ox-i-TOE-sin

Pitocin

Therapeutic class: Oxytocics
Pharmacologic class: Exogenous hormones

AVAILABLE FORMS
Injection: 10 units/mL in 1-mL ampule; 1-mL, 3-mL, 10-mL, 30-mL, and 50-mL vials

INDICATIONS & DOSAGES
➤ **To induce or stimulate labor**
Adults: Initially, 10 units in 1,000 mL of D5W injection, lactated Ringer, or NSS I.V. infused at 0.5 to 2 milliunits/minute. Increase rate by 1 to 2 milliunits/minute at 30- to 60-minute intervals until normal

contraction pattern is established. Decrease rate when labor is firmly established. Rates exceeding 9 to 10 milliunits/minute are rarely required.

➤ **To reduce postpartum bleeding after expulsion of placenta**
Adults: 10 to 40 units in 1,000 mL of D5W injection, lactated Ringer, or NSS I.V. infused at rate needed to control bleeding, which is usually 20 to 40 milliunits/minute. Also, 10 units may be given I.M. after delivery of placenta.

➤ **Incomplete or inevitable abortion**
Adults: 10 units I.V. in 500 mL of NSS, lactated Ringer, or dextrose 5% in NSS. Infuse at 10 to 20 milliunits (20 to 40 drops)/minute. Don't exceed 30 units in 12 hours.

ADMINISTRATION
I.V.
▼ Never give drug simultaneously by more than one route.
▼ To induce or stimulate labor, dilute drug by adding 10 units to 1 L of NSS, lactated Ringer solution, or D5W solution.
▼ To produce intense uterine contractions and reduce postpartum bleeding, dilute drug by adding 10 units to 1,000 mL of NSS, lactated Ringer solution, or D5W solution.
▼ Don't give bolus injection; use an infusion pump. Give drug only by piggyback infusion so that it may be stopped without interrupting I.V. line.
▼ **Incompatibilities:** Pantoprazole.
I.M.
• Drug isn't recommended for routine I.M. use, but 10 units may be given I.M. after delivery of placenta to control postpartum uterine bleeding.
• Never give drug simultaneously by more than one route.

ACTION
Causes potent and selective stimulation of uterine and mammary gland smooth muscle.

Route	Onset	Peak	Duration
I.V.	Immediate	Unknown	1 hr
I.M.	3–5 min	Unknown	2–3 hr

Half-life: 3 to 5 minutes.

ADVERSE REACTIONS
Maternal

CNS: *subarachnoid hemorrhage, seizures, coma.*

CV: *arrhythmias,* hypertension, PVCs.

GI: nausea, vomiting.

GU: *abruptio placentae,* tetanic uterine contractions, *postpartum hemorrhage, uterine rupture,* impaired uterine blood flow, pelvic hematoma, increased uterine motility.

Hematologic: *afibrinogenemia, possibly related to postpartum bleeding.*

Other: *anaphylaxis, death from oxytocin-induced water intoxication,* hypersensitivity reactions.

Fetal

CNS: *infant brain damage, seizures.*

CV: *bradycardia, arrhythmias,* PVCs.

EENT: neonatal retinal hemorrhage.

Hepatic: neonatal jaundice.

Other: *low Apgar scores at 5 minutes, death.*

INTERACTIONS
Drug-drug. *Cyclopropane anesthetics:* May cause less pronounced bradycardia and hypotension. Use together cautiously.

Drugs that prolong QT interval: May increase risk of life-threatening cardiac arrhythmias, including torsades de pointes. Use together cautiously.

Misoprostol: May increase oxytocin adverse effects. Don't use together.

Vasoconstrictors: May cause severe hypertension if oxytocin is given within 3 to 4 hours of vasoconstrictor in patient receiving caudal block anesthetic. Avoid using together.

EFFECTS ON LAB TEST RESULTS
None reported.

CONTRAINDICATIONS & CAUTIONS
• Contraindicated in patients hypersensitive to drug.

• Contraindicated when vaginal delivery isn't advised (placenta previa, vasa previa, invasive cervical carcinoma, genital herpes), when cephalopelvic disproportion is present, or when delivery requires conversion, as in transverse lie.

• Contraindicated in fetal distress when delivery isn't imminent, in prematurity, in other obstetric emergencies, and in patients with severe toxemia or hypertonic uterine patterns.

• Use cautiously, if at all, in patients with invasive cervical cancer and in those with previous cervical or uterine surgery (including cesarean section), grand multiparity, uterine sepsis, traumatic delivery, or overdistended uterus.

⊙ Alert: May cause antidiuretic effect and risk of severe water intoxication, seizures, or death, particularly with large doses or when given by slow infusion over 24 hours and if patient is receiving fluids by mouth.

Dialyzable drug: Unknown.

⚠ Overdose S&S: Uterine hypersensitivity, tumultuous labor, uterine rupture, cervical and vaginal lacerations, postpartum hemorrhage, uteroplacental hypoperfusion, variable deceleration of fetal HR, fetal hypoxia, hypercapnia, perinatal hepatic necrosis, water intoxication, seizures, death.

PREGNANCY-LACTATION-REPRODUCTION
Black Box Warning Drug is only indicated for the medical, rather than the elective, induction of labor. ∎

• Use cautiously during first and second stages of labor because uterine hypertonicity, tetanic contraction, cervical laceration, uterine rupture, and maternal and fetal death have been reported.

• Drug wouldn't be expected to cause fetal abnormalities when used as indicated. Use cautiously in pregnant or breast-feeding women.

NURSING CONSIDERATIONS
⊙ Alert: All patients receiving oxytocin I.V. must be under continuous observation by trained personnel who have a thorough knowledge of the drug and are qualified to identify complications.

⊙ Alert: Discontinue oxytocin infusion immediately if uterine hyperactivity or fetal distress occurs. Administer oxygen to the mother. Mother and fetus must be evaluated by the responsible physician.

• Drug is used to induce or reinforce labor only when pelvis is known to be adequate, when vaginal delivery is indicated, when

---

Reactions in bold italics are *life-threatening*. Interactions may have a *rapid onset* or a *delayed onset*.

fetal maturity is assured, and when fetal position is favorable. Use drug only in hospital where critical care facilities and prescriber are immediately available.
• Monitor fluid intake and output. Antidiuretic effect may lead to fluid overload, seizures, and coma from water intoxication.
• Monitor and record uterine contractions, HR, BP, intrauterine pressure, fetal HR, and character of blood loss at least every 15 minutes.

PATIENT TEACHING
• Explain use and administration of drug to patient and family.
• Instruct patient to promptly report adverse reactions (site irritation, nausea, bleeding, blurred vision, difficulty speaking, wheezing, itching, swelling).

SAFETY ALERT!

paclitaxel
pak-leh-TAX-ell

Taxol

Therapeutic class: Antineoplastics
Pharmacologic class: Taxoids

AVAILABLE FORMS
Injection: 6 mg/mL in 5-mL, 16.7-mL, 25-mL, 50-mL vials

INDICATIONS & DOSAGES
➤ **AIDS-related Kaposi sarcoma**
Adults: 135 mg/m^2 I.V. over 3 hours every 3 weeks, or 100 mg/m^2 I.V. over 3 hours every 2 weeks.
Adjust-a-dose: Don't give drug if baseline or subsequent neutrophil counts are less than 1,000/mm^3. Reduce subsequent doses by 20% for patients who experience neutrophil count less than 500/mm^3 for 1 week or longer. Patient also may need reduction in dexamethasone premedication dose (10 mg P.O. instead of 20 mg P.O.) and start of a hematopoietic growth factor. For patients with hepatic impairment, reduce first 3-hour dose based on transaminase and bilirubin levels. If transaminase levels are less than 10 × ULN and bilirubin levels are 1.25 × ULN or less, give 175 mg/m^2. If

transaminase levels are less than 10 × ULN and bilirubin levels are 1.26 to 2 × ULN, give 135 mg/m^2. If transaminase levels are less than 10 × ULN and bilirubin levels are 2.01 to 5 × ULN, give 90 mg/m^2. If transaminase levels are 10 × ULN or more or bilirubin levels are more than 5 × ULN, don't use drug. For subsequent courses, base dosage adjustment on individual tolerance.
➤ **First-line and subsequent therapy for advanced ovarian cancer**
Adults (previously untreated): 175 mg/m^2 I.V. over 3 hours every 3 weeks, followed by cisplatin 75 mg/m^2; or, 135 mg/m^2 I.V. over 24 hours every 3 weeks, followed by cisplatin 75 mg/m^2, every 3 weeks.
Adults (previously treated): 135 or 175 mg/m^2 I.V. over 3 hours every 3 weeks.
Adjust-a-dose: For patients with hepatic impairment, reduce first 3-hour dose based on transaminase and bilirubin levels. If transaminase levels are less than 10 × ULN and bilirubin levels are 1.25 × ULN or less, give 175 mg/m^2. If transaminase levels are less than 10 × ULN and bilirubin levels are 1.26 to 2 × ULN, give 135 mg/m^2. If transaminase levels are less than 10 × ULN and bilirubin levels are 2.01 to 5 × ULN, give 90 mg/m^2. If transaminase levels are 10 × ULN or more or bilirubin levels are more than 5 × ULN, don't use drug. For subsequent courses, base dosage adjustment on individual tolerance.
➤ **Breast cancer after failure of combination chemotherapy for metastatic disease or relapse within 6 months of adjuvant chemotherapy (previous therapy should have included an anthracycline unless contraindicated); adjuvant therapy for node-positive breast cancer given sequentially to standard doxorubicin-containing combination chemotherapy**
Adults: 175 mg/m^2 I.V. over 3 hours every 3 weeks for four cycles.
Adjust-a-dose: For patients with hepatic impairment, reduce first 3-hour dose based on transaminase and bilirubin levels. If transaminase levels are less than 10 × ULN and bilirubin levels are 1.25 × ULN or less, give 175 mg/m^2. If transaminase levels are less than 10 × ULN and bilirubin levels are 1.26 to 2 × ULN, give 135 mg/m^2. If transaminase levels are less than 10 × ULN

P

and bilirubin levels are 2.01 to 5 × ULN, give 90 mg/m^2. If transaminase levels are 10 × ULN or more or bilirubin levels are more than 5 × ULN, don't use drug. For subsequent courses, base dosage adjustment on individual tolerance.

➤ **First treatment of advanced non–small-cell lung cancer for patients who aren't candidates for curative surgery or radiation**

Adults: 135 mg/m^2 I.V. infusion over 24 hours, followed by cisplatin 75 mg/m^2. Repeat cycle every 3 weeks.

Adjust-a-dose: Subsequent courses shouldn't be repeated until neutrophil count is at least 1,500/mm^3 and platelet count is at least 100,000/mm^3. Reduce subsequent doses by 20% for patients who experience neutrophil count less than 500/mm^3 for a week or longer or severe peripheral neuropathy. For patients with hepatic impairment, adjust doses for the first courses of therapy as follows: For first 24-hour infusion if transaminase levels are less than 2 × ULN and bilirubin levels are 1.5 mg/dL or less, give 135 mg/m^2. If transaminase levels are 2 to less than 10 × ULN and bilirubin levels are 1.5 mg/dL or less, give 100 mg/m^2. If transaminase levels are less than 10 × ULN and bilirubin levels are 1.6 to 7.5 mg/dL, give 50 mg/m^2. If transaminase levels are 10 × ULN or more, or bilirubin levels are more than 7.5 mg/dL, don't use drug.

ADMINISTRATION

I.V.

🜂 *Alert:* Preparing and giving drug may be mutagenic, teratogenic, or carcinogenic. Follow institutional safe handling and disposal policies to reduce risks. Mark all waste materials with CHEMOTHERAPY HAZARD labels.

▼ Prepare and store infusion solutions in glass containers. Undiluted concentrate shouldn't contact polyvinyl chloride I.V. bags or tubing.

▼ Dilute concentrate before infusion. Compatible solutions include NSS for injection, D$_5$W, 5% dextrose in NSS for injection, and 5% dextrose in lactated Ringer injection. Dilute to yield 0.3 to 1.2 mg/mL. Diluted solutions are stable for

27 hours at room temperature. Prepared solution may appear hazy.

▼ Give through polyethylene-lined administration sets, and use an in-line 0.22-micron filter.

🜂 *Alert:* Watch for irritation and infiltration; extravasation can cause tissue damage and necrosis. Administration of hyaluronidase may be needed.

▼ Closely monitor patient and vital signs during infusion, especially during the first hour.

▼ Store diluted solution in glass or polypropylene bottles, or use polypropylene or polyolefin bags.

▼ **Incompatibilities:** Amphotericin B, chlorpromazine, doxorubicin liposomal, hydroxyzine hydrochloride, methylprednisolone sodium succinate, mitoxantrone.

ACTION

Prevents depolymerization of cellular microtubules, inhibiting normal reorganization of microtubule network needed for mitosis and other vital cellular functions.

Route	Onset	Peak	Duration
I.V.	Unknown	Unknown	Unknown

Half-life: 13 to 53 hours.

ADVERSE REACTIONS

CNS: peripheral neuropathy, asthenia.
CV: *bradycardia,* hypotension, abnormal ECG.
GI: nausea, vomiting, diarrhea, mucositis.
Hematologic: *neutropenia, leukopenia, thrombocytopenia,* anemia, *bleeding.*
Musculoskeletal: myalgia, arthralgia.
Skin: alopecia, cellulitis and phlebitis at injection site.
Other: hypersensitivity reactions, *anaphylaxis,* infections.

INTERACTIONS

Drug-drug. *Carbamazepine, phenobarbital:* May increase metabolism and may decrease paclitaxel levels. Use together cautiously.
Cisplatin: May cause additive myelosuppressive effects. Give paclitaxel before cisplatin.

Doxorubicin: May increase plasma levels of doxorubicin and its active metabolite, doxorubicinol. Use together cautiously.
*Drugs that inhibit CYP450 (cyclosporine, dexamethasone, diazepam, etoposide, felodipine, **ketoconazole**, quinidine, retinoic acid, teniposide, testosterone, verapamil, vincristine):* May increase paclitaxel level. Monitor patient for toxicity.
Live-virus vaccines: May increase risk of vaccine-induced adverse reactions. Use together isn't recommended. Patients with malignancies who are in remission can receive live-virus vaccines 3 months after completion of chemotherapy.

EFFECTS ON LAB TEST RESULTS
• May increase alkaline phosphatase, AST, bilirubin, and triglyceride levels.
• May decrease Hb level and neutrophil, WBC, and platelet counts.

CONTRAINDICATIONS & CAUTIONS
• Contraindicated in patients hypersensitive to drug or polyoxyethylated castor oil (also known as Cremophor EL, a vehicle used in drug solution).
Black Box Warning Contraindicated in those with baseline neutrophil counts below 1,500/mm^3 and platelet counts below 100,000/mm^3, or in those with AIDS-related Kaposi sarcoma with baseline neutrophil counts below 1,000/mm^3. ■
• Use cautiously in patients with hepatic impairment.
Dialyzable drug: No.
⚠ **Overdose S&S:** Bone marrow suppression, sensory neurotoxicity, mucositis, acute ethanol toxicity (in children), CNS toxicity (in children).

PREGNANCY-LACTATION-REPRODUCTION
• There are no adequate studies in pregnant women and drug may cause fetal harm. Safe use during pregnancy hasn't been established.
• Women of childbearing potential should avoid becoming pregnant during therapy. Men shouldn't father a child during therapy.
• It isn't known if drug appears in breast milk. Patient should discontinue breast-feeding or discontinue drug.

NURSING CONSIDERATIONS
Black Box Warning Administer drug under the supervision of a physician experienced with cancer chemotherapeutic agents. ■
• Patient may experience peripheral neuropathies, which may be cumulative and dose related. Patients with severe symptoms may need dosage reduction.
Black Box Warning To reduce risk or severity of hypersensitivity, patients must receive pretreatment with corticosteroids, such as dexamethasone, and antihistamines. Both H$_1$-receptor antagonists, such as diphenhydramine, and H$_2$-receptor antagonists, such as cimetidine or ranitidine, may be used. Fatal reactions have occurred despite premedication. ■
Black Box Warning Monitor blood counts before therapy is initiated and often during therapy. Bone marrow toxicity is the most common and dose-limiting toxicity. Institute bleeding precautions, as indicated. ■
• Avoid all I.M. injections when platelet count is below 50,000/mm^3.
• If patient develops significant cardiac conduction abnormalities, use indicated therapy and continuous cardiac monitoring during therapy and subsequent infusions.
❸ *Alert:* When indicated, cisplatin dose should follow dose of paclitaxel.
• *Look alike–sound alike:* Don't confuse paclitaxel with paroxetine.

PATIENT TEACHING
• Advise patient to report any pain or burning at site of injection during or after administration.
• Urge patient to report all adverse reactions and to watch for fever, sore throat, fatigue, easy bruising, nosebleeds, bleeding gums, or tarry stools. Tell patient to take temperature daily.
• Teach patient symptoms of peripheral neuropathy, such as a tingling or burning sensation or numbness in limbs, and to report these symptoms immediately.
• Warn patient that reversible hair loss will probably occur.
• Caution female patient of childbearing potential to avoid becoming pregnant during therapy. Recommend that she consult prescriber before becoming pregnant.

P

paclitaxel protein-bound particles
pak-leh-TAX-ell

Abraxane

Therapeutic class: Antineoplastics
Pharmacologic class: Taxoids

AVAILABLE FORMS
Lyophilized powder for injection: 100 mg in single-use vials

INDICATIONS & DOSAGES
➤ **Metastatic breast cancer after failure of combination chemotherapy or relapse within 6 months of adjuvant chemotherapy (previous therapy should have included an anthracycline unless clinically contraindicated at the time)**
Adults: 260 mg/m^2 I.V. over 30 minutes every 3 weeks.
Adjust-a-dose: For patients with severe sensory neuropathy or a neutrophil count less than 500/mm^3 for a week or longer, reduce dose to 220 mg/m^2. For recurring severe sensory neuropathy or severe neutropenia, reduce dose to 180 mg/m^2. For grade 3 (severe) sensory neuropathy, stop drug until condition improves to grade 1 or 2 (mild to moderate); then restart at a reduced dose for the rest of treatment.

For patients with moderate hepatic impairment (serum bilirubin level greater than 1.5 to 3 × ULN and AST level 1 to 10 × ULN) and patients with severe hepatic impairment (serum bilirubin level greater than 3 to 5 × ULN and AST level 1 to 10 × ULN), recommended dosage is 200 mg/m^2/dose initially; may increase dosage to 260 mg/m^2/dose in subsequent courses if patient tolerates reduced dosage for two cycles. Don't give to patients with very severe hepatic impairment (serum bilirubin level more than 5 × ULN or AST level more than 10 × ULN).
➤ **Non-small-cell lung cancer (NSCLC) as first-line treatment in combination with carboplatin in patients who aren't candidates for surgery or radiation therapy**

Adults: 100 mg/m^2 I.V. over 30 minutes on days 1, 8, and 15 of each 21-day cycle. Give carboplatin immediately after paclitaxel protein-bound particles dose on day 1 of each 21-day cycle. Refer to manufacturer's instructions for carboplatin dosage.
Adjust-a-dose: For patients with moderate hepatic impairment (serum bilirubin level greater than 1.5 to 3 × ULN and AST level 1 to 10 × ULN) and severe hepatic impairment (serum bilirubin level greater than 3 to 5 × ULN and AST level 1 to 10 × ULN), recommended dosage is 80 mg/m^2/dose; may increase dosage to 100 mg/m^2/dose in subsequent courses if patient tolerates reduced dosage for two cycles. Don't give to patients with very severe hepatic impairment (serum bilirubin level more than 5 × ULN or AST level more than 10 × ULN).

Don't administer paclitaxel on day 1 of a cycle until ANC is at least 1,500/mm^3 and platelet count is at least 100,000/mm^3. In patients who develop severe neutropenia or thrombocytopenia, withhold treatment until counts recover to an ANC of at least 1,500/mm^3 and platelet count of at least 100,000/mm^3 on day 1 or to an ANC of at least 500/mm^3 and platelet count of at least 50,000/mm^3 on days 8 or 15 of the cycle. Upon resumption of dosing, permanently reduce paclitaxel and carboplatin doses per manufacturer's instructions.

Withhold paclitaxel for grade 3 to 4 peripheral neuropathy. Resume paclitaxel and carboplatin at reduced doses when peripheral neuropathy improves to grade 1 or completely resolves.
➤ **Metastatic pancreatic adenocarcinoma as first-line treatment in combination with gemcitabine**
Adults: 125 mg/m^2 I.V. over 30 to 40 minutes on days 1, 8, and 15 of each 28-day cycle. Give gemcitabine 1,000 mg/m^2 I.V. immediately after each paclitaxel dose.
Adjust-a-dose: For patients with mild hepatic impairment (bilirubin level greater than ULN to 1.5 × ULN and AST less than 10 × ULN), no dosage adjustment is needed. Drug isn't recommended for patients with moderate to severe hepatic impairment.

If necessary, dose level reductions for paclitaxel and gemcitabine are as follows: First dose level reduction consists

---

of paclitaxel 100 mg/m² and gemcitabine 800 mg/m²; second dose level reduction consists of paclitaxel 75 mg/m² and gemcitabine to 600 mg/m². If further dosage reductions are needed, discontinue both drugs.

On day 1, if ANC is less than 1,500/mm³ or platelet count is less than 100,000/mm³, delay doses until recovery. On day 8, if ANC is 500 to less than 1,000/mm³ or platelet count is 50,000 to less than 75,000/mm³, reduce one dose level. If day 8 ANC is less than 500/mm³ or platelet count is less than 50,000/mm³, withhold doses. On day 15, if day 8 doses were given or reduced and ANC is 500 to less than 1,000/mm³, or platelet count is 50,000 to less than 75,000/mm³, reduce one dose level from day 8; if ANC is less than 500/mm³ or platelet count is less than 50,000/mm³, withhold doses. On day 15, if day 8 doses were withheld and ANC is 1,000/mm³ or more or platelet count is 75,000/mm³ or more, reduce one dose level from day 1; if ANC is 500 to less than 1,000/mm³ or platelet count is 50,000 to less than 75,000/mm³, reduce two dose levels from day 1; if ANC is less than 500/mm³ or platelet count is less than 50,000/mm³, withhold doses.

For grade 3 or 4 febrile neutropenia, withhold paclitaxel and gemcitabine doses until fever resolves and ANC is 1,500/mm³ or more; then resume at next lower dose level. For grade 3 or 4 peripheral neuropathy, withhold paclitaxel until improvement to grade 1 or better; then resume at next lower dose level, continuing gemcitabine without dosage reduction. For grade 2 or 3 cutaneous toxicity, reduce paclitaxel and gemcitabine doses to next lower dose level; discontinue treatment if toxicity persists. For grade 3 mucositis or diarrhea, withhold both drugs until improvement to grade 1 or better; then resume at next lower dose level.

ADMINISTRATION

I.V.

▼ Because of drug's cytotoxicity, handle it cautiously and wear gloves. If drug contacts skin, wash area thoroughly with soap and water. If drug contacts mucous membranes, flush thoroughly with water.

▼ Reconstitute the vial with 20 mL of NSS to yield 5 mg/mL of drug. Direct the stream slowly, over at least 1 minute, onto the inside wall of the vial to avoid foaming. Let the vial sit for 5 minutes to ensure proper wetting of the powder. Gently swirl or turn the vial for at least 2 minutes until completely dissolved. If foaming occurs, let the solution stand for 15 minutes for the foam to subside. If particles are visible, gently invert the vial again to ensure complete resuspension. The solution should appear milky and uniform. Inject the correct dose into an empty polyvinyl chloride-type I.V. bag and use immediately.

▼ Give drug over 30 minutes.

▼ The suspension for infusion, when prepared in an infusion bag, can be stored at 36° to 46° F (2° to 8° C), protected from bright light, for up to 24 hours.

▼ Store unopened vials at room temperature in the original package. Store reconstituted vials at 36° to 46° F (2° to 8° C) for up to 24 hours, protected from light.

▼ The total combined refrigerated storage time of reconstituted solution in vial and infusion bag is 24 hours. This may be followed by storage in infusion bag at ambient temperature and lighting conditions for a maximum of 4 hours.

▼ **Incompatibilities:** None known.

ACTION

Prevents depolymerization of cellular microtubules, inhibiting reorganization of the microtubule network and disrupting mitosis and other vital cell functions.

Route	Onset	Peak	Duration
I.V.	Unknown	Unknown	Unknown

Half-life: 13 to 27 hours.

ADVERSE REACTIONS

CNS: asthenia, sensory neuropathy.
CV: abnormal ECG, edema, *cardiac arrest,* chest pain, *supraventricular tachycardia, thromboembolism,* thrombosis, hypertension, hypotension.
EENT: visual disturbances.
GI: diarrhea, nausea, oral candidiasis, vomiting, intestinal obstruction, *ischemic colitis, pancreatitis, perforation,* mucositis.

P

GU: *renal failure.*
Hematologic: anemia, *neutropenia, thrombocytopenia, bleeding, myelosuppression.*
Hepatic: *hepatic encephalopathy, hepatic necrosis.*
Musculoskeletal: arthralgia, myalgia.
Respiratory: *PE,* cough, dyspnea, pneumonia, respiratory tract infection.
Skin: alopecia, injection-site reactions.
Other: infections, hypersensitivity reactions.

INTERACTIONS

Drug-drug. *Clozapine:* May increase risk of agranulocytosis. Avoid use together.
CYP450 inhibitors: May decrease paclitaxel metabolism. Use together cautiously.
Live-virus vaccines: May increase vaccine-related adverse effects. Avoid use together. Don't give vaccines for at least 3 months after immunosuppressants.
Vaccines (inactivated): May diminish vaccine therapeutic effects. Monitor therapy.

EFFECTS ON LAB TEST RESULTS

• May increase alkaline phosphatase, AST, bilirubin, creatinine, and GGT levels. May decrease Hb level.
• May decrease neutrophil and platelet counts.

CONTRAINDICATIONS & CAUTIONS

Black Box Warning Contraindicated in patients with baseline neutrophil count of less than 1,500/mm^3. ∎
• Contraindicated in patients hypersensitive to drug or its components; severe and sometimes fatal hypersensitivity reactions can occur. Don't rechallenge patients who experience a hypersensitivity reaction.
• Don't repeat dose until neutrophil counts recover to more than 1,500/mm^3 and platelet count recovers to more than 100,000/mm^3.
• Use hasn't been studied in patients with creatinine level over 2 mg/dL or bilirubin level over 1.5 mg/dL.
Dialyzable drug: Unknown.
⚠ *Overdose S&S:* Bone marrow suppression, sensory neurotoxicity, acute ethanol toxicity (in children), CNS toxicity (in children).

PREGNANCY-LACTATION-REPRODUCTION

• Drug may cause fetal harm. Women of childbearing potential should avoid becoming pregnant during therapy. Males shouldn't father a child during therapy.
• Drug appears in breast milk. Consider discontinuing breast-feeding or drug.

NURSING CONSIDERATIONS

⊘ *Alert:* Give only under supervision of practitioner experienced in using chemotherapy in a facility that can manage complications of therapy.
Black Box Warning Don't substitute Abraxane for other forms of paclitaxel. ∎
Black Box Warning Monitor CBC frequently to evaluate for neutropenia, which may be severe and may result in infection. ∎
⊘ *Alert:* Obtain CBC before dosing on day 1 for metastatic breast cancer and before days 1, 8, and 15 for NSCLC or pancreatic cancer.
⊘ *Alert:* If patient becomes febrile (regardless of ANC), initiate treatment with broad-spectrum antibiotics.
⊘ *Alert:* Watch for pneumonitis in patients receiving drug in combination with gemcitabine. If pneumonitis is suspected, interrupt treatment. If pneumonitis is diagnosed, permanently discontinue treatment with paclitaxel and gemcitabine.
• Dosage reductions or drug discontinuation may be needed based on severe hematologic, neurologic, cutaneous, or GI toxicities.
• Because drug contains human albumin, a remote risk exists of transmitting viruses and Creutzfeldt-Jakob disease.
• Assess patient for symptoms of sensory neuropathy and severe neutropenia.
• Monitor LFT and renal function test results.
• Monitor infusion site closely.

PATIENT TEACHING

• Warn patient that alopecia commonly occurs but is reversible after therapy.
• Teach patient to recognize signs of neuropathy, such as tingling, burning, and numbness in arms and legs.
• Tell patient to report fever or other signs of infection, severe abdominal pain, or severe diarrhea.

• Advise patient to contact prescriber if nausea and vomiting persist or interfere with adequate nutrition. Reassure patient that an antiemetic can be prescribed.

• Explain that many patients experience weakness and fatigue, so it's important to rest. Tiredness, paleness, and shortness of breath may result from low blood counts, and patient may need a transfusion.

• To reduce or prevent mouth sores, remind patient to perform proper oral hygiene.

• Tell female patient to avoid becoming pregnant and not to breast-feed. Advise male patient to avoid fathering a child during therapy.

SAFETY ALERT!

palbociclib
pal-boe-SYE-klib

Ibrance

Therapeutic class: Antineoplastics
Pharmacologic class: Kinase inhibitors

AVAILABLE FORMS
Capsules ⓞ: 75 mg, 100 mg, 125 mg

INDICATIONS & DOSAGES
➤ **Postmenopausal women with estrogen receptor (ER)–positive, human epidermal growth factor receptor 2 (HER2)–negative metastatic breast cancer, as initial endocrine-based therapy in combination with letrozole or in combination with fulvestrant in women with disease progression after endocrine therapy**
Adults: 125 mg P.O. daily for 21 consecutive days followed by 7 days off, in combination with continuous letrozole 2.5 mg P.O. daily throughout the 28-day cycle.
Adjust-a-dose: First dosage reduction for adverse reactions is to 100 mg/day; second dosage reduction is to 75 mg/day. If further dosage reduction is needed, discontinue treatment. For grade 3 hematologic toxicity, no dosage reduction is needed; however, consider repeating CBC monitoring 1 week later and withhold start of next cycle until recovery to grade 2 or better. For grade 3 hematologic toxicity with ANC less than 500 to 1,000/mm³, temperature of 101.3° F

(38.5° C) or more, or infection, withhold drug and delay start of next cycle until recovery to grade 2 or better with ANC 1,000/mm³ or more; then resume at next lower dose. For grade 4 hematologic toxicity, except lymphopenia unless associated with clinical events such as opportunistic infections, withhold drug and start of next cycle until recovery to grade 2 or better; then resume at next lower dose. For non-hematologic toxicities of grade 3 or greater and persisting despite medical treatment, withhold drug until symptoms resolve to grade 1 or less, or to grade 2 if toxicity isn't considered a safety risk for patient; then resume at next lower dose.

ADMINISTRATION
P.O.
• Drug is hazardous; use appropriate safe handling and disposal precautions.
• Give capsule whole with food.
• Ensure patient doesn't ingest capsule that's broken, cracked, or otherwise not intact.
• Give dose at same time each day.
• If patient vomits after taking a dose or misses a dose, don't give an additional dose that day; patient should take next prescribed dose at the usual time.

ACTION
Inhibits cyclin-dependent kinase 4 and 6. Reduces cellular proliferation of ER-positive breast cancer cell line by blocking progression of cell from G_1 to S phase of the cell cycle, resulting in decreased phosphorylation and decreased tumor growth.

Route	Onset	Peak	Duration
P.O.	N/A	6–12 hr	N/A

Half-life: 24 to 34 hours.

ADVERSE REACTIONS
CNS: peripheral neuropathy, asthenia, fatigue.
EENT: epistaxis.
GI: decreased appetite, stomatitis, nausea, diarrhea, vomiting.
Hematologic: *neutropenia, leukopenia,* anemia, *thrombocytopenia.*
Respiratory: URI, *PE.*
Skin: alopecia.

P

INTERACTIONS

Drug-drug. *Alfentanil, cyclosporine, dihydroergotamine, ergotamine, everolimus, fentanyl, midazolam, pimozide, quinidine, sirolimus, tacrolimus:* May increase concentrations of these drugs. Dosages of these drugs may need to be decreased.

Strong or moderate CYP3A inducers (bosentan, carbamazepine, efavirenz, etravirine, modafinil, nafcillin, phenytoin, rifampin): May decrease palbociclib concentration. Avoid concurrent use.

Strong CYP3A inhibitors (clarithromycin, indinavir, itraconazole, ketoconazole, lopinavir–ritonavir, nefazodone, nelfinavir, posaconazole, ritonavir, saquinavir, telithromycin, verapamil, voriconazole): May increase palbociclib concentration. Avoid use together. If use together can't be avoided, decrease palbociclib dosage to 75 mg daily. If strong inhibitor is discontinued, increase palbociclib dosage after three to five half-lives have passed from CYP3A dose.

Drug-herb. *St. John's wort:* May decrease palbociclib concentration. Discourage use together.

Drug-food. *Grapefruit, grapefruit juice:* May increase palbociclib concentration. Discourage use together.

EFFECTS ON LAB TEST RESULTS

● May decrease Hb level and WBC, neutrophil, lymphocyte, and platelet counts.

CONTRAINDICATIONS & CAUTIONS

● Contraindicated in patients hypersensitive to drug or its components.
● May cause neutropenia and risk of infection.
● May increase risk of PE.
● Drug hasn't been studied in children.
● Use cautiously in elderly patients, who may experience a greater sensitivity to drug's effects.
Dialyzable drug: Unknown.

PREGNANCY-LACTATION-REPRODUCTION

● Drug has caused fetal harm in animal studies and is contraindicated in pregnant women. Women of childbearing potential should use effective contraception during treatment and for at least 2 weeks after last dose.
● It isn't known if drug appears in breast milk. Contraindicated in breast-feeding women.
● Although drug isn't indicated for men, animal studies suggest drug may affect male fertility.

NURSING CONSIDERATIONS

● Monitor CBC before start of therapy, at beginning of each cycle, on day 14 of first two cycles, and as clinically indicated. Interrupt therapy and adjust dosage as necessary.
● Monitor patient for myelosuppression or infection (fever, chills, dizziness, shortness of breath, weakness, increased tendency to bleed or bruise); treat appropriately.
● Monitor patient for PE (shortness of breath, chest pain, tachypnea, tachycardia); treat appropriately.

PATIENT TEACHING

● Instruct patient to take with food and to swallow capsules whole.
● Advise patient that if vomiting occurs after taking a dose or if patient misses a dose not to make it up but to take the next prescribed dose at the usual time.
● Teach patient to report signs and symptoms of decreased bone marrow function and infection, such as fever, chills, dizziness, and increased tendency to bleed or bruise.
● Tell patient to report shortness of breath, chest pain, or rapid heartbeat.
● Warn female patient to avoid becoming pregnant and to use effective contraception during therapy and for at least 2 weeks after last dose. Advise patient to contact prescriber as soon as pregnancy occurs or is suspected.
● Instruct patient to tell prescriber of all medications he or she is taking, including prescription and OTC drugs and herbal products.
● Caution patient to avoid grapefruit and grapefruit juice.

paliperidone
pahl-ee-PEHR-ih-dohn

Invega

paliperidone palmitate
Invega Sustenna, Invega Trinza

Therapeutic class: Antipsychotics
Pharmacologic class: Benzisoxazole derivatives

AVAILABLE FORMS
Injection: 39 mg, 78 mg, 117 mg, 156 mg, 234 mg, 273 mg, 410 mg, 546 mg, 819 mg
Tablets (extended-release) ⓓ: 1.5 mg, 3 mg, 6 mg, 9 mg

INDICATIONS & DOSAGES
Adjust-a-dose (for all indications): In patients with CrCl of 50 to 80 mL/minute, initial dosage is 3 mg P.O. once daily and maximum dosage is 6 mg once daily; for patients with CrCl of 10 to 49 mL/minute, initial dosage is 1.5 mg P.O. once daily and maximum dosage is 3 mg once daily. If using injectable form (Invega Sustenna) and CrCl is 50 to 80 mL/minute, give 156 mg I.M. on day 1 and 117 mg I.M. 1 week later, followed by monthly injections of 78 mg I.M. If using injectable 3-month form (Invega Trinza) and CrCl is 50 to less than 80 mL/minute, adjust dosage and stabilize patient using the monthly I.M. injection, then transition to the 3-month I.M. injection.

➤ **Schizophrenia and schizoaffective disorder**
Adults: 6 mg P.O. once daily in the morning; may increase or decrease dose in 3-mg increments to a range of 3 to 12 mg daily; maximum dose is 12 mg/day. Or, 234 mg I.M. on treatment day 1 and 156 mg I.M. 1 week later, both administered in deltoid muscle. Recommended maintenance dosage is 117 mg I.M. monthly (range, 39 to 234 mg based on tolerability and efficacy). Adjustments may be made monthly. Maximum recommended monthly dose is 234 mg. See manufacturer's instructions for missed dosage schedules.

Use 3-month I.M. paliperidone only after monthly I.M. paliperidone (Invega Sustenna) has been established as adequate treatment for at least 4 months. The last two doses of monthly I.M. paliperidone should be the same dosage strength before starting 3-month I.M. paliperidone (Invega Trinza). Initiate 3-month I.M. paliperidone when next monthly I.M. paliperidone dose is scheduled. Base 3-month dose on the previous monthly dose, using the equivalent 3.5 times higher dose. May adjust dosage of 3-month paliperidone every 3 months in increments ranging from 273 to 819 mg based on response and tolerability. Because of long-acting nature of Invega Trinza, patient's response to an adjusted dose may not be apparent for several months.

➤ **Schizophrenia**
Adolescents ages 12 to 17: Initially, 3 mg P.O. daily. Dosage may be increased by 3 mg/day every 5 days based on clinical response. Maximum dose is 12 mg/day for patients weighing 51 kg or more and 6 mg/day for patients weighing less than 51 kg.

ADMINISTRATION
P.O.
• Give with or without food.
• Don't crush or break or allow patient to chew tablets.
I.M.
• Inspect for particulate matter and discoloration.
• For Invega Sustenna, shake syringe vigorously for at least 10 seconds to ensure a homogenous suspension before administration.
• For Invega Trinza, shake syringe vigorously for at least 15 seconds within 5 minutes before administration to ensure a homogenous suspension before administration.
• Inject slowly and deeply into muscle.
• Don't give I.V. or subcutaneously.
• Administer first two doses of Invega Sustenna into deltoid muscle. After second dose, monthly maintenance doses can be given in deltoid or gluteal muscle.
• Injection is for single use only. Don't administer dose in divided injections.
• May give monthly or 3-month I.M. paliperidone maintenance doses within

P

7 days before or after next monthly dose date.

ACTION

May antagonize both central dopamine (D_2) and serotonin type 2 receptors, as well as $alpha_1$, $alpha_2$, and H_1 receptors. Drug is a major active metabolite of risperidone.

Route	Onset	Peak	Duration
P.O.	Unknown	24 hr	Unknown
I.M.	24 hr	13 days	126 days

Half-life: 23 hours; 25 to 49 days for I.M.

ADVERSE REACTIONS

CNS: akathisia, headache, parkinsonism, somnolence, anxiety, asthenia, dizziness, dystonia, extrapyramidal disorder, fatigue, hypertonia, pyrexia, tremor, dyskinesia, hyperkinesia, insomnia, *suicidal ideation.*
CV: abnormal T waves, hypertension, orthostatic hypotension, palpitations, sinus arrhythmia, tachycardia, *AV block,* bundle branch block, *prolonged QTc interval.*
EENT: blurred vision, nasopharyngitis.
GI: abdominal pain, dry mouth, dyspepsia, nausea, salivary hypersecretion, vomiting, diarrhea, constipation, dry mouth.
Metabolic: blood insulin increases, hyperprolactinemia.
Musculoskeletal: back pain, extremity pain, musculoskeletal stiffness, myalgia.
Respiratory: cough, URI.
Skin: injection-site reaction.

INTERACTIONS

Drug-drug. *Anticholinergics:* May worsen side effects. Use cautiously together.
Antihypertensives: May worsen orthostatic hypotension. Avoid using together.
Centrally acting drugs: May worsen CNS side effects. Use cautiously together.
Drugs that prolong QTc interval, such as antiarrhythmics (amiodarone, procainamide, quinidine, sotalol), antipsychotics (chlorpromazine, thioridazine), quinolone antibiotics (moxifloxacin): May further prolong QTc interval. Avoid using together.
Levodopa, other dopamine agonists: May antagonize effects of these drugs. Use cautiously together.

Black Box Warning *Opioids:* May cause slow or difficult breathing, sedation, and death. Avoid use together. If use together is necessary, limit dosage and duration of each drug to minimum necessary for desired effect. ■
Risperidone: May increase toxic effects of paliperidone. Use alternative combination if possible.
Serotonin modulators: May increase risk of neuroleptic malignant syndrome and serotonin syndrome. Monitor therapy.
Strong CYP3A and P-glycoprotein inducers: May decrease paliperidone concentration. Dosage may need to be increased or decreased depending on use. Avoid use of Invega Trinza during 3-month dosing interval, if possible.
Drug-herb. *St. John's wort:* May increase serum concentration of paliperidone. Consider therapy modification.
Drug-lifestyle. *Alcohol use:* May worsen CNS side effects. Discourage use together.

EFFECTS ON LAB TEST RESULTS

● May increase insulin and prolactin levels.

CONTRAINDICATIONS & CAUTIONS

● Contraindicated in patients hypersensitive to paliperidone or risperidone.
Black Box Warning Elderly patients with dementia-related psychosis treated with atypical or conventional antipsychotics are at increased risk for death. Antipsychotics aren't approved for the treatment of dementia-related psychosis. ■
Black Box Warning Opioids should only be prescribed with benzodiazepines or other CNS depressants to patients for whom alternative treatment options are inadequate. ■
● Contraindicated in patients with congenital long QT syndrome or history of cardiac arrhythmias.
● Contraindicated in patients with preexisting severe GI narrowing (esophageal motility disorders, small-bowel inflammatory disease, short gut syndrome).
● Use cautiously in patients with a history of seizures, diabetes, or Parkinson disease; in those at risk for aspiration pneumonia or impaired temperature regulation; and in those with bradycardia, hypokalemia,

---

hypomagnesemia, CV disease, cerebrovascular disease, dehydration, or hypovolemia.

• Use cautiously in patients taking antihypertensives and drugs that lower the seizure threshold.

• Use cautiously in patients with history of suicide attempts.

• Rare cases of priapism (requiring surgery) have been reported.

Dialyzable drug: Unknown.

⚠ *Overdose S&S:* Extrapyramidal symptoms, unsteady gait, drowsiness, sedation, tachycardia, hypotension, prolonged QT interval.

PREGNANCY-LACTATION-REPRODUCTION

• Use in pregnancy only if potential benefit justifies fetal risk.

• Pregnant women exposed to drug should enroll in the National Pregnancy Registry for Atypical Antipsychotics (1-866-961-2388).

⟐ *Alert:* Neonates exposed to antipsychotics during the third trimester are at increased risk for developing extrapyramidal signs and symptoms (repetitive muscle movements of the face and body) and withdrawal signs and symptoms (agitation, abnormally increased or decreased muscle tone, tremors, sleepiness, severe difficulty breathing, difficulty feeding) after delivery.

• Drug appears in breast milk. Patient should discontinue breast-feeding or discontinue drug.

NURSING CONSIDERATIONS

• Establish tolerability with oral paliperidone or oral risperidone before initiating treatment with paliperidone injection.

⟐ *Alert:* Monitor patient for atypical ventricular tachycardia, such as torsades de pointes, and ECG changes, particularly lengthening of the QT interval.

• Obtain baseline BP before starting therapy, and monitor BP regularly. Watch for orthostatic hypotension.

⟐ *Alert:* Watch for evidence of neuroleptic malignant syndrome (extrapyramidal effects, hyperthermia, autonomic disturbance), which is rare but deadly.

• Monitor patient for tardive dyskinesia; it may disappear spontaneously or persist for life despite discontinuing drug. Seek

smallest dosage and shortest duration of treatment that produce a satisfactory clinical response. Periodically reassess need for continued treatment.

⟐ *Alert:* Drug may cause hyperglycemia. Monitor patient with diabetes regularly. In patient with risk factors for diabetes, obtain fasting blood glucose test results at baseline and periodically.

• Monitor patient for seizure activity, especially if patient has conditions that lower the seizure threshold.

• Monitor patient for dysphagia that can lead to aspiration and aspiration pneumonia.

• Monitor patient for abnormal body temperature regulation, especially if he exercises, is exposed to extreme heat, takes anticholinergics, or is dehydrated.

• Monitor patient for somnolence and sedation. Antipsychotics, including paliperidone, have the potential to impair judgment, thinking, or motor skills.

• Dispense lowest appropriate quantity of drug, to reduce risk of overdose.

PATIENT TEACHING

Black Box Warning Caution patient or caregiver of patient taking an opioid with a benzodiazepine, CNS depressant, or alcohol to seek immediate medical attention if patient experiences dizziness, light-headedness, extreme sleepiness, slowed or difficult breathing, or unresponsiveness. ∎

• Tell patient that remains of the tablet may appear in feces.

• Tell patient to swallow whole with liquids and not to chew, crush, or break tablets.

• Instruct patient not to perform activities that require mental alertness until effects of drug are known.

• Warn patient to use caution in performing excessively strenuous activities because his body temperature may be disrupted.

• Advise patient that drug may lower BP and to change positions slowly.

• Advise patient to seek medical attention if he experiences an erection lasting more than 4 hours.

• Instruct patient to contact prescriber before taking any other drugs to avoid potential interactions.

• Advise patient to avoid alcohol while taking this medication.

P

• Advise patient to contact prescriber if she becomes pregnant or wants to breast-feed.

palonosetron hydrochloride
pal-on-OS-e-tron

Aloxi

Therapeutic class: Antiemetics
Pharmacologic class: Selective serotonin (5-HT$_3$) receptor antagonists

AVAILABLE FORMS
Injection: 0.25 mg in 5-mL single-use vial

INDICATIONS & DOSAGES
➤ **To prevent acute nausea and vomiting from moderately or highly emetogenic chemotherapy or delayed nausea and vomiting from moderately emetogenic chemotherapy**
Adults: 0.25 mg given I.V. over 30 seconds, 30 minutes before chemotherapy starts.
➤ **To prevent acute nausea and vomiting associated with initial and repeat courses of emetogenic, including highly emetogenic, cancer chemotherapy**
Children age 1 month to younger than 17 years: Infuse 20 mcg/kg I.V. over 15 minutes beginning approximately 30 minutes before chemotherapy starts. Maximum dose is 1.5 mg.
➤ **To prevent postoperative nausea and vomiting for up to 24 hours following surgery**
Adults: 0.075 mg I.V. over 10 seconds immediately before anesthesia induction.

ADMINISTRATION
I.V.
▼ Flush with NSS before and after injection.
▼ Give by rapid I.V. injection through a peripheral or central I.V. line.
▼ **Incompatibilities:** fosaprepitant, methylprednisolone sodium succinate.

ACTION
Antagonizes 5-HT$_3$ receptors in the GI tract and brain, which inhibits emesis caused by chemotherapy.

Route	Onset	Peak	Duration
I.V.	30 min	Unknown	5 days

Half-life: I.V., 40 hours (adults); 20 to 30 hours (children).

ADVERSE REACTIONS
CNS: anxiety, dizziness, headache, weakness.
CV: ***bradycardia, nonsustained ventricular tachycardia,*** hypotension, ***QT-interval prolongation.***
GI: constipation, diarrhea.
GU: urine retention.
Metabolic: *hyperkalemia.*
Skin: pruritus.

INTERACTIONS
Drug-drug. *Antiarrhythmics or other drugs that prolong the QTc interval, diuretics that induce electrolyte abnormalities, high-dose anthracycline:* May increase risk of prolonged QTc interval. Use together cautiously.
Apomorphine: May cause profound hypotension and loss of consciousness. Use together is contraindicated.

EFFECTS ON LAB TEST RESULTS
• May increase potassium level.
• May increase serum ALT or AST level.

CONTRAINDICATIONS & CAUTIONS
• Contraindicated in patients hypersensitive to palonosetron or its ingredients.
• Use cautiously in patients hypersensitive to other 5-HT$_3$ antagonists, in those taking drugs that affect cardiac conduction, and in those with cardiac conduction abnormalities, hypokalemia, or hypomagnesemia.
Dialyzable drug: Unlikely.

PREGNANCY-LACTATION-REPRODUCTION
• Use in pregnancy only if clearly needed.
• It isn't known if drug appears in breast milk. Patient should discontinue breast-feeding or discontinue drug.

NURSING CONSIDERATIONS
• Before giving this drug, check patient's potassium level.
• Consider adding corticosteroids to the antiemetic regimen, particularly for patients receiving highly emetogenic chemotherapy.

Reactions in bold italics are *life-threatening*. Interactions may have a *rapid onset* or a *delayed onset*.

- Make sure patient has additional antiemetics to take for breakthrough nausea or vomiting.
- If patient has cardiac conduction abnormalities, check the ECG before giving drug.

PATIENT TEACHING

- Advise patient to take a different antiemetic for breakthrough nausea or vomiting at the first sign of nausea rather than waiting until symptoms are severe.
- Urge patient with a history of cardiac conduction abnormalities to report any changes in drug regimen, such as adding or stopping an antiarrhythmic.

pamidronate disodium
pah-MIH-dro-nate

Aredia

Therapeutic class: Antiosteoporotics
Pharmacologic class: Bisphosphonates

AVAILABLE FORMS
Powder for injection: 30 mg/vial, 90 mg/vial
Solution for injection: 3 mg/mL, 6 mg/mL, 9 mg/mL in 10-mL vials

INDICATIONS & DOSAGES
➤ **Moderate to severe hypercalcemia from cancer (with or without bone metastases)**
Adults: Dosage depends on severity of hypercalcemia. Correct calcium level for albumin. Corrected calcium (CCa) level is calculated using this formula:

$$\frac{CCa}{(mg/dL)} = \frac{serum}{calcium} + \frac{0.8\,(4 - serum}{albumin)}$$
$$\text{(mg/dL)} \quad \text{(g/dL)}$$

Give patients with CCa levels of 12 to 13.5 mg/dL 60 to 90 mg by I.V. infusion as a single dose over 2 to 24 hours. Give patients with CCa levels greater than 13.5 mg/dL 90 mg by I.V. infusion over 2 to 24 hours. Allow at least 7 days before retreatment to permit full response to first dose.
➤ **Moderate to severe Paget disease**
Adults: 30 mg I.V. as a 4-hour infusion on 3 consecutive days for total dose of 90 mg. Repeat cycle as needed.

➤ **Osteolytic bone metastases of breast cancer with standard antineoplastic therapy**
Adults: 90 mg I.V. infusion over 2 hours every 3 to 4 weeks.
➤ **Osteolytic bone lesions of multiple myeloma**
Adults: 90 mg I.V. over 4 hours once monthly.

ADMINISTRATION
I.V.
▼ Hazardous drug; use safe handling and disposal precautions.
▼ Reconstitute drug with 10 mL of sterile water for injection. After drug is completely dissolved, add to 250 mL (2-hour infusion), 500 mL (4-hour infusion), or 1,000 mL (up to 24-hour infusion) of half-NSS or NSS for injection or D_5W.
▼ Inspect solution for precipitate before use.
▼ Give drug only by I.V. infusion. Injecting a bolus may cause nephropathy.
▼ Infusions longer than 2 hours may reduce the risk of renal toxicity, particularly in patients with preexisting renal insufficiency.
▼ Solution is stable for 24 hours at room temperature.
▼ Store reconstituted drug at 36° to 46° F (2° to 8° C) for up to 24 hours.
▼ **Incompatibilities:** Calcium-containing infusion solutions, such as Ringer injection.

ACTION
An antihypercalcemic that inhibits resorption of bone but apparently not bone formation. Adsorbs to hydroxyapatite crystals in bone and may directly block calcium phosphate dissolution and mature osteoclast formation.

Route	Onset	Peak	Duration
I.V.	Unknown	Unknown	Unknown

Half-life: 21 to 35 hours.

ADVERSE REACTIONS
CNS: *seizures,* fatigue, somnolence, fever, headache, psychosis.
CV: atrial fibrillation, tachycardia, hypertension, fluid overload, syncope.

EENT: sinusitis, rhinitis.
GI: abdominal pain, anorexia, constipation, nausea, vomiting, *GI hemorrhage.*
GU: renal dysfunction, UTI, *renal failure.*
Hematologic: *leukopenia, thrombocytopenia,* anemia.
Metabolic: hypophosphatemia, *hypokalemia, hypomagnesemia, hypocalcemia.*
Musculoskeletal: arthralgia, back pain, myalgia, osteonecrosis of the jaw.
Respiratory: cough, dyspnea, pleural effusions, URI, crackles.
Skin: infusion-site reaction, pain at infusion site.

INTERACTIONS
None significant.

EFFECTS ON LAB TEST RESULTS
- May increase creatinine level.
- May decrease phosphate, potassium, magnesium, calcium, and Hb levels.
- May decrease WBC and platelet counts.
- May interfere with technetium-99m diphosphonate imaging agents used in bone scans.

CONTRAINDICATIONS & CAUTIONS
- Contraindicated in patients hypersensitive to drug or other bisphosphonates such as etidronate.
- ❸ *Alert:* There may be an increased risk of atypical fractures of the thigh in patients treated with bisphosphonates.
- Use with caution, considering risks versus benefits, in patients with renal impairment.
Dialyzable drug: Yes.
⚠ *Overdose S&S:* High fever, hypotension, taste perversion, hypocalcemia.

PREGNANCY-LACTATION-REPRODUCTION
- May cause fetal harm. Contraindicated in pregnant women.
- It isn't known if drug appears in breast milk. Patient should discontinue breast-feeding or discontinue drug.

NURSING CONSIDERATIONS
- Assess hydration before treatment. Use drug only after patient has been vigorously hydrated with NSS. In patients with mild to moderate hypercalcemia, hydration alone may be sufficient.
- Because drug can cause electrolyte disturbances, carefully monitor electrolyte levels, especially calcium, phosphate, and magnesium. Short-term use of calcium may be needed in patients with severe hypocalcemia. Also monitor CBC and differential count, creatinine and Hb levels, and hematocrit.
- Carefully monitor patients with preexisting anemia, leukopenia, or thrombocytopenia during first 2 weeks of therapy.
- Monitor patient's temperature. Patient may experience a slight elevation for 24 to 48 hours after therapy.
- ❸ *Alert:* Because renal dysfunction may lead to renal failure, single doses shouldn't exceed 90 mg.
- Monitor creatinine level before each treatment.
- In patients treated for bone metastases who have renal dysfunction, withhold dose until renal function returns to baseline. Treating bone metastases in patients with severe renal impairment isn't recommended. For other indications, determine whether the potential benefit outweighs the potential risk.
- Severe musculoskeletal pain has been associated with bisphosphonate use and may occur within days, months, or years of start of therapy. When drug is stopped, symptoms may resolve partially or completely.
- Bisphosphonates can interfere with bone-imaging agents.
- ❸ *Alert:* Patients should have a dental examination with appropriate preventive dentistry before taking drug, especially those with risk factors, including cancer, chemotherapy, corticosteroid therapy, and poor oral hygiene. These patients should avoid dental procedures, if possible, during therapy.

PATIENT TEACHING
- Explain use and administration of drug to patient and family.
- Instruct patient to report adverse reactions promptly.
- Advise female patient to alert health care provider if pregnant or breast-feeding.

---

pancrelipase
pan-kre-LYE-pase

Creon, Pancreaze, Pertzye, Ultrase, Ultresa, Viokace, Zenpep

Therapeutic class: Digestive enzymes
Pharmacologic class: Pancreatic enzymes

AVAILABLE FORMS
Creon
Capsules (delayed-release) 🔘: 3,000 units lipase, 9,500 units protease, 15,000 units amylase; 6,000 units lipase, 19,000 units protease, 30,000 units amylase; 12,000 units lipase, 38,000 units protease, 60,000 units amylase; 24,000 units lipase, 76,000 units protease, 120,000 units amylase; 36,000 units lipase, 114,000 units protease, 180,000 units amylase

Pancreaze
Capsules (delayed-release) 🔘: 2,600 units lipase, 6,200 units protease, 10,850 units amylase; 4,200 units lipase, 10,000 units protease, 17,500 units amylase; 10,500 units lipase, 25,000 units protease, 43,750 units amylase; 16,800 units lipase, 40,000 units protease, 70,000 units amylase; 21,000 units lipase, 37,000 units protease, 61,000 units amylase

Pertzye
Capsules (delayed-release) 🔘: 8,000 units lipase, 28,750 units protease, 30,250 units amylase; 16,000 units lipase, 57,500 units protease, 60,500 units amylase

Ultresa
Capsules (delayed-release) 🔘: 13,800 units lipase, 27,600 units protease, 27,600 units amylase; 20,700 units lipase, 41,400 units protease, 41,400 units amylase; 23,000 units lipase, 46,000 units protease, 46,000 units amylase

Viokace
Tablets: 10,440 units lipase, 39,150 units protease, 39,150 units amylase; 20,880 units lipase, 78,300 units protease, 78,300 units amylase

Zenpep
Capsules (enteric-coated beads) 🔘: 3,000 units lipase, 10,000 units protease, 16,000 units amylase; 5,000 units lipase, 17,000 units protease, 27,000 units amylase; 10,000 units lipase, 34,000 units protease, 55,000 units amylase; 15,000 units lipase, 51,000 units protease, 82,000 units amylase; 20,000 units lipase, 68,000 units protease, 109,000 units amylase; 25,000 units lipase, 85,000 units protease, 136,000 units amylase; 40,000 units lipase, 136,000 units protease, 218,000 units amylase

INDICATIONS & DOSAGES
➤ **Exocrine pancreatic secretion insufficiency; cystic fibrosis in adults and children; steatorrhea and other disorders of fat metabolism caused by insufficient pancreatic enzymes**
Adults and children older than age 4: 500 lipase units/kg P.O. per meal (up to the maximum dose).
Children older than age 12 months to 4 years: 1,000 lipase units/kg P.O. per meal up to maximum dose of 2,500 lipase units/kg per meal, 10,000 lipase units/kg daily, or 4,000 lipase units/g of fat ingested daily.
Infants up to age 12 months: 2,000 to 4,000 lipase units P.O. per 120 mL of formula or per breast-feeding.
➤ **Exocrine pancreatic insufficiency due to chronic pancreatitis or pancreatectomy (Creon)**
Adults: 72,000 lipase units P.O. per meal while consuming at least 100 g of fat per day. Or, 500 lipase units/kg per meal. Adjust dosage to patient's response.
➤ **Exocrine pancreatic insufficiency due to chronic pancreatitis or pancreatectomy, with a PPI (Viokace)**
Adults: 500 lipase units/kg P.O. per meal to a maximum of 2,500 lipase units/kg per meal (or 10,000 lipase units/kg/day) or less than 4,000 lipase units/g fat ingested per day. Adjust dosage to patient's response.
➤ **Exocrine pancreatic insufficiency due to cystic fibrosis or other conditions**
Adults and children age 4 and older weighing 16 kg or more: Pertzye: 500 lipase units/kg P.O. per meal to a maximum of 2,500 lipase units/kg per meal (or 10,000 lipase units/kg or less per day), or less than 4,000 lipase units/g fat ingested per day.
Adults and children age 4 and older: Ultresa: 500 lipase units/kg P.O. per meal

P

to a maximum of 2,500 lipase units/kg per meal (or 10,000 lipase units/kg or less per day) or less than 4,000 lipase units/g fat ingested per day.

Children age 12 months to 4 years weighing 8 kg or more: Pertzye: 1,000 lipase units/kg P.O. per meal to a maximum of 2,500 lipase units/kg per meal (or 10,000 lipase units/kg or less per day), or less than 4,000 lipase units/g fat ingested per day.

Children older than age 12 months to younger than 4 years: Ultresa: 1,000 lipase units/kg per meal to a maximum of 2,500 lipase units/kg per meal (or 10,000 lipase units/kg or less per day), or less than 4,000 lipase units/g fat per day.

ADMINISTRATION

P.O.

● Give drug before or with meals and snacks.

● Don't crush or allow patient to chew capsules. Capsules containing enteric-coated microspheres may be opened and sprinkled on a small quantity of soft food at room temperature. Have patient swallow immediately, without chewing, and follow dose with glass of water or juice.

● For infants, mix powder with applesauce and give with meals. Avoid contact with or inhalation of powder because it may be highly irritating. Older children may swallow capsules with food.

● Don't mix Zenpep capsule contents directly into formula or breast milk before administration. Capsule contents may be administered directly into the infant's mouth before feeding.

● Viokace tablets aren't enteric-coated; patient should take with a PPI.

ACTION

Replaces endogenous exocrine pancreatic enzymes and aids digestion of starches, fats, and proteins.

Route	Onset	Peak	Duration
P.O.	Variable	Variable	Variable

Half-life: Unknown.

ADVERSE REACTIONS

CNS: headache, dizziness.

EENT: nasopharyngitis, pharyngolaryngeal pain, epistaxis.

GI: abdominal pain, nausea, cramping, diarrhea with high doses, dyspepsia, vomiting, weight loss.

Metabolic: hyperglycemia, *hypoglycemia.*

Respiratory: cough.

Other: biliary tract stones, anal pruritus.

INTERACTIONS

Drug-drug. *Antacids:* May destroy enteric coating and enhance degradation of pancrelipase. Avoid using together.

Oral iron supplement: May decrease iron response. Monitor patient for decreased effectiveness.

EFFECTS ON LAB TEST RESULTS

● May increase uric acid level.

CONTRAINDICATIONS & CAUTIONS

● Contraindicated in patients with severe hypersensitivity to pork and in those with acute pancreatitis or acute worsening of chronic pancreatic diseases.

● Use Ultresa, Viokace, and Pertzye cautiously in patients with gout, renal impairment, or hyperuricemia.

● Viokace isn't approved for use in children. Ultresa and Pertzye aren't approved for use in children younger than age 1.

Dialyzable drug: Unknown.

⚠ **Overdose S&S:** Transient intestinal upset, diarrhea.

PREGNANCY-LACTATION-REPRODUCTION

● Use cautiously in pregnant women and only if clearly needed. Nutrition should be optimized during pregnancy; pancreatic enzyme replacement isn't considered to pose a risk in pregnant women.

● Use cautiously in breast-feeding women.

NURSING CONSIDERATIONS

◑ *Alert:* Use drug only for confirmed exocrine pancreatic insufficiency. It isn't effective in GI disorders unrelated to enzyme deficiency.

◑ *Alert:* Fibrosing colonopathy is associated with high-dose use of pancreatic enzymes. Use cautiously when doses exceed 2,500 lipase units/kg per meal (or are greater than 10,000 lipase units/kg per day).

Reactions in bold italics are *life-threatening*. Interactions may have a *rapid onset* or a *delayed onset*.

• Lipase activity is greater than with other pancreatic enzymes.
• Monitor patient's stools. Adequate replacement decreases number of bowel movements and improves stool consistency.
• Individual products aren't bioequivalent and shouldn't be interchanged without prescriber supervision.
• Dosage varies with degree of maldigestion and malabsorption, amount of fat in diet, and enzyme activity of individual preparations.
• Enteric coating on some products may reduce available enzyme in upper portion of jejunum.
• Viokace tablets aren't enteric-coated and should be taken with a PPI.

PATIENT TEACHING
• Instruct patient to take drug before or with meals and snacks, but always with food and generous amounts of liquid.
• Advise patient not to crush or chew capsules; retention of a capsule in the mouth before swallowing may cause mucosal irritation and stomatitis.
• Capsules containing enteric-coated microspheres may be opened and sprinkled on a small quantity of soft food at room temperature. Stress importance of swallowing immediately, without chewing, and following with glass of water or juice.
• Warn patient not to inhale powder form or powder from capsules; it may irritate skin or mucous membranes.
• Tell patient to store drug in airtight container at room temperature.
• Instruct patient not to change brands without consulting prescriber.

SAFETY ALERT!

pancuronium bromide
pan-kyoo-ROW-nee-uhm

Therapeutic class: Skeletal muscle relaxants
Pharmacologic class: Nondepolarizing neuromuscular blockers

AVAILABLE FORMS
Injection: 1 mg/mL, 2 mg/mL

INDICATIONS & DOSAGES
➤ **Adjunct to anesthesia to relax skeletal muscle, facilitate intubation, and assist with mechanical ventilation**
Adults and children age 1 month and older: Initially, 0.04 to 0.1 mg/kg I.V.; then 0.01 mg/kg I.V. every 30 to 60 minutes. For endotracheal intubation, a bolus dose of 0.06 to 0.1 mg/kg I.V. is recommended. Conditions satisfactory for intubation are usually present within 2 to 3 minutes.
Neonates: Individualize dosage. It's recommended that a test dose of 0.02 mg/kg I.V. be given first to measure responsiveness.

ADMINISTRATION
I.V.
Black Box Warning This drug should be administered by adequately trained individuals familiar with its actions, characteristics, and hazards. ▪
▼ Only staff skilled in airway management should use drug.
▼ Drug has no known effect on consciousness, pain threshold, or cerebration. To avoid patient distress, don't induce neuromuscular blockade before unconsciousness.
▼ Keep endotracheal equipment, ventilator, oxygen, atropine, edrophonium, epinephrine, and neostigmine immediately available.
▼ Store in refrigerator. The 10-mL vial will maintain full clinical potency for up to 6 months at room temperature.
▼ Compatible in solution with NSS, dextrose 5%, dextrose 5% and sodium chloride, and lactated Ringer solution.
▼ When mixed with approved solutions in glass or plastic containers, drug will remain stable in solution for 48 hours with no alteration in potency or pH.
▼ **Incompatibilities:** Alkaline solutions, barbiturates, diazepam, thiopental sodium.

ACTION
Prevents acetylcholine from binding to receptors on the motor end plate, blocking neuromuscular transmission.

Route	Onset	Peak	Duration
I.V.	30–45 sec	3–4½ min	35–65 min

Half-life: 89 to 161 minutes.

ADVERSE REACTIONS
CV: tachycardia, increased BP.
EENT: excessive salivation.
Musculoskeletal: residual muscle weakness.
Respiratory: *prolonged respiratory insufficiency or apnea.*
Skin: transient rashes.
Other: allergic or idiosyncratic hypersensitivity reactions.

INTERACTIONS
Drug-drug. *Aminoglycosides (amikacin, gentamicin, neomycin, streptomycin, tobramycin), magnesium salts:* May increase the effects of pancuronium, including prolonged respiratory depression. Use together only when necessary. Dose of pancuronium may need to be reduced.
Azathioprine: May reverse neuromuscular blockade induced by pancuronium. Monitor patient.
Beta blockers, clindamycin, general anesthetics (enflurane, halothane, isoflurane), ketamine, lincomycin, magnesium sulfate, polymyxin antibiotics (colistin, polymyxin B sulfate), quinidine, quinine, verapamil: May enhance neuromuscular blockade, increasing skeletal muscle relaxation and prolonging effect of pancuronium. Use together cautiously during and after surgery.
Carbamazepine, phenytoin: May decrease effects of pancuronium. May need to increase pancuronium dose.
Diuretics: May cause electrolyte imbalance or alter neuromuscular blockade. Monitor electrolytes before giving drug.
Lithium, opioid analgesics: May enhance neuromuscular blockade, increasing skeletal muscle relaxation and possibly causing respiratory paralysis. Use cautiously, and reduce dose of pancuronium.
Succinylcholine: May increase intensity and duration of neuromuscular blockade. Allow effects of succinylcholine to subside before giving pancuronium.
TCAs: May increase risk of ventricular arrhythmias in patients anesthetized with both halothane and pancuronium. Monitor ECG closely in patients taking TCAs before surgery.
Theophylline: May produce a dose-dependent reversal of neuromuscular blocking effects. Monitor patient for clinical effect.

EFFECTS ON LAB TEST RESULTS
None reported.

CONTRAINDICATIONS & CAUTIONS
● Contraindicated in patients hypersensitive to bromides, those with tachycardia, and those for whom even a minor increase in HR is undesirable.
● Use cautiously in elderly or debilitated patients; in patients with renal, hepatic, or pulmonary impairment; and in those with respiratory depression, myasthenia gravis, myasthenic syndrome related to lung cancer, dehydration, thyroid disorders, CV disease, collagen diseases, porphyria, electrolyte disturbances, hyperthermia, severe obesity, and toxemic states. Also, use large doses cautiously in patients undergoing cesarean section.
Dialyzable drug: Unknown.
⚠ *Overdose S&S:* Residual neuromuscular blockade (skeletal muscle weakness, decreased respiratory reserve, low tidal volume, apnea).

PREGNANCY-LACTATION-REPRODUCTION
● It isn't known if drug can cause fetal harm. Use during pregnancy only if benefit justifies risk to the fetus.
● There is no information on the use of drug in breast-feeding women.

NURSING CONSIDERATIONS
● Dosage depends on anesthetic used, individual needs, and response. Dosages are representative and must be adjusted.
● Allow succinylcholine effects to subside before giving this drug.
● Monitor baseline electrolyte determinations (electrolyte imbalance can potentiate neuromuscular effects) and vital signs, especially respirations and HR.
● Measure fluid intake and output; renal dysfunction may prolong duration of action because 25% of drug is excreted unchanged in the urine.
● A nerve stimulator and train-of-four monitoring are recommended to confirm antagonism of neuromuscular blockade and recovery of muscle strength. Make

---

Reactions in bold italics are *life-threatening*. Interactions may have a *rapid onset* or a *delayed onset*.

sure there's some evidence of spontaneous recovery before attempting pharmacologic reversal with neostigmine.

• Monitor respirations closely until patient recovers fully from neuromuscular blockade, as indicated by tests of muscle strength (hand grip, head lift, and ability to cough).

• After spontaneous recovery starts, neuromuscular blockade may be reversed with an anticholinesterase (such as neostigmine or edrophonium), which is usually given with an anticholinergic (such as atropine).

• Drug doesn't cause histamine release or hypotension, but it may raise HR and BP.

• Give analgesics for pain.

🟡 *Alert:* Careful dosage calculation is essential. Always verify dosage with another health care professional.

PATIENT TEACHING

• Explain all events and procedures to patient because he can still hear.

pantoprazole sodium
pan-TOE-pray-zol

Panto IV✤, Pantoloc✤, Protonix✐, Protonix I.V.

Therapeutic class: Antiulcer drugs
Pharmacologic class: PPIs

AVAILABLE FORMS
Injection: 40 mg/vial
Suspension (delayed-release) ⓞⓝⓒ*:* 40 mg
Tablets (delayed-release) ⓞⓝⓒ*:* 20 mg, 40 mg
Tablets (enteric-coated) ⓞⓝⓒ*:* 20 mg✤, 40 mg✤

INDICATIONS & DOSAGES
➤ **Maintenance of healing of erosive esophagitis**
Adults: 40 mg P.O. once daily.
➤ **Short-term treatment of erosive esophagitis associated with GERD**
Adults: 40 mg P.O. once daily for up to 8 weeks. For patients who haven't healed after 8 weeks of treatment, another 8-week course may be considered. Or, 40 mg I.V. once daily for 7 to 10 days. Switch to P.O. form as soon as patient is able to take orally.

Children age 5 and older weighing 40 kg) or more: 40 mg P.O. once daily for up to 8 weeks.
Children age 5 and older weighing 15 to less than 40 kg: 20 mg P.O. once daily for up to 8 weeks.
Adjust-a-dose: Consider dosage reduction in children who are poor CYP2C19 metabolizers.
➤ **Long-term maintenance of healing erosive esophagitis and reduction in relapse rates of daytime and nighttime heartburn symptoms in patients with GERD**
Adults: 40 mg P.O. once daily.
➤ **Treatment of pathologic hypersecretion caused by Zollinger-Ellison syndrome**
Adults: Individualize dosage. Usual dosage is 40 mg P.O. b.i.d. Usual I.V. dose is 80 mg I.V. every 12 hours for no more than 6 days. For those needing a higher dose, 80 mg every 8 hours is expected to maintain acid output below 10 mEq/hour. Maximum daily dose is 240 mg/day. When converting from I.V. to P.O. form, ensure continuity of suppression of acid secretion.

ADMINISTRATION
P.O.
• Give tablets without regard for food and make sure patient swallows them whole.
• May give with antacids.
• Don't crush or split tablets.
• Give delayed-release suspension in applesauce or apple juice 30 minutes prior to a meal. Don't give in water or other liquids or foods.
• Don't split, crush, or allow patient to chew granules for delayed-release oral suspension.
I.V.
▼ Safety and effectiveness of the I.V. form to start therapy for GERD are unknown.
▼ Reconstitute each vial with 10 mL of NSS.
▼ Compatible diluents for infusion include NSS, D₅W, and lactated Ringer solution for injection.
▼ For patients with GERD, further dilute with 100 mL of diluent to yield 0.4 mg/mL.

P

▼ For patients with hypersecretion, combine two reconstituted vials and further dilute with 80 mL of diluent to a total volume of 100 mL, to yield 0.8 mg/mL.
▼ Infuse diluted solutions over 15 minutes at a rate of about 7 mL/minute.
▼ For a 2-minute infusion, give the reconstituted vials (final yield of about 4 mg/mL) over at least 2 minutes.
▼ Reconstituted 15-minute infusion (0.4 mg/mL) may be stored for up to 6 hours and the diluted solutions for up to 24 hours at room temperature.
▼ Reconstituted 2-minute solution (4 mg/mL) may be stored for up to 24 hours at room temperature before infusion.
▼ **Incompatibilities:** Midazolam, zinc-containing products or solutions. Don't give another infusion simultaneously through the same line.

ACTION
Inhibits proton pump activity by binding to hydrogen-potassium adenosine triphosphatase, located at secretory surface of gastric parietal cells, to suppress gastric acid secretion.

Route	Onset	Peak	Duration
P.O.	Unknown	2½ hr	>24 hr
I.V.	15–30 min	Unknown	24 hr

Half-life: 1 hour.

ADVERSE REACTIONS
CNS: anxiety, asthenia, dizziness, headache, insomnia, migraine, pain, depression.
CV: chest pain.
EENT: pharyngitis, rhinitis, sinusitis.
GI: abdominal pain, constipation, diarrhea, dyspepsia, eructation, flatulence, gastroenteritis, GI disorder, nausea, rectal disorder, vomiting.
GU: urinary frequency, UTI.
Metabolic: hyperglycemia, hyperlipidemia.
Musculoskeletal: arthralgia, back pain, hypertonia, neck pain.
Respiratory: bronchitis, dyspnea, increased cough, URI.
Skin: rash, pruritus, urticaria.

Other: flulike syndrome, infection, injection-site reaction, photosensitivity reactions.

INTERACTIONS
Drug-drug. *Ampicillin esters, iron salts, ketoconazole, mycophenolate:* May decrease absorption of these drugs. Monitor patient closely and separate doses.
Azole antifungals (itraconazole, ketoconazole): May decrease plasma levels of these drugs. Avoid this combination if possible.
Protease inhibitors (atazanavir, indinavir, nelfinavir): May reduce antiviral activity of these drugs. Adjust dosage as needed; administration of atazanavir with pantoprazole isn't recommended.
Salicylates: Enteric-coated salicylates may dissolve more rapidly, increasing gastric adverse reactions. Monitor patient.
Warfarin: May increase INR and PT. Monitor patient and laboratory values.
Drug-herb. *St. John's wort:* May increase risk of sunburn. Advise patient to avoid excessive sunlight exposure.
Drug-lifestyle. *Sun exposure:* May increase risk of sunburn. Advise patient to avoid excessive sunlight exposure.

EFFECTS ON LAB TEST RESULTS
• May increase glucose and lipid levels.
• May increase LFT result values.
• May cause false-positive urine screen test for tetrahydrocannabinol.

CONTRAINDICATIONS & CAUTIONS
• Contraindicated in patients hypersensitive to any component of the formulation.
• PPI therapy may be associated with an increased risk of osteoporosis-related fractures. Patients should use lowest dose and shortest duration of therapy appropriate to condition being treated.
Dialyzable drug: No.

PREGNANCY-LACTATION-REPRODUCTION
• There are no adequate studies in pregnant women. Use cautiously and only if clearly needed.
• Drug appears in breast milk. Patient should discontinue breast-feeding or discontinue drug.

Reactions in bold italics are *life-threatening*. Interactions may have a *rapid onset* or a *delayed onset*.

NURSING CONSIDERATIONS

● Symptomatic response to therapy doesn't preclude the presence of gastric malignancy.
❸ *Alert:* Prolonged use of PPIs may cause low magnesium levels. Monitor magnesium levels before start of treatment and periodically thereafter.
❸ *Alert:* Monitor patient for signs and symptoms of low magnesium level, such as abnormal HR or rhythm, palpitations, muscle spasms, tremor, or seizures. In children, abnormal HR may present as fatigue, upset stomach, dizziness, and light-headedness. Magnesium supplementation or drug discontinuation may be required.
❸ *Alert:* May increase risk of CDAD. Evaluate for CDAD in patients who develop diarrhea that doesn't improve.
● *Look alike–sound alike:* Don't confuse Protonix with Prilosec, Prozac, or Prevacid. Don't confuse pantoprazole with aripiprazole.

PATIENT TEACHING

● Instruct patient to take exactly as prescribed and at about the same time every day.
● Advise patient that drug can be taken without regard to meals.
● Tell patient to swallow tablet whole and not to crush, split, or chew it.
● Tell patient that antacids don't affect drug absorption.
● Teach patient to report all adverse reactions and to recognize and report signs and symptoms of low magnesium levels.

---

paroxetine hydrochloride
pah-ROX-a-teen

Paxil, Paxil CR

paroxetine mesylate
Brisdelle, Pexeva

Therapeutic class: Antidepressants
Pharmacologic class: SSRIs

AVAILABLE FORMS
paroxetine hydrochloride
Suspension: 10 mg/5 mL
Tablets ⓓ: 10 mg, 20 mg, 30 mg, 40 mg

Tablets (controlled-release) ⓓ: 12.5 mg, 25 mg, 37.5 mg
paroxetine mesylate
Capsules: 7.5 mg
Tablets ⓓ: 10 mg, 20 mg, 30 mg, 40 mg

INDICATIONS & DOSAGES
Adjust-a-dose (for all indications): For elderly and debilitated patients and those with renal or hepatic impairment taking immediate-release form, initially, 10 mg P.O. daily, preferably in morning. If patient doesn't respond after full antidepressant effect has occurred, increase dose in 10-mg/day increments at intervals of at least 1 week to a maximum of 40 mg daily. If using controlled-release form, start therapy at 12.5 mg daily. Don't exceed 50 mg daily.

➤ **Depression (excluding Brisdelle)**
Adults: Initially, 20 mg P.O. daily, preferably in morning, as indicated. If patient doesn't improve, increase dose by 10 mg daily at intervals of at least 1 week to a maximum of 50 mg daily. If using controlled-release form, initially, 25 mg P.O. daily. Increase dose in 12.5-mg/day increments at intervals of at least 1 week to a maximum of 62.5 mg daily.
Elderly patients: Initially, 10 mg P.O. daily, preferably in morning, as indicated. If patient doesn't improve, increase dose by 10 mg daily at weekly intervals, to a maximum of 40 mg daily. If using controlled-release form, start therapy at 12.5 mg P.O. daily. Don't exceed 50 mg daily.

➤ **Obsessive-compulsive disorder (OCD) (Paxil and Pexeva only)**
Adults: Initially, 20 mg P.O. daily, preferably in morning. Increase dose in 10-mg day increments at intervals of at least 1 week. Recommended daily dose is 40 mg. Maximum daily dose is 60 mg.

➤ **Panic disorder (excluding Brisdelle)**
Adults: Initially, 10 mg P.O. daily. Increase dose in 10-mg/day increments at intervals of at least 1 week, up to a maximum of 60 mg daily. Or, 12.5 mg Paxil CR P.O. as a single daily dose. Increase dose in 12.5-mg/day increments at intervals of at least 1 week, up to a maximum of 75 mg daily.

➤ **Social anxiety disorder (Paxil and Paxil CR only)**

P

Adults: Initially, 20 mg P.O. daily. Dosage range is 20 to 60 mg daily. Adjust dosage to maintain patient on lowest effective dose. Or, 12.5 mg Paxil CR P.O. as a single daily dose. Increase dose in 12.5-mg/day increments at intervals of at least 1 week, up to a maximum of 37.5 mg daily.

➤ **Generalized anxiety disorder (Paxil and Pexeva only)**
Adults: 20 mg P.O. daily initially. Increase dose in 10-mg/day increments at intervals of at least 1 week, up to a maximum of 50 mg daily.

➤ **Posttraumatic stress disorder (Paxil only)**
Adults: Initially, 20 mg P.O. daily. Increase dose in 10-mg/day increments at intervals of at least 1 week. Maximum daily dose is 50 mg P.O.

➤ **Premenstrual dysphoric disorder (PMDD) (Paxil CR only)**
Adults: Initially, 12.5 mg Paxil CR P.O. as a single daily dose. May be given daily throughout menstrual cycle or daily during the luteal phase of menstrual cycle. Dose changes should occur at intervals of at least 1 week. Maximum dose is 25 mg P.O. daily.

➤ **Moderate to severe vasomotor symptoms associated with menopause (Brisdelle only)**
Adults: 7.5 mg P.O. daily at bedtime.

ADMINISTRATION
P.O.
● Give drug in the morning without regard for food.
● Don't split or crush controlled-release tablets.

ACTION
Thought to be linked to drug's inhibition of CNS neuronal uptake of serotonin.

Route	Onset	Peak	Duration
P.O.	Unknown	2–8 hr	Unknown
P.O. (controlled-release)	Unknown	6–10 hr	Unknown

Half-life: Paroxetine, 21 hours; controlled-release, 15 to 20 hours; paroxetine mesylate, 33.2 hours.

ADVERSE REACTIONS
CNS: asthenia, dizziness, headache, insomnia, somnolence, tremor, nervousness, ***suicidal behavior,*** anxiety, paresthesia, confusion, agitation.
CV: palpitations, vasodilation, hypertension, tachycardia, chest pain.
EENT: blurred vision, tinnitus, lump or tightness in throat, pharyngitis, rhinitis, sinusitis.
GI: dry mouth, nausea, constipation, diarrhea, flatulence, vomiting, dyspepsia, dysgeusia, increased or decreased appetite, abdominal pain.
GU: ejaculatory disturbances, sexual dysfunction, urinary frequency, other urinary disorders, dysmenorrhea, female genital tract disease.
Musculoskeletal: myopathy, myalgia, myasthenia, back pain.
Skin: diaphoresis, rash, pruritus.
Respiratory: dyspnea.
Other: decreased libido, yawning.

INTERACTIONS
Drug-drug. *Atomoxetine:* May alter atomoxetine level. Initiate atomoxetine at a reduced dosage.
Barbiturates (phenobarbital), phenytoin: May alter pharmacokinetics of both drugs. Dosage adjustments may be needed.
Cimetidine: May decrease hepatic metabolism of paroxetine, leading to risk of adverse reactions. Dosage adjustments may be needed.
Cyclosporine: May increase cyclosporine level and toxicity. Monitor cyclosporine level when adding or discontinuing paroxetine; adjust cyclosporine dosage as needed.
Digoxin: May decrease digoxin level. Use together cautiously.
Drugs that prolong QT interval (antiarrhythmics [amiodarone, bretylium, disopyramide, dofetilide, procainamide, quinidine, sotalol], arsenic trioxide, chlorpromazine, cisapride, dolasetron, droperidol, mefloquine, mesoridazine, moxifloxacin, pentamidine, pimozide, tacrolimus, thioridazine, ziprasidone): May increase risk of life-threatening cardiac arrhythmias, including torsades de pointes. Monitor patient closely.
Fosamprenavir, ritonavir: May decrease paroxetine plasma level. Adjust dosage as needed.
Galantamine: May alter oral bioavailability of galantamine. Use together cautiously.

Linezolid: May cause serotonin syndrome. Allow at least 2 weeks after stopping linezolid before giving paroxetine.

Lithium: May enhance serotonergic effects of paroxetine. Use with caution.

MAO inhibitors (phenelzine, selegiline, tranylcypromine): May cause serotonin syndrome and signs and symptoms resembling neuroleptic malignant syndrome. Avoid using within 14 days of MAO inhibitor therapy.

Metoclopramide, sibutramine, L-*tryptophan, sympathomimetics:* May increase risk of serotonin syndrome. Monitor patient closely.

NSAIDs: May increase risk of GI bleeding. If possible, avoid concurrent use. If coadministration can't be avoided, consider shortening NSAID treatment duration, decreasing dosage, or switching to acetaminophen or a TCA.

Phenothiazines (thioridazine): May increase phenothiazine plasma level, increasing pharmacologic and adverse reactions of phenothiazine. Use together is contraindicated.

Pimozide: May increase pimozide level. Use together is contraindicated.

Procyclidine: May increase procyclidine level. Reduce procyclidine dosage if anticholinergic effects occur.

Risperidone: May increase risperidone level, increasing risk of adverse reactions; serotonin syndrome may occur. Use together cautiously.

Sympathomimetics: May increase sensitivity to the effect of sympathomimetics and increase risk of serotonin syndrome. Monitor patient.

Drug-herb. *SAM-e:* May increase risk of serotonin syndrome. Avoid use together.

St. John's wort: May increase sedative-hypnotic effects. Discourage use together.

Drug-lifestyle. *Alcohol use:* May alter psychomotor function. Discourage use together.

EFFECTS ON LAB TEST RESULTS

None reported.

CONTRAINDICATIONS & CAUTIONS

● Contraindicated in patients hypersensitive to drug, within 14 days of MAO inhibitor therapy, and in those taking thioridazine.

Black Box Warning Contraindicated in children and adolescents younger than age 18 because of increased risk of suicidal thinking and behavior. ■

❸ Alert: Use with linezolid or methylene blue can cause serotonin syndrome (fever, mental status changes, muscle twitching, excessive sweating, shivering or shaking, diarrhea, loss of coordination). Use drug with linezolid or methylene blue only for life-threatening or urgent conditions when the potential benefits outweigh the risks of toxicity.

● Use cautiously in patients with history of seizure disorders or mania and in those with other severe, systemic illness.

● Use cautiously in patients at risk for volume depletion and monitor them appropriately.

Dialyzable drug: Unlikely.

⚠ Overdose S&S: Coma, confusion, dizziness, nausea, somnolence, tachycardia, tremor, vomiting, acute renal failure, aggressive reactions, bradycardia, dystonia, hepatic necrosis, hypertension, hypotension, jaundice, manic reactions, mydriasis, myoclonus, rhabdomyolysis, seizures, serotonin syndrome, stupor, hepatic impairment, syncope, urine retention, ventricular arrhythmias.

PREGNANCY-LACTATION-REPRODUCTION

● Drug can cause fetal harm. Manufacturer suggests discontinuing drug or switching to another antidepressant unless benefits justify continuing treatment. Consider other treatment options for women who are planning to become pregnant.

● Contraindicated for treatment of vasomotor symptoms in pregnant women.

● Drug appears in breast milk. Use in breast-feeding women only if benefit of treating postpartum depression with this drug outweighs risk. Monitor infants for growth.

P

NURSING CONSIDERATIONS

• Patients taking Paxil CR for PMDD should be periodically reassessed to determine the need for continued treatment.

• If signs or symptoms of psychosis occur or increase, expect prescriber to reduce dosage. Record mood changes. Monitor patient for suicidal tendencies, and allow only a minimum supply of drug.

Black Box Warning Drug may increase the risk of suicidal thinking and behavior in children, adolescents, and young adults ages 18 to 24 during the first 2 months of treatment, especially in those with major depressive disorder or other psychiatric disorder. ■

☯ Alert: If linezolid or methylene blue must be given, stop paroxetine and monitor patient for serotonin toxicity for 2 weeks or until 24 hours after the last dose of methylene blue or linezolid, whichever comes first. Treatment with paroxetine may be resumed 24 hours after the last dose of methylene blue or linezolid.

• Monitor patient for complaints of sexual dysfunction. In men, they include anorgasmia, erectile difficulties, delayed ejaculation or orgasm; in women, they include anorgasmia or difficulty with orgasm.

☯ Alert: Don't stop drug abruptly. Withdrawal or discontinuation syndrome may occur if drug is stopped abruptly. Symptoms include headache, myalgia, lethargy, and general flulike symptoms. Taper drug slowly over 1 to 2 weeks.

☯ Alert: Combining triptans with an SSRI or an SSNRI may cause serotonin syndrome or neuroleptic malignant syndrome-like reactions. Signs and symptoms of serotonin syndrome may include restlessness, hallucinations, loss of coordination, fast heartbeat, rapid changes in BP, increased body temperature, overactive reflexes, nausea, vomiting, and diarrhea. Serotonin syndrome may be more likely to occur when starting or increasing the dose of triptan, SSRI, or SSNRI.

• **Look alike–sound alike:** Don't confuse paroxetine with fluoxetine or paclitaxel. Don't confuse Paxil with Doxil, paclitaxel, Plavix, or Taxol.

PATIENT TEACHING

Black Box Warning Advise families and caregivers to closely observe patient for increased suicidal thinking and behavior. ■

☯ Alert: Teach patient to recognize and immediately report signs and symptoms of serotonin toxicity.

• Tell patient that drug may be taken with or without food, usually in morning.

• Tell patient not to break, crush, or chew controlled-release tablets.

• Warn patient to avoid activities that require alertness and good coordination until effects of drug are known.

• Advise woman of childbearing potential to contact prescriber if she becomes pregnant or plans to become pregnant during therapy or if she's currently breast-feeding.

• Tell patient to avoid alcohol and to consult prescriber before taking other prescription or OTC drugs or herbal medicines.

• Instruct patient not to stop taking drug abruptly.

SAFETY ALERT!

pegaspargase (PEG-L-asparaginase)
peg-AHS-per-jays

Oncaspar

Therapeutic class: Antineoplastics
Pharmacologic class: Modified L-asparaginases

AVAILABLE FORMS
Injection: 3,750 international units/5-mL solution in single-use vial (750 international units/mL)

INDICATIONS & DOSAGES
➤ **As part of a multidrug chemotherapy regimen in the treatment of acute lymphoblastic leukemia, and acute lymphoblastic leukemia with hypersensitivity to native forms of L-asparaginase**
Adults and children older than age 1: 2,500 international units/m^2 I.V. or I.M. every 14 days.

ADMINISTRATION
I.V.
▼ Give I.V. only if I.M. route is contraindicated. Don't administer by I.V. push.

▼ Give I.V. over 1 to 2 hours in 100 mL of NSS or D$_5$W injection through an infusion that's already running.

▼ Drug may be a contact irritant, and solution must be handled and given with care. Wear gloves. Avoid inhalation of vapors and contact with skin or mucous membranes, especially in the eyes. If contact occurs, wash with generous amounts of water for at least 15 minutes.

▼ Don't use if cloudy or contains precipitate. Avoid excessive agitation of drug; don't shake.

▼ Don't freeze or use drug that has been frozen because freezing destroys drug's effectiveness.

▼ Discard unused portions. Use only one dose per vial; don't reenter vial.

▼ Don't use if stored at room temperature for longer than 48 hours. Keep refrigerated at 36° to 46° F (2° to 8° C). Protect infusion bags from light.

▼ **Incompatibilities:** None reported, but don't mix with other I.V. drugs.
I.M.
● I.M. is the preferred route and is associated with lower incidence of adverse effects.
● When giving I.M., limit volume given at a single injection site to 2 mL. If volume to be given exceeds 2 mL, use multiple injection sites.
● Administer as deep I.M. injection into a large muscle.

ACTION
A modified version of the enzyme L-asparaginase that exerts cytotoxic effects by inactivating the amino acid asparagine, which tumor cells need to synthesize proteins.

Route	Onset	Peak	Duration
I.V.	Unknown	Unknown	2–4 wk
I.M.	Unknown	3–4 days	21 days

Half-life: I.V., about 7 days; I.M., about 6 days.

ADVERSE REACTIONS
CNS: *stroke.*
GI: *pancreatitis.*

Hematologic: *coagulopathy.*
Hepatic: abnormal LFT values, hyperbilirubinemia.
Metabolic: hyperglycemia.
Other: hypersensitivity reactions.

INTERACTIONS
Drug-drug. *Aspirin, dipyridamole, heparin, NSAIDs, warfarin:* May cause imbalances in coagulation factors, predisposing patient to bleeding or thrombosis. Use together cautiously.
Live-virus vaccines: May increase adverse or toxic effects of vaccines; may diminish vaccines' therapeutic effects. Avoid use together. Don't give live vaccines for at least 3 months after drug.
Protein-bound drugs: May increase toxicity of other drugs that bind to proteins and may interfere with enzymatic detoxification of other drugs, especially in the liver. Check for toxicity, and use together cautiously.
Vaccines (inactivated): May diminish therapeutic effect of vaccines. Monitor therapy.

EFFECTS ON LAB TEST RESULTS
● May increase BUN, creatinine, amylase, lipase, bilirubin, ALT, AST, uric acid, and ammonia levels. May decrease sodium and protein levels. May increase or decrease glucose level.
● May prolong PT and aPTT, and increase INR and thromboplastin.
● May decrease Hb level and antithrombin III, WBC, RBC, platelet, and granulocyte counts.

CONTRAINDICATIONS & CAUTIONS
● Contraindicated in patients with pancreatitis or history of pancreatitis, in those who have had significant hemorrhagic events related to previous treatment with L-asparaginase, and in those with history of serious allergic reactions to drug, such as generalized urticaria, bronchospasm, laryngeal edema, hypotension, or other unacceptable adverse reactions.
● Discontinue drug in patients with serious thrombotic events.
● Use cautiously in patients with hepatic impairment.
● Use cautiously in patients with a history of diabetes.

Dialyzable drug: Unknown.
⚠ *Overdose S&S:* Elevated liver enzyme levels, rash.

PREGNANCY-LACTATION-REPRODUCTION
● It isn't known if drug causes fetal harm. Use only if clearly needed.
● It isn't known if drug appears in breast milk. Patient should discontinue breast-feeding or discontinue drug.

NURSING CONSIDERATIONS
● Take preventive measures (including adequate hydration) before starting treatment. Hyperuricemia may result from rapid lysis of leukemic cells.
◐ *Alert:* Monitor patients closely for hypersensitivity (including life-threatening anaphylaxis), especially those hypersensitive to other forms of L-asparaginase. Observe patient for 1 hour after giving drug and have emergency equipment and other drugs needed to treat anaphylaxis readily available. Moderate to life-threatening hypersensitivity requires stopping L-asparaginase.
● To assess effects of therapy, monitor patient's peripheral blood count and bone marrow. A drop in circulating lymphoblasts is often noted after therapy starts, sometimes accompanied by a marked rise in uric acid level.
● Obtain frequent amylase and lipase determinations to detect pancreatitis. Monitor patient's glucose level during therapy to detect hyperglycemia.
● Monitor patient for liver dysfunction when drug is used with hepatotoxic chemotherapeutic drugs.
● Drug may affect several plasma proteins; monitor fibrinogen, PT, INR, and PTT at baseline and periodically during and after treatment.
● *Look alike–sound alike:* Don't confuse pegaspargase with asparaginase.

PATIENT TEACHING
● Inform patient of risk of hypersensitivity reactions and importance of reporting them immediately.
● Tell patient not to take other drugs, including OTC preparations, until approved by prescriber because risk of bleeding is higher when pegaspargase is given with drugs such as aspirin. Drug may also increase toxicity of other drugs.
● Urge patient to report all adverse reactions and signs and symptoms of infection (fever, chills, and malaise); drug may suppress the immune system.
● Caution woman of childbearing potential to avoid pregnancy and breast-feeding during therapy.

SAFETY ALERT!

pegfilgrastim
peg-fill-GRASS-tim

Neulasta, Neulasta Delivery Kit

Therapeutic class: Colony stimulating factors
Pharmacologic class: Hematopoietics

AVAILABLE FORMS
Injection: 6 mg/0.6-mL syringe

INDICATIONS & DOSAGES
➤ **To reduce frequency of infection in patients with nonmyeloid malignancies receiving myelosuppressive chemotherapy that may cause febrile neutropenia**
Adults weighing more than 45 kg: 6 mg subcutaneously once per chemotherapy cycle. Don't give in period between 14 days before and 24 hours after administration of cytotoxic chemotherapy.
Children: Give once per chemotherapy cycle, beginning 24 hours after completion of chemotherapy. If weight is 31 to 44 kg, give 4 mg subcutaneously. If weight is 21 to 30 kg, give 2.5 mg subcutaneously. If weight is 10 to 20 kg, give 1.5 mg subcutaneously. If weight is less than 10 kg, give 0.1 mg/kg subcutaneously.
➤ **To increase survival in patients acutely exposed to myelosuppressive doses of radiation greater than 2 gray (Gy)**
Adults and children weighing 45 kg or more: 6 mg subcutaneously as soon as possible after suspected or confirmed exposure. Repeat 1 week after first dose.
Children weighing 31 to 44 kg: 4 mg (0.4 mL) subcutaneously as soon as possible after suspected or confirmed exposure. Repeat 1 week after first dose.

Reactions in bold italics are *life-threatening*. Interactions may have a *rapid onset* or a *delayed onset*.

Children weighing 21 to 30 kg: 2.5 mg (0.25 mL) subcutaneously as soon as possible after suspected or confirmed exposure. Repeat 1 week after first dose.
Children weighing 10 to 20 kg: 1.5 mg (0.15mL) subcutaneously as soon as possible after suspected or confirmed exposure. Repeat 1 week after first dose.
Children weighing less than 10 kg: 0.1 mg/kg (0.01 mL/kg) subcutaneously as soon as possible after suspected or confirmed exposure. Repeat 1 week after first dose.

ADMINISTRATION
Subcutaneous
• Allow drug to come to room temperature before giving; protect from light.
• Don't shake.
• Don't use if discoloration or particulate matter is seen.
• Refer to manufacturer's instructors for administering drug using the On-body injector and for its removal and disposal.
• Discard drug if left at room temperature for more than 48 hours.
⊕ *Alert:* Don't use prefilled syringe for patients requiring less than 6 mg (0.6 mL) as syringe doesn't have graduated markings for smaller doses. Transfer drug to appropriately marked syringe to measure dose less than 0.6 mL.

ACTION
Binds cell receptors to stimulate proliferation, differentiation, commitment, and end-cell function of neutrophils.

Route	Onset	Peak	Duration
Subcut.	Unknown	Unknown	Unknown

Half-life: 15 to 80 hours.

ADVERSE REACTIONS
CNS: dizziness, fatigue, fever, headache, insomnia, asthenia.
GI: abdominal pain, anorexia, constipation, diarrhea, dyspepsia, mucositis, nausea, stomatitis, taste perversion, vomiting.
Hematologic: *granulocytopenia, neutropenic fever.*
Musculoskeletal: arthralgia, bone pain, generalized weakness, myalgia, skeletal pain.

Skin: alopecia.
Other: peripheral edema.

INTERACTIONS
Drug-drug. *Lithium:* May increase the release of neutrophils. Monitor neutrophil counts closely.

EFFECTS ON LAB TEST RESULTS
• May increase LDH, alkaline phosphatase, and uric acid levels.
• May decrease granulocyte, platelet, and RBC counts.

CONTRAINDICATIONS & CAUTIONS
• Contraindicated in patients hypersensitive to *Escherichia coli*–derived proteins, filgrastim, or any component of the drug. Don't use for peripheral blood progenitor cell mobilization.
• Use cautiously in patients with sickle cell disease, those receiving chemotherapy causing delayed myelosuppression, those receiving radiation therapy and during breast-feeding.
• Infants, children, and adolescents who weigh less than 45 kg shouldn't receive the 6-mg single-use syringe dose.
Dialyzable drug: Unknown.
⚠ *Overdose S&S:* Leukocytosis.

PREGNANCY-LACTATION-REPRODUCTION
• There are no adequate studies in pregnant women. Use only if potential benefit justifies potential fetal risk.
• Women who become pregnant during treatment should enroll in Amgen's Pregnancy Surveillance Program (1-800-772-6436).
• It isn't known if drug appears in in breast milk. Use cautiously in breast-feeding women.

NURSING CONSIDERATIONS
⊕ *Alert:* Splenic rupture may occur rarely. Assess patient who experiences signs or symptoms of left upper abdominal or shoulder pain for an enlarged spleen or splenic rupture.
• Obtain CBC and platelet count before therapy.
• Monitor patient's Hb level, hematocrit, CBC, and platelet count, as well as LDH,

alkaline phosphatase, and uric acid levels during therapy.

• Monitor patient for allergic-type reactions, including anaphylaxis, skin rash, and urticaria, which can occur with first or subsequent treatment.

• Evaluate patient with fever, lung infiltrates, or respiratory distress for adult respiratory distress syndrome. Notify prescriber if respiratory status worsens.

• Keep patient with sickle cell disease well hydrated, and monitor him for symptoms of sickle cell crisis.

• Monitor patient for capillary leak syndrome (hypotension, hypoalbuminemia, edema, hemoconcentration) and manage with symptomatic treatment, if necessary.

• Pegfilgrastim may act as a growth factor for tumors.

◑ **Alert:** After acute radiation exposure, obtain a baseline CBC but don't delay drug administration if a CBC isn't readily available. Estimate patient's absorbed radiation dose (level of radiation exposure) based on information from public health authorities, biodosimetry if available, or clinical findings, such as time to onset of vomiting or lymphocyte depletion kinetics.

• **Look alike–sound alike:** Don't confuse Neulasta with Neumega, Neupogen, or Lunesta.

PATIENT TEACHING

• Advise patient to report all adverse reactions.

• Tell patient to report signs and symptoms of allergic reactions, fever, or breathing problems.

◑ **Alert:** Rarely, splenic rupture may occur. Advise patient to immediately report upper left abdominal or shoulder tip pain.

• Tell patient with sickle cell disease to keep drinking fluids and report signs or symptoms of sickle cell crisis.

• Instruct patient or caregiver how to give drug if it's to be given at home.

peginterferon alfa-2a
peg-in-ter-FEER-on

Pegasys, Pegasys ProClick

Therapeutic class: Antivirals
Pharmacologic class: Biological response modifiers

AVAILABLE FORMS
Injection: 180 mcg/1 mL single-dose vials; 180 mcg/0.5 mL prefilled syringe; 135 mcg/0.5 mL, 180 mcg/0.5 mL autoinjector

INDICATIONS & DOSAGES
Adjust-a-dose (for all indications): For adults who experience moderate adverse reactions, decrease dose to 135 mcg subcutaneously once a week; for severe adverse reactions, decrease to 90 mcg subcutaneously once a week.

Refer to manufacturer's instructions for dosage adjustments for neutropenia, thrombocytopenia, and ALT elevations in adults and children. In adults and children with CrCl less than 30 mL/minute or ESRD requiring hemodialysis, decrease dose to 135 mcg subcutaneously once a week. If severe laboratory abnormalities or severe adverse reactions occur, may further reduce dose to 90 mg once weekly until reactions resolve; if intolerance persists, discontinue drug.

In patients with moderate clinical depression, decrease dose to 135 mcg weekly for adults and 135 mcg/$1.73 \text{ m}^2 \times$ BSA or 90 mcg/$1.73 \text{ m}^2 \times$ BSA once weekly for children. For severe depression, discontinue therapy and obtain an immediate psychiatric consultation.

➤ **Chronic HCV infection with compensated hepatic disease in patients not previously treated with interferon alfa, in combination with other HCV antiviral drugs**
Adults with HCV genotype 1 or 4: 180 mcg subcutaneously in abdomen or thigh once weekly. Refer to prescribing information of the other HCV antiviral for duration of entire treatment regimen. If used with

---

Reactions in bold italics are *life-threatening*. Interactions may have a *rapid onset* or a *delayed onset*.

ribavirin with or without other HCV antivirals, treatment duration is 48 weeks.

Adults with HCV genotype 2 or 3: 180 mcg subcutaneously in abdomen or thigh once weekly. Refer to prescribing information of the other HCV antiviral for duration of entire treatment regimen. If used with ribavirin with or without other HCV antivirals, treatment duration is 24 weeks.

Children age 5 and older: 180 mcg/ 1.73 m^2 × BSA subcutaneously once weekly in combination with ribavirin. Treat patients with genotype 2 or 3 for 24 weeks, other genotypes for 48 weeks. Maximum dose is 180 mcg once weekly.

➤ **Chronic HCV infection (regardless of genotype) in HIV-infected patients who haven't previously been treated with interferon alfa**

Adults: 180 mcg subcutaneously in abdomen or thigh once weekly. When used with ribavirin, treatment duration is 48 weeks. When used with other HCV antivirals, refer to prescribing information of the other HCV antiviral for treatment duration.

➤ **Chronic HBV infection in patients with compensated liver disease and evidence of viral replication and liver inflammation**

Adults: 180 mcg subcutaneously in abdomen or thigh once weekly for 48 weeks.

ADMINISTRATION

Subcutaneous

● Vials and prefilled syringes are for single use only. Discard unused portion.

● Don't shake. Allow to reach room temperature before use, but don't leave out of refrigerator for more than 24 hours. Don't freeze.

● Protect from light.

● Visually inspect drug for particulate matter and discoloration before administration; don't use if particulate matter is visible or product is discolored.

ACTION

Causes reversible decreases in leukocyte and platelet counts, partially through stimulation of production of effector proteins in vitro.

Route	Onset	Peak	Duration
Subcut.	Unknown	3–4 days	<1 wk

Half-life: 160 hours (range 84 to 353 hours).

ADVERSE REACTIONS

CNS: depression, dizziness, fatigue, headache, insomnia, irritability, pain, pyrexia, anxiety, asthenia, concentration impairment, memory impairment, mood alteration, nervousness.

GI: abdominal pain, anorexia, diarrhea, nausea, dry mouth, vomiting.

Hematologic: *neutropenia, thrombocytopenia,* anemia, *lymphopenia.*

Musculoskeletal: arthralgia, myalgia, back pain.

Respiratory: cough, dyspnea.

Skin: alopecia, pruritus, dermatitis, increased sweating, rash, dry skin, eczema.

Other: injection-site reaction, rigors.

INTERACTIONS

Drug-drug. *Methadone:* May increase methadone level. Monitor patient closely and decrease methadone dosage as needed.

Nucleoside reverse transcriptase inhibitors (NRTIs): May cause severe and potentially fatal hepatic decompensation. If used together in patients coinfected with HIV who are taking NRTIs, monitor for toxicities.

Ribavirin: May cause additive hematologic toxicity. Monitor hematologic function.

Telbivudine: May increase risk of peripheral neuropathy. Avoid use together.

Theophylline, other drugs metabolized by CYP1A2: May increase theophylline level and may interact with other drugs metabolized by this enzyme system. Monitor theophylline level and adjust dosage as needed.

EFFECTS ON LAB TEST RESULTS

● May increase triglyceride and ALT levels. May decrease Hb level and hematocrit.

● May decrease ANC, WBC, and platelet counts. May increase or decrease thyroid function test values.

CONTRAINDICATIONS & CAUTIONS

● Contraindicated in patients hypersensitive to interferon alfa-2a or any components of formulation.

P

• Contraindicated in patients with autoimmune hepatitis or decompensated liver disease (with monoinfection or coinfection with HIV) before or during treatment with drug and in neonates and infants.

• Use cautiously in patients with a history of depression.

• Use cautiously in patients with baseline neutrophil counts less than $1,500/mm^3$, baseline platelet counts less than $90,000/mm^3$, or baseline Hb level less than 10 g/dL.

• Use cautiously in patients with CrCl less than 50 mL/minute.

• Use cautiously in patients with cardiac disease or hypertension, thyroid disease, autoimmune disorders, pulmonary disorders, colitis, pancreatitis, and ophthalmologic disorders.

• Use cautiously in elderly patients because they may be at increased risk for adverse reactions.

🖖 *Alert:* Use cautiously in patients also taking ribavirin. Ribavirin is also known to cause hemolytic anemia, which may worsen cardiac disease.

• Safety and effectiveness haven't been established in patients who have failed to respond to other interferon alfa treatments, in solid organ transplant recipients, and in patients also infected with HBV.

Dialyzable drug: No.

⚠ *Overdose S&S:* Fatigue, elevated liver enzyme levels, neutropenia, thrombocytopenia.

PREGNANCY-LACTATION-REPRODUCTION
• There are no adequate studies of drug used as monotherapy in pregnant women. Manufacturer advises using drug as monotherapy only if potential benefit justifies potential fetal risk and only in women of childbearing potential when they are using effective contraception. Some professional guidelines recommend that drug not be used during pregnancy.

• Combination therapy with ribavirin may cause fetal birth defects or death; combination therapy with ribavirin in pregnant women is contraindicated. Patient must have a confirmed negative pregnancy test immediately before start of combination treatment. Monthly pregnancy tests must be performed. Women of childbearing potential and men must use two forms of effective contraception during therapy and for at least 6 months after therapy ends.

• It isn't known if drug appears in breast milk. Patient should discontinue breast-feeding or discontinue drug.

NURSING CONSIDERATIONS
Black Box Warning Alpha interferons may cause or aggravate fatal or life-threatening neuropsychiatric, autoimmune, ischemic, and infectious disorders. Monitor patients closely with periodic clinical and laboratory evaluations. Withdraw patients with persistently severe or worsening signs or symptoms of these conditions from therapy. ▮

• Obtain CBC before treatment and monitor counts routinely during therapy. Stop drug in patients who develop severe decrease in neutrophil or platelet counts.

• Stop drug if uncontrollable thyroid disease, hyperglycemia, hypoglycemia, or diabetes mellitus occurs during treatment.

• If persistent or unexplained pulmonary infiltrates or pulmonary dysfunction occur, stop drug.

• Stop drug if signs and symptoms of colitis occur, such as abdominal pain, bloody diarrhea, and fever. Symptoms should resolve within 1 to 3 weeks.

• Stop drug if signs and symptoms of pancreatitis occur, including fever, malaise, and abdominal pain.

• Obtain baseline eye examination and periodically monitor eye examinations during treatment. Stop drug if new or worsening eye disorders occur.

• Monitor patient with impaired renal function for interferon toxicity.

• Use in women of childbearing potential only when effective contraception is being used.

• *Look alike–sound alike:* Don't confuse peginterferon alfa-2a with interferon alfa-2a, interferon alfa-2b, interferon alfa-n3, or peginterferon alfa-2b.

PATIENT TEACHING
• Advise patient to read medication guide that comes with drug.

• Teach patient proper way to give drug and dispose of needles and syringes.

Reactions in bold italics are *life-threatening*. Interactions may have a *rapid onset* or a *delayed onset*.

• Tell patient to immediately report depression or suicidal ideation.

• Tell patient to report signs and symptoms of pancreatitis, colitis, eye disorders, or respiratory disorders.

• Advise patient to avoid driving or operating machinery if he feels dizzy, tired, confused, or sleepy.

• Advise patient not to switch to another brand of interferon without consulting health care provider.

• Advise female patient that drug may alter menstrual cycles and impaired fertility is possible.

❸ Alert: When drug is used with ribavirin, tell male and female patients and their partners to take extreme care to avoid pregnancy during treatment with ribavirin and for 6 months after treatment ends.

SAFETY ALERT!

peginterferon alfa-2b
peg-in-ter-FEER-on

PegIntron, PegIntron Redipen, Sylatron

Therapeutic class: Antivirals
Pharmacologic class: Biological
response modifiers

AVAILABLE FORMS
Injection: 50 mcg/0.5 mL, 80 mcg/0.5 mL, 120 mcg/0.5 mL, 150 mcg/0.5 mL
Powder for injection: 200-mcg, 300-mcg, 600-mcg pens

INDICATIONS & DOSAGES
➤ **Chronic HCV infection, as monotherapy in patients with compensated liver disease not previously treated with interferon alfa (PegIntron, PegIntron Redipen)**
Adults: 1 mcg/kg subcutaneously once weekly for up to 1 year on same day each week. Volume to be injected depends on the strength of drug and patient's body weight. Refer to manufacturer's instructions for weight-based tables.
Adjust-a-dose: Decrease peginterferon alfa-2b dose by 50% in patients with WBC count of 1,000 to less than 1,500/mm³, neu-

trophil count of 500 to less than 750/mm³, or platelet count of 25,000 to less than 50,000/mm³. Discontinue treatment for WBC count less than 1,000/mm³, neutrophil count less than 500/mm³, or platelet count less than 25,000/mm³.

For patients with stable CV disease, decrease peginterferon alfa-2b dose by 50% if Hb level drops more than 2 g/dL in any 4-week period and stop drug if Hb level falls below 8.5 g/dL or 12 g/dL after 4 weeks of reduced dosages. In patients without history of cardiac disease, stop drug if Hb level is less than 8.5 g/dL.

For patients with renal impairment at start of treatment, decrease dosage by 25% for CrCl of 30 to 50 mL/minute and by 50% for CrCl of 10 to 29 mL/minute (including patients on hemodialysis). If renal function decreases during treatment, discontinue drug.

For patients who develop mild depression, continue peginterferon alfa-2b, but evaluate patient once weekly for 4 to 8 weeks. For adults with moderate depression, reduce peginterferon alfa-2b dosage by 50% for 4 to 8 weeks; evaluate patient every week and consider psychiatric consultation. In severe depression, stop peginterferon alfa-2b and obtain immediate psychiatric evaluation.

➤ **Chronic HCV infection in patients with compensated liver disease, combined with ribavirin (PegIntron, PegIntron Redipen)**
Adults: 1.5 mcg/kg subcutaneously once weekly for 24 to 48 weeks on same day every week. Treatment duration depends on genotype and treatment status (naive versus prior treatment failures). For interferon alfa–naive patients with HCV genotype 1, treatment duration is 48 weeks; for patients with HCV genotypes 2 and 3, treatment duration is 24 weeks. Treatment duration for patients who previously failed therapy is 48 weeks, regardless of HCV genotype. For patients with HCV genotype 1 who previously failed therapy, PegIntron and ribavirin without an HCV NS3/4A protease inhibitor should only be used if there are contraindications, significant intolerance, or other clinical factors that wouldn't warrant use of an HCV NS3/4A protease inhibitor. Volume

P

to be injected depends on the strength of PegIntron and patient's body weight. Refer to manufacturer's instructions for weight-based tables and for ribavirin dosages.

Adjust-a-dose: Patients with a history of significant or unstable cardiac disease or CrCl of less than 50 mL/minute shouldn't be treated with PegIntron/ribavirin combination. If dosage reductions are needed, first dosage reduction of PegIntron is to 1 mcg/kg/week and second dosage reduction of PegIntron is to 0.5 mcg/kg/week.

Reduce peginterferon alfa-2b dose in patients with WBC count of 1,000 to less than 1,500/mm³, neutrophil count of 500 to less than 750/mm³, or platelet count of 25,000 to less than 50,000/mm³. Discontinue treatment if Hb level is less than 8.5 g/dL (patients without history of cardiac disease), WBC count is less than 1,000/mm³, neutrophil count is less than 500/mm³, or platelet count is less than 25,000/mm³. Refer to manufacturer's instructions for ribavirin dosage adjustments.

For patients who develop mild depression, continue peginterferon alfa-2b, but evaluate patient once weekly for 4 to 8 weeks. For adults with moderate depression, reduce peginterferon alfa-2b dosage by 50% for 4 to 8 weeks; evaluate patient every week and consider psychiatric consultation. For severe depression, stop peginterferon alfa-2b and obtain immediate psychiatric evaluation.

Children ages 3 to 17: 60 mcg/m² subcutaneously on same day every week. Treatment duration for patients with HCV genotype 1 is 48 weeks; patients with HCV genotypes 2 and 3 should be treated for 24 weeks. Refer to manufacturer's instructions for ribavirin weight-based dosage tables. Patients who reach age 18 while receiving combination therapy should remain on the pediatric dosing regimen.

Adjust-a-dose: Patients with a history of significant or unstable cardiac disease or CrCl of less than 50 mL/minute shouldn't be treated with PegIntron/ribavirin combination. If dosage reductions are needed, first dosage reduction of PegIntron is to 40 mcg/m²/week and second dosage reduction of PegIntron is to 20 mcg/m²/week. Reduce peginterferon alfa-2b dose in pa-

tients with WBC count of 1,000 to less than 1,500/mm³, neutrophil count of 500 to less than 750/mm³, or platelet count of 50,000 to less than 70,000/mm³. Discontinue treatment if Hb level is less than 8.5 g/dL (patients without history of cardiac disease), WBC count is less than 1,000/mm³, neutrophil count is less than 500/mm³, or platelet count is less than 25,000/mm³. Refer to manufacturer's instructions for ribavirin dosage adjustments.

For patients who develop mild depression, continue peginterferon alfa-2b, but evaluate patient once weekly for 4 to 8 weeks. In children with moderate depression, reduce peginterferon alfa-2b dose to 40 mcg/m²/week, then to 20 mcg/m²/week if needed for 4 to 8 weeks; evaluate patient every week and consider psychiatric consultation. In severe depression, stop peginterferon alfa-2b and obtain immediate psychiatric evaluation.

➤ **For adjuvant treatment of melanoma with microscopic or gross nodal involvement within 84 days of definitive surgical resection including complete lymphadenectomy (Sylatron only)**

Adults: 6 mcg/kg/week subcutaneously for 8 doses, followed by 3 mcg/kg/week subcutaneously for up to 5 years. Premedicate with acetaminophen 500 to 1,000 mg P.O. 30 minutes before the first dose and as needed for subsequent doses.

Adjust-a-dose: Refer to manufacturer's instructions for initial and follow-up dosages in renal impairment and dosage adjustments for hematologic and nonhematologic adverse events. Permanently discontinue drug for persistent or worsening severe neuropsychiatric disorders, grade 4 nonhematologic toxicity, inability to tolerate a dose of 1 mcg/kg/week, or new or worsening retinopathy.

ADMINISTRATION
Subcutaneous
- To reconstitute the lyophilized peginterferon alfa-2b in the Redipen, hold the Redipen upright (dose button down), and press the two halves of the pen together until there is an audible click.
- Gently invert the pen to mix the solution. Don't shake.

• Keeping the pen upright, attach the supplied needle, and select the appropriate peginterferon alfa-2b dose by pulling back on the dosing button until the dark bands are visible and turning the button until the dark band is aligned with the correct dose.

• The Redipen is for single use only.

• Reconstitute the peginterferon alfa-2b lyophilized product with only 0.7 mL of supplied diluent (sterile water for injection). Discard the remaining diluent.

• Swirl gently to dissolve completely.

• Before mixing, store PegIntron Redipen in refrigerator between 36° and 46° F (2° and 8° C) and store vials at room temperature between 68° and 77° F (20° and 25° C).

• **Incompatibilities:** Don't add any other medication to solutions containing peginterferon alfa-2b.

ACTION

Binds to specific membrane receptors on the cell surface, inducing certain enzymes, suppressing cell proliferation and immunomodulating activities, and inhibiting virus replication in virus-infected cells. Increases levels of effector proteins and body temperature, and decreases leukocyte and platelet counts.

Route	Onset	Peak	Duration
Subcut.	Unknown	15–44 hr	Unknown

Half-life: PegIntron, 40 hours; Sylatron, 43 to 51 hours.

ADVERSE REACTIONS

CNS: anxiety, depression, dizziness, emotional lability, fatigue, fever, headache, insomnia, irritability, *suicidal behavior,* hypertonia, malaise, agitation, nervousness.
CV: flushing, chest pain.
EENT: pharyngitis, sinusitis, rhinitis, conjunctivitis, blurred vision, dry mouth, taste perversion.
GI: abdominal pain, anorexia, diarrhea, nausea, dyspepsia, right upper quadrant pain, vomiting.
GU: menstrual disorder.
Hematologic: *neutropenia, thrombocytopenia,* anemia.
Hepatic: hepatomegaly.
Metabolic: weight loss, hypothyroidism.

Musculoskeletal: musculoskeletal pain, myalgia, arthralgia.
Respiratory: cough, dyspnea.
Skin: alopecia, dry skin, increased sweating, injection-site inflammation or reaction, pruritus, rash, injection-site pain.
Other: flulike symptoms, rigors, viral infection.

INTERACTIONS

Drugs metabolized by CYP2C8, CYP2C9 (phenytoin, warfarin), or CYP2D6 (flecainide): May decrease serum levels of these drugs. Monitor patient response and drug levels; adjust dosage as needed.
Methadone: May increase methadone level. Monitor patient closely and decrease methadone dosage as needed.
Nucleoside reverse transcriptase inhibitors (NRTIs): May cause severe and potentially fatal hepatic decompensation. If used together in patient coinfected with HIV, monitor patient for toxicities.
Ribavirin: May cause additive hematologic toxicity. Monitor therapy.
Telbivudine: May increase risk of peripheral neuropathy. Avoid use together.

EFFECTS ON LAB TEST RESULTS

• May increase serum bilirubin, uric acid, triglyceride, and ALT levels. May increase or decrease TSH level.

• May decrease Hb level.

• May decrease neutrophil and platelet counts.

CONTRAINDICATIONS & CAUTIONS

• Contraindicated in patients hypersensitive to drug or any of its components, in patients with autoimmune hepatitis or decompensated liver disease, in those with diabetes or thyroid disorders that can't be controlled with medication, in patients who have failed to respond to other alpha interferon treatment or have had an organ transplant, and in those with HIV or HBV.

• Use cautiously in patients with psychiatric disorders, diabetes mellitus, CV disease, CrCl less than 50 mL/minute, pulmonary infiltrates, pulmonary function impairment, or autoimmune, ischemic, or infectious disorders.

Dialyzable drug: No.

P

PREGNANCY-LACTATION-REPRODUCTION

Black Box Warning Use of drug with ribavirin may cause birth defects and fetal death. Combination use is contraindicated in women who are pregnant and in male partners of women who are pregnant. ■

• Combination therapy with ribavirin should begin only after obtaining a negative pregnancy test immediately before start of therapy. Obtain pregnancy tests monthly during therapy and for 6 months after therapy ends. Patients should use two effective forms of contraception.

• There are no adequate studies of drug used as monotherapy in pregnancy. Manufacturer recommends that drug be used in pregnancy only if potential benefit justifies potential fetal risks and that women of childbearing potential use effective contraception during treatment. Some professional guidelines recommend that drug not be used in pregnant women.

• It isn't known if drug appears in breast milk. Patient should discontinue breastfeeding or discontinue drug.

NURSING CONSIDERATIONS

• Obtain eye examination in patient with diabetes or hypertension before starting drug. Retinal hemorrhages, cotton-wool spots, and retinal artery or vein obstruction may occur.

Black Box Warning Drug may cause or aggravate fatal or life-threatening neuropsychiatric, autoimmune, ischemic, and infectious disorders. Monitor patients closely with periodic clinical and laboratory evaluations. In patient with persistently severe or worsening signs or symptoms of these conditions from therapy, withhold drug. In many but not all cases, these disorders resolve after stopping PegIntron therapy. ■

Black Box Warning The risk of serious depression with suicidal ideation, completed suicides, and other neuropsychiatric disorders increases with use of alpha interferons, including Sylatron. Permanently discontinue Sylatron in patients with persistently severe or worsening signs or symptoms of depression, psychosis, or encephalopathy. These disorders may not resolve after stopping Sylatron. ■

• Combination therapy with ribavirin for HCV infection is preferred over monotherapy because of better response rates, unless contraindication or intolerance exists. Monotherapy is only indicated for previously untreated adults.

Black Box Warning If used in combination therapy with ribavirin, monitor patient for worsening cardiac disease secondary to anemia. ■

• Drug may cause or aggravate hypothyroidism, hyperthyroidism, or diabetes.

• Perform ECG on patient with history of MI or arrhythmias before starting drug.

• Start treatment in patient who is well hydrated.

• Monitor patient with history of MI or arrhythmias closely for hypotension, arrhythmias, tachycardia, cardiomyopathy, and signs and symptoms of MI.

• Monitor patient for depression and other mental health disorders. If symptoms are severe, stop drug and refer patient for psychiatric care.

• Monitor patient for signs and symptoms of colitis, such as abdominal pain, bloody diarrhea, and fever. Stop drug if colitis occurs. Symptoms should resolve 1 to 3 weeks after stopping drug.

• Monitor patient for signs and symptoms of pancreatitis (due to elevated triglyceride levels) or hypersensitivity reactions, and stop drug if these occur.

• Monitor patient with pulmonary disease for dyspnea, pulmonary infiltrates, pneumonitis, and pneumonia.

• Monitor patient with renal disease for signs and symptoms of toxicity.

• Monitor CBC count, platelet count, and AST, ALT, bilirubin, and TSH levels before starting drug and periodically during treatment.

• Notify prescriber if severe neutropenia or thrombocytopenia occurs.

• Children may experience growth delays in height and weight.

• *Look alike–sound alike:* Don't confuse peginterferon alfa-2b with interferon alfa-2a, interferon alfa-2b, interferon alfa-n3, or peginterferon alfa-2a. Don't confuse PEG-Intron with Intron A.

PATIENT TEACHING

• Teach patient the appropriate use of the drug and the benefits and risks of treatment. Tell patient that adverse reactions may continue for several months after treatment is stopped.
• Tell patient to immediately report symptoms of depression or suicidal thoughts.
• Instruct patient on importance of proper disposal of needles and syringes, and caution him against reuse of old needles and syringes.
• Tell patient that drug won't prevent transmission of HCV to others and may not cure HCV infection or prevent cirrhosis, liver failure, or liver cancer that may result from HCV infection.
• Advise patient that laboratory tests are needed before starting therapy and periodically thereafter.
• Tell patient to take drug at bedtime and to use fever-reducing drugs to decrease risk of flulike signs and symptoms.
• Inform breast-feeding patient of the potential for adverse reactions in infants. Tell her to either stop using drug or stop breast-feeding.
• Advise patient to brush teeth thoroughly at least twice a day, have regular dental examinations, and rinse mouth thoroughly after emesis.
Black Box Warning Tell patient using combination therapy to avoid pregnancy. ∎

pegloticase
peg-LOE-tih-kase

Krystexxa

Therapeutic class: Antigout agents
Pharmacologic class: Uric acid–specific enzymes

AVAILABLE FORMS
Injection: 8 mg/mL in 2-mL single-use vial

INDICATIONS & DOSAGES
➤ **Treatment of chronic gout in patients refractory to conventional therapy**
Adults: 8 mg by I.V. infusion every 2 weeks over at least 120 minutes.

ADMINISTRATION
I.V.
▼ Keep drug refrigerated until ready to use.
▼ Inspect vial for particulate matter and discoloration. Don't use unless solution is clear and colorless.
▼ Withdraw 8 mg (1 mL) and place into 250 mL NSS or half-NSS. Invert bag several times to ensure mixing; don't shake. After mixing, drug is stable for 4 hours at room temperature or refrigerated. Use within 4 hours of dilution.
▼ Protect from light.
▼ Don't administer diluted drug until it's at room temperature.
▼ Don't administer as I.V. push or bolus. Give drug via gravity feed, syringe-type pump, or infusion pump.
Black Box Warning Premedicate with antihistamine and corticosteroid. ∎
▼ **Incompatibilities:** Solutions other than NSS or half-NSS.

ACTION
Enables oxidation of uric acid to allantoin, thereby lowering serum uric acid level.

Route	Onset	Peak	Duration
I.V.	Unknown	Unknown	Unknown

Half-life: 14 days.

ADVERSE REACTIONS
CV: chest pain.
EENT: nasopharyngitis.
GI: nausea, constipation, vomiting.
Musculoskeletal: gout flare.
Skin: contusion, ecchymosis, urticaria.
Other: *infusion reaction, anaphylaxis.*

INTERACTIONS
Drug-drug. *Febuxostat:* May increase pegloticase-related adverse effects. Avoid use together.
Other pegylated drugs (pegylated interferon, pegylated liposomal doxorubicin): May cause excessive binding. Avoid use together.

EFFECTS ON LAB TEST RESULTS
• May increase or decrease uric acid levels.

P

CONTRAINDICATIONS & CAUTIONS

Black Box Warning Contraindicated in patients with G6PD deficiency because of risk of hemolysis and methemoglobinemia. Screen patients at risk for G6PD deficiency before initiating therapy. ■

• Contraindicated in patients hypersensitivity to pegloticase.

• Use cautiously in patients with HF and in those with history of anaphylactic or infusion reactions.

• Drug isn't recommended for treatment of asymptomatic hyperuricemia.

• Safety and effectiveness in children haven't been established.

Dialyzable drug: Unknown.

PREGNANCY-LACTATION-REPRODUCTION

• Use cautiously in pregnant women and only if potential benefit justifies potential fetal risk.

• It isn't known if drug appears in breast milk. Breast-feeding isn't recommended unless potential benefit outweighs possible risk to the infant.

NURSING CONSIDERATIONS

Black Box Warning Screen high-risk patients, such as those with African or Mediterranean ancestry, for G6PD deficiency because of increased risk of hemolysis and methemoglobinemia. ■

Black Box Warning Administer drug in health care setting. Monitor patient for anaphylactic and infusion reactions. Anaphylaxis may occur with any infusion (including the first one) and at any time, although most reactions have occurred within 2 hours of initiation. Premedicate with antihistamine and corticosteroid. If reaction occurs, slow or stop infusion at physician discretion. ■

Black Box Warning Monitor patient for anaphylactic and infusion reactions for at least 1 hour after administration; realize that hypersensitivity reaction may be delayed. ■

Black Box Warning Monitor uric acid levels and discontinue drug if levels are greater than 6 mg/dL, especially after two successive readings, because risk of anaphylaxis rises with increases in uric acid levels and loss of therapeutic response. ■

• Monitor patient for gout flares and treat with an NSAID or colchicine for at least

1 week before initiation of infusion. Gout flare prophylaxis is recommended for at least the first 6 months of therapy unless medically contraindicated or not tolerated. Drug may still be given during gout flare.

• Carefully monitor patient who requires retreatment after 4-week drug-free interval because he may be at higher risk for infusion reaction or anaphylaxis.

• Monitor patient for signs and symptoms of HF (peripheral edema, shortness of breath, chest pain).

PATIENT TEACHING

• Tell patient to immediately report signs and symptoms of allergic reaction (wheezing, shortness of breath, cough, chest tightness, trouble breathing, reddening of skin or face, tongue swelling, trouble swallowing).

• Caution patient with G6PD deficiency to report it to prescriber because patient shouldn't take drug.

• Tell patient that drug shouldn't be given for high uric acid levels with no symptoms.

• Instruct patient to notify prescriber if he has HF.

• Before treatment begins, tell female patient to inform prescriber if she is pregnant, plans to become pregnant, or is breast-feeding.

• Teach patient to report gout flares during treatment.

• Instruct patient that periodic monitoring of serum uric acid levels will be needed during and after treatment.

SAFETY ALERT!

pemetrexed disodium
peh-meh-TREX-ed

Alimta

Therapeutic class: Antineoplastics
Pharmacologic class: Folate antagonists

AVAILABLE FORMS

Injection: 100 mg, 500 mg in single-use vials

INDICATIONS & DOSAGES

Adjust-a-dose (for all indications): In patients who develop toxic reactions, adjust dosage according to the table.

Toxic reaction	Dosage change
− Grade 3 (severe or undesirable) or grade 4 (life-threatening or disabling) diarrhea or diarrhea requiring hospitalization − Any grade 3 toxicity (except mucositis and increased transaminase levels) − Any grade 4 toxicity (except mucositis) − Platelet count ≥ 50,000/mm³ and ANC < 500/mm³	Give 75% of previous pemetrexed and cisplatin doses.
− Platelet count < 50,000/mm³ without bleeding	
− Platelet count < 50,000/mm³ with bleeding	Give 50% of previous pemetrexed and cisplatin doses.
Grade 3 or 4 mucositis	Give 50% of previous pemetrexed dose and 100% of previous cisplatin dose.
Grade 2 (moderate) neurotoxicity	Give 100% of previous pemetrexed dose and 50% of previous cisplatin dose.
− Grade 3 or 4 neurotoxicity − Any grade 3 or 4 toxicity (except increased transaminase levels) present after two dose reductions	Stop therapy.

➤ **Malignant pleural mesothelioma in patients whose disease is unresectable or who aren't candidates for curative surgery, in combination with cisplatin; locally advanced or metastatic non-small-cell (nonsquamous) lung cancer (NSCLC) as initial treatment, in combination with cisplatin**
Adults: 500 mg/m² I.V. over 10 minutes on day 1 of each 21-day cycle. Starting 30 minutes after pemetrexed infusion ends, give cisplatin 75 mg/m² I.V. over 2 hours.
➤ **Locally advanced or metastatic NSCLC after prior chemotherapy; as maintenance therapy for patients whose disease hasn't progressed after four cycles of platinum-based first-line chemotherapy, as single-agent therapy**
Adults: 500 mg/m² I.V. over 10 minutes on day 1 of each 21-day cycle.

ADMINISTRATION

I.V.
▼ Hazardous drug; use safe handling and disposal precautions.
▼ Premedicate with folic acid 400 to 1,000 mcg P.O. once daily beginning 7 days before first dose of drug and continued during therapy and for 21 days after last dose. Administer vitamin B_{12} 1 mg I.M. 1 week before first dose of pemetrexed and every three cycles thereafter. Administer dexamethasone 4 mg P.O. b.i.d. the day before, the day of, and the day after pemetrexed administration.
▼ Reconstitute 100-mg vial with 4.2 mL or 500-mg vial with 20 mL of preservative-free NSS to yield 25 mg/mL.
▼ Swirl vial gently until powder is completely dissolved. Solution should be clear and colorless to yellow or yellow-green.
▼ Calculate appropriate dose, and further dilute with NSS so total volume of solution is 100 mL.
▼ Give over 10 minutes.
▼ Reconstituted solution and dilution are stable for 24 hours refrigerated.
▼ **Incompatibilities:** Calcium-containing diluents, including Ringer or lactated Ringer for injection; other drugs or diluents.

ACTION

Disturbs cell replication by inhibiting several folate-dependent enzymes involved in nucleotide synthesis. When given with other antineoplastics, drug inhibits growth of mesothelioma cell lines.

Route	Onset	Peak	Duration
I.V.	Unknown	Unknown	Unknown

Half-life: 3½ hours.

ADVERSE REACTIONS

CNS: depression, fatigue, fever, neuropathy.
CV: *cardiac ischemia,* chest pain, edema, *emboli,* thrombosis.
EENT: pharyngitis, conjunctivitis.

GI: anorexia, constipation, diarrhea, nausea, stomatitis, vomiting, esophagitis, painful, difficult swallowing, taste disturbance.
GU: *renal failure.*
Hematologic: anemia, *leukopenia, neutropenia, thrombocytopenia.*
Metabolic: dehydration.
Musculoskeletal: arthralgia, myalgia.
Respiratory: dyspnea.
Skin: alopecia, rash.
Other: allergic reaction, infection.

INTERACTIONS

Drug-drug. *Nephrotoxic drugs, probenecid:* May delay pemetrexed clearance. Monitor patient.
NSAIDs: May decrease pemetrexed clearance in patients with mild to moderate renal insufficiency. For NSAIDs with short half-lives, avoid use for 2 days before, during, and 2 days after pemetrexed therapy. For NSAIDs with long half-lives, avoid use for 5 days before, during, and 2 days after pemetrexed therapy.

EFFECTS ON LAB TEST RESULTS

● May increase ALT, AST, and creatinine levels. May decrease Hb level and hematocrit.
● May decrease absolute neutrophil, platelet, and WBC counts.

CONTRAINDICATIONS & CAUTIONS

● Contraindicated in patients with a history of severe hypersensitivity reaction to drug.
● Don't use in patients with CrCl of less than 45 mL/minute.
Dialyzable drug: Unknown.
⚠ *Overdose S&S:* Neutropenia, anemia, thrombocytopenia, mucositis, rash, infection with or without fever, diarrhea.

PREGNANCY-LACTATION-REPRODUCTION

● There are no adequate studies in pregnant women. Drug can cause fetal harm. Advise women to avoid becoming pregnant and to use effective contraception during therapy. If drug is used during pregnancy or if patient becomes pregnant during therapy, apprise her of potential fetal harm.

● It isn't known if drug appears in breast milk. Patient should discontinue breastfeeding or discontinue drug.

NURSING CONSIDERATIONS

● Patient shouldn't start a new cycle of treatment unless ANC is 1,500/mm³ or more, platelet count is 100,000/mm³ or more, and CrCl is 45 mL/minute or more.
● Patients with pleural effusion and ascites may need to have effusion drained before therapy.
● Monitor renal function, CBC, platelet count, Hb level, hematocrit, and LFT values.
● Assess patient for neurotoxicity, mucositis, and diarrhea. Severe symptoms may warrant dosage adjustment.
⊙ *Alert:* To reduce the occurrence and severity of cutaneous reactions, give a corticosteroid, such as dexamethasone 4 mg P.O. b.i.d., the day before, the day of, and the day after giving this drug.
⊙ *Alert:* To reduce toxicity, patient should take 350 to 1,000 mcg of folic acid daily, 5 days before therapy until 21 days after therapy.
⊙ *Alert:* Give vitamin B$_{12}$ 1,000 mcg I.M. once during the week before the first dose and every three cycles thereafter. After the first cycle, vitamin injections may be given on the first day of the cycle.
● *Look alike–sound alike:* Don't confuse pemetrexed with methotrexate or pralatrexate.

PATIENT TEACHING

● Inform patient that corticosteroids and vitamins will be given before pemetrexed to help minimize its adverse effects.
● Tell patient to avoid NSAIDs for several days before, during, and after treatment.
● Urge patient to report adverse effects, especially fever, sore throat, infection, diarrhea, fatigue, and limb pain.

---

penicillin G benzathine
(benzathine benzylpenicillin)
pen-i-SILL-in

Bicillin L-A, Permapen

Therapeutic class: Antibiotics
Pharmacologic class: Natural penicillins

AVAILABLE FORMS
Injection: 300,000 units/mL, 600,000
units/mL

INDICATIONS & DOSAGES
➤ **Congenital syphilis**
Children ages 2 to 12: Adjust dosage based
on adult dosage schedule.
Children younger than age 2: 50,000
units/kg (up to 2.4 million units) I.M. as
a single dose.
➤ **Group A streptococcal URIs**
Adults: 1.2 million units I.M. as a single
injection.
Children weighing 27 kg or more: 900,000
units I.M. as a single injection.
*Infants and children weighing less than
27 kg:* 300,000 to 600,000 units I.M. as a
single injection.
➤ **To prevent poststreptococcal
rheumatic fever and glomerulonephritis**
Adults and children: 1.2 million units I.M.
once monthly or 600,000 units I.M. every
2 weeks.
➤ **Syphilis (primary, secondary, and
latent)**
Adults: 2.4 million units I.M. as a single
dose.
➤ **Syphilis (tertiary and neurosyphilis)**
Adults: 2.4 million units I.M. once every
7 days for 3 weeks.
➤ **Yaws, bejel, and pinta**
Adults: 1.2 million units I.M. as a single
injection.

ADMINISTRATION
I.M.
Black Box Warning Inadvertent I.V. use
may cause cardiac arrest and death. ■
● Before giving drug, ask patient about
allergic reactions to penicillin.

● Obtain specimen for culture and sensitivity tests before giving first dose. Begin
therapy while awaiting results.
● Shake well before injecting.
● Inject deep into upper outer quadrant of
buttocks in adults and in midlateral thigh
in infants and small children. Rotate injection sites. Avoid injection into or near
major nerves or blood vessels to prevent
permanent neurovascular damage.
● Injection may be painful, but ice applied
to the site may ease discomfort.
● Store in refrigerator at 36° to 46 °F (2° to
8° C); don't freeze.

ACTION
Inhibits cell-wall synthesis during bacterial
multiplication.

Route	Onset	Peak	Duration
I.M.	Unknown	13–24 hr	1–4 wk

Half-life: 30 to 60 minutes.

ADVERSE REACTIONS
CNS: neuropathy.
GI: *pseudomembranous colitis,* enterocoli-
tis, nausea, vomiting.
GU: nephropathy.
Hematologic: *agranulocytosis, leukopenia,
thrombocytopenia,* eosinophilia, hemolytic
anemia.
Skin: exfoliative dermatitis, maculopapular
rash.
Other: *anaphylaxis,* hypersensitivity reac-
tions, sterile abscess at injection site.

INTERACTIONS
Drug-drug. *Aminoglycosides:* Physical and
chemical incompatibility. Give separately.
Anticoagulants (warfarin): May increase or
decrease anticoagulant effects of warfarin.
Monitor coagulation studies and adjust
warfarin dosages as needed.
Hormonal contraceptives: May decrease
hormonal contraceptive effectiveness. Advise use of additional form of contraception
during therapy.
Live-virus vaccines: May decrease effectiveness of live-virus vaccines. Avoid concurrent use.
Methotrexate: May increase risk of
methotrexate toxicity. Monitor patient
closely.

P

Probenecid: May increase penicillin level. Probenecid may be used for this purpose.
Tetracycline: May antagonize penicillin G benzathine effects. Avoid using together.

EFFECTS ON LAB TEST RESULTS
• May increase BUN, creatinine, and AST levels.
• May decrease Hb level.
• May increase eosinophil count. May decrease platelet, WBC, and granulocyte counts. May cause positive Coombs test results.
• May falsely decrease aminoglycoside level. May cause false-positive CSF protein test results. May alter urine glucose testing using cupric sulfate (Benedict reagent).

CONTRAINDICATIONS & CAUTIONS
• Contraindicated in patients hypersensitive to drug or other penicillins.
• Inadvertent intravascular administration has resulted in severe neurovascular damage, including transverse myelitis with permanent paralysis and gangrene.
• Use cautiously in patients allergic to other drugs, especially to cephalosporins, because of possible cross-sensitivity.
• Use cautiously in patients with a history of significant allergies or asthma.
• Drug may cause CDAD ranging in severity from mild diarrhea to fatal colitis. If CDAD is suspected or confirmed, drug may need to be discontinued and treatment initiated.
Dialyzable drug: Unknown.
⚠ *Overdose S&S:* Neuromuscular hyperexcitability, seizures.

PREGNANCY-LACTATION-REPRODUCTION
• There are no adequate studies in pregnant women, and animal studies have shown no adverse fetal effects. Use during pregnancy only if clearly needed.
• Use cautiously in breast-feeding women.

NURSING CONSIDERATIONS
🕒 *Alert:* Bicillin L-A is the only penicillin G benzathine product indicated for sexually transmitted infections. Don't substitute Bicillin C-R because it may not be effective.
• Monitor patient for diarrhea. Drug may need to be stopped.

• Drug's extremely slow absorption time makes allergic reactions difficult to treat.
• If large doses are given or if therapy is prolonged, bacterial or fungal superinfection may occur, especially in elderly, debilitated or immunosuppressed patients.
• *Look alike–sound alike:* Don't confuse penicillin G benzathine with Polycillin, penicillamine, or the various other types of penicillin.

PATIENT TEACHING
• Tell patient to report adverse reactions promptly.
• Inform patient that fever and increased WBC count are the most common reactions.
• Warn patient that I.M. injection may be painful but that ice applied to the site may ease discomfort.

penicillin G potassium (benzylpenicillin potassium)
pen-i-SILL-in

Pfizerpen

Therapeutic class: Antibiotics
Pharmacologic class: Natural penicillins

AVAILABLE FORMS
Injection: 1 million units, 5 million units, 20 million units
Premixed injection: 1 million units/50 mL, 2 million units/50 mL, 3 million units/50 mL

INDICATIONS & DOSAGES
Adjust-a-dose (for all indications): If CrCl is greater than 10 mL/minute/1.73 m², give full loading dose followed by one-half of loading dose every 4 to 5 hours.
➤ **Actinomycosis**
Adults: For cervicofacial infections, 1 to 6 million units/day in divided doses I.M. or I.V. every 4 to 6 hours. For thoracic or abdominal infections, 10 to 20 million units/day in divided doses I.M. or I.V. every 4 to 6 hours or by continuous I.V. infusion.
➤ **Anthrax**
Adults: 8 million units/day in divided doses I.M. or I.V. every 6 hours; higher doses may

be required depending on susceptibility of the organism.

➤ **Clostridial infections**
Adults: 20 million units/day in divided doses I.M. or I.V. every 4 to 6 hours.

➤ **Diphtheria**
Adults: 2 to 3 million units/day in divided doses I.M. or I.V. every 4 to 6 hours for 10 to 12 days.
Children: 150,000 to 250,000 units/kg/day in equal doses I.M. or I.V. every 6 hours for 7 to 10 days.

➤ **Disseminated gonococcal infections**
Adults: 10 million units/day in divided doses I.M. or I.V. every 4 to 6 hours.
Children weighing 45 kg or more with arthritis, endocarditis, or meningitis: 10 million units/day in four equally divided doses I.M. or I.V., with duration of therapy depending on type of infection.
Children weighing less than 45 kg with arthritis: 100,000 units/kg/day in four equally divided doses I.M. or I.V. for 7 to 10 days.
Children weighing less than 45 kg with endocarditis: 250,000 units/kg/day in equal doses I.M. or I.V. every 4 hours for 4 weeks.
Children weighing less than 45 kg with meningitis: 250,000 units/kg/day in equal doses I.M. or I.V. every 4 hours for 10 to 14 days.

➤ *Erysipelothrix* **endocarditis**
Adults: 12 to 20 million units/day in divided doses I.M. or I.V. every 4 to 6 hours for 4 to 6 weeks.

➤ **Fusospirochetosis**
Adults: 5 to 10 million units/day in divided doses I.M. or I.V. every 4 to 6 hours.

➤ **Gram-negative bacillary bacteremia**
Adults: 20 to 80 million units/day by continuous I.V. infusion. Penicillin G isn't drug of choice for treatment of gram-negative bacillary infections.

➤ **Haverhill fever; rat bite fever**
Adults: 12 to 20 million units/day in divided doses I.M. or I.V. every 4 to 6 hours for 3 to 4 weeks.

➤ **Haverhill fever (with endocarditis caused by** *Streptobacillus moniliformis***); rat bite fever**
Children: 150,000 to 250,000 units/kg/day in equal doses every 4 hours for 4 weeks.

➤ *Listeria monocytogenes* **endocarditis or meningitis**
Adults: 15 to 20 million units/day in divided doses I.M. or I.V. every 4 to 6 hours. Treat for 2 weeks for meningitis and 4 weeks for endocarditis.
Neonates: 500,000 to 1 million units I.M. or I.V. daily in divided doses.

➤ **Meningococcal meningitis or septicemia**
Adults: 24 million units/day as 2 million units I.M. or I.V. every 2 hours. Or, a continuous I.V. infusion of 20 to 30 million units/day.

➤ **Neurosyphilis**
Adults: 12 to 24 million units/day (2 to 4 million units every 4 hours) I.M. or I.V. for 10 to 14 days. Many experts recommend benzathine penicillin G 2.4 million units I.M. weekly for 3 weeks following completion of this regimen.

➤ *Pasteurella multocida* **bacteremia or meningitis**
Adults: 4 to 6 million units/day in divided doses I.M. or I.V. every 4 to 6 hours for 2 weeks.

➤ **Serious staphylococcal infections**
Adults: 5 to 24 million units/day in equally divided doses I.M. or I.V. every 4 to 6 hours.

➤ **Serious streptococcal infections**
Adults: 12 to 24 million units/day in equally divided doses I.M. or I.V. every 4 to 6 hours.

➤ **Meningitis caused by susceptible strains of pneumococcus and meningococcus**
Children: 250,000 units/kg/day in equal doses I.M. or I.V. every 4 hours for 7 to 14 days, depending on infecting organism. Maximum dosage is 12 to 20 million units/day.

➤ **Serious streptococcal infections, such as pneumonia and endocarditis (***Streptococcus pneumoniae***), and meningococcal infections**
Children: 150,000 to 300,000 units/kg/day in equal doses I.M. or I.V. every 4 to 6 hours. Duration of therapy depends on infecting organism and type of infection.

➤ **Syphilis (congenital and neurosyphilis) after newborn period**
Children: 200,000 to 300,000 units/kg/day (administered as 50,000 units/kg I.V. every 4 to 6 hours) for 10 to 14 days.

P

ADMINISTRATION
I.V.
▼ Before giving drug, ask patient about allergic reactions to penicillin.

▼ Obtain specimen for culture and sensitivity tests before giving first dose. Begin therapy while awaiting results.

▼ Reconstitute drug with sterile water for injection, D_5W, or NSS for injection. Volume of diluent varies with manufacturer.

▼ Reconstituted solution may be stored in refrigerator for up to 7 days.

▼ For intermittent infusion in adults, give drug over 1 to 2 hours. For intermittent infusion in infants, give drug over 15 to 30 minutes.

⚠ **Alert:** Don't use in children requiring less than 1 million units/dose.

▼ For continuous infusion, add reconstituted drug to 1 to 2 L of compatible solution. Determine how much fluid is needed and what the rate should be for a 24-hour period; then, add the drug to this fluid.

▼ Don't administer premixed solutions to patients requiring less than 1 million units per dose.

▼ **Incompatibilities:** Other drugs.

I.M.
● Before giving drug, ask patient about allergic reactions to penicillin.

● Obtain specimen for culture and sensitivity tests before giving first dose. Begin therapy while awaiting results.

⚠ **Alert:** Don't use in children requiring less than 1 million units/dose.

● I.M. is the preferred route. Keep total volume of injection small.

● Give deep into large muscle; injection may be extremely painful.

● I.M. injection may be painful, but ice applied to the site may help alleviate discomfort.

ACTION
Inhibits cell-wall synthesis during bacterial multiplication.

Route	Onset	Peak	Duration
I.V.	Immediate	Immediate	Unknown
I.M.	Unknown	15–30 min	Unknown

Half-life: 30 to 60 minutes.

ADVERSE REACTIONS
CNS: *seizures,* agitation, anxiety, confusion, depression, dizziness, fatigue, hallucinations, lethargy, neuropathy.
CV: thrombophlebitis, *cardiac arrest, arrhythmias.*
GI: *pseudomembranous colitis,* enterocolitis, nausea, vomiting.
GU: interstitial nephritis, nephropathy.
Hematologic: *agranulocytosis, leukopenia, thrombocytopenia,* anemia, eosinophilia, hemolytic anemia.
Metabolic: *severe potassium poisoning.*
Skin: exfoliative dermatitis, maculopapular eruptions, pain at injection site.
Other: *anaphylaxis,* hypersensitivity reactions, overgrowth of nonsusceptible organisms.

INTERACTIONS
Drug-drug. *Aminoglycosides:* Physically and chemically incompatible. Administer separately.
Aspirin, furosemide, indomethacin, sulfonamides, thiazide diuretics: May compete with penicillin for renal tubular secretion, prolonging penicillin half-life. Monitor patient.
Bacteriostatic antibacterial agents (chloramphenicol, macrolide antibiotics, sulfonamides, tetracyclines): Physically and chemically incompatible. Give separately.
Heparin: May increase risk of bleeding. Closely monitor patient and adjust heparin dose as needed.
Hormonal contraceptives: May decrease hormonal contraceptive effectiveness. Advise use of additional form of contraception during therapy.
Live-virus vaccines: May decrease effectiveness of live-virus vaccines. Don't use together.
Methotrexate: May increase risk of methotrexate toxicity. Monitor patient closely.
Oral anticoagulants: May increase or decrease anticoagulant effects. Monitor PT and INR.
Potassium-sparing diuretics: May increase risk of hyperkalemia. Avoid using together.
Probenecid: May increase penicillin level. Probenecid may be used for this purpose.

Reactions in bold italics are *life-threatening*. Interactions may have a *rapid onset* or a **delayed onset**.

EFFECTS ON LAB TEST RESULTS
• May increase potassium level. May decrease Hb level.
• May increase eosinophil count. May decrease platelet, WBC, and granulocyte counts.
• May cause positive Coombs test result.
• May falsely decrease aminoglycoside levels. May cause false-positive CSF protein test result. May alter urine glucose testing using cupric sulfate (Benedict reagent).

CONTRAINDICATIONS & CAUTIONS
• Contraindicated in patients hypersensitive to drug or other penicillins.
• Use cautiously in patients with other drug allergies, especially to cephalosporins, because of possible cross-sensitivity.
• Use cautiously in patients with renal impairment.
• Drug may cause CDAD ranging in severity from mild diarrhea to fatal colitis. If CDAD is suspected or confirmed, drug may need to be discontinued and treatment initiated.
Dialyzable drug: Yes.
⚠ *Overdose S&S:* Agitation, confusion, asterixis, hallucinations, stupor, coma, multifocal myoclonus, seizures, encephalopathy, hyperkalemia.

PREGNANCY-LACTATION-REPRODUCTION
• There are no adequate studies in pregnant women. Animal studies reveal no evidence of fetal harm. Use during pregnancy only if clearly needed.
• Use cautiously in breast-feeding women.

NURSING CONSIDERATIONS
• Before starting drug, obtain culture and susceptibility tests to identify organisms causing infection.
• Monitor renal function closely. Patients with poor renal function may have increased levels of penicillin and are at increased risk for adverse effects.
• Due to increased risk of electrolyte imbalances, monitor potassium and sodium levels closely in patients receiving more than 10 million units I.V. daily.
• Observe patient closely. With large doses and prolonged therapy, bacterial or fungal superinfection may occur, especially in elderly, debilitated, or immunosuppressed patients.
• *Look alike–sound alike:* Don't confuse penicillin G potassium with Polycillin, penicillamine, or the various other types of penicillin.

PATIENT TEACHING
• Tell patient to notify prescriber if rash, fever, or chills develop. A rash is the most common allergic reaction.
• Warn patient that I.M. injection may be painful but that ice applied to the site may help alleviate discomfort.

penicillin G procaine (benzylpenicillin procaine)
pen-i-SILL-in

Therapeutic class: Antibiotics
Pharmacologic class: Natural penicillins

AVAILABLE FORMS
Injection: 300,000 units/mL, 600,000 units/mL

INDICATIONS & DOSAGES
➤ **Cutaneous anthrax**
Adults: 600,000 to 1 million units/day I.M.
➤ **Inhalational anthrax (postexposure)**
Adults: 1.2 million units I.M. every 12 hours. Available safety data for penicillin G procaine at this dose would best support a duration of therapy of 2 weeks or less.
Children: 25,000 units/kg (maximum, 1.2 million units) I.M. every 12 hours.
Note: Treatment of inhalational anthrax (postexposure) must be continued for a total of 60 days. Consider risks and benefits of continuing administration of penicillin G procaine for more than 2 weeks or switching to an effective alternative treatment.
➤ **Bacterial endocarditis (group A streptococci), only in extremely sensitive infections**
Adults: 600,000 to 1 million units/day I.M.
➤ **Adjunctive therapy for diphtheria with antitoxin**
Adults: 300,000 to 600,000 units/day I.M. for 14 days.

P

➤ **Diphtheria carrier state**
Adults: 300,000 units/day I.M. for 10 days.
➤ **Erysipeloid**
Adults: 600,000 to 1 million units/day I.M.
➤ **Fusospirochetosis (Vincent infection)**
Adults: 600,000 to 1 million units/day I.M.
➤ **Pneumonia (pneumococcal), moderately severe (uncomplicated)**
Adults and children weighing 27.3 kg or more: 600,000 to 1 million units/day I.M. for a minimum of 10 days.
Children weighing less than 27.3 kg: 300,000 units/day I.M.
➤ **Rat bite fever (*Streptobacillus moniliformis* and *Spirillum minus*)**
Adults: 600,000 to 1 million units/day I.M.
➤ **Staphylococcal infections, moderately severe to severe**
Adults and children weighing 27.3 kg or more: 600,000 to 1 million units/day I.M. for a minimum of 10 days.
Children weighing less than 27.3 kg: 300,000 units/day I.M.
➤ **Streptococcal infections (group A), including moderately severe to severe tonsillitis, erysipelas, scarlet fever, URI, and skin and soft-tissue infections**
Adults and children weighing 27.3 kg or more: 600,000 to 1 million units/day I.M. for minimum of 10 days.
Children weighing less than 27.3 kg: 300,000 units/day I.M.
➤ **Syphilis (primary, secondary, and latent syphilis with negative spinal fluid)**
Adults and children older than age 12: 600,000 units/day I.M. for 8 days; total, 4.8 million units.
➤ **Late syphilis (tertiary syphilis, neurosyphilis, and latent syphilis with positive spinal fluid examination or no spinal fluid examination)**
Adults: 600,000 units/day I.M. for 10 to 15 days; total, 6 to 9 million units.
➤ **Yaws, bejel, pinta**
Adults: Treatment as for syphilis in the corresponding stage of disease.

ADMINISTRATION
I.M.
● Before giving drug, ask patient about allergic reactions to penicillin.

● Obtain specimen for culture and sensitivity tests before giving first dose. Begin therapy while awaiting results.
● Give deep in upper outer quadrant of buttocks in adults and in midlateral thigh in small children. Rotate injection sites. Don't give subcutaneously. Don't massage injection site. Avoid injection near major nerves or blood vessels.
🕔 *Alert:* Inadvertent I.V., intravascular, or intra-arterial administration may cause severe or permanent neurovascular damage.
● I.M. injection may be painful, but ice applied to the site may help alleviate discomfort.

ACTION
Inhibits cell-wall synthesis during bacterial multiplication.

Route	Onset	Peak	Duration
I.M.	Unknown	1–4 hr	1–5 days

Half-life: 30 to 60 minutes.

ADVERSE REACTIONS
CNS: *seizures,* agitation, anxiety, confusion, depression, dizziness, fatigue, hallucinations, lethargy.
GI: *pseudomembranous colitis,* enterocolitis, nausea, vomiting.
GU: interstitial nephritis, nephropathy.
Hematologic: *agranulocytosis, thrombocytopenia,* hemolytic anemia, *leukopenia,* anemia, eosinophilia.
Musculoskeletal: arthralgia.
Other: *anaphylaxis,* hypersensitivity reactions, overgrowth of nonsusceptible organisms.

INTERACTIONS
Drug-drug. *Aminoglycosides:* Physically and chemically incompatible. Give separately.
Hormonal contraceptives: May decrease hormonal contraceptive effectiveness. Advise use of additional form of contraception during therapy.
Live-virus vaccines: May decrease vaccine effectiveness. Avoid concurrent use.
Methotrexate: May increase risk of methotrexate toxicity. Monitor patient closely.

Reactions in bold italics are *life-threatening*. Interactions may have a *rapid onset* or a *delayed onset*.

Oral anticoagulants (warfarin): May increase or decrease effects of warfarin. Monitor coagulation status and adjust warfarin dosage as needed.
Probenecid: May increase penicillin level. Probenecid may be used for this purpose.

EFFECTS ON LAB TEST RESULTS
• May decrease Hb level.
• May increase eosinophil count. May decrease platelet, WBC, and granulocyte counts.

CONTRAINDICATIONS & CAUTIONS
• Contraindicated in patients hypersensitive to drug or other penicillins.
• Use cautiously in patients with other drug allergies, especially to cephalosporins, because of possible cross-sensitivity. Some formulations contain sulfites, which may cause allergic reactions in sensitive people.
• In patients with a history of hypersensitivity to procaine, administer test with 0.1 mL of 1% or 2% procaine solution and observe for wheal, flare, or eruption. If these occur, don't use drug and treat sensitivity supportively.
• Use cautiously in patients with a history of seizure disorders and renal impairment.
• Drug may cause CDAD ranging in severity from mild diarrhea to fatal colitis. If CDAD is suspected or confirmed, drug may need to be discontinued and treatment initiated.
Dialyzable drug: Yes.
⚠ *Overdose S&S:* Neuromuscular hyperexcitability, seizures.

PREGNANCY-LACTATION-REPRODUCTION
• There are no adequate studies in pregnant women. Drug crosses placental barrier. Use during pregnancy only when clearly needed.
• Use cautiously in breast-feeding women.

NURSING CONSIDERATIONS
🔹 *Alert:* Continue postexposure treatment for inhalation anthrax for 60 days. Prescriber should consider the risk-benefit ratio of continuing penicillin longer than 2 weeks, compared with switching to another drug.
• Monitor patient for diarrhea and initiate therapeutic measures as needed. Drug may need to be stopped.

• Allergic reactions are hard to treat because of drug's slow absorption rate.
• Monitor renal and hematopoietic function periodically.
• If large doses are given or if therapy is prolonged, bacterial or fungal superinfection may occur, especially in elderly, debilitated, or immunosuppressed patients.
• Treatment duration depends on site and cause of infection.
• *Look alike–sound alike:* Don't confuse penicillin G procaine with Polycillin, penicillamine, or the various other types of penicillin.

PATIENT TEACHING
• Tell patient to report adverse reactions promptly. A rash is the most common allergic reaction.
• Warn patient that I.M. injection may be painful but that ice applied to the site may help alleviate discomfort.

penicillin G sodium (benzylpenicillin sodium)
pen-i-SILL-in

Crystapen✦

Therapeutic class: Antibiotics
Pharmacologic class: Natural penicillins

P

AVAILABLE FORMS
Injection: 5 million-unit vial

INDICATIONS & DOSAGES
Adjust-a-dose (for all indications): If CrCl is less than 10 mL/minute, give the full loading dose followed by 50% of the loading dose every 8 to 10 hours. If patient is uremic and CrCl is more than 10 mL/minute, give full loading dose; then give half the loading dose every 4 to 5 hours for additional doses.
➤ **Actinomycosis**
Adults: For cervicofacial infections, 1 to 6 million units/day in divided doses I.M. or I.V. every 4 to 6 hours. For thoracic or abdominal infections, 10 to 20 million units/day in divided doses every 4 to 6 hours.

➤ **Anthrax**
Adults: 8 million units/day in divided doses I.M. or I.V. every 6 hours; higher dosages may be required depending on susceptibility of the organism.

➤ **Clostridial infections**
Adults: 20 million units/day in divided doses I.M. or I.V. every 4 to 6 hours.

➤ **Diphtheria**
Adults: 2 to 3 million units/day in divided doses I.M. or I.V. every 4 to 6 hours for 10 to 12 days.

➤ **Disseminated gonococcal infection**
Adults: 10 million units/day I.M. or I.V. in divided doses every 4 to 6 hours.
Children weighing 45 kg or more with arthritis, endocarditis, or meningitis: 10 million units/day I.M. or I.V. in four equally divided doses, with duration of therapy depending on type of infection.
Children weighing less than 45 kg with arthritis: 100,000 units/kg/day I.M. or I.V. in four equally divided doses for 7 to 10 days.
Children weighing less than 45 kg with endocarditis: 250,000 units/kg/day I.M. or I.V. in equal doses every 4 hours for 4 weeks.
Children weighing less than 45 kg with meningitis: 250,000 units/kg/day I.M. or I.V. in equal doses every 4 hours for 10 to 14 days.

➤ *Erysipelothrix* **endocarditis**
Adults: 12 to 20 million units/day I.M. in divided doses I.M. or I.V. every 4 to 6 hours for 4 to 6 weeks.

➤ **Fusospirochetosis**
Adults: 5 to 10 million units/day in divided doses I.M. or I.V. every 4 to 6 hours.

➤ **Haverhill fever; rat bite fever**
Adults: 12 to 20 million units/day in divided doses I.M. or I.V. every 4 to 6 hours for 3 to 4 weeks.

➤ **Haverhill fever with endocarditis caused by** *Streptobacillus moniliformis;* **rat bite fever**
Children: 150,000 to 250,000 units/kg/day I.M. or I.V. in equal doses every 4 to 6 hours for 4 weeks.

➤ *Listeria monocytogenes* **endocarditis or meningitis**
Adults: 15 to 20 million units/day in divided doses I.M. or I.V. every 4 to 6 hours. Treat for 2 weeks for meningitis and 4 weeks for endocarditis.

➤ **Meningococcal meningitis or septicemia**
Adults: 24 million units/day as 2 million units I.M. or I.V. every 2 hours.

➤ **Neurosyphilis**
Adults: 12 to 24 million units/day (2 to 4 million units I.M. or I.V. every 4 hours) for 10 to 14 days. Many experts recommend benzathine penicillin G 2.4 million units I.M. weekly for 3 weeks following completion of this regimen.

➤ *Pasteurella multocida* **bacteremia or meningitis**
Adults: 4 to 6 million units/day in divided doses I.M. or I.V. every 4 to 6 hours for 2 weeks.

➤ **Serious staphylococcal and streptococcal infections**
Adults: 5 to 24 million units/day in equally divided doses I.M. or I.V. every 4 to 6 hours.

➤ **Diphtheria (adjunctive therapy to antitoxin and for prevention of carrier state)**
Children: 150,000 to 250,000 units/kg/day in equal doses I.M. or I.V. every 6 hours for 7 to 10 days.

➤ **Meningitis caused by susceptible strains of pneumococcus and meningococcus**
Children: 250,000 units/kg/day in equal doses I.M. or I.V. every 4 hours for 7 to 14 days, depending on infecting organism. Maximum dosage is 12 to 20 million units/day.

➤ **Serious streptococcal infections, such as pneumonia and endocarditis (***Streptococcus pneumoniae***), and meningococcal infections**
Children: 150,000 units/kg/day in equal doses I.M. or I.V. every 4 to 6 hours. Duration of therapy depends on infecting organism and type of infection.

➤ **Syphilis (congenital and neurosyphilis) after newborn period**
Children: 200,000 to 300,000 units/kg/day (administered as 50,000 units/kg I.M. or I.V. every 4 to 6 hours) for 10 to 14 days.

Reactions in bold italics are *life-threatening*. Interactions may have a *rapid onset* or a **delayed onset**.

ADMINISTRATION
I.V.

▼ Before giving drug, ask patient about allergic reactions to penicillin.

▼ Obtain specimen for culture and sensitivity tests before giving first dose. Begin therapy while awaiting results.

▼ Reconstitute drug with sterile water for injection, NSS for injection, or D_5W. Check manufacturer's instructions for volume of diluent necessary to produce desired drug level.

▼ Give by intermittent infusion: Dilute drug in 50 to 100 mL, and give over 30 minutes to 2 hours every 4 to 6 hours.

☉ Alert: Don't use in children requiring less than 1 million units/dose.

▼ In infants and children, give divided doses over 15 to 30 minutes.

▼ Sterile reconstituted solution may be kept in refrigerator for up to 3 days.

▼ **Incompatibilities:** Other drugs.

I.M.

☉ Alert: Before giving drug, ask patient about allergic reactions to penicillin and cephalosporin.

● I.M. is the preferred route.

● Obtain specimen for culture and sensitivity tests before giving first dose. Begin therapy while awaiting results.

☉ Alert: Don't use in children requiring less than 1 million units/dose.

● Injection may be painful, but ice applied to site may help alleviate discomfort.

ACTION

Inhibits cell-wall synthesis during bacterial multiplication.

Route	Onset	Peak	Duration
I.V.	Immediate	Immediate	Unknown
I.M.	Unknown	15–30 min	Unknown

Half-life: 30 to 60 minutes.

ADVERSE REACTIONS

CNS: neuropathy, *seizures,* agitation, anxiety, confusion, depression, dizziness, fatigue, hallucinations, lethargy.

CV: *HF,* thrombophlebitis.

GI: enterocolitis, ischemic colitis, nausea, vomiting, *pseudomembranous colitis.*

GU: nephropathy, interstitial nephritis.

Hematologic: hemolytic anemia, *agranulocytosis, leukopenia, thrombocytopenia,* anemia, eosinophilia.

Musculoskeletal: arthralgia.

Other: hypersensitivity reactions, *anaphylaxis,* overgrowth of nonsusceptible organisms, injection-site pain, vein irritation.

INTERACTIONS

Drug-drug. *Aminoglycosides:* Physically and chemically incompatible. Give separately.

Aspirin, furosemide, indomethacin, sulfonamides, thiazide diuretics: May compete with penicillin for renal tubular secretion, prolonging the half-life of penicillin. Monitor patient.

Bacteriostatic antibacterial agents (chloramphenicol, macrolide antibiotics, sulfonamides, tetracyclines): May antagonize bactericidal effect of penicillin. Avoid concomitant use.

Heparin: May increase risk of bleeding. Closely monitor coagulation status. Adjust heparin dose as needed.

Hormonal contraceptives: May decrease hormonal contraceptive effectiveness. Advise use of additional form of contraception during penicillin therapy.

Live-virus vaccines: May decrease effectiveness of live-virus vaccines. Avoid concurrent use.

Oral anticoagulants: May increase or decrease anticoagulant effects. Monitor PT and INR.

Probenecid: May increase penicillin level. Probenecid may be used for this purpose.

EFFECTS ON LAB TEST RESULTS

● May decrease Hb level.

● May cause positive Coombs test result. May increase eosinophil count. May decrease platelet, WBC, granulocyte, and RBC counts.

● May cause false-positive CSF protein test result. May falsely decrease aminoglycoside level. May alter urine glucose testing using cupric sulfate (Benedict reagent).

P

CONTRAINDICATIONS & CAUTIONS
• Contraindicated in patients hypersensitive to drug or other penicillins and in those on sodium-restricted diets.
• Drug may cause CDAD ranging in severity from mild diarrhea to fatal colitis. If CDAD is suspected or confirmed, drug may need to be discontinued and treatment initiated.
• Use cautiously in patients with other drug allergies, especially to cephalosporins, because of possible cross-sensitivity.
Dialyzable drug: Yes.
⚠ *Overdose S&S:* Neuromuscular hyperexcitability, seizures.

PREGNANCY-LACTATION-REPRODUCTION
• There are no adequate studies in pregnant women but experience hasn't shown evidence of adverse fetal effects. Use during pregnancy only if clearly needed.
• Drug appears in breast milk. Use cautiously in breast-feeding women.

NURSING CONSIDERATIONS
• Drug may alter normal colon flora. Monitor patient for diarrhea, and initiate therapeutic measures as needed. Drug may need to be stopped.
• Observe patient closely. With large doses and prolonged therapy, bacterial or fungal superinfection may occur, especially in elderly, debilitated, or immunosuppressed patients.
• Antibiotic use can cause overgrowth of nonsusceptible organisms (superinfection). Monitor patient for infection.
• *Look alike–sound alike:* Don't confuse penicillin G sodium with Polycillin, penicillamine, or the various other types of penicillin.

PATIENT TEACHING
• Tell patient to report adverse reactions promptly, especially hypersensitivity reactions and diarrhea.
• Instruct patient to report discomfort at I.V. site.
• Warn patient receiving I.M. injection that the injection may be painful but that ice applied to site may help alleviate discomfort.

penicillin V potassium (phenoxymethyl penicillin potassium)
pen-i-SILL-in

Apo-Pen VK✤, Novo-Pen-VK✤, Penicillin-VK, Pen-VK✤

Therapeutic class: Antibiotics
Pharmacologic class: Natural penicillins

AVAILABLE FORMS
Oral suspension: 125 mg/5 mL, 250 mg/5 mL (after reconstitution)
Tablets: 250 mg, 500 mg

INDICATIONS & DOSAGES
➤ **Fusospirochetosis (Vincent infection) and staphylococcal infections**
Adults and children age 12 and older: 250 to 500 mg P.O. every 6 to 8 hours.
➤ **Pneumococcal infections**
Adults and children age 12 and older: 250 to 500 mg P.O. every 6 hours until patient has been afebrile for at least 2 days.
➤ **Streptococcal infections**
Adults and children age 12 and older: 125 to 250 mg P.O. every 6 to 8 hours for 10 days.
➤ **To prevent recurrent rheumatic fever**
Adults and children age 12 and older: 125 to 250 mg P.O. b.i.d.

ADMINISTRATION
P.O.
• Before giving drug, ask patient about allergic reactions to penicillins.
• Obtain specimen for culture and sensitivity tests before giving first dose. Begin therapy while awaiting results.
• Give drug with food if patient has stomach upset.
• Store oral solution in refrigerator. Discard any portion after 14 days.

ACTION
Inhibits cell-wall synthesis during bacterial multiplication.

Route	Onset	Peak	Duration
P.O.	Unknown	30–60 min	Unknown

Half-life: 30 minutes.

ADVERSE REACTIONS

GI: epigastric distress, nausea, diarrhea, black hairy tongue, vomiting.
Hematologic: *leukopenia, thrombocytopenia,* eosinophilia, hemolytic anemia.
Other: *anaphylaxis,* hypersensitivity reactions, overgrowth of nonsusceptible organisms.

INTERACTIONS

Drug-drug. *Hormonal contraceptives:*
May decrease hormonal contraceptive effectiveness. Advise use of another form of contraception during therapy.
Methotrexate: May increase risk of methotrexate toxicity. Monitor patient closely.
Probenecid: May increase penicillin level. Probenecid may be used for this purpose.
Tetracyclines: May impair bactericidal effects of penicillin V. Avoid use together.

EFFECTS ON LAB TEST RESULTS

● May decrease Hb level.
● May increase eosinophil count. May decrease platelet, WBC, and granulocyte counts.
● May alter results of turbidimetric test methods using sulfosalicylic acid, acetic acid, trichloroacetic acid, and nitric acid.

CONTRAINDICATIONS & CAUTIONS

● Contraindicated in patients hypersensitive to drug or other penicillins.
● Drug may cause CDAD ranging in severity from mild diarrhea to fatal colitis. If CDAD is suspected or confirmed, drug may need to be discontinued and treatment initiated.
● Use cautiously in patients with GI disturbances, seizure disorders, or renal impairment and in those with other drug allergies, especially to cephalosporins, because of possible cross-sensitivity.
Dialyzable drug: Unknown.
⚠ **Overdose S&S:** Neuromuscular hyperexcitability, seizures.

PREGNANCY-LACTATION-REPRODUCTION

● May use cautiously in pregnant and breast-feeding women.

NURSING CONSIDERATIONS

● Drug may alter normal colon flora. Monitor patient for diarrhea, and initiate therapeutic measures as needed. Drug may need to be stopped.
● Periodically assess renal and hematopoietic function in patients receiving long-term therapy.
● If large doses are given or if therapy is prolonged, bacterial or fungal superinfection may occur, especially in elderly, debilitated, or immunosuppressed patients.
● After treatment for streptococcal infections, reculture patient to determine whether streptococci have been eradicated.
● Amoxicillin is the preferred drug to prevent endocarditis because GI absorption is better and drug levels are sustained longer. Penicillin V is considered an alternative drug.
● *Look alike–sound alike:* Don't confuse penicillin V potassium with Polycillin, penicillamine, or the various other types of penicillin.

PATIENT TEACHING

● Instruct patient to take entire quantity of drug exactly as prescribed, even after he feels better.
● Tell patient to take drug with food if stomach upset occurs.
● Advise patient to discard any unused reconstituted suspension after 14 days.
● Advise patient to notify prescriber if rash, fever, or chills develop. A rash is the most common allergic reaction.

pentamidine isethionate
pen-TA-ma-deen

NebuPent, Pentam

Therapeutic class: Antiprotozoals
Pharmacologic class: Diamidine derivatives

AVAILABLE FORMS

Aerosol, injection, powder for injection:
300-mg vial

P

INDICATIONS & DOSAGES

➤ *Pneumocystis jiroveci* pneumonia
Adults and children age 4 months and older:
4 mg/kg I.V. or I.M. once daily for 14 to
21 days.
➤ To prevent *P. jiroveci* pneumonia in
high-risk patients
Adults: 300 mg by inhalation using a Respirgard II nebulizer once every 4 weeks.

ADMINISTRATION

I.V.
▼ Reconstitute drug with 3 to 5 mL sterile
water for injection or D_5W.
▼ Dilute reconstituted drug in 50 to
250 mL D_5W.
▼ Infuse over 60 to 120 minutes.
▼ I.V. infusion solutions prepared in D_5W
are stable at room temperature for up to
24 hours.
▼ To minimize risk of hypotension, infuse drug slowly with patient lying down.
Closely monitor BP.
🔂 *Alert:* Closely monitor infusion. Extravasation may cause ulceration, tissue
necrosis, or sloughing and may require
surgical debridement and skin grafting. If
extravasation occurs, discontinue infusion
immediately and manage symptoms.
▼ **Incompatibilities:** Aldesleukin,
cephalosporins, fluconazole, foscarnet,
linezolid.
I.M.
● Reconstitute drug with 3 mL sterile water
for a solution containing 100 mg/mL.
● Give deep into muscle.
● Patient may have pain and induration at
injection site.
● Rotate injection sites.
Inhalational
● Drug is considered a biohazardous agent.
Follow safe-handling procedures.
● Give aerosol form only by Respirgard II
nebulizer. Dosage recommendations are
based on particle size and delivery rate of
this device. Deliver dose until nebulizer
chamber is empty (about 30 to 45 minutes).
● To give aerosol, mix contents of one vial
in 6 mL sterile water for injection. Don't use
NSS. Don't mix with other drugs.
● Don't use the Respirgard II to administer
a bronchodilator because there may be an
incompatibility between pentamidine and
the bronchodilator.
● Don't use low-pressure (less than
20 pounds per square inch [psi]) compressors. The flow rate should be 5 to 7 L/minute
from 40- to 50-psi air or oxygen source.

ACTION

May interfere with biosynthesis of DNA,
RNA, phospholipids, and proteins in susceptible organisms.

Route	Onset	Peak	Duration
I.V.	Unknown	1 hr	Unknown
I.M.	Unknown	30 min	Unknown
Inhalation	Unknown	Unknown	Unknown

Half-life: I.M., 9 to 13 hours; I.V., about 6½ hours;
inhalation, unknown.

ADVERSE REACTIONS

CNS: confusion, hallucinations, headache.
CV: chest pain, hypotension.
GI: nausea, metallic taste, diarrhea,
anorexia.
Hematologic: *leukopenia, thrombocytopenia,* anemia.
Metabolic: *hypoglycemia.*
Respiratory: cough, wheezing.
Skin: rash; sterile abscess or necrosis, pain,
or induration at site of I.M. injection.
Other: night sweats, infection.

INTERACTIONS

Drug-drug. *Aminoglycosides, amphotericin
B, capreomycin, cisplatin, methoxyflurane,
polymyxin B, vancomycin:* May increase
risk of nephrotoxicity. Monitor renal function test results closely.
Antineoplastics: May cause additive bone
marrow suppression. Use together cautiously; monitor hematologic study results.
*Drugs that prolong the QT interval (antipsychotics; antiarrhythmics, such as amiodarone, disopyramide, procainamide, quinidine, sotalol; fluoroquinolones; macrolides;
TCAs):* May cause additive effect. Use
together cautiously; monitor patient for
adverse cardiac effects.

EFFECTS ON LAB TEST RESULTS

● May increase BUN, creatinine, and potassium levels and LFT values. May decrease

Hb level and hematocrit. May increase or decrease glucose level.
• May decrease WBC and platelet counts.

CONTRAINDICATIONS & CAUTIONS
• Contraindicated in patients with history of anaphylactic reaction to drug.
• Use cautiously in patients with hypertension, hypotension, hypoglycemia, hypocalcemia, leukopenia, thrombocytopenia, anemia, diabetes, pancreatitis, Stevens-Johnson syndrome, or hepatic or renal dysfunction.
⚠ *Alert:* Severe hypotension may occur after a single I.V. or I.M. dose. Monitor patients closely.
Dialyzable drug: No.
⚠ *Overdose S&S:* Renal and hepatic impairment, hypotension, cardiopulmonary arrest.

PREGNANCY-LACTATION-REPRODUCTION
• It isn't known if drug causes fetal harm. Use in pregnant women only if potential benefits justify unknown risks.
• Use cautiously in breast-feeding women and only if potential benefits justify unknown risks.

NURSING CONSIDERATIONS
⚠ *Alert:* Monitor glucose, creatinine, and BUN levels daily. After parenteral administration, glucose level may decrease initially; hypoglycemia may be severe in 5% to 10% of patients. After several months of therapy, this may be followed by hyperglycemia and type 1 diabetes mellitus, which may be permanent.
• Monitor CBC, platelet count, LFT, calcium level, and ECG before, during, and after therapy.
⚠ *Alert:* Monitor BP during and after infusion because of increased risk of severe hypotension with I.V. or I.M. administration.
• Extravasation can lead to ulceration, tissue necrosis, or sloughing at injection site. Monitor I.V. site closely.
• Inhalation drug may cause bronchospasm or cough, especially in patients with a history of asthma or smoking. Use of an inhaled bronchodilator before each inhaled pentamidine dose may minimize symptom recurrence.

• Use of aerosolized drug has been associated with acute pancreatitis. Discontinue drug if signs or symptoms of acute pancreatitis occur.
• Obtain the following tests before, during, and after therapy: CBC, platelet count, LFT, serum calcium level, and ECG.
• In patients with AIDS, drug may produce less severe adverse reactions than sulfamethoxazole–trimethoprim.

PATIENT TEACHING
• Instruct patient to use the aerosol device until the chamber is empty, which may take up to 45 minutes.
• Warn patient that I.M. injection is painful.
• Instruct patient to complete the full course, even if he's feeling better.
• Tell patient to report signs and symptoms of pulmonary infection, such as shortness of breath, fever, or cough.

SAFETY ALERT!

pentazocine hydrochloride
pen-TAZ-oh-seen

Talwin✱

pentazocine lactate
Talwin

Therapeutic class: Analgesics
Pharmacologic class: Opioid agonist-antagonists–opioid partial agonists
Controlled substance schedule: IV

P

AVAILABLE FORMS
pentazocine hydrochloride
Tablets: 50 mg ✱
pentazocine lactate
Injection: 30 mg/mL

INDICATIONS & DOSAGES
➤ **Moderate to severe pain; preoperative or preanesthetic supplement to surgical anesthesia**
Adults and children older than age 12:
30 mg I.M., I.V., or subcutaneously every 3 to 4 hours p.r.n. Maximum parenteral dose is 360 mg/day. Single doses above 30 mg I.V. or 60 mg I.M. or subcutaneously aren't recommended.

➤ **Labor**
Adults and children older than age 12:
30 mg I.M. as a single dose or 20 mg I.V.
every 2 to 3 hours when contractions become regular for two to three doses.

ADMINISTRATION
P.O.
● Give drug with aspirin or acetaminophen for additive analgesic effect.
I.V.
▼ Give drug slowly by direct I.V. injection.
▼ **Incompatibilities:** Soluble barbiturates in same syringe.
I.M.
● Rotate injection sites to minimize tissue irritation.
Subcutaneous
● Rotate injection sites to minimize tissue irritation. Use subcutaneous route only when necessary to avoid risk of severe tissue damage at injection site.

ACTION
Unknown. Binds with opioid receptors in the CNS, altering perception of and emotional response to pain.

Route	Onset	Peak	Duration
P.O.	15–30 min	1–3 hr	2–3 hr
I.V.	2–3 min	15–30 min	2–3 hr
I.M., subcut.	15–20 min	30–60 min	2–3 hr

Half-life: 2 to 3 hours.

ADVERSE REACTIONS
CNS: dizziness, euphoria, light-headedness, sedation, confusion, drowsiness, hallucinations, headache, psychotomimetic effects, visual disturbances.
CV: *shock, circulatory depression,* hypertension, hypotension.
EENT: dry mouth.
GI: nausea, vomiting, constipation.
GU: urine retention.
Respiratory: *apnea, respiratory depression,* dyspnea.
Skin: diaphoresis, induration, nodules, sclerosis at injection site, pruritus, sloughing.
Other: *anaphylaxis,* hypersensitivity reactions, physical/psychological dependence.

INTERACTIONS
Drug-drug. **Black Box Warning** *Benzodiazepines, CNS depressants:* May cause slow or difficult breathing, sedation, and death. Avoid use together. If use together is necessary, limit dosage and duration of each drug to minimum necessary for desired effect. ■
Fluoxetine: May cause additive effects resulting in serotonin syndrome. Use together cautiously.
◐ *Alert:* Serotonergic drugs (amoxapine, antiemetics [dolasetron, granisetron, ondansetron, palonosetron], antimigraine drugs, buspirone, cyclobenzaprine, dextromethorphan, linezolid, lithium, MAO inhibitors, maprotiline, methylene blue, mirtazapine, nefazodone, SNRIs, SSRIs, TCAs, trazodone, tryptophan, vilazodone): May increase risk of serotonin syndrome. Use together cautiously and monitor patient for serotonin syndrome.
Drug-herb. ◐ *Alert: St. John's wort:* May increase risk of serotonin syndrome. Use together cautiously and monitor patient for serotonin syndrome.
Drug-lifestyle. *Alcohol use:* May cause additive effects. Discourage use together. *Smoking:* May increase requirements for pentazocine. Monitor drug's effectiveness.

EFFECTS ON LAB TEST RESULTS
● May interfere with laboratory tests for urinary 17-hydroxycorticosteroids.

CONTRAINDICATIONS & CAUTIONS
● Contraindicated in patients hypersensitive to drug or its components and in children younger than age 12.
● Use cautiously in patients with hepatic or renal disease, acute MI, hypertension, head injury, increased ICP, and respiratory depression.
◐ *Alert:* Drug may lead to rare but serious decrease in adrenal gland cortisol production.
◐ *Alert:* Drug may cause decreased sex hormone levels with long-term use.
Black Box Warning Opioids should only be prescribed with benzodiazepines or other CNS depressants to patients for whom alternative treatment options are inadequate. ■
Dialyzable drug: Unknown.

Reactions in bold italics are *life-threatening*. Interactions may have a *rapid onset* or a *delayed onset*.

PREGNANCY-LACTATION-REPRODUCTION

• Drug is approved for use in labor. Use in pregnant women other than during labor only if potential benefits justify possible hazards.

• Drug may cause neonatal abstinence syndrome (fever, temperature instability, diarrhea, vomiting, poor feeding, high-pitched crying, increased muscle tone, seizure, tremor) with prolonged use during pregnancy.

• It isn't known if drug appears in breast milk. Monitor breast-feeding patient and infant for psychotomimetic reactions (psychological and behavioral changes similar to those of psychosis). Monitor breast-feeding infants exposed to large doses of drug for apnea and sedation.

NURSING CONSIDERATIONS

• Reassess patient's pain level at least 15 and 30 minutes after parenteral administration and 30 minutes after giving orally.

❸ *Alert:* If patient is taking opioids with serotonergic drugs, watch for signs and symptoms of serotonin syndrome (agitation, hallucinations, rapid HR, fever, excessive sweating, shivering or shaking, muscle twitching or stiffness, trouble with coordination, nausea, vomiting, diarrhea), especially at start of treatment or dosage increases. Signs and symptoms may occur within several hours of coadministration but may also occur later, especially after dosage increase. Discontinue opioid, serotonergic drug, or both if serotonin syndrome is suspected.

❸ *Alert:* Monitor patient for signs and symptoms of adrenal insufficiency (nausea, vomiting, loss of appetite, fatigue, weakness, dizziness, low BP). Perform diagnostic testing if adrenal insufficiency is suspected. If adrenal insufficiency is confirmed, treat with corticosteroids and wean patient off opioids if appropriate. Discontinue corticosteroids when clinically appropriate.

❸ *Alert:* Monitor patient for signs and symptoms of decreased sex hormone levels (low libido, erectile dysfunction, amenorrhea, infertility). If signs and symptoms occur, evaluate patient and obtain laboratory testing.

• Drug may cause constipation. Assess bowel function and need for stool softeners or stimulant laxatives. Encourage fluids.

• Have naloxone readily available to reverse respiratory depression.

• Drug has opioid antagonist properties. May cause withdrawal syndrome in opioid-dependent patients.

• Psychological and physical dependence may occur with prolonged use.

PATIENT TEACHING

❸ *Alert:* Encourage patient to report all medications being taken, including prescription and OTC medications and supplements.

❸ *Alert:* Caution patient to immediately report signs and symptoms of serotonin syndrome, adrenal insufficiency, and decreased sex hormone levels.

Black Box Warning Caution patient or caregiver of patient taking an opioid with a benzodiazepine, CNS depressant, or alcohol to seek immediate medical attention if patient experiences dizziness, light-headedness, extreme sleepiness, slowed or difficult breathing, or unresponsiveness. ∎

• Instruct patient to ask for drug before pain is intense.

• Caution ambulatory patient about getting out of bed or walking. Warn outpatient to avoid driving and other hazardous activities that require mental alertness until drug's CNS effects are known.

• Advise patient to avoid alcohol during therapy.

• Instruct patient or family to report rash, disorientation, or confusion to prescriber.

SAFETY ALERT!

pertuzumab
per-TOO-zoo-mab

Perjeta

Therapeutic class: Antineoplastics
Pharmacologic class: Monoclonal antibodies

AVAILABLE FORMS

Injection: 420 mg/14 mL (30 mg/mL) in single-use vials

INDICATIONS & DOSAGES
Adjust-a-dose (for all indications): If a dose is missed or delayed and the time between infusions is less than 6 weeks, give 420-mg dose when possible; don't wait until the next planned dose. If the time between the two infusions is 6 weeks or more, give 840 mg loading dose followed by maintenance dose 3 weeks later. Withhold drug for at least 3 weeks if LVEF is less than 45% or is 45% to 49% with a 10% or more decrease below pretreatment values. Repeat LVEF assessment in 3 weeks. Discontinue both pertuzumab and trastuzumab if LVEF isn't improved or is worse, unless benefit outweighs risk. Dosage reductions aren't recommended for pertuzumab.

➤ **HER2-positive metastatic breast cancer with trastuzumab and docetaxel in patients who haven't received prior anti-HER2 therapy or chemotherapy for metastatic disease**
Adults: Initial loading dose of 840 mg I.V. as a 60-minute infusion in combination with trastuzumab 8 mg/kg and docetaxel 75 mg/m². Administer a maintenance regimen every 3 weeks with pertuzumab 420 mg I.V. as a 30- to 60-minute infusion in combination with trastuzumab 6 mg/kg and docetaxel (may increase docetaxel dose to 100 mg/m² if initial dose is tolerated).

➤ **Neoadjuvant treatment of HER2-positive, locally advanced, inflammatory, or early-stage breast cancer (either greater than 2 cm in diameter or node positive) in combination with other drugs**
Adults: Initial loading dose of 840 mg I.V. as a 60-minute infusion, then a maintenance regimen every 3 weeks with pertuzumab 420 mg I.V. as a 30- to 60-minute infusion in combination with either 4 preoperative cycles with trastuzumab and docetaxel followed by 3 postoperative cycles of 5-FU, epirubicin, and cyclophosphamide (FEC); or 3 preoperative cycles of FEC alone followed by 3 postoperative cycles of pertuzumab in combination with docetaxel and trastuzumab; or 6 preoperative cycles of pertuzumab in combination with docetaxel, carboplatin, and trastuzumab (TCH). Following surgery, continue trastuzumab to complete 1 year of treatment regardless of regimen used.

ADMINISTRATION
I.V.
▼ Hazardous drug; use safe handling and disposal precautions.
▼ Don't administer as I.V. push or bolus.
▼ Refrigerate vials. Store in outer carton to protect from light.
▼ Inspect solution for particulates and discoloration. Solution should be clear to slightly opalescent and colorless to pale brown.
▼ Withdraw appropriate amount of pertuzumab and dilute in 250 mL NSS in a PVC or non-PVC polyolefin infusion bag.
▼ Invert bag gently to mix solution; don't shake. Administer immediately.
▼ May store diluted solution, refrigerated, for up to 24 hours.
▼ Administer pertuzumab sequentially. Pertuzumab and trastuzumab can be given in any order. Give docetaxel after pertuzumab and trastuzumab. Wait 30 to 60 minutes after infusing pertuzumab before administering the other drugs.
▼ **Incompatibilities:** Other drugs. Only mix with NSS.

ACTION
Binds to HER2 protein receptor, causing inhibition of signaling pathways, which results in cell growth arrest and apoptosis. The combination of pertuzumab and trastuzumab synergistically increases their antitumor activity.

Route	Onset	Peak	Duration
I.V.	Unknown	Unknown	Unknown

Half-life: 18 days.

ADVERSE REACTIONS
CNS: fatigue, asthenia, pyrexia, peripheral neuropathy, headache, dizziness, insomnia.
CV: peripheral edema, *left ventricular dysfunction.*
EENT: nasopharyngitis, increased tearing.
GI: diarrhea, nausea, vomiting, constipation, stomatitis, dysgeusia, decreased appetite, abdominal pain.
Hematologic: *neutropenia,* anemia, *leukopenia, febrile neutropenia.*
Musculoskeletal: myalgia, arthralgia.
Respiratory: URI, dyspnea, pleural effusion.

Reactions in bold italics are *life-threatening*. Interactions may have a *rapid onset* or a *delayed onset*.

Skin: alopecia, rash, pruritus, dry skin, paronychia, nail disorder.

Other: mucosal inflammation, infusion-related hypersensitivity, immunogenicity.

INTERACTIONS

Drug-drug. *Abciximab:* May enhance potential for allergic or hypersensitivity reactions to monoclonal antibodies. Also may cause thrombocytopenia or diminished therapeutic effects. Monitor therapy.

Anthracyclines: Prior exposure to anthracyclines may increase risk of left ventricular dysfunction. Use pertuzumab cautiously.

Belimumab: Monoclonal antibodies may enhance adverse or toxic effect of belimumab. Avoid combination.

EFFECTS ON LAB TEST RESULTS

• May decrease WBC and RBC counts.

CONTRAINDICATIONS & CAUTIONS

Black Box Warning Pertuzumab can cause subclinical and clinical cardiac failure. Evaluate LVEF in all patients before and during treatment. Discontinue drug treatment for a confirmed clinically significant decrease in left ventricular function. ∎

۞ Alert: The safe use of pertuzumab with a doxorubicin-containing regimen or administration of more than 6 cycles for early breast cancer has not been established.

• Contraindicated in patients hypersensitive to drug or its components.

• Use cautiously in patients with a history of HF or reduced LVEF and in those with severe renal impairment. Prior exposure to radiotherapy may increase risk of left ventricular dysfunction.

Dialyzable drug: Unknown.

PREGNANCY-LACTATION-REPRODUCTION

Black Box Warning Exposure to drug during pregnancy can result in embryo or fetal death, delayed renal development, and other birth defects. Verify pregnancy status before starting drug. Advise patients of risks and the need for effective contraception during therapy and for 7 months after therapy ends. ∎

• Women exposed to drug during pregnancy or within 7 months before conception should be enrolled in the MotHER Preg-

nancy Registry (1-800-690-6720) and the exposure reported to the Genentech Adverse Event Line (1-888-835-2555).

• If patient becomes pregnant during therapy, monitor closely. If oligohydramnios occurs, perform fetal testing.

• It isn't known if drug appears in breast milk. Patient should discontinue breast-feeding or discontinue drug. Consider drug's extended half-life when making breast-feeding decisions after therapy ends.

NURSING CONSIDERATIONS

• Verify HER2 status with reputable laboratory. Drug is only useful in patients with HER2 protein overexpression.

• Assess LVEF before starting treatment and every 3 months during treatment for metastatic disease or every 6 weeks during neoadjuvant treatment and every 6 months after therapy ends, up to 24 months after last dose.

• Withhold or discontinue pertuzumab if trastuzumab is withheld or discontinued. If docetaxel is discontinued, treatment with pertuzumab and trastuzumab may continue.

• Monitor patient for hypersensitivity or infusion reactions for 60 minutes after first infusion and for 30 minutes after subsequent infusions. For significant infusion-related reactions, slow or interrupt infusion and treat symptoms. If severe reactions occur, consider permanently discontinuing drug.

• Monitor CBC regularly.

• Monitor patients for fever or infection.

• An increased incidence of febrile neutropenia has occurred in Asian patients.

• Assess LVEF before starting treatment and every 3 months during treatment.

PATIENT TEACHING

Black Box Warning Inform women of childbearing potential that drug may cause fetal harm. Counsel patient to use reliable birth control methods while taking this drug and for 7 months after therapy ends. ∎

• Teach patient that hair loss (alopecia) and skin and nail adverse reactions are common during treatment.

• Instruct patient to immediately report fever or other signs and symptoms of infection.

• Caution patient to immediately report shortness of breath, unusual edema, weight gain, or excessive fatigue.
• Tell patient that laboratory monitoring of cardiac function will be needed.

phentermine hydrochloride
FEN-ter-meen

Adipex-P, Lomaira

Therapeutic class: Anorexiants
Pharmacologic class: Sympathomimetic amines
Controlled substance schedule: IV

AVAILABLE FORMS
Capsules: 15 mg, 30 mg, 37.5 mg
Tablets: 8 mg, 37.5 mg

INDICATIONS & DOSAGES
➤ **Short-term adjunct in exogenous obesity for patients with an initial BMI of 30 kg/m² or more, or of 27 kg/m² or more in the presence of other risk factors (e.g., controlled hypertension, diabetes, hyperlipidemia)**
Adults and children age 17 and older: 15 to 37.5 mg P.O. daily as a single dose before breakfast or 1 to 2 hours after breakfast. Or, 8 mg (Lomaira) P.O. three times/day 30 minutes before meals. Individualize dose to obtain an adequate response with the lowest effective dose.

ADMINISTRATION
P.O.
• Adipex-P tablets may be split and given in two divided doses if desired.
• Avoid giving drug in the late evening, to prevent insomnia.

ACTION
Unknown. Probably promotes nerve impulse transmission by releasing stored norepinephrine from nerve terminals in the brain, especially in the cerebral cortex and reticular activating system.

Route	Onset	Peak	Duration
P.O.	Unknown	Unknown	12–14 hr

Half-life: 19 to 24 hours.

ADVERSE REACTIONS
CNS: insomnia, overstimulation, headache, restlessness, euphoria, dysphoria, dizziness, tremor.
CV: palpitations, tachycardia, ischemic events, increased BP, *primary pulmonary hypertension.*
GI: dry mouth, dysgeusia, constipation, diarrhea, unpleasant taste, other GI disturbances.
GU: erectile dysfunction.
Skin: urticaria.
Other: altered libido.

INTERACTIONS
Drug-drug. *Acetazolamide, antacids, sodium bicarbonate:* May increase renal reabsorption. Monitor patient for enhanced effects.
Ammonium chloride, ascorbic acid: May decrease level and increase renal excretion of phentermine. Monitor patient for decreased phentermine effects.
Hormonal contraceptives: May reduce effectiveness of hormonal contraceptives. Advise patient to use alternative methods of contraception during treatment and for 1 month after discontinuation of therapy.
Insulin, oral antidiabetics: May alter antidiabetic requirements. Monitor glucose level.
MAO inhibitors: May cause severe hypertension or hypertensive crisis. Avoid using within 14 days of MAO inhibitor therapy.
Serotonin uptake inhibitors (fluoxetine, fluvoxamine, paroxetine, sertraline): May increase risk of serotonin syndrome. Use together isn't recommended.
Drug-food. *Alcohol use:* May increase risk of adverse drug reactions. Monitor patient.
Caffeine: May increase CNS stimulation. Discourage use together.

EFFECTS ON LAB TEST RESULTS
None reported.

CONTRAINDICATIONS & CAUTIONS
• Contraindicated in patients hypersensitive to sympathomimetic amines, in those with idiosyncratic reactions to them, in agitated patients, and in those with hyperthyroidism, moderate to severe or uncontrolled

---

Reactions in bold italics are *life-threatening*. Interactions may have a *rapid onset* or a ***delayed onset***.

hypertension, advanced arteriosclerosis, symptomatic CV disease, or glaucoma.
• Rare cases of valvular heart disease have been reported in patients who have taken phentermine alone.
• Use cautiously in patients with mild hypertension or seizure disorders.
Dialyzable drug: Unknown.
⚠ *Overdose S&S:* Restlessness, tremor, hyperreflexia, rapid respiration, confusion, assaultiveness, hallucinations, panic states, fatigue, depression, arrhythmias, hypertension, hypotension, circulatory collapse, nausea, vomiting, diarrhea, abdominal cramps, seizures, coma.

PREGNANCY-LACTATION-REPRODUCTION
• Contraindicated in pregnant and breast-feeding women.

NURSING CONSIDERATIONS
• Use drug with a weight-reduction program.
• Monitor patient for tolerance, dependence, or potential abuse. Drug is chemically related to amphetamines, which carry a high abuse potential.
• *Look alike–sound alike:* Don't confuse phentermine with phentolamine or phenytoin.

PATIENT TEACHING
• Counsel patient in use of effective contraception. Advise her to inform prescriber immediately if pregnancy occurs.
• Instruct patient to immediately report shortness of breath or dyspnea, which could be an early sign of a serious adverse effect such as primary pulmonary hypertension.
• Tell patient to take sustained-release drug at least 10 to 14 hours before bedtime to avoid sleep interference.
• Advise patient to avoid products that contain caffeine. Tell him to report evidence of excessive stimulation.
• Warn patient that fatigue may result as drug effects wear off and that he'll need more rest.
• Warn patient that drug may lose its effectiveness over time.

phentermine hydrochloride–topiramate
FEN-ter-meen/toe-PIE-rah-mate

Qsymia

Therapeutic class: Anorexiants–anticonvulsants
Pharmacologic class: Sympatho-mimetic amines–sulfamate-substituted monosaccharides
Controlled substance schedule: IV

AVAILABLE FORMS
Capsules: 3.75 mg phentermine and 23 mg topiramate extended-release, 7.5 mg phentermine and 46 mg topiramate extended-release, 11.25 mg phentermine and 69 mg topiramate extended-release, 15 mg phentermine and 92 mg topiramate extended-release

INDICATIONS & DOSAGES
➤ **Chronic weight management, as an adjunct to diet and increased physical activity in patients with initial BMI of 30 kg/m^2 or greater (obese) or 27 kg/m^2 or greater (overweight) and at least one weight-related comorbidity, such as hypertension, type 2 diabetes mellitus, or dyslipidemia**
Adults: Initially, 3.75 mg phentermine/23 mg topiramate extended-release P.O. every morning for 14 days; then increase to 7.5 mg phentermine/46 mg topiramate extended-release every morning. Evaluate weight loss after 12 weeks of treatment. If patient hasn't lost at least 3% of baseline body weight, discontinue drug or escalate dosage to 11.25 mg phentermine/69 mg topiramate extended-release every morning for 14 days, followed by 15 mg phentermine/92 mg topiramate extended-release every morning. Evaluate weight loss 12 weeks after dosage escalation. If patient hasn't lost at least 5% of baseline body weight, discontinue drug by decreasing dosage to every other day for at least 1 week before stopping treatment altogether.
Adjust-a-dose: For patients with moderate renal impairment (CrCl of 30 to less than 50 mL/minute), severe renal impairment

P

(CrCl less than 30 mL/minute), or moderate hepatic impairment (Child-Pugh class B), don't exceed 7.5 mg phentermine/46 mg topiramate once daily. Drug isn't for use in patients with ESRD on dialysis or those with severe hepatic impairment.

ADMINISTRATION
P.O.
● Give drug in morning with or without food. Don't give in evening due to risk of insomnia.

ACTION
Phentermine: Unknown. May be mediated by release of catecholamines in hypothalamus, resulting in decreased appetite and decreased food consumption. Topiramate: Unknown in weight management. May involve appetite suppression and satiety enhancement via a variety of neurotransmitter or enzymatic effects.

Route	Onset	Peak	Duration
P.O.	Unknown	6 hr (phentermine); 9 hr (topiramate)	Unknown

Half-life: Phentermine, 20 hours; topiramate, 65 hours.

ADVERSE REACTIONS
CNS: paresthesia, headache, dizziness, dysgeusia, hypoesthesia, disturbance in attention or memory, cognitive disorder, insomnia, depression, anxiety, fatigue, irritability.
CV: palpitations, chest discomfort, palpitations.
EENT: blurred vision, eye pain, dry eye, dry mouth, nasopharyngitis, sinusitis, sinus congestion, pharyngolaryngeal pain, nasal congestion.
GI: constipation, nausea, diarrhea, dyspepsia, GERD, oral paresthesia, gastroenteritis, decreased appetite, thirst.
GU: UTI, kidney stones, dysmenorrhea.
Metabolic: *hypokalemia, metabolic acidosis.*
Musculoskeletal: back pain, extremity pain, muscle spasms, musculoskeletal pain, neck pain.
Respiratory: cough, bronchitis, URI.
Skin: alopecia, rash.
Other: procedural pain, flulike symptoms.

INTERACTIONS
Drug-drug. *Amitriptyline:* May increase amitriptyline level. Adjust amitriptyline dosage based on patient clinical response.
Anticholinergics (atropine, benztropine): May increase risk of heat-related disorders, such as decreased sweating and increased body temperature. Use together cautiously.
Carbamazepine, phenytoin: May decrease topiramate plasma concentration. Use together cautiously.
Carbonic anhydrase inhibitors (acetazolamide, methazolamide, zonisamide): May increase risk of metabolic acidosis and kidney stones. May also increase risk of heat-related disorders, such as decreased sweating and increased body temperature. Avoid concurrent use.
CNS depressants (barbiturates, benzodiazepines, sleep medications): May increase CNS depressant effects. Avoid use together.
Diltiazem: May decrease diltiazem level and increase topiramate level. Use together cautiously.
Lithium: High topiramate dosage may increase lithium level. Monitor lithium level.
MAO inhibitors: May increase risk of hypertensive crisis. Use is contraindicated during or within 14 days of MAO inhibitor administration.
Non-potassium-sparing diuretics (loop and thiazide diuretics): May increase risk of hypokalemia. Monitor potassium level.
Oral antidiabetics, insulin: May increase risk of hypoglycemia. Monitor glucose level closely.
Oral contraceptives(progestins): May decrease contraceptive effectiveness. Consider therapy modification and adding an additional, nonhormonal contraceptive method.
Other weight-loss drugs: Use with other weight-loss drugs hasn't been studied. Avoid use together.
Serotonin uptake inhibitors (fluoxetine, fluvoxamine, paroxetine, sertraline): May increase risk of serotonin syndrome. Use together isn't recommended.
Valproic acid: May increase risk of hyperammonemia and encephalopathy. Monitor patient and measure blood ammonia level if symptoms develop.

Reactions in bold italics are *life-threatening*. Interactions may have a *rapid onset* or a **delayed onset**.

Drug-herb. *Weight-loss supplements:* Use with other weight-loss products hasn't been studied. Avoid use together.

Drug-food. *Ketogenic diet (high-protein, low-carbohydrate):* May increase risk of kidney stones. Use together cautiously.

Drug-lifestyle. *Alcohol use:* May increase CNS depressant effects. Discourage use together.

EFFECTS ON LAB TEST RESULTS

● May increase creatinine level. May decrease sodium bicarbonate, potassium, and glucose levels.

CONTRAINDICATIONS & CAUTIONS

● Contraindicated in patients hypersensitive to drug or its components; in those with glaucoma, hyperthyroidism, severe hepatic dysfunction, or ESRD; and in patients with a history of or active suicidal ideation or attempts.

● Use cautiously in patients with increased resting HR, especially those with cardiac or cerebrovascular disease (history of MI or stroke in the past 6 months, life-threatening arrhythmias, HF); in patients with depression or suicidal thoughts; in elderly patients; and in those at risk for development of metabolic acidosis or kidney stones.

Black Box Warning Drug is a controlled substance because it can be abused, leading to drug dependence. ■

● The safety and effectiveness of this drug in combination with other products intended for weight loss, including prescription and OTC drugs and herbal preparations, haven't been established.

● Drug is only available through certified pharmacies that are enrolled in the Qsymia certified pharmacy network; see www.qsymiarems.com or call 1-888-998-4887.

Dialyzable drug: Unknown.

⚠ *Overdose S&S:* Phentermine: Restlessness, tremor, rapid respiration, confusion, hallucinations, arrhythmias, changes in BP, nausea, vomiting, diarrhea. Topiramate: Metabolic acidosis, seizures, drowsiness, speech disturbance, blurred vision, hypotension, abdominal pain, agitation, dizziness, depression.

PREGNANCY-LACTATION-REPRODUCTION

● Contraindicated in pregnant and breast-feeding women.

● Assess for pregnancy before and monthly during treatment. Women of childbearing potential should use effective contraception during therapy.

● Prescribers and patients should report pregnancies that occur during therapy to the Qsymia Pregnancy Surveillance Program (1-888-998-4887).

NURSING CONSIDERATIONS

● Gradually decrease dosage when discontinuing drug to lower risk of seizures. If it's necessary to stop drug immediately, monitor patient closely.

● Monitor patient for mood disorders and insomnia; if present, decrease dosage or discontinue drug.

● Monitor patient for emergence or worsening of depression, suicidal thoughts or behavior, or unusual changes in mood or behavior. Discontinue drug in patients who experience suicidal thoughts or behaviors.

● Monitor resting HR. If sustained tachycardia occurs, decrease dosage or stop drug.

● Assess electrolyte, glucose, and bicarbonate levels before and periodically during treatment.

● Drug causes decreased sweating, which can predispose patients to heat-related disorders. Monitor fluid loss, especially in hot weather.

● Monitor BP regularly, especially in patients with history of hypertension.

● Monitor patient for ocular changes (acute myopia, severe and persistent eye pain, vision changes, anterior chamber shallowing, redness, increased IOP, mydriasis). Discontinue drug immediately if any of these symptoms occur.

● Monitor patient for potential abuse of drug. Phentermine has a known potential for abuse.

● Phentermine is related chemically and pharmacologically to amphetamines.

PATIENT TEACHING

● Advise patient to take drug once daily in the morning and to avoid nighttime dosing because of insomnia.

P

• Inform patient that drug is only available through certified pharmacies that are enrolled in the Qsymia certified pharmacy network. Pharmacies can be found at www.qsymiarems.com or by calling 1-888-998-4887.

Black Box Warning Tell patient to keep drug in a safe place and protect it from theft. Advise patient never to give drug to anyone else because it can cause harm or death and is against the law. ■

• Warn patient not to increase dosage without first discussing with prescriber.

• Advise woman of childbearing potential that pregnancy testing will be done before start of therapy and monthly during therapy.

• Counsel patient to use effective contraception. Advise her to inform prescriber immediately if pregnancy occurs.

• Instruct patient to tell all health care providers about all medications, nutritional supplements, and vitamins (including weight-loss products) that are being taken or may be taken during therapy.

• Caution patient to report sustained periods of heart pounding or racing while at rest; mood changes, depression, or suicidal ideation; prolonged diarrhea; scheduled surgery; occurrence or history of seizures; or use of a high-protein, low-carbohydrate diet.

• Teach patient to immediately report severe and persistent eye pain or significant vision changes.

• Instruct patient to report changes in attention, concentration, memory, or difficulty finding words.

• Tell patient to avoid operating hazardous machinery, including automobiles, until effects of drug are known.

• Advise diabetic patient to monitor glucose level closely and to report episodes of hypoglycemia. Medication regimen may need adjustment.

• Caution patient to watch for decreased sweating or increased body temperature during physical activity, especially during hot weather.

• Warn patient not to stop drug abruptly as seizures may result.

• Advise patient to increase fluid intake to avoid kidney stones and to report severe side or back pain or blood in urine.

phenylephrine hydrochloride (ophthalmic)
fen-ill-EF-rin

Mydfrin✱

Therapeutic class: Mydriatics
Pharmacologic class: Sympathomimetic amines–adrenergics

AVAILABLE FORMS
Ophthalmic solution: 2.5%, 10%

INDICATIONS & DOSAGES
➤ **Mydriasis**
Adults and children age 1 and older: Instill 1 drop of 2.5% or 10% solution every 3 to 5 minutes, up to 3 drops per eye. May repeat dose.
Children younger than age 1: Instill 1 drop of 2.5% solution every 3 to 5 minutes, up to 3 drops per eye.

ADMINISTRATION
Ophthalmic
• Don't touch tip of dropper to eye or surrounding tissue.
• Apply light finger pressure on lacrimal sac for 1 minute after instilling drug to minimize systemic absorption.
• Don't use brown solution or solution that contains precipitate.

ACTION
Dilates the pupil by contracting the dilator muscle.

Route	Onset	Peak	Duration
Ophthalmic	Rapid	20–90 min	3–7 hr

Half-life: Unknown.

ADVERSE REACTIONS
CNS: brow ache, headache.
CV: hypertension with 10% solution, *MI,* palpitations, PVCs, tachycardia.
EENT: allergic conjunctivitis, blurred vision, IOP, keratitis, lacrimation, reactive hyperemia of eye, rebound miosis, transient eye burning or stinging on instillation, photophobia.
Skin: dermatitis, diaphoresis, pallor.
Other: trembling.

Reactions in bold italics are *life-threatening*. Interactions may have a *rapid onset* or a *delayed onset*.

INTERACTIONS
Drug-drug. *Atropine (topical), cyclopentolate, homatropine, scopolamine:* May increase pupil dilation. Use together cautiously.
Beta blockers, MAO inhibitors: May cause arrhythmias because of increased pressor effect. Use together cautiously.
Levodopa: May reduce mydriatic effect of phenylephrine. Use together cautiously.
TCAs: May increase cardiac effects of epinephrine. Use together cautiously.
Drug-lifestyle. *Sun exposure:* May cause photophobia. Advise patient to wear sunglasses.

EFFECTS ON LAB TEST RESULTS
● May lower IOP in normal eyes or in angle-closure glaucoma.
● May cause false-normal tonometry readings.

CONTRAINDICATIONS & CAUTIONS
● Contraindicated in patients hypersensitive to drug, in those with angle-closure glaucoma, and in those who wear soft contact lenses.
● Use cautiously in patients with marked hypertension, cardiac disorders, or advanced arteriosclerotic changes; in children with low body weight; and in elderly patients.
● The 10% solution is contraindicated in patients younger than age 1 due to increased risk of systemic toxicity.
Dialyzable drug: Unknown.

PREGNANCY-LACTATION-REPRODUCTION
● It isn't known if drug can cause fetal harm. Use during pregnancy only if clearly needed.
● It isn't known if drug appears in breast milk. Use cautiously in breast-feeding women.

NURSING CONSIDERATIONS
● Systemic adverse reactions are least likely with 2.5% solution and most likely with 10% solution.

PATIENT TEACHING
● Teach patient how to instill drug. Advise him to wash hands before and after instillation and to apply light finger pressure on lacrimal sac for 1 minute after drops are instilled. Warn him not to touch tip of dropper to eye or surrounding tissue.
● Warn patient not to exceed recommended dosage because systemic effects can result. Monitor BP and pulse rate.
● Tell patient not to use brown solution or solution that contains precipitate.
● Warn patient to avoid hazardous activities, such as operating machinery or driving, until temporary blurring subsides.
● Advise patient to contact prescriber if condition persists longer than 12 hours after stopping drug.
● Advise patient to ease photophobia by wearing dark glasses.

phenytoin (diphenylhydantoin)
FEN-i-toe-in

Dilantin 125, Dilantin Infatabs

phenytoin sodium (extended)
Dilantin, Phenytek

Therapeutic class: Anticonvulsants
Pharmacologic class: Hydantoin derivatives

AVAILABLE FORMS
phenytoin
Oral suspension: 125 mg/5 mL*
Tablets (chewable): 50 mg
phenytoin sodium
Injection: 50 mg/mL (46 mg base)
phenytoin sodium (extended)
Capsules (extended-release): 30 mg (27.6 mg base), 100 mg (92 mg base), 200 mg (184 mg base), 300 mg (276 mg base)

INDICATIONS & DOSAGES
➤ **To control tonic-clonic (grand mal) and complex partial (temporal lobe) seizures**
Adults: Highly individualized. Initially, 100 mg (immediate-release, extended-release) P.O. t.i.d. Adjust dosage at no less than 7- to 10-day intervals until desired response is obtained. Usual range is 300 to 600 mg daily. If patient is stabilized on

100-mg extended-release capsules t.i.d., once-daily dosing with 300-mg extended-release capsules is possible as an alternative. Or, 125 mg oral solution t.i.d. in patients without previous treatment. May increase to 625 mg daily.

Children: 5 mg/kg/day in two to three equally divided doses. Adjust dosage at no less than 7- to 10-day intervals. Usual maintenance dose range is 4 to 8 mg/kg daily. Maximum dose is 300 mg/day.

➤ **To control tonic-clonic (grand mal) and complex partial (temporal lobe) seizures in patients requiring a loading dose**

Adults: Initially, 1 g (extended release) P.O. divided into three doses, which are given at 2-hour intervals with careful monitoring. Begin maintenance dosage of 100 mg (extended-release) P.O. t.i.d. to q.i.d. 24 hours after loading dose.

➤ **To prevent and treat seizures occurring during neurosurgery**

Adults: 100 to 200 mg I.M. every 4 hours during and after surgery.

➤ **Status epilepticus**

Adults: Loading dose of 10 to 15 mg/kg I.V. (1 to 1.5 g may be needed) at a rate not exceeding 50 mg/minute; then maintenance dosage of 100 mg P.O. or I.V. every 6 to 8 hours.

Children: Loading dose of 15 to 20 mg/kg I.V., at a rate not exceeding 1 to 3 mg/kg/minute; then highly individualized maintenance dosages.

Elderly patients: May need lower dosages.

ADMINISTRATION
P.O.
● Give divided doses with or after meals to decrease adverse GI reactions.
● For chewable tablets, patient may chew thoroughly before swallowing or may swallow whole.
● Shake suspension well before use. Administer dose using a calibrated oral dosing syringe.

I.V.
▼ Clear tubing with NSS. Use only clear solution for injection. A slight yellow color is acceptable.
▼ Mix with NSS, if needed, and give as an infusion over 30 minutes to 1 hour when possible. Don't exceed 50 mg/minute in adults or 1 to 3 mg/kg/minute in neonates.
▼ Infusion must begin within 1 hour after preparation and should run through an in-line filter.
▼ Check patency of catheter before giving. Monitor site for extravasation because it can cause severe tissue damage.

Black Box Warning Drug must be administered slowly. In adults, don't exceed 50 mg/minute I.V. In neonates, administer drug at a rate not exceeding 1 to 3 mg/kg/minute. ■

▼ Follow each injection with injection of sterile NSS through the same needle or catheter.
▼ If possible, don't give by I.V. push into veins on back of hand to avoid purple glove syndrome. Inject into larger veins or central venous catheter, if available.
▼ Continuous monitoring of BP and ECG during I.V. administration is essential.
▼ Discard 4 hours after preparation. Don't refrigerate.
▼ **Incompatibilities:** Amikacin, aminophylline, amphotericin B, bretylium, cephapirin, ciprofloxacin, D_5W, diltiazem, dobutamine, enalaprilat, fat emulsions, hydromorphone, insulin (regular), levorphanol, lidocaine, lincomycin, meperidine, morphine sulfate, nitroglycerin, norepinephrine, other I.V. drugs or infusion solutions, pentobarbital sodium, potassium chloride, procaine, propofol, streptomycin, sufentanil citrate, theophylline, vitamin B complex with C. If giving as an infusion, don't mix drug with D_5W because it will precipitate.

I.M.
● Give I.M. only if dosage adjustments are made; I.M. dose is 50% greater than oral dose.
● Be aware that drug may precipitate at injection site, cause pain, and be absorbed erratically.
● Don't give by I.M. route for treatment of status epilepticus as peak plasma levels may not be attained for up to 24 hours.

ACTION
May stabilize neuronal membranes and limit seizure activity either by increasing efflux or decreasing influx of sodium ions across

cell membranes in the motor cortex during generation of nerve impulses.

Route	Onset	Peak	Duration
PO	Unknown	1½–12hr	Unknown
P.O. (extended-release)	Unknown	4–12 hr	Unknown
I.V.	Immediate	1–2 hr	Unknown
I.M.	Unknown	Unknown	Unknown

Half-life: Varies with dose and concentration changes.

ADVERSE REACTIONS
CNS: ataxia, decreased coordination, mental confusion, slurred speech, dizziness, headache, insomnia, nervousness, twitching, peripheral neuropathy.
CV: *bradycardia,* periarteritis nodosa, hypotension.
EENT: diplopia, nystagmus, blurred vision, thickening of facial features.
GI: gingival hyperplasia, nausea, vomiting, constipation.
Hematologic: *agranulocytosis, leukopenia, pancytopenia, thrombocytopenia,* macrocythemia, megaloblastic anemia.
Hepatic: *toxic hepatitis.*
Metabolic: hyperglycemia.
Musculoskeletal: osteomalacia.
Skin: *Stevens-Johnson syndrome, toxic epidermal necrolysis,* bullous or purpuric dermatitis, discoloration of skin if given by I.V. push in back of hand, exfoliative dermatitis, hypertrichosis, inflammation at injection site, necrosis, pain, photosensitivity reactions, scarlatiniform or morbilliform rash.
Other: lymphadenopathy, systemic lupus erythematosus.

INTERACTIONS
Drug-drug. *Acetaminophen:* May decrease the therapeutic effects of acetaminophen and increase the incidence of hepatotoxicity. Monitor for toxicity.
Amiodarone, antihistamines, chloramphenicol, **cimetidine,** *cycloserine, diazepam,* **fluconazole, isoniazid,** *metronidazole, omeprazole, phenylbutazone, salicylates,* **sulfonamides, ticlopidine,** *valproate:* May increase phenytoin activity and toxicity. Monitor patient for toxicity and adjust dose as needed.

Atracurium, cisatracurium, pancuronium, rocuronium, vecuronium: May decrease the effects of nondepolarizing muscle relaxant. May need to increase the nondepolarizing muscle relaxant dose.
Barbiturates, carbamazepine, dexamethasone, diazoxide, folic acid, rifampin: May decrease phenytoin activity. Monitor phenytoin level.
Carbamazepine, cardiac glycosides, doxycycline, quinidine, theophylline, valproic acid: May decrease effects of these drugs. Monitor patient.
Colesevelam: May impair phenytoin absorption. Administer phenytoin 4 hours prior to colesevelam.
Corticosteroids: May decrease phenytoin level and corticosteroid effects. Measure phenytoin level and adjust phenytoin and corticosteroid dosages as needed.
Cyclosporine: May decrease cyclosporine levels, risking organ rejection. Monitor cyclosporine levels closely and adjust dose as needed.
Delavirdine: May cause loss of virologic response. Use together is contraindicated.
Disulfiram: May increase toxic effects of phenytoin. Monitor phenytoin level closely and adjust dose as needed.
Efavirenz: May increase phenytoin level and decrease efavirenz level. Monitor patient and adjust dosages of either or both drugs if needed.
Erlotinib: May increase phenytoin level and decrease erlotinib level. Monitor patient response.
Hormonal contraceptives: May increase phenytoin level and decrease contraceptive effectiveness. Monitor phenytoin level and adjust dosage if needed. Alternative form of contraception is recommended during therapy.
Isoniazid: May increase phenytoin level. Monitor phenytoin level and patient for toxicity.
Lithium: May increase toxicity of lithium, despite normal lithium levels. Monitor patient for adverse effects.
Methylphenidate: May increase phenytoin level. Monitor phenytoin level and adjust phenytoin dosage as needed.

P

Protease inhibitors (fosamprenavir, lopinavir–ritonavir): May decrease levels of both drugs. Measure phenytoin level and adjust dosage of phenytoin or protease inhibitor as needed.

Warfarin: May increase effects of warfarin. Monitor patient for bleeding.

Drug-food. *Enteral tube feedings:* May interfere with absorption of oral drug. Stop enteral feedings for 2 hours before and 2 hours after drug use.

Drug-lifestyle. *Alcohol use (long-term):* May decrease drug's activity. Strongly discourage use together.

EFFECTS ON LAB TEST RESULTS
• May increase alkaline phosphatase, GGT, and glucose levels. May decrease urinary 17-hydroxysteroid, 17-ketosteroid, and Hb levels and hematocrit.
• May decrease platelet, WBC, RBC, and granulocyte counts.
• May increase urine 6-hydroxycortisol excretion. May decrease dexamethasone suppression and metyrapone test results.
• May falsely reduce protein-bound iodine or free T_4 level test results.

CONTRAINDICATIONS & CAUTIONS
• Contraindicated in patients hypersensitive to hydantoin, in those taking delavirdine, and in those with sinus bradycardia, SA block, second- or third-degree AV block, or Adams-Stokes syndrome.
• Use cautiously in patients with hepatic dysfunction, hypotension, myocardial insufficiency, diabetes, or respiratory depression; in elderly or debilitated patients; and in those receiving other hydantoin derivatives.
• Elderly patients tend to metabolize drug slowly and may need reduced dosages.
Dialyzable drug: Yes.
⚠ Overdose S&S: Ataxia, dysarthria, nystagmus, hyperreflexia, lethargy, nausea, slurred speech, tremor, vomiting, coma, hypotension, circulatory and respiratory depression.

PREGNANCY-LACTATION-REPRODUCTION
• Drug may cause fetal harm. Avoid use during pregnancy when possible and monotherapy is recommended.
• If drug is necessary, pregnant women may need dosage adjustments to maintain clinical response. Therapeutic dose needs usually increase during pregnancy.
• Drug may interact with hormone-containing contraceptives; use of nonhormonal contraceptives is recommended.
• Women exposed to drug during pregnancy should enroll in the Antiepileptic Drug Pregnancy Registry (1-888-233-2334).
• Drug appears in breast milk. Breastfeeding isn't recommended.

NURSING CONSIDERATIONS
• Asian patients who have tested positive for the allele HLA-B*1502 have a potentially increased risk of serious skin reactions, including Stevens-Johnson syndrome and toxic epidermal necrolysis. Monitor these patients carefully.
• If rash appears, stop drug. If rash is scarlatiniform or morbilliform, resume drug after rash clears. If rash reappears, stop therapy. If rash is exfoliative, purpuric, or bullous, don't resume drug.
• Don't stop drug suddenly because this may worsen seizures. Call prescriber immediately if adverse reactions develop.
• Monitor drug level. Therapeutic level of total phenytoin is 10 to 20 mcg/mL in adults and children and 8 to 15 mcg/mL in neonates. Therapeutic range of free phenytoin is 1 to 2 mcg/mL.
• Long-term use may decrease bone mineral density. Vitamin D and calcium supplements may be needed.
• Because of the risks of cardiac and local toxicity with parenteral phenytoin, use oral form when possible.
• Monitor CBC and calcium level every 6 months, and periodically monitor hepatic function. If megaloblastic anemia is evident, prescriber may order folic acid and vitamin B_{12}.
• Maintain seizure precautions, as needed.
• Mononucleosis may decrease level. Watch for increased seizures.
⚡ Alert: Closely monitor all patients for changes in behavior that may indicate worsening of suicidal thoughts or behavior or depression.

- Watch for gingival hyperplasia, especially in children.
- **Alert:** Doubling the dose doesn't double the level but may cause toxicity. Consult pharmacist for specific dosing recommendations.
- If seizure control is established with divided doses, once-daily dosing may be considered.
- **Look alike–sound alike:** Don't confuse phenytoin with mephenytoin, fosphenytoin, phenelzine, phentermine, or phenobarbital. Don't confuse Dilantin with Dilaudid, diltiazem, or Dipentum.

PATIENT TEACHING

- Tell patient to notify prescriber if skin rash develops.
- Advise patient to avoid driving and other potentially hazardous activities that require mental alertness until drug's CNS effects are known.
- Advise patient not to change brands or dosage forms once he's stabilized on therapy.
- Dilantin capsules are the only oral form that can be given once daily. Toxic levels may result if any other brand or form is given once daily. Dilantin tablets and oral suspension should never be taken once daily.
- Tell patient not to use capsules that are discolored.
- Advise patient to avoid alcohol.
- Warn patient and parents not to stop drug abruptly.
- Stress importance of good oral hygiene and regular dental examinations. Surgical removal of excess gum tissue may be needed periodically if dental hygiene is poor.
- Caution patient that drug may color urine pink, red, or reddish brown.

pilocarpine hydrochloride (ophthalmic)
pie-low-KAR-peen

Akarpine✽, Diocarpine✽, Isopto Carpine, Pilopine HS

Therapeutic class: Miotics
Pharmacologic class: Direct-acting parasympathomimetics

AVAILABLE FORMS
Ophthalmic solution: 1%, 2%, 4%

INDICATIONS & DOSAGES
➤ **Primary open-angle glaucoma or ocular hypertension**
Adults and children: Instill 1 or 2 drops every 6 to 8 hours; adjust concentration and frequency to control IOP. Start pilocarpine-naive patients on the 1% concentration.
➤ **Management of acute angle-closure glaucoma**
Adults and children age 2 and older: Instill 1 drop of 1% or 2% solution in affected eye up to three times in a 30-minute period.
➤ **Prevention of postoperative elevated IOP associated with laser surgery**
Adults and children age 2 and older: Instill 1 drop of 1%, 2%, or 4% solution in affected eye 15 to 60 minutes before surgery. May give 2 drops, but give them at least 5 minutes apart.
➤ **Induction of miosis**
Adults and children age 2 and older: Instill 1 drop of 1%, 2%, or 4% solution in eye. May give 2 drops, but give them at least 5 minutes apart.
Children younger than age 2: Instill 1 drop of 1% solution in eye t.i.d.
➤ **Induction of miosis before goniotomy or trabeculotomy**
Children: Instill 1 drop of 1% or 2% solution in eye 15 to 60 minutes before surgery.
➤ **Mydriasis caused by mydriatic or cycloplegic drugs**
Adults and children: Instill 1 drop of 1% solution.

P

ADMINISTRATION
Ophthalmic
- Don't touch tip of dropper to eye or surrounding tissue.
- Apply light finger pressure on lacrimal sac for 1 minute after instilling to minimize systemic absorption.
- Patient should remove lenses before instillation and wait 10 to 15 minutes after dosing before reinserting lenses.

ACTION
A cholinergic that causes contraction of iris sphincter muscles, resulting in miosis, and that produces ciliary spasm, deepening of the anterior chamber, and vasodilation of conjunctival vessels of the outflow tract.

Route	Onset	Peak	Duration
Ophthalmic	10–30 min	30–85 min	4–8 hr

Half-life: Unknown.

ADVERSE REACTIONS
EENT: blurred vision, brow pain, myopia, changes in visual field, ciliary spasm, conjunctival irritation, keratitis, lacrimation, lens opacity, periorbital or supraorbital headache, retinal detachment, transient stinging and burning.
GI: diarrhea, nausea, vomiting.
Other: diaphoresis.

INTERACTIONS
Drug-drug. *Carbachol, echothiophate:* May cause additive effects. Avoid using together.
Cyclopentolate, ophthalmic belladonna alkaloids such as atropine, scopolamine: May decrease pilocarpine's antiglaucoma effect and block mydriatic effects of these drugs. Avoid using together.
Phenylephrine: May decrease dilation by phenylephrine. Avoid using together.

EFFECTS ON LAB TEST RESULTS
None reported.

CONTRAINDICATIONS & CAUTIONS
- Contraindicated in patients hypersensitive to drug and in conditions in which cholinergic effects, such as constriction, are undesirable (acute iritis, some forms of secondary glaucoma, pupillary block glaucoma, or acute inflammatory disease of the anterior chamber).
- Use cautiously in patients with acute cardiac failure, bronchial asthma, peptic ulcer, hyperthyroidism, GI spasm, urinary tract obstruction, and Parkinson disease.
Dialyzable drug: Unknown.
⚠ *Overdose S&S:* Excess salivation, tearing, sweating, nausea, vomiting, diarrhea, bronchial constriction, tremors, bradycardia, hypotension.

PREGNANCY-LACTATION-REPRODUCTION
- It isn't known if drug causes fetal harm. Use in pregnancy only if clearly needed.
- It isn't known if drug appears in breast milk. Use cautiously in breast-feeding women.

NURSING CONSIDERATIONS
- Drug may be used in combination with beta blockers, carbonic anhydrase inhibitors, sympathomimetics, or hyperosmotic agents. If more than one topical ophthalmic drug is being used, the drugs should be administered at least 5 minutes apart.
❸ *Alert:* Patients with hazel or brown irises may need stronger solutions or more frequent instillation because eye pigment may absorb drug.
- *Look alike–sound alike:* Don't confuse Isopto Carpine with Isopto Carbachol.

PATIENT TEACHING
- Teach patient how to instill drug. Advise patient to wash hands before and after instillation and to apply light finger pressure on lacrimal sac for 1 minute after drops are instilled. Warn patient not to touch applicator tip to eye or surrounding tissue.
- Instruct patient who wears contact lenses to remove lenses before instilling drug and to wait 10 minutes after dosing before reinserting lenses.
- Warn patient that transient brow pain and nearsightedness are common at first but usually disappear in 10 to 14 days.
- Advise patient to carry medical identification at all times during therapy.

pilocarpine hydrochloride (oral)
pye-loe-CAR-peen

Salagen

Therapeutic class: Cholinergic agonists
Pharmacologic class: Cholinergic agonists

AVAILABLE FORMS
Tablets: 5 mg, 7.5 mg

INDICATIONS & DOSAGES
Adjust-a-dose (for all indications): For patients with moderate hepatic impairment, initial dose is 5 mg P.O. b.i.d. Adjust dosage based on tolerance.
➤ **Xerostomia from salivary gland hypofunction caused by radiotherapy for cancer of head and neck**
Adults: 5 mg P.O. t.i.d.; may increase to 10 mg P.O. t.i.d., as needed.
➤ **Dry mouth in patients with Sjögren syndrome**
Adults: 5 mg P.O. q.i.d.

ADMINISTRATION
P.O.
● Don't give drug with a high-fat meal.

ACTION
Cholinergic parasympathomimetic that increases secretion of salivary glands, eliminating dryness.

Route	Onset	Peak	Duration
P.O.	20 min	1 hr	3–5 hr

Half-life: 45 minutes to 1½ hours.

ADVERSE REACTIONS
CNS: asthenia, dizziness, headache, tremor.
CV: flushing, hypertension, tachycardia, edema.
EENT: abnormal vision, rhinitis, sinusitis, lacrimation, amblyopia, pharyngitis, voice alteration, conjunctivitis, epistaxis.
GI: nausea, dyspepsia, diarrhea, abdominal pain, vomiting, dysphagia, taste perversion.
GU: urinary frequency.
Musculoskeletal: myalgia.

Skin: sweating, rash, pruritus.
Other: chills.

INTERACTIONS
Drug-drug. *Beta blockers:* May increase risk of conduction disturbances. Use together cautiously.
Drugs with anticholinergic effects: May antagonize anticholinergic effects. Use together cautiously.
Drugs with parasympathomimetic effects: May result in additive pharmacologic effects. Monitor patient closely.
Drug-food. *High-fat meals:* May reduce drug absorption. Discourage patient from eating high-fat meals.

EFFECTS ON LAB TEST RESULTS
None reported.

CONTRAINDICATIONS & CAUTIONS
● Contraindicated in patients hypersensitive to pilocarpine, in those with uncontrolled asthma, and in those for whom miosis is undesirable, as in acute iritis or angle-closure glaucoma.
● Use in severe hepatic impairment isn't recommended.
● Use cautiously in patients with CV disease, controlled asthma, chronic bronchitis, COPD, cholelithiasis, biliary tract disease, nephrolithiasis, or cognitive or psychiatric disturbances.
● Safety and effectiveness in children haven't been established.
Dialyzable drug: Unknown.
⚠ *Overdose S&S:* Exaggerated parasympathetic effects, CV depression, bronchoconstriction, death.

PREGNANCY-LACTATION-REPRODUCTION
● There are no adequate studies in pregnant women. Use only if potential benefit justifies potential fetal risk.
● It isn't known if drug appears in breast milk. Patient should discontinue breast-feeding or discontinue drug.

NURSING CONSIDERATIONS
● Examine patient's fundus carefully before beginning therapy because retinal detachment may occur in patients with retinal disease.

P

• Monitor patient for signs and symptoms of toxicity: headache, visual disturbance, lacrimation, sweating, respiratory distress, GI spasm, nausea, vomiting, diarrhea, AV block, tachycardia, bradycardia, hypotension, hypertension, shock, mental confusion, arrhythmia, and tremors. Immediately notify prescriber of suspected toxicity.

• *Look alike–sound alike:* Don't confuse Salagen with selegiline.

PATIENT TEACHING
• Warn patient that driving ability may be impaired, especially at night, by drug-induced visual disturbances.
• Advise patient to drink plenty of fluids to prevent dehydration.
• Tell elderly patient with Sjögren syndrome that he may be especially prone to urinary frequency, diarrhea, and dizziness.
• Advise patient not to take drug with a high-fat meal.

---

pimavanserin tartrate
See NEW DRUGS for information.

---

pimecrolimus
py-meck-roh-LY-mus

Elidel

Therapeutic class: Immunosuppressants (topical)
Pharmacologic class: Topical immunomodulators

AVAILABLE FORMS
Cream: 1%*

INDICATIONS & DOSAGES
➤ **Second-line therapy for short and noncontinuous prolonged treatment of mild to moderate atopic dermatitis in nonimmunocompromised patients in whom use of other conventional therapies is deemed inadvisable, or in patients with inadequate response to or intolerance of conventional therapies**
Adults and children age 2 and older: Apply a thin layer to the affected skin b.i.d. and rub in gently and completely. Discontinue therapy when signs and symptoms (itch, rash, redness) resolve.

ADMINISTRATION
Topical
• Drug may be used on all skin surfaces, including the head, neck, and intertriginous areas.
• Clear infections at treatment sites before using.
• Don't use with occlusive dressing.

ACTION
Unknown. Inhibits T-cell activation and prevents the release of inflammatory cytokines and mediators from mast cells.

Route	Onset	Peak	Duration
Topical	Unknown	Unknown	Unknown

Half-life: Unknown.

ADVERSE REACTIONS
CNS: headache, fever.
EENT: nasopharyngitis, otitis media, sinusitis, pharyngitis, tonsillitis, eye infection, nasal congestion, rhinorrhea, sinus congestion, rhinitis, epistaxis, conjunctivitis, earache.
GI: gastroenteritis, abdominal pain, vomiting, diarrhea, nausea, constipation, loose stools.
GU: dysmenorrhea.
Musculoskeletal: back pain, arthralgias.
Respiratory: URI, bronchitis, cough, *asthma,* pneumonia, wheezing, dyspnea.
Skin: application-site reaction (burning, irritation, erythema, pruritus), skin infections, impetigo, folliculitis, molluscum contagiosum, herpes simplex, varicella, papilloma, urticaria, acne.
Other: flulike illness, hypersensitivity, toothache, bacterial infection, staphylococcal infection, viral infection.

INTERACTIONS
Drug-drug. *CYP3A4 inhibitors (calcium channel blockers, erythromycin, fluconazole, itraconazole, ketoconazole):* May affect metabolism of pimecrolimus. Use together cautiously.
Immunosuppressants (except cytarabine [liposomal]): May enhance adverse or toxic effect of immunosuppressants. Avoid use together.
Drug-lifestyle. *Natural or artificial sun exposure:* May worsen atopic dermatitis.

Reactions in bold italics are *life-threatening*. Interactions may have a *rapid onset* or a *delayed onset*.

Advise patient to avoid or minimize sunlight exposure.

EFFECTS ON LAB TEST RESULTS
None reported.

CONTRAINDICATIONS & CAUTIONS
• Contraindicated in patients hypersensitive to drug or its components, in patients with Netherton syndrome, and in immunocompromised patients.

Black Box Warning Long-term safety of topical calcineurin inhibitors hasn't been established. ∎

Black Box Warning Although a causal relationship hasn't been established, rare cases of malignancy (e.g., skin malignancy, lymphoma) have been reported in patients treated with topical calcineurin inhibitors, including pimecrolimus. ∎

• Contraindicated in patients with active cutaneous viral infections or infected atopic dermatitis.

Black Box Warning Contraindicated in children younger than age 2. ∎

• Use cautiously in patients with varicella zoster virus infection, HSV infection, or eczema herpeticum.

Dialyzable drug: Unknown.

PREGNANCY-LACTATION-REPRODUCTION
• There are no adequate studies in pregnant women. Use only if potential benefit justifies potential fetal risk.
• It's unknown if drug appears in breast milk. Serious adverse reactions may occur in breast-feeding infants exposed to drug. Patient should discontinue breast-feeding or discontinue drug.

NURSING CONSIDERATIONS
❸ *Alert:* Use drug only after other therapies have failed because of the risk of cancer.

Black Box Warning Long-term safety hasn't been established. Avoid continuous long-term use of drug and limit application to areas of involvement of atopic dermatitis. ∎

• If symptoms persist longer than 6 weeks, reevaluate patient.
• May cause local symptoms such as skin burning. Most local reactions start within 1 to 5 days after treatment, are mild to

moderately severe, and last no longer than 5 days.
• Monitor patient for lymphadenopathy. If lymphadenopathy occurs and its cause is unknown, or if patient develops acute infectious mononucleosis, consider stopping drug.
• Drug use may cause papillomas or warts. Consider stopping drug if papillomas worsen or don't respond to conventional treatment.
• *Look alike–sound alike:* Don't confuse pimecrolimus with tacrolimus.

PATIENT TEACHING
• Inform patient that this drug is for external use only and that he should use it as directed.
• Tell patient to report adverse reactions.
• Tell patient not to use with an occlusive dressing.
• Instruct patient to wash hands after application if hands are not treated.
• Tell patient to stop therapy after signs and symptoms have resolved. If symptoms persist longer than 6 weeks, tell him to contact his prescriber.
• Tell patient to resume treatment at first signs of recurrence.
• Stress that patient should minimize or avoid exposure to natural or artificial sunlight (including tanning beds and UVA-UVB treatment) while using this drug.
• Tell patient to expect application-site reactions but to notify his prescriber if reaction is severe or persists for longer than 1 week.

SAFETY ALERT!

pioglitazone hydrochloride
pie-oh-GLIT-ah-zohn

Actos♦

Therapeutic class: Antidiabetics
Pharmacologic class:
Thiazolidinediones

AVAILABLE FORMS
Tablets: 15 mg, 30 mg, 45 mg

P

INDICATIONS & DOSAGES
➤ **Type 2 diabetes mellitus, alone or with a sulfonylurea, metformin, or insulin as an adjunct to diet and exercise to improve glycemic control**
Adults: Initially, 15 or 30 mg P.O. once daily. Maximum daily dose, if used alone or in combination therapy, is 45 mg.
Adjust-a-dose: For patients taking pioglitazone with insulin, reduce insulin by 10% to 25% if patient reports hypoglycemia. Maximum recommended dose of pioglitazone is 15 mg when used with gemfibrozil or other strong CYP2C8 inhibitors. Start with 15 mg in patients with New York Heart Association (NYHA) class I or II HF.

ADMINISTRATION
P.O.
● Give drug without regard for meals.

ACTION
Lowers glucose level by decreasing insulin resistance and hepatic glucose production. Improves sensitivity of insulin in muscle and adipose tissue.

Route	Onset	Peak	Duration
P.O.	30 min	≤2 hr	Unknown

Half-life: 3 to 7 hours.

ADVERSE REACTIONS
CNS: headache.
CV: edema, *HF.*
EENT: sinusitis, pharyngitis, macular edema.
Hematologic: anemia.
Metabolic: *hypoglycemia,* weight gain.
Musculoskeletal: myalgia, fractures.
Respiratory: URI.
Other: tooth disorder.

INTERACTIONS
Drug-drug. *Atorvastatin:* May decrease atorvastatin and pioglitazone levels. Monitor patient and glucose level.
CYP2C8 inducers (rifampin): May decrease pioglitazone concentration. Don't exceed maximum recommended pioglitazone dose.
Hormonal contraceptives: May decrease level of hormonal contraceptives, reducing contraceptive effectiveness. Advise patient taking drug and hormonal contraceptives to consider additional birth control measures.
Insulin: May increase incidence of edema and HF and may cause additive or synergistic pharmacologic effects. If hypoglycemia occurs, decrease insulin dosage.
Ketoconazole: May inhibit pioglitazone metabolism. Monitor glucose level more frequently.
Strong CYP2C8 inhibitors (gemfibrozil): May increase pioglitazone level. Monitor patient and glucose level. Maximum pioglitazone dose is 15 mg.
Sulfonylureas: May increase risk of hypoglycemia. If hypoglycemia occurs, reduce sulfonylurea dosage.
Drug-herb. *Eucalyptus:* May increase hypoglycemic effects. Discourage use together.
Drug-lifestyle. *Alcohol use:* May alter glycemic control and increase risk of hypoglycemia. Discourage use together.

EFFECTS ON LAB TEST RESULTS
● May increase CK, ALT, HDL, LDL, and total cholesterol levels.
● May decrease glucose, triglyceride, and Hb levels and hematocrit.

CONTRAINDICATIONS & CAUTIONS
Black Box Warning Contraindicated in patients with symptomatic HF and in those with NYHA class III or IV HF. ■
● Contraindicated in patients hypersensitive to drug or its components and in those with active bladder disease, type 1 diabetes mellitus, diabetic ketoacidosis, active liver disease, ALT level greater than 2½ × ULN, and in those who experienced jaundice while taking troglitazone.
Black Box Warning Use cautiously in patients with edema or HF or patients at risk for HF. ■
● Use cautiously in patients with a history of bladder cancer.
● Safety and effectiveness in children haven't been established.
Dialyzable drug: Unknown.

PREGNANCY-LACTATION-REPRODUCTION
● Use during pregnancy only if benefit justifies risk to the fetus. Insulin is preferred antidiabetic during pregnancy.

• It isn't known if drug appears in breast milk. Patient should discontinue breast-feeding or discontinue drug.

NURSING CONSIDERATIONS

⚕ *Alert:* Measure liver enzyme levels at start of therapy, every 2 months for first year of therapy, and periodically thereafter. Obtain LFT results in patients who develop signs and symptoms of liver dysfunction, such as nausea, vomiting, abdominal pain, fatigue, anorexia, or dark urine. Stop drug if patient develops jaundice or if LFT results show ALT level greater than 3 × ULN.

Black Box Warning Drug can cause fluid retention, leading to or worsening HF. Observe patients carefully for signs and symptoms of HF (including excessive, rapid weight gain; dyspnea; and edema). If these signs and symptoms develop, the HF should be managed according to the current standards of care. Also, stopping or reducing dose of pioglitazone must be considered. ▪

• Hb level and hematocrit may drop, usually during first 4 to 12 weeks of therapy.

• Management of type 2 diabetes should include diet control. Because caloric restrictions, weight loss, and exercise help improve insulin sensitivity and help make drug therapy effective, these measures are essential for proper diabetes management.

⚕ *Alert:* Watch for hypoglycemia, especially in patients receiving combination therapy. Dosage adjustments of these drugs may be needed.

• Monitor glucose level regularly, especially during situations of increased stress, such as infection, fever, surgery, and trauma.

⚕ *Alert:* Drug may be associated with an increased risk of bladder cancer when used for more than 1 year. Monitor patients for signs and symptoms of bladder cancer (such as blood in urine or abdominal pain). If considering use in patients with a history of bladder cancer, weigh benefits of blood glucose control with drug against unknown risks of cancer recurrence.

• Risk of fractures (forearm, hand, wrist, foot, ankle, fibula, and tibia) in female patients receiving long-term treatment is increased. Give only if risk outweighs benefits.

• *Look alike–sound alike:* Don't confuse pioglitazone with rosiglitazone. Don't confuse Actos with Actidose or Actonel.

PATIENT TEACHING

• Instruct patient to adhere to dietary instructions and to have glucose and HbA$_{1c}$ levels tested regularly.

• Teach patient taking pioglitazone with insulin or oral antidiabetics the signs and symptoms of hypoglycemia.

• Advise patient to notify prescriber during periods of stress, such as fever, trauma, infection, or surgery, because dosage may need adjustment.

• Instruct patient how and when to monitor glucose level.

• Notify patient that blood tests of liver function will be performed before therapy starts, every 2 months for the first year, and periodically thereafter.

• Tell patient to report unexplained nausea, vomiting, abdominal pain, fatigue, anorexia, and dark urine immediately because these symptoms may indicate liver problems.

• Warn patient to contact his health care provider if he has signs or symptoms of HF (unusually rapid increase in weight, swelling, or shortness of breath).

• Advise anovulatory, premenopausal women with insulin resistance that therapy may cause resumption of ovulation; recommend using contraception.

• Tell patient to have regular eye examinations and to report any visual changes immediately.

P

---

piperacillin sodium–tazobactam sodium
pie-PER-us-sil-in/taz-oh-BAK-tem

Zosyn

Therapeutic class: Antibiotics
Pharmacologic class: Extended-spectrum penicillins–beta-lactamase inhibitors

AVAILABLE FORMS

Powder for injection: 2 g piperacillin and 0.25 g tazobactam per vial, 3 g piperacillin

---

and 0.375 g tazobactam per vial, 4 g piperacillin and 0.5 g tazobactam per vial
Premixed, frozen solution for injection:
2 g piperacillin and 0.25 g tazobactam per 50-mL container, 3 g piperacillin and 0.375 g tazobactam per 50-mL container, 4 g piperacillin and 0.5 g tazobactam per 100-mL container

INDICATIONS & DOSAGES
➤ **Moderate to severe infections from piperacillin-resistant, piperacillin-tazobactam–susceptible, beta-lactamase–producing strains of microorganisms in appendicitis (complicated by rupture or abscess) and peritonitis caused by** *Escherichia coli, Bacteroides fragilis, B. ovatus, B. thetaiotaomicron,* **or** *B. vulgatus;* **skin and skin-structure infections caused by** *Staphylococcus aureus;* **postpartum endometritis or pelvic inflammatory disease caused by** *E. coli;* **moderately severe community-acquired pneumonia caused by** *Haemophilus influenzae*
Adults: 3.375 g (3 g piperacillin/0.375 g tazobactam) every 6 hours by I.V. infusion for 7 to 10 days.
Adjust-a-dose: If CrCl is 20 to 40 mL/minute, give 2.25 g (2 g piperacillin/0.25 g tazobactam) every 6 hours; if CrCl is less than 20 mL/minute, give 2.25 g (2 g piperacillin/0.25 g tazobactam) every 8 hours. In continuous ambulatory peritoneal dialysis (CAPD) patients, give 2.25 g (2 g piperacillin/0.25 g tazobactam) every 12 hours. In hemodialysis patients, give 2.25 g (2 g piperacillin/0.25 g tazobactam) every 12 hours with a supplemental dose of 0.75 g (0.67 g piperacillin/0.08 g tazobactam) after each dialysis period.
➤ **Appendicitis, peritonitis**
Children weighing more than 40 kg with normal renal function: 3.375 g (3 g piperacillin/0.375 g tazobactam) every 6 hours by I.V. infusion for 7 to 10 days.
Children age 9 months and older weighing 40 kg or less with normal renal function: 100 mg piperacillin/12.5 mg tazobactam per kg of body weight every 8 hours by I.V. infusion for 7 to 10 days.
Children age 2 to 9 months: 80 mg piperacillin/10 mg tazobactam per kg of

body weight every 8 hours by I.V. infusion for 7 to 10 days.
➤ **Moderate to severe nosocomial pneumonia caused by piperacillin-resistant, beta-lactamase–producing strains of** *S. aureus* **or by piperacillin-tazobactam–susceptible** *Acinetobacter baumannii, H. influenzae, Klebsiella pneumoniae,* **and** *Pseudomonas aeruginosa*
Adults: 4.5 g (4 g piperacillin/0.5 g tazobactam) I.V. every 6 hours with aminoglycoside. Patients with *P. aeruginosa* should continue aminoglycoside or antipseudomonal fluoroquinolone treatment; if *P. aeruginosa* isn't isolated, aminoglycoside or fluoroquinolone treatment may be stopped. Duration of treatment is usually 7 to 14 days.

ADMINISTRATION
I.V.
▼ Before giving drug, ask patient about allergic reactions to penicillins.
▼ Obtain specimen for culture and sensitivity tests before giving first dose. Therapy may begin while awaiting results.
▼ Reconstitute each gram with 5 mL of diluent, such as sterile or bacteriostatic water for injection, NSS for injection, bacteriostatic NSS for injection, D₅W, dextrose 5% in NSS for injection, or dextran 6% in NSS for injection.
▼ Shake until dissolved.
▼ Further dilute to 50 to 150 mL before infusion.
▼ Use drug immediately after reconstitution.
▼ Stop any primary infusion during administration, if possible.
▼ Infuse over at least 30 minutes.
▼ Discard unused drug in single-dose vials after 24 hours if stored at room temperature or 48 hours if refrigerated.
▼ Change I.V. site every 48 hours.
▼ Diluted drug is stable in I.V. bags for 24 hours at room temperature or for 1 week refrigerated.
▼ Store premixed, frozen solution containers at or below –4° F (–20° C).
▼ Thaw frozen container at room temperature (68° to 77° F [20° to 25° C]) or under refrigeration (36° to 46° F [2° to 8° C]).

Don't force-thaw by immersion in water baths or by microwave irradiation.

▼ Check for minute leaks by squeezing container firmly. If leaks are detected, discard solution as sterility may be impaired.

▼ Visually inspect solution, which may precipitate while frozen but will dissolve upon reaching room temperature with little or no agitation. If, after visual inspection, solution remains cloudy, an insoluble precipitate is noted, or if any seals or outlet ports aren't intact, discard container.

▼ Don't use plastic containers in series connections.

▼ **Incompatibilities:** Acyclovir sodium, amiodarone, amphotericin B, amphotericin B cholesteryl sulfate complex, azithromycin, caspofungin (EDTA-formulated product only), chlorpromazine, cisatracurium, cisplatin, dacarbazine, daunorubicin, dobutamine, doxorubicin, doxycycline hyclate, droperidol, famotidine, ganciclovir, gemcitabine, haloperidol lactate, hydroxyzine hydrochloride, idarubicin, lactated Ringer solution, minocycline, mitomycin, mitoxantrone, nalbuphine, pantoprazole (EDTA-formulated product only), prochlorperazine edisylate, promethazine hydrochloride, streptozocin, tobramycin, vancomycin.

ACTION
Inhibits cell-wall synthesis during bacterial multiplication.

Route	Onset	Peak	Duration
I.V.	Immediate	Immediate	Unknown

Half-life: About 1 hour.

ADVERSE REACTIONS
CNS: headache, insomnia, fever, *seizures,* agitation, anxiety, dizziness, pain.
CV: *arrhythmia,* chest pain, edema, hypertension, tachycardia.
EENT: rhinitis.
GI: diarrhea, constipation, nausea, *pseudomembranous colitis,* abdominal pain, dyspepsia, stool changes, vomiting.
GU: candidiasis, interstitial nephritis.
Hematologic: *leukopenia, neutropenia, thrombocytopenia,* anemia, eosinophilia.
Respiratory: dyspnea.
Skin: pruritus, rash.

Other: *anaphylaxis,* hypersensitivity reactions, inflammation, phlebitis at I.V. site.

INTERACTIONS
Drug-drug. *Aminoglycosides:* Penicillins may decrease serum concentration of aminoglycosides. Consider therapy modification.
Anticoagulants, heparin: May prolong effectiveness and increase risk of bleeding. Monitor PT and INR closely.
Hormonal contraceptives: May decrease contraceptive effectiveness. Advise using another form of contraception.
Live-virus vaccines: May decrease vaccine effectiveness. Don't use together.
Methotrexate: May increase risk of methotrexate toxicity. Monitor closely.
Probenecid: May increase piperacillin level. Probenecid may be used for this purpose.
Vancomycin: May increase nephrotoxicity. Monitor therapy.
Vecuronium: May prolong neuromuscular blockade. Monitor patient closely.

EFFECTS ON LAB TEST RESULTS
● May increase serum sodium level because of increased sodium in drug.
● May decrease Hb level.
● May increase eosinophil count. May decrease neutrophil, platelet, and WBC counts.
● May cause false-positive result for urine glucose tests using copper reduction method such as Clinitest. May cause false-positive test for *Aspergillus.*

CONTRAINDICATIONS & CAUTIONS
● Contraindicated in patients hypersensitive to drug or other penicillins.
● Use cautiously in patients with bleeding tendencies, uremia, hypokalemia, and allergies to other drugs, especially cephalosporins, because of possible cross-sensitivity.
Dialyzable drug: Yes.
⚠ **Overdose S&S:** Neuromuscular hyperexcitability, seizures.

PREGNANCY-LACTATION-REPRODUCTION
● There are no adequate studies in pregnant women. Use only if clearly needed.

P

• Drug appears in low concentrations in breast milk. Use cautiously if breast-feeding.

NURSING CONSIDERATIONS
• Drug may cause CDAD ranging in severity from mild diarrhea to fatal colitis. Monitor patient for diarrhea and initiate therapeutic measures as needed. Drug may need to be stopped.
• Serious skin reactions can occur. If rash develops, monitor patient closely and discontinue if lesion progresses.
• Because peritoneal dialysis removes 6% of the piperacillin dose and 21% of the tazobactam dose, and hemodialysis removes 30% to 40% of a dose in 4 hours, additional doses may be needed after each dialysis period.
• If large doses are given or if therapy is prolonged, bacterial or fungal superinfection may occur, especially in elderly, debilitated, or immunosuppressed patients.
• Drug contains 2.84 mEq (65 mg) sodium per gram of piperacillin. Monitor patient's sodium intake and electrolyte levels.
• Monitor hematologic and coagulation parameters.
• Patients with cystic fibrosis may have a higher rate of fever and rash. Monitor these patients closely.
• *Look alike–sound alike:* Don't confuse Zosyn with Zofran or Zyvox.

PATIENT TEACHING
• Tell patient to report adverse reactions promptly.
• Tell patient to report discomfort at the I.V. site.

pitavastatin
pih-tav-a-STAT-in

Livalo

Therapeutic class: Antilipemics
Pharmacologic class: HMG-CoA reductase inhibitors

AVAILABLE FORMS
Tablets: 1 mg, 2 mg, 4 mg

INDICATIONS & DOSAGES
➤ **Adjunctive therapy with diet to decrease total cholesterol, LDL cholesterol, and apolipoprotein B triglyceride levels, and to increase HDL cholesterol level in patients with primary hyperlipidemia and mixed dyslipidemia**
Adults: Initially, 2 mg P.O. daily. May increase dosage as needed, to maximum of 4 mg P.O. daily.
Adjust-a-dose: For patients with CrCl of 15 to 59 mL/minute who aren't receiving hemodialysis and for those with ESRD who are receiving hemodialysis, start with 1 mg P.O. daily; maximum dosage is 2 mg daily. For persistent AST or ALT level 3 × ULN, reduce dosage or discontinue drug.

ADMINISTRATION
P.O.
• May be given without regard to food.

ACTION
Inhibits HMG-CoA reductase, a hepatic enzyme that's needed for cholesterol biosynthesis.

Route	Onset	Peak	Duration
P.O.	Unknown	1 hr	Unknown

Half-life: 12 hours.

ADVERSE REACTIONS
GI: constipation, diarrhea.
Musculoskeletal: back pain, myalgia, extremity pain, *rhabdomyolysis.*

INTERACTIONS
Drug-drug. ❸ *Alert: Atazanavir, atazanavir and ritonavir, darunavir and ritonavir, lopinavir–ritonavir:* May increase statin level and risk of myopathy and rhabdomyolysis. Avoid concurrent use with lopinavir–ritonavir combination; use together cautiously with other agents.
Cyclosporine: May increase pitavastatin level. Use together is contraindicated.
Erythromycin: May increase pitavastatin levels. Don't exceed 1 mg pitavastatin daily.
Fibrates (gemfibrozil, niacin): May increase risk of myopathy. Use together cautiously; consider reducing pitavastatin dosage when combined with niacin.

Reactions in bold italics are *life-threatening*. Interactions may have a *rapid onset* or a *delayed onset*.

Rifampin: May increase pitavastatin levels. Don't exceed 2 mg pitavastatin daily.
Vitamin K antagonists (warfarin): May enhance anticoagulant effect. Monitor therapy.

Drug-herb. *Herbal cholesterol-lowering products:* May increase pitavastatin levels. Discourage using together.

Drug-food. *Grapefruit juice:* May increase pitavastatin levels and increase risk of adverse effects, including rhabdomyolysis and myopathy. Avoid using together.

EFFECTS ON LAB TEST RESULTS
• May increase AST, ALT, CK, bilirubin, and glucose levels.

CONTRAINDICATIONS & CAUTIONS
• Contraindicated in patients hypersensitive to drug or its components and in those with active liver disease.
• Use cautiously in elderly patients and in those with renal impairment, inadequately treated hypothyroidism, or a history of myopathy or rhabdomyolysis.
• Statin therapy should be interrupted if patient shows signs of serious liver injury, hyperbilirubinemia, or jaundice. The drug shouldn't be restarted if another cause can't be found.
• Safety and effectiveness in children haven't been established.
Dialyzable drug: Unlikely.

PREGNANCY-LACTATION-REPRODUCTION
• Drug may cause fetal harm. Contraindicated in women who are or may become pregnant.
• It isn't known if drug appears in breast milk. Patient should discontinue breastfeeding or discontinue drug.

NURSING CONSIDERATIONS
• Start pitavastatin only after diet and other nondrug therapies have proved ineffective.
• Monitor PT and INR in patients taking warfarin when pitavastatin is added.
• Monitor LFT results and CK levels before therapy is started, 12 weeks after therapy is initiated, after a dosage change, and periodically thereafter.
• Discontinue drug if myopathy develops or if CK level markedly increases.

• Temporarily withhold drug if patient develops sepsis; hypotension; dehydration; severe metabolic, endocrine, or electrolyte disorders; uncontrolled seizures; or trauma or if patient requires major surgery. These conditions may predispose patient to myopathy or rhabdomyolysis.
• Adjust dosage about every 4 weeks.
• *Look alike–sound alike:* Don't confuse pitavastatin with atorvastatin, fluvastatin, lovastatin, nystatin, pravastatin, rosuvastatin, or simvastatin.

PATIENT TEACHING
• Tell patient that drug may be taken without regard to meals.
• Explain the importance of controlling serum lipid levels. Teach appropriate dietary management (restricting total fat and cholesterol intake), weight control, and exercise.
• Advise woman of childbearing potential to use birth control while taking pitavastatin and to discuss future pregnancy and breastfeeding plans with health care provider.
• Advise patient to report unexplained muscle pain, tenderness, or weakness, especially if accompanied by fever or malaise.
• Advise patient that blood tests to check liver enzyme levels will be needed at 12 weeks after the start of therapy, after a dosage increase, and periodically thereafter.
• Tell patient that the drug may increase blood sugar levels; however, the CV benefits are thought to outweigh the slight increase in risk.

---

posaconazole
pahs-ah-KON-ah-zall

Noxafil, Posanol ❦

Therapeutic class: Antifungals
Pharmacologic class: Triazole antifungals

AVAILABLE FORMS
Injection: 18 mg/mL
Oral suspension: 40 mg/mL
Tablets (delayed-release) ⓒ: 100 mg

INDICATIONS & DOSAGES
➤ **Prevention of invasive *Aspergillus* and *Candida* infections in high-risk immuno-compromised patients**
Adults: 200 mg (5 mL) oral suspension P.O. t.i.d. with a full meal or a liquid nutritional supplement. Or, 300 mg delayed-release tablet P.O. with food b.i.d. on first day, then 300 mg once daily. Or, 300 mg I.V. b.i.d. on first day, then 300 mg once daily. Duration of therapy is based on recovery from neutropenia or immunosuppression.
Children ages 13 to 17: 200 mg (5 mL) oral suspension P.O. t.i.d. with a full meal or a liquid nutritional supplement. Or, 300 mg delayed-release tablet P.O. b.i.d. with food on first day, then 300 mg once daily. Duration of therapy is based on recovery from neutropenia or immuno-suppression.
➤ **Oropharyngeal candidiasis**
Adults and children age 13 and older: 100 mg (2.5 mL) P.O. b.i.d. on first day, then 100 mg (2.5 mL) once daily for 13 days with a full meal or a liquid nutritional supplement.
➤ **Oropharyngeal candidiasis resistant to itraconazole or fluconazole treatment**
Adults and children age 13 and older: 400 mg (10 mL) P.O. b.i.d. with a full meal or a liquid nutritional supplement; duration of treatment is based on severity of underlying disease and patient response.

ADMINISTRATION
P.O.
• Delayed-release tablets and oral suspension aren't to be used interchangeably because of differences in the dosing of each formulation.
P.O. (suspension)
• Give with a full meal, liquid nutritional supplement, or an acidic carbonated beverage (e.g., ginger ale).
• Shake well before giving it.
• Measure doses using calibrated spoon provided with the drug, which has two markings, one for 2.5 mL and one for 5 mL. After patient takes dose, fill spoon with water and have him drink it to ensure a full dose.
• Store at room temperature.

P.O. (delayed-release tablets)
• Patient should swallow tablets whole; don't divide, crush, or allow patient to chew tablets.
• Administer with food.
• Delayed-release oral formulation is preferred for prophylaxis due to higher plasma drug exposures.
I.V.
▼ Bring refrigerated vial to room temperature.
▼ To prepare, transfer one vial of drug to I.V. bag or bottle of half-NSS, NSS, D_5W, D_5W half-NSS, D_5W NSS, or D_5W with 20 mEq potassium chloride to achieve a final concentration that's between 1 and 2 mg/mL. Solution may be colorless to yellow.
▼ Use mixture immediately after preparation, or it can be stored up to 24 hours refrigerated (36° to 46° F [2° to 8° C]).
🜂 *Alert:* Infuse over 90 minutes via central venous line. When multiple dosing is required, administer via central venous line. Don't give by I.V. push or bolus.
▼ If a central venous line isn't available, administer only once through peripheral venous catheter over 30 minutes in advance of central venous line placement or to bridge period during which central venous line is replaced or is in use for other I.V. treatment; multiple peripheral infusions given through the same vein have resulted in infusion-site reactions.
▼ An in-line filter (0.22-micron polyethersulfone or polyvinylidene difluoride) must be used during infusion.
▼ **Incompatibilities:** None reported.

ACTION
Blocks the synthesis of ergosterol, a vital component of the fungal cell membrane.

Route	Onset	Peak	Duration
P.O. (suspension)	Unknown	3–5 hr	Unknown
P.O. (tablets)	Unknown	4–5 hr	Unknown
I.V.	Unknown	Unknown	Unknown

Half-life: Suspension, 20 to 66 hours; tablets, 26 to 31 hours; injection, 27 hours.

ADVERSE REACTIONS
CNS: anxiety, dizziness, fatigue, fever, headache, insomnia, weakness.

CV: edema, hypertension, hypotension, tachycardia.
EENT: epistaxis, pharyngitis, altered taste, blurred vision.
GI: abdominal pain, constipation, diarrhea, dyspepsia, mucositis, nausea, vomiting.
GU: *vaginal hemorrhage.*
Hematologic: anemia, petechiae, *febrile neutropenia, neutropenia, thrombocytopenia.*
Hepatic: bilirubinemia.
Metabolic: anorexia, hyperglycemia, *hypokalemia, hypomagnesemia, hypocalcemia.*
Musculoskeletal: arthralgia, back pain, musculoskeletal pain.
Respiratory: cough, dyspnea, URI.
Skin: pruritus, rash, diaphoresis.
Other: bacteremia, CMV infection, herpes simplex, rigors.

INTERACTIONS
Drug-drug. *Atazanavir, ritonavir:* May increase plasma concentrations of these drugs. Frequently monitor for adverse effects and toxicity during coadministration.
Calcium channel blockers, cyclosporine, phenytoin, tacrolimus, vinca alkaloids: May increase levels of these drugs. Reduce dosages, increase monitoring of levels, and observe patient for adverse effects.
Cimetidine, phenytoin: May decrease level and effectiveness of posaconazole. Avoid using together.
CYP3A4 substrates (astemizole, cisapride, halofantrine, pimozide, quinidine, terfenadine): May lead to QT-interval prolongation and torsades de pointes. Use together is contraindicated.
Efavirenz: May significantly decrease posaconazole plasma concentration. Avoid use together unless benefit outweighs risks.
Ergot alkaloids (dihydroergotamine, ergotamine): May increase ergot level. Use together is contraindicated.
Fosamprenavir: May decrease posaconazole level. Monitor patient closely for breakthrough fungal infection.
HMG-CoA reductase inhibitors metabolized through CYP3A4, sirolimus: May increase levels of these drugs. Use with posaconazole is contraindicated.

Midazolam: May significantly increase midazolam concentration and potentiate or prolong sedative or hypnotic effects. Reversal agents should be readily available.
PPIs: May decrease posaconazole level. Consider therapy modification.
QTc interval–prolonging drugs: May enhance prolongation of QTc interval. When used with moderate QTc interval–prolonging drugs, monitor therapy. Avoid use with high-risk QTc interval–prolonging drugs; if use together is unavoidable, monitor QTc interval and cardiac rhythm closely.
Rifabutin: May decrease level and effectiveness of posaconazole while increasing rifabutin level and risk of toxicity. Avoid using together. If unavoidable, monitor patient for uveitis, leukopenia, and other adverse effects.
Drug-food. *Any food, liquid nutritional supplements:* May greatly enhance absorption of drug. Always give drug with liquid supplement or food.

EFFECTS ON LAB TEST RESULTS
● May increase AST, ALT, bilirubin, creatinine, alkaline phosphatase, and glucose levels.
● May decrease potassium, magnesium, and calcium levels.
● May decrease WBC, RBC, and platelet counts.

CONTRAINDICATIONS & CAUTIONS
● Contraindicated in patients hypersensitive to drug or its components and in patients taking sirolimus, HMG-CoA reductase inhibitors that are primarily metabolized through CYP3A4 (atorvastatin, lovastatin, simvastatin), CYP3A4 substrates that prolong the QT interval (pimozide, quinidine), other antifungal agents, or ergot derivatives.
● Use cautiously in patients hypersensitive to other azole antifungals, patients with potentially proarrhythmic conditions, and patients with hepatic or renal insufficiency.
● Safety in children younger than age 13 hasn't been established.
🕩 *Alert:* Drug may prolong QT interval and increase risk of torsades de pointes.
Dialyzable drug: No.

PREGNANCY-LACTATION-REPRODUCTION
- There are no adequate studies in pregnant women. Drug may cause fetal harm. Use during pregnancy only if potential benefit outweighs potential risk to the fetus.
- It isn't known if drug appears in breast milk. Patient should discontinue breast-feeding or discontinue drug.

NURSING CONSIDERATIONS
- Use I.V. route only when oral administration isn't possible.
- Don't use delayed-release tablets and oral suspension interchangeably.
- Correct electrolyte imbalances, especially potassium, magnesium, and calcium imbalances, before therapy.
- Monitor patient for signs and symptoms of electrolyte imbalance, including a slow, weak, or irregular pulse; ECG change; nausea; neuromuscular irritability; and tetany.
- Obtain baseline LFTs, including bilirubin level, before therapy and periodically during treatment. Notify prescriber if patient develops signs or symptoms of hepatic dysfunction.
- Monitor patient weighing more than 120 kg closely for breakthrough fungal infections because of lower plasma drug exposure.
- Monitor patient who has severe vomiting or diarrhea for breakthrough fungal infection.
- *Look alike–sound alike:* Don't confuse Noxafil with minoxidil.

PATIENT TEACHING
- If patient can't take a liquid supplement or eat a full meal, instruct him to notify prescriber. A different anti-infective may be needed, or monitoring may need to be increased.
- Tell patient to notify prescriber about an irregular heartbeat, fainting, or severe diarrhea or vomiting.
- Explain the signs and symptoms of liver dysfunction, including abdominal pain, yellowing skin or eyes, pale stools, and dark urine.
- Urge patient to contact the prescriber or pharmacist before taking other prescription

or OTC drugs, herbal supplements, or dietary supplements.
- Tell patient to shake the suspension well before taking it.
- Instruct patient to measure doses using the spoon provided with the drug. Household spoons vary in size and may yield an incorrect dose.
- Point out that the calibrated spoon has two markings: one for 2.5 mL and one for 5 mL. Make sure patient understands which mark to use for his prescribed dose.
- After patient takes dose, tell him to fill the spoon with water and drink it, to ensure a full dose. Tell him to clean the spoon with water before putting it away.
- Tell patient not to break, crush, or chew delayed-release tablets.

potassium acetate

Therapeutic class: Potassium supplements
Pharmacologic class: Potassium salts

AVAILABLE FORMS
Injection: 2 mEq/mL in 20-mL, 50-mL, and 100-mL vials; 4 mEq/mL in 50-mL vial

INDICATIONS & DOSAGES
➤ **Hypokalemia**
Adults age 19 and older: Individualize dosage; 40 to 80 mEq/24 hours by I.V. infusion.
Children: Individualize dosage; 2 to 3 mEq/kg/24 hours by I.V. infusion. For newborns, normal daily requirement is 2 to 6 mEq/kg/hour.

ADMINISTRATION
I.V.
▼ Use only in life-threatening hypokalemia or when oral replacement isn't feasible.
▼ Don't give undiluted potassium. Maximum infusion rate is 1 mEq/kg/hour.
▼ Don't add potassium to a hanging bag. Mix well to avoid layering.
▼ To prevent pain, use largest peripheral vein and a well-placed small-bore needle.
▼ Give only by infusion, never I.V. push or I.M. Watch for pain and redness at infusion site.

▼ Give slowly as diluted solution; rapid infusion may cause fatal hyperkalemia.
▼ **Incompatibilities:** None reported.

ACTION
Replaces potassium and maintains potassium level.

Route	Onset	Peak	Duration
I.V.	Immediate	Immediate	Unknown

Half-life: Unknown.

ADVERSE REACTIONS
CNS: paresthesia of limbs, listlessness, mental confusion, weakness or heaviness of legs, flaccid paralysis, pain, fever.
CV: *arrhythmias, cardiac arrest, heart block,* ECG changes, hypotension.
GI: nausea, vomiting, abdominal pain, diarrhea.
Metabolic: *hyperkalemia.*
Respiratory: *respiratory paralysis.*
Skin: redness at infusion site.

INTERACTIONS
Drug-drug. *ACE inhibitors, aldosterone blockers, ARBs, potassium-sparing diuretics:* May increase risk of hyperkalemia. Use together with caution.
Digoxin: May cause digoxin toxicity from hypokalemia if drug is stopped. Stop potassium cautiously if patient is taking digoxin.
Eplerenone: May increase hyperkalemia risk. Use together is contraindicated when eplerenone is used to treat hypertension.
Drug-food. *Potassium-containing salt substitutes:* May increase risk of hyperkalemia. Use together cautiously.

EFFECTS ON LAB TEST RESULTS
• May increase potassium level.

CONTRAINDICATIONS & CAUTIONS
• Contraindicated in patients with severe renal impairment with oliguria, anuria, or azotemia.
• Contraindicated in those with untreated Addison disease, acute dehydration, heat cramps, hyperkalemia, hyperkalemic form of familial periodic paralysis, or conditions linked to extensive tissue breakdown.
• Use cautiously in patients with cardiac disease or renal impairment.

Dialyzable drug: Unknown.
⚠ *Overdose S&S:* Paresthesia, flaccid paralysis, listlessness, confusion, weakness and heaviness of legs, hypotension, cardiac arrhythmias, heart block, ECG changes, cardiac arrest.

PREGNANCY-LACTATION-REPRODUCTION
• Safe use in pregnant women hasn't been established. Use only if benefit justifies potential risk to the fetus.
• It isn't known if drug appears in breast milk. Use cautiously in breast-feeding women.

NURSING CONSIDERATIONS
• During therapy, monitor ECG, renal function, fluid intake and output, and potassium, creatinine, and BUN levels. Never give potassium postoperatively until urine flow is established.
• Many adverse reactions may reflect hyperkalemia.
🔔 *Alert:* Consider a separate storage area for concentrated I.V. potassium. Fatal outcomes are possible if concentrated potassium is administered by I.V. push.
• *Look alike–sound alike:* Potassium preparations aren't interchangeable; verify preparation before use.

PATIENT TEACHING
• Explain use and administration to patient and family.
• Tell patient to report adverse effects, especially pain at insertion site.

SAFETY ALERT!

potassium chloride
Cena-K, Gen-K, Kaon, Kaon-Cl 20%, Kaylixir, K-Dur 10, K-Dur 20, K-Lor, Klor-Con, Klor-Con 8, Klor-Con 10, Klor-Con/25, Klor-Con/EF, Klor-Con M10, Klor-Con M15, Klor-Con M20, Klorvess, Klotrix, K-Lyte/Cl, K-Tab, K-Vescent, Micro-K, Micro-K 10, Potasalan, Twin-K

Therapeutic class: Potassium supplements
Pharmacologic class: Potassium salts

AVAILABLE FORMS
Capsules (controlled-release) ⬤: 8 mEq, 10 mEq
Injection concentrate: 1.5 mEq/mL, 2 mEq/mL
Injection for I.V. infusion: 0.1 mEq/mL, 0.2 mEq/mL, 0.3 mEq/mL, 0.4 mEq/mL
Oral liquid: 20 mEq/15 mL, 40 mEq/15 mL
Powder for oral administration: 20 mEq/packet, 25 mEq/packet
Tablets (controlled-release) ⬤: 8 mEq, 10 mEq, 20 mEq
Tablets (extended-release) ⬤: 8 mEq, 10 mEq, 15 mEq, 20 mEq
Tablets for solution (effervescent): 10 mEq, 20 mEq, 25 mEq, 50 mEq

INDICATIONS & DOSAGES
➤ **To prevent hypokalemia**
Adults: Initially, 16 to 24 mEq of potassium supplement P.O. daily, in divided doses. Adjust dosage, as needed, based on potassium levels. Patient should take no more than 20 or 25 mEq at a single dose.
➤ **Hypokalemia**
Adults: 40 to 100 mEq P.O. in two to five divided doses daily. Patient should take no more than 20 or 25 mEq at a single dose. Maximum dose of diluted I.V. potassium chloride is 40 mEq/L at 10 mEq/hour. Don't exceed 200 mEq daily. Further doses are based on potassium levels and blood pH. Give I.V. potassium replacement only with monitoring of ECG and potassium level.

➤ **Severe hypokalemia**
Adults: Dilute potassium chloride in a suitable I.V. solution of less than 80 mEq/L, and give at no more than 40 mEq/hour.
   Further doses are based on potassium level. Don't exceed 400 mEq I.V. daily. Give I.V. potassium replacement only with monitoring of ECG and potassium level.

ADMINISTRATION
P.O.
● Make sure powders are completely dissolved before giving.
● Enteric-coated tablets are not recommended because of increased risk of GI bleeding and small-bowel ulcerations.
● Patient should take with meals and a full glass of water or other liquid to minimize risk of GI irritation.
● Tablets in wax matrix may lodge in the esophagus and cause ulceration in cardiac patients with esophageal compression from an enlarged left atrium. Use sugar-free liquid form in these patients and in those with esophageal stasis or obstruction. Have patient sip slowly to minimize GI irritation.
● Don't crush controlled-release or extended-release forms.
I.V.
▼ Use only when oral replacement isn't feasible or when hypokalemia is life-threatening.
▼ Give by infusion only, never I.V. push or I.M. Give slowly as dilute solution; rapid infusion may cause fatal hyperkalemia.
▼ Administer high concentrations (300 and 400 mEq/L) exclusively via a central route.
▼ If burning occurs during infusion, decrease rate.
▼ **Incompatibilities:** Amikacin, amoxicillin, amphotericin B, azithromycin, diazepam, dobutamine, ergotamine, etoposide with cisplatin and mannitol, fat emulsion 10%, methylprednisolone, penicillin G, phenytoin, promethazine.

ACTION
Replaces potassium and maintains potassium level.

Route	Onset	Peak	Duration
P.O.	Unknown	Unknown	Unknown
I.V.	Immediate	Immediate	Unknown

Half-life: Unknown.

ADVERSE REACTIONS
CNS: paresthesia of limbs, listlessness, confusion, weakness or heaviness of limbs, flaccid paralysis.
CV: postinfusion phlebitis, *arrhythmias, heart block, cardiac arrest,* ECG changes, hypotension.
GI: nausea, vomiting, abdominal pain, diarrhea.
Metabolic: *hyperkalemia.*
Respiratory: *respiratory paralysis.*
Skin: injection-site reactions.

INTERACTIONS
Drug-drug. *ACE inhibitors, ARBs, digoxin, heparins, potassium-sparing diuretics:* May cause hyperkalemia. Use together with extreme caution. Monitor potassium level.
Eplerenone: May increase hyperkalemia risk. Use together is contraindicated when eplerenone is used to treat hypertension.

EFFECTS ON LAB TEST RESULTS
• May increase potassium level.

CONTRAINDICATIONS & CAUTIONS
• Contraindicated in patients with severe renal impairment with oliguria, anuria, or azotemia; with untreated Addison disease; or with acute dehydration, heat cramps, hyperkalemia, hyperkalemic form of familial periodic paralysis, or other conditions linked to extensive tissue breakdown.
• Use cautiously in patients with cardiac disease, renal impairment, and acid-base disorders.
Dialyzable drug: Yes.
⚠ **Overdose S&S:** ECG changes, weakness, flaccidity, respiratory paralysis, cardiac arrhythmias, death.

PREGNANCY-LACTATION-REPRODUCTION
• It isn't known if drug causes fetal harm. Use only if clearly needed.
• It isn't known if drug appears in breast milk. Use cautiously in breast-feeding women.

NURSING CONSIDERATIONS
• Patients at an increased risk of GI lesions include those with scleroderma, diabetes, mitral valve replacement, cardiomegaly, or esophageal strictures, and elderly or immobile patients.
• Drug is commonly used orally with potassium-wasting diuretics to maintain potassium levels.
• Monitor continuous ECG and electrolyte levels during therapy.
• Monitor renal function. After surgery, don't give drug until urine flow is established.
• Many adverse reactions may reflect hyperkalemia.
• Patient may be sensitive to tartrazine in some of these products.
⚠ *Alert:* Consider a separate storage area for concentrated I.V. potassium. Fatal outcomes are possible if concentrated potassium is administered by I.V. push.
• *Look alike–sound alike:* Potassium preparations aren't interchangeable; verify preparation before use and don't switch products. Don't confuse Kaon-Cl-10 with Kaolin, KCl with HCl, KlorCon with Klaron, or Micro-K with Macrobid or Micronase.

PATIENT TEACHING
• Teach patient how to prepare powders and how to take drug. Tell patient to take with or after meals with full glass of water or fruit juice to lessen GI distress.
• Teach patient signs and symptoms of hyperkalemia, and tell patient to notify prescriber if they occur.
• Tell patient to report discomfort at I.V. insertion site.
• Warn patient not to use salt substitutes concurrently, except with prescriber's permission.
• Tell patient not to be concerned if wax matrix appears in stool because the drug has already been absorbed.

pramipexole dihydrochloride
pram-ah-PEX-ole

Mirapex, Mirapex ER

Therapeutic class: Antiparkinsonians
Pharmacologic class: Nonergot
dopamine agonists

AVAILABLE FORMS
Tablets: 0.125 mg, 0.25 mg, 0.5 mg,
0.75 mg, 1 mg, 1.5 mg
Tablets (extended-release) ⓄⓃⒸ: 0.375 mg,
0.75 mg, 1.5 mg, 2.25 mg, 3 mg, 3.75 mg,
4.5 mg

INDICATIONS & DOSAGES
➤ **Signs and symptoms of idiopathic
Parkinson disease**
Adults: Initially, 0.375 mg P.O. daily in
three divided doses. Adjust doses slowly
(not more often than every 5 to 7 days) over
several weeks until desired therapeutic
effect is achieved. Maintenance dosage is
1.5 to 4.5 mg daily in three divided doses.
Or, 0.375 mg (extended-release form) P.O.
once daily. May titrate dosage gradually
(not more often than every 5 to 7 days),
first to 0.75 mg P.O. daily, then by 0.75-mg
increments to maximum recommended
dosage of 4.5 mg/day.
Adjust-a-dose: For patients with CrCl over
50 mL/minute, first dosage of immediate-
release tablets is 0.125 mg P.O. t.i.d., up to
1.5 mg t.i.d. For those with CrCl of 30 to
50 mL/minute, first dosage is 0.125 mg
P.O. b.i.d., up to 0.75 mg t.i.d. For those
with CrCl of 15 mL/minute to less than
30 mL/minute, first dosage is 0.125 mg P.O.
daily, up to 1.5 mg daily. If using extended-
release tablets, in patients with CrCl of
30 to 50 mL/minute, initially give dose
every other day. Use caution and assess response and tolerability before increasing to
daily dosing after 1 week and before titration. Titrate dosage in 0.375-mg increments
up to 2.25 mg/day, no more frequently than
at weekly intervals. Don't use extended-
release tablets in patients with CrCl of
less than 30 mL/minute or in hemodialysis
patients.

➤ **Moderate to severe primary restless
leg syndrome (immediate-release only)**
Adults: 0.125 mg P.O. daily, 2 to 3 hours
before bedtime. May increase after 4 to
7 days to 0.25 mg P.O. daily, as needed. May
increase again after 4 to 7 days to 0.5 mg
P.O. daily, if needed.
Adjust-a-dose: For patients with CrCl of
20 to 60 mL/minute, increase the duration
between titration steps to 14 days.

ADMINISTRATION
P.O.
● Give drug with or without food; giving
with food may reduce nausea.
● Patient must swallow extended-release
tablets whole; tablets shouldn't be chewed,
crushed, or divided.
● If a significant interruption in therapy
occurs, retitration of therapy may be warranted.

ACTION
Thought to stimulate dopamine receptors.

Route	Onset	Peak	Duration
P.O.	Rapid	2–6 hr	8–12 hr

Half-life: Approximately 8.5 hours.

ADVERSE REACTIONS
CNS: asthenia, confusion, dizziness, dream
abnormalities, dyskinesia, extrapyramidal
syndrome, hallucinations, insomnia, somnolence, amnesia, akathisia, drowsiness,
delusions, dystonia, gait abnormalities, hypoesthesia, hypertonia, myoclonus, paranoid
reaction, malaise, sleep disorders, thought
abnormalities, fever.
CV: orthostatic hypotension, chest pain,
peripheral edema.
EENT: accommodation abnormalities,
diplopia, rhinitis, vision abnormalities.
GI: constipation, nausea, dry mouth,
anorexia, dysphagia, vomiting.
GU: erectile dysfunction, urinary frequency,
UTI, urinary incontinence.
Metabolic: weight loss.
Musculoskeletal: arthritis, bursitis, myas-
thenia, twitching.
Respiratory: dyspnea, cough, pneumonia.
Skin: skin disorders.
Other: accidental injury, decreased libido,
general edema.

INTERACTIONS
Drug-drug. *Antipsychotics:* May diminish therapeutic effects of pramipexole. Avoid use together if possible; if use together is unavoidable, monitor therapy carefully.
Cimetidine, diltiazem, quinidine, quinine, ranitidine, triamterene, verapamil: May decrease pramipexole clearance. Adjust dosage as needed.
Dopamine antagonists: May reduce pramipexole effectiveness. Monitor patient closely.
Drug-lifestyle. *Alcohol use:* May increase sedative effects. Tell patient to avoid alcohol.

EFFECTS ON LAB TEST RESULTS
● May increase CK level.

CONTRAINDICATIONS & CAUTIONS
● Contraindicated in patients hypersensitive to drug or its components.
● Use cautiously in patients with renal impairment.
● Use cautiously in patients with a known major psychotic disorder due to risk of exacerbating psychosis.
Dialyzable drug: Unknown.

PREGNANCY-LACTATION-REPRODUCTION
● There are no studies in pregnant women. Animal studies suggest drug may cause fetal harm. Use only if benefit clearly justifies potential risk to the fetus.
● It isn't known if drug appears in breast milk. Patient should discontinue breast-feeding or discontinue drug.

NURSING CONSIDERATIONS
● Drug should be tapered off at a rate of 0.75 mg/day until daily dose has been reduced to 0.75 mg. Thereafter, dose may be reduced by 0.375 mg/day.
● Drug may cause orthostatic hypotension, especially during dosage increases. Monitor patient carefully.
● Drug may cause intense impulse control and compulsive behaviors. Monitor patient for problems with impulse control (such as gambling urges, intense sexual urges, binge eating).
● Adjust dosage gradually to achieve maximal therapeutic effect, balanced against the

main adverse effects of dyskinesia, hallucinations, somnolence, and dry mouth.
● **Look alike–sound alike:** Don't confuse Mirapex with Hiprex, Mifeprex, or MiraLax.

PATIENT TEACHING
● Instruct patient not to rise rapidly after sitting or lying down because of risk of dizziness.
● Caution patient to avoid hazardous activities until CNS response to drug is known.
● Tell patient to use caution before taking drug with other CNS depressants.
● Tell patient (especially elderly patient) that hallucinations may occur.
● Advise patient to take drug with food if nausea develops.
● Tell woman to notify prescriber if she is or will be breast-feeding.
● Advise patient that it may take 4 weeks for effects of drug to be noticed because of slow adjustment schedule.
● Instruct patient that drug should be tapered gradually and not stopped abruptly.

SAFETY ALERT!

pramlintide acetate
PRAM-lin-tyde

SymlinPen 60, SymlinPen 120

Therapeutic class: Antidiabetics
Pharmacologic class: Human amylin analogues

AVAILABLE FORMS
Injection: 1 mg/mL in 1.5-mL and 2.7-mL multidose pen injectors

INDICATIONS & DOSAGES
➤ **Adjunct to insulin in patients with type 1 diabetes mellitus**
Adults: Initially, 15 mcg subcutaneously before major meals (more than 250 calories or 30 g of carbohydrates). Reduce preprandial rapid-acting or short-acting insulin dose, including fixed-mix insulin such as 70/30, by 50%. Increase pramlintide dose by 15-mcg increments every 3 days if no nausea occurs, to a maintenance dose of 30 to 60 mcg. Adjust insulin dose as needed.

Adjust-a-dose: If significant nausea at 45 or 60 mcg persists, decrease to 30 mcg. If nausea persists at 30 mcg, consider stopping.

➤ **Adjunct to insulin in patients with type 2 diabetes mellitus, with or without a sulfonylurea or metformin**
Adults: Initially, 60 mcg subcutaneously immediately before major meals. Reduce preprandial rapid-acting or short-acting insulin dose, including fixed-mix insulin, by 50%. Increase pramlintide dose to 120 mcg if no significant nausea occurs for at least 3 days. Adjust insulin dose as needed.
Adjust-a-dose: If significant nausea persists at 120 mcg, decrease to 60 mcg.

ADMINISTRATION
Subcutaneous
• Before starting drug, review patient's HbA$_{1c}$ level, recent blood glucose monitoring data, hypoglycemic episodes, current insulin regimen, and body weight. Reduce preprandial, rapid-acting or short-acting insulin dosages, including fixed-mix insulins, by 50%.
• Allow medication to reach room temperature before injecting.
• Give each dose subcutaneously into abdomen or thigh. Rotate injection sites.
• Administer immediately before each major meal consisting of 250 kcal or more or containing 30 g or more of carbohydrates.
• Always administer pramlintide and insulin as separate injections. The injection site for pramlintide should be distinct from the site for concomitant insulin injection.
• Don't transfer drug to syringe for administration. Don't mix with any type of insulin.
❸ Alert: Multidose pens are for single patient use only. Pens should never be shared, even if the needle is changed. Clearly label with patient identifying information where it won't obstruct the dosing window, warning, or other product information.
• After initial use, may keep refrigerated or at room temperature (86° F [30° C]).
• Discard after 30 days; protect from light.

ACTION
Slows rate at which food leaves the stomach, reducing the initial postprandial increase in glucose level. Decreases hyperglycemia by reducing postprandial glucagon level and reduces total caloric intake by reducing appetite.

Route	Onset	Peak	Duration
Subcut.	Unknown	19–21 min	3 hr

Half-life: Parent drug and metabolite, about 48 minutes each.

ADVERSE REACTIONS
CNS: dizziness, fatigue, headache.
EENT: pharyngitis.
GI: abdominal pain, anorexia, nausea, vomiting.
Metabolic: *hypoglycemia.*
Musculoskeletal: arthralgia.
Respiratory: cough.
Skin: injection-site reaction.
Other: allergic reaction, accidental injury.

INTERACTIONS
Drug-drug. *ACE inhibitors, disopyramide, fibrates, fluoxetine, MAO inhibitors, oral antidiabetics, pentoxifylline, propoxyphene, salicylates, sulfonamide antibiotics:* May increase risk of hypoglycemia. Monitor glucose level closely.
Alpha-glucosidase inhibitors (acarbose), anticholinergics (atropine, benztropine, TCAs): May alter GI motility and slow intestinal absorption. Avoid using together.
Beta blockers, clonidine, guanethidine, reserpine: May mask signs of hypoglycemia. Monitor glucose level closely.
Oral drugs dependent on rapid onset of action (such as analgesics): May delay absorption because of slowed gastric emptying. If rapid effect is needed, give oral drug 1 hour before or 2 hours after pramlintide.

EFFECTS ON LAB TEST RESULTS
None reported.

CONTRAINDICATIONS & CAUTIONS
• Contraindicated in patients hypersensitive to drug or its components, including metacresol, and in patients with gastroparesis or hypoglycemia unawareness.
• Don't use in patients noncompliant with current insulin and glucose monitoring regimen, patients with an HbA$_{1c}$ level greater than 9%, patients with severe hypoglycemia during the previous 6 months, patients who take drugs that stimulate GI motility.

• Safe use in children hasn't been established.
• Use cautiously in elderly patients.
Dialyzable drug: Unknown.
⚠ *Overdose S&S:* Severe nausea, vomiting, diarrhea, vasodilation, dizziness.

PREGNANCY-LACTATION-REPRODUCTION
• There are no adequate studies in pregnant women. Use only if potential benefit justifies potential risk to the fetus. Other agents are currently recommended to treat diabetes in pregnant women.
• It isn't known if drug appears in breast milk. Use in breast-feeding women only if benefit clearly outweighs risk to infant.

NURSING CONSIDERATIONS
Black Box Warning When used with insulin, drug may increase risk of insulin-induced severe hypoglycemia, particularly in patients with type 1 diabetes. Risk of severe hypoglycemia is highest within first 3 hours after an injection. Serious injuries may occur if severe hypoglycemia develops while patient is operating a motor vehicle or heavy machinery or engaging in other high-risk activities. ■
Black Box Warning Appropriate patient selection, careful patient instruction, and insulin dosage adjustments are critical elements for reducing risk of hypoglycemia. ■
• Symptoms of hypoglycemia may be masked in patients with a long history of diabetes, diabetic nerve disease, or intensified diabetes control.
• Notify prescriber of severe nausea and vomiting. A reduced dose may be needed.
• If patient has persistent nausea or recurrent, unexplained hypoglycemia that requires medical assistance, stop drug.
• If patient doesn't comply with glucose monitoring or drug dosage adjustments, stop drug.

PATIENT TEACHING
• Teach patient how to take drug exactly as prescribed, at mealtimes. Explain that it doesn't replace daily insulin but may lower the amount of insulin needed.
• Explain that a meal is considered more than 250 calories or 30 g of carbohydrates.

• Caution patient not to mix drug with insulin; instruct him to give the injections at separate sites.
• Instruct patient not to change doses of pramlintide or insulin without consulting prescriber.
• Instruct patient not to transfer drug from pen injector to syringe.
❸ *Alert:* Warn patient not to share the multidose pen with other people, even if the needle is changed, because of the risk of bloodborne pathogen transmission, including HIV and hepatitis virus.
Black Box Warning Tell patient to refrain from driving, operating heavy machinery, or performing other risky activities where he could hurt himself or others until it's known how drug affects his glucose level. ■
Black Box Warning Caution patient about possibility of severe hypoglycemia, particularly within 3 hours after injection. ■
• Teach patient and family members the signs and symptoms of hypoglycemia, including hunger, headache, sweating, tremor, irritability, and difficulty concentrating.
• Instruct patient and family members what to do if patient develops hypoglycemia.
• Tell patient to report severe nausea and vomiting to prescriber.
• Advise women of childbearing potential to tell the prescriber if they are, could be, or are planning to become pregnant.
• Teach patient how to handle unplanned situations, such as illness or stress, low or forgotten insulin dose, accidental use of too much insulin or drug, not enough food, or missed meals.
• Tell patient injector pens can be refrigerated or kept at room temperature.

P

prasugrel hydrochloride
PRAH-soo-grel

Effient✐

Therapeutic class: Antiplatelet drugs
Pharmacologic class: Adenosine
diphosphate–induced platelet
aggregation inhibitors

AVAILABLE FORMS
Tablets: 5 mg, 10 mg

INDICATIONS & DOSAGES
➤ **To reduce thrombotic events in patients with acute coronary syndrome (ACS) (unstable angina and non-ST-elevation MI) managed with PCI; to reduce thrombotic events in patients with ACS (ST-elevation MI) managed with primary or delayed PCI**
Adults: Initially, single 60-mg loading dose; then 10 mg P.O. once daily. Patient should also take aspirin 75 to 325 mg P.O. daily.
Adjust-a-dose: For adults weighing less than 60 kg, consider reducing dosage to 5 mg P.O. once daily.

ADMINISTRATION
P.O.
● May give drug with or without food.
● Don't break tablets.

ACTION
Inhibits platelet activation and aggregation through irreversible binding of its active metabolite to the P2Y12 class of adenosine diphosphate receptors on platelets.

Route	Onset	Peak	Duration
P.O.	Rapid	30 min	5–9 days

Half-life: 7 hours (range, 2 to 15 hours).

ADVERSE REACTIONS
CNS: dizziness, fatigue, headache, fever.
CV: atrial fibrillation, bradycardia, hypertension or hypotension, peripheral edema.
GI: *GI bleeding,* nausea, diarrhea.
EENT: epistaxis.
Hematologic: *bleeding,* leukopenia, ***thrombotic thrombocytopenic purpura.***

Metabolic: hypercholesterolemia, hyperlipidemia.
Musculoskeletal: back pain, extremity pain.
Respiratory: cough, dyspnea.
Skin: rash.
Other: noncardiac chest pain.

INTERACTIONS
Drug-drug. *Direct factor Xa inhibitors (rivaroxaban), direct thrombin inhibitors (dabigatran, desirudin), fibrinolytics (tenecteplase), heparin, NSAIDs (long-term use), warfarin:* May increase the risk of bleeding. Use together cautiously.

EFFECTS ON LAB TEST RESULTS
● May increase cholesterol and lipid levels.
● May decrease WBC and platelet counts.

CONTRAINDICATIONS & CAUTIONS
Black Box Warning Contraindicated in patients with pathologic bleeding (such as peptic ulcer or intracranial hemorrhage) and in those with a history of TIA or stroke. ■
Black Box Warning Prasugrel is generally not recommended in patients age 75 and older because of the increased risk of intracranial and fatal bleeding and uncertain benefit, except in high-risk situations (patients with diabetes or a history of prior MI). In these situations, drug's effect appears to be greater and its use may be considered. ■
Black Box Warning Use cautiously in patients who weigh less than 60 kg and in those with a propensity to bleed or who are using drugs that increase bleeding risk (warfarin, heparin, fibrinolytic therapy, long-term NSAID use) because of increased risk of bleeding. ■
● Contraindicated in patients with hypersensitivity to prasugrel or its components.
● Use cautiously in patients at risk for increased bleeding from trauma, surgery, or other pathologic conditions and in those with severe hepatic impairment.
Dialyzable drug: Unlikely.
⚠ ***Overdose S&S:*** Bleeding due to impaired clotting ability.

PREGNANCY-LACTATION-REPRODUCTION
● There are no adequate studies in pregnant women. Use during pregnancy and

---

breast-feeding only if potential maternal benefit justifies potential fetal risk.

NURSING CONSIDERATIONS

Black Box Warning Drug may cause significant, sometimes fatal, bleeding. Suspect bleeding in patient who is hypotensive and has recently undergone PCI, CABG, or other surgical procedure. Manage bleeding without stopping drug, if possible. Stopping drug within first few weeks after ACS occurrence increases the risk of further CV events. ■

● Monitor patient for unusual bleeding or bruising.

● Drug should be taken with aspirin (75 to 325 mg daily).

Black Box Warning Discontinue drug 7 days before CABG or any surgery. Don't start drug if patient is likely to undergo urgent CABG. ■

● Bleeding associated with CABG may be treated with transfusion of blood products, such as RBCs and platelets; however, platelets may be ineffective if given within 6 hours of loading dose or within 4 hours of maintenance dose.

🕔 *Alert:* Drug may cause fatal thrombotic thrombocytopenic purpura (thrombocytopenia, hemolytic anemia, neurologic signs and symptoms, renal dysfunction, and fever) that requires urgent treatment, including plasmapheresis.

● *Look alike–sound alike:* Don't confuse prasugrel with pravastatin or propranolol.

PATIENT TEACHING

● Advise patient that drug can be taken without regard to food and not to break tablets.

● Inform patient that he will bruise more easily and that it may take longer than usual to stop bleeding.

● Instruct patient to report prolonged or excessive bleeding or blood in his stool or urine.

● Advise patient to inform health care providers that he's taking prasugrel before scheduling surgery or taking new drugs.

● Advise patient that duration of therapy may be determined by the type of stent used.

pravastatin sodium (eptastatin)
prah-va-STA-tin

Pravachol🔊

Therapeutic class: Antilipemics
Pharmacologic class: HMG-CoA reductase inhibitors

AVAILABLE FORMS
Tablets: 10 mg, 20 mg, 40 mg, 80 mg

INDICATIONS & DOSAGES
Adjust-a-dose (for all indications): In patients with renal dysfunction, start with 10 mg P.O. daily. In patients taking immunosuppressants, begin with 10 mg P.O. at bedtime and adjust to higher dosages with caution. Most patients treated with the combination of immunosuppressants and pravastatin receive up to 20 mg pravastatin daily. In patients taking clarithromycin, limit dose to 40 mg once daily.

➤ **Primary and secondary prevention of coronary events; hyperlipidemia**
Adults: Initially, 40 mg P.O. once daily at the same time each day, with or without food. Adjust dosage every 4 weeks, based on patient tolerance and response; maximum daily dose is 80 mg.

➤ **Heterozygous familial hypercholesterolemia**
Adolescents ages 14 to 18: Give 40 mg P.O. once daily. Maximum dose is 40 mg daily.
Children ages 8 to 13: Give 20 mg P.O. once daily. Maximum dose is 20 mg daily.

ADMINISTRATION
P.O.
● Give drug without regard for meals.
● If patient is also taking a bile acid resin (cholestyramine), administer pravastatin 1 hour before or 4 hours after the resin.

ACTION
Inhibits HMG-CoA reductase, an early (and rate-limiting) step in cholesterol biosynthesis.

P

Route	Onset	Peak	Duration
P.O.	Unknown	60–90 min	Unknown

Half-life: 1¼ to 2¼ hours.

ADVERSE REACTIONS

CNS: dizziness, fatigue, headache.
CV: chest pain.
EENT: rhinitis.
GI: nausea, abdominal pain, constipation, diarrhea, flatulence, heartburn, vomiting.
GU: *renal failure caused by myoglobinuria,* urinary abnormality.
Musculoskeletal: localized muscle pain, *rhabdomyolysis,* myalgia, myopathy, myositis.
Respiratory: common cold, cough.
Skin: rash.
Other: flulike symptoms, influenza.

INTERACTIONS

Drug-drug. *Azole antifungals (fluconazole, ketoconazole), erythromycin, fibric acid derivatives (gemfibrozil), niacin:* May increase risk of severe myopathy or rhabdomyolysis. Avoid using together.
Cholestyramine, colestipol: May decrease pravastatin level. Give pravastatin 1 hour before or 4 hours after these drugs.
Clarithromycin: May increase pravastatin level. Limit pravastatin to 40 mg once daily.
Colchicine: May increase risk of myopathy/rhabdomyolysis. Consider therapy modification.
Cyclosporine: May increase pravastatin level and pravastatin-related adverse reactions. If concomitant use can't be avoided, begin therapy with pravastatin 10 mg once daily at bedtime and titrate to higher doses with caution. Most patients received a maximum dose of pravastatin 20 mg daily.
U *Alert: Darunavir and ritonavir, lopinavir–ritonavir:* May increase pravastatin level and risk of myopathy and rhabdomyolysis. Use together cautiously.
Hepatotoxic drugs: May increase risk of hepatotoxicity. Avoid using together.
Protease inhibitors (ritonavir, saquinavir): May reduce pravastatin level. Monitor clinical response.
Rifamycins: May increase or decrease pravastatin levels. Carefully monitor clinical response.

Drug-herb. *Kava kava:* May increase risk of hepatotoxicity. Discourage use together.
Red yeast rice: May increase risk of adverse reactions because herb contains compounds similar to those in drug. Discourage use together.
Drug-food. *Oat bran:* May decrease effectiveness of pravastatin. Separate administration times as much as possible.
Drug-lifestyle. *Alcohol use:* May increase risk of hepatotoxicity. Discourage use together.

EFFECTS ON LAB TEST RESULTS

● May increase ALT, AST, CK, alkaline phosphatase, HbA$_{1c}$, fasting glucose, and bilirubin levels.
● May alter thyroid function test values.

CONTRAINDICATIONS & CAUTIONS

● Contraindicated in patients hypersensitive to drug and in those with active liver disease or conditions that cause unexplained, persistent elevations of transaminase levels.
● Use cautiously in patients who consume large quantities of alcohol or have history of liver disease.
● Statin therapy should be interrupted if patient shows signs of serious liver injury, hyperbilirubinemia, or jaundice. The drug shouldn't be restarted if another cause can't be found.
● Safety and effectiveness in children younger than age 8 haven't been established.
Dialyzable drug: Unknown.

PREGNANCY-LACTATION-REPRODUCTION

● Contraindicated in pregnant and breast-feeding women and in women of childbearing potential.

NURSING CONSIDERATIONS

● Patient should follow a diet restricted in saturated fat and cholesterol during therapy.
● Use in children with heterozygous familial hypercholesterolemia if LDL cholesterol level is at least 190 mg/dL, or if LDL cholesterol is at least 160 mg/dL and patient has either a positive family history of premature CV disease or two or more other CV disease risk factors.
● Obtain LFT results at start of therapy and then periodically. A liver biopsy may be

---

performed if elevated liver enzyme levels persist.

• *Look alike–sound alike:* Don't confuse Pravachol with Prevacid, Prinivil, or propranolol. Don't confuse pravastatin with nystatin, pitavastatin, or prasugrel.

PATIENT TEACHING

• Advise patient who is also taking a bile acid resin such as cholestyramine to take pravastatin at least 1 hour before or 4 hours after taking resin.

• Tell patient to notify prescriber of adverse reactions, particularly muscle aches and pains.

• Inform patient that LFTs will be performed before and periodically throughout treatment.

• Tell patient to promptly report signs and symptoms of liver injury, including fatigue, anorexia, right upper quadrant discomfort, dark urine, or jaundice.

• Tell patient to promptly report any unexplained muscle pain, tenderness, or weakness, especially if accompanied by malaise or fever or if symptoms persist after discontinuing drug.

• Tell patient that the drug may increase blood sugar levels; however, the CV benefits are thought to outweigh the slight increase in risk.

• Teach patient about proper dietary management of cholesterol and triglycerides. When appropriate, recommend weight control, exercise, and smoking cessation programs.

• Inform patient that it will take up to 4 weeks to achieve full therapeutic effect.

🜚 *Alert:* Tell female patient of childbearing potential to stop drug and notify prescriber immediately if she is or may be pregnant or if she's breast-feeding.

prazosin hydrochloride
PRA-zo-sin

Minipress

Therapeutic class: Antihypertensives
Pharmacologic class: Alpha blockers

AVAILABLE FORMS
Capsules: 1 mg, 2 mg, 5 mg

INDICATIONS & DOSAGES
➤ **Mild to moderate hypertension**
Adults: Test dose is 1 mg P.O. at bedtime to prevent first-dose syncope (severe syncope with loss of consciousness). First dosage is 1 mg P.O. b.i.d. or t.i.d. Dosage may be increased slowly. Maximum daily dose is 20 mg. Maintenance dosage is 6 to 15 mg daily in divided doses. Some patients need larger dosages (up to 40 mg daily).

If other antihypertensives or diuretics are added to therapy, decrease prazosin dosage to 1 to 2 mg t.i.d. and readjust to maintenance dosage.

ADMINISTRATION
P.O.
• Give drug without regard for meals.

ACTION
Unknown. Thought to act by blocking alpha-adrenergic receptors.

Route	Onset	Peak	Duration
P.O.	30–90 min	2–4 hr	7–10 hr

Half-life: 2 to 3 hours.

ADVERSE REACTIONS
CNS: dizziness, first-dose syncope, headache, drowsiness, nervousness, paresthesia, weakness, depression, vertigo, lack of energy.
CV: orthostatic hypotension, palpitations, edema.
EENT: blurred vision, conjunctivitis, epistaxis, nasal congestion.
GI: vomiting, diarrhea, abdominal cramps, nausea, constipation.
GU: urinary frequency.
Musculoskeletal: arthralgia, myalgia.
Respiratory: dyspnea.
Skin: rash.

INTERACTIONS
Drug-drug. *Acebutolol, atenolol, betaxolol, carteolol, esmolol, metoprolol, nadolol, pindolol, propranolol, sotalol, timolol:* May increase the risk of orthostatic hypotension in the early phases of use together. Help patient stand slowly until effects are known.
Diuretics, PDE5 inhibitors: May increase frequency of hypotensive effect or syncope

P

with loss of consciousness. Advise patient to sit or lie down if dizziness occurs.
Verapamil: May increase prazosin level. Monitor patient closely.
Drug-herb. *Butcher's broom:* May reduce prazosin effect. Discourage use together.
Ma huang: May decrease antihypertensive effects. Discourage use together.

EFFECTS ON LAB TEST RESULTS
• May increase levels of BUN, uric acid, and urinary metabolite of norepinephrine and vanillylmandelic acid.
• May increase LFT values. May alter results of screening tests for pheochromocytoma.
• May cause positive ANA titer.

CONTRAINDICATIONS & CAUTIONS
• Contraindicated in patients hypersensitive to drug or other alpha blockers.
• Use cautiously in patients receiving other antihypertensives.
• Not approved for use in children.
Dialyzable drug: No.
⚠ **Overdose S&S:** Profound drowsiness, depressed reflexes, hypotension.

PREGNANCY-LACTATION-REPRODUCTION
• There are no adequate studies in pregnant women. Use during pregnancy only if maternal benefits justify potential maternal and fetal risk.
• Drug appears in breast milk. Use cautiously in breast-feeding women.

NURSING CONSIDERATIONS
• Monitor patient's BP and pulse rate frequently.
• Elderly patients may be more sensitive to drug's hypotensive effects.
• Compliance might be improved with twice-daily dosing. Discuss dosing change with prescriber if compliance problems are suspected.
🌓 **Alert:** If first dose is more than 1 mg, first-dose syncope may occur.
• **Look alike–sound alike:** Don't confuse prazosin with prednisone.

PATIENT TEACHING
• Warn patient that dizziness may occur with first dose. If he experiences dizziness,

tell him to sit or lie down. Reassure him that this effect disappears with continued dosing.
• Caution patient to avoid driving or performing hazardous tasks for the first 24 hours after starting this drug or increasing the dose.
• Tell patient not to suddenly stop taking drug, but to notify prescriber if unpleasant adverse reactions occur.
• Advise patient to minimize low BP and dizziness upon standing by rising slowly and avoiding sudden position changes. Dry mouth can be relieved by chewing gum or sucking on hard candy or ice chips.

---

prednisoLONE
pred-NISS-oh-lone

Prelone

prednisoLONE sodium phosphate
Orapred ODT, Pediapred

Therapeutic class: Corticosteroids
Pharmacologic class: Glucocorticoids–mineralocorticoids

AVAILABLE FORMS
prednisolone
Syrup: 15 mg/5 mL*
Tablets: 5 mg
prednisolone sodium phosphate
ODTs 🆔: 10 mg, 15 mg, 30 mg
Oral solution: 5 mg/5 mL, 10 mg/5 mL, 15 mg/5 mL, 25 mg/5 mL

INDICATIONS & DOSAGES
➤ **Severe inflammation, immunosuppression**
Adults: 5 to 60 mg P.O. daily.
Children: 0.1 to 2 mg/kg/day P.O. in three or four divided doses (4 to 60 mg/m^2/day).
➤ **Uncontrolled asthma in those taking inhaled corticosteroids and long-acting bronchodilators**
Children: 1 to 2 mg/kg/day prednisolone sodium phosphate in single or divided doses. Continue short course (or "burst" therapy) until child achieves a peak expiratory flow rate of 80% of his personal best,

---

or until symptoms resolve. This usually requires 3 to 10 days of treatment but can take longer. Tapering the dose after improvement doesn't necessarily prevent relapse.

➤ **Acute exacerbations of MS**
Adults and children: 200 mg/day prednisolone sodium phosphate P.O. as single or divided dose for 7 days; then 80 mg every other day for 1 month.

➤ **Nephrotic syndrome**
Children: 60 mg/m² prednisolone sodium phosphate P.O. in three divided doses daily for 4 weeks, followed by 4 weeks of single-dose alternate-day therapy at 40 mg/m²/day.

ADMINISTRATION
P.O.
● Give drug with food or milk to reduce GI irritation. Patient may need another drug to prevent GI irritation.
● Don't cut or crush ODTs.
● Don't remove ODTs from blister pack until right before dosing.
● Patient may swallow ODT whole or allow to dissolve in mouth with or without water.

ACTION
Not clearly defined. Decreases inflammation, mainly by stabilizing leukocyte lysosomal membranes; suppresses immune response; stimulates bone marrow; and influences protein, fat, and carbohydrate metabolism.

Route	Onset	Peak	Duration
P.O.	Rapid	1–2 hr	3–36 hr

Half-life: 2 to 4 hours.

ADVERSE REACTIONS
CNS: euphoria, insomnia, *pseudotumor cerebri, seizures,* psychotic behavior, vertigo, headache, paresthesia.
CV: *arrhythmias, HF, thromboembolism,* hypertension, edema, thrombophlebitis.
EENT: cataracts, glaucoma.
GI: peptic ulceration, *pancreatitis,* GI irritation, increased appetite, nausea, vomiting.
GU: menstrual irregularities, increased urine calcium levels.
Metabolic: *hypokalemia,* hyperglycemia, carbohydrate intolerance, hypercholesterolemia, *hypocalcemia.*

Musculoskeletal: growth suppression in children, muscle weakness, osteoporosis.
Skin: hirsutism, delayed wound healing, acne, various skin eruptions.
Other: after increased stress—*acute adrenal insufficiency,* susceptibility to infections, cushingoid state; after abrupt withdrawal—rebound inflammation, fatigue, weakness, arthralgia, fever, dizziness, lethargy, depression, fainting, orthostatic hypotension, dyspnea, anorexia, *hypoglycemia;* after prolonged use followed by sudden withdrawal—*possible death.*

INTERACTIONS
Drug-drug. *Aspirin, indomethacin, other NSAIDs:* May increase risk of GI distress and bleeding. Use together cautiously.
Azole antifungals (fluconazole, ketoconazole): May increase antifungal toxicity. Reduce steroid dosage as needed.
Barbiturates, carbamazepine, fosphenytoin, phenytoin, rifampin: May decrease corticosteroid effect. Increase corticosteroid dosage.
Cyclosporine: May increase toxicity and risk of seizures. Monitor patient closely.
Drugs that deplete potassium, such as thiazide diuretics and amphotericin B: May enhance potassium-wasting effects of prednisolone. Monitor potassium level.
Estrogens: May increase pharmacologic and toxic effects of prednisolone. Monitor patient closely.
Oral anticoagulants: May alter dosage requirements. Monitor PT and INR closely.
Salicylates: May decrease salicylate level. Monitor patient for lack of salicylate effectiveness.
Skin-test antigens: May decrease response. Postpone skin testing until therapy is completed.
Toxoids, vaccines: May decrease antibody response and may increase risk of neurologic complications. Avoid using together.

EFFECTS ON LAB TEST RESULTS
● May increase glucose and cholesterol levels. May decrease T₃, T₄, potassium, and calcium levels.
● May decrease ¹³¹I uptake and protein-bound iodine levels in thyroid function tests. May alter skin-test results. May cause

false-negative results in nitroblue tetra-zolium test for systemic bacterial infections.

CONTRAINDICATIONS & CAUTIONS

• Contraindicated in patients hypersensitive to drug or its ingredients, in those with systemic fungal infections, and in those receiving immunosuppressive doses together with live-virus vaccines.

• Use cautiously in patients with recent MI, GI ulcer, renal disease, hypertension, osteoporosis, diabetes mellitus, hypothyroidism, cirrhosis, active hepatitis, diverticulitis, nonspecific ulcerative colitis, recent intestinal anastomoses, thromboembolic disorders, seizures, myasthenia gravis, HF, TB, ocular herpes simplex, emotional instability, and psychotic tendencies.

◊ *Alert:* Prolonged use can increase incidence of secondary infection, activate latent infections, prolong viral infections, and mask infections.

• Drug can suppress HPA axis, which can lead to adrenal crisis. Always withdraw drug slowly and carefully.

Dialyzable drug: Unknown.

⚠ *Overdose S&S:* Abnormal fat deposits, accentuated menopausal symptoms, acne, adrenal insufficiency, decreased glucose tolerance, decreased resistance to infection, dry scaly skin, ecchymosis, excessive appetite, fluid retention, fractures, headache, hypertrichosis, hypokalemia, increased BP, increased sweating, menstrual disorder, mental symptoms, moon face, negative nitrogen balance with delayed bone and wound healing, neuropathy, osteoporosis, peptic ulcer, pigmentation, striae, tachycardia, thinning scalp hair, thrombophlebitis, weakness, weight gain; hepatomegaly, abdominal distention (in children).

PREGNANCY-LACTATION-REPRODUCTION

• Not recommended during pregnancy. Refer to individual manufacturer's instructions for each product.

• Use cautiously in breast-feeding women. Refer to individual manufacturer's instructions for each product.

NURSING CONSIDERATIONS

• Determine whether patient is sensitive to other corticosteroids.

• Always adjust to lowest effective dose.

• Drug may be used for alternate-day therapy.

• Most adverse reactions to corticosteroids are dose- or duration-dependent.

• Monitor patient's weight, BP, and electrolyte level.

• Monitor patient for cushingoid effects, including moon face, buffalo hump, central obesity, thinning hair, hypertension, and increased susceptibility to infection.

• Watch for depression or psychotic episodes, especially during high-dose therapy.

• Diabetic patient may need increased insulin; monitor glucose level.

• Give patient low-sodium diet that's high in potassium and protein. Give potassium supplements as needed.

• Elderly patients may be more susceptible to osteoporosis with long-term use.

• Gradually reduce dosage after long-term therapy.

• *Look alike–sound alike:* Don't confuse prednisolone with prednisone. Don't confuse Prelone with Prozac.

PATIENT TEACHING

• Tell patient not to stop drug abruptly or without prescriber's consent.

• Instruct patient to take oral form of drug with food or milk.

• Teach patient signs and symptoms of early adrenal insufficiency: fatigue, muscle weakness, joint pain, fever, anorexia, nausea, shortness of breath, dizziness, and fainting.

• Instruct patient to carry medical identification that includes prescriber's name and name and dosage of drug and indicates his need for supplemental systemic glucocorticoids during stress.

• Warn patient on long-term therapy about cushingoid effects and the need to notify prescriber about sudden weight gain or swelling.

• Tell patient to report slow healing.

• Advise patient receiving long-term therapy to consider exercise or physical therapy. Also, tell him to ask prescriber about vitamin D or calcium supplement.

• Instruct patient to avoid exposure to infections and to notify prescriber if exposure occurs.

Reactions in bold italics are *life-threatening*. Interactions may have a *rapid onset* or a *delayed onset*.

• Tell patient to avoid immunizations while taking drug.

🜂 **Alert:** Tell patient not to cut, crush, or chew ODTs.

• Instruct patient not to remove the ODT from the blister pack until he's ready to take it. The tablet can be swallowed whole or allowed to dissolve on the tongue with or without water.

predniso**LONE** acetate (ophthalmic suspension)
pred-NISS-oh-lone

Omnipred, Pred Forte, Pred Mild

predniso**LONE** sodium phosphate (solution)

Therapeutic class: Anti-inflammatory drugs (ophthalmic)
Pharmacologic class: Corticosteroids

AVAILABLE FORMS
prednisolone acetate
Ophthalmic suspension: 0.12%, 1%
prednisolone sodium phosphate
Ophthalmic solution: 1%

INDICATIONS & DOSAGES
➤ **Inflammation of palpebral and bulbar conjunctiva, cornea, and anterior segment of globe**
Prednisolone acetate
Adults: 1 or 2 drops into affected eye b.i.d. to q.i.d. In severe conditions, may increase dosing frequency if needed. If signs and symptoms fail to improve after 2 days, reevaluate. In chronic conditions, taper doses gradually.
Prednisolone sodium phosphate
Adults: 1 or 2 drops into conjunctival sac hourly during the day and every 2 hours at night until response is observed. May reduce to 1 drop every 4 hours, then 1 drop t.i.d. to q.i.d. as needed for adequate response. In chronic conditions, taper doses gradually.

ADMINISTRATION
Ophthalmic
• Shake suspension and check dosage before giving to ensure correct strength. Store in tightly covered container.

• Apply light finger pressure on lacrimal sac for 1 minute after instillation.
• Don't touch dropper tip to eyelids or other surfaces when placing drops in eyes.

ACTION
Suppresses edema, fibrin deposition, capillary dilation, leukocyte migration, capillary proliferation, and collagen deposition.

Route	Onset	Peak	Duration
Ophthalmic	Unknown	Unknown	Unknown

Half-life: Unknown.

ADVERSE REACTIONS
EENT: cataracts, corneal ulceration, discharge, discomfort, foreign body sensation, glaucoma worsening, increased IOP, increased susceptibility to viral or fungal corneal infection, interference with corneal wound healing, optic nerve damage with excessive or long-term use, visual acuity and visual field defects.
Other: adrenal suppression with excessive or long-term use, systemic effects.

INTERACTIONS
None significant.

EFFECTS ON LAB TEST RESULTS
None reported.

CONTRAINDICATIONS & CAUTIONS
• Contraindicated in patients hypersensitive to prednisolone or components of the formulation and in patients with acute, untreated, purulent ocular infections; acute superficial herpes simplex (dendritic keratitis); vaccinia, varicella, or other viral or fungal eye diseases; or ocular TB.
• Use cautiously in patients with corneal thinning or corneal abrasions that may be contaminated (especially with herpes).
• Withdraw drug by gradually tapering dosage in patients with chronic conditions.
Dialyzable drug: Unknown.

PREGNANCY-LACTATION-REPRODUCTION
• There are no adequate studies in pregnant women. The amount of drug that crosses placental barrier through ophthalmic drops isn't known. Use during pregnancy only

if potential benefit justifies potential risks to the fetus.
• It isn't known if drug appears in breast milk. Patient should discontinue breast-feeding or discontinue drug.

NURSING CONSIDERATIONS
• IOP can increase with prolonged use. Use cautiously in patients with glaucoma. Monitor IOP and visual acuity in patients receiving treatment for 10 days or longer.
• *Look alike–sound alike:* Don't confuse prednisolone with prednisone.

PATIENT TEACHING
• Teach patient how to instill drops. Advise him to wash hands before and after instillation, and warn him not to touch tip of dropper to eye or surrounding area.
• Advise patient to apply light finger pressure on lacrimal sac for 1 minute after instillation.
• Tell patient on long-term therapy to have IOP tested frequently.
• Tell patient not to share drug, washcloths, or towels with family members and to notify prescriber if anyone develops the same signs or symptoms.
• Stress importance of compliance with recommended therapy.
• Tell patient to notify prescriber if improvement doesn't occur within several days or if pain, itching, or swelling of eye occurs.
• Warn patient not to use leftover drug for new eye inflammation because serious problems may occur.

---

predniSONE
PRED-ni-sone

Prednisone Intensol*, Rayos, Winpred✦

Therapeutic class: Corticosteroids
Pharmacologic class: Adrenocorticoids

AVAILABLE FORMS
Oral solution: 5 mg/5 mL*, 5 mg/mL (concentrate)*
Tablets: 1 mg, 2.5 mg, 5 mg, 10 mg, 20 mg, 50 mg
Tablets (delayed-release) ⊙: 1 mg, 2 mg, 5 mg

INDICATIONS & DOSAGES
➤ **Severe inflammation, immunosuppression, endocrine disorders (immediate-release, delayed-release)**
Adults and children: Initially, 5 to 60 mg P.O. daily in single dose or as two to four divided doses. Maintenance dose given daily or every other day (immediate-release only). Use lowest dose that will maintain adequate clinical response. Dosage must be individualized, and constant monitoring is needed.
➤ **Acute exacerbations of MS (immediate-release)**
Adults: 200 mg P.O. daily for 7 days; then 80 mg P.O. every other day for 1 month.

ADMINISTRATION
P.O.
• Unless contraindicated, give drug with food to reduce GI irritation. Patient may need another drug to prevent GI irritation.
• Solution may be diluted in juice or other flavored diluent or semisolid food such as applesauce before using.
• Make sure patient swallows delayed-release tablets whole and doesn't break, chew, or divide them.
• Discard opened bottle of solution after 90 days. Administer only using the provided calibrated dropper.

ACTION
Not clearly defined. Decreases inflammation, mainly by stabilizing leukocyte lysosomal membranes; suppresses immune response; stimulates bone marrow; and influences protein, fat, and carbohydrate metabolism.

Route	Onset	Peak	Duration
P.O. (immediate-release)	Variable	2 hr	Variable
P.O. (delayed-release)	4 hr	6–6½ hr	Unknown

Half-life: 2 to 3 hours.

ADVERSE REACTIONS
CNS: euphoria, insomnia, psychotic behavior, *pseudotumor cerebri,* vertigo, headache, paresthesia, *seizures.*
CV: *HF,* hypertension, edema, *arrhythmias,* thrombophlebitis, *thromboembolism.*

Reactions in bold italics are *life-threatening*. Interactions may have a *rapid onset* or a *delayed onset*.

EENT: cataracts, glaucoma.
GI: peptic ulceration, *pancreatitis,* GI irritation, increased appetite, nausea, vomiting.
GU: menstrual irregularities, increased urine calcium level.
Metabolic: *hypokalemia,* hyperglycemia, carbohydrate intolerance, hypercholesterolemia, *hypocalcemia.*
Musculoskeletal: growth suppression in children, muscle weakness, osteoporosis.
Skin: hirsutism, delayed wound healing, acne, various skin eruptions.
Other: cushingoid state, susceptibility to infections, *acute adrenal insufficiency* after increased stress or abrupt withdrawal after long-term therapy.
After abrupt withdrawal: rebound inflammation, fatigue, weakness, arthralgia, fever, dizziness, lethargy, depression, fainting, orthostatic hypotension, dyspnea, anorexia, *hypoglycemia. After prolonged use, sudden withdrawal may be fatal.*

INTERACTIONS
Drug-drug. *Aspirin, indomethacin, other NSAIDs:* May increase risk of GI distress and bleeding. Use together cautiously.
Barbiturates, carbamazepine, fosphenytoin, phenobarbital, phenytoin, rifampin: May decrease corticosteroid effect. Increase corticosteroid dosage.
Cyclosporine: May increase toxicity and cause seizures. Monitor patient closely.
Ketoconazole, troleandomycin: May inhibit the metabolism of corticosteroids and decrease their clearance. Titrate the dose of corticosteroid to avoid toxicity.
Oral anticoagulants: May alter dosage requirements. Monitor PT and INR closely.
Potassium-depleting drugs, such as thiazide diuretics and amphotericin B: May enhance potassium-wasting effects of prednisone. Monitor potassium level.
Salicylates: May decrease salicylate level. Monitor patient for lack of salicylate effectiveness.
Skin-test antigens: May decrease response. Postpone skin testing until therapy is completed.
Toxoids, vaccines: May decrease antibody response and may increase risk of neurologic complications. Avoid using together.

EFFECTS ON LAB TEST RESULTS
• May increase glucose and cholesterol levels. May decrease T_3, T_4, potassium, and calcium levels.
• May decrease ^{131}I uptake and protein-bound iodine values in thyroid function tests. May cause false-negative results in nitroblue tetrazolium test for systemic bacterial infections. May alter reactions to skin tests.

CONTRAINDICATIONS & CAUTIONS
• Contraindicated in patients hypersensitive to drug or its components; in those with systemic fungal infections (immediate-release only), cerebral malaria, or active ocular herpes simplex; and in those receiving immunosuppressive doses together with live-virus vaccines.
• Use cautiously in patients with recent MI, GI ulcer, renal disease, hypertension, osteoporosis, diabetes mellitus, hypothyroidism, cirrhosis, active hepatitis, diverticulitis, nonspecific ulcerative colitis, recent intestinal anastomoses, thromboembolic disorders, seizures, myasthenia gravis, HF, TB, ocular herpes simplex, emotional instability, and psychotic tendencies.
🔆 *Alert:* Patients are more susceptible to infections (from mild to fatal) during therapy. Drug can also mask signs and symptoms of infection.
• Drug can cause cataracts or glaucoma.
🔆 *Alert:* High-dose therapy is associated with acute myopathy that most often occurs in patients receiving neuromuscular drugs or in those with diseases such as myasthenia gravis.
Dialyzable drug: Unknown.

PREGNANCY-LACTATION-REPRODUCTION
• There are no adequate studies in pregnant women. Use only if potential benefits justify potential risks to the fetus.
• Monitor infants born to mothers who received substantial amounts of drug during pregnancy for signs and symptoms of hypoadrenalism.
• Drug appears in breast milk. Patient should discontinue breast-feeding or discontinue drug.
• Drug may increase or decrease motility and number of sperm.

P

NURSING CONSIDERATIONS

- Determine if patient is sensitive to other corticosteroids.
- Immediate-release drug may be used for alternate-day therapy.
- Always adjust to lowest effective dose.
- Most adverse reactions to corticosteroids are dose- or duration-dependent.
- For better results and less toxicity, give a once-daily dose in the morning.
- Drug may be used in conjunction with mineralocorticoids when needed.
- Monitor patient's BP, sleep patterns, and potassium level.
- If therapy lasts 6 weeks, monitor IOP.
- Weigh patient daily; report sudden weight gain to prescriber.
- Drug can cause HPA axis suppression and result in corticosteroid insufficiency if withdrawn. Reduce dosage gradually and reinstitute corticosteroid therapy if needed.
- Monitor patient for HPA axis suppression and cushingoid effects, including moon face, buffalo hump, central obesity, thinning hair, hypertension, and increased susceptibility to infection.
- Watch for depression or psychotic episodes, especially during high-dose therapy.
- Diabetic patient may need increased insulin; monitor glucose level.
- Elderly patients may be more susceptible to osteoporosis with long-term use.
- Patients with thyroid status changes may need dosage adjustment.
- Drug can cause osteoporosis at any age. Monitor bone density in patients on long-term therapy and bone growth in children. Institute bone-loss prevention measures if therapy is expected to last 3 months or more.
- Monitor patient for signs and symptoms of infection. Drug may mask or worsen infections, including latent amebiasis.
- Unless contraindicated, give low-sodium diet that's high in potassium and protein. Give potassium supplements as needed.
- Gradually reduce dosage after long-term therapy.
- *Look alike–sound alike:* Don't confuse prednisone with prednisolone or primidone.

PATIENT TEACHING

- Tell patient not to stop drug abruptly or without prescriber's consent.
- Instruct patient to take drug with food or milk and to swallow delayed-release tablets whole.
- Teach patient signs and symptoms of early adrenal insufficiency: fatigue, muscle weakness, joint pain, fever, anorexia, nausea, shortness of breath, dizziness, and fainting.
- Instruct patient to carry or wear medical identification indicating his need for supplemental systemic glucocorticoids during stress. It should include prescriber's name and name and dosage of drug.
- Warn patient on long-term therapy about cushingoid effects (moon face, buffalo hump) and the need to notify prescriber about sudden weight gain or swelling.
- Advise patient receiving long-term therapy to consider exercise or physical therapy. Also, tell patient to ask prescriber about vitamin D or calcium supplement.
- Tell patient to report slow healing.
- Advise patient receiving long-term therapy to have periodic eye examinations.
- Instruct patient to report infection, to avoid exposure to infections, and to contact prescriber if exposure occurs.

pregabalin
pray-GAB-ah-lin

Lyrica⬥

Therapeutic class: Anticonvulsants
Pharmacologic class: CNS drugs
Controlled substance schedule: V

AVAILABLE FORMS
Capsules: 25 mg, 50 mg, 75 mg, 100 mg, 150 mg, 200 mg, 225 mg, 300 mg
Oral solution: 20 mg/mL

INDICATIONS & DOSAGES
Adjust-a-dose (for all indications): If CrCl is 30 to 60 mL/minute, give 75 to 300 mg/day in two or three divided doses. If CrCl is 15 to 30 mL/minute, give 25 to 150 mg/day in one dose or divided into two doses. If CrCl is less than 15 mL/minute, give 25 to 75 mg/day in one dose. If patient undergoes

---

Reactions in bold italics are *life-threatening*. Interactions may have a *rapid onset* or a ***delayed onset***.

hemodialysis, give one supplemental dose according to these guidelines. If patient takes 25 mg daily, give 25 or 50 mg. If patient takes 25 to 50 mg daily, give 50 or 75 mg. If patient takes 50 to 75 mg daily, give 75 or 100 mg. If patient takes 75 mg daily, give 100 or 150 mg.

➤ **Fibromyalgia**
Adults: 75 mg P.O. b.i.d. (150 mg/day). May increase to 150 mg b.i.d. (300 mg/day) within 1 week, based on patient response. If pain relief insufficient with 300 mg/day, increase to 225 mg b.i.d. (450 mg/day).

➤ **Diabetic peripheral neuropathy**
Adults: Initially, 50 mg P.O. t.i.d. May increase to 100 mg P.O. t.i.d. within 1 week based on patient response.

➤ **Neuropathic pain associated with spinal cord injury**
Adults: Initially, 75 mg P.O. b.i.d. (150 mg/day). May increase to 150 mg b.i.d. (300 mg/day) within 1 week based on patient response. If pain relief is insufficient after 2 to 3 weeks, increase to 300 mg b.i.d. Maximum dose is 600 mg/day.

➤ **Postherpetic neuralgia**
Adults: Initially, 75 mg P.O. b.i.d. or 50 mg P.O. t.i.d. May increase to 300 mg/day in two or three equally divided doses within 1 week based on patient response. If pain relief insufficient after 2 to 3 weeks, may increase to 300 mg b.i.d. or 200 mg t.i.d.

➤ **Partial onset seizures**
Adults: Initially, 75 mg P.O. b.i.d. or 50 mg P.O. t.i.d. Range, 150 to 600 mg/day. Dosage may be increased to maximum 600 mg/day.

ADMINISTRATION
P.O.
• Give drug without regard for food.
• Don't stop drug abruptly. Instead, taper gradually over at least 1 week.

ACTION
May contribute to analgesic and anticonvulsant effects by binding to sites in CNS.

Route	Onset	Peak	Duration
P.O.	Unknown	1½–3 hr	Unknown

Half-life: 6 hours.

ADVERSE REACTIONS
CNS: ataxia, dizziness, somnolence, tremor, abnormal gait, abnormal thinking, amnesia, anxiety, asthenia, confusion, depersonalization, euphoria, headache, hypesthesia, hypertonia, incoordination, myoclonus, nervousness, nystagmus, pain, paresthesia, stupor, twitching, vertigo.
CV: edema, PR-interval prolongation.
EENT: blurred or abnormal vision, conjunctivitis, diplopia, eye disorder, otitis media, tinnitus.
GI: dry mouth, abdominal pain, constipation, flatulence, gastroenteritis, vomiting.
GU: anorgasmia, impotence, urinary incontinence, urinary frequency.
Metabolic: *hypoglycemia,* weight gain, increased or decreased appetite.
Musculoskeletal: arthralgia, back and chest pain, leg cramps, myalgia, myasthenia, neuropathy, tremor.
Respiratory: bronchitis, dyspnea.
Skin: ecchymosis, pruritus.
Other: accidental injury, infection, allergic reaction, decreased libido, flu syndrome.

INTERACTIONS
Drug-drug. *ACE inhibitors:* May increase risk of swelling and hives with concomitant use. Monitor patient.
CNS depressants: May have additive effects on cognitive and gross motor function. Monitor patient for increased dizziness and somnolence.
Pioglitazone, rosiglitazone: May cause additive fluid retention and weight gain. Monitor patient closely.
Drug-lifestyle. *Alcohol use:* May have additive depressant effects on cognitive and gross motor function. Discourage alcohol use.

EFFECTS ON LAB TEST RESULTS
• May increase CK level.
• May decrease platelet count.

CONTRAINDICATIONS & CAUTIONS
• Contraindicated in patients hypersensitive to drug or its components.
• Use cautiously in patients with New York Heart Association class III or IV HF.
🔴 *Alert:* Drug may increase risk of suicidal thoughts or behavior.

Dialyzable drug: Yes.

⚠ *Overdose S&S:* Exaggerated adverse effects.

PREGNANCY-LACTATION-REPRODUCTION

• There are no adequate studies in pregnant women. Drug may cause fetal harm. Use in pregnancy only if potential benefit clearly justifies risk to the fetus.

• Patients exposed to drug during pregnancy should enroll in the Antiepileptic Drug Pregnancy Registry (1-888-233-2334).

• Drug appears in breast milk. Patient should discontinue breast-feeding or discontinue drug.

NURSING CONSIDERATIONS

❸ *Alert:* Monitor patient for signs and symptoms of angioedema (including swelling of face, mouth, and neck), which may compromise breathing. Discontinue drug immediately if angioedema occurs.

❸ *Alert:* Monitor patient for worsening depression, suicidal thoughts or behavior, or unusual mood or behavior changes.

• Monitor patient's weight and fluid status, especially if patient has HF.

• Monitor patient for depression, suicidal thoughts or behavior, and unusual mood changes.

• Check for changes in vision.

• Withdraw drug gradually over 1 week, especially in patients with seizure disorder.

❸ *Alert:* Watch for signs of rhabdomyolysis, such as dark, red, or cola-colored urine; muscle tenderness; generalized weakness; or muscle stiffness or aching.

• *Look alike–sound alike:* Don't confuse Lyrica with Lopressor or Hydrea.

PATIENT TEACHING

• Explain that drug may be taken without regard to food.

• Warn patient not to stop drug abruptly and that it should be tapered over at least 1 week.

• Advise patient that drug may cause angioedema, with swelling of the face, mouth (lip, gum, and tongue), and neck (larynx and pharynx) that can lead to life-threatening respiratory compromise. Instruct patient to discontinue drug and immediately seek medical care if these symptoms occur.

• Tell patient to seek immediate medical care for a hypersensitivity reaction, such as blisters, dyspnea, hives, rash, or wheezing.

❸ *Alert:* Counsel patient, caregiver, and family about risk of suicidal thoughts and behaviors. Advise them of the need to be alert for the emergence or worsening of symptoms of depression, unusual changes in mood or behavior, or the emergence of suicidal thoughts, behavior, or thoughts about self-harm and to immediately report behaviors of concern to health care provider.

• Caution patient to avoid hazardous activities until drug's effects are known.

• Instruct patient to watch for weight changes and water retention.

• Advise patient to report vision changes and malaise or fever accompanied by muscle pain, tenderness, or weakness.

• Tell male patient taking pregabalin who plans to father a child to consult prescriber about potential risk to a fetus because of male-mediated teratogenicity.

• Urge patient with diabetes to inspect skin closely for ulcer formation.

• Advise patient to avoid alcohol.

primaquine phosphate
PRIM-uh-kween

Therapeutic class: Antimalarials
Pharmacologic class: Aminoquinolines

AVAILABLE FORMS
Tablets: 26.3 mg (equivalent to 15-mg base)

INDICATIONS & DOSAGES
➤ **Relapsing *Plasmodium vivax* malaria, eliminating symptoms and infection completely; to prevent relapse**
Adults: 15 mg base P.O. daily for 14 days. Begin therapy during the last 2 weeks of, or after, a course of suppression with chloroquine or comparable drug.

ADMINISTRATION
P.O.

❸ *Alert:* Drug dosage may be discussed in "mg" or "mg base"; be aware of the difference.

• Give drug with or without food. Give with a meal if stomach irritation occurs.

Reactions in bold italics are *life-threatening*. Interactions may have a *rapid onset* or a ***delayed onset***.

ACTION

May bind to and alter the properties of DNA in susceptible parasites.

Route	Onset	Peak	Duration
P.O.	Unknown	1–3 hr	Unknown

Half-life: 3 to 6 hours.

ADVERSE REACTIONS

GI: nausea, vomiting, epigastric distress, abdominal cramps.
Hematologic: *hemolytic anemia, leukopenia, methemoglobinemia.*

INTERACTIONS

Drug-drug. *QTc interval–prolonging drugs:* May increase QTc interval and risk of ventricular arrhythmias. Monitor therapy.
Quinacrine: May increase risk of toxicity. Avoid concomitant use.
Vaccine (rabies): May decrease antibody response to rabies vaccine. International travelers should complete a three-dose rabies vaccination series before starting primaquine. If this isn't possible, the rabies vaccine should be given intramuscularly and not intradermally.
Drug-food. *Grapefruit juice:* May increase drug plasma concentration and toxic effects. Advise patient to avoid grapefruit products.

EFFECTS ON LAB TEST RESULTS

● May decrease Hb level.
● May decrease RBC count. May increase or decrease WBC count.

CONTRAINDICATIONS & CAUTIONS

● Contraindicated in patients with systemic diseases in which agranulocytosis may develop, such as lupus erythematosus or RA, and in those taking a bone marrow suppressant, quinacrine, or hemolytic drugs.
● Use cautiously in patients with previous idiosyncratic reaction involving hemolytic anemia, methemoglobinemia, or leukopenia; in those with a family or personal history of favism; and in those with erythrocytic G6PD or nicotinamide-adenine-dinucleotide (NADH) methemoglobin reductase deficiency.
● May prolong QTc interval. Monitor ECG in patients with risk factors for QTc-interval prolongation.

Dialyzable drug: Unknown.
⚠ Overdose S&S: Abdominal cramps, anemia, burning epigastric distress, CNS and CV disturbances, cyanosis, methemoglobinemia, moderate leukocytosis or leukopenia, vomiting, granulocytopenia, acute hemolytic anemia, acute hemolysis.

PREGNANCY-LACTATION-REPRODUCTION

● Drug isn't recommended in pregnant women as safe use hasn't been established.
● It isn't known if drug appears in breast milk. If drug is needed, test mother and infant for G6PD deficiency; may use drug in breast-feeding patients and infants with normal G6PD levels.

NURSING CONSIDERATIONS

● Use drug with a fast-acting antimalarial such as chloroquine to reduce possibility of drug-resistant strains.
● Monitor CBC and glucose and electrolyte levels. Patients with G6PD deficiency will need more frequent monitoring.
● Monitor patient for markedly darkened urine and for suddenly reduced Hb level or RBC or WBC count, which suggest impending hemolytic reactions. Stop drug immediately and notify prescriber.
● *Look alike–sound alike:* Don't confuse primaquine with primidone.

PATIENT TEACHING

● Instruct patient to take drug with meals to minimize stomach upset. If nausea, vomiting, or stomach pain persists, tell patient to notify prescriber.
● Tell patient to report to prescriber chills, fever, chest pain, and bluish skin discoloration; these signs and symptoms may suggest a hemolytic reaction.
● Tell patient to stop drug and notify prescriber immediately if urine darkens markedly.
● Stress importance of completing full course of therapy.

procainamide hydrochloride
proe-KANE-a-myed

Therapeutic class: Antiarrhythmics
Pharmacologic class: Procaine
derivatives

AVAILABLE FORMS
Injection: 100 mg/mL, 500 mg/mL

INDICATIONS & DOSAGES
➤ **Life-threatening ventricular arrhythmias**
Adults: 100 mg every 5 minutes by slow I.V. push, no faster than 25 to 50 mg/minute, until arrhythmias disappear, adverse effects develop, or 500 mg has been given. Or, give a loading dose of 500 to 600 mg I.V. infusion over 25 to 30 minutes. Maximum total dose given by repeated bolus injections or loading infusion is 1 g. To maintain therapeutic levels, give continuous infusion of 2 to 6 mg/minute based on clinical response and patient condition; monitor closely.

For patients with less-threatening arrhythmias but who are nauseated, vomiting, or are ordered to receive nothing by mouth, give 50 mg/kg I.M. divided into fractional doses of ⅛ to ¼ every 3 to 6 hours until an oral antiarrhythmic is possible. For arrhythmias occurring during surgery, give 100 to 500 mg I.M.
Adjust-a-dose: For patients with renal or hepatic dysfunction, decrease dosage or increase dosing interval, as needed.

ADMINISTRATION
I.V.
▼ Vials for I.V. injection contain 1 g of drug: 100 mg/mL (10 mL) or 500 mg/mL (2 mL).
▼ Direct injection into a vein or into tubing of an established I.V. should be done slowly at a rate not to exceed 50 mg/minute.
▼ For loading dose infusion, dilute with compatible I.V. solution, such as D$_5$W injection (1 g diluted to 50 mL), and give with patient supine at a rate not exceeding 25 to 50 mg/minute. Keep patient supine during I.V. administration.

▼ For I.V. infusion to maintain therapeutic levels, dilute 1 g procainamide in 500 or 250 mL D$_5$W and administer at 2 to 6 mg/minute based on patient response and clinical condition.
▼ Attend patient receiving infusion at all times. Use an infusion-control device to give infusion precisely.
❸ *Alert:* Monitor BP and ECG continuously during I.V. administration. Watch for prolonged QTc intervals and QRS complexes, heart block, or increased arrhythmias. If such reactions occur, withhold drug, obtain rhythm strip, and notify prescriber immediately. If drug is given too rapidly, hypotension can occur. Watch closely for adverse reactions during infusion, and notify prescriber if they occur.
▼ Solution may turn slightly yellow upon standing. Discard solutions that are slightly darker than yellow or discolored in any other way.
▼ **Incompatibilities:** Bretylium, esmolol, ethacrynate, milrinone, phenytoin sodium.
I.M.
● I.M. injections are a substitute for oral administration in patients who aren't allowed anything by mouth. Oral dosing should be resumed as soon as possible.

ACTION
Decreases excitability, conduction velocity, automaticity, and membrane responsiveness with prolonged refractory period. Larger than usual doses may induce AV block.

Route	Onset	Peak	Duration
I.V.	Immediate	Immediate	Unknown
I.M.	10–30 min	15–60 min	Unknown

Half-life: About 2½ to 4¾ hours.

ADVERSE REACTIONS
CNS: fever, *seizures,* hallucinations, psychosis, giddiness, confusion, depression, dizziness.
CV: hypotension, *bradycardia, AV block, ventricular fibrillation, ventricular asystole.*
GI: abdominal pain, nausea, vomiting, anorexia, diarrhea, bitter taste.
Skin: maculopapular rash, urticaria, pruritus, flushing.

Reactions in bold italics are *life-threatening*. Interactions may have a *rapid onset* or a *delayed onset*.

Other: lupuslike syndrome, *angioneurotic edema.*

INTERACTIONS

Drug-drug. *Amiodarone:* May increase procainamide level and toxicity and have additive effects on QTc interval and QRS complex. Avoid using together.

Antiarrhythmics: May enhance antiarrhythmic and hypotensive effects. Avoid using together.

Anticholinergics: May increase antivagal effects. Monitor patient closely.

Beta blockers, ranitidine, trimethoprim: May increase procainamide level. Watch for toxicity.

Cimetidine, ranitidine: May increase procainamide level. Avoid using together if possible. Monitor procainamide level closely and adjust the dosage as necessary.

Macrolides and related antibiotics (azithromycin, clarithromycin, erythromycin, telithromycin): May prolong the QT interval. Use with caution. Avoid use with telithromycin.

Neuromuscular blockers: May increase skeletal muscle relaxant effect. May need to decrease dosage of neuromuscular blocker.

Quinolones: Life-threatening arrhythmias, including torsades de pointes, can occur. Avoid using together; sparfloxacin is contraindicated.

Thioridazine, ziprasidone: May prolong QTc interval. Avoid using together.

Drug-herb. *Jimsonweed:* May adversely affect CV function. Discourage use together.

Licorice: May prolong QTc interval. Urge caution.

Drug-lifestyle. *Alcohol use:* May reduce drug level. Discourage use together.

EFFECTS ON LAB TEST RESULTS

● May increase ALT, AST, alkaline phosphatase, LDH, and bilirubin levels.

● May decrease Hb level, hematocrit, and WBC and platelet counts.

● May cause positive ANA titers and positive direct antiglobulin (Coombs) tests.

CONTRAINDICATIONS & CAUTIONS

● Contraindicated in patients hypersensitive to this drug and related drugs.

● Drug contains sulfite, which can cause allergic-type reactions, including anaphylaxis. Sensitivity to sulfites may be more frequent in patients with asthma.

● Contraindicated in those with complete second- or third-degree heart block in the absence of an artificial pacemaker. Also contraindicated in those with myasthenia gravis, systemic lupus erythematosus, or atypical ventricular tachycardia (torsades de pointes).

● Use with extreme caution in patients with ventricular tachycardia during coronary occlusion.

● Use cautiously in patients with HF or other conduction disturbances, such as bundle-branch heart block, sinus bradycardia, or digoxin intoxication, and in those with hepatic or renal insufficiency.

Black Box Warning Use cautiously in patients with blood dyscrasias or bone marrow suppression. ■

Dialyzable drug: Procainamide, 20 to 50%; metabolite *N*-acetylprocainamide (NAPA), less than 5%.

⚠ Overdose S&S: Progressive widening of QRS complex, prolonged QT and PR intervals, lowered R and T waves, increasing AV block, ventricular ectopy, ventricular tachycardia, hypotension, CNS depression, tremor, respiratory depression.

PREGNANCY-LACTATION-REPRODUCTION

● Use during pregnancy only if clearly needed.

● Procainamide and metabolite NAPA appear in breast milk. Patient should discontinue breast-feeding or discontinue drug.

NURSING CONSIDERATIONS

Black Box Warning Because of its proarrhythmic effects, procainamide should be reserved for patients with life-threatening ventricular arrhythmias. ■

● Digitalize or cardiovert patients with atrial flutter or fibrillation before therapy with procainamide to prevent ventricular rate acceleration in patient.

● Monitor level of drug and its active metabolite NAPA.

● Monitor ECG closely. If QRS widens more than 25% or marked prolongation of

the QTc interval occurs, check for overdosage.
• Hypokalemia predisposes patient to arrhythmias. Monitor electrolytes, especially potassium level.
• Elderly patients may be more likely to develop hypotension. Monitor BP carefully.

Black Box Warning Agranulocytosis, bone marrow depression, neutropenia, hypoplastic anemia, and thrombocytopenia have been noted in patients during the first 12 weeks of therapy. It is recommended that CBCs be performed at weekly intervals for the first 3 months of therapy and periodically thereafter. ■

Black Box Warning Perform CBCs promptly if patient develops signs of infection, bruising, or bleeding. If hematologic disorder is identified, discontinue drug. Blood counts usually return to normal within 1 month of discontinuation. ■

Black Box Warning Positive ANA titer is common in about 60% of patients who don't have symptoms of lupuslike syndrome. This response seems to be related to prolonged use, not dosage. If positive ANA titer develops, assess the benefits and risks of continued therapy. ■

• Discontinue I.V. therapy if persistent conduction disturbances or hypotension develops. As soon as cardiac rhythm is stabilized, start oral antiarrhythmic maintenance therapy 3 to 4 hours after last I.V. dose.

PATIENT TEACHING
• Instruct patient to report fever, rash, muscle pain, diarrhea, bleeding, bruises, pleuritic chest pain, or signs and symptoms of infection.
• Instruct patient to report sulfite sensitivity before receiving drug.

procarbazine hydrochloride
proe-KAR-buh-zeen

Matulane

Therapeutic class: Antineoplastics
Pharmacologic class: Methylhydrazine derivatives

AVAILABLE FORMS
Capsules: 50 mg

INDICATIONS & DOSAGES
➤ **Single-agent therapy or adjunctive treatment of Hodgkin lymphoma (stages III and IV) and other cancers using nitrogen mustard, vincristine, procarbazine, prednisone (MOPP) regimen**
Adults: For single-agent therapy, give 2 to 4 mg/kg/day P.O. in single dose or divided doses for first week. Then, 4 to 6 mg/kg/day until WBC count falls below 4,000/mm^3, platelet count falls below 100,000/mm^3, or maximum response is obtained. Maintenance dose is 1 to 2 mg/kg/day after bone marrow recovery. For MOPP regimen, 100 mg/m^2 daily P.O. for first 14 days of 28-day cycle.
Children: For single-agent therapy, give 50 mg/m^2/day P.O. for first week; then 100 mg/m^2/day until response or toxicity occurs. Maintenance dose is 50 mg/m^2/day P.O. after bone marrow recovery.
Adjust-a-dose: If serum bilirubin level is 5 mg/dL or less and AST or ALT level is 1.6 to 6 × ULN, give 75% of usual dose. If serum bilirubin level is 5 mg/dL or less and AST or ALT level is more than 6 × ULN, use clinical judgment to determine dose. Don't give if serum bilirubin level is greater than 5 mg/dL.

ADMINISTRATION
P.O.
• Give drug with or after meals. May give once daily or in two to three divided doses.
• For patient unable to swallow capsules whole, empty capsule contents into sterile water for injection. Stir until dissolved; then have patient drink the mixture immediately.

Rinse the container with additional water and have patient drink.

ACTION
Unknown. Thought to inhibit DNA, RNA, and protein synthesis.

Route	Onset	Peak	Duration
P.O.	Unknown	Unknown	Unknown

Half-life: 10 minutes.

ADVERSE REACTIONS
CNS: ataxia, hallucinations, *coma,* confusion, depression, dizziness, headache, insomnia, nervousness, neuropathy, nightmares, paresthesia, syncope, *seizures.*
CV: flushing, hypotension, tachycardia.
EENT: nystagmus, photophobia, retinal hemorrhage, diplopia, hearing loss.
GI: nausea, vomiting, abdominal pain, anorexia, constipation, diarrhea, dry mouth, dysphagia, *hematemesis, melena,* stomatitis.
GU: hematuria, nocturia, urinary frequency.
Hematologic: *anemia, bleeding tendency, leukopenia, thrombocytopenia,* eosinophilia, hemolytic anemia.
Hepatic: *hepatotoxicity,* jaundice.
Respiratory: pleural effusion, cough, pneumonitis.
Skin: dermatitis, hyperpigmentation, pruritus, rash, reversible alopecia.
Other: *secondary malignancies,* allergic reaction, gynecomastia, herpes outbreak.

INTERACTIONS
Drug-drug. *Anticoagulants (warfarin):* May increase anticoagulant effect. Monitor coagulation status (PT and INR) and adjust dosage as needed.
CNS depressants: May cause additive depressant effects. Avoid using together.
Digoxin: May decrease digoxin level. Monitor digoxin level closely.
Drugs high in tyramine, local anesthetics, MAO inhibitors, sympathomimetics, TCAs: May cause tremor, palpitations, and increased BP. Monitor patient closely.
Methotrexate: The nephrotoxicity of methotrexate may be increased. Wait 72 hours or longer between giving the final dose of procarbazine and starting a high-dose methotrexate infusion.

Drug-food. *Caffeine:* May result in arrhythmias and severe hypertension. Discourage caffeine intake.
Foods high in tyramine (cheese, Chianti): May cause tremor, palpitations, and increased BP. Monitor patient closely; advise him to avoid or limit intake.
Drug-lifestyle. ◑ *Alert: Alcohol use:* Mild disulfiram-like reaction may cause flushing, headache, nausea, and hypotension. Warn patient to avoid alcoholic beverages.

EFFECTS ON LAB TEST RESULTS
- May decrease Hb level.
- May increase eosinophil count. May decrease platelet, RBC, and WBC counts.

CONTRAINDICATIONS & CAUTIONS
- Contraindicated in patients hypersensitive to drug and in those with inadequate bone marrow reserve as shown by bone marrow aspiration.
- Use cautiously in patients with impaired hepatic or renal function.
Dialyzable drug: 25% to 49%.
⚠ *Overdose S&S:* Nausea, vomiting, diarrhea, enteritis, hypotension, tremors, seizures, coma.

PREGNANCY-LACTATION-REPRODUCTION
- Drug can cause fetal harm. Women should avoid becoming pregnant during therapy.
- Women shouldn't breast-feed during therapy.

NURSING CONSIDERATIONS
Black Box Warning Give drug only under the supervision of a physician experienced with potent antineoplastic drugs. Adequate clinical and laboratory facilities should be available. ■
- Monitor CBC and platelet counts.
◑ *Alert:* Prompt discontinuation of therapy is recommended if patient develops CNS signs or symptoms, such as paresthesia, neuropathies, or confusion; leukopenia (WBC count less than 4,000 cell/mm^3); thrombocytopenia (platelet count less than 100,000/mm^3); hypersensitivity reaction; stomatitis; diarrhea; or hemorrhage or bleeding tendencies.
- Bone marrow depression begins 2 to 8 weeks after the start of treatment.

P

• Avoid all I.M. injections when platelet count is below 50,000/mm^3.
• Drug has high emetic potential; give antiemetics to prevent nausea and vomiting.
• The manufacturer recommends that if radiation or chemotherapeutic agents with bone marrow depressant activity have been used, give patient a 1-month interval without such therapy before beginning procarbazine therapy.
• **Look alike–sound alike:** Don't confuse procarbazine with dacarbazine.

PATIENT TEACHING
• To decrease nausea and vomiting, advise patient to take drug at bedtime and in divided doses and to take antiemetics as prescribed.
• Tell patient to watch for fever, sore throat, fatigue, easy bruising, nosebleeds, bleeding gums, or tarry stools. Tell patient to take temperature daily
• Tell patient not to consume alcohol or alcohol-containing products during therapy.
• Instruct patient to avoid OTC medications that contain antihistamines and sympathomimetics and to avoid foods and drinks high in tyramine, such as wine, tea, coffee, cola, cheese, and bananas.
• Warn patient to avoid hazardous activities that require alertness and good motor coordination until CNS effects of drug are known.
• Caution female patient of childbearing potential to avoid becoming pregnant during therapy and to consult prescriber before becoming pregnant.

prochlorperazine
proe-klor-PER-a-zeen

Compro

prochlorperazine edisylate

prochlorperazine maleate
Procomp

Therapeutic class: Antiemetics
Pharmacologic class: Dopamine antagonists

AVAILABLE FORMS
prochlorperazine
Suppositories: 10 mg✲, 25 mg
prochlorperazine edisylate
Injection: 5 mg/mL
prochlorperazine maleate
Tablets: 5 mg, 10 mg

INDICATIONS & DOSAGES
➤ **To control preoperative nausea**
Adults: 5 to 10 mg I.M. 1 to 2 hours before induction of anesthesia; repeat once in 30 minutes, if needed. Or, 5 to 10 mg I.V. at no more than 5 mg/minute 15 to 30 minutes before induction of anesthesia; repeat once, if needed. Maximum I.M. and I.V. dose is 40 mg/day.
➤ **Severe nausea and vomiting**
Adults: 5 to 10 mg P.O. t.i.d. or q.i.d.; 25 mg P.R. b.i.d.; or 5 to 10 mg I.M., repeated every 3 to 4 hours, as needed. Maximum I.M. dose is 40 mg daily. Or, 2.5 to 10 mg I.V. at no more than 5 mg/minute. Maximum I.V. dose is 40 mg daily.
Children weighing 18 to 39 kg: 2.5 mg P.O. t.i.d.; or 5 mg P.O. b.i.d. Maximum, 15 mg daily. Or, 0.132 mg/kg by deep I.M. injection. Control is usually achieved with one dose.
Children weighing 14 to 17 kg: 2.5 mg P.O. b.i.d. or t.i.d. Maximum, 10 mg daily. Or, 0.132 mg/kg by deep I.M. injection. Control is usually achieved with one dose.
Children weighing 9 to 13 kg: 2.5 mg P.O. once daily or b.i.d. Maximum, 7.5 mg daily. Or, 0.132 mg/kg by deep I.M. injection. Control is usually achieved with one dose.

➤ **Schizophrenia**

Adults: For mild conditions, 5 or 10 mg P.O. t.i.d. or q.i.d. For moderate to severe conditions, start with 10 mg P.O. t.i.d. or q.i.d.; increase by small increments every 2 or 3 days until symptoms are controlled or adverse reactions become bothersome. Patients may respond on 50 to 75 mg/day in divided doses. For severe conditions, 100 to 150 mg P.O. daily. Or, for severe symptoms, 10 to 20 mg by deep I.M. injection. Repeat the initial I.M. dose every 2 to 4 hours (or, in resistant cases, every hour) to gain control of patient, as necessary. More than three or four I.M. doses are seldom necessary. If, in rare cases, parenteral therapy is needed for a prolonged period, give 10 to 20 mg I.M. every 4 to 6 hours. After control is achieved, switch patient to an oral form of drug at same dosage level or higher.

Children ages 2 to 12: Initially, 2.5 mg P.O. b.i.d. or t.i.d., not to exceed 10 mg on the first day. Increase dosage according to patient's response. Maximum dose is 20 mg/day (ages 2 to 5) or 25 mg/day (ages 6 to 12). Or, give 0.132 mg/kg (0.06 mg/lb) by deep I.M. injection. Control is usually achieved with one I.M. dose. After control is achieved, switch patient to an oral form of drug at same dosage level or higher.

➤ **Nonpsychotic anxiety**

Adults: 5 mg P.O. t.i.d. or q.i.d. Maximum dose is 20 mg/day for no longer than 12 weeks.

ADMINISTRATION
P.O.
- Protect from light.
- Administer without regard to meals.

I.V.
▼ Add 20 mg of drug per liter of NSS 15 to 30 minutes before induction of anesthesia.
▼ Infuse slowly; rate shouldn't exceed 5 mg/minute. Maximum parenteral dose is 40 mg daily.
▼ To prevent contact dermatitis, avoid getting injection solution on hands or clothing.
▼ Protect from light.
▼ **Incompatibilities:** Other I.V. drugs.

I.M.
- For I.M. use, inject deeply into upper outer quadrant of gluteal region.

- Don't give by subcutaneous route or mix in syringe with another drug.
- To prevent contact dermatitis, avoid getting injection solution on hands or clothing.
- Store in light-resistant container. Slight yellowing doesn't affect potency; discard extremely discolored solutions.

Rectal
- Don't remove from wrapper until ready to use. Protect unwrapped suppository from light.

ACTION
Acts on the chemoreceptor trigger zone to inhibit nausea and vomiting; in larger doses, it partially depresses vomiting center.

Route	Onset	Peak	Duration
P.O.	30–40 min	Unknown	3–12 hr
I.V.	Unknown	Unknown	Unknown
I.M.	10–20 min	Unknown	3–4 hr
P.R.	1 hr	Unknown	3–4 hr

Half-life: Unknown.

ADVERSE REACTIONS
CNS: extrapyramidal reactions, dizziness, EEG changes, pseudoparkinsonism, sedation, drowsiness, motor restlessness, dystonia, tardive dyskinesia.
CV: orthostatic hypotension, ECG changes, tachycardia.
EENT: blurred vision, ocular changes.
GI: constipation, dry mouth, increased appetite.
GU: urine retention, dark urine, inhibited ejaculation, menstrual irregularities.
Hematologic: *agranulocytosis, transient leukopenia.*
Hepatic: cholestatic jaundice.
Metabolic: weight gain.
Skin: mild photosensitivity reactions, allergic reactions, exfoliative dermatitis.
Other: gynecomastia, hyperprolactinemia.

INTERACTIONS
Drug-drug. *Antacids:* May inhibit absorption of oral phenothiazines. Separate antacid and phenothiazine doses by at least 2 hours.
Anticholinergics, including antidepressants and antiparkinsonians: May increase anticholinergic activity and may aggravate parkinsonian symptoms. Use together cautiously.

Anticoagulants: May decrease anticoagulant effects. Monitor PT and INR, and adjust dosage as needed.

Anticonvulsants: May lower seizure threshold; dosage adjustments of anticonvulsants may be needed.

Barbiturates: May decrease phenothiazine effect. Monitor patient for decreased antiemetic effect.

CNS depressants (anesthetics, opioids): May intensify or prolong action of these drugs. Monitor patient.

Loop diuretics, thiazides: May add to orthostatic hypotension caused by prochlorperazine. Monitor BP.

Propranolol: May increase plasma levels of both drugs. Observe for increased adverse effects.

Drug-herb. *Dong quai, St. John's wort:* May increase risk of photosensitivity. Advise patient to avoid excessive sun exposure.

Kava: May increase risk of dystonic reactions. Discourage use together.

Drug-lifestyle. *Alcohol use:* May increase CNS depression, particularly psychomotor skills. Strongly discourage use together.

EFFECTS ON LAB TEST RESULTS
● May decrease WBC and granulocyte counts.
● May cause false-positive results for phenylketonuria and pregnancy tests. May cause abnormal LFT results.

CONTRAINDICATIONS & CAUTIONS
● Contraindicated in patients hypersensitive to phenothiazines and in patients with CNS depression, including those in a coma.
● Contraindicated during pediatric surgery, when using spinal or epidural anesthetic or adrenergic blockers, and in children younger than age 2.

Black Box Warning Drug isn't approved for the treatment of elderly patients with dementia-related psychosis due to an increased risk of death. ■

● Use cautiously in patients with impaired CV function, glaucoma, seizure disorders, and Parkinson disease; in those who have been exposed to extreme heat; and in children with acute illness.

● *Alert:* Potentially irreversible tardive dyskinesia and potentially fatal neuroleptic malignant syndrome have been reported with antipsychotic use.

▲ *Overdose S&S:* Dystonic reactions, CNS depression, agitation, restlessness, seizures, ECG changes, cardiac arrhythmias, fever, hypotension, dry mouth, ileus.

Dialyzable drug: No.

PREGNANCY-LACTATION-REPRODUCTION
● Safe use in pregnant women hasn't been established. Use during pregnancy only if potential benefit justifies potential risks to the fetus.
● *Alert:* Neonates exposed to antipsychotics in the third trimester are at risk for extrapyramidal or withdrawal symptoms after delivery that may range in severity from mild to severe and may require intensive care support.
● Drug may appear in breast milk. Use cautiously in breast-feeding women.

NURSING CONSIDERATIONS
Black Box Warning Elderly patients with dementia-related psychosis treated with antipsychotics are at an increased risk for death. ■
● Watch for orthostatic hypotension, especially when giving drug I.V.
● Monitor CBC and LFTs during long-term therapy.
● *Alert:* Use drug only when vomiting can't be controlled by other measures or when only a few doses are needed. If more than four doses are needed in 24 hours, notify prescriber.
● Immediately report signs and symptoms of tardive dyskinesia (involuntary rhythmic movements of the face, tongue, or jaw) as drug may need to be discontinued.
● Immediately report signs and symptoms of neuroleptic malignant syndrome (high fever, confusion, muscle rigidity, unstable vital signs) as drug should be discontinued and supportive therapy begun.
● *Look alike–sound alike:* Don't confuse prochlorperazine with chlorpromazine.

PATIENT TEACHING
● Advise patient to report all adverse reactions and to immediately report signs and symptoms of tardive dyskinesia and neuroleptic malignant syndrome.

• Tell patient to avoid extreme heat because drug may interfere with the body's thermoregulatory mechanisms.

• Advise patient to avoid alcohol while taking drug because of increased CNS depression.

• Tell patient to call prescriber if more than four doses are needed within 24 hours.

promethazine hydrochloride
proe-METH-a-zeen

Promethazine Plain, Promethegan

Therapeutic class: Antiemetics
Pharmacologic class: Phenothiazines

AVAILABLE FORMS
Injection: 25 mg/mL, 50 mg/mL
Suppositories: 12.5 mg, 25 mg, 50 mg
Syrup: 6.25 mg/5 mL*
Tablets: 12.5 mg, 25 mg, 50 mg

INDICATIONS & DOSAGES
➤ **Motion sickness**
Adults: 25 mg P.O. or P.R. taken 30 minutes to 1 hour before departure. May repeat dose 8 to 12 hours later p.r.n. Then, 25 mg P.O. b.i.d. on successive travel days.
Children older than age 2: 12.5 to 25 mg P.O. or P.R. 30 minutes to 1 hour before departure. May repeat dose 8 to 12 hours later p.r.n.
➤ **Nausea and vomiting**
Adults: 12.5 to 25 mg P.O., I.M., I.V., or P.R. every 4 to 6 hours p.r.n.
Children older than age 2: 12.5 to 25 mg P.O. or P.R. every 4 to 6 hours p.r.n. Or, 6.25 to 12.5 mg I.M. every 4 to 6 hours p.r.n.
➤ **Rhinitis, allergy symptoms**
Adults: 25 mg P.O. or P.R. at bedtime; or, 12.5 mg P.O. or P.R. t.i.d. Or, 25 mg deep I.M. or I.V. May repeat dose within 2 hours if needed. Use oral dosing as soon as possible.
Children older than age 2: 25 mg P.O. or P.R. at bedtime; or, 6.25 to 12.5 mg P.O. or P.R. t.i.d.
➤ **Nighttime sedation**
Adults: 25 to 50 mg P.O., I.M., or P.R. at bedtime. Or, 25 mg I.V. at bedtime.

Children older than age 2: 12.5 to 25 mg P.O., I.M., or P.R. at bedtime.
➤ **Adjunct to analgesics for routine preoperative or postoperative sedation**
Adults: 25 to 50 mg I.M., P.O., or P.R. Or, 25 mg I.V. with reduced dosage of concomitant analgesic or hypnotic.
Children older than age 2: 0.5 to 1.1 mg/kg P.O., I.M., or P.R.
➤ **Obstetric sedation**
Adults: 50 mg deep I.M. or I.V. in the early stages of labor. When labor is definitely established, may give 25 to 75 mg I.M. or I.V. with an appropriately reduced dose of desired opioid. If necessary, may repeat once or twice at 4-hour intervals. Maximum dose is 100 mg/24 hours.

ADMINISTRATION
P.O.
• Reduce GI distress by giving drug with food or milk.
I.V.
▼ If solution is discolored or contains a precipitate, discard.
▼ Give injection through a free-flowing I.V. line; consider giving over 10 to 15 minutes to minimize risk of phlebitis.
Black Box Warning Be alert for extravasation. Severe chemical irritation and damage can result. ■
🕓 *Alert:* Don't give at a concentration above 25 mg/mL or a rate above 25 mg/minute.
Black Box Warning Don't give I.V. solution subcutaneously or intra-arterially. ■
▼ **Incompatibilities:** Alkaline substances, allopurinol, amphotericin B cholesteryl complex, cefepime, cefotetan, ceftriaxone, dimenhydrinate, doxorubicin liposome, foscarnet, furosemide, heparin, hydromorphone, ketamine, morphine, piperacillin–tazobactam, nalbuphine, some contrast media, parenteral nutrient solutions.
I.M.
Black Box Warning I.M. injection is the preferred parenteral route. Inject deep I.M. into large muscle mass. ■
• Rotate injection sites.
Rectal
• If suppository is too soft, place wrapped in refrigerator for 15 minutes or run under cold water.

P

● Store in refrigerator between 36° and 46° F (2° and 8° C).

ACTION

Phenothiazine derivative that competes with histamine for H_1-receptor sites on effector cells. Prevents, but doesn't reverse, histamine-mediated responses. At high doses, drug also has local anesthetic effects.

Route	Onset	Peak	Duration
P.O.	15–60 min	Unknown	<12 hr
I.V.	3–5 min	Unknown	<12 hr
I.M., P.R.	20 min	Unknown	<12 hr

Half-life: Unknown.

ADVERSE REACTIONS

CNS: drowsiness, sedation, confusion, sleepiness, dizziness, disorientation, extrapyramidal symptoms.
CV: hypotension, hypertension.
EENT: dry mouth, blurred vision.
GI: nausea, vomiting.
GU: urine retention.
Hematologic: *leukopenia, agranulocytosis, thrombocytopenia.*
Metabolic: hyperglycemia.
Respiratory: *respiratory depression, apnea.*
Skin: photosensitivity, rash.

INTERACTIONS

Drug-drug. *Anticholinergics, TCAs:* May increase anticholinergic effects. Avoid using together.
Antipsychotics: May increase risk of neuroleptic malignant syndrome. Monitor patient; discontinue promethazine if interaction is suspected.
CNS depressants: May increase sedation. Use together cautiously. If used together, reduce opiate dose by at least 25% to 50%, and reduce barbiturate dose by at least 50%.
Epinephrine: May block or reverse effects of epinephrine. Use other pressor drugs instead.
Levodopa: May decrease antiparkinsonian action of levodopa. Avoid using together.
Lithium: May reduce GI absorption or enhance renal elimination of lithium. Avoid using together.
MAO inhibitors: May increase extrapyramidal effects. Avoid using together.

Drug-lifestyle. *Alcohol use:* May increase sedation. Discourage use together.
Sun exposure: May cause photosensitivity reactions. Advise patient to avoid extensive sunlight exposure and to use sun block.

EFFECTS ON LAB TEST RESULTS

● May increase Hb level and hematocrit and blood glucose level.
● May decrease WBC, platelet, and granulocyte counts.
● May prevent, reduce, or mask positive result in diagnostic skin test. May cause false-positive or false-negative pregnancy test result. May interfere with blood grouping in the ABO system.
● May cause false-positive or false-negative with urine detection of amphetamine/methamphetamine.

CONTRAINDICATIONS & CAUTIONS

● Contraindicated in patients hypersensitive to drug, those who have experienced adverse reactions to phenothiazines, breast-feeding women, comatose patients, and acutely ill or dehydrated children.
Black Box Warning Contraindicated in children younger than age 2 because of the potential for fatal respiratory depression. Use the lowest effective dose in children older than age 2 and avoid administering with drugs that can cause respiratory depression. ∎
● Use cautiously in patients with a history of seizures and in those taking drugs that affect the seizure threshold as drug can lower the seizure threshold.
● Use cautiously in patients with asthma or pulmonary, hepatic, or CV disease and in those with intestinal obstruction, prostatic hyperplasia, bladder-neck obstruction, angle-closure glaucoma, seizure disorders, CNS depression, and stenosing or peptic ulcerations.
Dialyzable drug: No.
⚠ **Overdose S&S:** Hypotension, respiratory depression, ataxia, athetosis, positive Babinski reflex, unconsciousness, hyperreflexia, hypertonia, dry mouth, fixed dilated pupils, flushing, GI symptoms, seizures, sudden death; hyperexcitability, nightmares (in children).

Reactions in bold italics are *life-threatening.* Interactions may have a *rapid onset* or a ***delayed onset***.

PREGNANCY-LACTATION-REPRODUCTION

- There are no adequate studies in pregnant women. Use only if potential benefit justifies risks to the fetus.
- Use of drug within 2 weeks of delivery may inhibit platelet aggregation in the newborn.
- It isn't known if drug appears in breast milk. Patient should discontinue breast-feeding or discontinue drug.

NURSING CONSIDERATIONS

Black Box Warning Perivascular extravasation, unintentional intra-arterial injection, or intraneuronal or perineuronal infiltration of the drug may result in irritation and tissue damage. Adverse reactions include burning, pain, thrombophlebitis, tissue necrosis, and gangrene. ∎

- Monitor patient for neuroleptic malignant syndrome: altered mental status, autonomic instability, muscle rigidity, and hyperpyrexia.
- Stop drug 4 days before diagnostic skin testing because antihistamines can prevent, reduce, or mask positive skin test response.
- Drug is used as an adjunct to analgesics, usually to increase sedation; it has no analgesic activity.
- *Look alike–sound alike:* Don't confuse promethazine with chlorpromazine or prednisone.

PATIENT TEACHING

- Tell patient to take oral form with food or milk.
- When treating motion sickness, tell patient to take first dose 30 to 60 minutes before travel; dose may be repeated in 8 to 12 hours, if necessary. On succeeding days of travel, patient should take dose upon arising and with evening meal.
- Warn patient to avoid alcohol and hazardous activities that require alertness until CNS effects of drug are known.
- Tell patient to report all adverse reactions promptly.
- Warn patient about possible photosensitivity reactions. Advise use of a sun block.
- Advise patient to report discomfort at I.V. site immediately.

---

propafenone hydrochloride
proe-PAF-a-non

Rythmol, Rythmol SR

Therapeutic class: Antiarrhythmics
Pharmacologic class: Sodium channel antagonists

AVAILABLE FORMS

Capsules (extended-release) ⊜: 225 mg, 325 mg, 425 mg
Tablets (immediate-release): 150 mg, 225 mg, 300 mg

INDICATIONS & DOSAGES

Adjust-a-dose (for all indications): For patients with hepatic impairment, reduce initial dose of immediate-release tablets by 70% to 80%. Reduce dosages in elderly patients.

➤ **To treat life-threatening ventricular arrhythmias such as sustained ventricular tachycardia; to prolong time to recurrence of paroxysmal supraventricular tachycardia (PSVT) and paroxysmal atrial fibrillation or flutter in patients without structural heart disease**
Adults: Initially, 150 mg immediate-release tablet P.O. every 8 hours. May increase dosage every 3 or 4 days to 225 mg every 8 hours. If needed, may increase dosage to 300 mg every 8 hours. Maximum daily dose, 900 mg.

➤ **To prolong time until recurrence of symptomatic atrial fibrillation (AF) in patients with episodic AF who don't have structural heart disease**
Adults: Initially, 150-mg immediate-release tablet P.O. every 8 hours. May increase dosage after 3 to 4 days to 225- to 300-mg immediate-release tablet P.O. every 8 hours. Maximum dosage is 900 mg/day. Or, 225 mg extended-release capsule P.O. every 12 hours. May increase dose after 5 days to 325 mg P.O. every 12 hours. May increase dose to 425 mg every 12 hours.
Adjust-a-dose: Reduce dosage in patients with hepatic impairment, significant QRS complex widening, or second- or third-degree AV block.

P

ADMINISTRATION
P.O.
- Give without regard to food.
- Don't crush or open the extended-release capsules.

ACTION
Reduces inward sodium current in cardiac cells, prolongs refractory period in AV node, and decreases excitability, conduction velocity, and automaticity in cardiac tissue.

Route	Onset	Peak	Duration
P.O. (immediate-release)	Unknown	3½ hr	Unknown
P.O. (extended-release)	Unknown	3–8 hr	Unknown

Half-life: Estimated at 10 to 32 hours.

ADVERSE REACTIONS
CNS: dizziness, anxiety, ataxia, drowsiness, fatigue, headache, insomnia, syncope, tremor, weakness.
CV: *HF, bradycardia, arrhythmias, ventricular tachycardia, PVCs, ventricular fibrillation,* AF, bundle-branch block, angina, chest pain, edema, first-degree AV block, hypotension, prolonged QRS complex, intraventricular conduction delay, palpitations.
EENT: blurred vision.
GI: nausea, vomiting, abdominal pain or cramps, constipation, diarrhea, dyspepsia, anorexia, flatulence, dry mouth, unusual taste.
Musculoskeletal: arthralgia.
Respiratory: dyspnea.
Skin: rash, diaphoresis.

INTERACTIONS
Drug-drug. *Antiarrhythmics, fluoxetine, paroxetine, sertraline:* May increase risk of prolonged QTc interval and arrhythmias. Avoid use together.
Beta blockers (metoprolol, propranolol): May decrease metabolism of these drugs. Adjust dosage of beta blocker as needed and monitor therapy.
Cimetidine: May increase propafenone levels. Monitor patient for adverse effects and toxicity.
*Cyclosporine, **digoxin:*** May increase levels of these drugs, causing toxicity. Monitor

patient closely; dosage adjustment may be necessary.
CYP2D6 inhibitors (paroxetine, ritonavir, sertraline), CYP3A4 inhibitors (erythromycin, ketoconazole, saquinavir): May increase propafenone level. Avoide use together.
Desipramine, haloperidol, imipramine, venlafaxine: May decrease metabolism of these drugs. Monitor patient closely.
Lidocaine: May decrease lidocaine metabolism. Monitor patient for increased CNS adverse effects and lidocaine toxicity.
Local anesthetics: May increase risk of CNS toxicity. Monitor patient closely.
Mexiletine: May decrease mexiletine metabolism, increasing level and adverse reactions. Monitor mexiletine level and patient closely.
Orlistat: May reduce fraction of propafenone available for absorption. Abrupt discontinuation of orlistat can result in severe adverse events. Use together with caution.
Phenobarbital, rifampin: May increase propafenone clearance. Watch for decreased antiarrhythmic effect.
QTc interval–prolonging drugs: Use together may enhance QTc-interval prolongation and risk of ventricular arrhythmias. Monitor patient closely and consider therapy modification.
Quinidine: May decrease propafenone metabolism. Avoid use together.
Ritonavir: May increase propafenone level, causing life-threatening arrhythmias. Avoid using together.
SSRIs, TCAs: May increase risk of cardiac arrhythmias. Avoid use together.
Theophylline: May decrease theophylline metabolism. Monitor theophylline level and ECG closely.
Warfarin: May increase warfarin level. Monitor PT and INR closely, and adjust warfarin dose as needed.
Drug-food. *Grapefruit, grapefruit juice:* May increase drug level. Discourage use together.
Drug-lifestyle. *Smoking:* May increase propafenone level and risk of cardiac arrhythmias.

Reactions in bold italics are *life-threatening*. Interactions may have a *rapid onset* or a *delayed onset*.

EFFECTS ON LAB TEST RESULTS
• May increase alkaline phosphatase, ALT, and AST levels.
• May cause positive ANA titers.

CONTRAINDICATIONS & CAUTIONS
• Contraindicated in patients hypersensitive to drug and in those with severe or uncontrolled HF; cardiogenic shock; SA, AV, or intraventricular disorders of impulse conduction without a pacemaker; bradycardia; Brugada syndrome; marked hypotension; bronchospastic disorders; or electrolyte imbalances.
• Drug has caused new or worsened arrhythmias. ECG monitoring is essential before and during therapy.
• Use cautiously in patients with a history of HF because drug may weaken the contraction of the heart.
• Use cautiously in patients taking other cardiac depressants and in those with hepatic or renal impairment.
• Use cautiously in patients with myasthenia gravis; may cause exacerbation.
Dialyzable drug: Unlikely.
⚠ *Overdose S&S:* Hypotension, somnolence, bradycardia, intra-atrial and intraventricular conduction disturbance.

PREGNANCY-LACTATION-REPRODUCTION
• There are no adequate studies in pregnant women. Use only if potential benefit justifies potential risk to the fetus.
• Drug appears in breast milk. Patient should discontinue breast-feeding or discontinue drug.

NURSING CONSIDERATIONS
Black Box Warning Because of its proarrhythmic effects, propafenone should be reserved for patients with life-threatening ventricular arrhythmias. ■
❸ *Alert:* Perform continuous cardiac monitoring at start of therapy and during dosage adjustments. If PR interval or QRS complex increases by more than 25%, reduce dosage.
• If using with digoxin, frequently monitor ECG and digoxin level.
• Pacing and sensing thresholds of artificial pacemakers may change; monitor pacemaker function.

• Agranulocytosis may develop during first 2 to 3 months of therapy. If patient has an unexplained fever, monitor leukocyte count. WBC count usually normalizes 14 days after drug is discontinued.

PATIENT TEACHING
• Stress importance of taking drug exactly as prescribed.
• Tell patient not to double the dose if he misses one, but to take the next dose at the usual time.
• Tell patient to report all adverse reactions promptly, including fever, sore throat, chills, and other signs and symptoms of infection.
• Tell patient to report palpitations, dizziness, passing out, swelling in arms or legs, trouble breathing, or sudden weight gain.
• Instruct patient to notify prescriber if prolonged diarrhea, sweating, vomiting, or loss of appetite or thirst occurs; these may cause an electrolyte imbalance.
• Tell patient not to crush, chew, or open the extended-release capsules.
• Tell patient to avoid grapefruit juice.

SAFETY ALERT!

propofol
PRO-puh-fole

Diprivan

Therapeutic class: Hypnotics
Pharmacologic class: Phenol derivatives

AVAILABLE FORMS
Injection*: 10 mg/mL in ampules, vials, and prefilled syringes

INDICATIONS & DOSAGES
➤ **To induce general anesthesia**
Adults younger than age 55 classified as American Society of Anesthesiologists (ASA) Physical Status (PS) category I or II: 2 to 2.5 mg/kg I.V. Give in 40-mg boluses every 10 seconds until desired response is achieved.
Children ages 3 to 16 classified as ASA PS I or II: 2.5 to 3.5 mg/kg I.V. over 20 to 30 seconds.
Adjust-a-dose: In geriatric, debilitated, hypovolemic, or ASA PS III or IV patients,

give half the usual induction dose, in 20-mg boluses, every 10 seconds. For cardiac anesthesia, give 20 mg (0.5 to 1.5 mg/kg) every 10 seconds until desired response is achieved. For neurosurgical patients, give 20 mg (1 to 2 mg/kg) every 10 seconds until desired response is achieved.

➤ **To maintain anesthesia**
Healthy adults younger than age 55: 0.1 to 0.2 mg/kg/minute (6 to 12 mg/kg/hour) I.V. Or, 20- to 50-mg intermittent boluses, p.r.n.
Healthy children ages 2 months to 16 years: Initially, 200 to 300 mcg/kg/minute for 30 minutes, then 125 to 150 mcg/kg/minute (7.5 to 9 mg/kg/hour) I.V. titrated to achieve desired clinical effect. Younger children may require higher maintenance infusion rates than older children.
Adjust-a-dose: In elderly, debilitated, hypovolemic, or ASA PS III or IV patients, give half the usual maintenance dose (0.05 to 0.1 mg/kg/minute or 3 to 6 mg/kg/hour). For cardiac anesthesia with secondary opioid, 100 to 150 mcg/kg/minute; low dose with primary opioid, 50 to 100 mcg/kg/minute. For neurosurgical patients, 100 to 200 mcg/kg/minute (6 to 12 mg/kg/hour).

➤ **Monitored anesthesia care**
Healthy adults younger than age 55: Initially, 100 to 150 mcg/kg/minute (6 to 9 mg/kg/hour) I.V. for 3 to 5 minutes or a slow injection of 0.5 mg/kg over 3 to 5 minutes. For maintenance dose, give infusion of 25 to 75 mcg/kg/minute (1.5 to 4.5 mg/kg/hour) for first 10 to 15 minutes, then reduce dosage to 25 to 50 mcg/kg/minute or incremental 10- or 20-mg boluses.
Adjust-a-dose: In elderly, debilitated, or ASA PS III or IV patients, give 80% of usual adult maintenance dose. Don't use rapid bolus.

➤ **To sedate intubated ICU patients**
Adults: Initially, 5 mcg/kg/minute (0.3 mg/kg/hour) I.V. for 5 minutes. Increments of 5 to 10 mcg/kg/minute (0.3 to 0.6 mg/kg/hour) over 5 to 10 minutes may be used until desired sedation is achieved. Maintenance rate, 5 to 50 mcg/kg/minute (0.3 to 3 mg/kg/hour).

ADMINISTRATION
I.V.
▼ Maintain aseptic technique when handling solution. Drug can support growth of microorganisms; don't use if solution might be contaminated. Don't access vial more than once or use on multiple patients.
▼ Shake well.
▼ Dilute only with D_5W. Don't dilute to less than 2 mg/mL.
▼ Don't use if emulsion shows evidence of separation.
▼ Don't infuse through a filter with a pore size smaller than 5 microns. Give via larger veins in arms to decrease injection-site pain.
▼ Titrate drug daily to maintain minimum effective level. Allow 3 to 5 minutes between dosage adjustments to assess effects.
▼ Discard tubing and unused portions of drug after 12 hours.
▼ Store between 40° and 77° F (4° and 25° C); don't freeze. Protect from light.
▼ **Incompatibilities:** Other I.V. drugs, blood and plasma.

ACTION
Unknown. Rapid-acting I.V. sedative-hypnotic.

Route	Onset	Peak	Duration
I.V.	<40 sec	Unknown	10–15 min

Half-life: Initial (distribution) phase, about 2 to 10 minutes; second (redistribution) phase, 21 to 70 minutes; terminal (elimination) phase, 1½ to 31 hours.

ADVERSE REACTIONS
CNS: dystonic or choreiform movement.
CV: *bradycardia,* hypotension, hypertension, decreased cardiac output.
Metabolic: hyperlipidemia.
Respiratory: *apnea, respiratory acidosis.*
Skin: rash, pruritus.
Other: burning or stinging at injection site.

INTERACTIONS
Drug-drug. *Inhaled anesthetics (enflurane, halothane, isoflurane), opioids (alfentanil, fentanyl, meperidine, morphine), sedatives (barbiturates, benzodiazepines, chloral hydrate, droperidol):* May increase anesthetic

---

Reactions in bold italics are ***life-threatening.*** Interactions may have a *rapid onset* or a ***delayed onset.***

and sedative effects and further decrease BP and cardiac output. Monitor patient closely.

EFFECTS ON LAB TEST RESULTS
● May increase serum triglyceride levels.

CONTRAINDICATIONS & CAUTIONS
● Contraindicated in patients hypersensitive to drug or its components (including egg lecithin, soybean oil, and glycerol) and in those unable to undergo general anesthesia or sedation.
● Drug isn't recommended for obstetric surgery, including cesarean deliveries, because of potential neonatal depression.
● Use cautiously in patients who are hemodynamically unstable or who have seizures, disorders of lipid metabolism, or increased ICP.
Dialyzable drug: Unknown.
⚠ *Overdose S&S:* Cardiorespiratory depression.

PREGNANCY-LACTATION-REPRODUCTION
● There are no adequate studies in pregnant women. Use only if clearly needed.
● Drug isn't recommended for obstetric uses as it may cause neonatal depression.
● Drug appears in breast milk. Avoid use in breast-feeding women.

NURSING CONSIDERATIONS
● If drug is used for prolonged sedation in ICU, urine may turn green.
● For general anesthesia or monitored anesthesia care sedation, trained staff not involved in the surgical or diagnostic procedure should give drug. For ICU sedation, persons skilled in managing critically ill patients and trained in cardiopulmonary resuscitation and airway management should give drug.
● Continuously monitor vital signs.
● *Alert:* The FDA issued an alert after receiving reports of chills, fever, and body aches in several clusters of patients shortly after patients received propofol for sedation or general anesthesia. Various lots of the drug were tested, but no toxins, bacteria, or other signs of contamination were found. The FDA advises all health care providers to carefully follow the handling and use sections of the prescribing information for this

drug. They recommend that all patients be evaluated for possible reactions following use of the drug, and that anyone experiencing signs of acute febrile reactions be evaluated for possible bacterial sepsis. They ask that any adverse events following the use of propofol be reported to MedWatch.
● Monitor patient at risk for hyperlipidemia for elevated triglyceride levels.
● Drug contains 0.1 g of fat (1.1 kcal)/mL. Reduce other lipid products if given together.
● Some formulations contain ethylenediaminetetraacetic acid, a strong metal chelator. Consider supplemental zinc during prolonged therapy and in patients predisposed to zinc deficiency (those with burns, sepsis, or diarrhea).
● When giving drug in the ICU, assess patient's CNS function daily to determine minimum dose needed.
● Stop drug gradually to prevent abrupt awakening and increased agitation.
● Drug may be misused. Manage drug to prevent risk of diversion.
● *Look alike–sound alike:* Don't confuse Diprivan with Ditropan or Diflucan.

PATIENT TEACHING
● Advise patient that performance of activities requiring mental alertness may be impaired for some time after drug use.
● Tell patient that abnormal dreams or anesthesia awareness may occur.

SAFETY ALERT!

propranolol hydrochloride
proe-PRAN-oh-lol

Hemangeol, Inderal🐾, Inderal LA🐾, InnoPran XL

Therapeutic class: Antihypertensives
Pharmacologic class: Nonselective beta blockers

AVAILABLE FORMS
Capsules (extended-release) 🚫*:* 60 mg, 80 mg, 120 mg, 160 mg
Injection: 1 mg/mL

Oral solution: 4 mg/mL, 4.28 mg/mL, 8 mg/mL
Tablets: 10 mg, 20 mg, 40 mg, 60 mg, 80 mg

INDICATIONS & DOSAGES

➤ **Angina pectoris**
Adults: Total daily doses of 80 to 320 mg (immediate-release) P.O. in two to four divided doses. Or, one 80-mg extended-release capsule daily. Increase dosage at 3- to 7-day intervals until optimal response is obtained or a maximum of 320 mg P.O. daily has been given.

➤ **To decrease risk of death after MI**
Adults: Initially, 40 mg P.O. t.i.d. After 1 month, titrate to 60 to 80 mg t.i.d. as tolerated. Maintenance dose is 180 to 240 mg/day in divided doses b.i.d., t.i.d., or q.i.d.

➤ **Supraventricular, ventricular, and atrial arrhythmias; tachyarrhythmias caused by excessive catecholamine action during anesthesia, hyperthyroidism, or pheochromocytoma**
Adults: 1 to 3 mg by slow I.V. push, not to exceed 1 mg/minute. After 3 mg have been given, another dose may be given in 2 minutes; subsequent doses, no sooner than every 4 hours. Usual maintenance dose is 10 to 30 mg P.O. t.i.d. or q.i.d.

➤ **Hypertension**
Adults: Initially, 80 mg P.O. daily in two divided doses or extended-release form once daily. Increase at 3- to 7-day intervals to maximum daily dose of 640 mg. Usual maintenance dose is 120 to 240 mg daily or 120 to 160 mg daily as extended-release. For InnoPran XL, dose is 80 mg P.O. once daily at bedtime. Give consistently with or without food. Adjust to maximum of 120 mg daily if needed. Full effects are seen in about 2 to 3 weeks.

➤ **Essential tremor**
Adults: 40 mg (tablets or oral solution) P.O. b.i.d. Usual maintenance dose is 120 to 320 mg daily in three divided doses.

➤ **Hypertrophic subaortic stenosis**
Adults: 20 to 40 mg P.O. t.i.d. or q.i.d., or 80 to 160 mg extended-release capsules once daily.

➤ **Adjunctive therapy in pheochromocytoma**

Adults: 60 mg P.O. daily in divided doses with an alpha blocker 3 days before surgery.

➤ **Prevention of migraine**
Adults: Initially, 80 mg P.O. daily in divided doses. May increase to 160 to 240 mg/day.

➤ **Proliferating infantile hemangioma requiring systemic therapy (Hemangeol)**
Infants ages 5 weeks to 5 months: Initially, 0.63 mg/kg P.O. b.i.d. for 1 week. Increase to 1.1 mg/kg P.O. b.i.d. after 1 week. Increase to maintenance dose of 1.7 mg/kg P.O. b.i.d. after 2 weeks of treatment and maintain for 6 months. Administer doses at least 9 hours apart during or after feeding.
Adjust-a-dose: Readjust dosage periodically for changes in child's weight.

➤ **Gastroesophageal varices ◆**
Adults: Initially, 20 mg P.O. b.i.d. Titrate to maximum tolerable dose.

ADMINISTRATION
P.O.
● Give immediate-release tablets on an empty stomach. Give extended-release capsules with or without food, but patient should always take consistently (with or without food). Food may increase absorption of propranolol.
● Compliance may be improved by giving drug twice daily or as extended-release capsules. Check with prescriber.
● Check BP and apical pulse before giving drug. If hypotension or extremes in pulse rate occur, withhold drug and notify prescriber.
● Monitor HR and BP for 2 hours after first dose and when increasing Hemangeol dosage.
● Give Hemangeol during or right after a feeding. Skip dose if child isn't eating or is vomiting. Don't shake before use.
● Give Hemangeol directly into child's mouth using the oral dosing syringe. If needed, may dilute with a small quantity of milk or fruit juice and give in baby's bottle.
● Don't substitute extended-release form for immediate-release on a milligram-for-milligram basis. Retitration may be necessary.
I.V.
▼ For direct injection, give into a large vessel or into the tubing of a free-flowing,

---

compatible I.V. solution; don't give by continuous I.V. infusion.

▼ Drug is compatible with D_5W, half-NSS, NSS, and lactated Ringer solution.

▼ Infusion rate shouldn't exceed 1 mg/minute.

▼ Double-check dose and route. I.V. doses are much smaller than oral doses.

▼ Monitor BP, ECG, central venous pressure, and HR and rhythm frequently, especially during I.V. administration. If patient develops severe hypotension, notify prescriber; a vasopressor may be prescribed.

▼ For overdose, give I.V. isoproterenol, I.V. atropine, or glucagon; refractory cases may require a pacemaker.

▼ **Incompatibilities:** Amphotericin B, diazoxide.

ACTION

Reduces cardiac oxygen demand by blocking catecholamine-induced increases in HR, BP, and force of myocardial contraction. Drug depresses renin secretion and prevents vasodilation of cerebral arteries.

Route	Onset	Peak	Duration
P.O.	30 min	1–4 hr	12 hr
P.O. (Hemangeol)	Rapid	≤2 hr	Unknown
P.O. (extended-release)	Unknown	6–14 hr	24 hr
I.V.	Immediate	1 min	5 min

Half-life: About 3 to 6 hours; 8 hours for InnoPran XL; 3½ hours for Hemangeol.

ADVERSE REACTIONS

CNS: fatigue, lethargy, fever, vivid dreams, hallucinations, mental depression, lightheadedness, dizziness, insomnia.
CV: hypotension, *bradycardia, HF, intensification of AV block,* intermittent claudication.
GI: abdominal cramping, constipation, diarrhea, nausea, vomiting.
Hematologic: *agranulocytosis.*
Respiratory: *bronchospasm.*
Skin: rash.

INTERACTIONS

Drug-drug. *Aminophylline:* May antagonize beta-blocking effects of propranolol. Use together cautiously.

Amiodarone, diltiazem, verapamil: May cause hypotension, bradycardia, and increased depressant effect on myocardium. Use together cautiously.
Cardiac glycosides: May reduce the positive inotrope effect of the glycoside. Monitor patient for clinical effect.
Cimetidine, ciprofloxacin, fluconazole, fluoxetine, paroxetine: May inhibit metabolism of propranolol. Watch for increased beta-blocking effect.
Epinephrine: May cause severe vasoconstriction. Monitor BP and observe patient carefully.
Glucagon, isoproterenol: May antagonize propranolol effect. May be used therapeutically and in emergencies.
Haloperidol: May cause cardiac arrest. Avoid using together.
Insulin, oral antidiabetics: May alter requirements for these drugs in previously stabilized diabetics. Monitor patient for hypoglycemia.
Lidocaine: May reduce clearance of lidocaine. Monitor lidocaine level closely.
Phenothiazines (chlorpromazine, thioridazine): May increase risk of serious adverse reactions to either drug. Use with thioridazine is contraindicated. If chlorpromazine must be used, monitor patient's pulse and BP; decrease propranolol dose as needed.
Propafenone, quinidine: May increase propranolol level. Monitor cardiac function, and adjust propranolol dose as needed.
Theophylline derivatives: May decrease theophylline clearance by 30% to 52% and diminish their bronchodilatory effect. Consider therapy modification.
Drug-herb. *Betel palm:* May decrease temperature-elevating effects and enhanced CNS effects. Discourage use together.
Ma huang: May decrease antihypertensive effects. Discourage use together.
Drug-lifestyle. *Alcohol use:* May increase or decrease propranolol level. Discourage alcohol use.
Smoking: May decrease propranolol level. Monitor clinical response and adjust dosage as needed.

P

EFFECTS ON LAB TEST RESULTS
- May increase T_4, BUN, transaminase, alkaline phosphatase, potassium, and LDH levels. May decrease T_3 level.
- May decrease granulocyte count.

CONTRAINDICATIONS & CAUTIONS
Black Box Warning Abrupt withdrawal of drug may cause exacerbation of angina or MI. To discontinue drug, gradually reduce dosage over 1 to 2 weeks. If angina worsens or acute coronary insufficiency develops, resume therapy at least temporarily. Because CAD may be unrecognized, don't discontinue drug abruptly, even when taken for other indications. ■

- Contraindicated in patients with known hypersensitivity to drug, bronchial asthma, sinus bradycardia and heart block greater than first-degree, cardiogenic shock, and overt and decompensated HF (unless failure is secondary to a tachyarrhythmia that can be treated with propranolol).
- Hemangeol is contraindicated in infants weighing less than 2 kg, premature infants with corrected age younger than 5 weeks, infants with an HR less than 80 beats/minute or BP less than 50/30 mm Hg, and in infants with pheochromocytoma or history of bronchospasm.
- Use cautiously in patients with hepatic or renal impairment, Wolff-Parkinson-White syndrome, nonallergic bronchospastic diseases, or hepatic disease and in those taking other antihypertensives.
- Use cautiously in patients who have diabetes mellitus because drug masks some symptoms of hypoglycemia.
- In patients with thyrotoxicosis, use drug cautiously because it may mask the signs and symptoms. Abrupt withdrawal may exacerbate symptoms of hyperthyroidism, including thyroid storm.
- Elderly patients may experience enhanced adverse reactions and may need dosage adjustment.
Dialyzable drug: No.
⚠ *Overdose S&S:* Bradycardia, cardiac failure, hypotension, bronchospasm.

PREGNANCY-LACTATION-REPRODUCTION
- There are no adequate studies in pregnant women. Use only if potential benefit justifies potential risk to the fetus.
- Drug is associated with fetal intrauterine growth retardation and neonatal bradycardia, hypoglycemia, and respiratory depression. If drug is used during pregnancy, ensure adequate monitoring of infants is available at birth.
- Drug appears in breast milk, with peak concentrations occurring 2 to 3 hours after oral doses. Use cautiously in breast-feeding women. Monitor infants for signs and symptoms of beta blockade.

NURSING CONSIDERATIONS
- Drug masks common signs and symptoms of shock and hypoglycemia.
- Monitor black patients for expected therapeutic effects; dosage adjustments may be necessary.
🔔 *Alert:* Don't stop drug before surgery for pheochromocytoma. Before any surgical procedure, tell anesthesiologist that patient is receiving propranolol.
- *Look alike–sound alike:* Don't confuse propranolol with prasugrel or Pravachol. Don't confuse Inderal with Isordil, Adderall, or Imuran.

PATIENT TEACHING
- Caution patient to continue taking drug as prescribed, even if feeling well, and to promptly report adverse reactions.
- Instruct patient to take immediate-release product without food and extended-release product consistently with or without food.
- Advise patient that propranolol may interfere with glaucoma screening because it can reduce IOP.
- Teach caregiver to skip Hemangeol dose if child isn't eating or is vomiting.
Black Box Warning Caution patient not to stop drug without advice from prescriber because abruptly stopping drug can worsen chest pain or cause an MI. ■
- Advise patient to avoid smoking and alcohol.

pyridostigmine bromide
peer-id-oh-STIG-meen

Mestinon*, Mestinon-SR♣, Regonol*

Therapeutic class: Muscle stimulants
Pharmacologic class: Cholinesterase inhibitors

AVAILABLE FORMS
Injection: 5 mg/mL
Syrup: 60 mg/5 mL*
Tablets: 60 mg
Tablets (extended-release) ⓓ: 180 mg

INDICATIONS & DOSAGES
Adjust-a-dose (for all indications): Smaller doses may be required in patients with renal disease. Adjust dosage to achieve desired effect.
➤ **Antidote for nondepolarizing neuromuscular blockers**
Adults: 0.1 to 0.25 mg/kg I.V. Immediately before or with dose, also give atropine sulfate 0.6 to 1.2 mg I.V. or an equipotent dose of glycopyrrolate.
➤ **Myasthenia gravis**
Adults: 60 to 120 mg immediate-release P.O. every 3 or 4 hours. Average dosage is 600 mg daily, but dosages up to 1,500 mg daily may be needed. Dosage must be adjusted for each patient, based on response and tolerance. Or, 180 to 540 mg extended-release tablets P.O. daily or b.i.d., with at least 6 hours between doses.

ADMINISTRATION
P.O.
● Don't crush extended-release tablets.
● If patient has trouble swallowing, give syrup form. If patient can't tolerate sweet flavor, give over ice chips.
I.V.
⊕ *Alert:* Drug should only be administered by individuals familiar with its actions, characteristics, and hazards.
▼ Don't use solution if it contains particulate matter or is discolored.
▼ Position patient to ease breathing. Keep atropine injection available, and be prepared to give it immediately.

▼ Monitor vital signs frequently, especially respirations. Provide respiratory support as needed.
▼ Give injection no faster than 1 mg/minute. Rapid infusion may cause bradycardia and seizures.
▼ **Incompatibilities:** Alkaline solutions.

ACTION
Inhibits acetylcholinesterase, blocking destruction of acetylcholine from the parasympathetic and somatic efferent nerves. Acetylcholine accumulates, promoting increased stimulation of the receptors.

Route	Onset	Peak	Duration
P.O.	20–30 min	2 hr	3–6 hr
P.O. (extended-release)	30–60 min	1–2 hr	6–12 hr
I.V.	2–5 min	Unknown	2–4 hr

Half-life: 1 to 3 hours, depending on route.

ADVERSE REACTIONS
CNS: headache with high doses, weakness, syncope.
CV: *bradycardia, cardiac arrest,* hypotension, thrombophlebitis.
EENT: miosis, rhinorrhea.
GI: nausea, vomiting, abdominal cramps, diarrhea, excessive salivation, increased peristalsis.
GU: urinary frequency, urinary urgency.
Musculoskeletal: muscle cramps, muscle fasciculations, muscle weakness, tingling in extremities.
Respiratory: *bronchospasm, bronchoconstriction,* increased bronchial secretions.
Skin: rash, diaphoresis.

INTERACTIONS
Drug-drug. *Anticholinergics, atropine, corticosteroids, general or local anesthetics, magnesium, procainamide, quinidine:* May antagonize cholinergic effects. Observe patient for lack of drug effect.
Beta blockers: May increase bradycardia risk. Monitor therapy.
Ganglionic blockers: May increase risk of hypotension. Monitor patient closely.
Succinylcholine: May prolong the phase I block of the depolarizing muscle relaxant. Avoid using together.

P

EFFECTS ON LAB TEST RESULTS
None reported.

CONTRAINDICATIONS & CAUTIONS
• Contraindicated in patients hypersensitive to anticholinesterases or bromides and in those with mechanical obstruction of the intestinal or urinary tract.
• Use cautiously in patients with bronchial asthma, bradycardia, arrhythmias, epilepsy, recent coronary occlusion, vagotonia, renal impairment, hyperthyroidism, glaucoma, or peptic ulcer.
• Use cautiously in patients taking beta blockers for hypertension or glaucoma.
Dialyzable drug: Unknown.

PREGNANCY-LACTATION-REPRODUCTION
• Drug may cross placental barrier. Use during pregnancy only if potential benefits justify potential maternal and fetal hazards.
• Drug appears in breast milk. Use cautiously in breast-feeding women.

NURSING CONSIDERATIONS
• Stop all other cholinergics before giving this drug.
• Monitor and document patient's response after each dose. Optimum dosage is difficult to judge.
❸ *Alert:* Regonol contains benzyl ethanol preservative, which may cause toxicity in neonates if given in high doses.
• *Look alike–sound alike:* Don't confuse pyridostigmine with physostigmine. Don't confuse Regonol with Reglan or Renagel.

PATIENT TEACHING
• When giving drug for myasthenia gravis, stress importance of taking exactly as prescribed, on time, in evenly spaced doses. For extended-release tablets, tell patient to take at same time each day, at least 6 hours apart.
• Advise patient not to crush or chew extended-release tablets.
• Explain that patient may have to take drug for life.
• Advise patient to wear or carry medical identification that identifies his myasthenia gravis.

quetiapine fumarate
kwe-TIE-ah-peen

Seroquel✿, Seroquel XR

Therapeutic class: Antipsychotics
Pharmacologic class: Dibenzothiazepine derivatives

AVAILABLE FORMS
Tablets: 25 mg, 50 mg, 100 mg, 150 mg, 200 mg, 300 mg, 400 mg
Tablets (extended-release) ⓄⓉⒸ: 50 mg, 150 mg, 200 mg, 300 mg, 400 mg

INDICATIONS & DOSAGES
➤ **Schizophrenia**
Adults: Initially, 25 mg (immediate-release) P.O. b.i.d., with increases in increments of 25 to 50 mg b.i.d. or t.i.d. on days 2 and 3, as tolerated. Target range is 300 to 400 mg daily divided into two or three doses by day 4. Further dosage adjustments, if indicated, should occur at intervals of not less than 2 days. Dosage can be increased or decreased by 25 to 50 mg b.i.d. Effect generally occurs at 150 to 750 mg daily. Maximum dosage is 750 mg/day.
  Or, initially, 300 mg/day extended-release tablets P.O. once daily, preferably in the evening. Titrate within a dose range of 400 to 800 mg/day, depending on the response and tolerance of the individual. Increase at intervals as short as 1 day and in increments of up to 300 mg/day.
Adolescents ages 13 to 17: For immediate-release tablets, usual dosage is 400 to 800 mg/day, which may be divided into three doses per day depending on response and tolerability; maximum dosage, 800 mg/day. Initially, 25 mg P.O. b.i.d. on day 1; 50 mg b.i.d. on day 2; 100 mg b.i.d. on day 3; 150 mg b.i.d. on day 4; and 200 mg b.i.d. on day 5. Adjust dosage by no more than 100 mg/day. For extended-release tablets, usual dosage is 400 to 800 mg/day; maximum dosage, 800 mg/day. Initially, 50 mg/day P.O. on day 1; 100 mg/day on day 2; 200 mg/day on day 3; 300 mg/day on day 4; and 400 mg/day on day 5. Make adjustments in increments of no greater than 100 mg/day.

Adjust-a-dose: Elderly patients: For both formulations, use slow titration and regular monitoring. Begin extended-release formula at 50 mg/day; may increase dosage in increments of 50 mg/day depending on clinical response and tolerance. In patients with hepatic impairment, initial dose (immediate-release) is 25 mg daily. Increase daily in increments of 25 to 50 mg daily to an effective dose. Or, begin extended-release formula at 50 mg/day; may increase dosage in increments of 50 mg/day depending on clinical response and tolerance. For debilitated patients and those with hypotension, consider lower dosages and slower adjustment.

➤ **Monotherapy and adjunctive therapy with lithium or divalproex for the short-term treatment of acute manic episodes associated with bipolar I disorder; adjunctive maintenance therapy with lithium or divalproex**

Adults: Initially, 50 mg (immediate-release) P.O. b.i.d. on day 1; 100 mg b.i.d. on day 2; 150 mg b.i.d. on day 3; and 200 mg b.i.d. on day 4. Further dosage adjustments after day 4 should be no greater than 200 mg daily up to 800 mg daily. Usual dose is 400 to 800 mg daily. For maintenance therapy with lithium or divalproex, continue treatment at the dosage required to maintain symptom remission.

Or, start with 300 mg (extended-release) P.O. on day 1 and 600 mg P.O. on day 2 once daily in the evening. Dosage may be adjusted between 400 and 800 mg beginning on day 3.

Adjust-a-dose: Elderly patients: For immediate-release formula, use slow titration and regular monitoring. Or, begin extended-release formula at 50 mg/day; may increase dosage in increments of 50 mg/day depending on clinical response and tolerance. In patients with hepatic impairment, initial dose (immediate-release) is 25 mg daily. Increase daily in increments of 25 to 50 mg daily to an effective dose. Or, begin extended-release formula at 50 mg/day; may increase dosage in increments of 50 mg/day depending on clinical response and tolerance. For debilitated patients and those with hypotension, consider lower dosages and slower adjustment.

➤ **Bipolar I disorder, acute manic episodes (immediate-release)**

Children ages 10 to 17: Total daily dosage for initial 5 days of therapy is 50 mg P.O. on day 1, then 100 mg on day 2, then 200 mg on day 3, then 300 mg on day 4, and 400 mg on day 5, usually given in divided doses b.i.d. After day 5, adjust dosage within recommended range of 400 to 600 mg/day.

➤ **Depression associated with bipolar disorder**

Adults: Initially, 50 mg P.O. once daily at bedtime; increase on day 2 to 100 mg; increase on day 3 to 200 mg; increase on day 4 to maintenance dose of 300 mg.

Adjust-a-dose: Elderly patients: For immediate-release formula, use slow titration and regular monitoring. Or, begin extended-release formula at 50 mg/day; may increase dosage in increments of 50 mg/day depending on clinical response and tolerance. In patients with hepatic impairment, initial dose (immediate-release) is 25 mg daily. Increase daily in increments of 25 to 50 mg daily to an effective dose. Or, begin extended-release formula at 50 mg/day; may increase dosage in increments of 50 mg/day depending on clinical response and tolerance. For debilitated patients and those with hypotension, consider lower dosages and slower adjustment.

➤ **Major depressive disorder, adjunctive therapy**

Adults: 50 mg P.O. (extended-release) once daily in the evening. On day 3, may increase dosage to 150 mg P.O. once daily in the evening. Dosages ranging from 150 to 300 mg/day have proved effective.

ADMINISTRATION
P.O.
• Don't break or crush extended-release tablets.
• Give drug without regard for food; give extended-release tablets without food or with a light meal (about 300 calories).
• Patients with schizophrenia who are currently being treated with divided doses of the immediate-release form may be switched to extended-release tablets at the equivalent total daily dose taken once daily. Individual dosage adjustments may

be necessary. Those requiring less than 200 mg/dose should remain on the immediate-release form.

ACTION

Blocks dopamine and serotonin 5-HT$_2$ receptors. Its action may be mediated through this antagonism.

Route	Onset	Peak	Duration
P.O.	Unknown	1½ hr	Unknown
P.O. (extended-release)	Unknown	6 hr	Unknown

Half-life: 6 hours; extended-release, 7 to 12 hours.

ADVERSE REACTIONS

CNS: dizziness, headache, somnolence, *neuroleptic malignant syndrome, seizures,* hypertonia, dysarthria, asthenia, agitation, extrapyramidal reaction.
CV: orthostatic hypotension, tachycardia, palpitations, peripheral edema.
EENT: ear pain, epistaxis, nasal congestion, pharyngitis, rhinitis.
GI: dry mouth, dyspepsia, abdominal pain, constipation, nausea, anorexia, xerostomia, vomiting.
Hematologic: *leukopenia.*
Metabolic: weight gain, hyperglycemia.
Musculoskeletal: back pain.
Respiratory: increased cough, dyspnea.
Skin: rash, diaphoresis.
Other: flulike syndrome.

INTERACTIONS

Drug-drug. *Antihypertensives:* May increase effects of antihypertensives. Monitor BP.
Carbamazepine, glucocorticoids, phenobarbital, phenytoin, rifampin, thioridazine: May increase quetiapine clearance. May need to adjust quetiapine dosage.
CNS depressants: May increase CNS effects. Use together cautiously.
Dopamine agonists, levodopa: May antagonize the effects of these drugs. Monitor patient.
Erythromycin, fluconazole, itraconazole, ketoconazole: May decrease quetiapine clearance. Use together cautiously.
Lorazepam: May decrease lorazepam clearance. Monitor patient for increased CNS effects.

Black Box Warning *Opioids:* May cause slow or difficult breathing, sedation, and death. Avoid use together. If use together is necessary, limit dosage and duration of each drug to minimum necessary for desired effect. ■
QTc interval–prolonging drugs: May enhance QTc-interval prolongation and risk of ventricular arrhythmias. Consider therapy modification.
Drug-herb. *St. John's wort:* May increase risk of serotonin syndrome and decrease quetiapine serum concentration. Consider therapy modification.
Drug-lifestyle. *Alcohol use:* May increase CNS effects. Discourage use together.

EFFECTS ON LAB TEST RESULTS

● May increase liver enzyme, cholesterol, triglyceride, and glucose levels. May decrease T$_4$ and TSH levels.
● May decrease WBC count.
● May cause false-positive results in urine enzyme immunoassays for methadone and TCAs.

CONTRAINDICATIONS & CAUTIONS

● Contraindicated in patients hypersensitive to drug or its ingredients.
Black Box Warning Opioids should only be prescribed with benzodiazepines or other CNS depressants to patients for whom alternative treatment options are inadequate. ■
● Use cautiously in patients with CV disease, cerebrovascular disease, conditions that predispose to hypotension, a history of seizures or conditions that lower the seizure threshold, and conditions in which core body temperature may be elevated.
● Use cautiously in patients at risk for aspiration pneumonia.
● Drug isn't approved for use in children younger than age 10 (immediate-release or extended-release) due to increased risk of suicidal thoughts and behavior in children, adolescents, and young adults (younger than age 24).
Dialyzable drug: Unknown.
⚠ *Overdose S&S:* Drowsiness, hypotension, sedation, tachycardia, hypokalemia, QTc-interval prolongation, first-degree heart block.

Reactions in bold italics are *life-threatening.* Interactions may have a *rapid onset* or a *delayed onset.*

PREGNANCY-LACTATION-REPRODUCTION

⚠ *Alert:* Neonates exposed to antipsychotics during the third trimester are at risk for developing extrapyramidal signs and symptoms (repetitive muscle movements of the face and body) and withdrawal signs and symptoms (agitation, abnormally increased or decreased muscle tone, tremors, sleepiness, severe difficulty breathing, difficulty feeding) after delivery. Use in pregnancy only if potential benefit justifies fetal risk.

• Women exposed to drug during pregnancy should be enrolled in the National Pregnancy Registry for Atypical Antipsychotics (1-866-961-2388).

• Drug appears in breast milk. Breastfeeding isn't recommended.

NURSING CONSIDERATIONS

• Dispense lowest appropriate quantity of drug to reduce risk of overdose.

Black Box Warning Drug isn't indicated for use in elderly patients with dementia-related psychosis because of increased risk of death from CV disease or infection. ∎

⚠ *Alert:* Watch for evidence of neuroleptic malignant syndrome (extrapyramidal effects, hyperthermia, autonomic disturbance), which is rare but deadly.

• Monitor patient for tardive dyskinesia, which may occur after prolonged use. It may not appear until months or years later and may disappear spontaneously or persist for life, despite ending drug.

• Hyperglycemia may occur in patients taking drug. Monitor patients with diabetes regularly.

• Monitor patient for weight gain.

⚠ *Alert:* Monitor patient for symptoms of metabolic syndrome (significant weight gain and increased BMI, hypertension, hyperglycemia, hypercholesterolemia, and hypertriglyceridemia).

• Drug use may cause cataract formation.

• Obtain baseline ophthalmologic examination and reassess every 6 months.

Black Box Warning Drug may increase the risk of suicidal thinking and behavior in children, adolescents, and young adults ages 18 to 24, especially during the first few months of treatment, especially in those with major depressive or other psychiatric disorder. ∎

• *Look alike–sound alike:* Don't confuse Seroquel with Serzone.

PATIENT TEACHING

Black Box Warning Caution patient or caregiver of patient taking an opioid with a benzodiazepine, CNS depressant, or alcohol to seek immediate medical attention if patient experiences dizziness, light-headedness, extreme sleepiness, slowed or difficult breathing, or unresponsiveness. ∎

• Warn patient about risk of dizziness when standing up quickly. The risk is greatest during the 3- to 5-day period of first dosage adjustment, when resuming treatment, and when increasing dosages.

• Tell patient to avoid becoming overheated or dehydrated.

• Warn patient to avoid activities that require mental alertness until effects of drug are known, especially during first dosage adjustment or dosage increases.

• Remind patient to have an eye examination at start of therapy and every 6 months during therapy to check for cataracts.

• Tell patient to notify prescriber about other prescription or OTC drugs he's taking or plans to take.

• Tell female patient of childbearing potential to notify prescriber about planned, suspected, or known pregnancy.

• Advise female patient not to breast-feed during therapy.

• Advise patient to avoid alcohol while taking drug.

• Tell patient to take immediate-release drug with or without food.

• Tell patient not to crush, chew, or break extended-release tablets.

• Tell patient to take extended-release tablets once daily without food or with a light meal, preferably in the evening.

• Tell patient and caregivers to report all adverse reactions and to be alert for fever, muscle rigidity, repetitive muscle movements of the face, anxiety, agitation, panic attacks, insomnia, irritability, hostility, aggressiveness, impulsivity, motor restlessness, hypomania, mania, other unusual changes in behavior, worsening of depression, and suicidal thoughts.

• Tell patient not to stop medication abruptly.

Q

---

quinapril hydrochloride
KWIN-ah-pril

Accupril⬧

Therapeutic class: Antihypertensives
Pharmacologic class: ACE inhibitors

AVAILABLE FORMS
Tablets: 5 mg, 10 mg, 20 mg, 40 mg

INDICATIONS & DOSAGES
➤ **Hypertension**
Adults: Initially, 10 to 20 mg P.O. daily.
Dosage may be adjusted based on patient
response at intervals of about 2 weeks. Most
patients are controlled at 20, 40, or 80 mg
daily as a single dose or in two divided
doses. If patient is taking a diuretic, start
therapy with 5 mg daily.
Elderly patients: For patients older than age
65, start therapy at 10 mg P.O. daily.
Adjust-a-dose: For adults with CrCl over
60 mL/minute, initially, 10 mg maximum
daily; for CrCl of 30 to 60 mL/minute, 5 mg;
for CrCl of 10 to 30 mL/minute, 2.5 mg.
➤ **HF**
Adults: 5 mg P.O. b.i.d. initially. Dosage
may be increased at weekly intervals. Usual
effective dose is 20 to 40 mg daily in two
equally divided doses.
Adjust-a-dose: For patients with CrCl over
30 mL/minute, first dose is 5 mg P.O. daily;
if CrCl is 10 to 30 mL/minute, 2.5 mg.

ADMINISTRATION
P.O.
• Don't give drug with a high-fat meal
because this may decrease absorption of
drug.

ACTION
Prevents conversion of angiotensin I to
angiotensin II, a potent vasoconstrictor. Less
angiotensin II decreases peripheral arterial
resistance, decreasing aldosterone secretion,
which reduces sodium and water retention
and lowers BP.

Route	Onset	Peak	Duration
P.O.	1 hr	2–6 hr	24 hr

Half-life: 25 hours.

ADVERSE REACTIONS
CNS: headache, dizziness, fatigue, depression.
CV: *hypertensive crisis,* hypotension, chest
pain.
GI: abdominal pain, vomiting, nausea,
diarrhea.
GU: erectile dysfunction, UTI, *acute renal
failure.*
Metabolic: *hyperkalemia.*
Musculoskeletal: back pain, myalgia.
Respiratory: dry, persistent, tickling,
nonproductive cough; dyspnea.
Skin: rash.

INTERACTIONS
Drug-drug. ⊗ *Alert: Aliskiren:* May increase risk of renal impairment, hypotension, and hyperkalemia in diabetic patients
and those with moderate to severe renal impairment (GFR less than 60 mL/minute).
Concomitant use is contraindicated in diabetic patients. Avoid concomitant use in
those with moderate to severe renal impairment.
Diuretics, other antihypertensives: May
cause excessive hypotension. Stop diuretic
or reduce dose of quinapril, as needed.
Lithium: May increase lithium level and
lithium toxicity. Monitor lithium level.
NSAIDs: May decrease antihypertensive
effects. Monitor BP.
*Potassium-sparing diuretics, potassium
supplements:* May cause hyperkalemia.
Monitor patient closely.
Tetracycline: May decrease absorption if
taken with quinapril. Avoid using together.
Drug-herb. *Yohimbe:* May decrease antihypertensive effects. Avoid use together.
Drug-food. *Salt substitutes containing
potassium:* May cause hyperkalemia. Discourage use together.

EFFECTS ON LAB TEST RESULTS
• May increase potassium, BUN, and creati-
nine levels.
• May increase LFT values.

CONTRAINDICATIONS & CAUTIONS
• Contraindicated in patients hypersensitive
to ACE inhibitors and in those with a history
of angioedema related to treatment with an
ACE inhibitor.

Reactions in bold italics are *life-threatening*. Interactions may have a *rapid onset* or a *delayed onset*.

- Use cautiously in patients with impaired renal function.

Dialyzable drug: No.

⚠ Overdose S&S: Hypotension.

PREGNANCY-LACTATION-REPRODUCTION

Black Box Warning Use during pregnancy can cause injury and death to the developing fetus. When pregnancy is detected, stop drug as soon as possible. ∎

- Drug appears in breast milk. Use cautiously in breast-feeding women.

NURSING CONSIDERATIONS

- Assess renal and hepatic function before and periodically throughout therapy.
- Monitor BP for effectiveness of therapy. When adjusting dosage, measure BP before giving dose (trough) and 2 to 6 hours after dosing (peak).
- Monitor potassium level. Risk factors for the development of hyperkalemia include renal insufficiency, diabetes, and concomitant use of drugs that raise potassium level.
- Although ACE inhibitors reduce BP in all races, they reduce it less in blacks taking an ACE inhibitor alone. Black patients should take drug with a thiazide diuretic for a better response.
- ACE inhibitors appear to increase risk of angioedema in black patients.
- Other ACE inhibitors have caused agranulocytosis and neutropenia. Monitor CBC with differential counts before therapy and periodically thereafter.

PATIENT TEACHING

- Advise patient to report signs of infection, such as fever and sore throat.

🕭 Alert: Facial and throat swelling (including swelling of the tongue and larynx) may occur, especially after first dose. Advise patient to report signs or symptoms of breathing difficulty or swelling of face, eyes, lips, or tongue.

- Light-headedness can occur, especially during first few days of therapy. Tell patient to rise slowly to minimize effect and to report signs and symptoms to prescriber. If he faints, patient should stop taking drug and call prescriber immediately.
- Inform patient that inadequate fluid intake, vomiting, diarrhea, and excessive

perspiration can lead to light-headedness and fainting. Tell him to use caution in hot weather and during exercise.

- Tell patient to avoid salt substitutes. These products may contain potassium, which can cause high potassium level in patients taking quinapril.
- Advise female patient of childbearing potential about potential fetal hazards and to notify prescriber at once if pregnancy occurs. Drug will need to be stopped.
- Tell patient to avoid taking with a high-fat meal because this may decrease absorption of drug.

SAFETY ALERT!

quinidine gluconate
KWIN-i-deen

quinidine sulfate

Therapeutic class: Antiarrhythmics
Pharmacologic class: Cinchona alkaloids

AVAILABLE FORMS

quinidine gluconate (62% quinidine base)
Injection: 80 mg/mL
Tablets (extended-release) ⊕: 324 mg
quinidine sulfate (83% quinidine base)
Injection: 190 mg/mL ✤
Tablets: 200 mg, 300 mg
Tablets (extended-release) ⊕: 300 mg

INDICATIONS & DOSAGES

Adjust-a-dose (for all indications): In patients with hepatic impairment or HF, reduce dosage.

➤ **Atrial flutter or fibrillation**
Adults: 400 mg quinidine sulfate (immediate-release) or equivalent base P.O. every 6 hours. Or, 300 mg quinidine sulfate (extended-release) P.O. every 8 to 12 hours. Or, quinidine gluconate 648 mg (2 tablets) P.O. every 8 hours. Or, begin quinidine gluconate I.V. infusion no faster than 0.25 mg/kg/minute (1 mL/kg/hour).

Discontinue infusion if patient hasn't converted to sinus rhythm after receiving 10 mg/kg. Discontinue drug if QRS complex widens to 130% of pretreatment duration, QTc interval widens to 130% of pretreatment duration and is longer than 50 msec, P waves disappear, or patient develops significant tachycardia, symptomatic bradycardia, or hypotension.

➤ **Severe *Plasmodium falciparum* malaria**
Adults: 10 mg/kg quinidine gluconate I.V. diluted in 250 mL NSS and infused over 1 to 2 hours; then begin a continuous infusion of 0.02 mg/kg/minute. In patients able to swallow, discontinue infusion and give oral quinine sulfate every 8 hours. Continue quinidine/quinine therapy for 72 hours or until parasitemia is reduced to less than 1%, whichever occurs first. Or, give a loading dose of 24 mg/kg of quinidine gluconate I.V. diluted in 250 mL of NSS and infused over 4 hours; 4 hours later, give maintenance dose of 12 mg/kg of quinidine gluconate by I.V. infusion over 4 hours at 8-hour intervals until three maintenance doses have been given and parasitemia is reduced to less than 1% and oral quinidine sulfate can be initiated.
Children: 10 mg/kg gluconate I.V. over 1 to 2 hours; then continuous infusion of 0.02 mg/kg/minute for up to 72 hours or until parasitemia is reduced to 1% or less, whichever comes first. For patients able to swallow pills, maintenance therapy may be given P.O. with quinine sulfate every 8 hours in divided doses of same quinine base amount.

ADMINISTRATION
P.O.
● Give drug with food to avoid adverse GI reactions.
● Don't crush extended-release tablets. If necessary, scored tablets may be broken in half to adjust quinidine dose.
● Don't give drug with grapefruit juice.

I.V.
▼ For quinidine gluconate infusion to treat atrial fibrillation or flutter in adults, dilute 800 mg (10 mL of injection) with 40 mL D₅W and infuse at up to 0.25 mg/kg/minute using a volumetric pump.
▼ For quinidine gluconate infusion to treat malaria, dilute in 5 mL/kg (usually 250 mL) NSS and infuse over 1 to 2 hours, followed by a continuous maintenance infusion.

▼ During infusion, continuously monitor patient's BP and ECG.
▼ Adjust rate so that the arrhythmia is corrected without disturbing the normal mechanism of the heartbeat.
▼ Never use discolored (brownish) quinidine solution.
▼ Store drug away from heat and direct light.
▼ **Incompatibilities:** Alkalies, amiodarone, atracurium besylate, furosemide, heparin sodium, iodides.

ACTION
A class IA antiarrhythmic with direct and indirect (anticholinergic) effects on cardiac tissue. Decreases automaticity, conduction velocity, and membrane responsiveness; prolongs effective refractory period; and reduces vagal tone.

Route	Onset	Peak	Duration
P.O.	1–3 hr	1–6 hr	6–8 hr
I.V.	Immediate	Immediate	Unknown

Half-life: 5 to 12 hours.

ADVERSE REACTIONS
CNS: syncope, headache, light-headedness, sleep disturbance, tremor, incoordination.
CV: ECG changes, tachycardia, *PVCs, ventricular tachycardia, atypical ventricular tachycardia, complete AV block, aggravated HF,* angina, palpitations, hypotension.
EENT: tinnitus, blurred vision, diplopia.
GI: diarrhea, nausea, vomiting, anorexia, excessive salivation, abdominal pain.
Hematologic: *thrombocytopenia, agranulocytosis,* hemolytic anemia.
Hepatic: *hepatotoxicity.*
Respiratory: *acute asthmatic attack, respiratory arrest.*
Skin: rash, petechial hemorrhage of buccal mucosa.
Other: cinchonism, *angioedema,* lupus erythematosus.

INTERACTIONS
Drug-drug. *Amiloride:* May increase the risk of arrhythmias. If use together can't be avoided, monitor ECG closely.
Amiodarone: May increase quinidine level, producing life-threatening cardiac arrhythmias. Monitor quinidine level closely if use

---

Reactions in bold italics are *life-threatening*. Interactions may have a *rapid onset* or a *delayed onset*.

together can't be avoided. Adjust quinidine as needed.

Antacids, sodium bicarbonate: May increase quinidine level. Monitor patient for increased effect.

Azole antifungals: May increase the risk of CV events. Use together is contraindicated.

Barbiturates, phenytoin, rifampin: May decrease quinidine level. Monitor patient for decreased effect.

Cimetidine: May increase quinidine level. Monitor patient for increased arrhythmias.

Digoxin: May increase digoxin level after starting quinidine therapy. Monitor digoxin level.

Drugs that prolong the QT interval (antipsychotics, disopyramide, procainamide, sotalol, TCAs): May have additive effect with quinidine and cause life-threatening cardiac arrhythmias. Avoid using together when possible.

Fluvoxamine, nefazodone, TCAs: May increase antidepressant level, thus increasing its effect. Monitor patient for adverse reactions.

Macrolides and related antibiotics (azithromycin, clarithromycin, erythromycin, telithromycin): May cause additive effects or prolongation of the QT interval. Use with caution. Avoid use with telithromycin.

Neuromuscular blockers: May potentiate effects of these drugs. Avoid use of quinidine immediately after surgery.

Nifedipine: May decrease quinidine level. May need to adjust dosage.

Other antiarrhythmics (lidocaine, procainamide, propranolol): May increase risk of toxicity. Use together cautiously.

Protease inhibitors (nelfinavir, ritonavir): May significantly increase quinidine levels and toxicity. Use together is contraindicated.

Quinolones: May cause life-threatening arrhythmias, including torsades de pointes. Avoid using together.

Verapamil: May decrease quinidine clearance and cause hypotension, bradycardia, AV block, or pulmonary edema. Avoid use together.

Warfarin: May increase anticoagulant effect. Monitor patient closely.

Drug-herb. *Licorice:* May decrease potassium level and increase risk for arrhythmias. Don't use together.

Drug-food. *Grapefruit:* May delay absorption and onset of action of drug. Discourage use together.

EFFECTS ON LAB TEST RESULTS
● May decrease Hb level.
● May decrease platelet and granulocyte counts.

CONTRAINDICATIONS & CAUTIONS
● Contraindicated in patients with idiosyncrasy or hypersensitivity to quinidine or related cinchona derivatives.
● Contraindicated in patients with myasthenia gravis, intraventricular conduction defects, digoxin toxicity when AV conduction is grossly impaired, abnormal rhythms caused by escape mechanisms, complete AV block, history of drug-induced torsades de pointes, or history of prolonged QT interval syndrome and in patients whose cardiac rhythm depends on a junctional or idioventricular pacemaker.
● Contraindicated in patients who developed thrombocytopenia after exposure to quinidine or quinine.
■ **Black Box Warning** In many trials of antiarrhythmic therapy for non-life-threatening arrhythmias, active antiarrhythmic therapy has resulted in increased mortality. Risk of active therapy is probably greatest in patients with structural heart disease. ■
● Use cautiously in patients with HF, asthma, muscle weakness, or infection accompanied by fever because hypersensitivity reactions to drug may be masked.
● Use cautiously in patients with hepatic or renal impairment because systemic accumulation may occur.
● Avoid use during breast-feeding.
Dialyzable drug: No.
⚠ **Overdose S&S:** Depressed mental function, headache, nausea, vomiting, diarrhea, abdominal pain, tachyarrhythmias, depressed cardiac automaticity and conduction, hypotension, HF, hypokalemia, acidosis.

Q

PREGNANCY-LACTATION-REPRODUCTION
- There are no adequate studies in pregnant women. Use only if clearly needed.
- Drug appears in breast milk. Avoid use in breast-feeding women.

NURSING CONSIDERATIONS
- Check apical pulse rate and BP before therapy. If extremes in pulse rate are detected, withhold drug and notify prescriber at once.
- Anticoagulant therapy is commonly advised before quinidine therapy in longstanding atrial fibrillation because restoration of normal sinus rhythm may result in thromboembolism caused by dislodgment of thrombi from atrial wall.
- Monitor patient for atypical ventricular tachycardia, such as torsades de pointes and ECG changes, particularly widening of QRS complex and widened QT and PR intervals.
- ☼ *Alert:* When changing route of administration or oral salt form, prescriber should alter dosage to compensate for variations in quinidine base content.
- ☼ *Alert:* Hospitalize patients with severe malaria in an intensive care setting, with continuous monitoring. Decrease infusion rate if quinidine level exceeds 6 mcg/mL, uncorrected QT interval exceeds 0.6 second, or QRS complex widening exceeds 25% of baseline.
- Monitor LFT results during first 4 to 8 weeks of therapy.
- Monitor quinidine level. Therapeutic levels for antiarrhythmic effects are 2 to 6 mcg/mL.
- Correct electrolyte imbalances before and during therapy.
- Monitor patient response carefully. If adverse GI reactions occur, especially diarrhea, notify prescriber as these may be symptoms of quinidine toxicity.
- *Look alike–sound alike:* Don't confuse quinidine with quinine or clonidine.

PATIENT TEACHING
- Stress importance of taking drug exactly as prescribed and taking it with food if adverse GI reactions occur.
- ☼ *Alert:* Instruct patient not to crush or chew extended-release tablets. If necessary, he may break scored tablets in half to adjust quinidine dose.
- Tell patient to avoid grapefruit juice because it may delay drug absorption and inhibit drug metabolism.
- Advise patient to report all adverse reactions promptly, especially signs and symptoms of quinidine toxicity (ringing in the ears, visual disturbances, dizziness, headache, nausea), palpitations, chest pain, and slow or fast heartbeat.

rabeprazole sodium
rah-BEH-pray-zol

Aciphex✦, Aciphex Sprinkle

Therapeutic class: Antiulcer drugs
Pharmacologic class: PPIs

AVAILABLE FORMS
Capsules (delayed-release) ⓞⓣⓒ: 5 mg, 10 mg
Tablets (delayed-release) ⓞⓣⓒ: 20 mg

INDICATIONS & DOSAGES
➤ **Healing of erosive or ulcerative GERD**
Adults: 20 mg P.O. daily for 4 to 8 weeks. Additional 8-week course may be considered, if needed.
➤ **Maintenance of healing of erosive or ulcerative GERD**
Adults: 20 mg P.O. daily for up to 12 months.
➤ **Healing of duodenal ulcers**
Adults: 20 mg P.O. daily after morning meal for up to 4 weeks.
➤ **Pathologic hypersecretory conditions, including Zollinger-Ellison syndrome**
Adults: Initially, 60 mg P.O. daily; may increase, as needed, to 100 mg P.O. daily or 60 mg P.O. b.i.d.
➤ **Symptomatic GERD, including daytime and nighttime heartburn**
Adults: 20 mg P.O. daily for 4 weeks. May consider additional 4-week course, if needed.
Children age 12 and older: 20 mg P.O. daily for up to 8 weeks.
➤ **GERD (Aciphex Sprinkle)**
Children ages 1 to 11 weighing 15 kg or more: 10 mg P.O. once daily for up to 12 weeks.

Children ages 1 to 11 weighing less than 15 kg: 5 mg P.O. once daily for up to 12 weeks. May increase to 10 mg once daily if inadequate response.

➤ **Helicobacter pylori eradication, to reduce risk of duodenal ulcer recurrence**
Adults: 20 mg P.O. b.i.d., combined with amoxicillin 1,000 mg P.O. b.i.d. and clarithromycin 500 mg P.O. b.i.d., for 7 days with morning and evening meals.

ADMINISTRATION
P.O.
- Don't crush, split, or allow patient to chew tablets.
- Give tablets without regard for food but if used for treatment of duodenal ulcers, give after a meal; when used for *H. pylori* eradication, give with food.
- Open Aciphex Sprinkle delayed-release capsules and empty onto a spoonful of soft food (applesauce) or liquid that's at or below room temperature.
- Give whole dose within 15 minutes of sprinkling and 30 minutes before a meal.
- Sprinkle granules shouldn't be chewed or crushed.

ACTION
Blocks proton pump activity and gastric acid secretion by inhibiting gastric hydrogen–potassium adenosine triphosphatase (an enzyme) at secretory surface of gastric parietal cells.

Route	Onset	Peak	Duration
P.O.	<1 hr	1–6½ hr	24 hr

Half-life: 1 to 2 hours.

ADVERSE REACTIONS
CNS: headache, pain.
EENT: pharyngitis.
GI: abdominal pain, constipation, diarrhea, flatulence, nausea, vomiting.
Hepatic: elevated liver enzyme levels, *hepatitis, hepatic encephalopathy.*
Musculoskeletal: arthralgia, myalgia.
Other: infection.

INTERACTIONS
Drug-drug. *Clarithromycin:* May increase rabeprazole level. Monitor patient closely.

Cyclosporine: May inhibit cyclosporine metabolism. Use together cautiously.
Digoxin, ketoconazole, other gastric pH-dependent drugs: May decrease or increase drug absorption at increased pH values. Monitor patient closely.
Methotrexate: May increase methotrexate concentration and risk of toxicity. Closely monitor methotrexate concentration, and watch for signs and symptoms of methotrexate toxicity. Rabeprazole may need to be suspended or stopped in patients taking high-dose methotrexate.
Protease inhibitors (atazanavir, indinavir, nelfinavir, saquinavir): May decrease levels of these drugs. Monitor clinical response. Contraindicated with atazanavir.
Rilpivirine-containing products: May reduce antiviral effect and promote drug resistance. Use together is contraindicated.
Salicylates (aspirin): May increase release of salicylate from enteric coating, increasing gastric side effects. Use together cautiously.
Warfarin: May inhibit warfarin metabolism. Monitor PT and INR.

EFFECTS ON LAB TEST RESULTS
- May decrease magnesium level.

CONTRAINDICATIONS & CAUTIONS
- Contraindicated in patients hypersensitive to drug, other benzimidazoles (lansoprazole, omeprazole), or components of these formulations and with rilpivirine-containing products.
- In *H. pylori* eradication, clarithromycin is contraindicated in patients hypersensitive to macrolides and in those taking pimozide; amoxicillin is contraindicated in patients hypersensitive to penicillin or cephalosporins.
- Use cautiously in patients with severe hepatic impairment.
- Long-term (1 year or more) and multiple daily-dose rabeprazole therapy may be associated with an increased risk of osteoporosis-related fractures of the hip, wrist, or spine. Use lowest dosage and shortest duration of therapy appropriate to condition being treated. May consider vitamin D and calcium supplementation and following appropriate guidelines to reduce risk of fractures in patients at risk.

R

• Acute interstitial nephritis has been observed in patients taking rabeprazole and may occur at any point during therapy. Discontinue drug if this condition develops.
• Vitamin B_{12} malabsorption and deficiency have been reported in patients receiving prolonged daily treatment (longer than 3 years) with acid suppressants.
Dialyzable drug: No.

PREGNANCY-LACTATION-REPRODUCTION
• There are no adequate studies in pregnant women. Use during pregnancy only if potential benefit justifies potential fetal risk.
• In *H. pylori* eradication, clarithromycin is contraindicated in pregnant women.
• It isn't known if drug appears in breast milk. Use cautiously in breast-feeding women.

NURSING CONSIDERATIONS
• Consider additional courses of therapy if duodenal ulcer or GERD isn't healed after first course of therapy.
• If *H. pylori* eradication is unsuccessful, do susceptibility testing. If patient is resistant to clarithromycin or susceptibility testing isn't possible, expect to start therapy using a different antimicrobial.
❷ *Alert:* Prolonged use of PPIs (longer than 3 months) may cause low magnesium levels. Monitor magnesium levels before starting treatment and periodically thereafter.
❷ *Alert:* Monitor patients for signs and symptoms of low magnesium level, such as abnormal HR or rhythm, palpitations, muscle spasms, tremor, or seizures. In children, abnormal HR may present as fatigue, upset stomach, dizziness, and light-headedness. Magnesium supplementation or drug discontinuation may be needed.
• Symptomatic response to therapy doesn't preclude presence of gastric malignancy.
❷ *Alert:* Patients treated for *H. pylori* eradication have developed pseudomembranous colitis with nearly all antibiotics, including clarithromycin and amoxicillin. Monitor patient closely.
❷ *Alert:* May increase CDAD. Evaluate for CDAD in patients who develop diarrhea that doesn't improve. Use lowest dosage and shortest duration appropriate to condition being treated.

• *Look alike–sound alike:* Don't confuse Aciphex with Accupril or Aricept. Don't confuse rabeprazole with aripiprazole.

PATIENT TEACHING
• Explain importance of taking drug exactly as prescribed.
• Advise patient to swallow delayed-release tablet whole and not to crush, chew, or split the tablet.
• Inform patient that delayed-release tablet may be taken without regard to meals.
• Tell patient or caregiver to open Aciphex Sprinkle delayed-release capsules and empty onto a spoonful of soft food (applesauce) or liquid that's at or below room temperature, and to take the whole dose within 15 minutes of sprinkling and 30 minutes before a meal.
• Advise patient or caregiver that Aciphex Sprinkle granules shouldn't be chewed or crushed.
• Inform patient that drug may increase the risk of osteoporosis-related fractures of the hip, wrist, or spine with multiple daily doses that are continued for longer than 1 year.
• Teach patient to recognize and report signs and symptoms of low magnesium levels.

raloxifene hydrochloride
rah-LOX-i-feen

Evista⬩

Therapeutic class: Antiosteoporotics
Pharmacologic class: Selective estrogen receptor modulators

AVAILABLE FORMS
Tablets: 60 mg

INDICATIONS & DOSAGES
➤ **To prevent or treat osteoporosis; to reduce risk of invasive breast cancer in postmenopausal women with osteoporosis and postmenopausal women at high risk for invasive breast cancer**
Postmenopausal women: 60 mg P.O. once daily.

ADMINISTRATION
P.O.
- Give drug without regard for food.
- Stop drug at least 72 hours before pro-longed immobilization and resume only after patient is fully mobilized.

ACTION
Reduces resorption of bone and decreases overall bone turnover. These effects on bone are manifested as reductions in serum and urine levels of bone turnover markers and increases in bone mineral density.

Route	Onset	Peak	Duration
P.O.	Unknown	Unknown	Unknown

Half-life: 27½ to 32½ hours.

ADVERSE REACTIONS
CNS: depression, insomnia, fever, mi-graine.
CV: chest pain.
EENT: sinusitis, pharyngitis, laryngitis.
GI: nausea, dyspepsia, vomiting, flatulence, gastroenteritis.
GU: vaginitis, UTI, cystitis, leukorrhea, endometrial disorder, vaginal bleeding.
Metabolic: weight gain.
Musculoskeletal: arthralgia, myalgia, arthritis, leg cramps.
Respiratory: increased cough, pneumonia.
Skin: rash, diaphoresis.
Other: infection, flulike syndrome, hot flashes, peripheral edema.

INTERACTIONS
Drug-drug. *Bile acid sequestrants (cholestyramine):* May cause significant reduction in absorption of raloxifene. Avoid using together.
Highly protein-bound drugs (clofibrate, diazepam, diazoxide, ibuprofen, in-domethacin, naproxen): May interfere with binding sites. Use together cautiously.
Levothyroxine: May decrease levothyroxine absorption. Consider therapy modification.
Ospemifene: May increase adverse toxic effects of raloxifene. Avoid combination.
Systemic estrogens: Safety of concomitant use hasn't been established. Use together isn't recommended.
Warfarin: May cause a decrease in PT. Monitor PT and INR closely.

EFFECTS ON LAB TEST RESULTS
- May increase triglyceride level.

CONTRAINDICATIONS & CAUTIONS
Black Box Warning Increased risk of venous thromboembolism and death from stroke. Contraindicated in women with a history of, or active, venous thromboem-bolism, including DVT, PE, and retinal vein thrombosis. Consider risk-benefit bal-ance in women at risk for stroke, including those with documented CAD or who are at increased risk for major coronary events. ■
- Raloxifene shouldn't be used for primary or secondary prevention of CV disease.
- Use cautiously in patients with severe hepatic or renal impairment.
- Safety and effectiveness of drug haven't been evaluated in men.
Dialyzable drug: Unknown.
⚠ Overdose S&S: Leg cramps, dizziness, ataxia, flushing, rash, tremors, vomiting, elevated alkaline phosphatase level.

PREGNANCY-LACTATION-REPRODUCTION
- Contraindicated during pregnancy and in women who may become pregnant; drug may cause fetal harm. If drug is used during pregnancy or if patient becomes pregnant during therapy, apprise her of potential hazard to the fetus.
- Contraindicated in breast-feeding women.

NURSING CONSIDERATIONS
- Watch for signs of blood clots. Great-est risk of thromboembolic events occurs during first 4 months of treatment.
- Watch for breast abnormalities; drug doesn't eliminate risk of breast cancer.
- Conduct breast examinations and mam-mograms before starting, and regularly during, therapy.
- Effect on bone mineral density beyond 2 years of drug treatment isn't known.
- For osteoporosis treatment, add supple-mental calcium (average of 1,500 mg daily) and vitamin D (400 to 800 units daily) to the diet if daily intake is inadequate.
- Monitor triglyceride level if previous treatment with estrogen caused elevation.

R

PATIENT TEACHING

● Advise patient to avoid long periods of restricted movement (such as during traveling) because of increased risk of venous thromboembolic events.

● Inform patient that hot flashes or flushing may occur and that drug doesn't aid in reducing them.

● Instruct patient to practice other bone loss-prevention measures, including taking supplemental calcium and vitamin D if dietary intake is inadequate, performing weight-bearing exercises, and stopping alcohol consumption and smoking.

● Tell patient that drug may be taken without regard for food.

● Advise patient to report unexplained uterine bleeding or breast abnormalities during therapy.

● Explain adverse reactions and instruct patient to read patient package insert before starting therapy and each time prescription is renewed.

---

raltegravir potassium
ral-TEG-rah-veer

Isentress

Therapeutic class: Antiretrovirals
Pharmacologic class: HIV integrase strand transfer inhibitors

AVAILABLE FORMS
Powder for oral suspension: 100 mg
Tablets (chewable): 25 mg, 100 mg
Tablets (film-coated) ⒹⓃⒸ *:* 400 mg

INDICATIONS & DOSAGES
➤ **HIV-1 infection, with other antiretrovirals, in patients age 4 weeks and older weighing at least 3 kg**
Adults and children weighing at least 25 kg: 400 mg tablet P.O. b.i.d.
Adults and children age 18 and older: When administered concomitantly with rifampin, give 800 mg tablet P.O. b.i.d.
Children unable to swallow tablets and weighing at least 40 kg: 300 mg chewable tablets P.O. b.i.d.

Children unable to swallow tablets and weighing 28 to less than 40 kg: 200 mg chewable tablets P.O. b.i.d.
Children unable to swallow tablets and weighing 25 to less than 28 kg: 150 mg chewable tablets P.O. b.i.d.
Children weighing 20 to less than 25 kg: 150 mg chewable tablets P.O. b.i.d.
Children weighing 14 to less than 20 kg: 100 mg chewable tablets or 100 mg oral suspension (5 mL) P.O. b.i.d.
Children at least age 4 weeks weighing 11 to less than 14 kg: 75 mg chewable tablets or 80 mg oral suspension (4 mL) P.O. b.i.d.
Children at least age 4 weeks weighing 8 to less than 11 kg: 60 mg oral suspension (3 mL) P.O. b.i.d.
Children at least age 4 weeks weighing 6 to less than 8 kg: 40 mg oral suspension (2 mL) P.O. b.i.d.
Children at least age 4 weeks weighing 4 to less than 6 kg: 30 mg oral suspension (1.5 mL) P.O. b.i.d.
Children at least age 4 weeks weighing 3 to less than 4 kg: 20 mg oral suspension (1 mL) P.O. b.i.d.

ADMINISTRATION
P.O.
● Don't substitute chewable tablets or oral suspension for film-coated tablets.
● Give drug without regard for meals.
Tablets and chewable tablets
● Maximum dosage of chewable tablets is 300 mg b.i.d.
● Patient must swallow film-coated tablets whole.
● The 100-mg chewable tablet can be broken into two equal halves.
● Chewable tablets can be chewed or swallowed whole.
Oral suspension
● Maximum dosage of oral suspension is 100 mg b.i.d.
● To administer, open foil packet of drug (100 mg). Measure 5 mL of water in provided mixing cup. Pour packet contents into the water, close lid, and swirl for 30 to 60 seconds. Don't turn mixing cup upside down.
● When mixed, measure recommended suspension dose into an oral syringe.

Reactions in bold italics are ***life-threatening***. Interactions may have a *rapid onset* or a ***delayed onset***.

• Give within 30 minutes of mixing with water. Discard any remaining suspension in the trash.
• See detailed "Instructions for Use" that come with the oral suspension.

ACTION

Inhibits HIV-1 integrase, an enzyme required for HIV-1 replication.

Route	Onset	Peak	Duration
P.O.	Rapid	3 hr	Unknown

Half-life: About 9 hours.

ADVERSE REACTIONS

CNS: headache, fatigue, dizziness, insomnia.
GI: nausea, abdominal pain, vomiting.
Hematologic: anemia, *neutropenia, thrombocytopenia.*
Metabolic: hyperglycemia.
Musculoskeletal: asthenia, myopathy, *rhabdomyolysis.*
Skin: lipodystrophy, rash, *Stevens-Johnson syndrome, toxic epidermal necrolysis.*
Other: immune reconstitution syndrome.

INTERACTIONS

Drug-drug. *Antacids containing aluminum or magnesium:* Ingestion within 2 hours of raltegravir administration significantly decreases raltegravir plasma level. Use alternative antacids, such as those containing calcium carbonate.
Fibric acid derivatives, HMG-CoA reductase inhibitors: May increase risk of rhabdomyolysis. Monitor therapy.
UGT1A1 inducers (rifampin): May decrease raltegravir level. Adjust raltegravir dosage to 800 mg b.i.d. when administering with rifampin.

EFFECTS ON LAB TEST RESULTS

• May increase bilirubin, AST, ALT, alkaline phosphatase, amylase, lipase, glucose, and CK levels. May decrease Hb level.
• May decrease neutrophil and platelet counts.

CONTRAINDICATIONS & CAUTIONS

⚠ Alert: Severe, potentially life-threatening and fatal skin reactions have been reported, including Stevens-Johnson syndrome and

toxic epidermal necrolysis. Hypersensitivity reactions, including rash; organ dysfunction, including hepatic failure; and general malaise, muscle or joint aches, edema, conjunctivitis, facial edema, angioedema, oral blisters, and eosinophilia have also been reported. Discontinue drug immediately if signs or symptoms of severe skin reactions or hypersensitivity reactions occur.
• Patient can remain on the oral suspension as long as patient's weight is less than 20 kg.
• Use cautiously in elderly patients, especially those with hepatic, renal, and cardiac insufficiency.
• Safety and effectiveness haven't been established in children younger than age 4 weeks.
Dialyzable drug: Unknown.

PREGNANCY-LACTATION-REPRODUCTION

• There are no adequate studies in pregnant women. Use during pregnancy only if potential benefit justifies potential fetal risk.
• Enroll pregnant women exposed to drug in the Antiretroviral Pregnancy Registry (1-800-258-4263).
• Mothers with HIV-1 infection shouldn't breast-feed to avoid risking postnatal HIV-1 transmission.

NURSING CONSIDERATIONS

• Perform laboratory tests, including CBC, platelet count, and LFTs, before therapy and regularly throughout therapy.
• Use drug with at least one other antiretroviral.
• Watch for signs of myopathy or rash.
• Monitor patient for immune reconstitution syndrome. During initial phase of treatment, patients responding to antiretroviral therapy may develop an inflammatory response to indolent or residual opportunistic infections (CMV, *Mycobacterium avium* complex, *Pneumocystis jiroveci* pneumonia, TB), which may necessitate further evaluation and treatment. Autoimmune disorders (such as Graves disease, polymyositis, and Guillain-Barré syndrome) have also been reported in the setting of immune reconstitution; however, time to onset is more variable, and can occur many months after initiation of antiretroviral treatment.

R

PATIENT TEACHING

• Inform patient that drug doesn't cure HIV infection. He may continue to develop opportunistic infections and other complications of HIV infection, and transmission of HIV to others through sexual contact or blood contamination is still possible.

• Advise patient to use barrier protection during sexual intercourse.

• Tell women that breast-feeding isn't recommended.

• Advise patient to immediately report worsening symptoms or unexplained muscle pain, tenderness, or weakness while taking the drug.

• Instruct patient to avoid missing any doses to decrease the risk of developing HIV resistance.

• Inform patient that severe and potentially life-threatening rash has been reported and to immediately contact the health care provider if a rash develops. Instruct patient to immediately stop taking raltegravir and seek medical attention if the rash is associated with any of the following signs or symptoms: fever; generally ill feeling; extreme tiredness; muscle or joint aches; blisters; oral lesions; eye inflammation; facial swelling; swelling of the eyes, lips, or mouth; breathing difficulty; or signs and symptoms of liver problems (such as yellowing of the skin or whites of the eyes, dark or tea-colored urine, pale-colored stools or bowel movements, nausea, vomiting, loss of appetite, pain, aching or sensitivity on the right side below the ribs).

• Advise patient with phenylketonuria that the 25-mg and 100-mg chewable tablets contain phenylalanine.

• Tell patient if a dose is missed to take the next dose as soon as possible and not to double the next dose.

• Advise patient to report use of other drugs, including OTC drugs; this drug interacts with other drugs.

• Tell patient that drug may be taken without regard for meals.

• Tell patient or caregiver to carefully follow directions in manufacturer's "Instructions for Use" when preparing and administering oral solution. Use calibrated syringe to administer dose.

• Tell patient or caregiver to administer oral solution within 30 minutes of mixing.

• Instruct patient to swallow film-coated tablets whole.

• Inform patient that chewable tablets or oral suspension can't be substituted for film-coated tablets.

ramelteon
rah-MELL-tee-on

Rozerem

Therapeutic class: Hypnotics
Pharmacologic class: Melatonin receptor agonists

AVAILABLE FORMS
Tablets ⓞⓣⓒ: 8 mg

INDICATIONS & DOSAGES
➤ **Insomnia characterized by trouble falling asleep**
Adults: 8 mg P.O. within 30 minutes of bedtime. Maximum dose is 8 mg daily.

ADMINISTRATION
P.O.
• Don't give drug with or immediately after a high-fat meal.

• Give drug within 30 minutes of bedtime.

• Don't break, crush, or allow patient to chew tablets. Patient should swallow tablets whole.

ACTION
Acts on receptors believed to maintain the circadian rhythm underlying the normal sleep-wake cycle.

Route	Onset	Peak	Duration
P.O.	Rapid	½–1½ hr	Unknown

Half-life: Parent compound, 1 to 2½ hours; metabolite M-II, 2 to 5 hours.

ADVERSE REACTIONS
CNS: complex sleep-related behaviors, depression, dizziness, fatigue, headache, somnolence, worsened insomnia.
GI: nausea.

Reactions in bold italics are *life-threatening*. Interactions may have a *rapid onset* or a *delayed onset*.

INTERACTIONS

Drug-drug. *CNS depressants:* May cause excessive CNS depression. Use together cautiously.

Donepezil, doxepin: May increase ramelteon level. Monitor patient closely.

Black Box Warning *Opioids:* May cause slow or difficult breathing, sedation, and death. Avoid use together. If use together is necessary, limit dosage and duration of each drug to minimum necessary for desired effect. ∎

Strong CYP enzyme inducer (rifampin): May decrease ramelteon level. Monitor patient for lack of effect.

Strong CYP1A2 inhibitor (fluvoxamine): May increase ramelteon level. Don't use together.

Strong CYP2C9 inhibitor (fluconazole), strong CYP3A4 inhibitor (ketoconazole), weak CYP1A2 inhibitors: May increase ramelteon level. Use together cautiously.

Drug-food. *Food (especially high-fat meals):* May delay time to peak drug effect. Tell patient to take drug on an empty stomach.

Drug-lifestyle. *Alcohol use:* May cause excessive CNS depression. Discourage alcohol use.

EFFECTS ON LAB TEST RESULTS

• May increase prolactin level.
• May decrease testosterone level.

CONTRAINDICATIONS & CAUTIONS

• Contraindicated in patients hypersensitive to drug or its components. Don't use in patients taking fluvoxamine or in those with severe hepatic impairment, severe sleep apnea, or severe COPD.

Black Box Warning Opioids should only be prescribed with benzodiazepines or other CNS depressants to patients for whom alternative treatment options are inadequate. ∎

• Use cautiously in patients with depression or moderate hepatic impairment.

Dialyzable drug: No.

PREGNANCY-LACTATION-REPRODUCTION

• There are no adequate studies in pregnant women. Drug may cause fetal harm. Use during pregnancy only if clearly needed and potential benefit justifies potential fetal risk.

• It isn't known if drug appears in breast milk. Use cautiously in breast-feeding women.

NURSING CONSIDERATIONS

⚠ *Alert:* Anaphylaxis and angioedema may occur as early as the first dose. Monitor patient closely. Emergency treatment may be needed.

• Thoroughly evaluate the cause of insomnia before starting drug.

• Assess patient for behavioral or cognitive disorders.

• Drug doesn't cause physical dependence.

• *Look alike–sound alike:* Don't confuse Rozerem with Razadyne. Don't confuse ramelteon with Remeron.

PATIENT TEACHING

Black Box Warning Caution patient or caregiver of patient taking an opioid with a benzodiazepine, CNS depressant, or alcohol to seek immediate medical attention if patient experiences dizziness, light-headedness, extreme sleepiness, slowed or difficult breathing, or unresponsiveness. ∎

⚠ *Alert:* Warn patient that drug may cause allergic reactions, facial swelling, and complex sleep-related behaviors, such as driving, eating, and making phone calls while asleep. Advise patient to report these and all adverse effects.

• Instruct patient to take dose within 30 minutes of bedtime.

• Tell patient not to take drug with or after a heavy meal.

• Tell patient not to break, chew, or crush tablets. Tablets must be swallowed whole.

• Caution against performing activities that require mental alertness or physical coordination after taking drug.

• Caution patient to avoid alcohol while taking drug.

• Tell patient to consult prescriber if insomnia worsens or behavior changes.

• Urge female patient to consult prescriber if menses stops or, for both genders, if libido decreases or galactorrhea or fertility problems develop.

R

---

ramipril
ra-MI-pril

Altace

Therapeutic class: Antihypertensives
Pharmacologic class: ACE inhibitors

AVAILABLE FORMS
Capsules ⓄⓃⒸ: 1.25 mg, 2.5 mg, 5 mg, 10 mg
Tablets ⓄⓃⒸ: 1.25 mg, 2.5 mg, 5 mg, 10 mg

INDICATIONS & DOSAGES
➤ **Hypertension**
Adults: Initially, 2.5 mg P.O. once daily for patients not taking a diuretic, and 1.25 mg P.O. once daily for patients taking a diuretic. Increase dosage, if needed, based on patient response. Maintenance dose is 2.5 to 20 mg daily as a single dose or in divided doses.
Adjust-a-dose: For patients with CrCl less than 40 mL/minute, give 1.25 mg P.O. daily. Adjust dosage gradually based on response. Maximum daily dose is 5 mg.
➤ **HF after MI**
Adults: Initially, 2.5 mg P.O. b.i.d. If hypotension occurs, decrease dosage to 1.25 mg P.O. b.i.d. Adjust as tolerated, with dosage increase (as tolerated) at 1 week and subsequent increases about 3 weeks apart, to target dosage of 5 mg P.O. b.i.d.
Adjust-a-dose: For patients with CrCl less than 40 mL/minute, give 1.25 mg P.O. daily. Adjust dosage gradually based on response. Maximum dosage is 2.5 mg b.i.d.
➤ **To reduce risk of MI, stroke, and death from CV causes**
Adults age 55 and older: 2.5 mg P.O. once daily for 1 week, then 5 mg P.O. once daily for 3 weeks. Increase as tolerated to a maintenance dose of 10 mg P.O. once daily.
Adjust-a-dose: In patients who are hypertensive or who have recently had an MI, daily dose may be divided.

ADMINISTRATION
P.O.
● Give drug without regard for meals.
● Patient should swallow tablets or capsules whole.
● If patient can't swallow tablets or capsules, open capsule and sprinkle contents on a small amount of applesauce or mix with 118 mL of water or apple juice. May store for up to 24 hours at room temperature or up to 48 hours under refrigeration if not given immediately.

ACTION
Prevents conversion of angiotensin I to angiotensin II, a potent vasoconstrictor. Less angiotensin II decreases peripheral arterial resistance, decreasing aldosterone secretion, which reduces sodium and water retention and lowers BP.

Route	Onset	Peak	Duration
P.O.	1–2 hr	1–3 hr	24 hr

Half-life: 13 to 17 hours.

ADVERSE REACTIONS
CNS: headache, dizziness, fatigue, asthenia, malaise, light-headedness, vertigo, syncope.
CV: *HF,* MI, orthostatic hypotension, angina pectoris, chest pain, edema.
GI: nausea, vomiting, diarrhea.
Metabolic: *hyperkalemia.*
Respiratory: dyspnea; dry, persistent, tickling, nonproductive cough.

INTERACTIONS
Drug-drug. ❸ *Alert: Aliskiren:* May increase risk of renal impairment, hypotension, and hyperkalemia in diabetic patients and those with moderate to severe renal impairment (GFR less than 60 mL/minute). Concomitant use is contraindicated in diabetic patients. Avoid concomitant use in those with moderate to severe renal impairment.
Diuretics: May cause excessive hypotension, especially at start of therapy. Stop diuretic at least 3 days before therapy begins, increase sodium intake, or reduce starting dose of ramipril.
Insulin, oral antidiabetics: May cause hypoglycemia, especially at start of ramipril therapy. Monitor glucose level closely.
Lithium: May increase lithium level. Use together cautiously and monitor lithium level.
NSAIDs: May decrease antihypertensive effects. Monitor BP.
Potassium-sparing diuretics, potassium supplements: May cause hyperkalemia;

ramipril attenuates potassium loss. Monitor potassium level closely.

Salicylates (aspirin): May decrease antihypertensive effects of ramipril. Ramipril dosage increase or aspirin dosage decrease may be needed.

Telmisartan: May increase risk of renal dysfunction. Avoid use together.

Tizanidine: May cause severe hypotension. Use cautiously and monitor BP closely.

Drug-herb. *Capsaicin:* May cause cough. Discourage use together.

Ma huang: May decrease antihypertensive effects. Discourage use together.

Drug-food. *Salt substitutes containing potassium:* May cause hyperkalemia; ramipril attenuates potassium loss. Discourage use of salt substitutes during therapy.

EFFECTS ON LAB TEST RESULTS

● May increase BUN, creatinine, bilirubin, liver enzyme, glucose, and potassium levels.
● May decrease Hb level and hematocrit.
● May decrease RBC and platelet counts.

CONTRAINDICATIONS & CAUTIONS

● Contraindicated in patients hypersensitive to ACE inhibitors and in those with a history of angioedema related to treatment with an ACE inhibitor.
● Use cautiously in patients with renal impairment.
● Anaphylactoid reactions have been reported in patients dialyzed with high-flux membranes and also treated with ACE inhibitors and in those undergoing LDL apheresis with dextran sulfate absorption.
Dialyzable drug: Unknown.
⚠ *Overdose S&S:* Hypotension.

PREGNANCY-LACTATION-REPRODUCTION

Black Box Warning Use during pregnancy can cause injury and death to the developing fetus. When pregnancy is detected, stop drug as soon as possible. ∎
● Drug may appear in breast milk. Use in breast-feeding women isn't recommended.

NURSING CONSIDERATIONS

● Monitor BP regularly for drug effectiveness.
● Correct fluid and electrolyte imbalances before starting therapy.

● Closely assess renal function in patients during first few weeks of therapy. Regular assessment of renal function is advisable. Patients with severe HF whose renal function depends on the RAAS have experienced acute renal failure during ACE inhibitor therapy. Hypertensive patients with unilateral or bilateral renal artery stenosis also may show signs of worsening renal function during first few days of therapy. Dose reduction or drug stoppage may be necessary.
● Although ACE inhibitors reduce BP in all races, they reduce it less in blacks taking the ACE inhibitor alone. Black patients should use drug in combination therapy for a more favorable response.
● ACE inhibitors appear to increase risk of angioedema in black patients.
● Discontinue drug if patient develops jaundice or significant hepatic enzyme elevation (rare).
● Monitor CBC with differential counts before therapy and periodically thereafter.
● Drug may reduce Hb and WBC, RBC, and platelet counts, especially in patients with impaired renal function or collagen vascular diseases (systemic lupus erythematosus or scleroderma).
● Monitor potassium level. Risk factors for the development of hyperkalemia include renal insufficiency, diabetes, and concomitant use of drugs that raise potassium level.

PATIENT TEACHING

● Tell patient to notify prescriber if any adverse reactions occur. Dosage adjustment or stoppage of drug may be needed.
⟳ *Alert:* Rarely, swelling of the face and throat (including swelling of the larynx) may occur, especially after first dose. Advise patient to report signs or symptoms of breathing difficulty or swelling of face, eyes, lips, or tongue.
● Inform patient that light-headedness can occur, especially during the first few days of therapy. Tell him to rise slowly to minimize this effect and to report signs and symptoms to prescriber. If he faints, patient should stop taking drug and call prescriber immediately.
● Tell patient that if he has difficulty swallowing drug, he can open capsules and sprinkle contents on a small amount of

R

applesauce (about 4 oz [120 mL]) or mix in 4 oz of water or apple juice.

• Advise patient to report signs and symptoms of infection, such as fever and sore throat.

• Tell patient to avoid salt substitutes. These products may contain potassium, which can cause high potassium level in patients taking ramipril.

Black Box Warning Tell women of childbearing potential to notify prescriber if pregnancy occurs. Drug will need to be stopped. ∎

SAFETY ALERT!

ramucirumab
RA-mue-SIR-ue-mab

Cyramza

Therapeutic class: Antineoplastics
Pharmacologic class: Monoclonal antibodies

AVAILABLE FORMS
Injection: 10-mg/mL single-dose vial

INDICATIONS & DOSAGES
Adjust-a-dose (for all indications): For grade 1 or 2 infusion-related reaction (IRR), reduce infusion rate by 50%; for grade 3 or 4 IRR, permanently discontinue drug. For severe hypertension, interrupt treatment until hypertension is controlled with medical management. If severe hypertension can't be controlled, permanently discontinue drug. If urine protein level is 2 g/24 hours or more, withhold drug; once urine protein level returns to less than 2 g/24 hours, reduce dose by 2 mg/kg and restart drug. If urine protein level of 2 g/24 hours or more recurs, withhold drug; once urine protein level returns to less than 2 g/24 hours, restart drug at 6 mg/kg if initial dose was 10 mg/kg or 5 mg/kg if initial dose was 8 mg/kg. For urine protein level of 3 g/24 hours or more or if nephrotic syndrome occurs, permanently discontinue drug. If arterial thromboembolic event (ATE) occurs, permanently discontinue drug. There are no manufacturer dosage adjustment recommendations for hepatic impairment.

Black Box Warning If GI perforation or severe bleeding occurs, permanently discontinue drug. ∎

Black Box Warning Withhold drug before surgery and discontinue if patient develops wound-healing complications. ∎

➤ **Advanced gastric cancer or gastroesophageal junction adenocarcinoma, as a single agent or in combination with paclitaxel, after prior fluoropyrimidine- or platinum-containing chemotherapy**
Adults: 8 mg/kg I.V. over 60 minutes every 2 weeks. Continue until disease progression or unacceptable toxicity. When given in combination, administer ramucirumab before paclitaxel.

➤ **Metastatic non-small-cell lung cancer in combination with docetaxel in patients with disease progression on or after platinum-based chemotherapy. (Patients with *EGFR* or *ALK* genomic tumor aberrations should have shown disease progression on FDA-approved therapy for these before treatment with ramucirumab.)**
Adults: 10 mg/kg I.V. over 60 minutes on day 1 of a 21-day cycle before docetaxel infusion. Continue until disease progression or unacceptable toxicity.

➤ **Colorectal cancer in combination with FOLFIRI (irinotecan, folinic acid, and 5-FU) in patients with disease progression on or after therapy with bevacizumab, oxaliplatin, and a fluoropyrimidine**
Adults: 8 mg/kg I.V. over 60 minutes every 2 weeks before FOLFIRI administration. Continue until disease progression or unacceptable toxicity.

ADMINISTRATION
I.V.
▼ Administer as I.V. infusion only, not as I.V. push or bolus.
▼ For each infusion, premedicate with I.V. histamine (H_1) antagonist (diphenhydramine). For patients with prior grade 1 or 2 IRR, also premedicate with dexamethasone or equivalent and acetaminophen before each infusion.
▼ Dilute drug with NSS to final volume of 250 mL. Diluted solution is stable for 24 hours if refrigerated or 4 hours at room

---

Reactions in bold italics are *life-threatening*. Interactions may have a *rapid onset* or a **delayed onset**.

temperature. Gently invert container; don't shake.

▼ Inspect solution for particles and discoloration before administration.

▼ Give infusion through separate infusion line using a protein-sparing 0.22-micron filter. Flush line with NSS at end of infusion.

▼ Store vials in refrigerator at 36° to 46° F (2° to 8° C) until ready to use. Keep vial in outer carton to protect from light. Don't freeze or shake vial.

▼ Drug is a hazardous agent; use appropriate handling and disposal precautions.

▼ **Incompatibilities:** Dextrose solutions, electrolytes, other medications.

ACTION

A vascular endothelial growth factor receptor 2 antagonist that inhibits proliferation and migration of human endothelial cells, angiogenesis, and tumor growth.

Route	Onset	Peak	Duration
I.V.	Unknown	Unknown	Unknown

Half-life: 14 days.

ADVERSE REACTIONS

CNS: headache.
CV: hypertension, *arterial thromboembolic events, hemorrhage.*
EENT: epistaxis.
GI: diarrhea, intestinal obstruction.
GU: proteinuria.
Hematologic: anemia, hyponatremia, *neutropenia.*
Skin: rash.
Other: infusion-related reaction, antibody development, hypothyroidism.

INTERACTIONS

None reported.

EFFECTS ON LAB TEST RESULTS

• May increase urine protein level and decrease serum sodium level.
• May decrease RBC count.

CONTRAINDICATIONS & CAUTIONS

Black Box Warning Drug increases risk of hemorrhage and GI hemorrhage, including severe and sometimes fatal hemorrhagic

events. Permanently discontinue drug in patients who experience severe bleeding. ∎
Black Box Warning Withhold drug before surgery. Resume after the surgical intervention based on clinical judgment of adequate wound healing. If patient develops wound-healing complications during therapy, discontinue drug until wound is fully healed. ∎
Black Box Warning Permanently discontinue drug in patients who experience GI perforation, a potentially fatal event. ∎
• Contraindicated in patients hypersensitive to drug or its components.
• Use cautiously in patients with cirrhosis (Child-Pugh class B or C). Use in patients with hepatic impairment (Child-Pugh class B or C) only if potential benefits outweigh potential risks.
⊕ Alert: Rare and sometimes fatal reversible posterior leukoencephalopathy syndrome (RPLS) has been reported.
• Safety and effectiveness in children haven't been established.
Dialyzable drug: Unknown.

PREGNANCY-LACTATION-REPRODUCTION

• Drug may cause fetal harm. Women of childbearing potential should use effective contraception during and for at least 3 months after last ramucirumab dose.
• It isn't known if drug appears in breast milk. Because of the potential risk of serious adverse reactions in breast-feeding infants, breast-feeding isn't recommended during treatment.
• Based on animal data, drug may impair fertility in women.

NURSING CONSIDERATIONS

⊕ Alert: Serious, sometimes fatal, ATEs, including MI, cardiac arrest, stroke, and cerebral ischemia, have occurred. Monitor patient closely, and permanently discontinue drug in patients who experience a severe ATE.
• Assess BP every 2 weeks or more frequently as clinically indicated. Control hypertension before start of therapy. If severe hypertension occurs, withhold drug until controlled. Discontinue drug permanently if hypertension can't be controlled,

R

in hypertensive crisis, or in hypertensive encephalopathy.
● Premedicate patient before each infusion, and monitor patient for IRR.
⊕ *Alert:* Assess patient for signs and symptoms of GI perforation (severe abdominal pain, nausea, vomiting, fever).
⊕ *Alert:* Monitor recent wounds for complications during therapy. For wound healing complications, withhold drug until wound is fully healed.
● Monitor patients with cirrhosis (Child-Pugh class B or C) for new-onset or worsening encephalopathy, ascites, or hepatorenal syndrome.
● Monitor patient for signs and symptoms of RPLS (hypertension, headache, visual disturbances, altered consciousness, seizures). Confirm diagnosis with MRI; discontinue drug and provide supportive care.
● Monitor thyroid function because of risk of hypothyroidism.

PATIENT TEACHING
⊕ *Alert:* Inform patient that drug can cause severe bleeding. Advise patient to contact prescriber for bleeding or symptoms of bleeding, including light-headedness.
● Warn patient of increased risk of arterial thromboembolic event.
● Advise patient to undergo routine BP monitoring and to contact health care provider if BP is elevated or if signs and symptoms of hypertension (severe headache, light-headedness, or neurologic symptoms) occur.
⊕ *Alert:* Caution patient to notify health care provider for severe diarrhea, vomiting, or severe abdominal pain.
⊕ *Alert:* Warn patient that drug may impair wound healing. Instruct patient not to undergo surgery without first discussing potential risk with health care provider.
● Teach patient about potential risk of maintaining pregnancy, risk to fetus, and risk to postnatal infant development during and after treatment with ramucirumab. Discuss the need to avoid pregnancy, including use of adequate contraception, for at least 3 months after last dose.
● Advise female patient of childbearing potential that drug may impair fertility.

● Counsel patient on the need to discontinue breast-feeding during treatment.

ranibizumab
RA-ni-BIZ-oo-mab

Lucentis

Therapeutic class: Vascular endothelial growth factor A inhibitors
Pharmacologic class: Monoclonal antibodies

AVAILABLE FORMS
Intravitreal injection: 6 mg/mL, 10 mg/mL

INDICATIONS & DOSAGES
➤ **Neovascular (wet) age-related macular degeneration or macular edema after retinal vein occlusion**
Adults: 0.5 mg (0.05 mL of 10-mg/mL solution) by intravitreal injection once a month (approximately 28 days between doses), or 0.5 mg administered by intravitreal injection once a month for 4 months followed by 0.5 mg every 3 months thereafter, although this dosing may be less effective.
➤ **Diabetic macular edema**
Adults: 0.3 mg (0.05 mL of 6-mg/mL solution) by intravitreal injection once a month (approximately 28 days between doses).
➤ **Diabetic retinopathy in patients with diabetic macular edema**
Adults: 0.3 mg (0.05 mL of 6-mg/mL solution) by intravitreal injection once a month (approximately 28 days between doses).

ADMINISTRATION
Ophthalmic intravitreal injection
● Store vials in original carton under refrigeration until use. Don't freeze.
● Protect from light.
● Withdraw vial contents through a 5-micron, 19G filter needle attached to a 1-mL tuberculin syringe; discard filter needle after withdrawal of vial contents.
● Replace filter needle with a sterile 30G × ½-inch needle for the intravitreal injection. Expel contents until 0.05 mL remains in syringe.

Reactions in bold italics are *life-threatening*. Interactions may have a *rapid onset* or a *delayed onset*.

ACTION

Binds to the receptor-binding site of active forms of vascular endothelial growth factor A, reducing endothelial cell proliferation, vascular leakage, and new blood vessel formation.

Route	Onset	Peak	Duration
Intravitreal injection	Unknown	1 day	Unknown

Half-life: 9 days.

ADVERSE REACTIONS

CNS: headache, peripheral neuropathy.
CV: atrial fibrillation, peripheral edema, *arterial thromboembolic events.*
EENT: conjunctival hemorrhage, eye pain, vitreous floaters, increased IOP, vitreous detachment, intraocular inflammation, cataract, foreign body sensation in eyes, eye irritation, increased lacrimation, blepharitis, dry eye, visual disturbance or blurred vision, eye pruritus, ocular hyperemia, retinal disorder, maculopathy, retinal degeneration, ocular discomfort, conjunctival hyperemia, posterior capsule opacification, injection-site hemorrhage, nasopharyngitis, sinusitis.
GI: nausea, constipation, GERD.
GU: renal failure, chronic renal failure.
Hematologic: anemia.
Metabolic: hypercholesterolemia.
Musculoskeletal: arthralgia.
Respiratory: URI, bronchitis, COPD, cough.
Skin: wound healing complications.
Other: seasonal allergy, flulike symptoms, antibody formation.

INTERACTIONS

None reported.

EFFECTS ON LAB TEST RESULTS

None reported.

CONTRAINDICATIONS & CAUTIONS

• Contraindicated in patients with known hypersensitivity to drug or its components and in patients with ocular or periocular infections.
• May increase risk of arterial thromboembolic events (nonfatal stroke, nonfatal MI, vascular death, or death of unknown cause), especially in diabetic patients.

• May cause serious intraocular inflammation if drug is given within 9 days after verteporfin photodynamic therapy.
Dialyzable drug: Unknown.

PREGNANCY-LACTATION-REPRODUCTION

• There are no studies in pregnant women, and it isn't known if drug can cause fetal harm. Based on its mechanism of action, drug may pose a risk to embryo-fetal development (including teratogenicity) and reproductive capacity. Use during pregnancy only if clearly needed.
• It isn't known if drug appears in breast milk. Use cautiously in breast-feeding women.

NURSING CONSIDERATIONS

• Carry out intravitreal injection procedure under aseptic conditions with adequate anesthesia and a broad-spectrum microbicide given before injection.
• Before and 30 minutes after intravitreal injection, monitor patient for elevated IOP using tonometry.
• Check for perfusion of the optic nerve head immediately after injection.
• Use one vial per treatment of a single eye. If second eye treatment is necessary, use new vial and reestablish sterile field.
• Monitor patient for hypersensitivity reactions, which may present as severe intraocular inflammation.
• Monitor patient for signs and symptoms suggestive of endophthalmitis (eye redness, sensitivity to light, eye pain, vision changes).
• Monitor patient for arterial thromboembolic events.

PATIENT TEACHING

• Instruct patient to seek immediate care from the ophthalmologist for eye redness, sensitivity to light, eye pain, or vision changes.

R

ranitidine hydrochloride
ra-NYE-te-deen

Acid Reducer❋ ◇, Zantac✎,
Zantac 75 ◇, Zantac 150 ◇,
Zantac 300

Therapeutic class: Antiulcer drugs
Pharmacologic class: H$_2$-receptor
antagonists

AVAILABLE FORMS
Capsules: 150 mg, 300 mg
Injection: 25 mg/mL
Syrup: 15 mg/mL*
Tablets: 75 mg ◇, 150 mg ◇, 300 mg

INDICATIONS & DOSAGES
Adjust-a-dose (for all indications): For patients with CrCl below 50 mL/minute,
150 mg P.O. every 24 hours or 50 mg I.V.
every 18 to 24 hours.
➤ **Active duodenal and gastric ulcer**
Adults: 150 mg P.O. b.i.d. or 300 mg daily
after evening meal or at bedtime. Or, 50 mg
I.V. or I.M. every 6 to 8 hours. Maximum
daily I.V. dose, 400 mg. Or, 150 mg by
continuous infusion at 6.25 mg/hour over
24 hours.
Children ages 1 month to 16 years: For
duodenal and gastric ulcers only, 2 to
4 mg/kg P.O. b.i.d., up to 300 mg/day. Or,
2 to 4 mg/kg/day I.V., divided every 6 to
8 hours, up to a maximum of 50 mg every
6 to 8 hours.
➤ **Maintenance therapy for duodenal or
gastric ulcer**
Adults: 150 mg P.O. at bedtime.
Children ages 1 month to 16 years: 2 to
4 mg/kg P.O. daily, up to 150 mg daily.
➤ **Pathologic hypersecretory conditions,
such as Zollinger-Ellison syndrome**
Adults: 150 mg P.O. b.i.d.; doses up to 6 g
or more frequent intervals may be needed
in patients with severe disease. Or, infuse
continuously at 1 mg/kg/hour. After 4 hours,
if patient remains symptomatic or gastric
acid output is greater than 10 mEq/hour, increase dose in increments of 0.5 mg/kg/hour
and recheck gastric acid output. Doses up
to 2.5 mg/kg/hour and infusion rates up to
220 mg/hour have been used.

➤ **GERD**
Adults: 150 mg P.O. b.i.d.
Children ages 1 month to 16 years: 5 to
10 mg/kg P.O. daily given as two divided
doses.
➤ **Erosive esophagitis**
Adults: 150 mg P.O. q.i.d. Maintenance
dosage is 150 mg P.O. b.i.d.
Children ages 1 month to 16 years: 5 to
10 mg/kg P.O. daily given as two divided
doses.
➤ **Heartburn**
Adults and children age 12 and older: 75 to
150 mg (OTC only) P.O. 30 to 60 minutes
before food or beverages that cause heartburn or as symptoms occur, up to 300 mg
daily. Don't use more than twice daily or
exceed 2 weeks of continuous treatment.

ADMINISTRATION
P.O.
● Give once-daily dose after evening meal
or at bedtime.
I.M.
● Administer undiluted.
I.V.
▼ To prepare I.V. injection, dilute 2 mL
(50 mg) ranitidine with compatible I.V.
solution to a total volume of 20 mL, and
inject over at least 5 minutes. Compatible
solutions include sterile water for injection,
NSS for injection, D$_5$W, and lactated
Ringer injection.
▼ To give drug by intermittent I.V. infusion, dilute 50 mg (2 mL) in 100 mL
compatible solution and infuse at a rate
of 5 to 7 mL/minute. Infuse over 15 to
20 minutes.
▼ For continuous infusion to treat active
duodenal or gastric ulcer, dilute 150 mg in
250 mL of D$_5$W. For hypersecretory conditions such as Zollinger-Ellison syndrome,
dilute with D$_5$W or other compatible solution to no more than 2.5 mg/mL.
▼ Administer continuous I.V. infusion at 6.25 mg/hour. For patients with
Zollinger-Ellison syndrome, administer
at 1 mg/kg/hour. Rapid I.V. administration has been associated with bradycardia
(rarely), particularly in patients predisposed to cardiac rhythm disturbances.
Don't exceed recommended infusion rates.

Reactions in bold italics are *life-threatening*. Interactions may have a *rapid onset* or a **delayed onset**.

▼ After dilution, solution is stable for 48 hours at room temperature.

▼ Store I.V. injection at 39° to 86° F (4° to 30° C).

▼ **Incompatibilities:** Amphotericin B, atracurium, cefazolin, cefoxitin, ceftazidime, cefuroxime, chlorpromazine, clindamycin phosphate, diazepam, ethacrynate sodium, hetastarch, hydroxyzine, insulin (regular), methotrimeprazine, midazolam, norepinephrine, pantoprazole, pentobarbital sodium, phenobarbital, phytonadione.

ACTION
Competitively inhibits action of histamine at H_2-receptor sites of parietal cells, decreasing gastric acid secretion.

Route	Onset	Peak	Duration
P.O.	1 hr	1–3 hr	13 hr
I.V.	Unknown	Unknown	Unknown

Half-life: 2 to 3 hours.

ADVERSE REACTIONS
CNS: headache, malaise, vertigo.
EENT: blurred vision.
Hepatic: jaundice.
Other: *anaphylaxis, angioedema,* burning and itching at injection site.

INTERACTIONS
Drug-drug. *Glipizide:* May increase hypoglycemic effect. Adjust glipizide dosage, as directed.
Iron salts: May reduce absorption of iron salts. Monitor therapy.
Ketoconazole: May decrease ketoconazole serum concentration. Give at least 2 hours before ranitidine.
Methylphenidate: May decrease absorption and interfere with normal release of extended-release formulations of methylphenidate. Monitor therapy.
Midazolam, triazolam: May prolong sedation. Monitor patient for excessive sedation.
Procainamide: May decrease renal clearance of procainamide. Monitor patient closely for toxicity.
Warfarin: May interfere with warfarin clearance. Monitor patient closely.

EFFECTS ON LAB TEST RESULTS
● May increase creatinine and ALT levels.
● May cause false-positive results in urine protein tests using Multistix.

CONTRAINDICATIONS & CAUTIONS
● Contraindicated in patients hypersensitive to drug and in those with acute porphyria.
● Use cautiously in patients with hepatic dysfunction. Adjust dosage in patients with impaired renal function.
● Rarely, drug may cause confusion; risk is greater in elderly or severely ill patients and in those with renal or hepatic impairment.
● Prolonged treatment (at least 2 years) may lead to vitamin B_{12} malabsorption and deficiency. The magnitude of deficiency is dose-related and association is stronger in women and those younger than age 30.
Dialyzable drug: Yes.
⚠ *Overdose S&S:* Exaggeration of adverse reactions, abnormal gait, hypotension.

PREGNANCY-LACTATION-REPRODUCTION
● There are no adequate studies in pregnant women. Use during pregnancy only if clearly needed.
● Drug appears in breast milk. Use cautiously in breast-feeding women.

NURSING CONSIDERATIONS
● Assess patient for abdominal pain. Note presence of blood in emesis, stool, or gastric aspirate.
● Drug may be added to total parenteral nutrition solutions.
● High doses (100 mg or more) or prolonged I.V. therapy (5 days or longer) may increase ALT level. Monitor ALT level daily for remainder of treatment.
● *Look alike–sound alike:* Don't confuse ranitidine with rimantadine. Don't confuse Zantac with Xanax or Zyrtec.

PATIENT TEACHING
● Instruct patient on proper use of OTC preparation, as indicated.
● Remind patient to take once-daily prescription drug at bedtime for best results.
● Instruct patient to take without regard to meals because absorption isn't affected by food.

R

● Urge patient to avoid cigarette smoking because this may increase gastric acid secretion and worsen disease.
● Advise patient to report abdominal pain, blood in stool or emesis, black, tarry stools, or coffee-ground emesis.

ranolazine
ran-OH-lah-zeen

Ranexa♦

Therapeutic class: Antianginals
Pharmacologic class: Cardiovascular drugs

AVAILABLE FORMS
Tablets (extended-release) ⓝ: 500 mg, 1,000 mg

INDICATIONS & DOSAGES
➤ **Chronic angina**
Adults: Initially, 500 mg P.O. b.i.d. Increase, if needed, to maximum of 1,000 mg b.i.d.
Adjust-a-dose: Limit maximum dose to 500 mg b.i.d. in patients on moderate CYP3A inhibitors, such as diltiazem, verapamil, and erythromycin.

ADMINISTRATION
P.O.
● Give drug without regard for meals.
● Give drug whole; don't crush or cut tablets.
● Don't give drug with grapefruit juice.
● If a dose is missed, give at next scheduled time; don't double a dose.

ACTION
May result from increased efficiency of myocardial oxygen use when myocardial metabolism is shifted away from fatty acid oxidation toward glucose oxidation. Antianginal and anti-ischemic properties don't decrease HR or BP and don't increase myocardial work.

Route	Onset	Peak	Duration
P.O.	Rapid	2–5 hr	Unknown

Half-life: 7 hours.

ADVERSE REACTIONS
CNS: dizziness, headache.
CV: palpitations, peripheral edema, syncope.
EENT: tinnitus, vertigo.
GI: abdominal pain, constipation, dry mouth, nausea, vomiting.
Respiratory: dyspnea.

INTERACTIONS
Drug-drug. *Antipsychotics or TCAs metabolized by CYP2D6:* May increase levels of these drugs. Dosage reduction may be needed.
Clarithromycin, nefazodone, protease inhibitors: May cause QTc prolongation. Use together is contraindicated.
Cyclosporine, paroxetine, ritonavir: May increase ranolazine level. Use cautiously together, and monitor patient for increased adverse effects.
Digoxin: May increase digoxin level. Monitor digoxin level periodically; digoxin dosage may need to be reduced.
Diltiazem, ketoconazole and other azole antifungals, macrolide antibiotics (azithromycin, erythromycin), verapamil, other CYP3A inhibitors: May increase ranolazine level and prolong QT interval. Avoid using together.
Drugs that prolong the QT interval (antiarrhythmics, such as dofetilide, quinidine, sotalol), antipsychotics (chlorpromazine, ziprasidone): May increase risk of prolonged QT interval and ventricular arrhythmia. Use cautiously together.
Rifabutin, rifampin, rifapentine, other CYP3A inducers (carbamazepine, phenobarbital, phenytoin): May reduce plasma concentration of ranolazine to subtherapeutic levels. Don't use together.
Simvastatin: May increase simvastatin level. Limit simvastatin dosage to 20 mg once daily, and monitor patient for adverse effects.
Drug-herb. *St. John's wort:* May reduce plasma concentration of ranolazine to subtherapeutic levels. Don't use together.
Drug-food. *Grapefruit:* May increase drug level and prolong QT interval. Discourage use together.

EFFECTS ON LAB TEST RESULTS
• May increase creatinine and BUN levels. May decrease Hb and HbA$_{1c}$ levels and hematocrit.
• May increase eosinophil count.

CONTRAINDICATIONS & CAUTIONS
• Contraindicated in patients taking QT interval–prolonging drugs, CYP3A inducers (rifampin, phenobarbital), or strong CYP3A inhibitors (clarithromycin, ketoconazole, nelfinavir), and in patients with ventricular tachycardia, hepatic impairment, or prolonged QT interval.
• Use cautiously in patients with renal impairment.
Dialyzable drug: Unlikely.

PREGNANCY-LACTATION-REPRODUCTION
• There are no adequate studies in pregnant women. Use during pregnancy only if potential benefit justifies potential risk to the fetus.
• It isn't known if drug appears breast milk. Patient should discontinue breast-feeding or discontinue drug.

NURSING CONSIDERATIONS
🔆 *Alert:* Drug prolongs the QT interval according to the dose. If drug is given with other drugs that prolong the QTc interval, torsades de pointes or sudden death may occur. Don't exceed maximum dosage.
• Obtain baseline ECG and monitor subsequent ECG for prolonged QT interval. Measure the QTc interval regularly.
• If patient has renal insufficiency, monitor BP closely.

PATIENT TEACHING
• Teach patient about this drug's potential to affect the heart's rhythm. Advise patient to immediately report palpitations or fainting.
• Urge patient to tell prescriber about all other prescription or OTC drugs or herbal supplements he takes.
• Tell patient that he should keep taking other drugs prescribed for angina.
• Tell patient that drug may be taken with or without food.
• Advise patient to avoid grapefruit juice while taking this drug.

🔆 *Alert:* Warn patient that tablets must be swallowed whole and not crushed, broken, or chewed.
• Explain that drug won't stop a sudden anginal attack; advise him to keep other treatments, such as S.L. nitroglycerin, readily available.
• Tell patient to avoid activities that require mental alertness until effects of the drug are known.

rasagiline mesylate
reh-SAH-jih-leen

Azilect𝒪

Therapeutic class: Antiparkinsonians
Pharmacologic class: Irreversible, selective MAO inhibitors type B

AVAILABLE FORMS
Tablets: 0.5 mg, 1 mg

INDICATIONS & DOSAGES
➤ **Idiopathic Parkinson disease, as monotherapy or with levodopa**
Adults: As monotherapy, 1 mg P.O. once daily. As adjunctive therapy, initial dose is 0.5 mg P.O. once daily. May increase to 1 mg P.O. once daily.
Adjust-a-dose: If patient has mild hepatic impairment or takes a CYP1A2 inhibitor such as ciprofloxacin, give 0.5 mg once daily.

ADMINISTRATION
P.O.
• Give drug without regard to meals.

ACTION
Unknown. May increase extracellular dopamine level in the CNS, improving neurotransmission and relieving signs and symptoms of Parkinson disease.

Route	Onset	Peak	Duration
P.O.	Variable	1 hr	1 wk

Half-life: 3 hours.

R

ADVERSE REACTIONS
Monotherapy
CNS: dizziness, falls, headache, depression, fever, hallucinations, malaise, paresthesia, syncope, vertigo.
CV: chest pain, angina pectoris, postural hypotension.
EENT: gingivitis.
GI: anorexia, diarrhea, dyspepsia, gastroenteritis, vomiting.
GU: albuminuria, impotence.
Hematologic: *leukopenia.*
Musculoskeletal: arthralgia, arthritis, neck pain.
Respiratory: asthma, flu syndrome, rhinitis.
Skin: alopecia, *carcinoma,* ecchymosis, vesiculobullous rash.
Other: allergic reaction, decreased libido.
Combined with levodopa
CNS: confusion, falls, headache, abnormal dreams, amnesia, ataxia, dyskinesia, dystonia, hallucinations, paresthesia, somnolence, sweating, abnormal gait, anxiety, asthenia, hyperkinesia, hypertonia, neuropathy, tremor.
CV: bundle-branch block, orthostatic hypotension.
EENT: epistaxis, gingivitis.
GI: nausea, abdominal pain, anorexia, constipation, diarrhea, dry mouth, dyspepsia, dysphagia, vomiting, weight loss, *GI hemorrhage.*
GU: albuminuria, hematuria, urinary incontinence.
Hematologic: *hemorrhage,* anemia.
Musculoskeletal: arthralgia, arthritis, bursitis, hernia, leg cramps, myasthenia, neck pain, tenosynovitis.
Respiratory: dyspnea, increased cough.
Skin: *carcinoma,* ecchymosis, pruritus, rash, ulcer.
Other: infection.

INTERACTIONS
Drug-drug. *Ciprofloxacin and other CYP1A2 inhibitors:* May double rasagiline level. Decrease rasagiline dosage to 0.5 mg daily.
Dextromethorphan: May cause episodes of psychosis or bizarre behavior. Concomitant use is contraindicated.

Levodopa: May increase rasagiline level. Watch for dyskinesia, dystonia, hallucinations, and hypotension, and reduce levodopa dosage if needed.
MAO inhibitors: May cause hypertensive crisis. Contraindicated with other MAO inhibitors.
Opiate agonists (meperidine, methadone, tramadol): May cause severe, sometimes fatal, serotonin syndrome. Concomitant use is contraindicated.
SSRIs, SNRIs, TCAs: May cause severe or fatal CNS toxicity. Stop rasagiline for at least 14 days before starting an antidepressant. Stop fluoxetine for 5 weeks before starting rasagiline.
Drug-herb. *St. John's wort:* May cause severe reaction. Use together is contraindicated.
Drug-food. *Foods with very high levels of tyramine (more than 150 mg), such as aged cheeses, cured meats, fava beans:* May cause hypertensive reaction. Urge patient to avoid foods high in tyramine.

EFFECTS ON LAB TEST RESULTS
• May increase liver enzyme levels.
• May decrease WBC count.

CONTRAINDICATIONS & CAUTIONS
• Contraindicated in patients with pheochromocytoma, those with moderate to severe hepatic impairment, and those taking amphetamines, cold products, dextromethorphan, ephedrine, MAO inhibitors, meperidine, methadone, phenylephrine, pseudoephedrine, St. John's wort, sympathomimetic amines, or tramadol.
• Exacerbation of hypertension may occur during treatment, which may require medication adjustment if sustained.
• Potentially life-threatening serotonin syndrome has been reported in patients treated with antidepressants concomitantly with rasagiline. Use together isn't recommended.
• Somnolence and falling asleep without prior warning while engaged in activities of daily living (including operating motor vehicles) have been reported in some patients. Evaluate patient for factors that may increase these risks.
• Use cautiously in patients with mild hepatic impairment. Dosage reduction may be

---

needed. Avoid use in patients with moderate to severe hepatic impairment.

Dialyzable drug: Unknown.

⚠ *Overdose S&S:* Drowsiness, dizziness, faintness, irritability, hyperactivity, agitation, severe headache, hallucinations, trismus, opisthotonos, seizures, coma, rapid and irregular pulse, hypertension, hypotension and vascular collapse, precordial pain, respiratory depression and failure, hyperpyrexia, diaphoresis, cool and clammy skin.

PREGNANCY-LACTATION-REPRODUCTION

• There are no adequate studies in pregnant women. Use during pregnancy only if potential benefit justifies potential risk to the fetus.

• It isn't known if drug appears in breast milk. Use cautiously in breast-feeding women.

NURSING CONSIDERATIONS

• Orthostatic hypotension may occur during first 2 months of therapy; help patient to rise from a reclining position.

• Monitor patient for new-onset hypertension or hypertension that isn't adequately controlled after starting drug.

• Monitor patient taking antidepressants and rasagiline concomitantly for serotonin syndrome.

• Monitor patient for drowsiness, significant daytime sleepiness, or episodes of falling asleep during activities that require active participation. Discontinue drug if these symptoms occur.

• Ask patient or caregiver about development or worsening of impulsive or compulsive behaviors, such as new or increased gambling urges, sexual urges, uncontrolled spending, or other urges; patient may not recognize these behaviors as abnormal.

• Notify prescriber if patient experiences adverse effects; levodopa dose may need to be reduced.

• Examine patient's skin periodically for possible melanoma because of drug's associated risk of skin cancer.

• Notify prescriber if patient is having elective surgery; drug should be stopped at least 2 weeks before.

• *Look alike–sound alike:* Don't confuse Azilect with Aricept.

PATIENT TEACHING

• Explain the risk of hypertensive crisis if patient ingests foods containing very high levels of tyramine while taking rasagiline. Give patient a list of these foods and products.

• Advise patient to rise slowly after prolonged sitting or lying down.

• Advise patient taking antidepressants concomitantly with rasagiline to immediately report confusion, hallucinations, agitation, delirium, syncope, shivering, sweating, high fever, tachycardia, nausea, diarrhea, muscle rigidity or twitching, or tremors.

• Advise patient that drug may cause patient to fall asleep during activities that require active participation and to report if drowsiness, significant daytime sleepiness, or episodes of falling asleep during such activities occur.

• Tell patient to report difficulty controlling impulsive or compulsive behaviors, such as new or increased gambling urges, sexual urges, uncontrolled spending, or other urges.

• Urge patient to watch for skin changes that could suggest melanoma and to have periodic skin examinations.

• Instruct patient to maintain usual dosage schedule if a dose is missed and not to double the next dose.

• Tell female patient to inform prescriber if she plans to become pregnant or breast-feed.

• Advise patient to contact prescriber before discontinuing rasagiline.

SAFETY ALERT!

repaglinide
re-PAG-lah-nyde

Prandin

Therapeutic class: Antidiabetics
Pharmacologic class: Meglitinides

AVAILABLE FORMS

Tablets: 0.5 mg, 1 mg, 2 mg

INDICATIONS & DOSAGES

➤ **Type 2 diabetes alone or with metformin or a thiazolidinedione**

Adults: For patients not previously treated or whose HbA$_{1c}$ level is below 8%, starting dose is 0.5 mg P.O. taken about 15 minutes before each meal. For patients previously treated with glucose-lowering drugs and whose HbA_{1c} is 8% or more, first dose is 1 to 2 mg P.O. before each meal. Recommended dosage range is 0.5 to 4 mg before meals b.i.d., t.i.d., or q.i.d. Maximum daily dose is 16 mg.

Determine dosage by glucose response. May double dosage up to 4 mg before each meal until satisfactory glucose response is achieved. At least 1 week should elapse between dosage adjustments to assess response to each dose.

Metformin or a thiazolidinedione may be added if repaglinide monotherapy is inadequate; no initial repaglinide dosage adjustment is necessary; however, dosage adjustment may be needed if patient experiences hypoglycemic episodes.

Adjust-a-dose: In patients with severe renal impairment, starting dosage is 0.5 mg P.O. before meals. Use cautiously in patients with impaired liver function and allow longer intervals between dosage adjustments to allow full assessment of response.

ADMINISTRATION
P.O.
● Give drug before meals, usually 15 minutes before start of meal; however, time can vary from immediately preceding meal to up to 30 minutes before meal.

ACTION
Stimulates insulin release from beta cells in the pancreas by closing adenosine triphosphate (ATP)-dependent potassium channels in beta cell membranes, which causes calcium channels to open. Increased calcium influx induces insulin secretion; the overall effect is to lower glucose level.

Route	Onset	Peak	Duration
P.O.	15–60 min	1 hr	6 hr

Half-life: 1 hour.

ADVERSE REACTIONS
CNS: headache, paresthesia.
CV: angina.
EENT: rhinitis, sinusitis.
GI: constipation, diarrhea, dyspepsia, nausea, vomiting.

GU: UTI.
Metabolic: *hypoglycemia,* hyperglycemia.
Musculoskeletal: arthralgia, back pain.
Respiratory: bronchitis, URI.
Other: tooth disorder.

INTERACTIONS
Drug-drug. *Barbiturates, carbamazepine, rifampin:* May increase repaglinide metabolism. Monitor glucose level.
Beta blockers, chloramphenicol, coumarin derivatives, MAO inhibitors, NSAIDs, other drugs that are highly protein bound, probenecid, salicylates, sulfonamides: May increase hypoglycemic action of repaglinide. Monitor glucose level.
Calcium channel blockers, corticosteroids, estrogens, fosphenytoin, hormonal contraceptives, isoniazid, nicotinic acid, phenothiazines, phenytoin, sympathomimetics, thiazides and other diuretics, thyroid products: May produce hyperglycemia, resulting in a loss of glycemic control. Monitor glucose level.
Clarithromycin: May increase repaglinide levels. Adjust repaglinide dosage.
Erythromycin, itraconazole, ketoconazole, miconazole, similar inhibitors of CYP3A4: May inhibit repaglinide metabolism. Monitor glucose level.
Gemfibrozil: Significantly increases repaglinide level. Use together is contraindicated.
Drug-herb. *Burdock:* May increase hypoglycemic effects. Discourage use together.
St. John's wort: May decrease repaglinide level and its therapeutic effect. Don't use together.
Drug-food. *Grapefruit juice:* May inhibit metabolism of drug. Discourage use together.
Drug-lifestyle. *Alcohol use:* May alter glycemic control, most commonly causing hypoglycemia. Discourage use together.

EFFECTS ON LAB TEST RESULTS
● May increase or decrease glucose level.

CONTRAINDICATIONS & CAUTIONS
● Contraindicated in patients hypersensitive to drug or its inactive ingredients and in those with type 1 diabetes or diabetic ketoacidosis with or without coma.

Reactions in bold italics are *life-threatening*. Interactions may have a *rapid onset* or a *delayed onset*.

• Drug isn't indicated for use in combination with NPH insulin.

• Use cautiously in elderly, debilitated, or malnourished patients and in those with hepatic, adrenal, or pituitary insufficiency.

Dialyzable drug: Unknown.

⚠ *Overdose S&S:* Hypoglycemia, severe hypoglycemic reactions (coma, seizures, neurologic impairment).

PREGNANCY-LACTATION-REPRODUCTION

• Safety in pregnancy hasn't been established. Use only if clearly needed.

• Abnormal blood glucose levels during pregnancy may cause fetal harm. Most experts recommend that insulin be used during pregnancy to maintain blood glucose levels as close to normal as possible.

• It isn't known if drug appears in breast milk. Patient should discontinue breast-feeding or discontinue drug.

NURSING CONSIDERATIONS

• Increase dosage carefully in patients with impaired renal function or renal failure requiring dialysis.

• Metformin may be added if repaglinide alone is inadequate.

• Monitor glucose and HbA_{1c} levels for loss of glycemic control, especially during stress.

• Hypoglycemia may be difficult to recognize in elderly patients and in patients taking beta blockers.

• When switching to a different oral antidiabetic, begin new drug on day after last dose of repaglinide.

• *Look alike–sound alike:* Don't confuse Prandin with Avandia.

PATIENT TEACHING

• Stress importance of diet and exercise with drug therapy.

• Discuss symptoms of hypoglycemia with patient and family.

• Encourage patient to keep regular appointments and have his HbA_{1c} level checked every 3 months to determine long-term glucose control.

• Tell patient to take drug before meals, usually 15 minutes before start of meal; however, time can vary from immediately preceding meal to up to 30 minutes before meal.

• Tell patient that, if a meal is skipped or added, he should skip dose or add an extra dose of drug for that meal, respectively.

• Instruct patient to monitor glucose level carefully and tell him what to do when he's ill, undergoing surgery, or under stress.

• Advise women planning pregnancy to first consult prescriber. Insulin may be needed during pregnancy and breast-feeding.

• Teach patient to carry candy or other simple sugars to treat mild hypoglycemia episodes. Patient experiencing severe episode may need emergency treatment.

• Advise patient to avoid alcohol, which lowers glucose level.

reslizumab
See NEW DRUGS for information.

ribavirin
rye-ba-VYE-rin

Copegus, Ibavyr✥, Moderiba, Rebetol, Ribasphere, Ribasphere RibaPak, Ribavarin, Virazole

Therapeutic class: Antivirals
Pharmacologic class: Nucleosides–nucleotides

AVAILABLE FORMS
Capsules ⊙: 200 mg
Oral solution: 40 mg/mL
Powder to be reconstituted for inhalation: 6 g in 100-mL glass vial
Tablets: 200 mg, 400 mg, 500 mg, 600 mg

INDICATIONS & DOSAGES
Adjust-a-dose (for all indications): Refer to manufacturer's instructions for each formulation for dosage adjustments in patients with impaired renal function or hematologic toxicities. Some formulations are contraindicated in patients with CrCl of less than 50 mL/minute or in patients with hepatic decompensation (Child-Pugh classes B and C).

Black Box Warning Ribavirin alone isn't effective for treatment of chronic HCV infection. ■

R

➤ **Hospitalized infants and young children infected by RSV**

Infants and young children: Solution in concentration of 20 mg/mL delivered via the Viratek Small Particle Aerosol Generator (SPAG-2) and mechanical ventilator or oxygen hood, face mask, or oxygen tent at a rate of about 12.5 L of mist/minute. Treatment is given for 12 to 18 hours/day for at least 3 days, and no longer than 7 days.

➤ **Chronic HCV infection (monoinfection), in combination with peginterferon alfa-2b (capsules, oral solution)**

Adults weighing more than 105 kg: 1,400 mg P.O. daily in two divided doses, 600 mg in the morning and 800 mg in the evening.

Adults weighing 81 to 105 kg: 1,200 mg P.O. daily in two divided doses, 600 mg in the morning and 600 mg in the evening.

Adults weighing 66 to 80 kg: 1,000 mg P.O. daily in two divided doses, 400 mg in the morning and 600 mg in the evening.

Adults weighing less than 66 kg: 800 mg P.O. daily in two divided doses, 400 mg in the morning and 400 mg in the evening.

For HCV genotype 1, treatment duration is 48 weeks; for HCV genotypes 2 and 3, treatment duration is 24 weeks. Recommended treatment duration for patients of any genotype who previously failed therapy is 48 weeks.

➤ **Chronic HCV infection (monoinfection), in combination with interferon alfa-2b (capsules)**

Adults weighing more than 75 kg: 1,200 mg P.O. daily in two divided doses, 600 mg in the morning and 600 mg in the evening. Individualize therapy duration (24 to 48 weeks).

Adults weighing 75 kg or less: 1,000 mg P.O. daily in two divided doses, 400 mg in the morning and 600 mg in the evening. Individualize therapy duration (24 to 48 weeks).

➤ **Chronic HCV infection (monoinfection) in children, in combination with peginterferon alfa-2b or interferon alfa-2b (capsules, oral solution)**

Children age 3 and older weighing more than 73 kg: 1,200 mg P.O. daily in two divided doses, 600 mg in the morning and 600 mg in the evening.

Children age 3 and older weighing 60 to 73 kg: 1,000 mg P.O. daily in two divided doses, 400 mg in the morning and 600 mg in the evening.

Children age 3 and older weighing 47 to 59 kg: 800 mg P.O. daily in two divided doses, 400 mg in the morning and 400 mg in the evening.

Children age 3 and older weighing less than 47 kg: 15 mg/kg/day (oral solution) P.O. in two divided doses, in the morning and evening.

For children with HCV genotypes 2 or 3, recommended therapy duration is 24 weeks; for all other genotypes, therapy duration is 48 weeks.

➤ **Chronic HCV infection (monoinfection), in combination with peginterferon alfa-2a (tablets)**

Adults with genotype 1 or 4 weighing 75 kg or more: 1,200 mg P.O. daily in two divided doses for 48 weeks.

Adults with genotype 1 or 4 weighing less than 75 kg: 1,000 mg daily in two divided doses for 48 weeks.

Adults with genotype 2 or 3: 800 mg P.O. daily in two divided doses for 24 weeks.

Adolescents and children age 5 and older weighing 75 kg or more: 1,200 mg P.O. daily in two divided doses, 600 mg in the morning and 600 mg in the evening.

Adolescents and children age 5 and older weighing 60 to 74 kg: 1,000 mg P.O. daily in two divided doses, 400 mg in the morning and 600 mg in the evening.

Adolescents and children age 5 and older weighing 47 to 59 kg: 800 mg P.O. daily in two divided doses, 400 mg in the morning and 400 mg in the evening.

Adolescents and children age 5 and older weighing 34 to 46 kg: 600 mg P.O. daily in two divided doses, 200 mg in the morning and 400 mg in the evening.

Adolescents and children age 5 and older who weigh 23 to 33 kg: 400 mg P.O. daily in two divided doses, 200 mg in the morning and 200 mg in the evening.

Treatment duration for children and adolescents with genotype 2 or 3 is 24 weeks and for all other genotypes is 48 weeks.

➤ **Chronic HCV infection (regardless of genotype) in HIV-infected patients, in combination with peginterferon alfa-2a**
Adults: 800 mg (tablets) P.O. daily in two divided doses for 48 weeks.

ADMINISTRATION
🜂 *Alert:* Drug is a hazardous agent. Use appropriate precautions for handling and disposal.
Inhalational
• Give by the Viratek SPAG-2 only. Don't use any other aerosol-generating device.
• Use sterile USP water for injection, not bacteriostatic water. Water used to reconstitute this drug must not contain any antimicrobial product.
• Discard solutions placed in the SPAG-2 unit at least every 24 hours before adding newly reconstituted solution.
• Store reconstituted solutions at room temperature for 24 hours.
P.O.
• Give drug with food and at the same time every day.
🜂 *Alert:* Capsules should never be opened, crushed, or broken.

ACTION
Inhibits viral activity by an unknown mechanism, possibly by inhibiting RNA and DNA synthesis by depleting intracellular nucleotide pools.

Route	Onset	Peak	Duration
Inhalation	Unknown	Unknown	Unknown
P.O.	Unknown	2 hr	Unknown

Half-life: First phase, 9¼ hours; second phase, 40 hours.

ADVERSE REACTIONS
CNS: fatigue, anxiety, depression, dizziness, headache, insomnia, agitation, rigors, irritability, nervousness, fever.
CV: *bradycardia, cardiac arrest.*
EENT: blurred vision, conjunctivitis, rhinitis, sinusitis, taste perversion.
GI: anorexia, diarrhea, nausea, vomiting, weight loss, abdominal pain.
Hematologic: anemia, hemolytic anemia, *leukopenia, neutropenia, thrombocytopenia,* reticulocytosis.
Musculoskeletal: myalgia, arthralgia.

Respiratory: *apnea, bronchospasm,* bacterial pneumonia, *pneumothorax, pulmonary edema,* worsening respiratory state, cough.
Skin: flushing, alopecia, pruritus, rash, dry skin, diaphoresis, injection-site reaction.
Other: chills, flulike illness, pain, homicidal ideation, *suicidal ideation.*

INTERACTIONS
Drug-drug. *Azathioprine:* May induce severe pancytopenia and increase risk of myelotoxicity (neutropenia, thrombocytopenia, anemia). Monitor closely for signs of myelosuppression. Consider an alternative agent if possible.
Didanosine: May increase toxicity. Coadministration is contraindicated.
Lamivudine, stavudine, zidovudine: May decrease antiretroviral activity and enhance hepatotoxic effects. Use together cautiously; consider therapy modification.

EFFECTS ON LAB TEST RESULTS
• May increase ALT, AST, and bilirubin levels. May decrease Hb level.
• May increase reticulocyte count. May decrease WBC and platelet counts.

CONTRAINDICATIONS & CAUTIONS
Black Box Warning Monotherapy is ineffective for treatment of chronic HCV infection; drug shouldn't be used alone for this indication. ■
Black Box Warning Aerosol form isn't indicated for use in adults. ■
Black Box Warning Ribavirin may cause hemolytic anemia and worsen cardiac disease, leading to potentially fatal MI. Patients with a history of significant or unstable cardiac disease shouldn't be treated with ribavirin. ■
Black Box Warning Ribavirin has been shown to be teratogenic in all animal species in which adequate studies have been conducted (rodents and rabbits). ■
• Aerosol form is contraindicated in patients hypersensitive to drug.
• Oral form is contraindicated in patients with known hypersensitivity reactions to ribavirin or its components; in patients with autoimmune hepatitis, hemoglobinopathies, or CrCl of less than 50 mL/minute; and when administered with didanosine.

R

• Ribavirin tablets and peginterferon alfa-2a combination therapy is contraindicated in hepatic decompensation (Child-Pugh score greater than 6; class B and C) in cirrhotic chronic HCV monoinfected patients before treatment and in hepatic decompensation (Child-Pugh score of 6 or greater) in cirrhotic chronic HCV patients coinfected with HIV before treatment.

Black Box Warning In infants, aerosolized ribavirin has been associated with sudden deterioration of respiratory function. Monitor respiratory function carefully and stop treatment if sudden respiratory deterioration occurs. Reinstitute only with extreme caution, continuous monitoring, and consideration of concomitant administration of bronchodilators. ■

• Use cautiously in elderly patients and patients with hepatic or renal insufficiency.

• Patients who initiate oral treatment before their 18th birthday should maintain pediatric dosing through completion of therapy.

Dialyzable drug: 50%.

⚠ *Overdose S&S:* Increased severity of adverse reactions.

PREGNANCY-LACTATION-REPRODUCTION
Black Box Warning Contraindicated in pregnant women and in men whose partners are pregnant; significant teratogenic and embryocidal effects have occurred in all animal species exposed to ribavirin. ■

Black Box Warning Women receiving ribavirin and female partners of men receiving ribavirin should use extreme care to avoid pregnancy during therapy and for 6 months after therapy ends and should use at least two reliable forms of effective contraception during therapy and during 6-month posttreatment follow-up. ■

• If pregnancy occurs during therapy or during 6 months after therapy ends, patient must be advised of teratogenic fetal risk.

• Women of childbearing potential must have a negative pregnancy test immediately before start of therapy. Pregnancy tests must be performed monthly during therapy and for 6 months after therapy ends.

• Advise pregnant health care workers to avoid unnecessary exposure to aerosol form.

• Report pregnancies that occur during therapy to the Ribavirin Pregnancy Registry (1-800-593-2214).

• It isn't known if drug appears in breast milk. Patient should discontinue breastfeeding or discontinue drug, taking into account importance of drug to the mother.

NURSING CONSIDERATIONS
Aerosol form
🛈 *Alert:* The long-term and cumulative effects in health care personnel exposed to this form aren't known. Eye irritation and headache may occur.

Black Box Warning Use in mechanically ventilated patients should only be undertaken by health care providers and staff familiar with this mode of administration and the specific ventilator used. Experienced providers and staff should use procedures that minimize accumulation of drug precipitate, which can result in ventilator dysfunction and increases in pulmonary pressures. ■

• This form is indicated only for severe lower respiratory tract infection caused by RSV. Although you should begin treatment while awaiting test results, an RSV infection must be documented eventually.

• Most infants and children with RSV infection don't require treatment with antivirals because the disease is commonly mild and self-limiting. Premature infants or those with cardiopulmonary disease experience RSV in its severest form and benefit most from treatment with ribavirin aerosol.

Oral form
• Don't start therapy until a negative pregnancy test is confirmed in patient or partner of patient; they should take a pregnancy test every month during therapy and for 6 months afterward.

• Monitor hematologic status, liver and renal function, and TSH level at baseline and throughout therapy.

• Combination therapy has been observed to inhibit growth in children ages 5 to 17. Monitor child's height and weight during therapy.

🛈 *Alert:* Monitor patient for suicidal ideation, severe depression, hemolytic anemia, bone marrow suppression, autoimmune and infective disorders,

---

Reactions in bold italics are *life-threatening*. Interactions may have a *rapid onset* or a *delayed onset*.

pulmonary dysfunction, pancreatitis, and diabetes.

• Stop drug if pulmonary infiltrates or severe pulmonary impairment or pancreatitis occurs.

• In patients receiving azathioprine with ribavirin, monitor CBC, including platelet counts, weekly for first month, twice monthly for second and third months of treatment, then monthly or more frequently if dosage or other therapy changes are necessary.

PATIENT TEACHING

• Inform parents of need for drug, and answer any questions.

• Tell patient not to crush, chew, or open capsules.

• Encourage parents to immediately report any subtle change in child.

• Inform patient that oral form may be taken without regard to meals but should be taken in a consistent manner.

• Warn patient of childbearing potential that drug is a teratogen, and provide contraception counseling. Advise patient that extreme care must be taken to avoid pregnancy during therapy and for 6 months after completion of treatment.

• Advise female patient to immediately report a pregnancy.

rifampin (rifampicin)
rif-AM-pin

Rifadin, Rimactane, Rofact ✦

Therapeutic class: Antituberculotics
Pharmacologic class: Semisynthetic rifamycins

AVAILABLE FORMS
Capsules: 150 mg, 300 mg
Powder for injection: 600 mg/vial

INDICATIONS & DOSAGES
➤ **Pulmonary TB, with other antituberculotics**
Adults: 10 mg/kg P.O. or I.V. daily in single dose. Give oral doses 1 hour before or 2 hours after meals with a full glass of water. Maximum daily dose is 600 mg.

Children: 10 to 20 mg/kg P.O. or I.V. daily in single dose. Give oral doses 1 hour before or 2 hours after meals with a full glass of water. Maximum daily dose is 600 mg. Give with other antituberculotics.

➤ **Meningococcal carriers**
Adults: 600 mg P.O. or I.V. every 12 hours for 2 days.
Children ages 1 month to 12 years: 10 mg/kg P.O. or I.V. every 12 hours for 2 days, not to exceed 600 mg/day.
Neonates: 5 mg/kg P.O. or I.V. every 12 hours for 2 days.

➤ **Cholestatic pruritus ✦**
Adults: 150 mg/day P.O. if bilirubin level is less than 3 mg/dL or 150 mg P.O. b.i.d. if bilirubin level is 3 mg/dL or higher.

ADMINISTRATION
P.O.

• Give drug with at least one other antituberculotic.

• For best absorption, give capsules 1 hour before or 2 hours after a meal with a full glass of water.

• For patients who can't tolerate capsules on an empty stomach or those who have difficulty swallowing capsules or when lower doses are needed, consult pharmacist for preparation of an oral suspension.

I.V.

▼ Reconstitute drug with 10 mL of sterile water for injection to yield 60 mg/mL.

▼ Add to 100 mL of D_5W and infuse over 30 minutes, or add to 500 mL of D_5W and infuse over 3 hours.

▼ When dextrose is contraindicated, dilute with NSS for injection. Once prepared, dilutions in D_5W are stable for up to 4 hours and dilutions in NSS are stable for up to 24 hours at room temperature.

▼ **Incompatibilities:** Diltiazem, minocycline, other I.V. solutions.

ACTION
Inhibits DNA-dependent RNA polymerase, which impairs RNA synthesis; bactericidal.

Route	Onset	Peak	Duration
P.O.	Unknown	2–4 hr	Unknown
I.V.	Unknown	Unknown	Unknown

Half-life: 1¼ to 5 hours.

R

ADVERSE REACTIONS

CNS: headache, fatigue, drowsiness, behavioral changes, dizziness, mental confusion, generalized numbness, ataxia.
CV: *shock.*
EENT: visual disturbances, exudative conjunctivitis.
GI: *pancreatitis, pseudomembranous colitis,* epigastric distress, anorexia, nausea, vomiting, abdominal pain, diarrhea, flatulence, sore mouth and tongue.
GU: *acute renal failure,* hemoglobinuria, hematuria, menstrual disturbances.
Hematologic: *thrombocytopenia, transient leukopenia,* eosinophilia, hemolytic anemia.
Hepatic: *hepatotoxicity.*
Metabolic: hyperuricemia.
Musculoskeletal: muscular weakness, pain in extremities.
Respiratory: shortness of breath, wheezing.
Skin: pruritus, urticaria, rash.
Other: flulike syndrome, discoloration of body fluids, porphyria exacerbation.

INTERACTIONS

Drug-drug. *Amiodarone, analgesics, anticonvulsants, barbiturates, beta blockers, cardiac glycosides, chloramphenicol, clofibrate,* **corticosteroids,** **cyclosporine,** *dapsone, delavirdine, diazepam, digoxin, disopyramide, doxycycline, enalapril, fluoroquinolones, hormonal contraceptives, hydantoins, losartan, methadone, mexiletine, midazolam, nifedipine, ondansetron, opioids, progestins, propafenone, quinidine,* **ritonavir,** *sulfonylureas,* **tacrolimus,** *TCAs, theophylline, tocainide, triazolam, verapamil, zidovudine, zolpidem:* May decrease effectiveness of these drugs. Monitor effectiveness.
Anticoagulants: May increase requirements for anticoagulant. Monitor PT and INR closely, and adjust dosage of anticoagulants.
Atazanavir, darunavir, fosamprenavir, tipranavir: May decrease plasma concentrations of antivirals, resulting in loss of antiviral efficacy or development of viral resistance. Use together is contraindicated.
Halothane: May increase risk of hepatotoxicity. Monitor LFT results.
Isoniazid: May increase risk of hepatotoxicity. Monitor LFT results.
Ketoconazole, para-aminosalicylate sodium: May interfere with absorption of rifampin. Separate doses by 8 to 12 hours.
Macrolide antibiotics, protease inhibitors: May inhibit rifampin metabolism but increase metabolism of other drug. Monitor patient for clinical and adverse effects.
Probenecid: May increase rifampin levels. Use together cautiously.
Saquinavir: May increase risk of severe hepatocellular toxicity. Use together is contraindicated.
Voriconazole: May decrease voriconazole's therapeutic effects while increasing the risk of rifampin adverse effects. Use together is contraindicated.
Drug-lifestyle. *Alcohol use:* May increase risk of hepatotoxicity. Discourage use together.

EFFECTS ON LAB TEST RESULTS

● May increase ALT, AST, alkaline phosphatase, bilirubin, and uric acid levels. May decrease Hb level.
● May increase eosinophil counts. May decrease platelet and WBC counts.
● May alter standard folate and vitamin B_{12} assay results.

CONTRAINDICATIONS & CAUTIONS

● Contraindicated in patients hypersensitive to rifampin or related drugs.
● Use cautiously in patients with liver disease or diabetes.
Dialyzable drug: Poorly.
⚠ **Overdose S&S:** Nausea; vomiting; abdominal pain; pruritus; headache; increasing lethargy; unconsciousness; transient increases in liver enzyme or bilirubin levels; brownish red or orange discoloration of skin, urine, sweat, saliva, tears, and feces; facial or periorbital edema; hypotension; tachycardia; ventricular arrhythmias; seizures; cardiac arrest; liver enlargement; jaundice.

PREGNANCY-LACTATION-REPRODUCTION

● There are no adequate studies in pregnant women. Use during pregnancy only if clearly needed and potential benefit justifies potential risk to the fetus.
● Reportedly, drug can cause postnatal hemorrhages in the mother and infant when

given during last few weeks of pregnancy; treatment with vitamin K may be indicated.
• Drug appears in breast milk. Patient should discontinue breast-feeding or discontinue drug.

NURSING CONSIDERATIONS
• Monitor hepatic function, hematopoietic studies, and uric acid levels. Drug's systemic effects may asymptomatically raise LFT results and uric acid level.
• Watch for and report to prescriber signs and symptoms of hepatic impairment.
• *Look alike–sound alike:* Don't confuse rifampin with rifabutin, rifaximin, rifapentine, or Rifamate.

PATIENT TEACHING
• Advise patient who is unable to swallow capsules whole or can't tolerate capsules on an empty stomach that an oral suspension can be prepared by the pharmacist.
• Warn patient that drowsiness may occur and that drug can turn body fluids red-orange and permanently stain contact lenses.
• Advise female patient using hormonal contraceptives to consider another form of contraception.
• Advise patient to report fever, loss of appetite, malaise, nausea, vomiting, dark urine, or yellowing of eyes or skin.
• Advise patient to avoid alcohol during drug therapy.
• Instruct patient on importance of not missing any doses and completing full course of therapy.

rifapentine
RIF-a-PEN-teen

Priftin

Therapeutic class: Antituberculotics
Pharmacologic class: Synthetic rifamycins

AVAILABLE FORMS
Tablets (film-coated): 150 mg

INDICATIONS & DOSAGES
➤ *Alert:* Give drug as directly observed therapy for all indications.

➤ **Pulmonary TB, with at least one other antituberculotic to which the isolate is susceptible**
Adults and children age 12 and older: During intensive phase of short-course therapy, 600 mg P.O. twice weekly for 2 months, with an interval between doses of at least 3 days (72 hours). During continuation phase of short-course therapy, 600 mg P.O. once weekly for 4 months, combined with isoniazid or another drug to which the isolate is susceptible.
Elderly patients: Begin therapy at low end of dosing range.
➤ **Latent TB infection caused by *Mycobacterium tuberculosis*, in combination with isoniazid, in patients at high risk for progression to TB disease**
Adults and children age 12 and older: Rifapentine dosage is based on patient's weight and administered P.O. once weekly. If patient weighs more than 50 kg, give 900 mg; if weight is 32.1 to 50 kg, give 750 mg; if weight is 25.1 to 32 kg, give 600 mg; if weight is 14.1 to 25 kg, give 450 mg; if weight is 10 to 14 kg, give 300 mg. Maximum dose is 900 mg once weekly. Recommended isoniazid dose is 15 mg/kg (rounded to nearest 50 or 100 mg) up to maximum of 900 mg once weekly for 12 weeks.
Children ages 2 to 11: Rifapentine dosage is based on patient's weight and administered P.O. once weekly. If patient weighs more than 50 kg, give 900 mg; if weight is 32.1 to 50 kg, give 750 mg; if weight is 25.1 to 32 kg, give 600 mg; if weight is 14.1 to 25 kg, give 450 mg; if weight is 10 to 14 kg, give 300 mg. Maximum dose is 900 mg once weekly. Recommended isoniazid dose is 25 mg/kg (rounded to nearest 50 or 100 mg) up to maximum of 900 mg once weekly for 12 weeks.

ADMINISTRATION
P.O.
• Give drug with pyridoxine (vitamin B_6) in malnourished patients; in those predisposed to neuropathy, such as alcoholics and diabetics; and in adolescents.
• Give drug with meals to increase oral bioavailability and possibly reduce the incidence of GI upset, nausea, and vomiting.

R

● For patients who can't swallow tablets, tablets may be crushed and added to small amount of semisolid food and consumed immediately.

◑ *Alert:* Give drug with appropriate daily companion drugs. Compliance with all drug regimens, especially with daily companion drugs on the days when rifapentine isn't given, is crucial for early sputum conversion and protection from relapse of TB.

ACTION

Inhibits DNA-dependent RNA polymerase in susceptible strains of *M. tuberculosis.* Demonstrates bactericidal activity against the organism both intracellularly and extra-cellularly.

Route	Onset	Peak	Duration
P.O.	Unknown	3–10 hr	Unknown

Half-life: 17 hours.

ADVERSE REACTIONS

CNS: headache, dizziness, pain.
GI: anorexia, nausea, vomiting, dyspepsia, diarrhea.
GU: hyperuricemia, pyuria, proteinuria, hematuria, urinary casts.
Hematologic: *leukopenia, neutropenia,* anemia, *thrombocytosis.*
Metabolic: hyperuricemia.
Musculoskeletal: arthralgia.
Respiratory: hemoptysis.
Skin: rash, pruritus, acne, maculopapular rash.

INTERACTIONS

Drug-drug. *Antiarrhythmics (disopyramide, mexiletine, quinidine, tocainide), antibiotics (chloramphenicol, clarithromycin, dapsone, doxycycline, fluoroquinolones), anticonvulsants (phenytoin), antifungals (fluconazole, itraconazole, ketoconazole), barbiturates, benzodiazepines (diazepam), beta blockers, calcium channel blockers (diltiazem, nifedipine, verapamil), cardiac glycosides, clofibrate, **corticosteroids**, haloperidol, HIV protease inhibitors (indinavir, nelfinavir, ritonavir, saquinavir), hormonal contraceptives, **immunosuppressants (cyclosporine, tacrolimus)**, levothyroxine, opioid analgesics (methadone), oral anticoagulants (warfarin), oral antidiabetics (sulfonylureas), progestins, quinine, reverse transcriptase inhibitors (delavirdine, zidovudine), sildenafil, TCAs (amitriptyline, nortriptyline), theophylline:* May decrease activity of these drugs because of cytochrome P-450 enzyme metabolism. May need to adjust dosage.
Ritonavir: May decrease ritonavir levels. Carefully monitor patient's response.

EFFECTS ON LAB TEST RESULTS

● May increase uric acid, ALT, and AST levels.
● May increase platelet count. May decrease Hb level and neutrophil and WBC counts.
● May alter folate and vitamin B_{12} assay results.

CONTRAINDICATIONS & CAUTIONS

● Contraindicated in patients hypersensitive to rifamycins (rifapentine, rifampin, or rifabutin).
● May cause hypersensitivity reactions, including anaphylaxis (flulike illness, hypotension, urticaria, angioedema, bronchospasm, conjunctivitis, thrombocytopenia, neutropenia). If signs or symptoms occur, stop drug and notify prescriber.
● Patients with abnormal LFT values or liver disease and those initiating treatment for active pulmonary TB should receive rifapentine only in cases of necessity and under strict medical supervision.
● For HIV-infected patients with active pulmonary TB, don't use drug once weekly in the continuation phase regimen in combination with isoniazid because of a higher rate of failure or relapse with rifampin-resistant organisms. Rifapentine hasn't been studied as part of the initial phase treatment regimen in HIV-infected patients with active pulmonary TB.
● Rule out active TB disease before starting treatment for latent TB infection.
● Patients considered at high risk for progression to TB disease include those in close contact with patients with active TB or recent conversion to a positive result on tuberculin skin test, patients with pulmonary fibrosis on X-ray, and HIV-infected patients.
● Rifapentine in combination with isoniazid isn't recommended for patients presumed

---

Reactions in bold italics are *life-threatening*. Interactions may have a *rapid onset* or a **delayed onset**.

to be exposed to rifamycin- or isoniazid-resistant *M. tuberculosis.*

• CDAD has been reported, ranging from mild diarrhea to fatal colitis, and can occur more than 2 months after therapy ends. Drug may need to be discontinued and appropriate measures initiated.

• Avoid using drug in patients with porphyria.

Dialyzable drug: Unlikely.

⚠ *Overdose S&S:* Hematuria, neutropenia, hyperglycemia, hyperuricemia, arthritis, increased ALT level, pruritus.

PREGNANCY-LACTATION-REPRODUCTION

• There are no adequate studies in pregnant women. Use during pregnancy only if potential benefit justifies potential fetal risk.

• Reportedly, postnatal hemorrhages in the mother and infant have occurred when another rifamycin (rifampin) was given during last few weeks of pregnancy. Monitor PT of pregnant women and neonates exposed to rifapentine during last few weeks of pregnancy. Treatment with vitamin K may be indicated.

• It isn't known if drug appears in breast milk. Patient should discontinue breastfeeding or discontinue drug.

NURSING CONSIDERATIONS

• Monitor patient for signs and symptoms of hypersensitivity reaction; if they occur, use supportive measures and discontinue drug.

• Rifamycin antibiotics may cause hepatotoxicity. In patients with abnormal LFT values or liver disease and patients starting treatment for active pulmonary TB, obtain serum transaminase levels before start of therapy and every 2 to 4 weeks during therapy. Discontinue drug if evidence of liver injury occurs.

• *Look alike–sound alike:* Don't confuse rifapentine with rifabutin or rifampin.

PATIENT TEACHING

• Stress importance of strict compliance with this drug regimen and that of daily companion drugs, as well as needed follow-up visits and laboratory tests.

• Advise female patient to use nonhormonal contraceptive methods.

• Tell patient to take drug with meals to increase oral bioavailability and possibly reduce the incidence of GI upset, nausea, and vomiting.

• Instruct patient to report all adverse reactions, especially fever, appetite loss, malaise, nausea, vomiting, darkened urine, yellowish skin and eyes, joint pain or swelling, or excessive loose stools or diarrhea.

• Instruct patient to protect pills from excessive heat.

• Tell patient that drug may turn body fluids red-orange and permanently stain contact lenses.

---

rifaximin
reh-FACKS-ah-men

Xifaxan

Therapeutic class: Antibiotics
Pharmacologic class: Rifamycin antibacterials

AVAILABLE FORMS
Tablets: 200 mg, 550 mg

INDICATIONS & DOSAGES
➤ **Traveler's diarrhea from noninvasive strains of *Escherichia coli***
Adults and children age 12 and older: 200 mg P.O. t.i.d. for 3 days.
➤ **Hepatic encephalopathy**
Adults: 550 mg P.O. b.i.d.
➤ **Irritable bowel syndrome with diarrhea**
Adults: 550 mg P.O. t.i.d. for 14 days.

ADMINISTRATION
P.O.
• Give drug without regard for food.

ACTION
Binds to the beta-subunit of bacterial DNA-dependent RNA polymerase, which inhibits bacterial RNA synthesis and kills *E. coli.*

Route	Onset	Peak	Duration
P.O.	Unknown	½–4 hr	Unknown

Half-life: 1.8 to 6 hours.

R

ADVERSE REACTIONS
CNS: depression, dizziness, fatigue, fever, headache, insomnia.
CV: peripheral edema.
EENT: nasopharyngitis.
GI: ascites, abdominal pain, constipation, defecation urgency, flatulence, nausea, rectal tenesmus, vomiting.
Hematologic: anemia.
Musculoskeletal: arthralgia, muscle spasms, myalgia.
Respiratory: dyspnea.
Skin: rash, pruritus.

INTERACTIONS
Drug-drug. *BCG (intravesical):* May diminish therapeutic effect of BCG. Avoid combination.
Cyclosporine: May increase systemic exposure of rifaximin. Monitor therapy.

EFFECTS ON LAB TEST RESULTS
● May increase CK level.

CONTRAINDICATIONS & CAUTIONS
● Contraindicated in patients hypersensitive to rifaximin or any rifamycin antibacterial.
● Use with caution in patients with severe hepatic impairment.
Dialyzable drug: Unknown.

PREGNANCY-LACTATION-REPRODUCTION
● Safety in pregnant women hasn't been established; some animal studies have demonstrated adverse events. Because of limited absorption of rifaximin in patients with normal hepatic function, fetal exposure to drug is expected to be low.
● It isn't known if drug appears in breast milk. Patient should discontinue breast-feeding or discontinue drug.

NURSING CONSIDERATIONS
● Don't use drug in patients whose illness may be caused by *Campylobacter jejuni, Shigella,* or *Salmonella.*
◑ **Alert:** Don't use drug in patients with blood in the stool, diarrhea with fever, or diarrhea from pathogens other than *E. coli.*
● Stop drug if diarrhea worsens or lasts longer than 24 to 48 hours. Patient may need a different antibiotic.

● Patients who have diarrhea after antibiotic therapy may have CDAD, which may range from mild to life-threatening.
● Monitor patient for overgrowth of nonsusceptible organisms.

PATIENT TEACHING
● Explain that drug may be taken with or without food.
● Tell patient to take all the prescribed drug, even if feeling better before drug is finished.
● Advise patient to notify prescriber if diarrhea worsens or lasts longer than 1 or 2 days after starting treatment. A different treatment may be needed.
● Tell patient to report fever or bloody stool.
● Explain that this drug is only for treating diarrhea caused by contaminated foods or beverages while traveling and not for any other type of infection.
● Caution patient not to share drug with others.

rilpivirine hydrochloride
ril-pi-VIR-een

Edurant

Therapeutic class: Antiretrovirals
Pharmacologic class: NNRTIs

AVAILABLE FORMS
Tablets: 25 mg

INDICATIONS & DOSAGES
➤ **Treatment of HIV-1 infection in antiretroviral-naive patients with HIV-1 RNA 100,000 copies/mL or less at start of therapy, in combination with other antiretrovirals**
Adults and children age 12 and older weighing at least 35 kg: 25 mg P.O. once daily.
Adjust-a-dose: For patients concomitantly receiving rifabutin, increase rilpivirine dosage to 50 mg once daily. When rifabutin is stopped, decrease rilpivirine to 25 mg once daily.

ADMINISTRATION
P.O.
● Give drug with a normal to high-calorie meal.

● Patient should swallow tablets whole with water.
● Store tablets at room temperature and in the original bottle to protect from light.

ACTION
Inhibits HIV-1 replication by noncompetitive inhibition of HIV-1 reverse transcriptase but doesn't inhibit the human cellular DNA polymerases alpha, beta, and gamma.

Route	Onset	Peak	Duration
P.O.	Rapid	4–5 hr	Unknown

Half-life: 50 hours.

ADVERSE REACTIONS
CNS: abnormal dreams, dizziness, fatigue, headache, insomnia, depression.
GI: nausea, vomiting, abdominal pain.
Skin: rash.

INTERACTIONS
Drug-drug. *Antacids (aluminum or magnesium hydroxide, calcium carbonate):* May significantly decrease rilpivirine level. Give antacids either 2 hours before or at least 4 hours after rilpivirine.
Anticonvulsants (carbamazepine, oxcarbazepine, phenobarbital, phenytoin): May decrease rilpivirine level, decrease response, and increase risk of resistance to NNRTIs. Use together is contraindicated.
Azole antifungals (fluconazole, itraconazole, ketoconazole, posaconazole, voriconazole): May increase rilpivirine level and decrease antifungal level. Monitor effectiveness of antifungal.
Delavirdine: May increase rilpivirine level. Don't use together.
Dexamethasone (more than a single dose): May decrease rilpivirine level and virologic response, and increase risk of resistance to NNRTIs. Use together is contraindicated.
Didanosine (buffered): May decrease rilpivirine level. Administer didanosine at least 2 hours before or 4 hours after rilpivirine.
Drugs that prolong QT interval: May increase risk of torsades de pointes. Use together cautiously.
H_2-receptor antagonists (cimetidine, famotidine, nizatidine, ranitidine): May significantly decrease rilpivirine level. Give H_2-receptor antagonists at least 12 hours before or 4 hours after rilpivirine.
Macrolide antibiotics (clarithromycin, erythromycin, troleandomycin): May increase rilpivirine level. When possible, consider an alternative such as azithromycin.
Methadone: May decrease levels of both drugs. Monitor effectiveness of methadone and adjust methadone dosage as needed.
Other NNRTIs (efavirenz, etravirine, nevirapine): May decrease rilpivirine level. Don't use together.
PPIs (esomeprazole, lansoprazole, pantoprazole, rabeprazole): May decrease rilpivirine level, decrease virologic response, and increase risk of resistance to NNRTIs. Use together is contraindicated.
Rifamycins (rifampin, rifapentine): May decrease rilpivirine level, decrease virologic response, and increase risk of resistance to NNRTIs. Use together is contraindicated.
Systemic glucocorticoids (dexamethasone): May decrease rilpivirine level if more than one dose of dexamethasone is administered. Use together is contraindicated.
Drug-herb. *St. John's wort:* May decrease rilpivirine level, decrease virologic response, and increase risk of resistance to NNRTIs. Use together is contraindicated.

EFFECTS ON LAB TEST RESULTS
● May increase AST, ALT, bilirubin, creatinine, total cholesterol, and LDL and triglyceride levels.

CONTRAINDICATIONS & CAUTIONS
● Contraindicated in patients hypersensitive to drug or its components.
● Use cautiously when administering with drugs known to prolong QT interval, in elderly patients, and in those with severe renal impairment, ESRD, or severe hepatic impairment.
● Redistribution or accumulation of body fat, including central obesity, dorsocervical fat enlargement (buffalo hump), peripheral wasting, facial wasting, breast enlargement, and "cushingoid appearance," has occurred in patients receiving antiretroviral therapy. The mechanism and long-term consequences of these events are currently unknown. A causal relationship hasn't been established.

• Hepatic adverse events have been reported. Patients with underlying HBV or HCV infection or marked elevations in transaminase levels before treatment may be at increased risk for worsening or development of transaminase elevations. A few cases of hepatotoxicity have been reported in patients who had no preexisting hepatic disease or other identifiable risk factors.

• Severe skin and hypersensitivity reactions have been reported, including severe rash or rash accompanied by fever, blisters, mucosal involvement, conjunctivitis, facial edema, angioedema, hepatitis, eosinophilia, or drug reaction with eosinophilia and systemic symptoms (DRESS). Most rashes occurred within first 4 to 6 weeks of therapy. Discontinue drug if hypersensitivity reaction or rash develops.

Dialyzable drug: Unlikely.

PREGNANCY-LACTATION-REPRODUCTION

• There are no adequate studies in pregnant women. Use during pregnancy only if potential benefit justifies potential risk to the fetus.

• Enroll pregnant women exposed to drug in the Antiretroviral Pregnancy Registry (1-800-258-4263).

• It isn't known if drug appears in breast milk. Patients shouldn't breast-feed during therapy.

• The CDC recommends that an HIV-infected mother not breast-feed to avoid postnatal transmission of HIV.

NURSING CONSIDERATIONS

• Patients should take drug with a regular meal and not with a protein drink; taking drug with a protein-rich nutritional drink alone may lower the exposure of rilpivirine by 50%.

• Always use rilpivirine in combination with other antiretrovirals.

• Drug isn't a cure for HIV infection. Patients must stay on continuous HIV therapy to control HIV infection and decrease HIV-related illnesses.

• Monitor patient for severe rash or rash accompanied by fever, blisters, mucosal involvement, conjunctivitis, facial edema, angioedema, hepatitis, eosinophilia, or DRESS. Discontinue drug if hypersensi-

tivity reaction or rash develops; initiate appropriate therapy.

• Assess patient for redistribution or accumulation of body fat.

• Monitor patients for reemergence of infections, such as *Mycobacterium avium*, cytomegalovirus, *Pneumocystis jiroveci* pneumonia, and TB, during initial phase of combination treatment. Treat infections appropriately.

• Monitor patients for depressive disorders (depressed mood, dysphoria, negative thoughts, suicidal ideation or attempt). Weigh risks of continued therapy against benefits of treatment.

• Monitor liver enzyme levels before and during treatment for patients with underlying hepatic disease, including HBV or HCV infection, and for patients with marked transaminase elevations. Consider monitoring liver enzyme levels for patients without preexisting hepatic dysfunction or other risk factors. Monitor patients with severe renal impairment or ESRD for adverse reactions during treatment.

PATIENT TEACHING

• Advise patient that rilpivirine isn't a cure for HIV infection or AIDS and that patient must stay on continuous antiretroviral therapy so that the HIV infection can be controlled.

• Tell patient to report all medications and supplements being taken because many of them interact with rilpivirine.

• Instruct patient to take rilpivirine once daily with a full meal and to keep tablets in the original container to protect them from light.

• Inform patient that if a dose is missed, not to take the missed dose if the next scheduled dose is within 12 hours.

• Warn patient that rilpivirine may cause depressed or altered mood and to report mood changes or symptoms of depression immediately.

• Advise patient to immediately report hypersensitivity reaction or rash.

• Tell female patient to report pregnancy immediately. Also advise patient not to breast-feed.

Reactions in bold italics are *life-threatening*. Interactions may have a *rapid onset* or a **delayed onset**.

risedronate sodium
rah-SED-ro-nate

Actonel🖊, Atelvia

Therapeutic class: Antiosteoporotics
Pharmacologic class: Bisphosphonates

AVAILABLE FORMS
Tablets 🔵: 5 mg, 30 mg, 35 mg, 150 mg
Tablets (delayed-release) 🔵: 35 mg

INDICATIONS & DOSAGES
Adjust-a-dose (for all indications): Don't use
if CrCl is less than 30 mL/minute.
➤ **To prevent and treat postmenopausal
osteoporosis**
Women: 5-mg immediate-release tablet P.O.
once daily, or 35-mg immediate-release
tablet P.O. once weekly.
➤ **To treat postmenopausal osteoporosis**
Women: 35-mg delayed-release tablet P.O.
once weekly.
➤ **To prevent or treat postmenopausal
osteoporosis when fewer dosing days are
desirable**
Adults: 75 mg P.O. on 2 consecutive days for
a total of two immediate-release tablets each
month. Or, one 150-mg immediate-release
tablet P.O. once each month.
➤ **To increase bone mass in men with
osteoporosis**
Men: One 35-mg immediate-release tablet
P.O. once weekly.
➤ **Glucocorticoid-induced osteoporosis in patients taking 7.5 mg or more of
prednisone or equivalent glucocorticoid
daily**
Adults: 5 mg immediate-release tablet P.O.
daily.
➤ **Paget disease (immediate-release)**
Adults: 30 mg P.O. daily for 2 months. If
relapse occurs or alkaline phosphatase level
doesn't normalize, may repeat treatment
course 2 months or more after completing
first treatment course.

ADMINISTRATION
P.O.
● Give immediate-release tablets at least
30 minutes before the first food, drink, or
medication of the day, other than water.

Give with 6 to 8 oz (177 to 236 mL) of plain
water while patient is sitting or standing.
● Give delayed-release tablet in the morning
immediately after breakfast and not under
fasting conditions because of a higher risk
of abdominal pain if taken when fasting.
Give with at least 120 mL of plain water
while patient is sitting or standing.
● Warn patient against lying down for
30 minutes after taking drug.
● Make sure patient doesn't chew, crush,
cut, or suck tablets.

ACTION
Reverses the loss of bone mineral density by
reducing bone turnover and bone resorption.
In patients with Paget disease, drug causes
bone turnover to return to normal.

Route	Onset	Peak	Duration
P.O.	1 hr	1 hr	Unknown
P.O. (delayed-release)	Unknown	3 hr	Unknown

Half-life: Immediate-release, 23 hours; delayed-
release, 561 hours.

ADVERSE REACTIONS
CNS: asthenia, headache, depression, dizziness, insomnia, anxiety, neuralgia, vertigo,
hypertonia, paresthesia, pain.
CV: hypertension, CV disorder, angina
pectoris, chest pain, peripheral edema.
EENT: pharyngitis, rhinitis, sinusitis,
cataract, conjunctivitis, otitis media, am-
blyopia, tinnitus.
GI: nausea, diarrhea, abdominal pain, flatu-
lence, gastritis, rectal disorder, constipation.
GU: UTI, cystitis.
Hematologic: ecchymosis, anemia.
Musculoskeletal: arthralgia, neck pain,
back pain, myalgia, bone pain, leg cramps,
bursitis, tendon disorder.
Respiratory: URI, bronchitis, increased
cough.
Skin: rash, pruritus.
Other: infection, tooth disorder.

INTERACTIONS
Drug-drug. *Aspirin, NSAIDs:* May increase risk of gastric ulcers. Use cautiously
together.
*Calcium supplements; antacids that contain
calcium, magnesium, or aluminum:* May

R

interfere with risedronate absorption. Advise patient to separate dosing times.

H₂ antagonists, PPIs: May affect enteric coating on delayed-release tablets, decreasing bioavailability. Use together isn't recommended.

Drug-food. *Any food:* May interfere with absorption of drug. Advise patient to take immediate-release tablets at least 30 minutes before first food or drink of the day (other than water).

EFFECTS ON LAB TEST RESULTS
• May decrease calcium and phosphorus levels.

CONTRAINDICATIONS & CAUTIONS
• Contraindicated in patients hypersensitive to any component of the product, in hypocalcemic patients, in patients with conditions that delay esophageal emptying, in patients with CrCl less than 30 mL/minute, and in those who can't stand or sit upright for 30 minutes after administration.
• Hypersensitivity and skin reactions have been reported, including angioedema, generalized rash, bullous skin reactions, Stevens-Johnson syndrome, and toxic epidermal necrolysis.
◑ Alert: There may be an increased risk of fractures of the thigh in patients treated with bisphosphonates.
• Drug increases risk of osteonecrosis of the jaw, which can occur spontaneously. For patients requiring invasive dental procedures, discontinuing bisphosphonate treatment may reduce risk.
• Use cautiously in patients with upper GI disorders, such as dysphagia, esophagitis, and esophageal or gastric ulcers.
• Treat hypocalcemia and other disturbances of bone and mineral metabolism before starting treatment.
• Immediate-release and delayed-release formulations contain the same active ingredient and must not be given together.
Dialyzable drug: Unknown.
⚠ Overdose S&S: Hypocalcemia, hypophosphatemia.

PREGNANCY-LACTATION-REPRODUCTION
• There are no adequate studies in pregnant women. Use during pregnancy only if potential benefit justifies potential risk to the fetus.
• It isn't known if drug appears in breast milk. Patient should discontinue breastfeeding or discontinue drug.

NURSING CONSIDERATIONS
• Risk factors for the development of osteoporosis include family history, previous fracture, smoking, a decrease in bone mineral density below the premenopausal mean, a thin body frame, White or Asian race, and early menopause.
• Monitor patient for osteonecrosis of the jaw. Associated risk factors include invasive dental procedures, cancer diagnosis, concomitant treatment such as chemotherapy and steroids, poor oral hygiene, and preexisting dental disease. If signs or symptoms occur, stop drug and refer patient to oral surgeon.
◑ Alert: Drug may cause dysphagia, esophagitis, and esophageal or gastric ulcers. Monitor patient for symptoms of esophageal disease.
• Severe musculoskeletal pain has been associated with bisphosphonate use and may occur within days, months, or years of start of therapy. When drug is stopped, symptoms may resolve partially or completely.
• Give supplemental calcium and vitamin D if dietary intake is inadequate. Because calcium supplements and drugs containing calcium, aluminum, or magnesium may interfere with risedronate absorption, separate dosing times.
• Periodically evaluate need for continued therapy in all patients. Consider discontinuation of therapy in patients at low risk for fracture after 3 to 5 years of use. Periodically evaluate risk of fracture in patients who discontinue therapy.
• Bisphosphonates can interfere with bone-imaging agents.
• Look alike–sound alike: Don't confuse Actonel with Actos.

PATIENT TEACHING
• Explain that drug may reverse bone loss by stopping more bone loss and increasing bone strength.
• Caution patient about the importance of adhering to special dosing instructions,

including staying in an upright position for 30 minutes after taking drug with plain water.

• Tell patient not to chew, cut, crush, or suck the tablet because doing so may irritate the mouth.

• Advise patient to immediately report GI discomfort (such as difficulty or pain when swallowing, retrosternal pain, or severe heartburn).

• Tell patient that Actonel and Atelvia contain the same active ingredient and must not be taken together.

• Advise patient to take calcium and vitamin D if dietary intake is inadequate, but to take them at a different time than risedronate.

• Advise patient to stop smoking and drinking alcohol, as appropriate. Also, advise patient to perform weight-bearing exercise.

• Tell patient to store drug in a cool, dry place, at room temperature, and away from children.

• Tell patient that if a dose of the 35-mg delayed-release tablet is missed, to take one tablet on the morning after patient remembers and return to taking one tablet once a week, as originally scheduled, on chosen day. Patient shouldn't take two tablets on the same day.

---

risperiDONE
ris-PEER-i-dohn

Risperdal✔, Risperdal Consta, Risperdal M-TAB

Therapeutic class: Antipsychotics
Pharmacologic class: Benzisoxazole derivatives

AVAILABLE FORMS
Injection: 12.5 mg, 25 mg, 37.5 mg, 50 mg
ODTs: 0.25 mg, 0.5 mg, 1 mg, 2 mg, 3 mg, 4 mg
Oral solution: 1 mg/mL
Tablets: 0.25 mg, 0.5 mg, 1 mg, 2 mg, 3 mg, 4 mg

INDICATIONS & DOSAGES
Adjust-a-dose (for all indications): When oral formulations are administered with an enzyme inducer, such as carbamazepine, phenytoin, rifampin, or phenobarbital, increase risperidone dosage up to double patient's usual dosage; decrease dosage when the enzyme inducer is discontinued. When administered with an enzyme inhibitor, such as fluoxetine or paroxetine, reduce risperidone dosage; titrate slowly and don't exceed 8 mg/day in adults. It may be necessary to increase risperidone dosage when the enzyme inhibitor is discontinued.

➤ **Schizophrenia**
Adults: Drug may be given once daily or b.i.d. Initial dosing is generally 2 mg P.O. daily. Increase dosage at intervals not less than 24 hours, in increments of 1 to 2 mg/day, as tolerated, to a recommended dose of 4 to 8 mg/day. Periodically reassess to determine the need for maintenance treatment with an appropriate dose. Maximum dose is 16 mg/day.

Adjust-a-dose: In elderly or hypotensive patients and in those with CrCl of less than 30 mL/minute or severe hepatic impairment, use lower starting dosage of 0.5 mg P.O. b.i.d. May increase in increments of 0.5 mg or less b.i.d. Increase to dosages above 1.5 mg b.i.d. at intervals of at least 1 week.

Adolescents ages 13 to 17: Start treatment with 0.5 mg P.O. once daily, given as a single daily dose in either the morning or evening. Adjust dose, if indicated, at intervals of not less than 24 hours, in increments of 0.5 or 1 mg/day, as tolerated, to a recommended dose of 3 mg/day. Reassess periodically to determine need for maintenance treatment with an appropriate dose.

➤ **Parenteral maintenance therapy for schizophrenia or bipolar I disorder (as monotherapy or as combination therapy with lithium or valproate)**
Adults: Establish tolerance to oral risperidone before giving I.M. Give 25 mg deep I.M. into the buttock every 2 weeks, alternating injections between the two buttocks.

Adjust dose no sooner than every 4 weeks. Maximum, 50 mg I.M. every 2 weeks. Continue oral antipsychotic for 3 weeks after first I.M. injection, then stop oral therapy. Continue therapy at lowest dose needed. Periodically reevaluate long-term risks and benefits of drug for the individual patient.

R

Adjust-a-dose: In patients with hepatic or renal impairment, titrate slowly to 2 mg P.O. daily for 1 week. If tolerated, give 25 mg I.M. every 2 weeks, or may consider initial dose of 12.5 mg I.M. Continue oral form of risperidone (or another antipsychotic) with the first injection and for 3 subsequent weeks to maintain therapeutic drug levels.

At initiation of therapy with carbamazepine or other known CYP3A4 hepatic enzyme inducers, closely monitor patient during first 4 to 8 weeks. A dosage increase or additional oral risperidone may need to be considered. On discontinuation of carbamazepine or other CYP3A4 hepatic enzyme inducers, reevaluate risperidone injection dosage and, if necessary, decrease dosage. Patients may be placed on a lower risperidone injection dosage between 2 and 4 weeks before the planned discontinuation of carbamazepine or other CYP3A4 inducers to adjust for the expected increase in risperidone plasma concentration.

➤ **Monotherapy or combination therapy with lithium or valproate for 3-week treatment of acute manic or mixed episodes from bipolar I disorder**
Adults: Initially, 2 to 3 mg P.O. once daily. Adjust dose by 1 mg daily. Dosage range is 1 to 6 mg daily. Or, 25 mg I.M. every 2 weeks. Some patients may benefit from a higher dose of 37.5 or 50 mg.
Adjust-a-dose: In elderly or hypotensive patients, or those with severe renal or hepatic impairment, start with 0.5 mg P.O. b.i.d. Increase dosage by 0.5 mg b.i.d. Increase in dosages above 1.5 mg b.i.d. should occur at least 1 week apart. Subsequent switches to once-daily dosing may be made after patient is on a twice-daily regimen for 2 to 3 days at the target dose.
Children and adolescents ages 10 to 17: 0.5 mg P.O. as a single daily dose in either the morning or evening. Adjust dose, if indicated, at intervals not less than 24 hours, in increments of 0.5 or 1 mg/day, as tolerated, to a recommended dose of 2.5 mg/day.
➤ **Irritability, including aggression, self-injury, and temper tantrums, associated with an autistic disorder**
Adolescents and children ages 5 to 17 weighing 20 kg or more: Initially, 0.5 mg P.O. once daily or in two divided doses.

After 4 days, increase dose to 1 mg. Increase dosage further in 0.5-mg increments at intervals of at least 2 weeks.
Children ages 5 to 17 weighing more than 15 and less than 20 kg: Initially, 0.25 mg P.O. once daily or in two divided doses. After 4 days, increase dose to 0.5 mg. Increase dosage further in 0.25-mg increments at intervals of at least 2 weeks.

ADMINISTRATION
P.O.
● Give drug without regard for meals.
● Oral solution isn't compatible with cola or tea.
● Open package for ODTs immediately before giving by peeling off foil backing with dry hands. Don't push tablets through the foil. ODTs can be swallowed with or without liquid.
● Phenylalanine contents of ODTs are as follows: 0.5-mg tablet contains 0.14 mg phenylalanine; 1-mg tablet contains 0.28 mg phenylalanine; 2-mg tablet contains 0.42 mg phenylalanine; 3-mg tablet contains 0.63 mg phenylalanine; 4-mg tablet contains 0.84 mg phenylalanine.
I.M.
● Continue oral therapy for the first 3 weeks of I.M. injection therapy until injections take effect, then stop oral therapy.
● To reconstitute I.M. injection, inject premeasured diluent into vial and shake vigorously for at least 10 seconds. Suspension appears uniform, thick, and milky; particles are visible, but no dry particles remain. Use drug immediately, or refrigerate for up to 6 hours after reconstitution. If more than 2 minutes pass before injection, shake vigorously again. See manufacturer's package insert for more detailed instructions.
● Refrigerate I.M. injection kit and protect it from light. Drug can be stored at temperature less than 77° F (25° C) for no more than 7 days before administration.

ACTION
Blocks dopamine, 5-HT$_2$, alpha 1 and alpha 2 adrenergic, and H$_1$ histaminergic receptors in the brain.

Reactions in bold italics are *life-threatening*. Interactions may have a *rapid onset* or a ***delayed onset***.

Route	Onset	Peak	Duration
P.O.	Unknown	1 hr	Unknown
I.M.	3 wk	4–6 wk	7 wk

Half-life: P.O., 3 to 20 hours; I.M., 3 to 6 days.

ADVERSE REACTIONS
CNS: akathisia, somnolence, dystonia, headache, insomnia, agitation, anxiety, pain, parkinsonism, *neuroleptic malignant syndrome, suicide attempt,* dizziness, fever, hallucination, mania, impaired concentration, abnormal thinking and dreaming, tremor, hypoesthesia, fatigue, depression, nervousness, parkinsonism.
CV: tachycardia, chest pain, orthostatic hypotension, peripheral edema, syncope, hypertension.
EENT: rhinitis, sinusitis, pharyngitis, abnormal vision, ear disorder (I.M.).
GI: constipation, nausea, vomiting, dyspepsia, abdominal pain, anorexia, dry mouth, increased saliva, diarrhea.
GU: urinary incontinence, increased urination, abnormal orgasm, decreased libido, vaginal dryness, amenorrhea.
Metabolic: weight gain or loss, hyperglycemia, gynecomastia.
Musculoskeletal: arthralgia, back pain, leg pain, myalgia.
Respiratory: coughing, dyspnea, URI.
Skin: rash, dry skin, photosensitivity reactions, acne, injection-site pain (I.M.).
Other: tooth disorder, toothache, injury, decreased libido.

INTERACTIONS
Drug-drug. *Antihypertensives:* May enhance hypotensive effects. Monitor BP.
Carbamazepine, phenobarbital, phenytoin, rifampin: May increase risperidone clearance and decrease effectiveness. Monitor patient closely.
Clozapine: May decrease risperidone clearance, increasing toxicity. Monitor patient closely.
CNS depressants: May cause additive CNS depression. Use together cautiously.
Dopamine agonists, levodopa: May antagonize effects of these drugs. Use together cautiously and monitor patient.
Fluoxetine, paroxetine: May increase the risk of risperidone's adverse effects, including

serotonin syndrome. Monitor patient closely and decrease risperidone dose as needed.
Black Box Warning *Opioids:* May cause slow or difficult breathing, sedation, and death. Avoid use together. If use together is necessary, limit dosage and duration of each drug to minimum necessary for desired effect. ∎

QTc interval–prolonging drugs: May increase risk of QTc-interval prolongation and risk of life-threatening ventricular arrhythmias. Use together cautiously unless contraindicated.
Drug-lifestyle. *Alcohol use:* May cause additive CNS depression. Discourage use together.

EFFECTS ON LAB TEST RESULTS
• May increase AST, ALT, blood glucose, and prolactin levels.
• May decrease Hb level, hematocrit, and WBC count.

CONTRAINDICATIONS & CAUTIONS
• Contraindicated in patients hypersensitive to drug.
Black Box Warning Opioids should only be prescribed with benzodiazepines or other CNS depressants to patients for whom alternative treatment options are inadequate. ∎
• Use cautiously in patients with prolonged QT interval, CV disease, cerebrovascular disease, dehydration, hypovolemia, history of seizures, or conditions that could affect metabolism or hemodynamic responses.
• Use cautiously in patients exposed to extreme heat.
• Use caution in patients at risk for aspiration pneumonia.
• Use I.M. injection cautiously in those with hepatic or renal impairment.
Dialyzable drug: Unknown.
⚠ **Overdose S&S:** Drowsiness, sedation, tachycardia, hypotension, extrapyramidal symptoms, QT-interval prolongation, seizures, torsades de pointes.

PREGNANCY-LACTATION-REPRODUCTION
🕐 *Alert:* Neonates exposed to antipsychotics during the third trimester are at risk for developing extrapyramidal signs and symptoms (repetitive muscle movements of the face and body) and withdrawal signs and

R

symptoms (agitation, abnormally increased or decreased muscle tone, tremors, sleepiness, severe difficulty breathing, difficulty feeding) after delivery. Use in pregnant women only if potential benefit justifies fetal risk.

• Enroll women exposed to drug during pregnancy in the National Pregnancy Registry for Atypical Antipsychotics (1-866-961-2388).

• Drug appears in breast milk. Patient should discontinue breast-feeding or discontinue drug.

• Breast-feeding is contraindicated for 12 weeks after last I.M. injection.

• Drug may cause hyperprolactinemia, which may decrease reproductive function in both men and women.

NURSING CONSIDERATIONS

❸ Alert: Obtain baseline BP measurements before starting therapy, and monitor pressure regularly. Watch for orthostatic hypotension, especially during first dosage adjustment.

Black Box Warning Elderly patients with dementia-related psychosis treated with antipsychotics are at increased risk for death. Drug isn't approved to treat elderly patients with dementia-related psychosis. ∎

• Monitor patient for tardive dyskinesia, which may occur after prolonged use. It may not appear until months or years later and may disappear spontaneously or persist for life, despite stopping drug.

❸ Alert: Watch for evidence of neuroleptic malignant syndrome (extrapyramidal effects, hyperthermia, autonomic disturbance), which is rare but can be fatal.

• Life-threatening hyperglycemia may occur in patients taking atypical antipsychotics. Monitor patients with diabetes regularly.

❸ Alert: Monitor patient for symptoms of metabolic syndrome (significant weight gain and increased BMI, hypertension, hyperglycemia, hypercholesterolemia, and hypertriglyceridemia).

• Periodically reevaluate drug's risks and benefits, especially during prolonged use.

• Patients experiencing persistent somnolence may benefit from administering half the daily P.O. dose b.i.d.

• Monitor patient for weight gain.

• **Look alike–sound alike:** Don't confuse risperidone with reserpine or ropinirole. Don't confuse Risperdal with Restoril.

PATIENT TEACHING

• Warn patient to avoid activities that require alertness until effects of drug are known.

Black Box Warning Caution patient or caregiver of patient taking an opioid with a benzodiazepine, CNS depressant, or alcohol to seek immediate medical attention if patient experiences dizziness, light-headedness, extreme sleepiness, slowed or difficult breathing, or unresponsiveness. ∎

• Warn patient to rise slowly, and use other precautions to avoid fainting when starting therapy.

• Advise patient to use caution in hot weather to prevent heatstroke.

• Tell patient to take drug with or without food.

• Instruct patient to keep the ODT in the blister pack until just before taking it. After opening the pack, he should dissolve the tablet on tongue without cutting or chewing. Tell patient to use dry hands to peel apart the foil to expose the tablet; he shouldn't attempt to push it through the foil.

• Advise women not to become pregnant or to breast-feed for 12 weeks after the last I.M. injection.

• Advise patient to avoid alcohol during therapy.

ritonavir
ri-TON-ah-veer

Norvir

Therapeutic class: Antiretrovirals
Pharmacologic class: Protease inhibitors

AVAILABLE FORMS
Capsules: 100 mg
Oral solution: 80 mg/mL*
Tablets ⓞⓝⓒ: 100 mg

INDICATIONS & DOSAGES
➤ **HIV infection, with other antiretrovirals**
Adults: 600 mg P.O. b.i.d. with meals.
To reduce adverse GI effects, begin with
300 mg P.O. b.i.d. and increase by 100 mg
b.i.d. at 2- to 3-day intervals.
Children older than age 1 month: 350 to
400 mg/m^2 P.O. b.i.d.; don't exceed 600 mg
P.O. b.i.d. Initially, start with 250 mg/m^2
b.i.d. and increase by 50 mg/m^2 P.O. every
12 hours at 2- to 3-day intervals. If children
can't reach b.i.d. doses of 400 mg/m^2 because of adverse effects, consider alternative
therapy.

ADMINISTRATION
P.O.
● Give drug with meals.
● Oral solution may be mixed with choco-
late milk or enteral nutrition therapy liquids
within 1 hour of dosing. Shake well.
● When giving oral solution to children, use
a calibrated dosing syringe, if possible.
● Make sure patient swallows tablets whole
and doesn't break, crush, or chew them.

ACTION
An HIV-1 and HIV-2 protease inhibitor.
Drug binds to the protease-active site and
inhibits activity of the enzyme, preventing
cleavage of the viral polyproteins and causing formation of immature, noninfectious
viral particles.

Route	Onset	Peak	Duration
P.O.	Unknown	2–4 hr	Unknown

Half-life: 3 to 5 hours.

ADVERSE REACTIONS
CNS: asthenia, *generalized tonic-clonic
seizure,* anxiety, circumoral paresthesia,
confusion, depression, dizziness, fever,
headache, insomnia, malaise, pain, paresthesia, peripheral paresthesia, somnolence,
thinking abnormality.
CV: syncope, vasodilation.
EENT: blurred vision, pharyngitis.
GI: diarrhea, nausea, taste perversion, vomiting, *pancreatitis, pseudomembranous
colitis,* abdominal pain, anorexia, constipation, dyspepsia, flatulence.

Hematologic: anemia, *leukopenia, throm-
bocytopenia.*
Hepatic: *hepatitis.*
Metabolic: *diabetes mellitus,* weight loss,
lipid disorders.
Musculoskeletal: arthralgia, myalgia.
Skin: sweating, flushing.
Other: hypersensitivity reactions, fat redis-
tribution or accumulation, immune reconsti-
tution syndrome.

INTERACTIONS
Drug-drug. ▬**Black Box Warning**▬ *Alfuzosin,
amiodarone, bepridil, ergot derivatives, flecainide, lurasidone, methylergonovine, oral
midazolam, pimozide, propafenone, quinidine, sildenafil (Revatio when used to treat
pulmonary arterial hypertension), simvastatin, triazolam:* May cause life-threatening
adverse reactions due to possible effects of
ritonavir on the hepatic metabolism of these
drugs. Use together is contraindicated. ▮
❂ *Alert: Atorvastatin, pitavastatin, pravastatin, rosuvastatin:* May increase statin level
and risk of myopathy and rhabdomyolysis.
Use together cautiously at the recommended
dosage for the statin given in combination
with ritonavir. Refer to prescribing information for statin drug dosage limitations.
*Atovaquone, divalproex, lamotrigine,
phenytoin:* May decrease levels of these
drugs. Use together cautiously and monitor
drug levels closely.
*Beta blockers, disopyramide, fluoxetine,
mexiletine, nefazodone:* May increase levels
of these drugs, causing cardiac and neurologic events. Use together cautiously.
*Bupropion, buspirone, calcium channel
blockers, carbamazepine, clonazepam, clorazepate, cyclosporine, desipramine, dexamethasone, diazepam,* **digoxin,** *dronabinol,
estazolam, ethosuximide, flurazepam, lidocaine, methamphetamine, metoprolol,
perphenazine, prednisone, quinine, risperidone, sirolimus, SSRIs, tacrolimus, TCAs,
thioridazine, timolol, tramadol, zolpidem:*
May increase levels of these drugs. Use
cautiously together and consider decreasing
the dosage of these drugs by almost 50%.
Monitor therapeutic levels.
Clarithromycin: May increase clarithromycin level. If CrCl is 30 to
60 mL/minute, reduce clarithromycin

R

dosage by 50%. If CrCl is less than 30 mL/minute, reduce clarithromycin dosage by 75%.

Clozapine, piroxicam: May increase levels and toxicity of these drugs. Avoid using together.

Delavirdine: May increase ritonavir level. Adjusted dose recommendations aren't established. Use together cautiously.

Didanosine: May decrease didanosine absorption. Separate doses by 2½ hours.

Disulfiram, metronidazole: May increase risk of disulfiram-like reactions because ritonavir formulations contain alcohol. Monitor patient.

Ethinyl estradiol: May decrease ethinyl estradiol level. Use an alternative or additional method of birth control.

Fluticasone: May significantly increase fluticasone exposure, significantly decreasing cortisol concentrations and causing systemic corticosteroid effects (including Cushing syndrome). Don't use together, if possible.

HMG-CoA reductase inhibitors: May cause large increase in statin levels, resulting in myopathy. Use cautiously with atorvastatin and rosuvastatin, using lowest doses possible; monitor patient carefully. Consider using fluvastatin or pravastatin.

Indinavir: May increase indinavir levels. Use together cautiously.

Itraconazole, ketoconazole: May increase levels of these drugs. Don't exceed 200 mg/day of these drugs.

❸ *Alert: Lovastatin, simvastatin:* May increase statin level and risk of myopathy and rhabdomyolysis. Use together is contraindicated.

Meperidine: May decrease meperidine level and increase level of its metabolite. Dosage increases and long-term use together aren't recommended because of CNS effects. Use cautiously together.

Methadone: May decrease methadone levels. Consider increasing methadone dosage.

PDE5 inhibitors (sildenafil, tadalafil, vardenafil): May increase levels of PDE5 inhibitor, causing hypotension, syncope, visual changes, or prolonged erection. Use together cautiously and increase monitoring for adverse reactions. Tell patient not to ex-

ceed 25 mg of sildenafil in a 48-hour period, 10 mg of tadalafil in a 72-hour period, or 2.5 mg of vardenafil in a 72-hour period.

Rifabutin: May increase rifabutin levels. Monitor patient and reduce rifabutin daily dosage by at least 75% of usual dose.

Rifampin, rifapentine: May decrease ritonavir levels. Consider using rifabutin.

Saquinavir: May increase saquinavir plasma levels. Adjust dose by taking saquinavir 400 mg b.i.d. and ritonavir 400 mg b.i.d.

Saquinavir: May prolong QT and PR intervals. Avoid concomitant use in patients with history of prolonged QT interval and in those already receiving drugs known to prolong QT interval (class I or class III antiarrhythmics).

Theophylline: May decrease theophylline levels. Increase dose based on blood levels.

Trazodone: May increase trazodone level, causing nausea, dizziness, hypotension, and syncope. Avoid using together. If unavoidable, use cautiously and lower trazodone dose.

Voriconazole: Decreases voriconazole level and reduces antifungal response. Voriconazole is contraindicated with ritonavir doses of 400 mg every 12 hours or greater.

Warfarin: May affect INR. Monitor patient frequently after initiating coadministration and adjust warfarin dosage as needed.

Drug-herb. St. John's wort: May substantially reduce drug levels. Use together is contraindicated.

Drug-lifestyle. *Smoking:* May decrease drug levels. Discourage smoking.

EFFECTS ON LAB TEST RESULTS
● May increase ALT, AST, GGT, glucose, triglyceride, lipid, CK, and uric acid levels. May decrease Hb level and hematocrit.
● May decrease WBC, RBC, platelet, and neutrophil counts.

CONTRAINDICATIONS & CAUTIONS
● Contraindicated in patients hypersensitive to drug or its components.
❸ *Alert:* Consult full prescribing information before and during treatment for potential drug interactions.
● Use cautiously in patients with hepatic disease, liver enzyme abnormalities, or hepatitis.

Alert: Patients with advanced HIV infection may have increased risk of elevated triglyceride levels and in some cases fatal pancreatitis.

• In postmarketing surveillance, hyperglycemia requiring treatment has been reported. A causal relationship with ritonavir hasn't been established.

• Safety and effectiveness in children younger than age 1 month haven't been established.

• May cause toxicity in preterm neonates. Don't use oral solution in preterm neonates in the immediate postnatal period. A safe and effective dose in this patient population hasn't been established.

Dialyzable drug: Unlikely.

⚠ Overdose S&S: Paresthesia, renal failure with eosinophilia, alcohol-related toxicity with oral solution.

PREGNANCY-LACTATION-REPRODUCTION

• There are no adequate studies in pregnant women. Use only if potential benefit justifies potential risk to the fetus.

• Enroll pregnant women exposed to drug in the Antiretroviral Pregnancy Registry (1-800-258-4263).

• Once-daily dosing isn't recommended during pregnancy. Avoid using oral solution during pregnancy because it contains alcohol.

• Breast-feeding is contraindicated because of the potential for postnatal HIV-1 transmission.

NURSING CONSIDERATIONS

Black Box Warning Administration with sedative-hypnotics, antiarrhythmics, or ergot alkaloid preparations may result in potentially serious or life-threatening adverse events because of possible effects on the hepatic metabolism of certain drugs. Review medications taken by patients before administering ritonavir or when administering other medications to patients already taking ritonavir. ∎

• Monitor patient for immune reconstitution syndrome. During initial phase of treatment, patients responding to antiretroviral therapy may develop an inflammatory response to indolent or residual opportunistic infections (CMV, *Mycobacterium avium* complex,

Pneumocystis jiroveci pneumonia, TB), which may necessitate further evaluation and treatment. Autoimmune disorders (such as Graves disease, polymyositis, and Guillain-Barré syndrome) have also been reported in the setting of immune reconstitution; however, time to onset is more variable, and can occur many months after initiation of antiretroviral treatment.

• Patients beginning regimens with ritonavir and nucleosides may improve GI tolerance by starting ritonavir alone and then adding nucleosides before completing 2 weeks of ritonavir.

• Patients who switch from soft gel capsule to tablet formulation may experience increased GI adverse effects because of greater maximum plasma concentration achieved with the tablet formulation relative to the capsule.

• In patients with liver disease, monitor liver enzyme and triglyceride levels frequently, especially during the first 3 months of treatment.

• Monitor patient for redistribution or accumulation of body fat, which has been observed with antiretroviral therapy.

• Monitor total amounts of alcohol and propylene glycol from all drugs given to children ages 1 to 6 months, to avoid alcohol-related toxicity.

• **Look alike–sound alike:** Don't confuse Norvir with Norvasc.

PATIENT TEACHING

• Inform patient that drug doesn't cure HIV infection. He may continue to develop opportunistic infections and other complications of HIV infection. Drug hasn't been shown to reduce the risk of transmitting HIV to others through sexual contact or blood contamination.

• Caution patient to take drug as prescribed and not to adjust dosage or stop therapy without first consulting prescriber.

• Advise patient who is experiencing increased GI adverse effects, such as nausea, vomiting, abdominal pain, or diarrhea, after switching from soft gel capsule to tablet formulation that these effects may diminish as therapy continues.

• Tell patient that taste of oral solution may be improved by mixing it with chocolate

R

♣Canada   ◇OTC   ♦ Off-label use   𝒫 Photoguide   ⊕ Do not crush   *Liquid contains alcohol.

milk, Ensure, or Advera within 1 hour of the scheduled dose.

• Advise patient not to chew, crush, or break tablets.

• Instruct patient to take drug with a meal.

• Tell patient that if a dose is missed, to take the next dose as soon as possible. Advise patient not to double the next dose.

• Advise patient taking a PDE5 inhibitor for erectile dysfunction to promptly report hypotension, dizziness, visual changes, and prolonged erection to prescriber. Caution against exceeding the recommended reduced dosage.

• Advise patient using estrogen-based contraceptives to use an alternative contraceptive method during therapy.

• Caution patient to report signs and symptoms of pancreatitis (nausea, vomiting, and abdominal pain) immediately.

• Counsel patient that ritonavir must always be taken in combination with other antiretrovirals.

• Advise patient to report use of other drugs, including OTC drugs; this drug interacts with many drugs.

SAFETY ALERT!

rituximab
ri-TUX-i-mab

Rituxan

Therapeutic class: Antineoplastics
Pharmacologic class: Monoclonal antibodies

AVAILABLE FORMS
Injection: 10 mg/mL in 10-mL and 50-mL single-use, sterile vials

INDICATIONS & DOSAGES
➤ **Maintenance therapy for patients with previously untreated follicular, CD20-positive, B-cell non-Hodgkin lymphoma (NHL) who achieve response to rituximab in combination with chemotherapy**
Adults: 375 mg/m^2 I.V. as single agent every 8 weeks for 12 doses beginning 8 weeks after completion of combination therapy.

➤ **Wegener granulomatosis (WG); microscopic polyangiitis (MPA) in combination with glucocorticoids**
Adults: 375 mg/m^2 I.V. once weekly for 4 weeks. Give methylprednisolone 1,000 mg/day I.V. for 1 to 3 days followed by oral prednisone 1 mg/kg/day (not to exceed 80 mg/day and tapered per clinical need) to treat severe vasculitis symptoms. This regimen should begin within 14 days before or with the initiation of rituximab and may continue during and after the 4-week course of rituximab treatment.

➤ **Previously untreated, follicular CD20-positive, B-cell NHL with cyclophosphamide-vincristine-prednisolone (CVP) chemotherapy regimen**
Adults: 375 mg/m^2 I.V. given on day 1 of each CVP cycle, for up to eight doses.

➤ **Previously untreated low-grade, CD20-positive, B-cell NHL following first-line treatment with CVP chemotherapy**
Adults: For patients who fail to progress after six to eight cycles of CVP chemotherapy, give 375 mg/m^2 I.V. once weekly for 4 doses every 6 months for up to 16 doses.

➤ **CD20-positive chronic lymphocytic leukemia (CLL) in combination with fludarabine and cyclophosphamide**
Adults: 375 mg/m^2 I.V. given day before combination treatment. Then give 500 mg/m^2 I.V. on day 1 of cycles two through six in combination with fludarabine and cyclophosphamide (every 28 days).

➤ **Relapsed or refractory low-grade or follicular, CD20-positive, B-cell NHL**
Adults: Initially, 375 mg/m^2 I.V. once weekly for four or eight doses. Retreatment for patients with progressive disease, 375 mg/m^2 I.V. infusion once weekly for four doses.

➤ **With ibritumomab tiuxetan (Zevalin) for relapsed or refractory low-grade, follicular or transformed B-cell NHL**
Adults: 250 mg/m^2 I.V. 4 hours before indium-111 Zevalin infusion. Repeat in 7 to 9 days, 4 hours before yttrium-90 Zevalin infusion.

➤ **With methotrexate to reduce the signs and symptoms of moderate to severely active RA in patients who have had an**

---

inadequate response to one or more TNF antagonists

Adults: Two 1,000-mg I.V. infusions 2 weeks apart. To reduce the incidence and severity of infusion reactions, give methylprednisolone 100 mg I.V., or its equivalent, 30 minutes before each infusion.

➤ **Diffuse large B-cell, CD20-positive NHL, given with cyclophosphamide-Adriamycin (doxorubicin)-Oncovin (vincristine)-prednisone (CHOP) chemotherapy regimen or other anthracycline-based chemotherapy regimens**

Adults: 375 mg/m^2 I.V. on day 1 of each chemotherapy cycle for up to eight infusions.

ADMINISTRATION
I.V.
▼ Give acetaminophen and diphenhydramine before each infusion.
▼ Protect vials from direct sunlight.
▼ Give as an infusion; don't give as I.V. push or bolus.
▼ Begin infusion at rate of 50 mg/hour. If no hypersensitivity or infusion-related events occur, increase rate by 50 mg/hour every 30 minutes, to maximum of 400 mg/hour. Start subsequent infusions at 100 mg/hour and increase by 100 mg/hour every 30 minutes, to maximum of 400 mg/hour as tolerated.
▼ Dilute to yield 1 to 4 mg/mL in bag of D$_5$W or NSS. Gently invert bag to mix solution.
▼ Discard unused portion left in vial.
▼ Store diluted solutions in refrigerator at 36° to 46° F (2° to 8° C) because they don't contain a preservative.
▼ **Incompatibilities:** Other I.V. drugs.

ACTION
A murine and human monoclonal antibody directed against CD20 antigen found on the surface of normal and malignant B lymphocytes. Binding to this antigen mediates the lysis of the B cells.

Route	Onset	Peak	Duration
I.V.	Variable	Variable	6–12 mo

Half-life: Varies widely, possibly because of differences in tumor burden among patients and changes in CD-positive B-cell populations on repeated therapy.

ADVERSE REACTIONS
CNS: asthenia, fever, headache, agitation, dizziness, fatigue, hypesthesia, hypertonia, insomnia, malaise, nervousness, pain, paresthesia, somnolence, vertigo.
CV: hypotension, *arrhythmias, bradycardia,* chest pain, edema, flushing, hypertension, peripheral edema, tachycardia, *HF.*
EENT: conjunctivitis, lacrimation disorder, rhinitis, sinusitis, sore throat.
GI: nausea, abdominal pain or enlargement, anorexia, diarrhea, dyspepsia, taste perversion, vomiting, *bowel perforation.*
GU: *acute renal failure.*
Hematologic: *leukopenia, neutropenia, thrombocytopenia, lymphopenia,* anemia.
Metabolic: hyperglycemia, hypocalcemia, weight gain.
Musculoskeletal: arthritis, back pain, myalgia.
Respiratory: *bronchospasm,* bronchitis, cough increase, dyspnea.
Skin: pruritus, rash, *severe mucocutaneous reactions,* pain at injection site, urticaria.
Other: chills, rigors, *angioedema, infusion reaction,* infection, *serious infection, tumor lysis syndrome (TLS),* tumor pain.

INTERACTIONS
Drug-drug. *Cisplatin:* May cause renal toxicity. Monitor renal function tests.
⊙ Alert: *Live-virus vaccines:* Virus replication may occur. Avoid vaccination with live-virus vaccines.
Tocilizumab: May increase risk of serious infection. Avoid use together.

EFFECTS ON LAB TEST RESULTS
● May increase glucose and LDH levels. May decrease calcium and phosphate levels.
● May decrease Hb level and WBC, platelet, and neutrophil counts.

CONTRAINDICATIONS & CAUTIONS
Black Box Warning HBV reactivation, including fulminant hepatitis, hepatic failure,

R

and death, may occur in patients treated with rituximab. ■

⚠ Alert: Consult hepatitis expert when screening identifies patients at risk for HBV reactivation due to prior HBV infection.

Dialyzable drug: Unknown.

PREGNANCY-LACTATION-REPRODUCTION

• There are no adequate studies in pregnant women. Use only if potential benefit justifies potential fetal risk.

• Women of childbearing potential should use effective contraception during therapy and for 12 months after therapy ends.

• Enroll women with RA exposed to rituximab during pregnancy in the MotherToBaby Autoimmune Diseases in Pregnancy Study (1-877-311-8972).

• It isn't known if drug appears in breast milk. Patient should discontinue breastfeeding or discontinue drug, taking into account importance of drug to the mother.

NURSING CONSIDERATIONS

Black Box Warning Deaths from infusion reactions have occurred; 80% of fatal reactions are associated with the first infusion. Monitor patient for infusion reaction complex, including hypoxia, pulmonary infiltrates, ARDS, MI, or cardiogenic shock. Discontinue rituximab infusion for severe reactions and administer medical treatment for grade 3 or 4 infusion reactions. ■

• Monitor patient closely for signs and symptoms of hypersensitivity. Have drugs, such as epinephrine, antihistamines, and corticosteroids, on hand for emergency treatment.

• Monitor patient's BP closely during infusion. If hypotension, bronchospasm, or angioedema occurs, stop infusion and restart at half the rate when symptoms resolve.

• Withhold antihypertensives 12 hours before infusion because transient hypotension may occur.

• If serious or life-threatening arrhythmias occur, stop infusion. If patient develops significant arrhythmias, monitor cardiac function during and after subsequent infusions.

• *Pneumocystis jiroveci* pneumonia and antiherpetic viral prophylaxis is recommended

for patients with CLL during and for up to 12 months after treatment ends.

Black Box Warning Screen all patients for HBV infection before treatment by measuring hepatitis B surface antigen and hepatitis B core antibody. Monitor patients with evidence of current or prior HBV infection during and for several months after therapy. If HBV reactivation occurs, discontinue rituximab and concomitant chemotherapy and begin appropriate treatment. ■

• Monitor patients with WG and MPA carefully for signs and symptoms of infection (fever, pain, cold or flu symptoms, erythema) if biological agents or DMARDs are used concomitantly.

⚠ Alert: Prophylaxis for *P. jiroveci* pneumonia is recommended for patients with WG and MPA during treatment with rituximab and for at least 6 months after the last infusion.

Black Box Warning Severe mucocutaneous reactions (including toxic epidermal necrolysis, Stevens-Johnson syndrome, paraneoplastic pemphigus, and lichenoid or vesiculobullous dermatitis) may occur 1 to 13 weeks after administration. Avoid further infusions and promptly start treatment of the skin reaction. ■

• Infusion-related reactions are most severe with the first infusion. Subsequent infusions are generally well tolerated.

⚠ Alert: Acute renal failure requiring dialysis has been reported in the setting of TLS after treatment of patients with NHL.

• Patients at high risk for TLS may receive prophylactic allopurinol and hydration to correct hyperuricemia. Monitor renal function and fluid balance, and correct electrolyte abnormalities.

Black Box Warning JC virus infection resulting in progressive multifocal leukoencephalopathy has been reported in patients within 12 months of their last rituximab infusion. Monitor patient for new-onset neurologic manifestations. ■

• Obtain CBC at regular intervals and more frequently in patients in whom cytopenias develop.

• Monitor patients at risk for HBV infection closely. Discontinue drug at first sign of HBV infection.

• Monitor patient for abdominal pain. Bowel obstruction and perforation have occurred with chemotherapy.

PATIENT TEACHING

• Provide patient with medication guide to read before each treatment session.
• Tell patient to report symptoms of hypersensitivity, such as itching, rash, chills, or rigor, during and after infusion.
• Urge patient to watch for fever, sore throat, fatigue, easy bruising, nosebleeds, bleeding gums, abdominal pain, or tarry stools and to take temperature daily.
• Advise breast-feeding patient to stop breast-feeding until drug levels are undetectable.

rivaroxaban
ri-va-ROX-a-ban

Xarelto✔

Therapeutic class: Anticoagulants
Pharmacologic class: Factor Xa inhibitors

AVAILABLE FORMS
Tablets: 10 mg, 15 mg, 20 mg

INDICATIONS & DOSAGES
➤ **Prophylaxis of DVT that may lead to PE in patients undergoing knee or hip replacement surgery**
Adults: 10 mg P.O. once daily, 6 to 10 hours after surgery once hemostasis has been established. Treat for 35 days after hip replacement surgery and 12 days after knee replacement surgery.
Adjust-a-dose: If CrCl is less than 30 mL/minute, avoid use. Use cautiously in patients with moderate renal impairment (CrCl ranging from 30 to less than 50 mL/minute).
➤ **Treatment of DVT or PE**
Adults: 15 mg P.O. b.i.d. with food for 21 days; then 20 mg P.O. once daily for remainder of treatment.
Adjust-a-dose: If CrCl is less than 30 mL/minute, avoid use.

➤ **To decrease risk of recurrent DVT or PE**
Adults: 20 mg P.O. once daily with food.
Adjust-a-dose: If CrCl is less than 30 mL/minute, avoid use.
➤ **Stroke and systemic embolism risk reduction in patients with nonvalvular atrial fibrillation**
Adults: 20 mg once daily with evening meal.
Adjust-a-dose: In patients with CrCl of 15 to 50 mL/minute, reduce dosage to 15 mg once daily with evening meal. Avoid use in patients with CrCl less than 15 mL/minute.

ADMINISTRATION
P.O.
• Give 10-mg tablets without regard for food. Give 15- and 20-mg tablets with food. For nonvalvular atrial fibrillation, give with evening meal.
• For patients unable to swallow tablets whole, crush tablet and mix with applesauce immediately before use; administer orally. Immediately follow administration of a crushed 15- or 20-mg tablet with food.
• For administration via NG or gastric feeding tube, crush tablet and suspend in 50 mL of water; confirm gastric placement and administer within 4 hours. Delivery of drug into the small intestine will result in reduced absorption. Immediately follow administration of a crushed 15- or 20-mg tablet with an enteral feeding.

ACTION
Selectively blocks the active site of factor Xa, which is necessary for coagulation.

Route	Onset	Peak	Duration
P.O.	Unknown	2–4 hr	Unknown

Half-life: 5 to 9 hours.

ADVERSE REACTIONS
CNS: syncope, fatigue.
EENT: oropharyngeal pain, sinusitis.
GI: abdominal pain, dyspepsia, *GI hemorrhage.*
GU: UTI.
Hematologic: *bleeding events (including hemorrhage).*
Musculoskeletal: extremity pain, muscle spasm, back pain, osteoarthritis.
Skin: wound secretion, pruritus, blister.

R

INTERACTIONS
Drug-drug. *Anticoagulants (warfarin), antithrombotic agents, aspirin, fibrinolytics, NSAIDs, P2Y12 platelet aggregation inhibitors, thienopyridines, SNRIs, SSRIs:* May increase bleeding risk. Avoid use together. Monitor patient carefully for bleeding if drugs must be given together.
Combined P-glycoprotein (P-gp) and strong CYP3A4 inducers (carbamazepine, phenytoin, rifampin): May significantly decrease rivaroxaban level. Avoid use together.
Combined P-gp and strong CYP3A4 inhibitors (clarithromycin, conivaptan, indinavir–ritonavir, itraconazole, ketoconazole, lopinavir–ritonavir, ritonavir): May significantly increase rivaroxaban level. Avoid use together.
Combined P-gp and weak or moderate CYP3A4 inhibitors (amiodarone, azithromycin, diltiazem, dronedarone, erythromycin, felodipine, quinidine, ranolazine, verapamil): May increase rivaroxaban level. Use together only if benefit outweighs risk.
Drug-herb. *St. John's wort:* May significantly decrease rivaroxaban level. Avoid use together.

EFFECTS ON LAB TEST RESULTS
● May increase AST, ALT, total bilirubin, and GGT levels.

CONTRAINDICATIONS & CAUTIONS
Black Box Warning There is an increased risk of epidural or spinal hematomas, possibly resulting in long-term or permanent paralysis, in patients who have received anticoagulants and are receiving neuraxial anesthesia or undergoing spinal puncture. Factors that can increase the risk of epidural or spinal hematomas in these patients include use of indwelling epidural catheters; concomitant use of other drugs that affect hemostasis, such as NSAIDs, platelet inhibitors, and other anticoagulants; history of traumatic or repeated epidural or spinal punctures; and history of spinal deformity or spinal surgery. Monitor patients frequently for neurologic impairment. If neurologic compromise is noted, urgent treatment is necessary. Consider risks and benefits before neuraxial procedures in patients who have received anticoagulants for thromboprophylaxis. ■
Black Box Warning Discontinuing rivaroxaban places patients at increased risk for thrombotic events. If anticoagulation with rivaroxaban must be discontinued for a reason other than pathological bleeding or completion of a course of therapy, consider coverage with another anticoagulant. ■
● Contraindicated in patients hypersensitive to drug and in those with active major bleeding.
● Use isn't recommended in patients with prosthetic heart valves.
● Use cautiously in conditions associated with increased risk of hemorrhage, with concurrent use of drugs affecting hemostasis (platelet aggregation inhibitors, other antithrombotic agents, fibrinolytics, thienopyridines, long-term NSAIDs, SNRIs, SSRIs), and in elderly patients.
● Avoid use in patients with CrCl of less than 30 mL/minute who are taking drug for PE or DVT treatment or recurrence prophylaxis or prophylaxis of DVT after hip or knee replacement surgery.
● In patients with nonvalvular atrial fibrillation, assess renal function more frequently in situations in which renal function may decline and adjust therapy accordingly. Consider dosage adjustment or drug discontinuation in patients who develop acute renal failure.
● Avoid use in patients with moderate or severe hepatic impairment (Child-Pugh class B or C) and in those with hepatic disease associated with coagulopathy.
● Avoid use in patients receiving drugs that are concurrent P-gp and strong CYP3A4 inhibitors or inducers.
● Use cautiously in Japanese patients because drug exposure in these patients may be increased up to 40% when compared to other ethnicities but differences are reduced when values are corrected for body weight.
● Safety and efficacy in children haven't been established.
Dialyzable drug: Unlikely.
⚠ ***Overdose S&S:*** Hemorrhage.

PREGNANCY-LACTATION-REPRODUCTION
● There are no adequate studies in pregnant women. Use cautiously and only if potential

---

benefit justifies potential fetal risk because of the potential for pregnancy-related hemorrhage or emergent delivery with use of an anticoagulant that isn't readily reversible.
• It isn't known if drug appears in breast milk. Patient should discontinue breast-feeding or discontinue drug.

NURSING CONSIDERATIONS
Black Box Warning Monitor patient frequently for signs and symptoms of neurologic impairment. If neurologic compromise is noted, urgent treatment is necessary. ■
Black Box Warning Consider the benefits and risks before neuraxial intervention in patients anticoagulated or to be anticoagulated for thromboprophylaxis. Optimal timing between rivaroxaban administration and neuroaxial procedures isn't known. ■
• Don't remove an epidural catheter earlier than 18 hours after last administration of drug, and don't give next dose until 6 hours after catheter removal unless traumatic puncture occurred; if puncture has occurred, wait 24 hours before giving next dose.
• Monitor patient carefully for bleeding, which can occur at any site during therapy.
• If an anticoagulant must be discontinued to reduce risk of bleeding with surgical or other procedures, stop drug at least 24 hours before procedure. When deciding whether to delay a procedure until 24 hours after last dose, weigh the increased risk of bleeding against the urgency of intervention. Restart drug after procedure when adequate hemostasis has been established, as the time to onset of therapeutic effect is short.
🖲 *Alert:* Watch for signs and symptoms of blood loss. Search for a bleeding site if an unexplained fall in hematocrit or BP occurs. Patients with moderate renal failure (CrCl ranging from 30 to less than 50 mL/minute) are at increased risk.

PATIENT TEACHING
• Instruct patient to take drug only as directed and not to discontinue drug without consulting prescriber.
• Tell patient on once-daily dosing that if a dose is missed, to take dose as soon as patient remembers and to resume normal regimen the following day.

🖲 *Alert:* If patient has had neuraxial anesthesia or spinal puncture, especially if taking concomitant NSAIDs or platelet inhibitors, advise patient to watch for signs and symptoms of spinal or epidural hematoma (midline back pain, tingling, numbness of the limbs, muscular weakness, bowel or bladder dysfunction). If any of these signs and symptoms occur, advise patient to contact prescriber immediately.
• Advise patient to watch for bleeding risks, especially if patient had a spinal catheter or is currently taking drugs or supplements that increase bleeding risk.
• Instruct female patient to consult prescriber if she is pregnant, plans to become pregnant, or intends to breast-feed.
• Caution patient to report changes in medications or herbal supplements or unusual bleeding or bruising.
• Advise patient who can't swallow the tablet whole to crush tablet and combine with a small amount of applesauce followed by food.
• Instruct patient with an NG or gastric feeding tube to crush the tablet and mix it with 50 mL of water before administering via the tube and to follow administration of 15- or 20-mg tablet with an enteral feeding.
• Instruct patient to inform all health care providers that patient is taking rivaroxaban before any invasive procedure (including dental procedures) is scheduled.

rivastigmine
riv-ah-STIG-meen

Exelon Patch

rivastigmine tartrate🖉
Exelon

Therapeutic class: Anti-Alzheimer drugs
Pharmacologic class: Cholinesterase inhibitors

AVAILABLE FORMS
Capsules 🖲: 1.5 mg, 3 mg, 4.5 mg, 6 mg
Transdermal patch: 4.6 mg/24 hours, 9.5 mg/24 hours, 13.3 mg/24 hours

R

INDICATIONS & DOSAGES
Adjust-a-dose (for all indications): Patients with moderate to severe renal impairment (GFR less than 50 mL/minute) or mild to moderate hepatic impairment (Child-Pugh score of 5 to 9) may be able to only tolerate lower doses of oral drug. For patients with mild to moderate hepatic impairment, consider using 4.6 mg/24 hours transdermal patch for both initial and maintenance dose. For patients weighing less than 50 kg, watch for toxicities (nausea, vomiting) and if they occur, consider reducing maintenance dose; reduce dose of transdermal patch to 4.6 mg/24 hours.

➤ **Mild to moderate Alzheimer dementia**
Adults: Initially, 1.5 mg P.O. b.i.d. with food. If tolerated, may increase to 3 mg b.i.d. after 2 weeks. After 2 weeks at this dose, may increase to 4.5 mg b.i.d. and to 6 mg b.i.d., as tolerated. Effective dosage range is 6 to 12 mg daily; maximum, 12 mg daily. Or, 4.6 mg/24 hours transdermal patch. After 4 weeks, if tolerated, increase to 9.5 mg/24 hours transdermal patch for as long as therapeutic benefit persists; if needed after at least 4 weeks, increase to 13.3 mg/24 hours transdermal patch. Maximum dose is 13.3 mg/24 hours.

➤ **Severe Alzheimer dementia (transdermal patch only)**
Adults: Initially, 4.6 mg/24 hours transdermal patch once daily. After 4 weeks, if tolerated, increase to 9.5 mg/24 hours transdermal patch; then, if tolerated after an additional 4 weeks, increase to 13.3 mg/24 hours transdermal patch.

➤ **Mild to moderate dementia associated with Parkinson disease**
Adults: Initially, 1.5 mg P.O. b.i.d. May increase, as tolerated, to 3 mg b.i.d., then to 4.5 mg b.i.d., and finally to 6 mg b.i.d. after a minimum of 4 weeks at each dose. Or, 4.6 mg/24 hours transdermal patch. After 4 weeks, if tolerated, increase to 9.5 mg/24 hours transdermal patch for as long as therapeutic benefit persists; if needed after at least 4 weeks, increase to 13.3 mg/24 hours transdermal patch. Maximum dose is 13.3 mg/24 hours.

➤ **Treatment of neuropsychiatric symptoms associated with Lewy body dementia** ◆

Adults: Initially, 1.5 mg P.O. b.i.d.; increase as tolerated by 1.5 mg b.i.d. every 2 weeks to a maximum of 6 mg b.i.d. Ongoing therapy is required.

ADMINISTRATION
P.O.
● Give drug with food in the morning and evening.
● Patient should swallow capsule whole.
Transdermal
● Apply patch once daily to clean, dry, hairless skin on the upper or lower back, upper arm, or chest, in a place not rubbed by tight clothing.
● Change the site daily, and don't use the same site within 14 days. Avoid exposing patch to external heat sources (sauna, excess sunlight).
● Press patch firmly into place until the edges stick well.
● Avoid eye contact; wash hands with soap and water after removing patch. In case of contact with eyes or if eyes become red after handling patch, rinse immediately with plenty of water. Seek medical advice if symptoms don't resolve.

ACTION
Thought to increase acetylcholine level by inhibiting cholinesterase enzyme, which causes acetylcholine hydrolysis.

Route	Onset	Peak	Duration
P.O.	Unknown	1 hr	8–10 hr
Transdermal	Unknown	8–16 hr	24 hr

Half-life: Oral, 1½ hours; transdermal, 3 hours.

ADVERSE REACTIONS
CNS: headache, dizziness, syncope, fatigue, asthenia, malaise, somnolence, tremor, insomnia, confusion, depression, anxiety, hallucinations, aggressive reaction, vertigo, agitation, nervousness, delusion, paranoid reaction, pain.
CV: hypertension, chest pain, peripheral edema, *bradycardia.*
EENT: rhinitis, pharyngitis.
GI: nausea, vomiting, diarrhea, anorexia, abdominal pain, dyspepsia, constipation, flatulence, eructation, GI bleeding.
GU: UTI, incontinence, hematuria.
Metabolic: weight loss.

Reactions in bold italics are *life-threatening*. Interactions may have a *rapid onset* or a *delayed onset*.

Musculoskeletal: bradykinesia, dyskinesia, hypokinesia, weakness.
Respiratory: URI, cough, bronchitis.
Skin: increased sweating, rash.
Other: accidental trauma, flulike symptoms.

INTERACTIONS

Drug-drug. *Anticholinergics:* May decrease effectiveness of anticholinergic. Monitor patient for expected therapeutic effects.
Bethanechol, succinylcholine, other neuromuscular-blocking drugs or cholinergic antagonists: May have synergistic effect. Monitor patient closely.
NSAIDs: May increase gastric acid secretions. Monitor patient for symptoms of active or occult GI bleeding.
Drug-lifestyle. *Smoking:* May increase drug clearance. Discourage smoking.

EFFECTS ON LAB TEST RESULTS
None reported.

CONTRAINDICATIONS & CAUTIONS
● Contraindicated in patients hypersensitive to drug, other carbamate derivatives, or other components of drug.
● Isolated cases of disseminated allergic dermatitis, irrespective of administration route (oral or transdermal), have been noted in postmarketing reports. Discontinue drug if disseminated allergic dermatitis occurs.
● Contraindicated in patients with history of transdermal patch application-site reaction suggestive of allergic contact dermatitis.
● Use cautiously in patients with history of CV disease, GI bleeding, seizure disorder, genitourinary conditions, asthma, or obstructive pulmonary disease.
Dialyzable drug: No.
⚠ **Overdose S&S:** Nausea, vomiting, excessive salivation, sweating, bradycardia, hypotension, respiratory depression, syncope, seizures, muscle weakness.

PREGNANCY-LACTATION-REPRODUCTION
● There are no adequate studies in pregnant women. Use during pregnancy only if clearly needed.
● It isn't know if drug appears in breast milk. Patient should discontinue breast-feeding or discontinue drug.

NURSING CONSIDERATIONS
● Expect significant GI adverse effects (such as nausea, vomiting, anorexia, and weight loss). These effects are less common during maintenance doses.
● Monitor patient for evidence of active or occult GI bleeding.
● Dramatic memory improvement is unlikely. As disease progresses, the benefits of drug may decline.
● Monitor patient for severe nausea, vomiting, and diarrhea, which may lead to dehydration and weight loss.
● Carefully monitor patient with a history of GI bleeding, NSAID use, arrhythmias, seizures, or pulmonary conditions for adverse effects.
● If adverse reactions, such as diarrhea, loss of appetite, nausea, or vomiting, occur with transdermal patch, stop use for several days, then restart at the same or lower dose. If treatment is interrupted for more than several days, restart patch at the lowest dose and retitrate.
● Patients weighing less than 50 kg may experience more adverse reactions when using the transdermal patch.
● Application-site reactions may occur with the transdermal patch. Discontinue treatment if application-site reaction spreads beyond the patch size, if there's evidence of a more intense local reaction (increasing erythema, edema, papules, vesicles), and if symptoms don't significantly improve within 48 hours after patch removal.
● When switching from oral form to the transdermal patch, patients on a total daily dose of less than 6 mg can be switched to 4.6 mg/24 hours. Patients taking 6 to 12 mg P.O. can switch to the 9.5 mg/24 hour patch. The patch should be applied on the day after the last oral dose.

PATIENT TEACHING
● Tell caregiver to give drug with food in the morning and evening.
● Advise patient that memory improvement may be subtle and that drug more likely slows future memory loss.
● Tell patient to report nausea, vomiting, or diarrhea.
● Tell patient to consult prescriber before using OTC drugs.

R

• Tell patient to apply patch once daily to clean, dry, hairless skin in a place not rubbed by tight clothing and to retain pouch for disposal.
• Teach patient that the recommended sites for patch placement include the upper or lower back, upper arm, or chest.
• Tell patient to change the site daily and not to use the same site within 14 days.
• Tell patient to press the patch firmly into place until the edges stick well.
• Advise patient to remove used patch, place in previously saved pouch and discard in trash (away from pets or children), and then wash hands with soap and water. In case of contact with eyes or if eyes become red after handling patch, tell patient to rinse immediately with plenty of water and seek medical advice if symptoms don't resolve.

---

roflumilast
roe-FLUE-mi-last

Daliresp

Therapeutic class: Miscellaneous respiratory drugs
Pharmacologic class: Selective phosphodiesterase inhibitors

AVAILABLE FORMS
Tablets: 500 mcg

INDICATIONS & DOSAGES
➤ **To reduce risk of COPD exacerbations in patients with severe COPD associated with chronic bronchitis and a history of exacerbations**
Adults: 500 mcg P.O. daily.

ADMINISTRATION
P.O.
• Give drug without regard to food.

ACTION
Selectively inhibits phosphodiesterase-4 (PDE_4), which is a cAMP-metabolizing enzyme in the lung tissue. Inhibition of PDE_4 leads to accumulation of intracellular cAMP. Effects of drug are thought to be related to the increased intracellular cAMP in lung cells.

Route	Onset	Peak	Duration
P.O.	Unknown	1–2 hr	Unknown

Half-life: 17 hours.

ADVERSE REACTIONS
CNS: headache, insomnia, dizziness, tremor, anxiety, depression.
EENT: rhinitis, sinusitis.
GI: diarrhea, nausea, decreased appetite, abdominal pain, dyspepsia, gastritis, vomiting.
GU: UTI.
Metabolic: weight loss.
Musculoskeletal: back pain, muscle spasms.
Other: flulike symptoms.

INTERACTIONS
Drug-drug. *CYP450 inducers (carbamazepine, phenobarbital, phenytoin, rifampin):* May decrease the effectiveness of roflumilast. Avoid use together.
CYP450 inhibitors (cimetidine, enoxacin, erythromycin, fluvoxamine, ketoconazole), hormonal contraceptives containing gestodene and ethinyl estradiol: May increase roflumilast concentration and risk of adverse reactions. Use together cautiously.

EFFECTS ON LAB TEST RESULTS
None reported.

CONTRAINDICATIONS & CAUTIONS
• Contraindicated in patients hypersensitive to drug or its components and in those with moderate to severe hepatic impairment (Child-Pugh class B or C).
• Use cautiously in patients with history of depression or suicidal thoughts and behaviors.
Dialyzable drug: Unlikely.

PREGNANCY-LACTATION-REPRODUCTION
• There are no adequate studies in pregnant women. Use only if potential benefit justifies potential risk to the fetus.
• Don't use during labor and delivery.
• Drug may appear in breast milk. Patient should discontinue breast-feeding or discontinue drug.

---

ns in bold italics are *life-threatening*. Interactions may have a *rapid onset* or a **delayed onset**.

NURSING CONSIDERATIONS
- Drug isn't a bronchodilator and isn't indicated for the relief of acute bronchospasm.
- Monitor patients for signs and symptoms of psychiatric adverse events, including insomnia, anxiety, depression, suicidal ideation, and suicide attempts. If events occur, evaluate the risks versus benefits of continuing drug.
- Monitor weight regularly; if unexplained or significant weight loss occurs, evaluate cause and consider stopping drug.

PATIENT TEACHING
- Educate patient that drug isn't a bronchodilator and isn't to be used for the relief of acute bronchospasm.
- Advise patient, family, and caregivers to watch for signs and symptoms of psychiatric adverse events, including insomnia, anxiety, depression, suicidal ideation, and suicide attempts, and to report any occurrences to the health care provider.
- Tell patient to report unexplained or significant weight loss.

rolapitant hydrochloride
roe-LA-pi-tant

Varubi

Therapeutic class: Antiemetics
Pharmacologic class: Substance P and neurokinin-1 receptor antagonists

AVAILABLE FORMS
Tablets: 90 mg

INDICATIONS & DOSAGES
➤ **Prevention of delayed nausea and vomiting associated with cisplatin-based or highly emetogenic chemotherapy, in combination with other antiemetics**
Adults: 180 mg P.O. 1 to 2 hours before chemotherapy on day 1. Give dexamethasone 20 mg on day 1, 30 minutes before chemotherapy and then 8 mg P.O. b.i.d. on days 2, 3, and 4. Also give a 5-HT$_3$ receptor antagonist on day 1. Refer to manufacturer's instructions for appropriate dosing information.

➤ **Prevention of delayed nausea and vomiting associated with anthracycline and cyclophosphamide–based or moderately emetogenic chemotherapy, in combination with other antiemetics**
Adults: 180 mg P.O. 1 to 2 hours before chemotherapy on day 1. Give dexamethasone 20 mg P.O. 30 minutes before chemotherapy on day 1. Also give a 5-HT$_3$ receptor antagonist on day 1. Refer to manufacturer's instructions for appropriate dosing information.

ADMINISTRATION
P.O.
- Give drug before each scheduled chemotherapy cycle, but at no less than 2-week intervals.
- Give without regard to meals.
- Store at room temperature.

ACTION
A selective and competitive antagonist of human substance P/neurokinin-1 receptors in the brain. Appears to be synergistic with 5-HT$_3$ antagonists and corticosteroids.

Route	Onset	Peak	Duration
P.O.	30 min	4 hr	Unknown

Half-life: About 7 days.

ADVERSE REACTIONS
CNS: dizziness.
GI: abdominal pain, decreased appetite, dyspepsia, stomatitis.
GU: UTI.
Hematologic: *neutropenia,* anemia.
Respiratory: hiccups.

INTERACTIONS
Drug-drug. *Breast cancer resistance protein (BCRP) substrates with a narrow therapeutic index (irinotecan, methotrexate, rosuvastatin, topotecan):* May increase plasma concentrations of BCRP substrates and risk of BCRP-related adverse reactions. Monitor patient for increased adverse effects. Use lowest effective rosuvastatin dose.
CYP2D6 substrates with a narrow therapeutic index (dextromethorphan, TCAs, thioridazine): May increase plasma concentrations of CYP2D6 substrates. Monitor

R

patient closely for increased adverse effects. Use with thioridazine is contraindicated.

P-glycoprotein (P-gp) substrates with a narrow therapeutic index (digoxin): May increase plasma concentrations of P-gp substrates and risk of P-gp–related adverse reactions. Monitor drug levels and watch for increased adverse reactions if concomitant use can't be avoided.

Pimozide: May increase pimozide level and risk of QT-interval prolongation. Monitor patient closely for QT-interval prolongation if concomitant use can't be avoided.

Strong CYP3A4 inducers (rifampin): May decrease plasma concentration and therapeutic effect of rolapitant. Avoid concomitant use, if possible.

EFFECTS ON LAB TEST RESULTS
● May decrease Hb level and neutrophil count.

CONTRAINDICATIONS & CAUTIONS
● Contraindicated in patients receiving thioridazine because of risk of QT-interval prolongation and torsades de pointes.
● Use cautiously in patients receiving drugs that affect the CYP2D6 enzyme system. Inhibitory effects of rolapitant on CYP2D6 may last for 7 days or longer.
● Drug hasn't been studied in patients with severe hepatic impairment (Child-Pugh class C); avoid use. Monitor closely for adverse reactions if use can't be avoided.
● Safety and effectiveness in children haven't been established.
Dialyzable drug: Unlikely.

PREGNANCY-LACTATION-REPRODUCTION
● There are no data regarding use of rolapitant in pregnant women. Use cautiously.
● It isn't known if drug appears in breast milk. Give only if benefits outweigh potential risks to breast-fed infant.

NURSING CONSIDERATIONS
◐ **Alert:** Before giving drug, assess patient's current drug list for potential drug-drug interactions.
● Drug is used to prevent, not treat, nausea and vomiting.
● Always use drug in combination with a corticosteroid and a 5-HT$_3$ inhibitor.

● *Look alike–sound alike:* Don't confuse rolapitant with aprepitant or fosaprepitant.

PATIENT TEACHING
● Remind patient that rolapitant is taken in combination with a corticosteroid and a 5-HT$_3$ inhibitor.
● Instruct patient to take breakthrough antiemetics rather than taking more rolapitant if nausea or vomiting isn't controlled.
● Remind patient to take drug 1 to 2 hours before scheduled chemotherapy.
● Inform patient that rolapitant is associated with drug-drug interactions and that it's important to report all medications being taken, including OTC drugs and supplements, before starting therapy.
● Advise patient to inform prescriber and pharmacist of dosage changes or new prescription drug therapy because drug interactions can be delayed after rolapitant is discontinued.
● Advise female patient to inform prescriber if she is or plans to become pregnant or is breast-feeding.

r*O*PINIRole hydrochloride
row-PIN-ah-roll

Requip, Requip XL

Therapeutic class: Antiparkinsonians
Pharmacologic class: Nonergot dopamine agonists

AVAILABLE FORMS
Tablets: 0.25 mg, 0.5 mg, 1 mg, 2 mg, 3 mg, 4 mg, 5 mg
Tablets (extended-release) ⓞ: 2 mg, 4 mg, 6 mg, 8 mg, 12 mg

INDICATIONS & DOSAGES
Adjust-a-dose (for all indications): For patients with ESRD on hemodialysis using immediate-release formula, give 0.25 mg P.O. t.i.d. Base further dosage escalations on tolerability and need for efficacy. Recommended maximum total daily dose is 18 mg/day in patients receiving regular dialysis. Supplemental doses after dialysis aren't required. No dosage adjustment is

necessary in patients with moderate renal impairment (CrCl of 30 to 50 mL/minute).

For patients with ESRD on hemodialysis using extended-release formula, give 2 mg once daily initially. May titrate dosage upward for a maximum dose of 18 mg/day if needed. Supplemental doses after dialysis aren't required.

➤ **Idiopathic Parkinson disease**
Adults: Initially, 0.25 mg P.O. t.i.d. Increase dose by 0.25 mg t.i.d. at weekly intervals for 4 weeks. After week 4, daily dosage may be increased by 1.5 mg/day on a weekly basis up to a dose of 9 mg/day, and then by up to 3 mg/day weekly to a total dose of 24 mg/day. For extended-release form, starting dosage is 2 mg P.O. once daily for 1 to 2 weeks. May increase by 2 mg/day at 1-week or longer intervals. Maximum dosage is 24 mg/day. To switch from immediate-release to extended-release tablets, refer to manufacturer's instructions.
Elderly patients: Adjust dosages individually, according to patient response; clearance may be reduced in these patients.

➤ **Moderate to severe restless legs syndrome (immediate-release)**
Adults: Initially, 0.25 mg P.O. 1 to 3 hours before bedtime. May increase dose as needed and tolerated after 2 days to 0.5 mg, then to 1 mg by the end of the first week. May further increase dose as needed and tolerated as follows: Week 2, give 1 mg once daily. Week 3, give 1.5 mg once daily. Week 4, give 2 mg once daily. Week 5, give 2.5 mg once daily. Week 6, give 3 mg once daily. Week 7, give 4 mg once daily. Maximum dosage is 4 mg/day. Patient should take all doses 1 to 2 hours before bedtime.

ADMINISTRATION
P.O.
● Give drug with food if nausea occurs.
● Patient must swallow extended-release tablets whole; they mustn't be chewed, crushed, or divided.

ACTION
Thought to stimulate dopamine (D2) receptors.

Route	Onset	Peak	Duration
P.O. (immediate release)	Unknown	1–2 hr	6 hr
P.O. (extended-release)	Unknown	6–10 hr	Unknown

Half-life: 6 hours.

ADVERSE REACTIONS
Early Parkinson disease (without levodopa)
CNS: dizziness, fatigue, somnolence, syncope, hallucinations, aggravated Parkinson disease, headache, confusion, hyperkinesia, hypoesthesia, vertigo, amnesia, impaired concentration, malaise, asthenia, pain.
CV: orthostatic hypotension, orthostatic symptoms, hypertension, edema, chest pain, extrasystoles, atrial fibrillation, palpitations, tachycardia, flushing.
EENT: pharyngitis, abnormal vision, eye abnormality, xerophthalmia, rhinitis, sinusitis.
GI: nausea, vomiting, dyspepsia, dry mouth, flatulence, abdominal pain, anorexia, constipation.
GU: UTI, erectile dysfunction.
Respiratory: bronchitis, dyspnea, yawning.
Other: viral infection, increased sweating, peripheral ischemia.

Advanced Parkinson disease (with levodopa)
CNS: dizziness, somnolence, headache, hallucinations, aggravated Parkinsonism, insomnia, abnormal dreaming, confusion, tremor, anxiety, nervousness, amnesia, paresis, paresthesia, syncope, pain.
CV: hypotension.
EENT: diplopia.
GI: nausea, abdominal pain, dry mouth, vomiting, constipation, diarrhea, dysphagia, flatulence, increased saliva.
GU: UTI, pyuria, urinary incontinence.
Hematologic: anemia.
Metabolic: weight decrease, suppressed prolactin.
Musculoskeletal: dyskinesia, arthralgia, arthritis, hypokinesia.
Respiratory: URI, dyspnea.
Skin: increased sweating.
Other: falls, injury, viral infection.

Restless legs syndrome
CNS: fatigue, somnolence, dizziness, vertigo, paresthesia.

R

CV: peripheral edema.
EENT: nasopharyngitis, nasal congestion.
GI: nausea, vomiting, diarrhea, dyspepsia, dry mouth.
Musculoskeletal: arthralgia, muscle cramps, extremity pain.
Respiratory: cough.
Skin: increased sweating.
Other: influenza.

INTERACTIONS

Drug-drug. *BP-lowering agents:* May enhance hypotensive effect. Monitor BP carefully.
Cimetidine, ciprofloxacin, fluvoxamine, inhibitors or substrates of CYP1A2, ritonavir: May alter ropinirole clearance. Adjust ropinirole dose if other drugs are started or stopped during treatment.
CNS depressants: May increase CNS effects. Use together cautiously.
Dopamine antagonists (neuroleptics), metoclopramide: May decrease ropinirole effects. Avoid using together.
Estrogens: May decrease ropinirole clearance. Adjust ropinirole dosage if estrogen therapy is started or stopped during treatment.
Warfarin: May increase anticoagulation. Monitor coagulation parameters and adjust warfarin dosage as needed.
Drug-lifestyle. *Alcohol use:* May increase sedative effect. Discourage use together.
Smoking: May increase drug clearance. Discourage use together.

EFFECTS ON LAB TEST RESULTS

● May increase BUN and alkaline phosphatase levels. May decrease Hb level.

CONTRAINDICATIONS & CAUTIONS

● Contraindicated in patients hypersensitive to drug.
● Use cautiously in patients with severe hepatic or renal impairment.
Dialyzable drug: 30%.
⚠ **Overdose S&S:** Nausea, dizziness, visual hallucinations, hyperhidrosis, claustrophobia, chorea, palpitations, asthenia, nightmares, vomiting, increased coughing, fatigue, syncope, vasovagal syncope, dyskinesia, agitation, chest pain, orthostatic hypotension, somnolence, confusion.

PREGNANCY-LACTATION-REPRODUCTION

● There are no adequate studies in pregnant women. Use only if potential benefit justifies potential risk to the fetus.
● Drug inhibits prolactin secretion and could potentially inhibit lactation. It isn't known if drug appears in breast milk. Use cautiously in breast-feeding women.

NURSING CONSIDERATIONS

⟳ **Alert:** Monitor patient carefully for orthostatic hypotension, especially during dosage increases.
● Drug may potentiate the adverse effects of levodopa and may cause or worsen dyskinesia. Dosage may be decreased.
● Although not reported with ropinirole, other adverse reactions reported with dopaminergic therapy include hyperpyrexia, fibrotic complications, and confusion, which may occur with rapid dosage reduction or withdrawal of drug.
● Patient may have syncope, with or without bradycardia. Monitor patient carefully, especially for 4 weeks after start of therapy and with dosage increases.
● When used for Parkinson disease, withdraw drug gradually over 7 days.
● When used for restless legs syndrome, stop drug without tapering.
● Drug can cause somnolence and sudden episodes of falling asleep. Continually reassess patient for drowsiness or sleepiness and for factors that could contribute to sleepiness.
● Avoid use in patients with major psychotic disorders. Drug may cause changes in or worsening of mental status, abnormal thinking, and behavioral changes, which may be severe and include paranoid ideation, delusions, hallucinations, confusion, psychotic-like behavior, disorientation, aggressive behavior, agitation, and delirium.
● Augmentation (an increase in symptoms or earlier onset of symptoms in the evening or even the afternoon, or spread of symptoms to other extremities) and early-morning rebound symptoms (onset of symptoms in the early morning) have been observed in a postmarketing trial in restless legs syndrome. Review use of drug, adjust dosage, or discontinue treatment if

---

Reactions in bold italics are *life-threatening*. Interactions may have a *rapid onset* or a *delayed onset*.

augmentation or early-morning rebound symptoms occur.

• Ask patient about development or worsening of impulsive or compulsive behaviors, such as new or increased gambling urges, sexual urges, uncontrolled spending, or other urges, because patient may not recognize these behaviors as abnormal.

• Patients with Parkinson disease have an increased risk of melanoma. Monitor patient for melanoma development during periodic dermatologic screenings.

• **Look alike–sound alike:** Don't confuse ropinirole with risperidone.

PATIENT TEACHING
• Advise patient to take drug with food if nausea occurs.

• Tell patient not to crush, chew, or divide extended-release tablets.

• Advise patient to inform prescriber if starting or stopping medications, OTC drugs or herbs, or smoking.

• Tell patient (especially elderly patient) to contact prescriber if paranoid ideation, delusions, hallucinations, confusion, psychotic-like behavior, disorientation, aggressive behavior, agitation, or delirium occurs.

• Instruct patient not to rise rapidly after sitting or lying down because of risk of dizziness, which may occur more frequently early in therapy or when dosage increases.

• Sleepiness and sudden episodes of falling asleep can occur, sometimes without warning. Warn patient to minimize hazardous activities until CNS effects of drug are known.

• Tell patient to contact prescriber if experiencing difficulty controlling impulsive or compulsive behaviors, such as new or increased gambling urges, sexual urges, uncontrolled spending, or other urges.

• Teach patient about melanoma and to report skin changes to prescriber.

• Advise patient to avoid alcohol.

• Tell woman to notify prescriber about planned, suspected, or known pregnancy; also tell her to inform prescriber if she's breast-feeding.

rosiglitazone maleate
roh-zee-GLIT-ah-zohn

Avandia♦

Therapeutic class: Antidiabetics
Pharmacologic class:
Thiazolidinediones

AVAILABLE FORMS
Tablets: 2 mg, 4 mg, 8 mg

INDICATIONS & DOSAGES
➤ **Type 2 diabetes mellitus, alone or with a sulfonylurea or metformin, in patients currently benefiting from therapy or in patients unable to achieve glucose control with other medications**
Adults: Initially, 4 mg P.O. daily in the morning or in two divided doses (morning and evening). Increase to 8 mg P.O. daily or in two divided doses if fasting glucose level doesn't improve after 8 to 12 weeks of treatment. Maximum dose is 8 mg/day.

ADMINISTRATION
P.O.
Alert: Check liver enzyme levels before therapy starts. Don't use drug in patients with increased baseline liver enzyme levels (ALT level greater than 2.5 × ULN).
• Give drug without regard for food.

ACTION
Lowers glucose level by improving insulin sensitivity.

Route	Onset	Peak	Duration
P.O.	Unknown	1 hr	Unknown

Half-life: 3 to 4 hours.

ADVERSE REACTIONS
CNS: headache, fatigue.
CV: edema, *worsening HF, MI*, angina.
EENT: blurred vision, sinusitis.
GI: diarrhea.
Hematologic: anemia.
Metabolic: hyperglycemia, weight gain.
Musculoskeletal: back pain, fractures.
Respiratory: URI.
Other: accidental injury.

INTERACTIONS

Drug-drug. *Atazanavir, fluvoxamine, gemfibrozil, ketoconazole, trimethoprim:* May increase rosiglitazone levels, increasing hypoglycemic effects and adverse reactions. Monitor glucose; dosage adjustment may be necessary.

Insulin: May increase incidence of edema and risk of MI. Use together isn't recommended.

MAO inhibitors, salicylates, SSRIs, sulfonylureas: May enhance hypoglycemic effects. Monitor therapy.

Quinolone antibiotics: May enhance hypoglycemic effect or diminish therapeutic blood glucose–lowering effect of rosiglitazone. Carefully monitor therapy and glucose level.

Rifampin: May decrease rosiglitazone levels. Monitor glucose; dosage adjustment may be necessary.

EFFECTS ON LAB TEST RESULTS

- May increase glucose, HDL, LDL, total cholesterol, and ALT levels.
- May decrease Hb level and hematocrit.
- May decrease free fatty acid levels.

CONTRAINDICATIONS & CAUTIONS

- Don't use for treatment of diabetic ketoacidosis or type 1 diabetes mellitus.
- Administration with insulin isn't recommended.
- Contraindicated in patients hypersensitive to drug or its components.

Black Box Warning Drug isn't recommended in patients with symptomatic HF. Initiating drug in patients with established New York Heart Association class III or IV HF is contraindicated. ∎

- Contraindicated in patients with active liver disease, increased baseline liver enzyme levels (ALT level greater than 2½ × ULN), type 1 diabetes, or diabetic ketoacidosis and in those who experienced jaundice while taking troglitazone.
- Don't start drug in patients experiencing acute coronary syndrome.
- Use cautiously in patients with edema or HF.

Dialyzable drug: No.

PREGNANCY-LACTATION-REPRODUCTION

- There are no adequate studies in pregnant women. Use only if potential benefit justifies potential risk to the fetus.
- Careful monitoring of glucose control is essential during pregnancy. Insulin monotherapy is recommended to maintain blood glucose levels as close to normal as possible.
- Drug can cause ovulation in some premenopausal anovulatory women and increase risk of pregnancy. Premenopausal women should use adequate contraception.
- It isn't known if drug appears in breast milk. Patient should discontinue breastfeeding or discontinue drug.

NURSING CONSIDERATIONS

❸ *Alert:* Monitor liver enzyme levels every 2 months for first 12 months and periodically thereafter. If ALT level becomes elevated, recheck as soon as possible. Stop drug if levels remain elevated.

Black Box Warning Drug may cause or exacerbate congestive HF in some patients. After drug initiation and after dosage increases, observe patient carefully for signs and symptoms of HF (excessive, rapid weight gain, dyspnea, edema). If these develop, manage HF according to current standards of care. Consider discontinuing drug or reducing dosage. ∎

- Management of type 2 diabetes should include diet control. Because caloric restriction, weight loss, and exercise help improve insulin sensitivity and effectiveness of drug therapy, these measures are essential to proper diabetes treatment.
- Check glucose and HbA$_{1c}$ levels periodically to monitor therapeutic response to drug.
- Hb level and hematocrit may drop during therapy, usually during first 4 to 8 weeks. Increases in total cholesterol, LDL, and HDL levels and decreases in free fatty acid level also may occur.
- For patients inadequately controlled with a maximum dose of a sulfonylurea or metformin, add rosiglitazone to, rather than substituting it for, the sulfonylurea or metformin.

Reactions in bold italics are *life-threatening*. Interactions may have a *rapid onset* or a *delayed onset*.

• Drug may increase the incidence of bone fractures (most common in the arm, hand, and foot) in women.

• *Look alike–sound alike:* Don't confuse rosiglitazone with pioglitazone. Don't confuse Avandia with Prandin.

PATIENT TEACHING

• Advise patient that drug can be taken with or without food.

• Notify patient that blood will be tested to check liver function before therapy starts, every 2 months for first 12 months, and then periodically thereafter.

• Tell patient to immediately notify prescriber about unexplained signs and symptoms, such as nausea, vomiting, abdominal pain, fatigue, anorexia, or dark urine; these may indicate liver problems.

• Tell patient to immediately notify prescriber of changes in vision as this may indicate macular edema.

• Warn patient to report signs or symptoms of HF (unusually rapid increase in weight or swelling, shortness of breath) or MI (chest pain or pressure, dyspnea).

• Recommend use of contraceptives to premenopausal, anovulatory female patient with insulin resistance because ovulation may resume with therapy.

• Advise patient that management of diabetes includes diet control, calorie restriction, weight loss, and exercise, and that these measures improve effectiveness of drug therapy.

• Instruct patient to monitor glucose level carefully. Tell patient what to do if ill, undergoing surgery, or under added stress.

---

rosuvastatin calcium
row-SUE-va-sta-tin

Crestor⚘

Therapeutic class: Antilipemics
Pharmacologic class: HMG-CoA reductase inhibitors

AVAILABLE FORMS
Tablets: 5 mg, 10 mg, 20 mg, 40 mg

INDICATIONS & DOSAGES
Adjust-a-dose (for all indications): If CrCl is less than 30 mL/minute, initially, 5 mg once daily; don't exceed 10 mg once daily. For Asian patients, initial dose is 5 mg. For patients also taking cyclosporine, limit rosuvastatin dose to 5 mg once daily. For patients taking atazanavir and ritonavir, lopinavir and ritonavir, or simeprevir, initially, 5 mg once daily; don't exceed 10 mg once daily. Avoid concomitant use with gemfibrozil. If concomitant use can't be avoided, initially give 5 mg once daily; don't exceed 10 mg once daily.

➤ **Risk reduction in patients without clinical evidence of CAD but with multiple risk factors**
Adults: Initially, 10 mg P.O. once daily; 5 mg P.O. once daily in patients needing less aggressive LDL cholesterol reduction. For aggressive lipid reduction (LDL greater than 190 mg/dL) initially, 20 mg P.O. once daily. Increase as needed to maximum of 40 mg P.O. daily. Dosage may be titrated every 2 to 4 weeks, based on lipid levels.

➤ **Children with heterozygous familial hypercholesterolemia to reduce total cholesterol, LDL cholesterol, and apolipoprotein B levels after failing an adequate trial of diet therapy when LDL cholesterol is more than 190 mg/dL, or more than 160 mg/dL and there is a positive family history of premature CV disease or two or more other CV disease risk factors**
Children ages 10 to 17: 5 to 20 mg P.O. daily.
Children ages 8 to younger than 10: 5 to 10 mg P.O. daily.
Adjust-a-dose: May titrate dosage every 4 weeks or more, based on lipid levels.

➤ **Children with homozygous familial hypercholesterolemia to reduce LDL cholesterol, total cholesterol, non-HDL cholesterol, and apolipoprotein B levels after failing an adequate trial of diet therapy**
Children ages 7 to 17: 20 mg P.O. once daily either alone or with other lipid-lowering treatments.

➤ **Adjunct to diet to reduce LDL cholesterol, total cholesterol, apolipoprotein B, non-HDL cholesterol, and triglyceride**

R

(TG) levels and to increase HDL cholesterol level in patients with primary hypercholesterolemia (heterozygous familial and nonfamilial) and mixed dyslipidemia (Fredrickson types IIa and IIb); adjunct to diet to treat elevated TG level (Fredrickson type IV); adjunct to diet to treat primary dysbetalipoproteinemia

Adults: Initially, 10 mg P.O. once daily; 5 mg P.O. once daily in patients needing less aggressive LDL cholesterol reduction or those predisposed to myopathy. For aggressive lipid lowering when LDL is greater than 190 mg/dL, initially, 20 mg P.O. once daily. Increase as needed to maximum of 40 mg P.O. daily. Dosage may be titrated every 2 to 4 weeks, based on lipid levels.

➤ **Adjunct to diet to slow atherosclerosis progression in patients with elevated cholesterol**

Adults: Initially, 10 mg P.O. daily. Increase as needed every 2 to 4 weeks based on lipid levels, to maximum of 40 mg daily.

➤ **Adjunct to lipid-lowering therapies; to reduce LDL cholesterol, apolipoprotein B, and total cholesterol levels in homozygous familial hypercholesterolemia**

Adults: Initially, 20 mg P.O. once daily. Maximum, 40 mg once daily.

ADMINISTRATION
P.O.
● Give drug without regard for meals.
● Wait 2 hours after giving dose to give aluminum- or magnesium-containing antacid.

ACTION
Inhibits HMG-CoA reductase, increases LDL receptors on liver cells, and inhibits hepatic synthesis of very–low-density lipoprotein.

Route	Onset	Peak	Duration
P.O.	1 wk	3–5 hr	Unknown

Half-life: About 19 hours.

ADVERSE REACTIONS
CNS: asthenia, dizziness, headache, insomnia.
GI: abdominal pain, constipation, diarrhea, dyspepsia, nausea, vomiting.
GU: hematuria.

Hematologic: anemia, ecchymosis.
Metabolic: diabetes mellitus.
Musculoskeletal: arthralgia, myalgia, neck pain.
Skin: pruritus, rash.

INTERACTIONS
Drug-drug. *Antacids:* May decrease rosuvastatin level. Give antacids at least 2 hours after rosuvastatin.

Atazanavir, atazanavir–ritonavir, lopinavir–ritonavir, simeprevir: May increase rosuvastatin level and risk of myopathy and rhabdomyolysis. Rosuvastatin dosage shouldn't exceed 10 mg daily.

Bile acid sequestrants (cholestyramine, colestipol): May decrease GI absorption of rosuvastatin. Separate doses by at least 4 hours.

Colchicine: May increase risk of myopathy and rhabdomyolysis. Avoid use together. If use together is necessary, monitor patient for signs and symptoms of myopathy and elevated CK level during use and after dosage increases.

Cyclosporine: May increase rosuvastatin level and risk of myopathy or rhabdomyolysis. Don't exceed 5 mg of rosuvastatin daily. Watch for evidence of toxicity.

Daptomycin: May increase risk of rhabdomyolysis. Withhold rosuvastatin temporarily or monitor patient and CK level closely during coadministration.

Eltrombopag: May increase rosuvastatin level and risk of toxicity. Consider reducing rosuvastatin dosage.

Fenofibrate: May increase rosuvastatin level and risk of myopathy or rhabdomyolysis. Use together cautiously.

Gemfibrozil: May significantly increase rosuvastatin level and risk of myopathy or rhabdomyolysis. Avoid use together. If used together, don't exceed 10 mg/day of rosuvastatin.

Hormonal contraceptives: May increase ethinyl estradiol and norgestrel levels. Watch for adverse effects.

Niacin: May increase risk of myopathy or rhabdomyolysis. Decrease rosuvastatin dosage and monitor patient closely.

Warfarin: May increase INR and risk of bleeding. Monitor INR, and watch for evidence of increased bleeding.

Reactions in bold italics are *life-threatening*. Interactions may have a *rapid onset* or a ***delayed onset***.

Drug-lifestyle. *Alcohol use:* May increase risk of hepatotoxicity. Discourage use together.

EFFECTS ON LAB TEST RESULTS
● May increase HbA_{1c}, fasting blood sugar, CK, ALT, AST, glucose, glutamyl transpeptidase, alkaline phosphatase, and bilirubin levels.
● May cause thyroid function abnormalities, dipstick-positive proteinuria, and microscopic hematuria.

CONTRAINDICATIONS & CAUTIONS
● Contraindicated in patients hypersensitive to rosuvastatin or its components, patients with active liver disease, and those with unexplained persistently increased transaminase levels.
● Use cautiously in patients who drink substantial amounts of alcohol or have a history of liver disease and in those at increased risk for myopathies, such as those with renal impairment, advanced age, or hypothyroidism.
● Use cautiously in Asian patients because they have a greater risk of elevated drug levels.
● Rare postmarketing reports of cognitive impairment (memory loss, forgetfulness, amnesia, memory impairment, confusion) have been associated with statin use. These reported symptoms are generally not serious and are reversible upon statin discontinuation, with variable times to symptom onset (1 day to years) and symptom resolution (median of 3 weeks).
Dialyzable drug: No.
⚠ Overdose S&S: Unexplained muscle pain, tenderness, or weakness, especially with malaise or fever.

PREGNANCY-LACTATION-REPRODUCTION
● May cause fetal harm when given to pregnant women. Use during pregnancy is contraindicated. Discontinue drug before conception. If patient becomes pregnant during therapy, apprise her of potential fetal risks and the lack of known clinical benefit with continued use during pregnancy.
  Drug may appear in breast milk. Use while breast-feeding is contraindicated.

NURSING CONSIDERATIONS
● Before therapy starts, assess patient for underlying causes of hypercholesterolemia, including poorly controlled diabetes, hypothyroidism, nephrotic syndrome, dyslipoproteinemias, obstructive liver disease, drug interaction, and alcoholism.
● Before therapy starts, advise patient to control hypercholesterolemia with diet, exercise, and weight reduction.
● Interrupt statin therapy if patient shows signs or symptoms of serious liver injury, hyperbilirubinemia, or jaundice. Don't restart drug if another cause can't be found.
● Monitor LFTs at baseline and with any indication of hepatotoxicity.
⊙ Alert: Rarely, rhabdomyolysis with acute renal failure has developed in patients taking drugs in this class, including rosuvastatin.
● Monitor lipid panel at baseline and a fasting lipid profile within 4 to 12 weeks after initiation or dosage adjustment and every 3 to 12 months thereafter.
● Patients who are age 65 or older, have hypothyroidism, or have renal insufficiency may be at a greater risk for developing myopathy while receiving a statin.
● Notify prescriber if CK level becomes markedly elevated or myopathy is suspected, or if routine urinalysis shows persistent proteinuria and patient is taking 40 mg daily.
● Withhold drug temporarily if patient becomes predisposed to myopathy or rhabdomyolysis because of sepsis, hypotension, major surgery, trauma, uncontrolled seizures, or severe metabolic, endocrine, or electrolyte disorders.

PATIENT TEACHING
● Instruct patient to take drug exactly as prescribed.
● Teach patient about diet, exercise, and weight control.
● Inform patient that rare instances of memory loss and confusion have occurred with statin use. These reported events were generally not serious and resolved when drug was discontinued.
● Tell patient that drug may increase blood sugar level but that the CV benefits are thought to outweigh the slight increase in risk.

R

• Tell patient to immediately report unexplained muscle pain, tenderness, or weakness (especially if accompanied by malaise or fever) and loss of appetite, upper abdominal pain, dark-colored urine, or yellowing of skin or eyes.

• Instruct patient to take drug at least 2 hours before taking aluminum- or magnesium-containing antacids.

◑ **Alert:** Tell female patient to stop drug and notify prescriber immediately if she is or may be pregnant or if she's breast-feeding.

SAFETY ALERT!

ruxolitinib phosphate
RUX-oh-LI-ti-nib

Jakafi

Therapeutic class: Antineoplastics
Pharmacologic class: Janus-associated kinase inhibitors

AVAILABLE FORMS
Tablets: 5 mg, 10 mg, 15 mg, 20 mg, 25 mg

INDICATIONS & DOSAGES
➤ **Treatment of patients with intermediate or high-risk myelofibrosis, including primary myelofibrosis, post–polycythemia vera myelofibrosis, and post–essential thrombocythemia myelofibrosis**
Adults: Initially, 20 mg P.O. b.i.d. if platelet count is greater than 200×10^9/L, 15 mg P.O. b.i.d. if platelet count is 100 to 200 $\times$ 10^9/L, or 5 mg P.O. b.i.d. if platelet count is 50 to less than 100×10^9/L. May increase in 5-mg increments b.i.d. to a maximum of 25 mg b.i.d. Don't increase during the first 4 weeks of therapy and not more frequently than every 2 weeks. Consider dosage increases in patients who meet all of the following conditions: failure to achieve either a 50% reduction from pretreatment baseline in palpable spleen length or a 35% reduction in spleen volume as measured by CT scan or MRI; platelet count greater than 125×10^9/L at 4 weeks and never below 100×10^9/L; and ANC greater than 0.75 $\times$ 10^9/L. Long-term maintenance at a 5-mg b.i.d. dosage hasn't shown response; limit

continued use at this dosage to patients in whom benefits outweigh risks. Discontinue drug after 6 months if there is no spleen reduction or symptom improvement. If drug needs to be stopped for any reason except thrombocytopenia, taper gradually by 5 mg b.i.d. each week.

Adjust-a-dose: To avoid thrombocytopenia, reduce dosage if platelet count begins to fall. If platelet count is 100 to less than 125×10^9/L and current dosage is 25 mg b.i.d., decrease to 20 mg b.i.d.; if current dosage is 20 mg b.i.d., decrease to 15 mg b.i.d. If platelet count is 75 to less than 100×10^9/L and current dosage is 15 to 25 mg b.i.d., decrease to 10 mg b.i.d. If platelet count is 50 to less than 75×10^9/L and current dosage is 10 to 25 mg b.i.d., decrease to 5 mg b.i.d. If platelet count is less than 50×10^9/L, withhold drug. When platelet count begins to recover, refer to manufacturer's dosing instructions to restart drug.

For moderate to severe renal impairment (CrCl of 15 to 59 mL/minute) and platelet count between 100 and 150×10^9/L, initial dose is 10 mg b.i.d. For patients with ESRD on dialysis and with platelet count between 100 and 200×10^9/L, initial dose is 15 mg once after dialysis. For patients with ESRD on dialysis and with platelet count greater than 200×10^9/L, initial dose is 20 mg once after dialysis. Give subsequent doses on dialysis days after each dialysis session. Avoid use in patients with ESRD not requiring dialysis.

For patients with hepatic impairment and platelet count between 100 and 150 $\times$ 10^9/L, initial dose is 10 mg b.i.d.

Modify dosage when giving concomitantly with strong CYP3A4 inhibitors and fluconazole. Avoid use with fluconazole doses greater than 200 mg daily.

➤ **Polycythemia vera in patients with an inadequate response to or who are intolerant of hydroxyurea**
Adults: Initially, 10 mg P.O. b.i.d. If response is inadequate and platelet count is 140×10^9 or greater, Hb level is 12 g/dL or greater, and ANC is 1.5×10^9/L or greater, may increase dose by 5 mg b.i.d. to a maximum of 25 mg b.i.d. (Maximum is 50 mg/day.) Doses shouldn't be increased

---

Reactions in bold italics are *life-threatening*. Interactions may have a *rapid onset* or a ***delayed onset***.

during first 4 weeks of therapy and not more frequently than every 2 weeks. Inadequate response is defined as one of the following: continued need for phlebotomy, WBC count higher than ULN, platelet count greater than ULN, or palpable spleen that's reduced by less than 25% from baseline.

Adjust-a-dose: Consider dosage reduction if Hb level and platelet count decrease. If Hb level is 12 g/dL or greater AND platelet count is 100×10^9/L or more, no dosage change is required. If Hb level is 10 to less than 12 g/dL AND platelet count is 75 to less than 100×10^9/L, consider dosage reduction with the goal of avoiding dose interruptions for anemia and thrombocytopenia. If Hb level is 8 to less than 10 g/dL OR platelet count is 50 to less than 75 $\times$ 10^9/L, reduce dosage by 5 mg b.i.d. For patients on 5 mg b.i.d., decrease dosage to 5 mg once daily. If Hb level is less than 8 g/dL OR platelet count is less than 50 $\times$ 10^9/L, interrupt dosing. Refer to manufacturer's instructions for restarting drug after interruption for hematologic conditions.

Modify dosage when giving concomitantly with strong CYP3A4 inhibitors and fluconazole. Avoid use with fluconazole doses greater than 200 mg daily.

Recommended starting dose in patients with ESRD on dialysis is 10 mg. Avoid use in those with ESRD not requiring dialysis.

Recommended starting dose in patients with any degree of hepatic impairment is 5 mg b.i.d.

ADMINISTRATION
P.O.
● May give without regard to food.
● To give through an NG tube (8 French or greater), place one tablet in approximately 40 mL water and stir for 10 minutes to dissolve. Give within 6 hours of preparing the suspension, using an appropriate syringe. Rinse NG tube with 75 mL water.

Drug is a hazardous agent; use safe handling precautions.

ACTION
Inhibits signaling of cytokines and growth factors important for hematopoiesis and immune functions. Prevents splenomegaly

by decreasing circulating inflammatory cytokines.

Route	Onset	Peak	Duration
P.O.	Rapid	1–2 hr	10 hr

Half-life: 3 hours.

ADVERSE REACTIONS
CNS: dizziness, headache, insomnia.
EENT: nasopharyngitis, epistaxis.
GI: flatulence, abdominal pain, diarrhea, constipation.
GU: UTI.
Hematologic: *neutropenia, thrombocytopenia,* anemia.
Hepatic: increased AST/ALT levels.
Metabolic: hypercholesterolemia, hypertriglyceridemia, weight gain.
Musculoskeletal: muscle spasm, weakness.
Respiratory: dyspnea, cough.
Skin: bruising, pruritus.
Other: serious bacterial, mycobacterial, fungal, or viral infections.

INTERACTIONS
Drug-drug. *CYP3A4 inducers (rifampin):* May decrease ruxolitinib level. No initial dosage adjustment is necessary. Monitor patients closely and titrate dosage if necessary.
Fluconazole (doses of 200 mg or less): May increase ruxolitinib level. Avoid using fluconazole doses greater than 200 mg daily concomitantly with ruxolitinib. If patient with myelofibrosis is taking fluconazole 200 mg or less daily and platelet count is 100×10^9/L or more, start ruxolitinib at 10 mg b.i.d. If patient is taking fluconazole 200 mg or less daily and platelet count is 50 to less than 100×10^9/L, start ruxolitinib at 5 mg once daily. If patient is taking fluconazole 200 mg or less daily and is on stable ruxolitinib dose of 10 mg or more b.i.d., reduce ruxolitinib dosage by 50% (rounded up to closest available tablet strength). If patient is taking fluconazole 200 mg or less and is on stable ruxolitinib dose of 5 mg b.i.d., reduce ruxolitinib dosage to 5 mg once daily. If patient is on stable ruxolitinib dose of 5 mg once daily, avoid use of fluconazole or interrupt ruxolitinib treatment for duration of fluconazole use. For concomitant administration during

R

polycythemia vera treatment, decrease ruxolitinib dose by 50%; if dose is 5 mg daily, avoid concomitant administration. Make additional dosage modifications with careful monitoring of safety and effectiveness.

Strong CYP3A4 inhibitors (clarithromycin, conivaptan, indinavir, itraconazole, ketoconazole, lopinavir–ritonavir, mibefradil, nefazodone, nelfinavir, posaconazole, ritonavir, saquinavir, telithromycin, voriconazole): May increase ruxolitinib level. If patient with myelofibrosis is taking a strong CYP3A4 inhibitor and platelet count is 100×10^9/L or more, start ruxolitinib at 10 mg b.i.d. If patient is taking a strong CYP3A4 inhibitor and platelet count is 50 to less than 100×10^9/L, start ruxolitinib at 5 mg once daily. If patient is taking a strong CYP3A4 inhibitor and is on stable ruxolitinib dose of 10 mg or more b.i.d., reduce ruxolitinib dosage by 50% (rounded up to closest available tablet strength). If patient is taking a strong CYP3A4 inhibitor and is on stable ruxolitinib dose of 5 mg b.i.d., reduce ruxolitinib dosage to 5 mg once daily. If patient is on stable ruxolitinib dose of 5 mg once daily, avoid use of strong CYP3A4 inhibitor or interrupt ruxolitinib treatment for duration of strong CYP3A4 inhibitor use. For concomitant administration during polycythemia vera treatment, decrease ruxolitinib dose by 50%; if dose is 5 mg daily, avoid concomitant administration. Make additional dosage modifications with careful monitoring of safety and effectiveness.

Drug-food. *Grapefruit juice:* May increase ruxolitinib level. Don't use together.

EFFECTS ON LAB TEST RESULTS
• May increase total cholesterol, LDL cholesterol, triglyceride, AST, and ALT levels.
• May decrease platelet and neutrophil counts.
• May decrease Hb level.

CONTRAINDICATIONS & CAUTIONS
• Contraindicated in patients hypersensitive to drug and in those with ESRD not requiring dialysis, moderate to severe renal failure and platelet count less than 100×10^9/L, or

hepatic impairment with platelet count less than 100×10^9/L.
• Use cautiously in patients with thrombocytopenia, anemia, or neutropenia.
• Serious bacterial, mycobacterial (including TB), fungal, or viral infections (such as herpes zoster) have occurred. Evaluate patient for TB before treatment. Serious infections should be resolved before start of treatment. Progressive multifocal leukoencephalopathy (PML) has been reported; discontinue drug and evaluate patient if suspected.
• Myelofibrosis signs and symptoms commonly return to pretreatment levels about 1 week after ruxolitinib is discontinued, with some patients experiencing one or more adverse effects, including fever, respiratory distress, hypotension, DIC, and multiorgan failure. Evaluate and treat any illness, and consider restarting or increasing dosage of ruxolitinib.
• Drug may increase risk of nonmelanoma skin cancer.
Dialyzable drug: Unlikely.

PREGNANCY-LACTATION-REPRODUCTION
• There are no adequate studies in pregnant women. Use during pregnancy only if potential benefit justifies potential risk to the fetus.
• It isn't known if drug appears in breast milk. Patient should discontinue breastfeeding or discontinue drug.

NURSING CONSIDERATIONS
• Obtain platelet, RBC, and WBC counts before starting drug, every 2 to 4 weeks until dosage is stabilized, then as needed.
• Resolve active infections before starting therapy.
• Blood transfusions may be necessary to manage anemia.
• Monitor patient for signs and symptoms of serious bacterial, mycobacterial, fungal, or viral infections (such as herpes zoster) during therapy; begin treatment for infection, if necessary, as soon as possible.
• Monitor patient for skin cancer.
• Monitor lipid levels 8 to 12 weeks after start of therapy and treat according to clinical guidelines for management of hyperlipidemia.

• To discontinue drug, consider tapering dosage gradually rather than stopping drug abruptly unless drug is being discontinued because of thrombocytopenia or neutropenia.

PATIENT TEACHING

• Inform patient that drug must be taken daily and not to change dosage or stop drug without consulting prescriber. Myelofibrosis and related signs and symptoms will return if drug is discontinued.
• Instruct patient not to drink grapefruit juice.
• Instruct patient that if a dose is missed, not to take an additional dose but to take the next usual prescribed dose.
• Inform patient on dialysis to not take a dose before dialysis, but to wait and take it after dialysis.
• Inform patient that blood tests will be needed to monitor for adverse effects and possible dosage adjustment.
• Inform patient of increased risk of infection. Advise patient to immediately report signs and symptoms of illness (fever, cough, malaise, skin eruptions).
• Tell patient that drug can cause low blood cell counts and to report bleeding, bruising, fatigue, or shortness of breath.
• Warn patient that skin cancers have occurred in those taking drug and to report new or changing skin lesions.

sacubitril–valsartan
sak-UE-bi-tril/val-SAR-tan

Entresto

Therapeutic class: Antihypertensives
Pharmacologic class: Neprilysin inhibitors–ARBs

AVAILABLE FORMS
Tablets: 24 mg sacubitril/26 mg valsartan, 49 mg sacubitril/51 mg valsartan, 97 mg sacubitril/103 mg valsartan

INDICATIONS & DOSAGES
➤ **To reduce risk of CV death and hospitalization for HF in patients with chronic HF (New York Heart Association class II to IV) and reduced ejection fraction, usually in conjunction with other HF therapies, in place of an ACE inhibitor or other ARB**
Adults: Initially, 49 mg sacubitril/51 mg valsartan P.O. b.i.d. Increase after 2 to 4 weeks to target maintenance dose of 97 mg sacubitril/103 mg valsartan, as tolerated.
Adjust-a-dose: In patients not currently taking an ACE inhibitor or ARB or previously taking a low dose of these agents and in patients with severe renal impairment (estimated GFR less than 30 mL/minute/1.73 m^2) or moderate hepatic impairment (Child-Pugh class B), reduce starting dose to 24 mg sacubitril/26 mg valsartan b.i.d. Double the dose every 2 to 4 weeks to target maintenance dose of 97 mg sacubitril/103 mg valsartan, as tolerated.

ADMINISTRATION
P.O.
• If patient is switching to or from an ACE inhibitor, allow a washout period of 36 hours between giving the two drugs.
• May give with or without food.
• Store at room temperature; protect tablets from moisture.
• If a dose is missed, give as soon as possible on the same day, then resume twice-daily dosing. If missed dose is close to the scheduled next dose, omit it.

ACTION
Inhibits neprilysin and angiotensin II, enhancing the protective neurohormonal systems of the heart (naturetic peptide system) while suppressing the harmful RAAS.

Route	Onset	Peak	Duration
P.O.	Unknown	½–2 hr	Unknown

Half-life: Sacubitril, 1.4 hours; valsartan, 9.9 hours.

ADVERSE REACTIONS
CNS: dizziness.
CV: *hypotension.*
GU: *renal failure.*
Hematologic: anemia.
Metabolic: *hyperkalemia.*
Respiratory: cough.
Other: *angioedema (black patients),* falls.

S

INTERACTIONS
Drug-drug. *ACE inhibitors:* May increase risk of angioedema. Use together is contraindicated. Don't give sacubitril–valsartan within 36 hours of switching from or to an ACE inhibitor.
Aliskiren: May increase risk of renal failure. Contraindicated for use together in patients with diabetes. Avoid use in patients with renal impairment (GFR less than 60 mL/minute/1.73 m^2).
ARBs: Will cause dual blockade of the RAAS. Avoid concurrent use as product contains valsartan.
Cyclooxygenase-2 inhibitors, NSAIDs: May increase risk of renal failure, especially in patients who are elderly, volume-depleted, or with prior impaired renal function. Monitor renal function closely.
Lithium: May increase lithium level and risk of lithium toxicity. Monitor serum lithium level.
Potassium-sparing diuretics (amiloride, spironolactone, triamterene), potassium supplements: May increase serum potassium level. Use cautiously and monitor patient closely.

EFFECTS ON LAB TEST RESULTS
● May increase serum creatinine, urea, and potassium levels.
● May decrease Hb level and hematocrit.

CONTRAINDICATIONS & CAUTIONS
● Contraindicated in patients hypersensitive to either drug or its components, in patients with a history of angioedema related to previous ACE or ARB therapy, in patients currently receiving ACE inhibitors or within 36 hours of using an ACE inhibitor, and in patients with diabetes who are using aliskiren.
● Use in patients with severe hepatic impairment (Child-Pugh class C) isn't recommended.
◔ *Alert:* Drug may cause angioedema requiring emergency treatment and which can be fatal. Risk is greater in black than in non-black patients.
● Drug lowers BP and may cause symptomatic hypotension.
● ACE inhibitors and ARBs have been associated with oliguria, progressive azotemia,

acute renal failure, and death. Monitor patient closely.
● Safety and effectiveness in children haven't been established.
Dialyzable drug: Unlikely.
⚠ *Overdose S&S:* Hypotension.

PREGNANCY-LACTATION-REPRODUCTION
Black Box Warning Use during pregnancy can cause injury and death to the developing fetus. Stop drug as soon as pregnancy is detected. ■
● Use during pregnancy only if there is no appropriate alternative therapy and if drug is considered lifesaving for the mother. Advise pregnant women of potential risk to the fetus.
● It isn't known if drug appears in breast milk. Because of the potential for serious reactions in breast-fed infants, breast-feeding isn't recommended during therapy.

NURSING CONSIDERATIONS
● Drug is usually given with other HF therapies, in place of an ACE inhibitor or other ARB.
● Don't give with or within 36 hours of an ACE inhibitor.
● To help prevent hypotension, correct volume- or salt-depletion before start of therapy.
● Monitor patients for hypotension. Patients who are volume- or salt-depleted, such as those on high-dose diuretics, may be at increased risk. Consider dosage adjustment of diuretics and concomitant antihypertensives and treat other cause of hypotension such as hypovolemia. Reduce dosage or temporarily discontinue sacubitril–valsartan for persistent hypotension.
● Monitor patients for angioedema (swelling of the face, tongue, throat, and lips; airway compromise; dyspnea). Discontinue drug and treat emergently.
● Monitor renal function and reduce dosage or temporarily interrupt therapy in patients who develop clinically significant decreased renal function.
● Monitor serum potassium level periodically and treat appropriately. Patients with severe renal impairment, diabetes, hypoaldosteronism, or a high-potassium diet may be at increased risk for hyperkalemia.

Reduce dosage or interrupt therapy as clinically indicated.

PATIENT TEACHING
• Explain to patient that drug is usually used with other HF therapies, in place of an ACE inhibitor or other ARB therapy.
• Advise patient to report all adverse reactions, especially signs and symptoms of an allergic reaction (swelling of the face, lips, or tongue or trouble breathing).
• Instruct patient to take drug exactly as prescribed and not to take within 36 hours of an ACE inhibitor.
• Tell female patient to notify prescriber if she becomes pregnant. Drug will need to be stopped. Caution patient not to breast-feed during therapy.
• Caution patient to contact prescriber if dizziness, light-headedness, or extreme fatigue occurs.
• Inform patient that blood tests will be needed to monitor drug's effects.

---

salmeterol xinafoate
sal-MEE-ter-ol

Serevent Diskus

Therapeutic class: Bronchodilators
Pharmacologic class: Long-acting selective beta$_2$ agonists

AVAILABLE FORMS
Inhalation powder: 50 mcg/blister

INDICATIONS & DOSAGES
➤ **Long-term maintenance of asthma; to prevent bronchospasm in patients with nocturnal asthma or reversible obstructive airway disease as concomitant therapy with a long-term asthma control medication such as an inhaled corticosteroid**
Adults and children age 4 and older:
1 inhalation (50 mcg) b.i.d. in the morning and evening, about 12 hours apart.
➤ **To prevent exercise-induced bronchospasm**
Adults and children age 4 and older:
1 inhalation (50 mcg) at least 30 minutes before exercise. Additional doses shouldn't be taken for at least 12 hours.
➤ **COPD, emphysema, or chronic bronchitis**
Adults: 1 inhalation (50 mcg) b.i.d. in the morning and evening, about 12 hours apart.

ADMINISTRATION
Inhalational
• Give drug 30 to 60 minutes before exercise to prevent exercise-induced bronchospasm.
• Don't use a spacer device with this drug.

ACTION
Unclear. Selectively activates beta$_2$ receptors, which results in bronchodilation; also, blocks the release of allergic mediators from mast cells lining the respiratory tract.

Route	Onset	Peak	Duration
Inhalation	30–120 min	2–5 hr	12 hr

Half-life: 5½ hours.

ADVERSE REACTIONS
CNS: anxiety, headache, dizziness, tremor, nervousness, paresthesia, sleep disturbance, fever.
CV: tachycardia, palpitations.
EENT: conjunctivitis, keratitis, nasopharyngitis, pharyngitis, hoarseness, nasal cavity or sinus disorder, candidiasis of mouth/throat, hyposalivation.
GI: nausea, vomiting, diarrhea, heartburn.
Musculoskeletal: joint and back pain, myalgia.
Respiratory: URI, cough, lower respiratory tract infection.
Other: hypersensitivity reactions, rash, urticaria, flulike symptoms, photodermatitis.

INTERACTIONS
Drug-drug. *Antiarrhythmics (amiodarone, disopyramide, sotalol), chlorpromazine, dolasetron, droperidol, moxifloxacin, pentamidine, pimozide, tacrolimus, thioridazine, ziprasidone:* May prolong QT interval and increase risk of life-threatening cardiac arrhythmias. Monitor QT interval closely.
Beta agonists, other methylxanthines, theophylline: May cause adverse cardiac effects with excessive use. Monitor patient.

S

CYP3A4 inhibitors (atazanavir, clar-ithromycin, itraconazole, ketoconazole, ritonavir): May increase cardiac effects. Avoid use together.

Diuretics (non-potassium-sparing): May worsen hypokalemia and ECG changes. Use cautiously together.

MAO inhibitors: May cause risk of severe adverse CV effects. Avoid use within 14 days of MAO inhibitor therapy.

TCAs: May cause risk of moderate to severe adverse CV effects. Avoid use together within 14 days.

EFFECTS ON LAB TEST RESULTS
None reported.

CONTRAINDICATIONS & CAUTIONS
• Contraindicated in patients hypersensitive to drug or its ingredients.

Black Box Warning Contraindicated for treatment of asthma without a concomitant long-term asthma control medication such as an inhaled corticosteroid. ∎

🔾 *Alert:* Don't use drug with other medications containing long-acting beta$_2$ agonists.

• Use cautiously in patients unusually responsive to sympathomimetics and those with coronary insufficiency, arrhythmias, hypertension, other CV disorders, thyrotoxicosis, hepatic impairment, or seizure disorders.

Dialyzable drug: Unknown.

⚠ *Overdose S&S:* Exaggeration of adverse reactions, hypokalemia, seizures, angina, hypertension, hypotension, dry mouth, muscle cramps, dizziness, fatigue, insomnia, tachycardia, ventricular arrhythmias, cardiac arrest, sudden death.

PREGNANCY-LACTATION-REPRODUCTION
• There are no adequate studies in pregnant women, but drug may be teratogenic. Use during pregnancy only if potential benefit justifies potential risk to the fetus.

• It isn't known if drug appears in breast milk. Use cautiously in breast-feeding women.

NURSING CONSIDERATIONS
Black Box Warning Drug may increase the risk of asthma-related death. Only use salmeterol as additional therapy for pa-

tients whose condition is not adequately controlled on other medications or patients whose disease severity warrants initiation of treatment with two maintenance therapies. ∎

Black Box Warning Once asthma control is achieved and maintained, assess patient at regular intervals; step down therapy (e.g., discontinue salmeterol) if possible without loss of asthma control and maintain patient on a long-term asthma control medication such as an inhaled corticosteroid. Don't use salmeterol for patients whose asthma is adequately controlled on low- or medium-dose inhaled corticosteroids. ∎

Black Box Warning Long-acting beta$_2$-adrenergic agonists may increase risk of asthma-related hospitalization in children and adolescents. For children and adolescents with asthma who require addition of a long-acting beta$_2$-adrenergic agonist to an inhaled corticosteroid, a fixed-dose combination product containing both an inhaled corticosteroid and a long-acting beta$_2$-adrenergic agonist should ordinarily be used to ensure adherence with both drugs. In cases in which use of a separate long-term asthma-control medication (such as an inhaled corticosteroid) and a long-acting beta$_2$-adrenergic agonist is clinically indicated, appropriate steps must be taken to ensure adherence with both treatment components. If adherence can't be ensured, a fixed-dose combination product containing both an inhaled corticosteroid and a long-acting beta$_2$-adrenergic agonist is recommended. ∎

• Drug isn't indicated for acute bronchospasm.

🔾 *Alert:* Monitor patient for rash and urticaria, which may signal a hypersensitivity reaction.

• Rarely, potentially life-threatening paradoxical bronchospasm can occur. Distinguish this symptom from inadequate response.

PATIENT TEACHING
Black Box Warning Teach parents of child or adolescent who requires the use of a separate long-term asthma-control medication (such as an inhaled corticosteroid) and a long-acting beta$_2$-adrenergic agonist that appropriate steps must be taken to ensure

adherence with both treatment components. If adherence can't be ensured, a fixed-dose combination product containing both an inhaled corticosteroid and a long-acting beta$_2$-adrenergic agonist is recommended. ∎

• Remind patient to take drug at about 12-hour intervals for optimal effect and to take drug even when feeling better.

• If patient is taking drug to prevent exercise-induced bronchospasm, tell patient to take it 30 to 60 minutes before exercise.

◐ *Alert:* Tell patient drug shouldn't be used to treat acute bronchospasm. Patient must use a short-acting beta$_2$ agonist, such as albuterol, to treat worsening symptoms.

◐ *Alert:* Rare serious asthma episodes or asthma-related deaths may occur in patients using salmeterol. Black patients may be at greater risk.

• Tell patient to contact prescriber if the short-acting agonist no longer provides sufficient relief or if patient needs more than 4 inhalations daily. This may be a sign that the asthma symptoms are worsening. Tell patient not to increase the dosage of salmeterol.

• If patient takes an inhaled corticosteroid, patient should continue to use it regularly. Warn patient not to take other drugs without prescriber's consent.

• If patient takes the inhalation powder (in a multidose inhaler), instruct patient not to exhale into the device. Patient should activate and use it only in a level, horizontal position.

• Tell patient not to use dry-powder multi-dose inhaler with a spacer.

• Instruct patient never to wash mouthpiece or any part of dry-powder multidose inhaler; it must be kept dry.

• Advise female patient to contact physician if she becomes pregnant during therapy.

SAFETY ALERT!

sargramostim (GM-CSF; granulocyte-macrophage colony-stimulating factor)
sar-GRAM-oh-stim

Leukine

Therapeutic class: Hematopoietics
Pharmacologic class: Colony-stimulating factors

AVAILABLE FORMS
Powder for injection: 250 mcg
Solution for injection: 500 mcg/mL*

INDICATIONS & DOSAGES
➤ **To accelerate hematopoietic reconstitution after autologous or allogeneic bone marrow transplantation in patients with malignant lymphoma or acute lymphoblastic leukemia or in patients with Hodgkin lymphoma**
Adults: 250 mcg/m^2 daily given as 2-hour I.V. infusion beginning 2 to 4 hours after bone marrow transplantation and not less than 24 hours after last dose of chemotherapy or radiotherapy. Don't give until post–marrow infusion ANC is less than 500 cells/mm^3. Continue until ANC is more than 1,500/mm^3 for 3 consecutive days.
Adjust-a-dose: Discontinue immediately if blast cells appear or disease progression occurs. Temporarily discontinue or reduce dosage by 50% if a severe adverse reaction occurs. Interrupt therapy or reduce dosage by 50% if ANC exceeds 20,000 cells/mm^3.
➤ **Neutrophil recovery following chemotherapy in acute myelogenous leukemia**
Adults age 55 and older: Initially, 250 mcg/m^2 I.V. once daily over 4 hours beginning day 11 or 4 days after completion of induction therapy; initiate only if bone marrow is hypoplastic with less than 5% blasts on day 10. If a second induction cycle is needed, begin sargramostim 4 days after completing chemotherapy and only if bone marrow is hypoplastic with less than 5% blasts. Continue until the ANC is more than 1,500/mm^3 for 3 consecutive days or for a maximum of 42 days.

S

Adjust-a-dose: Discontinue immediately if leukemic regrowth occurs. Reduce dosage by 50% or temporarily discontinue if a severe adverse reaction occurs. Interrupt therapy or reduce dosage by 50% if ANC exceeds 20,000 cells/mm³.

➤ **Mobilization of peripheral blood progenitor cells (PBPCs)**
Adults: 250 mcg/m² by continuous I.V. infusion over 24 hours or by subcutaneous injection once daily. Continue through PBPC collection.
Adjust-a-dose: If WBC count is more than 50,000/mm³, reduce dosage by 50%. If adequate numbers of cells aren't collected, consider other mobilization therapy.

➤ **Post-PBPC transplantation**
Adults: 250 mcg/m² by continuous I.V. infusion over 24 hours or by subcutaneous injection once daily beginning immediately after PBPC infusion; continue until ANC is more than 1,500/mm³ for 3 consecutive days.

➤ **Bone marrow transplantation failure or engraftment delay**
Adults: 250 mcg/m² as a 2-hour I.V. infusion daily for 14 days. This course of therapy may be repeated after 7 days of no therapy. If engraftment still hasn't occurred, a third course of 500 mcg/m² daily I.V. for 14 days may be attempted after another therapy-free 7 days.
Adjust-a-dose: Stimulation of marrow precursors may result in rapid rise of WBC count. If blast cells appear or increase to 10% or more of WBC count or if the underlying disease progresses, stop therapy. If ANC is above 20,000/mm³ or if platelet count is above 500,000/mm³, temporarily stop drug or reduce dose by 50%.

ADMINISTRATION
I.V.
▼ Reconstitute powder for injection with 1 mL of sterile or bacteriostatic water for injection. Direct stream of sterile water against side of vial and gently swirl contents to minimize foaming. Avoid excessive or vigorous agitation or shaking.
▼ Dilute in NSS. If drug yield is below 10 mcg/mL, add human albumin at final concentration of 0.1% to NSS before adding sargramostim to prevent adsorption to components of the delivery system. To yield 0.1% human albumin, add 1 mg human albumin to each milliliter of NSS (dilute 1 mL of 5% human albumin in 50 mL of NSS).
▼ Don't use in-line filter.
▼ Give as soon as possible after mixing and no later than 6 hours after reconstituting.
▼ **Incompatibilities:** Other I.V. drugs, unless specific compatibility data are available.
Subcutaneous
● Further dilution of injection or reconstituted solution isn't needed.

ACTION
Induces cellular responses by binding to specific receptors on surfaces of target cells.

Route	Onset	Peak	Duration
I.V.	15 min	1–3 hr	Unknown
Subcut.	15 min	1–3 hr	Unknown

Half-life: I.V., about 1 hour; subcutaneous, about 3 hours.

ADVERSE REACTIONS
CNS: asthenia, CNS disorders, fever, headache, malaise.
CV: *hemorrhage,* edema, peripheral edema, hypertension, supraventricular arrhythmias, pericardial effusion.
GI: anorexia, diarrhea, GI disorders, nausea, stomatitis, vomiting, *GI hemorrhage.*
GU: urinary tract disorder, abnormal kidney function.
Hematologic: blood dyscrasias.
Hepatic: liver damage, bilirubinemia.
Musculoskeletal: arthralgias.
Respiratory: dyspnea, lung disorders, pleural effusion.
Skin: alopecia, pruritus, rash.
Other: *sepsis,* mucous membrane disorder, chills.

INTERACTIONS
Drug-drug. *Corticosteroids, lithium:* May increase myeloproliferative effects of sargramostim. Use cautiously together.

EFFECTS ON LAB TEST RESULTS
● May increase BUN, creatinine, AST, ALT, alkaline phosphatase, bilirubin, glucose, and cholesterol levels.
● May decrease calcium and albumin levels.

CONTRAINDICATIONS & CAUTIONS
● Contraindicated in patients hypersensitive to drug or its components or to yeast-derived products and in those with excessive leukemic myeloid blasts in bone marrow or peripheral blood.
● Giving within 24 hours of chemotherapy or radiation is contraindicated.
● Use cautiously in patients with cardiac disease, hypoxia, fluid retention, pulmonary infiltrates, HF, or impaired renal or hepatic function because these conditions may be worsened.
● Drug may interfere with bone imaging studies; increased hematopoietic activity of the bone marrow may appear as transient positive bone imaging changes.
● Safety and effectiveness haven't been established in children.
Dialyzable drug: Unknown.
⚠ Overdose S&S: Dyspnea, malaise, nausea, fever, rash, sinus tachycardia, headache, chills.

PREGNANCY-LACTATION-REPRODUCTION
● There are no adequate studies in pregnant women. Use during pregnancy only if clearly needed.
● It isn't known if drug appears in breast milk. Use in breast-feeding women only if clearly needed.

NURSING CONSIDERATIONS
● If severe adverse reactions occur, reduce dose by 50% or temporarily stop drug and notify prescriber. Resume therapy when reactions decrease. Transient rash and local reactions at injection site may occur.
● Solution for injection contains benzyl alcohol, which has been associated with fatal "gasping syndrome" in neonates. Don't administer to neonates.
● Rapidly dividing progenitor cells may be sensitive to cytotoxic therapies, making the drug ineffective; don't give within 24 hours of last dose of chemotherapy or radiotherapy.

● Monitor CBC with differential, including examination for presence of blast cells, biweekly.
● Drug accelerates myeloid recovery in patients receiving bone marrow that is either unpurged or purged by anti-B cell monoclonal antibodies more than in those who receive bone marrow that is chemically purged.
● Drug may produce a limited response in transplant patients who have received extensive radiotherapy or who have received other myelotoxic drugs.
● Drug can act as a growth factor for any tumor type, particularly myeloid malignant disease.

PATIENT TEACHING
● Review administration schedule with patient and caregivers, and address their concerns.
● Urge patient to report adverse reactions promptly.

SAFETY ALERT!

saxagliptin
sax-ah-GLIP-ten

Onglyza⌀

Therapeutic class: Antidiabetics
Pharmacologic class: DPP-4 enzyme inhibitors

AVAILABLE FORMS
Tablets: 2.5 mg, 5 mg

INDICATIONS & DOSAGES
➤ **Adjunct to diet and exercise to improve glycemic control in type 2 diabetes**
Adults: 2.5 or 5 mg P.O. once daily.
Adjust-a-dose: For patient with CrCl of 50 mL/minute or less, give 2.5 mg P.O. once daily; if patient requires hemodialysis, give 2.5 mg once daily after treatment.

ADMINISTRATION
P.O.
● Give drug with or without food.
● Don't split or cut tablets.

S

ACTION

Inhibits DPP-4, an enzyme that rapidly inactivates incretin hormones, which play a part in the body's regulation of glucose. By increasing active incretin levels, drug helps to increase insulin release and decrease circulating glucose.

Route	Onset	Peak	Duration
P.O.	Unknown	2 hr	24 hr

Half-life: 2½ hours.

ADVERSE REACTIONS

CNS: headache.
CV: facial edema, peripheral edema.
EENT: sinusitis.
GI: abdominal pain, gastroenteritis, vomiting.
GU: UTI.
Metabolic: *hypoglycemia.*
Respiratory: URI.
Skin: urticaria.

INTERACTIONS

Drug-drug. *Strong CYP3A4/5 inhibitors (atazanavir, clarithromycin, indinavir, itraconazole, ketoconazole, nefazodone, nelfinavir, ritonavir, saquinavir, telithromycin):* May increase saxagliptin level. Reduce dosage to 2.5 mg P.O. daily.

EFFECTS ON LAB TEST RESULTS

● May decrease lymphocyte count.

CONTRAINDICATIONS & CAUTIONS

● Contraindicated in patients hypersensitive to drug or its components.
● Hypersensitivity reactions, including anaphylaxis, angioedema, and exfoliative skin conditions, have occurred within first 3 months of therapy. Discontinue drug if hypersensitivity is suspected.
● **Alert:** Use cautiously in patients with a history of HF or renal disease. Drug may increase risk of HF in these patients.
● Use cautiously in patients taking secretagogues (such as sulfonylureas) because of increased risk of hypoglycemia.
● Discontinue drug if pancreatitis is suspected.
● Drug isn't indicated to treat type 1 diabetes or diabetic ketoacidosis.

● Safety and effectiveness in children haven't been established.
Dialyzable drug: 23%.

PREGNANCY-LACTATION-REPRODUCTION

● There are no adequate studies in pregnant women. Use during pregnancy only if clearly needed.
● It isn't known if drug appears in breast milk. Use cautiously in breast-feeding women.

NURSING CONSIDERATIONS

● **Alert:** Drug may cause joint pain that can be severe and disabling. Report severe and persistent joint pain to prescriber as drug may need to be discontinued.
● **Alert:** Monitor patient for signs and symptoms of HF (dyspnea, orthopnea, tiredness, weakness, fatigue, weight gain, peripheral or abdominal edema). Drug may need to be discontinued and other antidiabetic drugs may be required.
● Monitor blood glucose level and watch for signs and symptoms of hypoglycemia.
● Monitor HbA$_{1c}$ level periodically to assess long-term glycemic control.
● Monitor patient for signs and symptoms of pancreatitis. If pancreatitis is suspected, discontinue drug and initiate appropriate management.
● Assess renal function before starting drug and periodically thereafter.
● Management of type 2 diabetes should also include diet control and exercise. Because calorie restriction, weight loss, and exercise help improve insulin sensitivity and help make drug therapy effective, these measures are essential for proper diabetes management.
● **Look alike–sound alike:** Don't confuse saxagliptin with sitagliptin.

PATIENT TEACHING

● Tell patient drug may be taken with or without food.
● Instruct patient not to split or cut tablets.
● Tell patient to stop drug and seek immediate medical attention for signs and symptoms of hypersensitivity, including rash, flaking or peeling skin, itching, or swelling of the skin, face, lips, tongue, or throat.

Reactions in bold italics are *life-threatening*. Interactions may have a *rapid onset* or a *delayed onset*.

❸ *Alert:* Instruct patient to immediately report signs and symptoms of HF to prescriber. Patient should not stop drug without first discussing with prescriber.

• Advise patient that drug isn't a substitute for diet and exercise and that it's important to follow prescribed diet and physical activity and to monitor glucose levels.

• Inform patient and family members of the signs and symptoms of hypoglycemia and hyperglycemia and the steps to take should these occur.

• Tell patient to notify prescriber during periods of stress because dosage may need adjustment.

• Tell patient to stop drug if signs and symptoms of pancreatitis (persistent severe abdominal pain, sometimes radiating to the back; vomiting) occur.

sebelipase alfa
See NEW DRUGS for information.

selegiline
se-LEH-ge-leen

Emsam

selegiline hydrochloride (L-deprenyl hydrochloride)
Eldepryl, Zelapar

Therapeutic class: Antiparkinsonians
Pharmacologic class: MAO inhibitors

AVAILABLE FORMS
selegiline
Transdermal system: 6 mg/24 hours, 9 mg/24 hours, 12 mg/24 hours
selegiline hydrochloride
Capsules: 5 mg
ODTs: 1.25 mg
Tablets: 5 mg

INDICATIONS & DOSAGES
➤ **Adjunctive treatment with levodopa–carbidopa in managing signs and symptoms of Parkinson disease**
Adults: For capsules and tablets, 10 mg P.O. daily divided as 5 mg at breakfast and 5 mg at lunch. After 2 or 3 days, gradual decrease of levodopa–carbidopa dosage may

be needed. Or, if using ODTs, start with 1.25 mg P.O. once daily before breakfast and without liquid. Increase to 2.5 mg daily after at least 6 weeks, if tolerated and needed. Maximum dose is 10 mg/day for tablets and capsules and 2.5 mg once daily for ODTs.
➤ **Major depressive disorder**
Adults: Apply one patch daily to dry intact skin on the upper torso, upper thigh, or upper arm. Initially, use 6 mg/day. Increase, if needed, in increments of 3 mg/day at intervals of 2 or more weeks. Maximum daily dose, 12 mg.
Elderly patients: 6 mg transdermal patch daily.

ADMINISTRATION
P.O.
• Don't give food or liquids for 5 minutes before and after giving ODTs.
• Don't push ODTs through the foil backing; peel backing and gently remove the tablet.
Transdermal
• Apply patch to dry, intact skin on the upper torso, upper thigh, or outer surface of the upper arm once every 24 hours.
• Don't cut the transdermal patch into smaller pieces.

ACTION
May inhibit MAO type B (mainly found in the brain) and dopamine metabolism. At higher-than-recommended doses, drug nonselectively inhibits MAO, including MAO type A (mainly found in the intestine). May also directly increase dopaminergic activity by decreasing the reuptake of dopamine into nerve cells.

Route	Onset	Peak	Duration
P.O. (tablet, capsule)	Unknown	40–90 min	Unknown
P.O. (ODT)	5 min	10–15 min	Unknown
Transdermal	Unknown	Unknown	24 hr

Half-life: Selegiline, 2 to 10 hours; N-desmethyl-deprenyl, 2 hours; L-amphetamine, 17¾ hours; L-methamphetamine, 20½ hours.

ADVERSE REACTIONS
Oral form
CNS: dizziness, agitation, delusions, loss of balance, depression, increased bradykinesia, involuntary movements, headache,

S

confusion, hallucinations, vivid dreams, insomnia, syncope, pain.
CV: *arrhythmias,* orthostatic hypotension, hypertension, new or increased angina.
EENT: pharyngitis, rhinitis.
GI: nausea, dry mouth, abdominal pain, diarrhea.
Musculoskeletal: leg cramps, myalgia, back pain.
Respiratory: dyspnea.
Skin: rash, ecchymosis.
Transdermal form
CNS: headache, insomnia.
CV: chest pain, hypotension, orthostatic BP.
GI: diarrhea, dry mouth, dyspepsia.
Metabolic: weight gain, weight loss.
Respiratory: pharyngitis, sinusitis.
Skin: application-site reaction, rash.

INTERACTIONS
Drug-drug. *Bupropion, cyclobenzaprine, dextromethorphan, meperidine, methadone, mirtazapine, MAO inhibitors, sympathomimetic amines (including amphetamines, cold products, and weight-loss preparations containing vasoconstrictors), TCAs, tramadol:* May cause hypertensive crisis. Separate use by at least 2 weeks.
Carbamazepine, oxcarbazepine: May increase selegiline levels. Use together is contraindicated.
Citalopram, duloxetine, fluoxetine, fluvoxamine, nefazodone, paroxetine, sertraline, venlafaxine: May cause serotonin syndrome (CNS irritability, shivering, and altered consciousness). Separate use by at least 2 weeks (5 weeks if switching to or from fluoxetine).
Hormonal contraceptives: May increase plasma selegiline level and increase adverse reactions. Monitor patient closely.
Linezolid, methylene blue: May cause serotonin syndrome. Don't administer within 14 days of each other.
Drug-herb. *St. John's wort:* May cause increased serotonergic effects. Warn against using together.
Drug-food. ❸ *Alert: Foods high in tyramine:* May cause hypertensive crisis, especially at increased doses. Provide patient with a list of foods to avoid.

EFFECTS ON LAB TEST RESULTS
● May cause positive result for amphetamine on urine drug screen.

CONTRAINDICATIONS & CAUTIONS
● Contraindicated in patients hypersensitive to drug, in patients with pheochromocytoma, and in those taking bupropion, carbamazepine, cyclobenzaprine, dextromethorphan, duloxetine, methadone, meperidine, mirtazapine, MAO inhibitors, oxcarbazepine, SSRIs, sympathomimetics, tramadol, TCAs, or venlafaxine.
❸ *Alert:* Concomitant use with linezolid or methylene blue can cause serotonin syndrome (fever, mental status changes, muscle twitching, excessive sweating, shivering or shaking, diarrhea, loss of coordination). Use drug with linezolid or methylene blue only for life-threatening or urgent conditions when the potential benefits outweigh the risks of toxicity.
● Don't use oral drug with the transdermal system.
● Don't use ODTs at daily doses exceeding 2.5 mg/day.
● Orthostatic hypotension may occur during first 2 months of therapy or after dosage increases, especially in older patients.
● Potentially life-threatening serotonin syndrome and hyperpyrexia have been reported in patients taking antidepressants concomitantly with selegiline. Use together isn't recommended.
● Somnolence and falling asleep without prior warning while engaged in activities of daily living (including operating motor vehicles) have been reported in some patients. Evaluate patients for factors that may increase these risks, such as elderly patients with sleep disorders and those taking sedatives.
● Avoid use in patients with major psychotic disorders. Drug may cause changes in or worsening of mental status, abnormal thinking, and behavioral changes, which may be severe and include paranoid ideation, delusions, hallucinations, confusion, psychotic-like behavior, disorientation, aggressive behavior, agitation, and delirium. Drug isn't approved for bipolar depression.
Dialyzable drug: Unknown.

⚠ Overdose S&S: Drowsiness, dizziness, faintness, irritability, hyperactivity, agitation, severe headache, hallucinations, trismus, opisthotonos, seizures, coma, rapid and irregular pulse, hypertension, hypotension and vascular collapse, precordial pain, respiratory depression and failure, hyperpyrexia, diaphoresis, cool and clammy skin.

PREGNANCY-LACTATION-REPRODUCTION
• There are no adequate studies in pregnant women. Use during pregnancy only if potential benefit justifies potential fetal risk.
• It isn't known if drug appears in breast milk. Use cautiously in breast-feeding women.

NURSING CONSIDERATIONS
🔆 **Alert:** Some patients experience new or increased adverse reactions to levodopa, such as dyskinesia, when it's used with selegiline. These patients need a 10% to 30% reduction of levodopa–carbidopa dosage.
Black Box Warning Drug may increase risk of suicidal thinking and behavior in children, adolescents, and young adults ages 18 to 24, especially during the first few months of treatment, especially in those with major depressive or other psychiatric disorder. Contraindicated in patients younger than age 12 because of risk of hypertensive crisis. ■
🔆 **Alert:** If linezolid or methylene blue must be given, stop selegiline and monitor patient for serotonin toxicity for 2 weeks, or until 24 hours after the last dose of methylene blue or linezolid, whichever comes first. May resume selegiline 24 hours after last dose of methylene blue or linezolid.
• Monitor patients with major depressive disorder for worsening of symptoms and of suicidal behavior, especially during the first few weeks of treatment and during dosage changes.
🔆 **Alert:** Monitor patient carefully for orthostatic hypotension, especially during first 2 months of treatment and after dosage increases. Help patient rise from a reclining position.
• Monitor patient for new-onset hypertension or hypertension that isn't adequately controlled after starting drug.

• Monitor patient taking antidepressants and selegiline concomitantly for serotonin syndrome and hyperpyrexia.
• Monitor patient for drowsiness, significant daytime sleepiness, or episodes of falling asleep during activities that require active participation. Discontinue drug if present.
• Monitor patient for psychotic-like behavior, changes in or worsening of mental status, abnormal thinking, and behavioral changes.
• Ask patient about the development or worsening of impulsive or compulsive behaviors, such as new or increased gambling urges, sexual urges, binge eating, uncontrolled spending, or other urges, because patient may not recognize these behaviors as abnormal.
• Examine patient's skin periodically for possible melanoma, because of risk of skin cancer associated with drug and with Parkinson disease.
• Examine patient's mouth for irritation or ulceration; be aware of patient complaints of swallowing or mouth pain when taking ODTs.
• **Look alike–sound alike:** Don't confuse Eldepryl with enalapril.

PATIENT TEACHING
🔆 **Alert:** Teach patient to recognize and immediately report signs and symptoms of serotonin toxicity (fever, mental status changes, muscle twitching, excessive sweating, shivering or shaking, diarrhea, loss of coordination).
• Advise patient not to take drug in the evening because doing so may cause insomnia.
• Explain risk of hypertensive crisis if patient ingests foods or beverages containing tyramine during therapy; if using a 9-mg/day or higher transdermal system, patient should avoid these products altogether. Give patient a list of tyramine-containing foods and products.
• Advise patient to avoid liquids for 5 minutes before and after taking ODTs.
🔆 **Alert:** Warn patient about the many drugs, including OTC drugs, that may interact with this drug and about the need to consult a pharmacist or his prescriber before using them.

● Teach patient and family the signs and symptoms of hypertensive crisis, including severe headache, sore or stiff neck, nausea, vomiting, sweating, rapid heartbeat, dilated pupils, and photophobia.

● Instruct patient not to rise rapidly after sitting or lying down because of risk of dizziness, which may occur more frequently early in therapy or after dosage increases.

● Advise patient taking antidepressants concomitantly with selegiline to immediately report such signs and symptoms as confusion, hallucinations, agitation, delirium, syncope, shivering, sweating, high fever, tachycardia, nausea, diarrhea, muscle rigidity or twitching, or tremors.

● Advise patient that drug may cause him to fall asleep during activities that require active participation and to contact prescriber if drowsiness, significant daytime sleepiness, or episodes of falling asleep during such activities occur.

● Tell patient to report paranoid ideation, delusions, hallucinations, confusion, psychotic-like behavior, disorientation, aggressive behavior, agitation, or delirium.

● Tell patient to contact prescriber if experiencing difficulty controlling impulsive or compulsive behaviors, such as new or increased gambling urges, sexual urges, binge eating or uncontrolled spending.

● Urge patient to watch for skin changes that could suggest melanoma and to have periodic skin examinations.

● Advise patient taking ODTs to report mouth pain, pain when swallowing, or ulcerations.

● Advise patient to contact prescriber before discontinuing selegiline.

● Tell patient that each ODT contains 1.25 mg phenylalanine.

Black Box Warning Advise family members to watch patient for anxiety, agitation, insomnia, irritability, hostility, and aggressiveness and to report these immediately to prescriber. ■

● Tell patient to avoid exposing transdermal system to direct external heat sources, such as heating pads, electric blankets, hot tubs, heated water beds, and prolonged sunlight.

● Tell patient to stop using the transdermal system 10 days before having surgery requiring general anesthesia.

● Tell patient not to cut the transdermal system into smaller pieces.

● Advise women planning pregnancy or breast-feeding to first contact prescriber.

selexipag
See NEW DRUGS for information.

sertraline hydrochloride
SIR-trah-leen

Apo-Sertraline✽, Zoloft♦

Therapeutic class: Antidepressants
Pharmacologic class: SSRIs

AVAILABLE FORMS
Capsules ⊕*:* 25 mg, 50 mg, 100 mg
Oral concentrate*: 20 mg/mL
Tablets: 25 mg, 50 mg, 100 mg, 150 mg, 200 mg

INDICATIONS & DOSAGES
Adjust-a-dose (for all indications): Dosage changes shouldn't occur at intervals of less than 1 week. For patients with hepatic disease, use lower or less-frequent dosages.

➤ **Depression**
Adults: 50 mg P.O. daily. Adjust dosage as needed and tolerated; dosage range is 50 to 200 mg daily.

➤ **Obsessive-compulsive disorder**
Adults: 50 mg P.O. once daily. If patient doesn't improve, increase dosage, up to 200 mg daily.
Children ages 6 to 17: Initially, 25 mg P.O. daily in children ages 6 to 12, or 50 mg P.O. daily in adolescents ages 13 to 17. Increase dosage, as needed, up to 200 mg daily at intervals of no less than 1 week.

➤ **Panic disorder**
Adults: Initially, 25 mg P.O. daily. After 1 week, increase dose to 50 mg P.O. daily. If patient doesn't improve, increase dose to maximum of 200 mg daily.

➤ **Posttraumatic stress disorder**
Adults: Initially, 25 mg P.O. once daily. Increase dosage to 50 mg P.O. once daily after 1 week. Increase at weekly intervals to a maximum of 200 mg daily. Maintain patient on lowest effective dose.

Reactions in bold italics are *life-threatening*. Interactions may have a *rapid onset* or a ***delayed onset***.

➤ **Premenstrual dysphoric disorder**
Adults: Initially, 50 mg P.O. daily either continuously or only during the luteal phase of the menstrual cycle. If patient doesn't respond, dose may be increased 50 mg per menstrual cycle, up to 150 mg daily for use throughout the menstrual cycle or 100 mg daily for luteal-phase doses. If a 100-mg daily dose has been established with luteal-phase dose, use a 50-mg daily adjustment for 3 days at the beginning of each luteal phase.

➤ **Social anxiety disorder**
Adults: Initially, 25 mg P.O. once daily. Increase dosage to 50 mg P.O. once daily after 1 week of therapy. Dose range is 50 to 200 mg daily. Adjust to the lowest effective dosage and periodically reassess patient to determine the need for long-term treatment.

ADMINISTRATION
P.O.
- Give drug without regard for food.
- Don't use oral concentrate dropper, which is made of rubber, for patient with latex allergy.
- Mix oral concentrate with 4 oz (118 mL) of water, ginger ale, lemon-lime soda, lemonade, or orange juice only, and give immediately.

ACTION
Thought to be linked to drug's inhibition of CNS neuronal uptake of serotonin.

Route	Onset	Peak	Duration
P.O.	1 wk	4–8 hr	Unknown

Half-life: 26 hours.

ADVERSE REACTIONS
CNS: fatigue, headache, tremor, dizziness, insomnia, somnolence, *suicidal behavior,* paresthesia, hypesthesia, nervousness, anxiety, agitation, hypertonia, pain.
CV: palpitations, chest pain, hot flashes.
GI: dry mouth, nausea, diarrhea, loose stools, dyspepsia, vomiting, constipation, thirst, flatulence, anorexia, abdominal pain, increased appetite.
GU: male sexual dysfunction.
Musculoskeletal: myalgia.
Skin: rash, pruritus, diaphoresis.

INTERACTIONS
Drug-drug. *Agents with antiplatelet properties (P2Y12 inhibitors, NSAIDs, SSRIs):* May enhance antiplatelet effect. Monitor therapy.
Amphetamines, buspirone, dextromethorphan, dihydroergotamine, lithium salts, meperidine, other SSRIs or SSNRIs (duloxetine, venlafaxine), sumatriptan, TCAs, **tramadol,** *trazodone, tryptophan:* May increase the risk of serotonin syndrome. Avoid combinations of drugs that increase the availability of serotonin in the CNS; monitor patient closely if used together.
Benzodiazepines, tolbutamide: May decrease clearance of these drugs. Significance unknown; monitor patient for increased drug effects.
Cimetidine: May decrease clearance of sertraline. Monitor patient closely.
Disulfiram: Oral concentrate contains alcohol, which may react with drug. Avoid using together.
Linezolid, methylene blue: May cause serotonin syndrome. Use extreme caution and monitor patient closely.
MAO inhibitors (phenelzine, selegiline, tranylcypromine): May cause serotonin syndrome or signs and symptoms resembling neuroleptic malignant syndrome. Avoid using within 14 days of MAO inhibitor therapy.
Pimozide: May increase pimozide level. Avoid using together.
Triptans: May cause serotonin syndrome (restlessness, hallucinations, loss of coordination, fast heartbeat, rapid changes in BP, increased body temperature, hyperreflexia, nausea, vomiting, and diarrhea) or neuroleptic malignant syndrome–like reactions. Use cautiously, with close monitoring, especially at the start of treatment and during dosage adjustments.
Warfarin, other highly protein-bound drugs: May increase level of sertraline or other highly protein-bound drug. May prolong PT, or INR may increase by 8%. Monitor patient closely; monitor PT and INR.
Drug-herb. *St. John's wort:* May cause additive effects and serotonin syndrome. Discourage use together.

S

EFFECTS ON LAB TEST RESULTS
● May increase ALT and AST levels.
● May show false-positive urine immunoassay screening tests for benzodiazepines.

CONTRAINDICATIONS & CAUTIONS
● Contraindicated in patients hypersensitive to drug or its components.
🜂 *Alert:* Concomitant use with linezolid or methylene blue can cause serotonin syndrome (fever, mental status changes, muscle twitching, excessive sweating, shivering or shaking, diarrhea, loss of coordination). Use drug with linezolid or methylene blue only for life-threatening or urgent conditions when the potential benefits outweigh the risks of toxicity.
● Contraindicated in patients taking pimozide or MAO inhibitors or within 14 days of MAO inhibitor therapy.
🜂 *Alert:* Oral concentrate is contraindicated with disulfiram because it contains alcohol.
● Use cautiously in patients at risk for suicide and in those with seizure disorders, major affective disorder, or diseases or conditions that affect metabolism or hemodynamic responses.
Black Box Warning Sertraline isn't approved for use in children except those with obsessive-compulsive disorder. ■
Dialyzable drug: Unknown.
⚠ *Overdose S&S:* Somnolence, vomiting, tachycardia, nausea, dizziness, agitation, tremor, bradycardia, bundle-branch block, coma, seizures, delirium, hallucinations, hypertension, hypotension, manic reactions, pancreatitis, prolonged QT interval, serotonin syndrome, stupor, syncope.

PREGNANCY-LACTATION-REPRODUCTION
● There are no adequate studies in pregnant women. Use only if potential benefit justifies potential risk to the fetus.
● Neonates exposed to sertraline and other SSRIs or SNRIs late in the third trimester have developed complications requiring prolonged hospitalization, respiratory support, and tube feeding.
● Neonates exposed to SSRIs during pregnancy may be at increased risk for persistent pulmonary hypertension of the newborn.

● It isn't known if drug appears in breast milk. Use cautiously in breast-feeding women.

NURSING CONSIDERATIONS
● Give sertraline once daily, either in morning or evening, with or without food.
● Make dosage adjustments at intervals of no less than 1 week.
● Record mood changes. Monitor patient for suicidal tendencies, and allow only a minimum supply of drug.
Black Box Warning Drug may increase the risk of suicidal thinking and behavior in children, adolescents, and young adults with major depressive disorder or other psychiatric disorder. ■
🜂 *Alert:* If linezolid or methylene blue must be given, stop sertraline and monitor patient for serotonin toxicity for 2 weeks, or until 24 hours after the last dose of methylene blue or linezolid, whichever comes first. May resume selegiline 24 hours after last dose of methylene blue or linezolid.
● Don't use the oral concentrate dropper, which is made of rubber, for patient with latex allergy.
🜂 *Alert:* Combining triptans with an SSRI or an SSNRI may cause serotonin syndrome or neuroleptic malignant syndrome–like reactions. Signs and symptoms of serotonin syndrome may include restlessness, hallucinations, loss of coordination, fast heartbeat, rapid changes in BP, increased body temperature, overactive reflexes, nausea, vomiting, and diarrhea. Serotonin syndrome may be more likely to occur when starting or increasing the dose of triptan, SSRI, or SSNRI.
● *Look alike–sound alike:* Don't confuse sertraline with cetirizine or Soriatane.

PATIENT TEACHING
Black Box Warning Advise families and caregivers to closely observe patient for increased suicidal thinking and behavior. ■
🜂 *Alert:* Teach patient to recognize and immediately report signs and symptoms of serotonin toxicity (fever, mental status changes, muscle twitching, excessive sweating, shivering or shaking, diarrhea, loss of coordination).

- Advise patient to use caution when performing hazardous tasks that require alertness.
- Tell patient to avoid alcohol and to consult prescriber before taking OTC drugs.
- Advise patient to mix the oral concentrate with 4 oz (½ cup; 118 mL) of water, ginger ale, lemon-lime soda, lemonade, or orange juice only, and to take the dose right away.
- Instruct patient to avoid stopping drug abruptly.

sevelamer carbonate
seh-VELL-ah-meer

Renvela

sevelamer hydrochloride
Renagel

Therapeutic class: Hypophosphatemics
Pharmacologic class: Polymeric phosphate binders

AVAILABLE FORMS
sevelamer carbonate
Oral suspension: 0.8-g, 2.4-g packets
Tablets (film-coated) ⓓ: 800 mg
sevelamer hydrochloride
Tablets (film-coated) ⓓ: 400 mg, 800 mg

INDICATIONS & DOSAGES
➤ **To control phosphorus level in chronic kidney disease patients on dialysis**
Adults not taking a phosphate binder: Initially, 800 to 1,600 mg (one to two 800-mg tablets or two to four 400-mg tablets) P.O. with each meal, based on phosphorus level. If phosphorus level is greater than 5.5 mg/dL and less than 7.5 mg/dL, start with 800 mg t.i.d. with meals. If phosphorus level is greater than or equal to 7.5 mg/dL and less than 9 mg/dL, start with two 800-mg tablets t.i.d., or three 400-mg tablets t.i.d. with meals. If phosphorus level is greater than or equal to 9 mg/dL, start with 1,600 mg t.i.d. (two 800-mg tablets or four 400-mg tablets) with meals.
Adults switching from calcium acetate: Initially, if taking one 667-mg calcium acetate tablet per meal, start with 800 mg P.O. per meal. If taking two 667-mg calcium

acetate tablets per meal, start with two 800-mg tablets or three 400-mg tablets per meal. If taking three 667-mg calcium acetate tablets per meal, start with three 800-mg tablets or five 400-mg tablets per meal.
Adjust-a-dose: If phosphorus level is greater than 5.5 mg/dL, increase by one tablet per meal at 2-week intervals. If phosphorus level is 3.5 to 5.5 mg/dL, maintain current dose. If phosphorus level is less than 3.5 mg/dL, decrease dose by one tablet per meal.

ADMINISTRATION
P.O.
- Don't cut, crush, or allow patient to chew tablets.
- Mix powder packets with appropriate amount of water as directed. Stir mixture vigorously (it doesn't dissolve) and have patient drink entire preparation within 30 minutes.
- Give drug with meals.
- Drug may bind to other drugs and decrease their bioavailability. Give other drugs 1 hour before or 3 hours after this drug.
- Take special precautions when using antiarrhythmics or anticonvulsants with this drug.

ACTION
Inhibits intestinal phosphate absorption and decreases phosphorus levels.

Route	Onset	Peak	Duration
P.O.	Unknown	Unknown	Unknown

Half-life: Unknown.

ADVERSE REACTIONS
CNS: headache, pain, fever.
CV: hypertension.
GI: diarrhea, dyspepsia, vomiting, nausea, constipation, flatulence.
Metabolic: hypercalcemia.
Musculoskeletal: limb pain, arthralgia.
Skin: pruritus.

INTERACTIONS
Drug-drug. *Ciprofloxacin:* May decrease effectiveness of ciprofloxacin. Give ciprofloxacin either 2 hours before or 6 hours after sevelamer.

S

Mycophenolate: May decrease mycophenolic acid plasma concentration, decreasing effectiveness. Administer sevelamer 2 hours after mycophenolate.

Thyroid hormones (levothyroxine): May decrease effectiveness of hormones. Separate administration times by at least several hours. Consider therapy modification.

EFFECTS ON LAB TEST RESULTS
None reported.

CONTRAINDICATIONS & CAUTIONS
• Contraindicated in patients hypersensitive to drug or its components and in those with hypophosphatemia or bowel obstruction.
• Use cautiously in patient with dysphagia, swallowing disorders, severe GI motility disorders, or major GI tract surgery.
• May reduce absorption of vitamins D, E, and K and folic acid.
Dialyzable drug: Unknown.

PREGNANCY-LACTATION-REPRODUCTION
• There are no adequate studies in pregnant women. Use only if potential benefit justifies potential risk to the fetus.
• No information is available regarding use in breast-feeding women.

NURSING CONSIDERATIONS
• Monitor calcium, bicarbonate, and chloride levels.
• *Look alike–sound alike:* Don't confuse Renvela with Renagel.

PATIENT TEACHING
• Instruct patient to take with meals and to adhere to prescribed diet.
• **Alert:** Inform patient that tablets must be taken whole because contents expand in water. Tell him not to cut, crush, or chew.
• Tell patient to take other drugs as directed, but they must be taken either 2 hours before or 4 hours after sevelamer.
• Inform patient about common adverse reactions, including constipation that, if left untreated, may lead to severe complications.

sildenafil citrate
sill-DEN-ah-fill

Revatio, Viagra✦

Therapeutic class: Erectile dysfunction drugs–pulmonary vasodilators
Pharmacologic class: PDE5 inhibitors

AVAILABLE FORMS
Injection: 10 mg/12.5 mL single-use vials
Oral suspension (Revatio): 10 mg/mL
Tablets (Revatio): 20 mg
Tablets (Viagra): 25 mg, 50 mg, 100 mg

INDICATIONS & DOSAGES
➤ **Erectile dysfunction (Viagra only)**
Adult men younger than age 65: About 1 hour before sexual activity, 50 mg P.O., as needed. Dosage range is 25 to 100 mg based on effectiveness and tolerance. Maximum is 100 mg daily.
Elderly male patients (age 65 and older): 25 mg P.O., as needed, about 1 hour before sexual activity. Dosage may be adjusted based on patient response.
Adjust-a-dose: For adults with hepatic or severe renal impairment, 25 mg P.O. about 1 hour before sexual activity. Dosage may be adjusted based on patient response.
➤ **To improve exercise ability and delay clinical worsening in patients with World Health Organization group I pulmonary arterial hypertension (PAH) (Revatio only)**
Adults: 5 or 20 mg P.O. t.i.d., 4 to 6 hours apart. Or, 2.5 or 10 mg I.V. bolus t.i.d.

ADMINISTRATION
P.O.
• When used for erectile dysfunction, give on empty stomach for rapid absorption.
• When used for PAH, give without regard for food.
• Don't give to patients taking nitrates.
• Follow manufacturer's directions for reconstitution of powder for oral suspension.
• Label suspension with expiration date, which is 60 days from date of reconstitution.

I.V.

▼ Inspect solution visually for particulate matter and discoloration before administering.

▼ Don't give to patients taking nitrates.

▼ Ten-mg I.V. dose is equivalent to 20-mg oral dose (Revatio).

ACTION

When used for erectile dysfunction, drug increases effect of nitric oxide by inhibiting PDE5, which is responsible for degradation of cyclic guanosine monophosphate (cGMP) in the corpus cavernosum. When sexual stimulation causes local release of nitric oxide, inhibition of PDE5 by sildenafil causes increased levels of cGMP in the corpus cavernosum, resulting in smooth muscle relaxation and inflow of blood to the corpus cavernosum. In PAH, drug increases cyclic guanosine monophosphate level by preventing its breakdown by phosphodiesterase, prolonging smooth muscle relaxation of the pulmonary vasculature, which leads to vasodilation.

Route	Onset	Peak	Duration
P.O.	15–30 min	30–120 min	4 hr
I.V.	Unknown	Unknown	Unknown

Half-life: 4 hours.

ADVERSE REACTIONS

CNS: headache, *seizures,* anxiety, dizziness, insomnia, somnolence, vertigo, paresthesia, fever.
CV: flushing.
EENT: diplopia, temporary vision loss, photophobia, altered color perception, blurred vision, nasal congestion, epistaxis, rhinitis, sinusitis.
GI: dyspepsia, diarrhea, gastritis.
GU: UTI.
Musculoskeletal: back pain, myalgia.
Respiratory: dyspnea.
Skin: erythema, rash.

INTERACTIONS

Drug-drug. *Alpha blockers:* May cause symptomatic hypotension. Consider dosage reduction.
Amyl nitrate: May increase vasodilatory effects. Don't use together.

Antihypertensives: May increase hypotension. Use cautiously.
Bosentan: May decrease sildenafil level and increase bosentan level. Monitor patient closely for bosentan adverse reactions.
CYP3A inhibitors (ritonavir): May increase sildenafil level, increasing risk of adverse events, including hypotension, visual changes, and priapism. Reduce initial Viagra dose to 25 mg in a 48-hour period. Use with Revatio isn't recommended.
CYP450 inducers, rifampin: May reduce sildenafil level. Monitor effect.
Guanylate cyclase (GC) stimulators (riociguat): May potentiate hypotensive effects of GC stimulators. Use together is contraindicated.
Hepatic isoenzyme inhibitors (cimetidine, erythromycin, itraconazole, ketoconazole): May reduce sildenafil clearance. Avoid using together.
Isosorbide, nitroglycerin: May cause severe hypotension. Use of nitrates in any form with sildenafil is contraindicated.
Other PDE5 inhibitors: May increase risk of hypotension. Don't use together.
Vitamin K antagonists: May increase risk of bleeding (primarily epistaxis). Monitor patient.
Drug-food. *Grapefruit:* May increase drug level, while delaying absorption. Advise patient to avoid using together.
Drug-herb. *St. John's wort:* May decrease sildenafil level. Don't use together.
Drug-lifestyle. *Alcohol use:* Excessive alcohol intake may increase risk of hypotension. Advise patient to avoid or limit alcohol consumption.

EFFECTS ON LAB TEST RESULTS

● May increase liver enzyme levels.

CONTRAINDICATIONS & CAUTIONS

● Contraindicated in patients hypersensitive to drug or its components and in those taking organic nitrates or GC stimulators.
● Use cautiously in patients age 65 and older; in patients with hepatic or severe renal impairment, retinitis pigmentosa, bleeding disorders, or active peptic ulcer disease; in those who have suffered an MI, stroke, or life-threatening arrhythmia within past 6 months; in those with history

of cardiac failure, CAD, uncontrolled high or low BP, or anatomic deformation of the penis (such as angulation, cavernosal fibrosis, or Peyronie disease); and in those with conditions that may predispose them to priapism (such as sickle cell anemia, multiple myeloma, or leukemia).

• Vision loss, including permanent loss of vision, has been reported in patients taking drug for erectile dysfunction and may be a sign of nonarteritic anterior ischemic optic neuropathy (NAION). Risk may increase with history of vision loss. Other risk factors for NAION include low cup-to-disk ratio ("crowded disk"), CAD, diabetes, hypertension, hyperlipidemia, smoking, and age older than 50.

• Pulmonary vasodilators used to treat PAH can worsen the CV status of patients with pulmonary venoocclusive disease (PVOD). Use in patients with PVOD isn't recommended. If pulmonary edema occurs after drug is administered for PAH, consider the possibility of PVOD.

• Safe and effective use of drug to treat PAH in patients with sickle cell anemia hasn't been established.

• Safe use of drug to treat PAH in children hasn't been established.

• Decreased hearing and hearing loss have been reported. Obtain prompt medical attention for hearing loss.

Dialyzable drug: Unlikely.

PREGNANCY-LACTATION-REPRODUCTION

• Viagra isn't indicated for use in women. There are no adequate studies of use in pregnant or breast-feeding women.

• Information regarding use of drug to treat PAH in pregnant women is limited. Current guidelines recommend that women with PAH use effective contraception and avoid pregnancy.

• It isn't known if Revatio appears in breast milk. Use cautiously in breast-feeding women.

NURSING CONSIDERATIONS

🔹 *Alert:* Systemic vasodilatory properties cause transient decreases in supine BP and cardiac output (about 2 hours after ingestion).

• The serious CV events linked to this drug's use in erectile dysfunction mainly involve patients with underlying CV disease who are at increased risk for cardiac effects related to sexual activity.

• Patients with PAH caused by connective tissue disease are more prone to epistaxis during therapy than those with primary pulmonary hypertension.

• Oral Revatio and I.V. Revatio doses aren't equivalent: A 10-mg I.V. dose is predicted to provide pharmacologic effect equivalent to that of a 20-mg oral dose.

• I.V. use is for patients with PAH currently unable to take oral medications.

🔹 *Alert:* Don't substitute Viagra for Revatio because there isn't an equivalent dose.

• *Look alike–sound alike:* Don't confuse Viagra with Allegra.

PATIENT TEACHING

• Advise patient that drug shouldn't be used with nitrates or GC stimulators under any circumstances. Revatio and Viagra or other PDE5 inhibitors used for erectile dysfunction shouldn't be used together.

• Advise patient of potential cardiac risk of sexual activity, especially in presence of CV risk factors. Instruct patient to notify prescriber and refrain from further activity if such symptoms as chest pain, dizziness, or nausea occur when starting sexual activity.

• Warn patient that erections lasting longer than 4 hours and priapism (painful erections lasting longer than 6 hours) may occur, and tell him to seek immediate medical attention. Penile tissue damage and permanent loss of potency may result if priapism isn't treated immediately.

• Inform patient that drug used for erectile dysfunction doesn't protect against sexually transmitted diseases; advise patient to use protective measures such as condoms.

• Tell patient receiving HIV medications that he's at increased risk for sildenafil adverse events, including low BP, visual changes, and priapism, and that he should promptly report such symptoms to his prescriber. Tell him not to exceed 25 mg of sildenafil in 48 hours.

• Instruct patient to take drug for erectile dysfunction 30 minutes to 4 hours before

---

Reactions in bold italics are *life-threatening*. Interactions may have a *rapid onset* or a *delayed onset*.

sexual activity; maximum benefit can be expected less than 2 hours after ingestion.
• Advise patient that drug for erectile dysfunction is most rapidly absorbed if taken on an empty stomach.
• Inform patient that impairment of color discrimination (blue, green) may occur and to avoid hazardous activities that rely on color discrimination.
• Instruct patient to immediately notify prescriber of vision or hearing changes.
• Caution patient to take drug only as prescribed.

silodosin
sigh-low-DOSE-in

Rapaflo

Therapeutic class: BPH drugs
Pharmacologic class: Alpha₁ blockers

AVAILABLE FORMS
Capsules 🅞🅝🅒: 4 mg, 8 mg

INDICATIONS & DOSAGES
➤ **To improve symptoms of BPH**
Men: 8 mg P.O. once daily.
Adjust-a-dose: For patients with CrCl of 30 to 50 mL/minute, give 4 mg once daily.

ADMINISTRATION
P.O.
• Give drug once daily with a meal.
• For patients who can't swallow capsules, contents of capsule may be sprinkled on a tablespoonful of applesauce (not hot), swallowed within 5 minutes without chewing, and followed with 8 oz of cool water to ensure complete swallowing of the powder. Don't store for future use.

ACTION
Causes relaxation of smooth muscles in the prostate and bladder tissues by antagonizing postsynaptic alpha₁ adrenoreceptors, thereby improving urine flow and reducing signs and symptoms of BPH.

Route	Onset	Peak	Duration
P.O.	Unknown	3 hr	Unknown

Half-life: About 13 hours.

ADVERSE REACTIONS
CNS: asthenia, dizziness, headache, insomnia.
CV: orthostatic hypotension.
EENT: nasal congestion, nasopharyngitis, rhinorrhea, sinusitis.
GI: abdominal pain, diarrhea.
GU: retrograde ejaculation.

INTERACTIONS
Drug-drug. *Alpha blockers:* May cause interactions. Avoid use together.
Antihypertensives: May cause dizziness and orthostatic hypotension. Use together cautiously and monitor patient for adverse reactions.
Moderate CYP3A4 inhibitors (diltiazem, erythromycin, verapamil): May increase silodosin level. Use together cautiously.
Strong CYP3A4 inhibitors (clarithromycin, itraconazole, ketoconazole, ritonavir): May increase silodosin level. Use together is contraindicated.
Strong P-glycoprotein inhibitors (cyclosporine, ketoconazole): May increase silodosin levels. Don't use together.
Drug-herb. *St. John's wort:* May decrease silodosin level and its effects. Consider modifying therapy.

EFFECTS ON LAB TEST RESULTS
None reported.

CONTRAINDICATIONS & CAUTIONS
• Contraindicated in patients hypersensitive to drug or its components, in those with severe renal or hepatic impairment, and in those taking strong CYP3A4 inhibitors.
Dialyzable drug: Unlikely.
⚠ **Overdose S&S:** Orthostatic hypotension.

PREGNANCY-LACTATION-REPRODUCTION
• Drug isn't approved for use in women.

NURSING CONSIDERATIONS
• Because BPH and prostate cancer cause similar signs and symptoms, prostate cancer should be ruled out before the start of silodosin therapy.
• Monitor patient for orthostatic hypotension. Carefully monitor older patients for hypotension because risk of orthostatic hypotension increases with age.

S

• Don't use drug to treat hypertension.
• Current or previous use of an alpha blocker may predispose patient to floppy-iris syndrome during cataract surgery.

PATIENT TEACHING
• Tell patient to take silodosin with the same meal each day.
• Advise patient who can't swallow capsules to sprinkle contents of capsule on a tablespoonful of applesauce (not hot), swallow within 5 minutes without chewing, and follow with 8 oz of cool water to ensure complete swallowing of the powder. Tell patient not to store for future use.
• Warn patient about possible hypotension, and explain that it may cause dizziness.
• Caution patient against driving or operating hazardous machinery until drug's effects are known.
• If patient needs cataract surgery, advise him to inform ophthalmologist that he is taking or has taken silodosin.

---

simeprevir sodium
sim-E-pre-vir

Olysio

Therapeutic class: Antivirals
Pharmacologic class: NS3/4A protease inhibitors

AVAILABLE FORMS
Capsules ⬤: 150 mg

INDICATIONS & DOSAGES
Adjust-a-dose (for all indications): To prevent treatment failure, don't reduce dosage or interrupt simeprevir dosing. If treatment is discontinued because of adverse reactions or inadequate on-treatment virologic response to simeprevir, don't restart. Treatment-experienced patients include prior relapsers, prior partial responders, and prior null-responders who failed prior interferon-based therapy.

If HCV-RNA is 25 international units/mL or greater at 4 weeks, stop simeprevir, peginterferon alfa, and ribavirin. If HCV-RNA is 25 international units/mL or greater at 12 or 24 weeks, stop peginterferon alfa

and ribavirin; treatment with simeprevir is complete at week 12. No treatment-stopping rules apply to the combination of simeprevir with sofosbuvir.

If adverse reactions related to peginterferon alfa, ribavirin, or sofosbuvir occur that require dosage adjustment or interruption of any of the drugs, refer to manufacturer's prescribing information for the specific drug. If any of the other antivirals used in combination with simeprevir are permanently discontinued for any reason, discontinue simeprevir.

➤ **Treatment-naive and treatment-experienced patients with chronic HCV genotype 1 infection, without cirrhosis or with compensated cirrhosis (Child-Pugh class A), in combination with sofosbuvir**
Adults: 150 mg P.O. once daily with sofosbuvir for 12 weeks in patients without cirrhosis or 24 weeks in patients with cirrhosis.

✳ *NEW INDICATION:* **Treatment-naive patients and prior relapsers with chronic HCV genotype 1 or 4 monoinfection, without cirrhosis or with compensated cirrhosis (Child-Pugh class A), in combination with peginterferon alfa and ribavirin**
Adults: 150 mg P.O. once daily with peginterferon alfa and ribavirin for 12 weeks, followed by 12 additional weeks of peginterferon alfa and ribavirin.

✳ *NEW INDICATION:* **Treatment-naive patients and prior relapsers with chronic HCV genotype 1 or 4 infection with HIV-1 coinfection, without cirrhosis or with compensated cirrhosis (Child-Pugh class A), in combination with peginterferon alfa and ribavirin**
Adults: 150 mg P.O. once daily with peginterferon alfa and ribavirin for 12 weeks, followed by 12 additional weeks of peginterferon alfa and ribavirin in patients without cirrhosis or an additional 36 weeks in patients with cirrhosis.

✳ *NEW INDICATION:* **Prior nonresponders (including partial and null responders) with chronic HCV genotype 1 or 4 monoinfection or HIV-1 coinfection, without cirrhosis or with compensated cirrhosis (Child-Pugh class A), in**

combination with peginterferon alfa and ribavirin

Adults: 150 mg P.O. once daily with peginterferon alfa and ribavirin for 12 weeks, followed by 36 additional weeks of peginterferon alfa and ribavirin.

ADMINISTRATION
P.O.
- Give with food to enhance absorption; maintain adequate hydration.
- Administer concurrently with peginterferon alfa and ribavirin or sofosbuvir.
- If dose is missed within 12 hours of time it's usually taken, administer dose as soon as possible. If more than 12 hours have passed since dose is usually taken, don't administer missed dose and resume usual schedule.
- Treatment as monotherapy isn't recommended.
- Patient must swallow capsule whole. Capsules shouldn't be chewed, crushed, broken, cut, or dissolved.
- Keep in original container.

ACTION
Inhibits HCV NS3/4A protease, halting viral replication.

Route	Onset	Peak	Duration
P.O.	Unknown	4–6 hr	Unknown

Half-life: 41 hours in HCV-infected patients receiving 200 mg.

ADVERSE REACTIONS
CNS: fatigue, headache, dizziness.
GI: nausea, diarrhea.
Hepatic: hyperbilirubinemia.
Musculoskeletal: myalgia.
Respiratory: dyspnea.
Skin: rash, photosensitivity, pruritus.

INTERACTIONS
Drug-drug. *Amiodarone:* May cause symptomatic bradycardia. Coadministration isn't recommended. If combination is required, cardiac monitoring in inpatient setting for 48 hours is recommended followed by outpatient HR monitoring for at least 2 weeks.
Atorvastatin: May increase statin level. Start at lowest atorvastatin dosage; don't exceed 40 mg if given concurrently.

Calcium channel blockers (amlodipine, diltiazem, felodipine, nicardipine, nifedipine, nisoldipine, verapamil): May increase levels of calcium channel blockers. Monitor patient carefully.
CYP3A inducers (carbamazepine, dexamethasone [systemic], efavirenz, etravirine, nevirapine, oxcarbazepine, phenobarbital, phenytoin, rifabutin, rifampin, rifapentine): May decrease simeprevir level. Avoid use together.
CYP3A inhibitors (clarithromycin, cobicistat, erythromycin, fluconazole, itraconazole, ketoconazole, posaconazole, ritonavir, telithromycin, voriconazole): May increase simeprevir level. Avoid use together systemically.
Digoxin: May increase digoxin level. Monitor digoxin level.
Disopyramide, flecainide, mexiletine, propafenone, quinidine: May increase levels of these drugs. Monitor patient carefully and obtain drug levels as appropriate.
Erythromycin: May increase erythromycin level. Avoid use together.
Midazolam, triazolam: May increase levels of these drugs when taken orally. Monitor patient carefully.
NNRTIs (delavirdine, efavirenz, etravirine, nevirapine): May increase or decrease simeprevir level. Use together isn't recommended.
PDE5 inhibitors (sildenafil, tadalafil, vardenafil): May increase levels of these drugs. No dosage adjustment needed when prescribed for erectile dysfunction. Monitor patients with pulmonary arterial hypertension closely and use lowest dosage necessary.
Protease inhibitors: May increase simeprevir level. Avoid use together.
Rosuvastatin: May increase statin level. Start rosuvastatin at 5-mg dose; don't exceed 10 mg if given concurrently.
Statins (lovastatin, pitavastatin, pravastatin, simvastatin): May increase statin level. Start at lowest statin dose. Titrate carefully to lowest dosage necessary. Monitor patient closely.
Drug-herb. *Milk thistle:* May increase simeprevir concentration. Don't use together.

S

St. John's wort: May decrease simeprevir level. Use together isn't recommended.
Drug-food. *Any food:* Increases bioavailability. Encourage taking with food.
Drug-lifestyle. *Sun exposure:* May increase risk of serious photosensitivity reactions. Discourage sun exposure.

EFFECTS ON LAB TEST RESULTS
● May increase alkaline phosphatase, amylase, lipase, and bilirubin levels.

CONTRAINDICATIONS & CAUTIONS
● Contraindicated in patients hypersensitive to drug or its components and in those with decompensated cirrhosis receiving drug with peginterferon alfa and ribavirin.
● Use as monotherapy isn't recommended.
● Contraindications to peginterferon alfa and ribavirin or sofosbuvir also apply when these drugs are given with simeprevir.
Black Box Warning Reactivation of HBV may occur in HCV-coinfected patients, and result in fulminant hepatitis, hepatic failure, and death. Screen all patients for current or prior HBV infection before treatment; if patient is positive for HBV infection, assess baseline HBV DNA. ■
● Not recommended in patients who have previously failed therapy with a treatment regimen that included simeprevir or other HCV protease inhibitors.
● Symptomatic bradycardia and cases requiring pacemaker intervention have been reported when amiodarone is given with sofosbuvir in combination with simeprevir. Bradycardia has generally occurred within hours to days of administration, but cases have been reported up to 2 weeks after treatment initiation. Coadministration isn't recommended.
● Not recommended in patients with moderate or severe hepatic impairment (Child-Pugh class B or C) because of reports of hepatic decompensation, hepatic failure, and death in patients with advanced or decompensated cirrhosis who have received this drug combination.
● Use cautiously in patients with history of sulfa allergy. Increased incidence and severity of adverse reactions may occur.
● Use cautiously in patients of East Asian ancestry because serum drug levels may be higher in these patients, increasing risk of adverse events.
Dialyzable drug: Unlikely.

PREGNANCY-LACTATION-REPRODUCTION
● There are no adequate studies in pregnant women. Use only if potential benefit justifies potential risk to the fetus.
● Women of childbearing potential should use an effective contraceptive method.
● Refer to prescribing information for coadministered drugs regarding their use during pregnancy, including contraindications and precautions.
● It isn't known if drug or its metabolites appear in breast milk. Patient should discontinue breast-feeding or discontinue drug.

NURSING CONSIDERATIONS
◑ *Alert:* If peginterferon alfa, ribavirin, or sofosbuvir is discontinued, simeprevir must also be discontinued.
Black Box Warning Monitor patient with current or prior HBV infection for hepatitis flare or HBV reactivation with laboratory testing; watch for signs and symptoms of liver injury during active and posttreatment follow-up. ■
● There is a risk of serious symptomatic bradycardia in patients taking amiodarone who have no alternative treatment options and who will be taking simeprevir and sofosbuvir. Cardiac monitoring in an inpatient setting for the first 48 hours of coadministration is recommended, after which outpatient monitoring or self-monitoring of HR should occur on a daily basis through at least the first 2 weeks of treatment. Patients discontinuing amiodarone just before starting treatment combination should also undergo similar cardiac monitoring; monitor patient for signs and symptoms of bradycardia.
● Screen patients with HCV genotype 1a infections before starting simeprevir with peginterferon alfa and ribavirin for NS3 Q80K polymorphism at baseline. Effectiveness of drug is reduced in these patients; consider alternative therapy. Also consider screening for patients starting simeprevir with sofosbuvir.
● Refer to prescribing information for the antivirals used in combination with simeprevir for recommendations on dosage

---

Reactions in bold italics are *life-threatening*. Interactions may have a *rapid onset* or a *delayed onset*.

adjustment or therapy interruption needed because of adverse reactions potentially related to their use.

• Monitor bilirubin, liver enzyme, and uric acid levels at baseline, then periodically (and when clinically indicated). Closely monitor patients who experience an increase in total bilirubin level to greater than 2.5 × ULN.

• Discontinue drug if increased bilirubin level is accompanied by liver transaminase increases or clinical signs and symptoms of hepatic decompensation develop.

• For patients taking simeprevir with peginterferon alfa and ribavirin, monitor serum HCV-RNA level at baseline; at weeks 4, 12, and 24; at end of treatment; during treatment follow-up; and when clinically indicated.

• Monitor patients for serious photosensitivity reactions (severe rash or exaggerated sunburn, burning erythema, exudation, blistering, edema) during combination therapy with peginterferon alfa and ribavirin. Consider drug discontinuation if photosensitivity reaction occurs.

• Monitor patients for severe rash (oral lesions, conjunctivitis, systemic symptoms); discontinue drug if these symptoms occur.

PATIENT TEACHING
Black Box Warning Warn patient to immediately report signs and symptoms of liver injury (fatigue, weakness, loss of appetite, nausea, vomiting, yellowing of skin or eyes, light-colored stool). ▪

• Caution patient that drug isn't for use as monotherapy and that it's always part of a regimen containing peginterferon alfa and ribavirin or sofosbuvir.

• Instruct patient to swallow capsule whole and not to chew, crush, break, cut, or dissolve it in liquid.

• Instruct patient not to interrupt treatment without first discussing with prescriber.

• Tell patient that laboratory values will be monitored before and during treatment.

• Advise patient taking amiodarone with simeprevir and sofosbuvir to seek immediate medical evaluation if fainting or near-fainting, dizziness or light-headedness, malaise, weakness, excessive tiredness, shortness of breath, chest pain, confusion, or memory problems occur.

• Counsel patient to seek immediate medical attention for signs or symptoms of significant reaction (wheezing, chest tightness, fever, itching, heavy cough, blue-colored skin, seizures, or swelling of face, lips, tongue, or throat).

• Tell patient to seek medical attention for fatigue, weakness, lack of appetite, nausea or vomiting, jaundice, or discolored feces.

• Advise female patient to contact prescriber immediately if she becomes pregnant.

• Warn patient to use sun-protection measures and limit sun exposure, and to contact prescriber immediately if photosensitivity reaction occurs.

• Tell patient to report adverse reactions (such as nausea, dyspepsia, and rash) to prescriber.

• Counsel patient to use precautions to prevent HCV transmission.

simvastatin (synvinolin)
sim-va-STAH-tin

Zocor✐

Therapeutic class: Antilipemics
Pharmacologic class: HMG-CoA reductase inhibitors

AVAILABLE FORMS
Tablets: 5 mg, 10 mg, 20 mg, 40 mg, 80 mg

INDICATIONS & DOSAGES
Adjust-a-dose (for all indications): In patients taking fibrates or niacin, maximum is 10 mg P.O. daily. In patients taking dronedarone, diltiazem, or verapamil, maximum is 10 mg P.O. daily. In patients taking amiodarone, amlodipine, lomitapide, or ranolazine, maximum is 20 mg P.O. daily. In patients with severe renal insufficiency, start with 5 mg P.O. daily.

➤ **To reduce risk of death from CV disease and CV events in patients at high risk for coronary events; to reduce total and LDL cholesterol, apolipoprotein B, and triglyceride levels and increase HDL cholesterol level in patients with primary hyperlipidemia and mixed dyslipidemia; to reduce triglyceride levels; to reduce**

S

triglyceride levels and VLDL cholesterol level in patients with dysbetalipoproteinemia

Adults: Initially, 10 to 20 mg P.O. daily in evening. In patients at high risk for a CAD event due to existing CAD, diabetes, peripheral vascular disease, or history of stroke, the recommended initial dose is 40 mg P.O. daily. Adjust dosage every 4 weeks based on patient tolerance and response. Patients unable to achieve their LDL-cholesterol goals utilizing simvastatin 40 mg shouldn't be titrated to 80-mg dose but should be placed on alternative LDL-cholesterol lowering treatment.

➤ **To reduce total and LDL cholesterol levels in patients with homozygous familial hypercholesterolemia**

Adults: 40 mg P.O. daily in evening.

➤ **Heterozygous familial hypercholesterolemia in boys and postmenarchal girls**

Children ages 10 to 17: Give 10 mg P.O. once daily in the evening. Maximum, 40 mg daily.

ADMINISTRATION
P.O.

● Give drug in the evening.

ACTION

Inhibits HMG-CoA reductase, an early (and rate-limiting) step in cholesterol biosynthesis.

Route	Onset	Peak	Duration
P.O.	Unknown	1–2 hr	Unknown

Half-life: Unknown.

ADVERSE REACTIONS

CNS: asthenia, headache.
GI: abdominal pain, constipation, diarrhea, dyspepsia, flatulence, nausea, vomiting.
Respiratory: URI.

INTERACTIONS

Drug-drug. *Amiodarone, amlodipine, lomitapide, ranolazine:* May increase risk of myopathy and rhabdomyolysis. Don't exceed 20 mg simvastatin daily.
Azole antifungals (fluconazole, itraconazole, ketoconazole), **macrolides (azithromycin, clarithromycin, erythro-**

mycin, telithromycin): May increase simvastatin level and adverse effects. Avoid using together or, if it can't be avoided, suspend simvastatin therapy for course of treatment.
Bile acid sequestrants (cholestyramine, colestipol): May decrease GI absorption of simvastatin. Separate administration times by at least 4 hours.
Cyclosporine, *danazol, gemfibrozil:* May increase risk of myopathy and rhabdomyolysis. Use together is contraindicated.
Digoxin: May slightly increase digoxin level. Closely monitor digoxin levels at the start of simvastatin therapy.
Dronedarone, diltiazem, **verapamil:** May increase risk of myopathy and rhabdomyolysis. Don't exceed 10 mg simvastatin daily.
Efavirenz, rifampin: May decrease simvastatin level. Monitor effectiveness.
Fibrates (other than gemfibrozil): Increase risk of myopathy. Use cautiously together.
Hepatotoxic drugs: May increase risk for hepatotoxicity. Avoid using together.
Nefazodone, protease inhibitors (amprenavir, atazanavir, darunavir, fosamprenavir, indinavir, lopinavir–ritonavir, nelfinavir, ritonavir, saquinavir): May inhibit metabolism of simvastatin and increase the risk of adverse effects, including rhabdomyolysis. Use together is contraindicated.
Niacin: May increase risk of myopathy and rhabdomyolysis with niacin dose of 1 g/day or more. Use cautiously in Chinese patients when administering with simvastatin doses exceeding 20 mg/day. Chinese patients and possibly others of Asian descent shouldn't receive simvastatin 80 mg with lipid-modifying dose of niacin-containing products.
Warfarin: May slightly enhance anticoagulant effect. Monitor PT and INR when therapy starts or dose is adjusted.
Drug-herb. *Eucalyptus, kava kava:* May increase risk of hepatotoxicity. Discourage use together.
Red yeast rice: May increase risk of rhabdomyolysis. Discourage use together.
St. John's wort: May decrease simvastatin level. Discourage use together.
Drug-food. *Grapefruit juice:* Large amounts (greater than 1 quart/day [1 L/day]) may increase drug levels, increasing risk of

---

Reactions in bold italics are *life-threatening*. Interactions may have a *rapid onset* or a ***delayed onset***.

adverse effects, including myopathy and rhabdomyolysis. Discourage use together.
Drug-lifestyle. *Alcohol use:* May increase risk of hepatotoxicity. Discourage use together.

EFFECTS ON LAB TEST RESULTS
• May increase HbA$_{1c}$, fasting blood glucose, ALT, AST, and CK levels.

CONTRAINDICATIONS & CAUTIONS
• Simvastatin occasionally causes myopathy manifested as muscle pain, tenderness, or weakness, with CK level more than 10 × ULN. Myopathy sometimes takes the form of rhabdomyolysis with or without acute renal failure secondary to myoglobinuria, and rare fatalities have occurred. The risk of myopathy, including rhabdomyolysis, is dose related. Predisposing factors for myopathy include advanced age (age 65 and older), female gender, uncontrolled hypothyroidism, and renal impairment.
• Contraindicated in patients hypersensitive to drug and in those with active liver disease or conditions that cause unexplained persistent elevations of transaminase levels.
• Contraindicated for use at its highest dosage (80 mg/day) in patients not previously prescribed simvastatin or in patients who have had prior muscle toxicity. Patients who can't reach their goal LDL cholesterol level on 40-mg dose should be switched to an alternative agent. Only patients who have tolerated the 80-mg dose without muscle toxicity for more than 12 months should continue taking 80 mg daily.
• Use cautiously in patients who consume large amounts of alcohol or have a history of liver disease.
• Rare reports of cognitive impairment (memory loss, forgetfulness, amnesia, memory impairment, confusion) have been associated with statin use. These reported symptoms are generally not serious and are reversible upon statin discontinuation, with variable times to symptom onset (1 day to years) and symptom resolution (median of 3 weeks).
• Use cautiously when treating Chinese patients with simvastatin dosages exceeding 20 mg/day administered with lipid-modifying doses of niacin-containing products (niacin 1 g/day or more) because of the increased risk of myopathy. Don't give Chinese patients simvastatin 80 mg with lipid-modifying doses of niacin-containing products. It's unknown whether this increased risk of myopathy also applies to other Asian patients.
Dialyzable drug: Unknown.

PREGNANCY-LACTATION-REPRODUCTION
• Contraindicated in women who are pregnant or may become pregnant; drug may cause fetal harm. Use in women of childbearing potential only when they are highly unlikely to conceive.
• Discontinue drug immediately if pregnancy occurs. Apprise patient of potential hazard to the fetus.
• Contraindicated in breast-feeding women.

NURSING CONSIDERATIONS
• Obtain LFT results before initiation of treatment and thereafter when clinically indicated. Obtain lipid determinations after 4 weeks of therapy and periodically thereafter.
• Monitor all patients for myopathy (unexplained muscle pain, weakness, or tenderness). Periodic CK determinations may be considered in patients starting therapy or in patients whose dosage is being increased, but there's no assurance that such monitoring will prevent myopathy.
• Patient should follow a diet restricted in saturated fat and cholesterol during therapy.
• Interrupt statin therapy if patient shows signs or symptoms of serious liver injury, hyperbilirubinemia, or jaundice. Don't restart drug if another cause can't be found.
• A daily dose of 40 mg significantly reduces risk of death from CAD, nonfatal MI, stroke, and revascularization procedures.
• *Look alike–sound alike:* Don't confuse Zocor with Cozaar.

PATIENT TEACHING
• Instruct patient to take drug in the evening.
• Teach patient about proper dietary management of cholesterol and triglycerides. When appropriate, recommend weight control, exercise, and smoking cessation programs.

• Inform patient that rare instances of memory loss and confusion have occurred with statin use. These reported events were generally not serious and resolved when drug was discontinued.

• Tell patient that drug may increase blood glucose level, but the CV benefits are thought to outweigh the slight increase in risk.

• Tell patient to immediately report unexplained muscle pain, tenderness, or weakness (especially if accompanied by malaise or fever) and loss of appetite, upper abdominal pain, dark-colored urine, or yellowing of skin or eyes.

❸ **Alert:** Tell woman to stop drug and notify prescriber immediately if she is or may be pregnant or if she's breast-feeding.

SAFETY ALERT!

sirolimus
sir-AH-lih-mus

Rapamune

Therapeutic class: Immunosuppressants
Pharmacologic class:
Immunosuppressants

AVAILABLE FORMS
Oral solution: 1 mg/mL
Tablets ⓄⓉⒸ: 0.5 mg, 1 mg, 2 mg

INDICATIONS & DOSAGES
➤ **With cyclosporine and corticosteroids, to prevent organ rejection in patients receiving renal transplants**
Adults and adolescents: Initially, 6 mg P.O. for patients with low to moderate immunologic risk weighing 40 kg or more or 3 mg/m² for patients weighing less than 40 kg as one-time dose as soon as possible after transplantation; then maintenance dose of 2 mg P.O. once daily for patients weighing 40 kg or more or 1 mg/m² P.O. once daily for patients weighing less than 40 kg. For patients with high immunologic risk, may give up to 15 mg P.O. on day 1 after transplantation, then 5 mg/day P.O. beginning on day 2 after transplantation.

Maximum daily dose shouldn't exceed 40 mg. If a daily dose exceeds 40 mg due to

a loading dose, give the loading dose over 2 days. Monitor trough concentrations at least 3 to 4 days after a loading dose.
Children age 13 and older weighing less than 40 kg: First dose is 3 mg/m² P.O. as one-time dose after transplantation; then 1 mg/m² P.O. once daily.

Adjust-a-dose: For patients with mild to moderate hepatic impairment, reduce maintenance dose by about one-third, and by about one-half in patients with severe hepatic impairment. It isn't necessary to reduce loading dose. Two to 4 months after transplant in patients with low to moderate risk of graft rejection, taper off cyclosporine over 4 to 8 weeks. While tapering cyclosporine, adjust sirolimus dose every 1 to 2 weeks to obtain levels between 16 and 24 nanograms/mL. Base dosage adjustments on clinical status, tissue biopsies, and laboratory findings.

➤ **Lymphangioleiomyomatosis**
Adults: Initially, 2 mg P.O. daily consistently with or without food at same time each day. Measure trough concentration in 10 to 20 days and adjust dosage to achieve sirolimus trough level of between 5 and 15 nanograms/mL, allowing at least 7 to 14 days on new dose before further dosage adjustment. Once a stable dosage is achieved, perform therapeutic drug monitoring at least every 3 months.

ADMINISTRATION
P.O.
• Follow safe-handling procedures when preparing, administering, and dispensing drug.

• Give drug consistently either with or without food.

• Patients should swallow tablets whole. Don't crush or split tablets.

• Dilute oral solution before use. After dilution, use immediately and discard oral solution syringe.

• When diluting oral solution, empty correct amount into glass or plastic (not Styrofoam) container holding at least ¼ cup (60 mL) of either water or orange juice. Don't use grapefruit juice or any other liquid. Stir vigorously and have patient drink immediately. Refill container with at least ½ cup (120 mL) of water or orange juice, stir again, and have patient drink all contents.

• A slight haze may develop during refrigeration, which doesn't affect potency of drug. If haze develops, bring to room temperature and shake until haze disappears.

• Store away from light, and refrigerate at 36° to 46° F (2° to 8° C). After opening bottle, use contents within 1 month. If needed, store bottles and pouches at room temperature (up to 77° F [25° C]) for several days. Drug may be kept in oral syringe for 24 hours at room temperature.

• Store tablets between 68° and 77° F (20° and 25° C).

ACTION

Inhibits T-cell activation and proliferation that occurs in response to antigenic and cytokine stimulation. Also inhibits antibody formation.

Route	Onset	Peak	Duration
P.O.	Unknown	1–3 hr (solution); 1–6 hr (tablet)	Unknown

Half-life: About 46 to 78 hours.

ADVERSE REACTIONS

CNS: fever, headache.
CV: chest pain, edema, hypertension, peripheral edema, tachycardia, *thrombosis.*
EENT: epistaxis.
GI: abdominal pain, constipation, diarrhea, nausea, ascites.
GU: UTI, *toxic nephropathy,* dysuria, glycosuria, hematuria, hemolytic-uremic syndrome, polynephritis.
Hematologic: anemia, *thrombocytopenia, leukopenia, thrombotic thrombocytopenic purpura,* ecchymosis.
Hepatic: *hepatic artery thrombosis, hepatotoxicity.*
Metabolic: hypercholesteremia, *hyperkalemia,* hyperlipidemia, hypokalemia, hypophosphatemia, *hypoglycemia, acidosis, diabetes mellitus,* dehydration, hypercalcemia, hyperglycemia.
Musculoskeletal: arthralgia, back pain, bone necrosis, myalgia.
Respiratory: atelectasis, cough, dyspnea, URI, *interstitial lung disease, asthma,* bronchitis, *hypoxia,* lung edema, pleural effusion, pneumonia.

Skin: acne, rash, fungal dermatitis, pruritus, *melanoma, squamous cell carcinoma, basal cell carcinoma.*
Other: *sepsis;* abnormal healing, including fascial dehiscence and anastomotic disruption (wound, vascular, airway, ureteral, biliary); abscess; flu syndrome; infection; lymphadenopathy; lymphocele; hypersensitivity reactions; *angioedema;* herpes simplex; herpes zoster.

INTERACTIONS

Drug-drug. *Aminoglycosides, amphotericin B, other nephrotoxic drugs:* May increase risk of nephrotoxicity. Use with caution.
Amiodarone, bromocriptine, cimetidine, clarithromycin, clotrimazole, danazol, erythromycin, fluconazole, indinavir, itraconazole, metoclopramide, nicardipine, posaconazole, ritonavir, verapamil, voriconazole, other drugs that inhibit CYP3A4: May increase blood levels of sirolimus. Monitor sirolimus levels closely.
Carbamazepine, phenobarbital, phenytoin, rifabutin, rifapentine, other drugs that induce CYP3A4: May decrease blood levels of sirolimus. Monitor patient closely.
Cyclosporine: May increase sirolimus level and toxicity. Give sirolimus 4 hours after cyclosporine; monitor levels and adjust dose, as needed.
Diltiazem: May increase sirolimus levels. Monitor sirolimus level, as needed.
HMG-CoA reductase inhibitors or fibrates: May increase risk of rhabdomyolysis with the combination of sirolimus and cyclosporine. Monitor patient closely.
Ketoconazole: May increase rate and extent of sirolimus absorption. Avoid using together.
Live-virus vaccines: May reduce vaccine effectiveness. Avoid using together.
Rifampin: May decrease sirolimus level. Alternative therapy to rifampin may be prescribed.
Drug-herb. *St. John's wort:* May decrease sirolimus levels. Discourage use together.
Drug-food. *Grapefruit juice:* May decrease drug metabolism. Discourage use together.
Drug-lifestyle. *Sun exposure:* May increase risk of skin cancer. Advise patient to avoid sunlight exposure.

S

EFFECTS ON LAB TEST RESULTS

• May increase BUN, creatinine, liver enzyme, cholesterol, and lipid levels. May increase or decrease phosphate, potassium, and glucose levels.

• May increase RBC count. May decrease platelet count. May increase or decrease WBC count.

CONTRAINDICATIONS & CAUTIONS

• Contraindicated in patients hypersensitive to active drug, its derivatives, or components of product.

• Use cautiously in patients with hyperlipidemia and impaired liver or renal function.

• Cases of interstitial lung disease (ILD), including pneumonitis, bronchiolitis obliterans organizing pneumonia, and pulmonary fibrosis (some fatal), have occurred. ILD may be associated with pulmonary hypertension and risk may increase with higher trough levels. ILD may resolve with reduced doses or with drug discontinuation.

Black Box Warning Fatal bronchial anastomotic dehiscence has been reported in lung transplant patients when sirolimus has been used as part of an immunosuppressive regimen. Safety and effectiveness of sirolimus as immunosuppressive therapy haven't been established in liver or lung transplant patients. Use in these patients isn't recommended. ∎

Dialyzable drug: No.

⚠ *Overdose S&S:* Exaggerated adverse effects.

PREGNANCY-LACTATION-REPRODUCTION

• There are no adequate studies in pregnant women; drug may cause fetal harm. Patient must use effective contraception before and during therapy and for 12 weeks after therapy ends. Use during pregnancy only if potential benefit outweighs potential risk to the fetus.

• It isn't known if drug appears in breast milk. Patient should discontinue breast-feeding or discontinue drug.

NURSING CONSIDERATIONS

Black Box Warning Using this drug with tacrolimus or cyclosporine may cause hepatic artery thrombosis, leading to graft loss and death in liver transplant patients. ∎

Black Box Warning Only those experienced in immunosuppressive therapy and management of kidney transplant patients should prescribe drug. Manage patients receiving drug in facilities equipped and staffed with adequate laboratory and supportive medical resources. ∎

Black Box Warning Patients taking drug are more susceptible to infection and lymphoma. ∎

◑ *Alert:* Drugs causing immunosuppression increase the risk of opportunistic infections, including activation of latent viral infections such as BK virus-associated neuropathy, which may lead to serious outcomes, including kidney graft loss.

◑ *Alert:* This drug has been associated with angioedema; using it with ACE inhibitors increases the risk. Monitor patient closely.

• Use drug in regimen with cyclosporine and corticosteroids; have patient take drug 4 hours after cyclosporine dose.

• Dosage adjustment more often than every 7 to 14 days may result in overdose due to the long half-life of sirolimus.

• Cyclosporine withdrawal in patients with high risk of graft rejection isn't recommended. This includes patients with Banff grade III acute rejection or vascular rejection before cyclosporine withdrawal, those who are dialysis dependent, those with serum creatinine level greater than 4.5 mg/dL, black patients, patients with retransplants or multiorgan transplants, and patients with high panel of reactive antibodies.

• After transplantation, give antimicrobial prophylaxis for *Pneumocystis jiroveci* for 1 year and for cytomegalovirus for 3 months.

• Monitor renal function tests because use with cyclosporine may cause creatinine level to increase. Adjustment of immunosuppressive regimen may be needed.

• Monitor cholesterol and triglyceride levels. Treatment with lipid-lowering drugs during therapy isn't uncommon. If hyperlipidemia is detected, additional interventions, such as diet and exercise, should begin.

• Check for rhabdomyolysis.

• Monitor drug levels in patients age 13 and older who weigh less than 40 kg, patients

with hepatic impairment, those also receiving drugs that induce or inhibit CYP3A4, and patients in whom cyclosporine dosing is markedly reduced or stopped.
• Monitor patient for impaired or delayed wound healing, including wound dehiscence, and fluid accumulation, including edema, lymphedema, pleural effusion, ascites, and pericardial effusion.

PATIENT TEACHING
• Teach patient how to properly store, dilute, and give drug.
• Advise female patient about risks during pregnancy. Tell her to use effective contraception before and during therapy and for 12 weeks after stopping therapy.
• Tell patient to take drug consistently with or without food to minimize absorption variability.
• Tell patient to take drug 4 hours after cyclosporine to avoid drug interactions.
• Advise patient to wash area with soap and water if drug solution touches skin or mucous membranes.
• Advise patient to limit ultraviolet light and sun exposure because of the increased risk of skin cancer.

SAFETY ALERT!

sitagliptin phosphate
sit-ah-GLIP-ten

Januvia✐

Therapeutic class: Antidiabetics
Pharmacologic class: DPP-4 enzyme inhibitors

AVAILABLE FORMS
Tablets: 25 mg, 50 mg, 100 mg

INDICATIONS & DOSAGES
➤ **To improve glycemic control in addition to diet and exercise in patients with type 2 diabetes, alone or in combination therapy**
Adults: 100 mg P.O. once daily.
Adjust-a-dose: For patients with CrCl of 30 to 49 mL/minute, give 50 mg once daily; for patients with CrCl less than

30 mL/minute or ESRD with hemodialysis or peritoneal dialysis, give 25 mg once daily. Give without regard to timing of dialysis session.

ADMINISTRATION
P.O.
• Give drug without regard for food.

ACTION
Inhibits DPP-4, an enzyme that rapidly inactivates incretin hormones, which play a part in the body's regulation of glucose. By increasing and prolonging active incretin levels, the drug helps to increase insulin release and decrease circulating glucose.

Route	Onset	Peak	Duration
P.O.	Rapid	1–4 hr	Unknown

Half-life: About 12½ hours.

ADVERSE REACTIONS
CNS: headache.
EENT: nasopharyngitis.
GI: abdominal pain, nausea, diarrhea.
Metabolic: *hypoglycemia.*
Respiratory: URI.

INTERACTIONS
None significant.

EFFECTS ON LAB TEST RESULTS
• May increase creatinine level.
• May increase WBC count.

CONTRAINDICATIONS & CAUTIONS
• Contraindicated in patients with type 1 diabetes or diabetic ketoacidosis.
• Contraindicated in patients with a history of hypersensitivity to sitagliptin. Angioedema, anaphylaxis, and exfoliative skin conditions have been reported, some after first dose or up to 3 months after drug initiation.
• Use cautiously in patients with moderate to severe renal insufficiency or a history of pancreatitis and in those taking other antidiabetics.
• Safety and effectiveness in children haven't been evaluated.
Dialyzable drug: 13.5%.

S

PREGNANCY-LACTATION-REPRODUCTION

● There are no adequate studies in pregnant women. Use only if clearly needed.
● Report prenatal exposure to the Januvia Pregnancy Registry (1-800-986-8999).
● It isn't known if drug appears in breast milk. Use cautiously in breast-feeding women.

NURSING CONSIDERATIONS

● In elderly patients and those at risk for renal insufficiency, periodically assess renal function.
● Assess renal function before start of therapy and periodically thereafter.
● Monitor HbA$_{1c}$ level periodically to assess long-term glycemic control.
● Management of type 2 diabetes should include diet control. Because caloric restrictions, weight loss, and exercise help improve insulin sensitivity and help make drug therapy effective, these measures are essential for proper diabetes management.
● Watch for hypoglycemia, especially in patients receiving combination therapy.
● Monitor patient for pancreatitis (persistent abdominal pain with or without vomiting). Discontinue drug if pancreatitis is suspected.
● **Alert:** Drug may cause joint pain that can be severe and disabling. Report severe and persistent joint pain to prescriber; drug may need to be discontinued.
● **Look alike–sound alike:** Don't confuse sitagliptin with saxagliptin.

PATIENT TEACHING

● Tell patient that drug isn't a substitute for diet and exercise and that it's important to follow a prescribed dietary and physical activity routine and to monitor his glucose levels.
● Instruct patient to immediately report persistent, severe abdominal pain that may radiate to the back, with or without vomiting.
● Inform patient and family members of the signs and symptoms of hyperglycemia and hypoglycemia and the steps to take if these symptoms occur.
● Advise patient to report all adverse reactions, and to immediately report signs and symptoms of hypersensitivity (rash,

swelling of the face) or new or worsening joint pain.
● Provide patient with information on complications associated with diabetes and ways to assess for them.
● Tell patient to notify prescriber during periods of stress, such as fever, infection, or surgery; dosage may need adjustment.
● Tell patient drug may be taken without regard to food.

sodium ferric gluconate complex
Ferrlecit

Therapeutic class: Iron supplements
Pharmacologic class: Macromolecular iron complexes–hematinics

AVAILABLE FORMS
Injection: 62.5 mg elemental iron (12.5 mg/mL) in 5-mL ampules

INDICATIONS & DOSAGES
➤ **Iron deficiency anemia in patients receiving long-term hemodialysis and supplemental erythropoietin**
Adults and children age 15 and older: 10 mL (125 mg elemental iron) I.V. over 1 hour. Most patients need minimum cumulative dose of 1 g elemental iron given over more than eight sequential dialysis treatments to achieve a favorable Hb or hematocrit response.
Children age 6 and older: 1.5 mg/kg (maximum 125 mg/dose) I.V. over 1 hour during 8 consecutive hemodialysis treatments.

ADMINISTRATION
I.V.
▼ Drug contains benzyl alcohol. Don't use in neonates.
▼ For adults, dilute in 100 mL NSS; for children, dilute in 25 mL NSS. Give immediately over 1 hour.
▼ Alternatively, give undiluted at a rate not to exceed 1 mL/minute (12.5 mg/minute) at the end of dialysis.
▼ Life-threatening hypersensitivity reactions, such as CV collapse, cardiac arrest, bronchospasm, oral or pharyngeal edema, dyspnea, angioedema, urticaria,

and pruritus—sometimes linked to pain and muscle spasm of chest or back—may occur during infusion. Have adequate supportive measures readily available. Monitor patient closely during infusion.

▼ After administration, profound hypotension with flushing, light-headedness, malaise, fatigue, weakness, or severe chest, back, flank, or groin pain may occur; these symptoms aren't hypersensitivity reactions. Monitor patient closely during infusion.

▼ **Incompatibilities:** Other I.V. drugs. Don't add drug to parenteral nutrition solutions for infusion.

ACTION

Restores total body iron content, which is critical for normal Hb synthesis and oxygen transport.

Route	Onset	Peak	Duration
I.V.	Unknown	Varies	Unknown

Half-life: 1 hour in healthy, iron-deficient adults.

ADVERSE REACTIONS

CNS: asthenia, headache, fatigue, malaise, dizziness, paresthesia, agitation, insomnia, somnolence, syncope, pain, chills, fever.
CV: hypotension, hypertension, tachycardia, *bradycardia,* angina, chest pain, *MI,* edema, flushing.
EENT: conjunctivitis, abnormal vision, rhinitis.
GI: nausea, vomiting, diarrhea, rectal disorder, dyspepsia, eructation, flatulence, melena, abdominal pain.
GU: UTI.
Hematologic: anemia.
Metabolic: *hyperkalemia, hypoglycemia, hypokalemia,* hypervolemia.
Musculoskeletal: myalgia, arthralgia, back pain, arm pain, cramps.
Respiratory: dyspnea, coughing, URI, pneumonia, pulmonary edema.
Skin: pruritus, increased sweating, rash, injection-site reaction.
Other: infection, rigors, flu syndrome, *sepsis, carcinoma,* hypersensitivity reactions, lymphadenopathy.

INTERACTIONS

Drug-drug. *ACE inhibitors:* May cause sensitivity reactions. Stop I.V. iron if sensitivity reactions occur.
Oral iron preparations: May reduce absorption of oral iron preparations. Avoid using together.

EFFECTS ON LAB TEST RESULTS

● May decrease glucose and Hb levels. May increase or decrease potassium level.

CONTRAINDICATIONS & CAUTIONS

● Contraindicated in patients hypersensitive to drug or its components (such as benzyl alcohol) and in those with iron overload or anemias not related to iron deficiency.
● Don't use in patients with ferritin levels greater than 1,000 nanograms/mL.
● Use cautiously in elderly patients.
Dialyzable drug: No.
⚠ *Overdose S&S:* Abdominal pain, diarrhea, vomiting, pallor or cyanosis, lassitude, drowsiness, hyperventilation, CV collapse.

PREGNANCY-LACTATION-REPRODUCTION

● There are no adequate studies in pregnant women. Use only if clearly needed.
● It isn't known if drug appears in breast milk. Use cautiously in breast-feeding women.

NURSING CONSIDERATIONS

❸ *Alert:* Dosage is expressed in milligrams of elemental iron.
● Drug shouldn't be used in patients with iron overload, which often occurs in hemoglobinopathies and other refractory anemias.
● Monitor ferritin level, iron saturation, Hb level, and hematocrit.
● In hemodialysis patients, adverse reactions may be related to dialysis itself or to chronic renal failure.
● Check with patient about other potential sources of iron, such as OTC iron preparations and iron-containing multiple vitamins with minerals.

PATIENT TEACHING

● Abdominal pain, diarrhea, vomiting, drowsiness, and rapid breathing may indicate iron poisoning. Urge patient to notify prescriber immediately.

S

sofosbuvir
soe-FOS-bue-vir

Sovaldi

Therapeutic class: Antivirals
Pharmacologic class: Nucleotide
analogue NS5B polymerase inhibitors

AVAILABLE FORMS
Tablets: 400 mg

INDICATIONS & DOSAGES
Adjust-a-dose (for all indications): Sofosbuvir dosage reduction isn't recommended.
Discontinue sofosbuvir if concomitant antivirals are stopped. Adjust concomitant ribavirin or peginterferon alfa dosage if GFR
is less than 50 mL/minute or hepatic decompensation occurs. Refer to manufacturer's
instructions for ribavirin or peginterferon
alfa dosage adjustments.

➤ **Chronic HCV infection (genotype
1 or 4) with or without HIV coinfection,
as component of combination antiviral
regimen**
Adults: 400 mg P.O. daily with peginterferon
alfa and ribavirin for 12 weeks. For patients
with HCV genotype 1 who can't receive
interferon, give 400 mg P.O. daily with
ribavirin for 24 weeks.

➤ **Chronic HCV infection (genotype 2)
with or without HIV coinfection, as part
of combination antiviral regimen**
Adults: 400 mg P.O. daily with ribavirin for
12 weeks.

➤ **Chronic HCV infection (genotype 3)
with or without HIV coinfection, as part
of combination antiviral regimen**
Adults: 400 mg P.O. daily with ribavirin for
24 weeks.

➤ **Chronic HCV infection with hepatocellular carcinoma in patients awaiting
liver transplant**
Adults: 400 mg P.O. daily with ribavirin for
48 weeks or until liver transplant.

ADMINISTRATION
P.O.
● Give without regard for food.

ACTION
Inhibits HCV NS5B RNA polymerase,
inhibiting viral replication.

Route	Onset	Peak	Duration
P.O.	Unknown	0.5–2 hr	Unknown

Half-life: 0.4 hour.

ADVERSE REACTIONS
CNS: headache, insomnia, asthenia,
pyrexia, fatigue.
GI: nausea, diarrhea.
Hematologic: anemia, ***neutropenia.***
Metabolic: decreased appetite, chills.
Musculoskeletal: myalgia.
Skin: pruritus, rash.
Other: flulike illness, irritability.

INTERACTIONS
Drug-drug. ✪ *Alert: Amiodarone:* May
increase risk of symptomatic bradycardia,
including cardiac arrest and cases requiring
pacemaker intervention. Avoid use together.
If use together can't be avoided, advise
patient of risk and monitor carefully.
*Anticonvulsants (carbamazepine, oxcar-
bazepine, phenobarbital, phenytoin),
antimycobacterials (rifabutin, rifampin,
rifapentine), HIV protease inhibitors
(tipranavir, ritonavir):* May decrease sofosbuvir level. Avoid use together.
Drug-herb. *St. John's wort:* May decrease
sofosbuvir plasma concentration. Don't use
together.

EFFECTS ON LAB TEST RESULTS
● May increase CK, bilirubin, and lipase
levels.
● May decrease Hb level and neutrophil and
platelet counts.

CONTRAINDICATIONS & CAUTIONS
● Contraindicated in patients hypersensitive to drug or its components. When used
in combination with other drugs, the contraindications applicable to those agents also
apply to combination therapies.
Black Box Warning Reactivation of HBV
may occur in HCV coinfected patients and
result in fulminant hepatitis, hepatic failure,
and death. Screen all patients for current
or prior HBV infection before treatment;

if patient is positive for HBV infection, assess baseline HBV DNA. ■

🌢 *Alert:* Symptomatic bradycardia, including fatal cardiac arrest and cases requiring pacemaker intervention, has been reported when sofosbuvir is administered with amiodarone. Patients taking amiodarone who are also taking beta blockers or who have underlying cardiac comorbidities or advanced liver disease may be at increased risk. Signs and symptoms may occur within hours to up to 2 weeks after start of HCV therapy.

• Safety and effectiveness of drug haven't been studied in patients with estimated GFR of less than 30 mL/minute, ESRD, or decompensated cirrhosis.

• Using Sovaldi with other products containing sofosbuvir isn't recommended.

• Refer to prescribing information for peginterferon alfa and ribavirin for contraindications when drug is given in these combination regimens.

Dialyzable drug: 18%.

PREGNANCY-LACTATION-REPRODUCTION

• Contraindicated in pregnant women and in men whose female partners are pregnant. Obtain baseline negative pregnancy test before start of therapy.

• Women of childbearing potential and their male partners must use two forms of effective nonhormonal contraception while receiving treatment regimens that include ribavirin and for 6 months after therapy ends.

• Men whose partners are exposed to ribavirin through sexual intercourse while pregnant and pregnant women who are themselves exposed to ribavirin should enroll in the Ribavirin Pregnancy Registry (1-800-593-2214).

• Pregnant patients coinfected with HCV/HIV-1 who are taking concomitant antiretrovirals should enroll in the Antiretroviral Pregnancy Registry (1-800-258-4263).

• Contraindicated in breast-feeding women. Patients must discontinue breast-feeding or discontinue drug.

NURSING CONSIDERATIONS

• Sofosbuvir isn't recommended as monotherapy. Always use as part of combination regimen.

Black Box Warning Monitor patient with current or prior HBV infection for hepatitis flare or HBV reactivation with laboratory testing; watch for signs and symptoms of liver injury during active and posttreatment follow-up. ■

🌢 *Alert:* Monitor patients who must take amiodarone and those who must start amiodarone or who recently discontinued amiodarone for signs and symptoms of bradycardia (near-fainting or fainting, dizziness, light-headedness, malaise, weakness, excessive fatigue, shortness of breath, chest pain, confusion or memory problems). Inpatient cardiac monitoring should be utilized for first 48 hours, then outpatient monitoring or self-monitoring of HR for bradycardia should continue daily through at least first 2 weeks of treatment. Discontinue HCV treatment if signs or symptoms occur.

• Refer to ribavirin or peginterferon alfa prescribing information for complete guidance on their concomitant use.

• Monitor blood counts and bilirubin, liver enzyme, and serum creatinine levels at baseline and periodically when clinically indicated.

• Monitor serum HCV-RNA level at baseline, during treatment, at end of treatment, during treatment follow-up, and when clinically indicated.

• Obtain baseline negative pregnancy test before initiation of therapy and monthly thereafter until 6 months after treatment is discontinued.

• Treatment response varies based on patient and viral factors. Monitor patient carefully.

PATIENT TEACHING

• Advise patient that using drug as single agent isn't recommended. Sofosbuvir must always be used as part of combination regimen with ribavirin or peginterferon and ribavirin.

Black Box Warning Warn patient to immediately report signs and symptoms of liver injury (fatigue, weakness, loss of appetite, nausea, vomiting, yellowing of skin or eyes, light-colored stool). ■

● Teach patient to report signs and symptoms of hypersensitivity reaction (wheezing, chest tightness, fever, itching, heavy cough, blue-colored skin, seizures, or swelling of face, lips, tongue, or throat) and to seek medical attention.

◑ **Alert:** Caution patient to seek immediate medical attention for signs and symptoms of bradycardia.

● Instruct patient in risk of birth defects, contraception requirements, and pregnancy testing related to therapy.

● Teach patient to report all signs and symptoms of adverse reactions, such as headache, dyspepsia, and insomnia.

● Caution patient not to use other medications while taking this drug without first notifying prescriber.

● Advise patient to report liver problems (other than HCV infection), history of liver transplant, severe kidney problems or dialysis, positive HIV status, or other medical conditions.

● Warn female patient not to breast-feed while taking drug.

● Instruct patient not to discontinue drug without first discussing with prescriber.

---

sofosbuvir–velpatasvir
See NEW DRUGS for information.

---

solifenacin succinate
sole-ah-FEN-ah-sin

VESIcare✦

Therapeutic class: Urinary antispasmodics
Pharmacologic class: Antimuscarinics

AVAILABLE FORMS
Tablets (film-coated) ⊙⊙: 5 mg, 10 mg

INDICATIONS & DOSAGES
➤ **Overactive bladder with urinary urgency, frequency, and urge incontinence**
Adults: 5 mg P.O. once daily. May increase to 10 mg once daily if 5-mg dose is well tolerated.

Adjust-a-dose: If CrCl is less than 30 mL/minute or patient has moderate liver impairment (Child-Pugh class B), or if drug is taken concurrently with CYP3A4 inhibitors, maintain the dose at 5 mg.

ADMINISTRATION
P.O.
● Give drug without regard for food.
● Drug should be swallowed whole with liquid.

ACTION
Relaxes smooth muscle of bladder by antagonizing muscarinic receptors, relieving symptoms of overactive bladder.

Route	Onset	Peak	Duration
P.O.	Unknown	3–8 hr	Unknown

Half-life: About 45 to 68 hours.

ADVERSE REACTIONS
CNS: depression, dizziness, fatigue.
CV: hypertension, leg swelling.
EENT: blurred vision, dry eyes, pharyngitis.
GI: constipation, dry mouth, dyspepsia, nausea, upper abdominal pain, vomiting.
GU: urine retention, UTI.
Respiratory: cough.
Other: influenza.

INTERACTIONS
Drug-drug. *Drugs that prolong QT interval:* May increase risk of serious cardiac arrhythmias. Monitor patient and ECG closely.
Potent CYP3A4 inducers (carbamazepine, phenobarbital, phenytoin, rifampin): May decrease solifenacin concentration. Monitor effectiveness. Some drugs may be contraindicated.
Potent CYP3A4 inhibitors (ketoconazole): May increase solifenacin level. Don't exceed solifenacin dose of 5 mg daily when used together.

EFFECTS ON LAB TEST RESULTS
None reported.

CONTRAINDICATIONS & CAUTIONS
● Contraindicated in patients hypersensitive to drug or its components and in patients

---

with urine or gastric retention or uncontrolled narrow-angle glaucoma. Don't use in patients with severe hepatic impairment (Child-Pugh class C). Angioedema has been reported after first dose.

• Use cautiously in patients with a history of prolonged QT interval, those being treated for angle-closure glaucoma, and those with bladder outflow obstruction, decreased GI motility, renal insufficiency, or moderate liver impairment.

Dialyzable drug: Unknown.

⚠ *Overdose S&S:* Anticholinergic effects (fixed and dilated pupils, blurred vision, failure of heel-to-toe examination, tremors, dry skin).

PREGNANCY-LACTATION-REPRODUCTION

• There are no adequate studies in pregnant women. Use only if potential benefit justifies potential risk to the fetus.

• It isn't known if drug appears in breast milk. Patient should discontinue breastfeeding or discontinue drug.

NURSING CONSIDERATIONS

• Assess bladder function, and monitor drug effects.

• If patient has bladder outlet obstruction, watch for urine retention.

• Monitor patient for decreased gastric motility and constipation.

• Safety and effectiveness are similar in older and younger adults, but levels and half-life may be increased in the elderly.

• *Look alike–sound alike:* Don't confuse VESIcare with Vesanoid.

PATIENT TEACHING

• Explain that drug may cause blurred vision. Tell patient to use caution when performing hazardous activities or tasks that require clear vision until effects of the drug are known.

• Discourage use of other drugs that may cause dry mouth, constipation, urine retention, or blurred vision.

• Urge patient to report all adverse reactions, especially swelling in the face, lips, or tongue or abdominal pain or constipation that lasts 3 days or longer.

• Tell patient that drug decreases the ability to sweat normally, and advise cautious use

in hot environments or during strenuous activity.

• Tell patient to swallow tablet whole with liquid.

• Inform patient that drug may be taken with or without food.

somatropin
soe-ma-TROE-pin

Genotropin, Genotropin MiniQuick, Humatrope, Norditropin FlexPro, Nutropin AQ NuSpin, Nutropin AQ Pen, Omnitrope, Saizen, Serostim, Zomacton, Zorbtive

Therapeutic class: Growth hormones
Pharmacologic class: Anterior pituitary hormones

AVAILABLE FORMS

Genotropin injection: 5 mg and 12 mg in two-chamber cartridges

Genotropin MiniQuick injection: 0.2 mg/vial, 0.4 mg/vial, 0.6 mg/vial, 0.8 mg/vial, 1 mg/vial, 1.2 mg/vial, 1.4 mg/vial, 1.6 mg/vial, 1.8 mg/vial, 2 mg/vial

Humatrope injection: 5 mg (about 15 international units/vial), 6 mg (18 international units/cartridge), 12 mg (36 international units/cartridge), 24 mg (72 international units/cartridge)

Norditropin injection: 5 mg/1.5 mL, 10 mg/1.5 mL, 15 mg/1.5 mL, 30 mg/3 mL cartridges

Nutropin AQ injection: 5 mg (about 15 international units)/2-mL device, 10 mg (about 30 international units)/2-mL device or pen, 20 mg (about 60 international units)/2-mL device or pen

Omnitrope injection: 5.8 mg/vial, 5 mg/1.5 mL injection cartridge, 10 mg/1.5 mL injection cartridge

Saizen injection: 5 mg (about 15 international units/vial), 8.8 mg (about 26.4 international units/vial)

Serostim injection: 4 mg (about 12 international units/vial), 5 mg (about 15 international units/vial), 6 mg (about 18 international units/vial)

Zomacton* injection: 5-mg and 10-mg vials

S

Zorbtive injection: 8.8 mg (approximately 26.4 international units/vial)

INDICATIONS & DOSAGES

➤ **Long-term treatment of growth failure in children with inadequate secretion of endogenous growth hormone (GH)**

Children: 0.18 to 0.3 mg/kg/week Humatrope subcutaneously, divided equally and given six times weekly or once daily. Or, up to 0.3 mg/kg Nutropin AQ subcutaneously weekly in daily divided doses; in pubertal patients, a weekly dosage of up to 0.7 mg/kg (Nutropin AQ) in daily divided doses may be used. Or, Saizen 0.18 mg/kg/week subcutaneously divided into equal doses given on 3 alternate days, 6 times per week, or daily. Or, 0.024 to 0.034 mg/kg Norditropin subcutaneously six or seven times weekly. Or, 0.16 to 0.24 mg/kg Genotropin or Omnitrope subcutaneously weekly, divided into six or seven doses. Or, up to 0.1 mg/kg Zomacton subcutaneously three times per week (up to 0.3 mg/kg/week).

➤ **Growth failure from chronic renal insufficiency up to time of renal transplantation**

Children: Up to 0.35 mg/kg/week Nutropin AQ subcutaneously divided into daily doses.

➤ **Long-term treatment of short stature from Turner syndrome**

Children: Up to 0.375 mg/kg/week Humatrope or Nutropin AQ subcutaneously, divided into equal doses given three to seven times weekly. Or, up to 0.067 mg/kg/day Norditropin subcutaneously. Or, 0.33 mg/kg/week Genotropin or Omnitrope divided into six or seven once-daily subcutaneous injections per week.

➤ **Short stature in children with Noonan syndrome**

Children: Up to 0.066 mg/kg/day Norditropin subcutaneously.

➤ **Long-term treatment of growth failure in children with Prader-Willi syndrome diagnosed by genetic testing**

Children: 0.24 mg/kg Genotropin or Omnitrope subcutaneously weekly, divided into six or seven doses.

➤ **Replacement of endogenous GH in adult patients with GH deficiency**

Adults: Initially, not more than 0.006 mg/kg Humatrope or Nutropin AQ subcutaneously

daily. May be increased to maximum of 0.0125 mg/kg Humatrope daily. Or initially not more than 0.004 mg/kg or 0.15 to 0.3 mg Norditropin subcutaneously daily.

Nutropin AQ dosages may be increased to maximum of 0.025 mg/kg daily in patients younger than age 35 or 0.0125 mg/kg daily in patients older than age 35. Or, starting dosages not exceeding 0.04 mg/kg Genotropin or Omnitrope subcutaneously weekly, divided into six or seven doses, may be increased at 4- to 8-week intervals to a maximum dose of 0.08 mg/kg subcutaneously weekly, divided into six or seven doses. Initially, not more than 0.005 mg/kg Saizen daily. May increase after 4 weeks to a maximum dose of 0.01 mg/kg daily based on patient tolerance and clinical response. Norditropin may be increased to maximum of 0.016 mg/kg daily after about 6 weeks. Or increase by 0.1 to 0.2 mg/day every 1 to 2 months based on clinical response and insulin-like growth factor-1 concentration.

➤ **AIDS wasting or cachexia**

Adults and children weighing more than 55 kg: 6 mg Serostim subcutaneously at bedtime.

Adults and children weighing 45 to 55 kg: 5 mg Serostim subcutaneously at bedtime.

Adults and children weighing 35 to 45 kg: 4 mg Serostim subcutaneously at bedtime.

Adults and children weighing less than 35 kg: 0.1 mg/kg/day Serostim subcutaneously at bedtime.

➤ **Long-term treatment of growth failure in children born small for gestational age (SGA) who don't catch up by age 2**

Children: 0.48 mg/kg Genotropin or Omnitrope subcutaneously weekly, divided into six or seven doses.

➤ **Short stature in children born SGA who don't catch up by age 2 to 4**

Children: Up to 0.067 mg/kg/day Norditropin or Humatrope subcutaneously.

➤ **Idiopathic short stature**

Children: Up to 0.37 mg/kg Humatrope subcutaneously weekly, divided into six or seven equal doses. Or, up to 0.47 mg/kg/week Genotropin or Omnitrope subcutaneously, divided into six or seven equal doses.

> **Short bowel syndrome**
Adults: 0.1 mg/kg/day Zorbtive subcutaneously daily for 4 weeks. Maximum dosage, 8 mg/day.

ADMINISTRATION
• Refer to product insert for brand-specific reconstitution instructions.
I.M.
• To prepare solution, inject supplied diluent into vial containing drug by aiming stream of liquid against wall of glass vial. Then swirl vial gently until contents are completely dissolved. Don't shake vial.
• After reconstitution, make sure solution is clear. Don't inject solution if it's cloudy or contains particles.
• For patients on hemodialysis, give drug before bedtime or 3 to 4 hours after dialysis. For long-term cycling peritoneal dialysis, give drug in the morning after completion of dialysis. For long-term ambulatory peritoneal dialysis, give drug in the evening at the time of the overnight exchange.
• Store reconstituted drug in refrigerator; use within manufacturer's recommended time frame for each drug.
• If patient develops sensitivity to diluent, reconstitute drug with sterile water for injection. When drug is reconstituted in this way, use only one reconstituted dose per vial, refrigerate solution if it isn't used immediately after reconstitution, use reconstituted dose within 24 hours, and discard unused portion.
☉ Alert: When administering to newborn, reconstitute with sterile water for injection.
Subcutaneous
• To prepare solution, inject supplied diluent into vial containing drug by aiming stream of liquid against wall of glass vial. Then swirl vial gently until contents are completely dissolved. Don't shake vial.
☉ Alert: Don't use Zomacton 5-mg vials if patient has a known benzyl alcohol sensitivity.
• After reconstitution, make sure solution is clear. Don't inject solution if it's cloudy or contains particles.
• For patients on hemodialysis, give drug before bedtime or 3 to 4 hours after dialysis. For long-term cycling peritoneal dialysis, give drug in the morning after completion of dialysis. For long-term ambulatory peri-

toneal dialysis, give drug in the evening at the time of the overnight exchange.
• Rotate injection sites.
• Store reconstituted drug in refrigerator; use within manufacturer's recommended time frame for each drug.
• If patient develops sensitivity to diluent, reconstitute drug with sterile water for injection. When drug is reconstituted in this way, use only one reconstituted dose per vial, refrigerate solution if it isn't used immediately after reconstitution, use reconstituted dose within 24 hours, and discard unused portion.
☉ Alert: When administering to newborn, reconstitute with sterile water for injection.

ACTION
Purified GH of recombinant DNA origin that stimulates skeletal, linear, muscle, and organ growth.

Route	Onset	Peak	Duration
I.M., subcut.	Unknown	Varies by route and brand	18–20 hr

Half-life: Varies by route and brand. Refer to manufacturer's drug label.

ADVERSE REACTIONS
CNS: headache, weakness, paresthesia, fatigue.
CV: mild, transient edema; peripheral edema.
EENT: otitis media.
Hematologic: *leukemia.*
Metabolic: mild hyperglycemia, hypothyroidism.
Musculoskeletal: localized muscle pain, arthralgia, stiffness of extremities.
Respiratory: URI.
Skin: injection-site pain.
Other: antibodies to GH.

INTERACTIONS
Drug-drug. *Corticotropin, corticosteroids:* Long-term use may inhibit growth response to GH. Monitor patient for lack of effect.
Estrogen replacement: May decrease somatropin level in adult women. Increase somatropin dosage as necessary.
Insulin, oral antidiabetic agents: Somatropin may decrease insulin sensitivity. Antidiabetic agent dosage may need adjustment.

S

♣Canada   ◇OTC   ◆Off-label use   ✎Photoguide   ⓞ Do not crush   *Liquid contains alcohol.

EFFECTS ON LAB TEST RESULTS

- May increase glucose, serum phosphorus, alkaline phosphatase, and parathyroid hormone levels.

CONTRAINDICATIONS & CAUTIONS

- Contraindicated in patients with hypersensitivity to somatropin or its excipients.
- Contraindicated in patients with closed epiphyses, active proliferative or severe nonproliferative diabetic retinopathy, or an active underlying intracranial lesion.
- Contraindicated in patients with active malignancy. An increased risk of second neoplasm has been reported in childhood cancer survivors treated with somatropin. Patients with HIV and children with short stature (genetic cause) have increased baseline risk of developing malignancies. Consider risk and benefits before initiating therapy; monitor these patients carefully.
- Contraindicated in patients with Prader-Willi syndrome who are severely obese, have a history of upper airway obstruction or sleep apnea, or have severe respiratory impairment.
- For patients hypersensitive to either metacresol or glycerin, don't use supplied diluent to reconstitute Humatrope.
- Don't begin therapy in patients with acute critical illness due to complications following open heart or abdominal surgery, trauma, or acute respiratory failure.
- Use cautiously in children with hypothyroidism and in those with GH deficiency caused by intracranial lesion.
- Use cautiously in patients with diabetes.
- May increase risk of pancreatitis. Monitor patient for persistent abdominal pain with or without vomiting.

Dialyzable drug: Unknown.

⚠ *Overdose S&S:* Fluid retention, hypoglycemia followed by hyperglycemia, glucose intolerance, gigantism, acromegaly.

PREGNANCY-LACTATION-REPRODUCTION

- There are no adequate studies in pregnant women. Use only if clearly needed.
- It isn't known if drug appears in breast milk. Use cautiously in breast-feeding women.

NURSING CONSIDERATIONS

- Frequently examine children with hypothyroidism and those whose GH deficiency is caused by an intracranial lesion for progression or recurrence of underlying disease.
- ✪ *Alert:* In patients with Prader-Willi syndrome who are morbidly obese and in those with a history of respiratory impairment, sleep apnea, or unidentified respiratory infection, therapy may be life-threatening. Assess patients with Prader-Willi syndrome for sleep apnea and upper airway obstruction before treatment. Interrupt treatment if signs of upper airway obstruction occur.
- Monitor patient with Prader-Willi syndrome for signs of respiratory infection.
- Monitor child's height regularly. Regular checkups, including monitoring of blood and radiologic studies, are also needed.
- Monitor patient's glucose level regularly because GH may induce a state of insulin resistance or new-onset diabetes mellitus.
- Excessive glucocorticoid therapy inhibits somatropin's growth-promoting effect. Patients with coexisting corticotropin deficiency should have their glucocorticoid replacement dosage carefully adjusted to avoid growth inhibition.
- Watch for slipped capital femoral epiphysis or progression of scoliosis in patients with rapid growth.
- Monitor results of periodic thyroid function tests for hypothyroidism; condition may need thyroid hormone treatment.
- Patient should have ophthalmic examinations to monitor for intracranial hypertension before therapy (to establish baseline) and periodically thereafter.
- Monitor patients with preexisting tumors or growth failure secondary to an intracranial lesion for recurrence or progression of underlying disease; discontinue therapy with evidence of recurrence.
- Monitor all patients for increased growth, or potential malignant changes, of skin lesions.
- Only adults with GH deficiency alone or together with multiple hormone deficiencies from pituitary or hypothalamic disease, surgery, radiation, or trauma or those who were GH deficient as children and have been

---

confirmed GH deficient as adults can take Saizen.
● **Look alike–sound alike:** Don't confuse somatropin with somatrem or sumatriptan.

PATIENT TEACHING
● Inform parents that child with endocrine disorders (including GH deficiency) may have an increased risk of slipped capital epiphyses. Tell parents to notify prescriber if they notice their child limping.
● Instruct patients with diabetes to monitor glucose level closely and report changes to prescriber.
● Instruct patient or parents in appropriate injection technique and needle disposal. Tell them to rotate injection sites.
● Stress importance of close follow-up care and of reporting all adverse reactions.

sotalol hydrochloride
SOH-ta-lol

Betapace, Betapace AF, Sorine, Sotylize

Therapeutic class: Antiarrhythmics
Pharmacologic class: Nonselective beta blockers

AVAILABLE FORMS
Solution for injection: 15 mg/mL
Betapace
Tablets: 80 mg, 120 mg, 160 mg, 240 mg
Betapace AF
Tablets: 80 mg, 120 mg, 160 mg
Sorine
Tablets: 80 mg, 120 mg, 160 mg, 240 mg
Sotylize
Oral solution: 5 mg/mL

INDICATIONS & DOSAGES
▪**Black Box Warning** Calculate CrCl before dosing. Don't initiate therapy with I.V. sotalol or oral solution if baseline QTc is longer than 450 msec. ▪
▪**Black Box Warning** Don't substitute sotalol for sotalol AF. ▪
➤ **Documented, life-threatening ventricular arrhythmias (Betapace, Sorine, Sotylize)**

Adults: Initially, 80 mg P.O. b.i.d. Increase dosage gradually (increments of 80 mg/day for Sotylize) every 3 days as needed and tolerated. Most patients respond to 160 to 320 mg/day, although some patients with refractory arrhythmias need up to 640 mg/day. Or, 75 mg I.V. once daily or b.i.d. based on CrCl. After 3 days, dosage may be increased to 75 to 150 mg I.V. once daily or every 12 hours based on CrCl. For refractory life-threatening arrhythmias, dosage may be increased to 225 to 300 mg I.V. once daily or every 12 hours.
Children age 2 and older with normal renal function: Initially, 30 mg/m² P.O. t.i.d. Titrate dosage to a maximum of 60 mg/m² (equivalent to 360 mg total daily dose for adults). Guide titration by clinical response, HR, and QTc interval. Allow at least 36 hours between dose increments.
Children younger than age 2 with normal renal function: Initially, 30 mg/m² P.O. t.i.d. multiplied by age factor plotted on a logarithmic scale found in manufacturer's instructions.
Adjust-a-dose: Adults: For oral route, if CrCl is 30 to 60 mL/minute, increase dosage interval to every 24 hours; if CrCl is 10 to 29 mL/minute, increase interval to every 36 to 48 hours; and if CrCl is less than 10 mL/minute, individualize dosage. For I.V. route, if CrCl is 40 to 59 mL/minute, give I.V. drug once daily; don't give if CrCl is less than 40 mL/minute.
Children: Use in any age-group with decreased renal function should be at lower dosages or at increased intervals between doses. Use of sotalol in children with renal impairment hasn't been investigated. Use with particular caution in children if QTc interval is greater than 500 msec on therapy; seriously consider reducing dosage or discontinuing therapy when QTc interval exceeds 550 msec.
➤ **To maintain normal sinus rhythm or to delay recurrence of atrial fibrillation or atrial flutter in patients with symptomatic atrial fibrillation or flutter who are currently in sinus rhythm (Betapace AF, Sotylize, sotalol I.V.)**
Adults: 80 mg P.O. b.i.d. (Don't use if baseline QT interval is greater than 450 msec.) Increase dosage as needed to 120 mg P.O.

S

b.i.d. after 3 days if the QTc interval is less than 500 msec. Maximum dose is 160 mg P.O. b.i.d. Or, 75 mg I.V. once daily or every 12 hours based on CrCl. After 3 days, dosage may be increased to 112.5 to 150 mg I.V. once daily or every 12 hours based on clearance.

Children age 2 and older with normal renal function: Initially, 30 mg/m^2 P.O. t.i.d. Titrate dosage to a maximum of 60 mg/m^2 (equivalent to 360 mg total daily dose for adults). Guide titration by clinical response, HR, and QTc interval. Allow at least 36 hours between dose increments.

Children younger than age 2 with normal renal function: Initially, 30 mg/m^2 P.O. t.i.d. multiplied by age factor plotted on a logarithmic scale found in manufacturer's instructions.

Adjust-a-dose: *Adults:* For oral route, if CrCl is 40 to 60 mL/minute, increase dosage interval to every 24 hours; if CrCl is less than 40 mL/minute, use is contraindicated. For I.V. route, if CrCl is 40 to 59 mL/minute, give I.V. drug once daily; don't give if CrCl is less than 40 mL/minute.

Children: Use in any age-group with decreased renal function should be at lower dosages or at increased intervals between doses. Use of sotalol in children with renal impairment hasn't been investigated. Use with particular caution in children if QTc interval is greater than 500 msec on therapy; seriously consider reducing dosage or discontinuing therapy when QTc interval exceeds 550 msec.

ADMINISTRATION

P.O.

● Give 1 hour before or 2 hours after antacids.

● May give without regard for food, but patient should take the same way each time.

I.V.

▼ Dilute drug with NSS, D$_5$W, or lactated Ringer solution in a volume of 120 to 300 mL to compensate for dead space in the infusion set.

▼ Use an infusion pump to administer drug at a constant rate over 5 hours.

ACTION

Depresses sinus HR, slows AV conduction, decreases cardiac output, and lowers systolic and diastolic BP. Drug also has class III antiarrhythmic properties and can prolong duration of the cardiac action potential.

Route	Onset	Peak	Duration
P.O.	1–2 hr	2–4 hr	Unknown
I.V.	5–10 min	Unknown	Unknown

Half-life: Adults, 12 hours; children, 9½ hours.

ADVERSE REACTIONS

CNS: asthenia, headache, dizziness, weakness, fatigue, light-headedness, sleep problems, anxiety, confusion, paresthesia, mood changes, fever.

EENT: visual disturbance.

CV: chest pain, palpitations, ***bradycardia, arrhythmias, HF, AV block, proarrhythmic events (including polymorphic ventricular tachycardia, PVCs, ventricular fibrillation)***, edema, ECG abnormalities, hypotension.

GI: nausea, vomiting, diarrhea, dyspepsia, abdominal pain.

GU: erectile dysfunction.

Metabolic: hyperglycemia, decreased appetite.

Musculoskeletal: pain.

Respiratory: dyspnea, URI, ***bronchospasm.***

Skin: hyperhidrosis, rash.

Other: infection, influenza.

INTERACTIONS

Drug-drug. *Antacids containing aluminum oxide and magnesium hydroxide:* May reduce bradycardic effect. Avoid sotalol administration within 2 hours of antacid.

Antiarrhythmics: May increase drug effects. Avoid using together.

Antihypertensives, catecholamine-depleting drugs (guanethidine, reserpine): May increase hypotensive effects or cause marked bradycardia. Monitor BP and pulse closely.

Calcium channel blockers: May increase myocardial depression. Avoid using together.

Clonidine: May enhance rebound effect after withdrawal of clonidine. Stop sotalol several days before withdrawing clonidine.

Reactions in bold italics are *life-threatening*. Interactions may have a *rapid onset* or a ***delayed onset***.

Drugs that prolong the QT interval (class I and III antiarrhythmics, bepridil, phenothiazines, TCAs): May cause excessive QT prolongation. Monitor QT interval.

General anesthetics: May increase myocardial depression. Monitor patient closely.

Insulin, oral antidiabetics: May cause hyperglycemia and may mask signs and symptoms of hypoglycemia. Adjust dosage accordingly.

Macrolides and related antibiotics (azithromycin, clarithromycin, erythromycin, telithromycin), quinolones, TCAs: May cause additive effects or prolong the QT interval. Use with caution. Avoid use with telithromycin.

Prazosin: May increase the risk of orthostatic hypotension. Assist patient to stand slowly until effects are known.

Theophylline: May decrease bronchodilating effects. Avoid using together.

Drug-lifestyle. *Cocaine:* May increase cardiotoxic effects of cocaine. Don't use with cocaine-associated myocardial ischemia or infarction.

EFFECTS ON LAB TEST RESULTS
• May increase glucose level.
• May cause false-positive catecholamine level.

CONTRAINDICATIONS & CAUTIONS
• Contraindicated in patients hypersensitive to drug.
• Contraindicated in those with severe sinus node dysfunction, sinus bradycardia, second- and third-degree AV block unless patient has a pacemaker, congenital or acquired long QT-interval syndrome, cardiogenic shock, uncontrolled HF, CrCl of less than 40 mL/minute, serum potassium level of less than 4 mEq/L, and bronchial asthma.
• Contraindicated in patients with hypomagnesemia before correction of imbalance.
Black Box Warning Sotalol can cause life-threatening ventricular tachycardia associated with QT-interval prolongation. ∎
• Use cautiously in patients with renal impairment or diabetes mellitus (beta blockers may mask signs and symptoms of hypoglycemia).

Dialyzable drug: Yes.

⚠ *Overdose S&S:* Bradycardia, bronchospasm, HF, hypoglycemia, hypotension, asystole, QT-interval prolongation, torsades de pointes, ventricular tachycardia, death.

PREGNANCY-LACTATION-REPRODUCTION
• There are no adequate studies in pregnant women. Use only if potential benefit justifies potential risk to the fetus. Drug crosses placental barrier and appears in amniotic fluid.
• Drug appears in breast milk. Patient should discontinue breast-feeding or discontinue drug.

NURSING CONSIDERATIONS
Black Box Warning Because proarrhythmic events may occur at the start of therapy and during dosage adjustments, patients should be hospitalized for a minimum of 3 days in a facility that can provide calculations of CrCl, continuous ECG monitoring, and cardiac resuscitation. Calculate CrCl before dosing. ∎
Black Box Warning The baseline QTc interval must be less than or equal to 450 msec before starting sotalol I.V. or oral suspension. If QT interval is 500 msec or more, dosage or frequency must be decreased or drug discontinued. ∎
• Assess patient for new or worsened symptoms of HF.
• Although patients receiving I.V. lidocaine may start sotalol therapy without ill effects, withdraw other antiarrhythmics before therapy begins. Sotalol therapy typically is delayed until two or three half-lives of the withdrawn drug have elapsed. After withdrawing amiodarone, give sotalol only after QT interval normalizes.
• Adjust dosage slowly, allowing 3 days between dosage increments for adequate monitoring of QT intervals and for drug levels to reach a steady-state level.
• Monitor electrolytes regularly, especially if patient is receiving diuretics. Electrolyte imbalances, such as hypokalemia or hypomagnesemia, may enhance QT-interval prolongation and increase the risk of serious arrhythmias such as torsades de pointes.
• *Look alike–sound alike:* Don't confuse sotalol with Sudafed.

S

PATIENT TEACHING

• Explain to patient that he will need to be hospitalized for initiation of drug therapy.
• Stress need to take drug as prescribed, even when he is feeling well. Caution patient against stopping drug suddenly.
• Caution patient against using OTC drugs and decongestants while taking drug.
• Advise patient to take drug consistently with or without food.
• Because antacids can interfere with absorption, tell patient to take drug 2 hours before or after antacids.
• Warn patient not to double the next dose if a dose is missed.

---

spironolactone
speer-on-oh-LAK-tone

Aldactone✇

Therapeutic class: Diuretics
Pharmacologic class: Potassium-sparing diuretics–aldosterone receptor antagonists

AVAILABLE FORMS
Tablets: 25 mg, 50 mg, 100 mg

INDICATIONS & DOSAGES
Black Box Warning Use spironolactone only for those conditions for which it's indicated. Drug has been shown to be tumorigenic in long-term toxicity studies in rats. Avoid unnecessary use. ■
➤ **Edema due to HF, hepatic cirrhosis, or nephrotic syndrome**
Adults: Initially, 100 mg P.O. daily given as a single dose or in divided doses. Usual range is 25 to 200 mg P.O. daily.
➤ **Hypertension**
Adults: 50 to 100 mg P.O. daily or in divided doses. Some practitioners use a lower dosage range of 25 to 50 mg daily and add another antihypertensive to the regimen, rather than continually increasing this drug.
➤ **Diuretic-induced hypokalemia**
Adults: 25 to 100 mg P.O. daily.
➤ **To detect primary hyperaldosteronism**
Adults: 400 mg P.O. daily for 4 days (short test) or 3 to 4 weeks (long test). If hypokalemia and hypertension are corrected, a presumptive diagnosis of primary hyperaldosteronism is made.
➤ **To manage primary hyperaldosteronism**
Adults: 100 to 400 mg P.O. daily. Use lowest effective dose.
➤ **Severe HF (class III or IV), as adjunct to ACE inhibitor or loop diuretic, with or without cardiac glycoside**
Adults: 25 mg P.O. daily if serum potassium level is 5 mEq/L or less and serum creatinine level is 2.5 mg/dL or less. May increase to 50 mg P.O. daily as clinically indicated.
Adjust-a-dose: Patients who don't tolerate 25 mg daily may have dosage decreased to every other day.

ADMINISTRATION
P.O.
• To enhance absorption, give drug with meals.
• Give drug in morning to prevent nocturia. If second dose is needed, give it with food in early afternoon.
• Protect tablets from light.

ACTION
Antagonizes aldosterone in the distal tubules, increasing sodium and water excretion.

Route	Onset	Peak	Duration
P.O.	Unknown	3–4 hr	2–3 days

Half-life: 1¼ hours.

ADVERSE REACTIONS
CNS: headache, drowsiness, lethargy, confusion, ataxia.
GI: diarrhea, *gastric bleeding*, ulceration, cramping, gastritis, vomiting.
GU: inability to maintain erection, menstrual disturbances.
Hematologic: *agranulocytosis.*
Metabolic: *hyperkalemia,* dehydration, hyponatremia, mild acidosis.
Skin: urticaria, hirsutism, maculopapular eruptions.
Other: *anaphylaxis,* gynecomastia, breast soreness, drug fever.

Reactions in bold italics are *life-threatening*. Interactions may have a *rapid onset* or a *delayed onset*.

INTERACTIONS

Drug-drug. *ACE inhibitors, ARBs:* May increase risk of severe hyperkalemia. Use together with caution.

Anticoagulants: May decrease anticoagulant effects. Monitor PT and INR.

Aspirin and other salicylates: May block diuretic effect of spironolactone. Watch for diminished spironolactone response.

Digoxin: May alter digoxin clearance, increasing risk of toxicity. Monitor digoxin level.

⊘ Alert: *Eplerenone:* May increase risk of severe hyperkalemia. Use together is contraindicated.

Lithium: May reduce lithium renal clearance and increase risk of lithium toxicity. Monitor patient closely.

NSAIDs, potassium-sparing diuretics, potassium supplements: May result in hyperkalemia. Avoid use together.

Drug-herb. *Licorice:* May block ulcer-healing and aldosterone-like effects of herb; may increase risk of hypokalemia. Discourage use together.

Drug-food. *Potassium-rich foods, such as citrus fruits and tomatoes, salt substitutes containing potassium:* May increase risk of hyperkalemia. Urge caution.

EFFECTS ON LAB TEST RESULTS

- May increase BUN and potassium levels. May decrease sodium level.
- May decrease granulocyte count.
- May alter fluorometric determinations of plasma and urinary 17-hydroxycorticosteroid levels.

CONTRAINDICATIONS & CAUTIONS

- Contraindicated in patients hypersensitive to drug and in those with anuria, acute or progressive renal insufficiency, Addison disease, or hyperkalemia.
- Use cautiously in patients with fluid or electrolyte imbalances and in those with impaired renal or hepatic function.
- Safety and effectiveness in children haven't been established.

⚠ Overdose S&S: Drowsiness, confusion, rash, nausea, vomiting, dizziness, diarrhea, hyperkalemia.

PREGNANCY-LACTATION-REPRODUCTION

- Use of diuretics to treat edema during normal pregnancies isn't appropriate. Drug may cause fetal harm because of its antiandrogenic activity; avoid use in the first trimester. Use during pregnancy only if clearly needed and potential benefit justifies potential risk to the fetus.
- A major metabolite of drug appears in breast milk. Patient should discontinue breast-feeding or discontinue drug, taking into account importance of drug to the mother.

NURSING CONSIDERATIONS

- Monitor electrolyte levels, fluid intake and output, weight, and BP.
- Monitor elderly patients closely, who are more susceptible to excessive diuresis.
- Inform laboratory that patient is taking spironolactone because drug may interfere with tests that measure digoxin level.
- Drug is less potent than thiazide and loop diuretics and is useful as an adjunct to other diuretic therapy. Diuretic effect is delayed 2 to 3 days when used alone.
- Maximum antihypertensive response may be delayed for up to 2 weeks.
- Watch for hyperchloremic metabolic acidosis, especially in patients with hepatic cirrhosis.
- **Look alike–sound alike:** Don't confuse Aldactone with Aldactazide.

PATIENT TEACHING

- Instruct patient to take drug in morning to prevent need to urinate at night. If second dose is needed, tell him to take it with food in early afternoon.
- **⊘ Alert:** To prevent serious hyperkalemia, warn patient to avoid excessive ingestion of potassium-rich foods (such as citrus fruits, tomatoes, bananas, dates, and apricots), salt substitutes containing potassium, and potassium supplements.
- Caution patient not to perform hazardous activities if adverse CNS reactions occur.
- Advise patient about possible breast tenderness or enlargement.

stavudine (2′ 3′-didehydro-3-deoxythymidine, d4T)
STAV-yoo-deen

Zerit

Therapeutic class: Antiretrovirals
Pharmacologic class: Nucleosides–nucleotide reverse transcriptase inhibitors

AVAILABLE FORMS
Capsules: 15 mg, 20 mg, 30 mg, 40 mg
Oral solution: 1 mg/mL

INDICATIONS & DOSAGES
➤ **HIV infection, with other antiretrovirals**
Adults weighing 60 kg or more: 40 mg P.O. every 12 hours.
Adults weighing less than 60 kg: 30 mg P.O. every 12 hours.
Children weighing 60 kg or more: 40 mg P.O. every 12 hours.
Children weighing 30 to 60 kg: 30 mg P.O. every 12 hours.
Neonates age 14 days and older and children weighing less than 30 kg: 1 mg/kg P.O. every 12 hours.
Neonates age 13 days and younger: 0.5 mg/kg P.O. every 12 hours.
Adjust-a-dose: For patients experiencing peripheral neuropathy, stop therapy and consider permanent discontinuation. For adults with CrCl of 26 to 50 mL/minute, adjust dosage to 20 mg (if weight exceeds 60 kg) or 15 mg (if weight is less than 60 kg) P.O. every 12 hours; if CrCl is 10 to 25 mL/minute or in adults undergoing dialysis, 20 mg (if weight exceeds 60 kg) or 15 mg (if weight is less than 60 kg) P.O. every 24 hours. There are insufficient data to recommend a specific dosage adjustment in children.

ADMINISTRATION
P.O.
● Give drug without regard for meals.
● Reconstitute oral solution with 202 mL of purified water. Shake solution well before giving.
● Give drug after hemodialysis on hemodialysis treatment days.
● Discard unused solution after 30 days.

ACTION
A thymidine nucleoside analogue that prevents replication of retroviruses, including HIV, by inhibiting the enzyme reverse transcriptase and causing termination of DNA chain growth.

Route	Onset	Peak	Duration
P.O.	Unknown	1 hr	Unknown

Half-life: 1 to 2 hours.

ADVERSE REACTIONS
CNS: asthenia, fever, anxiety, headache, insomnia, malaise, motor weakness, nervousness, peripheral neuropathy.
GI: abdominal pain, anorexia, diarrhea, nausea, vomiting, *pancreatitis.*
Hematologic: *neutropenia, thrombocytopenia,* anemia.
Hepatic: *hepatotoxicity,* severe hepatomegaly with steatosis.
Metabolic: *lactic acidosis,* lipodystrophy, lipoatrophy, weight loss, diabetes mellitus, hyperglycemia.
Musculoskeletal: myalgia.
Respiratory: dyspnea.
Skin: pruritus, rash.
Other: chills.

INTERACTIONS
Drug-drug. *Didanosine, hydroxyurea:* Coadministration may increase risk for lactic acidosis, hepatotoxicity, pancreatitis, or peripheral neuropathy. Consider therapy modification.
Doxorubicin, ribavirin: May decrease effectiveness of stavudine. Use together cautiously.
Zidovudine: May inhibit phosphorylation of stavudine. Avoid using together.

EFFECTS ON LAB TEST RESULTS
● May increase amylase, lipase, bilirubin, ALT, and AST levels. May decrease Hb level.
● May decrease neutrophil and platelet count.

Reactions in bold italics are *life-threatening*. Interactions may have a *rapid onset* or a *delayed onset*.

CONTRAINDICATIONS & CAUTIONS

• Contraindicated in patients hypersensitive to drug.

Black Box Warning Lactic acidosis and severe hepatomegaly with steatosis, including fatal cases, have been reported. ∎

Black Box Warning Fatal and nonfatal cases of pancreatitis have occurred in combination therapy with didanosine. ∎

• Use cautiously in patients with renal impairment or history of peripheral neuropathy. Adjust dosage for CrCl of less than 50 mL/minute; stop drug in patients with peripheral neuropathy.

Dialyzable drug: Yes.

⚠ *Overdose S&S:* Peripheral neuropathy, hepatotoxicity.

PREGNANCY-LACTATION-REPRODUCTION

Black Box Warning Use cautiously in pregnant women and only if potential benefit clearly outweighs potential risk; fatal lactic acidosis may occur in pregnant women who receive stavudine and didanosine with other antiretrovirals. ∎

• Register patients in the Antiretroviral Pregnancy Registry (1-800-258-4263).

• The CDC recommends that mothers infected with HIV-1 not breast-feed, to avoid risking postnatal transmission of HIV-1.

NURSING CONSIDERATIONS

Black Box Warning Due to increased risk of pancreatic toxicity, monitor patient for signs and symptoms of pancreatitis, especially if he takes stavudine with didanosine. ∎

🔷 *Alert:* Hepatotoxicity and fatal hepatic failure have been reported in patients treated with hydroxyurea and other antiretrovirals. Fatal hepatic events were most often reported in patients treated with combination of hydroxyurea, didanosine, and stavudine. Avoid using together and monitor LFTs.

🔷 *Alert:* Motor weakness mimicking the signs and symptoms of Guillain-Barré syndrome (including respiratory failure) in HIV patients taking stavudine with other antiretrovirals may occur, especially in patients with lactic acidosis. Monitor patient for characteristics of lactic acidosis, including generalized fatigue, GI problems, tachypnea, and dyspnea. Patients with these symptoms should promptly interrupt an-

tiretroviral therapy and rapidly receive a full medical workup. Consider permanently stopping drug. Symptoms may continue or worsen when drug is stopped.

• Monitor patient for lipoatrophy and lipodystrophy, and consider the risk and benefit of treatment.

🔷 *Alert:* Peripheral neuropathy may be the major dose-limiting adverse effect; it may or may not resolve after drug is stopped.

• Monitor CBC results and creatinine.

PATIENT TEACHING

• Tell patient that drug may be taken without regard to meals.

• Warn patient not to take other drugs for HIV or AIDS unless prescriber has approved them.

• Inform patient that drug doesn't cure HIV infection, that opportunistic infections and other complications of HIV infection may still occur, and that transmission of HIV to others through sexual contact or blood contamination is still possible.

• Teach patient signs and symptoms of peripheral neuropathy (pain, burning, aching, weakness, or pins and needles in the limbs), and tell him to report these immediately.

• Tell patient to report symptoms of lactic acidosis, including fatigue, GI problems, dyspnea, or tachypnea.

• Tell patient to report symptoms of pancreatitis, including abdominal pain, nausea, vomiting, weight loss, or fatty stools.

• Tell patient to monitor weight patterns and report weight loss or gain.

• Tell patient to discard unused solution after 30 days.

SAFETY ALERT!

succinylcholine chloride (suxamethonium chloride)
SUK-seh-nil-KOH-leen

Anectine, Quelicin

Therapeutic class: Skeletal muscle relaxants
Pharmacologic class: Depolarizing neuromuscular blockers

AVAILABLE FORMS
Injection: 20 mg/mL

INDICATIONS & DOSAGES

➤ **Adjunct to anesthesia to facilitate tracheal intubation; to provide skeletal muscle relaxation during surgery or mechanical ventilation**

Adults: 0.6 mg/kg I.V. given over 10 to 30 seconds. Dosage range is 0.3 to 1.1 mg/kg. For longer response, give 1 mg/mL solution as a continuous infusion at 0.5 to 10 mg/minute, or give an initial I.V. injection of 0.3 to 1.1 mg/kg followed by further injections of 0.04 to 0.07 mg/kg, as needed, to maintain relaxation. Or, 3 to 4 mg/kg I.M. Maximum I.M. dose is 150 mg.

Children: 1 to 2 mg/kg I.V. or 3 to 4 mg/kg I.M. Maximum I.M. dose is 150 mg.

ADMINISTRATION

I.V.

▼ Only staff skilled in airway management should use drug.

▼ Give test dose of 5 to 10 mg after patient has been anesthetized. If no respiratory depression occurs or transient depression lasts for up to 5 minutes, then patient can metabolize drug, and it is safe to continue. Don't give if patient develops respiratory paralysis sufficient to need endotracheal intubation. (Recovery should occur within 30 to 60 minutes.)

▼ Use within 24 hours after reconstitution.

▼ Store injectable form in refrigerator.

▼ **Incompatibilities:** Alkaline solutions, barbiturates, nafcillin, sodium bicarbonate, solutions with pH above 8.5, thiopental sodium.

I.M.

● Inject deeply, preferably high into deltoid muscle. Use I.M. route only when I.V. access isn't available.

● Store injectable form in refrigerator.

ACTION

Binds with a high affinity to cholinergic receptors, prolonging depolarization of the motor end plate and ultimately producing muscle paralysis.

Route	Onset	Peak	Duration
I.V.	30–60 sec	1–2 min	4–6 min
I.M.	2–3 min	Unknown	Unknown

Half-life: Unknown.

ADVERSE REACTIONS

CV: *arrhythmias, bradycardia, cardiac arrest,* tachycardia, hypertension, hypotension, flushing.

EENT: increased IOP.

GI: excessive salivation.

Metabolic: *hyperkalemia.*

Musculoskeletal: postoperative muscle pain, muscle fasciculation, jaw rigidity, *rhabdomyolysis with acute renal failure.*

Respiratory: *apnea, bronchoconstriction, prolonged respiratory depression.*

Skin: rash.

Other: allergic or idiosyncratic hypersensitivity reactions, *anaphylaxis, malignant hyperthermia.*

INTERACTIONS

Drug-drug. *Aminoglycosides, anticholinesterases (echothiophate, edrophonium, neostigmine, physostigmine, pyridostigmine), aprotinin, general anesthetics (enflurane, halothane, isoflurane), glucocorticoids, hormonal contraceptives, lidocaine, lithium, magnesium, metoclopramide, oxytocin, polymyxin antibiotics (colistin, polymyxin B sulfate), procainamide, quinine:* May enhance neuromuscular blockade, increasing skeletal muscle relaxation and potentiating effect. Use together cautiously during and after surgery.

Cardiac glycosides: May cause arrhythmias. Use together cautiously.

Cyclophosphamide, lithium, MAO inhibitors: May enhance neuromuscular blockade and prolong apnea. Use together cautiously.

Opioid analgesics: May enhance neuromuscular blockade, increasing skeletal muscle relaxation and possibly causing respiratory paralysis. Use together cautiously.

Parenteral magnesium sulfate: May enhance neuromuscular blockade, may increase skeletal muscle relaxation, and may cause respiratory paralysis. Use together cautiously, preferably at reduced doses.

EFFECTS ON LAB TEST RESULTS

● May increase myoglobin and potassium levels.

Reactions in bold italics are *life-threatening*. Interactions may have a *rapid onset* or a *delayed onset*.

CONTRAINDICATIONS & CAUTIONS

● Contraindicated in patients hypersensitive to drug and in those with personal or family history of malignant hyperthermia.
● Contraindicated in patients with skeletal muscle myopathies and after the acute phase of injury following acute major burns, multiple trauma, skeletal muscle denervation, or upper motor neuron injury.
● Drug increases IOP. Use only when potential benefit outweighs potential risk when an increase in IOP is undesirable, such as in narrow-angle glaucoma or penetrating eye injury.
● Use carefully in patients with reduced plasma cholinesterase activity due to risk of prolonged neuromuscular block. Plasma cholinesterase activity may be diminished in the presence of genetic abnormalities of plasma cholinesterase, pregnancy, severe liver or kidney disease, malignant tumors, infections, burns, anemia, decompensated heart disease, peptic ulcer, myxedema, and certain drugs and chemicals.
● Use cautiously in elderly or debilitated patients; in patients receiving quinidine or cardiac glycoside therapy; in patients with hepatic, renal, or pulmonary impairment; and in those with respiratory depression, severe burns or trauma, electrolyte imbalances, hyperkalemia, paraplegia, spinal CNS injury, stroke, degenerative or dystrophic neuromuscular disease, myasthenia gravis, myasthenic syndrome related to lung cancer, dehydration, thyroid disorders, collagen diseases, porphyria, fractures, muscle spasms, dislocations, eye surgery, and pheochromocytoma.
Dialyzable drug: Unknown.
⚠ **Overdose S&S:** Prolonged neuromuscular blockade.

PREGNANCY-LACTATION-REPRODUCTION

● There are no adequate studies in pregnant women. Use during pregnancy only if clearly needed.
● Use large doses cautiously in patients undergoing cesarean section.
● It isn't known if drug appears in breast milk. Use cautiously in breast-feeding women.

NURSING CONSIDERATIONS

● Drug has no known effect on consciousness, pain threshold, or cerebration. To avoid patient distress, don't induce neuromuscular blockade before unconsciousness.
● Dosage depends on anesthetic used, individual needs, and response. Recommended dosages must be individually adjusted.
Black Box Warning Drug may cause acute rhabdomyolysis with hyperkalemia followed by ventricular arrhythmias, cardiac arrest, and death after administration to apparently healthy children who have undiagnosed skeletal muscle myopathy, most frequently Duchenne muscular dystrophy. Institute treatment for hyperkalemia when a healthy-appearing infant or child develops cardiac arrest soon after administration of succinylcholine. In children, drug should be reserved for use in emergency intubation, for instances when securing the airway is necessary, or for I.M. use when a suitable vein is inaccessible. ■
● Children may be less sensitive to drug than adults.
● May cause a transient increase in ICP, and may increase intragastric pressure, which could result in regurgitation and possible aspiration of stomach contents.
● Monitor baseline electrolyte determinations and vital signs. Check respirations every 5 to 10 minutes during infusion.
● Monitor respirations closely until tests of muscle strength (hand grip, head lift, and ability to cough) indicate full recovery from neuromuscular blockade.
🕓 **Alert:** Don't use reversing drugs. Unlike nondepolarizing drugs, neostigmine or edrophonium may worsen neuromuscular blockade if given before succinylcholine is metabolized by cholinesterase.
● Repeated or continuous infusions aren't advisable; they may cause reduced response or prolonged muscle relaxation and apnea.
● Give analgesics for pain.
● Keep airway clear. Have emergency respiratory support equipment (endotracheal equipment, ventilator, oxygen, atropine, and epinephrine) immediately available.
🕓 **Alert:** Careful dosage calculation is essential. Always verify dosage with another health care professional.

S

PATIENT TEACHING
- Explain all events and procedures to patient because he can still hear.
- Reassure patient that postoperative stiffness is normal and will soon subside.

---

sucralfate
soo-KRAL-fayt

Carafate♦

Therapeutic class: Antiulcer drugs
Pharmacologic class: GI protectants

AVAILABLE FORMS
Suspension: 1 g/10 mL
Tablets: 1 g

INDICATIONS & DOSAGES
➤ **Short-term (up to 8 weeks) treatment of duodenal ulcer**
Adults: 1 g P.O. q.i.d. 1 hour before meals and at bedtime for 4 to 8 weeks unless healing has been demonstrated by X-ray or endoscopic examination.
➤ **Maintenance therapy for duodenal ulcer**
Adults: 1 g P.O. b.i.d.

ADMINISTRATION
P.O.
- Shake suspension well before pouring.
- After administration, flush NG tube with water to ensure passage into stomach.
- Give drug on an empty stomach 1 hour before meals.

ACTION
Probably adheres to and protects surface of ulcer by forming a barrier.

Route	Onset	Peak	Duration
P.O.	Unknown	Unknown	6 hr

Half-life: Unknown.

ADVERSE REACTIONS
GI: constipation.

INTERACTIONS
Drug-drug. *Antacids:* May decrease binding of drug to gastroduodenal mucosa, impairing effectiveness. Separate doses by 30 minutes.
Cimetidine, digoxin, fosphenytoin, ketoconazole, phenytoin, quinidine, ranitidine, tetracycline, theophylline: May decrease absorption. Separate doses by at least 2 hours.
Ciprofloxacin, levofloxacin, moxifloxacin, ofloxacin: May decrease absorption of these drugs, reducing anti-infective response. If use together can't be avoided, give at least 6 hours apart.
Diclofenac: May decrease effectiveness of diclofenac. Monitor patient response.
Warfarin: May decrease anticoagulant effect. Monitor effectiveness and adjust dosage as necessary.

EFFECTS ON LAB TEST RESULTS
None reported.

CONTRAINDICATIONS & CAUTIONS
- Use cautiously in patients with chronic renal failure.
- Safety and effectiveness in children haven't been established.
Dialyzable drug: Unknown.
⚠ *Overdose S&S:* Dyspepsia, abdominal pain, nausea, vomiting.

PREGNANCY-LACTATION-REPRODUCTION
- There are no adequate studies in pregnant women. Use during pregnancy only if clearly needed.
- It isn't known if drug appears in breast milk. Use cautiously in breast-feeding women.

NURSING CONSIDERATIONS
- Drug is minimally absorbed and causes few adverse reactions.
- Monitor patient for severe, persistent constipation.
- Drug is as effective as cimetidine in healing duodenal ulcer.
- Drug contains aluminum but isn't classified as an antacid. Monitor patient with renal insufficiency for aluminum toxicity.

PATIENT TEACHING
- Tell patient to take sucralfate on an empty stomach, 1 hour before each meal and at bedtime.

Reactions in bold italics are *life-threatening*. Interactions may have a *rapid onset* or a *delayed onset*.

• Instruct patient to continue prescribed regimen to ensure complete healing. Pain and other ulcer signs and symptoms may subside within first few weeks of therapy.
• Urge patient to avoid cigarette smoking, which may increase gastric acid secretion and worsen disease.
• Antacids may be used while taking drug, but separate doses by 30 minutes.

sulfacetamide sodium 10%
sul-fah-SEE-tah-mide

Bleph-10

Therapeutic class: Antibiotics
Pharmacologic class: Sulfonamides

AVAILABLE FORMS
Ophthalmic ointment: 10%
Ophthalmic solution: 10%

INDICATIONS & DOSAGES
➤ **Treatment of conjunctivitis and other superficial ocular infections due to susceptible microorganisms**
Adults and children age 2 months and older: 1 or 2 drops into lower conjunctival sac every 2 to 3 hours. Increase interval as condition responds. Or, apply ½ inch of 10% ointment into conjunctival sac every 3 to 4 hours and at bedtime. Ointment may be used at night along with drops during the day. Usual duration of treatment is 7 to 10 days.
➤ **Trachoma**
Adults and children age 2 months and older: 2 drops into lower conjunctival sac every 2 hours with systemic sulfonamide or tetracycline.

ADMINISTRATION
Ophthalmic
• Store drug away from heat in tightly closed, light-resistant container.
• Avoid contacting tube or bottle tip with skin or eye.
• Apply light finger pressure on lacrimal sac for 1 minute after drops are instilled.
• Wait at least 5 to 10 minutes before instilling other eyedrops.

ACTION
Bacteriostatic; bactericidal in high concentrations. Prevents uptake of PABA, a metabolite of bacterial folic acid synthesis.

Route	Onset	Peak	Duration
Ophthalmic	Unknown	Unknown	Unknown

Half-life: Unknown.

ADVERSE REACTIONS
EENT: burning, eye itching, headache or brow pain, pain on instillation of drops, slowed corneal wound healing with ointment, bacterial and fungal corneal ulcers.
Other: overgrowth of nonsusceptible organisms, hypersensitivity reactions, *anaphylaxis.*

INTERACTIONS
Drug-drug. *Silver preparations:* May cause precipitate formation. Avoid using together.
Drug-lifestyle. *Sun exposure:* May cause photophobia. Advise patient to avoid excessive sunlight exposure.

EFFECTS ON LAB TEST RESULTS
None reported.

CONTRAINDICATIONS & CAUTIONS
• Contraindicated in patients hypersensitive to sulfonamides and in children younger than age 2 months.
◑ *Alert:* Fatalities have occurred rarely due to severe reactions to sulfonamides, including Stevens-Johnson syndrome, toxic epidermal necrolysis, fulminant hepatic necrosis, agranulocytosis, aplastic anemia, and other blood dyscrasias. Sensitizations may recur when a sulfonamide is readministered, irrespective of the route of administration. Sensitivity reactions have been reported in individuals with no prior history of sulfonamide hypersensitivity. At the first sign or symptom of hypersensitivity, rash, or other serious reaction, discontinue use.
• Use cautiously in patients with severe dry eye. Ointment may have a negative effect on corneal epithelial healing.
• Prolonged use can increase overgrowth of nonsusceptible organisms (superinfection).
Dialyzable drug: Unknown.

S

PREGNANCY-LACTATION-REPRODUCTION
• It isn't known if topically applied ophthalmic sulfonamides can cause fetal harm when used in pregnant women. Use during pregnancy only if potential benefit justifies potential risk to the fetus.
• Because of the potential for development of kernicterus in neonates, patient should discontinue breast-feeding or discontinue drug.

NURSING CONSIDERATIONS
• Drug is often used with oral tetracycline to treat trachoma and inclusion conjunctivitis.
• Concomitant use with topical corticosteroids may mask clinical signs and symptoms of infection and ineffective treatment. Monitor patient closely.
• *Look alike–sound alike:* Don't confuse Bleph-10 (sulfacetamide sodium) with Blephamide (sulfacetamide sodium and prednisolone acetate).

PATIENT TEACHING
• Tell patient to clean excessive discharge from eye area before application.
• Teach patient how to instill drops or apply ointment. Advise him to wash hands before and after applying ointment or solution and not to touch tip of dropper to eye or surrounding tissue.
• Instruct patient to apply light finger pressure on lacrimal sac for 1 minute after drops are instilled.
• Warn patient that eyedrops burn slightly.
• Advise patient to watch for and report signs and symptoms of sensitivity (itching lids, swelling, or constant burning).
• Tell patient to wait at least 5 to 10 minutes before instilling other eyedrops.
• Warn patient that solution may stain clothing.
• Tell patient to minimize sensitivity to sunlight by wearing sunglasses and avoiding prolonged exposure to sunlight.
• Advise patient not to use discolored solution.
• Tell patient not to share drug, washcloths, or towels with family members and to notify prescriber if anyone develops same signs or symptoms.

• Stress importance of compliance with recommended therapy.
• Advise patient to alert prescriber if no improvement occurs.

sulfamethoxazole–trimethoprim
sul-fa-meth-OX-a-zole/tri-meth-O-prim

Apo-Sulfatrim✤, Bactrim, Bactrim DS✐, Protrin DF✤, Septra, Septra DS, Sulfatrim Pediatric*

Therapeutic class: Antibiotics
Pharmacologic class: Sulfonamides–folate antagonists

AVAILABLE FORMS
Injection: sulfamethoxazole 80 mg/mL and trimethoprim 16 mg/mL in 5-mL vials*
Oral suspension: sulfamethoxazole 200 mg and trimethoprim 40 mg/5 mL*
Tablets (double-strength): sulfamethoxazole 800 mg and trimethoprim 160 mg
Tablets (single-strength): sulfamethoxazole 400 mg and trimethoprim 80 mg

INDICATIONS & DOSAGES
Adjust-a-dose (for all indications): For patients with CrCl of 15 to 30 mL/minute, reduce daily dose by 50%. Don't give to those with CrCl less than 15 mL/minute.
➤ **Shigellosis or UTIs caused by susceptible strains of *Escherichia coli*, *Proteus* (indole positive or negative), *Klebsiella*, *Morganella morganii*, or *Enterobacter* species**
Adults: 800 mg sulfamethoxazole/160 mg trimethoprim P.O. every 12 hours for 10 to 14 days in UTIs and for 5 days in shigellosis. If indicated, give 8 to 10 mg/kg/day I.V., based on trimethoprim component, in two to four divided doses every 6, 8, or 12 hours for 5 days for shigellosis or up to 14 days for severe UTIs. Maximum daily dose is 960 mg trimethoprim.
Children age 2 months and older: 8 mg/kg/day P.O., based on trimethoprim component, in two divided doses every 12 hours for 10 days for UTIs and 5 days for shigellosis. If indicated, give 8 to 10 mg/kg/day I.V., based on trimethoprim

component, in two to four divided doses every 6, 8, or 12 hours for up to 14 days for severe UTIs and 5 days for shigellosis. Don't exceed adult dose.

➤ **Otitis media in patients with penicillin allergy or penicillin-resistant infection**
Children age 2 months and older:
8 mg/kg/day P.O., based on trimethoprim component, in two divided doses every 12 hours for 10 days.

➤ **Chronic bronchitis, URIs**
Adults: 800 mg sulfamethoxazole/160 mg trimethoprim P.O. every 12 hours for 14 days.

➤ **Traveler's diarrhea**
Adults: 800 mg sulfamethoxazole/160 mg trimethoprim P.O. b.i.d. for 5 days.

➤ *Pneumocystis jiroveci* **pneumonia treatment**
Adults and children older than age 2 months: 15 to 20 mg/kg/day I.V. or P.O., based on trimethoprim component, in three or four divided doses for 14 to 21 days.

➤ *P. jiroveci* **pneumonia prophylaxis**
Adults: 800 mg sulfamethoxazole/160 mg trimethoprim every 24 hours.
Children older than age 2 months:
750 mg/m² sulfamethoxazole with trimethoprim 150 mg/m² daily in equally divided doses b.i.d., on 3 consecutive days per week.

➤ **Community-acquired pneumonia ◆**
Adults: 800 mg sulfamethoxazole/160 mg trimethoprim P.O. b.i.d. for 10 to 14 days.

ADMINISTRATION
P.O.
● Before giving drug, ask patient if he's allergic to sulfa drugs.
● Obtain specimen for culture and sensitivity tests before giving. Begin therapy while awaiting results.
● Shake suspension well before using.
● Give drug with 8 oz (240 mL) of water.

I.V.
▼ Before giving drug, ask patient if he's allergic to sulfa drugs.
▼ Obtain specimen for culture and sensitivity tests before giving. Begin therapy while awaiting results.
▼ Don't give by rapid infusion or bolus injection.

▼ Dilute each 5 mL of concentrate in 75 to 125 mL of D₅W. Don't mix with other drugs or solutions.
▼ Infuse slowly over 60 to 90 minutes.
▼ Don't refrigerate; use within 6 hours if diluted in 125 mL, within 4 hours if diluted in 100 mL, and within 2 hours if diluted in 75 mL.
▼ Discard solution if it's cloudy or crystallized.
▼ Never give drug I.M.
▼ **Incompatibilities:** Other drugs.

ACTION
Sulfamethoxazole inhibits formation of dihydrofolic acid from PABA; trimethoprim inhibits dihydrofolate reductase formation. Both decrease bacterial folic acid synthesis and are bactericidal.

Route	Onset	Peak	Duration
P.O.	Unknown	1–4 hr	Unknown
I.V.	Immediate	Unknown	Unknown

Half-life: Sulfamethoxazole, 10 to 13 hours; trimethoprim, 8 to 11 hours.

ADVERSE REACTIONS
CNS: *seizures,* apathy, aseptic meningitis, ataxia, depression, fatigue, hallucinations, headache, insomnia, nervousness, tinnitus, vertigo.
CV: thrombophlebitis.
GI: *pancreatitis, pseudomembranous colitis,* diarrhea, nausea, vomiting, abdominal pain, anorexia, stomatitis.
GU: *toxic nephrosis with oliguria and anuria,* crystalluria, hematuria, interstitial nephritis.
Hematologic: *agranulocytosis, aplastic anemia, leukopenia, thrombocytopenia,* hemolytic anemia, megaloblastic anemia.
Hepatic: *hepatic necrosis,* jaundice.
Musculoskeletal: arthralgia, muscle weakness, myalgia.
Respiratory: pulmonary infiltrates.
Skin: generalized skin eruption, *erythema multiforme, Stevens-Johnson syndrome, toxic epidermal necrolysis,* exfoliative dermatitis, photosensitivity reactions, pruritus, urticaria.
Other: *anaphylaxis,* drug fever, hypersensitivity reactions, serum sickness.

S

INTERACTIONS
Drug-drug. *Cyclosporine:* May decrease cyclosporine level and increase nephrotoxicity risk. Avoid using together.
Digoxin: May increase digoxin level. Monitor digoxin level.
Dofetilide: May increase dofetilide level and effects. May increase risk of prolonged QT-interval syndrome and fatal ventricular arrhythmias. Avoid using together.
Methotrexate: May increase methotrexate level. Monitor methotrexate level.
Oral antidiabetics: May increase hypoglycemic effect. Monitor glucose level.
Phenytoin: May inhibit hepatic metabolism of phenytoin. Monitor phenytoin level.
Warfarin: May increase anticoagulant effect. Monitor patient for bleeding; monitor PT and INR.
Drug-herb. *St. John's wort:* May decrease drug level. Consider therapy modification.
Drug-lifestyle. *Sun exposure:* May cause photosensitivity reactions. Advise patient to avoid excessive sunlight exposure.

EFFECTS ON LAB TEST RESULTS
• May increase aminotransferase, bilirubin, BUN, and creatinine levels. May decrease Hb level.
• May decrease granulocyte, platelet, and WBC counts.

CONTRAINDICATIONS & CAUTIONS
• Contraindicated in patients hypersensitive to trimethoprim or sulfonamides.
• Contraindicated in those with CrCl less than 15 mL/minute, porphyria, megaloblastic anemia from folate deficiency, or marked hepatic damage.
• Contraindicated in infants younger than age 2 months.
• Some forms may contain benzyl alcohol, which, in newborn infants, has been associated with an increased incidence of neurologic and other complications that are sometimes fatal. Avoid use in neonates.
• Use cautiously and in reduced dosages in patients with CrCl of 15 to 30 mL/minute, severe allergy or bronchial asthma, G6PD deficiency, or blood dyscrasia.
• May cause CDAD ranging from mild diarrhea to fatal colitis.

• Using sulfamethoxazole–trimethoprim with antiarrhythmics (amiodarone, bretylium, disopyramide, dofetilide, procainamide, quinidine, sotalol), arsenic trioxide, chlorpromazine, dolasetron, droperidol, mefloquine, mesoridazine, moxifloxacin, pentamidine, pimozide, tacrolimus, thioridazine, and ziprasidone may prolong QT interval and increase the risk of life-threatening cardiac arrhythmias, including torsades de pointes.
Dialyzable drug: Moderately.
⚠ **Overdose S&S:** Headache, drowsiness, unconsciousness, pyrexia, depression, confusion, anorexia, colic, nausea, vomiting, diarrhea, hematuria, crystalluria; blood dyscrasias and jaundice (late signs).

PREGNANCY-LACTATION-REPRODUCTION
• There are no well-controlled studies in pregnant women; drug may cause fetal harm. Use only if potential benefit justifies potential risk to the fetus.
• Contraindicated in breast-feeding women because of potential risk of bilirubin displacement and kernicterus.

NURSING CONSIDERATIONS
🕛 **Alert:** Double-check dosage, which may be written as trimethoprim component.
🕛 **Alert:** "DS" product means "double strength."
• Monitor renal function test and LFT results.
• Promptly report rash, sore throat, fever, cough, mouth sores, or iris lesions—early signs and symptoms of erythema multiforme, which may progress to life-threatening Stevens-Johnson syndrome, or blood dyscrasias.
• Watch for signs and symptoms of superinfection, such as fever, chills, and increased pulse.
🕛 **Alert:** Adverse reactions—especially hypersensitivity reactions, rash, and fever—occur much more frequently in patients with AIDS.

PATIENT TEACHING
• Tell patient to take drug as prescribed, even if he feels better.

Reactions in bold italics are *life-threatening*. Interactions may have a *rapid onset* or a *delayed onset*.

- Encourage patient to drink plenty of fluids to prevent crystalluria and kidney stone formation.
- Tell patient to report adverse reactions promptly.
- Instruct patient receiving drug I.V. to report discomfort at I.V. insertion site.
- Advise patient to avoid prolonged sun exposure, wear protective clothing, and use sunscreen.
- Instruct patient to take oral form with 8 oz (240 mL) of water.

sulfasalazine (salazosulfapyridine, sulphasalazine)
sul-fuh-SAL-uh-zeen

Azulfidine, Azulfidine EN-tabs, Salazopyrin✚, Salazopyrin EN-Tabs✚

Therapeutic class: Anti-inflammatory drugs
Pharmacologic class: Sulfonamide salicylates

AVAILABLE FORMS
Tablets: 500 mg
Tablets (delayed-release) ⓓⓝⓒ: 500 mg

INDICATIONS & DOSAGES
➤ **Mild to moderate ulcerative colitis, adjunctive therapy in severe ulcerative colitis, prolongation of remission period between acute ulcerative colitis attacks**
Adults: Initially, 3 to 4 g P.O. daily in evenly divided doses not exceeding 8 hours apart; may start with 1 to 2 g, with gradual increase to minimize adverse effects. Usual maintenance dose is 2 g P.O. daily.
Children age 6 and older: Initially, 40 to 60 mg/kg P.O. daily, divided into three to six doses; may start at lower dose if GI intolerance occurs. Maintenance dose is 30 mg/kg in each 24-hour period, divided into four doses.
➤ **RA in patients who have responded inadequately to salicylates or NSAIDs**
Adults (delayed-release tablets): 2 g P.O. daily in two evenly divided doses. To reduce

possible GI intolerance, start at 0.5 to 1 g daily.
➤ **Polyarticular-course juvenile RA in patients who have responded inadequately to salicylates or other NSAIDs**
Children age 6 and older (delayed-release tablets): 30 to 50 mg/kg P.O. daily in two evenly divided doses. Maximum dose is 2 g daily. To reduce possible GI intolerance, start with one-quarter to one-third of planned maintenance dose and increase weekly until reaching maintenance dose at 1 month.

ADMINISTRATION
P.O.
- Give drug with food to decrease GI irritation.
- Patient must swallow delayed-release tablets whole and mustn't crush, chew, or split them.

ACTION
Unknown.

Route	Onset	Peak	Duration
P.O.	Unknown	3–12 hr	Unknown

Half-life: 10 to 15 hours.

ADVERSE REACTIONS
CNS: *seizures,* dizziness, headache, depression, hallucinations.
GI: nausea, vomiting, diarrhea, abdominal pain, anorexia, stomatitis.
GU: oligospermia, infertility.
Hematologic: *agranulocytosis, leukopenia, thrombocytopenia, aplastic anemia,* megaloblastic anemia, *hemolytic anemia.*
Hepatic: *hepatotoxicity,* urticaria, pruritus.
Other: drug fever.

INTERACTIONS
Drug-drug. *Antibiotics:* May alter action of sulfasalazine by changing intestinal flora. Monitor patient closely.
Cyclosporine: May reduce cyclosporine efficacy and increase nephrotoxicity. Monitor cyclosporine level and renal function.
Digoxin: May reduce absorption of digoxin. Monitor patient closely.
Folic acid: May decrease absorption of folic acid. Monitor patient.

Heparin, oral anticoagulants: May increase anticoagulant effect. Watch for bleeding.
Methotrexate: May enhance hepatotoxic effect of methotrexate. Monitor patient for hematologic toxicity and adverse GI events, especially nausea.
Prilocaine: May increase risk of significant methemoglobinemia. Monitor patient. Avoid lidocaine and prilocaine in infants receiving such agents.
Thiopurines (azathioprine, mercaptopurine): May increase leukopenia. Monitor WBC count closely.
Drug-herb. *Dong quai, St. John's wort:* May also cause photosensitization. Avoid use together.

EFFECTS ON LAB TEST RESULTS
● May increase ALT and AST levels. May decrease Hb level.
● May decrease granulocyte, platelet, and WBC counts.
● May interfere with measurements, by liquid chromatography, of urinary normetanephrine and cause false-positive test results in patients exposed to sulfasalazine or its metabolite.

CONTRAINDICATIONS & CAUTIONS
● Contraindicated in patients hypersensitive to drug, its metabolites, sulfonamides, or salicylates and in those with porphyria or intestinal and urinary obstruction.
● Use cautiously and in reduced doses in patients with impaired hepatic or renal function, severe allergy, bronchial asthma, or G6PD deficiency. Deaths have occurred from renal damage.
● Serious skin reactions, some fatal, including exfoliative dermatitis, Stevens-Johnson syndrome, and toxic epidermal necrolysis, have been reported. Patients are at highest risk for these events early in therapy, with most events occurring within the first month of treatment. Discontinue drug at the first appearance of rash or mucosal lesions.
● Serious CNS reactions can occur, including seizures, meningitis, spinal cord disorders, peripheral neuropathy, hearing loss, ataxia, and hallucinations.
Dialyzable drug: Yes.
⚠ **Overdose S&S:** Nausea, gastric distress, abdominal pain, drowsiness, seizures.

PREGNANCY-LACTATION-REPRODUCTION
● There are no adequate studies in pregnant women. Use only if clearly needed.
● Drug and its active metabolite appear in breast milk. Use cautiously in breast-feeding women; monitor infant for kernicterus and diarrhea or bloody stools.

NURSING CONSIDERATIONS
● Therapeutic response in patients with RA may occur as soon as 4 weeks after starting therapy, but it may take up to 12 weeks in others.
● Drug may cause urine discoloration.
⚠ **Alert:** Stop drug immediately and notify prescriber if patient shows signs and symptoms of hypersensitivity.
● Maintain adequate fluid intake to prevent crystalluria and stone formation.
● Obtain CBCs, including differential WBC count and LFTs, before start of treatment and every second week during first 3 months of therapy. During second 3 months, do the same tests once monthly and thereafter once every 3 months and as clinically indicated. Obtain a urinalysis with careful microscopic examination and an assessment of renal function periodically during treatment.
● Serum sulfapyridine levels greater than 50 mcg/mL appear to be associated with an increased incidence of adverse reactions.
● Observe patients with G6PD deficiency closely for signs and symptoms of hemolytic anemia.
● *Look alike–sound alike:* Don't confuse sulfasalazine with sulfisoxazole, salsalate, or sulfadiazine.

PATIENT TEACHING
● Instruct patient to take drug after eating and to space doses evenly.
● Warn patient to avoid ultraviolet light; drug may increase risk of sunburn. Advise patient to use sunscreen and wear protective clothing and to avoid sunlamps and tanning booths.
● Advise patient that drug may produce an orange-yellow discoloration of skin and urine and may cause contact lenses to turn yellow.
● Teach patient about adverse reactions and to report them. Advise patient of the need for careful medical supervision. A sore

---

throat, fever, pallor, purpura, or jaundice may indicate a serious blood disorder.
● Tell patient to drink plenty of water and to swallow tablets whole without crushing or chewing.
● Advise patient that blood and urine tests will be needed to monitor treatment and that it's important to keep laboratory and physician appointments.

sumatriptan succinate
sue-mah-TRIP-tan

Alsuma, Imitrex✒, Imitrex STATdose, Onzetra Xsail, Sumavel DosePro, Zembrace SymTouch

Therapeutic class: Antimigraine drugs
Pharmacologic class: Serotonin 5-HT$_1$ receptor agonists

AVAILABLE FORMS
Injection: 4 mg/0.5 mL, 6 mg/0.5 mL prefilled syringes; 6 mg/0.5 mL vials; 3 mg/0.5 mL, 6 mg/0.5 mL single-dose autoinjector
Nasal powder: 11 mg (base)/disposable nosepiece
Nasal solution: 5 mg/0.1 mL, 20 mg/0.1 mL
Tablets 🅞🅝🅖: 25 mg, 50 mg, 100 mg (base)

INDICATIONS & DOSAGES
➤ **Acute migraine attacks (with or without aura)**
Adults: 6 mg subcutaneously; maximum dose is two 6-mg injections in 24 hours, separated by at least 1 hour. Or 25 to 100 mg P.O., initially. If desired response isn't achieved in 2 hours, may give second dose of 25 to 100 mg. Additional doses may be used in at least 2-hour intervals. Maximum daily oral dose, 200 mg.
  For nasal spray, give 5 mg, 10 mg, or 20 mg once in one nostril; may repeat once after 2 hours, for maximum daily dose of 40 mg.
  For nasal powder, one 11 mg nosepiece in each nostril (22 mg total), using the Xsail breath-powered delivery device. If desired response isn't achieved in 2 hours, or migraine returns after a transient improvement, may give second dose of 22 mg. Maximum

recommended dose within 24 hours is two doses (44 mg/4 nosepieces) or one dose of 22 mg and one dose of another sumatriptan product, separated by at least 2 hours.
Adjust-a-dose: In patients with hepatic impairment, the maximum single oral dose shouldn't exceed 50 mg.
➤ **Cluster headache (except Zembrace)**
Adults: 6 mg subcutaneously. Maximum recommended dose is two 6-mg injections in 24 hours, separated by at least 1 hour.

ADMINISTRATION
P.O.
● Give drug without regard for food.
● Give drug whole; don't crush or break tablet.
Subcutaneous
● Redness or pain at injection site should subside within 1 hour after injection.
● Use injection site with adequate skin and subcutaneous tissue thickness to accommodate length of needle.
● Use only the abdomen or thigh for needle-free injection system.
Intranasal spray
● Have patient blow his nose before use.
● Give medication on inhalation in one nostril, while blocking the other nostril.
Intranasal powder
● Use with the Xsail device only; insert disposable nosepiece into the device body.
● Pierce capsule inside nosepiece by pressing and releasing the white piercing button one time on the device body.
● Insert nosepiece into one nostril, ensuring a tight seal; rotate device, place mouthpiece into mouth, and blow forcefully through mouthpiece for 2 to 3 seconds to deliver powder into the nasal cavity.
● Remove and discard nosepiece; repeat in other nostril, using a second nosepiece.

ACTION
May act as an agonist at serotonin receptors on extracerebral intracranial blood vessels, which constricts the affected vessels, inhibits neuropeptide release, and reduces pain transmission in the trigeminal pathways.

S

Route	Onset	Peak	Duration
P.O.	30 min	2–2½ hr	Unknown
Subcut.	10 min	12 min	Unknown
Intranasal spray	15–30 min	1–2 hr	Unknown
Intranasal powder	Unknown	45 min	Unknown

Half-life: About 2 hours; intranasal, about 3 hours.

ADVERSE REACTIONS

CNS: dizziness, vertigo, drowsiness, headache, anxiety, malaise, fatigue.
CV: *atrial fibrillation, ventricular fibrillation, ventricular tachycardia, coronary artery vasospasm, transient myocardial ischemia, MI,* pressure or tightness in chest.
EENT: discomfort of throat, nasal cavity or sinus, mouth, jaw, or tongue; altered vision.
GI: abdominal discomfort, dysphagia, diarrhea, nausea, vomiting, unusual or bad taste (nasal spray).
Musculoskeletal: myalgia, muscle cramps, neck pain.
Respiratory: upper respiratory tract inflammation and dyspnea (P.O.).
Skin: injection-site or application-site reaction, tingling, diaphoresis, flushing.
Other: warm or hot sensation, burning sensation, heaviness, pressure or tightness, tight feeling in head, cold sensation, numbness.

INTERACTIONS

Drug-drug. *Antipsychotics, metoclopramide, serotonin modulators:* May enhance adverse or toxic effect of other serotonin modulators, increasing risk of serotonin syndrome. Monitor therapy.
Ergot and ergot derivatives, other 5-HT₁ agonists: May prolong vasospastic effects. Don't use within 24 hours of sumatriptan therapy.
MAO inhibitors: May reduce sumatriptan clearance. Avoid using within 2 weeks of MAO inhibitor. Use injection cautiously and decrease sumatriptan dose.
Methylene blue, SSRIs: May cause serotonin syndrome. Monitor patient closely for weakness, hyperreflexia, and incoordination if use together can't be avoided.
Drug-herb. *St. John's wort:* May increase serotonin levels. Use together cautiously.

EFFECTS ON LAB TEST RESULTS

● May increase liver enzyme levels.

CONTRAINDICATIONS & CAUTIONS

● Contraindicated in patients with hypersensitivity to drug or its components and in those with history, symptoms, or signs of ischemic cardiac, cerebrovascular (such as stroke or TIA), or peripheral vascular syndromes (such as ischemic bowel disease); significant underlying CV diseases, including angina pectoris, MI, and silent myocardial ischemia; Wolff-Parkinson-White syndrome or arrhythmias associated with other cardiac accessory conduction pathway disorders; uncontrolled hypertension; or severe hepatic impairment.
● Contraindicated within 24 hours of another 5-HT agonist or drug containing ergotamine and within 2 weeks of MAO inhibitor.
● Use cautiously in patient with risk factors for CAD, such as postmenopausal women, men older than age 40, or patients with hypertension, hypercholesterolemia, obesity, diabetes, smoking, or family history of CAD.
● Safety and effectiveness of using more than four transdermal patches in 1 month haven't been established.
Dialyzable drug: Unknown.

PREGNANCY-LACTATION-REPRODUCTION

● There are no adequate studies in pregnant women. Use only if potential benefit justifies potential risk to the fetus.
● Drug appears in breast milk after subcutaneous administration. Patients should minimize infant exposure by avoiding breast-feeding for 12 hours after treatment with oral and subcutaneous forms. Some manufacturers recommend that patients not breast-feed.
● Refer to individual manufacturer's instructions regarding breast-feeding. Some manufacturers don't recommend breast-feeding and other sources note that patient doesn't have to discontinue breast-feeding.

NURSING CONSIDERATIONS

🕒 *Alert:* When giving drug to patient at risk for CAD, give first dose in presence of other

---

medical personnel. Rarely, serious adverse cardiac effects can follow administration.

☉ Alert: Combining drug with an SSRI or an SSNRI may cause serotonin syndrome. Symptoms include restlessness, hallucinations, loss of coordination, fast heartbeat, rapid changes in BP, increased body temperature, hyperreflexia, nausea, vomiting, and diarrhea. Serotonin syndrome may occur when starting or increasing the dose of drug, SSRI, or SSNRI.

• Monitor patient for seizures. Seizures have been reported in patients with and without a history of seizures.

• After subcutaneous injection, most patients experience relief in 1 to 2 hours.

• **Look alike–sound alike:** Don't confuse sumatriptan with somatropin.

PATIENT TEACHING

• Inform patient that drug is intended only to treat migraine attacks, not to prevent them or reduce their occurrence.

• If patient is pregnant or may become pregnant, tell her not to use drug but to discuss with prescriber the risks and benefits of using drug during pregnancy.

• Tell patient that drug may be taken at any time during a migraine attack, as soon as signs or symptoms appear.

• Review information about drug's injectable form, which is available in a spring-loaded injector system for easier patient use. Make sure patient understands how to load the injector, give the injection, and dispose of used syringes.

• Teach patient to select subcutaneous administration sites with adequate subcutaneous tissue thickness.

• Teach patient using intranasal powder how to use Xsail device correctly.

• Teach patient to blow his nose before using nasal spray. Patient should block other nostril while inhaling gently during administration and should keep head upright and breathe gently for 10 to 20 seconds after dose is given.

☉ Alert: Tell patient to report all adverse reactions and to immediately report persistent or severe chest pain. Warn patient to stop using drug and to call prescriber if pain or tightness in the throat, wheezing, heart throbbing, rash, lumps, hives, or swollen eyelids, face, or lips develop.

SAFETY ALERT!

sunitinib malate
soo-NIH-tih-nib

Sutent⬦

Therapeutic class: Antineoplastics
Pharmacologic class: Protein-tyrosine kinase inhibitors

AVAILABLE FORMS
Capsules: 12.5 mg, 25 mg, 37.5 mg, 50 mg

INDICATIONS & DOSAGES
➤ **GI stromal tumor that's progressing despite imatinib therapy or because patient is intolerant of imatinib; advanced renal cell carcinoma**
Adults: 50 mg P.O. once daily for 4 weeks, followed by 2 weeks off the drug. Repeat cycle.
Adjust-a-dose: Increase or decrease dosage in 12.5-mg increments based on individual safety and tolerability. If drug must be administered with a strong CYP3A4 inhibitor such as ketoconazole, reduce dosage to a minimum of 37.5 mg/day. If drug must be administered with a CYP3A4 inducer such as rifampin, consider increasing dosage to 87.5 mg daily; carefully monitor patient for toxicity. Refer to package insert for dosage adjustments for toxicities.
➤ **Progressive, well-differentiated pancreatic neuroendocrine tumors in patients with unresectable, locally advanced, or metastatic disease**
Adults: 37.5 mg P.O. once daily given continuously without a scheduled off-treatment period. Maximum recommended dosage is 50 mg daily.
Adjust-a-dose: Increase or decrease in 12.5-mg increments based on patient tolerance and safety. If drug must be administered with a strong CYP3A4 inhibitor such as ketoconazole, consider decreasing dosage to 25 mg daily. If drug must be administered with a CYP3A4 inducer such as rifampin, consider increasing dosage to 62.5 mg daily and carefully monitor patient for toxicity.

S

Refer to manufacturer's instructions for dosage adjustments for toxicities.

ADMINISTRATION

P.O.

• Hazardous agent; use safe handling and disposal precautions according to facility policy. Avoid contact with broken capsules.
• Give drug without regard for meals.

ACTION

A multi-kinase inhibitor targeting several receptor tyrosine kinases, which are involved in tumor growth, pathologic angiogenesis, and metastatic progression of cancer.

Route	Onset	Peak	Duration
P.O.	Unknown	6–12 hr	Unknown

Half-life: 40 to 60 hours; primary metabolite, 80 to 110 hours.

ADVERSE REACTIONS

CNS: asthenia, dizziness, fatigue, fever, headache, peripheral neuropathy.
CV: *decreased LVEF, thromboembolic events,* hypertension, peripheral edema.
EENT: increased lacrimation, periorbital edema.
GI: *GI perforation, pancreatitis,* abdominal pain, altered taste, anorexia, appetite disturbance, burning sensation in mouth, constipation, diarrhea, dyspepsia, flatulence, mucositis, nausea, oral pain, stomatitis, vomiting.
Hematologic: *bleeding, leukopenia, lymphopenia, neutropenia, thrombocytopenia,* anemia.
Metabolic: dehydration, hypernatremia, hyperuricemia, hypokalemia, *hyperkalemia,* hyponatremia, hypophosphatemia, hypothyroidism.
Musculoskeletal: arthralgia, back pain, limb pain, myalgia.
Respiratory: cough, dyspnea.
Skin: alopecia, dry skin, hair color changes, hand-foot syndrome, rash, skin discoloration, skin blistering.
Other: *adrenal insufficiency.*

INTERACTIONS

Drug-drug. *Azole antifungals, CYP3A4 inducers (carbamazepine, dexamethasone, phenobarbital, phenytoin, rifabutin,*

rifampin, rifapentine): May decrease sunitinib level and effects. If use together can't be avoided, increase sunitinib dosage.
Bevacizumab: May enhance hypertensive effect of sunitinib and increase risk of microangiopathic hemolytic anemia. Avoid use together.
QTc interval–prolonging drugs: May increase risk of QTc interval prolongation and ventricular arrhythmias. Carefully monitor ECG and QT interval. Consider therapy modification.
Strong CYP3A4 inhibitors (atazanavir, clarithromycin, indinavir, itraconazole, ketoconazole, nefazodone, nelfinavir, ritonavir, saquinavir, telithromycin, voriconazole): May increase sunitinib level and toxicity. If use together can't be avoided, decrease sunitinib dosage.
Drug-herb. *St. John's wort:* May cause an unpredictable decrease in drug level. Discourage use together.
Drug-food. *Grapefruit:* May increase drug level. Discourage use together.

EFFECTS ON LAB TEST RESULTS

• May increase AST, ALT, alkaline phosphatase, total and indirect bilirubin, amylase, lipase, creatinine, uric acid, and TSH levels.
• May decrease phosphorus and Hb levels and hematocrit.
• May increase or decrease potassium and sodium levels.
• May decrease RBC, neutrophil, lymphocyte, WBC, and platelet counts.

CONTRAINDICATIONS & CAUTIONS

• Contraindicated in patients hypersensitive to drug or its components.
• Use cautiously in patients with electrolyte imbalance or a history of hypertension, QT-interval prolongation, concurrent antiarrhythmic use, bradycardia, MI, angina, CABG, symptomatic HF, stroke, TIA, or PE.
• Thrombotic microangiopathy (TMA), including thrombotic thrombocytopenic purpura and hemolytic-uremic syndrome, sometimes leading to renal failure or a fatal outcome, has been reported. Discontinue if TMA develops.

Reactions in bold italics are *life-threatening*. Interactions may have a *rapid onset* or a *delayed onset*.

• Proteinuria and nephrotic syndrome have been reported, and some cases have resulted in renal failure and fatal outcomes. Monitor patient for development or worsening of proteinuria. Obtain urinalysis at baseline and periodically during treatment, with follow-up measurement of 24-hour urine protein as clinically indicated.

• Severe cutaneous reactions have been reported, including erythema multiforme, Stevens-Johnson syndrome (SJS), and toxic epidermal necrolysis (TEN), some of which were fatal. If patient develops signs or symptoms of a progressive rash, often with blisters or mucosal lesions, discontinue drug. If a diagnosis of SJS or TEN is suspected, don't restart drug.

• Necrotizing fasciitis, including of the perineum and secondary to fistula formation, sometimes fatal, has been reported. Discontinue drug if necrotizing fasciitis develops.

• Drug has been associated with symptomatic hypoglycemia, which may result in loss of consciousness or require hospitalization. Blood glucose level reductions may be worse in patients with diabetes. Check blood glucose levels regularly during and after discontinuation of treatment. Assess if antidiabetic drug dosage needs adjustment to minimize risk of hypoglycemia.

• Using sunitinib malate with antiarrhythmics (amiodarone, bretylium, disopyramide, dofetilide, procainamide, quinidine, sotalol), arsenic trioxide, chlorpromazine, cisapride, dolasetron, droperidol, mefloquine, mesoridazine, moxifloxacin, pentamidine, pimozide, tacrolimus, thioridazine, and ziprasidone may prolong QT interval and increase the risk of life-threatening cardiac arrhythmias, including torsades de pointes. *Dialyzable drug:* No.

PREGNANCY-LACTATION-REPRODUCTION

• Drug can cause fetal harm when used in pregnant women. Women of childbearing potential should avoid becoming pregnant during therapy. If drug is used during pregnancy, or if patient becomes pregnant while taking drug, apprise her of potential hazard to the fetus.

• It isn't known if drug appears in breast milk. Patient should discontinue breastfeeding or discontinue drug.

NURSING CONSIDERATIONS

Black Box Warning Drug may cause severe, sometimes fatal, hepatotoxicity. Monitor liver function before and during each cycle of therapy. ■

✺ *Alert:* Drug may cause CV events, including HF, myocardial disorders, and cardiomyopathy, which may be fatal. Monitor CV status closely.

• Obtain CBC with platelet count and serum chemistries, including phosphate level, before each treatment cycle.

• Obtain LFTs at baseline, before each treatment cycle, and when clinically indicated.

• Obtain baseline evaluation of LVEF in all patients before treatment. If patient had a cardiac event in the year before treatment, check LVEF periodically.

• Interrupt therapy or decrease dosage in patients with LVEF less than 50% and more than 20% below baseline.

• Monitor patient's BP closely. If severe hypertension occurs, notify prescriber. Drug may need to be withheld until BP is controlled.

• Monitor patient for signs and symptoms of HF, especially if there is a history of heart disease.

• If patient has seizures, he may have reversible posterior leukoencephalopathy syndrome. Signs and symptoms include hypertension, headache, decreased alertness, altered mental functioning, and vision loss. Stop treatment temporarily.

• Impaired wound healing has been reported during therapy. Temporarily interrupt therapy in patients undergoing major surgical procedures. May resume drug when health care provider determines patient has recovered.

• If patient will be undergoing surgery or suffers trauma or severe infection, assess him for adrenal insufficiency (muscle weakness, weight loss, depression, salt craving, low BP).

• Provide antiemetics or antidiarrheals as needed for adverse GI effects.

• Monitor patient with renal cell carcinoma or GI stromal tumor with high tumor burden closely and treat as clinically indicated because of the risk of tumor lysis syndrome. Correct dehydration and high uric acid levels before treatment.

• Osteonecrosis of the jaw has been reported. Consider preventive dentistry before treatment with sunitinib. If possible, avoid invasive dental procedures, particularly in patients receiving I.V. bisphosphonate therapy.

🟊 **Alert:** Drug may cause bleeding in GI tract, urinary tract, respiratory tract, and brain, which may be fatal. Monitor patient and CBC closely.

PATIENT TEACHING

• Advise patient to keep appointments for blood tests and periodic heart function evaluations.

• Tell patient about common adverse effects, such as diarrhea, nausea, vomiting, fatigue, mouth pain, and taste disturbance, and to report all adverse reactions.

• Inform patient about changes that may occur in skin and hair, including color changes and dry, red, blistering skin of the hands and feet.

• Urge patient to tell prescriber about all prescribed and OTC drugs or herbal supplements.

• Warn patient not to consume grapefruit during therapy.

• Tell patient to notify prescriber about unusual bleeding, trouble breathing, wheezing, severe or prolonged diarrhea or vomiting, or swelling of the hands or lower legs.

• Advise female patient of childbearing potential to avoid becoming pregnant during therapy.

suvorexant
soo-voe-REX-ant

Belsomra

Therapeutic class: Hypnotics
Pharmacologic class: Orexin receptor antagonists
Controlled substance schedule: IV

AVAILABLE FORMS
Tablets: 5 mg, 10 mg, 15 mg, 20 mg

INDICATIONS & DOSAGES
➤ **Insomnia characterized by difficulties with sleep onset or sleep maintenance**
Adults: 10 mg P.O. daily within 30 minutes of going to bed. If 10-mg dose is tolerated but not effective, increase to a maximum of 20 mg P.O. daily. Don't exceed more than one dose per night.
Adjust-a-dose: For patients taking concomitant moderate CYP3A4 inhibitors, give 5 mg P.O. daily at night. Maximum dose is 10 mg daily.

ADMINISTRATION
P.O.
• Give drug within 30 minutes of bedtime and ensure at least 7 hours remain before planned time of awakening.
• May give with or without food; however, the time to drug's effect is delayed if drug is taken with or soon after a meal.

ACTION
Blocks orexin receptors, suppressing the system responsible for promoting wakefulness.

Route	Onset	Peak	Duration
P.O.	30 min	2 hr	Unknown

Half-life: 12 hours.

ADVERSE REACTIONS
CNS: somnolence, behavioral changes, headache, dizziness, abnormal dreams.
EENT: dry mouth.
GI: diarrhea.
Respiratory: cough, URI.

Reactions in bold italics are *life-threatening*. Interactions may have a *rapid onset* or a ***delayed onset***.

INTERACTIONS
Drug-drug. *CNS depressants, including other drugs that treat insomnia:* May cause excessive CNS depression. Use together isn't recommended.
Digoxin: May decrease digoxin metabolism. Monitor digoxin level.
Moderate CYP3A4 inhibitors (amprenavir, aprepitant, atazanavir, ciprofloxacin, diltiazem, erythromycin, fluconazole, fosamprenavir, imatinib, verapamil): May decrease suvorexant metabolism. Decrease initial suvorexant daily dose to 5 mg; don't exceed a dose of 10 mg.
Black Box Warning *Opioids:* May cause slow or difficult breathing, sedation, and death. Avoid use together. If use together is necessary, limit dosage and duration of each drug to minimum necessary for desired effect. ∎
Strong CYP3A4 inducers (carbamazepine, phenytoin, rifampin): May decrease clinical effect of suvorexant. Monitor patient for reduced therapeutic effect.
Strong CYP3A4 inhibitors (clarithromycin, conivaptan, indinavir, itraconazole, ketoconazole, nefazodone, nelfinavir, posaconazole, ritonavir, saquinavir, telithromycin): May increase risk of additive toxicity. Avoid use together.
Drug-food. *Grapefruit juice:* May decrease drug metabolism and increase drug level. Decrease suvorexant dosage.
Drug-lifestyle. *Alcohol use:* May cause excessive CNS depression. Discourage use together.

EFFECTS ON LAB TEST RESULTS
● May increase cholesterol level.

CONTRAINDICATIONS & CAUTIONS
● Contraindicated in patients hypersensitive to drug or its components and in those with narcolepsy.
Black Box Warning Opioids should only be prescribed with benzodiazepines or other CNS depressants to patients for whom alternative treatment options are inadequate. ∎
● Not recommended for use in patients with severe hepatic impairment.
⚠ *Alert:* Drug may increase risk of suicidal ideation. Immediately evaluate patients

who report suicidal ideation or exhibit new behavioral signs or symptoms.
● Use cautiously in patients with compromised respiratory status (obstructive sleep apnea, COPD) or a history of drug abuse or dependence.
● Safety and effectiveness in children haven't been studied.
Dialyzable drug: Unknown.
⚠ *Overdose S&S:* Increased frequency and duration of somnolence.

PREGNANCY-LACTATION-REPRODUCTION
● Drug hasn't been studied in pregnant women. Use cautiously during pregnancy and only if benefits outweigh risk to the fetus.
● It isn't known if drug appears in breast milk. Use cautiously in breast-feeding women.

NURSING CONSIDERATIONS
● Use the smallest effective dosage in all patients. Lower dosages may be necessary in obese or female patients because a higher incidence of adverse effects have been observed.
● Complex behaviors, such as "sleep driving" (driving while not fully awake), preparing and eating food, making phone calls, or having sex with subsequent amnesia of the event, have been reported with therapeutic doses; use of alcohol and other CNS depressants increases the risk. Discontinue drug for complex sleep behavior.
● Monitor patient for daytime somnolence. Decrease dosage or discontinue drug if daytime somnolence develops in patients who drive.
● Carefully evaluate patient for physical or psychiatric causes of sleep disturbances before drug is prescribed. If insomnia persists for more than 7 to 10 days, reevaluate patient.
● Monitor patients for sleep paralysis (inability to move or speak during sleep-wake transitions), hallucinations, and mild cataplexy signs and symptoms (periods of leg weakness).
⊙ *Alert:* Worsening of depression or suicidal thinking may occur. Be alert for signs and symptoms of depression or behavioral changes.

S

• *Look alike–sound alike:* Don't confuse suvorexant with Serevent.

PATIENT TEACHING

Black Box Warning Caution patient or caregiver of patient taking an opioid with a benzodiazepine, CNS depressant, or alcohol to seek immediate medical attention if patient experiences dizziness, light-headedness, extreme sleepiness, slowed or difficult breathing, or unresponsiveness. ■

• Teach patient to take drug immediately before going to bed and to allow at least 7 hours for sleep before planned awakening.

• Inform patient that drug may be taken with or without food but, for more rapid sleep onset, to avoid taking drug with or after meals.

• Advise patient to avoid alcohol and other drugs that cause sleepiness while taking suvorexant.

• Tell patient to notify prescriber if abnormal thoughts and behavior, symptoms of depression (changes in mood, excessive tiredness), or insomnia that persists for more than 7 to 10 days occurs.

❸ Alert: Caution patient to immediately report suicidal ideation or new behavioral signs or symptoms.

• Inform patient that sleep paralysis (inability to move or speak during sleep-wake transitions), vivid and disturbing perceptions, and temporary leg weakness can occur.

• Warn patient that daytime somnolence can occur and to avoid performing activities that require mental alertness or physical coordination (such as driving) until fully awake.

• Warn patient of the risk of performing complex behaviors, such as driving, eating, and making phone calls, while asleep and to report if these symptoms occur.

• Instruct patient not to increase dosage without first consulting prescriber.

• Advise female patient to inform prescriber if she's pregnant, intends to become pregnant, or is breast-feeding.

tacrolimus
tack-ROW-lim-us

Astagraf XL, Envarsus XR, Prograf

Therapeutic class: Immunosuppressants
Pharmacologic class: Calcineurin inhibitors

AVAILABLE FORMS

Capsules ⓞⓝⓒ*:* 0.5 mg, 1 mg, 5 mg
Capsules (extended-release) ⓞⓝⓒ*:* 0.5 mg, 1 mg, 5 mg
Injection: 5 mg/mL
Tablets (extended-release) ⓞⓝⓒ*:* 0.75 mg, 1 mg, 4 mg

INDICATIONS & DOSAGES

❸ Alert: Individualizing dosing regimen is necessary for optimal therapy. Frequently monitor trough concentrations in the early transplant period to ensure adequate drug exposure.

➤ **To prevent organ rejection in allogenic liver, kidney, or heart transplant (with corticosteroids)**
Adults: For patients who can't take drug P.O., 0.03 to 0.05 mg/kg/day (liver or kidney) or 0.01 mg/kg/day (heart) I.V. as continuous infusion at least 6 hours after transplant. Switch to oral therapy as soon as possible, with first dose 8 to 12 hours after stopping I.V. infusion. For renal transplant, give oral dose within 24 hours of transplantation after renal function has recovered. Initial oral dosages: For liver transplant, 0.1 to 0.15 mg/kg P.O. daily in two divided doses every 12 hours; for kidney transplant, 0.2 mg/kg P.O. daily (in combination with azathioprine) or 0.1 mg/kg P.O. daily (in combination with mycophenolate mofetil and interleukin-2 receptor agonist) in two divided doses every 12 hours; for heart transplant, 0.075 mg/kg P.O. daily in two divided doses every 12 hours. Adjust dosages based on patient response.

For Astagraf XL extended-release (ER) form (renal transplant only): When using with basiliximab induction, mycophenolate mofetil, and corticosteroids, administer initial dose of 0.15 mg/kg/day P.O. before or within 48 hours of completion of transplant procedure, but may delay until renal function has recovered. When using without basiliximab induction, give 0.1 mg/kg/day P.O. (preoperative); 0.2 mg/kg/day P.O. (postoperative). When using with mycophenolate mofetil and corticosteroids, give preoperative dose as one dose within 12 hours before reperfusion; give initial postoperative dose not less than 4 hours after preoperative dose and within 12 hours after reperfusion.

To convert from immediate-release form to Astagraf XL, initiate ER treatment in a 1:1 ratio (mg:mg) using previously established total daily dose of immediate-release form. Give once daily. To convert from immediate-release form to Envarsus XR, initiate ER treatment with a once-daily dose that's 80% of the total daily dose of the immediate-release product.

Children (liver transplant only): Initially, 0.03 to 0.05 mg/kg I.V. daily as continuous infusion; then 0.15 to 0.2 mg/kg P.O. daily on schedule similar to that of adults, adjusted as needed.

Adjust-a-dose: Give lowest recommended oral and I.V. dosages to patients with renal or hepatic impairment. Black patients with renal transplants may need higher dosages than white patients to attain comparable trough concentrations.

➤ **Immunosuppression (maintenance) after lung transplant ♦**

Adults: 0.05 to 0.3 mg/kg/day (immediate-release) P.O. or by NG tube in two divided doses every 12 hours (usual dose, 0.05 mg/kg every 12 hours); titrate to target trough concentrations. May also administer sublingually at approximately 50% of the oral/NG dose. Usually used in combination regimen that contains a corticosteroid and either azathioprine or mycophenolate. May convert to once-daily dosing (on a mg-per-mg basis) using extended-release formulation (Astagraf XL) in stable lung transplant recipients.

ADMINISTRATION

P.O.
● Give drug 1 hour before or 2 hours after a meal.

● Make sure patient swallows capsules whole and doesn't chew, divide, or crush them.
● Don't give with grapefruit juice.

I.V.
▼ Dilute drug with NSS for injection or D_5W injection to 0.004 to 0.02 mg/mL before use.
▼ Monitor patient continuously during first 30 minutes and frequently thereafter for signs and symptoms of anaphylaxis.
● *Alert:* Because of risk of anaphylaxis, give injection only to patients who can't take oral form. Keep epinephrine 1:1,000 and oxygen available.
▼ Store diluted infusion solution for up to 24 hours in glass or polyethylene containers. Don't store drug in a polyvinyl chloride container because of decreased stability and potential for extraction of phthalates.
▼ **Incompatibilities:** Solutions or I.V. drugs with a pH above 9, such as acyclovir and ganciclovir.

ACTION

Exact mechanism unknown. Inhibits T-cell activation, which results in immunosuppression.

Route	Onset	Peak	Duration
P.O., I.V.	Unknown	½–6 hr	Unknown

Half-life: Immediate-release: variable—23 to 46 hours in healthy volunteers; 2.1 to 36 hours in transplant patients. Extended-release: 35 to 41 hours.

ADVERSE REACTIONS

CNS: asthenia, delirium, fever, headache, insomnia, pain, paresthesia, tremor, *coma.*
CV: peripheral edema, hypertension.
GI: abdominal pain, anorexia, ascites, constipation, diarrhea, nausea, vomiting.
GU: abnormal renal function, oliguria, UTI.
Hematologic: *thrombocytopenia,* anemia, leukocytosis.
Metabolic: hyperglycemia, *hyperkalemia,* hypokalemia, *hypomagnesemia.*
Musculoskeletal: back pain.
Respiratory: atelectasis, dyspnea, pleural effusion.
Skin: burning, photosensitivity, pruritus, rash, alopecia.

T

INTERACTIONS
Drug-drug. *Antacids (aluminum and magnesium hydroxide):* May increase tacrolimus level and risk of serious adverse reactions. Monitor patient closely; adjust dosage as needed.

Cyclosporine: May increase risk of excess nephrotoxicity. Avoid using together.

CYP450 inducers (carbamazepine, phenobarbital, phenytoin, **rifamycins [rifampin]):** May decrease tacrolimus level. Monitor effectiveness of tacrolimus.

CYP450 inhibitors, **(azole antifungals,** *bromocriptine, cimetidine, clarithromycin, cyclosporine, danazol, diltiazem, erythromycin, methylprednisolone, metoclopramide, nicardipine, protease inhibitors [nelfinavir, ritonavir], PPIs [lansoprazole, omeprazole], verapamil):* May increase tacrolimus level. Watch for adverse effects. Dosage adjustment may be needed.

Drugs that prolong QT interval (amiodarone, moxifloxacin), ziprasidone: May cause cardiac arrhythmias, including torsades de pointes. Use together is contraindicated.

Immunosuppressants (except adrenal corticosteroids): May oversuppress immune system. Monitor patient closely, especially during times of stress. Dosage adjustment may be needed.

Live-virus vaccines: May interfere with immune response to live-virus vaccines. Postpone routine immunizations.

Nephrotoxic drugs, such as aminoglycosides, amphotericin B, cisplatin, cyclosporine: May cause additive or synergistic effects. Monitor patient closely. Don't use tacrolimus simultaneously with cyclosporine. Stop cyclosporine at least 24 hours before starting tacrolimus.

Potassium-sparing diuretics: May cause severe hyperkalemia. Don't use together.

Sirolimus: May decrease tacrolimus level and increase risk of wound-healing complications, renal impairment, and insulin-dependent posttransplant diabetes mellitus in heart transplant patients. Avoid using together.

Strong CYP3A inducers (rifabutin, rifampin): May increase metabolism of CYP3A4 substrates. Some combinations may be contraindicated; check manufacturer's labeling. Tacrolimus dosage adjustments and subsequent frequent monitoring of tacrolimus whole blood trough concentrations and tacrolimus-associated adverse reactions are recommended when used concurrently.

Strong CYP3A4 inhibitors (clarithromycin, itraconazole, ketoconazole, ritonavir, voriconazole): May decrease metabolism of CYP3A4 substrates. Tacrolimus dosage adjustments and subsequent frequent monitoring of tacrolimus whole blood trough concentrations and tacrolimus-associated adverse reactions are recommended when used concurrently.

Drug-herb. *Echinacea,* **St. John's wort:** May decrease drug level and desired effects. Avoid use together.

Drug-food. *Any food:* May inhibit drug absorption. Urge patient to take drug on empty stomach.

Grapefruit, grapefruit juice: May increase drug level. Discourage patient from taking together.

Drug-lifestyle. *Alcohol use:* May modify rate of tacrolimus release. Avoid use together.

EFFECTS ON LAB TEST RESULTS
- May increase BUN, creatinine, and glucose levels. May decrease magnesium and Hb levels.
- May increase or decrease potassium level and cause abnormal LFT values.
- May decrease WBC and platelet counts.

CONTRAINDICATIONS & CAUTIONS
- Contraindicated in patients hypersensitive to drug. Serious hypersensitivity reactions, including anaphylaxis, have been reported.
- I.V. form is contraindicated in patients hypersensitive to castor oil derivatives.

Black Box Warning Use of extended-release form (Astagraf XL) in liver transplantation isn't approved because of increased mortality rate in female liver transplant recipients. ∎

⚠ *Alert:* May prolong QT/QTc interval and cause torsades de pointes. Avoid use in patients with congenital long QT syndrome. In patients with congestive HF or bradyarrhythmias, those taking certain antiarrhythmic medications or other medicina

---

Reactions in bold italics are *life-threatening*. Interactions may have a *rapid onset* or a *delayed onset*.

products that lead to QT prolongation, and those with electrolyte disturbances, such as hypokalemia, hypocalcemia, or hypomagnesemia, consider obtaining ECGs and periodically monitoring magnesium, potassium, and calcium levels during treatment.

• GI perforation has been reported in patients treated with tacrolimus; institute appropriate medical/surgical management promptly.

Dialyzable drug: Unlikely.

⚠ *Overdose S&S:* Exaggerated adverse effects.

PREGNANCY-LACTATION-REPRODUCTION

• There are no adequate studies in pregnant women. Use only if potential benefit justifies potential risk to the fetus.

• Drug appears in breast milk. Patient should discontinue breast-feeding or discontinue drug.

NURSING CONSIDERATIONS

Black Box Warning Drug increases risk of infections, lymphomas, and other malignant diseases. Only health care providers experienced in immunosuppressive therapy and management of organ transplant patients should prescribe this drug. Manage patients in facilities equipped and staffed with adequate laboratory and supportive medical resources. ▌

🖐 *Alert:* Drugs causing immunosuppression increase the risk of opportunistic infections, including activation of latent viral infections (such as BK virus-associated neuropathy and JC virus-associated progressive multifocal leukoencephalopathy), which may lead to serious, even fatal outcomes.

• Children with normal renal and hepatic function may need higher dosages than adults.

• Patients with hepatic or renal dysfunction should receive lowest dosage possible.

• Use with adrenocorticosteroids for all indications. For heart transplant patients, also use with azathioprine or mycophenolate mofetil.

• Don't use tacrolimus simultaneously with cyclosporine. Stop either drug at least 24 hours before initiating the other.

• Monitor patient for signs and symptoms of neurotoxicity and nephrotoxicity, especially if patient is receiving a high dose or has renal or hepatic dysfunction.

• Monitor patient for signs and symptoms of hyperkalemia, such as palpitations and muscle weakness or cramping. Obtain potassium levels regularly. Avoid potassium-sparing diuretics during drug therapy.

• Monitor patient's glucose level regularly. Also monitor patient for signs and symptoms of hyperglycemia, such as dizziness, confusion, and frequent urination. Insulin-dependent posttransplant diabetes may occur; Black and Hispanic renal transplant patients are at increased risk.

PATIENT TEACHING

• Advise patient to check with prescriber before taking other drugs during therapy.

• Urge patient to report adverse reactions promptly.

• Tell patient that glucose levels may increase and monitoring is needed.

• Advise patient taking extended-release capsules that if a dose is missed, the dose may be taken up to 14 hours (for Astagraf) or 15 hours (for Envarsus XR) after the scheduled time. Beyond the 14- or 15-hour time frame, patient should wait until the usual scheduled time the following morning to take the next regular daily dose. It isn't recommended to double the dose to make up for the missed dose.

tacrolimus (topical)
tack-ROW-lim-us

Protopic

Therapeutic class: Immunosuppressants
Pharmacologic class: Calcineurin inhibitors

AVAILABLE FORMS
Ointment: 0.03%, 0.1%

INDICATIONS & DOSAGES
➤ **Moderate to severe atopic dermatitis in patients unresponsive to other therapies or unable to use other therapies because of potential risks**

Adults: Thin layer of 0.03% or 0.1%
strength applied to affected areas b.i.d.
and rubbed in completely.
Children age 16 and older: Thin layer of
0.1% strength applied to affected areas b.i.d.
and rubbed in completely.
Children ages 2 to 15: Thin layer of 0.03%
strength applied to affected areas b.i.d. and
rubbed in completely.

ADMINISTRATION
Topical
● In patients with infected atopic dermatitis,
clear infections at treatment site before
using drug.
● Don't use with occlusive dressings.

ACTION
Unknown. Probably acts as an immune
system modulator in the skin by inhibiting
T-lymphocyte activation, which causes
immunosuppression. Drug also inhibits the
release of mediators from mast cells and
basophils in skin.

Route	Onset	Peak	Duration
Topical	Unknown	Unknown	Unknown

Half-life: Unknown.

ADVERSE REACTIONS
CNS: headache, hyperesthesia, asthenia,
insomnia, fever, pain.
CV: peripheral edema.
EENT: otitis media, pharyngitis, rhinitis,
sinusitis, conjunctivitis.
GI: diarrhea, vomiting, nausea, abdominal
pain, gastroenteritis, dyspepsia.
GU: dysmenorrhea.
Musculoskeletal: back pain, myalgia.
Respiratory: increased cough, *asthma,*
pneumonia, bronchitis.
Skin: burning, pruritus, erythema, infection, herpes simplex, eczema herpeticum,
pustular rash, folliculitis, urticaria, maculopapular rash, fungal dermatitis, acne,
sunburn, tingling, benign skin neoplasm,
vesiculobullous rash, dry skin, varicella
zoster, herpes zoster, eczema, exfoliative
dermatitis, contact dermatitis.
Other: flulike symptoms, accidental injury,
infection, facial edema, alcohol intolerance,
periodontal abscess, cyst, allergic reaction.

INTERACTIONS
Drug-drug. *Calcium channel blockers,
cimetidine, CYP3A4 inhibitors (erythromycin, itraconazole, ketoconazole, fluconazole):* May increase tacrolimus level if
systemic absorption occurs. Use together
cautiously.
Tacrolimus (systemic): May increase toxicity. Use together cautiously and decrease
dosage as needed.
Drug-lifestyle. *Alcohol use:* May cause
flushing. Discourage use together.
Sun exposure: May cause phototoxicity.
Advise patient to avoid excessive sunlight or
artificial ultraviolet light exposure.

EFFECTS ON LAB TEST RESULTS
None reported.

CONTRAINDICATIONS & CAUTIONS
● Contraindicated in patients hypersensitive
to drug.
Black Box Warning Long-term safety
of topical calcineurin inhibitors such as
tacrolimus hasn't been established. ■
Black Box Warning Don't use in children
younger than age 2. Only 0.03% ointment is
indicated for children ages 2 to 15. ■
● Don't use in immunocompromised patients or in patients with Netherton syndrome or generalized erythroderma.
۞ Alert: Use only after other therapies have
failed because of the risk of cancer.
Dialyzable drug: Unknown.

PREGNANCY-LACTATION-REPRODUCTION
● There are no adequate studies of topical
tacrolimus use in pregnant women, and
experience is too limited for assessment of
its safe use during pregnancy. Use only if
potential benefit justifies potential risk to the
fetus.
● Drug appears in breast milk. Patient
should discontinue breast-feeding or discontinue drug.

NURSING CONSIDERATIONS
Black Box Warning Use drug only for
short-term or intermittent long-term therapy. Limit application to areas of involvement with atopic dermatitis. Rare cases of
malignancy have been reported. ■

- If signs and symptoms of atopic dermatitis don't improve within 6 weeks, reevaluate patient to confirm the diagnosis.
- Use of this drug may increase the risk of varicella zoster, HSV, and eczema herpeticum.
- Consider stopping drug in patients with lymphadenopathy if cause is unknown or acute mononucleosis is diagnosed.
- Monitor all cases of lymphadenopathy until resolution.
- Local adverse effects are most common during the first few days of treatment.

PATIENT TEACHING

- Advise patient to read medication guide that comes with drug.
- Tell patient to wash hands before and after applying drug and to avoid applying drug to wet skin.
- Urge patient not to use bandages or other occlusive dressings.
- Tell patient not to bathe, shower, or swim immediately after application because doing so could wash the ointment off.
- Tell patient to stop treatment when the signs and symptoms resolve.
- Advise patient to avoid or minimize exposure to natural or artificial sunlight.
- Caution patient not to use drug for any disorder other than that for which it was prescribed.
- Encourage patient to report adverse reactions.
- Tell patient to store the ointment at room temperature.

tadalafil
tah-DAL-ah-fill

Adcirca, Cialis⋙

Therapeutic class: Erectile dysfunction drugs
Pharmacologic class: PDE5 inhibitors

AVAILABLE FORMS
Tablets (film-coated): 2.5 mg, 5 mg, 10 mg, 20 mg

INDICATIONS & DOSAGES
➤ **Erectile dysfunction (Cialis)**
Adults: 10 mg P.O. as a single dose, as needed, before sexual activity. Range is 5 to 20 mg, based on effectiveness and tolerance. Maximum is one dose daily. Or 2.5 mg P.O. once daily without regard to timing of sexual activity. May increase to 5 mg P.O. daily.
Adjust-a-dose: If CrCl is 31 to 50 mL/minute, starting dosage is 5 mg once daily and maximum is 10 mg once every 48 hours. If CrCl is 30 mL/minute or less, maximum is 5 mg once every 72 hours as needed; daily use isn't recommended. Use cautiously in patients with mild or moderate hepatic impairment (Child-Pugh class A or B); don't exceed 10 mg daily. Patients taking potent CYP450 inhibitors (erythromycin, itraconazole, ketoconazole, ritonavir) shouldn't exceed one 10-mg dose every 72 hours; the once-daily dose shouldn't exceed 2.5 mg.
➤ **Pulmonary arterial hypertension (Adcirca)**
Adults: 40 mg (two 20-mg tablets) P.O. once daily. Dividing dose over course of the day isn't recommended.
Adjust-a-dose: For patients with CrCl of 31 to 80 mL/minute, start with 20 mg P.O. once daily. Increase to 40 mg once daily if tolerated. Avoid use in patients with CrCl less than 30 mL/minute. Consider starting dose of 20 mg P.O. once daily in patients with Child-Pugh class A or B. In patients receiving ritonavir for at least 1 week, start at 20 mg P.O. once daily and increase to 40 mg as tolerated. Don't use Adcirca when starting ritonavir; stop Adcirca at least 24 hours before starting ritonavir. After at least 1 week, may give 20 mg P.O. once daily and increase to 40 mg as tolerated.
➤ **BPH (Cialis)**
Adults: 5 mg P.O. once daily taken at approximately the same time every day. When used with finasteride, recommended dose of Cialis is 5 mg once daily taken at approximately the same time every day for up to 26 weeks.
Adjust-a-dose: In patients with CrCl of 30 to 50 mL/minute, starting dose is 2.5 mg P.O. daily. May increase to 5 mg P.O. daily based on individual response. Not

T

recommended for patients with CrCl less than 30 mL/minute or in patients on hemodialysis.

➤ **BPH and erectile dysfunction (Cialis)**
Adults: 5 mg P.O. once daily taken at approximately the same time every day, without regard to the timing of sexual activity.

Adjust-a-dose: In patients with CrCl of 30 to 50 mL/minute, starting dose is 2.5 mg P.O. daily. May increase to 5 mg P.O. daily based on individual response. Not recommended for patients with CrCl less than 30 mL/minute or in patients on hemodialysis.

ADMINISTRATION
P.O.
● Give drug without regard for food.

ACTION
Increases cyclic guanosine monophosphate levels, prolongs smooth muscle relaxation, and promotes blood flow into the corpus cavernosum.

Route	Onset	Peak	Duration
P.O.	Within 1 hr	½–6 hr	Up to 36 hr

Half-life: 15 to 17½ hours; pulmonary arterial hypertension (in patients not receiving bosentan), 35 hours.

ADVERSE REACTIONS
CNS: dizziness, headache.
CV: flushing, hypertension.
EENT: decrease or loss of hearing, nasal congestion, tinnitus, nasopharyngitis.
GI: dyspepsia, abdominal pain, diarrhea, gastroesophageal reflux, gastroenteritis, nausea.
Musculoskeletal: back pain, limb pain, myalgia.
Respiratory: bronchitis, cough, URI.

INTERACTIONS
Drug-drug. *Alpha blockers:* May increase risk of hypotension. Patient should be on stable dose before starting tadalafil at lowest recommended dosage. Use with tadalafil for BPH treatment isn't recommended. Stop alpha blocker at least 1 day before starting tadalafil.

Guanylate cyclase (GC) stimulators (riociguat): May increase hypotension. Use together is contraindicated.
Nitrates: May enhance hypotensive effects. Use together is contraindicated.
Potent CYP450 inhibitors (erythromycin, itraconazole, ketoconazole, ritonavir): May increase tadalafil level. Don't exceed a 10-mg dose of Cialis every 72 hours.
Rifampin, other CYP450 inducers: May decrease tadalafil level. Monitor patient closely.
Drug-food. *Grapefruit:* May increase drug level. Discourage use together.
Drug-lifestyle. *Alcohol use:* May increase risk of headache, dizziness, orthostatic hypotension, and increased HR. Discourage use together.

EFFECTS ON LAB TEST RESULTS
None reported.

CONTRAINDICATIONS & CAUTIONS
● Contraindicated in patients hypersensitive to drug or its components and in those taking nitrates or GC stimulators.
● Use cautiously in patients with mild or moderate hepatic impairment (Child-Pugh class A or B).
● Drug isn't recommended for patients with severe hepatic impairment (Child-Pugh class C), unstable angina, angina that occurs during sexual intercourse, New York Heart Association class II or greater HF within past 6 months, uncontrolled arrhythmias, hypotension (lower than 90/50 mm Hg), uncontrolled hypertension (higher than 170/100 mm Hg), stroke within past 6 months, or an MI within past 90 days.
● Use cautiously in patients with left ventricular outflow obstruction. Use in patients with pulmonary veno-occlusive disease isn't recommended.
● Drug isn't recommended for patients whose cardiac status makes sexual activity inadvisable or for those with hereditary degenerative retinal disorders.
● Use cautiously in patients with bleeding disorders, significant peptic ulceration, or renal or hepatic impairment.
● Use cautiously in patients with conditions predisposing them to priapism (sickle cell

anemia, multiple myeloma, and leukemia) and in those with anatomic penis abnormalities.

● Use cautiously in elderly patients.
Dialyzable drug: No.

PREGNANCY-LACTATION-REPRODUCTION
● There are no adequate studies in pregnant women. Use only if clearly needed.
● It isn't known if drug appears in breast milk. Use cautiously in breast-feeding women.

NURSING CONSIDERATIONS
⚊ *Alert:* Sexual activity may increase cardiac risk. Evaluate patient's cardiac risk before he starts taking drug.
● Before patient starts drug, assess him for underlying causes of erectile dysfunction.
● Transient decreases in supine BP may occur.
● Prolonged erections and priapism may occur.
● Monitor patients for (rare) vision or hearing loss and report immediately.

PATIENT TEACHING
● Warn patient that taking drug with nitrates could cause a serious drop in BP, which increases the risk of heart attack or stroke.
● Tell patient to seek immediate medical attention if chest pain develops after taking the drug.
● Tell patient that drug doesn't protect against sexually transmitted diseases and that he should use protective measures.
● Urge patient to seek emergency medical care if his erection lasts more than 4 hours.
● Tell patient to take drug about 60 minutes before anticipated sexual activity. Explain that drug has no effect without sexual stimulation.
● Warn patient not to change dosage unless directed by prescriber.
● Caution patient against drinking large amounts of alcohol while taking drug.
● Instruct patient to notify prescriber of vision or hearing changes.

tafluprost
TA-floo-prost

Zioptan

Therapeutic class: Antiglaucoma drugs
Pharmacologic class: Prostaglandin analogues

AVAILABLE FORMS
Ophthalmic solution: 0.0015%

INDICATIONS & DOSAGES
➤ **Increased IOP in patients with open-angle glaucoma or ocular hypertension**
Adults: 1 drop instilled in conjunctival sac of affected eye once daily in the evening.

ADMINISTRATION
Ophthalmic
● Store drug in original pouch in refrigerator at 36° to 46° F (2° to 8° C).
● After pouch is opened, the single-use containers may be stored at room temperature (68° to 77° F [20° to 25° C]) for up to 28 days. Date pouch in space provided once it has been opened. Discard unused single units after 28 days.
● Discard single-use unit immediately after use; sterility can't be maintained.
● If patient is receiving more than one ophthalmic drug, give drugs at least 5 minutes apart.

ACTION
Exact mechanism unknown; believed to reduce IOP by increasing uveoscleral outflow.

Route	Onset	Peak	Duration
Ophthalmic	Rapid	10 min	Unknown

Half-life: Unknown.

ADVERSE REACTIONS
CNS: headache.
EENT: ocular stinging or irritation, ocular pruritus, conjunctivitis, cataract, dry eye, ocular pain, eyelash darkening, eyelash growth, blurred vision, conjunctival redness.
GU: UTI.
Respiratory: cough.
Other: common cold.

INTERACTIONS
None reported.

EFFECTS ON LAB TEST RESULTS
None reported.

CONTRAINDICATIONS & CAUTIONS
• Contraindicated in patients hypersensitive to drug or its components.
• Use cautiously in patients with intraocular inflammation, aphakic eyes (lens has been removed), pseudophakic eyes (presence of artificial lens), or torn posterior lens capsule.
Dialyzable drug: Unknown.

PREGNANCY-LACTATION-REPRODUCTION
• There are no adequate studies in pregnant women. Use only if potential benefit justifies potential risk to the fetus.
• It isn't known if drug appears in breast milk. Use cautiously in breast-feeding women.

NURSING CONSIDERATIONS
• Drug shouldn't be given more than once daily because more frequent administration of prostaglandin analogues may lessen the IOP-lowering effect.
• May use concomitantly with other topical ophthalmic drugs to lower IOP. If more than one topical ophthalmic drug is being used, separate administration times by at least 5 minutes.
• After opening individual unit for one or both eyes, use immediately because sterility can't be maintained. Discard remaining contents after administration.
• Drug can cause changes to pigmented tissues of the iris, periorbital tissue, and eyelashes. Pigmentation increases for as long as tafluprost is administered. After drug discontinuation, pigmentation of the iris is most likely permanent; however, pigmentation of the periorbital tissue and eyelash changes may be reversible. Long-term effects are unknown.
• Drug may gradually change eyelashes and vellus hair in the treated eye. Changes include increased length and number of eyelashes and changes in color, thickness, and shape. Usually these changes are reversible after drug discontinuation.

PATIENT TEACHING
• Inform patient of once-daily nighttime dosing. More frequent dosing may decrease drug's effectiveness.
• Inform patient that drug comes in single-use containers and that unused portions must be discarded because containers don't contain a preservative.
• Caution patient that brown iris pigmentation may not be reversible but that eyelid skin darkening may be reversible.
• Inform patient of the possibility of eyelash and vellus hair changes, which may be reversible.
• Advise patient to report all adverse reactions and to immediately report new ocular conditions (such as trauma or infection), sudden decrease in visual acuity, or ocular surgery.
• Instruct patient taking more than one topical ophthalmic drug to separate administration times by 5 minutes.
• Show patient how to store medication properly.

SAFETY ALERT!

tamoxifen citrate
ta-MOX-i-fen

APO-Tamox ✤, Nolvadex-D ✤, Soltamox

Therapeutic class: Antineoplastics
Pharmacologic class: Nonsteroidal antiestrogens

AVAILABLE FORMS
Oral solution: 10 mg/5 mL
Tablets: 10 mg, 20 mg

INDICATIONS & DOSAGES
➤ **Advanced breast cancer in women and men**
Adults: 20 to 40 mg P.O. daily; divide doses of more than 20 mg/day into two doses.
➤ **Adjuvant treatment of breast cancer**
Women: 20 to 40 mg P.O. daily for 5 years; divide doses of more than 20 mg/day into two doses.
➤ **To reduce breast cancer occurrence**
High-risk women: 20 mg P.O. daily for 5 years.

➤ **Ductal carcinoma in situ (DCIS) after breast surgery and radiation**
Adults: 20 mg P.O. daily for 5 years.
➤ **Gynecomastia** ◆
Adults: 20 mg P.O. daily for 1 to 12 months.
➤ **Mastalgia** ◆
Adults: 10 to 20 mg/day P.O. for 3 to 6 months.

ADMINISTRATION
P.O.
• Drug is a hormonal agent and is considered a potential teratogen. Follow safe-handling procedures.
• Give drug without regard to food.
• Store between 68° and 77° F (20° and 25° C). Protect from light.
• Don't freeze or refrigerate oral solution; use within 3 months of opening.

ACTION
Unknown. Drug is selective estrogen-receptor modulator.

Route	Onset	Peak	Duration
P.O.	1 mo–several mo	5 hr	Several wk

Half-life: Distribution phase, 7 to 14 hours; terminal phase, 5 to 7 days.

ADVERSE REACTIONS
CNS: *stroke,* confusion, weakness, sleepiness, headache.
CV: fluid retention, hot flashes, *thromboembolism.*
EENT: corneal changes, cataracts, retinopathy.
GI: nausea, vomiting, diarrhea.
GU: amenorrhea, irregular menses, vaginal discharge, *endometrial cancer, uterine sarcoma,* vaginal bleeding.
Hematologic: *leukopenia, thrombocytopenia.*
Metabolic: hypercalcemia, weight gain or loss.
Musculoskeletal: brief worsening of pain from osseous metastases.
Respiratory: *PE.*
Skin: skin changes, rash, alopecia.
Other: temporary bone or tumor pain.

INTERACTIONS
Drug-drug. *Bromocriptine:* May elevate tamoxifen level. Monitor patient closely.

Coumarin-type anticoagulants: May significantly increase anticoagulant effect. Monitor patient, PT, and INR closely. Use is contraindicated when tamoxifen is used to reduce risk of breast cancer in high-risk women and women with DCIS.
CYP3A4 inducers (such as rifampin): May increase tamoxifen metabolism and may lower drug levels. Monitor patient for clinical effects.
Cytotoxic drugs: May increase risk of thromboembolic events. Monitor patient.
Drug-herb. *St. John's wort:* May increase serotonin levels. Use together cautiously.

EFFECTS ON LAB TEST RESULTS
• May increase BUN, calcium, T_4, and liver enzyme levels.
• May decrease WBC and platelet counts.

CONTRAINDICATIONS & CAUTIONS
• Contraindicated in patients hypersensitive to drug.
• Contraindicated as therapy to reduce risk of breast cancer in high-risk women and women with DCIS who also need coumarin-type anticoagulants or in women with history of DVT or PE.
Black Box Warning Serious and life-threatening events associated with tamoxifen have occurred in the risk-reduction setting (women at high risk for cancer and women with DCIS) and include uterine malignancies, stroke, and PE). ▮
• Use cautiously in patients with leukopenia or thrombocytopenia.
Dialyzable drug: No.
⚠ *Overdose S&S:* Tremors, hyperreflexia, unsteady gait, dizziness, seizures, prolonged QT interval.

PREGNANCY-LACTATION-REPRODUCTION
• May cause fetal harm when used in pregnant women. Advise women not to become pregnant during therapy or within 2 months of stopping drug and to use barrier or non-hormonal contraceptive measures if sexually active.
• Breast-feeding is contraindicated during therapy.

T

NURSING CONSIDERATIONS

• Monitor lipid levels during long-term therapy in patients with hyperlipidemia.
• Monitor calcium level. At start of therapy, drug may compound hypercalcemia related to bone metastases.
• Women should have baseline and periodic gynecologic examinations because of a slight increased risk of endometrial cancer.
• Women should have periodic eye examinations because of increased risk of cataracts, retinal vein thrombosis, and retinopathy.
• Monitor CBC closely in patients with leukopenia or thrombocytopenia.
• Rule out pregnancy before therapy.
• Patient may initially experience worsening symptoms.
• Adverse reactions are usually minor and well tolerated.
• In postmenopausal women, karyopyknotic index of vaginal smears and various degrees of estrogen effect of Papanicolaou smears may vary.

Black Box Warning Discuss potential benefits versus potential risks with women at high risk for breast cancer and women with DCIS who are considering tamoxifen to reduce their risks of developing breast cancer. Benefits of drug outweigh its risks in women already diagnosed with breast cancer. ■

PATIENT TEACHING

• Reassure patient that acute worsening of bone pain during therapy usually indicates drug will produce good response. Give analgesics to relieve pain.
• Strongly encourage women who are taking or have taken drug to have regular gynecologic examinations because drug may increase risk of uterine cancer.
• Encourage women to have annual mammograms and breast examinations.
• Advise patient to use a barrier form of contraception because short-term therapy induces ovulation in premenopausal women.
• Instruct patient to report vaginal bleeding or changes in menstrual cycle.
• Caution women to avoid becoming pregnant during therapy and for first 2 months after stopping drug. Advise consulting prescriber before becoming pregnant.

• Tell patient to report all adverse reactions, especially signs and symptoms of stroke (headache, vision changes, confusion, difficulty speaking, weakness of face, arm, or leg, especially on one side of the body) and PE (chest pain, difficulty breathing, rapid breathing, sweating, fainting).
• Advise patient to report vision changes.
• Tell patient not to freeze or refrigerate oral solution, to protect solution from light, and to use it within 3 months of opening.

tamsulosin hydrochloride
tam-soo-LOE-sin

Flomax✧

Therapeutic class: BPH drugs
Pharmacologic class: Alpha blockers

AVAILABLE FORMS
Capsules ⊙*:* 0.4 mg

INDICATIONS & DOSAGES
➤ **BPH**
Adults: 0.4 mg P.O. once daily, given 30 minutes after same meal each day. If no response after 2 to 4 weeks, increase dosage to 0.8 mg P.O. once daily.
➤ **Adjunctive treatment of ureteral stones ◆**
Adults: 0.4 mg P.O. daily at bedtime for up to 6 weeks or until expulsion.

ADMINISTRATION
P.O.
• Don't crush or open capsules.
• Give drug 30 minutes after same meal each day.

ACTION
Selectively blocks alpha receptors in the prostate, leading to relaxation of smooth muscles in the bladder neck and prostate, improving urine flow and reducing symptoms of BPH.

Route	Onset	Peak	Duration
P.O.	Unknown	4–7 hr	9–15 hr

Half-life: 9 to 13 hours.

Reactions in bold italics are *life-threatening*. Interactions may have a *rapid onset* or a *delayed onset*.

ADVERSE REACTIONS

CNS: dizziness, headache, asthenia, insomnia, somnolence, syncope, vertigo.
CV: chest pain, orthostatic hypotension.
EENT: rhinitis, amblyopia, pharyngitis, sinusitis.
GI: diarrhea, nausea.
GU: decreased libido, abnormal ejaculation, priapism.
Musculoskeletal: back pain.
Respiratory: increased cough.
Other: infection, tooth disorder.

INTERACTIONS

Drug-drug. *Alpha blockers:* May interact with tamsulosin. Avoid using together.
Cimetidine: May decrease tamsulosin clearance. Use together cautiously.
CYP3A4 inducers (strong): May increase metabolism of CYP3A4 substrates. Consider therapy modification. Some combinations may be specifically contraindicated. Consult appropriate manufacturer labeling.
CYP3A4 inhibitors (moderate): May decrease metabolism of CYP3A4 substrates. Use cautiously and monitor therapy.
CYP3A4 inhibitors (strong): May increase tamsulosin serum concentration. Avoid combination.
PDE5 inhibitors: May cause symptomatic hypotension. Use together cautiously.
Warfarin: Limited studies are inconclusive. Use together cautiously.
Drug-herb. *St. John's wort:* May decrease serum concentration of CYP3A4 substrates. Consider therapy modification.

EFFECTS ON LAB TEST RESULTS

None reported.

CONTRAINDICATIONS & CAUTIONS

• Contraindicated in patients hypersensitive to drug or its components.
• Use cautiously in patients with serious or life-threatening sulfa allergy.
• Intraoperative floppy iris syndrome has been observed during cataract and glaucoma surgery in some patients who are taking or had previously taken alpha$_1$ blockers, including tamsulosin, which may increase risk of eye complications during and after surgery. Initiation of drug in patients for whom cataract or glaucoma surgery is scheduled isn't recommended.
Dialyzable drug: Unlikely.
⚠ **Overdose S&S:** Severe headache.

PREGNANCY-LACTATION-REPRODUCTION

• Drug isn't indicated for use in women.
• Don't use drug for off-label indication in pregnant or breast-feeding women.

NURSING CONSIDERATIONS

• Monitor patient for decreases in BP.
• Symptoms of BPH and prostate cancer are similar; rule out prostate cancer before starting therapy.
• If treatment is interrupted for several days or more, restart therapy at the 0.4-mg P.O. once-daily dose.
• ***Look alike–sound alike:*** Don't confuse Flomax with Fosamax.

PATIENT TEACHING

• Instruct patient not to crush, chew, or open capsules.
• Advise patient that drug may cause sudden drop in BP, especially after first dose or when changing doses. Tell patient to rise slowly from a chair or bed when starting therapy and to avoid situations in which injury could occur as a result of fainting.
• Warn patient that priapism can occur and to report it immediately.
• Instruct patient not to drive or perform hazardous tasks for 12 hours after first dose or changes in dose until response can be monitored.
• Tell patient to take drug about 30 minutes after same meal each day.
• Advise patient considering cataract or glaucoma surgery to inform the ophthalmologist that he is taking the drug.

tapentadol hydrochloride
tah-PEN-tah-dol

Nucynta✦, Nucynta ER✦

Therapeutic class: Opioid analgesics
Pharmacologic class: Centrally acting synthetic opioid analgesics
Controlled substance schedule: II

AVAILABLE FORMS
Oral solution: 20 mg/mL
Tablets: 50 mg, 75 mg, 100 mg
Tablets (extended-release) ⓞⓝⓒ*:* 50 mg, 100 mg, 150 mg, 200 mg, 250 mg

INDICATIONS & DOSAGES
➤ **Moderate to severe acute pain (immediate-release only)**
Adults: 50 to 100 mg P.O. every 4 to 6 hours, as needed, for pain. On day 1, may give second dose in 1 hour if first dose is ineffective. Adjust subsequent dosing to maintain adequate pain control. Maximum daily dose, 700 mg on day 1; 600 mg on subsequent days.
Adjust-a-dose: For patients with moderate hepatic impairment, initially give 50 mg P.O. every 8 hours. Maximum, three doses (150 mg) in 24 hours; the interval between doses should be no less than 8 hours.
➤ **Severe chronic pain when continuous, around-the-clock opioid analgesia is needed for an extended period (extended-release)**
Adults: Initially, 50 mg P.O. every 12 hours. Titrate with dose increases of 50 mg no more than b.i.d. every 3 days. Therapeutic range is 100 to 250 mg P.O. b.i.d.
Adjust-a-dose: For patients with moderate hepatic impairment, initially 50 mg (extended-release) P.O. once every 24 hours. Maximum dose is 100 mg (extended-release) once daily.
➤ **Neuropathic pain associated with diabetic peripheral neuropathy (extended-release)**
Adults: Initially, 50 mg P.O. every 12 hours. Titrate with dose increases of 50 mg no more than twice a day every 3 days. Therapeutic range is 100 to 250 mg P.O. b.i.d.

Adjust-a-dose: In patients with moderate hepatic impairment, initially give 50 mg (extended-release) once every 24 hours. Maximum dosage is 100 mg once daily.

ADMINISTRATION
P.O.
• Give drug with or without food.
• Always use calibrated oral syringe enclosed with oral solution to ensure dose is measured and administered accurately.
Black Box Warning Patients must swallow extended-release tablets whole. Taking split, broken, chewed, dissolved, or crushed tablets could lead to rapid release and a potentially fatal overdose. ∎

ACTION
Unknown. Thought to work by possessing mu-opioid agonist activity and inhibiting norepinephrine reuptake in the brain.

Route	Onset	Peak	Duration
P.O.	Rapid	1¼ hr	Unknown
P.O. (extended-release)	Rapid	3–6 hr	Unknown

Half-life: Immediate-release, 4 hours; extended-release, 5 hours.

ADVERSE REACTIONS
CNS: abnormal dreams, anxiety, *CNS depression,* confusion, dizziness, fatigue, insomnia, lethargy, somnolence, tremor.
EENT: nasopharyngitis.
GI: constipation, decreased appetite, dry mouth, dyspepsia, nausea, vomiting.
GU: UTI.
Musculoskeletal: arthralgia.
Respiratory: *respiratory depression,* URI.
Skin: hot flushes, hyperhidrosis, pruritus, rash.

INTERACTIONS
Drug-drug. Black Box Warning *Benzodiazepines, CNS depressants:* May cause slow or difficult breathing, sedation, and death. Avoid use together. If use together is necessary, limit dosage and duration of each drug to minimum necessary for desired effect. ∎
MAO inhibitors: May cause adverse CV events. Avoid use together. Avoid giving drug within 14 days of MAO inhibitor use.

Reactions in bold italics are *life-threatening*. Interactions may have a *rapid onset* or a *delayed onset*.

MAO inhibitors, SSNRIs, SSRIs, TCAs, triptans: May cause serotonin syndrome (mental changes, tachycardia, labile BP, hyperthermia, hyperreflexia, incoordination, nausea, vomiting, diarrhea). Avoid use together.

⊕ *Alert:* *Serotonergic drugs (antiemetics [dolasetron, granisetron, ondansetron, palonosetron], antimigraine drugs, amoxapine, buspirone, cyclobenzaprine, dextromethorphan, linezolid, lithium, MAO inhibitors, maprotiline, methylene blue, mirtazapine, nefazodone, SNRIs, SSRIs, TCAs, trazodone, tryptophan, vilazodone):* May increase risk of serotonin syndrome. Use together cautiously. Monitor patient for serotonin syndrome.

Drug-herb. ⊕ *Alert:* *St. John's wort:* May increase risk of serotonin syndrome. Use together cautiously. Monitor patient for serotonin syndrome.

Drug-lifestyle. **Black Box Warning** *Alcohol use:* May result in a potentially fatal overdose of tapentadol, if alcohol, including prescription or OTC drugs that contain alcohol, is used with extended-release form. Don't use together. ∎

EFFECTS ON LAB TEST RESULTS
None reported.

CONTRAINDICATIONS & CAUTIONS
• Contraindicated in patients with hypersensitivity (anaphylaxis, angioedema) to tapentadol or to ingredients of the product.
Black Box Warning Opioids should only be prescribed with benzodiazepines or other CNS depressants to patients for whom alternative treatment options are inadequate. ∎
⊕ *Alert:* Drug may lead to a rare but serious decrease in adrenal gland cortisol production.
⊕ *Alert:* Drug may cause decreased sex hormone levels with long-term use.
• Extended-release tapentadol is indicated for the management of severe pain or neuropathic pain associated with diabetic peripheral neuropathy in adults severe enough to require daily, around-the-clock, long-term opioid treatment and for which alternative treatment options are inadequate.
• Extended-release tapentadol should be prescribed only by health care professionals

knowledgeable in the use of potent opioids for the management of chronic pain.
⊕ *Alert:* Patients are at increased risk for oversedation and respiratory depression if they snore or have a history of sleep apnea, haven't used opioids recently or are first-time opioid users, have increased opioid dosage requirements or opioid habituation, have received general anesthesia for longer lengths of time or received other sedating drugs, have preexisting pulmonary or cardiac disease, or have thoracic or other surgical incisions that may impair breathing. Monitor patients carefully.
• Contraindicated in patients with significant respiratory depression, acute or severe bronchial asthma, or hypercarbia in unmonitored settings or when resuscitative equipment isn't available.
Black Box Warning Extended-release tapentadol must not be used as an as-needed analgesic or to treat acute or postoperative pain. ∎
Black Box Warning Schedule II opioids have the highest potential for abuse and risk of fatal overdose due to respiratory depression. ∎
• Contraindicated in patients who have or are suspected of having paralytic ileus and in those receiving MAO inhibitors or who have used MAO inhibitors within the past 14 days.
• Don't use in patients with head injury, increased ICP, or severe renal or severe hepatic impairment.
• Use cautiously in patients with conditions accompanied by hypoxia, hypercapnia, or decreased respiratory reserve (such as asthma, COPD, cor pulmonale, severe obesity, sleep apnea syndrome, myxedema, kyphoscoliosis, CNS depression, coma, or upper airway obstruction).
• Use cautiously in patients with a history of seizures, mild to moderate hepatic impairment, or biliary tract disease, including acute pancreatitis, and in elderly and debilitated patients.
Dialyzable drug: Unknown.
⚠ *Overdose S&S:* CNS and respiratory depression, hypotension, bradycardia, hypothermia, shock, apnea, cardiopulmonary arrest.

T

PREGNANCY-LACTATION-REPRODUCTION

• Safety and effectiveness in pregnant women haven't been established. Use only if benefits outweigh potential risk to the fetus.

Black Box Warning Prolonged use of extended-release form during pregnancy can result in neonatal opioid withdrawal syndrome, which may be life-threatening if not recognized and treated and requires management according to protocols developed by neonatology experts. ■

• It isn't known if drug appears in breast milk. However, because of risk of serious adverse reactions, breast-feeding isn't recommended.

NURSING CONSIDERATIONS

• Keep opioid antagonist (naloxone) available.

Black Box Warning Caution patient or caregiver of patient taking an opioid with a benzodiazepine, CNS depressant, or alcohol to seek immediate medical attention if patient experiences dizziness, light-headedness, extreme sleepiness, slowed or difficult breathing, or unresponsiveness. ■

◑ *Alert:* Carefully monitor vital signs, pain level, respiratory status, and sedation level in all patients receiving opioids, especially those receiving I.V. drugs, even those given postoperatively.

• Monitor vital signs, respiratory status, and level of consciousness closely, especially in elderly, cachectic, or debilitated patients and in those with chronic pulmonary disease, particularly during first 24 to 72 hours after initiating therapy; drug may cause hypotension and respiratory depression. If respiratory rate drops below 12 breaths/minute, withhold dose and notify prescriber.

• Reassess patient's pain level 15 to 30 minutes after giving dose.

• Avoid using drug immediately before and during labor and delivery. Watch for respiratory depression in newborns of mothers who have been taking drug.

Black Box Warning Assess patient's risk of opioid addiction, abuse, and misuse before prescribing extended-release tapentadol. ■

Black Box Warning Drug has the potential for addiction and abuse. Chewing, crushing, snorting, or injecting it can lead to overdose

and death. Monitor patients for signs and symptoms of abuse or addiction. ■

Black Box Warning Monitor patient for respiratory depression, especially during initiation of extended-release tapentadol and after a dosage increase. ■

• Taper dosage gradually to prevent withdrawal symptoms (anxiety, sweating, insomnia, rigors, pain, nausea, tremors, diarrhea, upper respiratory symptoms, piloerection, and hallucinations).

• Consider dosage reduction of one or both drugs if taken with another opioid, sedative, or illicit drug because of additive effects.

• Prevent constipation with the use of stool softeners or senna preparations at the start of therapy.

• Drug may cause spasm of the sphincter of Oddi and may worsen pain in patients with biliary disease, including pancreatitis.

◑ *Alert:* If patient is taking opioids with serotonergic drugs, watch for signs and symptoms of serotonin syndrome (agitation, hallucinations, rapid HR, fever, excessive sweating, shivering or shaking, muscle twitching or stiffness, trouble with coordination, nausea, vomiting, diarrhea), especially when starting treatment or increasing dosages. Signs and symptoms may occur within several hours of coadministration but may also occur later, especially after dosage increase. Discontinue the opioid, serotonergic drug, or both if serotonin syndrome is suspected.

◑ *Alert:* Monitor patient for signs and symptoms of adrenal insufficiency (nausea, vomiting, loss of appetite, fatigue, weakness, dizziness, low BP). Perform diagnostic testing if adrenal insufficiency is suspected. If adrenal insufficiency is confirmed, treat with corticosteroids and wean patient off opioids if appropriate. Discontinue corticosteroids when clinically appropriate.

◑ *Alert:* Monitor patient for signs and symptoms of decreased sex hormone levels (low libido, erectile dysfunction, amenorrhea, infertility). If signs and symptoms occur, evaluate patient and obtain laboratory testing.

Black Box Warning Accidental ingestion of even one dose of extended-release form may cause fatal overdose, especially in children. ■

Reactions in bold italics are *life-threatening*. Interactions may have a *rapid onset* or a *delayed onset*.

PATIENT TEACHING

• Instruct patient to ask for drug before pain is intense and to report episodes of breakthrough pain.

• Explain assessment and monitoring process to patient and family. Instruct them to immediately report difficulty breathing or other signs or symptoms of a potential adverse opioid-related reaction.

• Advise ambulatory patients to use caution when getting out of bed or walking.

• Warn patient to avoid driving and other hazardous activities that require mental alertness until drug's CNS effects are known.

Black Box Warning Warn patient not to crush, break, chew, or dissolve tablets. ■

Black Box Warning Instruct patient to keep tablets in a child-resistant container in a safe place because accidental ingestion by a child can result in death. ■

Black Box Warning If a pregnant woman must use an opioid for a prolonged period, advise her of risk of neonatal opioid withdrawal syndrome; ensure her that appropriate treatment will be available. ■

Black Box Warning Caution patient not to consume alcohol or take drugs containing alcohol; doing so may lead to fatal overdose. ■

• Inform patient that drug has the potential for abuse. Advise patient to protect drug from theft.

☙ *Alert:* Encourage patient to report all medications being taken, including prescription and OTC medications and supplements.

☙ *Alert:* Caution patient to immediately report all adverse reactions and signs and symptoms of serotonin syndrome, adrenal insufficiency, and decreased sex hormone levels.

• Tell female patient of childbearing potential to consult prescriber if pregnant or considering becoming pregnant.

Advise female patient who is breast-feeding to choose an alternative feeding method during therapy.

Advise patient not to stop drug abruptly.

tedizolid phosphate
TED-eye-zoe-lid

Sivextro

Therapeutic class: Antibiotics
Pharmacologic class: Oxazolidinones

AVAILABLE FORMS
Injection: 200 mg/vial
Tablets: 200 mg

INDICATIONS & DOSAGES
➤ **Acute bacterial skin and skin-structure infections (ABSSSI) caused by susceptible gram-positive isolates (*Staphylococcus aureus* [including MRSA and methicillin-susceptible strains], *Streptococcus pyogenes, Streptococcus agalactiae, Streptococcus anginosus* group [including *S. anginosus, S. intermedius,* and *S. constellatus*], and *Enterococcus faecalis*)**
Adults: 200 mg P.O. or I.V. once daily for 6 days.

ADMINISTRATION
• Drug is used only to treat ABSSSI that's proven or strongly suspected to be caused by susceptible bacteria.
P.O.
• May give with or without food.
• Store at room temperature.
I.V.
▼ Vial contains no preservatives.
▼ Reconstitute with 4 mL sterile water for injection. Gently swirl contents and let stand until cake has dissolved completely and foam has dispersed.
▼ Inspect vial for particulate matter, remaining cake, or powder. Invert vial to dissolve any remaining powder, if necessary, and swirl gently to prevent foaming.
▼ Reconstituted solution should appear clear and colorless to pale yellow.
▼ Further dilute 4 mL of reconstituted solution in 250 mL of NSS. Invert bag gently to mix. Don't shake.
▼ Inspect I.V. bag for particulate matter before administering.

T

▼ Time from reconstitution to administration shouldn't exceed 24 hours at room temperature or under refrigeration.

▼ Administer infusion over 1 hour. Don't administer as an I.V. push or bolus; don't give intra-arterially, I.M., intrathecally, intraperitoneally, or subcutaneously.

▼ Don't mix with other drugs while administering.

▼ **Incompatibilities:** Lactated Ringer solution, Hartmann solution, additives, or other medications shouldn't be added to or infused with tedizolid phosphate.

ACTION

Binds to bacterial ribosome, resulting in inhibition of bacterial protein synthesis. This mechanism of action differs from that of other nonoxazolidinone-class antibacterial drugs; therefore, cross-resistance is unlikely.

Route	Onset	Peak	Duration
P.O.	Unknown	3 hr	Unknown
I.V.	Unknown	1 hr	Unknown

Half-life: 12 hours.

ADVERSE REACTIONS

CNS: headache, dizziness, hypoesthesia, paresthesia, cranial nerve VII paralysis, insomnia, peripheral neuropathy.
CV: palpitations, tachycardia, flushing, hypertension.
EENT: asthenopia, blurred vision, visual impairment, vitreous floaters, vitreous opacity, optic neuropathy, oral candidiasis.
GI: nausea, vomiting, diarrhea, CDAD, colitis.
GU: vulvovaginal mycotic infection.
Hematologic: anemia, decreased WBC and RBC counts.
Hepatic: increased transaminase levels.
Skin: pruritus, urticaria, dermatitis.
Other: infusion-related reactions, hypersensitivity.

INTERACTIONS

None reported.

EFFECTS ON LAB TEST RESULTS

• May increase hepatic transaminase levels.
• May decrease Hb level and WBC and RBC counts.
• May decrease ANC and platelet count.

CONTRAINDICATIONS & CAUTIONS

• Contraindicated in patients hypersensitive to drug or its components.
• Safety and effectiveness in patients with neutropenia (neutrophil count less than $1,000/mm^3$) haven't been adequately evaluated. Consider alternative therapies when treating patients with neutropenia.
Dialyzable drug: No.

PREGNANCY-LACTATION-REPRODUCTION

• There are no adequate studies in pregnant women. Use only if potential benefit justifies potential risk to the fetus.
• It isn't known if drug appears in breast milk. Use cautiously in breast-feeding women.

NURSING CONSIDERATIONS

❸ *Alert:* Severe, persistent diarrhea may indicate CDAD, which can range in severity from mild diarrhea to fatal colitis and can occur up to 2 months after treatment. Monitor patient closely. Drug may need to be discontinued and treatment begun.
• *Look alike–sound alike:* Don't confuse tedizolid with linezolid. Don't confuse Sivextro with Stalevo.

PATIENT TEACHING

• Explain to patient that antibiotics are used to treat bacterial infections only and aren't used to treat viral infections.
• Inform patient that it's common to feel better early in treatment but to continue to take medication exactly as directed.
• Teach patient to take medication with or without food.
• Advise patient that antibiotic therapy may cause diarrhea, but that diarrhea usually resolves when drug is discontinued. Advise patient to contact prescriber immediately if watery or bloody stools occur, as this may indicate CDAD; drug may need to be discontinued and other treatment begun.
• Instruct patient that if a dose is missed, to take missed dose as soon as possible up to 8 hours before next scheduled dose. If less than 8 hours remain before next dose, advise patient to wait until next scheduled dose.

Reactions in bold italics are *life-threatening*. Interactions may have a *rapid onset* or a *delayed onset*.

telavancin
tell-uh-VAN-sin

Vibativ

Therapeutic class: Antibiotics
Pharmacologic class: Lipoglycopeptides

AVAILABLE FORMS
Lyophilized powder for injection: 250-mg,
750-mg single-use vials

INDICATIONS & DOSAGES
⚠ *Alert:* Drug should be used to prevent
or treat bacterial infections only. Reserve
use for when alternative treatments aren't
suitable.
Adjust-a-dose (for all indications): For patients with CrCl of 30 to 50 mL/minute, give
7.5 mg/kg every 24 hours; if CrCl is 10 to
29 mL/minute, give 10 mg/kg every
48 hours.
➤ **Complicated skin and skin-structure
infections caused by susceptible gram-
positive organisms, such as *Staphylococcus aureus*, MRSA, *Streptococcus pyogenes*, *Streptococcus agalactiae*, *Streptococcus anginosus* group, or *Enterococcus
faecalis* (vancomycin-susceptible isolates
only)**
Adults: 10 mg/kg I.V. infusion once every
24 hours for 7 to 14 days.
➤ **Hospital-acquired and ventilator-
associated bacterial pneumonia caused by
susceptible isolates of *S. aureus* (including
methicillin-susceptible and methicillin-
resistant isolates)**
Adults: 10 mg/kg I.V. once every 24 hours
for 7 to 21 days.

ADMINISTRATION
I.V.
▼ Reconstitute 250-mg vial with 15 mL
sterile water for injection and 750-mg vial
with 45 mL sterile water for injection. Solutions of D_5W and NSS for injection also
may be used. Mix thoroughly; reconstitution may take up to 20 minutes.
▼ Further dilute doses of 150 to 800 mg in
100 to 250 mL of D_5W, NSS, or lactated
Ringer solution before infusion. Further
dilute doses less than 150 mg or greater

than 800 mg to a final concentration of
0.6 to 8 mg/mL.
▼ Inspect for particulate matter before
infusion.
▼ Infuse drug over 60 minutes.
▼ Reconstituted solution is stable for
4 hours at room temperature or 72 hours if
refrigerated.
▼ Diluted I.V. solution is stable for 4 hours
at room temperature or 72 hours if refrigerated (includes reconstituted time).
▼ **Incompatibilities:** Other I.V. drugs. If
line is used for other I.V. drugs, flush with
D_5W, NSS, or lactated Ringer solution
before and after infusion.

ACTION
Inhibits bacterial cell-wall synthesis by
binding to the bacterial cell membrane and
disrupting its function.

Route	Onset	Peak	Duration
I.V.	Unknown	Unknown	Unknown

Half-life: About 6½ to 9½ hours.

ADVERSE REACTIONS
CNS: dizziness.
GI: abdominal pain, decreased appetite, di-
arrhea, nausea, taste disturbance, vomiting,
CDAD.
GU: foamy urine, new-onset or worsening
renal impairment.
Skin: generalized pruritus, infusion-site
pain, infusion-site erythema, rash.
Other: rigors.

INTERACTIONS
Drug-drug. *Drugs that prolong QTc interval:* May enhance QTc-prolonging effect
of highest-risk QTc-prolonging drugs.
Avoid combination. May enhance QTc-
prolonging effect of other moderate-risk
QTc-prolonging drugs. Avoid such combinations when possible. Use should be
accompanied by close monitoring for evidence of QT prolongation or other cardiac
rhythm alterations.

EFFECTS ON LAB TEST RESULTS
• May falsely prolong PT, PTT, and acti-
vated clotting time, and may increase factor
Xa and INR.

T

• May falsely affect urine qualitative dipstick protein assays and quantitative dye methods, such as pyrogallol red-molybdate.

CONTRAINDICATIONS & CAUTIONS

◑ *Alert:* Serious and potentially fatal hypersensitivity reactions, including anaphylactic reactions, may occur after first or subsequent doses. Use cautiously in patients with known hypersensitivity to vancomycin.

◑ *Alert:* Concomitant use of I.V. unfractionated heparin sodium is contraindicated because aPTT test results are expected to be artificially prolonged for 0 to 18 hours after administration.

• Avoid use in patients with prolonged QTc interval, uncompensated HF, or severe left ventricular hypertrophy and in those taking other drugs known to prolong QTc interval.

Black Box Warning Drug may cause nephrotoxicity. Monitor renal function in all patients. Use drug in patients with preexisting moderate to severe renal impairment (CrCl of 50 mL/minute or less) only when anticipated benefit outweighs potential risk. ■

Black Box Warning Decreased effectiveness has occurred among patients with moderate to severe preexisting renal impairment being treated for skin and skin-structure infections. Consider alternative drug when selecting antibacterial therapy for patients with baseline CrCl of 50 mL/minute or less. ■

• Safety and effectiveness in children haven't been established.

Dialyzable drug: 5.9%.

PREGNANCY-LACTATION-REPRODUCTION

Black Box Warning Women of childbearing potential should have a pregnancy test before therapy. Avoid use during pregnancy unless benefits outweigh potential risks to the fetus. ■

Black Box Warning Adverse developmental outcomes observed in three animal species at clinically relevant doses raise concerns about potential adverse developmental outcomes in humans. ■

• Register pregnant women exposed to drug in the Vibativ Pregnancy Registry (1-855-633-8479).

• It isn't known if drug appears in breast milk. Use cautiously in breast-feeding women.

NURSING CONSIDERATIONS

Black Box Warning Monitor renal function before and during therapy. ■

◑ *Alert:* Rapid I.V. infusion may cause "red-man syndrome" (flushing of the upper body, urticaria, pruritus, or rash). Infuse over at least 60 minutes.

• If diarrhea develops, test patient for CDAD, which can be fatal and can occur up to 2 months after last dose.

• Watch for signs and symptoms of superinfection, such as continued fever, chills, and increased pulse rate.

• Reduce dosage in elderly patients who have diminished renal function.

PATIENT TEACHING

• Advise women of childbearing potential to use an effective method of contraception during therapy.

• Advise women not to breast-feed while taking drug.

• Tell patient to notify prescriber if he has a history of kidney problems, heart problems (including QTc-interval prolongation), or diabetes before starting drug.

• Tell patient not to skip doses or to stop treatment without notifying prescriber.

• Tell patient to notify prescriber of all adverse reactions, especially if diarrhea develops during treatment or within 2 months of completing treatment.

telbivudine
tell-BIV-you-deen

Sebivo✦, Tyzeka

Therapeutic class: Antivirals
Pharmacologic class: Nucleosides–nucleotides

AVAILABLE FORMS
Tablets: 600 mg

INDICATIONS & DOSAGES
➤ **Chronic HBV infection**
Adults and children age 16 or older: 600 mg P.O. daily.
Adjust-a-dose: If CrCl is 30 to 49 mL/minute, give 600-mg tablet every 48 hours; if CrCl is less than 30 mL/minute and patient doesn't require dialysis, give 600-mg tablet every 72 hours. For patients with ESRD, give 600-mg tablet every 96 hours after dialysis.

ADMINISTRATION
P.O.
● Give drug without regard for meals.

ACTION
Inhibits HBV replication by interrupting DNA polymerase activity.

Route	Onset	Peak	Duration
P.O.	Immediate	1–4 hr	Unknown

Half-life: 40 to 49 hours.

ADVERSE REACTIONS
CNS: dizziness, insomnia, fatigue, headache, pyrexia.
EENT: pharyngolaryngeal pain.
GI: abdominal pain, abdominal distention, diarrhea, dyspepsia, nausea.
Hematologic: *neutropenia.*
Musculoskeletal: myalgia, arthralgia, back pain, myopathy.
Respiratory: cough.
Other: pruritus, rash.

INTERACTIONS
Drug-drug. *Drugs associated with myopathy (azole antifungals, chloroquine, corticosteroids, cyclosporine, erythromycin, fibric acid derivatives, HMG-CoA reductase inhibitors, niacin):* It isn't known if use together increases risk of myopathy. Monitor patient closely.
Drugs that alter renal function (aminoglycosides, cyclosporine, NSAIDs, tacrolimus, vancomycin): May increase risk of nephrotoxicity. Monitor renal function closely.
Peginterferon alfa-2a, other interferons: May increase risk and severity of peripheral neuropathy. Avoid use together.

EFFECTS ON LAB TEST RESULTS
● May increase CK, ALT, AST, lipase, creatinine, and lactate levels.
● May decrease neutrophil and platelet counts.

CONTRAINDICATIONS & CAUTIONS
● Contraindicated in patients hypersensitive to drug or its components.
● Use cautiously in patients with renal impairment or with lamivudine-resistant HBV infection.
● Safety and effectiveness in children haven't been established.
Dialyzable drug: 23%.

PREGNANCY-LACTATION-REPRODUCTION
● There are no adequate studies in pregnant women. Use only if potential benefit justifies potential risks to the fetus.
● Register pregnant patients in the Antiretroviral Pregnancy Registry (1-800-258-4263) to monitor fetal outcomes.
● Drug may appear in breast milk. Don't use in breast-feeding women.

NURSING CONSIDERATIONS
● Monitor renal function tests and LFTs.
Black Box Warning Patient may develop lactic acidosis and severe hepatomegaly with steatosis during treatment. Risk factors include female gender, obesity, and concurrent antiretroviral therapy. ■
● Monitor patient for symptoms of myopathy.
Black Box Warning Stopping telbivudine may cause worsening of HBV infection. Monitor hepatic function closely during therapy and for several months after stopping the drug. Therapy may need to be restarted. ■

PATIENT TEACHING
● Teach patient to report all adverse reactions and to immediately report signs and symptoms of lactic acidosis (weakness, muscle pain, difficulty breathing, nausea and vomiting, coldness in arms and legs, dizziness, light-headedness, and fast or irregular heartbeat).
● Advise patient not to change the dose or stop the drug because symptoms may worsen.

T

• Teach patient to report signs and symptoms of worsening liver disease (jaundice, dark urine, light-colored stool, decreased appetite, nausea, and abdominal pain).
• Remind patient that telbivudine won't cure HBV and doesn't stop the spread of HBV to others.

telmisartan
tell-mah-SAR-tan

Micardis✍

Therapeutic class: Antihypertensives
Pharmacologic class: Angiotensin II receptor antagonists

AVAILABLE FORMS
Tablets: 20 mg, 40 mg, 80 mg

INDICATIONS & DOSAGES
➤ **Hypertension (used alone or with other antihypertensives)**
Adults: 40 mg P.O. daily. BP response is dose-related over a range of 20 to 80 mg daily.
➤ **CV risk reduction in patients at high risk and unable to take ACE inhibitors**
Adults age 55 and older: 80 mg P.O. once daily.

ADMINISTRATION
P.O.
• Give drug without regard to meals.

ACTION
Blocks vasoconstricting and aldosterone-secreting effects of angiotensin II by preventing angiotensin II from binding to the angiotensin I receptor.

Route	Onset	Peak	Duration
P.O.	3 hr	30–60 min	24 hr

Half-life: 24 hours.

ADVERSE REACTIONS
CNS: dizziness, pain, fatigue, headache.
CV: chest pain, hypertension, peripheral edema.
EENT: pharyngitis, sinusitis.
GI: nausea, abdominal pain, diarrhea, dyspepsia.

GU: UTI.
Musculoskeletal: back pain, myalgia.
Respiratory: cough, URI.
Other: flulike symptoms.

INTERACTIONS
Drug-drug. *ACE inhibitors:* May affect renal function and cause acute renal failure. Consider therapy modification.
Aliskiren: Increases risk of renal impairment, hypotension, and hyperkalemia in diabetic patients. Use together is contraindicated. Also avoid coadministration in patients with moderate to severe renal impairment (GFR less than 60 mL/minute).
COX-2 inhibitors, NSAIDs: May result in worsening renal function. Monitor renal function periodically.
Digoxin: May increase digoxin level. Monitor digoxin level closely.
Heparin, low-molecular-weight heparin, potassium-sparing diuretics, potassium supplements, trimethoprim: May increase risk of hyperkalemia. Closely monitor serum potassium concentration. Adjust treatment as needed.
Lithium: May cause reversible increase in lithium level and toxicity. Monitor lithium level, and adjust lithium dose as needed.
Ramipril, ramiprilat: May increase levels of these drugs and decrease telmisartan level. Avoid use together.
Drug-food. *Salt substitutes containing potassium:* May cause hyperkalemia. Discourage use together.

EFFECTS ON LAB TEST RESULTS
• May increase serum creatinine or BUN level and liver enzyme levels.
• May decrease HB level.

CONTRAINDICATIONS & CAUTIONS
• Contraindicated in patients hypersensitive to drug or its components.
• Use cautiously in patients with biliary obstruction disorders or renal and hepatic insufficiency and in those with an activated RAAS, such as volume- or sodium-depleted patients (for example, those being treated with high doses of diuretics).
Dialyzable drug: No.
⚠ *Overdose S&S:* Hypotension, dizziness, tachycardia, bradycardia.

Reactions in bold italics are *life-threatening*. Interactions may have a *rapid onset* or a *delayed onset*.

PREGNANCY-LACTATION-REPRODUCTION
Black Box Warning Use during pregnancy can cause injury and death to a developing fetus because drug acts directly on the RAAS. When pregnancy is detected, stop drug as soon as possible. ■
• It isn't known if drug appears in breast milk. Patient should discontinue breast-feeding or discontinue drug.

NURSING CONSIDERATIONS
• Monitor patient for hypotension after starting drug. Place patient supine if hypotension occurs, and give I.V. NSS, if needed.
• Most of the antihypertensive effect occurs within 2 weeks. Maximal BP reduction is usually reached after 4 weeks. Diuretic may be added if BP isn't controlled by drug alone.
⟳ Alert: In patients whose renal function may depend on the activity of the RAAS (such as those with severe HF), drug may cause oliguria or progressive azotemia and (rarely) acute renal failure or death.
• Drug isn't removed by hemodialysis. Patients undergoing dialysis may develop orthostatic hypotension. Closely monitor BP.
• Monitor patients with impaired hepatic function or biliary obstruction carefully. Start telmisartan at low dose and titrate slowly.

PATIENT TEACHING
• Inform female patient of childbearing potential of the consequences of second- and third-trimester exposure to drug and to immediately report pregnancy.
• Advise breast-feeding patient that she will need to stop breast-feeding or stop drug.
• Tell patient that if dizziness or low BP occurs on standing, to lie down, rise slowly from a lying to standing position, and climb stairs slowly.
• Tell patient that drug may be taken without regard to meals.
• Tell patient not to remove drug from blister-sealed packet until just before use.
• Tell patient to report all OTC drugs being taken before starting drug and to report all adverse reactions.

temazepam
te-MAZ-e-pam

Restoril⟋

Therapeutic class: Hypnotics
Pharmacologic class: Benzodiazepines
Controlled substance schedule: IV

AVAILABLE FORMS
Capsules: 7.5 mg, 15 mg, 22.5 mg, 30 mg

INDICATIONS & DOSAGES
➤ **Short-term treatment (7 to 10 days) of insomnia**
Adults: 7.5 to 30 mg P.O. at bedtime.
Elderly or debilitated patients: 7.5 mg P.O. at bedtime until individualized response is determined.

ADMINISTRATION
P.O.
• Give drug 15 to 30 minutes before bedtime.
• Give drug without regard for food.

ACTION
Potentiates GABA neuronal inhibition in the CNS.

Route	Onset	Peak	Duration
P.O.	10–20 min	1½ hr	Unknown

Half-life: Terminal, 3½ to 18 hours.

ADVERSE REACTIONS
CNS: complex sleep-related behaviors, drowsiness, dizziness, lethargy, disturbed coordination, daytime sedation, confusion, nightmares, vertigo, euphoria, weakness, headache, fatigue, nervousness, anxiety, depression, minor changes in EEG patterns (usually low-voltage fast activity).
EENT: blurred vision.
GI: abdominal discomfort, diarrhea, nausea, dry mouth.
Other: physical and psychological dependence.

INTERACTIONS
Drug-drug. *Antacids (aluminum hydroxide–containing):* May decrease or

T

delay sedative effects. Monitor patient closely.

Clozapine: May cause delirium, sedation, sialorrhea, and ataxia. Don't start drugs simultaneously, and monitor patient carefully.

CNS depressants: May increase CNS depression. Use together cautiously.

Digoxin: May increase digoxin level. Monitor patient carefully for digoxin toxicity.

Diphenhydramine: May increase effects of both drugs. Use together cautiously.

Hormonal contraceptives: May increase temazepam clearance. Monitor patient closely.

Black Box Warning *Opioids:* May cause slow or difficult breathing, sedation, and death. Avoid use together. If use together is necessary, limit dosage and duration of each drug to minimum necessary for desired effect. ■

Probenecid: May cause rapid or prolonged temazepam effects. Monitor patient for increased sedation or lethargy with concurrent use.

Theophylline: May decrease sedative effects. Monitor patient closely.

Drug-herb. *Calendula, kava, lemon balm, passion flower, skullcap, valerian:* May enhance sedation. Don't use together.

Drug-lifestyle. *Alcohol use:* May cause additive CNS effects. Discourage use together.

EFFECTS ON LAB TEST RESULTS
• May increase LFT values.

CONTRAINDICATIONS & CAUTIONS
• Contraindicated in patients hypersensitive to drug or other benzodiazepines.

Black Box Warning Opioids should only be prescribed with benzodiazepines or other CNS depressants to patients for whom alternative treatment options are inadequate. ■

• Use cautiously in patients with chronic pulmonary insufficiency, impaired hepatic or renal function, severe or latent depression, suicidal tendencies, and history of drug abuse. Abrupt discontinuation can result in withdrawal symptoms.

Dialyzable drug: Unknown.

⚠ *Overdose S&S:* Somnolence, impaired coordination, slurred speech, confusion, coma, decreased reflexes, hypotension, seizures, respiratory depression, apnea.

PREGNANCY-LACTATION-REPRODUCTION
• Contraindicated in women who are or may become pregnant; may cause fetal harm. If used during pregnancy, or if patient becomes pregnant during therapy, apprise her of potential hazard to the fetus.

• It isn't known if drug appears in breast milk. Use cautiously in breast-feeding women; monitor infants for possible drowsiness, lethargy, or weight loss.

NURSING CONSIDERATIONS
❂ *Alert:* Monitor patient closely. Anaphylaxis and angioedema may occur as early as the first dose (rare).

• Assess mental status before starting therapy and reduce doses in elderly patients; these patients may be more sensitive to drug's adverse CNS effects.

• Take precautions to prevent drug hoarding by patients who are depressed, suicidal, or drug-dependent or who have a history of drug abuse.

• Don't stop drug abruptly as this may cause withdrawal symptoms (cramps, seizures, tremor, and sweating). To discontinue drug, follow a gradual dosage-tapering schedule.

• Consider possibility that a woman of childbearing potential may be pregnant at start of therapy.

• *Look alike–sound alike:* Don't confuse Restoril with Risperdal or Vistaril.

PATIENT TEACHING
❂ *Alert:* Warn patient that drug may cause allergic reactions (rare), facial swelling (rare), and complex sleep-related behaviors, such as driving, eating, and making phone calls while asleep. Advise patient to report these adverse effects.

Black Box Warning Caution patient or caregiver of patient taking an opioid with a benzodiazepine, CNS depressant, or alcohol to seek immediate medical attention if patient experiences dizziness, light-headedness, extreme sleepiness, slowed or difficult breathing, or unresponsiveness. ■

• Tell patient to avoid alcohol.

• Caution patient to avoid performing activities that require mental alertness or physical coordination.

- Instruct patient to stop drug before becoming pregnant.
- Warn patient not to stop drug abruptly.

temozolomide
teh-moh-ZOH-loh-mide

Temodar

Therapeutic class: Antineoplastics
Pharmacologic class: Alkylating drugs

AVAILABLE FORMS
Capsules ⓓ: 5 mg, 20 mg, 100 mg, 140 mg, 180 mg, 250 mg
Injection: 100 mg/vial

INDICATIONS & DOSAGES
➤ **Newly diagnosed glioblastoma in combination with radiation therapy**
Adults: Initially, 75 mg/m^2 I.V. infusion or P.O. daily for 42 days. Maintenance dose is 150 mg/m^2 I.V. infusion or P.O. on days 1 to 5 of a 28-day cycle for six cycles; may increase dose to 200 mg/m^2 for cycles two to six if CTCAE is grade 2 or less, ANC is 1.5×10^9/L or more, and platelet count is 100×10^9/L or more. If dose was increased in cycle two, maintain dose at 200 mg/m^2 for days 1 to 5 of subsequent cycles, unless toxicity occurs. If dose wasn't increased in cycle two, don't increase in subsequent cycles.
➤ **Refractory anaplastic astrocytoma**
Adults: Initially, 150 mg/m^2 I.V. infusion or P.O. daily for 5 days of a 28-day treatment cycle. May increase dose to 200 mg/m^2 for 5 days of a 28-day treatment cycle, if nadir and day 1 of next cycle ANC is 1.5×10^9/L or more and platelet count is 100×10^9/L or more.
Adjust-a-dose: For CTCAE grade 2, ANC 0.5 to 1.4×10^9/L, or platelet count 10 to 99×10^9/L during concurrent radiation therapy, interrupt therapy until CTCAE is grade 1 or less, ANC is 1.5×10^9/L or more, and platelet count is 100×10^9/L or more. For CTCAE grade 3, ANC less than 1×10^9/L, or platelet count less than 50×10^9/L, reduce maintenance dose by 50 mg/m^2; however, don't reduce below 100 mg/m^2. Discontinue therapy if CTCAE is grade 3 or 4, ANC is less than 0.5×10^9/L, or platelet count is less than 10×10^9/L.

ADMINISTRATION
- Use of gloves and safety glasses is recommended to avoid exposure due to vial or capsule breakage.
P.O.
- There are no dietary restrictions with drug; however, consistency of administration with respect to food is recommended because food reduces rate and extent of temozolomide absorption.
- Give drug on an empty stomach to reduce nausea or vomiting. Bedtime administration may be advised.
- An antiemetic may be administered before or after giving drug.
- Don't open capsules or allow patient to chew them. If capsules are accidentally opened or damaged, use precautions to avoid inhalation or contact with skin or mucous membranes.
I.V.
▼ Preparing and giving parenteral drug may be mutagenic, teratogenic, or carcinogenic. Follow facility policy to reduce risks.
▼ Reconstitute vial with 41 mL sterile water for injection and gently swirl vial.
▼ For infusion, withdraw proper dose of solution using aseptic technique; then transfer it into an empty 250-mL PVC infusion bag. Administer by I.V. infusion over 90 minutes using an infusion pump.
▼ Discard cloudy, particulate solution. Reconstituted solution is stable at room temperature for 14 hours (including the 90-minute infusion time).
▼ **Incompatibilities:** Other I.V. diluents, medications, and additives.

ACTION
Undergoes rapid nonenzymatic conversion to a reactive compound. This compound alkalizes the cell's DNA, causing cell death.

Route	Onset	Peak	Duration
P.O., I.V.	Unknown	1 hr	7 days

Half-life: About 2 hours.

T

ADVERSE REACTIONS

CNS: amnesia, anxiety, confusion, depression, dizziness, fatigue, headache, hemiparesis, insomnia, memory impairment, paresthesia, paresis, *seizures,* somnolence, weakness.

CV: peripheral edema.

EENT: abnormal vision, blurred vision, diplopia, pharyngitis, sinusitis, taste perversion.

GI: abdominal pain, anorexia, constipation, diarrhea, dysphagia, nausea, stomatitis, vomiting.

GU: incontinence, UTI.

Hematologic: decreased Hb, *leukopenia, lymphopenia, neutropenia, thrombocytopenia.*

Metabolic: adrenal hypercorticism, weight gain.

Musculoskeletal: abnormal coordination, abnormal gait, arthralgia, asthenia, back pain, myalgia.

Respiratory: cough, dyspnea, URI.

Skin: alopecia, dry skin, itching, rash.

Other: breast pain, viral infection, fever.

INTERACTIONS

Drug-drug. *Valproic acid:* May increase temozolomide drug levels. Use together cautiously.

Drug-food. *Any food:* May decrease drug absorption. Advise patient to take drug on an empty stomach.

EFFECTS ON LAB TEST RESULTS

● May decrease Hb level and WBC, neutrophil, lymphocyte, and platelet counts.

CONTRAINDICATIONS & CAUTIONS

● Contraindicated in patients hypersensitive to drug, its components, or dacarbazine (because both drugs are metabolized to the same reactive compound).

● Use cautiously in patients taking other drugs that cause myelosuppression, such as carbamazepine, phenytoin, and sulfamethoxazole–trimethoprim.

● Use cautiously in patients with a history of *Pneumocystis jiroveci* pneumonia, myelodysplastic syndrome, secondary malignancies, or severe renal or hepatic impairment.

● Fatal or severe hepatotoxicity has been reported in patients receiving temozolomide.

Dialyzable drug: Unknown.

⚠ *Overdose S&S:* Pancytopenia, fever, multisystem organ failure, death.

PREGNANCY-LACTATION-REPRODUCTION

● Drug can cause fetal harm if used in pregnant women. If used during pregnancy or if patient becomes pregnant during therapy, apprise her of potential fetal hazard. Women of childbearing potential should avoid becoming pregnant during therapy.

● It isn't known if drug appears in breast milk. Patient should discontinue breastfeeding or discontinue drug.

● Drug may impair male fertility by causing immature sperm formation or testicular atrophy.

NURSING CONSIDERATIONS

● Monitor vital signs and intake and output.

● Monitor CBC with differential before and after each cycle and at least weekly during therapy.

● Prophylaxis against *P. jiroveci* pneumonia is required for all patients receiving concomitant temozolomide and radiotherapy for the 42-day treatment regimen for newly diagnosed glioblastoma multiforme because of higher occurrence during longer dosing regimen.

● Monitor patients, especially those receiving corticosteroids, for lymphopenia and *P. jiroveci* pneumonia.

● Obtain LFT values at baseline, midway through first cycle, before each subsequent cycle, and approximately 2 to 4 weeks after last dose.

● Oral and I.V. doses are equivalent when I.V. dose is infused over 90 minutes.

● Give antiemetic as prescribed to prevent nausea and vomiting.

● Monitor patients for signs and symptoms of another malignancy.

PATIENT TEACHING

● Tell patient to swallow capsule whole with a glass of water and not to open or chew capsule. If capsule opens accidentally, caution patient to avoid inhaling the powder or getting it on the skin or mucous membranes. If powder contacts the skin or

---

Reactions in bold italics are *life-threatening*. Interactions may have a *rapid onset* or a *delayed onset*.

mucous membranes, advise patient to flush the area with water immediately.
- Instruct female patient of childbearing potential to use contraceptive measures while taking drug or if male partner is receiving therapy.
- Inform patient that common side effects include nausea, vomiting, diarrhea, constipation, and hair loss.
- Advise patient to avoid exposure to people with infections.
- Tell patient to report all adverse reactions and signs and symptoms of infection (fever, sore throat, fatigue) and bleeding (easy bruising, bleeding gums, nosebleeds, tarry stools).

SAFETY ALERT!

tenecteplase
teh-NEK-ti-plaze

TNKase

Therapeutic class: Thrombolytics
Pharmacologic class: Recombinant tissue plasminogen activators

AVAILABLE FORMS
Injection: 50 mg/vial

INDICATIONS & DOSAGES
➤ **To reduce risk of death from an acute MI**
Adults weighing 90 kg or more: 50 mg (10 mL) by I.V. bolus over 5 seconds.
Adults weighing 80 to less than 90 kg: 45 mg (9 mL) by I.V. bolus over 5 seconds.
Adults weighing 70 to just under 80 kg: 40 mg (8 mL) by I.V. bolus over 5 seconds.
Adults weighing 60 to just under 70 kg: 35 mg (7 mL) by I.V. bolus over 5 seconds.
Adults weighing less than 60 kg: 30 mg (6 mL) by I.V. bolus over 5 seconds. Maximum dose is 50 mg.

ADMINISTRATION
I.V.
▼ Use syringe prefilled with 10 mL sterile water for injection, and inject the entire contents into drug vial. Gently swirl solution once mixed. Don't shake. Visually inspect product for particulate matter before administration.
▼ Draw up the appropriate dose needed from the reconstituted vial with the syringe and discard any unused portion. Give drug immediately, or refrigerate and use within 8 hours.
▼ Give drug in a designated line. Flush dextrose-containing lines with NSS before administration.
▼ Give the drug rapidly over 5 seconds.
▼ **Incompatibilities:** Solutions containing dextrose, other I.V. drugs.

ACTION
Binds to fibrin and converts plasminogen to plasmin. The specificity to fibrin decreases systemic activation of plasminogen and the resulting breakdown of circulating fibrinogen.

Route	Onset	Peak	Duration
I.V.	Immediate	Immediate	Unknown

Half-life: 90 to 130 minutes.

ADVERSE REACTIONS
CNS: *stroke, intracranial hemorrhage.*
EENT: pharyngeal bleeding, epistaxis.
GI: *GI bleeding.*
GU: hematuria.
Skin: hematoma.
Other: bleeding at puncture site.

INTERACTIONS
Drug-drug. *Anticoagulants (heparin, vitamin K antagonists), drugs that alter platelet function (aspirin, dipyridamole, glycoprotein IIb/IIIa inhibitors, NSAIDs):* May increase risk of bleeding when used before, during, or after tenecteplase use. Use together cautiously.

EFFECTS ON LAB TEST RESULTS
- May prolong PT and PTT, and increase INR.

CONTRAINDICATIONS & CAUTIONS
- Contraindicated in patients with hypersensitivity to drug; active internal bleeding; history of stroke; intracranial or intraspinal surgery or trauma during previous 2 months; intracranial neoplasm, aneurysm, or

arteriovenous malformation; severe uncontrolled hypertension; or bleeding diathesis.
• Use cautiously in patients who have had recent major surgery (such as CABG), organ biopsy, obstetric delivery, or previous puncture of noncompressible vessels.
• Use cautiously in patients age 75 and older and patients with recent trauma, recent GI or GU bleeding, high risk of left ventricular thrombus, acute pericarditis, systolic BP 180 mm Hg or higher or diastolic BP 110 mm Hg or higher, severe hepatic dysfunction, hemostatic defects, subacute bacterial endocarditis, septic thrombophlebitis, diabetic hemorrhagic retinopathy, or cerebrovascular disease.
Dialyzable drug: Unknown.

PREGNANCY-LACTATION-REPRODUCTION
• There are no adequate studies in pregnant women. Use only if potential benefit justifies potential risk to the fetus.
• It isn't known if drug appears in breast milk. Use cautiously in breast-feeding women.

NURSING CONSIDERATIONS
• Begin therapy as soon as possible after onset of MI symptoms.
• Avoid noncompressible arterial punctures and internal jugular and subclavian venous punctures. Minimize all arterial and venous punctures during treatment.
• Avoid I.M. use.
• Give heparin but not in the same I.V. line.
• Monitor patient for bleeding. If serious bleeding occurs, stop heparin and antiplatelet drugs immediately.
⚠ Alert: Use exact patient weight for dosage. An overestimation in patient weight can lead to significant increase in bleeding or intracerebral hemorrhage.
• Monitor ECG for reperfusion arrhythmias.
• Life-threatening cholesterol embolism has been rarely reported in patients treated with thrombolytics. Signs and symptoms may include livedo reticularis (blue toe syndrome), acute renal failure, gangrenous digits, hypertension, pancreatitis, MI, cerebral infarction, spinal cord infarction, retinal artery occlusion, bowel infarction, and rhabdomyolysis.

PATIENT TEACHING
• Tell patient to report all adverse reactions or excessive bleeding immediately.
• Explain use of drug to patient and family.

tenofovir disoproxil fumarate
te-NOE-fo-veer

Viread✦

Therapeutic class: Antiretrovirals
Pharmacologic class: Nucleoside–nucleotide reverse transcriptase inhibitors

AVAILABLE FORMS
Oral powder: 40 mg. One level scoop delivers 1 g of powder containing tenofovir 40 mg
Tablets: 150 mg, 200 mg, 250 mg, 300 mg

INDICATIONS & DOSAGES
Adjust-a-dose (for all indications): For adults with CrCl of 30 to 49 mL/minute, 300 mg P.O. every 48 hours. For CrCl of 10 to 29 mL/minute, 300 mg P.O. every 72 to 96 hours. For patients receiving hemodialysis, 300 mg P.O. every 7 days or after a total of about 12 hours of hemodialysis. Give dose after session. There are no recommendations for patients with CrCl of less than 10 mL/minute not receiving hemodialysis.
➤ **HIV-1 infection, with other antiretrovirals**
Adults and children age 12 and older weighing 35 kg or more: 300 mg P.O. once daily. For adults weighing more than 60 kg who are taking didanosine concomitantly, reduce didanosine dose to 250 mg once daily; for those weighing less than 60 kg, reduce didanosine dose to 200 mg once daily.
Children ages 2 to 11: 8 mg/kg P.O. once daily. Maximum dosage is 300 mg/day. See product insert for weight-based oral powder scoop dosing recommendations.
➤ **Chronic HBV infection**
Adults: 300 mg P.O. once daily.
Children age 12 and older weighing 35 kg or more: 300 mg P.O. once daily.
Adjust-a-dose: There are no recommendations for children with renal impairment.

ADMINISTRATION
P.O.
● Give without regard to food.
● For patients receiving tenofovir and didanosine (enteric-coated form), give under
fasting conditions or with a light meal (less
than 400 kcal, 20% fat). Buffered form of
didanosine taken with tenofovir should be
given under fasting conditions.
● For patients receiving tenofovir powder,
measure only with supplied dosing scoop.
Mix in container with 2 to 4 oz of soft food
not requiring chewing (such as applesauce,
baby food, or yogurt). Patient should ingest
entire mixture immediately to avoid bitter
taste. Don't administer tenofovir in a liquid
because the powder may float on top of the
liquid, even after stirring.

ACTION
Hydrolyzed to produce tenofovir, a nucleoside analogue of adenosine monophosphate
that yields tenofovir diphosphate. Tenofovir
diphosphate inhibits HIV replication.

Route	Onset	Peak	Duration
P.O.	Unknown	36–144 min	Unknown

Half-life: 17 hours.

ADVERSE REACTIONS
CNS: asthenia, headache, pain, fever, pe-
ripheral neuropathy, insomnia, dizziness,
depression, anxiety.
GI: nausea, abdominal pain, dyspepsia,
diarrhea, vomiting.
Hematologic: *neutropenia.*
Hepatic: hepatomegaly, *hepatitis.*
Metabolic: hyperglycemia, *lactic acidosis.*
Musculoskeletal: arthralgia, back pain,
myalgia.
Skin: rash.

INTERACTIONS
Drug-drug. *Atazanavir:* May decrease
atazanavir level, causing resistance. Give
both drugs with ritonavir.
*Atazanavir with ritonavir, darunavir with
ritonavir, lopinavir–ritonavir:* May increase
tenofovir-associated adverse reactions.
Monitor patient carefully.
*Didanosine (buffered or enteric-coated
form):* May increase didanosine bioavailability. Use together cautiously and monitor

patient closely for didanosine-associated
adverse reactions.
*Drugs that reduce renal function or com-
pete for renal tubular secretion (acyclovir,
cidofovir, ganciclovir, valacyclovir, valganciclovir):* May increase levels of tenofovir
or other renally eliminated drugs. Monitor
patient for adverse effects.

EFFECTS ON LAB TEST RESULTS
● May increase amylase, AST, ALT, CK,
serum and urine glucose, creatinine, phosphate, cholesterol, and triglyceride levels.
● May decrease neutrophil count.

CONTRAINDICATIONS & CAUTIONS
● Contraindicated in patients hypersensitive
to components of drug.
● Use very cautiously in patients with risk
factors for liver disease or with hepatic
impairment.
● Don't use tenofovir in combination with
the fixed-dose combination products that
also contain tenofovir. Don't administer
tenofovir with adefovir.
● Monitor patients receiving tenofovir concomitantly with ledipasvir–sofosbuvir without an HIV-1 protease inhibitor/ritonavir
or an HIV-1 protease inhibitor/cobicistat
combination for adverse reactions associated with tenofovir. In patients receiving
tenofovir concomitantly with ledipasvir–
sofosbuvir and an HIV-1 protease inhibitor/
ritonavir or an HIV-1 protease inhibitor/
cobicistat combination, consider an alternative HCV or antiretroviral therapy, as the
safety of increased tenofovir concentrations
in this setting hasn't been established. If
coadministration is necessary, monitor patient for adverse reactions associated with
tenofovir.
● Don't use triple antiretroviral therapy with
abacavir, lamivudine, and tenofovir as new
regimen for treatment-naive or pretreated
patient with HIV infection because of high
rate of early virologic resistance.
Dialyzable drug: Yes.

PREGNANCY-LACTATION-REPRODUCTION
● There are no adequate studies in pregnant
women. Use only if clearly needed.

• Register pregnant women exposed to drug in the Antiretroviral Pregnancy Registry (1-800-258-4263).
• The CDC recommends that mothers with HIV-1 infection not breast-feed to avoid risking postnatal transmission of HIV-1. Advise women not to breast-feed.

NURSING CONSIDERATIONS

Black Box Warning Drug may cause lactic acidosis and hepatomegaly with steatosis, even fatal cases. These effects may occur without elevated transaminase levels. Risk factors include long-term antiretroviral use, obesity, and being female. Monitor all patients closely. ■

Black Box Warning Severe acute exacerbations of hepatitis have been reported in HBV-infected patients after anti-HBV therapy has stopped. Monitor hepatic function closely for at least several months. Resumption of therapy may be warranted. ■

• Drug may cause body fat to accumulate and be redistributed, resulting in central obesity, peripheral wasting, and buffalo hump. Monitor patient for changes.
• Drug may be linked to osteomalacia and decreased bone mineral density, increased creatinine and BUN levels, and phosphaturia. Monitor patient carefully.
• Drug may lead to decreased HIV-RNA level and CD4$^+$ cell counts.
• In elderly patients, use drug cautiously as they may be at higher risk for decreased renal function.
• Because of a high rate of early virologic resistance, triple antiretroviral therapy with abacavir, lamivudine, and tenofovir shouldn't be used as new regimen for treatment-naive or pretreated patient with HIV infection. Monitor patients carefully and consider a different therapy.

PATIENT TEACHING

• Instruct patient to take drug with a meal to enhance bioavailability.
• Inform patient that drug doesn't cure HIV infection, that opportunistic infections and other complications of HIV infection may still occur, and that transmission of HIV to others through sexual contact or blood contamination is still possible.

• Instruct patient taking tenofovir and didanosine (buffered or enteric-coated form) to take these drugs on an empty stomach or with a light meal (less than 400 kcal, 20% fat).
• Tell patient to report adverse effects, including nausea, vomiting, diarrhea, flatulence, and headache.

terazosin hydrochloride
ter-AY-zoe-sin

Therapeutic class: Antihypertensives
Pharmacologic class: Alpha blockers

AVAILABLE FORMS
Capsules: 1 mg, 2 mg, 5 mg, 10 mg

INDICATIONS & DOSAGES
➤ **Hypertension**
Adults: Initially, 1 mg P.O. at bedtime. Dosage may be increased gradually based on response. Usual dosage range is 1 to 5 mg daily. Maximum recommended dose is 20 mg daily.
➤ **Symptomatic BPH**
Adults: Initially, 1 mg P.O. at bedtime. Dosage may be titrated to 2, 5, or 10 mg once daily to achieve optimal response. Most patients need 10 mg daily for optimal response. Maximum recommended dosage is 20 mg/day.

ADMINISTRATION
P.O.
• Give drug without regard for meals.
• If drug is discontinued for several days or longer, restart drug with the initial dosing regimen.

ACTION
Improves urine flow in patients with BPH by blocking alpha-adrenergic receptors in the bladder neck and prostate, relieving urethral pressure. Drug also reduces peripheral vascular resistance and BP via arterial and venous dilation.

Route	Onset	Peak	Duration
P.O.	1–2 hr	1 hr	24 hr

Half-life: About 12 hours.

Reactions in bold italics are *life-threatening*. Interactions may have a *rapid onset* or a *delayed onset*.

ADVERSE REACTIONS

CNS: headache, dizziness, asthenia, first-dose syncope, nervousness, paresthesia, somnolence.
CV: peripheral edema, palpitations, orthostatic hypotension, tachycardia, atrial fibrillation.
EENT: conjunctivitis, blurred vision, tinnitus, nasal congestion, sinusitis.
GI: nausea, constipation, dyspepsia, vomiting.
GU: erectile dysfunction.
Hematologic: *thrombocytopenia.*
Musculoskeletal: back pain, muscle pain.
Respiratory: dyspnea, flulike symptoms, cough.
Skin: pruritus, rash.

INTERACTIONS

Drug-drug. *Antihypertensives, antipsychotics, calcium channel blockers (verapamil), tadalafil, vardenafil:* May cause excessive hypotension. Use together cautiously.

EFFECTS ON LAB TEST RESULTS

● May decrease total protein and albumin levels. May decrease Hb level and hematocrit.
● May decrease WBC and platelet counts.

CONTRAINDICATIONS & CAUTIONS

● Contraindicated in patients hypersensitive to drug.
● May cause marked lowering of BP, especially orthostatic hypotension, and syncope in association with first dose or first few days of therapy. A similar effect can be expected if therapy is interrupted for several days, then restarted.
● Intraoperative floppy iris syndrome has been observed during cataract and glaucoma surgery in some patients who are taking or had previously taken alpha₁ blockers, which may increase risk of eye complications during and after surgery. Initiation of drug in patients for whom cataract or glaucoma surgery is scheduled isn't recommended.
Dialyzable drug: Unlikely.
⚠ *Overdose S&S:* Hypotension.

PREGNANCY-LACTATION-REPRODUCTION

● There are no adequate studies in pregnant women and safety in pregnancy hasn't been established. Use only if potential benefit justifies potential risk to the fetus.
● It isn't known if drug appears in breast milk. Use cautiously in breast-feeding women.

NURSING CONSIDERATIONS

● Monitor BP frequently.
● Symptoms of BPH and prostate cancer are similar. Rule out prostate cancer before start of therapy.

PATIENT TEACHING

● Tell patient not to stop drug suddenly but to notify prescriber if adverse reactions occur.
● Inform patient about the rare but serious possibility of priapism and to report it immediately.
● Warn patient to avoid hazardous activities that require mental alertness, such as driving or operating heavy machinery, for 12 hours after first dose.
● Tell patient that light-headedness from hypotension can occur. Advise patient to rise slowly and to report signs and symptoms to prescriber.
● Advise patient considering cataract or glaucoma surgery to inform ophthalmologist about taking terazosin.

---

terbinafine hydrochloride
ter-BIN-ah-fin

Lamisil

Therapeutic class: Antifungals
Pharmacologic class: Synthetic allylamine derivatives

AVAILABLE FORMS
Oral granules (packets): 125 mg, 187.5 mg
Tablets: 250 mg

INDICATIONS & DOSAGES
➤ **Fingernail and toenail onychomycosis caused by dermatophytes (tinea unguium)**

Adults: 250 mg P.O. once daily for 6 weeks for fingernail infection and 12 weeks for toenail infection.

➤ **Tinea capitis**
Adults: 250 mg P.O. once daily for 6 weeks (granules only).
Children age 4 and older: One dose of granules daily for 2 to 8 weeks based on body weight. If less than 25 kg, give 125 mg; if 25 to 35 kg, give 187.5 mg; if more than 35 kg, give 250 mg.

ADMINISTRATION
P.O.
● Obtain pretreatment transaminase levels for all patients taking drug. Tablets aren't recommended for patients with acute or chronic liver disease.
● Give tablets without regard for food.
● Sprinkle entire contents of granule packet on a spoonful of nonacidic food, such as pudding or mashed potatoes; don't use applesauce or fruit-based foods. Have patient swallow spoonful without chewing.

ACTION
Prevents biosynthesis of ergosterol, causing a deficiency of this essential component of fungal cell membranes.

Route	Onset	Peak	Duration
P.O.	Unknown	2 hr	Unknown

Half-life: 26 to 30 hours.

ADVERSE REACTIONS
CNS: headache, pyrexia.
EENT: vision disturbances, smell disturbances, nasopharyngitis.
GI: taste disturbances, diarrhea, dyspepsia, abdominal pain, nausea, flatulence.
Hematologic: *neutropenia, thrombocytopenia.*
Hepatic: liver enzyme elevations.
Skin: rash, pruritus, urticaria.

INTERACTIONS
Drug-drug. *Antiarrhythmics class 1C (flecainide) and beta blockers:* Inhibit drugs metabolized by CYP2D6 isozyme. Monitor patient carefully and decrease dosage as necessary.
Caffeine: May decrease caffeine clearance. Use cautiously together.

Cimetidine: May decrease clearance of terbinafine by one-third. Avoid using together.
Cyclosporine: May increase cyclosporine clearance. Monitor cyclosporine level.
CYP2C9, CYP3A4 enzyme inhibitors (amiodarone, fluconazole): May substantially increase systemic exposure of terbinafine. Use together cautiously.
Rifampin: Increases terbinafine clearance by 100%. Avoid use together.
SSRIs (paroxetine, venlafaxine): May increase SSRI levels. Monitor patient carefully and adjust SSRI dosage as necessary.

EFFECTS ON LAB TEST RESULTS
● May increase AST and ALT levels.
● May decrease neutrophil and lymphocyte counts.

CONTRAINDICATIONS & CAUTIONS
● Contraindicated in patients hypersensitive to drug or its components and in those with chronic or active liver disease.
● Serious skin reactions (Stevens-Johnson syndrome, toxic epidermal necrolysis, and others) and hypersensitivity reactions have occurred. If these occur, discontinue drug should.
Dialyzable drug: Unknown.
⚠ *Overdose S&S:* Abdominal pain, dizziness, frequent urination, headache, nausea, rash, vomiting.

PREGNANCY-LACTATION-REPRODUCTION
● There are no adequate studies in pregnant women. Because treatment can be postponed until after pregnancy is completed, it's recommended that terbinafine not be initiated during pregnancy.
● Drug appears in breast milk. Use in breast-feeding women isn't recommended.

NURSING CONSIDERATIONS
🕭 *Alert:* Rarely, patients may suffer life-threatening liver failure.
● Monitor CBC and hepatic enzyme levels in patients receiving drug for longer than 6 weeks. Stop drug if hepatobiliary dysfunction or cholestatic hepatitis develops.
● *Look alike–sound alike:* Don't confuse terbinafine with terbutaline. Don't confuse Lamisil with Lamictal.

PATIENT TEACHING
• Inform patient that successful treatment may take 12 weeks for toenail infections and 6 weeks for fingernail infections.
• Tell patient to immediately report depression; smell, taste, or vision disturbances (changes in the ocular lens and retina may occur); and persistent nausea, anorexia, fatigue, vomiting, right upper quadrant pain, jaundice, dark urine, or pale stools.
• Teach patient to sprinkle entire contents of granule packet on spoonful of nonacidic food, such as pudding or mashed potatoes, and to swallow without chewing. Tell patient not to use applesauce or fruit-based food.

terbutaline sulfate
ter-BYOO-ta-leen

Therapeutic class: Bronchodilators
Pharmacologic class: Beta$_2$ agonists

AVAILABLE FORMS
Injection: 1 mg/mL
Tablets: 2.5 mg, 5 mg

INDICATIONS & DOSAGES
➤ **Bronchospasm in patients with reversible obstructive airway disease**
Adults and children age 12 and older:
0.25 mg subcutaneously. If needed, repeat in 15 to 30 minutes. Maximum, 0.5 mg in 4 hours. If patient fails to respond to second dose, consider other measures.
Adults and adolescents older than age 15:
2.5 to 5 mg P.O. t.i.d. every 6 hours while awake. Maximum, 15 mg daily.
Children ages 12 to 15: 2.5 mg P.O. t.i.d. every 6 hours while awake. Maximum, 7.5 mg daily.

ADMINISTRATION
P.O.
• Give drug without regard for food.
Subcutaneous
• Give subcutaneous injections into the side of the deltoid.
• Protect drug from light. Don't use if discolored.

ACTION
Relaxes bronchial smooth muscle by stimulating beta$_2$ receptors.

Route	Onset	Peak	Duration
P.O.	30 min	2–3 hr	4–8 hr
Subcut.	6–15 min	30 min	1½–4 hr

Half-life: Oral, 3.4 hours; subcutaneous, 2.9 to 14 hours.

ADVERSE REACTIONS
CNS: nervousness, tremor, drowsiness, dizziness, headache, weakness.
CV: palpitations, *arrhythmias,* tachycardia, flushing.
GI: vomiting, nausea, heartburn.
Metabolic: hypokalemia.
Respiratory: *paradoxical bronchospasm with prolonged use,* dyspnea.
Skin: diaphoresis.

INTERACTIONS
Drug-drug. *Cardiac glycosides, cyclopropane, halogenated inhaled anesthetics, levodopa:* May increase risk of arrhythmias. Monitor patient closely, and avoid using together with levodopa.
CNS stimulants: May increase CNS stimulation. Avoid using together.
MAO inhibitors: When given with sympathomimetics, may cause severe hypertension (hypertensive crisis). Avoid using together.
Propranolol, other beta blockers: May block bronchodilating effects of terbutaline. Avoid using together.
Sympathomimetics (ephedrine): May result in additive CV effects. Monitor HR and rhythm.

EFFECTS ON LAB TEST RESULTS
• May decrease potassium level.

CONTRAINDICATIONS & CAUTIONS
• Contraindicated in patients hypersensitive to drug or sympathomimetic amines.
• Use cautiously in patient with CV disorders, hyperthyroidism, diabetes, or seizure disorders.
Dialyzable drug: Unknown.
⚠ *Overdose S&S:* Seizures, angina, hypertension, hypotension, tachycardia, arrhythmias, nervousness, headache, tremors, dry

mouth, palpitations, nausea, dizziness, fatigue, insomnia, hypokalemia.

PREGNANCY-LACTATION-REPRODUCTION
• There are no adequate studies in pregnant women. Use only if potential benefit justifies potential risk to the fetus.
Black Box Warning Don't use injectable form in pregnant women for prevention or prolonged treatment (beyond 48 to 72 hours) of preterm labor in either the hospital or outpatient setting because of the potential for serious maternal heart problems and death. Oral terbutaline shouldn't be used for prevention or for any treatment of preterm labor. ■
• It isn't known if drug appears in breast milk. Use during breast-feeding only if potential benefit justifies potential risk to the infant.

NURSING CONSIDERATIONS
• Drug may reduce the sensitivity of spirometry for the diagnosis of bronchospasm.
• Monitor pulmonary function and CV effects (HR, BP, ECG, QTc-interval prolongation).
• *Look alike–sound alike:* Don't confuse terbutaline with tolbutamide or terbinafine.

PATIENT TEACHING
• Ensure patient and caregivers understand drug's use.
• Instruct patient to immediately report changes in HR or rhythm, which patient may experience as feeling anxious, palpitations, or a racing heart.

---

terconazole
ter-CONE-uh-zole

Terazol 3, Terazol 7

Therapeutic class: Antifungals
Pharmacologic class: Triazole derivatives

AVAILABLE FORMS
Vaginal cream: 0.4%, 0.8%
Vaginal suppositories: 80 mg

INDICATIONS & DOSAGES
➤ **Vulvovaginal candidiasis**
Adults: One applicatorful of cream or 1 suppository inserted into vagina at bedtime; 0.4% cream used for 7 consecutive days; 0.8% cream or 80-mg suppository for 3 consecutive days. Repeat course, if needed, after reconfirmation by smear or culture.

ADMINISTRATION
Vaginal
• Insert drug high in vagina (unless patient is pregnant).
• Store drug at room temperature.

ACTION
May increase *Candida* cell membrane permeability.

Route	Onset	Peak	Duration
Vaginal	Unknown	5–10 hr	Unknown

Half-life: 6.4 to 8.5 hours.

ADVERSE REACTIONS
CNS: headache, fever.
GI: abdominal pain.
GU: dysmenorrhea, genital pain, vulvovaginal burning.
Skin: pruritus, irritation, photosensitivity.
Other: body aches.

INTERACTIONS
None significant.

EFFECTS ON LAB TEST RESULTS
None reported.

CONTRAINDICATIONS & CAUTIONS
• Contraindicated in patients hypersensitive to drug or its inactive ingredients.
Dialyzable drug: Unknown.

PREGNANCY-LACTATION-REPRODUCTION
• Because drug is absorbed from the vagina, it shouldn't be used in the first trimester unless prescriber considers it essential to patient's welfare.
• May use during the second and third trimesters if potential benefit outweighs potential risks to the fetus.
• It isn't known if drug appears in breast milk. Patient should discontinue breast-feeding or discontinue drug.

Reactions in bold italics are *life-threatening*. Interactions may have a *rapid onset* or a *delayed onset*.

NURSING CONSIDERATIONS

• Therapeutic effect of drug is unaffected by menstruation or hormonal contraceptive use.

• *Look alike–sound alike:* Don't confuse terconazole with tioconazole.

PATIENT TEACHING

• Advise patient to administer drug at bedtime.

• Advise patient to continue treatment during menstrual period. However, tell her not to use tampons.

• Instruct patient to insert drug high in vagina (except during pregnancy).

• Tell patient to use drug for full treatment period prescribed. Explain how to prevent reinfection.

• Instruct patient to notify prescriber and stop drug if fever, chills, other flulike signs and symptoms, or sensitivity develops.

• Caution patient to refrain from sexual intercourse during treatment.

• Tell patient that drug base may react with latex, causing decreased effectiveness of condoms and diaphragms (for up to 72 hours after treatment is completed).

• Advise patient that her partner also may need treatment if he has symptoms.

• Instruct patient to wash applicator after each use and to allow it to dry thoroughly.

---

teriparatide (rDNA origin)
tehr-ih-PAHR-uh-tide

Forteo

Therapeutic class: Antiosteoporotics
Pharmacologic class: Recombinant human parathyroid hormones

AVAILABLE FORMS
Injection: 20 mcg/dose in multidose prefilled pen

INDICATIONS & DOSAGES
➤ **Osteoporosis in postmenopausal women at high risk for fracture; primary or hypogonadal osteoporosis in men at high risk for fracture; glucocorticoid-induced osteoporosis in men and women**

Adults: 20 mcg subcutaneously in thigh or abdominal wall once daily for up to 2 years.

ADMINISTRATION
Subcutaneous
• Inspect solution before giving.
• Drug is a colorless, clear liquid.
• Don't use if solid particles are present or if the solution is cloudy or colored.
• Give while patient is in a sitting position to avoid orthostatic hypotension.
• Discard the pen after the 28-day use period, even if some unused solution still remains.

ACTION
Promotes new bone formation, skeletal bone mass, and bone strength by regulating calcium and phosphorus metabolism in bones and kidneys.

Route	Onset	Peak	Duration
Subcut.	Rapid	30 min	3 hr

Half-life: 1 hour.

ADVERSE REACTIONS
CNS: asthenia, depression, dizziness, headache, insomnia, pain, syncope, vertigo.
CV: angina pectoris, hypertension, orthostatic hypotension.
EENT: pharyngitis, rhinitis.
GI: constipation, diarrhea, dyspepsia, nausea, tooth disorder, vomiting.
Metabolic: hypercalcemia.
Musculoskeletal: arthralgia, leg cramps, neck pain.
Respiratory: dyspnea, increased cough, pneumonia.
Skin: rash, sweating.

INTERACTIONS
Drug-drug. *Calcium supplements:* May increase urinary calcium excretion. Dosage may need adjustment.
Digoxin: May predispose hypercalcemic patient to digitalis toxicity. Use together cautiously.

EFFECTS ON LAB TEST RESULTS
• May increase calcium and uric acid levels. May decrease phosphorus level.

T

• May increase urinary calcium and phosphorus excretion.

CONTRAINDICATIONS & CAUTIONS
• Contraindicated in patients hypersensitive to drug or its components.

Black Box Warning Drug increases risk of osteosarcoma and is contraindicated in patients at increased risk for osteosarcoma, such as those with Paget disease or unexplained alkaline phosphatase elevations, children and young adults with open epiphyses, and patients who have had skeletal radiation. ■

• Contraindicated in patients with bone metastases; a history of skeletal malignancies, hypercalcemia, or metabolic bone diseases other than osteoporosis; and in patients with hypercalcemia.
• Use cautiously in patients with active or recent urolithiasis; hepatic, renal, or cardiac disease; or hypotension.
Dialyzable drug: Unknown.
⚠ Overdose S&S: Hypercalcemia, orthostatic hypotension, nausea, vomiting, dizziness, headache.

PREGNANCY-LACTATION-REPRODUCTION
• There are no adequate studies in pregnant women. Use only if potential benefit justifies potential risk to the fetus.
• There are no indications for use in pregnant or premenopausal women.
• It isn't known if drug appears in breast milk. Patient should discontinue breastfeeding or discontinue drug.

NURSING CONSIDERATIONS
• Treatment shouldn't exceed 2 years.
• If patient may have urolithiasis or hypercalciuria, measure urinary calcium excretion before treatment.
• Monitor patient for orthostatic hypotension.
• Monitor calcium level. If persistent hypercalcemia develops, stop drug and evaluate possible cause.

PATIENT TEACHING
• Instruct patient on proper use and disposal of prefilled pen.
• Tell patient not to share pen with others.

• Advise patient to remain in a sitting position while taking drug to prevent orthostatic hypotension.
• Advise patient to sit or lie down if drug causes a fast heartbeat, light-headedness, or dizziness. Tell patient to report persistent or worsening symptoms.
• Urge patient to report persistent symptoms of hypercalcemia, which include nausea, vomiting, constipation, lethargy, and muscle weakness.
• Tell patient to discard pen after 28-day use period, even if some unused solution remains.

testosterone
tes-TOS-te-rone

Natesto, Striant, Testopel

testosterone cypionate
Depo-Testosterone

testosterone enanthate
Delatestryl

testosterone undecanoate
Aveed

Therapeutic class: Androgens
Pharmacologic class: Androgens
Controlled substance schedule: III

AVAILABLE FORMS
testosterone
Blister packs (buccal; extended-release) **OTC**: 30 mg
Nasal gel (metered): 5.5 mg/actuation
Pellets (subcutaneous implant): 75 mg
testosterone cypionate
Injection (in oil): 100 mg/mL, 200 mg/mL
testosterone enanthate
Injection (in oil): 200 mg/mL
testosterone undecanoate
Injection (in oil): 250 mg/mL

INDICATIONS & DOSAGES
➤ **Hypogonadism**
Men: 50 to 400 mg cypionate or enanthate I.M. every 2 to 4 weeks. Or, 750 mg undecanoate I.M., followed by 750 mg I.M. 4 weeks later, then 750 mg I.M. every

10 weeks thereafter. Or, 150 to 450 mg (2 to 6 pellets) implanted subcutaneously every 3 to 6 months. Or, apply 1 buccal system (30 mg) to the gum region just above the incisor tooth on either side of the mouth b.i.d. (morning and evening) about 12 hours apart. Alternate sides of the mouth with each application. Or, 11 mg (2 pump actuations; 1 actuation per nostril) intranasally t.i.d., once in the morning, once in the afternoon, and once in the evening (6 to 8 hours apart), preferably at same time each day for a total daily dose of 33 mg.

Adjust-a-dose: When total testosterone concentration consistently exceeds 1,050 ng/dL, discontinue Natesto. If total testosterone concentration is consistently below 300 ng/dL, consider alternative treatment.

➤ **Delayed puberty**
Men and boys: 50 to 200 mg enanthate I.M. every 2 to 4 weeks for 4 to 6 months. Or, 150 to 450 mg (2 to 6 pellets) implanted subcutaneously every 3 to 6 months for a limited duration (e.g., 4 to 6 months).

➤ **Metastatic breast cancer**
Women 1 to 5 years after menopause: 200 to 400 mg enanthate I.M. every 2 to 4 weeks.

ADMINISTRATION
I.M.
● Store I.M. preparations at room temperature. If crystals appear, warm and shake bottle to disperse them.
● Inject deep into upper outer quadrant of gluteal muscle. Rotate injection sites; report soreness at site.
Subcutaneous
● In most men, the pellets are implanted in an area on the anterior abdominal wall.
Buccal
● The buccal system should be placed in the gum region just above the incisor tooth on either side of the mouth.
● Have patient rotate sides of the mouth with each administration.
● Make sure patient doesn't chew or swallow the buccal system.
● The buccal system should remain in place until the next dosing. Check placement after toothbrushing, mouthwash use, eating, and drinking.
● To remove the system, gently slide it downward from the gum toward the tooth.

Intranasal
● Prime pump before first use by inverting then depressing pump 10 times (discard this portion of product into sink).
● Have patient blow nose before application.
● To administer, insert actuator into nostril until pump reaches base of nose; tilt so tip is in contact with lateral wall of nostril. Depress slowly until pump stops, then remove from nose while wiping tip to transfer gel to lateral side of nostril.
● After administration, press on nostrils just below bridge of nose and lightly massage.
● Make sure patient refrains from blowing nose or sniffing for 1 hour after administration.
● If gel gets on hands, wash with warm soap and water.

ACTION
Stimulates target tissues to develop normally in androgen-deficient men. May have some antiestrogen properties, making it useful in treating certain estrogen-dependent breast cancers.

Route	Onset	Peak	Duration
I.M.	Unknown	10–100 min	Unknown
Subcut.	Unknown	Unknown	3–6 mo
Buccal	Unknown	10–12 hr	2–4 hr
Intranasal	Unknown	40 min	Unknown

Half-life: 10 to 100 minutes.

ADVERSE REACTIONS
CNS: headache, anxiety, depression, paresthesia, sleep apnea.
CV: edema.
EENT: nasal discomfort, nasopharyngitis, rhinorrhea, epistaxis, parosmia, nasal dryness or congestion, nasal scabbing.
GI: nausea; gum or mouth irritation; bitter taste; gum pain, tenderness, or edema; taste perversion (with buccal application).
GU: amenorrhea, oligospermia, decreased ejaculatory volume, priapism.
Hematologic: polycythemia, *suppression of clotting factors.*
Hepatic: reversible jaundice, *cholestatic hepatitis.*
Metabolic: hypernatremia, *hyperkalemia,* hypercalcemia, hyperphosphatemia, hypercholesterolemia.
Respiratory: URI.

T

Skin: pain, induration at injection site, local edema, acne.

Other: androgenic effects in women, gynecomastia, hypersensitivity reactions, hypoestrogenic effects in women, excessive hormonal effects in men, male pattern baldness.

INTERACTIONS

Drug-drug. *Corticosteroids:* May increase risk of edema. Use together cautiously, especially in patients with cardiac or hepatic disease.

Hepatotoxic drugs: May increase risk of hepatotoxicity. Monitor liver function closely.

Insulin, oral antidiabetics: May decrease glucose level; may alter dosage requirements. Monitor glucose level in diabetic patients.

Oral anticoagulants: May increase sensitivity; may alter dosage requirements. Monitor PT and INR; decrease anticoagulant dose if necessary.

Oxyphenbutazone: May increase oxyphenbutazone level. Monitor patient.

Drug-food. *Licorice:* May decrease testosterone level. Avoid use.

EFFECTS ON LAB TEST RESULTS

• May increase sodium, potassium, phosphate, cholesterol, liver enzyme, calcium, creatinine, and serum PSA levels.

• May decrease thyroxine-binding globulin, total T_4 levels, serum creatinine, and 17-ketosteroid levels.

• May increase RBC count and resin uptake of T_3 and T_4.

• May cause abnormal glucose tolerance test results.

CONTRAINDICATIONS & CAUTIONS

• Contraindicated in patients hypersensitive to drug and in those with hypercalcemia or cardiac, hepatic, or renal decompensation.

• Contraindicated in men with breast or prostate cancer.

• Venous thromboembolic events (VTEs), including DVT and PE, have been reported in patients using testosterone products.

Black Box Warning Serious pulmonary oil microembolism reactions, involving urge to cough, dyspnea, throat tightening, chest pain, dizziness, and syncope, and episodes of anaphylaxis, including life-threatening reactions, have been reported to occur during or immediately after administration of testosterone undecanoate injection. These reactions can occur after any injection of testosterone undecanoate during the course of therapy, including after first dose. Observe patients for 30 minutes after each dose. Drug is available only through a restricted program under a risk evaluation and mitigation strategy (REMS) called the Aveed REMS Program. ▪

❸ **Alert:** Contraindicated in men with age-related low testosterone signs and symptoms only. Testosterone replacement therapy is only approved for men with primary or secondary hypogonadism resulting from certain medical conditions and with low testosterone levels confirmed by laboratory testing.

❸ **Alert:** Drug may increase risk of heart attack and stroke.

• Prolonged use of high doses of androgens has been associated with the development of peliosis hepatis and hepatic neoplasms, including hepatocellular carcinoma.

• Use cautiously in elderly patients.

• Intranasal form isn't recommended for use with nasally administered drugs other than sympathomimetic decongestants or for use in patients with mucosal inflammatory disorders, sinus disease. or history of nasal disorders, nasal or sinus surgery, nasal fracture within previous 6 months, or nasal fracture that caused a deviated anterior nasal septum.

Dialyzable drug: Unknown.

⚠ *Overdose S&S:* Stroke (with enanthate injection).

PREGNANCY-LACTATION-REPRODUCTION

• Drug is teratogenic and may cause fetal harm. Use is contraindicated in pregnant women and women who may become pregnant. If a woman becomes pregnant during therapy, apprise her of potential fetal hazard.

• Contraindicated in breast-feeding women because of potential for virilization in breast-fed infants.

NURSING CONSIDERATIONS

● Unless contraindicated, use with high-calorie, high-protein diet. Give small, frequent meals to help avoid nausea.

● Don't give to women of childbearing potential until pregnancy is ruled out.

● Cypionate, enanthate, and undecanoate are long-acting solutions.

● If patient experiences severe rhinitis, temporarily discontinue intranasal therapy until signs and symptoms resolve. If signs and symptoms persist, an alternative testosterone replacement therapy is recommended.

● Monitor patient's liver function, and check PSA, cholesterol, and HDL levels periodically.

● Check Hb and hematocrit levels periodically.

● **Alert:** Confirm low testosterone levels on at least two mornings before initiating therapy. Avoid measuring testosterone level later in the day when levels can be low, even in men who don't have hypogonadism.

● Evaluate patients who report pain, edema, or warmth and erythema in lower extremity for DVT; evaluate those who present with acute shortness of breath for PE. If a VTE is suspected, discontinue drug and initiate appropriate workup and management.

● In patients with metastatic breast cancer, hypercalcemia usually indicates progression of bone metastases. Report signs and symptoms of hypercalcemia.

● Report evidence of virilization in women. Androgenic effects include acne, edema, weight gain, increased hair growth, hoarseness, clitoral enlargement, decreased breast size, changes in libido, male pattern baldness, and oily skin or hair.

● Watch for hypoestrogenic effects in women (flushing; diaphoresis; vaginitis, including itching, drying, and burning; vaginal bleeding; menstrual irregularities).

● Watch for excessive hormonal effects in men and boys. In prepubertal boy, watch for premature epiphyseal closure, acne, priapism, growth of body and facial hair, and phallic enlargement. In postpubertal men, watch for testicular atrophy, oligospermia, decreased ejaculatory volume, impotence, gynecomastia, and epididymitis.

● Monitor patient's weight and BP routinely.

● Monitor prepubertal boys by X-ray for rate of bone maturation.

● The treatment of hypogonadal men with testosterone esters may potentiate sleep apnea. Monitor patients with risk factors such as obesity or chronic lung diseases.

● **Alert:** Therapeutic response in breast cancer is usually apparent within 3 months. If disease progresses, stop drug.

● Androgens may alter results of laboratory studies during therapy and for 2 to 3 weeks after therapy ends.

● **Alert:** Testosterone salts aren't interchangeable.

● **Look alike–sound alike:** Don't confuse testosterone with testolactone.

PATIENT TEACHING

● Make sure patient understands importance of using an effective nonhormonal contraceptive during therapy.

● **Alert:** Warn patient to seek immediate medical attention for signs and symptoms of heart attack (chest pain, shortness of breath, trouble breathing) or stroke (weakness in one part or side of the body, slurred speech).

● Instruct patient to stop drug immediately and notify prescriber if pregnancy is suspected.

● Review signs and symptoms of virilization with female patient, and instruct her to notify prescriber if they occur.

● Advise female patient to wear cotton underwear and to wash after intercourse to decrease risk of vaginitis.

● Instruct male patient to report priapism, reduced ejaculatory volume, or gynecomastia.

● Warn diabetic patient to be alert for hypoglycemia and to notify prescriber if it occurs.

● Instruct boys using testosterone for delayed puberty to have X-rays of hand and wrist obtained every 6 months during treatment.

● Tell patient to report sudden weight gain.

● Warn patient that drug shouldn't be used to enhance athletic performance.

● Instruct patient how to use the buccal system.

● Advise patient to avoid dislodging buccal system and ensure that the system is in place

after toothbrushing, use of mouthwash, and eating or drinking.
• Tell male patient not to chew or swallow buccal system.
• Show patient how to administer drug intranasally.

testosterone transdermal
Androderm, AndroGel, Axiron, Fortesta, Testim, Vogelxo

Therapeutic class: Androgens
Pharmacologic class: Androgens
Controlled substance schedule: III

AVAILABLE FORMS
1% gel: 25 mg, 50 mg per unit dose; 12.5 mg per pump actuation
1.62% gel: 20.25 mg per pump actuation
2% gel: 10 mg per pump actuation
Transdermal solution: 30 mg per metered-dose pump
Transdermal system: 2 mg/day, 4 mg/day

INDICATIONS & DOSAGES
➤ **Primary or hypogonadotropic hypogonadism**
Men: One Androderm 4 mg/day system applied to back, abdomen, arm, or thigh nightly for total dosage of 4 mg daily. Dose may be increased to 6 mg once daily or decreased to 2 mg once daily, depending on morning serum testosterone levels.

Or, initially, 50 mg of AndroGel 1% (two 25-mg packets or one 50-mg packet) or Testim (one tube) applied every morning to shoulders, upper arms, or abdomen. Don't apply Testim to abdomen. Check testosterone level after about 2 weeks. If response is inadequate, may increase AndroGel to 75 mg daily. Then, adjust to 100 mg (either gel) if needed. Or, for AndroGel pump, 50 mg (4 pump actuations) applied every morning to shoulders, upper arms, or abdomen. Check testosterone level after about 2 weeks. If response is inadequate, may increase to 75 mg (6 pumps) daily or from 75 to 100 mg (8 pumps) daily. Or, initially, 40.5 mg (2 pumps) of AndroGel 1.62% daily to upper arms or shoulders. May adjust dosage between a minimum of 20.25 mg (1 pump) and a maximum of 81 mg

(4 pumps) titrated based on the predose morning serum testosterone concentration at about 14 days and 28 days after starting treatment or the last dosage adjustment.

Or, initially 40 mg (4 pumps) of Fortesta once daily to the thighs in the morning. May adjust dosage between 10 mg and maximum of 70 mg based on testosterone concentration drawn 2 hours after application approximately 14 days and 35 days after start of treatment and the last dosage adjustment.

Or, initially 60 mg (2 pumps) of Axiron solution, one actuation to each axilla, once daily. May adjust dosage between 30 mg (1 pump) and a maximum of 120 mg (4 pumps) based on serum testosterone concentration drawn 2 to 8 hours after application and at least 14 days after starting treatment or the last dosage adjustment.

Or, 50 mg of Vogelxo once daily to shoulders or upper arms. If serum testosterone concentration is below normal range, increase dose to 100 mg of testosterone.

ADMINISTRATION
Transdermal
• Wear gloves when handling patches. Fold used patches with adhesive sides together to discard.
• Apply patch nightly to clean, dry, intact skin of the back, abdomen, upper arms, or thighs only and not to the genitals or bony prominences.
Topical
• AndroGel 1.62% and AndroGel 1% and topical solution aren't interchangeable.
• Fully prime the pumps by pumping three times before first use. Discard that gel.
• Wear gloves to apply gel to clean, dry, intact skin of shoulders, upper arms, or abdomen only and not to the genitals or bony prominences. Don't apply Testim and Vogelxo to the abdomen.
• Application in the morning is preferable. Allow application sites to dry before dressing. Cover the application sites with clothing.
• Patient should avoid swimming or washing the administration site for 2 hours after application.
• Apply Fortesta to clean, dry, intact skin of the front and inner thighs only.

• Gel contains alcohol and is flammable. Patient should avoid fire, flames, or smoking until gel has dried.

• Apply topical solution, using the applicator provided, to clean, dry, intact skin of the axilla as directed. Don't use the fingers or hand to rub the solution into the skin.

• Patient should apply deodorants before applying the solution.

ACTION

Releases testosterone, which stimulates target tissues to develop normally in androgen-deficient men.

Route	Onset	Peak	Duration
Transdermal, topical	Unknown	2–4 hr	2 hr after removal

Half-life: 10 to 100 minutes.

ADVERSE REACTIONS

CNS: *stroke,* asthenia, depression, headache, sleep apnea.
GI: *GI bleeding.*
GU: prostatitis, prostate abnormalities, UTI.
Hepatic: *cholestatic hepatitis,* reversible jaundice.
Metabolic: hypernatremia, hyperkalemia, hypercalcemia, hyperphosphatemia, hypercholesterolemia.
Skin: pruritus, blister under patch, acne irritation, allergic contact dermatitis, burning.
Other: gynecomastia, breast tenderness, flulike syndrome.

INTERACTIONS

Drug-drug. *Corticosteroids:* May increase risk of edema. Use together cautiously, especially in patients with cardiac or hepatic disease.
Hepatotoxic drugs: May increase risk of hepatotoxicity. Monitor liver function closely.
Insulin: May alter insulin dosage requirements. Monitor glucose level.
Oral anticoagulants: May alter anticoagulant dosage requirements. Monitor PT and INR.
Oxyphenbutazone: May increase oxyphenbutazone level. Monitor patient.

EFFECTS ON LAB TEST RESULTS

• May increase sodium, potassium, phosphate, cholesterol, liver enzyme, calcium, and creatinine levels and resin uptake of T_3 and T_4. May decrease total T_4 levels.

• May increase glucose level and RBC count.

CONTRAINDICATIONS & CAUTIONS

• Contraindicated in patients hypersensitive to drug, in women, in men with known or suspected breast or prostate cancer, and in patients with CV, renal, or hepatic disease.

⚠ *Alert:* Contraindicated in men with age-related low testosterone symptoms only. Testosterone replacement therapy is only approved for men with primary or secondary hypogonadism resulting from certain medical conditions and with low testosterone levels confirmed by laboratory testing.

⚠ *Alert:* Drug may increase risk of heart attack and stroke.

• Venous thromboembolic events (VTEs), including DVT and PE, have been reported in patients using testosterone products.

• Prolonged use of high doses of androgens has been associated with development of peliosis hepatis and hepatic neoplasms, including hepatocellular carcinoma.

• Use cautiously in elderly men.

Dialyzable drug: Unknown.

PREGNANCY-LACTATION-REPRODUCTION

• Drug is teratogenic; may cause fetal harm. Use is contraindicated in pregnant women and women who may become pregnant. If a woman becomes pregnant during therapy, apprise her of potential fetal hazard.

• Contraindicated in women who are breastfeeding because of potential for virilization in breast-fed infants.

NURSING CONSIDERATIONS

Black Box Warning Virilization in children and women can occur after secondary exposure to transdermal application sites on men. Women and children should avoid contact with application sites. ∎

• Treatment of hypogonadal men with testosterone esters may potentiate sleep apnea. Monitor patients with risk factors, such as obesity or chronic lung diseases.

T

- Periodically assess LFT results, lipid profiles, Hb level, hematocrit (with long-term use), and levels of prostatic acid phosphatase and PSA.
🌓 *Alert:* Confirm low testosterone levels on at least two mornings before initiating therapy. Avoid measuring testosterone level later in the day when levels can be low, even in men who don't have hypogonadism.
- Watch for excessive hormonal effects.
- Evaluate patients who report pain, edema, or warmth and erythema in lower extremity for DVT; evaluate those who present with acute shortness of breath for PE. If a VTE is suspected, discontinue treatment and initiate appropriate workup and management.

PATIENT TEACHING
- Tell patient to fully prime the AndroGel, Vogelxo, or Fortesta pump by pumping three times before first use and to discard that gel.
Black Box Warning Instruct patient to strictly adhere to recommended instructions for use. ∎
- Instruct patient to thoroughly wash the application site with soap and water before situations in which direct skin-to-skin contact is anticipated.
- Tell patient using patch to apply it at night.
- Tell patient using gel to apply in the morning.
Black Box Warning Tell patient to wash his hands thoroughly after using product and to cover treated area with clothing. ∎
- Instruct patient that patch must be changed every 24 hours.
- For best results, advise patient not to swim or shower for at least 2 hours after applying gel. Showering or swimming at least 1 hour after applying, if done infrequently, should have minimal effects on drug absorption.
- Tell patient that if the patch falls off, it may be reapplied. If patch falls off and can't be reapplied, and it has been worn at least 12 hours, a new patch may be applied at the next application time.
- Warn diabetic patient that drug may decrease glucose level and to be alert for hypoglycemia.
🌓 *Alert:* Warn patient to seek immediate medical attention for signs and symptoms of heart attack (chest pain, shortness of breath,

trouble breathing) or stroke (weakness in one part or side of the body, slurred speech).
- Advise patient to report persistent erections, nausea, vomiting, changes in skin color, ankle swelling, or sudden weight gain to prescriber.
- Tell patient that women and children should avoid contact with his application sites.
- Tell patient that Androderm doesn't have to be removed during sexual intercourse or while showering.
- Tell patient undergoing an MRI to alert the facility that he is using a transdermal patch.

tetracycline hydrochloride
tet-ra-SYE-kleen

Achromycin V

Therapeutic class: Antibiotics
Pharmacologic class: Tetracyclines

AVAILABLE FORMS
Capsules: 250 mg, 500 mg

INDICATIONS & DOSAGES
Adjust-a-dose (for all indications): Decrease recommended dosages or extend dosing intervals in patients with renal impairment.
➤ **Infections caused by susceptible gram-negative and gram-positive organisms, such as *Haemophilus ducreyi, Yersinia pestis, Campylobacter fetus, Rickettsiae* species, *Mycoplasma pneumoniae, Chlamydia trachomatis, Entamoeba histolytica, Actinomyces* species, *Bacillus anthracis, Vibrio cholerae, Listeria monocytogenes, Fusobacterium fusiforme*, and *Treponema* species; *Francisella tularensis;* psittacosis; granuloma inguinale**
Adults: 1 to 2 g/day P.O. in two or four divided doses depending on the severity of infection.
Children older than age 8: 25 to 50 mg/kg P.O. daily, in divided doses every 6 hours.
➤ **Uncomplicated urethral, endocervical, or rectal infections caused by *C. trachomatis***
Adults: 500 mg P.O. q.i.d. for at least 7 days.

➤ **Brucellosis**
Adults: 500 mg P.O. every 6 hours for
3 weeks in combination with streptomycin.
➤ **Uncomplicated gonorrhea in patients
allergic to penicillin**
Adults: 500 mg P.O. every 6 hours for
7 days.
➤ **Syphilis in patients allergic to
penicillin**
Adults and adolescents: 500 mg P.O. q.i.d.
for 15 days. If infection has lasted 1 year or
longer, treat for 30 days.
➤ **Acne (severe; long-term therapy)**
Adults and adolescents: Initially, 1 g daily
in divided doses. For maintenance, 125 to
500 mg daily. (Alternate-day or intermittent
therapy may be adequate in some patients.)

ADMINISTRATION
P.O.
● Obtain specimen for culture and sensitivity tests before giving first dose. Begin
therapy while awaiting results.
● Effectiveness is reduced when drug is
given with milk or other dairy products,
antacids, or iron products. For best drug
absorption, give drug with a full glass of
water on an empty stomach, at least 1 hour
before or 2 hours after meals.
● Give drug at least 1 hour before bedtime
to prevent esophageal irritation or ulceration.
🟢 *Alert:* Be careful not to administer outdated drug because of the highly increased
risk of nephrotoxicity and Fanconi syndrome.

ACTION
May exert bacteriostatic effect by binding to the 30S and possibly 50S ribosomal
subunits of microorganisms, thus inhibiting protein synthesis. May also alter the
cytoplasmic membrane of susceptible microorganisms.

Route	Onset	Peak	Duration
P.O.	Unknown	2–4 hr	Unknown

Half-life: 8 to 11 hours.

ADVERSE REACTIONS
CNS: *intracranial hypertension,* dizziness,
headache.
CV: pericarditis.

EENT: sore throat.
GI: diarrhea, epigastric distress, nausea, anorexia, dysphagia, enterocolitis,
esophagitis, glossitis, oral candidiasis, stomatitis, vomiting.
GU: inflammatory lesions in anogenital
region.
Hematologic: *neutropenia, thrombocytopenia,* eosinophilia.
Musculoskeletal: bone growth retardation
in children younger than age 8.
Skin: candidal superinfection, increased
pigmentation, maculopapular and erythematous rash, photosensitivity reactions,
urticaria.
Other: enamel defects, hypersensitivity
reactions, permanent discoloration of teeth.

INTERACTIONS
Drug-drug. *Antacids and laxatives containing aluminum, magnesium, or calcium;*
*antidiarrheals containing kaolin, pectin,
or bismuth subsalicylate:* May decrease
antibiotic absorption. Give antibiotic 1 hour
before or 2 hours after these drugs.
Digoxin: May increase digoxin absorption.
Monitor digoxin levels and monitor patient
for signs of toxicity.
*Ferrous sulfate and other iron products,
zinc:* May decrease antibiotic absorption.
Give tetracycline 2 hours before or 3 hours
after these products.
Hormonal contraceptives: May decrease
contraceptive effectiveness and increase risk
of breakthrough bleeding. Advise patient to
use nonhormonal contraceptive.
Isotretinoin: May increase risk of pseudotumor cerebri. Avoid use together.
🟢 *Alert: Methoxyflurane:* May cause fatal
nephrotoxicity. Avoid using together.
Oral anticoagulants: May increase anticoagulant effects. Monitor PT and INR, and
adjust anticoagulant dosage.
Penicillins: May interfere with bactericidal
action of penicillins. Avoid using together.
Drug-food. *Dairy products:* May decrease
antibiotic absorption. Give antibiotic 1 hour
before or 2 hours after eating or drinking
dairy products.
Drug-lifestyle. *Sun exposure:* May cause
photosensitivity reactions. Advise patient to
avoid excessive sunlight exposure.

T

EFFECTS ON LAB TEST RESULTS

- May increase BUN and liver enzyme levels.
- May increase eosinophil count. May decrease platelet and neutrophil counts.

CONTRAINDICATIONS & CAUTIONS

- Contraindicated in patients hypersensitive to drug or other tetracyclines.
- Some tetracyclines may contain sulfites and are contraindicated in patients with sulfite hypersensitivity.
- CDAD, ranging in severity from mild diarrhea to fatal colitis, has been reported with use of nearly all antibacterial drugs, including tetracyclines.
- Use cautiously in patients with renal or hepatic impairment. Avoid using or use cautiously in children younger than age 8 because drug may cause permanent discoloration of teeth, enamel defects, and bone growth retardation.

Dialyzable drug: No.

⚠ *Overdose S&S:* Dizziness, nausea, vomiting.

PREGNANCY-LACTATION-REPRODUCTION

- Don't use during pregnancy unless absolutely necessary. May have toxic effects on the developing fetus (often related to retardation of skeletal development) and teeth. If used during pregnancy or if patient becomes pregnant during therapy, apprise her of potential fetal hazard.
- Pregnant women with renal disease may be more prone to developing tetracycline-associated liver failure.
- Drug appears in breast milk. Patient should discontinue breast-feeding or discontinue drug.

NURSING CONSIDERATIONS

- ❸ *Alert:* Check expiration date. Using outdated or deteriorated drug has been linked to severe reversible nephrotoxicity (Fanconi syndrome).
- Don't expose drug to light or heat.
- If CDAD is suspected or confirmed, discontinue ongoing use of antibacterial drugs not directed at *Clostridium difficile.* Institute appropriate fluid and electrolyte management, protein supplementation, and antibacterial treatment of *C. difficile.*

- If large doses are given, therapy is prolonged, or patient is at high risk, monitor patient for signs and symptoms of superinfection.
- Pseudotumor cerebri (benign intracranial hypertension) in adults has been associated with tetracycline use. Monitor patient for clinical manifestations, including headache, blurred vision, diplopia, and vision loss; papilledema can be found on funduscopy.
- In patients with renal or hepatic impairment, monitor renal function tests and LFT results if drug is used.
- Check patient's tongue for signs of candidal infection. Emphasize good oral hygiene.
- Drug isn't indicated for treatment of neurosyphilis.
- Photosensitivity reactions may occur within a few minutes to several hours after sun exposure. Photosensitivity lasts after therapy ends.

PATIENT TEACHING

- Tell patient to take drug exactly as prescribed, even after feeling better, and to take entire amount prescribed.
- Tell patient to check drug's expiration date and not to use if outdated.
- Advise patient to promptly report all adverse reactions and to immediately report headache, blurred vision, diplopia, vision loss, watery diarrhea, abdominal cramping and pain, fever, or blood or pus in the stool.
- Warn patient that use of tetracyclines with oral contraceptives may make contraceptives less effective.
- Explain that effectiveness is reduced when drug is taken within 2 hours before or after ingestion of milk or other dairy products, antacids, laxatives, or iron products. For best drug absorption, tell patient to take each dose with a full glass of water on an empty stomach, at least 1 hour before or 2 hours after meals. Also tell patient to take it at least 1 hour before bedtime to prevent esophageal irritation or ulceration.
- Warn patient to avoid direct sunlight and ultraviolet light and to use sun protection.

Reactions in bold italics are *life-threatening*. Interactions may have a *rapid onset* or a ***delayed onset***.

tetrahydrozoline hydrochloride (intranasal)
tet-rah-hi-DRAZ-oh-leen

Tyzine

Therapeutic class: Decongestants
Pharmacologic class:
Sympathomimetics

AVAILABLE FORMS
Nasal solution: 0.05%, 0.1%
Nasal spray: 0.1%

INDICATIONS & DOSAGES
➤ **Nasal congestion**
Adults and children age 6 and older: 2 to 4 drops or 3 to 4 sprays of 0.1% solution in each nostril no more often than every 3 hours, p.r.n.
Children ages 2 to 5: Give 2 to 3 drops of 0.05% solution in each nostril no more often than every 3 hours, p.r.n.

ADMINISTRATION
Intranasal
● Instill nose drops with patient in lateral head-low position.
● Give nasal spray with patient's head tilted back slightly. Wait 1 to 2 minutes between sprays.
● Rinse spray tip in hot water and dry with a clean tissue.

ACTION
Thought to cause local vasoconstriction of dilated arterioles, reducing blood flow and nasal congestion.

Route	Onset	Peak	Duration
Intranasal	Few min	Unknown	4–8 hr

Half-life: Unknown.

ADVERSE REACTIONS
EENT: rebound nasal congestion, sneezing, transient burning or stinging, mucosal dryness.

INTERACTIONS
Drug-drug. *Bromocriptine, catechol-O-methyltransferase inhibitors, such as tolcapone:* May increase the effects of these drugs. Monitor patient for increased clinical response and adverse effects.
MAO inhibitors: May cause headache, hypertension, and hyperpyrexia. Use together or within 14 days of stopping an MAO inhibitor is contraindicated.
TCAs: May decrease the effects of tetrahydrozoline. Monitor patient for clinical effect.
Drug-herb. *St. John's wort:* May increase adverse effects of herb. Discourage use together.

EFFECTS ON LAB TEST RESULTS
None reported.

CONTRAINDICATIONS & CAUTIONS
● Contraindicated in patients hypersensitive to drug and in children younger than age 2. The 0.1% solution is contraindicated in children younger than age 6.
● Contraindicated in patients being treated with MAO inhibitors or within 14 days of treatment with MAO inhibitors.
● Use cautiously in patients with hyperthyroidism, hypertension, or diabetes mellitus.
Dialyzable drug: Unknown.
⚠ *Overdose S&S:* Hypertension, bradycardia, drowsiness, rebound hypotension, shock, profuse sweating.

PREGNANCY-LACTATION-REPRODUCTION
● It isn't known if drug can cause fetal harm when used in pregnant women or if it can affect reproduction capacity. Use during pregnancy only if clearly needed.
● It isn't known if drug appears in breast milk. Use cautiously in breast-feeding women.

NURSING CONSIDERATIONS
● Drug should be used for only 3 to 5 days.
● Overdose in young children may cause oversedation.

PATIENT TEACHING
● Teach patient how to use drug.
● Advise patient to keep drug out of reach of small children. Accidental ingestion of even a small amount (1 to 2 mL) may result in bradycardia, respiratory depression, sedation, or coma. Tell patient to contact a poison control center and immediately

T

seek emergency medical care for accidental ingestion.

• Caution patient not to share drug because this could spread infection.

• Tell patient not to exceed recommended dosage and to use only as needed for 3 to 5 days.

thiotepa (TESPA, tri-ethylenethiophosphoramide, TSPA)
thye-oh-TEE-pa

Therapeutic class: Antineoplastics
Pharmacologic class: Alkylating drugs

AVAILABLE FORMS
Injection: 15 mg/vial

INDICATIONS & DOSAGES
➤ **Breast and ovarian cancers, lymphoma, Hodgkin lymphoma**
Adults: 0.3 to 0.4 mg/kg I.V. every 1 to 4 weeks.
➤ **Bladder tumor**
Adults: 30 to 60 mg in 30 to 60 mL of NSS instilled in bladder for 2 hours once weekly for 4 weeks.
➤ **Neoplastic effusions**
Adults: 0.6 to 0.8 mg/kg intracavitarily every 1 to 4 weeks.

ADMINISTRATION
I.V.
▼ Preparing and giving drug may be mutagenic, teratogenic, or carcinogenic. Follow facility policy to reduce risks.
▼ Reconstitute with 1.5 mL of sterile water for injection in 15-mg vial to yield 10 mg/mL. Don't reconstitute with other solutions.
▼ Further dilute with NSS for injection. If larger volume is desired, further dilute with sodium chloride solution, D_5W, dextrose 5% in NSS for injection, Ringer injection, or lactated Ringer injection.
▼ If solution appears grossly opaque or has a precipitate, discard it. Make sure solutions are clear to slightly opaque. To eliminate haze, filter solutions through a 0.22-micron filter before use.

▼ If pain occurs at insertion site, dilute drug further or use a local anesthetic to reduce pain. Make sure drug doesn't infiltrate.
▼ Use solutions within 8 hours.
▼ Refrigerate and protect dry powder from direct sunlight to avoid possible drug breakdown.
▼ **Incompatibilities:** Cisplatin, filgrastim, minocycline, vinorelbine.
Intravesical
• Preparing and giving drug may be mutagenic, teratogenic, or carcinogenic. Follow facility policy to reduce risks.
• For bladder instillation, dehydrate patient 8 to 10 hours before therapy. Instill drug into bladder by catheter; ask patient to retain solution for 2 hours. If discomfort is too great with 60 mL, reduce volume to 30 mL. Reposition patient every 15 minutes for maximum area contact.
Intracavitary
• Preparing and giving drug may be mutagenic, teratogenic, or carcinogenic. Follow facility policy to reduce risks.
• For intracavitary instillation, drug may be given through the same tubing used to remove the fluid from the cavity involved.

ACTION
Cross-links strands of cellular DNA and interferes with RNA transcription, causing an imbalance of growth that leads to cell death. Not specific to cell cycle.

Route	Onset	Peak	Duration
I.V., topical	Unknown	Unknown	Unknown

Half-life: 2¼ hours.

ADVERSE REACTIONS
CNS: headache, dizziness, fatigue, weakness, fever.
EENT: blurred vision, conjunctivitis.
GI: nausea, vomiting, abdominal pain, anorexia, stomatitis.
GU: amenorrhea, decreased spermatogenesis, dysuria, increased urine levels of uric acid, urine retention, hemorrhagic cystitis (with intravesical administration).
Hematologic: *leukopenia, thrombocytopenia, neutropenia,* anemia.
Respiratory: *laryngeal edema.*

Reactions in bold italics are *life-threatening*. Interactions may have a *rapid onset* or a *delayed onset*.

Skin: dermatitis, alopecia, injection-site pain, urticaria, rash.
Other: hypersensitivity reactions, including *anaphylaxis.*

INTERACTIONS

Drug-drug. *Anticoagulants, aspirin, NSAIDs:* May increase risk of bleeding. Avoid using together.
Live-virus vaccines: May increase risk of infection. Avoid using together.
Myelosuppressive agents: May increase myelosuppression. Monitor patient.
Neuromuscular blockers: May prolong muscular paralysis. Monitor patient.
Other alkylating drugs, irradiation therapy: May intensify toxicity rather than enhance therapeutic response. Avoid using together.

EFFECTS ON LAB TEST RESULTS

● May increase uric acid level. May decrease pseudocholinesterase and Hb levels.
● May decrease lymphocyte, platelet, WBC, RBC, and neutrophil counts.

CONTRAINDICATIONS & CAUTIONS

● Contraindicated in patients hypersensitive to drug.
● Generally contraindicated in patients with existing hepatic or renal dysfunction or bone marrow suppression. However, if need outweighs risk in such patients, may use drug cautiously in low dosage, and accompanied by hepatic, renal, and hematopoietic function tests.
● Myelodysplastic syndromes and acute nonlymphocytic leukemia have been reported in patients treated with thiotepa.
● Death has occurred after intravesical administration, caused by bone marrow depression from systemically absorbed drug, and from septicemia and hemorrhage as a direct result of hematopoietic depression.
Dialyzable drug: Yes.
⚠ **Overdose S&S:** Hematopoietic toxicity, bleeding.

PREGNANCY-LACTATION-REPRODUCTION

● Drug can cause fetal harm when used in pregnant women. If used during pregnancy, or if pregnancy occurs during therapy, apprise patient and patient's partner of potential fetal hazard.
● Effective contraception should be used during therapy if either patient or patient's partner is of childbearing potential.
● It isn't known if drug appears in breast milk. Patient should discontinue breast-feeding or discontinue drug.
● May interfere with spermatogenesis.

NURSING CONSIDERATIONS

● Monitor CBC weekly for at least 3 weeks after last dose.
● If patient's WBC count drops below 3,000/mm^3 or if platelet count falls below 150,000/mm^3, stop drug and notify prescriber. If WBC count falls below 2,000/mm^3 or granulocyte count falls below 1,000/mm^3, follow institutional policy for infection control in immunocompromised patients.
● Monitor uric acid level. To prevent hyperuricemia with resulting uric acid nephropathy, give allopurinol along with adequate hydration.
● Therapeutic effects are commonly accompanied by toxicity.
● To prevent bleeding, avoid all I.M. injections when platelet count is below 50,000/mm^3.
● Give blood transfusions for cumulative anemia.
● Doses of 300 mg/m^2 or greater are associated with high emetic potential in children. Antiemetics are recommended to prevent nausea and vomiting.

PATIENT TEACHING

● Advise patient to watch for signs and symptoms of infection (fever, sore throat, fatigue) and bleeding (easy bruising, nosebleeds, bleeding gums, tarry stools). Tell patient to take temperature daily and to report even mild infections.
● Instruct patient to avoid OTC products containing aspirin or NSAIDs.
● Advise female patient to stop breast-feeding during therapy because of risk of toxicity to infant.
● Caution female patient of childbearing potential to consult prescriber before becoming pregnant.

T

---

tiagabine hydrochloride
tye-AG-ah-been

Gabitril Filmtabs

Therapeutic class: Anticonvulsants
Pharmacologic class: GABA enhancers

AVAILABLE FORMS
Tablets: 2 mg, 4 mg, 12 mg, 16 mg

INDICATIONS & DOSAGES
➤ **Adjunctive treatment of partial seizures in patients taking enzyme-inducing anticonvulsants**
Adults: Initially, 4 mg P.O. once daily. Total daily dose may be increased by 4 to 8 mg at weekly intervals until clinical response or up to 56 mg daily. Give total daily dose in two to four divided doses.
Children ages 12 to 18: Initially, 4 mg P.O. once daily. Total daily dose may be increased by 4 mg at beginning of week 2 and thereafter by 4 to 8 mg per week until clinical response or up to 32 mg daily. Give total daily dose in two to four divided doses.
Adjust-a-dose: For patients with hepatic impairment, reduce first and maintenance doses or increase dosing intervals.

ADMINISTRATION
P.O.
● Give drug with food.
● If patient doesn't take a dose at the scheduled time, don't attempt to make up for the missed dose by increasing the next dose. If more than one dose has been missed, drug may need to be retitrated.

ACTION
Unknown. May act by facilitating the effects of the inhibitory neurotransmitter GABA. By binding to recognition sites linked to GABA uptake carrier, drug may make more GABA available.

Route	Onset	Peak	Duration
P.O.	Rapid	45 min	7–9 hr

Half-life: 2 to 5 hours when given with enzyme inducers; 7 to 9 hours when given without enzyme inducers.

ADVERSE REACTIONS
CNS: asthenia, dizziness, nervousness, somnolence, abnormal gait, agitation, ataxia, confusion, depression, difficulty with concentration and attention, difficulty with memory, emotional lability, hostility, insomnia, language problems, paresthesia, speech disorder, tremor, pain, malaise, syncope, paranoia, migraine.
CV: vasodilation, chest pain, hypertension, palpitations, tachycardia, edema.
EENT: amblyopia, nystagmus, abnormal vision, ear pain, otitis media, tinnitus, epistaxis, pharyngitis.
GI: nausea, abdominal pain, diarrhea, increased appetite, mouth ulceration, vomiting, gingivitis.
GU: UTI, dysmenorrhea, dysuria, metrorrhagia, urinary incontinence, vaginitis.
Hematologic: lymphadenopathy.
Metabolic: weight gain or loss.
Musculoskeletal: generalized weakness, myasthenia, neck pain, arthralgia.
Respiratory: increased cough, bronchitis, dyspnea, pneumonia.
Skin: pruritus, rash, ecchymoses, alopecia, dry skin, sweating.
Other: accidental injury, flulike syndrome, infection.

INTERACTIONS
Drug-drug. *Carbamazepine, phenobarbital, phenytoin:* May increase tiagabine clearance. Monitor patient closely.
CNS depressants: May enhance CNS effects. Use together cautiously.
Drug-herb. *St. John's wort:* May enhance tiagabine metabolism. Monitor patient closely.
Drug-lifestyle. *Alcohol use:* May enhance CNS effects. Discourage use together.

EFFECTS ON LAB TEST RESULTS
None reported.

CONTRAINDICATIONS & CAUTIONS
● Contraindicated in patients hypersensitive to drug or its components.
۞ Alert: Drug may cause new-onset seizures and status epilepticus in patients without a history of epilepsy. In these patients, stop drug and evaluate for underlying seizure

---

Reactions in bold italics are *life-threatening*. Interactions may have a *rapid onset* or a *delayed onset*.

disorder. Drug shouldn't be used for off-label uses.
• Use cautiously in patients with psychiatric symptoms.
• Safety and effectiveness haven't been established for any indication other than as adjunctive therapy for partial seizures in adults and children age 12 and older.
Dialyzable drug: Unlikely.
⚠ ***Overdose S&S:*** Somnolence, impaired consciousness, agitation, confusion, speech difficulty, hostility, depression, weakness, seizures.

PREGNANCY-LACTATION-REPRODUCTION
• Drug may cause fetal harm, but there are no adequate studies in pregnant women. Use during pregnancy only if clearly needed.
• Pregnant women taking drug should enroll in the North American Antiepileptic Drug Pregnancy Registry (1-888-233-2334).
• It isn't known if drug or its metabolites appear in breast milk. Use in breast-feeding women only if benefit clearly outweighs risks.

NURSING CONSIDERATIONS
Alert: Closely monitor all patients taking or starting antiepileptic drugs for changes in behavior indicating worsening of suicidal thoughts or behavior or depression. Symptoms such as anxiety, agitation, hostility, mania, and hypomania may be precursors to emerging suicidality.
• Withdraw drug gradually unless safety concerns require a more rapid withdrawal because sudden withdrawal may cause more frequent seizures.
Alert: Use of anticonvulsants, including tiagabine, may cause status epilepticus and sudden unexpected death in patients with and without epilepsy.
• Patients who aren't receiving at least one enzyme-inducing anticonvulsant when starting tiagabine may need lower doses or slower dosage adjustment.
• Monitor patient for cognitive and neuropsychiatric symptoms, including impaired concentration, speech or language problems, confusion, somnolence, and fatigue.
• Drug may cause moderately severe to incapacitating generalized weakness, which resolves after dosage is reduced or drug stopped.
• ***Look alike–sound alike:*** Don't confuse tiagabine with tizanidine; both have 4-mg starting doses.

PATIENT TEACHING
• Advise patient to take drug only as prescribed.
• Tell patient to take drug with food.
• Warn patient that drug may cause dizziness, somnolence, and other signs and symptoms of CNS depression. Advise patient to avoid driving and other potentially hazardous activities that require mental alertness until drug's CNS effects are known.
• Tell female patient of childbearing potential to call prescriber if she becomes pregnant or plans to become pregnant during therapy.
• Instruct female patient of childbearing potential to notify prescriber if she's planning to breast-feed because drug may appear in breast milk.

SAFETY ALERT!

ticagrelor
TYE-ka-GREL-or

Brilinta

Therapeutic class: Antiplatelet drugs
Pharmacologic class: $P2Y_{12}$ platelet inhibitors

AVAILABLE FORMS
Tablets: 60 mg, 90 mg

INDICATIONS & DOSAGES
➤ **Acute coronary syndrome (ACS) or a history of MI to reduce rate of CV death, MI, and stroke; after stent placement for treatment of ACS to reduce rate of thrombosis**
Adults: Initially, 180 mg P.O. as a loading dose; then, a maintenance dose of 90 mg P.O. b.i.d. during first year after an ACS event. After 1 year, give 60 mg b.i.d. Give daily maintenance dose with 75 to 100 mg of aspirin daily.

ADMINISTRATION
P.O.
• Give drug without regard to food.
• For patients unable to swallow tablets whole, tablets can be crushed, mixed with water, and drunk. The mixture can also be given via an NG tube.
• Store at room temperature in the original container. Keep away from moisture and humidity.

ACTION
Inhibits platelet aggregation by reversibly interacting with the $P2Y_{12}$ adenosine diphosphate receptor.

Route	Onset	Peak	Duration
P.O.	Rapid	1–4 hr	8 hr

Half-life: 9 hours (active metabolite).

ADVERSE REACTIONS
CNS: headache, dizziness, fatigue, syncope, loss of consciousness.
CV: *bleeding,* atrial fibrillation, hypertension, hypotension, chest pain, bradyarrhythmias.
GI: nausea, diarrhea.
Musculoskeletal: back pain, noncardiac chest pain.
Respiratory: cough, dyspnea.

INTERACTIONS
Drug-drug. *Anticoagulants, fibrinolytics, long-term NSAIDs:* May increase risk of bleeding. Use cautiously together.
Black Box Warning *Aspirin:* Maintenance doses of aspirin greater than 100 mg/day may decrease ticagrelor effectiveness and increase risk of bleeding. Maintenance doses of aspirin shouldn't exceed 100 mg/day. ∎
CYP3A strong inducers (carbamazepine, dexamethasone, phenobarbital, phenytoin, rifampin): May significantly decrease ticagrelor level and therapeutic effect. Avoid use together.
CYP3A strong inhibitors (atazanavir, clarithromycin, indinavir, itraconazole, ketoconazole, nefazodone, nelfinavir, ritonavir, saquinavir, telithromycin, voriconazole): May significantly increase ticagrelor level and risk of adverse reactions. Avoid use together.

Digoxin: May increase digoxin level. Monitor digoxin level at start of treatment and with any changes to treatment.
Other $P2Y_{12}$ platelet inhibitors: Increases risk of bleeding. Use together is contraindicated.
Statins: May increase levels of these drugs. Don't exceed 40 mg of simvastatin or lovastatin with concurrent ticagrelor use.

EFFECTS ON LAB TEST RESULTS
• May increase uric acid and creatinine levels.

CONTRAINDICATIONS & CAUTIONS
Black Box Warning Drug can cause serious, sometimes fatal bleeding. Contraindicated in patients with history of intracranial hemorrhage or active pathologic bleeding (including peptic ulcer) because of risk of bleeding. ∎
Black Box Warning Don't start ticagrelor in patients who will undergo planned urgent CABG. If possible, discontinue ticagrelor at least 5 days before any surgery. ∎
• Don't give drug with another oral $P2Y_{12}$ platelet inhibitor.
• Contraindicated in patients hypersensitive to drug and in those with severe hepatic impairment.
• Use cautiously in patients with moderate hepatic failure, elderly patients, patients with history of a bleeding disorder, and patients who have had percutaneous invasive procedures.
Dialyzable drug: No.

PREGNANCY-LACTATION-REPRODUCTION
• There are no adequate studies in pregnant women. Use only if potential benefit justifies potential risk to the fetus.
• It isn't known if drug or its active metabolites appear in breast milk. Patient should discontinue breast-feeding or discontinue drug.

NURSING CONSIDERATIONS
Black Box Warning If possible, manage bleeding without discontinuing ticagrelor; premature discontinuation of treatment increases risk of MI, stent thrombosis, or death. If drug must be temporarily stopped, restart as soon as possible. ∎

• Monitor patient for bleeding.

• Monitor patient for dyspnea and rule out underlying conditions that require treatment in patients with new, prolonged, or worsened difficulty breathing. Dyspnea secondary to ticagrelor therapy is usually mild to moderate, and often self-limiting with continued treatment. If ticagrelor is discontinued for intolerable dyspnea, consider another antiplatelet agent.

• Ticagrelor can be given to patients with ACS who have already been given a loading dose of clopidogrel.

• *Look alike–sound alike:* Don't confuse Brilinta and Brintellix.

PATIENT TEACHING
Black Box Warning Tell patient not to take more than 100 mg of aspirin per day. Warn that other OTC products may also contain aspirin. ■

• Inform patient that bleeding or bruising may occur more easily and it will take longer for the bleeding to stop. Tell patient to immediately report unexpected, prolonged, or excessive bleeding, or blood in the urine or stool.

• Warn patient not to stop drug without consulting prescriber.

• Instruct patient that, before any scheduled surgery or dental appointment, to notify all health care providers that he is taking ticagrelor. Advise patient to discuss with original prescriber recommendations by other providers to stop taking ticagrelor.

• Tell patient that ticagrelor may cause mild to moderate shortness of breath and to report unexpected shortness of breath, especially if it's severe.

• Advise patient that if a dose is missed to take the next dose at its scheduled time and not to take extra medication to make up for the missed dose.

• Tell female patient who is pregnant or planning to become pregnant to consult her primary health care provider before using this medication.

• Warn female patient taking drug not to breast-feed.

tigecycline
tye-gah-SYE-klin

Tygacil

Therapeutic class: Antibiotics
Pharmacologic class: Glycylcycline antibacterials

AVAILABLE FORMS
Lyophilized powder: 50-mg vial

INDICATIONS & DOSAGES
Black Box Warning Compared to other drugs used to treat serious infections, tigecycline has an increased mortality risk. Consider using an alternative drug when possible. ■

Adjust-a-dose (for all indications): For patients with severe hepatic impairment, give initial dose of 100 mg I.V. and then 25 mg I.V. every 12 hours.

➤ **Community-acquired bacterial pneumonia**
Adults: Initially, 100 mg I.V.; then 50 mg I.V. every 12 hours for 7 to 14 days. Infuse drug over 30 to 60 minutes.

➤ **Complicated skin or skin-structure infection; complicated intra-abdominal infection**
Adults: Initially 100 mg I.V.; then 50 mg every 12 hours for 5 to 14 days. Infuse drug over 30 to 60 minutes.

ADMINISTRATION
I.V.
▼ Assess patient for tetracycline allergy before therapy.

▼ Obtain specimen for culture and sensitivity tests before first dose. Begin therapy while awaiting results.

▼ Reconstitute powder with 5.3 mL of NSS or D_5W to yield 10 mg/mL. Gently swirl the vial until the powder dissolves.

▼ Inspect solution for particulates and discoloration (green or black) before giving. Reconstituted solution should be yellow or orange.

▼ Immediately withdraw the dose from the vial and add it to 100 mL of NSS or D_5W. The maximum concentration is 1 mg/mL.

▼ Immediately dilute reconstituted drug.

▼ Use a dedicated I.V. line or a Y-site, and flush the line with NSS or D_5W before and after infusion.

▼ Infuse the drug over 30 to 60 minutes.

▼ Store unopened vials at room temperature in the original package. Store diluted solution at room temperature for up to 24 hours—6 hours in the vial and the remaining time in the I.V. bag or up to 48 hours in the I.V. bag if refrigerated.

▼ **Incompatibilities:** Amphotericin B, amphotericin B lipid complex, diazepam, esomeprazole, omeprazole.

ACTION

Inhibits protein translation in bacteria by binding to the 30S ribosomal unit.

Route	Onset	Peak	Duration
I.V.	Unknown	Unknown	Unknown

Half-life: 27 to 42 hours.

ADVERSE REACTIONS

CNS: asthenia, dizziness, fever, headache, insomnia, pain.

CV: phlebitis.

GI: diarrhea, nausea, vomiting, abdominal pain, constipation, dyspepsia, acute pancreatitis, *Clostridium difficile*–related colitis, hepatic cholestasis, jaundice.

Hematologic: *thrombocytopenia,* anemia, leukocytosis.

Metabolic: hyperglycemia, hypokalemia, hypoproteinemia.

Musculoskeletal: back pain.

Respiratory: cough, dyspnea.

Skin: local reaction, pruritus, rash, sweating.

Other: *sepsis,* abnormal healing, abscess, allergic reaction, infection.

INTERACTIONS

Drug-drug. *Hormonal contraceptives:* May decrease contraceptive's effectiveness. Advise patient to use nonhormonal form of contraception during treatment.

Warfarin: May increase risk of bleeding. Monitor INR.

EFFECTS ON LAB TEST RESULTS

● May increase alkaline phosphatase, amylase, bilirubin, BUN, creatinine, LDH, and AST and ALT levels.

● May decrease potassium, protein, calcium, sodium, and Hb levels and hematocrit.

● May increase or decrease glucose levels.

● May increase WBC count and INR. May prolong aPTT and PT. May decrease platelet count.

CONTRAINDICATIONS & CAUTIONS

● Contraindicated in patients hypersensitive to drug.

● Drug isn't indicated to treat diabetic foot infections, hospital-acquired pneumonia, or ventilator-assisted pneumonia.

● Use cautiously in patients with severe hepatic impairment and in those hypersensitive to tetracycline antibiotics. Also use cautiously as monotherapy in patients with complicated intra-abdominal infections caused by intestinal perforation.

Dialyzable drug: No.

⚠ *Overdose S&S:* Nausea, vomiting.

PREGNANCY-LACTATION-REPRODUCTION

● There are no adequate studies in pregnant women. Use only if potential benefit justifies potential risk to the fetus.

● Use of drug during fetal tooth development may cause permanent tooth discoloration.

● It isn't known if drug appears in breast milk. Use cautiously in breast-feeding women.

NURSING CONSIDERATIONS

● Drug can cause superinfection, including CDAD, which can occur up to 2 months after therapy ends. Monitor patient for diarrhea as drug may need to be stopped and other therapy begun.

● If patient has abdominal infection caused by intestinal perforation, monitor for sepsis.

● Monitor LFTs.

● Monitor patient for symptoms of dangerous toxicities of tetracyclines, such as photosensitivity, pseudotumor cerebri, pancreatitis, and antianabolic action (increased BUN level, azotemia, acidosis, and hypophosphatemia).

Reactions in bold italics are *life-threatening*. Interactions may have a *rapid onset* or a ***delayed onset***.

PATIENT TEACHING
• Tell patient that drug is used to treat only bacterial infections, not viral, and to report all adverse reactions promptly.
• Tell patient to report burning or pain at the I.V. site.
• Tell female patient of childbearing potential to avoid becoming pregnant during treatment and to notify health care provider if pregnancy is suspected or confirmed.
• Urge patient who uses hormonal contraception to also use an alternative contraceptive method during treatment.

timolol maleate
tye-MOE-lol

Betimol, Istalol, Timoptic, Timoptic in Ocudose, Timoptic-XE

Therapeutic class: Antiglaucoma drugs
Pharmacologic class: Nonselective beta blockers

AVAILABLE FORMS
Ophthalmic gel-forming solution: 0.25%, 0.5%
Ophthalmic solution: 0.25%, 0.5%
Ophthalmic solution (preservative-free): 0.25%, 0.5%

INDICATIONS & DOSAGES
➤ **To reduce IOP in ocular hypertension or open-angle glaucoma**
Adults: Initially, 1 drop of 0.25% solution in each affected eye b.i.d.; maintenance dosage is 1 drop once daily. If no response, instill 1 drop of 0.5% solution in each affected eye b.i.d. If IOP is controlled, reduce dosage to 1 drop daily. Or, 1 drop of gel-forming solution (0.25% or 0.5%) in each affected eye once daily. Or, for Istalol, initially 1 drop 0.5% solution in each affected eye once daily in the morning. If response is unsatisfactory, concomitant therapy may be considered.

ADMINISTRATION
Ophthalmic
• Don't touch tip of dropper to eye or surrounding tissue.

• Apply light finger pressure on lacrimal sac for 1 minute after instilling drug to minimize systemic absorption.
• Invert closed container of gel-forming solution and shake once before each use.
• Give other ophthalmic drugs at least 10 minutes before giving gel form of drug.

ACTION
Thought to reduce formation, and possibly increase outflow, of aqueous humor.

Route	Onset	Peak	Duration
Ophthalmic	30 min	1–2 hr	24 hr

Half-life: 4 hours.

ADVERSE REACTIONS
CNS: syncope, confusion, depression, dizziness, fatigue, hallucinations, lethargy, headache.
CV: hypotension, *arrhythmia, bradycardia, cardiac arrest, heart block, HF,* worsening of angina, palpitations, slight reduction in resting HR, hypertension.
EENT: burning and stinging, blepharitis, conjunctivitis, decreased corneal sensitivity with long-term use, diplopia, keratitis, minor eye irritation, ptosis, visual disturbances, discharge, tearing, ocular pain, itching.
Metabolic: hyperglycemia, hyperuricemia.
Respiratory: *bronchospasm in patients with history of asthma,* dyspnea, respiratory infection.

INTERACTIONS
Drug-drug. *Calcium channel blockers, cardiac glycosides, quinidine:* May increase risk of adverse cardiac effects if large amounts of timolol are systemically absorbed. Use together cautiously.
Epinephrine: May cause a hypertensive episode, followed by bradycardia. Stop beta blocker 3 days before starting epinephrine. Monitor patient closely.
Insulin, oral antidiabetic agents: May mask symptoms of hypoglycemia (such as tachycardia) as a result of beta blockade. Use together cautiously in patients with diabetes.
Oral beta blockers: May increase ocular and systemic effects. Use together cautiously.
Prazosin: May increase risk of orthostatic hypotension in early phases of use together.

Assist patient to stand slowly until effects are known.

Reserpine, other catecholamine-depleting drugs: May increase hypotensive and bradycardia-induced effects. Avoid using together.

Theophylline: May act antagonistically, reducing effects of one or both drugs. Consider therapy modification.

EFFECTS ON LAB TEST RESULTS
• May increase BUN, potassium, glucose, and uric acid levels.

CONTRAINDICATIONS & CAUTIONS
• Contraindicated in patients hypersensitive to drug and in those with bronchial asthma, sinus bradycardia, second- or third-degree AV block, cardiac failure, cardiogenic shock, or history of bronchial asthma or severe COPD.
• Use cautiously in patients with nonallergic bronchospasm, chronic bronchitis, emphysema, diabetes mellitus, hyperthyroidism, or cerebrovascular insufficiency.
Dialyzable drug: Unknown.
⚠ *Overdose S&S:* Bradycardia, bronchospasm, dizziness, headache, shortness of breath, cardiac arrest.

PREGNANCY-LACTATION-REPRODUCTION
• There are no adequate studies in pregnant women. Use only if potential benefit justifies potential risk to the fetus.
• Drug appears in breast milk. Patient should discontinue breast-feeding or discontinue drug.

NURSING CONSIDERATIONS
• Monitor diabetic patients carefully. Systemic beta-blocking effects can mask some signs and symptoms of hypoglycemia.
• Some patients may need a few weeks of treatment to stabilize pressure-lowering response. Determine IOP after 4 weeks of treatment.
• *Look alike–sound alike:* Don't confuse timolol with atenolol. Don't confuse Timoptic with Viroptic.

PATIENT TEACHING
• Teach patient how to instill drops. Warn patient not to touch tip of dropper to eye or surrounding tissue.
• Instruct patient using gel-forming solution to invert container and shake once before each use. Also tell patient to use other ophthalmic drugs at least 10 minutes before applying gel.
• Tell patient to instill drug without contact lenses in place. Lenses may be reinserted about 15 minutes after drug use.
• Drug may be absorbed systemically and produce signs and symptoms of beta blockade. Advise patient to monitor pulse rate and report slow rate to prescriber.
• Tell patient to report difficulty breathing or chest pain to prescriber.

SAFETY ALERT!

tinidazole
teh-NID-ah-zol

Tindamax

Therapeutic class: Antiprotozoals
Pharmacologic class: Antiprotozoals

AVAILABLE FORMS
Tablets: 250 mg, 500 mg

INDICATIONS & DOSAGES
Black Box Warning Use tinidazole only for the conditions for which it's indicated. ■
Adjust-a-dose (for all indications): For patients receiving hemodialysis, give an additional dose equal to one-half the recommended dose after the hemodialysis session.
➤ **Bacterial vaginosis in nonpregnant adult women**
Adults: 2 g once daily for 2 days with food, or 1 g once daily for 5 days with food.
➤ **Trichomoniasis caused by *Trichomonas vaginalis***
Adults: 2 g P.O. as a single dose taken with food. Sexual partners should be treated at the same time with the same dose.
➤ **Giardiasis caused by *Giardia lamblia* (*G. duodenalis*)**
Adults: 2 g P.O. as a single dose taken with food.

Children age 3 and older: Give 50 mg/kg (up to 2 g) as a single dose taken with food.

➤ **Intestinal amebiasis caused by *Entamoeba histolytica***

Adults: 2 g P.O. daily for 3 days, taken with food.

Children age 3 and older: Give 50 mg/kg (up to 2 g) P.O. daily for 3 days, taken with food.

➤ **Amebic liver abscess (amebiasis)**

Adults: 2 g P.O. daily for 3 to 5 days, taken with food.

Children age 3 and older: Give 50 mg/kg (up to 2 g) P.O. daily for 3 to 5 days, taken with food.

ADMINISTRATION

P.O.

• Give drug with food to minimize adverse GI effects.

• For children who can't swallow pills, drug can be compounded by the pharmacy by crushing tablets into fine powder and mixing with 10 mL of artificial cherry syrup. Suspension is stable at room temperature for 7 days. Shake well before administration.

ACTION

For *Trichomonas*, cell extracts of *Trichomonas* reduce the compound's nitro group into a free nitro radical that may be responsible for the antiprotozoal activity. Mechanism of action against *Giardia* and *Entamoeba* is unknown.

Route	Onset	Peak	Duration
P.O.	Unknown	1½ hr	Unknown

Half-life: 12 to 14 hours.

ADVERSE REACTIONS

CNS: *seizures,* dizziness, fatigue, headache, malaise, weakness.

GI: anorexia, constipation, cramps, dyspepsia, metallic taste, nausea, vomiting.

INTERACTIONS

Drug-drug. *Cyclosporine, tacrolimus:* May increase cyclosporine or tacrolimus level. Monitor closely for toxicity, including headache, nausea, vomiting, nephrotoxicity, and electrolyte abnormalities.

Disulfiram: May cause psychotic reactions and may increase abdominal cramping,

nausea, vomiting, headaches, and flushing. Separate doses by 2 weeks.

CYP450 inducers (fosphenytoin, phenobarbital, phenytoin, rifampin): May increase tinidazole elimination. Monitor patient.

CYP450 inhibitors (cimetidine, ketoconazole): May prolong tinidazole half-life and decrease clearance. Monitor patient.

5-FU: May decrease 5-FU clearance, increasing adverse effects without added benefit. Monitor patient for rash, nausea, vomiting, stomatitis, and leukopenia.

Fosphenytoin, phenytoin: May prolong phenytoin half-life and decrease clearance of I.V. drug. Monitor patient for toxicity.

Lithium: May increase lithium level. Monitor patient; monitor lithium and creatinine levels.

Warfarin, other oral anticoagulants: May increase anticoagulant effect. Anticoagulant dosage may need adjustment during and for up to 8 days after tinidazole therapy.

Drug-herb. *St. John's wort:* May increase or decrease drug level. Discourage use together.

Drug-lifestyle. *Use of alcohol and alcohol-containing products:* May increase abdominal cramps, nausea, vomiting, headaches, and flushing. Avoid using together and for 3 days after stopping drug.

EFFECTS ON LAB TEST RESULTS

• May increase AST, ALT, glucose, LDH, and triglyceride levels.

• May decrease WBC count.

CONTRAINDICATIONS & CAUTIONS

• Contraindicated in patients hypersensitive to drug, its component, or other nitroimidazole derivatives.

Black Box Warning Carcinogenicity has been seen in mice and rats treated long-term with metronidazole, another nitroimidazole agent. Although such data haven't been reported for tinidazole, both drugs are structurally related and have similar biologic effects. ∎

• Use cautiously in patients with CNS disorders, the elderly, and in those with blood dyscrasias or hepatic dysfunction.

Dialyzable drug: 43% in 6 hours.

T

PREGNANCY-LACTATION-REPRODUCTION
• Drug crosses placental barrier and enters fetal circulation; contraindicated in pregnant women during the first trimester. Use after the first trimester requires that potential benefits be weighed against potential risks to both mother and fetus.
• Drug appears in breast milk for up to 72 hours after administration. Patient shouldn't breast-feeding during therapy and for 3 days after last dose.

NURSING CONSIDERATIONS
• If therapy exceeds 3 days, monitor children closely.
• Patient should take drug with food to minimize adverse GI effects.
⊙ **Alert:** If abnormal neurologic signs, such as seizures or paresthesia of the arms or legs, occur, stop drug immediately.
• Superinfection and CDAD can occur up to 2 months after therapy ends. Monitor patient for diarrhea.
• If candidiasis develops during therapy, patient may need an antifungal.
• Use cautiously in elderly patients, who may have decreased liver or kidney function.

PATIENT TEACHING
• Tell patient to take drug with food.
⊙ **Alert:** Tell patient to report to prescriber seizures and numbness in arms or legs.
• Warn patient not to drink alcohol or use alcohol-containing products while taking drug and for 3 days afterward.
• Advise female patient to immediately notify prescriber if she becomes pregnant.
• Tell female patient to stop breast-feeding during therapy and for 3 days after last dose.
• If patient is being treated for a sexually transmitted infection, explain that patient's sexual partners should be treated at the same time.

tiotropium bromide
tye-oh-TROH-pee-um

Spiriva, Spiriva Respimat

Therapeutic class: Bronchodilators
Pharmacologic class: Anticholinergics

AVAILABLE FORMS
Capsules (powder for inhalation): 18 mcg
Spray inhaler (Respimat): 1.25 mcg/actuation, 2.5 mcg/actuation

INDICATIONS & DOSAGES
Adjust-a-dose (for all indications): Closely monitor patients with moderate to severe renal impairment for anticholinergic effects.
➤ **To reduce COPD exacerbations; maintenance treatment of bronchospasm in COPD, including chronic bronchitis and emphysema**
Adults: 2 oral inhalations of 1 capsule (18 mcg) once daily using HandiHaler inhalation device. Or, 2 inhalations (2.5 mcg each) of spray once daily.
➤ **Long-term maintenance treatment of asthma (Spiriva Respimat)**
Adults and adolescents age 12 and older: 2 inhalations of 1.25 mcg/actuation spray once daily; total dose equals 2.5 mcg of tiotropium. Maximum benefits in lung function may take up to 4 to 8 weeks of dosing.

ADMINISTRATION
Inhalational
Capsules
• Give capsules only by oral inhalation with the HandiHaler device.
• Open capsule blister immediately before use.
• Capsules aren't for oral ingestion.
Respimat spray inhaler
• Before first use, insert cartridge into the inhaler.
• Prime the unit before using it for the first time by actuating the inhaler toward the ground until an aerosol cloud is visible; then repeat the process three more times.
• If not used for more than 3 days, the inhaler should be actuated once to prepare it for use. If not used for more than 21 days,

the inhaler should be actuated until an aerosol cloud is visible; then repeat the process three more times.

ACTION
Competitive, reversible inhibition of muscarinic receptors leads to bronchodilation.

Route	Onset	Peak	Duration
Inhalation	Unknown	5–7 min	>24 hr

Half-life: 5 to 6 days.

ADVERSE REACTIONS
CNS: depression, paresthesia, headache.
CV: *angina pectoris,* chest pain, edema.
EENT: sinusitis, cataract, dysphonia, epistaxis, glaucoma, laryngitis, pharyngitis, rhinitis.
GI: dry mouth, abdominal pain, constipation, dyspepsia, gastroesophageal reflux, stomatitis, vomiting.
GU: UTI.
Metabolic: hypercholesterolemia, hyperglycemia.
Musculoskeletal: arthritis, leg pain, myalgia, skeletal pain.
Respiratory: URI, cough, bronchitis.
Skin: rash.
Other: accidental injury, allergic reaction, candidiasis, flulike syndrome, herpes zoster, infections.

INTERACTIONS
Drug-drug. *Anticholinergics:* May increase the risk of adverse reactions. Avoid using together.

EFFECTS ON LAB TEST RESULTS
• May increase cholesterol and glucose levels.

CONTRAINDICATIONS & CAUTIONS
• Contraindicated in patients hypersensitive to atropine, its derivatives, ipratropium, or components of the product.
• Use cautiously in patients with CrCl of 50 mL/minute or less, or patients with angle-closure glaucoma, prostatic hyperplasia, or bladder neck obstruction.
• Use cautiously in patients with severe hypersensitivity to milk protein.
Dialyzable drug: Unknown.

⚠ Overdose S&S: Change in mental status, tremors, abdominal pain, severe constipation.

PREGNANCY-LACTATION-REPRODUCTION
• There are no adequate studies in pregnant women. Use only if potential benefit justifies potential risk to the fetus.
• It isn't known if drug appears in breast milk. Use cautiously in breast-feeding women.

NURSING CONSIDERATIONS
⊕ *Alert:* Use drug for maintenance treatment of COPD or asthma, not for acute bronchospasm.
• Watch for evidence of hypersensitivity (especially angioedema) and paradoxical bronchospasm.
• *Look alike–sound alike:* Don't confuse Spiriva with Inspra.

PATIENT TEACHING
• Inform patient that drug is for maintenance treatment of COPD or asthma and not for immediate relief of breathing problems.
⊕ *Alert:* Explain that capsules are for inhalation and shouldn't be swallowed.
• Provide full instructions for the Handi-Haler device or the Respimat spray inhaler. Demonstrate use and observe return demonstration from patient.
• Tell patient not to get powder or spray in eyes.
• Tell patient not to take more than one dose (2 inhalations) in 24 hours.
• Review signs and symptoms of hypersensitivity (especially angioedema) and paradoxical bronchospasm. Tell patient to stop the drug and contact prescriber if they occur.
• Advise patient to report eye pain, blurred vision, visual halos, colored images, or red eyes immediately.
• Tell patient to keep capsules in sealed blisters and to remove each capsule just before use. Caution against storing capsules in the HandiHaler device.
• Instruct patient to store capsules and cartridges at 77° F (25° C) and not to expose them to extreme temperatures or moisture.
• Advise patient that when the labeled number of actuations (28 or 60) has been

T

dispensed from the Respimat inhaler, a locking mechanism will be engaged and no more actuations can be dispensed.

tipranavir
tih-PRAN-uh-veer

Aptivus

Therapeutic class: Antiretrovirals
Pharmacologic class: Protease inhibitors

AVAILABLE FORMS
Capsules ⒪ⓉⒸ: 250 mg
Oral solution: 100 mg/mL

INDICATIONS & DOSAGES
➤ **HIV-1 in patients with viral replication who are highly treatment-experienced or have HIV-1 strains resistant to multiple protease inhibitors**
Adults: 500 mg P.O. b.i.d. with 200 mg of ritonavir b.i.d.
Children ages 2 to 18: 14 mg/kg with ritonavir 6 mg/kg (or tipranavir 375 mg/m² with ritonavir 150 mg/m²) b.i.d., not to exceed dosage of tipranavir 500 mg with ritonavir 200 mg b.i.d. For children who develop intolerance or toxicity, prescribers may consider decreasing dosage to tipranavir 12 mg/kg with ritonavir 5 mg/kg b.i.d. provided the virus isn't resistant to multiple protease inhibitors.
Adjust-a-dose: Discontinue if asymptomatic AST or ALT elevations greater than 10 × ULN occur. Also discontinue if AST or ALT elevations greater than 5 to 10 × ULN occur concurrently with total bilirubin level greater than 2.5 × ULN.

ADMINISTRATION
P.O.
• Give with 200 mg ritonavir and other antiretrovirals.
• Make sure patient swallows capsules whole and doesn't break, crush, or chew them.
• When given with ritonavir tablets, drug must only be taken with meals; when given with ritonavir capsules or solution, drug can be taken with or without meals.
• Don't freeze or refrigerate oral solution.

• Store unopened capsule bottle in refrigerator; after bottle is opened, store at room temperature.
• Use within 60 days of opening capsule or oral solution bottle.

ACTION
Inhibits virus-specific processing of polyproteins in HIV-1 infected cells, preventing formation of mature virions.

Route	Onset	Peak	Duration
P.O.	Unknown	3 hr	Unknown

Half-life: Adults, 6 hours; children age 2 to younger than 6, 8 hours; children age 6 to younger than 12, 7 hours; children age 12 to 18, 5 hours.

ADVERSE REACTIONS
CNS: dizziness, fatigue, headache, insomnia, malaise, peripheral neuropathy, pyrexia, sleep disorder, somnolence.
GI: diarrhea, *pancreatitis,* abdominal distention, abdominal pain, dyspepsia, flatulence, GERD, nausea, vomiting.
GU: renal insufficiency.
Hematologic: *neutropenia, thrombocytopenia,* anemia.
Hepatic: *hepatic failure, hepatitis.*
Metabolic: anorexia, decreased appetite, dehydration, diabetes mellitus, facial wasting, hyperglycemia, hyperlipidemia, hypertriglyceridemia, weight loss.
Musculoskeletal: muscle cramps, myalgia.
Respiratory: cough, dyspnea.
Skin: rash, acquired lipodystrophy, exanthem, lipoatrophy, lipohypertrophy, pruritus.
Other: flulike illness, hypersensitivity, reactivation of herpes simplex and varicella zoster.

INTERACTIONS
Drug-drug. *Amiodarone, bepridil, flecainide, propafenone, quinidine:* May increase levels of these drugs and risk of life-threatening arrhythmias. Use together is contraindicated.
⊘ *Alert: Atorvastatin:* May increase levels of both drugs and risk of myopathy and rhabdomyolysis. Avoid use together.
Clarithromycin: May increase levels of both drugs. If CrCl is 30 to 60 mL/minute, decrease clarithromycin dose by 50%. If

---

Reactions in bold italics are *life-threatening*. Interactions may have a *rapid onset* or a ***delayed onset***.

CrCl is less than 30 mL/minute, decrease clarithromycin dose by 75%.
Colchicine: May increase risk of life-threatening and fatal colchicine toxicity. In patients with healthy renal and hepatic function, reduce colchicine dosage to no more than 0.3 mg b.i.d.; monitor patient carefully for colchicine-related adverse effects. Avoid coadministration in patients with hepatic or renal impairment.
Cyclosporine, sirolimus, tacrolimus: May cause unpredictable interaction. Monitor drug levels closely until they've stabilized.
Desipramine: May increase desipramine level. Decrease dose and monitor desipramine level.
Didanosine: May decrease didanosine level. Separate dosing by at least 2 hours.
Diltiazem, felodipine, nicardipine, nisoldipine, verapamil: May cause unpredictable interaction. Use together cautiously, and monitor patient closely.
Disulfiram, metronidazole: May cause disulfiram-like reaction. Use together cautiously.
Ergot derivatives (dihydroergotamine, ergonovine, ergotamine, methylergonovine): May cause acute ergot toxicity, including peripheral vasospasm and ischemia of extremities. Use together is contraindicated.
Estrogen-based hormone therapy: May decrease estrogen level, and rash may occur. Monitor patient carefully. Advise using nonhormonal contraception.
Fluoxetine, paroxetine, sertraline: May increase levels of these drugs. Adjust dosages as needed.
Glimepiride, glipizide, glyburide, pioglitazone, repaglinide, tolbutamide: May affect glucose levels. Monitor glucose level carefully.
🜄 *Alert: Lovastatin, simvastatin:* May increase risk of myopathy and rhabdomyolysis. Use together is contraindicated.
Meperidine: May increase normeperidine metabolite. Avoid using together.
Methadone: May decrease methadone level by 50%. Consider increased methadone dose.
Midazolam, triazolam: May cause prolonged or increased sedation or respiratory depression. Use together is contraindicated.

Pimozide: May cause life-threatening arrhythmias. Use together is contraindicated.
Rifabutin: May increase rifabutin level. Decrease rifabutin dose by 75%.
Rifampin: May lead to loss of virologic response and resistance to tipranavir and other protease inhibitors. Use together is contraindicated.
Sildenafil, tadalafil, vardenafil: May increase levels of these drugs. Use together cautiously. Tell patient not to exceed 25 mg sildenafil in 48 hours, 10 mg tadalafil every 72 hours, or 2.5 mg vardenafil every 72 hours. Use of sildenafil (Revatio) for treatment of pulmonary arterial hypertension is contraindicated.
Valproic acid: May reduce valproic acid plasma level. Use with caution.
Warfarin: May cause unpredictable reaction. Check INR often.
Drug-herb. *St. John's wort:* May lead to loss of virologic response and resistance to tipranavir and other antiretrovirals. Don't use together.

EFFECTS ON LAB TEST RESULTS
• May increase total cholesterol, triglyceride, blood glucose, amylase, lipase, ALT, and AST levels.
• May decrease WBC count.

CONTRAINDICATIONS & CAUTIONS
Black Box Warning Administration of tipranavir has been associated with fatal and nonfatal intracranial hemorrhage, clinical hepatitis, and hepatic decompensation. ∎
• Contraindicated in patients hypersensitive to ingredients of the product, patients with moderate (Child-Pugh class B) or severe (Child-Pugh class C) hepatic insufficiency, and patients taking drugs that are potent CYP3A inducers or that depend on CYP3A for clearance plus ritonavir.
• Use cautiously in patients with sulfonamide allergy, diabetes, liver disease, HBV or HCV infection, or hemophilia A or B.
Dialyzable drug: No.

PREGNANCY-LACTATION-REPRODUCTION
• There are no adequate studies in pregnant women. Use only if potential benefit justifies potential risk to the fetus.

• To monitor maternal-fetal outcomes, register patients exposed to drug in the Antiretroviral Pregnancy Registry (1-800-258-4263).

• The CDC recommends that mothers with HIV-1 infection not breast-feed to avoid risking postnatal transmission of HIV-1.

NURSING CONSIDERATIONS

❶ *Alert:* Don't give drug to treatment-naive patients.

• To be effective, drug must be given with ritonavir and with other antiretrovirals.

❶ *Alert:* Monitor patient for signs and symptoms of intracranial hemorrhage, including headache, nausea and vomiting, change in mental status, speech or balance difficulties, and seizures.

❶ *Alert:* Obtain thorough patient drug history. Many drugs may interact with tipranavir. Consider potential for drug interactions before and during therapy; review concomitant medications during therapy; and monitor patient for adverse reactions associated with concomitant medications.

• Monitor LFTs at start of treatment and often during treatment.

• Assess for evidence of hepatitis, such as fatigue, malaise, anorexia, nausea, jaundice, bilirubinemia, acholic stools, liver tenderness, and hepatomegaly.

• If patient develops signs or symptoms of hepatitis, notify prescriber.

Black Box Warning Patients with chronic HBV or HCV infection are at increased risk for hepatotoxicity; fatalities have been reported. ∎

• In diabetic patients, monitor glucose level closely; hyperglycemia may occur.

• Obtain baseline cholesterol and triglyceride levels at start of and periodically during therapy.

• Monitor patient for cushingoid symptoms, such as central obesity, buffalo hump, peripheral wasting, facial wasting, and breast enlargement.

• Use cautiously in elderly patients because they are more likely to have decreased organ function, multidrug therapy, and other illnesses.

PATIENT TEACHING

• Explain that drug doesn't cure HIV infection and doesn't reduce the risk of transmitting the virus to others.

❶ *Alert:* Many drugs may interfere with this drug. Urge patient to report all prescription and OTC drugs and herbal products being taken.

• Tell patient that drug is effective only when taken with ritonavir and other antiretrovirals.

• Instruct patient taking ritonavir tablets to take them with meals; patient taking ritonavir capsules or solution can take them with or without meals.

• Tell patient to store unopened capsule bottle in refrigerator and to store at room temperature after bottle is opened. Advise patient not to freeze or refrigerate oral solution.

• Tell patient to swallow capsules whole and to not break, crush, or chew them.

• Instruct patient taking oral solution not to take supplemental vitamin E in an amount greater than a standard multivitamin.

• Urge patient to stop drug and contact prescriber if signs and symptoms of hepatitis or intracranial hemorrhage occur.

• If female patient uses hormonal contraceptives, advise use of barrier contraception.

• Tell patient that redistribution or accumulation of body fat may occur.

• Advise female patient that breast-feeding isn't recommended during therapy.

SAFETY ALERT!

tirofiban hydrochloride
tye-row-FYE-ban

Aggrastat

Therapeutic class: Antiplatelet drugs
Pharmacologic class: Glycoprotein IIb/IIIa receptor antagonists

AVAILABLE FORMS
Injection (premixed bag): 50 mcg/mL in 100 mL or 250 mL

INDICATIONS & DOSAGES
➤ **In patients with non-ST elevation acute coronary syndrome to reduce the**

---

rate of thrombotic CV events (combined endpoint of death, MI, or refractory ischemia/repeat cardiac procedure)
Adults: I.V. loading dose of 25 mcg/kg administered within 5 minutes, followed by 0.15 mcg/kg/minute for up to 18 hours.
Adjust-a-dose: If CrCl is 60 mL/minute or less, use an I.V. loading dose of 25 mcg/kg administered within 5 minutes, followed by 0.075 mcg/kg/minute for up to 18 hours.

➤ **To support PCI (administered at the time of PCI) for ST-elevation MI ◆**
Adults: Loading dose of 25 mcg/kg I.V. administered over 5 minutes or less at the time of PCI, followed by maintenance infusion of 0.15 mcg/kg/minute in combination with heparin or bivalirudin in selected patients; was continued for 18 to 24 hours in clinical trials.

ADMINISTRATION
I.V.
▼ Inspect solution for particulate matter before giving, and check for leaks by squeezing the inner bag firmly. If bag leaks or particles are visible, discard solution.
▼ Avoid use of noncompressible sites (such as subclavian or jugular veins).
▼ Don't use plastic containers in series connections; may result in air embolism by drawing air from the first bag if it's empty of solution.
▼ May give tirofiban through same I.V. line as heparin, atropine sulfate, epinephrine hydrochloride, furosemide, midazolam hydrochloride, morphine sulfate, nitroglycerin, propranolol hydrochloride, dopamine, lidocaine, potassium chloride, and famotidine.
▼ Discard unused solution 24 hours after the start of infusion.
▼ Store drug at room temperature. Protect from light.
▼ **Incompatibilities:** Diazepam.

ACTION
Reversibly binds to the glycoprotein IIb/IIIa receptor on human platelets and inhibits platelet aggregation.

Route	Onset	Peak	Duration
I.V.	Immediate	Immediate	4–6 hr

Half-life: About 2 hours.

ADVERSE REACTIONS
CNS: dizziness.
CV: *bradycardia, coronary artery dissection,* edema, vasovagal reaction.
GI: occult bleeding, nausea.
Hematologic: bleeding, *thrombocytopenia.*
Musculoskeletal: leg pain.
Skin: sweating.
Other: bleeding at arterial access site, pelvic pain.

INTERACTIONS
Drug-drug. ✪ *Alert:* Anticoagulants such as aspirin, clopidogrel, dipyridamole, fibrinolytics, heparin, NSAIDs, ticlopidine warfarin: May increase risk of bleeding. Monitor patient closely.
Levothyroxine, omeprazole: May increase tirofiban renal clearance. Monitor patient.

EFFECTS ON LAB TEST RESULTS
● May decrease Hb level and hematocrit.
● May decrease platelet count.

CONTRAINDICATIONS & CAUTIONS
● Contraindicated in patients hypersensitive to drug or its components.
● Contraindicated in patients with active internal bleeding or history of bleeding diathesis within previous 30 days, major surgical procedure or physical trauma within previous month, thrombocytopenia after previous exposure to drug, and severe hypertension.
● Use cautiously in patients with renal impairment and those with increased risk of bleeding, including patients with hemorrhagic retinopathy or platelet count less than 150,000/mm^3.
● Safety and effectiveness haven't been studied in patients younger than age 18.
Dialyzable drug: Yes.
⚠ *Overdose S&S:* Bleeding.

PREGNANCY-LACTATION-REPRODUCTION
● There are no adequate studies in pregnant women; adverse events haven't been observed in animal reproduction studies.
● It isn't known if drug appears in breast milk. Patient should discontinue breastfeeding or discontinue drug.

T

NURSING CONSIDERATIONS

● Monitor Hb level, hematocrit, and platelet count before starting therapy, 6 hours after loading dose, and at least daily during therapy. If thrombocytopenia occurs, notify prescriber.

● Monitor aPTT before treatment and 6 hours after the start of heparin infusion.

● Monitor patient for bleeding.

❸ **Alert:** The most common adverse effect is bleeding at the arterial access site for cardiac catheterization.

● Minimize use of arterial and venous punctures, I.M. injections, urinary catheters, and nasotracheal and NG tubes.

● Elderly patients have a higher risk of bleeding complications.

● **Look alike–sound alike:** Don't confuse Aggrastat with argatroban.

PATIENT TEACHING

● Explain that drug is used to prevent chest pain and heart attack.

● Explain that the benefits of the drug far outweigh the risk of serious bleeding.

● Instruct patient to report chest discomfort or other adverse effects immediately.

● Tell patient that frequent blood sampling may be needed to evaluate therapy.

---

tizanidine hydrochloride
tis-AN-i-deen

Zanaflex

Therapeutic class: Skeletal muscle relaxants
Pharmacologic class: Centrally acting alpha$_2$-adrenergic agonists

AVAILABLE FORMS
Capsules: 2 mg, 4 mg, 6 mg
Tablets: 2 mg, 4 mg

INDICATIONS & DOSAGES

➤ **Acute and intermittent management of increased muscle tone with spasticity**
Adults: Initially, 2 mg P.O. every 6 to 8 hours, as needed, to maximum of three doses in 24 hours. Dosage can be increased gradually in 2- to 4-mg increments, with 1 to

4 days between increases. Maximum, 36 mg daily.

Adjust-a-dose: Use cautiously and reduce dosage in patients with any hepatic impairment or renal insufficiency (CrCl of less than 25 mL/minute). If higher dosages are needed, increase individual doses rather than frequency.

ADMINISTRATION
P.O.

● Give drug consistently as either tablets or capsules and with or without food for same absorption rate and effect.

ACTION

Unknown. Acts as an alpha$_2$ agonist. May reduce spasticity by increasing presynaptic inhibition of motor neurons at the level of the spinal cord.

Route	Onset	Peak	Duration
P.O.	Unknown	1–2 hr	3–6 hr

Half-life: 2½ hours; metabolites, 20 to 40 hours.

ADVERSE REACTIONS

CNS: somnolence, sedation, asthenia, dizziness, speech disorder, dyskinesia, nervousness, hallucinations.
CV: hypotension, *bradycardia.*
EENT: amblyopia, pharyngitis, rhinitis.
GI: dry mouth, constipation, vomiting.
GU: UTI, urinary frequency.
Hepatic: hepatic injury.
Other: infection, flulike syndrome.

INTERACTIONS

Drug-drug. *Acetaminophen:* May delay acetaminophen absorption time. Monitor patient for clinical effect.
Antihypertensives, other alpha agonists (such as clonidine): May cause hypotension; monitor patient closely. Avoid using together.
Baclofen, benzodiazepines, other CNS depressants: May have additive CNS depressant effects. Avoid using together.
CYP1A2 inhibitors (amiodarone, acyclovir, cimetidine, ciprofloxacin, famotidine, fluoroquinolones, fluvoxamine, mexiletine, propafenone, ticlopidine, verapamil, zileuton): May cause significant increases in tizanidine levels. Use together should be

---

avoided; use of ciprofloxacin or fluvoxamine with tizanidine is contraindicated.

Black Box Warning *Opioids:* May cause slow or difficult breathing, sedation, and death. Avoid use together. If use together is necessary, limit dosage and duration of each drug to minimum necessary for desired effect. ■

Oral contraceptives: May decrease tizanidine clearance. Reduce tizanidine dosage.

Drug-lifestyle. *Alcohol use:* May increase CNS depression. Discourage use together.

EFFECTS ON LAB TEST RESULTS
● May increase AST and ALT levels.

CONTRAINDICATIONS & CAUTIONS
● Contraindicated in patients hypersensitive to drug.

Black Box Warning Opioids should only be prescribed with benzodiazepines or other CNS depressants to patients for whom alternative treatment options are inadequate. ■

● Use cautiously in patients who are taking antihypertensives, in those with renal and hepatic impairment, and in elderly patients.

● Safety and effectiveness in children haven't been established.

Dialyzable drug: Unlikely.

⚠ *Overdose S&S:* Lethargy, somnolence, confusion, coma, bradycardia, hypotension, respiratory depression, depressed cardiac function.

PREGNANCY-LACTATION-REPRODUCTION
● Drug hasn't been studied in pregnant women. Use only if potential benefit justifies potential risk to the fetus.

● It isn't known if drug appears in breast milk. Use cautiously in breast-feeding women.

NURSING CONSIDERATIONS
🔹 *Alert:* The capsules and tablets are bioequivalent only if taken on an empty stomach.

● Obtain LFT results before treatment; during treatment at 1, 3, and 6 months; and then periodically thereafter.

● May prolong QT interval and cause bradycardia and hypotension. Closely monitor vital signs, especially in patients receiving

maximum recommended dosa— taking other drugs that prolong use

● Monitor patient for signs and s l. of excess sedation if patient is tak along with another CNS depressan

● Consider discontinuing drug in pa who develop hallucinations.

🔹 *Alert:* Stop drug gradually, especially patients taking high doses for a prolong period. Decrease dose slowly to minimiz the potential for rebound hypertension, tachycardia, and hypertonia.

● *Look alike–sound alike:* Don't confuse tizanidine with tiagabine; both have 4-mg starting doses.

PATIENT TEACHING
Black Box Warning Caution patient or caregiver of patient taking an opioid with a benzodiazepine, CNS depressant, or alcohol to seek immediate medical attention if patient experiences dizziness, light-headedness, extreme sleepiness, slowed or difficult breathing, or unresponsiveness. ■

● Caution patient to avoid alcohol and activities that require alertness. Drug may cause drowsiness.

● Inform patient that dizziness upon standing quickly can be minimized by rising slowly.

🔹 *Alert:* Advise patient that tizanidine absorption varies depending on whether drug is taken with or without food and that it should always be taken the same way to reduce risk of changes in efficacy and adverse reactions.

● Instruct patient to inform the health care provider and pharmacist when any medication is added or removed from his regimen.

● Advise patient not to suddenly stop taking medication.

T

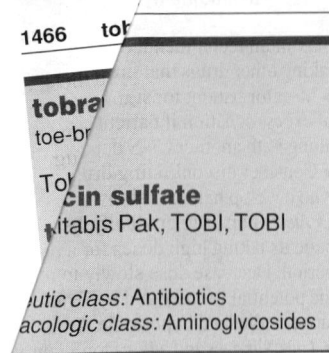

tobra
toe-br

Tob
cin sulfate
itabis Pak, TOBI, TOBI

utic class: Antibiotics
acologic class: Aminoglycosides

LABLE FORMS
ules (for inhalation): 28 mg
tidose vials (pediatric): 10 mg/mL,
mg/mL
Nebulizer solution (for inhalation):
300 mg/4 mL, 300 mg/5 mL
Ophthalmic ointment: 0.3%
Ophthalmic solution: 0.3%
Prefilled syringe (pediatric): 40 mg/mL
Premixed parenteral injection for infusion:
60 mg or 80 mg in 100 mL NSS

INDICATIONS & DOSAGES
➤ **Serious infection by sensitive strains
of *Escherichia coli*, *Proteus*, *Klebsiella*,
Enterobacter, *Serratia*, *Morganella morganii*, *Staphylococcus aureus*, *Citrobacter*,
Pseudomonas, or *Providencia***
Adults: 3 mg/kg/day I.M. or I.V. in
three equal doses every 8 hours. For
life-threatening infections, give up to
5 mg/kg/day in divided doses every 6 to
8 hours; reduce to 3 mg/kg daily as soon as
clinically indicated.
Children older than age 1 week: 6 to
7.5 mg/kg/day I.M. or I.V., in three or four
divided doses.
*Neonates younger than age 1 week or
preterm infants:* Up to 4 mg/kg/day I.V.
or I.M. in two equal doses every 12 hours.
Adjust-a-dose: For patients with renal impairment, give loading dose of 1 mg/kg;
then give decreased doses at 8-hour intervals or same dose at prolonged intervals.
For hemodialysis patients, give 50% of the
normal dose after dialysis and adjust according to serum concentrations. For patients
with severe cystic fibrosis, initial dose is
10 mg/kg/day I.V. or I.M., in four divided
doses.

➤ **To manage cystic fibrosis patients with
Pseudomonas aeruginosa infection**
Adults and children age 6 and older:
300 mg via nebulizer every 12 hours for
28 days. Continue cycle of 28 days on drug
and 28 days off. Or, using TOBI Podhaler
device, have patient inhale contents of four
28-mg capsules every 12 hours for 28 days,
stop therapy for 28 days, then repeat and
continue cycles of 28 days on drug and
28 days off.
➤ **External ocular infections by susceptible bacteria**
Adults and children age 2 months and older:
In mild to moderate infections, instill 1 or
2 drops into affected eye every 4 hours,
or apply ½-inch (1.27-cm) ribbon of ointment every 8 to 12 hours. In severe infections, instill 2 drops into infected eye every
60 minutes until condition improves; then
reduce frequency. Or, apply ½-inch ribbon
of ointment every 3 to 4 hours until condition improves; then reduce frequency to
b.i.d. to t.i.d.

ADMINISTRATION
I.V.
▼ Obtain specimen for culture and sensitiv-
ity tests before giving. Begin therapy while
awaiting results.
▼ For adults, dilute in 50 to 100 mL of NSS
or D₅W; use a smaller volume for children.
▼ Keep reconstituted solution in refrigerator and use within 96 hours.
▼ Infuse over 20 to 60 minutes.
▼ After infusion, flush line with NSS or
D₅W.
▼ Obtain blood for peak level 30 minutes
after infusion stops; draw blood for trough
level just before next dose. Don't collect
blood in a heparinized tube because of
incompatibility.
▼ **Incompatibilities:** Allopurinol; amphotericin B; azithromycin; beta-lactam
antibiotics; cefepime; clindamycin; dextrose 5% in Isolyte E, M, or P; heparin
sodium; hetastarch; indomethacin; propofol; sargramostim; solutions containing
alcohol.
I.M.
● Obtain specimen for culture and sensitivity tests before giving. Begin therapy while
awaiting results.

Reactions in bold italics are *life-threatening*. Interactions may have a *rapid onset* or a ***delayed onset***.

• Obtain blood for peak level 1 hour after I.M. injection; draw blood for trough level just before next dose. Don't collect blood in a heparinized tube because of incompatibility.

Inhalational

• Obtain specimen for culture and sensitivity tests before giving. Begin therapy while awaiting results.

• Give nebulizer solution over 10 to 15 minutes using handheld Pari LC Plus reusable nebulizer with DeVilbiss Pulmo-Aide compressor.

• Capsules aren't for oral ingestion.

• Give capsules only by oral inhalation using Podhaler device.

• Store capsules in blister packs at room temperature and remove immediately before use.

• Give doses as close to 12 hours apart as possible. Doses shouldn't be taken less than 6 hours apart.

Ophthalmic

• When two different ophthalmic solutions are used, allow at least 10 minutes between instillations.

• Apply light finger pressure on lacrimal sac for 1 minute after drops are instilled.

• Apply ointment to conjunctiva. Don't let tube touch eye.

ACTION

Generally bactericidal. Inhibits protein synthesis by binding directly to the 30S ribosomal subunit.

Route	Onset	Peak	Duration
I.V.	Immediate	30 min	8 hr
I.M.	Unknown	30–60 min	8 hr
Inhalation	Unknown	Unknown	Unknown
Ophthalmic	Unknown	Unknown	Unknown

Half-life: Adults: I.V., 2 to 3 hours; inhalation, 4 hours; ophthalmic, 2 to 3 hours; adults with impaired renal function, 5 to 70 hours. Neonates weighing 1,200 g or less, 11 hours; neonates weighing more than 1,200 g, 2 to 9 hours.

ADVERSE REACTIONS

CNS: *seizures,* headache, lethargy, confusion, disorientation, fever.

CENT: blurred vision (ophthalmic); ototoxicity, hoarseness, pharyngitis.

GI: vomiting, nausea, diarrhea.

GU: *nephrotoxicity,* possible increase in urinary excretion of casts.

Hematologic: anemia, eosinophilia, *leukopenia, thrombocytopenia, agranulocytosis.*

Metabolic: electrolyte imbalances.

Musculoskeletal: muscle twitching.

Respiratory: *bronchospasm.*

Skin: rash, urticaria, pruritus.

INTERACTIONS

Drug-drug. **Black Box Warning** *Acyclovir, amphotericin B, cephalosporins, cidofovir, cisplatin, methoxyflurane, vancomycin, other aminoglycosides:* May increase nephrotoxicity when used with injectable tobramycin formulation. Monitor renal function. ∎

Atracurium, pancuronium, rocuronium, vecuronium: May increase effects of nondepolarizing muscle relaxants, including prolonged respiratory depression. Use together only when necessary, and expect to reduce dosage of nondepolarizing muscle relaxant.

Dimenhydrinate: May mask symptoms of ototoxicity. Monitor patient's hearing.

General anesthetics: May increase neuromuscular blockade. Monitor patient for increased clinical effects.

Black Box Warning *I.V. loop diuretics such as furosemide:* May increase ototoxicity when used with injectable tobramycin. Monitor patient's hearing. ∎

Parenteral penicillins: May inactivate tobramycin in vitro. Don't mix together.

EFFECTS ON LAB TEST RESULTS

• May increase AST, ALT, LDH, bilirubin, BUN, creatinine, nonprotein nitrogen, and urine urea levels. May decrease calcium, magnesium, and potassium levels.

• May increase eosinophil count. May decrease WBC and platelet counts.

CONTRAINDICATIONS & CAUTIONS

• Contraindicated in patients hypersensitive to drug or other aminoglycosides.

Black Box Warning Use tobramycin injection cautiously in premature infants and neonates because of their renal immaturity and resulting prolongation of drug's serum half-life. ∎

Black Box Warning For injectable tobramycin, neurotoxicity manifested as both auditory and vestibular ototoxicity can occur. Auditory changes are irreversible, are usually bilateral, and may be partial or total. Other manifestations of neurotoxicity may include numbness, skin tingling, muscle twitching, and seizures. Risk of hearing loss increases with degree of exposure to either high peak or high trough serum concentrations; other factors that may increase patient risk are advanced age and dehydration. Patients who develop cochlear damage may not have symptoms during therapy to warn them of eighth-nerve toxicity, and partial or total irreversible bilateral deafness may continue to develop after drug discontinuation. ■

• Use cautiously in patients with impaired renal function or neuromuscular disorders and in elderly patients.
Dialyzable drug: Yes.
⚠ *Overdose S&S:* Nephrotoxicity, dizziness, tinnitus, vertigo, loss of high-tone hearing acuity, neuromuscular blockade, respiratory failure, respiratory paralysis (systemic); punctate keratitis, erythema, tearing, edema, eyelid itching (ophthalmic).

PREGNANCY-LACTATION-REPRODUCTION
Black Box Warning Aminoglycosides can cause fetal harm when given to pregnant women. ■
• There are no adequate studies in pregnant women. If used during pregnancy, or if patient becomes pregnant during therapy, apprise her of potential fetal hazard.
• Amount of drug that appears in breast milk isn't known. Because of the potential for adverse effects in breast-fed infants, patient should discontinue breast-feeding or discontinue drug.

NURSING CONSIDERATIONS
• It's recommended that dosage be determined by appropriate pharmacokinetic methods and patient-specific parameters.
⊕ *Alert:* Tobramycin ophthalmic solution isn't for injection.
• If topical ocular tobramycin is given with systemic tobramycin, carefully monitor levels.

• Weigh patient and review renal function studies before therapy.
⊕ *Alert:* If patient complains of tinnitus, vertigo, or hearing loss, notify prescriber.
Black Box Warning If possible, obtain serial audiograms in patients old enough to be tested, particularly high-risk patients. Evidence of impairment of renal, vestibular, or auditory function requires drug discontinuation or dosage adjustment. ■
• Don't dilute or mix with dornase alfa in a nebulizer.
• Unrefrigerated drug, which is normally slightly yellow, may darken with age. This doesn't affect product quality.
• Avoid exposing ampules to intense light.
Black Box Warning Peak levels over 12 mcg/mL and trough levels over 2 mcg/mL may increase risk of toxicity. Periodically monitor peak and trough serum concentrations during therapy to ensure adequate levels and to avoid potentially toxic levels. ■
Black Box Warning Due to increased risk of nephrotoxicity, monitor renal function: urine output, specific gravity, urinalysis, CrCl, and BUN, serum creatinine, and CrCl. Notify prescriber about signs and symptoms of decreasing renal function. ■
Black Box Warning Closely monitor patient treated with tobramycin injection because of the inherent potential for ototoxicity and nephrotoxicity. ■
Black Box Warning Monitor patient for manifestations of neurotoxicity, including numbness, skin tingling, muscle twitching, and seizures. ■
• Carefully monitor peak and trough levels in order to determine appropriate dosage in patients with burns or cystic fibrosis as altered pharmacokinetics may cause reduced drug serum concentrations. Reserve higher peak levels for patients with cystic fibrosis, who need a greater lung penetration.
• Watch for signs and symptoms of superinfection, such as continued fever, chills, and increased pulse rate.
• If no response occurs in 3 to 5 days, therapy may be stopped and new specimens obtained for culture and sensitivity testing.
• *Look alike–sound alike:* Don't confuse Tobrex with TobraDex.

Reactions in bold italics are *life-threatening*. Interactions may have a *rapid onset* or a *delayed onset*.

PATIENT TEACHING

⚠ *Alert:* Explain that capsules are for inhalation only and shouldn't be swallowed.

• Provide full instructions for the Podhaler device and tell patient to always use the new Podhaler device provided with each weekly pack.

• Advise patient not to get powder in eyes.

• Tell patient to keep capsules in sealed blisters and to remove each capsule immediately before use.

• Instruct patient to store capsules at room temperature.

• Instruct patient to report all adverse reactions promptly.

• Caution patient not to perform hazardous activities if adverse CNS reactions occur.

• Encourage patient to maintain adequate fluid intake.

• Teach patient how to use and maintain nebulizer.

• Tell patient using several inhaled therapies to use this drug last.

• Instruct patient not to use if the inhalation solution is cloudy or contains particles or if it has been stored at room temperature for longer than 28 days.

• Tell patient to clean excessive discharge from eye area before applying ocular tobramycin.

• Tell patient to remove contact lenses before using ocular tobramycin and not to wear contact lenses when signs or symptoms of ocular infection are present.

• Teach patient how to instill drops or apply ointment. Advise patient to wash hands before and after applying and to avoid touching tip of dropper to eye or surrounding tissue.

• Instruct patient to apply light finger pressure on lacrimal sac for 1 minute after drops are instilled.

• Tell patient to wait at least 10 minutes before instilling other eyedrops.

tocilizumab
toe sih-LIZ-oo-mab

Actemra

Therapeutic class: Antiarthritics
Pharmacologic class: Interleukin-6 receptor inhibitors

AVAILABLE FORMS

Injection (for I.V. use): 80 mg/4 mL, 200 mg/10 mL, 400 mg/20 mL in single-use vials
Injection (for subcutaneous use): 162 mg/0.9-mL prefilled syringe

INDICATIONS & DOSAGES

Adjust-a-dose (for all indications): For patients with ANC of 500 to 1,000/mm³, interrupt drug until ANC is greater than 1,000/mm³ and then resume drug at 4 mg/kg. May increase to 8 mg/kg if appropriate. If ANC is less than 500/mm³, discontinue drug. If platelet count is 50,000 to 100,000/mm³, interrupt drug until platelet count is greater than 100,000/mm³, and then resume drug at 4 mg/kg. May increase to 8 mg/kg if appropriate. If platelet count is less than 50,000/mm³, discontinue drug. For patients with liver enzyme levels greater than 1 to 3 × ULN, reduce dosage to 4 mg/kg or interrupt drug until levels normalize. For liver enzyme levels greater than 3 to 5 × ULN, stop drug until levels are less than 3 × ULN and then restart at 4 mg/kg. Discontinue drug for persistent levels greater than 3 × ULN.

➤ **Systemic juvenile idiopathic arthritis (SJIA) alone or in combination with methotrexate**

Children age 2 and older weighing 30 kg or more: 8 mg/kg I.V. infusion over 60 minutes once every 2 weeks.

Children age 2 and older weighing less than 30 kg: 12 mg/kg I.V. infusion over 60 minutes once every 2 weeks.

Adjust-a-dose: If appropriate, concomitant methotrexate or other medications should be dose-modified or stopped and tocilizumab dosage adjusted until the clinical situation has been evaluated. In SJIA, the decision to discontinue tocilizumab for a laboratory abnormality should be based on medical assessment of the individual patient.

➤ **As monotherapy or with methotrexate or other DMARDs, for moderately to severely active RA when response to one or more DMARDs is inadequate**

Adults: Initially, 4 mg/kg I.V. over 60 minutes every 4 weeks. May increase dosage to 8 mg/kg based on clinical response. Maximum dose is 800 mg per infusion. Or, for patients weighing 100 kg or more, 162 mg subcutaneously once each week. Or, for patients weighing less than 100 kg, 162 mg subcutaneously every other week, followed by an increase to every week based on clinical response.

➤ **Polyarticular juvenile idiopathic arthritis (PJIA) alone or in combination with methotrexate**

Children age 2 and older weighing 30 kg or more: 8 mg/kg I.V. infusion over 60 minutes once every 4 weeks.

Children age 2 and older weighing less than 30 kg: 10 mg/kg I.V. over 60 minutes once every 4 weeks.

Adjust-a-dose: If appropriate, concomitant methotrexate or other medications should be dose-modified or stopped and tocilizumab dosage adjusted until the clinical situation has been evaluated. In PJIA, the decision to discontinue tocilizumab for a laboratory abnormality should be based on medical assessment of the individual patient.

ADMINISTRATION

I.V.

▼ Check body weight before calculating each dose. Withdraw NSS from 100-mL container in volume equal to drug dose, slowly add drug to infusion bag, then gently invert bag to mix solution. Use a 50-mL infusion bag or bottle for SJIA or PJIA patients who weigh less than 30 kg. Allow diluted solution to reach room temperature before infusing.

▼ Don't use solution if it's discolored or contains particulate matter.

▼ Store diluted solution at 36° to 46° F (2° to 8° C) or at room temperature for up to 24 hours; protect from light.

▼ Administer infusion over 60 minutes; infusion must be administered with infusion set. Don't administer as I.V. push or bolus.

▼ **Incompatibilities:** Don't infuse in same line with other I.V. drugs.

Subcutaneous

● When transitioning from I.V. therapy to subcutaneous administration, administer the first subcutaneous dose instead of the next scheduled I.V. dose.

● Interruption of dose or reduction in frequency of administration of subcutaneous dose from every week to every other week dosing is recommended for management of certain dose-related laboratory changes, including elevated liver enzymes, neutropenia, and thrombocytopenia.

● Subcutaneous administration isn't approved for SJIA or PJIA.

● Inject full amount in the syringe (0.9 mL).

● Rotate injection sites with each injection; never give into moles, scars, or areas where skin is tender, bruised, red, hard, or not intact.

ACTION

Inhibits interleukin-6–mediated inflammatory processes by decreasing inflammatory markers such as C-reactive protein, rheumatoid factor, and erythrocyte sedimentation rate.

Route	Onset	Peak	Duration
I.V.	Unknown	Unknown	Unknown
Subcut.	Unknown	Unknown	Unknown

Half-life: I.V., 11 to 13 days; subcutaneous, 5 to 13 days.

ADVERSE REACTIONS

CNS: dizziness, headache.
CV: hypertension.
EENT: nasopharyngitis.
GI: gastritis, mouth ulceration, upper abdominal pain.
Hematologic: *thrombocytopenia, neutropenia.*
Respiratory: bronchitis, URI.
Skin: pruritus, rash, urticaria.
Other: *antibody development, malignancy,* infection.

INTERACTIONS

Drug-drug. *Biological DMARDs (anti-CD20 monoclonal antibodies, interleukin-1 receptor antagonists, TNF*

Reactions in bold italics are *life-threatening*. Interactions may have a *rapid onset* or a *delayed onset*.

antagonists): May increase risk of serious infection. Don't use together.

Cyclosporine, theophylline, warfarin: May decrease drug levels. Monitor levels closely and adjust dosage as needed.

CYP3A4 substrates (atorvastatin, lovastatin, omeprazole, simvastatin): May affect levels of these drugs. Avoid use together.

Hormonal contraceptives: May decrease effects of contraceptives. Consider nonhormonal alternatives for contraception.

Live-virus vaccines: No data are available on secondary transmission of infection from live-virus vaccine. Avoid using together.

EFFECTS ON LAB TEST RESULTS
● May increase ALT, AST, and lipid levels.
● May decrease platelet and neutrophil counts.

CONTRAINDICATIONS & CAUTIONS
Black Box Warning Risks and benefits of treatment with tocilizumab should be carefully considered before start of therapy in patients with chronic or recurrent infection. ■

Black Box Warning Patients treated with tocilizumab are at increased risk for developing serious infections (active pulmonary or extrapulmonary TB; invasive fungal infections [candidiasis, aspergillosis, pneumocystis]; or bacterial, viral, and other infections caused by opportunistic pathogens) that may lead to hospitalization or death. Most patients who developed these infections were taking concomitant immunosuppressants, such as methotrexate or corticosteroids. ■

● Don't initiate drug in patients with ANC less than 2,000/mm^3 or platelet count less than 100,000/mm^3, or in those with ALT or AST level more than 1.5 × ULN.

● Contraindicated in patients hypersensitive to drug or its components. Avoid use in those with active infection, active hepatic disease, or hepatic impairment.

◐ Alert: Use cautiously in patients who have been exposed to TB, in those with history of chronic or recurrent infection, serious or opportunistic infection, or underlying conditions that increase risk of infection. Use cautiously in those who have resided

or traveled in areas with endemic TB or mycosis.

● Use cautiously in patients at risk for GI perforation.

● For patients older than age 65 being treated with tocilizumab, give drug cautiously because serious infections are more common in this population.

Dialyzable drug: Unknown.

PREGNANCY-LACTATION-REPRODUCTION
● Use in pregnant women only if benefit outweighs risk to the fetus.

● Encourage pregnant patients taking drug to register with the MotherToBaby Autoimmune Diseases in Pregnancy registry (1-877-311-8972).

● It isn't known if drug appears in breast milk. Patient should discontinue breastfeeding or discontinue drug.

NURSING CONSIDERATIONS
Black Box Warning Sepsis or serious infections, including TB and bacterial, invasive fungal, viral, and other opportunistic infections, may occur. Monitor patient closely for signs and symptoms of infection during and after treatment. Drug may need to be discontinued if infection occurs during treatment. ■

Black Box Warning Patient should be evaluated and treated, if necessary, for latent TB before start of therapy. Monitor patient for possible TB development during therapy, even if he tested negative before therapy. ■

● Suspect GI perforation in patient with new-onset abdominal symptoms.

● Monitor LFTs, lipid levels, and neutrophil and platelet counts every 4 to 8 weeks during therapy.

● Ensure availability of appropriate supportive measures to treat possible hypersensitivity reaction.

● Drug may increase risk of malignancy.

● Monitor patient closely for signs and symptoms of demyelinating disorders.

● Recommended immunizations (except live-virus vaccines) should be brought up-to-date before beginning therapy.

PATIENT TEACHING

🔔 *Alert:* Warn patient to seek immediate medical attention if abdominal pain or signs and symptoms of infection occur.

● Instruct patient to have TB screening before therapy.

● Advise female patient to consult prescriber if she becomes pregnant or plans to breast-feed.

● Tell patient to avoid exposure to infections.

● Remind patient to contact prescriber before scheduling surgery.

● Advise patient to avoid live-virus vaccines during therapy.

● Recommend that patient use nonhormonal contraception during therapy.

tofacitinib citrate
TOE-fa-SYE-ti-nib

Xeljanz, Xeljanz XR

Therapeutic class: Antirheumatics
Pharmacologic class: Janus kinase inhibitors

AVAILABLE FORMS
Tablets: 5 mg
Tablets (extended-release) ⓄⓉⒸ: 11 mg

INDICATIONS & DOSAGES
➤ **Moderately to severely active RA in patients who have had an inadequate response or intolerance to methotrexate, as monotherapy or in combination with methotrexate or other nonbiological DMARDs**
Adults: 5 mg (immediate-release) P.O. b.i.d. Or, 11 mg (extended-release) once daily.
Adjust-a-dose: Reduce dosage to 5 mg (immediate-release) once daily in patients with moderate or severe renal insufficiency or moderate hepatic impairment, in those receiving concurrent potent CYP3A4 inhibitors (such as ketoconazole), and in those receiving a drug that moderates inhibition of CYP3A4 and acts as a potent inhibitor of CYP2C19 (such as fluconazole). Interrupt therapy if ANC is 500 to 1,000/mm^3; resume at 5 mg b.i.d. or 11 mg once daily when ANC is greater than 1,000/mm^3.

Interrupt therapy if Hb level drops more than 2 g/dL or if Hb level is less than 8 g/dL during therapy until Hb values have normalized. Discontinue drug based on confirmed lymphocyte count of less than 500/mm^3 or if confirmed ANC is less than 500/mm^3.

ADMINISTRATION
P.O.
● May give with or without food.
● Make sure patient swallows extended-release tablets whole and intact. Don't crush, split, or allow patient to chew tablets.
● Store at room temperature.

ACTION
Inhibits activity of Janus kinases, preventing activation of certain intracellular activities that influence immune cell function.

Route	Onset	Peak	Duration
P.O. (immediate-release)	Unknown	½–1 hr	Unknown
P.O. (extended-release)	Unknown	4 hr	Unknown

Half-life: Immediate-release, 3 hours; extended-release, 6 hours.

ADVERSE REACTIONS
CNS: headache, paresthesia, insomnia, fever, fatigue.
CV: hypertension, edema.
EENT: nasopharyngitis.
GI: diarrhea, abdominal pain, dyspepsia, vomiting, gastritis, nausea.
Hematologic: anemia.
Metabolic: dehydration.
Musculoskeletal: muscle and bone pain, arthralgia, tendon disorder, joint swelling.
Respiratory: URI, dyspnea, cough.
Skin: rash, erythema, pruritus.
Other: infection.

INTERACTIONS
Drug-drug. ▌Black Box Warning▐ *Immunosuppressants (corticosteroids, methotrexate):* May increase risk of serious infection. If infection occurs, discontinue tofacitinib until infection is controlled. ▌
Moderate inhibitors of CYP3A4 plus potent inhibitors of CYP2C19 (fluconazole), potent inhibitors of CYP3A4 (ketoconazole): May increase tofacitinib plasma level. Decrease tofacitinib dosage to 5 mg daily.

Reactions in bold italics are *life-threatening*. Interactions may have a *rapid onset* or a *delayed onset*.

Potent immunosuppressants (abatacept, adalimumab, anakinra, azathioprine, certolizumab, cyclosporine, etanercept, golimumab, infliximab, rituximab, tacrolimus, tocilizumab): May significantly increase risk of immunosuppression and infection. Don't use together.

Potent inducers of CYP3A4 (rifampin): May decrease tofacitinib plasma level. Use together isn't recommended.

EFFECTS ON LAB TEST RESULTS
● May increase creatinine, liver enzyme, and lipid levels.
● May decrease Hb level.
● May decrease lymphocyte and neutrophil counts.

CONTRAINDICATIONS & CAUTIONS
● Contraindicated in patients hypersensitive to drug or its components.
● Use in patients with severe hepatic impairment isn't recommended.
● **Alert:** Use cautiously in patients at risk for serious infection (including those who have resided or traveled in areas of endemic TB or mycoses), those at risk for GI perforation (history of diverticulitis), and those with known malignancy.

Black Box Warning Serious infections leading to hospitalization or death, including TB and bacterial, invasive fungal, viral, and other opportunistic infections, have occurred in patients receiving tofacitinib, especially patients on concomitant immunosuppressants, such as methotrexate or corticosteroids. Weigh risk before starting therapy in patients with chronic or recurrent infection. If a serious infection develops, interrupt therapy until infection is controlled. ∎

Black Box Warning Lymphoma and other malignancies have been observed in patients treated with tofacitinib. ∎

Black Box Warning Epstein-Barr virus–associated post-transplant lymphoproliferative disorder has been increasingly observed in renal transplant patients treated with tofacitinib and concomitant immunosuppressants. ∎

● Patients shouldn't receive live-virus vaccines during therapy. Update immunizations according to current guidelines before starting drug.
● Use in combination with biological DMARDs or with potent immunosuppressants, such as azathioprine and cyclosporine, isn't recommended.
● Use cautiously when giving extended-release formulation to patients with preexisting severe GI narrowing (pathologic or iatrogenic). There have been rare reports of obstructive signs and symptoms in patients with known strictures in association with ingestion of other drugs utilizing a nondeformable extended-release formulation.
● Safety and effectiveness in children haven't been established.
● Use cautiously in patients with diabetes and in patients older than age 65 because of increased risk of serious infection.
Dialyzable drug: Unknown.

PREGNANCY-LACTATION-REPRODUCTION
● There are no adequate studies in pregnant women, but drug may cause fetal harm. Use only if clearly needed and potential benefit justifies potential risk to the fetus.
● Encourage pregnant patients taking drug to register with the MotherToBaby Autoimmune Diseases in Pregnancy registry (1-877-311-8972).
● It isn't known if drug appears in breast milk. Patient should discontinue breastfeeding or discontinue drug.

NURSING CONSIDERATIONS
Black Box Warning Before therapy, patients should be tested for latent TB. If test is positive, treatment for TB should begin before start of tofacitinib therapy. Monitor all patients for active TB during treatment, even if initial latent TB test is negative. ∎
● Drug may reactivate viral infections such as herpes zoster. Risk of reactivation of herpes zoster appears to be higher in patients treated in Japan.
● The impact of drug on chronic viral hepatitis reactivation is unknown. Screen for viral hepatitis in accordance with clinical guidelines before starting therapy.
● Patients treated with Xeljanz 5 mg twice daily may be switched to Xeljanz XR 11 mg once daily the day after last dose of Xeljanz 5 mg.

T

• Interrupt treatment if serious infection occurs; don't restart until infection is resolved.
• Monitor lymphocyte count at baseline and every 3 months thereafter.
• Monitor neutrophil count and Hb level at baseline, after 4 to 8 weeks of treatment, and every 3 months thereafter.
• Don't initiate therapy if lymphocyte count is less than 500/mm^3, ANC is less than 1,000/mm^3, or Hb level is less than 9 g/dL.
• Monitor LFT results regularly, especially in patients with history of taking DMARDs such as methotrexate. If drug-induced liver injury is suspected, stop drug until drug cause is ruled out.
• Assess lipid levels 4 to 8 weeks after drug initiation; manage appropriately as needed.
• Monitor patients for GI perforation. Promptly evaluate patients with sudden new-onset abdominal pain or other GI signs and symptoms.
• Perform periodic skin examination of patients who are at increased risk for skin cancer.

PATIENT TEACHING
• Advise patient to inform prescriber of all adverse reactions, especially signs and symptoms of infection, abdominal pain, or illness.
• Caution patient to obtain laboratory tests (CBC, liver enzymes, lipids) regularly as directed.
• Instruct female patient to contact prescriber if she becomes pregnant or plans to become pregnant.
• Warn patient to avoid live-virus vaccines.

tolcapone
toll-KAP-own

Tasmar

Therapeutic class: Antiparkinsonians
Pharmacologic class: Catechol-O-methyltransferase inhibitors

AVAILABLE FORMS
Tablets: 100 mg

INDICATIONS & DOSAGES
➤ **Adjunct to levodopa–carbidopa for signs and symptoms of idiopathic Parkinson disease in patients who have symptom fluctuation or haven't responded to other adjunctive treatment**
Adults: Initially, 100 mg P.O. t.i.d. with levodopa–carbidopa. Recommended daily dosage is 100 mg P.O. t.i.d. Levodopa dosage may need to be reduced by 20% to 30% to minimize risk of dyskinesias, especially when levodopa dose is over 600 mg daily. Stop drug if patient shows no benefit within 3 weeks.

ADMINISTRATION
P.O.
• Give drug without regard for food.
• Give first dose of the day with first daily dose of levodopa–carbidopa.

ACTION
May reversibly inhibit catechol-O-methyltransferase when given with levodopa–carbidopa, increasing levodopa bioavailability. This causes a more constant dopaminergic stimulation in the brain.

Route	Onset	Peak	Duration
P.O.	Unknown	2 hr	Unknown

Half-life: 2 to 3 hours.

ADVERSE REACTIONS
CNS: dyskinesia, sleep disorder, dystonia, excessive dreaming, somnolence, confusion, headache, hallucinations, dizziness, fever, hyperkinesia, hypertonia, fatigue, falling, syncope, balance loss, depression, tremor, speech disorder, paresthesia, agitation, irritability, mental deficiency, hyperactivity, hypokinesia.
CV: orthostatic complaints, chest pain, chest discomfort, palpitations, hypotension.
EENT: pharyngitis, tinnitus, sinus congestion.
GI: nausea, anorexia, diarrhea, vomiting, flatulence, constipation, abdominal pain, dyspepsia, dry mouth.
GU: UTI, urine discoloration, hematuria, micturition disorder, urinary incontinence, impotence.
Hepatic: *hepatotoxicity.*

Reactions in bold italics are *life-threatening*. Interactions may have a *rapid onset* or a *delayed onset*.

Musculoskeletal: muscle cramps, stiffness, arthritis, neck pain.
Respiratory: bronchitis, dyspnea, URI.
Skin: increased sweating, rash.
Other: influenza, hyperpyrexia.

INTERACTIONS

Drug-drug. *CNS depressants:* May cause additive effects. Monitor patient closely.
Nonselective MAO inhibitors (phenelzine, tranylcypromine): May cause hypertensive crisis. Avoid using together.
Phenytoin, tolbutamide: May increase serum concentrations of these drugs. Monitor patient closely.
SSRIs, TCAs: May increase risk of adverse effects. Use together cautiously.
Warfarin: May cause increased warfarin level. Monitor INR and adjust warfarin dosage as needed.

EFFECTS ON LAB TEST RESULTS

● May increase LFT values.

CONTRAINDICATIONS & CAUTIONS

● Contraindicated in patients with liver disease, in those who were withdrawn from tolcapone because of evidence of drug-induced hepatocellular injury, in those who have demonstrated hypersensitivity to drug or its components, and in those with history of drug-related confusion and hyperpyrexia or nontraumatic rhabdomyolysis.
Black Box Warning Don't initiate tolcapone therapy if patient exhibits clinical evidence of liver disease or two ALT or AST values greater than ULN. ■
Black Box Warning Use cautiously in patients with severe dyskinesia or dystonia. ■
Black Box Warning Cases of severe hepatocellular injury, including fulminant liver failure resulting in death, have been reported. ■
● Use cautiously in patients with severe renal impairment.
● May cause new or worsening mental status and behavioral changes, which may be severe and include psychotic-like behavior, hallucinations, paranoid ideation, delusions, confusion, disorientation, aggressive behavior, agitation, and delirium.
● Reports suggest that patients may experience an intense urge to gamble, increased

sexual urges, intense urge to spend money, binge eating, or other intense urges, and the inability to control these urges.
Dialyzable drug: Unlikely.
⚠ Overdose S&S: Nausea, vomiting, dizziness.

PREGNANCY-LACTATION-REPRODUCTION

● There are no adequate studies in pregnant women. Use only if potential benefit justifies potential risk to the fetus.
● It isn't known if drug appears in breast milk. Use cautiously in breast-feeding women.

NURSING CONSIDERATIONS

Black Box Warning Because of risk of hepatotoxicity, stop treatment if patient shows no benefit within 3 weeks. ■
Black Box Warning Because of risk of fatal hepatic failure, use drug only in patients taking levodopa–carbidopa who don't respond to or who aren't appropriate candidates for other adjunctive therapies. If drug is discontinued because of hepatocellular injury, don't reintroduce. ■
● Drug shouldn't be used by patient until there has been a complete discussion of the risks; make sure patient provides written informed consent before taking drug.
Black Box Warning Prescribers who elect to use drug in the face of the increased risk of liver injury are strongly advised to monitor patients for evidence of emergent liver injury. ■
Black Box Warning Monitor LFT results before starting drug, every 2 weeks for first year of therapy, every 4 weeks for next 6 months, and then every 8 weeks thereafter. If dose is increased to 200 mg t.i.d., obtain liver enzyme levels before increasing dose and then resume monitoring as described. Also, discontinue treatment if ALT or AST level exceeds 2 × ULN or if clinical signs and symptoms suggest onset of hepatic failure. Frequent laboratory monitoring may not prevent fulminant liver failure. Early detection of hepatic injury along with immediate withdrawal of the suspect drug may enhance likelihood for recovery. ■
● Monitor patient for orthostatic hypotension and syncope.

T

PATIENT TEACHING

● Advise patient to take drug exactly as prescribed.

Black Box Warning Teach patient to immediately report signs and symptoms of liver injury (clay-colored stools, yellow eyes or skin, fatigue, loss of appetite, persistent nausea, itching, dark urine, right upper abdominal tenderness, lethargy). ■

● Warn patient about risk of dizziness upon standing up quickly; tell him to stand up cautiously.

● Advise patient to avoid hazardous activities until CNS effects of drug are known.

● Tell patient that nausea may occur early in therapy.

● Inform patient that diarrhea is common, sometimes occurring 2 to 12 weeks after therapy begins, and usually resolves when therapy stops.

● Advise patient about risk of increased problems making voluntary movements or impaired muscle tone.

● Inform patient and caregivers that drug may cause new or worsening mental status and behavioral changes, which may be severe and include psychotic-like behavior, hallucinations, paranoid ideation, delusions, confusion, disorientation, aggressive behavior, agitation, and delirium.

● Instruct patient and caregivers to report intense urges to gamble, increased sexual urges, increased urge to spend money, binge eating, and other intense urges as well as the inability to control these urges.

● Tell female patient to notify prescriber about planned, suspected, or known pregnancy.

● Inform patient that drug may be taken without regard to meals.

tolterodine tartrate
toll-TEAR-oh-deen

Detrol✧, Detrol LA

Therapeutic class: Urinary antispasmodics
Pharmacologic class: Antimuscarinics

AVAILABLE FORMS

Capsules (extended-release) ⓞⓝⓒ: 2 mg, 4 mg
Tablets: 1 mg, 2 mg

INDICATIONS & DOSAGES

➤ **Overactive bladder in patients with symptoms of urinary frequency, urgency, or urge incontinence**

Adults: 2-mg tablet P.O. b.i.d. or 4-mg extended-release capsule P.O. daily. Dose may be reduced to 1-mg tablet P.O. b.i.d. or 2-mg extended-release capsule P.O. daily, based on patient response and tolerance.

Adjust-a-dose: For patients with mild to moderate hepatic impairment (Child-Pugh class A or B) or significantly reduced renal function (CrCl of 10 to 30 mL/minute) or those taking a potent CYP3A4 inhibitor, such as ketoconazole, clarithromycin, or ritonavir, give 1-mg tablet P.O. b.i.d. or 2-mg extended-release capsule P.O. daily.

ADMINISTRATION
P.O.

● Give extended-release capsules with liquid because they must be swallowed whole.

ACTION

Relaxes smooth muscle of bladder by antagonizing muscarinic receptors, relieving symptoms of overactive bladder.

Route	Onset	Peak	Duration
P.O.	Unknown	1–2 hr	Unknown
P.O. (extended-release)	Unknown	2–6 hr	Unknown

Half-life: 2 to 4 hours; about 8 hours with hepatic impairment.

ADVERSE REACTIONS

CNS: headache, fatigue, paresthesia, vertigo, dizziness, nervousness, somnolence.
CV: chest pain.
EENT: abnormal vision, xerophthalmia, pharyngitis, sinusitis.
GI: dry mouth, abdominal pain, constipation, diarrhea, dyspepsia, flatulence, nausea, vomiting.
GU: dysuria, urine retention, UTI.
Metabolic: weight gain.
Musculoskeletal: arthralgia, back pain.
Respiratory: bronchitis, coughing, URI.
Skin: dry skin.
Other: flulike syndrome, infection.

Reactions in bold italics are *life-threatening*. Interactions may have a *rapid onset* or a *delayed onset*.

INTERACTIONS

Drug-drug. *Anticholinergics (ipratropium, tiotropium):* Coadministration may increase frequency or severity of anticholinergic adverse reactions (such as blurred vision, constipation, dry mouth, or somnolence). Monitor patient closely.

Antifungals (itraconazole, ketoconazole, miconazole), CYP3A4 inhibitors (clarithromycin, erythromycin): May increase tolterodine level. Don't give more than 1-mg tablet b.i.d. or 2-mg extended-release capsule daily of tolterodine if used together.

Fluoxetine: May increase tolterodine level. Monitor patient. No dosage adjustment is needed.

EFFECTS ON LAB TEST RESULTS
None reported.

CONTRAINDICATIONS & CAUTIONS

• Contraindicated in patients hypersensitive to drug or its components or to fesoterodine fumarate and in those with uncontrolled angle-closure glaucoma or urine or gastric retention.

• Use cautiously in patients with significant bladder outflow obstruction, GI obstructive disorders (such as pyloric stenosis), controlled angle-closure glaucoma, myasthenia gravis, and hepatic or renal impairment.

☉ Alert: Anaphylaxis and angioedema requiring hospitalization and emergency medical treatment have occurred with the first or subsequent doses of tolterodine. Discontinue drug and promptly initiate appropriate therapy if difficulty breathing, upper airway obstruction, or fall in BP occurs.

• An additive effect of tolterodine with other drugs that prolong the QT interval cannot be excluded, which increases risk of life-threatening cardiac arrhythmias. Consider this when tolterodine is prescribed to patients with known history of QT-interval prolongation or those who are taking other drugs that prolong the QT interval, such as Class IA (procainamide, quinidine) or Class III (amiodarone, sotalol) antiarrhythmics.

• Extended-release capsules aren't recommended for use in patients with severe hepatic impairment (Child-Pugh

class C) or those with CrCl of less than 10 mL/minute.

• Effectiveness in children hasn't been established.

Dialyzable drug: Unknown.

⚠ Overdose S&S: Dry mouth, severe central anticholinergic effects, QT-interval prolongation.

PREGNANCY-LACTATION-REPRODUCTION

• There are no adequate studies in pregnant women. Use only if potential benefit justifies potential risk to the fetus.

• It isn't known if drug appears in breast milk. Patient should discontinue breastfeeding or discontinue drug.

NURSING CONSIDERATIONS

• Assess baseline bladder function and monitor therapeutic effects.

• Monitor patient for residual urine after voiding.

PATIENT TEACHING

• Advise patient to avoid driving or other potentially hazardous activities until effects of drug are known.

• Instruct patient to immediately report all adverse reactions and signs and symptoms of infection, urine retention, GI problems, or difficulty breathing.

• Tell patient taking extended-release form to swallow capsule whole and to take with liquids.

• Advise female patient to stop breastfeeding during therapy.

tolvaptan
tol-VAP-tan

Samsca

Therapeutic class: Vasopressin antagonists
Pharmacologic class: Selective vasopressin receptor antagonists

AVAILABLE FORMS
Tablets: 15 mg, 30 mg

T

INDICATIONS & DOSAGES

➤ **Hypervolemic and euvolemic hyponatremia (serum sodium level less than 125 mEq/L and symptomatic hyponatremia) in hospitalized patients, including those with HF, cirrhosis, or SIADH**
Adults: Initially, 15 mg P.O. once daily. After 24 hours, may increase to 30 mg P.O. once daily, to maximum dosage of 60 mg P.O. once daily for no more than 30 days.

ADMINISTRATION
P.O.
● Give drug with or without food.
● Avoid restricting fluids during the first 24 hours of therapy.
● Patient should avoid grapefruit and grapefruit juice during therapy.

ACTION
Antagonizes the effect of vasopressin, causing an increase in urine excretion, which results in an increase in free water clearance, a decrease in urine osmolality, and ultimately an increase in serum sodium level.

Route	Onset	Peak	Duration
P.O.	2–4 hr	2–4 hr	Unknown

Half-life: 12 hours.

ADVERSE REACTIONS
CNS: asthenia, fever, *stroke.*
CV: *intracardiac thrombus, PE, ventricular fibrillation, DVT.*
EENT: dry mouth, thirst.
GI: anorexia, constipation, nausea.
GU: polyuria, urinary frequency, urethral hemorrhage, vaginal hemorrhage.
Hematologic: *DIC.*
Metabolic: hyperglycemia, *diabetic ketoacidosis.*
Musculoskeletal: *rhabdomyolysis.*
Respiratory: *respiratory failure.*

INTERACTIONS
Drug-drug. *CYP3A inducers (barbiturates, carbamazepine, phenytoin, rifabutin, rifampin, rifapentine):* May decrease tolvaptan level. Avoid using together.
Moderate CYP3A inhibitors (aprepitant, diltiazem, erythromycin, fluconazole, verap-

amil): May increase tolvaptan level. Don't use together.
P-glycoprotein (P-gp) inhibitors (such as cyclosporine): May increase tolvaptan levels. Reduce tolvaptan dosage.
P-gp substrates (digoxin): May increase digoxin level. Monitor patient, and adjust digoxin dosage as needed.
Drug-herb. *St John's wort:* May decrease drug level. Don't use together.
Drug-food. *Grapefruit juice:* May increase drug level. Don't use together.

EFFECTS ON LAB TEST RESULTS
● May increase glucose level.
● May prolong PT.

CONTRAINDICATIONS & CAUTIONS
● Contraindicated in patients hypersensitive to drug or its components.
● Contraindicated in patients with hypovolemic hyponatremia and in those who require urgent rise in serum sodium level, are anuric, or are unable to sense or appropriately respond to thirst.
● Contraindicated in patients receiving strong CYP3A inhibitors.
● Use cautiously in patients with dehydration and in those receiving hypertonic saline solution.
Dialyzable drug: Unlikely.
⚠ *Overdose S&S:* Polyuria, thirst, dehydration, hypovolemia.

PREGNANCY-LACTATION-REPRODUCTION
● There are no adequate studies in pregnant women. Use only if potential benefit justifies potential risk to the fetus.
● It isn't known if drug appears in breast milk. Patient shouldn't breast-feed during therapy.

NURSING CONSIDERATIONS
Black Box Warning Initiate and reinitiate drug in hospital setting where serum sodium level can be monitored closely. ■
Black Box Warning Don't correct hyponatremia (for example, more than 12 mEq/L/24 hours) too rapidly; doing so may cause osmotic demyelination resulting in dysarthria, mutism, dysphagia, lethargy, affective changes, spastic quadriparesis, seizures, coma, and death. Slower correction

---

Reactions in bold italics are *life-threatening*. Interactions may have a *rapid onset* or a *delayed onset*.

may be necessary in patients with severe malnutrition, alcoholism, or advanced liver disease. ■

⦿ *Alert:* Drug may increase risk of irreversible and potentially fatal liver injury. Assess liver function promptly in patients reporting fatigue, anorexia, right upper abdominal discomfort, dark urine, or jaundice. If liver injury is suspected, stop drug immediately, initiate treatment, and investigate cause. Don't reinitiate drug unless cause for the observed liver injury is definitively established to be unrelated to tolvaptan treatment.

• Monitor sodium level and neurologic status regularly during therapy.

• Monitor potassium level in patients with potassium level greater than 5 mEq/L who are taking drugs known to increase potassium level.

PATIENT TEACHING

• Advise patient to promptly report all adverse reactions, especially difficulty speaking or swallowing, drowsiness, mood changes, trouble controlling body movement, seizures, fatigue, anorexia, right upper abdominal discomfort, dark urine, or jaundice.

• Advise patient to inform prescriber of all drugs and supplements being taken because of the potential for interactions.

• Advise patient to continue ingestion of fluid in response to thirst during therapy and to resume fluid intake after tolvaptan is discontinued.

• Advise patient to prevent dehydration.

• Tell patient not to stop or restart drug on his own; drug should only be restarted in the hospital where sodium level can be monitored closely.

• Advise female patient not to breast-feed.

topiramate
toe-PIE-rah-mate

Qudexy XR, Topamax✒,
Trokendi XR

Therapeutic class: Anticonvulsants
Pharmacologic class: Sulfamate-substituted monosaccharides

AVAILABLE FORMS
Capsules, sprinkles: 15 mg, 25 mg
Capsules (extended-release) ⓓⓝⓒ: 25 mg, 50 mg, 100 mg, 150 mg, 200 mg
Tablets ⓓⓝⓒ: 25 mg, 50 mg, 100 mg, 200 mg

INDICATIONS & DOSAGES
Adjust-a-dose (for all indications): For adults, if CrCl is less than 70 mL/minute/1.73 m², reduce dosage by 50%. For patients at high risk for renal insufficiency, obtain an estimated CrCl before dosing. For hemodialysis patients, supplemental doses may be needed to avoid rapid drops in drug level during prolonged dialysis treatment.

➤ **Initial monotherapy for partial-onset or primary generalized tonic-clonic seizures**
Adults and children age 10 or older: Recommended daily dose is 400 mg (immediate-release) P.O. in two divided doses (morning and evening). To achieve this dosage, adjust as follows: first week, 25 mg P.O. b.i.d.; second week, 50 mg P.O. b.i.d.; third week, 75 mg P.O. b.i.d.; fourth week, 100 mg P.O. b.i.d.; fifth week, 150 mg P.O. b.i.d.; and sixth week, 200 mg P.O. b.i.d. Or, using extended-release capsules, initially 50 mg P.O. daily. Increase dosage weekly by increments of 50 mg for first 4 weeks, then 100 mg for weeks 5 and 6 to recommended 400 mg daily.
Children ages 2 to younger than 10 (immediate-release and Qudexy XR extended-release) or children ages 6 to younger than 10 (Trokendi XR extended-release): During titration period, initially 25 mg/day (immediate-release or extended-release) P.O. nightly for first week. Based on tolerability, can increase to 50 mg/day (once daily for extended-release or 25 mg P.O. b.i.d. for immediate-release) in the

second week. Can increase by 25 to 50 mg/day each subsequent week as tolerated. Attempt titration to the minimum maintenance dosage over 5 to 7 weeks of the total titration period. Based on tolerability and seizure control, can attempt additional titration to a higher dosage (up to the maximum maintenance dosage) at 25 to 50 mg/day in weekly increments. Total daily dosage shouldn't exceed the maximum maintenance dosage for each range of body weight.

Give maintenance doses of extended-release form once daily; give maintenance doses of immediate-release form in two equally divided P.O. doses daily. If patient weighs up to 11 kg, maintenance dosage range is 150 mg/day to a maximum of 250 mg/day. If patient weighs 12 to 22 kg, maintenance dosage range is 200 mg/day to a maximum of 300 mg/day. If patient weighs 23 to 31 kg, maintenance dosage range is 200 mg/day to a maximum of 350 mg/day. If patient weighs 32 to 38 kg, maintenance dosage range is 250 mg/day to a maximum of 350 mg/day. If patient weighs more than 38 kg, maintenance dosage range is 250 mg/day to a maximum of 400 mg/day.

➤ **Adjunctive treatment for partial-onset or primary generalized tonic-clonic seizures or Lennox-Gastaut syndrome**
Adults and children age 17 and older: Initially, 25 to 50 mg P.O. daily; increase gradually by 25 to 50 mg/week until an effective daily dose is reached. Adjust to recommended daily dose of 200 to 400 mg P.O. in two divided doses of immediate-release or once daily of extended-release for adults with partial-onset seizures or Lennox-Gastaut syndrome, or 400 mg P.O. in two divided doses of immediate-release or once daily of extended-release for adults with primary generalized tonic-clonic seizures.
Children ages 6 to 16 (Trokendi) or ages 2 to 16 (Qudexy XR): Initially, 25 mg P.O. daily at bedtime (based on range of 1 to 3 mg/kg once daily) for first week. Increase dosage at 1- or 2-week intervals by increments of 1 to 3 mg/kg daily. Guide dosage titration by clinical outcome. Recommended daily dose is 5 to 9 mg/kg once daily.
Children ages 2 to 16 (immediate-release): Initially, 25 mg/day (or less, based on a range of 1 to 3 mg/kg/day) P.O. given at

bedtime for 1 week. Increase at 1- or 2-week intervals by 1 to 3 mg/kg daily (given in two divided doses) to achieve optimal response. Guide titration by clinical outcome. Recommended daily dose is 5 to 9 mg/kg, in two divided doses.
➤ **To prevent migraine headache**
Adults and adolescents age 12 and older (immediate-release): Initially, 25 mg P.O. daily in evening for first week. Then, 25 mg P.O. b.i.d. in morning and evening for second week. For third week, 25 mg P.O. in morning and 50 mg P.O. in evening. For fourth week, 50 mg P.O. b.i.d. in morning and evening.

ADMINISTRATION
P.O.
● Give drug without regard for food.
● Immediate-release and Qudexy XR capsules may be opened and contents sprinkled on a teaspoon of soft food. Patient should swallow immediately without chewing.
● Patient should swallow Trokendi XR capsules whole and intact. Don't sprinkle capsule contents on food or allow patient to chew or crush capsules; doing so may disrupt the triphasic release properties.

ACTION
Unknown. May block a sodium channel, potentiate the activity of GABA, and inhibit kainate's ability to activate an amino acid receptor.

Route	Onset	Peak	Duration
P.O.	Unknown	2 hr	Unknown

Half-life: 21 hours.

ADVERSE REACTIONS
CNS: anxiety, asthenia, ataxia, confusion, difficulty with memory, dizziness, fatigue, nervousness, paresthesia, psychomotor slowing, somnolence, speech disorders, tremor, *generalized tonic-clonic seizures, suicide attempts,* abnormal coordination, aggressive reaction, agitation, apathy, depression, depersonalization, emotional lability, euphoria, fever, hallucination, hyperkinesia, hypertonia, hypoesthesia, hypokinesia, insomnia, malaise, mood problems, personality disorder, psychosis,

---

Reactions in bold italics are *life-threatening*. Interactions may have a *rapid onset* or a *delayed onset*.

stupor, vertigo; difficulty with concentration, attention, or language.
CV: chest pain, edema, palpitations, vasodilation.
EENT: abnormal vision, diplopia, nystagmus, conjunctivitis, epistaxis, eye pain, hearing problems, pharyngitis, sinusitis, tinnitus.
GI: anorexia, nausea, abdominal pain, constipation, diarrhea, dry mouth, dyspepsia, flatulence, gastroenteritis, gingivitis, taste perversion, vomiting.
GU: amenorrhea, dysuria, dysmenorrhea, hematuria, impotence, intermenstrual bleeding, leukorrhea, menstrual disorder, menorrhagia, urinary frequency, renal calculi, urinary incontinence, UTI, vaginitis.
Hematologic: *leukopenia,* anemia.
Metabolic: decreased weight, increased weight.
Musculoskeletal: arthralgia, back or leg pain, muscle weakness, myalgia, rigors.
Respiratory: URI, bronchitis, coughing, dyspnea.
Skin: acne, alopecia, increased sweating, pruritus, rash.
Other: body odor, breast pain, decreased libido, flulike syndrome, hot flashes, lymphadenopathy.

INTERACTIONS
Drug-drug. *Carbamazepine:* May decrease topiramate level. Monitor patient.
Carbonic anhydrase inhibitors (acetazolamide, dichlorphenamide): May cause renal calculus formation. Avoid using together.
CNS depressants: May cause CNS depression and other adverse cognitive and neuropsychiatric events. Use together cautiously.
Hormonal contraceptives: May decrease effectiveness. Report changes in menstrual patterns. Advise patient to use another contraceptive method.
Phenytoin: May decrease topiramate level and increase phenytoin level. Monitor levels.
Valproic acid: May decrease valproic acid and topiramate level. Monitor patient.
Drug-lifestyle. *Alcohol use:* May cause CNS depression and other adverse cognitive

and neuropsychiatric events. Discourage use together.

EFFECTS ON LAB TEST RESULTS
• May increase liver enzyme levels. May decrease bicarbonate and Hb levels and hematocrit.
• May decrease WBC count.

CONTRAINDICATIONS & CAUTIONS
• Contraindicated in patients hypersensitive to drug or its components.
• Use cautiously in patients with hepatic impairment.
❸ *Alert:* Alcohol use is contraindicated within 6 hours before and 6 hours after taking Trokendi XR.
• Contraindicated in patients with metabolic acidosis who are taking concomitant metformin.
• Bioequivalence hasn't been demonstrated between Trokendi XR and Qudexy XR.
• Acute myopia associated with secondary angle-closure glaucoma has been reported in adults and children receiving topiramate. Such symptoms as acute-onset decreased visual acuity or ocular pain typically occur within 1 month of therapy initiation. Discontinue drug as rapidly as possible, according to judgment of health care provider.
• Use cautiously with other drugs that predispose patients to heat-related disorders, including other carbonic anhydrase inhibitors and anticholinergics.
Dialyzable drug: Yes.
⚠ **Overdose S&S:** Abdominal pain, abnormal coordination, agitation, blurred vision, seizures, depression, diplopia, dizziness, drowsiness, hypotension, lethargy, impaired mentation, speech disturbance, stupor, severe metabolic acidosis.

PREGNANCY-LACTATION-REPRODUCTION
❸ *Alert:* Drug is associated with increased risk of oral clefts (cleft lip or palate) in infants born to women treated with topiramate during pregnancy. Use in pregnant women only if potential benefit outweighs risk to the fetus. Consider alternative medications with a lower risk of adverse outcomes for these patients.
❸ *Alert:* Women who become pregnant during therapy should register with the

Antiepileptic Drug Pregnancy Registry (1-888-233-2334).

• Although drug's effect on labor and delivery hasn't been established, development of topiramate-induced metabolic acidosis in the mother or fetus may result in adverse effects and fetal death.

• Tell women of childbearing potential that drug may decrease effectiveness of hormonal contraceptives. Advise women using hormonal contraceptives to report change in menstrual patterns.

• Drug appears in breast milk, but effect of exposure in infants isn't known. Use cautiously in breast-feeding women.

NURSING CONSIDERATIONS

☞ *Alert:* Closely monitor all patients taking or starting antiepileptic drugs for changes in behavior indicating worsening of suicidal thoughts or behavior or depression. Symptoms such as anxiety, agitation, hostility, mania, and hypomania may be precursors to emerging suicidality.

• If needed, withdraw anticonvulsant (including topiramate) gradually to minimize risk of increased seizure activity.

• Monitoring topiramate level isn't necessary.

• Drug may infrequently cause oligohidrosis and hyperthermia, mainly in children. Monitor patient closely, especially in hot weather.

• Drug may cause hyperchloremic, nonanion gap metabolic acidosis from renal bicarbonate loss. Factors that may predispose patients to acidosis, such as renal disease, severe respiratory disorders, status epilepticus, diarrhea, surgery, ketogenic diet, or drugs, may add to topiramate's bicarbonate-lowering effects.

• Measure baseline and periodic bicarbonate levels. If metabolic acidosis develops and persists, consider reducing the dose, gradually stopping the drug, or offering alkali treatment.

• Drug is rapidly cleared by dialysis. A prolonged period of dialysis may cause low drug level and seizures. A supplemental dose may be needed.

• Stop drug if patient experiences acute myopia and secondary angle-closure glaucoma.

• *Look alike–sound alike:* Don't confuse Topamax with Toprol-XL, Tegretol, or Tegretol-XR.

PATIENT TEACHING

• Tell patient not to consume alcohol within 6 hours before to 6 hours after taking Trokendi XR form.

• Instruct patient to report all adverse reactions and to immediately seek medical attention if blurred vision, visual disturbances, or eye pain occurs, to reduce risk of permanent vision loss.

• Advise patient to immediately report high or persistent fever or decreased sweating.

• Tell patient to use appropriate caution when engaging in activities in which loss of consciousness could result in serious danger to patient or others nearby. Some patients with epilepsy will continue to have unpredictable seizures and may need to avoid such activities entirely.

• Tell patient to drink plenty of fluids during therapy to minimize risk of forming kidney stones.

• Advise patient not to drive or operate hazardous machinery until CNS effects of drug are known. Drug can cause sleepiness, dizziness, confusion, and concentration problems.

☞ *Alert:* Teach female patient of childbearing potential to use effective contraceptive while taking topiramate, and explain about the drug's effect on fetal development. Tell her to contact prescriber if she becomes pregnant or plans to become pregnant during therapy.

• Inform patient that drug can be taken without regard to food.

• Tell patient taking Trokendi XR to swallow capsules whole and intact and not to chew or crush capsules or sprinkle capsule contents on food.

• Tell patient taking Qudexy XR that capsules may be swallowed whole or opened and the contents sprinkled on a spoonful of soft food; patient should swallow immediately and not chew.

• Tell patient that immediate-release capsules may either be swallowed whole or carefully opened and contents sprinkled on a teaspoonful of soft food. Tell patient to swallow immediately without chewing.

topotecan hydrochloride
toh-poh-TEE-ken

Hycamtin

Therapeutic class: Antineoplastics
Pharmacologic class: DNA topoisomerase inhibitors

AVAILABLE FORMS
Capsules ⦿: 0.25 mg, 1 mg
Injection: 4-mg single-dose vial (preservative-free)

INDICATIONS & DOSAGES
🔵 *Alert:* Verify dosage using BSA before dispensing. Recommended I.V. dosage should generally not exceed 4 mg.

➤ **Relapsed small-cell lung cancer (SCLC) in patients with a prior complete or partial response who are at least 45 days from the end of first-line chemotherapy**
Adults: 2.3 mg/m^2/day P.O. once daily for 5 consecutive days. Repeat every 21 days. Round the calculated dose to the nearest 0.25 mg.

Adjust-a-dose: For patients with moderate renal impairment (CrCl 30 to 49 mL/minute), give 1.5 mg/m^2/day. For patients with severe renal impairment (CrCl less than 30 mL/minute), give 0.6 mg/m^2/day. For all patients with dosage adjustment due to renal impairment, dosage can be increased after the first course by 0.4 mg/m^2/day if no severe hematologic or GI toxicities occur.

Withhold subsequent courses until neutrophil count is greater than 1,000/mm^3, platelet count is greater than 100,000/mm^3, and Hb is 9 g/dL or more. Reduce dose for subsequent courses to 0.4 mg/m^2/day for patients who experience severe neutropenia (neutrophil count less than 500/mm^3 associated with fever or infection or lasting 7 days or more), neutropenia (neutrophil count 500 to 1,000/mm^3 lasting beyond day 21 of the treatment course), platelet count below 25,000/mm^3, or grade 3 or 4 diarrhea. After recovery to grade 1 or less, reduce dose by 0.4 mg/m^2/day for subsequent courses.

➤ **With cisplatin, stage-IVB recurrent or persistent cervical cancer unresponsive to surgery or radiation**
Adults: 0.75 mg/m^2 by I.V. infusion on days 1, 2, and 3, followed by 50 mg/m^2 cisplatin by I.V. infusion on day 1. Repeat cycle every 21 days. Adjust subsequent doses of drug based on hematologic toxicities.

➤ **Metastatic carcinoma of the ovary after failure of first or subsequent chemotherapy; SCLC in patients with platinum-sensitive disease who progressed at least 60 days after initiation of first-line chemotherapy**
Adults: 1.5 mg/m^2 I.V. infusion daily for 5 consecutive days, starting on day 1 of a 21-day cycle. Give a minimum of four cycles.

Adjust-a-dose: For patients with CrCl of 20 to 39 mL/minute, decrease dosage to 0.75 mg/m^2. If severe neutropenia occurs, decrease dosage by 0.25 mg/m^2 for subsequent courses or give granulocyte colony-stimulating factor (G-CSF) after subsequent course (before resorting to dosage reduction) starting from day 6 of course (24 hours after completion of topotecan administration).

ADMINISTRATION
P.O.
● Hazardous drug; avoid direct contact with capsule contents.
● Give drug without regard to food.
● Don't crush or divide capsules.
● If patient vomits after taking dose, don't give a replacement dose.

I.V.
▼ Hazardous drug; use safe handling and disposal precautions.
▼ Reconstitute each 4-mg vial with 4 mL sterile water for injection. Dilute appropriate volume of reconstituted solution in either NSS or D$_5$W before giving.
▼ Lyophilized form contains no antibacterial preservative; use reconstituted product immediately.
▼ Infuse over 30 minutes and monitor insertion site during infusion. Extravasation has been linked to mild local reactions, such as erythema and bruising.
▼ When giving topotecan with cisplatin, always give topotecan first.

▼ If stored at 68° to 77° F (20° to 25° C) and exposed to normal lighting, reconstituted drug is stable for 24 hours. Protect unopened vials from light.

▼ **Incompatibilities:** Dexamethasone, 5-FU, mitomycin, ticarcillin disodium–clavulanate potassium.

ACTION

Interacts with topoisomerase I, inducing reversible single-strand DNA breaks. Drug binds to the topoisomerase I–DNA complex and prevents repair of these single-strand breaks.

Route	Onset	Peak	Duration
I.V.	Unknown	Unknown	Unknown
P.O.	Unknown	1–2 hr	Unknown

Half-life: I.V., 2 to 3 hours; oral, 3 to 6 hours.

ADVERSE REACTIONS

CNS: asthenia, fatigue, fever, headache.
GI: abdominal pain, anorexia, constipation, *severe diarrhea,* nausea, stomatitis, vomiting.
Hematologic: anemia, *leukopenia, neutropenia, thrombocytopenia.*
Hepatic: *hepatotoxicity.*
Musculoskeletal: back and skeletal pain.
Respiratory: coughing, dyspnea, pneumonia.
Skin: alopecia, rash.
Other: *sepsis.*

INTERACTIONS

Drug-drug. *Breast cancer resistance protein inhibitors (cyclosporine, eltrombopag), P-glycoprotein inhibitors (cyclosporine, ketoconazole, ritonavir):* May increase systemic exposure to oral topotecan. Avoid concomitant use.
Cisplatin, cytotoxic agents: May increase severity of myelosuppression. Use together with extreme caution. Dosage reductions may be needed.
G-CSF: May prolong duration of neutropenia. If G-CSF is to be used, don't start it until day 6 of the course, 24 hours after completion of I.V. topotecan treatment.

EFFECTS ON LAB TEST RESULTS

● May increase ALT, AST, and bilirubin levels. May decrease Hb level.

● May decrease WBC, platelet, and neutrophil counts.

CONTRAINDICATIONS & CAUTIONS

❸ *Alert:* Administer drug under the supervision of a health care provider experienced in the use of chemotherapeutic agents. Ensure that appropriate diagnostic and treatment facilities are readily available.
● Contraindicated in patients hypersensitive to drug or its components.
● Safety and effectiveness of drug in children haven't been established.
Dialyzable drug: Unknown.
⚠ *Overdose S&S:* Bone marrow suppression.

PREGNANCY-LACTATION-REPRODUCTION

● Drug can cause fetal harm. If used during pregnancy, or if patient becomes pregnant during therapy, apprise her of potential hazard to a fetus.
● Highly effective contraception should be used during treatment and for at least 1 month after therapy ends.
● Drug may damage spermatozoa, possibly resulting in genetic and fetal abnormalities. Advise males with a female partner of childbearing potential to use effective contraception during and for 3 months after therapy ends.
● It isn't known if drug appears in breast milk. Patient should discontinue breast-feeding or discontinue drug.
● In females of childbearing potential, drug may have both acute and long-term effects on fertility. Because of potential risk of impaired fertility, males should seek counseling on fertility and family planning options before starting treatment.

NURSING CONSIDERATIONS

Black Box Warning Before first course of therapy is started, patient must have baseline neutrophil count of 1,500/mm^3 or more and platelet count of 100,000/mm^3 or more. Perform peripheral blood counts frequently to monitor patient for bone marrow suppression, primarily neutropenia, which may be severe and result in infection and death. ∎
● Don't give subsequent courses until neutrophil count recovers to more than 1,000/mm^3, platelet count recovers to more than 100,000/mm^3, and Hb level recovers

---

Reactions in bold italics are *life-threatening*. Interactions may have a *rapid onset* or a *delayed onset*.

to more than 9 mg/dL (with transfusion, if needed).

• Bone marrow suppression indicates toxic levels of topotecan. The nadir occurs at about 11 days. Neutropenia isn't cumulative over time.

• Duration of thrombocytopenia is about 5 days, with nadir at 15 days. The nadir for anemia is 15 days. Blood or platelet transfusions may be needed.

• WBC colony-stimulating factors may promote cell growth and decrease risk for infection.

🌓 *Alert:* Fatalities due to neutropenic colitis have been reported. Consider possibility of neutropenic colitis in patients presenting with fever, neutropenia, and a compatible pattern of abdominal pain.

🌓 *Alert:* Drug may cause interstitial lung disease, which may be fatal. Monitor patient for cough, fever, dyspnea, and hypoxia; stop drug if they occur.

PATIENT TEACHING

• Urge patient to promptly report all adverse reactions, especially sore throat, fever, chills, or unusual bleeding or bruising.

• Advise patient that although diarrhea is common, it may become severe and should be reported to health care provider.

• Caution patient to avoid contact with people with infections.

• Inform patient of potential hazard to the fetus if drug is used during pregnancy, or if patient becomes pregnant while taking drug.

• Advise female patient to use highly ef- fective contraception during treatment and for at least 1 month after last dose and to contact health care provider if she becomes pregnant or suspects she is pregnant during therapy.

• Advise male patient with a female partner of childbearing potential to use effective contraception during and for 3 months after therapy ends.

• Caution female patient to avoid breast- feeding during therapy.

• Teach patient and family about drug's adverse reactions and need for frequent monitoring of blood counts.

• Advise patient that capsules can be taken without regard to food.

• Tell patient not to chew, crush, or divide capsules; they should be swallowed whole.

---

torsemide
TOR-seh-mide

Demadex🔧

Therapeutic class: Diuretics
Pharmacologic class: Loop diuretics

AVAILABLE FORMS
Injection: 10 mg/mL in 2- and 5-mL single- dose vials
Tablets: 5 mg, 10 mg, 20 mg, 100 mg

INDICATIONS & DOSAGES
➤ **Diuresis in patients with HF**
Adults: Initially, 10 to 20 mg P.O. or I.V. once daily. If response is inadequate, dou- ble dose until desired effect is achieved. Maximum, 200 mg daily.
➤ **Diuresis in patients with chronic renal failure**
Adults: Initially, 20 mg P.O. or I.V. once daily. If response is inadequate, double dose until response is obtained. Maximum, 200 mg daily.
➤ **Diuresis in patients with hepatic cirrhosis**
Adults: Initially, 5 to 10 mg P.O. or I.V. once daily with an aldosterone antagonist or a potassium-sparing diuretic. If response is inadequate, double dose until desired effect is achieved. Maximum, 40 mg daily.
➤ **Hypertension**
Adults: Initially, 5 mg P.O. or I.V. daily. In- crease to 10 mg if needed and tolerated after 4 to 6 weeks. Add another antihypertensive if response is still inadequate.

ADMINISTRATION
P.O.
• To prevent nocturia, give drug in the morning.
I.V.
▼ Inspect ampules for precipitate or discol- oration before use.
▼ Give by direct injection over at least 2 minutes. Rapid injection may cause ototoxicity. Don't give more than 200 mg at a time.

T

▼ Drug may be given as a continuous infusion.

▼ If drug is given through an I.V. line, flush with NSS before and after administration.

▼ Drug remains stable for 24 hours at room temperature when mixed in D_5W, NSS, or half-NSS.

▼ **Incompatibilities:** Solutions with pH below 8.3. Flush line with NSS before and after administration to avoid incompatibility.

ACTION

Enhances excretion of sodium, chloride, and water by acting on the ascending loop of Henle.

Route	Onset	Peak	Duration
P.O.	1 hr	1–2 hr	6–8 hr
I.V.	10 min	1 hr	6–8 hr

Half-life: 3½ hours.

ADVERSE REACTIONS

CNS: asthenia, dizziness, headache, nervousness, insomnia.

CV: ECG abnormalities, chest pain, edema, orthostatic hypotension.

EENT: rhinitis, sore throat.

GI: excessive thirst, diarrhea, constipation, nausea, dyspepsia.

GU: excessive urination, impotence.

Metabolic: electrolyte imbalances, including hypokalemia and *hypomagnesemia; dehydration;* hypochloremic alkalosis; hyperuricemia; hypercholesterolemia.

Musculoskeletal: arthralgia, myalgia.

Respiratory: cough.

INTERACTIONS

Drug-drug. *Aminoglycoside antibiotics, cisplatin:* May increase ototoxicity. Use together cautiously.

Amphotericin B, corticosteroids, metolazone: May increase risk of hypokalemia. Monitor potassium level.

Anticoagulants: May enhance anticoagulant activity. Use together cautiously.

Antidiabetics: May decrease hypoglycemic effect, resulting in higher glucose level. Monitor glucose level.

Chlorothiazide, chlorthalidone, hydrochlorothiazide, indapamide, metolazone: May cause excessive diuretic response, resulting in serious electrolyte abnormalities or dehydration. Adjust doses carefully, and monitor patient closely for signs and symptoms of excessive diuretic response.

Cholestyramine: May decrease absorption of torsemide. Separate doses by at least 3 hours.

Digoxin: Electrolyte imbalance caused by diuretic may lead to digoxin-induced arrhythmia. Use together cautiously.

Lithium: May increase lithium level and cause toxicity. Use together cautiously and monitor lithium level.

NSAIDs: May decrease effects of loop diuretics. Use together cautiously.

Probenecid: May decrease diuretic effect. Avoid using together.

Salicylates: May decrease excretion, possibly leading to salicylate toxicity. Avoid using together.

Drug-herb. *Licorice:* May cause unexpected rapid potassium loss. Discourage use together.

EFFECTS ON LAB TEST RESULTS

● May increase BUN, creatinine, cholesterol, glucose, and uric acid levels.

● May decrease potassium and magnesium levels.

CONTRAINDICATIONS & CAUTIONS

● Contraindicated in patients hypersensitive to drug or other sulfonamide derivatives and in those with anuria.

● Use cautiously in patients with hepatic disease and related cirrhosis and ascites; sudden changes in fluid and electrolyte balance may precipitate hepatic coma in these patients.

● Serious skin reactions, including Stevens-Johnson syndrome and toxic epidermal necrolysis, leukopenia, thrombocytopenia, pancreatitis, and ototoxicity have been reported in association with torsemide use.

Dialyzable drug: No.

⚠ *Overdose S&S:* Dehydration, hypovolemia, hypotension, hypokalemia, hypochloremic alkalosis, hemoconcentration.

PREGNANCY-LACTATION-REPRODUCTION

● There are no adequate studies in pregnant women. Use only if clearly needed.

Reactions in bold italics are *life-threatening*. Interactions may have a *rapid onset* or a *delayed onset*.

• It isn't known if drug appears in breast milk. Use cautiously in breast-feeding women.

NURSING CONSIDERATIONS

• Monitor fluid intake and output, electrolyte levels, BP, weight, and pulse rate during rapid diuresis and routinely with long-term use. Drug can cause profound diuresis and water and electrolyte depletion.
• Watch for signs of hypokalemia, such as muscle weakness and cramps.
• Consult prescriber and dietitian about providing a high-potassium diet or potassium supplement. Foods rich in potassium include citrus fruits, bananas, and dates.
• Monitor elderly patients, who are especially susceptible to excessive diuresis with potential for circulatory collapse and thromboembolic complications.
• *Look alike–sound alike:* Don't confuse torsemide with furosemide. Don't confuse Demadex with Denorex.

PATIENT TEACHING

• Tell patient to take drug in morning to prevent the need to urinate at night.
• Advise patient to change positions slowly to prevent dizziness and to limit alcohol intake and strenuous exercise in hot weather to prevent dizziness.
• Advise patient to immediately report ringing in ears because it may indicate toxicity.
• Tell patient to report weakness, cramping, nausea, and dizziness.
• Tell patient to check with prescriber or pharmacist before taking OTC drugs.

---

tramadol hydrochloride
TRAM-uh-dohl

ConZip, Ultram, Ultram ER

Therapeutic class: Analgesics
Pharmacologic class: Synthetic centrally active analgesics
Controlled substance schedule: IV

AVAILABLE FORMS
Capsules (extended-release) ⓞ: 100 mg, 150 mg, 200 mg, 300 mg

Tablets: 50 mg
Tablets (extended-release) ⓞ: 100 mg, 200 mg, 300 mg

INDICATIONS & DOSAGES
➤ **Moderate to moderately severe chronic pain**
Adults age 17 and older: Initially, 25 mg P.O. in the morning. Adjust by 25 mg every 3 days to 100 mg/day (25 mg q.i.d.). Thereafter, adjust by 50 mg every 3 days to reach 200 mg/day (50 mg q.i.d.). Thereafter, give 50 to 100 mg P.O. every 4 to 6 hours p.r.n. Maximum, 400 mg daily.
Adults age 18 and older not taking immediate-release tablets: 100 mg extended-release form P.O. once daily. Titrate by 100 mg every 5 days to relieve pain. Do not exceed 300 mg/day.
Adults age 18 and older currently taking immediate-release tablets: Calculate the 24-hour tramadol immediate-release dose and initiate a total daily dose of extended-release product rounded down to the next lowest 100-mg increment. Subsequently, individualize according to patient need. Maximum dose is 300 mg daily.
Adjust-a-dose: For immediate-release form, if CrCl is less than 30 mL/minute, increase dose interval to every 12 hours; maximum is 200 mg daily. For patients with cirrhosis, give 50 mg (immediate-release) every 12 hours. For patients older than age 75, maximum is 300 mg daily in divided doses. Don't use extended-release form in patients with severe hepatic or renal impairment.

ADMINISTRATION
P.O.
• Give drug without regard for meals.
• Extended-release capsules and tablets must be swallowed whole; don't break or crush tablets.

ACTION
Unknown. Thought to bind to opioid receptors and inhibit reuptake of norepinephrine and serotonin.

T

Route	Onset	Peak	Duration
P.O.	1 hr	2 hr	9 hr
P.O. (extended-release)	Unknown	10–12 hr	Unknown

Half-life: 6 to 7 hours; extended-release, 8 to 9 hours.

ADVERSE REACTIONS
CNS: dizziness, headache, somnolence, vertigo, *seizures,* anxiety, asthenia, CNS stimulation, confusion, coordination disturbance, euphoria, malaise, nervousness, sleep disorder.
CV: vasodilation.
EENT: visual disturbances.
GI: constipation, nausea, vomiting, abdominal pain, anorexia, diarrhea, dry mouth, dyspepsia, flatulence.
GU: menopausal symptoms, proteinuria, urinary frequency, urine retention.
Musculoskeletal: hypertonia.
Respiratory: *respiratory depression.*
Skin: diaphoresis, pruritus, rash.

INTERACTIONS
Drug-drug. **Black Box Warning** *Benzodiazepines, CNS depressants:* May cause slow or difficult breathing, sedation, and death. Avoid use together. If use together is necessary, limit dosage and duration of each drug to minimum necessary for desired effect. ∎
Carbamazepine: May increase tramadol metabolism. Patients receiving long-term carbamazepine therapy up to 800 mg daily may need up to twice the recommended tramadol dose.
CNS depressants, opioids: May cause additive effects. Use together cautiously; tramadol dosage may need to be reduced.
Cyclobenzaprine, MAO inhibitors, neuroleptics, other opioids, TCAs: May increase risk of seizures. Monitor patient closely.
Quinidine: May increase level of tramadol. Monitor patient closely.
❸ *Alert:* *Serotonergic drugs (amoxapine, antiemetics [dolasetron, granisetron, ondansetron, palonosetron], antimigraine drugs, buspirone, cyclobenzaprine, dextromethorphan, linezolid, lithium, MAO inhibitors, maprotiline, methylene blue, mirtazapine, nefazodone, SNRIs, SSRIs, TCAs, trazodone, tryptophan, vilazodone):* May

increase risk of serotonin syndrome. Use together cautiously and monitor patient for serotonin syndrome.
Drug-herb. ❸ *Alert:* *St. John's wort:* May increase risk of serotonin syndrome. Use together cautiously and monitor patient for serotonin syndrome.
Drug-lifestyle. *Alcohol, illicit drug use:* May have additive effects. Use cautiously together.

EFFECTS ON LAB TEST RESULTS
● May increase creatinine, GGT, and liver enzyme levels.
● May decrease creatinine and Hb levels.

CONTRAINDICATIONS & CAUTIONS
● Contraindicated in patients hypersensitive to drug or opioids, in patients with severe renal impairment, suicidal patients, and in those with acute intoxication from alcohol, hypnotics, centrally acting analgesics, opioids, or psychotropic drugs.
● Contraindicated in patients with significant respiratory depression or acute or severe bronchial asthma or hypercapnia in unmonitored settings or where resuscitative equipment isn't available.
Black Box Warning Opioids should only be prescribed with benzodiazepines or other CNS depressants to patients for whom alternative treatment options are inadequate. ∎
❸ *Alert:* Serious hypersensitivity reactions can occur, usually after the first dose. Patients with history of anaphylactic reaction to codeine and opioids may be at increased risk.
❸ *Alert:* Patients are at increased risk for oversedation and respiratory depression if they snore or have a history of sleep apnea, haven't used opioids recently or are first-time opioid users, have increased opioid dosage requirements or opioid habituation, have received general anesthesia for longer lengths of time or received other sedating drugs, have preexisting pulmonary or cardiac disease, or have thoracic or other surgical incisions that may impair breathing. Monitor patients carefully.
● Use cautiously in patients at risk for seizures or respiratory depression; in patients with increased ICP or head injury, acute abdominal conditions, or renal or

hepatic impairment; and in patients with physical dependence on opioids. Withdrawal symptoms may occur if drug is abruptly discontinued.

🌓 *Alert:* Drug can cause life-threatening serotonin syndrome.

🌓 *Alert:* Use cautiously in patients suffer from depression or emotional disturbance because of the increased risk of suicide.

🌓 *Alert:* Drug isn't approved for use in children and when used off label; may increase risk of rare but serious slowed or difficult breathing.

🌓 *Alert:* Drug may lead to rare but serious decrease in adrenal gland cortisol production.

🌓 *Alert:* Drug may cause decreased sex hormone levels with long-term use.

Dialyzable drug: 7%.

⚠ *Overdose S&S:* Lethargy, somnolence, stupor, coma, seizures, skeletal muscle flaccidity, respiratory depression, cool clammy skin, miosis, bradycardia, hypotension, cardiac arrest, death.

PREGNANCY-LACTATION-REPRODUCTION
● Safe use in pregnant women hasn't been established. Use only if potential benefit justifies potential fetal risk.

● Prolonged use during pregnancy may lead to physical dependence and postpartum withdrawal symptoms in the neonate. Neonatal seizures, neonatal withdrawal syndrome, fetal death, and stillbirth have been reported.

● Drug isn't recommended for postdelivery analgesia in women who plan to breast-feed because its safety in infants and neonates hasn't been studied. It isn't known if drug appears in breast milk.

NURSING CONSIDERATIONS
Black Box Warning Caution patient or caregiver of patient taking an opioid with a benzodiazepine, CNS depressant, or alcohol to seek immediate medical attention if patient experiences dizziness, light-headedness, extreme sleepiness, slowed or difficult breathing, or unresponsiveness. ■

● Reassess patient's level of pain at least 30 minutes after administration.

● Monitor CV and respiratory status. Withhold dose and notify prescriber if

respirations are shallow or rate is below 12 breaths/minute.

🌓 *Alert:* Carefully monitor vital signs, pain level, respiratory status, and sedation level in all patients receiving opioids, especially those receiving I.V. drugs, even those given postoperatively.

● Monitor bowel and bladder function. Anticipate need for stimulant laxative.

● For better analgesic effect, give drug before onset of intense pain.

● Monitor patients at risk for seizures. Drug may reduce seizure threshold.

● In the case of an overdose, naloxone may also increase risk of seizures.

● Monitor patient for drug dependence. Drug can produce dependence similar to that of codeine and thus has potential for abuse.

● Withdrawal symptoms may occur if drug is stopped abruptly. Reduce dosage gradually.

🌓 *Alert:* If patient is taking opioids with serotonergic drugs, watch for signs and symptoms of serotonin syndrome (agitation, hallucinations, rapid HR, fever, excessive sweating, shivering or shaking, muscle twitching or stiffness, trouble with coordination, nausea, vomiting, diarrhea), especially when starting treatment or increasing dosages. Signs and symptoms may occur within several hours of coadministration but may also occur later, especially after dosage increase. Discontinue the opioid, serotonergic drug, or both if serotonin syndrome is suspected.

🌓 *Alert:* Monitor patient for signs and symptoms of adrenal insufficiency (nausea, vomiting, loss of appetite, fatigue, weakness, dizziness, low BP). Perform diagnostic testing if adrenal insufficiency is suspected. If adrenal insufficiency is confirmed, treat with corticosteroids and wean patient off opioids if appropriate. Discontinue corticosteroids when clinically appropriate.

🌓 *Alert:* Monitor patient for signs and symptoms of decreased sex hormone levels (low libido, erectile dysfunction, amenorrhea, infertility). If signs and symptoms occur, evaluate patient and obtain laboratory testing.

● *Look alike–sound alike:* Don't confuse tramadol with trazodone or trandolapril.

PATIENT TEACHING

Black Box Warning Caution patient or caregiver of patient taking an opioid with a benzodiazepine, CNS depressant, or alcohol to seek immediate medical attention if patient experiences dizziness, light-headedness, extreme sleepiness, slowed or difficult breathing, or unresponsiveness. ■

• Explain assessment and monitoring process to patient and family. Instruct them to immediately report difficulty breathing or other signs or symptoms of a potential adverse opioid-related reaction.

• Tell patient to take drug as prescribed and not to increase dose or dosage interval unless ordered by prescriber.

• Caution ambulatory patient to be careful when rising and walking. Warn outpatient to avoid driving and other potentially hazardous activities that require mental alertness until drug's CNS effects are known.

• Advise patient to check with prescriber before taking OTC drugs because drug interactions can occur.

• Warn patient not to stop the drug abruptly.

❸ *Alert:* Encourage patient to report all medications being taken, including prescription and OTC medications and supplements.

❸ *Alert:* Caution patient to immediately report signs and symptoms of serotonin syndrome, adrenal insufficiency, and decreased sex hormone levels.

SAFETY ALERT!

trastuzumab
trass-too-ZOO-mab

Herceptin

Therapeutic class: Antineoplastics
Pharmacologic class: Monoclonal antibodies

AVAILABLE FORMS
Lyophilized powder for injection: 440 mg/vial

INDICATIONS & DOSAGES
Adjust-a-dose (for all indications): If patient misses a dose by 1 week or less, give usual maintenance dose as soon as possible. Don't wait until next planned cycle. Give subsequent maintenance doses 7 or 21 days later according to the weekly or 3-weekly schedules, respectively. If patient misses a dose by more than 1 week, give a reloading dose as soon as possible followed by maintenance doses 7 or 21 days later according to the weekly or 3-weekly schedules.

➤ **Human epidermal growth factor receptor 2 (HER2)-overexpressing metastatic gastric or gastroesophageal junction adenocarcinoma in patients not previously treated for metastatic disease in combination with cisplatin and capecitabine or 5-FU**
Adults: Initially, 8 mg/kg I.V. Then, 6 mg/kg I.V. every 3 weeks until disease progression or intolerable toxicity develops.

➤ **Metastatic breast cancer in patients whose tumors overexpress HER2 protein**
Adults: Loading dose of 4 mg/kg I.V. over 90 minutes. If tolerated, continue with 2 mg/kg I.V. weekly. If patient hasn't previously received one or more chemotherapy regimens for their metastatic disease, drug is given with paclitaxel.

➤ **After surgical resection of HER2-overexpressing node-positive or node-negative breast cancer**
Adults: During treatment with paclitaxel, docetaxel, or docetaxel–carboplatin, give loading dose of 4 mg/kg I.V. Then, 2 mg/kg I.V. weekly during chemotherapy for the first 12 weeks (paclitaxel or docetaxel) or 18 weeks (docetaxel–carboplatin). Continue trastuzumab 6 mg/kg I.V. every 3 weeks for a total of 52 weeks.

➤ **As single agent after surgical resection of HER2-overexpressing breast cancer within 3 weeks of completion of multimodality, anthracycline-based chemotherapy**
Adults: Initial dose, 8 mg/kg I.V. Then, 6 mg/kg I.V. every 3 weeks for a total of 52 weeks.

➤ **Neoadjuvant treatment of HER2-positive locally advanced, inflammatory, or early breast cancer ◆**
Adults: Initially, 8 mg/kg I.V. (cycle 1) followed by 6 mg/kg I.V. every 3 weeks for a total of four neoadjuvant cycles; postoperatively, administer three cycles of adjuvant FEC [5-FU, epirubicin, and cyclophosphamide] chemotherapy and

---

Reactions in bold italics are *life-threatening*. Interactions may have a *rapid onset* or a *delayed onset*.

continue trastuzumab to complete 1 year of treatment.

➤ **HER2-positive metastatic breast cancer (in combination with pertuzumab and docetaxel) in patients without prior anti-HER2 therapy or chemotherapy to treat metastatic disease** ◆

Adults: Initially, 8 mg/kg I.V. followed by a maintenance dose of 6 mg/kg I.V. every 3 weeks until disease progression or unacceptable toxicity.

➤ **HER2-positive metastatic breast cancer (in combination with either docetaxel or vinorelbine)** ◆

Adults: Initially, 8 mg/kg I.V. followed by a maintenance dose of 6 mg/kg I.V. every 3 weeks until disease progression or unacceptable toxicity (in combination with docetaxel or vinorelbine), or 4 mg/kg I.V. loading dose followed by a maintenance dose of 2 mg/kg I.V. weekly until disease progression (in combination with docetaxel).

➤ **HER2-overexpressing metastatic breast cancer (in combination with lapatinib) that had progressed on prior trastuzumab-containing therapy** ◆

Adults: Initially, 4 mg/kg I.V. followed by a maintenance dose of 2 mg/kg I.V. every week.

ADMINISTRATION

I.V.

▼ Hazardous drug; use safe handling and disposal precautions.

▼ Reconstitute drug in each vial with 20 mL of bacteriostatic water for injection, 1.1% benzyl alcohol preserved, as supplied, to yield a multidose solution containing 21 mg/mL. Don't shake vial during reconstitution. Make sure reconstituted preparation is colorless to pale yellow and free of particulates. Immediately after reconstitution, label vial with expiration 28 days from date of reconstitution.

▼ If patient is hypersensitive to benzyl alcohol, reconstitute drug with sterile water for injection, use immediately, and discard unused portion. Avoid use of other reconstitution diluents.

▼ Calculate volume of 21-mg/mL solution, and withdraw this amount from vial and add it to an infusion bag containing 250 mL of NSS. Don't use D₅W or dextrose-containing solutions. Gently invert bag to mix solution.

▼ Don't give as I.V. push or bolus.

▼ Infuse loading dose over 90 minutes. If well tolerated, infuse maintenance doses over 30 minutes.

▼ Vials are stable at 36° to 46° F (2° to 8° C). Discard reconstituted solution after 28 days. Don't freeze. Store solution of drug diluted in NSS for injection at 36° to 46° F (2° to 8° C) before use; it's stable for up to 24 hours.

▼ **Incompatibilities:** Other I.V. drugs or dextrose solutions.

ACTION

A recombinant DNA-derived monoclonal antibody that selectively binds to HER2, inhibiting proliferation of tumor cells that overexpress HER2.

Route	Onset	Peak	Duration
I.V.	Unknown	Unknown	Unknown

Half-life: Unknown.

ADVERSE REACTIONS

CNS: asthenia, dizziness, fever, headache, insomnia, pain, depression, neuropathy, paresthesia, peripheral neuritis.
CV: peripheral edema, *HF,* hypotension, tachycardia.
EENT: pharyngitis, rhinitis, sinusitis.
GI: abdominal pain, anorexia, diarrhea, nausea, vomiting.
GU: UTI.
Hematologic: *leukopenia,* anemia, *neutropenia.*
Musculoskeletal: back pain, arthralgia, bone pain.
Respiratory: dyspnea, increased cough.
Skin: rash, acne.
Other: *anaphylaxis,* chills, flulike syndrome, infection, allergic reaction, herpes simplex.

INTERACTIONS

Drug-drug. *Anthracyclines, cyclophosphamide:* May increase cardiotoxicity, even if started after trastuzumab is discontinued. Consider therapy modification.

T

EFFECTS ON LAB TEST RESULTS
• May decrease Hb level and WBC count.

CONTRAINDICATIONS & CAUTIONS
• Contraindicated in patients hypersensitive to the drug.
• Use cautiously in elderly patients, in patients hypersensitive to drug or its components, and in those with cardiac dysfunction.
• Use with extreme caution in patients with pulmonary compromise, symptomatic intrinsic pulmonary disease (such as asthma, COPD), or extensive tumor involvement of the lungs.
• Patients who receive anthracycline after stopping trastuzumab may be at increased risk for cardiac dysfunction. If possible, avoid anthracycline-based therapy for up to 7 months after stopping trastuzumab. Carefully monitor patient's cardiac function.
• Safety and effectiveness in children haven't been established.
Dialyzable drug: Unknown.

PREGNANCY-LACTATION-REPRODUCTION
Black Box Warning Exposure to drug during pregnancy can result in oligohydramnios, in some cases complicated by pulmonary hypoplasia, skeletal abnormalities, and neonatal death. Patient must use effective contraception. ■
• If drug is used during pregnancy, or if patient becomes pregnant during therapy or within 7 months after last dose, fetal harm can occur. Immediately report exposure to the Genentech Adverse Event Line (1-888-835-2555).
• Encourage women who may be exposed to drug during pregnancy or within 7 months after last dose to enroll in the MotHER Pregnancy Registry (1-800-690-6720).
• It isn't known if drug appears in breast milk. Patient should discontinue breastfeeding or discontinue drug.

NURSING CONSIDERATIONS
Black Box Warning Drug can cause HF, especially when used with anthracycline-containing chemotherapy regimens. Evaluate LVEF before and during treatment. Discontinue drug in patients receiving adjuvant therapy and withhold drug in those

with metastatic disease for clinically significant decreases in LVEF. ■
• Assess LVEF before therapy, every 3 months during therapy, and when therapy ends. If decreased LVEF occurs, assess LVEF every month; assess LVEF every 6 months for 2 years after therapy ends when drug is used in adjuvant therapy.
• Monitor patient receiving both drug and chemotherapy closely for cardiac dysfunction or failure, anemia, renal toxicity, leukopenia, diarrhea, and infection.
• When used in metastatic breast cancer, drug is only indicated in tumors with HER2 protein overexpression.
• Extending adjuvant treatment beyond 1 year isn't recommended.
Black Box Warning Drug can cause serious infusion reactions and pulmonary toxicity. Interrupt infusion if patient experiences dyspnea or clinically significant hypotension. Strongly consider discontinuation for patients who develop anaphylaxis, angioedema, pneumonitis, or ARDS. ■
• Check for first-infusion symptom complex, commonly consisting of chills or fever. Give acetaminophen, diphenhydramine, and meperidine (with or without reducing rate of infusion). Other signs or symptoms include nausea, vomiting, pain, rigors, headache, dizziness, dyspnea, hypotension, rash, and asthenia and occur infrequently with subsequent infusions.
• ***Look alike–sound alike:*** Don't confuse trastuzumab with ado-trastuzumab emtansine.

PATIENT TEACHING
• Tell patient about risk of first-dose infusion-related adverse reactions and to report all adverse reactions to prescriber.
• Urge patient to notify prescriber immediately if signs or symptoms of heart problems occur, such as shortness of breath, increased cough, or swelling in arms or legs. Tell patient that these effects can occur after therapy ends.
• Advise female patient to stop breastfeeding during therapy and for 7 months after last dose.
• Tell patient to avoid pregnancy during therapy and for 7 months after last dose

and to notify prescriber immediately if pregnancy occurs during this time.

travoprost
TRA-voe-prost

Travatan Z

Therapeutic class: Antiglaucoma drugs
Pharmacologic class: Prostaglandin analogues

AVAILABLE FORMS
Ophthalmic solution: 0.004%

INDICATIONS & DOSAGES
➤ **To reduce IOP in patients with open-angle glaucoma or ocular hypertension**
Adults and children age 16 and older: One drop in each affected eye once daily at bedtime.

ADMINISTRATION
Ophthalmic
• Don't touch tip of dropper to eye or surrounding tissue.
• Apply light finger pressure on lacrimal sac for 1 minute after instilling drug to minimize systemic absorption.
• If using more than one ophthalmic drug, give them at least 5 minutes apart.
• Store drug between 36° and 77° F (2° and 25° C).

ACTION
Thought to reduce IOP by increasing uveoscleral outflow.

Route	Onset	Peak	Duration
Ophthalmic	2 hr	30 min	Unknown

Half-life: 45 minutes.

ADVERSE REACTIONS
CNS: anxiety, depression, headache, pain.
CV: *bradycardia,* angina pectoris, chest pain, hypertension, hypotension.
EENT: eye discomfort, eye pain, eye pruritus, decreased visual acuity, foreign body sensation, ocular hyperemia, abnormal vision, blepharitis, blurred vision, cataract, conjunctival hyperemia, conjunctivitis, dry eye, eye disorder, iris discoloration, keratitis, lid margin crusting, photophobia, sinusitis, subconjunctival hemorrhage, tearing.
GI: dyspepsia, GI disorder.
GU: prostate disorder, urinary incontinence, UTI.
Metabolic: hypercholesterolemia.
Musculoskeletal: arthritis, back pain.
Respiratory: bronchitis.
Other: accidental injury, cold syndrome, infection.

INTERACTIONS
Drug-drug. *NSAIDs:* May increase or decrease effects of travoprost. Monitor therapy.

EFFECTS ON LAB TEST RESULTS
• May increase cholesterol level.

CONTRAINDICATIONS & CAUTIONS
• Contraindicated in patients hypersensitive to drug or its components. Safe use hasn't been established in those with angle-closure, inflammatory, or neovascular glaucoma.
• Use cautiously in patients with active intraocular inflammation (iritis, uveitis), in aphakic and pseudophakic patients, and in those with risk factors for macular edema.
Dialyzable drug: Unknown.

PREGNANCY-LACTATION-REPRODUCTION
• There are no adequate studies in pregnant women. Use only if potential benefit justifies potential risks to the fetus.
• It isn't known if drug appears in breast milk. Use cautiously in breast-feeding women.

NURSING CONSIDERATIONS
• Temporary or permanent increased pigmentation of the iris and eyelid may occur as well as increased pigmentation and growth of eyelashes.
• *Look alike–sound alike:* Don't confuse Travatan Z with Xalatan.

PATIENT TEACHING
• Teach patient how to instill drops, and advise him to wash hands before and after instilling solution. Warn him not to touch tip of dropper to eye or surrounding tissue.

- Advise patient to apply light finger pressure on lacrimal sac for 1 minute after instillation to minimize systemic absorption of drug.
- Tell patient to remove contact lenses before administration and explain that he can reinsert them 15 minutes afterward.
- Tell patient receiving treatment in only one eye about potential for increased iris pigmentation, eyelid darkening, and increased length, thickness, pigmentation, or number of lashes in the treated eye.
- If eye trauma or infection occurs or if eye surgery is needed, advise patient to seek medical advice before continuing to use the multidose container.
- Advise patient to immediately report eye inflammation or lid reactions.
- If patient is using more than one ophthalmic drug, tell patient to apply them at least 5 minutes apart.

trazodone hydrochloride
TRAYZ-oh-dohn

Therapeutic class: Antidepressants
Pharmacologic class: Triazolopyridine derivatives

AVAILABLE FORMS
Tablets (OTC): 50 mg, 100 mg, 150 mg, 300 mg

INDICATIONS & DOSAGES
➤ **Depression**
Adults: Initially, 150 mg P.O. daily in divided doses; then increased by 50 mg daily every 3 to 4 days, as needed. Dose ranges from 150 to 400 mg daily. Maximum, 600 mg daily for inpatients and 400 mg daily for outpatients.

ADMINISTRATION
P.O.
- Give drug after meals or a light snack for optimal absorption and to decrease risk of dizziness.
- Make sure patient swallows tablets whole or breaks them along the score lines. Tablets shouldn't be chewed or crushed.

ACTION
Unknown. Inhibits CNS neuronal uptake of serotonin; not a tricyclic derivative.

Route	Onset	Peak	Duration
P.O.	Unknown	1–2 hr	Unknown

Half-life: 10 hours.

ADVERSE REACTIONS
CNS: drowsiness, dizziness, nervousness, fatigue, confusion, tremor, weakness, hostility, anger, nightmares, vivid dreams, headache, insomnia, syncope.
CV: orthostatic hypotension, tachycardia, hypertension, shortness of breath, ECG changes.
EENT: blurred vision, tinnitus, nasal congestion.
GI: dry mouth, dysgeusia, constipation, nausea, vomiting, anorexia.
GU: urine retention, priapism possibly leading to impotence, hematuria.
Hematologic: anemia.
Skin: rash, urticaria, diaphoresis.
Other: decreased libido.

INTERACTIONS
Drug-drug. *Amphetamines, buspirone, dextromethorphan, dihydroergotamine, lithium salts, meperidine, SSRIs or SSNRIs (duloxetine, venlafaxine), sumatriptan, TCAs, tramadol, tryptophan:* May increase the risk of serotonin syndrome. Avoid combining drugs that increase the availability of serotonin in the CNS; monitor patient closely if used together.
Antihypertensives: May increase hypotensive effect of trazodone. Antihypertensive dosage may need to be decreased.
Clonidine, CNS depressants: May enhance CNS depression. Avoid using together.
CYP3A4 inducers (carbamazepine): May reduce trazodone level. Monitor patient closely; may need to increase trazodone dose.
CYP3A4 inhibitors (ketoconazole): May slow the clearance of trazodone and increase trazodone level. May cause nausea, hypotension, and fainting. Consider decreasing trazodone dose.
Digoxin, phenytoin: May increase levels of these drugs. Watch for toxicity.

Linezolid, methylene blue: May cause sero-tonin syndrome. Don't use together.

❸ Alert: *MAO inhibitors:* Serious and some-times fatal reactions have occurred. Allow at least 14 days between discontinuing an MAO inhibitor and starting trazodone and at least 14 days after stopping trazodone before starting an MAO inhibitor.

Protease inhibitors (amprenavir, atazanavir, fosamprenavir, indinavir, lopinavir–ritonavir, nelfinavir, ritonavir, saquinavir): May increase trazodone levels and ad-verse effects. Monitor patient and adjust trazodone dose, as needed.

Warfarin: May increase PT. Adjust warfarin dosage as needed.

Drug-herb. *Ginkgo biloba:* May cause sedation. Discourage use together.

St. John's wort: May cause serotonin syn-drome. Discourage use together.

Drug-lifestyle. *Alcohol use:* May enhance CNS depression. Discourage use together.

EFFECTS ON LAB TEST RESULTS
● May increase ALT and AST levels. May decrease Hb level.

CONTRAINDICATIONS & CAUTIONS
● Contraindicated in patients hypersensitive to drug.

❸ Alert: Concomitant use with linezolid or methylene blue can cause serotonin syn-drome. Use drug with linezolid or methy-lene blue only for life-threatening or urgent conditions when the potential benefits out-weigh the risks of toxicity.

● Use cautiously in patients with cardiac disease or in the initial recovery phase of MI, as drug can prolong QTc interval, and in patients at risk for suicide.

● May cause mild pupillary dilation, which may trigger an angle-closure attack in pa-tient with anatomically narrow angles who doesn't have a patent iridectomy.

Dialyzable drug: Unlikely.

⚠ Overdose S&S: Priapism, respiratory arrest, seizures, ECG changes, drowsiness, vomiting.

PREGNANCY-LACTATION-REPRODUCTION
● There are no adequate studies in pregnant women. Use only if clearly needed and potential benefit justifies potential fetal risk.

● Drug may appears in breast milk. Use cautiously in breast-feeding women.

NURSING CONSIDERATIONS
● Monitor patient for signs and symptoms of serotonin syndrome (mental status changes, tachycardia, labile BP, hyper-reflexia, incoordination, nausea, vomiting, diarrhea) or neuroleptic malignant syn-drome (hyperthermia, muscle rigidity, rapidly fluctuating vital signs, mental status change). If these signs and symptoms occur, immediately discontinue trazodone and any other serotonergic, antidopaminergic, or antipsychotic drugs.

❸ Alert: If linezolid or methylene blue must be given, stop trazodone and monitor patient for serotonin toxicity for 2 weeks, or until 24 hours after the last dose of methylene blue or linezolid, whichever comes first. May resume trazodone 24 hours after last dose of methylene blue or linezolid.

● Record mood changes. Monitor patient for suicidal tendencies and allow only minimum supply of drug.

Black Box Warning Drug may increase the risk of suicidal thinking and behavior in children, adolescents, and young adults ages 18 to 24, especially during the first few months of treatment, especially those with major depressive disorder or other psychiatric disorder. Drug isn't approved for use in children. ■

● Consider evaluating patients who haven't had an iridectomy for narrow-angle glau-coma risk factors.

● *Look alike–sound alike:* Don't confuse trazodone hydrochloride with tramadol hydrochloride.

PATIENT TEACHING
❸ Alert: Tell patient to report a persistent, painful erection (priapism); immediate intervention may be needed.

❸ Alert: Tell patient to immediately report signs and symptoms of serotonin toxicity and neuroleptic malignant syndrome.

● Warn patient to avoid activities that re-quire alertness and good coordination until effects of drug are known.

Black Box Warning Teach caregivers to recognize and report signs and symptoms of suicidal tendency or suicidal thoughts. ■

• Tell patient to take extended-release tablets at bedtime on an empty stomach.
• Advise patient not to crush or chew tablets. Tell patient that if needed, tablets can be broken in half along the score line.

treprostinil
tra-PROS-tin-ill

Remodulin, Tyvaso

treprostinil diolamine
Orenitram

Therapeutic class: Antihypertensives
Pharmacologic class: Vasodilators

AVAILABLE FORMS
Injection: 1 mg/mL, 2.5 mg/mL, 5 mg/mL, 10 mg/mL in 20-mL vials
Solution for inhalation: 1.74 mg/2.9-mL ampule
Tablets (extended-release) ⓞ*:* 0.125 mg, 0.25 mg, 1 mg, 2.5 mg

INDICATIONS & DOSAGES
➤ **To reduce symptoms caused by exercise in patients with New York Heart Association class II to IV pulmonary arterial hypertension (PAH)**
Adults: Initially, 1.25 nanograms/kg/minute by continuous subcutaneous infusion. If patient doesn't tolerate initial dose, reduce infusion rate to 0.625 nanogram/kg/minute. Increase by 1.25 nanograms/kg/minute each week for the first 4 weeks and then by no more than 2.5 nanograms/kg/minute each week for the remaining duration of infusion. Experience with treprostinil dosages exceeding 40 nanograms/kg/minute is limited. May be given I.V. through a central venous catheter if subcutaneous route isn't tolerated. Or, initially, 3 breaths (18 mcg) per treatment session q.i.d., approximately 4 hours apart. Dosage should be increased by 3 breaths in 1- to 2-week intervals as tolerated to target maintenance dosage of 9 breaths (54 mcg) q.i.d. If 3 breaths aren't tolerated initially, decrease to 1 or 2 breaths and increase as tolerated.
Adjust-a-dose: For patients with mild or moderate hepatic insufficiency, initially,

0.625 nanogram/kg ideal body weight per minute by continuous I.V. infusion, and increase cautiously.
➤ **To decrease the rate of clinical deterioration in patients requiring transition from epoprostenol sodium (Flolan)**
Adults: Start treprostinil at 10% of the current epoprostenol dose; increase dose as the epoprostenol dose is reduced. Decrease epoprostenol dose in 20% increments and increase treprostinil in 20% increments, always maintaining a total dose of 110% of epoprostenol starting dose. Once epoprostenol is at 20% of starting dose and treprostinil is at 90%, decrease epoprostenol to 5% and increase treprostinil to 110%. Finally, stop epoprostenol and maintain treprostinil dose at 110% of epoprostenol starting dose plus an additional 5% to 10% as needed. Change rate based on individual patient response. Treat worsening of PAH symptoms with increases in treprostinil dose. Treat adverse effects associated with prostacyclin and prostacyclin analogues with decreases in epoprostenol dose.
➤ **Treatment of PAH in patients with WHO functional class II to III signs and symptoms to improve exercise capacity**
Adults: 0.25 mg P.O. every 12 hours or 0.125 mg P.O. every 8 hours. May increase in increments of 0.25 or 0.5 mg every 12 hours or 0.125 mg every 8 hours every 3 to 4 days as tolerated to achieve optimal clinical response. If incremental increases aren't tolerated, consider slower titration. Maximum dose is determined by tolerability. If patient is taking strong CYP2C8 inhibitors (such as gemfibrozil), initiate at 0.125 mg P.O. every 12 hours; increase in increments of 0.125 mg every 12 hours every 3 to 4 days.
  To transition from subcutaneous or I.V. to P.O. administration, refer to manufacturer's instructions.
Adjust-a-dose: If intolerable adverse effects occur, decrease dose in 0.25-mg increments. To discontinue therapy, reduce dose in steps of 0.5 to 1 mg/day; avoid discontinuing drug abruptly. If patient is unable to continue oral treatment, consider a temporary infusion of subcutaneous or I.V. treprostinil. For patients with mild hepatic impairment, initiate drug at 0.125 mg every 12 hours and

increase in increments of 0.125 mg every 12 hours every 3 to 4 days. Avoid use in patients with moderate hepatic impairment.

ADMINISTRATION
P.O.
● Give with food.
● Make sure patient swallows tablets whole and doesn't split, crush, or chew them.
● If a dose is missed, patient should take missed dose as soon as possible. If more than two doses are missed, drug must be restarted at a lower dosage and retitrated.
I.V.
▼ Give I.V. through a central venous catheter only if subcutaneous route isn't tolerated.
▼ Dilute with either sterile water for injection or NSS.
▼ Inspect for particulate matter and discoloration before giving.
▼ Give by continuous infusion through a surgically placed indwelling central venous catheter, using an infusion pump designed for I.V. drug delivery.
▼ To avoid potential interruptions in drug delivery, make sure patient has immediate access to a backup infusion pump and infusion sets.
▼ Diluted drug is stable at room temperature for up to 48 hours.
▼ **Incompatibilities:** Other I.V. drugs.
Subcutaneous
● Preferred route is continuous subcutaneous infusion via a self-inserted subcutaneous catheter, using an infusion pump designed for subcutaneous drug delivery.
● The infusion pump should be small and lightweight; adjustable to about 0.002 mL/hour; have occlusion/no delivery, low-battery, programming-error, and motor-malfunction alarms; have delivery accuracy of $\pm 6\%$ or better; and be positive-pressure driven.
● The reservoir should be made of polyvinyl chloride, polypropylene, or glass.
Inhalational
● One ampule contains sufficient volume for all four treatment sessions in a single day.
● Oral inhalation is intended for use with the Optineb-ir Model ON-100/7.

● Before the first treatment of the day, empty entire ampule into medicine cup of inhalation device.
● Cap the device and store upright between treatments.
● Clean the medicine cup and discard any remaining drug at the end of the day. Clean device daily.
● Avoid skin and eye contact with treprostinil.
● Drug shouldn't be ingested orally.
● Don't mix treprostinil with other medications in the nebulizer.
● To avoid potential interruptions in drug therapy, make sure patient has access to backup Optineb-ir device.

ACTION
Directly vasodilates pulmonary and systemic arterial vascular beds and inhibits platelet aggregation.

Route	Onset	Peak	Duration
I.V.	Unknown	Unknown	Unknown
P.O.	Unknown	4–6 hr	Unknown
Subcut.	Rapid	Unknown	Unknown
Inhalation	Rapid	Unknown	Unknown

Half-life: I.V. and subcutaneous, 2 to 4 hours; P.O., unknown; inhalation, 4 hours.

ADVERSE REACTIONS
CNS: dizziness, fatigue, headache.
CV: vasodilation, *right ventricular HF,* chest pain, edema, hypotension.
EENT: pharyngeal pain, epistaxis (inhalation).
GI: diarrhea, nausea.
Musculoskeletal: jaw pain.
Respiratory: dyspnea, cough, wheezing, hemoptysis, pneumonia.
Skin: infusion-site pain, infusion-site reaction, rash, flushing, pallor, pruritus.

INTERACTIONS
Drug-drug. *Anticoagulants, NSAIDs, thrombolytics:* May increase risk of bleeding. Monitor patient closely for bleeding. *Antihypertensives, diuretics, vasodilators:* May worsen reduction in BP. Monitor BP. *QTc interval–prolonging drugs:* May increase QTc interval and risk of ventricular arrhythmia. Consider therapy modification.

T

Drug-lifestyle. *Alcohol use:* May cause drug to be released from tablet faster than intended. Don't use together.

EFFECTS ON LAB TEST RESULTS
None reported.

CONTRAINDICATIONS & CAUTIONS
• Contraindicated in patients hypersensitive to drug or structurally related compounds. Oral form is contraindicated in patients with severe hepatic impairment.
• Use cautiously in patients with hepatic or renal impairment and in elderly patients.
• Drug should be used only by clinicians experienced in diagnosis and treatment of PAH.
• Drug may increase risk of bleeding.
• Abrupt discontinuation of drug or sudden large dosage reductions may worsen PAH signs and symptoms.
• Continuous subcutaneous infusion (undiluted) is the preferred mode of administration because infusion via an indwelling central venous catheter is associated with risk of bloodstream infections and sepsis, which may be fatal.
Dialyzable drug: No.
⚠ *Overdose S&S:* Diarrhea, flushing, headache, hypotension, nausea, vomiting.

PREGNANCY-LACTATION-REPRODUCTION
• There are no adequate studies in pregnant women. Women with PAH are encouraged to avoid pregnancy.
• It isn't known if drug appears in breast milk. Patient should discontinue breastfeeding or discontinue drug.

NURSING CONSIDERATIONS
• Assess patient's ability to accept, place, and care for a subcutaneous catheter and to use an infusion pump.
• During use, a single reservoir syringe can be given for up to 72 hours at 98.6° F (37° C).
• Don't use a single vial longer than 14 days after the initial introduction to the vial.
• Start treatment in setting where adequate monitoring and emergency care are available.
• Increase dose if patient doesn't improve or symptoms worsen, and decrease if drug

effects become excessive or unacceptable infusion-site symptoms develop.
• Avoid abrupt withdrawal or sudden large dose reductions because PAH symptoms may worsen.
• Monitor patient for bleeding.

PATIENT TEACHING
• Inform patient that he'll need to continue therapy for a prolonged period, possibly years.
• Tell patient that subsequent disease management may require I.V. therapy.
• Inform patient that tablets must be swallowed whole and intact.
• Tell patient to report side effects, such as labored breathing, wheezing, fatigue, jaw pain, chest pain, flushing, nausea, diarrhea, pharyngitis, blue skin color, or facial swelling, which may be related to the underlying disease or a drug reaction.
• Tell patient that the most common local reactions are pain, redness, tissue hardening, and rash at the infusion site.
• Tell patient that a backup infusion pump or Optineb-ir device must be available to avoid interruption in therapy.
• Instruct patient in proper administration of inhalation solution and use and cleaning of device.
• Advise patient to coordinate with pharmacy to have next dose always available.

tretinoin (retinoic acid, vitamin A acid)
TRET-i-noyn

Atralin, Avita, ReFissa, Renova, Retin-A, Retin-A Micro, StieVA-A ✲

Therapeutic class: Antiacne drugs
Pharmacologic class: Retinoids

AVAILABLE FORMS
Cream: 0.01%✲, 0.02%, 0.025%, 0.0375%, 0.05%, 0.075%, 0.1%
Gel: 0.04%, 0.05%, 0.01%, 0.025%
Microsphere gel: 0.04%, 0.08%, 0.1%
Solution: 0.05%

INDICATIONS & DOSAGES
➤ **Acne vulgaris (except ReFissa and Renova)**
Adults: Clean affected area and lightly apply once daily at bedtime.
Children age 12 and older (Retin-A Micro): Clean affected area and lightly apply once daily at bedtime.
Children age 10 and older (Atralin): Clean affected area and lightly apply once daily at bedtime.
➤ **Adjunctive use in the mitigation of fine facial wrinkles in patients who use comprehensive skin care and sunlight avoidance programs (Renova); adjunctive treatment for mitigation of fine wrinkles, mottled hyperpigmentation, and tactile roughness of facial skin in patients who don't achieve such palliation using comprehensive skin care and sun avoidance programs alone (ReFissa)**
Adults: Apply a small, pea-sized amount (¼ inch or 5 mm in diameter) to cover the entire face lightly, once daily in the evening.

ADMINISTRATION
Topical
● Clean area thoroughly before application, and avoid getting drug in eyes, mouth, or mucous membranes.
● Patients using ReFissa or Renova should gently wash their faces with a mild soap, pat the skin dry, and wait 20 to 30 minutes before applying medication.

ACTION
Inhibits comedones by increasing epidermal cell mitosis and turnover.

Route	Onset	Peak	Duration
Topical	Unknown	Unknown	Unknown

Half-life: Unknown.

ADVERSE REACTIONS
Skin: feeling of warmth, slight stinging, local erythema, peeling, chapping, swelling, blistering, crusting, temporary hyperpigmentation or hypopigmentation.

INTERACTIONS
Drug-drug. *Topical drugs containing benzoyl peroxide, resorcinol, salicylic acid, or sulfur:* May increase risk of skin irritation. Avoid using together.
Topical minoxidil or photosensitizing drugs (fluoroquinolones, phenothiazines, sulfonamides, tetracyclines, thiazides): May increase risk of skin irritation. Avoid using together.
Drug-lifestyle. *Abrasive cleansers, cream depilatories, medicated cosmetics, skin preparations containing alcohol, waxes:* May increase risk of skin irritation. Discourage use together.
Sun exposure: May increase photosensitivity reaction. Advise patient to avoid excessive sunlight exposure.

EFFECTS ON LAB TEST RESULTS
None reported.

CONTRAINDICATIONS & CAUTIONS
● Contraindicated in patients hypersensitive to drug or its components and in those with sunburn.
● Use cautiously in patients with eczema.
● Use Atralin gel with caution in patients with known sensitivities or allergies to fish because gel contains soluble fish proteins.
● Don't use ReFissa or Renova if patient is sunburned or has eczema or other chronic skin conditions of the face, is inherently sensitive to sunlight, or is also taking drugs known to be photosensitizers, because of the possibility of augmented phototoxicity.
Dialyzable drug: Unknown.
⚠ *Overdose S&S:* Marked redness, skin peeling, skin discomfort.

PREGNANCY-LACTATION-REPRODUCTION
⊕ *Alert:* Don't use ReFissa or Renova if patient is pregnant, is attempting to become pregnant, or is at high risk for pregnancy.
● There are no adequate studies in pregnant women. Use only if potential benefit justifies potential risk to the fetus.
● It isn't known if drug appears in breast milk. Use cautiously in breast-feeding women.

NURSING CONSIDERATIONS
● Initially, drug may be applied every 2 to 3 days using a lower concentration to reduce irritation.

T

• Relapses typically occur within 3 to 6 weeks after therapy is stopped.
• **Look alike–sound alike:** Don't confuse tretinoin with trientine or isotretinoin.

PATIENT TEACHING
• Instruct patient to clean area thoroughly before application and to avoid getting drug in eyes, mouth, or mucous membranes.
• Tell patient to apply with fingertips, gauze pad, or cotton swab.
• Tell patient to wash hands after application.
• Tell patient to wash face with mild soap no more than b.i.d. or t.i.d. Warn patient against using strong or medicated cosmetics, soaps, or other skin cleansers. Also advise him to avoid topical products containing alcohol, astringents, spices, and lime because they may interfere with drug's actions.
• Caution patient not to apply to sunburned skin.
• Tell patient using drug for treatment of fine wrinkles to wait 20 to 30 minutes after washing face to apply drug, and to avoid washing face or applying another skin product or cosmetic for 1 hour after application.
• Tell patient that normal use of cosmetics is allowed.
• Advise patient not to stop drug if temporary worsening of inflammatory lesions occurs. If severe local irritation develops, advise patient to stop drug temporarily and notify prescriber. Dosage will be readjusted when application is resumed. Some redness and scaling are normal reactions.
• Warn patient that he may experience increased sensitivity to wind or cold temperatures.
• Instruct patient to minimize exposure to sunlight or ultraviolet rays during treatment. If he becomes sunburned, he should delay therapy until sunburn subsides. Tell patient who can't avoid exposure to sunlight to use SPF-15 sunblock and to wear protective clothing.
• Warn patient that he may have a temporary increase in lesions, which will improve in 2 to 3 weeks.
• Tell patient not to use ReFissa or Renova if she is pregnant or trying to become pregnant. Advise patient to stop use and notify prescriber if pregnancy is suspected.

---

triamcinolone acetonide (injection)
trye-am-SIN-oh-lone

Kenalog-10, Kenalog-40, Triesence

triamcinolone hexacetonide
Aristospan Intra-articular, Aristospan Intralesional

Therapeutic class: Corticosteroids
Pharmacologic class: Glucocorticoids

AVAILABLE FORMS
triamcinolone acetonide
Injection (suspension): 10 mg/mL, 40 mg/mL
Injection (intravitreal): 40 mg/mL
triamcinolone hexacetonide
Injection (suspension): 5 mg/mL (intralesional); 20 mg/mL (intra-articular)

INDICATIONS & DOSAGES
➤ **Severe inflammation, immunosuppression**
Adults: 60 mg acetonide I.M., then 20 to 100 mg acetonide I.M. as needed every 6 weeks, if possible. Or, 1 mg acetonide into lesions. Or, initially, 2.5 to 15 mg acetonide into joints (depending on joint size) or soft tissue; then may increase to 40 mg for larger areas. A local anesthetic is commonly injected with triamcinolone into the joint. For hexacetonide, up to 0.5 mg (of 5 mg/mL suspension) intralesional or sublesional injection per square inch of affected skin. Additional injections based on patient's response. Or, 2 to 20 mg (using the 20 mg/mL suspension) via intra-articular injection. Repeat every 3 to 4 weeks.
Children older than age 12: Initially, 60 mg acetonide I.M.; repeat with additional I.M. doses of 20 to 100 mg, as needed, at 6-week intervals, if possible.
Children ages 6 to 12: 0.03 to 0.2 mg/kg acetonide, or 1 to 6.25 mg/m^2 I.M. at 1- to 7-day intervals.

➤ **Ophthalmic diseases (sympathetic ophthalmia, temporal arteritis, uveitis, ocular inflammatory conditions unresponsive to topical corticosteroids)**
Adults and children: 4 mg/0.1 mL injected intravitreally, with subsequent doses as needed during the course of treatment.

➤ **Visualization during vitrectomy**
Adults and children: 1 to 4 mg (25 to 100 mcL of 40 mg/mL suspension) injected intravitreally.

ADMINISTRATION
I.M.
● Give deep into gluteal muscle. Rotate injection sites to prevent muscle atrophy.
● Don't use 10 mg/mL strength for this route.

Intra-articular
● Strict aseptic technique is mandatory.
● Prior use of a local anesthetic may be desirable.

Intralesional
● Strict aseptic technique is mandatory.
● Inject directly into the lesion intradermally or subcutaneously.
● It is preferable to use a tuberculin syringe and small-bore needle (not smaller than 24G).

Intravitreal
● Before injecting, give adequate anesthesia and a broad-spectrum microbicide.
● Shake vial vigorously for 10 seconds to ensure a uniform suspension. Inspect suspension for clumping or granules. If present, don't use.
● Inject drug without delay under controlled aseptic conditions.
● Each vial is for the treatment of a single eye only.
● Protect from light. Don't freeze. Store between 39° and 77° F (4° and 25° C).

ACTION
Not clearly defined. Decreases inflammation, mainly by stabilizing leukocyte lysosomal membranes; suppresses immune response; stimulates bone marrow; and influences protein, fat, and carbohydrate metabolism.

Route	Onset	Peak	Duration
I.M., intra-articular, intralesional	Variable	Variable	Variable
Intravitreal	Unknown	Unknown	Unknown

Half-life: 18 to 36 hours; intravitreal, 13 to 24 days.

ADVERSE REACTIONS
CNS: euphoria, insomnia, ***pseudotumor cerebri, seizures,*** headache, paresthesia, psychotic behavior, vertigo.
CV: ***arrhythmias, HF, thromboembolism,*** hypertension, edema, thrombophlebitis.
EENT: cataracts, glaucoma.
GI: ***pancreatitis,*** peptic ulceration, GI irritation, increased appetite, nausea, vomiting.
GU: menstrual irregularities, increased urine calcium level.
Metabolic: ***hypokalemia,*** hyperglycemia and carbohydrate intolerance, hypercholesterolemia, hypocalcemia.
Musculoskeletal: growth suppression in children, muscle weakness, osteoporosis.
Skin: hirsutism, delayed wound healing, acne, various skin eruptions.
Other: ***acute adrenal insufficiency,*** cushingoid state, susceptibility to infections after increased stress or abrupt withdrawal after long-term therapy.

INTERACTIONS
Drug-drug. *Antidiabetics:* May increase blood glucose level. Adjust dosage of antidiabetics as needed.
Aspirin, indomethacin, other NSAIDs: May increase risk of GI distress and bleeding. Use together cautiously.
Barbiturates, carbamazepine, fosphenytoin, phenytoin, rifampin: May decrease corticosteroid effect. Increase corticosteroid dosage.
Cyclosporine: May increase toxicity and seizures. Monitor patient closely.
Ketoconazole, macrolide antibiotics: May decrease metabolism or clearance of triamcinolone, respectively. Decrease triamcinolone dose or dosage interval if needed.
Oral anticoagulants: May alter dosage requirements. Monitor PT and INR closely.
Potassium-depleting drugs, such as thiazide diuretics and amphotericin B: May enhance potassium-wasting effects of triamcinolone. Monitor potassium level.

T

Salicylates: May decrease salicylate level. Monitor patient for lack of salicylate effectiveness.

Skin-test antigens: May decrease response. Postpone skin testing until after therapy.

Toxoids, vaccines: May decrease antibody response and increase risk of neurologic complications. Defer routine administration of vaccines or toxoids until corticosteroid therapy is discontinued, if possible.

EFFECTS ON LAB TEST RESULTS
● May increase glucose and cholesterol levels. May decrease potassium and calcium levels.
● May alter thyroid function tests. May alter reactions to skin tests.

CONTRAINDICATIONS & CAUTIONS
● Contraindicated in patients hypersensitive to drug or its ingredients, in patients with cerebral malaria, in those with systemic fungal infections, and in those receiving immunosuppressive doses together with live-virus vaccines.
● Intravitreal injections are also contraindicated in patients with active ocular HSV.
● Use cautiously in patients with recent MI, GI ulcer, renal disease, hypertension, osteoporosis, diabetes mellitus, hypothyroidism, cirrhosis, diverticulitis, nonspecific ulcerative colitis, recent intestinal anastomoses, thromboembolic disorders, seizures, myasthenia gravis, active hepatitis, lactation, HF, TB, ocular herpes simplex, emotional instability, or psychotic tendencies.
◑ Alert: Use of corticosteroids increases risk of cataracts.
Dialyzable drug: Unknown.

PREGNANCY-LACTATION-REPRODUCTION
● There are no adequate studies in pregnant women. Use only if potential benefit justifies potential fetal risk.
● Carefully observe infants born to mothers who have received corticosteroids during pregnancy for signs and symptoms of hypoadrenalism.
● Drug may appear in breast milk and could suppress infant growth, interfere with endogenous corticosteroid production, or cause other untoward effects. Use cautiously in breast-feeding women.

NURSING CONSIDERATIONS
● Determine whether patient is sensitive to other corticosteroids.
● Drug isn't used for alternate-day therapy.
● Always adjust to lowest effective dose.
● Most adverse reactions to corticosteroids are dose- or duration-dependent.
● Monitor patient's weight, BP, and electrolyte levels.
● Monitor patient for cushingoid effects, such as moon face, buffalo hump, central obesity, thinning hair, hypertension, and increased susceptibility to infection.
● Watch for allergic reaction to tartrazine in patients sensitive to aspirin.
● Watch for depression or psychotic episodes, especially during high-dose therapy.
● Diabetic patient may need increased insulin dosage; monitor glucose level.
● Drug may mask or worsen infections, including latent amebiasis.
● Elderly patients may be more susceptible to osteoporosis with long-term use.
● Unless contraindicated, give low-sodium diet that's high in potassium and protein. Give potassium supplements as needed.
● Gradually reduce dosage after long-term therapy. Drug may affect patient's sleep.
◑ Alert: Intravitreal injections must be performed under mandatory aseptic technique, which includes the use of sterile gloves, sterile drape, and sterile eyelid speculum.
◑ Alert: Monitor patients receiving intravitreal injections for increased IOP, which can lead to glaucoma and damage to the optic nerve.
● *Look alike–sound alike:* Don't confuse triamcinolone with Triaminic.

PATIENT TEACHING
● Tell patient not to stop drug abruptly or without prescriber's consent.
● Teach patient signs and symptoms of early adrenal insufficiency: fatigue, muscle weakness, joint pain, fever, anorexia, nausea, shortness of breath, dizziness, and fainting.
● Instruct patient to carry medical identification that includes prescriber's name and drug's name and dosage and indicates his need for supplemental systemic glucocorticoids during stress.

Reactions in bold italics are *life-threatening*. Interactions may have a *rapid onset* or a ***delayed onset***.

• Warn patient on long-term therapy about cushingoid effects (moon face, buffalo hump) and the need to notify prescriber about sudden weight gain and swelling.
• Tell patient to report slow healing.
• Advise patient receiving long-term therapy to consider exercise or physical therapy. Also, tell patient to ask prescriber about vitamin D or calcium supplement.
• Instruct patient to avoid exposure to infections and to notify prescriber if exposure occurs.
• Tell patient to report ophthalmic signs and symptoms (eye pain, redness, sensitivity to light, vision loss or disturbance) to prescriber and to seek immediate care from an ophthalmologist if these occur.

---

triamcinolone acetonide (intranasal)
trye-am-SIN-oh-lone

Children's Nasacort Allergy 24 Hour ◊, Nasacort Allergy 24 Hour ◊

Therapeutic class: Corticosteroids
Pharmacologic class: Corticosteroids

AVAILABLE FORMS
Nasal spray: 55 mcg/spray

INDICATIONS & DOSAGES
➤ **Treatment of nasal symptoms of seasonal and perennial allergic rhinitis**
Adults and children age 12 and older:
2 sprays in each nostril daily; may decrease to 1 spray in each nostril daily for allergic disorders. Adjust to minimum effective dosage.
Children ages 6 to 11: 1 spray in each nostril daily. Maximum dosage is 2 sprays in each nostril daily. Adjust to minimum effective dosage.
Children ages 2 to 5: 1 spray in each nostril daily.
Adjust-a-dose: Start elderly patients at lower end of dosing range.

ADMINISTRATION
Intranasal
• Shake well before each use.

• Release 5 sprays into the air to prime before first use. Reprime with 1 spray if not used for 2 weeks or more.
• Insert nozzle into nostril, pointing away from septum. Hold other nostril closed and have patient inhale gently while spraying.

ACTION
Unknown. A glucocorticoid with anti-inflammatory properties.

Route	Onset	Peak	Duration
Intranasal	Unknown	1½–4 hr	Unknown

Half-life: About 3 hours.

ADVERSE REACTIONS
CNS: headache, fever.
EENT: nasal irritation, burning, dry mucous membranes, epistaxis, irritation, nasal and sinus congestion, otitis media, pharyngitis, rhinitis, sinusitis, sneezing, stinging, throat discomfort.
GI: dyspepsia, nausea, vomiting.
Respiratory: *asthma symptoms,* cough.

INTERACTIONS
None significant.

EFFECTS ON LAB TEST RESULTS
None reported.

CONTRAINDICATIONS & CAUTIONS
• Contraindicated in patients hypersensitive to drug or its components and in those with untreated mucosal infection.
• Use with caution, if at all, in patients with active or quiescent tuberculous infection of respiratory tract and in patients with untreated fungal, bacterial, or systemic viral infection or ocular herpes simplex.
• Use cautiously in patients already receiving systemic corticosteroids because of increased likelihood of HPA axis suppression.
• Use cautiously in patients with recent nasal septal ulcers, nasal surgery, or trauma because drug may inhibit wound healing.
Dialyzable drug: Unknown.
⚠ **Overdose S&S:** GI upset, nasal irritation, headache.

T

PREGNANCY-LACTATION-REPRODUCTION

• There are no adequate studies in pregnant women. Use only if potential benefit justifies potential risk to the fetus.
• It isn't known if drug appears in breast milk. Use cautiously in breast-feeding women.

NURSING CONSIDERATIONS

🌢 **Alert:** Excessive doses may cause signs and symptoms of hyperadrenocorticism and adrenal axis suppression; stop drug slowly.
• To decrease risk of adverse effects, individualize drug dosage and titrate to minimum effective dosage.
• Discontinue drug if symptom relief hasn't occurred after 3 weeks of treatment.
• *Look alike–sound alike:* Don't confuse triamcinolone with Triaminicin.

PATIENT TEACHING

• Teach patient to prime pump before first use and how to use nasal spray.
• Instruct patient to avoid getting aerosol in eyes. If this occurs, tell him to rinse with copious amounts of cool tap water.
• Stress importance of using drug on a regular schedule because its effectiveness depends on regular use. Warn patient not to exceed prescribed dosage.
• Tell patient to notify prescriber if signs and symptoms don't diminish or if condition worsens in 2 to 3 weeks.
• Warn patient to avoid exposure to chickenpox or measles and, if exposed, to notify prescriber.
• Instruct patient to watch for and report signs and symptoms of nasal infection. Drug may need to be stopped.

triamcinolone acetonide (topical)
trye-am-SIN-oh-lone

Kenalog, Trianex, Triderm

Therapeutic class: Corticosteroids
Pharmacologic class: Corticosteroids

AVAILABLE FORMS
Aerosol: 0.2 mg/2-second spray
Cream: 0.025%, 0.1%, 0.5%

Dental paste: 0.1%
Lotion: 0.025%, 0.1%
Ointment: 0.025%, 0.05%, 0.1%, 0.5%

INDICATIONS & DOSAGES
➤ **Inflammation and pruritus from corticosteroid-responsive dermatoses**
Adults and children: Clean area; apply aerosol, cream, lotion, or ointment sparingly b.i.d. to q.i.d. Rub in lightly. Or, 3 or 4 applications of spray daily.
➤ **Inflammation from oral lesions**
Adults and children: Apply paste at bedtime and, if needed, b.i.d. or t.i.d., preferably after meals. Apply small amount without rubbing; press to lesion in mouth until thin film develops.

ADMINISTRATION
Topical
• Gently wash skin before applying. To avoid skin damage, rub in gently, leaving a thin coat. When treating hairy sites, part hair and apply directly to lesions.
• Don't apply near eyes or in ear canal.
• When using aerosol near the face, cover patient's eyes and warn against inhaling spray. Aerosol contains alcohol and may cause irritation or burning when used on open lesions. Don't spray longer than 3 seconds or from closer than 6 inches (15 cm) to avoid freezing tissues.
• Occlusive dressings may be used in severe or resistant dermatoses.

ACTION
Unclear. Diffuses across cell membranes to form complexes with cytoplasmic receptors, showing anti-inflammatory, antipruritic, vasoconstrictive, and antiproliferative activity. Considered a medium-potency (0.025% and 0.1% cream, ointment, lotion) and high-potency (0.5% cream, ointment) drug, according to vasoconstrictive properties.

Route	Onset	Peak	Duration
Topical	Several hr	Unknown	1 wk

Half-life: Unknown.

ADVERSE REACTIONS
GU: glycosuria.
Metabolic: hyperglycemia.

Skin: burning, pruritus, irritation, dryness, erythema, folliculitis, hypertrichosis, hypopigmentation, acneiform eruptions, perioral dermatitis, allergic contact dermatitis, maceration, secondary infection, atrophy, striae, miliaria with occlusive dressings.

Other: *HPA axis suppression,* Cushing syndrome.

INTERACTIONS
None significant.

EFFECTS ON LAB TEST RESULTS
• May increase glucose level.

CONTRAINDICATIONS & CAUTIONS
• Contraindicated in patients hypersensitive to drug or its components.
• Contraindicated in the presence of fungal, viral, or bacterial infections of the mouth or throat (paste).
• Don't use as monotherapy in primary bacterial infections (impetigo, paronychia, erysipelas, cellulitis, angular cheilitis), treatment of rosacea, perioral dermatitis, or acne.
• Don't use very-high-potency or high-potency agents on the face, groin, or axilla areas.
• Drug isn't for ophthalmic use.
Dialyzable drug: Unknown.
⚠ **Overdose S&S:** Systemic effects (including reversible HPA axis suppression, Cushing syndrome, hyperglycemia, glycosuria).

PREGNANCY-LACTATION-REPRODUCTION
• There are no adequate studies in pregnant women. Use only if potential benefit justifies potential risk to the fetus. Drug shouldn't be used extensively in pregnant patients in large amounts or for prolonged periods.
• It isn't known if drug appears in breast milk. Use cautiously in breast-feeding women.

NURSING CONSIDERATIONS
• Stop drug and tell prescriber if skin infection, striae, or atrophy occur.
• If antifungal or antibiotic combined with corticosteroid fails to provide prompt improvement, stop corticosteroid until infection is controlled.

• Systemic absorption is more likely with the use of occlusive dressings, prolonged treatment, or extensive body surface treatment.
• Avoid using plastic pants or tight-fitting diapers on treated areas in young children. Children may absorb larger amounts of drug and be more susceptible to systemic toxicity.

PATIENT TEACHING
• Teach patient or family member how to apply drug.
• Advise patient not to use an occlusive dressing unless instructed to. If an occlusive dressing is ordered, advise patient to leave it in place for no longer than 12 hours each day and not to use the dressing on infected or weeping lesions.
• Instruct patient spray is flammable.
• Tell patient to stop drug and report signs of systemic absorption, skin irritation or ulceration, hypersensitivity, infection, or lack of improvement.

triamterene– hydrochlorothiazide
try-AM-tur-een/hye-droe-klor-oh-THYE-a-zide

Dyazide, Maxzide

Therapeutic class: Antihypertensives–diuretics
Pharmacologic class: Thiazide diuretics–potassium-sparing diuretics

AVAILABLE FORMS
Capsules: triamterene 37.5 mg and hydrochlorothiazide 25 mg, triamterene 50 mg and hydrochlorothiazide 25 mg
Tablets: triamterene 37.5 mg and hydrochlorothiazide 25 mg, triamterene 75 mg and hydrochlorothiazide 50 mg

INDICATIONS & DOSAGES
➤ **Hypertension or edema in patients who develop hypokalemia on hydrochlorothiazide alone, or who require a thiazide diuretic and in whom development of hypokalemia can't be risked**
Adults: Triamterene 37.5 mg/hydrochlorothiazide 25 mg, or triamterene

50 mg/hydrochlorothiazide 25 mg P.O. once daily or b.i.d., or triamterene 75 mg/ hydrochlorothiazide 50 mg P.O. once daily.

ADMINISTRATION
P.O.
● Give drug with food to minimize GI upset.
● To prevent nocturia, give drug in morning. If second dose is needed, give in early afternoon.

ACTION
Triamterene works on distal tubule to inhibit reabsorption of sodium in exchange for potassium and hydrogen; hydrochlorothiazide increases excretion of sodium, chloride, and water by inhibiting reabsorption in distal segment of the nephron.

Route	Onset	Peak	Duration
P.O. (triamterene)	2 hr	1 hr	6–12 hr
P.O. (hydrochlorothiazide)	2 hr	2 hr	6–12 hr

Half-life: Triamterene, 1½ to 2½ hours; hydrochlorothiazide, 5.6 to 15 hours.

ADVERSE REACTIONS
CNS: weakness, fatigue, dizziness, headache, drowsiness, insomnia, depression, anxiety, vertigo, restlessness, paresthesia.
CV: arrhythmia, orthostatic hypotension, chest pain.
EENT: xanthopsia, transient blurred vision, dry mouth, sialadenitis.
GI: diarrhea, nausea, vomiting, constipation, abdominal pain, pancreatitis, change in appetite, taste alteration, anorexia, gastric irritation, cramping.
GU: erectile dysfunction, *acute renal failure,* interstitial nephritis, renal calculi.
Hematologic: *leukopenia, thrombocytopenia,* purpura, anemia, agranulocytosis.
Hepatic: jaundice, altered LFT results.
Metabolic: diabetes mellitus, *hyperkalemia,* hyperglycemia, glycosuria, hyperuricemia, *hypokalemia,* hyponatremia, *metabolic acidosis,* hypochloremic alkalosis.
Musculoskeletal: muscle cramps.
Respiratory: shortness of breath, *pulmonary edema.*
Skin: rash, urticaria, photosensitivity.

Other: hypersensitivity reaction, anaphylaxis.

INTERACTIONS
Drug-drug. *ACE inhibitors, potassium-containing medications (such as penicillin G potassium), potassium supplements:* May increase risk of hyperkalemia. Avoid concurrent use.
Adrenocorticotropic hormone, amphotericin B, corticosteroids: May increase electrolyte depletion, particularly potassium. Use together carefully.
Amiloride, spironolactone, triamterene-containing agents: May increase risk of hyperkalemia. Use together is contraindicated.
Antidiabetics (oral agents and insulin): May increase or decrease blood glucose level. Dosage adjustment of antidiabetic may be required.
Antigout drugs: May increase uric acid level. Increase dosage of antigout medication if indicated.
Barbiturates, opioids: May increase risk of orthostatic hypotension. Use together cautiously.
Laxatives: May increase potassium loss. Avoid use together.
Lithium: May increase lithium level, especially in patients with renal insufficiency. Avoid use together.
NSAIDs: May diminish antihypertensive effects and increase risk of acute renal failure. Use together cautiously.
Oral anticoagulants: May decrease anticoagulant effect. Adjust anticoagulant dosage as necessary.
Other antihypertensives: May increase risk of hypotension. Use together carefully and adjust dosage as appropriate.
Polystyrene, other exchange resins: May reduce potassium level, increase sodium retention, and increase edema. Avoid use together unless in setting of hyperkalemia.
Skeletal muscle relaxants, nondepolarizing (tubocurarine): May increase responsiveness to muscle relaxant. Avoid concurrent use.
Drug-food. *Salt substitutes with potassium:* May increase risk of hyperkalemia. Discourage use together.

Reactions in bold italics are *life-threatening.* Interactions may have a *rapid onset* or a *delayed onset.*

Drug-lifestyle. *Alcohol use:* May increase risk of orthostatic hypotension. Discourage use together.

Sun exposure: May increase risk of photosensitivity. Discourage sun exposure.

EFFECTS ON LAB TEST RESULTS

● May increase BUN, creatinine, liver enzyme, calcium, uric acid, cholesterol, and triglyceride levels.

● May decrease sodium, chloride, magnesium, and phosphate levels.

● May increase or decrease potassium or glucose level.

● May decrease protein-bound iodine level without signs of thyroid imbalance.

● May decrease leukocyte and platelet counts.

● May interfere with quinidine assays and parathyroid function tests.

CONTRAINDICATIONS & CAUTIONS

Black Box Warning Abnormal elevation of serum potassium levels (5.5 mEq/L or more) can occur and is more likely in patients with renal impairment or diabetes (even without concurrent renal impairment) and in elderly and severely ill patients. ■

● Contraindicated in patients hypersensitive to either drug or to sulfonamides; in those with preexisting hyperkalemia, anuria, acute and chronic renal insufficiency or significant renal impairment, or severe hepatic disease; and in those at risk for metabolic or respiratory acidosis.

● Use cautiously in patients with impaired hepatic function, electrolyte imbalance, or lupus and in those with a history of kidney stones.

Dialyzable drug: Unlikely.

⚠ **Overdose S&S:** Hyperkalemia or hypokalemia, dehydration, nausea, vomiting, weakness, hypotension, lethargy, GI irritation, coma.

PREGNANCY-LACTATION-REPRODUCTION

● There are no adequate studies in pregnant women. Use only if potential benefit justifies potential risk to the fetus.

● Both drugs may appear in breast milk. Patient should discontinue breast-feeding or discontinue drug.

NURSING CONSIDERATIONS

Black Box Warning Monitor potassium level at initiation of therapy, with dosage changes, and with any illness that may influence renal function. ■

● Warning signs and symptoms of hyperkalemia include paresthesia, muscular weakness, fatigue, flaccid paralysis, bradycardia, and shock.

● Fixed-dose combinations aren't to be used for initial therapy except in patients in whom development of hyperkalemia can't be risked (patients taking cardiac glycosides and those with history of cardiac arrhythmias).

● Monitor potassium level carefully in patients using this combination; if hyperkalemia is suspected, obtain ECG and monitor levels.

● If hyperkalemia is present, stop combination and use thiazide alone.

● If potassium level is greater than 6.5 mEq/L, consider I.V. calcium chloride, sodium bicarbonate, glucose, or sodium polystyrene sulfonate; consider dialysis if no improvement.

● Monitor patient for infection (sore throat, fever), which could be a sign of leukopenia, or for bruising, which could be a sign of thrombocytopenia.

● Monitor patient for acute myopia and secondary angle-closure glaucoma (acute vision changes, ocular pain usually within hours to weeks of drug ingestion), especially in patient with a history of possible sulfonamide or penicillin allergy. Discontinue drug as soon as possible if symptoms occur.

● Monitor patient for hyperuricemia or acute gout.

● Thiazides may alter calcium and phosphate levels. Discontinue drug before testing parathyroid function.

● Monitor diabetic patients for changes in antidiabetic agent or insulin requirements. Patients with latent diabetes may become fully diabetic during therapy.

PATIENT TEACHING

● Teach patient to report light-headedness, especially during first few days of therapy. Warn patient to discontinue drug and notify prescriber if syncope occurs.

- Caution patient to notify prescriber if fluid loss occurs from excessive perspiration, dehydration, vomiting, or diarrhea.
- Advise patient not to use salt substitutes containing potassium.
- Instruct patient to promptly report signs and symptoms of infection (sore throat, fever) or bruising.
- Inform patient that to be effective, drug must be taken daily as prescribed, and to continue to take drug even if feeling well.
- Advise patient to avoid taking drug at bedtime, to prevent nighttime diuresis.
- Teach patient the warning signs and symptoms of fluid and electrolyte imbalance (decreased urine production, drowsiness, dry mouth, fast HR, fatigue, low BP, muscular fatigue, muscle pain or cramps, restlessness, stomach disturbances, thirst, and weakness).
- Advise patient to keep follow-up appointments to monitor electrolyte levels.
- Warn patient to avoid sun exposure.
- Caution patient to avoid alcohol, to decrease risk of a sudden drop in BP.

SAFETY ALERT!

triazolam
trye-AY-zoe-lam

Halcion

Therapeutic class: Hypnotics
Pharmacologic class: Benzodiazepines
Controlled substance schedule: IV

AVAILABLE FORMS
Tablets: 0.125 mg, 0.25 mg

INDICATIONS & DOSAGES
➤ **Short-term treatment (7 to 10 days) of insomnia**
Adults: 0.125 to 0.5 mg P.O. at bedtime.
Elderly or debilitated patients: 0.125 mg P.O. at bedtime. Maximum dose is 0.25 mg.

ADMINISTRATION
P.O.
- Give drug without regard for food.

ACTION
Unknown. Probably acts on the limbic system, thalamus, and hypothalamus of the CNS to produce hypnotic effects.

Route	Onset	Peak	Duration
P.O.	15–30 min	1–2 hr	Unknown

Half-life: 1½ to 5½ hours.

ADVERSE REACTIONS
CNS: drowsiness, ataxia, dizziness, headache, nervousness.
GI: nausea, vomiting.

INTERACTIONS
Drug-drug. **Black Box Warning** *Benzodiazepines, CNS depressants:* May cause slow or difficult breathing, sedation, and death. Avoid use together. If use together is necessary, limit dosage and duration of each drug to minimum necessary for desired effect. ∎
Cimetidine, erythromycin, fluoxetine, fluvoxamine, isoniazid, nefazodone, ranitidine: May increase triazolam level. Avoid using with azole antifungals or nefazodone. Watch for increased sedation if used with other drugs.
CNS depressants: May cause excessive CNS depression. Use together cautiously.
Diltiazem: May increase CNS depression and prolong effects of triazolam. Reduce triazolam dose.
Fluconazole, itraconazole, ketoconazole, miconazole: May increase and prolong drug level, CNS depression, and psychomotor impairment. Avoid using together.
Drug-herb. *Calendula, hops, kava, lemon balm, passion flower, skullcap, valerian:* May enhance sedative effect of drug. Discourage use together.
Drug-food. *Grapefruit:* May delay onset and increase drug effects. Discourage use together.
Drug-lifestyle. *Alcohol use:* May cause additive CNS effects. Discourage use together.

EFFECTS ON LAB TEST RESULTS
- May increase LFT values.

CONTRAINDICATIONS & CAUTIONS
- Contraindicated in patients hypersensitive to benzodiazepines.

Reactions in bold italics are *life-threatening*. Interactions may have a *rapid onset* or a *delayed onset*.

Black Box Warning Opioids should only be prescribed with benzodiazepines or other CNS depressants to patients for whom alternative treatment options are inadequate. ∎
• Use cautiously in patients with impaired hepatic or renal function, chronic pulmonary insufficiency, sleep apnea, mental depression, suicidal tendencies, or history of drug abuse.
Dialyzable drug: Unlikely.
⚠ *Overdose S&S:* Somnolence, impaired coordination, slurred speech, confusion, coma, decreased reflexes, hypotension, seizures, respiratory depression, apnea.

PREGNANCY-LACTATION-REPRODUCTION
• Drug may cause fetal harm and is contraindicated in pregnant women.
• Patient should stop drug before becoming pregnant. If patient becomes pregnant, apprise her of risk to the fetus.
• Drug may appear in breast milk. Use in breast-feeding women isn't recommended.

NURSING CONSIDERATIONS
❸ *Alert:* Anaphylaxis and angioedema may occur as early as the first dose; monitor patient closely.
• Assess mental status before starting therapy, and reduce doses in elderly patients.
• Take precautions to prevent hoarding or overdosing by patients who are depressed, suicidal, or drug-dependent or who have history of drug abuse.
• Minor changes in EEG patterns (usually low-voltage fast activity) may occur during and after therapy.
• *Look alike–sound alike:* Don't confuse Halcion with Haldol or halcinonide.

PATIENT TEACHING
Black Box Warning Caution patient or caregiver of patient taking an opioid with a benzodiazepine, CNS depressant, or alcohol to seek immediate medical attention if patient experiences dizziness, light-headedness, extreme sleepiness, slowed or difficult breathing, or unresponsiveness. ∎
❸ *Alert:* Warn patient that drug may cause allergic reactions, facial swelling, and complex sleep-related behaviors (driving, eating, and making phone calls while asleep). Advise patient to report these effects.

• Warn patient not to take more than prescribed amount; overdose can occur at total daily dose of 2 mg (or four times highest recommended amount).
• Tell patient to avoid alcohol use while taking drug.
• Warn patient not to stop drug abruptly after taking for 2 weeks or longer.
• Caution patient to avoid performing activities that require mental alertness or physical coordination.
• Inform patient that drug doesn't tend to cause morning drowsiness.
• Tell patient that rebound insomnia may occur for 1 or 2 nights after stopping therapy.
• Tell patient to avoid pregnancy and breast-feeding while taking drug.

trospium chloride
TROZ-pee-um

Therapeutic class: Urinary antispasmodics
Pharmacologic class: Antimuscarinics

AVAILABLE FORMS
Capsules (extended-release): 60 mg
Tablets: 20 mg

INDICATIONS & DOSAGES
➤ **Overactive bladder (urinary urge incontinence, urgency, frequency)**
Adults younger than age 75: 20 mg P.O. b.i.d. taken on an empty stomach or at least 1 hour before a meal. Or 60 mg extended-release capsule P.O. daily in morning.
Adjust-a-dose: For adults age 75 and older, reduce dosage to 20 mg P.O. once daily based on patient tolerance. For CrCl of less than 30 mL/minute, give 20 mg (immediate-release) P.O. once daily at bedtime. Extended-release form isn't recommended if CrCl is less than 30 mL/minute.

ADMINISTRATION
P.O.
• Give at least 1 hour before meals or on an empty stomach.
• Give extended-release form with water on an empty stomach at least 1 hour before meal.

ACTION

Relaxes smooth muscle of bladder by antagonizing muscarinic receptors, relieving symptoms of overactive bladder.

Route	Onset	Peak	Duration
P.O.	Unknown	5–6 hr	Unknown

Half-life: About 20 hours.

ADVERSE REACTIONS

CNS: fatigue, headache.
EENT: dry eyes and nose.
GI: constipation, dry mouth, abdominal pain, dyspepsia, flatulence, nausea.
GU: urine retention, UTI.
Other: flulike symptoms.

INTERACTIONS

Drug-drug. *Anticholinergics:* May increase dry mouth, constipation, or other adverse effects. Monitor patient.
Metformin, morphine, procainamide, pancuronium, tenofovir, vancomycin: May alter elimination of these drugs or trospium, increasing levels. Monitor patient closely.
Drug-food. *High-fat foods:* May significantly decrease absorption. Give drug at least 1 hour before meals or on an empty stomach.
Drug-lifestyle. *Alcohol use:* May increase drowsiness. Discourage use together.

EFFECTS ON LAB TEST RESULTS

None reported.

CONTRAINDICATIONS & CAUTIONS

● Contraindicated in patients hypersensitive to the drug or any of its ingredients and in those with or at risk for urine retention, gastric retention, or uncontrolled angle-closure glaucoma.
● Use cautiously in patients with significant bladder outflow obstruction, obstructive GI disorders, ulcerative colitis, intestinal atony, myasthenia gravis, renal insufficiency, moderate or severe hepatic impairment, or controlled angle-closure glaucoma.
Dialyzable drug: Unknown.
⚠ *Overdose S&S:* Severe anticholinergic effects, tachycardia, mydriasis.

PREGNANCY-LACTATION-REPRODUCTION

● There are no adequate studies in pregnant women. Use only if potential benefit justifies potential risk to the fetus.
● It isn't known if drug appears in breast milk. Use during breast-feeding only if potential benefit justifies potential risk to the infant.

NURSING CONSIDERATIONS

● Assess patient to determine baseline bladder function, and monitor patient for therapeutic effects.
● Angioedema of the face, lips, tongue, or larynx, which may be life-threatening, can occur after first dose. Discontinue drug and promptly provide treatment to ensure a patent airway.
● Various CNS anticholinergic effects have been reported, including dizziness, confusion, hallucinations, and somnolence. Monitor patients for signs and symptoms of anticholinergic CNS effects, particularly after beginning treatment or increasing dosage. Dosage may need to be reduced or drug discontinued.
● If patient has bladder outflow obstruction, watch for evidence of urine retention.
● Monitor patient for decreased gastric motility and constipation.

PATIENT TEACHING

● Tell patient to take drug on an empty stomach or at least 1 hour before meals.
● Tell patient to take extended-release form with water in the morning on an empty stomach, at least 1 hour before a meal.
● Discourage use of other drugs that may cause dry mouth, constipation, blurred vision, or urine retention.
● Tell patient that alcohol may increase drowsiness and fatigue. Discourage alcohol consumption.
● Explain that drug may decrease sweating and increase the risk of heatstroke when used in hot environments or during strenuous activities.
● Urge patient to avoid activities that are hazardous or require mental alertness until he knows how the drug affects him.

Reactions in bold italics are *life-threatening*. Interactions may have a *rapid onset* or a ***delayed onset***.

ulipristal acetate
UE-li-PRIS-tal

ella

Therapeutic class: Contraceptives
Pharmacologic class: Progesterone
agonists–antagonists

AVAILABLE FORMS
Tablets: 30 mg

INDICATIONS & DOSAGES
➤ **Prevention of pregnancy following
unprotected intercourse or a known or
suspected contraceptive failure**
Women and postmenarchal adolescents:
30 mg (1 tablet) P.O. as soon as possible
within 120 hours (5 days) after unprotected
intercourse or a known or suspected contraceptive failure.

ADMINISTRATION
P.O.
● May give without regard for food.
● May give at any time during the menstrual
cycle.

ACTION
Inhibits or delays ovulation and alters endometrium to avoid egg implantation.

Route	Onset	Peak	Duration
P.O.	1 hr	Unknown	Unknown

Half-life: 32 to 38 hours.

ADVERSE REACTIONS
CNS: headache, fatigue, dizziness.
GI: nausea, abdominal pain.
GU: dysmenorrhea, intermenstrual
bleeding.
Skin: acne.

INTERACTIONS
Drug-drug. *CYP3A4 inducers (barbiturates, bosentan, carbamazepine, felbamate,
griseofulvin, oxcarbazepine, phenytoin,
rifampin, topiramate):* May decrease effectiveness of contraceptive. Avoid concurrent
use.
*CYP3A4 inhibitors (itraconazole, ketocona-
zole):* May increase serum uliprital levels

and risk of adverse reactions. Monitor clinical response and adjust dosage if needed.
Hormonal contraceptives: May impair
ability of uliprital to delay ovulation or
decrease effectiveness of regular hormonal
contraceptives. Avoid coadministration.
Drug-herb. *St. John's wort:* May decrease
effectiveness of contraceptive. Avoid concurrent use.

EFFECTS ON LAB TEST RESULTS
None reported.

CONTRAINDICATIONS & CAUTIONS
● Contraindicated for use as routine contraception.
● Contraindicated in prepubescent and
postmenopausal females.
● Safety and effectiveness of repeated use
within the same menstrual cycle aren't
known.
● Drug exposure in South Asian patients
may exceed that in white and black patients;
however, no difference in efficacy and safety
was observed.
Dialyzable drug: Unknown.

PREGNANCY-LACTATION-REPRODUCTION
● There are no adequate studies in pregnant
women. Drug is contraindicated in women
who are pregnant or may be pregnant.
● Effect of drug exposure on newborns or
infants hasn't been studied; risk to breast-
fed infants can't be excluded. Use by breast-
feeding women isn't recommended.

NURSING CONSIDERATIONS
● If vomiting occurs within 3 hours of
taking drug, prescriber should consider
repeating dose.
● Rule out pregnancy by obtaining history
and physical examination before drug administration. If pregnancy isn't ruled out,
perform pregnancy test.
● Perform follow-up physical and pelvic examination if there is concern about patient's
health or pregnancy status following drug
administration.
● Uliprital won't terminate existing pregnancy.
● Rule out ectopic pregnancy in those who
become pregnant or complain of lower

U

abdominal pain 3 to 5 weeks after ulipristal use.

• Fertility returns rapidly after drug administration; routine contraceptives should be initiated or continued as soon as possible but not sooner than 5 days.

• Drug may reduce efficacy of regular hormonal contraceptives; additional use of a barrier method is recommended for subsequent intercourse during the same menstrual cycle.

• After drug administration, menses can occur a few days earlier or later than usual. If menses is late (beyond 1 week), rule out pregnancy.

• Drug doesn't protect against HIV infection (AIDS) or other sexually transmitted infections.

• *Look alike–sound alike:* Don't confuse ulipristal with ursodiol.

PATIENT TEACHING

• Educate patient that drug isn't intended for routine use as a contraceptive, won't terminate an existing pregnancy, and should only be used once per menstrual cycle.

• Warn patient not to use ulipristal if she suspects she is pregnant or is breast-feeding because potential risks to the infant are unknown.

• Tell patient to report lower abdominal pain immediately.

• Instruct patient to resume routine contraceptives no sooner than 5 days after ulipristal, and to use a barrier method during the same menstrual cycle.

• Advise patient that after drug administration, menses can occur a few days earlier or later than usual and that she should report if menses is late (beyond 1 week) because pregnancy will have to be ruled out.

• Warn patient that drug doesn't protect against HIV infection (AIDS) or other sexually transmitted infections.

ustekinumab
US-te-KIN-ue-mab

Stelara

Therapeutic class: Immunomodulators
Pharmacologic class: Monoclonal antibodies

AVAILABLE FORMS
Injection: 45 mg/0.5 mL, 90 mg/mL single-use vials or prefilled syringes

INDICATIONS & DOSAGES

➤ **Moderate to severe plaque psoriasis in patients who are candidates for phototherapy or systemic therapy**
Adults weighing more than 100 kg: Initially, 90 mg subcutaneously; repeat dose in 4 weeks, followed by maintenance dose of 90 mg subcutaneously every 12 weeks.
Adults weighing 100 kg or less: Initially, 45 mg subcutaneously; repeat dose in 4 weeks, followed by maintenance dose of 45 mg subcutaneously every 12 weeks.

➤ **Psoriatic arthritis as monotherapy or in combination with methotrexate**
Adults: Initially, 45 mg subcutaneously; repeat in 4 weeks. Then maintenance dose of 45 mg subcutaneously every 12 weeks.

➤ **Psoriatic arthritis with coexistent moderate to severe plaque psoriasis as monotherapy or in combination with methotrexate**
Adults weighing more than 100 kg: Initially, 90 mg subcutaneously; repeat dose in 4 weeks. Then maintenance dose of 90 mg subcutaneously every 12 weeks.

✴ *NEW INDICATION:* **Crohn disease**
Adults: For induction as a single dose: If patient weighs more than 85 kg, 520 mg I.V.; if patient weighs more than 55 to less than 85 kg, 390 mg I.V.; if patient weighs 55 kg or less, 260 mg I.V. Begin maintenance dose 8 weeks after induction. Maintenance dose is 90 mg subcutaneously every 8 weeks.

ADMINISTRATION
I.V.
▼ After calculating dosage and volume, withdraw an equal amount of fluid from

250-mL bag of NSS and discard. Add drug to the NSS bag and gently mix.

▼ Infuse over 1 hour using an in-line, low-protein-binding filter (0.2 micrometer).

▼ **Incompatibilities:** Don't infuse in same I.V. line with other drugs.

Subcutaneous

● Before administration, inspect ustekinumab for particulate matter and discoloration. Drug is colorless to light yellow and may contain a few small translucent or white particles. Don't use if discolored or cloudy or if other particulate matter is present.

◑ *Alert:* The needle cover on the prefilled syringe contains dry natural rubber (a derivative of latex). Persons sensitive to latex shouldn't handle needle cover.

● Each subcutaneous injection should be administered at a different anatomic location (such as upper arms, gluteal regions, thighs, or any quadrant of abdomen) than the previous injection; drug shouldn't be administered into areas where the skin is tender, bruised, erythematous, or indurated.

● Drug should only be administered under the guidance and supervision of a health care provider and to patients who will be closely monitored and have regular follow-up visits with a health care provider.

ACTION

Antagonizes interleukin 12 and 23 cytokines by binding to an interleukin-specific P40 protein subunit that disrupts interleukin-based inflammatory and immune responses.

Route	Onset	Peak	Duration
Subcut.	Unknown	7–13½ days	Unknown

Half-life: 10 to 126 days.

ADVERSE REACTIONS

CNS: depression, dizziness, fatigue, headache.
EENT: nasopharyngitis, pharyngolaryngeal pain.
GI: diarrhea, nausea.
Musculoskeletal: back pain, myalgia.
Respiratory: URI.
Skin: injection-site erythema, pruritus.
Other: *severe infection.*

INTERACTIONS

Drug-drug. *CYP450 substrates (cyclosporine, warfarin):* May alter drug concentrations. Monitor patient for clinical effects and adjust dosage as needed.
Live-virus vaccines: May transmit infection. Use together is contraindicated.

EFFECTS ON LAB TEST RESULTS
None reported.

CONTRAINDICATIONS & CAUTIONS
◑ *Alert:* Don't administer live-virus vaccines during or after treatment.

● Contraindicated in patients with clinically significant hypersensitivity to drug or its components. Hypersensitivity reactions, including anaphylaxis and angioedema, have been reported.

● Drug may increase risk of infections and reactivation of latent infections, including serious bacterial, fungal, and viral infections.

● Drug is contraindicated in patients with a clinically important active infection. Don't administer ustekinumab until the infection resolves or is adequately treated. Instruct patients to seek medical advice if signs or symptoms suggestive of an infection occur. Exercise caution when considering the use of ustekinumab in patients with a chronic infection or a history of recurrent infection.

● Don't administer to patients with active TB. Initiate treatment of latent TB before administering ustekinumab. Consider anti-TB therapy before initiation of ustekinumab in patients with a history of latent or active TB in which an adequate course of treatment can't be confirmed.

● Drug may increase the risk of malignancy. Safety of ustekinumab hasn't been evaluated in patients with a history of malignancy or a known malignancy.

● Safety of use in combination with other immunosuppressants or phototherapy hasn't been evaluated in psoriasis studies.

● Drug may decrease the protective effect of allergen immunotherapy, which may increase the risk of an allergic reaction to a dose of allergen immunotherapy. Use cautiously in patients receiving or who have received allergen immunotherapy, particularly for anaphylaxis.

U

• The rapid appearance of multiple cutaneous squamous cell carcinomas in patients with preexisting risk factors for developing nonmelanoma skin cancer has been reported.

• Drug may cause reversible posterior leukoencephalopathy syndrome (RPLS). Signs and symptoms include headache, seizures, confusion, and visual disturbances. If RPLS is suspected, discontinue drug and administer appropriate treatment.

Dialyzable drug: Unknown.

PREGNANCY-LACTATION-REPRODUCTION

• Drug hasn't been studied in pregnant women. Use only if potential benefit outweighs potential risk to the fetus.

• Encourage women exposed to ustekinumab during pregnancy to enroll in the MotherToBaby Autoimmune Diseases in Pregnancy registry (1-877-311-8972).

• It isn't known if drug appears in breast milk. Use cautiously in breast-feeding women.

NURSING CONSIDERATIONS

• Evaluate patients for TB before initiating drug. Closely monitor patients receiving drug for signs and symptoms of active TB (fever, cough, night sweats, fatigue, and unexplained weight loss) during and after treatment.

• Patients should receive all immunizations appropriate for age as recommended by current immunization guidelines before starting treatment. Patients being treated with ustekinumab shouldn't receive live-virus vaccines. Don't give bacillus Calmette-Guérin vaccines for 1 year before initiating treatment, during treatment, or for 1 year after discontinuation of treatment.

• Use caution when administering live-virus vaccines to household contacts of patient receiving drug because of the potential risk of shedding from the household contact and transmission to patient.

• Non-live-virus vaccinations received by patient during a course of ustekinumab may not elicit an immune response sufficient to prevent disease.

• Monitor patients for signs and symptoms of infection (fever, fatigue, sore throat, erythema, pain, cough). If infection develops, withhold drug and treat infection.

• Monitor patient for signs and symptoms of RPLS (headache, seizures, confusion, visual disturbances).

• Monitor all patients for the appearance of nonmelanoma skin cancer. Patients older than age 60, those with a medical history of prolonged immunosuppressive therapy, and those with a history of psoralen-ultraviolet A treatment should be followed closely.

• After proper training in subcutaneous injection technique, patient may self-inject.

PATIENT TEACHING

• Instruct patient to immediately report signs or symptoms of RPLS.

• Inform patient that drug may lower the ability of the immune system to fight infections. Stress importance of communicating any history of infections to health care provider and reporting signs or symptoms of infection.

• Advise patient to seek immediate medical attention if signs or symptoms of serious allergic reactions occur (wheezing, chest tightness, fever, itching, cough, blue skin color, seizures, facial swelling).

• Instruct patient or caregiver in injection techniques. Assess their ability to inject subcutaneously to ensure proper administration. The first self-injection should be performed under the supervision of a qualified health care professional.

• Advise patient that the needle cover on the prefilled syringe contains dry natural rubber (a derivative of latex), which may cause allergic reactions in latex-sensitive individuals.

• Instruct patient or caregiver in proper technique for syringe and needle disposal. Advise patient not to reuse or share needles or syringes.

• Caution patient to avoid live-virus vaccines during and after therapy.

• Warn patient that drug may increase the risk of malignancy.

valacyclovir hydrochloride
val-ah-SYE-kloe-vir

Valtrex⬧

Therapeutic class: Antivirals
Pharmacologic class: Nucleosides–
nucleotides

AVAILABLE FORMS
Tablets: 500 mg, 1 g

INDICATIONS & DOSAGES
➤ **Herpes zoster infection (shingles)**
Adults: 1 g P.O. t.i.d. for 7 days.
Adjust-a-dose: For patients with CrCl of
30 to 49 mL/minute, give 1 g P.O. every
12 hours; if CrCl is 10 to 29 mL/minute,
give 1 g P.O. every 24 hours; if CrCl is less
than 10 mL/minute, give 500 mg P.O. every
24 hours.
➤ **First episode of genital herpes**
Adults: 1 g P.O. b.i.d. for 10 days.
Adjust-a-dose: For patients with CrCl of
10 to 29 mL/minute, give 1 g P.O. every
24 hours; if CrCl is less than 10 mL/minute,
give 500 mg P.O. every 24 hours.
➤ **Recurrent genital herpes in immunocompetent patients**
Adults: 500 mg P.O. b.i.d. for 3 days, given
at the first sign or symptom of an episode.
Adjust-a-dose: For patients with CrCl of
29 mL/minute or less, give 500 mg P.O.
every 24 hours.
➤ **Long-term suppression of recurrent
genital herpes**
Adults: 1 g P.O. once daily. In patients with
a history of nine or fewer recurrences per
year, use alternative dose of 500 mg once
daily.
Adjust-a-dose: For patients with CrCl of
29 mL/minute or less, give 500 mg P.O.
every 24 hours (every 48 hours if patient has
nine or fewer occurrences per year).
➤ **Long-term suppression of recurrent
genital herpes in patients with HIV and
CD4$^+$ cell count of 100/mm^3**
Adults: 500 mg P.O. b.i.d.
Adjust-a-dose: For patients with CrCl of
29 mL/minute or less, give 500 mg P.O.
every 24 hours (every 48 hours if patient has
nine or fewer occurrences per year).

➤ **Cold sores (herpes labialis)**
Adults and children age 12 and older: 2 g
P.O. b.i.d. for 1 day taken 12 hours apart.
Adjust-a-dose: For patients with CrCl of
30 to 49 mL/minute, give 1 g every 12 hours
for two doses; if CrCl is 10 to 29 mL/minute,
give 500 mg every 12 hours for two doses;
if CrCl is less than 10 mL/minute, give
500 mg as a single dose.
➤ **To reduce transmission of genital
herpes in patients with history of nine or
fewer occurrences per year**
Adults: 500 mg P.O. daily for source partner.
➤ **Chickenpox**
Children ages 2 to 18: 20 mg/kg P.O. t.i.d.
for 5 days. Maximum dose is 1 g t.i.d.

ADMINISTRATION
P.O.
● Give drug without regard for meals.
● An oral suspension may be compounded
by a pharmacist if needed.
● Suspension must be refrigerated then
shaken before each dose. Discard unused
portion after 28 days.

ACTION
Rapidly converts to acyclovir, which in
turn becomes incorporated into viral DNA,
thereby terminating growth of the DNA
chain; inhibits viral DNA polymerase,
causing inhibition of viral replication.

Route	Onset	Peak	Duration
P.O.	30 min	Unknown	Unknown

Half-life: 2½ to 3¼ hours.

ADVERSE REACTIONS
CNS: headache, depression, dizziness.
EENT: nasopharyngitis, rhinorrhea.
GI: nausea, abdominal pain, diarrhea,
vomiting.
GU: dysmenorrhea.
Hematologic: *thrombocytopenia.*
Musculoskeletal: arthralgia.
Skin: rash.

INTERACTIONS
Drug-drug. *Foscarnet:* May increase risk of
nephrotoxicity. Avoid use together.

V

EFFECTS ON LAB TEST RESULTS
• May increase alkaline phosphatase, ALT, AST, and creatinine levels. May decrease Hb level.
• May decrease platelet and WBC counts.

CONTRAINDICATIONS & CAUTIONS
• Contraindicated in patients hypersensitive to or intolerant of valacyclovir, acyclovir, or components of the formulation.
◐ **Alert:** Thrombotic thrombocytopenic purpura (TTP) and hemolytic-uremic syndrome (HUS) may occur in allogeneic bone marrow or renal transplant recipients and patients with advanced HIV at doses of 8 g/day. Discontinue drug if signs or symptoms or laboratory findings of TTP or HUS occur.
• Use cautiously in elderly or dehydrated patients, in those with renal impairment, and in those receiving other nephrotoxic drugs.
• Safety and effectiveness in prepubertal children haven't been established.
Dialyzable drug: 33%.
⚠ **Overdose S&S:** Precipitation of acyclovir in renal tubules.

PREGNANCY-LACTATION-REPRODUCTION
• There are no adequate studies in pregnant women. Use in pregnant women only if potential benefits outweigh potential risk to the fetus.
• Drug appears in breast milk. Use cautiously in breast-feeding women.

NURSING CONSIDERATIONS
• Safety and effectiveness of therapy beyond 12 months (beyond 6 months in HIV-1–infected patients) haven't been established.
• Start treatment for herpes zoster infection at earliest signs or symptoms. It's most effective when started within 48 hours of onset of rash.
• Monitor renal function; give appropriate dose adjusted for renal status.
• If renal failure and anuria occur, hemodialysis may be beneficial until renal function returns.
• Monitor patient for CNS changes (agitation, hallucinations, confusion, delirium, seizures, and encephalopathy). Discontinue drug if changes occur.

• *Look alike–sound alike:* Don't confuse valacyclovir (Valtrex) with valganciclovir (Valcyte) or acyclovir. Don't confuse Valtrex with Keflex or Zovirax.

PATIENT TEACHING
• Inform patient that drug may be taken without regard for meals.
• Teach patient the signs and symptoms of herpes infection (rash, tingling, itching, and pain), and advise him to notify prescriber immediately if they occur. Treatment should begin as soon as possible after symptoms appear, preferably within 48 hours of the onset of zoster rash.
• Caution patient to immediately report CNS changes and other adverse reactions.
• Tell patient that drug isn't a cure for herpes but may decrease length and severity of symptoms.
• Advise patient with genital herpes to use safe sex practices in combination with suppressive therapy, even if no symptoms are apparent.
• Advise patient to maintain adequate hydration.

valganciclovir hydrochloride
val-gan-SYE-kloe-veer

Valcyte

Therapeutic class: Antivirals
Pharmacologic class: Nucleosides—nucleotides

AVAILABLE FORMS
Oral solution: 50 mg/mL
Tablets ⊙*:* 450 mg

INDICATIONS & DOSAGES
Adjust-a-dose (for all indications): For adult patients with CrCl of 40 to 59 mL/minute, induction dosage is 450 mg b.i.d.; maintenance dosage is 450 mg daily. If CrCl is 25 to 39 mL/minute, induction dosage is 450 mg daily; maintenance dosage is 450 mg every 2 days. If CrCl is 10 to 24 mL/minute, induction dosage is 450 mg every 2 days; maintenance dosage is 450 m twice weekly. Drug isn't recommended

for patients with CrCl of less than 10 mL/minute.

➤ **To prevent CMV disease in heart, kidney, and kidney-pancreas transplantation in patients at high risk (donor CMV-seropositive or recipient CMV-seronegative)**

Adults: For patients with a heart or kidney-pancreas transplant, give 900 mg P.O. once daily starting within 10 days of transplantation until 100 days posttransplantation. For patients with a kidney transplant, give 900 mg P.O. daily starting within 10 days of transplantation until 200 days post-transplantation.

➤ **To prevent CMV disease in pediatric kidney transplant patients at high risk**

Children age 4 months to 16 years: Give dose once daily starting within 10 days of transplantation until 200 days posttransplantation of kidney, based on BSA and CrCl (modified Schwartz formula):

$$\text{Dose (mg)} = 7 \times \text{BSA} \times \text{CrCl}$$

Adjust-a-dose: For pediatric patients, the maximum calculated CrCl (modified Schwartz formula) to be used is 150 mL/minute/1.73 m^2, even if the calculated value is greater. The maximum pediatric dose is 900 mg, even if the calculated dose is greater.

➤ **To prevent CMV disease in pediatric heart transplant patients at high risk**

Children age 1 month to 16 years: Give dose once daily starting within 10 days of transplantation until 100 days posttransplantation of heart, based on BSA and CrCl (modified Schwartz formula):

$$\text{Dose (mg)} = 7 \times \text{BSA} \times \text{CrCl}$$

Maximum dose is 900 mg once daily.

➤ **CMV retinitis in patients with AIDS**

Adults: For active disease, give 900 mg P.O. b.i.d. with food for 21 days; maintenance dose is 900 mg P.O. daily with food. For inactive disease, give 900 mg P.O. once daily.

ADMINISTRATION

P.O.

Give drug with food.

● *Alert:* Handle and dispose of drug according to safe handling guidelines.

● Don't crush tablets. Avoid direct contact with broken or crushed tablets, powder for oral solution, and oral solution. If contact with skin or mucous membranes occurs, wash thoroughly with soap and water, and rinse eyes with plain water.

● Adults should use tablets, not oral solution.

● Refrigerate oral solution; discard unused portion after 49 days.

ACTION

Converted to the active drug ganciclovir, which inhibits replication of CMV.

Route	Onset	Peak	Duration
P.O.	Unknown	1–3 hr	Unknown

Half-life: 4 hours.

ADVERSE REACTIONS

CNS: pyrexia, headache, insomnia, peripheral neuropathy, paresthesia, tremors, *seizures,* fatigue, pain, weakness, depression, psychosis, hallucinations, confusion, agitation.

CV: hypertension, edema, peripheral edema, hypotension.

EENT: retinal detachment, pharyngitis, nasopharyngitis.

GI: diarrhea, nausea, vomiting, constipation, abdominal pain, dyspepsia, abdominal distention, ascites.

GU: UTI, renal impairment, dysuria, decreased CrCl.

Hematologic: *neutropenia,* anemia, *thrombocytopenia, bleeding, pancytopenia, bone marrow depression, aplastic anemia.*

Hepatic: abnormal hepatic function.

Metabolic: *hyperkalemia, hypokalemia, hypomagnesemia,* hyperglycemia, decreased appetite, dehydration, hypophosphatemia, *hypocalcemia.*

Musculoskeletal: back pain, arthralgia, muscle cramps, limb pain.

Respiratory: URI, cough, dyspnea, pleural effusion.

Skin: dermatitis, pruritus, acne.

Other: graft rejection, catheter-related infections, hypersensitivity reactions, local and systemic infections, *sepsis,* postoperative wound infection, increased wound drainage, wound dehiscence.

V

INTERACTIONS

Drug-drug. *Imipenem:* May increase risk of seizures. Don't use together.

Mycophenolate mofetil: May increase levels of both drugs in renally impaired patients. Monitor therapy.

NRTIs (didanosine, zidovudine): May cause hematologic toxicity. Consider therapy modification.

Probenecid: May decrease renal clearance of ganciclovir. Monitor patient for ganciclovir toxicity.

Tenofovir: May increase serum levels of both drugs. Monitor therapy.

Drug-food. *Any food:* May increase drug absorption. Give drug with food.

EFFECTS ON LAB TEST RESULTS

• May increase creatinine level.
• May decrease Hb level and hematocrit and neutrophil, platelet, RBC, and WBC counts.

CONTRAINDICATIONS & CAUTIONS

• Contraindicated in patients hypersensitive to valganciclovir or ganciclovir. Don't use in patients receiving hemodialysis.

Black Box Warning In animal studies, drug was carcinogenic and mutagenic; consider it a potential carcinogen in humans. ■

• Drug isn't indicated for use in liver transplant patients.

• Acute renal failure can occur. Use cautiously in elderly or dehydrated patients, in those with renal impairment, and in those receiving other nephrotoxic drugs.

• The safety and effectiveness of drug for the prevention of CMV disease in other solid organ transplant patients, such as lung transplant patients, haven't been established.

• Use cautiously in patients with cytopenias and in those who have received immunosuppressants or radiation.

Dialyzable drug: Yes.

⚠ *Overdose S&S:* Bone marrow depression, renal toxicity.

PREGNANCY-LACTATION-REPRODUCTION

Black Box Warning Based on findings in animal studies, drug may cause fetal toxicity. ■

• Females of childbearing potential should use effective contraception during and for at least 30 days after therapy. Males should use barrier contraceptives during and for at least 90 days after therapy.

• Breast-feeding isn't recommended during therapy because of potential for serious adverse events in the infant and potential for postnatal HIV transmission.

Black Box Warning Based on animal data, drug may temporarily or permanently inhibit spermatogenesis in males, and may suppress fertility in females. ■

NURSING CONSIDERATIONS

• Adhere to dosing guidelines for valganciclovir because ganciclovir and valganciclovir aren't interchangeable and overdose may occur.

Black Box Warning Toxicities include severe leukopenia, neutropenia, anemia, pancytopenia, bone marrow depression, aplastic anemia, and thrombocytopenia. ■

• Don't use if ANC is less than $500/mm^3$, platelet count is less than $25,000/mm^3$, or Hb level is less than 8 g/dL.

• Monitor CBC, platelet counts, and creatinine level or CrCl values frequently during treatment.

• Cytopenia may occur at any time during treatment and may increase with continued use. Counts usually recover 3 to 7 days after stopping drug.

• Perform pregnancy testing before starting drug in females of childbearing potential.

• No drug interaction studies have been conducted but, because drug is converted to ganciclovir, assume that drug interactions will be similar.

• *Look alike–sound alike:* Don't confuse valganciclovir hydrochloride (Valcyte) with valacyclovir (Valtrex). Don't confuse Valcyte with Valium.

PATIENT TEACHING

• Tell patient to take drug with food.

• Tell patient to follow dosage instructions precisely. Ganciclovir capsules and valganciclovir tablets aren't interchangeable.

• Advise patient that blood tests are needed during treatment. Doses may need to be adjusted based on blood counts.

• Tell woman of childbearing potential to use contraception during treatment and for 30 days after therapy. Tell man to use barrier

---

Reactions in bold italics are *life-threatening*. Interactions may have a *rapid onset* or a ***delayed onset***.

contraception during and for 90 days after therapy.

• Advise patient that drug may temporarily or permanently impair fertility.

• Advise patient that ganciclovir is a carcinogen.

• Tell patient to report all adverse effects. Advise patient that CNS effects (seizures, ataxia, dizziness) can occur and to use care when driving or operating machinery.

• Advise patient that this drug isn't a cure for CMV retinitis and that the condition may recur. Tell patient to see an ophthalmologist at least every 4 to 6 weeks during treatment.

---

valproate sodium
val-PROH-ayt

Depacon

valproic acid
Depakene

divalproex sodium
Depakote✐, Depakote ER, Depakote Sprinkle✐

Therapeutic class: Anticonvulsants
Pharmacologic class: Carboxylic acid derivatives

AVAILABLE FORMS
valproate sodium
Injection: 100 mg/mL
valproic acid
Capsules ⓞⓝⓒ: 250 mg
Syrup: 250 mg/5 mL
divalproex sodium
Capsules (sprinkle) ⓞⓝⓒ: 125 mg
Tablets (delayed-release) ⓞⓝⓒ: 125 mg, 250 mg, 500 mg
Tablets (extended-release) ⓞⓝⓒ: 250 mg, 500 mg

INDICATIONS & DOSAGES
Adjust-a-dose (for all indications): For elderly patients, start at lower dosage. Increase dosage more slowly and with regular monitoring of fluid and nutritional intake, and watch for dehydration, somnolence, and other adverse reactions.

➤ **Simple and complex absence seizures, mixed seizure types (including absence seizures)**
Adults and children age 2 and older: Initially, 15 mg/kg P.O. or I.V. daily; then increase by 5 to 10 mg/kg daily at weekly intervals up to maximum of 60 mg/kg daily. Don't use Depakote ER in children younger than age 10.

➤ **Complex partial seizures**
Adults and children age 10 and older: 10 to 15 mg/kg Depakote or Depakote ER P.O. or valproate sodium I.V. daily; then increase by 5 to 10 mg/kg daily at weekly intervals, up to 60 mg/kg daily.

➤ **Mania**
Adults: Initially, 750 mg Depakote P.O. daily in divided doses, or 25 mg/kg Depakote ER P.O. once daily. Adjust dosage based on patient's response; maximum dose for either form is 60 mg/kg daily. Maximum recommended dosage is 60 mg/kg/day.

➤ **To prevent migraine headache**
Adults: Initially, 250 mg delayed-release divalproex sodium P.O. b.i.d. Some patients may need up to 1,000 mg daily. Or, 500 mg Depakote ER P.O. daily for 1 week; then 1,000 mg P.O. daily. Maximum recommended dosage is 60 mg/kg/day.

ADMINISTRATION
P.O.
• Don't crush delayed- or extended-release tablets.

• Give drug with food or milk to reduce adverse GI effects.

• Don't mix syrup with carbonated beverages; mixture may be irritating to oral mucosa.

• Don't give syrup to patients who need sodium restriction. Check with prescriber.

• Sprinkle capsules may be swallowed whole or opened and contents sprinkled on a teaspoonful of soft food. Patient should swallow immediately without chewing.

I.V.
▼ I.V. use is indicated only in patients who can't take drug orally. Switch patient to oral form as soon as feasible; effects of I.V. use for longer than 14 days are unknown.

▼ Dilute valproate sodium injection with at least 50 mL of a compatible diluent. It's physically compatible and chemically

V

---

stable in D_5W, NSS, and lactated Ringer solution for 24 hours.
▼ Infuse drug over 60 minutes at no more than 20 mg/minute and at the same frequency as oral dosage.
▼ Monitor drug level, and adjust dosage as needed.
▼ **Incompatibilities:** None reported.

ACTION

Unknown. Probably facilitates the effects of the inhibitory neurotransmitter GABA.

Route	Onset	Peak	Duration
P.O.	Unknown	15 min–4 hr	Unknown
I.V.	Unknown	1 hr	Unknown

Half-life: 6 to 16 hours.

ADVERSE REACTIONS

CNS: asthenia, dizziness, drowsiness, headache, insomnia, nervousness, somnolence, tremor, abnormal thinking, amnesia, ataxia, depression, emotional upset, fever.
CV: chest pain, edema, hypertension, hypotension, tachycardia.
EENT: blurred vision, diplopia, nystagmus, pharyngitis, rhinitis, tinnitus.
GI: abdominal pain, anorexia, diarrhea, dyspepsia, nausea, vomiting, *pancreatitis,* constipation, increased appetite.
Hematologic: *bone marrow suppression, hemorrhage, thrombocytopenia,* bruising, petechiae.
Hepatic: *hepatotoxicity.*
Metabolic: hyperammonemia, weight gain or loss.
Musculoskeletal: back and neck pain.
Respiratory: bronchitis, dyspnea.
Skin: alopecia, *erythema multiforme, hypersensitivity reactions, Stevens-Johnson syndrome,* rash, photosensitivity reactions, pruritus.
Other: flulike syndrome, infection.

INTERACTIONS

Drug-drug. *Aspirin, erythromycin, felbamate:* May cause valproic acid toxicity. Use together cautiously and monitor drug level.
Benzodiazepines, other CNS depressants: May cause excessive CNS depression. Avoid using together.
Carbamazepine: May cause carbamazepine CNS toxicity; may decrease valproic acid

level and cause loss of seizure control. Use together cautiously, if at all. Monitor patient for seizure activity and toxicity during therapy and for at least 1 month after stopping either drug.
Carbapenem antibiotics (ertapenem, imipenem, meropenem): May decrease valproic acid level and cause loss of seizure control. Consider alternative antimicrobial agent. Monitor levels closely.
Lamotrigine: May increase lamotrigine level and decrease valproate level; serious skin reactions may occur. Monitor levels closely.
Phenobarbital: May increase phenobarbital level; may increase clearance of valproate. Monitor patient closely.
Phenytoin: May increase or decrease phenytoin level; may decrease valproate level. Monitor patient closely.
Rifampin: May decrease valproate level. Monitor level of valproate.
Rufinamide: May increase rufinamide serum concentration. Begin valproate therapy at a low dosage, and titrate to a clinically effective dosage.
TCAs (amitriptyline, nortriptyline): May increase TCA level. Monitor drug level.
Topiramate: May cause hyperammonemia with and without encephalopathy. Concomitant use has been associated with hypothermia. Check blood ammonia levels in patients reporting hypothermia.
Warfarin: May displace warfarin from binding sites. Monitor PT and INR.
Zidovudine: May decrease zidovudine clearance. Avoid using together.
Drug-lifestyle. *Alcohol use:* May cause excessive CNS depression. Discourage use together.

EFFECTS ON LAB TEST RESULTS

• May increase ammonia, ALT, AST, and bilirubin levels.
• May increase eosinophil count and bleeding time. May decrease platelet, RBC, and WBC counts.
• May cause false-positive results for urine ketone levels.

CONTRAINDICATIONS & CAUTIONS

• Contraindicated in patients hypersensitive to drug and in those with hepatic disease or significant hepatic dysfunction, and in patients with a urea cycle disorder (UCD). **Black Box Warning** Patients with hereditary neurometabolic syndromes caused by DNA mutations of the mitochondrial DNA polymerase gamma (*POLG*) gene such as Alpers-Huttenlocher syndrome are at high risk for acute liver failure and fatalities. Drug is contraindicated in patients known to have mitochondrial disorders caused by *POLG* mutations and in children younger than age 2 who are suspected of having a mitochondrial disorder. In patients older than age 2 who are clinically suspected of having a hereditary mitochondrial disease, use only after other anticonvulsants have failed. ■

• Safety and effectiveness of Depakote ER in children younger than age 10 haven't been established.

☉ Alert: Drug is associated with a rare but serious reaction known as DRESS (drug reaction with eosinophilia and systemic symptoms), which may be fatal. DRESS is the presence of three or more symptoms, including cutaneous reactions (rash, exfoliative dermatitis), eosinophilia, fever, lymphadenopathy, and one or more systemic complications (hepatitis, nephritis, pneumonitis, myocarditis, pericarditis). Immediately discontinue drug if DRESS is suspected.

Dialyzable drug: 20%.

⚠ Overdose S&S: Somnolence, heart block, deep coma, hypernatremia.

PREGNANCY-LACTATION-REPRODUCTION
Black Box Warning Avoid use in women who may become pregnant. Valproate can cause teratogenic effects, such as neural tube defects and other organ system malformations. Drug is contraindicated for use in pregnancy for the prevention of migraines. ■

☉ Alert: There is an increased risk of lower cognitive test scores in children born to mothers who took drug during pregnancy. Consider alternative medication in pregnant women unless use of drug is essential. Women of childbearing potential should use effective contraception during therapy.

• Use in pregnant women with epilepsy or bipolar disorder only if other drugs

have failed to control symptoms. Drug is contraindicated for use in pregnancy for reversible conditions not associated with permanent injury or death.

• To prevent major seizures, pregnant women with epilepsy shouldn't discontinue drug abruptly.

• Pregnant patients should enroll in the North American Antiepileptic Drug Pregnancy Registry (1-888-233-2334).

• Drug appears in breast milk. Use cautiously in breast-feeding women.

NURSING CONSIDERATIONS
• Obtain LFT results before starting therapy, and monitor periodically.

☉ Alert: Closely monitor all patients taking or starting antiepileptic drugs for changes in behavior indicating worsening of suicidal thoughts or behavior or depression. Symptoms such as anxiety, agitation, hostility, mania, and hypomania may be precursors to emerging suicidality.

☉ Alert: Dose-related thrombocytopenia can occur. Monitor CBC, platelet count, PT, and INR before starting therapy and at frequent intervals. Decrease dose or discontinue drug if hemorrhage, bruising, or coagulation disorder occurs.

☉ Alert: Monitor patients and immediately report symptoms of DRESS (rash, fever, swollen glands). Discontinue drug if DRESS is suspected.

• Adverse reactions may not be caused by valproic acid alone because it's usually used with other anticonvulsants.

• When converting adults and children age 10 and older with seizures from Depakote to Depakote ER, make sure the extended-release dose is 8% to 20% higher than the regular dose taken previously. See manufacturer's package insert for more details.

• Never withdraw drug suddenly because sudden withdrawal may worsen seizures. Call prescriber at once if adverse reactions develop.

Black Box Warning During treatment, closely monitor patients older than age 2 who are suspected of having a mitochondrial disorder for development of acute liver injury; perform regular clinical assessments and serum liver testing. Perform *POLG* mutation screening in accordance with current clinical practice. ∎

Black Box Warning Fatal hepatotoxicity may follow nonspecific symptoms, such as malaise, fever, anorexia, facial edema, vomiting, weakness, and lethargy. If these symptoms occur during therapy, notify prescriber at once because patient who might be developing hepatic dysfunction must stop taking drug. Perform LFTs before initiating therapy and at frequent intervals, especially during the first 6 months. ∎

Black Box Warning Patients at high risk for fatal hepatotoxicity include those with congenital metabolic disorders, mental retardation, or organic brain disease; those taking multiple anticonvulsants; and children younger than age 2. In children younger than age 2, use with extreme caution and as a sole agent, weighing benefits of therapy against risks. ∎

• Notify prescriber if tremors occur; a dosage reduction may be needed.

• Monitor drug level. Therapeutic level is commonly considered to be 50 to 100 mcg/mL.

• When converting patients from a brand-name drug to a generic drug, use caution because breakthrough seizures may occur.

🕚 **Alert:** Sometimes fatal, hyperammonemic encephalopathy may occur when starting valproate therapy in patients with UCD. Evaluate patients with UCD risk factors before starting valproate therapy. Patients who develop symptoms of unexplained hyperammonemic encephalopathy during valproate therapy should stop drug, undergo prompt appropriate treatment, and be evaluated for underlying UCD.

• **Look alike–sound alike:** Don't confuse Depakote with Depakote ER or Depakene.

PATIENT TEACHING

• Tell patient to take drug with food or milk to reduce adverse GI effects.

• Advise patient not to chew capsules; irritation of mouth and throat may result.

• Tell patient that sprinkle capsules may be either swallowed whole or carefully opened and contents sprinkled on a teaspoonful of soft food. Tell patient to swallow immediately without chewing.

• Tell patient and parents that syrup shouldn't be mixed with carbonated beverages; mixture may be irritating to mouth and throat.

• Tell patient and parents to keep drug out of children's reach.

• Warn patient and parents not to stop drug therapy abruptly.

🕚 **Alert:** Tell patient to immediately report rash (with or without blisters), fever, swollen lymph nodes, mouth ulcers, or skin shedding.

Black Box Warning Cases of life-threatening pancreatitis have been reported in children and adults receiving valproate shortly after initial use, as well as after several years of use. Warn patients and guardians that abdominal pain, nausea, vomiting, and anorexia can be symptoms of pancreatitis that require prompt medical evaluation. ∎

• Advise patient to avoid driving and other potentially hazardous activities that require mental alertness until drug's CNS effects are known.

• Instruct patient or parents to call prescriber if malaise, weakness, lethargy, facial swelling, loss of appetite, or vomiting occurs.

• Tell female patient to call prescriber if she becomes pregnant or plans to become pregnant during therapy.

valsartan
val-SAR-tan

Diovan◊

Therapeutic class: Antihypertensives
Pharmacologic class: Angiotensin II receptor antagonists

AVAILABLE FORMS
Tablets: 40 mg, 80 mg, 160 mg, 320 mg

INDICATIONS & DOSAGES
➤ **Hypertension (used alone or with other antihypertensives)**
Adults: Initially, 80 or 160 mg P.O. once daily. Expect to see a reduction in BP in 2 to 4 weeks. If additional antihypertensive effect is needed, dose may be increased to

---

160 or 320 mg daily, or a diuretic may be added. (Addition of a diuretic has a greater effect than dosage increases beyond 80 mg.) Usual dosage range is 80 to 320 mg daily. *Children ages 6 to 16:* Initially, 1.3 mg/kg P.O. daily (up to 40 mg total). Adjust according to patient response up to 2.7 mg/kg or 160 mg daily.

➤ **New York Heart Association class II to IV HF**
Adults: Initially, 40 mg P.O. b.i.d.; increase as tolerated to 80 mg b.i.d., and then to target dose of 160 mg b.i.d.

➤ **To reduce CV death in stable post-MI patients with left ventricular failure or dysfunction**
Adults: 20 mg P.O. b.i.d. Initial dose may be given as soon as 12 hours after MI. Increase dose to 40 mg b.i.d. within 7 days. Increase subsequent doses, as tolerated, to target dose of 160 mg b.i.d.

ADMINISTRATION
P.O.
● Give drug without regard for food.
● Pharmacists may prepare suspension for children unable to swallow pills.
● Shake suspension at least 10 seconds before pouring. Store suspension at room temperature for 30 days or in refrigerator for 75 days.

ACTION
Blocks the binding of angiotensin II to receptor sites in vascular smooth muscle and the adrenal gland, which inhibits the pressor effects of the RAAS.

Route	Onset	Peak	Duration
P.O.	2 hr	2–4 hr	24 hr

Half-life: 6 hours.

ADVERSE REACTIONS
CNS: dizziness, headache, insomnia, fatigue, vertigo.
CV: edema, hypotension, orthostatic hypotension, syncope.
EENT: rhinitis, sinusitis, pharyngitis, blurred vision.
GI: abdominal pain, diarrhea, nausea, dyspepsia.
GU: renal impairment.
Hematologic: *neutropenia.*

Metabolic: hyperkalemia.
Musculoskeletal: arthralgia, back pain.
Respiratory: URI, cough.
Other: viral infection.

INTERACTIONS
Drug-drug. *ACE inhibitors:* May increase risk of renal dysfunction, hypotension, and hyperkalemia. Avoid use together but, if necessary, closely monitor BP, serum potassium level, and renal function.
Aliskiren: May increase risk of renal impairment, hypotension, and hyperkalemia in diabetic patients and those with moderate to severe renal impairment (GFR less than 60 mL/minute). Concomitant use is contraindicated in diabetic patients. Avoid concomitant use in those with moderate to severe renal impairment.
Canagliflozin: May increase risk of hyperkalemia and hypotension. Monitor therapy.
Lithium: May increase lithium level. Monitor lithium level and patient for toxicity.
NSAIDs: May result in deterioration of renal function in patients who are elderly or volume-depleted or in those with compromised renal function. Monitor renal function. May also decrease antihypertensive effect. Monitor BP.
Potassium supplements, potassium-sparing diuretics, other angiotensin II blockers: May increase potassium level. May also increase creatinine level in HF patients. Avoid using together.
Trimethoprim: May increase risk of hyperkalemia, especially in elderly patients. Closely monitor serum potassium level.
Drug-herb. *Ma huang:* May decrease antihypertensive effects. Discourage use together.
Drug-food. *Salt substitutes containing potassium:* May increase potassium level. May also increase creatinine level in HF patients. Discourage use together.

EFFECTS ON LAB TEST RESULTS
● May increase potassium, BUN, and creatinine levels.
● May decrease neutrophil count.

CONTRAINDICATIONS & CAUTIONS
● Contraindicated in patients hypersensitive to drug or its components.

V

• Angioedema, a rare life-threatening re-action, has been reported. Discontinue drug immediately and treat emergently if angioedema occurs. Don't give drug to patients with history of angioedema.
• Use cautiously in patients with renal or hepatic disease.
• Safety and effectiveness haven't been established in children younger than age 6 and in children of any age with GFR less than 30 mL/minute/1.73 m².
Dialyzable drug: No.
⚠ *Overdose S&S:* Hypotension, tachycardia, bradycardia, decreased level of consciousness, circulatory collapse.

PREGNANCY-LACTATION-REPRODUCTION
Black Box Warning Drugs that act directly on the RAAS can cause injury and even death to the developing fetus. When pregnancy is detected, stop drug as soon as possible. ∎
• It isn't known if drug appears in breast milk. Patient should discontinue breast-feeding or discontinue drug.

NURSING CONSIDERATIONS
• Watch for hypotension. Excessive hypotension can occur when drug is given with high doses of diuretics.
• Correct volume and sodium depletions before starting drug.
• Suspension has 1.6 times greater exposure than tablets. Patients may require a higher dose if switched to tablets.
• Monitor serum BUN, creatinine, and potassium levels.
• *Look alike–sound alike:* Don't confuse Diovan with Zyban.

PATIENT TEACHING
• Tell women of childbearing potential to notify prescriber if pregnancy occurs. Drug will need to be stopped.
• Advise patient that drug may be taken without regard for food.
• Advise patient to report all adverse effects, especially dizziness upon standing or other signs and symptoms of hypotension.

vancomycin hydrochloride
van-koh-MYE-sin

Vancocin

Therapeutic class: Antibiotics
Pharmacologic class: Glycopeptides

AVAILABLE FORMS
Capsules: 125 mg, 250 mg
Powder for injection: 500-mg vials, 750-mg vials, 1-g vials
Premixed: 500 mg/100 mL, 750 mg/150 mL, 1 g/200 mL

INDICATIONS & DOSAGES
Adjust-a-dose (for all indications): In renal insufficiency, adjust dosage based on degree of renal impairment, drug level, severity of infection, and susceptibility of causative organism. Initially, give 15 mg/kg, and adjust subsequent doses as needed.
➤ **Serious or severe infections when other antibiotics are ineffective or contraindicated, including those caused by MRSA, *Staphylococcus epidermidis*, or diphtheroid organisms**
Adults: 500 mg I.V. every 6 hours or 1 g I.V. every 12 hours.
Children: 10 mg/kg I.V. every 6 hours.
Neonates and young infants: 15 mg/kg I.V. loading dose; then 10 mg/kg I.V. every 12 hours if child is younger than age 1 week or 10 mg/kg I.V. every 8 hours if older than 1 week but younger than 1 month.
Elderly patients: 15 mg/kg I.V. loading dose. Subsequent doses are based on renal function and drug levels.
➤ **CDAD**
Adults: 125 mg P.O. every 6 hours for 10 days.
Children: 40 mg/kg/day P.O. in three or four divided doses for 7 to 10 days. Maximum daily dose is 2 g.
➤ **Staphylococcal enterocolitis**
Adults: 500 mg to 2 g P.O. in three or four divided doses daily for 7 to 10 days.
Children: 40 mg/kg/day P.O. in divided doses every 6 hours for 7 to 10 days. Maximum daily dose is 2 g.

ADMINISTRATION

P.O.

● Obtain specimen for culture and sensitivity tests before giving. Because of the emergence of vancomycin-resistant enterococci, reserve use of drug for treatment of serious infections caused by gram-positive bacteria resistant to beta-lactam anti-infectives.

🔴 *Alert:* Oral form is ineffective for systemic infections.

● Oral solution is stable for 2 weeks if refrigerated.

I.V.

🔴 *Alert:* Obtain specimen for culture and sensitivity tests before giving. Because of the emergence of vancomycin-resistant enterococci, reserve use of drug for treatment of serious infections caused by gram-positive bacteria resistant to beta-lactam anti-infectives.

▼ This form is ineffective for CDAD. Reconstitute 500-mg vial with 10 mL or 1-g vial with 20 mL sterile water for injection to provide a solution containing 50 mg/mL.

▼ For infusion, further dilute 500 mg in 100 mL or 1 g in 200 mL NSS for injection or D_5W, and infuse over 60 minutes; if dose is greater than 1 g, infuse over 90 minutes.

🔴 *Alert:* Rapid infusion (over several minutes) has been associated with hypotension, shock and, rarely, cardiac arrest. Check site daily for phlebitis and irritation. Severe irritation and necrosis can result from extravasation.

▼ Refrigerate solution after reconstitution and use within 14 days.

▼ **Incompatibilities:** Beta-lactam antibiotics, many other drugs (vancomycin has a low pH).

ACTION

Hinders bacterial cell-wall synthesis, damaging the bacterial plasma membrane and making the cell more vulnerable to osmotic pressure. Also interferes with RNA synthesis.

Route	Onset	Peak	Duration
P.O.	Unknown	Unknown	Unknown
I.V.	Immediate	Immediate	Unknown

Half-life: 6 hours.

ADVERSE REACTIONS

CNS: fever, pain, headache, fatigue.
CV: hypotension, thrombophlebitis at injection site.
EENT: ototoxicity, tinnitus.
GI: *pseudomembranous colitis,* nausea, abdominal pain, vomiting, diarrhea, flatulence.
GU: *nephrotoxicity.*
Hematologic: *leukopenia, neutropenia,* eosinophilia.
Metabolic: hypokalemia.
Respiratory: dyspnea, wheezing.
Skin: red-man syndrome (with rapid I.V. infusion).
Other: *anaphylaxis,* chills, superinfection.

INTERACTIONS

Drug-drug. *Aminoglycosides, amphotericin B, cisplatin, pentamidine:* May increase risk of nephrotoxicity and ototoxicity. Monitor renal function and hearing function tests.
Nondepolarizing muscle relaxants: May enhance neuromuscular blockade. Monitor patient closely.
NSAIDs: May increase vancomycin serum concentration. Monitor therapy.

EFFECTS ON LAB TEST RESULTS

● May increase BUN and creatinine levels. May decrease potassium level.
● May increase eosinophil count. May decrease neutrophil and WBC counts.

CONTRAINDICATIONS & CAUTIONS

● Contraindicated in patients hypersensitive to drug or its components.
● Use cautiously in patients receiving other neurotoxic, nephrotoxic, or ototoxic drugs; in patients older than age 60; and in those with impaired hepatic or renal function, hearing loss, or allergies to other antibiotics.
Dialyzable drug: No.

PREGNANCY-LACTATION-REPRODUCTION

● It isn't known if drug causes fetal harm. Use during pregnancy only if clearly needed.
● Drug appears in breast milk. Patient should discontinue breast-feeding or discontinue drug.

V

NURSING CONSIDERATIONS

• Obtain hearing evaluation before and during prolonged therapy.
• Monitor patient's fluid balance and watch for oliguria and cloudy urine.
• Monitor patient carefully for red-man syndrome, which can occur if drug is infused too rapidly. Signs and symptoms include maculopapular rash on face, neck, trunk, and limbs and pruritus and hypotension caused by histamine release. If wheezing, urticaria, or pain and muscle spasm of the chest and back occur, stop infusion and notify prescriber.
• Don't give drug I.M.
• Assess renal function (BUN, creatinine level and CrCl, urinalysis, and urine output) before and during therapy.
• Patients with renal dysfunction need dosage adjustment. Monitor peak and trough blood levels to adjust I.V. dosage requirements.
• Monitor patient for signs and symptoms of superinfection. CDAD can occur up to 2 months after therapy ends.
• For staphylococcal endocarditis, give for at least 4 weeks.
• *Look alike–sound alike:* Don't confuse vancomycin with clindamycin, gentamicin, or Vibramycin.

PATIENT TEACHING

• Tell patient to take entire amount of drug exactly as directed, even after he feels better.
• Instruct patient receiving drug I.V. to report discomfort at I.V. insertion site.
• Tell patient to report ringing in ears.
• Tell patient to report adverse reactions to prescriber immediately.

vardenafil hydrochloride
var-DEN-ah-fill

Levitra✥, Staxyn

Therapeutic class: Erectile dysfunction drugs
Pharmacologic class: PDE5 inhibitors

AVAILABLE FORMS

ODTs 🆑: 10 mg
Tablets (film-coated): 2.5 mg, 5 mg, 10 mg, 20 mg

INDICATIONS & DOSAGES

➤ **Erectile dysfunction**
Adults: 10 mg P.O. as a single dose, as needed, 1 hour before sexual activity. Dosage range is 5 to 20 mg, based on effectiveness and tolerance. Maximum, 10 mg/day (Staxyn) or 20 mg once daily (Levitra).
Adjust-a-dose: For patients with moderate hepatic impairment (Child-Pugh class B) and patients age 65 and older, first dose of Levitra is 5 mg daily, as needed. Don't exceed 10 mg daily in patients with hepatic impairment. Don't use Staxyn in patients with moderate or severe hepatic impairment (Child-Pugh class B or C).

ADMINISTRATION
P.O.
• Give drug without regard for food.
• Don't split or crush ODTs.
• Place ODT on the tongue to disintegrate. Have patient take without water.

ACTION

Increases cyclic guanosine monophosphate levels, prolongs smooth muscle relaxation, and promotes blood flow into the corpus cavernosum.

Route	Onset	Peak	Duration
P.O.	60 min	30–120 min	Unknown

Half-life: 4 to 6 hours.

ADVERSE REACTIONS

CNS: headache, dizziness.
CV: flushing, hypotension, tachycardia.
EENT: blurred vision, decrease or loss of hearing, tinnitus, rhinitis, sinusitis, nasal congestion.
GI: dyspepsia, nausea.
Musculoskeletal: back pain.
Other: flulike syndrome.

INTERACTIONS

Drug-drug. *Alpha blockers:* May enhance hypotensive effects. Start concomitant treatment only if patient is stable on alpha-blocker therapy.
Antiarrhythmics of class IA (quinidine, procainamide) and class III (amiodarone, sotalol): May prolong QTc interval. Avoid using together.

Reactions in bold italics are *life-threatening*. Interactions may have a *rapid onset* or a *delayed onset*.

Guanylate cyclase stimulators (riociguat), nitrates: May enhance hypotensive effects. Use together is contraindicated.

Potent and moderate CYP3A4 inhibitors (erythromycin, indinavir, itraconazole, ketoconazole, ritonavir): May increase vardenafil level. Reduce vardenafil dosage. If taken with ritonavir, reduce dose and extend dosing interval to once every 72 hours.

Drug-food. *Grapefruit, grapefruit juice:* May increase vardenafil level. Avoid use together.

High-fat meals: May reduce peak level of drug. Discourage use with a high-fat meal.

Drug-lifestyle. *Alcohol use:* May increase risk of hypotension and orthostasis. Discourage use together.

EFFECTS ON LAB TEST RESULTS

● May increase CK and liver transaminase levels.

CONTRAINDICATIONS & CAUTIONS

● Contraindicated in patients hypersensitive to drug or its components and in those taking nitrates.

● Contraindicated in patients with unstable angina, hypotension (systolic less than 90 mm Hg), uncontrolled hypertension (over 170/110 mm Hg), stroke, life-threatening arrhythmia, an MI within past 6 months, severe cardiac failure, severe hepatic impairment (Child-Pugh class C), ESRD requiring dialysis, congenital QTc-interval prolongation, or hereditary degenerative retinal disorders.

● Use cautiously in patients with bleeding disorders or significant peptic ulceration.

● Use cautiously in those with anatomic penis abnormalities or conditions that predispose patient to priapism (such as sickle cell anemia, multiple myeloma, or leukemia).

● May cause vision loss and visual disturbances. Use cautiously in patients with or at increased risk for nonarteritic ischemic optic neuropathy, "crowded optic disc."

Dialyzable drug: Unlikely.

⚠ *Overdose S&S:* Back pain or myalgia, abnormal vision.

PREGNANCY-LACTATION-REPRODUCTION

● Drug isn't indicated for use in women.

NURSING CONSIDERATIONS

⚠ *Alert:* Sexual activity may increase cardiac risk. Evaluate patient's cardiac risk before he starts taking drug.

● Before patient starts drug, assess for underlying causes of erectile dysfunction.

● Transient decreases in supine BP may occur.

● Prolonged erections and priapism may occur.

PATIENT TEACHING

● Tell patient that drug doesn't protect against sexually transmitted diseases and that he should use protective measures.

● Tell patient to notify prescriber about vision or hearing changes.

● Urge patient to seek immediate medical care if erection lasts more than 4 hours.

● Tell patient to take drug 60 minutes before anticipated sexual activity. Explain that drug has no effect without sexual stimulation.

● Warn patient not to change dosage unless directed by prescriber.

● Tell patient to stop drug and seek medical attention if he experiences sudden vision loss in one or both eyes or sudden decrease in or loss of hearing.

● Tell patient not to split, crush, or chew ODTs.

varenicline tartrate
vah-RENN-ih-kleen

Chantix✐

Therapeutic class: Smoking cessation aids
Pharmacologic class: Nicotinic acetylcholine receptor partial agonists

AVAILABLE FORMS
Tablets: 0.5 mg, 1 mg

INDICATIONS & DOSAGES
➤ **Smoking cessation**
Adults: Starting 1 week before patient stops smoking, give 0.5 mg P.O. once daily on days 1 through 3. Days 4 through 7, give 0.5 mg P.O. b.i.d. Day 8 through the end of week 12, give 1 mg P.O. b.i.d. If patient successfully stops smoking, give an additional

12-week course to help with long-term success.

Adjust-a-dose: In patient with severe renal impairment, 0.5 mg P.O. once daily. Adjust as needed to maximum of 0.5 mg b.i.d. In patient with ESRD who is undergoing dialysis, 0.5 mg once daily.

ADMINISTRATION

P.O.

● Give drug with full glass of water after a meal.

ACTION

Blocks the effects of nicotine by binding at alpha$_4$ beta$_2$ neuronal nicotinic acetylcholine receptors. Drug also provides some of nicotine's effects to ease withdrawal.

Route	Onset	Peak	Duration
P.O.	4 days	3–4 hr	24 hr

Half-life: 24 hours.

ADVERSE REACTIONS

CNS: abnormal dreams, headache, insomnia, altered attention or emotions, asthenia, depression, drowsiness, fatigue, irritability, lethargy, malaise, nightmares, sleep disorder, somnolence, suicidal ideation.
CV: chest pain, edema, hot flush, hypertension.
EENT: altered taste.
GI: nausea, abdominal pain, constipation, diarrhea, dry mouth, dyspepsia, flatulence, vomiting, GERD.
Metabolic: increased appetite, increased appetite.
Respiratory: dyspnea, URI.
Skin: rash.

INTERACTIONS

Drug-drug. *Cimetidine:* May decrease renal clearance of varenicline. Monitor patient closely.
Nicotine-replacement therapy: May increase nausea, vomiting, dizziness, dyspepsia, and fatigue. Monitor patient closely.
Drug-lifestyle. ◑ *Alert: Alcohol use:* May decrease alcohol tolerance, with symptoms of increased drunkenness, unusual or aggressive behavior, or amnesia. Caution patient to reduce amount of alcohol con-

sumed until ability to tolerate alcohol is known.

EFFECTS ON LAB TEST RESULTS

● May increase LFT values.

CONTRAINDICATIONS & CAUTIONS

● Contraindicated in patients hypersensitive to drug or its components.
Black Box Warning Consider risks versus benefits before use. Drug increases the likelihood of abstinence from smoking for as long as 1 year. Health benefits of quitting smoking are immediate and substantial. ■
Black Box Warning Serious neuropsychiatric events have been reported with use of this drug. Carefully weigh risks versus benefits of smoking cessation. ■
◑ *Alert:* Drug may be associated with increased risk of CV events (angina, MI, need for coronary revascularization, new diagnosis of peripheral vascular disease [PVD], or admission for a procedure to treat PVD) in patients who have CV disease. Consider risks and benefits before prescribing.
◑ *Alert:* Drug may increase risk of seizures. Use cautiously in patients with a history of seizures or who are at increased risk for seizures.
● Use cautiously in elderly patients and in patients with severe renal impairment or preexisting psychiatric illness.
● Not recommended for use in children younger than age 18.
Dialyzable drug: Yes.

PREGNANCY-LACTATION-REPRODUCTION

● There are no adequate studies in pregnant women. Use during pregnancy only if potential benefit justifies potential fetal risk.
● It isn't known if drug appears in breast milk. Patient should discontinue breastfeeding or discontinue drug.

NURSING CONSIDERATIONS

● Assess patient's readiness and motivation to stop smoking.
● Encourage patient who is motivated to quit but didn't succeed during prior therapy or who relapsed after treatment, to make another attempt once factors contributing to the failed attempt have been identified and addressed.

Reactions in bold italics are *life-threatening*. Interactions may have a *rapid onset* or a *delayed onset*.

Black Box Warning Monitor patient for changes in behavior, agitation, depressed mood, hostility, suicidal ideation, suicidal behavior, and worsening of preexisting psychiatric illness and report immediately. ■

● Notify prescriber if patient develops intolerable adverse reactions such as nausea; dosage reduction may be needed.

● Life-threatening angioedema and serious skin reactions have been reported. Discontinue drug for such signs and symptoms as swelling of the face, mouth, neck, or extremities or rash with mucosal lesions.

● Temporarily monitor levels of drugs (theophylline, warfarin, and insulin) after patient stops smoking to be sure levels are still within therapeutic range.

PATIENT TEACHING

● Provide patient with educational materials and needed counseling.

● Instruct patient to choose a date to stop smoking and to begin treatment 1 week before this date. Or, patient can begin drug, then quit smoking between days 8 and 35.

● Advise patient to take each dose with a full glass of water after eating.

● Teach patient to gradually increase the dose over the first week to a target of 1 mg in the morning and 1 mg in the evening.

🟉 **Alert:** Caution patient that drug can affect reaction to alcohol. Advise patient to reduce amount of alcohol consumed until his or her alcohol tolerance is known.

🟉 **Alert:** Warn patient to stop drug and seek medical attention if seizures occur.

● Advise patient to discontinue drug and seek immediate medical care if swelling of the face, mouth, extremities, and neck or a rash with mucosal lesions develops.

● Explain that nausea and insomnia are common and usually temporary. Urge patient to contact prescriber if adverse effects are persistently troubling; a dosage reduction may help.

● Urge patient to continue trying to abstain from smoking if early lapses occur after successfully quitting.

Tell patient that dosages of other drugs being taken may need adjustment when patient stops smoking.

● Advise patient to use caution when driving or operating machinery until effects of drug are known.

Black Box Warning Instruct patient and family to monitor patient for changes in behavior and mood, including agitation, depression, hostility, suicidal ideation or behavior, and worsening of preexisting psychiatric illness; stop drug and report changes to health care provider immediately. ■

● If female patient plans to become pregnant or to breast-feed, explain the risks of smoking and the risks and benefits of taking drug to aid smoking cessation.

venetoclax
See NEW DRUGS for information.

venlafaxine hydrochloride
vin-lah-FACKS-in

Effexor XR🖉

Therapeutic class: Antidepressants
Pharmacologic class: SSNRIs

AVAILABLE FORMS
Capsules (extended-release) 🔵: 37.5 mg, 75 mg, 150 mg
Tablets: 25 mg, 37.5 mg, 50 mg, 75 mg, 100 mg
Tablets (extended-release) 🔵: 37.5 mg, 75 mg, 150 mg, 225 mg

INDICATIONS & DOSAGES
Adjust-a-dose (for all indications): For patients with mild to moderate renal impairment (CrCl 30 to 89 mL/minute), reduce daily amount by 25% in patients taking immediate-release tablets. Reduce by 25% to 50% in those taking extended-release form. For those with severe renal impairment (CrCl less than 30 mL/minute) or on hemodialysis, reduce total daily dose by 50% or more and withhold dose until dialysis is completed. For patients with mild to moderate hepatic impairment (Child-Pugh score 5 to 9), reduce daily amount by 50%. For patients with severe hepatic impairment (Child-Pugh score 10 to 15) or cirrhosis, reduce total daily dose by 50% or more.

V

🍁Canada   ◇OTC   ◆ Off-label use   🖉 Photoguide   🔵 Do not crush   *Liquid contains alcohol.

➤ Depression
Adults: Initially, 75 mg (immediate-release) P.O. daily in two or three divided doses with food. Increase as tolerated and needed by 75 mg daily every 4 days. For moderately depressed outpatients, usual maximum is 225 mg daily; in certain severely depressed patients, dose may be as high as 375 mg daily. For extended-release capsules, 75 mg P.O. daily in a single dose. For some patients, it may be desirable to start at 37.5 mg P.O. daily for 4 to 7 days before increasing to 75 mg daily. Dosage may be increased by 75 mg daily every 4 days to maximum of 225 mg daily.

➤ Generalized anxiety disorder
Adults: Initially, 75 mg extended-release capsule P.O. daily in a single dose. For some patients, it may be desirable to start at 37.5 mg P.O. daily for 4 to 7 days before increasing to 75 mg daily. Dosage may be increased by 75 mg daily every 4 days to maximum of 225 mg daily.

➤ Panic disorder
Adults: Initially, 37.5 mg extended-release capsule P.O. daily for 1 week, then increase dose to 75 mg daily. If patient isn't responding, may increase dose by up to 75 mg/day in no less than weekly intervals, as needed, to a maximum dose of 225 mg daily.

➤ Social anxiety disorder
Adults: Initially, 75 mg extended-release capsule P.O. daily as a single dose.

➤ Hot flashes ♦
Adults: 37.5 to 150 mg P.O. daily in one dose or in two divided doses (immediate or extended-release).

ADMINISTRATION
P.O.
- Give drug with food and a full glass of water.
- May give pellet-filled capsules by carefully opening capsule and sprinkling the pellets on a spoonful of applesauce. Patient should swallow applesauce immediately without chewing, then follow with a glass of cool water to ensure that all pellets are swallowed.

ACTION
May increase the amount of norepinephrine, serotonin, or both in the CNS by blocking their reuptake by the presynaptic neurons.

Route	Onset	Peak	Duration
P.O. (immediate-release)	Unknown	2 hr	Unknown
P.O. (extended-release)	Unknown	5½ hr	Unknown

Half-life: 3 to 7 hours.

ADVERSE REACTIONS
CNS: asthenia, headache, palpitations, somnolence, dizziness, nervousness, insomnia, *suicidal behavior,* anxiety, tremor, abnormal dreams, paresthesia, agitation.
CV: hypertension, tachycardia, vasodilation, chest pain.
EENT: blurred vision, mydriasis.
GI: nausea, constipation, dry mouth, anorexia, vomiting, diarrhea, dyspepsia, flatulence.
GU: abnormal ejaculation, erectile dysfunction, anorgasmia, urinary frequency, impaired urination.
Metabolic: decreased libido, weight gain, weight loss, increased appetite, hypercholesterolemia.
Skin: diaphoresis, ecchymosis, rash.
Other: yawning, chills, weakness.

INTERACTIONS
Drug-drug. *Aspirin, NSAIDs:* May increase antiplatelet effect of aspirin and NSAIDs. Monitor patient for increased risk of bleeding.
Lithium: May increase serotonergic effect of drug. Serotonin syndrome (restlessness, hallucinations, loss of coordination, fast heartbeat, rapid changes in BP, increased body temperature, hyperreflexia, nausea, vomiting, and diarrhea) may occur. Monitor patient closely.
MAO inhibitors, such as phenelzine, selegiline, tranylcypromine: May cause serotonin syndrome and signs and symptoms resembling neuroleptic malignant syndrome. Avoid using within 14 days of MAO inhibitor therapy.
Methylene blue, linezolid: May cause serotonin syndrome. Use with extreme caution and monitor patient closely.

Reactions in bold italics are *life-threatening*. Interactions may have a *rapid onset* or a *delayed onset*.

*Other serotonergic drugs (fentanyl, meperidine, **tramadol**, trazodone):* May cause serotonin syndrome. Monitor patient closely.

Triptans: May cause serotonin syndrome or neuroleptic malignant syndrome–like reactions. Use cautiously and with increased monitoring at the start of therapy and with dose increase.

Warfarin: May increase PT, PTT, or INR. Monitor these lab values and patient closely.

Drug-herb. *St. John's wort:* May cause serotonin syndrome. Monitor patient closely.

Drug-lifestyle. *Alcohol use:* May increase mental and psychomotor impairment. Avoid alcohol.

EFFECTS ON LAB TEST RESULTS
• May cause false-positive urine immunoassay screening tests for phencyclidine and amphetamine.
• May increase cholesterol and triglyceride levels.

CONTRAINDICATIONS & CAUTIONS
• Contraindicated in patients hypersensitive to drug or within 14 days of stopping MAO inhibitor therapy. Don't start MAO inhibitor less than 7 days after stopping venlafaxine.
Black Box Warning Venlafaxine isn't approved for use in children. ■
◑ Alert: Concomitant use with serotonergic drugs, linezolid, or methylene blue can cause serotonin syndrome. Use drug with linezolid or methylene blue only for life-threatening or urgent conditions when the potential benefits outweigh the risks of toxicity.

Use cautiously in patients with renal impairment, diseases or conditions that could affect hemodynamic responses or metabolism, and in those with history of mania or seizures.

May trigger an angle-closure attack. Use cautiously in patients at risk for acute narrow-angle glaucoma.

Hyponatremia can occur, which may be a result of SIADH. Elderly, volume-depleted patients and those taking diuretics are at increased risk. Discontinue drug if patient develops symptomatic hyponatremia.
Dialyzable drug: Unlikely.

⚠ Overdose S&S: Altered level of consciousness, tachycardia, mydriasis, seizures, vomiting, ECG changes, hypotension, liver necrosis, rhabdomyolysis, serotonin syndrome, vertigo, death.

PREGNANCY-LACTATION-REPRODUCTION
• There are no adequate studies in pregnant women. Use during pregnancy only if clearly needed and potential benefit justifies potential risks.
◑ Alert: Neonates exposed to drug during the late third trimester have developed complications (sometimes immediately upon delivery) that require respiratory support, tube feedings, and prolonged hospitalization.
• Drug may appear in breast milk. Patient should discontinue breast-feeding or discontinue drug.

NURSING CONSIDERATIONS
◑ Alert: Closely monitor patients being treated for depression for signs and symptoms of clinical worsening and suicidal ideation, especially at the beginning of therapy and with dosage adjustments. Symptoms may include agitation, insomnia, anxiety, aggressiveness, or panic attacks.
Black Box Warning Drug may increase the risk of suicidal thinking and behavior in children, adolescents, and young adults ages 18 to 24, especially during the first few months of treatment, especially those with major depressive disorder or other psychiatric disorder. ■
◑ Alert: Sudden discontinuation or abrupt decrease in venlafaxine dose can lead to serotonin withdrawal (agitation, confusion, flulike symptoms, sensory disturbances, tremor). Reduce dose gradually and watch for symptoms.
◑ Alert: If linezolid or methylene blue must be given, stop venlafaxine and monitor patient for serotonin toxicity for 2 weeks or until 24 hours after last dose of methylene blue or linezolid, whichever comes first. May resume serotonergic psychiatric drugs 24 hours after last dose of methylene blue or linezolid.
• Carefully monitor BP. Drug therapy may cause sustained, dose-dependent increases in BP.

V

• Monitor patient's weight, particularly underweight, depressed patients.

⚠ *Alert:* Combining triptans with an SSRI or an SSNRI may cause serotonin syndrome or neuroleptic malignant syndrome-like reactions. Signs and symptoms of serotonin syndrome may include restlessness, hallucinations, loss of coordination, fast heartbeat, rapid changes in BP, increased body temperature, overactive reflexes, nausea, vomiting, and diarrhea. Serotonin syndrome may be more likely to occur when starting or increasing the dose of triptan, SSRI, or SSNRI.

PATIENT TEACHING

• If medication is to be stopped, inform patient who has received drug for 6 weeks or longer that drug will be stopped gradually by tapering dosage over a 2-week period, as instructed by prescriber. Patient shouldn't abruptly stop taking the drug.

Black Box Warning Warn family members to closely monitor patient for signs of worsening condition or suicidal ideation. ∎

• Warn patient to avoid hazardous activities that require alertness and good coordination until effects of drug are known.

• Tell patient to avoid alcohol and to consult prescriber before taking other prescription or OTC drugs.

• Teach patient to recognize and immediately report signs and symptoms of serotonin toxicity (fever, mental status changes, muscle twitching, excessive sweating, shivering or shaking, diarrhea, loss of coordination).

• Advise female patient of childbearing potential to contact prescriber if she becomes pregnant or intends to become pregnant during therapy or if she's breast-feeding.

• Tell patient to take each dose with food and a full glass of water.

• Tell patient not to crush, chew, or place extended-release capsules or tablets in water. If patient can't swallow capsule whole, advise patient to carefully open capsule and sprinkle contents on a spoonful of applesauce, mix and take immediately without chewing pellets, then follow with a full glass of water.

verapamil hydrochloride
ver-AP-a-mill

Apo-Verap✶, Calan⬦, Calan SR, Covera-HS, Isoptin SR✶, Novo-Veramil✶, Verelan⬦, Verelan PM

Therapeutic class: Antihypertensives
Pharmacologic class: Calcium channel blockers

AVAILABLE FORMS

Capsules (extended-release) ⓞⓝⓒ: 100 mg, 120 mg, 180 mg, 200 mg, 240 mg, 300 mg
Capsules (sustained-release) ⓞⓝⓒ: 120 mg, 180 mg, 240 mg, 360 mg
Injection: 2.5 mg/mL
Tablets: 40 mg, 80 mg, 120 mg
Tablets (extended-release) ⓞⓝⓒ: 120 mg, 180 mg, 240 mg
Tablets (sustained-release) ⓞⓝⓒ: 120 mg, 180 mg, 240 mg

INDICATIONS & DOSAGES

Adjust-a-dose (for all indications): In patients with severe liver dysfunction, give 30% of dose.

➤ **Vasospastic angina (Prinzmetal or variant angina); unstable angina; classic chronic, stable angina pectoris; chronic atrial fibrillation**
Adults: Starting dose is 80 to 120 mg P.O. t.i.d. Increase dosage at daily or weekly intervals as needed. Some patients may require up to 480 mg daily. Don't exceed 480 mg/day. For Covera-HS, initial dose is 180 mg/day P.O. at bedtime. Dosage range i 180 to 540 mg/day P.O. at bedtime.

➤ **To prevent paroxysmal supraventricular tachycardia**
Adults: 80 to 120 mg (immediate-release) P.O. t.i.d. or q.i.d.

➤ **Atrial flutter/atrial fibrillation; supraventricular arrhythmias**
Adults: 0.075 to 0.15 mg/kg (5 to 10 mg) by I.V. push over 2 minutes with ECG and BP monitoring. Repeat dose of 0.15 mg/kg (10 mg) in 30 minutes if response is inadequate.
Children ages 1 to 15: Give 0.1 to 0.3 mg/l as I.V. bolus over 2 minutes; not to exceed

5 mg. Repeat dose in 30 minutes if response is inadequate.

Children younger than age 1: Give 0.1 to 0.2 mg/kg as I.V. bolus over 2 minutes with continuous ECG monitoring. Repeat dose in 30 minutes if response is inadequate.

➤ **Digitalized patients with chronic atrial fibrillation or flutter**

Adults: 240 to 320 mg P.O. daily, in three or four divided doses.

➤ **Hypertension**

Adults: 240 mg extended-release tablet (Verelan) P.O. once daily in the morning. If response isn't adequate, may increase by 120 mg daily (maximum, 480 mg). If using Verelan PM, 200 mg P.O. daily at bedtime. May increase to 300 mg at bedtime if response is inadequate. Maximum dose is 400 mg. If using Covera-HS, 180 mg P.O. daily at bedtime. May increase to 240 mg daily if response is inadequate. Subsequent dosage adjustments may be made in 120-mg increments up to a maximum of 480 mg at bedtime. If using Calan SR, give 180 mg P.O. in the morning. Evaluate weekly and approximately 24 hours after previous dose. May increase as follows: 240 mg each morning, 180 mg each morning plus 180 mg each evening, or 240 mg each morning plus 120 mg each evening; 240 mg every 12 hours. For immediate-release, 80 mg P.O. t.i.d.

ADMINISTRATION

P.O.

● Pellet-filled capsules may be given by carefully opening the capsule and sprinkling the pellets on a spoonful of applesauce. This should be swallowed immediately without chewing, followed by a glass of cool water to ensure that all the pellets are swallowed.

● Give long-acting forms of the drug whole; don't crush or break tablet.

I.V.

▼ This form is contraindicated in patients receiving I.V. beta blockers and in those with ventricular tachycardia.

▼ Inject directly into a vein or into the tubing of a free-flowing, compatible solution, such as D5W, half-NSS, NSS, Ringer solution, or lactated Ringer solution.

▼ Give doses over at least 2 minutes (3 minutes in elderly patients) to minimize the risk of adverse reactions.

▼ Monitor ECG and BP continuously.

▼ **Incompatibilities:** Albumin, amphotericin B, hydralazine, sodium bicarbonate, solutions with a pH greater than 6, sulfamethoxazole–trimethoprim.

ACTION

Not clearly defined. A calcium channel blocker that inhibits calcium ion influx across cardiac and smooth-muscle cells, thus decreasing myocardial contractility and oxygen demand; it also dilates coronary arteries and arterioles.

Route	Onset	Peak	Duration
P.O.	30 min	1–2 hr	8–10 hr
P.O. (extended)	30 min	5–9 hr	24 hr
I.V.	Immediate	1–5 min	1–6 hr

Half-life: 6 to 12 hours.

ADVERSE REACTIONS

CNS: dizziness, headache, asthenia, fatigue, sleep disturbances.

CV: transient hypotension, *HF, bradycardia, AV block, ventricular asystole, ventricular fibrillation,* peripheral edema.

GI: constipation, nausea, diarrhea, dyspepsia.

Respiratory: dyspnea, pharyngitis, *pulmonary edema,* rhinitis, sinusitis, URI.

Skin: rash.

INTERACTIONS

Drug-drug. *Beta blockers, digoxin:* May increase digoxin level and effects of both drugs. Monitor digoxin level and cardiac function closely and decrease doses as needed.

Amiodarone: May cause bradycardia and decrease cardiac output. Monitor patient closely.

Antihypertensives, quinidine: May cause hypotension. Monitor BP.

Barbiturates (phenobarbital): May increase verapamil clearance. Monitor response and adjust verapamil dose as needed.

Carbamazepine: May increase levels of carbamazepine. Monitor patient for toxicity and adjust dosage as needed.

V

Cyclosporine: May increase cyclosporine level. Monitor cyclosporine level.

Disopyramide, flecainide: May cause HF. Avoid using together.

Dofetilide: May increase dofetilide level. Avoid using together.

HMG-CoA reductase inhibitors (atorvastatin, lovastatin, simvastatin): May elevate plasma concentrations of these drugs. If coadministration can't be avoided, administer conservative dose of the HMG-CoA reductase inhibitor.

Inhalation anesthetics (enflurane): May potentiate cardiac effects. Titrate doses carefully to avoid excessive CV depression.

Lithium: May decrease or increase lithium level. Monitor lithium level.

Macrolide antibiotics (clarithromycin, erythromycin): May increase erythromycin and verapamil levels. Monitor cardiac function closely and adjust doses as needed.

Neuromuscular blockers: May potentiate the activity of these drugs. Monitor neuromuscular function, and adjust dosages of either drug as needed.

Phenytoin: May decrease effects of verapamil. Monitor patient closely and adjust dose as needed.

Rifampin: May decrease oral bioavailability of verapamil. Monitor patient for lack of effect.

Sirolimus, tacrolimus: May increase levels of these drugs. Monitor drug levels closely and adjust dosage as needed.

Theophylline: May decrease clearance of theophylline. Monitor for signs of theophylline toxicity.

Drug-herb. *St. John's wort:* May decrease drug level and effect. Discourage use together.

Drug-food. *Grapefruit juice:* May increase drug level. Discourage use together.

Drug-lifestyle. *Alcohol use:* May increase serum concentration of alcohol. Discourage use together.

EFFECTS ON LAB TEST RESULTS
● May increase ALT, AST, alkaline phosphatase, and bilirubin levels.

CONTRAINDICATIONS & CAUTIONS
● Contraindicated in patients hypersensitive to drug and in those with severe left ventricular dysfunction, cardiogenic shock, second- or third-degree AV block or sick sinus syndrome except in presence of functioning pacemaker, atrial flutter or fibrillation and accessory bypass tract syndrome, severe HF (unless secondary to therapy), and severe hypotension.

● I.V. form is contraindicated in patients receiving I.V. beta blockers and in those with ventricular tachycardia.

● Use cautiously in elderly patients and in those with increased ICP or hepatic or renal disease.

Dialyzable drug: No.

⚠ **Overdose S&S:** Hypotension, bradycardia, arrhythmias, hyperglycemia, depressed mental status, noncardiogenic pulmonary edema, increasing AV block.

PREGNANCY-LACTATION-REPRODUCTION
● There are no adequate studies in pregnant women. Use during pregnancy only if clearly needed. Fetal monitoring is recommended.

● Drug appears in breast milk. Some manufacturers recommend that patients stop breast-feeding.

NURSING CONSIDERATIONS
● Patients receiving beta blockers should receive lower doses of this drug. Monitor these patients closely.

● Frequently monitor PR interval.

● Monitor BP at the start of therapy and during dosage adjustments. Assist patient with walking because dizziness may occur.

● If signs and symptoms of HF occur, such as swelling of hands and feet and shortness of breath, notify prescriber.

● Monitor renal function test and LFT results during prolonged treatment.

● *Look alike–sound alike:* Don't confuse Verelan with Vivarin or Voltaren.

PATIENT TEACHING
● Instruct patient to take oral form of drug exactly as prescribed.

● Tell patient that long-acting forms shouldn't be crushed or chewed.

● Caution patient against abruptly stopping drug.

● If patient continues nitrate therapy during oral verapamil dosage adjustment, urge

continued compliance. S.L. nitroglycerin may be taken, as needed, for acute chest pain.
• Drug significantly inhibits alcohol elimination. Advise patient to avoid or severely limit alcohol use.
• Inform patient taking Covera-HS that the outer shell of the drug may be excreted in feces.

vigabatrin
veye-gah-BA-trin

Sabril

Therapeutic class: Anticonvulsants
Pharmacologic class: GABA transaminase inhibitors

AVAILABLE FORMS
Powder for oral solution: 500 mg
Tablets: 500 mg

INDICATIONS & DOSAGES
➤ **Refractory complex partial seizures in patients with inadequate response to several alternative treatments**
Adults and children age 17 and older and children ages 10 to 16 weighing more than 60 kg: Initially, 500 mg P.O. b.i.d. May increase dosage by 500 mg weekly to maximum of 1,500 mg P.O. b.i.d.
Children ages 10 to 16 weighing 25 to 60 kg: Initially, 250 mg P.O. b.i.d. Increase weekly in 500-mg/day (250 mg b.i.d.) increments to a total maintenance dose of 2,000 mg b.i.d.
Adjust-a-dose: For patients with CrCl of 51 to 80 mL/minute, reduce dosage by 25%; for CrCl of 31 to 50 mL/minute, decrease dosage by 50%; for CrCl of 11 to 30 mL/minute, decrease dosage by 75%.
➤ **Infantile spasms**
Infants and children ages 1 month to 2 years: 50 mg/kg/day P.O. given in two divided doses. Titrate in 25- to 50-mg/kg/day increments every 3 days as needed. Maximum dose is 150 mg/kg/day.

ADMINISTRATION
P.O.
• Drug may be given with or without food.

• The entire contents of the appropriate number of packets (500 mg/packet) of powder should be emptied into an empty cup, and should be dissolved in 10 mL of cold or room-temperature water per packet using the 10-mL oral syringe supplied with the medication. The concentration of the final solution is 50 mg/mL.

ACTION
Precise mechanism unknown. Thought to control seizures by inhibiting GABA transaminase, the enzyme responsible for metabolizing the inhibitory neurotransmitter GABA, thereby increasing GABA levels in the CNS.

Route	Onset	Peak	Duration
P.O.	Unknown	1–2½ hr	Unknown

Half-life: 5½ to 10½ hours.

ADVERSE REACTIONS
CNS: abnormal behavior, abnormal coordination, abnormal dreams, abnormal thinking, anxiety, asthenia, attention disturbance, confusion, *seizures,* depression, dizziness, dysarthria, expressive language disorder, fatigue, fever, headache, hyperreflexia, hypoesthesia, hyporeflexia, insomnia, irritability, lethargy, malaise, memory impairment, nervousness, paresthesia, peripheral neuropathy, postictal state, sedation, sensory disturbance, sensory loss, sinus headache, somnolence, ***status epilepticus,*** tremor, vertigo.
CV: chest pain, peripheral edema.
EENT: asthenopia, blurred vision, diplopia, nystagmus, eye pain, nasopharyngitis, pharyngolaryngeal pain, tinnitus, toothache, visual field defect.
GI: abdominal distention, constipation, diarrhea, dyspepsia, nausea, stomach discomfort, upper abdominal pain, vomiting.
GU: dysmenorrhea, erectile dysfunction, UTI.
Metabolic: increased appetite, weight gain.
Musculoskeletal: arthralgia, back pain, contusion, extremity pain, gait disturbance, joint sprain, myalgia, muscle spasm, muscle twitching.
Respiratory: bronchitis, cough, influenza, pulmonary congestion, URI.

V

Skin: rash, wound secretion.
Other: thirst.

INTERACTIONS
Drug-drug. *Clonazepam:* May increase clonazepam level. Use together cautiously. *Drugs associated with serious adverse ophthalmic effects, such as retinopathy (hydroxychloroquine) or glaucoma (corticosteroids, TCAs):* May increase risk of serious adverse ophthalmic effects. Avoid coadministration unless benefits clearly outweigh risks. *Phenytoin:* May decrease phenytoin level, especially when drug is started or stopped. Monitor drug levels.
Drug-lifestyle. *Alcohol use:* May increase CNS depression. Patient should avoid alcohol.

EFFECTS ON LAB TEST RESULTS
• May decrease Hb level, hematocrit, and RBC count.
• May decrease ALT and AST levels. May increase amino acid levels in urine.

CONTRAINDICATIONS & CAUTIONS
• Contraindicated in patients hypersensitive to drug or its components and as first-line therapy for complex partial seizures.
Black Box Warning Drug may cause progressive and permanent bilateral concentric visual field constriction and may reduce visual acuity. Risk of visual impairment increases with use and may continue after drug is discontinued. Because of risk of permanent vision loss, drug is available only through the SHARE program. Prescribers, pharmacists, and patients must enroll by calling 1-888-45-SHARE (1-888-457-4273). A visual examination should be performed before, every 3 months during, and 3 to 6 months after therapy. ■
Black Box Warning Due to risk of vision loss, withdraw drug in patients who don't show substantial benefit within 3 months of initiation for refractory complex partial seizures and within 2 to 4 weeks of initiation in patients with infantile spasms, or sooner if treatment failure becomes obvious. Periodically reassess patient response to and continued need for drug. Use drug at lowest dosage with shortest exposure time as clinically necessary. ■

Black Box Warning Don't use drug in patients who have or are at high risk for other types of irreversible vision loss unless benefits clearly outweigh risks. Don't use vigabatrin with other drugs associated with serious ophthalmic effects, such as retinopathy or glaucoma, unless benefits clearly outweigh risks. ■
• Use cautiously in patients with a history of abnormalities noted on MRI, neurotoxicity, depression, suicidal behavior or ideation, or anemia.
Dialyzable drug: Unknown.
⚠ Overdose S&S: Unconsciousness, coma, drowsiness, vertigo, psychosis, apnea, respiratory depression, bradycardia, agitation, irritability, confusion, headache, hypotension, abnormal behavior, increased seizure activity, status epilepticus, speech disorder.

PREGNANCY-LACTATION-REPRODUCTION
• There are no adequate studies in pregnant women; animal studies suggest drug may cause fetal harm. Use during pregnancy only if potential benefit justifies potential risk to the fetus.
• Pregnant patients taking drug should enroll in the North American Antiepileptic Drug Pregnancy Registry (1-888-233-2334).
• Drug appears in breast milk. Patient should discontinue breast-feeding or discontinue drug.

NURSING CONSIDERATIONS
☉ Alert: Closely monitor all patients taking or starting therapy with antiepileptics for changes in behavior indicating worsening suicidal thoughts or behavior or depression. Symptoms such as anxiety, agitation, hostility, mania, and hypomania may be precursors to emerging suicidality.
• Discontinue drug if patient fails to comply with therapy.
• Discontinue drug within 3 months if patient shows no improvement.
☉ Alert: Don't withdraw drug suddenly. For adults, taper by decreasing daily dose by 1,000 mg/day weekly until discontinued. For children with complex partial seizures, taper daily dose by one-third every week for 3 weeks. For infantile spasms, decrease daily dose at a rate of 25 to 50 mg/kg every 3 to 4 days.

• Monitor patient closely for such adverse effects as dizziness, which may lead to falls.
• Drug may cause anemia, somnolence, fatigue, peripheral neuropathy, peripheral edema, and weight gain. Monitor patient closely.
• Monitor ALT and AST levels; drug decreases levels, making these measurements unreliable for detecting early hepatic injury.

PATIENT TEACHING

• Advise patient that drug may be taken without regard to food.
• Instruct patient to read the manufacturer's medication guide before starting treatment and before each prescription refill.
• Warn patient that drug may cause dizziness and somnolence and that he should avoid driving or other hazardous activities until drug's effects are known.
■ Black Box Warning ■ Inform patient that drug may cause vision loss, and explain the importance of regular eye examinations and of the need for immediately reporting vision changes. Counsel patient that signs and symptoms of vision loss may be difficult to recognize before vision loss is severe. ■
• Advise patient to call prescriber and not to stop drug suddenly if adverse reactions occur.
• Tell woman of childbearing potential to notify prescriber if she becomes pregnant or plans to become pregnant during therapy.
• Inform patient who is breast-feeding that drug appears in breast milk and that she shouldn't breast-feed.

vilazodone hydrochloride
vil-AZ-oh-dohne

Viibryd⬦

Therapeutic class: Antidepressants
Pharmacologic class: SSRIs—partial
5-HT$_{1A}$ receptor agonists

AVAILABLE FORMS
Tablets: 10 mg, 20 mg, 40 mg

INDICATIONS & DOSAGES
➤ **Major depressive disorder**
Adults: Initially,10 mg P.O. daily for 7 days, then 20 mg P.O. daily for 7 days, then 40 mg P.O. daily thereafter.

ADMINISTRATION
P.O.
• Give drug with food.

ACTION
Binds to serotonin reuptake sites and 5-HT$_{1A}$ receptors; is a partial agonist at serotonergic 5-HT$_{1A}$ receptors.

Route	Onset	Peak	Duration
P.O.	Unknown	4–5 hr	Unknown

Half-life: 25 hours.

ADVERSE REACTIONS
CNS: dizziness, headache, somnolence, paresthesia, insomnia, abnormal dreams, restlessness, fatigue.
CV: palpitations.
GI: abdominal pain, diarrhea, nausea, dry mouth, vomiting, dyspepsia, flatulence, gastroenteritis, increased appetite.
GU: delayed ejaculation, erectile dysfunction, sexual dysfunction, abnormal orgasm.
Musculoskeletal: arthralgia.
Other: decreased libido.

INTERACTIONS
Drug-drug. *Aspirin, NSAIDs, warfarin:* May increase risk of bleeding. Monitor patient closely; adjust dosages of these drugs, or discontinue them.
CNS drugs: May cause additive effects. Use together cautiously.
CYP3A4 inducers: May decrease vilazodone level. Monitor patient for effectiveness.
CYP3A4 inhibitors (moderate to strong, such as erythromycin, ketoconazole): May increase vilazodone level. Reduce vilazodone dosage to 20 mg daily.
Digoxin: May increase digoxin level. Monitor levels before and during use with vilazodone. Reduce digoxin dose as necessary.
Drugs metabolized by CYP2C8 (thiazolidinedione class of antidiabetics, such as pioglitazone, rosiglitazone): May

V

increase levels of these drugs. Monitor patient closely.

Highly protein-bound drugs (aripiprazole, diazepam, fluoxetine): May increase levels of these drugs. Monitor patient closely.

MAO inhibitors, linezolid, methylene blue: May increase risk of serious or fatal adverse effects. Don't use concurrently with MAO inhibitor or within 14 days of starting or discontinuing an MAO inhibitor.

Serotonergics (buspirone, MAO inhibitors, SSNRIs, SSRIs, tramadol, triptans): May cause serotonin syndrome. Use together with extreme caution.

Triptans (almotriptan, sumatriptan): May increase risk of serotonin syndrome or neuroleptic malignant syndrome (NMS). Use together isn't recommended. If coadministration can't be avoided, closely monitor patient for emergence of serotonin syndrome or NMS-like signs or symptoms. If signs or symptoms occur, discontinue both drugs immediately and initiate supportive symptomatic treatment.

Drug-herb. *St. John's wort:* May increase risk of serotonin syndrome. Avoid use together.

Drug-lifestyle. *Alcohol use:* May increase bioavailability of vilazodone. Discourage use together.

EFFECTS ON LAB TEST RESULTS
• May decrease sodium level.

CONTRAINDICATIONS & CAUTIONS
◐ *Alert:* Life-threatening serotonin syndrome (fever, mental status changes, muscle twitching, excessive sweating, shivering or shaking, diarrhea, loss of coordination) and NMS (hyperthermia, muscle rigidity, autonomic instability with possible rapid fluctuation of vital signs, mental status changes) have been reported with antidepressant use.

◐ *Alert:* Concomitant use with methylene blue or linezolid can cause serotonin syndrome. Don't initiate drug in patients receiving linezolid or methylene blue.

• Contraindicated in patients hypersensitive to drug or its inactive components and with concurrent use or within 14 days of starting or stopping MAO inhibitor therapy.

• Use cautiously in patients with history or family history of depression, hypomania,

severe hepatic dysfunction, seizure disorder, acute-angle glaucoma, or hyponatremia and in patients taking NSAIDs, aspirin, or warfarin.

Dialyzable drug: Unlikely.

⚠ *Overdose S&S:* Serotonin syndrome, lethargy, restlessness, hallucinations, disorientation.

PREGNANCY-LACTATION-REPRODUCTION
• Neonates born to women who used drug in the third trimester can develop complications (including persistent pulmonary hypertension of the newborn) upon delivery requiring prolonged hospitalization, respiratory support, and tube feedings. Use drug during pregnancy only if potential benefits outweigh risks to the fetus.

• Drug may appear in breast milk. Use only when benefit to mother outweighs risk to infant.

NURSING CONSIDERATIONS
• Evaluate patients for the diagnosis of major depressive disorder according to established guidelines.

Black Box Warning Drug may increase the risk of suicidal thinking and behavior in children, adolescents, and young adults with major depressive disorder or other psychiatric disorders. Drug isn't approved for use in children. ■

• Screen patients for risk of bipolar disorder. Vilazodone isn't approved for treatment of bipolar depression. Use of an antidepressant in bipolar patients may precipitate mixed or manic episodes.

◐ *Alert:* If linezolid or methylene blue must be given concurrently with vilazodone (or other serotonergic drug), stop serotonergic drug and monitor patient for serotonin toxicity for 2 weeks (5 weeks if fluoxetine was taken) or until 24 hours after the last dose of methylene blue or linezolid, whichever comes first. May resume vilazodone 24 hours after last dose of methylene blue or linezolid.

• Evaluate patient for history of drug abuse, and watch closely for signs and symptoms of misuse or abuse (increased tolerance, drug-seeking behavior, requests for dosage increase).

• If patient had recently been taking MAO inhibitors, monitor him closely for tremor, myoclonus, diaphoresis, nausea, vomiting, flushing, dizziness, hyperthermia with features that resemble NMS, seizures, rigidity, autonomic instability with possible rapid fluctuations of vital signs, and mental status changes that include extreme agitation progressing to delirium and coma.

• Monitor patient for signs and symptoms of NMS (hyperthermia, rigidity, autonomic instability with possible rapid fluctuations of vital signs, mental status changes).

• Drug hasn't been studied in patients with severe hepatic dysfunction. Closely monitor patient with hepatic impairment for excessive fatigue or yellowing of the eyes or skin.

• Monitor patients taking aspirin, NSAIDs, or warfarin for signs and symptoms of bleeding.

• When discontinuing vilazodone, avoid abrupt discontinuation. Gradually reduce dosage and monitor patient for adverse events. If withdrawal symptoms are intolerable, consider resuming the previous prescribed dosage and decreasing the dosage at a more gradual rate. Wait at least 14 days before starting an MAO inhibitor.

• Hyponatremia, which may be life-threatening, has occurred as a result of treatment with other SSRIs and SSNRIs, especially in elderly patients and in patients taking diuretics or who are otherwise volume-depleted. Discontinue vilazodone in patients with symptomatic hyponatremia and treat appropriately. Monitor patient for signs and symptoms of hyponatremia, such as headache, difficulty concentrating, memory impairment, confusion, weakness, unsteadiness, hallucinations, syncope, seizures, coma, and respiratory arrest.

• Monitor patients for acute-angle glaucoma. Many antidepressants, including vilazodone, may trigger an angle-closure attack in patients with anatomically narrow angles who don't have a patent iridectomy.

PATIENT TEACHING
Black Box Warning Advise families and caregivers to closely observe patient for increased suicidal thinking and behavior. ∎

🚺 *Alert:* Teach patient to recognize and immediately report signs and symptoms of serotonin toxicity (fever, mental status changes, muscle twitching, excessive sweating, shivering or shaking, diarrhea, and loss of coordination) and NMS (hyperthermia, rigidity, autonomic instability with possible rapid fluctuations of vital signs, and mental status changes).

• Teach patient to take drug with food.

• Warn patient not to stop drug abruptly.

• Instruct patient to inform prescriber of all other medicines he is taking to avoid dangerous interactions.

• Tell patient to immediately seek medical attention if fever, rigidity, rapid changes in pulse rate or BP, sweating, or confusion occurs.

• Counsel patient to keep all appointments for monitoring blood work and for follow-up care.

• Advise patient to use caution when driving or operating hazardous equipment until effects of drug are known; drug may impair judgment, thinking, and motor skills.

• Advise patient and caregivers to watch for signs and symptoms of the onset of manic or hypomanic episodes.

• Warn patient to avoid alcohol during drug therapy.

• Advise female patient to notify her health care provider if she becomes pregnant or intends to become pregnant during therapy. Counsel her to consult prescriber before breast-feeding.

SAFETY ALERT!

vinBLAStine sulfate (VLB)
vin-BLAS-teen

Therapeutic class: Antineoplastics
Pharmacologic class: Vinca alkaloids

AVAILABLE FORMS
Injection: 1 mg/mL in 10-mL vials

INDICATIONS & DOSAGES
Adjust-a-dose (for all indications): For patients with serum bilirubin level of 1.5 to 3 mg/dL and AST level of 60 to 180 units/L, give 50% of usual dose. For patients with serum bilirubin level of 3 to 5 mg/dL, give

V

25% of usual dose. For patients with serum bilirubin level greater than 5 mg/dL and AST level greater than 180 units/L, don't administer. For patients with recent exposure to radiation therapy or chemotherapy, single doses usually don't exceed 5.5 mg/m². Once a dose is determined to produce a WBC count below 3,000/mm³, give maintenance doses of one increment less than this amount at weekly intervals.

➤ **Breast or testicular cancer, Hodgkin and malignant lymphoma, choriocarcinoma, lymphosarcoma, mycosis fungoides, Kaposi sarcoma, histiocytosis**
Adults: 3.7 mg/m² I.V. weekly. May increase to maximum dose of 18.5 mg/m² I.V. weekly based on response. Don't repeat dose if WBC count is below 4,000/mm³. Increase dosage at weekly intervals in increments of 1.8 mg/m² until desired therapeutic response is obtained, WBC count decreases to 3,000/mm³, or maximum weekly dose of 18.5 mg/m² is reached.

➤ **Hodgkin disease**
Children: 6 mg/m² I.V. in combination with other chemotherapeutic drugs.

➤ **Letterer-Siwe disease (histiocytosis X)**
Children: 6.5 mg/m² I.V. as a single agent.

➤ **Testicular germ-cell carcinomas**
Children: 3 mg/m²/day I.V. on days 1 through 5 of each cycle in combination with other chemotherapeutic drugs.

ADMINISTRATION
I.V.
▼ Preparing and giving drug may be mutagenic, teratogenic, or carcinogenic. Follow institutional policy to reduce risks.
Black Box Warning Drug is fatal if given intrathecally; it's for intravenous use only. ∎
🕭 *Alert:* When drug is dispensed in other than the original container, it must be packaged in the overwrap provided and labeled, using the auxiliary sticker provided and must state "Do not remove covering until moment of injection. For intravenous use only. Fatal if given by other routes." A syringe containing a specific dose must be labeled, using the auxiliary sticker provided to state: "For intravenous use only. Fatal if given by other routes."

▼ Inject drug directly into tubing of running I.V. line over 1 minute.
Black Box Warning Make sure catheter is properly positioned in vein. Drug is a vesicant; if extravasation occurs, stop infusion immediately and notify prescriber. The manufacturer recommends that moderate heat be applied to area of leakage. Local injection of hyaluronidase may help disperse drug. ∎
▼ Warm compresses may be applied to the area for 15 minutes every 6 hours for 48 hours.
▼ **Incompatibilities:** Cefepime, doxorubicin, furosemide, heparin.

ACTION
Arrests mitosis in metaphase, blocking cell division.

Route	Onset	Peak	Duration
I.V.	Unknown	Unknown	Unknown

Half-life: Initial phase, 3½ minutes; second phase, 1½ hours; terminal phase, 25 hours.

ADVERSE REACTIONS
CNS: numbness, paresthesia, peripheral neuropathy and neuritis, *seizures, stroke,* depression, headache.
CV: *MI,* hypertension.
EENT: pharyngitis.
GI: anorexia, constipation, ileus, nausea, stomatitis, vomiting, abdominal pain, bleeding ulcer, diarrhea.
Hematologic: anemia, *leukopenia, thrombocytopenia.*
Musculoskeletal: loss of deep tendon reflexes, muscle pain and weakness, jaw pain.
Respiratory: *acute bronchospasm,* shortness of breath.
Skin: irritation, phlebitis, cellulitis, reversible alopecia, vesiculation and necrosis with extravasation.
Other: SIADH.

INTERACTIONS
Drug-drug. *Azole antifungals, erythromycin, other drugs that inhibit cytochrome P-450 pathway:* May increase toxicity of vinblastine. Monitor patient closely for toxicity.

Reactions in bold italics are *life-threatening*. Interactions may have a *rapid onset* or a *delayed onset*.

Mitomycin: May increase risk of bronchospasm and shortness of breath. Monitor patient's respiratory status.
Ototoxic drugs, such as platinum-containing antineoplastics: May cause temporary or permanent hearing impairment. Monitor hearing function.
Phenytoin: May decrease plasma phenytoin level. Monitor phenytoin level closely.

EFFECTS ON LAB TEST RESULTS
• May decrease Hb level and WBC and platelet counts.

CONTRAINDICATIONS & CAUTIONS
• Contraindicated in patients hypersensitive to drug and in those with severe leukopenia or bacterial infection or significant granulocytopenia unless it's a result of the disease being treated.
• Use cautiously in patients with hepatic dysfunction or CV disease.
Dialyzable drug: No.
⚠ Overdose S&S: Exaggerated effects, neurotoxicity.

PREGNANCY-LACTATION-REPRODUCTION
• There are no adequate studies in pregnant women, but drug can cause fetal harm. If drug is used during pregnancy or if patient becomes pregnant during therapy, inform her of potential hazard to the fetus. Women of childbearing potential should avoid becoming pregnant during therapy.
• It isn't known if drug appears in breast milk. Patient should discontinue breastfeeding or discontinue drug.

NURSING CONSIDERATIONS
• To reduce nausea, give antiemetic before drug.
• Don't give drug into a limb with compromised circulation.
❸ Alert: After giving drug, be alert for development of life-threatening acute bronchospasm. If this occurs, notify prescriber immediately. Reaction is most likely to occur in patients who are also receiving mitomycin.
• Monitor patient for stomatitis. If stomatitis occurs, stop drug and notify prescriber.

• Assess bowel activity. Give laxatives as indicated. Stool softeners may be used prophylactically.
• Don't repeat dosage more frequently than every 7 days or severe leukopenia will occur. Nadir occurs on days 5 to 10. Recovery of WBC count is fairly rapid and usually complete within another 7 to 14 days.
• Assess patient for numbness and tingling in hands and feet. Assess gait for early evidence of footdrop.
• Drug is less neurotoxic than related drug vincristine.
• Stop drugs known to cause urine retention for first few days after therapy, particularly in elderly patients.
• **Look alike–sound alike:** Don't confuse vinblastine with vincristine or vinorelbine.

PATIENT TEACHING
• Tell patient to report evidence of infection (fever, sore throat, fatigue) and bleeding (easy bruising, nosebleeds, bleeding gums, tarry stools). Tell patient to take temperature daily.
• Urge patient to report pain, swelling, burning, or any unusual feeling at injection site during infusion.
• Warn patient that hair loss may occur but that it's usually temporary.
• Caution female patient to avoid pregnancy during therapy.
• Tell patient that pain may occur in jaw and in the organ with the tumor.

SAFETY ALERT!

vinCRIStine sulfate (VCR)
vin-KRIS-teen

Therapeutic class: Antineoplastics
Pharmacologic class: Vinca alkaloids

AVAILABLE FORMS
Injection: 1 mg/mL in 1-mL, 2-mL preservative-free vials

INDICATIONS & DOSAGES
➤ **Acute lymphoblastic and other leukemias, Hodgkin lymphoma, malignant lymphoma, neuroblastoma, rhabdomyosarcoma, Wilms tumor**

V

Adults: 1.4 mg/m² I.V. weekly. Typical weekly dose is 2 mg.

Children weighing more than 10 kg: 1 to 2 mg/m² I.V. weekly.

Children weighing 10 kg and less or with BSA less than 1 m²: Initially, 0.05 mg/kg I.V. weekly. Titrate dosage as tolerated, up to 2 mg/dose.

Adjust-a-dose: For patients with direct bilirubin level of 1.5 to 3 mg/dL, reduce dose by 50%. If serum bilirubin level is 3 to less than 5 mg/dL, give 25% of usual dose. If bilirubin level is greater than 5 mg/dL, don't give drug.

ADMINISTRATION

I.V.

▼ Preparing and giving drug may be mutagenic, teratogenic, or carcinogenic. Follow institutional policy to reduce risks.

▼ Inject directly into tube of running I.V. line of NSS or D₅W only, slowly over 1 minute.

☉ Alert: To prevent inadvertent intrathecal administration, the World Health Organization and the Institute For Safe Medication Practices strongly recommend dispensing vincristine in a minibag (not in a syringe).

Black Box Warning Make sure catheter is positioned correctly in vein. Drug is a vesicant; if it extravasates, stop infusion immediately and notify prescriber. Apply heat on and off every 2 hours for 24 hours. ∎

Black Box Warning Drug is fatal if given intrathecally; it's for I.V. use only. ∎

Black Box Warning Syringes containing this product should be labeled, using the auxiliary sticker provided, to state, "For intravenous use only. Fatal if given by other routes." Extemporaneously prepared syringes containing this product must be packaged in an overwrap that's labeled, "Do not remove covering until moment of injection. For intravenous use only. Fatal if given by other routes." ∎

▼ If protocol requires a continuous infusion, use a central line. Give as a short 5- to 10-minute infusion in 25 to 50 mL of NSS or D₅W.

▼ All vials contain 1 mg/mL solution; refrigerate them.

▼ **Incompatibilities:** Cefepime, furosemide, idarubicin, sodium bicarbonate.

ACTION

Arrests mitosis in metaphase, blocking cell division.

Route	Onset	Peak	Duration
I.V.	Unknown	Unknown	Unknown

Half-life: Initial phase, 5 minutes; second phase, 2¼ hours; terminal phase, 3½ days.

ADVERSE REACTIONS

CNS: loss of deep tendon reflexes, paresthesia, peripheral neuropathy, *coma, seizures,* ataxia, cranial nerve palsies, fever, headache, sensory loss.

CV: hypertension, hypotension.

EENT: blindness, diplopia, hoarseness, optic and extraocular neuropathy, photophobia, ptosis, visual disturbances, vocal cord paralysis.

GI: constipation, cramps, nausea, stomatitis, vomiting, *intestinal necrosis,* anorexia, diarrhea, dysphagia, ileus that mimics surgical paralytic ileus.

GU: dysuria, polyuria, urine retention.

Hematologic: *leukopenia, thrombocytopenia,* anemia.

Metabolic: hyponatremia, weight loss.

Musculoskeletal: cramps, jaw pain, muscle weakness.

Respiratory: *acute bronchospasm,* dyspnea.

Skin: phlebitis, cellulitis at injection site, rash, reversible alopecia, severe local reaction following extravasation.

Other: SIADH.

INTERACTIONS

Drug-drug. *Digoxin:* May decrease digoxin's effects. Monitor digoxin level.

HIV protease inhibitors (atazanavir, ritonavir): May increase pharmacologic effects of vinblastine. Monitor patient for profound neutropenia and severe neuropathy. Temporarily suspend HIV protease inhibitor or reduce vincristine dosage if significant hematologic or GI toxicity occurs.

Mitomycin: May increase frequency of bronchospasm and acute pulmonary reactions. Monitor patient's respiratory status.

Reactions in bold italics are *life-threatening.* Interactions may have a *rapid onset* or a *delayed onset.*

Ototoxic drugs: May potentiate loss of hearing. Use together with caution.
Phenytoin: May reduce phenytoin level. Monitor phenytoin level closely.
Triazole antifungals (itraconazole, posaconazole, voriconazole): Concomitant use may increase risk of neurotoxicity. Monitor patient closely.
Warfarin: May increase anticoagulant effects. Monitor INR and adjust warfarin dose as needed.

EFFECTS ON LAB TEST RESULTS
● May decrease sodium and Hb levels. May increase uric acid level.
● May decrease WBC and platelet counts.

CONTRAINDICATIONS & CAUTIONS
● Contraindicated in patients hypersensitive to drug and in those with demyelinating form of Charcot-Marie-Tooth syndrome.
● Don't give to patients who are receiving radiation therapy through ports that include the liver.
● Use cautiously in patients with hepatic dysfunction, neuromuscular disease, or infection.
Dialyzable drug: No.
⚠ *Overdose S&S:* Exaggerated effects, death.

PREGNANCY-LACTATION-REPRODUCTION
● There are no adequate studies in pregnant women, but drug may cause fetal harm. If drug is used during pregnancy or if patient becomes pregnant during therapy, inform her of potential fetal hazard. Women of childbearing potential should use effective contraception during therapy.
● It isn't known if drug appears in breast milk. Patient should discontinue breastfeeding or discontinue drug.

NURSING CONSIDERATIONS
⚠ *Alert:* Patient also taking mitomycin has a higher risk of life-threatening bronchospasm. Monitor him after dose, and notify prescriber immediately if it occurs.
⚠ *Alert:* Drug is considered a vesicant. If signs or symptoms of extravasation occur, stop infusion immediately and notify prescriber. Extravasation site may need to be injected with hyaluronidase.

● Watch for hyperuricemia, especially in patients with leukemia or lymphoma. Maintain hydration and give allopurinol to prevent uric acid nephropathy. Watch for toxicity.
● If SIADH develops, fluid restriction may be needed. Monitor fluid intake and output.
● Because of risk of neurotoxicity, don't give drug more often than once weekly. Children are more resistant to neurotoxicity than adults. Neurotoxicity is dose related and usually reversible.
● Elderly patients and those with underlying neurologic disease may be more susceptible to neurotoxic effects.
● Monitor patient for Achilles tendon reflex depression, numbness, tingling, footdrop or wristdrop, difficulty walking, ataxia, and slapping gait. Monitor his ability to walk on heels. Support him while walking.
● Monitor bowel function. Give stool softener, laxative, or water before giving dose. Constipation may be an early sign of neurotoxicity.
● Stop drugs known to cause urine retention, particularly in elderly patients, for first few days after therapy.
● *Look alike–sound alike:* Don't confuse vincristine with vinblastine or vinorelbine.

PATIENT TEACHING
● Advise patient to report pain or burning at injection site during or after administration.
● Tell patient to report increased shortness of breath and evidence of infection (fever, sore throat, fatigue) and bleeding (easy bruising, nosebleeds, bleeding gums, tarry stools). Tell patient to take temperature daily.
● Warn patient that hair loss may occur, but explain that it's usually temporary.
● Caution female patient to avoid becoming pregnant during therapy and to consult prescriber before becoming pregnant.

V

SAFETY ALERT!

vinorelbine tartrate
vin-oh-REL-been

Navelbine

Therapeutic class: Antineoplastics
Pharmacologic class: Semisynthetic vinca alkaloids

AVAILABLE FORMS
Injection: 10 mg/mL, 50 mg/5 mL

INDICATIONS & DOSAGES
➤ **Alone or as adjunctive therapy with cisplatin for first-line treatment of ambulatory patients with nonresectable advanced non–small-cell lung cancer (NSCLC); alone or with cisplatin in stage IV NSCLC; with cisplatin in stage III NSCLC**
Adults: 30 mg/m^2 I.V. weekly as monotherapy. In combination treatment, 25 mg/m^2 I.V. weekly with cisplatin 100 mg/m^2 given every 4 weeks. Or, 30 mg/m^2 I.V. weekly in combination with cisplatin 120 mg/m^2 given on days 1 and 29, then every 6 weeks.
Adjust-a-dose: If granulocyte count is 1,000/mm^3 to 1,499/mm^3, give 50% of dose. If less than 1,000/mm^3, withhold dose. Repeat granulocyte count in 1 week. If three consecutive doses are withheld, discontinue drug. For patients who develop fever or sepsis while granulocytopenic or had two consecutive doses withheld due to granulocytopenia, give 75% of dose if granulocyte count is 1,500/mm^3 or more, or 37.5% if granulocyte count is 1,000 to 1,499/mm^3. If granulocyte count is less than 1,000/mm^3, don't give dose. Repeat granulocyte count in 1 week. If three consecutive doses are withheld, discontinue drug. For patients who develop hyperbilirubinemia, adjust dosage as follows: If total bilirubin is 2.1 to 3 mg/dL, give 50% of starting dose; if total bilirubin is greater than 3 mg/dL, give 25% of starting dose.

ADMINISTRATION
I.V.
▼ Drug may be a contact irritant; handle and give with care. Wear gloves. Avoid inhaling vapors and allowing contact with skin or mucous membranes, especially those of the eyes. In case of contact, wash with generous amounts of water for at least 15 minutes.
▼ Dilute drug before use to 1.5 to 3 mg/mL with D$_5$W or NSS in a syringe. Or, dilute to 0.5 to 2 mg/mL in an I.V. bag of D$_5$W, NSS, half-NSS, or D$_5$W half-NSS.
▼ Give drug I.V. over 6 to 10 minutes into side port of a free-flowing I.V. line that is closest to I.V. bag; then flush with 75 to 125 mL or more of D$_5$W or NSS.
▼ Monitor site for irritation and infiltration because drug can cause localized tissue damage, necrosis, and thrombophlebitis.
Black Box Warning Make sure catheter is properly positioned in vein. If extravasation occurs, stop drug immediately and inject remaining dose into a different vein; notify prescriber. ■
Black Box Warning Drug is fatal if given intrathecally; it's for I.V. use only. Syringes containing this product should be labeled "Warning: For I.V. use only. Fatal if given intrathecally." ■
▼ Diluted drug may be stored for up to 24 hours at room temperature.
▼ **Incompatibilities:** Acyclovir, allopurinol, aminophylline, amphotericin B, ampicillin sodium, cefazolin, ceftriaxone, cefuroxime, 5-FU, furosemide, ganciclovir, methylprednisolone, mitomycin, piperacillin, sodium bicarbonate, sulfamethoxazole–trimethoprim, thiotepa.

ACTION
Exerts its primary antineoplastic effect by disrupting microtubule assembly, which in turn disrupts spindle formation and prevents mitosis.

Route	Onset	Peak	Duration
I.V.	Unknown	Unknown	Unknown

Half-life: About 27 to 43½ hours.

ADVERSE REACTIONS
CNS: asthenia, fatigue, peripheral neuropathy.
CV: chest pain, phlebitis.
GI: anorexia, constipation, diarrhea, nausea, stomatitis, vomiting.

Reactions in bold italics are *life-threatening*. Interactions may have a *rapid onset* or a ***delayed onset***.

Hematologic: anemia, *agranulocytosis, bone marrow suppression, granulocytopenia, thrombocytopenia, leukopenia.*
Hepatic: hyperbilirubinemia.
Musculoskeletal: arthralgia, jaw pain, loss of deep tendon reflexes, myalgia.
Respiratory: dyspnea.
Skin: alopecia, injection-site pain or reaction, rash.

INTERACTIONS
Drug-drug. *Cisplatin:* May increase risk of bone marrow suppression when used with cisplatin. Monitor hematologic status closely.
Cyclosporine: May increase therapeutic and toxic effects of vinorelbine. Close clinical and laboratory monitoring is indicated.
Cytochrome P-450 inhibitors: May decrease metabolism of vinorelbine. Watch for increased adverse effects.
Mitomycin: May cause pulmonary reactions. Monitor respiratory status closely.
Paclitaxel: May increase risk of neuropathy. Monitor patient closely.
Triazole antifungals: May increase risk of neurotoxicity. Monitor patient closely.
Vaccines, live-virus: May increase risk of live-virus vaccine–induced adverse reactions. Concurrent use isn't recommended.

EFFECTS ON LAB TEST RESULTS
• May increase bilirubin level. May decrease Hb level.
• May increase LFT values. May decrease granulocyte, WBC, and platelet counts.

CONTRAINDICATIONS & CAUTIONS
• Contraindicated in patients with pretreatment granulocyte count below 1,000/mm^3 and in patients hypersensitive to the drug.
• Use with caution in patients whose bone marrow may have been compromised by previous exposure to radiation therapy or chemotherapy or whose bone marrow is still recovering from chemotherapy.
• Use with caution in patients with hepatic impairment.
• Safety and effectiveness in children haven't been established.
Dialyzable drug: 0% to 24%.

⚠ *Overdose S&S:* Paralytic ileus, stomatitis, esophagitis, bone marrow aplasia, sepsis, paresis, death.

PREGNANCY-LACTATION-REPRODUCTION
• Drug can cause fetal harm when used during pregnancy. Advise women of childbearing potential to use highly effective contraception during therapy. If drug is used during pregnancy or patient becomes pregnant during therapy, inform her of potential fetal hazard.
• It isn't known if drug appears in breast milk. Patient should discontinue breastfeeding or discontinue drug.

NURSING CONSIDERATIONS
Black Box Warning Severe myelosuppression resulting in serious infection, septic shock, hospitalization, and death may occur. ∎
Black Box Warning Decrease dose or withhold drug in accordance with recommended dose modifications. Granulocyte count should be 1,000/mm^3 or more before administration. ∎
• If granulocyte count is less than 1,000/mm^3, withhold drug and notify prescriber. Granulocyte count nadir occurs between days 7 and 10.
• In patients with hepatic impairment, monitor liver enzyme levels.
• Patient may receive injections of WBC colony-stimulating factors to promote cell growth and decrease risk of infection.
⚕ *Alert:* Monitor deep tendon reflexes; loss may represent cumulative toxicity.
• Monitor patients closely for hypersensitivity and new or worsening signs and symptoms of neuropathy in those with prior history of or preexisting neuropathy.
• Severe acute bronchospasm, interstitial pneumonitis, and ARDS have been reported. Monitor patient for unexplained dyspnea or other signs and symptoms of pulmonary toxicity.
• As a guide to the effects of therapy, monitor patient's peripheral blood count and bone marrow.
• *Look alike–sound alike:* Don't confuse vinorelbine with vinblastine or vincristine.

V

PATIENT TEACHING
● Advise patient to report any pain or burning at site of injection.
● Instruct patient not to take other drugs, including OTC preparations, until approved by prescriber.
● Tell patient to report all adverse reactions, especially evidence of infection (fever, sore throat, fatigue) and bleeding (easy bruising, nosebleeds, bleeding gums, tarry stools). Tell patient to take temperature daily.
● Advise patient to report increased shortness of breath, cough, abdominal pain, or constipation.
● Caution female patient to avoid becoming pregnant during therapy.

vismodegib
VIS-moe-DEG-ib

Erivedge

Therapeutic class: Antineoplastics
Pharmacologic class: Hedgehog
pathway inhibitors

AVAILABLE FORMS
Capsules ⓞⓣⓒ: 150 mg

INDICATIONS & DOSAGES
➤ **Metastatic basal cell carcinoma; locally advanced basal cell carcinoma that has recurred following surgery or in patients who aren't candidates for surgery or radiation**
Adults: 150 mg P.O. once daily until disease progression or unacceptable toxicity.

ADMINISTRATION
P.O.
● Hazardous agent; use safe handling precautions.
● May give with or without food.
● Store capsules at room temperature.
● Don't open, crush, or allow patient to chew capsules.

ACTION
Inhibits Hedgehog signaling pathway by binding to and inhibiting Smoothened, a transmembrane protein involved in Hedge-hog signal transmission. Inhibition of this protein slows pathway for tumor growth.

Route	Onset	Peak	Duration
P.O.	Unknown	Unknown	Unknown

Half-life: 4 days with continued dosing; 12 days after one dose.

ADVERSE REACTIONS
CNS: fatigue.
GI: nausea, diarrhea, vomiting, constipation, taste perversion, absence of taste, decreased appetite.
GU: azotemia, amenorrhea.
Metabolic: hyponatremia, *hypokalemia.*
Musculoskeletal: muscle spasms, arthralgia.
Skin: alopecia.
Other: weight loss.

INTERACTIONS
Drug-drug. *Antacids, H₂-receptor antagonists, PPIs:* May decrease vismodegib exposure and its effects. Avoid use together.
P-glycoprotein inhibitors (macrolides such as azithromycin, clarithromycin, erythromycin): May increase vismodegib exposure and adverse effects. Avoid use together.

EFFECTS ON LAB TEST RESULTS
● May increase BUN and creatinine levels.
● May decrease sodium and potassium levels.

CONTRAINDICATIONS & CAUTIONS
● Contraindicated in patients hypersensitive to drug.
Dialyzable drug: Unknown.

PREGNANCY-LACTATION-REPRODUCTION
Black Box Warning Contraindicated in pregnant women. Drug can cause embryo-fetal death or severe birth defects. ▮
Black Box Warning Verify pregnancy status within 7 days before start of therapy. ▮
Black Box Warning Females of childbearing potential should use effective contraception during therapy and for 7 months after final dose; male patients should use condoms, even after a vasectomy, to avoid drug exposure to pregnant partners and female

---

Reactions in bold italics are *life-threatening*. Interactions may have a *rapid onset* or a *delayed onset*.

partners of childbearing potential during therapy and for 3 months after final dose. ∎
• Report exposure during pregnancy (directly or from seminal fluid) or within 7 months after treatment ends to Genentech at 1-888-835-2555.
• It isn't known if drug appears in breast milk. Breast-feeding isn't recommended during therapy and for 7 months after final dose.
• Drug may cause amenorrhea, which may be irreversible.

NURSING CONSIDERATIONS
Black Box Warning Advise male and female patients of the risks to an embryo or fetus, the need for contraception, and the potential risk of drug exposure through semen. ∎
• **Look alike–sound alike:** Don't confuse vismodegib with vemurafenib or vandetanib.

PATIENT TEACHING
Black Box Warning Counsel all patients of childbearing potential and their partners about risk of embryo-fetal death or severe birth defects and in the use of contraception during and after drug therapy. ∎
• Tell female patient to use highly effective contraception during therapy and for 7 months after last dose; advise male patient to use condoms, even after a vasectomy, to avoid drug exposure to pregnant partners and female partners of childbearing potential during therapy and for 3 months after final dose.
• If patient misses a dose, instruct him not to make up that dose but to resume dosing with the next scheduled dose.
• Instruct patient to immediately contact health care provider if pregnancy occurs or is suspected after exposure to drug, or if patient has unprotected sex.
• Advise women experiencing drug-induced amenorrhea that it's unknown if amenorrhea will be reversed after drug discontinuation.
• Caution patient not to donate blood or blood products while taking drug and for at least 7 months (or semen for 3 months) after last dose.
• Teach patient to swallow capsules whole and not to crush, chew, or open them.

vorapaxar sulfate
VOR-a-PAX-ar

Zontivity

Therapeutic class: Antiplatelet drugs
Pharmacologic class: Platelet aggregation inhibitors

AVAILABLE FORMS
Tablets: 2.08 mg

INDICATIONS & DOSAGES
➤ **To reduce thrombotic CV events in patients with history of MI or peripheral arterial disease, in combination with aspirin or clopidogrel**
Adults: 1 tablet P.O. once daily.

ADMINISTRATION
P.O.
• Store tablets in original package at room temperature.
• Give drug in addition to aspirin and clopidogrel, as indicated.
• May give with or without food.

ACTION
Inhibits platelet aggregation. Drug is a reversible antagonist of the protease-activated receptor-1 expressed on platelets.

Route	Onset	Peak	Duration
P.O.	Unknown	1 hr	Unknown

Half-life: 8 days.

ADVERSE REACTIONS
CNS: depression, *intracranial bleeding.*
EENT: retinopathy, retinal disorders.
GI: *GI bleeding.*
Hematologic: *hemorrhage,* anemia, iron deficiency.
Skin: rash, eruption, exanthemas.

INTERACTIONS
Drug-drug. *Drugs known to cause bleeding (anticoagulants, fibrinolytics, NSAIDs [long-term], SNRIs, SSRIs, warfarin):* Increase risk of bleeding, including intracranial hemorrhage and fatal bleeding. Avoid use together.

V

Strong CYP3A inducers (carbamazepine, phenytoin, rifampin): May decrease vorapaxar level. Avoid use together.
Strong CYP3A inhibitors (clarithromycin, ketoconazole, nefazodone, ritonavir): May increase vorapaxar level. Avoid use together.
Drug-herb. *St. John's wort:* May decrease vorapaxar level. Avoid use together.

EFFECTS ON LAB TEST RESULTS
• May decrease RBC count.

CONTRAINDICATIONS & CAUTIONS
Black Box Warning Don't use in patients with history of intracranial hemorrhage, pathological bleeding, stroke, or TIA. Antiplatelet drugs, including vorapaxar, increase risk of bleeding, including intracranial hemorrhage and fatal bleeding. ■
• Drug has only been studied in combination with aspirin or clopidogrel.
• Use cautiously in elderly patients; in those with low body weight, reduced renal or hepatic function, or history of bleeding disorder; and in patients concomitantly using drugs known to increase bleeding.
• Use isn't recommended in patients with severe hepatic impairment.
• There are no overall differences in safety or effectiveness between younger and older patients. Since elderly patients are at higher risk for bleeding, consider patient's age before administering drug.
• Safety and effectiveness in children haven't been established.
Dialyzable drug: Unlikely.

PREGNANCY-LACTATION-REPRODUCTION
• Use cautiously in pregnant women and only if potential benefits outweigh risk to the fetus.
• It isn't known if drug appears in breast milk. Use in breast-feeding women isn't recommended.

NURSING CONSIDERATIONS
☻ *Alert:* Stopping drug briefly during an episode of acute bleeding won't be useful in managing bleeding, because of drug's long half-life. There's no known treatment to reverse the antiplatelet effect; drug will significantly inhibit platelet aggregation for 4 weeks after discontinuation.

• Discontinue drug if patient experiences a stroke, TIA, or intracranial hemorrhage.
• Monitor Hb level and hematocrit periodically. Monitor patient for bleeding.
• Evaluate hypotensive patients who have had recent coronary angiography, PCI, CABG, or other surgical procedure for possible bleeding.

PATIENT TEACHING
Black Box Warning Caution patient that drug increases risk of bleeding, including intracranial hemorrhage and fatal bleeding. ■
• Advise patient to tell other providers that he or she is taking drug, especially before any surgery or dental procedure.
• Instruct patient to take drug exactly as prescribed in addition to aspirin or clopidogrel, and not to discontinue drug without first consulting prescriber.
• Instruct patient to report bruising or severe prolonged or excessive unexplained bleeding (blood in stool, vomit, or urine and coughing up blood or blood clots).
• Advise patient to report all prescription drugs, OTC medications, vitamins, herbs, and other dietary supplements he is taking to prescriber and pharmacist so that they are aware of other treatment that may affect bleeding risk.
• Warn female patient that drug is used during pregnancy only if potential benefits outweigh risks.
• Tell female patient that breast-feeding isn't recommended during therapy.

voriconazole
vor-ah-KON-ah-zole

Vfend

Therapeutic class: Antifungals
Pharmacologic class: Synthetic triazoles

AVAILABLE FORMS
Oral suspension: 40 mg/mL (after reconstitution)
Powder for injection: 200 mg/vial
Tablets: 50 mg, 200 mg

INDICATIONS & DOSAGES

Adjust-a-dose (for all indications): For patients with mild or moderate hepatic impairment (Child-Pugh class A or B), decrease the maintenance dosage by 50%. In patients with a CrCl of less than 50 mL/minute, use oral form instead of I.V. form to prevent accumulation of a component of the I.V. mixture. In patients also receiving phenytoin, increase maintenance dose of voriconazole to 5 mg/kg I.V. every 12 hours, or increase P.O. dose from 100 mg to 200 mg (in patients weighing 40 kg or less) or from 200 mg to 400 mg (in patients weighing more than 40 kg). In patients also receiving efavirenz, increase voriconazole dosage to 400 mg P.O. every 12 hours and decrease efavirenz dosage to 300 mg P.O. every 24 hours. When treatment with voriconazole is stopped, restore initial dosage of efavirenz.

➤ **Esophageal candidiasis**
Adults and children age 12 and older weighing 40 kg or more: 200 mg P.O. every 12 hours. Treat for a minimum of 14 days and for at least 7 days after symptoms resolve.
Adults and children age 12 and older weighing less than 40 kg: 100 mg P.O. every 12 hours. Treat for a minimum of 14 days and for at least 7 days after symptoms resolve.

➤ **Invasive aspergillosis; serious infections caused by *Fusarium* species and *Scedosporium apiospermum* in patients intolerant of or refractory to other therapy**
Adults and children age 12 and older: Initially, 6 mg/kg I.V. every 12 hours for two doses; then maintenance dose of 4 mg/kg I.V. every 12 hours. If patient can't tolerate 4-mg/kg dose, decrease to 3 mg/kg. Switch to P.O. form as tolerated, using the maintenance dosages shown here.
Adults and children age 12 and older weighing 40 kg or more: 200 mg P.O. every 12 hours. May increase to 300 mg P.O. every 12 hours, if needed. If unable to tolerate the 300-mg dose, reduce dose in 50-mg decrements to a minimum of 200 mg every 12 hours.
Adults and children age 12 and older weighing less than 40 kg: 100 mg P.O. every 12 hours. May increase to 150 mg P.O. every

12 hours, if needed. If unable to tolerate the 150-mg dose, reduce dose to 100 mg every 12 hours.

➤ **Candidemia in nonneutropenic patients; *Candida* infections of the kidney, abdomen, bladder wall, or wounds and disseminated skin infections**
Adults and children age 12 and older: Initially, 6 mg/kg I.V. every 12 hours for two doses, then 3 to 4 mg/kg I.V. every 12 hours for maintenance, depending on severity of the infection. If patient can't tolerate 4-mg/kg dose, decrease to 3 mg/kg. Switch to P.O. form as tolerated, using the maintenance dosages shown here.
Adults and children age 12 and older weighing 40 kg or more: 200 mg P.O. every 12 hours. May increase to 300 mg P.O. every 12 hours, if needed. If unable to tolerate the 300-mg dose, reduce dose in 50-mg decrements to a minimum of 200 mg every 12 hours.
Adults and children age 12 and older weighing less than 40 kg: 100 mg P.O. every 12 hours. May increase to 150 mg P.O. every 12 hours, if needed. If unable to tolerate the 150-mg dose, reduce dose to 100 mg every 12 hours.

Treat patients with candidemia for at least 14 days after symptoms resolve or after the last positive culture result, whichever is longer.

ADMINISTRATION
P.O.
● Give tablets or oral suspension at least 1 hour before or 1 hour after a meal.
● For the oral suspension, use only the dispenser provided in the medication package.
● Don't mix oral suspension with other drugs or beverages.
● Shake suspension for 10 seconds before each use. May store at room temperature. Discard unused portion of suspension after 14 days.

I.V.
▼ In patients with CrCl less than 50 mL/minute, use I.V. form cautiously. Change to oral form is recommended.
▼ Reconstitute the powder with 19 mL of water for injection to obtain a volume of 20 mL of clear concentrate containing 10 mg/mL of drug. Discard the vial if a

V

vacuum doesn't pull the diluent into the vial. Shake the vial until all the powder is dissolved. Use the reconstituted solution immediately.

▼ Further dilute the 10-mg/mL solution to 5 mg/mL or less. Follow manufacturer's instructions for diluting. Stable in NSS, lactated Ringer solution, and D₅W.

▼ Infuse over 1 to 2 hours at 5 mg/mL or less and a maximum hourly rate of 3 mg/kg/hour.

▼ **Incompatibilities:** Blood products, electrolyte supplements, 4.2% sodium bicarbonate infusion.

ACTION

Inhibits the cytochrome P-450–dependent synthesis of ergosterol, a vital component of fungal cell membranes.

Route	Onset	Peak	Duration
P.O., I.V.	Immediate	1–2 hr	12 hr

Half-life: Depends on dose.

ADVERSE REACTIONS

CNS: fever, headache, hallucinations.
CV: tachycardia.
EENT: abnormal vision, photophobia, chromatopsia.
GI: nausea, vomiting.
GU: renal dysfunction.
Hepatic: cholestatic jaundice.
Metabolic: *hypokalemia.*
Skin: rash.
Other: chills.

INTERACTIONS

Drug-drug. *Benzodiazepines, calcium channel blockers, methadone, NSAIDs, sulfonylureas, vinca alkaloids:* May increase levels of these drugs. Adjust dosages of these drugs; monitor patient for adverse reactions.

Carbamazepine, long-acting barbiturates, rifabutin, rifampin, *ritonavir (high-dose therapy):* May decrease voriconazole level. Use together is contraindicated.

Cyclosporine, tacrolimus: May increase levels of these drugs. Adjust dosages; monitor levels.

Efavirenz: May significantly decrease voriconazole level while significantly increasing efavirenz level. Adjust dosage of both drugs. Use of voriconazole when efavirenz dosage is 400 mg or more/day is contraindicated.

Ergot alkaloids (such as ergotamine), sirolimus: May increase levels of these drugs. Use together is contraindicated.

Fluconazole: May increase voriconazole level. Avoid use together. Monitor patient for adverse effects 24 hours after last fluconazole.

HIV protease inhibitors (amprenavir, nelfinavir, saquinavir), NNRTIs (delavirdine): May increase levels of both drugs. Monitor patient for adverse reactions and toxicity.

HMG-CoA reductase inhibitors (atorvastatin, fluvastatin, lovastatin, pravastatin, rosuvastatin, simvastatin): May increase levels and adverse effects, including rhabdomyolysis, of these drugs. Monitor patient closely and reduce dose of HMG-CoA reductase inhibitor as needed.

Omeprazole: May increase omeprazole level. When initiating voriconazole therapy in patients already receiving omeprazole doses of 40 mg or greater, reduce omeprazole dose by one-half.

Opioids, long-acting (fentanyl, oxycodone): May increase levels of these drugs. Adjust doses of these drugs; monitor patient for adverse reactions.

Oral contraceptives containing ethinyl estradiol and norethindrone: May increase levels and adverse effects of these drugs. Monitor patient closely.

Phenytoin: May decrease voriconazole level and increase phenytoin level. Increase voriconazole maintenance dose; monitor phenytoin level.

Pimozide, quinidine: May increase levels of these drugs, leading to torsades de pointes and prolonged QT interval. Use together is contraindicated.

Ritonavir: May decrease voriconazole level. Use with ritonavir dosages of 400 mg b.i.d. is contraindicated. Avoid using with low-dose ritonavir (100 mg b.i.d.) unless benefits outweigh risks.

Warfarin: May significantly increase PT and INR. Monitor PT, INR, and bleeding.

Drug-herb. *St. John's wort:* May increase drug level. Avoid use together.

Reactions in bold italics are *life-threatening*. Interactions may have a *rapid onset* or a **delayed onset**.

Drug-lifestyle. *Sun exposure:* May cause photosensitivity. Advise patient to avoid excessive sunlight exposure.

EFFECTS ON LAB TEST RESULTS
• May increase alkaline phosphatase, AST, ALT, bilirubin, and creatinine levels. May decrease potassium level.
• May decrease Hb level, hematocrit, and platelet, WBC, and RBC counts.

CONTRAINDICATIONS & CAUTIONS
• Contraindicated in patients hypersensitive to drug or its components; in those with rare hereditary galactose intolerance, Lapp lactase deficiency, or glucose-galactose malabsorption; and in those taking carbamazepine, efavirenz (400-mg dose or higher), ergot alkaloid, a long-acting barbiturate, pimozide, quinidine, rifabutin, rifampin, ritonavir (high dose, 400 mg b.i.d.), terfenadine, or sirolimus.
• May prolong QT interval. Rare cases of torsades de pointes, cardiac arrest, and sudden death have been reported. Use cautiously in patients with proarrhythmic conditions and in those taking concomitant drugs that can prolong QT interval.
• Use cautiously in patients hypersensitive to other azoles.
• Serious reactions, including Stevens-Johnson syndrome, toxic epidermal necrolysis, and erythema multiforme, have been reported. Discontinue drug for exfoliative cutaneous reactions.
Dializable drug: Unlikely.
⚠ **Overdose S&S:** Photophobia.

PREGNANCY-LACTATION-REPRODUCTION
• Drug can cause fetal harm when used in pregnant women. Use during pregnancy only if benefit to mother clearly outweighs potential risk to the fetus. If used during pregnancy, inform patient of potential fetal hazard.
• It isn't known if drug appears in breast milk. Patient should discontinue breast-feeding or discontinue drug.

NURSING CONSIDERATIONS
• Correct electrolyte disturbances before initiating therapy.

• Infusion reactions, including flushing, fever, sweating, tachycardia, chest tightness, dyspnea, faintness, nausea, pruritus, and rash, may occur as soon as infusion starts. If reaction occurs, notify prescriber; infusion may need to be stopped.
• Monitor LFT results at start of and during therapy. Monitor patients who develop abnormal LFT results for more severe hepatic injury. If patient develops signs and symptoms of liver disease, drug may need to be stopped.
• Monitor patient for serious exfoliative cutaneous reactions and photosensitivity skin reactions that could lead to melanoma or squamous cell carcinoma of the skin. Discontinue drug if patient develops a skin lesion consistent with squamous cell carcinoma or melanoma.
• If treatment lasts longer than 28 days, vision changes may occur.
• **Look alike–sound alike:** Don't confuse voriconazole with fluconazole.

PATIENT TEACHING
• Tell patient to take oral form at least 1 hour before or 1 hour after a meal.
• Tell patient taking the oral suspension to only use the dispenser provided with the medication pack.
• Advise patient not to mix oral suspension with other drugs or beverages.
• Tell patient to discard any unused portion of suspension after 14 days.
• Advise patient to avoid driving or operating machinery while taking drug, especially at night, because vision changes, including blurring, photophobia, and changes in color perception, may occur.
• Tell patient to avoid strong, direct sunlight and to use sun-protective measures.
• Advise female patient to avoid becoming pregnant during therapy because of the risk of fetal harm.

V

vortioxetine hydrobromide
vor-tie-OX-e-teen

Trintellix

Therapeutic class: Antidepressants
Pharmacologic class: Multimodal antidepressants

AVAILABLE FORMS
Tablets: 5 mg, 10 mg, 15 mg, 20 mg

INDICATIONS & DOSAGES
➤ **Major depressive disorder**
Adults: 10 mg P.O. once daily. Increase as tolerated to targeted dose of 20 mg once daily.
Adjust-a-dose: If 10 mg once daily isn't tolerated, decrease dosage to 5 mg once daily. If discontinuing drug when patient is taking 15 or 20 mg daily, first decrease dosage to 10 mg daily for 1 week, then stop drug to avoid adverse reactions. For CYP2D6 poor metabolizers, maximum recommended dose is 10 mg daily.

ADMINISTRATION
P.O.
- Give drug without regard to meals.
- Store tablets at room temperature.

ACTION
Antidepressant effect of vortioxetine isn't fully understood, but is thought to be related to its enhancement of serotonergic activity in the CNS through inhibition of the reuptake of serotonin (5-HT), as well as 5-HT_3 receptor antagonism and 5-HT_{1A} receptor agonism.

Route	Onset	Peak	Duration
P.O.	2–4 wk	7–11 hr	Unknown

Half-life: 66 hours.

ADVERSE REACTIONS
CNS: dizziness, abnormal dreams.
GI: nausea, diarrhea, dry mouth, constipation, vomiting, flatulence, xerostomia.
Skin: pruritus.
Other: sexual dysfunction.

INTERACTIONS
Drug-drug. *Aspirin, NSAIDs, warfarin:* May increase risk of upper GI bleeding. Use together cautiously.
Diuretics: May increase risk of hyponatremia. Monitor patient carefully.
Linezolid, methylene blue: May increase risk of serotonin syndrome. Don't use together. Monitor patient for serotonin syndrome for 21 days or until 24 hours after last dose of linezolid or methylene blue, whichever comes first. Resume vortioxetine 24 hours after last dose of linezolid or methylene blue.
MAO inhibitors: May cause severe adverse effects from impaired serotonin metabolism. Concurrent use is contraindicated. Don't restart MAO inhibitor for at least 21 days after vortioxetine has been stopped. Start vortioxetine at least 14 days after MAO inhibitor has been stopped.
Serotonergics (buspirone, fentanyl, lithium, SSNRIs, SSRIs, TCAs, tramadol, triptans, tryptophan products): May increase risk of serotonin syndrome. Monitor patient carefully.
Strong CYP inducers (carbamazepine, phenytoin, rifampin): May decrease vortioxetine level if coadministered for more than 14 days. Consider increasing vortioxetine dosage with concurrent use, to maximum of three times original dose. Decrease vortioxetine dosage to original level within 14 days when strong CYP inducer is discontinued.
Strong CYP2D6 inhibitors (bupropion, fluoxetine, paroxetine, quinidine): May increase vortioxetine level. Decrease vortioxetine dosage by half when given together. Increase vortioxetine dosage to original level when CYP2D6 inhibitor is discontinued.
Drug-herb. *St. John's wort:* May increase risk of serotonin syndrome. Don't use together.

EFFECTS ON LAB TEST RESULTS
- May decrease sodium level.

CONTRAINDICATIONS & CAUTIONS
- Contraindicated in patients hypersensitive to drug or its components.
- **Black Box Warning** Safety and efficacy haven't been established in children. ∎

- Use cautiously in patients with a history or family history of bipolar disorder, mania, or hypomania.
- Use cautiously in patients taking diuretics or who are otherwise volume-depleted because of increased risk of hyponatremia.
- Drug hasn't been studied in patients with severe hepatic impairment.
- Drug may increase bleeding risk, particularly if used with aspirin, NSAIDs, warfarin, or other anticoagulants.
- Drug may cause withdrawal syndrome (dysphoric mood, irritability, agitation, dizziness, sensory disturbances, anxiety, confusion, headache, lethargy, emotional lability, insomnia, hypomania, tinnitus, and seizures). At discontinuation of therapy, it's recommended that dosages of 15 mg once daily or more be decreased to 10 mg once daily for 1 week before full discontinuation to prevent withdrawal signs and symptoms. If intolerable signs and symptoms occur after a dosage decrease or upon discontinuation of therapy, consider resuming previous dosage with a more gradual taper.

Dialyzable drug: Unknown.

⚠ *Overdose S&S:* Dizziness, diarrhea, abdominal discomfort, generalized pruritus, somnolence, flushing.

PREGNANCY-LACTATION-REPRODUCTION
- Drug's effects during pregnancy are unknown. Use only if potential benefits outweigh potential risks.
- It isn't known if drug appears in breast milk. Patient should discontinue breastfeeding or discontinue drug.

NURSING CONSIDERATIONS
- Abrupt discontinuation is possible, but may cause headache, muscle tension, mood swings, and outbursts of anger.

Black Box Warning Drug increases risk of suicidal thoughts and behavior in children, adolescents, and young adults.

Black Box Warning Monitor patients for signs and symptoms of worsening depression, emergence of suicidal ideation and behavior (suicidality), or unusual changes in behavior, especially during initial treatment or with dosage changes, either increases or decreases. ∎

- Screen patients for bipolar disorder before drug initiation. Drug isn't approved for use in bipolar depression.
- Monitor patients for signs and symptoms of hyponatremia and SIADH (headache, difficulty concentrating, memory impairment, confusion, weakness, unsteadiness, hallucination, syncope, seizure, coma, respiratory arrest, death). Discontinue drug if hyponatremia occurs.
- Monitor patients for signs and symptoms of serotonin syndrome, including mental status changes (agitation, hallucinations, delirium, coma), autonomic instability (tachycardia, labile blood pressure, dizziness, diaphoresis, flushing, hyperthermia), neuromuscular symptoms (tremor, rigidity, myoclonus, hyperreflexia, incoordination), seizures, or severe GI symptoms (nausea, vomiting, diarrhea). Discontinue drug immediately if signs and symptoms occur.

PATIENT TEACHING
Black Box Warning Advise patient and caregivers to watch for signs and symptoms of suicidal ideation and behavior, especially when dosage is being adjusted. ∎
- Tell patient to report all adverse reactions to prescriber.
- Warn patient about signs and symptoms of serotonin syndrome or autonomic instability.
- Advise patient that nausea, xerostomia, dizziness, constipation, diarrhea, or sexual dysfunction may occur.
- Tell patient to immediately report behavioral changes, insomnia, or signs and symptoms of hyponatremia, hemorrhaging, or serotonin syndrome.
- Warn patient not to stop drug abruptly or without discussing with prescriber.
- Caution patient about operating machinery or doing tasks that require alertness while taking drug.

warfarin sodium
WAR-far-in

Coumadin✒, Jantoven

Therapeutic class: Anticoagulants
Pharmacologic class: Coumarin
derivatives

AVAILABLE FORMS
Tablets: 1 mg, 2 mg, 2.5 mg, 3 mg, 4 mg,
5 mg, 6 mg, 7.5 mg, 10 mg

INDICATIONS & DOSAGES
➤ **PE, DVT, MI, rheumatic heart disease
with heart valve damage, prosthetic heart
valves, chronic atrial fibrillation**
Adults: 2 to 5 mg P.O. daily for 2 to 4 days;
then dosage based on daily PT and INR.
Usual maintenance dosage is 2 to 10 mg
P.O. daily. Base dosages on INR target goals
and other clinical factors. Consider lower
initiation and maintenance doses for Asian
and elderly patients and those with CYP2C9
and VKORC1 genotypes.

ADMINISTRATION
P.O.
• Establish baseline coagulation parameters
before therapy. PT and INR determinations
are essential for proper control. Recommended INR range is usually 2 to 3 for most
patients. Target INR in patients with tilting
disk valves and bileaflet mechanical valves
in mitral position or caged ball or caged disk
valves is 2.5 to 3.5.
• Give drug at same time daily.

ACTION
Inhibits vitamin K-dependent activation of
clotting factors II, VII, IX, and X, formed
in the liver. Also inhibits anticoagulant
proteins C and S.

Route	Onset	Peak	Duration
P.O.	Within 24 hr	4 hr	2–5 days

Half-life: 20 to 60 hours.

ADVERSE REACTIONS
CV: vasculitis.
GI: abdominal pain, diarrhea, flatulence,
bloating, nausea, taste perversion, vomiting.
Hematologic: *hemorrhage.*
Hepatic: hepatitis.
Skin: alopecia, pruritus, rash, dermatitis,
bullous eruptions.
Other: chills, hypersensitivity or allergic
reactions, including *anaphylactic reactions*
and urticaria.

INTERACTIONS
Drug-drug. *Acetaminophen:* May increase
bleeding with long-term therapy (more than
2 weeks) at high doses (more than 2 g/day)
of acetaminophen. Monitor therapy.
Allopurinol, **amiodarone**, **anabolic steroids**,
anticoagulants (argatroban, bivalirudin),
azole antifungals, *aspirin, beta blockers
(atenolol, propranolol), cephalosporins,
chloramphenicol, cimetidine,* **danazol**,
*diazoxide, diflunisal, disulfiram, eryth-
romycin, ethacrynic acid, felbamate,* **fibric
acids**, **fluoxymesterone**, **fluoroquinolones**,
*furosemide, glucagon, HMG-CoA reductase
inhibitors (fluvastatin, lovastatin, simvastatin), heparin, influenza virus vaccine,
isoniazid,* **lansoprazole**, *macrolide antibiotics (azithromycin, clarithromycin, erythromycin), meclofenamate, methimazole,
methyldopa, methylphenidate,* **methyltestosterone**, **metronidazole**, **nalidixic acid**,
neomycin (oral), **NSAIDs**, *omeprazole,*
oxandrolone, *pentoxifylline, propafenone,
propoxyphene, propylthiouracil, quinidine,
quinolones (ciprofloxacin, levofloxacin,
norfloxacin, ofloxacin),* **salicylates**, *selective
cyclo-oxygenase-2 inhibitors (celecoxib, ro-
fecoxib, valdecoxib), SSRIs,* **sulfinpyrazone**,
sulfamethoxazole–trimethoprim, **sulfonamides**, *tamoxifen, tetracyclines, thiazides,
thrombolytics,* **thyroid drugs**, *ticlopidine,
tramadol, vitamin E, valproic acid, zafirlukast:* May increase anticoagulant effect.
Monitor patient carefully for bleeding. Reduce anticoagulant dosage as directed.
Aprepitant, ascorbic acid, **barbiturates**,
*bosentan, carbamazepine, clozapine, cor-
ticosteroids, corticotropin, cyclosporine,
dicloxacillin, ethchlorvynol, griseofulvin,
haloperidol, meprobamate, mercaptopurine,
nafcillin, oral contraceptives containing
estrogen, protease inhibitors (indinavir,
ritonavir), raloxifene, ribavirin, rifampin,
spironolactone, sucralfate, thiazide diuretics, trazodone, vitamin K:* May reduce the

PT and thereby decrease the INR, which reduces the anticoagulant effect. Monitor PT and INR carefully. Increase warfarin dosage, as needed.

Cyclophosphamide, phenytoin, propylthiouracil, ranitidine: May affect PT and INR. Monitor PT and INR carefully.

Sulfonylureas (oral antidiabetics): May increase hypoglycemic response. Monitor glucose levels.

Drug-herb. *Coenzyme Q10, ginseng, St. John's wort:* May reduce action of warfarin. Modify therapy.

Green tea: May decrease anticoagulant effect caused by vitamin K content of green tea. Advise patient to minimize variable consumption of green tea.

*Herbs with anticoagulant properties (such as dong quai, fenugreek, feverfew, garlic, ginger, **ginkgo**, willow bark):* May increase risk of bleeding. Discourage use together.

Drug-food. *Cranberry juice:* May increase risk of severe bleeding. Discourage use together.

Foods, multivitamins, and other enteral products containing vitamin K: May impair anticoagulation. Tell patient to maintain consistent daily intake of foods containing vitamin K.

Drug-lifestyle. *Alcohol use:* May enhance anticoagulant effects. Tell patient to avoid large amounts of alcohol.

EFFECTS ON LAB TEST RESULTS

- May increase ALT and AST levels.
- May increase INR, and prolong PT and PTT.
- May falsely decrease theophylline level.

CONTRAINDICATIONS & CAUTIONS

Black Box Warning Drugs, dietary changes, and other factors affect INR levels achieved with warfarin therapy. ∎

- Contraindicated in patients hypersensitive to drug and in those with bleeding from the GI, GU, or respiratory tract; aneurysm; cerebrovascular hemorrhage; severe or malignant hypertension; severe renal or hepatic disease; subacute bacterial endocarditis, pericarditis, or pericardial effusion; or blood dyscrasias or hemorrhagic tendencies.
- Contraindicated after recent surgery involving large open areas, eye, brain, or

spinal cord; recent prostatectomy; or major regional lumbar block anesthesia, spinal puncture, or diagnostic or therapeutic invasive procedures.

- Fatal and serious calciphylaxis (calcium uremic arteriolopathy) has been reported in patients with and without ESRD. If calciphylaxis is diagnosed, stop drug and treat calciphylaxis. Consider alternative anticoagulation.
- Avoid using in patients with a history of warfarin-induced necrosis; in unsupervised patients with senility, alcoholism, or psychosis; or in situations in which there are inadequate laboratory facilities for coagulation testing.
- Use cautiously in patients with diverticulitis, colitis, mild or moderate hypertension, or mild or moderate hepatic or renal disease; with drainage tubes in any orifice; with regional or lumbar block anesthesia; with heparin-induced thrombocytopenia and deep venous thrombosis; or in conditions that increase risk of hemorrhage.

Dialyzable drug: Unknown.

⚠ ***Overdose S&S:*** Blood in stools or urine, excessive bruising, persistent oozing from superficial injuries, excessive menstrual bleeding, melena, petechiae.

PREGNANCY-LACTATION-REPRODUCTION

- Drug can cause fetal harm. Contraindicated in pregnant women except those with mechanical heart valves, who are at high risk for thromboembolism and for whom benefits of warfarin may outweigh risks.
- Women of childbearing potential should use effective contraception during therapy and for 1 month after final dose.
- Drug hasn't been detected in breast milk. Use cautiously in breast-feeding women. Monitor breast-fed infants for bruising or bleeding.

NURSING CONSIDERATIONS

Black Box Warning Warfarin can cause major or fatal bleeding, which is more likely to occur during the starting period and with a higher dose. Regularly monitor INR in all patients. Consider more frequent INR monitoring in those at high risk for bleeding. ∎

- Avoid all I.M. injections.

W

• Regularly inspect patient for bleeding gums, bruises on arms or legs, petechiae, nosebleeds, melena, tarry stools, hematuria, and hematemesis.

• Check for unexpected bleeding in breast-fed children of women who take this drug.

• Monitor patient for purple-toes syndrome, characterized by a dark purple or mottled color of the toes; may occur 3 to 10 weeks, or even later, after start of therapy.

◑ **Alert:** Withhold drug and call prescriber at once in the event of fever or rash (signs of severe adverse reactions).

• Effect can be neutralized by oral or parenteral vitamin K.

• Elderly patients and patients with renal or hepatic failure are especially sensitive to drug's effect.

• **Look alike–sound alike:** Don't confuse Coumadin with Avandia or Cardura. Don't confuse Jantoven with Janumet or Januvia.

PATIENT TEACHING

• Stress importance of complying with pre-scribed dosage and follow-up appointments. Tell patient to carry a card that identifies his increased risk of bleeding.

Black Box Warning Tell patient and family about measures to prevent bleeding, to watch for signs of bleeding or abnormal bruising, and to call prescriber at once if they occur. ∎

• Warn patient to avoid OTC products containing aspirin, other salicylates, or drugs that may interact with warfarin unless ordered by prescriber.

◑ **Alert:** Advise patient to consult prescriber before initiating any herbal therapy as many herbs have anticoagulant, antiplatelet, or fibrinolytic properties.

• Tell patient to consult prescriber before using miconazole vaginal cream or supposi-tories. Abnormal bleeding and bruising have occurred.

• Instruct female patient to notify prescriber if menstruation is heavier than usual; she may need dosage adjustment.

• Tell patient to use electric razor when shaving and to use a soft toothbrush.

• Tell patient to read food labels. Food, nu-tritional supplements, and multivitamins that contain vitamin K may impair anticoag-ulation.

• Tell patient to eat a daily, consistent diet of food and drinks containing vitamin K, because eating varied amounts may alter anticoagulant effects.

• Tell patient to inform all health care providers about taking warfarin and to inform warfarin prescriber of upcoming surgeries or procedures.

zafirlukast
zah-FUR-luh-kast

Accolate

Therapeutic class: Antiasthmatics
Pharmacologic class: Leukotriene receptor antagonists

AVAILABLE FORMS
Tablets: 10 mg, 20 mg

INDICATIONS & DOSAGES
➤ **Prevention and long-term treatment of asthma**
Adults and children age 12 and older: 20 mg P.O. b.i.d.
Children ages 5 to 11: 10 mg P.O. b.i.d.

ADMINISTRATION
P.O.
• Give drug 1 hour before or 2 hours after meals.

ACTION
Selectively competes for leukotriene recep-tor sites, blocking inflammatory action.

Route	Onset	Peak	Duration
P.O.	Rapid	3 hr	Unknown

Half-life: 10 hours.

ADVERSE REACTIONS
CNS: headache, asthenia, dizziness, pain, fever.
GI: abdominal pain, diarrhea, dyspepsia, gastritis, nausea, vomiting.
Musculoskeletal: back pain, myalgia.
Other: accidental injury, infection.

INTERACTIONS
Drug-drug. *Aspirin:* May increase zafir-lukast level. Monitor patient for adverse effects.

Reactions in bold italics are *life-threatening*. Interactions may have a *rapid onset* or a *delayed onset*.

Erythromycin, theophylline: May decrease zafirlukast level. Monitor patient for decreased effectiveness.

Warfarin: May prolong PT. Monitor PT and INR, and adjust anticoagulant dosage.

Drug-food. *Any food:* May reduce rate and extent of drug absorption. Advise patient to take drug 1 hour before or 2 hours after a meal.

EFFECTS ON LAB TEST RESULTS
• May increase liver enzyme levels.

CONTRAINDICATIONS & CAUTIONS
• Contraindicated in patients hypersensitive to drug and in those with hepatic impairment, including hepatic cirrhosis.
• Use cautiously in elderly patients.
Dialyzable drug: Unknown.
⚠ *Overdose S&S:* Rash, upset stomach.

PREGNANCY-LACTATION-REPRODUCTION
• There are no adequate studies in pregnant women. Use during pregnancy only if clearly needed.
• Drug appears in breast milk. Don't use in breast-feeding women because of potential for tumorigenicity shown in animal studies.

NURSING CONSIDERATIONS
🔆 *Alert:* Reducing oral corticosteroid dose has been followed in rare cases by eosinophilia, vasculitic rash, worsening pulmonary symptoms, cardiac complications, or neuropathy, sometimes as Churg-Strauss syndrome.
• Drug isn't indicated to reverse bronchospasm in acute asthma attacks, including status asthmaticus.
🔆 *Alert:* Drug may cause behavior and mood changes, including agitation, depression, insomnia, and suicidal thinking and behavior. Monitor patient and consider discontinuing drug if neuropsychiatric symptoms develop.
• *Look alike–sound alike:* Don't confuse Accolate with Accupril or Accutane.

PATIENT TEACHING
• Tell patient that drug is used for long-term treatment of asthma and to keep taking it even if symptoms resolve.
• Advise patient that drug isn't indicated for use in reversal of bronchospasm in acute asthma attacks, including status asthmaticus.
• Advise patient to continue taking other antiasthmatics, as prescribed.
• Instruct patient to take drug 1 hour before or 2 hours after meals.
• Warn patient that drug may cause behavior and mood changes (agitation, insomnia, depression, suicidal thinking and behavior), and to report development of these symptoms to prescriber.
• Teach patient to report rare but serious signs and symptoms of hepatic dysfunction (right upper quadrant abdominal pain, nausea, fatigue, lethargy, pruritus, jaundice, flulike symptoms, anorexia).

---

zaleplon
ZAL-ah-plon

Sonata

Therapeutic class: Hypnotics
Pharmacologic class:
Pyrazolopyrimidines
Controlled substance schedule: IV

AVAILABLE FORMS
Capsules: 5 mg, 10 mg

INDICATIONS & DOSAGES
➤ **Short-term treatment (7 to 10 days) of insomnia**
Adults: 10 mg P.O. daily at bedtime; may increase to 20 mg as needed. Low-weight adults may respond to 5-mg dose. Limit use to 7 to 10 days. Reevaluate patient if drug is used for more than 2 to 3 weeks.
Adjust-a-dose: For elderly or debilitated patients, initially, 5 mg P.O. daily at bedtime; doses of more than 10 mg aren't recommended. For patients with mild to moderate hepatic impairment or those also taking cimetidine, 5 mg P.O. daily at bedtime.

ADMINISTRATION
P.O.
• Give drug immediately before bed or after patient has gone to bed and has experienced difficulty falling asleep.
• Don't give drug after a high-fat or heavy meal (may delay onset).

Z

ACTION

A hypnotic with chemical structure unrelated to benzodiazepines that interacts with the GABA–benzodiazepine receptor complex in the CNS. Modulation of this complex is thought to be responsible for sedative, anxiolytic, muscle relaxant, and anticonvulsant effects of benzodiazepines.

Route	Onset	Peak	Duration
P.O.	Rapid	1 hr	Unknown

Half-life: 1 hour.

ADVERSE REACTIONS

CNS: complex sleep-related behaviors, amnesia, anxiety, asthenia, confusion, depersonalization, depression, difficulty concentrating, dizziness, drowsiness, fever, hallucinations, hypertonia, hypoesthesia, malaise, migraine, nervousness, paresthesia, somnolence, tremor, vertigo.
CV: chest pain, peripheral edema.
EENT: abnormal vision, conjunctivitis, eye discomfort, ear discomfort, hyperacusis, epistaxis, smell alteration.
GI: abdominal pain, anorexia, colitis, constipation, dry mouth, dysgeusia, dyspepsia, nausea, taste perversion.
GU: dysmenorrhea.
Musculoskeletal: arthralgia, arthritis, back pain, myalgia.
Respiratory: bronchitis.
Skin: photosensitivity reactions, pruritus, rash.

INTERACTIONS

Drug-drug. *Carbamazepine, phenobarbital, phenytoin, rifampin, other CYP3A4 inducers:* May reduce zaleplon bioavailability and peak level by 80%. Consider using a different hypnotic.
Cimetidine: May increase zaleplon bioavailability and peak level by 85%. Use an initial zaleplon dose of 5 mg.
CNS depressants (imipramine, thioridazine): May cause additive CNS effects. Use together cautiously.
Black Box Warning *Opioids:* May cause slow or difficult breathing, sedation, and death. Avoid use together. If use together is necessary, limit dosage and duration of each drug to minimum necessary for desired effect. ∎

Drug-food. *Heavy meals, high-fat foods:* May prolong absorption, delaying peak drug level by about 2 hours; may delay sleep onset. Advise patient not to take with meals.
Drug-lifestyle. *Alcohol use:* May increase CNS effects. Discourage use together.

EFFECTS ON LAB TEST RESULTS

None reported.

CONTRAINDICATIONS & CAUTIONS

• Contraindicated in patients hypersensitive to drug or its components and in those with severe hepatic impairment.
• If hypersensitivity reactions occur, don't rechallenge patient.
Black Box Warning Opioids should only be prescribed with benzodiazepines or other CNS depressants to patients for whom alternative treatment options are inadequate. ∎
• Avoid use in patients with sensitivity to tartrazine (FD&C Yellow No. 5), which is contained in capsules. Reactions may occur more frequently in patients with aspirin hypersensitivity.
• Use cautiously in elderly, depressed, or debilitated patients; in patients with history of drug dependence, benzodiazepine abuse, or benzodiazepine-like hypnotic abuse; and in patients with compromised respiratory function or asthma.
Dialyzable drug: Unknown.
⚠ Overdose S&S: Drowsiness, confusion, lethargy, ataxia, hypotension, respiratory depression, coma, death.

PREGNANCY-LACTATION-REPRODUCTION

• There are no adequate studies in pregnant women. Use during pregnancy isn't recommended.
• Drug appears in breast milk in a small amount, with highest amount occurring during a feeding at about 1 hour after administration. Use in breast-feeding women isn't recommended.

NURSING CONSIDERATIONS

• Closely monitor patients who have compromised respiratory function caused by illness or who are elderly or debilitated because they are more sensitive to respiratory depression.

Reactions in bold italics are *life-threatening*. Interactions may have a *rapid onset* or a *delayed onset*.

• Start treatment only after carefully evaluating patient because sleep disturbances may be a symptom of an underlying physical or psychiatric disorder.

• Adverse reactions are usually dose-related. Consult prescriber about dose reduction if adverse reactions occur.

• *Look alike–sound alike:* Don't confuse zaleplon with Zelapar, Zemplar, or zolpidem.

PATIENT TEACHING

Black Box Warning Caution patient or caregiver of patient taking an opioid with a benzodiazepine, CNS depressant, or alcohol to seek immediate medical attention if patient experiences dizziness, light-headedness, extreme sleepiness, slowed or difficult breathing, or unresponsiveness. ■

۩ Alert: Warn patient that drug may cause allergic reactions, facial swelling, and complex sleep-related behaviors, such as driving, eating, and making phone calls while asleep. Advise patient to report these adverse effects.

• Advise patient that drug works rapidly and should only be taken immediately before bedtime or after he has gone to bed and has had trouble falling asleep.

• Advise patient to take drug only if he will be able to sleep for at least 4 undisturbed hours.

• Caution patient that drowsiness, dizziness, light-headedness, and coordination problems occur most often within 1 hour after taking drug.

• Advise patient to avoid alcohol use while taking drug and to notify prescriber before taking other prescription or OTC drugs.

• Tell patient not to take drug after a high-fat or heavy meal.

• Advise patient to report sleep problems that continue despite use of drug.

• Notify patient that dependence can occur and that drug is recommended for short-term use only.

• Warn patient not to abruptly stop drug because of risk of withdrawal symptoms, including unpleasant feelings, stomach and muscle cramps, vomiting, sweating, shakiness, and seizures.

• Notify patient that insomnia may recur for a few nights after stopping drug but should resolve on its own.

• Warn patient that drug may cause changes in behavior and thinking, including outgoing or aggressive behavior, loss of personal identity, confusion, strange behavior, agitation, hallucinations, worsening of depression, or suicidal thoughts. Tell patient to notify prescriber immediately if these symptoms occur.

• Advise female patient to consult prescriber before becoming pregnant or breast-feeding.

zidovudine (azidothymidine, AZT, Compound S)
zid-oh-VEW-den

Novo-AZT ✽, Retrovir⌀

Therapeutic class: Antiretrovirals
Pharmacologic class: Nucleoside–nucleotide reverse transcriptase inhibitors

AVAILABLE FORMS

Capsules ⓓ: 100 mg
Injection: 10 mg/mL
Syrup: 50 mg/5 mL
Tablets ⓓ: 300 mg

INDICATIONS & DOSAGES

Adjust-a-dose (for all indications): In patients with significant anemia (Hb level less than 7.5 g/dL or more than 25% below baseline) or significant neutropenia (granulocyte count less than 750/mm^3 or more than 50% below baseline), interrupt therapy until evidence proves marrow has recovered. In patients receiving hemodialysis or peritoneal dialysis, or with CrCl less than 15 mL/minute, give 100 mg P.O. or 1 mg/kg I.V. every 6 to 8 hours. For patients with mild to moderate hepatic dysfunction or liver cirrhosis, daily dose may need to be reduced.

➤ **HIV infection, with other antiretrovirals**

Adults: 300 mg P.O. b.i.d. with other antiretrovirals. If patient is unable to tolerate oral drug, give 1 mg/kg I.V. infused over 1 hour every 4 hours until oral form can be given.

Z

Children ages 4 weeks to less than 18 years: Do not exceed the recommended adult dose. For patients weighing 30 kg or more, 300 mg P.O. b.i.d. or 200 mg P.O. t.i.d. For patients weighing 9 to less than 30 kg, 9 mg/kg P.O. b.i.d. or 6 mg/kg P.O. t.i.d. For patients weighing 4 to less than 9 kg, 12 mg/kg P.O. b.i.d. or 8 mg/kg P.O. t.i.d.

➤ **To prevent maternal-fetal transmission of HIV**

Pregnant women at more than 14 weeks' gestation: 100 mg P.O. five times daily until the start of labor. Then, 2 mg/kg I.V. over 1 hour followed by a continuous I.V. infusion of 1 mg/kg/hour until the umbilical cord is clamped.

Neonates: 2 mg/kg P.O. every 6 hours starting within 12 hours after birth and continuing until 6 weeks old. Or, give 1.5 mg/kg via I.V. infusion over 30 minutes every 6 hours.

ADMINISTRATION
P.O.
● Give drug orally without regard to meals.
● Capsules shouldn't be kept in places that may be damp or hot. Heat and moisture may cause the drug to break down.
● Drug is considered hazardous; use safe handling precautions.

I.V.
▼ Give by this route only until oral drug can be tolerated.
▼ Remove the calculated dose from the vial; add to D_5W to achieve a concentration no greater than 4 mg/mL.
▼ Infuse drug over 1 hour (adults) or 30 minutes (neonates) at a constant rate. Avoid rapid infusion or bolus injection.
▼ Don't give by I.M. injection.
▼ Protect undiluted vials from light.
▼ After dilution, solution is physically and chemically stable for 24 hours at room temperature and for 48 hours if refrigerated at 36° to 46° F (2° to 8° C). Administer diluted solution within 8 hours if stored at 77° F (25° C) or within 24 hours if refrigerated at 36° to 46° F.
▼ **Incompatibilities:** Biological or colloidal solutions, such as blood products or protein-containing solutions; meropenem.

ACTION
Nucleoside reverse transcriptase inhibitor that inhibits replication of HIV by blocking DNA synthesis.

Route	Onset	Peak	Duration
P.O., I.V.	Unknown	30–90 min	Unknown

Half-life: ½ to 3 hours.

ADVERSE REACTIONS
CNS: asthenia, dizziness, fever, fatigue, headache, malaise, neuropathy, *seizures,* insomnia, paresthesia, somnolence.
GI: anorexia, nausea, vomiting, *pancreatitis,* abdominal pain, constipation, diarrhea, dyspepsia, taste perversion.
Hematologic: *agranulocytosis, neutropenia, severe bone marrow suppression, thrombocytopenia,* anemia.
Hepatic: altered LFT values, hepatomegaly.
Metabolic: *lactic acidosis.*
Musculoskeletal: arthralgia, myalgia, myopathy.
Respiratory: cough, wheezing.
Skin: rash, diaphoresis.

INTERACTIONS
Drug-drug. *Atovaquone, fluconazole, methadone, probenecid, trimethoprim, valproic acid:* May increase bioavailability of zidovudine. May need to adjust dosage.
Doxorubicin, ribavirin, stavudine: May have antagonistic effects. Avoid using together.
Ganciclovir, interferon alfa, other bone marrow suppressive or cytotoxic drugs: May increase hematologic toxicity of zidovudine. Use together cautiously.
Phenytoin: May alter phenytoin level and decrease zidovudine clearance by 30%. Monitor patient closely.
Zidovudine-containing products (such as Combivir, Trizivir): May increase risk of zidovudine toxicity. Don't use together.

EFFECTS ON LAB TEST RESULTS
● May increase ALT, AST, alkaline phosphatase, and LDH levels.
● May decrease RBC, WBC, granulocyte, neutrophil, and platelet counts and Hb level.

CONTRAINDICATIONS & CAUTIONS

• Contraindicated in patients who have had a potentially life-threatening hypersensitivity reaction to drug or its components.

Black Box Warning Use cautiously and with close monitoring in patients with advanced symptomatic HIV infection and in those with severe bone marrow depression. Use of this drug has been associated with hematologic toxicity, including neutropenia and severe anemia. ∎

• Use cautiously in patients with hepatomegaly, hepatitis, or other risk factors for liver disease and in those with renal insufficiency. Monitor renal function tests and LFTs.

• Use cautiously in patients with granulocyte count less than 1,000 cells/mm^3 or Hb level less than 9.5 g/dL.

Black Box Warning Prolonged use has been associated with myopathy. ∎

Dialyzable drug: Unlikely.

⚠ *Overdose S&S:* Fatigue, headache, vomiting, hematologic disturbances.

PREGNANCY-LACTATION-REPRODUCTION

• U.S. Department of Health and Human Services Perinatal HIV Guidelines consider zidovudine in combination with lamivudine to be a preferred nucleoside reverse transcriptase inhibitor for use in antiretroviral-naive pregnant women.

• Administer zidovudine I.V. near delivery regardless of antepartum regimen or mode of delivery in women with HIV RNA greater than 1,000 copies/mL or unknown HIV RNA status.

• Register patients in the Antiretroviral Pregnancy Registry (1-800-258-4263) that monitors pregnant women exposed to zidovudine.

• Drug appears in breast milk. Because of potential for postnatal HIV-1 transmission, breast-feeding is contraindicated.

• In couples who want to conceive, the HIV-infected partner should attain maximum viral suppression before conception.

NURSING CONSIDERATIONS

Black Box Warning Although rare, lactic acidosis without hypoxemia and severe hepatomegaly with steatosis may occur. Notify prescriber if patient develops unexplained tachypnea, dyspnea, or a decrease in bicarbonate level. Therapy may need to be suspended until lactic acidosis is ruled out. ∎

• Frequently monitor blood studies to detect anemia or agranulocytosis or hepatic decompensation. Patients may need reduced dosage or temporary stop to therapy.

• Drug may temporarily decrease morbidity and mortality in certain patients with AIDS.

• *Look alike–sound alike:* Don't confuse Retrovir with ritonavir.

PATIENT TEACHING

• Tell patient to take drug without regard to meals.

• Tell patient to take drug exactly as directed and not to share it with others.

• Remind patient to comply with the dosage schedule. Suggest ways to avoid missing doses, perhaps by using an alarm clock.

• Tell patient that dosages vary among patients and not to change his dosing instructions unless directed to do so by his prescriber.

• Warn patient not to take other drugs for AIDS unless prescriber has approved them.

• Advise patient that monotherapy isn't recommended and to discuss any questions with prescriber.

• Advise patient that blood transfusions may be needed during therapy because of drug-related anemia.

• Advise pregnant, HIV-infected patient that drug therapy only reduces the risk of HIV transmission to her newborn. Long-term risks to infants are unknown.

• Inform pregnant patient considering use of zidovudine for prevention of HIV-1 transmission to her infant that transmission may still occur in some cases despite therapy.

• Advise pregnant patient infected with HIV-1 not to breast-feed, to avoid postnatal transmission of HIV.

• Tell patient not to keep capsules in the kitchen, bathroom, or other places that may be damp or hot. Heat and moisture may cause the drug to break down and affect the intended results.

• Advise health care worker considering prophylactic use after occupational exposure (such as needlestick injury) that drug's safety and effectiveness haven't been established.

Z

- Tell patient that drug may change how fat is distributed in the body and may change body shape.
- Advise patient to report signs and symptoms of lactic acidosis (nausea, vomiting, shortness of breath, weakness).

ziprasidone hydrochloride
zih-PRAZ-i-done

Geodon◆, Zeldox❧

ziprasidone mesylate
Geodon

Therapeutic class: Antipsychotics
Pharmacologic class: Benzisoxazole derivatives

AVAILABLE FORMS
Capsules ⓞⓣⓒ: 20 mg, 40 mg, 60 mg, 80 mg
I.M. injection: 20 mg/mL single-dose vials (after reconstitution)

INDICATIONS & DOSAGES
➤ **Symptomatic treatment of schizophrenia**
Adults: Initially, 20 mg P.O. b.i.d. with food. Dosages are highly individualized. Adjust dosage, if necessary, no more frequently than every 2 days; to allow for lowest possible doses, the interval should be several weeks to assess symptom response. Effective dosage range is usually 20 to 100 mg b.i.d., but an increase to a dosage greater than 80 mg b.i.d. generally isn't recommended.
➤ **Rapid control of acute agitation in schizophrenic patients**
Adults: 10 to 20 mg I.M. as needed, up to a maximum dose of 40 mg daily. Doses of 10 mg may be given every 2 hours; doses of 20 mg may be given every 4 hours.
➤ **Acute bipolar I mania, including manic and mixed episodes, as monotherapy; maintenance treatment of bipolar I disorder as an adjunct to lithium or valproate**
Adults: 40 mg P.O. b.i.d. with food on day 1. Increase to 60 to 80 mg P.O. b.i.d. with food on day 2; then adjust dosage based on

patient response from 40 to 80 mg b.i.d. with food.

ADMINISTRATION
P.O.
- Always give drug with food (at least 500 calories) for optimal effect.
- Capsules must be swallowed whole.
I.M.
- To prepare I.M. ziprasidone, add 1.2 mL of sterile water for injection to the vial and shake vigorously until drug is completely dissolved. Each milliliter of reconstituted solution contains 20 mg ziprasidone.
- Don't mix injection with other medicinal products or solvents other than sterile water for injection.
- Inspect parenteral drug products for particulate matter and discoloration before administration. Discard unused portion of reconstituted solution.
- The effects of giving I.M. for more than 3 consecutive days are unknown. If long-term therapy of drug is necessary, switch to P.O. as soon as possible.
- Store injection at controlled room temperature of 77° F (25° C), excursions permitted to 59° to 86° F (15° to 30° C) in dry form, and protect from light. After reconstituting, it may be stored away from light for up to 24 hours at 59° to 86° F (15° to 30° C) or up to 7 days refrigerated, 36° to 46° F (2° to 8° C).

ACTION
May inhibit dopamine and serotonin-2 receptors, causing reduction in schizophrenia symptoms.

Route	Onset	Peak	Duration
P.O.	Unknown	6–8 hr	12 hr
I.M.	Unknown	1 hr	Unknown

Half-life: P.O., about 7 hours; I.M., 2 to 5 hours.

ADVERSE REACTIONS
CNS: confusion, headache, somnolence, *suicide attempt,* akathisia, dizziness, extrapyramidal symptoms, hypertonia, asthenia, dystonia (P.O.); tremor, twitching, fever, hypoesthesia, ataxia, amnesia, delirium, akinesia, dysarthria, choreoathetosis, incoordination, neuropathy, anxiety, insomnia, hypertonia, agitation, cogwheel rigidity,

---

Reactions in bold italics are *life-threatening*. Interactions may have a *rapid onset* or a *delayed onset*.

paresthesia, personality disorder, psychosis, speech disorder (I.M.).

CV: ***bradycardia, QT-interval prolongation,*** orthostatic hypotension, tachycardia, chest pain (P.O.); hypertension, vasodilation (I.M.).

EENT: rhinitis, abnormal vision (P.O.).

GI: nausea, constipation, dyspepsia, diarrhea, dry mouth, anorexia, abdominal pain, ***rectal hemorrhage,*** vomiting, tooth disorder (I.M.).

GU: dysmenorrhea, priapism (I.M.).

Metabolic: hyperglycemia.

Musculoskeletal: myalgia (P.O.), back pain (I.M.).

Respiratory: cough (P.O.).

Skin: rash (P.O.); injection-site pain, furunculosis, sweating (I.M.).

Other: flulike syndrome (I.M.).

INTERACTIONS

Drug-drug. *Antihypertensives:* May enhance hypotensive effects. Monitor BP.

Carbamazepine: May decrease ziprasidone level. May need to increase ziprasidone dose to achieve desired effect.

CYP3A4 inhibitors (itraconazole, ketoconazole): May increase ziprasidone level. Ziprasidone dosage reduction may be needed to achieve desired effect.

Drugs that decrease potassium or magnesium, such as diuretics: May increase risk of arrhythmias. Monitor potassium and magnesium levels if using these drugs together.

Black Box Warning *Opioids:* May cause slow or difficult breathing, sedation, and death. Avoid use together. If use together is necessary, limit dosage and duration of each drug to minimum necessary for desired effect. ∎

QT interval–prolonging drugs such as antiarrhythmics (amiodarone, bretylium, disopyramide, dofetilide, procainamide, quinidine, sotalol), arsenic trioxide, dolasetron, droperidol, levomethadyl, mefloquine, pentamidine, phenothiazines, pimozide, quinolones, tacrolimus: May increase risk of life-threatening arrhythmias. Use together is contraindicated.

Serotonin modulators (nefazodone, trazodone, vilazodone, vortioxetine): May increase risk of serotonin syndrome and

neuroleptic malignant syndrome. Monitor therapy.

Drug-lifestyle. *Alcohol use:* May increase dizziness, drowsiness, confusion, and difficulty concentrating. Don't use together.

EFFECTS ON LAB TEST RESULTS
- May increase glucose and lipid levels.
- May decrease WBC count.

CONTRAINDICATIONS & CAUTIONS
- Contraindicated in patients hypersensitive to drug and in those with recent MI or uncompensated HF.
- Contraindicated in patients with history of prolonged QT interval or congenital long QT syndrome and in those taking other drugs that prolong QT interval, such as dofetilide, sotalol, quinidine, other class IA and III antiarrhythmics, mesoridazine, thioridazine, chlorpromazine, droperidol, pimozide, sparfloxacin, gatifloxacin, moxifloxacin, halofantrine, mefloquine, pentamidine, arsenic trioxide, levomethadyl acetate, dolasetron mesylate, and tacrolimus.

Black Box Warning Opioids should only be prescribed with benzodiazepines or other CNS depressants to patients for whom alternative treatment options are inadequate. ∎

⊕ *Alert:* Drug is associated with a rare but serious skin reaction known as DRESS (drug reaction with eosinophilia and systemic symptoms), which may be fatal. DRESS is the presence of three or more symptoms, including cutaneous reactions (rash, exfoliative dermatitis), eosinophilia, fever, lymphadenopathy, and one or more systemic complications (hepatitis, nephritis, pneumonitis, myocarditis, pericarditis). Immediately discontinue drug if DRESS is suspected.

- Use cautiously in patients with history of seizures, bradycardia, hypokalemia, or hypomagnesemia; in those with acute diarrhea; and in those with conditions that may lower the seizure threshold (such as Alzheimer dementia).
- Use cautiously in patients at risk for aspiration pneumonia.

I.M.
- Don't use I.M. form in schizophrenic patients already taking oral ziprasidone.

✤ Canada   ◇ OTC   ◆ Off-label use   ✐ Photoguide   ⊕ Do not crush   *Liquid contains alcohol.

Z

• Use cautiously in elderly patients and in patients with renal or hepatic impairment.
Dialyzable drug: No.
⚠ *Overdose S&S:* Sedation, slurred speech, transitory hypertension, anxiety, extrapyramidal symptoms, somnolence, tremor.

PREGNANCY-LACTATION-REPRODUCTION

• There are no adequate studies in pregnant women. Use in pregnancy only if potential benefit justifies potential fetal risk.
☻ *Alert:* Neonates exposed to antipsychotics during the third trimester are at risk for developing extrapyramidal signs and symptoms (repetitive movements of the face and body) and withdrawal symptoms (agitation, abnormally increased or decreased muscle tone, tremors, sleepiness, severe difficulty breathing, difficulty feeding) after delivery.
• Enroll women ages 18 to 45 exposed to drug during pregnancy in the Atypical Antipsychotics Pregnancy Registry (1-866-961-2388).
• It isn't known if drug or its metabolites appear in breast milk. Breast-feeding isn't recommended.

NURSING CONSIDERATIONS

Black Box Warning In elderly patients with dementia-related psychosis, drug isn't indicated for use because of increased risk of death from CV events or infection. ∎
☻ *Alert:* Monitor patients and immediately report signs and symptoms of DRESS (rash, fever, swollen glands), as drug will be discontinued if DRESS is suspected.
☻ *Alert:* Severe and sometimes fatal cutaneous adverse reactions, such as Stevens-Johnson syndrome, have been reported in patients taking ziprasidone. Discontinue drug if a severe cutaneous adverse reaction is suspected.
☻ *Alert:* Hyperglycemia may occur. Monitor patients with diabetes regularly. Patients with risk factors for diabetes should undergo fasting blood glucose testing at baseline and periodically. Monitor all patients for symptoms of hyperglycemia, including excessive hunger or thirst, frequent urination, and weakness. Hyperglycemia may be reversible when drug is stopped.
☻ *Alert:* Monitor patient for symptoms of metabolic syndrome (significant weight gain and increased BMI, hypertension, hyperglycemia, hypercholesterolemia, and hypertriglyceridemia).
• Stop drug in patients with a QTc interval longer than 500 msec.
• Dizziness, palpitations, or syncope may be symptoms of a life-threatening arrhythmia such as torsades de pointes. Provide CV evaluation and monitoring in patients who experience these symptoms.
• Don't give to patients with electrolyte disturbances, such as hypokalemia or hypomagnesemia, because these increase the risk of arrhythmia. Monitor serum electrolyte levels periodically.
☻ *Alert:* Patient taking an antipsychotic may develop life-threatening neuroleptic malignant syndrome (hyperpyrexia, muscle rigidity, altered mental status, and autonomic instability) or tardive dyskinesia. Assess abnormal involuntary movement before starting therapy, at dosage changes, and periodically thereafter, to monitor patient for tardive dyskinesia.
• Monitor patient for abnormal body temperature regulation, especially if he is exercising strenuously, is exposed to extreme heat, is also receiving anticholinergics, or is subject to dehydration.
• Symptoms may not improve for 4 to 6 weeks.
• *Look alike–sound alike:* Don't confuse ziprasidone with trazodone, zafirlukast, zidovudine, zonisamide, or Zyprexa.

PATIENT TEACHING

Black Box Warning Caution patient or caregiver of patient taking an opioid with a benzodiazepine, CNS depressant, or alcohol to seek immediate medical attention if patient experiences dizziness, light-headedness, extreme sleepiness, slowed or difficult breathing, or unresponsiveness. ∎
• Tell patient to take drug with food and to swallow capsules whole.
• Tell patient to immediately report signs or symptoms of dizziness, fainting, irregular heartbeat, or relevant heart problems.
• Advise patient to report recent episodes of diarrhea, abnormal movements, sudden fever, muscle rigidity, or change in mental status.

◑ *Alert:* Tell patient to immediately report rash (with or without blisters), fever, swollen lymph nodes, mouth ulcers, skin shedding, or targetlike spots in the skin.

• Advise female patient to consult prescriber if she is pregnant or plans to become pregnant.

• Tell female patient that breast-feeding isn't recommended during therapy.

• Advise patient that drug can cause sleepiness and to use care when operating machinery or driving a motor vehicle.

• Advise patient that symptoms may not improve for 4 to 6 weeks.

zoledronic acid
zoh-leh-DROH-nik

Reclast, Zometa

Therapeutic class: Antiosteoporotics
Pharmacologic class: Bisphosphonates

AVAILABLE FORMS
Injection as ready-to-infuse solution:
5 mg/100 mL (Reclast), 4 mg/100 mL (Zometa)
Injection (Zometa): 4 mg/5-mL vial

INDICATIONS & DOSAGES
➤ **Hypercalcemia caused by malignancy**
Adults: 4 mg (Zometa) by I.V. infusion over at least 15 minutes. If albumin-corrected calcium level doesn't return to normal, may repeat 4 mg. Let at least 7 days pass before retreatment to allow a full response to the first dose.
Adjust-a-dose: Zometa: Assess serum creatinine level before each treatment or retreatment. Dosage adjustments aren't necessary for patients presenting with mild to moderate renal impairment before initiation of therapy (serum creatinine level less than 400 micromol/L or less than 4.5 mg/dL).
➤ **Multiple myeloma and bone metastases of solid tumors in conjunction with standard antineoplastics**
Adults: 4 mg (Zometa) I.V. infused over at least 15 minutes every 3 to 4 weeks. Treatment duration depends on type of cancer. Use for prostate cancer only after it has progressed after treatment with at

least one course of hormonal therapy. Give patients an oral calcium supplement of 500 mg and a multiple vitamin containing 400 international units of vitamin D daily.
Adjust-a-dose: Zometa: For patients with CrCl of 50 to 60 mL/minute, give 3.5 mg. If 40 to 49 mL/minute, give 3.3 mg. If 30 to 39 mL/minute, give 3 mg. For patients with normal baseline creatinine level but an increase of 0.5 mg/dL and in those with abnormal baseline creatinine level who have an increase of 1 mg/dL, withhold drug. Resume treatment at the same dose as that before treatment interruption only when creatinine level has returned to within 10% of baseline value. If CrCl is less than 30 mL/minute, don't give drug.
➤ **Paget disease of bone (osteitis deformans)**
Adults: 5 mg (Reclast) by I.V. infusion over at least 15 minutes. Give through a vented infusion line. May repeat if relapse occurs. Patient also needs 1,500 mg elemental calcium in divided doses (750 mg b.i.d. or 500 mg t.i.d.) and 800 international units vitamin D daily, especially during the 2 weeks after dosing.
➤ **Treatment of osteoporosis in men; to reduce incidence of fractures in postmenopausal women with osteoporosis, diagnosed by bone mineral density or prevalent vertebral fracture, and in those at high risk for fracture, defined as a recent low-trauma hip fracture; to treat and prevent glucocorticoid-induced osteoporosis in patients taking a daily dosage equivalent to 7.5 mg or greater of prednisone and who are expected to remain on glucocorticoids for at least 12 months**
Adults: 5 mg (Reclast) by I.V. infusion over no less than 15 minutes once a year.
➤ **Prevention of osteoporosis**
Postmenopausal women: 5 mg (Reclast) by I.V. infusion over no less than 15 minutes once every 2 years.
➤ **Osteopenia secondary to androgen-deprivation therapy in prostate cancer ◆**
Adults: 4 mg (Zometa) I.V. infused over 15 minutes every 3 months or once yearly for the duration of 1 year.
➤ **Osteopenia in estrogen-deprived breast cancer ◆**

Z

Adults: 4 mg (Zometa) I.V. infused over 15 minutes every 6 months for up to 5 years.

ADMINISTRATION

I.V.
Zometa

▼ For patient with CrCl greater than 60 mL/minute, withdraw 5 mL to obtain 4 mg of drug and mix in 100 mL of NSS or D_5W. For ready-to-use bottles, if reduced doses are needed for patients with renal impairment, withdraw appropriate volume of solution and replace with an equal amount of NSS or D_5W and refer to manufacturer's instructions.

▼ Give as I.V. infusion over at least 15 minutes.

▼ If drug isn't used immediately after reconstitution, refrigerate solution and give within 24 hours. Bring refrigerated solution to room temperature before administering.

Reclast

▼ Reclast is infused over not less than 15 minutes at a constant infusion rate. Give as a single I.V. solution through a separate vented infusion line.

▼ Flush I.V. line with 10 mL NSS after infusion.

▼ If refrigerated, allow the refrigerated solution to reach room temperature before administration.

▼ After opening, solution is stable for 24 hours at 36° to 46° F (2° to 8° C).

▼ **Incompatibilities (Zometa and Reclast):** Solutions containing calcium (such as lactated Ringer solution) or other I.V. drugs.

ACTION

Inhibits bone resorption, probably by inhibiting osteoclast activity and osteoclastic resorption of mineralized bone and cartilage. Decreases calcium release induced by the stimulatory factors produced by tumors.

Route	Onset	Peak	Duration
I.V. (Zometa)	Unknown	Unknown	228 days
I.V. (Reclast)	Unknown	Unknown	Unknown

Half-life: Triphasic with terminal half-life, 146 hours.

ADVERSE REACTIONS

CNS: headache, anxiety, somnolence, insomnia, confusion, agitation, depression, paresthesia, hypoesthesia, fatigue, weakness, dizziness, fever, asthenia, malaise, vertigo, lethargy, fever.

CV: hypotension, hypertension, atrial fibrillation, leg edema, chest pain, palpitations.

GI: nausea, constipation, diarrhea, abdominal pain, vomiting, anorexia, dysphagia, decreased appetite, dyspepsia, abdominal distention, mucositis, stomatitis.

EENT: eye pain.

GU: *increased creatinine level,* urinary infection, moniliasis.

Hematologic: anemia, *granulocytopenia, neutropenia, thrombocytopenia, pancytopenia.*

Metabolic: dehydration, weight decrease.

Musculoskeletal: skeletal pain, arthralgia, myalgia, back pain, osteonecrosis of the jaw, osteoarthritis, muscle spasms, bone pain, neck pain, shoulder pain, extremity pain.

Respiratory: dyspnea, cough.

Skin: alopecia, dermatitis, rash, pruritus.

Other: *progression of cancer,* rigors, infection, influenza, hyperhidrosis.

INTERACTIONS

Drug-drug. *Aminoglycosides, loop diuretics:* May have additive effects that lower calcium level. Use together cautiously, and monitor calcium level.

Nephrotoxic drugs, such as NSAIDs: Renal toxicity may be greater in patients with renal impairment. Use Reclast cautiously with other potentially nephrotoxic drugs. Monitor serum creatinine before each dose.

Thalidomide: May increase risk of renal dysfunction in patients with multiple myeloma. Use together cautiously.

EFFECTS ON LAB TEST RESULTS

● May increase creatinine level.

● May decrease calcium, phosphorus, magnesium, potassium, and Hb levels and hematocrit.

● May decrease RBC, WBC, and platelet counts.

CONTRAINDICATIONS & CAUTIONS

● Contraindicated in patients hypersensitive to drug, other bisphosphonates, or any of

---

Reactions in bold italics are *life-threatening*. Interactions may have a *rapid onset* or a *delayed onset*.

drug's ingredients; Zometa is contraindicated in patients with hypercalcemia of malignancy whose creatinine level is more than 4.5 mg/dL and in patients with bone metastases and a creatinine level of more than 3 mg/dL.

❸ Alert: There may be an increased risk of fractures of the thigh in patients treated with bisphosphonates.

• Reclast is contraindicated in patients with hypocalcemia. Patients must be adequately supplemented with calcium and vitamin D.

❸ Alert: Reclast may increase risk of renal failure, especially in patients with underlying renal impairment, dehydration, and increased age. Screen patients before use and monitor carefully.

❸ Alert: Reclast is contraindicated in patients with CrCl less than 35 mL/minute and in patients with evidence of acute renal failure.

• Use cautiously in elderly patients and those with aspirin-sensitive asthma because other bisphosphonates have been linked to bronchoconstriction in aspirin-sensitive patients with asthma.

Dialyzable drug: Unknown.

⚠ Overdose S&S: Hypocalcemia, hypophosphatemia, hypomagnesemia, renal impairment.

PREGNANCY-LACTATION-REPRODUCTION

• Drug shouldn't be used during pregnancy. Women should avoid becoming pregnant during therapy. Drug may cause fetal harm if used during pregnancy or if patient becomes pregnant after completing therapy because drug binds to bone long term and may be released over weeks to years. Inform patient of potential fetal hazard.

• It isn't known if drug appears in breast milk. Patient should discontinue breast-feeding or discontinue drug.

NURSING CONSIDERATIONS

• Reclast contains the same active ingredient found in Zometa, used for oncology indications. Patient being treated with Zometa shouldn't be treated with Reclast.

• Hydrate patient adequately before giving; urine output should be about 2 L daily.

• Each vial of Zometa contains 220 mg mannitol and 24 mg sodium citrate.

❸ Alert: Because of the risk of decreased renal function progressing to renal failure, don't exceed 4 mg as a single dose of Zometa and always infuse over at least 15 minutes.

• Monitor calcium, phosphate, magnesium, and creatinine levels carefully. Correct decreased calcium, phosphorus, and magnesium levels using I.V. calcium gluconate, potassium and sodium phosphate, and magnesium sulfate.

• Monitor renal function closely. Patients with renal impairment may be at a greater risk for adverse reactions.

❸ Alert: Patients, especially those who have cancer or poor oral hygiene or who are receiving chemotherapy or corticosteroids, should have a dental examination with appropriate preventive dentistry before therapy.

• Osteonecrosis of the jaw has been reported rarely in postmenopausal osteoporosis patients treated with bisphosphonates, including zoledronic acid. All patients should have a routine oral examination before treatment and should be monitored while on therapy.

• Severe incapacitating bone, joint, and muscle pain may occur. Withhold future doses of Reclast if severe symptoms occur. When drug is stopped, symptoms may resolve partially or completely.

• *Look alike–sound alike:* Don't confuse Zometa with Zofran or Zoladex.

PATIENT TEACHING

• Review use and administration of drug with patient and family.

• Instruct patient to report adverse effects promptly (such as fever, flulike symptoms, myalgia, arthralgia, headache, muscle cramps, numbness, tingling, difficulty swallowing, palpitations, jaw pain, thigh and bone pain, edema).

• Explain importance of periodic laboratory tests to monitor therapy and renal function.

• If female patient becomes pregnant or is breast-feeding, advise her to alert prescriber.

• On day of Reclast treatment, instruct patient to drink at least 2 glasses of fluid such as water within a few hours before infusion. Advise patient of importance of calcium and vitamin D supplementation.

Z

• Advise patient to report persistent pain or nonhealing sore of the mouth or jaw and to maintain good oral hygiene and receive routine dental checkups.

zolmitriptan
zohl-mah-TRIP-tan

Zomig, Zomig-ZMT

Therapeutic class: Antimigraine drugs
Pharmacologic class: Serotonin 5-HT$_1$ receptor agonists

AVAILABLE FORMS
Nasal spray: 2.5 mg, 5 mg
ODTs 🆕: 2.5 mg, 5 mg
Tablets (immediate-release): 2.5 mg, 5 mg

INDICATIONS & DOSAGES
➤ **Acute migraine headaches**
Adults: Initially, 2.5 mg or less P.O. Break a 2.5-mg immediate-release tablet in half if a lower dose is needed. Increase to 5 mg per dosage, as needed. If using ODTs, initially, 2.5 mg P.O. Maximum dosage is 10 mg in 24 hours.
Adjust-a-dose: In patients with moderate to severe hepatic impairment, give 1.25 mg (one-half of one 2.5-mg tablet. Don't use ODTs because they shouldn't be broken in half.) Limit total daily dose in patients with severe hepatic impairment to no more than 5 mg/day. In patients taking cimetidine, limit maximum single dose to 2.5 mg, not to exceed 5 mg in any 24-hour period.
Adults and children age 12 and older: Initially, 1 spray (2.5 mg) into nostril; may increase to maximum 5-mg single dose if needed. If headache returns after first dose, give a second dose no sooner than 2 hours after first dose. Maximum dose is 10 mg in 24 hours.
Adjust-a-dose: Nasal spray isn't recommended in patients with moderate or severe hepatic impairment. In patients taking cimetidine, limit maximum single dose to 2.5 mg, not to exceed 5 mg in any 24-hour period.

ADMINISTRATION
P.O.
• Give ODT immediately after opening.
• Don't break or crush ODT.
• ODT dissolves on tongue and is swallowed with saliva; fluid isn't needed.
Intranasal
• Patient should gently blow his nose before use.
• Remove cap and insert device into nostril and block the opposite nostril.
• Press plunger device while patient breathes gently in through the nose. Patient should then breathe gently through the mouth for 5 to 10 seconds.
• Don't test or prime spray before use; nasal sprayer contains only one dose.
• Discard after use.

ACTION
May act as an agonist at serotonin receptors on extracerebral intracranial blood vessels, which constricts the affected vessels, inhibits neuropeptide release, and reduces pain transmission in the trigeminal pathways.

Route	Onset	Peak	Duration
P.O.	Unknown	1½–3 hr	Unknown
Intranasal	5 min	3 hr	Unknown

Half-life: 3 hours.

ADVERSE REACTIONS
CNS: dizziness, somnolence, vertigo, paresthesia, asthenia, pain, drowsiness, depersonalization, headache, chills, insomnia.
CV: palpitations; chest pain, pressure, tightness, or heaviness; facial edema.
EENT: pain, tightness, or pressure in the neck, throat, or jaw; nasal irritation.
GI: dry mouth, dysgeusia, dyspepsia, dysphagia, nausea, abdominal pain, vomiting.
Musculoskeletal: myalgia, myasthenia.
Skin: sweating.
Other: warm or cold sensations, hypersensitivity reaction.

INTERACTIONS
Drug-drug. *Cimetidine:* May double half-life of zolmitriptan. Limit maximum single dose of zolmitriptan to 2.5 mg, not to exceed 5 mg in any 24-hour period. Monitor patient closely.

Reactions in bold italics are *life-threatening*. Interactions may have a *rapid onset* or a *delayed onset*.

Ergot-containing drugs, other triptans: May exacerbate headaches and increase vasoconstricting effects. Avoid using within 24 hours of zolmitriptan.

Hormonal contraceptives, propranolol: May increase zolmitriptan level. Monitor patient closely.

MAO inhibitors: May increase zolmitriptan level. Avoid using within 2 weeks of MAO inhibitor.

SSRIs: May cause additive serotonin effects, resulting in weakness, hyperreflexia, or incoordination. Monitor patient closely.

EFFECTS ON LAB TEST RESULTS
● May increase alkaline phosphatase level.

CONTRAINDICATIONS & CAUTIONS
● Contraindicated in patients hypersensitive to drug or its components, within 24 hours of treatment with another 5-HT$_1$ agonist or ergot-type drug, and in patients with uncontrolled hypertension, hemiplegic or basilar migraine, stroke, TIA history, peripheral vascular disease, ischemic bowel disease, Wolff-Parkinson-White syndrome or arrhythmias associated with other cardiac accessory conduction pathway disorders, ischemic heart disease (angina pectoris, history of MI or documented silent ischemia), symptoms of ischemic heart disease (coronary artery vasospasm, including Prinzmetal variant angina), or other significant heart disease.
● Contraindicated within 2 weeks of stopping MAO inhibitor.
● Use cautiously in patients with liver disease and in those who may be at risk for CAD (such as postmenopausal women or men older than age 40) or those with risk factors, such as hypertension, hypercholesterolemia, obesity, diabetes, smoking, or family history.

Dialyzable drug: Unknown.
⚠ *Overdose S&S:* Sedation.

PREGNANCY-LACTATION-REPRODUCTION
● Drug has caused fetal harm in animal studies, but there are no adequate studies in pregnant women. Use during pregnancy only if clearly needed and potential benefit justifies potential risk to the fetus.

● It isn't known if drug appears in breast milk. Patient should discontinue breastfeeding or discontinue drug.

NURSING CONSIDERATIONS
● Drug isn't intended for preventing migraines or treating hemiplegic or basilar migraines.
● Safety of drug hasn't been established for cluster headaches or for treatment of an average of more than three headaches (oral formulation) or four headaches (intranasal formulation) in a 30-day period.
● *Alert:* Combining drug with an SSRI or an SSNRI may cause serotonin syndrome. Signs and symptoms may include restlessness, hallucinations, loss of coordination, fast heartbeat, rapid changes in BP, increased body temperature, overactive reflexes, nausea, vomiting, and diarrhea. Serotonin syndrome may be more likely to occur when starting or increasing the dose of drug, SSRI, or SSNRI.
● Watch for serotonin syndrome in patients taking other drugs that increase serotonin level.
● Zomig ODT tablets contain phenylalanine, which can be harmful to patients with phenylketonuria.
● *Look alike–sound alike:* Don't confuse Zomig with Zoloft or Zonegran. Don't confuse zolmitriptan with rizatriptan, sumatriptan, or zolpidem.

PATIENT TEACHING
● Tell patient that drug is intended to relieve, not prevent, signs and symptoms of migraine. It isn't used to treat other types of headaches, and misuse of drug to treat more than 10 headaches per month may lead to worsening of headaches.
● Advise patient to take drug as prescribed and not to take a second dose unless instructed by prescriber. Tell patient if a second dose is indicated and permitted, he should take it 2 hours after first dose.
● Warn patient that maximum total daily dose is 10 mg.
● Instruct patient to release the ODTs from the blister pack just before taking; tablet should dissolve on tongue.
● Advise patient not to chew or break ODTs in half.

Z

• Advise patient to immediately report pain or tightness in the chest or throat, heart throbbing, rash, skin lumps, or swelling of the face, lips, or eyelids.
• Tell female patient not to take drug if she is or may become pregnant or is breast-feeding.
• Warn patient that serotonin syndrome may occur if drug is used in combination with other drugs that increase serotonin level (SSRIs, SSNRIs).

SAFETY ALERT!

zolpidem tartrate
ZOL-pih-dem

Ambien✒, Ambien CR, Edluar, Intermezzo, Zolpimist

Therapeutic class: Hypnotics
Pharmacologic class: Imidazopyridines
Controlled substance schedule: IV

AVAILABLE FORMS
Oral spray: 5 mg/actuation
Tablets: 5 mg, 10 mg
Tablets (extended-release) ⓒ: 6.25 mg, 12.5 mg
Tablets (S.L.): 1.75 mg, 3.5 mg, 5 mg, 10 mg

INDICATIONS & DOSAGES
➤ **Short-term management of insomnia**
Adults: 5 or 10 mg (men) or 5 mg (women) immediate-release or 6.25 or 12.5 mg (men) or 6.25 mg (women) extended-release P.O. immediately before bedtime. Or, Intermezzo 3.5 mg (men) or 1.75 mg (women) S.L. once per night as needed for middle-of-the-night waking and difficulty returning to sleep, only if at least 4 hours of bedtime remain. Or, Zolpimist 5 or 10 mg (men) or 5 mg (women) once per night immediately before bedtime with at least 7 to 8 hours remaining before planned time of awakening. May increase to 10 mg as needed.
Adjust-a-dose: For elderly or debilitated patients and those with hepatic insufficiency, 5 mg P.O. immediately before bedtime. Or, 6.25 mg of extended-release form. Or, 1.75 mg P.O. Intermezzo if needed in men and women older than age 65. Maximum

daily dose is 10 mg immediate-release and 12.5 mg extended-release.

ADMINISTRATION
P.O.
• For rapid sleep onset, drug should not be taken with or immediately after meals.
• Don't crush, break, or divide extended-release tablets.
• Place S.L. tablet under tongue to disintegrate. Patient shouldn't swallow tablet whole or take with water.
• Prime oral spray pump with 5 sprays before first use or with 1 spray if pump hasn't been used for 14 days.
• Pump spray directly over tongue. Have patient press down fully to make sure full dose is delivered.

ACTION
Although drug interacts with one of three identified GABA–benzodiazepine receptor complexes, it isn't a benzodiazepine. It exhibits hypnotic activity and minimal muscle relaxant and anticonvulsant properties.

Route	Onset	Peak	Duration
P.O.	Rapid	30–120 min	6–8 hr

Half-life: 1½ to 8½ hours.

ADVERSE REACTIONS
CNS: headache, amnesia, abnormal dreams, complex sleep-related behaviors, drowsiness, depression, dizziness, drugged feeling, lethargy, light-headedness, nervousness, sleep disorder, euphoria, mood swings, memory disorder.
CV: palpitations, chest pain.
EENT: pharyngitis, sinusitis.
GI: abdominal pain, constipation, diarrhea, dry mouth, dyspepsia, nausea, vomiting, dry mouth.
Musculoskeletal: arthralgia, myalgia, back pain.
Skin: rash, urticaria.
Other: flulike syndrome, hypersensitivity reactions.

INTERACTIONS
Drug-drug. *CNS depressants:* May cause excessive CNS depression. Use together cautiously.

Reactions in bold italics are *life-threatening*. Interactions may have a *rapid onset* or a *delayed onset*.

CYP3A4 inducers (rifampin): May decrease effects of zolpidem. Avoid use together.

CYP3A4 inhibitors (itraconazole, ketoconazole, verapamil): May increase zolpidem level. Use a low zolpidem dosage and monitor therapy.

Black Box Warning *Opioids:* May cause slow or difficult breathing, sedation, and death. Avoid use together. If use together is necessary, limit dosage and duration of each drug to minimum necessary for desired effect. ■

Drug-herb. *Calendula, chamomile, gotu kola, kava, valerian:* May increase risk of CNS depression. Avoid concomitant use.

St. John's wort: May decrease zolpidem level and effects. Avoid concomitant use.

Drug-food. *Grapefruit juice:* May decrease zolpidem metabolism. Avoid grapefruit juice.

Drug-lifestyle. *Alcohol use:* May cause excessive CNS depression. Discourage use together.

EFFECTS ON LAB TEST RESULTS

- May increase ALT, AST, and bilirubin levels.
- May decrease radioactive iodine uptake.

CONTRAINDICATIONS & CAUTIONS

- Contraindicated in patients hypersensitive to drug or its components.

Black Box Warning Opioids should only be prescribed with benzodiazepines or other CNS depressants to patients for whom alternative treatment options are inadequate. ■

- Use cautiously in patients with compromised respiratory status or a history of depression or worsening depression.
- Complex behaviors such as "sleep driving" (driving while not fully awake after taking a sedative-hypnotic with subsequent amnesia of the event) have been reported. These can occur with therapeutic doses, although the use of alcohol and other CNS depressants appears to increase the risk. Strongly consider discontinuing drug if patient reports such an event.

❸ *Alert:* Drug level may remain elevated the day after drug use, impairing mental alertness. Risk increases if patient sleeps for less than 7 hours, takes drug with other CNS depressants including alcohol, or takes higher than recommended dose.

❸ *Alert:* Patients taking extended-release formulation shouldn't drive or engage in other activities that require complete mental alertness the day after taking drug because drug level can remain high enough to impair these activities.

❸ *Alert:* Drug can cause drowsiness and decreased level of consciousness, which may lead to falls and severe injuries, such as hip fractures and intracranial hemorrhage.

Dialyzable drug: No.

⚠ *Overdose S&S:* Impaired consciousness, somnolence, coma, CV or respiratory compromise, death.

PREGNANCY-LACTATION-REPRODUCTION

- There are no adequate studies in pregnant women, but drug may cause fetal or neonatal harm. Use during pregnancy only if potential benefit outweighs potential risk to the fetus.
- Drug appears in breast milk. Use cautiously in breast-feeding women.

NURSING CONSIDERATIONS

❸ *Alert:* Anaphylaxis and angioedema may occur as early as the first dose. Monitor patient closely. Discontinue drug and don't restart if these occur.

- Use drug only for short-term management of insomnia, usually 7 to 10 days.
- Use the smallest effective dose in all patients.
- Take precautions to prevent hoarding by patients who are depressed, suicidal, or drug-dependent, or who have a history of drug abuse.
- *Look alike–sound alike:* Don't confuse Ambien with Abilify, Ativan, or Coumadin. Don't confuse zolpidem with lorazepam, zaleplon, or zolmitriptan.

PATIENT TEACHING

Black Box Warning Caution patient or caregiver of patient taking an opioid with a benzodiazepine, CNS depressant, or alcohol to seek immediate medical attention if patient experiences dizziness, light-headedness, extreme sleepiness, slowed or difficult breathing, or unresponsiveness. ■

Z

⊙ *Alert:* Warn patient that drug may cause allergic reactions, facial swelling, and complex sleep-related behaviors, such as driving, eating, and making phone calls while asleep. Advise patient to immediately report these adverse effects.

⊙ *Alert:* Tell patient that drug has the potential to cause next-day impairment, and that this risk increases if dosing instructions aren't carefully followed. Tell patient to wait for at least 8 hours after dosing before driving or engaging in other activities requiring full mental alertness. Inform patient that impairment can be present even though he may feel fully awake.

⊙ *Alert:* Tell patient that drug can cause drowsiness and decreased level of consciousness, which may lead to falls and severe injuries.

• For rapid sleep onset, instruct patient not to take drug with or immediately after meals.

• Instruct patient to take drug immediately before going to bed; onset of action is rapid.

• Tell patient to take Intermezzo in bed when he awakens in the middle of the night and has difficulty returning to sleep, and only if he has at least 4 hours of bedtime remaining.

• Tell patient to avoid alcohol use while taking drug.

• Tell patient to place the S.L. tablet under the tongue and allow the tablet to disintegrate. Tell patient not to swallow, chew, break, or split the tablet, or take the tablet with water.

⊙ *Alert:* Tell patient not to crush, chew, or divide the extended-release tablets.

• Instruct patient to prime spray pump with 5 sprays before first use or with 1 spray if pump hasn't been used for 14 days.

• Tell patient to aim the spray directly over the tongue and press down fully to make sure the full dose is delivered.

• Caution patient to avoid performing activities that require mental alertness or physical coordination during therapy.

zonisamide
zoh-NISS-a-mide

Zonegran

Therapeutic class: Anticonvulsants
Pharmacologic class: Sulfonamides

AVAILABLE FORMS
Capsules 🅾: 25 mg, 50 mg, 100 mg

INDICATIONS & DOSAGES
➤ **Adjunctive therapy for partial seizures in adults with epilepsy**
Adults and children older than age 16:
Initially, 100 mg P.O. as a single daily dose for 2 weeks. Then, dosage may be increased to 200 mg daily for at least 2 weeks. Dosage can be increased to 300 mg and then to 400 mg P.O. daily, with the dose stable for at least 2 weeks to achieve steady state at each level. Doses can be given once or twice daily, except for the daily dose of 100 mg at start of therapy. Maximum recommended dose is 600 mg daily.

Adjust-a-dose: For patients with renal or hepatic impairment, titrate dosages more slowly and monitor patients more frequently. Use isn't recommended in patients with GFR of less than 50 mL/minute.

ADMINISTRATION
P.O.
• Give drug without regard for food.
• Don't crush or open capsule.

ACTION
May stabilize neuronal membranes and suppress neuronal hypersynchronization, which prevents seizures.

Route	Onset	Peak	Duration
P.O.	Unknown	2–6 hr	Unknown

Half-life: 63 hours.

ADVERSE REACTIONS
CNS: dizziness, headache, somnolence, *seizures, status epilepticus,* agitation or irritability, anxiety, asthenia, ataxia, confusion, depression, difficulties in concentration or memory, difficulties in verbal expression, fatigue, hyperesthesia, incoordination,

---

insomnia, mental slowing, nervousness, paresthesia, schizophrenic or schizophreniform behavior, speech disorders, tremor.
EENT: amblyopia, diplopia, pharyngitis, rhinitis, taste perversion, tinnitus, nystagmus.
GI: anorexia, abdominal pain, constipation, diarrhea, dry mouth, dyspepsia, nausea, vomiting.
GU: kidney stones.
Hematologic: ecchymoses.
Metabolic: weight loss.
Respiratory: cough.
Skin: pruritus, rash.
Other: accidental injury, flulike syndrome.

INTERACTIONS
Drug-drug. *Drugs that induce or inhibit CYP3A4:* May change zonisamide level; phenytoin, carbamazepine, phenobarbital, and valproate increase zonisamide clearance. Monitor patient closely.

EFFECTS ON LAB TEST RESULTS
• May increase BUN and creatinine levels.

CONTRAINDICATIONS & CAUTIONS
• According to manufacturer, drug is contraindicated in patients hypersensitive to drug or to sulfonamides.
• Use cautiously in patients with renal and hepatic dysfunction or kidney stones.
• Use cautiously in patients with history of psychiatric symptoms.
• Use cautiously with other drugs that predispose patients to heat-related disorders, including but not limited to carbonic anhydrase inhibitors and drugs with anticholinergic activity.
• Safety and effectiveness in children younger than age 16 haven't been established; children are at increased risk for oligohidrosis and hyperthermia.
Dialyzable drug: Yes.
⚠ *Overdose S&S:* CNS symptoms, coma, bradycardia, hypotension, respiratory depression.

PREGNANCY-LACTATION-REPRODUCTION
• Use during pregnancy may present a significant fetal risk; a variety of fetal abnormalities can occur. Use in pregnant women only if potential benefit justifies potential

fetal risk. Women of childbearing potential should use effective contraception.
• Encourage pregnant patients taking drug to enroll in the North American Antiepileptic Drug Pregnancy Registry (1-888-233-2334).
• Drug appears in breast milk. Patient should discontinue breast-feeding or discontinue drug.

NURSING CONSIDERATIONS
❸ *Alert:* Rarely, patients receiving sulfonamides have died because of severe reactions, such as Stevens-Johnson syndrome, fulminant hepatic necrosis, aplastic anemia, otherwise unexplained rashes, and agranulocytosis. If signs and symptoms of hypersensitivity or other serious reactions occur, stop drug immediately and notify prescriber.
❸ *Alert:* Closely monitor all patients taking or starting antiepileptic drugs for changes in behavior indicating worsening of suicidal thoughts or behavior or depression. Symptoms such as anxiety, agitation, hostility, mania, and hypomania may be precursors to emerging suicidality.
• If patient develops acute renal failure or a significant sustained increase in creatinine or BUN level, stop drug and notify prescriber. Periodically monitor renal function.
• Drug can cause metabolic acidosis, especially in those with predisposing conditions or therapies. This risk is more frequent and severe in younger patients. Measure serum bicarbonate level before starting treatment and periodically during treatment, even in the absence of symptoms.
• Don't stop drug abruptly because this may cause increased seizures or status epilepticus; reduce dosage or stop drug gradually.
• Achieving steady-state levels may take 2 weeks.
• Monitor patient for signs and symptoms of hypersensitivity.
• Increase fluid intake and urine output to help prevent kidney stones, especially in patients with predisposing factors.
• Monitor patient for cognitive and neuropsychiatric adverse reactions, including psychomotor slowing, difficulty with concentration, speech or language problems (especially word-finding difficulties),

Z

somnolence or fatigue, depression, and psychosis.

PATIENT TEACHING

• Tell patient to take drug with or without food and to swallow capsule whole.

• Advise patient to call prescriber immediately if rash develops or seizures worsen.

• Tell patient to contact prescriber immediately if he develops sudden back or abdominal pain, pain when urinating, bloody or dark urine, fever, sore throat, mouth sores or easy bruising, decreased sweating, fever, depression, or speech or language problems.

• Tell patient to avoid dehydration and to maintain adequate fluid intake.

• Caution patient that this drug can cause drowsiness and not to drive or operate dangerous machinery until drug's effects are known.

• Advise patient not to stop taking drug without prescriber's approval because abrupt withdrawal can cause seizures.

• Instruct female patient of childbearing potential to inform prescriber if she is pregnant, plans to become pregnant, or is breast-feeding and to use contraception during therapy.

---

alectinib hydrochloride
al-EK-ti-nib

Alecensa

Therapeutic class: Antineoplastics
Pharmacologic class: Tyrosine kinase inhibitors

AVAILABLE FORMS
Capsules ⊙⊙: 150 mg

INDICATIONS & DOSAGES
➤ **Anaplastic lymphoma kinase (ALK)-positive, metastatic non-small-cell lung cancer in patients who have progressed on or are intolerant to crizotinib**
Adults: 600 mg P.O. b.i.d. until disease progression or unacceptable toxicity.
Adjust-a-dose: For dosage modifications for adverse reactions, first reduce dosage to 450 mg b.i.d. If a second dosage reduction is needed, reduce dosage to 300 mg b.i.d. Discontinue drug if patient is unable to tolerate 300-mg b.i.d. dose. For ALT or AST level greater than $5 \times$ ULN with total bilirubin level $2 \times$ ULN or less, withhold drug until recovery to baseline or to $3 \times$ ULN or less, then resume at reduced dosage. For ALT or AST level greater than $3 \times$ ULN with total bilirubin level greater than $2 \times$ ULN without cholestasis or hemolysis, permanently discontinue drug. For total bilirubin level greater than $3 \times$ ULN, withhold drug until recover to baseline or to $1.5 \times$ ULN or less, then resume at reduced dose.

For treatment-related interstitial lung disease (ILD) or pneumonitis, permanently discontinue drug.

For symptomatic bradycardia and after a contributing concomitant medication is identified and discontinued or its dosage adjusted, resume alectinib at the previous dosage upon recovery to asymptomatic bradycardia or to HR of 60 beats per minute (bpm) or higher. For symptomatic bradycardia with no contributing concomitant drug identified or, if the contributing concomitant drug isn't discontinued or its dosage adjusted, resume alectinib at a reduced dosage upon recovery to asymptomatic bradycardia or to HR of 60 bpm or higher. If life-threatening (requires urgent intervention) bradycardia occurs and no contributing concomitant drug is identified, permanently discontinue alectinib. If life-threatening bradycardia occurs, and a contributing concomitant drug is identified and discontinued or its dosage adjusted, resume alectinib at a reduced dosage upon recovery to asymptomatic bradycardia or to HR of 60 bpm or higher, with frequent patient monitoring. If bradycardia recurs, permanently discontinue alectinib.

For CK level greater than $5 \times$ ULN, withhold drug until recovery to baseline or to $2.5 \times$ ULN or less, then resume at same dosage. For CK level greater than

$10 \times$ ULN, or for a second occurrence of CK level greater than $5 \times$ ULN, withhold drug until recovery to baseline or to $2.5 \times$ ULN or less, then resume at reduced dosage.

ADMINISTRATION
P.O.
• Hazardous drug; use safe handling and disposal precautions according to facility policy.
• Give with food.
• Don't open or dissolve contents of capsule.
• If a dose is missed or vomiting occurs after taking a dose, give next dose at the scheduled time.
• Don't store above 86° F (30° C). Store in the original container to protect from light and moisture.

ACTION
A tyrosine kinase inhibitor that targets ALK and RET ALK gene abnormalities that alter signaling and expression and result in increased cellular proliferation and survival in tumors that express these fusion proteins. Inhibiting ALK signaling decreases tumor cell viability.

Route	Onset	Peak	Duration
P.O.	Unknown	4 hr	Unknown

Half-life: 33 hours (parent drug).

ADVERSE REACTIONS
CNS: fatigue, headache.
CV: *bradycardia, PE,* edema.
EENT: vision disorder.
GI: vomiting, constipation, nausea, diarrhea.
Hematologic: anemia, *lymphopenia.*
Hepatic: hyperbilirubinemia, elevated AST and ALT levels.
Metabolic: increased weight.
Musculoskeletal: myalgia, back pain.
Respiratory: dyspnea, cough.
Skin: rash, photosensitivity.

INTERACTIONS
Drug-drug. *Bradycardia-causing drugs:* May increase risk of bradycardia. Monitor patient closely.
Drug-lifestyle. *Sun exposure:* May increase risk of photosensitivity. Discourage sun exposure and recommend use of broad-spectrum sunscreen and lip balm.

EFFECTS ON LAB TEST RESULTS
• May increase AST, ALT, alkaline phosphatase, CK, bilirubin, glucose, and creatinine levels. May decrease calcium, potassium, phosphorus, and sodium levels.
• May decrease WBC and RBC counts.

CONTRAINDICATIONS & CAUTIONS
• Safety and effectiveness in children haven't been determined.
• Drug may increase risk of hepatotoxicity, pulmonary toxicity (ILD or pneumonitis), intestinal perforation, endocarditis, and hemorrhage.
Dialyzable drug: Unlikely.

PREGNANCY-LACTATION-REPRODUCTION
• Drug may cause fetal harm. Women of childbearing potential should use effective contraception during treatment and for 1 week after therapy ends.
• Males with female partners of childbearing potential should use effective contraception during treatment and for 3 months after final dose.
• It's unknown if drug appears in breast milk. Due to the potential for serious adverse reactions in breast-fed infants, breast-feeding isn't recommended during treatment and for 1 week after therapy ends.

NURSING CONSIDERATIONS
• Monitor LFTs (ALT, AST, and total bilirubin levels) every 2 weeks during first 2 months of treatment, then periodically during treatment, with more frequent testing as clinically indicated. Monitor patients for signs and symptoms of hepatotoxicity (dark urine, abdominal pain, nausea, vomiting, malaise) and intestinal perforation (severe abdominal pain, fever, nausea, vomiting).
• Monitor patients for signs and symptoms of ILD or pneumonitis (worsening of respiratory symptoms, cough, dyspnea, fever). Withhold drug if patients are diagnosed with ILD or pneumonitis and permanently discontinue drug if it's the causative factor.
• Monitor patients for myalgia or musculoskeletal pain.
• Assess CK level every 2 weeks for first month of treatment and as clinically indicated Drug may need to be withheld or dosage reduced.
• Monitor patients for chest pain and monitor HR and BP regularly. Dosage modification isn't required in cases of asymptomatic bradycardia. Adjust dosage for non-life-threatening, symptomatic bradycardia and assess for concomitant bradycardia-contributing drugs. Treat life-threatening bradycardia appropriately.
• Monitor patients for abnormal bleeding.
• Monitor patients for signs and symptoms of photosensitivity.

PATIENT TEACHING
• Advise patient to report all drugs and supplements being taken before beginning therapy.
• Teach patient to report signs and symptoms of liver injury or intestinal perforation (tiredness, anorexia, jaundice, dark urine, pruritus, nausea, vomiting, right-sided stomach pain, sharp abdominal pain, fever, easy bleeding or bruising); explain the need for blood tests throughout treatment.
• Inform patient of the risks of severe ILD or pneumonitis. Advise patient to contact prescriber immediately for new or worsening respiratory symptoms.
• Educate patient about the possibility of muscle pain, tenderness, and weakness and to immediately report new, worsening, or persistent signs and symptoms of muscle pain or weakness.
• Counsel patient that drug may cause dizziness, light-headedness, syncope, and rarely chest pain and to immediately report these symptoms to prescriber.
• Advise patient to report abnormal bleeding.

• Advise patient to avoid prolonged sun exposure while taking drug and for at least 7 days after last dose. Advise patient to use broad-spectrum sunscreen and lip balm to protect from potential sunburn.
• Advise patient that if a dose is missed or if patient vomits after taking a dose, not to take an extra dose, but to take the next dose at the regular time.
• Caution female patient of childbearing potential of possible fetal harm if drug is taken during pregnancy. Advise her to use effective contraception during treatment and for 1 week after last dose and to inform health care provider immediately if she is or may be pregnant.
• Explain to male patient with female partners of childbearing potential the need to use effective contraception during and for 3 months after treatment ends.
• Warn female patient not to breast-feed during treatment and for 1 week after treatment ends.

SAFETY ALERT!

atezolizumab
A-te-zoe-liz-ue-mab

Tecentriq

Therapeutic class: Antineoplastics
Pharmacologic class: Monoclonal antibodies

AVAILABLE FORMS
Injection: 1,200 mg/20 mL single-dose vial

INDICATIONS & DOSAGES
➤**Locally advanced or metastatic urothelial carcinoma in patients who have disease progression during or after platinum-containing chemotherapy or disease progression within 12 months of neoadjuvant or adjuvant treatment with platinum-containing chemotherapy; patients with metastatic non-small-cell lung cancer with disease progression during or after platinum-containing chemotherapy**
Adults: 1,200 mg I.V. over 60 minutes every 3 weeks until disease progression or unacceptable toxicity.
Adjust-a-dose: For grade 2 pneumonitis, ocular inflammatory toxicity, or infusion-related reactions; grade 2 or 3 diarrhea, colitis, or pancreatitis; grade 3 or 4 infection; increased amylase or lipase level to greater than 2 × ULN; hyperglycemia or symptomatic hypophysitis, adrenal insufficiency, hypothyroidism, or hyperthyroidism; increased AST or ALT level to 3 to 5 × ULN or total bilirubin level to 1.5 to 3 × ULN; or grade 3 rash, withhold drug and restart when reactions recover to grade 0 to 1.

For grade 3 or 4 pneumonitis, ocular inflammatory toxicity, or infusion-related reactions; grade 4 diarrhea or colitis; hypophysitis; rash; AST or ALT level more than 5 × ULN or total bilirubin level more than 3 × ULN; myasthenic syndrome, myasthenia gravis, Guillain-Barré syndrome, or meningoencephalitis; or grade 4 or any grade of recurrent pancreatitis, permanently discontinue drug.

ADMINISTRATION

I.V.
▼ Visually inspect vial for particulate matter and discoloration. Discard vial if solution is cloudy or discolored or if particles are present. Don't shake vial.
▼ Withdraw 20 mL of atezolizumab and dilute in 250 mL polyvinyl chloride, polyethylene, or polyolefin infusion bag containing NSS.
▼ Mix diluted solution by gentle inversion; don't shake.
▼ Vial doesn't contain a preservative; administer immediately once prepared and discard unused solution in vial.
▼ May give through I.V. tubing with or without a sterile, nonpyrogenic, low-protein-binding in-line filter (pore size 0.2 to 0.22 micron).
▼ Don't give as I.V. push or bolus. Administer as I.V. infusion over 60 minutes. If first infusion is tolerated, may give subsequent infusions over 30 minutes.
▼ If necessary, prepared solution can be stored up to 6 hours at room temperature, including administration time, or up to 24 hours in refrigerator at 36° to 46° F (2° to 8° C).
▼ Store at 36° to 46° F (2° to 8° C), don't freeze. Store in original carton and protect from light.
▼ **Incompatibilities:** Don't dilute in any solution other than NSS, or administer other drugs in same I.V. line.

ACTION

A monoclonal antibody that binds to PD-1, allowing activation of the antitumor immune response without inducing antibody-dependent cellular cytotoxicity.

Route	Onset	Peak	Duration
I.V.	Unknown	Unknown	Unknown

Half-life: 27 days.

ADVERSE REACTIONS

CNS: fatigue, pyrexia, confusion.
CV: peripheral edema, dehydration, *venous thromboembolism.*
GI: nausea, constipation, abdominal pain, vomiting, decreased appetite, intestinal obstruction, immune-mediated colitis, diarrhea.
GU: UTI, hematuria, urinary obstruction, acute kidney injury.
Hematologic: anemia, *lymphopenia.*
Hepatic: *immune-mediated hepatitis,* increased liver enzyme levels.
Musculoskeletal: back pain, neck pain, arthralgia.
Respiratory: dyspnea, cough, pneumonia, *immune-mediated pneumonitis, interstitial lung disease.*
Skin: rash, pruritus.
Other: severe infection (*sepsis,* herpes encephalitis, mycobacterial infection), infusion-related reaction, hypothyroidism, hyperthyroidism.

INTERACTIONS
None reported.

EFFECTS ON LAB TEST RESULTS
• May increase glucose, AST, ALT, alkaline phosphatase, and creatinine levels. May decrease sodium and albumin levels.
• May decrease hematocrit and lymphocyte count.

CONTRAINDICATIONS & CAUTIONS
• Drug increases risk of immune-mediated reactions, including pneumonitis, hepatitis, colitis, endocrinopathy (thyroid disorders, pituitary gland inflammation, adrenal insufficiency), meningitis, and encephalitis.
• Initiating drug in patients with moderate or severe hepatic impairment hasn't been studied.
• Safe and effective use in children hasn't been established.
Dialyzable drug: Unknown.

PREGNANCY-LACTATION-REPRODUCTION
• Based on its mechanism of action, drug can cause fetal harm. If drug is used during pregnancy, or patient becomes pregnant during treatment, advise her of potential risk to the fetus.
• Women should use effective contraception during treatment and for at least 5 months after last dose.
• Drug may impair fertility in females of childbearing potential who are receiving treatment.
• It isn't known if drug appears in breast milk. Patients shouldn't breast-feed during treatment and for at least 5 months after last dose.

NURSING CONSIDERATIONS
• Monitor patient for infusion reactions (rash, pruritus, chills, flushing, dyspnea, wheezing, dizziness, pain, facial swelling); if a mild or moderate reaction occurs, interrupt or slow infusion rate. Permanently discontinue drug in patients with grade 3 or 4 reactions.
• Monitor patient for immune-related pneumonitis with radiographic imaging and assess for signs and symptoms (new or worsening cough, chest pain, dyspnea). Give 1 to 2 mg/kg/day of prednisone or equivalent for grade 2 or greater pneumonitis, followed by corticosteroid taper. Withhold drug until resolution for grade 2 pneumonitis; discontinue drug for grade 3 or 4.
• Monitor patient for immune-mediated hepatitis (jaundice, severe nausea, vomiting, right quadrant abdominal pain, lethargy, easy bruising, bleeding). Obtain baseline AST, ALT, and bilirubin levels and monitor periodically during treatment. Give 1 to 2 mg/kg/day of prednisone or equivalent for grade 2 or greater transaminase elevations, with or without elevation in total bilirubin level, followed by corticosteroid taper. Withhold drug for grade 2 transaminase elevations and permanently discontinue drug for grade 3 or 4 immune-mediated hepatitis.
• Monitor patient for immune-related colitis or diarrhea (frequent or bloody stools, abdominal pain).

Withhold drug for grade 2 symptoms. If symptoms persist for more than 5 days or recur, give 1 to 2 mg/kg/day of prednisone or equivalent. For grade 3 symptoms, withhold drug and treat with 1 to 2 mg/kg/day of I.V. methylprednisolone, then convert to oral steroids once patient improves. For grade 2 or 3 diarrhea or colitis, when symptoms improve to grade 1, taper steroids over 1 month or more. Resume drug if symptoms improve to grade 0 or 1 within 12 weeks and steroids have been tapered to 10 mg or less of oral prednisone per day. Permanently discontinue drug for grade 4 diarrhea or colitis.
• Monitor patient for immune-related hypophysitis (pituitary gland inflammation). Treat with corticosteroids and hormone replacement as clinically indicated. Withhold drug for grade 2 or 3 hypophysitis and permanently discontinue for grade 4.
• Assess baseline thyroid levels and monitor thyroid function periodically during treatment. For symptomatic hypothyroidism (tiredness, feeling cold, dizziness, mood changes), give replacement therapy. Manage isolated hypothyroidism with replacement therapy without corticosteroids. For symptomatic hyperthyroidism (poor concentration, heat intolerance, tremors, palpitations), withhold drug and start antithyroid drugs as needed. Resume drug when symptoms are controlled and thyroid function improves.
• Monitor patient for adrenal insufficiency (fatigue, arthralgia, myalgia, nausea, vomiting, weakness, low BP, dizziness). For symptomatic adrenal insufficiency, withhold drug and give I.V. methylprednisolone 1 to 2 mg/kg/day followed by oral prednisone 1 to 2 mg/kg/day or equivalent once symptoms improve. Begin steroid taper when symptoms improve to grade 1 or less and taper over at least 1 month. May restart drug if symptoms improve to grade 1 or less within 12 weeks, corticosteroids have been reduced to 10 mg of oral prednisone per day or less, and patient is stable on replacement therapy.
• Monitor patient for new-onset diabetes with ketoacidosis (decreased alertness, dry skin, flushing, frequent urination or thirst, headache, fruity-smelling breath, nausea, vomiting). Initiate treatment with insulin. For grade 3 or more hyperglycemia, withhold drug. Resume drug when glucose metabolic control is achieved on insulin replacement therapy.
• Monitor patient for immune-related meningitis or encephalitis and permanently discontinue drug if these conditions occur. Treat with I.V. steroids and convert to oral steroids once patient has improved.
• Monitor patient for myasthenic syndrome, myasthenia gravis, Guillain-Barré syndrome, and signs and symptoms of sensory and motor neuropathy (severe muscle weakness, numbness or tingling of the hands or feet, confusion, mood changes, neck stiffness, photosensitivity). Permanently discontinue drug if these occur. Treat as appropriate, and consider systemic prednisone 1 to 2 mg/kg/day.
• Monitor patient for acute pancreatitis (severe epigastric pain, nausea, vomiting, diarrhea, chills, tachycardia). Withhold drug for grade 3 or higher amylase or lipase levels (greater than $2 \times$ ULN) or grade 2 or 3 pancreatitis. Give I.V. methylprednisolone or equivalent per day and follow with oral prednisone or equivalent when symptoms improve. May resume drug if serum amylase and lipase levels improve to grade 1 or better within 12 weeks, symptoms have resolved, and corticosteroids have been reduced to 10 mg of oral prednisone or less. Permanently discontinue drug for grade 4 pancreatitis or any grade recurrent pancreatitis.
• Monitor patient for signs and symptoms of infection (fever, cough, pain while urinating, flulike symptoms), including sepsis, herpes encephalitis, and mycobacterial infections. UTI and pneumonia are the most common serious infections. Treat as clinically indicated for suspected or confirmed infection. Withhold drug for grade 3 or greater infection.

PATIENT TEACHING
• Teach patient signs and symptoms of immune-mediated reactions and that they may require corticosteroid treatment and interruption or discontinuation of therapy.
• Advise patient to immediately report infusion-related and hypersensitivity reactions.
• Caution patient to immediately report all adverse effects to health care provider.
• Instruct patient to immediately report signs and symptoms of infection to health care provider.
• Instruct patient that laboratory testing will be needed to monitor for adverse reactions related to treatment.
• Advise female patient that drug causes fetal harm if used during pregnancy.
• Caution female patient not to breast-feed during therapy and for at least 5 months after last dose.
• Counsel female patient of childbearing potential to use effective contraception during therapy and for at least 5 months after last dose.

brivaracetam
BRIV-a-re-se-tam

Briviact

Therapeutic class: Anticonvulsants
Pharmacologic class: Anticonvulsants
Controlled substance schedule: V

AVAILABLE FORMS
Tablets ⊞: 10 mg, 25 mg, 50 mg, 75 mg, 100 mg
Injection: 50 mg/5 mL single-dose vial
Oral solution: 10 mg/mL

INDICATIONS & DOSAGES
➤ **Adjunctive therapy of partial-onset seizures in patients with epilepsy**
Adults and children age 16 and older: Initially, 50 mg P.O. or I.V. b.i.d. Titrate dosage to individual patient

---

Reactions in bold italics are *life-threatening.* Interactions may have a *rapid onset* or a ***delayed onset.***

tolerability and therapeutic response to a minimum dose of 25 mg b.i.d. and a maximum dose of 100 mg b.i.d.

Adjust-a-dose: For all stages of hepatic impairment, recommended starting dosage is 25 mg b.i.d.; maximum dosage is 75 mg b.i.d.

ADMINISTRATION
P.O.
- May give with or without food.
- Patients should swallow tablets whole and not chew or crush them.
- Use a calibrated measuring device for measuring oral solution. Don't use a household teaspoon.
- May give oral solution via NG or gastrostomy tube.
- Discard any unused oral solution that remains 5 months after first opening the bottle.
- Store between 59° and 86° F (15° and 30° C). Don't freeze oral solution.

I.V.
▼ Visually inspect vial. Don't administer if particulate matter or discoloration is present.
▼ May give I.V. without further dilution.
▼ If further dilution is required, use NSS or lactated Ringer or 5% dextrose solution.
▼ Administer I.V. over 2 to 15 minutes.
▼ Diluted solution shouldn't be stored for more than 4 hours at room temperature and may be stored in polyvinyl chloride bags. Don't freeze.
▼ Discard any unused portion of the injection vial contents.

ACTION
Exact mechanism unknown. Anticonvulsant effect may be related to affinity for synaptic vesicle protein 2A in the brain.

Route	Onset	Peak	Duration
P.O.	Unknown	1 hr	Unknown
I.V.	Unknown	Unknown	Unknown

Half-life: About 9 hours.

ADVERSE REACTIONS
CNS: somnolence, sedation, ataxia, balance disorder, abnormal coordination, nystagmus, dizziness, fatigue, irritability, euphoric mood, feeling drunk, anxiety, aggression, anger, agitation, restlessness, depression, apathy, mood swings, psychotic disorder.
GI: nausea, vomiting, constipation, dysgeusia.
Other: infusion-site pain.

INTERACTIONS
Drug-drug. *Azelastine (nasal), orphenadrine, paraldehyde, thalidomide:* May increase CNS depressant effect of these drugs. Avoid use together.
Cannabis: May enhance CNS depressant effect. Monitor therapy.
Carbamazepine: May increase exposure to active metabolite carbamazepine epoxide. Decrease carbamazepine dosage if intolerance occurs.

CNS depressants, magnesium sulfate: May enhance CNS depressant effects. Monitor therapy.
Orlistat: May decrease brivaracetam level. Monitor therapy.
Phenytoin: May increase phenytoin plasma concentration. Monitor phenytoin level when brivaracetam is started or stopped, and adjust dosage as needed.
Rifampin: May decrease brivaracetam level. Increase brivaracetam dosage by up to 100%.
Drug-herb. *Kava kava:* May enhance adverse effects of brivaracetam. Monitor therapy.
Drug-lifestyle. *Alcohol use:* May increase CNS depression. Monitor therapy.

EFFECTS ON LAB TEST RESULTS
- May decrease WBC count.

CONTRAINDICATIONS & CAUTIONS
- Contraindicated in patients hypersensitive to drug or its components.
- Hypersensitivity reactions and drug rash, eosinophilia, and systemic symptoms (DRESS) have been reported.
- Antiepileptics may increase risk of suicidal behavior and ideation. Consider risk before prescribing and administering.
- Use in patients with ESRD undergoing dialysis isn't recommended.
- Safety and effectiveness in children younger than age 16 years haven't been established.
- Start elderly patients on the lowest dose possible, taking into consideration hepatic, kidney, or cardiac function and other concomitant disease and drugs.
Dialyzable drug: Unlikely.
⚠ **Overdose S&S:** Vertigo, balance disorder, fatigue, nausea, diplopia, anxiety, bradycardia.

PREGNANCY-LACTATION-REPRODUCTION
- There are no adequate and well-controlled studies in pregnant women. Use in pregnancy only if potential benefit justifies risk to the fetus.
- Pregnant patients exposed to drug should enroll in the North American Antiepileptic Drug Pregnancy Registry (1-888-233-2334).
- It isn't known if drug appears in breast milk. Patient should discontinue breast-feeding or discontinue drug.

NURSING CONSIDERATIONS
- Monitor patients for signs and symptoms of hypersensitivity reactions (bronchospasm, angioedema) and DRESS (fever, rash, eosinophilia, lymphadenopathy, hepatitis, nephritis, myocarditis). Discontinue drug and treat appropriately if signs and symptoms of hypersensitivity or DRESS occur.
- Abrupt withdrawal of drug may increase risk of increased seizure frequency and status epilepticus. Withdraw drug gradually.
- Monitor patients for new or worsening of depression, suicidal thoughts or behaviors, or unusual changes in mood or behavior during therapy.

NEW DRUGS

• Monitor patients for neurologic effects (somnolence, fatigue, asthenia, malaise, hypersomnia, sedation, lethargy, dizziness, vertigo, balance disorder, ataxia, nystagmus, gait disturbance, and abnormal coordination). Patients shouldn't drive or operate machinery until drug's effects are known.

PATIENT TEACHING

• Counsel family member or caregivers to watch for changes in patient's behavior and to immediately report suicidal thoughts or behaviors, or thoughts about self-harm.
• Warn patient not to drive or operate machinery until drug's effects are known.
• Advise patient to immediately report behavioral changes, including irritability, depression, aggressive behavior, anxiety, and psychotic symptoms (hallucinations, paranoia).
• Warn patient to seek immediate medical care if signs or symptoms of hypersensitivity reactions, including bronchospasm and angioedema, occur.
• Instruct patient not to discontinue drug abruptly without first consulting prescriber.

SAFETY ALERT!

cobimetinib fumarate
koe-bi-ME-ti-nib

Cotellic

Therapeutic class: Antineoplastics
Pharmacologic class: Tyrosine kinase inhibitors

AVAILABLE FORMS

Tablets ⊕: 20 mg

INDICATIONS & DOSAGES

➤ **Unresectable or metastatic melanoma with a *BRAF V600E* or *V600K* mutation in combination with vemurafenib**

Adults: 60 mg P.O. once daily for first 21 days of each 28-day treatment cycle until disease progression or unacceptable toxicity.

Adjust-a-dose: For adverse events, first dosage reduction is to 40 mg P.O. once daily; second dosage reduction is to 20 mg P.O. daily. Permanently discontinue drug if patient is unable to tolerate 20 mg.

For grade 3 hemorrhage, withhold drug for up to 4 weeks; if improved to grade 0 or 1, resume at next lower dosage level. If no improvement within 4 weeks or grade 4 hemorrhage develops, permanently discontinue drug.

For asymptomatic, absolute decrease in LVEF from baseline of 10% or more and less than the institutional lower level of normal (LLN), withhold drug for 2 weeks and repeat LVEF. Resume at next lower dosage level if LVEF is at or above LLN and absolute decrease from baseline LVEF is 10% or less. If LVEF

is less than LLN or absolute decrease from baseline LVEF is more than 10%, permanently discontinue drug.

For symptomatic LVEF decrease from baseline, withhold drug for up to 4 weeks and repeat LVEF. Resume at next lower dosage level if symptoms resolve and LVEF is at or above LLN and absolute decrease from baseline LVEF is 10% or less. If symptoms persist or LVEF is less than LLN or absolute decrease from baseline LVEF is more than 10%, permanently discontinue drug.

For grade 3 or 4 or intolerable grade 2 dermatologic reactions, withhold drug or reduce dosage.

For serious retinopathy, withhold drug for up to 4 weeks. If signs and symptoms improve, resume at next lower dosage level. If signs and symptoms aren't improved or recur within 4 weeks or retinal vein occlusion occurs, permanently discontinue drug.

For grade 4 hepatotoxicity, withhold drug for up to 4 weeks. If improved to grade 0 or 1, resume at next lower dosage. If not improved within 4 weeks, or grade 4 hepatotoxicity recurs after resuming treatment, permanently discontinue drug.

For grade 4 CK elevation, or any CK elevation with myalgia, withhold drug for up to 4 weeks. If improved to grade 3 or lower, resume at next lower dosage. If not improved within 4 weeks, permanently discontinue drug.

For intolerable grade 2, or grade 3 or 4 photosensitivity, withhold drug for up to 4 weeks. If improved to grade 0 or 1, resume at next lower dosage level. If not improved within 4 weeks, permanently discontinue drug.

For other intolerable grade 2 or any grade 3 toxicity, withhold drug for up to 4 weeks. If improved to grade 0 or 1, resume at next lower dosage. If not improved within 4 weeks, permanently discontinue drug. At first occurrence of any grade 4 adverse reaction, withhold drug until improved to grade 0 or 1; then resume at next lower dosage level or permanently discontinue drug. Discontinue drug for any recurrent grade 4 adverse reaction.

ADMINISTRATION

P.O.

• Hazardous drug; use safe handling and disposal precautions according to facility policy.
• May give without regard for food. Patient should swallow tablets whole with water.
• If dose is missed or vomiting occurs when dose is taken, resume dosing with the next scheduled dose.
• Store at room temperature below 86° F (30° C).

ACTION

A potent and selective inhibitor of the mitogen-activated extracellular kinase (MEK) pathway; reversibly inhibits MEK1 and MEK2, regulators of the extracellular signal-related kinase (ERK) pathway. The ERK pathway promotes cellular proliferation. MEK1 and MEK2 are part of the BRAF pathway, which is activated by *BRAF V600E* and *V600K* mutations. When used with vemurafenib, apoptosis increases and tumor growth is reduced.

Route	Onset	Peak	Duration
P.O.	Unknown	2.4 hr	Unknown

Half-life: 44 hours (mean).

ADVERSE REACTIONS

CNS: fever, chills.
CV: decreased LVEF, hypertension, *hemorrhage.*
EENT: vision impairment, chorioretinopathy, retinal detachment.
GI: diarrhea, nausea, vomiting, stomatitis.
Hematologic: anemia, *lymphocytopenia, thrombocytopenia.*
Hepatic: elevated liver enzyme and bilirubin levels.
Metabolic: *hyperkalemia,* hypokalemia, *hypocalcemia,* hypophosphatemia, hyponatremia.
Musculoskeletal: *rhabdomyolysis.*
Respiratory: pneumonitis.
Skin: rash, photosensitivity reactions, acneiform dermatitis, basal cell carcinoma, squamous cell carcinoma, keratoacanthoma.

INTERACTIONS

Drug-drug. *Strong or moderate CYP3A inducers (carbamazepine, efavirenz, phenytoin, rifampin):* May significantly decrease level and efficacy of cobimetinib. Avoid concurrent use.
Strong or moderate CYP3A inhibitors (ciprofloxacin, erythromycin): May increase cobimetinib level. Avoid use together. If concurrent short-term use together of 14 days or less is unavoidable, reduce 60-mg dose to 20 mg daily. Resume previous dose after discontinuing CYP3A inhibitor. Use an alternative CYP3A inhibitor in patients taking less than 60 mg.
Drug-herb. *St. John's wort:* May significantly decrease efficacy of cobimetinib. Discourage use together.

EFFECTS ON LAB TEST RESULTS

• May increase creatinine, AST, ALT, alkaline phosphatase, CK, GGT, and bilirubin levels. May decrease phosphate, albumin, sodium, and calcium levels. May increase or decrease potassium level.
• May decrease Hb level and lymphocyte and platelet counts.

CONTRAINDICATIONS & CAUTIONS

• Drug isn't indicated for wild-type BRAF melanoma. Confirm presence of *BRAF V600E* or *V600K* with an approved test before start of treatment.
• New primary cutaneous and noncutaneous malignancies and hypertension, hemorrhage, cardiomyopathy, severe dermatologic reactions, serous retinopathy, retinal vein occlusion, hepatotoxicity, rhabdomyolysis, and severe photosensitivity may occur with treatment.
• Safety and effectiveness in children haven't been established.
Dialyzable drug: Unknown.

PREGNANCY-LACTATION-REPRODUCTION

• Drug may cause fetal harm and is contraindicated in pregnant women. Women should avoid pregnancy and use contraception during therapy and for 2 weeks after last dose.
• May decrease fertility in both males and females of reproductive potential.
• Patient should avoid breast-feeding during therapy and for 2 weeks after last dose.

NURSING CONSIDERATIONS

• Monitor patients for bleeding, including GI, GU, lung, brain, and pulmonary hemorrhage.
• Evaluate LVEF before drug initiation by echocardiogram or MUGA scan, 1 month after initiation, and every 3 months until discontinuation. In patients restarting after dosage reduction or drug interruption, evaluate LVEF at 2, 4, 10, and 16 weeks, then as clinically indicated.
• Monitor LFTs before drug initiation and monthly during treatment, or more frequently as indicated.
• Monitor patients for visual disturbances. Patients should have an ophthalmologic evaluation at regular intervals and with new or worsening symptoms.
• Obtain CK and creatinine levels before start of therapy, periodically during treatment, and as clinically indicated. If CK level is elevated, evaluate for signs and symptoms of rhabdomyolysis.
• Monitor ECG and electrolyte levels before and periodically during treatment when drug is given with vemurafenib. Monitor BP regularly.
• Monitor patients for severe rash and other skin reactions. Patients should have dermatologic evaluations before start of therapy, every 2 months during therapy, and for 6 months after therapy ends. Suspicious skin lesions should be excised and a pathologic evaluation performed.

PATIENT TEACHING

• Caution patient to immediately report change in or new skin lesions (new wart, skin sore, or reddish bump that bleeds or doesn't heal; change in size or color of a mole; rash, blisters, peeling skin).
• Explain importance of obtaining laboratory blood work as ordered.
• Teach patient to immediately report signs and symptoms of heart problems (shortness of breath, coughing, wheezing, swelling of feet and ankles, fast heartbeat), unusual bleeding or signs and symptoms of bleeding (red or black stools, blood in urine, headache, dizziness, stomach pain, unusual vaginal bleeding), signs and symptoms of rhabdomyolysis (muscle pain or spasms, weakness, dark and reddish urine), vision changes (blurred or distorted vision, loss of visual field, halos), or signs and symptoms of liver toxicity (yellowing of skin or eyes, dark or brown urine, nausea, vomiting, fatigue, loss of appetite).
• Instruct patient to avoid sun exposure and to wear protective clothing and use broad-spectrum UVA/UVB sunscreen and lip balm (30 SPF or higher) when outdoors.

NEW DRUGS

- Caution patient to report photosensitivity reactions (red, painful, itchy skin that's hot to the touch; sun rash; skin irritation; bumps or tiny pimples; thickened, dry, wrinkled skin).
- Inform female patient of risk to the fetus. Advise her to use contraception during and for 2 weeks after therapy ends.
- Warn female patient to contact health care provider if she suspects she's pregnant or becomes pregnant during treatment.
- Advise female patient not to breast-feed during therapy and for 2 weeks after last dose.
- Caution male and female patient that drug can affect fertility.

daclizumab
dah-KLIH-zyoo-mab

Zinbryta

Therapeutic class: Immunomodulators
Pharmacologic class: Interleukin-2 receptor blocking antibodies

AVAILABLE FORMS
Injection: 150 mg/mL in single-dose, prefilled syringe

INDICATIONS & DOSAGES
➤ **Relapsing forms of MS in patients who have had an inadequate response to two or more drugs**
Adults: 150 mg subcutaneously once monthly.
Adjust-a-dose: If ALT or AST level is more than 5 × ULN, or total bilirubin level is more than 2 × ULN, or ALT or AST level is 3 × ULN to less than 5 × ULN and total bilirubin level is more than 1.5 × ULN but less than 2 × ULN, interrupt therapy and look for other etiologies of abnormal laboratory values. If no other etiologies are identified, discontinue drug. If other etiologies are identified, reassess the overall risk-benefit profile of drug and consider whether to resume drug when both AST and ALT levels are less than 2 × ULN and total bilirubin level is ULN or less.

ADMINISTRATION
Subcutaneous
- Store drug in refrigerator at 36° to 46° F (2° to 8° C) until use. May also store protected from light at room temperature for up to 30 days.
- Allow syringe to warm to room temperature for 30 minutes before use. Don't use hot water or external heat sources to warm drug. Don't return drug to refrigerator after it has warmed to room temperature.
- Don't use drug if it's cloudy or if visible particles are noted.
- Inject into thigh, abdomen, or back of upper arm.
- Give a missed dose as soon as possible but no more than 2 weeks late. If missed dose is more than 2 weeks late, skip missed dose and give next dose as scheduled. Give only one dose at a time.

ACTION
Unknown. Thought to involve modulation of interleukin-2-mediated activation of lymphocytes.

Route	Onset	Peak	Duration
Subcut.	Unknown	5–7 days	Unknown

Half-life: 21 days.

ADVERSE REACTIONS
CNS: depression, pyrexia, *seizures.*
EENT: nasopharyngitis, rhinitis, tonsillitis, pharyngitis, oropharyngeal pain, laryngitis.
GI: diarrhea.
GU: UTI.
Hematologic: anemia.
Hepatic: *hepatic injury,* abnormal hepatic enzyme levels.
Respiratory: URI, bronchitis, pneumonia.
Skin: rash, allergic skin reaction, dermatitis, eczema, acne, dry skin, erythema, folliculitis, pruritus, psoriasis, *exfoliation, toxic skin eruption.*
Other: infection, flulike symptoms, viral infection, lymphadenopathy, lymphadenitis, *immune-mediated disorders, acute hypersensitivity.*

INTERACTIONS
Drug-drug. *Hepatotoxic drugs (acetaminophen, chlorpromazine, methyldopa, NSAIDs, phenytoin, sertraline, statins):* May increase risk of hepatic injury. Avoid use together.
Live-virus vaccines: Safe use of live-virus vaccines during treatment hasn't been studied. Give necessary live-virus vaccines before treatment. Use of live-virus vaccines isn't recommended during therapy and for up to 4 months after therapy ends.
Drug-herb. *Dietary supplements or herbal products such as kava that can cause hepatotoxicity:* May increase risk of hepatic injury. Avoid use together.

EFFECTS ON LAB TEST RESULTS
- May increase bilirubin, ALT, and AST levels.
- May decrease Hb level and hematocrit and lymphocyte count.

CONTRAINDICATIONS & CAUTIONS
- Contraindicated in patients hypersensitive to drug or its components.
- **Black Box Warning** Contraindicated in patients with preexisting hepatic disease or hepatic impairment, including ALT or AST level at least 2 × ULN, and in those with a history of autoimmune hepatitis or other autoimmune condition involving the liver. Drug can cause severe liver injury, including life-threatening events, liver failure, and autoimmune hepatitis. Liver injury can occur at any time during therapy and for up to 4 months after last dose. ■
- **Black Box Warning** Immune-mediated disorders, such as skin reactions, lymphadenopathy, and noninfectious colitis, can occur. If patient develops a serious immune-mediated disorder, drug may need to be stopped and patient referred to a specialist to ensure

---

Reactions in bold italics are *life-threatening*. Interactions may have a *rapid onset* or a *delayed onset*.

comprehensive diagnostic evaluation and appropriate treatment. Some patients may need systemic corticosteroids or other immunosuppressive therapy for autoimmune hepatitis or other immune-mediated disorders during therapy; treatment may need to continue after therapy ends. ■

Black Box Warning Because of risks of hepatic injury and other immune-mediated disorders, drug is available only through the ZINBRYTA REMS Program. Pharmacies and prescribers must be certified, and patients must be enrolled. Information is available at 1-800-456-2255. ■

• Use cautiously in patients with previous or current depressive disorders. Drug may need to be stopped if severe depression or suicidal ideation occurs.
• Don't start drug in patients with severe active infection.
• Safety and effectiveness in children younger than age 17 haven't been established.
Dialyzable drug: Unknown.

PREGNANCY-LACTATION-REPRODUCTION
• Use in pregnant women hasn't been studied, but adverse events were noted in animal studies. Use of similar agents to treat MS in pregnant women isn't recommended.
• It isn't known if drug appears in breast milk. Use in breast-feeding women only if benefits to the mother outweigh risks to the infant.

NURSING CONSIDERATIONS
Black Box Warning Obtain serum transaminase levels (ALT, AST) and total bilirubin level before starting therapy. During therapy, monitor transaminase and total bilirubin levels monthly before next dose and continue to follow monthly for up to 6 months after last dose. ■
• Screen patients for HBV, HBC, and other preexisting hepatic disease before treatment.
• Monitor patient for hepatic dysfunction (nausea, vomiting, abdominal pain, fatigue, anorexia, jaundice, dark urine). Assess serum transaminase and total bilirubin levels if signs or symptoms occur and interrupt or discontinue treatment as clinically indicated.
• Monitor patient for hypersensitivity reactions, anaphylaxis, angioedema, and urticaria. Discontinue drug and don't restart if anaphylaxis or other allergic reactions occur.
• Monitor patient for skin reactions. If patient develops a serious diffuse or inflammatory rash, consider having a dermatologist evaluate patient before next dose, as discontinuation may be appropriate.
• Monitor patient for lymphadenopathy and lymphadenitis (infections, benign salivary neoplasm, skin reactions, thrombocytopenia, interstitial lung changes). Refer patient to specialist for full diagnostic evaluation if these signs or symptoms occur.
• Monitor patient for noninfectious colitis (abdominal pain, fever, prolonged diarrhea). Consider referral to a specialist if colitis occurs.
• Evaluate patient at high risk for TB before starting treatment. Treat TB before starting drug.

• Assess patient for active infection before treatment. Don't start therapy until infection cleared.
• Monitor patient for severe active infections during therapy. If serious infection develops, consider withholding drug until infection resolves.

PATIENT TEACHING
• Explain to patient the need to be enrolled in the REMS program and to comply with necessary laboratory monitoring.
• Caution patient to carry a Zinbryta Patient Wallet Card at all times. The card describes signs and symptoms for which patient should immediately seek medical evaluation.
• Advise patient to report all current drugs, herbal products, and other supplements being taken to prescriber before starting therapy.
• Advise patient of the need to obtain frequent LFTs during therapy and for up to 6 months after last dose.
• Teach patient proper technique for self-administration.
• Advise patient and caregivers to immediately report signs and symptoms of new or worsening depression or suicidal ideation.
• Advise patient to report all adverse reactions and to immediately report signs and symptoms of allergic reaction (fever, hives, difficulty breathing, nausea, facial swelling), infection (fever, pain, cough, difficulty breathing, painful urination), diarrhea, abdominal pain, or swollen lymph nodes.
• Caution patient of risk of skin reactions ranging from mild to serious and that may require hospitalization. Instruct patient to seek immediate medical attention for dermatologic reactions.
• Inform patient of risk of hepatic injury and to immediately report signs and symptoms of hepatic dysfunction (abdominal pain, nausea, yellowing of skin or eyes, dark urine).
• Instruct patient to inject a missed dose as soon as possible and only if dose is no more than 2 weeks late. After 2 weeks, advise patient to skip the missed dose and to take the next dose on schedule. Caution patient to administer only one dose at a time.

SAFETY ALERT!

daratumumab
DAR-a-toom-ue-mab

Darzalex

Therapeutic class: Antineoplastics
Pharmacologic class: Monoclonal antibodies

AVAILABLE FORMS
Injection: 100 mg/5 mL, 400 mg/20 mL single-dose vials

NEW DRUGS

INDICATIONS & DOSAGES

Adjust-a-dose (for all indications): For infusion reaction of any severity, immediately stop infusion and manage symptoms. For grade 1 to 2 infusion reactions, once symptoms resolve, restart infusion at no more than half the rate at which the reaction occurred; may increase rate as tolerated at increments and intervals as appropriate, up to a maximum of 200 mL/hour. For grade 3 reaction, once reaction resolves, may consider restarting infusion at no more than half the rate at which the reaction occurred; if patient doesn't experience additional symptoms, may increase rate as tolerated at increments and intervals as appropriate. Repeat procedure above if grade 3 symptoms recur. For a third occurrence of a grade 3 symptom or any grade 4 symptoms, permanently discontinue drug.

➤ **Multiple myeloma monotherapy in patients who received at least three prior lines of therapy, including a proteasome inhibitor (PI) and an immunomodulatory agent or who are double refractory to a PI and an immunomodulatory agent; multiple myeloma in combination with lenalidomide and low-dose dexamethasone in patients who have received at least one prior therapy**

Adults: Initially, 16 mg/kg (actual body weight) I.V. infusion once weekly for weeks 1 through 8 (total of eight doses); then for weeks 9 through 24, give 16 mg/kg I.V. infusion every 2 weeks (total of eight doses). Then, beginning week 25 onwards, give 16 mg/kg I.V. infusion every 4 weeks until disease progression. Refer to manufacturer's instructions for dosing instructions for combination agents.

➤ **Multiple myeloma in combination with bortezomib and dexamethasone in patients who have received at least one prior therapy**

Adults: Initially, 16 mg/kg (actual body weight) I.V. infusion once weekly for weeks 1 through 9 (total of nine doses); then give 16 mg/kg I.V. infusion every 3 weeks beginning week 10 through week 24 (total of five doses); then give 16 mg/kg I.V. infusion every 4 weeks beginning week 25 onwards until disease progression. Refer to manufacturer's instructions for dosing instructions for combination agents.

ADMINISTRATION

I.V.

▼ One to three hours before each infusion, premedicate with I.V. corticosteroid (methylprednisolone 100 mg or equivalent dose of an intermediate-acting or long-acting corticosteroid for monotherapy or 20 mg dexamethasone for combination therapy), an oral antipyretic (acetaminophen 650 to 1,000 mg), and an oral or I.V. antihistamine (diphenhydramine 25 to 50 mg or equivalent). After second monotherapy infusion, may reduce methylprednisolone dose to 60 mg P.O. or I.V. In combination therapy, after first infusion, may consider dexamethasone 20 mg P.O. before subsequent infusions.

▼ On first and second day after monotherapy infusions, administer an oral corticosteroid (20 mg methylprednisolone or equivalent dose of a corticosteroid). For combination therapy, may consider methylprednisolone 20 mg or less P.O. or equivalent the day after infusion.

▼ For patients with a history of obstructive pulmonary disorder, postinfusion medications, such as short- and long-acting bronchodilators and inhaled corticosteroids, may be indicated. After first four infusions, if patient has no major infusion reactions, the additional postinfusion drugs may be discontinued.

▼ Solution should be colorless to pale yellow; don't use if vials contain opaque particles, discoloration, or other foreign particles.

▼ Remove volume of NSS from infusion bag that's equal to the volume of drug. Infusion bags should be made of polyvinyl chloride (PVC), polypropylene (PP), polyethylene (PE), or polyolefin blend.

▼ Withdraw medication from vial and add to infusion bag. Discard unused solution.

▼ Gently invert bag; don't shake.

▼ May store infusion bag up to 24 hours in refrigerator at 36° to 46° F (2° to 8° C). Protect from light; don't freeze.

▼ Allow infusion bag to come to room temperature; then use immediately, as the solution doesn't contain a preservative.

▼ Administer with infusion set with flow regulator and in-line, sterile, nonpyrogenic, low-protein-binding polyethersulfone filter (pore size 0.22 or 0.2 micron). Polyurethane, polybutadiene, PVC, PP, or PE administration sets must be used.

▼ Give first infusion of 1,000 mL initially at 50 mL/hour; may increase by 50 mL/hour every hour to maximum rate of 200 mL/hr. Consider escalating infusion rate only in the absence of infusion reactions. If there are no grade 1 or greater infusion reactions during first 3 hours of first infusion, may decrease second infusion dilution volume to 500 mL and begin infusion at 50 mL/hour and increase by 50 mL/hour to a maximum of 200 mL/hour. Otherwise, continue the dilution volume of 1,000 mL and instructions for the first infusion. If there are no grade 1 or greater infusion reactions during final infusion rate of 100 mL/hour or more in first two infusions, may give subsequent infusions in 500 mL at an initial rate of 100 mL/hour; may increase by 50 mL/hour every hour to maximum rate of 200 mL/hour. Otherwise, continue to use instructions for the second infusion.

▼ Complete infusion within 15 hours.

▼ Give missed dose as soon as possible and adjust dosing schedule accordingly to maintain treatment interval.

▼ **Incompatibilities:** Don't infuse in same I.V. line with other agents.

ACTION

An IgG1 kappa human monoclonal antibody that binds to CD38 and inhibits growth of CD38-expressing tumor cells by inducing apoptosis.

Route	Onset	Peak	Duration
I.V.	Unknown	Unknown	Unknown

Half-life: 9 to 27 days.

ADVERSE REACTIONS
CNS: fatigue, pyrexia, headache.
CV: hypertension.
EENT: nasal congestion, nasopharyngitis.
GI: nausea, vomiting, diarrhea, constipation, decreased appetite.
Hematologic: anemia, *thrombocytopenia, neutropenia, lymphopenia.*
Musculoskeletal: back pain, arthralgia, extremity pain, musculoskeletal chest pain.
Respiratory: cough, dyspnea, URI, pneumonia.
Other: infusion reactions, chills, herpes zoster reactivation.

INTERACTIONS
None reported.

EFFECTS ON LAB TEST RESULTS
• May decrease RBC, platelet, neutrophil, and lymphocyte counts.
• May cause positive indirect antiglobulin tests (Coombs' test), interfering with cross-matching and RBC antibody screening that may persist for up to 6 months after last daratumumab infusion.
• May cause false-positive serum protein electrophoresis and immunofixation assay results in patients with IgG kappa myeloma protein affecting assessment of compete response by International Myeloma Working Group criteria.

CONTRAINDICATIONS & CAUTIONS
⚠ *Alert:* Drug should only be given by health care professional with immediate access to emergency equipment and medical support to manage severe infusion reactions. Approximately half of all patients may experience an infusion reaction, and most occur during the first infusion. Infusion reactions can occur with subsequent infusions and within 4 hours of completing an infusion.
• Drug may increase risk of herpes zoster reactivation. Initiate antiviral prophylaxis within 1 week of starting treatment and continue for 3 months after treatment ends.
• Safety and efficacy in children haven't been established.
Dialyzable drug: Unknown.

PREGNANCY-LACTATION-REPRODUCTION
• Risk during pregnancy is unknown. Patient should use contraception during therapy and for up to 3 months after therapy ends.
• Based on the mechanism of action, drug may cause fetal myeloid- or lymphoid-cell depletion and decrease bone density with in utero exposure. Delay administering live vaccines to neonates and infants exposed to drug in utero until hematology evaluation is completed.
• It isn't known if drug appears in breast milk. Discuss risk and benefits with patient who plans to breast-feed.

NURSING CONSIDERATIONS
⚠ *Alert:* Be sure to premedicate patient and frequently monitor for signs and symptoms of infusion reaction (bronchospasm, hypoxia, dyspnea, hypertension or hypotension, cough, wheezing, larynx and throat tightness or irritation, laryngeal edema, pulmonary edema, nasal congestion, allergic rhinitis, headache, rash, urticaria, pruritus, nausea, vomiting, chills). Emergency treatment may be needed for severe infusion reactions.
• Patients should be typed and screened for blood transfusions before start of therapy because drug can interfere with cross-matching and antibody screening. Inform blood bank that patient is taking drug if typed and screened after initiating therapy.

PATIENT TEACHING
• Advise patient to immediately report signs and symptoms of infusion reaction.
• Explain to patient that blood test results to match blood type for transfusions may be affected for up to 6 months after last dose. Advise patient to inform all health care providers he or she is taking drug in the event of a planned transfusion.
• Inform patient that drug may occasionally affect results of some tests used to determine complete response and additional tests may be needed.
• Advise patient to report all adverse reactions and to immediately report fever or signs and symptoms of bruising or bleeding.
• Instruct female patient to avoid pregnancy and to use effective contraception during therapy and for up to 3 months after last dose.
• Warn female patient who wants to breast-feed that it isn't known if drug appears in breast milk.
• Caution patient to take postinfusion medications and antiviral prophylaxis, as prescribed.

SAFETY ALERT!

defibrotide sodium
dee-FYE-broe-tide

Defitelio

Therapeutic class: Thrombolytics
Pharmacologic class: Thrombolytics

AVAILABLE FORMS
Injection: 200 mg/2.5 mL (80 mg/mL)

INDICATIONS & DOSAGES
➤ **Hepatic veno-occlusive disease (VOD), also known as sinusoidal obstruction syndrome, with renal or pulmonary dysfunction after hematopoietic stem-cell transplantation (HSCT)**
Adults and children: 6.25 mg/kg I.V. given as a 2-hour infusion every 6 hours. Administer for a minimum of 21 days; if after 21 days, signs and symptoms of hepatic VOD haven't resolved, continue until resolution of VOD or to a maximum of 60 days.

NEW DRUGS

Adjust-a-dose: For severe or life-threatening (anaphylaxis) hypersensitivity reaction, discontinue drug permanently. For persistent, severe or potentially life-threatening bleeding, withhold drug, treat the cause of the bleeding, and provide appropriate supportive care. Consider resuming treatment at the same dose and infusion volume when bleeding has stopped and patient is hemodynamically stable. For recurrent, significant bleeding, permanently discontinue drug.

ADMINISTRATION

I.V.

▼ Base dose on patient's body weight before the preparative regimen for HSCT.

▼ Add calculated dose to sufficient D₅W or NSS to a make a final concentration of 4 to 20 mg/mL.

▼ Gently mix solution.

▼ Visually inspect solution for particulate matter and discoloration before administration. Use only clear solutions without visible particles. Depending on the type and amount of diluent, the color of the diluted solution may range from colorless to light yellow.

▼ Flush I.V. line with D₅W or NSS immediately before and after administration.

▼ Administer through a 0.2-micron in-line filter over 2 hours.

▼ Use diluted solution within 4 hours if stored at room temperature or within 24 hours if refrigerated. Up to four doses may be prepared at one time if refrigerated.

▼ Vials contain no antimicrobial preservatives. Discard partially used vials.

▼ Store at 68° to 77° F (20° to 25° C); excursions between 59° and 86° F (15° and 30° C) are permitted.

▼ **Incompatibilities:** Don't give with other I.V. drugs in the same line.

ACTION

Enhances the enzymatic activity of plasmin to hydrolyze fibrin clots and protects endothelial cells from damage caused by chemotherapy, tumor necrosis factor-α, serum starvation, and perfusion.

Route	Onset	Peak	Duration
I.V.	Unknown	End of each infusion	Unknown

Half-life: Less than 2 hours.

ADVERSE REACTIONS

CNS: *cerebral hemorrhage.*
CV: *hypotension, catheter-site hemorrhage.*
EENT: epistaxis.
GI: diarrhea, nausea, vomiting, *GI hemorrhage.*
GU: hyperuricemia.
Respiratory: *pulmonary alveolar hemorrhage, pulmonary hemorrhage,* lung infiltration, pneumonia.
Skin: rash, urticaria, *angioedema.*
Other: *anaphylaxis, sepsis, GVHD, multiorgan failure,* infection.

INTERACTIONS

Drug-drug. *Anticoagulants (heparin), fibrinolytics (alteplase):* May increase risk of hemorrhage. Use together is contraindicated. Discontinue these drugs before treatment with defibrotide; consider delaying treatment until effects of other drugs have resolved.

EFFECTS ON LAB TEST RESULTS

• May increase uric acid level.

CONTRAINDICATIONS & CAUTIONS

• Contraindicated in patients also receiving anticoagulants or fibrinolytics (not including those used for maintenance or reopening of central venous lines) and in patients who are actively bleeding.

• Contraindicated in patients hypersensitive to drug or its components.

Dialyzable drug: No.

PREGNANCY-LACTATION-REPRODUCTION

• Use in pregnant women hasn't been studied. Use during pregnancy only if benefit to mother outweighs risk to the fetus. Advise women of potential miscarriage risk based on animal studies.

• It isn't known if drug appears in breast milk, and drug's effects on breast-fed infants or on milk production haven't been determined. Breast-feeding isn't recommended during treatment.

NURSING CONSIDERATIONS

• Before administration, confirm that patients have no significant bleeding and are hemodynamically stable on no more than one vasopressor.

• Monitor patients for bleeding. Withhold infusion if bleeding occurs, treat the underlying cause, and provide supportive care until bleeding has stopped.

• Monitor patients for signs and symptoms of a hypersensitivity reaction (rash, urticaria, angioedema), especially if there is a history of previous exposure to defibrotide. Discontinue infusion if a severe reaction occurs and treat appropriately. Continue monitoring until signs and symptoms of the reaction resolve.

🛈 *Alert:* There's no known reversal agent for the profibrinolytic effects of defibrotide. For patients undergoing an invasive procedure, discontinue infusion at least 2 hours before the procedure. May resume treatment as soon as any procedure-related risk of bleeding is resolved.

• *Look alike–sound alike:* Don't confuse defibrotide with eptifibatide.

PATIENT TEACHING

• Advise patient to report all adverse reactions and to immediately report signs or symptoms of bleeding (unusual bleeding, easy bruising, blood in urine or stool, headache, confusion, slurred speech, altered vision).

• Teach patient signs and symptoms of an allergic reaction and to seek immediate medical attention if they occur.

Reactions in bold italics are *life-threatening.* Interactions may have a *rapid onset* or a ***delayed onset.***

elbasvir–grazoprevir
EL-bas-vir/graz-OH-pre-vir

Zepatier

Therapeutic class: Antivirals
Pharmacologic class: HCV NS5A
inhibitors/HCV NS3/4A protease inhibitors

AVAILABLE FORMS
Tablets: elbasvir 50 mg/grazoprevir 100 mg

INDICATIONS & DOSAGES
➤ **Chronic HCV genotypes 1 or 4 infection, with or without ribavirin**
Adults: One tablet P.O. once daily. For patients with genotype 1a treatment-naive or PegINF/RBV-experienced without baseline NS5A polymorphisms; genotype 1b treatment-naive or PegINF/RBV-experienced; genotype 1a or 1b PegINF/RBV/PI-experienced; or genotype 4 treatment-naive, continue treatment for 12 weeks. For patients with genotype 1a treatment-naive or PegINF/RBV-experienced with baseline NS5A polymorphisms, or genotype 4 PegINF/RBV-experienced, continue treatment for 16 weeks.
Adjust-a-dose: If ALT level is greater than 10 × ULN, consider discontinuing drug. If ALT level is elevated and accompanied by signs or symptoms of liver inflammation or increased bilirubin or alkaline phosphatase level or INR, discontinue drug.

ADMINISTRATION
P.O.
• May give without regard to food.
• Store at 68° to 77° F (20° to 25° C). Protect from moisture.

ACTION
Elbasvir inhibits HCV NS5A, an enzyme needed for viral RNA replication and assembly of virions. Grazoprevir inhibits HCV NS3/4A protease, an enzyme essential for viral replication and responsible for HCV protein cleavage.

Route	Onset	Peak	Duration
P.O. (elbasvir)	Unknown	3 hr	Unknown
P.O. (grazoprevir)	Unknown	2 hr	Unknown

Half-life: 24 hours (elbasvir); 31 hours (grazoprevir).

ADVERSE REACTIONS
CNS: headache, fatigue, insomnia, irritability, depression.
GI: nausea, diarrhea, abdominal pain (with ribavirin).
Hematologic: anemia (with ribavirin).
Hepatic: ALT elevations, bilirubin elevations (with ribavirin).
Musculoskeletal: arthralgia (with ribavirin).
Respiratory: dyspnea (with ribavirin).
Skin: rash, pruritus (with ribavirin).

INTERACTIONS
Drug-drug. *Antibiotics (nafcillin):* May decrease concentrations of elbasvir and grazoprevir and therapeutic effects. Use together isn't recommended.
HIV medications (cobicistat, elvitegravir, emtricitabine, tenofovir): May increase elbasvir–grazoprevir concentrations. Use together isn't recommended.
HMG-CoA reductase inhibitors (atorvastatin, rosuvastatin): May increase atorvastatin and rosuvastatin concentrations. Maximum recommended doses are atorvastatin 20 mg/day and rosuvastatin 10 mg/day.
HMG-CoA reductase inhibitors (fluvastatin, lovastatin, simvastatin): May increase concentrations of these drugs. Use lowest necessary dose of the statin and monitor patient closely for statin-associated adverse effects such as myopathy.
Immunosuppressants (tacrolimus): May increase tacrolimus concentration. Frequently monitor renal function and tacrolimus level, and watch for tacrolimus-associated adverse effects.
Moderate CYP3A inducers (bosentan, etravirine, modafinil): May decrease elbasvir and grazoprevir plasma concentrations. Use together isn't recommended.
OATP1B1/3 inhibitors (atazanavir, cyclosporine, darunavir, lopinavir, saquinavir, tipranavir): May increase risk of ALT elevation. Use together is contraindicated.
Strong CYP3A inducers (carbamazepine, efavirenz, phenytoin, rifampin): May cause loss of virologic response. Use together is contraindicated.
Strong CYP3A inhibitors (atazanavir, clarithromycin, darunavir, indinavir, itraconazole, ketoconazole, lopinavir, nefazodone, nelfinavir, ritonavir, saquinavir, telithromycin, tipranavir): May increase elbasvir and grazoprevir concentrations. Use together isn't recommended.
Drug-herb. *St. John's wort:* May cause loss of virologic response. Use together is contraindicated.
Drug-food. *Grapefruit juice:* May increase elbasvir and grazoprevir concentrations. Discourage use together.

EFFECTS ON LAB TEST RESULTS
• May increase ALT and bilirubin levels. May decrease Hb level.

CONTRAINDICATIONS & CAUTIONS
• Patients with HCV genotype 1a infection should undergo testing for NS5A resistance-associated polymorphisms before starting treatment, to determine the need for ribavirin and treatment duration.
• If elbasvir–grazoprevir is administered with ribavirin, the contraindications with ribavirin also apply.
Black Box Warning Reactivation of HBV may occur in HCV coinfected patients, and result in fulminant hepatitis, hepatic failure, and death. Screen all patients for current or prior HBV infection before treatment and if positive for HBV infection, assess baseline HBV DNA. ∎

NEW DRUGS

• Contraindicated in patients with moderate or severe hepatic impairment (Child-Pugh class B or C).
• Female patients, Asian patients, and patients age 65 and older are at increased risk for elevated ALT level.
• Safe use in children, liver transplant recipients, and patients with HBV/HCV coinfection hasn't been established.
Dialyzable drug: No.

PREGNANCY-LACTATION-REPRODUCTION
• There are no human data regarding use in pregnant women, and safe use during pregnancy hasn't been established. If drug is used with ribavirin, the combination regimen is contraindicated in pregnant women and in men whose female partners are pregnant.
• It isn't known if elbasvir or grazoprevir appears in breast milk. Use cautiously in breast-feeding women.

NURSING CONSIDERATIONS
Black Box Warning Monitor patient with current or prior HBV infection for hepatitis flare or HBV reactivation with laboratory testing, and watch for signs and symptoms of liver injury during active and posttreatment follow-up. ■
• Obtain LFTs before start of therapy, at treatment week 8, at week 12 in patients receiving 16 weeks of treatment, and as clinically indicated.
• Drug is approved for patients with or without cirrhosis.
• Monitor patients for signs and symptoms of liver inflammation (fatigue, weakness, lack of appetite, abdominal pain, nausea, vomiting, jaundice, and discolored feces).

PATIENT TEACHING
Black Box Warning Warn patient to immediately report signs and symptoms of liver injury (fatigue, weakness, loss of appetite, nausea, vomiting, yellowing of skin or eyes, light-colored stool). ■
• Instruct patient to report current or new prescription or OTC medications or supplements being taken before starting therapy because of possible interactions.
• Explain importance of taking drug around the same time every day, without missing or skipping doses. Advise patient to contact health care provider if a dose is missed and not to double a dose.
• Teach patient importance of adherence and regular follow-up with health care provider during therapy.
• Advise female patient to avoid pregnancy during and for 6 months after treatment ends when drug is used concomitantly with ribavirin.
• Warn patient to watch for and immediately report signs and symptoms of hepatotoxicity (tiredness, nausea and vomiting, lack of appetite, jaundice, and discolored stools).

elotuzumab
EL-oh-tooz-ue-mab

Empliciti

Therapeutic class: Antineoplastics
Pharmacologic class: Monoclonal antibodies

AVAILABLE FORMS
Injection: 300 mg, 400 mg single-dose vials

INDICATIONS & DOSAGES
➤ **Multiple myeloma in combination with lenalidomide and dexamethasone in patients who have received one to three prior therapies**
Adults: 10 mg/kg I.V. every week for first two 28-day cycles, then every 2 weeks thereafter in combination with lenalidomide 25 mg P.O. on days 1 through 21 of every cycle until disease progression or unacceptable toxicity. Between 3 and 24 hours before elotuzumab is given, administer dexamethasone 28 mg P.O. Additionally, give dexamethasone 8 mg I.V. between 45 and 90 minutes before elotuzumab is administered. On days that elotuzumab isn't administered (days 8 and 22 of cycle 3 and all subsequent cycles), give dexamethasone 40 mg P.O. Elotuzumab must be given with premedications (dexamethasone, diphenhydramine, ranitidine, and acetaminophen).
Adjust-a-dose: If the dose of one drug in the regimen is delayed or interrupted or the drug is discontinued, treatment with the other drugs may continue as scheduled. However, if dexamethasone is delayed or discontinued, base the decision whether to administer drug on clinical judgment for the risk of hypersensitivity. For grade 2 or higher infusion reaction, interrupt infusion and institute appropriate medical and supportive measures; upon resolution to grade 1 or lower, restart drug at 0.5 mL/minute and gradually increase at a rate of 0.5 mL/minute every 30 minutes as tolerated to rate at which the infusion reaction occurred. Resume the escalation regimen if there's no recurrence of the infusion reaction. If the infusion reaction recurs, stop the infusion and don't restart on that day; severe infusion reactions may require permanent discontinuation of drug and emergency treatment.
   Delay and modify dosage of dexamethasone and lenalidomide as recommended in their prescribing information.

ADMINISTRATION
I.V.
▼ Premedicate patient 45 to 90 minutes before infusion with diphenhydramine 25 to 50 mg P.O. or I.V., or equivalent H_1 blocker; ranitidine 50 mg I.V. or 150 mg P.O., or equivalent H_2 blocker; and acetaminophen 650 to 1,000 mg P.O.

▼ Reconstitute each vial with sterile water for injection, with 13 mL for 300-mg vial and 17 mL for 400-mg vial for a final concentration of either vial of 25 mg/mL.

▼ Hold vial upright and swirl solution by rotating vial to dissolve the lyophilized cake. Invert vial a few times to dissolve any powder that may be present on top of vial or stopper; don't shake. Powder should dissolve in less than 10 minutes. After dissolution, allow reconstituted solution to stand for 5 to 10 minutes.

▼ Solution should be colorless to slightly yellow, clear to slightly opalescent. Discard solution if particulate matter or discoloration is observed.

▼ After reconstitution, withdraw necessary volume for the calculated dose from each vial, up to a maximum of 16 mL from 400-mg vial and 12 mL from 300-mg vial, and further dilute with 230 mL of either NSS or D₅W into an infusion bag made of polyvinyl chloride or polyolefin. Volume of NSS or D₅W can be adjusted so as not to exceed 5 mL/kg of patient weight at any given dose of drug.

▼ Complete infusion within 24 hours of reconstitution. If not used immediately, store under refrigeration at 36° F to 46° F (2° to 8° C) and protected from light for up to 24 hours. A maximum of 8 hours of the total 24 hours can be at room temperature and room light.

▼ Administer infusion through a nonpyrogenic low-protein-binding filter (with a pore size of 0.2 to 1.2 microns) using an automated infusion pump.

▼ Initiate infusion at a rate of 0.5 mL/minute and increase in stepwise fashion as follows: if no infusion reactions develop: For cycle 1/dose 1, infuse at 0.5 mL/minute for first 30 minutes, then increase to 1 mL/minute for next 30 minutes, then increase to 2 mL/minute until infusion is completed. For cycle 1/dose 2, for first 30 minutes, infuse at 1 mL/minute, then 2 mL/minute from 30 minutes until finished; all infusions after this may be infused at 2 mL/minute. Maximum infusion rate usually shouldn't exceed 2 mL/minute, but if patient has received four cycles of drug, may increase to maximum rate of 5 mL/minute. Adjust infusion rate after any grade 2 or higher infusion reaction.

▼ Keep unopened vials under refrigeration.

▼ **Incompatibilities:** Administer alone; don't mix or infuse in same line with other drugs.

ACTION

A humanized IgG1 monoclonal antibody that specifically targets the SLAMF7 signaling protein, activating natural killer cells and targeting the SLAMF7 protein on myeloma cells to kill the cells.

Route	Onset	Peak	Duration
I.V.	Unknown	Unknown	Unknown

Half-life: Unknown.

ADVERSE REACTIONS

CNS: peripheral neuropathy, headache, hypoesthesia, fatigue, pyrexia, altered mood.

CV: chest pain, hypertension, hypotension, tachycardia, *bradycardia.*
EENT: cataracts, nasopharyngitis, oropharyngeal pain.
GI: diarrhea, constipation, vomiting, decreased appetite.
GU: *acute renal failure.*
Hematologic: anemia, *leukopenia, thrombocytopenia.*
Hepatic: *hepatotoxicity.*
Metabolic: decreased weight.
Musculoskeletal: pain in extremities.
Respiratory: cough, URI, pneumonia, *PE.*
Skin: night sweats.
Other: hypersensitivity, infusion reactions.

INTERACTIONS
None reported.

EFFECTS ON LAB TEST RESULTS
• May increase transaminase, bilirubin, alkaline phosphatase, glucose, and potassium levels. May decrease albumin, calcium, and bicarbonate levels.
• May decrease lymphocyte, leukocyte, and platelet counts.
• May interfere with gamma region serum protein electrophoresis and immunofixation assay results.

CONTRAINDICATIONS & CAUTIONS
• May cause hypersensitivity reactions. Patient must be premedicated with dexamethasone, diphenhydramine, ranitidine, and acetaminophen.
• Safety and effectiveness in children haven't been established.
Dialyzable drug: No.

PREGNANCY-LACTATION-REPRODUCTION
• There are no studies of elotuzumab use in pregnant women. Drug may cause fetal harm. Lenalidomide is contraindicated for use during pregnancy.
• Males and females of reproductive potential must use effective contraception during treatment and for a significant amount of time after final dose. Follow lenalidomide prescribing information for specific details on pregnancy testing and contraception.
• It isn't known if drug appears in breast milk. Breast-feeding isn't recommended.

NURSING CONSIDERATIONS
• Monitor patients for development of infusion reactions (fever, chills, hypertension or hypotension, bradycardia). Interrupt infusion for grade 2 or higher infusion reactions and treat appropriately.
• In patients who experience an infusion reaction, monitor vital signs every 30 minutes for 2 hours after end of infusion.
• Ensure patient has taken premedications before infusion.
• Monitor patients for development of infection, which can be fatal, and treat promptly.
• Monitor patients for second primary malignancies.

NEW DRUGS

- Obtain baseline liver enzyme levels and monitor periodically during treatment. Stop drug for grade 3 or higher liver enzyme elevations. May consider continuing treatment after results return to baseline.

PATIENT TEACHING
- Advise patient that lenalidomide used in combination with elotuzumab can cause fetal harm and has specific requirements regarding contraception, pregnancy testing, blood and sperm donation, and transmission in sperm.
- Inform patient of risk of liver toxicity during treatment and to report signs and symptoms (tiredness, weakness, loss of appetite, confusion, jaundice, change in stool color, abdominal pain, swelling of stomach area).
- Advise patient to immediately report signs and symptoms of infusion reactions (fever, chills, rash, breathing problems, dizziness, light-headedness) that could occur within 24 hours of infusion.
- Instruct patient to take oral dexamethasone, an H_1 blocker, an H_2 blocker, and acetaminophen before infusions to reduce risk of infusion reactions.
- Caution patient about risk of developing infections during treatment and to report signs and symptoms of infection (fever, flulike symptoms, cough, shortness of breath, burning with urination, painful rash).
- Warn patient of risk of developing second primary malignancies during treatment.
- Advise patient that laboratory testing will be needed to monitor treatment.

---

emtricitabine–rilpivirine–tenofovir alafenamide fumarate
em-tra-SYE-ta-ben/ril-pi-VIR-een/te-NOE-fo-veer

Odefsey

Therapeutic class: Antiretrovirals
Pharmacologic class: NRTIs–NNRTIs

AVAILABLE FORMS
Tablets: 200 mg emtricitabine, 25 mg rilpivirine, and 25 mg tenofovir alafenamide fumarate

INDICATIONS & DOSAGES
➤ **HIV-1 infection as initial therapy in patients with no antiretroviral treatment history with HIV-1 RNA 100,000 copies/mL or less; to replace a stable antiretroviral regimen in patients who are virologically suppressed (HIV-1 RNA less than 50 copies/mL) for at least 6 months with no history of treatment failure and no known substitutions associated with resistance to the individual components**
Adults and children age 12 and older weighing 35 kg or more with CrCl of 30 mL/minute or more: One tablet P.O. once daily with a meal.

ADMINISTRATION
P.O.
- Give drug with a meal.
- Store below 86° F (30° C).
- Keep only in tightly closed, original container.

ACTION
Each drug interferes with HIV viral RNA-dependent DNA polymerase activities, resulting in inhibition of viral replication.

Route	Onset	Peak	Duration
P.O. (emtricitabine)	Unknown	3 hr	Unknown
P.O. (rilpivirine)	Unknown	4 hr	Unknown
P.O. (tenofovir)	Unknown	1 hr	Unknown

Half-life: Emtricitabine, 10 hours; rilpivirine, 50 hours; tenofovir, 0.51 hour.

ADVERSE REACTIONS
CNS: headache, insomnia, depression, somnolence, dizziness.
GI: nausea, vomiting, abdominal pain.
GU: *acute renal failure,* Fanconi syndrome, nephrotic syndrome.
Hepatic: *lactic acidosis, severe hepatomegaly with steatosis.*
Metabolic: fat redistribution, weight increase, hypophosphatemia.
Musculoskeletal: bone loss, osteomalacia.
Skin: rash.
Other: hypersensitivity reaction, drug reaction with eosinophilia and systemic symptoms (DRESS) syndrome, autoimmune disorders, opportunistic infections.

INTERACTIONS
Drug-drug. *Acyclovir, aminoglycosides, cidofovir, ganciclovir, valacyclovir, valganciclovir:* May increase Odefsey concentration. Monitor patient for Odefsey-related increased adverse effects.
Antacids (aluminum, magnesium hydroxide, calcium carbonate): May decrease Odefsey serum concentration. Give antacids at least 2 hours before or at least 4 hours after Odefsey.
Anticonvulsants (carbamazepine, oxcarbazepine, phenobarbital, phenytoin): May decrease Odefsey serum concentration, resulting in loss of virologic response and possible drug resistance. Use together is contraindicated.
Antimycobacterial drugs (rifabutin, rifampin, rifapentine): May decrease Odefsey serum concentration, resulting in loss of virologic response and possible drug resistance. Use together is contraindicated.
Azole antifungals (fluconazole, itraconazole, ketoconazole): May increase azole level. Monitor patient for breakthrough fungal infections.
CYP3A inducers: May decrease Odefsey serum concentration, resulting in loss of virologic response and possible drug resistance. Use together is contraindicated.

Reactions in bold italics are *life-threatening.* Interactions may have a *rapid onset* or a *delayed onset.*

CYP3A inhibitors: May increase Odefsey plasma concentration and possible Odefsey-related adverse events. Monitor therapy.

Dexamethasone (systemic): May decrease Odefsey serum concentration, resulting in loss of virologic response and possible drug resistance. Use of more than a single dose of dexamethasone with Odefsey is contraindicated.

H₂-receptor antagonists (cimetidine, famotidine, nizatidine, ranitidine): May decrease Odefsey serum concentration. Administer H₂-receptor antagonist at least 12 hours before or 4 hours after Odefsey. Consider therapy modification.

Ketolide or macrolide antibiotics (clarithromycin, erythromycin, telithromycin): May increase Odefsey serum concentration. Consider using an alternative antibiotic.

Methadone: May increase methadone metabolism. Adjust methadone dosage as clinically indicated.

NSAIDs: May increase risk of nephrotoxicity and adverse effects, especially at high doses. Use alternatives to these combinations if possible.

P-glycoprotein (P-gp) inhibitors: May increase Odefsey absorption and plasma concentration. Monitor patient for increased Odefsey-related adverse effects.

P-gp inducers: May decrease Odefsey absorption and plasma concentration, which may lead to loss of therapeutic effect and resistance. Monitor patient closely.

PPIs (dexlansoprazole, esomeprazole, lansoprazole, omeprazole, pantoprazole, rabeprazole): May decrease Odefsey serum concentration, resulting in loss of virologic response and possible drug resistance. Use together is contraindicated.

QTc interval–prolonging agents: May enhance QTc interval–prolonging effect. Consider alternative medications to Odefsey in patients with known risk of torsade de pointes.

Drug-herb. *St. John's wort:* May decrease Odefsey serum concentration, resulting in loss of virologic response and possible resistance to drug combination. Don't use together.

EFFECTS ON LAB TEST RESULTS

- May increase triglyceride and lipid levels.
- May decrease urine protein-to-creatinine ratio.

CONTRAINDICATIONS & CAUTIONS

Black Box Warning Drug may cause lactic acidosis and hepatomegaly with steatosis, including fatal cases. These effects may occur without elevated transaminase levels and in patients with no known risk factors. Risk factors include long-term antiretroviral use, obesity, and being female. Monitor all patients closely. ■

Black Box Warning Use very cautiously in patients with risk factors for liver disease. ■

Black Box Warning Odefsey isn't approved for treatment of chronic HBV infection, and safety and effectiveness haven't been established in patients coinfected with HIV-1 and HBV. Severe acute exacerbations of HBV infection have been reported in

patients coinfected with HIV-1 and HBV after discontinuation of antiretroviral therapy. Monitor hepatic function during and for several months after discontinuation of treatment. If appropriate, initiate anti-HBV therapy. ■

- Contraindicated in patients hypersensitive to drug or its components.
- Consider alternative therapy in patients at high risk for torsades de pointes or when administered with medications known to increase risk of torsades de pointes. Supratherapeutic dosages of Odefsey have been shown to prolong QTc interval and may increase risk of ventricular arrhythmias.
- May increase risk of immune reconstitution syndrome, resulting in an inflammatory response to an indolent or opportunistic infection or activation of autoimmune disorders (*Mycobacterium avium* infection, CMV, *Pneumocystis jirovecii* pneumonia, TB, Graves disease, polymyositis, Guillain-Barré syndrome).
- Use isn't recommended in patients with CrCl of less than 30 mL/minute.
- Use cautiously in patients with history of pathologic bone fracture or with risk factors for osteoporosis or bone loss. Components of drug have been associated with decreases in bone mineral density and increases in bone metabolism markers. Monitor bone density in patients with risk factors for bone loss or osteoporosis.
- Use cautiously in patients at risk for renal dysfunction. Osteomalacia and hypophosphatemia have been reported secondary to proximal renal tubulopathy.
- Use in patients with severe hepatic impairment hasn't been studied.

Dialyzable drug: Emtricitabine, 30%; rilpivirine, unlikely; tenofovir, 54%.

PREGNANCY-LACTATION-REPRODUCTION

- There are no well-controlled studies in pregnant women. Use cautiously during pregnancy.
- Some components of drug appear in breast milk. It isn't known if Odefsey affects lactation or has effects on an infant. The CDC recommends that HIV-infected mothers not breast-feed, to avoid HIV transmission to the infant.
- To monitor pregnancy outcomes, health care providers are encouraged to register patients in the Antiretroviral Pregnancy Registry (1-800-258-4263).

NURSING CONSIDERATIONS

- Discontinue Odefsey if clinical or laboratory findings suggestive of lactic acidosis or hepatotoxicity develop.
- Test for HBV before initiation of antiretroviral therapy in all patients.
- Assess CD4 count, HIV RNA plasma levels, LFT values, serum creatinine, urine glucose, and urine protein before initiation and during therapy.
- In virologically suppressed patients, additional monitoring of HIV-1 RNA and regimen tolerability is recommended after replacing therapy to assess for potential virologic failure or rebound.

NEW DRUGS

• Monitor patient for hypersensitivity, rash, and severe skin reactions, including drug reaction with eosinophilia and systemic symptoms (DRESS); (severe rash or rash accompanied by fever, blisters, mucosal involvement, conjunctivitis, facial edema, angioedema, hepatitis, eosinophilia). Most rashes occurred within first 4 to 6 weeks of therapy. Monitor laboratory parameters and clinical status. Stop drug immediately if hypersensitivity or rash develops.
• Monitor serum phosphorus level in patients with chronic kidney disease. Odefsey may increase risk of Fanconi syndrome. Discontinue drug for significantly decreased renal function or evidence of Fanconi syndrome.
• Monitor bone density in patients with a history of bone fracture or risk factors for bone loss. Calcium and vitamin D supplementation may be beneficial for all patients.
• Monitor patient for redistribution or accumulation of body fat (central obesity, dorsocervical fat enlargement [buffalo hump], peripheral wasting, facial wasting, breast enlargement, cushingoid appearance). Long-term consequences are unknown.
• Monitor patient for depression, dysphoria, mood changes, negative thoughts, suicide attempts, or suicidal ideation. Patients who develop these symptoms should be promptly evaluated; consider risks versus benefits of continued treatment.

PATIENT TEACHING
🚱 *Alert:* Counsel patient, family members, or caregivers to watch for signs and symptoms of depression and to immediately report depression, negative thoughts, dysphoria, or suicidal thoughts or behaviors to prescriber.
`Black Box Warning` Advise patient that Odefsey can cause buildup of lactic acid in the blood. Instruct patient to seek immediate medical attention for weakness, fatigue, muscle pain, trouble breathing, stomachache with nausea and vomiting, dizziness, chills, or fast or irregular heartbeat. ■
`Black Box Warning` Caution patient that Odefsey may cause liver problems. Instruct patient to seek immediate medical attention for yellowing of the skin or eyes, dark-colored urine, loss of appetite, light-colored stool, nausea, or pain or tenderness on right side of the stomach. ■
🚱 *Alert:* Warn patient to stop taking drug and immediately seek medical attention for allergic reactions (rash, fever, blisters, mucosal involvement, eye inflammation; swelling of the face eyes, lips, mouth, tongue, or throat, which may lead to difficulty swallowing or breathing).
• Caution patient not to discontinue drug combination without first discussing with prescriber. Advise patient of the importance of not running out of the medications and of not missing doses. Severe acute exacerbations of hepatitis B have been reported in coinfected patients.
• Advise patient to take calcium and vitamin D supplements as directed by prescriber.

• Remind patient to notify prescriber about other prescription or OTC drugs, including herbal and vitamin supplements, patient is taking or plans to take.
• Inform patient that blood tests will be needed to check for effectiveness and adverse effects of therapy.
• Advise patient to immediately report signs and symptoms of infection.
• Explain that patient may notice an increased amount of fat in the upper back and neck, breast, and around the middle of the body trunk and a loss of fat from the legs, arms, and face.
• Tell female patient of childbearing potential to notify prescriber about planned, suspected, or known pregnancy and that there is a pregnancy registry for women who take antivirals during pregnancy.
• Advise female patient not to breast-feed during therapy.

emtricitabine–tenofovir alafenamide fumarate
em-tra-SYE-tah-ben/te-NOE-fo-veer

Descovy

Therapeutic class: Antiretrovirals
Pharmacologic class: NNRTIs

AVAILABLE FORMS
Tablets: Emtricitabine 200 mg and tenofovir alafenamide fumarate 25 mg

INDICATIONS & DOSAGES
➤ **Treatment of HIV-1 infection in combination with other antiretrovirals**
Adults and children age 12 and older weighing 35 kg or more, with CrCl of 30 mL/minute or more: One tablet P.O. once daily.

ADMINISTRATION
P.O.
• May give with or without food.
• Store below 86° F (30° C). Keep container tightly closed.
• Give a missed dose as soon possible. If it's close to the time for the next dose, skip missed dose. Don't give two doses at the same time or extra doses.

ACTION
Interferes with HIV viral RNA-dependent DNA polymerase activities, resulting in inhibition of viral replication.

Route	Onset	Peak	Duration
P.O. (emtricitabine)	Unknown	3 hr	Unknown
P.O. (tenofovir)	Unknown	1 hr	Unknown

Half-life: Emtricitabine, 10 hours; tenofovir, ½ hour.

Reactions in bold italics are *life-threatening.* Interactions may have a *rapid onset* or a ***delayed onset.***

ADVERSE REACTIONS

CNS: dizziness, asthenia, headache, pain, fever, peripheral neuropathy, neuritis, paresthesia, insomnia, abnormal dreams, depression, anxiety, fatigue.
CV: chest pain.
EENT: otitis media, rhinitis, sinusitis, pharyngitis.
GI: nausea, diarrhea, vomiting, abdominal pain, dyspepsia, gastroenteritis.
GU: renal disease, hematuria.
Hematologic: *neutropenia*, anemia.
Metabolic: hyperglycemia.
Musculoskeletal: arthralgia, myalgia, decreased bone mineral density, increased CK level, back pain.
Respiratory: cough, pneumonia, URI.
Skin: hyperpigmentation, rash, allergic skin reaction, pruritus.

INTERACTIONS

Drug-drug. *Acyclovir, valacyclovir:* May increase serum concentration of tenofovir products. Tenofovir products may increase serum concentration of acyclovir or valacyclovir. Monitor therapy.
Adefovir: May diminish therapeutic effect of tenofovir products. Adefovir may increase serum concentration of tenofovir products. Tenofovir products may increase adefovir serum concentration. Avoid use together.
Aminoglycosides: May increase serum concentration of tenofovir products. Tenofovir products may increase serum concentration of aminoglycosides. Monitor therapy.
Anticonvulsants (carbamazepine, oxcarbazepine, phenobarbital, phenytoin): May decrease tenofovir serum concentration. Consider alternative anticonvulsant.
Antimycobacterial drugs (rifabutin, rifampin, rifapentine): May decrease tenofovir level. Use together isn't recommended.
Cidofovir: May increase serum concentration of tenofovir products. Tenofovir products may increase cidofovir serum concentration. Monitor therapy.
Cobicistat: May increase risk of adverse effects of tenofovir. Monitor therapy.
Ganciclovir, valganciclovir: May increase emtricitabine–tenofovir serum concentration and risk of adverse effects. Monitor patients closely.
Lamivudine: May increase risk of adverse effects of emtricitabine. Avoid use together.
NSAIDs: May enhance nephrotoxic effect of tenofovir. Seek alternatives to this combination whenever possible. Avoid use of tenofovir with multiple NSAIDs or with any NSAID given at a high dose.
P-glycoprotein (P-gp) inducers: May decrease tenofovir absorption, causing loss of therapeutic effect and development of resistance.
P-gp inhibitors: May increase tenofovir level. Use cautiously together.
Primidone: May decrease tenofovir serum concentration. Avoid combination.
Ribavirin (oral inhalation, systemic): May increase risk of hepatotoxicity. Use together cautiously.

Protease inhibitors (ritonavir, tipranavir): May decrease tenofovir serum concentration. Use together isn't recommended.
Drug-herb. *St John's wort:* May decrease tenofovir serum concentration. Use together isn't recommended.

EFFECTS ON LAB TEST RESULTS

• May increase total cholesterol, LDL, HDL, triglyceride, ALT, amylase, AST, bilirubin, CK, lipase, and glucose levels. May decrease phosphate level.
• May decrease neutrophil count.

CONTRAINDICATIONS & CAUTIONS

Black Box Warning Lactic acidosis and severe hepatomegaly with steatosis, including fatal cases, have been reported with nucleoside analogues (tenofovir) in combination with other antiretrovirals. Interrupt treatment in patients who develop clinical or laboratory findings suggestive of lactic acidosis or hepatotoxicity (hepatomegaly and steatosis with or without transaminase elevations). Some cases of hepatotoxicity have occurred in patients with no hepatic disease before treatment. ■
• Use cautiously in women, obese patients, patients with risk factors for liver disease, and those with prolonged nucleoside exposure.
Black Box Warning Drug isn't approved for treatment of chronic HBV infection. Safety and efficacy haven't been established for patients coinfected with HIV and HBV; acute, severe exacerbations of HBV infection (liver decompensation and liver failure) have been reported after discontinuation of antiretroviral therapy. ■
• Descovy isn't indicated for preexposure prophylaxis to reduce risk of sexually acquired HIV-1 in high-risk adults.
• Descovy isn't recommended for patients with CrCl of less than 30 mL/minute.
• Immune reconstitution syndrome may occur, resulting in an inflammatory response to an indolent or residual opportunistic infection (*Mycobacterium avium* infection, CMV, *Pneumocystis jirovecii* pneumonia, TB) or an autoimmune disorder (Graves disease, polymyositis, Guillain-Barré syndrome); evaluate and treat appropriately.
• Use cautiously in patients at risk for renal dysfunction. Evaluate patients with persistent or worsening bone or muscle symptoms for renal dysfunction, hypophosphatemia, and osteomalacia.
• Drug may increase risk of acute renal failure and Fanconi syndrome. Patients with preexisting renal impairment and those taking nephrotoxic agents (including NSAIDs) are at increased risk.
• Use in patients with severe hepatic impairment (Child-Pugh class C) hasn't been studied.
• Drug may increase risk of decreased bone mineral density. Consider monitoring bone density in adults and children with a history of pathologic fractures or with other risk factors for bone loss or osteoporosis. If abnormalities are suspected, expert assessment is

NEW DRUGS

recommended. Calcium and vitamin D supplements may be beneficial for all patients.

• Drug may cause redistribution of fat, resulting in buffalo hump, peripheral wasting, facial wasting, increased abdominal girth, breast enlargement, and cushingoid appearance.

• Safety and effectiveness in children younger than age 12 or weighing less than 35 kg haven't been established.

Dialyzable drug: Emtricitabine, 30%; tenofovir alafenamide fumarate, 54%.

PREGNANCY-LACTATION-REPRODUCTION

• If indicated, drug shouldn't be withheld because of pregnancy.

• Emtricitabine and tenofovir appear in breast milk. Emtricitabine and tenofovir are contraindicated in breast-feeding women.

• The CDC recommends that HIV-infected mothers shouldn't breast-feed, to avoid risking postnatal transmission of HIV.

• To monitor pregnancy outcomes, health care providers are encouraged to register patients in the Antiretroviral Pregnancy Registry (1-800-258- 4263).

NURSING CONSIDERATIONS

• Test for HBV before initiation of antiretroviral therapy. Drug isn't approved for the treatment of chronic HBV infection.

• Descovy must be given as part of a regimen with other antiretrovirals.

• Monitor CD4 counts and HIV RNA plasma levels to evaluate effectiveness of treatment.

• Assess estimated CrCl, urine protein, and urine glucose before initiation and during therapy. Monitor serum phosphorus level in patients with chronic kidney disease due to increased risk of developing Fanconi syndrome. Discontinue drug in patients who develop clinically significant decreases in renal function or evidence of Fanconi syndrome.

• Monitor lipid levels periodically.

Black Box Warning Monitor patients with HIV and HBV coinfection for several months after therapy discontinuation for acute exacerbations of HBV infection. Monitor hepatic function by clinical assessment and laboratory testing. Start anti–hepatitis B therapy as clinically indicated, especially in patients with advanced liver disease or cirrhosis. ■

• Monitor bone mineral density in patients at risk for bone less.

PATIENT TEACHING

Black Box Warning Caution patient that drug may cause liver enlargement and increased acid in the blood; risk may be higher in women, overweight people, and in people who have taken similar drugs for a long time. ■

• Advise patient that hepatitis B sometimes worsens when drug is stopped in patients with hepatitis B and that close follow-up for a few months is needed when therapy is stopped.

• Caution patient not to stop drug without first discussing with prescriber.

• Advise patient of importance of taking drug without missing doses, to avoid loss of treatment effectiveness.

• Warn patient to report signs and symptoms of kidney problems (inability to pass urine, change in how much urine is passed, blood in the urine, weight gain).

Black Box Warning Instruct patient to report signs and symptoms of liver problems (dark urine, loss of appetite, nausea, right upper quadrant abdominal pain, achiness or tenderness, light-colored stools, vomiting, yellowing of skin or eyes). ■

Black Box Warning Advise patient to report signs and symptoms of lactic acidosis (trouble breathing, fast or irregular heartbeat, stomach pain with nausea or vomiting, fatigue, shortness of breath, weakness, dizziness or light-headedness, feeling cold, muscle pain, or cramps). ■

• Advise patient to report bone pain and change in body fat distribution.

• Instruct patient to report signs and symptoms of infection (fever, sore throat, weakness, cough, shortness of breath).

• Teach patient to avoid behaviors that can spread HIV-1 infection to others, including sharing or reusing needles, sharing razors or toothbrushes, or having sex without using a latex or polyurethane condom.

• Caution female patient not to breast feed, to avoid transmitting HIV-1 to her infant.

• Inform patient that there is an antiretroviral pregnancy registry to monitor fetal outcomes of pregnant women exposed to Descovy.

---

etanercept-szzs
ee-tan-ER-sept

Erelzi

Therapeutic class: Antiarthritics– antipsoriatics
Pharmacologic class: TNF blockers

AVAILABLE FORMS
Prefilled single-dose Sensoready pen: 50 mg/mL
Prefilled single-dose syringe: 25 mg/0.5 mL, 50 mg/mL

INDICATIONS & DOSAGES
➤ **Moderately to severely active RA with or without methotrexate; psoriatic arthritis with or without methotrexate; ankylosing spondylitis**
Adults: 50 mg subcutaneously once weekly. Methotrexate, glucocorticoids, salicylates, NSAIDs, or analgesics may be continued during treatment.

➤ **Moderately to severely active polyarticular juvenile idiopathic arthritis (JIA)**
Children weighing more than 63 kg: 50 mg subcutaneously once weekly. Glucocorticoids, NSAIDs, or analgesics may be continued during treatment.

➤ **Chronic, moderate to severe plaque psoriasis in patients who are candidates for systemic therapy or phototherapy**
Adults: Initially, 50 mg subcutaneously twice weekly for 3 months, then a maintenance dose of 50 mg subcutaneously once weekly. Or, initially, may give 25 or 50 mg subcutaneously once a week for 3 months.

ADMINISTRATION
Subcutaneous
🜂 *Alert:* Components of the Sensoready pen contain natural rubber and may cause allergic reactions in individuals sensitive to latex.
• Store in refrigerator between 36° and 46° F (2° and 8° C). Don't freeze. Allow drug to reach room temperature for 15 to 30 minutes before use. Don't remove needle cover until ready to inject.
• For convenience, may store syringe or pen at room temperature between 68° and 77° F (20° and 25° C) for up to 28 days; once drug has reached room temperature, don't put it back in refrigerator. Discard drug that has been stored at room temperature after 28 days.
• Visually inspect solution for particulate matter and discoloration before administering. Small white particles of protein may be present in solution. Don't give if solution is discolored or cloudy, or if foreign particles are present.
• Give injection into thigh (preferred), lower abdomen at least 2 inches (5 cm) from the navel, or outer upper area of the arm.
• Don't inject into tender, bruised, red, hardened, raised, thick, or scaly skin or into scars or stretch marks.
• If a dose is missed, give missed dose as soon as possible; then give next dose as scheduled.

ACTION
TNF, a cytokine involved in normal inflammatory and immune responses, is bound by the drug and becomes biologically inactive.

Route	Onset	Peak	Duration
Subcut.	Unknown	Unknown	Unknown

Half-life: 72 to 132 hours.

ADVERSE REACTIONS
CNS: pyrexia, headache.
GI: diarrhea.
Respiratory: URI, pneumonia.
Skin: injection-site reactions, urticaria, pruritus, rash.
Other: serious infections, hypersensitivity.

INTERACTIONS
Drug-drug. *Antidiabetic medications:* May increase risk of hypoglycemia. Monitor blood glucose level and reduce antidiabetic medication dosage if needed.
Cyclophosphamide: May increase risk of malignancy. Use together isn't recommended.
Live-virus vaccines: May increase risk of secondary infection transmission. Don't give together.
Other immune-modulating biological products (abatacept, anakinra): May increase risk of serious infection. Avoid use together.

Sulfasalazine: May decrease neutrophil count. Monitor patient closely.

EFFECTS ON LAB TEST RESULTS
• May increase ANA level.

CONTRAINDICATIONS & CAUTIONS
Black Box Warning Patients with TB have frequently presented with disseminated or extrapulmonary disease; test for latent TB before use and periodically during therapy. Begin treatment for latent infection before therapy begins. ■
• Consider anti-TB therapy in patients with a history of latent or active TB when an adequate course of treatment can't be confirmed, and in patients with a negative test for latent TB but with risk factors for TB infection. Consultation with an infectious disease specialist is recommended.
Black Box Warning Use cautiously in patients with chronic or recurrent infection. ■
• Use cautiously in patients with underlying conditions that may predispose them to infection, including advanced or poorly controlled diabetes and age over 65.
• TNF blockers may increase risk of leukemia, lymphoma, skin cancer, and other malignancies.
Black Box Warning Lymphoma and other malignancies, some fatal, have been reported in children and adolescents treated with TNF blockers, including etanercept. ■
• Rare cases of new-onset or exacerbations of CNS and peripheral nervous system demyelinating disorders (transverse myelitis, optic neuritis, MS, Guillain-Barré syndrome) and seizure disorders have occurred. Monitor patient closely.
• Use cautiously in patients with a history of HF and moderate to severe alcoholic hepatitis.
• Don't start drug in patients with an active infection, including clinically important localized infections.
• Use cautiously in patients previously infected with HBV. Evaluate patients at increased risk for HBV infection before treatment and monitor patients for reactivation during and for several months after therapy ends. If reactivation occurs, drug may need to be stopped and antiviral therapy begun.
• Avoid use in patients with Wegener granulomatosis who are receiving immunosuppressants; drug may increase risk of malignancy.
• Temporarily interrupt treatment in patients with varicella virus exposure and consider prophylactic treatment with varicella zoster immune globulin.
• Children should be up to date with all immunizations before start of therapy.
Dialyzable drug: Unknown.

PREGNANCY-LACTATION-REPRODUCTION
• Use during pregnancy only if clearly needed.
• Drug appears in breast milk in low levels and is minimally absorbed by the breast-fed infant. Use cautiously in breast-feeding women.

NEW DRUGS

🍁Canada   ◇ OTC   ◆ Off-label use   ✐Photoguide   ⓒⓡⓤDo not crush   *Liquid contains alcohol.

NURSING CONSIDERATIONS

• Etanercept-szzs is biosimilar to the FDA-approved reference product etanercept. There are no clinically meaningful differences between the biosimilar product and the reference product based on the conditions of its use.

Black Box Warning Patients treated with etanercept products are at increased risk for developing serious, sometimes fatal, infections, such as TB, invasive fungal infections, viral and bacterial infections, and *Legionella* and *Listeria* infections. Most patients who developed serious infections were also receiving immunosuppressants, such as methotrexate or corticosteroids. If serious infection occurs, stop therapy and notify prescriber. ∎

Black Box Warning Closely monitor patients for signs and symptoms of infection during therapy and after treatment ends, including the possible development of TB in patients who tested negative for latent TB infection before start of therapy. ∎

Black Box Warning Histoplasmosis, coccidioidomycosis, candidiasis, aspergillosis, blastomycosis, and pneumocystosis have been reported. Consider empirical antifungal therapy in patients at risk for invasive fungal infections who develop severe systemic illness. ∎

• Rare cases of pancytopenia and aplastic anemia have occurred. Monitor patient for persistent fever, bruising, bleeding, or pallor. If hematologic abnormalities occur, drug may need to be stopped.

• Monitor patient for signs and symptoms of infection during and after treatment ends. Obtain prompt diagnostic workup and begin antimicrobial therapy if infection occurs. Discontinue drug for serious infection or sepsis.

• Monitor patient for anaphylaxis or serious allergic reactions, signs and symptoms of new or worsening HF, hypoglycemia (in diabetic patients), and injection-site reactions (redness, swelling, itching, bleeding, bruising, pain), which usually resolve in 3 to 5 days.

• Monitor patient for autoimmune disorders, such as lupuslike syndrome or autoimmune hepatitis. Drug may cause formation of autoantibodies. Discontinue drug if autoimmune disorder occurs.

• Skin cancers have been reported. Perform periodic skin examinations in patients at increased risk for skin cancer.

• Ensure that immunizations are up to date before start of therapy.

PATIENT TEACHING

Black Box Warning Warn patient of increased risk of serious infection and to immediately report active infection or signs and symptoms suggesting infection (fever, sweats or chills, cough or flulike symptoms, shortness of breath, blood in phlegm, weight loss, muscle aches; warm, red, or painful areas on skin; sores on body; diarrhea or stomach pain; burning upon urination or urinating more often than normal; fatigue). ∎

Black Box Warning Counsel patient about risk of lymphoma and other malignancies during therapy. ∎

• Advise patient to report signs or symptoms of pancytopenia, such as bruising, bleeding, persistent fever, or pallor.

• Instruct patient on proper administration of injection and provide written educational materials.

• Advise patient to report signs or symptoms of new or worsening medical conditions, such as CNS demyelinating disorders (numbness, tingling, vision changes, weakness of arms and legs, dizziness), seizures, or HF.

• Warn patient to notify prescriber if he has diabetes, HIV, hepatitis B, or a weak immune system as these conditions increase chance of infection.

• Tell patient to notify prescriber if he has TB, has been in close contact with someone with TB, or was born in, lived in, or traveled to countries where there is a risk of contracting TB.

• Instruct patient to notify prescriber if he lives in, has lived in, or has traveled to certain parts of the country (such as the Ohio and Mississippi River valleys or the Southwest) where there is a greater risk of contracting certain kinds of fungal infections.

eteplirsen
e-TEP-lir-sen

Exondys 51

Therapeutic class: Muscular dystrophy drugs
Pharmacologic class: Antisense oligonucleotide

AVAILABLE FORMS
Injection: 50 mg/mL single-dose vials

INDICATIONS & DOSAGES
➤ **Treatment of Duchenne muscular dystrophy (DMD) in patients with confirmed mutation of the DMD gene that's amenable to exon 51 skipping**
Adults and children: 30 mg/kg I.V. infusion once weekly.

ADMINISTRATION
I.V.
▼ Allow vials to warm to room temperature before giving. Mix contents by gently inverting two or three times. Don't shake.
▼ Dilute in NSS to make a total volume of 100 to 150 mL. Visually inspect for particulates. Drug is a preservative-free clear and colorless solution that may have some opalescence. Flush I.V. access line with NSS before and after infusion.
▼ May use topical anesthetic cream at infusion site before administration.
▼ Administer immediately after dilution by I.V. infusion over 35 to 60 minutes. Complete infusion within 4 hours of dilution. If not used immediately, may store

diluted solution for up to 24 hours at 36° to 46° F (2° to 8° C). Don't freeze. Discard unused solution.

▼ Give missed dose as soon as possible.

▼ Store vial at 36° to 46° F (2° to 8° C). Don't freeze. Protect from light and store in original carton until ready for use.

▼ **Incompatibilities:** Don't mix or infuse with other drugs concomitantly in the same I.V. line.

ACTION
Binds to exon 51 of dystrophin pre-mRNA, resulting in exclusion of this exon during mRNA processing in patients with genetic mutations that are amenable to exon 51 skipping. Exon skipping allows for production of a dystrophin protein thought to increase muscle strength.

Route	Onset	Peak	Duration
I.V.	Unknown	1.1–1.2 hr	Unknown

Half-life: 3 to 4 hours.

ADVERSE REACTIONS
CNS: balance disorder, fever.
CV: facial flushing.
GI: vomiting.
Hematologic: contusion.
Musculoskeletal: arthralgia.
Respiratory: URI.
Skin: contact dermatitis, rash, transient erythema, excoriation.
Other: I.V. catheter-site pain.

INTERACTIONS
None reported.

EFFECTS ON LAB TEST RESULTS
None reported.

CONTRAINDICATIONS & CAUTIONS
• A clinical benefit of drug hasn't been established. Continued FDA approval may be contingent upon verification of a clinical benefit in confirmatory trials.
• Drug hasn't been studied in patients with renal or hepatic impairment.
Dialyzable drug: Unknown.

PREGNANCY-LACTATION-REPRODUCTION
• There are no data regarding safe use in pregnant women or drug's impact on fertility. Drug hasn't been studied in women.
• There are no data regarding safe use in breast-feeding women. Consider benefits of breast-feeding, clinical need for drug, and risk to the infant.

NURSING CONSIDERATIONS
• Treatment of DMD must be managed individually. Other treatment options include physical and occupational therapy, braces and other mobilization tools, and psychosocial, mental, and educational evaluation and care.

PATIENT TEACHING
• Explain to patient and caregivers that drug is infused I.V. weekly and if a dose is missed, to schedule an infusion as soon as possible.
• Advise patient and caregivers to report all adverse events, such as balance disorder, vomiting, and injection-site reactions or pain.

---

infliximab-dyyb
in-FLICKS-ih-mab

Inflectra

Therapeutic class: Anti-inflammatory drugs
Pharmacologic class: TNF blockers

AVAILABLE FORMS
Lyophilized powder for injection: 100 mg/20 mL vial

INDICATIONS & DOSAGES
➤ **Moderately to severely active Crohn disease or fistulizing Crohn disease in patients with inadequate response to conventional therapy**
Adults: 5 mg/kg I.V. infusion at weeks 0, 2, and 6, then every 8 weeks thereafter. For patients who respond and then lose their response, consider 10 mg/kg. Patients who don't respond by week 14 are unlikely to respond with continued therapy; consider stopping drug in those patients.
Children ages 6 to 17: For Crohn disease, 5 mg/kg I.V. infusion at weeks 0, 2, and 6, and then every 8 weeks thereafter.
➤ **Moderately to severely active ulcerative colitis in patients with inadequate response to conventional therapy; psoriatic arthritis, with or without methotrexate; chronic severe plaque psoriasis when other systemic therapies are medically less appropriate**
Adults: 5 mg/kg I.V. infusion at weeks 0, 2, and 6, then every 8 weeks thereafter.
➤ **Moderately to severely active RA, with methotrexate**
Adults: 3 mg/kg I.V. infusion at weeks 0, 2, and 6, then every 8 weeks thereafter. For patients with an incomplete response, adjust dosage up to 10 mg/kg or give as often as every 4 weeks.
➤ **Ankylosing spondylitis**
Adults: 5 mg/kg I.V. infusion at weeks 0, 2, and 6, then every 6 weeks thereafter.

ADMINISTRATION
I.V.
▼ Store vials in refrigerator at 36° to 46° F (2° to 8° C). Product doesn't contain preservative.
▼ Reconstitute with 10 mL sterile water for injection using syringe with a 21G or smaller needle. Don't shake; gently swirl to dissolve powder. Allow solution to stand for 5 minutes. Solution should be colorless to light yellow and opalescent; a few translucent

---

particles may develop. Don't use if solution isn't fully dissolved or is discolored, or if other foreign particles are present.

▼ Dilute reconstituted solution to total volume 250 mL using NSS only. Gently mix. Infusion concentration range is 0.4 to 4 mg/mL.

▼ Use an infusion set with an in-line, sterile, nonpyrogenic, low-protein-binding filter (pore size of 1.2 microns or less).

▼ Begin infusion within 3 hours of preparation and give over at least 2 hours. Discard unused portion of infusion solution.

▼ **Incompatibilities:** Don't infuse with other drugs or solutions.

ACTION
Binds to human TNF-alpha to neutralize its activity and inhibit its binding to receptors, thereby reducing the infiltration of inflammatory cells and TNF-alpha production in inflamed areas.

Route	Onset	Peak	Duration
I.V.	Unknown	Unknown	Unknown

Half-life: 7.7 to 9.5 days.

ADVERSE REACTIONS
CNS: fatigue, fever, chills, headache, pain.
CV: hypertension, flushing, chest pain, hypotension.
EENT: sinusitis, pharyngitis.
GI: nausea, abdominal pain, diarrhea, dyspepsia.
GU: UTI.
Hematologic: anemia, *leukopenia, neutropenia.*
Hepatic: elevated ALT and AST levels.
Musculoskeletal: arthralgia, bone fracture.
Respiratory: URI, cough, bronchitis, pneumonia, respiratory tract allergic reaction.
Skin: rash, pruritus, cellulitis, abscess, skin ulceration.
Other: infusion reactions, hypersensitivity reactions, development of antibodies to infliximab, bacterial infection, *sepsis,* viral infections, candidiasis.

INTERACTIONS
Drug-drug. *Abatacept, anakinra:* May increase risk of serious infections. Use together isn't recommended.
CYP450 substrates with narrow therapeutic index (cyclosporine, theophylline, warfarin): May alter levels of these drugs. Monitor levels and effects of these drugs, and adjust dosages as needed when infliximab-dyyb is begun or discontinued.
Methotrexate: May increase infliximab-dyyb level and decrease incidence of anti-inflammatory antibody production. Use together may be favorable.
Other biological therapeutics: May increase risk of infection. Use together isn't recommended.
Therapeutic infectious agents (BCG bladder instillation), vaccines (live): May increase risk of infections. Avoid use together. Also avoid administration of live vaccine to infants with in utero infliximab-dyyb exposure for at least 6 months after birth.
Tocilizumab: May increase immunosuppression and risk of infection. Avoid use together.

EFFECTS ON LAB TEST RESULTS
• May increase ALT and AST levels.
• May decrease RBC, WBC, and neutrophil counts.
• May produce false-negative TB test results.
• May develop positive ANA and detectable antibodies to infliximab products.

CONTRAINDICATIONS & CAUTIONS
• Contraindicated at doses greater than 5 mg/kg in patients with moderate to severe HF (New York Heart Association functional class III/IV) due to risk of worsening HF and death.
• Contraindicated in patients with a known hypersensitivity or who develop a severe hypersensitivity reaction to components of drug or to murine proteins.
• Contraindicated in patients with active infection, including clinically important localized infection.
Black Box Warning Drug may increase risk of development of serious infections leading to hospitalization or death, especially in patients taking concomitant immunosuppressants, such as methotrexate or corticosteroids. Discontinue drug if serious infection or sepsis occur. ▪
Black Box Warning Carefully consider risks and benefits of treatment in patients with chronic or recurrent infection. ▪
Black Box Warning Lymphoma and other malignancies, some fatal, have occurred in children and adolescents treated with TNF blockers, including infliximab products. ▪
Black Box Warning Hepatosplenic T-cell lymphoma, a rare, aggressive lymphoma with fatalities, has occurred in patients treated with TNF blockers. The majority of cases occurred in adolescent or young adult males treated for Crohn disease or ulcerative colitis, and almost all had received treatment with azathioprine or 6-mercaptopurine concomitantly with a TNF blocker at or before diagnosis. ▪
• TNF blockers may increase risk of reactivation of HBV in patients who are chronic carriers. Patients taking concomitant immunosuppressants are at increased risk. Test for HBV infection before therapy begins.
• Use cautiously in patients with COPD due to increased risk of lung, head, or neck cancer.
• Use cautiously in patients with a history of malignancy, when continuing treatment in patients who develop malignancy, and in those with seizure disorder.
• Use cautiously in patients with HF and only after considering other treatment options. Closely monitor patients during therapy; discontinue drug if new or worsening symptoms of HF appear.
• Use cautiously in patients with current or past significant hematologic abnormalities (leukopenia, neutropenia, thrombocytopenia, pancytopenia). Monitor patients for blood dyscrasias and infection. Discontinue drug if serious abnormalities occur.
• Use cautiously in patients with CNS demyelination disorders (MS, optic neuritis) and peripheral demyelinating disorders (Guillain-Barré syndrome). Discontinue drug if exacerbation of disorder occurs.

Reactions in bold italics are *life-threatening.* Interactions may have a *rapid onset* or a *delayed onset.*

- Use cautiously in patients older than age 65, in patients with comorbid conditions, and in patients taking concomitant immunosuppressants (corticosteroids, methotrexate) due to increased risk of infection.
- Use cautiously in patients with chronic or recurrent infections, exposure to TB, residence or travel in areas of endemic TB or mycoses, history of an opportunistic infection, and underlying conditions that predispose them to infection. Consider risks and benefits before starting therapy.
- Rare cases of severe hepatic reactions (acute liver failure, jaundice, hepatitis, cholestasis) with or without elevations in aminotransferase levels have been reported in postmarketing data. Discontinue drug if signs and symptoms of liver injury occur.
- Safety and effectiveness in children younger than age 6 with disorders other than Crohn disease and ulcerative colitis haven't been established.
Dialyzable drug: Unknown.

PREGNANCY-LACTATION-REPRODUCTION

- It isn't known if drug causes fetal harm or affects reproductive capacity. Use cautiously in pregnant women and only if clearly needed.
- Drug crosses placental barrier and may be present in the serum of infants up to 6 months after birth. Exposed infants may be at increased risk for infection.
- It isn't known if drug appears in breast milk. Patient should discontinue breast-feeding or discontinue drug.

NURSING CONSIDERATIONS

- Infliximab-dyyb is biosimilar to the FDA-approved reference product infliximab for the indications listed. There are no clinically meaningful differences between the biosimilar product and the reference product.
- **Black Box Warning** Don't initiate treatment in individuals with active infection. Discontinue drug if serious infection (active or reactivated latent disseminated or extrapulmonary TB, invasive fungal infections, bacterial, viral, or other infections) or sepsis occurs. ∎
- **Black Box Warning** Consider empirical antifungal therapy while a diagnostic workup is being performed in patients at risk for invasive fungal infections who develop severe systemic illness. ∎
- **Black Box Warning** Closely monitor patients for signs and symptoms of infection during and after treatment, including the possible development of TB in patients who tested negative for latent TB before therapy. ∎
- **Black Box Warning** Evaluate patients for latent TB before initiating and periodically during therapy. Treatment for latent infection should begin before start of therapy. ∎
- Closely monitor patients who develop a new infection, including a prompt and complete workup and initiation of appropriate antimicrobial therapy.
- Patients may be premedicated with antihistamines, acetaminophen, or corticosteroids to prevent or lower severity of infusion reactions.

- Monitor patients for infusion reactions (flulike symptoms, headache, dyspnea, hypotension, transient fever, chills, GI symptoms, rash). Mild to moderate reactions may improve by slowing infusion rate, or by withholding drug and upon resolution of reaction, reinitiating at a slower rate or administering antihistamines, acetaminophen, or corticosteroids. Discontinue drug in patients who don't tolerate the infusion after these interventions. Discontinue drug in patients with severe infusion-related hypersensitivity reactions and anaphylaxis; treat symptomatically.
- **Black Box Warning** Watch for development of lymphoma and other malignancies, especially in children, adolescents, and young adults. ∎
- Before start of therapy, test patients for HBV; consult specialist if tests are positive. Monitor patients for signs and symptoms of HBV reactivation throughout therapy and for several months after therapy ends. If reactivation occurs, discontinue drug and begin antiviral therapy. Monitor patients closely if drug is resumed.
- Monitor patient for hepatotoxicity (jaundice, liver enzyme elevations $5 \times$ ULN or more). Discontinue drug and evaluate patient closely.
- Monitor patient for signs and symptoms of hypersensitivity reactions (urticaria, dyspnea, hypotension), which may occur during or within 2 hours of infusion and may be severe. Discontinue drug for severe reactions and treat appropriately.
- Monitor patient for serum sickness–like reaction (fever, rash, headache, sore throat, myalgia, polyarthralgia, hand and facial edema, dysphagia), especially during initial therapy and when drug is reinstituted after an extended period without treatment.
- Monitor patient for worsening or new onset of CNS adverse reactions (systemic vasculitis, seizures, MS, optic neuritis, Guillain-Barré syndrome). Drug may need to be discontinued.
- Treatment may result in autoantibody formation and, rarely, a lupuslike syndrome. Discontinue drug if lupuslike signs and symptoms occur.
- Ensure children are up to date with all vaccinations before start of therapy.
- *Look alike–sound alike:* Don't confuse infliximab-dyyb with reference drug infliximab or rituximab. Don't confuse Inflectra with Entyvio, Enbrel, Infergen, or Injectafer.

PATIENT TEACHING

- **Black Box Warning** Tell patient that testing for TB will be done before therapy and to immediately report signs and symptoms of infection. ∎
- **Black Box Warning** Counsel patient about risk of lymphoma and other malignancies. ∎
- Instruct patient to immediately report chest pain, shortness of breath, rash, fever, chills, and signs and symptoms of new or worsening conditions, such as allergic reactions, heart disease, CNS disease, malignancy, liver disease, COPD, or autoimmune disorders.
- Teach patient to report signs and symptoms of cytopenia, including bruising, bleeding, or persistent fever.

NEW DRUGS

♣Canada   ◇ OTC   ◆ Off-label use   ✐ Photoguide   ⊕Do not crush   *Liquid contains alcohol.

• Advise female patient to report if she is or plans to become pregnant before start of therapy. Tell female patient not to breast-feed during therapy.
• Warn patient to avoid live-virus vaccine immunizations during therapy.

SAFETY ALERT!

ixazomib citrate
ix-AZ-oh-mib

Ninlaro

Therapeutic class: Antineoplastics
Pharmacologic class: Proteasome inhibitors

AVAILABLE FORMS
Capsules ⊙: 2.3 mg, 3 mg, 4 mg

INDICATIONS & DOSAGES
➤ **Multiple myeloma in combination with lenalidomide and dexamethasone in patients who have received at least one prior therapy**
Adults: 4 mg P.O. once a week on days 1, 8, and 15 of a 28-day treatment cycle, in combination with lenalidomide 25 mg on days 1 through 21 and dexamethasone 40 mg on days 1, 8, 15, and 22 of a 28-day treatment cycle. Before initiating a new cycle of therapy, ANC should be at least 1,000/mm³, platelet count should be at least 75,000/mm³, and nonhematologic toxicities should generally be recovered to patient's baseline or grade 1 or lower. Continue treatment until disease progression or unacceptable toxicity.
Adjust-a-dose: For adverse reactions, first dosage reduction of ixazomib should be to 3 mg; second reduction should be to 2.3 mg; for a third occurrence, discontinue drug. Refer to lenalidomide and dexamethasone prescribing information for dosage adjustments.

For platelet count less than 30,000/mm³, withhold ixazomib and lenalidomide until platelet count is at least 30,000/mm³. After recovery, resume lenalidomide at the next lower dose according to its prescribing information and resume ixazomib at its most recent dose. If platelet count falls to less than 30,000/mm³ again, withhold ixazomib and lenalidomide until platelet count is at least 30,000/mm³. After recovery, resume ixazomib at the next lower dose and resume lenalidomide at its most recent dose. For additional occurrence, alternate dosage modifications of ixazomib and lenalidomide.

For ANC less than 500/mm³, withhold ixazomib and lenalidomide until ANC is at least 500/mm³; consider adding granulocyte-colony stimulating factor as per clinical guidelines. After recovery, resume lenalidomide at the next lower dose according to its prescribing information and resume ixazomib at its most recent dose. If ANC falls to less than 500/mm³ again, withhold ixazomib and lenalidomide until ANC

is at least 500/mm³. After recovery, resume ixazomib at the next lower dose and resume lenalidomide at its most recent dose. For additional occurrence, alternate dosage modifications of ixazomib and lenalidomide.

For grade 2 or 3 rash, withhold lenalidomide until rash recovers to grade 1 or lower. After recovery, resume lenalidomide at the next lower dose according to its prescribing information. If grade 2 or 3 rash recurs, withhold ixazomib and lenalidomide until rash recovers to grade 1 or lower. After recovery, resume ixazomib at the next lower dose and resume lenalidomide at its most recent dose. For additional occurrence, alternate dosage modifications of ixazomib and lenalidomide. If grade 4 rash occurs, discontinue entire regimen.

For grade 1 peripheral neuropathy with pain or grade 2 peripheral neuropathy, withhold drug until peripheral neuropathy recovers to grade 1 or lower without pain or to patient's baseline. After recovery, resume ixazomib at its most recent dose. If grade 2 peripheral neuropathy with pain or grade 3 peripheral neuropathy occurs, withhold ixazomib. If neuropathy, at the physician's discretion, recovers to patient's baseline or grade 1 or lower, may resume ixazomib at the next lower dose. If grade 4 peripheral neuropathy occurs, discontinue entire regimen.

For other grade 3 or 4 nonhematologic toxicities, withhold drug; toxicities should, at the physician's discretion, generally recover to patient's baseline condition or grade 1 or lower before resuming drug. If toxicities are attributable to ixazomib, resume at the next lower dose after recovery.

Reduce starting dose of drug to 3 mg in patients with moderate (total bilirubin level greater than 1.5 to 3 × ULN) or severe (total bilirubin level greater than 3 × ULN) hepatic impairment and in patients with severe renal impairment (CrCl of less than 30 mL/minute) or ESRD requiring dialysis. Refer to lenalidomide prescribing information for dosing recommendation in patients with renal impairment.

ADMINISTRATION
P.O.
• Hazardous drug: use safe handling and disposal precautions according to facility policy. Use gloves to administer intact capsules.
• Give drug once weekly on the same day, at approximately the same time.
• Give at least 1 hour before or at least 2 hours after food.
• Patient should swallow capsules whole with water and shouldn't chew them. Don't crush or open capsules.
• May give without regard to timing of dialysis.
• If dose is delayed or missed, give only if the next scheduled dose is 72 hours or more away; don't double-dose. Don't repeat dose if patient vomits after taking a dose; resume dosing at the time of the next scheduled dose.
• Store at room temperature. Don't store above 86° F (30° C). Don't freeze.

Reactions in bold italics are *life-threatening*. Interactions may have a *rapid onset* or a ***delayed onset***.

• Store capsules in original packaging until immediately before use.

ACTION

A reversible proteasome inhibitor that binds and inhibits the chymotrypsin-like activity of the beta 5 subunit of the 20S proteasome, thereby inducing death of multiple myeloma cell lines.

Route	Onset	Peak	Duration
P.O.	Unknown	1 hr	Unknown

Half-life: 9½ days.

ADVERSE REACTIONS

CNS: peripheral neuropathy.
CV: peripheral edema.
EENT: blurred vision, dry eyes, conjunctivitis.
GI: diarrhea, constipation, nausea, vomiting.
Hematologic: *thrombocytopenia, neutropenia.*
Hepatic: liver impairment, *tumor lysis syndrome.*
Musculoskeletal: back pain.
Respiratory: URI.
Skin: rash.

INTERACTIONS

Drug-drug. *Strong CYP3A inducers (carbamazepine, phenytoin, rifampin):* May decrease ixazomib concentration. Avoid use together.
Drug-herb. *St. John's wort:* May decrease ixazomib concentration. Avoid use together.
Drug-food. *High-fat meals:* May decrease ixazomib concentration. Patient should take drug at least 1 hour before or at least 2 hours after food.

EFFECTS ON LAB TEST RESULTS

• May decrease platelet and neutrophil counts.

CONTRAINDICATIONS & CAUTIONS

• Bone marrow suppression was commonly reported in clinical trials.
• Thrombocytopenia purpura and tumor lysis syndrome can occur rarely.
• Drug isn't indicated for use in children.
Dialyzable drug: No.

PREGNANCY-LACTATION-REPRODUCTION

• Drug may cause fetal harm; advise women of risk. Lenalidomide is contraindicated during pregnancy.
• Males and females of reproductive potential must use effective contraception during treatment and for 90 days after final dose.
• It isn't known if drug appears in breast milk. Breast-feeding isn't recommended.

NURSING CONSIDERATIONS

• Monitor patients for signs and symptoms of thrombocytopenia (bleeding, bruising). Adjust dosage and consider platelet transfusions as per standard medical guidelines if indicated.
• Monitor patients for thrombocytopenia. Platelet nadirs typically occur between days 14 and 21 of each

28-day cycle and recover to baseline by the start of the next cycle. Monitor platelet count at least monthly; consider more frequent monitoring during the first three cycles.
• Monitor patients for GI adverse effects (severe diarrhea, constipation, nausea, vomiting); provide antidiarrheals, antiemetics, and supportive care as needed. Adjust dosage for grade 3 or 4 symptoms.
• Monitor patients for new or worsening peripheral neuropathy. Adjust dosage as clinically indicated.
• Monitor patients for rash; Stevens-Johnson syndrome can occur rarely. Provide supportive care or adjust dosage as clinically indicated.
• Monitor patients for peripheral edema. Evaluate for underlying causes and provide supportive care as clinically indicated. Adjust dexamethasone dosage per prescribing information or ixazomib dosage for grade 3 or 4 symptoms.
• Monitor liver enzyme levels regularly and adjust dosage for grade 3 or 4 symptoms.
• *Look alike–sound alike:* Don't confuse Teflaro with Ninlaro.

PATIENT TEACHING

• Advise patient to take drug once a week on the same day and at approximately the same time for the first 3 weeks of a 4-week cycle.
• Remind patient to take drug at least 1 hour before or at least 2 hours after food.
• Explain that capsules must be stored in original packaging until immediately before use.
• Warn patient not to open or crush capsules.
• Advise patient to avoid direct contact with the capsule contents: In case of capsule breakage, avoid direct contact of contents with the skin or eyes. If skin contact occurs, wash thoroughly with soap and water. If eye contact occurs, flush thoroughly with water.
• Teach patient to report all adverse reactions and to immediately report bleeding and easy bruising, diarrhea, constipation, nausea and vomiting, rash, abdominal pain, or yellowing of the skin.
• Advise patient to report new or worsening peripheral neuropathy signs and symptoms (tingling, numbness, pain, burning feeling in the feet or hands, weakness in the arms or legs).
• Instruct patient to report unusual extremity swelling or weight gain due to swelling.
• Remind male and female patient of reproductive potential that they must use effective contraception during treatment and for 90 days after final dose.
• Inform female patient of risk to fetus with ixazomib use during pregnancy. Instruct her to immediately report suspected pregnancy.
• Caution female patient not to breast-feed during treatment.

ixekizumab
IX-e-kiz-ue-mab

Taltz

Therapeutic class: Immunomodulators
Pharmacologic class: Humanized
interleukin-17A antagonists

AVAILABLE FORMS
Injection: 80 mg/mL autoinjector or prefilled syringe

INDICATIONS & DOSAGES
➤ **Moderate to severe plaque psoriasis in patients
who are candidates for systemic therapy or phototherapy**
Adults: Initially, 160 mg (two 80-mg injections)
subcutaneously followed by 80 mg subcutaneously
at weeks 2, 4, 6, 8, 10, and 12; then 80 mg every
4 weeks.

ADMINISTRATION
Subcutaneous
- Allow medication to reach room temperature for
30 minutes before injection without removing needle
cap.
- Inspect solution for particulate matter and discoloration before administration. Solution should be clear
and colorless to slightly yellow. Don't use if solution
contains particles or is discolored or cloudy. Don't
shake.
- Inject the full 1 mL of medication in the autoinjector
or prefilled syringe.
- Discard unused portion if any medication remains
in the autoinjector or prefilled syringe after injection.
Drug doesn't contain preservatives.
- Give each injection in a different location (upper
arm, thigh, or abdomen) than previous injection.
- Don't inject into skin that is tender, bruised,
erythematous, indurated, or affected by psoriasis.
- If a dose is missed, give as soon as possible; then
resume dosing at the regularly scheduled time.
- Store in refrigerator at 36° to 46° F (2° to 8° C).
Protect from light. Don't freeze.

ACTION
A humanized monoclonal IgG antibody that binds
selectively to IL-17A receptors and inhibits release of
proinflammatory cytokines and chemokines.

Route	Onset	Peak	Duration
Subcut.	Unknown	4 days	Unknown

Half-life: 13 days.

ADVERSE REACTIONS
GI: nausea.
Hematologic: *neutropenia, thrombocytopenia.*
Respiratory: URI.
Skin: injection-site reaction.

Other: tinea infection, infection, development of neutralizing antibodies.

INTERACTIONS
Drug-drug. *CYP450 substrates (cyclosporine, warfarin):* May affect substrate levels, especially those with
narrow therapeutic index. Monitor patient for effect
and consider dosage modification of substrate.
Live-virus vaccines: May reduce effectiveness of
live-virus vaccine. Immunocompromised patients may
be at increased risk for vaccine-induced infection.
Avoid use of live-virus vaccines.

EFFECTS ON LAB TEST RESULTS
- May decrease WBC and platelet counts.

CONTRAINDICATIONS & CAUTIONS
- Contraindicated in patients hypersensitive to drug
or its components. Rarely, angioedema and urticaria
were reported.
- Contraindicated in patients with active TB. Evaluate
patients for TB before initiating treatment and consider providing TB treatment in patients with a history of
latent or active TB in whom adequate treatment can't
be confirmed.
- Use cautiously in patients at risk for serious infections
and in those with Crohn disease or ulcerative colitis.
- Safety in children hasn't been established.
Dialyzable drug: Unknown.

PREGNANCY-LACTATION-REPRODUCTION
- No data exist on the use of drug during pregnancy.
Human IgG is known to cross the placental barrier
so it's possible that ixekizumab, a humanized IgG
monoclonal antibody, may be transmitted from mother
to fetus. Other agents are preferred for treatment of
plaque psoriasis in pregnant women.
- It isn't known if drug appears in breast milk. Weigh
benefits to mother against potential risk to the infant.

NURSING CONSIDERATIONS
- Monitor patients for signs and symptoms of infection,
including TB, during and after treatment.
- Monitor patients for hypersensitivity reactions
(angioedema, urticaria). If serious reaction occurs,
discontinue drug and initiate treatment.
- Monitor patients for onset or exacerbation of Crohn
disease and ulcerative colitis.
- Before start of therapy, consider completion of all
appropriate immunizations. Avoid live-virus vaccines.
- *Look alike–sound alike:* Don't confuse ixekizumab with infliximab, reslizumab, or rituximab.

PATIENT TEACHING
- Advise patient to report all adverse reactions and
to promptly report signs or symptoms of infection
(because drug may lower patient's ability to fight
infection).
- Warn patient to seek immediate medical attention if
signs or symptoms of severe hypersensitivity reaction
occur.

Reactions in bold italics are *life-threatening.* Interactions may have a *rapid onset* or a *delayed onset.*

• Teach patient and caregivers how to safely use auto-injectors or prefilled syringes.

lesinurad
le-SIN-ure-ad

Zurampic

Therapeutic class: Antigout drugs
Pharmacologic class: Uric acid transporter 1 inhibitors

AVAILABLE FORMS
Tablets: 200 mg

INDICATIONS & DOSAGES
Black Box Warning Don't use as monotherapy. Drug should only be used in combination with a xanthine oxidase inhibitor. ∎
➤ **Hyperuricemia associated with gout in combination with a xanthine oxidase inhibitor in patients who haven't achieved target serum uric acid levels with a xanthine oxidase inhibitor alone**
Adults: 200 mg P.O. once daily.
Adjust-a-dose: If creatinine level increases to more than 2 × baseline level, withhold drug. If lesinurad is found to be cause of creatinine elevation or when CrCl is persistently less than 45 mL/minute, discontinue drug. If treatment with xanthine oxidase inhibitor is interrupted, drug should also be withheld.

ADMINISTRATION
P.O.
• Give in the morning with food and water.
• Give at the same time as the morning dose of the xanthine oxidase inhibitor. If treatment with the xanthine oxidase inhibitor is interrupted, lesinurad should also be interrupted.
• Don't give a missed dose; give the next day.
• Store at room temperature. Protect from light.

ACTION
A uric acid transporter 1 inhibitor that reduces serum uric acid levels by inhibiting the function of transporter proteins involved in renal uric acid reabsorption.

Route	Onset	Peak	Duration
P.O.	Rapid	1–4 hr	Unknown

Half-life: 5 hours.

ADVERSE REACTIONS
CNS: headache.
CV: *major adverse CV event (MI, stroke, death).*
GI: GERD.
GU: elevated creatinine levels, *renal failure,* nephrolithiasis.
Other: flulike symptoms.

INTERACTIONS
Drug-drug. *Aspirin:* May decrease efficacy of lesinurad in combination with allopurinol. Avoid use together unless aspirin dose is 325 mg or less per day.
CYP2C9 inducers (carbamazepine, rifampin): May decrease lesinurad level. Monitor patient for decreased therapeutic effect.
CYP2C9 inhibitors (amiodarone, fluconazole): May increase lesinurad level. Use lesinurad cautiously in patients taking moderate CYP2C9 inhibitors and in CYP2C9 poor metabolizers.
CYP3A4 substrates (amlodipine, HMG-CoA reductase inhibitors, sildenafil): May decrease levels of CYP3A4 substrates. Monitor efficacy of sensitive CYP3A4 substrates when used with lesinurad.
Epoxide hydrolase inhibitors (valproic acid): May interfere with lesinurad metabolism. Don't use together.
Hormonal contraceptives: Oral, injectable, transdermal, and implantable forms of hormonal contraceptives may not be reliable when used with lesinurad. Females should use additional methods of contraception.

EFFECTS ON LAB TEST RESULTS
• May increase creatinine level.

CONTRAINDICATIONS & CAUTIONS
• Contraindicated in patients with severe renal impairment (CrCl of less than 30 mL/minute) or ESRD, in kidney transplant recipients, and in patients on dialysis.
• Contraindicated in patients with tumor lysis syndrome or Lesch-Nyhan syndrome.
Black Box Warning Use only in combination with a xanthine oxidase inhibitor. Acute renal failure has occurred with lesinurad use and was more common when drug was given alone. ∎
• Drug isn't recommended for treatment of asymptomatic hyperuricemia.
• Drug isn't recommended for patients taking daily doses of allopurinol less than 300 mg (or less than 200 mg in patients with CrCl of less than 60 mL/minute).
• Drug may increase risk of major adverse CV events (death, nonfatal MI, nonfatal strokes). Monitor patients as clinically appropriate.
• Safety and effectiveness in children younger than age 18 haven't been established.
Dialyzable drug: No.

PREGNANCY-LACTATION-REPRODUCTION
• Drug hasn't been studied in pregnant women. Use cautiously during pregnancy and only if benefit outweighs possible risk to the fetus.
• Hormonal contraceptives may not be reliable when used with drug. Females should use additional methods of contraception.
• It isn't known if drug appears in breast milk. Use cautiously in breast-feeding women and only if benefit to the mother outweighs risk to the infant.

NEW DRUGS

NURSING CONSIDERATIONS
• Don't start treatment in patients with CrCl of less than 45 mL/minute. Monitor renal function before start of therapy and periodically thereafter as clinically indicated. More frequent renal function monitoring is recommended in patients with CrCl of less than 60 mL/minute or serum creatinine level of 1.5 to 2 × baseline level.
• Monitor patients for signs and symptoms of acute uric acid nephropathy (flank pain, nausea, vomiting). Withhold drug and assess serum creatinine level if signs and symptoms occur.
• Monitor fluid intake. Patient should maintain adequate hydration of at least 68 oz (2 L) of liquid per day.
• Gout flares may occur after start of therapy and gout flare prophylaxis is recommended. Drug doesn't need to be stopped if a gout flare occurs. ∎

PATIENT TEACHING
• Advise patient to take medication with food and water. Recommend that patient drink 68 oz (2 L) of fluid each day to stay hydrated.
Black Box Warning Warn patient not to take drug by itself. Drug should always be taken with a xanthine oxidase inhibitor, such as allopurinol or febuxostat. ∎
• Counsel patient that if a dose is missed in the morning, not to take the missed dose later in the day but to wait until the next day to take a dose. Advise patient not to double the dose.
• Inform patient that renal events, including increases in blood creatinine level and acute renal failure, may occur.
• Advise patient that periodic monitoring of blood creatinine levels is recommended.
• Teach patient that gout flares may occur after starting therapy and that gout flare prophylaxis medication is recommended to prevent gout flares. Advise patient not to discontinue drug if a gout flare occurs during treatment.
• Educate female patient to tell prescriber if she is pregnant, plans to become pregnant, or is breast-feeding.
• Caution female patient using hormonal contraceptives to use a back-up contraceptive method during treatment.

lifitegrast
LIF-i-teg-rast

Xiidra

Therapeutic class: Anti-inflammatory drugs (ophthalmic)
Pharmacologic class: Lymphocyte function-associated antigen 1 antagonist

AVAILABLE FORMS
Ophthalmic solution: 5% (50 mg/mL)

INDICATIONS & DOSAGES
➤ **Dry eye disease**
Adults: Instill 1 drop into each eye b.i.d., approximately 12 hours apart.

ADMINISTRATION
Ophthalmic
• Use solution immediately after opening.
• May use single-use container to dose both eyes.
• Discard container and any remaining solution after use.
• Have patient remove contact lenses before administration; may reinsert 15 minutes later.
• Store at 68° to 77° F (20° to 25° C) in original foil pouch.

ACTION
Exact mechanism unknown. May inhibit T-cell activation and migration to target tissues.

Route	Onset	Peak	Duration
Ophthalmic	Unknown	Unknown	Unknown

Half-life: Unknown.

ADVERSE REACTIONS
CNS: headache.
EENT: eye irritation, reduced visual acuity, blurred vision, conjunctival hyperemia, increased lacrimation, eye discharge, eye discomfort, eye pruritus, sinusitis.
GI: dysgeusia.

INTERACTIONS
None reported.

EFFECTS ON LAB TEST RESULTS
None reported.

CONTRAINDICATIONS & CAUTIONS
• Safety and effectiveness in children haven't been established.
Dialyzable drug: Unknown.

PREGNANCY-LACTATION-REPRODUCTION
• There are no data in pregnant women concerning drug-associated risks.
• Use in breast-feeding women hasn't been studied. Drug has low systemic exposure; use only if potential benefit justifies potential risk to infant.

NURSING CONSIDERATIONS
• Monitor patient for adverse reactions to the eye.
• *Look alike–sound alike:* Don't confuse Xiidra with Xalatan. Don't confuse lifitegrast with Lumigan.

PATIENT TEACHING
• Remind patient to wash hands thoroughly before using drug.
• Advise patient not to touch tip of single-use container to eye or to any surface, to avoid eye injury or contamination of the solution.

Reactions in bold italics are *life-threatening*. Interactions may have a *rapid onset* or a *delayed onset*.

• Instruct patient to discard single-use container after using in each eye.
• Caution patient to remove contact lenses before administration; may reinsert 15 minutes later.
• Instruct patient to store single-use containers in their original foil pouch.

SAFETY ALERT!

lixisenatide
lix-i-SEN-a-tide

Adlyxin

Therapeutic class: Antidiabetics
Pharmacologic class: Glucagon-like peptide-1 receptor antagonists

AVAILABLE FORMS
Injection: 10 mcg/dose in 3-mL prefilled pen (14 doses); 20 mcg/dose in 3-mL prefilled pen (14 doses)

INDICATIONS & DOSAGES
➤ **Adjunct to diet and exercise to improve glycemic control in patients with type 2 diabetes**
Adults: Initially, 10 mcg subcutaneously once daily for 14 days; then on day 15, increase to maintenance dose of 20 mcg subcutaneously once daily.

ADMINISTRATION
Subcutaneous
• Inspect pen before each use; it should be clear and colorless. Don't use if there is particulate matter or discoloration.
• Administer subcutaneous injection in abdomen, thigh, or upper arm once daily. Rotate injection site with every use.
• Give within 1 hour before first meal of the day, preferably the same meal every day. If a dose is missed, give dose 1 hour before next meal.
• Replace cap after each use. Don't store pen with needle attached.
• Store unused pen in refrigerator at 36° to 46° F (2° to 8° C) in original package; protect from light. After first dose, may store pen at room temperature, below 86° F (30° C). Discard pen after 14 days.
✪ Alert: Use a new needle for each dose. Pens are for single patient use; don't share among patients even if needle is changed, because of risk of blood-borne pathogen transmission.

ACTION
A glucagon-like peptide-1 (GLP-1) receptor antagonist that increases glucose-dependent insulin release, decreases glucagon secretion, and slows gastric emptying.

Route	Onset	Peak	Duration
Subcut.	Unknown	1–3½ hr	Unknown

Half-life: 3 hours.

ADVERSE REACTIONS
CNS: headache, dizziness.
GI: nausea, vomiting, diarrhea, dyspepsia, constipation, abdominal distention, abdominal pain.
Metabolic: *hypoglycemia.*
Skin: injection-site reactions.
Other: immunogenicity.

INTERACTIONS
Drug-drug. *Basal insulin, sulfonylurea:* May increase risk of hypoglycemia. Reduce basal insulin or sulfonylurea dosage as needed.
Oral contraceptives: May alter concentration of contraceptive. Patient should take contraceptive at least 1 hour before or at least 11 hours after lixisenatide injection.
Oral drugs dependent on threshold concentrations for efficacy (antibiotics) or for which a delay in effect is undesirable (acetaminophen): Lixisenatide causes delayed gastric emptying, which may affect concentrations of other drugs or cause delays in effects. Use together cautiously and give oral drugs 1 hour before lixisenatide injection.

EFFECTS ON LAB TEST RESULTS
• May decrease glucose level.

CONTRAINDICATIONS & CAUTIONS
• Contraindicated in patients hypersensitive to drug or its components. Hypersensitivity, including anaphylaxis, has occurred.
• Use cautiously in patients with a history of anaphylaxis or angioedema after receiving another GLP-1 receptor antagonist.
• May increase risk of pancreatitis, especially in patients with history of cholelithiasis or alcohol abuse.
• Drug hasn't been studied in patients with chronic pancreatitis or a history of unexplained pancreatitis. Consider other antidiabetic therapies.
• May increase risk of acute kidney injury or worsening of renal impairment, especially in patients with nausea, vomiting, diarrhea, or dehydration. Use isn't recommended in patients with ESRD.
• Drug isn't indicated to treat type 1 diabetes or diabetic ketoacidosis.
• Use with short-acting insulin hasn't been studied. Use together isn't recommended.
• Drug hasn't been studied in patients with gastroparesis. Use isn't recommended.
• Antibodies to drug may develop, decreasing glycemic control and increasing risk of injection-site or allergic reactions. Consider alternative therapy if antibodies develop.
• Safety and effectiveness in children haven't been established.
Dialyzable drug: Unknown.
⚠ Overdose S&S: Increased GI disorders.

PREGNANCY-LACTATION-REPRODUCTION
• Data are limited concerning use in pregnant women. Use during pregnancy only if benefits outweigh risks.

- It isn't known if drug appears in breast milk. Before use, consider clinical needs of the mother and potential adverse effects on the infant.

NURSING CONSIDERATIONS

- Monitor patient for hypersensitivity reactions, including anaphylaxis and angioedema. Discontinue drug and treat appropriately if reaction occurs.
- Monitor glucose level closely to evaluate effectiveness.
- Monitor renal function at beginning of therapy and at dosage escalations in patients with renal impairment or severe GI reactions.
- Monitor patient for signs and symptoms of pancreatitis. Discontinue drug and manage signs and symptoms clinically if pancreatitis is suspected. If pancreatitis is confirmed, don't restart drug.
- **Look alike–sound alike:** Don't confuse lixisenatide with liraglutide.

PATIENT TEACHING

- Tell patient to report all medications being taken before start of therapy.
- Teach patient how to prepare pen, to always use a new needle, and to administer drug according to manufacturer's instructions.
- Instruct patient to store pen in original container without the needle at room temperature, and to discard pen 14 days after first use.
- **Alert:** Teach patient not to share pens even if the needle is changed, because of risk of blood-borne pathogen transmission.
- Caution patient to report all adverse reactions, especially signs and symptoms of hypoglycemia (dizziness, confusion, weakness, feeling jittery, sweating), particularly if patient is taking a sulfonylurea or basal insulin, and pancreatitis (persistent, severe abdominal pain that may radiate to the back, with or without vomiting).
- Warn patient to watch for signs and symptoms of hypersensitivity reactions (fever, nausea, difficulty breathing, rash; swelling of the face, lips, or tongue) and to stop drug and seek immediate medical attention if they occur.
- Teach patient to report nausea, vomiting, diarrhea, and dehydration promptly, because of risk of kidney injury.
- Advise female patient to inform prescriber if she is or plans to become pregnant or to breast-feed before start of therapy.

SAFETY ALERT!

necitumumab
NE-si-toom-oo-mab

Portrazza

Therapeutic class: Antineoplastics
Pharmacologic class: Epidermal growth factor receptor antagonists

AVAILABLE FORMS
Injection: 800 mg/50 mL single-dose vial

INDICATIONS & DOSAGES
➤ **First-line treatment of metastatic squamous cell non-small cell lung cancer in combination with gemcitabine and cisplatin**
Adults: 800 mg I.V. infusion over 60 minutes on days 1 and 8 of each 3-week cycle given before gemcitabine and cisplatin infusions. Continue until disease progression or unacceptable toxicity.
Adjust-a-dose: For grade 1 infusion reaction, reduce infusion rate by 50%. For grade 2 infusion reaction, interrupt infusion until signs and symptoms have resolved to grade 0 or 1, then resume at infusion rate reduced by 50% for all subsequent infusions. For grade 3 or 4 infusion reaction, permanently discontinue drug.

For grade 1 or 2 infusion reaction with prior doses, premedicate patient with diphenhydramine (or equivalent) before all subsequent infusions. For a second grade 1 or 2 infusion reaction, premedicate patient with diphenhydramine, acetaminophen, and dexamethasone before each subsequent infusion.

For grade 3 rash or acneiform rash, withhold drug until signs and symptoms resolve to grade 2 or less and decrease dosage to 400 mg for at least one cycle. If signs and symptoms don't worsen, may increase to 600 mg and then 800 mg in subsequent cycles. Permanently discontinue drug for grade 3 rash or acneiform rash that doesn't resolve to grade 2 or less within 6 weeks or if reactions worsen or become intolerable at 400-mg dose. Discontinue drug for grade 4 skin reactions or for grade 3 skin induration or fibrosis.
Black Box Warning For grade 3 or 4 electrolyte abnormalities, withhold drug and replace electrolytes as medically indicated. Resume subsequent cycles after electrolyte abnormalities improve to grade 2 or less. ∎

ADMINISTRATION
I.V.
▼ Inspect solution for particulate matter and discoloration. If present, discard solution.
▼ Dilute to a final volume of 250 mL in NSS. Don't use solutions containing dextrose.
▼ Gently invert to ensure mixing; don't shake.
▼ Store diluted infusions up to 24 hours at 36° to 46° F (2° to 8° C) or up to 4 hours at room temperature (up to 77° F [25° C]).
▼ Discard vial with any unused portion.
▼ Administer via infusion pump over 60 minutes through a separate infusion line. Flush line with NSS at end of infusion.
▼ Refrigerate vials at 36° to 46° F (2° to 8° C); don't freeze. Protect from light.
▼ **Incompatibilities:** Dextrose, electrolytes, other drugs.

ACTION
A recombinant human IgG1 monoclonal antibody that binds to human epidermal growth factor receptor (EGFR) and blocks binding of EGFR to ligands, inhibiting angiogenesis and malignant progression, and allowing apoptosis.

Route	Onset	Peak	Duration
I.V.	Unknown	Unknown	Unknown

Half-life: 14 days.

ADVERSE REACTIONS
CNS: headache, *stroke, cerebral ischemia.*
CV: *cardiopulmonary arrest, sudden death, MI, arterial thromboembolism, PE, venous thromboembolism.*
EENT: conjunctivitis, oropharyngeal pain.
GI: vomiting, diarrhea, stomatitis, dysphagia.
Metabolic: weight loss, *hypomagnesemia, hypokalemia, hypocalcemia,* hypophosphatemia.
Musculoskeletal: muscle spasms.
Respiratory: hemoptysis.
Skin: rash, dermatitis, acneiform rash, acne, pruritus, dry skin, skin fissures, erythema, skin toxicity.
Other: paronychia, infusion reaction.

INTERACTIONS
Drug-lifestyle. *Sun exposure:* May increase photosensitivity. Patient should avoid sun exposure.

EFFECTS ON LAB TEST RESULTS
• May decrease magnesium, potassium, calcium, and phosphorus levels.

CONTRAINDICATIONS & CAUTIONS
Black Box Warning Drug may increase risk of cardiopulmonary arrest and sudden death when used in combination with gemcitabine and cisplatin. Closely monitor electrolyte levels, including magnesium, potassium, and calcium. ■
Black Box Warning May increase risk of hypomagnesemia. Monitor electrolyte levels and replace electrolytes as needed. ■
• Drug isn't indicated for nonsquamous non-small-cell lung cancer.
• Drug increases risk of venous thromboembolism (VTE) and arterial thromboembolism (ATE), which can be fatal. Discontinue drug for serious or life-threatening VTE or ATE.
• Safety and effectiveness in children haven't been established.
• Use cautiously in elderly patients, because they may have increased risk of adverse reactions.
Dialyzable drug: Unknown.

PREGNANCY-LACTATION-REPRODUCTION
• Contraindicated for use in pregnancy; drug may cause fetal harm. Advise women to use effective contraception during therapy and for 3 months after therapy ends.
• There are no data about breast-feeding. Women shouldn't breast-feed during treatment and for 3 months after last dose.

NURSING CONSIDERATIONS
Black Box Warning Closely monitor electrolyte levels, including magnesium, potassium, and calcium,

before each dose and for at least 8 weeks after last dose. ■
Black Box Warning Aggressively replace electrolytes as indicated. ■
• Monitor patients for infusion reaction.
• Monitor patients for skin reactions, which may be severe and usually develop within first 2 weeks of treatment; drug may need to be withheld or discontinued, or dosage reduced.
• Monitor patients for signs and symptoms of ATE (pain, pallor, pulselessness, loss of function, coldness) and VTE (pain, swelling, erythema, dyspnea, hypotension, tachycardia).

PATIENT TEACHING
• Teach patient about adverse reactions and to immediately report them.
• Explain that drug may reduce blood levels of magnesium, calcium, and potassium and that these levels must be carefully monitored. Advise patient to take any supplements prescribed.
• Advise patient that laboratory monitoring will be needed to monitor for adverse reactions to treatment.
• Teach patient signs and symptoms of infusion reactions (fever, chills, difficulty breathing) and to report them immediately.
• Warn female patient of childbearing potential to use contraception during therapy and up to 3 months after last dose.
• Instruct female patient not to breast-feed during therapy and for up to 3 months after last dose.
• Caution patient to minimize sun exposure, wear protective clothing, and use sunscreen.

obeticholic acid
oh-BET-i-kol-ik

Ocaliva

Therapeutic class: Miscellaneous GI drugs
Pharmacologic class: Farnesoid X receptor agonists

AVAILABLE FORMS
Tablets: 5 mg, 10 mg

INDICATIONS & DOSAGES
➤ **Primary biliary cholangitis in combination with ursodeoxycholic acid (UDCA) in adults with an inadequate response to UDCA, or as monotherapy in adults unable to tolerate UDCA**
Adults: 5 mg P.O. once daily in patients who haven't achieved an adequate biochemical response to an appropriate dosage of UDCA for at least 1 year, or are intolerant to UDCA. If an adequate reduction in alkaline phosphatase (ALP) or total bilirubin level hasn't been achieved after 3 months, and patient is tolerating drug, increase to maximum dosage of 10 mg once daily.

Adjust-a-dose: For moderate (Child-Pugh class B) and severe (Child-Pugh class C) hepatic impairment, initial dosage is 5 mg once weekly; if an adequate reduction in ALP or total bilirubin level hasn't been achieved after 3 months at 5 mg once weekly, and patient is tolerating drug, increase dosage to 5 mg twice weekly (at least 3 days apart) and subsequently to 10 mg twice weekly (at least 3 days apart) depending on response and tolerability.

For patients with intolerable pruritus, add an antihistamine or bile acid–binding resin, reduce dosage to 5 mg every other day (for patients intolerant to 5 mg once daily) or 5 mg once daily (for patients intolerant to 10 mg once daily); or temporarily interrupt dosing for up to 2 weeks, then restart at a reduced dosage. Increase dosage to 10 mg once daily, as tolerated, to achieve optimal response. Drug may need to be discontinued in patients who continue to experience persistent, intolerable pruritus.

ADMINISTRATION
P.O.
- May give without regard for food.
- Store at controlled room temperature.

ACTION
An agonist for farnesoid X receptor (FXR), a nuclear receptor expressed in the liver and intestine. FXR activation decreases the intracellular hepatocyte concentrations of bile acids while promoting bile secretion and reducing hepatic exposure to bile acids.

Route	Onset	Peak	Duration
P.O.	Unknown	1½ hr	Unknown

Half-life: Unknown.

ADVERSE REACTIONS
CNS: dizziness, fatigue, fever.
CV: palpitations, peripheral edema.
EENT: oropharyngeal pain.
GI: abdominal pain and discomfort, constipation.
Hepatic: elevated LFT values, jaundice, worsening ascites, primary biliary cholangitis flare, ***hepatic encephalopathy.***
Musculoskeletal: arthralgia.
Skin: pruritus, rash, eczema.
Other: thyroid function abnormality.

INTERACTIONS
Drug-drug. *Bile acid–binding resins (cholestyramine, colesevelam, colestipol):* May reduce absorption and efficacy of obeticholic acid. If necessary to continue bile acid–binding resin, give obeticholic acid at least 4 hours before or 4 hours after giving bile acid–binding resin, or at as great an interval as possible.
Caffeine: May increase caffeine concentration. Use cautiously together.
CYP1A2 substrates with narrow therapeutic index (theophylline, tizanidine): May increase concentrations of substrates. Monitor patient closely.

Warfarin: May decrease INR. Monitor INR and adjust warfarin dosage to maintain target INR range.

EFFECTS ON LAB TEST RESULTS
- May decrease HDL cholesterol and alkaline phosphatase levels. May increase liver enzyme levels.

CONTRAINDICATIONS & CAUTIONS
- Contraindicated in patients with complete biliary obstruction.
- May increase risk of liver-related adverse reactions. Monitor patients during treatment for elevations in LFT values and for development of liver-related adverse reactions. Weigh risks against benefits of continuing treatment in patients who have experienced clinically significant liver-related adverse reactions.
- Safety and effectiveness in children haven't been established.
- Use cautiously in elderly patients, as greater sensitivity to drug is possible.
Dialyzable drug: Unknown.
⚠ ***Overdose S&S:*** Elevated LFT values, liver-related adverse reactions (such as ascites, jaundice, portal hypertension, flare of primary biliary cholangitis).

PREGNANCY-LACTATION-REPRODUCTION
- Use in pregnant women hasn't been studied. Data are insufficient concerning drug-associated risk.
- It isn't known if drug appears in breast milk. The decision to breast-feed should weigh benefits of breast-feeding and risks to the infant.

NURSING CONSIDERATIONS
- Monitor patients for development of or worsening liver disease. Discontinue drug for complete biliary obstruction.
- Monitor LFTs periodically during treatment.
- Monitor patients for changes in serum lipid levels during treatment. Weigh risks and benefits of continued treatment in patients who don't respond after 1 year at the highest recommended dosage that can be tolerated and who experience a reduction in HDL cholesterol.
- Assess patients for pruritus. If pruritus occurs, consider addition of bile acid resins or antihistamines, dosage reduction, or temporary interruption of drug until pruritus is resolved. Drug may need to be discontinued in patients who continue to experience persistent, intolerable pruritus.

PATIENT TEACHING
- Warn patient to report all adverse reactions, including pruritus, and especially signs and symptoms of worsening liver disease (abdominal pain, nausea, yellowing of skin or eyes, dark urine), as liver function evaluation may be needed.
- Inform patient that laboratory testing will be needed to evaluate treatment and to check for changes in liver function and lipid levels.

Reactions in bold italics are ***life-threatening.*** Interactions may have a *rapid onset* or a ***delayed onset.***

obiltoxaximab
OH-bil-tox-AX-i-mab

Anthim

Therapeutic class: Antibodies
Pharmacologic class: Monoclonal
antibodies

AVAILABLE FORMS
Injection: 600 mg/6 mL single-dose vial

INDICATIONS & DOSAGES
➤ **Inhalational anthrax due to *Bacillus anthracis* in combination with appropriate antibacterial drugs; prophylaxis of inhalational anthrax due to *B. anthracis* when alternative therapies aren't available or not appropriate**
Adults weighing more than 40 kg: 16 mg/kg/dose I.V. over 90 minutes as a single dose.
Adults and children weighing between 15 and 40 kg: 24 mg/kg/dose I.V. over 90 minutes as a single dose.
Children weighing 15 kg or less: 32 mg/kg/dose I.V. over 90 minutes as a single dose.

ADMINISTRATION
I.V.
🔾 *Alert:* Premedicate with diphenhydramine before administration.
▼ Dilute injection in NSS according to prescribing information.
▼ Drug is a clear to opalescent, colorless to pale yellow/pale brownish yellow solution that may contain a few translucent-to-white particulates.
▼ Discard vial if solution is discolored or contains particulates other than a few translucent-to-white particles. Vials contain no preservative.
▼ Preparation for I.V. bag infusion:
— Select an appropriate-sized bag of NSS.
— Withdraw a volume of solution from the bag equal to the calculated volume in milliliters of obiltoxaximab.
— Discard solution that was withdrawn from the bag.
— Withdraw required volume of drug from the obiltoxaximab vials.
— Discard any unused portion remaining in vials.
— Transfer required volume of drug to infusion bag.
— Gently invert bag to mix solution. Don't shake.
— The prepared solution is stable for 4 hours stored at room temperature or for 4 hours stored in refrigerator at 36° to 46° F (2° to 8° C).
▼ Preparation for syringe infusion:
— Select an appropriate-sized syringe for the total volume of infusion to be administered.
— Withdraw required volume of obiltoxaximab injection.
— Discard any unused portion remaining in vials.

— Withdraw an appropriate amount of NSS to prepare the total infusion volume.
— Gently mix solution. Don't shake.
— Once a diluted solution of obiltoxaximab has been prepared, administer immediately. Don't store solution in syringe. Discard unused product.
🔾 *Alert:* After preparation of the bag or syringe for infusion, administer the infusion solution using a 0.22-micron inline filter.
▼ Flush line with NSS at the end of the I.V. infusion.
▼ Store vials in refrigerator at 36° to 46° F (2° to 8° C) in original carton to protect from light. Don't freeze or shake vials.

ACTION
A monoclonal antibody that binds to and inhibits the protective antigen of anthrax (*B. anthracis*), preventing the entry of anthrax toxins (lethal factor and edema factor) into healthy cells. Drug doesn't have direct antibacterial activity.

Route	Onset	Peak	Duration
I.V.	Unknown	Unknown	Unknown

Half-life: Unknown.

ADVERSE REACTIONS
CNS: dizziness, headache, fatigue, pyrexia.
CV: chest discomfort, chest pain, palpitations, cyanosis.
EENT: rhinorrhea, nasal congestion, sinus congestion, oropharyngeal pain, dysphonia, throat irritation.
GI: vomiting, dry mouth.
Hematologic: *lymphopenia, leukopenia, neutropenia.*
Musculoskeletal: extremity pain, musculoskeletal pain, myalgia.
Respiratory: URI.
Skin: urticaria, rash, pruritus, infusion-site pain, injection-site swelling.
Other: hypersensitivity reaction, *anaphylaxis*, antibody development.

INTERACTIONS
None reported.

EFFECTS ON LAB TEST RESULTS
• May increase CK level.
• May decrease lymphocyte, neutrophil, and WBC counts.

CONTRAINDICATIONS & CAUTIONS
Black Box Warning Hypersensitivity and anaphylaxis have been reported during the I.V. infusion of drug. ∎
🔾 *Alert:* Drug should only be used for prophylaxis when its benefit for prevention of inhalational anthrax outweighs risk of hypersensitivity and anaphylaxis.
• Drug should be used in combination with appropriate antibacterial drugs.
• Drug doesn't prevent or treat meningitis and isn't expected to cross the blood-brain barrier.

NEW DRUGS

• No studies of the safety or pharmacokinetics in children have been conducted. Dosing recommendations are derived from simulations using a population pharmacokinetics approach.
Dialyzable drug: Unknown.

PREGNANCY-LACTATION-REPRODUCTION
• There are no well-controlled studies in pregnant women. Use during pregnancy only if clearly needed.
• Drug hasn't been evaluated in breast-feeding women. Effects of exposure to drug on the breast-fed infant are unknown.

NURSING CONSIDERATIONS
Black Box Warning Administer drug in appropriately monitored settings equipped to manage anaphylaxis.■
Black Box Warning Monitor patient closely for signs and symptoms of hypersensitivity (rash, urticaria, pruritus, cough, throat irritation, dysphonia, dyspnea, cyanosis, postural dizziness, chest discomfort) throughout infusion and for a period of time after administration.■
Black Box Warning If hypersensitivity or anaphylaxis occurs, stop infusion immediately and treat appropriately.■

PATIENT TEACHING
Black Box Warning Inform patient that hypersensitivity reactions, including anaphylaxis, have occurred. Instruct patient to notify prescriber for itching, hives, rash, throat irritation, cough, dizziness, shortness of breath, or chest discomfort that occurs during or after drug administration.■
• Determine if patient is allergic to or has contraindications for diphenhydramine, and explain that this drug will be given before infusion.
• Caution patient that diphenhydramine may cause sleepiness.
• Inform patient that drug will be given in combination with antibiotics.
• Advise female patient to notify prescriber if she is pregnant or breast-feeding before start of therapy.

SAFETY ALERT!

osimertinib
OH-si-mer-ti-nib

Tagrisso

Therapeutic class: Antineoplastics
Pharmacologic class: Tyrosine kinase inhibitors

AVAILABLE FORMS
Tablets ⊙: 40 mg, 80 mg

INDICATIONS & DOSAGES
➤ **Metastatic epidermal growth factor receptor (EGFR) T790M mutation-positive non-small-cell lung cancer in patients who have progressed on or after EGFR tyrosine kinase inhibitor therapy**
Adults: 80 mg P.O. once daily until disease progression or unacceptable toxicity.
Adjust-a-dose: If interstitial lung disease (ILD) or pneumonitis occurs, permanently discontinue drug. If QTc interval is greater than 500 msec on at least two separate ECGs, withhold drug until QTc interval is less than 481 msec or recovers to baseline if the baseline QTc interval was 481 msec or more, then resume at 40 mg once daily. If QTc-interval prolongation with signs or symptoms of life-threatening arrhythmia or symptomatic HF occurs, permanently discontinue drug. If patient has an asymptomatic, absolute decrease in LVEF of 10% from baseline and below 50%, withhold drug for up to 4 weeks. If LVEF improves to baseline, resume drug. If LVEF doesn't improve to baseline, permanently discontinue drug.

If other grade 3 or higher adverse reactions occur, withhold drug for up to 3 weeks. If other adverse reactions improve to grade 0 to 2 within 3 weeks, resume drug at 80 or 40 mg daily; if no improvement occurs within 3 weeks, permanently discontinue drug.

If drug must be given with a strong CYP3A4 inducer, increase osimertinib dosage to 160 mg daily. Resume osimertinib at 80 mg daily 3 weeks after discontinuing the strong CYP3A4 inducer.

ADMINISTRATION
P.O.
• Hazardous drug; use safe handling and disposal precautions. Use single gloves to administer intact tablets. Avoid exposure to crushed tablets.
• May give with or without food.
• Don't make up for a missed dose. Resume dosing at next scheduled dose.
• If patient is unable to swallow solids, disperse tablet in approximately 50 mL of noncarbonated water. Stir until tablet is completely dispersed and have patient swallow, or give through an NG tube immediately. Rinse container with 120 to 240 mL of water and give to patient immediately or administer through an NG tube.
• Prepare oral liquid in a controlled device using double gloves and protective gown. Don't crush, heat, or ultrasonicate during preparation.
• Store at room temperature (68° to 77° F [20° to 25° C]).

ACTION
A kinase inhibitor of EGFR that binds irreversibly to select mutant forms of EGFR. It's selective for sensitizing mutations and the T790M resistance mutation, which is the most common resistance to EGFR tyrosine kinase inhibitors.

Route	Onset	Peak	Duration
P.O.	Unknown	6 hr	Unknown

Half-life: 48 hours.

Reactions in bold italics are *life-threatening*. Interactions may have a *rapid onset* or a *delayed onset*.

ADVERSE REACTIONS

CNS: headache, fatigue, *stroke.*
CV: *venous thromboembolism, QTc-interval prolongation*, reduced LVEF.
EENT: eye disorders.
GI: diarrhea, nausea, decreased appetite, constipation, stomatitis.
Hematologic: *lymphopenia, thrombocytopenia,* anemia, *neutropenia.*
Metabolic: hypermagnesemia, hyponatremia.
Musculoskeletal: back pain.
Respiratory: cough, pneumonia, interstitial pneumonitis, *PE.*
Skin: rash, dry skin, pruritus, nail toxicity.

INTERACTIONS

Drug-drug. *Breast cancer resistance protein (BCRP) substrate (rosuvastatin, sulfasalazine, topotecan):* Use together may increase exposure to the BCRP substrate and risk of exposure-related toxicity. Monitor patient for BCRP substrate–related adverse reactions.
CYP1A2 drugs with narrow therapeutic indices (carbamazepine, phenytoin), sensitive substrates of CYP3A (cyclosporine, ergot alkaloids, fentanyl, quinidine): May decrease plasma concentrations of these drugs. Avoid use together.
Strong CYP3A inducers (carbamazepine, phenytoin, rifampin): May decrease osimertinib plasma concentration. Avoid use together.
Strong CYP3A inhibitors (antifungals [itraconazole], antivirals [ritonavir], macrolide antibiotics [telithromycin], nefazodone): May increase osimertinib level. Avoid concomitant administration. If no alternative exists, monitor patient closely for adverse reactions.
Drug-herb. *St. John's wort:* May decrease osimertinib plasma concentration. Discourage use together.

EFFECTS ON LAB TEST RESULTS

• May increase magnesium level. May decrease sodium level.
• May decrease Hb level and lymphocyte, platelet, and neutrophil counts.

CONTRAINDICATIONS & CAUTIONS

• Use cautiously in patients with congenital long QTc syndrome, HF, or electrolyte abnormalities and in those taking medications known to prolong QTc interval.
• ILD, cardiomyopathy (cardiac failure, pulmonary edema, decreased ejection fraction, stress cardiomyopathy) may occur with treatment.
• Safety and effectiveness in children haven't been established.
Dialyzable drug: Unknown.

PREGNANCY-LACTATION-REPRODUCTION

• Based on animal study data, drug may cause fetal harm. Advise women of childbearing potential of potential fetal risk and to use effective contraception during therapy and for up to 6 weeks after last dose.

• Men should use contraception during therapy and for up to 4 months after last dose.
• It isn't known if drug appears in breast milk. Because of potential for adverse effects in the infant, women shouldn't breast-feed during therapy and for 2 weeks after last dose.
• Drug may impair fertility in men and women of reproductive potential. It isn't known if the effects are reversible.

NURSING CONSIDERATIONS

• Confirm *T790M* EGFR mutation before initiation of treatment.
• Assess LVEF by echocardiogram or multigated acquisition scan before therapy begins and every 3 months during therapy.
• Monitor ECG and electrolyte levels in patients with congenital long QTc syndrome, HF, or electrolyte abnormalities and in those taking medications known to prolong QTc interval.
• Monitor patient for signs and symptom of ILD (dyspnea, cough, fever, worsening respiratory symptoms). Interrupt treatment and promptly evaluate for ILD. Discontinue drug if ILD is confirmed.

PATIENT TEACHING

• Teach patient to promptly report all adverse reactions, especially new or worsening cough, trouble breathing, shortness of breath, or fever.
• Teach patient to seek medical attention for rapid heartbeat or heart pounding, swollen feet or ankles, dizziness, light-headedness, or faintness.
• Advise female patient not to breast-feed during therapy and for up to 2 weeks after therapy ends.
• Warn female patient of fetal risk, and to use contraception during therapy and for 6 weeks after therapy ends. Teach men to use contraception during therapy and for 4 months after therapy ends.
• Caution female patient to contact prescriber if she becomes pregnant or suspects she is pregnant during treatment.
• Instruct patient to swallow tablets whole and not to crush or chew them. Tell patient to report difficulty swallowing tablets to prescriber.

pimavanserin tartrate
pim-a-VAN-ser-in

Nuplazid

Therapeutic class: Antipsychotics
Pharmacologic class: 5-HT receptor inverse agonist and antagonists

AVAILABLE FORMS
Tablets: 17 mg

NEW DRUGS

INDICATIONS & DOSAGES
➤ **Hallucinations and delusions associated with Parkinson disease psychosis**
Adults: 34 mg P.O. once daily.
Adjust-a-dose: If drug is used with strong CYP3A4 inhibitors, reduce pimavanserin dosage to 17 mg once daily.

ADMINISTRATION
P.O.
• May give with or without food.
• Store at 68° to 77° F (20° to 25° C).

ACTION
Unknown. Effects may be mediated through inverse agonist and antagonist activity at serotonin receptors.

Route	Onset	Peak	Duration
P.O.	Unknown	6 hr (mean)	Unknown

Half-life: Pimavanserin, 57 hours; N-desmethylated metabolite, 200 hours.

ADVERSE REACTIONS
CNS: confusion, hallucinations, fatigue, gait disturbance.
CV: peripheral edema, *QT-interval prolongation.*
GI: nausea, constipation.
GU: UTI.

INTERACTIONS
Drug-drug. *Drugs that prolong QT interval (amiodarone, chlorpromazine, disopyramide, gatifloxacin, moxifloxacin, procainamide, quinidine, sotalol, thioridazine, ziprasidone):* May cause additive QT-interval prolongation and increased risk of cardiac arrhythmia. Avoid use together.
Black Box Warning *Opioids:* May cause slow or difficult breathing, sedation, and death. Avoid use together. If use together is necessary, limit dosage and duration of each drug to minimum necessary for desired effect. ∎
Strong CYP3A4 inducers (carbamazepine, phenytoin, rifampin): May decrease pimavanserin level and therapeutic effects. Monitor patient for reduced response and increase pimavanserin dosage as appropriate.
Strong CYP3A4 inhibitors (clarithromycin, indinavir, itraconazole, ketoconazole): May increase pimavanserin level. If used together, reduce pimavanserin dose to 17 mg once daily.
Drug-herb. *St. John's wort:* May decrease pimavanserin level and therapeutic response. Monitor patient and increase pimavanserin dosage if needed.

EFFECTS ON LAB TEST RESULTS
None reported.

CONTRAINDICATIONS & CAUTIONS
Black Box Warning Elderly patients with dementia-related psychosis treated with antipsychotics are at an increased risk for death. Pimavanserin isn't approved for the treatment of patients with dementia-related psychosis unrelated to hallucinations and delusions associated with Parkinson disease psychosis. ∎
Black Box Warning Opioids should only be prescribed with benzodiazepines or other CNS depressants to patients for whom alternative treatment options are inadequate. ∎
• Drug prolongs QT interval. Avoid use with drugs that prolong QT interval, in patients with a history of cardiac arrhythmias, and in those with other conditions that increase risk of torsades de pointes ventricular arrhythmia or sudden death, including symptomatic bradycardia, hypokalemia or hypomagnesemia, and the presence of congenital prolongation of QT interval.
• Drug may cause orthostatic hypotension. Use cautiously in patients at risk for hypotension and in patients who wouldn't tolerate transient hypotension.
• Use isn't recommended in patients with severe renal impairment or any degree of hepatic impairment.
• Safety and effectiveness in children haven't been established.
Dialyzable drug: Unknown.
⚠ Overdose S&S: Nausea and vomiting, QT-interval prolongation.

PREGNANCY-LACTATION-REPRODUCTION
• There are no data concerning drug risks in pregnant or breast-feeding women.

NURSING CONSIDERATIONS
• Monitor patient for QT-interval prolongation.
• Monitor patient for orthostatic hypotension.
• ***Look alike–sound alike:*** Don't confuse pimavanserin with palivizumab, pamidronate, or pitavastatin.

PATIENT TEACHING
• Counsel patient to report changes in medications or supplements, because of potential for drug interactions.
Black Box Warning Caution patient or caregiver of patient taking an opioid with a benzodiazepine, CNS depressant, or alcohol to seek immediate medical attention if patient experiences dizziness, lightheadedness, extreme sleepiness, slowed or difficult breathing, or unresponsiveness. ∎
• Warn patient to immediately report signs and symptoms of ventricular arrhythmia (dizziness or fainting, rapid or irregular heartbeat) or hypotension (dizziness, weakness).
• Advise patient to report swelling in the arms or legs.
• Instruct patient to report confusion or hallucinations that are new or worse after start of therapy.

---

reslizumab
res-li-ZOO-mab

Cinqair

Therapeutic class: Immunomodulators
Pharmacologic class: Interleukin-5
antagonist monoclonal antibodies

AVAILABLE FORMS
Injection: 100 mg/10 mL single-use vial

INDICATIONS & DOSAGES
➤ **Add-on maintenance treatment of patients with severe asthma with an eosinophilic phenotype**
Adults: 3 mg/kg I.V. every 4 weeks.

ADMINISTRATION
I.V.
▼ Don't give as I.V. push or bolus.
▼ Visually inspect for particulate matter and discoloration. Solution should be clear to slightly hazy/opalescent, colorless to slightly yellow. Particles that appear as translucent-to-white amorphous particulates may be present. Discard if solution is discolored or if other foreign particulates are present.
▼ To minimize foaming, don't shake.
▼ Discard any unused portion. Drug doesn't contain preservative.
▼ Slowly inject required volume into a 50-mL NSS infusion bag of polyvinyl chloride or polyolefin. Gently invert bag. Don't shake. Don't mix or dilute with other drugs.
▼ Time between preparation and administration shouldn't exceed 16 hours. If not used immediately, store diluted reslizumab solution in refrigerator at 36° to 46° F (2° to 8° C) or at room temperature (up to 77° F [25° C]), protected from light, for up to 16 hours.
▼ If refrigerated before administration, allow diluted solution to warm to room temperature.
▼ Use an infusion set with an in-line, low-protein-binding, 0.2-micron polyethersulfone, polyvinylidene fluoride nylon, or cellulose acetate in-line infusion filter.
▼ Infuse over 20 to 50 minutes; then flush I.V. administration set with NSS to ensure that all reslizumab has been administered.
▼ **Incompatibilities:** Physical and biochemical compatibility studies haven't been conducted. Don't infuse with other drugs or solutions other than NSS.

ACTION
Binds to interleukin-5, reducing production and survival of eosinophils, which limits inflammation, a component of the pathogenesis of asthma; however, its exact mechanism in asthma hasn't been established.

Route	Onset	Peak	Duration
I.V.	Unknown	End of infusion	Unknown

Half-life: 24 days.

ADVERSE REACTIONS
EENT: oropharyngeal pain.
Musculoskeletal: myalgia, musculoskeletal chest pain, neck pain, muscle spasm, extremity pain, muscle fatigue, musculoskeletal pain.
Other: antibody development.

INTERACTIONS
None reported.

EFFECTS ON LAB TEST RESULTS
• May increase CK level.
• May decrease blood eosinophil count.

CONTRAINDICATIONS & CAUTIONS
Black Box Warning Anaphylaxis has occurred in patients receiving reslizumab. Give only in a health care setting prepared to manage anaphylactic reactions. ■
Black Box Warning Contraindicated in patients hypersensitive to drug or its components. ■
• Drug isn't indicated for status asthmaticus, acute bronchospasm, or acute asthma exacerbations.
• Drug isn't indicated for eosinophilic conditions other than severe asthma with an eosinophilic phenotype.
• Safety and effectiveness in children haven't been established.
Dialyzable drug: Unlikely.

PREGNANCY-LACTATION-REPRODUCTION
• Use in pregnancy hasn't been studied. Weigh risks to the developing fetus against risks of the mother's poorly controlled asthma.
• Monoclonal antibodies such as reslizumab are known to cross the placental barrier, so drug may affect a fetus. The possibility is likely to be greater during the second and third trimesters.
• It isn't known if reslizumab appears in breast milk; however, human IgG is known to appear in breast milk. Closely monitor the level of asthma control in pregnant women and adjust reslizumab dosage as necessary to maintain optimal control. Weigh risks to the breast-fed infant against the mother's need for the drug.

NURSING CONSIDERATIONS
⚠ *Alert:* Monitor patient for signs and symptoms of anaphylaxis (dyspnea, decreased oxygen saturation, wheezing, vomiting, urticaria) during infusion and for an appropriate amount of time after infusion has been completed. Discontinue drug immediately if severe systemic reaction occurs.
• If patient has preexisting helminth infection, treat infection before initiating reslizumab. If patient becomes infected with parasites while receiving drug and doesn't respond to antihelminth treatment, discontinue reslizumab until infection resolves.

NEW DRUGS

• Don't abruptly discontinue systemic or inhaled corticosteroids upon initiation of reslizumab. If appropriate, decrease corticosteroid dosage gradually.
• *Look alike–sound alike:* Don't confuse reslizumab with infliximab, ixekizumab, or rituximab.

PATIENT TEACHING
Black Box Warning Teach patient signs and symptoms of hypersensitivity and anaphylaxis (mucosal swelling, airway compromise, reduced BP, rash, hives, itching). Instruct patient to immediately report signs and symptoms of an allergic reaction that occur during or after receiving a reslizumab infusion. ∎
• Explain to patient that reslizumab doesn't treat acute asthma symptoms or exacerbations. Advise patient to seek medical attention if asthma remains uncontrolled or worsens after initiation of reslizumab.
• Inform patient that there is a small risk of malignancy associated with reslizumab therapy.
• Warn patient not to discontinue systemic or inhaled corticosteroids except under medical supervision. Inform patient that reducing corticosteroid dosage may be associated with signs and symptoms of systemic withdrawal or may unmask conditions previously suppressed by corticosteroid therapy.
• Tell patient to notify health care provider for an existing or developing parasitic infection.
• Teach patient to report all adverse reactions to prescriber.

sebelipase alfa
se-BEL-ip-ase

Kanuma

Therapeutic class: Replacement enzymes
Pharmacologic class: Recombinant human lysosomal acid lipases

AVAILABLE FORMS
Injection: 20 mg/10 mL single-use vial

INDICATIONS & DOSAGES
➤Lysosomal acid lipase (LAL) deficiency
Adults and children age 6 months and older: 1 mg/kg I.V. infusion once every other week.
Children age 6 months or younger with rapidly progressing disease: 1 mg/kg I.V. infusion once weekly. May increase to 3 mg/kg once weekly for patients who don't achieve an optimal clinical response.

ADMINISTRATION
I.V.
▼ Allow vials to warm to room temperature before diluting.
▼ Dilute with NSS according to dose and patient's weight. See manufacturer's instructions.
▼ Gently invert vial to mix; don't shake vial.

▼ Inspect for particulate matter or discoloration; solution should be a clear to slightly opalescent, colorless to slightly colored solution. Thin, translucent particles or fibers may be present in vials or diluted solution. Don't use if cloudy or vial contains particulate matter.
▼ Use immediately after dilution. If not possible, store diluted solution in refrigerator for up to 24 hours.
▼ Discard unused product.
▼ Administer diluted solution using a low-protein-binding infusion set with an in-line, low-protein-binding 0.2-micron filter.
▼ Infuse over at least 2 hours. Consider prolonging infusion time for patients receiving 3-mg/kg dose and for those who have experienced hypersensitivity reactions. Consider a 1-hour infusion for patients receiving 1-mg/kg dose who tolerate the 2-hour infusion.
▼ Solution is preservative-free. Store vials in refrigerator at 36° to 46° F (2° to 8° C). Don't freeze. Protect from light.
▼ **Incompatibilities:** None reported.

ACTION
Catalyzes the hydrolysis of cholesteryl esters and triglycerides to free cholesterol and fatty acids, and the hydrolysis of triglycerides to glycerol and free fatty acids, reversing the accumulation of lipids that affects multiple organs in the body in patients with LAL enzyme deficiency.

Route	Onset	Peak	Duration
I.V.	Immediate	1.3 hr	Unknown

Half-life: 5.4 to 6.6 minutes.

ADVERSE REACTIONS
CNS: fever, headache, weakness.
EENT: rhinitis, nasopharyngitis, oropharyngeal pain.
GI: diarrhea, vomiting, constipation, nausea.
Hematologic: anemia.
Metabolic: hyperlipidemia.
Respiratory: cough.
Skin: urticaria.
Other: immunogenicity, hypersensitivity reactions, *anaphylaxis.*

INTERACTIONS
None reported.

EFFECTS ON LAB TEST RESULTS
• May increase LDL and triglyceride levels. May decrease ALT level.
• May decrease RBC count.

CONTRAINDICATIONS & CAUTIONS
• Use cautiously in patients hypersensitive to eggs or egg products.
• Safety and effectiveness in children younger than age 1 month haven't been established.
Dializable drug: Unknown.

Reactions in bold italics are *life-threatening.* Interactions may have a *rapid onset* or a *delayed onset.*

PREGNANCY-LACTATION-REPRODUCTION
• There are no data concerning drug-associated risk during pregnancy or breast-feeding. Use cautiously in pregnant and breast-feeding women.

NURSING CONSIDERATIONS
• Monitor patient for hypersensitivity reactions, including anaphylaxis (chest discomfort, conjunctival injection, dyspnea, rash, hyperemia, swelling of eyelids, rhinorrhea, severe respiratory distress, tachycardia, tachypnea, urticaria). Reactions generally occur during or within 4 hours of infusion, and may have early or late onset up to 1 year after start of treatment.
• If hypersensitivity reaction occurs, consider interrupting infusion or lowering infusion rate, based on severity of the reaction. May resume infusion at a slower rate with increases as tolerated. If a severe hypersensitivity reaction occurs, immediately stop infusion and initiate appropriate treatment.
• Pretreat patients who had hypersensitivity reactions to drug with antipyretics, antihistamines, or both as appropriate.
• Have emergency medical equipment readily available during drug administration, because of risk of anaphylaxis.
• Consider risk and benefits of readministering drug after a severe hypersensitivity reaction. Closely monitor patient if readministering.
• During first 2 to 4 weeks of treatment, LDL cholesterol and triglyceride levels may increase due to initial breakdown of accumulated lipids. After 8 weeks of treatment, these parameters should decrease to below pretreatment values.

PATIENT TEACHING
• Warn patient about potential for hypersensitivity reactions, especially anaphylaxis, and to report signs and symptoms immediately.
• Tell patient to report all adverse reactions promptly.
• Explain to patient and caregivers the importance of keeping appointments for infusions.
• Warn patient to report allergy to eggs before starting treatment.

selexipag
se-LEX-i-pag

Uptravi

Therapeutic class: Vasodilators
Pharmacologic class: Prostacyclin receptor agonists

AVAILABLE FORMS
Tablets (extended-release) ⓜ: 200 mcg, 400 mcg, 600 mcg, 800 mcg, 1,000 mcg, 1,200 mcg, 1,400 mcg, 1,600 mcg

INDICATIONS & DOSAGES
➤ **Pulmonary arterial hypertension (PAH, World Health Organization Group I) to delay disease progression and reduce risk of hospitalization**
Adults: Initially, 200 mcg P.O. b.i.d. Increase dosage by increments of 200 mcg b.i.d. at weekly intervals to the highest tolerated dose. If dose isn't tolerated, decrease dose to the previous tolerated dose. Maximum dose is 1,600 mcg b.i.d.
Adjust-a-dose: For patients with moderate hepatic impairment (Child-Pugh class B), initiate therapy at 200 mcg once daily and increase by 200-mcg increments once daily at weekly intervals, as tolerated. Avoid use in patients with severe hepatic impairment (Child-Pugh class C).

ADMINISTRATION
P.O.
• Giving with food may improve tolerability.
• If a dose is missed, give as soon as possible. If next scheduled dose is due within 6 hours, skip the missed dose and give next dose at the regular time.
• If 3 or more days of medication are missed, restart medication at a lower dose and retitrate to maximum tolerated dose.
• Don't split, crush, or allow patient to chew tablets.
• Store at 68° to 77° F (20° to 25° C).

ACTION
A selective prostacyclin receptor agonist. Prostacyclin is produced in the endothelial cells and induces vasodilation and inhibits platelet aggregation.

Route	Onset	Peak	Duration
P.O.	Rapid	1–4 hr	Unknown

Half-life: 0.8 to 2.5 hours. Active metabolite, 6.2 to 13.5 hours.

ADVERSE REACTIONS
CNS: headache.
CV: flushing.
GI: diarrhea, nausea, vomiting, decreased appetite.
Hematologic: anemia.
Metabolic: hyperthyroidism.
Musculoskeletal: myalgia, arthralgia, limb pain, jaw pain.
Skin: rash.

INTERACTIONS
Drug-drug. *Strong inhibitors of CYP2C8 (gemfibrozil):* May increase levels of selexipag and its active metabolite. Avoid use together.

EFFECTS ON LAB TEST RESULTS
• May decrease Hb and TSH levels.

CONTRAINDICATIONS & CAUTIONS
• Use cautiously in patients with moderate hepatic impairment. Avoid use in patients with severe hepatic impairment.
• Drug hasn't been studied in patients with ESRD.

NEW DRUGS

- Safety and effectiveness in children haven't been established.
Dialyzable drug: No.
⚠ *Overdose S&S:* Mild, transient nausea.

PREGNANCY-LACTATION-REPRODUCTION

- There are no adequate well-controlled studies in pregnant women.
- Women with PAH are encouraged to avoid pregnancy.
- Women shouldn't breast-feed while taking drug. Patient should discontinue breast-feeding or discontinue drug.

NURSING CONSIDERATIONS

- Monitor patient for signs and symptoms of pulmonary edema (dyspnea, cough with pink foamy sputum, fatigue, tachycardia). If signs and symptoms occur, evaluate patient for pulmonary veno-occlusive disease. If confirmed, discontinue drug.
- *Look alike–sound alike:* Don't confuse selexipag with Celexa or Lexapro.

PATIENT TEACHING

- Teach patient to report all adverse reactions and to immediately report signs and symptoms of pulmonary edema.
- Instruct patient to take with food to improve tolerance.
- Warn patient not to split, crush, or chew tablets.
- Advise patient to take drug exactly as prescribed and not to discontinue drug without first discussing with prescriber.
- Counsel female patient not to breast-feed while taking drug.
- Advise female patient to inform prescriber if she is pregnant or plans to become pregnant.

---

sofosbuvir–velpatasvir
soe-FOS-bue-vir/vel-PAT-as-vir

Epclusa

Therapeutic class: Antivirals
Pharmacologic class: Nucleotide analogue NS5B polymerase inhibitors/HCV NS5A inhibitors

---

AVAILABLE FORMS

Tablets: 400 mg sofosbuvir and 100 mg velpatasvir

INDICATIONS & DOSAGES

➤ **Chronic HCV genotype 1, 2, 3, 4, 5, or 6 infection without cirrhosis or with compensated cirrhosis (Child-Pugh class A) or with decompensated cirrhosis (Child-Pugh class B or C) in combination with ribavirin**
Adults: One tablet P.O. once daily for 12 weeks.

ADMINISTRATION
P.O.
- Keep drug in original container.
- May give with or without food.
- Store below 86° F (30° C).

ACTION

Sofosbuvir and velpatasvir are direct-acting antivirals that inhibit viral replication of HCV.

Route	Onset	Peak	Duration
P.O. (sofosbuvir)	Unknown	½–1 hr	Unknown
P.O. (velpatasvir)	Unknown	3 hr	Unknown

Half-life: Sofosbuvir, ½ hour; velpatasvir, 15 hours.

ADVERSE REACTIONS

CNS: headache, fatigue, asthenia, insomnia, irritability, depression.
GI: nausea, diarrhea, lipase elevations.
Hematologic: anemia.
Metabolic: CK elevations.
Skin: rash.

INTERACTIONS

Drug-drug. *Antacids (aluminum hydroxide, magnesium hydroxide):* May decrease velpatasvir level. Separate antacid and drug administration by 4 hours.
❸ *Alert: Amiodarone:* May result in serious symptomatic bradycardia. Use together isn't recommended but if coadministration is necessary, cardiac monitoring is recommended.
Anticonvulsants (carbamazepine, oxcarbazepine, phenobarbital, phenytoin), antimycobacterial drugs (rifabutin, rifampin, rifapentine): May decrease levels of both antivirals. Avoid use together.
Atorvastatin, rosuvastatin: May significantly increase statin level and increase risk of rhabdomyolysis. Use together cautiously and monitor patient closely.
Digoxin: May increase digoxin level. Monitor digoxin level and adjust digoxin dosage as needed.
Efavirenz: May decrease velpatasvir level. Use together isn't recommended.
H_2 antagonists (famotidine): May decrease velpatasvir level. Give H_2 antagonist simultaneously or 12 hours apart from drug at a dose that doesn't exceed an equivalent of famotidine 40 mg b.i.d.
Moderate to potent CYP2B6, CYP2C8, or CYP3A4 inducers (carbamazepine, rifampin), P-glycoprotein inducers: May significantly decrease sofosbuvir or velpatasvir level, reducing therapeutic effect. Use together isn't recommended.
Omeprazole: May decrease velpatasvir level. Avoid use together, but if coadministration is necessary, give drug 4 hours before omeprazole 20 mg.
Tenofovir: May increase tenofovir level. Monitor patient for tenofovir-associated adverse reactions.
Tipranavir; ritonavir: May decrease levels of both antivirals. Avoid use together.
Topotecan: May increase topotecan level. Avoid use together.

Reactions in bold italics are *life-threatening*. Interactions may have a *rapid onset* or a *delayed onset*.

Drug-herb. *St. John's wort:* May decrease antiviral levels and therapeutic effects. Use together isn't recommended.

EFFECTS ON LAB TEST RESULTS
• May increase lipase, CK, and indirect bilirubin levels.
• May decrease Hb level.

CONTRAINDICATIONS & CAUTIONS
• Combination regimen with ribavirin is contraindicated in patients for whom ribavirin is contraindicated. Refer to ribavirin manufacturer's instructions for contraindications.
• Warnings and precautions for ribavirin apply when used in combination with Epclusa. Refer to ribavirin prescribing information.
Black Box Warning Reactivation of HBV infection may occur in HCV coinfected patients, and result in fulminant hepatitis, hepatic failure, and death. Screen all patients for current or prior HBV infection before treatment and if positive for HBV infection, assess baseline HBV DNA. ■
⚠ Alert: Serious symptomatic bradycardia may occur in patients taking amiodarone, particularly in patients also taking beta blockers, in those with underlying cardiac comorbidities, and in patients with advanced liver disease.
• Safety and effectiveness in children haven't been established.
Dialyzable drug: Sofosbuvir, 53%; velpatasvir, unlikely.

PREGNANCY-LACTATION-REPRODUCTION
• Use of sofosbuvir and velpatasvir in pregnancy hasn't been studied.
• Combination regimen with ribavirin is contraindicated in pregnant women and in men whose female partners are pregnant.
• Advise patients using combination treatment with ribavirin to use two effective forms of contraception during treatment and for 6 months after therapy ends. Refer to ribavirin manufacturer's instructions for pregnancy testing before, during, and after therapy and for information about breast-feeding.
• It isn't known if sofosbuvir and velpatasvir and their metabolites appear in breast milk, affect human milk production, or have effects on the breast-fed infant. Use cautiously, weighing benefits for the mother and risk of breast-feeding for the infant.

NURSING CONSIDERATIONS
Black Box Warning Monitor patient with current or prior HBV infection for hepatitis flare or HBV reactivation with laboratory testing; watch for signs and symptoms of liver injury during active and posttreatment follow-up. ■
⚠ Alert: For patients taking amiodarone (with or without beta blockers) who have no other treatment options and must begin Epclusa, cardiac monitoring

in an inpatient setting for first 48 hours of coadministration is recommended, followed by outpatient or self-monitoring of HR daily for at least 2 weeks. Patients who discontinue amiodarone just before starting Epclusa and those who must begin amiodarone while taking Epclusa should also undergo similar cardiac monitoring.
• Monitor patient for bradycardia (near-fainting, syncope, dizziness, light-headedness, malaise, weakness, excessive fatigue, shortness of breath, chest pain, confusion, memory problems) and report it immediately.
• Clinical and hepatic laboratory monitoring, including direct bilirubin, is recommended for patients with decompensated cirrhosis taking Epclusa plus ribavirin.
• Monitor patient for anemia.

PATIENT TEACHING
Black Box Warning Warn patient to immediately report signs and symptoms of liver injury (fatigue, weakness, loss of appetite, nausea, vomiting, yellowing of skin or eyes, and light-colored stool). ■
• Advise patient to report other prescription or OTC medications or herbal products being taken, including St. John's wort.
• Inform patient that it's important not to miss or skip doses and to take this medication for as long as recommended by prescriber.
• Advise patient to avoid pregnancy during combination treatment with ribavirin and to contact prescriber immediately if pregnancy occurs.
⚠ Alert: Counsel patient who is also taking amiodarone about the risk of symptomatic bradycardia. Teach patient to self-monitor HR.
• Caution patient to seek medical attention for signs and symptoms of bradycardia.

SAFETY ALERT!

venetoclax
ven-ET-oh-klax

Venclexta

Therapeutic class: Antineoplastics
Pharmacologic class: BCL-2 inhibitors

AVAILABLE FORMS
Tablets ⓞⓝⓒ: 10 mg, 50 mg, 100 mg

INDICATIONS & DOSAGES
➤ **Chronic lymphocytic leukemia (CLL) with 17p deletion after at least one prior therapy**
Adults: Initially, 20 mg P.O. once daily week 1; increase to 50 mg P.O. once daily week 2; increase to 100 mg P.O. once daily week 3; increase to 200 mg P.O. once daily week 4; then increase to 400 mg P.O. once daily week 5 and thereafter. Continue until disease progression or unacceptable toxicity.

NEW DRUGS

Adjust-a-dose: Dosage adjustments for toxicity during treatment are as follows: If dose interrupted is 400 mg, restart at 300 mg; if dose interrupted is 300 mg, restart at 200 mg; if dose interrupted is 200 mg, restart at 100 mg; if dose interrupted is 100 mg, restart at 50 mg; if dose interrupted is 50 mg, restart at 20 mg; if dose interrupted is 20 mg, restart at 10 mg. During the ramp-up phase, continue the reduced dose for 1 week before increasing the dose. Consider discontinuing drug in patients who require dosage reduction to less than 100 mg for more than 2 weeks. For patients who have had a dosing interruption greater than 1 week during first 5 weeks of the ramp-up phase or greater than 2 weeks at the maintenance dose of 400 mg, reassess for risk of tumor lysis syndrome (TLS) to determine if reinitiation with a reduced dose is necessary.

For serum chemistry changes or signs and symptoms of TLS (acute renal failure, cardiac arrhythmias, seizures), withhold next day's dose. If resolved within 24 to 48 hours, resume at same dose; if more than 48 hours is required to resolve, then resume at a reduced dose after resolution.

For first occurrence of grade 3 or 4 nonhematologic toxicities, interrupt treatment until resolved to grade 1 or baseline, then resume at the same dose without dosage modification. For second or subsequent occurrence of grade 3 or 4 nonhematologic toxicity, interrupt therapy until resolved, then resume at a modified dose (a larger dosage reduction may occur at prescriber's discretion). For first occurrence of grade 3 or 4 neutropenia with infection or fever, or grade 4 hematologic toxicity (except lymphopenia), give granulocyte-colony stimulating factor (G-CSF) for neutropenia, if clinically indicated, and interrupt treatment until resolved to grade 1 or baseline, then resume at the same dose. For second or subsequent hematologic toxicity, give G-CSF as clinically indicated and interrupt therapy until resolved, then resume at a modified dose (a larger dosage reduction may occur at prescriber's discretion).

ADMINISTRATION
P.O.
☉ *Alert:* Hazardous drug; use safe handling and disposal precautions. Wear gloves to handle tablet.
• Give with a meal and water at approximately the same time each day.
• If a dose is missed and it's within 8 hours of the usual dosing time, give missed dose as soon as possible and resume normal daily dosing schedule. If it's more than 8 hours, don't give missed dose and resume usual dosing schedule the next day.
• If patient vomits after administration of a dose, don't give additional doses that day; give next dose at the usual time.
• Tablets must be swallowed whole; don't crush, break, or allow patient to chew tablets.
• Store at or below 86° F (30° C).

ACTION
An inhibitor of BCL-2 (B cell lymphoma 2), an anti-apoptotic protein. Overexpression of BCL-2 has been demonstrated in CLL cells and has been associated with resistance to chemotherapeutic agents. Venetoclax helps restore apoptosis by binding directly to the BCL-2 protein, displacing proapoptotic proteins and restoring the apoptotic process.

Route	Onset	Peak	Duration
P.O.	Unknown	5–8 hr	Unknown

Half-life: 26 hours.

ADVERSE REACTIONS
CNS: fatigue, headache, fever.
CV: peripheral edema.
GI: diarrhea, nausea, vomiting, constipation.
Hematologic: *neutropenia*, anemia, *thrombocytopenia, febrile neutropenia, autoimmune hemolytic anemia.*
Metabolic: *hyperkalemia*, hyperphosphatemia, *hypokalemia, hypocalcemia,* hyperuricemia, *TLS.*
Musculoskeletal: back pain.
Respiratory: URI, cough, pneumonia.

INTERACTIONS
Drug-drug. *Live attenuated vaccines:* Safety and efficacy haven't been studied and vaccines may be less effective. Don't give vaccines before, during, or after treatment until B-cell recovery occurs.
Moderate CYP3A inducers (bosentan, efavirenz, etravirine, modafinil, nafcillin), strong CYP3A inducers (carbamazepine, phenytoin, rifampin): May decrease venetoclax level. Consider alternative treatments.
Moderate CYP3A inhibitors (ciprofloxacin, diltiazem, dronedarone, erythromycin, fluconazole), P-glycoprotein (P-gp) inhibitors (amiodarone, azithromycin, captopril, carvedilol, cyclosporine, felodipine, quercetin, quinidine, ranolazine, ticagrelor): May increase venetoclax level and risk of TLS. Consider alternative treatments. If a moderate inhibitor must be used, reduce venetoclax dosage by at least 50%; monitor patient closely. Resume venetoclax dose that was used before initiating the inhibitor 2 to 3 days after discontinuing inhibitor.
P-gp substrates (digoxin, everolimus, sirolimus): May inhibit absorption of P-gp substrates. Coadministration of narrow therapeutic index P-gp substrates with venetoclax should be avoided. If substrate must be used, patient should take it at least 6 hours before venetoclax.
Strong CYP3A inhibitors (clarithromycin, conivaptan, indinavir, itraconazole, ketoconazole, lopinavir, posaconazole, ritonavir, telaprevir, voriconazole): May increase venetoclax level and risk of TLS. Use during initiation and ramp-up phase is contraindicated. For patients who have completed ramp-up phase and are on a steady daily dose of venetoclax, reduce venetoclax dosage by at least 75% when used concomitantly with strong CYP3A inhibitors. Resume venetoclax

---

Reactions in bold italics are *life-threatening.* Interactions may have a *rapid onset* or a *delayed onset.*

dose that was used before initiating the CYP3A inhibitor 2 to 3 days after discontinuing inhibitor.
Warfarin: May increase INR. Monitor INR closely.
Drug-herb. *St. John's wort:* May decrease venetoclax level. Don't use together.
Drug-food. *Grapefruit products, Seville oranges, starfruit:* May increase venetoclax level. Avoid use together

EFFECTS ON LAB TEST RESULTS
• May increase phosphate and uric acid levels. May decrease calcium level. May increase or decrease potassium level.
• May decrease Hb, hematocrit, and neutrophil and platelet counts.

CONTRAINDICATIONS & CAUTIONS
• Contraindicated in patients hypersensitive to drug or its components.
🕒 *Alert:* Drug may cause a rapid reduction in tumor volume and increases the risk of TLS and renal failure (requiring dialysis); fatalities have been reported. Risk of TLS increases with high tumor burden, concomitant use of CYP3A or P-gp inhibitors, and comorbidities. The 5-week ramp-up dosing schedule is designed to gradually reduce tumor burden and decrease risk of TLS.
• Use cautiously in patients with hepatic impairment. Adverse events may be increased in patients with moderate impairment; monitor patients closely for toxicity, especially during initiation and ramp-up period. Use hasn't been studied in patients with severe impairment.
• Use cautiously in patients with renal impairment. Patients with decreased renal function (CrCl of less than 80 mL/minute) are at increased risk for TLS and may require more intensive TLS prophylaxis and monitoring during treatment initiation and dosage escalation.
• Safety and effectiveness in children haven't been established.
Dialyzable drug: Unlikely.

PREGNANCY-LACTATION-REPRODUCTION
• Drug may cause fetal harm. Women of childbearing potential should have pregnancy testing before therapy, and use effective contraception during and for at least 30 days after treatment ends. Women who become pregnant while taking venetoclax should be made aware of fetal risk.
• Based on animal data, venetoclax may compromise fertility in males.
• It isn't known if drug appears in breast milk. Because of potential for serious adverse reactions in the breast-fed infant, patient should discontinue breast-feeding.

NURSING CONSIDERATIONS
• Patients without 17p deletion at diagnosis should be retested at relapse because acquisition of 17p deletion

can occur, making patient eligible for treatment with venetoclax.
• Patients at high risk for TLS may require hospitalization at treatment initiation.
• Assess patient for risk of TLS before treatment (radiographic evaluation; assessment of potassium, uric acid, phosphorus, calcium, and creatinine levels and renal function). Give prophylactic hydration and antihyperuricemics as clinically indicated. See prescribing information for recommended TLS prophylaxis and monitoring.
• Monitor serum chemistry values. Changes due to TLS can occur as soon as 6 to 8 hours after first dose and at each dosage increase.
• Monitor CBC with differential throughout treatment; treatment interruption and dosage reduction may be required. Consider WBC growth factor support as clinically indicated.
• Monitor patient for infection, including neutropenic fever. Treat with antimicrobials as appropriate.
• *Look alike–sound alike:* Don't confuse venetoclax with vandetanib, vemurafenib, venlafaxine, or vismodegib. Don't confuse Venclexta with venlafaxine.

PATIENT TEACHING
• Teach patient that treatment may be interrupted, dosage decreased, or treatment stopped due to adverse effects. Tell patient to report all adverse reactions promptly.
• Advise patient of risk of TLS, particularly at treatment initiation and during ramp-up phase, and to immediately report TLS signs and symptoms (fever, chills, nausea, vomiting, confusion, shortness of breath, seizures, irregular heartbeat, dark or cloudy urine, unusual tiredness, muscle pain, joint discomfort).
• Inform patient that it may be necessary to take drug under direct medical supervision to allow for monitoring for TLS.
• Advise patient to maintain adequate hydration to reduce risk of TLS. Recommended intake is 6 to 8 glasses (56 oz) beginning 2 days before treatment, on first day of treatment, and each time dosage is increased.
• Warn patient to immediately report fever or signs and symptoms of infection.
• Remind patient of importance of keeping scheduled appointments for blood work or other laboratory tests to monitor for adverse effects.
• Caution patient that venetoclax may interact with other drugs. Advise patient to report the use of prescription and OTC medications and supplements and not to start new medications or supplements without first discussing with prescriber.
• Instruct patient to avoid consuming grapefruit products, Seville oranges, or starfruit during treatment.
• Advise patient to avoid vaccination with live vaccines during treatment.

• Teach patient that if a dose is missed by less than 8 hours, to take missed dose right away and take the next dose as usual.

• Advise patient that if vomiting occurs after taking venetoclax, not to take an additional dose that day, but to take the next dose at the usual time the following day.

• Caution female patient of childbearing potential to use effective contraception during and for at least 30 days after therapy.

• Instruct female patient to immediately contact prescriber if she becomes pregnant, is planning a pregnancy, or suspects she is pregnant.

• Warn female patient not to breast-feed during treatment.

• Advise male patient of risk of infertility due to treatment and of the option of sperm banking.

Appendices

Avoiding common drug errors:
Best practices and prevention

In addition to following your institution's administration policies, you can help prevent errors in drug administration by reviewing these common errors and ways to prevent them. The Joint Commission, the Institute for Safe Medication Practices (ISMP), and the FDA also maintain resources to help improve drug safety.

Topic	Error	Best practices and prevention
Drug orders		
Pharmacy computer system	The system may not detect all unsafe orders.	• Don't rely on the pharmacy computer system to detect all unsafe orders. • Before giving a drug, understand the correct indication, dosage, and potential adverse effects. • Consult the pharmacist if there is any question, and verify the information using a current drug reference.
Confusing drug names	Many drugs have names that look alike–sound alike and may easily be mistaken one for the other.	• Be aware of the drugs your patient takes regularly, and question any deviations from his routine. • Take your time and read the label carefully. • Consult the ISMP list of look alike–sound alike drugs. • Be aware of tall man lettering, which helps differentiate similar drug names.
Abbreviations	Using dangerous abbreviations can result in giving the wrong drug or wrong dose, by the wrong route, or at the wrong time.	• Don't abbreviate drug names. • Be aware of The Joint Commission's official "Do Not Use" list of drug abbreviations to avoid (see *Appendix 4: Abbreviations to avoid [The Joint Commission]*, page 1625). • Consult your facility's list of approved abbreviations and the ISMP's "List of Error-Prone Abbreviations, Symbols, and Dose Designations" (www.ismp.org/tools/errorproneabbreviations.pdf).
Unclear order	A drug order with incomplete or unclear information can result in giving the wrong drug or wrong dose, by the wrong route, or at the wrong time.	• Keep in mind that each order should specify the correct drug name, concentration, dosage, route, and frequency of administration. • Clarify all incomplete or unclear orders with the prescriber. Utilize read-back and verify when taking phone and verbal orders.
Inadvertent overdose	A prescriber may write an order for a combination drug such as acetaminophen–opioid analgesic tablets without realizing the total acetaminophen dose could be toxic (exceed 4 g).	• Note the amount of acetaminophen in each combined formulation. • Warn patients not to take additional drugs that contain acetaminophen. • Verify any "as needed" pain or fever medication orders to check if they contain acetaminophen. Monitor patient's use of "as needed" drugs as prescribed.

Topic	Error	Best practices and prevention
Anticoagulants	Lack of standardization for drug naming, labeling, and packaging can create confusion. Dosing regimens, assay methods, narrow therapeutic ranges, complex drug interactions, and drug monitoring methods create high potential for complications.	• Keep current with the different dosing regimens, assay methods and their standardized range of normal values, drug interactions, monitoring methods, and reversal regimens for each anticoagulant given. • Be especially aware of the correct doses and indications for neonates and children. • Teach patients to manage their therapy appropriately.

Drug preparation

Crushing drugs for oral or enteral administration	Crushing certain oral or enteral drugs may: • alter the drug's effects, causing overdose or other adverse reactions • result in skin irritation or other adverse reactions for the preparer • produce teratogenic effects in pregnant women.	• Use a liquid formulation instead of crushing a drug whenever possible. • Before crushing a drug, always check with the pharmacist and established references, such as the ISMP's list of "Oral Dosage Forms That Should Not Be Crushed" (www.ismp.org/tools/donotcrush.pdf).
Solution color change or particulate matter	Unusual appearance may indicate that: • the drug has been improperly stored or manufactured • the drug has expired • the wrong drug has been provided by the pharmacy • the wrong liquid was chosen out of patient's medication supply.	• Closely examine all solutions before giving them, and know what their appearance should be. • If you note a color change, contact the pharmacist who dispensed the solution and report it. • Don't give a drug until verifying that the drug has been correctly labeled and that it is safe to give. • Verify you have chosen the correct solution from patient's supply if patient is on more than one liquid drug.
Incorrect drug storage	Incorrect storage may change a drug's physical properties or result in its being inadvertently administered.	• Follow your facility's policy for storing drugs. • Always store drugs in the appropriate container, in the appropriate place, at the appropriate temperature.
Incomplete or incorrect drug labels	Incorrect or incomplete labeling can result in giving the wrong drug, formulation, or dose.	• Never give a drug whose label is incomplete or incorrect. Notify the pharmacy immediately and obtain the correctly labeled drug. • Label all medications, medication containers, and other solutions on and off the sterile field.

Drug administration

Using a parenteral syringe for oral or enteral drugs	Using a parenteral syringe with a luer-lock to prepare small amounts of oral or enteral drugs can result in misadministration because the drug could be accidentally injected into an I.V. line.	• Always use special oral syringes to give oral or enteral drugs. Their hubs won't support a needle and they don't have a luer-lock, so they can't be attached to I.V. lines. • Always label syringes (if they aren't thrown away immediately).
Infusion pump safety problems	Problems with infusion pumps (used to deliver controlled fluids, drugs, and nutrients) can cause fluid overload or administration of inaccurate doses.	• Make sure you know how to safely operate an infusion pump. Consult your facility's policy on proper usage. • Before beginning an infusion, always verify that the pump is working properly. Make sure all alarms are functional and never bypass them. • Double-check all dosing. • Always double-check that the correct medication bag is hanging in the pump.

Topic	Error	Best practices and prevention
Calculation errors	Dosage calculation errors can cause significant patient harm, especially with "high alert" medications, and in neonates and children.	• Be aware of medications that are considered high alert. • Write out the mg/kg or mg/m^2 dose and the calculated dose as a safeguard. • Whenever a prescriber provides a calculation, double-check it and document that the dose was verified in the medical record. • Use only approved abbreviations, and be aware of the placement of decimal points.
OTC products/supplements (herbal supplements and vitamins)	Because OTC products, herbal supplements, and vitamins aren't subject to the same quality assurance standards as drugs, their labels may be misrepresented and their effects and interactions with drugs may not be well studied.	• Always assess and document all OTC drugs, herbal supplements, and vitamins patient is taking in patient's medical record. • Monitor patient carefully, and report unusual adverse reactions. • Consult an evidence-based drug reference for known drug-herb interactions.

Pregnancy risk categories: The FDA's Final Rule

In December 2014, the FDA published a final rule that set new standards for how information about using medications during pregnancy and breast-feeding will be presented in the labels of biological products and prescription drugs. These new standards went into effect June 30, 2015, for all newly approved drug and biological products; the new labeling requirements are being phased in gradually for previously approved products.

The final rule recognizes that decisions for medication use during pregnancy and breast-feeding involve complex risk-benefit considerations and must be individualized because many pregnant and breast-feeding patients need medications to manage acute and chronic conditions. According to the final rule, the letter category system was often misinterpreted as a grading system and provided oversimplified information about a drug's risk. Consequently, the current pregnancy risk categories (A, B, C, D, X) will be replaced with three labeled subsections titled "Pregnancy," "Lactation," and "Females and Males of Reproductive Potential." These subsections will provide more consistent, relevant explanations and information about a drug's risks and benefits in the real-world context of caring for patients. Pregnant and breast-feeding women should always consult their health care professionals before taking any prescription or OTC medication or supplements.

Controlled substance schedules

Drugs regulated under the jurisdiction of the Controlled Substances Act of 1970 are divided into the following groups or schedules:

- Schedule I (C-I): High abuse potential, lack of accepted safety, and no accepted medical use. Examples include heroin and LSD.
- Schedule II (C-II): High abuse potential with severe dependence liability. Has an accepted medical use for treatment in the U.S., but use maybe be severely restricted. Examples include opioids, amphetamines, and some barbiturates.
- Schedule III (C-III): Less abuse potential than Schedule I or II drugs; abuse may cause moderate to low physical dependence or high psychological dependence. Has an accepted medical use for treatment in the U.S. Examples include nonbarbiturate sedatives, nonamphetamine stimulants, anabolic steroids, and limited amounts of certain opioids.
- Schedule IV (C-IV): Less abuse potential than Schedule III drugs and limited dependence liability. Has an accepted medical use for treatment in the U.S. Examples include some sedatives, anxiolytics, and nonopioid analgesics.
- Schedule V (C-V): Low abuse potential with limited physical or psychological dependence compared to Schedule IV drugs. Has an accepted medical use for treatment in the U.S. This category mainly includes small amounts of opioids, such as codeine, used in antitussives or antidiarrheals. Under federal law, limited quantities of certain Schedule V drugs may be purchased without a prescription directly from a pharmacist if allowed under specific state statutes. Legal purchasing age is generally age 18 with valid identification. All such transactions and relevant personal information must be recorded by the dispensing pharmacist.

Abbreviations to avoid (The Joint Commission)

The Joint Commission requires every health care facility to develop a list of approved abbreviations for staff use. Certain abbreviations should be avoided because they're easily misunderstood, especially when handwritten. The Joint Commission has identified a minimum list of dangerous abbreviations, acronyms, and symbols. This do-not-use list includes the following items.

Official "Do Not Use" List[1]		
Do not use	**Potential problem**	**Use instead**
U, u (unit)	Mistaken for "0" (zero), the number "4" (four), or "cc"	Write "unit"
IU (International Unit)	Mistaken for "IV" (intravenous) or the number "10" (ten)	Write "International Unit"
Q.D., QD, q.d., qd (daily)	Mistaken for each other	Write "daily"
Q.O.D., QOD, q.o.d, qod (every other day)	Period after the Q mistaken for "I" and the "O" mistaken for "I"	Write "every other day"
Trailing zero (X.0 mg)* Lack of leading zero (.X mg)	Decimal point is missed	Write "X mg" Write "0.X mg"
MS	Can mean morphine sulfate or magnesium sulfate	Write "morphine sulfate"
MSO_4 and $MgSO_4$	Confused for one another	Write "magnesium sulfate"

[1]Applies to all orders and all medication-related documentation that is handwritten (including free-text computer entry) or on preprinted forms.

***Exception:** A "trailing zero" may be used only where required to demonstrate the level of precision of the value being reported, such as for laboratory results, imaging studies that report size of lesions, or catheter/tube size. It may not be used in medication orders or other medication-related documentation.

Additional Abbreviations, Acronyms, and Symbols
(For <u>possible</u> future inclusion in the Official "Do Not Use" List)

Do not use	**Potential problem**	**Use instead**
> (greater than) < (less than)	Misinterpreted as the number "7" (seven) or the letter "L" Confused for one another	Write "greater than" Write "less than"
Abbreviations for drug names	Misinterpreted due to similar abbreviations for multiple drugs	Write drug names in full
Apothecary units	Unfamiliar to many practitioners Confused with metric units	Use metric units
@	Mistaken for the number "2" (two)	Write "at"
cc	Mistaken for "U" (units) when poorly written	Write "mL" or "ml" or "milliliters" ("mL" is preferred)
μg	Mistaken for "mg" (milligrams) resulting in one thousand-fold overdose	Write "mcg" or "micrograms"

SOURCE: The Joint Commission: Information Management (IM) Standard IM.02.02.01. 2016 *Comprehensive Accreditation Manual for Hospitals.* Oakbrook Terrace, IL: The Joint Commission, 2016.

Pediatric drugs commonly involved in drug errors

According to The Joint Commission, the rate of medication errors for pediatric and adult inpatients is similar, but potentially harmful errors occur almost three times as frequently in children. One of the most common errors that occur in hospitalized children is administering the incorrect pediatric dosage. Here are some of the medications most commonly involved in medication errors as reported to the national voluntary medication error reporting system, MEDMARX, with their FDA-approved dosages.

Medication	Indication	Route	Usual dosage
albuterol sulfate	Bronchospasm in children with reversible obstructive airway disease	P.O. (immediate-release tablets and extended-release tablets)	• *Children older than age 12:* Initially, 2 or 4 mg (immediate-release tablets) P.O. t.i.d. or q.i.d. If patient fails to respond, may increase dosage to maximum of 8 mg P.O. q.i.d. Or, 8 mg (extended-release tablets) P.O. every 12 hours. If patient fails to respond, increase dosage cautiously to maximum of 16 mg P.O. every 12 hours. • *Children ages 6 to 12:* Initially, 2 mg (immediate-release tablets) P.O. t.i.d. or q.i.d. May increase dosage cautiously, but total daily dosage shouldn't exceed 24 mg/day (given in divided doses). Or, 4 mg (extended-release tablets) P.O. every 12 hours. If control of reversible airway isn't achieved with optimized asthma therapy, may cautiously increase dosage to maximum of 12 mg P.O. every 12 hours.
	Bronchospasm in children with reversible obstructive airway disease	P.O. (syrup)	• *Children older than age 14:* Initially, 2 mg (1 teaspoonful) or 4 mg (2 teaspoonfuls) P.O. t.i.d. or q.i.d. If patient fails to respond, dosage may be cautiously increased to maximum of 8 mg P.O. q.i.d. • *Children ages 6 to 14:* Initially, 2 mg (1 teaspoonful) P.O. t.i.d. or q.i.d. If patient fails to respond, dosage may be increased to maximum of 24 mg/day given in divided doses. • *Children ages 2 to younger than 6:* Initially, 0.1 mg/kg P.O. t.i.d. Initial dose shouldn't exceed 2 mg (1 teaspoonful) P.O. t.i.d. If patient fails to respond, may increase dosage to 0.2 mg/kg P.O. t.i.d. Maximum dosage is 4 mg (2 teaspoonfuls) P.O. t.i.d.

Medication	Indication	Route	Usual dosage
ceftriaxone sodium	Acute bacterial otitis media in children younger than age 12	I.M.	• *Children:* Give single dose of 50 mg/kg I.M. Maximum dosage is 1 g.
	Serious infections (including skin and skin-structure infections) other than meningitis	I.V. infusion over at least 30 minutes or I.M.	• *Children:* 50 to 75 mg/kg I.M. or I.V. once daily or in divided doses every 12 hours. Continue for at least 2 days after signs and symptoms of infection have disappeared. Usual duration of therapy is 4 to 14 days. Maximum dosage is 2 g/day.
	Meningitis	I.V. infusion over at least 30 minutes or I.M.	• *Children:* Initially, 100 mg/kg (not to exceed 4 g) I.M. or I.V. Thereafter, give total daily dose of 100 mg/kg/day I.M. or I.V. for 7 to 14 days. Maximum dosage is 4 g daily. Daily dose may be administered once a day or in equally divided doses every 12 hours.
fentanyl	To manage persistent, chronic pain only in opioid-tolerant patients (children receiving at least 60 mg/day of morphine P.O.)	Transdermal	• *Children age 2 and older:* When converting to transdermal system, base first dose on the daily dose, potency, and characteristics of the current opioid therapy; reliability of the relative potency estimates used to calculate the needed dose; degree of opioid tolerance; and patient's condition. Each patch is worn for 72 hours; dosage may be increased 3 days after first dose and then no sooner than every 6 days thereafter.
gentamicin sulfate	Serious infections caused by sensitive strains of *Pseudomonas aeruginosa, Escherichia coli, Proteus, Klebsiella, Serratia,* or *Staphylococcus*	I.V. infusion over 30 minutes to 2 hours or I.M.	• *Children:* 2 to 2.5 mg/kg I.V. or I.M. every 8 hours usually for 7 to 10 days. • *Infants and neonates:* 2.5 mg/kg I.V. or I.M. every 8 hours usually for 7 to 10 days. • *Premature or full-term neonates age 1 week or younger:* 2.5 mg/kg I.V. or I.M. every 12 hours usually for 7 to 10 days.
heparin sodium (unfractionated)	Thrombosis	I.V.	• *Children:* Initially, 75 to 100 units/kg I.V. bolus over 10 minutes, followed by continuous I.V. infusion of 25 to 30 units/kg/hour (infants) or 18 to 20 units/kg/hour (children older than age 1). Adjust dosage to maintain aPTT of 60 to 85 seconds.
vancomycin	Treatment of serious or severe infections caused by susceptible strains of methicillin-resistant (beta-lactam-resistant) staphylococci	I.V.	• *Children age 1 month and older:* 10 mg/kg/dose I.V. every 6 hours. Administer over at least 60 minutes.
	Treatment of serious or severe infections caused by susceptible strains of methicillin-resistant (beta-lactam-resistant) staphylococci	I.V.	• *Neonates:* Initially, 15 mg/kg I.V., followed by 10 mg/kg I.V. every 12 hours for neonates in the first week of life and every 8 hours thereafter up to the age of 1 month. Administer over 60 minutes. In premature infants, longer dosing intervals may be necessary.
	Pseudomembranous colitis or staphylococcal enterocolitis	P.O.	• *Children:* 40 mg/kg/day P.O. in three or four divided doses for 7 to 10 days. Maximum dosage is 2 g/day.

Elder care medication tips

Age-related changes can alter the way older people absorb, distribute, metabolize, and eliminate medications compared to younger adults or children. Medication dosages and routes may need adjustment to optimize the patient's response to medication and help prevent adverse reactions. Understanding how age-related factors can alter how an older patient's body uses medication will help you plan and implement your patient's medication regimen and monitor his response appropriately. The table below describes how age-related factors can change the pharmacokinetics of medications in older adults.

Pharmacokinetics	Age-related change	Effect on pharmacokinetics
Absorption	Diminished quality and quantity of digestive enzymes	▼
	Increased gastric pH	▲ or ▼
	Decreased GI motility and emptying time	▼
	Decreased GI blood flow	▼
	Diminished number of absorbing cells	▼
Distribution	Diminished cardiac output and reserve	▼
	Diminished blood flow to target organs and tissues	▼
	Decreased lean body mass	▼
	Increased adipose tissue	▲ or ▼
	Decreased circulating plasma proteins	▼
	Decreased total body water	▼
Metabolism	Decreased liver size	▼
	Diminished intestinal and portal vein blood flow	▼
Excretion	Decreased GFR	▼
	Decreased renal tubular secretion	▼
	Decreased renal blood flow from renovascular occlusive disease, microvascular nephropathy, or HF	▼

Prescription drug abuse: Identifying and treating toxicity

Prescription drugs have CNS effects that can be used or altered in order to achieve stimulant, euphoric, or mind-altering effects. Commonly used preparations (e.g., tablets and capsules) can be crushed, inhaled, or injected to produce quicker results. The table below lists commonly abused prescription drugs with examples of brand names, along with signs and symptoms of toxicity, potential adverse health effects, and treatment/reversal care. Not all drugs have reversal agents that can be used to rapidly counteract adverse effects. General supportive care measures (respiratory and cardiac function support and I.V. fluids) are needed to improve clinical outcomes when prescription drugs are abused.

Substance	Toxicity signs & symptoms	Possible health effects	Toxicity care and treatment
Anesthetics			
cocaine • Medical uses: topical (ENT) anesthesia • Generic/brand names: cocaine • Routes: inhalation (nasal/oral), injection	↑Increased HR, ↑BP, arrhythmias, chest pain, nosebleeds, vomiting, ↓appetite, dilated pupils, euphoria, insomnia, restlessness, anxiety, erratic behavior, paranoia, seizures	MI, stroke, cardiomyopathy, coma, ↑HIV risk from shared needles, ↓birth weight/premature delivery (if used during pregnancy), psychosis	General supportive care; seizure control with I.V. benzodiazepines (e.g., diazepam, lorazepam). Dialysis and hemoperfusion are ineffective.
propofol • Medical uses: general anesthesia/sedation • Generic/brand names: propofol (Diprivan) • Routes: injection	Hyperthermia, ↓HR, ↓BP, ↑LFTs, nausea, vomiting, itching, wheezing, hypoxia, ↓consciousness, stupor, anxiety, confusion, delirium, seizures	HF, metabolic acidosis, pancreatitis, liver damage, renal failure, respiratory depression, ↑HIV risk from shared needles	General supportive care; seizure control with I.V. benzodiazepines (e.g., diazepam, lorazepam). May consider hemofiltration for metabolic acidosis. Monitor urine output (urine may be rusty, tea-colored, or green/olive).
ketamine • Medical uses: anesthesia, analgesia, sedation • Generic/brand names: ketamine (Ketalar) • Routes: injection, inhalation (nasal/oral)	↑HR, ↑BP, ↓respiratory rate, dysuria, diplopia, nystagmus, abnormal dreams, ↓consciousness, hallucinations, dysphoria, sedation, confusion, inability to speak, ↓coordination, seizures	Renal impairment, bladder dysfunction, depression, loss of memory, ↑HIV risk from shared needles	General supportive care; seizure control with I.V. benzodiazepines (e.g., diazepam, lorazepam)

(continued)

Substance	Toxicity signs & symptoms	Possible health effects	Toxicity care and treatment
Opioid analgesics			
• Medical uses: pain treatment • Generic/brand names: codeine, fentanyl (Duragesic), hydrocodone bitartrate–acetaminophen (Norco), hydromorphone hydrochloride (Dilaudid), meperidine (Demerol), methadone hydrochloride (Methadose), morphine sulfate (MS Contin), oxycodone hydrochloride (Roxicodone), oxycodone hydrochloride–acetaminophen (Percocet), oxycodone–aspirin (Percodan), oxymorphone hydrochloride (Opana), tapentadol (Nucynta), tramadol hydrochloride (Ultram) • Routes: oral, inhalation (nasal), injection	↓BP, ↓HR, ↓respiratory rate, nausea, vomiting, constipation, drowsiness, euphoria, sedation, seizures	Apnea, hypoxia, coma, CNS depression, respiratory depression, liver function abnormality/liver damage (associated with long-term acetaminophen use), death	General supportive care; seizure control with I.V. benzodiazepines (e.g., diazepam, lorazepam). Naloxone is the preferred reversal agent for opioids. Activated charcoal isn't recommended due to risk of CNS depression and aspiration.
Stimulants			
Amphetamines • Medical uses: ADHD, narcolepsy • Generic/brand names: dextroamphetamine (Dexedrine), amphetamine–dextroamphetamine (Adderall XR), lisdexamfetamine (Vyvanse) • Routes: oral, inhalation (nasal/oral), injection	Hyperthermia, ↑HR, ↑BP, arrhythmias, palpitations, chest pain, diaphoresis, flushing, paranoia, agitation, abnormal behavior, seizures	HF, MI, psychosis, renal/hepatic failure, serotonin syndrome, coma, ↑HIV risk from shared needles	General supportive care; seizure control with I.V. benzodiazepines (e.g., diazepam, lorazepam). Consider activated charcoal (most effective within 1 hour of toxic ingestion); dialysis and hemoperfusion are ineffective.
methylphenidate • Medical uses: ADHD, narcolepsy • Generic/brand names: methylphenidate (Ritalin LA/SR) • Routes: oral, inhalation (nasal/oral), injection	Hyperthermia, ↑HR, ↑BP, arrhythmias, palpitations, chest pain, diaphoresis, flushing, nausea, headache, tremor, paranoia, agitation, abnormal behavior, seizures, serotonin syndrome	HF, MI, pulmonary hypertension, psychosis, renal/hepatic failure, coma, ↑HIV risk from shared needles, sudden death	General supportive care; seizure control with I.V. benzodiazepines (e.g., diazepam, lorazepam). Consider activated charcoal (most effective within 1 hour of toxic ingestion); dialysis and hemoperfusion are ineffective.
Sedatives			
Barbiturates • Medical uses: sedation, seizures, hypnotic • Generic/brand names: pentobarbital (Nembutal) • Routes: oral, injection	Hypothermia, ↓BP, ↓respiratory rate, ↓reflexes, drowsiness, slurred speech, nystagmus, confusion, ataxia	Respiratory failure, CV collapse, coma	General supportive care. Activated charcoal, urine alkalinization, hemoperfusion/hemofiltration, and dialysis have all been used with some success to increase elimination of barbiturates.

Substance	Toxicity signs & symptoms	Possible health effects	Toxicity care and treatment

Sedatives (continued)

Benzodiazepines • Medical uses: alcohol withdrawal, anxiety/panic disorder, insomnia, preoperative/moderate sedation, seizure disorder • Generic/brand names: alprazolam (Xanax), chlordiazepoxide (Librium), clonazepam (Klonopin), diazepam (Valium), lorazepam (Ativan), oxazepam, temazepam (Restoril), midazolam, triazolam (Halcion) • Routes: oral, injection	Hypothermia, ↓BP, ↓respiratory rate, sedation, confusion, slurred speech, ataxia	Metabolic acidosis (from propylene glycol diluent used in Valium and Ativan injection preparations), respiratory failure, coma, rhabdomyolysis	General supportive care. Consider activated charcoal (most effective within 1 hour of toxic oral ingestion); hemodialysis and forced/enhanced diuresis are ineffective. Flumazenil is the reversal agent for benzodiazepines.
Sleep drugs • Medical uses: insomnia • Generic/brand names: zolpidem (Ambien CR), zaleplon (Sonata), eszopiclone (Lunesta) • Routes: oral	↓BP, ↓respiratory rate, nausea, vomiting, abdominal pain, dizziness, confusion, ↓coordination, delusions, headache, sleep-eating/sleep-driving, slurred speech, somnolence	Respiratory depression, CV collapse, coma	General supportive care. Consider activated charcoal (most effective within 1 hour of toxic oral ingestion); hemodialysis is ineffective.

Miscellaneous drugs

Cannabinoids • Medical uses: treatment of nausea/vomiting, appetite stimulant, epilepsy • Generic/brand names: nabilone (Cesamet), dronabinol (Marinol) • Routes: oral, inhalation (oral), injection (rare)	Lethargy, ataxia, muscle tremors, pulmonary irritation, sore throat, rhinitis, coughing, mydriasis, somnolence, euphoria, depersonalization, alteration of time sense, loss of social inhibition, mood alterations	• Oral: significant altered mental status, hypotonia, coma • Injection (extract or oil): shock, DIC, rhabdomyolysis, acute renal failure, death	General supportive care; seizure control with I.V. benzodiazepines (e.g., diazepam, lorazepam). Absorption/elimination techniques (e.g., activated charcoal, hemodialysis, hemoperfusion, urine alkalinization) are ineffective.
Anabolic steroids • Medical uses: breast cancer, delayed puberty, hypogonadism • Generic/brand names: testosterone cypionate/enanthate (Aveed), oxandrolone (Oxandrin), oxymetholone (Anadrol) • Routes: oral, injection	↑BP, acne, fluid retention, ↑lipid levels, jaundice, tendon rupture, breast enlargement (men), male-pattern baldness, changes in sex organs, infertility, libido changes, rage, aggression, mania, delusions, insomnia	Short stature, MI, hepatitis, hepatic tumors, hepatic failure, thrombosis, stroke, ↑HIV risk from shared needles	General supportive care. Absorption/elimination techniques (e.g., activated charcoal, hemodialysis, hemoperfusion, urine alkalinization) are ineffective.

Understanding biosimilar drugs

What are nonbiologic drug products and how are they approved?

Most drugs on the market are nonbiologic drugs, which are made from chemicals with known structures that can be identically re-created. Brand-name nonbiologic drugs are first approved by the FDA through a New Drug Application approval process that requires evidence of safety and effectiveness of the drug, the quality of the product, and the accuracy of its labeling. Pharmaceutical companies file for patents or exclusive marketing rights with the FDA for each drug.

Once these patents expire, other pharmaceutical companies can manufacture the brand-name nonbiologic drug by making an identical (bioequivalent), less expensive, generic formulation (called an "innovator drug" by the FDA) of the same brand-name drug. Generic formulations are less expensive because the pharmaceutical companies file for an Abbreviated New Drug Application (ANDA) approval process, which doesn't require the pharmaceutical company to perform clinical trials and submit evidence of safety and effectiveness of the generic drug. The FDA's *Approved Drug Products with Therapeutic Equivalence Evaluations* (also known as the Orange Book) contains all of the FDA-approved drugs and identifies which drugs are therapeutically equivalent. If drugs are deemed therapeutically equivalent, a less costly drug may be able to be substituted for a higher-cost drug.

What are biological drug products?

In contrast to conventional drug products, which are pure chemical substances, biological drugs are made from living organisms (human or animal cells or tissues, proteins, microorganisms), and their manufacturing processes are more complex than those for conventional drugs and are also proprietary. Examples of biological products include vaccines, blood and blood products, and recombinant therapeutic proteins. Biological drugs work by targeting a certain biological structure, enzyme, pathway, or other mechanism; for example, they may change the way the immune system reacts to a virus or change cells and proteins involved in inflammation.

What are biosimilar drugs and how are they approved?

Just as nonbiologic drugs have brand-name and generic forms, biological drugs have brand-name and biosimilar drugs. Unlike generic drugs, which are chemical replicas of the original brand-name drug, biosimilar drugs are similar to but not exact duplicates of the brand-name drug (biological reference product) because they are made from tissues and other nonchemical components. Each pharmaceutical company must demonstrate that its biosimilar drug is highly similar to a biological reference product that has already been FDA-approved. According to the FDA, biosimilar drugs must demonstrate they have "no clinically meaningful differences in terms of safety and effectiveness from the reference product. Minor differences in clinically inactive components are allowed."

As with nonbiologic drugs, brand-name biological drugs are approved by the FDA through a biologics license application, which requires evidence of safety, purity, potency, and effectiveness of the biological drug.

An abbreviated licensure pathway for biological products is described in The Patient Protection and Affordable Care Act (Affordable Care Act) of 2010. Similar to the ANDA approval process, biological drugs have an abbreviated licensure pathway for biological products that are demonstrated to be "biosimilar" to or "interchangeable" with an FDA-licensed biological product. The Biologics Price Competition and Innovation Act (BPCI Act), part of the Affordable Care Act, provides this licensure pathway. According to the BPCI Act, an interchangeable biological drug may be substituted for the reference product by a pharmacist without the consultation or intervention of the prescriber.

Similar to the Orange Book for nonbiologic drugs, the FDA's *Lists of Licensed Biological Products with Reference Product Exclusivity and Biosimilarity or Interchangeability Evaluations* (also known as the Purple Book) states whether a biological product has been determined by the FDA to be biosimilar to or interchangeable with a biological reference product.

Why are biosimilar drugs important?

The FDA is expected to approve an increasing number of biosimilar drugs, as these drugs are expected to compete with each other in the medical marketplace and decrease consumer costs. The first approved biosimilar drug, Zarxio, cost 15% less than its biological reference drug, Neupogen. Some pharmaceutical companies have embraced the new technology of biosimilar drugs and have a pipeline of biosimilar drugs in the development or approval stage. Just like generics, biosimilar drugs can be made by more than one pharmaceutical company, thereby increasing competition and hopefully lowering overall health care costs.

What is important to know about biosimilar and biological reference drugs?

Biosimilarity is based on the product being highly similar to the biological reference product as determined by toxicity studies in animals and one or more clinical studies demonstrating the safety, purity, and potency of the product.

Biosimilar drugs:
• may be approved for the same or fewer indications as the biological reference drug. The number of approved indications may not exceed the number of approved indications for the reference drug.
• must have the same mechanism of action, route of administration, dosage forms, and strength as the reference drug.
• are expected to have no differences in safety and effectiveness compared to the reference drug.

How are biosimilar drug names determined?

Biological products and their biosimilar drugs share a nonproprietary name (also referred to as a "proper name"). Biosimilar drugs use the nonproprietary name plus a suffix composed of four lowercase letters.

These four letters represent the name of the pharmaceutical company that holds the biosimilar drug's licensing agreement. On March 6, 2015, the FDA approved the very first biosimilar drug, which is named filgrastim-sndz (Zarxio); Zarxio is licensed by the Sandoz Company. It's a biosimilar drug to the biological reference product filgrastim (Neupogen).

Nursing process: Patient safety during drug therapy

Drug therapy is a complex process that can easily lead to adverse patient events. In 2007, the Institute of Medicine (IOM) released its report on the drug safety system, *The Future of Drug Safety: Promoting and Protecting the Health of the Public.* The IOM reported that approximately 400,000 preventable adverse drug events occurred each year in the United States. The IOM also estimated that preventable hospital medication errors occurred at a rate of one/patient/day and contributed to 7,000 patient deaths/year. Although much progress has been made, problems with using medications safely remain. Medication errors are one of the top 10 most frequently reviewed sentinel events by The Joint Commission. Applying the nursing process (assessment, nursing diagnosis, planning, intervention, and evaluation) during drug therapy enables the nurse to systematically identify the drug therapy needs of each patient, thereby reducing the number of adverse events and providing safe patient care.

Nursing process step	Key points

Assessment	• Collect data—subjective and objective
	  ○ Current/previous health status
	  ○ Cultural considerations
	  ○ Lab values
	  ○ Allergies
	  ○ Physical assessment
	  ○ Medication history
	    ■ Prescriptions/OTCs
	    ■ Herbal supplements
	    ■ Response to medications
	    ■ Knowledge of medications.

Nursing diagnosis/problem	• Identify all associated nursing diagnoses.
Planning	• Review prescribed medications. • Identify possible adverse effects of medications. • Identify potential interactions with other medications. • Determine route of administration. • Determine time of administration. • Develop patient education regarding medication administration. • Review patient allergies.

Intervention	• Administer medication utilizing the "eight rights"
	  ○ Right patient
	  ○ Right drug
	  ○ Right dose
	  ○ Right time
	  ○ Right route
	  ○ Right reason
	  ○ Right response
	  ○ Right documentation.
	• Educate patient about each medication at time of administration.

Evaluation	• Monitor patient's response to medication. • Monitor for possible adverse effects of medication. • Monitor for unexpected effects of medication. • Document medication administration.

Serotonin syndrome: What you should know to protect your patient

Serotonin is a neurotransmitter involved in the conduction of nerve impulses. Serotonin syndrome is a drug reaction resulting from an increase in plasma serotonin levels and can range in severity from mild to life-threatening to fatal. It occurs when drugs that affect serotonin levels are given together, causing serotonin levels to rise. Serotonin syndrome can occur within minutes or hours of drug administration and may cause acute respiratory distress syndrome, DIC, liver and renal failure, rhabdomyolysis, intractable myoclonus, and seizures. Identifying the symptoms and initiating prompt treatment can prevent a potentially fatal outcome. Some drugs commonly associated with serotonin syndrome include SSRIs (fluoxetine), SSNRIs (duloxetine), MAO inhibitors (phenelzine), opiates (methadone), antiemetics (ondansetron), antibiotics (linezolid), antiretrovirals (ritonavir), dextromethorphan, and dietary supplements (St. John's wort).

Key points	What you need to know or do
Risk factors	• Coadministration of medications that affect serotonin levels • Overdose of medications that affect serotonin levels
Signs and symptoms	• Agitation, restlessness, mental status changes, hallucinations • Headache, muscle pain • Loss of muscle coordination, muscle rigidity, seizures, muscle spasms, tremor • Fever, shivering, goose bumps, hypertension, tachycardia, arrhythmia • Profound diaphoresis • Nausea, vomiting, diarrhea
Preventive measures	• Review medication history and drug therapy for potential interactions. • Identify patients at risk for serotonin syndrome. • Perform thorough baseline assessment.
Monitoring	• Monitor patient's condition closely. • Monitor temperature, HR (continuous cardiac monitoring), BP, fluid status, and urine output frequently. • Monitor oxygenation, mental status, and pain levels. • Monitor serum serotonin levels. • Monitor electrolyte and CK levels.
Treatment and interventions	• Discontinue drugs associated with serotonin syndrome. • Administer oxygen therapy, ventilation, and paralytics (succinylcholine chloride) as needed to maintain adequate ventilation. • Institute cooling measures (i.e., cooling baths) for fever. • Administer I.V. fluids to maintain hydration. • Administer medications to block serotonin production (antihistamines [cyproheptadine hydrochloride]), to control seizures and myoclonus (benzodiazepines [diazepam]), and to control hypertension (nitroprusside), tachycardia (beta blockers [esmolol]), and pain (opioids if needed).

Tumor lysis syndrome: A life-threatening emergency

Tumor lysis syndrome (TLS) is a potentially life-threatening oncologic emergency caused by a rapid and massive breakdown of tumor cells, either immediately or within 48 to 72 hours after chemotherapy administration. The release of tumor cell debris into the bloodstream causes an array of metabolic disturbances, such as hyperkalemia, hyperphosphatemia, hyperuricemia, and hypocalcemia, which can lead to seizures, acute kidney injury, fluid overload, cardiac arrhythmias, cardiopulmonary arrest, and death. TLS is associated with treatment for acute leukemias, chronic lymphocytic leukemia, non-Hodgkin lymphomas such as Burkitt lymphoma, small-cell lung cancer, testicular cancer, rhabdomyosarcoma, neuroblastoma, and breast cancer and with the use of such chemotherapeutic drugs as paclitaxel, fludarabine, etoposide, bortezomib, zoledronic acid, and hydroxyurea.

Key considerations	What you need to know or do
Risk factors	• Disease with high tumor-cell proliferation rate • Chemosensitivity of the malignancy, bulky tumor, or extensive metastasis; organ infiltration; bone marrow involvement • Pretreatment hyperuricemia, elevated LDH levels, renal insufficiency, nephrotoxic drugs
Signs and symptoms	• Lethargy, syncope, seizures, altered mental state • HF, arrhythmias, sudden death • Edema, weight gain, fluid overload • Renal failure, metabolic acidosis, decreased or absent urine output, urine sediment, flank pain, hematuria • Anorexia, nausea, vomiting, constipation, diarrhea • Muscle cramping, tetany • Hyperkalemia, hypocalcemia, hyperphosphatemia, hyperuricemia
Preventive measures	• Identify at-risk patients as soon as possible. • Obtain central venous access. • Obtain baseline ECG, vital signs, and hemodynamic status. • Administer I.V. hydration to improve renal perfusion and GFR. • Administer sodium bicarbonate for metabolic acidosis and to promote alkaline urine diuresis. • Administer pretreatment hypouricemics (allopurinol or rasburicase). • Avoid potassium-sparing diuretics.
Treatment and monitoring	• Monitor mental status. • Monitor respiratory status and oxygenation. Administer oxygen therapy as prescribed. • Institute continuous cardiac monitoring. • Closely monitor vital signs and fluid volume status (fluid intake, urine output, weight, edema). • Monitor serial electrolytes, acid-base balance, BUN, creatinine, and uric acid levels every 4 to 6 hours. Monitor calcium, phosphate, and LDH levels. Correct abnormalities. • Monitor fluid volume and administer diuretics. • Administer low-dose dopamine to increase renal perfusion. • Possible renal replacement therapy or hemodialysis may be needed.

Antidiarrheals: Indications and dosages

Refer to manufacturer's instructions for complete prescribing and safety information.

bismuth subsalicylate
BIS-mith sub-sal-LISS-so-late

Bismatrol ◊, Diotame ◊, Kaopectate ◊, Kao-Tin ◊, Peptic Relief ◊, Pepto-Bismol ◊, Pink Bismuth ◊, Stomach Relief ◊, Stomak-care❧ ◊

Therapeutic class: Antidiarrheals
Pharmacologic class: Adsorbents

AVAILABLE FORMS
Caplets ⓄⓉⒸ: 262 mg ◊
Oral suspension: 262 mg/15 mL (regular strength), 525 mg/15 mL (maximum strength)
Tablets (chewable): 262 mg ◊

INDICATIONS & DOSAGES
➤ **Mild, nonspecific diarrhea; gas, indigestion, heartburn, nausea**
Adults and children age 12 and older: 525 mg P.O. every 30 to 60 minutes or 1,050 mg P.O. every 60 minutes as needed for up to 2 days. Maximum, 4,200 mg/24 hours.

crofelemer
kro-FEL-e-mer

Fulyzaq

Therapeutic class: Antidiarrheals
Pharmacologic class: Antidiarrheals

AVAILABLE FORMS
Tablets (delayed-release) ⓄⓉⒸ: 125 mg

INDICATIONS & DOSAGES
➤ **Noninfectious diarrhea in patients with HIV/AIDS on antiretroviral therapy**
Adults: 125 mg P.O. b.i.d.

diphenoxylate hydrochloride–atropine sulfate
dye-fen-OKS-ul-ate/A-troe-peen

Lomotil*

Therapeutic class: Antidiarrheals
Pharmacologic class: Opioids
Controlled substance schedule: V

AVAILABLE FORMS
Liquid: 2.5 mg/5 mL (with atropine sulfate 0.025 mg/5 mL)*
Tablets: 2.5 mg (with atropine sulfate 0.025 mg)

INDICATIONS & DOSAGES
➤ **Acute, nonspecific diarrhea**
Adults and children older than age 12: Initially, 5 mg P.O. q.i.d.; reduce dosage as soon as initial control of symptoms is achieved. Maximum dosage, 20 mg/day.
Children ages 2 to 12: 0.3 to 0.4 mg/kg liquid form P.O. daily in four divided doses. For maintenance, reduce dose when initial control of symptoms is achieved. Dosage may be reduced by as much as 75%. Maximum, 10 mg/day.

loperamide hydrochloride
loe-PER-a-mide

Diamode ◊, Imodium A-D ◊

Therapeutic class: Antidiarrheals
Pharmacologic class: Piperidine derivatives

AVAILABLE FORMS
Capsules: 2 mg
Oral liquid: 1 mg/5 mL ◊, 1 mg/7.5 mL ◊
Tablets: 2 mg ◊
Tablets (chewable): 2 mg ◊

INDICATIONS & DOSAGES
Black Box Warning Use of higher-than-recommended doses can cause death. Capsules are contraindicated in children younger than age 2. ∎
➤ **Acute, nonspecific diarrhea; reducing volume of discharge from ileostomies**
Adults and children older than age 12: Initially, give 4 mg P.O.; then 2 mg after each unformed stool. Maximum, 16 mg/day (prescription strength) or 8 mg/day (OTC) unless otherwise directed.
Children ages 8 to 12 weighing more than 30 kg: 2 mg P.O. t.i.d. on first day. Maximum, 6 mg daily. If diarrhea persists, contact prescriber.
Children ages 6 to younger than 8 weighing 20 to 30 kg: 2 mg P.O. b.i.d. on first day. If diarrhea persists, contact prescriber. Maximum, 4 mg daily.
Children ages 2 to 5 weighing 13 to 20 kg: 1 mg P.O. t.i.d. for first day. After first day, give 1 mg/10 kg body weight only after a loose stool. Maximum, 3 mg/day.
➤ **Chronic diarrhea associated with inflammatory bowel disease**
Adults: Initially, 4 mg P.O.; then 2 mg after each unformed stool until diarrhea subsides. Adjust dosage to individual response. Maximum, 16 mg/day (prescription strength).
➤ **Traveler's diarrhea**
Adults: 4 mg P.O. followed by 2 mg after each unformed stool for a maximum of 16 mg/day (prescription strength).

Antidotes: Indications and dosages

Refer to manufacturer's instructions for complete prescribing and safety information.

activated charcoal

Actidose-Aqua ◇, Actidose with Sorbitol ◇, Char-Flo with Sorbitol ◇, Charac-25 ✤◇, Charactol-25 ✤◇, Charcodote TFS ✤◇, Kerr Insta-Char ◇

Therapeutic class: Antidotes
Pharmacologic class: Adsorbents

AVAILABLE FORMS
Capsules: 260 mg ◇
Liquid: 15 g ◇*, 25 g ◇*, 50 g ◇*
Oral suspension: 15 g ◇, 25 g ◇

INDICATIONS & DOSAGES
➤Poisoning
Adults and children age 13 and older weighing more than 32 kg: 50 to 60 g (sorbitol base) P.O.
Children ages 1 to 12 weighing 16 to less than 32 kg: 25 to 30 g P.O. (sorbitol base).
Adults and children older than age 1: 5 to 60 g P.O. (aqueous base). Dosage should be 10 times by volume the amount of poison ingested, if known. If amount of poison ingested isn't known, a dosage of at least 20 to 30 g should be given.

deferasirox
deh-fir-A-si-rocks
Exjade, Jadenu

Therapeutic class: Chelating agents
Pharmacologic class: Heavy metal antagonists

AVAILABLE FORMS
Tablets: 90 mg, 180 mg, 360 mg
Tablets for oral suspension ⒹⓈⒸ 125 mg, 250 mg, 500 mg

INDICATIONS & DOSAGES
Black Box Warning Drug can cause fatal renal failure, hepatic failure, and GI hemorrhage. Monitor patient carefully. ∎
*Adjust-a-dose (for all indications):*When converting therapy from Exjade to Jadenu, the dose of Jadenu should be approximately 30% lower (rounded to the nearest whole tablet) than the current dose of Exjade.

Contraindicated in patients with serum creatinine level greater than 2 × the age-appropriate ULN or CrCl less than 40 mL/minute. Discontinue drug if necessary. Start elderly patients at low end of dosing range. Avoid use in patients with severe (Child-Pugh class C) hepatic impairment. Reduce starting dose by 50% in patients with moderate (Child-Pugh class B) hepatic impairment. Closely monitor all patients with mild (Child-Pugh class A) or moderate hepatic impairment for effectiveness and adverse reactions.
➤Chronic iron overload caused by blood transfusions (transfusional hemosiderosis)
Adults and children age 2 and older: Exjade: Initially, 20 mg/kg P.O. daily on an empty stomach 30 minutes before eating. Monitor serum ferritin level monthly, and adjust dose every 3 to 6 months by 5 or 10 mg/kg based on ferritin trends. Don't exceed 40 mg/kg daily. Consider stopping therapy if serum ferritin level drops below 500 mcg/L.

Jadenu: Initially, 14 mg/kg P.O. once daily on an empty stomach or with a light meal. Monitor serum ferritin level monthly, and adjust dose every 3 to 6 months by increments of 3.5 or 7 mg/kg, based on serum ferritin trends. Don't exceed 28 mg/kg. Consider stopping therapy if serum ferritin level drops below 500 mcg/L.
*Adjust-a-dose:*For adults and adolescents age 16 and older with serum creatinine level more than 33% above average baseline seen at two consecutive visits within 1 week that isn't attributable to other causes, decrease daily dosage by 10 mg/kg of Exjade or 7 mg/kg of Jadenu. For children ages 2 to 15 with serum creatinine level more than 33% above average baseline measurement and greater than the age-appropriate ULN, decrease dosage by 10 mg/kg of Exjade or 7 mg/kg of Jadenu.
➤Chronic iron overload in patients with non-transfusion-dependent thalassemia syndromes and with a liver iron (Fe) concentration (LIC) of at least 5 mg Fe per gram of dry weight (dw) and a serum ferritin level greater than 300 mcg/L
Adults and children age 10 and older: Exjade: Initially, 10 mg/kg P.O. once daily. Calculate dose to the nearest whole tablet. If baseline LIC is greater than 15 mg Fe/g dw, may increase to 20 mg/kg/day after 4 weeks. Interrupt treatment when serum ferritin level is less than 300 mcg/L, and obtain LIC to determine if LIC is less than 3 mg Fe/g dw. If LIC remains greater than 7 mg Fe/g dw after 6 months of therapy, increase dosage to maximum of 20 mg/kg/day. If LIC is 3 to 7 mg Fe/g dw after 6 months, continue treatment at maximum of 10 mg/kg/day. If LIC is less than 3 mg Fe/g dw, stop treatment. Continue to monitor LIC, and restart treatment when LIC rises again to more than 5 mg Fe/g dw.

Jadenu: Initially, 7 mg/kg P.O. once daily. Calculate dose to the nearest whole tablet. If baseline LIC is greater than 15 mg Fe/g dw, may increase to 14 mg/kg/day after 4 weeks. Interrupt treatment when serum ferritin level is less than 300 mcg/L, and obtain LIC to determine if LIC is less than 3 mg Fe/g dw. If LIC remains greater than 7 mg Fe/g dw after 6 months of therapy, increase dosage to maximum of 14 mg/kg/day. If LIC is 3 to 7 mg Fe/g dw after 6 months, continue treatment at maximum of 7 mg/kg/day. If LIC is less than 3 mg Fe/g dw, stop treatment. Continue to monitor LIC and restart treatment when LIC rises again to more than 5 mg Fe/g dw.

Adjust-a-dose: For adults and adolescents age 16 and older: If serum creatinine level increases by 33% or more above the average baseline measurement, repeat serum creatinine within 1 week and, if still elevated by 33% or more, interrupt Exjade therapy if dose is 5 mg/kg, or reduce by 50% if dose is 10 or 20 mg/kg; interrupt Jadenu therapy if the dose is 3.5 mg/kg, or reduce by 50% if the dose is 7 or 14 mg/kg. For children ages 10 to 15: Reduce Exjade dose by 5 mg/kg or Jadenu dose by 3.5 mg/kg if serum creatinine level increases to greater than 33% above the average baseline measurement and greater than the age-appropriate ULN.

deferiprone
de-FER-i-prone

Ferriprox

Therapeutic class: Chelating drugs
Pharmacologic class: Heavy metal antagonists

AVAILABLE FORMS
Solution: 100 mg/mL
Tablets: 500 mg

INDICATIONS & DOSAGES
Black Box Warning Drug can cause agranulocytosis that can lead to serious infections and death. Measure ANC before therapy and weekly during therapy. Interrupt therapy for neutropenia or infection. ∎
➤**Treatment of transfusional iron overload due to thalassemia syndromes when current chelation therapy is inadequate**
Adults: Initially, 25 mg/kg P.O. t.i.d. for a total of 75 mg/kg/day. May titrate to maximum dosage of 33 mg/kg t.i.d. for a total of 99 mg/kg/day based on patient response and therapeutic goals. Round dose to nearest 250 mg (half tablet).
Adjust-a-dose: Withhold drug for ANC less than 1,500/mm^3 or if serum ferritin level is consistently below 500 mcg/L.

digoxin immune Fab (ovine)
di-JOX-in

DigiFab

Therapeutic class: Antidotes
Pharmacologic class: Antibody fragments

AVAILABLE FORMS
Injection: 40-mg vial

INDICATIONS & DOSAGES
➤**Life-threatening digoxin toxicity**
Adults and children: Base dosage on ingested amount or level of digoxin. When calculating amount of antidote, round up to the nearest whole number. For digoxin tablets, calculate number of antidote vials as

follows: multiply ingested amount by 0.8; then divide answer by 0.5. For example, if patient takes 25 tablets of 0.25 mg digoxin, the ingested amount is 6.25 mg. Multiply 6.25 mg by 0.8 and divide answer by 0.5 to obtain 10 vials of antidote. If digoxin level is known, determine the number of antidote vials as follows: multiply the digoxin level in nanograms per milliliter by patient's weight in kilograms; then divide by 100.
➤**Acute toxicity or if estimated ingested amount or digoxin level is unknown**
Adults and children: Consider giving 10 vials of digoxin immune Fab and observing patient's response. Follow with another 10 vials if indicated. Dosage should be effective in most life-threatening cases in adults and children but may cause volume overload in young children.

dimercaprol
dye-mer-KAP-rawl

BAL in Oil

Therapeutic class: Chelating drugs
Pharmacologic class: Heavy metal antagonists

AVAILABLE FORMS
Injection: 100 mg/mL

INDICATIONS & DOSAGES
➤**Severe arsenic or gold poisoning**
Adults and children: 3 mg/kg deep I.M. every 4 hours for 2 days; then q.i.d. on third day; then b.i.d. for 10 days.
➤**Mild arsenic or gold poisoning**
Adults and children: 2.5 mg/kg deep I.M. q.i.d. for 2 days; then b.i.d. on third day; then once daily for 10 days.
➤**Mercury poisoning**
Adults and children: Initially, 5 mg/kg deep I.M.; then 2.5 mg/kg daily or b.i.d. for 10 days.
➤**Acute lead encephalopathy or lead level greater than 100 mcg/mL**
Adults and children: 4 mg/kg given alone by deep I.M.; then every 4 hours with edetate calcium disodium administered at a separate site for 2 to 7 days. For less severe poisoning, reduce dose to 3 mg/kg after first dose.

doxapram hydrochloride
DOCKS-a-pram

Dopram

Therapeutic class: CNS stimulants
Pharmacologic class: Analeptics

AVAILABLE FORMS
Injection: 20 mg/mL (benzyl alcohol 0.9%)

INDICATIONS & DOSAGES
➤ **Postanesthesia respiratory stimulation**
Adults: 0.5 to 1 mg/kg as a single I.V. injection (not to exceed 1.5 mg/kg) or as multiple injections every 5 minutes, total not to exceed 2 mg/kg or 3 g daily. Or, 250 mg in 250 mL of NSS or D_5W infused at initial rate of 5 mg/minute I.V. until satisfactory response is achieved. Maintain at 1 to 3 mg/minute. Don't exceed total dose for infusion of 4 mg/kg or 3 g daily.
➤ **Drug-induced CNS depression**
Adults: For injection, priming dose of 1 to 2 mg/kg I.V., repeated in 5 minutes and again every 1 to 2 hours until patient awakens (and if relapse occurs). Maximum daily dose is 3 g.

For infusion, priming dose of 1 to 2 mg/kg I.V., repeated in 5 minutes and again in 1 to 2 hours, if needed. If response occurs, give I.V. infusion (1 mg/mL) at 1 to 3 mg/minute until patient awakens. Don't infuse for longer than 2 hours or give more than 3 g/day. May resume I.V. infusion after rest period of 30 minutes to 2 hours, if needed.
➤ **COPD related to acute hypercapnia**
Adults: 1 to 2 mg/minute by I.V. infusion using 2 mg/mL solution. Maximum, 3 mg/minute. Don't infuse for longer than 2 hours.

---

edetate calcium disodium
ED-e-tate

Calcium Disodium Versenate

Therapeutic class: Chelating drugs
Pharmacologic class: Heavy metal antagonists

AVAILABLE FORMS
Injection: 200 mg/mL

INDICATIONS & DOSAGES
Black Box Warning Toxic effects of drug can be fatal. Never exceed the recommended daily dosage. ■
➤ **Acute lead encephalopathy or lead level greater than 70 mcg/dL**
Adults and children: Use in conjunction with dimercaprol. Consult published protocols and specialized references for dosage recommendations.
➤ **Lead poisoning without encephalopathy or asymptomatic with lead level less than 70 mcg/dL but greater than 20 mcg/dL**
Adults and children: 1 g/m²/day I.V. infused over 8 to 12 hours once daily or 1 g/m² I.M. daily in divided doses spaced 8 to 12 hours apart for 5 days. Or, for adults with lead nephropathy, give as follows: If serum creatinine level is 2 to 3 mg/dL, give 500 mg/m² every 24 hours for 5 days; if serum creatinine level is 3 to 4 mg/dL, give 500 mg/m² every 48 hours for three doses; if serum creatinine level is more than 4 mg/dL, give 500 mg/m² once weekly.

---

flumazenil
floo-MAZ-eh-nill

Therapeutic class: Antidotes
Pharmacologic class: Benzodiazepine antagonists

AVAILABLE FORMS
Injection: 0.1 mg/mL in 5-mL and 10-mL multiple-dose vials

INDICATIONS & DOSAGES
Black Box Warning Seizures can occur, and precautions are recommended. ■
➤ **Complete or partial reversal of sedative effects of benzodiazepines after anesthesia or conscious sedation**
Adults: Initially, 0.2 mg I.V. over 15 seconds. If patient doesn't reach desired level of consciousness after 45 seconds, give 0.2 mg and repeat at 1-minute intervals to a maximum total dose of 1 mg.
Children age 1 year and older: 0.01 mg/kg (up to 0.2 mg) I.V. over 15 seconds. If patient doesn't reach desired level of consciousness after 45 seconds, repeat dose. Repeat at 1-minute intervals, if needed, until cumulative dose of 0.05 mg/kg or 1 mg, whichever is lower, has been given.
➤ **Suspected benzodiazepine overdose**
Adults: Initially, 0.2 mg I.V. over 30 seconds. If patient doesn't reach desired level of consciousness after 30 seconds, give 0.3 mg over 30 seconds. If patient still doesn't respond adequately, give 0.5 mg over 30 seconds. Repeat 0.5-mg doses, as needed, at 1-minute intervals until cumulative dose of 3 mg has been given. Most patients with benzodiazepine overdose respond to cumulative doses between 1 and 3 mg; rarely, patients who respond partially after 3 mg may need additional doses, up to 5 mg total. If patient doesn't respond in 5 minutes after receiving 5 mg, sedation is unlikely to be caused by benzodiazepines. In case of resedation, dosage may be repeated after 20 minutes, but never give more than 1 mg at any one time or exceed 3 mg in any 1 hour.

---

glucarpidase
gloo-CAR-pi-daze

Voraxaze

Therapeutic class: Antidotes
Pharmacologic class: Recombinant bacterial enzymes

AVAILABLE FORMS
Powder for injection: 1,000 units/vial

INDICATIONS & DOSAGES
➤ **Methotrexate toxicity (more than 1 micromole/L) in patients with impaired renal function**
Adults and children age 1 month and older: 50 units/kg as a single I.V. injection over 5 minutes.

---

lanthanum carbonate
LAN-thah-num

Fosrenol

Therapeutic class: Antihyperphosphatemics
Pharmacologic class: Non-calcium, non-aluminum phosphate binders

AVAILABLE FORMS
Oral powder: 750 mg, 1,000 mg
Tablets (chewable): 500 mg, 750 mg, 1 g

INDICATIONS & DOSAGES
➤ **To reduce phosphate level in patients with ESRD**
Adults: Initially, 500 mg P.O. t.i.d. with meals. Adjust every 2 to 3 weeks by 750 mg daily until reaching desired phosphate level. Reducing phosphate level to less than 6 mg/dL usually requires 1,500 to 3,000 mg daily. Maximum daily dose is 4,500 mg.

naloxegol oxalate
nal-OX-ee-gol

Movantik

Therapeutic class: Antidotes
Pharmacologic class: Opioid antagonists
Controlled substance schedule: II

AVAILABLE FORMS
Tablets Ⓓ: 12.5 mg, 25 mg

INDICATIONS & DOSAGES
➤ **Opioid-induced constipation in patients with chronic noncancer pain**
Adults: 25 mg P.O. once daily in the morning.
Adjust-a-dose: For CrCl of less than 60 mL/minute, decrease starting dose to 12.5 mg; if tolerated, may increase to 25 mg if needed. If use with CYP3A4 inhibitors is necessary, decrease dosage to 12.5 mg daily.

naloxone hydrochloride
nal-OX-one

Evzio

Therapeutic class: Antidotes
Pharmacologic class: Opioid antagonists

AVAILABLE FORMS
Injection: 0.4 mg/mL, 1 mg/mL
Nasal spray: 4 mg/0.1 mL
Prefilled auto-injector: 0.4 mg/0.4 mL

INDICATIONS & DOSAGES
➤ **Known or suspected opioid-induced respiratory depression, including that caused by pentazocine, methadone, nalbuphine, and butorphanol**
Adults: 0.4 to 2 mg I.V., I.M., or subcutaneously. Repeat dose every 2 to 3 minutes, p.r.n. If patient doesn't respond after 10 mg have been given, question

diagnosis of opioid-induced toxicity. After reversal, additional dose(s) may be needed at a later interval (e.g., 20 to 60 minutes) depending on type and duration of opioid. May also give via endotracheal tube at 2 to 2.5 times initial I.V. dose (e.g., 0.8 to 5 mg).
Children age 1 month and older: 0.01 mg/kg I.V.; then, second dose of 0.1 mg/kg I.V., if needed. If I.V. route isn't available, drug may be given I.M. or subcutaneously in divided doses.
Neonates: 0.01 mg/kg I.V., I.M., or subcutaneously. Repeat dose every 2 to 3 minutes, p.r.n.
➤ **Postoperative opioid depression**
Adults: 0.1 to 0.2 mg I.V. every 2 to 3 minutes, p.r.n. Repeat doses may be required within 1- or 2-hour intervals depending on amount, type (short- or long-acting), and time interval since last administration. Supplemental I.M. doses have produced a longer-lasting effect.
➤ **Emergency treatment of known or suspected opioid overdose**
Adults and children: 0.4 mg I.M. or subcutaneously or one spray of nasal spray into one nostril. If desired response isn't obtained after 2 or 3 minutes, may give another dose. If there is still no response and additional doses are available, give 0.4 mg I.M. or subcutaneously or one spray of nasal spray every 2 or 3 minutes until emergency medical assistance arrives.

phentolamine mesylate
fen-TOLE-a-meen

OraVerse, Regitine, Rogitine ✢

Therapeutic class: Antihypertensives
Pharmacologic class: Alpha blockers

AVAILABLE FORMS
Injection: 0.4 mg/1.7 mL, 5 mg/mL, 10 mg/mL ✢

INDICATIONS & DOSAGES
➤ **To aid in diagnosis of pheochromocytoma, to control or prevent hypertension before or during pheochromocytomectomy (except OraVerse)**
Adults: I.V. or I.M. diagnostic dose is 5 mg with close monitoring of BP. Give 5 mg I.V. or I.M. 1 to 2 hours before surgical removal of tumor. During surgery, patient may need an additional 5 mg I.V.
Children: I.V. diagnostic dose is 1 mg, and I.M. diagnostic dose is 3 mg with close monitoring of BP. Give 1 mg I.V. or I.M. 1 to 2 hours before surgical removal of tumor. During surgery, patient may need an additional 1 mg I.V.
➤ **To prevent dermal necrosis from norepinephrine extravasation (except OraVerse)**
Adults: Add 10 mg of phentolamine to each liter of solution containing norepinephrine; the pressor effect of norepinephrine is unaffected.
➤ **Dermal necrosis and sloughing after I.V. extravasation of norepinephrine or dopamine (except OraVerse)**
Adults: Infiltrate area with 5 to 10 mg phentolamine in 10 mL of NSS within 12 hours of extravasation.

➤ **Reversal of soft-tissue anesthesia (OraVerse only)**
Adults and children age 6 and older weighing more than 30 kg: Dosage depends on amount of anesthetic used. Refer to manufacturer's instructions.

pralidoxime chloride (2-PAM chloride, 2-pyridine-aldoxime methochloride)
pra-li-DOX-eem

Protopam Chloride

Therapeutic class: Antidotes
Pharmacologic class: Quaternary ammonium oximes

AVAILABLE FORMS
Injection: 1 g/20 mL in 20-mL vial
Injection (for I.M. use): 300 mg/mL

INDICATIONS & DOSAGES
➤ **Antidote for organophosphate poisoning in combination with atropine**
Adults: 1 to 2 g in 100 mL of NSS by I.V. infusion over 15 to 30 minutes. If not practical or if pulmonary edema is present, give dose as a 5% solution in sterile water by slow I.V. push over at least 5 minutes. Repeat in 1 hour if muscle weakness persists. Additional doses may be given cautiously. I.M. or subcutaneous injection may be used if I.V. isn't feasible

For I.M. dosing: *For mild symptoms,* give 600 mg (2 mL) I.M. Wait 15 minutes; if symptoms persist, give a second dose. A third dose may be given after an additional 15 minutes. If at any time after the first dose patient develops severe symptoms, give two additional 600-mg doses in rapid succession for a total cumulative dose of 1,800 mg. *For severe symptoms,* give three 600-mg doses (three doses of 2 mL each) in rapid succession. If symptoms persist after the complete 1,800-mg regimen (three injections of 600 mg each), the series may be repeated beginning approximately 1 hour after the last injection.
Children age 16 and younger (I.V. dosing): Give loading dose of 20 to 50 mg/kg (maximum 2 g) I.V. over 15 to 30 minutes, followed by 10 to 20 mg/kg/hour by continuous I.V. infusion. Or, give initial dose of 20 to 50 mg/kg I.V. over 15 to 30 minutes, then give second dose of 20 to 50 mg/kg I.V. in 1 hour if muscle weakness persists. May repeat dose every 10 to 12 hours p.r.n. Maximum is 2 g/dose. Or, if pulmonary edema is present or it isn't practical to give intermittent or continuous I.V. infusions, give dose of 20 to 50 mg/kg as 50-mg/mL solution in water by I.V. push slowly over 5 minutes. If muscle weakness persists, additional doses may be given every 10 to 12 hours.
Children age 16 and younger with mild symptoms who weigh 40 kg or more (I.M. dosing): Give 600 mg I.M. If symptoms persist after 15 minutes, give second dose of 600 mg I.M. If symptoms persist 15 minutes after second dose, give third dose of 600 mg I.M. Maximum combined dose for three injections is 1,800 mg. If patient develops severe symptoms at any time after

first dose, administer second and third doses in rapid succession. For severe symptoms, give all three doses of 600 mg I.M. each in rapid succession for total combined dose of 1,800 mg.
Children age 16 and younger with mild symptoms who weigh less than 40 kg (I.M. dosing): Give 15 mg/kg I.M. in anterolateral thigh. If symptoms persist after 15 minutes, give second dose of 15 mg/kg I.M. If symptoms persist after second dose, give third dose of 15 mg/kg I.M. If patient develops severe symptoms at any time after first dose, give second and third doses in rapid succession. For severe symptoms, give all three doses of 15 mg/kg I.M. each in rapid succession. Maximum combined dose for three injections is 45 mg/kg.
➤ **Cholinergic crisis in myasthenia gravis**
Adults: 1 to 2 g I.V.; then 250 mg I.V. every 5 minutes, p.r.n.

protamine sulfate
PROE-ta-meen

Therapeutic class: Antidotes
Pharmacologic class: Heparin antagonists

AVAILABLE FORMS
Injection: 10 mg/mL

INDICATIONS & DOSAGES
Black Box Warning Drug can cause severe hypotension, CV collapse, noncardiogenic pulmonary edema, catastrophic pulmonary vasoconstriction, and pulmonary hypertension. Keep vasopressors and resuscitation equipment immediately available. ■
➤ **Heparin overdose**
Adults: Base dosage on venous blood coagulation studies; usually 1 mg neutralizes not less than 100 units of heparin. Give by slow I.V. injection over 10 minutes in doses not to exceed 50 mg.

sodium polystyrene sulfonate
pol-ee-STYE-reen

Kalexate, Kayexalate, Kionex, SPS

Therapeutic class: Potassium-removing resins
Pharmacologic class: Cation-exchange resins

AVAILABLE FORMS
Powder: 1-lb jar (3.5 g/tsp)
Suspension: 15 g/60 mL*

INDICATIONS & DOSAGES
➤ **Hyperkalemia**
Adults: 15 g P.O. daily to q.i.d. in water or syrup (3 to 4 mL/g of resin). Or, mix powder with appropriate medium—aqueous suspension or diet appropriate for renal failure—and instill through NG tube. Or, 30 to 50 g in 100 mL of an aqueous vehicle every 6 hours as warm emulsion (at body temperature) deep into sigmoid colon (20 cm).

succimer
SUX-i-mer

Chemet

Therapeutic class: Chelating drugs
Pharmacologic class: Heavy metal chelators

AVAILABLE FORMS
Capsules: 100 mg

INDICATIONS & DOSAGES
➤ **Lead poisoning in children with lead levels greater than 45 mcg/dL**
Children age 12 months and older: Initially, 10 mg/kg or 350 mg/m^2 P.O. every 8 hours for 5 days. Then reduce to 10 mg/kg or 350 mg/m^2 P.O. every 12 hours for additional 14 days.

Selected biologicals and blood derivatives: Indications and dosages

albumin 5%
al-BYOO-min

Albuked-5, Albuminar-5, AlbuRx 5%, Albutein 5%, Buminate 5%, Flexbumin 5%, Plasbumin-5

albumin 25%
Albuked-25, Albuminar-25, Albutein 25%, Buminate 25%, Flexbumin 25%, Kedbumin 25%, Plasbumin-25

Therapeutic class: Plasma volume expanders
Pharmacologic class: Blood derivatives

AVAILABLE FORMS
albumin 5%
Injection: 50 mg/mL in 50-mL, 250-mL, 500-mL, 1,000-mL vials
albumin 25%
Injection: 250 mg/mL in 20-mL, 50-mL, 100-mL vials

INDICATIONS & DOSAGES
➤ **Hypovolemic shock**
Adults: Initially, 12.5 to 25 g (250 to 500 mL) of 5% solution by I.V. infusion, repeated every 15 to 30 minutes, as needed. As plasma volume approaches normal, rate of infusion of 5% solution shouldn't exceed 2 to 4 mL/minute. Dosage of 25% solution varies with patient's condition and response. As plasma volume approaches normal, rate of infusion of 25% solution shouldn't exceed 1 mL/minute.
Infants and younger children: Initially, 0.5 to 1 g/kg/dose I.V. (10 to 20 mL/kg/dose of albumin 5%); repeat in 30-minute intervals as needed.
Older children and adolescents: Initially, 12.5 to 25 g I.V. (250 to 500 mL of albumin 5%); repeat in 30-minute intervals as needed.
➤ **Burns**
Adults: 25% solution infused no faster than 2 to 3 mL/minute to maintain plasma albumin concentration at approximately 2.5 ± 0.5 g/100 mL with a plasma oncotic pressure of 20 mm Hg (equal to a total plasma protein concentration of 5.2 g/100 mL). The duration of therapy is determined by the loss of protein from burned areas and in the urine.
➤ **Hypoproteinemia**
Adults: 200 to 300 mL of 25% albumin. Dosage varies with patient's condition and response. Usual daily dose is 50 to 75 g. Rate of infusion shouldn't exceed 2 mL/minute.

Children: Usual daily dosage is 25 g or 25% albumin. Rate of infusion shouldn't exceed 2 mL/minute.
➤ **Acute nephrosis**
Adults: 100 mL of 25% albumin daily for 7 to 10 days in combination with a loop diuretic.
➤ **Neonatal hemolytic disease**
Children: 1 g/kg body weight of 25% albumin I.V. before or during exchange transfusion.

antihemophilic factor (AHF factor VIII)
Advate, Adynovate, Eloctate, Helixate FS, Hemofil M, Koate-DVI, Kogenate FS, Kovaltry, Monoclate-P, Novoeight, Nuwiq, Obizur, Recombinate, ReFacto, Xyntha

Therapeutic class: Clotting factors
Pharmacologic class: Plasma proteins

AVAILABLE FORMS
Injection: Vials, with diluent; units specified on label

INDICATIONS & DOSAGES
Drug provides hemostasis in factor VIII deficiency, hemophilia A. Specific dosage depends on patient's weight, severity of hemorrhage, and presence of inhibitors. Mild bleeding episodes require a circulating factor VIII level 20% to 40% of normal; moderate to major bleeding episodes and minor surgery, a level 30% to 60% of normal; severe bleeding or major surgery, a level 60% to 100% of normal depending on product used. Refer to specific brand for actual dosage.

anti-inhibitor coagulant complex
Feiba, Feiba NF✜

Therapeutic class: Clotting factors
Pharmacologic class: Plasma proteins

AVAILABLE FORMS
Black Box Warning Thrombotic and thromboembolic events have been reported during postmarketing surveillance. ■
Injection: Number of units of factor VIII correctional activity indicated on label of vial

INDICATIONS & DOSAGES
➤ **To prevent or control hemorrhagic episodes in some patients with hemophilia A and B in whom inhibitor antibodies to antihemophilic factor have**

developed; to manage bleeding in patients with acquired hemophilia who have spontaneously acquired inhibitors to factor VIII, XI, and XII
Adults and children: Drug controls hemorrhage in hemophilia A patients who have a factor VIII inhibitor level above 10 Bethesda units. Patients with a level of 5 to 10 Bethesda units may receive the drug if they have severe hemorrhage or respond poorly to factor VIII infusion.
Adults and children age 31 days and older: Dosage is highly individualized and varies among manufacturers. Maximum daily dose is 200 units/kg/day. Maximum infusion rate is 2 units/kg/minute.
➤ **Joint hemorrhage**
Adults and children age 31 days and older: 50 to 100 units/kg I.V. every 12 hours until patient's condition improves.
➤ **Mucous membrane hemorrhage**
Adults and children age 31 days and older: 50 units/kg I.V. every 6 hours, increasing to 100 units/kg every 6 hours if hemorrhage continues.
➤ **Soft-tissue hemorrhage**
Adults and children age 31 days and older: 100 units/kg I.V. every 12 hours. Maximum daily dose, 200 units/kg.
➤ **Other severe hemorrhage**
Adults and children age 31 days and older: 100 units/kg I.V. every 6 to 12 hours.
➤ **Perioperative management**
Adults and children age 31 days and older: 50 to 100 units/kg I.V. immediately before surgery. For postoperative management, give 50 to 100 units/kg I.V. every 6 to 12 hours.
➤ **Routine prophylaxis**
Adults and children age 31 days and older: 85 units/kg I.V. every other day.

beractant (natural lung surfactant)
ber-AK-tant

Survanta

Therapeutic class: Lung surfactants
Pharmacologic class: Bovine lung extracts

AVAILABLE FORMS
Suspension for intratracheal instillation: 25 mg/mL

INDICATIONS & DOSAGES
➤ **To prevent respiratory distress syndrome (RDS), also known as hyaline membrane disease, in premature neonates weighing 1,250 g (2 lb, 12 oz) or less at birth or having symptoms consistent with surfactant deficiency**
Neonates: 4 mL/kg intratracheally. Divide each dose into four quarter-doses and give each quarter-dose with infant in a different position to ensure even distribution of drug; between quarter-doses, use a handheld resuscitation bag at 60 breaths/minute and suffi-

cient oxygen to prevent cyanosis. Give drug as soon as possible, preferably within 15 minutes of birth. Repeat in 6 hours if respiratory distress continues. Give no more than four doses in 48 hours.
➤ **Rescue treatment of RDS in premature infants**
Neonates: 4 mL/kg intratracheally; before giving, increase ventilator rate to 60 breaths/minute with an inspiratory time of 0.5 second and a fraction of inspired oxygen of 1. Divide each dose into four quarter-doses and give each quarter-dose with infant in a different position to ensure even distribution of drug; between quarter doses, continue mechanical ventilation for at least 30 seconds or until stable. Give dose as soon as RDS is confirmed by X-ray, preferably within 8 hours of birth. Repeat in 6 hours if respiratory distress continues. Give no more than four doses in 48 hours.

calfactant
kal-FAK-tant

Infasurf

Therapeutic class: Lung surfactants
Pharmacologic class: Bovine lung extracts

AVAILABLE FORMS
Intratracheal suspension: 35 mg phospholipids and 0.7 mg proteins/mL in 3-mL, 6-mL vials

INDICATIONS & DOSAGES
➤ **To prevent respiratory distress syndrome (RDS) in premature infants younger than 29 weeks' gestational age at high risk for RDS; to treat infants younger than age 72 hours who develop RDS (confirmed by clinical and radiologic findings) and need an endotracheal tube**
Neonates: 3 mL/kg of body weight at birth intratracheally, given in two aliquots of 1.5 mL/kg each, every 12 hours for a total of up to three doses.

eltrombopag
ell-trom-BOW-pag

Promacta

Therapeutic class: Hematopoietics
Pharmacologic class: Thrombopoietin receptor agonists

AVAILABLE FORMS
Powder for oral suspension: 25-mg packet
Tablets: 12.5 mg, 25 mg, 50 mg, 75 mg, 100 mg

INDICATIONS & DOSAGES
Black Box Warning Drug increases risk of hepatotoxicity when used for HCV. Consult prescribing information for specific monitoring guidelines. ∎
➤ **Thrombocytopenia associated with chronic immune thrombocytopenic purpura when response to**

corticosteroids, immunoglobulins, or splenectomy is inadequate

Adults and children age 6 and older: Initially, 50 mg P.O. once daily.

Children ages 1 to 5: Initially, 25 mg P.O. once daily.

Adjust-a-dose: Adjust dosage as necessary to achieve and maintain platelet count at 50×10^9/L or greater; maximum dosage is 75 mg daily. For patients older than age 6 and of East Asian descent or those with mild, moderate, or severe hepatic impairment, reduce dosage to 25 mg once daily. For patients of East Asian descent and any hepatic impairment, reduce dosage to 12.5 mg once daily. Refer to manufacturer's instructions for dosage adjustments based on hematologic parameters.

➤ **Thrombocytopenia in patients with chronic HCV infection to allow use of interferon-based therapy**

Adults: Initially, 25 mg P.O. once daily. Increase by 25-mg increments every 2 weeks as necessary to achieve target platelet count required to initiate antiviral therapy. Maximum dose is 100 mg daily.

Adjust-a-dose: During antiviral therapy, adjust dosage to avoid dose reduction of peginterferon. Refer to manufacturer's instruction for dosage adjustments based on hematologic parameters. Discontinue drug when antiviral treatment is stopped.

➤ **Severe aplastic anemia when response to immunosuppressive therapy is insufficient**

Adults: Initially, 50 mg P.O. once daily. Adjust dosage as necessary in 50-mg increments every 2 weeks to achieve target platelet count of 50×10^9/L or greater. Maximum dosage is 150 mg daily.

Adjust-a-dose: In patients of East Asian descent or those with mild, moderate, or severe hepatic impairment, reduce initial dosage to 25 mg once daily. Refer to manufacturer's instructions for dosage adjustments based on hematologic parameters.

If no hematologic response has occurred after 16 weeks of therapy, or new cytogenetic abnormalities are observed, discontinue drug.

factor IX complex
Bebulin VH, Profilnine SD

factor IX (human)
AlphaNine SD, Mononine

factor IX (recombinant)
Alprolix, BeneFIX, Ixinity, Rixubis

Therapeutic class: Clotting factors
Pharmacologic class: Plasma proteins

AVAILABLE FORMS
Injection: Vials, with diluent; international units specified on label

INDICATIONS & DOSAGES
➤ **Factor IX deficiency (also called hemophilia B or Christmas disease), anticoagulant overdose**

Adults and children: To calculate international units of factor IX needed, use the following equations:

Human product

$$\text{1 international unit/kg} \times \text{body weight in kg} \times \text{percentage of desired increase of factor IX level}$$

Recombinant product

$$\text{reciprocal of observed recovery (units/kg per units/dL)} \times \text{body weight in kg} \times \text{percentage of desired increase of factor IX level}$$

Infusion rates vary with product and patient comfort. Dosage is highly individualized, depending on degree of deficiency, level of factor IX desired, patient weight, and severity of bleeding.

hepatitis B immune globulin (human)
hep-ah-TYE-tis

HepaGam B, HyperHEP BS/D, Nabi-HB

Therapeutic class: Prophylaxis drugs
Pharmacologic class: Immune serums

AVAILABLE FORMS
Injection: 1-mL, 5-mL vials; 0.5-mL neonatal single-dose syringe; 1-mL single-dose syringe

INDICATIONS & DOSAGES
➤ **HBV exposure in high-risk patients**

Adults and children: 0.06 mL/kg (usual dose is 3 to 5 mL) I.M. as soon as possible (within 24 hours if possible) but within 7 days after exposure (within 14 days if sexual exposure). Repeat dose 28 days after exposure if patient doesn't elect to receive the hepatitis B vaccine.

Neonates born to hepatitis B surface antigen (HBsAg)-positive patients: 0.5 mL I.M. within 12 hours of birth. Active vaccination with hepatitis B vaccine may begin at the same time.

➤ **To prevent recurrence of HBV infection after liver transplantation in HBsAg-positive liver transplant patients (HepaGam B only)**

Adults: 20,000 international units I.V. at rate of 2 mL/minute. Give first dose simultaneously with the grafting of the transplanted liver (anhepatic phase); then give daily on days 1 through 7, every 2 weeks from day 14 through 12 weeks, and monthly from month 4 onward.

Adjust-a-dose: Adjust dosage in patients who don't reach anti-HBs levels of 500 international units/L within the first week after transplantation. Give 10,000 international units I.V. until target level is reached.

immune globulin intramuscular (gamma globulin, IG, IGIM)
GamaSTAN S/D

immune globulin intravenous (IGIV)
Bivigam, Carimune NF, Flebogamma DIF, Gammagard Liquid, Gammagard S/D, Gammaked, Gammaplex, Gamunex-C, Octagam, Privigen

immune globulin subcutaneous (IGSC, SCIG)
Gammagard, Gamunex-C, Hizentra, HyQvia

Therapeutic class: Antibodies
Pharmacologic class: Immune serums

AVAILABLE FORMS
immune globulin intramuscular
Injection: 15% to 18% in 2-mL, 10-mL single-dose vials
immune globulin intravenous
Powder for injection (preservative free): 2.5-g, 3-g, 5-g, 6-g, 10-g, 12-g vials
Solution, injection (preservative free): 5% in 10-mL, 25-mL, 50-mL, 100-mL, 200-mL, 400-mL, 500-mL vials; 10% in 10-mL, 20-mL, 50-mL, 100-mL, 200-mL, 300-mL, 400-mL vials
immune globulin subcutaneous
Solution, injection (kit): 10% in 25-mL, 50-mL, 200-mL, 300-mL vials
Solution, injection (preservative free): 20% in 5-mL, 10-mL, 20-mL, 50-mL vials.

INDICATIONS & DOSAGES
Black Box Warning Increases risk of thrombosis; don't exceed recommended dose. ■
➤ **Primary immunodeficiency**
Bivigam
Adults and children age 6 and older: 300 to 800 mg/kg I.V. every 3 to 4 weeks. Begin I.V. infusion at a rate of 0.5 mg/kg/minute for the first 10 minutes. Increase every 20 minutes, if tolerated, by 0.8 mg/kg/minute, up to a maximum rate of 6 mg/kg/minute.
Carimune NF
Adults and children: 400 to 800 mg/kg I.V. every 3 to 4 weeks. First infusion in previously untreated patients must be given as a 3% immunoglobulin solution at initial infusion rate of 0.5 mg/kg/minute. If tolerated, after 30 minutes the rate may be increased to 1 mg/kg/minute for the next 30 minutes, then gradually increased in a stepwise manner up to a maximum of 3 mg/kg/minute as tolerated. See package insert for infusion rates in mL/kg/minute.

Flebogamma DIF
Adults: 300 to 600 mg/kg I.V. every 3 to 4 weeks. Infuse 5% solution at 0.5 mg/kg/minute and increase after 30 minutes to 5 mg/kg/minute.
Gammagard Liquid
Adults and children age 2 and older: 300 to 600 mg/kg I.V. every 3 to 4 weeks. Infuse at 0.8 mg/kg/minute and increase every 30 minutes to 8 mg/kg/minute. Maintenance therapy may be given subcutaneously starting 1 week after last IGIV infusion. Initial subcutaneous dose is 1.37 × current I.V. dose in mg/kg ÷ number of weeks between I.V. doses.
Gammagard S/D
Adults and children age 2 and older: 300 to 600 mg/kg I.V. every 3 to 4 weeks depending on patient response, initially infused in a 5% solution at 0.5 mL/kg/hour that may be increased gradually if patient doesn't experience distress to a maximum rate of 4 mL/kg/hour for patients with no history of adverse reactions to IGIV and no significant risk factors for renal dysfunction or thrombotic complications. See package insert for subsequent solution concentration and infusion-rate increases.
Gammaked
Adults, children, and adolescents: 300 to 600 mg/kg I.V. every 3 to 4 weeks. Initially (first 30 minutes), 1 mg/kg/minute (0.6 mL/kg/hour), increased gradually (if tolerated) up to 8 mg/kg/minute (4.8 mL/kg/hour). Maintenance therapy may be given subcutaneously starting 1 week after last IGIV infusion. Initial subcutaneous dose is 1.37 × current I.V. dose in mg/kg ÷ number of weeks between I.V. doses.
Gammaplex
Adults: 300 to 800 mg/kg I.V. every 3 to 4 weeks. Initially (first 15 minutes), 0.5 mg/kg/minute (0.6 mL/kg/hour), increased every 15 minutes (if tolerated) up to 4 mg/kg/minute (4.8 mL/kg/hour).
Gamunex-C
Adults: 300 to 600 mg/kg I.V. every 3 to 4 weeks. Maintenance therapy may be given subcutaneously starting 1 week after last IGIV infusion. Initial subcutaneous dose is 1.37 × current I.V. dose in mg/kg ÷ number of weeks between I.V. doses.
Hizentra
Adults and children: Initial weekly dose is the previous IGIV dose in grams ÷ number of weeks between IGIV doses × 1.37.
  When switching to biweekly dosing, multiply the calculated Hizentra weekly dose by 2. Adjust dose based on clinical response and IgG trough levels to goal of 1.3 times trough level before last IGIV treatment. Give by subcutaneous infusion weekly. See package insert for full dosage adjustment guidelines. Infusion shouldn't exceed 25 mL/hour per site.
HyQvia
Adults: See manufacturer's labeling for initial ramp-up schedule.
Patients naive to IgG therapy or switching from IG subcutaneous therapy: 300 to 600 mg/kg subcutaneous infusion every 3 to 4 weeks, after the initial dose ramp-up.

Patients switching from IGIV therapy: Administer the same dose and frequency as the previous IGIV therapy by subcutaneous infusion every 3 to 4 weeks after the initial dose ramp-up. For subsequent dose adjustments, refer to manufacturer's instructions.

Octagam (5%)
Adults and children age 6 and older: 300 to 600 mg/kg I.V. every 3 to 4 weeks. Start infusion at 30 mg/kg/hour for 30 minutes.

Privigen
Adults: 200 to 800 mg/kg I.V. every 3 to 4 weeks. Start infusion at 0.5 mg/kg/minute and increase slowly to 8 mg/kg/minute.

➤ **Chronic inflammatory demyelinating polyneuropathy**
Gamunex-C, Gammaked
Adults: 2,000 mg/kg I.V. in divided doses over 2 to 4 days every 3 weeks. Or, 1,000 mg/kg I.V. over 1 day every 3 weeks or 500 mg/kg I.V. on 2 consecutive days every 3 weeks.

➤ **ITP**
Carimune NF
Adults and children: 400 mg/kg I.V. for 2 to 5 consecutive days, depending on platelet count and immune response.

Gammagard S/D
Adults: 1,000 mg/kg I.V. May give up to three separate doses on alternate days, if needed, as determined by clinical response and platelet count.

Gamunex-C, Gammaked
Adults: 2,000 mg/kg I.V. in divided doses over 2 days or 400 mg/kg I.V. in five doses over 5 days.

Octagam (10%)
Adults: 1,000 mg/kg/day for 2 consecutive days. Administer total dose of 2 g/kg, divided into two doses of 1 g/kg given on 2 consecutive days.

Privigen
Adults: 1,000 mg/kg I.V. for 2 days.

➤ **Multifocal motor neuropathy**
Gammagard Liquid
Adults: 500 to 2,400 mg/kg/month I.V. based on response.

➤ **Kawasaki syndrome**
Children: 400 mg/kg I.V. daily over 2 hours for 4 consecutive days, or a single dose of 1,000 mg/kg over 10 hours. Start within 10 days of disease onset. Give with aspirin (100 mg/kg P.O. daily through day 14; then 3 to 5 mg/kg P.O. daily for 5 weeks).

➤ **Hepatitis A exposure (IGIM)**
Adults and children: 0.02 mL/kg I.M. as soon as possible after exposure. Up to 0.06 mL/kg may be given for prolonged or intense exposure.

➤ **Measles exposure (IGIM)**
Adults and children: 0.25 mL/kg I.M. within 6 days after exposure.

➤ **Measles postexposure prophylaxis (IGIM)**
Immunocompromised children: 0.5 mL/kg I.M. (maximum 15 mL) immediately after exposure.

➤ **Chickenpox exposure (IGIM)**
Adults and children: 0.6 to 1.2 mL/kg I.M. as soon as possible after exposure.

➤ **Rubella exposure in first trimester of pregnancy (IGIM)**
Women: 0.55 mL/kg I.M. as soon as possible after exposure (within 72 hours).

➤ **B-cell chronic lymphocytic leukemia**
Adults and children: 400 mg/kg I.V. Gammagard S/D every 3 to 4 weeks for patients with hypogammaglobulinemia or recurrent bacterial infections.

➤ **Guillain-Barré syndrome (IGIV) ◆**
Adults: 2,000 mg/kg I.V. over 2 to 5 days within 2 to 4 weeks of onset.
Children: 2,000 mg/kg I.V. over 2 days within 2 to 4 weeks of onset.

lymphocyte immune globulin (antithymocyte globulin [equine], ATG, LIG)
LIM-foh-site

Atgam

Therapeutic class: Immunosuppressants
Pharmacologic class: Immunoglobulins

AVAILABLE FORMS
Injection: 50 mg of equine IgG/mL in 5-mL ampules

INDICATIONS & DOSAGES
Black Box Warning Drug can cause anaphylaxis. Only use drug in facilities with adequate laboratory and supportive medical resources. ■

➤ **Acute renal allograft rejection**
Adults and children: 10 to 15 mg/kg I.V. daily for 14 days. Additional alternate-day therapy to total of 21 doses can be given. Start therapy when rejection is diagnosed.

➤ **Aplastic anemia**
Adults and children: 10 to 20 mg/kg I.V. daily for 8 to 14 days. Additional alternate-day therapy to total of 21 doses can be given.

plasma protein fractions
Plasmanate, Plasma-Plex, Protenate

Therapeutic class: Plasma volume expanders
Pharmacologic class: Plasma proteins

AVAILABLE FORMS
Injection: 5% (50 mg/mL) solution in 50-mL, 250-mL, 500-mL vials

INDICATIONS & DOSAGES
➤ **Shock**
Adults: Dosage varies with patient's condition and response, but usual dosage is 250 to 500 mL I.V. (12.5 to 25 g protein), usually no faster than 10 mL/minute.

protein C concentrate
Ceprotin

Therapeutic class: Anticoagulants
Pharmacologic class: Protein C
replacements

AVAILABLE FORMS
Vials: 500 international units, 1,000 international units

INDICATIONS & DOSAGES
Adjust-a-dose (for all indications): Dose is adjusted based on severity of protein C deficiency, plasma level of protein C, and patient's age and condition.
➤ **Venous thrombosis and purpura fulminans in patients with severe congenital protein C deficiency**
Adults, neonates, and pediatric patients: Initially for acute episodes and short-term prophylaxis, 100 to 120 international units/kg I.V.; then, 60 to 80 international units/kg I.V. every 6 hours for subsequent three doses to maintain peak protein C activity of 100%. Maintenance dose of 45 to 60 international units/kg I.V. every 6 to 12 hours to maintain trough protein C activity levels above 25%.
➤ **Long-term prevention of venous thrombosis and purpura fulminans**
Adults, neonates, and pediatric patients: 45 to 60 international units/kg I.V. every 12 hours to maintain trough protein C activity levels above 25%.

rabies immune globulin (human)
RAY-beez

HyperRAB S/D, Imogam Rabies-HT

Therapeutic class: Antibodies
Pharmacologic class: Immunoglobulins

AVAILABLE FORMS
Injection: 150 international units/mL in 2-mL, 10-mL vials

INDICATIONS & DOSAGES
➤ **Rabies exposure**
Adults and children: 20 international units/kg I.M. at time of first dose of rabies vaccine. If anatomically feasible, up to the full dose is used to infiltrate wound area; remainder is given I.M. in a different site.

Rho(D) immune globulin intramuscular (human) (IGIM)
HyperRHO S/D Full Dose, HyperRHO S/D Mini-Dose, MICRhoGAM, RhoGAM

Rho(D) immune globulin intravenous (human) (IGIV)
Rhophylac, WinRho SDF

Therapeutic class: Immune globulins
Pharmacologic class: Immunoglobulins

AVAILABLE FORMS
IGIM
Injection: 300 mcg vial (standard dose); 50 mcg vial (microdose)
IGIV
Injection: 120-mcg (600 international units), 300-mcg (1,500 international units), 500-mcg (2,500 international units), 1,000-mcg (5,000 international units), 3,000-mcg (15,000 international units) vials

INDICATIONS & DOSAGES
Black Box Warning Intravascular hemolysis leading to acute respiratory distress syndrome and death has been reported in patients treated for ITP with IGIV. ■
➤ **Rh exposure after abortion, miscarriage, ectopic pregnancy, or childbirth**
Adults: Transfusion unit or blood bank determines fetal packed RBC volume entering patient's blood; one vial IGIM is given I.M. if fetal packed RBC volume is less than 15 mL. More than one vial I.M. may be needed if severe fetomaternal hemorrhage occurs; must be given within 72 hours after delivery or miscarriage.
➤ **To prevent Rh antibody formation after abortion or miscarriage**
Adults: Consult transfusion unit or blood bank. Up to and including 12 weeks' gestation, one IGIM microdose vial I.M. will suppress immune reaction to 2.5 mL Rho(D)-positive RBCs. At 13 weeks' gestation and later, use one vial IGIM standard dose. Ideally, give within 3 hours, but may be given up to 72 hours after abortion or miscarriage.
➤ **Rh exposure after abortion, amniocentesis after 34 weeks' gestation, or other manipulations past 34 weeks' gestation with increased risk of Rh isoimmunization**
Adults: 120 mcg IGIV, given I.V. or I.M. within 72 hours of delivery, miscarriage, or manipulation.
➤ **To suppress Rh isoimmunization during pregnancy**
Adults: 300 mcg I.V. or I.M. at 28 weeks' gestation. If given early in pregnancy, give additional doses at 12-week intervals to maintain adequate levels of passively acquired anti-Rh antibodies. Then, within 72 hours of delivery, give 120 mcg WinRho or 300 mcg HyperRHO, RhoGAM, or Rhophylac I.M. or I.V. If

72 hours have elapsed, give drug as soon as possible, up to 28 days.

➤ **Incompatible blood transfusion**

Adults: 600 mcg I.V. every 8 hours or 1,200 mcg I.M. every 12 hours until total dose given. Total dose depends on volume of packed RBCs or whole blood infused. Consult blood bank or transfusion unit at once; must be given within 72 hours.

➤ **Rho(D) antigen–positive patients with chronic idiopathic thrombocytopenic purpura (ITP); ITP secondary to HIV; children with acute ITP**

Adults and children: Initially, 50 mcg/kg I.V. as single dose or divided into two doses on separate days. If Hb level is less than 10 g/dL, reduce first dose to 25 to 40 mcg/kg. Then, give 25 to 60 mcg/kg I.V. as needed to elevate platelet count with specific individually determined dosage.

romiplostim
roh-mih-PLOH-stim

Nplate

Therapeutic class: Hematopoietics
Pharmacologic class: Thrombopoietin receptor agonists

AVAILABLE FORMS
Injection: 250-mcg, 500-mcg single-use vials

INDICATIONS & DOSAGES
➤ **Thrombocytopenia in patients with chronic immune ITP who have had an insufficient response to corticosteroids, immunoglobulins, or splenectomy**

Adults: Initially, 1 mcg/kg subcutaneously once weekly. Adjust dosage in increments of 1 mcg/kg to maintain platelet count of 50×10^9/L or higher, as needed, to reduce the risk of bleeding. Maximum dosage is 10 mcg/kg weekly. Refer to manufacturer's instructions for dosage adjustments for platelet counts. Discontinue if platelet count doesn't increase after 4 weeks at maximum dosage.

tetanus immune globulin (human)
HyperTET S/D

Therapeutic class: Prophylaxis drugs
Pharmacologic class: Immunoglobulins

AVAILABLE FORMS
Injection: 250-unit vial or syringe

INDICATIONS & DOSAGES
➤ **Postexposure prevention of tetanus after injury, in patients whose immunization is incomplete or unknown**

Adults and children: 250 units deep I.M. injection.

Common combination drugs: Indications and dosages

Refer to manufacturer's instructions for complete prescribing and safety information.

Analgesics

Duexis

GENERIC COMPONENTS
ibuprofen–famotidine
Tablets
800 mg ibuprofen and 26.6 mg famotidine
DOSAGES
Black Box Warning NSAIDs are contraindicated after CABG surgery and may cause an increased risk of serious CV thrombotic events, MI, stroke, and GI adverse reactions, which can be fatal. ■
RA and osteoarthritis; to decrease risk of upper GI ulcers
Adults: 1 tablet P.O. t.i.d. Elderly patients may need reduced dosages.

Fioricet with Codeine

Controlled Substance Schedule III
GENERIC COMPONENTS
acetaminophen–butalbital–caffeine–codeine phosphate
Capsules
300 mg acetaminophen, 50 mg butalbital, 40 mg caffeine, and 30 mg codeine phosphate
325 mg acetaminophen, 50 mg butalbital, 40 mg caffeine, and 30 mg codeine phosphate
DOSAGES
Black Box Warning Acetaminophen has been associated with cases of acute liver failure and death. Codeine can cause respiratory depression and death in children. Opioids combined with benzodiazepines or CNS depressants can cause death. ■
Tension headache
Adults: 1 to 2 capsules P.O. every 4 hours. Maximum dosage, 6 capsules in 24 hours.

Fiorinal with Codeine

Controlled Substance Schedule III
GENERIC COMPONENTS
codeine phosphate–aspirin–butalbital–caffeine
Capsules
30 mg codeine phosphate, 325 mg aspirin, 50 mg butalbital, and 40 mg caffeine
DOSAGES
Black Box Warning Opioids combined with benzodiazepines or CNS depressants can cause death. ■
Headache, mild to moderate pain
Adults: 1 to 2 capsules P.O. every 4 hours. Maximum dosage, 6 capsules in 24 hours.

pentazocine–naloxone hydrochloride

Controlled Substance Schedule IV
GENERIC COMPONENTS
pentazocine–naloxone hydrochloride
Tablets
50 mg pentazocine and 0.5 mg naloxone hydrochloride
DOSAGES
Black Box Warning Drug is for oral use only; severe, potentially lethal, reactions may result from misuse by injection. Opioids combined with benzodiazepines or CNS depressants can cause death. ■
Moderate to severe pain
Adults and children age 12 and older: 1 tablet P.O. every 3 to 4 hours. May increase to 2 tablets if necessary. Maximum dosage, 12 tablets in 24 hours.

Percodan

Controlled Substance Schedule II
GENERIC COMPONENTS
oxycodone hydrochloride–aspirin
Tablets
4.835 mg oxycodone hydrochloride and 325 mg aspirin
DOSAGES
Black Box Warning Opioids combined with benzodiazepines or CNS depressants can cause death. ■
Moderate to moderately severe pain
Adults: 1 tablet P.O. every 6 hours. Maximum dosage, 12 tablets in 24 hours.

Reprexain

Controlled Substance Schedule II
GENERIC COMPONENTS
hydrocodone bitartrate–ibuprofen
Tablets
2.5 mg hydrocodone bitartrate and 200 mg ibuprofen
5 mg hydrocodone bitartrate and 200 mg ibuprofen
10 mg hydrocodone bitartrate and 200 mg ibuprofen
DOSAGES
Black Box Warning Opioids combined with benzodiazepines or CNS depressants can cause death. ■
Acute pain (short-term)
1 tablet P.O. every 4 to 6 hours p.r.n. Maximum dosage, 5 tablets in 24 hours.

Ultracet✐

Controlled Substance Schedule IV
GENERIC COMPONENTS
tramadol hydrochloride–acetaminophen
Tablets
37.5 mg tramadol hydrochloride and 325 mg acetaminophen

DOSAGES

Black Box Warning Acetaminophen has been associated with acute liver failure and death. Opioids combined with benzodiazepines or CNS depressants can cause death. ∎

Acute pain

Adults: 2 tablets P.O. every 4 to 6 hours as needed for up to 5 days. Maximum dosage, 8 tablets in 24 hours.

Vicoprofen

Controlled Substance Schedule II

GENERIC COMPONENTS

hydrocodone–ibuprofen

Tablets

7.5 mg hydrocodone and 200 mg ibuprofen

DOSAGES

Acute pain (short-term)

Adults and children age 16 and older: 1 tablet P.O. every 4 to 6 hours p.r.n. Maximum dosage, 5 tablets in 24 hours.

Vimovo

GENERIC COMPONENTS

naproxen–esomeprazole

Tablets Ⓓ

375 mg naproxen and 20 mg esomeprazole 500 mg naproxen and 20 mg esomeprazole

DOSAGES

Black Box Warning Contraindicated for use in CABG surgery. Drug may cause an increased risk of serious CV thrombotic events, MI, stroke, and GI adverse reactions, which can be fatal. ∎

Osteoarthritis, RA, ankylosing spondylitis; to decrease risk of gastric ulcer development

Adults: 1 tablet P.O. b.i.d.

Antiacne drugs

Epiduo
Epiduo Forte

GENERIC COMPONENTS

benzoyl peroxide–adapalene

Topical gel

2.5% benzoyl peroxide and 0.1% adapalene
2.5% benzoyl peroxide and 0.3% adapalene

DOSAGES

Acne vulgaris

Adults and children age 9 and older (Epiduo): Apply a thin film to affected areas of face or trunk once daily after washing.

Adults and children age 12 and older (Epiduo Forte): Apply a thin film to affected areas of face or trunk once daily after washing.

Estrostep Fe

GENERIC COMPONENTS

norethindrone–ethinyl estradiol
norethindrone–ethinyl estradiol–ferrous fumarate

Tablets

1 mg norethindrone and 20 mcg ethinyl estradiol
1 mg norethindrone and 30 mcg ethinyl estradiol
1 mg norethindrone and 35 mcg ethinyl estradiol and 75 mg ferrous fumarate

DOSAGES

Black Box Warning Risk of serious CV events; not for use by women older than age 35 who smoke. ∎

Acne vulgaris

Women older than age 15: 1 tablet P.O. daily.

Ortho Tri-Cyclen

GENERIC COMPONENTS

norgestimate–ethinyl estradiol

Tablets

0.18 mg norgestimate and 35 mcg ethinyl estradiol
0.215 mg norgestimate and 35 mcg ethinyl estradiol
0.25 mg norgestimate and 35 mcg ethinyl estradiol

DOSAGES

Black Box Warning Risk of serious CV events; not for use by women older than age 35 who smoke. ∎

Acne vulgaris

Women older than age 15: 1 tablet P.O. daily.

Veltin
Ziana

GENERIC COMPONENTS

clindamycin phosphate–tretinoin

Topical gel

Clindamycin phosphate 1.2% and tretinoin 0.025%

DOSAGES

Acne vulgaris

Adults and children age 12 and older: Apply pea-size amount to cover entire affected area once daily in the evening. Avoid eyes, lips, and mucous membranes.

Antidiabetics

ActoPlus Met
ActoPlus Met XR

GENERIC COMPONENTS

pioglitazone–metformin hydrochloride

Tablets

15 mg pioglitazone and 500 mg metformin hydrochloride
15 mg pioglitazone and 850 mg metformin hydrochloride

Tablets (extended-release) Ⓓ

15 mg pioglitazone and 1,000 mg extended-release metformin hydrochloride
30 mg pioglitazone and 1,000 mg extended-release metformin hydrochloride

DOSAGES

Black Box Warning May cause or exacerbate HF in some patients; lactic acidosis can occur and may require hospitalization. ∎

Adjunct to diet and exercise to improve glycemic control in adults with type 2 diabetes

Adults: 15 mg pioglitazone/500 mg metformin or 15 mg pioglitazone/850 mg metformin P.O. once daily or b.i.d. with food. Maximum dosage, 45 mg pioglitazone/2,550 mg metformin per day. Or, 15 mg pioglitazone/1,000 mg extended-release metformin or 30 mg pioglitazone/1,000 mg extended-release metformin P.O. once daily with evening meal. Maximum dosage

of extended-release formula, 45 mg pioglitazone and 2,000 mg extended-release metformin per day.
Adjust-a-dose: Discontinue drug if estimated GFR falls below 30 mL/minute/1.73 m².

glipizide–metformin hydrochloride
GENRIC COMPONENTS
glipizide–metformin hydrochloride
Tablets
2.5 mg glipizide and 250 mg metformin hydrochloride
2.5 mg glipizide and 500 mg metformin hydrochloride
5 mg glipizide and 500 mg metformin hydrochloride
DOSAGES
Black Box Warning Serious and sometimes fatal lactic acidosis can occur. ■
Adjust-a-dose (for all indications): Discontinue drug if estimated GFR falls below 30 mL/minute/1.73 m².
As initial adjunctive therapy to diet and exercise to improve glycemic control in type 2 diabetes
Adults: Initially, glipizide 2.5 mg/metformin 250 mg once a day with a meal. May increase dosage every 2 weeks per glycemic response to maximum daily dose of 10 mg glipizide with 2,000 mg metformin in divided doses.
Second-line therapy when diet, exercise, and initial treatment with a sulfonylurea or metformin don't achieve glycemic control
Adults: Initially, 2.5 mg glipizide/500 mg metformin or 5 mg glipizide/500 mg metformin P.O. b.i.d. Increase dosage in increments of no more than glipizide 5 mg/metformin 500 mg up to a maximum daily dose of glipizide 20 mg/metformin 2,000 mg.

Glucovance
GENERIC COMPONENTS
glyburide–metformin hydrochloride
Tablets
1.25 mg glyburide and 250 mg metformin hydrochloride
2.5 mg glyburide and 500 mg metformin hydrochloride
5 mg glyburide and 500 mg metformin hydrochloride
DOSAGES
Black Box Warning Serious and sometimes fatal lactic acidosis can occur. ■
As initial adjunctive therapy to diet and exercise to improve glycemic control in type 2 diabetes; as second-line therapy when diet, exercise, and initial treatment with a sulfonylurea or metformin don't achieve glycemic control
Adults: 1 or 2 tablets P.O. daily or b.i.d. with meals. Maximum dosage, glyburide 20 mg and metformin 2,000 mg for treatment of type 2 diabetes, as second-line therapy.
Adjust-a-dose: Discontinue drug if estimated GFR falls below 30 mL/minute/1.73 m².

Invokamet
GENERIC COMPONENTS
canagliflozin–metformin
Tablets
50 mg canagliflozin and 500 mg metformin

50 mg canagliflozin and 1,000 mg metformin
150 mg canagliflozin and 500 mg metformin
150 mg canagliflozin and 1,000 mg metformin
DOSAGES
Black Box Warning Serious and sometimes fatal lactic acidosis can occur. ■
Adjunct to diet and exercise to improve glycemic control in type 2 diabetes when treatment with both canagliflozin and metformin is appropriate
Adults already on metformin: 50 mg canagliflozin plus previously prescribed dose of metformin P.O. b.i.d. with meals.
Adults already on canagliflozin: 500 mg metformin plus previously prescribed dose of canagliflozin P.O. b.i.d. with meals.
Adults already on canagliflozin and metformin: Switch to the same total daily doses of each component P.O. b.i.d. with meals.
Adjust-a-dose: Increase dosage gradually if needed to reduce metformin's GI adverse effects. Don't exceed maximum daily dose of 2,000 mg of metformin and 300 mg of canagliflozin. Limit dose of the canagliflozin component to 50 mg b.i.d. in patients with moderate renal impairment with an estimated GFR (eGFR) of 45 to less than 60 mL/minute/1.73 m². Discontinue drug if eGFR falls below 30 mL/minute/1.73 m².

Janumet
GENERIC COMPONENTS
sitagliptin–metformin hydrochloride
Tablets
50 mg sitagliptin and 500 mg metformin hydrochloride
50 mg sitagliptin and 1,000 mg metformin hydrochloride
DOSAGES
Black Box Warning Serious and sometimes fatal lactic acidosis can occur. ■
Adjunct to diet and exercise to improve glycemic control in type 2 diabetes when treatment with both sitagliptin and metformin is appropriate
Adults already on metformin: 50 mg sitagliptin P.O. b.i.d. plus the dose of metformin already being taken. For patients taking 850 mg metformin P.O. b.i.d., recommended starting dosage is 50 mg sitagliptin/1,000 mg metformin P.O. b.i.d.
Adults not on metformin: 50 mg sitagliptin/500 mg metformin P.O. b.i.d.
Adjust-a-dose: Discontinue drug if estimated GFR falls below 30 mL/minute/1.73 m².

Janumet XR
GENERIC COMPONENTS
sitagliptin–metformin hydrochloride
Tablets (extended-release) ⓓⓝⓒ
50 mg sitagliptin and 500 mg extended-release metformin hydrochloride
50 mg sitagliptin and 1,000 mg extended-release metformin hydrochloride
100 mg sitagliptin and 1,000 mg extended-release metformin hydrochloride

DOSAGES
Black Box Warning Serious and sometimes fatal lactic acidosis can occur. ∎

Adjunct to diet and exercise to improve glycemic control in type 2 diabetes when treatment with both sitagliptin and metformin is appropriate

Adults already on metformin: 100 mg/day sitagliptin plus previously prescribed dose of metformin. For patients taking 850 mg immediate-release metformin P.O. b.i.d. or 1,000 mg metformin P.O. b.i.d., recommended starting dosage is 100 mg sitagliptin/2,000 mg extended-release metformin P.O. once daily.

Adults not on metformin: 100 mg sitagliptin/1,000 mg extended-release metformin P.O. once daily.

Adjust-a-dose: Discontinue drug if estimated GFR falls below 30 mL/minute/1.73 m^2.

Jentadueto
Jentadueto XR

GENERIC COMPONENTS
linagliptin–metformin hydrochloride
Tablets
2.5 mg linagliptin and 500 mg metformin hydrochloride
2.5 mg linagliptin and 850 mg metformin hydrochloride
2.5 mg linagliptin and 1,000 mg metformin hydrochloride

Tablets (extended-release) ⓒ
2.5 mg linagliptin and 1,000 mg metformin hydrochloride extended-release
5 mg linagliptin and 1,000 mg metformin hydrochloride extended-release

DOSAGES
Black Box Warning Serious and sometimes fatal lactic acidosis can occur. ∎

Adjunct to diet and exercise to improve glycemic control in type 2 diabetes when treatment with both linagliptin and metformin is appropriate

Adults already on metformin: 2.5 mg linagliptin P.O. b.i.d. or linagliptin 5 mg extended-release once daily plus current dose of metformin already being taken.

Adults not on metformin: 2.5 mg linagliptin/500 mg metformin P.O. b.i.d. or 5 mg linagliptin/1,000 mg metformin extended-release P.O. once daily. Maximum dose, 2.5 mg linagliptin and 1,000 mg metformin b.i.d.

Adjust-a-dose: Discontinue drug if estimated GFR falls below 30 mL/minute/1.73 m^2.

Kazano

GENERIC COMPONENTS
alogliptin benzoate–metformin
Tablets
12.5 mg alogliptin benzoate and 500 mg metformin
12.5 mg alogliptin benzoate and 1,000 mg metformin

DOSAGES
Black Box Warning Serious and sometimes fatal lactic acidosis can occur. ∎

Adjunct to diet and exercise to improve glycemic control in type 2 diabetes

Adults: 1 tablet P.O. b.i.d. with food. Adjust dosage based on effectiveness and tolerability. Maximum daily dose, 25 mg alogliptin and 2,000 mg metformin.

Adjust-a-dose: Discontinue drug if estimated GFR falls below 30 mL/minute/1.73 m^2.

Oseni

GENERIC COMPONENTS
alogliptin benzoate–pioglitazone hydrochloride
Tablets
12.5 mg alogliptin benzoate and 15 mg pioglitazone hydrochloride
12.5 mg alogliptin benzoate and 30 mg pioglitazone hydrochloride
12.5 mg alogliptin benzoate and 45 mg pioglitazone hydrochloride
25 mg alogliptin benzoate and 15 mg pioglitazone hydrochloride
25 mg alogliptin benzoate and 30 mg pioglitazone hydrochloride
25 mg alogliptin benzoate and 45 mg pioglitazone hydrochloride

DOSAGES
Black Box Warning May cause or exacerbate HF in some patients. ∎

Adjunct to diet and exercise to improve glycemic control in type 2 diabetes mellitus when treatment with both alogliptin and pioglitazone is appropriate

Adults inadequately controlled on diet and exercise, inadequately controlled on metformin monotherapy, or who require additional glycemic control on alogliptin: Alogliptin 25 mg/pioglitazone 15 mg or alogliptin 25 mg/pioglitazone 30 mg P.O. once daily. May titrate to a maximum of alogliptin 25 mg/pioglitazone 45 mg once daily based on glycemic response as determined by HbA_{1c}.

Adults who require additional glycemic control on pioglitazone: Alogliptin 25 mg/pioglitazone 15 mg, alogliptin 25 mg/pioglitazone 30 mg, or alogliptin 25 mg/pioglitazone 45 mg P.O. once daily as appropriate based on current therapy. May titrate to a maximum of alogliptin 25 mg/pioglitazone 45 mg once daily based on glycemic response as determined by HbA_{1c}.

Adults switching from alogliptin administered with pioglitazone: Initiate at the dosage of alogliptin and pioglitazone based on current therapy. May titrate to a maximum of alogliptin 25 mg/pioglitazone 45 mg once daily based on glycemic response as determined by HbA_{1c}.

Adults with HF (New York Heart Association class I or II): Alogliptin 25 mg/pioglitazone 15 mg P.O. once daily. May titrate to a maximum of alogliptin 25 mg/pioglitazone 45 mg once daily based on glycemic response as determined by HbA_{1c}.

PrandiMet

GENERIC COMPONENTS
repaglinide–metformin
Tablets
1 mg repaglinide and 500 mg metformin
2 mg repaglinide and 500 mg metformin

DOSAGES

Black Box Warning Serious and sometimes fatal lactic acidosis can occur. ∎

Adjunct to diet and exercise to improve glycemic control in type 2 diabetes

Adults: Individualize dosage based on patient's current regimen. Can be administered b.i.d. to t.i.d. with meals. Maximum daily dose, 10 mg repaglinide and 2,500 mg metformin.

Adjust-a-dose: Discontinue drug if estimated GFR falls below 30 mL/minute/1.73 m^2.

rosiglitazone maleate–metformin hydrochloride

GENERIC COMPONENTS
rosiglitazone maleate–metformin hydrochloride
Tablets
2 mg rosiglitazone and 500 mg metformin
2 mg rosiglitazone and 1 g metformin
4 mg rosiglitazone and 500 mg metformin
4 mg rosiglitazone and 1 g metformin
DOSAGES

Black Box Warning May cause or exacerbate HF in some patients; lactic acidosis can occur and require hospitalization. ∎

Adjunct to diet and exercise to improve glycemic control in adults with type 2 diabetes

Adults inadequately controlled on diet and exercise in whom combination therapy is appropriate: Initially, 2 mg rosiglitazone with 500 mg metformin P.O. once daily or b.i.d. with meals

Adults inadequately controlled on rosiglitazone monotherapy: Initially, the current dose of rosiglitazone with 1,000 mg metformin P.O. b.i.d.

Adults inadequately controlled on metformin monotherapy: 4 mg rosiglitazone with current metformin dose P.O. b.i.d. Titrate gradually based on individual response and tolerance. Rosiglitazone dosage may be increased by 4-mg increments every 8 to 12 weeks and metformin by 500-mg increments every 1 to 2 weeks. Maximum dose, 8 mg rosiglitazone and 2,000 mg metformin per day.

Adjust-a-dose: Discontinue drug if estimated GFR falls below 30 mL/minute/1.73 m^2.

Antigout drugs

Col-Probenecid

GENERIC COMPONENTS
probenecid–colchicine
Tablets
500 mg probenecid and 0.5 mg colchicine
DOSAGES
Chronic gouty arthritis
Adults: 1 tablet P.O. daily for 1 week, then 1 tablet P.O. b.i.d. Adjust dosage based on symptoms and uric acid levels. Maximum dosage, 4 tablets daily.

Antihypertensives

Accuretic
Quinaretic

GENERIC COMPONENTS
quinapril–hydrochlorothiazide
Tablets
10 mg quinapril and 12.5 mg hydrochlorothiazide
20 mg quinapril and 12.5 mg hydrochlorothiazide
20 mg quinapril and 25 mg hydrochlorothiazide
DOSAGES
Black Box Warning Can cause fetal harm; when pregnancy is detected, discontinue drug as soon as possible. ∎
Hypertension
Adults: 1 tablet P.O. per day in the morning. Adjust drug using the individual products, then switch to appropriate dosage of the combination product.

Atacand HCT
GENERIC COMPONENTS
candesartan cilexetil–hydrochlorothiazide
Tablets
16 mg candesartan cilexetil and 12.5 mg hydrochlorothiazide
32 mg candesartan cilexetil and 12.5 mg hydrochlorothiazide
32 mg candesartan cilexetil and 25 mg hydrochlorothiazide
DOSAGES
Black Box Warning Can cause fetal harm; when pregnancy is detected, discontinue drug as soon as possible. ∎
Hypertension
Adults: Initially, 16 mg candesartan/12.5 mg hydrochlorothiazide P.O. daily in patients who aren't volume-depleted. Adjust dosage using individual products, then switch to appropriate dosage of combination product.

Avalide
GENERIC COMPONENTS
irbesartan–hydrochlorothiazide
Tablets
150 mg irbesartan and 12.5 mg hydrochlorothiazide
300 mg irbesartan and 12.5 mg hydrochlorothiazide
DOSAGES
Black Box Warning Can cause fetal harm; when pregnancy is detected, discontinue drug as soon as possible. ∎
Hypertension
Adults: Initially, 150 mg irbesartan/12.5 mg hydrochlorothiazide tablet P.O. daily. Adjust dosage with individual products, then switch to combination product when patient's condition is stabilized. Maximum daily dose, 300 mg irbesartan and 25 mg hydrochlorothiazide.

Azor

GENERIC COMPONENTS
amlodipine besylate–olmesartan medoxomil
Tablets
5 mg amlodipine besylate and 20 mg olmesartan medoxomil
5 mg amlodipine besylate and 40 mg olmesartan medoxomil
10 mg amlodipine besylate and 20 mg olmesartan medoxomil
10 mg amlodipine besylate and 40 mg olmesartan medoxomil
DOSAGES
Black Box Warning Can cause fetal harm; when pregnancy is detected, discontinue drug as soon as possible. ■
Hypertension
Adults: Initially, 5 mg amlodipine/20 mg olmesartan P.O. once daily for 1 to 2 weeks. Titrate as needed up to maximum of 10 mg amlodipine/40 mg olmesartan once daily.

Benicar HCT 🖉

GENERIC COMPONENTS
olmesartan medoxomil–hydrochlorothiazide
Tablets
20 mg olmesartan medoxomil and 12.5 mg hydrochlorothiazide
40 mg olmesartan and 12.5 mg hydrochlorothiazide
40 mg olmesartan and 25 mg hydrochlorothiazide
DOSAGES
Black Box Warning Can cause fetal harm; when pregnancy is detected, discontinue drug as soon as possible. ■
Hypertension
Adults: 1 tablet P.O. daily in the morning. Adjust dosage using individual products, then switch to combination product when patient's adjustment schedule is stable. Dosage may be titrated at 2- to 4-week intervals. Maximum dosage, 40 mg olmesartan/25 mg hydrochlorothiazide.

captopril and hydrochlorothiazide

GENERIC COMPONENTS
captopril–hydrochlorothiazide
Tablets
25 mg captopril and 15 mg hydrochlorothiazide
50 mg captopril and 15 mg hydrochlorothiazide
25 mg captopril and 25 mg hydrochlorothiazide
50 mg captopril and 25 mg hydrochlorothiazide
DOSAGES
Black Box Warning Can cause fetal harm; when pregnancy is detected, discontinue drug as soon as possible. ■
Hypertension
Adults: Initially, 25 mg captopril/15 mg hydrochlorothiazide P.O. daily. Adjust dosage using individual products, then switch to combination product when patient's adjustment schedule is stable. Maximum daily dose, 150 mg captopril or 50 mg hydrochlorothiazide.

Clorpres

GENERIC COMPONENTS
chlorthalidone–clonidine hydrochloride
Tablets
15 mg chlorthalidone and 0.1 mg clonidine hydrochloride
15 mg chlorthalidone and 0.2 mg clonidine hydrochloride
15 mg chlorthalidone and 0.3 mg clonidine hydrochloride
DOSAGES
Hypertension
Adults: 1 to 2 tablets P.O. daily in the morning or b.i.d. Maximum dosage, 30 mg chlorthalidone and 0.6 mg clonidine.

Corzide

GENERIC COMPONENTS
nadolol–bendroflumethiazide
Tablets
40 mg nadolol and 5 mg bendroflumethiazide
80 mg nadolol and 5 mg bendroflumethiazide
DOSAGES
Black Box Warning May exacerbate ischemic heart disease if withdrawn abruptly. ■
Hypertension
Adults: 1 tablet P.O. daily in the morning. Adjust dosage using individual products, then switch to combination product when patient's adjustment schedule is stable.
Adjust-a-dose: Adjust dosing frequency for CrCl less than 50 mL/minute per manufacturer's instructions.

Diovan HCT 🖉

GENERIC COMPONENTS
valsartan–hydrochlorothiazide
Tablets
80 mg valsartan and 12.5 mg hydrochlorothiazide
160 mg valsartan and 12.5 mg hydrochlorothiazide
160 mg valsartan and 25 mg hydrochlorothiazide
320 mg valsartan and 12.5 mg hydrochlorothiazide
320 mg valsartan and 25 mg hydrochlorothiazide
DOSAGES
Black Box Warning Can cause fetal harm; when pregnancy is detected, discontinue drug as soon as possible. ■
Hypertension
Adults: Initially, 160 mg valsartan/12.5 mg hydrochlorothiazide P.O. daily. Titrate to desired effect after 1 to 2 weeks. Maximum dose, 320 mg valsartan/25 mg hydrochlorothiazide.

Dutoprol

GENERIC COMPONENTS
metoprolol succinate–hydrochlorothiazide
Tablets (extended-release)
25 mg metoprolol succinate and 12.5 mg hydrochlorothiazide
50 mg metoprolol succinate and 12.5 mg hydrochlorothiazide

100 mg metoprolol succinate and 12.5 mg hydrochlorothiazide
DOSAGES
Black Box Warning May exacerbate ischemic heart disease if withdrawn abruptly. ∎
Hypertension
Adults: Initially, 25 mg metoprolol/12.5 mg hydrochlorothiazide P.O. per day. Adjust dosage using the individual products, then switch to appropriate combination product. Maximum dose, 200 mg metoprolol succinate and 25 mg hydrochlorothiazide.

Exforge
GENERIC COMPONENTS
amlodipine besylate–valsartan
Tablets
5 mg amlodipine besylate and 160 mg valsartan
5 mg amlodipine besylate and 320 mg valsartan
10 mg amlodipine besylate and 160 mg valsartan
10 mg amlodipine besylate and 320 mg valsartan
DOSAGES
Black Box Warning Can cause fetal harm; when pregnancy is detected, discontinue drug as soon as possible. ∎
Hypertension
Adults: Initially, 5 mg amlodipine/160 mg valsartan P.O. once daily. Increase after 1 to 2 weeks to desired effect or a maximum of 10 mg amlodipine/320 mg valsartan daily.

Exforge HCT
GENERIC COMPONENTS
amlodipine besylate–valsartan–hydrochlorothiazide
Tablets
5 mg amlodipine besylate, 160 mg valsartan, and 12.5 mg hydrochlorothiazide
10 mg amlodipine besylate, 160 mg valsartan, and 12.5 mg hydrochlorothiazide
5 mg amlodipine besylate, 160 mg valsartan, and 25 mg hydrochlorothiazide
10 mg amlodipine besylate, 160 mg valsartan, and 25 mg hydrochlorothiazide
10 mg amlodipine besylate, 320 mg valsartan, and 25 mg hydrochlorothiazide
DOSAGES
Black Box Warning Can cause fetal harm; when pregnancy is detected, discontinue drug as soon as possible. ∎
Hypertension
Adults: Give 1 tablet P.O. once daily. Dosage may be increased after 2 weeks. Maximum recommended dosage, 10 mg amlodipine/320 mg valsartan/25 mg hydrochlorothiazide.
Adjust-a-dose: In elderly patients and patients with hepatic impairment, initiate drug with lower doses and titrate cautiously.

fosinopril and hydrochlorothiazide
GENERIC COMPONENTS
fosinopril–hydrochlorothiazide
Tablets
10 mg fosinopril and 12.5 mg hydrochlorothiazide
20 mg fosinopril and 12.5 mg hydrochlorothiazide
DOSAGES
Black Box Warning Can cause fetal harm; when pregnancy is detected, discontinue drug as soon as possible. ∎
Hypertension
Adults: 1 tablet P.O. per day in the morning. Adjust dosage using individual products, then switch to appropriate combination product.

Hyzaar
GENERIC COMPONENTS
losartan–hydrochlorothiazide
Tablets
50 mg losartan and 12.5 mg hydrochlorothiazide
100 mg losartan and 12.5 mg hydrochlorothiazide
100 mg losartan and 25 mg hydrochlorothiazide
DOSAGES
Black Box Warning Can cause fetal harm; when pregnancy is detected, discontinue drug as soon as possible. ∎
Hypertension
Adults: 1 tablet P.O. daily as a substitute for individual titrated components in patients not adequately controlled with monotherapy with either of the component products. May use as initial therapy in severe hypertension when benefits outweigh risk. Maximum dosage, 100 mg losartan/25 mg hydrochlorothiazide daily.

Lopressor HCT
GENERIC COMPONENTS
metoprolol tartrate–hydrochlorothiazide
Tablets
50 mg metoprolol tartrate and 25 mg hydrochlorothiazide
100 mg metoprolol tartrate and 25 mg hydrochlorothiazide
DOSAGES
Black Box Warning May exacerbate ischemic heart disease if withdrawn abruptly. ∎
Hypertension
Adults: 100 to 200 mg metoprolol/25 to 50 mg hydrochlorothiazide P.O. once daily or 50 to 100 mg metoprolol/12.5 to 50 mg hydrochlorothiazide P.O. b.i.d. Adjust dosage using individual products, then switch to appropriate combination product.

Lotensin HCT
GENERIC COMPONENTS
benazepril–hydrochlorothiazide
Tablets
5 mg benazepril and 6.25 mg hydrochlorothiazide
10 mg benazepril and 12.5 mg hydrochlorothiazide
20 mg benazepril and 12.5 mg hydrochlorothiazide
20 mg benazepril and 25 mg hydrochlorothiazide

DOSAGES

Black Box Warning Can cause fetal harm; when pregnancy is detected, discontinue drug as soon as possible. ■

Hypertension

Adults: 1 tablet P.O. daily in the morning. Adjust dosage using individual products, then switch to appropriate combination product. Wait 2 to 3 weeks before increasing hydrochlorothiazide dose.

Lotrel

GENERIC COMPONENTS

amlodipine besylate–benazepril hydrochloride

Capsules

2.5 mg amlodipine besylate and 10 mg benazepril hydrochloride

5 mg amlodipine besylate and 10 mg benazepril hydrochloride

5 mg amlodipine besylate and 20 mg benazepril hydrochloride

5 mg amlodipine besylate and 40 mg benazepril hydrochloride

10 mg amlodipine besylate and 20 mg benazepril hydrochloride

10 mg amlodipine besylate and 40 mg benazepril hydrochloride

DOSAGES

Black Box Warning Can cause fetal harm; when pregnancy is detected, discontinue drug as soon as possible. ■

Hypertension

Adults: 1 tablet P.O. daily in morning. Monitor for hypertension and adverse effects closely over first 2 weeks and regularly thereafter. Maximum dosage, 10 mg amlodipine and 40 mg benazepril.

Adjust-a-dose: Consider lower initial doses for elderly patients and patients with hepatic impairment.

methyldopa and hydrochlorothiazide

GENERIC COMPONENTS

methyldopa–hydrochlorothiazide

Tablets

250 mg methyldopa and 15 mg hydrochlorothiazide

250 mg methyldopa and 25 mg hydrochlorothiazide

DOSAGES

Black Box Warning Not indicated for initial therapy of hypertension. ■

Hypertension

Adults: Initially, 250 mg methyldopa/15 mg hydrochlorothiazide P.O. b.i.d. or t.i.d. or 250 mg methyldopa/25 mg hydrochlorothiazide P.O. b.i.d. Adjust dosage using individual products, then switch to appropriate combination product. Maximum dosage, 3,000 mg methyldopa and 50 mg hydrochlorothiazide daily.

Micardis HCT

GENERIC COMPONENTS

telmisartan–hydrochlorothiazide

Tablets

40 mg telmisartan and 12.5 mg hydrochlorothiazide

80 mg telmisartan and 12.5 mg hydrochlorothiazide

80 mg telmisartan and 25 mg hydrochlorothiazide

DOSAGES

Black Box Warning Can cause fetal harm; when pregnancy is detected, discontinue drug as soon as possible. ■

Hypertension

Adults: Initially, 80 mg telmisartan/12.5 mg hydrochlorothiazide P.O. per day; may be adjusted up to 160 mg telmisartan and 25 mg hydrochlorothiazide, based on patient's response.

Adjust-a-dose: In mild to moderate hepatic impairment or biliary obstructive disorders, begin therapy with 40 mg telmisartan/12.5 mg hydrochlorothiazide P.O. once daily.

moexipril hydrochloride–hydrochlorothiazide

GENERIC COMPONENTS

moexipril hydrochloride–hydrochlorothiazide

Tablets

7.5 mg moexipril hydrochloride and 12.5 mg hydrochlorothiazide

15 mg moexipril hydrochloride and 12.5 mg hydrochlorothiazide

15 mg moexipril hydrochloride and 25 mg hydrochlorothiazide

DOSAGES

Black Box Warning Can cause fetal harm; when pregnancy is detected, discontinue drug as soon as possible. ■

Hypertension

Adults: Initially, 7.5 mg moexipril/12.5 mg hydrochlorothiazide, or 15 mg moexipril/12.5 mg hydrochlorothiazide, or 15 mg moexipril/25 mg hydrochlorothiazide P.O. once daily. Not for initial therapy. Adjust dosage after 2 to 3 weeks to maintain appropriate BP.

propranolol and hydrochlorothiazide

GENERIC COMPONENTS

propranolol hydrochloride–hydrochlorothiazide

Tablets

40 mg propranolol hydrochloride and 25 mg hydrochlorothiazide

80 mg propranolol hydrochloride and 25 mg hydrochlorothiazide

DOSAGES

Black Box Warning May exacerbate angina and, in some cases, MI if withdrawn abruptly. ■

Hypertension

Adults: 1 tablet P.O. b.i.d. Adjust dosage using individual products, then switch to appropriate combination product. Maximum daily dose, 160 mg propranolol and 50 mg hydrochlorothiazide.

Tarka

GENERIC COMPONENTS

trandolapril–verapamil hydrochloride

Tablets (extended-release)

1 mg trandolapril and 240 mg verapamil hydrochloride

2 mg trandolapril and 180 mg verapamil hydrochloride

2 mg trandolapril and 240 mg verapamil hydrochloride

4 mg trandolapril and 240 mg verapamil hydrochloride

DOSAGES

Black Box Warning Can cause fetal harm; when pregnancy is detected, discontinue drug as soon as possible. ■

Hypertension

Adults: 1 tablet P.O. per day, taken with food. Adjust dosage using the individual products, then switch to appropriate combination product.

Adjust-a-dose: In hepatic impairment and renal impairment (CrCl of less than 30 mL/minute), lower doses are recommended.

Tekturna HCT

GENERIC COMPONENTS
aliskiren hemifumarate–hydrochlorothiazide
Tablets
150 mg aliskiren hemifumarate and 12.5 mg hydrochlorothiazide
150 mg aliskiren hemifumarate and 25 mg hydrochlorothiazide
300 mg aliskiren hemifumarate and 12.5 mg hydrochlorothiazide
300 mg aliskiren hemifumarate and 25 mg hydrochlorothiazide

DOSAGES
Black Box Warning Can cause fetal harm; when pregnancy is detected, discontinue drug as soon as possible. ■

Hypertension

Adults: Initially, 150 mg aliskiren/12.5 mg hydrochlorothiazide. Titrate up as needed after 2 to 4 weeks to a maximum of 300 mg aliskiren/25 mg hydrochlorothiazide.

Tenoretic

GENERIC COMPONENTS
atenolol–chlorthalidone
Tablets
50 mg atenolol and 25 mg chlorthalidone
100 mg atenolol and 25 mg chlorthalidone

DOSAGES
Hypertension

Adults: Initially, 50 mg atenolol/25 mg chlorthalidone P.O. daily. Adjust dosage using individual products, then switch to appropriate combination product.

Adjust-a-dose: If CrCl is 15 to 35 mL/minute/1.73 m², maximum dose is 50 mg atenolol/25 mg chlorthalidone daily. If CrCl is less than 15 mL/minute/1.73 m², maximum dose is 50 mg atenolol/25 mg chlorthalidone every other day.

Tribenzor

GENERIC COMPONENTS
amlodipine besylate–hydrochlorothiazide–olmesartan medoxomil
Tablets
5 mg amlodipine besylate, 12.5 mg hydrochlorothiazide, and 20 mg olmesartan medoxomil
5 mg amlodipine besylate, 12.5 mg hydrochlorothiazide, and 40 mg olmesartan medoxomil
5 mg amlodipine besylate, 25 mg hydrochlorothiazide, and 40 mg olmesartan medoxomil
10 mg amlodipine besylate, 12.5 mg hydrochlorothiazide, and 40 mg olmesartan medoxomil
10 mg amlodipine besylate, 25 mg hydrochlorothiazide, and 40 mg olmesartan medoxomil

DOSAGES
Black Box Warning Can cause fetal harm; when pregnancy is detected, discontinue drug as soon as possible. ■

Hypertension

Adults: 1 tablet P.O. daily. Adjust dosage of individual products; then switch to appropriate combination product. May increase dosage after 2 weeks. Maximum recommended dose, 10 mg amlodipine/25 mg hydrochlorothiazide/40 mg olmesartan.

Twynsta

GENERIC COMPONENTS
amlodipine besylate–telmisartan
Tablets
5 mg amlodipine besylate and 40 mg telmisartan
5 mg amlodipine besylate and 80 mg telmisartan
10 mg amlodipine besylate and 40 mg telmisartan
10 mg amlodipine besylate and 80 mg telmisartan

DOSAGES
Black Box Warning Can cause fetal harm; when pregnancy is detected, discontinue drug as soon as possible. ■

Hypertension

Adults: 1 tablet P.O. daily. Substitute for its individually titrated components or initiate therapy with 5 mg amlodipine/40 mg telmisartan or 5 mg amlodipine/80 mg telmisartan. May increase dosage after at least 2 weeks to maximum dose of 10 mg amlodipine/80 mg telmisartan.

Vaseretic

GENERIC COMPONENTS
enalapril maleate–hydrochlorothiazide
Tablets
5 mg enalapril maleate and 12.5 mg hydrochlorothiazide
10 mg enalapril maleate and 25 mg hydrochlorothiazide

DOSAGES
Black Box Warning Can cause fetal harm; when pregnancy is detected, discontinue drug as soon as possible. ■

Hypertension

Adults: Initially, 10 mg enalapril/25 mg hydrochlorothiazide P.O. daily. Adjust dosage using individual products, then switch to appropriate combination product. Maximum dosage, 20 mg enalapril and 50 mg hydrochlorothiazide daily.

Ziac

GENERIC COMPONENTS
bisoprolol fumarate–hydrochlorothiazide
Tablets
2.5 mg bisoprolol fumarate and 6.25 mg hydrochlorothiazide
5 mg bisoprolol fumarate and 6.25 mg hydrochlorothiazide
10 mg bisoprolol fumarate and 6.25 mg hydrochlorothiazide
DOSAGES
Hypertension
Adults: Initially, 2.5 mg bisoprolol/6.25 mg hydrochlorothiazide P.O. daily. Increase dosage in 14-day intervals; optimal antihypertensive effect may require 2 to 3 weeks. Maximum dosage, 20 mg bisoprolol and 12.5 mg hydrochlorothiazide daily.
Adjust-a-dose: Use caution when titrating drug in patients with renal or hepatic impairment. Drug is contraindicated with anuria.

Antimigraine drugs

Cafergot
Migergot
GENERIC COMPONENTS
ergotamine tartrate–caffeine
Tablets
1 mg ergotamine tartrate and 100 mg caffeine
Suppositories
2 mg ergotamine tartrate and 100 mg caffeine
DOSAGES
Black Box Warning Use with potent CYP3A4 inhibitors, including protease inhibitors and macrolide antibiotics, can cause serious vasospasm and is contraindicated. ■
Prevention and treatment of migraine headache
Adults: 2 tablets P.O. at the first sign of attack. Follow with 1 tablet every 30 minutes, if needed. Maximum dose is 6 tablets per attack. Don't exceed 10 tablets per week. Or, 1 suppository P.R. at first sign of attack; follow with second dose after 1 hour, if needed. Maximum dose is 2 suppositories per attack. Don't exceed 5 suppositories per week.

Treximet

GENERIC COMPONENTS
sumatriptan succinate–naproxen sodium
Tablets
85 mg sumatriptan succinate and 500 mg naproxen sodium
10 mg sumatriptan succinate and 60 mg naproxen sodium

DOSAGES
Black Box Warning NSAIDs may cause an increased risk of serious and sometimes fatal CV thrombotic events, MI, stroke, and GI adverse reactions. ■
Migraine headache
Adults: One 85 mg sumatriptan/500 mg naproxen tablet P.O. at first sign of migraine. May follow with a second dose 2 hours later. Maximum dosage, 2 tablets in 24 hours.
Children age 12 and older: 10 mg sumatriptan/60 mg naproxen P.O. at first sign of migraine. Maximum dose, 85 mg/500 mg tablet in 24 hours.
Adjust-a-dose: In mild to moderate hepatic impairment, give no more than 10 mg sumatriptan/60 mg naproxen in 24 hours.

Antiplatelet drugs

Aggrenox
GENERIC COMPONENTS
dipyridamole–aspirin
Capsules (ⓄⓃⒸ)
200 mg dipyridamole and 25 mg aspirin
DOSAGES
Reduce stroke risk
Adults: 1 capsule P.O. b.i.d. in morning and evening.

Antiretrovirals

Atripla
GENERIC COMPONENTS
efavirenz–emtricitabine–tenofovir disoproxil fumarate
600 mg efavirenz, 200 mg emtricitabine, and 300 mg tenofovir disoproxil fumarate
DOSAGES
Black Box Warning Lactic acidosis and severe hepatomegaly with steatosis, including fatal cases, have been reported. Not approved for treatment of chronic HBV infection. ■
Treatment of HIV infection
Adults and children older than age 12 weighing at least 40 kg: 1 tablet P.O. daily on empty stomach. Dosing at bedtime may improve tolerability of nervous system symptoms.

Combivir ✐
GENERIC COMPONENTS
lamivudine–zidovudine
Tablets
150 mg lamivudine and 300 mg zidovudine
DOSAGES
Black Box Warning Hematologic toxicity, myopathy, lactic acidosis, and severe hepatomegaly, including fatal cases, and exacerbations of HBV infection have been reported. ■
Treatment of HIV infection
Adults and children weighing 30 kg or more: 1 tablet P.O. b.i.d.

Complera

GENERIC COMPONENTS
emtricitabine–rilpivirine–tenofovir disoproxil fumarate
Tablets
200 mg emtricitabine, 25 mg rilpivirine, and 300 mg tenofovir disoproxil fumarate
DOSAGES
Black Box Warning Lactic acidosis and severe hepatomegaly with steatosis, including fatal cases, have been reported. Not approved for treatment of chronic HBV infection. ■
Treatment of HIV infection
Adults and children age 12 and older weighing 35 kg or more: 1 tablet P.O. once daily with food.

Epzicom

GENERIC COMPONENTS
abacavir sulfate–lamivudine
Tablets
600 mg abacavir and 300 mg lamivudine
DOSAGES
Black Box Warning Contraindicated in patients with prior hypersensitivity reaction to abacavir and in HLA-B*5701-positive patients; screen for the HLA-B*5701 allele before starting drug. Lactic acidosis and severe hepatomegaly with steatosis, including fatal cases, and exacerbations of HBV infection have been reported. ■
Treatment of HIV infection
Adults and children weighing 25 kg or more: 1 tablet P.O. daily in combination with other antiretrovirals.

Trizivir

GENERIC COMPONENTS
abacavir sulfate–lamivudine–zidovudine
Tablets
300 mg abacavir sulfate, 150 mg lamivudine, and 300 mg zidovudine
DOSAGES
Black Box Warning Contraindicated in patients with prior hypersensitivity reaction to abacavir and in HLA-B*5701-positive patients; screen for the HLA-B*5701 allele before starting drug. Hematologic toxicity, myopathy, lactic acidosis, and severe hepatomegaly with steatosis, including fatal cases and exacerbations of HBV infection have been reported. ■
Treatment of HIV infection
Adults and children weighing 40 kg or more: 1 tablet P.O. b.i.d., alone or with other antiretrovirals.

Truvada

GENERIC COMPONENTS
emtricitabine–tenofovir disoproxil fumarate
Tablets
100 mg emtricitabine and 150 mg tenofovir disoproxil fumarate
133 mg emtricitabine and 200 mg tenofovir disoproxil fumarate
167 mg emtricitabine and 250 mg tenofovir disoproxil fumarate
200 mg emtricitabine and 300 mg tenofovir disoproxil fumarate
DOSAGES
Black Box Warning Lactic acidosis and severe hepatomegaly with steatosis have been reported with use of drug. Not approved for treatment of chronic HBV infection. For preexposure prophylaxis, confirm that patient is HIV-negative immediately before initiating and periodically during use. ■
Preexposure prophylaxis (adults) and treatment of HIV infection (adults and children) in combination with other retrovirals
Adults and children weighing 35 kg or more: 200 mg emtricitabine/300 mg tenofovir disoproxil fumarate P.O. daily.
Children weighing 28 to less than 35 kg: 167 mg emtricitabine/250 mg tenofovir disoproxil fumarate P.O. daily.
Children weighing 22 to less than 28 kg: 133 mg emtricitabine/200 mg tenofovir disoproxil fumarate P.O. daily.
Children weighing 17 to less than 22 kg: 100 mg emtricitabine/150 mg tenofovir disoproxil fumarate P.O. daily.
Adjust-a-dose: For CrCl of 30 to 49 mL/minute, give dose every 48 hours. Withhold drug for CrCl of less than 30 mL/minute.

Antiulcer drugs

Prevpac

GENERIC COMPONENTS
lansoprazole–amoxicillin–clarithromycin
Daily administration pack
Two 30-mg lansoprazole capsules, four 500-mg amoxicillin capsules, and two 500-mg clarithromycin tablets
DOSAGES
Eradication of *Helicobacter pylori* infection
Adults: Divide pack equally to take in two equal doses, morning and evening, for 10 to 14 days.

Pylera

GENERIC COMPONENTS
bismuth subcitrate potassium–metronidazole–tetracycline hydrochloride
Capsules
140 mg bismuth subcitrate potassium, 125 mg metronidazole, and 125 mg tetracycline hydrochloride
DOSAGES
Eradication of *Helicobacter pylori* infection; active duodenal ulcers associated with *H. pylori* infection
Adults: Give each dose (which includes all 3 capsules) P.O. q.i.d. after meals and at bedtime for 10 days with omeprazole 20 mg P.O. b.i.d. (after the morning and evening meals) for 10 days.

Benign prostatic hyperplasia drugs

Jalyn
GENERIC COMPONENTS
dutasteride–tamsulosin hydrochloride
Capsules ⓞⓝⓒ
0.5 mg dutasteride and 0.4 mg tamsulosin hydrochloride
DOSAGES
Treatment of symptomatic benign prostatic hyperplasia
Adult men: 1 capsule P.O. daily 30 minutes after same meal each day.

Diuretics

Aldactazide
GENERIC COMPONENTS
spironolactone–hydrochlorothiazide
Tablets
25 mg spironolactone and 25 mg hydrochlorothiazide
50 mg spironolactone and 50 mg hydrochlorothiazide
DOSAGES
Black Box Warning May be tumorigenic; use only as prescribed and avoid unnecessary use. Not indicated for initial therapy of edema or hypertension. ∎
Edema or hypertension
Adults: 1 to 8 25-mg spironolactone and 25-mg hydrochlorothiazide tablets P.O. daily. Or, 1 to 4 50-mg spironolactone and 50-mg hydrochlorothiazide tablets P.O. daily. May give daily dosage as single or divided doses.
Adjust-a-dose: In elderly patients, initiate with lowest available dose. Avoid spironolactone doses of more than 25 mg/day in elderly patients with HF or renal impairment.

amiloride and hydrochlorothiazide
GENERIC COMPONENTS
amiloride hydrochloride–hydrochlorothiazide
Tablets
5 mg amiloride hydrochloride and 50 mg hydrochlorothiazide
DOSAGES
Black Box Warning May cause potentially fatal hyperkalemia; monitor serum potassium levels carefully. ∎
Edema or hypertension
Adults: 1 to 2 tablets P.O. per day with food.

Heart failure drugs

BiDil
GENERIC COMPONENTS
isosorbide dinitrate–hydralazine
Tablets
20 mg isosorbide dinitrate and 37.5 mg hydralazine
DOSAGES
Adjunct to standard HF therapy
Adults: 1 to 2 tablets P.O. t.i.d.

Lipid-lowering drugs

Vytorin ✐
GENERIC COMPONENTS
ezetimibe–simvastatin
Tablets
10 mg ezetimibe with 10, 20, 40, or 80 mg simvastatin
DOSAGES
Homozygous familial hypercholesterolemia and primary hyperlipidemia
Adults: 1 tablet P.O. daily, taken in the evening in combination with a cholesterol-lowering diet and exercise. May adjust dosage of simvastatin in combination based on patient response.

Only use 10 mg ezetimibe/80 mg simvastatin in patients who have been taking drug long-term without evidence of muscle toxicity. In patients unable to achieve their LDL cholesterol goal using 10 mg ezetimibe/40 mg simvastatin, don't titrate to the 10 mg ezetimibe/80 mg simvastatin dose; use an alternative therapy.

If drug is given with a bile acid sequestrant, drug must be given at least 2 hours before or 4 hours after the bile acid sequestrant.

Adjust-a-dose: For patients with moderate to severe renal impairment, give 10 mg ezetimibe/20 mg simvastatin once daily. If patient is also taking diltiazem, dronedarone, or verapamil, don't exceed 10 mg ezetimibe/10 mg simvastatin daily. If patient is also taking amiodarone, amlodipine, or ranolazine, don't exceed 10 mg ezetimibe/20 mg simvastatin daily. If patient is also taking lomitapide, reduce simvastatin dosage by 50%.

Menopause drugs

Duavee
GENERIC COMPONENTS
conjugated estrogens–bazedoxifene acetate
Tablets
0.45 mg conjugated estrogens and 20 mg bazedoxifene acetate
DOSAGES
Black Box Warning Risk of endometrial cancer and CV disease; not for preventing dementia; use at lowest effective doses, for the shortest duration, consistent with treatment goals and risks for the individual woman. ∎
Vasomotor symptoms; postmenopausal osteoporosis prevention
Adults: 1 tablet P.O. once daily.

Premphase
GENERIC COMPONENTS
conjugated estrogens/conjugated estrogens–medroxyprogesterone
Tablets
0.625 mg conjugated estrogens; 0.625 mg conjugated estrogens and 5 mg medroxyprogesterone
DOSAGES
Black Box Warning Risk of endometrial and breast cancer and CV disease; not for preventing dementia; use at lowest effective doses, for the

shortest duration, consistent with treatment goals and risks for the individual woman. ■

Moderate to severe symptoms of menopause; to prevent osteoporosis
Women with intact uterus: 1 tablet P.O. per day. Use estrogen alone on days 1 to 14 and estrogen–medroxy-progesterone tablet on days 15 to 28.

Prempro

GENERIC COMPONENTS
conjugated estrogens–medroxyprogesterone
Tablets
0.3 mg conjugated estrogens and 1.5 mg medroxy-progesterone
0.45 mg conjugated estrogens and 1.5 mg medroxy-progesterone
0.625 mg conjugated estrogens and 2.5 mg medroxy-progesterone
0.625 mg conjugated estrogens and 5 mg medroxy-progesterone
DOSAGES
Black Box Warning Risk of endometrial and breast cancer and CV disease; not for preventing dementia; use at lowest effective doses, for the shortest duration, consistent with treatment goals and risks for the individual woman. ■

Symptoms of menopause; to prevent osteoporosis
Women with intact uterus: 1 tablet P.O. per day.

Miscellaneous cardiac drugs

Caduet

GENERIC COMPONENTS
amlodipine besylate–atorvastatin calcium
Tablets
2.5 mg amlodipine besylate with 10 mg, 20 mg, or 40 mg atorvastatin calcium
5 mg amlodipine besylate with 10 mg, 20 mg, 40 mg, or 80 mg atorvastatin calcium
10 mg amlodipine besylate with 10 mg, 20 mg, 40 mg, or 80 mg atorvastatin calcium
DOSAGES
Adjust-a-dose (for all indications): For small or fragile patients, initially, amlodipine 2.5 mg once daily. Atorvastatin is contraindicated in patients with active liver disease or unexplained of LFT elevations. Refer to manufacturer's instructions for dosage adjustments when used with concomitant drugs.

Treatment of hypertension, chronic stable angina, or suspected vasospastic angina in patients with primary hypercholesterolemia and mixed dyslipidemia or hypertriglyceridemia
Adults: Determine the most effective dose for each component. Then select the most appropriate combination product. Maximum dose, amlodipine 10 mg and atorvastatin 80 mg/day.

Treatment of hypertension, adjunct to diet to reduce total cholesterol, LDL cholesterol in children with heterozygous familial hypercholesterolemia
Boys and postmenarchal girls age 10 and older: Initially 2.5 amlodipine /10 mg atorvastatin P.O. once daily. Maintenance dosage is 2.5 to 5 mg amlodipine P.O.

once daily. Atorvastatin maximum dose, 20 mg/day. When titrating amlodipine, wait 7 to 14 days between titration steps. When titrating atorvastatin, adjust dosage at intervals of 4 weeks or more.

Opioid agonists

Bunavail
Suboxone
Zubsolv
Controlled Substance Schedule III
GENERIC COMPONENTS
buprenorphine–naloxone
Sublingual tablets
2 mg buprenorphine and 0.5 mg naloxone
8 mg buprenorphine and 2 mg naloxone
Sublingual tablets (Zubsolv)
1.4 mg buprenorphine and 0.36 mg naloxone
2.9 buprenorphine and 0.71 mg naloxone
5.7 mg buprenorphine and 1.4 mg naloxone
8.6 buprenorphine and 2.1 mg naloxone
11.4 buprenorphine and 2.9 mg naloxone
Sublingual film
2 mg buprenorphine and 0.5 mg naloxone
4 mg buprenorphine and 1 mg naloxone
8 mg buprenorphine and 2 mg naloxone
12 mg buprenorphine and 3 mg naloxone
Buccal film
2 mg buprenorphine and 0.5 mg naloxone
2.1 mg buprenorphine and 0.3 mg naloxone
4 mg buprenorphine and 1 mg naloxone
4.2 mg buprenorphine and 0.7 mg naloxone
6.3 mg buprenorphine and 1 mg naloxone
8 mg buprenorphine and 2 mg naloxone
12 mg buprenorphine and 3 mg naloxone
DOSAGES
Black Box Warning Opioids combined with benzodiazepines or CNS depressants can cause death. ■

Induction of opioid dependence treatment
Adults: On day 1, when objective and clear signs of moderate withdrawal are evident, initial dose is 1.4 mg buprenorphine/0.36 mg naloxone sublingually. Remainder of day 1 dose of up to 4.2 mg buprenorphine/1.08 mg naloxone should be divided into doses of 1 to 2 tablets of 1.4 mg buprenorphine/0.36 mg naloxone sublingually at 1.5- to 2-hour intervals up to a total day 1 dosage of 5.7 mg buprenorphine/1.4 mg naloxone. On day 2, give up to 11.4 mg buprenorphine/2.9 mg naloxone sublingually as a single dose. Maintenance treatment is 11.4 mg buprenorphine/2.9 mg naloxone sublingually daily. Adjust dosage based on clinical need to control acute withdrawal symptoms.

Opioid dependence
Adults and children age 16 and older: Maintenance dose is based on buprenorphine. Give 12 to 16 mg (buprenorphine) S.L. tablet once daily, after induction with S.L. buprenorphine (one Zubsolv 5.7-mg buprenorphine/1.4-mg naloxone sublingual tablet is equivalent to one 8-mg buprenorphine/2-mg naloxone tablet). Or, buprenorphine 4 to 24 mg with naloxone

1 to 6 mg S.L. film as a single daily maintenance dose after buprenorphine induction. Or, buprenorphine 2.1 to 12.6 mg with naloxone 0.3- to 2-mg buccal film as a single daily maintenance dose after S.L. buprenorphine induction (4.2-mg buprenorphine/0.7-mg naloxone buccal film is equivalent to one 8-mg buprenorphine/2-mg naloxone tablet).

Psychotherapeutics

chlordiazepoxide–amitriptyline
Controlled Substance Schedule IV
GENERIC COMPONENTS
chlordiazepoxide–amitriptyline
Tablets
5 mg chlordiazepoxide and 12.5 mg amitriptyline
10 mg chlordiazepoxide and 25 mg amitriptyline
DOSAGES
Black Box Warning Not approved for use in children because of suicide risk. Opioids combined with benzodiazepines or CNS depressants can cause death. ■
Severe depression
Adults: 10 mg chlordiazepoxide/25 mg amitriptyline P.O. t.i.d. to up to six times daily. For patients who don't tolerate higher doses, 5 mg chlordiazepoxide/12.5 mg amitriptyline P.O. t.i.d. to q.i.d. Reduce dosage after initial response.
Adjust-a-dose: Elderly patients may need lower dosages.

perphenazine and amitriptyline
GENERIC COMPONENTS
perphenazine–amitriptyline
Tablets
2 mg perphenazine and 10 mg amitriptyline
2 mg perphenazine and 25 mg amitriptyline
4 mg perphenazine and 10 mg amitriptyline
4 mg perphenazine and 25 mg amitriptyline
4 mg perphenazine and 50 mg amitriptyline
DOSAGES
Black Box Warning Not approved for use in children because of suicide risk or in patients with dementia-related psychosis because of increased risk of death. Opioids combined with benzodiazepines or CNS depressants can cause death. ■
Treatment of anxiety, agitation, or depression
Adults: 2 to 4 mg perphenazine/10 to 25 mg amitriptyline P.O. t.i.d. to q.i.d. or 4 mg perphenazine/50 mg amitriptyline P.O. b.i.d. Reduce dosage after initial response.

Symbyax
GENERIC COMPONENTS
olanzapine–fluoxetine
Capsules
3 mg olanzapine and 25 mg fluoxetine
6 mg olanzapine and 25 mg fluoxetine
6 mg olanzapine and 50 mg fluoxetine
12 mg olanzapine and 25 mg fluoxetine
12 mg olanzapine and 50 mg fluoxetine

DOSAGES
Black Box Warning Not approved for use in children younger than age 10 because of suicide risk or in patients with dementia-related psychosis because of increased risk of death. ■
Treatment of bipolar I disorder or depression
Adults: 1 capsule P.O. daily in the evening. Begin with 6 mg/25 mg capsule and adjust according to effectiveness and tolerability.
Children age 10 and older with bipolar depression: Initially, olanzapine 3 mg/fluoxetine 25 mg P.O. daily in the evening, adjusted according to effectiveness and tolerability.

Respiratory tract drugs

Claritin-D ◇
Claritin-D 24 Hour ◇
GENERIC COMPONENTS
loratadine–pseudoephedrine
Tablets (extended-release) DNC
5 mg loratadine and 120 mg pseudoephedrine
10 mg loratadine and 240 mg pseudoephedrine
DOSAGES
Seasonal allergic rhinitis
Adults and children age 12 and older: 5 mg loratadine/120 mg pseudoephedrine P.O. b.i.d., or 10 mg loratadine/240 mg pseudoephedrine P.O. daily.

Combivent Respimat
GENERIC COMPONENTS
ipratropium bromide–albuterol
Metered-dose inhaler
20 mcg ipratropium bromide and 100 mcg albuterol
DOSAGES
Bronchospasm with COPD in patients who require more than a single bronchodilator
Adults: 1 inhalation q.i.d. May take additional doses as needed up to maximum of 6 total inhalations in 24 hours.

Dulera
GENERIC COMPONENTS
mometasone furoate–formoterol fumarate dihydrate
Oral inhalation
100 mcg mometasone furoate and 5 mcg formoterol fumarate dihydrate
200 mcg mometasone furoate and 5 mcg formoterol fumarate dihydrate
DOSAGES
Black Box Warning Increases the risk of asthma-related death; don't use if patient is controlled on low- or medium-dose inhaled corticosteroids. ■
Asthma
Adults and children over age 12: 2 inhalations b.i.d. Starting dose based on prior asthma therapy.

Symbicort

GENERIC COMPONENTS
budesonide–formoterol fumarate dihydrate
Aerosol inhalation
80 mcg budesonide and 4.5 mcg formoterol fumarate
dihydrate per actuation
160 mcg budesonide and 4.5 mcg formoterol fumarate
dihydrate per actuation
DOSAGES
Black Box Warning Increases the risk of asthma-
related death; don't use if patient controlled on
low- or medium-dose inhaled corticosteroids. ∎
Asthma, COPD
Adults and children age 12 and older: Initially, 2 inhalations b.i.d. approximately 12 hours apart.

Tussionex Pennkinetic ER

Controlled Substance Schedule II
GENERIC COMPONENTS
chlorpheniramine polistirex–hydrocodone
bitartrate
Oral solution (extended-release)
8 mg chlorpheniramine polisterix and 10 mg hydrocodone bitartrate/5 mL
DOSAGES
Black Box Warning Opioids combined with
benzodiazepines or CNS depressants can cause
death. ∎
**Cough and upper respiratory tract infection signs
and symptoms**
Adults and children age 12 and older: 8 mg chlorpheniramine polisterix/10 mg hydrocodone P.O. every
12 hours. Maximum dose, 16 mg chlorpheniramine
polisterix and 20 mg hydrocodone in 24 hours.
Children ages 6 to 11: 4 mg chlorpheniramine polis-
terix/5 mg hydrocodone P.O. every 12 hours. Maximum dose is 8 mg chlorpheniramine maleate/10 mg
hydrocodone in 24 hours.

Vaccines and toxoids: Indications and dosages

Refer to manufacturer's instructions for complete prescribing and safety information.

anthrax vaccine, adsorbed
BioThrax

Pharmacologic class: Vaccines

AVAILABLE FORMS
Injection: 0.5 mL/dose in 5-mL multidose vial

INDICATIONS & DOSAGES
Pre-exposure prophylaxis of disease caused by *Bacillus anthracis* in persons at high risk of exposure
Adults ages 18 through 65: 0.5 mL I.M. at day 0, month 1, and then 6, 12, and 18 months. Yearly booster injections of 0.5 mL I.M. are recommended for those who remain at risk. Or, 0.5 mL subcutaneously at 0, 2, and 4 weeks and 6 months, with booster doses at 12 and 18 months and at 1-year intervals thereafter.
Postexposure prophylaxis of disease following suspected or confirmed *Bacillus anthracis* exposure, in conjunction with recommended antibacterial drugs
Adults ages 18 through 65: 0.5 mL subcutaneously 0, 2, and 4 weeks after exposure.

Haemophilus b conjugate vaccines

Haemophilus b conjugate vaccine, meningococcal protein conjugate (PRP-OMP)
PedvaxHIB

Haemophilus b conjugate, tetanus toxoid conjugate (PRP-T)
ActHIB, Hiberix

Pharmacologic class: Vaccines

AVAILABLE FORMS
HIB conjugate vaccine, hepatitis B
Injection: 7.5 mcg of HIB capsular polysaccharide and 5 mcg hepatitis B surface antigen (HBsAg) per 0.5 mL
HIB conjugate vaccine, meningococcal protein conjugate
Injection: 7.5 mcg of HIB PRP and 125 mcg *N. meningitides* OMPC per 0.5 mL
HIB conjugate vaccine, tetanus toxoid conjugate
Injection: 10 mcg HIB capsular polysaccharide and 24 mcg tetanus toxoid (ActHIB) or 10 mcg HIB capsular polysaccharide and 24 mcg tetanus toxoid (Hiberix)

INDICATIONS & DOSAGES
Conjugate vaccine, hepatitis B
Infants born to HBsAg-negative mothers: 0.5 mL I.M. at ages 2, 4, and 12 to 15 months for a total of three doses.
Conjugate vaccine, meningococcal protein conjugate
Infants: 0.5 mL I.M. at age 2 months; repeat at age 4 months. Give booster dose at age 12 months.
Previously unvaccinated children ages 15 months to 6 years: 0.5 mL I.M. Booster dose isn't needed. Premature infants follow same schedule as full-term infants.
Previously unvaccinated infants ages 12 to 14 months: 0.5 mL I.M. Give booster dose at age 15 months (but no sooner than 2 months after first vaccination).
Previously unvaccinated infants ages 7 to 11 months: 0.5 mL I.M.; repeat in 2 months. Give booster dose at age 15 months (but no sooner than 2 months after last vaccination).
Previously unvaccinated infants ages 2 to 6 months: 0.5 mL I.M.; repeat in 2 months. Give booster dose at age 12 months.
Conjugate vaccine, tetanus toxoid conjugate
Infants: 0.5 mL I.M. at age 2 months. Repeat at ages 4 and 6 months. Give booster doses at ages 15 to 18 months.
Previously unvaccinated infants ages 7 to 11 months: 0.5 mL I.M. Repeat in 2 months, for a total of two doses. Give booster doses at ages 15 to 18 months.
Previously unvaccinated infants ages 12 to 14 months: 0.5 mL I.M. Repeat in 2 months, for a total of two doses.

diphtheria and tetanus toxoids and acellular pertussis vaccine adsorbed (DTaP)
Daptacel, Infanrix

tetanus toxoid and reduced diphtheria toxoid and acellular pertussis vaccine adsorbed (Tdap)
Adacel, Boostrix

Pharmacologic class: Vaccines/toxoids

AVAILABLE FORMS
DTaP
Daptacel
Injection: 15 limit flocculation (Lf) units diphtheria toxoid, 5 Lf units tetanus toxoid, and 10 mcg pertussis toxoid adsorbed per 0.5 mL
Infanrix
Injection: 25 Lf units diphtheria toxoid, 10 Lf units tetanus toxoid, and 58 mcg inactivated pertussis toxins adsorbed per 0.5 mL

Tdap
Adacel
Injection: 5 Lf units tetanus toxoid, 2 Lf units diphtheria toxoid, and 15.5 mcg detoxified pertussis toxins adsorbed per 0.5 mL
Boostrix
Injection: 5 Lf units tetanus toxoid, 2.5 Lf units diphtheria toxoid, and 18.5 mcg inactivated pertussis toxins adsorbed per 0.5 mL

INDICATIONS & DOSAGES
➤ **Primary immunization (Daptacel, Infanrix)**
Children ages 6 weeks to 6 years (prior to 7th birthday): 0.5 mL I.M. 4 to 8 weeks apart for three doses (6 to 8 weeks for Daptacel) and a fourth dose at least 6 months after the third dose.
➤ **Booster immunization**
Children ages 6 weeks to 7 years: Daptacel may be given to complete the immunization series in children who have received at least one dose of whole-cell DTP vaccine.

Infanrix is indicated as a fifth dose in children ages 4 to 6 before entering school in those who received at least one dose of whole-cell DTP vaccine, unless the fourth dose was given after the fourth birthday.

If Tripedia was used for the first four doses, a fifth dose is recommended at age 4 to 6 before entering school. If the fourth dose was given after age 4, a fifth dose isn't needed.
Adults and children ages 10 to 64 (Adacel): 0.5 mL I.M. as a single dose at least 5 years after the last DTaP vaccination.
Adults and children age 10 and older (Boostrix): 0.5 mL I.M. as a single dose at least 5 years after the last DTaP vaccination.

diphtheria and tetanus toxoids, acellular pertussis adsorbed, hepatitis B (recombinant), and inactivated poliovirus vaccine combined
Pediarix

Pharmacologic class: Vaccines/toxoids

AVAILABLE FORMS
Injection: 0.5-mL single-dose vials and disposable, prefilled Tip-Lok syringes

INDICATIONS & DOSAGES
➤ **Active immunization**
Children ages 6 weeks to 7 years: Primary series is three 0.5-mL doses I.M. at 6- to 8-week intervals (preferably 8), usually starting at age 2 months; may start at age 6 weeks.

diphtheria and tetanus toxoids, acellular pertussis adsorbed, and inactivated poliovirus combination vaccine (DTaP/IPV)
Kinrix

Pharmacologic class: Vaccines/toxoids

AVAILABLE FORMS
Injection: 25 limit flocculation (Lf) units diphtheria toxoid, 10 Lf tetanus toxoid, 25 mcg inactivated pertussis toxin (PT), 25 mcg filamentous hemagglutinin, 8 mcg pertactin, 40 D-antigen units type 1 poliovirus (Mahoney), 8 D-antigen units type 2 poliovirus (MEF-1), and 32 D-antigen units/0.5 mL type 3 poliovirus (Saukett)

INDICATIONS & DOSAGES
➤ **Active immunization against diphtheria, tetanus, pertussis, and poliomyelitis as the fifth dose in the DTaP vaccine series and the fourth dose in the IPV series in those whose previous DTaP vaccine doses have been with Infanrix (diphtheria and tetanus toxoids and acellular pertussis vaccine adsorbed) or Pediarix (diphtheria and tetanus toxoids, acellular pertussis adsorbed, hepatitis B [recombinant], and IPV vaccine combined) for first three doses and Infanrix for fourth dose**
Children ages 4 through 6: 0.5 mL I.M., preferably in the deltoid muscle of the upper arm.

diphtheria and tetanus toxoids, acellular pertussis adsorbed, inactivated poliovirus, and *Haemophilus influenzae* type b conjugate vaccine combined
Pentacel

Pharmacologic class: Vaccines/toxoids

AVAILABLE FORMS
Injection: 15 limit flocculation (Lf) diphtheria toxoid, 5 Lf tetanus toxoid, 20 mcg pertussis toxin detoxified, 20 mcg filamentous hemagglutinin, 3 mcg pertactin, 5 mcg fimbriae types 2 and 3, 40 D-antigen units type 1 inactivated poliovirus (Mahoney), 8 D-antigen units type 2 inactivated poliovirus (MEF-1), 32 D-antigen units type 3 inactivated poliovirus (Saukett), and 10 mcg lyophilized polyribosyl-ribitol-phosphate of *H. influenzae* type b bound to tetanus toxoid 24 mcg per 0.5 mL

INDICATIONS & DOSAGES
➤ **Active immunization against diphtheria, tetanus, pertussis, poliomyelitis, and invasive disease caused by *H. influenzae* type b**
Children ages 6 weeks to 4 years (prior to 5th birthday): 0.5 mL I.M. Approved for administration as a four-dose

series at ages 2, 4, 6, and 15 through 18 months. The first dose may be given as early as age 6 weeks.

hepatitis A vaccine, inactivated
Havrix, Vaqta

Pharmacologic class: Vaccines

AVAILABLE FORMS
Havrix
Injection: 720 enzyme-linked immunosorbent assay (ELISA) units (ELU)/0.5 mL; 1,440 ELU/mL
Vaqta
Injection: 25 units/0.5 mL, 50 units/mL

INDICATIONS & DOSAGES
➤ **Active immunization against hepatitis A virus; with immune globulin, to prevent hepatitis A in those exposed to virus or who travel to endemic areas**
Adults: 1,440 ELU Havrix or 50 units Vaqta I.M. as single dose. For booster dose, give 1,440 ELU Havrix 6 to 12 months after first dose or 50 units Vaqta I.M. 6 to 18 months after first dose. Booster is recommended for prolonged immunity.
Children ages 12 months to 18 years: 720 ELU Havrix or 25 units Vaqta I.M. as single dose. Then, give booster dose of 720 ELU Havrix 6 to 12 months after first dose or 25 units Vaqta I.M. 6 to 18 months after first dose. Booster is recommended for prolonged immunity.

hepatitis B vaccine, recombinant
Engerix-B, Recombivax HB, Recombivax HB Dialysis Formulation

Pharmacologic class: Vaccines

AVAILABLE FORMS
Injection: 5 mcg hepatitis B surface antigen (HBsAg)/ 0.5 mL (Recombivax HB, pediatric and adolescent form with or without preservative); 10 mcg HBsAg/ 0.5 mL (Engerix-B, pediatric and adolescent form); 10 mcg HBsAg/mL (Recombivax HB, adult form); 20 mcg HBsAg/mL (Engerix-B, adult form); 40 mcg HBsAg/mL (Recombivax HB Dialysis Formulation)

INDICATIONS & DOSAGES
➤ **Immunization against infection from all known subtypes of HBV, primary preexposure prophylaxis against HBV, postexposure prophylaxis when given with hepatitis B immune globulin (HBIG)**
Engerix-B
Adults age 20 and older: Initially, 20 mcg I.M.; then second dose of 20 mcg I.M. after 30 days. A third dose of 20 mcg I.M. is given 6 months after the first dose.

Adjust-a-dose: For adults undergoing dialysis or receiving immunosuppressants, initially, 40 mcg I.M. (divided into two 20-mcg doses and given at different sites). Then second dose of 40 mcg I.M. in 30 days, a third dose after 2 months, and final dose of 40 mcg I.M. 6 months after first dose.
Adolescents ages 11 to 19: Initially, 10 mcg (pediatric and adolescent form) I.M.; then second dose of 10 mcg I.M. 30 days later. Give third dose of 10 mcg I.M. 6 months after first dose. Or, 20 mcg (adult form) I.M.; then second dose of 20 mcg I.M. 30 days later. Give third dose of 20 mcg I.M. 6 months after first dose.
Neonates and children up to age 10: Initially, 10 mcg I.M.; then second dose of 10 mcg I.M. 30 days later. Give third dose of 10 mcg I.M. 6 months after first dose.
Recombivax HB
Adults age 20 and older: Initially, 10 mcg I.M.; then second dose of 10 mcg I.M. after 30 days. Give third dose of 10 mcg I.M. 6 months after first dose. For adults undergoing dialysis, initially, 40 mcg I.M. (use dialysis form, which contains 40 mcg/mL); then second dose of 40 mcg I.M. in 30 days, and final dose of 40 mcg I.M. 6 months after first dose. A booster or revaccination may be indicated if anti-HBs titer is below 10 mIU/mL 1 to 2 months after third dose.
Infants, children, and adolescents age 19 or younger: Initially, 5 mcg I.M.; then second dose of 5 mcg I.M. after 30 days. Give third dose of 5 mcg I.M. 6 months after first dose. Or, in adolescents ages 11 to 15, give 10 mcg (1 mL adult form) I.M.; then second dose of 10 mcg 4 to 6 months later.
Infants born of HBsAg-positive mothers or mothers of unknown HbsAg status: Initially, 5 mcg I.M.; then second dose of 5 mcg I.M. after 30 days. Give third dose of 5 mcg I.M. 6 months after first dose.
Infants born of HBsAg-negative mothers: Initially, 5 mcg I.M.; then second dose of 5 mcg I.M. after 30 days. Give third dose of 5 mcg I.M. 6 months after first dose.
Note: If the mother is found to be HbsAg-positive within 7 days of delivery, also give the infant a dose of HBIG (0.5 mL) in the opposite anterolateral thigh.

human papillomavirus recombinant vaccine, bivalent
Cervarix

Pharmacologic class: Vaccines

AVAILABLE FORMS
Injection: 0.5 mL single-dose vial

INDICATIONS & DOSAGES
➤ **To prevent cervical cancer, cervical intraepithelial neoplasia (CIN) grade 2 or worse and adenocarcinoma in situ, and CIN grade 1 caused by human papillomavirus types 16 and 18**
Women and girls ages 9 to 25: 0.5 mL I.M. given as three doses at 0, 1, and 6 months.

human papillomavirus recombinant vaccine, quadrivalent
Gardasil

human papillomavirus recombinant vaccine, 9-valent
Gardasil 9

Pharmacologic class: Virus antigens

AVAILABLE FORMS
Injection: 0.5 mL single-dose vial, prefilled syringe

INDICATIONS & DOSAGES
➤ **To prevent cervical cancer, genital warts, cervical adenocarcinoma in situ, and cervical, vulval, vaginal, and anal intraepithelial neoplasias caused by human papillomavirus types 6, 11, 16, and 18 (Gardasil, Gardasil 9) and 31, 33, 45, 52, and 58 (Gardasil 9)**
Women and girls ages 9 to 26: Three separate I.M. injections of 0.5 mL each. Give second injection 2 months after first, then give third injection 6 months after the first.
➤ **To prevent genital warts, anal cancer, and anal intraepithelial neoplasia caused by human papillomavirus types 6, 11, 16, and 18 (Gardasil, Gardasil 9) and 31, 33, 45, 52, and 58 (Gardasil 9)**
Men and boys ages 9 to 26: Three separate I.M. injections of 0.5 mL each. Give second injection 2 months after first, then give third injection 6 months after first.

influenza virus vaccine, live
Afluria, Fluarix, Fluarix Quadrivalent, Flublok, Flucelvax, FluLaval, FluLaval Quadrivalent, Fluvirin, Fluzone High-Dose, Fluzone Intradermal, Fluzone Quadrivalent

Pharmacologic class: Vaccines

AVAILABLE FORMS
Injection: 0.25 mL single-dose syringes (FluLaval Quadrivalent, Fluzone Quadrivalent); 0.1 mL single-dose microinjection system (Fluzone Intradermal); 0.5 mL single-dose syringes (Afluria, Fluarix, Fluarix Quadrivalent, Flublok, Flucelvax, FluLaval Quadrivalent, Fluvirin, Fluzone High-Dose, Fluzone Quadrivalent); 5-mL multidose vials (Afluria, FluLaval, Fluvirin)

INDICATIONS & DOSAGES
➤ **Active immunization to prevent disease caused by influenza A and B viruses**

Adults ages 18 to 64: 0.5 mL I.M. as a single dose or 0.1 mL intradermally as a single dose (Fluzone Intradermal).
Children age 9 and older: 0.5 mL I.M. as a single dose (Afluria, Fluarix, Fluarix Quadrivalent, FluLaval, FluLaval Quadrivalent, Fluvirin, Fluzone Quadrivalent).
Children ages 3 to 8: 0.5 mL I.M. as a single dose (Fluarix, Fluarix Quadrivalent, FluLaval Quadrivalent, Fluzone Quadrivalent). Repeat at least 1 month later for those receiving influenza vaccine for first time or who were vaccinated for first time last season with only one dose.
Children ages 4 to 8: 0.5 mL I.M. as a single dose (Fluvirin). Repeat at least 1 month later for those receiving influenza vaccine for first time or who were vaccinated for first time last season with only one dose.
Children ages 5 to 8: 0.5 mL (Afluria) I.M. as a single dose.
Children ages 6 to 35 months: 0.25 mL I.M. as a single dose (Fluzone Quadrivalent). Repeat at least 1 month later for those receiving influenza vaccine for first time or who were vaccinated for first time last season with only one dose.
Elderly patients (age 65 and older): 0.5 mL I.M. as a single dose (Fluzone High-Dose, Fluzone Quadrivalent).

influenza virus vaccine, live, intranasal
FluMist Quadrivalent

Pharmacologic class: Vaccines

AVAILABLE FORMS
Intranasal spray: 0.2 mL

INDICATIONS & DOSAGES
➤ **Active immunization to prevent disease caused by influenza A and B viruses**
Adults younger than age 50 and children older than age 9: 0.2-mL intranasal dose (0.1 mL in each nostril) once each season.
Children ages 2 through 8 not previously vaccinated with FluMist: Two intranasal doses of 0.2 mL (0.1 mL in each nostril) at least 1 month apart for the first season.
Children ages 2 through 8 previously vaccinated with FluMist: 0.2-mL intranasal dose (0.1 mL in each nostril) once each season.

Japanese encephalitis virus vaccine
Ixiaro

Pharmacologic class: Vaccines

AVAILABLE FORMS
Injection: 6 mcg/0.5 mL

INDICATIONS & DOSAGES

➤ **To prevent disease caused by Japanese encephalitis virus**

Adults and children age 3 and older: Two doses of 0.5 mL I.M. 28 days apart. Complete immunization at least 1 week before exposure. If primary series of two doses was completed more than a year previously, may give a booster dose if ongoing exposure or reexposure is expected.

Children ages 2 months to younger than 3 years: Two doses of 0.25 mL I.M. 28 days apart.

measles, mumps, and rubella virus vaccine, live
M-M-R II

Pharmacologic class: Vaccines

AVAILABLE FORMS

Injection: Single-dose vial containing at least 1,000 tissue culture infective doses ($TCID_{50}$), 20,000 $TCID_{50}$ of mumps strain, and 1,000 $TCID_{50}$ rubella virus per 0.5-mL dose

INDICATIONS & DOSAGES

➤ **Routine immunization**

Adults: 0.5 mL subcutaneously.

Children age 12 months and older: 0.5 mL subcutaneously. A two-dose schedule is recommended, with first dose given between ages 12 and 15 months (between ages 6 and 12 months in high-risk areas) and second dose given at ages 4 to 6 before elementary school entry.

measles, mumps, rubella, and varicella (MMRV) virus vaccine, live, attenuated
ProQuad

Pharmacologic class: Vaccines

AVAILABLE FORMS

Injection: Single-dose vial containing at least 3.00 log_{10} measles tissue culture infective doses ($TCID_{50}$), 4.30 log_{10} mumps $TCID_{50}$, 3.00 log_{10} rubella $TCID_{50}$, and at least 3.99 log_{10} varicella plaque-forming units (PFU) per 0.5-mL dose

INDICATIONS & DOSAGES

➤ **Routine immunization**

Children ages 12 months to 12 years: 0.5 mL subcutaneously. The first dose is usually given between ages 12 and 15 months but may be given anytime through age 12. A second dose, if needed, is usually given between ages 4 and 6. At least 1 month should elapse between a dose of a measles-containing vaccine and a dose of MMRV vaccine. If a second dose of a varicella-containing vaccine is required, at least 3 months should elapse between administration of the two doses.

meningococcal (groups A, C, Y, and W-135) polysaccharide diphtheria toxoid conjugate vaccine (MCV4)
Menactra

meningococcal polysaccharide vaccine, groups A, C, Y, and W-135 combined (MPSV4)
Menomune A/C/Y/W-135, Menveo (Men ACWY-CRM)

meningococcal (group B) vaccine
Bexsero, Trumemba

Pharmacologic class: Vaccines

AVAILABLE FORMS

Injection: 0.5 mL single-dose vials and prefilled syringes

INDICATIONS & DOSAGES

➤ **Active immunization for the prevention of invasive meningococcal disease caused by *Neisseria meningitidis* serogroups A, C, Y, and W-135**

Adults and children ages 2 to 55: 0.5 mL MCV4 I.M. as a single dose, preferably in the deltoid muscle.

Adults and children ages 15 to 55 who are at continued risk for meningococcal disease: 0.5 mL Menactra as a booster at least 4 years after prior dose.

Children ages 9 to 23 months: 0.5 mL Menactra I.M. given as a two-dose series 3 months apart.

Adults and children older than age 2: 0.5 mL MPSV4 subcutaneously as a single dose, preferably in the upper-outer triceps area.

Adults and children ages 2 to 55: 0.5 mL Menveo I.M. as single dose, preferably into deltoid muscle. For children ages 2 to 5 at continued high risk for meningococcal disease, a second dose may be given 2 months after the first dose.

Children ages 7 to 23 months: 0.5 mL Menveo I.M. given as a two-dose series with second dose in the second year of life and at least 3 months after first dose.

Infants: 0.5 mL Menveo I.M. given as a four-dose series at 2, 4, 6, and 12 months.

➤ **Active immunization for the prevention of invasive meningococcal disease caused by *N. meningitidis* serogroup B**

Adults and children age 10 and older: 0.5 mL/dose (Bexsero) I.M. as a two-dose series at least 1 month apart. Or, 0.5 mL/dose (Trumemba) I.M. at 0 and 6 months (two-dose schedule), or at 0 and then a second dose at either 1 or 2 months and then a third dose at 6 months (three-dose schedule).

meningococcal (groups C and Y) and *Haemophilus* b tetanus toxoid conjugate
MenHibrix

Pharmacologic class: Vaccines

AVAILABLE FORMS
Injection: Single-dose vials containing 5 mcg *Neisseria meningitidis* C capsular polysaccharide, 5 mcg *N. meningitidis* Y capsular polysaccharide, and 2.5 mcg *Haemophilus influenzae* b capsular polysaccharide in 0.5 mL

INDICATIONS & DOSAGES
➤ **To prevent invasive disease caused by *N. meningitidis* serogroups C and Y and *H. influenzae* type b**
Children ages 6 weeks through 18 months: 0.5 mL I.M. at age 2, 4, 6, and 12 through 15 months. May give first dose as early as age 6 weeks. May give fourth dose as late as age 18 months.

palivizumab
Synagis

Pharmacologic class: Monoclonal antibodies

AVAILABLE FORMS
Injection: 50-mg, 100-mg vials

INDICATIONS & DOSAGES
➤ **Prevention of serious lower respiratory tract disease caused by RSV**
High-risk infants age 24 months and younger: 15 mg/kg I.M. monthly throughout RSV season. Give first dose before commencement of RSV season.

pneumococcal vaccine, polyvalent
Pneumovax 23

13-valent conjugate vaccine
Prevnar 13

Pharmacologic class: Vaccines

AVAILABLE FORMS
Injection: 25 mcg each of 23 polysaccharide isolates/0.5 mL (Pneumovax 23); 2.2 mcg each of *Streptococcus pneumoniae* serotypes 1, 3, 4, 5, 6A, 7f, 9v, 14, 18C, 19a, 19f, and 23f saccharides and 4.4 mcg of serotype 6B saccharides (Prevnar 13)

INDICATIONS & DOSAGES
➤ **Pneumococcal immunization**
Adults age 50 and older; children age 2 and older at high risk: 0.5 mL Pneumovax I.M. or subcutaneously. Adults younger than age 50 who are at high risk may be immunized following Advisory Committee on Immunization Practices guidelines.
➤ **Immunization against *S. pneumoniae* and otitis media (Prevnar 13)**
Infants ages 6 weeks to 15 months: 0.5 mL I.M. for a total of four doses at ages 2, 4, 6, and 12 to 15 months.
Children ages 7 to 11 months, previously unvaccinated: 0.5 mL I.M.; three doses with at least 4 weeks between first and second doses, and 8 weeks between second and third doses.
Children ages 12 to 23 months, previously unvaccinated: Two doses of 0.5 mL I.M. at least 2 months apart.
Children ages 24 months to 5 years, previously unvaccinated: 0.5 mL I.M. as a single dose.
Children ages 6 to 17 (before the 18th birthday): 0.5 mL I.M. as a single dose. For children previously vaccinated with PCV7, wait at least 8 weeks.
Children who have received one or more doses of Prevnar (7-valent conjugate vaccine): Complete the four-dose immunization series with 13-valent conjugate vaccine.
Children ages 15 months through 5 years who have previously received four doses of Prevnar: 0.5 mL I.M. as a single dose.
➤ **Immunization against *S. pneumoniae* (Prevnar 13)**
Adults age 50 and older: 0.5 mL I.M. as a single dose.

poliovirus vaccine, inactivated (IPV)
IPOL

Pharmacologic class: Vaccines

AVAILABLE FORMS
0.5-mL prefilled syringe: Mixture of three types of poliovirus (types 1, 2, and 3) grown in tissue culture

INDICATIONS & DOSAGES
➤ **Poliovirus immunization**
Unvaccinated adults: 0.5 mL subcutaneously or I.M.; give second dose 4 to 8 weeks later. Give third dose 6 to 12 months later.
Children: 0.5 mL subcutaneously or I.M. at ages 2 months and 4 months. Give third dose at ages 6 to 18 months. Give a reinforcing dose of 0.5 mL subcutaneously before entry into school at ages 4 to 6.

rabies vaccine, human diploid cell (HDCV)
Imovax Rabies, RabAvert

Pharmacologic class: Vaccines

AVAILABLE FORMS
I.M. injection: 2.5 international units rabies antigen/mL, in single-dose vial with diluent

INDICATIONS & DOSAGES
➤ **Postexposure antirabies immunization**
Adults and children: Five 1-mL doses of HDCV I.M. Give first dose as soon as possible after exposure; give additional doses on days 3, 7, 14, and 28 after first dose. If no antibody response occurs after this primary series, booster dose is recommended.
➤ **Postexposure antirabies immunization in previously immunized people**
Adults and children: 1 mL I.M. immediately and 1 mL I.M. 3 days later.
➤ **Preexposure preventive immunization for persons in high-risk groups**
Adults and children: Three 1-mL injections I.M. Give first dose on day 0 (first day of therapy), second dose on day 7, and third dose on day 21 or 28.

rotavirus, live
Rotarix, RotaTeq

Pharmacologic class: Vaccines

AVAILABLE FORMS
Lyophilized powder for oral suspension: Rotavirus human 89-12 strain (G1P[8] type); $\geq 10^6$ cell culture infective dose per 1 mL (after reconstitution)
Oral suspension: Rotavirus outer capsid protein (2.2×10^6 infectious units of G1, 2.8×10^6 infectious units of G2, 2.2×10^6 infectious units of G3, 2×10^6 infectious units of G4, and 2.3×10^6 infectious units of rotavirus attachment protein P1A[8]) per 2 mL

INDICATIONS & DOSAGES
➤ **Prevention of rotavirus gastroenteritis**
RotaTeq
Children ages 6 to 32 weeks: 2 mL P.O. Give second dose 4 weeks later, followed by third dose at 10 weeks. Do not give third dose after the patient reaches age 32 weeks.
Rotarix
Infants ages 6 to 24 weeks: Give first dose of 1 mL P.O. at age 6 weeks. Give another 1-mL dose P.O. after at least 4 weeks. The two-dose series should be completed by age 24 weeks.

tetanus toxoid, adsorbed

Pharmacologic class: Vaccines

AVAILABLE FORMS
tetanus toxoid, adsorbed
Injection: 5 limit flocculation (Lf) units inactivated tetanus/0.5-mL dose, in 0.5-mL syringes and 5-mL vials

INDICATIONS & DOSAGES
➤ **Primary immunization to prevent tetanus**
Adults and children age 7 and older: 0.5 mL (adsorbed) I.M. 4 to 8 weeks apart for two doses; then give third dose 6 to 12 months after second.
➤ **Booster dose to prevent tetanus**
Adults and children age 7 and older: 0.5 mL I.M. at 10-year intervals.
➤ **Postexposure prevention of tetanus**
Adults and children age 7 and older: For a clean, minor wound, give emergency booster dose if more than 10 years have elapsed since last dose. For all other wounds, give booster dose if more than 5 years have elapsed since last dose.

varicella virus vaccine
Varivax

Pharmacologic class: Vaccines

AVAILABLE FORMS
Injection: Single-dose vial containing 1,350 plaque-forming units of Oka/Merck varicella virus (live)

INDICATIONS & DOSAGES
➤ **To prevent varicella zoster (chickenpox) infections**
Adults and children age 13 and older: 0.5 mL subcutaneously; then, second 0.5-mL dose 4 to 8 weeks later.
Children ages 1 to 12: 0.5 mL subcutaneously. If a second dose is given, allow a minimum interval of 3 months between doses.

zoster vaccine, live
Zostavax

Pharmacologic class: Vaccines, live attenuated

AVAILABLE FORMS
Injection: Lyophilized vaccine of 19,400 plaque-forming units/0.65 mL

INDICATIONS & DOSAGES
➤ **Prevention of herpes zoster (shingles)**
Adults age 50 and older: 0.65 mL subcutaneously as a single dose, preferably in the upper arm.

Vitamins and minerals: Indications and dosages

Refer to manufacturer's instructions for complete prescribing and safety information.

ferrous fumarate
FAIR-us

Femiron ◇, Feostat✚ ◇, Ferretts ◇, Ferrocite ◇, Hemocyte ◇, Iron ◇, Nephro-Fer ◇

Therapeutic class: Iron supplements
Pharmacologic class: Hematinics

AVAILABLE FORMS
Each 100 mg of ferrous fumarate provides 33 mg of elemental iron.
Tablets ⓄⓉⒸ: 29 mg ◇, 90 mg ◇, 150 mg ◇, 200 mg ◇, 324 mg ◇, 325 mg ◇, 350 mg ◇
Tablets (extended-release) ⓄⓉⒸ: 18 mg ◇

INDICATIONS & DOSAGES
➤ **Iron deficiency**
Adults: 1 or 2 tablets P.O. daily between meals or as directed by prescriber. For extended-release tablets, give 1 tablet P.O. daily.
Children: 3 to 6 mg/kg/day P.O. in three divided doses.
➤ **As a supplement during pregnancy**
Women: 27 mg elemental iron P.O. daily.

ferrous gluconate
FAIR-us

Fergon✚ ◇

Therapeutic class: Iron supplements
Pharmacologic class: Hematinics

AVAILABLE FORMS
Each 100 mg of ferrous gluconate provides 11.6 mg of elemental iron.
Tablets ⓄⓉⒸ: 225 mg ◇, 240 mg ◇, 324 mg ◇, 325 mg ◇

INDICATIONS & DOSAGES
➤ **Iron deficiency**
Adults: 100 to 200 mg P.O. daily in two to three divided doses.
Children: 3 to 6 mg/kg/day P.O. in three divided doses.

ferrous sulfate
FAIR-us

Feosol ◇ *, FeroSul ◇, Fer-Iron ◇

ferrous sulfate (dried)
Feosol ◇, Feratab ◇, Slow FE ◇, Slow Release Iron ◇

Therapeutic class: Iron supplements
Pharmacologic class: Hematinics

AVAILABLE FORMS
Each 100 mg of ferrous sulfate provides 20 mg of elemental iron or 30 mg of elemental iron in ferrous sulfate dried products.
Caplets (extended-release) ⓄⓉⒸ: 160 mg (dried) ◇
Capsules: 190 mg (dried)
Drops: 125 mg/mL ◇
Elixir: 220 mg/5 mL ◇ *
Liquid: 300 mg/5 mL ◇
Tablets: 195 mg ◇, 200 mg (dried) ◇, 300 mg (dried) ◇, 325 mg ◇
Tablets (slow-release) ⓄⓉⒸ: 142 mg ◇, 160 mg (dried) ◇

INDICATIONS & DOSAGES
➤ **Iron deficiency**
Adults: 100 to 200 mg P.O. daily in two or three divided doses. Extended- or slow-release tablets are intended for once-daily use.
Children: 3 to 6 mg/kg/day P.O. in three divided doses.

vitamin A (retinol)
Aquasol A, Vitamin A Palmitate ◇

AVAILABLE FORMS
Capsules: 7,500 international units ◇, 8,000 international units ◇, 10,000 international units ◇, 25,000 international units
Injection: 2-mL vials (50,000 international units/mL)
Tablets: 10,000 international units ◇, 15,000 international units ◇

INDICATIONS & DOSAGES
➤ **RDA**
Men and boys older than age 14: 900 mcg retinol equivalent (RE) or 3,000 international units.
Women and girls older than age 14: 700 mcg RE or 2,330 international units.
Children ages 9 to 13: 600 mcg RE or 2,000 international units.
Children ages 4 to 8: 400 mcg RE or 1,330 international units.
Children ages 1 to 3: 300 mcg RE or 1,000 international units.

Infants ages 7 to 12 months: 500 mcg RE or 1,665 international units.
Neonates and infants younger than age 6 months: 400 mcg RE or 1,330 international units.
Pregnant women ages 14 to 18: 750 mcg RE or 2,500 international units.
Pregnant women ages 19 to 50: 770 mcg RE or 2,564 international units.
Breast-feeding women ages 14 to 18: 1,200 mcg RE or 4,000 international units.
Breast-feeding women ages 19 to 50: 1,300 mcg RE or 4,330 international units.
➤ **Severe vitamin A deficiency**
Adults and children older than age 8: 100,000 international units I.M. or 100,000 to 500,000 international units P.O. for 3 days; then 50,000 international units P.O. or I.M. daily for 2 weeks, followed by 10,000 to 20,000 international units P.O. for 2 months. Follow with adequate dietary nutrition and RE vitamin A supplements.
Children ages 1 to 8: 17,500 to 35,000 international units I.M. daily for 10 days.
Infants: 7,500 to 15,000 international units I.M. daily for 10 days.
➤ **Maintenance dose to prevent recurrence of vitamin A deficiency**
Adults and children older than age 8: 10,000 to 20,000 international units P.O. daily for 2 months.
Children infants to age 8: Give 5,000 to 10,000 international units P.O. daily for 2 months; then adequate dietary nutrition and RE vitamin A supplements.

---

vitamin B complex
cyanocobalamin (vitamin B₁₂)
Nascobal, Rapid B-12 Energy ◇

hydroxocobalamin
(vitamin B₁₂)

AVAILABLE FORMS
cyanocobalamin
Capsules: 1,000 mcg ◇, 3,000 mcg ◇
Injection: 1,000 mcg/mL
Intranasal spray: 500 mcg/spray
Liquid: 1,000 mcg ◇, 3,000 mcg ◇, 5,000 mcg ◇
Lozenges: 50 mcg ◇, 100 mcg ◇, 250 mcg ◇, 500 mcg ◇, 1,000 mcg ◇, 3,000 mcg ◇, 5,000 mcg ◇
Oral spray: 200 mcg/spray ◇
Tablets: 50 mcg ◇, 100 mcg ◇, 250 mcg ◇, 500 mcg ◇, 1,000 mcg ◇, 5,000 mcg ◇
Tablets (extended-release): 1,000 mcg ◇, 1,500 mcg ◇
Tablets (S.L.): 500 mcg ◇, 1,000 mcg ◇, 1,500 mcg ◇, 2,500 mcg ◇, 3,000 mcg ◇, 5,000 mcg ◇, 6,000 mcg ◇
hydroxocobalamin
Injection: 1,000 mcg/mL

INDICATIONS & DOSAGES
➤ **RDA for cyanocobalamin**
Adults and children age 14 and older: 2.4 mcg.
Children ages 9 to 13: 1.8 mcg.

Children ages 4 to 8: 1.2 mcg.
Children ages 1 to 3: 0.9 mcg.
Infants ages 6 months to 1 year: 0.5 mcg.
Neonates and infants younger than age 6 months: 0.4 mcg.
Pregnant women: 2.6 mcg.
Breast-feeding women: 2.8 mcg.
➤ **Vitamin B₁₂ deficiency from inadequate diet, subtotal gastrectomy, or other condition, disorder, or disease, except malabsorption, related to pernicious anemia or other GI disease**
Adults: 30 mcg hydroxocobalamin I.M. daily for 5 to 10 days, depending on severity of deficiency. Maintenance dose is 100 to 200 mcg I.M. once monthly or 500 mcg gel intranasally once weekly. For subsequent prophylaxis, advise adequate nutrition and daily RDA vitamin B₁₂ supplements.
Children: 1 to 5 mg hydroxocobalamin in single doses of 100 mcg I.M. over 2 or more weeks, depending on severity of deficiency. Maintenance dose is 30 to 50 mcg I.M. every 4 weeks. For subsequent prophylaxis, advise adequate nutrition and daily RDA vitamin B₁₂ supplements.
➤ **Pernicious anemia or vitamin B₁₂ malabsorption**
Adults: Initially, 100 mcg cyanocobalamin I.M. or subcutaneously daily for 6 to 7 days. If response is observed, 100 mcg I.M. or subcutaneously every other day for 7 doses, then 100 mcg every 3 to 4 days for 2 to 3 weeks; then 100 mcg I.M. or subcutaneously once monthly.
➤ **Maintenance therapy for remission of pernicious anemia after I.M. vitamin B₁₂ therapy in patients without nervous system involvement; dietary deficiency, malabsorption disorders, and inadequate secretion of intrinsic factor**
Adults: Initially, 1 spray in one nostril once weekly (Nascobal). Give at least 1 hour before or after hot foods or liquids. Or 1 spray in each nostril daily. May increase to 1 spray in each nostril b.i.d. (total daily dose of 100 mcg) as needed.
➤ **Schilling test flushing dose**
Adults and children: 1,000 mcg hydroxocobalamin I.M. as single dose.
➤ **Cyanide poisoning**
Adults: Initially, 5 g hydroxocobalamin I.V. over 15 minutes. Based on patient's condition, may repeat 5 g dose I.V. over 15 minutes to 2 hours.

---

coenzyme Q10
Chew Q ◇, CoQ10 ◇, H₂Q ◇, LiQsorb ◇, Qunol Mega CoQ10 ◇, Vitaline CoQ10 ◇

AVAILABLE FORMS
Capsules: 10 mg ◇, 30 mg ◇, 50 mg ◇, 60 mg ◇, 75 mg ◇, 100 mg ◇, 120 mg ◇, 150 mg ◇, 200 mg ◇, 400 mg ◇
Capsules (extended-release): 100 mg ◇
Oral liquid: 2.5 mg/drop ◇, 6 mg/mL ◇, 20 mg/mL ◇, 100 mg/mL ◇

Tablets: 50 mg ◊, 60 mg ◊, 100 mg ◊
Tablets (chewable): 30 mg ◊, 100 mg ◊
Wafers: 60 mg ◊, 100 mg ◊, 300 mg ◊, 400 mg ◊, 600 mg ◊

INDICATIONS & DOSAGES
➤ **Dietary supplement for conditions associated with coenzyme Q10 deficiency**
Adults: 10 to 300 mg/day P.O. in one or divided doses. Higher doses (up to 3,000 mg/day) have been used.

folic acid (vitamin B₉)
FA-8 ◊

AVAILABLE FORMS
Injection: 10-mL vials (5 mg/mL with 1.5% benzyl alcohol, 5 mg/mL with 1.5% benzyl alcohol and 0.2% ethylenediaminetetraacetic acid)
Capsules: 5 mg ◊, 20 mg ◊
Tablets: 0.4 mg ◊, 0.8 mg ◊, 1 mg

INDICATIONS & DOSAGES
➤ **RDA**
Adults and children age 14 and older: 400 mcg.
Children ages 9 to 13: 300 mcg.
Children ages 4 to 8: 200 mcg.
Children ages 1 to 3: 150 mcg.
Infants ages 7 months to 1 year: 80 mcg.
Neonates and infants younger than age 6 months: 65 mcg.
Pregnant women: 600 mcg.
Breast-feeding women: 500 mcg.
➤ **Megaloblastic or macrocytic anemia from folic acid or other nutritional deficiency, hepatic disease, alcoholism, intestinal obstruction, or excessive hemolysis**
Adults and children age 4 and older: 0.4 to 1 mg P.O., I.M., or subcutaneously daily. After anemia caused by folic acid deficiency is corrected, proper diet and RDA supplements are needed to prevent recurrence.
Children younger than age 4: Up to 0.3 mg P.O., I.M., or subcutaneously daily.
Pregnant and breast-feeding women: 0.8 mg P.O., I.M., or subcutaneously daily.
➤ **To prevent fetal neural tube defects during pregnancy** ♦
Adults: 400 to 800 mcg P.O. daily before conception through at least first 4 to 12 weeks of fetal formation. For women at high risk, recommended dosage is 4 mg daily starting up to 3 months before conception and through first 3 months of pregnancy.

leucovorin calcium (citrovorum factor, folinic acid)

AVAILABLE FORMS
Injection: 50-mg, 100-mg, 200-mg, 350-mg, 500-mg vials for reconstitution (contains no preservatives)
Tablets: 5 mg, 10 mg, 15 mg, 25 mg

INDICATIONS & DOSAGES
➤ **Leucovorin rescue after high-dose methotrexate therapy**
Adults: 15 mg (approximately 10 mg/m²) P.O., I.M., or I.V. every 6 hours for 10 doses starting 24 hours after start of methotrexate infusion. Maximum, 25 mg/dose. Continue treatment until methotrexate level is less than 5×10^{-8} M. See manufacturer's instructions for dosage adjustment guidelines for methotrexate toxicity.
➤ **Impaired methotrexate elimination or inadvertent overdose**
Adults: 10 mg/m² P.O., I.M., or I.V. every 6 hours until serum methotrexate level is less than 10^{-8} M. If 24-hour serum creatinine level increases 50% over baseline or if 24-hour methotrexate level is greater than 5×10^{-6} M or 48-hour level is greater than 9×10^{-7} M, increase dosage to 100 mg/m² I.V. every 3 hours until methotrexate level is less than 10^{-8} M.
➤ **Folate-deficient megaloblastic anemia**
Adults and children: Up to 1 mg I.M. daily.
➤ **Palliative treatment of advanced colorectal cancer**
Adults: 20 mg/m² I.V. daily followed by 5-FU 425 mg/m² I.V. Or, 200 mg/m² I.V. daily for 5 days (over 3 minutes or longer) followed by 5-FU 370 mg/m² daily for 5 consecutive days. Repeat at 4-week intervals for two additional courses; then at intervals of 4 to 5 weeks, if tolerated.

niacin (nicotinic acid, vitamin B₃)
Endur-Acin ◊, Niacor, Niaspan, Slo-Niacin ◊

niacinamide ◊ (nicotinamide ◊)

AVAILABLE FORMS
niacin
Capsules (timed-release): 250 mg ◊, 500 mg
Tablets: 50 mg ◊, 100 mg ◊, 250 mg ◊, 500 mg
Tablets (extended-release): 250 mg ◊, 400 mg ◊, 500 mg ◊, 750 mg ◊, 1,000 mg ◊
niacinamide
Tablets: 100 mg ◊, 500 mg ◊
Tablets (extended-release): 500 mg ◊

INDICATIONS & DOSAGES
➤ **RDA**
Adult men and boys ages 14 to 18: 16 mg.
Adult women and girls ages 14 to 18: 14 mg.
Children ages 9 to 13: 12 mg.
Children ages 4 to 8: 8 mg.
Children ages 1 to 3: 6 mg.
Infants ages 7 months to 1 year: 4 mg.
Neonates and infants younger than age 6 months: 2 mg.
Pregnant women: 18 mg.
Breast-feeding women: 17 mg.

✦Canada   ◊ OTC   ♦ Off-label use   ⓓⓝⓒDo not crush   *Liquid contains alcohol.

➤ **Pellagra**

Adults: Initially, 500 mg Niaspan P.O. daily at bedtime. Titrate to patient response and tolerance. Maximum dose is 2,000 mg daily.

➤ **Niacin deficiency**

Adults: Up to 100 mg P.O. daily.

➤ **Hyperlipidemias, especially with hypercholesterolemia**

Adults: 250 mg Niacor P.O. daily after evening meal. Increase at 4- to 7-day intervals up to 1 to 2 g P.O. daily in two or three divided doses. Maximum 6 g daily. Or, 1 to 2 g extended-release tablets P.O. daily at bedtime.

paricalcitol
Zemplar

AVAILABLE FORMS
Capsules: 1 mcg, 2 mcg, 4 mcg
Injection: 2 mcg/mL, 5 mcg/mL

INDICATIONS & DOSAGES
➤ **To prevent or treat secondary hyperparathyroidism in patients with stage 3 or 4 chronic kidney disease**

Adults: Initial dose is based on baseline intact parathyroid hormone (iPTH) levels. If iPTH is less than or equal to 500 picograms (pg)/mL, give 1 mcg P.O. daily or 2 mcg P.O. three times weekly, no more often than every other day. If iPTH is greater than 500 pg/mL, give 2 mcg P.O. daily or 4 mcg P.O. three times weekly, no more often than every other day. Adjust dose at 2- to 4-week intervals, based on iPTH levels.

➤ **To prevent or treat secondary hyperparathyroidism in patients with chronic renal failure**

Adults: 0.04 to 0.1 mcg/kg (2.8 to 7 mcg) I.V. no more often than every other day during dialysis. Doses as high as 0.24 mcg/kg (16.8 mcg) may be safely given. If satisfactory response isn't observed, increase dosage by 2 to 4 mcg at 2- to 4-week intervals.

pyridoxine hydrochloride (vitamin B$_6$)
B-6 ◇, B-Natal ◇, Vitamin B-6 ◇, Vitamin B-6 ER ◇

AVAILABLE FORMS
Capsules: 250 mg ◇
Injection: 100 mg/mL
Tablets: 25 mg ◇, 50 mg ◇, 100 mg ◇, 200 mg ◇, 250 mg ◇, 500 mg ◇
Tablets (extended-release): 200 mg ◇

INDICATIONS & DOSAGES
➤ **RDA**

Adults ages 19 to 50: 1.3 mg.
Men age 51 and older: 1.7 mg.
Women age 51 and older: 1.5 mg.
Boys ages 14 to 18: 1.3 mg.
Girls ages 14 to 18: 1.2 mg.

Children ages 9 to 13: 1 mg.
Children ages 4 to 8: 0.6 mg.
Children ages 1 to 3: 0.5 mg.
Infants ages 7 months to 1 year: 0.3 mg.
Neonates and infants younger than age 6 months: 0.1 mg.
Pregnant women: 1.9 mg.
Breast-feeding women: 2 mg.

➤ **Dietary vitamin B$_6$ deficiency**

Adults: 100 to 200 mg P.O. daily. Or, 10 to 20 mg I.M. or I.V. daily for 3 weeks; then maintenance dose is 2 to 5 mg P.O. daily for several weeks.

➤ **Antidote for isoniazid poisoning**

Adults: 4 g I.V.; then 1 g I.M. every 30 minutes until amount of pyridoxine given equals amount of isoniazid ingested.

sodium fluoride
Fluor-A-Day, Fluoritab, Flura, Flura-Loz, Karidium, Ludent, Luride Lozi-Flur, Pharmaflur df, Pharmaflur 1.1, Phos-Flur ◇

sodium fluoride, topical
ACT ◇, Denta5000 Plus, EtheDent, Fluorigard ◇, Fluorinse, Gel-Kam, Gel-Tin ◇, Just For Kids ◇, Karigel, Karigel-N, Listerine Tooth Defense ◇, Luride, MouthKote F/R ◇, Point-Two, Prevident, SF 5000 Plus, Stop Gel ◇, Thera-Flur, Thera-Flur-N

AVAILABLE FORMS
sodium fluoride
Drops: 0.125 mg/drop, 0.25 mg/drop, 0.2 mg/mL, 0.5 mg/mL
Lozenges: 1 mg
Tablets: 1 mg
Tablets (chewable): 0.25 mg, 0.5 mg, 1 mg
sodium fluoride, topical
Cream: 1.1%
Gel: 0.1% ◇, 0.5%, 1.1%, 1.2%, 1.23%
Rinse: 0.02% ◇, 0.04% ◇

INDICATIONS & DOSAGES
➤ **To prevent dental caries**

Adults and children older than age 6: 5 to 10 mL of rinse once or twice daily (see product instructions), or thin ribbon of gel applied to teeth with toothbrush or mouth trays.

If fluoride ion level in drinking water is less than 0.3 parts/million (ppm)

Children ages 6 to 16: 1 mg P.O. daily.
Children ages 3 to 5: 0.5 mg P.O. daily.
Infants and children ages 6 months to 2 years: 0.25 mg P.O. daily.

If fluoride ion level in drinking water is 0.3 to 0.6 ppm

Children ages 6 to 16: 0.5 mg P.O. daily.
Children ages 3 to 5: 0.25 mg P.O. daily.

thiamine hydrochloride (vitamin B₁)
Betaxin✤, Thiamiject✤

AVAILABLE FORMS
Capsules: 50 mg
Injection: 100 mg/mL
Tablets: 50 mg ◇, 100 mg ◇, 250 mg ◇, 500 mg

INDICATIONS & DOSAGES
➤ **RDA**
Adult men: 1.2 mg.
Adult women: 1.1 mg.
Boys ages 14 to 18: 1.2 mg.
Girls ages 14 to 18: 1 mg.
Children ages 9 to 13: 0.9 mg.
Children ages 4 to 8: 0.6 mg.
Children ages 1 to 3: 0.5 mg.
Infants ages 7 months to 1 year: 0.3 mg.
Neonates and infants younger than age 6 months: 0.2 mg.
Pregnant women: 1.4 mg.
Breast-feeding women: 1.4 mg.
➤ **Beriberi**
Adults: Depending on severity, 10 to 20 mg I.M. t.i.d. for 2 weeks; then dietary correction and multivitamin supplement containing 5 to 10 mg thiamine daily for 1 month.
Children: 25 mg I.V. daily.
➤ **Wet beriberi with myocardial failure**
Adults and children: 10 to 20 mg I.V. t.i.d.
➤ **Wernicke encephalopathy**
Adults: Initially, 100 mg I.V.; then 50 to 100 mg I.M. daily until patient is consuming a regular balanced diet.
➤ **Thiamine deficiency**
Adults: 100 mg/L I.V. as rapidly as possible. Continue daily parenteral doses at RDA if GI disturbances prevent adequate oral absorption. Or, 1 tablet or capsule P.O. daily.
➤ **Neuritis of pregnancy in patients unable to take adequate oral therapy due to vomiting**
Adults: 5 to 10 mg I.M. daily.

vitamin C (ascorbic acid)
Acerola ◇, Ascocid ◇, Ascor L 500, Asco-Tabs ◇, C-Caps ◇, Cemill ◇, Chew-C ◇, Halls Defense Vitamin C Drops ◇

AVAILABLE FORMS
Capsules: 500 mg ◇
Capsules (timed-release): 500 mg ◇
Crystals: 1,000 mg/¼ tsp
Injection: 500 mg/mL
Lozenges: 60 mg ◇
Oral solution: 100 mg/mL ◇, 500 mg/15 mL ◇
Powder: 60 mg/¼ tsp ◇, 1,060 mg/¼ tsp ◇
Tablets: 250 mg ◇, 500 mg ◇, 1,000 mg ◇, 1,500 mg ◇

Tablets (chewable): 100 mg ◇, 250 mg ◇, 500 mg ◇
Tablets (timed-release): 500 mg ◇
Wafer: 500 mg ◇

INDICATIONS & DOSAGES
➤ **RDA**
Men age 19 and older: 90 mg.
Women age 19 and older: 75 mg.
Boys ages 14 to 18: 75 mg.
Girls ages 14 to 18: 65 mg.
Children ages 9 to 13: 45 mg.
Children ages 4 to 8: 25 mg.
Children ages 1 to 3: 15 mg.
Infants ages 7 months to 1 year: 50 mg.
Neonates and infants up to age 6 months: 40 mg.
Pregnant women: 80 to 85 mg.
Breast-feeding women: 115 to 120 mg.
➤ **Frank and subclinical scurvy**
Adults: Depending on severity, 100 to 300 mg P.O. or 300 to 1,000 mg I.V., I.M., or subcutaneously daily.
Children: Depending on severity, 100 to 300 mg P.O. daily.
➤ **Extensive burns, delayed fracture or wound healing, postoperative wound healing, severe febrile or chronic disease states**
Adults: 200 to 500 mg I.V., I.M., or subcutaneously daily for 7 to 10 days; 1 to 2 g daily for extensive burns.

vitamin D cholecalciferol (vitamin D₃)
Baby Ddrops ◇, Bio-D-Mulsion ◇, Decara, Delta-D ◇, D-Vi-Sol ◇, D-Vita ◇, JustD ◇, Replesta ◇, VitaMelts ◇

ergocalciferol (vitamin D₂)
Calcidol ◇, Calciferol, Drisdol

AVAILABLE FORMS
cholecalciferol
Capsules: 10 mcg (400 international units), 25 mcg (1,000 international units), 50 mcg (2,000 international units), 125 mcg (5,000 international units), 250 mcg (10,000 international units), 625 mcg (25,000 international units), 1.25 mg (50,000 international units)
Liquid: 400 international units/mL ◇, 400 international units/0.03 mL ◇, 1,000 international units/0.03 mL ◇, 2,000 international units/0.03 mL ◇, 1,000 international units/spray ◇, 1,000 international units/10 mL ◇, 5,000 international units/mL ◇
Tablets: 10 mcg (400 international units) ◇, 25 mcg (1,000 international units) ◇, 50 mcg (2,000 international units) ◇, 75 mcg (3,000 international units) ◇, 125 mcg (5,000 international units) ◇
Tablets (chewable): 10 mcg (400 international units) ◇, 25 mcg (1,000 international units) ◇, 50 mcg (2,000 international units) ◇, 125 mcg (5,000 international units) ◇

Tablets (dispersible): 25 mcg (1,000 international units)
Wafers: 350 mcg (14,000 international units) ◇ , 1.25 mg (50,000 international units) ◇
ergocalciferol
Capsules: 1.25 mg (50,000 international units)
Oral liquid: 200 mcg (8,000 international units)/mL in 60-mL dropper bottle ◇
Tablets: 10 mcg (400 international units) ◇ , 50 mcg (2,000 international units) ◇

INDICATIONS & DOSAGES
➤ **RDA for cholecalciferol**
Adults older than age 70: 15 mcg (800 international units).
Adults ages 51 to 70: 10 mcg (600 international units).
Infants, children, and adults up to age 50: 5 mcg (200 international units).
Pregnant or breast-feeding women: 5 mcg (200 international units).
➤ **RDA for ergocalciferol**
Adults older than age 70: 20 mcg (800 international units).
Adults up to age 70 and children age 1 and older: 15 mcg (600 international units).
Children from birth to less than 12 months: 10 mcg (400 international units).
➤ **Rickets and other vitamin D deficiency diseases**
Adults and children: Initially, 12,000 international units P.O. daily; expect to increase, based on response, to maximum of 500,000 international units daily. After correction of deficiency, maintenance includes adequate diet and RDA supplements.
➤ **Hypoparathyroidism**
Adults and children: 1.25 to 5 mg (50,000 to 200,000 international units) ergocalciferol P.O. daily with calcium supplement.

vitamin D analogue
doxercalciferol
Hectorol

AVAILABLE FORMS
Capsules: 0.5 mcg, 1 mcg, 2.5 mcg
Injection: 2 mcg/mL

INDICATIONS & DOSAGES
➤ **Secondary hyperparathyroidism in dialysis patients with chronic kidney disease**
Adults: Initially, 10 mcg P.O. three times weekly at dialysis. Adjust dosage as needed to lower intact parathyroid hormone (iPTH) levels to 150 to 300 picograms (pg)/mL. Increase dose by 2.5 mcg at 8-week intervals if iPTH level hasn't decreased by 50% and fails to reach target range. Maximum dose is 20 mcg P.O. three times weekly. If iPTH levels fall below 100 pg/mL, suspend drug for 1 week; then give dose of at least 2.5 mcg less than last dose. Or, 4 mcg I.V. bolus three times a week at the end of dialysis, about every other day. Adjust dose as needed to lower iPTH levels to 150 to 300 pg/mL. Dosage may be increased by 1

to 2 mcg at 8-week intervals if the iPTH level isn't decreased by 50% and fails to reach target range. Maximum dose is 18 mcg weekly. If iPTH levels go below 100 pg/mL, suspend drug for 1 week, then resume at a dose that's at least 1 mcg P.O. lower than the last dose.
➤ **Secondary hyperparathyroidism in predialysis patients with stage 3 or 4 chronic kidney disease**
Adults: 1 mcg P.O. daily. Adjust dosage as needed to lower iPTH levels to 35 to 70 pg/mL for stage 3 or 70 to 110 pg/mL for stage 4. Increase dosage at 2-week intervals by 0.5 mcg if levels are above 70 pg/mL for stage 3 or above 110 pg/mL for stage 4. If level falls below 35 pg/mL for stage 3 or 70 pg/mL for stage 4, suspend treatment for 1 week, then give dose at least 0.5 mcg lower than last dose. Maximum dose, 3.5 mcg daily.

vitamin E (tocopherols)
Alpha-E ◇ , E 1000 ◇ , Nutr-E-Sol ◇

AVAILABLE FORMS
Capsules: 100 international units ◇ , 200 international units ◇ , 400 international units ◇ , 600 international units ◇ , 1,000 international units ◇
Liquid: 15 international units/0.3 mL ◇ , 100 international units/0.25 mL ◇ , 400 international units/15 mL ◇
Tablets: 100 international units ◇ , 200 international units ◇ , 400 international units ◇

INDICATIONS & DOSAGES
Note: RDAs for vitamin E have been converted to α-tocopherol equivalents (α-TE). One α-TE equals 1 mg of D-α tocopherol, or 1.49 international units.
➤ **RDA**
Adults and children ages 14 to 18: 15 mg.
Children ages 9 to 13: 11 mg.
Children ages 4 to 8: 7 mg.
Children ages 1 to 3: 6 mg.
Infants ages 7 months to 1 year: 5 mg.
Neonates and infants younger than age 6 months: 4 mg.
Pregnant women: 15 mg.
Breast-feeding women: 19 mg.

vitamin K analogue
phytonadione (vitamin K₁)
K-100 ◇ , Mephyton, Phytonadione, Vitamin K₁

AVAILABLE FORMS
Injection (emulsion): 1 mg/0.5 mL, 10 mg/mL
Tablets: 100 mcg ◇ , 5 mg

INDICATIONS & DOSAGES
Black Box Warning Risk of severe and even fatal reactions using I.V. or I.M. routes; restrict their use to situations where the subcutaneous route isn't feasible and the serious risk involved is considered justified. ∎

➤ **RDA**

Men age 19 and older: 120 mcg.
Women age 19 and older, including pregnant and breast-feeding women: 90 mcg.
Children ages 14 to 18: 75 mcg.
Children ages 9 to 13: 60 mcg.
Children ages 4 to 8: 55 mcg.
Children ages 1 to 3: 30 mcg.
Infants ages 7 months to 1 year: 2.5 mcg.
Neonates and infants younger than age 6 months: 2 mcg.

➤ **Hypoprothrombinemia caused by vitamin K malabsorption, drug therapy, or excessive vitamin A dosage**

Adults: Depending on severity, 2.5 to 25 mg P.O., I.M., or subcutaneously, repeated and increased up to 50 mg as needed.

➤ **Hypoprothrombinemia caused by effect of oral anticoagulants**

Adults: 2.5 to 10 mg P.O., I.M., or subcutaneously, based on PT and INR; repeat if needed within 12 to 48 hours after oral dose or within 6 to 8 hours after parenteral dose.

➤ **To prevent hemorrhagic disease of newborn**

Neonates: 0.5 to 1 mg I.M. within 1 hour after birth.

➤ **Hemorrhagic disease of newborn**

Neonates: 1 mg subcutaneously or I.M. Higher doses may be needed if mother has been receiving oral anticoagulants.

Antacids: Indications and dosages

Refer to manufacturer's instructions for complete prescribing and safety information.

aluminum hydroxide
a-LOO-mi-num

aluminum hydroxide gel ◇
Therapeutic class: Antacids
Pharmacologic class: Aluminum salts

AVAILABLE FORMS
Oral suspension: 320 mg/5 mL

INDICATIONS & DOSAGES
➤ **Acid indigestion**
Adults: 10 mL (640 mg) of oral suspension five to six times daily after meals and at bedtime or as directed by prescriber. Maximum dose is 3,840 mg/day.

aluminum hydroxide–magnesium carbonate
a-LOO-mi-num

Acid Gone ◇ , Gaviscon ◇ ,
Gaviscon Extra Relief Formula ◇ ,
Gaviscon Extra Strength ◇

Therapeutic class: Antacids
Pharmacologic class: Aluminum salts

AVAILABLE FORMS
Oral suspension: 95 mg aluminum hydroxide/358 mg magnesium carbonate in 15 mL; 254 mg aluminum hydroxide/237.5 mg magnesium carbonate in 5 mL; 508 mg aluminum hydroxide/475 mg magnesium carbonate in 10 mL
Tablets (chewable): 160 mg aluminum hydroxide/ 105 mg magnesium carbonate

INDICATIONS & DOSAGES
➤ **Acid indigestion, heartburn, sour stomach, GI upset**
Adults: 2 to 4 chewable tablets P.O. q.i.d.; maximum dose, 16 tablets/24 hours.
Adults and children age 12 and older: 15 to 30 mL (31.7 mg aluminum hydroxide/119.3 mg magnesium carbonate/5 mL) P.O. q.i.d.; maximum dose, 120 mL/ 24 hours. Or, 10 to 20 mL (254 mg aluminum hydroxide/237.5 mg magnesium carbonate/5 mL) P.O. q.i.d.; maximum dose, 80 mL/24 hours.

calcium carbonate
KAL-see-um

Alcalak ◇ , Cal-Carb Forte ◇ ,
Calci-Chew ◇ , Cal-Gest ◇ ,
Cal-Mint ◇ , Caltrate ◇ , Children's
Mylanta ◇ , Children's Pepto ◇ ,
Maalox ◇ , Oystercal ◇ , Rolaids ◇ ,
Tums ◇ , Tums Smoothies ◇

Therapeutic class: Antacids
Pharmacologic class: Calcium salts

AVAILABLE FORMS
Calcium carbonate contains 40% calcium; 20 mEq calcium per gram.
Capsules: 1,250 mg ◇
Oral suspension: 1,250 mg/5 mL ◇
Tablets: 600 mg ◇ , 648 mg ◇ , 650 mg ◇ , 1,250 mg ◇ , 1,500 mg ◇
Tablets (chewable): 260 mg ◇ , 400 mg ◇ , 420 mg ◇ , 500 mg ◇ , 600 mg ◇ , 750 mg ◇ , 1,000 mg ◇ , 1,177 mg ◇ , 1,250 mg

INDICATIONS & DOSAGES
➤ **Acid indigestion, calcium supplement**
Adults and children age 12 and older: 1 to 4 tablets P.O. as symptoms occur for indigestion. Maximum dose is 8,000 mg daily for up to 2 weeks. For calcium supplement use, 500 mg to 4 g daily in one to three divided doses. Dosing recommendations vary by product.
Children ages 6 to 11 and weighing at least 21.8 kg: 750 to 800 mg P.O. as symptoms occur. Maximum dose is 3,000 mg daily for up to 2 weeks.
Children ages 4 to 11 (calcium supplementation): 750 mg P.O. t.i.d. Dosage varies by product.
Children ages 2 to 5 and weighing 10.9 to 21.3 kg: 375 to 400 mg P.O. as symptoms occur. Maximum dose is 1,500 mg daily for up to 2 weeks. For calcium supplement use, give 750 mg b.i.d. Dosage varies by product.

magnesium oxide
mag-NEE-see-um

Mag-Ox 400 ◇ , Maox 420 ◇ ,
Uro-Mag ◇

Therapeutic class: Antacids
Pharmacologic class: Magnesium salts

AVAILABLE FORMS
Capsules: 140 mg
Tablets: 400 mg, 420 mg, 500 mg

INDICATIONS & DOSAGES
➤ **Acid indigestion**
Adults: 1 tablet P.O. one or two times daily. Maximum dosage, 2 tablets/day.
➤ **Dietary supplement**
Adults: 1 to 2 tablets or 1 to 5 capsules P.O. daily.

Laxatives: Indications and dosages

Refer to manufacturer's instructions for complete prescribing and safety information.

bisacodyl
bye-suh-KOH-dil

Bisac-Evac ◇, Bisacodyl EC ◇,
Biscolax ◇, Carter's Little Pills ◇,
Codulax ✤ ◇, Correctol ◇,
Dulcolax ◇, Ex-Lax Ultra ◇,
Feen-a-Mint ◇, Fleet Bisacodyl ◇,
Fleet Laxative ◇, Silver Bullet ✤ ◇,
Soflax EX ✤ ◇, The Magic Bullet ◇,
Woman's Laxative ◇

Therapeutic class: Laxatives
Pharmacologic class: Diphenylmethane
derivatives

AVAILABLE FORMS
Enema: 10 mg/30 mL ◇
Suppositories: 10 mg ◇
Tablets (enteric-coated) ⓞⓝⓒ: 5 mg ◇

INDICATIONS & DOSAGES
➤ **Chronic constipation; preparation for childbirth, surgery, or rectal or bowel examination**
Adults and children age 12 and older: 5 to 15 mg P.O. in evening or before breakfast. Or, 10 mg P.R. for evacuation before examination or surgery. Enema may be given as a single daily dose.
Children ages 6 to 11: 5 mg P.O. or P.R. (suppository) at bedtime or before breakfast. Oral dose isn't recommended if child can't swallow tablet whole. Don't give enema in children younger than age 12.

calcium polycarbophil
KAL-see-um

FiberCon ◇, Fiber-Lax ◇,
Konsyl Fiber ◇

Therapeutic class: Laxatives
Pharmacologic class: Hydrophilic drugs

AVAILABLE FORMS
Tablets: 625 mg ◇

INDICATIONS & DOSAGES
➤ **Constipation**
Adults and children older than age 12: 2 tablets (1,250 mg) P.O. once daily to q.i.d., p.r.n.
Children ages 6 to 12: 1 tablet (625 mg) P.O. once daily to t.i.d., p.r.n.

docusate calcium (dioctyl calcium sulfosuccinate)
DOK-yoo-sayt

Calax ✤ ◇, Kao-Tin ◇, Soflax C ✤ ◇,
Surfak ◇, Sur-Q-Lax ◇

docusate sodium (dioctyl sodium sulfosuccinate)
Colace ◇, Correctol Extra Gentle ◇,
Diocto ◇, DocQLace ◇,
Docuprene ◇, Docusoft-S ◇,
DocuSol Kids Enema ◇, DOK ◇,
D.O.S. ◇, Dosolax ✤ ◇, DSS ◇,
Dulcocomfort ✤ ◇, Dulcolax Stool
Softener ◇, Enemeez Mini ◇,
Pedia-Lax ◇, Phillips Stool
Softener ◇, Promolaxin ◇, Selax ✤ ◇,
Silace ◇, Sof-Lax ◇

Therapeutic class: Laxatives
Pharmacologic class: Surfactants

AVAILABLE FORMS
docusate calcium
Capsules: 240 mg ◇
docusate sodium
Capsules: 50 mg ◇, 100 mg ◇, 200 mg ◇
Oral liquid: 50 mg/15 mL ◇, 150 mg/15 mL ◇
Rectal suspension: 100 mg/5 mL ◇, 283 mg/4 mL ◇
Syrup: 20 mg/5 mL ✤ ◇, 60 mg/15 mL ◇
Tablets: 100 mg ◇

INDICATIONS & DOSAGES
➤ **Constipation (stool softener)**
Adults and children older than age 12: 50 to 300 mg docusate calcium or sodium P.O. daily until bowel movements are normal. Or, give enema. Administer contents of 1 bottle P.R. as a single dose.
Children ages 2 to 12: 20 to 150 mg docusate sodium P.O. daily as a single dose or in divided doses.

glycerin
GLI-ser-in

Fleet ◇, Fleet Babylax ◇,
Pedia-Lax ◇, Sani-Supp ◇

Therapeutic class: Laxatives
Pharmacologic class: Trihydric alcohols

AVAILABLE FORMS
Enema: 5.4 g
Enema (pediatric): 4 mL/applicator ◇
Suppositories: Adult, children, and infant sizes ◇

INDICATIONS & DOSAGES
➤ **Constipation**
Adults and children age 6 and older: 1 rectal suppository/
day, or 5 to 15 mL as enema.
Children ages 2 to 6: 1 rectal suppository/day, or 2 mL
as enema.

linaclotide
LIN-a-KLOE-tide

Constella ✤, Linzess

Therapeutic class: Laxatives
Pharmacologic class: Guanylate cyclase-C
agonists

AVAILABLE FORMS
Capsules ⓓⓝⓒ: 145 mcg, 290 mcg

INDICATIONS & DOSAGES
Black Box Warning Safety and effectiveness
hasn't been established in patients under age 18. ■
➤ **Irritable bowel syndrome with constipation**
Adults: 290 mcg P.O. once daily on an empty stomach
at least 30 minutes before first meal of the day.
➤ **Chronic idiopathic constipation**
Adults: 145 mcg P.O. once daily on an empty stomach
at least 30 minutes before first meal of the day.

lactulose
LAK-tyoo-lose

Cholac, Constilac, Constulose,
Enulose, Generlac, Kristalose

Therapeutic class: Laxatives
Pharmacologic class: Disaccharides

AVAILABLE FORMS
Oral solution: 10 g/15 mL
Packets: 10 g, 20 g
Rectal solution: 10 g/15 mL

INDICATIONS & DOSAGES
➤ **Constipation**
Adults: 10 to 20 g or 15 to 30 mL P.O. daily, increased
to 60 mL/day, if needed.
➤ **To prevent and treat hepatic encephalopathy, including hepatic precoma and coma in patients with
severe hepatic disease**
Adults: Initially, 20 to 30 g or 30 to 45 mL P.O. t.i.d. or
q.i.d., until two or three soft stools are produced daily.
Usual dose is 60 to 100 g daily in divided doses. Or,
200 g or 300 mL diluted with 700 mL of water or NSS
and given as retention enema P.R. every 4 to 6 hours,
as needed.
Infants: Initially, 2.5 to 10 mL/day P.O. in divided doses to produce two or three soft stools daily.

Older children and adolescents: 40 to 90 mL/day P.O.
in divided doses to produce two or three soft stools
daily.
➤ **Treatment of subclinical hepatic encephalopathy ◆**
Adults: 30 to 60 mL/day P.O. in two to three divided
doses to maintain two or three daily bowel movements
for up to 3 months.

lubiprostone
loo-bee-PRAHS-tohn

Amitiza ✐

Therapeutic class: Laxatives
Pharmacologic class: Chloride channel
activators

AVAILABLE FORMS
Capsules ⓓⓝⓒ: 8 mcg, 24 mcg

INDICATIONS & DOSAGES
➤ **Chronic idiopathic constipation**
Adults: 24 mcg P.O. b.i.d. with food.
Adjust-a-dose: For patients with moderately impaired hepatic function (Child-Pugh class B), starting
dose is 16 mcg b.i.d.; for those with severely impaired
hepatic function (Child-Pugh class C), starting dose is
8 mcg b.i.d. May increase to full dose after appropriate
interval if tolerated and an adequate response hasn't
been obtained at initial dose. Monitor patient response.
➤ **Irritable bowel syndrome with constipation**
Women age 18 and older: 8 mcg P.O. b.i.d. with food
and water.
Adjust-a-dose: For patients with severely impaired
hepatic function (Child-Pugh class C), starting dose
is 8 mcg once daily. May increase to full dose after
appropriate interval if tolerated and an adequate response hasn't been obtained at initial dose. Monitor
patient response.
➤ **Opioid-induced constipation in patients with
chronic, noncancer pain**
Adults: 24 mcg P.O. b.i.d. with food and water.
Adjust-a-dose: For patients with moderately impaired hepatic function (Child-Pugh class B), starting
dose is 16 mcg b.i.d.; for those with severely impaired
hepatic function (Child-Pugh class C), starting dose is
8 mcg b.i.d. May increase to full dose after appropriate
interval if tolerated and an adequate response hasn't
been obtained at initial dose. Monitor patient response.

---

magnesium citrate (citrate of magnesia)

magnesium hydroxide (milk of magnesia)

Dulcolax Milk of Magnesia ◇, Milk of Magnesia ◇, Milk of Magnesia-Concentrated ◇, Phillips' Milk of Magnesia ◇

magnesium sulfate ◇ (Epsom salts ◇)

Therapeutic class: Laxatives
Pharmacologic class: Magnesium salts

AVAILABLE FORMS
magnesium citrate
Oral solution: 1.75 g/30 mL ◇
Tablets: 100 mg
magnesium hydroxide
Chewable tablets: 311 mg ◇, 400 mg ◇
Oral suspension: 400 mg/5 mL ◇, 800 mg/5 mL ◇, 1,200 mg/15 mL ◇, 2,400 mg/10 mL ◇
magnesium sulfate
Granules: About 40 mEq magnesium/5 g ◇

INDICATIONS & DOSAGES
➤ **Constipation; to evacuate bowel before surgery**
Adults and children age 12 and older: 6.5 to 10 fluid oz magnesium citrate with 8 oz water P.O. in single or divided doses in 24 hours. Or, 2 to 4 tablets magnesium citrate P.O. daily at bedtime or in divided doses. Or, 8 chewable magnesium hydroxide tablets P.O. at bedtime or in divided doses. Or, 30 to 60 mL magnesium hydroxide liquid (400 mg/5 mL) P.O. as a single daily dose at bedtime or in divided doses. Or, 15 to 30 mL magnesium hydroxide liquid (800 mg/5 mL) P.O. as a single daily dose at bedtime or in divided doses. Or, 10 to 20 mL magnesium hydroxide (1,200 mg/5 mL) P.O. as a single daily dose at bedtime or in divided doses. Or, 10 to 30 g magnesium sulfate granules dissolved in 8 fluid oz water P.O. daily as a single dose or divided doses.
Children ages 6 to 11: 3 to 7 fluid oz magnesium citrate with 8 oz water P.O. in 24 hours as a single daily dose or in divided doses. Or, 4 chewable tablets magnesium hydroxide P.O. as a single daily dose at bedtime or in divided doses. Or, 15 to 30 mL magnesium hydroxide liquid (400 mg/5 mL) as a single daily dose at bedtime or in divided doses. Or, 7.5 to 15 mL magnesium hydroxide liquid (800 mg/5 mL) P.O. as a single daily dose at bedtime or in divided doses. Or, 5 to 10 mL magnesium hydroxide liquid (1,200 mg/5 mL) P.O. as a single daily dose at bedtime or in divided doses. Or, 5 to 10 g magnesium sulfate dissolved in 8 fluid oz water P.O. daily as a single dose or in divided doses.
Children ages 3 to 5: 2 magnesium hydroxide chewable tablets P.O. as a single daily dose or in divided

doses. Or, 5 to 15 mL magnesium hydroxide liquid (400 mg/5 mL) P.O. as a single daily dose or in two to four divided doses. Or, 2.5 to 7.5 mL magnesium hydroxide liquid (800 mg/5 mL) P.O. as a single daily dose at bedtime or in divided doses.

polyethylene glycol (PEG)
pol-ee-ETH-ih-leen

Clearlax❧ ◇, GaviLAX ◇, GlycoLax, Lax-A-Day❧ ◇, MiraLax ◇, PEG 3350❧ ◇, Pegalax❧ ◇, Polylax❧ ◇, Relaxa❧ ◇, Restoralax❧ ◇

Therapeutic class: Laxatives
Pharmacologic class: Osmotic drugs

AVAILABLE FORMS
Powder: 17 g in single-dose packets

INDICATIONS & DOSAGES
➤ **Short-term treatment of occasional constipation**
Adults: 17 g (about 1 heaping tablespoon or one individual dose packet) powder P.O. dissolved in 120 to 240 mL beverage once daily.

polyethylene glycol (PEG)–electrolyte solution
pol-ee-ETH-ih-leen

Colyte, GaviLyte-C, GaviLyte-G, GaviLyte-N, GoLYTELY, MoviPrep, NuLYTELY, Suclear, TriLyte

Therapeutic class: Laxatives
Pharmacologic class: Osmotic laxatives

AVAILABLE FORMS
Oral solution: PEG 3350 (refer to individual manufacturer for strength and dosage of electrolytes)
Powder for oral solution: 4-L dose of solution contains PEG 3350 (refer to individual manufacturer for strength and dosage of electrolytes)

INDICATIONS & DOSAGES
➤ **Bowel preparation before GI examination**
Adults: 240 mL P.O. every 10 minutes until 4 L are consumed or rectal effluent is clear. Typically, give 4 hours before examination, allowing 3 hours for drinking and 1 hour for bowel evacuation. May give via NG tube: 20 to 30 mL/minute (1.2 to 1.8 L/hour) until 4 L is administered or rectal effluent is clear. Or, for MoviPrep and Suclear, refer to package instructions for split-dose or full-dose regimen.
Children age 6 months and older (GaviLyte-N, NuLYTELY, TriLyte): 25 mL/kg/hour P.O. or via NG tube until rectal effluent is clear and free of solid matter.

sodium phosphate monobasic monohydrate–sodium phosphate dibasic anhydrous
OsmoPrep

Therapeutic class: Laxatives
Pharmacologic class: Osmotic laxatives

AVAILABLE FORMS
Tablets: 1.5 g sodium phosphate (1.102 g sodium phosphate monobasic monohydrate and 0.398 g sodium phosphate dibasic anhydrous)

INDICATIONS & DOSAGES
Black Box Warning Acute phosphate nephropathy has been reported. Use the dose and dosing regimen as recommended (p.m./a.m. split dose). ▪
➤ **To cleanse bowel before colonoscopy**
Adults age 18 and older: 32 tablets taken in the following manner: The evening before the procedure, 4 tablets P.O. with 8 oz of clear liquid every 15 minutes for a total of 20 tablets; 3 to 5 hours before the procedure, 4 tablets P.O. with at least 8 oz of clear liquid every 15 minutes for a total of 12 tablets.

sodium phosphates
Fleet Enema ◇ , Fleet Enema Extra ◇ ,
Fleet For Children ◇ , LaCrosse
Complete ◇ , Pedia-Lax ◇

Therapeutic class: Laxatives
Pharmacologic class: Acid salts

AVAILABLE FORMS
Enema solution (pediatric use): 9.5 g monobasic sodium phosphate monohydrate and 3.5 g dibasic sodium phosphate heptahydrate/59 mL ◇
Enema solution: 19 g monobasic sodium phosphate monohydrate and 7 g dibasic sodium phosphate heptahydrate/118 mL ◇ , 19 g monobasic sodium phosphate monohydrate and 7 g dibasic sodium phosphate heptahydrate/197 mL ◇

INDICATIONS & DOSAGES
➤ **Constipation**
Adults and children age 12 and older: 1 bottle P.R. as an enema once in 24 hours.
Children ages 5 to 11: 66 mL (1 bottle enema for pediatric use) P.R. as an enema once in 24 hours.
Children ages 2 to younger than 5: 33 mL (½ bottle enema for pediatric use) P.R. as an enema once in 24 hours.

sodium picosulfate–magnesium oxide–anhydrous citric acid
Prepopik

Therapeutic class: Laxatives
Pharmacologic class: Peristaltic stimulants–osmotic agents

AVAILABLE FORMS
Powder for oral solution (16.1 g/packet, 2 packets/dosing carton): 10 mg sodium picosulfate, 3.5 g magnesium oxide, and 12 g anhydrous citric acid

INDICATIONS & DOSAGES
➤ **To cleanse colon in preparation for colonoscopy**
Adults: The split-dose method is preferred. Give first dose during the evening before colonoscopy (5 p.m. to 9 p.m.) followed by five 8-oz drinks of clear liquids within 5 hours and before bed. Give second dose next day, during the morning approximately 5 hours before colonoscopy. Follow dose with at least three 8-oz drinks of clear liquids before colonoscopy; continue with clear liquids within 5 hours and up to 2 hours before colonoscopy. If split-dose method isn't appropriate, use the "day before" method: Give first dose in the afternoon or early evening (4 p.m. to 6 p.m.) before colonoscopy followed by five 8-oz drinks of clear liquids within 5 hours and before next dose. Give second dose approximately 6 hours later in the late evening (10 p.m. to 12 a.m.) the night before colonoscopy, followed by three 8-oz drinks of clear liquids within 5 hours and before bed.

Additional OTC drugs: Indications and dosages

Refer to manufacturer's instructions for complete prescribing and safety information.

benzocaine
ben-ZOH-cane

Anacaine ◇, Cepacol Extra Strength Sore Throat ◇, Dermoplast ◇, Hurricaine ◇, Ivy-Rid, Trocaine Throat ◇

Therapeutic class: Dermatologic agents
Pharmacologic class: Topical anesthetics

AVAILABLE FORMS
Lozenge: 10 mg ◇, 15 mg ◇
Spray (aerosol): 5% ◇, 20% ◇
Spray (dental): 5% ◇, 20% ◇

INDICATIONS & DOSAGES
Refer to individual manufacturer's instructions for use.
➤ **Sore throat**
Adults and children age 5 and older: Allow 1 lozenge to dissolve slowly in mouth. May repeat every 2 hours as needed.
➤ **Mouth and gum irritation**
Adults: 1 spray in the mouth up to four times daily as needed.
➤ **Dermal irritation**
Adults and children age 2 and older: 1 spray up to four times daily.

cetirizine hydrochloride
se-TEER-i-zeen

All Day Allergy ◇, Zyrtec ◇, Zyrtec Children's Allergy ◇

Therapeutic class: Antihistamines
Pharmacologic class: Piperazine derivatives

AVAILABLE FORMS
Capsules: 10 mg ◇
ODTs: 10 mg ◇
Syrup: 5 mg/5 mL ◇
Tablets: 5 mg ◇, 10 mg ◇
Tablets (chewable): 5 mg ◇, 10 mg ◇

INDICATIONS & DOSAGES
Adjust-a-dose (for all indications): For adults and children age 6 and older receiving hemodialysis, those with hepatic impairment, those with CrCl less than 31 mL/minute, and patients age 65 and older, give 5 mg P.O. daily. Don't use in children younger than age 6 with renal or hepatic impairment.

➤ **Seasonal allergic rhinitis**
Adults and children age 6 and older: 5 to 10 mg P.O. once daily.
Children ages 2 to 5: 2.5 mg P.O. once daily. Maximum daily dose is 5 mg.
➤ **Perennial allergic rhinitis, chronic urticaria**
Adults and children age 6 and older: 5 to 10 mg P.O. once daily.
Children ages 1 to 5 years: 2.5 mg P.O. once daily; increase to maximum of 5 mg daily. Children ages 12 to 23 months should receive the 5-mg dose as two divided doses.
Children ages 6 to 11 months: 2.5 mg P.O. once daily.

chlorpheniramine maleate
klor-fen-IR-a-meen

Allergy Time ◇, ChlorTabs ◇, Chlor-Trimeton ◇, Chlor-Trimeton Allergy 12 Hour ◇, Diabetic Tussin Allergy ◇

Therapeutic class: Antihistamines
Pharmacologic class: Alkylamines

AVAILABLE FORMS
Liquid: 2 mg/mL ◇
Syrup: 2 mg/5 mL ◇ *
Tablets: 4 mg ◇
Tablets (extended-release) **OTC**: 8 mg ◇, 12 mg ◇

INDICATIONS & DOSAGES
➤ **Allergic rhinitis**
Adults and children age 12 and older: 4 mg P.O. every 4 to 6 hours, not to exceed 24 mg daily. Or, 8 to 12 mg extended-release P.O. every 8 to 12 hours, not to exceed 24 mg daily.
Children ages 6 to 12: 2 mg P.O. every 4 to 6 hours, not to exceed 12 mg daily.
Children ages 2 to 6: 1 mg P.O. every 4 to 6 hours, not to exceed 6 mg daily.

dextromethorphan hydrobromide

dex-troe-meth-OR-fan

Balminil DM✿ ◇, Buckley's Cough Mixture ◇, Creomulsion ◇, Creo-Terpin ◇ *, Delsym ◇, ElixSure Cough ◇, Hold DM ◇, Koffex DM✿ ◇, Little Colds Cough Formula ◇, PediaCare ◇, PediaCare Long-Acting Cough Freezer Pops ◇, Robitussin ◇, Robitussin Pediatric ◇, Scot-Tussin ◇, Simply Cough ◇, St. Joseph Cough Suppressant ◇, Sucrets Cough ◇, Triaminic Long Acting Cough ◇ *, Trocal ◇, Vicks Formula 44 ◇

Therapeutic class: Antitussives
Pharmacologic class: Levorphanol derivatives

AVAILABLE FORMS
Gelcaps: 5 mg ◇, 30 mg ◇
Liquid (extended-release): 30 mg/5 mL ◇
Lozenges: 5 mg ◇, 7.5 mg ◇, 10 mg ◇
Solution: 3 mg/mL✿ ◇, 3.5 mg/5 mL ◇, 5 mg/5 mL ◇ *, 7.5 mg/5 mL ◇, 10 mg/5 mL ◇ *, 12.5 mg/5 mL ◇, 15 mg/5 mL ◇ *, 15 mg/15 mL ◇ *
Strips (orally disintegrating): 7.5 mg ◇ *

INDICATIONS & DOSAGES
➤ **Nonproductive cough**
Adults and children age 12 and older: 10 to 20 mg P.O. every 4 hours, or 30 mg every 6 to 8 hours. Or, 60 mg extended-release liquid P.O. b.i.d. Maximum, 120 mg daily. Or 5 to 15 mg lozenges P.O. every 1 to 4 hours, up to 120 mg/day.
Children ages 6 to 11: 5 to 10 mg P.O. every 4 hours, or 15 mg every 6 to 8 hours. Or, 30 mg extended-release liquid P.O. b.i.d. Maximum, 60 mg daily. Or 5 to 10 mg lozenges P.O. every 1 to 4 hours, up to 60 mg/day. Don't exceed four doses in 24 hours.
Children ages 2 to 5: 2.5 to 5 mg P.O. every 4 hours, or 7.5 mg every 6 to 8 hours. Or, 15 mg extended-release liquid P.O. b.i.d. Maximum, 30 mg daily.

fexofenadine hydrochloride

fecks-oh-FEN-a-deen

Allegra 12 Hour✿ ◇, Allegra 24 Hour✿ ◇, Allegra Allergy ◇, Allegra Allergy Children's ◇, Mucinex Allergy ◇

Therapeutic class: Antihistamines
Pharmacologic class: Piperidines

AVAILABLE FORMS
ODTs: 30 mg ◇
Oral suspension: 30 mg/5 mL ◇
Tablets: 30 mg ◇, 60 mg ◇, 120 mg✿ ◇, 180 mg ◇

INDICATIONS & DOSAGES
Adjust-a-dose (for all indications): For patients with impaired renal function or need for dialysis, give adults and children age 12 and older 60 mg P.O. daily, children ages 2 to 11, 30 mg daily, and children ages 6 months to 2 years, 15 mg daily.
➤ **Seasonal allergies/hay fever**
Adults and children age 12 and older: 60 mg P.O. b.i.d. or 180 mg P.O. once daily.
Children ages 2 to 11: 30 mg P.O. every 12 hours. Maximum, 60 mg daily.

guaifenesin (glyceryl guaiacolate)

gwye-FEN-e-sin

Altarussin ◇, Balminil✿ ◇, Benylin E✿ ◇, Diabetic Tussin ◇, Fenesin IR ◇, Geri-Tussin ◇, Liquibid ◇, Liquituss GG ◇, Mucinex ◇, Mucinex Maximum Strength ◇, Mucosa ◇, Mucus Relief ◇, Organ-I NR ◇, Q-Tussin ◇, Refenesen ◇, Robafen ◇, Robitussin Chest Congestion ◇, Tussin ◇

Therapeutic class: Expectorants
Pharmacologic class: Propanediol derivatives

AVAILABLE FORMS
Capsules: 200 mg ◇
Liquid: 100 mg/5 mL ◇ *, 200 mg/10 mL ◇
Syrup: 100 mg/5 mL ◇
Tablets: 100 mg ◇, 200 mg ◇, 400 mg
Tablets (extended-release) 🚫: 600 mg ◇, 1,200 mg ◇

INDICATIONS & DOSAGES
➤ Expectorant
Adults and children age 12 and older: 200 to 400 mg
P.O. every 4 hours, or 600 to 1,200 mg (extended-release tablets) P.O. every 12 hours. Maximum,
2,400 mg daily.
Children ages 6 to 11: 100 to 200 mg P.O. every
4 hours. Maximum, 1,200 mg daily.
Children ages 2 to 5: 50 to 100 mg P.O. every 4 hours.
Maximum, 600 mg daily.

ketotifen fumarate
kee-toe-TYE-fen

Alaway ◊ , Zaditor ◊

Therapeutic class: Antihistamines
(ophthalmic)
Pharmacologic class: H_1-receptor
antagonists–mast cell stabilizers

AVAILABLE FORMS
Ophthalmic solution: 0.025%

INDICATIONS & DOSAGES
➤ To temporarily prevent eye itching from allergic
conjunctivitis or temporarily relieve itchy eyes due
to pollen, ragweed, grass, animal hair, and dander
Adults and children age 3 and older: Instill 1 drop in
each affected eye every 8 to 12 hours but not more
than b.i.d.

loratadine
lor-AT-a-deen

Alavert Allergy ◊ , Children's Claritin
Allergy ◊ , Children's Loratadine ◊ ,
Claritin ◊ , Claritin 24-Hour Allergy ◊ ,
Claritin Liqui-Gels ◊ , Claritin
RediTabs ◊

Therapeutic class: Antihistamines
Pharmacologic class: Piperidines

AVAILABLE FORMS
Capsules: 10 mg ◊
ODTs: 5 mg ◊ , 10 mg ◊
Syrup: 1 mg/mL ◊
Tablets: 10 mg ◊
Tablets (chewable): 5 mg ◊

INDICATIONS & DOSAGES
➤ Allergic rhinitis
Adults and children age 6 and older: 10 mg P.O. daily.
Or, 5 mg Claritin RediTabs every 12 hours.
Children ages 2 to 5: 5 mg chewable tablets or syrup
P.O. daily.
➤ To relieve itching due to hives (urticaria)
Adults and children age 6 and older: 10 mg P.O. daily.

meclizine hydrochloride (meclozine hydrochloride)
MEK-li-zeen

ABonine ◊ , Dramamine Less Drowsy
Formula ◊ , Motion-Time ◊ , Travel
Sickness ◊

Therapeutic class: Antivertigo drugs
Pharmacologic class: Anticholinergics

AVAILABLE FORMS
Tablets: 12.5 mg, 25 mg ◊ , 50 mg
Tablets (chewable): 25 mg ◊

INDICATIONS & DOSAGES
➤ Vertigo
Adults and children age 12 and older: 25 to 100 mg
P.O. daily in divided doses. Dosage varies with re-
sponse.
➤ Motion sickness
Adults and children age 12 and older: 25 to 50 mg P.O.
1 hour before travel; then daily for duration of trip.

minoxidil (topical)
mi-NOX-i-dill

Men's Rogaine ◊ , Minoxidil Extra
Strength for Men ◊ , Rogaine Extra
Strength for Men ◊ , Theroxidil ◊ ,
Women's Rogaine ◊

Therapeutic class: Hair-growth stimulants
Pharmacologic class: Direct-acting
vasodilators

AVAILABLE FORMS
Topical foam: 5% ◊
Topical solution: 2% ◊ , 5% ◊

INDICATIONS & DOSAGES
➤ Androgenetic alopecia
Adults: 1 mL of solution or half a capful of foam
applied to affected area b.i.d. Maximum daily dose is
2 mL of solution.

oxymetazoline hydrochloride (intranasal)
ox-i-met-AZ-oh-leen

Afrin Sinus ◇, Dristan ◇, Duration Spray ◇, Mucinex Sinus-Max Full Force ◇, Nasal Spray ◇, Neo-Synephrine 12 Hour Spray ◇, Vicks Sinex 12 Hour Decongestant ◇

Therapeutic class: Decongestants
Pharmacologic class: Sympathomimetics

AVAILABLE FORMS
Nasal solution: 0.05% ◇

INDICATIONS & DOSAGES
➤ **Nasal congestion**
Adults and children age 6 and older: 2 to 3 sprays of 0.05% solution in each nostril b.i.d. Don't use for more than 3 days.

oxymetazoline hydrochloride (ophthalmic)
ox-i-met-AZ-oh-leen

Therapeutic class: Vasoconstrictors
Pharmacologic class: Direct-acting sympathomimetic amines

AVAILABLE FORMS
Ophthalmic solution: 0.025%

INDICATIONS & DOSAGES
➤ **Relief from eye redness caused by minor eye irritation**
Adults and children age 6 and older: Instill 1 to 2 drops in affected eye every 6 hours, as needed.

phenylephrine hydrochloride (intranasal)
fen-ill-EF-rin

4-Way Fast Acting ◇, 4-Way Menthol ◇, Afrin Children's ◇, Contac-D ◇, Little Noses Decongestant ◇, Neo-Synephrine ◇, Rhinall ◇, Sudafed PE Maximum Strength ◇, Sudafed PE Children's ◇, Sudogest PE ◇

Therapeutic class: Vasoconstrictors
Pharmacologic class: Adrenergics

AVAILABLE FORMS
Nasal solution: 0.125% ◇, 0.25% ◇, 0.5% ◇, 1% ◇

INDICATIONS & DOSAGES
➤ **Nasal congestion**
Adults and children age 12 and older: 2 to 3 drops or 2 to 3 sprays of 0.25% to 1% solution in each nostril every 4 hours, p.r.n. Don't use for longer than 3 days.
Children ages 6 to 11: 2 to 3 drops or 2 to 3 sprays of 0.25% solution in each nostril every 4 hours, p.r.n. Don't use for longer than 3 days.
Children ages 2 to 5: 2 to 3 drops of 0.125% solution every 4 hours, p.r.n. Don't use for longer than 3 days.

pseudoephedrine hydrochloride
soo-dow-e-FED-rin

CongestAid ◇, ElixSure Congestion ◇, Genaphed ◇, Sudafed ◇, SudoGest ◇, Nexafed ◇, Zephrex-D ◇

Therapeutic class: Decongestants
Pharmacologic class: Adrenergics

AVAILABLE FORMS
Oral solution: 15 mg/5 mL ◇, 30 mg/5 mL ◇
Syrup: 15 mg/5 mL ◇, 30 mg/5 mL ◇
Tablets: 30 mg ◇, 60 mg ◇
Tablets (abuse-deterrent): 30 mg ◇
Tablets (extended-release) ⓓⓝⓒ*:* 120 mg ◇, 240 mg ◇

INDICATIONS & DOSAGES
➤ **Nasal decongestant**
Adults and children older than age 12: 60 mg P.O. every 4 to 6 hours; or 120 mg extended-release tablet P.O. every 12 hours; or 240 mg extended-release tablet P.O. once daily. Maximum dosage, 240 mg daily.
Children ages 6 to 12 (immediate-release products only): 30 mg P.O. every 4 to 6 hours. Maximum dosage, 120 mg daily.
Children ages 2 to 5 (immediate-release products only): 15 mg P.O. every 4 to 6 hours. Maximum dosage, 60 mg daily.

pyrethrins–piperonyl butoxide
pi-RETH-rinz/PI-per-oh-nel

Lice Shampoo❧ ◇, Licide ◇, RID ◇

Therapeutic class: Pediculicides
Pharmacologic class: Pyrethrins

AVAILABLE FORMS
Lotion: pyrethrins 0.3% and piperonyl butoxide 2% ◇
Mousse: pyrethrins 0.33% and piperonyl butoxide 4% ◇
Shampoo: pyrethrins 0.33% and piperonyl butoxide 4% ◇
Topical gel: pyrethrins 0.3% and piperonyl butoxide 3% ◇

❧ Canada   ◇ OTC   ⓓⓝⓒ Do not crush   *Liquid contains alcohol.

INDICATIONS & DOSAGES
➤ **Treatment of *Pediculus humanus* infestations**
Adults and children age 2 years and older: Apply to hair, scalp, or other infested areas until entirely wet. Allow to remain for 10 minutes but no longer. Wash thoroughly with warm water and soap or shampoo. Remove dead lice and eggs with fine-toothed comb. Repeat treatment in 7 to 10 days to kill newly hatched lice.

simethicone
sye-METH-ih-kone

Gas Relief ◊ , Gas-X ◊ , Gas-X Extra Strength ◊ , Gas-X Infant Drops ◊ , Infacol ✦ , Mylanta Gas ◊ , Mylanta Gas Relief Maximum Strength ◊ , Mylicon ◊ , Ovol ✦◊ , Ovol Drops ✦◊ , Pediacol ✦◊ , Phazyme Maximum Strength ◊

Therapeutic class: Antiflatulents
Pharmacologic class:
Polydimethylsiloxanes

AVAILABLE FORMS
Capsules: 125 mg ◊ , 180 mg ◊ , 250 mg ◊
Drops: 40 mg/0.6 mL ◊
Liquid: 20 mg/0.3 mL ◊
Strips (orally disintegrating): 40 mg ◊ , 62.5 mg ◊
Tablets: 60 mg ◊ , 80 mg ◊ , 125 mg ◊
Tablets (chewable): 40 mg ◊ , 80 mg ◊ , 125 mg ◊

INDICATIONS & DOSAGES
➤ **Flatulence, functional gastric bloating**
Adults and children older than age 12: 40 to 360 mg P.O. q.i.d. as needed after each meal and at bedtime, up to 500 mg daily. For drops, 40 to 80 mg P.O. as needed after each meal and at bedtime, up to 500 mg daily.
Children ages 2 to 12 or weighing more than 11 kg: 40 mg P.O. q.i.d. as needed after meals and at bedtime, up to 480 mg daily.
Children younger than age 2 or weighing less than 11 kg: 20 mg P.O. q.i.d. as needed after meals and at bedtime, up to 240 mg daily.

terbinafine hydrochloride (topical)
ter-BIN-ah-fin

Antifungal Foot ◊ , Lamisil ◊ , Lamisil AT ◊

Therapeutic class: Antifungals
Pharmacologic class: Allylamine derivatives

AVAILABLE FORMS
Cream: 1% ◊
Gel: 1% ◊

Solution: 1% ◊
Spray: 1% ◊

INDICATIONS & DOSAGES
➤ **Athlete's foot**
Adults and children age 12 and older: For athlete's foot between the toes, apply b.i.d. or as directed by prescriber. For athlete's foot on the bottom or sides of the foot, apply b.i.d. for 2 weeks or as directed by prescriber.
➤ **Jock itch, ringworm**
Adults and children age 12 and older: Apply once daily for 1 week or as directed by prescriber.

tetrahydrozoline hydrochloride (ophthalmic)
tet-rah-hi-DRAZ-oh-leen

Clear Eyes Triple Action ◊ , Murine Tears Plus ◊ , Opti-Clear ◊ , Visine ◊

Therapeutic class: Vasoconstrictors
Pharmacologic class: Sympathomimetics

AVAILABLE FORMS
Ophthalmic solution: 0.05% ◊

INDICATIONS & DOSAGES
➤ **Conjunctival congestion, irritation, and allergic conditions**
Adults: Instill 1 to 2 drops in affected eye up to q.i.d., or as directed by prescriber.

witch hazel
wich HA-zel

Preparation H ◊ , Tucks ◊

Therapeutic class: Dermatologic agents
Pharmacologic class: Astringents

AVAILABLE FORMS
External pads: 50% ◊ , 86% ◊

INDICATIONS & DOSAGES
➤ **Anal or vaginal irritation**
Adults and children age 12 and older: Apply to affected area up to six times daily or after each bowel movement.

Do not use: Dangerous abbreviations, symbols, and dose designations (ISMP Canada)

The abbreviations, symbols, and dose designations found in this table have been reported as being frequently misinterpreted and involved in harmful medication errors. They should NEVER be used when communicating medication information.

Abbreviation	Intended meaning	Problem	Correction
U	unit	Mistaken for "0" (zero), "4" (four), or cc	Use "unit."
IU	international unit	Mistaken for "IV" (intravenous) or "10" (ten)	Use "unit."
Abbreviations for drug names		Misinterpreted because of similar abbreviations for multiple drugs; e.g., MS, MSO_4 (morphine sulphate), $MgSO_4$ (magnesium sulphate) may be confused for one another	Do not abbreviate drug names.
QD	every day	Mistaken for each other, or as "qid."	Use "daily" and "every other day."
QOD	every other day	Q has also been misinterpreted as "2" (two)	
OD	every day	Mistaken for "right eye" (OD = oculus dexter)	Use "daily."
OS, OD, OU	left eye, right eye, both eyes	May be confused with one another	Use "left eye," "right eye" or "both eyes."
D/C	discharge	Interpreted as "discontinue whatever medications follow" (typically discharge medications)	Use "discharge."
cc	cubic centimetre	Mistaken for "u" (units)	Use "mL" or "millilitre."
µg	microgram	Mistaken for "mg" (milligram) resulting in one thousand-fold overdose	Use "mcg."

Symbol	Intended meaning	Potential problem	Correction
@	at	Mistaken for "2" (two) or "5" (five)	Use "at."
>	greater than	Mistaken for "7"(seven) or the letter "L"	Use "greater than"/"more than" or "less than"/"lower than."
<	less than	Confused with each other	

Dose designation	Intended meaning	Potential problem	Correction
Trailing zero	X.0 mg	Decimal point is overlooked, resulting in 10-fold dose error	Never use a zero by itself after a decimal point. Use "X mg."
Lack of leading zero	.X mg	Decimal point is overlooked, resulting in 10-fold dose error	Always use a zero before a decimal point. Use "0.X mg."

Adapted from ISMP's *List of Error-Prone Abbreviations, Symbols, and Dose Designations 2006*.
Available from: https://www.ismp-canada.org/download/ISMPCanadaListOfDangerousAbbreviations.pdf
Reprinted with permission from ISMP Canada 2016.

Decision tree: Deciding about medication administration

Use this tool to help you determine whether or not to administer a medication. Be sure to consider all of the phases of medication administration in this document.

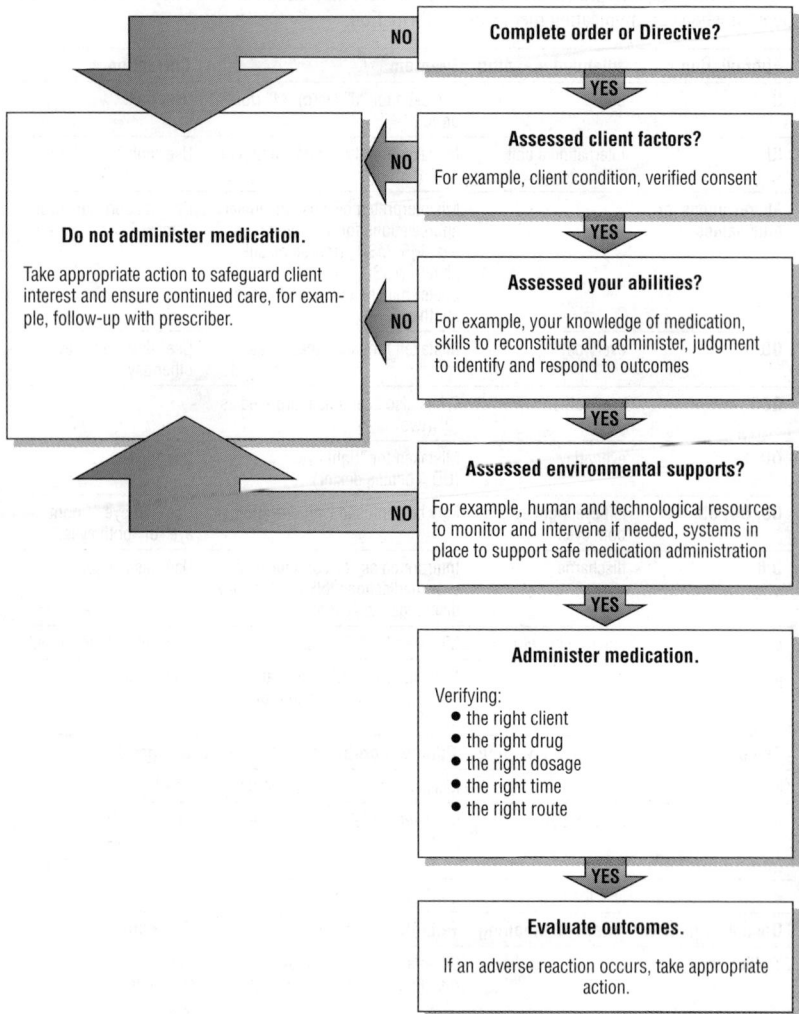

Complete order or Directive?

NO → YES

Assessed client factors?

For example, client condition, verified consent

NO → YES

Do not administer medication.

Take appropriate action to safeguard client interest and ensure continued care, for example, follow-up with prescriber.

Assessed your abilities?

For example, your knowledge of medication, skills to reconstitute and administer, judgment to identify and respond to outcomes

NO → YES

Assessed environmental supports?

For example, human and technological resources to monitor and intervene if needed, systems in place to support safe medication administration

NO → YES

Administer medication.

Verifying:
- the right client
- the right drug
- the right dosage
- the right time
- the right route

YES

Evaluate outcomes.

If an adverse reaction occurs, take appropriate action.

Note: Document during and/or after administering medication, according to documentation standards.
© Nurses Association of New Brunswick. Reproduced with permission. Further reproduction prohibited.

Canadian National Drug Schedules

The Canadian National Drug Schedules (NDS), issued by the National Association of Pharmacy Regulatory Authorities (NAPRA), is the regulatory model that defines the conditions of sale for all drug products sold in Canada. NAPRA assigns each drug product to one of four categories (Schedule I, II, III, or Unscheduled) depending on various factors, including the level of professional intervention required, public safety, and the drug's level of toxicity. The NDS is based on a cascading structure that allows regulators to use clinical judgment to determine market placement of the drug product: Schedule I products are considered the most highly regulated, and Unscheduled products have the least restrictions at point of sale.

Schedule	Description of regulatory drug categories
Schedule I drugs	• Drug requires a prescription by a licensed practitioner. • Ongoing drug monitoring and evaluation is required. • Appropriate drug use may cause dependency. • Serious drug reactions may occur at normal therapeutic dosages. • Narrow margin of safety exists between therapeutic and toxic dosages. • Serious drug interactions are known or may occur. • Drug's use may promote development of resistant strains of microorganisms. • Drug is new or the indication isn't appropriate for self-treatment and its safe use hasn't been established.
Schedule II drugs	• Drug isn't included in Schedule I and the initial need for the drug is identified or confirmed by a regulated health professional (i.e., pharmacist, physician). • Drug should be administered in a health care setting or under the direction of a regulated health professional. • Drug must be readily available under exceptional circumstances when a prescription isn't practical, but must be physically located behind the counter to prevent self-selection by the public. • Chronic therapy or subsequent retreatment requires monitoring by a pharmacist. • Drug requires intervention by a pharmacist to confirm that the patient has made an appropriate self-assessment, the condition is new to patient self-assessment, or the condition generally isn't appropriate for patient self-assessment. • Drug has significant potential for abuse or misuse. • Drug may cause serious adverse reactions not completely addressed in product label. • Safe use of drug requires a pharmacist to provide more detailed information and education than appear on the product label. • Drug may mask or delay signs and symptoms of a serious disease. • Drug is new or is in a new drug delivery system, for self-medication.
Schedule III drugs	• Drug isn't in Schedule I or II and is a new ingredient for self-medication, and advice from a pharmacist can support safe use. • Drug is used to treat a chronic or persistent condition, and advice from a pharmacist can support safe use. • There is potential for abuse or misuse. • Drug may mask or delay signs and symptoms of a serious disease. • Advice from a pharmacist to explain, reinforce, or expand on product labeling information, or when product selection is likely to cause confusion, can promote safe use of drug. • Products may be located in the self-selection area of the pharmacy but must be under direct supervision of the pharmacist and clearly identified as the "professional services area" of the pharmacy.
Unscheduled drugs	• Drug can be sold from any retail outlet without professional supervision. • Acceptable and adequate label information is available for patients to make a safe drug choice. • Drug isn't included in Schedules I, II, or III.

Safe disposal of unused drugs: What patients need to know

Why is the safe disposal of unused drugs important?

The FDA reported that in 2014, Americans filled approximately 4.3 billion prescriptions, and many new drugs are approved each year. More available drugs and the saving of unused drugs create an increased potential for drug abuse, misuse, dependence, overdose, and accidental poisoning.

According to data from the 2015 National Survey on Drug Use and Health, almost 19 million Americans age 12 and older have misused prescription psychotherapeutic drugs (pain relievers, tranquilizers, stimulants, and sedatives); of these, 12.5 million people misused pain relievers. The Substance Abuse and Mental Health Services Administration reports that over 50% of opioid abusers are first exposed by trying someone else's medication. Presently, steps are being taken to combat the growing epidemic of opioid abuse, dependence, and overdose in the United States: An FDA advisory committee will assess New Drug Applications for opioids that don't have abuse-deterrent formulations; the pharmaceutical industry is developing technologies to develop abuse-deterrent formulations; prescribers will have more training on long-acting and immediate-release opioid use and prescribing; immediate-release opioids will have stronger warnings similar to the warnings enacted for the long-acting formulations; and the FDA will require more postmarketing data to assess misuse and abuse of long-acting opioids and is researching how to make the life-saving drug naloxone more readily available to the consumer (e.g., OTC programs).

Other important drug safety considerations include unused drugs leading to harmful drug misuse and abuse, and accidental drug exposure and poisoning, particularly in children and pets. The U.S. Poison Control Center reported that in 2014, 79.4% of all reported poison exposures were unintentional. The most common substance linked to poison exposure in adults age 20 or older is pain medication, followed by sedatives and sleeping medications, antidepressants, and CV medications. Over the past 20 years, the FDA has documented more than 30 cases of accidental exposure to transdermal fentanyl pain patches. Most of these cases occurred in children younger than age 2; almost half of these exposures resulted in death. Child-resistant containers are no guarantee that the container is child-proof; one study reported that 45% of accidental drug exposures in children were to drugs stored in child-resistant containers.

Now, more than ever, it's important for you as a health care provider to discuss the critical issue of safe disposal of prescribed drugs with all patients. Be sure to remind patients about the safe disposal of unused drugs at follow-up visits. Teaching patients to safely dispose of unused drugs is an important strategy to protect household members and pets from accidental drug exposure and poisoning.

Patient-teaching points

Here are some important patient-teaching points about safe disposal of unused drugs:
- Tell patients that the FDA doesn't recommend the reuse or redistribution of an unused drug, because the safety and effectiveness of the drug can't be guaranteed once it's dispensed. Such factors as improper drug storage and possible drug tampering can alter the drug's safety and effectiveness.
- Counsel patients, caregivers, or family members to dispose of all unused drugs as soon as they are no longer needed.
- Advise patients to check for community drug take-back programs. These programs are especially important for the convenient disposal of drugs that can be harmful to others, such as psychotherapeutic drugs. Drug take-back programs were designed by the U.S. Drug Enforcement Administration and are administered in conjunction with local law enforcement. Patients can mail in their unused drugs or drop them off in person to local law enforcement personnel. Or, they can dispose of the drugs in a special receptacle (known as a "drop-box") located in local

clinics or retail pharmacies. If drug take-back programs aren't locally available, advise patients to check with community resources or their pharmacist or prescriber to see if they may dispose of drugs themselves.
• Instruct patients that certain drugs considered harmful if ingested by others may be flushed down the sink or toilet and to check the following resources to see if flushing is appropriate:

   ○ Medicines Recommended for Disposal by Flushing: www.fda.gov/downloads/Drugs/ResourcesForYou/Consumers/BuyingUsingMedicineSafely/EnsuringSafeUseofMedicine/SafeDisposalofMedicines/UCM337803.pdf

   ○ DailyMed (official FDA drug label information and package inserts): https://dailymed.nlm.nih.gov/dailymed/index.cfm. Search for the drug's name; then look for the following sections within the label:

      – Information for Patients and Caregivers
      – Patient Information
      – Patient Counseling Information
      – Safety and Handling Instructions
      – Medication Guide.

• Advise patients that nonharmful drugs may be disposed of by placing them intact (don't crush capsules or tablets) in a plastic bag or container filled with an undesirable substance, such as dirt, cat litter, or coffee grounds, and then placing the container in the household trash. Tell patients to make sure that children and pets can't access the trash receptacle.
• Warn patients to remove and destroy all labels from medication containers before recycling or disposing of them, to maintain privacy.
• Instruct patients to safely dispose of transdermal drug patches by folding them in half (sticky sides together) while avoiding contact with the sticky sides. Fentanyl patches should be immediately flushed down the toilet. Patches containing nitroglycerin or testosterone may be placed in the household trash.

Additional resources

Here are additional resources to find out more information about safe drug disposal of unused drugs:

• DEA Diversion Control Division–Drug disposal information: www.deadiversion.usdoj.gov/drug_disposal/index.html
• DEA Diversion Control Division–Controlled substance public disposal locations: https:/apps.deadiversion.usdoj.gov/pubdispsearch/spring/main?execution=e1s1
• DEA Diversion Control Division–Registration call center: 1-800-882-9539
• FDA. How to dispose of unused medicines: www.fda.gov/ForConsumers/ConsumerUpdates/ucm101653.htm
• FDA. Medication disposal: Questions and answers: www.fda.gov/Drugs/ResourcesForYou/Consumers/BuyingUsingMedicineSafely/EnsuringSafeUseofMedicine/SafeDisposalofMedicines/ucm186188.htm
• FDA. Contact number: 1-888-INFO-FDA (1-888-463-6332).

Therapeutic drug monitoring guidelines

Laboratory value ranges may vary among laboratories. Be sure to compare test results with the normal values of the laboratory that did the test.

Drug	Laboratory test monitored	Therapeutic ranges of test
ACE inhibitors (benazepril, captopril, enalapril, enala-prilat, fosinopril, lisinopril, moexipril, quinapril, ramipril, trandolapril)	Creatinine BUN Potassium WBC with differential	Men: 0.9–1.3 mg/dL Women: 0.6–1.1 mg/dL 6–20 mg/dL 3.5–5.2 mEq/L *****
aminoglycoside antibiotics (amikacin, gentamicin, tobramycin)	Amikacin peak Amikacin trough Creatinine Gentamicin peak Tobramycin peak Gentamicin, tobramycin trough	20–30 mcg/mL 1–8 mcg/mL Men: 0.9–1.3 mg/dL Women: 0.6–1.1 mg/dL 6–10 mcg/mL 5–10 mcg/mL <2 mcg/mL
amphotericin B	BUN CBC with differential and platelets Creatinine Electrolytes (especially potassium and magnesium) Liver function	6–20 mg/dL ***** Men: 0.9–1.3 mg/dL Women: 0.6–1.1 mg/dL Potassium: 3.5–5.2 mEq/L Magnesium: 1.3–2.2 mEq/L Sodium: 135–147 mEq/L Chloride: 95–110 mEq/L *
antibiotics	Cultures and sensitivities WBC with differential	*****
biguanides (metformin)	CBC Creatinine Fasting glucose HbA$_{1c}$	***** Men: 0.9–1.3 mg/dL Women: 0.6–1.1 mg/dL ≤100 mg/dL 5.0–7.0% of total hemoglobin
carbamazepine	BUN Carbamazepine CBC with differential Liver function Platelet count	6–20 mg/dL 4–12 mcg/mL ***** * 140–400 × 10³/mm³
corticosteroids (betametha-sone, cortisone, dexametha-sone, hydrocortisone, methylPREDNISolone, predniSONE, prednisoLONE, triamcinolone)	Electrolytes (especially potassium) Fasting glucose	Potassium: 3.5–5.2 mEq/L Magnesium: 1.8–2.6 mEq/L Sodium: 136–145 mEq/L Chloride: 96–106 mEq/L Calcium: 8.8–10.4 mg/dL ≤100/dL

***** For those areas marked with asterisks, the following values can be used:

Hb: Women: 12–16 g/dL
　　Men: 14–18 g/dL
Hematocrit: Women: 37%–48%
　　Men: 42%–52%
RBCs: 4–5.5 × 10⁶/mm³
WBCs: 5–10 × 10³/mm³

Differential: Neutrophils: 45%–74%
Bands: 0%–8%
Lymphocytes: 16%–45%
Monocytes: 4%–10%
Eosinophils: 0%–7%
Basophils: 0%–2%

Monitoring guidelines

Monitor WBC with differential before therapy, monthly during first 3 months, then periodically for first year. Monitor renal function and potassium level closely at start of therapy, after dosage changes, and periodically during therapy.

Wait until after third dose is given to check drug levels. Obtain blood for peak level 30 minutes after I.V. infusion ends or 60 minutes after I.M. administration. For trough levels, draw blood just before next dose. Dosage may need to be adjusted accordingly. Recheck after three doses. Monitor creatinine and BUN levels and urine output for signs of decreasing renal function. Monitor urine for increased proteins, cells, and casts.

Monitor creatinine, BUN, and electrolyte levels at least daily at start of therapy, then as clinically indicated. Regularly monitor blood counts and LFT results during therapy.

Monitor WBC with differential weekly during therapy. Specimen cultures and sensitivities will determine cause of the infection and the best treatment.

Check renal function and hematologic values before starting therapy and at least annually thereafter. If patient has impaired renal function, don't use metformin because it may cause lactic acidosis. Monitor response to therapy by periodically evaluating fasting glucose and HbA_{1c} levels. A patient's home monitoring of glucose levels helps monitor compliance and response.

Monitor blood counts and platelets before therapy; monitor closely during therapy. Check LFTs and BUN before and periodically during therapy.

Monitor electrolyte and glucose levels regularly during long-term therapy.

(continued)

* For those areas marked with one asterisk, the following values can be used:
ALT: 7–56 units/L
AST: 5–40 units/L
Alkaline phosphatase: 17–142 units/L
LDH: 140–280 units/L
GGT: <40 units/L
Total bilirubin: 0.2–1 mg/dL

Drug	Laboratory test monitored	Therapeutic ranges of test
digoxin	Creatinine	Men: 0.9–1.3 mg/dL Women: 0.6–1.1 mg/dL
	Digoxin	0.8–2 nanograms/mL
	Electrolytes	Potassium: 3.5–5.2 mEq/L Magnesium: 1.8–2.6 mEq/L Sodium: 136–145 mEq/L Chloride: 96–106 mEq/L Calcium: 8.8–10.4 mg/dL
epoetin alfa	CBC with differential	*****
	Hematocrit	Women: 36%–48% Men: 42%–52%
	Platelet count	140–400 × 10^3/mm^3
	Serum ferritin	18–270 nanograms/mL
	Transferrin	250–425 mg/dL
ethosuximide	CBC with differential	******
	Ethosuximide	40–100 mcg/mL
	Liver function	*
gemfibrozil	CBC	*****
	Lipids	Total cholesterol: <200 mg/dL LDL: <130 mg/dL HDL: ≥35 mg/dL Triglycerides: <150 mg/dL
	Liver function	*
	Serum glucose	<100 mg/dL
	CK	26–174 units/L
heparin (unfractionated)	aPTT	1.5–2 × control
	Hematocrit	*****
	Platelet count	140–400 × 10^3/mm^3
HMG-CoA reductase inhibitors (atorvastatin, fluvastatin, lovastatin, pravastatin, rosuvastatin, simvastatin)	Lipids	Total cholesterol: <200 mg/dL LDL: <130 mg/dL HDL: ≥35 mg/dL Triglycerides: <150 mg/dL
	Liver function	*
insulin	Fasting glucose	≤100 mg/dL
	HbA$_{1c}$	<5%–7% of total Hb
isotretinoin	CBC with differential	*****
	Liver function	*
	Lipids	Total cholesterol: <200 mg/dL LDL: <130 mg/dL HDL: ≥35 mg/dL Triglycerides: <150 mg/dL
	Platelet count	140–400 × 10^3/mm^3
	Pregnancy test	Negative

***** For those areas marked with asterisks, the following values can be used:

Hb: Women: 12–16 g/dL
    Men: 14–18 g/dL
Hematocrit: Women: 37%–48%
            Men: 42%–52%
RBCs: 4–5.5 × 10^6/mm^3
WBCs: 5–10 × 10^3/mm^3

Differential: Neutrophils: 45%–74%
              Bands: 0%–8%
              Lymphocytes: 16%–45%
              Monocytes: 4%–10%
              Eosinophils: 0%–7%
              Basophils: 0%–2%

Monitoring guidelines

Check digoxin levels just before next dose or at least 6 to 8 hours after last dose. To monitor maintenance therapy, check drug levels at least 1 to 2 weeks after therapy is initiated or changed. Make any adjustments in therapy based on entire clinical picture, not solely on drug levels. Also, check electrolyte levels and renal function periodically during therapy.

After therapy is initiated or changed, monitor hematocrit twice weekly for 2 to 6 weeks until stabilized in target range and a maintenance dose has been determined. Monitor hematocrit regularly thereafter.

Check drug level 8 to 10 days after therapy is initiated or changed. Periodically monitor CBC with differential and LFTs.

Therapy is usually withdrawn after 3 months if response is inadequate. Patient must be fasting to measure triglyceride levels. Periodically obtain blood counts, LFT values during first 12 months. Obtain CK for muscle pain or weakness.

When drug is given by continuous I.V. infusion, check aPTT every 4 hours and according to facility policy in early stages of therapy, and daily thereafter. Check platelet counts and hematocrit and test for occult blood in stools periodically during therapy.

Perform LFTs at baseline, 2 to 4 weeks after therapy is initiated or changed (depending on drug), and periodically thereafter.

A patient's home monitoring of glucose levels helps measure compliance and response. HbA$_{1c}$ level is a good measure of long-term control.

Use a serum or urine pregnancy test with a sensitivity of at least 25 milli-international units/mL. Perform one test before therapy and a second test during first 5 days of the menstrual cycle before therapy begins or at least 11 days after last unprotected act of sexual intercourse, whichever is later. Repeat pregnancy tests monthly. Obtain baseline LFTs and lipid levels; repeat every 1 to 2 weeks until response to treatment is established (usually 4 weeks).

(continued)

---

* For those areas marked with one asterisk, the following values can be used:
ALT: 7–56 units/L
AST: 5–40 units/L
Alkaline phosphatase: 17–142 units/L
LDH: 140–280 units/L
GGT: <40 units/L
Total bilirubin: 0.2–1 mg/dL

Drug	Laboratory test monitored	Therapeutic ranges of test
linezolid	Amylase	25–125 international units/L
	CBC with differential	*****
	Cultures and sensitivities	
	Liver function	*
	Lipase	10–140 units/L
	Platelet count	140–400 × 10³/mm³
lithium	Creatinine	Men: 0.9–1.3 mg/dL
		Women: 0.6–1.1 mg/dL
	CBC	*****
	Electrolytes (especially potassium and sodium)	Potassium: 3.5–5.2 mEq/L
		Magnesium: 1.8–2.6 mEq/L
		Sodium: 136–145 mEq/L
		Chloride: 96–106 mEq/L
	Fasting glucose	≤100 mg/dL
	Lithium	0.6–1.2 mEq/L
	Thyroid function tests	TSH: 0.45–4.5 microunits/mL
		T₃: 80–200 nanograms/dL
		T₄: 5.4–11.5 mcg/dL
methotrexate	CBC with differential	*****
	Creatinine	Men: 0.9–1.3 mg/dL
		Women: 0.6–1.1 mg/dL
	Liver function	*
	Methotrexate	Normal elimination:
		~ 5 micromol/L 24 hours postdose
		~ 0.5 micromol/L 48 hours postdose
		~ <0.2 micromol/L 72 hours postdose
	Platelet count	140–400 × 10³/mm³
NNRTIs (delavirdine, efavirenz, nevirapine)	Amylase	25–125 international units/L
	CBC with differential and platelets	*****
	Liver function	*
	Lipids (efavirenz)	Total cholesterol: <200 mg/dL
		LDL: <130 mg/dL
		HDL: ≥35 mg/dL
		Triglycerides: <150 mg/dL
phenytoin	Albumin	3.5–5.2 g/dL
	CBC	*****
	Phenytoin	10–20 mcg/mL
procainamide	ANA titer	Negative
	CBC	*****
	Liver function	*
	N-acetylprocainamide (NAPA)	15–25 mcg/mL
	Procainamide	4–8 mcg/mL

***** For those areas marked with asterisks, the following values can be used:

Hb: Women: 12–16 g/dL	Differential: Neutrophils: 45%–74%
Men: 14–18 g/dL	Bands: 0%–8%
Hematocrit: Women: 37%–48%	Lymphocytes: 16%–45%
Men: 42%–52%	Monocytes: 4%–10%
RBCs: 4–5.5 × 10⁶/mm³	Eosinophils: 0%–7%
WBCs: 5–10 × 10³/mm³	Basophils: 0%–2%

Monitoring guidelines

Obtain baseline CBC with differential and platelet count weekly during therapy. Monitor LFTs and amylase and lipase levels during therapy.

Checking drug levels is crucial to safe use of drug. Obtain level immediately before next dose. Monitor level twice weekly until stable. Once at steady state, check level weekly; when patient is on appropriate maintenance dose, check level every 2 or 3 months. Monitor CBC; creatinine, electrolyte, and fasting glucose levels; and thyroid function test results before therapy starts and periodically thereafter.

Monitor drug level according to dosing protocol. Monitor CBC with differential, platelet count, and LFT and renal function test results more frequently when therapy starts or changes, and when methotrexate levels may be elevated, such as when patient is dehydrated.

Obtain baseline LFTs and monitor closely during first 12 weeks of therapy. Continue to monitor regularly during therapy. Check CBC with differential and platelet count before therapy and periodically during therapy. Monitor lipid levels during efavirenz therapy. Monitor amylase level during efavirenz and delavirdine therapy.

Monitor drug level immediately before next dose and 7 to 10 days after therapy starts or changes. Obtain a CBC at baseline and monthly early in therapy. Watch for toxic effects at therapeutic levels. Adjust the measured level for hypoalbuminemia or renal impairment, which can increase free drug levels.

Measure drug levels 6 to 12 hours after a continuous infusion is started or immediately before next oral dose. Combined procainamide and NAPA levels can be used as an index of toxicity when renal impairment exists. Obtain CBC, LFTs, and ANA titer periodically during longer-term therapy.

(continued)

---

* For those areas marked with one asterisk, the following values can be used:
ALT: 7–56 units/L
AST: 5–40 units/L
Alkaline phosphatase: 17–142 units/L
LDH: 140–280 units/L
GGT: <40 units/L
Total bilirubin: 0.2–1 mg/dL

Drug	Laboratory test monitored	Therapeutic ranges of test
quinidine	CBC	*****
	Creatinine	Men: 0.9–1.3 mg/dL
		Women: 0.6–1.1 mg/dL
	Electrolytes (especially potassium)	Potassium: 3.5–5.2 mEq/L
		Magnesium: 1.8–2.6 mEq/L
		Sodium: 136–145 mEq/L
		Chloride: 96–106 mEq/L
	Liver function	*
	Quinidine	2–5 mcg/mL
sulfonylureas	Fasting glucose	≤100 mg/dL
	HbA$_{1c}$	5%–7% of total Hb
theophylline	Theophylline	10–20 mcg/mL
thiazolidinediones (pioglitazone, rosiglitazone)	Fasting glucose	≤100 mg/dL
	HbA$_{1c}$	5%–7% of total Hb
	Liver function	*
thyroid hormones	Thyroid function tests	TSH: 0.45–5.4 microunits/mL
		T_3: 80–200 nanograms/dL
		T_4: 5.4–11.5 mcg/dL
valproate sodium, valproic acid, divalproex sodium	Ammonia	15–45 mcg/dL
	Amylase	25–125 international units/L
	BUN	8–25 mg/dL
	CBC with differential	*****
	Creatinine	Men: 0.9–1.3 mg/dL
		Women: 0.6-1.1 mg/dL
	Liver function	*
	Platelet count	140–400 × 10^3/mm^3
	PT	11–13 seconds
	Valproic acid	50–120 mcg/mL
vancomycin	Creatinine	Men: 0.9–1.3 mg/dL
		Women: 0.6–1.1 mg/dL
	Vancomycin	25–40 mcg/mL (peak)
		10–20 mcg/mL (trough)
warfarin	INR	For an acute MI, atrial fibrillation, treatment of pulmonary embolism, prevention of systemic embolism, tissue heart valves, valvular heart disease, or prophylaxis or treatment of venous thrombosis: 2–3
		For mechanical prosthetic valves or recurrent systemic embolism: 2.5–3.5

***** For those areas marked with asterisks, the following values can be used:

Hb: Women: 12–16 g/dL	Differential: Neutrophils: 45%–74%
Men: 14–18 g/dL	Bands: 0%–8%
Hematocrit: Women: 37%–48%	Lymphocytes: 16%–45%
Men: 42%–52%	Monocytes: 4%–10%
RBCs: 4–5.5 × 10^6/mm^3	Eosinophils: 0%–7%
WBCs: 5–10 × 10^3/mm^3	Basophils: 0%–2%

Monitoring guidelines

Obtain levels immediately before next oral dose and 30 to 35 hours after therapy starts or changes. Periodically obtain blood counts, LFT and renal function test results, and electrolyte levels.

Monitor response to therapy by periodically evaluating fasting glucose and HbA_{1c} levels. Patient should monitor glucose levels at home to help measure compliance and response.

Obtain drug levels right before next dose of sustained-release oral product and at least 2 days after therapy starts or changes.

Monitor response by evaluating fasting glucose and HbA_{1c} levels. Obtain baseline LFT results, and repeat tests periodically during therapy. Don't initiate therapy with pioglitazone or rosiglitazone if ALT is more than $2.5 \times$ ULN.

Monitor thyroid function test results every 2 to 3 weeks until appropriate maintenance dose is determined and annually thereafter.

Monitor LFT results, ammonia level, coagulation test results, renal function test results, CBC, and platelet count at baseline and periodically during therapy. LFT results should be closely monitored during first 6 months.

Drug levels may be checked with third dose administered, at the earliest. Draw peak levels 1.5 to 2.5 hours after a 1-hour infusion or I.V. infusion is complete. Draw trough levels within 1 hour of next dose administered. Renal function can be used to adjust dosing and intervals.

Check INR daily, beginning 3 days after therapy starts. Continue checking it until therapeutic goal is achieved, and monitor it periodically thereafter. Also, check level 7 days after change in dose or start of a potentially interacting therapy.

* For those areas marked with one asterisk, the following values can be used:
ALT: 7–56 units/L
AST: 5–40 units/L
Alkaline phosphatase: 17–142 units/L
LDH: 140–280 units/L
GGT: <40 units/L
Total bilirubin: 0.2–1 mg/dL

Less commonly used drugs: Indications and dosages

Refer to manufacturer's instructions for complete prescribing and safety information.

SAFETY ALERT!

abciximab
ab-SIX-ah-mab

ReoPro

Therapeutic class: Antiplatelet drugs
Pharmacologic class: Glycoprotein IIb/IIIa inhibitors

AVAILABLE FORMS
Injection: 2 mg/mL

INDICATIONS & DOSAGES
➤ **Adjunct to PCI to prevent acute cardiac ischemic complications**
Adults: 0.25 mg/kg as I.V. bolus given 10 to 60 minutes before start of PCI; then, continuous I.V. infusion of 0.125 mcg/kg/minute to maximum 10 mcg/minute for 12 hours.
➤ **Unstable angina not responding to conventional medical therapy in patients scheduled for PCI within 24 hours**
Adults: 0.25 mg/kg as I.V. bolus; then 18- to 24-hour infusion of 10 mcg/minute concluding 1 hour after PCI.

SAFETY ALERT!

acarbose
a-KAR-boz

Glucobay✦, Precose

Therapeutic class: Antidiabetics
Pharmacologic class: Alpha-glucosidase inhibitors

AVAILABLE FORMS
Tablets: 25 mg, 50 mg, 100 mg

INDICATIONS & DOSAGES
➤ **Adjunct to diet and exercise as monotherapy or with a sulfonylurea, metformin, or insulin to lower glucose level in patients with type 2 diabetes**
Adults: Individualized. Initially, 25 mg P.O. t.i.d. with first bite of each main meal. Adjust dosage every 4 to 8 weeks, based on 1-hour postprandial glucose level or HbA$_{1c}$ levels and tolerance. Maintenance dosage is 50 to 100 mg P.O. t.i.d. To minimize GI adverse effects, may initiate treatment at 25 mg P.O. once daily and increase to 25 mg P.O. t.i.d. For patients who weigh less than 60 kg, don't exceed 50 mg P.O. t.i.d. For patients who weigh more than 60 kg, don't exceed 100 mg P.O. t.i.d.

acetaZOLAMIDE
ah-set-a-ZOLE-ah-mide

Acetazolam✦, Diamox, Diamox Sequels

acetaZOLAMIDE sodium
Therapeutic class: Diuretics
Pharmacologic class: Carbonic anhydrase inhibitors

AVAILABLE FORMS
acetazolamide
Capsules (extended-release) ⓄⓃⒸ: 500 mg
Tablets: 125 mg, 250 mg
acetazolamide sodium
Powder for injection: 500-mg vial

INDICATIONS & DOSAGES
➤ **Secondary glaucoma; preoperative treatment of acute angle-closure glaucoma**
Adults: 250 mg P.O. every 4 hours or 250 mg P.O. b.i.d. for short-term therapy. In acute cases, 500 mg P.O.; then 125 to 250 mg P.O. every 4 hours. Or, for extended-release capsules, 500 mg P.O. b.i.d. To rapidly lower IOP, initially, 500 mg I.V.; may repeat in 2 to 4 hours, if needed, followed by 125 to 250 mg P.O. every 4 to 6 hours.
➤ **Chronic open-angle glaucoma**
Adults: 250 mg to 1 g P.O. daily in divided doses q.i.d., or 250 mg I.V. every 4 hours, or 500 mg extended-release P.O. b.i.d.
➤ **To prevent or treat acute mountain sickness (high-altitude sickness)**
Adults and children age 12 and older: 500 mg to 1 g (regular or extended-release) P.O. daily in divided doses every 12 hours. Start 24 to 48 hours before ascent and continue for 48 hours while at high altitude. When rapid ascent is required, start with 1,000 mg P.O. daily.
➤ **Adjunct for epilepsy and myoclonic, refractory, generalized tonic-clonic, absence, or mixed seizures**
Adults: 8 to 30 mg/kg P.O. or I.V. daily in divided doses; optimum range is 375 mg to 1 g daily. If given with other anticonvulsants, start at 250 mg P.O. or I.V. once daily, and increase to 375 mg to 1 g daily.
➤ **Edema caused by HF; drug-induced edema**
Adults: 250 to 375 mg (5 mg/kg) P.O. daily in the morning. For best results, use every other day or 2 days on followed by 1 to 2 days off. Or, 250 to 375 mg I.V. once daily for 1 or 2 days, alternating with a day of rest.

afatinib dimaleate
a-FA-ti-nib

Gilotrif, Giotrif✤

Therapeutic class: Antineoplastics
Pharmacologic class: Tyrosine kinase inhibitors

AVAILABLE FORMS
Tablets: 20 mg, 30 mg, 40 mg

INDICATIONS & DOSAGES
➤ **First-line treatment of patients with metastatic non–small-cell lung cancer whose tumors have epidermal growth factor receptor exon 19 deletions or exon 21 (*L858R*) substitution mutations as detected by an FDA-approved test**
Adults: 40 mg P.O. once a day on an empty stomach until disease progression or intolerability occurs.
Adjust-a-dose: Withhold drug for grade 3 or higher adverse reactions, diarrhea of grade 2 lasting for 2 or more consecutive days while patient is taking antidiarrheals, cutaneous reactions of grade 2 lasting more than 7 days or that are intolerable, or renal dysfunction of grade 2 or higher. If adverse reactions improve to grade 1, restart afatinib at a reduced dosage at 10 mg/day less than the dosage at which the adverse reaction occurred. Discontinue drug for severe or intolerable adverse reactions occurring at a dosage of 20 mg/day.

aflibercept
a-FLIB-er-sept

Eylea

Therapeutic class: Vascular endothelial growth factor inhibitors
Pharmacologic class: Antiangiogenetic drugs

AVAILABLE FORMS
Intravitreal injection: 40 mg/mL in 0.05-mL single-use vial

INDICATIONS & DOSAGES
➤ **Neovascular (wet) age-related macular degeneration**
Adults: 2 mg (0.05 mL) intravitreal injection every 4 weeks for first 12 weeks; then 2 mg (0.05 mL) once every 8 weeks.
➤ **Macular edema following retinal vein occlusion**
Adults: 2 mg (0.05 mL) intravitreal injection once every 4 weeks.
➤ **Diabetic macular edema (DME) and diabetic retinopathy in patients with DME**
Adults: 2 mg (0.05 mL) intravitreal injection every 4 weeks for first 5 injections; then 2 mg (0.05 mL) every 8 weeks.

albiglutide
al-bi-GLOO-tide

Eperzan✤, Tanzeum

Therapeutic class: Antidiabetics
Pharmacologic class: GLP-1 receptor agonists

AVAILABLE FORMS
Injection: 30-mg, 50-mg single-dose pen

INDICATIONS & DOSAGES
Black Box Warning Other GLP-1 receptor agonists have caused thyroid C-cell tumors in rodent studies. It isn't known whether this drug causes thyroid C-cell tumors in humans. ■
➤ **Adjunct to diet and exercise to improve glycemic control in adults with type 2 diabetes mellitus**
Adults: 30 mg subcutaneously once weekly in the abdomen, thigh, or upper arm. May increase to 50 mg once weekly if glycemic response is inadequate.

alcaftadine
al-CAFF-tuh-deen

Lastacaft

Therapeutic class: Antihistamines
Pharmacologic class: Histamine$_1$-receptor antagonists

AVAILABLE FORMS
Ophthalmic solution: 0.25% (2.5 mg/mL)

INDICATIONS & DOSAGES
➤ **Prevention of itching associated with allergic conjunctivitis**
Adults and children age 2 and older: Instill 1 drop in each eye once daily.

alglucosidase alfa
AL-gloo-KOH-sih-dase

Lumizyme, Myozyme

Therapeutic class: Metabolic agents
Pharmacologic class: Lysosomal glycogen-specific enzymes

AVAILABLE FORMS
Powder for I.V. infusion: 50 mg/vial

INDICATIONS & DOSAGES
Black Box Warning Life-threatening anaphylactic reactions and severe hypersensitivity reactions may occur. Supportive measures should be readily available. Patients with infantile-onset Pompe disease and compromised cardiac or respiratory function require additional monitoring. ■

✤Canada   ◇ OTC   ◆ Off-label use   ✐Photoguide   ⓓⓝⓒDo not crush   *Liquid contains alcohol.

➤ **Pompe disease (alpha-glucosidase deficiency)**
Adults and children weighing 1.25 kg or more: 20 mg/kg by I.V. infusion over 4 hours every 2 weeks. Initial infusion rate is 1 mg/kg/hour; may increase in stepwise manner by 2 mg/kg/hour every 30 minutes, if tolerated, to maximum rate of 7 mg/kg/hour. Obtain vital signs at each step increase. May stop or slow infusion rate temporarily if infusion reactions occur.

alosetron hydrochloride
ah-LOSS-e-tron

Lotronex

Therapeutic class: Anti-IBS drugs
Pharmacologic class: Selective 5-HT$_3$ receptor antagonists

AVAILABLE FORMS
Tablets: 0.5 mg, 1 mg

INDICATIONS & DOSAGES
Black Box Warning Drug is only appropriate for women with severe diarrhea-predominant irritable bowel syndrome (IBS) who haven't responded to conventional therapy. ■
➤ **Severe diarrhea-predominant IBS**
Women: 0.5 mg P.O. b.i.d. If, after 4 weeks, drug is well tolerated but doesn't adequately control IBS symptoms, increase to 1 mg b.i.d. After 4 weeks at this dosage, if symptoms aren't controlled, stop drug.

alprostadil (intracavernosal injection; urogenital suppository)
al-PROSS-ta-dil

Caverject, Caverject Impulse, Edex, Muse

Therapeutic class: Erectile dysfunction drugs
Pharmacologic class: Prostaglandins

AVAILABLE FORMS
Intracavernosal injection: 5 mcg/vial, 10 mcg/vial, 20 mcg/vial, 40 mcg/vial
Urethral suppository: 125 mcg, 250 mcg, 500 mcg, 1,000 mcg

INDICATIONS & DOSAGES
➤ **Erectile dysfunction of vasculogenic, psychogenic, or mixed causes**
Injection
Men: Dosages highly individualized; initially, inject 2.5 mcg intracavernosally. If partial response occurs, give second dose of 2.5 mcg; increase by 5 to 10 mcg until patient achieves erection suitable for intercourse lasting no longer than 1 hour. If no response to first dose, increase second dose to 7.5 mcg within 1 hour; then increase by 5 to 10 mcg until patient achieves suitable erection. After initial doses, patient must remain in prescriber's office until complete detumescence occurs. Don't repeat for at least 24 hours. For

Edex, give 1 to 40 mcg by intracavernosal injection over 5 to 10 seconds. Use the lowest effective dose no more than three times per week with at least 24 hours between doses.
Urethral suppository
Men: Initially, 125 to 250 mcg, under supervision of prescriber. Adjust dosage as needed until response is sufficient for sexual intercourse. Maximum of two administrations in 24 hours; maximum dose is 1,000 mcg.
➤ **Erectile dysfunction of neurogenic cause (spinal cord injury)**
Men: Dosages highly individualized; initially, inject 1.25 mcg intracavernosally. If partial response occurs, give second dose of 1.25 mcg. Increase in increments of 2.5 mcg, to dose of 5 mcg; then increase in increments of 5 mcg until patient achieves erection suitable for intercourse lasting no longer than 1 hour. If no response to first dose, give next higher dose within 1 hour. After initial doses, patient must remain in prescriber's office until complete detumescence occurs. Don't repeat procedure for at least 24 hours. For Edex, give 1 to 40 mcg by intracavernosal injection over 5 to 10 seconds. Use the lowest effective dose no more than three times per week with at least 24 hours between doses.

apomorphine hydrochloride
ah-poe-MORE-feen

Apokyn

Therapeutic class: Antiparkinsonians
Pharmacologic class: Nonergot-derivative dopamine agonists

AVAILABLE FORMS
Solution for injection: 10 mg/mL (contains benzyl alcohol)

INDICATIONS & DOSAGES
➤ **Intermittent hypomobility, "off" episodes caused by advanced Parkinson disease (given with an antiemetic)**
Adults: Initially, give a 2-mg subcutaneous test dose when patient is in an "off" episode. Measure supine and standing BP every 20 minutes for first hour. If patient tolerates and responds to drug, start with 2 mg subcutaneously as needed as outpatient. Separate doses by at least 2 hours. Increase by 1 mg every few days, if needed.

If initial 2-mg dose is ineffective but tolerated, give 4 mg at next "off" period, but no sooner than 2 hours after the initial test dose of 2 mg. Measure supine and standing BP every 20 minutes for first hour. If drug is tolerated, start with 3 mg subcutaneously as outpatient. If needed, increase by 1 mg every few days.

If patient doesn't tolerate 4-mg dose, give 3 mg as test dose at next "off" period, measuring supine and standing BP every 20 minutes for first hour. If drug is tolerated, give 2 mg as outpatient. Increase by 1 mg every few days, as needed; doses higher than 4 mg usually not tolerated if 2 mg is starting dose.

Maximum recommended dose is usually 6 mg as needed. Most patients use drug t.i.d. Experience is limited at more than five times daily or more than 20 mg daily.

Adjust-a-dose: In patients with mild to moderate renal impairment, give test and starting doses of 1 mg subcutaneously.

artemether–lumefantrine
art-TEM-mah-ther/loo-meh-FAN-treen

Coartem

Therapeutic class: Antimalarials
Pharmacologic class: Schizontocides

AVAILABLE FORMS
Tablets: artemether 20 mg and lumefantrine 120 mg

INDICATIONS & DOSAGES
➤ **Uncomplicated malaria caused by *Plasmodium falciparum***
Adults and children weighing 35 kg or more: Initially, 4 tablets P.O., followed by 4 tablets in 8 hours, and then 4 tablets b.i.d. for the next 2 days. Total course is 24 tablets.
Children weighing 25 to 34 kg): Initially, 3 tablets P.O., followed by 3 tablets in 8 hours, and then 3 tablets b.i.d. on each of the next 2 days. Total course is 18 tablets.
Children weighing 15 to 24 kg): Initially, 2 tablets P.O., followed by 2 tablets in 8 hours, and then 2 tablets b.i.d. on each of the next 2 days. Total course is 12 tablets.
Children weighing 5 to 14 kg): Initially, 1 tablet P.O., followed by 1 tablet in 8 hours, and then 1 tablet b.i.d. on each of the next 2 days. Total course is 6 tablets.

asfotase alfa
AZ-fo-tase

Strensiq

Therapeutic class: Enzyme therapies
Pharmacologic class: Enzyme therapies

AVAILABLE FORMS
Injection: 18 mg/0.45 mL, 28 mg/0.7 mL, 40 mg/mL, 80 mg/0.8 mL

INDICATIONS & DOSAGES
➤ **Treatment of perinatal/infantile and juvenile-onset hypophosphatasia**
Children: 2 mg/kg subcutaneously three times weekly, or 1 mg/kg subcutaneously six times weekly. Maximum dose is 9 mg/kg/week.

SAFETY ALERT!

asparaginase *Erwinia chrysanthemi*
as-PAR-a-jin-ase er-WIN-ee-uh chris-AN-tha-me

Erwinase ✦, Erwinaze

Therapeutic class: Antineoplastics
Pharmacologic class: Enzyme inhibitors

AVAILABLE FORMS
Powder for injection: 10,000 international units/vial

INDICATIONS & DOSAGES
➤ **Acute lymphoblastic leukemia in patients who have developed hypersensitivity to *Escherichia coli*–derived asparaginase as part of a multiagent chemotherapy regimen**
Adults and children age 1 and older: When substituting for pegaspargase, give 25,000 international units/m^2 I.M. or I.V. three times a week (Monday/Wednesday/Friday) for six doses. When substituting for native *E. coli* asparaginase, give 25,000 international units/m^2 I.M. or I.V. for each scheduled dose of native *E. coli* asparaginase within a treatment. When giving I.V., consider monitoring nadir serum asparaginase activity (NSAA) levels and switching to I.M. administration if desired NSAA levels aren't achieved.

SAFETY ALERT!

atracurium besylate
at-truh-KYOO-ree-um

Therapeutic class: Skeletal muscle relaxants
Pharmacologic class: Nondepolarizing neuromuscular blockers

AVAILABLE FORMS
Injection: 10 mg/mL

INDICATIONS & DOSAGES
➤ **Adjunct to general anesthesia to facilitate endotracheal intubation and relax skeletal muscles during surgery or mechanical ventilation**
Adults and children age 2 and older: 0.4 to 0.5 mg/kg by I.V. bolus. Give maintenance dose of 0.08 to 0.1 mg/kg within 20 to 45 minutes during prolonged surgery. Give maintenance doses every 15 to 25 minutes in patients receiving balanced anesthesia. For prolonged procedures, use a constant infusion at an initial rate of 9 to 10 mcg/kg/minute; then reduce to 5 to 9 mcg/kg/minute. For infusion in the ICU, an infusion rate of 11 to 13 mcg/kg/minute should provide adequate neuromuscular blockade.
Children ages 1 month to 2 years: First dose, 0.3 to 0.4 mg/kg I.V. for children under halothane anesthesia. Frequent maintenance doses may be needed.

Adjust-a-dose: In adults, adolescents, children, or infants with significant CV disease or history suggesting a greater risk of histamine release (anaphylactic reaction, asthma), give initial dose of 0.3 to 0.4 mg/kg slowly or in divided doses over 1 minute. In adults receiving enflurane or isoflurane at the same time, reduce initial atracurium dose by 33% (0.25 to 0.35 mg/kg). In adults receiving atracurium following succinylcholine, initial dose is 0.3 to 0.4 mg/kg.

auranofin
or-RAIN-oh-fin

Ridaura

Therapeutic class: Antiarthritics
Pharmacologic class: Gold compounds

AVAILABLE FORMS
Capsules: 3 mg

INDICATIONS & DOSAGES
Black Box Warning   May cause gold toxicity. Review laboratory study results before each new prescription. Advise patients of risk, teach them toxicity symptoms, and tell them to promptly report any adverse effects. ■
➤ **RA in patients who have had an insufficient response to or are intolerant of trial doses of one or more NSAIDs**
Adults: 3 mg P.O. b.i.d. or 6 mg P.O. once daily. After 6 months, may increase to 3 mg P.O. t.i.d. If response is inadequate after 3 months of 9 mg/day, stop use.

azelaic acid
aze-eh-LAY-ik

Azelex, Finacea

Therapeutic class: Antiacne drugs
Pharmacologic class: Dicarboxylic acids

AVAILABLE FORMS
Cream: 20%
Foam: 15%
Gel: 15%

INDICATIONS & DOSAGES
➤ **Mild to moderate inflammatory acne vulgaris**
Adults and children age 12 and older: Apply thin film of cream (Azelex) and gently but thoroughly massage into affected areas b.i.d., in morning and evening.
➤ **Mild to moderate rosacea**
Adults: Apply thin film of foam or gel (Finacea) and gently but thoroughly massage into affected areas b.i.d., in morning and evening. Reassess if no improvement in 12 weeks.

basiliximab
ba-sil-IK-si-mab

Simulect

Therapeutic class: Immunosuppressants
Pharmacologic class: Monoclonal antibodies

AVAILABLE FORMS
Injection: 10-mg, 20-mg vials

INDICATIONS & DOSAGES
Black Box Warning   Drug should only be prescribed by physicians experienced in management of organ transplant and immunosuppression therapy and only in facilities equipped and staffed with adequate laboratory and supportive medical resources. ■
➤ **To prevent acute organ rejection in patients receiving renal transplantation when used as part of an immunosuppressive regimen that includes cyclosporine and corticosteroids**
Adults and children weighing 35 kg or more: 20 mg I.V. given within 2 hours before transplant surgery and 20 mg I.V. given 4 days after transplantation.
Children weighing less than 35 kg: 10 mg I.V. given within 2 hours before transplant surgery and 10 mg I.V. given 4 days after transplantation.

SAFETY ALERT!

bendamustine hydrochloride
ben-dah-MOO-steen

Bendeka, Treanda

Therapeutic class: Antineoplastics
Pharmacologic class: Mechlorethamine derivatives

AVAILABLE FORMS
Injection solution: 100 mg/4-mL vial
Lyophilized powder for injection: 25 mg, 100 mg in single-use vials

INDICATIONS & DOSAGES
↻ *Alert:* Available formulations have different concentrations; don't mix or combine. See manufacturer's instructions for preparation.
➤ **Chronic lymphocytic leukemia**
Adults: 100 mg/m^2 I.V. over 30 minutes on days 1 and 2 of a 28-day cycle, given for up to six cycles.
Adjust-a-dose: Refer to manufacturer's instructions for dosage adjustments for hematologic and nonhematologic toxicities.
➤ **Indolent B-cell non-Hodgkin lymphoma that has progressed during or within 6 months of treatment with rituximab or a rituximab-containing regimen**
Adults: 120 mg/m^2 I.V. over 60 minutes on days 1 and 2 of a 21-day cycle, given in up to eight cycles.

Adjust-a-dose: Refer to manufacturer's instructions for dosage adjustments for hematologic and nonhematologic toxicities.

benzonatate
ben-ZOE-na-tate

Tessalon

Therapeutic class: Antitussives
Pharmacologic class: Local anesthetics

AVAILABLE FORMS
Capsules 🚫: 100 mg, 150 mg, 200 mg

INDICATIONS & DOSAGES
➤ **Symptomatic relief of cough**
Adults and children older than age 10: 100 to 200 mg P.O. t.i.d.; up to 600 mg daily.

benzyl alcohol
ben-zill AL-ko-hall

Ulesfia

Therapeutic class: Scabicides–pediculicides
Pharmacologic class: Topical alcohols

AVAILABLE FORMS
Lotion: 5%

INDICATIONS & DOSAGES
➤ **Head lice infestation**
Adults age 60 and younger and children age 6 months and older: Apply to hair and scalp until completely saturated. Allow to remain for 10 minutes; then rinse thoroughly with water. Remove dead lice and nits with fine-toothed comb. Repeat treatment after 7 days. For each treatment, refer to manufacturer's instructions for the appropriate volume to use based on hair length.

bepotastine besilate
beh-POT-uh-steen

Bepreve

Therapeutic class: Antihistamines (ophthalmic)
Pharmacologic class: Histamine₁-receptor antagonists

AVAILABLE FORMS
Ophthalmic solution: 1.5%

INDICATIONS & DOSAGES
➤ **Itching associated with conjunctivitis**
Adults and children age 2 and older: Instill 1 drop into affected eye(s) b.i.d.

betaxolol hydrochloride
beh-TAX-oh-lol

Betoptic, Betoptic S

Therapeutic class: Antiglaucoma drugs–antihypertensives
Pharmacologic class: Beta blockers

AVAILABLE FORMS
Ophthalmic solution: 0.5%
Ophthalmic suspension: 0.25%
Tablets: 10 mg, 20 mg

INDICATIONS & DOSAGES
➤ **Chronic open-angle glaucoma, ocular hypertension (ophthalmic only)**
Adults: Instill 1 or 2 drops in the affected eye(s) b.i.d.
➤ **Hypertension with or without diuretic therapy**
Adults: 10 mg P.O. once daily. May increase dose to 20 mg if desired response isn't achieved after 7 to 14 days.
Adjust-a-dose: To prevent bradycardia, reduce starting dose to 5 mg in elderly patients. In patients with severe renal impairment and those on dialysis, reduce initial dose to 5 mg daily. May increase dosage by 5 mg/day every 2 weeks to a maximum dose of 20 mg/day.

SAFETY ALERT!

bexarotene
bex-AR-oh-teen

Targretin

Therapeutic class: Antineoplastics
Pharmacologic class: Retinoids

AVAILABLE FORMS
Capsules: 75 mg
Topical gel: 1%

INDICATIONS & DOSAGES
➤ **Cutaneous manifestations of cutaneous T-cell lymphoma (CTCL) in patients refractory to at least one prior systemic therapy**
Adults: Initially, 300 mg/m² P.O. once daily. If no tumor response after 8 weeks and if initial dose of 300 mg/m²/day is well tolerated, may increase dosage to 400 mg/m²/day with careful monitoring. Continue until disease progression or unacceptable toxicity.
Adjust-a-dose: If toxicity occurs, decrease dosage to 200 mg/m²/day then to 100 mg/m²/day, or temporarily withhold. When toxicity is controlled, may carefully titrate doses upward. Interrupt or discontinue therapy if AST, ALT, or bilirubin level exceeds 3 × ULN.
➤ **Cutaneous lesions in patients with CTCL (Stage IA and IB) with refractory or persistent**

disease after other therapies or who haven't tolerated other therapies

Adults: Apply sufficient gel to cover lesion with a generous coating. Initially apply once every other day for first week. Increase application frequency at weekly intervals to once daily, then b.i.d., then t.i.d., and finally q.i.d. according to individual lesion tolerance; continue as long as patient derives benefits. Most patients can tolerate a dosing frequency of two to four times per day.

Adjust-a-dose: If application-site toxicity occurs, application frequency can be reduced. Should severe irritation occur, application can be temporarily discontinued for a few days until symptoms subside.

SAFETY ALERT!

bicalutamide

bye-ka-LOO-ta-mide

Casodex

Therapeutic class: Antineoplastics
Pharmacologic class: Androgen receptor inhibitors

AVAILABLE FORMS
Tablets: 50 mg

INDICATIONS & DOSAGES
➤ **Metastatic prostate cancer in combination with a luteinizing hormone-releasing hormone (LHRH) analogue**
Adult males: 50 mg P.O. once daily.

blinatumomab

BLIN-a-TOOM-oh-mab

Blincyto

Therapeutic class: Antineoplastics
Pharmacologic class: Monoclonal antibodies

AVAILABLE FORMS
Injection: 35-mcg single-use vial

INDICATIONS & DOSAGES
Black Box Warning   Drug can cause fatal cytokine release syndrome (CRS) and neurologic toxicities. ∎
➤ **Philadelphia chromosome–negative relapsed or refractory B-cell precursor acute lymphoblastic leukemia (ALL)**
Adults weighing at least 45 kg: A treatment course consists of up to two induction cycles followed by three additional consolidation cycles (up to a total of five cycles) with at least a 2-week treatment-free interval between cycles. For cycle 1, initially give 9 mcg/day by continuous I.V. infusion on days 1 through 7, then 28 mcg/day by continuous I.V. infusion on days 8 through 28. For subsequent cycles, give 28 mcg/day on days 1 through 28.

Adjust-a-dose: If the interruption after an adverse event is no longer than 7 days, continue the same cycle to a total of 28 days of infusion inclusive of days before and after the interruption in that cycle. If an interruption due to an adverse event is longer than 7 days, start a new cycle. Refer to manufacturer's instructions for dosage adjustments for CRS, neurotoxicity, and hepatotoxicity.

bosutinib

boe-SUE-ti-nib

Bosulif

Therapeutic class: Antineoplastics
Pharmacologic class: Kinase inhibitors

AVAILABLE FORMS
Tablets ⓒ*:* 100 mg, 500 mg

INDICATIONS & DOSAGES
➤ **Chronic myelogenous leukemia with resistance or intolerance to prior therapy**
Adults: 500 mg P.O. once daily. Consider dosage escalation to 600 mg once daily in patients who don't reach complete hematologic response by week 8 or a complete cytogenetic response by week 12, who didn't have grade 3 or higher adverse reactions, and who are currently taking 500 mg daily.

Adjust-a-dose: If CrCl is 30 to 50 mL/minute at start of therapy, give 400 mg once daily; if CrCl is less than 30 mL/minute, give 300 mg once daily. For preexisting hepatic impairment (Child-Pugh class A, B, or C) at start of therapy, give 200 mg once daily. Refer to manufacturer's instructions for dosage adjustments based on hematologic and nonhematologic toxicities.

brinzolamide–brimonidine tartrate

brin-ZOL-ah-mide/brih-MOE-neh-deen

Simbrinza

Therapeutic class: Antiglaucoma drugs
Pharmacologic class: Carbonic anhydrase inhibitors–alpha$_2$ adrenergic receptor agonists

AVAILABLE FORMS
Ophthalmic suspension: brinzolamide 1% and brimonidine 0.2%

INDICATIONS & DOSAGES
➤ **Reduction of IOP in patients with open-angle glaucoma or ocular hypertension**
Adults and children age 2 and older: Instill 1 drop into affected eye(s) t.i.d.

busulfan
byoo-SUL-fan

Busulfex, Myleran

Therapeutic class: Antineoplastics
Pharmacologic class: Alkyl sulfonates

AVAILABLE FORMS
Injection: 6 mg/mL
Tablets: 2 mg

INDICATIONS & DOSAGES
Black Box Warning Injection causes severe and prolonged myelosuppression at recommended dosage. Hematopoietic progenitor cell transplantation is required to prevent potentially fatal complications. Drug may cause secondary malignancies. ■
➤ **Chronic myelocytic (granulocytic) leukemia**
Adults: 4 to 8 mg P.O. daily until WBC count falls to 15,000/mm³; stop drug until WBC count rises to 50,000/mm³, then resume dosage as before. When remission is shorter than 3 months, may give maintenance therapy of 1 to 3 mg P.O. daily. Or, 0.8 mg/kg I.V. (ideal or actual body weight, whichever is lower) every 6 hours for 4 days (a total of 16 doses) beginning 7 days before transplant. Give cyclophosphamide 60 mg/kg I.V. over 1 hour daily for 2 days beginning 6 hours after the 16th dose of busulfan injection.
Children: 0.06 to 0.12 mg/kg daily or 1.8 to 4.6 mg/m² daily P.O. until WBC count falls to 15,000/mm³; stop drug until WBC count rises to 50,000/mm³, then resume dosage as before.

cabazitaxel
ka-baz-ih-TAX-el

Jevtana

Therapeutic class: Antineoplastics
Pharmacologic class: Taxoids

AVAILABLE FORMS
Injection: 60 mg/1.5 mL

INDICATIONS & DOSAGES
Black Box Warning Drug is associated with severe hypersensitivity and neutropenic deaths. Monitor patient and blood cell counts closely and provide appropriate therapy. ■
➤ **In combination with prednisone for hormone-refractory metastatic prostate cancer previously treated with docetaxel-containing treatment regimen**
Adults: 25 mg/m² I.V. over 1 hour every 3 weeks. Give oral prednisone 10 mg daily throughout cabazitaxel therapy. Premedicate at least 30 minutes before each dose of cabazitaxel with the following I.V. medications to reduce risk or severity of hypersensitivity: antihistamine (5 mg dexchlorpheniramine, or 25 mg diphen-

hydramine or equivalent antihistamine), corticosteroid (8 mg dexamethasone or equivalent steroid), and H₂ antagonist (50 mg ranitidine or equivalent H₂ antagonist). Antiemetic prophylaxis is recommended and can be given P.O. or I.V. as needed.
Adjust-a-dose: Refer to manufacturer's instructions for dosage adjustments due to hematologic and nonhematologic toxicities; hepatic impairment, and use with strong CYP3A inhibitors.

canakinumab
kan-ah-KIN-yoo-mab

Ilaris

Therapeutic class: Anti-autoimmune agents
Pharmacologic class: Monoclonal antibodies

AVAILABLE FORMS
Injection: 180-mg single-use vial

INDICATIONS & DOSAGES
➤ **Cryopyrin-associated periodic syndromes (familial cold autoinflammatory syndrome and Muckle-Wells syndrome)**
Adults and children age 4 and older weighing more than 40 kg: 150 mg subcutaneously every 8 weeks.
Adults and children age 4 and older weighing 15 to 40 kg: 2 mg/kg subcutaneously every 8 weeks; may increase dosage to 3 mg/kg in children weighing 15 to 40 kg who have an inadequate response.
➤ **Active systemic juvenile idiopathic arthritis**
Children age 2 and older weighing at least 7.5 kg): 4 mg/kg subcutaneously every 4 weeks. Maximum dose is 300 mg.
Adults and children age 2 and older weighing 15 to 40 kg: Initially, 2 mg/kg subcutaneously every 4 weeks. May increase to 4 mg/kg every 4 weeks if clinical response is inadequate.
✱ ***NEW INDICATION:*** **TNF receptor-associated periodic syndrome; hyperimmunoglobulin D syndrome/mevalonate kinase deficiency; familial Mediterranean fever**
Adults and children age 2 and older weighing more than 40 kg: Initially, 150 mg subcutaneously every 4 weeks; may increase to 300 mg every 4 weeks if clinical response is inadequate.

carboprost tromethamine
KAR-boe-prost

Hemabate

Therapeutic class: Oxytocics
Pharmacologic class: Prostaglandins

AVAILABLE FORMS
Injection: 250 mcg/mL

INDICATIONS & DOSAGES
Black Box Warning Strictly adhere to recommended dosages and only use in a hospital that can

provide immediate intensive and acute surgical care. ■

➤ **To terminate pregnancy between weeks 13 and 20 of gestation**
Adults: Initially, 250 mcg deep I.M.; optionally, a 100-mcg I.M. test dose may be given. Give subsequent doses of 250 mcg at intervals of 1½ to 3½ hours, depending on uterine response. Dosage may be increased in increments to 500 mcg if contractility is inadequate after several 250-mcg doses. Total dose shouldn't exceed 12 mg or continuous administration for more than 2 days.

➤ **Refractory postpartum hemorrhage**
Adults: 250 mcg by deep I.M. injection. Repeat doses every 15 to 90 minutes as needed. Maximum total dose is 2 mg (eight doses).

SAFETY ALERT!

carfilzomib
car-FIL-zoe-mib

Kyprolis

Therapeutic class: Antineoplastics
Pharmacologic class: Proteasome inhibitors

AVAILABLE FORMS
Powder for injection: 30-mg, 60-mg single-use vial

INDICATIONS & DOSAGES
❸ *Alert:* See manufacturer's instructions for administration precautions.

➤ **Multiple myeloma (monotherapy) in patients who have received at least two prior therapies, including bortezomib and an immunomodulatory agent, and have demonstrated disease progression on or within 60 days of completion of the last therapy; multiple myeloma in combination with lenalidomide and dexamethasone in patients who have received one to three prior therapies**
Adults: For monotherapy, 20 mg/m^2 I.V. over 2 to 10 minutes on 2 consecutive days each week for 3 weeks (days 1, 2, 8, 9, 15, and 16), followed by 12-day rest period (days 17 to 28). If tolerated, may increase to 27 mg/m^2 in cycle 2 and to 27 mg/m^2 for subsequent cycles. For the combination regimen, administer carfilzomib I.V. as a 10-minute infusion on 2 consecutive days, each week for 3 weeks followed by a 12-day rest period. See manufacturer's instructions for other dosing and schedules. Each 28-day period is considered one treatment cycle. The recommended starting dose is 20 mg/m^2 on days 1 and 2 of cycle 1. If tolerated, escalate to a target dose of 27 mg/m^2 on days 8, 9, 15, and 16 of cycles 1 to 12. From cycle 13 on, omit day 8 and 9 doses. Discontinue drug after cycle 18. Maximum dosage is based on BSA of 2.2 m^2. See manufacturer's instructions for other dosing and schedules.
Adjust-a-dose: Adjust dosage for weight change of more than 20% from baseline. Refer to manufacturer's instructions for dosage adjustments based on toxicities.

carglumic acid
kar-GLOO-mik as-id

Carbaglu

Therapeutic class: Antihyperammonemics
Pharmacologic class: Ammonia detoxicants

AVAILABLE FORMS
Tablets ⓓⓝⓒ: 200 mg

INDICATIONS & DOSAGES
➤ **Acute or chronic hyperammonemia in patients with N-acetylglutamate synthetase deficiency**
Adults and children: Initially, 100 to 250 mg/kg/day P.O., divided into two to four doses, immediately before meals. Disperse tablets in 2.5 mL of water. Round each dose to nearest 100 mg. Titrate dosage according to ammonia level and symptoms.

SAFETY ALERT!

ceritinib
se-RI-ti-nib

Zykadia

Therapeutic class: Antineoplastics
Pharmacologic class: Kinase inhibitors

AVAILABLE FORMS
Capsules: 150 mg

INDICATIONS & DOSAGES
➤ **Anaplastic lymphoma kinase-positive metastatic non–small-cell lung cancer in patients who have progressed on or are intolerant to crizotinib**
Adults: 750 mg P.O. once daily until disease progression or unacceptable toxicity occurs.
Adjust-a-dose: Refer to manufacturer's instructions for dosage adjustments for symptomatic bradycardia, QTc interval prolongation, persistent hyperglycemia, GI adverse reactions, and hepatotoxicity. Permanently discontinue drug if patient is unable to tolerate 300-mg dose daily after dosage adjustments. If any grade of treatment-related interstitial lung disease or pneumonitis occurs, permanently discontinue drug.

cetrorelix acetate
SE-troe-REL-ix

Cetrotide

Therapeutic class: Infertility drugs
Pharmacologic class: Gonadotropin-releasing hormone antagonists

AVAILABLE FORMS
Powder for injection: 0.25 mg

INDICATIONS & DOSAGES

➤ **To inhibit premature luteinizing hormone surges in women undergoing controlled ovarian stimulation**
Women: Ovarian stimulation therapy with gonadotropins is started on cycle day 2 or 3. Give cetrorelix acetate 0.25 mg subcutaneously on stimulation day 5 (morning or evening) or day 6 (morning), and continue once daily until day of hCG administration.

cevimeline hydrochloride
seh-vih-MEH-leen

Evoxac

Therapeutic class: Cholinergic agonists
Pharmacologic class: Cholinergic agonists

AVAILABLE FORMS
Capsules: 30 mg

INDICATIONS & DOSAGES
➤ **Dry mouth in patients with Sjögren syndrome**
Adults: 30 mg P.O. t.i.d.

SAFETY ALERT!

chlorambucil
klor-AM-byoo-sill

Leukeran

Therapeutic class: Antineoplastics
Pharmacologic class: Nitrogen mustards

AVAILABLE FORMS
Tablets: 2 mg

INDICATIONS & DOSAGES
Black Box Warning Drug can severely suppress bone marrow function; is a carcinogen, and probably mutagenic and teratogenic; and produces human infertility. ■
➤ **Chronic lymphocytic leukemia; malignant lymphomas, including lymphosarcoma, giant follicular lymphoma, and Hodgkin lymphoma**
Adults: For initiation of therapy or for short courses of treatment, give 0.1 to 0.2 mg/kg P.O. daily for 3 to 6 weeks (usually 4 to 10 mg daily). Maintenance dosage shouldn't exceed 0.1 mg/kg/day and may be as low as 0.03 mg/kg/day. Adjust dosage according to patient response; reduce when WBC count falls abruptly. For pulse dosage, give initial single dose of 0.4 mg/kg. Then give doses at biweekly or monthly intervals, increasing by 0.1-mg/kg increments until lymphocytosis is controlled or toxicity occurs.
Adjust-a-dose: Reduce first dose if given within 4 weeks after a full course of radiation therapy or myelosuppressive drugs, or if pretreatment WBC or platelet count is depressed from bone marrow disease.

chloramphenicol sodium succinate
klor-am-FEN-i-kole

Therapeutic class: Antibiotics
Pharmacologic class: Dichloroacetic acid derivatives

AVAILABLE FORMS
Injection: 1-g vial

INDICATIONS & DOSAGES
Black Box Warning Drug is associated with serious and fatal blood dyscrasias. Use alternative therapies when possible. Patient should be hospitalized during therapy to closely monitor blood laboratory levels. ■
➤ *Haemophilus influenzae* **meningitis, acute** *Salmonella typhi* **infection, and meningitis, bacteremia, or other severe infections caused by sensitive** *Salmonella* **species, rickettsia, lymphogranuloma, psittacosis, or various sensitive gram-negative organisms**
Adults: 50 to 100 mg/kg I.V. daily, divided every 6 hours. Maximum dosage, 100 mg/kg daily.
Full-term infants older than age 2 weeks with normal metabolic processes and children: Up to 50 mg/kg I.V. daily, divided every 6 hours. May use up to 100 mg/kg/day in four divided doses for meningitis.
Preterm infants, neonates age 2 weeks and younger, and children and infants with suspected immature metabolic processes: 25 mg/kg I.V. once daily.
Adjust-a-dose: For patients with renal or hepatic impairment, excessive blood levels may result from administration of the recommended dosage. Determine drug blood concentration at appropriate intervals and adjust dosage accordingly.

SAFETY ALERT!

chlordiazepoxide hydrochloride
klor-dye-az-e-POX-ide

Therapeutic class: Anxiolytics
Pharmacologic class: Benzodiazepines
Controlled substance schedule: IV

AVAILABLE FORMS
Capsules: 5 mg, 10 mg, 25 mg

INDICATIONS & DOSAGES
Black Box Warning Opioids combined with benzodiazepines or CNS depressants can cause death. ■
Adjust-a-dose (for all indications): In elderly or debilitated patients, give 5 mg P.O. b.i.d. to q.i.d. Use smallest effective dose, to prevent oversedation or ataxia.
➤ **Mild to moderate anxiety**
Adults: 5 to 10 mg P.O. t.i.d. or q.i.d.

Children older than age 6: 5 mg P.O. b.i.d. to q.i.d. Maximum, 10 mg P.O. b.i.d. or t.i.d.
➤ **Severe anxiety**
Adults: 20 to 25 mg P.O. t.i.d. or q.i.d.
➤ **Withdrawal symptoms of acute alcoholism**
Adults: 50 to 100 mg P.O. Repeat as needed, up to 300 mg daily.
➤ **Preoperative apprehension and anxiety**
Adults: 5 to 10 mg P.O. t.i.d. or q.i.d. on days before surgery.

chlorproMAZINE hydrochloride
klor-PROE-ma-zeen

Therapeutic class: Antipsychotics
Pharmacologic class: Phenothiazines

AVAILABLE FORMS
Injection: 25 mg/mL
Tablets: 10 mg, 25 mg, 50 mg, 100 mg, 200 mg

INDICATIONS & DOSAGES
➤ **Psychosis, mania**
Adults and children older than age 12: For hospitalized patients with acute disease, 25 mg I.M.; may give an additional 25 to 50 mg I.M. in 1 hour if needed. Increase over several days to 400 mg every 4 to 6 hours. Switch to oral therapy as soon as possible. Or, 25 mg P.O. t.i.d. initially; then gradually increase to 500 mg (400 mg in less acutely disturbed patients) daily in divided doses. For outpatients, 30 to 75 mg daily in two to four divided doses. Increase dosage by 20 to 50 mg twice weekly until symptoms are controlled.
➤ **Nausea and vomiting**
Adults and children older than age 12: 10 to 25 mg P.O. every 4 to 6 hours, p.r.n. Or, 25 mg I.M. initially. If no hypotension occurs, 25 to 50 mg I.M. every 3 to 4 hours may be given, p.r.n., until vomiting stops.
Children ages 6 months to 12 years: 0.55 mg/kg P.O. every 4 to 6 hours or I.M. every 6 to 8 hours. Maximum I.M. dose in children younger than age 5 or weighing less than 23 kg is 40 mg. Maximum I.M. dose in children ages 5 to 12 or weighing 23 to 45 kg is 75 mg.
➤ **Acute intermittent porphyria, intractable hiccups**
Adults and children older than age 12: 25 to 50 mg P.O. t.i.d. or q.i.d. If hiccups persist for 2 to 3 days, 25 to 50 mg I.M. If hiccups still persist, 25 to 50 mg diluted in 500 to 1,000 mL of NSS and infused slowly with patient in supine position. For porphyria, 25 mg I.M. t.i.d. or q.i.d. until patient can take oral therapy.
➤ **Tetanus**
Adults and children older than age 12: 25 to 50 mg I.V. or I.M. t.i.d. or q.i.d.
Children ages 6 months to 12 years: 0.55 mg/kg I.M. or I.V. every 6 to 8 hours. Maximum parenteral dosage in children weighing less than 23 kg is 40 mg daily; for children weighing 23 to 45 kg, 75 mg, except in severe cases. If giving I.V., dilute to 1 mg/mL with NSS and give at a rate of 0.5 mg/minute.

➤ **Behavioral disorders; hyperactivity**
Children ages 6 months to 12 years: For outpatients: 0.55 mg/kg P.O. every 4 to 6 hours or I.M. every 6 to 8 hours, as needed. For hospitalized patients, start with low oral doses and increase gradually. In severe behavioral disorders, 50 to 100 mg P.O. daily or, in older children, 200 mg/day or more P.O. may be necessary. There is little evidence that improvement in severely disturbed mentally retarded patients is enhanced by doses beyond 500 mg/day. In hospitalized patients age 5 or younger or weighing less than 23 kg, don't exceed 40 mg/day I.M. In children ages 5 to 12 weighing 23 to 45 kg, don't exceed 75 mg/day I.M., except in unmanageable cases.
➤ **Surgery**
Adults and children older than age 12: Preoperatively, 25 to 50 mg P.O. 2 to 3 hours before surgery or 12.5 to 25 mg I.M. 1 to 2 hours before surgery; during surgery, 12.5 mg I.M., repeated in 30 minutes, if needed, or fractional 2-mg doses I.V. at 2-minute intervals to maximum dose of 25 mg.
Children ages 6 months to 12 years: Preoperatively, 0.55 mg/kg P.O. 2 to 3 hours before surgery or I.M. 1 to 2 hours before surgery. During surgery, 0.25 mg/kg I.M., repeated in 30 minutes if needed, or fractional 1-mg doses I.V. at 2-minute intervals to maximum of 0.25 mg/kg. May repeat fractional I.V. regimen in 30 minutes if needed.
Elderly patients: Lower dosages are sufficient; dosage increments should be more gradual than in adults.

chlorthalidone
klor-THAL-i-done

Therapeutic class: Antihypertensives
Pharmacologic class: Thiazide diuretics

AVAILABLE FORMS
Tablets: 25 mg, 50 mg

INDICATIONS & DOSAGES
➤ **Edema**
Adults: 50 to 100 mg P.O. daily, or 100 mg P.O. on alternating days.
➤ **Hypertension**
Adults: 25 mg P.O. daily. May increase to 50 mg, then 100 mg daily as needed.

cholic acid
koe-lik acid

Cholbam

Therapeutic class: Bile acids
Pharmacologic class: Bile acids

AVAILABLE FORMS
Capsules : 50 mg, 250 mg

INDICATIONS & DOSAGES
Adjust-a-dose (for all indications): For patients with concomitant familial hypertriglyceridemia, give 11 to

17 mg/kg P.O. once daily or in two divided doses. Interrupt treatment for persistent clinical or laboratory indicators of worsening liver function or cholestasis. Consider restarting at lower dose when the parameters return to baseline.

➤ **Treatment of bile acid synthesis disorders due to single enzyme defects; adjunctive treatment of peroxisomal disorders, including Zellweger spectrum disorders, in patients who exhibit manifestations of liver disease, steatorrhea, or complications from decreased fat-soluble vitamin absorption**
Adults and children: 10 to 15 mg/kg P.O. once daily or in two divided doses.

clomiPHENE citrate
KLOE-mi-feen

Clomid

Therapeutic class: Ovulation stimulants
Pharmacologic class: Chlortrianisene derivatives

AVAILABLE FORMS
Tablets: 50 mg

INDICATIONS & DOSAGES
➤ **To induce ovulation**
Women: 50 mg P.O. daily for 5 days, starting on day 5 of menstrual cycle (first day of menstrual flow is day 1) if bleeding occurs, or at any time if patient hasn't had recent uterine bleeding. If ovulation doesn't occur, may increase dose to 100 mg P.O. daily for 5 days as soon as 30 days after previous course. Repeat until conception occurs or until three courses of therapy are completed.

clomiPRAMINE hydrochloride
kloe-MI-pra-meen

Anafranil

Therapeutic class: Antidepressants
Pharmacologic class: TCAs

AVAILABLE FORMS
Capsules: 25 mg, 50 mg, 75 mg

INDICATIONS & DOSAGES
➤ **Obsessive-compulsive disorder**
Adults: Initially, 25 mg P.O. daily with meals, gradually increased to 100 mg/day in divided doses during first 2 weeks. Thereafter, increase to maximum dose of 250 mg/day in divided doses with meals, as needed. After adjustment, may give total daily dose at bedtime. *Children age 10 and older and adolescents:* Initially, 25 mg P.O. daily with meals, gradually increased over first 2 weeks to maximum of 3 mg/kg daily or 100 mg P.O. daily in divided doses, whichever is smaller. Maximum daily dose is 3 mg/kg or 200 mg, whichever is smaller; give at bedtime after adjustment. Reassess and adjust dosage periodically.

➤ **Panic disorder** ◆
Adults: Initially, 10 mg P.O. daily and increased to a maximum dosage of 150 mg P.O. daily, given in divided doses.

collagenase *Clostridium histolyticum*
kuh-LAJ-eh-nase kloss-TRID-ee-um hiss-toe-LIH-teh-kum

Xiaflex

Therapeutic class: Anticollagen drugs
Pharmacologic class: Enzymes

AVAILABLE FORMS
Injection: 0.9-mg single-use vial

INDICATIONS & DOSAGES
Black Box Warning Drug is associated with penile fracture and other related penile injuries, which may require surgery. ∎
➤ **Dupuytren contracture with palpable cord**
Adults: 0.58 mg injected into palpable cord with contracture of metacarpophalangeal joint or proximal interphalangeal joint. May repeat up to three times per cord at 4-week intervals.
➤ **Peyronie disease with palpable plaque and curvature deformity of at least 30 degrees at start of therapy**
Adults: Initially, 0.58 mg injected into the target plaque once; then repeat injection 1 to 3 days later. May repeat up to four treatment cycles of two injections approximately every 6 weeks. Discontinue treatment if curvature deformity is less than 15 degrees after any cycle.

crotamiton
kroe-TAM-ih-tuhn

Eurax

Therapeutic class: Scabicides–pediculicides
Pharmacologic class: Scabicides

AVAILABLE FORMS
Cream: 10%
Lotion: 10%

INDICATIONS & DOSAGES
➤ **Parasitic infestation (scabies)**
Adults: Scrub entire body with soap and water. Remove scales or crusts. Then apply thin layer of cream over entire body, from chin down (with special attention to skinfolds, creases, interdigital spaces, and genital area). Apply second coat in 24 hours. Change clothing and bed linen the next morning. Wait another 48 hours after last application; then wash off. If retreatment is needed, use an alternative regimen.
➤ **Itching**
Adults: Apply locally, massaging gently into affected area until completely absorbed; repeat p.r.n.

---

cycloSERINE
sye-kloe-SER-een

Seromycin

Therapeutic class: Antituberculotics
Pharmacologic class: Isoxazolidine
derivatives, D-alanine analogues

AVAILABLE FORMS
Capsules: 250 mg

INDICATIONS & DOSAGES
➤ **Adjunctive treatment for pulmonary or extrapulmonary TB**
Adults: Initially, 250 mg P.O. every 12 hours for 2 weeks. Maintenance dose is 500 mg to 1 g daily in divided doses monitored by blood levels. Dosage shouldn't exceed 1 g daily.

dalfampridine
dal-FAM-prih-deen

Ampyra

Therapeutic class: MS drugs
Pharmacologic class: Potassium channel blockers

AVAILABLE FORMS
Tablets (extended-release) ⓃⒸ*:* 10 mg

INDICATIONS & DOSAGES
➤ **To improve walking in patients with MS**
Adults: 10 mg P.O. every 12 hours.

dantrolene sodium
DAN-troe-leen

Dantrium, Dantrium I.V., Revonto, Ryanodex

Therapeutic class: Skeletal muscle relaxants
Pharmacologic class: Hydantoin derivatives

AVAILABLE FORMS
Capsules: 25 mg, 50 mg, 100 mg
Injection: 20 mg/vial, 250 mg/vial

INDICATIONS & DOSAGES
Black Box Warning   Opioids combined with benzodiazepines or CNS depressants can cause death. ∎
➤ **Spasticity and sequelae from severe chronic disorders, such as MS, cerebral palsy, spinal cord injury, and stroke**
Adults: Initially, 25 mg P.O. daily; then 25 mg t.i.d., 50 mg t.i.d., and finally,100 mg t.i.d. Maintain each dosage level for 7 days to determine response. May increase t.i.d. to q.i.d. if necessary. Maximum, 400 mg daily.

Children age 5 and older: Initially, 0.5 mg/kg P.O. daily; then 0.5 mg/kg t.i.d., 1 mg/kg t.i.d., and finally, 2 mg/kg t.i.d. Maintain each dosage level for 7 days to determine response. May increase t.i.d. to q.i.d. if necessary. Maximum, 100 mg q.i.d.
Adjust-a-dose: If no further benefit is observed at the next higher dose, decrease dosage to the previous lower dose. Stop drug if benefits aren't evident within 45 days.
➤ **To manage malignant hyperthermic crisis**
Adults and children: Initially, 1 mg/kg I.V. push. Repeat, as needed, up to cumulative dose of 10 mg/kg.
➤ **To prevent or attenuate malignant hyperthermic crisis in susceptible patients who need surgery**
Adults and children age 5 and older: 4 to 8 mg/kg P.O. daily in three or four divided doses for 1 or 2 days before procedure. Give final dose 3 or 4 hours before procedure. Or, 2.5 mg/kg I.V. about 1.25 hours before anesthesia; infuse Dantrium or Revonto over 1 hour or Ryanodex over at least 1 minute.
➤ **To prevent recurrence of malignant hyperthermic crisis**
Adults and children age 5 and older: 4 to 8 mg/kg P.O. daily in four divided doses for up to 3 days after hyperthermic crisis.

darunavir ethanolate
duh-ROO-nah-veer

Prezista

Therapeutic class: Antiretrovirals
Pharmacologic class: Protease inhibitors

AVAILABLE FORMS
Oral suspension: 100 mg/mL
Tablets ⓃⒸ*:* 75 mg, 150 mg, 600 mg, 800 mg

INDICATIONS & DOSAGES
➤ **HIV infection, with ritonavir and other antiretrovirals**
Adults who are treatment-experienced with at least one darunavir resistance–associated substitution or when genotypic testing isn't feasible (testing is recommended): 600 mg P.O. b.i.d., given with 100 mg ritonavir P.O. b.i.d. and food.
Adults who are treatment-naive or treatment-experienced with no darunavir resistance–associated substitutions: 800 mg P.O. once daily, given with ritonavir 100 mg P.O. once daily and food.
Children ages 3 to younger than 18 who are treatment-naive or treatment-experienced with no darunavir resistance–associated substitutions: Don't exceed recommended dosage for treatment-experienced adults. For those weighing 40 kg or more, 800 mg P.O. once daily with ritonavir 100 mg once daily and food; for those weighing 30 to less than 40 kg, 675 mg (may round dose to 680 mg for oral suspension) P.O. once daily with ritonavir 100 mg once daily and food; for those weighing 15 to less than 30 kg, 600 mg P.O. once daily with ritonavir 100 mg once daily and food; for those weighing 14 to less than 15 kg, 490 mg

(may round dose to 500 mg for oral suspension) P.O. once daily with ritonavir 96 mg once daily and food; for those weighing 13 to less than 14 kg, 455 mg (may round dose to 460 mg for oral suspension) P.O. once daily with ritonavir 80 mg once daily and food; for those weighing 12 to less than 13 kg, 420 mg P.O. once daily with ritonavir 80 mg once daily and food; for those weighing 11 to less than 12 kg, 385 mg (may round dose to 400 mg for oral suspension) P.O. once daily with ritonavir 64 mg once daily and food; for those weighing 10 to less than 11 kg, 350 mg (may round dose to 360 mg for oral suspension) P.O. once daily with ritonavir 64 mg once daily and food. *Children ages 3 to younger than 18 who are treatment-experienced with at least one darunavir resistance–associated substitution:* Don't exceed recommended dosage for treatment-experienced adults. For those weighing 40 kg or more, 600 mg P.O. b.i.d. with ritonavir 100 mg b.i.d. and food; for those weighing 30 to less than 40 kg, 450 mg (may round dose to 460 mg for oral suspension) P.O. b.i.d. with ritonavir 60 mg b.i.d. and food; for those weighing 15 to less than 30 kg, 375 mg (may round dose to 380 mg for oral suspension) P.O. b.i.d. with ritonavir 48 mg b.i.d. and food; for those weighing 14 to less than 15 kg, 280 mg P.O. b.i.d. with ritonavir 48 mg b.i.d. and food; for those weighing 13 to less than 14 kg, 260 mg P.O. b.i.d. with ritonavir 40 mg b.i.d. and food; for those weighing 12 to less than 13 kg, 240 mg P.O. b.i.d. with ritonavir 40 mg b.i.d. and food; for those weighing 11 to less than 12 kg, 220 mg P.O. b.i.d. with ritonavir 32 mg b.i.d. and food; for those weighing 10 to less than 11 kg, 200 mg P.O. b.i.d. with ritonavir 32 mg b.i.d. and food.

SAFETY ALERT!

dasatinib
duh-SAH-tin-nib

Sprycel

Therapeutic class: Antineoplastics
Pharmacologic class: Protein–tyrosine kinase inhibitors

AVAILABLE FORMS
Tablets ⓓⓝⓒ: 20 mg, 50 mg, 70 mg, 80 mg, 100 mg, 140 mg

INDICATIONS & DOSAGES
Adjust-a-dose (for all indications): If patient has hematologic toxicity, such as neutropenia or thrombocytopenia, consider reducing dose or interrupting or stopping therapy. If patient has severe, nonhematologic toxicity, hold dose until condition resolves; then resume at previous or reduced dose as appropriate.
➤ **Accelerated, myeloid, or lymphoid blast-phase chronic myeloid leukemia (CML) with resistance or intolerance to earlier treatment, including imatinib; Philadelphia chromosome–positive acute lymphoblastic leukemia with resistance or intolerance to prior therapy**

Adults: 140 mg P.O. once daily. If patient tolerates this dose but fails to respond to treatment, increase to 180 mg P.O. once daily. Continue until disease progresses or intolerable adverse effects occur.
Adjust-a-dose: Refer to manufacturer's instructions for dosage adjustments for hematologic toxicities.
➤ **Newly diagnosed Philadelphia chromosome–positive chronic-phase CML or chronic-phase CML resistant or intolerant to previous therapy, including imatinib**
Adults: 100 mg P.O. daily. May increase to 140 mg daily.
Adjust-a-dose: Refer to manufacturer's instructions for dosage adjustments for hematologic toxicities.

SAFETY ALERT!

DAUNOrubicin hydrochloride
daw-nah-ROO-buh-sin

Cerubidine

Therapeutic class: Antineoplastics
Pharmacologic class: Anthracycline glycoside antibiotics

AVAILABLE FORMS
Injection: 5 mg/mL
Powder for injection: 20-mg vials

INDICATIONS & DOSAGES
Black Box Warning Inject into a rapidly flowing I.V. infusion; never by I.M. or subcutaneous route. Drug may cause severe myelosuppression or myocardial toxicity in the form of potentially fatal HF, during therapy or months to years afterward. Reduce dosage for renal or hepatic impairment. ∎
Adjust-a-dose (for all indications): For patients with impaired hepatic and renal function, reduce dosage as follows: If bilirubin level is 1.2 to 3 mg/dL, give ¾ normal dose; if bilirubin or creatinine level exceeds 3 mg/dL, give ½ normal dose. Dosages vary. Check treatment protocol with prescriber.
➤ **To induce remission in acute nonlymphocytic (myelogenous, monocytic, erythroid) leukemia**
Adults age 60 and older: In combination, 30 mg/m^2/day I.V. on days 1, 2, and 3 of first course and on days 1 and 2 of subsequent courses with cytarabine infusions. Maximum lifetime cumulative dose is 550 mg/m^2; in patients who received mediastinal radiation, maximum lifetime cumulative dose is 400 mg/m^2.
Adults younger than age 60: In combination, 45 mg/m^2/day I.V. on days 1, 2, and 3 of first course and on days 1 and 2 of subsequent courses with cytarabine infusions. Maximum lifetime cumulative dose is 500 mg/m^2; in patients who received mediastinal radiation, maximum lifetime cumulative dose is 400 mg/m^2.
➤ **To induce remission in acute lymphocytic leukemia (with combination therapy)**
Adults: 45 mg/m^2/day I.V. on days 1, 2, and 3 of first course. Maximum lifetime cumulative dose is 550 mg/m^2; in patients who received mediastinal

radiation, maximum lifetime cumulative dose is 400 mg/m².

Children age 2 and older: 25 mg/m² I.V. on day 1 every week for up to 6 weeks, if needed. Maximum lifetime cumulative dose is 300 mg/m².

Children younger than age 2 or with BSA less than 0.5 m²: 1 mg/kg/dose for 1 to 3 days (dose based on body weight, not BSA). Administration frequency is specific to each combination chemotherapy regimen. Maximum lifetime cumulative dose is 10 mg/kg.

deoxycholic acid
dee-OX-i-koe-lik

Kybella

Therapeutic class: Lipolytic agents
Pharmacologic class: Lipolytics

AVAILABLE FORMS
Injection: 10 mg/mL in 2-mL single-use vials*

INDICATIONS & DOSAGES
➤ **Improvement in appearance of moderate to severe convexity or fullness associated with submental fat**
Adults: Inject subcutaneously into the submental region using an area-adjusted dose of 2 mg/cm². A single treatment consists of a maximum of 50 injections (up to a total of 10 mL), 0.2 mL each, spaced 1 cm apart. A maximum of six single treatments may be administered at intervals no less than 1 month apart. Tailor the number of injections and the number of treatments to patient's submental fat distribution and treatment goals.

SAFETY ALERT!

desirudin
deh-SIHR-uh-din

Iprivask

Therapeutic class: Anticoagulants
Pharmacologic class: Thrombin inhibitors

AVAILABLE FORMS
Injection: 15 mg desirudin lyophilized powder and 0.6 mL mannitol (3%) diluent

INDICATIONS & DOSAGES
Black Box Warning Drug increases risk of epidural or spinal hematoma, which can result in long-term or permanent paralysis, if patient receives epidural or spinal anesthesia or spinal puncture. ∎
➤ **To prevent DVT in patients undergoing hip replacement surgery**
Adults: 15 mg subcutaneously every 12 hours for 9 to 12 days. Give first injection 5 to 15 minutes before surgery, after induction of regional block anesthesia, if used.

Adjust-a-dose: If CrCl is 31 to 60 mL/minute, give 5 mg subcutaneously every 12 hours. If CrCl is less than 31 mL/minute, give 1.7 mg subcutaneously every 12 hours. Check aPTT and creatinine daily. If aPTT exceeds 2 times control, stop therapy until it's within 2 times control; then resume at a reduced dose.

diflunisal
dye-FLOO-ni-sal

Therapeutic class: NSAIDs
Pharmacologic class: Salicylates–NSAIDs

AVAILABLE FORMS
Tablets ⊕: 500 mg

INDICATIONS & DOSAGES
Black Box Warning Drug may increase risk of serious CV thrombotic events, MI, stroke, and GI adverse reactions. Contraindicated for use in CABG surgery. ∎
➤ **Osteoarthritis, RA**
Adults: 500 to 1,000 mg P.O. daily in two divided doses, usually every 12 hours. Maximum, 1,500 mg daily.
Children age 12 and older: 250 to 1,000 mg P.O. daily in two divided doses. Maximum dose, 1,500 mg daily.
➤ **Mild to moderate pain**
Adults and children age 12 and older: 1,000 mg P.O., then 500 mg every 8 to 12 hours. A lower dosage of 500 mg P.O., then 250 mg every 8 to 12 hours, may be appropriate.

dimenhyDRINATE
dye-men-HYE-dri-nate

Children's Motion Sickness Liq✜ ◇, Dinate✜ ◇, Dramamine ◇, Gravol✜ ◇, Nauseatol✜ ◇, Travel Tabs✜ ◇

Therapeutic class: Antivertigo drugs
Pharmacologic class: Anticholinergics

AVAILABLE FORMS
Capsules: 50 mg✜ ◇
Injection: 50 mg/mL
Oral solution: 15 mg/5 mL✜ ◇
Tablets: 15 mg✜ ◇, 50 mg ◇
Tablets (chewable): 15 mg✜ ◇, 25 mg ◇, 50 mg ◇

INDICATIONS & DOSAGES
➤ **To prevent and treat motion sickness**
Adults and children age 12 and older: 50 to 100 mg P.O. every 4 to 6 hours; 50 mg I.M., as needed; or 50 mg I.V. diluted in 10 mL NSS for injection, injected over 2 minutes. Maximum, 400 mg daily. For prevention, use drug at least 30 minutes before motion exposure.
Children ages 6 to 11: 25 to 50 mg P.O. every 6 to 8 hours, not to exceed 150 mg in 24 hours. Or, 1.25 mg/kg or 37.5 mg/m² I.M. q.i.d.

Children ages 2 to 5: 12.5 to 25 mg P.O. every 6 to 8 hours, not to exceed 75 mg in 24 hours. Or, 1.25 mg/kg or 37.5 mg/m² I.M. q.i.d. Maximum, 300 mg daily.

dinoprostone
dye-noe-PROST-ohn

Cervidil, Prepidil, Prostin E2

Therapeutic class: Oxytocics
Pharmacologic class: Prostaglandins

AVAILABLE FORMS
Endocervical gel: 0.5 mg/application (2.5-mL syringe)
Vaginal insert: 10 mg
Vaginal suppositories: 20 mg

INDICATIONS & DOSAGES
Black Box Warning Strictly adhere to recommended dosages. ∎
➤ **To terminate second-trimester pregnancy; to evacuate uterine contents in missed abortion, intrauterine fetal death up to 28 weeks' gestation, or benign hydatidiform mole (vaginal suppository only)**
Women: Insert 20-mg suppository high into posterior vaginal fornix; repeat every 3 to 5 hours until abortion is complete, for a maximum of 2 days.
➤ **To ripen an unfavorable cervix in pregnant woman at or near term (endocervical gel and vaginal insert only)**
Women: Apply 0.5 mg endocervical gel intravaginally; if cervix remains unfavorable after 6 hours, repeat dose. Don't exceed 1.5 mg (three applications) within 24 hours. After obtaining desired response, wait 6 to 12 hours before giving I.V. oxytocin. Or, place 10-mg vaginal insert transversely in posterior vaginal fornix immediately after removing insert from foil. Take insert out when active labor begins or after 12 hours have passed, whichever occurs first. After insert removal, wait at least 30 minutes before giving oxytocin.

SAFETY ALERT!

dinutuximab
DIN-ue-TUX-i-mab

Unituxin

Therapeutic class: Antineoplastics
Pharmacologic class: GD2-binding monoclonal antibodies

AVAILABLE FORMS
Injection: 17.5 mg/5 mL (3.5 mg/mL) single-use vial

INDICATIONS & DOSAGES
Black Box Warning Life-threatening infusion reactions can occur. Give required prehydration and premedication before each infusion and monitor

patient for infusion reaction during and for at least 4 hours after infusion. Interrupt drug for infusion reaction and permanently discontinue for anaphylaxis. Drug causes severe neuropathic pain and requires I.V. opioids before, during, and after infusion. Discontinue drug for severe unresponsive pain, and severe sensory or motor neuropathy. ∎
➤ **High-risk neuroblastoma, in combination with granulocyte-macrophage colony-stimulating factor, interleukin-2, and 13-*cis*-retinoic acid, in patients who achieved at least a partial response to prior first-line multiagent, multimodality therapy**
Children: 17.5 mg/m²/day I.V. over 10 to 20 hours for 4 consecutive days for up to five cycles. Cycles 1, 3, and 5 are 24 days in duration, and drug is administered on days 4, 5, 6, and 7. Cycles 2 and 4 are 32 days in duration, and drug is administered on days 8, 9, 10, and 11.
Adjust-a dose: Refer to manufacturer's instructions for dosage modifications for mild to moderate or prolonged or severe infusion-related reactions; moderate to severe and life-threatening capillary leak syndrome; hypotension requiring medical intervention; severe systemic infection or sepsis; or neurologic disorders of the eye. Permanently discontinue drug for grade 3 or 4 anaphylaxis or serum sickness, grade 3 pain unresponsive to maximum supportive measures, grade 3 sensory neuropathy that interferes with daily activities for more than 2 weeks, grade 4 sensory neuropathy, grade 2 peripheral motor neuropathy, subtotal or total vision loss or first recurrence of neurologic disorders of the eye, grade 4 hyponatremia despite appropriate fluid management, second recurrence of prolonged or severe adverse reactions (mild bronchospasm without other symptoms or angioedema that doesn't affect the airway), or first recurrence of life-threatening capillary leak syndrome.

disulfiram
dye-SUL-fi-ram

Antabuse

Therapeutic class: Alcohol deterrents
Pharmacologic class: Aldehyde dehydrogenase inhibitors

AVAILABLE FORMS
Tablets: 250 mg, 500 mg

INDICATIONS & DOSAGES
Black Box Warning Never give drug to an intoxicated patient or without his full knowledge. ∎
➤ **Adjunct to management of alcohol abstinence**
Adults: 250 to 500 mg P.O. as single dose in morning for 1 to 2 weeks (or in evening if drowsiness occurs) after patient has abstained from alcohol for at least 12 hours. Maintenance dosage is 125 to 500 mg P.O. daily (average 250 mg) until permanent self-control is established. Treatment may continue for months or years.

doripenem
dor-eh-PEN-em

Doribax

Therapeutic class: Antibiotics
Pharmacologic class: Carbapenems

AVAILABLE FORMS
Injection: 250-mg, 500-mg vial

INDICATIONS & DOSAGES
Adjust-a-dose (for all indications): In patients
with CrCl of 30 to 50 mL/minute, give 250 mg I.V.
every 8 hours; with CrCl of more than 10 to less than
30 mL/minute, give 250 mg I.V. every 12 hours.
➤ **Complicated intra-abdominal infections caused
by *Escherichia coli, Klebsiella pneumoniae, Pseudomonas aeruginosa, Bacteroides caccae, B. fragilis,
B. thetaiotaomicron, B. uniformis, B. vulgatas,
Streptococcus intermedius, S. constellatus,* or
*Peptostreptococcus micros***
Adults: 500 mg I.V. every 8 hours for 5 to 14 days.
➤ **Complicated UTIs, including pyelonephritis
caused by *E. coli, K. pneumoniae, Proteus mirabilis, Pseudomonas aeruginosa,* or *Acinetobacter
baumannii***
Adults: 500 mg I.V. every 8 hours for 10 days. May be
given for 14 days to patient with concurrent bacteremia.

ecallantide
ee-KAL-lan-tide

Kalbitor

Therapeutic class: Protein inhibitors
Pharmacologic class: Human plasma
kallikrein inhibitors

AVAILABLE FORMS
Injection: 10 mg/mL vials

INDICATIONS & DOSAGES
Black Box Warning Anaphylaxis has been
reported after administration. ■
➤ **Acute attacks of hereditary angioedema**
Adults and adolescents age 12 and older: 30 mg subcutaneously given as three 10-mg injections; give additional 30-mg dose within 24 hours if attack persists.

econazole nitrate
ee-KOE-na-zole

Ecoza

Therapeutic class: Antifungals
Pharmacologic class: Imidazole derivatives

AVAILABLE FORMS
Cream: 1%
Foam: 1%

INDICATIONS & DOSAGES
➤ **Tinea corporis, tinea cruris, tinea pedis, tinea
versicolor**
Adults and children: Rub cream into affected areas
daily for at least 2 weeks (1 month for tinea pedis).
*Adults and children age 12 and older (tinea pedis
only):* Apply foam to affected areas daily for 4 weeks.
➤ **Cutaneous candidiasis**
Adults and children: Rub cream into affected areas
b.i.d. for 2 weeks.

SAFETY ALERT!

eculizumab
eck-u-LIZ-uh-mob

Soliris

Therapeutic class: Hemolysis inhibitors
Pharmacologic class: Monoclonal IgG
antibodies

AVAILABLE FORMS
Injection: 10 mg/mL in 300-mg single-use vial

INDICATIONS & DOSAGES
Black Box Warning Life-threatening and fatal
meningococcal infections have occurred. Meningococcal vaccine is required at least 2 weeks before
administration of eculizumab.
➤ **Hemolysis in patients with paroxysmal nocturnal hemoglobinuria**
Adults: 600 mg I.V. every 7 days for 4 weeks, 900 mg
7 days later, then 900 mg every 14 days thereafter.
➤ **Atypical hemolytic-uremic syndrome**
Adults and children weighing 40 kg) or more: 900 mg
I.V. weekly for 4 weeks, then 1,200 mg at week 5, then
1,200 mg every 2 weeks.
Children weighing 30 to 39 kg: 600 mg I.V. weekly
for 2 weeks, then 900 mg at week 3, then 900 mg
every 2 weeks.
Children weighing 20 to 29 kg: 600 mg I.V. weekly
for 2 weeks, then 600 mg at week 3, then 600 mg
every 2 weeks.
Children weighing 10 to 19 kg: 600 mg I.V. weekly
for one dose, then 300 mg at week 2, then 300 mg
every 2 weeks.
Children weighing 5 to 9 kg: 300 mg I.V. weekly for
one dose, then 300 mg at week 2, then 300 mg every
3 weeks.

efinaconazole
EF-in-a-KON-a-zole

Jublia

Therapeutic class: Antifungals
Pharmacologic class: Azole antifungals

AVAILABLE FORMS
Topical solution: 10%

INDICATIONS & DOSAGES

➤ **Toenail onychomycosis due to *Trichophyton rubrum* or *Trichophyton mentagrophytes***

Adults: Apply solution to affected toenails using the brush applicator once daily for 48 weeks.

eliglustat tartrate
EL-i-gloo-stat

Cerdelga

Therapeutic class: Protein inhibitors
Pharmacologic class: Glucosylceramide synthase inhibitors

AVAILABLE FORMS
Capsules ⓄⓃⒸ: 84 mg

INDICATIONS & DOSAGES

➤ **Long-term treatment of type 1 Gaucher disease in patients who are CYP2D6 extensive metabolizers (EMs), intermediate metabolizers (IMs), or poor metabolizers (PMs) as detected by an FDA-approved test**

Adults: After CYP2D6 metabolizer status is identified, recommended dosage is 84 mg P.O. b.i.d. in CYP2D6 EMs and IMs; recommended dosage in CYP2D6 PMs is 84 mg P.O. once daily.

Adjust-a-dose: Reduce dosage to 84 mg P.O. daily in CYP2D6 EMs and IMs taking strong or moderate CYP2D6 inhibitors, or CYP2D6 EMs taking strong or moderate CYP3A inhibitors.

elosulfase alfa
el-oh-SUL-fase

Vimizim

Therapeutic class: Human enzyme replacements
Pharmacologic class: Glycosaminoglycans reducers

AVAILABLE FORMS
Injection: 5 mg/5 mL in single-use vial

INDICATIONS & DOSAGES

Black Box Warning Drug has caused life-threatening anaphylactic reactions. ∎

➤ **Mucopolysaccharidosis type IVA (MPS IVA; Morquio A syndrome)**

Adults and children age 5 and older: 2 mg/kg I.V. weekly For patients weighing less than 25 kg, initially infuse at 3 mL/hour for first 15 minutes. If tolerated, increase to 6 mL/hour for next 15 minutes. If tolerated, increase every 15 minutes in 6-mL/hour increments, up to 36 mL/hour. Deliver total volume over a minimum of 3½ hours. For patients weighing 25 kg or more, initially infuse at 6 mL/hour for first 15 minutes. If tolerated, increase to 12 mL/hour for next 15 minutes. If tolerated, increase every 15 minutes in 12-mL/hour

increments, up to 72 mL/hour. Deliver total volume over a minimum of 4½ hours.

entacapone
en-tah-KAP-own

Comtan

Therapeutic class: Antiparkinsonians
Pharmacologic class: Catechol-O-methyltransferase inhibitors

AVAILABLE FORMS
Tablets ⓄⓃⒸ: 200 mg

INDICATIONS & DOSAGES

➤ **Adjunct to levodopa–carbidopa for treatment of idiopathic Parkinson disease in patients with signs and symptoms of end-of-dose wearing-off**

Adults: 200 mg P.O. with each dose of levodopa–carbidopa, up to eight times daily. Maximum, 1,600 mg daily. May need to reduce daily levodopa dose or extend the interval between doses to optimize patient's response.

SAFETY ALERT!

enzalutamide
EN-za-LOO-ta-mide

Xtandi

Therapeutic class: Antineoplastics
Pharmacologic class: Androgen receptor inhibitors

AVAILABLE FORMS
Capsules ⓄⓃⒸ: 40 mg

INDICATIONS & DOSAGES

➤ **Metastatic castration-resistant prostate cancer**

Adults: 160 mg P.O. once daily.

Adjust-a-dose: For grade 3 or 4 toxicity or an intolerable adverse effect, withhold drug for 1 week or until symptoms improve to grade 2 or less. Resume at same or reduced dosage as appropriate. If use with strong CYP3A4 inducers is unavoidable, increase dose to 240 mg once daily. If use with strong CYP2C8 inhibitors is unavoidable, reduce dosage to 80 mg once daily.

eprosartan mesylate
ep-row-SAR-tan

Teveten

Therapeutic class: Antihypertensives
Pharmacologic class: Angiotensin II receptor antagonists

AVAILABLE FORMS
Tablets: 400 mg, 600 mg

INDICATIONS & DOSAGES

Black Box Warning Can cause fetal harm; don't use during pregnancy.

➤ **Hypertension (alone or with other antihypertensives)**

Adults: Initially, 600 mg P.O. daily. Dosage ranges from 400 to 800 mg daily, given as single daily dose or two divided doses. Maximum dose is 800 mg/day.

SAFETY ALERT!

exemestane
ecks-eh-MES-tayn

Aromasin

Therapeutic class: Antineoplastics
Pharmacologic class: Aromatase inhibitors

AVAILABLE FORMS
Tablets: 25 mg

INDICATIONS & DOSAGES

Adjust-a-dose (for all indications): In patients also taking strong CYP3A4 inducers (rifampicin, phenytoin), increase daily dose to 50 mg.

➤ **Advanced breast cancer in postmenopausal women whose disease has progressed after treatment with tamoxifen**

Adults: 25 mg P.O. once daily after food.

➤ **Early-stage breast cancer in postmenopausal women who have taken tamoxifen for 2 to 3 years** ◆

Adults: 25 mg P.O. once daily after food to complete a 5-year course, unless cancer recurs or is found in the other breast.

---

fibrin sealant (human)
FYE-brin SEEL-ent

Raplixa

Therapeutic class: Dermatologic agents
Pharmacologic class: Fibrin sealants

AVAILABLE FORMS
Topical solution: 0.5-g, 1-g, 2-g vials

INDICATIONS & DOSAGES

➤ **Adjunct to hemostasis for mild to moderate surgical bleeding when control of bleeding by standard surgical techniques (such as suture, ligature, and cautery) is ineffective or impractical**

Adults: Required amount of drug needed to stop bleeding varies and is based on size of bleeding area to be treated; maximum total dose per surgery is 3 g. Using 0.5 g of drug covers up to a 25-cm² area when directly applied from vial or 50 cm² when applied using the RaplixaSpray device. Using 1 g of drug covers up to a 50-cm² area when applied directly from vial or 100 cm² when applied using the RaplixaSpray device. Using 2 g of drug covers a 100-cm² area when applied directly from vial or 200 cm² when applied using the

RaplixaSpray device. Use in conjunction with an absorbable gelatin sponge.

---

finafloxacin
fin-ah-FLOX-ah-sin

Xtoro

Therapeutic class: Antibacterials
Pharmacologic class: Fluoroquinolones

AVAILABLE FORMS
Otic suspension: 0.3%

INDICATIONS & DOSAGES

➤ **Acute otitis externa, with or without an otowick, caused by susceptible strains of *Pseudomonas aeruginosa* and *Staphylococcus aureus***

Adults and children age 1 and older: Instill 4 drops into affected ear(s) b.i.d. for 7 days. For patients requiring use of an otowick (a special sponge placed in the ear for medication delivery), can double initial dose (to 8 drops), followed by 4 drops into affected ear(s) b.i.d. for 7 days.

---

fludrocortisone acetate
floo-droe-KOR-ti-sone

Therapeutic class: Mineralocorticoids
Pharmacologic class: Mineralocorticoids

AVAILABLE FORMS
Tablets: 0.1 mg

INDICATIONS & DOSAGES

➤ **Salt-losing adrenogenital syndrome**
Adults: 0.1 to 0.2 mg P.O. daily.

➤ **Addison disease (adrenocortical insufficiency)**
Adults: 0.1 mg P.O. daily. Usual dosage range is 0.1 mg three times weekly to 0.2 mg daily. Decrease dosage to 0.05 mg daily if transient hypertension develops.

---

fluorometholone
flur-oh-METH-oh-lone

FML, FML Forte

fluorometholone acetate
Flarex

Therapeutic class: Anti-inflammatory drugs (ophthalmic)
Pharmacologic class: Corticosteroids

AVAILABLE FORMS
fluorometholone
Ophthalmic ointment: 0.1%
Ophthalmic suspension: 0.1%, 0.25%
fluorometholone acetate
Ophthalmic suspension: 0.1%

INDICATIONS & DOSAGES

➤ **Inflammatory and allergic conditions of cornea, conjunctiva, sclera, or anterior uvea**

Adults and children older than age 2 (acetate form not for use in children of any age): 1 drop b.i.d. to q.i.d. or ½-inch ointment once daily to t.i.d. For first 24 to 48 hours, may increase dosing frequency to every 4 hours. For fluorometholone acetate, 1 to 2 drops q.i.d.; may give 2 drops every 2 hours during the initial 24 to 48 hours of treatment.

---

fosamprenavir calcium
foss-am-PREN-ah-ver

Lexiva

Therapeutic class: Antiretrovirals
Pharmacologic class: Protease inhibitors

AVAILABLE FORMS
Oral suspension: 50 mg/mL
Tablets: 700 mg

INDICATIONS & DOSAGES

➤ **HIV infection, with other antiretrovirals**

Adults: In patients not previously treated, 1,400 mg P.O. b.i.d. (without ritonavir). Or, 1,400 mg P.O. once daily with ritonavir 200 mg P.O. once daily. Or, 1,400 mg P.O. once daily with ritonavir 100 mg P.O. once daily. Or, 700 mg P.O. b.i.d. with ritonavir 100 mg P.O. b.i.d. In patients previously treated with a protease inhibitor, 700 mg P.O. b.i.d. plus ritonavir 100 mg P.O. b.i.d.

Adjust-a-dose: If patient has mild hepatic impairment (Child-Pugh score of 5 to 6), reduce dosage to 700 mg P.O. b.i.d. without ritonavir (in therapy-naive patients) or 700 mg b.i.d. plus ritonavir 100 mg once daily (in therapy-naive or protease inhibitor–experienced patients). If patient has moderate hepatic impairment (Child-Pugh score of 7 to 9), reduce dosage to 700 mg b.i.d. (in therapy-naive patients) without ritonavir or 450 mg b.i.d. plus ritonavir 100 mg once daily (in therapy-naive or protease inhibitor–experienced patients). If patient has severe hepatic impairment (Child-Pugh score of 10 to 15), reduce dosage to 350 mg b.i.d. without ritonavir (in therapy-naive patients). Or, in therapy-naive or protease inhibitor–experienced patients, 300 mg P.O. b.i.d. plus ritonavir 100 mg once daily.

➤ **HIV infection with other antiretrovirals for protease inhibitor–naive children age 4 weeks and older**

Children ages 4 weeks to 18 years weighing 20 kg or more: 18 mg/kg P.O. with ritonavir 3 mg/kg b.i.d.
Children ages 4 weeks to 18 years weighing 15 to less than 20 kg: 23 mg/kg P.O. with ritonavir 3 mg/kg b.i.d.
Children ages 4 weeks to 18 years weighing 11 to less than 15 kg: 30 mg/kg P.O. with ritonavir 3 mg/kg b.i.d.
Children ages 4 weeks to 18 years weighing less than 11 kg: 45 mg/kg P.O. with ritonavir 7 mg/kg b.i.d.
Adjust-a-dose: There are no dosing recommendations for pediatric patients with hepatic impairment.

Dosage for pediatric patients shouldn't exceed recommended adult dosage of 700 mg fosamprenavir with ritonavir 100 mg b.i.d. Drug isn't approved for once-daily dosing in pediatric patients.

➤ **HIV infection with other antiretrovirals for protease inhibitor–experienced children age 6 months and older**

Children ages 6 months to 18 years weighing 20 kg or more: 18 mg/kg P.O. with ritonavir 3 mg/kg b.i.d.
Children ages 6 months to 18 years weighing 15 to less than 20 kg: 23 mg/kg P.O. with ritonavir 3 mg/kg b.i.d.
Children ages 6 months to 18 years weighing 11 to less than 15 kg: 30 mg/kg P.O. with ritonavir 3 mg/kg b.i.d.
Children ages 6 months to 18 years weighing less than 11 kg: 45 mg/kg P.O. with ritonavir 7 mg/kg b.i.d.
Adjust-a-dose: There are no dosing recommendations for pediatric patients with hepatic impairment. Dosage for pediatric patients shouldn't exceed recommended adult dosage of 700 mg fosamprenavir with ritonavir 100 mg b.i.d. Drug isn't approved for once-daily dosing in pediatric patients.

➤ **HIV infection without ritonavir in protease inhibitor–naive children**

Children age 2 years and older: 30 mg/kg P.O. b.i.d. Maximum dose is 1,400 mg b.i.d.
Adjust-a-dose: There are no dosing recommendations for pediatric patients with hepatic impairment. Drug isn't approved for once-daily dosing in pediatric patients.

---

glucagon
GLOO-ka-gon

GlucaGen Diagnostic Kit, GlucaGen HypoKit

Therapeutic class: Diagnostic agents
Pharmacologic class: Antihypoglycemics

AVAILABLE FORMS
Powder for injection: 1-mg (1-unit) vial

INDICATIONS & DOSAGES

➤ **Hypoglycemia**

Glucagon
Adults and children weighing more than 20 kg or older than age 6: 1 mg (1 unit) I.V., I.M., or subcutaneously. May repeat in 15 minutes, if needed. I.V. glucose must be given if patient fails to respond.
Children weighing 20 kg or less: 0.5 mg (0.5 units) or 20 to 30 mcg/kg I.V., I.M., or subcutaneously; maximum dose, 1 mg. May repeat in 15 minutes, if needed. I.V. glucose must be given if patient fails to respond.
GlucaGen
Adults and children weighing more than 25 kg and age 6 or older or when weight is unknown: 1 mL I.V., I.M., or subcutaneously.
Children weighing less than 25 kg or younger than age 6 when weight is unknown: 0.5 mL I.V., I.M., or subcutaneously.

➤ **Diagnostic aid for radiologic examination of the GI tract**
Adults: 0.25 to 0.75 mg I.V. or 1 to 2 mg I.M. before radiologic examination.

SAFETY ALERT!

goserelin acetate
GOE-se-REL-in

Zoladex

Therapeutic class: Antineoplastics
Pharmacologic class: Gonadotropin-releasing hormone analogues

AVAILABLE FORMS
Implants: 3.6 mg, 10.8 mg

INDICATIONS & DOSAGES
➤ **Endometriosis, including pain relief and lesion reduction**
Women: 3.6 mg subcutaneously every 28 days into the anterior abdominal wall below the navel. Maximum length of therapy is 6 months.
➤ **Endometrial thinning before endometrial ablation**
Women: 3.6 mg subcutaneously into the anterior abdominal wall below the navel. Give one or two implants, 4 weeks apart.
➤ **Palliative treatment of advanced breast cancer in premenopausal and postmenopausal women**
Women: 3.6 mg subcutaneously every 28 days into anterior abdominal wall below navel.
➤ **Palliative treatment of advanced prostate cancer**
Men: 3.6 mg subcutaneously every 28 days or 10.8 mg subcutaneously every 12 weeks into anterior abdominal wall below navel.
➤ **Stage B2-C prostate cancer in combination with radiotherapy and flutamide**
Men: Start 8 weeks before initiating radiotherapy and continue during radiation therapy. Give 3.6 mg subcutaneously into anterior abdominal wall below navel 8 weeks before radiotherapy, followed in 28 days by 10.8 mg subcutaneously. Or, give four injections of 3.6 mg at 28-day intervals, two injections preceding and two during radiotherapy.

guanfacine hydrochloride
GWAHN-fa-seen

Intuniv, Tenex

Therapeutic class: Antihypertensives
Pharmacologic class: Centrally acting antiadrenergics

AVAILABLE FORMS
Tablets: 1 mg, 2 mg
Tablets (extended-release) ⓄⓃⒸ: 1 mg, 2 mg, 3 mg, 4 mg

INDICATIONS & DOSAGES
➤ **Hypertension**
Adults and children age 12 and older: Initially, 1 mg immediate-release tablet P.O. once daily at bedtime. If response isn't adequate after 3 to 4 weeks, may increase dosage to 2 mg daily. Higher doses have been used, but adverse effects increase significantly with dosages of more than 3 mg/day.
➤ **Attention deficit hyperactivity disorder**
Children ages 6 to 17: Extended-release form only. Initially, 1 mg P.O. once daily in a.m. or p.m. at approximately same time each day. Adjust dosage in increments of 1 mg/week as needed. Dosage range is 1 to 4 mg/day. Or, initially, 0.05 to 0.08 mg/kg P.O. once daily. Adjust dosage up to 0.12 mg/kg once daily if well tolerated and necessary. Maximum total dose is 4 mg/day.

hydroxyprogesterone caproate
hye-drox-ee-proh-JESS-te-rone

Makena

Therapeutic class: Hormones
Pharmacologic class: Progestins

AVAILABLE FORMS
Injection: 250 mg/mL in multidose vial

INDICATIONS & DOSAGES
➤ **To reduce risk of preterm birth in women with singleton pregnancy and history of singleton spontaneous preterm birth**
Pregnant adolescents and women age 16 and older: 250 mg I.M. once weekly starting between 16 weeks, 0 days and 20 weeks, 6 days of gestation and continuing until week 37 (through 36 weeks, 6 days) of gestation or delivery, whichever occurs first.

icosapent ethyl
eye-KOE-sa-pent

Vascepa

Therapeutic class: Antilipemics
Pharmacologic class: Ethyl esters

AVAILABLE FORMS
Capsules ⓄⓃⒸ: 1 g

INDICATIONS & DOSAGES
➤ **Adjunct to diet to reduce triglyceride levels 500 mg/dL or more**
Adults: 2 g P.O. b.i.d. with food.

imiquimod
ih-mih-KWI-mahd

Aldara, Vyloma ✠, Zyclara

Therapeutic class: Immunosuppressants
(topical)
Pharmacologic class: Immune response
modifiers

AVAILABLE FORMS
Cream: 2.5%, 3.75%, 5% in single-use packets containing 12.5 mg imiquimod

INDICATIONS & DOSAGES
➤ **External genital and perianal warts**
Adults and adolescents age 12 and older: Apply thin layer of 3.75% cream once daily before sleep; leave on for 8 hours. Continue up to 8 weeks. Or, apply thin layer of 5% cream three times per week before sleep; leave on for 6 to 10 hours. Continue for up to 16 weeks.
➤ **Typical, nonhyperkeratotic, nonhypertrophic actinic keratoses on the face or scalp in immunocompetent adults**
Adults: Wash area with mild soap and water, and allow to dry for at least 10 minutes. Apply Aldara cream to face or scalp, but not both concurrently, twice weekly at bedtime; wash off after about 8 hours. Treat for 16 weeks. Or, apply Zyclara 3.75% cream once daily at bedtime for two 2-week cycles. Separate cycles by a 2-week no-treatment period.
➤ **Superficial basal cell carcinoma**
Adults: Wash area with mild soap and water, and allow to dry thoroughly. Apply a thin layer of 5% cream to the biopsy-confirmed area, including 1 cm of skin surrounding tumor, five times a week at bedtime; wash off after about 8 hours. Treat for 6 weeks.

indacaterol maleate–glycopyrrolate
in-da-KAT-er-ol/glye-koe-PIR-oh-late

Utibron Neohaler

Therapeutic class: Bronchodilators
Pharmacologic class: Beta$_2$ adrenergic
agonists–anticholinergics

AVAILABLE FORMS
Capsules (powder for inhalation): 27.5 mcg indacaterol maleate/15.6 mcg glycopyrrolate

INDICATIONS & DOSAGES
Black Box Warning Long-acting beta$_2$-adrenergic agonists increase the risk of asthma-related death. Drug isn't indicated for asthma treatment. ∎
➤ **Long-term maintenance treatment of airflow obstruction in patients with COPD, including chronic bronchitis and emphysema**
Adults: 1 capsule b.i.d. by oral inhalation.

interferon gamma-1b
in-ter-FEER-on

Actimmune

Therapeutic class: Immune response
modifiers
Pharmacologic class: Biological response
modifiers

AVAILABLE FORMS
Injection: 100 mcg (2 million international units) in 0.5-mL vial

INDICATIONS & DOSAGES
➤ **Chronic granulomatous disease in adults and children age 1 year and older, severe malignant osteopetrosis in adults and children age 1 month and older**
Adults and children with BSA greater than 0.5 m^2: Give 50 mcg/m^2 (1 million international units/m^2) subcutaneously three times weekly, preferably at bedtime.
Adults and children with a BSA of 0.5 m^2: or less: 1.5 mcg/kg subcutaneously three times weekly.
Adjust-a-dose: If patient has severe reaction, decrease dosage by 50% or stop drug until reaction subsides.

irinotecan liposome
eh-rin-OH-te-kan

Onivyde

Therapeutic class: Antineoplastics
Pharmacologic class: DNA topoisomerase
inhibitors

AVAILABLE FORMS
Injection: 43 mg/10 mL single-use vials

INDICATIONS & DOSAGES
Black Box Warning Withhold drug and initiate loperamide for late-onset diarrhea of any severity. Administer I.V. or subcutaneous atropine 0.25 to 1 mg (unless clinically contraindicated) for early-onset diarrhea of any severity. Drug may cause fatal neutropenic sepsis and severe or life-threatening neutropenic fever. Withhold drug for ANC below 1,500/mm^3 or neutropenic fever. Monitor CBC periodically during treatment. ∎
➤ **Metastatic adenocarcinoma of the pancreas after disease progression after gemcitabine-based therapy, in combination with 5-FU and leucovorin**
Adults: 70 mg/m^2 I.V. infusion over 90 minutes every 2 weeks. Premedicate with a corticosteroid and an antiemetic 30 minutes before infusion.

Adjust-a-dose: For patients known to be homozygous for the UGT1A1*28 allele, decrease initial dose to 50 mg/m^2; may increase to 70 mg/m^2 in subsequent cycles if tolerated. For first occurrence of grade 3 or 4 adverse reactions in patients homozygous for UGT1A1*28 without previous increase to 70 mg/m^2, withhold drug, and upon recovery to grade 1 or less, give 43 mg/m^2. For second occurrence of grade 3 or 4 reactions, withhold drug, and upon recovery to grade 1 or less, give 35 mg/m^2. For third occurrence, discontinue drug.

For other patients receiving 70 mg/m^2 and who develop grade 3 or 4 adverse reactions, withhold drug and upon recovery to grade 1 or less, give 50 mg/m^2. For second occurrence of grade 3 or 4 adverse reactions withhold drug, and upon recovery to grade 1 or less, give 43 mg/m^2. For third occurrence of grade 3 or 4 adverse reactions, discontinue drug.

With first occurrence of interstitial lung disease or anaphylactic reaction, discontinue drug.

isoproterenol hydrochloride
eye-soe-proe-TER-e-nole

Isuprel

Therapeutic class: Bronchodilators
Pharmacologic class: Nonselective beta-adrenergic agonists

AVAILABLE FORMS
Injection: 200 mcg/mL in 1-mL, 5-mL ampules

INDICATIONS & DOSAGES
➤ **Bronchospasm during anesthesia**
Adults: Dilute 1 mL (0.2 mg) with 10 mL of NSS or D$_5$W. Give 0.01 to 0.02 mg I.V. and repeat as necessary.
➤ **Heart block, ventricular arrhythmias**
Adults: Initially, 0.02 to 0.06 mg I.V.; then 0.01 to 0.2 mg I.V. or 5 mcg/minute I.V. Or, initially, 0.2 mg I.M. or subcutaneously; then 0.02 to 1 mg I.M. or 0.15 to 0.3 mg subcutaneously as needed.
➤ **Shock**
Adults: 0.5 to 5 mcg/minute by continuous I.V. infusion. Usual concentration is 1 mg in 500 mL D$_5$W. Titrate infusion rate according to HR, central venous pressure, BP, and urine flow.

ivacaftor
EYE-va-KAF-tor

Kalydeco

Therapeutic class: Metabolic agents
Pharmacologic class: Cystic fibrosis transmembrane conductance regulator potentiator

AVAILABLE FORMS
Granules: 50 mg/packet, 75 mg/packet
Tablets: 150 mg

INDICATIONS & DOSAGES
➤ **Cystic fibrosis in patients with *G551D, G1244E, G1349D, G178R, G551S, R117H, S1251N, S1255P, S549N,* or *S549R* mutation in the cystic fibrosis transmembrane conductance regulator gene as determined by an FDA-approved test**
Adults and children age 6 and older: 150 mg P.O. every 12 hours with fat-containing food.
Children age 2 to younger than 6: For those weighing 14 kg or more, give 75-mg granule packet mixed with 1 teaspoon (5 mL) of fat-containing soft food or liquid every 12 hours; if less than 14 kg, give 50-mg granule packet every 12 hours.
Adjust-a-dose: In patients with moderate hepatic insufficiency (Child-Pugh class B), give 1 tablet or 1 packet of granules once daily. In those with severe hepatic insufficiency (Child-Pugh class C), use cautiously at recommended dose once daily or less frequently. If hepatotoxicity develops during treatment (ALT or AST greater than 5 × ULN), hold drug. If elevated transaminases resolve, may resume after assessing benefits versus risks of continued treatment. In those taking strong CYP3A inhibitors (ketoconazole and others), give recommended dose twice a week. In those taking moderate CYP3A inhibitors (fluconazole and others), give recommended dose once daily.

SAFETY ALERT!

ixabepilone
ecks-ah-BEH-pill-own

Ixempra Kit

Therapeutic class: Antineoplastics
Pharmacologic class: Microtubule inhibitors

AVAILABLE FORMS
Injection: 15-mg, 45-mg vials

INDICATIONS & DOSAGES
Black Box Warning Drug is contraindicated in patients with AST or ALT greater than 2.5 × the ULN or bilirubin 1 × the ULN when used with capecitabine. ∎
➤ **With capecitabine for metastatic or locally advanced breast cancer, after failure of anthracycline and a taxane; or alone for metastatic or locally advanced breast cancer, after failure of anthracycline, taxanes, and capecitabine**
Adults: 40 mg/m^2 I.V. over 3 hours every 3 weeks. Doses for patients with BSA greater than 2.2 m^2 should be calculated based on 2.2 m^2. Premedicate with an H$_1$-receptor antagonist, such as diphenhydramine 50 mg P.O., and an H$_2$-receptor antagonist, such as ranitidine 150 to 300 mg P.O., 1 hour before ixabepilone infusion. For patients who experienced a prior hypersensitivity reaction, premedicate with corticosteroids (such as dexamethasone 20 mg I.V. 30 minutes before infusion or P.O. 60 minutes before infusion) in addition to the H$_1$- and H$_2$-receptor antagonists.

Adjust-a-dose: Refer to manufacturer's instructions for monotherapy and combination therapy dosage adjustments for toxicities and hepatic.

lactulose
LAK-tyoo-lose

Cholac, Constilac, Constulose, Enulose, Generlac, Kristalose

Therapeutic class: Laxatives
Pharmacologic class: Disaccharides

AVAILABLE FORMS
Oral solution: 10 g/15 mL
Packets: 10 g, 20 g
Rectal solution: 10 g/15 mL

INDICATIONS & DOSAGES
➤ **Constipation**
Adults: 10 to 20 g or 15 to 30 mL P.O. daily, increased to 60 mL/day, if needed.
➤ **To prevent and treat hepatic encephalopathy, including hepatic precoma and coma in patients with severe hepatic disease**
Adults: Initially, 20 to 30 g or 30 to 45 mL P.O. t.i.d. or q.i.d., until two or three soft stools are produced daily. Usual dose is 60 to 100 g daily in divided doses. Or, 200 g or 300 mL diluted with 700 mL of water or NSS and given as retention enema P.R. every 4 to 6 hours, as needed.
Infants: Initially, 2.5 to 10 mL/day P.O. in divided doses to produce two or three soft stools daily.
Older children and adolescents: 40 to 90 mL/day P.O. in divided doses to produce two or three soft stools daily.
➤ **Treatment of subclinical hepatic encephalopathy ◆**
Adults: 30 to 60 mL/day P.O. in two to three divided doses to maintain two or three daily bowel movements for up to 3 months.

SAFETY ALERT!

lapatinib
lah-PAH-tih-nihb

Tykerb

Therapeutic class: Antineoplastics
Pharmacologic class: Kinase inhibitors

AVAILABLE FORMS
Tablets: 250 mg

INDICATIONS & DOSAGES
Black Box Warning Severe and fatal hepatotoxicity has been observed in clinical trials and postmarketing experience. ■
Adjust-a-dose (for all indications): Refer to manufacturer's instructions for dosage adjustments for decreases in LVEF, hepatic impairment, diarrhea, other grade 2 or greater toxicities, and use with strong CYP34A4 inhibitors and CYP3A4 inducers.
➤ **Advanced or metastatic breast cancer with capecitabine when tumors overexpress HER2 and patient has had prior therapy, including an anthracycline, a taxane, and trastuzumab**
Adults: 1,250 mg (5 tablets) P.O. once daily as a single dose on days 1 through 21, with 2,000 mg/m^2/day capecitabine given P.O. in two doses 12 hours apart on days 1 to 14. Repeat 21-day cycle. Continue until disease progression or unacceptable toxicity occurs.
➤ **HER2-positive, hormone receptor–positive metastatic breast cancer in postmenopausal women**
Adults: 1,500 mg P.O. once daily with letrozole 2.5 mg once daily.

lenvatinib mesylate
len-VA-ti-nib

Lenvima

Therapeutic class: Antineoplastics
Pharmacologic class: Kinase inhibitors

AVAILABLE FORMS
Capsules: 4 mg, 10 mg

INDICATIONS & DOSAGES
Adjust-a-dose (for all indications): See manufacturer's instructions for toxicity-related dosage adjustments.
➤ **Locally recurrent or metastatic, progressive, radioactive iodine-refractory differentiated thyroid cancer**
Adults: 24 mg P.O. daily until disease progression or unacceptable toxicity occurs.
Adjust-a-dose: For preexisting severe renal impairment (CrCl less than 30 mL/minute) or severe hepatic impairment (Child-Pugh class C), decrease dosage to 14 mg P.O. daily. Initiate medical management for nausea, vomiting, or diarrhea before interruption or dosage reduction.
➤ **Advanced renal cell carcinoma after one prior antiangiogenic therapy, in combination with everolimus**
Adults: 18 mg P.O. once daily with everolimus 5 mg P.O. once daily until disease progression or unacceptable toxicity occurs.
Adjust-a-dose: For preexisting severe renal impairment (CrCl less than 30 mL/minute) or severe hepatic impairment (Child-Pugh class C), decrease lenvatinib dosage to 10 mg P.O. daily. Initiate medical management for nausea, vomiting, or diarrhea before interruption or dosage reduction.
For adverse reactions thought to be related to everolimus alone, discontinue, interrupt, or use alternate-day everolimus dosing according to everolimus prescribing information. For adverse reactions related to both lenvatinib and everolimus, first reduce lenvatinib dosage, then everolimus dosage.

lidocaine (intradermal, ophthalmic, topical)
LYE-doe-kane

Lidocaine, Lidoderm

lidocaine hydrochloride
Akten, AneCream◇, AneCream 5, Betacaine✷◇, Glydo, Larng-O-Jet Kit, LTA Kit II, Lidocaine Viscous, Lidodan✷◇, Maxilene✷◇, Predator◇, RectiCare◇, Regenecare HA◇, Solarcaine Aloe Extra Burn Relief◇, Xolido◇, Xylocaine, Zingo

Therapeutic class: Analgesics
Pharmacologic class: Local anesthetics

AVAILABLE FORMS
Cream: 2%◇, 4%◇, 5%◇
Gel: 2%◇, 5%◇
Jelly: 2%
Ointment: 5%
Ophthalmic gel: 3.5%
Patch: 5%
Powder for injection: 0.5-mg single-use intradermal injection system
Topical solution: 2%, 4%
Topical spray: 0.5%
Viscous oral solution: 2%, 4%

INDICATIONS & DOSAGES
Black Box Warning Postmarketing cases of seizures, cardiopulmonary arrest, and death in patients younger than age 3 have been reported with use of lidocaine 2% viscous solution when it wasn't administered in strict adherence to the dosing and administration recommendations. Lidocaine 2% viscous solution isn't approved for teething pain. ∎
Adjust-a- dose (for all indications): Decrease dosage as needed based on patient's age, weight, and physical condition.
➤ **Urethra anesthesia and treatment of painful urethritis**
Male adults and children: Slowly instill 15 mL (300 mg lidocaine) 2% jelly into urethra using an easy syringelike action, until patient has a feeling of tension or until about 15 mL is instilled. Apply penile clamp for 5 to 10 minutes at the corona then, if needed, an additional 15 mL may be instilled as needed for adequate anesthesia. Before catheterization, 5 to 10 mL (100 to 200 mg) is usually adequate. Maximum dose for adults is 600 g in any 12-hour period. Maximum dose for children is 4.5 mg/kg.
Female adults and children: Slowly instill 3 to 5 mL (60 to 100 mg) of 2% jelly to urethra. A small amount of jelly may be applied to cotton swab and deposited into the urethral opening before instillation. Allow several minutes for anesthetic effect to occur. Maximum dose for adults is 600 g in any 12-hour period. Maximum dose for children is 4.5 mg/kg.

➤ **Anesthetic lubricant for endotracheal intubation**
Adults and children: Apply moderate amount of 2% jelly to external surface of endotracheal tube shortly before use. Maximum adult dose is 30 mL (600 mg) in any 12-hour period. Maximum dose in children is 4.5 mg/kg. Or, apply up to 5 g per single application, approximately 6 inches, of 5% ointment to external surface of endotracheal tube shortly before use. Maximum adult dose of 5% ointment is 20 g of ointment (equivalent to lidocaine base 1,000 mg) per day. Maximum dose in children is 4.5 mg/kg.
➤ **Topical anesthesia of accessible mucous membranes of oral and nasal cavities and proximal portions of digestive tract**
Adults and children age 10 and older: Apply 1 to 5 mL (40 to 200 mg) 4% oral topical solution to affected area as a spray, applied with cotton applicators or packs, as when instilled into a cavity. Maximum dose is 4.5 mg/kg, not to exceed 300 mg/dose.
Children younger than age 10 who have a normal lean body mass and normal body development: Apply 4% oral topical solution to affected area as a spray, applied with cotton applicators or packs, as when instilled into a cavity. May determine dose by applying one of the standard pediatric drug formulas. Maximum dose is 4.5 mg/kg.
➤ **Oropharynx anesthetic**
Adults and children (used in dentistry): Apply 5% ointment to previously dried oral mucosa. For use in adults with the insertion of new dentures, apply to all denture surfaces with mucosal contact. Maximum dose for adults is 5 g/single application (equivalent to lidocaine base 250 mg or 6 inches of ointment) or 20 g of ointment (equivalent to 1,000 g lidocaine base) per day. Patient should consult a dentist at least every 48 hours throughout denture-fitting period. Maximum dose for children is 5 g/single application (equivalent to 250 mg lidocaine base or approximately 6 inches of ointment) or 4.5 mg/kg lidocaine base.
Adults: 15 mL 2% solution swished in the mouth and spit out or gargled and swallowed no more frequently than every 3 hours. Maximum dose for adults is 4.5 mg/kg/dose (or 300 mg/dose); eight doses per 24 hours.
Children age 3 and older: Don't exceed 4.5 mg/kg/dose (or 300 mg/dose) swished in the mouth and spit out no more frequently than every 3 hours (four doses in 12 hours).
Children younger than age 3: 1.2 mL 2% solution applied to immediate area with a cotton-tipped applicator no more frequently than every 3 hours. Maximum is four doses in 12 hours and 1.2 mL/dose.
➤ **Skin discomfort (irritation, itching, pain)**
↻ **Alert:** For children weighing less than 10 kg, a single application should be applied over an area no greater than 100 cm². For children weighing between 10 and 20 kg, a single application should be applied over an area no greater than 600 cm².
Adults and children (5% ointment): Apply ointment topically for adequate control of symptoms. Maximum dose for adults is 5 g/single application (equivalent to

---

✷Canada   ◇ OTC   ◆ Off-label use   ✐Photoguide   ⓞⓣⓒDo not crush   *Liquid contains alcohol.

lidocaine base 250 mg or approximately 6 inches of ointment) or 20 g of ointment (equivalent to lidocaine base 1,000 mg)/day. Maximum dose for children is 5 g/single application (equivalent to lidocaine base 250 mg or approximately 6 inches of ointment), or 4.5 mg/kg lidocaine base.

Adults and children age 2 and older (cream, gel, spray): Apply 4% cream or 4% gel or spray to affected areas t.i.d. to q.i.d. Or apply 2% gel to affected areas t.i.d. as needed.

➤ **Local analgesia for venipuncture (Zingo)**
Adults and children age 3 and older: Apply one intra-dermal lidocaine (0.5 mg) device to site planned for venipuncture 1 to 3 minutes before needle insertion.

➤ **Anorectal discomfort**
Adults and children age 12 and older: Apply 5% cream or 5% gel up to six times a day.

➤ **Postherpetic neuralgia**
Adults: Apply 5% patch to most painful area for up to 12 hours in any 24-hour period. Maximum dose is 3 patches in a single application.

➤ **Ocular surface anesthesia (Akten)**
Adults and children: Apply 2 drops to ocular surface in area of planned procedure. Reapply as needed to maintain anesthetic effect.

lindane
LIN-dayn

Therapeutic class: Scabicides–pediculicides
Pharmacologic class: Ectoparasiticides–ovicides

AVAILABLE FORMS
Lotion: 1%
Shampoo: 1%

INDICATIONS & DOSAGES
Black Box Warning   Only use drug for scabies in patients who can't tolerate or have failed first-line treatment with safer medications. Drug can cause seizures and death. ∎

➤ **Parasitic infestation (scabies, pediculosis) in patients who can't tolerate other therapies or have failed treatment with other therapies**
Adults and children: For scabies, apply thin layer of lotion over entire skin surface from the neck down (with special attention to skin folds, creases, under fingernails, interdigital spaces, and genital area) and rub in thoroughly; for pediculosis, apply thin layer of lotion to hairy areas. After 8 to 12 hours, wash drug off.

Apply undiluted shampoo to dry hair and work into lather for 4 minutes; small amounts of water may increase lathering. Most patients require 30 mL of shampoo. Based on length and density of hair, some patients may require 60 mL. Rinse thoroughly and rub dry with towel. Comb with a fine-toothed comb.
Elderly patients: May need to reduce dosage because of increased skin absorption.

liothyronine sodium (T₃)
lye-oh-THYE-roe-neen

Cytomel, Triostat

Therapeutic class: Thyroid hormone replacements
Pharmacologic class: Thyroid hormones

AVAILABLE FORMS
Injection: 10 mcg/mL in 1-mL vials*
Tablets: 5 mcg, 25 mcg, 50 mcg

INDICATIONS & DOSAGES
Black Box Warning   Large doses of drug are toxic, particularly in combination with sympathomimetic amines commonly used in treatment of obesity. Drug is ineffective in weight loss for patients who are euthyroid. ∎

➤ **Congenital hypothyroidism**
Children: Initially, 5 mcg P.O. daily; increase by 5 mcg every 3 to 4 days until desired response is achieved. For maintenance: Infants may require only 20 mcg daily; children ages 1 to 3 may require 50 mcg daily; and children older than age 3 may require full adult dosage.

➤ **Myxedema**
Adults: Initially, 5 mcg P.O. daily; increase by 5 to 10 mcg every 1 to 2 weeks until daily dose reaches 25 mcg. Then increase by 5 to 25 mcg daily every 1 to 2 weeks. Maintenance dosage, 50 to 100 mcg daily.

➤ **Myxedema coma, premyxedema coma**
Adults: Initially, 10 to 20 mcg I.V. for patients with CV disease; 25 to 50 mcg I.V. for patients who don't have CV disease. Adjust dosage based on patient's condition and response. Switch patient to oral therapy as soon as possible.

➤ **Simple (nontoxic) goiter**
Adults: Initially, 5 mcg P.O. daily; may increase by 5 to 10 mcg daily every 1 to 2 weeks until daily dose reaches 25 mcg. Then increase by 12.5 to 25 mcg daily every 1 to 2 weeks. Usual maintenance dosage, 75 mcg daily.
Patients older than age 65 and children: 5 mcg daily; increase by 5 mcg daily every 1 to 2 weeks.

➤ **Thyroid hormone replacement**
Adults: Initially, 25 mcg P.O. daily; increase by up to 25 mcg every 1 to 2 weeks until satisfactory response occurs. Usual maintenance dosage, 25 to 75 mcg daily.

➤ **T₃ suppression test to differentiate hyperthyroidism from euthyroidism**
Adults: 75 to 100 mcg P.O. daily for 7 days.

♣ Canada   ◇ OTC   ♦ Off-label use   ✐ Photoguide   (mc) Do not crush   *Liquid contains alcohol.

liotrix
LYE-oh-trix

Thyrolar

Therapeutic class: Thyroid hormone replacements
Pharmacologic class: Thyroid hormones

AVAILABLE FORMS
Tablets: levothyroxine sodium 12.5 mcg and liothyronine sodium 3.1 mcg (Thyrolar-0.25); levothyroxine sodium 25 mcg and liothyronine sodium 6.25 mcg (Thyrolar-0.5); levothyroxine sodium 50 mcg and liothyronine sodium 12.5 mcg (Thyrolar-1); levothyroxine sodium 100 mcg and liothyronine sodium 25 mcg (Thyrolar-2); levothyroxine sodium 150 mcg and liothyronine sodium 37.5 mcg (Thyrolar-3)

INDICATIONS & DOSAGES
Black Box Warning   Large doses of drug are toxic, particularly in combination with sympathomimetic amines commonly used in treatment of obesity. Drug is ineffective in weight loss for patients who are euthyroid. ■

Dosages are expressed in thyroid equivalents and must be individualized to approximate the deficit in patient's thyroid secretion.
➤ **Hypothyroidism**
Adults: Initially, a single daily dose of Thyrolar-0.5. Adjust dosage by 1 tablet of Thyrolar-0.25 at 2- to 3-week intervals. Maintenance dose is 1 tablet of Thyrolar-1 or Thyrolar-2 daily. Readjust dosage within the first 4 weeks of therapy after proper clinical and laboratory evaluations of T_4 and TSH.
Adjust-a-dose: For elderly patients and patients with long-standing myxedema with CV impairment, initial dose is 1 tablet of Thyrolar-0.25 daily. Reduce dosage if angina occurs.
➤ **Congenital hypothyroidism**
Children older than age 12: More than 18.75/75 (T_3/T_4) mcg P.O. daily.
Children ages 6 to 12: 12.5/50 (T_3/T_4) to 18.75/75 (T_3/T_4) mcg P.O. daily.
Children ages 1 to 5: 9.35/37.5 (T_3/T_4) to 12.5/50 (T_3/T_4) mcg P.O. daily.
Children ages 6 to 12 months: 6.25/25 (T_3/T_4) to 9.35/37.5 (T_3/T_4) mcg P.O. daily.
Newborns and infants from birth to 6 months: 3.1/12.5 (T_3/T_4) to 6.25/25 (T_3/T_4) mcg P.O. daily.

lomustine (CCNU)
loe-MUS-teen

Gleostine

Therapeutic class: Antineoplastics
Pharmacologic class: Nitrosoureas

AVAILABLE FORMS
Capsules: 5 mg, 10 mg, 40 mg, 100 mg

INDICATIONS & DOSAGES
Black Box Warning   Drug can cause severe and fatal myelosuppression. Monitor blood cell counts weekly for at least 6 weeks after a dose. Patient should take only a single dose every 6 weeks. ■
➤ **Brain tumor, Hodgkin lymphoma**
Adults and children: 130 mg/m² P.O. as single dose every 6 weeks. Round doses to nearest 5 mg.
Adjust-a-dose: Reduce dosage to 100 mg/m² once every 6 weeks in patients with compromised bone marrow function. Refer to manufacturer's instructions for dosage adjustments for hematologic toxicity or when used with other myelosuppressive drugs.

loxapine
LOX-a-peen

Adasuve

loxapine succinate
Therapeutic class: Antipsychotics
Pharmacologic class: Dibenzapine derivatives

AVAILABLE FORMS
Capsules: 5 mg, 10 mg, 25 mg, 50 mg
Oral inhalation: 10 mg

INDICATIONS & DOSAGES
Black Box Warning   Elderly patients with dementia-related psychosis treated with atypical antipsychotics are at an increased risk of death. Not approved for treatment of dementia-related psychosis. ■
Black Box Warning   Inhalation drug can cause bronchospasm and respiratory distress and arrest. Only give drug in a facility equipped to handle acute bronchospasm. ■
➤ **Schizophrenia**
Adults: Initially, 10 mg P.O. b.i.d. In severely disturbed patients, up to 50 mg daily may be desirable. Increase dosage fairly rapidly over the first 7 to 10 days until symptoms are controlled. Usual therapeutic and maintenance range is 60 to 100 mg daily. Maximum dose is 250 mg/day.
➤ **Agitation associated with schizophrenia or bipolar I disorder**
Adults: 10 mg by oral inhalation once daily. Maximum dose is 10 mg/day.

luliconazole
loo-li-KON-a-zole

Luzu

Therapeutic class: Antifungals
Pharmacologic class: Azole antifungals

AVAILABLE FORMS
Cream: 1%

INDICATIONS & DOSAGES
➤ **Interdigital tinea pedis (athlete's foot) caused by** *Trichophyton rubrum* **or** *Epidermophyton floccosum*
Adults: Apply thin layer to affected area and approximately 1 inch (2.5 cm) of surrounding area once daily for 2 weeks.
➤ **Tinea cruris (jock itch) and tinea corporis (ringworm) caused by** *T. rubrum* **or** *E. floccosum*
Adults: Apply thin layer to affected area and approximately 1 inch (2.5 cm) of surrounding area once daily for 1 week.

mecasermin
meh-KAH-sur-men

Increlex

Therapeutic class: Growth factors
Pharmacologic class: Human insulin growth factors

AVAILABLE FORMS
Injection: 10 mg/mL

INDICATIONS & DOSAGES
➤ **Growth failure in children with severe primary insulin growth factor-1 (IGF-1) deficiency or children with growth hormone gene deletion who have developed neutralizing antibodies to growth hormone**
Children age 2 and older: Initially, 0.04 to 0.08 mg/kg subcutaneously b.i.d. If well tolerated for at least 1 week, may increase by 0.04 mg/kg per dose, to the maximum dose of 0.12 mg/kg b.i.d.

meloxicam
mel-OX-i-kam

Mobic, Mobicox✢

Therapeutic class: Antirheumatics
Pharmacologic class: NSAIDs

AVAILABLE FORMS
Oral suspension: 7.5 mg/5 mL
Tablets: 7.5 mg, 15 mg

INDICATIONS & DOSAGES
Black Box Warning NSAIDs may increase risk of serious CV thrombotic events, MI, stroke, and GI adverse reactions. Contraindicated for use in CABG surgery. ■
➤ **To relieve signs and symptoms of osteoarthritis or RA**
Adults: 7.5 mg P.O. once daily. May increase as needed to maximum dosage of 15 mg daily.
➤ **To relieve signs and symptoms of pauciarticular or polyarticular course juvenile RA**
Children ages 2 to 17: 0.125 mg/kg P.O. once daily to a maximum dosage of 7.5 mg daily.

menotropins
men-oh-TROE-pins

Menopur

Therapeutic class: Ovulation stimulants
Pharmacologic class: Gonadotropins

AVAILABLE FORMS
Injection: 75 international units of luteinizing hormone and 75 international units of FSH activity per ampule

INDICATIONS & DOSAGES
➤ **Assisted reproductive technologies**
Adults: Initially, 225 units subcutaneously into lower abdomen starting on cycle day 2 or 3. Menopur may be used in combination with urofollitropin, but total initial dose of both shouldn't exceed 225 units (150 international units of menotropins and 75 international units of urofollitropin or 75 international units of menotropins and 150 international units of urofollitropin). Adjust dosage after 5 days, based on ovarian response. Don't make additional adjustments more frequently than every 2 days and not to exceed 150 units per adjustment. Maximum daily dosage is 450 units. Use for maximum of 20 days. Then, 5,000 to 10,000 units of human chorionic gonadotropin after adequate follicular development.

mepolizumab
meh-po-LIZZ-ue-mabb

Nucala

Therapeutic class: Miscellaneous respiratory drugs
Pharmacologic class: Monoclonal antibodies

AVAILABLE FORMS
Injection: 100-mg single-dose vial

INDICATIONS & DOSAGES
➤ **Add-on maintenance treatment of severe asthma in patients with an eosinophilic phenotype**
Adults and children age 12 and older: 100 mg subcutaneously every 4 weeks into upper arm, thigh, or abdomen.

✢Canada ◇ OTC ◆ Off-label use ✎Photoguide ⓓⓝⓒ Do not crush *Liquid contains alcohol.

methocarbamol
meth-oh-KAR-ba-mal

Robaxin, Robaxin-750

Therapeutic class: Skeletal muscle relaxants

Pharmacologic class: CNS depressants

AVAILABLE FORMS
Injection: 1,000 mg/10 mL vials
Tablets: 500 mg, 750 mg

INDICATIONS & DOSAGES
➤ **As adjunct to rest, physical therapy, and other measures for relief of discomfort associated with acute, painful musculoskeletal conditions**
Adults and children older than age 16: Initially 1,500 mg P.O. q.i.d. for first 48 to 72 hours. For severe conditions, may increase up to 8,000 mg/day P.O. in divided doses. For maintenance therapy, give 1,000 mg P.O. q.i.d., or 1,500 mg P.O. t.i.d., or 750 mg P.O. every 4 hours. Or, initially, 1,000 mg I.V. or I.M. every 8 hours, with maximum dose of 3,000 mg/day for no more than 3 consecutive days. May repeat course after a drug-free interval of 48 hours.
Adjust-a-dose: Base dosage adjustment and frequency of injection on severity of condition and therapeutic response. For moderate symptoms, one dose of 1 g I.V. or I.M. may be adequate.
➤ **Tetanus, in addition to standard treatment**
Adults: Initially, 1,000 to 2,000 mg by direct I.V. injection, which may be followed by an additional 1,000 to 2,000 mg I.V., with maximum initial dose of 3,000 mg total. May repeat initial dosage I.V. every 6 hours until NG tube or oral therapy is possible; total oral daily dose of up to 2,400 mg may be needed. Don't use injection for more than 3 consecutive days.
Children: Initially, give minimum dose of 15 mg/kg or 500 mg/m^2 I.V.; may repeat every 6 hours if needed. Maximum dose is 1.8 g/m^2/day I.V. for 3 consecutive days.

methylergonovine maleate
meth-ill-er-goe-NOE-veen

Methergine

Therapeutic class: Oxytocics
Pharmacologic class: Ergot alkaloids

AVAILABLE FORMS
Injection: 0.2 mg/mL in 1-mL ampules
Tablets: 0.2 mg

INDICATIONS & DOSAGES
➤ **To prevent and treat postpartum hemorrhage caused by uterine atony or subinvolution**
Adults: 0.2 mg I.M. or I.V. after delivery of the anterior shoulder, after delivery of the placenta, or during puerperium. May repeat every 2 to 4 hours as needed.
During life-threatening emergencies, 0.2 mg I.V. over at least 1 minute while monitoring BP and uterine contractions. After first I.M. or I.V. dose, 0.2 mg P.O. every 6 to 8 hours for up to 7 days. Decrease dosage if severe cramping occurs.

metreleptin
MET-re-LEP-tin

Myalept

Therapeutic class: Hormone replacements
Pharmacologic class: Leptin receptor agonists

AVAILABLE FORMS
Injection: 11.3-mg vial (5 mg/mL when reconstituted)

INDICATIONS & DOSAGES
Black Box Warning Drug is linked to risk of T-cell lymphoma and production of anti-metreleptin antibodies. Although complete significance is unknown, severe infection or loss of effectiveness could be associated with development of anti-metreleptin antibodies. ■
➤ **Adjunct to diet as replacement therapy to treat complications of leptin deficiency in patients with congenital or acquired generalized lipodystrophy**
Adults and children: For patients weighing 40 kg or less, starting dose is 0.06 mg/kg/day subcutaneously; increase or decrease based on clinical response by 0.02 mg/kg to maximum daily dose of 0.13 mg/kg. For males weighing more than 40 kg, starting dose is 2.5 mg/day subcutaneously; increase or decrease by 1.25 to 2.5 mg/day to maximum dose of 10 mg/day. For females weighing more than 40 kg, starting dose is 5 mg/day subcutaneously; increase or decrease by 1.25 to 2.5 mg/day to maximum dose of 10 mg/day.

miltefosine
mil-te-FOS-een

Impavido

Therapeutic class: Antiprotozoals
Pharmacologic class: Antileishmanials

AVAILABLE FORMS
Capsules ⓞⓝⓔ: 50 mg

INDICATIONS & DOSAGES
Black Box Warning Drug can cause fetal harm, including death. Don't use during pregnancy. Effective contraception is required during and for 5 months after therapy. ■
➤ **Visceral leishmaniasis caused by *Leishmania donovani*; cutaneous leishmaniasis caused by *L. braziliensis*, *L. guyanensis*, or *L. panamensis*; mucosal leishmaniasis caused by *L. braziliensis***
Adults and adolescents age 12 and older weighing 45 kg) or more: 50 mg P.O. t.i.d. with food (breakfast, lunch, and dinner) for 28 days.

Adults and adolescents age 12 and older weighing 30 to 44 kg: 50 mg P.O. b.i.d. with food (breakfast and dinner) for 28 days.

misoprostol
mye-soe-PROST-ole

Cytotec

Therapeutic class: Antiulcer drugs
Pharmacologic class: Prostaglandin E₁ analogues

AVAILABLE FORMS
Tablets: 100 mcg, 200 mcg

INDICATIONS & DOSAGES
Black Box Warning Drug can cause abortion, premature birth, birth defects, and uterine rupture and is contraindicated during pregnancy.
➤ **To prevent NSAID-induced gastric ulcer in patients at high risk for complications from gastric ulcer and in patients with history of NSAID-induced ulcer**
Adults: 200 mcg P.O. q.i.d. with food; if not tolerated, decrease to 100 mcg P.O. q.i.d. Give dosage for duration of NSAID therapy.

moexipril hydrochloride
moe-EX-eh-pril

Therapeutic class: Antihypertensives
Pharmacologic class: ACE inhibitors

AVAILABLE FORMS
Tablets: 7.5 mg, 15 mg

INDICATIONS & DOSAGES
Black Box Warning Drug can cause fetal harm; when pregnancy is detected, discontinue as soon as possible. ∎
➤ **Hypertension, alone or in combination with thiazide diuretics**
Adults: Initially, 7.5 mg P.O. once daily as monotherapy, given 1 hour before a meal. Or initially, 3.75 mg if diuretic therapy can't be discontinued. Increase dosage incrementally according to BP response. Maximum dosage is 60 mg daily in one or two divided doses.
Adjust-a-dose: For patients currently being treated with a diuretic, if possible stop diuretic 2 to 3 days before therapy is initiated to reduce likelihood of hypotension. If BP isn't adequately controlled with moexipril alone, may reinstitute diuretic therapy. For patients with CrCl of 40 mL/minute/1.73 m² or less, cautiously give initial dose of 3.75 mg once daily. May titrate dosage upward to a maximum daily dosage of 15 mg.

nabumetone
nah-BYOO-meh-tone

Therapeutic class: NSAIDs
Pharmacologic class: NSAIDs

AVAILABLE FORMS
Tablets: 500 mg, 750 mg

INDICATIONS & DOSAGES
Black Box Warning NSAIDs may increase risk of serious CV thrombotic events, MI, stroke, and GI adverse reactions. Contraindicated for use in CABG surgery. ∎
➤ **RA, osteoarthritis**
Adults: Initially, 1,000 mg P.O. daily as a single dose or in two divided doses. Maximum, 2,000 mg daily.
Adjust-a-dose: For patients with CrCl of 30 to 49 mL/minute, maximum starting dosage shouldn't exceed 750 mg P.O. once daily; with careful monitoring, daily doses may be increased to a maximum of 1,500 mg. For patients with CrCl less than 30 mL/minute, the maximum starting dosage shouldn't exceed 500 mg P.O. once daily; with careful monitoring, daily doses may be increased to a maximum of 1,000 mg.

nefazodone hydrochloride
ne-FAZ-oh-done

Therapeutic class: Antidepressants
Pharmacologic class: Antidepressants

AVAILABLE FORMS
Tablets: 50 mg, 100 mg, 150 mg, 200 mg, 250 mg

INDICATIONS & DOSAGES
➤ **Depression**
Adults: Initially, 100 mg/day P.O. b.i.d. Increase dosage in increments of 100 to 200 mg/day in two divided doses at intervals of no less than 1 week. Effective dosage range is 300 to 600 mg/day.
Adjust-a-dose: In elderly or debilitated patients, especially women, initially 50 mg P.O. b.i.d.

SAFETY ALERT!

nelarabine
neh-LAR-uh-been

Arranon, Atriance✤

Therapeutic class: Antineoplastics
Pharmacologic class: DNA demethylation agents; prodrugs of cytotoxic deoxyguanosine

AVAILABLE FORMS
Injection: 5 mg/mL in 50-mL vial

✤ Canada ◇ OTC ◆ Off-label use ✐ Photoguide ⒹⓄⒸ Do not crush *Liquid contains alcohol.

INDICATIONS & DOSAGES

Black Box Warning Severe neurologic adverse reactions have been reported, including altered mental states (e.g., severe somnolence), CNS effects (e.g., seizures), and peripheral neuropathy, ranging from numbness and paresthesia to motor weakness and paralysis. ∎

➤ **T-cell acute lymphoblastic leukemia and T-cell lymphoblastic lymphoma in patients whose disease hasn't responded to or has relapsed after treatment with at least two chemotherapy regimens**

Adults: 1,500 mg/m² I.V. over 2 hours on days 1, 3, and 5. Repeat every 21 days.

Children: 650 mg/m² I.V. over 1 hour daily for 5 consecutive days. Repeat every 21 days.

---

nimodipine
nye-MOE-dih-peen

Nymalize

Therapeutic class: Vasodilators
Pharmacologic class: Calcium channel blockers

AVAILABLE FORMS

Capsules: 30 mg
Oral solution: 60 mg/20 mL

INDICATIONS & DOSAGES

Black Box Warning Don't administer parenterally; may cause life-threatening reactions and death. ∎

➤ **To improve neurologic deficits after subarachnoid hemorrhage from ruptured intracranial berry aneurysm**

Adults: 60 mg P.O. every 4 hours for 21 days. Begin therapy within 96 hours after subarachnoid hemorrhage.

Adjust-a-dose: For patients with hepatic failure, 30 mg P.O. every 4 hours for 21 days.

---

nintedanib
nin-TED-a-nib

Ofev

Therapeutic class: Miscellaneous respiratory drugs
Pharmacologic class: Tyrosine kinase inhibitors

AVAILABLE FORMS

Capsules ⓓⓝⓒ: 100 mg, 150 mg

INDICATIONS & DOSAGES

➤ **Idiopathic pulmonary fibrosis**

Adults: 150 mg P.O. b.i.d. approximately 12 hours apart.

Adjust-a-dose: If adverse reactions occur, reduce dosage to 100 mg P.O. b.i.d. or temporarily interrupt treatment. If AST or ALT level is greater than 3 × ULN but less than 5 × ULN without signs or symptoms of severe liver damage, may reduce dosage to 100 mg P.O. b.i.d. or may interrupt treatment. Once

liver enzyme levels have returned to baseline values, may reinitiate at 100 mg b.i.d. and subsequently increase to full dosage of 150 mg b.i.d. If AST or ALT level is more than 5 × ULN or more than 3 × ULN with signs or symptoms of severe liver damage, discontinue drug.

---

nisoldipine
nye-SOHL-di-peen

Sular

Therapeutic class: Antihypertensives
Pharmacologic class: Calcium channel blockers

AVAILABLE FORMS

Tablets (extended-release) ⓓⓝⓒ: 8.5 mg, 17 mg, 20 mg, 25.5 mg, 30 mg, 34 mg, 40 mg

INDICATIONS & DOSAGES

➤ **Hypertension**

Adults: Initially, 17 mg (Sular) P.O. once daily, increased by 8.5 mg/week or at longer intervals, as needed. Usual maintenance dose is 17 to 34 mg daily. Doses of more than 34 mg daily aren't recommended. Or, initially, 20 mg (extended release) P.O. once daily, increased by 10 mg per week or at longer intervals as needed. Usual maintenance dose is 20 to 40 mg daily. Doses of more than 60 mg daily aren't recommended.

Patients older than age 65: Initially, 8.5 or 10 mg P.O. once daily; adjust dosage as for other adults.

Adjust-a-dose: For patients with hepatic impairment, initial dose shouldn't exceed 10 mg (extended release or 8.5 mg (Sular) P.O. once daily.

---

nitazoxanide
nye-te-ZOCKS-a-nide

Alinia

Therapeutic class: Antiprotozoals
Pharmacologic class: Antiprotozoals

AVAILABLE FORMS

Oral suspension: 100 mg/5 mL
Tablets: 500 mg

INDICATIONS & DOSAGES

➤ **Diarrhea caused by** *Cryptosporidium parvum* **or** *Giardia lamblia*

Adults and children age 12 and older: 500 mg P.O. with food every 12 hours for 3 days.

Children ages 4 to 11: 200 mg (10 mL) P.O. with food every 12 hours for 3 days.

Children ages 1 to 3: 100 mg (5 mL) P.O. with food every 12 hours for 3 days.

SAFETY ALERT!

olaparib
oh-LAP-a-rib

Lynparza

Therapeutic class: Antineoplastics
Pharmacologic class: Poly ADP-ribose
polymerase inhibitors

AVAILABLE FORMS
Capsules ⓒⓝⓒ: 50 mg

INDICATIONS & DOSAGES
➤ **Deleterious or suspected deleterious germline** *BRCA*-**mutated advanced ovarian cancer, as detected by FDA-approved test, in women who have been treated with three or more prior lines of chemotherapy**
Adults: 400 mg (eight 50-mg capsules) P.O. b.i.d. for a total daily dose of 800 mg. Continue treatment until disease progression or unacceptable toxicity occurs.
Adjust-a-dose: To manage adverse reactions, reduce dosage to 200 mg (four 50-mg capsules) P.O. b.i.d., for a total daily dose of 400 mg; if a further final dosage reduction is required, reduce to 100 mg (two 50-mg capsules) b.i.d., for a total daily dose of 200 mg. If drug must be given with a CYP3A inhibitor, reduce dosage to 150 mg (three 50-mg capsules) b.i.d. if patient is also taking a concurrent strong CYP3A inhibitor or 200 mg (four 50-mg capsules) b.i.d. if taking a concurrent moderate CYP3A inhibitor.

olopatadine hydrochloride
oh-loh-PAT-ah-dine

Pataday, Patanase, Patanol, Pazeo

Therapeutic class: Antihistamines
Pharmacologic class: H$_1$-receptor antagonists

AVAILABLE FORMS
Nasal spray: 0.6%
Ophthalmic solution: 0.1%, 0.2%, 0.7%

INDICATIONS & DOSAGES
➤ **Seasonal allergic rhinitis (nasal)**
Adults and children age 12 and older: 2 sprays into each nostril b.i.d.
Children ages 6 to 11: 1 spray into each nostril b.i.d.
➤ **Allergic conjunctivitis**
Adults and children age 3 and older (Patanol): 1 drop (0.1%) in each affected eye b.i.d. at an interval of 6 to 8 hours.
Adults and children age 2 and older (Pataday, Pazeo): 1 drop (0.2%, 0.7%) in each affected eye once a day.

oprelvekin
oh-PRELL-veh-kin

Neumega

Therapeutic class: Hematopoietics
Pharmacologic class: Recombinant human interleukins

AVAILABLE FORMS
Injection: 5-mg single-dose vial with diluent

INDICATIONS & DOSAGES
| **Black Box Warning** | May cause anaphylaxis. Permanently discontinue drug for any allergic or hypersensitivity reaction. ∎
➤ **To prevent severe thrombocytopenia and reduce need for platelet transfusions after myelosuppressive chemotherapy with nonmyeloid malignancies**
Adults: 50 mcg/kg as single daily subcutaneous injection until postnadir platelet count is at least 50,000/mm^3. Treatment beyond 21 days per course isn't recommended. Begin dosing 6 to 24 hours after completion of chemotherapy. Discontinue drug at least 2 days before the start of the next planned cycle of chemotherapy.
Adjust-a-dose: In patients with CrCl less than 30 mL/minute, recommended dosage is 25 mcg/kg daily.

orlistat
ORE-lah-stat

Alli ◇, Xenical

Therapeutic class: Antiobesity drugs
Pharmacologic class: Lipase inhibitors

AVAILABLE FORMS
Capsules: 60 mg ◇, 120 mg

INDICATIONS & DOSAGES
➤ **To manage obesity, including weight loss and weight maintenance with a reduced-calorie diet; to reduce risk of weight gain after previous weight loss**
Adults and children ages 12 and older: 120 mg P.O. t.i.d. with or up to 1 hour after each main meal containing fat.
➤ **Weight loss (OTC formulation)**
Adults age 18 and older: One 60-mg capsule P.O. with each meal containing fat. Dosage shouldn't exceed 3 capsules a day.

SAFETY ALERT!

panitumumab
pan-eh-TOO-moo-mab

Vectibix

Therapeutic class: Antineoplastics
Pharmacologic class: Monoclonal antibodies

AVAILABLE FORMS
Solution for infusion: 20 mg/mL

INDICATIONS & DOSAGES
Black Box Warning Dermatologic toxicities occur in 90% of patients and are severe in 15%. ■
➤ **Wild-type KRAS (exon 2 in codons 12 or 13) metastatic colorectal cancer as determined by FDA-approved test: as first-line therapy in combination with FOLFOX (5-FU, leucovorin, oxaliplatin); as monotherapy following disease progression during or after fluoropyrimidine-, oxaliplatin-, and irinotecan-containing regimens**
Adults: 6 mg/kg I.V. infusion over 60 minutes every 14 days as a single agent or in combination with FOLFOX. For doses greater than 1,000 mg, infuse over 90 minutes.
Adjust-a-dose: For patients with mild or moderate (grade 1 or 2) infusion reactions, reduce infusion rate by 50%. For patients with severe infusion reactions, stop drug permanently. Refer to manufacturer's instructions for dosage adjustments for dermatologic toxicity.

parathyroid hormone
par-a-THYE-roid

Natpara

Therapeutic class: Hormone replacements
Pharmacologic class: Parathyroid hormone analogues

AVAILABLE FORMS
Injection: 25 mcg, 50 mcg, 75 mcg, 100 mcg multidose cartridges

INDICATIONS & DOSAGES
➤ **Adjunct to calcium and vitamin D to control hypocalcemia in patients with hypoparathyroidism who can't be well controlled on calcium supplements and active forms of vitamin D alone**
Adults: Initially, 50 mcg subcutaneously once daily. Titrate maintenance dose to lowest dose that achieves a total albumin-corrected serum calcium level within the lower half of the normal total serum calcium range (between 8 and 9 mg/dL) without the need for active forms of vitamin D and with calcium supplementation sufficient to meet daily requirements.
Adjust-a-dose: If albumin-corrected serum calcium level can't be maintained above 8 mg/dL without an active form of vitamin D and/or oral calcium supple-

mentation, may increase Natpara dosage in increments of 25 mcg every 4 weeks to a maximum daily dose of 100 mcg. If total serum calcium level is repeatedly above 9 mg/dL after active form of vitamin D has been discontinued and calcium supplement has been decreased to a dosage sufficient to meet daily requirements, may decrease Natpara dosage to 25 mcg/day.

patiromer sorbitex calcium
pa-TIR-oh-mer

Veltassa

Therapeutic class: Potassium-removing resins
Pharmacologic class: Cation exchange polymers

AVAILABLE FORMS
Oral powder: 8.4-g, 16.8-g, 25.2-g packets

INDICATIONS & DOSAGES
Black Box Warning Patiromer may decrease GI absorption and cause loss of efficacy of other drugs when given close in time to other oral drugs. Give other oral drugs at least 6 hours before or 6 hours after patiromer. ■
➤ **Nonemergency treatment of hyperkalemia**
Adults: Initially, 8.4 g P.O. once daily. Monitor serum potassium level and adjust dosage based on potassium level at intervals of 1 week or longer, in increments of 8.4 g, to reach desired potassium concentration. Maximum dosage is 25.2 g once daily.

SAFETY ALERT!

pazopanib
paz-OH-pa-nib

Votrient

Therapeutic class: Antineoplastics
Pharmacologic class: Multi-tyrosine kinase inhibitors

AVAILABLE FORMS
Tablets: 200 mg

INDICATIONS & DOSAGES
Black Box Warning Severe and fatal hepatotoxicity has been observed in clinical trials. ■
➤ **Advanced renal cell carcinoma, soft-tissue sarcoma in patients who have received prior chemotherapy**
Adults: 800 mg P.O. daily at least 1 hour before or 2 hours after a meal.
Adjust-a-dose: For patients with moderate hepatic impairment, 200 mg P.O. daily. Drug isn't recommended for patients with severe hepatic impairment. When coadministration of strong CYP3A4 inhibitors (clarithromycin, ketoconazole, ritonavir) is necessary, decrease pazopanib dosage to 400 mg P.O. daily.

✤ Canada   ◇ OTC   ◆ Off-label use   ✐ Photoguide   ⓓⓒ Do not crush   *Liquid contains alcohol.

peginterferon beta-1a
peg-in-ter-FEER-on

Plegridy

Therapeutic class: Antivirals
Pharmacologic class: Biological response modifiers

AVAILABLE FORMS
Injection: 125 mcg/0.5 mL in single-dose prefilled pens or syringes

INDICATIONS & DOSAGES
➤ **Relapsing forms of MS**
Adults: On day 1, 63 mcg subcutaneously. On day 15, 94 mcg subcutaneously. On day 29 and every 14 days thereafter, 125 mcg subcutaneously.

SAFETY ALERT!

pembrolizumab
PEM-broe-liz-ue-mab

Keytruda

Therapeutic class: Antineoplastics
Pharmacologic class: Monoclonal antibodies

AVAILABLE FORMS
Injection: 50-mg single-use vial

INDICATIONS & DOSAGES
Adjust-a-dose (for all indications): Refer to manufacturer's instructions for toxicity-related dosage adjustments.
➤ **Unresectable or metastatic melanoma; metastatic non-small-cell lung cancer (NSCLC) in patients whose tumors express PD-L1 as determined by an FDA-approved test and who have disease progression on or after platinum-containing chemotherapy**
Adults: 2 mg/kg I.V. infusion over 30 minutes every 3 weeks until disease progression or unacceptable toxicity occurs.
✳ **NEW INDICATION: Recurrent or metastatic head and neck squamous cell carcinoma in patients with disease progression on or after platinum-containing chemotherapy; first-line treatment for metastatic NSCLC in patients whose tumors have high PD-L1 expression and don't have EGFR or ALK genomic tumor aberrations**
Adults: 200 mg I.V. infusion over 30 minutes every 3 weeks until disease progression or unacceptable toxicity, or up to 24 months in patients without disease progression on drug.

pentoxifylline
pen-tox-IH-fi-leen

Pentoxil

Therapeutic class: Hemorrheologic drugs
Pharmacologic class: Xanthine derivatives

AVAILABLE FORMS
Tablets (extended-release): 400 mg

INDICATIONS & DOSAGES
➤ **Intermittent claudication from chronic occlusive vascular disease**
Adults: 400 mg P.O. t.i.d. with meals for at least 8 weeks. May decrease to 400 mg b.i.d. if GI and CNS adverse effects occur. If adverse effects persist, discontinue drug.
Adjust-a-dose: For CrCl of 10 to 50 mL/minute, give usual dose every 12 to 24 hours. For CrCl of less than 10 mL/minute, give usual dose every 24 hours. For patients undergoing peritoneal dialysis, give usual dose every 24 hours.

peramivir
per-AM-i-vir

Rapivab

Therapeutic class: Antivirals
Pharmacologic class: Neuraminidase inhibitors

AVAILABLE FORMS
Injection: 200 mg/20 mL (10 mg/mL) vials

INDICATIONS & DOSAGES
➤ **Acute uncomplicated influenza in patients age 18 and older who have been symptomatic for no more than 2 days**
Adults: 600-mg I.V. infusion over 15 to 30 minutes as a single dose.
Adjust-a-dose: For patients with CrCl of 30 to 49 mL/minute, dose is 200 mg; for patients with CrCl of 10 to 29 mL/minute, dose is 100 mg. For patients with chronic kidney disease maintained on dialysis, give after dialysis session at a dose adjusted for renal function.

perindopril erbumine
pur-IN-doh-pril

Aceon, Coversyl ✤

Therapeutic class: Antihypertensives
Pharmacologic class: ACE inhibitors

AVAILABLE FORMS
Tablets: 2 mg, 4 mg, 8 mg

✤Canada   ◇ OTC   ◆ Off-label use   ✐Photoguide   ⓓⓝⓒDo not crush   *Liquid contains alcohol.

INDICATIONS & DOSAGES

Black Box Warning May cause fetal harm; when pregnancy is detected, discontinue drug as soon as possible. ∎

Adjust-a-dose (for all indications): For patients with renal insufficiency and CrCl of 30 mL/minute or greater, initially 2 mg P.O. daily. Maximum daily maintenance dose is 8 mg. Not recommended for patients with CrCl of less than 30 mL/minute. For inpatients taking diuretics, reduce the diuretic dose before initiating drug and monitor BP closely. Adjust dosage based on patient's BP response.

➤ **To reduce the risk of CV death or nonfatal MI in patients with stable CAD**

Adults age 70 or younger: 4 mg P.O. once daily for 2 weeks; then, increase as tolerated to 8 mg once daily. *Adults older than age 70:* Initially, 2 mg P.O. once daily for the first week; then, 4 mg once daily for the second week and 8 mg once daily after that, if tolerated.

➤ **Essential hypertension**

Adults: Initially, 4 mg P.O. once daily. Increase dosage until BP is controlled or to maximum of 16 mg/day; usual maintenance dosage is 4 to 8 mg once daily; may be given in two divided doses.

Adults older than age 65: Initially, 4 mg P.O. daily as one dose or in two divided doses. May increase dosage by more than 8 mg/day with careful BP monitoring.

permethrin
per-METH-rin

Elimite, Kwellada-P✚ ◇ , Nix ◇

Therapeutic class: Scabicides–pediculicides
Pharmacologic class: Pyrethroids

AVAILABLE FORMS
Cream: 5%
Lotion: 1% ◇

INDICATIONS & DOSAGES

➤ **Infestation with *Pediculus humanus capitis* (head louse) and its nits (lotion)**

Adults and children age 2 months and older: Use after hair has been washed with shampoo, rinsed with water, and towel dried. Apply 25 to 50 mL of liquid to saturate hair and scalp. Allow drug to remain on hair for 10 minutes before rinsing off with warm water. Remove remaining nits with comb. Usually only one application is needed. May repeat 7 days after first treatment if lice or nits are still present.

➤ **Infestation with *Sarcoptes scabiei* (cream)**

Adults and children age 2 months and older: Thoroughly massage into the skin from the head to the soles of feet. Treat infants on hairline, neck, scalp, temple, and forehead. Wash cream off after 8 to 14 hours. Usually one application is needed. May retreat if living mites are observed 14 days after first treatment.

perphenazine
per-FEN-uh-zeen

Therapeutic class: Antipsychotics
Pharmacologic class: Phenothiazines

AVAILABLE FORMS
Tablets: 2 mg, 4 mg, 8 mg, 16 mg

INDICATIONS & DOSAGES

Black Box Warning Not approved to treat patients with dementia-related psychosis. Use with opioids can cause death. ∎

➤ **Schizophrenia in nonhospitalized patients**

Adults and children older than age 12: Initially, 4 to 8 mg P.O. t.i.d.; reduce as soon as possible to minimum effective dose.

➤ **Schizophrenia in hospitalized patients**

Adults and children older than age 12: Initially, 8 to 16 mg P.O. b.i.d., t.i.d., or q.i.d.; increase to 64 mg daily, as needed.

➤ **Severe nausea and vomiting**

Adults: 8 to 16 mg P.O. daily in divided doses to maximum of 24 mg.

phenelzine sulfate
FEN-el-zeen

Nardil

Therapeutic class: Antidepressants
Pharmacologic class: MAO inhibitors

AVAILABLE FORMS
Tablets: 15 mg

INDICATIONS & DOSAGES

➤ **Depression clinically characterized as atypical, nonendogenous, or neurotic in patients who failed to respond to other therapy**

Adults: Initially, 15 mg P.O. t.i.d. Increase to at least 60 mg/day as tolerated. Many patients don't show a clinical response until treatment at 60 mg has been continued for at least 4 weeks. May increase to maximum dosage of 90 mg/day to achieve clinical response. After maximum benefit is achieved, slowly reduce dosage over several weeks as tolerated. Maintenance dose may be as low as 15 mg daily or every other day. Continue as long as needed.

pirfenidone
peer-FEH-nih-dohn

Esbriet

Therapeutic class: Miscellaneous respiratory drugs
Pharmacologic class: Antifibrotics

AVAILABLE FORMS
Capsules ⓒ*:* 267 mg

INDICATIONS & DOSAGES
➤ **Idiopathic pulmonary fibrosis**
Adults: Initially, 1 capsule P.O. t.i.d. with food for days 1 to 7 of therapy; then increase to 2 capsules (534 mg) P.O. t.i.d. with food for 7 more days (days 8 to 14); then increase to 3 capsules (801 mg) P.O. t.i.d. starting on day 15 of therapy. Maintenance dosage is 801 mg P.O. t.i.d. Maximum dosage is 9 capsules (2,403 mg)/day.
Adjust-a-dose: Refer to manufacturer's instructions for toxicity-related dosage adjustments.

plerixafor
pleh-RIX-uh-for

Mozobil

Therapeutic class: Hematopoietics
Pharmacologic class: CXCR4 chemokine receptor inhibitors

AVAILABLE FORMS
Injection: 24 mg/1.2 mL in single-use vial

INDICATIONS & DOSAGES
➤ **To mobilize hematopoietic stem cells for collection and subsequent autologous transplantation in patients with non-Hodgkin lymphoma and multiple myeloma**
Adults: For patients weighing 83 kg or less, 20 mg fixed dose or 0.24 mg/kg. Or, for patients weighing more than 83 kg, 0.24 mg/kg. Use actual body weight and administer subcutaneously once daily beginning about 11 hours before apheresis for up to 4 consecutive days. Begin treatment after patient receives 4 days of granulocyte-colony stimulating factor therapy. Don't exceed 40 mg/day.
Adjust-a-dose: For patients with CrCl of 50 mL/minute or less and weighing 83 kg or less, give 13 mg or 0.16 mg/kg once daily. For patients with CrCl of 50 mL/minute or less and weighing more than 83 kg and less than 160 kg, give 0.16 mg/kg once daily (not to exceed 27 mg/day).

potassium iodide
po-TASS-ee-um

Iosat ◇, ThyroSafe ◇, ThyroShield ◇

Therapeutic class: Antihyperthyroid drugs
Pharmacologic class: Salts of stable iodine

AVAILABLE FORMS
Oral solution: 65 mg/mL
Tablets: 65 mg, 130 mg

INDICATIONS & DOSAGES
➤ **Radiation protectant for thyroid gland (Iosat, ThyroSafe, ThyroShield)**
Adults and children ages 12 to 18 weighing at least 68 kg: 130 mg P.O. every 24 hours for 10 to 14 days as directed by public health authorities. Start no later

than 3 to 4 hours after exposure. Avoid repeat dosing in pregnant or breast-feeding women.
Children ages 3 to 12 or children ages 12 to 18 weighing less than 68 kg: 65 mg P.O. every 24 hours as directed by public health authorities. Start no later than 3 to 4 hours after exposure.
Children older than 1 month to 3 years: 32.5 mg P.O. every 24 hours as directed by public health authorities. Start no later than 3 to 4 hours after exposure.
Neonates from birth to 1 month: 16.25 mg P.O. every 24 hours as directed by public health authorities. Start no later than 3 to 4 hours after exposure. Avoid repeat dosing, if possible.

SAFETY ALERT!

pralatrexate
PRAL-ah-TREX-ate

Folotyn

Therapeutic class: Antineoplastics
Pharmacologic class: Folate analogue metabolic inhibitors

AVAILABLE FORMS
Injection: 20 mg/mL, 40 mg/2 mL in single-use vials

INDICATIONS & DOSAGES
➤ **Relapsed or refractory peripheral T-cell lymphoma**
Adults: 30 mg/m^2 I.V. push over 3 to 5 minutes weekly for 6 weeks in 7-week cycles until disease progresses or unacceptable toxicity develops.
Adjust-a-dose: Refer to manufacturer's instructions for dosage adjustments for hematologic and nonhematologic toxicities.

primidone
PRI-mi-done

Mysoline

Therapeutic class: Anticonvulsants
Pharmacologic class: Barbiturate analogues

AVAILABLE FORMS
Tablets: 50 mg, 250 mg

INDICATIONS & DOSAGES
➤ **Grand mal, psychomotor, and focal epileptic seizures**
Adults and children age 8 and older: Initially, 100 to 125 mg P.O. at bedtime on days 1 to 3; then 100 to 125 mg P.O. b.i.d. on days 4 to 6; then 100 to 125 mg P.O. t.i.d. on days 7 to 9, followed by maintenance dose of 250 mg P.O. t.i.d. May increase maintenance dose to 250 mg q.i.d., if needed. May increase dosage to maximum of 2 g daily in divided doses. See manufacturer's instructions for beginning therapy in patients already receiving other anticonvulsants.

Children younger than age 8: Initially, 50 mg P.O. at bedtime for 3 days; then 50 mg P.O. b.i.d. for days 4 to 6; then 100 mg P.O. b.i.d. for days 7 to 9, followed by maintenance dose of 125 to 250 mg P.O. t.i.d. or 10 to 25 mg/kg daily in divided doses.

probenecid
proe-BEN-e-sid

Benuryl ✤, Probalan

Therapeutic class: Uricosurics
Pharmacologic class: Sulfonamide derivatives

AVAILABLE FORMS
Tablets: 500 mg

INDICATIONS & DOSAGES
➤ **Adjunct to penicillin therapy**
Adults and children age 15 and older weighing more than 50 kg: 500 mg P.O. q.i.d.
Children ages 2 to 14 or weighing 50 kg or less: Initially, 25 mg/kg P.O.; then 40 mg/kg/day in four divided doses daily.
➤ **Hyperuricemia of gout, gouty arthritis**
Adults: 250 mg P.O. b.i.d. for first week; then 500 mg b.i.d. Review maintenance dose every 6 months and reduce daily dosage by increments of 500 mg, if indicated.

pyrimethamine
pihr-ih-METH-ah-meen

Daraprim

Therapeutic class: Antimalarials
Pharmacologic class: Folate antagonists

AVAILABLE FORMS
Tablets: 25 mg

INDICATIONS & DOSAGES
➤ **To prevent and control transmission of malaria**
Adults and children older than age 10: 25 mg P.O. once weekly.
Children ages 4 to 10: 12.5 mg P.O. once weekly.
Infants and children younger than age 4: 6.25 mg P.O. once weekly.
➤ **Acute attacks of malaria (in combination with a sulfonamide)**
Adults and children age 10 and older: 25 mg P.O. daily for 2 days with a sulfonamide. Clinical cure should be followed with 25 mg P.O. once weekly for at least 10 weeks. Or, 50 mg P.O. daily for 2 days; then 25 mg once weekly for at least 10 weeks if pyrimethamine must be used alone in people with semi-immunity.
Children ages 4 to 10: 25 mg P.O. once daily for 2 days; then 12.5 mg once weekly for at least 10 weeks.
➤ **Toxoplasmosis**
Adults: Initially, 50 to 75 mg P.O. with a sulfonamide and leucovorin calcium; continue for 1 to 3 weeks.

After 3 weeks, reduce dosage by half and continue for 4 to 5 weeks.
Children: Initially, 1 mg/kg/day P.O. in two equally divided doses for 2 to 4 days; then 0.5 mg/kg daily divided into two equal doses for 4 weeks, along with a sulfonamide at a pediatric dosage.

quinupristin–dalfopristin
QUIN-uh-pris-tin/DALF-oh-pris-tin

Synercid

Therapeutic class: Antibiotics
Pharmacologic class: Streptogramins

AVAILABLE FORMS
Injection: 500-mg vial (150 mg quinupristin and 350 mg dalfopristin)

INDICATIONS & DOSAGES
➤ **Complicated skin and skin-structure infections caused by methicillin-susceptible *Staphylococcus aureus* or *Streptococcus pyogenes***
Adults and adolescents age 12 and older: 7.5 mg/kg I.V. over 1 hour every 12 hours for at least 7 days.

SAFETY ALERT!

radioactive iodine (sodium iodide, ^{131}I)
Hicon, Sodium Iodide ^{131}I Therapeutic

Therapeutic class: Radiopharmaceuticals
Pharmacologic class: Antithyroid drugs

AVAILABLE FORMS
All radioactivity concentrations are determined at time of calibration.
Capsules: Radioactivity range, 0.75 to 100 mCi/capsule
Concentrated oral solution: 1,000 mCi/mL
Oral solution: Radioactivity range, 5 to 150 mCi/vial

INDICATIONS & DOSAGES
➤ **Hyperthyroidism**
Adults: Usual dosage is 4 to 10 mCi P.O. Dosage is based on estimated weight of thyroid gland and thyroid uptake. Repeat treatment after 6 weeks, based on T_4 level as needed.
➤ **Thyroid cancer**
Adults: Initially, 30 to 100 mCi P.O., with subsequent doses of 100 to 200 mCi for metastases. Dosage is based on estimated malignant thyroid tissue and metastatic tissue as determined by total body scan. Repeat treatment according to clinical status.
➤ **Thyroid function evaluation**
Adults: Dosage ranges from 5 to 100 mCi P.O. based on patient's weight and type of procedure.

regorafenib
RE-goe-RAF-e-nib

Stivarga

Therapeutic class: Antineoplastics
Pharmacologic class: Kinase inhibitors

AVAILABLE FORMS
Tablets: 40 mg

INDICATIONS & DOSAGES
Black Box Warning May cause severe or fatal hepatotoxicity. Monitor closely. ∎
Adjust-a-dose (for all indications): Refer to manufacturer's instructions for dosage modification due to adverse reactions. Discontinue drug permanently for failure to tolerate 80-mg dose; any occurrence of AST or ALT level more than 20 × ULN; any occurrence of AST or ALT level more than 3 × ULN with concurrent bilirubin level more than 2 × ULN; recurrence of AST or ALT level more than 5 × ULN despite dosage reduction to 120 mg; or any grade 4 adverse reaction.
➤ **Metastatic colorectal cancer previously treated with fluoropyrimidine-, oxaliplatin-, and irinotecan-based chemotherapy, an anti–vascular endothelial growth factor therapy and, if *KRAS* wild type, an anti–epidermal growth factor receptor therapy**
Adults: 160 mg P.O. once a day for first 21 days of each 28-day cycle. Continue therapy until disease progression or unacceptable toxicity occurs.
➤ **Locally advanced, unresectable, or metastatic GI stromal tumor previously treated with imatinib mesylate and sunitinib malate**
Adults: 160 mg P.O. once daily for first 21 days of each 28-day cycle. Continue therapy until disease progression or unacceptable toxicity occurs.

retapamulin
re-te-PAM-ue-lin

Altabax

Therapeutic class: Antibiotics
Pharmacologic class: Pleuromutilins

AVAILABLE FORMS
Topical ointment: 1%

INDICATIONS & DOSAGES
➤ **Impetigo due to *Staphylococcus aureus* (methicillin-susceptible isolates only) or *Streptococcus pyogenes***
Adults and children age 9 months and older: Apply a thin layer to affected area b.i.d. for 5 days.

reteplase (recombinant)
RET-ah-place

Retavase

Therapeutic class: Thrombolytics
Pharmacologic class: Tissue plasminogen activators

AVAILABLE FORMS
Injection: 10.4 units (18.1 mg)/vial, supplied in a kit with components for reconstitution for two single-use vials

INDICATIONS & DOSAGES
➤ **To manage acute MI**
Adults: Double-bolus injection of 10 + 10 units. Give each bolus I.V. over 2 minutes. If complications, such as serious bleeding or anaphylactoid reaction, don't occur after first bolus, give second bolus 30 minutes after start of first.

rifabutin
rif-ah-BYOO-tin

Mycobutin

Therapeutic class: Antituberculotics
Pharmacologic class: Semisynthetic ansamycins

AVAILABLE FORMS
Capsules: 150 mg

INDICATIONS & DOSAGES
Adjust-a-dose (for all indications): For patients with CrCl of less than 30 mL/minute, reduce rifabutin dosage by 50%.
➤ **To prevent disseminated *Mycobacterium avium* complex in patients with advanced HIV infection**
Adults: 300 mg P.O. daily as a single dose or in two divided doses.
➤ **To substitute for rifampin in patients with TB concurrently receiving medications that have unacceptable interactions with rifampin or who have intolerance to rifampin ◆**
Adults: 5 mg/kg P.O. two or three times weekly, not to exceed 300 mg/day.

riluzole
RILL-yoo-zole

Rilutek

Therapeutic class: Neuroprotectors
Pharmacologic class: Benzothiazoles

AVAILABLE FORMS
Tablets: 50 mg

INDICATIONS & DOSAGES
➤**Amyotrophic lateral sclerosis**
Adults: 50 mg P.O. every 12 hours, taken on empty stomach 1 hour before or 2 hours after a meal.

SAFETY ALERT!

romidepsin
roh-mih-DEP-sin

Istodax

Therapeutic class: Antineoplastics
Pharmacologic class: Histone deacetylase inhibitors

AVAILABLE FORMS
Injection: 10-mg vial

INDICATIONS & DOSAGES
*Adjust-a-dose (for all indications):*Refer to manufacturer's instructions for dosage adjustments for hematologic and nonhematologic toxicities.
➤**Cutaneous T-cell lymphoma in patients who have received at least one prior systemic therapy**
Adults: 14 mg/m^2 by I.V. infusion over 4 hours on days 1, 8, and 15 of 28-day cycle. Repeat every 28 days if effective and well tolerated.
➤**Treatment of peripheral T-cell lymphoma in patients who have received at least one prior therapy**
Adults: 14 mg/m^2 I.V. over 4 hours on days 1, 8, and 15 of a 28-day cycle. Repeat cycle every 28 days if effective and tolerated.

rufinamide
roo-FIN-ah-mide

Banzel

Therapeutic class: Anticonvulsants
Pharmacologic class: Triazole derivatives

AVAILABLE FORMS
Suspension: 40 mg/mL
Tablets: 200 mg, 400 mg

INDICATIONS & DOSAGES
➤**Adjunct treatment of seizures associated with Lennox-Gastaut syndrome**
Adults: Initially, 200 to 400 mg P.O. b.i.d. Increase dosage by 400 to 800 mg/day every 2 days to 3,200 mg P.O. daily in divided doses.
Children ages 1 to less than age 17: Initially, 5 mg/kg P.O. b.i.d. Increase dosage by 10 mg/kg every other day to 45 mg/kg or 3,200 mg (whichever is less) P.O. daily in divided doses.
*Adjust-a-dose:*Dialysis clears drug by 30%; dosage adjustment may be necessary. For patients taking valproate, start rufinamide at dosages less than 400 mg/day (adults) or less than 10 mg/kg/day (children).

sapropterin dihydrochloride
SAP-roh-TEHR-in

Kuvan

Therapeutic class: Phenylalanine reducers
Pharmacologic class: Enzyme cofactors

AVAILABLE FORMS
Powder for suspension: 100 mg/packet, 500 mg/packet
Tablets: 100 mg

INDICATIONS & DOSAGES
➤**Hyperphenylalaninemia caused by tetrahydrobiopterin-responsive phenylketonuria**
Adults and children age 7 and older: Initially, 10 to 20 mg/kg P.O. once daily with food.
Children ages 1 month to 6 years: Initially, 10 mg/kg P.O. once daily with food.
*Adjust-a-dose:*If a 10 mg/kg per day starting dose is used and phenylalanine level hasn't decreased from baseline after 4 weeks, increase dose to 20 mg/kg P.O. Stop treatment if patient has no response after 4 weeks at 20 mg/kg. If a 20 mg/kg per day starting dose is used, and phenylalanine level hasn't decreased from baseline after 4 weeks, discontinue treatment. Once responsiveness to drug has been established, adjust dosage within the range of 5 to 20 mg/kg per day according to response to therapy.

saquinavir mesylate
sa-KWEN-ah-veer

Invirase

Therapeutic class: Antiretrovirals
Pharmacologic class: Protease inhibitors

AVAILABLE FORMS
Capsules (hard gelatin): 200 mg
Tablets (film-coated): 500 mg

INDICATIONS & DOSAGES
➤**Adjunctive treatment of advanced HIV infection in selected patients, in combination with ritonavir**
Adults and adolescents age 16 and older: Initially, in treatment-naive patients or patients switching from a regimen containing delavirdine or rilpivirine, give 500 mg P.O. b.i.d. for first 7 days. In patients switching from a regimen that doesn't contain delavirdine or rilpivirine, give 1,000 mg P.O. b.i.d. Maintenance dosage is 1,000 mg P.O. b.i.d. given at the same time with 100 mg ritonavir P.O. b.i.d.

---

scopolamine (hyoscine)
skoe-POL-a-meen

Transderm-Scop

Therapeutic class: Antispasmodics
Pharmacologic class: Belladonna alkaloids–antimuscarinics

AVAILABLE FORMS
Transdermal patch: $1.5 \text{ mg}/2.5 \text{ cm}^2$ (1 mg/72 hours)

INDICATIONS & DOSAGES
Adjust-a-dose (for all indications): Elderly patients may require lower doses.
➤ **To prevent postoperative nausea and vomiting**
Adults: Apply 1 transdermal patch the evening before scheduled surgery. To minimize exposure to newborns, apply patch 1 hour before cesarean birth. Keep patch in place for 24 hours after surgery.
➤ **To prevent nausea and vomiting from motion sickness**
Adults: One transdermal patch, formulated to deliver 1 mg scopolamine over 3 days, applied to the skin behind the ear at least 4 hours before antiemetic is needed. Replace patch every 3 days if needed.

secukinumab
SEK-ue-KIN-ue-mab

Cosentyx, Cosentyx Sensoready Pen

Therapeutic class: Immunomodulators
Pharmacologic class: Human IgG1 monoclonal antibodies

AVAILABLE FORMS
Injection: 150 mg/mL auto-injector or prefilled syringe
Injection (lyophilized powder): 150 mg in single-use vial

INDICATIONS & DOSAGES
➤ **Moderate to severe plaque psoriasis in patients who are candidates for systemic therapy or phototherapy; psoriatic arthritis in patients with coexistent moderate to severe plaque psoriasis**
Adults: 300 mg as two subcutaneous injections of 150 mg each on weeks 0, 1, 2, 3, and 4; then 300 mg every 4 weeks thereafter. If clinically indicated, a 150-mg dose may be acceptable for some patients with plaque psoriasis.
➤ **Active psoriatic arthritis; ankylosing spondylitis**
Adults: To use with a loading dose, give 150 mg subcutaneously once weekly at weeks 0, 1, 2, 3, and 4; then 150 mg subcutaneously every 4 weeks. To use without a loading dose, give 150 mg subcutaneously every 4 weeks. For active psoriatic arthritis, may consider increasing dosage to 300 mg subcutaneously every 4 weeks.

sertaconazole nitrate
sir-tah-KAHN-uh-zole

Ertaczo

Therapeutic class: Antifungals
Pharmacologic class: Imidazoles

AVAILABLE FORMS
Topical cream: 2%

INDICATIONS & DOSAGES
➤ **Interdigital tinea pedis caused by *Trichophyton rubrum*, *Trichophyton mentagrophytes*, or *Epidermophyton floccosum* in immunocompetent patients**
Adults and children age 12 and older: Apply cream b.i.d. to affected areas between toes and healthy surrounding areas for 4 weeks.

siltuximab
sil-TUX-i-mab

Sylvant

Therapeutic class: Immune response modifiers
Pharmacologic class: Monoclonal antibodies

AVAILABLE FORMS
Injection: 100 mg, 400 mg lyophilized powder in single-use vials

INDICATIONS & DOSAGES
➤ **Multicentric Castleman disease in patients who are HIV-negative and human herpesvirus-8–negative**
Adults: 11 mg/kg I.V. over 1 hour every 3 weeks until treatment failure.
Adjust-a-dose: Consider delaying treatment if ANC is less than $1,000/\text{mm}^3$, Hb level is 17 g/dL or more, or platelet count is less than $50,000/\text{mm}^3$ before first dose.

silver sulfadiazine
sul-fa-DYE-a-zeen

Dermazin ✴, Flamazine ✴, Hydrogel Ag ◇, Silvadene, SSD, Thermazene

Therapeutic class: Antibacterials (topical)
Pharmacologic class: Broad-spectrum sulfonamides

AVAILABLE FORMS
Cream: 1%

INDICATIONS & DOSAGES
➤ **To prevent or treat wound infection in second- and third-degree burns**
Adults: Apply 1/16-inch ribbon of cream to clean, debrided wound daily or b.i.d. Burn areas should be

covered with cream at all times. Reapply to areas from which it has been removed by patient activity.

sodium bicarbonate

Therapeutic class: Antacids
Pharmacologic class: Alkalinizers

AVAILABLE FORMS
Injection: 7.5% (8.92 mEq/10 mL, 44.6 mEq/50 mL), 8.4% (10 mEq/10 mL, 50 mEq/50 mL)
Powder: 30 mg/½ tsp ◊
Tablets: 325 mg ◊, 650 mg ◊

INDICATIONS & DOSAGES
➤ **Metabolic acidosis**
Adults and children: Dosage depends on blood carbon dioxide content, pH, and patient's condition; usually, 2 to 5 mEq/kg I.V. infused over 4- to 8-hour period.
➤ **Urinary alkalinization**
Adults: Initially, 4,000 mg P.O.; then 1,000 to 2,000 mg P.O. every 4 hours; dosage based on urine pH.
Children: 84 to 840 mg/kg P.O. daily in four divided doses. Titrate based on urine pH.
➤ **Antacid**
Adults: 650 mg to 2,600 mg P.O. up to every 4 hours taken with glass of water.
Adults and children older than age 12: 30 mg (½ tsp) oral powder in 120 mL water P.O. every 2 hours up to six doses daily for patients under age 60, or three doses daily for patients over age 60.
➤ **Cardiac arrest**
Adults and children age 2 and older: Administer according to results of arterial blood pH, partial pressure of arterial carbon dioxide, and calculated base deficit. Usual dose is 200 to 300 mEq of bicarbonate given as 7.5% or 8.4% solution. Then redetermine serum pH and bicarbonate concentration.
Children younger than age 2: 1 mEq/kg (1 mL/kg of 8.4% solution) I.V. slowly followed by 1 mEq/kg every 10 minutes of arrest. Don't give more than 8 mEq/kg I.V. total; a 4.2% solution may be preferred.
➤ **Prevention of contrast media nephrotoxicity** ♦
Adults: 154 mEq/L in dextrose 5% infusion administered as an I.V. bolus of 3 mL/kg/hour I.V. for 1 hour immediately before contrast administration, followed by an infusion of 1 mL/kg/hour for 6 hours after the procedure.

sonidegib phosphate
SOE-ni-deg-ib

Odomzo

Therapeutic class: Antineoplastics
Pharmacologic class: Hedgehog pathway inhibitors

AVAILABLE FORMS
Capsules: 200 mg

INDICATIONS & DOSAGES
Black Box Warning Drug can cause birth defects or embryofetal death if used during pregnancy. Female patients must use contraception during therapy and for 20 months after last dose. Male patients must use condoms and shouldn't donate sperm during therapy and for at least 8 months after last dose. ∎
➤ **Locally advanced basal cell carcinoma that has recurred after surgery or radiation therapy, or in patients who aren't candidates for surgery or radiation therapy**
Adults: 200 mg P.O. once daily. Administer until disease progression or unacceptable toxicity occurs.
Adjust-a-dose: For first occurrence of serum CK elevation of 2.5 to 10 × ULN or recurrent serum CK levels between 2.5 and 5 × ULN or severe or intolerable musculoskeletal adverse reactions, interrupt therapy and resume at 200 mg/day upon resolution of toxicity. Permanently discontinue drug for serum CK level greater than 2.5 × ULN with worsening renal function or serum CK level greater than 10 × ULN or recurrent serum CK level greater than 5 × ULN or recurrent severe or intolerable musculoskeletal adverse reactions.

SAFETY ALERT!

sorafenib tosylate
sohr-uh-FEN-ib

Nexavar

Therapeutic class: Antineoplastics
Pharmacologic class: Multi-kinase inhibitors

AVAILABLE FORMS
Tablets: 200 mg

INDICATIONS & DOSAGES
➤ **Advanced renal cell carcinoma; unresectable hepatocellular carcinoma; locally advanced or metastatic, progressive, differentiated thyroid carcinoma refractory to radioactive iodine treatment**
Adults: 400 mg P.O. b.i.d. at least 1 hour before or 2 hours after eating. Continue until disease progresses or unacceptable toxicity occurs.
Adjust-a-dose: Refer to manufacturer's instructions for dosage adjustments for dermatologic and other toxicities.

spinosad
SPIN-oh-sad

Natroba

Therapeutic class: Scabicides–pediculicides
Pharmacologic class: Topical actinomycete bacterium derivatives

AVAILABLE FORMS
Topical solution: 0.9%*

✚Canada   ◊ OTC   ♦ Off-label use   ✒Photoguide   ⓓⓝⓒDo not crush   *Liquid contains alcohol.

INDICATIONS & DOSAGES
➤ **Head lice infestation**
Adults and children age 6 months and older: Apply only amount needed to adequately cover scalp and hair, up to 120 mL. Leave on for 10 minutes; then thoroughly rinse off with warm water. If live lice are seen 7 days after first treatment, apply a second treatment.

sulfADIAZINE
sul-fa-DYE-a-zeen

Therapeutic class: Antibiotics
Pharmacologic class: Sulfonamides

AVAILABLE FORMS
Tablets: 500 mg

INDICATIONS & DOSAGES
➤ **Acute otitis media due to *Haemophilus influenzae* in combination with penicillin; chancroid; meningococcal meningitis prophylaxis or treatment; *H. influenzae* meningitis in combination with streptomycin; inclusion conjunctivitis; trachoma; nocardiosis; adjunctive therapy for chloroquine-resistant malaria; toxoplasmosis encephalitis in combination with pyrimethamine**
Adults: Initially, 2 to 4 g P.O.; then 2 to 4 g P.O. divided into three to six doses daily.
Children age 2 months and older: Initially, 75 mg/kg P.O.; then 150 mg/kg or 4 g/m² P.O. divided into four to six doses daily. Maximum dosage is 6 g daily.
➤ **UTI due to *Escherichia coli*, *Klebsiella* or *Enterobacter* species, *Proteus mirabilis*, or *Proteus vulgaris* after failure of other sulfonamides**
Adults: Initially, 2 to 4 g P.O.; then 2 to 4 g P.O. divided into three to six doses daily.
➤ **To prevent rheumatic fever**
Children weighing more than 30 kg: 1 g P.O. daily.
Children weighing less than 30 kg: 500 mg P.O. daily.

taliglucerase alfa
TAL-i-GLOO-ser-ase

Elelyso

Therapeutic class: Metabolic agents
Pharmacologic class: Recombinant enzymes

AVAILABLE FORMS
Injection: 200 units/vial

INDICATIONS & DOSAGES
➤ **Long-term enzyme replacement in patients with confirmed type 1 Gaucher disease**
Adults and children age 4 and older: 60 units/kg I.V. infused over 60 to 120 minutes every other week. Initial rate of infusion for children should be 1 mL/minute; may be increased if tolerated, but not to exceed 2 mL/minute. Initial rate of infusion for adults should be 1.2 mL/minute; may be increased if tolerated, but not to exceed 2.2 mL/minute.
Adjust-a-dose: Adjust dosage based on achievement and maintenance of therapeutic goals.

tasimelteon
TAS-i-MEL-tee-on

Hetlioz

Therapeutic class: Hypnotics
Pharmacologic class: Melatonin receptor agonists

AVAILABLE FORMS
Capsules ⓄⓉⒸ: 20 mg

INDICATIONS & DOSAGES
➤ **Non-24-hour sleep-wake disorder**
Adults: 20 mg P.O. daily at the same time each night at bedtime.

tavaborole
tah-vah-BOR-ole

Kerydin

Therapeutic class: Antifungals
Pharmacologic class: Antifungals

AVAILABLE FORMS
Topical solution: 5%

INDICATIONS & DOSAGES
➤ **Onychomycosis of toenails due to *Trichophyton rubrum* or *Trichophyton mentagrophytes***
Adults: Apply once daily for 48 weeks to entire surface of affected toenail and under the tip of affected toenail.

tbo-filgrastim
fill-GRASS-tim

Granix

Therapeutic class: Colony stimulating factors
Pharmacologic class: Hematopoietics

AVAILABLE FORMS
Injection: 300 mcg/0.5 mL, 480 mcg/0.8 mL single-use prefilled syringes

INDICATIONS & DOSAGES
➤ **To reduce duration of severe neutropenia in myelosuppressive chemotherapy recipients with non-myeloid malignancies**
Adults: 5 mcg/kg subcutaneously daily. Give first dose no earlier than 24 hours after myelosuppressive chemotherapy. Don't give drug within 24 hours before chemotherapy. Continue daily dosing until expected neutrophil nadir is passed and neutrophil count has recovered to normal range.

temsirolimus
TEM-seer-OLE-ih-muss

Torisel

Therapeutic class: Antineoplastics
Pharmacologic class: Kinase inhibitors

AVAILABLE FORMS
I.V. solution: 25 mg/mL

INDICATIONS & DOSAGES
➤ **Advanced renal cell carcinoma**
Adults: 25 mg I.V. over 30 to 60 minutes once weekly until disease progresses or unacceptable toxicity occurs. Give diphenhydramine 25 to 50 mg I.V. 30 minutes before each dose.
Adjust-a-dose: In patients with an ANC of less than 1,000/mm^3, a platelet count of less than 75,000/mm^3, or National Cancer Institute CTCAE grade 3 or greater adverse reactions, hold dose. Once toxicities have resolved to grade 2 or less, may restart drug, with dosage reduced by 5 mg weekly to dosage no lower than 15 mg/week. With mild hepatic impairment (bilirubin level 1 to 1.5 × ULN or AST level greater than ULN but with bilirubin level less than or equal to ULN), reduce dosage to 15 mg/week.
   If use with a strong CYP3A4 inhibitor is necessary, consider a dosage reduction to 12.5 mg once weekly. If use wih a strong CYP3A4 inducer is necessary, increase dosage to 50 mg once weekly.

teriflunomide
TER-i-FLOO-noe-mide

Aubagio

Therapeutic class: Immunomodulators
Pharmacologic class: Pyrimidine synthesis inhibitors

AVAILABLE FORMS
Tablets: 7 mg, 14 mg

INDICATIONS & DOSAGES
Black Box Warning Severe and fatal liver injury can occur. May cause major birth defects. Contraindicated during pregnancy. ∎
➤ **Relapsing forms of MS**
Adults: 7 or 14 mg P.O. once daily.

tetrabenazine
TEH-tra-BEN-ah-zeen

Nitoman❧, Xenazine

Therapeutic class: Antichorea drugs
Pharmacologic class: Monoamine depleters

AVAILABLE FORMS
Tablets: 12.5 mg, 25 mg

INDICATIONS & DOSAGES
Black Box Warning Increases risk for depression and suicidal thoughts and behavior. Monitor closely. ∎
➤ **Chorea associated with Huntington disease**
Adults: Initially, 12.5 mg P.O. daily in the morning. After 1 week, increase dosage to 12.5 mg P.O. b.i.d. Titrate dosage by 12.5 mg at weekly intervals, as needed. Maximum single dose, 25 mg. If dosage of 37.5 to 50 mg/day is needed, administer in three divided doses. Patients requiring more than 50 mg/day should be genotyped for CYP2D6 metabolism.
Adjust-a-dose: In patients who are extensive or intermediate CYP2D6 metabolizers, slowly titrate dosages above 50 mg at weekly intervals by 12.5 mg as needed and tolerated. Maximum daily dosage is 100 mg; maximum single dose, 37.5 mg. In patients who are poor CYP2D6 metabolizers, maximum daily dosage is 50 mg; maximum single dose, 25 mg.

theophylline
thee-OFF-i-lin

Elixophyllin*, Pulmophylline ELX❧, Theo-24, Uniphyl

Therapeutic class: Bronchodilators
Pharmacologic class: Xanthine derivatives

AVAILABLE FORMS
Capsules (extended-release) ⓓⓝⓒ: 100 mg, 200 mg, 300 mg, 400 mg
D$_5$W injection: 200 mg in 50 mL or 100 mL; 400 mg in 100 mL, 250 mL, 500 mL, or 1,000 mL; 800 mg in 500 mL or 1,000 mL
Syrup: 80 mg/15 mL*
Tablets (extended-release) ⓓⓝⓒ: 100 mg, 200 mg, 300 mg, 400 mg, 450 mg, 600 mg

INDICATIONS & DOSAGES
Extended-release preparations shouldn't be used to treat acute bronchospasm.
➤ **Parenteral theophylline (preferred route) for acute bronchospasm in patients not currently receiving theophylline**
Loading dose: 4.6 mg/kg ideal body weight I.V. over 30 minutes; then maintenance infusion.
Nonsmoking adults younger than age 60 and children older than age 16: 0.4 mg/kg/hour I.V. (maximum 900 mg daily).

Nonsmoking children ages 12 to 16: 0.5 mg/kg/hour I.V. (maximum 900 mg daily).

Children ages 12 to 16 who smoke and children ages 9 to 12: 0.7 mg/kg/hour I.V.

Children ages 1 to 9: 0.8 mg/kg/hour I.V.

Infants ages 6 weeks to 1 year: Calculate mg/kg/hour I.V. dosage as follows. 0.008 × (age in weeks) + 0.21.

Neonates older than 24 days: 1.5 mg/kg I.V. every 12 hours to achieve target theophylline concentration of 7.5 mcg/mL.

Neonates 24 days old and younger: 1 mg/kg I.V. every 12 hours to achieve a target theophylline concentration of 7.5 mcg/mL.

Adjust-a-dose: For adults older than age 60, give 0.3 mg/kg/hour I.V., up to a maximum of 17 mg/hour. For adults with HF, cor pulmonale, liver disease, sepsis with multiorgan failure, or shock, give 0.2 mg/kg/hour I.V., up to a maximum infusion rate of 17 mg/hour unless serum theophylline concentrations are monitored at 24-hour intervals. Maximum daily dose is 400 mg.

➤ **Oral theophylline for acute bronchospasm in patients not currently receiving theophylline**

Adults age 60 and younger, children ages 16 and older, and children ages 1 to 15 weighing 45 kg or more: 5 mg/kg P.O., then 300 mg (immediate-release syrup) P.O. daily in divided doses every 6 to 8 hours for 3 days. If tolerated, increase to 400 mg P.O. daily in divided doses every 6 to 8 hours. If necessary, dosage may be increased after 3 days to 600 mg P.O. daily in divided doses every 6 to 8 hours.

Children ages 1 to 15 weighing less than 45 kg: 5 mg/kg P.O., then 12 to 14 mg/kg immediate-release (maximum 300 mg) P.O. daily in divided doses every 4 to 6 hours for 3 days. If tolerated, increase to 16 mg/kg (maximum 400 mg) P.O. daily in divided doses every 4 to 6 hours. After 3 days, if necessary, increase to 20 mg/kg (maximum 600 mg) P.O. daily in divided doses every 4 to 6 hours.

Adjust-a-dose: For children ages 1 to 15 with risk factors for reduced theophylline clearance or for whom serum concentrations can't be monitored, give 5 mg/kg P.O., then 12 to 14 mg/kg (maximum 300 mg) P.O. daily in divided doses every 4 to 6 hours for 3 days. If tolerated, increase to 16 mg/kg (maximum 400 mg) P.O. daily in divided doses every 4 to 6 hours. For children age 16 and older and adults with risk factors for reduced theophylline clearance or for whom serum concentrations can't be monitored, give 5 mg/kg P.O., then 300 mg P.O. daily in divided doses every 6 to 8 hours for 3 days. If tolerated, increase to 400 mg P.O. daily in divided doses every 6 to 8 hours.

➤ **Chronic bronchospasm using extended-release preparations**

Adults age 60 or younger, children age 16 and older, and children ages 6 to 15 weighing more than 45 kg: 300 mg P.O. daily in divided doses every 8 to 12 hours or 300 to 400 mg (24-hour extended-release capsule) P.O. daily for 3 days. If tolerated, increase to 400 mg P.O. in divided doses every 8 to 12 hours or 400 to 600 mg (24-hour extended-release capsule) P.O. daily. After 3 more days, if necessary, increase dose

to 600 mg P.O. daily in divided doses every 8 to 12 hours. Titrate dosages greater than 600 mg according to serum blood levels.

Children ages 6 to 15 weighing less than 45 kg: 12 to 14 mg/kg (maximum 300 mg extended-release tablet) daily in divided doses every 8 to 12 hours for 3 days. If tolerated, increase to 16 mg/kg (maximum 400 mg extended-release tablet) daily in divided doses every 8 to 12 hours. After 3 more days, if necessary, increase to 20 mg/kg (maximum 600 mg extended-release tablet) daily in divided doses every 8 to 12 hours.

Adjust-a-dose: For children ages 6 to 15 with risk factors for reduced theophylline clearance or for whom serum concentrations can't be monitored, give 12 to 14 mg/kg (maximum 300 mg) daily in divided doses for 3 days. If tolerated, increase to a maximum of 16 mg/kg (maximum 400 mg) P.O. daily in divided doses every 8 to 12 hours. For children 16 and older and adults age 60 or younger or for whom serum concentrations can't be monitored, give 300 mg P.O. daily in divided doses every 8 to 12 hours. After 3 days, if necessary, increase to maximum of 400 mg P.O. daily in divided doses every 8 to 12 hours. For adults older than age 60, the recommended maximum daily dose is 400 mg P.O. per day in divided doses every 8 to 12 hours unless symptoms continue and peak serum concentration is less than 10 mcg/mL. Administer dosages greater than 400 mg P.O. daily cautiously.

thioridazine hydrochloride
thye-oh-RYE-da-zeen

Therapeutic class: Antipsychotics
Pharmacologic class: Phenothiazines

AVAILABLE FORMS
Tablets: 10 mg, 25 mg, 50 mg, 100 mg

INDICATIONS & DOSAGES
Black Box Warning   Prolongs QTc interval and risk for life-threatening ventricular arrhythmias. Drug isn't approved to treat patients with dementia-related psychosis. Opioids combined with benzodiazepines or CNS depressants can cause death. ∎

➤ **Schizophrenia in patients who don't respond to treatment with at least two other antipsychotic drugs**

Adults: Initially, 50 to 100 mg P.O. t.i.d.; increase gradually to 800 mg daily in divided doses, as needed. Daily maintenance doses range from 200 to 800 mg divided into two to four doses.

Children: Initially, 0.5 mg/kg P.O. daily in divided doses. Increase gradually to optimal therapeutic effect; maximum dose is 3 mg/kg daily.

---

thiothixene
thye-oh-THIX-een

Navane

Therapeutic class: Antipsychotics
Pharmacologic class: Thioxanthenes

AVAILABLE FORMS
Capsules: 1 mg, 2 mg, 5 mg, 10 mg

INDICATIONS & DOSAGES
Black Box Warning   Drug isn't approved to treat patients with dementia-related psychosis. Opioids combined with benzodiazepines or CNS depressants can cause death. ■
➤ **Mild to moderate schizophrenia**
Adults and children age 12 and older: Initially, 2 mg P.O. t.i.d. Increase gradually to 15 mg daily, as needed.
➤ **Severe schizophrenia**
Adults and children age 12 and older: Initially, 5 mg P.O. b.i.d. Increase gradually to 20 to 30 mg daily, as needed. Maximum dose is 60 mg daily.

ticlopidine hydrochloride
tye-KLOH-pih-deen

Therapeutic class: Antiplatelet drugs
Pharmacologic class: Platelet aggregation inhibitors

AVAILABLE FORMS
Tablets: 250 mg

INDICATIONS & DOSAGES
Adjust-a-dose (for all indications): For patients with renal impairment, it may be necessary to reduce dosage or discontinue drug if hemorrhage or hematopoietic problems occur
➤ **To reduce risk of thrombotic stroke in patients who have had a stroke or stroke precursors**
Adults: 250 mg P.O. b.i.d. with meals.
➤ **Adjunct to aspirin to prevent subacute stent thrombosis in patients having coronary stent placement**
Adults: 250 mg P.O. b.i.d., combined with antiplatelet doses of aspirin. Start therapy after stent placement and continue for up to 30 days. If prescribed longer than 30 days, use is off-label.

toremifene citrate
tore-EM-ah-feen

Fareston

Therapeutic class: Antineoplastics
Pharmacologic class: Nonsteroidal antiestrogens

AVAILABLE FORMS
Tablets: 60 mg

INDICATIONS & DOSAGES
Black Box Warning   May prolong QTc interval and risk of fatal ventricular arrhythmias. ■
➤ **Metastatic breast cancer in postmenopausal women with estrogen receptor–positive or estrogen receptor–unknown tumors**
Adults: 60 mg P.O. once daily. Continue until disease progresses.

trandolapril
tran-DOLE-ah-pril

Mavik✐

Therapeutic class: Antihypertensives
Pharmacologic class: ACE inhibitors

AVAILABLE FORMS
Tablets: 1 mg, 2 mg, 4 mg

INDICATIONS & DOSAGES
Black Box Warning   May cause fetal harm; when pregnancy is detected, discontinue drug as soon as possible. ■
Adjust-a-dose (for all indications): If CrCl is below 30 mL/minute or patient has hepatic cirrhosis, first dose is 0.5 mg daily.
➤ **Hypertension**
Adults: For patients not taking a diuretic, initially 2 mg P.O. for a black patient and 1 mg P.O. for all other races, once daily. If control isn't adequate, increase dosage at intervals of at least 1 week. Maintenance doses for most patients: 2 to 4 mg daily. Some patients taking once-daily doses of 4 mg may need twice-daily doses. For patients also taking a diuretic, initially, 0.5 mg P.O. once daily. Subsequent dosage adjustment is based on BP response.
➤ **HF or left ventricular dysfunction after MI**
Adults: Initially, 1 mg P.O. daily, adjusted to 4 mg P.O. daily. If patient can't tolerate 4 mg, continue at highest tolerated dose.

tranylcypromine sulfate
TRAN-il-SIP-roe-meen

Parnate

Therapeutic class: Antidepressants
Pharmacologic class: MAO inhibitors

AVAILABLE FORMS
Tablets: 10 mg

INDICATIONS & DOSAGES
➤ **Major depressive episode without melancholia**
Adults: 30 mg P.O. daily given in two or three divided doses daily. If no signs of improvement after a reasonable period (up to 2 weeks), may increase dosage in 10-mg/day increments at intervals of 1 to 3 weeks. Maximum total daily dosage is 60 mg.

trifluoperazine hydrochloride
trye-floo-oh-PER-eh-zeen

Therapeutic class: Antipsychotics
Pharmacologic class: Phenothiazines

AVAILABLE FORMS
Tablets (regular and film-coated): 1 mg, 2 mg, 5 mg, 10 mg

INDICATIONS & DOSAGES
Black Box Warning Not approved to treat patients with dementia-related psychosis. ∎
➤ **Nonpsychotic anxiety**
Adults: 1 to 2 mg P.O. b.i.d. Maximum, 6 mg daily. Don't give drug for longer than 12 weeks for anxiety.
➤ **Schizophrenia, other psychotic disorders**
Adults and children older than age 12: 2 to 5 mg P.O. b.i.d., gradually increased until therapeutic response occurs. Most patients respond to 15 to 20 mg P.O. daily, although some may need 40 mg daily or more.
Children ages 6 to 12: For hospitalized or closely supervised patients, 1 mg P.O. daily or b.i.d.; may increase gradually to 15 mg daily, if needed.

trifluridine–tipiracil hydrochloride
trye-FLURE-i-deen/tye-PIR-a-sil

Lonsurf

Therapeutic class: Antineoplastics
Pharmacologic class: Pyrimidine analogues

AVAILABLE FORMS
Tablets: 15 mg trifluridine/6.14 mg tipiracil, 20 mg trifluridine/8.19 mg tipiracil

INDICATIONS & DOSAGES
➤ **Metastatic colorectal cancer in patients previously treated with fluoropyrimidine-, oxaliplatin-,** and irinotecan-based chemotherapy, an anti-VEGF biological therapy and, if RAS wild-type, an anti-EGFR therapy
Adults: 35 mg/m^2 P.O. b.i.d. up to a maximum of 80 mg/dose (based on trifluridine component) on days 1 through 5 and days 8 through 12 of a 28-day cycle. Round doses to nearest 5-mg increment. Continue until disease progression or unacceptable toxicity occurs. Before initiating each drug cycle, ensure that ANC is 1,500/mm^3 or more or febrile neutropenia is resolved, platelet count is 75,000/mm^3 or greater, and grade 3 or 4 nonhematologic adverse reactions are resolved to grade 0 or 1.
Adjust-a-dose: Refer to manufacturer's instructions for dosage adjustments for hematologic and nonhematologic toxicities.

trimethobenzamide hydrochloride
trye-meth-oh-BEN-za-mide

Tigan

Therapeutic class: Antiemetics
Pharmacologic class: Anticholinergics

AVAILABLE FORMS
Capsules: 300 mg
Injection: 100 mg/mL

INDICATIONS & DOSAGES
➤ **Postoperative nausea and vomiting; nausea associated with gastroenteritis**
Adults: 300 mg P.O. or 200 mg I.M. t.i.d. or q.i.d.

uridine triacetate
URE-i-deen

Xuriden, Vistogard

Therapeutic class: Replacement enzymes
Pharmacologic class: Uridine replacements

AVAILABLE FORMS
Oral granules ⓓⓝⓒ*:* 2-g, 10-g single-use packets

INDICATIONS & DOSAGES
➤ **Hereditary orotic aciduria (Xuriden)**
Adults and children: 60 mg/kg P.O. daily; may increase to 120 mg/kg daily for insufficient efficacy. Maximum dose is 8 g/day. See manufacturer's instructions for weight-based dosing tables.
➤ **Fluoropyrimidine overdose (emergency treatment of 5-FU or capecitabine overdose; or early-onset severe or life-threatening cardiac or CNS toxicity; or early-onset, unusually severe adverse reactions [e.g., GI toxicity or neutropenia] within 96 hours after end of 5-FU or capecitabine administration) (Vistogard)**
Adults: 10 g P.O. every 6 hours for a total of 20 doses beginning as soon as possible after overdose or early-onset toxicity within 96 hours after end of 5-FU or

capecitabine administration. Maximum, 10 g/dose.
Children: 6.2 g/m^2 P.O. not to exceed 10 g/dose every
6 hours for 20 doses beginning as soon as possible
after overdose or early-onset toxicity within 96 hours
after end of 5-FU or capecitabine administration. Refer to manufacturer's information for weight-based
dosing tables.

SAFETY ALERT!

vandetanib
van-DET-a-nib

Caprelsa

Therapeutic class: Antineoplastics
Pharmacologic class: Kinase inhibitors

AVAILABLE FORMS
Tablets: 100 mg, 300 mg

INDICATIONS & DOSAGES
Black Box Warning   May prolong QTc interval
and increase risk for fatal ventricular arrhythmias. ▪
➤ **Symptomatic or progressive medullary thyroid
cancer in patients with unresectable locally advanced or metastatic disease**
Adults: 300 mg P.O. daily until disease progression or
unacceptable toxicity occurs.
Adjust-a-dose: In patients with moderate to severe
renal impairment (CrCl of less than 50 mL/minute),
initiate therapy at 200 mg P.O. daily. In the event of
corrected QT interval (Fridericia [QTcF]) greater than
500 msec, interrupt therapy until QTcF returns to less
than 450 msec; then resume at a reduced dosage. In
patients with grade 3 or greater toxicity, stop drug until toxicity resolves or improves to grade 1; resume at
reduced dosage of 200 mg, then 100 mg, if necessary.

vedolizumab
VE-doe-LIZ-ue-mab

Entyvio

Therapeutic class: Immune response
modifiers
Pharmacologic class: Humanized IgG1
monoclonal antibodies

AVAILABLE FORMS
Injection: 300 mg/20 mL single-use vial

INDICATIONS & DOSAGES
➤ **Moderate to severe Crohn disease or ulcerative
colitis in patients with inadequate response to, loss
of response to, or intolerance to TNF blocker or
immunomodulator, or in patients with inadequate
response, intolerance to, or demonstrated dependence on corticosteroids**
Adults: 300 mg I.V. infusion over 30 minutes, administered at weeks 0, 2, and 6, then every 8 weeks there-

after. Discontinue use if no evidence of therapeutic
benefit by week 14.

velaglucerase alfa
vel-uh-GLOO-ser-ase

VPRIV

Therapeutic class: Metabolic agents
Pharmacologic class: Hydrolytic lysosomal
glucocerebroside-specific enzymes

AVAILABLE FORMS
Injection: 400 units/vial

INDICATIONS & DOSAGES
➤ **Long-term enzyme replacement in patients with
type 1 Gaucher disease**
Adults and children age 4 and older: 60 units/kg I.V.
infused over 60 minutes every other week. Adjust dosage to 15 to 60 units/kg, based on treatment goals.

SAFETY ALERT!

vemurafenib
VEM-ue-RAF-e-nib

Zelboraf

Therapeutic class: Antineoplastics
Pharmacologic class: Kinase inhibitors

AVAILABLE FORMS
Tablets ⬚: 240 mg

INDICATIONS & DOSAGES
➤ **Treatment of unresectable or metastatic melanoma with *BRAF*^{V600E} mutation**
Adults: Usual dosage is 960 mg P.O. b.i.d.
Adjust-a-dose: In patients with symptomatic adverse drug reactions or prolongation of QTc interval,
refer to manufacturer's instructions for dosage adjustment.

SAFETY ALERT!

vinCRIStine sulfate liposome
vin-KRIS-teen

Marqibo

Therapeutic class: Antineoplastics
Pharmacologic class: Vinca alkaloids

AVAILABLE FORMS
Injection: 5 mg/31 mL in single-dose vial

INDICATIONS & DOSAGES
Black Box Warning   Liposomal form has differ-
ent dosage recommendation than nonliposomal form.
To avoid overdose, verify drug name and dose before

preparation and administration. For I.V. use only; fatal if given by other routes. ■

➤ **Patients with Philadelphia chromosome–negative (Ph-) acute lymphoblastic leukemia (ALL) in second or greater relapse or whose disease has progressed following two or more antileukemia therapies**

Adults: 2.25 mg/m² I.V. over 1 hour every 7 days.

Adjust-a-dose: Refer to manufacturer's instruction for dosage adjustments for peripheral neuropathy toxicity.

---

zanamivir
zan-AM-ah-veer

Relenza

Therapeutic class: Antiretrovirals
Pharmacologic class: Selective neuraminidase inhibitors

AVAILABLE FORMS
Powder for inhalation: 5 mg/blister

INDICATIONS & DOSAGES
➤ **Uncomplicated acute illness caused by influenza virus A and B in patients who have had symptoms for no longer than 2 days; treatment of H1N1 influenza A**

Adults and children age 7 and older: 2 oral inhalations (one 5-mg blister per inhalation for total dose of 10 mg) b.i.d. using the dry-powder inhalation device for 5 days. Give two doses on first day of treatment, allowing at least 2 hours to elapse between doses. Give subsequent doses about 12 hours apart (in the morning and evening) at about the same time each day.

➤ **Prevention of influenza in a household setting; prevention of H1N1 influenza A**

Adults and children age 5 and older: 2 oral inhalations (one 5-mg blister per inhalation for total dose of 10 mg) once daily for 10 days.

➤ **Prevention of influenza in a community setting**

Adults and adolescents ages 12 to 16: 2 oral inhalations (one 5-mg blister per inhalation for total dose of 10 mg) once daily for 28 days.

SAFETY ALERT!

---

ziv-aflibercept
ZIV-a-FLIB-er-sept

Zaltrap

Therapeutic class: Antineoplastics
Pharmacologic class: Vascular endothelial growth factor inhibitors

AVAILABLE FORMS
Injection: 100 mg/4 mL (25 mg/mL), 200 mg/8 mL (25 mg/mL) in single-use vials

INDICATIONS & DOSAGES
Black Box Warning May cause severe and fatal GI adverse reactions and compromise wound healing. Don't use for 4 weeks before or after surgery. ■

➤ **Metastatic colorectal cancer that is resistant or has progressed following an oxaliplatin-containing regimen in combination with 5-FU, leucovorin, and irinotecan (FOLFIRI)**

Adults: 4 mg/kg I.V. over 1 hour every 2 weeks until disease progression or unacceptable toxicity occurs. Give before any component of FOLFIRI regimen on day of treatment.

Adjust-a-dose: For recurrent or severe hypertension, withhold drug until controlled; then permanently reduce dosage to 2 mg/kg. For proteinuria of 2 g/24 hours or greater, withhold drug until proteinuria is less than 2 g/24 hours; then permanently reduce dosage to 2 mg/kg. For neutropenia, delay treatment until ANC is greater than 1.5×10^9/L.

Additional new drugs: Indications and dosages

Refer to manufacturer for complete prescribing and safety information.

bezlotoxumab
bez-lo-TOX-u-mab

Zinplava

Therapeutic class: Immunomodulators
Pharmacologic class: Human monoclonal antibodies

AVAILABLE FORMS
Injection: 25 mg/mL single-dose vial

INDICATIONS & DOSAGE
➤ **To reduce recurrence of** *Clostridium difficile* **infection (CDI) in patients who are receiving antibacterial treatment of CDI and are at high risk for CDI recurrence**
Adults: 10 mg/kg I.V. infusion over 60 minutes as a single dose.

olaratumab
oh-la-RAH-too-mab

Lartruvo

Therapeutic class: Antineoplastics
Pharmacologic class: Recombinant human IgG1 monoclonal blocking antibodies

AVAILABLE FORMS
Injection: 500 mg/50 mL single-use vial

INDICATIONS & DOSAGES
➤ **Soft-tissue sarcoma with a histologic subtype that's appropriate for an anthracycline-containing regimen and when radiotherapy or surgery isn't a curative option**
Adults: 15 mg/kg I.V. over 60 minutes on days 1 and 8 of each 21-day cycle until disease progression or unacceptable toxicity occurs. For first eight cycles, give with doxorubicin.
Adjust-a-dose: For grade 1 or 2 infusion-related reactions, interrupt infusion. After resolution, resume infusion at 50% of initial infusion rate. For grade 3 or 4 infusion-related reactions, permanently discontinue drug. For neutropenic fever/infection or grade 4 neutropenia lasting longer than 1 week, discontinue drug until ANC is 1,000/µL or greater, then permanently reduce dosage to 12 mg/kg.

Index

A

abacavir sulfate, 52, 60–61
abacavir sulfate–lamivudine, 1661
abacavir sulfate–lamivudine–zidovudine, 1661
abatacept, 39, 61–63
abciximab, 37, 1704
Abelcet, 124–126
Abenol, 67–70
Abilify, 145–150, **C3**
Abilify Discmelt, 145–150
Abilify Maintena, 145–150
abiraterone acetate, 64–65
ABonine, 1688
Abraxane, 1158–1161
Absorica, 839–841
Abstral, 624–630
acamprosate calcium, 65–66
acarbose, 30–31, 1704
Accolate, 1556–1557
AccuNeb, 84–87
Accupril, 1276–1277, **C24**
Accuretic, 1655
ACE inhibitors, 33–34, 1696–1697
Aceon, 1737–1738
Acephen, 67–70
Acerola, 1677
ACET, 67–70
Acetadote, 70–73
acetaminophen, 67–70
acetaminophen–butalbital–caffeine–codeine phosphate, 1651
Acetazolam, 1704
acetaZOLAMIDE, 1704
acetaZOLAMIDE sodium, 1704
acetylcysteine, 70–73
acetylsalicylic acid, 154–157
Achromycin V, 1444–1446
Acid Gone, 1680
Acid Reducer, 1294–1296
Aciphex, 1280–1282, **C24**
Aciphex Sprinkle, 1280–1282

ACT, 1676
Actemra, 1469–1472
ActHIB, 1666
Acticlate, 490–494
Acticlate Cap, 490–494
Actidose-Aqua, 1638
Actidose with Sorbitol, 1638
ACT-Imatinib, 772–775
Actimmune, 1725
Actiq, 624–630
Activase, 102–104
activated charcoal, 1638
Activella, 591–596
Actonel, 1313–1315, **C25**
ActoPlus Met, 1652–1653
ActoPlus Met XR, 1652–1653
Actos, 1223–1225, **C23**
Acular, 852–853
Acular LS, 852–853
Acuvail, 852–853
acyclovir, 73–75
acyclovir sodium, 73–75
Adacel, 1666–1667
Adalat CC, 1072–1074
Adalat XL, 1072–1074
adalimumab, 39, 76–78
Adasuve, 1730
Adcetris, 224–226
Adcirca, 1409–1411
Adderall XR, 438–442, 1630
Addyi, 644–645
adefovir dipivoxil, 78–79
Adenocard, 79–81
adenosine, 26–27, 79–81
Adipex-P, 1210–1211
Adlyxin, 1605–1606
ado-trastuzumab emtansine, 81–84
Adrenaclick, 534–537
Adrenalin, 534–537
adrenaline, 534–537
Advair Diskus 100/50, 669–671
Advair Diskus 250/50, 669–671

Advair Diskus 500/50, 669–671
Advair HFA 45/21, 669–671
Advair HFA 115/21, 669–671
Advair HFA 230/21, 669–671
Advate, 1644
Adverse drug reactions, 3–4
Advil, 756–759
Advil Gel Caplets, 756–759
Advil Infants' Concentrated Drops, 756–759
Adynovate, 1644
AeroSpan HFA, 650–652
afatinib dimaleate, 1705
Afeditab CR, 1072–1074
Afinitor, 605–609
Afinitor Disperz, 605–609
aflibercept, 1705
Afluria, 1669
Afrezza, 803–809
Afrin Children's, 1689
Afrin Sinus, 1689
Aggrastat, 1462–1464
Aggrenox, 1660
AHF factor VIII, 1644
A-Hydrocort, 738–741
Airomir, 84–87
Akarpine, 1219–1220
Akten, 1728–1729
Ala-Cort, 741–743
Ala-Scalp, 741–743
Alavert Allergy, 1688
Alaway, 1688
Albalon, 1052–1053
albiglutide, 30–31, 1705
Albuked-5, 1644
Albuked-25, 1644
albumin 5%, 1644
albumin 25%, 1644
Albuminar-5, 1644
Albuminar-25, 1644
AlbuRx 5%, 1644
Albutein 5%, 1644
Albutein 25%, 1644
albuterol sulfate, 84–87, 1626
alcaftadine, 1705

Alcalak, 1680
Aldactazide, 1662
Aldactone, 1384–1385, **C27**
Aldara, 1725
Alecensa, 1575–1576
alectinib hydrochloride, 1575–1576
alefacept, 49
alendronate sodium, 87–89, **C3**
Aler-Cap, 464–466
Alertec, 1022–1024
Aleve, 1054–1056
alfuzosin hydrochloride, 22–23, 89–90, **C3**
alglucosidase alfa, 1705–1706
Alimta, 1190–1192
Alinia, 1734
alirocumab, 35, 90–91
aliskiren, 33–34
aliskiren hemifumarate, 92–93
aliskiren hemifumarate–hydrochlorothiazide, 1659
Alkeran, 949–952
Alkylating drugs, 22
All Clear, 1052–1053
All Day Allergy, 1686
Allegra Allergy, 1687
Allegra Allergy Children's, 1687
Allegra 12 Hour, 1687
Allegra 24 Hour, 1687
Allergy, drug, 3
Allergy Time, 1686
Alli, 1735
allopurinol, 93–95
allopurinol sodium, 93–95
almotriptan malate, 36, 95–97
alogliptin, 30–31
alogliptin benzoate, 97–98
alogliptin benzoate–metformin, 1654
alogliptin benzoate–pioglitazone hydrochloride, 1654
Aloprim, 93–95
Alora, 569–573
alosetron hydrochloride, 1706

Aloxi, 1166–1167
Alpha blockers
centrally acting, sympatholytics, 33–34
peripherally acting, 22–23, 33–34
Alpha-E, 1678
Alphagan P, 229–230
AlphaNine SD, 1646
alprazolam, 40, 98–100,1630, **C3**
Alprolix, 1646
alprostadil
injection, 100–102
intracavernosal injection, 1706
urogenital suppository, 1706
Alsuma, 1397–1399
Altabax, 1741
Altace, 1288–1290
Altarussin, 1687–1688
Altavera, 591–596
alteplase, 58–59, 102–104
Altoprev, 930–932
aluminum hydroxide, 25, 1680
gel, 1680
aluminum hydroxide–magnesium carbonate, 1680
Alvesco, 326–328
alvimopan, 104–105
Alyacen 1/35, 591–596
Alyacen 7/7/7, 591–596
Alyacen 777, 591–596
Alzheimer disease drugs, 23
amantadine hydrochloride, 36–37, 105–107
Amaryl, 711–713, **C13**
Ambien, 1570–1572, **C32**
Ambien CR, 1570–1572, 1631
AmBisome, 126–128
ambrisentan, 107–109
Amerge, 1056–1058
amethopterin, 971–975
amikacin, 1696–1697
amikacin sulfate, 23–24, 109–111

amiloride and hydrochlorothiazide, 1662
amiloride hydrochloride, 45–46, 111–112
Aminofen, 67–70
Aminoglycosides, 23–24, 1696–1697
Aminopenicillins, 53–54
amiodarone hydrochloride, 26–27, 112–115
Amitiza, 1683, **C18**
amitriptyline hydrochloride, 29–30, 116–118
amlodipine besylate, 25–26, 33–34, 41–42, 118–119, **C3**
amlodipine besylate–atorvastatin calcium, 1663
amlodipine besylate–benazepril hydrochloride, 1658
amlodipine besylate–hydrochlorothiazide–olmesartan medoxomil, 1659
amlodipine besylate–olmesartan medoxomil, 1656
amlodipine besylate–telmisartan, 1659
amlodipine besylate–valsartan, 1657
amlodipine besylate–valsartan–hydrochlorothiazide, 1657
Amox, 119–121
amoxicillin, 53–54, 119–121
amoxicillin–clavulanate potassium, 53–54, 121–124
Amoxil, 119–121
amphetamine–dextroamphetamine, 1630
Amphetamines, 1630
amphotericin B, 1696–1697

amphotericin B lipid complex,
    32–33, 124–126
amphotericin B liposomal,
    32–33, 126–128
amplcillin, 53–54, 128–130
ampicillin sodium, 128–130
ampicillin sodium–sulbactam
    sodium, 53–54, 131–132
ampicillin trihydrate, 53–54
Ampyra, 1716
Amrix, 384–386
Anabolic steroids, 1631
Anacaine, 1686
Anadrol, 1631
Anafranil, 1715
anakinra, 49, 132–134
Analgesics, 1651–1652
Anaprox, 1054–1056
Anaprox DS, 1054–1056
anastrozole, 134–135, **C3**
Ancef, 288–290
Androderm, 1442–1444
AndroGel, 1442–1444
Android, 987–988
AneCream, 1728–1729
AneCream 5, 1728–1729
Anectine, 1387–1390
Anesthetics, 1629
Angiomax, 215–216
Angiotensin-converting
    enzyme inhibitors, 24–25
Angiotensin II receptor
    blockers, 33–34
anidulafungin, 32–33,
    135–136
Antabuse, 1719
Antacids, 25
Antara, 621–623
Anthim, 1609–1610
anthrax vaccine, adsorbed,
    1666
Antiacne drugs, 1652
Antianginals, 25–26
Antiarrhythmics, 26–27
Antibiotic antineoplastics, 27
Antibiotics, 1635, 1696–1697
Anticholinergics, 27–28
Anticoagulants, 28–29
Anticonvulsants, 29

Antidepressants, tricyclic,
    29–30
Antidiabetics, 30–31,
    1652–1655
Antidiarrheals, 31–32, 1637
Antidotes, 1638–1643
Antiemetics, 32, 1635
Antifungal Foot, 1690
Antifungals, 32–33
Antigout drugs, 1655
antihemophilic factor, 1644
Antihistamines, 33
Antihypertensives, 33–34,
    1655–1660
Anti-infectives, macrolide, 50
anti-inhibitor coagulant
    complex, 1644–1645
Antilipemics, 35
Antimetabolite antineoplastics,
    35–36
Antimigraine drugs, 36, 1660
Antiparkinsonian drugs, 36–37
Antiplatelet drugs, 37, 1660
Antipsychotics, 38–39
Antiretrovirals, 1660
Antirheumatics, 39
antithymocyte globulin
    [equine], ATG, LIG, 1648
Antituberculotics, 39–40
Antiulcer drugs, 1661
Anusol HC, 741–743
Anzemet, 475–476
APAP, 67–70
APAP Extra Strength, 67–70
Aphen, 67–70
Apidra, 803–809
Apidra SoloStar, 803–809
apixaban, 28–29, 136–138
Aplenzin, 245–248
Apo-Alpraz, 98–100
Apo-Alpraz TS, 98–100
Apo-Amoxi, 119–121
Apo-Cephalex, 316–318
Apo-Diclo, 445–447
Apo-Diclo Rapide, 445–447
Apo-Digoxin, 456–460
Apo-Diltiaz, 460–462
Apo-Hydro, 728–730
Apo-Imatinib, 772–775

Apo-ISMN, 837–839
Apokyn, 1706–1707
Apo-Metoclop, 988–990
apomorphine hydrochloride,
    36–37, 1706–1707
Apo-Napro-Na, 1054–1056
Apo-Nifed PA-SRT, 1072–1074
Apo-Pen VK, 1202–1203
Apo-Sertraline, 1354–1357
Apo-Sulfatrim, 1392–1395
APO-Tamox, 1412–1414
Apo-Verap, 1532–1535
apremilast, 138–139
aprepitant, 32, 139–141
Apresoline, 726–728
Apriso, 961–963
Aptensio XR, 979–983
Aptiom, 559–561
Aptivus, 1460–1462
Aquasol A, 1673–1674
ara-C, 392–394
Aralen, 323–324
Aranelle, 591–596
Aranesp, 408–411
Arava, 873–875
Arcapta Neohaler, 779–780
Aredia, 1167–1168
arformoterol tartrate, 141–143
argatroban, 28–29, 143–145
Aricept, 476–477, **C9**
Aricept ODT, 476–477
Arimidex, 134–135, **C3**
aripiprazole, 38–39, 145–150,
    C3
aripiprazole lauroxil, 145–150
Aristada, 145–150
Aristospan Intra-articular,
    1500–1503
Aristospan Intralesional,
    1500–1503
Arixtra, 676–678
armodafinil, 43–44, 150–152
Arnuity Ellipta, 663–665
Aromasin, 1722
Arranon, 1733–1734
artemether–lumefantrine,
    1707
Arthritis Pain Relief, 67–70
ASA, 154–157

Asacol HD, 961–963
Asaphen, 154–157
Asatab, 154–157
Ascocid, 1677
ascorbic acid, 1677
Ascor L 500, 1677
Asco-Tabs, 1677
asenapine, 152–154
asenapine maleate, 38–39
asfotase alfa, 1707
Asmanex HFA, 1024–1027
Asmanex Twisthaler,
    1024–1027
asparaginase *Erwinia*
    chrysanthemi, 1707
Aspir-81, 154–157
aspirin, 51–52, 154–157
Aspir-Low, 154–157
Astagraf XL, 1404–1407
Astepro, 182–183
Astramorph PF, 1029–1034
Atacand, 261–263
Atacand HCT, 1655
Atarax, 751–752
Atasol Forte, 67–70
atazanavir sulfate, 55–56,
    157–163, **C4**
Atelvia, 1313–1315
atenolol, 25–26, 33–34,
    40–41, 163–165, **C4**
atenolol–chlorthalidone,
    1659
atezolizumab, 1576–1578
ATG, 1648
Atgam, 1648
Ativan, 924–926, 1631, **C17**
atomoxetine hydrochloride,
    165–167, **C4**
atorvastatin, 1698–1699
atorvastatin calcium, 35,
    167–169, **C4**
atovaquone, 169–170
atovaquone–proguanil
    hydrochloride, 170–172
atracurium besylate, 51,
    1707–1708
Atralin, 1498–1500
Atriance, 1733–1734
Atripla, 1660

AtroPen, 172–174
atropine sulfate, 27–28,
    172–174
Atrovent, 823–824
Atrovent HFA, 823–824
Aubagio, 1746
Augmentin, 121–124
Augmentin ES 600, 121–124
Augmentin XR, 121–124
auranofin, 39, 1708
Auvi-Q, 534–537
Avalide, 1655
avanafil, 174–175
Avandia, 1335–1337, **C26**
Avapro, 825–826, **C14**
Avastin, 209–212
Aveed, 1438–1442, 1631
Avelox, 1038–1041, **C20**
Avelox I.V., 1038–1041
Aviane-28, 591–596
Avita, 1498–1500
Avodart, 508–509, **C9**
Avonex, 816–818
Avycaz, 305–307
Axert, 95–97
Axiron, 1442–1444
axitinib, 175–177
Aygestin, 1088–1089
azacitidine, 177–179
Azactam, 190–192
Azasan, 180–182
AzaSite, 186–189
azathioprine, 49, 180–182
azathioprine sodium, 180–182
azelaic acid, 1708
azelastine hydrochloride,
    182–183
azelastine hydrochloride–
    fluticasone propionate,
    183–184
Azelex, 1708
azidothymidine, 1559–1562
Azilect, 1297–1299, **C25**
azilsartan medoxomil,
    185–186
azithromycin, 50, 186–189, **C4**
Azor, 1656
AZT, 1559–1562
aztreonam, 190–192

Azulfidine, 1395–1397
Azulfidine EN-tabs, 1395–1397

B

Baby Ddrops, 1677–1678
baclofen, 57, 192–194
Bactrim, 1392–1395
Bactrim DS, 1392–1395, **C28**
Bactroban, 1041–1042
BAL in Oil, 1639
Balminil, 1687–1688
Balminil DM, 1687
Balziva-28, 591–596
Banophen, 464–466
Banzel, 1742
Baraclude, 531–533
Barbiturates, 1630
basiliximab, 49, 1708
Bayer Aspirin, 154–157
BCNU, 278–281
Bebulin VH, 1646
beclomethasone dipropionate,
    44–45
  inhalation, 194–195
  intranasal, 195–197
Beconase AQ, 195–197
bedaquiline fumarate, 39–40,
    197–198
Beleodaq, 200–202
belimumab, 49, 198–200
belinostat, 200–202
Belsomra, 1402–1404
Belviq, 926–928
Benadryl, 464–466
Benadryl Allergy Childrens,
    464–466
benazepril, 1696–1697
benazepril–
    hydrochlorothiazide,
    1657–1658
benazepril hydrochloride,
    24–25, 33–34, 202–204,
    C5
bendamustine hydrochloride,
    22, 1708–1709
Bendeka, 1708–1709
BeneFIX, 1646
Benicar, 1106–1108, **C22**

Benicar HCT, 1656, **C22**
Benign prostatic hyperplasia
    drugs, 1662
Benlysta, 198–200
Bentyl, 450–452
Bentylol, 450–452
Benuryl, 1740
Benylin E, 1687–1688
benzathine benzylpenicillin,
    1193–1194
benzocaine, 1686
Benzodiazepines, 40, 1630
benzonatate, 1709
benzoyl peroxide–adapalene,
    1652
benztropine mesylate, 27–28,
    36–37, 204–206
benzyl alcohol, 1709
benzylpenicillin potassium,
    1194–1197
benzylpenicillin procaine,
    1197–1199
benzylpenicillin sodium,
    1199–1202
bepotastine besilate, 1709
Bepreve, 1709
beractant, 1645
besifloxacin hydrochloride,
    206
Besivance, 206
Beta blockers, 25–26, 33–34,
    40–41
Betacaine, 1728–1729
Betagan, 883–884
betamethasone, 44–45,
    1696–1697
betamethasone dipropionate,
    207–208
betamethasone valerate,
    207–208
Betapace, 1381–1384
Betapace AF, 1381–1384
Betaseron, 818–820
Beta Temp Childrens, 67–70
Beta-Val, 207–208
Betaxin, 1677
betaxolol, 40–41
betaxolol hydrochloride, 1709
bethanechol chloride, 208–209

Bethkis, 1466–1469
Betimol, 1455–1456
Betoptic, 1709
Betoptic S, 1709
bevacizumab, 209–212
bexarotene, 1709–1710
Bexsero, 1670
bezlotoxumab, 1752
Biaxin, 347–349, **C6**
bicalutamide, 1710
Bicillin L-A, 1193–1194
BiCNU, 278–281
BiDil, 1662
Biguanides, 1696–1697
bimatoprost, 212–213
Binosto, 87–89
Bio-D-Mulsion, 1677–1678
Biologicals, 1632–1633,
    1644–1650
Biosimilar drugs,
    understanding,
    1632–1633
BioThrax, 1666
Bisac-Evac, 1682
bisacodyl, 50, 1682
Bisacodyl EC, 1682
Biscolax, 1682
Bismatrol, 1637
bismuth subcitrate potassium–
    metronidazole–
    tetracycline
    hydrochloride, 1661
bismuth subsalicylate, 31–32,
    1637
bisoprolol fumarate, 25–26,
    33–34, 40–41, 213–215
bisoprolol fumarate–
    hydrochlorothiazide,
    1660
bivalirudin, 28–29, 215–216
Bivigam, 1647–1648
bleomycin sulfate, 27,
    217–219
Bleph-10, 1391–1392
blinatumomab, 1710
Blincyto, 1710
Blood derivatives, 1644–1650
B-Natal, 1676
Boniva, 752–754, **C14**

Boostrix, 1666–1667
bortezomib, 219–221, 1636
bosentan, 222–224
Bosulif, 1710
bosutinib, 1710
Botox, 1120–1124
Botox Cosmetic, 1120–1124
Breast-feeding, and drugs,
    7, 1624
brentuximab vedotin, 224–226
Breo Ellipta, 666–668
Brevibloc, 561–563
Brevicon 28-Day, 591–596
brexpiprazole, 38–39,
    226–229
Briellyn, 591–596
Brilinta, 1451–1453
brimonidine tartrate, 229–230
brinzolamide–brimonidine
    tartrate, 1710
Brisdelle, 1175–1178
brivaracetam, 1578–1580
Briviact, 1578–1580
bromfenac sodium, 230–231
bromocriptine mesylate,
    36–37, 232–234
Bromsite, 230–231
Brovana, 141–143
B-6, 1676
Buckley's Cough Mixture, 1687
budesonide, 44–45
    inhalation, 234–236
    intranasal, 234–236
    oral, 236–238
    rectal, 236–238
budesonide–formoterol
    fumarate dihydrate, 1665
Bulk-forming laxatives, 50
bumetanide, 45, 238–240
Bumex, 238–240
Buminate 5%, 1644
Buminate 25%, 1644
Bunavail, 1663–1664
Buprenex, 240–245
buprenorphine, 240–245
buprenorphine–naloxone,
    1663–1664
buprenorphine hydrochloride,
    240–245

buPROPion hydrobromide, 245–248

buPROPion hydrochloride, 245–248, **C5**

Burinex, 238–240

busPIRone hydrochloride, 248–249

busulfan, 22, 1711

Busulfex, 1711

butorphanol tartrate, 250–252

Butrans, 240–245

Bydureon, 610–613

Byetta, 610–613

Bystolic, 1061–1063, **C20**

C

cabazitaxel, 1711

Caduet, 1663

Cafergot, 1660

Calan, 1532–1535, **C31**

Calan SR, 1532–1535

Calax, 1682

Cal-Carb Forte, 1680

Calci-Chew, 1680

Calcidol, 1677–1678

Calciferol, 1677–1678

Calcionate, 256–259

calcitonin salmon, 252–254

calcitriol, 254–256

calcium acetate, 256–259

calcium carbonate, 25, 1680

Calcium channel blockers, 25–27, 33–34, 41–42

calcium chloride, 256–259

calcium citrate, 256–259

Calcium Disodium Versenate, 1640

calcium glubionate, 256–259

calcium gluconate, 256–259

calcium lactate, 256–259

calcium phosphate (tribasic), 256–259

calcium polycarbophil, 50, 1682

Caldolor, 756–759

calfactant, 1645

Cal-Gest, 1680

Cal-Mint, 1680

Calphron, 256–259

Caltrate, 1680

Cambia, 445–447

Camila, 1088–1089

Camptosar, 826–829

Canadian National Drug Schedules (NDS), 1693

canagliflozin, 30–31, 259–261

canagliflozin–metformin, 1653

canakinumab, 1711

Canasa, 961–963

Cancidas, 285–287

candesartan cilexetil, 33–34, 261–263

candesartan cilexetil–hydrochlorothiazide, 1655

Canesten, 366–367

cangrelor tetrasodium, 37, 263–264

Cannabinoids, 1631

capecitabine, 35–36, 264–267

Capex, 652–653

Capital and Codeine, 374–377

Caprelsa, 1750

captopril, 24–25, 33–34, 267–269, 1696–1697

captopril and hydrochlorothiazide, 1656

Carac, 655–657

Carafate, 1390–1391, **C28**

Carbaglu, 1712

carbamazepine, 29, 269–272, 1696–1697

Carbatrol, 269–272

Carbolith, 915–917

carboplatin, 22, 272–274

carboprost tromethamine, 1711–1712

Cardene, 1070–1072

Cardene I.V., 1070–1072

Cardiac drugs, miscellaneous, 1663

Cardizem, 460–462, **C8**

Cardizem CD, 460–462, **C8**

Cardizem LA, 460–462, **C8**

Cardura, 481–482, **C9**

Cardura XL, 481–482

carfilzomib, 1712

carglumic acid, 1712

Carimune NF, 1647–1648

cariprazine hydrochloride, 38–39, 274–277

carisoprodol, 57, 277–278, **C5**

carmustine, 22, 278–281

Carpine, 1219–1220

carteolol hydrochloride, 281–282

Carter's Little Pills, 1682

Cartia XT, 460–462

carvedilol, 33–34, 40–41, 282–285

carvedilol phosphate, 282–285

Casodex, 1710

caspofungin acetate, 32–33, 285–287

Cataflam, 445–447

Catapres, 361–364

Catapres-TTS, 361–364

Cathflo Activase, 102–104

Caverject, 1706

Caverject Impulse, 1706

Cayston, 190–192

C-Caps, 1677–1678

CCNU, 1730

CDDP, 342–344

cefadroxil, 42–43, 287–288

cefazolin sodium, 42–43, 288–290

cefdinir, 42–43, 290–291

cefepime hydrochloride, 42–43, 292–294

cefotaxime sodium, 42–43, 294–296

cefoxitin sodium, 42–43, 296–298

cefpodoxime proxetil, 42–43, 298–299

cefprozil, 42–43, 299–301

ceftaroline fosamil, 42–43, 301–303

ceftazidime, 42–43, 303–305

ceftazidime–avibactam, 305–307

Ceftin, 311–313

ceftolozane–tazobactam, 307–309

ceftriaxone sodium, 42–43, 309–311, 1627
cefuroxime axetil, 42–43, 311–313
cefuroxime sodium, 42–43, 311–313
Celebrex, 314–316, **C5**
celecoxib, 51–52, 314–316, **C5**
Celexa, 345–347, **C6**
CellCept, 1042–1045
CellCept Intravenous, 1042–1045
Cemill, 1677–1678
Cena-K, 1234–1235
Cenestin, 578–581
Centany, 1041–1042
Cepacol Extra Strength Sore Throat, 1686
cephalexin, 42–43, 316–318
Cephalosporins, 42–43
Ceprotin, 1649
Cerdelga, 1721
Cerebyx, 684–687
ceritinib, 1712
certolizumab pegol, 49, 318–320
Cerubidine, 1717–1718
Cervarix, 1668
Cervidil, 1719
C.E.S., 578–581
Cesamet, 1631
cetirizine hydrochloride, 33, 1686
Cetraxal, 339–340
cetrorelix acetate, 1712–1713
Cetrotide, 1712–1713
cetuximab, 320–323
cevimeline hydrochloride, 1713
Chantix, 1527–1529, **C31**
Charac-25, 1638
Charactol-25, 1638
Charcodote TFS, 1638
Char-Flo with Sorbitol, 1638
Chemet, 1643
Chew-C, 1677–1678
Chew Q, 1674–1675
Children, drug therapy in, 7–10, 1626–1627
Children's Advil, 756–759

Children's Claritin Allergy, 1688
Children's Loratadine, 1688
Children's Mapap Rapid Tabs, 67–70
Children's Motion Sickness Liq, 1718–1719
Children's Motrin Jr Strength, 756–759
Children's Mylanta, 1680
Children's Nasacort Allergy 24 Hour, 1503–1504
Children's Pepto, 1680
Children's Silapap, 67–70
chlorambucil, 22, 1713
chloramphenicol sodium succinate, 1713
Chloraseptic Sore Throat, 67–70
chlordiazepoxide–amitriptyline, 1664
chlordiazepoxide hydrochloride, 40, 1631, 1713–1714
chloroquine phosphate, 323–324
chlorpheniramine maleate, 33, 1686
chlorpheniramine polistirex–hydrocodone bitartrate, 1665
chlorproMAZINE hydrochloride, 38–39, 54–55, 1714
ChlorTabs, 1686
chlorthalidone, 1714
chlorthalidone–clonidine hydrochloride, 1656
Chlor-Trimeton, 1686
Chlor-Trimeton Allergy 12 Hour, 1686
Cholac, 1683, 1727
Cholbam, 1714–1715
cholestyramine, 35, 325–326
cholic acid, 1714–1715
Cialis, 1409–1411, **C28**
ciclesonide, 44–45
  inhalation, 326–328
  intranasal, 326–328
cidofovir, 328–330
cilostazol, 37, 330–331

Ciloxan, 339–340
cimetidine, 48–49, 331–333
cimetidine hydrochloride, 331–333
Cimzia, 318–320
cinacalcet hydrochloride, 333–335
Cinqair, 1613–1614
Cipro, 335–339, **C5**
ciprofloxacin, 47–48, 335–339, **C5**
ciprofloxacin hydrochloride
  ophthalmic, 339–340
  otic, 339–340
Cipro I.V., 335–339
Cipro XR, 335–339
cisatracurium besylate, 51, 340–342
cisplatin, 22, 342–344
citalopram hydrobromide, 56–57, 345–347, **C6**
Citracal, 256–259
Citracal Liquitab, 256–259
Citrate of magnesia, 1684
citrovorum factor, 1675
Claforan, 294–296
Claravis, 839–841
Clarinex, 420–421, **C7**
Clarinex RediTabs, 420–421
clarithromycin, 50, 347–349, **C6**
Claritin, 1688
Claritin-D, 1664
Claritin-D 24 Hour, 1664
Claritin Liqui-Gels, 1688
Claritin RediTabs, 1688
Claritin 24-Hour Allergy, 1688
Clavulin, 121–124
Clear Eyes, 1052–1053
Clear Eyes Triple Action, 1690
Clearlax, 1684
Cleocin, 353–354
Cleocin Hydrochloride, 351–353
Cleocin Pediatric, 351–353
Cleocin Phosphate, 351–353
Cleocin T, 353–354
clevidipine, 350–351
clevidipine butyrate, 41–42

Cleviprex, 350–351
Climara, 569–573
Clinda-Derm, 353–354
Clindagel, 353–354
clindamycin hydrochloride,
    351–353
clindamycin palmitate
    hydrochloride, 351–353
clindamycin phosphate
    injection, 351–353
    topical, 353–354
clindamycin phosphate–
    tretinoin, 1652
Clinda-T, 353–354
Clindesse, 353–354
Clindets, 353–354
clobazam, 29, 40, 354–356
clobetasol propionate, 357–358
Clobex, 357–358
Clomid, 1715
clomiPHENE citrate, 1715
clomiPRAMINE hydrochloride,
    29–30, 1715
clonazepam, 29, 40, 359–361,
    1631, **C6**
clonidine, 361–364
clonidine hydrochloride,
    33–34, 361–364
clopidogrel bisulfate, 37,
    364–365, **C6**
Clorpres, 1656
Clotrimaderm, 366–367
clotrimazole, 32–33, 366–367
clozapine, 38–39, 367–371, **C6**
Clozaril, 367–371, **C6**
CNS stimulants, 43–44
Coartem, 1707
cobimetinib fumarate,
    1580–1582
cocaine, 1629
codeine, 1630
codeine phosphate, 52–53,
    371–374
codeine phosphate–
    acetaminophen, 374–377,
    C6
codeine phosphate–aspirin–
    butalbital–caffeine, 1651

codeine sulfate, 52–53,
    371–374
Codulax, 1682
coenzyme Q10, 1674–1675
Cogentin, 204–206
Colace, 1682
colchicine, 377–379, **C7**
Colcrys, 377–379, **C7**
colesevelam hydrochloride,
    35, 379–380, **C7**
collagenase *Clostridium
    histolyticum*, 1715
Colocort, 738–741
Col-Probenecid, 1655
Colyte, 1684
CombiPatch, 573–576
Combivent Respimat, 1664
Combivir, 1660, **C15**
Complera, 1661
Compound S, 1559–1562
Compro, 1258–1261
Comtan, 1721
Concerta, 979–983, **C19**
CongestAid, 1689
conivaptan hydrochloride,
    380–382
Constella, 1683
Constilac, 1683, 1727
Constulose, 1683, 1727
Contac-D, 1689
Controlled substance
    schedules, 1624
ConZip, 1487–1490
Copaxone, 710–711
Copegus, 1301–1305
CoQ10, 1674–1675
Cordarone, 112–115
Coreg, 282–285
Coreg CR, 282–285
Corgard, 1045–1047
Corlanor, 844–848
Cormax, 357–358
Correctol, 1682
Correctol Extra Gentle,
    1682
Cortaid, 741–743
Cortef, 738–741
Cortenema, 738–741

Corticaine, 741–743
Corticosteroids, 44–45,
    1696–1697
Cortifoam, 741–743
cortisone, 1696–1697
Cortizone-5, 741–743
Cortizone-10, 741–743
Corvert, 759–761
Corzide, 1656
Cosentyx, 1743
Cosentyx Sensoready Pen,
    1743
Cotellic, 1580–1582
Coumadin, 1554–1556,
    C32
Coumarin derivative, 28–29
Covera-HS, 1532–1535
Coversyl, 1737–1738
Cozaar, 928–930, **C18**
Creomulsion, 1687
Creon, 1169–1171
Creo-Terpin, 1687
Cresemba, 832–835
Crestor, 1337–1340, **C26**
Crixivan, 782–784, **C14**
crizotinib, 382–384
crofelemer, 1637
crotamiton, 1715
Cruex, 366–367
Cryselle, 591–596
Crystapen, 1199–1202
Cubicin, 406–408
Cutivate, 668–669
cyanocobalamin, 1674
Cyclafem 1/35, 591–596
Cyclafem 7/7/7, 591–596
Cyclessa, 591–596
cyclobenzaprine hydrochloride,
    57, 384–386
cyclophosphamide, 22,
    386–388
cycloSERINE, 39–40,
    1716
Cycloset, 232–234
cycloSPORINE, 49, 388–392
cycloSPORINE (modified),
    388–392
Cymbalta, 506–508, **C9**

Cyramza, 1290–1292
cytarabine, 35–36, 392–394
Cytomel, 1729
Cytosar, 392–394
cytosine arabinoside, 392–394
Cytotec, 1733
Cytovene, 697–699

D

dabigatran etexilate mesylate,
    28–29, 394–396, **C7**
dacarbazine, 22, 396–398
daclatasvir dihydrochloride,
    398–400
daclizumab, 1582–1583
Daklinza, 398–400
Dalacin C, 351–353
Dalacin C Flavored Granules,
    351–353
Dalacin C Phosphate, 351–353
Dalacin T, 353–354
dalbavancin hydrochloride,
    400–402
dalfampridine, 1716
Daliresp, 1330–1331
dalteparin sodium, 28–29,
    402–405
Dalvance, 400–402
Dantrium, 1716
Dantrium I.V., 1716
dantrolene sodium, 57, 1716
dapagliflozin propanediol,
    30–31, 405–406
Daptacel, 1666–1667
daptomycin, 406–408
Daraprim, 1740
daratumumab, 1583–1585
darbepoetin alfa, 48, 408–411
darifenacin hydrobromide,
    411–412, **C7**
darunavir, 55–56
darunavir ethanolate,
    1716–1717
Darzalex, 1583–1585
dasatinib, 1717
Dasetta 1/35, 591–596
Dasetta 7/7/7, 591–596

DAUNOrubicin hydrochloride,
    27, 1717–1718
Daytrana, 979–983
DDAVP, 421–423
ddI, 452–454
Docara, 1677–1678
deferasirox, 1638–1639
deferiprone, 1639
defibrotide sodium, 58–59,
    1585–1586
Defitelio, 1585–1586
degarelix acetate, 412–414
Delatestryl, 1438–1442
delavirdine, 1700–1701
delavirdine mesylate, 414–416
Delestrogen, 569–573
Delsym, 1687
Delta-D, 1677–1678
delta-9-tetrahydrocannabinol,
    495–496
Delzicol, 961–963
Demadex, 1485–1487, **C30**
Demerol, 954–957, 1630, **C18**
denosumab, 416–418
Denta5000 Plus, 1676
deoxycholic acid, 1718
Depacon, 1519–1522
Depakene, 1519–1522
Depakote, 1519–1522, **C9**
Depakote ER, 1519–1522
Depakote Sprinkle, 1519–
    1522, **C9**
DepoCyt, 392–394
Depo-Estradiol, 569–573
Depo-Medrol, 984–986
Depo-Provera, 943–945
Depo-subQ Provera 104,
    943–945
Depo-Testosterone,
    1438–1442
Dermabet, 207–208
Derma-Smoothe/FS, 652–653
Dermazin, 1743–1744
Dermoplast, 1686
Dermotic, 652–653
Descovy, 1592–1594
Desenex, 366–367,
    1000–1002

desipramine hydrochloride,
    29–30, 418–420
desirudin, 28–29, 1718
desloratadine, 33, 420–421,
    C7
desmopressin acetate,
    421–423
Desogen, 591–596
desoximetasone, 423–425
desvenlafaxine, 425–427
desvenlafaxine fumarate,
    425–427
desvenlafaxine succinate,
    425–427, **C7**
Detrol, 1476–1477, **C29**
Detrol LA, 1476–1477
dexamethasone, 44–45,
    1696–1697
    ophthalmic, 427–429
    oral, 429–432
Dexamethasone Intensol,
    429–432
dexamethasone sodium
    phosphate, 44–45,
    427–429
    injection, 429–432
Dexedrine, 436–438, 1630
DexFerrum, 829–831
Dexilant, 432–434, **C7**
Dexilant Solutab, 432–434
DexIron, 829–831
dexlansoprazole, 56, 432–434,
    C7
dexmethylphenidate
    hydrochloride, 43–44,
    434–436, **C8**
dextroamphetamine sulfate,
    43–44, 436–438, 1630
dextroamphetamine sulfate–
    dextroamphetamine
    saccharate–amphetamine
    aspartate–amphetamine
    sulfate, 438–442
dextromethorphan
    hydrobromide, 1635,
    1687
d4T, 1386–1387
DHPG, 697–699

DiaBeta, 715–717, **C14**
Diabetic Tussin, 1687–1688
Diabetic Tussin Allergy, 1686
Diamode, 1637
Diamox, 1704
Diamox Sequels, 1704
Diastat, 442–444
Diastat Acudial, 442–444
diazepam, 29, 40, 442–444, 1631, **C8**
Diazepam Intensol, 442–444
Diclegis, 494–495
diclofenac, oral, 445–447
diclofenac epolamine, 51–52, 448–450
diclofenac potassium, 51–52, 445–447
diclofenac sodium, 51–52
    oral, 445–447
    topical, 448–450
dicyclomine hydrochloride, 27–28, 450–452
didanosine, 52, 452–454
dideoxyinosine, 452–454
Dietary supplements, 1635
Dificid, 632–633
Diflucan, 646–648, **C12**
diflunisal, 51–52, 1718
difluprednate, 454–455
DigiFab, 1639
digoxin, 49, 456–460, 1698–1699
digoxin immune Fab (ovine), 1639
dihydromorphinone hydrochloride, 743–747
Dilantin, 1215-1219
Dilantin 125, 1215–1219
Dilantin Infatabs, 1215–1219
Dilatrate-SR, 837–839
Dilaudid, 743–747, 1630
Dilaudid-HP, 743–747
diltiazem hydrochloride, 25–26, 26–27, 33–34, 41–42, 460–462, **C8**
Dilt XR, 460–462
Diltzac, 460–462
dimenhyDRINATE, 32, 1718–1719

dimercaprol, 1639
dimethyl fumarate, 462–464
Dinate, 1718–1719
dinoprostone, 1719
dinutuximab, 1719
Diocarpine, 1219–1220
Diocto, 1682
dioctyl calcium sulfosuccinate, 1682
dioctyl sodium sulfosuccinate, 1682
Diotame, 1637
Diovan, 1522–1524, **C30**
Diovan HCT, 1656, **C31**
Dipentum, 1110–1111
Diphenhist, 464–466
diphenhydrAMINE
    hydrochloride, 33, 36–37, 464–466
diphenoxylate hydrochloride–atropine sulfate, 31–32, 1637
diphenylhydantoin, 1215–1219
diphtherIa and tetanus toxoids, acellular pertussis adsorbed, and inactivated poliovirus combination vaccine, 1667
diphtheria and tetanus toxoids, acellular pertussis adsorbed, hepatitis B (recombinant), and inactivated poliovirus vaccine combined, 1667
diphtheria and tetanus toxoids, acellular pertussis adsorbed, inactivated poliovirus, and *Haemophilus influenzae* type b conjugate vaccine combined, 1667–1668
diphtheria and tetanus toxoids and acellular pertussis vaccine adsorbed, 1666–1667
Diprivan, 1265–1267
Diprolene, 207–208
Diprolene AF, 207–208
dipyridamole, 37, 466–467

dipyridamole–aspirin, 1660
Direct renin inhibitor, 33–34
disopyramide, 26–27
disulfiram, 1719
Ditropan XL, 1139–1141
Diuretics, 1662
    loop, 45
    potassium-sparing, 45–46
    thiazide and thiazide-like, 46
divalproex sodium, 1519–1522, 1702–1703, **C9**
Divigel, 569–573
Dixarit, 361–364
DOBUTamine hydrochloride, 59, 467–469
Docefrez, 469–472
docetaxel, 469–472
DocQLace, 1682
Docuprene, 1682
docusate calcium, 50, 1682
docusate sodium, 50, 1682
Docusoft-S, 1682
DocuSol Kids Enema, 1682
dofetilide, 26–27, 473–475
DOK, 1682
dolasetron mesylate, 32, 475–476
Dolophine, 966–970
Doloral, 1029–1034
donepezil hydrochloride, 23, 476–477, **C9**
DOPamine hydrochloride, 59, 478–479
Dopram, 1639–1640
Doribax, 1720
doripenem, 1720
Doryx, 490–494
dorzolamide hydrochloride, 479–480
D.O.S., 1682
Dosolax, 1682
doxapram hydrochloride, 43–44, 1639–1640
doxazosin mesylate, 22–23, 33–34, 481–482, **C9**
doxepin hydrochloride, 29–30, 482–484
Doxil, 487–490

DOXOrubicin hydrochloride, 27, 484–487
DOXOrubicin hydrochloride liposomal, 487–490
Doxy 100, 490–494
Doxy 200, 490–494
doxycycline, 58, 490–494
doxycycline calcium, 490–494
doxycycline hyclate, 58, 490–494
doxycycline monohydrate, 58, 490–494
doxylamine succinate–pyridoxine hydrochloride, 494–495
Dramamine, 1718–1719
Dramamine Less Drowsy Formula, 1688
Drisdol, 1677–1678
Dristan, 1689
dronabinol, 32, 495–496, 1631
dronedarone, 26–27, 496–498
drospirenone–ethinyl estradiole, 498–501
Droxia, 749–750
droxidopa, 501–502
Drug abuse, prescription drugs and, 1629–1631
Drug administration, safety of, 13–21
Drug classifications, 22–59
Drug errors
   avoiding, 1621–1623
   do not use list, 1625, 1691
   pediatric drugs in, 1626–1627
   prevention of, 1626
Drug interactions, 3–5
Drug properties, 1–3
Drug therapy, 6–12
   during pregnancy, 6–7
   in children, 7–10
   in elderly patients, 10–12, 1628
   patient safety during, 1634
DSS, 1682
DTaP, 1666–1667
DTaP/IPV, 1667
DTIC, 396–398

Duavee, 1662
Duexis, 1651
dulaglutide, 30–31, 503–505
Dulcocomfort, 1682
Dulcolax, 1682
Dulcolax Milk of Magnesia, 1684
Dulcolax Stool Softener, 1682
Dulera, 1664
duloxetine hydrochloride, 505–508, C9
Duopa, 886–889
Duraclon, 361–364
Duragesic-12, 624–630
Duragesic-25, 624–630
Duragesic-50, 624–630
Duragesic-75, 624–630
Duragesic-100, 624–630
Duramorph PF, 1029–1034
Duration Spray, 1689
Durezol, 454–455
Durlaza, 154–157
dutasteride, 508–509, C9
dutasteride–tamsulosin hydrochloride, 1662
Dutoprol, 1656–1657
Duvoid, 208–209
D-Vi-Sol, 1677–1678
D-Vita, 1677–1678
Dyazide, 1505–1508
Dymista, 183–184
Dynacin, 1010–1012

E

Ebixa, 952–954
ecallantide, 1720
EC-Naprosyn, 1054–1056
econazole nitrate, 32–33, 1720
Ecotrin, 154–157
Ecoza, 1720
EcPirin, 154–157
eculizumab, 1720
Ed-APAP, 67–70
Edarbi, 185–186
Edecrin, 588–590
Edex, 1706
edetate calcium disodium, 1640
Edluar, 1570–1572

edoxaban, 28–29
edoxaban tosylate, 509–511
Edurant, 1310–1312
E.E.S. Granules, 553–556
efavirenz, 511–514, 1700–1701
efavirenz–emtricitabine–tenofovir disoproxil fumarate, 1660
Effexor XR, 1529–1532, C31
Effient, 1240–1241, C23
efinaconazole, 32–33, 1720–1721
Efudex, 655–657
Elavil, 116–118
elbasvir–grazoprevir, 1587–1588
Eldepryl, 1351–1354
Elelyso, 1745
Elestat, 533–534
Elestrin, 569–573
eletriptan hydrobromide, 36, 514–516, C10
Elidel, 1222–1223
Eligard, 876–878
eliglustat tartrate, 1721
Elimite, 1738
Elinest, 591–596
Eliphos, 256–259
Eliquis, 136–138
Elixophyllin, 1746–1747
ElixSure Congestion, 1689
ElixSure Cough, 1687
ella, 1511–1512
Ellence, 537–539
Elocon, 1024–1027
Eloctate, 1644
elosulfase alfa, 1721
elotuzumab, 1588–1590
Eloxatin, 1132–1134
eltrombopag, 1645–1646
Eltroxin, 897–900
eluxadoline, 516–518
elvitegravir–cobicistat–emtricitabine–tenofovir disoproxil fumarate, 518–521
Embeda, 1034–1038
Embeline, 357–358

Embeline E, 357–358
Emend, 139–141
Emollient laxatives, 50
Emoquette, 591–596
empagliflozin, 30–31, 521–523
Empliciti, 1588–1590
Emsam, 1351–1354
emtricitabine, 52, 523–524
emtricitabine–rilpivirine
        tenofovir alafenamide
        fumarate, 1590–1592
emtricitabine–rilpivirine–
        tenofovir disoproxil
        fumarate, 1661
emtricitabine–tenofovir
        alafenamide fumarate,
        1592–1594
emtricitabine–tenofovir
        disoproxil fumarate, 1661
Emtriva, 523–524
Enablex, 411–412, **C7**
enalapril, 1696–1697
enalaprilat, 24–25, 33–34,
        524–526, 1696–1697
enalapril maleate, 24–25,
        33–34, 524–526, **C10**
enalapril maleate–
        hydrochlorothiazide,
        1659–1660
Enbrel, 586–588
Enbrel SureClick, 586–588
Endocet, 1145–1149
Endur-Acin, 1675–1676
Enemeez Mini, 1682
enfuvirtide, 527–528
Engerix-B, 1668
Enjuvia, 578–581
enoxaparin sodium, 28–29,
        528–531
Enpresse-28, 591–596
entacapone, 36–37, 1721
entecavir, 531–533
Entereg, 104–105
Entocort EC, 236–238
Entresto, 1343–1345
Entrophen, 154–157
Entyvio, 1750
Enulose, 1683, 1727
Envarsus XR, 1404–1407

enzalutamide, 1721
E 1000, 1678
Epaned Kit, 524–526
Epanova, 1116–1117
Epclusa, 1616–1617
Eperzan, 1705
ephedrine sulfate, 59
Epiduo, 1652
Epiduo Forte, 1652
epinastine hydrochloride,
        533–534
epinephrine, 534–537
epinephrine hydrochloride,
        534–537
EpiPen, 534–537
EpiPen Jr, 534–537
epirubicin hydrochloride, 27,
        537–539
Epitol, 269–272
Epivir, 860–863
Epivir-HBV, 860–863
eplerenone, 45–46, 539–541
epoetin alfa, 48, 541–544,
        1698–1699
Epogen, 541–544
Eprex, 541–544
eprosartan mesylate, 33–34,
        1721–1722
Epsom salts, 1684
eptastatin, 1241–1243
eptifibatide, 37, 544–545
Epzicom, 1661
Equetro, 269–272
Eraxis, 135–136
Erbitux, 320–323
Erelzi, 1594–1596
ergocalciferol, 1677–1678
ergotamine tartrate–caffeine,
        1660
eribulin mesylate, 545–547
Erivedge, 1546–1547
erlotinib, 547–549
Errin, 1088–1089
Ertaczo, 1743
ertapenem sodium, 549–552
Erwinase, 1707
Erwinaze, 1707
Erybid, 553–556
Eryc, 553–556, **C10**

Erygel, 552–553
EryPed, 553–556
Ery-Tab, 553–556, **C10**
Erythro Base, 553–556
Erythrocin, 553–556
Erythrocin Stearate, 553–556
Erythro-ES, 553–556
erythromycin
        ophthalmic, 552–553
        topical, 552–553
erythromycin base, 553–556,
        C10
erythromycin ethylsuccinate,
        50, 553–556
erythromycin lactobionate, 50,
        553–556
erythromycin stearate, 50,
        553–556
erythropoietin, 541–544
Erythro-S, 553–556
Esbriet, 1738–1739
escitalopram oxalate, 56–57,
        556–559, **C10**
eslicarbazepine acetate,
        559–561
esmolol hydrochloride, 26–27,
        40–41, 561–563
esomeprazole, 56
esomeprazole magnesium,
        563–566, **C10**
esomeprazole sodium,
        563–566
esterified estrogens, 46–47,
        566–568
Estrace Vaginal Cream,
        569–573
Estraderm, 569–573
estradiol, 46–47, 569–573
estradiol acetate, 569–573
estradiol cypionate, 46–47,
        569–573
estradiol gel, 569–573
estradiol hemihydrate, 46–47,
        569–573
estradiol–norethindrone
        acetate transdermal
        system, 573–576
estradiol valerate, 46–47,
        569–573

estradiol valerate–estradiol
    valerate with dienogest,
    576–578
Estragyn, 566–568
Estring Vaginal Ring, 569–573
EstroGel, 569–573
estrogenic substances
    conjugated, 578–581
estrogens, 46–47
    conjugated, 46–47, 578–581,
    C11
estrogens, conjugated–
    bazedoxifene acetate,
    1662
estrogens, conjugated/
    conjugated estrogens–
    medroxyprogesterone,
    1662–1663
estropipate, 46–47, 582–584
Estrostep Fe, 591–596, 1652
eszopiclone, 584–585, 1631,
    C11
etanercept, 49, 586–588
etanercept-szzs, 1594–1596
eteplirsen, 1596–1597
ethacrynate sodium, 45,
    588–590
ethacrynic acid, 45, 588–590
ethambutol hydrochloride,
    39–40, 590–591
EtheDent, 1676
ethinyl estradiol–desogestrel,
    591–594
ethinyl estradiol–ethynodiol
    diacetate, 591–596
ethinyl estradiol–
    levonorgestrel, 591–596
ethinyl estradiol–
    norethindrone, 591–596
ethinyl estradiol–norethindrone
    acetate, 591–596
ethinyl estradiol–
    norethindrone acetate–
    ferrous fumarate,
    591–596
ethinyl estradiol–norgestimate,
    591–596
ethinyl estradiol–norgestrel,
    591–596

ethosuximide, 1698–1699
Etibi, 590–591
etodolac, 51–52, 596–598
etonogestrel–ethinyl estradiol
    vaginal ring, 599–601
Etopophos, 601–603
etoposide, 601–603, 1636
etoposide phosphate, 601–603
etravirine, 603–605
Euglucon, 715–717
Eurax, 1715
Euthyrox, 897–900
Evamist, 569–573
everolimus, 605–609
Evista, 1282–1284, C25
Evoclin, 353–354
Evocin, 353–354
evolocumab, 35, 609–610
Evomela, 949–952
Evoxac, 1713
Evzio, 1641
Exalgo, 743–747
Exelon, 1327–1330
Exelon Patch, 1327–1330
exemestane, 1722
exetanide, 30–31, 610–613
Exforge, 1657
Exforge HCT, 1657
Exjade, 1638–1639
Ex-Lax Ultra, 1682
Exondys 51, 1596–1597
Extavia, 818–820
Extended-spectrum penicillins,
    53–54
Extina, 849–850
Eylea, 1705
ezetimibe, 35, 613–614, C11
ezetimibe–simvastatin, 1622
    C11
ezogabine, 29, 614–616

F

FA-8, 1675
Factive, 704–706
factor IX
    complex, 1646
    human, 1646
    recombinant, 1646
Falmina, 591–596
famciclovir, 616–617, C11

famotidine, 48–49, 617–619,
    C11
Famvir, 616–617, C11
Fanapt, 769–771
Fareston, 1748
Farxiga, 405–406
Faslodex, 688–690
FazaClo ODT, 367–371
Febrol, 67–70
febuxostat, 619–620
Feen-a-Mint, 1682
Feiba, 1644–1645
Feiba NF, 1644–1645
felbamate, 29
felodipine, 33–34, 41–42,
    620–621
Femara, 875–876
Femcon Fe, 591–596
Femhrt, 591–596
Femiron, 1673
Femring, 569–573
Fenesin IR, 1687–1688
fenofibrate, 35, 621–623
fenofibrate (choline), 621–623,
    C12
fenofibric acid, 621–623
Fenoglide, 621–623
fentanyl, 1627, 1630
fentanyl citrate, 52–53,
    624–630
fentanyl nasal spray, 624–630
fentanyl sublingual spray,
    624–630
fentanyl transdermal system,
    624–630
fentanyl transmucosal,
    624–630
Fentora, 624–630
Feosol, 1673
Feostat, 1673
Feratab, 1673
Fergon, 1673
Fer-Iron, 1673
FeroSul, 1673
Ferretts, 1673
ferric carboxymaltose,
    630–631
Ferriprox, 1639
Ferrlecit, 1372–1373

Ferrocite, 1673
ferrous fumarate, 1673
ferrous gluconate, 1673
ferrous sulfate, 1673
    dried, 1673
fesoterodine fumarate,
    631–632
Fetzima, 895–897
FeverAll Children's, 67–70
FeverAll Infant's, 67–70
fexofenadine hydrochloride,
    33, 1687
FiberCon, 1682
Fiber-Lax, 1682
Fibricor, 621–623
fibrin sealant (human), 1722
fidaxomicin, 50, 632–633
filgrastim, 633–635
filgrastim-sndz, 635–638
Finacea, 1708
finafloxacin, 1722
finasteride, 638–639, **C12**
fingolimod, 49, 639–642
Fioricet with Codeine, 1651
Fiorinal with Codeine, 1651
Firmagon, 412–414
5-fluorouracil, 655–657
5-FU, 655–657
Flagyl, 995–997
Flagyl ER, 995–997
Flagyl IV RTU, 995–997
Flamazine, 1743–1744
Flanax Pain Relief, 1054–1056
Flarex, 1722–1723
Flebogamma DIF, 1647–1648
flecainide acetate, 26–27,
    642–643
Flector, 448–450
Fleet, 1682–1683
Fleet Babylax, 1682–1683
Fleet Bisacodyl, 1682
Fleet Enema, 1685
Fleet Enema Extra, 1685
Fleet For Children, 1685
Fleet Laxative, 1682
Flexbumin 5%, 1644
Flexbumin 25%, 1644
flibanserin, 644–645
Flomax, 1414–1415, **C28**

Flonase, 663–665
Flovent Diskus, 663–665
Flovent HFA, 663–665
Fluarix, 1669
Fluarix Quadrivalent, 1669
Flublok, 1669
Flucelvax, 1669
fluconazole, 32–33, 646–648,
    C12
fludarabine phosphate, 35–36,
    648–650, 1636
fludrocortisone acetate,
    44–45, 1722
FluLaval, 1669
FluLaval Quadrivalent, 1669
flumazenil, 1640
FluMist Quadrivalent, 1669
flunisolide, 44–45
    inhalation, 650–652
    intranasal, 650–652
fluocinolone acetonide,
    652–653
fluocinonide, 653–654
Fluor-A-Day, 1676
Fluorigard, 1676
Fluorinse, 1676
Fluoritab, 1676
fluorometholone, 1722–1723
fluorometholone acetate,
    1722–1723
Fluoroplex, 655–657
Fluoroquinolones, 47–48
fluorouracil, 35–36, 655–657
fluoxetine hydrochloride,
    56–57, 657–659, 1635,
    C12
fluphenazine decanoate,
    38–39, 54–55, 660–662
fluphenazine hydrochloride,
    38–39, 660–662
Flura, 1676
Flura-Loz, 1676
flutamide, 662–663
fluticasone furoate, 663–665
fluticasone furoate–vilanterol
    trifenatate, 666–668
fluticasone propionate, 44–45,
    663–665
    topical, 668–669

fluticasone propionate–
    salmeterol inhalation
    powder, 669–671
fluvastatin, 1698–1699
fluvastatin sodium, 35,
    672–674, **C13**
Fluvirin, 1669
fluvoxamine maleate, 56–57,
    674–676
Fluzone High-Dose, 1669
Fluzone Intradermal, 1669
Fluzone Quadrivalent, 1669
FML, 1722–1723
FML Forte, 1722–1723
Focalin, 434–436
Focalin XR, 434–436, **C8**
folic acid, 1675
folinic acid, 1675
Folotyn, 1739
fondaparinux sodium, 28–29,
    676–678
Foradil Aerolizer, 678–680
Forfivo XL, 245–248
formoterol fumarate,
    678–680
Fortamet, 963–966
Fortaz, 303–305
Forteo, 1437–1438
Fortesta, 1442–1444
Fortical, 252–254
Fortolin, 67–70
Fosamax, 87–89, **C3**
fosamprenavir calcium, 55–56,
    1723
fosaprepitant dimeglumine,
    32, 139–141
foscarnet sodium, 680–682
Foscavir, 680–682
fosinopril, 1696–1697
fosinopril and
    hydrochlorothiazide,
    1657
fosinopril sodium, 24–25,
    33–34, 682–684
fosphenytoin sodium, 29,
    684–687
Fosrenol, 1641
4-Way Fast Acting, 1689
4-Way Menthol, 1689

Fragmin, 402–405
Frova, 687–688, **C13**
frovatriptan succinate, 36,
    687–688, **C13**
fulvestrant, 688–690
Fulyzaq, 1637
FungiCure Intensive NailGuard,
    366–367
Fungoid Tincture, 1000–1002
Furadantin, 1075–1076
furosemide, 45, 690–692,
    C13
Fuzeon, 527–528

G

gabapentin, 29, 692–695, **C13**
gabapentin enacarbil, 692–695
Gabitril Filmtabs, 1450–1451
Gablofen, 192–194
galantamine hydrobromide,
    23, 695–697
GamaSTAN S/D, 1647–1648
Gammagard, 1647–1648
Gammagard Liquid,
    1647–1648
Gammagard S/D, 1647–1648
Gammaked, 1647–1648
gamma globulins, 1647–1648
Gammaplex, 1647–1648
Gamunex-C, 1647–1648
ganciclovir, 697–699
Gardasil, 1669
Gardasil 9, 1669
Gas Relief, 1690
Gas-X, 1690
Gas-X Extra Strength, 1690
Gas-X Infant Drops, 1690
gatifloxacin, 47–48,
    699–700
GaviLAX, 1684
GaviLyte-C, 1684
GaviLyte-G, 1684
GaviLyte-N, 1684
Gaviscon, 1680
Gaviscon Extra Relief Formula,
    1680
Gaviscon Extra Strength, 1680
Gazyva, 1093–1096
G-CSF, 633–635

Gel-Kam, 1676
Gelnique, 1139–1141
Gelnique 3%, 1139–1141
Gel-Tin, 1676
gemcitabine, 35–36
gemcitabine hydrochloride,
    700–702
gemfibrozil, 35, 703–704,
    1698–1699, **C13**
gemifloxacin mesylate, 47–48,
    704–706
Gemzar, 700–702
Genaphed, 1689
Generlac, 1683, 1727
Gengraf, 388–392
Gen-K, 1234–1235
Genoptic, 708–709
Genotropin, 1377–1381
GenotropinMiniQuick,
    1377–1381
Gentak, 708–709
gentamicin, 1696–1697
gentamicin sulfate, 23–24,
    1627
  injection, 706–708
  ophthalmic, 708–709
  topical, 708–709
Geodon, 1562–1565, **C32**
Geri-Tussin, 1687–1688
Gildess Fe 1.5/30, 591–596
Gildess Fe 1/20, 591–596
Gilenya, 639–642
Gilotrif, 1705
Giotrif, 1705
glatiramer acetate, 49,
    710–711
Glatopa, 710–711
Gleevec, 772–775
Gleostine, 1730
Gliadel Wafer, 278–281
glibencamide, 715–717
glimepiride, 30–31, 711–713,
    C13
glipiZIDE, 30–31, 713–715, **C14**
glipiZIDE–metformin
    hydrochloride, 1653
GlucaGen Diagnostic Kit,
    1723–1724
GlucaGen HypoKit, 1723–1724

glucagon, 1723–1724
glucarpidase, 1640
Glucobay, 1704
Glucophage, 963–966, **C18**
Glucophage XR, 963–966, **C18**
Glucotrol, 713–715, **C14**
Glucotrol XL, 713–715, **C14**
Glucovance, 1653
Glumetza, 963–966
glyBURIDE 30–31, 715–717,
    C14
glyBURIDE–metformin
    hydrochloride, 1653
glycerin, 50, 1682–1683
glyceryl guaiacolate,
    1687–1688
glyceryl trinitrate, 1076–1079
GlycoLax, 1684
Glycon, 963–966
Glydo, 1728–1729
Glynase, 715–717
Glyset, 1005–1006
GM-CSF, 1347–1349
golimumab, 717–718
GoLYTELY, 1684
Gonitro, 1076–1079
goserelin acetate, 1724
Gralise, 692–695
granisetron, 718–720
granisetron hydrochloride, 32,
    718–720
Granix, 1745
granulocyte colony-stimulating
    factor, 633–635
granulocyte-macrophage
    colony-stimulating factor,
    1347–1349
Gravol, 1718–1719
guaifenesin, 1687–1688
guanfacine hydrochloride,
    33–34, 1724
Gynecort 10, 741–743
Gyne-Lotrimin, 366–367
Gyne-Lotrimin 3, 366–367

H

Haemophilus b conjugate,
    tetanus toxoid conjugate,
    1666

Haemophilus b conjugate
     vaccine, meningococcal
     protein conjugate, 1666
Haemophilus b conjugate
     vaccines, 1666
Halaven, 545–547
Halcion, 1508–1509, 1631
Haldol, 721–723
Haldol Decanoate, 721–723
Halls Defense Vitamin C
     Drops, 1677
haloperidol, 38–39, 721–723
haloperidol decanoate, 38–39,
     721–723
Haloperidol LA, 721–723
haloperidol lactate, 38–39,
     721–723
Harvoni, 871–873
Havrix, 1668
HDCV, 1672
Heart failure drugs, 1662
Heather, 1088–1089
Hectorol, 1678
Helixate FS, 1644
Hemabate, 1711–1712
Hemangeol, 1267–1270
Hematopoietic agents, 48
Hemocyte, 1673
Hemofil M, 1644
HepaGam B, 1646–1647
heparin (unfractionated),
     1698–1699
Heparin derivative, 28–29
Heparin Lock Flush Solution
     (with Tubex), 723–726
heparin sodium, 28–29,
     723–726
Heparin Sodium Injection,
     723–726
hepatitis A vaccine,
     inactivated, 1668
hepatitis B immune globulin
     (human), 1646–1647
hepatitis B vaccine,
     recombinant, 1668
Hepsera, 78–79
Heptovir, 860–863
Herceptin, 1490–1493
Hetlioz, 1745

Hiberix, 1666
Hicon, 1740
Histamine$_2$-receptor
     antagonists, 48–49
Hizentra, 1647–1648
HMG-CoA reductase inhibitors,
     1698–1699
Hold DM, 1687
Horizant, 692–695
H$_2$Q, 1674–1675
Humalog, 803–809
HumalogMix 50/50, 791–796
HumalogMix 75/25, 791–796
human papillomavirus
     recombinant vaccine
     bivalent, 1668
     quadrivalent, 1669
     q-valent, 1669
Humatrope, 1377–1381
Humira, 76–78
Humulin N, 796–799
Humulin N KwikPen,
     796–799
Humulin R, 809–813
Humulin R U-500
     (concentrated), 809–813
Humulin R U-500 KwikPen,
     809–813
Humulin 70/30, 791–796
Hurricaine, 1686
Hycamtin, 1483–1485
hydrALAZINE hydrochloride,
     33–34, 726–728
Hydrea, 749–750
hydrochlorothiazide, 46,
     728–730
hydrocodone–ibuprofen, 1652
hydrocodone bitartrate,
     730–734
hydrocodone bitartrate–
     acetaminophen, 734–737
hydrocodone bitartrate–
     ibuprofen, 1651
hydrocortisone, 44–45,
     1696–1697
     oral, 738–741
     injection, 738–741
     rectal, 738–741
     topical, 741–743

hydrocortisone acetate, 44–45
     rectal, 741–743
     topical, 741–743
hydrocortisone butyrate,
     44–45, 741–743
hydrocortisone cypionate,
     44–45, 738–741
hydrocortisone probutate,
     44–45, 741–743
hydrocortisone sodium
     succinate, 44–45,
     738–741
hydrocortisone valerate,
     44–45, 741–743
Hydrogel Ag, 1743–1744
hydromorphone hydrochloride,
     52–53, 743–747
hydroxocobalamin, 1674
hydroxychloroquine sulfate,
     747–748
hydroxyprogesterone
     caproate, 1724
hydroxyurea, 35–36, 749–750,
     1636
hydrOXYzine hydrochloride,
     751–752, 1630
hydrOXYzine pamoate,
     751–752
hyoscine, 1743
HyperHEP BS/D, 1646–1647
Hyperosmolar laxatives, 50
HyperRAB S/D, 1649
HyperRHO S/D Full Dose,
     1649–1650
HyperRHO S/D Mini-Dose,
     1649–1650
HyperTET S/D, 1650
HyQvia, 1647–1648
Hysingla ER, 730–734
Hyzaar, 1657

I

^{131}I, 1740
ibandronate sodium, 752–754,
     C14
Ibavyr, 1301–1305
Ibrance, 1161–1162
ibrutinib, 754–756
ibuprofen, 51–52, 756–759

ibuprofen–famotidine, 1651
ibuprofen lysine, 756–759
ibutilide fumarate, 26–27,
    759–761
icosapent ethyl, 1724
Idamycin PFS, 761–763
idarubicin hydrochloride, 27,
    761–763
idarucizumab, 763–764
idelalisib, 764–767
Ifex, 767–769
IFN-alpha 2b, 813–816
ifosfamide, 22, 767–769
IG, 1647–1648
IGIM, 1647–1648
IGIV, 1647–1648
IGSC, 1647–1648
Ilaris, 1711
iloperidone, 38–39, 769–771
iloprost, 771–772
imatinib mesylate, 772–775
Imbruvica, 754–756
Imdur, 837–839
imipenem–cilastatin sodium,
    775–777
imipramine hydrochloride,
    29–30, 777–779
imipramine pamoate, 29–30,
    777–779
Imiquimod, 1725
Imitrex, 1397–1399, **C28**
Imitrex STATdose, 1397–1399
immune globulin
    intramuscular,
    1647–1648
immune globulin intravenous,
    1647–1648
immune globulin
    subcutaneous,
    1647–1648
Immunosuppressants, 49
Imodium A-D, 1637
Imogam Rabies-HT, 1649
Imovax Rabies, 1672
Impavido, 1732–1733
Imuran, 180–182
Increlex, 1731
indacaterol maleate,
    779–780

indacaterol maleate–
    glycopyrrolate, 1725
indapamide, 46, 781–782
Inderal, 1267–1270, **C24**
Inderal LA, 1267–1270, **C24**
indinavir sulfate, 55–56,
    782–784, **C14**
Indocin, 784–787
Indocin I.V., 784–787
indomethacin, 51–52,
    784–787
indomethacin sodium, 51–52
indomethacin sodium
    trihydrate, 784–787
Infacol, 1690
Infanrix, 1666–1667
Infant's Advil, 756–759
Infant's Silapap, 67–70
Infasurf, 1645
InFeD, 829–831
Inflectra, 1597–1600
infliximab, 39, 49, 787–790
infliximab-dyyb, 1597–1600
influenza virus vaccine, live,
    1669
    intranasal, 1669
Infumorph, 1029–1034
ingenol mebutate, 790–791
INH, 835–837
Injectafer, 630–631
Inlyta, 175–177
InnoPran XL, 1267–1270
Inotropics, 49
Inspra, 539–541
insulin, 1698–1699
    human, 803–809
    lispro, 803–809
    regular, 809–813
insulin aspart (rDNA origin)
    injection, 803–809
insulin aspart (rDNA origin)
    protamine suspension–
    insulin aspart (rDNA
    origin) injection, 791–796
insulin degludec, 799–803
insulin degludec–insulin
    aspart, 791–796
insulin detemir (rDNA) origin
    injection, 799–803

insulin glargine (rDNA origin)
    injection, 799–803
insulin glulisine (rDNA origin)
    injection, 803–809
insulin lispro protamine–
    insulin lispro, 791–796
Insulins
    fixed combinations, 791–796
    intermediate-acting,
    796–799
    long-acting, 799–803
    rapid-acting, 803–809
    short-acting, 809–813
Integrilin, 544–545
Intelence, 603–605
interferon alfa-2b
    (recombinant), 813–816
interferon beta-1a, 816–818
interferon beta-1b
    (recombinant), 818–820
interferon gamma-1b, 1725
Intermezzo, 1570–1572
Intron A, 813–816
Introvale, 591–596
Intuniv, 1724
Invanz, 549–552
Invega, 1163–1166
Invega Sustenna, 1163–1166
Invega Trinza, 1163–1166
Invirase, 1742
Invokamet, 1653
Invokana, 259–261
Ionsys, 624–630
Iosat, 1739
ipilimumab, 820–823
IPOL, 1671
ipratropium bromide, 823–824
ipratropium bromide–
    albuterol, 1664
Iprivask, 1718
IPV, 1671
irbesartan, 33–34, 825–826,
    C14
irbesartan–
    hydrochlorothiazide, 1655
irinotecan hydrochloride,
    826–829
irinotecan liposome,
    1725–1726

Iron, 1673
iron dextran, 829–831
iron sucrose injection,
    831–832
isavuconazonium sulfate,
    32–33, 832–835
ISDN, 837–839
Isentress, 1284–1286
isoniazid, 39–40, 835–837
isonicotinic acid hydrazide,
    835–837
isophane insulin suspension
    (NPH), 796–799
isophane insulin suspension–
    insulin injection
    combinations, 791–796
isoproterenol hydrochloride,
    1726
Isoptin SR, 1532–1535
Isopto-Carpine, 1219–1220
Isordil, 837–839
isosorbide dinitrate, 25–26,
    837–839
isosorbide dinitrate–
    hydralazine, 1662
isosorbide mononitrate,
    25–26, 837–839
Isotamine, 835–837
isotretinoin, 839–841,
    1698–1699
isradipine, 41–42
Istalol, 1455–1456
Istodax, 1742
Isuprel, 1726
itraconazole, 32–33, 842–844
ivabradine, 844–846
Ivacaftor, 1726
Ivy-Rid, 1686
ixabepilone, 1726–1727
ixazomib citrate, 1600–1601
ixekizumab, 1602–1603
Ixempra Kit, 1726–1727
Ixiaro, 1669–1670
Ixinity, 1646

J

Jadenu, 1638–1639
Jakafi, 1340–1343
Jalyn, 1662

Jantoven, 1554–1556
Janumet, 1653
Janumet XR, 1653–1654
Januvia, 1371–1372, C27
Japanese encephalitis virus
    vaccine, 1669–1670
Jardiance, 521–523
Jencycla, 1088–1089
Jentadueto, 1654
Jentadueto XR, 1654
Jevtana, 1711
Jublia, 1720–1721
Junel 1/20, 591–596
Junel 1.5/30, 591–596
Junel Fe 1.5/30, 591–596
Junel Fe 1/20, 591–596
Junior Mapap, 67–70
Junior Strength Advil,
    756–759
JustD, 1677–1678
Just For Kids, 1676
Juxtapid, 917–920

K

Kadcyla, 81–84
Kadian, 1029–1034
Kalbitor, 1720
Kaletra, 920–924, C17
Kalexate, 1642
Kalydeco, 1726
Kanuma, 1614–1615
Kaon, 1234–1235
Kaon-Cl 20%, 1234–1235
Kaopectate, 1637
Kao-Tin, 1637, 1682
Kapvay, 361–364
Karidium, 1676
Karigel, 1676
Karigel-N, 1676
Kariva, 591–596
Kayexalate, 1642
Kaylixir, 1234–1235
Kazano, 1654
K-Dur 10, 1234–1235
K-Dur 20, 1234–1235
Kedbumin 25%, 1644
Keflex, 316–318
Kefzol, 288–290
Kelnor 1/35, 591–596

Kenalog, 1504–1505
Kenalog-10, 1500–1503
Kenalog-40, 1500–1503
Kengreal, 263–264
Keppra, 880–883
Keppra XR, 880–883
Kerr Insta-Char, 1638
Kerydin, 1745
ketamine, 1629
ketoconazole, 32–33
    oral, 846–849
    topical, 849–850
Ketoderm, 849–850
ketoprofen, 51–52, 850–852
ketorolac tromethamine,
    51–52
    injection, 853–856
    nasal, 853–856
    ophthalmic, 852–853
    oral, 853–856
ketotifen fumarate, 1688
Ketozole, 849–850
Keytruda, 1737
Khedezla, 425–427
Kineret, 132–134
Kinrix, 1667
Kionex, 1642
Kitabis Pak, 1466–1469
Klonopin, 359–361, 1631, C6
K-Lor, 1234–1235
Klor-Con, 1234–1235
Klor-Con/EF, 1234–1235
Klor-Con 8, 1234–1235
Klor-Con 10, 1234–1235
Klor-Con/25, 1234–1235
Klor-Con M10, 1234–1235
Klor-Con M15, 1234–1235
Klor-Con M20, 1234–1235
Klorvess, 1234–1235
Klotrix, 1234–1235
K-Lyte/Cl, 1234–1235
Koate-DVI, 1644
Koffex DM, 1687
Kogenate FS, 1644
K-100, 1678–1679
Konsyl Fiber, 1682
Kovaltry, 1644
Kristalose, 1683, 1727
Krystexxa, 1189–1190

K-Tab, 1234–1235
Kuvan, 1742
K-Vescent, 1234–1235
Kwellada-P, 1738
Kybella, 1718
Kynamro, 1012–1015
Kyprolis, 1712

L

labetalol hydrochloride, 33–34,
    40–41, 857–858
lacosamide, 29, 858–860
LaCrosse Complete, 1685
lactulose, 50, 1683, 1727
Lamictal, 863–867
Lamictal CD, 863–867
Lamictal ODT, 863–867
Lamictal XR, 863–867
Lamisil, 1433–1435, 1690
Lamisil AT, 1690
lamivudine, 52, 860–863, **C15**
lamivudine–zidovudine, 1660
lamotrigine, 29, 863–867
Lanoxin, 456–460
Lanoxin Pediatric, 456–460
lansoprazole, 56, 867–869,
    C15
lansoprazole–amoxicillin–
    clarithromycin, 1661
lanthanum carbonate, 1641
Lantus, 799–803
Lantus SoloStar, 799–803
lapatinib, 1727
Larin 1.5/30, 591–596
Larin 1/20, 591–596
Larin Fe 1.5/30, 591–596
Larin Fe 1/20, 591–596
Larin 24 Fe, 591–596
Larng-O-Jet Kit, 1728–1729
Larotid, 119–121
Lartruvo, 1752
Lasix, 690–692, **C13**
Lasix Special, 690–692
Lastacaft, 1705
latanoprost, 869–870
Latisse, 212–213
Latuda, 935–937, **C18**
Lax-A-Day, 1684
Laxatives, 50

Lazanda, 624–630
L-deprenyl hydrochloride,
    1351–1354
ledipasvir–sofosbuvir,
    871–873
leflunomide, 39, 873–875
lenvatinib mesylate, 1727
Lenvima, 1727
Lescol, 672–674, **C13**
Lescol XL, 672–674
lesinurad, 1603–1604
Lessina-28, 591–596
Letairis, 107–109
letrozole, 875–876
leucovorin calcium, 1675
Leukeran, 1713
Leukine, 1347–1349
leuprolide acetate, 876–878
levalbuterol hydrochloride,
    879–880
levalbuterol tartrate, 879–880
Levaquin, 891–895, **C15**
levarterenol bitartrate,
    1086–1088
Levate, 116–118
Levemir, 799–803
Levemir FlexTouch, 799–803
levetiracetam, 29, 880–883
Levitra, 1526–1527, **C31**
levobunolol hydrochloride,
    883–884
levocetirizine, 33
levocetirizine dihydrochloride,
    884–885
levodopa–carbidopa, 36–37,
    886–889, **C15**
levodopa–carbidopa–
    entacapone, 36–37,
    889–891, **C15**
levofloxacin, 47–48, 891–895,
    C15
levomilnacipran hydrochloride,
    895–897
Levonest, 591–596
Levophed, 1086–1088
Levora 0.15/30-28, 591–596
Levo-T, 897–900
levothyroxine sodium,
    897–900, **C16**

Levoxyl, 897–900, **C16**
Lexapro, 556–559, **C10**
Lexiva, 1723
Lialda, 961–963
Librium, 1631
Lice Shampoo, 1689–1690
Licide, 1689–1690
Lidocaine, 1728–1729
lidocaine
    intradermal, 1728–1729
    ophthalmic, 1728–1729
    topical, 1728–1729
lidocaine hydrochloride,
    26–27, 900–901,
    1728–1729
Lidocaine Viscous, 1728–1729
Lidodan, 1728–1729
Lidoderm, 1728–1729
lifitegrast, 1604–1605
LIG, 1648
linaclotide, 1683
linagliptin, 30–31, 902–903
linagliptin–metformin
    hydrochloride, 1654
lindane, 1729
linezolid, 903–905, 1635,
    1700–1701
Linzess, 1683
Lioresal Intrathecal, 192–194
liothyronine sodium, 1729
liotrix, 1730
Lipid-lowering drugs, 1662
Lipitor, 167–169, **C4**
Lipofen, 621–623
LiQsorb, 1674–1675
Liquibid, 1687–1688
Liquituss GG, 1687–1688
liraglutide, 30–31, 905–908
lisdexamfetamine dimesylate,
    43–44, 908–910, 1630,
    C17
lisinopril, 24–25, 33–34,
    910–912, 1696–1697,
    C17
lisinopril–hydrochlorothiazide,
    912–915
Listerine Tooth Defense, 1676
Lithane, 915–917
lithium, 1700–1701

lithium carbonate, 915–917
lithium citrate, 915–917
Lithobid, 915–917
Little Colds Cough Formula, 1687
Little Fevers Fever/Pain Reliever, 67–70
Little Noses Decongestant, 1689
Livalo, 1228–1229
lixisenatide, 1605–1606
Locoid, 741–743
Locoid Lipocream, 741–743
Loestrin Fe 1/20, 591–596
Loestrin Fe 1.5/30, 591–596
Loestrin 24 Fe, 591–596
Loestrin 21 1/20, 591–596
Loestrin 21 1.5/30, 591–596
Loestrin 24 Fe, 591–596
Lo Loestrin Fe, 591–596
Lomaira, 1210–1211
lomitapide mesylate, 917–920
Lomotil, 1637
lomustine, 22, 1730
Lonsurf, 1749
Lo/Ovral-28, 591–596
loperamide, 31–32
loperamide hydrochloride, 1637
Lopid, 703–704, **C13**
lopinavir–ritonavir, 55–56, 920–924, **C17**
Lopresor, 992–995
Lopresor SR, 992–995
Lopressor, 992–995, **C19**
Lopressor HCT, 1657
Lopurin, 93–95
loratadine, 33, 1688
loratadine–pseudoephedrine, 1664
lorazepam, 40, 924–926, 1631, **C17**
Lorazepam Intensol, 924–926
Lorazepam Preservative Free, 924–926
lorcaserin hydrochloride, 926–928
Loryna, 498–501

losartan–hydrochlorothiazide, 1657
losartan potassium, 33–34, 928–930, **C18**
Lo Seasonique, 591–596
Losec, 1117–1120
Lotensin, 202–204, **C5**
Lotensin HCT, 1657–1658
Lotrel, 1658
Lotrimin AF, 366–367, 1000–1002
Lotronex, 1706
lovastatin, 35, 930–932, 1698–1699
Lovaza, 1116–1117, **C22**
Lovenox, 528–531
Low-molecular-weight heparins, 28–29
Lowprin, 154–157
loxapine, 1730
loxapine hydrochloride, 38–39
loxapine succinate, 38–39, 1730
Lozide, 781–782
L-PAM, 949–952
LTA Kit II, 1728–1729
L-thyroxine sodium, 897–900
lubiprostone, 50, 1683, **C18**
Lucentis, 1292–1293
Ludent, 1676
luliconazole, 32–33, 1731
lumacaftor-ivacaftor, 932–935
Lumigan, 212–213
Lumizyme, 1705–1706
Lunesta, 584–585, 1631, **C11**
Lupron, 876–878
Lupron Depot, 876–878
Lupron Depot-Ped, 876–878
lurasidone hydrochloride, 38–39, 935–937, **C18**
Luride, 1676
Luride Lozi-Flur, 1676
Luvox, 674–676
Luvox CR, 674–676
Luxiq, 207–208
Luzu, 1731
lymphocyte immune globulin, 49, 1648

Lynparza, 1735
Lyrica, 1250–1252, **C23**

M

Maalox, 1680
Macrobid, 1075–1076
Macrodantin, 1075–1076, **C21**
Macrolide anti-infectives, 50
magnesium citrate, 50, 1684
magnesium hydroxide, 25, 50, 1684
magnesium oxide, 25, 1680–1681
magnesium sulfate, 29, 50, 937–939, 1684
Mag-Ox 400, 1680–1681
Makena, 1724
Malarone, 170–172
Malarone Pediatric, 170–172
mannitol, 939–941
Maox 420, 1680–1681
Mapap Arthritis Pain, 67–70
maraviroc, 941–943
Marinol, 495–496, 1631
Marlissa, 591–596
Marqibo, 1750–1751
Matulane, 1256–1258
Matzim LA, 460–462
Mavik, 1748, **C30**
Maxidex, 427–429
Maxidol, 1054–1056
Maxilene, 1728–1729
Maxipime, 292–294
Maxzide, 1505–1508
Mazepine, 269–272
MCV4, 1670
measles, mumps, and rubella virus vaccine, live, 1670
measles, mumps, rubella, and varicella (MMRV) virus vaccine, live, attenuated, 1670
mecasermin, 1731
meclizine hydrochloride, 32, 1688
meclozine hydrochloride, 1688
Medication administration, decision tree, 1692

Medication errors
  causes of, 14–16
  communication issues in,
    16–17
  definition of, 15
  lack of knowledge and, 17
  process and, 15–16
  reducing of, strategies for,
    19
  reporting of, 21
Medication reconciliation, 17
Mediproxen, 1054–1056
Medrol, 984–986, **C19**
medroxyPROGESTERone
  acetate, 55, 943–945,
    C18
mefloquine hydrochloride,
  945–948
Megace, 948–949
Megace ES, 948–949
Megace OS, 948–949
megestrol acetate, 948–949
meloxicam, 1731
melphalan, 22, 949–952
melphalan hydrochloride,
  949–952
memantine hydrochloride, 23,
  52–53, 952–954, **C18**
Menactra, 1670
Menest, 566–568
MenHibrix, 1671
meningococcal (groups
  A, C, Y, and W-135)
  polysaccharide diphtheria
  toxoid conjugate vaccine,
  1670
meningococcal (groups C and
  Y) and *Haemophilus* b
  tetanus toxoid conjugate,
  1671
meningococcal polysaccharide
  vaccine, groups A, C, Y,
  and W-135 combined,
  1670
meningococcal (group B)
  vaccine, 1670
Menomune A/C/Y/W-135,
  1670
Menopause drugs, 1662–1663

Menopur, 1731
Menostar, 569–573
menotropins, 1731
Men's Rogaine, 1688
Menveo (Men ACWY-CRM),
  1670
meperidine hydrochloride,
  52–53, 954–957, 1630,
  C18
Mephyton, 1678–1679
mepolizumab, 1731
Mepron, 169–170
mercaptopurine, 35–36,
  957–959
meropenem, 959–961
Merrem, 959–961
mesalamine, 961–963
Mesasal, 961–963
M-Eslon, 1029–1034
Mestinon, 1271–1272
Mestinon-SR, 1271–1272
mestranol–norethindrone,
  591–596
Metadate CD, 979–983
Metadate ER, 973–983
metformin, 1696–1697
metformin hydrochloride,
  30–31, 963–966, **C18**
methadone hydrochloride,
  52–53, 966–970, 1630,
  1635, **C19**
Methadose, 966–970, 1630
Methergine, 1732
methimazole, 970–971
methocarbamol, 57, 1732
methotrexate, 35–36,
  971–975, 1700–1701
methotrexate sodium,
  971–975
methyldopa, 33–34, 976–977
methyldopa and
  hydrochlorothiazide,
  1658
methyldopate hydrochloride,
  976–977
methylergonovine maleate, 1732
Methylin, 979–983
methylnaltrexone bromide,
  978–979

methylphenidate
  hydrochloride, 43–44,
    979–983, 1630, **C19**
methylphenidate transdermal
  system, 979–983
methylPREDNISolone, 44–45,
    984–986, 1696–1697,
    C19
methylPREDNISolone acetate,
    44–45, 984–986
methylPREDNISolone sodium
  succinate, 44–45,
    984–986
methylTESTOSTERone, 987–988
metoclopramide
  hydrochloride, 32,
    988–990
metolazone, 46, 991–992
Metonia, 988–980
metoprolol, 25–26
metoprolol succinate, 33–34,
    40–41, 992–995, **C19**
metoprolol succinate–
  hydrochlorothiazide,
    1656–1657
metoprolol tartrate, 33–34,
    40–41, 992–995, **C19**
metoprolol tartrate–
  hydrochlorothiazide,
    1657
Metozolv ODT, 988–990
metreleptin, 1732
MetroCream, 997–999
MetroGel, 997–999
MetroGel Vaginal, 997–999
Metro I.V. in Plastic Container,
    995–997
MetroLotion, 997–999
metronidazole
  injection, 995–997
  oral, 995–997
  topical, 997–999
  vaginal, 997–999
metronidazole hydrochloride,
    995–997
Mevacor, 930–932
mevinolin, 930–932
mexiletine hydrochloride,
    26–27

Mezavant, 961–963
Miacalcin, 252–254
micafungin sodium, 32–33, 999–1000
Micardis, 1424–1425, **C29**
Micardis HCT, 1658
Micatin, 1000–1002
miconazole, 1000–1002
miconazole nitrate, 32–33, 1000–1002
Micort-HC, 741–743
Micozole, 1000–1002
MICRhoGAM, 1649–1650
Microgestin 1.5/30, 591–596
Microgestin 1/20, 591–596
Microgestin Fe 1.5/30, 591–596
Microgestin Fe 1/20, 591–596
Micro-K, 1234–1235
Micro-K 10, 1234–1235
Micronor, 1088–1089
Microzide, 728–730
Midamor, 111–112
midazolam hydrochloride, 40, 1002–1005, 1631
Migergot, 1660
miglitol, 30–31, 1005–1006
milk of magnesia, 1684
Milk of Magnesia, 1684
Milk of Magnesia-Concentrated, 1684
milnacipran hydrochloride, 1006–1008, **C20**
milrinone, 49
milrinone lactate, 1008–1010
miltefosine, 1732–1733
mineral oil, 50
Minipress, 1243–1244
Minirin, 421–423
Miniprin Low Dose, 154–157
Minitran, 1076–1079
Minivelle, 569–573
Minocin, 1010–1012
minocycline hydrochloride, 58, 1010–1012
minoxidil (topical), 1688
Minoxidil Extra Strength for Men, 1688
mipomersen sodium, 35, 1012–1015

mirabegron, 1015–1016
MiraLax, 1684
Mirapex, 1236–1237
Mirapex ER, 1236–1237
mirtazapine, 1016–1018
Mirvaso, 229–230
misoprostol, 1733
Mitigare, 377–379
mitomycin, 27, 1018–1020
mitomycin-C, 1018–1020
mitoxantrone hydrochloride, 1020–1022
M-M-R II, 1670
Mobic, 1731
Mobicox, 1731
modafinil, 43–44, 1022–1024, **C20**
Modecate Concentrate, 660–662
Moderiba, 1301–1305
Modicon-28, 591–596
moexipril, 1696–1697
moexipril hydrochloride, 24–25, 33–34, 38–39, 1733
moexipril hydrochloride-hydrochlorothiazide, 1658
mometasone furoate, 44–45, 1024–1027
mometasone furoate monohydrate, 1024–1027
mometasone furoate-formoterol fumarate dihydrate, 1664
Monistat 1, 1000–1002
Monistat 3, 1000–1002
Monistat 7, 1000–1002
Monoamine oxidase inhibitors, 1635
Monoclate-P, 1644
Monodox, 490–494
Monoket, 837–839
Mono-Linyah, 591–596
Mononine, 1646
montelukast sodium, 1027–1029, **C20**
MorphaBond, 1029–1034
morphine hydrochloride, 1029–1034

Morphine LP Epidural, 1029–1034
morphine sulfate, 52–53, 1029–1034, 1630
morphine sulfate–naltrexone hydrochloride, 1034–1038
Motion-Time, 1688
Motrimax, 1054–1056
MouthKote F/R, 1676
Movantik, 1641
MoviPrep, 1684
Moxatag, 119–121
Moxeza, 1038–1041
moxifloxacin hydrochloride, 47–48, 1038–1041, **C20**
Mozobil, 1739
MPSV4, 1670
MS Contin, 1029–1034, 1630
MS.IR, 1029–1034
Mucinex, 1687–1688
Mucinex Allergy, 1687
Mucinex Maximum Strength, 1687–1688
Mucinex Sinus-Max Full Force, 1689
Mucosa, 1687–1688
Mucus Relief, 1687–1688
Multaq, 496–498
mupirocin, 1041–1042
Murine Tears Plus, 1690
muromonab-CD3, 49
Muse, 1706
Mya, 498–501
Myalept, 1732
Myambutol, 590–591
Mycamine, 999–1000
Mycelex, 366–367
Mycelex-7, 366–367
Mycobutin, 1741
mycophenolate mofetil, 49, 1042–1045
mycophenolate mofetil hydrochloride, 1042–1045
mycophenolate sodium, 1042–1045
mycophenolic acid, 1042–1045

Mydfrin, 1214–1215
Myfortic, 1042–1045
Mylanta Gas, 1690
Mylanta Gas Relief Maximum
    Strength, 1690
Myleran, 1711
Mylicon, 1690
Myorisan, 839–841
Myozyme, 1705–1706
Myrbetriq, 1015–1016
Mysoline, 1739–1740
Myzilra, 591–596
M-Zole 3, 1000–1002

N

Nabi-HB, 1646–1647
nabilone, 1631
nabumetone, 51–52, 1733
nadolol, 25–26, 33–34, 40–41,
    1045–1047
nadolol–bendroflumethiazide,
    1656
nafcillin sodium, 53–54,
    1047–1048
nalbuphine hydrochloride,
    52–53, 1048–1051
naloxegol oxalate, 1641
naloxone hydrochloride,
    1641
naltrexone, 1051–1052
naltrexone hydrochloride,
    1051–1052, 1641
Namenda, 952–954, **C18**
Namenda XR, 952–954
naphazoline hydrochloride,
    1052–1053
Naphcon-A, 1052–1053
Naphcon Forte, 1052–1053
Naprelan, 1054–1056
Naprosyn, 1054–1056, **C20**
naproxen, 51–52, 1054–1056,
    C20
Naproxen-EC, 1054–1056
naproxen–esomeprazole, 1652
naproxen sodium, 51–52,
    1054–1056
naratriptan hydrochloride, 36,
    1056–1058
Nardil, 1738

Nasacort Allergy 24 Hour,
    1503–1504
Nasal Spray, 1689
Nascobal, 1674
Nasonex, 1024–1027
natalizumab, 1058–1060
Natazia, 576–578
nateglinide, 30–31,
    1060–1061
Natesto, 1438–1442
Natpara, 1736
Natrecor, 1066–1067
Natroba, 1744–1745
natural lung surfactant, 1645
Natural penicillins, 53–54
Nauseatol, 1718–1719
Navane, 1748
Navelbine, 1544–1546
nebivolol hydrochloride,
    1061–1063, **C20**
NebuPent, 1203–1205
necitumumab, 1606–1607
nefazodone hydrochloride,
    1733
nelarabine, 1733–1734
nelfinavir mesylate, 55–56,
    1063–1064
Nembutal, 1630
Neo-Fradin, 1065–1066
neomycin sulfate, 23–24,
    1065–1066
NeoProfen, 756–759
Neoral, 388–392
Neo-Synephrine, 1689
Neo-Synephrine 12 Hour
    Spray, 1689
Nephro-Fer, 1673
Nesina, 97–98
nesiritide, 1066–1067
Neulasta, 1180–1182
Neulasta Delivery Kit,
    1180–1182
Neumega, 1735
Neupogen, 633–635
Neuromuscular blockers, 51
Neurontin, 692–695, **C13**
nevirapine, 1067–1070,
    1700–1701
Nexafed, 1689

Nexavar, 1744
Nexium, 563–566, **C10**
Nexium I.V., 563–566
Nexterone, 112–115
niacin, 1675–1676
niacinamide, 1675–1676
Niacor, 1675–1676
Niaspan, 1675–1676
niCARdipine hydrochloride,
    25–26, 33–34, 41–42,
    1070–1072
nicotinamide, 1675–1676
nicotinic acid, 1675–1676
NIFEdipine, 25–26, 33–34,
    41–42, 1072–1074,
    C21
Nikki, 498–501
Nimbex, 340–342
niMODipine, 41–42, 1734
Ninlaro, 1600–1601
nintedanib, 1734
Nipride, 1079–1081
nisoldipine, 33–34, 41–42,
    1734
nitazoxanide, 1734
Nitoman, 1746
Nitrates, 25–26
Nitro-Dur, 1076–1079
nitrofurantoin macrocrystals,
    1075–1076, **C21**
nitrofurantoin microcrystals,
    1075–1076
nitroglycerin, 25–26, 33–34,
    1076–1079, **C21**
Nitrolingual, 1076–1079
NitroMist, 1076–1079
Nitropress, 1079–1081
nitroprusside sodium, 33–34,
    1079–1081
Nitrostat, 1076–1079, **C21**
nivolumab, 1081–1084
Nix, 1738
nizatidine, 48–49
Nizoral, 849–850
Nizoral A-D, 849–850
NNRTIs, 1700–1701
Nolvadex-D, 1412–1414
Nonsteroidal anti-inflammatory
    drugs, 51–52

noradrenaline acid tartrate, 1086–1088
Norco, 734–737, 1630
Norditropin FlexPro, 1377–1381
norelgestromin–ethinyl estradiol transdermal system, 1084–1086
norepinephrine bitartrate, 59, 1086–1088
norethindrone, 55, 1088–1089
norethindrone–ethinyl estradiol, 1652
norethindrone–ethinyl estradiol–ferrous fumarate, 1652
norethindrone acetate, 55, 591–596, 1088–1089
norgestimate, 591–596
norgestimate–ethinyl estradiol, 1652
Norinyl 1+35, 591–596
Norinyl 1+50 28 Day, 591–596
Noritate, 997–999
Norpramin, 418–420
Nor-QD, 1088–1089
Nortemp Infants, 67–70
Northera, 501–502
Nortrel 0.5/35-28, 591–596
Nortrel 1/35, 591–596
Nortrel 7/7/7, 591–596
nortriptyline hydrochloride, 29–30, 1090–1092, **C21**
Norvasc, 118–119, **C3**
Norvir, 1318–1322
Norwich, 154–157
Novamoxin, 119–121
Novasen, 154–157
Novo-AZT, 1559–1562
Novoeight, 1644
Novo-Gesic, 67–70
Novolin N, 796–799
Novolin R, 809–813
Novolin 70/30, 791–796
NovoLog, 803–809
Novolog Mix 70/30, 791–796
Novo-Nidazol, 995–997
Novo-Pen-VK, 1202–1203
Novo-Peridol, 721–723

Novo-pramine, 777–779
Novo-Profen, 756–759
NovoRapid, 803–809
Novo-Veramil, 1532–1535
Novoxapam, 1135–1136
Noxafil, 1229–1232
Nplate, 1650
Nubain, 1048–1051
Nucala, 1731
Nucleoside reverse transcriptase inhibitors, 52
Nucynta, 1416–1419, 1630, **C29**
Nucynta ER, 1416–1419, **C29**
NuLYTELY, 1684
Nuplazid, 1611–1612
Nursing process, during drug therapy, 1634
Nutracort, 741–743
Nutr-E-Sol, 1678
Nutropin AQ NuSpin, 1377–1381
Nutropin AQ Pen, 1377–1381
NuvaRing, 599–601
Nuvessa, 997–999
Nuvigil, 150–152
Nuwiq, 1644
Nymalize, 1734
nystatin, 32–33, 1092–1093
Nystop, 1092–1093

O

obeticholic acid, 1607–1608
obiltoxaximab, 1609–1610, 1093–1096
obinutuzumab, 1093–1096
Obizur, 1644
Ocaliva, 1607–1608
Octagam, 1647–1648
octreotide acetate, 31–32, 1096–1098
Ocuflox, 1099–1100
Ocupress, 281–282
Odefsey, 1590–1592
Odomzo, 1744
oestradiol, 569–573
oestradiol valerate, 569–573

oestrogens, conjugated, 578–581
Ofev, 1734
Ofirmev, 67–70
ofloxacin, 47–48
   ophthalmic, 1099–1100
   oral, 1100–1102
   otic, 1099–1100
Ogen .625, 582–584
Ogen 5, 582–584
Ogen 1.25, 582–584
Ogen 2.5, 582–584
Ogestrel 0.5/50-28, 591–596
olanzapine, 38–39, 1103–1106, **C21**
olanzapine–fluoxetine, 1664
olanzapine pamoate, 38–39, 1103–1106
olaparib, 1735
olaratumab, 1752
Older adults, drug therapy in, 1628
olmesartan medoxomil, 33–34, 1106–1108, **C22**
olmesartan medoxomil–hydrochlorothiazide, 1656, **C22**
olodaterol, 1108–1110
olopatadine hydrochloride, 1735
olsalazine sodium, 1110–1111
Olux, 357–358
Olux-E, 357–358
Olysio, 1362–1365
omalizumab, 1111–1112
ombitasvir–paritaprevir–ritonavir–dasabuvir, 1113–1116
omega-3-acid ethyl esters, 1116–1117, **C22**
omeprazole, 56, 1117–1120
omeprazole magnesium, 1117–1120
Omnaris, 326–328
Omnipred, 1247–1248
Omnitrope, 1377–1381
Omtryg, 1116–1117
onabotulinumtoxinA, 1120–1124
   cosmetic, 1120–1124

Oncaspar, 1178–1180
ondansetron, 1124–1127,
    1635
ondansetron hydrochloride,
    32, 1124–1127
1,25-dihydroxycholecalciferol,
    254–256
Onfi, 354–356
Onglyza, 1349–1351, **C26**
Onivyde, 1725–1726
Onmel, 842–844
Onzetra Xsail, 1397–1399
Opana, 1149–1153, 1630
Opana ER, 1149–1153, 1630
Opdivo, 1081–1084
Opioid agonists, 1663–1664
Opioid analgesics, 1630, 1635
Opioids, 52–53
oprelvekin, 1735
Opti-Clear, 1690
Optivar, 182–183
Oracea, 490–494
Orapred ODT, 1244–1247
OraVerse, 1641–1642
Oravig, 1000–1002
Orbactiv, 1127–1128
Orencia, 61–63
Orenitram, 1496–1498
Oretic, 728–730
Organ-I NR, 1687–1688
oritavancin diphosphate,
    1127–1128
Orkambi, 932–935
orlistat, 1735
orphenadrine citrate, 57
Orsythia, 591–596
Ortho-Cyclen-28, 591–596
Ortho-Novum 1/35-28,
    591–596
Ortho-Novum 7/7/7-28,
    591–596
Ortho Tri-Cyclen, 591–596, 1652
OrthoTri-Cyclen Lo, 591–596
oseltamivir phosphate,
    1128–1130
Oseni, 1654
osimertinib, 1610–1611
Osmitrol, 939–941
OsmoPrep, 1685

ospemifene, 1130–1131
Osphena, 1130–1131
Otezla, 138–139
Otrexup, 971–975
Ovol, 1690
Ovol Drops, 1690
oxaliplatin, 22, 1132–1134
Oxandrine, 1631
oxandrolone, 1631
Oxaydo, 1142–1145
oxazepam, 40, 1135–1136, 1631
oxcarbazepine, 29, 1136–1139
Oxpam, 1135–1136
Oxtellar XR, 1136–1139
oxybutynin, 1139–1141
oxybutynin chloride,
    1139–1141
Oxycet, 1145–1149
oxycodone–aspirin, 1630
oxycodone hydrochloride,
    52–53, 1142–1145,
    1630, **C22**
oxycodone hydrochloride–
    acetaminophen,
    1145–1149, 1630
oxycodone hydrochloride–
    aspirin, 1651
OxyContin, 1142–1145, **C22**
Oxy IR, 1142–1145
oxymetazoline hydrochloride
    intranasal, 1689
    ophthalmic, 1689
oxymetholone, 1631
oxymorphone hydrochloride,
    52–53, 1149–1153
oxytocin (synthetic injection),
    1153–1155
Oxytrol, 1139–1141
Oxytrol for Women,
    1139–1141
Oystercal, 1680
Ozurdex, 427–429

P

Pacerone, 112–115
paclitaxel, 1155–1157, 1636
paclitaxel protein-bound
    particles, 1158–1161
palbociclib, 1161–1162

paliperidone, 38–39,
    1163–1166
paliperidone palmitate, 38–39,
    1163–1166
palivizumab, 1671
palonosetron hydrochloride,
    32, 1166–1167
Pamelor, 1090–1092, **C21**
pamidronate disodium,
    1167–1168
Pamprin All Day Relief,
    1054–1056
Pamprin Ibuprofen Formula,
    756–759
Pancreaze, 1169–1171
pancrelipase, 1169–1171
pancuronium bromide, 51,
    1171–1173
Pandel, 741–743
panitumumab, 1736
Panto IV, 1173–1175
Pantoloc, 1173–1175
pantoprazole, 56
pantoprazole sodium,
    1173–1175, **C22**
paracetamol, 67–70
parathyroid hormone, 1736
paricalcitol, 1676
Parlodel, 232–234
Parnate, 1749
paroxetine hydrochloride,
    56–57, 1175–1178
paroxetine mesylate,
    1175–1178
Parvolex, 70–73
Pataday, 1735
Patanase, 1735
Patanol, 1735
patiromer sorbitex calcium,
    1736
Paxil, 1175–1178
Paxil CR, 1175–1178
Pazeo, 1735
pazopanib, 1736
PCE, 553–556
PDP-Isoniazid, 835–837
PediaCare, 1687
PediaCare Childrens Allergy,
    464–466

PediaCare Long-Acting Cough Freezer Pops, 1687
Pediacol, 1690
Pedia-Lax, 1682–1683, 1685
Pediaphen, 67–70
Pediapred, 1244–1247
Pediarix, 1667
Pediatrix, 67–70
PedvaxHIB, 1666
PEG, 1684
PEG 3350, 1684
Pegalax, 1684
pegaspargase, 1178–1180
Pegasys, 1182–1185
Pegasys ProClick, 1182–1185
pegfilgrastim, 1180–1182
peginterferon alfa-2a, 1182–1185
peginterferon alfa-2b, 1185–1189
peginterferon beta-1a, 1737
PegIntron, 1185–1189
PegIntron Redipen, 1185–1189
PEG-L-asparaginase, 1178–1180
pegloticase, 1189–1190
pembrolizumab, 1737
pemetrexed, 35–36
pemetrexed disodium, 1190–1192
Penicillinase-resistant penicillins, 53–54
penicillin G benzathine, 53–54, 1193–1194
penicillin G potassium, 53–54, 1194–1197
penicillin G procaine, 53–54, 1197–1199
penicillin G sodium, 53–54, 1199–1202
Penicillins, 53–54
Penicillin-VK, 1202–1203
penicillin V potassium, 53–54, 1202–1203
Pennsaid, 448–450
Pentacel, 1667–1668
Pentam, 1203–1205

pentamidine isethionate, 1203–1205
Pentasa, 961–963
pentazocine–naloxone hydrochloride, 1651
pentazocine hydrochloride, 1205–1207
pentazocine lactate, 52–53, 1205–1207
pentobarbital, 1630
pentoxifylline, 1737
Pentoxil, 1737
Pen-VK, 1202–1203
Pepcid, 617–619, C11
Pepcid AC, 617–619
Peptic Relief, 1637
Pepto-Bismol, 1637
peramivir, 1737
Percocet, 1145–1149, 1630
Percodan, 1630, 1651
Perforomist, 678–680
perindopril erbumine, 24–25, 33–34, 1737–1738
Periostat, 490–494
Perjeta, 1207–1210
Permapen, 1193–1194
Permethrin, 1738
perphenazine, 38–39, 54–55, 1738
perphenazine and amitriptyline, 1664
Persantine, 466–467
pertuzumab, 1207–1210
Pertzye, 1169–1171
pethidine hydrochloride, 954–957
Pexeva, 1175–1178
PFA, 680–682
Pfizerpen, 1194–1197
Pharmaflur df, 1676
Pharmaflur 1.1, 1676
Phazyme Maximum Strength, 1690
phenelzine sulfate, 1635, 1738
Phenothiazines, 54–55
phenoxymethyl penicillin potassium, 1202–1203
phentermine hydrochloride, 43–44, 1210–1211

phentermine hydrochloride–topiramate, 1211–1214
phentolamine mesylate, 22–23, 1641–1642
phenylalanine mustard, 949–952
phenylephrine hydrochloride intranasal, 1689
ophthalmic, 1214–1215
Phenytek, 1215–1219
phenytoin, 1215–1219, 1700–1701
phenytoin sodium, 29
phenytoin sodium, extended, 29, 1215–1219
Philith, 591–596
Phillips' Milk of Magnesia, 1684
Phillips Stool Softener, 1682
PHL-Salbutamol, 84–87
Phos-Flur, 1676
PhosLo Gelcaps, 256–259
Phoslyra, 256–259
phosphonoformic acid, 680–682
Phytonadione, 1678–1679
Picato, 790–791
pilocarpine hydrochloride ophthalmic, 1219–1220
oral, 1221–1222
Pilopine HS, 1219–1220
pimavanserin tartrate, 1611–1612
Pimecrolimus, 1222–1223
pimozide, 38–39
Pink Bismuth, 1637
pioglitazone, 1702–1703
pioglitazone–metformin hydrochloride, 1652–1653
pioglitazone hydrochloride, 30–31, 1223–1225, C23
piperacillin sodium–tazobactam sodium, 53–54, 1225–1228
piperazine estrone sulfate, 582–584
pirfenidone, 1738–1739
pitavastatin, 35, 1228–1229

Pitocin, 1153–1155
Plaquenil, 747–748
Plasbumin-5, 1644
Plasbumin-25, 1644
Plasmanate, 1648
Plasma-Plex, 1648
plasma protein fractions, 1648
Plavix, 364–365, **C6**
Plegridy, 1737
Plendil, 620–621
plerixafor, 1739
Pletal, 330–331
pms-Ibuprofen, 756–759
PMS-Imipramine, 777–779
PMS-ISMN, 837–839
PMS-metronidazole, 995–997
PMS-nifedipine, 1072–1074
pneumococcal vaccine,
    polyvalent, 1671
Pneumovax 23, 1671
Point-Two, 1676
poliovirus vaccine, inactivated,
    1671
polyethylene glycol, 50, 1684
polyethylene glycol–electrolyte
    solution, 1684
Polylax, 1684
Polymorphisms, 5
Portia-28, 591–596
Portrazza, 1606–1607
posaconazole, 32–33,
    1229–1232
Posanol, 1229–1232
Potasalan, 1234–1235
potassium acetate, 1232–1233
potassium chloride,
    1234–1235
potassium iodide, 1739
Potiga, 614–615
Pradaxa, 394–396, **C7**
pralatrexate, 35–36, 1739
pralidoxime chloride, 1642
Praluent, 90–91
pramipexole dihydrochloride,
    36–37, 1236–1237
pramlintide acetate, 30–31,
    1237–1239
PrandiMet, 1654–1655
Prandin, 1299–1301

prasugrel, 37
prasugrel hydrochloride,
    1240–1241, **C23**
Pravachol, 1241–1243, **C23**
pravastatin, 1698–1699
pravastatin sodium, 35,
    1241–1243, **C23**
Praxbind, 763–764
prazosin hydrochloride, 22–23,
    33–34, 1243–1244
Precose, 1704
Predator, 1728–1729
Pred Forte, 1247–1248
Pred Mild, 1247–1248
prednisoLONE, 44–45,
    1244–1247, 1696–1697
prednisoLONE acetate, 44–45,
    1247–1248
    ophthalmic suspension,
    1247–1248
prednisoLONE sodium
    phosphate, 44–45,
    1244–1247, 1247–1248
    solution, 1247–1248
predniSONE, 44–45,
    1248–1250, 1696–1697
Prednisone Intensol,
    1248–1250
pregabalin, 1250–1252, **C23**
Pregnancy, drug therapy
    during, 6–7, 1624
Prelone, 1244–1247
Premarin, 578–581, **C11**
Premphase, 1662–1663
Prempro, 1663
Preparation H, 1690
Prepidil, 1719
Prepopik, 1685
Prescription drug abuse,
    identification and
    treatment toxicity,
    1629–1631
Prevacid, 867–869, **C15**
Prevacid SoluTab, 867–869
Prevacid 24 Hour, 867–869
Prevalite, 325–326
Prevident, 1676
Previfem, 591–596
Prevnar 13, 1671

Prevpac, 1661
Prezista, 1716–1717
Priftin, 1307–1309
Prilosec OTC, 1117–1120
primaquine phosphate,
    1252–1253
Primaxin 500, 775–777
Primaxin I.V., 775–777
primidone, 29, 1739–1740
Prinivil, 910–912, **C17**
Pristiq, 425–427, **C7**
Privigen, 1647–1648
ProAir HFA, 84–87
ProAir RespiClick, 84–87
Probalan, 1740
probenecid, 1740
probenecid–colchicine, 1655
Probuphine, 240–245
procainamide, 1700–1701
procainamide hydrochloride,
    26–27, 1254–1256
procarbazine hydrochloride,
    1256–1258
Procardia, 1072–1074
ProcardiaXL, 1072–1074, **C21**
Procentra, 436–438
prochlorperazine, 32,
    1258–1261
prochlorperazine edisylate,
    38–39, 1258–1261
prochlorperazine maleate,
    38–39, 54–55,
    1258–1261
Procomp, 1258–1261
Procort, 741–743
Procrit, 541–544
ProctoFoam-HC, 741–743
Procytox, 386–388
Profilnine SD, 1646
Progestins, 55
Prograf, 1404–1407
PRO-ISMN, 837–839
Prolensa, 230–231
Prolia, 416–418
Promacta, 1645–1646
promethazine hydrochloride,
    32, 33, 54–55,
    1261–1263
Promethazine Plain, 1261–1263

Promethegan, 1261–1263
Promolaxin, 1682
propafenone hydrochloride,
    26–27, 1263–1265
Propecia, 638–639
propofol, 1265–1267, 1629
propranolol and
    hydrochlorothiazide, 1658
propranolol hydrochloride,
    25–26, 33–34, 40–41,
    1267–1270, C24
ProQuad, 1670
Proscar, 638–639, C12
Prostin E2, 1719
Prostin VR Pediatric, 100–102
protamine sulfate, 1642
Protease inhibitors, 55–56
protein C concentrate, 1649
Protenate, 1648
Protonix, 1173–1175, C22
Protonix I.V., 1173–1175
Proton pump inhibitors, 56
Protopam Chloride, 1642
Protopic, 1407–1409
Protrin DF, 1392–1395
protriptyline hydrochloride,
    29–30
Protylol, 450–452
Proventil-HFA, 84–87
Provera, 943–945, C18
Provigil, 1022–1024, C20
Prozac, 657–659, C12
Prozac Weekly, 657–659, C12
PRP-OMP, 1666
PRP-T, 1666
pseudoephedrine
    hydrochloride, 1689
Psychotherapeutics, 1664
psyllium, 50
Pulmicort Flexhaler, 234–236
Pulmicort Respules, 234–236
Pulmicort Turbuhaler, 234–236
Pulmophylline ELX,
    1746–1747
Purixan, 957–959
Pylera, 1661
pyrazinamide, 39–40
pyrethrins–piperonyl butoxide,
    1689–1690

pyridostigmine bromide,
    1271–1272
pyridoxine hydrochloride,
    1676
pyrimethamine, 1740

Q

Qnasl, 195–197
Qoliana, 229–230
Q-PAP Infants, 67–70
Qsymia, 1211–1214
Q-Tussin, 1687–1688
Quasense, 591–596
Qudexy XR, 1479–1482
Quelicin, 1387–1390
quetiapine fumarate, 38–39,
    1272–1275, C24
QuilliChew ER, 979–983
Quillivant XR, 979–983
quinapril, 1696–1697
quinapril–hydrochlorothiazide,
    1655
quinapril hydrochloride, 24–25,
    33–34, 1276–1277, C24
Quinaretic, 1655
quinidine, 1702–1703
quinidine gluconate, 26–27,
    1277–1280
quinidine sulfate, 26–27,
    1277–1280
quinupristin–dalfopristin, 1740
Qunol Mega CoQ10,
    1674–1675
QVAR 40, 194–195
QVAR 80, 194–195

R

RabAvert, 1672
rabeprazole, 56
rabeprazole sodium,
    1280–1282, C24
rabies immune globulin
    (human), 1649
rabies vaccine, human diploid
    cell, 1672
radioactive iodine, 1740
raloxifene hydrochloride,
    1282–1284, C25

raltegravir potassium,
    1284–1286
ramelteon, 1286–1287
ramipril, 24–25, 33–34,
    1288–1290, 1696–1697
ramucirumab, 1290–1292
Ranexa, 1296–1297, C25
ranibizumab, 1292–1293
ranitidine hydrochloride,
    48–49, 1294–1296, C25
ranolazine, 25–26, 1296–1297,
    C25
Rapaflo, 1361–1362
Rapamune, 1368–1371
Rapid Action, 67–70
Rapid B-12 Energy, 1674
Rapivab, 1737
Raplixa, 1722
rasagiline mesylate, 36–37,
    1297–1299, C25
Rasilez, 92–93
Rasuvo, 971–975
Ratio-Indomethacin, 784–787
Ratio-Morphine, 1029–1034
Rayos, 1248–1250
Razadyne, 695–697
Razadyne ER, 695–697
Rebetol, 1301–1305
Rebif, 816–818
Reclast, 1565–1568
Recombinate, 1644
Recombivax HB, 1668
Recombivax HB Dialysis
    Formulation, 1668
RectiCare, 1728–1729
Rectiv, 1076–1079
ReFacto, 1644
Refenesen, 1687–1688
ReFissa, 1498–1500
Regenecare HA, 1728–1729
Regitine, 1641–1642
Reglan, 988–990
Regonol, 1271–1272
regorafenib, 1741
Relaxa, 1684
Relenza, 1751
Relief, 67–70
Relistor, 978–979
Relpax, 514–516, C10

Remeron, 1016–1018
RemeronSolTab, 1016–1018
Remicade, 787–790
Reminyl ER, 695–697
Remodulin, 1496–1498
Renagel, 1357–1358
Renova, 1498–1500
Renvela, 1357–1358
ReoPro, 1704
repaglinide, 30–31,
    1299–1301
repaglinide–metformin,
    1654–1655
Repatha, 609–610
Replesta, 1677–1678
Reprexain, 1651
Requip, 1332–1335
Requip XL, 1332–1335
Rescriptor, 414–416
reslizumab, 1613–1614
Respiratory tract drugs,
    1664–1665
Restoralax, 1684
Restoril, 1425–1427, 1631,
    C29
retapamulin, 1741
Retavase, 1741
reteplase, 58–59
reteplase (recombinant), 1741
Retin-A, 1498–1500
Retin-A Micro, 1498–1500
retinoic acid, 1498–1500
retinol, 1673–1674
Retrovir, 1559–1562, **C32**
Revatio, 1358–1361
ReVia, 1051–1052
Revonto, 1716
Rexulti, 226–229
Reyataz, 157–163, **C4**
Rhinall, 1689
Rhinocort Allergy, 234–236
Rhinocort Aqua, 234–236
Rho(D) immune globulin
    intramuscular (human),
    1649–1650
Rho(D) immune globulin
    intravenous (human),
    1649–1650
RhoGAM, 1649–1650

Rhophylac, 1649–1650
Ribasphere, 1301–1305
Ribasphere RibaPak,
    1301–1305
Ribavarin, 1301–1305
ribavirin, 1301–1305
RID, 1689–1690
Ridaura, 1708
rifabutin, 39–40, 1741
Rifadin, 1305–1307
rifampicin, 1305–1307
rifampin, 39–40, 1305–1307
rifapentine, 39–40,
    1307–1309
rifaximin, 1309–1310
rilpivirine hydrochloride,
    1310–1312
Rilutek, 1741–1742
riluzole, 1741–1742
Rimactane, 1305–1307
Riomet, 963–966
risedronate sodium,
    1313–1315, **C25**
Risperdal, 1315–1318, **C25**
Risperdal Consta, 1315–1318
Risperdal M-TAB, 1315–1318
risperiDONE, 38–39,
    1315–1318, **C25**
Ritalin, 979–983, **C19**
Ritalin LA, 979–983, 1630
Ritalin-SR, 979–983, 1630,
    C19
ritonavir, 55–56, 1318–1322,
    1635
Rituxan, 1322–1325
rituximab, 1322–1325
Rivanase AQ, 195–197
rivaroxaban, 28–29,
    1325–1327, **C26**
Rivasa, 154–157
rivastigmine, 1327–1330
rivastigmine tartrate, 23,
    1327–1330, **C26**
Rixubis, 1646
rizatriptan benzoate, 36
Robafen, 1687–1688
Robaxin, 1732
Robaxin-750, 1732
Robitussin, 1687

Robitussin Chest Congestion,
    1687–1688
Robitussin Pediatric, 1687
Rocaltrol, 254–256
Rocephin, 309–311
Rofact, 1305–1307
roflumilast, 1330–1331
Rogaine Extra Strength for
    Men, 1688
Rogitine, 1641–1642
Rolaids, 1680
rolapitant hydrochloride, 32,
    1331–1332
romidepsin, 1742
romiplostim, 1650
rOPINIRole hydrochloride,
    36–37, 1332–1335
rosiglitazone, 1702–1703
rosiglitazone maleate, 30–31,
    1335–1337, **C26**
rosiglitazone maleate–
    metformin hydrochloride,
    1655
rosuvastatin, 1698–1699
rosuvastatin calcium, 35,
    1337–1340, **C26**
Rotarix, 1672
RotaTeq, 1672
rotavirus, live, 1672
Rowasa, 961–963
Roxicet, 1145–1149
Roxicodone, 1142–1145, 1630
Rozerem, 1286–1287
rufinamide, 29, 1742
ruxolitinib phosphate,
    1340–1343
Ryanodex, 1716
Rytary, 886–889
Rythmol, 1263–1265
Rythmol SR, 1263–1265
Ryzodeg 70/30, 791–796

S

Sabril, 1535–1537
sacubitril–valsartan,
    1343–1345
Saizen, 1377–1381
Salagen, 1221–1222

Salazopyrin, 1395–1397
Salazopyrin EN-Tabs,
    1395–1397
salazosulfapyridine,
    1395–1397
Saline laxatives, 50
salmeterol xinafoate,
    1345–1347
Salofalk, 961–963
Samsca, 1477–1479
Sancuso, 718–720
Sandimmune, 388–392
Sandostatin, 1096–1098
Sandostatin LAR Depot,
    1096–1098
Sani-Supp, 1682–1683
Saphris, 152–154
sapropterin dihydrochloride,
    1742
saquinavir mesylate, 55–56,
    1742
Sarafem, 657–659, **C12**
sargramostim, 1347–1349
Savaysa, 509–511
Savella, 1006–1008, **C20**
saxagliptin, 30–31,
    1349–1351, **C26**
Saxenda, 905–908
Scalpicin, 741–743
SCIG, 1647–1648
scopolamine, 27–28, 32, 1743
Scot-Tussin, 1687
Seasonale, 591–596
Seasonique, 591–596
sebelipase alfa, 1614–1615
Sebivo, 1422–1424
secukinumab, 1743
Sedatives, 1630–1631
Selax, 1682
Selective factor Xa inhibitors,
    28–29
Selective serotonin and
    norepinephrine reuptake
    inhibitors,1635
Selective serotonin reuptake
    inhibitors, 56–57, 1635
selegiline, 1351–1354
selegiline hydrochloride,
    36–37, 1351–1354

selexipag, 1615–1616
Selzentry, 941–943
Sensipar, 333–335
Septra, 1392–1395
Septra DS, 1392–1395
Serevent Diskus, 1345–1347
Seromycin, 1716
Seroquel, 1272–1275, **C24**
Seroquel XR, 1272–1275
Serostim, 1377–1381
Serotonin syndrome, 1635
sertaconazole nitrate, 32–33,
    1743
sertraline hydrochloride,
    56–57, 1354–1357, **C27**
sevelamer carbonate,
    1357–1358
sevelamer hydrochloride,
    1357–1358
SF 5000 Plus, 1676
sfRowasa, 961–963
Silace, 1682
sildenafil citrate, 1358–1361,
    C27
Silenor, 482–484
silodosin, 22–23, 1361–1362
Silphen Cough, 464–466
siltuximab, 1743
Silvadene, 1743–1744
Silver Bullet, 1682
silver sulfadiazine, 1743–1744
Simbrinza, 1710
simeprevir sodium,
    1362–1365
simethicone, 1690
Simply Allergy, 464–466
Simply Cough, 1687
Simponi, 717–718
Simponi Aria, 717–718
Simulect, 1708
simvastatin, 35, 1365–1368,
    1698–1699, **C27**
Sinemet, 886–889, **C15**
Sinemet CR, 886–889, **C15**
Singulair, 1027–1029, **C20**
sirolimus, 49, 1368–1371
Sirturo, 197–198
sitagliptin–metformin
    hydrochloride, 1653–1654

sitagliptin phosphate, 30–31,
    1371–1372, **C27**
Sitavig, 73–75
Sivextro, 1419–1420
6-mercaptopurine, 957–959
6-MP, 957–959
Skeletal muscle relaxants, 57
Sleep drugs, 1631
Slo-Niacin, 1675–1676
Slow FE, 1673
Slow Release Iron, 1673
sodium bicarbonate, 25, 50,
    1744
sodium ferric gluconate
    complex, 1372–1373
sodium fluoride, 1676
    topical, 1676
sodium iodide, 1740
Sodium Iodide [131]I
    Therapeutic, 1740
sodium phosphate monobasic
    monohydrate–sodium
    phosphate dibasic
    anhydrous, 1685
sodium phosphates, 50,
    1685
sodium picosulfate–
    magnesium oxide–
    anhydrous citric acid,
    1685
sodium polystyrene sulfonate,
    1642
Sof-Lax, 1682
Soflax C, 1682
Soflax EX, 1682
sofosbuvir, 1374–1376
sofosbuvir–velpatasvir,
    1616–1617
Solaraze, 448–450
Solarcaine Aloe Extra Burn
    Relief, 1728–1729
solifenacin succinate,
    1376–1377, **C27**
Soliris, 1720
Solodyn, 1010–1012
Soltamox, 1412–1414
Solu-Cortef, 738–741
Solu-Medrol, 984–986
Soma, 277–278, **C5**

somatropin, 1377–1381
Sominex, 464–466
Sonata, 1557–1559, 1631
sonidegib phosphate, 1744
sorafenib tosylate, 1744
Sorine, 1381–1384
sotalol hydrochloride, 26–27,
    40–41, 1381–1384
Sotylize, 1381–1384
Sovaldi, 1374–1376
spinosad, 1744–1745
Spiriva, 1458–1460
Spiriva Respimat, 1458–1460
spironolactone, 45–46,
    1384–1385, **C27**
spironolactone–
    hydrochlorothiazide,
    1662
Sporanox, 842–844
Sprintec, 591–596
Spritam, 880–883
Sprix, 853–856
Sprycel, 1717
SPS, 1642
SSD, 1743–1744
Stalevo, 889–891, **C15**
Stanback Aspirin Free, 67–70
Starlix, 1060–1061
Statex, 1029–1034
Statex DPS, 1029–1034
stavudine, 52, 1386–1387
Staxyn, 1526–1527
Stelara, 1512–1514
Stendra, 174–175
StieVA-A, 1498–1500
Stimate, 421–423
Stimulant laxatives, 50
Stimulants, 1630
Stivarga, 1741
St. John's wort, 1635
St. Joseph Aspirin, 154–157
St. Joseph Cough
    Suppressant, 1687
Stomach Relief, 1637
Stomak-care, 1637
Stool softeners, 50
Stool surfactants, 50
Stop Gel, 1676
Strattera, 165–167, **C4**

Strensiq, 1707
Striant, 1438–1442
Stribild, 518–521
Striverdi Respimat,
    1108–1110
Sublimaze, 624–630
Suboxone, 1663–1664
SUBSYS, 624–630
succimer, 1643
succinylcholine chloride, 51,
    1387–1390
Suclear, 1684
sucralfate, 1390–1391, **C28**
Sucrets Cough, 1687
Sudafed, 1689
Sudafed PE Children's,
    1689
Sudafed PE Maximum
    Strength, 1689
SudoGest, 1689
Sudogest PE, 1689
Sular, 1734
sulfacetamide sodium 10%,
    1391–1392
sulfADIAZINE, 57–58, 1745
sulfamethoxazole–
    trimethoprim, 57–58,
    1392–1395, **C28**
sulfasalazine, 1395–1397
Sulfatrim Pediatric,
    1392–1395
Sulfonamides, 57–58
Sulfonylureas, 1702–1703
sulphasalazine, 1395–1397
sumatriptan succinate, 36,
    1397–1399, **C28**
sumatriptan succinate–
    naproxen sodium, 1660
Sumavel DosePro, 1397–1399
sunitinib malate, 1399–1402,
    C28
Supeudol, 1142–1145
Surfak, 1682
Sur-Q-Lax, 1682
Survanta, 1645
Sustiva, 511–514
Sustol, 718–720
Sutent, 1399–1402, **C28**
suvorexant, 1402–1404

suxamethonium chloride,
    1387–1390
Syeda, 498–501
Sylatron, 1185–1189
Sylvant, 1743
Symbicort, 1665
Symbyax, 1664
SymlinPen 60, 1237–1239
SymlinPen 120, 1237–1239
Synacort, 741–743
Synagis, 1671
Synalar, 652–653
Synercid, 1740
Synthroid, 897–900, **C16**
synvinolin, 1365–1368

T

tacrolimus, 49, 1404–1407
    topical, 1407–1409
tadalafil, 1409–1411, **C28**
tafluprost, 1411–1412
Tagamet, 331–333
Tagamet HB, 331–333
Tagrisso, 1610–1611
taliglucerase alfa, 1745
Taltz, 1602–1603
Talwin, 1205–1207
Tambocor, 642–643
Tamiflu, 1128–1130
Taminol, 67–70
tamoxifen citrate, 1412–1414
tamsulosin hydrochloride,
    22–23, 1414–1415, **C28**
Tanzeum, 1705
Tapazole, 970–971
tapentadol hydrochloride,
    1416–1419, 1630, **C29**
Tarceva, 547–549
Targretin, 1709–1710
Tarka, 1658–1659
tasimelteon, 1745
Tasmar, 1474–1476
tavaborole, 32–33
tavaborole, 1745
Taxol, 1155–1157
Taxotere, 469–472
Tazicef, 303–305
Taztia XT, 460–462
tbo-filgrastim, 1745

Tdap, 1666–1667
Tecentriq, 1576–1578
Tecfidera, 462–464
tedizolid phosphate,
    1419–1420
Teflaro, 301–303
Tegretol, 269–272
Tegretol-XR, 269–272
Tekturna, 92–93
Tekturna HCT, 1659
telavancin, 1421–1422
telbivudine, 1422–1424
telmisartan, 33–34,
    1424–1425, **C29**
telmisartan–
    hydrochlorothiazide,
    1658
temazepam, 40, 1425–1427,
    1631, **C29**
Temodar, 1427–1429
temozolomide, 22, 1427–1429
Tempra Children's Syrup,
    67–70
temsirolimus, 1746
tenecteplase, 58–59,
    1429–1430
Tenex, 1724
tenofovir disoproxil fumarate,
    52, 1430–1432, **C29**
Tenoretic, 1659
Tenormin, 163–165, **C4**
Terazol 3, 1436–1437
Terazol 7, 1436–1437
terazosin hydrochloride,
    22–23, 33–34,
    1432–1433
terbinafine hydrochloride,
    32–33, 1433–1435
    (topical), 1690
terbutaline sulfate, 1435–1436
terconazole, 1436–1437
teriflunomide, 1746
Teril, 269–272
teriparatide (rDNA origin),
    1437–1438
TESPA, 1448–1449
Tessalon, 1709
Testim, 1442–1444
Testopel, 1438–1442

testosterone, 1438–1442
testosterone cypionate,
    1438–1442
testosterone enanthate,
    1438–1442
testosterone transdermal,
    1442–1444
testosterone undecanoate,
    1438–1442
Testred, 987–988
tetanus immune globulin
    (human), 1650
tetanus toxoid, adsorbed, 1672
tetanus toxoid and reduced
    diphtheria toxoid and
    acellular pertussis
    vaccine adsorbed,
    1666–1667
tetrabenazine, 1746
tetracycline hydrochloride, 58,
    1444–1446
Tetracyclines, 58
tetrahydrozoline hydrochloride
    intranasal, 1447–1448
    ophthalmic, 1690
Tetterine, 1000–1002
Teva-Imatinib, 772–775
Teveten, 1721
Texacort, 741–743
T$_4$, 897–900
TH Allergy Relief, 464–466
TH Childrens Allergy, 464–466
The Magic Bullet, 1682
theophylline, 1702–1703,
    1746–1747
Theo-24, 1746–1747
TheraFlu Multi-Symptom,
    464–466
Thera-Flur, 1676
Thera-Flur-N, 1676
Thermazene, 1743–1744
Theroxidil, 1688
Thiamiject, 1677
thiamine hydrochloride, 1677
Thiazolidinediones, 1702–1703
thioridazine hydrochloride,
    38–39, 54–55, 1747
thiotepa, 22, 1448–1449
thiothixene, 54–55, 1748

thiothixene hydrochloride,
    38–39
13-valent conjugate vaccine,
    1671
3TC, 860–863
Thrombin inhibitors, 28–29
Thrombolytics, 58–59
Thyroid hormones, 1702–1703
Thyrolar, 1730
ThyroSafe, 1739
ThyroShield, 1739
tiagabine hydrochloride, 29,
    1450–1451
Tiazac, 460–462
Tiazac XC, 460–462
ticagrelor, 37, 1451–1453
ticarcillin disodium–
    clavulanate potassium,
    53–54
ticlopidine hydrochloride, 37,
    1748
Tigan, 1749
tigecycline, 1453–1455
Tikosyn, 473–475
timolol maleate, 40–41,
    1455–1456
Timoptic, 1455–1456
Timoptic in Ocudose,
    1455–1456
Timoptic-XE, 1455–1456
Tindamax, 1456–1458
tinidazole, 1456–1458
tiotropium bromide,
    1458–1460
tipranavir, 55–56, 1460–1462
tirofiban hydrochloride, 37,
    1462–1464
Tirosint, 897–900
Tivorbex, 784–787
tizanidine hydrochloride, 57,
    1464–1465
TNKase, 1429–1430
TOBI, 1466–1469
TOBI Podhaler, 1466–1469
tobramycin, 1466–1469,
    1696–1697
tobramycin sulfate, 23–24,
    1466–1469
Tobrex, 1466–1469

tocilizumab, 1469–1472
tocopherols, 1678
tofacitinib citrate, 1472–1474
Tofranil, 777–779
Tolak, 655–657
tolcapone, 36–37, 1474–1476
Toloxin, 456–460
tolterodine tartrate,
    1476–1477, **C29**
tolvaptan, 1477–1479
Topamax, 1479–1482, **C29**
Topicort, 423–425
topiramate, 29, 1479–1482,
    C29
topotecan hydrochloride,
    1483–1485
Toprol-XL, 992–995, **C19**
Toradol, 853–856
toremifene citrate, 1748
Torisel, 1746
torsemide, 45, 1485–1487,
    C30
Total Allergy, 464–466
Toujeo SoloStar, 799–803
Toviaz, 631–632
Tracleer, 222–224
Tradjenta, 902–903
tramadol hydrochloride,
    1487–1490
tramadol hydrochloride–
    acetaminophen,
    1651–1652, **C30**
Trandate, 857–858
trandolapril, 24–25, 33–34,
    1696–1697, 1748, **C30**
trandolapril–verapamil
    hydrochloride,
    1658–1659
Transderm-Scop, 1743
tranylcypromine sulfate, 1749
trastuzumab, 1490–1493
Travatan Z, 1493–1494
Travel Sickness, 1688
Travel Tabs, 1718–1719
travoprost, 1493–1494
trazodone hydrochloride,
    1494–1496
Treanda, 1708–1709
treprostinil, 1496–1498

treprostinil diolamine,
    1496–1498
Tresiba, 799–803
tretinoin, 1498–1500
Trexall, 971–975
Treximet, 1660
triamcinolone, 44–45,
    1696–1697
triamcinolone acetonide
    injection, 1500–1503
    intranasal, 1503–1504
    topical, 1504–1505
triamcinolone hexacetonide,
    1500–1503
Triaminic Fever Reducer,
    67–70
Triaminic Long Acting Cough,
    1687
Triaminic MultiSymptom,
    464–466
triamterene, 45–46
triamterene–
    hydrochlorothiazide,
    1505–1508
Trianex, 1504–1505
triazolam, 40, 1508–1509
Tribenzor, 1659
TriCor, 621–623, **C12**
Triderm, 1504–1505
Triesence, 1500–1503
triethylenethiophosphoramide,
    1448–1449
trifluoperazine hydrochloride,
    38–39, 54–55, 1749
trifluridine–tipiracil
    hydrochloride, 35–36,
    1749
Triglide, 621–623
Tri-Legest Fe, 591–596
Trileptal, 1136–1139
Tri-Linyah, 591–596
Trilipix, 621–623
TriLyte, 1684
trimethobenzamide
    hydrochloride, 32,
    1749
Trinipatch, 1076–1079
Tri-Norinyl 28-day, 591–596
Trintellix, 1552–1553

Triostat, 1729
Tri-Previfem, 591–596
Tri-Sprintec, 591–596
Trivagizole 3, 366–367
Trivora-28, 591–596
Trizivir, 1661
Trocaine Throat, 1686
Trocal, 1687
Trokendi XR, 1479–1482
trospium chloride, 1509–1510
Trulicity, 503–505
Trumemba, 1670
Trusopt, 479–480
Truvada, 1661
TSPA, 1448–1449
T_3, 1729
Tucks, 1690
Tumor lysis syndrome, 1636
Tums, 1680
Tums Smoothies, 1680
Tussin, 1687–1688
Tussionex Pennkinetic ER, 1665
Twin-K, 1234–1235
2-PAM chloride, 1642
2-pyridine-aldoxime
    methochloride, 1642
2′ 3′-didehydro-3-
    deoxythymidine,
    1386–1387
Twynsta, 1659
Tygacil, 1453–1455
Tykerb, 1727
Tylenol, 67–70
Tylenol Arthritis Pain, 67–70
Tylenol Extra Strength,
    67–70
Tylenol Go Tabs Extra
    Strength, 67–70
Tylenol Jr. Meltaways, 67–70
Tylenol Sore Throat Daytime,
    67–70
Tylenol with Codeine #3,
    374–377, **C6**
Tylenol with Codeine #4,
    374–377
Tysabri, 1058–1060
Tyvaso, 1496–1498
Tyzeka, 1422–1424
Tyzine, 1447–1448

U

Uceris, 236–238
U-cort, 741–743
Ulesfia, 1709
ulipristal acetate, 1511–1512
Uloric, 619–620
Ultracet, 1651–1652, **C30**
Ultram, 1487–1490
Ultram ER, 1487–1490
Ultrase, 1169–1171
Ultresa, 1169–1171
Unasyn, 131–132
Uniphyl, 1746–1747
Unisom SleepMelts, 464–466
Unithroid, 897–900
Unituxin, 1719
Unused drugs, safe disposal
    of, 1694–1695
Uptravi, 1615–1616
Urecholine, 208–209
uridine triacetate, 1749–1750
Uro-Mag, 1680–1681
Uroxatral, 89–90, **C3**
Urozide, 728–730
ustekinumab, 1512–1514
Utibron Neohaler, 1725

V

Vagifem, 569–573
Vagistat-3, 1000–1002
valacyclovir hydrochloride,
    1515–1516, **C30**
Valcyte, 1516–1519
valganciclovir hydrochloride,
    1516–1519
Valium, 442–444, 1631, **C8**
Valnac, 207–208
valproate sodium, 29,
    1519–1522,
    1702–1703
valproic acid, 29, 1519–1522,
    1702–1703
valsartan, 33–34, 1522–1524,
    C30
valsartan–hydrochlorothiazide,
    1656, **C31**
Valtrex, 1515–1516, **C30**
Vancocin, 1524–1526

vancomycin, 1627, 1702–1703
vancomycin hydrochloride,
    1524–1526
Vandazole, 997–999
vandetanib, 1750
Vanos, 653–654
Vaprisol, 380–382
Vaqta, 1668
vardenafil hydrochloride,
    1526–1527, **C31**
varenicline tartrate,
    1527–1529, **C31**
varicella virus vaccine, 1672
Varivax, 1672
Varubi, 1331–1332
Vascepa, 1116–1117, 1724
Vaseretic, 1659–1660
Vasodilators, 59, 33–34
Vasopressors, 59
Vasotec, 524–526, **C10**
VCR, 1541–1543
Vectibix, 1736
Vectical, 254–256
vedolizumab, 1750
velaglucerase alfa, 1750
Velcade, 219–221
Velivet, 591–596
Veltassa, 1736
Veltin, 1652
vemurafenib, 1750
Venclexta, 1617–1620
venetoclax, 1617–1620
venlafaxine hydrochloride,
    1529–1532, **C31**
Venofer, 831–832
Ventavis, 771–772
Ventolin HFA, 84–87
Veramyst, 663–665
verapamil hydrochloride,
    25–26, 26–27, 33–34,
    41–42, 1532–1535, **C31**
Verelan, 1532–1535, **C31**
Verelan PM, 1532–1535
Versacloz, 367–371
VESIcare, 1376–1377, **C27**
Vfend, 1548–1551
Viagra, 1358–1361, **C27**
Vibativ, 1421–1422
Viberzi, 516–518

Vibramycin, 490–494
Vicks Custom Care Body
    Aches, 67–70
Vicks Formula 44, 1687
Vicks Sinex 12 Hour
    Decongestant, 1689
Vicoprofen, 1652
Victoza, 905–908
Vidaza, 177–179
Videx, 452–454
Videx EC, 452–454
Viekira Pak, 1113–1116
Viekira XR, 1113–1116
vigabatrin, 29, 1535–1537
Vigamox, 1038–1041
Viibryd, 1537–1539, **C32**
vilazodone hydrochloride,
    1537–1539, **C32**
Vimizim, 1721
Vimovo, 1652
Vimpat, 858–860
vinBLAStine sulfate, 1539–1541
vinCRIStine sulfate, 1541–1543
vinCRIStine sulfate liposome,
    1750–1751
vinorelbine tartrate,
    1544–1546
Viokace, 1169–1171
Viorele, 591–596
Viracept, 1063–1064
Viramune, 1067–1070
Viramune XR, 1067–1070
Virazole, 1301–1305
Viread, 1430–1432, **C29**
Visine, 1690
vismodegib, 1546–1547
Vistaril, 751–752
Vistogard, 1749–1750
Vitaline CoQ10, 1674–1675
VitaMelts, 1677
vitamin A, 1673–1674
vitamin A acid, 1498–1500
Vitamin A Palmitate,
    1673–1674
vitamin B complex, 1674
vitamin B_1, 1677
Vitamin B-6, 1676
Vitamin B-6 ER, 1676
vitamin B_3, 1675–1676

vitamin B$_6$, 1676
vitamin B$_9$, 1675
vitamin B$_{12}$, 1674
vitamin C, 1677
vitamin D$_2$, 1677–1678
vitamin D$_3$, 1677–1678
vitamin D analogue
    doxercalciferol, 1678
vitamin D cholecalciferol,
    1677
vitamin E, 1678
vitamin K analogue
    phytonadione,
    1678–1679
vitamin K$_1$, 1678–1679
Vitamin K$_1$, 1678–1679
Vivelle, 569–573
Vivelle-Dot, 569–573
Vivitrol, 1051–1052
VLB, 1539–1541
Vogelxo, 1442–1444
Volibris, 107–109
Voltaren, 448–450
Voltaren Rapide, 445–447
Voltaren SR, 445–447
vorapaxar sulfate, 37,
    1547–1548
Voraxaze, 1640
voriconazole, 32–33,
    1548–1551
vortioxetine hydrobromide,
    1552–1553
VoSpire ER, 84–87
Votrient, 1736
VP-16-213, 601–603
VPRIV, 1750
Vraylar, 274–277
Vyloma, 1725
Vytorin, 1662, **C11**
Vyvanse, 908–910, 1630, **C17**

W

warfarin, 1702–1703
warfarin sodium, 28–29,
    1554–1556, **C32**
Welchol, 379–380, **C7**
Wellbutrin, 245–248, **C5**
Wellbutrin SR, 245–248, **C5**
Wellbutrin XL, 245–248

Wera, 591–596
Winpred, 1248–1250
WinRho SDF, 1649–1650
witch hazel, 1690
Woman's Laxative, 1682
Women's Rogaine, 1688

X

Xalatan, 869–870
Xalkori, 382–384
Xanax, 98–100, 1630, **C3**
Xanax XR, 98–100, 1630
Xarelto, 1325–1327, **C26**
Xartemis XR, 1145–1149
Xatral, 89–90
Xeljanz, 1472–1474
Xeljanz XR, 1472–1474
Xeloda, 264–267
Xenazine, 1746
Xenical, 1735
Xgeva, 416–418
Xiaflex, 1715
Xifaxan, 1309–1310
Xiidra, 1604–1605
Xolair, 1111–1112
Xolegel, 849–850
Xolido, 1728–1729
Xopenex, 879–880
Xopenex HFA, 879–880
Xtandi, 1721
Xtoro, 1722
Xulane, 1084–1086
Xuriden, 1749–1750
Xylocaine, 900–901,
    1728–1729
Xylocard, 900–901
Xyntha, 1644
Xyzal, 884–885

Y

Yasmin, 498–501
YAZ, 498–501
Yervoy, 820–823

Z

Zaditor, 1688
zafirlukast, 1556–1557

zaleplon, 1557–1559, 1631
Zaltrap, 1751
Zamine 21, 498–501
Zamine 28, 498–501
Zanaflex, 1464–1465
zanamivir, 1751
Zantac, 1294–1296, **C25**
Zantac 75, 1294–1296
Zantac 150, 1294–1296
Zantac 300, 1294–1296
Zaroxolyn, 991–992
Zarxio, 635–638
Zeasorb-AF, 1000–1002
Zebeta, 213–215
Zelapar, 1351–1354
Zelboraf, 1750
Zeldox, 1562–1565
Zembrace SymTouch,
    1397–1399
Zemplar, 1676
Zenatane, 839–841
Zenpep, 1169–1171
Zenzedi, 436–438
Zepatier, 1587–1588
Zephrex-D, 1689
Zerbaxa, 307–309
Zerit, 1386–1387
Zestoretic, 912–915
Zestril, 910–912, **C17**
Zetia, 613–614, **C11**
Zetonna, 326–328
Ziac, 1660
Ziagen, 60–61
Ziana, 1652
zidovudine, 52, 1559–1562,
    C32
Zinacef, 311–313
Zinbryta, 1582–1583
Zingo, 1728–1729
Zinplava, 1752
Zioptan, 1411–1412
ziprasidone hydrochloride,
    38–39, 1562–1565,
    C32
ziprasidone mesylate, 38–39,
    1562–1565
Zipsor, 445–447
Zirgan, 697–699
Zithromax, 186–189, **C4**

Boldface refers to full color photographs.

ziv-aflibercept, 1751
Zmax, 186–189
Zocor, 1365–1368, **C27**
Zofran, 1124–1127
Zofran ODT, 1124–1127
Zohydro ER, 730–734
Zoladex, 1724
zoledronic acid, 1565–1568, 1636
zolmitriptan, 36, 1568–1570
Zoloft, 1354–1357, **C27**
zolpidem tartrate, 1570–1572, 1631, **C32**
Zolpimist, 1570–1572
Zomacton, 1377–1381
Zometa, 1565–1568

Zomig, 1568–1570
Zomig-ZMT, 1568–1570
Zonegran, 1572–1574
zonisamide, 29, 1572–1574
Zontivity, 1547–1548
Zorbtive, 1377–1381
Zortress, 605–609
Zorvolex, 445–447
Zostavax, 1672
zoster vaccine, live, 1672
Zosyn, 1225–1228
Zovia 1/35E-28, 591–596
Zovia 1/50E-28, 591–596
Zovirax, 73–75
Zubsolv, 1663–1664
Zuplenz, 1124–1127

Zurampic, 1603–1604
Zyban, 245–248, **C5**
Zyclara, 1725
Zydelig, 764–767
Zykadia, 1712
Zyloprim, 93–95
Zymar, 699–700
Zymaxid, 699–700
Zyprexa, 1103–1106, **C21**
Zyprexa Relprevv, 1103–1106
Zyprexa Zydis, 1103–1106
Zyrtec, 1686
Zyrtec Children's Allergy, 1686
Zytiga, 64–65
Zyvox, 903–905